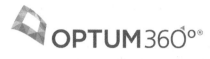

EXPERT

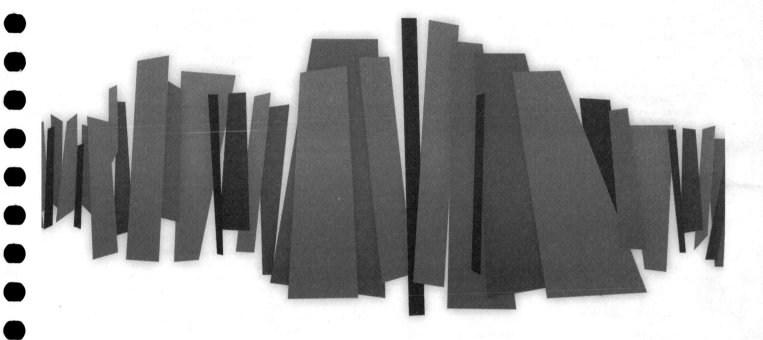

2017

Current Procedural Coding Expert

CPT® codes with Medicare essentials
enhanced for accuracy

Supports HIPAA Compliance

ICD-10 IS NOW. For more resources
and training visit **Optum360Coding.com.**

Notice

The *2017 Current Procedural Coding Expert* is designed to be an accurate and authoritative source of information about the CPT® coding system. Every effort has been made to verify the accuracy of the listings, and all information is believed reliable at the time of publication. Absolute accuracy cannot be guaranteed, however. This publication is made available with the understanding that the publisher is not engaged in rendering legal or other services that require a professional license.

American Medical Association Notice

CPT © 2016 American Medical Association. All rights reserved.

Fee schedules, relative value units, conversion factors and/or related components are not assigned by the AMA, are not part of CPT, and the AMA is not recommending their use. The AMA does not directly or indirectly practice medicine or dispense medical services. The AMA assumes no liability for data contained or not contained herein.

CPT is a registered trademark of the American Medical Association.

Our Commitment to Accuracy

Optum360 is committed to producing accurate and reliable materials.

To report corrections, please visit www.optumcoding.com/accuracy or email accuracy@optum360.com. You can also reach customer service by calling 1.800.464.3649, option 1.

Copyright

Acknowledgments

Marianne Randall, CPC, *Product Manager*
Karen Schmidt, BSN, *Technical Director*
Stacy Perry, *Manager, Desktop Publishing*
Lisa Singley, *Project Manager*
Karen H. Kachur, RN, CPC, *Clinical/Technical Editor*
Elizabeth Leibold, RHIT, *Clinical/Technical Editor*
Tracy Betzler, *Senior Desktop Publishing Specialist*
Hope M. Dunn, *Senior Desktop Publishing Specialist*
Katie Russell, *Desktop Publishing Specialist*
Kate Holden, *Editor*

About the Contributors

Karen H. Kachur, RN, CPC

Ms. Kachur has expertise in CPT/HCPCS and ICD-9-CM coding, in addition to physician billing, compliance, and fraud and abuse. Prior to joining Optum360, she worked for many years as a staff RN in a variety of clinical settings, including medicine, surgery, intensive care, and psychiatry. In addition to her clinical background, Ms. Kachur served as assistant director of a hospital utilization management and quality assurance department and has extensive experience as a nurse reviewer for Blue Cross/Blue Shield. She is an active member of the American Academy of Professional Coders (AAPC).

Elizabeth Leibold, RHIT

Ms. Leibold has more than 25 years of experience in the health care profession. She has served in a variety of roles, ranging from patient registration to billing and collections, and has an extensive background in both physician and hospital outpatient coding and compliance. She has worked for large health care systems and health information management services companies, and has wide-ranging experience in facility and professional component coding, along with CPT expertise in interventional procedures, infusion services, emergency department, observation, and ambulatory surgery coding. Her areas of expertise include chart-to-claim coding audits and providing staff education to both tenured and new coding staff. She is an active member of the American Health Information Management Association (AHIMA).

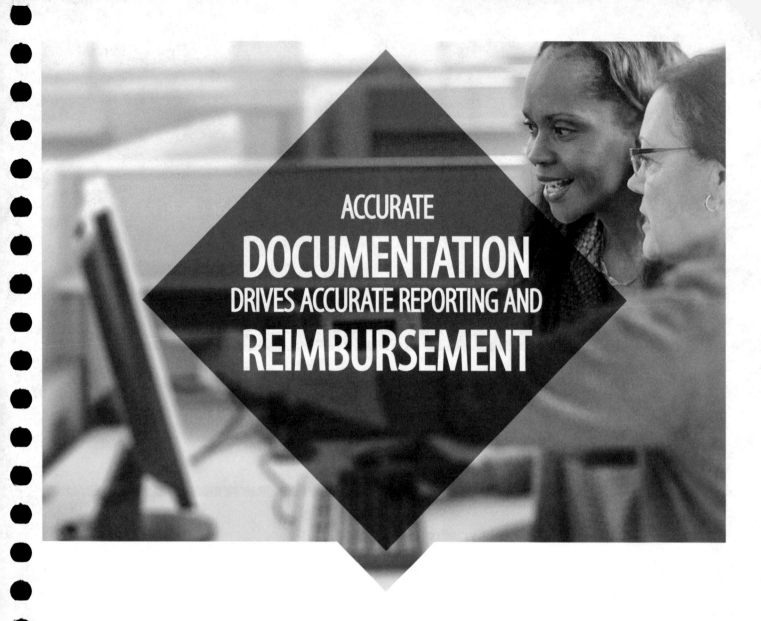

ACCURATE
DOCUMENTATION
DRIVES ACCURATE REPORTING AND
REIMBURSEMENT

Discover how breakthrough technology can strengthen your performance and provide unprecedented efficiencies to expand your CDI program. Using our clinically-based algorithms and patented LifeCode® NLP technology, Optum® CDI 3D reviews 100 percent of your records and automatically identifies those with documentation gaps and deficiencies. CDI 3D enables more timely documentation improvement, simplifies the CDI process, prepares your team for future industry demands, and positions your program for growth.

See how Optum CDI 3D can take your program to the next level.

Visit: optum360.com/CDI3D
Call: 1-866-223-4730
Email: optum360@optum.com

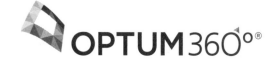

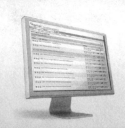
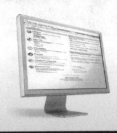

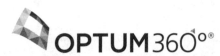

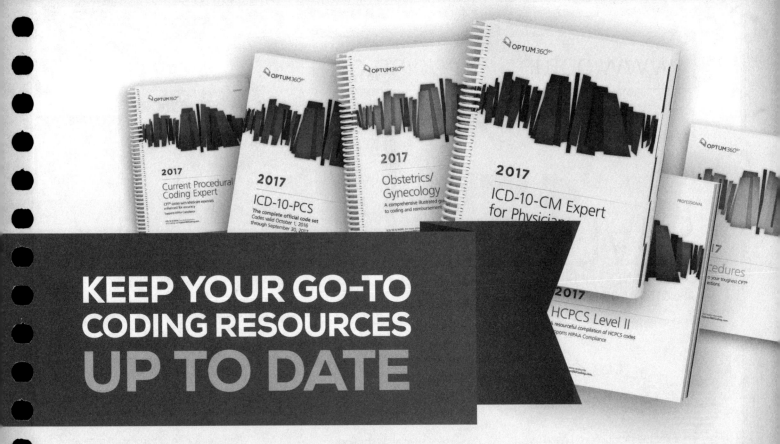

KEEP YOUR GO-TO CODING RESOURCES
UP TO DATE

Stay current and compliant with our 2017 edition code books. With more than 30 years in the coding industry, Optum360® is proud to be your trusted resource for coding, billing and reimbursement resources. Our 2017 editions include tools for ICD-10-CM/PCS, CPT®, HCPCS, DRG, specialty-specific coding and much more.

SAVE UP TO 25% ON ADDITIONAL CODING RESOURCES

 Visit us at optum360coding.com and enter promo code **FOBA17E4** to save 25%.

 Call 1-800-464-3649, option 1, and be sure to mention promo code **FOBA17E4** to save 20%.

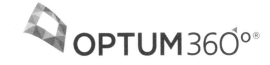

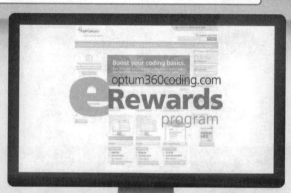
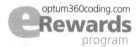
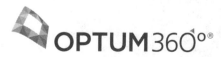

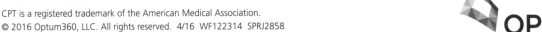
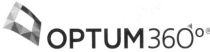

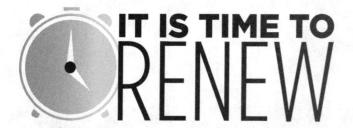

IT IS TIME TO RENEW

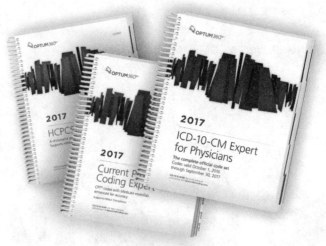

SAVE UP TO 25%*

when you renew your coding essentials.

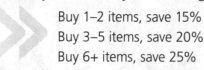

Buy 1–2 items, save 15%
Buy 3–5 items, save 20%
Buy 6+ items, save 25%

ITEM #	TITLE INDICATE THE ITEMS YOU WISH TO PURCHASE	QUANTITY	PRICE PER PRODUCT	TOTAL

	Subtotal	
(AK, DE, HI, MT, NH & OR are exempt)	Sales tax	
1 item $10.95 • 2–4 items $12.95 • 5+ CALL	Shipping & handling	
	TOTAL AMOUNT ENCLOSED	

Save up to 25% when you renew.

Visit **optum360coding.com** and enter the promo code below.

Call **1-800-464-3649, option 1,** and mention the promo code below.

Fax this order form with purchase order to **1-801-982-4033.** *Optum360 no longer accepts credit cards by fax.*

PROMO CODE
FOBA17R4

Mail this order form with payment and/or purchase order to:
Optum360, PO Box 88050, Chicago, IL 60680-9920.
Optum360 no longer accepts credit cards by mail.

Name _____

Address _____
_____

Customer number _____ Contact number _____

○ CHECK ENCLOSED (PAYABLE TO OPTUM360)

○ BILL ME ○ P.O.# _____

(___) _____
Telephone
(___) _____
Fax
_____ @ _____
Email

*Discount does not include digital coding solutions, workers' comp, custom fee or bookstore products.

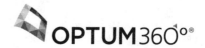

Contents

Introduction i
   Getting Started with *Current Procedural Coding Expert* i
   General Conventions i
   Resequencing of CPT Codes i
   Code Ranges for Medicare Billing ii
   Icons ii
   Appendixes iv

Anatomical Illustrations vii
   Integumentary System viii
      Skin and Subcutaneous Tissue viii
      Nail Anatomy viii
      Assessment of Burn Surface Area viii
   Musculoskeletal System ix
      Bones and Joints ix
      Muscles x
      Head and Facial Bones xi
      Nose xi
      Shoulder (Anterior View) xi
      Shoulder (Posterior View) xi
      Shoulder Muscles xi
      Elbow (Anterior View) xii
      Elbow (Posterior View) xii
      Elbow Muscles xii
      Elbow Joint xii
      Lower Arm xii
      Hand xii
      Hip (Anterior View) xiii
      Hip (Posterior View) xiii
      Knee (Anterior View) xiii
      Knee (Posterior View) xiii
      Knee Joint (Anterior View) xiii
      Knee Joint (Lateral View) xiii
      Lower Leg xiv
      Ankle Ligament (Lateral View) xiv
      Ankle Ligament (Posterior View) xiv
      Foot Tendons xiv
      Foot Bones xiv
   Respiratory System xv
      Upper Respiratory System xv
      Nasal Turbinates xv
      Paranasal Sinuses xvi
      Lower Respiratory System xvi
      Lung Segments xvi
      Alveoli xvi
   Arterial System xvii
      Internal Carotid and Arteries and Branches xviii
      External Carotid Arteries and Branches xviii
      Upper Extremity Arteries xviii
      Lower Extremity Arteries xviii
   Venous System xix
      Head and Neck Veins xx
      Upper Extremity Veins xx
      Venae Comitantes xx
      Venous Blood Flow xx
      Abdominal Veins xx
   Cardiovascular System xxi
      Coronary Veins xxi
      Anatomy of the Heart xxi
      Heart Cross Section xxi
      Heart Valves xxi
      Heart Conduction System xxii
      Coronary Arteries xxii

   Lymphatic System xxiii
      Axillary Lymph Nodes xxiv
      Lymphatic Capillaries xxiv
      Lymphatic System of Head and Neck xxiv
      Lymphatic Drainage xxiv
      Spleen Internal Structures xxv
      Spleen External Structures xxv
   Digestive System xxvi
      Gallbladder xxvi
      Stomach xxvi
      Mouth (Upper) xxvii
      Mouth (Lower) xxvii
      Pancreas xxvii
      Liver xxvii
      Anus xxvii
   Genitourinary System xxviii
      Urinary System xxviii
      Nephron xxix
      Male Genitourinary xxix
      Testis and Associate Structures xxix
      Male Genitourinary System xxix
      Female Genitourinary xxx
      Female Reproductive System xxx
      Female Bladder xxx
      Female Breast xxx
   Endocrine System xxxi
      Structure of an Ovary xxxi
      Thyroid and Parathyroid Glands xxxii
      Adrenal Gland xxxii
      Thyroid xxxii
      Thymus xxxii
   Nervous System xxxiii
      Brain xxxiv
      Cranial Nerves xxxiv
      Spinal Cord and Spinal Nerves xxxv
      Nerve Cell xxxvi
   Eye xxxvii
      Eye Structure xxxvii
      Posterior Pole of Globe/Flow of Aqueous Humor xxxvii
      Eye Musculature xxxvii
      Eyelid Structures xxxvii
   Ear and Lacrimal System xxxviii
      Ear Anatomy xxxviii
      Lacrimal System xxxviii

Index Index–1

Tabular 1
   Anesthesia 1
   Integumentary 15
   Musculoskeletal System 37
   Respiratory System 103
   Cardiovascular, Hemic, and Lymphatic 119
   Digestive System 169
   Urinary System 217
   Genital System 232
   Endocrine System 254
   Nervous System 257
   Eye, Ocular Adnexa, and Ear 285
   Radiology 303
   Pathology and Laboratory 339
   Medicine 409

Evaluation & Management 477
Category II Codes 503
Category III Codes 519

Appendix A — Modifiers 535
CPT Modifiers 535
Modifiers Approved for Ambulatory Surgery Center (ASC)
    Hospital Outpatient Use 537

Appendix B — New, Changed and Deleted Codes 543
New Codes 543
Changed Codes 547
Deleted Codes 548
Web Release New and Changed Codes 548
AMA Icon Only Changes 549

**Appendix C: Evaluation and Management
Extended Guidelines 551**

Appendix D — Crosswalk of Deleted Codes 569

Appendix E — Resequenced Codes 571

**Appendix F — Add-on Codes, Modifier 51 Exempt, Optum
Modifier 51 Exempt, Modifier 63 Exempt, and Modifier 95
Telemedicine Services 581**
Add-on Codes 581
AMA Modifer 51 Exempt Codes 581
Modifier 63 Exempt Codes 581
Optum Modifier 51 Exempt Codes 581
Telemedicine Services Codes 581

Appendix G — Medicare Internet-only Manuals (IOMs) 583
Medicare IOM references 583

Appendix H — Physician Quality Reporting System (PQRS) 685

Appendix I — Medically Unlikely Edits (MUEs) 687
Professional 687
OPPS 711

Appendix J — Inpatient Only Procedures 735

Appendix K — Place of Service and Type of Service 747

**Appendix L — Multianalyte Assays with Algorithmic
Analyses 751**

Appendix M — Glossary 753

**Appendix N — Listing of Sensory, Motor, and
Mixed Nerves 767**
Motor Nerves Assigned to Codes 95900 and
    95907-95913 767
Sensory and Mixed Nerves Assigned to Codes
    95907–95913 768

Appendix O — Vascular Families 769

Appendix P — Interventional Radiology Illustrations 773
Normal Aortic Arch and Branch Anatomy—Transfemoral
    Approach 773
Superior and Inferior Mesenteric Arteries and Branches 774
Portal System 775
Renal Artery Anatomy—Femoral Approach 776
Upper Extremity Arterial Anatomy—Transfemoral
    or Contralateral Approach 777
Lower Extremity Arterial Anatomy—Contralateral, Axillary
    or Brachial Approach 778
Portal System 779
Coronary Arteries Anterior View 780
Left Heart Catheterization 780
Heart Conduction System 781

Introduction

Welcome to Optum360's *Current Procedural Coding Expert*, an exciting Medicare coding and reimbursement tool and definitive procedure coding source that combines the work of the Centers for Medicare and Medicaid Services, American Medical Association, and Optum360 experts with the technical components you need for proper reimbursement and coding accuracy. Handy snap in tabs are included to indicate those sections used most often for easy reference.

This approach to CPT® Medicare coding utilizes innovative and intuitive ways of communicating the information you need to code claims accurately and efficiently. *Includes* and *Excludes* notes, similar to those found in the ICD-10-CM manual, help determine what services are related to the codes you are reporting. Icons help you crosswalk the code you are reporting to laboratory and radiology procedures necessary for proper reimbursement. CMS-mandated icons and relative value units (RVUs) help you determine which codes are most appropriate for the service you are reporting. Add to that additional information identifying age and sex edits, ambulatory surgery center (ASC) and ambulatory payment classification (APC) indicators, and Medicare coverage and payment rule citations, and *Current Procedural Coding Expert* provides the best in Medicare procedure reporting.

Current Procedural Coding Expert includes the information needed to submit claims to federal contractors and most commercial payers, and is correct at the time of printing. However, CMS, federal contractors, and commercial payers may change payment rules at any time throughout the year. *Current Procedural Coding Expert* includes effective codes that will not be published in the AMA's Physicians' Current Procedural Terminology (CPT) book until the following year. Commercial payers will announce changes through monthly news or information posted on their websites. CMS will post changes in policy on its website at http://www.cms.gov/transmittals. National and local coverage determinations (NCDs and LCDs) provide universal and individual contractor guidelines for specific services. The existence of a procedure code does not imply coverage under any given insurance plan.

Current Procedural Coding Expert is based on the AMA's Physicians' Current Procedural Terminology coding system, which is copyrighted and owned by the physician organization. The CPT codes are the nation's official, Health Information Portability and Accountability Act (HIPAA) compliant code set for procedures and services provided by physicians, ambulatory surgery centers (ASCs), and hospital outpatient services, as well as laboratories, imaging centers, physical therapy clinics, urgent care centers, and others.

For 2017, the AMA has deleted the moderate sedation icon ⊙ and removed it from all applicable CPT codes. These codes have all had the revised icon ▲ appended in the book. In appendix B, a list of these codes is provided without code descriptors. Codes where there were text changes to the code descriptor as well as removal of the icon, are listed with their descriptors in appendix B as usual. For moderate sedation services, see new codes 99151–99157.

For the 2017 update, the AMA deleted code 11752, which was an indented code under 11750 Excision of nail and nail matrix, partial or complete (eg, ingrown or deformed nail), for permanent removal. With the deletion of the single indented code 11752, the semicolon at the end of 11750 was no longer necessary and was removed. However, this official change is not identified with a change icon or in appendix B.

Getting Started with *Current Procedural Coding Expert*

Current Procedural Coding Expert is an exciting tool combining the most current material at the time of our publication from the AMA' CPT 2017, CMS's online manual system, the Correct Coding initiative, CMS fee schedules, official Medicare guidelines for reimbursement and coverage, the Integrated outpatient coding Editor (I/OCE), and Optum360's own coding expertise.

These coding rules and guidelines are incorporated into more specific section notes and code notes. Section notes are listed under a range of codes and apply to all codes in that range. Code notes are found under individual codes and apply to the single code.

Material is presented in a logical fashion for those billing Medicare, Medicaid, and many private payers. The format, based on customer comments, better addresses what customers tell us they need in a comprehensive Medicare procedure coding guide.

Designed to be easy to use and full of information, this product is an excellent companion to your AMA CPT manual, and other Optum360 and Medicare resources.

Note: The AMA releases code changes quarterly as well as errata or corrections to CPT codes and guidelines and posts them on their web site. Some of these changes will not appear in the AMA's CPT book until the following year. *Current Procedural Coding Expert* incorporates the most recent errata or release notes found on the AMA's web site at our publication time, including new, revised and deleted codes. *Current Procedural Coding Expert* identifies these new or revised codes from the AMA website errata or release notes with an icon similar to the AMA's current new ● and revised ▲ icons. For purposes of this publication, new CPT codes and revisions that won't be in the AMA book until the next edition are indicated with a ● and a ▲ icon. For the 2018 *Current Procedural Coding Expert*, these codes will appear with standard black new or revised icons, as appropriate, to correspond with those changes as indicated in the AMA CPT book. CPT codes that were new for 2016, and appeared in the 2016 *Current Procedural Coding Expert* but did not appear in the CPT code book until 2017 are identified in appendix B as "Web Release New and Changed Codes."

General Conventions

Many of the sources of information in this book can be determined by color.

- All CPT codes and descriptions and the Evaluation and Management guidelines from the American Medical Association are in **black text**.

- Includes, Excludes, and other notes appear in blue text. The resources used for this information are a variety of Medicare policy manuals, AMA resources and guidelines, and specialty association resources and our Optum360 clinical experts.

Resequencing of CPT Codes

The American Medical Association (AMA) uses a numbering methodology of resequencing, which is the practice of displaying codes outside of their numerical order according to the description relationship. According to the AMA, there are instances in which a new code is needed within an existing grouping of codes but an unused code number is not available. In these situations, the AMA will resequence the codes. In other words, it will assign a code that is not in numeric sequence with the related codes. However, the code and description will appear in the CPT manual with the other related codes.

Introduction

An example of resequencing from *Current Procedural Coding Expert* follows:

	21555	Excision, tumor, soft tissue of neck or anterior thorax, subcutaneous; less than 3 cm
#	21552	3 cm or greater
	21556	Excision, tumor, soft tissue of neck or anterior thorax, subfascial (eg, intramuscular); less than 5 cm
#	21554	5 cm or greater

Note that codes 21552 and 21554 are out of numeric sequence. However, as they are indented codes, they are in the correct place.

In *Current Procedural Coding Expert* the resequenced codes are listed twice. They appear in their resequenced position as shown above as well as in their original numeric position with a note indicating that the code is out of numerical sequence and where it can be found. (See example below.)

> **51797**   **Resequenced code. See code following 51729.**

This differs from the AMA CPT book, in which the coder is directed to a code range that contains the resequenced code and description, rather than to a specific location.

Resequenced codes will appear in brackets in the headers, section notes, and code ranges. For example:

> 27327-27329 [27337, 27339] Excision Soft Tissue Tumors Femur/Knee. Codes [27337, 27339] are included in section 27327-27329 in their resequenced positions.

> Code also toxoid/vaccine (90476-90750 [90620, 90621, 90625, 90630, 90644, 90672, 90673, 90674, 90750])

> This shows codes 90620, 90621, 90625, 90630, 90644, 90672, 90673, 90674, and 90750 are resequenced in this range of codes.

Code Ranges for Medicare Billing

Appendix E identifies all resequenced CPT codes. Optum360 will display the resequenced coding as assigned by the AMA in its CPT products so that the user may understand the code description relationships.

Each particular group of CPT codes in *Current Procedural Coding Expert* is organized in a more intuitive fashion for Medicare billing, being grouped by the Medicare rules and regulations as found in the official CMS online manuals, that govern payment of these particular procedures and services, as in this example:

> **99221-99233 Inpatient Hospital Visits: Initial and Subsequent**
> **CMS:** 100-4,11,40.1.3 Independent Attending Physician Services; 100-4,12,100.1.1 Teaching Physicians E/M Services; 100-4,12,30.6.10 Consultation Services; 100-4,12,30.6.15.1 Prolonged Services With Direct Face-to-Face Patient Contact; 100-4,12,30.6.4 Services Furnished Incident to Physician's Service; 100-4,12,30.6.9 Hospital Visit and Critical Care on Same Day

Icons

● **New Codes**
Codes that have been added since the last edition of the AMA CPT book was printed.

▲ **Revised Codes**
Codes that have been revised since the last edition of the AMA CPT book was printed.

● **New Web Release**
Codes that are new for the current year but will not be in the AMA CPT book until 2018.

▲ **Revised Web Release**
Codes that have been revised for the current year, but will not be in the AMA CPT book until 2018.

\# **Resequenced Codes**
Codes that are out of numeric order but apply to the appropriate category.

★ **Telemedicine Services**
Codes that may be reported for telemedicine services. Modifier 95 must be appended to code.

○ **Reinstated Code**
Codes that have been reinstated since the last edition of the book was printed.

Pink Color Bar—Not Covered by Medicare
Services and procedures identified by this color bar are never covered benefits under Medicare. Services and procedures that are not covered may be billed directly to the patient at the time of the service.

Yellow Color Bar—Unlisted Procedure
Unlisted CPT codes report procedures that have not been assigned a specific code number. An unlisted code delays payment due to the extra time necessary for review.

Green Color Bar—Resequenced Codes
Resequenced codes are codes that are out of numeric sequence—they are indicated with a green color bar. They are listed twice, in their resequenced position as well as in their original numeric position with a note that the code is out of numerical sequence and where the resequenced code and description can be found.

`INCLUDES` **Includes notes**
Includes notes identify procedures and services that would be bundled in the procedure code. These are derived from AMA, CMS, CCI, and Optum360 coding guidelines. This is not meant to be an all-inclusive list.

`EXCLUDES` **Excludes notes**
Excludes notes may lead the user to other codes. They may identify services that are not bundled and may be separately reported, OR may lead the user to another more appropriate code. These are derived from AMA, CMS, CCI, and Optum360 coding guidelines. This is not meant to be an all-inclusive list.

Code Also This note identifies an additional code that should be reported with the service and may relate to another CPT code or an appropriate HCPCS code(s) that should be reported along with the CPT code when appropriate.

Code First Found under add-on codes, this note identifies codes for primary procedures that should be reported first, with the add-on code reported as a secondary code.

◪ **Laboratory/Pathology Crosswalk**
This icon denotes CPT codes in the laboratory and pathology section of CPT that may be reported separately with the primary CPT code.

◈ **Radiology Crosswalk**
This icon denotes codes in the radiology section that may be used with the primary CPT code being reported.

`TC` **Technical Component Only**
Codes with this icon represent only the technical component (staff and equipment costs) of a procedure or service. Do not use either modifier 26 (physician component) or TC (technical component) with these codes.

`26` **Professional Component**
Only codes with this icon represent the physician's work or professional component of a procedure or service. Do not use either modifier 26 (physician component) or TC (technical component) with these codes.

`50` **Bilateral Procedure**
This icon identifies codes that can be reported bilaterally when the same surgeon provides the service for the same patient on the same date. Medicare allows payment for both procedures at 150 percent of the usual amount for one procedure. The modifier does not apply to bilateral procedures inclusive to one code.

80 **Assist-at-Surgery Allowed**
Services noted by this icon are allowed an assistant at surgery with a Medicare payment equal to 16 percent of the allowed amount for the global surgery for that procedure. No documentation is required.

80 **Assist-at-Surgery Allowed with Documentation**
Services noted by this icon are allowed an assistant at surgery with a Medicare payment equal to 16 percent of the allowed amount for the global surgery for that procedure. Documentation is required.

+ **Add-on Codes**
This icon identifies procedures reported in addition to the primary procedure. The icon "**+**" denotes add-on codes. An add-on code is neither a stand-alone code nor subject to multiple procedure rules since it describes work in addition to the primary procedure.

According to Medicare guidelines, add-on codes may be identified in the following ways:

- The code is found on Change Request (CR) 7501 or successive CRs as a Type I, Type II, or Type III add-on code.

- The add-on code most often has a global period of "ZZZ" in the Medicare Physician Fee Schedule Database.

- The code is found in the CPT book with the icon "**+**" appended. Add-on code descriptors typically include the phrases "each additional" or "(List separately in addition to primary procedure)."

⊘ **Modifier 51 Exempt**
Codes identified by this icon indicate that the procedure should not be reported with modifier 51 (Multiple procedures).

51 **Optum360 Modifier 51 Exempt**
Codes identified by this Optum360 icon indicate that the procedure should not be reported with modifier 51 (Multiple procedures). Any code with this icon is backed by official AMA guidelines but was not identified by the AMA with their modifier 51 exempt icon.

▢ **Correct Coding Initiative (CCI)**
Current Procedural Coding Expert identifies those codes with corresponding CCI edits. The CCI edits define correct coding practices that serve as the basis of the national Medicare policy for paying claims. The code noted is the major service/procedure. The code may represent a column 1 code within the column 1/column 2 correct coding edits table or a code pair that is mutually exclusive of each other.

✕ **CLIA Waived Test**
This symbol is used to distinguish those laboratory tests that can be performed using test systems that are waived from regulatory oversight established by the Clinical Laboratory Improvement Amendments of 1988 (CLIA). The applicable CPT code for a CLIA waived test may be reported by providers who perform the testing but do not hold a CLIA license.

63 **Modifier 63 Exempt**
This icon identifies procedures performed on infants that weigh less than 4 kg. Due to the complexity of performing procedures on infants less than 4 kg, modifier 63 may be added to the surgery codes to inform the payers of the special circumstances involved.

A2 – Z3 **ASC Payment Indicators**
This icon identifies ASC status payment indicators. They indicate how the ASC payment rate was derived and/or how the procedure, item, or service is treated under the revised ASC payment system. For more information about these indicators and how they affect billing, consult Optum360's *Outpatient Billing Editor.*

A2 Surgical procedure on ASC list in 2007; payment based on OPPS relative payment weight.

B5 Alternative code may be available; no payment made.

D5 Deleted/discontinued code; no payment made.

E4 Corneal tissue acquisition; hepatitis B vaccine; paid at reasonable cost.

G2 Non-office-based surgical procedure added in CY 2008 or later; payment based on OPPS relative payment weight.

H2 Brachytherapy source paid separately when provided integral to a surgical procedure on ASC list; payment based on OPPS rate.

J7 OPPS pass-through device paid separately when provided integral to a surgical procedure on ASC list; payment contractor-priced.

J8 Device-intensive procedure; paid at adjusted rate.

K2 Drugs and biologicals paid separately when provided integral to a surgical procedure on ASC list; payment based on OPPS rate.

K7 Unclassified drugs and biologicals; payment contractor-priced.

L1 Influenza vaccine; pneumococcal vaccine. Packaged item/service; no separate payment made.

L6 New technology intraocular lens (NTIOL); special payment.

N1 Packaged service/item; no separate payment made.

P2 Office-based surgical procedure added to ASC list in CY 2008 or later with MPFS nonfacility practice expense (PE) RVUs; payment based on OPPS relative payment weight.

P3 Office-based surgical procedure added to ASC list in CY 2008 or later with MPFS nonfacility PE RVUs; payment based on MPFS nonfacility PE RVUs.

R2 Office-based surgical procedure added to ASC list in CY 2008 or later without MPFS nonfacility PE RVUs; payment based on OPPS relative payment weight.

Z2 Radiology or diagnostic service paid separately when provided integral to a surgical procedure on ASC list; payment based on OPPS relative payment weight.

Z3 Radiology or diagnostic service paid separately when provided integral to a surgical procedure on ASC list; payment based on MPFS nonfacility PE RVUs.

A **Age Edit**
This icon denotes codes intended for use with a specific age group, such as neonate, newborn, pediatric, and adult. This edit is based on CMS I/OCE designations or age specifications in the CPT code descriptors. Carefully review the code description to ensure the code you report most appropriately reflects the patient's age.

M **Maternity**
This icon identifies procedures that by definition should be used only for maternity patients generally between 12 and 55 years of age based on CMS I/OCE designations.

♀ **Female Only**
This icon identifies procedures designated by CMS for females only based on CMS I/OCE designations.

♂ **Male Only**
This icon identifies procedures designated by CMS for males only based on CMS I/OCE designations.

⌨ **Facility RVU**
This icon precedes the facility RVU from CMS's 2016 physician fee schedule (PFS). It can be found under the code description.

New codes include no RVU information.

⌁ **Nonfacility RVU**
This icon precedes the nonfacility RVU from CMS's 2016 PFS. It can be found under the code description.

New codes include no RVU information.

FUD: Global days are sometimes referred to as "follow-up days" or FUDs. The global period is the time following surgery during which routine care by the physician is considered postoperative and included in the surgical fee. Office visits or other routine care related to the original surgery cannot be separately reported if provided during the global period. The statuses are:

000   No follow-up care included in this procedure

010   Normal postoperative care is included in this procedure for ten days

090   Normal postoperative care is included in the procedure for 90 days

MMM   Maternity codes; usual global period does not apply

XXX   The global concept does not apply to the code

YYY   The carrier is to determine whether the global concept applies and establishes postoperative period, if appropriate, at time of pricing

ZZZ   The code is related to another service and is always included in the global period of the other service

CMS: This notation indicates that there is a specific CMS guideline pertaining to this code in the CMS Online Manual System which includes the internet-only manual (IOM) *National Coverage Determinations Manual* (NCD). These CMS sources present the rules for submitting these services to the federal government or its contractors and are included in appendix G of this book.

AMA: This indicates discussion of the code in the American Medical Association's *CPT Assistant* newsletter. Use the citation to find the correct issue. This includes citations for the current year and the preceding six years. In the event no citations can be found during this time period, the most recent citations that can be found are used.

⚡   **Drug Not Approved by FDA**
The AMA CPT Editorial Panel is publishing new vaccine product codes prior to Food and Drug Administration approval. This symbol indicates which of these codes are pending FDA approval at press time.

Ⓐ–Ⓨ   **OPPS Status Indicators (OPSI)**
Status indicators identify how individual CPT codes are paid or not paid under the latest available hospital outpatient prospective payment system (OPPS). The same status indicator is assigned to all the codes within an ambulatory payment classification (APC). Consult your payer or other resource to learn which CPT codes fall within various APCs.

Ⓐ   Services furnished to a hospital outpatient that are paid under a fee schedule or payment system other than OPPS

- Ambulance Services
- Separately payable clinical diagnostic laboratory services
- Separately payable non-implantable prosthetics and orthotics
- Physical, occupational, and speech therapy
- Diagnostic mammography
- Screening mammography

Ⓑ   Codes that are not recognized by OPPS when submitted on an outpatient hospital Part B bill type (12x and 13x).

Ⓒ   Inpatient procedures

Ⓓ   Discontinued codes

Ⓔ¹   Items, codes, and services:

- Not covered by any Medicare outpatient benefit category
- Statutorily excluded by Medicare
- Not reasonable and necessary

Ⓔ²   Items and services for which pricing information and claims data are not available

Ⓕ   Corneal tissue acquisition; certain CRNA services and hepatitis B vaccines

Ⓖ   Pass-through drugs and biologicals

Ⓗ   Pass-through device categories

Ⓙ¹   Hospital Part B services paid through a comprehensive APC

Ⓙ²   Hospital Part B services that may be paid through a comprehensive APC

Ⓚ   Nonpass-through drugs and nonimplantable biologicals, including therapeutic radiopharmaceuticals

Ⓛ   Influenza vaccine; pneumococcal pneumonia vaccine

Ⓜ   Items and services not billable to the MAC

Ⓝ   Items and services packaged into APC rates

Ⓟ   Partial hospitalization

Ⓠ¹   STV-packaged codes

Ⓠ²   T-packaged codes

Ⓠ³   Codes that may be paid through a composite APC

Ⓠ⁴   Conditionally packaged laboratory tests

Ⓡ   Blood and blood products

Ⓢ   Procedure or service, not discounted when multiple

Ⓣ   Procedure or service, multiple procedure reduction applies

Ⓤ   Brachytherapy sources

Ⓥ   Clinic or emergency department visit

Ⓨ   Nonimplantable durable medical equipment

Appendixes

Appendix A: Modifiers—This appendix identifies modifiers. A modifier is a two-position alpha or numeric code that is appended to a CPT or HCPCS code to clarify the services being billed. Modifiers provide a means by which a service can be altered without changing the procedure code. They add more information, such as anatomical site, to the code. In addition, they help eliminate the appearance of duplicate billing and unbundling. Modifiers are used to increase the accuracy in reimbursement and coding consistency, ease editing, and capture payment data.

Appendix B: New, Changed, and Deleted Codes—This is a list of new, changed, and deleted CPT codes for the current year. This appendix also includes a list of codes for which the only change made for 2017 was the removal of the moderate sedation icon, and web release new and changed codes, which indicate official code changes in *Current Procedural Coding Expert* that will not be in the CPT code book until the following year.

Appendix C: Evaluation and Management Extended Guidelines—This appendix presents an overview of evaluation and management (E/M) services that augment the official AMA CPT E/M services. It includes tables that distinguish documentation components of each E/M code and the federal documentation guidelines (1995 and 1997) currently in use by the Centers for Medicare and Medicaid Services (CMS).

Appendix D: Crosswalk of Deleted Codes—This appendix is a cross-reference from a deleted CPT code to an active code when one is available. The deleted code cross-reference will also appear under the deleted code description in the tabular section of the book.

Appendix E: Resequenced Codes—This appendix contains a list of codes that are not in numeric order in the book. AMA resequenced some of the code numbers to relocate codes in the same category but not in numeric sequence.

Appendix F: Add-on, Modifier 51 Exempt, Optum360 Modifier 51 Exempt, Modifier 63 Exempt, and Modifier 95 Telemedicine Services codes—This list includes add-on codes that cannot be reported alone, codes that are exempt from modifier 51, codes that should not be reported with modifier 63, and codes identified by the ★ icon to which modifier 95 may be appended when the service is provided as a synchronous telemedicine service.

Appendix G: Medicare Internet-only Manual – IOM References (Pub 100)—This appendix contains a verbatim printout of the Medicare Internet Only Manual references that pertain to specific codes. The reference, when available, is listed after the header in the CPT section. For example:

93784-93790 Ambulatory Blood Pressure Monitoring
CMS: 100-3,20.19 Ambulatory Blood Pressure Monitoring (20.19); 100-4,32,10.1 Ambulatory Blood Pressure Monitoring Billing Requirements

Since appendix G contains these references from the *Medicare National Coverage Determinations (NCD) Manual*, Pub 100-3, chapter 20, section 20.19, and the *Medicare Claims Processing Manual*, Pub 100-4, chapter 32, section 10.1, there is no need to search the Medicare website for the applicable reference.

Appendix H: Physician Quality Reporting System (PQRS)—Previously, this appendix contained lists of the numerators and denominators applicable to Medicare PQRS. However, with the implementation of the Merit-based Incentive Payment System (MIPS), the PQRS system will be obsolete. For this year, the appendix contains information about MIPS but will be deleted for the 2018 edition. The full list of numerators and denominators associated with each individual measure can be found at www.OptumCoding.com/Product/Updates/PQRS16.

Appendix I: Medically Unlikely Edits—This appendix contains the published medically unlikely edits (MUEs). These edits establish maximum daily allowable units of service. The edits will be applied to the services provided to the same patient, for the same CPT code, on the same date of service when billed by the same provider. Included are the physician and facility edits.

Appendix J: Inpatient-Only Procedures—This appendix identifies services with the status indicator "C." Medicare will not pay an OPPS hospital or ASC when these procedures are performed on a Medicare patient as an outpatient. Physicians should refer to this list when scheduling Medicare patients for surgical procedures. CMS updates this list quarterly.

Appendix K: Place of Service and Type of Service—This appendix contains lists of place-of-service codes that should be used on professional claims and type-of-service codes used by the Medicare Common Working File.

Appendix L: Multianalyte Assays with Algorithmic Analyses—This appendix lists the administrative codes for multianalyte assays with algorithmic analyses. The AMA updates this list three times a year.

Appendix M: Glossary—This appendix contains general terms and definitions as well as those that would apply to or be helpful for billing and reimbursement.

Appendix N: Listing of Sensory, Motor, and Mixed Nerves—This appendix lists a summary of each sensory, motor, and mixed nerve with its appropriate nerve conduction study code.

Appendix O: Vascular Families—Appendix O contains a table of vascular families starting with the aorta. Additional information can be found in the interventional radiology illustrations located behind the index.

For more information about ongoing development of the CPT coding system, consult the AMA website at URL http://www.ama-assn.org/.

Appendix P: Interventional Radiology Illustrations—This appendix contains illustrations specific to interventional radiology procedures.

Note: All data current as of November 8, 2016.

Anatomical Illustrations

Body Planes and Movements

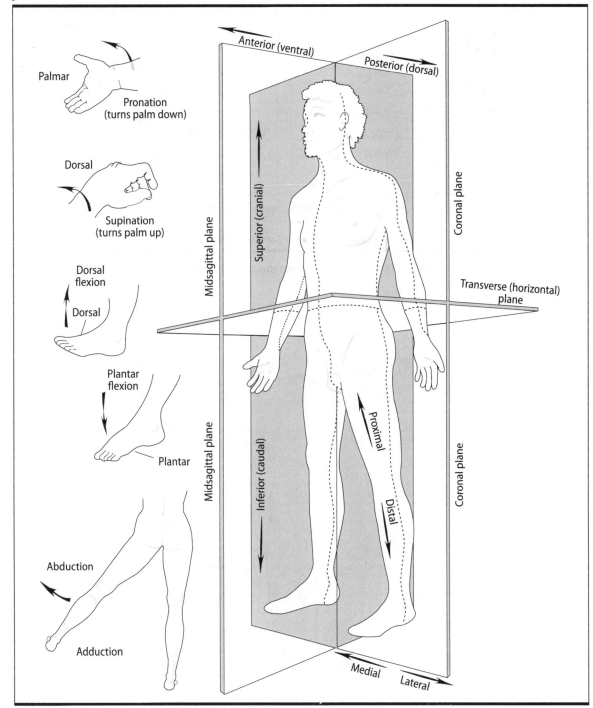

Integumentary System

Skin and Subcutaneous Tissue

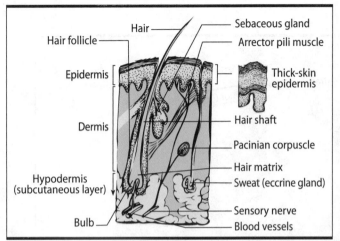

Nail Anatomy

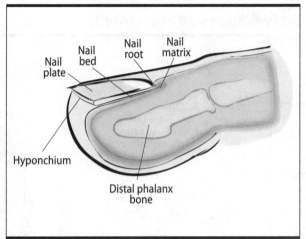

Assessment of Burn Surface Area

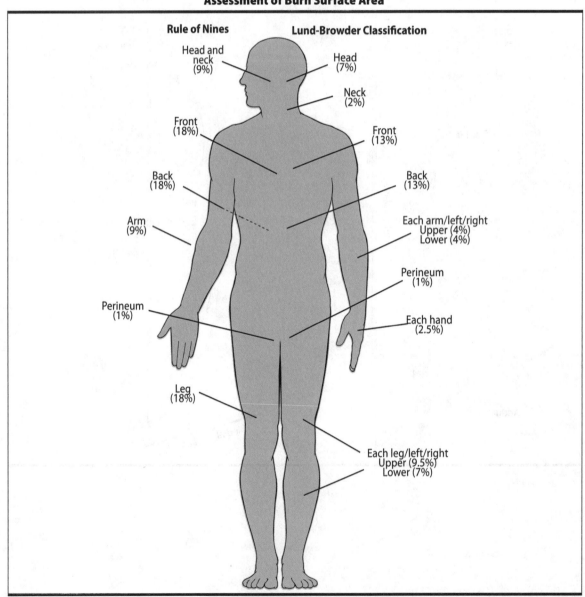

Musculoskeletal System

Bones and Joints

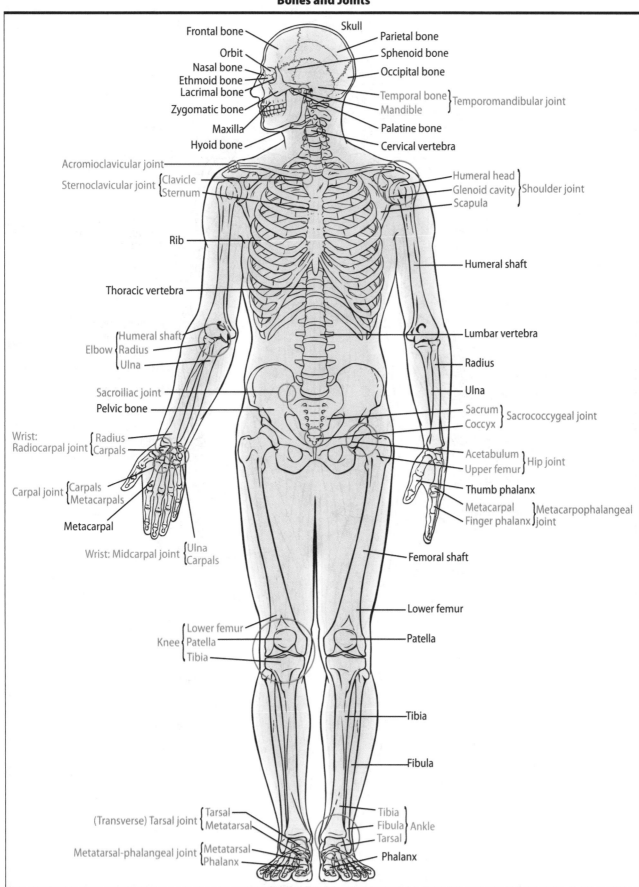

Muscles

Head and Facial Bones

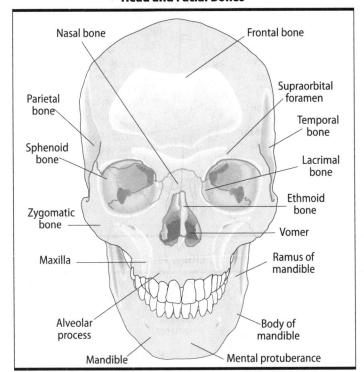

Nasal bone
Frontal bone
Parietal bone
Supraorbital foramen
Sphenoid bone
Temporal bone
Lacrimal bone
Zygomatic bone
Ethmoid bone
Vomer
Maxilla
Ramus of mandible
Alveolar process
Body of mandible
Mandible
Mental protuberance

Nose

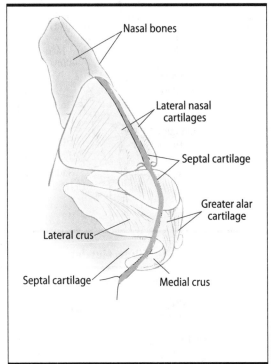

Nasal bones
Lateral nasal cartilages
Septal cartilage
Greater alar cartilage
Lateral crus
Septal cartilage
Medial crus

Shoulder (Anterior View)

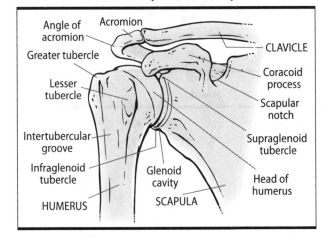

Angle of acromion
Acromion
Greater tubercle
CLAVICLE
Lesser tubercle
Coracoid process
Scapular notch
Intertubercular groove
Supraglenoid tubercle
Infraglenoid tubercle
Glenoid cavity
Head of humerus
HUMERUS
SCAPULA

Shoulder (Posterior View)

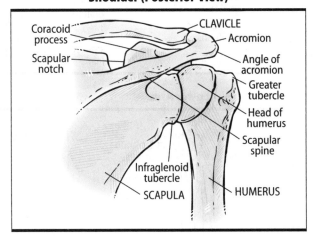

Coracoid process
CLAVICLE
Scapular notch
Acromion
Angle of acromion
Greater tubercle
Head of humerus
Scapular spine
Infraglenoid tubercle
SCAPULA
HUMERUS

Shoulder Muscles

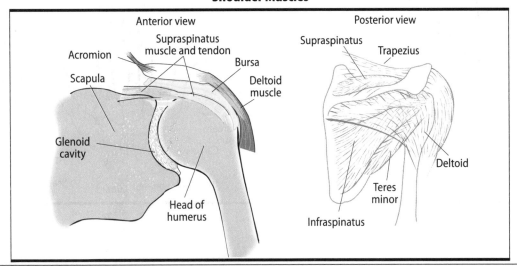

Anterior view
Supraspinatus muscle and tendon
Acromion
Bursa
Scapula
Deltoid muscle
Glenoid cavity
Head of humerus

Posterior view
Supraspinatus
Trapezius
Deltoid
Teres minor
Infraspinatus

Elbow (Anterior View)

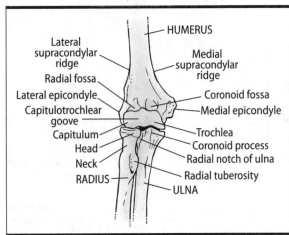

- HUMERUS
- Lateral supracondylar ridge
- Medial supracondylar ridge
- Radial fossa
- Lateral epicondyle
- Coronoid fossa
- Capitulotrochlear goove
- Medial epicondyle
- Capitulum
- Trochlea
- Head
- Coronoid process
- Neck
- Radial notch of ulna
- RADIUS
- Radial tuberosity
- ULNA

Elbow (Posterior View)

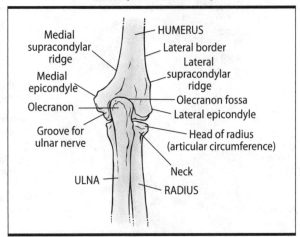

- HUMERUS
- Medial supracondylar ridge
- Lateral border
- Medial epicondyle
- Lateral supracondylar ridge
- Olecranon
- Olecranon fossa
- Lateral epicondyle
- Groove for ulnar nerve
- Head of radius (articular circumference)
- Neck
- ULNA
- RADIUS

Elbow Muscles

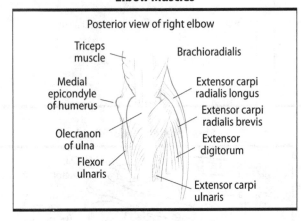

Posterior view of right elbow

- Triceps muscle
- Brachioradialis
- Medial epicondyle of humerus
- Extensor carpi radialis longus
- Extensor carpi radialis brevis
- Olecranon of ulna
- Extensor digitorum
- Flexor ulnaris
- Extensor carpi ulnaris

Elbow Joint

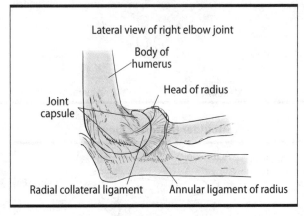

Lateral view of right elbow joint

- Body of humerus
- Head of radius
- Joint capsule
- Radial collateral ligament
- Annular ligament of radius

Lower Arm

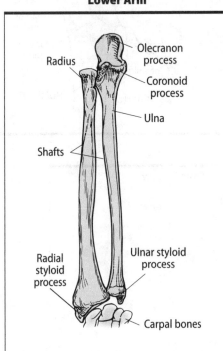

- Radius
- Olecranon process
- Coronoid process
- Ulna
- Shafts
- Radial styloid process
- Ulnar styloid process
- Carpal bones

Hand

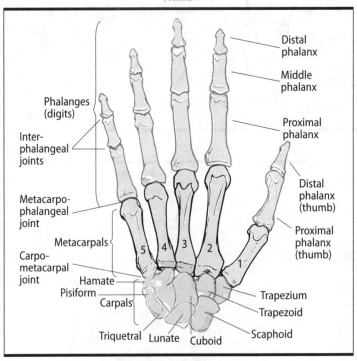

- Distal phalanx
- Middle phalanx
- Proximal phalanx
- Phalanges (digits)
- Inter-phalangeal joints
- Distal phalanx (thumb)
- Metacarpo-phalangeal joint
- Proximal phalanx (thumb)
- Metacarpals
- Carpo-metacarpal joint
- 5 4 3 2 1
- Hamate
- Pisiform
- Carpals
- Trapezium
- Trapezoid
- Scaphoid
- Triquetral
- Lunate
- Cuboid

Hip (Anterior View)

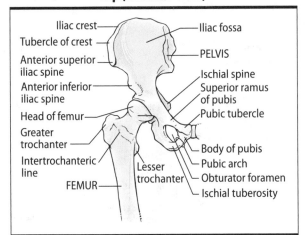

- Iliac crest
- Iliac fossa
- Tubercle of crest
- PELVIS
- Anterior superior iliac spine
- Ischial spine
- Anterior inferior iliac spine
- Superior ramus of pubis
- Pubic tubercle
- Head of femur
- Greater trochanter
- Body of pubis
- Pubic arch
- Intertrochanteric line
- Lesser trochanter
- Obturator foramen
- FEMUR
- Ischial tuberosity

Hip (Posterior View)

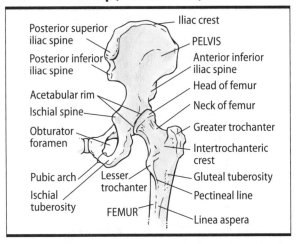

- Posterior superior iliac spine
- Iliac crest
- PELVIS
- Posterior inferior iliac spine
- Anterior inferior iliac spine
- Acetabular rim
- Head of femur
- Ischial spine
- Neck of femur
- Obturator foramen
- Greater trochanter
- Intertrochanteric crest
- Pubic arch
- Gluteal tuberosity
- Lesser trochanter
- Ischial tuberosity
- Pectineal line
- FEMUR
- Linea aspera

Knee (Anterior View)

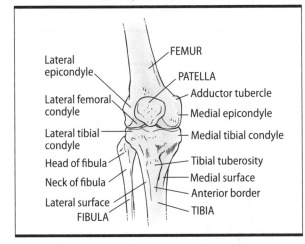

- FEMUR
- Lateral epicondyle
- PATELLA
- Adductor tubercle
- Lateral femoral condyle
- Medial epicondyle
- Lateral tibial condyle
- Medial tibial condyle
- Head of fibula
- Tibial tuberosity
- Neck of fibula
- Medial surface
- Lateral surface
- Anterior border
- FIBULA
- TIBIA

Knee (Posterior View)

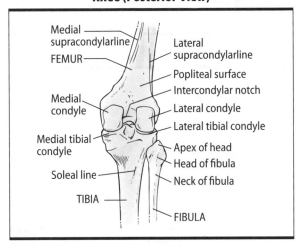

- Medial supracondylarline
- Lateral supracondylarline
- FEMUR
- Popliteal surface
- Intercondylar notch
- Medial condyle
- Lateral condyle
- Medial tibial condyle
- Lateral tibial condyle
- Apex of head
- Head of fibula
- Soleal line
- Neck of fibula
- TIBIA
- FIBULA

Knee Joint (Anterior View)

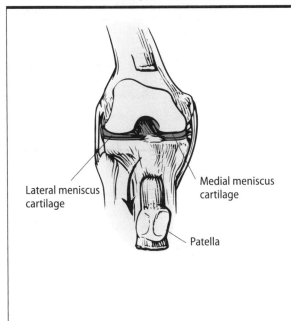

- Lateral meniscus cartilage
- Medial meniscus cartilage
- Patella

Knee Joint (Lateral View)

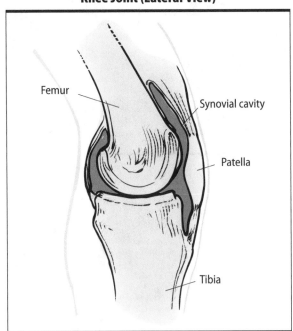

- Femur
- Synovial cavity
- Patella
- Tibia

Lower Leg

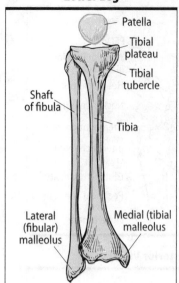

Patella
Tibial plateau
Tibial tubercle
Shaft of fibula
Tibia
Lateral (fibular) malleolus
Medial (tibial) malleolus

Ankle Ligament (Lateral View)

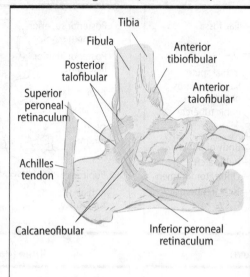

Tibia
Fibula
Posterior talofibular
Superior peroneal retinaculum
Anterior tibiofibular
Anterior talofibular
Achilles tendon
Calcaneofibular
Inferior peroneal retinaculum

Ankle Ligament (Posterior View)

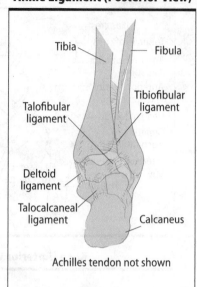

Tibia
Fibula
Talofibular ligament
Tibiofibular ligament
Deltoid ligament
Talocalcaneal ligament
Calcaneus

Achilles tendon not shown

Foot Tendons

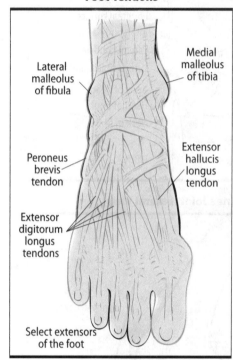

Lateral malleolus of fibula
Medial malleolus of tibia
Peroneus brevis tendon
Extensor hallucis longus tendon
Extensor digitorum longus tendons
Select extensors of the foot

Foot Bones

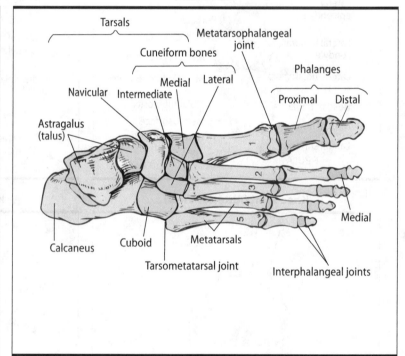

Tarsals
Metatarsophalangeal joint
Cuneiform bones
Phalanges
Navicular
Medial
Lateral
Intermediate
Proximal
Distal
Astragalus (talus)
Calcaneus
Cuboid
Metatarsals
Tarsometatarsal joint
Interphalangeal joints
Medial

Respiratory System

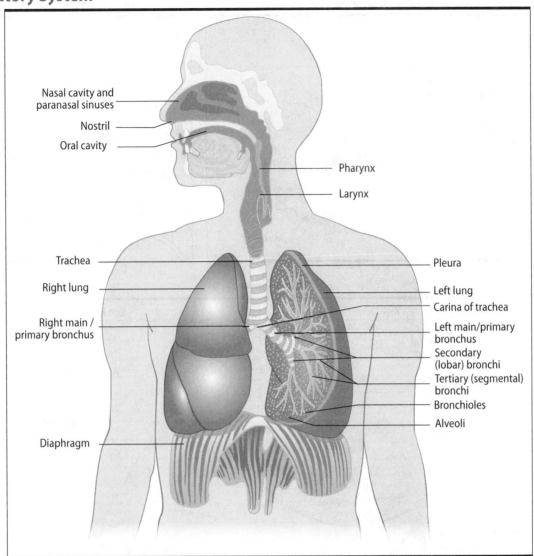

Nasal cavity and paranasal sinuses
Nostril
Oral cavity
Pharynx
Larynx
Trachea
Right lung
Right main / primary bronchus
Diaphragm
Pleura
Left lung
Carina of trachea
Left main/primary bronchus
Secondary (lobar) bronchi
Tertiary (segmental) bronchi
Bronchioles
Alveoli

Upper Respiratory System

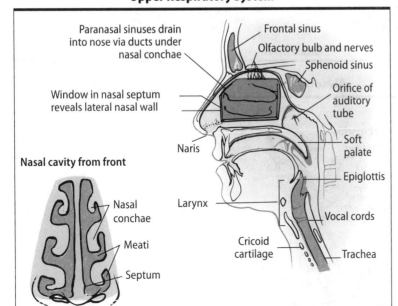

Paranasal sinuses drain into nose via ducts under nasal conchae
Window in nasal septum reveals lateral nasal wall
Frontal sinus
Olfactory bulb and nerves
Sphenoid sinus
Orifice of auditory tube
Naris
Soft palate
Epiglottis
Larynx
Vocal cords
Cricoid cartilage
Trachea

Nasal cavity from front
Nasal conchae
Meati
Septum

Nasal Turbinates

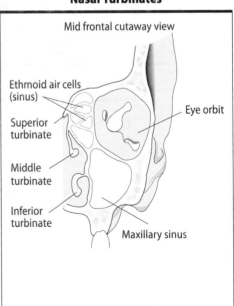

Mid frontal cutaway view
Ethmoid air cells (sinus)
Superior turbinate
Middle turbinate
Inferior turbinate
Eye orbit
Maxillary sinus

Paranasal Sinuses

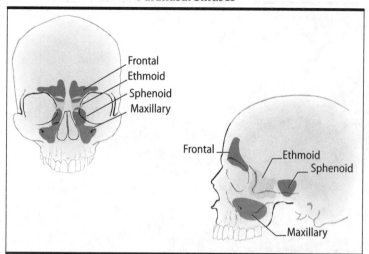

- Frontal
- Ethmoid
- Sphenoid
- Maxillary

Frontal
Ethmoid
Sphenoid
Maxillary

Lower Respiratory System

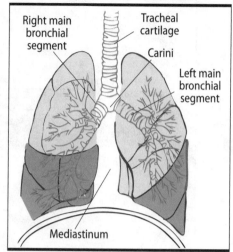

Right main bronchial segment
Tracheal cartilage
Carini
Left main bronchial segment
Mediastinum

Lung Segments

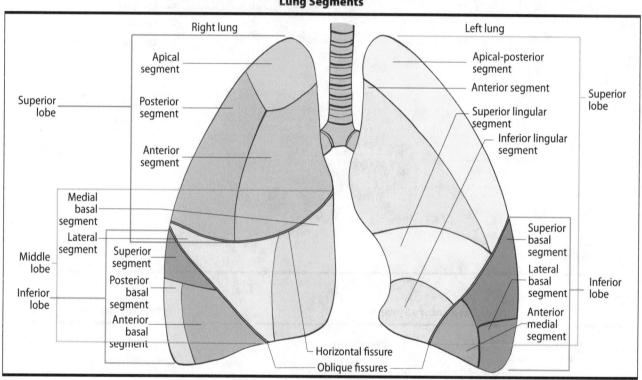

Right lung
Left lung

Apical segment
Posterior segment
Anterior segment

Superior lobe

Medial basal segment
Lateral segment

Middle lobe

Inferior lobe

Superior segment
Posterior basal segment
Anterior basal segment

Apical-posterior segment
Anterior segment
Superior lingular segment
Inferior lingular segment

Superior lobe

Superior basal segment
Lateral basal segment
Anterior medial segment

Inferior lobe

Horizontal fissure
Oblique fissures

Alveoli

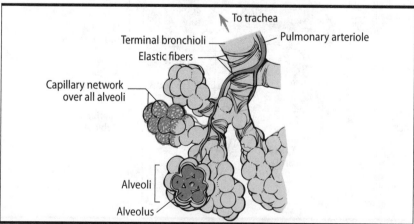

To trachea
Terminal bronchioli
Elastic fibers
Pulmonary arteriole
Capillary network over all alveoli
Alveoli
Alveolus

Arterial System

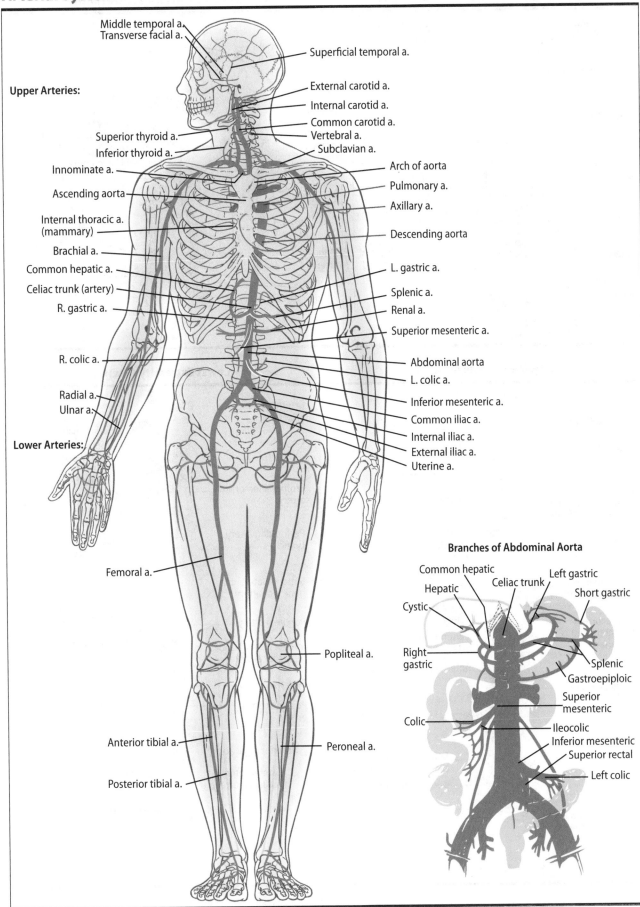

Upper Arteries:

Middle temporal a.
Transverse facial a.
Superficial temporal a.
External carotid a.
Internal carotid a.
Common carotid a.
Superior thyroid a.
Vertebral a.
Inferior thyroid a.
Subclavian a.
Innominate a.
Arch of aorta
Ascending aorta
Pulmonary a.
Axillary a.
Internal thoracic a. (mammary)
Descending aorta
Brachial a.
Common hepatic a.
L. gastric a.
Celiac trunk (artery)
Splenic a.
R. gastric a.
Renal a.
Superior mesenteric a.
R. colic a.
Abdominal aorta
L. colic a.
Radial a.
Inferior mesenteric a.
Ulnar a.
Common iliac a.
Internal iliac a.

Lower Arteries:

External iliac a.
Uterine a.

Femoral a.

Popliteal a.

Anterior tibial a.
Peroneal a.

Posterior tibial a.

Branches of Abdominal Aorta

Common hepatic
Left gastric
Hepatic
Celiac trunk
Short gastric
Cystic
Right gastric
Splenic
Gastroepiploic
Superior mesenteric
Colic
Ileocolic
Inferior mesenteric
Superior rectal
Left colic

Internal Carotid and Arteries and Branches

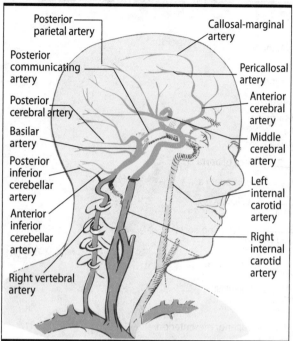

Posterior parietal artery
Callosal-marginal artery
Posterior communicating artery
Pericallosal artery
Anterior cerebral artery
Posterior cerebral artery
Middle cerebral artery
Basilar artery
Posterior inferior cerebellar artery
Left internal carotid artery
Anterior inferior cerebellar artery
Right internal carotid artery
Right vertebral artery

External Carotid Arteries and Branches

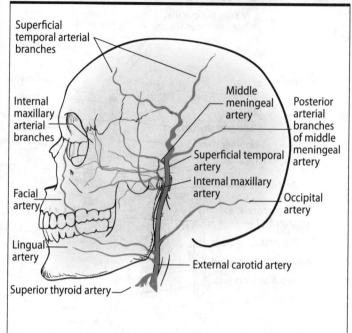

Superficial temporal arterial branches
Middle meningeal artery
Internal maxillary arterial branches
Posterior arterial branches of middle meningeal artery
Superficial temporal artery
Facial artery
Internal maxillary artery
Occipital artery
Lingual artery
External carotid artery
Superior thyroid artery

Upper Extremity Arteries

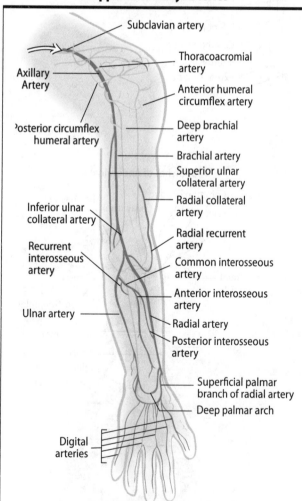

Subclavian artery
Thoracoacromial artery
Axillary Artery
Anterior humeral circumflex artery
Posterior circumflex humeral artery
Deep brachial artery
Brachial artery
Superior ulnar collateral artery
Radial collateral artery
Inferior ulnar collateral artery
Radial recurrent artery
Recurrent interosseous artery
Common interosseous artery
Anterior interosseous artery
Ulnar artery
Radial artery
Posterior interosseous artery
Superficial palmar branch of radial artery
Deep palmar arch
Digital arteries

Lower Extremity Arteries

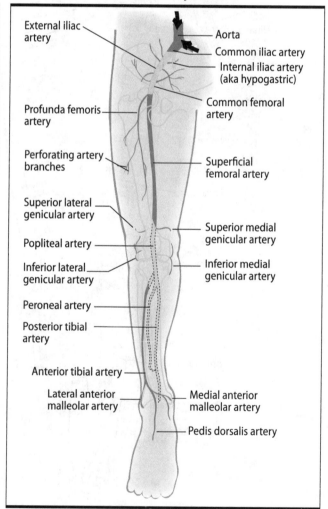

External iliac artery
Aorta
Common iliac artery
Internal iliac artery (aka hypogastric)
Profunda femoris artery
Common femoral artery
Perforating artery branches
Superficial femoral artery
Superior lateral genicular artery
Superior medial genicular artery
Popliteal artery
Inferior lateral genicular artery
Inferior medial genicular artery
Peroneal artery
Posterior tibial artery
Anterior tibial artery
Lateral anterior malleolar artery
Medial anterior malleolar artery
Pedis dorsalis artery

Venous System

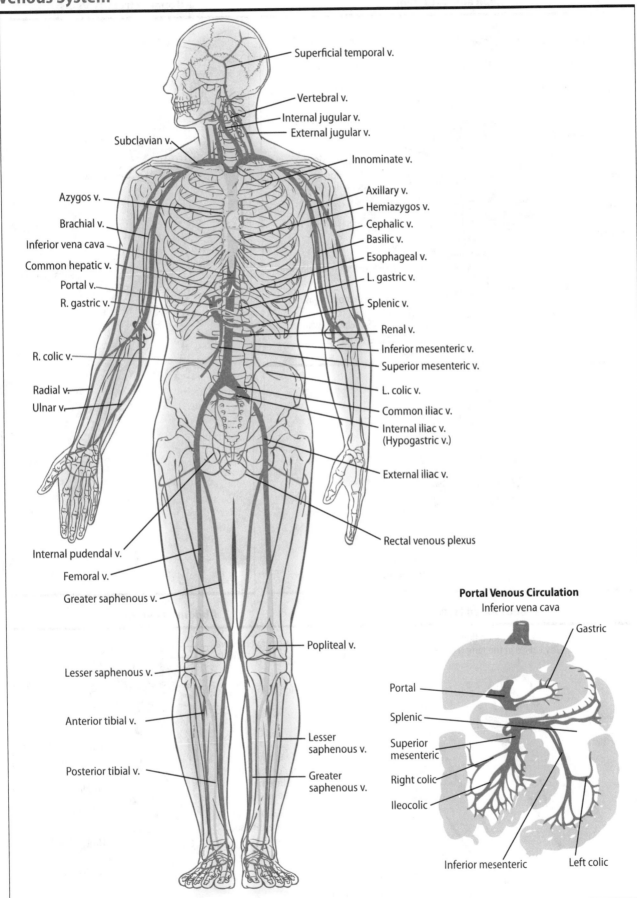

Superficial temporal v.

Vertebral v.

Internal jugular v.

External jugular v.

Subclavian v.

Innominate v.

Azygos v.

Axillary v.

Hemiazygos v.

Brachial v.

Cephalic v.

Inferior vena cava

Basilic v.

Common hepatic v.

Esophageal v.

Portal v.

L. gastric v.

R. gastric v.

Splenic v.

Renal v.

R. colic v.

Inferior mesenteric v.

Superior mesenteric v.

Radial v.

L. colic v.

Ulnar v.

Common iliac v.

Internal iliac v.
(Hypogastric v.)

External iliac v.

Rectal venous plexus

Internal pudendal v.

Femoral v.

Greater saphenous v.

Portal Venous Circulation

Inferior vena cava

Popliteal v.

Gastric

Lesser saphenous v.

Portal

Anterior tibial v.

Splenic

Lesser
saphenous v.

Superior
mesenteric

Posterior tibial v.

Right colic

Greater
saphenous v.

Ileocolic

Inferior mesenteric

Left colic

Head and Neck Veins

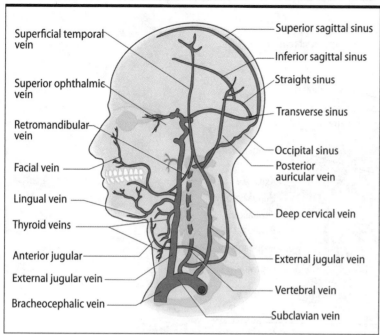

- Superficial temporal vein
- Superior ophthalmic vein
- Retromandibular vein
- Facial vein
- Lingual vein
- Thyroid veins
- Anterior jugular
- External jugular vein
- Bracheocephalic vein
- Superior sagittal sinus
- Inferior sagittal sinus
- Straight sinus
- Transverse sinus
- Occipital sinus
- Posterior auricular vein
- Deep cervical vein
- External jugular vein
- Vertebral vein
- Subclavian vein

Upper Extremity Veins

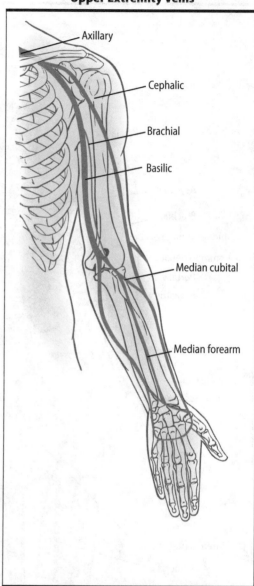

- Axillary
- Cephalic
- Brachial
- Basilic
- Median cubital
- Median forearm

Venae Comitantes

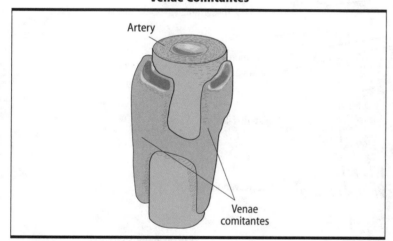

- Artery
- Venae comitantes

Venous Blood Flow

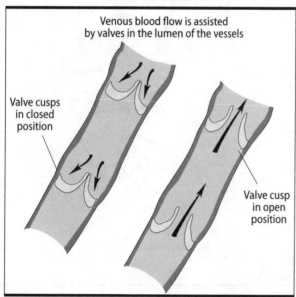

Venous blood flow is assisted by valves in the lumen of the vessels

- Valve cusps in closed position
- Valve cusp in open position

Abdominal Veins

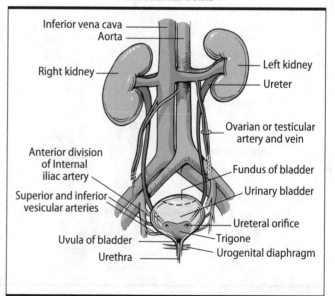

- Inferior vena cava
- Aorta
- Right kidney
- Left kidney
- Ureter
- Ovarian or testicular artery and vein
- Anterior division of Internal iliac artery
- Fundus of bladder
- Urinary bladder
- Superior and inferior vesicular arteries
- Ureteral orifice
- Uvula of bladder
- Trigone
- Urogenital diaphragm
- Urethra

Cardiovascular System

Coronary Veins

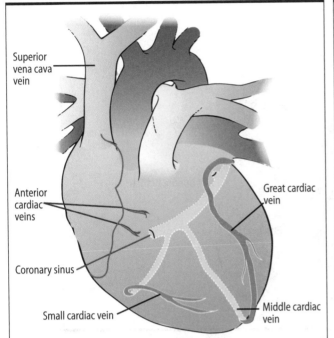

- Superior vena cava vein
- Anterior cardiac veins
- Coronary sinus
- Small cardiac vein
- Great cardiac vein
- Middle cardiac vein

Anatomy of the Heart

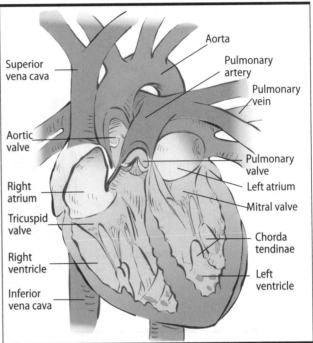

- Aorta
- Pulmonary artery
- Pulmonary vein
- Superior vena cava
- Aortic valve
- Right atrium
- Tricuspid valve
- Right ventricle
- Inferior vena cava
- Pulmonary valve
- Left atrium
- Mitral valve
- Chorda tendinae
- Left ventricle

Heart Cross Section

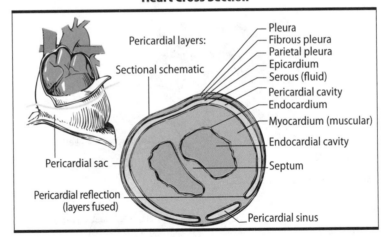

Pericardial layers:

- Sectional schematic
- Pleura
- Fibrous pleura
- Parietal pleura
- Epicardium
- Serous (fluid)
- Pericardial cavity
- Endocardium
- Myocardium (muscular)
- Endocardial cavity
- Septum
- Pericardial sac
- Pericardial reflection (layers fused)
- Pericardial sinus

Heart Valves

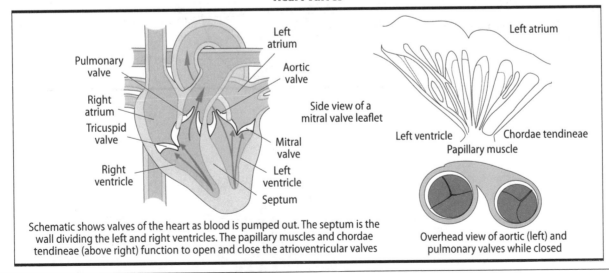

- Pulmonary valve
- Right atrium
- Tricuspid valve
- Right ventricle
- Left atrium
- Aortic valve
- Mitral valve
- Left ventricle
- Septum

- Left atrium
- Left ventricle
- Chordae tendineae
- Papillary muscle

Side view of a mitral valve leaflet

Schematic shows valves of the heart as blood is pumped out. The septum is the wall dividing the left and right ventricles. The papillary muscles and chordae tendineae (above right) function to open and close the atrioventricular valves

Overhead view of aortic (left) and pulmonary valves while closed

Anatomical Illustrations—Cardiovascular System

Heart Conduction System

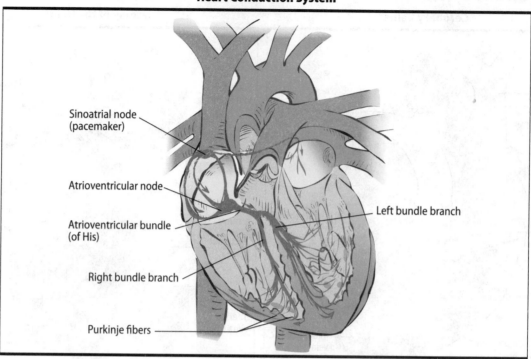

Sinoatrial node (pacemaker)

Atrioventricular node

Atrioventricular bundle (of His)

Right bundle branch

Left bundle branch

Purkinje fibers

Coronary Arteries

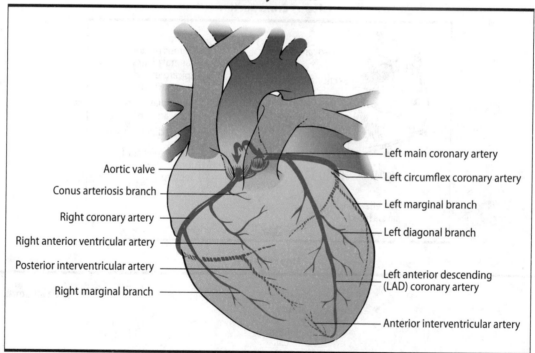

Aortic valve

Conus arteriosis branch

Right coronary artery

Right anterior ventricular artery

Posterior interventricular artery

Right marginal branch

Left main coronary artery

Left circumflex coronary artery

Left marginal branch

Left diagonal branch

Left anterior descending (LAD) coronary artery

Anterior interventricular artery

© 2016 Optum360, LLC

Lymphatic System

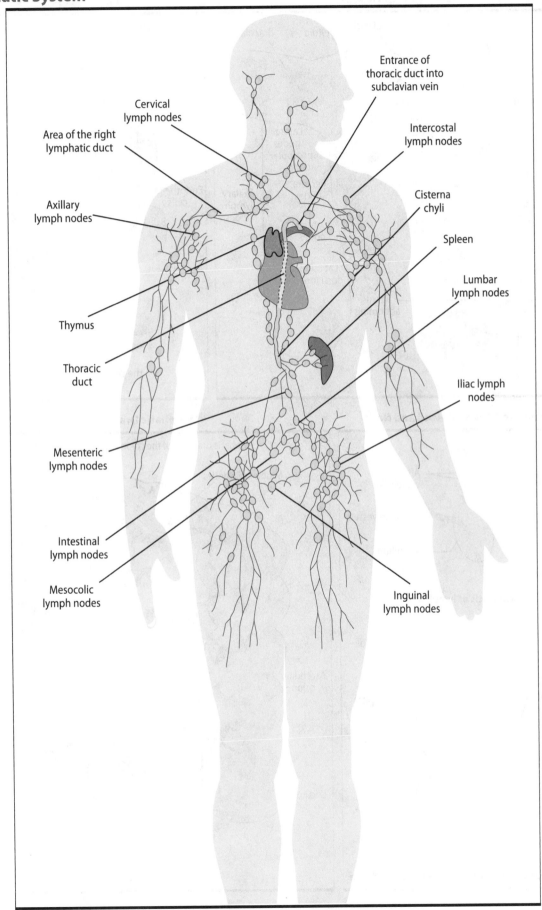

Cervical
lymph nodes

Entrance of
thoracic duct into
subclavian vein

Area of the right
lymphatic duct

Intercostal
lymph nodes

Axillary
lymph nodes

Cisterna
chyli

Spleen

Lumbar
lymph nodes

Thymus

Thoracic
duct

Iliac lymph
nodes

Mesenteric
lymph nodes

Intestinal
lymph nodes

Mesocolic
lymph nodes

Inguinal
lymph nodes

Axillary Lymph Nodes

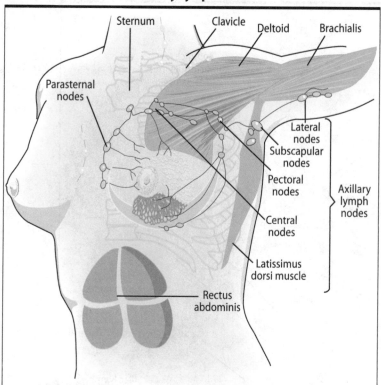

Lymphatic Capillaries

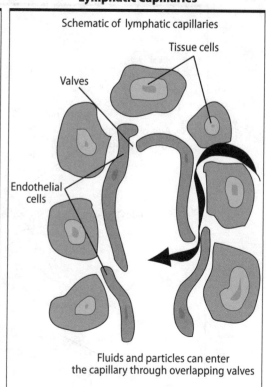

Schematic of lymphatic capillaries

Fluids and particles can enter
the capillary through overlapping valves

Lymphatic System of Head and Neck

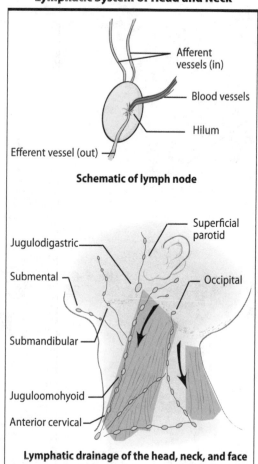

Schematic of lymph node

Lymphatic drainage of the head, neck, and face

Lymphatic Drainage

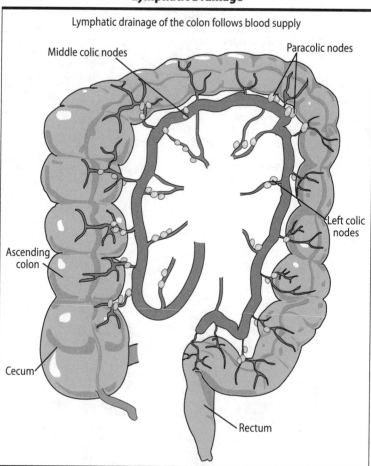

Lymphatic drainage of the colon follows blood supply

              © 2016 Optum360, LLC

Spleen Internal Structures

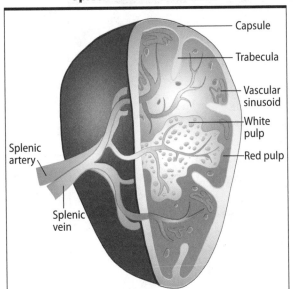

Capsule

Trabecula

Vascular sinusoid

White pulp

Red pulp

Splenic artery

Splenic vein

Spleen External Structures

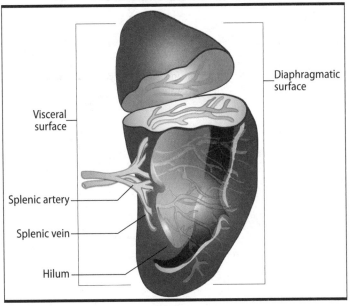

Diaphragmatic surface

Visceral surface

Splenic artery

Splenic vein

Hilum

Anatomical Illustrations—Lymphatic System

Digestive System

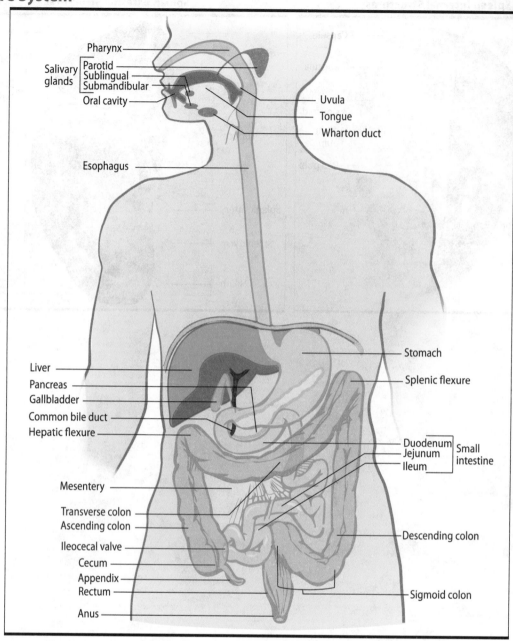

- Pharynx
- Salivary glands
  - Parotid
  - Sublingual
  - Submandibular
- Oral cavity
- Uvula
- Tongue
- Wharton duct
- Esophagus
- Liver
- Pancreas
- Gallbladder
- Common bile duct
- Hepatic flexure
- Stomach
- Splenic flexure
- Duodenum
- Jejunum — Small intestine
- Ileum
- Mesentery
- Transverse colon
- Ascending colon
- Descending colon
- Ileocecal valve
- Cecum
- Appendix
- Rectum
- Sigmoid colon
- Anus

Gallbladder

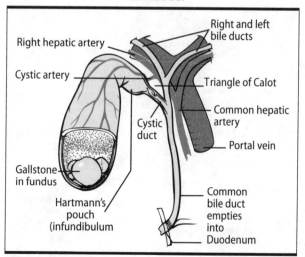

- Right hepatic artery
- Cystic artery
- Gallstone in fundus
- Hartmann's pouch (infundibulum
- Cystic duct
- Right and left bile ducts
- Triangle of Calot
- Common hepatic artery
- Portal vein
- Common bile duct empties into Duodenum

Stomach

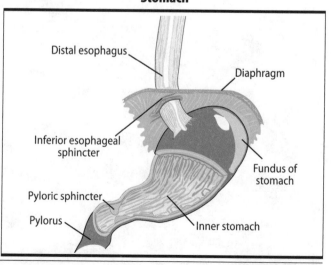

- Distal esophagus
- Inferior esophageal sphincter
- Pyloric sphincter
- Pylorus
- Diaphragm
- Fundus of stomach
- Inner stomach

Mouth (Upper)

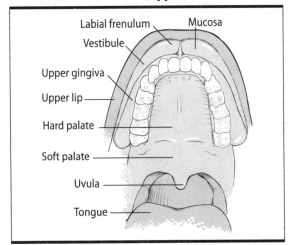

Labial frenulum
Mucosa
Vestibule
Upper gingiva
Upper lip
Hard palate
Soft palate
Uvula
Tongue

Mouth (Lower)

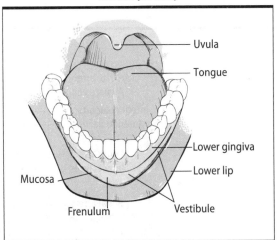

Uvula
Tongue
Lower gingiva
Lower lip
Mucosa
Vestibule
Frenulum

Pancreas

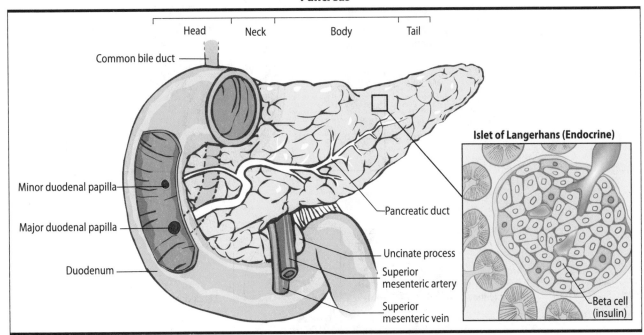

Head　Neck　Body　Tail

Common bile duct

Minor duodenal papilla

Major duodenal papilla

Duodenum

Pancreatic duct

Uncinate process

Superior mesenteric artery

Superior mesenteric vein

Islet of Langerhans (Endocrine)

Beta cell (insulin)

Liver

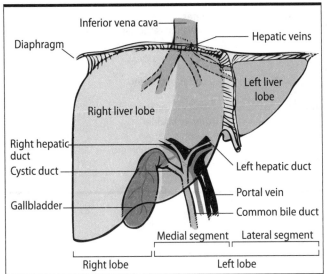

Inferior vena cava
Hepatic veins
Diaphragm
Left liver lobe
Right liver lobe
Right hepatic duct
Cystic duct
Gallbladder
Left hepatic duct
Portal vein
Common bile duct
Medial segment　Lateral segment
Right lobe　Left lobe

Anus

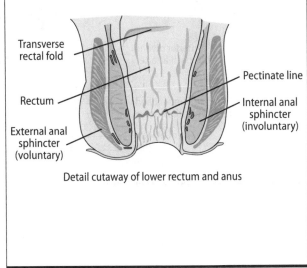

Transverse rectal fold
Rectum
External anal sphincter (voluntary)
Pectinate line
Internal anal sphincter (involuntary)

Detail cutaway of lower rectum and anus

Genitourinary System

Urinary System

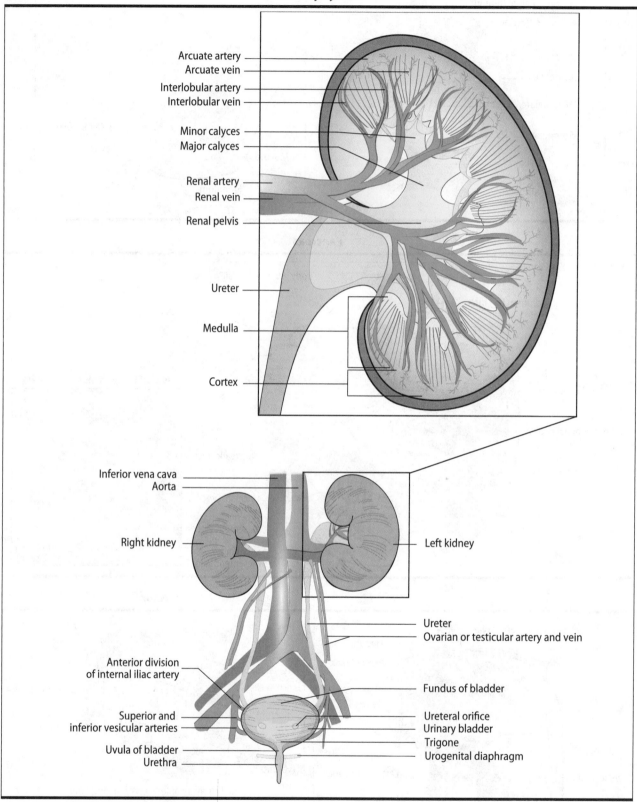

© 2016 Optum360, LLC

Nephron

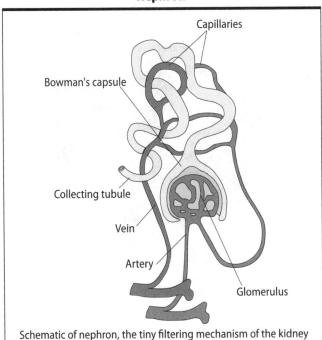

Schematic of nephron, the tiny filtering mechanism of the kidney

Male Genitourinary

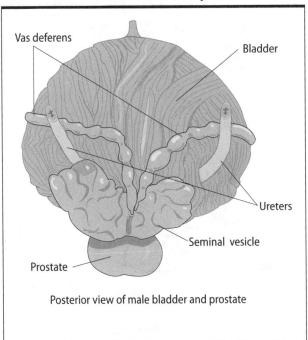

Posterior view of male bladder and prostate

Testis and Associate Structures

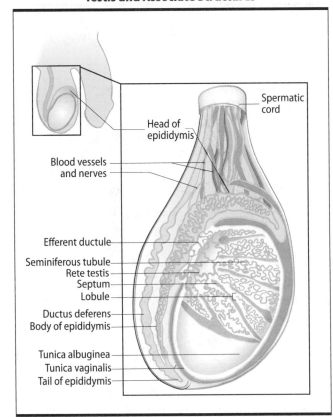

Male Genitourinary System

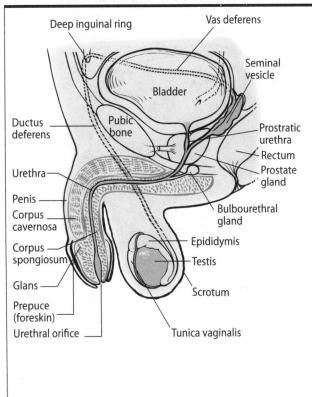

Female Genitourinary

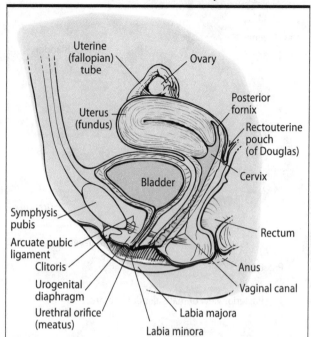

Female Reproductive System

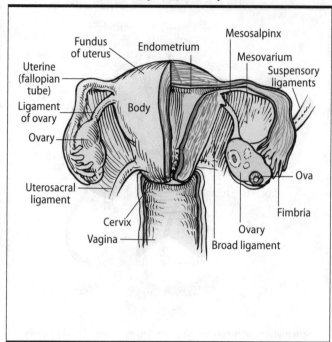

Female Bladder

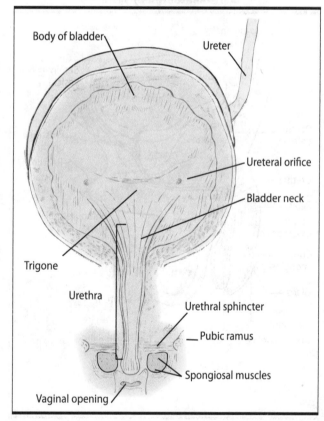

Female Breast

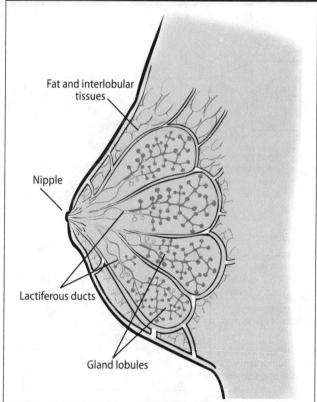

Endocrine System

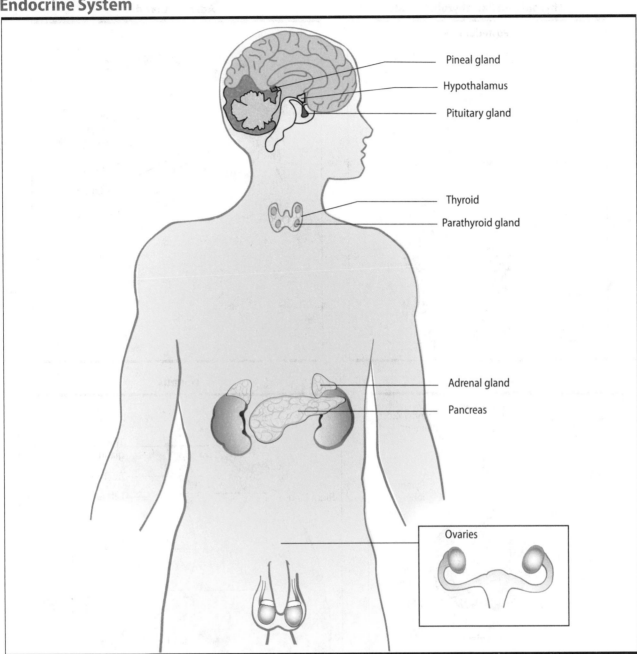

- Pineal gland
- Hypothalamus
- Pituitary gland
- Thyroid
- Parathyroid gland
- Adrenal gland
- Pancreas
- Ovaries

Structure of an Ovary

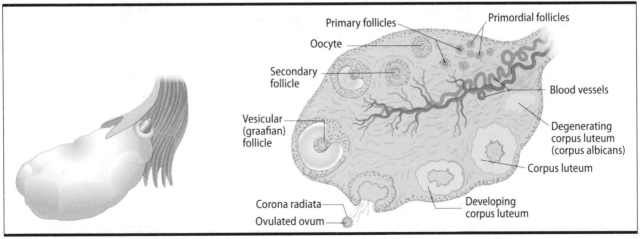

- Primary follicles
- Primordial follicles
- Oocyte
- Secondary follicle
- Vesicular (graafian) follicle
- Blood vessels
- Degenerating corpus luteum (corpus albicans)
- Corpus luteum
- Developing corpus luteum
- Corona radiata
- Ovulated ovum

Thyroid and Parathyroid Glands

Posterior view

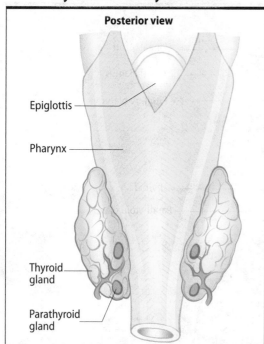

Epiglottis

Pharynx

Thyroid gland

Parathyroid gland

Adrenal Gland

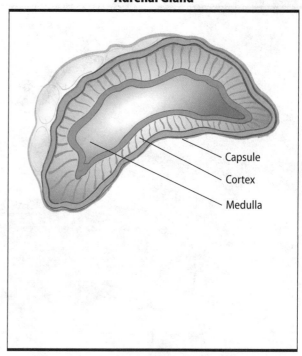

Capsule

Cortex

Medulla

Thyroid

Anterior view

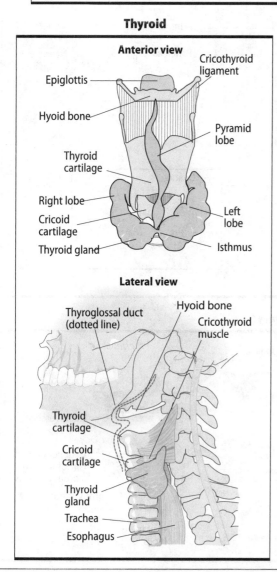

Epiglottis

Cricothyroid ligament

Hyoid bone

Pyramid lobe

Thyroid cartilage

Right lobe

Left lobe

Cricoid cartilage

Thyroid gland

Isthmus

Lateral view

Thyroglossal duct (dotted line)

Hyoid bone

Cricothyroid muscle

Thyroid cartilage

Cricoid cartilage

Thyroid gland

Trachea

Esophagus

Thymus

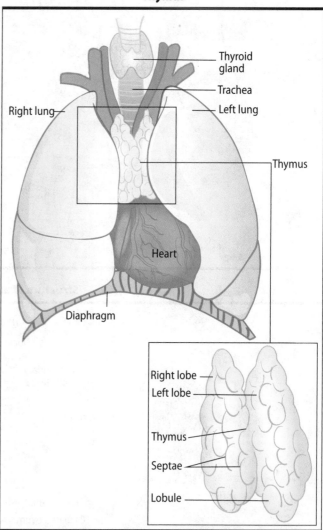

Right lung

Thyroid gland

Trachea

Left lung

Thymus

Heart

Diaphragm

Right lobe

Left lobe

Thymus

Septae

Lobule

Nervous System

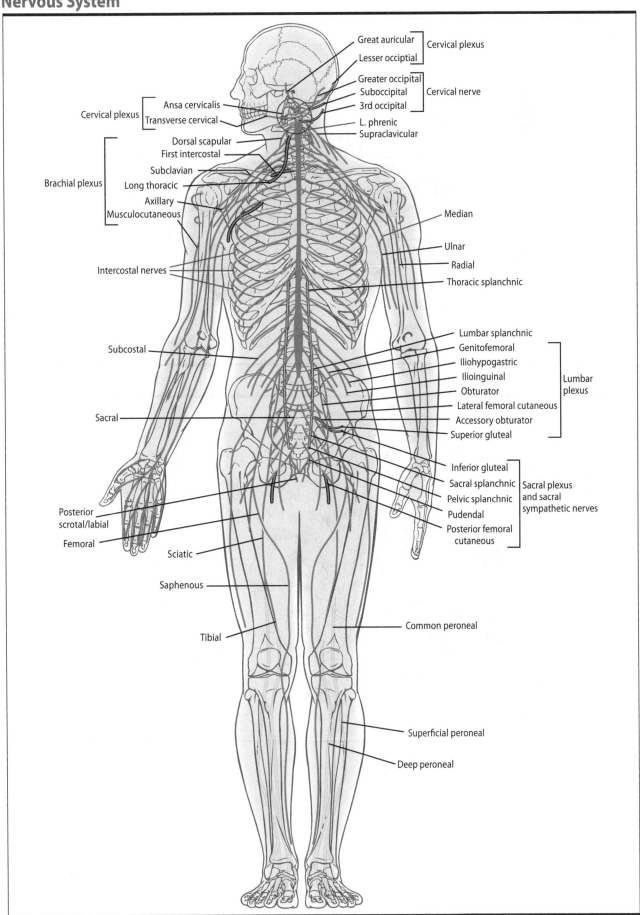

Anatomical Illustrations—Nervous System

Brain

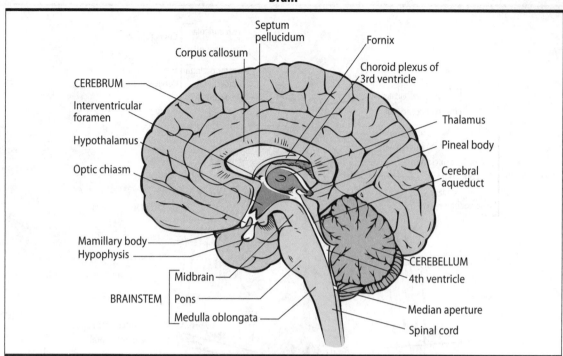

Septum pellucidum

Corpus callosum

Fornix

Choroid plexus of 3rd ventricle

CEREBRUM

Interventricular foramen

Hypothalamus

Optic chiasm

Thalamus

Pineal body

Cerebral aqueduct

Mamillary body
Hypophysis

Midbrain

BRAINSTEM   Pons

Medulla oblongata

CEREBELLUM

4th ventricle

Median aperture

Spinal cord

Cranial Nerves

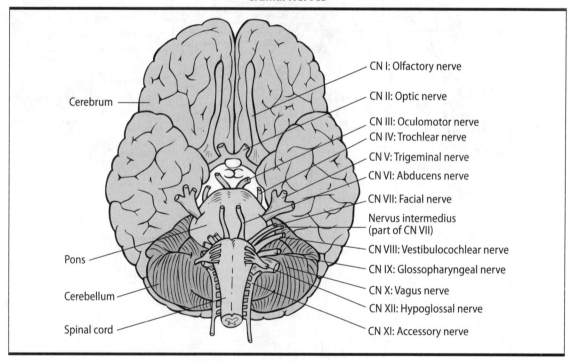

Cerebrum

Pons

Cerebellum

Spinal cord

CN I: Olfactory nerve

CN II: Optic nerve

CN III: Oculomotor nerve

CN IV: Trochlear nerve

CN V: Trigeminal nerve

CN VI: Abducens nerve

CN VII: Facial nerve

Nervus intermedius (part of CN VII)

CN VIII: Vestibulocochlear nerve

CN IX: Glossopharyngeal nerve

CN X: Vagus nerve

CN XII: Hypoglossal nerve

CN XI: Accessory nerve

Spinal Cord and Spinal Nerves

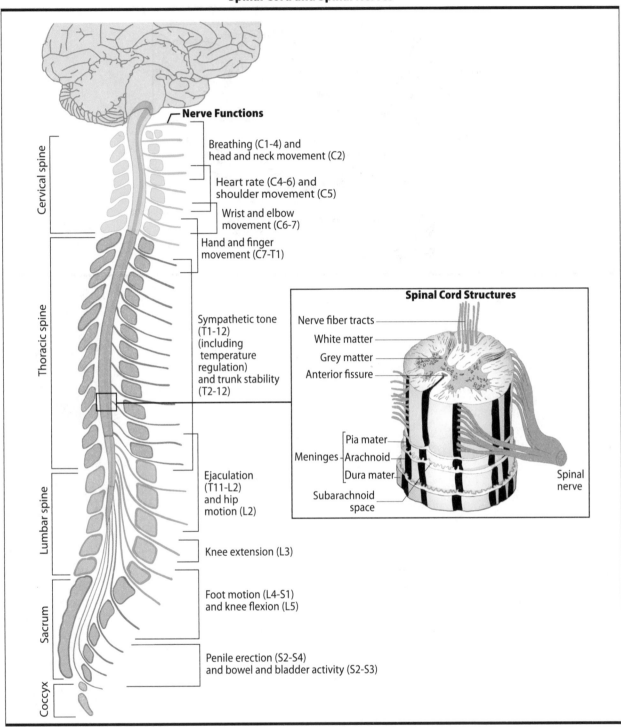

Nerve Functions

Breathing (C1-4) and head and neck movement (C2)

Heart rate (C4-6) and shoulder movement (C5)

Wrist and elbow movement (C6-7)

Hand and finger movement (C7-T1)

Sympathetic tone (T1-12) (including temperature regulation) and trunk stability (T2-12)

Ejaculation (T11-L2) and hip motion (L2)

Knee extension (L3)

Foot motion (L4-S1) and knee flexion (L5)

Penile erection (S2-S4) and bowel and bladder activity (S2-S3)

Cervical spine

Thoracic spine

Lumbar spine

Sacrum

Coccyx

Spinal Cord Structures

Nerve fiber tracts

White matter

Grey matter

Anterior fissure

Meninges
- Pia mater
- Arachnoid
- Dura mater

Subarachnoid space

Spinal nerve

Nerve Cell

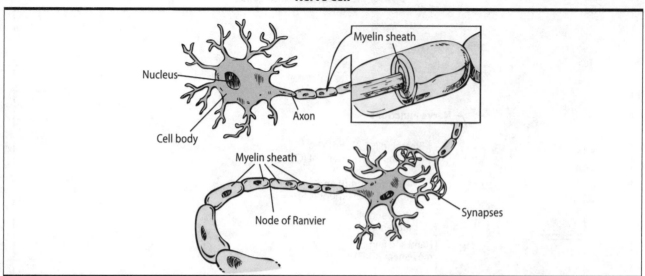

Eye

Eye Structure

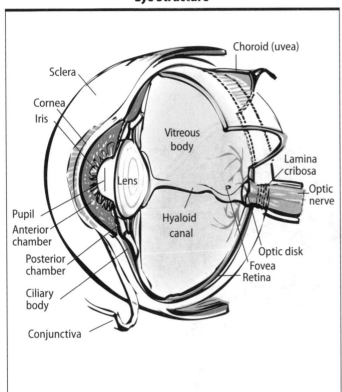

- Sclera
- Cornea
- Iris
- Choroid (uvea)
- Vitreous body
- Lens
- Lamina cribosa
- Optic nerve
- Pupil
- Anterior chamber
- Posterior chamber
- Ciliary body
- Conjunctiva
- Hyaloid canal
- Optic disk
- Fovea
- Retina

Posterior Pole of Globe/Flow of Aqueous Humor

Posterior Pole of Globe

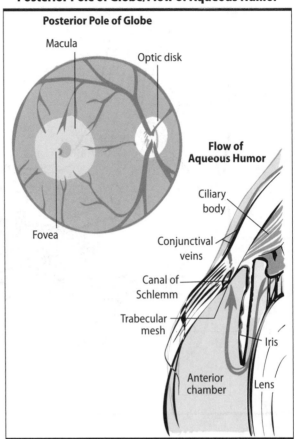

- Macula
- Optic disk
- Fovea

Flow of Aqueous Humor

- Ciliary body
- Conjunctival veins
- Canal of Schlemm
- Trabecular mesh
- Iris
- Anterior chamber
- Lens

Eye Musculature

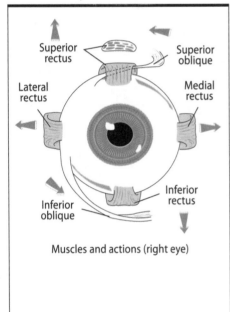

- Superior rectus
- Superior oblique
- Lateral rectus
- Medial rectus
- Inferior oblique
- Inferior rectus

Muscles and actions (right eye)

Eyelid Structures

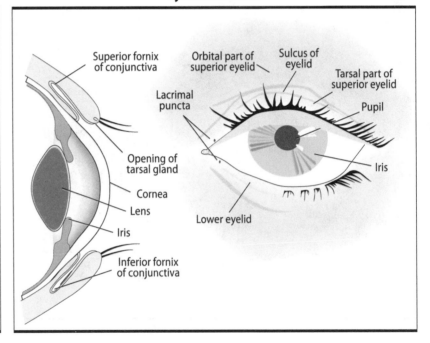

- Superior fornix of conjunctiva
- Lacrimal puncta
- Orbital part of superior eyelid
- Sulcus of eyelid
- Tarsal part of superior eyelid
- Pupil
- Opening of tarsal gland
- Cornea
- Lens
- Iris
- Lower eyelid
- Iris
- Inferior fornix of conjunctiva

Ear and Lacrimal System

Ear Anatomy

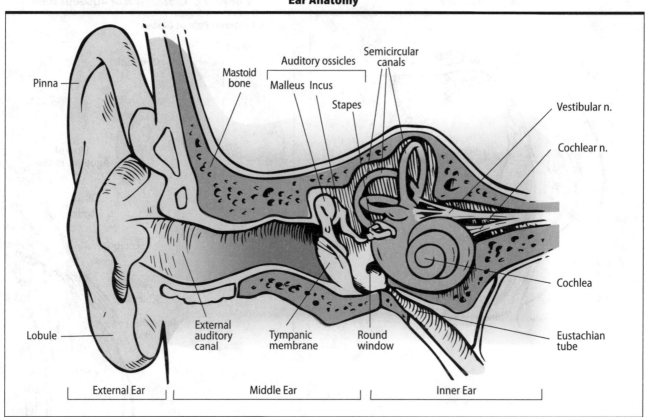

Lacrimal System

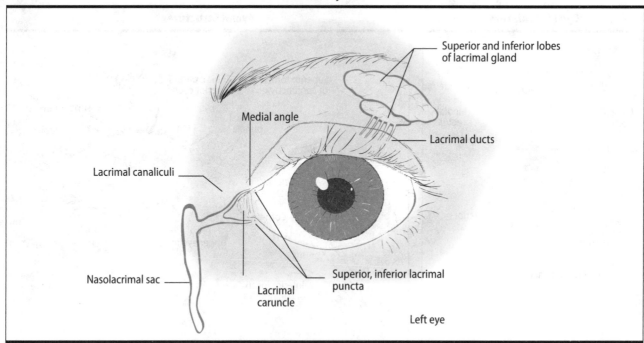

© 2016 Optum360, LLC

0-Numeric

3-Beta-Hydroxysteroid Dehydrogenase Type II Deficiency, 81404
3-Methylcrotonyl-CoA Carboxylase 1, 81406
5,10-Methylenetetrahydrofolate Reductase, 81291

A

Abbe–Estlander Procedure, 40527, 40761
ABBI Biopsy, 19081-19086
ABCA4, 81408
ABCC8, 81401, 81407
ABCD1, 81405
Abdomen, Abdominal
  Abscess, 49020, 49040
    Incision and Drainage
      Skin and Subcutaneous Tissue, 10060-10061
      Open, 49040
        Peritoneal, 49020
        Peritonitis, Localized, 49020
        Retroperitoneal, 49060
        Subdiaphragmatic, 49040
        Subphrenic, 49040
  Angiography, 74175, 75635
  Aorta
    Aneurysm, 34800-34805, 34825-34832, 34841-34848, 35081-35103, 75952, 75953
    Angiography, 75635
    Aortography, 75625, 75630
    Thromboendarterectomy, 35331
    Aortic Aneurysm, 34800-34805, 34825-34832, 34841-34848, 35081-35103, 75952, 75953
  Artery
    Ligation, 37617
  Biopsy
    Open, 49000
    Percutaneous, 49180
    Skin and Subcutaneous Tissue, 11100, 11101
  Bypass Graft, 35907
  Cannula/catheter
    Insertion, 49419, 49421
    Removal, 49422
  Catheter
    Removal, 49422
  Celiotomy
    for Staging, 49220
  CT Scan, 74150-74178, 75635
  Cyst
    Destruction/Excision, 49203-49205
    Sclerotherapy, 49185
  Delivery
    with Hysterectomy, 59525
    After Attempted Vaginal Delivery
      Delivery Only, 59620
        Postpartum Care, 59622
        Routine Care, 59618
    Delivery Only, 59514
    Peritoneal Abscess
      Open, 49020
      Peritonitis, localized, 49020
    Postpartum Care, 59515
    Routine Care, 59510
    Tubal Ligation at Time of, 58611
  Drainage, 49020, 49040
    Fluid, 49082-49083
    Retroperitoneal
      Open, 49060
    Skin and Subcutaneous Tissue, 10060-10061
    Subdiaphragmatic
      Open, 49040
    Subphrenic
      Open, 49040
  Ectopic Pregnancy, 59130
  Endometrioma, 49203-49205
    Destruction/Excision, 49203-49205
  Excision
    Excess Skin, 15830
    Tumor, Abdominal Wall, 22900
  Exploration, 49000-49084
    Blood Vessel, 35840

Abdomen, Abdominal — *continued*
  Exploration — *continued*
    Staging, 58960
  Hernia Repair, 49491-49590, 49650-49659
  Incision, 49000-49084
    Staging, 58960
  Incision and Drainage
    Pancreatitis, 48000
  Infraumbilical Panniculectomy, 15830
  Injection
    Air, 49400
    Contrast Material, 49400
  Insertion
    Catheter, 49324, 49418-49421
    Venous Shunt, 49425
  Intraperitoneal
    Catheter Exit Site, 49436
    Catheter Insertion, 49324, 49418-49421, 49425, 49435
    Catheter Removal, 49422
    Catheter Revision, 49325
    Shunt
      Insertion, 49425
      Ligation, 49428
      Removal, 49429
      Revision, 49426
  Laparoscopy, 49320-49329
  Laparotomy
    with Biopsy, 49000
    Exploration, 47015, 49000-49002, 58960
    Hemorrhage Control, 49002
    Reopening, 49002
    Second Look, 58960
    Staging, 49220, 58960
  Lymphangiogram, 75805, 75807
  Magnetic Resonance Imaging (MRI), 74181-74183
    Fetal, 74712-74713
  Needle Biopsy
    Mass, 49180
  Pancreatitis, 48000
  Paracentesis, 49082-49083
  Peritoneal Abscess, 49020
  Peritoneal Lavage, 49084
  Placement Guidance Devices, 49411-49412
  Radical Resection, 51597
  Removal Node(s), 49220
  Repair
    Blood Vessel, 35221
      with
        Other Graft, 35281
        Vein Graft, 35251
    Hernia, 49491-49590, 49650-49659
    Suture, 49900
  Revision
    Venous Shunt, 49426
  Suture, 49900
  Tumor
    Destruction/Excision, 49203-49205
  Tumor Staging, 58960
  Ultrasound, 76700, 76705, 76706
  Unlisted Services and Procedures, 49999
  Wall
    See Abdomen, X–Ray
    Debridement
      Infected, 11005-11006
    Implant
      Fascial Reinforcement, 0437T
    Reconstruction, 49905
    Removal
      Mesh, 11008
      Prosthesis, 11008
    Repair
      Hernia, 49491-49590
        by Laparoscopy, 49650-49651
    Surgery, 22999
    Tumor
      Excision, 22900-22905
  Wound Exploration
    Penetrating, 20102
  X–ray, 74000-74022
Abdominal Plane Block
  Bilateral, 64488-64489
  Unilateral, 64486-64487
Abdominohysterectomy
  Radical, 58210

Abdominohysterectomy — *continued*
  Resection of Ovarian Malignancy, 58951, 58953-58954, 58956
  Supracervical, 58180
  Total, 58150, 58200
    with Colpo-Urethrocystopexy, 58152
    with Omentectomy, 58956
    with Partial Vaginectomy, 58200
Abdominoplasty, 15830, 15847, 17999
ABG, 82803, 82805
ABL1, 81401
Ablation
  Anal
    Polyp, 46615
    Tumor, 46615
  Atria, 33257-33259
  Bone Tumor, 20982-20983
  Colon
    Polyp(s), [45346]
    Tumor, [45346]
  Cryosurgical
    Fibroadenoma, 19105
    Liver Tumor(s), 47381
    Renal mass, 50250
    Renal Tumor
      Percutaneous, 50593
  CT Scan Guidance, 77013
  Endometrial, 58353, 58356, 58563
  Endometrium
    Ultrasound Guidance, 58356
  Endoscopic
    Duodenum/Jejunum, [43270]
    Esophagus, 43229, [43270]
    Hepatobiliary System, [43278]
    Stomach, [43270]
  Heart
    Arrhythmogenic Focus, 93650-93657
      Intracardiac Catheter, 93650-93657
      Open, 33250-33261
    Intracardiac Pacing and Mapping, 93631
      Follow-up Study, 93624
      Stimulation and Pacing, 93623
  Liver
    Tumor, 47380-47383
      Ablation
        Cryoablation, 47381, 47383
        Radiofrequency, 47380, 47382
      Laparoscopic, 47370-47371
        Cryosurgical, 47371
      Open, 47380-47381
  Lung
    Tumor
      Radiofrequency, 32998
  Magnetic Resonance Guidance, 77022
  Nerve
    Cryoablation, 0440T-0442T
  Parenchymal Tissue
    CT Scan Guidance, 77013
    Magnetic Resonance Guidance, 77022
    Ultrasound Guidance, 76940
  Prostate, 55873
    Transurethral Waterjet, 0421T
  Pulmonary Tumor
    Cryoablation, 0340T
    Radiofrequency, 32998
  Radiofrequency
    Liver Tumor(s), 47382
    Lung Tumor(s), 32998
    Renal Tumor(s), 50592
    Tongue Base, 41530
  Renal
    Cyst, 50541
    Mass, 50542
      Radiofrequency, 50592
    Tumor, 50593
      Cryotherapy
        Percutaneous, 50593
  Supraventricular Arrhythmogenic Focus, 33250-33251
  Tongue Base
    Radiofrequency, 41530
  Turbinate Mucosa, 30801, 30802
  Ultrasound
    Guidance, 76940
    Ultrasound Focused, 0071T-0072T
    Uterine Tumor, 0071T-0072T

Ablation — *continued*
  Uterus
    Fibroids, 0404T, 58674
    Leiomyomata, 0071T-0072T
    Tumor
      Ultrasound, Focused, 0071T-0072T
  Vein
    Endovenous, 36473-36479
  Ventricular Arrhythmogenic Focus, 33261
ABLB Test, 92562
ABO, 86900
Abortion
  See Obstetrical Care
  Incomplete, 59812
  Induced by
    with Hysterotomy, 59100, 59852, 59857
    Amniocentesis Injection, 59850-59852
    Dilation and Curettage, 59840
    Dilation and Evacuation, 59841
    Saline, 59850, 59851
    Vaginal Suppositories, 59855, 59856
  Missed
    First Trimester, 59820
    Second Trimester, 59821
  Septic, 59830
  Spontaneous, 59812
  Therapeutic, 59840-59852
    by Saline, 59850
      with Dilatation and Curettage, 59851
      with Hysterotomy, 59852
ABR, 92585-92586
Abrasion, Skin
  Chemical Peel, 15788-15793
  Dermabrasion, 15780-15783
  Lesion, 15786, 15787
ABS, 86255, 86403, 86850
Abscess
  Abdomen, 49040
    Drainage, 49020, 49040
      Peritoneal
        Open, 49020
      Peritonitis, Localized, 49020
      Retroperitoneal
        Open, 49060
      Skin and Subcutaneous Tissue
        Complicated, 10061
        Multiple, 10061
        Simple, 10060
        Single, 10060
      Subdiaphragmatic
        Open, 49040
      Subphrenic, 49040
    Incision and Drainage
      Open, 49040
  Anal
    Incision and Drainage, 46045, 46050
  Ankle
    Incision and Drainage
      Bone Abscess, 27607
      Deep Abscess, 27603
      Hematoma, 27603
  Appendix
    Incision and Drainage, 44900
  Arm, Lower, 25028
    Bone Abscess, 25035
    Excision, 25145
    Incision and Drainage, 25035
    Sequestrectomy, 25145
  Arm, Upper
    Incision and Drainage, 23930-23935
  Auditory Canal, External, 69020
  Bartholin's Gland
    Incision and Drainage, 56420
  Bladder
    Incision and Drainage, 51080
  Brain
    Drainage by
      Burr Hole, 61150, 61151
      Craniotomy/Craniectomy, 61320, 61321
    Excision, 61514, 61522
    Incision and Drainage, 61320-61321
  Breast
    Incision and Drainage, 19020
  Carpals
    Incision, Deep, 25035

Abscess — *continued*
  Clavicle
    Sequestrectomy, 23170
  Drainage
    with X–ray, 75989, 76080
    Contrast Injection, 49424
  Ear, External
    Complicated, 69005
    Simple, 69000
  Elbow
    Incision and Drainage, 23930-23935
    Sequestrectomy, 24136-24138
  Epididymis
    Incision and Drainage, 54700
  Excision
    Olecranon Process, 24138
    Radius, 24136
    Ulna, 24138
  Eyelid
    Incision and Drainage, 67700
  Facial Bone(s)
    Excision, 21026
  Femur
    with Opening Bone Cortex, 27303
    Bursa, 27301
    Deep Abscess, 27301
    Hematoma, 27301
  Finger, 26010-26011
    Incision and Drainage, 26010, 26011, 26034
  Foot
    Incision, 28005
  Gums
    Incision and Drainage, 41800
  Hand
    Incision and Drainage, 26034
  Hematoma
    Incision and Drainage, 27603
  Hip
    Incision and Drainage, 26990-26992
  Humeral Head, 23174
  Humerus
    Excision, 24134
    Incision and Drainage, 23935
  Kidney
    Incision and Drainage
      Open, 50020
  Leg, Lower
    Incision and Drainage, 27603
      Bone Abscess, 27607
  Liver
    Incision and Drainage, 47010
      Open, 47010
    Injection, 47015
    Marsupialization, 47300
  Localization
    Nuclear Medicine, 78806, 78807
  Lung
    Open Drainage, 32200
  Lymph Node, 38300, 38305
    Incision and Drainage, 38300-38305
  Lymphocele
    Drainage, 49062
    Sclerotherapy, 49185
  Mandible
    Excision, 21025
  Mouth
    Dentoalveolar, 41800
    Floor of Mouth
      Extraoral, 41015-41018
      Intraoral, 41000-41009
    Incision and Drainage, 40800, 40801,
      41005-41009, 41015-41018
    Vestibule, 40800-40801
  Nasal
    Incision and Drainage, 30000, 30020
  Nasal Septum
    Incision and Drainage, 30020
  Neck
    Incision and Drainage, 21501, 21502
  Nose
    Incision and Drainage, 30000, 30020
  Olecranon Process
    Incision and Drainage, 23930-23935
    Sequestrectomy, 24138
  Ovarian
    Incision and Drainage, 58820-58822

Abscess — *continued*
  Ovarian — *continued*
    Incision and Drainage — *continued*
      Abdominal Approach, 58822
      Vaginal Approach, 58820
  Ovary
    Incision and Drainage
      Abdominal Approach, 58822
      Vaginal Approach, 58820
  Palate
    Incision and Drainage, 42000
  Paraurethral Gland
    Incision and Drainage, 53060
  Parotid Gland
    Drainage, 42300, 42305
  Pelvis
    Incision and Drainage, 26990-26992
    Transrectal, 45000
  Perineum
    Incision and Drainage, 56405
  Perirenal or Renal
    Drainage, 50020
  Peritoneum
    Incision and Drainage
      Open, 49020
  Pharynx, 42700-42725
  Posterior Spine, 22010, 22015
  Prostate
    Incision and Drainage, 55720-55725
      Prostatotomy, 55720, 55725
      Transurethral, 52700
  Radius
    Bone Abscess, 25035
    Incision and Drainage, 25028
    Incision, Deep, 25035
    Sequestrectomy, 24136
  Rectum
    Incision and Drainage, 45005, 45020,
      46040, 46060
  Retroperitoneal, 49060
    Drainage
      Open, 49060
  Salivary Gland
    Drainage, 42300-42320
  Scapula
    Sequestrectomy, 23172
  Scrotum
    Incision and Drainage, 54700, 55100
  Shoulder
    Bone Cortex, 23035
    Incision and Drainage, 23030
  Skene's Gland
    Incision and Drainage, 53060
  Skin
    Incision and Drainage, 10060-10061
      Complicated, 10061
      Multiple, 10061
      Simple, 10060
      Single, 10060
    Puncture Aspiration, 10160
  Soft Tissue
    Catheter Drainage, 10030
    Incision, 20005
  Spine
    Incision and Drainage, 22010-22015
  Subdiaphragmatic
    Incision and Drainage
      Open, 49040
  Sublingual Gland
    Drainage, 42310, 42320
  Submaxillary Gland
    Drainage, 42310, 42320
  Subphrenic, 49040
  Testis
    Incision and Drainage, 54700
  Thigh
    Incision and Drainage, 27301
      Bone Abscess, 27303
  Thoracostomy, 32551
  Thorax
    Bone Cortex, 21510
    Incision and Drainage, 21501, 21502
  Throat
    Incision and Drainage, 42700-42725
  Tongue
    Incision and Drainage, 41000-41006

Abscess — *continued*
  Tonsil
    Incision and Drainage, 42700
  Ulna
    Incision, Deep, 25035
  Urethra
    Incision and Drainage, 53040
  Uvula
    Incision and Drainage, 42000
  Vagina
    Incision and Drainage, 57010
  Visceral, 49405
  Vulva
    Incision and Drainage, 56405
  Wrist
    Excision, 25145
    Incision and Drainage, 25028, 25035
  X–ray, 76080
Absolute Neutrophil Count (ANC), 85048
Absorptiometry
  Dual Energy, 77080
    Bone
      Appendicular Skeleton, 77081
      Axial Skeleton, 77078, 77080
      Vertebral, 77080, [77086]
    Ordered and Documented (PQRS), 3095F-
      3096F
  Dual Photon
    Bone, 78351
  Single Photon
    Bone, 78350
Absorption Spectrophotometry, 82190
  Atomic, 82190
ACADM, 81400-81401
ACADS, 81404-81405
ACADVL, 81406
ACB, 82045
ACBE, 74280
Accelerometer Data Recording, 3-Axis, 0381T-
  0386T
Access
  Small Bowel via Biliary Tree, Percutaneous,
    47541
Accessory Nerve
  Incision, 63191
  Section, 63191
Accessory, Toes, 28344
ACD, 63075, 63076
ACE (Angiotensin Converting Enzyme)
  See Angiotensin
Acellular Immunization, 90700
Acetabuloplasty, 27120, 27122, [29915]
Acetabulum
  Fracture
    with Manipulation, 27222
    without Manipulation, 27220
    Closed Treatment, 27220, 27222
    Open Treatment, 27226-27228
  Reconstruction, 27120
    with Resection, Femoral Head, 27122
  Tumor
    Excision, 27076
Acetaminophen, [80329, 80330, 80331]
Acetic Anhydrides, 84600
Acetone
  Blood or Urine, 82009, 82010
Acetone Body, 82009, 82010
Acetylcholinesterase
  Blood or Urine, 82013
AcG, 85220
Achilles Tendon
  Incision, 27605, 27606
  Lengthening, 27612
  Repair, 27650-27654
Achillotomy, 27605-27606
ACI, 27412, 29870
Acid
  Adenylic, 82030
  Amino
    Blood or Urine, 82127-82139
  Aminolevulinic
    Urine or Blood, 82135
  Ascorbic
    Blood, 82180
  Bile, 82239
    Blood, 82240

Acid — *continued*
  Deoxyribonucleic
    Antibody, 86225-86226
  Diethylamide, Lysergic, 80299
  Fast Bacilli (AFB)
    Culture, 87116
    Fast Stain, 88312
  Fatty
    Blood, 82725
    Very Long Chain, 82726
  Folic, 82746
    RBC, 82747
  Gastric, 82930
  Glycocholic, 82240
  Lactic, 83605
  N-Acetylneuraminic, 84275
  Perfusion Test
    Esophagus, 91013, 91030
  Phenylethylbarbituric
    Assay, 80184
  Phosphatase, 84060-84066
  Probes, Nucleic
    See Nucleic Acid Probe
  Reflux Test, 91034-91038
  Salic, 84275
  Uric
    Blood, 84550
    Other Source, 84560
    Urine, 84560
Acidity/Alkalinity
  Blood Gasses, 82800-82805
  Body Fluid, Not Otherwise Specified, 83986
  Exhaled Breath Condensate, 83987
ACL Repair
  Arthroscopy aided, 29888
  Open, 27407, 27409
Acne Surgery
  Incision and Drainage
    Abscess, 10060, 10061
      Puncture Aspiration, 10160
    Bulla
      Puncture Aspiration, 10160
    Comedones, 10040
    Cyst, 10040
      Puncture Aspiration, 10160
    Milia, Multiple, 10040
    Pustules, 10040
Acne Treatment
  Abrasion, 15786, 15787
  Chemical Peel, 15788-15793
  Cryotherapy, 17340
  Dermabrasion, 15780-15783
  Exfoliation
    Chemical, 17360
Acoustic
  Evoked Brain Stem Potential, 92585, 92586
  Heart Sounds
    with Computer Analysis, 93799
  Immittance Testing, 92570
  Neuroma
    Brainstem
      Biopsy, 61575, 61576
      Decompression, 61575, 61576
      Evoked Potentials, 92585
      Lesion Excision, 61575, 61576
    Brain Tumor Excision, 61510, 61518, 61520,
      61521, 61526, 61530, 61545
    Mesencephalon
      Tractotomy, 61480
    Skull Base Surgery
      Anterior Cranial Fossa
        Bicoronal Approach, 61586
        Craniofacial Approach, 61580-
          61583
        Extradural, 61600, 61601
        LeFort I Osteotomy Approach,
          61586
        Orbitocranial Approach, 61584,
          61585
        Transzygomatic Approach, 61586
      Carotid Aneurysm, 61613
      Carotid Artery, 61610
      Transection
        Ligation, 61610-61612
      Craniotomy, 62121

Acoustic — *continued*
  Neuroma — *continued*
    Skull Base Surgery — *continued*
      Dura
        Repair of Cerebrospinal
          Fluid Leak, 61618, 61619
      Middle Cranial Fossa
        Extradural, 61605-61607
        Infratemporal Approach, 61590, 61591
        Intradural, 61606-61608
        Orbitocranial Zygomatic Approach, 61592
      Posterior Cranial Fossa
        Extradural, 61615
        Intradural, 61616
        Transcondylar Approach, 61596, 61597
        Transpetrosal Approach, 61598
        Transtemporal Approach, 61595
  Recording
    Heart Sounds, 93799
ACP, 84060-84066
Acromioclavicular Joint
  Arthrocentesis, 20605-20606
  Arthrotomy, 23044
    with Biopsy, 23101
  Dislocation, 23540-23552
    Open Treatment, 23550, 23552
  X–ray, 73050
Acromion
  Excision
    Shoulder, 23130
Acromionectomy
  Partial, 23130
Acromioplasty, 23415, 23420
  Partial, 23130
ACTA2, 81405, 81410
ACTC1, 81405
ACTH (Adrenocorticotropic Hormone), 80400-80406, 80412, 80418, 82024
ActHIB, 90648
ACTH Releasing Factor, 80412
Actigraphy, 95803
Actinomyces
  Antibody, 86602
Actinomycosis, 86000
Actinomycotic Infection
  See Actinomycosis
Actinotherapy, 96900
Activated Factor X, 85260
Activated Partial Thromboplastin Time, 85730, 85732
Activation, Lymphocyte, 86353
Activities of Daily Living (ADL), 97535, 99509
  See Physical Medicine/Therapy/ Occupational Therapy
  Training, 97535, 97537
Activity, Glomerular Procoagulant
  See Thromboplastin
ACTN4, 81406
Acupuncture
  One or More Needles
    with Electrical Stimulation, 97813-97814
    without Electrical Stimulation, 97810-97811
Acute Poliomyelitis
  See Polio
Acylcarnitines, 82016, 82017
Adacel, 90715
Adamantinoma, Pituitary
  See Craniopharyngioma
ADAMTS-13, 85397
Adaptive Behavior Assessments
  Behavior Identification, 0359T
  Exposure Behavioral Followup, 0362T-0363T
  Observational Followup, 0360T-0361T
Addam Operation, 26040-26045
Adductor Tenotomy of Hip
  See Tenotomy, Hip, Adductor
Adelson
  Crosby Immersion Method, 85999
Adenoidectomy
  with Tonsillectomy, 42820, 42821
  Primary
    Age 12 or Over, 42831
    Younger Than Age 12, 42830

Adenoidectomy — *continued*
  Secondary
    Age 12 or Over, 42836
    Younger Than Age 12, 42835
Adenoids
  Excision, 42830-42836
    with Tonsillectomy, 42820, 42821
  Unlisted Services and Procedures, 42999
Adenoma
  Pancreas
    Excision, 48120
  Parathyroid
    Injection for Localization, 78808
  Thyroid Gland
    Excision, 60200
Adenosine 3′, 5′ Monophosphate, 82030
Adenosine Diphosphate
  Blood, 82030
Adenosine Monophosphate (AMP)
  Blood, 82030
Adenovirus
  Antibody, 86603
  Antigen Detection
    Enzyme Immunoassay, 87301-87451
    Immunofluorescence, 87260
Adenovirus Vaccine, 90476-90477
ADH (Antidiuretic Hormone), 84588
ADHD Emotional/Behavioral Assessment, 96127
Adhesion, Adhesions
  Epidural, 62263, 62264
  Eye
    Corneovitreal, 65880
    Incision
      Anterior Segment, 65860-65870
      Posterior Segment, 65875
    Intermarginal
      Construction, 67880
      Transposition of Tarsal Plate, 67882
  Intestinal
    Enterolysis, 44005
      Laparoscopic, 44180
  Intracranial
    Lysis, 62161
  Intranasal Synechia, 30560
  Intrauterine
    Lysis, 58559
  Labial
    Lysis, 56441
  Lungs
    Pneumolysis, 32124, 32940
  Pelvic
    Lysis, 58660, 58662, 58740
  Penile
    Lysis
      Post–circumcision, 54162
  Preputial
    Lysis, 54450
  Urethral
    Lysis, 53500
Adipectomy, 15830-15839, 15876-15879
Adjustment
  External Fixation, 20693, 20696
ADL
  Activities of Daily Living, 97535, 97537
Administration
  Health Risk Assessment, 96160-96161
  Immunization
    with Counseling, 90460-90461
    without Counseling, 90471-90474
  Injection
    Intramuscular Antibiotic, 96372
    Therapeutic, Diagnostic, Prophylactic
      Intra–arterial, 96373
      Intramuscular, 96372
      Intravenous, 96374-96376
      Subcutaneous, 96372
  Occlusive Substance During Bronchoscopy, 31634
  Pharmacologic Agent w/Monitoring
    with Monitoring, 93463
    Endovascular Intracranial
      for Other Than Thrombolysis, 61650-61651
Administrative Codes for Multianalyte Assays with Algorithmic Analyses, 0001M-0004M, 0006M-0009M

ADP (Adenosine Diphosphate), 82030
ADRB2, 81401
Adrenal Cortex Hormone, 83491
Adrenalectomy, 60540
  with Excision Retroperitoneal Tumor, 60545
  Anesthesia, 00866
  Laparoscopic, 60650
Adrenal Gland
  Biopsy, 60540, 60545
  Excision
    Laparoscopy, 60650
    Retroperitoneal, 60545
  Exploration, 60540, 60545
  Nuclear Medicine
    Imaging, 78075
Adrenalin
  Blood, 82383, 82384
  Fractionated, 82384
  Urine, 82382, 82384
Adrenaline or Noradrenaline
  Testing, 82382-82384
Adrenal Medulla
  See Medulla
Adrenocorticotropic Hormone (ACTH), 80400-80406, 80412, 80418, 82024
  Blood or Urine, 82024
  Stimulation Panel, 80400-80406
Adrenogenital Syndrome, 56805, 57335
Adson Test, 95870
Adult T Cell Leukemia Lymphoma Virus I, 86687, 86689
Advance Care Planning, 99497-99498
Advance Directives, 99497-99498
Advanced Life Support
  Emergency Department Services, 99281-99288
  Physician Direction, 99288
Advancement
  Genioglossus, 21199
  Tendon
    Foot, 28238
    Genioglossus, 21199
Advancement Flap
  Skin, Adjacent Tissue Transfer, 14000-14350
AEP, 92585, 92586
Aerosol Inhalation
  Inhalation Treatment, 94640, 94664
  Pentamidine, 94642
AFB (Acid Fast Bacilli), 87116
AFBG, 35539, 35540, 35646
AFF2, 81401, 81404
Afferent Nerve
  See Sensory Nerve
AFG3L2, 81406
AFGE, 66020
AFI, 76815
Afluria, 90655-90658
AFP, 82105, 82106
After Hours Medical Services, 99050-99060
Afterloading Brachytherapy, 77767-77768, 77770-77772
Agents, Anticoagulant
  See Clotting Inhibitors
Agglutinin
  Cold, 86156, 86157
  Febrile, 86000
Aggregation
  Platelet, 85576
AGL, 81407
AGTR1, 81400
AGTT, 82951, 82952
AHG (Antihemophilic Globulin), 85240
AHI1, 81407
Ahmed Glaucoma Valve
  Insertion, 66180
  Removal, 67120
  Revision, 66185
AICD (Pacing Cardioverter–Defibrillator), 33223, 93282, 93289, 93292, 93295
  Heart
    Defibrillator, 33240-33249 *[33230, 33231, 33262, 33263, 33264]*, 93282, 93288, 93292, 93295
    Pacemaker, 33212-33214 *[33221]*, 33233-33237 *[33227, 33228, 33229]*
Aid, Hearing
  Bone Conduction, 69710-69711

Aid, Hearing — *continued*
  Check, 92590-92595
AIDS
  Antibodies, 86687-86689, 86701-86703
  Virus, 86701, 86703
A–II (Angiotensin II), 82163
Air Contrast Barium Enema (ACBE), 74280
AIRE, 81406
Airway
  Integrity Testing Car Seat/Bed Neonate, 94780-94781
  Resistance by pulse oscillometry, 94728
ALA (Aminolevulinic Acid), 82135
Alanine 2 Oxoglutarate Aminotransferase
  See Transaminase, Glutamic Pyruvic
Alanine Amino (ALT), 84460
Alanine Transaminase
  See Transaminase, Glutamic Pyruvic
Albumin
  Cobalt Binding (ACB), 82045
  Ischemia Modified, 82045
  Serum Plasma, 82040
  Urine, 82042-82044
  Whole Blood, 82040
Alcohol, *[80320]*
  Abuse Screening and Intervention, 99408-99409
  Biomarkers, *[80321, 80322]*
  Breath, 82075
  Ethylene Glycol, 82693
Alcohol Dehydrogenase
  See Antidiuretic Hormone
Alcohol, Isopropyl
  See Isopropyl Alcohol
Alcohol, Methyl
  See Methanol
ALDH7A1, 81406
Aldolase
  Blood, 82085
Aldosterone
  Blood, 82088
  Suppression Evaluation, 80408
  Urine, 82088
Alexander's Operation, 58400-58410
ALIF (Anterior Lumbar Interbody Fusion), 22558-22585
Alimentary Canal
  See Gastrointestinal Tract
ALK (Automated Lamellar Keratoplasty), 65710
Alkaline Phosphatase, 84075-84080
  Leukocyte, 85540
  WBC, 85540
Alkaloids, *[80323]*
  See Also Specific Drug
Allergen Bronchial Provocation Tests, 95070-95071
Allergen Challenge, Endobronchial, 95070-95071
Allergen Immunotherapy
  Allergen
    with Extract Supply, 95120-95134
    Injection Only, 95115-95117
  Allergenic Extracts
    Extract Supply with Injection, 95120-95134
    Injection, 95115, 95117
  Antigens, 95144-95165
  IgE, 86003, 86005
  IgG, 86001
  Injection
    with Extract Supply, 95120, 95125
    without Extract Supply, 95115, 95117
  Insect Venom
    Prescription
      Supply, 95145-95149
        Injection, 95130-95134
  Prescription
    Supply, 95165
      Insect, Whole Body, 95170
  Rapid Desensitization, 95180
  Unlisted Services and Procedures, 95199
Allergy Services/Procedures
  See Allergen Immunotherapy
Allergy Tests
  Challenge Test
    Bronchial, 95070, 95071
    Ingestion, 95076, 95079

Allergy Tests — *continued*
　Eye Allergy, 95060
　Food Allergy, 95076, 95079
　Intradermal
　　Allergen Extract, 95024, 95028
　　Biologicals or Drugs, 95018
　　Incremental, 95027
　　Venoms, 95017
　Nasal Mucous Membrane Test, 95065
　Nose Allergy, 95065
　Patch
　　Application Tests, 95044
　　Photo Patch, 95052
　Photosensitivity, 95056
　Skin Tests
　　Allergen Extract, 95004, 95024, 95027
　　Biologicals or Drugs, 95018
　　End Point Titration, 95027
　　Venoms, 95017
Allogeneic Donor
　Backbench Preparation
　　Intestine, 44715-44721
　　Kidney, 50323-50329
　　Liver, 47143-47147
　　Pancreas, 48551-48552
　Lymphocyte Infusion, 38242
Allogeneic Transplantation
　See Homograft
　Backbench Preparation, 44715-44721
　　Intestine, 44715-44721
　　Kidney, 50323-50329
　　Liver, 47143-47147
　　Pancreas, 48551-48552
　Hematopoietic Progenitor Cells, 38240
Allograft
　Aortic Valve, 33406, 33413
　Bone, Structural, 20931
　Cartilage
　　Knee, 27415
　Elbow, 24370-24371
　Lung Transplant, 32850
　Sacroiliac Joint (Stabilization), 27279
　Shoulder, 23473-23474
　Skin Substitute Graft, 15271-15278
　Spine Surgery
　　Morselized, 20930
　　Osteopromotive Material, 20930
　　Structural, 20931
Allograft Preparation
　Cornea, 65757
　Heart, 33933, 33944
　Intestines, 44715-44721
　Kidney, 50323-50329
　Liver, 47143-47147
　Lung, 32855-32856, 33933
　Pancreas, 48551-48552
　Renal, 50323-50329
Alloplastic Dressing
　Burns, 15002, 15004-15005
Allotransplantation
　Intestines, 44135, 44136
　Islets of Langerhans, 48999
　Renal, 50360, 50365
　　Removal, 50370
Almen Test
　Blood, Feces, 82270
ALP, 84075-84080, 85540
Alpha–2 Antiplasmin, 85410
Alpha–Fetoprotein
　AFP-L3 Fraction Isoform and Total AFP, 82107
　Amniotic Fluid, 82106
　Serum, 82105
Alpha Globin 1 and Alpha Globin 2 Gene Analysis, 81257
Alpha–1–Antitrypsin, 82103, 82104
Alphatocopherol, 84446
ALS, 99288
ALT, 84460
Altemeier Procedure
　Rectum Prolapse, Excision, 45130, 45135
Alternate Binaural Loudness Balance Test (ABLB), 92562
Aluminum
　Blood, 82108

Alveola
　Fracture
　　Closed Treatment, 21421
　　Open Treatment, 21422-21423
Alveolar Cleft
　Ungrafted Bilateral, 21147
　Ungrafted Unilateral, 21146
Alveolar Nerve
　Avulsion, 64738
　Incision, 64738
　Transection, 64738
Alveolar Ridge
　Fracture
　　Closed Treatment, 21440
　　Open Treatment, 21445
Alveolectomy, 41830
Alveoli
　Fracture
　　Closed Treatment, 21421
　　Open Treatment, 21422, 21423
Alveoloplasty, 41874
Alveolus
　Excision, 41830
Amide, Procaine, 80190-80192
Amikacin
　Assay, 80150
Amine
　Vaginal Fluid, 82120
Amino Acids
　Blood or Urine, 82127-82139
Aminolevulinic Acid (ALA)
　Blood or Urine, 82135
Aminotransferase
　Alanine (SGPT), 84460
　Aspartate (SGOT), 84450
Amitriptyline
　Assay, *[80335, 80336, 80337]*
Ammonia
　Blood, 82140
　Urine, 82140
Amniocentesis
　with Amniotic Fluid Reduction, 59001
　See Chromosome Analysis
　Diagnostic, 59000
　Induced Abortion, 59850
　　with Dilation and Curettage, 59851
　　with Dilation and Evacuation, 59851
　　with Hysterotomy, 59852
　Urine
　　with Amniotic Fluid Reduction, 59001
Amnioinfusion
　Transabdominal, 59070
Amnion
　Amniocentesis, 59000
　　with Amniotic Fluid Reduction, 59001
　Amnioinfusion
　　Transabdominal, 59070
　Membrane Placement
　　for Wound Healing, 65778-65779
Amniotic Fluid
　Alpha–Fetoprotein, 82106
　Index, 76815
　Scan, 82143
　Testing, 83661, 83663, 83664
Amniotic Membrane
　transplant (AMT), 65780
Amobarbital, *[80345]*
AMP (Adenosine Monophosphate), 82030
AMP, Cyclic, 82030
Amphetamine, *[80324, 80325, 80326]*
Amputation
　Ankle, 27888
　Arm and Shoulder, 23900-23921
　Arm, Lower, 25900, 25905, 25915
　　with Implant, 24931, 24935
　　Cineplasty, 24940
　　Revision, 25907, 25909
　Arm, Upper, 24900, 24920
　　with Implant, 24931, 24935
　　and Shoulder, 23900-23921
　　Revision, 24925, 24930
　Boyd, 27880-27889
　Cervix
　　Total, 57530
　Ear
　　Partial, 69110

Amputation — *continued*
　Ear — *continued*
　　Total, 69120
　Finger, 26910-26952
　Foot, 28800, 28805
　Hand
　　at Metacarpals, 25927
　　at Wrist, 25920
　　　Revision, 25922
　　Revision, 25924, 25929, 25931
　Interpelviabdominal, 27290
　Interthoracoscapular, 23900
　Knee joint Disarticulation, 27598
　Leg, Lower, 27598, 27880-27882
　　Revision, 27884, 27886
　Leg, Upper, 27590-27592
　　at Hip, 27290, 27295
　　Revision, 27594, 27596
　Metacarpal, 26910
　Metatarsal, 28810
　Penis
　　Partial, 54120
　　Radical, 54130, 54135
　　Total, 54125
　Thumb, 26910-26952
　Toe, 28810-28825
　Tuft of Distal Phalanx
　　Finger, 26236
　　Toe, 28124, 28160
　Upper Extremity
　　Cineplasty, 24940
Amputation, Nose
　See Resection, Nose
Amputation through Hand
　See Hand, Amputation
AMT, 65780
Amussat's Operation, 44025
Amygdalohippocampectomy, 61566
Amylase
　Blood, 82150
　Urine, 82150
ANA (Antinuclear Antibodies), 86038, 86039
Anabolic Steroid
　Androstenedione, 82160
Anal
　Abscess, 46045
　Bleeding, 46614
　Fissurectomy, 46200, 46261
　Fistula, 46262-46288, 46706-46707, 46715-46716
　Fistulectomy, 46270-46285
　Fistulotomy, 46270-46280
　Polyp, 46615
　Sphincter
　　Dilation, 45905
　　Incision, 46080
　Tumor, 46615
　Ulceration, 46200, 46261
Analgesia, 99151-99157
　See also Anesthesia, Sedation
Analgesic Cutaneous Electrostimulation
　See Application, Neurostimulation
Analysis
　Algorithmic
　　Electrocardiographic-derived Data, 0206T
　　Cardiovascular Monitoring System, 93290-93291, 93297, 93299
　　Chimerism (Engraftment), 81267-81268
　Comparative
　　Short Tandem Repeat Markers (STR), 81265-81266
　Computer Data, 99090
　　Multivariate Probability Assessment, 99199
　Electroencephalogram
　　Digital, 95957
　Electronic
　　Antitachycardia Pacemaker, 93724
　　Drug Infusion Pump, 62367-62370
　　Leads, 93640-93641
　　Pacemaker, 93288, 93293-93294
　　Pacing Cardio-Defibrillator
　　　Data Analysis, 93289, 93295-93296
　　　Initial Evaluation, 93640-93641
　　Pulse Generator, 64999, 95970-95982
　　Wearable Cardiac Device, 93288
　Gastric Acid, 82930

Analysis — *continued*
　Gene
　　3-Beta-Hydroxysteroid Dehydrogenase Type II Deficiency, 81404
　　3-Methylcrotonyl-CoA Carboxylase 1, 81406
　　5, 10-Methylenetetrahydrofolate Reductase, 81291
　　ABCA4, 81408, 81434
　　ABCC8, 81407
　　ABCCA8, 81401
　　ABCD1, 81405
　　ABL1 (ABL proto-oncogene 1, non-receptor tyrosine kinase), 81170, 81401
　　Abnormal Alleles (ATN1, ATXN 1-3,7,10, ATXN8OS), 81401
　　ACADM, 81400-81401
　　ACADS, 81404-81405
　　ACADVL, 81406
　　ACE, 81400
　　Achondroplasia, 81401, 81404
　　Acquired Imatinib Resistance, 81401
　　ACTA2, 81405, 81410
　　ACTC1, 81405
　　ACTN4, 81406
　　Acute Myeloid Leukemia, 81218
　　Acyl-CoA Dehydrogenase Deficiency
　　　Long Chain, 81406
　　　Short Chain, 81404-81405
　　Adenomatous Polyposis Coli (APC), 81201-81203
　　ADRB2, 81401
　　Adrenoleukodystrophy, 81405
　　AFF2, 81401, 81404
　　AFG3L2, 81406
　　AGL, 81407
　　AGTR1, 81400
　　AHI1, 81407
　　AIRE, 81406
　　Alagille Syndrome, 81406-81407
　　ALDH7A1, 81406
　　Alexander Disease, 81405
　　Allan-Herndon-Dudley Syndrome, 81404-81405
　　Alpers-Huttenlocher Syndrome, 81406
　　Alpha-1-Antitrypsin Deficiency, 81332
　　Alpha Globin 1 and Alpha Globin 2, 81257
　　Alport Syndrome, 81407-81408
　　Alveolar Rhabdomyosarcoma, 81401
　　Alzheimer Disease, 81401, 81405-81406
　　Amyotrophic Lateral Sclerosis, 81403-81405
　　Anaplastic Large Cell Lymphoma, 81401
　　Anderson-Tawil Syndrome, 81403
　　Androgen Insensitivity Syndrome, 81405
　　Aneurysms, Thoracic Aorta, 81405
　　ANG, 81403
　　Angelman Syndrome, 81331, 81402, 81406
　　ANK2, 81413
　　ANKRD1, 81405
　　ANO5, 81406
　　Aortic Dysfunction or Dilation, 81410-81411
　　Aortic Valve Disease, 81407
　　APC, 81201-81203, 81435
　　Apert Syndrome, 81404
　　APOB, 81401
　　APOE, 81401
　　APP, 81406
　　APTX, 81405
　　AQP1, 81403
　　AQP2, 81404
　　AR, 81401, 81405
　　Arrhythmogenic Right Ventricular Dysplasia/Cardiomyopathy, 81406, 81408
　　ARSA, 81405
　　ART4, 81403
　　ARX, 81403-81404
　　Arylsulfatase A Deficiency, 81405
　　Ashkenazi Jewish Associated Disorders, 81412
　　ASPA, 81200, 81412
　　Aspartoacylase (ASPA), 81200, 81412
　　ASPM, 81407
　　ASS1, 81406
　　Ataxia, 81404-81406, 81408
　　ATL1, 81406
　　ATM, 81408, 81432-81433
　　ATN1, 81401

Analysis — *continued*
Gene — *continued*
ATP1A2, 81406
ATP7B, 81406
ATXN10, 81401
ATXN1, 81401
ATXN2, 81401
ATXN3, 81401
ATXN7, 81401
ATXN8OS, 81401
Autism Spectrum Disorders, 81404-81405
Autoimmune Disorders
Polyendocrinopathy Syndrome, 81406
Rheumatoid Arthritis, 81490
Autosomal Disorders
Dominant Dopa-Responsive Dystonia, 81405
Dominant Hyper-IgE Syndrome, 81405
Dominant Progressive External Ophthalmoplegia, 81406
Recessive Nonsyndromic Hearing Impairment, 81405
AVPR2, 81404
Bardet-Biedel Syndrome, 81404, 81406
Barth Syndrome, 81406
Bartter Syndrome, 81404, 81406-81407
BBS10, 81404
BBS1, 81406
BBS2, 81406
BCAM, 81403
BCKDHA, 81400, 81405
BCKDHB, 81205, 81406
BCR/ABL1 (t(9;22)), 81206-81208
BCS1L, 81405
Beckwith-Wiedemann Syndrome, 81401
Berardinelli-Seip Congenital Lipodystrophy, 81406
Bernard-Soulier Syndrome Type B, 81404
BEST1, 81406
Biotinidase Deficiency, 81404
Blau Syndrome, 81401
BLM, 81209, 81412
Bloom Syndrome, RecQ Helicase-Like (BLM), 81209, 81412
BMPR1A, 81435
BMPR2, 81405-81406
BRAF (B-Raf proto-oncogene, serine/threonine kinase), 81210, 81406
Brain Small-Vessel Disease, 81408
Branched-Chain Keto Acid Dehydrogenase E1, Beta Polypeptide (BCKDHB), 81205, 81406
Branchio-Oto-Renal (BOR) Spectrum Disorders, 81405-81406
BRCA1, 81214-81215
BRCA1, BRCA2, 81211-81213, 81432-81433, *[81162]*
BRCA2, 81216-81217
Breast Cancer, 81402, 81406
Breast Cancer 1, 81214-81215
Breast Cancer 1 and 2, 81211-81213, 81432-81433, *[81162]*
Breast Cancer 2, 81216-81217
Breast Cancer Related Geonomic Sequence, Hereditary, 81432-81433
BRIP1, 81432-81433
Brugada Syndrome, 81404, 81406, 81413-81414
BSCL2, 81406
BTD, 81404
BTK, 81406
C10orf2, 81404
CACNA1A, 81401, 81407
CACNB2, 81406
CALR, 81219
Canavan Disease, 81200, 81412
CAPN3, 81406
Cardiofaciocutaneous Syndrome, 81406
Cardiomyopathy
Arrhythmogenic Right Ventricular, 81406, 81439
Dilated Hypertrophic, 81403, 81405-81407, 81439
Familial Hypertrophic, 81405-81407
Hypertrophic, 81439

Analysis — *continued*
Gene — *continued*
Carnitine-acylcarnitine Translocase Deficiency, 81404-81405
Carnitine Palmitoyltransferase II Deficiency, 81404, 81406
CASQ2, 81405, 81413
CASR, 81405
Catecholaminergic Polymorphic Ventricular Tachycardia, 81405, 81408, 81413-81414
CAV3, 81404, 81413
CBFB/MYH11, 81401
CBS, 81401, 81406
CCAAT/enhancer binding protein [C/EBP], alpha, 81218
CcEe Antigens, 81403
CCND1/IGH (BCL1/IgH, t(11;14)), 81401
CCR5, 81400
CD40LG, 81404
CDH1, 81406, 81432, 81435
CDH23, 81408, 81430
CDKL5, 81405-81406
CDKN2A, 81404
CDKNDA, 81445, 81455
C/EBP, 81218
CEBPA (CCAAT/enhancer binding protein [C/EBP]), 81218
CEL, 81403
CEP290, 81408
Cerebral Autosomal Dominant Arteriopathy, 81406
CFH/ARMS2, 81401
CFTR, 81220-81224, 81412
Charcot-Marie-Tooth, 81324-81326, 81403-81406
CHARGE Syndrome, 81407
CHD7, 81407
Chimerism Analysis, 81267-81268
Christianson Syndrome, 81406
CHRNA4, 81405
CHRNB2, 81405
Chromosome 1p-/19q, 18q, 81402
Citrullinemia Type I, 81406
CLCN1, 81406
CLCNKB, 81406
Clear Cell Sarcoma, 81401
CLRN1, 81400, 81404, 81430
CNBP, 81401
CNGA1, 81434
CNTNAP2, 81406
Coagulation Factor
F2 (Factor 2), 81240, 81400
F5 (Factor V), 81241, 81400
F7 (Factor VII), 81400
F8 (Factor VIII), 81403, 81406-81407
F9 (Factor IX), 81405
F11 (Factor XI), 81401
F12 (Factor XII), 81403
F13B (Factor XIII, B polypeptide), 81400
Cohen Syndrome, 81407-81408
COL1A1, 81408
COL1A1/PDGFB, 81402
COL1A2, 81408
COL3A1, 81410-81411
COL4A1, 81408
COL4A3, 81408
COL4A4, 81407
COL4A5, 81407-81408
COL6A1, 81407
COL6A2, 81406-81407
COL6A3, 81407
Collagen Related Disorders, 81406-81408
Colorectal Carcinoma, 81210, 81292-81301 *[81288]*, 81311, 81317-81319, 81401-81402, 81404
Combined Pituitary Hormone Deficiency, 81404-81405
Comparative Analysis Using Short Tandem Repeat (STR) Markers, 81265-81266
Cone-Rod Dystrophy 2, 81404
Congenital Adrenal Hyperplasia, 81402, 81405
Congenital Disorder Glycosylation 1b, 81405
Congenital Finnish Nephrosis, 81407

Analysis — *continued*
Gene — *continued*
Congenital Hypoventilation Syndrome, 81403-81404
Congenital/Infantile Fibrosarcoma, 81401
Coronary Artery Disease, 81493
Costello Syndrome, 81403-81404
Cowden Syndrome, 81321-81323
COX10, 81405
COX15, 81405
COX6B1, 81404
CPT1A, 81406
CPT2, 81404
Craniosynostosis, 81400, 81403-81404
CRB1, 81406, 81434
CREBBP, 81406-81407
Cri-du-chat Syndrome, 81422
Crohn's Disease, 81401
Crouzon Syndrome, 81404
CRX, 81404
CSTB, 81401, 81404
CTNNB1, 81403
Cutaneous Malignant Melanoma, CDKN2A Related, 81404
CYP11B1, 81405
CYP17A1, 81405
CYP1B1, 81404
CYP21A2, 81402, 81405
CYP2C19, 81225
CYP2C9, 81227
CYP2D6, 81226
CYP3A4, 81401
CYP3A5, 81401
Cystathionine Beta-synthase Deficiency, 81401
Cystic Fibrosis, 81412
Transmembrane Conductance Regulator (CFTR), 81220-81224
Cytochrome P450, Family 2, Subfamily C, Polypeptide 19 (CYP2C19), 81225
Cytochrome P450, Family 2, Subfamily C, Polypeptide 9 (CYP2C9), 81227
Cytochrome P450, Family 2, Subfamily D, Polypeptide 6 (CYP2D6), 81226
Cytogenomic Microarray Analysis, 81228-81229, 81405-81406
DARC, 81403
DAZ/SRY, 81403
DBT, 81405-81406
DCX, 81405
Deafness, Nonsyndromic Sensorineural, 81401
DEK/NUP214 (t(6;9)), 81401
Denys-Drash Syndrome, 81405
Dermatofibrosarcoma Protuberans, 81402
DES, 81405
Desmoid Tumors, 81403
Desmoplastic Small Round Cell Tumor, 81401
DFNB59, 81405
DGUOK, 81405
DHCR7, 81405
Diabetes Mellitus, 81401, 81404
Diamond-Blackfan Anemia, 81405
DiGeorge Syndrome, 81422
DLAT, 81406
DLD, 81406
DMD (dystrophin), 81408, *[81161]*
DMPK, 81401, 81404
DNMT3A, 81403
DPYD, 81400
DSC2, 81406
DSG2, 81406, 81439
DSP, 81406
Duplication/Deletion Panel
Alpha Thalassemia/Hb Bart/HbH Disease, 81257
Aortic Dysfunction/Dilation, 81411
APC (Adenomatous Polyposis Coli), 81203
BRCA1/BRCA2 (Breast Cancer), 81213, 81433
CFTR (Cystic Fibrois Transmembrane Conductance Regulator), 81222
FAP (Familial Adenomatosis Polyposis), 81203

Analysis — *continued*
Gene — *continued*
Duplication/Deletion Panel — *continued*
FLT3 (Fms-related tyrosine kinase 3), 81245
Hearing Loss, 81431
Hereditary Breast Cancer, 81433
Hereditary Colon Cancer, 81294, 81297, 81300, 81319, 81436
Hereditary Neuroendocrine Tumor, 81438
Long QT Syndrome, 81282
MECP2 (Rett Syndrome), 81304
Neuropathy (Charcot-Marie-Tooth), 81324
PTEN (Cowden Syndrome/Hamartoma Tumor Syndrome), 81323
DYSF, 81408
Dystrophin, *[81161]*
E2A/PBX1 (t(1;19)), 81401
Early Infantile Epileptic Encephalopathy, 81405-81406
Early-Onset Primary Dystonia, 81400
EAST Syndrome, 81404
EFHC1, 81406
EGFR, 81235
EGR2, 81404
Ehler Danlos Syndrome, 81410
EIF2B2, 81405
EIF2B3, 81405
EIF2B4, 81406
EIF2B5, 81406
EMD, 81404-81405
EML4/ALK, 81401
Endocrinology Biochemical Assays, 81506
EPCAM, 81403, 81436
Epidermal Growth Factor Receptor, 81235
Epileptic Encephalopathy, 81405-81406
EPM2A, 81404
ERMAP, 81403
ESR1/PGR, 81402
ETV6/NTRK3 (t(12;15)), 81401
ETV6/RUNX1 (t(12;21)), 81401
Ewing Sarcoma, 81401
EWSR1/ATF1 (t(12;22)), 81401
EWSR1/ERG (t(21;22)), 81401
EWSR1/FLI1 (t(11;22)), 81401
EWSR1/WT1 (t(11;22)), 81401
Exome, 81415-81417
EYA1, 81405
EYS, 81434
Fabry Disease, 81405
FAH, 81406
Familial Disorders/Variants
APC (Adenomatous Polyposis Coli), 81202
Atypical Mole-Malignant Melanoma, 81404
BRCA1, 81215
BRCA2, 81217
CFTR (Cystic Fibrosis Transmembrane Conductance Regulator), 81222
Dilated Hypertrophic Cardiomyopathy, 81403, 81405-81407
Dysautonomia, 81260, 81412
FAP (Familial Adenomatosis Polyposis), 81202
GJB2 (Gap Junction Protein), 81253
Hemiplegic Migraine, 81406-81407
Hereditary Colon Cancer, 81293, 81296, 81299, 81318, 81435
Hypercholesterolemia, 81401, 81405-81406
Hyperinsulinism, 81401, 81403, 81406-81407
Hypertrophic Cardiomyopathy, 81405-81407
Long QT Syndrome, 81413-81414
MECP2 (Rett Syndrome), 81303
Mediterranean Fever, 81402, 81404
Medullary Thyroid Carcinoma, 81404-81405
Neuropathy (Charcot-Marie-Tooth), 81326
Partial Lipodystrophy, 81406

Analysis — *continued*
  Gene — *continued*
    Familial Disorders/Variants — *continued*
      PTEN (Cowden Syndrome/Hamartoma Tumor Syndrome), 81322
      Transthyretin Amyloidosis, 81404
      Wilms Tumor, 81405
    FANCC, 81242, 81412
    Fanconi Anemia, Complementation Group C (FANCC), 81242, 81412
    FAP (Familial Adenomatosis Polyposis), 81201-81203
    FASTKD2, 81406
    FBN1, 81408, 81410
    Fetal Chromosomal Aneuploidy, 81420-81427, 81507
    Fetal Chromosomal Microdeletion, 81422
    Fetal Congenital Abnormalities, 81508-81512
    FGB, 81400
    FGF23, 81404
    FGFR1, 81400, 81405
    FGFR2, 81404
    FGFR3, 81400-81401, 81403-81404
    FG Syndrome, 81401
    FH, 81405
    FHL1, 81404
    FIG4, 81406
    FIP1L1/PDGFRA, 81401
    FKRP, 81404
    FKTN, 81400, 81405
    FLG, 81401
    FLT3, 81245-81246
    FMR1, 81243-81244
    Fms-Related Tyrosine Kinase 3 (FLT3), 81245-81246
    Follicular Lymphoma, 81401-81402
    Follicular Thyroid Carcinoma, 81401
    FOXG1, 81404
    FOXO1/PAX3 (t(2;13)), 81401
    FOXO1/PAX7 (t(1;13)), 81401
    Fragile X Mental Retardation 1 (FMR1), 81243-81244, 81401, 81404
    Friedreich Ataxia, 81401, 81404
    Frontotemporal Dementia, 81406
    FSHMD1A, 81404
    FTSJ1, 81405-81406
    Fumarate Hydratase Deficiency, 81405
    FUS, 81406
    FUS/DDIT3 (t(12;16)), 81401
    FXN, 81401, 81404
    G6PC, 81250
    GAA, 81406
    GABRG2, 81405
    Galactosemia, 81401, 81406
    GALC, 81401, 81406
    GALT, 81401, 81406
    Gap Junction Protein
      Beta 2, 26kDa, Connexin 26 (GJB2), 81252-81253
      Beta 6, 30kDa, Connexin 30 (GJB6), 81254
    GARS, 81406
    Gastrointestinal Stromal Tumor (GIST), 81272, 81314
    Gaucher Disease, 81412
    GBA, 81251, 81412
    GCDH, 81406
    GCH1, 81405
    GCK, 81406
    GDAP1, 81405
    Generalized Epilepsy with Febrile Seizures, 81405, 81407
    Genetic Prion Disease, 81404
    GFAP, 81405
    GH1, 81404
    GHR, 81405
    GHRHR, 81405
    Gingival Fibromatosis, 81406
    GIST, 81272, 81314
    Gitelman Syndrome, 81407
    GJB1, 81403
    GJB2, 81252-81253, 81430
    GJB6, 81254
    GLA, 81405

Analysis — *continued*
  Gene — *continued*
    Glial Tumors, 81402
    Glioblastoma Multiforme, [81287]
    Glioma, 81403
    Glomerulocystic Kidney Disease, 81406
    Glucose-6-Phosphatase, Catalytic Subunit, 81250
    Glucose Transporter Deficiency Syndrome (GLUT), 81405
    Glucosidase, Beta Acid, 81251
    GLUD1, 81406
    Glutaricacidemia, 81406
    Glycogen Storage Disease, 81406-81407
    GNAQ, 81403
    GNE, 81400, 81406
    Gonadal Dysgenesis, 81400
    GP1BB, 81404
    GPR98, 81430
    GRACILE Syndrome, 81405
    GRN, 81406
    Growth Hormone Deficiency, 81404-81405
    GYPA, 81403
    GYPB, 81403
    GYPE, 81403
    H19, 81401
    HADHA, 81406
    Hageman Factor, 81403
    Hamartoma Tumor Syndrome, 81321-81323
    HBA1/HBA2, 81257, 81404-81405
    HBB, 81401, 81403-81404
    Hb Bart Hydrops Fetalis Syndrome, 81257
    HbH Disease, 81257
    HDAHB, 81406
    Hearing Loss, 81404-81405, 81430-81431
    Hematopoietic Stem Cell Transplantation, 81403
    Hemochromatosis, 81256
    Hemolytic Diseease of Fetus/Newborn, 81403
    Hemolytic Transfusion Reaction, 81403
    Hemophilia, 81403, 81405-81407
    Hemorrhagic Telangiectasia Syndrome, 81405-81406
    Hepatocerebral Mitochondrial DNA Depletion Syndrome, 81405
    Hereditary Disorders
      Blood Pressure Regulation, 81400
      Breast Cancer, 81432-81433
      Colon Cancer, 81435-81436
      Diffuse Gastric Cancer, 81406
      Endometrial Cancer, 81432-81433
      Hemochromatosis, 81256
      Hemorrhagic Telangiectasia, 81405
      Hypercoagulability, 81291, 81400
      Leiomyomatosis with Renal Cell Cancer, 81405
      Neuroendocrine Tumor, 81437-81438
      Neuropathy, 81324-81326
      Non-polyposis Colorectal Cancer, 81292-81301 [81288]
      Ovarian Cancer, 81432-81433
      Pancreatitis, 81401, 81404
      Paraganglioma, 81404-81405
      Paraganglioma-Pheochromocytoma Syndrome, 81404-81405
      Pulmonary Arterial Hypertension, 81405-81406
      Retinal Disorders, 81434
    HEXA, 81255, 81406, 81412
    Hexosaminidase A (Alpha Polypeptide), 81255
    HFE, 81256
    Hirschsprung Disease, 81406
    HLA
      High Resolution
        Class I and II Typing, 81378
        Class II Typing, 81382-81383
        Class I Typing, 81379-81381
      Low Resolution
        Class I and II Typing, 81370-81371
        Class II Typing, 81375-81377
        Class I Typing, 81372-81374
    HLCS, 81406
    HNF1A, 81405

Analysis — *continued*
  Gene — *continued*
    HNF1B, 81404-81405
    HNF4A, 81406
    Holocarboxylase Synthetase Deficiency, 81406
    Holt-Oram Syndrome, 81405
    Homocystinuria, 81401, 81406
    HRAS, 81403-81404
    HSD11B2, 81404
    HSD3B2, 81404
    HSPB1, 81404
    HTRA1, 81405
    HTT, 81401
    Human Erythrocyte Antigen Gene Analyses, 81403
    Human Platelet Antigen 1-6, 9, 15, 81400
    Huntington Disease, 81401
    Hypercoagulability, 81240-81241, 81291, 81406
    Hyperkalemic Periodic Paralysis, 81406
    Hyperlipoproteinemia, Type III, 81401
    Hypocalcemia, 81406
    Hypochondroplasia, 81401, 81404
    Hypophosphatemic Rickets, 81404, 81406
    ICAM4, 81403
    Ichthyosis Vulgaria, 81401
    IDH1, 81403
    IDH2, 81403
    IDS, 81405
    IDUA, 81406
    IGH@, 81261-81263
    IGH@/BCL2 (t(14;18)), 81401-81402
    IGK@, 81264
    IKBKAP, 81260, 81412
    IL28B, 81400
    IL2RG, 81405
    Imatinib-Sensitive Chronic Eosinophilic Leukemia, 81401
    Immunoglobulin Heavy Chain Locus, 81261-81263
    Immunoglobulin Kappa Light Chain Locus, 81264
    Inclusion Body Myopathy, 81400, 81406
    INF2, 81406
    Inhibitor of Kappa Light Polypeptide Gene Enhancer in B-Cells, Kinase Complex-Associated Protein, 81260
    INS, 81404
    Intrauterine Growth Retardation, 81401
    Irinotecan Metabolism, 81350
    Isovalerice Acidemia, 81400, 81406
    ISPD, 81405
    ITPR1, 81408
    IVD, 81400, 81406
    JAG1, 81406-81407
    JAK2, 81270, 81403
    Joubert Syndrome, 81405-81408
    JUP, 81406
    Juvenile Myoclonic Epilepsy, 81406
    KAL1, 81406
    Kallmann Syndrome, 81405-81406
    KCNC3, 81403
    KCNE1, 81413
    KCNE2, 81413
    KCNH2, 81406, 81413-81414
    KCNJ10, 81404
    KCNJ1, 81404
    KCNJ11, 81403
    KCNJ2, 81413
    KCNQ1, 81406, 81413-81414
    KCNQ1OT1 (KNCQ1 overlapping transcript), 81401
    KCNQ2, 81406
    KDM5C, 81407
    Kennedy Disease, 81401
    KIAA0196, 81407
    Killer Cell Immunoglobulin-like Receptor (KIR), 81403
    KIT (v-kit Hardy-Zuckerman 4 feline sarcoma viral oncogene homolog), 81272
      D816 Variant, 81273
    Known Familial Variant Tier 1 or 2, NOS, 81403
    Krabbe Disease, 81401, 81406

Analysis — *continued*
  Gene — *continued*
    KRAS, 81275-81276, 81405
    L1CAM, 81407
    Lactic Acidosis, 81405-81406
    LAMA2, 81408
    LAMB2, 81407
    LAMP2, 81405
    Langer Mesomelic Dysplasia, 81405
    Laron Syndrome, 81405
    LCT (Lactose Intolerance), 81400
    LDB3, 81406
    LDLR, 81405-81406
    Leber Congenital Amaurosis, 81404, 81406
    Leber Hereditary Optic Neuropathy, 81401
    Legius Syndrome, 81406
    Leigh Syndrome, 81401, 81404-81406
    LEOPARD Syndrome, 81404, 81406, 81442
    LEPR, 81406
    Lethal Congenital Glycogen Storage Disease Heart, 81406
    Leukemia
      Acute Lymphoblastic, 81401
      Acute Lymphocytic, 81401
      Acute Myeloid, 81272, 81310, 81401, 81403
    Leukemias and Lymphomas, 81402
      B-cell, 81261-81264
      T-cell, 81340-81342
    Leukoencephalopathy, 81405-81406
    LHCGR, 81406
    Liddle Syndrome, 81406
    Li-Fraumeni Syndrome, 81405
    Lissencephaly, 81405-81406
    LITAF, 81404
    LMNA, 81406
    Loeys Dietz Syndrome, 81410
    Long QT Syndrome, 81413-81414
    LRP5, 81406
    LRRK2, 81401, 81408
    Lujan Syndrome, 81401
    Lynch Syndrome, 81292-81301 [81288], 81317-81319, 81403, 81435-81436
    Machado-Joseph Disease, 81401
    Macular Degeneration/Dystrophy, 81401, 81405-81406
    Male Infertility, 81403
    Malignant Hyperthermia, 81406, 81408
    Mantle Cell Lymphoma, 81401
    MAP2K1, 81406
    MAP2K2, 81406
    Maple Syrup Urine Disease, 81205, 81400, 81405-81406
    MAPT, 81406
    Marfan Syndrome, 81405, 81408, 81410
    Mastocytosis, 81273
    Maturity-Onset Diabetes of the Young (MODY), 81403-81404
    MAX, 81437
    MC4R, 81403
    McArdle Disease, 81401, 81406
    MCCC1, 81406
    MCCC2, 81406
    MCOLN1, 81290, 81412
    MECP2, 81302-81304
    MED12, 81401
    MEFV, 81402, 81404
    MEG3/DLK1, 81401
    Melanoma, 81272
      Uveal, 81403
    MEN1, 81404-81405
    Methylglutaconic Aciduria, 81406
    Methylmalonic Acidemia and Homocystinuria, 81404-81406
    MFN2, 81406
    MGMT, [81287]
    MHY11, 81408, 81410-81411
    MICA, 81403
    Microsatellite Instability Analysis, 81301
    Miller-Dieker Syndrome, 81405-81406
    Mineralocorticoid Excess Syndrome, 81404
    Mitochondrial Complex Deficiency, 81404-81406
    Mitochondrial DNA Depletion Syndrome, 81404-81405

Analysis — *continued*
  Gene — *continued*
    Mitochondrial Encephalopathy (MELAS), 81401
    Mitochondrial Respiratory Chain Complex IV Deficiency, 81404-81406
    MLH1, 81292-81294 *[81288]*, 81432-81433, 81435-81436
    MLL/AFF1 (t(4;11)), 81401
    MLL/MLLT3 (t(9;11)), 81401
    MMAA, 81405
    MMAB, 81405
    MMACHC, 81404
    Mowat-Wilson Syndrome, 81404-81405
    MPI, 81405
    MPL, 81402-81403
    MPV17, 81404-81405
    MPZ, 81405
    MSH2, 81295-81297, 81432-81433, 81435-81436
    MSH6, 81298-81300, 81432-81433, 81435
    MT-ATP6, 81401
    MTHFR, 81291
    MTM1, 81405-81406
    MT-ND4, 81401
    MT-ND5, 81401
    MT-ND6, 81401
    MT-RNR1, 81401, 81430
    MT-TL1, 81401
    MT-TS1, 81401, 81403
    Mucolipidosis, 81290
    Mucolipin 1, 81290
    Mucopolysaccharidosis, 81405-81406
    Muenke Syndrome, 81400
    Multiple Endocrine Neoplasia, 81404-81405
    Muscle-Eye-Brain Disease, 81405-81406
    Muscular Dystrophy
      Amyotrophic Lateral Sclerosis, 81404-81406
      Congenital, 81404, 81408
      Duchenne/Becker Muscular Dystrophy, 81408, *[81161]*
      Emery-Dreifuss, 81404-81406
      Facioscapulohumeral, 81404
      Fukuyama, 81400
      Limb-Girdle, 81404-81406, 81408
      Oculopharyngeal, 81401
      Spinal, 81400, 81403, 81405
    MUT, 81406
    MUTYH, 81401, 81406, 81435
    MYBPC3, 81407, 81439
    Myeloproliferative Disorders, 81219, 81270, 81402-81403
    MYH6, 81407
    MYH7, 81407, 81439
    MYH-associated Polyposis, 81401, 81406
    MYL2, 81405
    MYL3, 81405
    MYLK, 81410
    MYO15A, 81430
    MYO7A, 81407, 81430
    Myoclonic Dystonia, 81406
    Myoclonic Epilepsy (MERRF), 81401
    Myofibrillar Myopathy, 81405
    MYOT, 81405
    Myotonia Congenita, 81406
    Myotonic Dystrophy, 81401, 81404
    Myxoid Liposarcoma, 81401
    NBN, 81432
    NDP, 81403-81404
    NDUFA1, 81404
    NDUFAF2, 81404
    NDUFS1, 81406
    NDUFS4, 81404
    NDUFS7, 81405
    NDUFS8, 81405
    NDUFV1, 81405
    NEB, 81400, 81408
    NEFL, 81405
    Nemaline Myopathy, 81408
    Nephrogenic Diabetes Insipidus, 81404
    Nephrotic Syndrome, 81407
      Steroid Resistant, 81405
    Neurofibromatosis, 81405-81406
    NF1, 81408
    NF2, 81405-81406

Analysis — *continued*
  Gene — *continued*
    NHLRC1, 81403
    Niemann-Pick Disease, 81330, 81404, 81406
    NIPA1, 81404
    NLGN3, 81405
    NLGN4X, 81404-81405
    Nocturnal Frontal Lobe Epilepsy, 81405
    NOD2, 81401
    Nonaka Myopathy, 81400, 81406
    Non-small Cell Lung Cancer, 81401
    Nonsyndromic Hearing Loss, 81401, 81403, 81430-81431
    Noonan Spectrum Disorders, 81400, 81405-81406, 81442
    Norrie Disease, 81403-81404
    NOTCH1, 81407
    NOTCH3, 81406
    NPC1, 81404
    NPC2, 81406
    NPHP1, 81405-81406
    NPHS1, 81407
    NPHS2, 81405
    NPM1, 81310
    NPM1/ALK (t(2;5)), 81401
    NRAS, 81311
    NROB1, 81404
    NSD1, 81405-81406
    Nuclear Encoded Mitochondrial Genes, 81440
    Obesity, 81403, 81406
    Oculocutaneous Albinism (IA), 81404
    Oculomotor Apraxia, 81405
    Oncology
      Breast mRNA, 81519
      Cardiology (Heart Transplant), 81595
      Colon mRNA Screening, 81525
      Colorectal Screening, 81528
      Gynecologic
        Each Additional Single Drug or Drug Combination, 81536
        First Single Drug or Drug Combination, 81535
      Lung, 81538
      Ovary, 81500-81503
      Prostatic, 81539
      Thyroid, 81545
      Tissue of Origin, 81504
      Tumor, Unknown Origin, 81540
    OPA1, 81406-81407
    Optic Atrophy, 81406-81407
    OPTN, 81406
    Ornithine Transcarbamylase Deficiency, 81405
    Osteogenesis Imperfecta, 81408
    Osteoporosis, 81406
    OTC, 81405
    OTOF, 81430
    PABPN1, 81401
    PAFAH1B1, 81405-81406
    PAH, 81406
    PALB2, 81406, 81432
    Pancreatic Cancer, 81406
    PARK2, 81405-81406
    Parkinson Disease, 81401, 81405-81406, 81408
    Paroxysmal Nonkinesigenic Dyskinesia, 81406
    PAX2, 81406
    PAX8, 81401
    PC, 81406
    PCA3/KLK3, 81313
    PCCA, 81405-81406
    PCCB, 81406
    PCDH15, 81400, 81406-81407, 81430
    PCDH19, 81405
    PCSK9, 81406
    PDE6A, 81434
    PDE6B, 81434
    PDGFRA, 81314
    PDHA1, 81405-81406
    PDHB, 81405
    PDHX, 81406
    PDX1, 81404

Analysis — *continued*
  Gene — *continued*
    Pelizaeus-Merzbacher Disease, 81404-81405
    Pendred Syndrome, 81406, 81430-81431
    Peripheral Neuroectodermal Tumor, 81401
    Peutz-Jeghers Syndrome, 81405
    Pfeiffer Syndrome, Type 1, 81400
    Phenylketonuria, 81406
    PHEX, 81406
    PHOX2B, 81403-81404
    Pierson Syndrome, 81407
    PIK3CA, 81404
    PINK1, 81405
    Pitt-Hopkins Syndrome, 81405-81406
    PKD1, 81407
    PKD2, 81406
    PKHD1, 81408
    PKP2, 81406, 81439
    PLCE1, 81407
    PLN, 81403
    PLP1, 81404-81405
    PML/RARalpha, (t(15;17)), 81315-81316
    PMP22, 81324-81326
    PMS2, 81317-81319
    PNKD, 81406
    POLG, 81406
    Polycystic Kidney Disease, 81406-81408
    POMGNT1, 81406
    POMT1, 81406
    POMT2, 81406
    POU1F1, 81405
    PPARG (t(2;3)(q13;p25)), 81401
    PPP2R2B, 81401
    PQBP1, 81404-81405
    Prader-Willi Syndrome, 81331, 81402
    Precocious Male Puberty, 81406
    Primary Autosomal Recessive Microcephaly, 81407
    Primary Congenital Glaucoma, 81404
    Primary Microcephaly, 81407
    PRKAG2, 81406
    PRKCG, 81406
    PRNP, 81404
    Progressive External Ophthalmoplegia, 81404
    Progressive Myoclonus Epilepsy, 81403-81404
    Promyelocytic Leukemia, 81315-81316
    PROP1, 81404
    Propionic Acidemia, 81405-81406
    Prostate Cancer, 81313
    Prothrombin, Coagulation Factor II (F2), 81240
    PRPF31, 81434
    PRPH2, 81404, 81434
    PRSS1, 81401, 81404
    PRX, 81405
    PSEN1, 81405
    PSEN2, 81406
    Pseudohypoaldosteronism, 81406
    PTEN, 81321-81323, 81432, 81435
    PTPN11, 81406
    PYGM, 81401, 81406
    Pyridoxine-Dependent Epilepsy, 81406
    Pyruvate Dehydrogenase E2 Deficiency, 81406
    QT Syndrome
      Long, 81406, 81413-81414
      Short, 81406, 81413-81414
    RAB7A, 81405
    RAD51C, 81432
    RAF1, 81404, 81406
    RAI1, 81405
    RDH12, 81434
    Ready for Copy Edit, 81413
    Rearrangement
      T Cell Antigen Receptor, Beta, 81340-81341
      T Cell Antigen Receptor, Gamma, 81342
        TRB@, 81340-81341
        TRG@, 81342
    REEP1, 81405
    Renal Coloboma Syndrome, 81406
    Renpenning Syndrome, 81404-81405

Analysis — *continued*
  Gene — *continued*
    RET, 81404-81406
    Retinitis Pigmentosa, 81404, 81406
    Rett Syndrome, 81302-81304, 81404
    RHD, 81403
    Rheumatoid Arthritis, 81490
    Rh Maternal/Fetal Compatibility, 81403
    RHO, 81404, 81434
    RP1, 81404, 81434
    RP2, 81434
    RPE65, 81406, 81434
    RPGR, 81434
    RPS19, 81405
    RRM2B, 81405
    Rubinstein-Taybi Syndrome, 81406-81407
    RUNX1/RUNX1T1 (t(8;21)), 81401
    Russell-Silver Syndrome, 81402
    RYR1, 81406, 81408
    RYR2, 81408, 81413
    Saethre-Chotzen Syndrome, 81403-81404
    SCN1A, 81407
    SCN1B, 81404
    SCN4A, 81406
    SCN5A, 81407, 81413
    SCNN1A, 81406
    SCNN1B, 81406
    SCNN1G, 81406
    SCO1, 81405
    SCO2, 81404
    SDHA, 81406
    SDHB, 81405, 81437-81438
    SDHC, 81404-81405, 81437-81438
    SDHD, 81404, 81437-81438
    Segawa Syndrome, 81406
    Sensorineural Hearing Loss, 81404
    SEPT9, 81327
    SERPINA1, 81332
    SERPINE1, 81400
    SeSAME Syndrome, 81404
    SETX, 81406
    SGCA, 81405
    SGCB, 81405
    SGCD, 81405
    SGCE, 81405-81406
    SGCG, 81404-81405
    SH2D1A, 81403-81404
    SH3TC2, 81406
    SHOC2, 81400, 81405
    Short QT Syndrome, 81406, 81413-81414
    Short Tandem Repeat Markers (STR), 81265-81266
    SHOX, 81405
    Sickle Cell Anemia, 81401, 81403
    SIL1, 81405
    SLC12A1, 81407
    SLC12A3, 81407
    SLC14A1, 81403
    SLC16A2, 81404-81405
    SLC22A5, 81405
    SLC25A20, 81404-81405
    SLC25A4, 81404
    SLC26A4, 81406, 81430
    SLC2A10, 81410
    SLC2A1, 81405
    SLC37A4, 81406
    SLC4A1, 81403
    SLC9A6, 81406
    SLCO1B1, 81400
    SMAD3, 81410
    SMAD4, 81405-81406, 81435-81436
    Smith-Lemli-Opitz Syndrome, 81405
    Smith-Magenis Syndrome, 81405
    SMN1, 81400, 81403, 81405
    SMN1/SMN2, 81401
    SMPD1, 81330, 81412
    SNRPN/UBE3A, 81331
    SOD1, 81404
    Solid Organ Transplantation, 81403
    SOS1, 81406
    Sotos Syndrome, 81405-81406
    Spastic Paraplegia (SPAST), 81404-81407
    SPC11, 81407
    Specific Thyroid Hormone Cell Transporter Deficiency, 81404
    SPG7, 81405-81407

Analysis — *continued*
Gene — *continued*
Spinal Muscular Atrophy, 81401
SPINK1, 81404
Spinocerebellar Ataxia, 81401, 81406-81408
SPRED1, 81405
SPTBN2, 81407
SRY, 81400
SS18/SSX1, 81401
SS18/SSX2 (t(X;18)), 81401
Stargardt Disease, 81408
STAT3, 81405
STK11, 81404-81405, 81432-81433, 81435-81436
STR, 81265-81266
STXBP1, 81406
SURF1, 81405
Synovial Sarcoma, 81401
Systemic Primary Carnitine Deficiency, 81405
TACO1, 81404
TARDBP, 81405
Targeted Genomic Sequence Analysis Panel
Cardiac Ion Channelopathies, 81413-81414
Hematolymphoid Neoplasm or Disorder, 81450, 81455
Inherited Cardiomyopathy, 81439
Solid Organ Neoplasm, 81445, 81455
Tay-Sachs Disease, 81255, 81406, 81412
TAZ, 81406
TBP, 81401
TBX5, 81405
TCF4, 81405-81406
TGFBR1, 81405, 81410-81411
TGFBR2, 81405, 81410-81411
TH, 81406
Thalassemia, 81403-81405
Alpha, 81257, 81404
Beta, 81403-81404
THAP1, 81404
Thoracic Aortic Aneurysm/Dissection, 81408
THRB, 81405
Thrombocytopenia, 81400
Thrombophilia, 81400
Thyroid Hormone Deficiency, 81405
TK2, 81405
TMC1, 81430
TMEM127, 81437
TMEM43, 81406
TMEM67, 81407
TMPRSS3, 81430
TNNC1, 81405
TNNI3, 81405
TNNT2, 81406
TOR1A, 81400, 81404
Torsion Dystonia, 81404
TP53, 81404-81405, 81432
TPM1, 81405
TPMT, 81401
TRB@, 81340-81341
TRD@, 81402
TRG@, 81432
Trifunctional Protein Deficiency, 81406
TRPC6, 81406
TSC1, 81405-81407
TSC2, 81406-81407
TTN, 81439
TTPA, 81404
TTR, 81404
Tuberous Sclerosis, 81405-81407
TWIST1, 81403-81404
TYMP, 81405
TYMS, 81401
TYR, 81404
Tyrosinemia, 81406
UBA1, 81403
UBE3A, 81406
UDP Glucuronosyltransferase 1 Family, Polypeptide A1, 81350
UGT1A1, 81350
UMOD, 81406
Uniparental Disomy (UPD), 81402

Analysis — *continued*
Gene — *continued*
Unlisted Molecular Pathology Procedure, [81479]
Unlisted Multianalyte Assay, 81599
Unverricht-Lundborg Disease, 81401, 81404
USH1C, 81407, 81430
USH1G, 81404, 81430
USH2A, 81408, 81430, 81434
Usher Syndrome, 81400, 81404, 81406-81408, 81430-81431
Very Long Chain Acyl-Coenzyme A Dehydrogenase Deficiency, 81406
VHL, 81403-81404, 81437-81438
Vitamin K Epoxide Reductase Complex, Subunit 1, 81355
VKORC1, 81355
von Gierke Disease, 81250
von Hippel-Lindau Familial Cancer Syndrome, 81403-81404
von Willebrand Disease, 81401, 81403-81406, 81408
VPS13B, 81407-81408
VWF, 81401, 81403-81406, 81408
Walker-Warburg Syndrome, 81405-81406
Warfarin Metabolism, 81355
WAS, 81406
WDR62, 81407
Wermer Syndrome, 81404-81405
WFS1, 81430
Whole Mitochondrial Genome, 81460-81465
Wilson Disease, 81406
Wiskott-Aldrich Syndrome, 81406
WT1, 81405
X-linked Disorders
Agammaglobulinemia, 81406
Centronuclear Myopathy, 81405-81406
Hydrocephaly, 81407
Hyper IgM Syndrome, 81404
Intellectual Disability, 81470-81471
Lissencephaly with Ambiguous Genitalia, 81403-81405
Lymphoproliferative Syndrome, 81403-81404
Mental Retardation, 81403-81407
Severe Combined Immunodeficiency, 81405
ZEB2, 81404-81405
ZNF41, 81404
Genotype
by Nucleic Acid
Infectious Agent
Cytomegalovirus, [87910]
Hepatitis B Virus, [87912]
Hepatitis C Virus, 87902
HIV-1, [87906]
Protease/Reverse Transcriptase Regions, 87901
Implantable Defibrillator, 93282-93284, 93287, 93289-93290, 93292, 93295-93296
Loop Recorder, 93285, 93291, 93298-93299
Microarray
Cytogenomic Constitutional, 81228-81229
Microsatellite Instability, 81301
Multianalyte Assays with Algorithmic Analysis
Administrative, 0001M-0004M, 0006M-0009M
Categorical Result, 81545
Disease Activity, 81490
Drug Response Score, 81535-81536
Good vs Poor Overall Survival, 81538
Positive/Negative Result, 81528
Probability Predicted Main Cancer Type/Subtype, 81540
Recurrence Score, 81519, 81525
Rejection Risk Score, 81595
Risk Score, 81493, 81500, 81503-81504, 81506-81512
Tissue Similarity, 81504
Unlisted Assay, 81599
Multi-spectral, Skin Lesion, 0400T-0401T
Pacemaker, 93279-93281, 93288, 93293-93294
Patient Specific Findings, 99199
Physiologic Data, Remote, 99091

Analysis — *continued*
Prostate Tissue Fluorescence Spectroscopy, 0443T
Protein
Tissue
Western Blot, 88372
Semen, 89320-89322
Sperm Isolation, 89260, 89261
Skin Lesion, Multi-spectral, 0400T-0401T
Spectrum, 82190
Tear Osmolarity, 83861
Translocation
PML/RARalpha, 81315-81316
t(15;17), 81315-81316
t(9;22) (BCF/ABL1), 81206-81209

Anaspadias
See Epispadias

Anastomosis
Arteriovenous Fistula
with Bypass Graft, 35686
with Graft, 36825, 36830, 36832
with Thrombectomy, 36831
Direct, 36821
Revision, 36832, 36833
with Thrombectomy, 36833
without Thrombectomy, 36832
Artery
to Aorta, 33606
to Artery
Cranial, 61711
Bile Duct
to Bile Duct, 47800
to Intestines, 47760, 47780
Bile Duct to Gastrointestinal, 47760, 47780, 47785
Broncho-Bronchial, 32486
Caval to Mesenteric, 37160
Cavopulmonary, 33622, 33768
Colorectal, 44620, 44626
Epididymis
to Vas Deferens
Bilateral, 54901
Unilateral, 54900
Excision
Trachea, 31780, 31781
Cervical, 31780
Fallopian Tube, 58750
Gallbladder to Intestine, 47720-47740
Gallbladder to Pancreas, 47999
Hepatic Duct to Intestine, 47765, 47802
Ileo-Anal, 45113
Intestines
Colo-anal, 45119
Cystectomy, 51590
Enterocystoplasty, 51960
Enterostomy, 44620-44626
Ileoanal, 44157-44158
Resection
Laparoscopic, 44202-44205
Intestine to Intestine, 44130
Intrahepatic Portosystemic, 37182, 37183
Jejunum, 43820-43825
Microvascular
Free Transfer Jejunum, 43496
Nerve
Facial to Hypoglossal, 64868
Facial to Spinal Accessory, 64864, 64865
Oviduct, 58750
Pancreas to Intestines, 48520, 48540, 48548
Polya, 43632
Portocaval, 37140
Pulmonary, 33606
Renoportal, 37145
Splenorenal, 37180, 37181
Stomach, 43825
to Duodenum, 43810, 43855
Revision, 43850
to Jejunum, 43820, 43825, 43860, 43865
Tubotubal, 58750
Ureter
to Bladder, 50780-50785
to Colon, 50810, 50815
Removal, 50830
to Intestine, 50800, 50820, 50825
Removal, 50830
to Kidney, 50727-50750

Anastomosis — *continued*
Ureter — *continued*
to Ureter, 50725-50728, 50760, 50770
Vein
Saphenopopliteal, 34530
Vein to Vein, 37140-37183
Anastomosis, Aorta–Pulmonary Artery
See Aorta, Anastomosis, to Pulmonary Artery
Anastomosis, Bladder, to Intestine
See Enterocystoplasty
Anastomosis, Hepatic Duct
See Hepatic Duct, Anastomosis
Anastomosis of Lacrimal Sac to Conjunctival Sac
See Conjunctivorhinostomy
Anastomosis of Pancreas
See Pancreas, Anastomosis
ANC, 85048
Anderson Tibial Lengthening, 27715
Androstanediol Glucuronide, 82154
Androstanolone
See Dihydrotestosterone
Androstenedione
Blood or Urine, 82157
Androstenolone
See Dehydroepiandrosterone
Androsterone
Blood or Urine, 82160
Anesthesia
See also Analgesia
Abbe–Estlander Procedure, 00102
Abdomen
Abdominal Wall, 00700-00730, 00800, 00802, 00820-00836
Halsted Repair, 00750-00756
Blood Vessels, 00770, 00880-00882, 01930, 01931
Inferior Vena Cava Ligation, 00882
Transvenous Umbrella Insertion, 01930
Endoscopy, 00740, 00810
Extraperitoneal, 00860, 00862, 00866-00868, 00870
Hernia Repair, 00830-00836
Diaphragmatic, 00756
Halsted Repair, 00750-00756
Omphalocele, 00754
Intraperitoneal, 00790-00797, 00840-00851
Laparoscopy, 00790
Liver Transplant, 00796
Pancreatectomy, 00794
Renal Transplant, 00868
Abdominoperineal Resection, 00844
Abortion
Incomplete, 01965
Induced, 01966
Achilles Tendon Repair, 01472
Acromioclavicular Joint, 01620
Adrenalectomy, 00866
Amniocentesis, 00842
Amputation
Femur, 01232
Forequarter, 01636
Interthoracoscapular, 01636
Penis
Complete, 00932
Radical with Bilateral Inguinal and Iliac Lymphadenectomy, 00936
Radical with Bilateral Inguinal Lymphadenectomy, 00934
Aneurysm
Axillary–Brachial, 01652
Knee, 01444
Popliteal Artery, 01444
Angiography, 01920
Angioplasty, 01924-01926
Ankle, 00400, 01462-01522
Achilles Tendon, 01472
Nerves, Muscles, Tendons, 01470
Skin, 00400
Anorectal Procedure, 00902
Anus, 00902
Arm
Lower, 00400, 01810-01860
Arteries, 01842
Bones, Closed, 01820
Bones, Open, 01830
Cast Application, 01860

Anesthesia — *continued*
  Arm — *continued*
    Lower — *continued*
      Cast Removal, 01860
      Embolectomy, 01842
      Nerves, Muscle, Tendons, 01810
      Phleborrhaphy, 01852
      Shunt Revision, 01844
      Skin, 00400
      Total Wrist, 01832
      Veins, 01850
    Upper Arm, and Elbow, 00400, 01710-01782
      Nerves, Muscles, Tendons, 01710
        Tenodesis, 01716
        Tenoplasty, 01714
        Tenotomy, 01712
      Skin, 00400
  Arrhythmias, 00410
  Arteriograms, 01916
  Arteriography, 01916
  Arteriovenous (AV) Fistula, 01432
  Arthroplasty
    Hip, 01214, 01215
    Knee, 01402
  Arthroscopic Procedures
    Ankle, 01464
    Elbow, 01732-01740
    Foot, 01464
    Hip, 01202
    Knee, 01382, 01400, 01464
    Shoulder, 01610-01638
    Wrist, 01829-01830
  Auditory Canal, External
    Removal Foreign Body, 69205
  Axilla, 00400, 01610-01682
  Back Skin, 00300
  Batch–Spittler–McFaddin Operation, 01404
  Biopsy, 00100
    Anorectal, 00902
    Clavicle, 00454
    External Ear, 00120
    Inner Ear, 00120
    Intraoral, 00170
    Liver, 00702
    Middle Ear, 00120
    Nose, 00164
    Parotid Gland, 00100
    Salivary Gland, 00100
    Sinuses, Accessory, 00164
    Sublingual Gland, 00100
    Submandibular Gland, 00100
  Bladder, 00870, 00912
  Blepharoplasty, 00103
  Brain, 00210-00218, 00220-00222
  Breast, 00402-00406
    Augmentation Mammoplasty, 00402
    Breast Reduction, 00402
    Muscle Flaps, 00402
  Bronchi, 00542
    Intrathoracic Repair of Trauma, 00548
    Reconstruction, 00539
  Bronchoscopy, 00520
  Burns
    Debridement and/or Excision, 01951-01953
    Dressings and/or Debridement, 16020-16030
  Burr Hole, 00214
  Bypass Graft
    with pump oxygenator, younger than one year of age, 00561
    Coronary Artery without Pump Oxygenator, 00566
    Leg
      Lower, 01500
      Upper, 01270
    Shoulder, Axillary, 01654, 01656
  Cardiac Catheterization, 01920
  Cardioverter, 00534, 00560
  Cast
    Application
      Body Cast, 01130
      Forearm, 01860
      Hand, 01860
      Knee Joint, 01420
      Lower Leg, 01490

Anesthesia — *continued*
  Cast — *continued*
    Application — *continued*
      Pelvis, 01130
      Shoulder, 01680-01682
      Shoulder Spica, 01682
      Wrist, 01860
    Removal
      Forearm, 01860
      Hand, 01860
      Knee Joint, 01420
      Lower Leg, 01490
      Shoulder, 01680
      Shoulder Spica, 01682
    Repair
      Forearm, 01860
      Hand, 01860
      Knee Joint, 01420
      Lower Leg, 01490
      Shoulder, 01680
      Shoulder Spica, 01682
  Central Venous Circulation, 00532
  Cervical Cerclage, 00948
  Cervix, 00948
  Cesarean Section, 01961, 01963, 01968, 01969
  Chest, 00400-00410, 00470-00474, 00522, 00530-00539, 00542, 00546-00550
  Chest Skin, 00400
  Childbirth
    Cesarean Delivery, 01961, 01963, 01968, 01969
    External Cephalic Version, 01958
    Vaginal Delivery, 01960, 01967
  Clavicle, 00450, 00454
  Cleft Lip Repair, 00102
  Cleft Palate Repair, 00172
  Colpectomy, 00942
  Colporrhaphy, 00942
  Colpotomy, 00942
  Conscious Sedation, 99151-99157
  Corneal Transplant, 00144
  Coronary Procedures, 00560-00580
  Craniectomy, 00211
  Cranioplasty, 00215
  Craniotomy, 00211
  Culdoscopy, 00950
  Cystectomy, 00864
  Cystolithotomy, 00870
  Cystourethroscopy
    Local, 52265
    Spinal, 52260
  Decortication, 00542
  Defibrillator, 00534, 00560
  Diaphragm, 00540-00541
  Disarticulation
    Hip, 01212
    Knee, 01404
    Shoulder, 01634
  Discography, 01935-01936
  Donor
    Nephrectomy, 00862
  Dressing Change, 15852
  Drug Administration
    Epidural or Subarachnoid, 01996
  Ear, 00120-00126
  ECT, 00104
  Elbow, 00400, 01710-01782
  Electrocoagulation
    Intracranial Nerve, 00222
  Electroconvulsive Therapy (ECT), 00104
  Embolectomy
    Arm, Upper, 01772
    Femoral, 01274
    Femoral Artery, 01274
    Forearm, Wrist and Hand, 01842
    Leg, Lower, 01502
  Emergency, 99058, 99140
  Endoscopy
    Arm, Lower, 01830
    Gastrointestinal, 00740
    Intestines, 00810
    Uterus, 00952
    Vaginal, 00950
  Esophagoscopy, 00520
  Esophagus, 00320, 00500

Anesthesia — *continued*
  Excision
    Adrenal gland, 00866
    Bladder
      Total, 00864
    Gland
      Adrenal, 00866
    Iris, 00147
    Prostate, 00865
    Retropharyngeal tumor, 00174
    Testes
      Abdominal, 00928
      Inguinal, 00926
    Uterus
      Vaginal, 00944
    Vulva, 00906
  External Cephalic Version, 01958
  External Fixation System
    Adjustment/Revision, 20693
    Removal, 20694
  Eye, 00140-00148
    Corneal Transplant, 00144
    Iridectomy, 00147
    Iris, 00147
    Lens Surgery, 00142
    Ophthalmoscopy, 00148
    Vitrectomy, 00145
  Eyelid, 00103
  Facial Bones, 00190, 00192
    Mandibular, 00190
    Midface, 00190
    Zygomatic, 00190
  Fallopian Tube
    Ligation, 00851
  Femoral Artery
    Ligation, 01272
  Femur, 01220-01234, 01340, 01360
  Fibula, 01390, 01392
  Foot, 00400, 01462-01522
  Forearm, 00400, 01810-01860
  Fowler–Stephens Orchiopexy, 00930
  Gastrocnemius Recession, 01474
  Gastrointestinal Endoscopy, 00740
  Genitalia
    Female, 00940-00952, 01958-01969
    Male, 00920-00938
  Great Vessels of Chest, 00560-00563
  Hand, 00400, 01810-01860
  Harrington Rod Technique, 00670
  Head, 00210-00222, 00300
    Muscles, 00300
    Nerves, 00300
  Heart, 00560-00580
    Coronary Artery Bypass Grafting, 00566
    Electrophysiology/Ablation, 00537
    Grafting, 00566-00567
    Transplant, 00580
  Hepatectomy
    Partial, 00792
  Hernia Repair
    Abdomen
      Lower, 00830-00836
      Upper, 00750, 00752, 00756
    Hip, 01200-01215
  Humerus, 01620, 01730, 01740-01744, 01758
  Hysterectomy, 01962
    Cesarean, 01963, 01969
    Radical, 00846
    Vaginal, 00944
  Hysterosalpingography, 00952
  Hysteroscopy, 00952
  Implantable Defibrillator, 00534
  Incomplete Abortion, 01965
  Induced Abortion, 01966
  Inferior Vena Cava Ligation, 00882
  Injection procedures
    Discography
      Cervical, 01935-01936
      Lumbar, 01935-01936
    Myelography
      Cervical, 01935-01936
      Lumbar, 01935-01936
      Posterior Fossa, 01935-01936
    Nerve Blocks, 01991, 01992
    Neuroma
      Foot, 64455, 64632

Anesthesia — *continued*
  Injection procedures — *continued*
    Pneumoencephalography, 01935-01936
  Integumentary System
    Anterior Chest, 00400
    Anterior Pelvis, 00400
    Anterior Trunk, 00400
    Arm, Upper, 00400
    Axilla, 00400
    Elbow, 00400
    Extremity, 00400
    Forearm, 00400
    Hand, 00400
    Head, 00300
    Knee, 00400
    Leg, Lower, 00400
    Leg, Upper, 00400
    Neck, 00300
    Perineum, 00400
    Popliteal Area, 00400
    Posterior Chest, 00300
    Posterior Pelvis, 00300
    Posterior Trunk, 00300
    Shoulder, 00400
    Wrist, 00400
  Intestines
    Endoscopy, 00810
  Intracranial Procedures, 00210-00222
    Elevation of Depressed Skull Fracture, 00215
    Sitting Position, 00218
    Spinal Fluid Shunting, 00220
    Vascular Procedures, 00216
  Intrahepatic or Portal Circulation Shunt(s), 01931
  Intraoral Procedures, 00170-00176
    Radical Surgery, 00176
    Repair Cleft Palate, 00172
    Retropharyngeal Tumor Repair, 00174
  Intrathoracic Procedures
    Bronchi, 00539, 00548
    Trachea, 00539, 00548
  Intrathoracic System, 00500, 00520-00529, 00530-00548, 00550, 00560-00566, 00580
  Iridectomy, 00147
  Keen Operation, 00604
  Kidney, 00862, 00868, 00872, 00873
  Knee, 00400, 01320-01444
  Knee Skin, 00400
  Laminectomy, 00604
  Laparoscopy, 00790-00792, 00840
  Larynx, 00320, 00326
  Leg
    Lower, 00400, 01462-01522
    Upper, 01200-01274
  Lens, 00142
  Life Support for Organ Donor, 01990
  Ligation
    Fallopian Tube, 00851
  Lips
    Repair of Cleft, 00102
  Lithotripsy, 00872, 00873
  Liver, 00702, 00792, 00796
    Hemorrhage, 00792
    Percutaneous Biopsy, 00702
    Transplant, 00796, 01990
  Lumbar Puncture, 00635
  Lungs, 00522, 00539-00548
    Transplant, 00580
  Lymphadenectomy, 00934, 00936
    Bilateral, Inguinal and Iliac with Radical Amputation Penis, 00936
    Bilateral, Inguinal with Radical Amputation Penis, 00934
  Lymphatic System, 00320, 00322
  Malunion
    Humerus, 01744
  Mammoplasty, 00402
  Manipulation
    Spine, 22505
  Manipulation of Temporomandibular Joint(s) (TMJ)
    Therapeutic, 21073
  Marcellation Operation, 00944
  Mediastinoscopy, 00528-00529

Anesthesia — *continued*
- Mediastinum, 00528-00529, 00540-00541
- Mouth, 00170, 00172
- Myelography, 01935-01936
  - Cervical, 01935-01936
  - Injection Lumbar, 01935-01936
  - Posterior Fossa, 01935-01936
- Myringotomy, 69421
- Neck, 00300-00352
- Needle Biopsy
  - Pleura, 00522
  - Thyroid, 00322
- Nephrectomy, 00862
- Nerve Blocks, 01991-01992
- Neuraxial
  - Cesarean Delivery, 01968, 01969
  - Labor, 01967-01969
  - Vaginal Delivery, 01967
- Neurectomy, 01180, 01190
- Nose, 00160-00164
  - Removal
    - Foreign Body, 30310
- Omphalocele, 00754
- Ophthalmoscopy, 00148
- Orchiectomy, 00926-00928
  - Abdominal, 00928
  - Inguinal, 00926
- Orchiopexy, 00930
  - Torek Procedure, 00930
- Organ Harvesting
  - Brain–Dead Patient, 01990
- Osteoplasty
  - Tibia/Fibula, 01484
- Osteotomy
  - Humerus, 01742
  - Tibia/Fibula, 01484
- Other Procedures, 01990-01999
- Otoscopy, 00124
- Pacemaker Insertion, 00530
- Pacing Cardioverter/Defibrillator, 00534
- Pancreas, 00794
- Pancreatectomy, 00794
- Panniculectomy, 00802
- Parotid Gland, 00100
- Patella, 01390, 01392
- Pectus Excavatum, 00474
- Pelvic Exenteration, 00848
- Pelvis, 00400, 00865, 01112-01190
  - Amputation, 01140
  - Bone, 01120
  - Bone Marrow, 01112
  - Examination, 57400
  - Extraperitoneal, 00864
  - Intraperitoneal, 00844-00851
  - Repair, 01173
  - Skin, 00300, 00400
- Penis, 00932-00938
- Percutaneous
  - Liver Biopsy, 00702
  - Spine and Spinal Cord, 01935-01936
- Pericardial Sac, 00560-00563
- Pericardium, 00560-00563
- Perineum, 00904-00908
- Pharynx, 00174, 00176
- Phleborrhaphy
  - Arm, Upper, 01782
  - Forearm, Wrist and Hand, 01852
- Pleura, 00540-00541
  - Needle Biopsy, 00522
- Pleurectomy, 32310-32320, 32656
- Pneumocentesis, 00524
- Popliteal Area, 00400, 01320, 01430-01444
- Prognathism, 00192
- Prostate, 00865, 00908, 00914
- Prostatectomy
  - Perineal, 00908
  - Radical, 00865
    - Retropubic, 00865
    - Suprapubic, 00865
    - Walsh Modified Radical, 00865
- Ptosis Surgery, 00103
- Radical Surgery, Procedures, Resections
  - Ankle Resection, 01482
  - Breast, Radical or Modified, 00402
  - Breast with Internal Mammary Node Dissection, 00406

Anesthesia — *continued*
- Radical Surgery, Procedures, Resections — *continued*
  - Elbow, 01756
  - Facial Bones, 00192
  - Femur, 01234
  - Foot Resection, 01482
  - Hip Joint Resection, 01234
  - Humeral Head and Neck Resection, 01630
  - Humerus, 01756
  - Hysterectomy, 00846
  - Intraoral Procedures, 00176
  - Lower Leg Bone Resection, 01482
  - Nose, 00162
  - Orchiectomy, Abdominal, 00928
  - Orchiectomy, Inguinal, 00926
  - Pectus Excavatum, 00474
  - Pelvis, 01150
  - Penis Amputation with Bilateral Inguinal and Iliac Lymphadenectomy, 00936
  - Penis Amputation with Bilateral Inguinal Lymphadenectomy, 00934
  - Perineal, 00904
  - Prognathism, 00192
  - Prostatectomy, 00865
  - Shoulder Joint Resection, 01630-01638
  - Sinuses, Accessory, 00162
  - Sternoclavicular Joint resection, 01630
  - Testes
    - Abdominal, 00928
    - Inguinal, 00926
- Radiologic Procedures, 01916-01936
  - Arterial
    - Therapeutic, 01924-01926
  - Arteriograms
    - Needle, Carotid, Vertebral, 01916
    - Retrograde, Brachial, Femoral, 01916
  - Cardiac Catheterization, 01920
  - Discography Lumbar, 01935-01936
  - Injection Hysterosalpingography, 00952
  - Spine and Spinal Cord
    - Percutaneous Image, Guided, 01935-01936
  - Venous/Lymphatic, 01930-01933
    - Therapeutic, 01930-01933
- Reconstructive Procedures
  - Blepharoplasty, 00103
  - Breast, 00402
  - Ptosis Surgery, 00103
- Renal Procedures, 00862
- Repair
  - Achilles Tendon, Ruptured, with or without Graft, 01472
  - Cast
    - Forearm, 01860
    - Hand, 01860
    - Knee Joint, 01420
    - Lower Leg, 01490
    - Shoulder, 01680
    - Shoulder Spica, 01682
    - Wrist, 01860
  - Cleft Lip, 00102
  - Cleft Palate, 00172
  - Humerus
    - Malunion, 01744
    - Nonunion, 01744
  - Knee Joint, 01420
- Repair of Skull, 00215
- Repair, Plastic
  - Cleft Lip, 00102
  - Cleft Palate, 00172
- Replacement
  - Ankle, 01486
  - Elbow, 01760
  - Hip, 01212-01215
  - Knee, 01402
  - Shoulder, 01638
  - Wrist, 01832
- Restriction
  - Gastric
    - for Obesity, 00797
- Retropharyngeal Tumor Excision, 00174
- Rib Resection, 00470-00474
- Sacroiliac Joint, 01160, 01170, 27096
- Salivary Glands, 00100
- Scapula, 00450

Anesthesia — *continued*
- Scheie Procedure, 00147
- Second Degree Burn, 01953
- Sedation
  - Moderate, 99155-99157
    - with Independent Observation, 99151-99153
- Seminal Vesicles, 00922
- Shoulder, 00400-00454, 01610-01682
  - Dislocation
    - Closed Treatment, 23655
- Shunt
  - Spinal Fluid, 00220
- Sinuses
  - Accessory, 00160-00164
    - Biopsy, Soft Tissue, 00164
    - Radical Surgery, 00162
- Skin
  - Anterior Chest, 00400
  - Anterior Pelvis, 00400
  - Arm, Upper, 00400
  - Axilla, 00400
  - Elbow, 00400
  - Forearm, 00400
  - Hand, 00400
  - Head, 00300
  - Knee, 00400
  - Leg, Lower, 00400
  - Leg, Upper, 00400
  - Neck, 00300
  - Perineum, 00400
  - Popliteal Area, 00400
  - Posterior Chest, 00300
  - Posterior Pelvis, 00300
  - Shoulder, 00400
  - Wrist, 00400
- Skull, 00190
- Skull Fracture
  - Elevation, 00215
- Special Circumstances
  - Emergency, 99140
  - Extreme Age, 99100
  - Hypotension, 99135
  - Hypothermia, 99116
- Spinal Instrumentation, 00670
- Spinal Manipulation, 00640
- Spine and Spinal Cord, 00600-00670
  - Cervical, 00600-00604, 00640, 00670
  - Injection, 62320-62327
  - Lumbar, 00630-00635, 00640, 00670
  - Percutaneous Image Guided, 01935-01936
  - Thoracic, 00620-00626, 00640, 00670
  - Vascular, 00670
- Sternoclavicular Joint, 01620
- Sternum, 00550
- Stomach
  - Restriction
    - for Obesity, 00797
- Strayer Procedure, 01474
- Subcutaneous Tissue
  - Anterior Chest, 00400
  - Anterior Pelvis, 00400
  - Arm, Upper, 00400
  - Axilla, 00400
  - Elbow, 00400
  - Forearm, 00400
  - Hand, 00400
  - Head, 00100
  - Knee, 00400
  - Leg, Lower, 00400
  - Leg, Upper, 00400
  - Neck, 00300
  - Perineum, 00400
  - Popliteal Area, 00400
  - Posterior Chest, 00300
  - Posterior Pelvis, 00300
  - Shoulder, 00400
  - Wrist, 00400
- Subdural Taps, 00212
- Sublingual Gland, 00100
- Submandibular (Submaxillary) Gland, 00100
- Suture Removal, 15850-15851
- Sympathectomy
  - Lumbar, 00632
- Symphysis Pubis, 01160, 01170
- Temporomandibular Joint, 21073

Anesthesia — *continued*
- Tenodesis, 01716
- Tenoplasty, 01714
- Tenotomy, 01712
- Testis, 00924-00930
- Third Degree Burn, 01951-01953
- Thoracoplasty, 00472
- Thoracoscopy, 00528-00529, 00540-00541
- Thoracotomy, 00540-00541
- Thorax, 00400-00474
- Thromboendarterectomy, 01442
- Thyroid, 00320-00322
- Tibia, 01390, 01392, 01484
- TIPS, 01931
- Trachea, 00320, 00326, 00542, 00548
  - Reconstruction, 00539
- Transplant
  - Cornea, 00144
  - Heart, 00580
  - Kidney, 00868
  - Liver, 00796, 01990
  - Lungs, 00580
  - Organ Harvesting, 01990
- Transurethral Procedures, 00910-00918
  - Fragmentation
    - Removal Ureteral Calculus, 00918
  - Resection Bleeding, 00916
  - Resection of Bladder Tumors, 00912
  - Resection of Prostate, 00914
- Tubal Ligation, 00851
- Tuffier Vaginal Hysterectomy, 00944
- TURP, 00914
- Tympanostomy, 00120
- Tympanotomy, 00126
- Unlisted Services and Procedures, 01999
- Urethra, 00910, 00918, 00920, 00942
- Urethrocystoscopy, 00910
- Urinary Bladder, 00864, 00870, 00912
- Urinary Tract, 00860
- Uterus, 00952
- Vagina, 00940, 00942, 00950
  - Dilation, 57400
  - Removal
    - Foreign Body, 57415
- Vaginal Delivery, 01960
- Vascular Access, 00532
- Vascular Shunt, 01844
- Vascular Surgery
  - Abdomen, Lower, 00880, 00882
  - Abdomen, Upper, 00770
  - Arm, Lower, 01840-01852
  - Arm, Upper, 01770-01782
  - Brain, 00216
  - Elbow, 01770-01782
  - Hand, 01840-01852
  - Knee, 01430-01444
  - Leg, Lower, 01500-01522
  - Leg, Upper, 01260-01274
  - Neck, 00350, 00352
  - Shoulder, 01650-01670
  - Wrist, 01840-01852
- Vas Deferens
  - Excision, 00921
- Vasectomy, 00921
- VATS, 00520
- Venography, 01916
- Ventriculography, 00214, 01920
- Vertebral Process
  - Fracture/Dislocation
    - Closed Treatment, 22315
- Vertebroplasty, 01935-01936
- Vitrectomy, 00145
- Vitreoretinal Surgery, 00145
- Vitreous Body, 00145
- Vulva, 00906
- Vulvectomy, 00906
- Wertheim Operation, 00846
- Wound
  - Dehiscence
    - Abdomen
      - Upper, 00752
  - Wrist, 00400, 01810-01860

Aneurysm, Aorta, Abdominal
- *See* Aorta, Abdominal, Aneurysm
- Screening Study, 76706

Aneurysm, Artery, Femoral
  See Artery, Femoral, Aneurysm
Aneurysm, Artery, Radial
  See Artery, Radial, Aneurysm
Aneurysm, Artery, Renal
  See Artery, Renal, Aneurysm
Aneurysm, Basilar Artery
  See Artery, Basilar, Aneurysm
Aneurysm Repair
  Aorta
    Abdominal, 34800-34805, 34825-34832,
      34841-34848, 35081-35103, 75952,
      75953
    Thoracoabdominal, 33877
  Axillary Artery, 35011, 35013
  Basilar Artery, 61698, 61702
  Brachial Artery, 35011, 35013
  Carotid Artery, 35001, 35002, 61613, 61697,
    61700, 61703
  Celiac Artery, 35121, 35122
  Femoral Artery, 35141, 35142
  Hepatic Artery, 35121, 35122
  Iliac Artery, 34900, 35131-35132, 75953-75954
  Innominate Artery, 35021, 35022
  Intracranial Artery, 61705, 61708
  Mesenteric Artery, 35121, 35122
  Popliteal Artery, 35151, 35152
  Radial Artery, 35045
  Renal Artery, 35121, 35122
  Splenic Artery, 35111, 35112
  Subclavian Artery, 35001, 35002, 35021, 35022
  Thoracic Aorta, 33880-33889, 75956-75959
  Thoracoabdominal Aorta, 33877
  Ulnar Artery, 35045
  Vascular Malformation or Carotid Cavernous
    Fistula, 61710
  Vertebral Artery, 61698, 61702
ANG, 81403
Angel Dust, 83992
Anginal Symptoms and Level of Activity Assessment, 1002F
Angiocardiographies
  See Heart, Angiography
Angiography
  Abdomen, 74174-74175, 74185, 75726
  Abdominal Aorta, 75635, 75952, 75953
  Adrenal Artery, 75731, 75733
  Aortography, 75600-75630
    Injection, 93567
  Arm Artery, 73206, 75710, 75716
  Arteriovenous Shunt, 36901-36906
  Atrial, 93565-93566
  Brachial Artery, 75658
  Brain, 70496
  Bypass Graft, 93455, 93457, 93459-93461
  Carotid Artery, 36221-36228
  Cervico-Vertebral Arch, 36221-36226
  Chest, 71275, 71555
  Congenital Heart, 93563-93564
  Coronary Artery, 93454-93461, 93563
    Coronary Calcium Evaluation, 75571
    Flow Velocity Measurement During Angiography, 93571, 93572
  Dialysis Circuit, Diagnostic, 36901
    with Balloon Angioplasty, 36902
    with Mechanical Thrombectomy, 36904-36906
    with Stent Placement, 36903
  Endovascular Repair, 75952, 75953
  Extremity, Lower, 73725
  Extremity, Upper, 73225
  Fluorescein, 92235
  Head, 70496, 70544-70546
    with Catheterization, 93454-93461
  Heart Vessels
    Injection, 93454-93461, 93563, 93565-93566
  Indocyanine-Green, 92240
  Innominate Artery, 36222-36223, 36225
  Intracranail Administration Pharmacologic
    Agent
    Arterial, Other Than Thrombolysis, 61650-61651
  Intracranial Carotid, 36223-36224
  Left Heart
    Injection, 93458-93459, 93565

Angiography — *continued*
  Leg Artery, 73706, 75635, 75710, 75716
  Lung
    Injection pulmonary artery, 93568
      See Cardiac Catheterization, Injection
  Mammary Artery, 75756
  Neck, 70498, 70547-70549
  Non-Cardiac Vascular Flow Imaging, 78445
  Nuclear Medicine, 78445
  Other Artery, 75774
  Pelvic Artery, 72198, 75736
  Pelvis, 72191, 74174
  Pulmonary Artery, 75741-75746
  Right Heart
    Injection, 93456-93457, 93566
  Shunt, Dialysis, 36901-36906
  Spinal Artery, 75705
  Spinal Canal, 72159
  Subclavian Artery, 36225
  Thorax, 71275
  Transcatheter Therapy
    Embolization, 75894, 75898
    Infusion, 75898
  Ventricular, 93565-93566
  Vertebral Artery, 36221, 36225-36226, 36228
Angioma
  See Lesion, Skin
Angioplasty
  with Placement Intravascular Stent, 37217,
    37236-37239]
  Aorta, [37246, 37247]
  Axillary Artery, [37246, 37247]
  Blood Vessel Patch, 35201-35286
  Brachiocephalic Artery, [37246, 37247]
  Common Carotid Artery with Stent Placement,
    37217-37218
  Coronary Artery
    Percutaneous Transluminal, [92920, 92921]
      with Atherectomy, [92924, 92925],
        [92933, 92934, 92937, 92938,
        92941, 92943, 92944]
      with Stent, [92928, 92929, 92933,
        92934, 92937, 92938, 92941,
        92943, 92944]
  Dialysis Circuit, 36902-36903, 36905-36907
  Femoral Artery, 37224-37227
  for Revascularization
    Coronary, [92937, 92938], [92941, 92943,
      92944]
    Coronary Bypass Graft(s), [92937, 92938],
      [92941, 92943, 92944]
    Femoral, 37224-37227
    Iliac, 37220-37223
    Peroneal, 37228-37235
    Popliteal, 37224-37227
    Tibial, 37228-37235
  Iliac Artery, 37220-37223
  Innominate Artery with Stent Placement, 37217
  Intracranial, 61630, 61635
    Percutaneous, 61630
  Percutaneous Transluminal
    Coronary, [92920, 92921]
    Dialysis Circuit, 36905-36907
    Pulmonary, 92997-92998
  Peroneal Artery, 37228-37235
  Popliteal Artery, 37224-37227
  Pulmonary Artery
    Percutaneous Transluminal, 92997, 92998
  Renal or Visceral Artery, [37246, 37247]
  Subclavian Artery, [37246, 37247]
  Tibioperoneal Artery, 37228-37235
  Vein Patch Graft, 35879, 35884
  Venous, [37248, 37249]
  Visceral Artery, [37246, 37247]
    Endovascular, 34841-34848
Angioscopy
  Noncoronary vessels, 35400
Angiotensin
  A-I (Angiotensin I), 82164, 84244
  A-II (Angiotensin II), 82163
  Gene Analysis Receptor, 81400
  Performance Measures
    Angiotensin Converting Enzyme Inhibitor,
      4010F, 4480F-4481F
    Angiotensin Receptor Blocker, 4010F,
      4188F, 4210F, 4480F-4481F

Angiotensin — *continued*
  Renin, 80408, 80416-80417, 84244
  Riboflavin, 84252
Angiotensin Converting Enzyme (ACE)
  See Angiotensin
Angiotensin Forming Enzyme
  See Angiotensin
  See Renin
Angle Deformity
  Reconstruction
    Toe, 28313
Anhydride, Carbonic, 82374
Anhyrides, Acetic
  See Acetic Anhydrides
Animal Inoculation, 87003, 87250
Ankle
  See also Fibula, Leg, Lower; Tibia, Tibiofibular
    Joint
  Abscess
    Incision and Drainage, 27603
  Amputation, 27888
  Arthrocentesis, 20605-20606
  Arthrodesis, 27870
  Arthrography, 73615
  Arthroplasty, 27700, 27702, 27703
  Arthroscopy
    Surgical, 29891-29899
  Arthrotomy, 27610, 27612, 27620-27626
  Biopsy, 27613, 27614, 27620
  Bursa
    Incision and Drainage, 27604
  Disarticulation, 27889
  Dislocation
    Closed Treatment, 27840, 27842
    Open Treatment, 27846, 27848
  Exploration, 27610, 27620
  Fracture
    Bimalleolar, 27808-27814
    Lateral, 27786-27814
    Medial, 27760-27766, 27808-27814
    Posterior, 27767-27769, 27808-27814
    Trimalleolar, 27816-27823
  Fusion, 27870
  Hematoma
    Incision and Drainage, 27603
  Incision, 27607
  Injection
    Radiologic, 27648
  Lesion
    Excision, 27630
  Magnetic Resonance Imaging (MRI), 73721-73723
  Manipulation, 27860
  Removal
    Foreign Body, 27610, 27620
    Implant, 27704
    Loose Body, 27620
  Repair
    Achilles Tendon, 27650-27654
    Ligament, 27695-27698
    Tendon, 27612, 27680-27687
  Strapping, 29540
  Synovium
    Excision, 27625, 27626
  Tenotomy, 27605, 27606
  Tumor, 26535, 27615-27638 [27632, 27634],
    27645-27647
  Unlisted Services and Procedures, 27899
  X-ray, 73600, 73610
    with Contrast, 73615
ANKRD1, 81405
Ankylosis (Surgical)
  See Arthrodesis
Annuloplasty
  Percutaneous, Intradiscal, 22526-22527, 22899
ANO5, 81406
Anogenital Region
  See Perineum
Anoplasty
  Stricture, 46700, 46705
Anorectal
  Biofeedback, 90911
  Exam, 45990
  Myomectomy, 45108
  Repair
    Fistula, 46706-46707

Anorectovaginoplasty, 46744, 46746
Anoscopy
  with Delivery of Thermal Energy, 46999
  with Injection Bulking Agent, 0377T
  Ablation
    Polyp, 46615
    Tumor, 46615
  Biopsy, 46606-46607
  Dilation, 46604
  Exploration, 46600
  Hemorrhage, 46614
  High Resolution, 46601, 46607
  Removal
    Foreign Body, 46608
    Polyp, 46610-46612
    Tumor, 46610-46612
Antebrachium
  See Forearm
Antecedent, Plasma Thromboplastin, 85270
Antepartum Care
  Antepartum Care Only, 59425, 59426
  Cesarean Delivery, 59510
    Previous, 59610-59618
  Included with
    Cesarean Delivery, 59510
      Failed NSVD, Previous C-Section,
        59618
    Vaginal Delivery, 59400
      Previous C-Section, 59610
    Vaginal Delivery, 59425-59426
Anterior Ramus of Thoracic Nerve
  See Intercostal Nerve
Antesternal Esophagostomy, 43499
Anthrax Vaccine, 90581
Anthrogon, 80418, 80426, 83001
Antiactivator, Plasmin, 85410
Anti Australia Antigens
  See Antibody, Hepatitis B
Antibiotic Administration
  Injection, 96372-96379
  Prescribed or Dispensed, 4120F-4124F
Antibiotic Sensitivity, 87181, 87184, 87188
  Enzyme Detection, 87185
  Minimum Bactericidal Concentration, 87187
  Minimum Inhibitory Concentration, 87186
  Minimum Lethal Concentration, 87187
Antibodies, Thyroid-Stimulating, 84445
  See Immunoglobulin, Thyroid Stimulating
Antibodies, Viral
  See Viral Antibodies
Antibody
  Actinomyces, 86602
  Adenovirus, 86603
  Antinuclear, 86038, 86039
  Anti-Phosphatidylserine (Phospholipid), 86148
  Antistreptolysin 0, 86060, 86063
  Aspergillus, 86606
  Bacterium, 86609
  Bartonella, 86611
  Beta 2 Glycoprotein I, 86146
  Blastomyces, 86612
  Blood Crossmatch, 86920-86923
  Bordetella, 86615
  Borrelia, 86617-86619
  Brucella, 86622
  Campylobacter, 86625
  Candida, 86628
  Cardiolipin, 86147
  Chlamydia, 86631, 86632
  Coccidioides, 86635
  Coxiella Burnetii, 86638
  C-Reactive Protein (CRP), 86140-86141
  Cryptococcus, 86641
  Cyclic Citrullinated Peptide (CCP), 86200
  Cytomegalovirus, 86644, 86645
  Cytotoxic Screen, 86807, 86808
  Deoxyribonuclease, 86215
  Deoxyribonucleic Acid (DNA), 86225, 86226
  Diphtheria, 86648
  Ehrlichia, 86666
  Encephalitis, 86651-86654
  Enterovirus, 86658
  Epstein-Barr Virus, 86663-86665
  Fc Receptor, 86243
  Fluorescent, 86255, 86256
  Francisella Tularensis, 86668

Antibody — *continued*
  Fungus, 86671
  Giardia Lamblia, 86674
  Growth Hormone, 86277
  Helicobacter Pylori, 86677
  Helminth, 86682
  Hemoglobin, Fecal, 82274
  Hemophilus Influenza, 86684
  Hepatitis A, 86708, 86709
  Hepatitis B
    Core, 86704
    IgM, 86705
    Surface, 86706
  Hepatitis Be, 86707
  Hepatitis C, 86803, 86804
  Hepatitis, Delta Agent, 86692
  Herpes Simplex, 86694-86696
  Heterophile, 86308-86310
  Histoplasma, 86698
  HIV, 86689, 86701-86703
  HIV-1, 86701, 86703
  HIV-2, 86702, 86703
  HTLV-I, 86687, 86689
  HTLV-II, 86688
  Human Leukocyte Antigens (HLA), 86828-86835
  Influenza Virus, 86710
  Insulin, 86337
  Intrinsic Factor, 86340
  Islet Cell, 86341
  JC (John Cunningham) Virus, 86711
  Legionella, 86713
  Leishmania, 86717
  Leptospira, 86720
  Listeria Monocytogenes, 86723
  Lyme Disease, 86617
  Lymphocytic Choriomeningitis, 86727
  Lymphogranuloma Venereum, 86729
  Malaria, 86750
  Microsomal, 86376
  Mucormycosis, 86732
  Mumps, 86735
  Mycoplasma, 86738
  Neisseria Meningitidis, 86741
  Nocardia, 86744
  Nuclear Antigen, 86235
  Other Infectious Agent, 86317
  Other Virus, 86790
  Parvovirus, 86747
  Phospholipid
    Cofactor, 86849
    Neutralization, 85597-85598
  Plasmodium, 86750
  Platelet, 86022-86023
  Protozoa, 86753
  Red Blood Cell, 86850-86870
  Respiratory Syncytial Virus, 86756
  Rickettsia, 86757
  Rotavirus, 86759
  Rubella, 86762
  Rubeola, 86765
  Salmonella, 86768
  Screening, 86807-86808
  Shigella, 86771
  Sperm, 89325
  Streptokinase, 86590
  Tetanus, 86774
  Thyroglobulin, 86800
  Toxoplasma, 86777, 86778
  Treponema Pallidum, 86780
  Trichinella, 86784
  Tuberculosis, 86580
  Varicella-Zoster, 86787
  West Nile Virus, 86788-86789
  White Blood Cell, 86021
  Yersinia, 86793
Antibody Identification
  Fluorescent, 86255-86256
  Immunoassay, 83516, 83518-83520
  Immunochemistry, 88342, 88344, [88341]
  Immunoelectrophoresis, 86320, 86325, 86327, 86334-86335
  Leukocyte Antibodies, 86021, 86828-86835
  Platelet, 86022, 86023
  Red Blood Cell, 86850, 86860, 86870
    Pretreatment, 86970-86972, 86975-86978

Antibody Identification — *continued*
  Serum
    Pretreatment, 86975-86978
    Solid Phase Assay, 86828-86835
Antibody Neutralization Test, 86382
Antibody Receptor, 86243
Antibody Screening
  Cytotoxic Percent Reactive Antibody (PRA), 86807-86808
  Fluorescent Noninfectious Agent, 86255
Anticoagulant, 85300-85305, 85307
Anticoagulant Management, 99363-99364
Antidiabetic Hormone, 82943
Anti D Immunoglobulin, 90384-90386
Antidiuretic Hormone, 84588
Antidiuretic Hormone Measurement
  See Vasopressin
Anti–DNA Autoantibody, 86038-86039
Antigen
  Allergen Immunotherapy, 95144-95149, 95165, 95170
  Carcinoembryonic, 82378
  HIV, 87389
  Mononuclear Cell, 86356
  Prostate Specific
    Complexed, 84152
    Free, 84154
    Total, 84153
  Skin Test, 86486
Antigen, Australia
  See Hepatitis Antigen, B Surface
Antigen Bronchial Provocation Tests
  See Bronchial Challenge Test
Antigen, CD4, 86360
Antigen, CD8, 86360
Antigen Detection
  Direct Fluorescence, 87265-87272, 87276, 87278, 87280, 87285, 87290
    Bordetella, 87265
    Chlamydia Trachomatis, 87270
    Cryptosporidium, 87272
    Cytomegalovirus, 87271
    Enterovirus, 87267
    Giardia, 87269
    Influenza A, 87276
    Legionella Pneumophila, 87278
    Not Otherwise Specified, 87299
    Respiratory Syncytial Virus, 87280
    Treponema Pallidum, 87285
    Varicella Zoster, 87290
  Enzyme Immunoassay, 87301-87451
    Adenovirus, 87301
    Aspergillus, 87305
    Chlamydia Trachomatis, 87320
    Clostridium Difficile, 87324
    Cryptococcus Neoformans, 87327
    Cryptosporidium, 87328
    Cytomegalovirus, 87332
    Entamoeba Histolytica Dispar Group, 87336
    Entamoeba Histolytica Group, 87337
    Escherichia Coli 0157, 87335
    Giardia, 87329
    Helicobacter Pylori, 87338, 87339
    Hepatitis Be Antigen (HBeAg), 87350
    Hepatitis B Surface Antigen (HBsAg), 87340
    Hepatitis B Surface Antigen (HBsAg) Neu-tralization, 87341
    Hepatitis Delta Agent, 87380
    Histoplasma Capsulatum, 87385
    HIV-1, 87389-87390
    HIV-2, 87391
    Influenza A, 87400
    Influenza B, 87400
    Multiple Step Method, 87301-87449
    Polyvalent, 87451
    Not Otherwise Specified, 87449-87451
    Respiratory Syncytial Virus, 87420
    Rotavirus, 87425
    Shigella-like Toxin, 87427
    Single Step Method, 87450
    Streptococcus, Group A, 87430
  Immunoassay
    Direct Optical
      Clostridium Difficile Toxin A, 87803
      Influenza, 87804
      Respiratory Syncytial Virus, 87807

Antigen Detection — *continued*
  Immunoassay — *continued*
    Direct Optical — *continued*
      Streptococcus, Group B, 87802
      Trichomonas Vaginalis, 87808
    Immunofluorescence, 87260, 87273-87275, 87277, 87279, 87281, 87283, 87299, 87300
      Adenovirus, 87260
      Bordatella Pertussis, 87265
      Chlamydia Trachomatis, 87270
      Cryptosporidium, 87272
      Giardia, 87269
      Herpes Simplex, 87273, 87274
      Influenza A, 87276
      Influenza B, 87275
      Legionella Micdadei, 87277
      Legionella Pneumophila, 87278
      Not otherwise specified, 87299
      Parainfluenza Virus, 87279
      Pneumocystis Carinii, 87281
      Polyvalent, 87300
      Respiratory Syncytial Virus, 87280
      Rubeola, 87283
      Treponema Pallidum, 87285
      Varicella Zoster, 87290
Antigens, CD142
  See Thromboplastin
Antigens, CD143, 82164
Antigens, E, 87350
Antigens, Hepatitis
  See Hepatitis Antigen
Antigens, Hepatitis B, 87515-87517
Antihemophilic Factor B, 85250
Antihemophilic Factor C, 85270
Antihemophilic Globulin (AHG), 85240
Antihuman Globulin, 86880-86886
Anti–Human Globulin Consumption Test
  See Coombs Test
Anti–inflammatory/Analgesic Agent Prescribed, 4016F
Antimony, 83015
Antinuclear Antibodies (ANA), 86038, 86039
  Fluorescent Technique, 86255, 86256
Anti–Phosphatidylserine (Phospholipid) Anti-body, 86148
Anti–Phospholipid Antibody, 86147
Antiplasmin, Alpha–2, 85410
Antiprotease, Alpha 1
  See Alpha–1 Antitrypsin
Antistreptococcal Antibody, 86215
Antistreptokinase Titer, 86590
Antistreptolysin 0, 86060, 86063
Antithrombin III, 85300, 85301
Antithrombin VI, 85362-85380
Antitoxin Assay, 87230
Antiviral Antibody
  See Viral Antibodies
Antrostomy
  Sinus/Maxillary, 31256-31267
Antrotomy
  Sinus
    Maxillary, 31020-31032
    Transmastoid, 69501
Antrum of Highmore
  See Sinus, Maxillary
Antrum Puncture
  Sinus
    Maxillary, 31000
    Sphenoid, 31002
Anus
  Ablation, 46615
  Abscess
    Incision and Drainage, 46045, 46050
  Biofeedback, 90911
  Biopsy
    Endoscopic, 46606-46607
  Crypt
    Excision, 46999
  Dilation
    Endoscopy, 46604
  Endoscopy
    Biopsy, 46606-46607
    Dilation, 46604
    Exploration, 46600
    Hemorrhage, 46614

Anus — *continued*
  Endoscopy — *continued*
    High Resolution Anoscopy (HRA), 46601, 46607
    Removal
      Foreign Body, 46608
      Polyp, 46610, 46612
      Tumor, 46610, 46612
  Excision
    Tag, 46230, [46220]
  Exploration
    Endoscopic, 46600
    Surgical, 45990
  Fissure
    Destruction, 46940, 46942
    Excision, 46200
  Fistula
    Closure, 46288
    Excision, 46270-46285
    Repair, 46706-46707
  Hemorrhage
    Endoscopic Control, 46614
  Hemorrhoids
    Clot Excision, [46320]
    Destruction, 46930
    Excision, 46250-46262
    Injection, 46500
    Ligation, 0249T, 45350, 46221, [45398], [46945], [46946]
    Stapling, [46947]
    Suture, [46945], [46946]
  High Resolution Anoscopy, 46601, 46607
  Imperforated
    Repair, 46715-46742
  Incision
    Septum, 46070
    Sphincterotomy, 46200
  Lesion
    Destruction, 46900-46917, 46924
    Excision, 45108, 46922
  Manometry, 91122
  Placement
    Seton, 46020
  Polyp, 46615
  Reconstruction, 46742
    with Graft, 46753
    with Implant, 46762
    Congenital Absence, 46730-46740
    Sphincter, 46750, 46751, 46760-46762
  Removal
    Foreign Body, 46608
    Polyp(s), 46610, 46612
    Ablation, 46615
    Seton, 46030
    Suture, 46754
    Tumor(s), 46610, 46612
    Wire, 46754
  Repair
    Anovaginal Fistula, 46715, 46716
    Cloacal Anomaly, 46744-46748
    Fistula, 46706-46707
    Stricture, 46700, 46705
  Sphincter
    Chemodenervation, 46505
    Electromyography, 51784, 51785
    Needle, 51785
  Sphincterotomy, with Fissurectomy, 46200
  Thermal Energy Delivery, 46999
  Tumor, 46615
  Unlisted Procedure, 46999
Aorta
  Abdominal
    Aneurysm, 34800-34805, 34825-34832, 34841-34848, 35081-35103, 75952, 75953
      Screening Study, 76706
    Thromboendarterectomy, 35331
  Anastomosis
    to Pulmonary Artery, 33606
  Angiogram
    Injection, 93567
  Angioplasty, [37246, 37247, 37248, 37249]
  Aortography, 75600-75630
  Ascending
    Graft, 33864

Aorta — *continued*
Balloon
  Insertion, 33967, 33970, 33973
  Removal, 33968, 33971, 33974
Catheterization
  Catheter, 36200
  Intracatheter, 36160
  Needle, 36160
Circulation Assist
  Insertion, 33967, 33970, 33973
  Removal, 33968, 33971, 33974
Conduit to Heart, 33404
Excision
  Coarctation, 33840-33851
Graft, 33860-33864, 33875
Infrarenal
  Endovascular Repair, 34845-34848
Insertion
  Balloon Device, 33967, 33970, 33973
  Catheter, 36200
  Graft, 33330-33335, 33864
  Intracatheter, 36160
  Needle, 36160
Removal
  Balloon Assist Device, 33968, 33971, 33974
Repair, 33320-33322, 33802, 33803
  Aneurysm
    Abdominal, 34800-34805, 34832, 35081-35103
      Radiological S&I, 75952-75953
    Ascending, 33860, 33863-33864
    Sinus of Valsalva, 33720
    Thoracic, 33875, 33877
      Endovascular, 33880-33891
        Radiological S&I, 75956-75959
      Thoracoabdominal, 33877
      Transverse Arch, 33870
  Aortic Anomalies, 33800-33803
  Aortic Arch, 33852-33853
  Coarctation, 33840-33851
  Graft, 33860-33877
    Ascending, 33864
  Hypoplastic or Interrupted Aortic Arch
    with Cardiopulmonary Bypass, 33853
    without Cardiopulmonary Bypass, 33852
  Sinus of Valsalva, 33702-33720
  Thoracic Aneurysm with Graft, 33860-33877
    Endovascular, 33880-33891, 75956-75959
  Translocation Aortic Root, 33782-33783
  Transposition of the Great Vessels, 33770-33781
Suspension, 33800
Suture, 33320-33322
Thoracic
  Aneurysm, 33880-33889, 75956-75959
  Repair, 75956-75959
    Endovascular, 33880-33891
Thromboendarterectomy, 35331
Ultrasound, 76706, 76770, 76775
Valve
  Implantation, 33361-33369
  Incision, 33415
  Repair, 33390-33391
    Gusset Aortoplasty, 33417
    Left Ventricle, 33414
    Stenosis
      Idiopathic Hypertrophic, 33416
      Subvalvular, 33415
      Supravalvular, 33417
    Valvuloplasty
      Open
        with Cardiopulmonary Bypass, 33390
        Complex, 33391
  Replacement
    with Allograft Valve, 33406
    with Aortic Annulus Enlargement, 33411-33412
    with Cardiopulmonary Bypass, 33367-33369, 33405-33406, 33410
    with Prosthesis, 33361-33369, 33405
    with Stentless Tissue Valve, 33410

Aorta — *continued*
Valve — *continued*
  Replacement — *continued*
    with Translocation Pulmonary Valve, 33413
    Open, 33405-33413
    Transcatheter, 33361-33369
  Visceral
    Endovascular Repair, 34841-34848
  X–ray with Contrast, 75600-75630
Aorta–Pulmonary ART Transposition
  See Transposition, Great Arteries
Aortic Sinus
  See Sinus of Valsalva
Aortic Stenosis
  Repair, 33415
    Nikaidoh Procedure, 33782-33783
    Supravalvular, 33417
Aortic Valve
  See Heart, Aortic Valve
Aortic Valve Replacement
  See Replacement, Aortic Valve
Aortocoronary Bypass
  See Coronary Artery Bypass Graft (CABG)
Aortocoronary Bypass for Heart Revascularization
  See Artery, Coronary, Bypass
Aortography, 75600, 75605, 75630, 93567
  with Iliofemoral Artery, 75630, 75635
  See Angiography
  Serial, 75625
Aortoiliac
  Embolectomy, 34151, 34201
  Thrombectomy, 34151, 34201
Aortopexy, 33800
Aortoplasty
  Supravalvular Stenosis, 33417
AP, *[51797]*
APBI (Accelerated Partial Breast Irradiation), 19296-19298
APC, 81201-81203, 81435
Apendico-Vesicostomy, 50845
Apert–Gallais Syndrome
  See Adrenogenital Syndrome
Apexcardiogram, 93799
Aphasia Testing, 96105
Apheresis
  Therapeutic, 36511-36516
    with Selective HDL Delipidation and Plasma Reinfusion, 0342T
Apical–Aortic Conduit, 33404
Apicectomy
  with Mastoidectomy, 69530, 69605
    Petrous, 69530
Apicoectomy, 41899
Apnea
  Central
    Neurostimulator System, 0424T-0436T
Apoaminotransferase, Aspartate, 84550
APOB, 81401
APOE, 81401
Apolipoprotein
  Blood or Urine, 82172
APP, 81406
Appendectomy, 44950-44960
  Laparoscopic, 44970
Appendiceal Abscess
  See Abscess, Appendix
Appendico–Stomy, 44799
Appendico–Vesicostomy
  Cutaneous, 50845
Appendix
  Abscess
    Incision and Drainage, 44900
  Excision, 44950-44960
  Incision and Drainage
    Open, 44900
    Laparoscopic, 44970
Application
  Allergy Tests, 95044
  Bone Fixation Device
    Multiplane, 20692
    Stereo Computer Assisted, 20696-20697
    Uniplane, 20690
  Caliper, 20660
  Casts, 29000-29086, 29305-29450

Application — *continued*
  Compression System, 29581-29584
  Cranial Tongs, 20660
  Fixation Device
    Shoulder, 23700
  Halo
    Cranial, 20661
      Thin Skull Osteology, 20664
    Femoral, 20663
    Maxillofacial Fixation, 21100
    Pelvic, 20662
  Injector, 96377
    Subcutaneous, On-body, 96377
  Interbody Biomechanical Device, 22853
  Interdental Fixation Device, 21110
  Interlaminar/Interspinous Stabilization/Distraction Device, 22867-22870
  Intervertebral Biomechanical Device, 22854, 22859
  Multi-layer Compression System, 29581-29584
  Neurostimulation, 64550, 64566
    On-body Injector, 96377
  Pulmonary Artery Bands, 33620
  Radioelement
    with Ultrasound, 76965
    Interstitial or Intracavitary, 77761-77763, 77770-77772
    Surface, 77767-77768, 77789
  Skin Substitute, 15271-15278
  Splint, 29105-29131, 29505-29515
  Stereotactic Frame, 20660, 61800
  Topical Fluoride Varnish, 99188
Application of External Fixation Device
  See Fixation (Device), Application, External
APPT
  See Thromboplastin, Partial, Time
APPY, 44950-44960
APTT
  See Thromboplastin, Partial, Time
APTX, 81405
AQP1, 81403
AQP2, 81404
Aquatic Therapy
  with Exercises, 97113
Aqueous Shunt
  without Extraocular Reservoir, 0449T-0450T
  See also Drainage, Aqueous
  to Extraocular Reservoir, 66179-66180
    Revision, 66184-66185
AR, 81401, 81405
Archival Tissue Examination, 88363
Arch, Zygomatic
  See Zygomatic Arch
Arm
  See Radius; Ulna; Wrist
  Excision
    Excess Skin, 15836
    Lipectomy, Suction Assisted, 15878
  Lower
    Abscess, 25028
      Excision, 25145
      Incision and Drainage Bone, 25035
    Amputation, 25900, 25905, 25915
      Re-amputation, 25909
      Revision, 25907, 25909
    Angiography, 73206
    Artery
      Ligation, 37618
    Biopsy, 25065, 25066
    Bursa
      Incision and Drainage, 25031
    Bypass Graft, 35903
    Cast, 29075
    CT Scan, 73200-73206
    Decompression, 25020-25025
    Exploration
      Blood Vessel, 35860
    Fasciotomy, 24495, 25020-25025
    Hematoma, 25028
    Incision and Drainage, 23930
    Lesion, Tendon Sheath
      Excision, 25110
    Magnetic Resonance Imaging (MRI), 73218-73220, 73223
    Reconstruction
      Ulna, 25337

Arm — *continued*
Lower — *continued*
  Removal
    Foreign Body, 25248
  Repair
    Blood Vessel with Other Graft, 35266
    Blood Vessel with Vein Graft, 35236
    Decompression, 24495
    Muscle, 25260, 25263, 25270
      Secondary, 25265
    Secondary
      Muscle or Tendon, 25272, 25274
      Tendon, 25260-25274, 25280-25295, 25310-25316
        Secondary, 25265
      Tendon Sheath, 25275
  Replantation, 20805
  Splint, 29125, 29126
  Strapping, 29583-29584
  Tendon
    Excision, 25109
    Lengthening, 25280
    Shortening, 25280
    Transplantation, 25310-25312
  Tenotomy, 25290
  Tumor, 25075-25078 *[25071, 25073]*, 25120-25126
  Ultrasound, 76881-76882
  Unlisted Services and Procedures, 25999
  X–ray, 73090
    with Upper Arm, 73092
Removal
  Foreign Body
    Forearm or Wrist, 25248
Repair
  Muscle, 24341
  Tendon, 24341
Skin Graft
  Delay of Flap, 15610
  Full Thickness, 15220, 15221
  Muscle, Myocutaneous, or Fasciocutaneous Flaps, 15736
  Pedicle Flap, 15572
  Split, 15100-15111
Tendon
  Excision, 25109
Tissue Transfer, Adjacent, 14020, 14021
Upper
  Abscess
    Incision and Drainage, 23930
  Amputation, 23900-23921, 24900, 24920
    with Elongation Stump, 24935
    with Implant, 24931
    Cineplasty, 24940
    Revision, 24925
  Anesthesia, 00400, 01710-01782
  Angiography, 73206
  Artery
    Ligation, 37618
  Biopsy, 24065, 24066
  Bypass Graft, 35903
  Cast, 29065
  CT Scan, 73200-73206
  Exploration
    Blood Vessel, 35860
  Hematoma
    Incision and Drainage, 23930
  Magnetic Resonance Imaging (MRI), 73218-73220, 73223
  Muscle Revision, 24330, 24331
  Removal
    Cast, 29705
    Foreign Body, 24200, 24201
  Repair
    Blood Vessel with Other Graft, 35266
    Blood Vessel with Vein Graft, 35236
    Muscle Revision, 24301, 24320
    Muscle Transfer, 24301, 24320
    Tendon, 24332
    Tendon Lengthening, 24305
    Tendon Revision, 24320
    Tendon Transfer, 24301
    Tenotomy, 24310
  Replantation, 20802
  Splint, 29105
  Strapping, 29583-29584

Arm — *continued*
Upper — *continued*
Tumor, 24075-24079 *[24071, 24073]*
Ultrasound, 76881-76882
Unlisted Services and Procedures, 24999
Wound Exploration, 20103
Penetrating, 20103
X–ray, 73060
X–ray with Lower Arm
Infant, 73092
Arnold–Chiari Malformation Repair, 61343
AROM, 95851, 95852, 97110, 97530
Arrest, Epiphyseal
Femur, 20150, 27185, 27475, 27479, 27485, 27742
Fibula, 20150, 27477-27485, 27730-27742
Radius, 20150, 25450, 25455
Tibia, 20150, 27477-27485, 27730, 27734-27742
Ulna, 20150, 25450, 25455
Arrhythmias
Electrical Conversion Anesthesia, 00410
Induction, 93618
Arrhythmogenic Focus
Heart
Destruction, 33250-33251, 33261, 93653-93656
ARSA, 81405
Arsenic
Blood or Urine, 82175
Heavy Metal
Qualitative, Any Number of Analytes, 83015
Quantitative, Each, NEC, 82175, 83018
ART, 86592, 86593
ART4, 81403
Arterial Catheterization
See Cannulation, Arterial
Arterial Dilatation, Transluminal
See Angioplasty, Transluminal
Arterial Grafting for Coronary Artery Bypass
See Bypass Graft, Coronary Artery, Arterial
Arterial Pressure
See Blood Pressure
Non-invasive Waveform Analysis, 93050
Arterial Puncture, 36600
Arteriography, Aorta
See Aortography
Arteriosus, Ductus
Closure, Transcatheter, 93582
Repair, 33820-33824
Arteriosus, Truncus
Repair, 33786
Arteriotomy
See Incision, Artery; Transection, Artery
Arteriovenous Anastomosis, 36818-36821
Arteriovenous Fistula
Cannulization
Vein, 36815
Creation, 36825-36830
Hemodialysis via Fistula, 4052F
Referral, 4051F
Repair
Abdomen, 35182
Acquired or Traumatic, 35189
Head, 35180
Acquired or Traumatic, 35188
Lower Extremity, 35184
Acquired or Traumatic, 35190
Neck, 35180
Acquired or Traumatic, 35188
Thorax, 35182
Acquired or Traumatic, 35189
Upper Extremity, 35184
Acquired or Traumatic, 35190
Revision
Hemodialysis Graft or Fistula
with Thrombectomy, 36833
without Thrombectomy, 36832
Thrombectomy
Dialysis Circuit, 36904-36906
Arteriovenous Malformation
Carotid
Endovascular, 61623
Obliteration, 61613
Repair, 61705-61710

Arteriovenous Malformation — *continued*
Cranial
Balloon
Angioplasty, 61630
Dilatation for Vasospasm, 61640-61642
Endovascular, 61623-61624
Intravascular Stent(s), 61635
Repair, 61680-61692, 61705, 61708
Iliac Artery
Repair, 0254T, 34900
Spinal
Excision, 63250-63252
Injection, 62294
Repair, 63250-63252
Transcatheter, 61624
Vascular Embolization, 37241-37242
Arteriovenous Shunt
Angiography, 36901-36906
Aorta to Pulmonary Artery, 33755, 33762
Blalock-Taussig, 33750
Dialysis Circuit, 36901-36909
Intrahepatic Portosystemic
Insertion, 37182
Revision, 37183
Patency, 78291
Peritoneal-Venous
Evaluation, 49427
Insertion, 49425
Ligation, 49428
Removal, 49429
Revision, 49426
Potts-Smith Shunt, 33762
Subclavian to Pulmonary Artery, 33750
Thomas Shunt, 36835
Waterson Shunt, 33755
Artery
Abdomen
Angiography, 75726
Catheterization, 36245-36248
Ligation, 37617
Adrenal
Angiography, 75731, 75733
Anastomosis
Cranial, 61711
Angiography, Visceral, 75726
Angioplasty
Aorta
Aneurysm Screening Study, 76706
Angioplasty, *[37246, 37247]*
Aortobifemoral
Bypass Graft, 35540
Aortobi-iliac
Bypass Graft, 35538, 35638
Aortocarotid
Bypass Graft, 35526, 35626
Aortofemoral
Bypass Graft, 35539
Aortoiliac
Bypass Graft, 35537, 35637
Embolectomy, 34151, 34201
Thrombectomy, 34151, 34201
Aortoiliofemoral, 35363
Aortoinnominate
Bypass Graft, 35526, 35626
Aortosubclavian
Bypass Graft, 35526, 35626
Arm
Angiography, 75710, 75716
Harvest of Artery for Coronary Artery By-
pass Graft, 35600
Transluminal, 0234T-0238T
Assessment
Endothelial Function, 0337T
Atherectomy
Brachiocephalic, 0237T
Coronary, *[92924, 92925, 92928, 92929,
92933, 92934, 92937, 92938, 92941,
92943, 92944]*
Femoral, 37225, 37227
Iliac, 0238T
Peroneal, 37229, 37231, 37233, 37235
Popliteal, 37225, 37227
Renal, 0234T
Tibial, 37229, 37231, 37233, 37235

Artery — *continued*
Atherectomy — *continued*
Transluminal, 0234T-0238T, *[92924, 92925,
92928, 92929, 92933, 92934, 92937,
92938, 92941, 92943, 92944]*
Visceral, 0235T
Axillary
Aneurysm, 35011, 35013
Angioplasty, *[37246, 37247]*
Bypass Graft, 35516-35522, 35533, 35616-
35623, 35650, 35654
Embolectomy, 34101
Thrombectomy, 34101
Thromboendarterectomy, 35321
Basilar
Aneurysm, 61698, 61702
Biopsy
Transcatheter, 75970
Brachial
Aneurysm, 35011, 35013
Angiography, 75658
Bypass Graft, 35510, 35512, 35522, 35525
Catheterization, 36120
Embolectomy, 34101
Exploration, 24495
Exposure, 34834
Thrombectomy, 34101
Thromboendarterectomy, 35321
Brachiocephalic
Angioplasty, *[37246, 37247]*
Atherectomy, 0237T
Catheterization, 36215-36218
Bypass Graft
with Composite Graft, 35681-35683
Autogenous
Three or More Segments
Two Locations, 35683
Two Segments
Two Locations, 35682
Cannulization
for Extra Corporeal Circulation, 36823
to Vein, 36810-36821
Carotid
Aneurysm, 35001-35005, 61697-61710
Vascular Malformation or Carotid Cav-
ernous Fistula, 61710
Baroflex Activation Device
Implantation, 0266T-0268T
Interrogation Evaluation, 0272T-0273T
Removal, 0269T-0271T
Replacement, 0266T-0268T
Revision, 0269T-0271T
Bypass Graft, 35891, 35500-35510, 35526,
35601-35606, 35626, 35642
Catheterization, 36100, 36221-36224,
36227-36228
Cavernous Fistula, 61705, 61708, 61710
Decompression, 61590, 61591, 61595,
61596
Embolectomy, 34001
Excision, 60605
Exploration, 35701
Ligation, 37600-37606, 61611, 61612
Reimplantation, 35691, 35694-35695
Stenosis
Imaging Study Measurement, 3100F
Stent Placement
Transcatheter, 37215-37217
Transposition, 33889, 35691, 35694-
35695
Vascular Malformation, 61705, 61708,
61710
Thrombectomy, 34001
Thromboendarterectomy, 35301, 35390
Transection, 61611, 61612
Transposition, 33889, 35691, 35694-35695
Carotid Cavernous Fistula, 61705, 61708, 61710
Carotid, Common Intima–Media Thickness
Study, 0126T
Catheterization
Abdominal, 36245-36248
Aorta, 36200
Thoracic, Nonselective, 36221
Translumbar, 36160
AV Shunt, 36901-36902
with Stent Insertion, 36903

Artery — *continued*
Catheterization — *continued*
Brachial, 36120
Brachiocephalic Branch, 36215-36218
Carotid, 36100
Common Carotid, Selective, 36222,
36223
External Carotid, Selective, 36227
Internal Carotid, Selective, 36224
Each Intracranial Branch, 36228
Dialysis Circuit, 36901-36902
Extremity, 36140
Innominate, Selective, 36222-36223
Lower Extremity, 36245-36248
Pelvic, 36245-36248
Pulmonary, 36013-36015
Renal, 36251-36254
Thoracic Branch, 36215-36218
Vertebral, Selective
Each Intracranial Branch, 36228
Celiac
Aneurysm, 35121, 35122
Bypass Graft, 35531, 35631
Embolectomy, 34151
Endoprosthesis, 34841-34848
Thrombectomy, 34151
Thromboendarterectomy, 35341
Chest
Ligation, 37616
Coronary
Angiography, 93454-93461, *[92924, 92925],
[92933, 92934]*
Atherectomy, *[92924, 92925], [92933,
92934]*
Bypass
Arterial, 33533-33536
Internal Mammary Artery Graft,
4110F
Combined arterial and venous, 33517-
33523
Venous, 33510-33523
Graft, 33503-33505
Ligation, 33502
Obstruction Severity Assessment, 0206T
Repair, 33500-33507
Thrombectomy
Percutaneous, *[92973]*
Thrombolysis, *[92975], [92977]*
Translocation, 33506-33507
Unroofing, 33507
Digital
Sympathectomy, 64820
Endothelial Function Assessment Noninvasive,
0337T
Ethmoidal
Ligation, 30915
Extra Corporeal Circulation
for Regional Chemotherapy of Extremity,
36823
Extracranial
Anastomosis, 61711
Vascular Studies
Duplex Scan, 93880-93882
Extremities
Vascular Studies, 93922-93931
Bypass Grafts Extremities, 93925-93931
Extremity
Bypass Graft Revision, 35879-35884
Catheterization, 36140, 36245-36248
Ligation, 37618
Femoral
Aneurysm, 35141, 35142
Angiography, 73706
Angioplasty, 37224-37227
Atherectomy, 37225, 37227, 37229, 37231
Bypass Graft, 35521, 35533, 35539-35540,
35556-35558, 35566, 35621, 35646,
35647, 35650-35661, 35666, 35700
Bypass Graft Revision, 35883-35884
Bypass In Situ, 35583-35585
Embolectomy, 34201
Exploration, 35721
Exposure, 34812, 34813
Thrombectomy, 34201
Thromboendarterectomy, 35302, 35371-
35372

Artery — *continued*
Great Vessel Repair, 33770-33781
Hepatic
Aneurysm, 35121, 35122
Iliac
Aneurysm, 35131-35132, 75954
Angioplasty, 37220-37223
Atherectomy, 0238T
Bypass Graft, 35537-35538, 35563, 35565, 35632-35634, 35637-35638, 35663, 35665
Embolectomy, 34151, 34201
Endoprosthesis, 0254T-0255T
Exposure, 34820, 34833
Occlusion Device, 34808
Revascularization, 37220-37223
Thrombectomy, 34151, 34201
Thromboendarterectomy, 35351, 35361, 35363
Tube Endoprosthesis, 34900, 75954
Ilioceliac
Bypass Graft, 35632
Iliofemoral
Bypass Graft, 35565, 35665
Thromboendarterectomy, 35355, 35363
X–ray with Contrast, 75630
Iliomesenteric
Bypass Graft, 35633
Iliorenal
Bypass Graft, 35634
Innominate
Aneurysm, 35021, 35022
Catheterization, 36222-36223, 36225
Embolectomy, 34001, 34101
Stent Placement
Transcatheter, 37217
Thrombectomy, 34001, 34101
Thromboendarterectomy, 35311
Intracranial
Anastomosis, 33606
Aneurysm, 61705, 61708, 61710
Angioplasty, 61630
Infusion Thrombolysis, 61645
Thrombectomy, Percutaneous, 61645
Leg
Angiography, 75710, 75716
Catheterization, 36245-36248
Mammary
Angiography, 75756
Maxillary
Ligation, 30920
Mesenteric
Aneurysm, 35121, 35122
Bypass Graft, 35331, 35631
Embolectomy, 34151
Endoprosthesis, 34841-34848
Thrombectomy, 34151
Thromboendarterectomy, 35341
Middle Cerebral Artery, Fetal Vascular Studies, 76821
Neck
Ligation, 37615
Nose
Incision, 30915, 30920
Other Angiography, 75774
Other Artery
Angiography, 75774
Exploration, 35761
Pelvic
Angiography, 72198, 75736
Catheterization, 36245-36248
Peripheral Arterial Rehabilitation, 93668
Peroneal
Angioplasty, 37228-37235
Atherectomy, 37229, 37231, 37233, 37235
Bypass Graft, 35566, 35571, 35666, 35671
Bypass In Situ, 35585, 35587
Embolectomy, 34203
Thrombectomy, 34203
Thromboendarterectomy, 35305-35306
Popliteal
Aneurysm, 35151, 35152
Angioplasty, 37224-37227
Atherectomy, 37225, 37227
Bypass Graft, 35556, 35571, 35583, 35623, 35656, 35671, 35700

Artery — *continued*
Popliteal — *continued*
Bypass In Situ, 35583, 35587
Embolectomy, 34201-34203
Exploration, 35741
Thrombectomy, 34201-34203
Thromboendarterectomy, 35303
Pulmonary
Anastomosis, 33606
Angiography, 75741-75746
Angioplasty, 92997-92998
Banding, 33620, 33622, 33690
Embolectomy, 33910, 33915-33916
Endarterectomy, 33916
Ligation, 33924
Repair, 33690, 33925-33926
Arborization Anomalies, 33925-33926
Atresia, 33920
Stenosis, 33917
Radial
Aneurysm, 35045
Embolectomy, 34111
Sympathectomy, 64821
Thrombectomy, 34111
Rehabilitation, 93668
Reimplantation
Carotid, 35691, 35694, 35695
Subclavian, 35693-35695
Vertebral, 35691-35693
Visceral, 35697
Renal
Aneurysm, 35121, 35122
Angiography, 36251-36254
Angioplasty, [37246, 37247, 37248, 37249]
Atherectomy, 0234T
Bypass Graft, 35536, 35560, 35631, 35636
Catheterization, 36251-36254
Embolectomy, 34151
Endoprosthesis, 34841-34848
Thrombectomy, 34151
Thromboendarterectomy, 35341
Repair
with Other Graft, 35261-35286
with Vein Graft, 35231-35256
Aneurysm, 61697-61710
Angioplasty
Radiological Supervision, 36902, 36905
Direct, 35201-35226
Revision
Hemodialysis Graft or Fistula
Open without Revision, 36831
Revision
with Thrombectomy, 36833
without Thrombectomy, 36832
Spinal
Angiography, 75705
Splenic
Aneurysm, 35111, 35112
Angioplasty, [37246, 37247]
Bypass Graft, 35536, 35636
Stent Insertion
Dialysis Segment, 36903, 36906, 36908
Subclavian
Aneurysm, 35001-35002, 35021-35022
Angioplasty, [37246, 37247]
Bypass Graft, 35506, 35511-35516, 35526, 35606-35616, 35626, 35645
Catheterization, 36225
Embolectomy, 34001-34101
Reimplantation, 35693-35695
Thrombectomy, 34001-34101
Thromboendarterectomy, 35301, 35311
Transposition, 33889, 35693-35695
Unlisted Services and Procedures, 37799
Superficial Femoral
Thromboendarterectomy, 35302
Superficial Palmar Arch
Sympathectomy, 64823
Temporal
Biopsy, 37609
Ligation, 37609
Thoracic
Catheterization, 33621, 36215-36218
Thrombectomy, 37184-37186
Dialysis Circuit, 36904-36906
Hemodialysis Graft or Fistula, 36831

Artery — *continued*
Thrombectomy — *continued*
Intracranial, Percutaneous, 61645
Other than Hemodialysis Graft or Fistula, 35875, [37246, 37247]
Thrombolysis (Noncoronary), [37211], [37213, 37214]
Intracranial Infusion, 61645
Tibial
Angiography, 73706
Angioplasty, 37228
Atherectomy, 37229, 37231, 37233, 37235
Bypass Graft, 35566, 35571, 35623, 35666, 35671
Bypass In Situ, 35585, 35587
Embolectomy, 34203
Thrombectomy, 34203
Thromboendarterectomy, 35305-35306
Tibial/Peroneal Trunk-Tibial
Bypass Graft, 35570
Tibial-Tibial
Bypass Graft, 35570
Tibioperoneal
Angioplasty, 37228-37235
Atherectomy, 37229, 37231, 37233, 37235
Tibioperoneal Trunk Thromboendartectomy, 35304
Transcatheter Therapy, 75894, 75898
with Angiography, 75894, 75898
Transposition
Carotid, 33889, 35691, 35694, 35695
Subclavian, 33889, 35693-35695
Vertebral, 35691, 35693
Ulnar
Aneurysm, 35045
Bypass Graft, 35523
Embolectomy, 34111
Sympathectomy, 64822
Thrombectomy, 34111
Umbilical
Vascular Study, 76820
Unlisted Services and Procedures, 37799
Vascular Study
Extremities, 93922, 93923
Vertebral
Aneurysm, 35005, 61698, 61702
Bypass Graft, 35508, 35515, 35642, 35645
Catheterization, 36100
Decompression, 61597
Reimplantation, 35691-35693
Thromboendarterectomy, 35301
Transposition, 35691-35693
Visceral
Angioplasty, [37246, 37247]
Atherectomy, 0235T
Reimplantation, 35697
Artery Catheterization, Pulmonary
See Catheterization, Pulmonary Artery
Arthrectomy
Elbow, 24155
Arthrocentesis
Bursa
Intermediate joint, 20605-20606
Large joint, 20610-20611
Small joint, 20600-20604
Intermediate Joint, 20605-20606
Large Joint, 20610-20611
Small Joint, 20600-20604
Arthrodesis
Ankle, 27870
Tibiotalar and Fibulotalar Joints, 29899
Arthroscopy
Subtalar Joint, 29907
Atlas-axis, 22595
Blair, 27870
Campbell, 27870
Carpometacarpal Joint
Hand, 26843, 26844
Thumb, 26841, 26842
Cervical
Anterior, 22551-22552, 22554, 22585
Atlas-Axis, 22548, 22585, 22595
Below C2, 22551-22554, 22585, 22600
Clivus-C1-C2, 22548, 22585, 22595
Occiput-C2, 22590
Posterior, 22590, 22595, 22600, 22614

Arthrodesis — *continued*
Elbow, 24800, 24802
Finger Joint, 26850-26863
Interphalangeal, 26860-26863
Metacarpophalangeal, 26850
Foot Joint, 28705-28735, 28740
with Advancement, 28737
with Lengthening, 28737
Pantalar, 28705
Subtalar, 28725
with Stabilization Implant, 0335T
Triple, 28715
Grice, 28725
Hand Joint, 26843, 26844
Hip Joint, 27284, 27286
Intercarpal Joint, 25800-25825
Interphalangeal Joint, 26860-26863
Great Toe, 28755
with Tendon Transfer, 28760
Knee, 27580
Lumbar, 22612, 22614, 22630-22634
Metacarpophalangeal Joint, 26850-26852
Great Toe, 28750
Metatarsophalangeal Joint
Great Toe, 28750
Pre-Sacral Interbody, 0195T-0196T
With Instrumentation, 0309T
Pubic Symphysis, 27282
Radioulnar Joint, Distal, 25830
with Resection of Ulna, 25830
Sacroiliac Joint, 27280
with Stabilization, 27279
Presacral Interbody, 0195T
Shoulder
See Shoulder, Arthrodesis
Shoulder Joint, 23800
with Autogenous Graft, 23802
Smith-Robinson, 22808
Subtalar Joint, 29907
Talus
Pantalar, 28705
Subtalar, 28725
Triple, 28715
Tarsal Joint, 28730, 28735, 28737, 28740
with Advancement, 28737
with Lengthening, 28737
Tarsometatarsal Joint, 28730, 28735, 28740
Thumb Joint, 26841, 26842
Tibiofibular Joint, 27871
Vertebra, 22610
Additional Interspace
Anterior/Anterolateral Approach, 22585
Lateral Extracavitary, 22534
Posterior/Posterolateral and/or Lateral Transverse Process, 22632
Cervical
Anterior/Anterolateral Approach, 22548
Posterior/Posterolateral and/or Lateral Transverse Process, 22590-22600
Lumbar
Anterior/Anterolateral Approach, 22558, 22585
Lateral Extracavitary, 22533-22534
Posterior/Interbody, 22630-22632
Posterior/Posterolateral and/or Lateral Transverse Process, 22612, 22614, 22630
Presacral Interbody Technique, 0195T-0196T, 22586
Spinal Deformity
Anterior Approach, 22808-22812
Posterior Approach, 22800, 22802, 22804
Spinal Fusion
Exploration, 22830
Thoracic
Anterior/Anterolateral Approach, 22556
Lateral Extracavitary, 22532, 22534
Posterior/Posterolateral and/or Lateral Traverse Process, 22610
Transverse Technique, 22610, 22612

Arthrodesis — *continued*
  Vertebrae
    Additional Interspace
      Anterior/Anterolateral Approach,
        22585
      Lateral Extracavitary, 22534
      Posterior, 22632
      Posterior/Posterolateral with Posterior
        Interbody Technique, 22634
    Cervical
      Anterior/Anterolateral Approach,
        22548
      Posterior/Posterolateral and/or Lateral
        Transverse Process, 22590-
        22600
    Lumbar
      Anterior/Anterolateral Approach,
        22558
      Lateral Extracavitary, 22532-22534
      Posterior/Interbody, 22630
      Posterior/Posterolateral and/or Lateral
        Transverse Process, 22612
      Posterior/Posterolateral with Posterior
        Interbody Technique, 22633
      Pre-sacral Interbody, 0195T-0196T,
        0309T, 22586
      Transverse Process, 22612
    Spinal Deformity
      Anterior Approach, 22808-22812
      Kyphectomy, 22818-22819
      Posterior Approach, 22800-22804
      Smith-Robinson, 22808
    Spinal Fusion
      Exploration, 22830
    Thoracic
      Anterior/Anterolateral Approach,
        22556
      Lateral Extracavitary, 22532, 22534
      Posterior/Posterolateral and/or Lateral
        Transverse Process, 22610
  Wrist, 25800-25830
    with Graft, 25810
    with Sliding Graft, 25805
    Radioulnar Joint, Distal, 25820, 25830
Arthrography
  Ankle, 73615
    Injection, 27648
  Elbow, 73085
    Injection, 24220
    Revision, 24370-24371
  Hip, 73525
    Injection, 27093, 27095
  Knee, 73580
    Injection, 27370
  Sacroiliac Joint, 27096
  Shoulder, 73040
    Injection, 23350
  Temporomandibular Joint (TMJ), 70328-70332
    Injection, 21116
  Wrist, 73115
    Injection, 25246
Arthroplasty
  Ankle, 27700-27703
  Bower's, 25332
  Cervical, 0375T, 22856
  Elbow, 24360
    with Implant, 24361, 24362
    Revision, 24370-24371
    Total Replacement, 24363
  Hip, 27132
    Partial Replacement, 27125
    Revision, 27134-27138
    Total Replacement, 27130
  Interphalangeal Joint, 26535, 26536
  Intervertebral Disc
    Removal, 22864-22865, 0164T
    Revision, 22861-22862, 0165T
    Total Replacement, 0163T, 0375T, 22856-
      22857, [0376T]
    with Osteophytectomy, 22856
  Knee, 27437-27443, 27446, 27447
    with Prosthesis, 27438, 27445
    Implantation, 27445
    Intraoperative Balance Sensor, 0396T
    Revision, 27486, 27487
  Lumbar, 0163T, 22857

Arthroplasty — *continued*
  Lumbar — *continued*
    Removal, 0164T, 22865
    Revision, 0165T, 22862
  Metacarpophalangeal Joint, 26530, 26531
  Radius, 24365
    with Implant, 24366
  Reconstruction
    Prosthesis
      Hip, 27125
  Removal
    Cervical, 22864
    Each Additional Interspace, 0095T
    Lumbar, 22865
  Revision
    Cervical, 22861
    Each Additional Interspace, 0098T
    Lumbar, 22862
  Shoulder Joint
    with Implant, 23470, 23472
    Revision, 23473-23474
  Spine
    Cervical, 22856
    Lumbar, 22857
    Three or More Levels, 0375T
  Subtalar Joint
    Implant for Stabilization, 0335T
  Temporomandibular Joint, 21240-21243
  Vertebral Joint, 0200T-0202T
  Wrist, 25332, 25441-25447
    with Implant, 25441-25445
    Carpal, 25443
    Lunate, 25444
    Navicular, 25443
    Pseudarthrosis Type, 25332
    Radius, 25441
    Revision, 25449
    Total Replacement, 25446
    Trapezium, 25445
    Ulna, 25442
Arthropods
  Examination, 87168
Arthroscopy
  Diagnostic
    Elbow, 29830
    Hip, 29860
    Knee, 29870, 29871
    Metacarpophalangeal Joint, 29900
    Shoulder, 29805
    Temporomandibular Joint, 29800
    Wrist, 29840
  Surgical
    Ankle, 29891-29899
    Elbow, 29834-29838
    Foot, 29999
    Hip, 29861-29863 [29914, 29915, 29916]
    Knee, 29871-29889
      Cartilage Allograft, 29867
      Cartilage Autograft, 29866
      Debridement/Shaving, 29880-29881
        with Chondroplasty, 29880-29881
      Meniscal Transplantation, 29868
      Osteochondral Autograft, 29866
    Metacarpophalangeal Joint, 29901, 29902
    Shoulder, 29806-29828
      Biceps Tenodesis, 29828
    Subtalar Joint
      Arthrodesis, 29907
      Debridement, 29906
      Removal of Loose or Foreign Body,
        29904
      Synovectomy, 29905
    Temporomandibular Joint, 29804
    Toe, 29999
    Wrist, 29843-29848
  Unlisted Services and Procedures, 29999
Arthrotomy
  with Biopsy
    Acromioclavicular Joint, 23101
    Glenohumeral Joint, 23100
    Hip Joint, 27052
    Knee Joint, 27330
    Sacroiliac Joint
      Hip Joint, 27050
    Sternoclavicular Joint, 23101

Arthrotomy — *continued*
  with Synovectomy
    Glenohumeral Joint, 23105
    Sternoclavicular Joint, 23106
  Acromioclavicular Joint, 23044, 23101
  Ankle, 27610, 27612, 27620
  Ankle Joint, 27625, 27626
  Carpometacarpal Joint, 26070, 26100
    with Synovial Biopsy, 26100
  Elbow, 24000
    with Joint Exploration, 24101
    with Synovectomy, 24102
    with Synovial Biopsy, 24100
    Capsular Release, 24006
  Finger Joint, 26075
    Interphalangeal with Synovial Biopsy,
      26110
    Metacarpophalangeal with Biopsy, Synovi-
      um, 26105
  Glenohumeral Joint, 23040, 23100, 23105,
    23800-23802
  Hip, 27033
    with Synovectomy, 27054
    Exploration, 27033
    for Infection with Drainage, 27030
    Removal Loose or Foreign Body, 27033
  Interphalangeal Joint, 26080, 26110
    Toe, 28024, 28054
  Intertarsal Joint, 28020, 28050
  Knee, 27310, 27330-27335, 27403, 29868
  Metacarpophalangeal Joint, 26075, 26105
  Metatarsophalangeal Joint, 28022, 28052
  Sacroiliac Joint, 27050
  Shoulder, 23044, 23105-23107
  Shoulder Joint, 23100, 23101
    Exploration and/or Removal of Loose For-
      eign Body, 23107
  Sternoclavicular Joint, 23044, 23101, 23106
  Tarsometatarsal Joint, 28020, 28050, 28052
  Temporomandibular Joint, 21010
  Wrist, 25040, 25100-25107
Arthrotomy for Removal of Prosthesis of Ankle
  See Ankle, Removal, Implant
Arthrotomy for Removal of Prosthesis of Hip
  See Hip, Removal, Prosthesis
Arthrotomy for Removal of Prosthesis of Wrist
  See Prosthesis, Wrist, Removal
Articular Ligament
  See Ligament
Artificial Abortion
  See Abortion
Artificial Cardiac Pacemaker
  See Heart, Pacemaker
Artificial Eye
  Prosthesis
    Cornea, 65770
    Ocular, 21077, 65770, 66983-66985, 92358
Artificial Genitourinary Sphincter
  See Prosthesis, Urethral Sphincter
Artificial Insemination, 58976
  See In Vitro Fertilization
  Intra–Cervical, 58321
  Intra–Uterine, 58322
  In Vitro Fertilization
    Culture Oocyte, 89250, 89272
    Fertilize Oocyte, 89280, 89281
    Retrieve Oocyte, 58970
    Transfer Embryo, 58974, 58976
    Transfer Gamete, 58976
  Sperm Washing, 58323
Artificial Knee Joints
  See Prosthesis, Knee
Artificial Penis
  See Penile Prosthesis
Artificial Pneumothorax
  See Pneumothorax, Therapeutic
ARX, 81403-81404
Arytenoid
  Excision
    Endoscopic, 31560-31561
    External Approach, 31400
    Fixation, 31400
Arytenoid Cartilage
  Excision, 31400
  Repair, 31400
Arytenoidectomy, 31400

Arytenoidectomy — *continued*
  Endoscopic, 31560
Arytenoidopexy, 31400
ASAT, 84450
Ascorbic Acid
  Blood, 82180
ASO, 86060, 86063
ASPA, 81200, 81412
Aspartate Aminotransferase, 84450
Aspartoacylase Gene Analysis, 81200
Aspergillus
  Antibody, 86606
  Antigen Detection
    Enzyme Immunoassay, 87305
Aspiration
  See Puncture Aspiration
  Amniotic Fluid
    Diagnostic, 59000
    Therapeutic, 59001
  Bladder, 51100-51102
  Bone Marrow, 38220
  Brain Lesion
    Stereotactic, 61750, 61751
  Breast Cyst, 19000-19001
  Bronchi
    Endoscopy, 31629, 31633, 31645, 31646,
      31725
  Bronchus
    Nasotracheal, 31720
  Bursa, 20600-20611
  Catheter
    Nasotracheal, 31720
    Tracheobronchial, 31725
  Cyst
    Bone, 20615
    Breast, 19000-19001
    Fine Needle, 10021-10022, 67415
      Evaluation of Aspirate, 88172-88173,
        [88177]
    Ganglion, 20612
    Kidney, 50390
    Ovarian, 49322
    Pelvis, 50390
    Spinal Cord, 62268
    Thyroid, 60300
  Disc, 62267
  Duodenal, 43756-43757
  Fetal Fluid, 59074
  Fine Needle, 10021-10022
    Aspirate Evaluation, 88172-88173, [88177]
  Ganglion Cyst, 20612
  Gastric, 43753-43754
  Hydrocele
    Tunica Vaginalis, 55000
  Joint, 20600-20611
  Laryngoscopy
    Direct, 31515
  Lens Material, 66840
  Liver, 47015
  Nucleus of Disc
    Diagnostic, 62267
  Orbital Contents, 67415
  Pelvis
    Endoscopy, 49322
  Pericardium, 33010, 33011
  Puncture
    Cyst, Breast, 19000, 19001
  Spermatocele, 54699, 55899
  Spinal Cord
    Stereotaxis, 63615
  Stomach
    Diagnostic, 43754-43755
    Therapeutic, 43753
  Syrinx
    Spinal Cord, 62268
  Thyroid, 60300
  Trachea, 31612
    Nasotracheal, 31720
    Puncture, 31612
    Tracheobronchial, 31645-31646, 31725
    Transbronchial, 31629
  Tunica Vaginalis
    Hydrocele, 55000
  Vertebral
    Disc, 62267
    Nucleus Pulposus, 62267

Aspiration — *continued*
Vertebral — *continued*
Tissue, 62267
Vitreous, 67015
Aspiration, Chest, 32554-32555
Aspiration Lipectomies
See Liposuction
Aspiration, Lung Puncture
See Pneumocentesis
Aspiration, Nail
See Evacuation, Hematoma, Subungual
Aspiration of Bone Marrow from Donor for Transplant
See Bone Marrow Harvesting
Aspiration, Spinal Puncture
See Spinal Tap
ASPM, 81407
ASS1, 81406
Assay Tobramycin
See Tobramycin
Assay, Very Long Chain Fatty Acids
See Fatty Acid, Very Long Chain
Assessment
Adaptive Behavior, 0359T-0363T
Behavior Identification, 0359T
Exposure Behavioral Followup, 0362T-0363T
Observational Followup, 0360T-0361T
Asthma, 1005F
Emotional/Behavioral, 96127
Endothelial Function, 0337T
Heart Failure, 0001F
Level of Activity, 1003F
On-Line
Consult Physician, 99446-99449
Nonphysician, 98969
Physician, 99444
Osteoarthritis, 0005F, 1006F
Risk Factor
Coronary Heart Disease, 0126T
Gastrointestinal and Renal, 1008F
Telephone
Consult Physician, 99446-99449
Nonphysician, 98966-98968
Physician, 99441-99443
Use of Anti–inflammatory or analgesic (OTC) medications, 1007F
Volume Overload, 1004F, 2002F
Assisted
Circulation, 33946-33949, 33967, 33970, 33973, 33975-33976, 33979, 33990-33991, 92970-92971
Zonal Hatching (AZH), 89253
AST, 84450
Asthma, Long Term Control Medication, 4015F
Astragalectomy, 28130
Astragalus
See Talus
Asymmetry, Face
See Hemifacial Microsomia
Ataxia Telangiectasia
Chromosome Analysis, 88248
Ataxy, Telangiectasia, 88248
Atherectomy
Aorta, 0236T
Brachiocephalic, 0237T
Coronary, [92924, 92925] [92933, 92934, 92937, 92938, 92941, 92943, 92944]
Femoral, 37225, 37227
Iliac, 0238T
Peroneal, 37229, 37231, 37233, 37235
Popliteal, 37225, 37227, 37233, 37235
Renal, 0234T
Tibial, 37229, 37231, 37233, 37235
Tibioperoneal, 37229, 37231, 37233, 37235
Transluminal
Abdominal Aorta, 0236T
Brachiocephalic Trunk and Branches, 0237T
Coronary, [92924, 92925, 92928, 92929, 92933, 92934, 92937, 92938, 92941, 92943, 92944]
Iliac, 0238T
Renal, 0234T
Visceral, 0235T
Visceral, 0235T

Athletic Training Evaluation, [97169, 97170, 97171, 97172]
ATL1, 81406
ATLV, 86687, 86689
ATLV Antibodies, 86687, 86689
ATM, 81408, 81432
ATN1, 81401
Atomic Absorption Spectroscopy, 82190
ATP1A2, 81406
ATP7B, 81406
ATP Creatine Phosphotransferase, 82550, 82552
Atresia
Choanal, 30540-30545
Congenital
Auditory Canal, External, 69320
Bile Duct, 47700
Small Intestine, 44126-44127
Pulmonary Artery, 33920
Tetralogy of Fallot, 33697
Tricuspid, 33615
Atria
Ablation, 33254-33256, 33265-33266
Baffle Procedure, 33774
Blalock-Hanlon Operation, 33735
Cor Triatriatum Repair, 33732
Cuff Preparation, 32855-32856
Electrogram, 93615-93616
Endoscopy
Surgical, 33265-33266
Hemodynamic Monitor System, 0293T-0294T
Left Atrial Appendage Closure
with Implant, 33340
Membrane Resection, 33732
Rashkind Procedure, 92992
Reconstruction, 33254-33256, 33265-33266
Septectomy, 33735, 92992-92993
Septostomy, 33735, 92992-92993
Shunt, 62190, 62220
Surgical, 33265-33266
Thrombus, 33310
Atrial Electrogram
See Cardiology, Diagnostic
Esophageal Recording, 93615, 93616
Atrial Fibrillation
See Fibrillation, Atrial
Atrioseptopexy
See Heart, Repair, Atrial Septum
Atrioseptoplasty
See Heart, Repair, Atrial Septum
Attachment
See Fixation
Attendance and Resuscitation Services
Newborn, 99464
Attention Deficit Hyperactivity Disorder Assessment, 96127
Atticotomy, 69631, 69635
ATXN10, 81401
ATXN1, 81401
ATXN2, 81401
ATXN3, 81401
ATXN7, 81401
ATXN8OS, 81401
Audiologic Function Tests
Acoustic Immittance, 92570
Acoustic Reflex, 92568
Acoustic Reflex Decay, 92570
Audiometry
Automated, 0208T-0212T
Bekesy, 92560, 92561
Comprehensive, 0212T, 92557
Conditioning Play, 92582
Groups, 92559
Pure Tone, 0208T-0209T, 92552, 92553
Select Picture, 92583
Speech, 0210T-0211T, 92555, 92556
Visual Reinforcement, 92579
Auditory Brainstem Implant, 92640
Auditory Processing Treatment, 92507-92508
Central Auditory Function, 92620, 92621
Diagnostic Analysis
Auditory Brainstem Implant, 92640
Ear Protector Attenuation Measurement, 92596
Electrocochleography, 92584
Evoked Otoacoustic Emissions, 92587-92588, [92558]
Filtered Speech, 92571

Audiologic Function Tests — *continued*
Hearing Aid Evaluation, 92590-92595
Lombard Test, 92700
Loudness Balance, 92562
Screening, 92551
Sensorineural Acuity, 92575
Short Increment Sensitivity Index, 92564
Staggered Spondaic Word Test, 92572
Stenger Test, 92565, 92577
Synthetic Sentence Test, 92576
Tinnitus Assessment, 92625
Tone Decay, 92563
Tympanometry, 92550, 92567, 92570
Audiometry
Bekesy, 92560, 92561
Brainstem Evoked Response, 92585, 92586
Comprehensive, 0212T, 92557
Conditioning Play, 92582
Evoked Otoacoustic Emissions, 92587, 92588
Groups, 92559
Pure Tone, 92552, 92553
Automated
Air, 0208T
Air and Bone, 0209T
Select Picture, 92583
Speech, 0210T-0211T, 92555-92556
Tympanometry, 92550, 92567, 92570
Visual Reinforcement, 92579
Auditory Brain Stem Evoked Response, 92585-92586
Auditory Canal
Decompression, 61591
External
Abscess
Incision and Drainage, 69000, 69005, 69020
Atresia, Congenital, 69320
Biopsy, 69105
Hematoma, 69000, 69005
Lesion
Excision, 69140-69155
Reconstruction, 69310, 69320
for Congenital Atresia, 69320
for Stenosis, 69310
Removal
Cerumen, 69209, 69210
Ear Wax, 69209, 69210
Foreign Body, 69200, 69205
Internal
Decompression, 69960
Exploration, 69440
Auditory Canal Atresia, External
See Atresia, Congenital, Auditory Canal, External
Auditory Evoked Potentials, 92585, 92586
Auditory Labyrinth
See Ear, Inner
Auditory Meatus
X–ray, 70134
Auditory Tube
See Eustachian Tube
Augmentation
Chin, 21120, 21123
Cruciate Ligament, 29888-29889
Esophageal Sphincter
Laparoscopy, 43284-43285
Facial Bones, 21208
Knee Ligament, 27427, 27556-27558
Malar, 21210, 21270
Mammoplasty, 19324-19325
Mandibular Body
with Bone Graft, 21127
with Prosthesis, 21125
Osteoplasty
Facial Bones, 21208
Palate, 21082
Percutaneous
Spine, 0200T-0201T, 22513-22515
Pulmonary Valve Outflow, 33478
Sacral, 0200T-0201T
Spine, 22513-22515
Vertebral, 22513-22515
Augmented Histamine Test, 43755
Aural Rehabilitation Test, 92626-92633
Auricle (Heart)
See Atria

Auricular Fibrillation
See Fibrillation, Atrial
Auricular Prosthesis, 21086
Australia Antigen
Core, 86704
IgM, 86705
Surface, 86706
Autograft
Bone
Local, 20936
Morselized, 20937
Sacroiliac Joint for Stabilization, 27279
Structural, 20938
Chondrocytes
Knee, 27412
Dermal, 15130-15136
Epidermal, 15110-15111, 15115-15116
Osteochondral
Knee, 27416
Talus, 28446
Skin, 15150-15152, 15155-15157
Dermal, 15130-15136
Epidermal, 15110-15116
Harvesting
for Tissue Culture, 15040
Tissue Cultured, 15150-15157
Spine Surgery
Local, 20936
Morselized, 20937
Structural, 20938
Autologous Blood Transfusion
See Autotransfusion
Autologous Bone Marrow Cell Therapy
Complete
With Bone Marrow Harvest, 0263T
Without Bone Marrow Harvest, 0264T
Autologous Transplantation
See Autograft
Automated Lamellar Keratoplasty (ALK), 65710
Autonomic Nervous System Function
Heart Rate Response, 95921-95923
Pseudomotor Response, 95921-95923
Sympathetic and Parasympathetic, 95924 [95943]
Sympathetic Function, 95921-95923
AutoPap, 88152
Autoprothrombin C
See Thrombokinase
Autoprothrombin I
See Proconvertin
Autoprothrombin II
See Christmas Factor
Autoprothrombin III
See Stuart–Prower Factor
Autopsy
Coroner's Examination, 88045
Forensic Examination, 88040
Gross and Microscopic
Examination, 88020-88037
Infant with Brain, 88028
Stillborn or Newborn with Brain, 88029
Gross Examination, 88000-88016
Organ, 88037
Regional, 88036
Unlisted Services and Procedures, 88099
Autotransfusion
Blood, 86890, 86891
Autotransplant
See Autograft
Autotransplantation
Renal, 50380
AVF, 35180-35190, 36815
AV Fistula (Arteriovenous Fistula)
Cannulization
Vein, 36815
Repair
Abdomen, 35182
Acquired or Traumatic, 35189
Head, 35180
Acquired or Traumatic, 35188
Lower Extremity, 35184
Acquired or Traumatic, 35190
Neck, 35180
Acquired or Traumatic, 35188
Thorax, 35182
Acquired or Traumatic, 35189

AV Fistula (Arteriovenous Fistula) —
continued
  Repair — *continued*
    Upper Extremity, 35184
      Acquired or Traumatic, 35190
    Revision
      Hemodialysis Graft or Fistula
        with Thrombectomy, 36833
        without Thrombectomy, 36832
    Thrombectomy
      Dialysis Graft
        without Revision, 36831
A Vitamin, 84590
AVPR2, 81404
AV Shunt (Arteriovenous Shunt)
  Dialysis Circuit, 36901-36902
Avulsion
  Nails, 11730, 11732
  Nerves, 64732-64772
Axilla
  Skin Graft
    Delay of Flap, 15620
    Dermal, 15130-15131
    Full Thickness, 15200-15201, 15240-15241
    Pedicle Flap, 15574
    Tissue Cultured, 15150-15152
  Tissue Transfer
    Adjacent, 14040-14041
    Flap, 15574, 15620
  Wound Repair, 13131-13133
Axillary Arteries
  See Artery, Axillary
Axillary Nerve
  Injection
    Anesthetic, 64417
Axis, Dens
  See Odontoid Process
AZH (Assisted Zonal Hatching), 89253

B

Bacillus Calmette Guerin Vaccine
  See BCG Vaccine
Backbench Reconstruction Prior to Implant
  Intestine, 44715-44721
  Kidney, 50323-50329
  Liver, 47143-47147
  Pancreas, 48551-48552
  Wound Exploration, Penetrating, 20102
Backbone
  See Spine
Back/Flank
  Biopsy, 21920, 21925
  Repair
    Hernia, 49540
    Tumor, 21930-21936
  Wound Exploration
    Penetrating, 20102
Bacteria Culture
  Additional Methods, 87077
  Aerobic, 87040-87071, 87077
  Anaerobic, 87073-87076
  Blood, 87040
  Feces, 87045, 87046
  Mycobacteria, 87118
  Nose, 87070
  Other Source, 87070-87075
  Screening, 87081
  Stool, 87045-87046
  Throat, 87070
  Typing, 87140, 87143, 87147, 87149-87150,
    87152-87153, 87158
  Urine, 87086, 87088
Bacterial Endotoxins, 87176
Bacterial Overgrowth Breath Test, 91065
  Homogenization, Tissue, for Culture, 87176
Bactericidal Titer, Serum, 87197
Bacterium
  Antibody, 86609
BAEP (Brainstem Auditory Evoked Potential),
  92585-92586
BAER, 92585-92586
Baker's Cyst, 27345
Baker Tube
  Decompression of Bowel, 44021
Balanoplasty
  See Penis, Repair

Baldy–Webster Operation, 58400
Balkan Grippe, 86000, 86638
Balloon Angioplasty
  See Angioplasty
Balloon Assisted Device
  Aorta, 33967-33974
Balloon, Cardiac Catheter, Insertion, 33967
Banding
  Artery
    Fistula, 37607
    Pulmonary, 33690
      Application, 33620
      Removal, 33622
Band, Pulmonary Artery
  See Banding, Artery, Pulmonary
Bankart Procedure, 23455
Bank, Blood
  See Blood Banking
B Antibodies, Hepatitis
  See Antibody, Hepatitis B
B Antigens, Hepatitis
  See Hepatitis Antigen, B
Barany Caloric Test, 92533
Barbiturates, *[80345]*
Bardenheuer Operation, 37616
Bariatric Surgery, 43644-43645, 43770-43775,
  43842-43848, 43886-43888
Barium, 83015, 83018
Barium Enema, 74270, 74280
  Intussusception, 74283
Barker Operation, 28120
Baroreflex Activation Device
  Implantation/Replacement, 0266T-0268T
  Interrogation Evaluation, 0272T-0273T
  Revision/Removal, 0269T-0271T
Barr Bodies, 88130
Barrel–Stave Procedure, 61559
Barr Procedure, 27690-27692
Barsky's Procedures, 26580
Bartholin's Gland
  Abscess
    Incision and Drainage, 56420
  Cyst
    Repair, 56440
    Excision, 56740
    Marsupialization, 56440
Bartonella
  Antibody, 86611
  Nucleic Acid Probe, 87470-87472
Bartonella Detection
  Antibody, 86611
  Nucleic Acid Probe, 87470-87472
Basic Life Services, 99450
Basic Proteins, Myelin
  See Myelin Basic Protein
Basilar Arteries
  See Artery, Basilar
Bassett's Operation, 56630-56640
Batch–Spittler–McFaddin Operation, 27598
Battle's Operation, 44950, 44960
Bayley Scales of Infant Development
  Developmental Testing, 96110, 96111
BBS10, 81404
BBS1, 81406
BBS2, 81406
BCAM, 81403
B Cells
  Total Count, 86355
BCG Vaccine, 90585, 90586
BCKDHA, 81400, 81405
BCKDHB, 81205, 81406
B Complex Vitamins
  B–12 Absorption, 78270-78272
BCR/ABL1, 81206-81208
BCS1L, 81405
B–DNA
  See Deoxyribonucleic Acid
BE, 74270-74283
Be Antigens, Hepatitis
  See Hepatitis Antigen, Be
Bed
  Sore/Pressure Ulcer/Decubitus
    Excision, 15920-15999
    Testing, 94780-94781
Bekesy Audiometry
  See Audiometry, Bekesy

Belsey IV Procedure, 43280, 43327-43328
Bender–Gestalt Test, 96101-96103
Benedict Test for Urea, 81005
Benign Cystic Mucinous Tumor
  See Ganglion
Benign Neoplasm of Cranial Nerves
  See Cranial Nerve
Bennett Fracture
  Other Than Thumb
    Closed Treatment, 26670, 26675
    Open Treatment, 26685, 26686
    Percutaneous Treatment, 26676
  Thumb Fracture
    with Dislocation, 26645, 26650
    Open Treatment, 26665
Bennett Procedure, 27430
Bentall Procedure, 33863
Benzidine Test
  Blood, Feces, 82270, 82272
Benzodiazepines
  Assay, *[80335, 80336, 80337]*
Benzoyl Cholinesterase
  See Cholinesterase
Bernstein Test, 91030
Beryllium, 83015, 83018
BEST1, 81406
Beta 2 Glycoprotein I Antibody, 86146
Beta–2–Microglobulin
  Blood, 82232
  Urine, 82232
Beta Glucosidase, 82963
Beta–Hydroxydehydrogenase, 80406
Beta Hypophamine
  See Antidiuretic Hormone
Beta Lipoproteins
  See Lipoprotein, LDL
Beta Test, 96101-96103
  Psychiatric Diagnosis, Psychological Testing,
    96101-96103
Bethesda System, 88164-88167
Bevan's Operation, 54640
b-Hexosaminidase, 83080
Bicarbonate, 82374
Biceps Tendon
  Reinsertion, 24342
  Resection, 23440
  Tenodesis, 23430, 29828
  Transplantation, 23440
Bichloride, Methylene
  See Dichloromethane
Bicompartmental Knee Replacement, 27447
Bicuspid Valve
  Incision, 33420, 33422
  Repair, 33420-33427
  Replacement, 33430
Biesenberger Mammaplasty, 19318
Bifrontal Craniotomy, 61557
Bile Acids, 82239
  Blood, 82240
Bile Duct
  See Gallbladder
  Anastomosis
    with Intestines, 47760, 47780, 47785
  Biopsy
    Endoscopy, 47553
    Percutaneous, 47543
  Catheterization
    Drainage, 47533-47537
  Change Catheter Tube, 75984
  Cyst
    Excision, 47715
  Destruction
    Calculi (Stone), 43265
  Dilation
    Endoscopic, 47555, 47556, *[43277]*
    Percutaneous, 47542
  Drainage
    Catheter Insertion, 47533-47534
    Change Biliary Catheter, 47535-47536
    Radiological Supervision and Interpreta-
      tion, 75984
    Removal, 47537
  Endoscopy
    Biopsy, 47553
    Cannulation, 43273

Bile Duct — *continued*
  Endoscopy — *continued*
    Destruction
      Calculi (Stone), 43265
      Tumor, *[43278]*
    Dilation, 47555, 47556, *[43277]*
    Exploration, 47552
    Intraoperative, 47550
    Placement
      Stent, *[43274]*
    Removal
      Calculi, 43264, 47554
      Foreign Body, *[43275]*
      Stent, *[43275, 43276]*
    Specimen Collection, 43260
    Sphincterotomy, 43262, *[43274]*, *[43276]*,
      [43277]
    Sphincter Pressure, 43263
  Exploration
    Atresia, 47700
    Endoscopy, 47552
  Incision
    Sphincter, 43262, 47460
  Incision and Drainage, 47420, 47425
  Insertion
    Catheter, 47533-47534
      Revision, 47535-47536
    Stent, 47538-47540, 47801
  Nuclear Medicine
    Imaging, 78226-78227
  Placement
    Percutaneous, 47538-47540
    Stent, *[43274]*
  Reconstruction
    Anastomosis, 47800
  Removal
    Calculi (Stone), 43264, 47420, 47425
      Percutaneous, 47544
    Foreign Body, *[43275]*
    Stent, *[43275, 43276]*
  Repair, 47701
    with Intestines, 47760, 47780
    Gastrointestinal Tract, 47785
  Tumor
    Ablation, *[43278]*
    Destruction, *[43278]*
    Excision, 47711, 47712
  Unlisted Services and Procedures, Biliary Tract,
    47999
  X–ray
    with Contrast, 74300-74301
      Guide Catheter, 74328, 74330
      Guide Dilation, 74360
Bile Duct, Common, Cystic Dilatation
  See Cyst, Choledochal
Bilirubin
  Blood, 82247, 82248
  Feces, 82252
  Total
    Direct, 82247, 82248
    Transcutaneous, 88720
    Total Blood, 82247, 82248
Billroth I or II, 43631-43634
Bilobectomy, 32482, 32670
Bimone
  See Testosterone
Binding Globulin, Testosterone Estradiol
  See Globulin, Sex Hormone Binding
Binet–Simon Test, 96101-96103
Binet Test, 96101-96103
Binocular Microscopy, 92504
Bioelectrical Impedance Whole Body Analysis,
  0358T
Biofeedback
  Anorectal, 90911
  Blood–flow, 90901
  Blood Pressure, 90901
  Brainwaves, 90901
  EEG (Electroencephalogram), 90901
  Electromyogram, 90901
  Electro–Oculogram, 90901
  EMG (with Anorectal), 90911
  Eyelids, 90901
  Nerve Conduction, 90901
  Other (unlisted) biofeedback, 90901
  Perineal Muscles, 90911

Biofeedback — *continued*
  Psychiatric Treatment, 90875, 90876
  Urethral Sphincter, 90911
Bioimpedance
  Cardiovascular Analysis, 93701
  Extracellular fluid, 93702
  Whole Body Analysis, 0358T
Biological Skin Grafts
  See Allograft, Skin
Biometry
  Eye, 76516, 76519, 92136
Biopsies, Needle
  See Needle Biopsy
Biopsy
  with Arthrotomy
    Acromioclavicular Joint, 23101
    Glenohumeral Joint, 23100, 23105
    Sternoclavicular Joint, 23101, 23106
  with Cystourethroscopy, 52354
  See also Brush Biopsy; Needle Biopsy
  ABBI, 19081-19086
  Abdomen, 49000, 49321
    Mass, 49180
  Adenoids (and Tonsils), 42999
  Adrenal Gland, 60540-60545
    Laparoscopic, 60650
    Open, 60540, 60545, 60699
  Alveolus, 41899
  Anal
    Endoscopy, 46606-46607
  Ankle, 27613, 27614, 27620
  Arm, Lower, 25065, 25066
  Arm, Upper, 24065, 24066
  Artery
    Temporal, 37609
  Auditory Canal, External, 69105
  Back/Flank, 21920, 21925
  Bile Duct
    Endoscopic, 47553
    Percutaneous, 47543
  Bladder, 52354
    Cystourethroscope, 52204
    Cystourethroscopy, 52224, 52250
      with Fulguration, 52224
      with Insertion Transprostatic Implant, 52441-52442
      with Radioactive Substance, 52250
    Open, 53899
  Blood Vessel
    Transcatheter, 75970
  Bone, 20220-20245
  Bone Marrow, 38221, 88305
  Brain, 61140
    Stereotactic, 61750, 61751
  Brainstem, 61575-61576
  Breast, 19081-19086, 19100-19101
    with Magnetic Resonance Imaging, 19085-19086
    with Stereotactic Guidance, 19081-19082
    with Ultrasound Guidance, 19083-19084
    ABBI, 19081-19086
    Localization Clip Placement, 19081-19086
      with Magnetic Resonance Guidance, 19085-19086
      with Stereotactic Guidance, 19081-19082
      with Ultrasound Guidance, 19083-19084
    Stereotactic Localization, 77031
  Bronchi
    Catheterization, 31717
    Endoscopic, 31625-31629, 31632, 31633
    Open, 31899
  Brush
    with Cystourethroscopy, 52204
    Bronchi, 31717
    Renal Pelvis, 52007
    Ureter, 52007
  Carpometacarpal Joint
    Synovium, 26100
  Cervix, 57421, 57454-57455, 57460, 57500
  Chorionic Villus, 59015
  Colon, 44025, 44100
    Endoscopic, 44137, 44389, 45380, 45391-45392

Biopsy — *continued*
  Colon — *continued*
    Multiple
      with Colostomy, Cecostomy, 44322
  Colon–Sigmoid
    Endoscopic, 45305, 45331
  Conjunctiva, 68100
  Cornea, 65410
  Duodenum, 44010
  Ear
    External, 69100
    Inner, 69949
    Middle, 69799
  Elbow, 24065, 24066, 24101, 29830
    Synovium, 24100
  Embryo Blastomere, 89290, 89291
  Endometrium, 58100, 58110, 58558
  Epididymis, 54800, 54865
  Esophagus
    Endoscopic, 43193, 43198, 43202, 43238-43239, 43242
    Forceps, 3150F
    Open, 43499
  Eye
    Iris, Prolapsed, 66999
    Eyelid, [67810]
    Eye Muscle, 67346
  Fallopian Tube, 49321
  Foot
    Interphalangeal Joint, 28054
    Intertarsal Joint, 28050
    Metatarsophalangeal Joint, 28052
    Tarsometatarsal Joint, 28050
  Forearm, Soft Tissue, 25065, 25066
  Gallbladder
    Endoscopic, 43261
    Open, 47999
  Gastrointestinal, Upper
    Endoscopic, 43239
  Glenohumeral Joint, 23105
  Gum, 41899
  Hand
    Interphalangeal Joint, 26110
    Metacarpophalangeal Joint, 26105, 29900
    Synovium, 26100
  Heart, 93505
  Hip, 27040, 27041
    Joint, 27052
    Synovium, 29860
  Ileum
    Endoscopic, 44382
  Interphalangeal Joint
    Finger, 26110
    Finger Synovium, 26110
    Toe, 28054
  Intertarsal Joint
    Synovial, 28050
    Toe, 28050
  Intervertebral Disc, 62267
  Intestines, Small, 44010, 44020, 44100
    Endoscopic, 44361, 44377, 44382, 44386
  Intracranial Lesion, 61140, 61750
  Kidney, 50200-50205
    Endoluminal, Renal Pelvis, 50606
    Endoscopic, 50555-50557, 50574-50576, 52354
  Knee, 27323, 27324
    Synovium, 27330, 29870
  Knee Joint
    Synovium, 27330, 29870
  Lacrimal Gland, 68510
  Lacrimal Sac, 68525
  Larynx
    Endoscopy, 31510, 31535, 31536, 31576
  Leg
    Lower, 27613, 27614
    Upper, 27323, 27324
  Lip, 40490
  Liver, 47000, 47001, 47100, 47700
  Lung
    Needle, 32405
    Thoracoscopy, 32604-32608
    Thoracotomy, 32096-32097
  Lymph Nodes, 38500-38530, 38570
    Injection Procedure
      Identification of Sentinel Node, 38792

Biopsy — *continued*
  Lymph Nodes — *continued*
    Injection Procedure — *continued*
      Radioactive Tracer, 38792
    Laparoscopic, 38570-38572
    Mediastinum, 39000-39010, 39401-39402
    Needle, 38505
    Open, 38500, 38510-38530
      Superficial, 38500
    Para-aortic, 57109, 57112, 57531, 58210, 58548
    Prostate, 55812, 55842, 55862
  Mediastinum, 39401-39402
    Needle, 32405
  Metacarpophalangeal Joint, 26105, 29900
  Metatarsophalangeal Joint, 28052
  Mouth, 40808, 41108
  Muscle, 20200-20206
  Nail, 11755
  Nasopharynx, 42804, 42806
  Neck, 21550
  Needle
    Abdomen
      Mass, 49180
  Nerve, 64795
  Nose
    Endoscopic, 31237
    Intranasal, 30100
  Nucleus Pulposus, 62267
  Omentum, 49321
  Oocyte Polar Body, 89290, 89291
  Orbit, 61332
    Exploration, 67400, 67450
    Fine Needle Aspiration, 67415
  Oropharynx, 42800
  Ovary, 49321, 58900
  Palate, 42100
  Pancreas, 48100-48102
  Parathyroid Gland, 60699
  Paravertebral Tissue, 62267
  Pelvis, 27040, 27041
  Penis, 54100
    Cutaneous, 54100
    Deep Structures, 54105
  Percutaneous Needle
    Spinal Cord, 62269
  Pericardium, 32604
  Perineum, 56605, 56606
  Periprostatic Tissue, 54699, 55899
  Perirenal Tissue, 53899
  Peritoneum
    Endoscopic, 49321
  Periurethral Tissue, 53899
  Perivesical Tissue, 53899
  Pharynx, 42800-42806
  Pineal Gland, 60699
  Pituitary Gland, 60699
  Pleura, 32098, 32400, 32609
    Needle, 32400
    Thoracoscopy, 32609
    Thoracotomy, 32098
  Prostate, 55700, 55705, 55706
    with Fluorescence Spectroscopy, 0443T
    Lymph Nodes, 55812, 55842, 55862
  Rectum, 45100, 45305, 45331
  Renal Pelvis, 50606
  Retroperitoneal Area, 49010, 49180
  Sacroiliac Joint, 27050
  Salivary Gland, 42400, 42405
  Seminal Vesicles, 54699, 55899
  Shoulder
    Deep, 23066
    Glenohumeral Joint, 23105
    Joint, 23100-23101
    Soft Tissue, 23065
    Sternoclavicular Joint, 23106
    Synovium, 29805
  Sinus
    Sphenoid, 31050, 31051
  Skin Lesion, 11100, 11101
  Skull Base, 61575-61576
  Spinal Cord, 63275-63290
    Lesion, 63615
    Needle, 62269
    Percutaneous, 62269
    Stereotactic, 63615

Biopsy — *continued*
  Spinal Cord — *continued*
    Transoral, 61575-61576
  Spleen, 38999
  Stomach, 43605
  Tarsometatarsal Joint
    Synovial, 28050
  Temporomandibular Joint, 29800
  Testis, 54500, 54505
  Thigh, 27323-27324
  Thorax, 21550
  Throat, 42800, 42804-42806
  Thymus, 38999, 60699
  Thyroid, 60100
  Thyroid Gland, 60699
  Tongue, 41100, 41105
  Tonsils (and Adenoids), 42999
  Transcatheter, 37200
  Tunica Vaginalis, 54699, 55899
  Ureter, 52354
    Endoluminal, 50606
    Endoscopic, 50955-50957, 50974-50976
    Open, 53899
  Urethra, 52204, 52250, 52354, 53200
  Uterus
    Endometrial, 58100-58110
    Endoscopic, 58558
  Uvula, 42100
  Vagina, 57100, 57105, 57421
    Endocervical, 57454
  Vein, 37200
    Radiological Supervision and Interpretation, 75970
  Vertebral Body, 20250-20251
  Vulva, 56605, 56606, 56821
  Wrist, 25065-25066, 25100-25101, 29840
Biopsy, Skin
  See Skin, Biopsy
Biostatistics
  See Biometry
Biosterol
  See Vitamin, A
BIOTHRAX, 90581
Biotinidase, 82261
BiPAP, 94660
Birthing Room
  Attendance at Delivery, 99464
  Newborn Care, 99460, 99463-99465
  Resuscitation, 99465
Bischof Procedure
  Laminectomy, Surgical, 63170, 63172
Bismuth, 83015
Bizzozero's Corpuscle/Cell
  See Blood, Platelet
BKA, 27598, 27880-27882
Bladder
  Abscess
    Incision and Drainage, 51080
  Anastomosis
    with Intestine, 51960
    Ureter to Bladder, 50780, 50782
  Anesthesia, 00864, 00870, 00912
  Aspiration, 51100-51102
  Biopsy, 52204
    by Cystourethroscopy, 52204
  Catheterization, 51045, 51102, 51701-51703
  Change Tube, 51705, 51710
  Chemodenervation, 52287
  Creation/Stoma, 51980
  Cuff, 50234-50236, 50650
  Cyst
    Urachal
      Excision, 51500
  Cystometrogram (CMG), 51725-51729
  Cystostomy Tube, 51705-51710
  Cystourethroscopy, 52000
    with Urethrotomy, 52270-52276
    Biopsy, 52204, 52224, 52250, 52354
    Catheterization, 52005, 52010
    Destruction, 52214, 52224, 52400
    Dilation, 52260, 52265
      Urethra, 52281
    Diverticulum, 52305
    Evacuation
      Clot, 52001

Biofeedback — Bladder

Bladder — *continued*
  Cystourethroscopy — *continued*
    Excision
        Tumor, 52234-52240, 52355
      Exploration, 52351
      Fulguration, 52214-52224, 52234-52235,
          52240, 52250, 52400
      Injection, 52283
      Insertion of Stent, 52332, 52334
      Lithotripsy, 52353
      Radiotracer, 52250
      Removal
          Calculus, 52310, 52315, 52352
          Foreign Body, 52310, 52315
      Sphincter Surgery, 52277
      Tumor
          Excision, 52355
      Ureter Surgery, 52290, 52300
      Urethral Syndrome, 52285
  Destruction
    Endoscopic, 52214-52240, 52354
  Dilation
    Ureter, 52260, 52265
  Diverticulum
    Excision, 51525
    Incision, 52305
    Resection, 52305
  Endoscopy
    See Cystourethroscopy
  Excision
    Partial, 51550-51565
    Total, 51570, 51580, 51590-51597
        with Nodes, 51575, 51585, 51595
    Transurethral of Neck, 52640
    Tumor, 52234-52240
  Fulguration, 52214, 52250, 52400
    Tumor(s), 52224, 52234-52235, 52240
  Incision
    with
        Cryosurgery, 51030
        Destruction, 51020, 51030
        Fulguration, 51020
        Insertion Radioactive, 51020
        Radiotracer, 51020
    Catheter or Stent, 51045
  Incision and Drainage, 51040
  Injection
    Radiologic, 51600-51610
  Insertion
    Stent, 51045, 52282, 52334
  Instillation
    with Cystourethroscopy, 52005, 52010
    Anticarcinogenics, 51720
    Drugs, 51720
    Interstitial Cystitis, 52260-52265
  Irrigation, 51700, 52005, 52010
    Clot, 52001
  Laparoscopy, 51999
  Lesion
    Destruction, 51030
  Neck
    Endoscopy
        Injection of Implant Material, 51715
        Excision, 51520
      Remodeling for Incontinence, 53860
  Nuclear Medicine
    Residual Study, 78730
  Radiotracer, 51020, 52250
  Reconstruction
    with Intestines, 51960
    with Urethra, 51800, 51820
    Radiofrequency Micro-Remodeling, 53860
  Removal
    Calculus, 51050, 51065, 52310, 52315,
        52352
    Foreign Body, 52310, 52315
    Litholapaxy, 52317-52318
    Lithotripsy, 51065, 52353
    Urethral Stent, 52310, 52315
  Repair
    Diverticulum, 52305
    Exstrophy, 51940
    Fistula, 44660, 44661, 45800, 45805, 51880-
        51925
    Neck, 51845
    Wound, 51860, 51865

Bladder — *continued*
  Resection, 52500
  Residual Study, 78730
  Sphincter Surgery, 52277
  Suspension, 51990
  Suture
    Fistula, 44660, 44661, 45800, 45805, 51880-
        51925
    Wound, 51860, 51865
  Tumor
    Excision, 51530
    Fulguration, 52234-52240
    Resection, 52234-52240
  Unlisted Services and Procedures, 53899
  Ureterocele, 51535
  Urethrocystography, 74450, 74455
  Urethrotomy, 52270-52276
  Urinary Incontinence Procedures
    Laparoscopy, 51990, 51992
    Plan of Care Documented, 0509F
    Radiofrequency Micro-Remodeling, 53860
    Sling Operation, 51992
    Urethral Suspension, 51990
  Uroflowmetry, 51736-51741
  Voiding Pressure Studies, 51727-51729 *[51797]*
  X–ray, 74430
    with Contrast, 74450, 74455
Blair Arthrodesis, 27870
Blalock–Hanlon Procedure, 33735-33737
Blalock–Taussig Procedure, 33750
Blastocyst Transfer
  See Embryo Transfer
Blastogenesis, 86353
Blastomyces
  Antibody, 86612
Blastomycosis, European
  See Cryptococcus
Blast Transformation
  See Blastogenesis
Blatt Capsulodesis, 25320
Bleeding
  See Hemorrhage
Bleeding, Anal
  See Anus, Hemorrhage
Bleeding Disorder
  See Coagulopathy
Bleeding Time, 85002
Bleeding, Uterine
  See Hemorrhage, Uterus
Bleeding, Vaginal
  See Hemorrhage, Vagina
Blepharoplasty, 15820-15823
  See Canthoplasty
  Anesthesia, 00103
  Ectropion
      Excision Tarsal Wedge, 67916
      Extensive, 67917
  Entropion
      Excision Tarsal Wedge, 67923
      Extensive, 67924
Blepharoptosis
  Repair, 67901-67909
      Frontalis Muscle Technique, 67901
          with Fascial Sling, 67902
      Superior Rectus Technique with Fascial
          Sling, 67906
      Tarso Levator Resection
          Advancement
              External Approach, 67904
              Internal Approach, 67903
Blepharorrhaphy
  See Tarsorrhaphy
Blepharospasm
  Chemodenervation, 64612
Blepharotomy, 67700
Blister
  See Bulla
BLM, 81209, 81412
Blom–Singer Prosthesis, 31611
Blood
  Banking
    Frozen Blood Preparation, 86930-86932,
        88240
    Frozen Plasma Preparation, 86927
    Physician Services, 86077-86079
  Bleeding Time, 85002

Blood — *continued*
  Blood Clot
    Assay, 85396
    Clotting
        Factor, 85250-85293
        Factor Test, 85210
        Inhibitors, 85300-85301
    Coagulation Time, 85345-85348
    Lysis Time, 85175
    Retraction, 85170
    Thrombolytic Agents
        Tissue Plasminogen Activator (tPA),
            4077F
  Cell
    CD4 and CD8
        Including Ratio, 86360
    Enzyme Activity, 82657
    Exchange, 36511-36513
    Sedimentation Rate
        Automated, 85652
        Manual, 85651
  Cell Count
    Automated, 85049
    B–Cells, 86355
    Blood Smear, 85007, 85008
    Complete Blood Count (CBC), 85025, 85027
    Differential WBC Count, 85004-85007,
        85009
    Hematocrit, 85014
    Hemoglobin, 85018
    Hemogram
        Added Indices, 85025-85027
        Automated, 85025-85027
        Manual, 85032
    Microhematocrit, 85013
    Natural Killer (NK) Cells, 86357
    Red
        See Red Blood Cell (RBC), Count
    Red Blood Cells, 85032-85041
    Reticulocyte, 85044-85046
    Stem Cells, 86367
    T Cell, 86359-86361
    White
        See White Blood Cell, Count
    White Blood Cell, 85032, 85048, 89055
  Clot
    Assay, 85396
    Activity, 85397
        ADAMTS-13, 85397
    Clot Lysis Time, 85175
    Clot Retraction, 85170
    Clotting Factor, 85250-85293
    Clotting Factor Test, 85210-85244
    Clotting Inhibitors, 85300-85303, 85305-
        85307, 85335, 85337
    Coagulation Time, 85345-85348
    Factor Inhibitor Test, 85335
  Coagulation
    Factor I, 85384, 85385
    Factor II, 85210
    Factor III, 85730, 85732
    Factor IV, 82310
    Factor IX, 85250
    Factor V, 85220
    Factor VII, 85230
    Factor VIII, 85244, 85247
    Factor X, 85260
    Factor XI, 85270
    Factor XIII, 85290, 85291
  Collection, for Autotransfusion
    Intraoperative, 86891
    Preoperative, 86890
  Feces, 82270, 82272
    by Hemoglobin Immunoassay, 82274
  Flow Check
    Graft, 15860, 90940
  Gases
    by Pulse Oximetry, 94760
    CO2, 82803
    HCO3, 82803
    Hemoglobin–Oxygen Affinity, 82820
    O2, 82803-82810
    O2 Saturation, 82805, 82810
    pCO2, 82803
    pH, 82800, 82803
    pO2, 82803, 82820

Blood — *continued*
  Gastric Contents, 82271
  Harvesting of Stem Cells, 38205-38206
  Hemoglobin
    Concentration, 85046
    Quantitative, 88740
    Transcutaneous
        Carboxyhemoglobin, 88740
        Methemoglobin, 88741
  Hemoglobin A1c (HbA1c) Level, 3044F-3046F
  Injection
    Plasma, 0232T
  Nuclear Medicine
    Flow Imaging, 78445
    Red Cell, 78140
    Red Cell Survival, 78130, 78135
  Occult, 82270
  Osmolality, 83930
  Other Sources, 82271
  Patch, 62273
  Plasma
    Exchange, 36514-36516
    Frozen Preparation, 86927
    Injection, 0232T
    Volume, 78110-78111
  Platelet
    Aggregation, 85576
    Automated Count, 85049
    Count, 85008
    Manual Count, 85032
    Phospholipid Neutralization, 85597-85598
  Pool Imaging, 78472, 78473, 78481, 78483,
      78494, 78496
  Products
    Irradiation, 86945
    Pooling, 86965
    Splitting, 86985
    Volume Reduction, 86960
  Reticulocyte, 85046
  Sample
    Fetal, 59030
  Smear, 85060
    Microorganism Identification, 87205-87207
    Microscopic Examination, 85007-85008
    Peripheral, 85060
    Sex Chromatin, 88140
    Surgical Pathology, 88312-88313, 88319
  Stem Cell
    Count, 86367
    Donor Search, 38204
    Erythropoietin Therapy, 3160F, 4090F-
        4095F
    Harvesting, 38205-38206
    Preparation, 38207-38209
    Transplantation, 38240-38242
        Cell Concentration, 38215
        Cryopreservation, 38207, 88240
        Plasma Depletion, 38214
        Platelet Depletion, 38213
        Red Blood Cell Depletion, 38212
        T–cell Depletion, 38210
        Thawing, 38208-38209, 88241
        Tumor Cell Depletion, 38211
        Washing, 38209
  Test(s)
    Iron Stores, 3160F
    Kt/V, 3082F-3084F
    Nuclear Medicine
        Plasma Volume, 78110, 78111
        Platelet Survival, 78190, 78191
        Red Cell Survival, 78130, 78135
        Red Cell Volume, 78120, 78121
        Whole Blood Volume, 78122
    Panels
        Electrolyte, 80051
        General Health Panel, 80050
        Hepatic Function, 80076
        Hepatitis, Acute, 80074
        Lipid Panel, 80061
        Metabolic Panel, Basic
            Basic, 80047-80048
            Comprehensive, 80053
            Ionized Calcium, 80047
            Total Calcium, 80048
        Obstetric Panel, 80055, *[80081]*
        Renal Function, 80069

Blood — *continued*
  Test(s) — *continued*
    Volume Determination, 78122
  Transcutaneous
    Carboxyhemoglobin, 88740
    Methemoglobin, 88741
  Transfusion, 36430, 36440
    Exchange, 36455
      Newborn, 36450
        Partial, 36456
    Fetal, 36460
    Push
      Infant, 36440
  Typing
    ABO Only, 86900
    Antigen Testing, 86902, 86904
    Crossmatch, 86920-86923
    Other RBC Antigens, 86905
    Paternity Testing, 86910, 86911
    Rh(D), 86901
    Rh Phenotype, 86906
  Unlisted Services and Procedures, 85999
  Urea Nitrogen, 84520, 84525
  Urine, 83491
  Viscosity, 85810
  Volume
    Plasma, 78110-78111
    Red Blood Cells, 78120-78121
    Whole Blood, 78122
Blood Coagulation Defect
  See Coagulopathy
Blood Coagulation Disorders
  See Clot
Blood Coagulation Test
  See Coagulation
Blood Component Removal
  See Apheresis
Blood Count, Complete
  See Complete Blood Count (CBC)
Blood Letting
  See Phlebotomy
Blood Lipoprotein
  See Lipoprotein
Blood, Occult
  See Occult Blood
Blood Pressure
  Baroactivation Device, 0266T-0273T
  Central Arterial Analysis, Non-Invasive, 93050
  Diastolic, 3078F-3080F
  Monitoring, 24 hour, 93784-93990
  Systolic, 3074F-3075F
  Venous, 93770
Blood Serum
  See Serum
Blood Transfusion, Autologous
  See Autotransfusion
Blood Vessel(s)
  See Artery; Vein
  Angioscopy
    Noncoronary, 35400
  Endoscopy
    Surgical, 37500-37501
  Endothelial Function Assessment, 0337T
  Excision
    Arteriovenous
      Malformation, 63250-63252
  Exploration
    Abdomen, 35840
    Carotid Artery, 35701
    Chest, 35820
    Extremity, 35860
    Femoral Artery, 35721
    Neck, 35800
    Other Vessel, 35761
    Popliteal Artery, 35741
  Great
    Suture, 33320-33322
  Harvest
    Endoscopic, 33508
    Lower Extremity Vein, 35572
    Upper Extremity Artery, 35600
    Upper Extremity Vein, 35500
  Kidney
    Repair, 50100
  Repair
    Abdomen, 35221, 35251, 35281

Blood Vessel(s) — *continued*
  Repair — *continued*
    Abdomen — *continued*
      with Composite Graft, 35681-35683
      with Other Graft, 35281
      with Vein Graft, 35251
      See Aneurysm Repair; Fistula, Repair
    Aneurysm, 61705-61710
    Aorta, 33320-33322
    Arteriovenous Malformation, 61680-61692,
        61705-61710, 63250-63252
    Chest, 35211, 35216
      with Composite Graft, 35681-35683
      with Other Graft, 35271, 35276
      with Vein Graft, 35241, 35246
    Direct, 35201-35226
    Finger, 35207
    Graft Defect, 35870
    Great Vessels, 33320-33322
    Hand, 35207
    Intraabdominal, 35221, 35251, 35281
    Intrathoracic, 35211, 35216, 35241, 35246,
        35271, 35276
    Kidney, 50100
    Lower Extremity, 35226, 35256, 35286
      with Composite Graft, 35681-35683
      with Other Graft, 35281
      with Vein Graft, 35256
    Neck, 35201
      with Composite Graft, 35681-35683
      with Other Graft, 35261
      with Vein Graft, 35231
    Upper Extremity, 35206, 35236, 35266
      with Composite Graft, 35681-35683
      with Other Graft, 35266
      with Vein Graft, 35236
  Shunt Creation
    with Bypass Graft, 35686
    with Graft, 36825, 36830
    with Transposition, 36818-36820
    Direct, 36821
    Thomas Shunt, 36835
  Shunt Revision
    with Graft, 36832
  Suture Repair, Great Vessels, 33320-33322
Bloom Syndrome
  Chromosome Analysis, 88245
  Gene Analysis, 81209
  Genomic Sequencing Analysis, 81412
Blot Test, Ink
  See Inkblot Test
Blotting, Western
  See Western Blot
Blount Osteotomy, 27455, 27475-27485
Blow–Out Fracture
  Orbital Floor, 21385-21395
Blue, Dome Cyst
  See Breast, Cyst
BMAC (Breath Methylated Alkane Contour),
    0085T
BMPR1A, 81435
BMPR2, 81405-81406
BMT, 38240, 38241, 38242
Boarding Home Care, 99324-99337
Bodies, Acetone
  See Acetone Body
Bodies, Barr
  See Barr Bodies
Bodies, Carotid
  See Carotid Body
Bodies, Ciliary
  See Ciliary Body
Bodies, Heinz
  See Heinz Bodies
Bodies, Inclusion
  See Inclusion Bodies
Bodies, Ketone
  See Ketone Bodies
Body Cast
  Halo, 29000
  Removal, 29700, 29710
  Repair, 29720
  Risser Jacket, 29010, 29015
  Upper Body and One Leg, 29044
  Upper Body Only, 29035
  Upper Body with Head, 29040

Body Cast — *continued*
  Upper Body with Legs, 29046
Body Fluid
  Crystal Identification, 89060
Body of Vertebra
  See Vertebral Body
Body Section
  X–ray, 76100
    Motion, 76101, 76102
Body System, Neurologic
  See Nervous System
BOH, 93600
Bohler Procedure, 28405
Bohler Splinting, 29515
Boil
  See Furuncle
Boil, Vulva
  See Abscess, Vulva
Bone
  See Specific Bone
  Ablation
    Tumor, 20982-20983
  Biopsy, 20220-20245, 20250-20251
    with Vertebroplasty, 22510-22512
  Conduction Hearing Device
    Implantation, 69710
      Replacement, 69710
    Removal
      Repair, 69711
  CT Scan
    Density Study, 77078
  Cyst
    Drainage, 20615
    Injection, 20615
  Debridement, 11044 *[11047]*
  Density Study
    Appendicular Skeleton, 77081
    Axial Skeleton, 77078, 77080
    Ultrasound, 76977
    Vertebral Fracture Assessment, *[77085,
        77086]*
  Dual Energy X–ray
    Absorptiometry, 77080-77081, *[77085]*
  Excision
    Epiphyseal Bar, 20150
    Facial Bones, 21026
    Mandible, 21025
  Fixation
    Caliper, 20660
    Cranial Tong, 20660
    External, 20690
    Halo, 20661-20663, 21100
    Interdental, 21110
    Multiplane, 20692
    Pin
      Wire, 20650
    Skeletal
      Humeral Epicondyle
        Percutaneous, 24566
      Stereotactic Frame, 20660
      Uniplane, 20690
  Fracture
    Hyoid
      See Hyoid Bone
    Osteoporosis Screening, 5015F
  Graft
    Allograft
      Morselized, 20930
      Structural, 20931
    Any Donor Area, 20900-20902
    Augmentation
      Mandibular Body, 21127
    Autograft, 20936
      Morselized, 20937
      Structural, 20938
    Calcaneal Fracture, 28420
    Clavicle, 23485
    Craniofacial Separation, 21436
    Cranium, 61316, 61559, 62146-62148
    Femur, 27170, 27177, 27470
    Fracture
      Orbit, 21408
    Harvesting, 20900, 20902
    Knee Drilling, 29885
    Malar Area, 21210, 21366
    Mandible, 21127, 21194, 21215

Bone — *continued*
  Graft — *continued*
    Mandibular Ramus, 21194
    Maxilla, 21210
    Metacarpal, Nonunion, 26546
    Metatarsal Nonunion, 28322
    Microvascular Anastomosis
      Fibula, 20955
      Iliac Crest, 20956
      Metatarsal Bone, 20957
      Other, 20962
      Rib, 20962
    Midface, 21145-21147, 21150-21151,
        21154-21155, 21159-21160, 21182-
        21184, 21188
    Nasal Area, 21210
    Nasomaxillary Complex Fracture, 21348
    Open Treatment
      Craniofacial Separation, 21436
    Orbit
      Blowout Fracture, 21395
      Cleft Palate, 42210
      Fracture, 21408
      Hypertelorism, 21260
      Reconstruction, 21182-21184, 21256
      Repositioning, 21267
    Osteocutaneous Flap, 20969-20973
    Patella, 27599
    Reconstruction
      Mandibular Ramis, 21194
      Midface, 21145-21160
    Skull, 61316
      Excision, 62148
    Spine Surgery
      with Arthrodesis, Presacral Interbody
        Technique, 0195T-0196T,
        0309T, 22586
      Allograft
        Morselized, 20930
        Structural, 20931
      Autograft
        Local, 20936
        Morselized, 20937
        Structural, 20938
    Toe to Hand Transfer, 26551
    Ulna, 25830
    Vascular Pedicle, 25430
    Vertebra, 0222T
      Cervical, 0219T, 63051
      Lumbar, 0221T
      Thoracic, 0220T
    Wrist, 25805, 25810, 25825
  Healing
    Electrical Stimulation
      Invasive, 20975
      Noninvasive, 20974
    Ultrasound Stimulation, 20979
  Insertion
    Needle, 36680
    Osseointegrated Implant
      for External Speech Processor/Cochlear
        Stimulator, 69714-69718
  Marrow
    Aspiration, 38220
    Cell Preparation, 38207-38215
    Cell Therapy, 0263T-0265T
    Cytogenic Testing, 3155F
    Harvesting, 38230, 38232
      Allogeneic, 38230
      Autologous, 38232
    Intramuscular Therapy, 0263T, 0265T
    Magnetic Resonance Imaging (MRI), 77084
    Needle Biopsy, 38221
    Nuclear Medicine
      Imaging, 78102-78104
    Smear, 85097
    Surgical Pathology, 88305
    T–Cell
      Transplantation, 38240, 38241, 38242
    Trocar Biopsy, 38221
  Nuclear Medicine
    Density Study, 78350, 78351
    Imaging, 78300-78320
    SPECT, 78320
    Unlisted Services and Procedures, 78399
  Osseous Survey, 77074-77075

Bone — *continued*
Osteoporosis
Pharmacologic Therapy, 4005F
Plate
Mandible, 21244
Protein, 83937
Removal
Fixation Device, 20670, 20680
Replacement
Osseointegrated Implant
for External Speech Processor/Cochlear
Stimulator, 69717-69718
Spur, 28119
Wedge Reversal
Osteotomy, 21122
X-ray
Age Study, 77072
Dual Energy Absorptiometry (DEXA),
77080-77081
Joint Stress, 77071
Length Study, 77073
Osseous Survey, 77074-77077
Bone 4-Carboxyglutamic Protein
See Osteocalcin
Bone, Carpal
See Carpal Bone
Bone, Cheek
See Cheekbone
Bone, Facial
See Facial Bone
Bone, Hyoid
See Hyoid Bone
Bone Infection
See Osteomyelitis
Bone, Metatarsal
See Metatarsal
Bone, Nasal
See Nasal Bone
Bone, Navicular
See Navicular
Bone, Scan
See Bone, Nuclear Medicine; Nuclear Medicine
Bone, Semilunar
See Lunate
Bone, Sesamoid
See Sesamoid Bone
Bone, Tarsal
See Ankle Bone
Bone, Temporal
See Temporal, Bone
BOOSTRIX, 90715
Bordetella
Antibody, 86615
Antigen Detection
Direct Fluorescent Antibody, 87265
Borrelia (relapsing fever), 86619
Borrelia burgdorferi ab, 86617-86618
Borreliosis, Lyme, 86617-86618
Antigen/infectious agent, 87475-87477
Bost Fusion
Arthrodesis, Wrist, 25800-25810
Bosworth Operation, 23550, 23552
Bottle Type Procedure, 55060
Botulinum Toxin
Chemodenervation
Extraocular Muscle, 67345
Facial Muscle, 64612
Larynx, 64617
Neck Muscle, 64616
Boutonniere Deformity, 26426, 26428
Bowel
See Intestine(s)
Bower's Arthroplasty, 25332
Bowleg Repair, 27455, 27457
Boxer's Fracture Treatment, 26600-26615
Boyce Operation, 50040, 50045
Boyd Amputation, 27880-27889
Boyd Hip Disarticulation, 27590
Brace
See Cast
for Leg Cast, 29358
Vertebral Fracture, 22310, 22315
Brachial Arteries
See Artery, Brachial
Brachial Plexus
Decompression, 64713

Brachial Plexus — *continued*
Injection
Anesthetic, 64415, 64416
Neuroplasty, 64713
Release, 64713
Repair
Suture, 64861
Brachiocephalic Artery
See Artery, Brachiocephalic
Brachycephaly, 21175
Brachytherapy, 77761-77772, 77789
Dose Plan, 77316-77318
High Dose Electronic, 0394T-0395T
Heyman Capsule, 58346
Intracavitary, 77761-77763, 77770-77772
Placement of Device
Breast, 19296-19298
Genitalia, 55920
Head, 41019
Intraocular, 0190T
Neck, 41019
Pelvis, 55920
Uterus, 57155
Vagina, 57155-57156
Planning
Isodose Plan, 77316-77318
Prostate Volume Study, 76873
Radioelement Solution, 77750
Remote Afterloading
Intracavitary/Interstitial
1 Channel, 77770
2-12 Channels, 77771
Over 12 Channels, 77772
Skin Surface, 77767-77768
Surface Application, 77789-77790
Unlisted Services and Procedures, 77799
Vagina
Insertion
Afterloading Device, 57156
Ovoid, 57155
Tandem, 57155
Bradykinin
Blood or Urine, 82286
BRAF (B-Raf proto-oncogene, serine/threonine kinase), 81210, 81406
Brain
Abscess
Drainage, 61150, 61151
Excision, 61514, 61522
Incision and Drainage, 61320, 61321
Adhesions
Lysis, 62161
Anesthesia, 00210-00218, 00220-00222
Angiography, 36100, 70496
Biopsy, 61140
Stereotactic, 61750, 61751
Catheter
Insertion, 61210
Irrigation, 62194, 62225
Replacement, 62160, 62194, 62225
Catheter Placement
for Chemotherapy, 64999
for Radiation Source, 61770
Cisternography, 70015
Computer Assisted Procedure, 61781-61782
Cortex
Magnetic Stimulation, 0310T, 90867-90869
Mapping, 90867, 96020
Motor Function, 0310T
Coverings
Tumor
Excision, 61512, 61519
Craniopharyngioma, 61545
Excision, 61545
CT Scan, 0042T, 70450-70470, 70496
Cyst
Drainage, 61150, 61151, 62161, 62162
Excision, 61516, 61524, 62162
Death Determination, 95824
Debridement, 62010
Doppler Transcranial, 93886-93893
Electrocorticography, 61536, 61538, 61539
Electroencephalography
Cerebral Death Evaluation, 95824
Monitored, 95812-95813
Recorded, 95816, 95819, 95822, 95827

Brain — *continued*
Epileptogenic Focus
Excision, 61534, 61536
Monitoring, 61531, 61533, 61535, 61760
Excision
Amygdala, 61566
Choroid Plexus, 61544
Craniopharyngioma, 61545
Hemisphere, 61543
Hemispherectomy, 61543
Hippocampus, 61566
Meningioma, 61512, 61519
Other Lobe, 61323, 61539, 61540
Temporal Lobe, 61537, 61538
Exploration
Infratentorial, 61305
Supratentorial, 61304
Hematoma
Drainage, 61154
Incision and Drainage, 61312-61315
Implantation
Chemotherapeutic Agent, 61517
Electrode, 61210, 61850-61870
Pulse Generator, 61885, 61886
Receiver, 61885, 61886
Reservoir, 61210, 61215
Thermal Perfusion Probe, 61107, 61210
Incision
Corpus Callosum, 61541
Mesencephalic Tract, 61480
Subpial, 61567
Infusion, 64999, 95990-95991
Insertion
Catheter, 61210
Electrode, 61531, 61533, 61850-61870
Pulse Generator, 61885, 61886
Receiver, 61885, 61886
Reservoir, 61210, 61215
Lesion
Aspiration, Stereotactic, 61750, 61751
Excision, 61534, 61536, 61600-61608, 61615, 61616
Lobectomy, 61537-61540
Magnetic Resonance Imaging (MRI), 70551-70555
Intraoperative, 0398T
Magnetic Stimulation
Transcranial, 90867-90869
Magnetoencephalography, 95965-95967
Mapping, 90867-90869, 95961-95962, 96020
Meningioma
Excision, 61512, 61519
Myelography, 70010
Neurostimulation
Analysis, 95970-95982
Electrode
Implantation, 61210, 61850, 61860, 61863-61864, 61870
Removal, 61880
Revision, 61880
Pulse Generator
Insertion, 61885-61886
Removal, 61880
Revision, 61880
Nuclear Medicine
Blood Flow, 78610
Cerebrospinal Fluid, 78630-78650
Imaging, 78600-78607
Vascular Flow, 78610
Shunt Evaluation, 78645
Perfusion Analysis, 0042T
Positron Emission Tomography (PET), 78608, 78609
Radiosurgery
for Lesion, 61796-61800
Radiation Treatment Delivery, 77371-77373
Removal
Electrode, 61535, 61880
Foreign Body, 61570, 62163
Pulse Generator, 61888
Receiver, 61888
Shunt, 62256, 62258
Repair
Dura, 61618
Wound, 61571

Brain — *continued*
Shunt
Creation, 62180-62192, 62200-62223
Removal, 62256, 62258
Replacement, 62160, 62194, 62225-62258
Reprogramming, 62252
Skull
Transcochlear Approach, 61596
Transcondylar Approach, 61597
Transpetrosal Approach, 61598
Transtemporal Approach, 61595
Skull Base
Craniofacial Approach, 61580-61585
Infratemporal Approach, 61590, 61591
Orbitocranial Zygomatic Approach, 61592
Stem Auditory Evoked Potential, 92585-92586
Stereotactic
Aspiration, 61750, 61751
Biopsy, 61750, 61751
Catheter Placement, 64999
Computer Assisted Navigation, 61781-61782
Create Lesion, 61720, 61735, 61790, 61791
Localization for Placement Therapy Fields, 61770
Navigation, 61781-61782
Procedure, 61781-61782
Radiation Treatment, 77432
Radiosurgery, 61796-61800, 63620-63621, 77371-77373, 77435
Trigeminal Tract, 61791
Surface Electrode
Stimulation, 95961-95962
Transcranial Magnetic Stimulation (TMS), 90867-90869
Transection
Subpial, 61541, 61567
Tumor
Excision, 61510, 61518, 61520, 61521, 61526, 61530, 61545, 62164
Ventriculocisternostomy, 62200-62201
Torkildsen Type, 62180
X-ray with Contrast, 70010, 70015
Brainstem (Brain Stem)
See Brain
Auditory Implant, 92640
Biopsy, 61575, 61576
Decompression, 61575, 61576
Evoked Potentials, 92585, 92586
Lesion
Excision, 61575, 61576
Branched-Chain Keto Acid Dehydrogenase E1, Beta Polypeptide Gene Analysis, 81205
Branchial Cleft
Cyst
Excision, 42810, 42815
Branchioma
See Branchial Cleft, Cyst
Braun Procedure, 23405-23406
BRCA1, 81214-81215
BRCA1, BRCA 2, 81211-81213, 81432-81433, *[81162]*
BRCA2, 81216-81217
Breast
Ablation
Cryosurgery, 19105
Fibroadenoma, 19105
Abscess
Incision and Drainage, 19020
Augmentation, 19324, 19325
Biopsy, 19100-19101
with Localization Device Placement, 19081-19086
MRI Guided, 19085-19086
Stereotactic Guided, 19081-19082
Ultrasound Guided, 19083-19084
with Specimen Imaging, 19085-19086
ABBI, 19081-19086
Cancer Gene Analysis, 81211-81217, 81402, 81406, 81432-81433, *[81162]*
Catheter Placement
for Interstitial Radioelement Application, 19296-19298, 20555, 41019
Catheter Placement for Application Interstitial Radioelement, 19296-19298
Cryosurgical Ablation, 19105

CPT © 2016 American Medical Association. All Rights Reserved.

© 2016 Optum360, LLC

Breast — *continued*
Cyst
Excision, 19120
Puncture Aspiration, 19000, 19001
Excision
Biopsy, 19100-19101
Capsules, 19371
Chest Wall Tumor, 19260-19272
Cyst, 19120
Lactiferous Duct Fistula, 19112
Lesion, 19120-19126
Needle Localization, 19125-19126
Mastectomy, 19300-19307
Nipple Exploration, 19110
Tumors, 19120, 19260, 19271-19272
Exploration
Abscess, 19020
Nipple, 19110
Implants
Insertion, 19325, 19340, 19342
Preparation of Moulage, 19396
Removal, 19328, 19330
Soft Tissue Reinforcement, 15777
Supply, 19396
Incision
Capsules, 19370
Injection
Radiologic, 19030
Magnetic Resonance Imaging (MRI), 77058-77059
with Computer-aided Detection, 0159T
Mammography, 77065-77067
Bilateral, 77066-77067
Computer-Aided Detection, 77065-77067
Ductogram, 77053-77054
Galactogram, 77053-77054
Injection, 19030
Results Documented and Reviewed, 3014F
Screening, 3014F, 77067
Tactile Imaging, 0422T
Unilateral, 77066
Mammoplasty
Augmentation, 19324, 19325
Reduction, 19318
Mastectomy
Complete, 19303
Gynecomastia, 19300
Modified Radical, 19307
Partial, 19301-19302
Radical, 19303-19306
Subcutaneous, 19304
with Axillary Lymphadenectomy, 19302
Mastopexy, 19316
Metallic Localization Clip Placement, 19281-19288
Needle Biopsy, 19100
Needle Wire Placement, 19281-19288
Periprosthetic Capsulectomy, 19371
Periprosthetic Capsulotomy, 19370
Reconstruction, 19357-19369
with Free Flap, 19364
with Latissimus Dorsi Flap, 19361
with Other Techniques, 19366
with Tissue Expander, 19357
with Transverse Rectus Abdominis Myocutaneous (TRAM) Flap, 19367-19369
Augmentation, 19324, 19325
Mammoplasty, 19318-19325
Myocutaneous Flap, 19367-19369
Nipple, 19350-19355
Areola, 19350
Nipple and Areola, 19350
Correction Inverted Nipples, 19355
Revision, 19380
Reduction, 19318
Removal
Capsules, 19371
Modified Radical, 19307
Partial, 19300-19302
Radical, 19305-19306
Simple, Complete, 19303
Subcutaneous, 19304
Repair
Suspension, 19316
Stereotactic Localization, 19081, 19283

Breast — *continued*
Tactile Imaging, 0422T
Tomosynthesis, 77061-77063
TRAM, 19367-19369
Tumor
Excision
with Ribs, 19260, 19271-19272
Benign, 19120
Chest Wall, 19260, 19271-19272
Malignant, 19120
Microwave Thermotherapy, 0301T
Ultrasound, 76641-76642
Unlisted Services and Procedures, 19499
X-ray
with Computer-aided Detection, 77065-77067
Mammography
Bilateral, Diagnostic, 77065
Screening, 77067
Unilateral, Diagnostic, 77066
Placement Localization Device, 19281-19288
Breathing, Inspiratory Positive-Pressure
See Intermittent Positive Pressure Breathing (IPPB)
Breath Methylated Alkane Contour, 0085T
Breath Odor Alcohol
See Alcohol, Breath
Breath Test
Alcohol, Ethyl, 82075
Heart Transplant Rejection, 0085T
Helicobacter Pylori, 78267, 78268, 83013, 83014
Hydrogen, 91065
Methane, 91065
Urea, 78267-78268
Bricker Operation
Intestines Anastomosis, 50820
Brisement Injection, 20550-20551
Bristow Procedure, 23450-23462
Capsulorrhaphy, Anterior, 23450-23462
Brock Operation, 33470-33475
Valvotomy, Pulmonary Valve, 33470-33474
Broken, Nose
See Fracture, Nasal Bone
Bronchi
Allograft, 32855-32856
Aspiration
Catheter, 31720-31725
Endoscopic, 31629, 31633, 31645-31646
Biopsy
Endoscopic, 31625-31629, 31632, 31633
Bronchial Valve
Insertion, 31647, [31651]
Removal, 31648-31649
Bronchodilator
Home Care, 99503
Spirometry, 94012, 94060
Brushing
Protected Brushing, 31623
Catheterization
with Bronchial Brush Biopsy, 31717
Insertion
with Intracavitary Radioelement, 31643
Endoscopy
Ablation
Photodynamic Therapy, 96570-96571
Aspiration, 31645, 31646
Biopsy, 31625, 31628, 31629, 31632, 31633
Bronchial Valve Insertion, 31647, [31651]
Destruction
Tumor, 31641
Dilation, 31630-31631, 31636-31638
Excision
Lesion, 31640
Exploration, 31622
with Balloon Occlusion, 31634, 31647, [31651]
Foreign Body Removal, 31635
Fracture, 31630
Lesion, 31640, 31641
Stenosis, 31641
Tumor, 31640, 31641
Exploration
Endoscopic, 31622
Fracture
Endoscopy, 31630

Bronchi — *continued*
Needle Biopsy, 31629, 31633
Reconstruction
Anastomosis, 31775, 32486
Graft Repair, 31770
Stenosis, 31775
Removal
Foreign Body, 31635
Repair
Fistula, 32815, 32906
Stenosis, 31641, 96570-96571
Stenosis
Endoscopic Treatment, 31641
Stent
Placement, 31636-31637
Revision, 31638
Testing
Airway Sizing, 31647, [31651]
Assessment Air Leak, 31647, [31651]
Bronchospasm Evaluation, 94070, 94620
Tests
with Antigens, Gases, 95070
with Chemicals, 95071
Tumor
Excision, 31640
Unlisted Services and Procedures, 31899
Bronchial Allergen Challenge
See Bronchial Challenge Test
Bronchial Alveolar Lavage, 31624
Bronchial Brush Biopsy
with Catheterization, 31717
Bronchial Brushings
Protected Brushing, 31623
Bronchial Challenge Test
with Antigens or Gases, 95070
with Chemicals, 95071
See also Allergy Tests
Bronchial Provocation Test
See Allergy Tests, Challenge Test, Bronchial
Bronchoalveolar Lavage, 31624
Broncho-Bronchial Anastomosis, 32486
Bronchoplasty, 32501
Excision Stenosis and Anastomosis, 31775
Graft Repair, 31770
Reconstruction, Bronchi, 32501
Graft Repair, 31770
Stenosis, 31775
Bronchopneumonia, Hiberno-Vernal
See Q Fever
Bronchopulmonary Lavage, 31624
Bronchoscopy
Ablation
Photodynamic Therapy, 96570-96571
Airway Resizing, 31647, [31651]
Alveolar Lavage, 31624
Aspiration, 31629, 31633, 31645-31646, 31725
Assessment Airway Leak, 31647, [31651]
Balloon Occlusion, 31634, 31647, [31651]
Biopsy, 31625-31629, 31632, 31633
Brushing, Protected Brushing, 31623
Catheter Placement
Intracavity Radioelement, 31643
Computer-assisted Image-Guided Navigation, 31627
Diagnostic, 31622-31624, 31643
Dilation, 31630-31631, 31636-31638
Exploration, 31622
with Balloon Occlusion, 31634, 31647, [31651]
Fiducial Marker Placement, 31626
Foreign Body Removal, 31635
Fracture, 31630
Insertion Bronchial Valve(s), 31647, 31651
Needle Biopsy, 31629, 31633
Removal
Bronchial Valve(s), 31648-31649
Foreign Body, 31635
Tumor, 31640, 31641
Stenosis, 31641
Stent Placement, 31631, 31636-31637
Stent Revision, 31638
Thermoplasty, 31660-31661
Tumor
Destruction, 31641
Excision, 31640
via Existing Tracheostomy, 31615

Bronchospasm Evaluation, 94060, 94070
Pulmonology, Diagnostic, Spirometry, 94010-94070
Bronkodyl
See Theophylline
Browne's Operation, 54324
Brow Ptosis
Repair, 67900
Reduction of Overcorrection, 67909
Brucella, 86000
Antibody, 86622
Bruise
See Hematoma
Brunschwig Operation, 58240
Pelvis, Exenteration, 58240
Brush Biopsy
Bronchi, 31717
Brush Border ab
See Antibody, Heterophile
BSCL2, 81406
BSO, 58720
BTD, 81404
BTK, 81406
Bucca
See Cheek
Buccal Mucosa
See Mouth, Mucosa
Bulbourethral Gland
Excision, 53250
Bulla
Incision and Drainage
Puncture Aspiration, 10160
Lung
Excision-Plication, 32141
Endoscopic, 32655
BUN, 84520-84545
Bunionectomy
with First Metatarsal Medial Cuneiform Arthrodesis, 28297
with Implant, 28291
with Metatarsal Osteotomy, 28295, 28296
with Tendon Transplants, 28899
Phalanx Osteotomy, 28298-28299
Simple Exostectomy, 28292
Bunion Repair
with First Metatarsal Medial Cuneiform Arthrodesis, 28297
with Implant, 28291
with Metatarsal Osteotomy, 28295, 28296
with Tendon Transplants, 28899
Bunionectomy, 28299
Phalanx Osteotomy, 28298-28299
Simple Ostectomy, 28292
Bunnell Procedure, 24301
Burch Operation, 51840-51841
Laparoscopic, 58152
Burgess Amputation
Disarticulation, Ankle, 27889
Burhenne Procedure, 43500
Bile Duct, Removal of Calculus, 43264, 47420, 47425, 47554
Burkitt Herpes Virus
See Epstein-Barr Virus
Burns
Anesthesia, 01951-01953
Debridement, 01951-01953, 15002-15003, 15004-15005, 16020-16030
Dressing, 16020-16030
Escharotomy, 15002-15005, 16035-16036
Excision, 01951-01953, 15002, 15004-15005
First Degree Burn, Initial Treatment, 16000
Initial Treatment, 16000
Tissue Culture Skin Grafts, 15100-15157
Burr Hole
Anesthesia, 00214
Skull
with Injection, 61120
Aspiration
Cyst, 61156
Hematoma, 61156
Biopsy, Brain, 61140
Stereotactic, 61750-61751
Catheterization, 61210
Drainage
Abscess, 61150, 61151
Cyst, 61150, 61151

Burr Hole — *continued*
Skull — *continued*
Drainage — *continued*
Hematoma, 61154, 61156
Exploration
Infratentorial, 61253
Supratentorial, 61250
Implant
Catheter, 61210
Cerebral Monitoring Device, 61210
Cerebral Thermal Perfusion Probe, 61107, 61210
Device for Pressure Recording, 61210
EEG Electrode, 61210
Neurostimulator Array, 61850, 61863-61868
Strip Electrodes, 61531
Injection, Contrast Media, 61120
Insertion
Catheter, 61210
Pump, 61210
Reservoir, 61210
Lesion Creation, 61720
Stereotactic Localization, 61770
Ventricular Puncture, 61020
Contrast Media Injection, 61120
Diagnostic or Therapeutic Injection, 61026
Burrow's Operation, 14000-14350
Bursa
Ankle
Aspiration, 20605-20606
Incision and Drainage, 27604
Injection, 20605-20606
Arm, Lower
Aspiration, 20605-20606
Incision and Drainage, 25031
Injection, 20605-20606
Elbow
Aspiration, 20605-20606
Excision, 24105
Incision and Drainage, 23931
Injection, 20605-20606
Femur
Excision, 27062
Finger
Aspiration, 20600-20604
Injection, 20600-20604
Foot
Incision and Drainage, 28001
Hand
Incision and Drainage, 26025-26030
Hip
Aspiration, 20610-20611
Incision and Drainage, 26991
Injection, 20610-20611
Injection, 20600-20611
Ischial
Excision, 27060
Joint
Aspiration, 20600-20611
Drainage, 20600-20610
Injection, 20600-20611
Knee
Aspiration, 20610-20611
Excision, 27340
Incision and Drainage, 27301
Injection, 20610-20611
Leg
Lower, 27604
Upper, 27301
Palm
Incision and Drainage, 26025, 26030
Pelvis
Incision and Drainage, 26991
Shoulder
Aspiration, 20610-20611
Drainage, 23031
Injection, 20610-20611
Toe
Aspiration, 20600-20604
Injection, 20600-20604
Wrist
Aspiration, 20605-20606
Excision, 25115, 25116
Incision and Drainage, 25031

Bursa — *continued*
Wrist — *continued*
Injection, 20605-20606
Bursectomy
of Hand, 26989
Bursitis, Radiohumeral
See Tennis Elbow
Bursocentesis
See Aspiration, Bursa
Buttock
Excision
Excess Skin, 15835
Button
Bone Graft, 20900
Nasal Septal Prosthesis, 30220
Voice Prosthesis, 31611
Butyrylcholine Esterase
See Cholinesterase
B Vitamins
B–1 (Thiamine), 84425
B–2 (Riboflavin), 84252
B–6 (Pyridoxal Phosphate), 84207
B–12 (Cyanocobalamin), 82607, 82608
Absorption Study, 78270-78272
Bypass
Cardiopulmonary, 33510-33516
Bypass Graft
with Composite Graft, 35681-35683
Autogenous
Three or More Segments
Two Locations, 35683
Two Segments
Two Locations, 35682
Aortobifemoral, 35540, 35646
Aortobi-iliac, 35538, 35638
Aortocarotid, 35526, 35626
Aortoceliac, 35531, 35631
Aortofemoral, 35539, 35647
Aortoiliac, 35537, 35637
Aortoinnominate, 35526, 35626
Aortomesenteric, 35531, 35631
Aortorenal, 35560, 35631
Aortosubclavian, 35526, 35626
Axillary Artery, 35516-35522, 35533, 35616-35623, 35650, 35654
Brachial Artery, 35510, 35512, 35522-35525
Brachial-Ulnar or -Radial, 35523
Carotid Artery, 33891, 35501-35510, 35601, 35606, 35642
Celiac Artery, 35341, 35631-35632
Coronary Artery
Arterial, 33533-33536
Arterial-Venous, 33517-33519, 33521-33523, 33530
Venous Graft, 33510-33516
Excision
Abdomen, 35907
Extremity, 35903
Neck, 35901
Thorax, 35905
Femoral Artery, 35521, 35533, 35539, 35540, 35556, 35558, 35566, 35621, 35646, 35647, 35654-35661, 35666, 35700
Harvest
Endoscopic, Vein, 33508
Upper Extremity Artery, 35600
Upper Extremity Vein, 35500
Hepatorenal, 35535
Iliac Artery, 35537, 35538, 35563, 35637, 35638, 35663
Ilio-Celiac, 35632
Iliofemoral, 35565, 35665
Ilioiliac, 35563, 35663
Ilio-Mesenteric, 35633
Iliorenal, 35634
Mesenteric Artery, 35531, 35631
Peroneal Artery, 35566, 35570-35571, 35585, 35587, 35666, 35671
Peroneal-Tibial Vein, 35570
Placement
Vein Patch, 35685
Popliteal Artery, 35556, 35571, 35583, 35623, 35656, 35671, 35700
Renal Artery, 35536, 35560, 35631, 35636
Reoperation, 35700

Bypass Graft — *continued*
Repair
Abdomen, 35907
Extremity, 35903
Lower Extremity
with Composite Graft, 35681-35683
Neck, 35901
Thorax, 35905
Revascularization
Extremity, 35903
Neck, 35901
Thorax, 35905
Revision
Lower Extremity
with Angioplasty, 35879
with Vein Interposition, 35881
Femoral Artery, 35883-35884
Secondary Repair, 35870
Splenic Artery, 35536, 35636
Subclavian Artery, 35506, 35511-35516, 35526, 35606-35616, 35626, 35645, 35693-35694
Thrombectomy, 35875, 35876, 37184-37186
Other Than Hemodialysis Graft or Fistula, 35875-35876
Tibial Artery, 35566, 35571, 35623, 35666, 35671
Tibial-Tibial Vein, 35570
Vertebral Artery, 35508, 35515, 35642, 35645
Bypass In Situ
Femoral Artery, 35583-35585
Peroneal Artery, 35585, 35587
Popliteal Artery, 35583, 35587
Tibial Artery, 35585, 35587
Ventricular Restoration, 33548

<h1 style="text-align:center">C</h1>

C10orf2, 81404
C–13
Urea Breath Test, 83013, 83014
Urease Activity, 83013, 83014
C–14
Urea Breath Test, 78267, 78268
Urease Activity, 83013, 83014
CA, 82310-82340
CABG, 33503-33505, 33510-33536
CACNA1A, 81401, 81407
CACNB2, 81406
Cadmium
Urine, 82300
Caffeine
Assay, 80155
Caffeine Halothane Contracture Test (CHCT), 89049
Calcaneus
Bone Graft, 28420
Craterization, 28120
Cyst
Excision, 28100-28103
Diaphysectomy, 28120
Excision, 28118-28120
Fracture
with Bone Graft, 28420
with Manipulation, 28405, 28406
without Manipulation, 28400
Closed Treatment, 28400, 28405
Open Treatment, 28415, 28420
Percutaneous Fixation, 28406
Repair
Osteotomy, 28300
Saucerization, 28120
Sequestrectomy, 28120
Spur, 28119
Tumor
Excision, 28100-28103
Radical Resection, 27647
X-ray, 73650
Calcareous Deposits
Subdeltoid
Removal, 23000
Calcifediol
Blood Serum Level 25 Hydroxy, 82306
I, 25 Dihydroxy, [82652]
Calciferol
Blood Serum Level 25 Hydroxy, 82306

Calciferol — *continued*
I, 25 Dihydroxy, [82652]
Calcification
See Calcium, Deposits
Calciol
See Calcifediol
Calcitonin
Blood or Urine, 82308
Stimulation Panel, 80410
Calcium
Blood
Infusion Test, 82331
Deposits
Removal, Calculi–Stone
Bile Duct, 43264, 47420, 47425, 47554
Bladder, 51050, 52310-52318
Gallbladder, 47480
Hepatic Duct, 47400
Kidney, 50060-50081, 50130, 50561, 50580
Pancreas, 48020
Pancreatic Duct, 43264
Salivary Gland, 42330-42340
Ureter, 50610-50630, 50961, 50980, 51060, 51065, 52320-52330
Urethra, 52310, 52315
Ionized, 82330
Panel, 80047
Total, 82310
Panel, 80048
Urine, 82340
Calcium–Binding Protein, Vitamin K–Dependent
See Osteocalcin
Calcium–Pentagastrin Stimulation, 80410
Calculus
Analysis, 82355-82370
Destruction
Bile Duct, 43265
Kidney
Extracorporeal Shock Wave Lithotripsy, 50590
Pancreatic Duct, 43265
Ureter
Lithotripsy, 52353, [52356]
Removal
Bile Duct, 43264, 47554
Biliary Tract, 47400, 47420, 47425, 47480
Bladder, 51050, 52310-52318, 52352
Kidney, 50060-50081, 50130, 50561, 50580, 52352
Liver, 47400
Pancreatic Duct, 43264, 48020
Ureter, 50610-50630, 50945, 50961, 50980, 51060, 51065, 52310-52315, 52320, 52325, 52352
Urethra, 52310, 52315, 52352
Calculus of Kidney
See Calculus, Removal, Kidney
Caldwell–Luc Procedure(s), 21385, 31030, 31032
Orbital Floor Blowout Fracture, 21385
Sinusotomy, 31030, 31032
Caliper
Application
Removal, 20660
Callander Knee Disarticulation, 27598
Callosum, Corpus
See Corpus Callosum
Calmette Guerin Bacillus Vaccine
See BCG Vaccine
Caloric Vestibular Test, 92533, 92537-92538
Calprotectin
Fecal, 83993
Calycoplasty, 50405
Camey Enterocystoplasty, 50825
CAMP
See Cyclic AMP
Campbell Arthrodesis, 27870
Campbell Procedure, 27422
Campylobacter
Antibody, 86625
Antigen, 86628
Skin Test, 86485
Campylobacteri Pylori
Antibody, 86677
Antigen Detection Enzyme Immunoassay, 87338-87339

[Resequenced] © 2016 Optum360, LLC

Campylobacteri Pylori — *continued*
  Blood Test, 83009
  Breath Test, 78267-78268, 83013-83014
  Stool, 87338
  Urease Activity, 83009, 83013-83014
Canal, Ear
  See Auditory Canal
Canalith Repositioning Procedure, 95992
Canaloplasty, 69631, 69635
Canal, Semicircular
  See Semicircular Canal
Canavan Disease
  Geonomic Sequence Analysis, 81412
Candida
  Antibody, 86628
  Antigen, 87480-87482
  Skin Test, 86485
Cannulation
  Arterial, 36620, 36625
  Arteriovenous, 36810, 36815
  Endoscopic
    Common Bile Duct, 43273
    Pancreatic Duct, 43273
    Papilla, 43273
  Fallopian Tube, 58565
  Pancreatic Duct, 48999
  Sinus
    Maxillary, 31000
    Ostium, 31235
    Sphenoid, 31002
  Thoracic Duct, 38794
  Vas Deferens, 55200
  Vein to Vein, 36800
Cannulation, Renoportal
  See Anastomosis, Renoportal
Cannulization
  See Catheterization
  Arteriovenous (AV), 36810, 36815, 36901-36903
  Chemotherapy, 36823
  Declotting, 36593, 36860, 36861
  Dialysis Circuit, 36901-36903
  ECMO
    Insertion, 33951-33956
    Isolated with Chemotherapy Perfusion, 36823
    Removal, *[33965, 33966, 33969, 33984, 33985, 33986]*
    Repositioning, 33957-33959 *[33962, 33963, 33964]*
  External
    Declotting, 36860-36861
  Vas Deferens, 55200
  Vein to Vein, 36800
Canthocystostomy
  See Conjunctivorhinostomy
Canthopexy
  Lateral, 21282
  Medial, 21280
Canthoplasty, 67950
Canthorrhaphy, 67880, 67882
Canthotomy, 67715
Canthus
  Reconstruction, 67950
Cap, Cervical, 57170
CAPD, 90945, 90947
CAPN3, 81406
Capsule
  See Capsulodesis
  Ankle, 27612, 27630
  Biopsy of Intestine, 44100
  Elbow
    Arthrotomy, 24006
    Excision, 24006
  Endoscopy, 0355T, 91110-91111
  Eye, 66830
  Finger, 26160, 26520, 26525
  Foot, 28090, 28260-28264
  Heyman, 58346
  Hip, 27036
  Injection, 67515
  Interphalangeal Joint
    Foot, 28272
    Hand, 26525
  Knee, 27435
  Leg, 27630

Capsule — *continued*
  Metacarpophalangeal Joint
    Excision, 26160
    Incision, 26520
  Metatarsophalangeal Joint Release
    with Implant, 28291
    without Implant, 28289
  Shoulder, Incision, 23020
  Tenon's, 67515
  Toe, 28270, 28272
  Wrist
    Excision, 25320
Capsulectomy
  Breast, Periprosthetic, 19371
  Elbow, 24149
  Finger, 26160, 26525
  Foot, 28090
  Hand, 26160, 26520
  Hip, 27036
  Knee, 27347
Capsulodesis
  Blatt, 25320
  Metacarpophalangeal Joint, 26516-26518
Capsulorrhaphy
  Ankle, 27630
  Anterior, 23450-23462
  Bankart Procedure, 23455
  Bristow Procedure, 23460
  Glenohumeral Joint, 23465-23466
  Magnuson Type Procedure, 23450
  Multi–Directional Instability, 23466
  Posterior, 23465
  Putti-Platt Procedure, 23450
  Shoulder, Arthroscopic, 29806
  Thermal, 29999
  Wrist, 25320
Capsulotomy
  Breast
    Periprosthetic, 19370
  Eye, 66830
  Foot, 28260-28262, 28264
  Hip with Release, Flexor Muscles, 27036
  Interphalangeal Joint, 28272
  Knee, 27435
  Leg, 27630
  Metacarpophalangeal Joint, 26520
  Metatarsophalangeal Joint, 28270
  Shoulder, 23020
  Toe, 28270, 28272
  Wrist, 25085, 25320
Captopril, 80416, 80417
Carbamazepine
  Assay, 80156-80157
Carbazepin
  See Carbamazepine
Carbinol
  See Methanol
Carbohydrate Deficient Transferin, 82373
Carbon Dioxide
  Blood or Urine, 82374, 82803
Carboxycathepsin
  See Angiotensin Converting Enzyme (ACE)
Carboxyhemoglobin, 82375-82376, 88740
Carbuncle
  Incision and Drainage, 10060, 10061
Carcinoembryonal Antigen
  See Antigen, Carcinoembryonic
Carcinoembryonic Antigen, 82378
Cardiac Arrhythmia, Tachycardia
  See Tachycardia
Cardiac Atria
  See Atria
Cardiac Catheterization
  Angiography
    Bypass Graft(s), 93455, 93457, 93459, 93461
    Congenital Heart, 93563-93564
    Coronary, 93454-93461, 93563, 93571
    Left Atrium, 93565
    Left Ventricle, 93565
    Pulmonary, 93568
    Right Atrium, 93566
    Right Ventricle, 93566
    Combined Left and Right Heart, 93531-93533
      with Ventriculography, 93453, 93460-93461
    Congenital Anomalies, 93530-93533

Cardiac Catheterization — *continued*
  Flow Directed, 93503
  Flow Measurement, 93571-93572
  for Biopsy, 93505
  for Congenital Anomalies
    Right and Retrograde Left, 93531
    Transseptal and Retrograde Left, 93532, 93533
  for Dilution Studies, 93561, 93562
  for Measurement of O2 Cardiac Output, 93451
  for Opacification
    Bypass Grafts, 93564
  For Supravalvular Aortography, 93567
  Imaging, 93452-93461, 93563-93568
  Injection, 93461, 93563-93568
  Insertion Swan-Ganz, 93503
  Left Heart, 93452, 93458-93459
    with Ventriculography, 93452, 93458-93459, 93465
    By Transseptal Puncture, 93462
    for Transapical Puncture, 93462
  Right Heart, 93451, 93456-93457
    for Congenital Anomalies, 93530
Cardiac Contractility Modulation System, 0408T-0418T
Cardiac Electroversion
  See Cardioversion
Cardiac Event Recorder (wearable), 93224-93272
  Implantation, 33282
  Removal, 33284
Cardiac Magnetic Resonance Imaging (CMRI)
  with Contrast, 75561-75563
  without Contrast, 75557-75559
  Morphology and Function, 75557, 75559, 75561, 75563
  Stress Imaging, 75559, 75563
  Velocity Flow Mapping, 75565
Cardiac Massage
  Thoracotomy, 32160
Cardiac Output Measurement
  by Indicator Dilution, 93561, 93562
Cardiac Pacemaker
  See Heart, Pacemaker
Cardiac Rehabilitation, 93797, 93798
Cardiac Septal Defect
  See Septal Defect
Cardiac Transplantation
  See Heart, Transplantation
Cardiectomy
  Donor, 33930, 33940
Cardioassist, 92970, 92971
Cardio Defibrillator (Implantable)
  Transvenous Device
    Insertion
      Electrode, 33216-33217
      Pulse Generator, 33240, *[33230, 33231]*
      System, 33249
    Interrogation Device Evaluation, 93289
      Periprocedural, 93287
      Remote, 93295-93296
    Programming Device Evaluation, 93282-93284
    Relocation
      Skin Pocket, 33223
    Removal
      Electrode, 33243-33244
      Pulse Generator, 33241, *[33262, 33263, 33264]*
    Repair Electrode, 33218, 33220
    Reposition Electrode, 33215, 33226
  Wearable, 93745
    Data Analysis, 93292
Cardio-Fascio-Cutaneous Syndrome, 81442
Cardiolipin Antibody, 86147
Cardiology
  Diagnostic
    Atrial Electrogram
      Esophageal Recording, 93615, 93616
    Bioimpedence Analysis, 93701
    Echocardiography
      Doppler, 93303-93321, 93662
      Intracardiac, 93662
      Myocardial Contrast Perfusion, 0439T
      Strain Imaging, 0399T
      Transesophageal, 93318
      Transthoracic, 93303-93317, 93350

Cardiology — *continued*
  Diagnostic — *continued*
    Electrocardiogram
      Evaluation, 93000, 93010, 93660, 0178T-0180T
      Microvolt T–wave, Alternans, 93025
      Patient-Activated, 93268-93272
      Recording, 93000-93005, 93224-93229, 0178T-0179T
      Rhythm, 93040-93042
      Tracing, 93005
      Transmission, 93268, 93271
    Electrophysiologic
      with Myocardial Contrast Perfusion, 0439T
    Follow–Up Study, 93624
    Endoluminal Imaging, *[92978, 92979]*
    Ergonovine Provocation Test, 93024
    Evaluation
      Heart Device, 93640
    Heart
      Stimulation and Pacing, 93623
    Implantable Defibrillator
      Data Analysis, 93289, 93295-93296
      Evaluation of Programming, 93282-93284, 93287, 93289, 93292, 93295-93296, 93640-93642
    Implantable Monitor
      Data Analysis, 93290, 93297, 93299
    Intracardiac Pacing and Mapping, 93631
      3–D Mapping, 93613, 93654
      Follow–up Study, 93624
      Stimulation and Pacing, 93623
    Intracardiac Pacing and Recording
      Arrhythmia Induction, 93618, 93620-93622, 93624, 93640-93642, 93653-93656
      Bundle of His, 93600, 93619-93620, 93653-93654, 93656
      Comprehensive, 93619-93622
      Intra–Atrial, 93602, 93610, 93616, 93656
      Left Ventricle, 93654
      Right Ventricle, 93603, 93653, 93656
      Tachycardia Sites, 93609
      Ventricular, 93612
    Loop Recorder System
      Data Analysis, 93291, 93298-93299
      Evaluation and Programming, 93285
    M Mode and Real Time, 93307-93321
    Pacemaker Testing, 93642
      Antitachycardia System, 93724
      Data Analysis, 93288, 93293-93294
      Dual Chamber, 93280, 93288, 93293
      Evaluation of Device Programming, 93279-93281, 93286, 93288, 93290, 93293-93294, 93296
      Leads, 93641
      Single Chamber, 93279, 93288, 93294
    Perfusion Imaging, 78451-78454, 78491-78492
    Strain Imaging, 0399T
    Stress Tests
      Cardiovascular, 93015-93018
      Drug Induced, 93024
      MUGA (Multiple Gated Acquisition), 78483
    Temperature Gradient Studies, 93740
    Tilt Table Evaluation, 93660
    Vectorcardiogram
      Evaluation, 93799
      Tracing, 93799
    Venous Pressure Determination, 93784, 93786, 93788, 93790
  Therapeutic
    Ablation, 93650, 93653-93656
    Cardioassist, 92970, 92971
    Cardiopulmonary Resuscitation, 92950
    Cardioversion, 92960, 92961
    Endoluminal Imaging, *[92978, 92979]*
    Implantable Defibrillator
      Data Analysis, 93289, 93295-93296
      Evaluation of Device Programming, 93282-93284, 93287, 93289, 93292, 93295-93296
      Initial Set-up and Programming, 93745

Cardiology — continued
Therapeutic — continued
Pacing
Transcutaneous, Temporary, 92953
Rehabilitation, 93668, 93797-93798
Thrombolysis
Coronary Vessel, [92975, 92977]
Thrombolysis, Coronary, [92977]
Valvuloplasty
Open, 33390-33391
Percutaneous, 92986, 92990
Cardiomyotomy
See Esophagomyotomy
Cardioplasty, 43320
Cardioplegia, 33999
Cardiopulmonary Bypass
with Prosthetic Valve Repair, 33496
Aortic Valve Replacement, Transcatheter, 33367-33369
Lung Transplant with
Double, 32854
Single, 32852
Cardiopulmonary Resuscitation, 92950
Cardiotomy, 33310, 33315
Cardiovascular Stress Test
See Exercise Stress Tests
Cardioversion, 92960, 92961
Care, Custodial
See Nursing Facility Services
Care, Intensive
See Intensive Care
Care, Neonatal Intensive
See Intensive Care, Neonatal
Care Plan Oversight Services
Extracorporeal Liver Assist System, 0405T
Home Health Agency Care, 99374, 99375
Hospice, 99377, 99378
Nursing Facility, 99379, 99380
Care, Self
See Self Care
Carneous Mole
See Abortion
Carnitine Total and Free, 82379
Carotene, 82380
Carotid Artery
Aneurysm Repair
Vascular Malformation or Carotid Cavernous Fistula, 61710
Baroreflex Activation Device
Implantation/Replantation, 0266T-0268T
Interrogation Evaluation, 0272T-0273T
Revision/Removal, 0269T-0271T
Excision, 60605
Ligation, 37600-37606
Stenosis Imaging, 3100F
Stent, Transcatheter Placement, 0075T-0076T
Carotid Body
Lesion
Carotid Artery, 60605
Excision, 60600
Carotid Pulse Tracing
with ECG Lead, 93799
Carotid Sinus Baroreflex Activation Device
Implantation, 0266T-0268T
Interrogation Device Evaluation, 0272T, 0273T
Removal, 0269T-0271T
Replacement, 0266T-0268T
Carpal Bone
Arthroplasty
with Implant, 25441-25446
Cyst
Excision, 25130-25136
Dislocation
Closed Treatment, 25690
Open Treatment, 25695
Excision, 25210, 25215
Partial, 25145
Fracture, 25622-25628
with Manipulation, 25624, 25635
without Manipulation, 25630
Closed Treatment, 25622, 25630, 25635
Open Treatment, 25628, 25645
Incision and Drainage, 26034
Insertion
Vascular Pedicle, 25430
Ligament Release, 29848

Carpal Bone — continued
Navicular (Scaphoid)
Fracture, 25622-25624, 25628, 25630-25635, 25645
Nonunion, 25440
Osteoplasty, 25394
Prosthetic Replacement, 25443-25446
Repair, 25431-25440
with Fixation, 25628
with Styloidectomy, 25440
Nonunion, 25431, 25440
Sequestrectomy, 25145
Tumor
Excision, 25130-25136
Carpals
Incision and Drainage, 25035
Carpal Tunnel
Injection
Therapeutic, 20526
Carpal Tunnel Syndrome
Decompression, 64721
Arthroscopy, 29848
Injection, 20526
Median Nerve Neuroplasty, 64721
Carpectomy, 25210, 25215
Carpometacarpal Joint
Arthrodesis
Fingers, 26843-26844
Hand, 26843-26844
Thumb, 26841-26842
Wrist, 25800-25810
Arthrotomy, 26070, 26100
Biopsy
Synovium, 26100
Dislocation
Closed Treatment, 26670
with Manipulation, 26675, 26676
Open Treatment, 26685, 26686
Drainage, 26070
Exploration, 26070
Fusion
Hand, 26843, 26844
Thumb, 26841, 26842
Magnetic Resonance Imaging, 73221-73225
Removal
Foreign Body, 26070
Repair, 25447
Synovectomy, 26130
Carpue's Operation, 30400
Car Seat/Bed Neonatal Testing, 94780-94781
Car Seat Testing, 94780-94781
Cartilage, Arytenoid
See Arytenoid
Cartilage, Ear
See Ear Cartilage
Cartilage Graft
Costochondral, 20910
Ear to Face, 21235
Harvesting, 20910, 20912
Mandibular Condyle Reconstruction, 21247
Nasal Septum, 20912
Rib to Face, 21230
Zygomatic Arch Reconstruction, 21255
Cartilaginous Exostosis
See Exostosis
Case Management Services
Anticoagulation Management, 99363-99364
Online, 98969, 99444
Team Conferences, 99366-99368
Telephone Calls
Consult Physician, 99446-99449
Nonphysician, 98966-98968
Physician, 99441-99443
CASQ2, 81405
CASR, 81405
Cast
See Brace; Splint
Body
Halo, 29000
Risser Jacket, 29010, 29015
Upper Body and Head, 29040
Upper Body and Legs, 29046
Upper Body and One Leg, 29044
Upper Body Only, 29035
Clubfoot, 29450, 29750
Cylinder, 29365

Cast — continued
Figure-of-Eight, 29049
Finger, 29086
Gauntlet, 29085, 29750
Hand, 29085
Hip, 29305, 29325
Leg
Rigid Total Contact, 29445
Long Arm, 29065
Long Leg, 29345, 29355, 29365, 29450
Long Leg Brace, 29358
Minerva, 29040
Patellar Tendon Bearing (PTB), 29435
Removal, 29700-29710
Repair, 29720
Short Arm, 29075
Short Leg, 29405-29435, 29450
Shoulder, 29049-29058
Spica, 29055, 29305, 29325, 29720
Unlisted Services and Procedures, 29799
Velpeau, 29058
Walking, 29355, 29425
Revision, 29440
Wedging, 29740, 29750
Windowing, 29730
Wrist, 29085
Casting
Unlisted Services and Procedures, 29799
Castration
See Orchiectomy
Castration, Female
See Oophorectomy
Cataract
Dilated Fundus Evaluation Prior to Surgery, 2020F
Discission, 66820-66821
Excision, 66830
Incision, 66820-66821
Laser, 66821
Stab Incision, 66820
Presurgical Measurements, 3073F
Removal
Extraction
Extracapsular, 66982, 66984
Intracapsular, 66983
Catecholamines, 80424, 82382-82384
Blood, 82383
Fractionated, 82384
Pheochromocytoma Panel, 80424
Urine, 82382
Cathepsin-D, 82387
Catheter
See Cannulization; Venipuncture
Aspiration
Nasotracheal, 31720
Tracheobronchial, 31725
Biopsy, Transcatheter, 37200
Bladder, 51701-51703
Irrigation, 51700
Blood Specimen Collection, 36592, 37799
Breast
for Interstitial Radioelement Application, 19296-19298
Bronchus for Intracavitary Radioelement Application, 31643
Central Venous
Repair, 36575
Replacement, 36580, 36581, 36584
Repositioning, 36597
Cystourethroscopy, 52320-52353 [52356]
Declotting, 36593, 36861
Drainage
Biliary, 47533-47537
Peritoneal, 49406-49407
Pleural, 32556-32557
Retroperitoneal, 49406-49407
Spinal, 62272
Ventricular, 62162, 62164
Electrode Array, 63650
Embolectomy, 34001, 34051, 34101-34111, 34151, 34201, 34203
Embolization, 61624, 61626
Peritoneal, 49423
Enteral Alimentation, 44015
Exchange
Drainage, 49423

Catheter — continued
Exchange — continued
Nephrostomy, [50435]
Peritoneal, 49423
Flow Directed, 93503
Home Visit Catheter Care, 99507
Infusion
Brachial Plexus, 64416
Femoral Nerve, 64448
Lumbar Plexus, 64449
Saline, 58340
Sciatic Nerve, 64446
Vertebral, 62324-62327
Installation
Fibrinolysis, 32561-32562
Pleurodesis, 32560
Intracatheter
Irrigation, 99507
Obstruction Clearance, 36596
Intraperitoneal
Tunneled
Laparoscopic, 49324
Open, 49421
Percutaneous, 49418-49419
Pericatheter
Obstruction Clearance, 36595
Placement
Brain
Stereotactic, 64999
Breast
for Interstitial Radioelement Placement, 19296-19298, 20555
Bronchus
for Intracavitary Radioelement Placement, 31643
Head and/or Neck, 41019
Muscle and/or Soft Tissue, 20555
Nephrostomy, Percutaneous, [50432]
Nephroureteral, [50433, 50434]
Radiation Source, 61770
Stent, 33621, 61635
Wireless Physiologic Sensor, 34806
Removal
Central Venous, 36589
Foreign Body, 37197
Nephroureteral, Accessible, 50387
Obstruction, 36595-36596
Peritoneum, 49422
Pleural catheter, 32552
Spinal Cord, 62355
Repair
Central Venous, 36575
Intraperitoneal, 49325
Replacement
Central Venous, 36580-36581, 36584
Nephroureteral, Accessible, 50387
Shunt System, 62230
Subarachnoid, 62194
Subdural, 62194
Ventricular, 62225
Repositioning, 36597
Thrombectomy, 34001, 34051, 34101-34111, 34151, 34201, 34203, 34401, 34421, 34451, 61645
Transcatheter Therapy, 36640, 36660, 62320-62327, [37211, 37212, 37213, 37214]
Ureteral
Manometric Studies, 50396, 50686
Ureterography, 50684
Ureteropyelography, 50684
Catheterization
with Cholecystostomy, 47490
Abdomen, 49324, 49418-49419, 49421
Abdominal Artery, 36245-36248
Aorta, 36160-36215
Arterial
Aorta, 36200, 36221
Translumbar, 36160
Arteriovenous Shunt
Dialysis Circuit, 36901-36903
Cutdown, 36625
Intracatheter/Needle, 36100-36140
Percutaneous, 36620
Selective Placement, 36215-36218, 36222-36252
Superselective Placement, 36253-36254

Catheterization — *continued*
  Arteriovenous Shunt
    Dialysis Circuit, 36901-36903
  Bile Duct
    Change, 47535-47536
    Percutaneous, 47533-47534
    Removal, 47537
  Bladder, 51045, 51102
  Brachial Artery, Retrograde, 36120
  Brachiocephalic Artery, 36215-36218
  Brain, 61210
    Replacement, 62160, 62194, 62225
    Stereotactic, 64999
  Bronchus
    with Bronchial Brush Biopsy, 31717
    for Intracavitary Radioelement Application,
      31643
  Cardiac
    Combined Left and Right Heart, 93453,
      93460-93461
    Combined Right and Retrograde Left
      for Congenital Cardiac Anomalies,
        93531
    Combined Right and Transseptal Left
      for Congenital Cardiac Anomalies,
        93532-93533
    Flow Directed, 93503
    for Angiography
      Bypass Graft(s), 93455, 93457, 93459-
        93461
      Congenital Heart, 93563-93564
      Coronary, 93454-93461, 93563
      Left Atrial, 93565
      Left Ventricular, 93565
      Pulmonary, 93568
      Right Atrial, 93566
      Right Ventricular, 93566
    for Biopsy, 93505
    for Congenital Anomalies
      Right and Retrograde Left, 93531
      Transseptal and Retrograde Left,
        93532, 93533
    for Dilution Studies, 93561, 93562
    for Measurement O2, Cardiac Output,
      93451
    for Opacification
      Bypass Graft, 93564
    for Stent Placement, 33621
    for Supravalvular Aortography, 93567
    Injection, 93563-93568
    Left Heart, 93462
      with Ventriculography, 93452, 93458-
        93459, 93565
      by Transapical Puncture, 93462
      by Transseptal Puncture through Intact
        Septum, 93462
    Pacemaker, 33210
    Right Heart, 36013, 93451, 93530
      for Congenital Cardiac Anomalies,
        93530
  Carotid Artery, 36100, 36221-36224, 36227-
    36228
  Central, 36555-36566
  Cerebral Artery, 36215
  Cystourethroscopy
    with Insertion Transprostatic Implant,
      52441-52442
    Ejaculatory Duct, 52010
    Ureteral, 52005
  Dialysis, 49418-49419, 49421
  Dialysis Circuit, 36901-36903
  Electrode Array, 63650
  Extremity Artery, 36140
  Fallopian Tube, 58345, 74742
  Gastrointestinal, 43241
  Hepatic Vein, 37182-37183
  Innominate Artery, 36222-36223, 36225
  Interstitial Radioelement Application
    Breast, 19296-19298
    Genitalia, 55920
    Head, 41019
    Lung, 31643
    Muscle, 20555
    Neck, 41019
    Pelvic Organs, 55920
    Prostate, 55875

Catheterization — *continued*
  Interstitial Radioelement Application — *contin-
    ued*
    Soft Tissue, 20555
  Intracranial Neuroendoscopy, 62160
  Intraperitoneal Tunneled, 49324, 49421
  Jejunum
    for Enteral Therapy, 44015
  Legs, 36245-36248
  Nasotracheal, 31720
  Nasotracheobronchi, 31720
  Newborn
    Umbilical Vein, 36510
  Pelvic Artery, 36245-36248
  Peripheral, 36568-36571
  Placement
    Arterial Coronary Conduit without Left
      Heart Catheterization, 93455
    Coronary Artery without Left Heart
      Catheterization, 93455
    Venous Coronary Bypass Graft without Left
      Heart Catheterization, 93455
  Pleural Cavity, 32550-32552
  Portal Vein, 36481, 37182-37183
  Pulmonary Artery, 36013-36015
  Radioelement Application
    See Interstitial Radioelement Application
  Removal
    Obstructive Material
      Intracatheter, 36596
      Pericatheter, 36595
  Renal Artery, 36251-36254
  Salivary Duct, 42660
  Skull, 61107
  Spinal Cord, 62350, 62351
  Spinal Epidural or Intrathecal, 62350, 62351,
    62360-62362
    Removal, 62355
  Subclavian Artery, 36225
  Thoracic Artery, 36215-36218
  Tracheobronchi, 31725
  Umbilical Artery, 36660
  Umbilical Vein, 36510
  Ureter
    Endoscopic, 50553, 50572, 50953, 50972,
      52005
    Injection, 50684
    Manometric Studies, 50396, 50686
  Uterus, 58340
    Radiology, 58340
  Vena Cava, 36010
  Venous
    Central–Line, 36555, 36556, 36568, 36569,
      36580, 36584
    First Order, 36011
    Intracatheter, 36000
    Needle, 36000
    Organ Blood, 36500
    Second Order, 36012
    Umbilical Vein, 36510
  Ventricular, 61020, 61026, 61210, 61215, 62160-
    62162, 62164, 62225
  Vertebral Artery, 36100, 36221, 36225-36226,
    36228
CAT Scan
  See CT Scan
Cauda Equina
  See Spinal Cord
  Decompression, 63005, 63011-63012, 63017,
    63047-63048, 63056-63057
  Exploration, 63005, 63011, 63017
  Vertebral Corpectomy, 63087-63088
Cauterization
  Anus
    Bleeding Control, 46614
    Destruction of Hemorrhoid(s), 46930
    Fissure, 46940, 46942
    Removal
      Polyp
        Multiple, 46612
        Single, 46610
      Tumor
        Multiple, 46612
        Single, 46610
  Cervix, 57522
    Cryocautery, 57511

Cauterization — *continued*
  Cervix — *continued*
    Electro or Thermal, 57510
    Laser Ablation, 57513
  Chemical
    Corneal Epithelium, 65435-65436
    Granulation Tissue, 17250
  Colon
    Bleeding Control, 45334, 45382
    Removal Tumor, 45333, 45384
  Cornea, 65450
  Ectropion, 67915
  Entropion, 67922
  Esophagus
    Removal Tumor, 43216, 43250
  Everted Punctum, 68705
  Intrarenal Stricture, 52343, 52346
  Iris, 66155
  Lacrimal Punctum Closure, 68760
  Lower Esophageal Sphincter
    Thermal via Endoscopy, 43257
  Nasopharyngeal Hemorrhage, 42970
  Nose
    Hemorrhage, 30901-30906
  Prostate Resection, 52601
  Rectum
    Bleeding Control, 45317
    Removal Polyp
      Multiple, 45315
      Single, 45308
    Removal Tumor, 45308
      Multiple, 45315
      Single, 45308
  Skin Lesion
    Benign, 17000-17004
    Malignant, 17260-17286
    Pre–Malignant, 17000-17004
  Skin Tags, 11200, 11201
  Small Intestine
    Bleeding Control, 44366, 44378, 44391
    Removal Polyp(s), 44366, 44392
    Removal Tumor(s), 44365-44366, 44392
  Turbinate Mucosa, 30801, 30802
  Ureteral Stricture, 52341, 52344
  Ureteropelvic Junction Stricture, 52342, 52345
  Urethral Caruncle, 53265
CAV3, 81404
CAVB, 81650
Cavernitides, Fibrous
  See Peyronie Disease
Cavernosography
  Corpora, 54230
Cavernosometry, 54231
Cavities, Pleural
  See Pleural Cavity
Cavus Foot Correction, 28309
CBC (Complete Blood Count), 85025-85027
CBFB/MYH11, 81401
CBS, 81401, 81406
CcEe Antigens, 81403
CCND1/IGH, 81401
CCR5, 81400
CCU (Critical Care Unit)
  See Critical Care Services
CD142 Antigens, 85250
CD143 Antigens, 82164
CD4, 86360
CD40LG, 81404
CD8, 86360
CDH1, 81406, 81432, 81435
CDH23, 81408, 81430
CDKL5, 81405-81406
CDKN2A, 81404
CEA (Carcinoembryonic Antigen), 82378
C/EBP, 81218
**CEBPA (CCAAT/enhancer binding protein
  [C/EBP], alpha)**, 81218
Cecil Repair, 54318
Cecostomy
  with Colectomy, 44141
  Contrast, 49465
  Laparoscopic, 44188
  Obstructive Material Removal, 49460
  Radiological Evaluation, 49465
  Skin Level, 44320
  Tube Imaging, 49465

Cecostomy — *continued*
  Tube Insertion
    Open, 44300
    Percutaneous, 49442
  Tube Replacement, 49450
CEL, 81403
Celestin Procedure, 43510
Celiac Plexus
  Destruction, 64680
  Injection
    Anesthetic, 64530
    Neurolytic, 64680
Celiac Trunk Artery
  See Artery, Celiac
Celioscopy
  See Endoscopy, Peritoneum
Celiotomy, 49000
  Abdomen
    for Staging, 49220
Cell
  Blood
    See Blood Cell
    Count
      Bacterial Colony, 87086
      B Cells, 86355
      Body Fluid, 89050, 89051
      CD34, 86367
      CD4, 86360-86361
      CD8, 86360
      Natural Killer (NK), 86357
      Sperm, 89310, 89320, 89322
      Stem, 86367
      T Cells, 86359-86361
  Islet
    Antibody, 86341
  Mother
    See Stem Cell
  Stimulating Hormone, Interstitial
    See Luteinizing Hormone (LH)
Cellobiase, 82963
Cellular Function Assay, 86352
Cellular Inclusion
  See Inclusion Bodies
Central Shunt, 33764
Central Sleep Apnea
  Neurostimulator System, 0424T-0436T
Central Venous Catheter (CVC)
  Insertion
    Central, 36555-36558
    Non-tunneled, 36555-36556
    Peripheral, 36568, 36569
      with Port, 36570-36571
    Tunneled
      with Port, 36560-36561, 36566
      with Pump, 36563
      without Port or Pump, 36557-36558,
        36565
  Removal, 36589
  Repair, 36575-36576
  Replacement, 36580-36585
    Catheter Only, 36578
  Repositioning, 36597
Central Venous Catheter Removal, 36589
CEP290, 81408
Cephalic Version
  Anesthesia, 01958
  of Fetus
    External, 59412
Cephalocele
  See Encephalocele
Cephalogram, Orthodontic
  See Orthodontic Cephalogram
Cerclage
  Cervix, 57700
    Abdominal Approach, 59325
    Removal under Anesthesia, 59871
    Vaginal Approach, 59320
  McDonald, 57700
Cerebellopontine Angle Tumor
  Excision, 61510, 61518, 61520, 61521, 61526,
    61530, 61545
Cerebral Cortex Decortication
  See Decortication
Cerebral Death, 95824
Cerebral Hernia
  See Encephalocele

Index

Catheterization — Cerebral Hernia

Cerebral Perfusion Analysis, 0042T
Cerebral Ventriculographies
  See Ventriculography
Cerebral Vessel(s)
  Anastomosis, 61711
  Aneurysm
    Carotid Artery Occlusion, 61705, 61708, 61710
    Cervical Approach, 61703
    Intracranial Approach, 61697-61698, 61700, 61702
  Angioplasty, 61630
  Arteriovenous Malformation
    Dural, 61690, 61692
    Fistula, 61705, 61708
    Infratentorial, 61684, 61686
    Supratentorial, 61680, 61682
  Dilation
    Intracranial Vasospasm, 61640-61642
  Placement
    Stent, 61635
  Occlusion, 61623
  Stent Placement, 61635
  Thrombolysis, 37195
Cerebrose
  See Galactose
Cerebrospinal Fluid, 86325
  Drainage, Spinal Puncture, 62272
  Laboratory Tests
    Cell Count, 89050
    Immunoelectrophoresis, 86325
    Myelin Basic Protein, 83873
    Protein, Total, 84157
  Nuclear Imaging, 78630-78650
Cerebrospinal Fluid Leak
  Brain
    Repair, 61618, 61619, 62100
  Nasal
    Sinus Endoscopy Repair, 31290, 31291
  Spinal Cord
    Repair, 63707, 63709
Cerebrospinal Fluid Shunt, 63740-63746
  Creation, 62180-62192, 62200-62223
    Lumbar, 63740-63741
  Irrigation, 62194, 62225
  Removal, 62256, 62258, 63746
  Replacement, 62160, 62258, 63744
    Catheter, 62194, 62225, 62230
    Valve, 62230
  Reprogramming, 62252
  Torkildsen Operation, 62180
  Ventriculocisternostomy, 62180, 62200-62201
Ceruloplasmin, 82390
Cerumen
  Removal, 69209-69210
Cervical Canal
  Instrumental Dilation of, 57800
Cervical Cap, 57170
Cervical Cerclage
  Abdominal Approach, 59325
  Removal under Anesthesia, 59871
  Vaginal Approach, 59320
Cervical Lymphadenectomy, 38720, 38724
Cervical Mucus Penetration Test, 89330
Cervical Plexus
  Injection
    Anesthetic, 64413
Cervical Pregnancy, 59140
Cervical Puncture, 61050, 61055
Cervical Smears, 88141, 88155, 88164-88167, 88174-88175
  See Cytopathology
Cervical Spine
  See Vertebra, Cervical
Cervical Stump
  Dilation and Curettage of, 57558
Cervical Sympathectomy
  See Sympathectomy, Cervical
Cervicectomy
  Amputation Cervix, 57530
  Pelvic Exenteration, 45126, 58240
Cervicoplasty, 15819
Cervicothoracic Ganglia
  See Stellate Ganglion
Cervix
  See Cytopathology

Cervix — *continued*
  Amputation
    Total, 57530
  Biopsy, 57500, 57520
    Colposcopy, 57454, 57455, 57460
  Cauterization, 57522
    Cryocautery, 57511
    Electro or Thermal, 57510
    Laser Ablation, 57513
  Cerclage, 57700
    Abdominal, 59325
    Removal under Anesthesia, 59871
    Vaginal, 59320
  Colposcopy, 57452-57461
  Conization, 57461, 57520, 57522
  Curettage
    Endocervical, 57454, 57456, 57505
  Dilation
    Canal, 57800
    Stump, 57558
  Dilation and Curettage, 57520, 57558
  Ectopic Pregnancy, 59140
  Excision
    Electrode, 57460
    Radical, 57531
    Stump
      Abdominal Approach, 57540, 57545
      Vaginal Approach, 57550-57556
    Total, 57530
  Exploration
    Endoscopy, 57452
  Insertion
    Dilation, 59200
    Laminaria, 59200
    Prostaglandin, 59200
  Repair
    Cerclage, 57700
      Abdominal, 59325
      Vaginal, 59320
    Suture, 57720
  Stump, 57558
  Suture, 57720
  Unlisted Services and Procedures, 58999
Cesarean Delivery
  with Hysterectomy, 59525
  Antepartum Care, 59610, 59618
  Delivery
    After Attempted Vaginal Delivery, 59618
      Delivery Only, 59620
      Postpartum Care, 59622
      Routine Care, 59618
    Routine Care, 59610
  Delivery Only, 59514
  Postpartum Care, 59515
  Routine Care, 59510
  Tubal Ligation at Time of, 58611
  Vaginal after Prior Cesarean
    Delivery and Postpartum Care, 59614
    Delivery Only, 59612
    Routine Care, 59610
CFH/ARMS2, 81401
CFTR, 81220-81224, 81412
CGM (Continuous Glucose Monitoring System), 95250-95251
Chalazion
  Excision, 67800-67808
    Multiple
      Different Lids, 67805
      Same Lids, 67801
    Single, 67800
    Under Anesthesia, 67808
Challenge Tests
  Bronchial Inhalation, 95070-95071
  Cholinesterase Inhibitor, 95857
  Ingestion, 95076, 95079
Chambers Procedure, 28300
Change
  Catheter
    Percutaneous with Contrast, 75984
  Fetal Position
    by Manipulation, 59412
  Stent
    (Endoscopic), Bile or Pancreatic Duct, *[43275, 43276]*
    Ureteral, 50688

Change — *continued*
  Tube
    Gastrostomy, 43760
    Percutaneous, with Contrast Monitoring, 75984
    Tracheotomy, 31502
    Ureterostomy, 50688
Change, Gastrostomy Tube
  See Gastrostomy Tube, Change of
Change of, Dressing
  See Dressings, Change
CHCT (Caffeine Halothane Contracture Test), 89049
CHD7, 81407
Cheek
  Bone
    Excision, 21030, 21034
    Fracture
      Closed Treatment with Manipulation, 21355
      Open Treatment, 21360-21366
      Reconstruction, 21270
  Fascia Graft, 15840
  Muscle Graft, 15841-15845
  Muscle Transfer, 15845
  Rhytidectomy, 15828
  Skin Graft
    Delay of Flap, 15620
    Full Thickness, 15240, 15241
    Pedicle Flap, 15574
    Split, 15120-15121
  Tissue Transfer, Adjacent, 14040, 14041
  Wound Repair, 13131-13133
Cheekbone
  Fracture
    Closed Treatment Manipulation, 21355
    Open Treatment, 21360-21366
    Reconstruction, 21270
Cheilectomy
  Metatarsophalangeal Joint Release, 28289, 28291
Cheiloplasty
  See Lip, Repair
Cheiloschisis
  See Cleft, Lip
Cheilotomy
  See Incision, Lip
Chemical
  Cauterization
    Corneal Epithelium, 65435-65436
    Granulation Tissue, 17250
  Exfoliation, 15788-15793, 17360
  Peel, 15788-15793, 17360
Chemiluminescent Assay, 82397
Chemistry Tests
  Organ or Disease Oriented Panel
    Electrolyte, 80051
    General Health Panel, 80050
    Hepatic Function Panel, 80076
    Hepatitis Panel, Acute, 80074
    Lipid Panel, 80061
    Metabolic
      Basic, 80047-80048
      Calcium
        Ionized, 80047
        Total, 80048
      Comprehensive, 80053
    Obstetric Panel, 80055, *[80081]*
  Unlisted Services and Procedures, 84999
Chemocauterization
  Corneal Epithelium, 65435
    with Chelating Agent, 65436
Chemodenervation
  Anal Sphincter, 46505
  Bladder, 52287
  Eccrine Glands, 64650, 64653
  Electrical Stimulation for Guidance, 64617, 95873
  Extraocular Muscle, 67345
  Extremity Muscle, 64642-64645
  Facial Muscle, 64612, 64615
  Gland
    Eccrine, 64650, 64653
    Parotid, 64611
    Salivary, 64611
    Submandibular, 64611

Chemodenervation — *continued*
  Internal Anal Sphincter, 46505
  Larynx, 64617
  Muscle
    Extraocular, 67345
    Extremity, 64642-64645
    Facial, 64612
    Larynx, 64617
    Neck, 64616
    Trunk, 64646-64647
  Neck Muscle, 64615-64616
  Needle Electromyography Guidance, 95874
  Salivary Glands, 64611
  Trunk Muscle, 64646-64647
Chemonucleolysis, 62292
Chemosurgery
  Destruction
    Benign Lesion, 17110-17111
    Malignant Lesion, 17260-17266, 17270-17286
    Premalignant Lesion, 17000-17004
  Mohs Technique, 17311-17315
Chemotaxis Assay, 86155
Chemotherapy
  Arterial Catheterization, 36640
  Bladder Instillation, 51720
  Brain, 61517
  Cannulation, 36823
  Central Nervous System, 61517, 96450
  Extracorporeal Circulation Membrane Oxygenation
    Isolated with Chemotherapy Perfusion, 36823
  Home Infusion Procedures, 99601, 99602
  Intra–Arterial
    Cannulation, 36823
    Catheterization, 36640
    Infusion, 96422-96423, 96425
    Infusion Pump Insertion, 36260
    Push Technique, 96420
  Intralesional, 96405, 96406
  Intramuscular, 96401-96402
  Intravenous, 96409-96417
  Kidney Instillation, 50391
  Peritoneal Cavity, 96446
    Catheterization, 49418
  Pleural Cavity, 96440
  Pump Services
    Implantable, 96522
    Initiation, 96416
    Maintenance, 95990-95991, 96521-96522
    Portable, 96521
  Reservoir Filling, 96542
  Subcutaneous, 96401-96402
  Unlisted Services and Procedures, 96549
  Ureteral Instillation, 50391
Chest
  See Mediastinum; Thorax
  Angiography, 71275
  Artery
    Ligation, 37616
  Cavity
    Bypass Graft, 35905
    Thoracoscopy
      Exploration, 32601-32606
      Surgical, 32650-32665
      Therapeutic, 32654-32665
  CT Scan, 71250-71275
  Diagnostic Imaging
    Angiography, 71275
    CT, 71250, 71260, 71270
    CT Angiography, 71275
    Magnetic Resonance Angiography, 71555
    Magnetic Resonance Imaging (MRI), 71550-71552
    PET, 78811, 78814
    Ultrasound, 76604
  Exploration
    Blood Vessel, 35820
    Penetrating Wound, 20101
    Postoperative
      Hemorrhage, 35820
      Infection, 35820
      Thrombosis, 35820
  Flail, 21899

Chest — *continued*
Funnel
Anesthesia, 00474
Reconstructive Repair, 21740-21742
with Thoracoscopy, 21743
Magnetic Resonance Imaging (MRI), 71550-71552
Repair
Blood Vessel, 35211, 35216
with Other Graft, 35271, 35276
with Vein Graft, 35241, 35246
Tube, 32551
Ultrasound, 76604
Wound Exploration
Penetrating, 20101
X-ray, 71010-71035
with Computer-aided Detection, 0174T-0175T
Complete (four views) with Fluoroscopy, 71034
Partial (two views) with Fluoroscopy, 71023
Stereo, 71015
Chest Wall
Debridement, 11044, 11047
Manipulation, 94667-94669
Mechanical Oscillation, 94669
Reconstruction, 49904
Lung Tumor Resection, 32504
Trauma, 32820
Repair, 32905
Closure, 32810
Fistula, 32906
Lung Hernia, 32800
Resection, 32503
Tumor
Ablation, 32998
Excision, 19260-19272
Unlisted Services and Procedures, 32999
Chiari Osteotomy of the Pelvis
See Osteotomy, Pelvis
Chicken Pox (Varicella)
Immunization, 90716
Child Procedure, 48146
See also Excision, Pancreas, Partial
Chimerism (Engraftment) Analysis, 81267-81268
Chin
Cartilage Graft, 21230
Repair
Augmentation, 21120
Osteotomy, 21121-21123
Rhytidectomy, 15828
Skin Graft
Delay of Flap, 15620
Full Thickness, 15240, 15241
Pedicle Flap, 15574
Split, 15120-15121
Tissue Transfer, Adjacent, 14040, 14041
Wound Repair, 13131-13133
Chinidin, 80194
Chiropractic Manipulation
See Manipulation, Chiropractic
Chiropractic Treatment
Spinal
Extraspinal, 98940-98943
Chlamydia
Antibody, 86631, 86632
Antigen Detection
Direct
Optical Observation, 87810
Direct Fluorescent, 87270
Enzyme Immunoassay, 87320
Immunofluorescence, 87270
Nucleic Acid, 87485-87492
Culture, 87110
Chloramphenicol, 82415
Chlorhydrocarbon, 82441
Chloride
Blood, 82435
Other Source, 82438
Panels
Basic Metabolic, 80047-80048
Comprehensive Metabolic, 80053
Electrolyte, 80051
Renal Function, 80069
Spinal Fluid, 82438
Urine, 82436

Chloride, Methylene
See Dichloromethane
Chlorinated Hydrocarbons, 82441
Chlorohydrocarbon, 82441
Chlorpromazine, [80342, 80343, 80344]
Choanal Atresia
Repair, 30540, 30545
CHOL, 82465, 83718-83721
Cholangiogram
Intravenous, 76499
Cholangiography
with Cholecystectomy, 47563, 47605
Injection, 47531-47533
Intraoperative, 74300, 74301
Repair
with Bile Duct Exploration, 47700
with Cholecystectomy, 47620
Cholangiopancreatography
with Ablation, [43278]
with Biopsy, 43261
with Optical Endomicroscopy, 0397T
with Surgery, 43262-43265 [43274, 43275, 43276]
See Bile Duct, Pancreatic Duct
Destruction of Calculus, 43264-43265
Diagnostic, 43260
Exchange Stent, [43276]
Intraoperative, 74300-74301
Papillotomy, 43262
Pressure Measurement Sphincter of Oddi, 43263
Removal
Calculus, 43264-43265
Foreign Body, [43275, 43276]
Stent, [43275, 43276]
Specimen Collection, 43260
Sphincterotomy, 43262, 43266-43270 [43276, 43277], [43274]
Stent Placement, [43274]
Cholangiostomy
See Hepaticostomy
Cholangiotomy
See Hepaticostomy
Cholecalciferol
Blood Serum Level 25 Hydroxy, 82306
I, 25 Dyhydroxy, [82652]
Cholecystectomy
Donor Liver Preparation, 47143
Laparoscopic, 47562-47570
with Cholangiography, 47563
with Exploration Common Duct, 47564
Open Approach, 47600-47620
with Cholangiography, 47605, 47620
with Choledochoenterostomy, 47612
with Exploration Common Duct, 47610
Cholecystenterostomy
with Gastroenterostomy, 47721, 47741
Direct, 47720
Laparoscopic, 47570
Roux-en-Y, 47740-47741
Cholecystography, 74290
Cholecystostomy
with Placement Peripancreatic Drains, 48000
Open, 47480
Percutaneous, 47490
Cholecystotomy
with Choledochostomy, 47420
with Choledochotomy, 47420
Open, 47480
Percutaneous, 47490
Choledochoplasty
See Bile Duct, Repair
Choledochoscopy, 47550
Choledochostomy, 47420, 47425
Choledochotomy, 47420, 47425
Choledochus, Cyst
See Cyst, Choledochal
Cholera Vaccine
Injectable, Live Adult, [90625]
Cholesterol
Lipid Panel, 80061
Measurement
HDL, 83718
LDL, 83721
VLDL, 83719
Serum, 82465

Cholesterol — *continued*
Testing, 83718-83721
Choline Esterase I, 82013
Choline Esterase II, 82480, 82482
Cholinesterase
Blood, 82480, 82482
Cholinesterase Inhibitor Challenge Test, 95857
Cholylglycine
Blood, 82240
Chondroitin Sulfate, 82485
Chondromalacia Patella
Repair, 27418
Chondropathia Patellae
See Chondromalacia Patella
Chondroplasty, 29877, 29879
Chondrosteoma
See Exostosis
Chopart Procedure, 28800
Amputation, Foot, 28800, 28805
Chordotomies
See Cordotomy
Chorioangioma
See Lesion, Skin
Choriogonadotropin, 80414, 84702-84703
Stimulation, 80414-80415
Choriomeningitides, Lymphocytic, 86727
Chorionic Gonadotropin, 80414, 84702-84704
Stimulation, 80414, 80415
Chorionic Growth Hormone, 83632
Chorionic Tumor
See Hydatidiform Mole
Chorionic Villi, 59015
Chorionic Villus
Biopsy, 59015
Choroid
Aspiration, 67015
Destruction
Lesion, 67220-67225
Removal Neovascularization, 67043
Choroidopathy, 67208-67218
Choroid Plexus
Excision, 61544
Christmas Factor, 85250
CHRNA4, 81405
CHRNB2, 81405
Chromaffinoma, Medullary
See Pheochromocytoma
Chromatin, Sex
See Barr Bodies
Chromatography
Column
Mass Spectrometry, 82542
Drug Test, 80307
Gas–Liquid or HPLC
Typing, 87143
Hemoglobin, 83021, 83036
Sugars, 84375
Chromium, 82495
Chromogenic Substrate Assay, 85130
Chromosome 18q-, 81402
Chromosome 1p-/19q-, 81402
Chromosome Analysis
Added Study, 88280-88289
Amniotic Fluid, 88267, 88269
Culture, 88235
Biopsy Culture
Tissue, 88233
Bone Marrow Culture, 88237
Chorionic Villus, 88267
5 Cells, 88261
15–20 Cells, 88262
20–25 Cells, 88264
45 Cells, 88263
Culture, 88235
Cytogenomic Constitutional Microarray, 81228-81229
for Breakage Syndromes, 88245-88249
Ataxia Telangiectasia, 88248
Clastogen Stress, 88249
Fragile-X, 88248
Franconi Anemia, 88248
Fragile–X, 88248
In Situ Hybridization, 88272-88273
Lymphocyte Culture, 88230
Molecular Pathology, Level 5, 81404
Pregnancy Associated Plasma Protein A, 84163

Chromosome Analysis — *continued*
Skin Culture
Tissue, 88233
Tissue Culture, 88239
Amniotic Fluid Cells, 88325
Blood Cells, 88237
Bone Marrow Cells, 88237
Chorionic Villus Cells, 88235
Skin, 88233
Tumor, 88239
Unlisted Cytogenic Study, 88299
Unlisted Services and Procedures, 88299
Chromotubation
Oviduct, 58350
Chronic Erection
See Priapism
Chronic Interstitial Cystitides
See Cystitis, Interstitial
Ciliary Body
Cyst
Destruction
Cryotherapy, 66720
Cyclodialysis, 66740
Cyclophotocoagulation, 66710-66711
Diathermy, 66700
Nonexcisional, 66770
Destruction
Cyclophotcoagulation, 66710, 66711
Cyst or Lesion, 66770
Endoscopic, 66711
Lesion
Destruction, 66770
Repair, 66680
Cimino Type Procedure, 36821
Cinefluorographies
See Cineradiography
Cineplasty
Arm, Lower, 24940
Arm, Upper, 24940
Cineradiography
Esophagus, 74230
Pharynx, 70371, 74230
Speech Evaluation, 70371
Swallowing Evaluation, 74230
Unlisted Services and Procedures, 76120, 76125
Circulation Assist
Aortic, 33967, 33970
Counterpulsation
Ventricular, 0451T-0463T
Balloon Counterpulsation, 33967, 33970
Removal, 33971
Cardioassist Method
External, 92971
Internal, 92970
External, 33946-33949
Ventricular Assist
Aortic Counterpulsation, 0451T-0463T
Circulation, Extracorporeal
See Extracorporeal Circulation
Circulatory Assist
Aortic, 33967, 33970
Balloon, 33967, 33970
External, 33946-33949
Circumcision
with Clamp or Other Device, 54150
Adhesions, 54162
Incomplete, 54163
Repair, 54163
Surgical Excision
28 days or less, 54160
Older than 28 days, 54161
Cisternal Puncture, 61050, 61055
Cisternography, 70015
Nuclear, 78630
Citrate
Blood or Urine, 82507
CK, 82550-82554
Total, 82550
Cl, 82435-82438
Clagett Procedure
Chest Wall, Repair, Closure, 32810
Clavicle
Arthrocentesis, 20605
Arthrotomy
Acromioclavicular Joint, 23044, 23101
Sternoclavicular Joint, 23044, 23101, 23106

Clavicle — *continued*
Claviculectomy
Arthroscopic, 29824
Partial, 23120
Total, 23125
Craterization, 23180
Cyst
Excision, 23140
with Allograft, 23146
with Autograft, 23145
Diaphysectomy, 23180
Dislocation
without Manipulation, 23540
Acromioclavicular Joint
Closed Treatment, 23540, 23545
Open Treatment, 23550, 23552
Sternoclavicular Joint
Closed Treatment, 23520, 23525
Open Treatment, 23530, 23532
Excision, 23170
Partial, 23120, 23180
Total, 23125
Fracture
Closed Treatment
with Manipulation, 23505
without Manipulation, 23500
Open Treatment, 23515
Osteotomy, 23480
with Bone Graft, 23485
Pinning, Wiring, Etc., 23490
Prophylactic Treatment, 23490
Repair Osteotomy, 23480, 23485
Saucerization, 23180
Sequestrectomy, 23170
Tumor
Excision, 23140, 23146, 23200
with Allograft, 23146
with Autograft, 23145
Radical Resection, 23200
X–ray, 73000
Clavicula
See Clavicle
Claviculectomy
Arthroscopic, 29824
Partial, 23120
Total, 23125
Claw Finger Repair, 26499
Clayton Procedure, 28114
CLCN1, 81406
CLCNKB, 81406
Cleft, Branchial
See Branchial Cleft
Cleft Cyst, Branchial
See Branchial Cleft, Cyst
Cleft Foot
Reconstruction, 28360
Cleft Hand
Repair, 26580
Cleft Lip
Repair, 40700-40761
Rhinoplasty, 30460, 30462
Cleft Palate
Repair, 42200-42225
Rhinoplasty, 30460, 30462
Clinical Act of Insertion
See Insertion
Clitoroplasty
for Intersex State, 56805
Closed [Transurethral] Biopsy of Bladder
See Biopsy, Bladder , Cystourethroscopy
Clostridial Tetanus
See Tetanus
Clostridium Botulinum Toxin
See Chemodenervation
Clostridium Difficile Toxin
Amplified Probe Technique, 87493
Antigen Detection
Enzyme Immunoassay, 87324
by Immunoassay
with Direct Optical Observation, 87803
Tissue Culture, 87230
Clostridium Tetani ab
See Antibody, Tetanus
Closure
Anal Fistula, 46288
Appendiceal Fistula, 44799

Closure — *continued*
Atrial Appendage
with Implant, 33340
Atrial Septal Defect, 33641, 33647
Atrioventricular Valve, 33600
Cardiac Valve, 33600, 33602
Cystostomy, 51880
Diaphragm
Fistula, 39599
Enterostomy, 44620-44626
Laparoscopic, 44227
Esophagostomy, 43420-43425
Fistula
Anal, 46288, 46706
Anorectal, 46707
Bronchi, 32815
Carotid-Cavernous, 61710
Chest Wall, 32906
Enterovesical, 44660-44661
Ileoanal Pouch, 46710-46712
Kidney, 50520-50526
Lacrimal, 68770
Nose, 30580-30600
Oval Window, 69666
Rectovaginal, 57305-57308
Tracheoesophageal, 43305, 43312, 43314
Ureter, 50920-50930
Urethra, 53400-53405
Urethrovaginal, 57310-57311
Vesicouterine, 51920-51925
Vesicovaginal, 51900, 57320, 57330
Gastrostomy, 43870
Lacrimal Fistula, 68770
Lacrimal Punctum
Plug, 68761
Thermocauterization, Ligation, or Laser
Surgery, 68760
Meningocele, 63700-63702
Patent Ductus Arteriosus, 93582
Rectovaginal Fistula, 57300-57308
Semilunar Valve, 33602
Septal Defect, 33615
Ventricular, 33675-33677, 33681-33688,
93581
Skin
Abdomen
Complex, 13100-13102
Intermediate, 12031-12037
Layered, 12031-12037
Simple, 12001-12007
Superficial, 12001-12007
Arm, Arms
Complex, 13120-13122
Intermediate, 12031-12037
Layered, 12031-12037
Simple, 12001-12007
Superficial, 12001-12007
Axilla, Axillae
Complex, 13131-13133
Intermediate, 12031-12037
Layered, 12031-12037
Simple, 12001-12007
Superficial, 12001-12007
Back
Complex, 13100-13102
Intermediate, 12031-12037
Layered, 12031-12037
Simple, 12001-12007
Superficial, 12001-12007
Breast
Complex, 13100-13102
Intermediate, 12031-12037
Layered, 12031-12037
Simple, 12001-12007
Superficial, 12001-12007
Buttock
Complex, 13100-13102
Intermediate, 12031-12037
Layered, 12031-12037
Simple, 12001-12007
Superficial, 12001-12007
Cheek, Cheeks
Complex, 13131-13133
Intermediate, 12051-12057
Layered, 12051-12057
Simple, 12011-12018

Closure — *continued*
Skin — *continued*
Cheek, Cheeks — *continued*
Superficial, 12011-12018
Chest
Complex, 13100-13102
Intermediate, 12031-12037
Layered, 12031-12037
Simple, 12001-12007
Superficial, 12001-12007
Chin
Complex, 13131-13133
Intermediate, 12051-12057
Layered, 12051-12057
Simple, 12011-12018
Superficial, 12011-12018
Ear, Ears
Complex, 13151-13153
Intermediate, 12051-12057
Layered, 12051-12057
2.5 cm or less, 12051
Simple, 12011-12018
Superficial, 12011-12018
External
Genitalia
Intermediate, 12041-12047
Layered, 12041-12047
Simple, 12001-12007
Superficial, 12001-12007
Extremity, Extremities
Intermediate, 12031-12037
Layered, 12031-12037
Simple, 12001-12007
Superficial, 12001-12007
Eyelid, Eyelids
Complex, 13151-13153
Intermediate, 12051-12057
Layered, 12051-12057
Simple, 12011-12018
Superficial, 12011-12018
Face
Complex, 13131-13133
Intermediate, 12051-12057
Layered, 12051-12057
Simple, 12011-12018
Superficial, 12011-12018
Feet
Complex, 13131-13133
Intermediate, 12041-12047
Layered, 12041-12047
Simple, 12001-12007
Superficial, 12001-12007
Finger, Fingers
Complex, 13131-13133
Intermediate, 12041-12047
Layered, 12041-12047
Simple, 12001-12007
Superficial, 12001-12007
Foot
Complex, 13131-13133
Intermediate, 12041-12047
Layered, 12041-12047
Simple, 12001-12007
Superficial, 12001-12007
Forearm, Forearms
Complex, 13120-13122
Intermediate, 12031-12037
Layered, 12031-12037
Simple, 12001-12007
Superficial, 12001-12007
Forehead
Complex, 13131-13133
Intermediate, 12051-12057
Layered, 12051-12057
Simple, 12011-12018
Superficial, 12011-12018
Genitalia
Complex, 13131-13133
External
Intermediate, 12041-12047
Layered, 12041-12047
Simple, 12001-12007
Superficial, 12001-12007
Hand, Hands
Complex, 13131-13133
Intermediate, 12041-12047

Closure — *continued*
Skin — *continued*
Hand, Hands — *continued*
Layered, 12041-12047
Simple, 12001-12007
Superficial, 12001-12007
Leg, Legs
Complex, 13120-13122
Intermediate, 12031-12037
Layered, 12031-12037
Simple, 12001-12007
Superficial, 12001-12007
Lip, Lips
Complex, 13151-13153
Intermediate, 12051-12057
Layered, 12051-12057
Simple, 12011-12018
Superficial, 12011-12018
Lower
Arm, Arms
Complex, 13120-13122
Intermediate, 12031-12037
Layered, 12031-12037
Simple, 12001-12007
Superficial, 12001-12007
Extremity, Extremities
Intermediate, 12031-12037
Layered, 12031-12037
Simple, 12001-12007
Superficial, 12001-12007
Leg, Legs
Complex, 13120-13122
Intermediate, 12031-12037
Layered, 12031-12037
Simple, 12001-12007
Superficial, 12001-12007
Mouth
Complex, 13131-13133
Mucous Membrane, Mucous Membranes
Intermediate, 12051-12057
Layered, 12051-12057
Simple, 12011-12018
Superficial, 12011-12018
Neck
Complex, 13131-13133
Intermediate, 12041-12047
Layered, 12041-12047
Simple, 12001-12007
Superficial, 12001-12007
Nose
Complex, 13151-13153
Intermediate, 12051-12057
Layered, 12051-12057
Simple, 12011-12018
Superficial, 12011-12018
Palm, Palms
Complex, 13131-13133
Intermediate, 12041-12047
Layered, 12041-12047
Simple, 12001-12007
Superficial, 12001-12007
Scalp
Complex, 13120-13122
Intermediate, 12031-12037
Layered, 12031-12037
Simple, 12001-12007
Superficial, 12001-12007
Toe, Toes
Complex, 13131-13133
Intermediate, 12041-12047
Layered, 12041-12047
Simple, 12001-12007
Superficial, 12001-12007
Trunk
Complex, 13100-13102
Intermediate, 12031-12037
Layered, 12031-12037
Simple, 12001-12007
Superficial, 12001-12007
Upper
Arm, Arms
Complex, 13120-13122
Intermediate, 12031-12037
Layered, 12031-12037
Simple, 12001-12007
Superficial, 12001-12007

Closure — *continued*
  Skin — *continued*
    Upper — *continued*
      Extremity
        Intermediate, 12031-12037
        Layered, 12031-12037
        Simple, 12001-12007
        Superficial, 12001-12007
      Leg, Legs
        Complex, 13120-13122
        Intermediate, 12031-12037
        Layered, 12031-12037
        Simple, 12001-12007
        Superficial, 12001-12007
  Sternotomy, 21750
  Vagina, 57120
  Ventricular Septal Defect, 33675-33677, 33681-33688, 93581
  Ventricular Tunnel, 33722
Clot, 34001-34490, 35875, 35876, 50230
  Lysis Time, 85175
  Retraction, 85170
Clot Lysis Time
  Euglobin Lysis, 85360
  Whole Blood Dilution, 85175
Clotting, 85210-85293
  Disorder, 85390
  Factor, 85210-85293
    Factor II (Prothrombin), 85210
    Factor III (Thromboplastin) Inhibition, 85705
    Factor IX (Christmas Factor), 85250
    Factor VII, 85230
    Factor VIII
      AHG, 85240
      Related Antigen, 85244
      von Willebrand Factor, 85247
      VW Factor, 85245-85246
    Factor X (Thrombokinase), 85260
    Factor X (Stuart-Prower), 85260
    Factor XI, 85270
    Factor XII (Hageman Factor), 85280
    Factor XIII (Fibrin Stabilizing), 85290-85291
    Fitzgerald Factor Assay, 85293
    Fletcher Factor Assay, 85292
    High Molecular Weight Kininogen Assay, 85293
    Inhibition Test, 85347
    Partial Time, 85730-85732
    Plasma Thromboplastin Antecedent (TPA), 85270
    Prekallikrein Assay, 85292
  Inhibitors, 85300-85305, 85307
  Test
    Antithrombin III, 85300-85301
    Factor Inhibitor, 85335
    Mixed Screen, 85611, 85732
    Protein C, 85302-85303, 85307
    Protein S, 85305-85306
    Thrombomodulin, 85337
    Thromboplastin Inhibition, 85705
  Time, 85345-85348
Cloverleaf Skull
  Suture of, 61558
Clozapine
  Assay, 80159
CLRN1, 81400, 81404, 81430
Clubfoot Cast, 29450
  Wedging, 29750
CMG (Cystometrogram), 51725-51729
CMRI (Cardiac Magnetic Resonance Imaging)
  with Contrast, 75561-75563
  without Contrast, 75557-75559
  for Morphology and Function, 75557-75563
  Velocity Flow Mapping, 75565
CMV (Cytomegalovirus)
  Antibody, 86644, 86645
  Antigen Detection
    Enzyme Immunoassay, 87332
    Nucleic Acid, 87495-87497
CNBP, 81401
CNP, 94662
CNPB (Continuous Negative Pressure Breathing), 94662
CNTNAP2, 81406

CO₂
  See Carbon Dioxide
Coagulation
  Defect, 85390
    Assay, 85130
  Factor I, 85384, 85385
  Factor II, 85210
  Factor III, 85730, 85732
  Factor II, Prothrombin Gene Analysis, 81240
  Factor IV, 82310
  Factor IX, 85250
  Factor V, 85220
  Factor V Gene Analysis, 81241
  Factor VII, 85230
  Factor VIII, 85244, 85247
  Factor X, 85260
  Factor XI, 85270
  Factor XII, 85280
  Factor XIII, 85290, 85291
  Fibrinolysis, 85396-85397
  Time, 85345-85348
  Unlisted Services and Procedures, 85999
Coagulin
  See Thromboplastin
Coagulopathy, 85390
  Assay, 85130
Cocaine, [80305, 80306, 80307], [80353]
Coccidioides
  Antibody, 86635
Coccidioidin Test
  Streptokinase, Antibody, 86590
Coccidioidomycosis
  Skin Test, 86490
Coccygeal Spine Fracture
  See Coccyx, Fracture
Coccygectomy, 15920, 15922, 27080
Coccyx
  Excision, 27080
  Fracture
    Closed Treatment, 27200
    Open Treatment, 27202
  Pressure Ulcer, 15920, 15922
  Tumor
    Excision, 49215
  X–ray, 72220
Cochlear Device
  Analysis, 92601-92604
  Implantation Osseointegrated Implant, 69714-69715
    Replace Osseointegrated Implant, 69717-69718
  Insertion, 69930
  Programming, 92601-92604
Codeine Screen, [80305, 80306, 80307], [80361, 80362]
Co–Factor I, Heparin
  See Antithrombin III
Cofactor Protein S
  See Protein S
Coffey Operation
  Uterus, Repair, Suspension, 58400
    with Presacral Sympathectomy, 58410
Cognitive Function Tests, 96116, 96125
  See Neurology, Diagnostic
Cognitive Skills Development, 97532
  See Physical Medicine/Therapy/Occupational Therapy
COHB, 82375-82376
COL1A1, 81408
COL1A1/PDGFB, 81402
COL1A2, 81408
COL3A1, 81410-81411
COL4A1, 81408
COL4A3, 81408
COL4A4, 81407
COL4A5, 81408
COL6A2, 81406-81407
COL6A3, 81407
Cold Agglutinin, 86156, 86157
Cold Pack Treatment, 97010
Cold Preservation
  See Cryopreservation
Cold Therapies
  See Cryotherapy
Colectomy
  Miles', 44155

Colectomy — *continued*
  Partial, 44140
    with Anastomosis, 44140
      Laparoscopic, 44213
    with Coloproctostomy, 44145-44146
    with Colostomy, 44141-44144
      Laparoscopic, 44205
    with Ileocolostomy, Laparoscopic, 44205
    with Ileostomy, 44144
    with Mobilization Splenic Flexure, 44139
      Laparoscopic, 44213
    with Removal Ileum, 44160
    Transanal Approach, 44147
  Total
    without Proctectomy, 44210
    Laparoscopic
      Proctectomy and Ileostomy, 44211, 44212
      wthout Proctectomy, 44210
    Open
      with
        Complete Proctectomy, 45121
        Ileal Reservoir, 44211
        Ileoanal Anastomosis, 44211
        Ileoproctostomy, 44150, 44210
        Ileostomy, 44150-44151, 44210-44212
        Proctectomy, 44155-44158, 44211-44212
        Rectal Mucosectomy, 44211
Collagen Cross Links, 82523
Collagen Injection, 11950-11954
Collar Bone
  Craterization, 23180
  Cyst
    Excision, 23140
      with
        Allograft, 23146
        Autograft, 23145
  Diaphysectomy, 23180
  Dislocation
    with Manipulation, 23540
    Acromioclavicular Joint
      Closed Treatment, 23540, 23545
      Open Treatment, 23550, 23552
    Sternoclavicular Joint
      Closed Treatment, 23520, 23525
      Open Treatment, 23530, 23532
  Excision
    Partial, 23120, 23180
    Total, 23125
  Fracture
    Closed Treatment
      with Manipulation, 23505
      without Manipulation, 23500
    Open Treatment, 23515
  Osteotomy, 23480, 23485
  Pinning, Wiring, Etc., 23490
  Prophylactic Treatment, 23490
  Repair Osteotomy, 23480, 23485
  Saucerization, 23180
  Sequestrectomy, 23170
  Tumor
    Excision, 23140
      with Allograft, 23146
      with Autograft, 23145
    Radical Resection, 23200
  X–ray, 73000
Collateral Ligament
  Ankle
    Repair, 27695-27698
  Interphalangeal Joint, 26545
  Knee Joint
    Repair, 27409
  Knee Repair, 27405, 27409
  Metacarpophalangeal Joint Repair, 26540-26542
  Reconstruction
    Elbow, 24346
    Interphalangeal Joint, 26545
    Metacarpophalangeal Joint, 26541-26542
  Repair
    Ankle, 27695-27698
    Elbow, 24345
    Interphalangeal Joint, 26540
    Knee, 27405, 27409

Collateral Ligament — *continued*
  Repair — *continued*
    Metacarpophalangeal Joint, 26540
Collection and Processing
  Allogeneic Blood
    Harvesting of Stem Cells, 38205
  Autologous Blood
    Harvesting of Stem Cells, 38206
    Intraoperative, 86891
    Preoperative, 86890
  Brushings
    Abdomen, 49320
    Anus, 46600, 46601
    Biliary Tract, 47552
    Colon, 44388, 45300, 45330, 45378
    Duodenum, 43235, 44360, 44376
    Esophagus, 43197, 43200, 43235
    Hepatobiliary System, 43260
    Ileum, 44376, 44380
    Jejunum, 43235
    Omentum, 49320
    Peritoneum, 49320
    Rectum, 45300, 45330
    Small Intestine, 44385
    Stomach, 43235
  Radiological Guidance, 75989
  Specimen
    Capillary, 36416
    Duodenum, 43756-43757
    Ear, 36416
    for Dark Field Examination, 87164
    Hematoma, 10140
    Implantable Venous Access Device, 36591
    Sputum, 89220
    Stomach, 43754
    Sweat, 89230
    Tears, 83861
    Vein, 36415
    Venous Access Device, 36591
    Venous Blood, 36415, 36591-36592
    Venous Catheter, 36592
  Washings
    Abdomen, 49320
    Anus, 46600, 46601
    Biliary, 47552
    Bronchial, 31622
    Colon, 44388, 45300, 45330, 45378
    Duodenum, 43235, 44360, 44376
    ERCP, 43260
    Esophageal, 43197, 43200, 43235
    Hepatobiliary System, 43260
    Ileum, 44376, 44380
    Jejunum, 43235
    Omentum, 49320
    Peritoneal, 58943, 58960
    Peritoneum, 49320
    Small Intestine, 44360, 44376, 44380, 44385
    Stomach, 43235
    Upper GI, 43235
  Stem Cell Processing, 38210-38215
Colles Fracture, 25600-25609
Colles Fracture Reversed
  See Smith Fracture
Collins Syndrome, Treacher
  See Treacher–Collins Syndrome
Collis Procedure, 43338
Colon
  Biopsy, 44025, 44100, 44322
    by Colonoscopy, 45378
    Endoscopic, 44389, 45380, 45392
  Capsule Endoscopy, 0355T
  Colostomy, 44320, 44322
    Revision, 44340-44346
  Colotomy, 44322
    Colostomy, 44322
    Endoscopic, [45399]
  CT Scan
    Colonography, 74261-74263
    Virtual Colonoscopy, 74261-74263
  Destruction
    Lesion, [44401], [45388]
    Tumor, [44401], [45388]
  Endoscopy
    Band Ligation, [45398]
    Biopsy, 44389, 44407, 45380, 45392

Colon — *continued*
Endoscopy — *continued*
Collection of Specimen, 44388, 45378
Decompression, 44408, 45393
Destruction
Lesion, [44401], [45388]
Tumor, [44401], [45388]
Dilation, 44405, 45386
Exploration, 44388, 45378
Hemorrhage, 44391, 45382
Injection, Submucosal, 44404, 45381
Mucosal Resection, 44403, 45349, [45390]
Placement
Stent, 44402, 45389
Removal
Foreign Body, 44390, 45379
Polyp, 44392, 44394, 45384-45385
Tumor, 44392, 44394, 45384-45385
Ultrasound, 44406-44407, 45391-45392
via Stoma, 44388-44408 [44401]
Excision
Partial, 44140-44147, 44160
Laparoscopic, 44204-44208
Total, 44150-44158
Laparoscopic, 44210-44212
Exclusion, 44700
Exploration, 44025
Endoscopic, 44388, 45378, 45381, 45386
Hemorrhage
Endoscopic Control, 44391, 45382
Hernia, 44050
Incision
Creation
Stoma, 44320, 44322
Exploration, 44025
Revision
Stoma, 44340-44346
Intraluminal Imaging, 0355T
Lavage
Intraoperative, 44701
Lesion
Destruction, [44401], [45388]
Excision, 44110, 44111
Lysis
Adhesions, 44005
Motility Study, 91117
Obstruction, 44025, 44050
Reconstruction
Bladder from, 50810
Reduction
Hernia, 44050
Volvulus, 44050
Removal
Foreign Body, 44025, 44390, 45379
Polyp, 44392, 44394, 45384-45385
Tumor, 44392, 44394, 45384-45385
Repair
Diverticula, 44605
Fistula, 44650-44661
Hernia, 44050
Intussusception, 44050
Malrotation, 44055
Obstruction, 44050
Ulcer, 44605
Volvulus, 44050
Wound, 44605
Splenic Flexure Mobilization
Laparoscopic, 44213
Open, 44139
Stoma Closure, 44620, 44625-44626
Suture
Diverticula, 44605
Fistula, 44650-44661
Injury, 44604-44605
Plication, 44680
Rupture, 44604-44605
Stoma, 44620, 44625
Ulcer, 44605
Wound, 44604-44605
Tumor
Ablation, [44401], [45388]
Destruction, [44401], [45388]
Removal, 44392, 44394, 45384-45385
Ultrasound
Endoscopic, 45391-45392
via Colotomy, [45399]

Colon — *continued*
Ultrasound — *continued*
via Stoma, 44388-44408 [44401]
Unlisted Services and Procedures, 44799
X–ray with Contrast
Barium Enema, 74270, 74280
Colonna Procedure, 27120
Acetabulum, Reconstruction, 27120
with Resection, Femoral Head, 27122
Colonography
CT Scan
Diagnostic, 74261-74262
Screening, 74263
Colonoscopy
Ablation Lesions/Polyps/Tumors, [45388]
Band Ligation, [45398]
Biopsy, 45380, 45392
Collection of Specimen, 45378
via Colotomy, [45399]
Decompression, 45393
Destruction
Lesion, [45388]
Tumor, [45388]
Diagnostic, 45378
Dilation, 45386
Hemorrhage Control, 45382
Injection, Submucosal, 45381
Mucosal Resection, [45390]
Placement
Stent, 45389
Removal
Foreign Body, 45379
Polyp, 45384-45385
Tumor, 45384-45385
Surveillance Intervals, 0528F-0529F
Transabdominal, [45399]
Ultrasound, 45391-45392
via Stoma
Biopsy, 44389, 44407
Decompression, 44408
Destruction
Polyp, [44401]
Tumor, [44401]
Dilation, 44405
Exploration, 44388
Hemorrhage, 44391
Injection, Submucosal, 44404
Mucosal Resection, 44403
Placement
Stent, 44402
Removal
Foreign Body, 44390
Polyp, 44392, 44394
Tumor, 44392, 44394
Ultrasound, 44406-44407
Virtual, 74261-74263
Colon–Sigmoid
Biopsy
Endoscopy, 45331
Decompression, 45378
Volvulus, 45337
Dilation, 45340
Endoscopy
Ablation
Polyp, [45346]
Tumor, [45346]
Biopsy, 45331
Dilation, 45340
Exploration, 45330, 45335
Hemorrhage, 45334
Needle Biopsy, 45342
Placement
Stent, 45327, 45347
Removal
Foreign Body, 45332
Polyp, 45333, 45338
Tumor, 45333, 45338
Ultrasound, 45341, 45342
Volvulus, 45337
Exploration
Endoscopy, 45330, 45335
Hemorrhage
Endoscopy, 45334
Needle Biopsy
Endoscopy, 45342
Reconstruction Bladder Using Sigmoid, 50810

Colon–Sigmoid — *continued*
Removal
Foreign Body, 45332
Repair
Volvulus
Endoscopy, 45337
Ultrasound
Endoscopy, 45341, 45342
Colorrhaphy, 44604
Color Vision Examination, 92283
Colostomy
with Colorrhaphy, 44605
with Partial Colectomy, 44141, 44143-44144, 44146
Hartmann Type, 44143
Laparoscopic, 44206, 44208
with Pelvic Exenteration, 45126, 51597, 58240
with Proctectomy, 45110
Laparoscopic, 45395
with Rectal Repair, 45563, 45805, 45825
Abdominal
with Closure Rectovaginal Fistula, 57307
with Creation Sigmoid Bladder, 50810
Abdominoperineal, 51597, 58240
Delayed Opening, 44799
External Fistulization, 44320
Paracolostomy Hernia, 44346
Revision, 44340
Home Visit, 99505
Ileocolostomy, 44160, 44205
Intestine, Large
with Suture, 44605
Laparoscopic, 44188, 44206, 44208
Perineal, 50810
Revision, 44340
Paracolostomy Hernia, 44345, 44346
Colotomy, 44025
Colpectomy
with Hysterectomy, 58275
with Repair of Enterocele, 58280
Partial, 57106
Total, 57110
Colpoceliocentesis
See Colpocentesis
Colpocentesis, 57020
Colpocleisis, 57120
Colpocleisis Complete
See Vagina, Closure
Colpohysterectomies
See Excision, Uterus, Vaginal
Colpoperineorrhaphy, 57210
Colpopexy, 57280
Laparoscopic, 57425
Open, 57280
Vaginal, 57282-57283
Colpoplasty
See Repair, Vagina
Colporrhaphy
Anterior, 57240, 57289
with Insertion of Mesh, 57267
with Insertion of Prosthesis, 57267
Anteroposterior, 57260, 57265
with Enterocele Repair, 57265
with Insertion of Mesh, 57267
with Insertion of Prosthesis, 57267
Manchester, 58400
Nonobstetrical, 57200
Posterior, 57250
with Insertion of Mesh, 57267
with Insertion of Prosthesis, 57267
Colposcopy
Biopsy, 56821, 57421, 57454-57455, 57460
Endometrial, 58110
Cervix, 57420-57421, 57452-57461
Endometrium, 58110
Exploration, 57452
Loop Electrode Biopsy, 57460
Loop Electrode Conization, 57461
Perineum, 99170
Vagina, 57420-57421, 57452
Vulva, 56820
Biopsy, 56821
Colpotomy
Drainage
Abscess, 57010
Exploration, 57000

Colpo–Urethrocystopexy, 58152, 58267, 58293
Marshall–Marchetti–Krantz procedure, 58152, 58267, 58293
Pereyra Procedure, 58267, 58293
Colprosterone
See Progesterone
Columna Vertebralis
See Spine
Column Chromatography/Mass Spectrometry, 82542
Combined Heart–Lung Transplantation
See Transplantation, Heart–Lung
Combined Right and Left Heart Cardiac Catheterization
See Cardiac Catheterization, Combined Left and Right Heart
Combined Vaccine, 90710
Comedones
Opening or Removal of (Incision and Drainage)
Acne Surgery, 10040
Commando–Type Procedure, 41155
Commissurotomy
Right Ventricular, 33476, 33478
Common Sensory Nerve
Repair, Suture, 64834
Common Truncus
See Truncus, Arteriosus
Communication Device
Non–speech–generating, 92605-92606 [92618]
Speech–generating, 92607-92609
Community/Work Reintegration
See Physical Medicine/Therapy/ Occupational Therapy
Training, 97537
Comparative Analysis Using STR Markers, 81265-81266
Compatibility Test
Blood, 86920
Electronic, 86923
Specimen Pretreatment, 86970-86972
Complement
Antigen, 86160
Fixation Test, 86171
Functional Activity, 86161
Hemolytic
Total, 86162
Total, 86162
Complete Blood Count, 85025-85027
Complete Colectomy
See Colectomy, Total
Complete Pneumonectomy
See Pneumonectomy, Completion
Complete Transposition of Great Vessels
See Transposition, Great Arteries
Complex Chronic Care Management Services, 99487, 99489, [99490]
Complex, Factor IX
See Christmas Factor
Complex, Vitamin B
See B Complex Vitamins
Component Removal, Blood
See Apheresis
Composite Graft, 15760, 15770
Vein, 35681-35683
Autogenous
Three or More Segments
Two Locations, 35683
Two Segments
Two Locations, 35682
Compound B
See Corticosterone
Compound F
See Cortisol
Compression, Nerve, Median
See Carpal Tunnel Syndrome
Compression System Application, 29581-29584
Computed Tomographic Angiography
Abdomen, 74174-74175
Abdominal Aorta, 75635
Arm, 73206
Chest, 71275
Head, 70496
Heart, 75574
Leg, 73706
Neck, 70498
Pelvis, 72191, 74174

Index

Colon — Computed Tomographic Angiography

Computed Tomographic Scintigraphy
  See Emission Computerized Tomography
Computed Tomography (CT Scan)
  with Contrast
    Abdomen, 74160, 74175
    Arm, 73201, 73206
    Brain, 70460
    Cardiac Structure and Morphology, 75572-
      75573
    Chest, 71275
    Ear, 70481
    Face, 70487
    Head, 70460, 70496
    Heart, 75572-75574
    Leg, 73701, 73706
    Maxilla, 70487
    Neck, 70491, 70498
    Orbit, 70481
    Pelvis, 72191, 72193
    Sella Turcica, 70481
    Spine
      Cervical, 72126
      Lumbar, 72132
      Thoracic, 72129
    Thorax, 71260
  without Contrast
    Abdomen, 74150
    Arm, 73200
    Brain, 70450
    Ear, 70480
    Face, 70486
    Head, 70450
    Heart, 75571
    Leg, 73700
    Maxilla, 70486
    Neck, 70490
    Orbit, 70480
    Pelvis, 72192
    Sella Turcica, 70480
    Spine, Cervical, 72125
    Spine, Lumbar, 72131
    Spine, Thoracic, 72128
    Thorax, 71250
  without Contrast, followed by Contrast
    Abdomen, 74170
    Arm, 73202
    Brain, 70470
    Ear, 70482
    Face, 70488
    Leg, 73702
    Maxilla, 70488
    Neck, 70492
    Orbit, 70482
    Pelvis, 72194
    Sella Turcica, 70482
    Spine
      Cervical, 72127
      Lumbar, 72133
      Thoracic, 72130
    Thorax, 71270
  Bone
    Density Study, 77078
  Colon
    Colonography, 74261-74263
      Diagnostic, 74261-74262
      Screening, 74263
    Virtual Colonoscopy, 74261-74263
  Drainage, 75898
  Follow–up Study, 76380
  Guidance
    3D Rendering, 76376-76377
    Cyst Aspiration, 77012
    Localization, 77011
    Needle Biopsy, 77012
    Radiation Therapy, 77014
  Heart, 75571-75574
Computer
  Aided Animation and Analysis Retinal Images,
    0380T
  Aided Detection
    Chest Radiograph, 0174T-0175T
    Mammography
      Diagnostic, 77065-77066
      Magnetic Resonance Imaging (MRI),
        0159T
      Screening, 77067

Computer — *continued*
  Analysis
    Cardiac Electrical Data, 0206T
    Electrocardiographic Data, 93228
    Heart Sounds, Acoustic Recording, 93799
    Motion Analysis, 96000-96004
    Pediatric Home Apnea Monitor, 94776
    Probability Assessment
      Patient Specific Findings, 99199
    Stored Data, 99090
  Assisted Navigation
    Orthopedic Surgery, 20985, 0054T-0055T
  Assisted Testing
    Cytopathology, 88121
    Morphometric Analysis, 88121
    Neuropsychological, 96120
    Psychological, 96103
    Urinary Tract Specimen, 88121
Computerized Emission Tomography
  See Emission Computerized Tomography
COMVAX, 90748
Concentration, Hydrogen–Ion
  See pH
Concentration, Minimum Inhibitory
  See Minimum Inhibitory Concentration
Concentration of Specimen
  Cytopathology, 88108
  Electrophoretic Fractionation and Quantitation,
    84166
  Immunoelectrophoresis, 86325
  Immunofixation Electrophoresis, 86335
  Infectious Agent, 87015
  Ova and Parasites, 87177
Concha Bullosa Resection
  with Nasal/Sinus Endoscopy, 31240
Conchae Nasale
  See Nasal Turbinate
Conduction, Nerve
  See Nerve Conduction
Conduit, Ileal
  See Ileal Conduit
Condyle
  Femur
    Arthroplasty, 27442-27443, 27446-27447
    Fracture
      Closed, 27508, 27510
      Open, 27514
      Percutaneous, 27509
  Humerus
    Fracture
      Closed Treatment, 24576, 24577
      Open Treatment, 24579
      Percutaneous, 24582
  Mandible, Reconstruction, 21247
  Metatarsal
    Excision, 28288
  Phalanges
    Toe
      Excision, 28126
      Resection, 28153
Condylectomy
  with Skull Base Surgery, 61596, 61597
  Metatarsal Head, 28288
  Temporomandibular Joint, 21050
Condyle, Mandibular
  See Mandibular Condyle
Condyloma
  Destruction
    Anal, 46900-46924
    Penis, 54050-54065
    Vagina, 57061, 57065
    Vulva, 56501, 56515
Conference
  Interactive Videoconference, 0188T-0189T
  Medical
    with Interdisciplinary Team, 99366-99368

Confirmation
  Drug, *[80320, 80321, 80322, 80323, 80324,*
    80325, 80326, 80327, 80328, 80329,
    80330, 80331, 80332, 80333, 80334,
    80335, 80336, 80337, 80338, 80339,
    80340, 80341, 80342, 80343, 80344,
    80345, 80346, 80347, 80348, 80349,
    80350, 80351, 80352, 80353, 80354,
    80355, 80356, 80357, 80358, 80359,
    80360, 80361, 80362, 80363, 80364,
    80365, 80366, 80367, 80368, 80369,
    80370, 80371, 80372, 80373, 80374,
    80375, 80376, 80377, 83992]
Confocal Microscopy, 96931-96936
Congenital Arteriovenous Malformation
  See Arteriovenous Malformation
Congenital Elevation of Scapula
  See Sprengal's Deformity
Congenital Heart Anomaly
  Catheterization, 93530-93533
    Injection, 93563-93564
  Closure
    Interatrial Communication, 93580
    Ventricular Septal Defect, 93581
  Echocardiography
    Congenital Anomalies
      Transesophageal, 93315
      Transthoracic, 93303-93304
    Fetal, 76825-76826
      Doppler, 76827-76828
    Guidance for Intracardiac or Great Vessel
      Intervention, 93355
    Treatment Ventricular Ectopy, 93654
Congenital Heart Septum Defect
  See Septal Defect
Congenital Kidney Abnormality
  Nephrolithotomy, 50070
  Pyeloplasty, 50405
  Pyelotomy, 50135
Congenital Laryngocele
  See Laryngocele
Congenital Vascular Anomaly
  See Vascular Malformation
Conisation
  See Cervix, Conization
Conization
  Cervix, 57461, 57520, 57522
Conjoint Psychotherapy, 90847
Conjunctiva
  Biopsy, 68100
  Cyst
    Incision and Drainage, 68020
    Excision of Lesion, 68110, 68115
      with Adjacent Sclera, 68130
    Expression of Follicles, 68040
    Fistulize for Drainage
      with Tube, 68750
      without Tube, 68745
    Foreign Body Removal, 65205, 65210
  Graft, 65782
    Harvesting, 68371
    Insertion, 65150, 65782
  Injection, 68200
  Insertion Stent, 68750
  Lesion
    Destruction, 68135
    Excision, 68110-68130
      with Adjacent Sclera, 68130
      over 1 cm, 68115
    Reconstruction, 68320-68335
      with Flap
        Bridge or Partial, 68360
        Total, 68362
      Symblepharon
        with Graft, 68335
        without Graft, 68330
        Total, 68362
  Repair
    Symblepharon
      with Graft, 68335
      without Graft, 68330
      Division, 68340
    Wound
      with Eyelid Repair, 67961, 67966
      with Wound Repair, 65270, 65272-
        65273, 67930, 67935

Conjunctiva — *continued*
  Repair — *continued*
    Wound — *continued*
      Direct Closure, 65270
      Mobilization and Rearrangement,
        65272, 65273
  Unlisted Services and Procedure, 68399
Conjunctivocystorhinostomy
  See Conjunctivorhinostomy
Conjunctivodacryocystostomy
  See Conjunctivorhinostomy
Conjunctivoplasty, 68320-68330
  with Extensive Rearrangement, 68320
  with Graft, 68320
    Buccal Mucous Membrane, 68325
  Reconstruction Cul–de–Sac
    with Extensive Rearrangement, 68326
    with Graft, 68328
      Buccal Mucous Membrane, 68328
  Repair Symblepharon, 68330, 68335, 68340
Conjunctivorhinostomy
  with Tube, 68750
  without Tube, 68745
Conjunctivo–Tarso–Levator
  Resection, 67908
Conjunctivo–Tarso–Muller Resection, 67908
Conscious Sedation
  See Sedation
Construction
  Apical-Aortic Conduit, 33404
  Arterial
    Conduit, 33608, 33920
    Tunnel, 33505
  Bladder from Sigmoid Colon, 50810
  Eye Adhesions, 67880
  Finger
    Toe to Hand Transfer, 26551-26556
  Gastric Tube, 43832
  IMRT Device, 77332-77334
  Multi-leaf Collimator (MLC) Device, 77338
  Neobladder, 51596
  Tracheoesophageal Fistula, 31611
  Vagina
    with Graft, 57292
    without Graft, 57291
Consultation
  See Second Opinion; Third Opinion
  Clinical Pathology, 80500, 80502
  Initial Inpatient
    New or Established Patient, 99251-99255
  Interprofessional Via Telephone or Internet,
    99446-99449
  Office and/or Other Outpatient
    New or Established Patient, 99241-99245
  Pathology
    During Surgery, 88333-88334
  Psychiatric, with Family, 90887
  Radiation Therapy
    Radiation Physics, 77336, 77370
  Surgical Pathology, 88321-88325
    Intraoperation, 88329-88334
  X–ray, 76140
Consumption Test, Antiglobulin
  See Coombs Test
Contact Lens Services
  Fitting/Prescription, 92071-92072, 92310-92313
  Modification, 92325
  Prescription, 92314-92317
  Replacement, 92326
Continuous Epidural Analgesia, 01967-01969
Continuous Glucose Monitoring System (CGMS),
  95250-95251
Continuous Negative Pressure Breathing
  (CNPB), 94662
Continuous Positive Airway Pressure (CPAP),
  94660
  Intermittent Positive Pressure Breathing, 94660
Contouring
  Cranial
    Bones, 21181
    Sutures, 61559
  Forehead, 21137-21138
  Frontal Sinus Wall, 21139
  Septoplasty, 30520
  Silicone Injections, 11950-11954

Contouring — continued
Tumor
Facial Bone, 21029
Contraception
Cervical Cap
Fitting, 57170
Diaphragm
Fitting, 57170
Intrauterine Device (IUD)
Insertion, 58300
Removal, 58301
Contraceptive Capsules, Implantable
Insertion, 11981
Removal, 11976
Contraceptive Device, Intrauterine
See Intrauterine Device (IUD)
Contracture
Bladder Neck Resection, 52640
Elbow
Release with Radical Resection of Capsule, 24149
Finger Cast, 29086
Palm
Release, 26121-26125
Shoulder Capsule Release, 23020
Thumb
Release, 26508
Volkmann, 25315
Wrist Capsulotomy, 25085
Contracture of Palmar Fascia
See Dupuytren's Contracture
Contralateral Ligament
Repair, Knee, 27405
Contrast Aortogram
See Aortography
Contrast Bath Therapy, 97034
See Physical Medicine/ Therapy/Occupational Therapy
Contrast Material
Colonic Tube
Insertion, 49440-49442
Radiological Evaluation, 49465
Removal of Obstruction, 49460
Replacement, 49446, 49450-49452
Cranial
for Ventricular Puncture, 61120
Dacryocystography, 68850
Injection
Arteriovenous Dialysis Shunt
Dialysis Circuit, 36901-36903
Central Venous Access Device, 36598
Gastrostomy, Duodenostomy, Jejunostomy, Gastro-jejunostomy, or Cecostomy Tube, Percutaneous, 49465
via Peritoneal Catheter, 49424
Peritoneal
Assessment of Abscess or Cyst, 49424
Evaluation Venous Shunt, 49427
Tunneled Catheter Insertion, 49418
Peritoneal Cavity, 49400
Renal Angiography, 36251-36254
Saline Infusion Sonohysterography (SIS), 58340
Spine
Localization, 62263, 62320-62327
Urethrocystography, 51605
Contrast Phlebogram
See Venography
Contusion
See Hematoma
Converting Enzyme, Angiotensin
See Angiotensin Converting Enzyme (ACE)
Coombs Test
Direct, 86880
Indirect, 86885-86886
RBC Antibody Screen, 86850, 86860, 86870
Copper, 82525
Coprobilinogen
Feces, 84577
Coproporphyrin, 84119-84120
Coracoacromial Ligament Release, 23415, 29826
Coracoid Process Transfer, 23462
Cordectomy, 31300
Cordocentesis, 59012
Cordotomy, 63194-63199
Cord, Spermatic
See Spermatic Cord

Cord, Spinal
See Spinal Cord
Cord, Vocal
See Vocal Cords
Corectomy, 66500, 66505
Coreoplasty, 66762
Cornea
Biopsy, 65410
Collagen Cross-Linking (CXL), 0402T
Curettage, 65435, 65436
with Chelating Agent, 65436
Epithelium
Excision, 65435, 65436
with Chelating Agent, 65436
Hysteresis Determination, 92145
Incision
for Correction Astigmatism, 65772
for Keratoplasty, 0290T
Insertion
Intrastromal Corneal Ring Segment, 65785
Lesion
Destruction, 65450
Excision, 65400
with Graft, 65426
without Graft, 65420
Pachymetry, 76514
Prosthesis, 65770
Pterygium
with Graft, 65426
Excision, 65420
Puncture, 65600
Relaxing Incisions, 65772, 65775
Removal
Foreign Body, 65220, 65222
Lesion, 66600
Repair
with Amniotic Membrane, 65778-65780
with Glue, 65286
Astigmatism, 65772, 65775
Incision, 65772
Wedge Resection, 65775
Wound
Nonperforating, 65275
Perforating, 65280, 65285
Tissue Glue, 65286
Reshape
Epikeratoplasty, 65767
Keratomileusis, 65760
Keratophakia, 65765
Keratoprosthesis, 65767
Scraping
Smear, 65430
Tattoo, 65600
Tear Film Imaging, 0330T
Tear Osmolarity, 83861
Thickness Measurement, 76514
Topography, 92025
Transplantation
Amniotic Membrane, 65780
Autograft or Homograft
Allograft Preparation, 0290T, 65757
Endothelial, 65756
Lamellar, 65710
Penetrating, 65730-65755
Corneal Incisions by Laser
Recipient Cornea, 0290T
for Aphakia, 65750
Unlisted Procedure, 66999
Coronary
Thrombectomy
Percutaneous, [92973]
Coronary Angioplasty, Transluminal Balloon
See Percutaneous Transluminal Angioplasty
Coronary Arteriography
Anesthesia, 01920
Coronary Artery
Angiography, 93454-93461
Angioplasty
with Atherectomy, [92933, 92934], [92937, 92938], [92941], [92943, 92944]
with Placement Stent, [92928, 92929], [92933, 92934], [92937, 92938], [92941], [92943, 92944]
Atherectomy, [92924, 92925]
Bypass Graft (CABG), 33503-33505, 33510-33516

Coronary Artery — continued
Bypass Graft — continued
Arterial, 33533-33536
Arterial Graft
Spectroscopy, Catheter Based, 0205T
Arterial–Venous, 33517-33523
Beta Blocker Administered, 4115F
Harvest
Upper Extremity Artery, 35600
Upper Extremity Vein, 35500
Reoperation, 33530
Venous, 33510-33516
Ligation, 33502
Obstruction Severity Assessment, 0206T
Placement
Radiation Delivery Device, [92974]
Reconstruction, 33863-33864
Repair, 33500-33507
Revascularization, [92937, 92938], [92941], [92943, 92944]
Thrombectomy, [92973]
Thrombolysis, [92975], [92977]
Translocation, 33506-33507
Unroofing, 33507
Ventricular Restoration, 33548
Coronary Endarterectomy, 33572
Coroner's Exam, 88045
Coronoidectomy
Temporomandibular Joint, 21070
Corpectomy, 63101-63103
Corpora Cavernosa
Corpora Cavernosography, 74445
Injection, 54230
Corpus Spongiosum Shunt, 54430
Dynamic Cavernosometry, 54231
Glans Penis Fistulization, 54435
Injection
Peyronie Disease, 54200-54205
Pharmacologic Agent, 54235
Irrigation
Priapism, 54220
Peyronie Disease, 54200-54205
Priapism, 54220, 54430
Repair
Corporeal Tear, 54437
Saphenous Vein Shunt, 54420
X–ray with Contrast, 74445
Corpora Cavernosa, Plastic Induration
See Peyronie Disease
Corpora Cavernosography, 74445
Injection, 54230
Corpus Callosum
Transection, 61541
Corpus Uteri, 58100-58285
Corpus Vertebrae (Vertebrale)
See Vertebral Body
Correction of Cleft Palate
See Cleft Palate, Repair
Correction of Lid Retraction
See Repair, Eyelid, Retraction
Correction of Malrotation of Duodenum
See Ladd Procedure
Correction of Syndactyly, 26560-26562
Correction of Ureteropelvic Junction
See Pyeloplasty
Cortex Decortication, Cerebral
See Decortication
Cortical Mapping
Functional Mapping, 95961-95962
Noninvasive, 96020
TMS Treatment
Initial, 90867
Subsequent, 90868-90869
Corticoids
See Corticosteroids
Corticoliberin
See Corticotropic Releasing Hormone (CRH)
Corticosteroid Binding Globulin, 84449
Corticosteroid Binding Protein, 84449
Corticosteroids
Blood, 83491
Urine, 83491
Corticosterone
Blood or Urine, 82528
Corticotropic Releasing Hormone (CRH), 80412
Cortisol, 80400-80406, 80418, 80420, 80436, 82530

Cortisol — continued
Stimulation Panel, 80412
Total, 82533
Cortisol Binding Globulin, 84449
Costectomy
See Resection, Ribs
Costello Syndrome, 81442
Costen Syndrome
See Temporomandibular
Costotransversectomy, 21610
COTD (Cardiac Output Thermodilution), 93561-93562
Cothromboplastin
See Proconvertin
Cotte Operation, 58400, 58410
Repair, Uterus, Suspension, 58400, 58410
Cotting Operation
Excision, Nail Fold, 11765
Cotton (Bohler) Procedure, 28405
Cotton Scoop Procedure, 28118
Counseling
See Preventive Medicine
Smoking and Tobacco Use Cessation, 99406-99407
Counseling and /or Risk Factor Reduction Intervention – Preventive Medicine, Individual Counseling
Behavior Change Interventions, 0403T, 99406-99409
Caregiver-focused, 96161
Patient-focused, 96160
Preventive Medicine, 99411-99412
Counseling, Preventive
Group, 99411, 99412
Individual, 99401-99404
Other, 99429
Count, Blood Cell
See Blood Cell Count
Count, Blood Platelet
See Blood, Platelet, Count
Count, Cell
See Cell Count
Count, Complete Blood
See Complete Blood Count (CBC)
Counterimmunoelectrophoresis, 86185
Counters, Cell
See Cell Count
Countershock, Electric
See Cardioversion
Count, Erythrocyte
See Red Blood Cell (RBC), Count
Count, Leukocyte
See White Blood Cell, Count
Count, Reticulocyte
See Reticulocyte, Count
Coventry Tibial Wedge Osteotomy
See Osteotomy, Tibia
Cowper's Gland
Excision, 53250
COX10, 81405
COX15, 81405
COX6B1, 81404
Coxa
See Hip
Coxiella Brunetii
Antibody, 86638
Coxsackie
Antibody, 86658
CPAP (Continuous Positive Airway Pressure), 94660
CPB, 32852, 32854, 33496, 33503-33505, 33510-33523, 33533-33536
C–Peptide, 80432, 84681
CPK
Isoenzymes, 82252, 82552
Isoforms, 82554
MB Fraction Only, 82553
Total, 82550
CPR (Cardiopulmonary Resuscitation), 92950
CPT1A, 81406
CPT2, 81404
CR, 82565-82575
Cranial Bone
Frontal Bone Flap, 61556-61557
Halo
for Thin Skull Osteology, 20664

Cranial Bone — *continued*
  Parietal Bone Flap, 61556
  Reconstruction
    Extracranial, 21181-21184
  Temporal Bone
    Hearing Device, 69710-69711
    Implantation Cochlear Device, 69930
    Osseointegrated Implant, 69714-69715
    Removal Tumor, 69970
    Resection, 69535
    Unlisted Procedure, 69979
  Tumor
    Excision, 61563-61564
Cranial Halo, 20661
Cranial Nerve
  Avulsion, 64732-64760, 64771
  Decompression, 61458, 61460, 64716
  Implantation
    Electrode, 64553, 64568-64569
  Incision, 64732-64746, 64760
  Injection
    Anesthetic, 64400-64408
    Neurolytic, 64600-64610
  Insertion
    Electrode, 64553, 64568-64569
  Neuroplasty, 64716
  Release, 64716
  Repair
    Suture, with or without Graft, 64864, 64865
  Section, 61460
  Transection, 64732-64760, 64771
  Transposition, 64716
Cranial Nerve II
  See Optic Nerve
Cranial Nerve V
  See Trigeminal Nerve
Cranial Nerve VII
  See Facial Nerve
Cranial Nerve X
  See Vagus Nerve
Cranial Nerve XI
  See Accessory Nerve
Cranial Nerve XII
  See Hypoglossal Nerve
Cranial Tongs
  Application
    Removal, 20660
  Removal, 20665
Craniectomy
  with Craniotomy, 61530
  See Craniotomy
  Anesthesia, 00211
  Compression
    Sensory Root Gasserian Ganglion, 61450
  Craniosynostosis, 61558, 61559
    Multiple Sutures, 61552, 61558-61559
    Single Suture, 61550
  Decompression, 61322-61323, 61340-61343
    Cranial Nerves, 61458
    Sensory Root Gasserian Ganglion, 61450
  Drainage of Abscess, 61320-61321
  Electrode Placement
    Cortical, 61860, 61870
    Subcortical, 61863-61864, 61867-61868
  Excision
    for Osteomyelitis, 61501
    of Lesion or Tumor, 61500
  Exploratory, 61304-61305, 61458
  Section, 61450, 61460
  Stenosis Release, 61550-61552
  Surgical, 61312-61315, 61320-61323, 61450-
    61480, 61500-61522
  Tractotomy, 61480
  Wound Treatment, 61571
Craniofacial and Maxillofacial
  Unlisted Services and Procedures, 21299
Craniofacial Procedures
  Unlisted Services and Procedures, 21299
Craniofacial Separation
  Bone Graft, 21436
  Closed Treatment, 21431
  External Fixation, 21435
  Open Treatment, 21432-21436
  Wire Fixation, 21431-21432
Craniomegalic Skull
  Reduction, 62115-62117

Craniopharyngioma
  Excision, 61545
Cranioplasty, 62120
  with Autograft, 62146, 62147
  with Bone Graft, 61316, 62146, 62147
  Bone Graft Retrieval, 62148
  Encephalocele Repair, 62120
  for Defect, 62140, 62141, 62145
Craniostenosis
  See Craniosynostosis
Craniosynostosis
  Bifrontal Craniotomy, 61557
  Extensive Craniectomy, 61558, 61559
  Frontal, 61556
  Multiple Sutures, 61552
  Parietal, 61556
  Single Suture, 61550
Craniotomy
  with Bone Flap, 61510-61516, 61526, 61530,
    61533-61545, 61566-61567
    for Bone Lesion, 61500
  Abscess Drainage
    Infratentorial, 61321
    Supratentorial, 61320
  Anesthesia, 00211
  Barrel–Stave Procedure, 61559
  Bifrontal Bone Flap, 61557
  Cloverleaf Skull, 61558
  Craniosynostosis, 61556-61557
  Decompression, 61322-61323
    Orbit Only, 61330
    Other, Supratentorial, 61340
    Posterior Fossa, 61345
  Encephalocele, 62121
  Excision Brain Tumor
    Benign of Cranial Bone, 61563
      with Optic Nerve Decompression,
        61564
    Cerebellopontine Angle Tumor, 61520
    Cyst, Supratentorial, 61516
    Infratentorial or posterior fossa, 61518
    Meningioma, 61519
    Midline at Skull Base, 61521
    Supratentorial, 61510
  Excision Epileptogenic Focus
    with Electrocorticography, 61536
    without Electrocorticography, 61534
  Exploratory, 61304, 61305
    Orbit with Biopsy, 61332
    Removal
      Lesion, 61333
  Foreign Body, 61570
  Frontal Bone Flap, 61556
  Hematoma, 61312-61315
  Implantation Electrodes, 61531, 61533
    Stereotactic, 61760
  Implant of Neurostimulator, 61850-61870
  Lobectomy
    with Electrocorticography, 61538
  Meningioma, 61519
  Mesencephalic Tractotomy or Pedunculotomy,
    61480
  Multiple Osteotomies and Bone Autografts,
    61559
  Neurostimulators, 61850-61870
  Osteomyelitis, 61501
  Parietal Bone Flap, 61556
  Penetrating Wound, 61571
  Pituitary Tumor, 61546
  Recontouring, 61559
  Removal of Electrode Array, 61535
  Suboccipital
    with Cervical Laminectomy, 61343
    for Cranial Nerves, 61458
    Subtemporal, 61450
  Surgery, 61312-61323, 61546, 61570-61571,
    61582-61583, 61590, 61592, 61760,
    62120
  Transoral Approach, 61575
    requiring Splitting Tongue and/or
      Mandible, 61576
Cranium
  See Skull
Craterization
  Calcaneus, 28120
  Clavicle, 23180

Craterization — *continued*
  Femur, 27070, 27071, 27360
  Fibula, 27360, 27641
  Hip, 27070, 27071
  Humerus, 23184, 24140
  Ileum, 27070, 27071
  Metacarpal, 26230
  Metatarsal, 28122
  Olecranon Process, 24147
  Phalanges
    Finger, 26235, 26236
    Toe, 28124
  Pubis, 27070, 27071
  Radius, 24145, 25151
  Scapula, 23182
  Talus, 28120
  Tarsal, 28122
  Tibia, 27360, 27640
  Ulna, 24147, 25150
CRB1, 81406, 81434
C–Reactive Protein, 86140, 86141
Creatine, 82553-82554
  Blood or Urine, 82540
Creatine Kinase (Total), 82550
Creatine Phosphokinase
  Blood, 82552
  Total, 82550
Creatinine
  Blood, 82565
  Clearance, 82575
  Other Source, 82570
  Urine, 82570, 82575
Creation
  Arteriovenous
    Fistula, 35686, 36825, 36830
  Catheter Exit Site, 49436
  Cavopulmonary Anastomosis, 33622
  Colonic Reservoir, 45119
  Complete Heart Block, 93650
  Cutaneoperitoneal Fistula, 49999
  Defect, 40720
  Ileal Reservoir, 44158, 44211, 45113
  Iliac Artery Conduit, 34833
  Lesion
    Gasserian Ganglion, 61790
    Globus Pallidus, 61720
    Other Subcortical Structure, 61735
    Spinal Cord, 63600
    Thalamus, 61720
    Trigeminal Tract, 61791
  Mucofistula, 44144
  Pericardial Window, 32659, 33025
  Recipient Site, 15002-15003, 15004-15005
  Shunt
    Cerebrospinal Fluid, 62200
    Subarachnoid
      Lumbar–Peritoneal, 63740
    Subarachnoid–Subdural, 62190
    Ventriculo, 62220
  Sigmoid Bladder, 50810
  Speech Prosthesis, 31611
  Stoma
    Bladder, 51980
    Kidney, 50395
    Renal Pelvis, 50395
    Tympanic Membrane, 69433, 69436
    Ureter, 50860
  Ventral Hernia, 39503
CREBBP, 81406-81407
CRF, 80412
CRH (Corticotropic Releasing Hormone), 80412
Cricoid Cartilage Split, 31587
Cricothyroid Membrane
  Incision, 31605
Cristobalite
  See Silica
CRIT, 85013
Critical Care Services
  Cardiopulmonary Resuscitation, 92950
  Evaluation and Management, 99291-99292,
    99468-99476
  Interfacility Transport, 99466-99467 [99485]
    [99486]
  Ipecac Administration for Poison, 99175
  Neonatal
    Initial, 99468

Critical Care Services — *continued*
  Neonatal — *continued*
    Intensive, 99477
    Low Birth Weight Infant, 99478-99479
    Subsequent, 99469
  Pediatric
    Initial, 99471, 99475
    Interfacility Transport, 99466-99467 [99485,
      99486]
    Supervision, [99485, 99486]
    Subsequent, 99472, 99476
  Remote Interactive Videoconferenced, 0188T-
    0189T
Cross Finger Flap, 15574
Crossmatch, 86825-86826, 86920-86923
Crossmatching, Tissue
  See Tissue Typing
CRP, 86140
Cruciate Ligament
  Arthroscopic Repair, 29888-29889
  Repair, 27407, 27409
    Knee with Collateral Ligament, 27409
CRX, 81404
Cryoablation
  See Cryosurgery
Cryofibrinogen, 82585
Cryofixation
  Cells, 38207-38209, 88240-88241
  Embryo, 89258
  for Transplantation, 32850, 33930, 33940,
    44132, 47133, 47140, 48550, 50300-
    50320, 50547
  Freezing and Storage, 38207, 88240
  Oocyte, 89240
  Ovarian Tissue, 89240
  Sperm, 89259
  Testes, 89335
  Thawing
    Embryo, 89352
    Oocytes, 89353
    Reproductive Tissue, 89354
    Sperm, 89356
Cryoglobulin, 82595
Cryopreservation
  Bone Marrow, 38207-38209
  Cells, 38207-38208, 88240, 88241
  Embryo, 89258, 89352
  for Transplantation, 32850, 33930, 33940,
    44132-44133, 47140, 48550, 50300-
    50320, 50547
  Freezing and Storage
    Cells, 88240
    Embryo, 89258
    Reproductive Tissue
      Oocyte(s), 89337, [0357T]
      Ovarian, 0058T
      Sperm, 89259
      Testicular, 89335
    Stem Cells, 38207
  Oocyte, 89337, [0357T]
  Ovarian Tissue, 0058T
  Sperm, 89259
  Testes, 89335
    Embryo, 89352
    Oocytes, 89353
    Reproductive Tissue, 89354
    Sperm, 89356
  Thawing
    Cells, 88241
    Embryo, 89352
    Oocytes, 89356
    Reproductive Tissue, 89354
    Sperm, 89353
Cryosurgery, 17000-17286, 47371, 47381
  See Destruction
  Cervix, 57511
  Fibroadenoma
    Breast, 19105
  Lesion
    Anus, 46916, 46924
    Bladder, 51030, 52224
      Tumor(s), 52234-52235, 52240
    Ear, 17280-17284, 17286
    Eyelid, 17280-17284, 17286
    Face, 17280-17284, 17286
    Kidney, 50250

Cryosurgery — *continued*
Lesion — *continued*
Lips, 17280-17284, 17286
Liver, 47371, 47381
Mouth, 17280-17284, 17286, 40820
Nose, 17280-17284, 17286
Penis, 54056, 54065
Skin
Benign, 17000-17004, 17110-17111
Malignant, 17260-17286
Premalignant, 17000-17004
Vascular Proliferative, 17106-17108
Urethra, 52224
Vagina, 57061-57065
Vulva, 56501-56515
Nerve, Percutaneous, 0440T-0442T
Prostate, 52214, 55873
Trichiasis, 67825
Tumor
Bladder, 52234-52235, 52240
Rectum, 45190
Warts, flat, 17110, 17111
Cryotherapy
Ablation
Renal Tumor, 50593
Uterine Fibroid, Transcervical, 0404T
Acne, 17340
Destruction
Bronchial Tumor, 31641
Ciliary body, 66720
Retinopathy, 67227
Lesion
Cornea, 65450
Retina, 67208, 67227
Renal Tumor, 50593
Retinal Detachment
Prophylaxis, 67141
Repair, 67101, 67107-67108, 67113
Retinopathy, 67229
Destruction, 67227
Preterm Infant, 67229
Trichiasis
Correction, 67825
Crypectomy, 46999
Cryptococcus
Antibody, 86641
Antigen Detection
Enzyme Immunoassay, 87327
Cryptococcus Neoformans
Antigen Detection
Enzyme Immunoassay, 87327
Cryptorchism
See Testis, Undescended
Cryptosporidium
Antigen Detection
Direct Fluorescent Antibody, 87272
Enzyme Immunoassay, 87328
Crystal Identification
Any Body Fluid, 89060
Tissue, 89060
C–Section, 59510-59515, 59618-59622
See also Cesarean Delivery
CSF, 86325, 89050, 89051
CST, 59020
CSTB, 81401, 81404
CTNNB1, 81403
CTS, 29848, 64721
CT Scan
with Contrast
Abdomen, 74160, 74175
and Pelvis, 74177
Arm, 73201, 73206
Brain, 70460, 70496
Cerebral Blood Flow/Volume, 0042T
Chest, 71275
Ear, 70481
Face, 70487
Head, 70460, 70496
Leg, 73701, 73706
Maxilla, 70487
Neck, 70491
Orbit, 70481
Pelvis, 72191, 72193
and Abdomen, 74177
Sella Turcica, 70481

CT Scan — *continued*
with Contrast — *continued*
Spine
Cervical, 72126
Lumbar, 72132
Thoracic, 72129
Thorax, 71260
without Contrast
Abdomen, 74150
and Pelvis, 74176
Arm, 73200
Brain, 70450
Colon, 74261-74263
Ear, 70480
Face, 70480
Head, 70450
Leg, 73700
Maxilla, 70486
Neck, 70490
Orbit, 70480
Pelvis, 72192
and Abdomen, 74176
Sella Turcica, 70480
Spine
Cervical, 72125
Lumbar, 72131
Thoracic, 72128
Thorax, 71250
without Contrast, followed by Contrast
Abdomen, 74170
and Pelvis, 74178
Arm, 73202
Brain, 70470
Ear, 70482
Face, 70488
Head, 70470
Leg, 73702
Maxilla, 70488
Neck, 70492
Orbit, 70482
Pelvis, 72194
and Abdomen, 74178
Sella Turcica, 70482
Spine
Cervical, 72127
Lumbar, 72133
Thoracic, 72130
Thorax, 71270
3D Rendering, 76376-76377
Angiography
Abdomen, 74175
Abdomen and Pelvis, 74174
Aorta, 75635
Heart, 75574
Leg, 73706, 75635
Bone
Density Study, 77078
Brain, 70450-70470
Stroke Diagnosis, 3110F-3112F
Colon
Diagnostic, 74261-74262
Screening, 74263
Drainage, 75989
Follow–up Study, 76380
Guidance
Localization, 77011
Needle Biopsy, 77012
Parenchymal Tissue Ablation, 77013
Radiation Therapy, 77014
Tissue Ablation, 77013
Visceral Tissue Ablation, 77013
Heart
Evaluation
Angiography, 75574
Coronary Calcium, 75571
Structure and Morphology, 75572-75573
Hemorrhage Documented, 3110F
Infarction Documented, 3110F
Lesion Documented, 3110F
Optical Coherence Tomography, [92978, 92979]
Parathyroid Gland, 78072
Unlisted Procedure, 76497
CT Scan, Radionuclide
See Emission Computerized Tomography

Cuff, Rotator
See Rotator Cuff
Culdocentesis, 57020
Culdoplasty
McCall, 57283
Culdoscopy, 57452
Culdotomy, 57000
Culture
Acid Fast Bacilli, 87116
Amniotic Fluid
Chromosome Analysis, 88235
Bacteria
Aerobic, 87040-87071
Additional Methods, 87077
Anaerobic, 87073-87076
Blood, 87040
Feces, 87045-87046
Other, 87070-87073
Screening, 87081
Urine, 87086, 87088
Bone Marrow
Chromosome Analysis, 88237
Neoplastic Disorders, 88237
Chlamydia, 87110
Chorionic Villus
Chromosome Analysis, 88235
Fertilized Oocyte
for In Vitro Fertilization, 89250
with Co–Culture of Embryo, 89251
Assisted Microtechnique, 89280, 89281
Fungus
Blood, 87103
Hair, 87101
Identification, 87106
Nail, 87101
Other, 87102
Skin, 87101
Source Other Than Blood, 87102
Lymphocyte
Chromosome Analysis, 88230
HLA Typing, 86821-86822
Mold, 87107
Mycobacteria, 87116-87118
Mycoplasma, 87109
Oocyte/Embryo
Extended Culture, 89272
for In Vitro Fertilization, 89250
with Co–Culture of Embryo, 89251
Pathogen
by Kit, 87084
Screening Only, 87081
Skin
Chromosome Analysis, 88233
Stool, 87045-87046
Tissue
Drug Resistance, 87903-87904
Homogenization, 87176
Toxin
Antitoxin, 87230
Toxin Virus, 87252, 87253
Tubercle Bacilli, 87116
Tumor Tissue
Chromosome Analysis, 88239
Typing, 87140-87158
Culture, 87140-87158
Unlisted Services and Procedures, 87999
Yeast, 87106
Curettage
See Dilation and Curettage
Anal Fissure, 46940
Cervix
Endocervical, 57454, 57456, 57505
Cornea, 65435, 65436
Chelating Agent, 65436
Dentoalveolar, 41830
Hydatidiform Mole, 59870
Postpartum, 59160
Uterus
Endometrial, 58356
Postpartum, 59160
Curettage and Dilatation
See Dilation and Curettage
Curettage, Uterus
See Uterus, Curettage

Curettement
Skin Lesion, 11055-11057, 17004, 17110, 17270, 17280
Benign Hyperkeratotic Lesion, 11055-11057
Malignant, 17260-17264, 17266, 17270-17274, 17280-17284, 17286
Premalignant, 17000, 17003-17004, 17110-17111
Curietherapy
See Brachytherapy
Custodial Care
See Domiciliary Services; Nursing Facility Services
Cutaneolipectomy
See Lipectomy
Cutaneous Electrostimulation, Analgesic
See Application, Neurostimulation
Cutaneous Tag
See Skin, Tags
Cutaneous Tissue
See Integumentary System
Cutaneous–Vesicostomy
See Vesicostomy, Cutaneous
CVAD (Central Venous Access Device)
Insertion
Central, 36555-36558
Peripheral, 36568-36569
Removal, 36589
Repair, 36575
Replacement, 36580-36585
Repositioning, 36597
CVS, 59015
CXL, Collagen Cross-Linking, Cornea, 0402T
CXR, 71010-71035
Cyanide
Blood, 82600
Tissue, 82600
Cyanocobalamin, 82607, 82608
Cyclic AMP, 82030
Cyclic Citrullinated Peptide (CCP), Antibody, 86200
Cyclic Somatostatin
See Somatostatin
Cyclocryotherapy
See Cryotherapy, Destruction, Ciliary Body
Cyclodialysis
Destruction
Ciliary Body, 66740
Cyclophotocoagulation
Destruction
Ciliary Body, 66710, 66711
Cyclosporine
Assay, 80158
CYP11B1, 81405
CYP17A1, 81405
CYP1B1, 81404
CYP21A2, 81402, 81405
CYP2C19, 81225
CYP2C9, 81227
CYP2D6, 81226
CYP3A4, 81401
CYP3A5, 81401
Cyst
Abdomen
Destruction, 49203-49205
Excision, 49203-49205
Laparoscopy with Aspiration, 49322
Ankle
Capsule, 27630
Tendon Sheath, 27630
Bartholin's Gland
Excision, 56740
Marsupialization, 56440
Repair, 56440
Bile Duct
Excision, 47715
Bladder
Excision, 51500
Bone
Drainage, 20615
Injection, 20615
Brain
Drainage, 61150, 61151, 61156, 62161, 62162
Excision, 61516, 61524, 62162

Cyst — *continued*
- Branchial Cleft
  - Excision, 42810, 42815
- Breast
  - Excision, 19020
  - Puncture Aspiration, 19000, 19001
- Calcaneus, 28100-28103
- Carpal, 25130-25136
- Choledochal
  - Excision, 47715
- Ciliary Body
  - Destruction, 66770
- Clavicle
  - Excision, 23140-23146
- Conjunctiva, 68020
- Dermoid
  - Nose
    - Excision, 30124, 30125
- Drainage
  - Contrast Injection, 49424
    - with X–ray, 76080
  - Image-guided by catheter, 10030
- Enucleation
  - Mandible, 21040
  - Maxilla, 21030
  - Zygoma, 21030
- Excision
  - Cheekbone, 21030
  - Clavicle, 23140
    - with Allograft, 23146
    - with Autograft, 23145
  - Femur, 27065-27067, 27355-27358
  - Foot, 28090
  - Ganglion
    - *See* Ganglion
  - Hand
    - Capsule, 26160
    - Tendon Sheath, 26160
  - Humerus, 24120-24126
    - Proximal, 23150-23156
  - Hydatid
    - *See* Echinococcosis
  - Lymphatic
    - *See* Lymphocele
  - Maxilla, 21030
  - Mediastinum, 32662
  - Mouth
    - Dentoalveolar, 41800
    - Lingual, 41000
    - Masticator Space, 41009, 41018
    - Sublingual, 41005-41006, 41015
    - Submandibular, 41008, 41017
    - Submental, 41007, 41016
    - Vestibular, 40800-40801
  - Olecranon Process, 24120
    - with Allograft, 24126
    - with Autograft, 24125
  - Ovarian, 58925
  - Pancreas
    - Anastomosis, 48520, 48540
    - Excision, 48120
    - Marsupialization, 48500
  - Pericardial, 32661
    - Resection, 33050
  - Pilonidal, 11770-11772
  - Radius, 24120
    - with Allograft, 24126
    - with Autograft, 24125
  - Scapula, 23140
    - with Allograft, 23146
    - with Autograft, 23145
  - Symphysis Pubis, 27065-27067
  - Ulna, 24120, 25120
    - with Allograft, 24126, 25125
    - with Autograft, 24125, 25126
  - Wrist, 25111-25112, 25130, 25135-25136
  - Zygoma, 21030
- Facial Bones
  - Excision, 21030
- Femur
  - Excision, 27065-27067, 27355-27358
- Fibula, 27635-27638
- Finger, 26210, 26215
- Ganglion
  - Aspiration/Injection, 20612

Cyst — *continued*
- Gums
  - Incision and Drainage, 41800
- Hand
  - Capsule, 26160
  - Tendon Sheath, 26160
- Hip, 27065-27067
- Humerus
  - Excision, 23150-23156, 24110
    - with Allograft, 24116
    - with Autograft, 24115
- Ileum, 27065-27067
- Incision and Drainage, 10060, 10061
  - Mouth, 41800
    - Dentoalveolar, 41800
    - Lingual, 41000
    - Masticator Space, 41009, 41018
    - Sublingual, 41005-41006
    - Submandibular, 41008, 41017
    - Submental, 41007, 41016
    - Vestibular, 40800-40801
  - Pilonidal, 10080, 10081
  - Puncture Aspiration, 10160
- Iris
  - Destruction, 66770
- Kidney
  - Ablation, 50541
  - Aspiration, 50390
  - Excision, 50280, 50290
  - Injection, 50390
  - X–ray, 74470
- Knee
  - Baker's, 27345
  - Excision, 27347
- Leg, Lower
  - Capsule, 27630
  - Tendon Sheath, 27630
- Liver
  - Aspiration, 47015
  - Incision and Drainage
    - Open, 47010
  - Marsupialization, 47300
  - Repair, 47300
- Lung
  - Incision and Drainage, 32200
  - Removal, 32140
- Lymph Node
  - Axillary
    - Cervical
      - Excision, 38550, 38555
- Mandible
  - Excision, 21040, 21046, 21047
- Maxilla, 21030, 21048-21049
- Mediastinal
  - Excision, 32662
  - Resection, 39200
- Metacarpal, 26200, 26205
- Metatarsal, 28104-28107
- Mouth
  - Dentoalveolar, 41800
  - Lingual, 41000
  - Masticator Space, 41009, 41018
  - Sublingual, 41005-41006
  - Submandibular, 41008, 41017
  - Submental, 41007, 41016
  - Vestibular, 40800-40801
- Mullerian Duct
  - Excision, 55680
- Nose
  - Excision, 30124, 30125
- Olecranon, 24120, 24125-24126
- Opening or Removal of (Incision and Drainage)
  - Acne Surgery, 10040
- Ovarian
  - Excision, 58925
  - Incision and Drainage, 58800, 58805
- Pancreas
  - Anastomosis, 48520, 48540
  - Excision, 48120
  - Marsupialization, 48500
- Pelvis
  - Aspiration, 50390
  - Injection, 50390
- Pericardial
  - Excision, 33050

Cyst — *continued*
- Phalanges
  - Finger, 26210, 26215
  - Toe, 28092, 28108
- Pilonidal
  - Excision, 11770-11772
  - Incision and Drainage, 10080, 10081
- Pubis, 27065-27067
- Radius
  - Excision, 24120, 25120-25126
- Rathke's Pouch
  - *See* Craniopharyngioma
- Removal
  - Skin, 10040
- Retroperitoneum
  - Destruction, 49203-49205
  - Excision, 49203-49205
- Salivary Gland
  - Drainage, 42409
  - Excision, 42408
  - Marsupialization, 42409
- Scapula
  - Excision, 23140-23146
- Seminal Vesicles
  - Excision, 55680
- Skene's Gland
  - Destruction, 53270
  - Drainage, 53060
- Skin
  - Incision and Drainage, 10060-10061
  - Puncture Aspiration, 10160
  - Removal, 10040
- Spinal Cord
  - Aspiration, 62268
  - Incision and Drainage, 63172, 63173
- Sublingual Gland
  - Drainage, 42409
  - Excision, 42408
- Symphysis Pubis, 27065-27067
- Talus, 28100-28103
- Tarsal, 28104-28107
- Thyroglossal Duct
  - Excision, 60280, 60281
  - Incision and Drainage, 60000
- Thyroid Gland
  - Aspiration, 60300
  - Excision, 60200
  - Injection, 60300
- Tibia
  - Excision, 27635-27638
- Toe, 28108
- Tongue
  - Incision and Drainage, 41000-41009
- Ulna, 24120, 25120-25126
- Urachal
  - Bladder
    - Excision, 51500
- Vaginal
  - Biopsy, 57105
  - Excision, 57135
- Wrist, 25130-25136
  - Excision, 25111-25112
- Zygoma
  - Excision, 21030

Cystatin C, 82610
Cystatins, Kininogen
- *See* Kininogen
Cystectomy
- Complete, 51570
  - with Bilateral Pelvic Lymphadenectomy, 51575, 51585, 51595
  - with Continent Diversion, 51596
  - with Ureteroileal Conduit, 51590
  - with Ureterosigmoidostomy, 51580
- Ovarian
  - Laparoscopic, 58662
  - Open, 58925
- Partial, 51550
  - Complicated, 51555
  - Reimplantation of Ureters, 51565
  - Simple, 51550
Cystic Fibrosis
- Genomic Sequence Analysis, 81412
- Transmembrane Conductance Regulator Gene
  - Analysis, 81220-81224

Cystic Hygroma
- *See* Hygroma
Cystine
- Urine, 82615
Cystitis
- Interstitial, 52260, 52265
Cystography, 74430
- Injection, 52281
  - Radiologic, 51600, 74430
Cystolithotomy, 51050
Cystometrogram, 51725-51729
Cystoplasty, 51800
Cystorrhaphy, 51860, 51865
Cystoscopy, 52000
- with Ureteroneocystostomy, 50947
Cystoscopy, with Biopsy
- *See* Biopsy, Bladder, Cystourethroscopy
Cystostomy
- with Drainage, 51040
- with Fulguration, 51020
- with Insertion
  - Radioactive Material, 51020
- with Urethrectomy
  - Female, 53210
  - Male, 53215
- Change Tube, 51705, 51710
- Closure, 51880
- Destruction Intravesical Lesion, 51030
- Home Visit, 99505
Cystotomy
- with Calculus Basket Extraction, 51065
- with Destruction Intravesical Lesion, 51030
- with Drainage, 51040
- with Fulguration, 51020
- with Insertion
  - Radioactive Material, 51020
  - Urethral Catheter, 51045
- with Removal Calculus, 51050, 51065
- Excision
  - Bladder Diverticulum, 51525
  - Bladder Tumor, 51530
  - Diverticulum, 51525
  - Repair of Ureterocele, 51535
  - Vesical Neck, 51520
- Repair Ureterocele, 51535
Cystourethrogram, Retrograde, 51610
Cystourethropexy, 51840-51841
Cystourethroplasty, 51800, 51820
- Radiofrequency Micro-Remodeling, 53860
Cystourethroscopy, 52000, 52320-52355, 52601, 52647, 52648, 53500
- with Direct Vision Internal Urethrotomy, 52276
- with Duct Radiography, 52010
- with Ejaculatory Duct Catheterization, 52010
- with Fulguration, 52214, 52354
  - Congenital Obstructive Mucosal Folds, 52400
  - Lesion, 52224
  - Polyps, 52285
  - Tumor, 52234-52240
  - Ureterocele(s), 52300-52301
  - Urethral Valves, 52400
- with Internal Urethrotomy, 52630, 52647-52649
  - Female, 52270, 52285
  - Male, 52275
- with Prostate
  - Insertion Transprostatic Implant, 52441-52442
  - Laser Coagulation, 52647
  - Laser Enucleation, 52649
  - Laser Vaporization, 52648
- with Steroid Injection, 52283
- with Ureteropyelography, 52005
- with Ureteroscopy, 52351
- with Urethral Catheterization, 52005
- with Urethral Meatotomy, 52290, 52300, 52305
- Biopsy, 52204, 52224, 52250, 52354
- Brush, 52007
- Calibration and/or Dilation Urethral Stricture
  - or Stenosis, 52281, 52630, 52647-52649
- Catheterization
  - Ejaculatory Duct, 52010
  - Ureteral, 52005
- Chemodenervation of Bladder, 52287
- Destruction
  - Lesion, 52400

Cystourethroscopy — continued
Dilation
Bladder, 52260, 52265
Intra–Renal Stricture, 52343, 52346
Ureter, 52341, 52342, 52344, 52345
Urethra, 52281, 52285
Evacuation
Clot, 52001
Examination, 52000
Female Urethral Syndrome, 52285
Incision
Bladder Neck, 52285
Congenital Obstructive Mucosal Folds, 52400
Diverticulum, 52305
Ejaculatory Duct, 52402
Urethral Valves, 52400
Injection
for Cystography, 52281
Implant Material, 52327
Insertion
Indwelling Urethral Stent, 52282, 52332
Radioactive Substance, 52250
Ureteral Guide Wire, 52334
Urethral Stent, 52282
Instillation, 52005, 52010
Irrigation, 52005, 52010
Lithotripsy, 52353
with Ureteral Stent, [52356]
Lysis
Urethra, 53500
Urethrovaginal Septal Fibrosis, 52285
Manipulation of Ureteral Calculus, 52330, 52352
Meatotomy
Ureteral, 52290
Urethral, 52281, 52285, 52630, 52647-52649
Removal
Calculus, 52310, 52315, 52320, 52325, 52352
Foreign Body, 52310, 52315
Urethral Stent, 52310, 52315
Resection
Congenital Obstructive Mucosal Folds, 52400
Diverticulum, 52305
Ejaculatory Duct, 52402
External Sphincter, 52277
Prostate, 52601, 52630
Tumor, 52234-52235, 52240, 52355
Ureterocele(s), 52300-52301
Urethral Valves, 52400
Treatment
Lesion(s), 52224
Ureteral Stricture, 52341
Urethral Syndrome, 52285
Vasectomy
Transurethral, 52402, 52630, 52647-52649
Vasotomy
Transurethral, 52402
Cytochrome Gene Analysis, 81225-81227
Cytochrome, Reductase, Lactic
See Lactic Dehydrogenase
Cytogenetic Study
Bone Marrow
Breakage Syndromes
See Chromosome Analysis
Diagnostic, 3155F
Neoplastic Disorder, 88237
Interpretation and Report, 88291
Molecular DNA Probe, 88271-88275, 88291, 88365
Non-neoplastic Disorders
Amniotic Fluid, 88235
Chorionic Villus Cells, 88235
Lymphocyte, 88230
Skin or Tissue Biopsy, 88233
Unlisted Services and Procedures, 88299
Cytogenomic Constitutional Microarray Analysis, 81228-81229, 81406
Cytogenomic Microarray Analysis, 81406
Chromosome 22q13, 81405
X chromosome, 81405
Cytomegalovirus
Antibody, 86644, 86645

Cytomegalovirus — continued
Antigen Detection
Direct Fluorescence, 87271
Enzyme Immunoassay, 87332
Nucleic Acid, 87495-87497
Cytometries, Flow
See Flow Cytometry
Cytopathology
Cervical or Vaginal
Requiring Interpretation by Physician, 88141
Thin Layer Prep, 88142-88143, 88174-88175
Concentration Technique, 88108
Evaluation, 88172-88173, [88177]
Hormone Evaluation, 88155
Immediate Cytohistologic Study, 88172 [88177]
Fine Needle Aspirate, 88172-88173 [88177]
Fluids, Washings, Brushings, 88104-88108
Forensic, 88125
Other Source, 88160-88162
Pap, 88164-88167
Selective Cellular Enhancement Technique, 88112
Smears
Brushings, 88104
Cervical or Vaginal, 88141-88155, 88164-88167, 88174-88175
Manual Screen, 88150-88154, 88164-88167
Other Source, 88160-88162
Techniques
Concentration, 88108
In Situ Hybridization, 88120-88121, 88367-88368
Unlisted Services and Procedures, 88199
Urinary Tract
In Situ Hybridization Technique, 88120-88121
Cytoscopy
See Bladder, Endoscopy
Cytosol Aminopeptidase, 83670
Cytotoxic Screen
Lymphocyte, 86805, 86806
Percent Reactive Antibody (PRA), 86807, 86808
Serum Antibodies, 86807, 86808

D

D2, Vitamin
See Calciferol
Dacrocystogram
See Dacrocystography
Dacryoadenectomy
Partial, 68505
Total, 68500
Dacryocystectomy, 68520
Dacryocystography, 68850, 70170
with Nuclear Imaging, 78660
Dacryocystorhinostomy, 68720
Total
with Nasal
Sinus Endoscopy, 31239
Dacryocystostomy, 68420
Daily Living Activities
See Activities of Daily Living
D&C Yellow No. 7
See Fluorescein
Damus–Kaye–Stansel Procedure, 33606
Dana Operation, 63185, 63190
Rhizotomy, 63185, 63190
D and C (Dilation and Curettage), 59840
D and E (Dilation and Evacuation), 59841-59851
Dandy Operation, 62200
DAPTACEL, 90700
DARC, 81403
Dark Adaptation Examination, 92284
Dark Field Examination, 87164, 87166
Darrach Procedure, 25240
See Excision, Ulna, Partial
David Procedure, 33864
Day Test, 82270
DAZ/SRY, 81403
DBT, 81405-81406
DCP, 83951
DCR, 31239, 68720

DCX, 81405
DDST, 96101-96103
Death, Brain
See Brain Death
Debridement
Bone, 11044 [11047]
with Open Fracture and/or Dislocation, 11012
Brain, 62010
Burns, 16020-16030
Anesthesia, 01951-01953
Cartilage
Hip, 29862
Knee, 29877, 29880-29881, 29885
Elbow, 29837-29838
with Removal Prosthesis, 24160, 24164
Forearm, 25023, 25025
Infected Inflatable Urethral/Bladder Neck Sphincter, 53448
Infected Tissue, with Removal Penile Implant, 54411, 54417
Knee, 27441, 27443, 27497, 27499
Leg, 27892-27894
Liver, 47361
Mastoid Cavity
Complex, 69222
Simple, 69220
Metatarsophalangeal Joint, 28289, 28291, 29901-29902
Muscle, 11043-11044 [11046], 11044-11047 [11046]
with Open Fracture and/or Dislocation, 11011-11012
Infected, 11004-11006, 11008
Nails, 11720, 11721
Necrotizing Soft Tissue, 11004-11008
Nonviable Tissue, 25023, 25025, 27497, 27499, 27892-27894
Nose
Endoscopic, 31237
Pancreatic Tissue, 48105
Pathology Analysis, 88304-88305
Shoulder, 29822-29823
with Removal Prosthesis, 23334-23335
Skin
with Open Fracture and/or Dislocation, 11010-11012
Eczematous, 11000, 11001
Excision, 15920-15999
Infected, 11000-11006
Subcutaneous Tissue, 11042-11047 [11045, 11046]
Infected, 11004-11006, 11008
Necrotized, 49568
Sternum, 21627
Subcutaneous, 11042-11047 [11045, 11046]
Thigh, 27497, 27499
Wound
Non–Selective, 97602
Selective, 97597-97598
Wrist
Joint, 29846
Nonviable Tissue, 25023, 25025
Debulking Procedure
Ovary
Pelvis, 58952-58954
Decapsulation
of Kidney, 53899
DECAVAC, 90714
Declotting
Vascular Access Device, 36593
Decompression
with Nasal
Sinus Endoscopy
Optic Nerve, 31294
Orbit Wall, 31292, 31293
Arm, Lower, 24495, 25020-25025
Auditory Canal, Internal, 61591, 69960
Brainstem, 61575, 61576
Buttocks, 27057
Carotid Artery, 61590-61591
Carpal Tunnel, 64721
Cauda Equina, 63011, 63017, 63047, 63048, 63056, 63057, 63087-63091
Colon, 45378
Cranial Nerves, 61458

Decompression — continued
Esophagogastric Varices, 37181
Facial Nerve, 61590
Intratemporal
Lateral to Geniculate Ganglion, 69720, 69740
Medial to Geniculate Ganglion, 69725, 69745
Total, 69955
Transtemporal, 61595
Fasciotomy
Leg, 27892-27894
Pelvic/Buttock, 27027
with Debridement, 27057
Thigh/Knee, 27496-27499
Finger, 26035
Gasserian Ganglion
Sensory Root, 61450
Gill Type procedure, 63012
Hand, 26035, 26037
Intestines
Small, 44021
Jejunostomy
Laparoscopic, 44186-44187
Leg
Fasciotomy, 27600-27602
Nerve, 64702-64727
Laminotomy/Laminectomy, 0274T-0275T
Root, 22551-22552, 62380, 63020-63048, 63055-63103
Nucleus of Disc
Lumbar, 62287
Optic Nerve, 61564, 67570
Orbit, 61330
Removal of Bone, 67414, 67445
Pelvis/Buttock, 27027
with Debridement, 27057
Posterior Tibial Nerve, 28035
Shoulder, 29826-29828
Sigmoid Sinus, 61595
Skull, 61322-61323, 61340-61345
Spinal Cord, 0375T, 62287, 63001-63017, 63045-63103
with Arthrodesis, 22551-22552
Anterolateral Approach, 63075-63091
Endoscopic Lumbar, 62380
Osteophytectomy, 22551-22552, 22856
Posterior Approach, 63001-63048
Cauda Equina, 63001-63017
Cervical, 63001, 63015, 63020, 63035, 63045, 63048
Gill Type Procedure, 63012
Lumbar, 62380, 63005, 63017, 63030, 63042, 63047, 63048
Sacral, 63011
Thoracic, 63003, 63016, 63046, 63048
Transpedicular or Costovertebral Approach, 63055-63066
Tarsal Tunnel Release, 28035
Trachea, 33800
Volvulus, 45321, 45337
Wrist, 25020-25025
Decortication
Lung, 32220, 32225, 32320, 32651-32652
with Parietal Pleurectomy, 32320
Endoscopic, 32651, 32652
Partial, 32225
Total, 32220
Decubiti
See Decubitus Ulcers
Decubitus Ulcers
Coccygeal, 15920, 15922
Ischial, 15940-15941, 15944-15946
Sacral, 15931, 15933-15937
Trochanteric, 15950-15953, 15956, 15958
Unlisted Procedure, 15999
Deetjeen's Body
See Blood, Platelet
Defect, Coagulation
See Coagulopathy
Defect, Heart Septal
See Septal Defect
Defect, Septal Closure, Atrial
See Heart, Repair, Atrial Septum
Deferens, Ductus
See Vas Deferens

Defibrillation
See Cardioversion
Defibrillator/Defibrillator Pacemaker
Implantable
Data Analysis, 93285-93289 *[93260, 93261]*, 93289, 93295-93296
Evaluation, 93283, 93285-93289 *[93260, 93261]*, 93287, 93289, 93292, 93295-93296, 93640-93642, *[33270]*
Insertion, 33240, *[33230, 33231]*, *[33270]*
Electrodes, 33216-33217, 33224-33225, *[33271]*
Interrogation, 93289, 93295-93296, *[93261]*
Programming, 93282-93284, 93287, *[33270]*
Removal, 33233, 33241, *[33262, 33263, 33264]*
Electrode, 33243-33244, *[33272]*
Repair
Leads, Dual Chamber, 33220
Leads, Single Chamber, 33218
Replacement, 33249, *[33262]*, *[33264]*
Repositioning
Electrodes, 33215, 33226, *[33273]*
Revise Pocket Chest, 33223
Wearable Device, 93292, 93745
Deformity, Boutonniere
See Boutonniere Deformity
Deformity, Sprengel's
See Sprengel's Deformity
Degenerative, Articular Cartilage, Patella
See Chondromalacia Patella
Degradation Products, Fibrin
See Fibrin Degradation Products
Dehiscence
Suture
Abdominal Wall, 49900
Skin and Subcutaneous Tissue
Complex, 13160
Complicated, 13160
Extensive, 13160
Skin and Subcutaneous Tissue
Simple, 12020
with Packing, 12021
Superficial, 12020
with Packing, 12021
Wound
Abdominal Wall, 49900
Skin and Subcutaneous Tissue
Complex, 13160
Complicated, 13160
Extensive, 13160
Skin and Subcutaneous Tissue
Simple, 12020
with Packing, 12021
Superficial, 12020
with Packing, 12021
Dehydroepiandrosterone, 82626
Dehydroepiandrosterone–Sulfate, 82627
Dehydrogenase, 6–Phosphogluconate
See Phosphogluconate–6, Dehydrogenase
Dehydrogenase, Alcohol
See Antidiuretic Hormone
Dehydrogenase, Glucose–6–Phosphate
See Glucose–6–Phosphate, Dehydrogenase
Dehydrogenase, Glutamate
See Glutamate Dehydrogenase
Dehydrogenase, Isocitrate
See Isocitric Dehydrogenase
Dehydrogenase, Lactate
See Lactic Dehydrogenase
Dehydrogenase, Malate
See Malate Dehydrogenase
Dehydroisoandrosterone Sulfate
See Dehydroepiandrosterone Sulfate
DEK/NUP214, 81401
Delay of Flap, 15600-15630
Deligation
Ureter, 50940
Deliveries, Abdominal
See Cesarean Delivery
Delivery
See Cesarean Delivery, Vaginal Delivery
Pharmacologic Agent
Suprachoroidal, 67299
Delorme Operation, 33030

Denervation
Hip
Femoral Nerve, 27035
Obturator Nerve, 27035
Sciatic Nerve, 27035
Sympathetic
Chemodenervation, 64650, 64653
Neurolytic Agent, 64680-64681
Transcatheter Percutaneous, 0338T-0339T
Denervation, Sympathetic
See Excision, Nerve, Sympathetic
Dens Axis
See Odontoid Process
Denver Developmental Screening Test, 96101-96103
Denver Krupin Procedure, 66180
Denver Shunt
Patency Test, 78291
Deoxycorticosterone, 82633
Deoxycortisol, 80436, 82634
Deoxyephedrine
See Methamphetamine
Deoxyribonuclease
Antibody, 86215
Deoxyribonuclease I
See DNAse
Deoxyribonucleic Acid
Antibody, 86225, 86226
Depilation
See Removal, Hair
Depletion
Plasma, 38214
Platelet, 38213
T–Cell, 38210
Tumor Cell, 38211
Deposit Calcium
See Calcium, Deposits
Depression Inventory, 96127
Depth Electrode
Insertion, 61760
DeQuervain's Disease Treatment, 25000
Dermabrasion, 15780-15783
Derma–Fat–Fascia Graft, 15770
Dermatology
Actinotherapy, 96900
Examination of Hair
Microscopic, 96902
Laser Treatment for Psoriasis, 96920-96922
Photochemotherapy
Ultraviolet A Treatment, 96912-96913
Ultraviolet B Treatment, 96910, 96913
Ultraviolet A Treatment, 96912
Ultraviolet B Treatment, 96910-96913
Ultraviolet Light Treatment, 96900-96913
Unlisted Services and Procedures, 96999
Whole Body Photography, 96904
Dermatoplasty
Septal, 30620
Dermoid
See Cyst, Dermoid
Derrick–Burnet Disease
See Q Fever
DES, 81405
Descending Abdominal Aorta
See Aorta, Abdominal
Design
Collimator, 77338
IMRT Devices, 77332-77334
Desipramine
Assay, *[80335, 80336, 80337]*
Desmotomy
See Ligament, Release
Desoxycorticosterone, 82633
Desoxycortone
See Desoxycorticosterone
Desoxyephedrine
See Methamphetamine
Desoxynorephedrin
See Amphetamine
Desoxyphenobarbital
See Primidone
Desquamation
See Exfoliation
Destruction
with Cystourethroscopy, 52354
Acne, 17340, 17360

Destruction — *continued*
Acne — *continued*
Cryotherapy, 17340
Arrhythmogenic Focus
Heart, 33250, 33251, 33261
Bladder, 51020, 52214, 52224, 52354
Endoscopic, 52214
Large Tumors, 52240
Medium Tumors, 52235
Minor Lesions, 52224
Small Tumors, 52234
Calculus
Bile Duct, 43265
Kidney, 50590
Pancreatic Duct, 43265
Chemical Cauterization
Granulation Tissue, 17250
Chemosurgery, 17110-17111
Ciliary Body
Cryotherapy, 66720
Cyclodialysis, 66740
Cyclophotocoagulation, 66710, 66711
Diathermy, 66740
Endoscopic, 66711
Condyloma
Anal, 46900-46924
Penis, 54050-54065
Vagina, 57061-57065
Vulva, 56501-56515
Cryosurgery, 17110-17111
Curettement, 17110-17111
Cyst
Abdomen, 49203-49205
Ciliary Body, 66740, 66770
Iris, 66770
Retroperitoneal, 49203-49205
Electrosurgery, 17110-17111
Endometrial Ablation, 58356
Endometriomas
Abdomen, 49203-49205
Retroperitoneal, 49203-49205
Fissure
Anal, 46940, 46942
Hemorrhoids
Thermal, 46930
Kidney, 52354
Endoscopic, 50557, 50576
Laser Surgery, 17110-17111
Lesion
Anus, 46900-46917, 46924
Bladder, 51030
Choroid, 67220-67225
Ciliary Body, 66770
Colon, *[44401]*, *[45388]*
Conjunctiva, 68135
Cornea, 65450
Eyelid, 67850
Facial, 17000-17108, 17280-17286
Gastrointestinal, Upper, *[43270]*
Gums, 41850
Intestines
Large, *[44401]*, *[45388]*
Small, 44369
Iris, 66770
Mouth, 40820
Nerve
Celiac Plexus, 64680
Inferior Alveolar, 64600
Infraorbital, 64600
Intercostal, 64620
Mental, 64600
Other Peripheral, 64640
Paravertebral Facet Joint, *[64633, 64634, 64635, 64636]*
Plantar, 64632
Pudendal, 64630
Superior Hypogastric Plexus, 64681
Supraorbital, 64600
Trigeminal, 64600, 64605, 64610
Nose
Intranasal, 30117, 30118
Palate, 42160
Penis
Cryosurgery, 54056
Electrodesiccation, 54055
Extensive, 54065

Destruction — *continued*
Lesion — *continued*
Penis — *continued*
Laser Surgery, 54057
Simple, 54050-54060
Surgical Excision, 54060
Pharynx, 42808
Prostate, 45320
Thermotherapy, 53850-53852
Microwave, 53850
Radio Frequency, 53852
Rectum, 45320
Retina
Cryotherapy, Diathermy, 67208, 67227
Photocoagulation, 67210, 67228-67229
Radiation by Implantation of Source, 67218
Skin
Benign, 17110-17111
Cutaneous Vascular, 17106-17108
Malignant, 17260-17286
by Photodynamic Therapy, 96567
Photodynamic Therapy, 96567
Premalignant, 17000-17004
by Photodynamic Therapy, 96567
Spinal Cord, 62280-62282
Ureter, 52341, 52342, 52344, 52345
Urethra, 52400, 53265
Uvula, 42160
Vagina
Extensive, 57065
Simple, 57061
Vascular, Cutaneous, 17106-17108
Vulva
Extensive, 56515
Simple, 56501
Molluscum Contagiosum, 17110, 17111
Muscle Endplate
Extraocular, 67345
Extremity, 64642-64645
Facial, 64612
Neck Muscle, 64616
Trunk, 64646-64647
Nerve, 64600-64681 *[64633, 64634, 64635, 64636]*
Laryngeal, Recurrent, 31595
Paravertebral Facet, *[64633, 64634, 64635, 64636]*
Neurofibroma, 0419T-0420T
Plantar Common Digital Nerve, 64632
Polyp
Aural, 69540
Nasal, 30110, 30115
Rectum, 45320
Urethra, 53260
Prostate, 55873
Prostate Tissue
Transurethral
Thermotherapy, 53850-53852
Sinus
Frontal, 31080-31085
Skene's Gland, 53270
Skin Lesion
Benign
Fifteen Lesions or More, 17111
Fourteen Lesions or Less, 17110
Malignant, 17260-17286
by Photodynamic Therapy, 96567
Premalignant, 17000-17004
by Photodynamic Therapy, 96567
Fifteen or More Lesions, 17004
First Lesion, 17000
Two to Fourteen Lesions, 17003
Skin Tags, 11200, 11201
Tonsil
Lingual, 42870
Tumor
Abdomen, 49203-49205
Bile Duct, *[43278]*
Breast, 0301T
Chemosurgery, 17311-17315
Colon, *[44401]*, *[45388]*
Intestines
Large, *[44401]*, *[45388]*
Small, 44369
Mesentery, 49203-49205

Destruction — *continued*
 Tumor — *continued*
  Pancreatic Duct, *[43278]*
  Peritoneum, 49203-49205
  Rectum, 45190, 45320
  Retroperitoneal, 49203-49205
  Urethra, 53220
 Tumor or Polyp
  Rectum, 45320
 Turbinate Mucosa, 30801, 30802
 Unlisted Services and Procedures, 17999
 Ureter
  Endoscopic, 50957, 50976
 Urethra, 52214, 52224, 52354
  Prolapse, 53275
 Warts
  Flat, 17110, 17111
Determination
 Lung Volume, 94727-94728
Determination, Blood Pressure
 See Blood Pressure
Developmental
 Screening, 96110
 Testing, 96111
Device
 Adjustable Gastric Restrictive Device, 43770-43774
 Aortic Counterpulsation Ventricular Assist, 0451T-0463T
 Contraceptive, Intrauterine
  Insertion, 58300
  Removal, 58301
 Handling, 99002
 Iliac Artery Occlusion Device
  Insertion, 34808
 Intrauterine
  Insertion, 58300
  Removal, 58301
 Multi-leaf Collimator Design and Construction, 77338
 Programming, 93644, *[93260]*, *[93261]*
 Subcutaneous Port
  for Gastric Restrictive Device, 43770, 43774, 43886-43888
 Venous Access
  Collection of Blood Specimen, 36591-36592
   Implanted, 36591
   Venous Catheter, 36592
  Fluoroscopic Guidance, 77001
  Insertion
   Catheter, 36578
   Central, 36560-36566
   Imaging, 75901, 75902
   Obstruction Clearance, 36595, 36596
   Peripheral, 36570, 36571
   Removal, 36590
   Repair, 36576
   Replacement, 36582, 36583, 36585
  Irrigation, 96523
  Obstruction Clearance, 36595-36596
   Imaging, 75901-75902
  Removal, 36590
  Repair, 36576
  Replacement, 36582-36583, 36585
   Catheter, 36578
  Ventricular Assist, 0451T-0463T, 33975-33983, 33990-33993
Device, Orthotic
 See Orthotics
Dexamethasone
 Suppression Test, 80420
DFNB59, 81405
D Galactose
 See Galactose
D Glucose
 See Glucose
DGUOK, 81405
DHA Sulfate
 See Dehydroepiandrosterone Sulfate
DHCR7, 81405
DHEA (Dehydroepiandrosterone), 82626
DHEAS, 82627
DHT (Dihydrotestosterone), *[80327, 80328]*
Diagnosis, Psychiatric
 See Psychiatric Diagnosis

Diagnostic Amniocentesis
 See Amniocentesis
Diagnostic Aspiration of Anterior Chamber of Eye
 See Eye, Paracentesis, Anterior Chamber, with Diagnostic Aspiration of Aqueous
Dialysis
 Arteriovenous Fistula
  Revision
   without Thrombectomy, 36832
  Thrombectomy, 36831
 Arteriovenous Shunt, 36901-36909
  Revision
   with Thrombectomy, 36833
  Thrombectomy, 36831
 Dialysis Circuit, 36901-36909
 Documentation of Nephropathy Treatment, 3066F
 End Stage Renal Disease, 90951-90953, 90963, 90967
 Hemodialysis, 90935, 90937
  Blood Flow Study, 90940
  Plan of Care Documented, 0505F
 Hemoperfusion, 90997
 Hepatitis B Vaccine, 90740, 90747
 Kt/V Level, 3082F-3084F
 Patient Training
  Completed Course, 90989
  Per Session, 90993
 Peritoneal, 4055F, 90945, 90947
  Catheter Insertion, 49418-49421
  Catheter Removal, 49422
  Home Infusion, 99601-99602
  Plan of Care Documented, 0507F
 Unlisted Procedures, 90999
DI–Amphetamine
 See Amphetamine
Diaphragm
 Anesthesia, 00540
  Hernia Repair, 00756
 Assessment, 58943, 58960
 Imbrication for Eventration, 39545
 Repair
  Esophageal Hiatal, 43280-43282, 43325
  for Eventration, 39545
  Hernia, 39503-39541
   Neonatal, 39503
  Laceration, 39501
 Resection, 39560, 39561
 Unlisted Procedures, 39599
 Vagina
  Fitting, 57170
Diaphragm Contraception, 57170
Diaphysectomy
 Calcaneus, 28120
 Clavicle, 23180
 Femur, 27360
 Fibula, 27360, 27641
 Humerus, 23184, 24140
 Metacarpal, 26230
 Metatarsal, 28122
 Olecranon Process, 24147
 Phalanges
  Finger, 26235, 26236
  Toe, 28124
 Radius, 24145, 25151
 Scapula, 23182
 Talus, 28120
 Tarsal, 28122
 Tibia, 27360, 27640
 Ulna, 24147, 25150
Diastase
 See Amylase
Diastasis
 See Separation
Diathermy, 97024
 See Physical Medicine/ Therapy/Occupational
 Destruction
  Ciliary Body, 66700
 Lesion
  Retina, 67208, 67227
 Retinal Detachment
  Prophylaxis, 67141
 Treatment, 97024
Diathermy, Surgical
 See Electrocautery

Dibucaine Number, 82638
Dichloride, Methylene
 See Dichloromethane
Dichlorides, Ethylene
 See Dichloroethane
Dichloroethane, 82441
Dichloromethane, 82441
Diethylamide, Lysergic Acid
 See Lysergic Acid Diethylamide
Differential Count
 White Blood Cell Count, 85007, 85009, 85540
Differentiation Reversal Factor
 See Prothrombin
Diffusing Capacity, 94729
Diffusion Test, Gel
 See Immunodiffusion
Digestive Tract
 See Gastrointestinal Tract
Digit(s)
 See also Finger, Toe
 Nerve
  Destruction, 64632
  Injection, 64455
 Pinch Graft, 15050
 Replantation, 20816, 20822
 Skin Graft
  Split, 15120, 15121
Digital Artery Sympathectomy, 64820
Digital Slit–Beam Radiograph
 See Scanogram
Digoxin
 Assay, 80162-80163
 Blood or Urine, 80162
Dihydrocodeinone
 Definitive Testing, 80305-80307, *[80361]*
Dihydrohydroxycodeinone
 See Oxycodinone
Dihydromorphinone, 80305-80307, *[80361]*
Dihydrotestosterone, *[80327, 80328]*
Dihydroxyethanes
 See Ethylene Glycol
Dihydroxyvitamin D, *[82652]*
Dilation
 See Dilation and Curettage
 Anal
  Endoscopic, 46604
  Sphincter, 45905, 46940
 Aortic Valve, 33390-33391
 Aqueous Outflow Canal, 66174-66175
 Bile Duct
  Endoscopic, 47555, 47556, *[43277]*
  Percutaneous, 74363
  Stricture, 74363
 Bladder
  Cystourethroscopy, 52260, 52265
 Bronchi
  Endoscopy, 31630, 31636-31638
 Cerebral Vessels
  Intracranial Vasospasm, 61640-61642
 Cervix
  Canal, 57800
  Stump, 57558
 Colon
  Endoscopy, 45386
 Colon–Sigmoid
  Endoscopy, 45340
 Curettage, 57558
 Enterostomy Stoma, 44799
 Esophagus, 43450, 43453
  Endoscopic Balloon, 43195, 43220, 43249, *[43213, 43214]*, *[43233]*
  Endoscopy, 43195-43196, 43220, 43226, 43248-43249, *[43213, 43214]*, *[43233]*
  Surgical, 43510
 Frontonasal Duct, 30999
 Gastric/Duodenal Stricture, 43245
  Open, 43510
 Intestines, Small
  Endoscopy, 44370
  Open, 44615
  Stent Placement, 44379
 Intracranial Vasospasm, 61640-61642
 Kidney, 50080-50081, 50395
  Intra–Renal Stricture, 52343, 52346
 Lacrimal Punctum, 68801

Dilation — *continued*
 Larynx
  Endoscopy, 31528, 31529
 Nasolacrimal Duct
  Balloon Catheter, 68816
 Nose
  Balloon, 31295-31297
 Pancreatic Duct
  Endoscopy, *[43277]*
 Rectum
  Endoscopy, 45303
  Sphincter, 45910
 Salivary Duct, 42650, 42660
 Sinus Ostium, 31295-31297
 Trachea
  Endoscopic, 31630, 31631, 31636-31638
 Transluminal
  Aqueous Outflow Canal, 66174-66175
 Ureter, 50395, 50706, 52341-52342, 52344-52346
  Endoscopic, 50553, 50572, 50575, 50953, 50972
 Urethra, 52260, 52265
  with Prostatectomy, 55801, 55821
  with Prostate Resection, 52601, 52630, 52647-52649
  Female Urethral Syndrome, 52285
  General, 53665
  Suppository and/or Instillation, 53660-53661
 Urethral
  Stenosis, 52281
  Stricture, 52281, 53600-53621
 Vagina, 57400
Dilation and Curettage
 See Curettage; Dilation
 Cervical Stump, 57558
 Cervix, 57520, 57522, 57558, 57800
 Corpus Uteri, 58120
 Hysteroscopy, 58558
 Induced Abortion, 59840
  with Amniotic Injections, 59851
  with Vaginal Suppositories, 59856
 Postpartum, 59160
Dilation and Evacuation, 59841
 with Amniotic Injections, 59851
 with Vaginal Suppository, 59856
Dimethadione, *[80339, 80340, 80341]*
Dioxide, Carbon
 See Carbon Dioxide
Dioxide Silicon
 See Silica
Dipeptidyl Peptidase A
 See Angiotensin Converting Enzyme (ACE)
Diphenylhydantoin
 See Phenytoin
Diphosphate, Adenosine
 See Adenosine Diphosphate
Diphtheria
 Antibody, 86648
 Immunization, 90696-90698, 90700-90702, 90714-90715, 90723
Dipropylacetic Acid
 Assay, 80164
 See Also Valproic Acid
Direct Pedicle Flap
 Formation, 15570-15576
 Transfer, 15570-15576, 15650
Disability Evaluation Services
 Basic Life and/or Disability Evaluation, 99450
 Work–Related or Medical Disability Evaluation, 99455, 99456
Disarticulation
 Ankle, 27889
 Elbow, 20999
 Hip, 27295
 Knee, 27598
 Mandible, 61590
 Shoulder, 23920, 23921
 Wrist, 25920, 25924
  Revision, 25922
Disarticulation of Shoulder
 See Shoulder, Disarticulation
Disc Chemolyses, Intervertebral
 See Chemonucleolysis

Discectomies
  See Discectomy
Discectomies, Percutaneous
  See Discectomy, Percutaneous
Discectomy
  with Endplate Preparation, 22856
    with Osteophytectomy, 22856
  Additional Segment, 22226
  Anterior with Decompression
    Cervical Interspace, 63075
      Each Additional, 63076
    Thoracic Interspace, 63077
      Each Additional, 63078
  Arthrodesis
    Additional Interspace, 22534, 22585, 22634
    Cervical, 0375T, 22551-22552, 22554,
      22585, 22856, 63075-63076
    Lumbar, 0163T-0164T, 0195T-0196T, 0309T,
      22533, 22558, 22585, 22630, 22633-
      22634, 22857
    Sacral, 0195T, 22586
    Thoracic, 22532, 22534, 22556, 22585,
      63077-63078
    Vertebra
      Cervical, 22554
  Cervical, 22220
  Endoscopic Lumbar, 62380
  Lumbar, 22224, 22630, 62380
  Percutaneous, 0274T-0275T
  Sacral, 0195T, 22586
  Thoracic, 22222
    Additional Segment, 22226
Discharge, Body Substance
  See Drainage
Discharge Instructions
  Heart Failure, 4014F
Discharge Services
  See Hospital Services
  Hospital, 99238, 99239
  Newborn, 99463
  Nursing Facility, 99315, 99316
  Observation Care, 99217, 99234-99236
Disc, Intervertebral
  See Intervertebral Disc
Discission
  Cataract
    Laser Surgery, 66821
    Stab Incision, 66820
  Hyaloid Membrane, 65810
  Vitreous Strands, 67030
Discography
  Cervical Disc, 72285
  Injection, 62290, 62291
  Lumbar Disc, 62287, 72295
  Thoracic, 72285
Discolysis
  See Chemonucleolysis
Disease
  Durand–Nicolas–Favre
    See Lymphogranuloma Venereum
  Erb–Goldflam
    See Myasthenia Gravis
  Heine–Medin
    See Polio
  Hydatid
    See Echinococcosis
  Lyme
    See Lyme Disease
  Ormond
    See Retroperitoneal Fibrosis
  Peyronie
    See Peyronie Disease
  Posada–Wernicke
    See Coccidioidomycosis
Disease/Organ Panel
  See Organ/Disease Panel
Diskectomy
  See Discectomy
Dislocated Elbow
  See Dislocation, Elbow
Dislocated Hip
  See Dislocation, Hip Joint
Dislocated Jaw
  See Dislocation, Temporomandibular Joint
Dislocated Joint
  See Dislocation

Dislocated Shoulder
  See Dislocation, Shoulder
Dislocation
  with Debridement, 11010-11012
  Acromioclavicular Joint
    Closed Treatment, 23540, 23545
    Open Treatment, 23550, 23552
  Ankle Joint
    Closed Treatment, 27840, 27842
    Open Treatment, 27846, 27848
  Carpal
    Closed Treatment, 25690
    Open Treatment, 25695
  Carpometacarpal Joint
    Closed Treatment, 26641, 26645, 26670
      with Anesthesia, 26675
    Open Treatment, 26665, 26685, 26686
    Percutaneous Fixation, 26676
    Thumb, 26641
      Bennett Fracture, 26650, 26665
  Clavicle
    with Manipulation, 23545
    without Manipulation, 23540
    Closed Treatment, 23540, 23545
    Open Treatment, 23550, 23552
  Elbow
    with Manipulation, 24620, 24640
    Closed Treatment, 24600, 24605
      Monteggia, 24620, 24635
    Open Treatment, 24586-24587, 24615
  Finger(s)/Hand
    Interphalangeal, 26770-26785
    Metacarpal Except Thumb, 26670-26686
  Hand
    Carpal
      Closed, 25690
      Open, 25695
    Carpometacarpal
      Closed, 26670, 26675
      Open, 26685-26686
      Percutaneous, 26676
      Thumb, 26641, 26650, 26665
    Interphalangeal joint
      Closed, 26770, 26775
      Open, 26785
      Percutaneous, 26776
    Lunate
      Closed, 25690
      Open, 26715
      Percutaneous, 26705
    Metacarpophalangeal
      Closed, 26700-26705
      Open, 26715
      Percutaneous, 26705
    Radiocarpal
      Closed, 25660
      Open, 25670
    Thumb
      See Dislocation, thumb
    Wrist
      See Dislocation, Wrist
  Hip Joint
    without Trauma, 27265, 27266
    Closed Treatment, 27250, 27252, 27265,
      27266
    Congenital, 27256-27259
    Open Treatment, 27253, 27254, 27258,
      27259
  Interphalangeal Joint
    Finger(s)/Hand
      Closed Treatment, 26770, 26775
      Open Treatment, 26785
      Percutaneous Fixation, 26776
    Toe(s)/Foot, 28660-28675
      Closed Treatment, 28660, 28665
      Open Treatment, 28675
      Percutaneous Fixation, 28666
  Knee
    Closed Treatment, 27550, 27552
    Open Treatment, 27556-27558, 27566,
      27730
    Patella, 27560-27562
    Recurrent, 27420-27424
  Lunate
    with Manipulation, 25690, 26670-26676,
      26700-26706

Dislocation — continued
  Lunate — continued
    Closed Treatment, 25690
    Open Treatment, 25695
  Metacarpophalangeal Joint
    Closed Treatment, 26700-26706
    Open Treatment, 26715
  Metatarsophalangeal Joint
    Closed Treatment, 28630, 28635
    Open Treatment, 28645
    Percutaneous Fixation, 28636
  Patella
    Closed Treatment, 27560, 27562
    Open Treatment, 27566
    Recurrent, 27420-27424
  Pelvic Ring
    Closed Treatment, 27197-27198
    Open Treatment, 27217, 27218
    Percutaneous Fixation, 27216
  Percutaneous Fixation
    Metacarpophalangeal, 26705
  Peroneal Tendons, 27675, 27676
  Radiocarpal Joint
    Closed Treatment, 25660
    Open Treatment, 25670
  Radioulnar Joint
    Closed Treatment, 25675
      with Radial Fracture, 25520
    Galeazzi, 25520, 25525-25526
    Open Treatment, 25676
      with Radial Fracture, 25525, 25526
  Radius
    with Fracture, 24620, 24635
      Closed Treatment, 24620
      Open Treatment, 24635
    Closed Treatment, 24640
  Shoulder
    Closed Treatment
      with Manipulation, 23650, 23655
        with Fracture of Greater Humeral
          Tuberosity, 23665
        with Surgical or Anatomical Neck
          Fracture, 23675
    Open Treatment, 23660
    Recurrent, 23450-23466
  Sternoclavicular Joint
    Closed Treatment
      with Manipulation, 23525
      without Manipulation, 23520
    Open Treatment, 23530, 23532
  Talotarsal Joint
    Closed Treatment, 28570, 28575
    Open Treatment, 28546
    Percutaneous Fixation, 28576
  Tarsal
    Closed Treatment, 28540, 28545
    Open Treatment, 28555
    Percutaneous Fixation, 28545, 28546
  Tarsometatarsal Joint
    Closed Treatment, 28600, 28605
    Open Treatment, 28615
    Percutaneous Fixation, 28606
  Temporomandibular Joint
    Closed Treatment, 21480, 21485
    Open Treatment, 21490
  Thumb
    with Fracture, 26645
      Open Treatment, 26665
      Percutaneous Fixation, 26650, 26665
    with Manipulation, 26641-26650
    Closed Treatment, 26641, 26645
    Open Treatment, 26665
    Percutaneous Fixation, 26650
  Tibiofibular Joint
    Closed Treatment, 27830, 27831
    Open Treatment, 27832
  Toe
    Closed Treatment, 26770, 26775, 28630-
      28635
    Open Treatment, 28645
    Percutaneous Fixation, 26776, 28636
  Trans-scaphoperilunar, 25680
    Closed Treatment, 25680
    Open Treatment, 25685

Dislocation — continued
  Vertebrae
    Additional Segment, Any Level
      Open Treatment, 22328
    Cervical
      Open Treatment, 22318-22319, 22326
      Closed Treatment
        with Manipulation, Casting and/or
          Bracing, 22315
        without Manipulation, 22310
    Lumbar
      Open Treatment, 22325
    Thoracic
      Open Treatment, 22327
  Wrist
    with Fracture
      Closed Treatment, 25680
      Open Treatment, 25685
    Intercarpal
      Closed Treatment, 25660
      Open Treatment, 25670
    Percutaneous, 25671
    Radiocarpal
      Closed Treatment, 25660
      Open Treatment, 25670
    Radioulnar
      Closed Treatment, 25675
      Open Treatment, 25676
      Percutaneous Fixation, 25671
Disorder
  Blood Coagulation
    See Coagulopathy
  Penis
    See Penis
  Retinal
    See Retina
Displacement Therapy
  Nose, 30210
Dissection
  Axial Vessel for Island Pedicle Flap, 15740
  Cavernous Sinus, 61613
  Cranial Adhesions, 62161
  Donor Organs
    Heart, 33944
    Heart/Lung, 33933
    Kidney, 50323, 50325
    Liver, 47143
    Lung, 32855
    Pancreas, 48551
  for Debulking Malignancy, 58952-58954
  Hygroma, Cystic
    Axillary, 38550, 38555
    Cervical, 38550, 38555
  Infrarenal Aneurysm, 34800, 34802, 34825-
    34826, 34830-34832
  Lymph Nodes, 38542
  Mediastinal, 60521-60522
  Neurovascular, 32503
  Sclera, 67107
  Urethra, 54328, 54332, 54336, 54348, 54352
Dissection, Neck, Radical
  See Radical Neck Dissection
Distention
  See Dilation
Diverticulectomy, 44800
  Esophagus, 43130, 43135
Diverticulectomy, Meckel's
  See Meckel's Diverticulum, Excision
Diverticulopexy
  Esophagus, 43499
  Pharynx, 43499
Diverticulum
  Bladder
    See Bladder, Diverticulum
  Meckel's
    Excision, 44800
    Unlisted Procedure, 44899
  Repair
    Excision, 53230, 53235
    Large Intestine, 44604-44605
    Marsupialization, 53240
    Small Intestine, 44602-44603
    Urethroplasty, 53400, 53405
Division
  Anal Sphincter, 46080
  Flap, 15600, 15610, 15620, 15630

Index

Division — Drainage

Division — continued
Intrauterine Septum, 58560
Muscle
Foot, 28250
Neck
Scalenus Anticus, 21700, 21705
Sternocleidomastoid, 21720, 21725
Plantar Fascia
Foot, 28250
Rectal Stricture, 45150
Saphenous Vein, 37700, 37718, 37722, 37735
Division, Isthmus, Horseshoe Kidney
See Symphysiotomy, Horseshoe Kidney
Division, Scalenus Anticus Muscle
See Muscle Division, Scalenus Anticus
DLAT, 81406
DLD, 81406
DMD (Dystrophin), 81408, [81161]
DMO
See Dimethadione
DMPK, 81401, 81404
DNA Antibody, 86225, 86226
DNA Endonuclease
See DNAse
DNA Probe
See Cytogenetics Studies; Nucleic Acid Probe
DNAse, 86215
DNAse Antibody, 86215
DNMT3A, 81403
Domiciliary Services
See Nursing Facility Services
Assisted Living, 99339-99340
Care Plan Oversight, 99339-99340
Discharge Services, 99315, 99316
Established Patient, 99334-99337
New Patient, 99324-99328
Supervision, 99374-99375
Donor Procedures
Backbench Preparation Prior to Transplantation
Intestine, 44715-44721
Kidney, 50323-50329
Liver, 47143-47147
Pancreas, 48551-48552
Bone Harvesting, 20900-20902
Bone Marrow Harvesting, 38230, 38232
Conjunctival Graft, 68371
Heart Excision, 33940
Heart–Lung Excision, 33930
Intestine, 44132-44133
Kidney, 50300, 50320
Liver, 47133, 47140-47142
Lung, 32850
Mucosa of Vestibule of Mouth, 40818
Pancreas, 48550
Preparation Fecal Microbiota, 44705
Stem Cells
Donor Search, 38204
Dopamine
See Catecholamines
Blood, 82383, 82384
Urine, 82382, 82384
Doppler Echocardiography, 76827, 76828, 93320-93350
with Myocardial Contrast Perfusion, 0439T
Hemodialysis Access, 93990
Intracardiac, 93662
Strain Imaging, 0399T
Transesophageal, 93318
Transthoracic, 93303-93317
Doppler Scan
Arterial Studies
Coronary Flow Reserve, 93571-93572
Extracranial, 93880-93882
Extremities, 93922-93924
Fetal
Middle Cerebral Artery, 76821
Umbilical Artery, 76820
Intracranial, 93886-93893
Saline Infusion Sonohysterography (SIS), 76831
Transplanted Kidney, 76776
Dor Procedure, 33548
Dorsal Vertebra
See Vertebra, Thoracic
Dose Plan
Radiation Therapy, 77300, 77331, 77399

Dose Plan — continued
Radiation Therapy — continued
Brachytherapy, 77316-77318
Teletherapy, 77306-77307, 77321
Dosimetry
Radiation Therapy, 77300, 77331, 77399
Brachytherapy, 77316-77318
Dose Limits Established Before Therapy, 0520F
Intensity Modulation, 77301, 77338
Special, 77331
Teletherapy, 77306-77307, 77321
Unlisted Dosimetry Procedure, 77399
Double–J Stent, 52332
Cystourethroscopy, 52000, 52601, 52647, 52648
Double–Stranded DNA
See Deoxyribonucleic Acid
Douglas–Type Procedure, 41510
Doxepin
Assay, [80335, 80336, 80337]
DPH
See Phenytoin
DPYD, 81400
Drainage
See Excision; Incision; Incision and Drainage
Abdomen
Abdominal Fluid, 49082-49083
Paracentesis, 49082-49083
Peritoneal, 49020
Peritoneal Lavage, 49084
Peritonitis, Localized, 49020
Retroperitoneal, 49060
Subdiaphragmatic, 49040
Subphrenic, 49040
Wall
Skin and Subcutaneous Tissue, 10060, 10061
Complicated, 10061
Multiple, 10061
Simple, 10060
Single, 10060
Abscess
Abdomen, 49040
Peritoneal
Open, 49020
Peritonitis, localized, 49020
Retroperitoneal
Open, 49060
Skin and Subcutaneous Tissue
Complicated, 10061
Multiple, 10061
Simple, 10060
Single, 10060
Subdiaphragmatic, 49040
Subphrenic, 49040
Anal
Incision and Drainage, 46045, 46050, 46060
Ankle
Incision and Drainage, 27603
Appendix
Incision and Drainage, 44900
Arm, Lower, 25028
Incision and Drainage, 25035
Arm, Upper
Incision and Drainage, 23930-23935
Auditory Canal, External, 69020
Bartholin's Gland
Incision and Drainage, 56420
Biliary Tract, 47400, 47420, 47425, 47480, 47533-47536
Bladder
Cystotomy or Cystostomy, 51040
Incision and Drainage, 51080
Brain
by
Burrhole, 61150, 61151
Craniotomy/Craniectomy, 61320, 61321
Neuroendoscopy, 62160, 62162, 62164
Breast
Incision and Drainage, 19020
Carpals
Incision, Deep, 25035

Drainage — continued
Abscess — continued
Clavicle
Sequestrectomy, 23170
Contrast Injection, 49424
with X–ray, 75989, 76080
Dentoalveolar Structures, 41800
Ear, External
Complicated, 69005
Simple, 69000
Elbow
Incision and Drainage, 23930-23935
Epididymis
Incision and Drainage, 54700
Eyelid
Incision and Drainage, 67700
Facial Bone(s)
Excision, 21026
Finger
Incision and Drainage, 26010, 26011, 26034
Tendon Sheath, 26020
Foot
Incision, 28005
Ganglion Cyst, 20600-20605
Gums
Incision and Drainage, 41800
Hand
Incision and Drainage, 26034
Hematoma
Brain, 61154-61156
Incision and Drainage, 27603
Vagina, 57022, 57023
Hip
Incision and Drainage, 26990-26992
Humeral Head, 23174
Humerus
Incision and Drainage, 23935
Kidney
Incision and Drainage
Open, 50020
Knee, 27301
Leg, Lower, 27603
Incision and Drainage, 27603
Liver
Incision and Drainage
Open, 47010
Injection, 47015
Repair, 47300
Localization
Nuclear Medicine, 78806, 78807
Lung
Bronchoscopy, 31645-31646
Open Drainage, 32200, 32201
Lymph Node, 38300, 38305
Lymphocele, 49062, 49185
Mandible
Excision, 21025
Mouth
Lingual, 41000
Masticator Space, 41009, 41018
Sublingual, 41005-41006, 41015, 42310
Submandibular Space, 41008, 41017
Submaxillary, 42310, 42320
Submental Space, 41007, 41016
Nasal Septum
Incision and Drainage, 30020
Neck
Incision and Drainage, 21501, 21502
Nose
Incision and Drainage, 30000, 30020
Ovary
Incision and Drainage
Abdominal Approach, 58822
Vaginal Approach, 58820
Palate
Incision and Drainage, 42000
Paraurethral Gland
Incision and Drainage, 53060
Parotid Gland, 42300, 42305
Pelvic
Percutaneous, 49406
Supralevator, 45020
Transrectal, 49407
Transvaginal, 49407
Pelvis, 26990

Drainage — continued
Abscess — continued
Pelvis — continued
Incision and Drainage, 26990-26992, 45000
Perineum
Incision and Drainage, 56405
Perirenal or Renal
Open, 50020
Peritoneum
Open, 49020
Peritonsillar, 42700
Pharyngeal, 42720, 42725
Prostate
Incision and Drainage
Prostatotomy, 55720, 55725
Transurethral, 52700
Radius
Incision, Deep, 25035
Rectum
Incision and Drainage, 45005, 45020, 46040, 46060
Renal, 50020
Retroperitoneal
Laparoscopic, 49323
Open, 49060
Salivary Gland, 42300-42320
Scapula
Sequestrectomy, 23172
Scrotum
Incision and Drainage, 54700, 55100
Shoulder
Incision and Drainage, 23030
Skene's Gland
Incision and Drainage, 53060
Skin
Incision and Drainage
Complicated, 10061
Multiple, 10061
Simple, 10060
Single, 10060
Puncture Aspiration, 10160
Soft Tissue
Image-guided by catheter, 10030
Percutaneous, 10030
Subfascial, 20005, 22010, 22015
Spine, Subfascial, 22010, 22015
Subdiaphragmatic
Incision and Drainage, 49040
Sublingual Gland, 42310, 42320
Submaxillary Gland, 42310, 42320
Subphrenic, 49040
Testis
Incision and Drainage, 54700
Thigh, 27301
Thoracostomy, 32551
Thorax
Incision and Drainage, 21501, 21502
Throat
Incision and Drainage, 42700-42725
Tongue
Incision and Drainage, 41000-41006, 41015-41018
Tonsil
Incision and Drainage, 42700
Ulna
Incision, Deep, 25035
Urethra
Incision and Drainage, 53040
Uvula
Incision and Drainage, 42000
Vagina
Incision and Drainage, 57010
Vestibule of Mouth, 40800-40801
Visceral, 49405
Vulva
Incision and Drainage, 56405
Wrist
Incision and Drainage, 25028, 25035
X-ray, 75989, 76080
Amniotic Fluid
Diagnostic Aspiration, 59000
Therapeutic Aspiration, 59001
Aqueous, 0191T, 0449T-0450T, 66179-66180, 66183, [0253T]

Drainage — *continued*
  Bile Duct
    Transhepatic, 47533-47534
  Brain Fluid, 61070
  Bursa
    Arm, Lower, 25031
    Arm, Upper, 23931
    Arthrocentesis, 20600-20615
    Elbow, 23931
    Foot, 28001-28003
    Hip, 26991
    Knee, 27301
    Leg, 27604
    Palm, 26025, 26030
    Pelvis, 26991
    Shoulder, 23031
    Thigh, 27301
    Wrist, 25031
  Cerebrospinal Fluid, 61000-61020, 61050, 61070, 62272
  Cervical Fluid, 61050
  Cisternal Fluid, 61050
  Cyst
    Bone, 20615
    Brain, 61150, 61151, 62161, 62162
    Breast, 19000, 19001
    Conjunctiva, 68020
    Dentoalveolar Structures, 41800
    Ganglion, 20612
    Intramedullary, 63172-63173
    Liver, 47010
    Lung, 32200
    Mouth
      Lingual, 41000
      Masticator Space, 41009, 41018
      Sublingual, 41005-41006, 41015
      Submandibular Space, 41008, 41017
      Submental Space, 41007, 41016
      Vestibule, 40800-40801
    Ovary, 58800, 58805
    Pilonidal, 10080-10081
    Salivary Gland, 42409
    Skene's Gland, 53060
    Sublingual Gland, 42409
  Elbow, 23930
  Empyema, 32036, 32810
  Extraperitoneal Lymphocele
    Laparoscopic, 49323
    Open, 49062
    Percutaneous, Sclerotherapy, 49185
  Eye
    Anterior Chamber
      Aqueous Drainage Device, 66183
        Into Subconjunctival Space, 0449T-0450T
        Into Suprachoroidal Space, [0253T]
        Into Trabecular Meshwork, 0191T
      Paracentesis
        with Diagnostic Aspiration of Aqueous, 65800
      Removal Blood, 65815
      Removal Vitreous and/or Discission Anterior Hyaloid Membrane, 65810
    Lacrimal Gland, 68400
    Lacrimal Sac, 68420
  Fetal Fluid, 59074
  Fluid
    Abdominal, 49082-49083
    Amniotic Fluid, 59001
    Cerebrospinal, 62272
    Fetal, 59074
    Peritoneal
      Percutaneous, 49406
      Transrectal, 49407
      Transvaginal, 49407
    Retinal, 67108, 67113
    Retroperitoneal
      Percutaneous, 49406
      Transrectal, 49407
      Transvaginal, 49407
    Tendon Sheath Hand, 26020
    Visceral, 49405
  Ganglion Cyst, 20612
  Hematoma
    Ankle, 27603

Drainage — *continued*
  Hematoma — *continued*
    Arm, Lower, 25028
    Brain, 61108, 61154, 61156
    Dentoalveolar Structures, 41800
    Ear, External, 69000, 69005
    Joint, 20600-20610
    Mouth
      Lingual, 41000
      Masticator Space, 41009, 41018
      Sublingual, 41005-41006, 41015
      Submandibular Space, 41008, 41017
      Submental Space, 41007, 41016
      Vestibule, 40800-40801
    Subungual, 11740
    Superficial, 10140
    Vagina, 57022, 57023
    Wrist, 25028
  Joint
    Acromioclavicular, 23044
    Ankle, 27610
    Carpometacarpal, 26070
    Glenohumeral, 23040
    Hip, 26990, 27030
    Interphalangeal, 26080, 28024
    Intertarsal, 28020
    Knee, 27301, 29871
    Metacarpophalangeal, 26075
    Metatarsophalangeal, 28022
    Midcarpal, 25040
    Pelvis, 26990
    Radiocarpal, 25040
    Sternoclavicular, 23044
    Thigh, 27301
    Wrist, 29843
  Kidney, 50040
  Liver
    Abscess or Cyst, 47010
  Lymph Node, 38300-38305
  Lymphocele, 49062
    Endoscopic, 49323
    Percutaneous, Sclerotherapy, 49185
  Mediastinum, 39000-39010
  Onychia, 10060, 10061
  Orbit, 67405, 67440
  Pancreas
    See Anastomosis, Pancreas to Intestines
    Pseudocyst, 48510
  Paronychia, 10060, 10061
  Pelvis, 50125
  Penis, 54015
  Pericardial Sac, 32659
  Pericardium, 33025
  Peritonitis, 49020
  Pleura, 32556-32557
  Postoperative Wound Infection, 10180
  Pseudocyst
    Gastrointestinal, Upper
      Transmural Endoscopic, 43240
    Pancreas
      Open, 48510
  Radiologic Guidance, 75989
  Rectum Injury, 45562
  Seroma, 10140, 49185
  Sinus Venosus, 33645
  Skin, 10040-10180
  Spinal Cord
    Cerebrospinal Fluid, 62272
    Subdural Fluid, 61000, 61001
    Syrinx, 63172-63173
  Ureter, 50600, 53080-53085
  Urethra
    Extravasation, 53080, 53085
  Ventricular Fluid, 61020
  Via Tube Thoracostomy, 32551
Drainage Implant, Glaucoma
  See Aqueous Shunt
Dressings
  Burns, 16020-16030
  Change under Anesthesia, 15852
DREZ Procedure, 63170
Drill Hole
  Skull
    Catheter, 61107
    Drain Hematoma, 61108
    Exploration, 61105

Drill Hole — *continued*
  Skull — *continued*
    Implant
      Neurostimulator Electrode, 61850
      Neurostimulator Electrode Array, 61863-61864, 61867-61868
      Intracerebral Monitoring Device, 61107
      Pressure Recording Device, 61107
      Surgery, 61105-61108
Drug
  See also Drug Assay
  Administration For
    Cardiac Assessments, 93463
    Helicobacter Pylori Breath Test, 83014
    Infusion
      Epidural, 62360-62362
      Home Services, 99601-99602
      Intravenous, 4100F, 96365-96368, 96413-96417, 96422-96425
      Subcutaneous, 96369-96371
      Unlisted Infusion or Injection, 96379
  Antihistamines, [80375, 80376, 80377]
  Aspirin, 4084F, 4086F
  Confirmation, [80320, 80321, 80322, 80323, 80324, 80325, 80326, 80327, 80328, 80329, 80330, 80331, 80332, 80333, 80334, 80335, 80336, 80337, 80338, 80339, 80340, 80341, 80342, 80343, 80344, 80345, 80346, 80347, 80348, 80349, 80350, 80351, 80352, 80353, 80354, 80355, 80356, 80357, 80358, 80359, 80360, 80361, 80362, 80363, 80364, 80365, 80366, 80367, 80368, 80369, 80370, 80371, 80372, 80373, 80374, 80375, 80376, 80377, 83992]
  Implant Infusion Device, 62360-62362
  Infusion, 96365-96371, 96379, 96413-96417, 96422-96425
  Resistance Analysis HIV, 87903-87904
  Susceptibility Prediction, 87900
  Test, 80305-80307
Drug Assay
  Amikacin, 80150
  Amitriptyline, [80335, 80336, 80337]
  Benzodiazepine, [80346, 80347]
  Caffeine, 80155
  Carbamazepine, 80156, 80157
  Clozapine, 80159
  Cyclosporine, 80158
  Desipramine, [80335, 80336, 80337]
  Digoxin, 80162-80163
  Dipropylacetic Acid, 80164
  Doxepin, [80335, 80336, 80337]
  Ethosuximide, 80168
  Everolimus, 80169
  Gabapentin, 80171
  Gentamicin, 80170
  Gold, [80375]
  Haloperidol, 80173
  Imipramine, [80335, 80336, 80337]
  Lamotrigine, 80175
  Levetiracetam, 80177
  Lidocaine, 80176
  Lithium, 80178
  Mycophenolate (mycophenolic acid), 80180
  Nortriptyline, [80335, 80336, 80337]
  Oxcarbazepine, 80183
  Phenobarbital, 80184
  Phenytoin, 80185, 80186
  Primidone, 80188
  Procainamide, 80190, 80192
  Quantitative
    Other, 80299
  Quinidine, 80194
  Salicylate, [80329, 80330, 80331]
  Sirolimus, 80195
  Tacrolimus, 80197
  Theophylline, 80198
  Therapeutic, 80150-80299 [80164, 80165, 80171]
  Tiagabine, 80199
  Tobramycin, 80200
  Topiramate, 80201
  Vancomycin, 80202
  Zonisamide, 80203

Drug Confirmation, [80320, 80321, 80322, 80323, 80324, 80325, 80326, 80327, 80328, 80329, 80330, 80331, 80332, 80333, 80334, 80335, 80336, 80337, 80338, 80339, 80340, 80341, 80342, 80343, 80344, 80345, 80346, 80347, 80348, 80349, 80350, 80351, 80352, 80353, 80354, 80355, 80356, 80357, 80358, 80359, 80360, 80361, 80362, 80363, 80364, 80365, 80366, 80367, 80368, 80369, 80370, 80371, 80372, 80373, 80374, 80375, 80376, 80377, 83992]
Drug Delivery Implant
  Insertion, 11981
  Irrigation, 96523
  Maintenance
    Brain, 95990, 95991
    Epidural, 95990, 95991
    Intra–arterial, 96522
    Intrathecal, 95990, 95991
    Intravenous, 96522
    Intraventricular, 95990, 95991
  Removal, 11982, 11983
    with Reinsertion, 11983
Drug Instillation
  See Instillation, Drugs
Drug Management
  Pharmacist, 99605-99607
  Psychiatric, 90863
Drugs, Anticoagulant
  See Clotting Inhibitors
Drug Screen, 99408-99409
Drug Testing Definitive
  Alcohol Biomarkers, [80321, 80322]
  Alcohols, [80320]
  Alkaloids, Not Otherwise Specified, [80323]
  Amphetamines, [80324, 80325, 80326]
  Anabolic Steroids, [80327, 80328]
  Analgesics, Non Opioid, [80329, 80330, 80331]
  Antidepressants
    Not Otherwise Specified, [80338]
    Other Cyclicals, [80335, 80336, 80337]
    Serotonergic Class, [80332, 80333, 80334]
    Tricyclic, [80335, 80336, 80337]
  Antihistamines, [80375, 80376, 80377]
  Antipsychotics, [80342, 80343, 80344]
  Barbiturates, [80345]
  Benzodiazepines, [80346, 80347]
  Buprenorphine, [80348]
  Cannabinoids
    Natural, [80349]
    Synthetic, [80350, 80351, 80352]
  Cocaine, [80353]
  Drugs or Substances, Not Otherwise Specified, [80375, 80376, 80377]
  Fentanyl, [80354]
  Gabapentin, Non-Blood, [80355]
  Heroin Metabolite, [80356]
  Ketamine, [80357]
  MDA, [80359]
  MDEA, [80359]
  MDMA, [80359]
  Methadone, [80358]
  Methylenedioxyamphetamines (MDA, MDEA, MDMA), [80359]
  Methylphenidate, [80360]
  Norketamine, [80357]
  Opiates, [80361]
  Opioids and Opiate Analogs, [80362, 80363, 80364]
  Oxycodone, [80365]
  PCP, [83992]
  Phencyclidine (PCP), [83992]
  Phenobarbtital, [80345]
  Pregabalin, [80366]
  Presumptive, 80305-80307
  Propoxyphene, [80367]
  Sedative Hypnotics, [80368]
  Skeletal Muscle Relaxants, [80369, 80370]
  Stereoisomer (Enantiomer) Analysis Single Drug Class, [80374]
  Stimulants, Synthetic, [80371]
  Tapentadol, [80372]
  Tramadol, [80373]
DSC2, 81406
DSG2, 81406
DSP, 81406

DST, 80420
DT, 90702
DTaP, 90700
DTaP–HepB–IPV Immunization, 90723
DT Shots, 90702
Dual X–ray Absorptiometry (DXA)
 See Absorptiometry, Dual Photon
 Appendicular, 77081
 Axial Skeleton, 77080
Duct, Bile
 See Bile Duct
Duct, Hepatic
 See Hepatic Duct
Duct, Nasolacrimal
 See Nasolacrimal Duct
Ductogram, Mammary, 77053-77054
 Injection, 19030
Duct, Omphalomesenteric
 See Omphalomesenteric Duct
Duct, Pancreatic
 See Pancreatic Duct
Duct, Salivary
 See Salivary Duct
Duct, Stensen's
 See Parotid Duct
Duct, Thoracic
 See Thoracic Duct
Ductus Arteriosus
 Repair, 33820-33824
 Transcatheter Percutaneous Closure, 93582
Ductus Deferens
 See Vas Deferens
Duhamel Procedure, 45120
Dunn Operation, 28725
Duodenectomy
 Near Total, 48153, 48154
 Total, 48150, 48152
Duodenography, 74260
Duodenostomy
 Injection, 49465
 Insertion, 49441
 Obstructive Material Removal, 49460
 Replacement, 49451
Duodenotomy, 44010
Duodenum
 Biopsy, 44010
 Contrast Injection, 49465
 Correction Malrotation, 44055
 Donor Transplant, 48550
 Duodenography, 74260
 Endoscopy, 43235-43259 *[43233, 43266, 43270]*
  Diagnostic, 43235
  Dilation, 43245
  Placement Catheter or Tube, 43241
  Ultrasound, 43242, 43253, 43259
 Excision, 48150, 48152-48154
 Exclusion, 48547
 Exploration, 44010
 Incision, 44010
 Intubation, 43756-43757
 Motility Study, 91022
 Removal Foreign Body, 44010
 Repositioning Feeding Tube, 43761
 X–ray, 74260
Duplex Scan
 See Vascular Studies
 Arterial Studies
  Aorta, 93978, 93979
  Extracranial, 93880, 93882
  Lower Extremity, 93925, 93926
  Penile, 93980, 93981
  Upper Extremity, 93930, 93931
  Visceral, 93975-93979
 Hemodialysis Access, 93990
 Venous Studies
  Extremity, 93970, 93971
  Penile, 93980, 93981
Dupuy–Dutemp Operation, 67971
Dupuytren's Contracture
 Fasciotomy, 26040-26045
  Open, 26045
  Percutaneous, 26040
 Injection, 20527
 Manipulation, 26341
  Injection, 20527
  Manipulation, 26341

Dupuytren's Contracture — *continued*
 Palmar Fascial Cord, 26341
 Surgical Pathology, 88304
Durand–Nicolas–Favre Disease
 See Lymphogranuloma Venereum
Dust, Angel
 See Phencyclidine
Duvries Operation
 See Tenoplasty
D Vitamin
 See Vitamin, D
Dwyer Procedure, 28300
DXA (Dual Energy X–ray Absorptiometry), 77080-
  77081 *[77085, 77086]*
D–Xylose Absorption Test, 84620
Dynamometry
 See Osteotomy, Calcaneus
 Venous Studies
  with Ophthalmoscopy, 92260
DYSF, 81408

E

E1, 82679
E2, 82670
E2A/PBX1 (t(1;19)), 81401
E3, 82677
E Antigens
 See Hepatitis Antigen, Be
Ear
 Collection of Blood From, 36416
 Drum, 69420, 69421, 69424, 69433, 69436,
  69450, 69610, 69620
  See Tympanic Membrane
 External
  Abscess
   Incision and Drainage
    Complicated, 69005
    Simple, 69000
  Biopsy, 69100, 69105
  Customized Prosthesis, 21086
  Debridement Mastoidectomy Cavity,
   69220-69222
  Excision
   Exostosis, 69140
   Partial, 69110
   Soft Tissue, 69145
    with Neck Dissection, 69155
    without Neck Dissection, 69150
   Total, 69120
  Hematoma
   Incision and Drainage, 69000, 69005
  Reconstruction
   with Graft, 21230, 21235
   with Tissue Transfer, 14060-14061
   External Auditory Canal, 69310, 69320
   Protruding Ear(s), 69300
  Removal
   Cerumen, 69209-69210
   Foreign Body, 69200, 69205
  Repair
   Complex, 13151-13153
   Intermediate, 12051-12057
   Simple, 12011-12018
   Superficial, 12011-12018
  Unlisted Services and Procedures, 69399
 Inner
  CT Scan, 70480-70482
  Excision
   Labyrinth, 69905, 69910
  Exploration
   Endolymphatic Sac, 69805, 69806
  Incision
   Labyrinth, 69801
   Semicircular Canal, 69840
  Insertion
   Cochlear Device, 69930
  Labyrinthectomy, 69905, 69910
  Semicircular Canal, 69820, 69840
  Unlisted Services and Procedures, 69949
  Vestibular Nerve Section, 69915
 Meatoplasty, 69310
  for Congenital Atresia, 69320
 Middle
  CT Scan, 70480-70482
  Excision
   Aural Polyp, 69540

Ear — *continued*
 Middle — *continued*
  Excision — *continued*
   Glomus Tumor, 69550, 69552, 69554
   Polyp, 69540
  Exploration, 69440
  Facial Nerve
   Decompression, 69720, 69725
   Suture, 69740, 69745
  Lesion
   Excision, 69540
  Reconstruction
   Tympanoplasty with Antrotomy or
    Mastoidectomy, 69635-69637
   Tympanoplasty with Mastoidectomy,
    69641-69646
   Tympanoplasty without Mastoidecto-
    my, 69631-69633
  Removal
   Ventilating Tube, 69424
  Repair
   Fistula, 69666-69667
   Oval Window, 69666
   Round Window, 69667
  Revision
   Stapes, 69662
  Stapes
   Mobilization, 69650
   Stapedectomy, 69660-69662
   Stapedotomy, 69660-69662
  Tumor
   Excision, 69550-69554
  Unlisted Services and Procedures, 69799
 Outer
  CT Scan, 70480-70482
  Skin Graft
   Delay of Flap, 15630
   Full Thickness, 15260, 15261
   Pedicle Flap, 15576
   Split, 15120, 15121
   Tissue Transfer, Adjacent, 14060-14061
  Removal Skin Lesions
   Excision
    Benign, 11440-11446
    Malignant, 11640-11646
   Shaving, 11310-11313
  Temporal Bone
   Bone Conduction Hearing Device
    Implantation, 69710
    Removal, 69711
    Repair, 69711
   Osseointegrated Implant
    Implantation, 69714-69715
    Removal, 69717
    Replacement, 69717
   Resection, 69535
   Unlisted Service or Procedure, 69799
Ear Canal
 See Auditory Canal
Ear Cartilage
 Graft
  to Face, 21230
  to Nose or Ear, 21230, 21235
Ear Lobes
 Pierce, 69090
Ear, Nose, and Throat
 Acoustic, 92568
 Audiometric Group Testing, 92559
 Audiometry
  Conditioning Play, 92582
  Evoked Response, 92585-92586
  Groups, 92559
  Picture, 92583
  Pure Tone, 92552-92553, 0208T-0209T
  Select Picture, 92583
  Speech, 92555-92557, 0210T-0212T
  Tympanotomy and Reflex, 92550
  Visual Reinforcement, 92579
 Bekesy Screening, 92560-92561
 Binocular Microscopy, 92504
 Brainstem Evoked Response, 92585, 92586
 Central Auditory Function Evaluation, 92620-
  92621
 Comprehensive Audiometry Threshold Evalua-
  tion, 92557

Ear, Nose, and Throat — *continued*
 Diagnostic Analysis
  Auditory Brainstem Implant, 92640
  Cochlear Implant, 92601-92604
 Ear Protector Evaluation, 92596
 Electrocochleography, 92584
 Evaluation
  Auditory Rehabilitation Status, 92626-
   92627, 92630, 92633
  Communication Device
   Non-speech Generating, 92605,
    [92618]
   Speech Generating, 92607-92608
  Language Comprehensive and Expression,
   92523
  Laryngeal Sensory Testing, 92614-92617
  Speech Fluency, 92521
  Speech Sound Production, 92522
  Swallowing, 92610-92613, 92616
  Voice and Resonance Analysis, 92524
 Examination Under Anesthesia, 92502
 Facial Nerve Function Study, 92516
 Filtered Speech, 92571
 Hearing Aid Evaluation, 92590-92595
 Hearing, Language, and Speech Evaluation,
  92521-92524
 Immittance Testing, 92570
 Impedance Testing, 92567
 Laryngeal Function Study, 92520
 Lombard Test, 92700
 Loudness Balance, 92562
 Nasal Function Study, 92512
 Nasopharyngoscopy, 92511
 Reflex, 92568
 Screening Test, 92551
 Treatment
  Hearing, Language, Speech Disorder,
   92507-92508
  Oral Function for Feeding, 92526
  Swallowing Dysfunction, 92526
Ear Protector Attenuation, 92596
 See Hearing Aid Services
Ear Wax
 See Cerumen
Ebstein Anomaly Repair, 33468
EBV, 86663-86665
E B Virus
 See Epstein–Barr Virus
ECCE, 66840-66852, 66940
Eccrine Glands
 Chemodenervation
  Axillae, 64650
  Feet, 64999
  Hands, 64999
  Other Areas, 64653
ECG, 93000-93024, 93040-93278, 0178T-0180T,
  0295T-0298T
 External, 93224-93272, 0295T-0298T
 Signal-Averaged, 93278
Echinococcosis, 86171, 86280
ECHO, 0399T, 76825, 93303-93312, 93314, 93315,
  93317-93321, 93350
Echocardiography
 Cardiac, 93320-93350
  Intracardiac, 93662
  Strain Imaging, 0399T
  Transesophageal, 93318
  Transthoracic, 93303-93317
   with Myocardial Contrast Perfusion,
    0439T
   with Stress Test, 93350-93352
 Doppler, 93303-93321, 93350, 93662
 Fetal Heart, 76825-76828
  Doppler
   Complete, 76827
   Follow–up or Repeat Study, 76828
 for Assessment of Myocardial Ischemia/Viability,
  0439T
 for Congenital Anomalies
  Transesophageal, 93315-93317
  Transthoracic, 93303, 93304
 Intracardiac, 93662
 M Mode and Real Time, 93306
 Myocardial Contrast Perfusion, 0439T
 Strain Imaging, 0399T
 Stress Test, 93350-93351

[Resequenced]

Echocardiography — *continued*
  Stress Test — *continued*
    with Contrast, 93352
    with Myocardial Contrast Perfusion, 0439T
  Transesophageal, 93312-93318
    for Congenital Anomalies, 93315-93317
    for Guidance Intracardiac or Great Vessel
      Intervention, 93355
    for Monitoring Purposes, 93318
  Transthoracic, 93303-93308, 93350-93352
    with Stress Test, 93350-93352
    for Congenital Anomalies, 93303, 93304
Echoencephalography, 76506
Echography
  Abdomen, 76700-76705
  Arm
    Complete, 76881
    Limited, 76882
  Cardiac, 0439T, 93303-93317, 93320-93321,
    93350-93352, 93662
    Guidance for Biopsy, 76932
  Chest, 76604
  Extracranial Arteries, 93880, 93882
  Eyes, 76510-76529
  Follow–Up, 76970
  Head, 76536
  Heart, 0439T, 93303-93317, 93320-93321,
    93350-93352, 93662
    Guidance for Biopsy, 76932
  Hip
    Infant, 76885, 76886
  Intracranial Arteries, 93886-93893
  Intraoperative, 76998
  Kidney
    Transplant, 76776
  Leg
    Complete, 76881
    Limited, 76882
  Neck, 76536
  Pelvis, 76856, 76857
  Pregnant Uterus, 76801-76828
  Prostate, 76872-76873
  Retroperitoneal, 76770, 76775
  Scrotum, 76870
  Spine, 76800
  Transrectal, 76872, 76873
  Transvaginal, 76817, 76830
  Unlisted Ultrasound, 76999
  Vagina, 76817, 76830
Echotomography
  See Echography
ECLS (Extracorporeal Life Support Services)
  Cannulization
    Insertion, 33951-33956
    Removal, *[33965, 33966, 33969, 33984,*
      33985, 33986]
    Repositioning, 33957-33959 *[33962, 33963,*
      33964]
  Creation Graft Conduit, *[33987]*
  Daily Management, 33948-33949
  Initiation, 33946-33947
  Left Heart Vent Insertion, *[33988]*
  Left Heart Vent Removal, *[33989]*
ECMO (Extracorporeal Membrane Oxygenation)
  Cannulization
    Insertion, 33951-33956
    Isolated with Chemotherapy Perfusion,
      36823
    Removal, *[33965, 33966, 33969, 33984,*
      33985, 33986]
    Repositioning, 33957-33959 *[33962, 33963,*
      33964]
  Creation Graft Conduit, *[33987]*
  Daily Management, 33948-33949
  Initiation, 33946-33947
  Left Heart Vent Insertion, *[33988]*
  Left Heart Vent Removal, *[33989]*
ECS
  See Emission Computerized Tomography
ECSF (Erythrocyte Colony Stimulating Factor)
  See Erythropoietin
ECT (Emission Computerized Tomography),
  78607
ECT (Electroconvulsive Therapy), 90870
Ectasia
  See Dilation

Ectopic Pregnancy
  See Obstetrical Care
  Abdominal, 59130
  Cervix, 59140
  Interstitial
    Partial Resection Uterus, 59136
    Total Hysterectomy, 59135
  Laparoscopy, 59150
    with Salpingectomy and/or Oophorectomy,
      59151
  Ovarian
    with Salpingectomy and/or Oophorectomy,
      59120
    without Salpingectomy and/or Oophorec-
      tomy, 59121
  Tubal
    with Salpingectomy and/or Oophorectomy,
      59120
    without Salpingectomy and/or Oophorec-
      tomy, 59121
  Uterine
    with Hysterectomy, 59135
    with Partial Uterine Resection, 59136
Ectropion
  Repair
    Blepharoplasty
      Excision Tarsal Wedge, 67916
      Extensive, 67917
    Suture, 67914
    Thermocauterization, 67915
ED, 99281-99288
Education, 99078
  Patient
    Heart Failure, 4003F
    Pediatric Gastroenteritis to Caregiver,
      4058F
    Self-management by Nonphysician, 98960-
      98962
  Services (Group), 99078
  Supplies, 99071
EEG, 95812-95827, 95830, 95950-95953, 95955-
  95958
  See also Electroencephalography
EFHC1, 81406
EGD, 43235-43255 *[43233]*, 43257, 43259, *[43233]*,
  [43266], *[43270]*
EGFR, 81235
Egg
  See Ova
Eggers Procedure, 27100
EGR2, 81404
Ehrlichia, 86666
EIF2B2, 81405
EIF2B3, 81405-81406
EIF2B4, 81406
EIF2B5, 81406
EKG, 93000-93010
  64-Lead or Greater, 0178T-0180T
  External, 0295T-0298T, 93224-93272
  Rhythm Strips, 93040-93042
  Routine, 93000-93010
  Signal Averaged, 93278
Elastase, 82656
Elastography
  Liver, 91200
  Ultrasound, 0346T
Elbow
  See Humerus; Radius; Ulna
  Abscess
    Incision and Drainage, 23930, 23935
  Anesthesia, 00400, 01710-01782
  Arthrectomy, 24155
  Arthrocentesis, 20605-20606
  Arthrodesis, 24800, 24802
  Arthrography, 73085
    Contrast Injection, 24220
  Arthroplasty, 24360
    with Implant, 24361-24362
    Removal Prosthesis, 24160, 24164
    Revision, 24370-24371
    Total Replacement, 24363
  Arthroscopy
    Diagnostic, 29830
    Surgical, 29834-29838
  Arthrotomy, 24000
    with Joint Exploration, 24000, 24101

Elbow — *continued*
  Arthrotomy — *continued*
    with Synovectomy, 24102
    with Synovial Biopsy, 24100, 29830
    Capsular Release, 24006
    Drainage, 24000
    Foreign Body Removal, 24000
  Biopsy, 24065-24066, 24101
  Bone Cortex Incision, 23935
  Bursa
    Incision and Drainage, 23931
  Capsule
    Excision, 24006
    Radical Resection, 24149
  Contracture Release, 24149
  Dislocation
    Closed Treatment, 24600, 24605, 24640
    Nursemaid Elbow, 24640
    Open Treatment, 24615
    Partial, 24640
    Subluxate, 24640
  Epicondylitis
    Debridement, 24358-24359
    Percutaneous, 24357
  Excision, 24155
    Bursa, 24105
    Synovium, 24102, 29835-29836
    Tumor
      Soft Tissue, 24077-24079
        Subcutaneous, 24075, *[24071]*
        Subfascial, 24076, *[24073]*
  Exploration, 24000-24101 *[24071, 24073]*
  Fracture
    Monteggia, 24620, 24635
    Open Treatment, 24586, 24587
  Hematoma
    Incision and Drainage, 23930
  Incision and Drainage
    Abscess, Deep, 23930
    Bursa, 23931
    Hematoma, 23930
  Injection
    Arthrography (Radiologic), 24220
  Magnetic Resonance Imaging (MRI), 73221
  Manipulation, 24300
  Prosthesis
    Removal, 24160-24164
  Radical Resection
    Bone Tumor, 24150, 24152
    Capsule, Soft Tissue and Bone with Contrac-
      ture Release, 24149
    Soft Tissue Tumor, 24077-24079
  Removal
    Foreign Body, 24000, 24101, 24200, 24201,
      29834
    Implant, 24160-24164
    Loose Body, 24101, 29834
    Prosthesis, 24160
  Repair
    Advancement, 24330-24331
    Epicondylitis, 24357-24359
    Fasciotomy, 24357-24359
    Flexorplasty, 24330
    Graft, 24320
    Hemiepiphyseal Arrest, 24470
    Ligament, 24343-24346
    Muscle, 24341
    Muscle Transfer, 24301, 24320
    Tendon, 24340-24342
      Lengthening, 24305
      Release
        Debridement, 24358-24359
        Percutaneous, 24357
        Repair, 24359
      Repair, 24341, 24359
      Tenodesis, 24340
      Tenotomy, 24310, 24357-24359
    Tennis Elbow, 24357-24359
  Seddon-Brookes Procedure, 24320
  Steindler Advancement, 24330
  Strapping, 29260
  Tenotomy, 24357-24359
  Tumor
    Excision, 24075-24076 *[24071]*
    Radical Resection, 24077-24079
  Ulnar Neuroplasty, 64718

Elbow — *continued*
    Unlisted Services and Procedures, 24999
    X–ray, 73070, 73080
      with Contrast, 73085
Elbow, Golfer, 24357-24359
Elbow, Tennis, 24357-24359
Electrical Stimulation
  Acupuncture, 97813-97814
  Bone Healing
    Invasive, 20975
    Noninvasive, 20974
  Brain Surface, 95961, 95962
  Cardiac, 93623
    Induction of Arrhythmia, 93618
  Guidance
    Chemodenervation, 95873
  Physical Therapy
    Attended, Manual, 97032
    Unattended, 97014
  Spine, 63650, 63655, 63661-63664, 63685,
    63688
Electric Countershock
  See Cardioversion
Electric Modulation Pain Reprocessing
  Transcutaneous, 0278T
Electrocardiogram, 93000-93010
  64-Lead or Greater, 0178T-0180T
  See Electrocardiography
  External, 0295T-0298T, 93224-93272
  Rhythm Strips, 93040-93042
    with Interpretation and Report, 93040
    Interpretation and Report Only, 93042
    Tracing Only Without Interpretation and
      Report, 93041
  Routine 12-Lead, 93000-93010
  Signal-Averaged, 93278
Electrocardiography
  12-Lead ECG, 3120F, 93000
  24–hour Monitoring, 93224-93272
  48 Hours up to 21 Days, 0295T-0298T
  64 Leads or Greater, 0178T-0180T
    with Interpretation and Report, 0178T
    Interpretation and Report Only, 0180T
    Tracing and Graphics Only without Interpre-
      tation and Report, 0179T
  Evaluation, 0178T-0180T, 93000, 93010
  Event Monitors, 93268-93272
  External Recording
    48-Hours Duration, 93224-93229
    Auto Activated, 93268, 93270-93272
    Interpretation, 0295T, 0298T, 93272
    Mobile
      Greater than 24 Hours, 93228-93229
      Patient Activated, 93268, 93270-93272
      Transmission and Evaluation, 93268, 93270-
        93271
    Up to 30 Days Download, 93268, 93270-
      93272
  Holter Monitors, 93224-93227
  Microvolt T-Wave Alternans, 93025
  Mobile Telemetry, 93228-93229
  Monitoring
    with Attended Surveillance
      Cardiovascular Telemetry with Physi-
        cian Review and Report, 93228
      Technical Support, 93229
  Recording, 93224-93272
  Rhythm, 93040
    1-3 Leads, 93040
    Evaluation, 93042
    Interpretation and Report Only, 93042
    Microvolt T-Wave Alternans, 93025
    Recording, 0295T-0296T
    Scanning Analysis with Report, 0295T,
      0297T
    Tracing and Evaluation, 93040
    Tracing Only without Interpretation and
      Report, 93005, 93041
  Routine; at Least 12 Leads, 93000-93010
    with Interpretation and Report, 93000
    Interpretation and Report Only, 93010
    Tracing Only, without Interpretation and
      Report, 93005
  Signal Averaged, 93278
  Symptom-Related Memory Loop, 93268, 93270-
    93272

Electrocardiography — *continued*
  Tracing, 93005
Electrocautery, 17000-17286
  See Destruction
  Inferior Turbinates, 30801-30802
  Prostate Resection, 52601
  Ureteral Stricture, 52341-52346
Electrochemistry
  See Electrolysis
Electroconvulsive Therapy, 90870
Electrocorticogram
  Intraoperative, 61536, 61538, 95829
Electrode
  Array
    Intracranial, 61850-61868, 61885-61886, 64568-64570
    Peripheral Nerve, 64555, 64575
    Retinal, 0100T
    Spinal, 63650-63655
  Depth Electrode Implantation, 61760
Electrodesiccation, 17000-17286
  Lesion
    Penis, 54055
Electroejaculation, 55870
Electroencephalography (EEG)
  Brain Death, 95824
  Coma, 95822
  Digital Analysis, 95957
  Electrode Placement, 95830
  Intraoperative, 95955
  Monitoring, 95812, 95813, 95950-95953, 95956
    with Drug Activation, 95954
    with Physical Activation, 95954
    with WADA Activation, 95958
  Sleep, 95819, 95822, 95827
  Standard, 95816, 95819
Electrogastrography, 91132, 91133
Electrogram, Atrial
  Esophageal Recording, 93615, 93616
Electro–Hydraulic Procedure, 52325
Electrolysis, 17380
Electromyographs
  See Electromyography, Needle
Electromyography
  Anus
    Biofeedback, 90911
  Extremity, 95860-95872 *[95885, 95886]*
  Fine Wire, 96004
    Dynamic, 96004
  Guidance, 95874
    Chemodenervation, 95874
  Hemidiaphragm, 95866
  Larynx, 95865
  Needle
    Extremities, 95861-95872 *[95885, 95886, 95887]*
    Extremity, 95860
    Face and Neck Muscles, 95867, 95868
    Guidance
      Chemodenervation, 64617, 95874
    Hemidiaphragm, 95866
    Larynx, 95865
    Muscle Supplied by Cranial Nerve, 95867-95868
    Non-extremity, *[95887]*
    Ocular, 92265
    Other than Thoracic Paraspinal, 95870
    Single Fiber Electrode, 95872
    Thoracic Paraspinal Muscles, 95869
  Nonextremity, *[95887]*
  Rectum
    Biofeedback, 90911
  Sphincter Muscles
    Anus, 51784-51785
      Needle, 51785
    Urethra, 51784, 51785
      Needle, 51785
  Surface
    Dynamic, 96002-96004
Electronic Analysis
  Cardioverter–Defibrillator
    with Reprogramming, 93282-93284, 93287, 93642, 93644
    without Reprogramming, 93289, 93292, 93295, 93640-93641

Electronic Analysis — *continued*
  Cardioverter–Defibrillator — *continued*
    Evaluation
      in Person, 93289, 93640, 93642
      Remote, 93295-93296
  Data Analysis, 93289
  Defibrillator, 93282, 93289, 93292, 93295
  Drug Infusion Pump, 62367-62370, 95990-95991
  Loop Recorder System Implantable, 93285, 93291, 93298
    Data Analysis, 93291, 93298-93299
    Evaluation of Programming, 93285, 93291, 93298-93299
  Neurostimulator Pulse Generator, 95970-95975, 95978-95982
  Pulse Generator, 95970-95979
    Field Stimulation, 64999
    Gastric Neurostimulator, 95980-95982
Electron Microscopy, 88348
Electro–oculography, 92270
Electrophoresis
  Counterimmuno–, 86185
  Hemoglobin, 83020
  High Resolution, 83701
  Immuno–, 86320-86327
  Immunofixation, 86334-86335
  Protein, 84165-84166
  Unlisted Services and Procedures, 82664
Electrophysiology Procedure, 93600-93660
Electroretinography, 92275
Electrostimulation, Analgesic Cutaneous
  See Application, Neurostimulation
Electrosurgery
  Anal, 46924
  Penile, 54065
  Rectal Tumor, 45190
  Skin Lesion, 17000-17111, 17260-17286
  Skin Tags, 11200-11201
  Trichiasis
    Correction, 67825
  Vaginal, 57061, 57065
  Vulva, 56501, 56515
Electroversion, Cardiac
  See Cardioversion
Elevation, Scapula, Congenital
  See Sprengel's Deformity
Elliot Operation, 66130
  Excision, Lesion, Sclera, 66130
Eloesser Procedure, 32035, 32036
Eloesser Thoracoplasty, 32905
Embolectomy
  Aortoiliac Artery, 34151, 34201
  Axillary Artery, 34101
  Brachial Artery, 34101
  Carotid Artery, 34001
  Celiac Artery, 34151
  Femoral, 34201
  Iliac, 34151, 34201
  Innominate Artery, 34001-34101
  Mesentery Artery, 34151
  Peroneal Artery, 34203
  Popliteal Artery, 34201, 34203
  Pulmonary Artery, 33910-33916
  Radial Artery, 34111
  Renal Artery, 34151
  Subclavian Artery, 34001-34101
  Tibial Artery, 34203
  Ulnar Artery, 34111
Embolization
  Arterial (not hemorrhage or tumor), 37242
  Hemorrhage
    Arterial, 37244
    Venous, 37244
  Infarction, 37243
  Leiomyomata, 37243
  Lymphatic Extravasation, 37244
  Organ Ischemia, 37243
  Tumors, 37243
  Ureter, 50705
  Venous Malformations, 37241
Embryo
  Biopsy, 89290, 89291
  Carcinoembryonic Antigen, 82378
  Cryopreservation, 89258

Embryo — *continued*
  Cryopreserved
    Preparation/Thawing, 89352
  Culture, 89250
    with Co–Culture Oocyte, 89251
    Extended Culture, 89272
  Hatching
    Assisted Microtechnique, 89253
  Preparation for Transfer, 89255
  Storage, 89342
Embryo/Fetus Monitoring
  See Monitoring, Fetal
Embryo Implantation
  See Implantation
Embryonated Eggs
  Inoculation, 87250
Embryo Transfer
  In Vitro Fertilization, 58970, 58974, 58976
    Intrafallopian Transfer, 58976
    Intrauterine Transfer, 58974
    Preparation for Transfer, 89255
EMD, 81404-81405
Emergency Department Services, 99281-99288
  See Critical Care; Emergency Department
  Anesthesia, 99140
    in Office, 99058
  Physician Direction of Advanced Life Support, 99288
Emesis Induction, 99175
EMG (Electromyography, Needle), 51784, 51785, 92265, 95860-95872 *[95885, 95886, 95887]*
EMI Scan
  See CT Scan
Emission Computerized Tomography, 78607, 78647
Emission Computerized Tomography, Single–Photon
  See SPECT
EML4/ALK, 81401
Emmet Operation, 57720
Empyema
  Closure
    Chest Wall, 32810
  Empyemectomy, 32540
  Enucleation, 32540
  Thoracostomy, 32035, 32036, 32551
Empyemectomy, 32540
EMS, 99288
Encephalitis
  Antibody, 86651-86654
Encephalitis Virus Vaccine, 90738
Encephalocele
  Repair, 62120
    Craniotomy, 62121
Encephalography, A–Mode, 76506
Encephalon
  See Brain
Endarterectomy
  Coronary Artery, 33572
    Anomaly, 33500-33507
  Pulmonary, 33916
Endemic Flea–Borne Typhus
  See Murine Typhus
End–Expiratory Pressure, Positive
  See Pressure Breathing, Positive
Endobronchial Challenge Tests
  See Bronchial Challenge Test
Endocavitary Fulguration
  See Electrocautery
Endocrine, Pancreas
  See Islet Cell
Endocrine System
  Unlisted Services and Procedures, 60699, 78099
Endocrinology (Type 2 Diabetes) Biochemical Assays, 81506
Endolaser Photocoagulation
  Focal, 67039
  Panretinal, 67040
Endolymphatic Sac
  Exploration
    with Shunt, 69806
    without Shunt, 69805
Endometrial Ablation, 0404T, 58353, 58356, 58563
  Curettage, 58356
  Exploration via Hysteroscopy, 58563

Endometrioma
  Abdomen
    Destruction, 49203-49205
    Excision, 49203-49205
  Mesenteric
    Destruction, 49203-49205
    Excision, 49203-49205
  Peritoneal
    Destruction, 49203-49205
    Excision, 49203-49205
  Retroperitoneal
    Destruction, 49203-49205
    Excision, 49203-49205
Endometriosis, Adhesive
  See Adhesions, Intrauterine
Endometrium
  Ablation, 0404T, 58353, 58356, 58563
  Biopsy, 58100, 58110, 58558
  Curettage, 58356
Endomyocardial
  Biopsy, 93505
Endonuclease, DNA
  See DNAse
Endopyelotomy, 50575
Endorectal Pull–Through
  Proctectomy, Total, 45110, 45112, 45120, 45121
Endoscopic Retrograde Cannulation of Pancreatic Duct (ERCP)
  See Cholangiopancreatography
Endoscopic Retrograde Cholangiopancreatography
  with Optical Endomicroscopy, 0397T
  Ablation Lesion/Polyp/Tumor, *[43278]*
  Balloon Dilation, *[43277]*
  Destruction of Calculi, 43265
  Diagnostic, 43260
  Measure Pressure Sphincter of Oddi, 43263
  Placement
    Stent, *[43274]*
      with Removal and Replacement, *[43276]*
  Removal
    Calculi or Debris, 43264
    Foreign Body, *[43275]*
    Stent, *[43275]*
      with Stent Exchange, *[43276]*
  Removal Calculi or Debris, 43264
Endoscopies, Pleural
  See Thoracoscopy
Endoscopy
  See Arthroscopy; Thoracoscopy
  Adrenal Gland
    Biopsy, 60650
    Excision, 60650
  Anal
    Ablation
      Polyp, 46615
      Tumor, 46615
    Biopsy, 46606, 46607
    Collection of Specimen, 46600-46601
    Diagnostic, 46600-46601
    Dilation, 46604
    Exploration, 46600
    Hemorrhage, 46614
    High Resolution, 46601, 46607
    Removal
      Foreign Body, 46608
      Polyp, 46610, 46612
      Tumor, 46610, 46612
  Atria, 33265-33266
  Bile Duct
    Biopsy, 47553
    Cannulation, 43273
    Catheterization, 74328, 74330
    Destruction
      Calculi (Stone), 43265
      Tumor, *[43278]*
    Diagnostic, 43260
    Dilation, 47555, 47556, *[43277]*
    Exchange
      Stent, *[43276]*
    Exploration, 47552
    Intraoperative, 47550
    Percutaneous, 47552-47556
    Removal
      Calculi (Stone), 43264, 47554

Endoscopy — *continued*
Bile Duct — *continued*
Removal — *continued*
Foreign Body, [43275]
Stent, [43275]
Specimen Collection, 43260
Sphincterotomy, 43262, [43274]
Sphincter Pressure, 43263
Stent Placement, [43274]
Bladder
Biopsy, 52204, 52250, 52354
Catheterization, 52005, 52010
Destruction, 52354
with Fulguration, 52214
Lesion, 52400
Polyps, 52285
Diagnostic, 52000
Dilation, 52260, 52265
Evacuation
Clot, 52001
Excision
Tumor, 52355
Exploration, 52351
Insertion
Radioactive Substance, 52250
Stent, 52282, 53855
Instillation, 52010
Irrigation, 52010
Lesion, 52224, 52234-52235, 52240, 52400
Litholapaxy, 52317-52318
Lithotripsy, 52353
Neck, 51715
Removal
Calculus, 52310, 52315, 52352
Urethral Stent, 52310, 52315
Bladder Neck
Injection of Implant Material, 51715
Brain
Catheterization, 62160
Dissection
Adhesions, 62161
Cyst, 62162
Drainage, 62162
Excision
Brain Tumor, 62164
Cyst, 62162
Pituitary Tumor, 62165
Removal Foreign Body, 62163
Shunt Creation, 62201
Bronchi
Aspiration, 31645-31646
Biopsy, 31625, 31632, 31633
Computer-assisted Image Guidance, 31627
Destruction
Lesion, 31641, 96570-96571
Tumor, 31641, 96570-96571
Dilation, 31630-31631, 31636-31638
Excision Tumor, 31640
Exploration, 31622
Lavage, 31624
Lesion, 31641
Destruction, 31641, 96570-96571
Needle Biopsy, 31629, 31633
Occlusion, 31634
Placement
Fiducial Marker, 31626
Radioelement Catheter, 31643
Stent, 31631, 31636-31637
Removal
Foreign Body, 31635
Revision
Stent, 31638
Specimen Collection, 31623-31624
Stenosis, 31641
Tracheobronchoscopy, 31615
Tumor
Destruction, 31641, 96570-96571
Ultrasound
Destruction, 31641
Excision, 31640
Cannulization
Papilla, 43273
Capsule, 91111
Cervix
Biopsy, 57421, 57454, 57455, 57460
Curettage, 57454, 57456

Endoscopy — *continued*
Cervix — *continued*
Exploration, 57452
Loop Electrode Biopsy, 57460
Loop Electrode Conization, 57461
Chest Cavity
with Biopsy, 32607-32609
Diagnostic, 32601-32604
Exploration, 32601-32606
Surgical, 32650-32674
Colon
Ablation, [44401], [45388]
Band Ligation, [45398]
Biopsy, 44389, 44407, 45380, 45392
Collection of Specimen, 44388, 45378
Decompression, 44408, 45393
Destruction
Lesion, [44401], [45388]
Tumor, [44401], [45388]
Dilation, 44405, 45386
Exploration, 44388, 45378
Hemorrhage, 44391, 45382
Injection, Submucosal, 44404, 45381
Placement
Stent, 44402, 45389
Removal
Foreign Body, 44390, 45379
Polyp, 44392, 44394, 45384-45385
Tumor, 44392, 44394, 45384-45385
Ultrasound, 44406-44407, 45391-45392
via Colotomy, [45399]
via Stoma (Colostomy), 44388-44408
[44401]
Virtual, 74261-74263
Colon–Sigmoid
Ablation
Polyp, [45346]
Tumor, [45346]
Biopsy, 45331
Dilation, 45340
Exploration, 45330
Specimen Collection, 45331
Hemorrhage, 45334
Injection, 45335
Needle Biopsy, 45342
Placement
Stent, 45327, 45347
Removal
Foreign Body, 45332
Polyp, 45333, 45338
Tumor, 45333, 45338
Specimen Collection, 45330
Ultrasound, 45341, 45342
Volvulus, 45321, 45337
Duodenum Ultrasound, 43253
Endomicroscopy
Esophageal, 43206
Gastrointestinal, 43252
Esophagus
with Optical Endomicroscopy, 43206
Biopsy, 43193, 43198, 43202
Dilation, 43195-43196, 43220, 43220
[43212, 43213, 43214], 43226,
43229, 43248-43249 [43233],
[43233]
Exploration, 43191, 43197, 43200
Hemorrhage, 43227
Injection, 43192, 43201, 43204
Varices, 43243
Insertion Stent, [43212]
Mucosal Resection, [43211]
Needle Biopsy, 43232
Removal
Foreign Body, 43194, 43215
Polyp, 43216-43217, 43229
Tumor, 43216-43217, 43229
Specimen Collection, 43197, 43200
Ultrasound, 43231-43232, 43237-43238,
43242, 43253
Vein Ligation, 43205
Eye, 66990
Foot
Plantar Fasciotomy, 29893
Gastrointestinal
Ablation
Lesion, [43270]

Endoscopy — *continued*
Gastrointestinal — *continued*
Ablation — *continued*
Photodynamic Therapy, 96570-96571
Polyp, [43270]
Tumor, [43270]
Capsule, 91110-91111
Upper
with Optical Endomicroscopy, 43252
Biopsy, 43239
Catheterization, 43241
Destruction of Lesion, [43270]
Dilation, 43245, 43248, 43249, [43233]
Drainage of Pseudocyst, 43240
Exploration, 43235, 43252
Foreign Body, 43247
Gastric Bypass, 43644-43645
Gastroenterostomy, 43644-43645
Hemorrhage, 43255
Injection, 43236, 43253
Inject Varices, 43243
Mucosal Resection, 43254
Needle Biopsy, 43232, 43238, 43242
Performance Measures, 3130F-3132F,
3140F-3141F
Referral, 3132F
Removal, 43247, 43250, 43251
Roux–En–Y, 43644
Stent Placement, [43266]
Thermal Radiation, 43257
Tube Placement, 43246
Ultrasound, 43237-43242, 43253,
43259, 76975
Vein Ligation, 43244
Heart
Atria, 33265-33266
Ileum
Biopsy, 44382
Stent Insertion, 44384
via Stoma, 44384
Intestines, Small
Ablation
Polyp, 44369
Tumor, 44369
Biopsy, 44361, 44377
Destruction
Lesion, 44369
Tumor, 44369
Diagnostic, 44376
Exploration, 44360
Hemorrhage, 44366, 44378
Insertion
Stent, 44370, 44379
Tube, 44379
Pelvic Pouch, 44385, 44386
Placement
Stent, 44370, 44379
Tube, 44372-44373, 44379
Removal
Foreign Body, 44363
Lesion, 44365
Polyp, 44364, 44365
Tumor, 44364, 44365
Tube Placement, 44372
Tube Revision, 44373
via Stoma, 44380-44384 [44381]
Tumor, 44364, 44365
Intracranial, 62160-62165
Jejunum, 43253
Kidney
Biopsy, 50555, 50557, 50574-50576, 52354
Catheterization, 50553, 50572
Destruction, 50557, 50576, 52354
Dilation
Stricture, 52343, 52346
Excision
Tumor, 50562, 52355
Exploration, 52351
Lithotripsy, 52353
Removal
Calculus, 50561, 50580, 52352
Foreign Body, 50561, 50580
via Incision, 50562-50576, 50580
via Stoma, 50551-50557, 50561-50562
Larynx
with Injection, 31570

Endoscopy — *continued*
Larynx — *continued*
Arytenoidectomy, 31560-31561
Aspiration, 31515
Biopsy, 31510, 31535, 31536
Diagnostic, Newborn, 31525
Dilation, 31528-31529
Direct, 31515-31571
Diagnostic, 31520, 31525-31526
Operative, 31530-31531, 31535-31536,
31540-31541, 31545-31546,
31560-31561
Epiglottis Stripping, 31540-31541
Excision Tumor, 31540
Exploration, 31505, 31520-31526, 31575
Indirect, 31505-31513
Insertion Obturator, 31527
Operative, 31530-31561
Reconstruction, 31545-31546
Removal
Foreign Body, 31511, 31530, 31531
Lesion, 31512, 31545-31546
Telescopic, 31579
Telescopic, 31579
Vocal Cord
Injection, 31513, 31570-31571
Lesion Removal, 31545
Stripping, 31540-31541
Lung, Biopsy, 31628, 31632
Mediastinoscopy
Biopsy, 39401-39402
Esophagogastric Fundoplasty, [43210]
Exploration, 39401
Nasal
Diagnostic, 31231-31235
Surgical, 0406T-0407T, 31237-31297
Unlisted Procedure, Accessory Sinuses,
31299
Pancreatic Duct
Cannulation, 43273
Catheterization, 74329-74330
Destruction
Calculi (Stone), 43265
Tumor, [43278]
Dilation, [43277]
Removal
Calculi (Stone), 43264
Foreign Body, [43275]
Stent, [43275, 43276]
Specimen Collection, 43260
Sphincterotomy, 43262, [43274]
Sphincter Pressure, 43263
Stent Placement, [43274]
Pelvis
Aspiration, 49322
Destruction of Lesions, 52354, 58662
Lysis of Adhesions, 58660
Oviduct Surgery, 58670, 58671
Removal of Adnexal Structures, 58661
Peritoneum
Drainage Lymphocele, 49323, 54690
Pleural Cavity
Ablation
Photodynamic Therapy, 96570-96571
Prostate
Abscess Drainage, 52700
Destruction, 52214
Incision, 52450
Laser, 52647
Coagulation, 52647
Enucleation, 52649
Vaporization, 52647
Resection
Complete, 52601
Obstructive Tissue, 52630
Rectum
Ablation
Polyp, 45320
Tumor, 45320
Biopsy, 45305
Destruction
Tumor, 45320
Dilation, 45303
Exploration, 45300
Hemorrhage, 45317

[Resequenced]

Endoscopy — *continued*
    Rectum — *continued*
        Removal
            Foreign Body, 45307
            Polyp, 45308-45315
            Tumor, 45308-45315
        Volvulus, 45321
    Sinuses
        Diagnostic, 31233, 31235
        Surgical, 0406T-0407T, 31237-31240,
            31254-31256, 31267, 31276, 31287-
            31288, 31290-31297
        Unlisted Procedure, 31299
    Spleen
        Removal, 38120
    Stomach, Ultrasound Examination, 43253
    Testis
        Removal, 54690
    Trachea
        Biopsy, 31629
        Dilation, 31630-31631, 31636-31638
        Stent Placement, 31631
        via Tracheostomy, 31615
    Ureter
        With Endopyelotomy, 50575
        Biopsy, 50955-50957, 50974-50976, 52007,
            52354
        Catheterization, 50572, 50953, 50972,
            52005
        Destruction, 50957, 50976, 52354
        Uterocele, 52300-52301
        Diagnostic, 52351
        Dilation, 50572, 50575, 50953
            Stricture, 52341-52342, 52344-52345
        Excision
            Tumor, 52355
        Exploration, 52351
        Incision, 52290
        Injection of Implant Material, 52327
        Insertion Guide Wire, 52334
        Lithotripsy, 52325, 52353
        Manipulation of Ureteral Calculus, 52330
        Placement
            Stent, 50947, 52332
        Removal
            Calculus, 50961, 50980, 52310-52315,
                52320, 52352
            Foreign Body, 50961, 50980
        Resection, 52305, 52355
        via Incision, 50970-50976, 50980
        via Stoma, 50951-50957, 50961
        via Ureterotomy, 50970-50980
    Urethra, 52000, 52010
        Biopsy, 52204, 52354
        Catheterization, 52005, 52010
        Destruction, 52214, 52354
            Congenital Posterior Valves, 52400
            Lesion, 52214, 52224, 52234-52235,
                52240
            Polyps, 52285
        Evacuation
            Clot, 52001
        Excision
            Tumor, 52355
        Exploration, 52351
        Incision, 52285
            Congenital Posterior Valves, 52400
            Ejaculatory Duct, 52402
            Internal, 52270, 52275-52276
            Meatotomy, 52281, 52285
        Injection
            for Cystography, 52281
            Implant Material, 51715
            Steroid, 52283
        Insertion
            Radioactive Substance, 52250
            Stent, 52282
        Lithotripsy, 52353
        Lysis Fibrosis, 52285
        Removal
            Stent, 52310
        Resection
            Congenital Posterior Valves, 52400
            Ejaculatory Duct, 52402
            Sphincter, 52277
        Vasectomy, 52402

Endoscopy — *continued*
    Urethra — *continued*
        Vasotomy, 52402
    Uterus
        Anesthesia, 00952
        Hysteroscopy
            with Division
                Resection Intrauterine Septum,
                    58560
            with Lysis of Intrauterine Adhesions,
                58559
            Diagnostic, 58555
        Placement
            Fallopian Tube, 58565
        Removal
            Endometrial, 58563
            Impacted Foreign Body, 58562
            Leiomyomata, 58561
        Surgical with Biopsy, 58558
    Vagina, 57421
        Anesthesia, 00950
        Biopsy, 57421, 57454
        Exploration, 57452
    Vascular
        Surgical, 33508, 37500, 37501
    Virtual
        Colon, 74261-74263
    Vulva, 56820
        With Biopsy, 56821
Endosteal Implant
    Reconstruction
        Mandible, 21248, 21249
        Maxilla, 21248, 21249
Endothelial Function Assessment, 0337T
Endothelioma, Dural
    See Meningioma
Endotoxin
    Bacteria, 87176
Endotracheal Tube
    Intubation, 31500
Endovascular
    Repair
        Angiography, 75952-75959
        Aorta
            with Open Artery Exposure, 34833-
                34834
            Abdominal Aneurysm, 34812-34826
            Descending Thoracic, 33880-33891
            Open After Failed Endovascular Repair,
                34830-34832
            Visceral
                Fenestrated Endograft, 34841-
                    34848
                Modular Endograft, 34845-34848
                Unibody Endograft, 34845-34848
        Iliac Artery, 34900
        Iliac Artery Bifurcation, 0254T-0255T
        Imaging Neck, 75956-75959
        Infrarenal Abdominal Aorta
            with Endograft, 34845-34848
        Lower Extremity, 37220-37235
        Physician Planning 90 Minutes, 34839
        Vena Cava, 37191-37193
        Visceral Aorta
            with Endograft, 34841-34848
    Therapy
        Ablation
            Administration, Pharmacologic Agent,
                Other Than Thrombolysis,
                61650-61651
            Vein, 36473-36479
        Neurosurgery
            Balloon Angioplasty, 61630
            Intracranial Balloon Dilatation, 61640-
                61642
        Occlusion
            Balloon, Arterial, 61623
            Transcatheter, 61624, 61626
        Vascular Catheterization, 61630, 61635
End Stage Renal Disease Services, 90951-90962,
    90967-90970
    Home, 90963-90966
Enema
    Air Contrast, 74280
    Contrast, 74270
    Diagnostic, 74000, 74280

Enema — *continued*
    Home Visit for Fecal Impaction, 99511
    Intussusception, 74283
    Therapeutic
        for Intussusception, 74283
Energies, Electromagnetic
    See Irradiation
ENERGIX-B, 90744, 90746-90747
ENG, 81406
ENT
    See Ear, Nose, and Throat; Otorhinolaryngology,
        Diagnostic
    Therapeutic
        See Otorhinolaryngology
Entamoeba Histolytica
    Antigen Detection
        Enzyme Immunoassay, 87336, 87337
Enterectomy, 44126-44128, 44137
    with Enterostomy, 44125
    Donor, 44132, 44133
    for Congenital Atresia, 44126-44128
    Laparoscopic, 44202-44203
    Partial, 44133
    Resection, 44120, 44121
    Transplanted Allograft, 44137
Enterocele
    Repair
        with Colporrhaphy, 57265
        Abdominal Approach, 57270
        Hysterectomy, 58263, 58270, 58280, 58292,
            58294
        Vaginal Approach, 57268, 57556
Enterocystoplasty, 51960
    Camey, 50825
Enteroenterostomy, 44130
Enterolysis, 44005
    Laparoscopic, 44180
Enteropancreatostomy
    See Anastomosis, Pancreas to Intestines
Enterorrhaphy, 44602, 44603, 44615
Enteroscopy
    Intestines, Small
        Biopsy, 44361, 44377
        Control of Bleeding, 44378
        Destruction
            Lesion, 44369
            Tumor, 44369
        Diagnostic, 44376
        Exploration, 44360
        Hemorrhage, 44366
        Pelvic Pouch, 44385, 44386
        Removal
            Foreign Body, 44363
            Lesion, 44364, 44365
            Polyp, 44364, 44365
            Tumor, 44364, 44365
        Tube Placement, 44372
        Tube Revision, 44373
        via Stoma, 44380-44384 *[44381]*
        Tumor, 44364-44365
Enterostomy
    with Enterectomy
        Intestine, Small, 44125
    with Enteroenterostomy, 44130
    with Proctectomy, 45119, 45397
    Closure, 44227, 44620, 44625, 44626
    Tube Placement, 44300
Enterotomy
    Biopsy, 44020
    Decompression, 44021
    Excision of Lesion, 44110-44111
    Exploration, 44020
    Foreign Body Removal, 44020
    Intestinal Stricturoplasty, 44615
Enterovirus
    Antibody, 86658
    Antigen Detection
        Direct Fluorescence, 87265-87272, 87276,
            87278, 87280, 87285-87290
Entropion
    Repair, 67921-67924
        Blepharoplasty
            Excision Tarsal Wedge, 67923
            Extensive, 67923
        Suture, 67921
        Thermocauterization, 67922

Enucleation
    Cyst
        Mandible, 21040
        Maxilla, 21030
        Zygoma, 21030
    Eye
        with Implant, 65103
            Muscles Attached, 65105
        without Implant, 65101
    Pleural, 32540
    Prostate, 52649
    Tumor, Benign
        Mandible, 21040
        Maxilla, 21030
        Zygoma, 21030
Enucleation, Cyst, Ovarian
    See Cystectomy, Ovarian
Environmental Intervention
    for Psychiatric Patients, 90882
Enzyme Activity
    Constituents, 88319
    Detection, 87185
    Incubation, 86977
    Infectious Agent, 87905
    Nonradioactive Substrate, 82657
    Radioactive Substrate, 82658
Enzyme, Angiotensin Converting
    See Angiotensin Converting Enzyme (ACE)
Enzyme, Angiotensin–Forming
    See Renin
EOG (Electro–Oculography), 92270
Eosinocyte
    See Eosinophils
Eosinophils
    Nasal Smear, 89190
EPCAM, 81403, 81436
Epiandrosterone, *[80327, 80328]*
Epicondylitis, 24357-24359
Epidemic Parotitis
    See Mumps
Epididymectomy
    with Excision Spermatocele, 54840
    Bilateral, 54861
    Unilateral, 54860
Epididymis
    Abscess
        Incision and Drainage, 54700
    Anastomosis
        to Vas Deferens
            Bilateral, 54901
            Unilateral, 54900
    Biopsy, 54800, 54865
    Epididymography, 74440
    Excision
        Bilateral, 54861
        Unilateral, 54860
    Exploration
        Biopsy, 54865
    Hematoma
        Incision and Drainage, 54700
    Lesion
        Excision
            Local, 54830
            Spermatocele, 54840
    Needle Biopsy, 54800
    Repair, 54900, 54901
    Spermatocele
        Excision, 54840
    Unlisted Procedures, Male Genital, 54699, 55899
    X–ray with Contrast, 74440
Epididymograms, 55300
Epididymography, 74440
Epididymoplasty
    See Repair, Epididymis
Epididymovasostomy
    Bilateral, 54901
    Unilateral, 54900
Epidural
    With Disc Decompression, 62287
    Analgesia
        Continuous, 01967-01969
        Drug Administration, 01996
    Catheter
        Insertion, 62350-62351
        Removal, 62355
    Clot or Blood Patch, 62273

Epidural — *continued*
  Electrode
    Insertion, 63650, 63655
    Removal, 63661-63662
  Injection, 0228T-0231T, 62281, 62282, 62320-
    62327, 64479-64484
  Lysis, 62263, 62264
  Neurolytic Substance, 62281-62282
Epidurography, 72275
Epigastric
  Hernia Repair, 49570, 49572
    Laparoscopic, 49652
Epiglottidectomy, 31420
Epiglottis
  Excision, 31420
  Stripping, 31540-31541
Epikeratoplasty, 65767
Epilation, 17380
Epinephrine
  See Catecholamines
  Blood, 82383, 82384
  Urine, 82384
Epiphyseal Arrest
  Femur, 20150, 27185, 27475, 27479, 27485,
    27742
  Fibula, 20150, 27477-27485, 27730-27742
  Radius, 20150, 25450, 25455
  Tibia, 20150, 27477-27485, 27730, 27734-27742
  Ulna, 20150, 25450, 25455
Epiphyseal Separation
  Femur
    Closed Treatment, 27516-27517
    Open Treatment, 27519
    Percutaneous Treatment, 27509
  Radius
    Closed Treatment, 25600, 25605
    Open Treatment, 25607, 25608-25609
    Percutaneous Treatment, 25606
Epiphysiodesis
  See Epiphyseal Arrest
Epiphysis
  See Bone; Specific Bone
Epiploectomy, 49255
EPIS, 59300, 92585, 95925-95930 *[95938, 95939]*
Episiotomy, 59300, 59610, 59612
Epispadias
  Penis
    Reconstruction, 54385
  Repair, 54380-54390
    with Exstrophy of Bladder, 54390
    with Incontinence, 54385
Epistaxis
  with Nasal
    Sinus Endoscopy, 31238
  Control, 30901-30906
Epley Maneuver, 95992
EPM2A, 81404
EPO, 82668
EPS, 93600-93660
Epstein–Barr Virus
  Antibody, 86663-86665
Equina, Cauda
  Decompression, 63005, 63011, 63017, 63047-
    63048, 63055
  Exploration, 63005, 63011, 63017
ER, 99281-99288
ERCP (Cholangiopancreatography), 43260-43270
  [43274, 43275, 43276, 43277, 43278]
ERG (Electroretinography), 92275
Ergocalciferol
  See Calciferol
Ergocalciferols
  See Calciferol
Ergonovine Provocation Test, 93024
ERMAP, 81403
Erythrocyte
  See Red Blood Bell (RBC)
Erythrocyte ab
  See Antibody, Red Blood Cell
Erythrocyte Count
  See Red Blood Cell (RBC), Count
Erythropoietin, 82668
Escharotomy
  Burns, 16035, 16036
  Graft Site, 15002-15005

Escherichia Coli 0157
  Antigen Detection
    Enzyme Immunoassay, 87335
ESD
  See Endoscopy, Gastrointestinal, Upper
Esophageal Acid Infusion Test, 91030
Esophageal Polyp
  See Polyp, Esophagus
Esophageal Tumor
  See Tumor, Esophagus
Esophageal Varices
  Decompression, 37181
  Injection Sclerosis, 43204, 43243
  Ligation, 43205, 43244, 43400
  Repair/Transection, 43401
Esophagectomy
  Partial, 43116-43124
  Total, 43107-43113, 43124
Esophagoenterostomy
  with Total Gastrectomy, 43260
Esophagogastroduodenoscopy
  Ablation Lesions/Polyps/Tumors, *[43270]*
  Band Ligation of Varices, 43244
  Biopsy (single or multiple), 43239
  Collection of Specimen, 43235
  Control of Bleeding, 43255
  Delivery of Thermal Energy, 43257
  Diagnostic, 43235
  Dilation, 43245, 43248-43249, *[43233]*
  Directed Submucosal Injection(s), 43236
  Drainage of Pseudocyst, 43240
  Endoscopic Ultrasound Examination, 43237,
    43259
  Fine Needle Aspiration/Biopsy(s), 43238, 43242
  Guide Wire Insertion, 43248
  Injection
    Anesthetic Agent, 43253
    Diagnostic Substance(s), 43253
    Fiducial Marker(s), 43253
    Neurolytic Agent, 43253
    Sclerosis Agent, 43243
    Submucosal, 43236
    Therapeutic Substance(s), 43253
  Injection Varices, 43243
  Insertion Intraluminal Tube or Catheter, 43241
  Mucosal Resection, 43254
  Optical Endomicroscopy, 43252
  Placement
    Endoscopic Stent, *[43266]*
    Gastrostomy Tube, 43246
  Removal
    Foreign Body, 43247
    Lesion/Polyp/Tumor, 43250-43251
  Ultrasound Guided, 43237-43238, 43253, 43259
Esophagogastrostomy, 43320
Esophagojejunostomy, 43340, 43341
Esophagomyotomy, 32665, 43330, 43331
  With Fundoplasty, 43279
  Abdominal, 43330
  Heller Type, 32665, 43279, 43330
  Laparoscopic, 43279
  Thoracic Approach, 43331
  Thoracoscopic, 32665
Esophagoplasty, 43300-43312
Esophagorrphaphy
  See Esophagus, Suture
Esophagoscopies
  See Endoscopy, Esophagus
Esophagoscopy
  With Optical Endomicroscopy, 43206
  Operative By Incision, 43499
  Through Artificial Stoma, 43499
  Transnasal
    Biopsy, 43198
    Collection of Specimen, 43197
  Transoral
    With Diverticulectomy, 43180
    With Optical Endomicroscopy, 43206
    With Ultrasound Examination, 43231-43232
    Ablation of Lesion, 43229
    Biopsy, 43198
    Collection of Specimen, 43191, 43197,
      43202
    Dilation, 43195-43196, 43220, 43220
      [43212, 43213, 43214], 43226,
      43229, *[43233]*

Esophagoscopy — *continued*
  Transoral — *continued*
    Exploration, 43200
    Guide Wire Insertion, 43196, 43226, 43229,
      [43212]
    Hemorrhage, 43227
    Injection, 43192, 43201, 43204
    Ligation of Varices, 43205
    Mucosal Resection, *[43211]*
    Needle Biopsy, 43232
    Removal
      Foreign Body, 43194, 43215
      Polyp, 43216-43217, 43229
      Tumor, 43216-43217, 43229
    Stent Placement, *[43212]*
    Ultrasound, 43231-43232
    Vein Ligation, 43205
Esophagostomy
  With Esophagectomy, 43124
  Closure, 43420, 43425
  External Fistulization, 43351-43352
Esophagotomy, 43020, 43045
Esophagotracheal Fistula
  See Fistula, Tracheoesophageal
Esophagus
  Ablation
    Lesion, 43229
    Polyp, 43229
    Tumor, 43229
  Acid Perfusion Test, 91030
  Acid Reflux Tests, 91034-91035, 91037-91038
  Balloon Distension, 43249, *[43233]*
    Provocation Study, 91040
  Biopsy
    Endoscopy, 43198, 43202
    Forceps, 3150F
  Cineradiography, 74230
  Cricopharyngeal Myotomy, 43030
  Dilation, 43450, 43453
    Endoscopic, 43195-43196, 43220, 43220
      [43212, 43213, 43214], 43226,
      43229, 43248-43249, *[43213,
      43214]*, *[43233]*, *[43233]*
    Strictures
      Duodenal, 43245
      Gastric, 43245
      Surgical, 43510
  Endoscopy
    Biopsy, 43193, 43198, 43202
    Diagnostic, 43191, 43197, 43200
    Dilation, 43220, 43226
      Balloon, 43195, *[43214]*, *[43233]*
      Dilator over Guide Wire, 43196, 43226,
        43248
      Retrograde by Balloon or Dilator,
        [43213]
      Transendoscopic with Balloon, 43220,
        43249
    Exploration, 43200
    Hemorrhage, 43227
    Injection, 43192, 43201, 43204, 43243,
      43253
    Insertion Stent, *[43212]*
    Mucosal Resection, *[43211]*
    Needle Biopsy, 43232
    Removal
      Foreign Body, 43194, 43215
      Polyp, 43216-43217
      Tumor, 43216-43217
    Specimen Collection, 43191, 43197, 43200
    Ultrasound, 43231, 43232
    Vein Ligation, 43205
  Excision
    Diverticula, 43130, 43135
    Partial, 43116-43124
    Total, 43107-43113, 43124
  Exploration
    Endoscopy, 43200
  Hemorrhage, 43227
  Imaging Studies
    Motility, 78258
    Obstructions, 74360
    Reflux, 78262
    Removal Foreign Body, 74235
    Strictures, 74360

Esophagus — *continued*
  Imaging Studies — *continued*
    Swallowing Function Cineradiography,
      74230
    X-ray, 74210, 74220
  Incision, 43020, 43045
    Muscle, 43030
  Injection
    Sclerosis Agent, 43204
    Submucosal, 43192, 43201
  Insertion
    Sengstaken Tamponade, 43460
    Stent, *[43212]*
    Tamponade, 43460
    Tube, 43510
  Intraluminal Imaging, 91110-91111
  Intubation with Specimen Collection, 43753-
    43755
  Lengthening, 43283, 43338
  Lesion
    Excision, 43100, 43101
    Ligation, 43405
  Motility Study, 78258, 91010-91013
  Mucosal Resection, *[43211]*
  Needle Biopsy
    Endoscopy, 43232
  Nuclear Medicine
    Imaging (Motility), 78258
    Reflux Study, 78262
  Reconstruction, 43300, 43310, 43313
    Creation
      Stoma, 43351-43352
    Esophagostomy, 43351-43352
    Fistula, 43305, 43312, 43314
    Gastrointestinal, 43360, 43361
  Removal
    Foreign Bodies, 43020, 43045, 43194,
      43215, 74235
    Lesion, 43216-43217
    Polyp, 43216-43217
  Repair, 43300, 43310, 43313
    Esophagogastric Fundoplasty, 43325-43328
      Laparoscopic, 43280
    Esophagogastrostomy, 43320
    Esophagojejunostomy, 43340, 43341
    Esophagomyotomy, 43279
    Esophagoplasty, 43300, 43305, 43310,
      43312
    Fistula, 43305, 43312, 43314, 43420, 43425
    Heller Esophagomyotomy, 32665
    Muscle, 43330, 43331
    Nissan Procedure, 43280
    Paraesophageal Hernia
      Laparoscopic, 43281-43282
      Laparotomy, 43332-43333
      Thoracoabdominal Incision, 43336-
        43337
      Thoracotomy, 43334-43335
    Pre–existing Perforation, 43405
    Thal-Nissen Procedure, 43325
    Toupet Procedure, 43280
    Varices, 43401
    Wound, 43410, 43415
  Stapling Gastroesophageal Junction, 43405
  Suture
    Gastroesophageal Junction, 43405
    Wound, 43410, 43415
  Ultrasound, 43231, 43232
  Unlisted Services and Procedures, 43289, 43499
  Vein
    Ligation, 43205, 43400
  Video, 74230
  X–ray, 74220
Esophagus Neoplasm
  See Tumor, Esophagus
Esophagus, Varix
  See Esophageal Varices
ESR, 85651, 85652
ESR1/PGR, 81402
ESRD, 90951-90961, 90967-90970
  Home, 90963-90966
EST, 90870
Established Patient
  Checkout for Orthotic/Prosthetic Use, 97762
  Critical Care, 99291-99292

Established Patient — *continued*
    Domiciliary or Rest Home Visit, 99334-99337, 99339-99340
    Emergency Department Services, 99281-99285
    Evaluation Services
        Basic Life and/or Disability, 99450
        Work-related or Medical Disability, 99455
    Home Services, 99347-99350, 99601-99602
    Hospital Inpatient Services, 99221-99239
    Hospital Observation Services, 99217-99220, 99234-99236, [99224, 99225, 99226]
    Initial Inpatient Consultation, 99251-99255
    Nursing Facility, 99304-99310, 99315-99316, 99318
    Office and/or Other Outpatient Consultations, 99241-99245
    Office Visit, 99211-99215
    Online Evaluation and Management Services
        Nonphysician, 98969
        Physician, 99444
    Ophthalmological Services, 92012, 92014
    Outpatient Visit, 99211-99215
    Preventive Services, 99391-99397
    Prolonged Services
        With Patient Contact, 99354-99357
        Without Patient Contact, 99358-99359
    Telephone Services, 99441-99443, 98966-98968
Establishment
    Colostomy
        Abdominal, 50810
        Perineal, 50810
Estes Operation
    See Ovary, Transposition
Estlander Procedure, 40525, 40527
Estradiol, 82670
    Response, 80415
Estriol
    Blood or Urine, 82677
Estrogen
    Blood or Urine, 82671, 82672
    Receptor, 84233
Estrone
    Blood or Urine, 82679
ESWL, 50590
Ethanediols
    See Ethylene Glycol
Ethanol
    Alcohols and Biomarkers, [80320, 80321, 80322, 80323]
    Breath, 82075
Ethchlorvynol, [80320]
Ethmoid
    With Repair
        Cerebrospinal Fluid Leak, 31290
    Artery Ligation, 30915
    Fracture
        with Fixation, 21340
Ethmoidectomy
    with Nasal
        Sinus Endoscopy, 0406T-0407T, 31254, 31255
    Anterior, 31200
    Endoscopic, 0406T-0407T, 31254, 31255
    Partial, 31254
    Skull Base Surgery, 61580, 61581
    Total, 31201, 31205, 31255
Ethmoid, Sinus
    See Sinus, Ethmoid
Ethosuccimid
    See Ethosuximide
Ethosuximide
    Assay, 80168
Ethyl Alcohol (Ethanol)
    Alcohols and Biomarkers, [80320, 80321, 80322]
    Breath, 82075
Ethylene Dichlorides
    See Dichloroethane
Ethylene Glycol, 82693
Ethylmethylsuccimide
    See Ethosuximide
Etiocholanolone, 82696
Etiocholanolone Measurement
    See Etiocholanolone
ETOH, 82075, [80320, 80321, 80322]
ETV6/NTRK3 (t(t12;15)), 81401
ETV6/RUNX1 (t(t12;21)), 81401

EUA, 57410, 92018, 92019, 92502
Euglobulin Lysis, 85360
European Blastomycosis
    See Cryptococcus
Eustachian Tube
    Inflation
        Myringotomy, 69420
            Anesthesia, 69421
Eutelegenesis
    See Artificial Insemination
Evacuation
    Cervical Pregnancy, 59140
    Hematoma
        Bladder/Urethra, 52001
        Brain, 61108, 61154, 61312-61315
            Anesthesia, 00211
        Intraspinal Lesion, 63265
        Subungual, 11740
    Hydatidiform Mole, 59870
    Meibomian Glands, 0207T
    Stomach, 43753
Evaluation
    Aneurysm Pressure, 93982
    Asthma Symptoms, 1005F
    Athletic Training, [97169, 97170, 97171]
        Re-evaluation, 97172
    Central Auditory Function, 92620-92621
    Cine, 74230
    Electrophysiologic, 93653-93654, 93656
    Electrophysiologic Evaluation Implantable Defibrillator, [93260]
    for Prescription of Nonspeech Generating Device, 92605 [92618]
    Implantable Cardioverter-Defibrillator Device
        Interrogation, 93289, 93292, 93295, 93640-93641
        Programming, 93282-93284, 93287, 93642, 93644
    Integration Device Evaluation, 93289, 93292, 93295, 93640-93641
    Occupation Therapy, [97165, 97166, 97167]
        Re-evaluation, 97168
    Otoacoustic Emissions, 92587-92588
    Physical Therapy, [97161, 97162, 97163]
        Re-evaluation, 97164
    Scoliosis, Radiologic, 72081-72084
    Treatment of swallowing dysfunction, 92526
    Vestibular, basic, 92540
    Video, 74230
Evaluation and Management
    Alcohol and/or Substance Abuse, 99408-99409
    Anticoagulant Management, 99363-99364
    Assistive Technology Assessment, 97755
    Athletic Training, [97169], [97170], [97171]
        Re-evaluation, 97172
    Basic Life and/or Disability Evaluation Services, 99450
    Birthing Center, 99460, 99462-99465
    Care Plan Oversight Services, 99374-99380
        Extracorporeal Liver Assist System, 0405T
        Home, Domiciliary, or Rest Home Care, 99339-99340
        Home Health Agency Care, 99374
        Hospice, 99377
        Nursing Facility, 99379, 99380
    Case Management Services, 99366-99368
    Consultation, 99241-99255
    Critical Care, 99291, 99292
        Interfacility Pediatric Transport, 99466-99467
    Domiciliary or Rest Home
        Established Patient, 99334-99337
        New Patient, 99324-99328
    Emergency Department, 99281-99288
    Health Behavior
        Assessment, 96150
        Family Intervention, 96154, 96155
        Group Intervention, 0403T, 96153
        Individual Intervention, 96152
        Re-assessment, 96151
    Home Services, 99341-99350
    Hospital, 99221-99233
    Hospital Discharge, 99238, 99239
    Hospital Services
        Initial, 99221-99233, 99460-99463, 99477

Evaluation and Management — *continued*
    Hospital Services — *continued*
        Intensive Care
            Low Birth Weight, 99478-99480
            Neonate, 99477
        Observation Care, 99217-99220
        Subsequent, 99231, 99462-99463
    Insurance Examination, 99455-99456
    Internet Communication
        Consult Physician, 99446-99449
        Nonphysician, 98969
        Physician, 99444
    Low Birth Weight Infant, 99468-99469, 99478-99480
    Medical
        Team Conference, 99366-99368
    Neonatal
        Critical Care, 99468-99469
        Intensive Observation, 99477-99480
    Newborn Care, 99460-99465
    Nursing Facility, 99304-99318
        Annual Assessment, 99318
        Discharge, 99315-99316
        Initial Care, 99304-99306
        Subsequent Care, 99307-99310
    Observation Care, 99217-99220
    Occupation Therapy Evaluation, [97165, 97166, 97167]
        Re-evaluation, 97168
    Office and Other Outpatient, 99201-99215
    On-line Assessment
        Consult Physician, 99446-99449
        Nonphysician, 98969
        Physician, 99444
    Online Evaluation
        Consult Physician, 99446-99449
        Nonphysician, 98969
        Physician, 99444
    Pediatric
        Critical Care, 99471-99472
        Interfacility Transport, 99466-99467
    Physical Therapy Evaluation, [97161, 97162, 97163]
        Re-evaluation, 97164
    Physician Standby Services, 99360
    Preventive Services, 4000F-4001F, 99381-99429
    Prolonged Services, 99356, 99357
    Psychiatric/Records or Reports, 90885
    Smoking and Tobacco Cessation Counseling, 99406-99407
    Team Conference, 99366-99368
    Telephone Assessment
        Consult Physician, 99446-99449
        Nonphysician, 98966-98968
        Physician, 99441-99443
    Unlisted Service and Procedures, 99499
    Work-Related and/or Medical Disability Evaluation, 99455
Evaluation Studies, Drug, Preclinical
    See Drug Screen
EVAR (Endovascular Aortic Repair), 34800-34826
Everolimus
    Assay, 80169
Evisceration
    Ocular Contents
        with Implant, 65093
        without Implant, 65091
    Repair
        Abdominal Wall, 49900
    Suture
        Abdominal Wall, 49900
Evisceration, Pelvic
    See Exenteration, Pelvis
E Vitamin
    See Tocopherol
Evocative/Suppression Test, 80400-80439
    Stimulation Panel, 80410
Evoked Potential
    See Audiologic Function Tests
    Auditory Brainstem, 92585, 92586
    Central Motor
        Transcranial Motor Stimulation, 95928-95929
    Somatosensory Testing, 95925-95927 [95938]
    Visual, CNS, 95930

Ewart Procedure
    Palate, Reconstruction, Lengthening, 42226, 42227
EWSR1/ATF1 (t(12;22)), 81401
EWSR1/ERG (t(21;22)), 81401
EWSR1/FLI1 (t(11;22)), 81401
EWSR1/WT1 (t(11;22)), 81401
Examination
    Anorectal, 45990
    Involved Joint, 2004F
Excavatum, Pectus
    See Pectus Excavatum
Exchange
    Blood, 36450-36455
    Blood Components, 36511-36516
    Drainage Catheter
        under Radiologic Guidance, 49423
    External Fixation, 20697
    Intraocular Lens, 66986
Excision
    See Also Debridement; Destruction
    Abscess
        Brain, 61514, 61522
        Olecranon Process, 24138
        Radius, 24136
        Ulna, 24138
    Acromion, 23130
        Shoulder, 23130
    Adenoids
        with Tonsils, 42820, 42821
        Primary
            12 or over, 42831
            Younger Than Age 12, 42830
        Secondary
            12 or over, 42836
            Younger Than Age 12, 42835
    Adenoma
        Thyroid Gland, 60200
    Adrenal Gland, 60540
        with Excision Retroperitoneal Tumor, 60545
        Laparoscopic, 60650
    Alveolus, 41830
    Anal
        Crypt, 46999
        Fissure, 46200
        Tag, 46230 [46220]
    Aorta
        Coarctation, 33840-33851
    Appendix, 44950-44960
    Arteriovenous Malformation
        Spinal, 63250-63252
    Arytenoid Cartilage, 31400
        Endoscopic, 31560, 31561
    Atrial Septum, 33735-33737
    Bartholin's gland, 56740
    Bladder
        Diverticulum, 51525
        Neck, 51520
        Partial, 51550-51565
        Total, 51570, 51580, 51590-51597
            with Nodes, 51575, 51585, 51595
        Transurethral, 52640
        Tumor, 51530
    Bladder Neck Contracture, Postoperative, 52640
    Bone
        Abscess
            Facial, 21026
            Mandible, 21025
        Facial, 21026
        Femur, 20150
        Fibula, 20150
        Mandible, 21025
        Radius, 20150
        Tibia, 20150
        Ulna, 20150
    Brain
        Amygdala, 61566
        Epileptogenic Focus, 61536
        Hemisphere, 61543
        Hippocampus, 61566
        Other Lobe, 61323, 61539-61540
        Temporal Lobe, 61537, 61538
    Brain Lobe
        See Lobectomy, Brain
    Breast
        Biopsy, 19100-19101

Excision — *continued*
Breast — *continued*
Chest Wall Tumor, 19260-19272
Cyst, 19120-19126
Lactiferous Duct Fistula, 19112
Lesion, 19120-19126
by Needle Localization, 19125, 19126
Mastectomy, 19300-19307
Nipple Exploration, 19110
Bulbourethral Gland, 53250
Bullae
Lung, 32141
Endoscopic, 32655
Burns, 15002-15003, 15004-15005
Bursa
Elbow, 24105
Excision, 27060
Femur, 27062
Ischial, 27060
Knee, 27340
Wrist, 25115, 25116
Bypass Graft, 35901-35907
Calcaneus, 28118-28120
Calculi (Stone)
Parotid Gland, 42330, 42340
Salivary Gland, 42330-42340
Sublingual Gland, 42330, 42335
Submandibular Gland, 42330, 42335
Carotid Artery, 60605
Carpal, 25145, 25210, 25215
Cartilage
Knee Joint, 27332, 27333
Shoulder Joint, 23101
Temporomandibular Joint, 21060
Wrist, 25107
Caruncle, Urethra, 53265
Cataract
Secondary, 66830
Cervix
Electrode, 57460
Radical, 57531
Stump
Abdominal Approach, 57540, 57545
Vaginal Approach, 57550-57556
Total, 57530
Chalazion
with Anesthesia, 67808
Multiple
Different Lids, 67805
Same Lid, 67801
Single, 67800
Chest Wall Tumor, 19260-19272
Choroid Plexus, 61544
Clavicle
Partial, 23120, 23180
Sequestrectomy, 23170
Total, 23125
Tumor
Radical Resection, 23200
Coccyx, 27080
Colon
Excision
Partial, 44140-44147, 44160
with Anastomosis, 44140
Total, 44150-44156
Laparoscopic
with Anastomosis, 44204, 44207-44208
with Colostomy, 44206, 44208
with Ileocolostomy, 44205
Condyle
Temporomandibular Joint, 21050
Condylectomy, 21050
Constricting Ring
Finger, 26596
Cornea
Epithelium, 65435
with Chelating Agent, 65436
Scraping, 65430
Coronoidectomy, 21070
Cowper's gland, 53250
Cranial Bone
Tumor, 61563, 61564
Cyst
See Ganglion Cyst
Bile Duct, 47715
Bladder, 51500

Excision — *continued*
Cyst — *continued*
Brain, 61516, 61524, 62162
Branchial, 42810, 42815
Breast, 19120
Calcaneus, 28100-28103
Carpal, 25130-25136
Cheekbone, 21030
Clavicle, 23140
with Allograft, 23146
with Autograft, 23145
Facial Bone, 21030
Femur, 27065-27067, 27355-27358
Fibula, 27635-27638
Finger, 26034, 26160
Foot, 28090
Hand, 26160
Hip, 27065-27067
Humerus, 23150, 24110
with Allograft, 23156, 24116
with Autograft, 23155, 24115
Ileum, 27065-27067
Intra-abdominal, 49203-49205
Kidney, 50280, 50290
Knee, 27345, 27347
Lung, 32140
Mandible, 21040, 21046-21047
Maxilla, 21030, 21048-21049
Mediastinum, 32662
Metacarpal, 26200, 26205
Metatarsal, 28104-28107
Mullerian Duct, 55680
Nose, 30124-30125
Olecranon (Process), 24120
with Allograft, 24126
with Autograft, 24125
Ovarian, 58925
See Cystectomy, Ovarian
Pericardial, 33050
Endoscopic, 32661
Phalanges
Finger, 26210, 26215
Toe, 28108
Pilonidal, 11770-11772
Pubis, 27066, 27067
Radius, 24120, 25120-25126
with Allograft, 24126
with Autograft, 24125
Salivary Gland, 42408
Scapula, 23140
with Allograft, 23146
with Autograft, 23145
Seminal Vesicle, 55680
Sublingual Gland, 42408
Talus, 28100-28103
Tarsal, 28104-28107
Thyroglossal Duct, 60280, 60281
Thyroid Gland, 60200
Tibia, 27635-27638
Toe, 28092
Ulna, 24120, 25120
with Allograft, 24126
with Autograft, 24125
Urachal
Bladder, 51500
Vaginal, 57135
Destruction of the Vestibule of the Mouth
See Mouth, Vestibule of, Excision, Destruction
Diverticulum, Meckel's
See Meckel's Diverticulum, Excision
Ear, External
Partial, 69110
Total, 69120
Elbow Joint, 24155
Electrode, 57522
Embolectomy/Thrombectomy
Aortoiliac Artery, 34151, 34201
Axillary Artery, 34101
Brachial Artery, 34101
Carotid Artery, 34001
Celiac Artery, 34151
Femoral Artery, 34201
Heart, 33310-33315
Iliac Artery, 34151, 34201
Innominate Artery, 34001-34101

Excision — *continued*
Embolectomy/Thrombectomy — *continued*
Mesentery Artery, 34151
Peroneal Artery, 34203
Popliteal Artery, 34203
Radial Artery, 34111
Renal Artery, 34151
Subclavian Artery, 34001-34101
Tibial Artery, 34203
Ulnar Artery, 34111
Embolism
Pulmonary Artery, 33910-33916
Empyema
Lung, 32540
Pleural, 32540
Endometriomas
Intra-abdominal, 49203-49205
Epididymis
Bilateral, 54861
Unilateral, 54860
Epiglottis, 31420
Epikeratoplasty, 65767
Epiphyseal Bar, 20150
Esophagus
Diverticulum, 43130, 43135
Partial, 43116-43124
Total, 43107-43113, 43124
Excess Skin
Abdomen, 15830
Eye
See Enucleation, Eye
Fallopian Tubes
Salpingectomy, 58700
Salpingo–Oophorectomy, 58720
Fascia
See Fasciectomy
Femur, 27360
Partial, 27070, 27071
Fibula, 27360, 27455, 27457, 27641
Fistula
Anal, 46270-46285
Foot
Fasciectomy, 28060
Radical, 28062
Gallbladder
Open, 47600-47620
via Laparoscopy
Cholecystectomy, 47562
with Cholangiography, 47563
with Exploration Common Duct, 47564
Ganglion Cyst
Knee, 27347
Wrist, 25111, 25112
Gingiva, 41820
Gums, 41820
Alveolus, 41830
Operculum, 41821
Heart
Donor, 33940
Lung
Donor, 33930
Hemangioma, 11400-11446
Hemorrhoids, 46221, 46250
with Fissurectomy, 46257, 46258
Clot, [46320]
Complex, 46260-46262
Simple, 46255
Hip
Partial, 27070, 27071
Hippocampus, 61566
Humeral Head
Resection, 23195
Sequestrectomy, 23174
Humerus, 23184, 23220, 24134, 24140, 24150
Hydrocele
Spermatic Cord, 55500
Tunica Vaginalis, 55040, 55041
Bilateral, 55041
Unilateral, 55040
Hygroma, Cystic
Axillary
Cervical, 38550, 38555
Hymenotomy, 56700
See Hymen, Excision

Excision — *continued*
Ileum
Ileoanal Reservoir, 45136
Partial, 27070, 27071
Inner Ear
See Ear, Inner, Excision
Interphalangeal Joint
Toe, 28160
Intervertebral Disc
Decompression, 62380, 63075-63078
Hemilaminectomy, 63040, 63043, 63044
Herniated, 62380, 63020-63044, 63055-63066
Intestine
Laparoscopic
with Anastomosis, 44202, 44203
Intestines
Donor, 44132, 44133
Intestines, Small, 44120-44128
Transplantation, 44137
Iris
Iridectomy
with Corneoscleral or Corneal Section, 66600
with Cyclectomy, 66605
Optical, 66635
Peripheral, 66625
Sector, 66630
Kidney
with Ureters, 50220-50236
Donor, 50300, 50320, 50547
Partial, 50240
Recipient, 50340
Transplantation, 50370
Kneecap, 27350
Labyrinth
with Mastoidectomy, 69910
Transcanal, 69905
Lacrimal Gland
Partial, 68505
Total, 68500
Lacrimal Sac, 68520
Laparoscopy
Adrenalectomy, 60650
Larynx
with Pharynx, 31390, 31395
Endoscopic, 31545-31546
Partial, 31367-31382
Total, 31360-31365
Leg, 27630
Leg, Lower, 27630
Lesion
Anal, 45108, 46922
Ankle, 27630
Arthroscopic, 29891
Arm, 25110
Arthroscopic
Ankle, 29891
Talus, 29891
Tibia, 29891
Auditory Canal, External
Exostosis, 69140
Radical with Neck Dissection, 69155
Radical without Neck Dissection, 69150
Soft Tissue, 69145
Bladder, 52224
Brain, 61534, 61536-61540
Brainstem, 61575, 61576
Carotid Body, 60600, 60605
Colon, 44110, 44111
Conjunctiva, 68110-68130
with Adjacent Sclera, 68130
over One Centimeter, 68115
Cornea, 65400
without Graft, 65420
Ear, Middle, 69540
Epididymis
Local, 54830
Spermatocele, 54840
Esophagus, 43100, 43101
Eye, 65900
Eyelid
without Closure, 67840
Multiple, Different Lids, 67805
Multiple, Same Lid, 67801
Single, 67800

Excision — *continued*
Lesion — *continued*
Eyelid — *continued*
under Anesthesia, 67808
Femur, 27062
Finger, 26160
Foot, 28080, 28090
Gums, 41822-41828
Hand, 26160
Intestines, 44110
Small, 43250, 44111
Intraspinal, 63265-63273
Knee, 27347
Larynx
Endoscopic, 31545-31546
Meniscus, 27347
Mesentery, 44820
Mouth, 40810-40816, 41116
Nerve, 64774-64792
Neuroma, 64778
Orbit, 61333
Lateral Approach, 67420
Removal, 67412
Palate, 42104-42120
Pancreas, 48120
Penis, 54060
Plaque, 54110-54112
Pharynx, 42808
Rectum, 45108
Sclera, 66130
Skin
Benign, 11400-11471
Malignant, 11600-11646
Skull, 61500, 61615-61616
Spermatic Cord, 55520
Spinal Cord, 63300-63308
Stomach, 43611
Talus
Arthroscopic, 29891
Tendon Sheath
Arm, 25110
Foot, 28090
Hand/Finger, 26160
Leg/Ankle, 27630
Wrist, 25110
Testis, 54512
Tibia
Arthroscopic, 29891
Toe, 28092
Tongue, 41110-41114
Urethra, 52224, 53265
Uterus
Leiomyomata, 58140, 58545-58546, 58561
Uvula, 42104-42107
Wrist Tendon, 25110
Lip, 40500-40530
Frenum, 40819
Liver
Allotransplantation, 47135
Biopsy, wedge, 47100
Donor, 47133-47142
Extensive, 47122
Lobectomy, total
Left, 47125
Right, 47130
Resection
Partial, 47120, 47125, 47140-47142
Total, 47133
Trisegmentectomy, 47122
Lung, 32440-32445, 32488
Bronchus Resection, 32486
Bullae
Endoscopic, 32655
Completion, 32488
Emphysematous, 32491
Heart
Donor, 33930
Lobe, 32480, 32482
Pneumonectomy, 32440-32445
Segment, 32484
Total, 32440-32445
Tumor
with Reconstruction, 32504
with Resection, 32503
Wedge Resection, 32505-32507

Excision — *continued*
Lung — *continued*
Wedge Resection — *continued*
Endoscopic, 32666-32668
Lymph Nodes, 38500, 38510-38530
Abdominal, 38747
Axillary, 38740
Complete, 38745
Cervical, 38720, 38724
Cloquet's node, 38760
Deep
Axillary, 38525
Cervical, 38510, 38520
Mammary, 38530
Inguinofemoral, 38760, 38765
Limited, for Staging
Para–Aortic, 38562
Pelvic, 38562
Retroperitoneal, 38564
Mediastinal, 38746
Pelvic, 38770
Peritracheal, 38746
Radical
Axillary, 38740, 38745
Cervical, 38720, 38724
Suprahyoid, 38700
Retroperitoneal Transabdominal, 38780
Superficial
Needle, 38505
Open, 38500
Suprahyoid, 38700
Thoracic, 38746
Mandibular, Exostosis, 21031
Mastoid
Complete, 69502
Radical, 69511
Modified, 69505
Petrous Apicectomy, 69530
Simple, 69501
Maxilla
Exostosis, 21032
Maxillary Torus Palatinus, 21032
Meningioma
Brain, 61512, 61519
Meniscectomy
Temporomandibular Joint, 21060
Metacarpal, 26230
Metatarsal, 28110-28114, 28122, 28140
Condyle, 28288
Mucosa
Gums, 41828
Mouth, 40818
Mucous Membrane
Sphenoid Sinus, 31288
Nail Fold, 11765
Nails, 11750
Finger, 26236
Toe, 28124, 28160
Nasopharynx, 61586, 61600
Nerve
Foot, 28055
Hamstring, 27325
Leg, Upper, 27325
Popliteal, 27326
Sympathetic, 64802-64818
Neurofibroma, 64788, 64790
Neurolemmoma, 64788-64792
Neuroma, 64774-64786
Nose, 30117-30118
Dermoid Cyst
Complex, 30125
Simple, 30124
Polyp, 30110, 30115
Rhinectomy, 30150, 30160
Skin, 30120
Submucous Resection
Nasal Septum, 30520
Turbinate, 30140
Turbinate, 30130, 30140
Odontoid Process, 22548
Olecranon, 24147
Omentum, 49255
Orbit, 61333
Lateral Approach, 67420
Removal, 67412

Excision — *continued*
Ovary
Partial
Oophorectomy, 58940
Ovarian Malignancy, 58943
Peritoneal Malignancy, 58943
Tubal Malignancy, 58943
Wedge Resection, 58920
Total, 58940, 58943
Oviduct, 58720
Palate, 42104-42120, 42145
Pancreas, 48120
Ampulla of Vater, 48148
Duct, 48148
Lesion, 48120
Partial, 48140-48154, 48160
Peripancreatic Tissue, 48105
Total, 48155, 48160
Papilla
Anus, 46230 *[46220]*
Parathyroid Gland, 60500, 60502
Parotid Gland, 42340
Partial, 42410, 42415
Total, 42420-42426
Partial, 31367-31382
Patella, 27350
See Patellectomy
Penile Adhesions
Post–circumcision, 54162
Penis, 54110-54112
Frenulum, 54164
Partial, 54120
Penile Plaque, 54110-54112
Prepuce, 54150-54161, 54163
Radical, 54130, 54135
Total, 54125, 54135
Pericardium, 33030, 33031
Endoscopic, 32659
Petrous Temporal
Apex, 69530
Phalanges
Finger, 26235, 26236
Toe, 28124, 28126, 28150-28160
Pharynx, 42145
with Larynx, 31390, 31395
Lesion, 42808
Partial, 42890
Resection, 42892, 42894
Pituitary Gland, 61546, 61548
Pleura, 32310, 32320
Endoscopic, 32656
Polyp
Intestines, 43250
Nose
Extensive, 30115
Simple, 30110
Sinus, 31032
Urethra, 53260
Pressure Ulcers, 15920-15999
See Skin Graft and Flap
Coccygeal, 15920, 15922
Ischial, 15940-15946
Sacral, 15931-15936
Trochanteric, 15950-15958
Unlisted Procedure, Excision, 15999
Prostate
Abdominoperineal, 45119
Partial, 55801, 55821, 55831
Perineal, 55801-55815
Radical, 55810-55815, 55840-55845
Regrowth, 52630
Residual Obstructive Tissue, 52630
Retropubic, 55831-55845
Suprapubic, 55821
Transurethral, 52601
Pterygium
with Graft, 65426
Pubis
Partial, 27070, 27071
Radical Synovium
Wrist, 25115, 25116
Radius, 24130, 24136, 24145, 24152, 25145
Styloid Process, 25230
Rectum
with Colon, 45121
Partial, 45111, 45113-45116, 45123

Excision — *continued*
Rectum — *continued*
Prolapse, 45130, 45135
Stricture, 45150
Total, 45119, 45120
Tumor, 0184T
Redundant Skin of Eyelid
See Blepharoplasty
Ribs, 21600-21616, 32900
Scapula
Ostectomy, 23190
Partial, 23182
Sequestrectomy, 23172
Tumor
Radical Resection, 23210
Sclera, 66130, 66160
Scrotum, 55150
Semilunar Cartilage of Knee
See Knee, Meniscectomy
Seminal Vesicle, 55650
Sesamoid Bone
Foot, 28315
Sinus
Ethmoid, 31200-31205
Endoscopic, 0406T-0407T, 31254, 31255
Frontal
Endoscopic, 31276
Maxillary, 31225, 31230
Maxillectomy, 31230, 31255
Endoscopic, 31267
Unlisted Procedure, Accessory Sinuses, 31299
Skene's Gland, 53270
Skin
Excess, 15830-15839
Lesion
Benign, 11400-11471
Malignant, 11600-11646
Nose, 30120
Skin Graft
Preparation of Site, 15002-15003, 15004-15005
Skull, 61500-61501, 61615, 61616
Spermatic Veins, 55530-55540
with Hernia Repair, 55540
Abdominal Approach, 55535
Spleen, 38100-38102
Laparoscopic, 38120
Stapes
with Footplate Drill Out, 69661
without Foreign Material, 69660
Sternum, 21620, 21630, 21632
Stomach
Partial, 43631-43635, 43845
Total, 43620-43622, 43634
Tumor or ulcer, 43610-43611
Sublingual Gland, 42450
Submandibular Gland, 42440
Sweat Glands
Axillary, 11450, 11451
Inguinal, 11462, 11463
Perianal, 11470, 11471
Perineal, 11470, 11471
Umbilical, 11470, 11471
Synovium
Ankle, 27625, 27626
Carpometacarpal Joint, 26130
Elbow, 24102
Hip Joint, 27054
Interphalangeal Joint, Finger, 26140
Intertarsal Joint, 28070
Knee Joint, 27334, 27335
Metacarpophalangeal Joint, 26135
Metatarsophalangeal Joint, 28072
Shoulder, 23105, 23106
Tarsometatarsal Joint, 28070
Wrist, 25105, 25115-25119
Tag
Anus, 46230 *[46220]*
Skin, 11200-11201
Talus, 28120, 28130
Arthroscopic, 29891
Tarsal, 28116, 28122
Temporal Bone, 69535

Excision — *continued*
  Temporal, Petrous
    Apex, 69530
  Tendon
    Finger, 26180, 26390, 26415
    Forearm, 25109
    Hand, 26390, 26415
    Palm, 26170
    Wrist, 25109
  Tendon Sheath
    Finger, 26145
    Foot, 28086, 28088
    Forearm, 25110
    Palm, 26145
    Wrist, 25115, 25116
  Testis
    Extraparenchymal lesion, 54512
    Laparoscopic, 54690
    Partial, 54522
    Radical, 54530, 54535
    Simple, 54520
    Tumor, 54530, 54535
  Thrombectomy
    Axillary Vein, 34490
    Bypass Graft, 35875, 35876
    Femoropopliteal Vein, 34401-34451
    Iliac Vein, 34401-34451
    Subclavian Vein, 34471, 34490
    Vena Cava, 34401-34451
  Thromboendarterectomy
    Aorta, Abdominal, 35331
    Aortoiliac, 35361
    Aortoiliofemoral, 35363
    Axillary Artery, 35321
    Brachial Artery, 35321
    Carotid Artery, 35301, 35390
    Celiac Artery, 35341
    Femoral Artery, 35302, 35371, 35372
    Iliac, 35361, 35363
    Iliac Artery, 35351
    Iliofemoral Artery, 35355, 35363
    Innominate Artery, 35311
    Mesenteric Artery, 35341
    Peroneal Artery, 35305-35306
    Popliteal Artery, 35303
    Renal Artery, 35341
    Subclavian Artery, 35301, 35311, 35331,
      35390
    Superficial Femoral Artery, 35302
    Tibial Artery, 35305-35306
    Tibioperoneal Trunk, 35304
    Vertebral Artery, 35301, 35390
  Thymus Gland, 60521
  Thyroid Gland
    for Malignancy, 60252, 60254
      Limited Neck Dissection, 60252
      Radical Neck Dissection, 60254
    Partial, 60210-60225
    Removal All Thyroid Tissue, 60260
    Secondary, 60260
    Total, 60240
      Cervical Approach, 60271
      Sternal Split
        Transthoracic, 60270
  Tibia, 27360, 27640
    Arthroscopic, 29891
  Toe, 28092
  Tongue
    with Mouth Resection, 41150, 41153
    with Radical Neck Dissection, 41135, 41145-
      41155
    Complete, 41140-41155
    Frenum, 41115
    Partial, 41120-41135
  Tonsils
    Lingual, 42870
    Radical, 42842-42845
      Closure Local Flap, 42844, 42845
    Tag, 42860
    Tonsillectomy and Adenoidectomy
      Age 12 or Over, 42821
      Younger Than Age 12, 42820
    Tonsillectomy, Primary or Secondary
      Age 12 or Over, 42826
      Younger Than Age 12, 42825
  Torus Mandibularis, 21031

Excision — *continued*
  Total, 31360, 31365
  Trachea
    Stenosis, 31780, 31781
  Transcervical Approach, 60520
  Tricuspid Valve, 33460-33465
  Tumor
    Abdomen, 49203-49205
    Abdominal Wall, 22900-22905
    Acetabulum, 27076
    Ankle, 27615-27619 *[27632, 27634]*, 27647
    Arm, Lower, 25075-25078 *[25071, 25073]*,
      25120-25126, 25170
    Arm, Upper, 23220, 24075-24079 *[24071,
      24073]*, 24110-24126, 24150-24152
    Back
      Flank, 21930, 21935
    Bile Duct, 47711, 47712
    Bladder, 51530, 52234-52240, 52355
    Brain, 61510, 61518, 61520, 61521, 61526,
      61530, 61545, 62164
    Bronchi, 31640, 31641
    Calcaneus, 27647, 28100-28103
      with Allograft, 28103
      with Autograft, 28102
    Carpal, 25075-25078 *[25071, 25073]*, 25130-
      25136
    Cheekbone, 21030, 21034, 21048-21049
    Clavicle, 23075-23078 *[23071, 23073]*,
      23140, 23200
      with Allograft, 23146
      with Autograft, 23145
    Ear, Middle
      Extended, 69554
      Transcanal, 69550
      Transmastoid, 69552
    Elbow, 24075-24079 *[24071, 24073]*, 24120-
      24126, 24152
    Esophagus
      Endoscopic, 43216-43217
    Face or Scalp, 21011-21016
    Facial
      Bones, 21029, 21030, 21034, 21040,
        21046-21049
      Tissue, 21011-21016
    Femur, 27327-27328 *[27337, 27339]*, 27355-
      27358, 27364-27365 *[27329]*
    Fibula, 27615-27619 *[27632, 27634]*, 27635-
      27638, 27646
    Finger, 26115-26118 *[26111, 26113]*, 26210-
      26215, 26260-26262
    Foot, 28043-28047 *[28039, 28041]*, 28100-
      28107, 28171-28175
    Gums, 41825-41827
    Hand, 26115-26118 *[26111, 26113]*, 26200-
      26205, 26250
    Heart, 33120, 33130
    Hip, 27047-27049 *[27043, 27045, 27059]*,
      27065-27067, 27076-27078
    Humerus, 23150-23156, 23220, 24075-
      24079 *[24071, 24073]*, 24110, 24150
      with Allograft, 23156, 24116
      with Autograft, 23155, 24115
      Radial Head or Neck, 24152
    Ilium, 27047-27049 *[27043, 27045, 27059]*,
      27065-27067
    Innominate, 27047-27049 *[27043, 27045,
      27059]*, 27077
    Intestines
      Small, 43250
    Ischial, 27047-27049 *[27043, 27045, 27059]*,
      27078
    Kidney, 52355
    Knee, 27327-27328 *[27337, 27339]*, 27364-
      27365 *[27329]*
    Lacrimal Gland
      Frontal Approach, 68540
      Involving Osteotomy, 68550
    Larynx, 31300, 31320
      Endoscopic, 31540, 31541, 31578
    Leg, Lower, 27615-27619 *[27632, 27634]*,
      27635-27638, 27645-27647
    Leg, Upper, 27327-27328 *[27337, 27339]*,
      27355-27358, 27364-27365 *[27329]*
    Mandible, 21040-21047
    Maxilla, 21030, 21034, 21048, 21049

Excision — *continued*
  Tumor — *continued*
    Mediastinum, 32662
    Metacarpal, 26115-26118 *[26111, 26113]*,
      26200-26205
    Metatarsal, 28043-28047 *[28039, 28041]*,
      28100-28107, 28173
    Neck, 21555-21558 *[21552, 21554]*
    Olecranon Process, 24075-24079 *[24071,
      24073]*, 24120
      with Allograft, 24126
      with Autograft, 24125
    Parotid Gland, 42410-42426
    Pelvis, 27047-27049 *[27043, 27045, 27059]*,
      27065-27067
    Pericardium, 32661
    Phalanges
      Finger, 26115-26118 *[26111, 26113]*,
        26210, 26215, 26260-26262
      Toe, 28043-28047 *[28039, 28041]*,
        28108, 28175
    Pituitary Gland, 61546, 61548, 62165
    Presacral, 49215
    Pubis, 27065-27067
    Radius, 24152
    Rectum, 0184T, 45160, 45171-45172
      Transanal Endoscopic, 0184T
    Retropharyngeal
      Anesthesia, 00174
    Sacrococcygeal, 49215
    Scalp or Face, 21011-21014
    Scapula, 23140
      with Allograft, 23146
      with Autograft, 23145
    Shoulder, 23075-23078 *[23071, 23073]*
    Skull, 61500
    Spermatocele
      See Spermatocele, Excision
    Spinal Cord, 63275-63290
    Spleen, Total
      See Splenectomy, Total
    Sternum, 21630
    Stomach, 43610
    Talus, 27647
    Tarsal
      Benign, 28104
        with Allograft, 28107
        with Autograft, 28106
      Radical, 28171
    Thigh, 27327-27328 *[27337, 27339]*, 27355-
      27358, 27364-27365 *[27329]*
    Thorax, 21555-21558 *[21552, 21554]*
    Thyroid, 60200
    Tibia, 27615-27619 *[27632, 27634]*, 27635-
      27638, 27645
    Toe, 28043-28047 *[28039, 28041]*, 28108,
      28175
    Trachea
      Cervical, 31785
      Thoracic, 31786
    Ulna, 25075-25078 *[25071, 25073]*, 25120-
      25126, 25170
    Ureter, 52355
    Urethra, 52234, 52235, 52240, 52355, 53220
    Uterus
      Abdominal Approach, 58140, 58146
      Laparoscopic, 58541-58546, 58550
      Leiomyomata, 58546
      Vaginal Approach, 58145
    Uvula, 42120
    Vagina, 57135
    Vertebra
      Lumbar, 22102
      Thoracic, 22101
    Wrist, 25075-25078 *[25071, 25073]*, 25120-
      25126
    Zygoma, 21030, 21034
    Turbinate, 30130, 30140
    Tympanic Nerve, 69676
    Ulcer
      Stomach, 43610
    Ulna, 24147, 25145
      Complete, 25240
      Partial, 24147, 25150, 25240
      Radical, 25170
    Umbilicus, 49250

Excision — *continued*
  Ureter
    See Ureterectomy
  Ureterocele, 51535
  Urethra
    Diverticulum, 53230, 53235
    Prolapse, 53275
    Total
      Female, 53210
      Male, 53215
  Uterus
    with Colo-urethrocystopexy, 58267, 58293
    with Colpectomy, 58275-58280
    with Repair of Enterocele, 58270, 58292,
      58294
    Laparoscopic, 58550
    Partial, 58180
    Radical, 58210, 58285
    Removal Tubes and/or Ovaries, 58262-
      58263, 58291, 58552, 58554
    Total, 58150, 58152, 58200
    Vaginal, 58260, 58290-58294, 58550, 58553
      with Colpectomy, 58275-58280
      with Colpo-Urethrocystopexy, 58267,
        58293
      with Repair of Enterocele, 58270,
        58292, 58294
      Removal Tubes and
        or Ovaries, 58262, 58263, 58291,
          58552, 58554
  Uvula, 42104-42107, 42140, 42145
  Vagina
    with Hysterectomy, 58275, 58280
      with Colpectomy, 58275
      Repair of Enterocele, 58280
    Closure, 57120
    Complete
      with Removal of Paravaginal Tissue
        with Lymphadenectomy,
          57112
      with Removal of Paravaginal Tissue,
        57111
      with Removal of Vaginal Wall, 57110
    Partial
      with Removal of Paravaginal Tissue
        with Lymphadenectomy,
          57109
      with Removal of Paravaginal Tissue,
        57107
      with Removal of Vaginal Wall, 57106
    Septum, 57130
    Total, 57110
  Varicocele
    Spermatic Cord, 55530-55540
      with Hernia Repair, 55540
      Abdominal Approach, 55535
  Vascular Malformation
    Finger, 26115
    Hand, 26115
  Vas Deferens, 55250
  Vein
    Varicose, 37765, 37766
  Vertebra
    Additional Segment, 22103, 22116
    Cervical, 22110
      for Tumor, 22100, 22110
    Lumbar, 22102
      for Tumor, 22114
    Thoracic, 22112
      for Tumor, 22101
  Vertebral Body
    Decompression, 62380, 63081-63091
    Lesion, 63300-63308
  Vitreous
    with Retinal Surgery, 67108, 67113
    Applicator Placement, 0190T
    Mechanical, Pars Plana Approach, 67036-
      67043
  Vulva
    Radical
      Complete, 56633-56640
      Partial, 56630-56632
    Simple
      Complete, 56625
      Partial, 56620
  Wrist Tendon, 25110

Excision — Excision

Exclusion
Duodenum, 48547
Small Bowel, 44700
Exenteration
Eye
with Muscle or Myocutaneous Flap, 65114
Removal Orbital Contents, 65110
Therapeutic Removal of Bone, 65112
Pelvis, 45126, 58240
for Colorectal Malignancy, 45126
Exercise Stress Tests, 93015-93018, 93464
Exercise Test
See Electromyography, Needle
Ischemic Limb, 95875
Exercise Therapy, 97110-97113
See Physical Medicine/ Therapy/Occupational
Exfoliation
Chemical, 17360
Exhaled Breath Condensate pH, 83987
Exocrine, Pancreas
See Pancreas
Exomphalos
See Omphalocele
Exostectomy, 28288, 28292
Exostoses, Cartilaginous
See Exostosis
Exostosis
Excision, 69140
Expander, Tissue, Inflatable
Breast reconstruction with insertion, 19357
Skin
Insertion, 11960
Removal, 11971
Replacement, 11970
Expired Gas Analysis, 94680-94690, 94770
Nitrous Oxide, 95012
Exploration
Abdomen, 49000, 49002
Blood Vessel, 35840
Penetrating Wound, 20102
Staging, 58960
Adrenal Gland, 60540, 60545
Anal
Endoscopy, 46600
Surgical, 45990
Ankle, 27610, 27620
Arm, Lower, 25248
Artery
Brachial, 24495
Carotid, 35701
Femoral, 35721
Other, 35761
Popliteal, 35741
Unlisted Services and Procedures, 35761
Back, Penetrating Wound, 20102
Bile Duct
Atresia, 47700
Endoscopy, 47552, 47553
Blood Vessel
Abdomen, 35840
Chest, 35820
Extremity, 35860
Neck, 35800
Brain
Infratentorial, 61305
Supratentorial, 61304
via Burr Hole
Infratentorial, 61253
Supratentorial, 61250
Breast, 19020
Bronchi
Endoscopy, 31622
Bronchoscopy, 31622
Cauda Equina, 63005, 63011, 63017
Chest, Penetrating Wound, 20101
Colon
Endoscopic, 44388, 45378
Colon, Sigmoid
Endoscopy, 45330, 45335
Common Bile Duct
with Cholecystectomy, 47610
Duodenum, 44010
Ear, Inner
Endolymphatic Sac
with Shunt, 69806
without Shunt, 69805

Exploration — *continued*
Ear, Middle, 69440
Elbow, 24000-24101 *[24071, 24073]*
Epididymis, 54865
Exploration, 54865
Esophagus
Endoscopy, 43200
Extremity
Penetrating Wound, 20103
Finger Joint, 26075, 26080
Flank
Penetrating Wound, 20102
Gallbladder, 47480
Gastrointestinal Tract, Upper
Endoscopy, 43235
Hand Joint, 26070
Heart, 33310, 33315
Hepatic Duct, 47400
Hip, 27033
Interphalangeal Joint
Toe, 28024
Intertarsal Joint, 28020
Intestines, Small
Endoscopy, 43360
Enterotomy, 44020
Kidney, 50010, 50045, 50120, 50135
Knee, 27310, 27331
Lacrimal Duct, 68810
with Anesthesia, 68811
with Insertion Tube or Stent, 68815
Canaliculi, 68840
Laryngoscopy, 31575
Larynx, 31320, 31505, 31520-31526, 31575
Liver
Wound, 47361, 47362
Mediastinum, 39000, 39010
Metatarsophalangeal Joint, 28022
Nasolacrimal Duct, 68810
with Anesthesia, 68811
with Insertion Tube or Stent, 68815
Neck
Lymph Nodes, 38542
Penetrating Wound, 20100
Nipple, 19110
Nose
Endoscopy, 31231-31235
Orbit, 61332-61333
without Bone Flap, 67400
with/without Biopsy, 67450
Parathyroid Gland, 60500-60505
Pelvis, 49320
Peritoneum
Endoscopic, 49320
Prostate, 55860
with Nodes, 55862, 55865
Pterygomaxillary Fossa, 31040
Rectum
Endoscopic, 45300
Injury, 45562, 45563
Retroperitoneal Area, 49010
Scrotum, 55110
Shoulder Joint, 23040, 23044, 23107
Sinus
Frontal, 31070, 31075
Endoscopic, 31276
Transorbital, 31075
Maxillary, 31020, 31030
Sphenoid, 31050
Skull, Drill Hole, 61105
Spinal Cord, 63001-63011, 63015-63017, 63040-63044
Facetectomy, Foraminotomy
Partial Cervical, 63045
Additional Segments, 63048
Partial Lumbar, 62380, 63047
Additional Segments, 63048
Partial Thoracic, 63046
Additional Segments, 63048
Fusion, 22830
Hemilaminectomy (including partial Face-tectomy, Foraminotomy)
Cervical, 63045
Additional Segments, 63048
Lumbar, 63047
Additional Segments, 63048
Thoracic, 63046

Exploration — *continued*
Spinal Cord — *continued*
Hemilaminectomy — *continued*
Thoracic — *continued*
Additional Segments, 63048
Laminectomy
Cervical, 63001, 63015
Lumbar, 63005, 63017
Thoracic, 63003, 63016
Laminotomy
Endoscopic, Lumbar, 62380
Initial
Cervical, 63020
Each Additional Space, 63035
Lumbar, 63030
Reexploration
Cervical, 63040
Each Additional Space, 63043
Lumbar, 63042
Each Additional Interspace, 63044
Stomach, 43500
Tarsometatarsal Joint, 28020
Testis
Undescended, 54550, 54560
Toe Joint, 28024
Ureter, 50600, 50650, 50660
Vagina, 57000
Endoscopic Endocervical, 57452
Wrist, 25101, 25248
Joint, 25040
Exploration, Larynx by Incision
See Laryngotomy, Diagnostic
Exploratory Laparotomy
See Abdomen, Exploration
Expression
Lesion
Conjunctiva, 68040
Exteriorization, Small Intestine
See Enterostomy
External Auditory Canal
See Auditory Canal
External Cephalic Version, 59412
External Ear
See Ear, External
External Extoses
See Exostosis
External Fixation (System)
Adjustment/Revision, 20693
Application, 20690, 20692
Stereotactic Computer Assisted, 20696-20697
Mandibular Fracture
Open Treatment, 21454
Percutaneous Treatment, 21452
Removal, 20694
Extirpation, Lacrimal Sac
See Dacryocystectomy
Extracorporeal Circulation
Cannulization
Insertion, 33951-33956
Removal, *[33965, 33966, 33969, 33984, 33985, 33986]*
Repositioning, 33957-33959 *[33962, 33963, 33964]*
Daily Management, 33948-33949
Initiation, 33946-33947
Extracorporeal Dialysis
See Hemodialysis
Extracorporeal Life Support Services (ECLS)
Cannulization
Insertion, 33951-33956
Removal, *[33965, 33966, 33969, 33984, 33985, 33986]*
Repositioning, 33957-33959 *[33962, 33963, 33964]*
Daily Management, 33948-33949
Initiation, 33946-33947
Extracorporeal Membrane Oxygenation (ECMO)
Cannulization
Insertion, 33951-33956
Isolated with Chemotherapy Perfusion, 36823
Removal, *[33965, 33966, 33969, 33984, 33985, 33986]*

Extracorporeal Membrane Oxygenation (ECMO) — *continued*
Cannulization — *continued*
Repositioning, 33957-33959 *[33962, 33963, 33964]*
Daily Management, 33948-33949
Initiation, 33946-33947
Extracorporeal Photochemotherapies
See Photopheresis
Extracorporeal Shock Wave Therapy
See Lithotripsy
Lateral Humeral Epicondyle, 0102T
Musculoskeletal, 0101T, 20999
Plantar Fascia, 28890
Wound, 0299T-0300T
Extraction
Lens
Extracapsular, 66940
Intracapsular, 66920
Dislocated Lens, 66930
Extraction, Cataract
See Cataract, Excision
Extradural Anesthesia
See Anesthesia, Epidural
Extradural Injection
See Epidural, Injection
Extraocular Muscle
See Eye Muscles
Extrauterine Pregnancy
See Ectopic Pregnancy
Extravasation Blood
See Hemorrhage
Extremity
Lower
Harvest of Vein for Bypass Graft, 35500
Harvest of Vein for Vascular Reconstruction, 35572
Repair of Blood Vessel, 35286
Revision, 35879, 35881
Penetrating Wound, 20103
Testing
Physical Therapy, 97750
Vascular Diagnostics, 93924
Upper
Harvest of Artery for Coronary Artery By-pass Graft, 35600
Harvest of Vein for Bypass Graft, 35500
Repair of Blood Vessel, 35206
Wound Exploration, 20103
EYA1, 81405-81406
Eye
See Ciliary Body; Cornea; Iris; Lens; Retina; Sclera; Vitreous
Age Related Disease Study Counseling, 4171F
Biometry, 76516, 76519, 92136
Blood Flow Measurement, 0198T
Computerized Corneal Topography, 92025
Dilation
Aqueous Outflow Canal, 66174-66175
Discission of Secondary Membranous Cataract, 66821
Drainage
Anterior Chamber, 65800-65815
Diagnostic Aspiration of Aqueous, 65800
Removal of Blood, 65815
Therapeutic Drainage of Aqueous, 66183
Aqueous, 65800
Anterior Segment Device, 66183
Aqueous Shunt, 66179-66180
Insertion, Subconjunctival Space, 0449T-0450T
Revision of Aqueous Shunt, 66184-66185
Aspiration, 65800
Removal
Blood, 65815
Vitreous, 65810
Vitreous and/or Discission of Anterior Hyaloid Membrane, 65810
Drug Delivery
Suprachoroidal, 67299
Endoscopy, 66990
Enucleation, 65101-65105
Evisceration, 65091, 65093

Eye — *continued*
- Exam
  - with Anesthesia, 92018, 92019
  - Dilated Fundus, 2021F
  - Established Patient, 92012, 92014
  - New Patient, 92002, 92004
  - Radiologic, 70030
- Exenteration
  - with Muscle or Myocutaneous Flap, 65114
    - Muscles Attached, 65105
  - Ocular Contents
    - with Implant, 65093
    - without Implant, 65091
- Exercises
  - Training, 92065
- Goniotomy, 65820
- Implantation
  - Anterior Segment Drainage Device, 66183
  - Aqueous Shunt, 0449T-0450T, 66179-66180
  - Corneal Ring Segment, 65785
  - Drainage Device, 0191T, [0253T]
  - Drug Delivery System, 67027
  - Electrode Array, 0100T
  - Foreign Material for Reinforcement, 65155
  - Pharmacologic Agent, 68399
- Incision
  - Adhesions
    - Anterior Synechiae, 65860, 65870
    - Corneovitreal Adhesions, 65880
    - Goniosynechiae, 65865
    - Posterior Synechiae, 65875
  - Anterior Chamber, 65820
  - Trabecula, 65850
- Injection
  - Air, 66020
  - Medication, 66030
  - Suprachoroidal, 0465T
- Insertion
  - Corneal Ring Segment, 65785
  - Drainage Device, 0191T, 66180, 66183, [0253T]
  - Drug Delivery System, 67027
  - Electrode Array, 0100T
  - Foreign Material for Reinforcement, 65155
  - Ocular Implant
    - After
      - Enucleation
        - Muscles Attached to Implant, 65140
        - Muscles Not Attached to Implant, 65135
      - Evisceration, 65130
    - Pharmacologic Agent, 68399
    - Reinsertion, 65150
    - Scleral Shell, 65130
- Interferometry
  - Biometry, 92136
- Intraocular Pressure
  - Measurement Blood Flow, 0198T
  - Monitoring, 0329T
- Laser
  - Anterior Segment Adhesions, 65860
  - Corneovitreal Adhesions, 66821
  - Iridectomy, 66761
  - Iridotomy, 66761
  - Lacrimal Punctum, 68760
  - Posterior Lens, 66821
  - Secondary Cataract, 66821
  - Vitreous Strands/Adhesions, 67031
- Lesion
  - Excision, 65900
- Muscles
  - Biopsy, 67346
    - Extraocular muscle, 67346
  - Repair
    - Strabismus
      - with Scarring Extraocular Muscles, 67332
      - with Superior Oblique Muscle, 67318
      - Adjustable Sutures, 67335
      - Exploration and/or Repair Detached Extraocular Muscle, 67340
      - One Vertical Muscle, 67314

Eye — *continued*
- Muscles — *continued*
  - Repair — *continued*
    - Strabismus — *continued*
      - on Patient with Previous Surgery, 67331
      - Posterior Fixation Suture, 67334
      - Recession or Resection, 67311, 67312
      - Release of Scar Tissue without Detaching Extraocular Muscle, 67343
      - Two or More Vertical Muscles, 67316
    - Transposition, 67320
    - Unlisted Procedure, Ocular Muscle, 67399
- Nerve
  - Destruction, 67345
- Paracentesis
  - Anterior Chamber
    - with Diagnostic Aspiration of Aqueous, 65800
    - with Removal of Blood, 65815
    - Removal of Vitreous and/or Discission Anterior Hyaloid Membrane, 65810
- Photocoagulation
  - Iridoplasty, 66762
  - Lesion
    - Choroid, 67220
    - Cornea, 65450
    - Retina, 67210, 67227-67228
    - Retinal Detachment, 67105, 67107-67108, 67113, 67145
    - Retinopathy, 67228-67229
    - Vitrectomy, 67039-67040, 67043
  - Photodynamic Therapy Choroidal Lesions, 67221, 67225
- Placement
  - Pharmacologic Agent, 68399
- Prosthesis, 21077, 65770, 66982-66985
  - Loan, 92358
- Pupillometry, Quantitative, 0341T
- Radial Keratotomy, 65771
- Reconstruction
  - Amniotic Membrane, 65780
  - Conjunctiva, 65782
- Removal
  - Blood Clot, 65930
  - Bone, 65112
  - Foreign Body
    - Conjunctival Embedded, 65210
    - Conjunctival Superficial, 65205
    - Corneal without Slit Lamp, 65220
    - Corneal with Slit Lamp, 65222
    - Intraocular, 65235-65265
  - Implant, 65175
    - Anterior Segment, 65920
    - Muscles not Attached, 65103
    - Posterior Segment, 67120, 67121
- Repair
  - Conjunctiva
    - by Mobilization and Rearrangement with Hospitalization, 65273
    - by Mobilization and Rearrangement without Hospitalization, 65272
    - Direct Closure, 65270
  - Cornea
    - Nonperforating, 65275
    - Perforating, 65280, 65285
  - Muscles, 65290
  - Sclera
    - with Graft, 66225
    - with Tissue Glue, 65286
    - without Graft, 66220
    - Anterior Segment, 66250
  - Trabecular Meshwork, 65855
  - Wound
    - by Mobilization and Rearrangement, 65272, 65273
    - Direct Closure, 65270
- Shunt, Aqueous
  - into Subconjunctival Space, 0449T-0450T
  - to Extraocular Reservoir, 66179-66180
- Stem Cell Transplantation, 65781
- Tear Film Imaging, 0330T
- Tear Osmolarity, 83861

Eye — *continued*
- Transluminal Dilation
  - Aqueous Outflow Canal, 66174-66175
  - Ultrasound, 76510-76514
    - Biometry, 76516, 76519
    - Foreign Body, 76529
  - Unlisted Services and Procedures
    - Anterior Segment, 66999
    - Posterior Segment, 67299
  - X-ray, 70030
Eyebrow
- Repair
  - Ptosis, 67900
Eyeglasses
- *See* Spectacle Services
Eyelashes
- Repair Trichiasis
  - Epilation
    - by Forceps Only, 67820
    - by Other than Forceps, 67825
  - Incision of Lid Margin, 67830
    - with Free Mucous Membrane Graft, 67835
Eyelid
- Abscess
  - Incision and Drainage, 67700
- Biopsy, [67810]
- Blepharoplasty, 15820-15823
- Chalazion
  - Excision
    - with Anesthesia, 67808
    - Multiple, 67801, 67805
    - Single, 67800
- Closure by Suture, 67875
- Drug-eluting Ocular Insert Placement, 0444T-0445T
- Evacuation
  - Meibomian Glands, 0207T
- Incision
  - Canthus, 67715
- Injection
  - Subconjunctival, 68200
  - Sutures, 67710
- Lesion
  - Destruction, 67850
  - Excision
    - with Anesthesia, 67808
    - without Closure, 67840
    - Multiple, 67801, 67805
    - Single, 67800
- Meibomian Glands Evacuation, 0207T
- Placement, Drug-eluting Ocular Insert, 0444T-0445T
- Ptosis, 67901-67908
- Reconstruction
  - Canthus, 67950
  - Total Eyelid
    - Conjunctivo–Tarso–Muller's Muscle–Levator Resection, 67908
    - Lower, 67973
      - Second Stage, 67975
    - Upper, 67974
      - Second Stage, 67975
    - Full Thickness, 67973-67975
    - Transfer of Tarsoconjunctival Flap from Opposing Eyelid, 67971
- Removal
  - Foreign Body, 67938
- Repair, 21280, 21282
  - Blepharoptosis
    - Conjunctivo-Tarso-Muller's Muscle-Levator Resection, 67908
    - Frontalis Muscle Technique, 67901-67904
    - Reduction Overcorrection of Ptosis, 67909
    - Superior Rectus Technique with Fascial Sling, 67906
  - Ectropion
    - Excision Tarsal Wedge, 67916
    - Extensive, 67917
    - Suture, 67914
    - Thermocauterization, 67915
  - Entropion
    - Excision Tarsal Wedge, 67923

Eyelid — *continued*
- Repair — *continued*
  - Entropion — *continued*
    - Extensive, 67924
    - Frontalis Muscle Technique, 67901-67904
    - Suture, 67921
    - Thermocauterization, 67922
  - Excisional, 67961
    - over One–Fourth of Lid Margin, 67966
  - Lagophthalmos, 67912
  - Lashes
    - Epilation, by Forceps Only, 67820
    - Epilation by Other than Forceps, 67825
    - Lid Margin, 67830, 67835
  - Wound
    - Full Thickness, 67935
    - Partial Thickness, 67930
  - Skin Graft
    - Delay of Flap, 15630
    - Full Thickness, 15260, 15261, 67961
    - Pedicle Flap, 15576
    - Split, 15120, 15121, 67961
  - Suture, 67880
    - with Transposition of Tarsal Plate, 67882
  - Tissue Transfer, Adjacent, 14060, 14061, 67961
  - Unlisted Services and Procedures, 67999
Eye Socket
- *See* Orbit; Orbital Contents; Orbital Floor; Periorbital Region
EYS, 81434

F

F2, 81240, 81400
F5, 81241, 81400
F7, 81400
F8, 81403, 81406-81407
F9, 81405
F11, 81401
F12, 81403
F13B, 81400
Face
- CT Scan, 70486-70488
- Lesion
  - Destruction, 17000-17108, 17280-17286
- Magnetic Resonance Imaging (MRI), 70540-70543
- Skin Graft
  - Split, 15120, 15121
- Tumor Resection, 21011-21016
Face Lift, 15824-15828
Facial
- Bone
  - Abscess
    - Excision, 21026
  - Anesthesia, 00190, 00192
  - Reconstruction
    - Secondary, 21275
  - Repair, 21208, 21209
  - Tumor
    - Excision, 21029, 21030, 21034
    - Resection
      - Radical, 21015
  - X-ray
    - Complete, Minimum Three Views, 70150
    - Less than Three Views, 70140
    - Nasal Bones, 70160
- Nerve
  - Anastomosis
    - to Hypoglossal Nerve, 64868
    - to Spinal Accessory Nerve, 64866
  - Avulsion, 64742
  - Decompression, 61590, 61596
    - Intratemporal
      - Lateral to Geniculate Ganglion, 69720, 69740
      - Medial to Geniculate Ganglion, 69725, 69745
    - Total, 69955
  - Function Study, 92516
  - Incision, 64742
  - Injection
    - Anesthetic, 64402
  - Mobilization, 61590

Facial — continued
Nerve — continued
  Paralysis
    Graft, 15840-15845
    Repair, 15840-15845
  Paralysis Repair, 15840-15845
  Repair
    Lateral to Geniculate Ganglion, 69740
    Medial to Geniculate Ganglion, 69745
    Suture with or without Graft, 64864, 64865
  Suture
    Lateral to Geniculate Ganglion, 69740
    Medial to Geniculate Ganglion, 69745
  Transection, 64742
  Prosthesis, 21088

Facial Asymmetries
  See Hemifacial Microsomia

Facial Rhytidectomy
  See Face Lift

Factor
  ACTH Releasing, 80412
  Antinuclear, 86038-86039
  Blood Coagulation
    I, 85384, 85385
    II, 85210
    III, 85730, 85732
    IV, 82310
    IX, 85250
    V, 85220
    VII, 85230
    VIII, 85244, 85247
    X, 85260
    XI, 85270
    XIII, 85290, 85291
  Fitzgerald, 85293
  Fletcher, 85292
  Hyperglycemic-Glycogenolytic, 82943
  Inhibitor Test, 85335
  Intrinsic, 83528, 86340
  Rheumatoid, 86430-86431
  Sulfation, 84305

FAH, 81406

Fallopian Tube
  Anastomosis, 58750
  Catheterization, 58345, 74742
  Destruction
    Endoscopy, 58670
  Ectopic Pregnancy, 59121
    with Salpingectomy and/or Oophorectomy, 59120
  Excision, 58700, 58720
  Ligation, 58600-58611
  Lysis
    Adhesions, 58740
  Occlusion, 58615
    Endoscopy, 58671
  Placement
    Implant for Occlusion, 58565
  Repair, 58752
    Anastomosis, 58750
    Creation of Stoma, 58770
  Tumor
    Resection, 58950, 58952-58956
  Unlisted Procedure, Female Genital System, 58999
  X-ray, 74742

Fallopian Tube Pregnancy
  See Ectopic Pregnancy, Tubal

Fallot, Tetralogy of
  See Tetralogy of Fallot

Familial Dysautonomia Geonomic Sequence Analysis, 81412

Familial Hyperinsulinism, 81400

Family Psychotherapy
  See Psychotherapy, Family

FANCC, 81242, 81412

Fanconi Anemia, 88248
  Chromosome Analysis, 88248
  Complementation Group C Gene Analysis, 81242
  Geonomic Sequence Analysis, 81412

Fan Type Procedure, 40525

Farr Test, 82784, 82785

Fasanella–Servat Procedure, 67908

Fascia Graft, 15840

Fascia Graft — continued
  Free Microvascular Anastomosis, 15758
  Harvesting, 20920, 20922
  Open Treatment, Sternoclavicular Dislocation, 23532

Fascia Lata Graft
  Harvesting, 20920, 20922

Fascial Defect
  Repair, 50728

Fascial Graft
  Free
    Microvascular Anastomosis, 15758
  Open Treatment
    Sternoclavicular Dislocation, 23532

Fasciectomy
  Foot, 28060
    Radical, 28060, 28062
  Palm, 26121-26125

Fasciocutaneous Flap, 15732-15738
  Head and Neck, 15732
  Lower Extremity, 15738
  Trunk, 15734
  Upper Extremity, 15736

Fasciotomy
  Arm, Lower, 24495, 25020-25025
  Buttocks, 27027, 27057
  Elbow, 24357-24359
  Foot, 28008
  Hand, Decompression, 26037
  Hip, 27025
  Knee, 27305, 27496-27499
  Leg, Lower, 27600-27602, 27892-27894
  Leg, Upper, 27305, 27496-27499, 27892-27894
  Palm, 26040, 26045
  Pelvis, 27027, 27057
  Plantar
    Endoscopic, 29893
  Thigh, 27025
  Toe, 28008
  Wrist, 25020-25025

FAST
  See Allergen Immunotherapy

FASTKD2, 81406

Fat
  Feces, 82705-82715
  Removal
    Lipectomy, 15876-15879
  Respiratory Secretions, 89125

Fat Stain
  Feces, 89125
  Respiratory Secretions, 89125
  Sputum, 89125
  Urine, 89125

Fatty Acid
  Blood, 82725
  Long Chain Omega-3, 0111T
  Very Long Chain, 82726

Favre–Durand Disease
  See Lymphogranuloma Venereum

FBN1, 81408, 81410

FC Receptor, 86243

FDP (Fibrin Degradation Products), 85362-85379

Fe, 83540

Feedback, Psychophysiologic
  See Biofeedback; Training, Biofeedback

Female Castration
  See Oophorectomy

Female Gonad
  See Ovary

Femoral Artery
  See Artery, Femoral
  Embolectomy
    Anesthesia, 01274
  Ligation
    Anesthesia, 01272

Femoral Nerve
  Injection
    Anesthetic, 64447-64448

Femoral Stem Prosthesis
  Arthroplasty, Hip, 27132
    Partial Replacement, 27125
    Revision, 27134-27138
    Total Replacement, 27130
    Incision, 27303

Femoral Vein
  See Vein, Femoral

Femur
See Hip; Knee; Leg, Upper
Abscess
  Incision, 27303
Bursa
  Excision, 27062
Craterization, 27070, 27071, 27360
Cyst
  Excision, 27065-27067, 27355-27358
Diaphysectomy, 27360
Drainage, 27303
Excision, 27070, 27071, 27360
  Epiphyseal Bar, 20150
Femoroplasty, [29914]
Fracture
  Closed Treatment, 27501-27503
  Distal, 27508, 27510, 27514
  Distal, Medial or Lateral Condyle, 27509
  Epiphysis, 27516-27519
  Intertrochanteric, 27238-27245
    with Implant, 27245
    with Manipulation, 27240
    Closed Treatment, 27238
    Open Treatment, 27244
  Neck, 27230-27236
    Closed Treatment, 27230, 27232
    Open Treatment, 27236
    Percutaneous Fixation, 27235
  Open Treatment, 27244, 27245, 27506, 27507, 27511, 27513
  Percutaneous Fixation, 27509
  Peritrochanteric, 27238-27245
    with Intramedullary Implant, 27245
    with Manipulation, 27240
    Closed Treatment, 27238
    Open Treatment, 27244
  Proximal End
    Head
      Closed Treatment, 27267-27268
      Open Treatment, 27269
    Neck
      Closed Treatment, 27230-27232
      Open Treatment, 27236
      Percutaneous Treatment, 27235
  Shaft, 27500, 27502, 27506, 27507
  Subtrochanteric, 27238-27245
    with Implant, 27245
    with Manipulation, 27240
    Closed Treatment, 27238
    Open Treatment, 27244
  Supracondylar
    Closed, 27501, 27503
    Open, 27511, 27513
    Percutaneous, 27509
  Transcondylar
    Closed, 27501, 27503
    Open, 27511, 27513
    Percutaneous, 27509
  Trochanteric, 27246, 27248
    with Manipulation, 27503
    without Manipulation, 27501
    Closed Treatment, 27246
    Open Treatment, 27248
Halo, 20663
Lesion
  Excision, 27062
Neurectomy
  Hamstring, 27325
Osteoplasty
  Lengthening, 27466, 27468
  Shortening, 27465, 27468
Osteotomy
  without Fixation, 27448
  Prophylactic Treatment, 27187, 27495
  Realignment on Intramedullary Rod, 27454
Reconstruction, 27468
  at Knee, 27442, 27443, 27446
  Lengthening, 27466, 27468
  Shortening, 27465, 27468
Repair, 27470, 27472
  with Graft, 27170
  Epiphysis, 27181, 27742
    Arrest, 27185, 27475, 27479
  Muscle Transfer, 27110
  Osteotomy, 27448, 27450
    with Open Reduction, Hip, 27156

Femur — continued
Repair — continued
  Osteotomy — continued
    and Transfer of Greater Trochanter, 27140
    as part of other, 27151
    Femoral Neck, 27161
    Intertrochanteric or Subtrochanteric, 27165
    Multiple, Shaft, 27454
    Shaft or Supracondylar, 27448
  Saucerization, 27070, 27071, 27360
  Tumor
    Excision, 27065-27067, 27355-27358, 27365
  X-ray, 73551-73552

Fenestration, Pericardium
  See Pericardiostomy

Fenestration Procedure
  Lempert's, 69820
  Semicircular Canal, 69820
    Revision, 69840
  Tracheostomy, 31610

Fern Test
  Smear and Stain, Wet Mount, 87210

Ferric Chloride
  Urine, 81005

Ferrihemoglobin
  See Methemoglobin

Ferritin
  Blood or Urine, 82728

Ferroxidase
  See Ceruloplasmin

Fertility Control
  See Contraception

Fertility Test
  Semen Analysis, 89300-89322
  Sperm Evaluation
    Cervical Mucus Penetration Test, 89330
    Hamster Penetration, 89329

Fertilization
  Oocytes (Eggs)
    In Vitro, 89250-89251
      with Co–Culture of Embryo, 89251
    Assisted (Microtechnique), 89280, 89281

Fertilization in Vitro
  See In Vitro Fertilization

Fetal Aneuploidy, 81507

Fetal Biophysical Profile, 76818, 76819

Fetal Congenital Abnormalities Biochemical Assays, 81508-81512

Fetal Contraction Stress Test, 59020

Fetal Hemoglobin, 83030, 83033, 85460, 85461

Fetal Lung Maturity Assessment, Lecithin Sphingomyelin Ratio, 83661

Fetal Monitoring
  See Monitoring, Fetal

Fetal Non–Stress Test, 59025
  Ultrasound, 76818

Fetal Procedure
  Amnioinfusion, 59070
  Cord Occlusion, 59072
  Fluid Drainage, 59074
  Shunt Placement, 59076
  Unlisted Fetal Invasive Procedure, 59897
  Unlisted Laparoscopy Procedure Maternity and Delivery, 59898
  Unlisted Procedure Maternity and Delivery, 59899

Fetal Testing
  Amniotic Fluid Lung Maturity, 83661, 83663-83664
  Biophysical Profile, 76818-76819
    Lung Maturity, 83661, 83663, 83664
  Heart, 76825, 76826
    Doppler
      Complete, 76827
      Follow–up or Repeat Study, 76828
  Hemoglobin, 83030, 83033, 85460, 85461
  Scalp Blood Sampling, 59020
  Ultrasound, 76801-76828
    Heart, 76825
    Middle Cerebral Artery, 76821
    Umbilical Artery, 76820

Fetuin
  See Alpha–Fetoprotein

Fever, Australian Q
  See Q Fever
Fever, Japanese River
  See Scrub Typhus
FGB, 81400
FGF23, 81404
FGFR1, 81400, 81405
FGFR2, 81404
FGFR3, 81400-81401, 81403-81404
FH, 81405
FHL1, 81404
Fibrillation
  Atrial, 33254-33256
    Documentation, 1060F-1061F
Fibrillation, Heart
  See Heart, Fibrillation
Fibrinase
  See Plasmin
Fibrin Degradation Products, 85362-85380
Fibrin Deposit
  Removal, 32150
Fibrinogen, 85384, 85385
Fibrinolysin
  See Plasmin
Fibrinolysins, 85390
Fibrinolysis
  ADAMTS-13, 85397
  Alpha-2 Antiplasmin, 85410
  Assay, 85396
  Functional Activity, 85397
  Plasmin, 85400
  Plasminogen, 85420, 85421
  Plasminogen Activator, 85415
  Pleural Cavity
    Instillation of Agent, 32561-32562
Fibrin Stabilizing Factor, 85290, 85291
Fibroadenoma
  Ablation
    Cryosurgical, 19105
    Radiofrequency, 0404T
  Excision, 19120-19126
Fibroblastoma, Arachnoidal
  See Meningioma
Fibrocutaneous Tags
  Destruction, 11200, 11201
Fibroid Tumor of Uterus
  Ablation
    Radiofrequency, 0404T, 58674
    Ultrasound, 0071T-0072T
  Excision
    Abdominal Approach, 58140
    Vaginal Approach, 58145
Fibromatosis, Dupuytrens's
  See Dupuytren's Contracture
Fibromatosis, Penile
  See Peyronie Disease
Fibromyoma
  See Leiomyomata
Fibronectin, Fetal, 82731
Fibrosis, Penile
  See Peyronie Disease
Fibrosis, Retroperitoneal
  See Retroperitoneal Fibrosis
Fibrous Cavernitides
  See Peyronie Disease
Fibrous Dysplasia, 21029, 21181-21184
  Reconstruction
    Cranial, 21181
    Facial, 21029
    Orbital Walls, 21182
      40 cm to 80 cm, 21183
      80 cm or More, 21184
Fibula
  See Ankle; Knee; Tibia
  Bone Graft with Microvascular Anastomosis,
    20955
  Craterization, 27360, 27641
  Cyst
    Excision, 27635-27638
  Diaphysectomy, 27360, 27641
  Excision, 27360, 27641
    Epiphyseal Bar, 20150
  Fracture
    Malleolus
      Bimalleolar
        Closed Treatment, 27808

Fibula — *continued*
  Fracture — *continued*
    Malleolus — *continued*
      Bimalleolar — *continued*
        Closed Treatment — *contin-*
          ued
          with Manipulation, 27810
        Open Treatment, 27814
      Lateral
        Closed Treatment, 27786
          with Manipulation, 27788
        Open Treatment, 27792
      Medial
        Closed Treatment, 27760
          with Manipulation, 27762
        Open Treatment, 27766
      Trimalleolar
        Closed Treatment, 27816
          with Manipulation, 27818
        Open Treatment, 27822
          with Fixation, 27823
    Nonunion or Malunion, 27726
    Shaft
      Closed Treatment, 27780
        with Manipulation, 27781
      Open Treatment, 27784
  Incision, 27607
  Osteoplasty
    Lengthening, 27715
  Repair
    Epiphysis, 27477-27485, 27730-27742
    Nonunion or Malunion, 27726
    Osteotomy, 27707-27712
  Saucerization, 27360, 27641
  Tumor
    Excision, 27635-27638
    Radical Resection, 27615-27616, 27646
  X-ray, 73590
FIG4, 81406
Figure of Eight Cast, 29049
Filariasis, 86280
Filtering Operation
  Incision, Sclera, Fistulization
    with Iridectomy, 66160
    Sclerectomy with Punch or Scissors with
      Iridectomy, 66160
    Thermocauterization with Iridectomy,
      66155
    Trabeculectomy ab Externo in Absence
      Previous Surgery, 66170
    Trephination with Iridectomy, 66150
Filtration Implant, Glaucoma
  See Aqueous Shunt
Fimbrioplasty, 58760
  Laparoscopic, 58672
Fine Needle Aspiration, 10021, 10022
  Evaluation
    with Fluoroscence Spectroscopy, 0443T
    Abdominal Mass, 49180
    Bone, 20220, 20225
    Breast, 19081-19086
    Epididymis, 54800
    Evaluation, 88172-88173, [88177]
    General, 10021-10022
    Intervertebral Disc, 62267
    Kidney, 50200
    Lung, 32405
    Mediastinum, 32405
    Muscle, 20206
    Nucleus Pulposus, 62267
    Orbital Contents, 67415
    Pancreas, 48102
    Paravertebral Tissue, 62267
    Pleura, 32400
    Prostate, 55700, 55706
      with Fluorescence Spectroscopy, 0443T
    Retroperitoneal Mass, 49180
    Salivary Gland, 42400
    Soft Tissue Drainage, 10030
    Spinal Cord, 62269
    Testis, 54500
    Thyroid, 60100
    Transendoscopic
      Colon, 45392
      Esophagogastroduodenoscopy, 43238,
        43242

Fine Needle Aspiration — *continued*
  Evaluation — *continued*
    Transendoscopic — *continued*
      Esophagus, 43238
      Surgically Altered Stomach, 43242
Finger
  See Phalanx, Finger
  Abscess
    Bone
      Incision and Drainage, 26034
    Incision and Drainage, 26010, 26011
  Amputation, 26951
    with Exploration or Removal, 26910
  Arthrocentesis, 20600-20604
  Arthrodesis
    Interphalangeal Joint, 26860-26863
    Metacarpophalangeal Joint, 26850, 26852
  Bone
    Incision and Drainage, 26034
  Cast, 29086
  Collection of Blood, 36415, 36416
  Decompression, 26035
  Excision, 26235-26236
    Constricting Ring, 26596
    Tendon, 26180, 26390, 26415
  Flap
    Tissue Transfer, 14350
  Insertion
    Tendon Graft, 26392
  Magnetic Resonance Imaging (MRI), 73221
  Reconstruction
    Extra Digit, 26587
    Toe to Hand Transfer, 26551-26554, 26556
  Removal
    Implantation, 26320
    Tube, 26392, 26416
  Repair
    Blood Vessel, 35207
    Claw Finger, 26499
    Extra Digit, 26587
    Macrodactylia, 26590
    Tendon
      Dorsum, 26418, 26420
      Extensor, 26415-26434, 26445, 26449,
        26460
        Central Slip, 26426, 26428
        Distal Insertion, 26432, 26433
        Excision with Implantation, 26415
        Hand, 26410
        with Graft, 26412
        Realignment, Hand, 26437
      Flexor, 26356-26358, 26440, 26442,
        26455
      Flexor Excision with Implantation,
        26390
      Lengthening, 26476, 26478
      Opponensplasty, 26490-26496
      Profundus, 26370-26373
      Removal Tube or Rod
        Extensor, 26416
        Flexor, 26392
      Shortening, 26477, 26479
      Tenodesis, 26471, 26474
      Tenolysis, 26440-26449
      Tenotomy, 26450-26460
      Transfer or Transplant, 26485, 26489,
        26497, 26498
    Volar Plate, 26548
    Web Finger, 26560-26562
  Replantation, 20816, 20822
  Reposition, 26555
  Sesamoidectomy, 26185
  Splint, 29130, 29131
  Strapping, 29280
  Tendon Sheath
    Excision, 26145
    Incision, 26055
    Incision and Drainage, 26020
    Tenotomy, 26060, 26460
      Flexor, 26455
  Tumor
    Excision, 26115-26116 [26111] [26113]
    Radical Resection, 26117-26118
  Unlisted Services and Procedures/Hands or
    Fingers, 26989
  X-ray, 73140

Finger Joint
  See Intercarpal Joint
Finney Operation, 43850
FIP1L1/PDGFRA, 81401
FISH, 88365
Fissurectomy, 46200, 46261-46262
Fissure in Ano
  See Anus, Fissure
Fistula
  Anal
    Repair, 46262-46288, 46706
  Anorectal
    Repair, 46707
  Arteriovenous, 36831-36833
    Injection, 36901-36903
    Revision
      with Thrombectomy, 36831
      without Thrombectomy, 36832
    Thrombectomy without revision, 36831
  Autogenous Graft, 36825
  Bronchi
    Repair, 32815
  Carotid-Cavernous Repair, 61710
  Chest Wall
    Repair, 32906
  Conjunctiva
    with Tube or Stent, 68750
    without Tube, 68745
  Enterovesical
    Closure, 44660, 44661
  Ileoanal Pouch
    Repair, 46710-46712
  Kidney, 50520-50526
  Lacrimal Gland
    Closure, 68770
    Dacryocystorhinostomy, 68720
  Nose
    Repair, 30580, 30600
    Window, 69666
  Oval Window, 69666
  Postauricular, 69700
  Rectovaginal
    with Concomitant Colostomy, 57307
    Abdominal Approach, 57305
    Transperineal Approach, 57308
  Round Window, 69667
  Sclera
    Sclerectomy with Punch or Scissors with
      Iridectomy, 66160
    Thermocauterization with Iridectomy,
      66155
    Trabeculectomy ab Externo in Absence
      Previous Surgery, 66170
    Trabeculectomy ab Externo with Scarring,
      66172
    Trephination with Iridectomy, 66150
  Suture
    Kidney, 50520-50526
    Ureter, 50920, 50930
  Trachea, 31755
  Tracheoesophageal
    Repair, 43305, 43312, 43314
    Speech Prosthesis, 31611
  Transperineal Approach, 57308
  Ureter, 50920, 50930
  Urethra, 53400, 53405
  Urethrovaginal, 57310
    with Bulbocavernosus Transplant, 57311
  Vesicouterine
    Closure, 51920, 51925
  Vesicovaginal
    Closure, 51900
    Transvesical and Vaginal Approach, 57330
    Vaginal Approach, 57320
  X-ray, 76080
Fistula Arteriovenous
  See Arteriovenous Fistula
Fistulectomy
  Anal, 46060, 46262-46285
Fistulization
  Conjunction to Nasal Cavity, 68745
  Esophagus, 43351-43352
  Intestines, 44300-44346
  Lacrimal Sac to Nasal Cavity, 68720
  Penis, 54435
  Pharynx, 42955

Fistulization — *continued*
Tracheopharyngeal, 31755
Fistulization, Interatrial
See Septostomy, Atrial
Fistulotomy
Anal, 46270-46280
Fitting
Cervical Cap, 57170
Contact Lens, 92071-92072, 92310-92313
Diaphragm, 57170
Low Vision Aid, 92354, 92355
See Spectacle Services
Spectacle Prosthesis, 92352, 92353
Spectacles, 92340-92342
Fitzgerald Factor, 85293
Fixation (Device)
See Application; Bone; Fixation; Spinal Instrumentation
Application, External, 20690-20697
Insertion, 20690-20697, 22841-22844, 22853-22854, 22867-22870, [22859]
Reinsertion, 22849
Interdental without Fracture, 21497
Pelvic
Insertion, 22848
Removal
External, 20694
Internal, 20670, 20680
Sacrospinous Ligament
Vaginal Prolapse, 57282
Shoulder, 23700
Skeletal
Humeral Epicondyle
Percutaneous, 24566
Spinal
Insertion, 22841-22847, 22853-22854, 22867-22870, [22859]
Reinsertion, 22849
Fixation, External
See External Fixation
Fixation, Kidney
See Nephropexy
Fixation, Rectum
See Proctopexy
Fixation Test Complement
See Complement, Fixation Test
Fixation, Tongue
See Tongue, Fixation
FKRP, 81404
FKTN, 81400, 81405
Flank
See Back/Flank
Flap
See Skin Graft and Flap
Delay of Flap at Trunk, 15600
at Eyelids, Nose Ears, or Lips, 15630
at Forehead, Cheeks, Chin, Neck, Axillae, Genitalia, Hands, Feet, 15620
at Scalp, Arms, or Legs, 15610
Section Pedicle of Cross Finger, 15620
Free
Breast Reconstruction, 19364
Microvascular Transfer, 15756-15758
Grafts, 15574-15650, 15842
Composite, 15760
Derma–Fat–Fascia, 15770
Cross Finger Flap, 15574
Punch for Hair Transplant
Less than 15, 15775
More than 15, 15776
Island Pedicle, 15740
Neurovascular Pedicle, 15750
Latissimus Dorsi
Breast Reconstruction, 19361
Omentum
Free
with Microvascular Anastomosis, 49906
Transfer
Intermediate of Any Pedicle, 15650
Transverse Rectus Abdominis Myocutaneous
Breast Reconstruction, 19367-19369
Flatfoot Correction, 28735
Flea Typhus
See Murine Typhus
Fletcher Factor, 85292
FLG, 81401

Flick Method Testing, 93561-93562
Flow Cytometry, 86356, 88182-88189
Flow Volume Loop/Pulmonary, 94375
See Pulmonology, Diagnostic
FLT3, 81245-81246
FLUARIX, 90656
Flublok, [90673]
Flucelvax, 90661
Fluid, Amniotic
See Amniotic Fluid
Fluid, Body
See Body Fluid
Fluid, Cerebrospinal
See Cerebrospinal Fluid
Fluid Collection
Incision and Drainage
Skin, 10140
Fluid Drainage
Abdomen, 49082-49084
Flulaval, 90658, 90688
FluMist, 90660
Fluorescein
Angiography, Ocular, 92242, 92287
Intravenous Injection
Vascular Flow Check, Graft, 15860
Fluorescein, Angiography
See Angiography, Fluorescein
Fluorescent Antibody, 86255, 86256
Fluorescent In Situ Hybridization, 88365
Cytopathology, 88120-88121
Fluoride
Blood, 82735
Urine, 82735
Fluoride Varnish Application, 99188
Fluoroscopy
Bile Duct
Guide for Catheter, 74328, 74330
Chest
Bronchoscopy, 31622-31646
Complete (four views), 71034
Partial (two views), 71023
Drain Abscess, 75989
GI Tract
Guidance Intubation, 74340
Hourly, 76000, 76001
Introduction
GI Tube, 74340
Larynx, 70370
Nasogastric, 43752
Needle Biopsy, 77002
Orogastric, 43752
Pancreatic Duct
Catheter, 74329, 74330
Pharynx, 70370
Sacroiliac Joint
Injection Guidance, 27096
Spine/Paraspinous
Guide Catheter
Needle, 77003
Unlisted Procedure, 76496
Venous Access Device, 36598, 77001
Flurazepam, [80346, 80347]
Flu Vaccines, 90647-90648, 90651-90668 [90630, 90672, 90673], 90661 [90672, 90673], 90674, [90630]
Fluvirin, 90656, 90658
Fluzone, 90655-90658
Fluzone High Dose, 90662
FMR1, 81243-81244
FMRI (Functional MRI), 70554-70555
Fms-Related Tyrosine Kinase 3 Gene Analysis, 81245
FNA (Fine Needle Aspiration), 10021-10022
Foam Stability Test, 83662
FOBT (Fecal Occult Blood Test), 82270, 82272, 82274
Fold, Vocal
See Vocal Cords
Foley Operation Pyeloplasty
See Pyeloplasty
Foley Y–Pyeloplasty, 50400, 50405
Folic Acid, 82746
RBC, 82747
Follicle Stimulating Hormone (FSH), 80418, 80426, 83001

Folliculin
See Estrone
Follitropin
See Follicle Stimulating Hormone (FSH)
Follow–Up Services
See Hospital Services; Office and/or Other Outpatient Services
Post–Op, 99024
Fontan Procedure, 33615, 33617
Foot
See Metatarsal; Tarsal
Amputation, 28800, 28805
Bursa
Incision and Drainage, 28001
Capsulotomy, 28260-28264
Cast, 29450
Cock Up Fifth Toe, 28286
Fasciectomy, 28060
Radical, 28060, 28062
Fasciotomy, 28008
Endoscopic, 29893
Hammertoe Operation, 28285
Incision, 28002-28005
Joint
See Talotarsal Joint; Tarsometatarsal Joint
Magnetic Resonance Imaging (MRI), 73721-73723
Lesion
Excision, 28080, 28090
Magnetic Resonance Imaging (MRI), 73718-73720
Morton's
Destruction, 64632
Excision, 28080
Injection, 64455
Nerve
Destruction, 64632
Excision, 28055
Incision, 28035
Neurectomy, 28055
Neuroma
Destruction, 64632
Excision, 28080, 64782-64783
Injection, 64455
Ostectomy, Metatarsal Head, 28288
Reconstruction
Cleft Foot, 28360
Removal
Foreign Body, 28190-28193
Repair
Muscle, 28250
Tendon
Advancement Posterior Tibial, 28238
Capsulotomy; Metatarsophalangeal, 28270
Interphalangeal, 28272
Capsulotomy, Midfoot; Medial Release, 26820
Capsulotomy, Midtarsal (Heyman Type), 28264
Extensor, Single, 28208
Secondary with Free Graft, 28210
Flexor, Single, with Free Graft, 28200
Secondary with Free Graft, 28202
Tenolysis, Extensor
Multiple through Same Incision, 28226
Tenolysis, Flexor
Multiple through Same Incision, 28222
Single, 28220
Tenotomy, Open, Extensor
Foot or Toe, 28234
Tenotomy, Open, Flexor
Toe, Single Procedure, 28232
Replantation, 20838
Sesamoid
Excision, 28315
Skin Graft
Delay of Flap, 15620
Full Thickness, 15240, 15241
Pedicle Flap, 15574
Split, 15100, 15101
Suture
Tendon, 28200-28210

Foot — *continued*
Tendon Sheath
Excision, 28086, 28088
Tenolysis, 28220-28226
Tenotomy, 28230-28234
Tissue Transfer, Adjacent, 14040, 14041
Tumor, 28043-28047 [28039, 28041], 28100-28107, 28171-28173
Unlisted Services and Procedures, 28899
X–ray, 73620, 73630
Foot Abscess
See Abscess, Foot
Foot Navicular Bone
See Navicular
Forced Expiratory Flows, 94011-94012
Forearm
See Arm, Lower
Forehead
Reconstruction, 21179-21180, 21182-21184
Midface, 21159, 21160
Reduction, 21137-21139
Rhytidectomy, 15824, 15826
Skin Graft
Delay of Flap, 15620
Full Thickness, 15240, 15241
Pedicle Flap, 15574
Tissue Transfer, Adjacent, 14040, 14041
Forehead and Orbital Rim
Reconstruction, 21172-21180
Foreign Body
Removal
Adenoid, 42999
Anal, 46608
Ankle Joint, 27610, 27620
Arm
Lower, 25248
Upper, 24200, 24201
Auditory Canal, External, 69200
with Anesthesia, 69205
Bile Duct, [43275]
Bladder, 52310, 52315
Brain, 61570
Bronchi, 31635
Colon, 44025, 44390, 45379
Colon–Sigmoid, 45332
Conjunctival Embedded, 65210
Cornea
with Slip Lamp, 65222
without Slit Lamp, 65220
Duodenum, 44010
Elbow, 24000, 24101, 24200, 24201
Esophagus, 43020, 43045, 43194, 43215, 74235
External Eye, 65205
Eyelid, 67938
Finger, 26075, 26080
Foot, 28190-28193
Gastrointestinal, Upper, 43247
Gum, 41805
Hand, 26070
Hip, 27033, 27086, 27087
Hysteroscopy, 58562
Interphalangeal Joint
Toe, 28024
Intertarsal Joint, 28020
Intestines, Small, 44200, 44363
Intraocular, 65235
Kidney, 50561, 50580
Knee Joint, 27310, 27331, 27372
Lacrimal Duct, 68530
Lacrimal Gland, 68530
Larynx, 31511, 31530, 31531, 31577
Leg, Upper, 27372
Lung, 32151
Mandible, 41806
Maxillary Sinus, 31299
Mediastinum, 39000, 39010
Metatarsophalangeal Joint, 28022
Mouth, 40804, 40805
Muscle, 20520, 20525
Stimulator
Skeletal, 20999
Nose, 30300
Anesthesia, under, 30310
Lateral Rhinotomy, 30320
Orbit, 67413, 67430

Foreign Body — *continued*
  Removal — *continued*
    Orbit — *continued*
      with Bone Flap, 67430
      without Bone Flap, 67413
    Pancreatic Duct, [43275]
    Pelvis, 27086, 27087
    Penile Tissue, 54115
    Penis, 54115
    Pericardium, 33020
      Endoscopic, 32658
    Peritoneum, 49402
    Pharynx, 42809
    Pleura, 32150, 32151
      Endoscopic, 32653
    Posterior Segment
      Magnetic Extraction, 65260
      Nonmagnetic Extraction, 65265
    Rectum, 45307, 45915
    Scrotum, 55120
    Shoulder, 23040, 23044
      Deep, 23333
      Subcutaneous, 23330
    Skin
      with Debridement, 11010-11012
      Stomach, 43500
    Subcutaneous, 10120, 10121
      with Debridement, 11010-11012
    Tarsometatarsal Joint, 28020
    Tendon Sheath, 20520, 20525
    Toe, 28022
    Ureter, 50961, 50980
    Urethra, 52310, 52315
    Uterus, 58562
    Vagina, 57415
    Wrist, 25040, 25101, 25248
Forensic Exam, 88040
  Cytopathology, 88125
  Phosphatase, Acid, 84061
Foreskin of Penis
  See Penis, Prepuce
Formycin Diphosphate
  See Fibrin Degradation Products
Fournier's Gangrene
  See Debridement, Skin, Subcutaneous Tissue,
    Infected
Fowler Procedure
  Osteotomy, 28305
Fowler–Stephens Orchiopexy, 54650
FOXG1, 81404
FOXO1/PAX3 (t(2;13)), 81401
FOXO1/PAX7 (t(1;13)), 81401
Fox Operation, 67923
Fraction, Factor IX
  See Christmas Factor
Fracture Treatment
  Acetabulum
    with Manipulation, 27222
    without Manipulation, 27220
    Closed Treatment, 27220, 27222
    Open Treatment, 27226-27228
  Alveola
    Closed Treatment, 21421
    Open Treatment, 21422, 21423
  Alveolar Ridge
    Closed Treatment, 21440
    Open Treatment, 21445
  Ankle
    with Manipulation, 27818
    without Manipulation, 27816
    Closed Treatment, 27816, 27818
    Lateral, 27786, 27792, 27822
      Closed Treatment, 27786
        with Manipulation, 27788
      Open Treatment, 27792
    Malleolus
      Bimalleolar
        Closed Treatment, 27808
          with Manipulation, 27810
        Open Treatment, 27814
        Posterior, 27767-27769
      Medial, 27760-27766, 27808-27814
        Closed Treatment, 27760
          with Manipulation, 27762
        Open Treatment, 27766
      Open Treatment, 27822, 27823

Fracture Treatment — *continued*
  Ankle — *continued*
    Trimalleolar, 27816-27823
      Closed Treatment, 27816
        with Manipulation, 27818
      Open Treatment, 27822
        with Fixation, 27823
  Ankle Bone
    Medial, 27760, 27762
    Posterior, 27767-27769
  Bennett's
    See Thumb, Fracture
  Boxer's, 26600-26615
  Bronchi
    Endoscopy, 31630
  Calcaneus
    with Manipulation, 28405, 28406
    without Manipulation, 28400
    Closed Treatment, 28400, 28405
    Open Treatment, 28415, 28420
    Percutaneous Fixation, 28436
  Carpal, 25622-25628
    Closed Treatment
      with Manipulation, 25624, 25635
      without Manipulation, 25622, 25630
    Open Treatment, 25628, 25645
  Carpal Scaphoid
    Closed, 25622
    Open, 25628
  Carpometacarpal
    Closed Treatment, 26645
    Open Treatment, 26665
    Percutaneous Fixation, 26650
  Cheekbone
    with Manipulation, 21355
    Open Treatment, 21360-21366
  Clavicle
    Closed Treatment, 23500, 23505
      with Manipulation, 23505
      without Manipulation, 23500
    Open Treatment, 23515
  Coccyx
    Closed Treatment, 27200
    Open Treatment, 27202
  Colles–Reversed
    See Smith Fracture
  Craniofacial
    Closed Treatment, 21431
    Open Treatment, 21432-21435
  Debridement
    with Open Fracture, 11010-11012
  Elbow
    Closed, 24620, 24640
    Monteggia
      Closed, 24620
      Open, 24635
    Open, 24586-24587, 24635
  Femur
    with Manipulation, 27232, 27502, 27503,
      27510
    without Manipulation, 27230, 27238,
      27246, 27500, 27501, 27508, 27516,
      27517, 27520
    Closed Treatment, 27230, 27238, 27240,
      27246, 27500-27503, 27510, 27516,
      27517
    Distal, 27508, 27510, 27514
    Epiphysis, 27516-27519
    Intertrochanteric
      Closed Treatment, 27238
        with Manipulation, 27240
      Intramedullary Implant, 27245
      Open Treatment, 27244
        with Implant, 27245
    Neck
      Closed Treatment, 27230
        with Manipulation, 27232
      Open Treatment, 27236
      Percutaneous Fixation, 27235
    Open Treatment, 27244, 27245, 27248,
      27506, 27507, 27511-27514, 27519
    Percutaneous Fixation, 27235, 27509
    Peritrochanteric
      Closed Treatment, 27238
        with Manipulation, 27240

Fracture Treatment — *continued*
  Femur — *continued*
    Peritrochanteric — *continued*
      Intramedullary Implant Shaft, 27245,
        27500, 27502, 27506-27507
      Open Treatment, 27244, 27245
    Proximal
      Closed, 27267-27268
      Open, 27269
    Shaft, 27500, 27502, 27506, 27507
    Subtrochanteric
      Closed Treatment, 27238
        with Manipulation, 27240
      Intramedullary Implant, 27245
      Open Treatment, 27244, 27245
    Supracondylar, 27501-27503, 27509, 27511,
      27513
    Transcondylar, 27501-27503, 27509, 27511,
      27513
    Trochanteric
      Closed Treatment, 27246
      Open Treatment, 27248
  Fibula
    with Manipulation, 27781, 27788, 27810
    without Manipulation, 27780, 27786, 27808
    Bimalleolar
      Closed Treatment, 27808-27810
      Closed Treatment, 27780, 27781,
        27786, 27788, 27808, 27810
      Open Treatment, 27814
    Malleolus, 27786-27814
      Open Treatment, 27784, 27792, 27814
    Shaft, 27780-27786, 27808
  Frontal Sinus
    Open Treatment, 21343, 21344
  Great Toe
    Closed Treatment, 28490
      with Manipulation, 28490
  Heel
    Closed Treatment
      with Manipulation, 28405, 28406
      without Manipulation, 28400
    Open Treatment, 28415, 28420
  Humerus
    with Dislocation
      Closed Treatment, 23665
      Open Treatment, 23670
    with Shoulder Dislocation
      Closed Treatment, 23675
      Open Treatment, 23680
    Closed Treatment, 24500, 24505
      with Manipulation, 23605
      without Manipulation, 23600
    Condyle, 24582
      Closed Treatment, 24576, 24577
      Open Treatment, 24579
      Percutaneous, 24582
    Epicondyle
      Closed Treatment, 24560, 24565
      Open Treatment, 24575
      Percutaneous Fixation, 24566
    Greater Tuberosity Fracture
      Closed Treatment with Manipulation,
        23625
      Closed Treatment without Manipula-
        tion, 23620
      Open Treatment, 23630
    Open Treatment, 23615, 23616
    Shaft, 24500
      Open Treatment, 24515, 24516
    Supracondylar
      Closed Treatment, 24530, 24535
      Open Treatment, 24545, 24546
      Percutaneous Fixation, 24538
    Transcondylar
      Closed Treatment, 24530, 24535
      Open Treatment, 24545, 24546
      Percutaneous Fixation, 24538
  Hyoid Bone
    Open Treatment, 31584
  Ilium
    Open Treatment, 27215, 27218
    Percutaneous Fixation, 27216
  Knee, 27520
    Arthroscopic Treatment, 29850, 29851
    Open Treatment, 27524

Fracture Treatment — *continued*
  Larynx
    Open Treatment, 31584
  Leg
    Femur
      Closed Treatment
        With manipulation, 27502, 27503,
          27510, 27516
        Without manipulation, 27500,
          27501, 27508, 27517
      Open Treatment, 27506, 27507, 27511-
        27514, 27519
      Percutaneous fixation, 27509
    Fibula
      Closed Treatment
        With manipulation, 27752, 27781,
          27788
        Without manipulation, 27750,
          27780, 27786
      Open Treatment, 27758, 27759, 27784,
        27792, 27826-27832
    Tibia
      Closed Treatment
        With manipulation, 27752, 27825
        Without manipulation, 27750,
          27824, 27830, 27831
      Open Treatment, 27758, 27759, 27826-
        27829, 27832
      Percutaneous fixation, 27756
  Malar Area
    with Bone Graft, 21366
    with Manipulation, 21355
    Open Treatment, 21360-21366
  Mandible
    Closed Treatment
      with Manipulation, 21451
      without Manipulation, 21450
      Interdental Fixation, 21453
    Open Treatment, 21454-21470
      with Interdental Fixation, 21462
      without Interdental Fixation, 21461
      External Fixation, 21454
    Percutaneous Treatment, 21452
  Maxilla
    Closed Treatment, 21421
    Open Treatment, 21422, 21423
  Metacarpal
    with Manipulation, 26605, 26607
    without Manipulation, 26600
    Closed Treatment, 26600, 26605
      with Fixation, 26607
    Open Treatment, 26615
    Percutaneous Fixation, 26608
  Metatarsal
    with Manipulation, 28475, 28476
    without Manipulation, 28450, 28470
    Closed Treatment, 28470, 28475
    Open Treatment, 28485
    Percutaneous Fixation, 28476
  Monteggia
    Closed, 24620
    Open, 24635
  Nasal Bone
    with Manipulation, 21315, 21320
    without Manipulation, 21310
    Closed Treatment, 21310-21320
    Open Treatment, 21325-21335
  Nasal Septum
    Closed Treatment, 21337
    Open Treatment, 21336
  Nasal Turbinate
    Therapeutic, 30930
  Nasoethmoid
    with Fixation, 21340
    Open Treatment, 21338, 21339
    Percutaneous Treatment, 21340
  Nasomaxillary
    with Bone Grafting, 21348
    with Fixation, 21345-21347
    Closed Treatment, 21345
    Open Treatment, 21346-21348
  Navicular
    with Manipulation, 25624
    Closed Treatment, 25622
    Open Treatment, 25628

Fracture Treatment — *continued*
  Odontoid
    Open Treatment
      with Graft, 22319
      without Graft, 22318
  Orbit
    Closed Treatment, 21400
      with Manipulation, 21401
      without Manipulation, 21400
    Open Treatment, 21406-21408
      Blowout Fracture, 21385-21395
  Orbital Floor
    Blow Out, 21385-21395
  Palate
    Closed Treatment, 21421
    Open Treatment, 21422, 21423
  Patella
    Closed Treatment
      without Manipulation, 27520
    Open Treatment, 27524
  Pelvic Ring
    Closed Treatment, without Manipulation, 27197
      with Manipulation, 27198
    Open Treatment
      Anterior, 27217
      Posterior, 27218
    Percutaneous Fixation, 27216
  Phalanges
    Finger(s)
      Articular
        with Manipulation, 26742
        Closed Treatment, 26740
        Open Treatment, 26746
      Closed Treatment
        with Manipulation, 26725, 26742, 26755
        without Manipulation, 26720, 26740, 26750
      Distal, 26755, 26756
        Closed Treatment, 26750
        Open Treatment, 26765
        Percutaneous Fixation, 26756
    Finger/Thumb
      with Manipulation, 26725, 26727
      Bennett Fracture, 26650, 26665
      Closed Treatment, 26720, 26725
      Percutaneous Fixation, 26650, 26727, 26756
      Shaft, 26720-26727
    Great Toe, 28490
      Closed Treatment, 28490, 28495
      Open Treatment, 28505
      Percutaneous Fixation, 28496
        without Manipulation, 28496
    Open Treatment, 26735, 26746
    Distal, 26765
    Shaft
      Closed Treatment, 26725
      Open Treatment, 26735
      Percutaneous Fixation, 26727
    Toe
      with Manipulation, 28515
      without Manipulation, 28510
      Closed Treatment, 28515
      Open Treatment, 28525
  Radius
    with Manipulation, 25565, 25605
    with Ulna, 25560, 25565
      Open Treatment, 25575
    without Manipulation, 25560, 25600
    Closed Treatment, 24650, 24655, 25500, 25505, 25520, 25560, 25565, 25600, 25605
    Colles, 25600, 25605
    Distal, 25600-25609
      Open Treatment, 25607, 25608-25609
      Smith, 25600-25605, 25606, 25607, 25609
    Head/Neck
      Closed Treatment, 24650, 24655
      Open Treatment, 24665, 24666
      Open Treatment, 25515, 25607, 25608-25609
    Percutaneous Fixation, 25606
    Shaft, 25500, 25525, 25526

Fracture Treatment — *continued*
  Radius — *continued*
    Shaft — *continued*
      Closed Treatment, 25500, 25505, 25520
      Open Treatment, 25515, 25525, 25526, 25574
  Rib
    Closed Treatment
      See E&M codes
    Open Treatment, 21811-21813
  Scaphoid
    with Dislocation
      Closed Treatment, 25680
      Open Treatment, 25685
    with Manipulation, 25624
    Closed Treatment, 25622
    Open Treatment, 25628
  Scapula
    Closed Treatment
      with Manipulation, 23575
      without Manipulation, 23570
    Open Treatment, 23585
  Sesamoid
    Closed Treatment, 28530
    Foot, 28530, 28531
    Open Treatment, 28531
  Shoulder
    Closed Treatment
      with Greater Tuberosity Fracture, 23620, 23655
      with Surgical or Anatomical Neck Fracture, 23600, 23675
    Open Treatment, 23630, 23680
  Skin Debridement, 11010-11012
  Skull, 62000-62010
  Sternum
    Closed Treatment, 21820
    Open Treatment, 21825
  Talus
    with Manipulation, 28435, 28436
    without Manipulation, 28430
    Closed Treatment, 28430, 28435
    Open Treatment, 28445
  Tarsal
    with Manipulation, 28455, 28456
    without Manipulation, 28450
    Open Treatment, 28465
    Percutaneous Fixation, 28456
  Thigh
    Femur
      Closed Treatment
        with manipulation, 27502, 27503, 27510, 27517
        without manipulation, 27500, 27501, 27508, 27516, 27520
      Open Treatment, 27506, 27507, 27511, 27513, 27514, 27519, 27524
      Percutaneous fixation, 27509
  Thumb
    with Dislocation, 26645, 26650
      Open Treatment, 26665
    Closed Treatment, 26645, 26650
    Percutaneous Fixation, 26650
  Tibia
    with Manipulation, 27752, 27762, 27810
    without Manipulation, 27530, 27750, 27760, 27808, 27825
    Arthroscopic Treatment, 29855, 29856
    Closed Treatment, 27530, 27532, 27538, 27750, 27752, 27760, 27762, 27808, 27810, 27824, 27825
      with Traction, 27532, 27825
    Distal, 27824-27828
    Intercondylar Spines, 27538, 27540
    Malformation, 27810
    Malleolus, 27760-27766, 27808-27814
    Open Treatment, 27535, 27536, 27540, 27758, 27759, 27766, 27814, 27826-27828
    Percutaneous Fixation, 27756
      Bimalleolar
        Closed Treatment, 27808
          with Manipulation, 27810
        Open Treatment, 27814

Fracture Treatment — *continued*
  Tibia — *continued*
    Percutaneous Fixation — *continued*
      Lateral
        Closed Treatment, 27786
          with Manipulation, 27788
        Open Treatment, 27792
      Medial
        Closed Treatment, 27760
          with Manipulation, 27762
        Open Treatment, 27766
      Trimalleolar
        Closed Treatment, 27816
          with Manipulation, 27818
        Open Treatment, 27822
          with Fixation, 27823
      Plateau, 27530-27536, 29855, 29856
        Bicondylar, 29856
        Unicondylar, 29855
      Shaft, 27750-27759
        with Manipulation, 27752, 27762, 27825
        without Manipulation, 27530, 27750, 27760, 27824
  Tibia and Fibula
    Malleolar, 27808-27814
  Trachea
    Endoscopy Repair, 31630
  Turbinate
    Therapeutic, 30930
  Ulna
    with Dislocation, 24620, 24635
      Closed Treatment, 24620
      Monteggia, 24620, 24635
      Open Treatment, 24635
    with Manipulation, 25535, 25565
    with Radius, 25560, 25565
      Open Treatment, 25574-25575
    without Manipulation, 25530
    See Elbow; Humerus; Radius
    Closed Treatment, 25560, 25565
      Monteggia type, 24620
      of Shaft, 25530, 25535
        with Manipulation, 25535
        and Radial, 25560
          with Manipulation, 25565
      Proximal end, 24670
        with Manipulation, 24675
      Ulnar Styloid, 25650
    Olecranon
      Closed Treatment, 24670, 24675
        with Manipulation, 24675
      Open Treatment, 24685
    Open Treatment, 25574, 25575
      Proximal End, 24685
      Radial AND Ulnar Shaft, 25574, 25575
      Shaft, 25545
    Shaft
      Closed Treatment, 25530, 25535
      Open Treatment, 25545, 25574
    Styloid Process
      Closed Treatment, 25650
      Open Treatment, 25652
      Percutaneous Fixation, 25651
  Vertebra
    Additional Segment
      Open Treatment, 22328
    Cervical
      Open Treatment, 22326
    Closed Treatment
      with Manipulation, Casting and/or Bracing, 22315
      without Manipulation, 22310
    Lumbar
      Open Treatment, 22325
    Posterior
      Open Treatment, 22325-22327
    Thoracic
      Open Treatment, 22327
  Vertebral Process
    Closed Treatment
      See Evaluation and Management Codes
  Wrist
    with Dislocation, 25680, 25685
      Closed Treatment, 25680

Fracture Treatment — *continued*
  Wrist — *continued*
    with Dislocation — *continued*
      Open Treatment, 25685
    Zygomatic Arch
      Open Treatment, 21356, 21360-21366
        with Manipulation, 21355
Fragile–X
  Chromosome Analysis, 88248
  Mental Retardation 1 Gene Analysis, 81243-81244
Fragility
  Red Blood Cell
    Mechanical, 85547
    Osmotic, 85555, 85557
Frames, Stereotactic
  See Stereotactic Frame
Francisella, 86000
  Antibody, 86668
Frazier-Spiller Procedure, 61450
Fredet–Ramstedt Procedure, 43520
Free E3
  See Estriol
Free Skin Graft
  See Skin, Grafts, Free
Free T4
  See Thyroxine, Free
Frei Disease
  See Lymphogranuloma Venereum
Frenectomy, 40819, 41115
Frenoplasty, 41520
Frenotomy, 40806, 41010
Frenulectomy, 40819
Frenuloplasty, 41520
Frenum
  See Lip
  Lip
    Incision, 40806
Frenumectomy, 40819
Frickman Operation, 45550
Frontal Craniotomy, 61556
Frontal Sinus
  See Sinus, Frontal
Frontal Sinusotomy
  See Exploration, Sinus, Frontal
Frost Suture
  Eyelid
    Closure by Suture, 67875
Frozen Blood Preparation, 86930-86932
Fructose, 84375
  Semen, 82757
Fructose Intolerance Breath Test, 91065
Fruit Sugar
  See Fructose
FSF, 85290, 85291
FSH, 83001
  with Additional Tests, 80418, 80426
FSHMD1A, 81404
FSP, 85362-85380
FT–4, 84439
FTG, 15200-15261
FTI, 84439
FTSG, 15200-15261
FTSJ1, 81405-81406
Fulguration
  See Destruction
  Bladder, 51020
  Cystourethroscopy with, 52214
    Lesion, 52224
    Tumor, 52234-52240
  Ureter, 50957, 50976
  Ureterocele
    Ectopic, 52301
    Orthotopic, 52300
Fulguration, Endocavitary
  See Electrocautery
Full Thickness Graft, 15200-15261
Functional Ability
  See Activities of Daily Living
Functional MRI, 70554-70555
Function, Study, Nasal
  See Nasal Function Study
Function Test, Lung
  See Pulmonology, Diagnostic
Function Test, Vestibular
  See Vestibular Function Tests

Fundoplasty
  with Fundic Patch, 43325
  with Paraesophageal Hernia
    with Fundoplication
      Laparotomy, 43332-43333
        Thoracoabdominal Incisional, 43336-43337
        Thoracotomy, 43334-43335
      Laparoscopic, 43281-43282
    Esophagogastric
      with Gastroplasty, 43842-43843
      Laparoscopic, 43279-43280, 43283
      Laparotomy, 43327
      Thoracotomy, 43328
    Esophagomyotomy
      Laparoscopic, 43279
Fundoplication
  See Fundoplasty, Esophagogastric
Fungal Wet Prep, 87220
Fungus
  Antibody, 86671
  Culture
    Blood, 87103
    Hair, 87101
    Identification, 87106
    Nail, 87101
    Other, 87102
    Skin, 87101
  Tissue Exam, 87220
Funnel Chest
  See Pectus Excavatum
Furuncle
  Incision and Drainage, 10060, 10061
Furuncle, Vulva
  See Abscess, Vulva
FUS/DDIT3, 81401, 81406
Fusion
  See Arthrodesis
  Pleural Cavity, 32560
  Thumb
    in Opposition, 26820
Fusion, Epiphyseal–Diaphyseal
  See Epiphyseal Arrest
Fusion, Joint
  See Arthrodesis
Fusion, Joint, Ankle
  See Ankle, Arthrodesis
Fusion, Joint, Interphalangeal, Finger
  See Arthrodesis, Finger Joint, Interphalangeal
FXN, 81401, 81404

G

G6PC, 81250
GAA, 81406
Gabapentin
  Assay, 80171
GABRG2, 81405
Gago Procedure
  Repair, Tricuspid Valve, 33463-33465
Gait Training, 97116
Galactogram, 77053, 77054
  Injection, 19030
Galactokinase
  Blood, 82759
Galactose
  Blood, 82760
  Urine, 82760
Galactose–1–Phosphate
  Uridyl Transferase, 82775-82776
GALC, 81401, 81406
Galeazzi Dislocation
  Fracture
    Closed Treatment, 25520
    Open Treatment, 25525, 25526
Galectin-3, 82777
Gallbladder
  See Bile Duct
  Anastomosis
    with Intestines, 47720-47741
  Cholecystectomy, 47600
    Laparoscopic, 47562
      with Cholangiogram, 47564
    Open, 47600
      with Cholangiogram, 47605
      with Choledochoenterostomy, 47612
      with Exploration Common Duct, 47610

Gallbladder — *continued*
  Cholecystectomy — *continued*
    Open — *continued*
      with Transduodenal Sphincterotomy or Sphincteroplasty, 47620
  Cholecystostomy
    for Drainage, 47480
    for Exploration, 47480
    for Removal of Stone, 47480
    Percutaneous, 47490
  Excision, 47562-47564, 47600-47620
  Exploration, 47480
  Incision, 47490
  Incision and Drainage, 47480
  Nuclear Medicine
    Imaging, 78226-78227
  Removal Calculi, 47480
  Repair
    with Gastroenterostomy, 47741
    with Intestines, 47720-47740
  Unlisted Services and Procedures, 47999
  X–ray with Contrast, 74290
GALT, 81401, 81406
Galvanocautery
  See Electrocautery
Galvanoionization
  See Iontophoresis
Gamete Intrafallopian Transfer (GIFT), 58976
Gamete Transfer
  In Vitro Fertilization, 58976
Gamma Camera Imaging
  See Nuclear Medicine
Gammacorten
  See Dexamethasone
Gammaglobulin
  Blood, 82784-82787
Gamma Glutamyl Transferase, 82977
Gamma Seminoprotein
  See Antigen, Prostate Specific
Gamulin Rh
  See Immune Globulins, Rho (D)
Ganglia, Trigeminal
  See Gasserian Ganglion
Ganglion
  See Gasserian Ganglion
  Cyst
    Aspiration/Injection, 20612
    Drainage, 20612
    Wrist
      Excision, 25111, 25112
  Injection
    Anesthetic, 64505, 64510
Ganglion Cervicothoracicum
  See Stellate Ganglion
Ganglion, Gasser's
  See Gasserian Ganglion
Ganglion Pterygopalatinum
  See Sphenopalatine Ganglion
GARDASIL, 90649
Gardnerella Vaginalis Detection, 87510-87512
Gardner Operation, 63700, 63702
GARS, 81406
Gasser Ganglion
  See Gasserian Ganglion
Gasserian Ganglion
  Sensory Root
    Decompression, 61450
    Section, 61450
  Stereotactic, 61790
Gastrectomy
  Longitudinal, 43775
  Partial, 43631
    with Gastroduodenostomy, 43631
      with Roux–en–Y Reconstruction, 43633
    with Gastrojejunostomy, 43632
    with Intestinal Pouch, 43634
    Distal with Vagotomy, 43635
  Sleeve, 43775
  Total, 43621, 43622
    with Esophagoenterostomy, 43620
    with Intestinal Pouch, 43622
Gastric, 82930
  Acid, 82930
  Analysis Test, 43755-43757

Gastric — *continued*
  Electrodes
    Neurostimulator
      Implantation
        Laparoscopic, 43647
        Open, 43881
      Removal
        Laparoscopic, 43648
        Open, 43882
      Replacement
        Laparoscopic, 43647
        Open, 43881
      Revision
        Laparoscopic, 43648
        Open, 43882
  Intubation, 43753-43755
    Diagnostic, 43754-43757
    Therapeutic, 43753
  Lavage
    Therapeutic, 43753
  Restrictive Procedure
    Laparoscopy, 43770-43774
    Open, 43886-43888
  Tests
    Manometry, 91020
Gastric Ulcer Disease
  See Stomach, Ulcer
Gastrin, 82938, 82941
Gastrocnemius Recession
  Leg, Lower, 27687
Gastroduodenostomy, 43810
  with Gastrectomy, 43631, 43632
  Revision of Anastomosis with Reconstruction, 43850
  with Vagotomy, 43855
Gastroenterology, Diagnostic
  Breath Hydrogen Test, 91065
  Colon Motility Study, 91117
  Duodenal Intubation and Aspiration, 43756-43757
  Esophagus Tests
    Acid Perfusion, 91030
    Acid Reflux Test, 91034-91038
    Balloon Distension Provocation Study, 91040
    Intubation with Specimen Collection, 43754-43755
    Manometry, 91020
    Motility Study, 91010-91013
  Gastric Tests
    Manometry, 91020
  Gastroesophageal Reflux Test
    See Acid Reflux, 91034-91038
  Manometry, 91020
  Rectum
    Manometry, 91122
    Sensation, Tone, and Compliance Test, 91120
  Stomach
    Intubation with Specimen Collection, 43754-43755
    Manometry, 91020
    Stimulation of Secretion, 43755
  Unlisted Services and Procedures, 91299
Gastroenterostomy
  for Obesity, 43644-43645, 43842-43848
Gastroesophageal Reflux Test, 91034-91038
Gastrointestinal Endoscopies
  See Endoscopy, Gastrointestinal
Gastrointestinal Exam
  Nuclear Medicine
    Blood Loss Study, 78278
    Protein Loss Study, 78282
    Shunt Testing, 78291
    Unlisted Services and Procedures, 78299
Gastrointestinal Prophylaxis for NSAID Use Prescribed, 4017F
Gastrointestinal Tract
  Imaging Intraluminal
    Colon, 0355T
    Distal Ileum, 0355T
    Esophagus, 91111
    Esophagus Through Ileum, 91110
  Reconstruction, 43360, 43361
  Transit and Pressure Measurements, 91112

Gastrointestinal Tract — *continued*
  Upper
    Dilation, 43249
    X–ray, 74240-74245
      with Contrast, 74246-74249
    Guide Dilator, 74360
    Guide Intubation, 49440, 74340
Gastrointestinal, Upper
  Biopsy
    Endoscopy, 43239
  Dilation
    Endoscopy, 43245
    Esophagus, 43248
  Endoscopy
    Catheterization, 43241
    Destruction
      Lesion, [43270]
    Dilation, 43245
    Drainage
      Pseudocyst, 43240
    Exploration, 43235
    Hemorrhage, 43255
    Inject Varices, 43243
    Needle Biopsy, 43238, 43242
    Removal
      Foreign Body, 43247
      Lesion, 43250-43251
      Polyp, 43250-43251
      Tumor, 43250-43251
      Resection, Mucosa, 43254
    Stent Placement, [43266]
    Thermal Radiation, 43257
    Tube Placement, 43246
    Ultrasound, 43237, 43238, 43242, 43253, 76975
  Exploration
    Endoscopy, 43235
  Hemorrhage
    Endoscopic Control, 43255
  Injection
    Submucosal, 43236
    Varices, 43243
  Lesion
    Destruction, [43270]
    Ligation of Vein, 43244
  Needle Biopsy
    Endoscopy, 43238, 43242
  Removal
    Foreign body, 43247
    Lesion, 43250-43251
    Polyp, 43250-43251
    Tumor, 43250-43251
  Stent Placement, [43266]
  Tube Placement
    Endoscopy, 43237, 43238, 43246
  Ultrasound
    Endoscopy, 43237, 43238, 43242, 43259, 76975
Gastrojejunostomy, 43860, 43865
  with Duodenal Exclusion, 48547
  with Partial Gastrectomy, 43632
  with Vagotomy, 43825
  without Vagotomy, 43820
  Contrast Injection, 49465
  Conversion from Gastrostomy Tube, 49446
  Removal
    Obstructive Material, 49460
  Replacement
    Tube, 49452
  Revision, 43860
    with Vagotomy, 43865
Gastroplasty
  Collis, 43283, 43338
  Esophageal Lengthening Procedure, 43283, 43338
  Laparoscopic, 43283, 43644-43645
  Restrictive for Morbid Obesity, 43842-43843, 43845-43848
  Other than Vertical Banded, 43843
  Wedge, 43283, 43338
Gastrorrhaphy, 43840
Gastroschisis, 49605
Gastrostomy
  with Pancreatic Drain, 48001
  with Pyloroplasty, 43640
  with Vagotomy, 43640

Gastrostomy — *continued*
  Closure, 43870
  Laparoscopic
    Permanent, 43832
    Temporary, 43653
  Temporary, 43830
    Laparoscopic, 43653
    Neonatal, 43831
  Tube
    Change of, 43760
    Conversion to Gastro-jejunostomy Tube,
      49446
    Directed Placement
      Endoscopic, 43246
      Percutaneous, 49440
    Insertion
      Endoscopic, 43246
      Percutaneous, 49440
    Percutaneous, 49440
    Removal
      Obstructive Material, 49460
    Replacement, 49450
    Repositioning, 43761
Gastrotomy, 43500, 43501, 43510
Gaucher Disease Genomic Sequence Analysis,
  81412
GBA, 81251, 81412
GCDH, 81406
GCH1, 81405
GCK, 81406
GDAP1, 81405
GDH, 82965
GE
  Reflux, 78262
Gel Diffusion, 86331
Gene Analysis
  See Analysis, Gene
Genioplasty, 21120-21123
  Augmentation, 21120, 21123
  Osteotomy, 21121-21123
Genitalia
  Female
    Anesthesia, 00940-00952
  Male
    Anesthesia, 00920-00938
  Skin Graft
    Delay of Flap, 15620
    Full Thickness, 15240, 15241
    Pedicle Flap, 15574
    Split, 15120, 15121
    Tissue Transfer, Adjacent, 14040, 14041
Genitourinary Sphincter, Artificial
  See Prosthesis, Urethral Sphincter
Genotype Analysis
  See Analysis, Gene
Gentamicin, 80170
  Assay, 80170
Gentiobiase, 82963
Genus: Human Cytomegalovirus Group
  See Cytomegalovirus
GERD
  See Gastroesophageal Reflux Test
German Measles
  See Rubella
Gestational Trophoblastic Tumor
  See Hydatidiform Mole
GFAP, 81405
GGT, 82977
GH, 83003
GH1, 81404
GHb, 83036
GHR, 81405
GHRHR, 81405
Giardia
  Antigen Detection
    Enzyme Immunoassay, 87329
    Immunofluorescence, 87269
Giardia Lamblia
  Antibody, 86674
Gibbons Stent, 52332
GIF, 84307
GIFT, 58976
Gillies Approach
  Fracture
    Zygomatic Arch, 21356
Gill Operation, 63012

Gingiva
  See Gums
Gingiva, Abscess
  See Abscess
  Fracture
    See Abscess, Gums; Gums
    Zygomatic Arch
      See Abscess, Gums; Gums, Abscess
Gingivectomy, 41820
Gingivoplasty, 41872
Girdlestone Laminectomy
  See Laminectomy
Girdlestone Procedure
  Acetabulum, Reconstruction, 27120, 27122
GI Tract
  See Gastrointestinal Tract
  X-Rays, 74240-74249, 74340, 74360
GJB1, 81403
GJB2, 81252-81253, 81430
GJB6, 81254
GLA, 81405
Glabellar Frown Lines
  Rhytidectomy, 15826
Gland
  See Specific Gland
Gland, Adrenal
  See Adrenal Gland
Gland, Bartholin's
  See Bartholin's Gland
Gland, Bulbourethral
  See Bulbourethral Gland
Gland, Lacrimal
  See Lacrimal Gland
Gland, Mammary
  See Breast
Gland, Parathyroid
  See Parathyroid Gland
Gland, Parotid
  See Parotid Gland
Gland, Pituitary
  See Pituitary Gland
Gland, Salivary
  See Salivary Glands
Gland, Sublingual
  See Sublingual Gland
Gland, Sweat
  See Sweat Glands
Gland, Thymus
  See Thymus Gland
Gland, Thyroid
  See Thyroid Gland
Gla Protein (Bone)
  See Osteocalcin
Glasses
  See Spectacle Services
Glaucoma
  Cryotherapy, 66720
  Cyclophotocoagulation, 66710, 66711
  Diathermy, 66700
  Fistulization of Sclera, 66150
Glaucoma Drainage Implant
  See Aqueous Shunt
Glenn Procedure, 33622, 33766-33767
Glenohumeral Joint
  Arthrotomy, 23040
    with Biopsy, 23100
    with Synovectomy, 23105
  Exploration, 23107
  Removal
    Foreign or Loose Body, 23107
Glenoid Fossa
  Reconstruction, 21255
GLN, 82127-82131
Globulin
  Antihuman, 86880-86886
  Immune, 90281-90399
  Sex Hormone Binding, 84270
Globulin, Corticosteroid–Binding, 84449
Globulin, Rh Immune, 90384-90386
Globulin, Thyroxine–Binding, 84442
Glomerular Procoagulant Activity
  See Thromboplastin
Glomus Caroticum
  See Carotid Body
Glossectomies, 41120-41155
Glossectomy, 41120-41155

Glossopexy, 41500
Glossorrhaphy
  See Suture, Tongue
Glucagon, 82943
  Tolerance Panel, 80422, 80424
  Tolerance Test, 82946
Glucose, 80422, 80424, 80430-80435, 95250
  Blood Test, 82947-82950, 82962
  Body Fluid, 82945
  Hormone Panel, 80430
  Interstitial Fluid
    Continuous Monitoring, 95250
  Interstitial Sensor, 0446T-0448T
  Tolerance Test, 82951, 82952
Glucose-6-Phosphatase, Catalytic Subunit Gene
  Analysis, 81250
Glucose–6–Phosphate
  Dehydrogenase, 82955, 82960
Glucose Phosphate Isomerase, 84087
Glucose Phosphate Isomerase Measurement,
  84087
Glucosidase, 82963
  Beta Acid Gene Analysis, 81251
Glucuronide Androstanediol, 82154
GLUD1, 81406
Glue
  Cornea Wound, 65286
  Sclera Wound, 65286
Glukagon
  See Glucagon
Glutamate Dehydrogenase, 82965
Glutamate Pyruvate Transaminase, 84460
Glutamic Alanine Transaminase, 84460
Glutamic Aspartic Transaminase, 84450
Glutamic Dehydrogenase, 82965
Glutamine, 82127-82131
Glutamyltransferase, Gamma, 82977
Glutathione, 82978
  Glutathione Reductase, 82979
Glycanhydrolase, N–Acetylmuramide
  See Lysozyme
Glycated Hemoglobins
  See Glycohemoglobin
Glycated Protein, 82985
Glycerol, Phosphatidyl
  See Phosphatidylglycerol
Glycerol Phosphoglycerides
  See Phosphatidylglycerol
Glycerophosphatase
  See Alkaline Phosphatase
Glycinate, Theophylline Sodium
  See Theophylline
Glycocholic Acid
  See Cholylglycine
Glycohemoglobin, 83036-83037
Glycol, Ethylene
  See Ethylene Glycol
Glycols, Ethylene
  See Ethylene Glycol
Glycosaminoglycan
  See Mucopolysaccharides
GNAQ, 81403
GNE, 81400, 81406
Goeckerman Treatment
  Photochemotherapy, 96910-96913
Gold
  Assay, [80375]
Goldwaite Procedure
  Reconstruction, Patella, for Instability, 27422
Golfer's Elbow, 24357-24359
Gol–Vernet Operation, 50120
Gonadectomy, Female
  See Oophorectomy
Gonadectomy, Male
  See Excision, Testis
Gonadotropin
  Chorionic, 84702, 84703
  FSH, 83001
  ICSH, 83002
  LH, 83002
Gonadotropin Panel, 80426
Goniophotography, 92285
Gonioscopy, 92020
Goniotomy, 65820
Gonococcus
  See Neisseria Gonorrhoeae

Goodenough Harris Drawing Test, 96101-96103
GOTT
  See Transaminase, Glutamic Oxaloacetic
GP1BB, 81404
GPUT, 82775-82776
Graefe's Operation, 66830
Graft
  Anal, 46753
  Aorta, 33840, 33845, 33852, 33860-33877
  Artery
    Coronary, 33503-33505
  Bone
    See Bone Marrow, Transplantation
    Anastomosis, 20969-20973
    Harvesting, 20900, 20902
    Microvascular Anastomosis, 20955-20962
    Osteocutaneous Flap with Microvascular
      Anastomosis, 20969-20973
    Vascular Pedicle, 25430
    Vertebra, 0222T
      Cervical, 0219T
      Lumbar, 0221T
      Thoracic, 0220T
  Bone and Skin, 20969-20973
  Cartilage
    Costochondral, 20910
    Ear to Face, 21235
    Harvesting, 20910, 20912
      See Cartilage Graft
    Rib to Face, 21230
      Three or More Segments
      Two Locations, 35682, 35683
  Composite, 35681-35683
  Conjunctiva, 65782
    Harvesting, 68371
  Cornea
    with Lesion Excision, 65426
  Corneal Transplant
    Allograft Preparation, 0290T, 65757
    Endothelial, 65756
    in Aphakia, 65750
    in Pseudophakia, 65755
    Lamellar, 65710
    Penetrating, 65730
  Dura
    Spinal Cord, 63710
  Eye
    Amniotic Membrane, 65780
    Conjunctiva, 65782
      Harvesting, 68371
    Stem Cell, 65781
  Facial Nerve Paralysis, 15840-15845
  Fascia Graft
    Cheek, 15840
  Fascia Lata
    Harvesting, 20920, 20922
  Gum Mucosa, 41870
  Heart
    See Heart, Transplantation
  Heart Lung
    See Transplantation, Heart–Lung
  Hepatorenal, 35535
  Kidney
    See Kidney, Transplantation
  Liver
    See Liver, Transplantation
  Lung
    See Lung, Transplantation
  Muscle
    Cheek, 15841-15845
  Nail Bed Reconstruction, 11762
  Nerve, 64885-64907
  Oral Mucosa, 40818
  Organ
    See Transplantation
  Osteochondral
    Knee, 27415-27416
    Talus, 28446
  Pancreas
    See Pancreas, Transplantation
  Peroneal-Tibial, 35570
  Skin
    Autograft, 15150-15152, 15155-15157
    Biological, 15271-15278
    Blood Flow Check, Graft, 15860
    See Skin Graft and Flap

Graft — *continued*
  Skin — *continued*
    Check Vascular Flow Injection, 15860
    Composite, 15760, 15770
    Delayed Flap, 15600-15630
    Free Flap, 15757
    Full Thickness, Free
      Axillae, 15240, 15241
      Cheeks, Chin, 15240, 15241
      Ears, Eyelids, 15260, 15261
      Extremities (Excluding Hands/Feet), 15240, 15241
      Feet, Hands, 15240, 15241
      Forehead, 15240, 15241
      Genitalia, 15240, 15241
      Lips, Nose, 15260, 15261
      Mouth, Neck, 15240, 15241
      Scalp, 15220, 15221
      Trunk, 15200, 15201
    Harvesting
      for Tissue Culture, 15040
    Pedicle
      Direct, 15570, 15576
      Transfer, 15650
    Pinch Graft, 15050
    Preparation Recipient Site, 15002, 15004-15005
    Split Graft, 15100, 15101, 15120, 15121
    Substitute, 15271-15278
    Vascular Flow Check, Graft, 15860
  Tendon
    Finger, 26392
    Hand, 26392
    Harvesting, 20924
  Tibial/Peroneal Trunk-Tibial, 35570
  Tibial-Tibial, 35570
  Tissue
    Harvesting, 20926
  Vein
    Cross–Over, 34520
  Vertebra, 0222T
    Cervical, 0219T
    Lumbar, 0221T
    Thoracic, 0220T
Grain Alcohol
  See Alcohol, Ethyl
Granulation Tissue
  Cauterization, Chemical, 17250
Gravis, Myasthenia
  See Myasthenia Gravis
Gravities, Specific
  See Specific Gravity
Greater Tuberosity Fracture
  with Shoulder Dislocation
    Closed Treatment, 23665
    Open Treatment, 23670
Greater Vestibular Gland
  See Bartholin's Gland
Great Toe
  Free Osteocutaneous Flap with Microvascular Anastomosis, 20973
Great Vessel(s)
  Shunt
    Aorta to Pulmonary Artery
      Ascending, 33755
      Descending, 33762
    Central, 33764
    Subclavian to Pulmonary Artery, 33750
    Vena Cava to Pulmonary Artery, 33766, 33767
  Unlisted Services and Procedures, 33999
Great Vessels Transposition
  See Transposition, Great Arteries
Greenfield Filter Insertion, 37191
Green Operation
  See Scapulopexy
Grice Arthrodesis, 28725
Grippe. Balkan
  See Q Fever
Gritti Operation, 27590-27592
  See Amputation, Leg, Upper; Radical Resection; Replantation
GRN, 81406
Groin Area
  Repair
    Hernia, 49550-49557

Gross Type Procedure, 49610, 49611
Group Health Education, 99078
Grouping, Blood
  See Blood Typing
Growth Factors, Insulin–Like
  See Somatomedin
Growth Hormone, 83003
  with Arginine Tolerance Test, 80428
  Human, 80418, 80428, 80430, 86277
Growth Hormone Release Inhibiting Factor
  See Somatostatin
Growth Stimulation Expressed Gene, 83006
GTT, 82951, 82952
Guaiac Test
  Blood in Feces, 82270
Guanylic Acids
  See Guanosine Monophosphate
Guard Stain, 88313
Gullet
  See Esophagus
Gums
  Abscess
    Incision and Drainage, 41800
  Alveolus
    Excision, 41830
  Cyst
    Incision and Drainage, 41800
  Excision
    Gingiva, 41820
    Operculum, 41821
  Graft
    Mucosa, 41870
  Hematoma
    Incision and Drainage, 41800
  Lesion
    Destruction, 41850
    Excision, 41822-41828
  Mucosa
    Excision, 41828
  Reconstruction
    Alveolus, 41874
    Gingiva, 41872
  Removal
    Foreign Body, 41805
  Tumor
    Excision, 41825-41827
  Unlisted Services and Procedures, 41899
Gunning–Lieben Test, 82009, 82010
Gunther Tulip Filter Insertion, 37191
Guthrie Test, 84030
GYPA, 81403
GYPB, 81403
GYPE, 81403

H

H19, 81401
HAA (Hepatitis Associated Antigen), 87340-87380, 87515-87527
  See Hepatitis Antigen, B Surface
HAAb (Antibody, Hepatitis), 86708, 86709
HADHA, 81406
HADHB, 81406
Haemoglobin F
  See Fetal Hemoglobin
Haemorrhage
  See Hemorrhage
Haemorrhage Rectum
  See Hemorrhage, Rectum
Hageman Factor, 85280
  Clotting Factor, 85210-85293
Haglund's Deformity Repair, 28119
HAI (Hemagglutination Inhibition Test), 86280
Hair
  Electrolysis, 17380
  KOH Examination, 87220
  Microscopic Evaluation, 96902
  Transplant
    Punch Graft, 15775, 15776
    Strip Graft, 15220, 15221
Hair Removal
  See Removal, Hair
Hallux
  See Great Toe
Hallux Rigidus
  Correction with Cheilectomy, 28289, 28291
Hallux Valgus, 28292-28299

Halo
  Body Cast, 29000
  Cranial, 20661
    for Thin Skull Osteology, 20664
  Femur, 20663
  Maxillofacial, 21100
  Pelvic, 20662
  Removal, 20665
Haloperidol
  Assay, 80173
Halstead-Reitan Neuropsychological Battery, 96118
Halsted Mastectomy, 19305
Halsted Repair
  Hernia, 49495
Hammertoe Repair, 28285, 28286
Hamster Penetration Test, 89329
Ham Test
  Hemolysins, 85475
    with Agglutinins, 86940, 86941
Hand
  See Carpometacarpal Joint; Intercarpal Joint
  Abscess, 26034
  Amputation
    at Metacarpal, 25927
    at Wrist, 25920
      Revision, 25922
    Revision, 25924, 25929, 25931
  Arthrodesis
    Carpometacarpal Joint, 26843, 26844
    Intercarpal Joint, 25820, 25825
  Bone
    Incision and Drainage, 26034
  Cast, 29085
  Decompression, 26035, 26037
  Dislocation
    Carpal
      Closed, 25690
      Open, 25695
    Carpometacarpal
      Closed, 26670, 26675
      Open, 26685-26686
      Percutaneous, 26676
    Interphalangeal
      Closed, 26770, 26775
      Open, 26785
      Percutaneous, 26776
    Lunate
      Closed, 25690
      Open, 25695
    Metacarpalphalangeal
      Closed, 26700-26705
      Open, 26715
      Percutaneous, 26706
    Radiocarpal
      Closed, 25660
      Open, 25670
    Thumb
      See Dislocation Thumb
    Wrist
      See Dislocation, Wrist
  Dupuytren's Contracture(s)
    Fasciotomy
      Open Partial, 26045
      Percutaneous, 26040
    Injection
      Enzyme, 20527
    Manipulation, 26341
    Palmar Fascial Cord
      Injection
        Enzyme, 20527
      Manipulation, 26341
  Excision
    Excess Skin, 15837
  Fracture
    Carpometacarpal, 26641-26650
    Interphalangeal, 26740-26746
    Metacarpal, 26600
    Metacarpophalangeal, 26740-26746
    Phalangeal, 26720-26735, 26750-26765
  Implantation
    Removal, 26320
      Tube/Rod, 26392, 26416
    Tube/Rod, 26390
  Insertion
    Tendon Graft, 26392

Hand — *continued*
  Magnetic Resonance Imaging (MRI), 73218-73223
  Reconstruction
    Tendon Pulley, 26500-26502
  Removal
    Implant, 26320
  Repair
    Blood Vessel, 35207
    Cleft Hand, 26580
    Muscle, 26591, 26593
      Release, 26593
    Tendon
      Extensor, 26410-26416, 26426, 26428, 26433-26437
      Flexor, 26350-26358, 26440
      Profundus, 26370-26373
  Replantation, 20808
  Skin Graft
    Delay of Flap, 15620
    Full Thickness, 15240, 15241
    Pedicle Flap, 15574
    Split, 15100, 15101
  Strapping, 29280
  Tendon
    Excision, 26390
    Extensor, 26415
  Tenotomy, 26450, 26460
  Tissue Transfer, Adjacent, 14040, 14041
  Tumor
    Excision, 26115 [26111]
    Radical Resection, 26116-26118 [26113], 26250
  Unlisted Services and Procedures, 26989
  X–ray, 73120, 73130
Handling
  Device, 99002
  Radioelement, 77790
  Specimen, 99000, 99001
Hand Phalange
  See Finger, Bone
Hanganutziu Deicher Antibodies
  See Antibody, Heterophile
Haptoglobin, 83010, 83012
Hard Palate
  See Palate
Harelip Operation
  See Cleft Lip, Repair
Harrington Rod
  Insertion, 22840
  Removal, 22850
Hartley-Krause, 61450
Hartmann Procedure, 44143
  Laparoscopy
    Partial Colectomy with Colostomy, 44206
  Open, 44143
Harvesting
  Bone Graft, 20900, 20902
  Bone Marrow
    Allogeneic, 38230
    Autologous, 38232
  Cartilage, 20910, 20912
  Conjunctival Graft, 68371
  Eggs for In Vitro Fertilization, 58970
  Endoscopic
    Vein for Bypass Graft, 33508
  Fascia Lata Graft, 20920, 20922
  Intestines, 44132, 44133
  Kidney, 50300, 50320, 50547
  Liver, 47133, 47140-47142
  Lower Extremity Vein for Vascular Reconstruction, 35572
  Skin, 15040
  Stem Cell, 38205, 38206
  Tendon Graft, 20924
  Tissue Grafts, 20926
  Upper Extremity Artery
    for Coronary Artery Bypass Graft, 35600
  Upper Extremity Vein
    for Bypass Graft, 35500
Hauser Procedure
  Reconstruction, Patella, for Instability, 27420
HAVRIX, 90632-90634
Hayem's Elementary Corpuscle
  See Blood, Platelet
Haygroves Procedure, 27120, 27122

Graft — Haygroves Procedure

HBA1/HBA2, 81257, 81404-81405
HBB, 81401, 81403-81404
Hb Bart Hydrops Fetalis Syndrome, 81257
HBcAb, 86704, 86705
HBeAb, 86707
HBeAg, 87350
HbH Disease, 81257
HBsAb, 86706
HBsAg (Hepatitis B Surface Antigen), 87340
HCG, 84702-84704
HCO3
　　See Bicarbonate
Hct, 85013, 85014
HCV Antibodies
　　See Antibody, Hepatitis C
HD, 27295
HDL (High Density Lipoprotein), 83718
Head
　　Angiography, 70496, 70544-70546
　　CT Scan, 70450-70470, 70496
　　Excision, 21015-21070
　　Fracture and/or Dislocation, 21310-21497
　　Incision, 21010, 61316, 62148
　　Introduction, 21076-21116
　　Lipectomy, Suction Assisted, 15876
　　Magnetic Resonance Angiography (MRA),
　　　　70544-70546
　　Nerve
　　　　Graft, 64885, 64886
　　Other Procedures, 21299, 21499
　　Repair
　　　　Revision and/or Reconstruction, 21120-
　　　　　　21296
　　Ultrasound Examination, 76506, 76536
　　Unlisted Services and Procedures, 21499
　　X-ray, 70350
Head Brace
　　Application, 21100
　　Removal, 20661
Head Rings, Stereotactic
　　See Stereotactic Frame
Heaf Test
　　TB Test, 86580
Health Behavior
　　Alcohol and/or Substance Abuse, 99408-99409
　　Assessment, 96150
　　Family Intervention, 96154-96155
　　Group Intervention, 0403T, 96153
　　Individual Intervention, 96152
　　Re-assessment, 96151
　　Smoking and Tobacco Cessation, 99406-99407
Health Risk Assessment Instrument, 96160-96161
Hearing Aid
　　Bone Conduction
　　　　Implant, 69710
　　　　Removal, 69711
　　　　Repair, 69711
　　　　Replace, 69710
　　Check, 92592, 92593
Hearing Aid Services
　　Electroacoustic Test, 92594, 92595
　　Examination, 92590, 92591
Hearing Tests
　　See Audiologic Function Tests; Hearing Evalua-
　　　　tion
Hearing Therapy, 92507, 92601-92604
Heart
　　Ablation
　　　　Arrhythmogenic Focus
　　　　　　Intracardiac Catheter, 93650-93657
　　　　　　Open, 33250-33261
　　　　Ventricular Septum
　　　　　　Transcatheter Alcohol Septal Ablation,
　　　　　　　　93583
　　Acoustic Cardiography with Computer Analysis,
　　　　93799
　　Allograft Preparation, 33933, 33944
　　Angiography, 93454-93461
　　　　Injection, 93563-93568
　　Aortic Arch
　　　　with Cardiopulmonary Bypass, 33853
　　　　without Cardiopulmonary Bypass, 33852
　　Aortic Counterpulsation Ventricular Assist,
　　　　0451T-0463T
　　Aortic Valve
　　　　Implantation, 33361-33369, 33405-33413

Heart — continued
　　Aortic Valve — continued
　　　　Repair
　　　　　　Left Ventricle, 33414
　　　　　　Transcatheter Closure, 93591-93592
　　　　Replacement, 33405-33413
　　　　　　with Cardiopulmonary Bypass, 33405-
　　　　　　　　33406, 33410
　　　　　　Transcatheter, 33361-33369
　　Arrhythmogenic Focus
　　　　Destruction, 33250, 33251, 33261
　　Atria
　　　　See Atria
　　Biopsy, 93505
　　　　Radiologic Guidance, 76932
　　Blood Vessel
　　　　Repair, 33320-33322
　　Cardiac Output Measurements
　　　　by Indicator Dilution, 93561-93562
　　Cardiac Rehabilitation, 93797, 93798
　　Cardioassist, 92970, 92971
　　Cardiopulmonary Bypass
　　　　Lung Transplant, 32852, 32854
　　　　Replacement Ventricular Assist Device,
　　　　　　33983
　　Cardioverter-Defibrillator
　　　　Evaluation and Testing, 93640, 93641,
　　　　　　93642
　　Catheterization, 93451-93453, 93456-93462,
　　　　93530-93533
　　　　Combined Right and Retrograde Left for
　　　　　　Congenital Cardiac Anomalies,
　　　　　　93531
　　　　Combined Right and Transseptal Left for
　　　　　　Congenital Cardiac Anomalies,
　　　　　　93532, 93533
　　　　Flow-Directed, 93503
　　　　Right for Congenital Cardiac Anomalies,
　　　　　　93530
　　Closure
　　　　Patent Ductus Arteriosus, 93582
　　　　Septal Defect, 33615
　　　　　　Ventricular, 33675-33677, 33681-
　　　　　　　　33688, 33776, 33780, 93581
　　　　Valve
　　　　　　Atrioventricular, 33600
　　　　　　Semilunar, 33602
　　Commissurotomy, Right Ventricle, 33476, 33478
　　CT Scan, 75571-75573
　　　　Angiography, 75574
　　Defibrillator
　　　　Removal, 33243, 33244
　　　　　　Pulse Generator Only, 33241
　　　　Repair, 33218, 33220
　　　　Replacement, Leads, 33216, 33217, 33249
　　Destruction
　　　　Arrhythmogenic Focus, 33250, 33261
　　Electrical Recording
　　　　3-D Mapping, 93613
　　　　Acoustic Cardiography, 93799
　　　　Atria, 93602
　　　　Atrial Electrogram, Esophageal (or Trans-
　　　　　　esophageal), 93615, 93616
　　　　Bundle of His, 93600
　　　　Comprehensive, 93619-93622
　　　　External Heart Rate and 3-axis Accelerome-
　　　　　　ter Data, 0381T-0386T
　　　　Right Ventricle, 93603
　　　　Tachycardia Sites, 93609
　　Electroconversion, 92960, 92961
　　Electrode
　　　　Insertion, 33202-33203
　　Electrophysiologic Follow-Up Study, 93624
　　Electrophysiology Procedures, 93600-93660
　　Endoscopy
　　　　Atrial, 33265-33266
　　Evaluation of Device, 93640
　　Excision
　　　　Donor, 33930, 33940
　　　　Tricuspid Valve, 33460, 33465
　　Exploration, 33310, 33315
　　Fibrillation
　　　　Atrial, 33254, 33255-33256
　　Great Vessels
　　　　See Great Vessels

Heart — continued
　　Heart-Lung Bypass
　　　　See Cardiopulmonary Bypass
　　Heart-Lung Transplantation
　　　　See Transplantation, Heart-Lung
　　Hemodynamic Monitoring
　　　　with Pharmacologic Agent, 93463
　　　　with Physiologic Exercise Study, 93464
　　Implantable Defibrillator
　　　　Data Analysis, 93289, 93295-93296
　　　　Evaluation
　　　　　　In Person, 93282-93284, 93287, 93289-
　　　　　　　　93290, 93292
　　　　　　Remote, 93295-93297, 93299
　　　　Initial Setup and Programming, 93745
　　　　Insertion Electrodes, 33216, 33217, 33224-
　　　　　　33225, 33249
　　　　Pulse Generator, 33240
　　　　　　Insertion, 33240 [33230, 33231]
　　　　　　Removal, 33241
　　　　　　Replacement, [33262, 33263, 33264]
　　　　　　System, 33249, [33270]
　　　　Reposition Electrodes, 33215, 33226
　　　　Wearable Device, 93745
　　Implantation
　　　　Artificial Heart, Intracorporeal, 0051T
　　　　Intracorporeal, 33979
　　　　Total Replacement Heart System, Intracor-
　　　　　　poreal, 0051T
　　　　Ventricular Assist Device, 0451T-0452T,
　　　　　　0459T, 33976, 33990-33991
　　Incision
　　　　Atrial, 33254, 33255-33256
　　　　Exploration, 33310, 33315
　　Injection
　　　　Radiologic, 93565-93566
　　Insertion
　　　　Balloon Device, 33973
　　　　Defibrillator, 33212-33213
　　　　Electrode, 33210, 33211, 33214-33217,
　　　　　　33224-33225
　　　　Pacemaker, 33206-33208, 33212, 33213
　　　　　　Catheter, 33210
　　　　　　Pulse Generator, 33212-33214 [33221]
　　　　Ventricular Assist Device, 0451T-0452T,
　　　　　　0459T, 33975
　　Intraoperative Pacing and Mapping, 93631
　　Ligation
　　　　Fistula, 37607
　　Magnetic Resonance Imaging (MRI), 75557-
　　　　75565
　　　　with Contrast Material, 75561-75563
　　　　with Velocity Flow Mapping, 75565
　　　　without Contrast Material, 75557-75559
　　　　without Contrast Material, Followed by
　　　　　　Contrast Material, 75561-75563
　　Mitral Valve
　　　　See Mitral Valve
　　Muscle
　　　　See Myocardium
　　Myocardial Contrast Perfusion, 0439T
　　Myocardial Infarction tPA Administration Docu-
　　　　mented, 4077F
　　Myocardial Strain Imaging, 0399T
　　Myocardial Sympathetic Innervation Imaging,
　　　　0331T-0332T
　　Myocardium
　　　　Imaging, Nuclear, 78466-78469
　　　　Perfusion Study, 78451-78454
　　　　Sympathetic Innervation Imaging, 0331T-
　　　　　　0332T
　　Nuclear Medicine
　　　　Blood Flow Study, 78414
　　　　Blood Pool Imaging, 78472, 78473, 78481,
　　　　　　78483, 78494, 78496
　　　　Myocardial Imaging, 78466-78469
　　　　Myocardial Perfusion, 0439T, 78451-78454
　　　　Shunt Detection (Test), 78428
　　　　Unlisted Services and Procedures, 78499
　　Open Chest Massage, 32160
　　Output, 93561-93562
　　Pacemaker
　　　　Conversion, 33214
　　　　Evaluation
　　　　　　In Person, 93279-93281, 93286, 93288
　　　　　　Remote, 93293-93294, 93296

Heart — continued
　　Pacemaker — continued
　　　　Insertion, 33206-33208
　　　　　　Pulse Generator, 33212, 33213
　　　　Leadless, Ventricular
　　　　　　Device Evaluation, 0389T-0391T
　　　　　　Insertion, 0387T
　　　　　　Removal, 0388T
　　　　　　Replacement, 0387T
　　　　Removal, 33233-33237 [33227, 33228,
　　　　　　33229]
　　　　Replacement, 33206-33208
　　　　　　Catheter, 33210
　　　　Upgrade, 33214
　　Pacing
　　　　Arrhythmia Induction, 93618
　　　　Atria, 93610
　　　　Transcutaneous
　　　　　　Temporary, 92953
　　　　Ventricular, 93612
　　Positron Emission Tomography (PET), 78459
　　　　Perfusion Study, 78491, 78492
　　Pulmonary Valve
　　　　See Pulmonary Valve
　　Rate Increase
　　　　See Tachycardia
　　Reconstruction
　　　　Atrial Septum, 33735-33737
　　　　Vena Cava, 34502
　　Recording
　　　　Left Ventricle, 93622
　　　　Right Ventricle, 93603
　　　　Tachycardia Sites, 93609
　　Reduction
　　　　Ventricular Septum
　　　　　　Non-surgical, 93799
　　Removal
　　　　Balloon Device, 33974
　　　　Electrode, 33238
　　　　Ventricular Assist Device, 33977, 33978
　　　　　　Intracorporeal, 0455T-0458T, 33980
　　Removal Single/Dual Chamber
　　　　Electrodes, 33243, 33244
　　　　Pulse Generator, 33241
　　　　Repair, 33218, 33220
　　Repair
　　　　Anomaly, 33615, 33617
　　　　Aortic Sinus, 33702-33722
　　　　Aortic Valve, 93591-93592
　　　　Artificial Heart, Intracorporeal, 0052T,
　　　　　　0053T
　　　　Atrial Septum, 33254, 33255-33256, 33641,
　　　　　　33647, 93580
　　　　Atrioventricular Canal, 33660, 33665
　　　　　　Complete, 33670
　　　　　　Prosthetic Valve, 33670
　　　　Atrioventricular Valve, 33660, 33665
　　　　Cor Triatriatum, 33732
　　　　Electrode, 33218
　　　　Fenestration, 93580
　　　　　　Prosthetic Valve, 33670
　　　　Infundibular, 33476, 33478
　　　　Mitral Valve, 33420-33430, 93590-93592
　　　　Myocardium, 33542
　　　　Outflow Tract, 33476, 33478
　　　　Patent Ductus Arteriosus, 93582
　　　　Postinfarction, 33542, 33545
　　　　Prosthetic Valve Dysfunction, 33496
　　　　Septal Defect, 33608, 33610, 33660, 33813,
　　　　　　33814, 93581
　　　　Sinus of Valsalva, 33702-33722
　　　　Sinus Venosus, 33645
　　　　Tetralogy of Fallot, 33692-33697, 33924
　　　　Total Replacement Heart System, Intracor-
　　　　　　poreal, 0052T, 0053T
　　　　Tricuspid Valve, 33460-33468
　　　　Ventricle, 33611, 33612
　　　　　　Obstruction, 33619
　　　　Ventricular Septum, 33545, 33647, 33681-
　　　　　　33688, 33692-33697, 93581
　　　　Ventricular Tunnel, 33722
　　　　Wound, 33300, 33305
　　Replacement
　　　　Artificial Heart, Intracorporeal, 0052T,
　　　　　　0053T
　　　　Electrode, 33210, 33211, 33217

Heart — *continued*
  Replacement — *continued*
    Mitral Valve, 33430
    Total Replacement Heart System, Intracorporeal, 0052T, 0053T
    Tricuspid Valve, 33465
    Ventricular Assist Device, 0459T, 33981-33983
  Repositioning
    Aortic Counterpulsation, 0459T, 0460T-0461T
    Electrode, 33215, 33217, 33226
    Tricuspid Valve, 33468
  Resuscitation, 92950
  Septal Defect
    Repair, 33782-33783, 33813-33814
    Ventricular
      Closure, 33675-33688
      Open, 33675-33688
      Percutaneous, 93581
  Stimulation and Pacing, 93623
  Thrombectomy, 33310-33315
  Ventricular Assist Device, 33976
    Intracorporeal, 33979
  Transplantation, 33935, 33945
    Allograft Preparation, 33933, 33944
    Anesthesia, 00580
  Tricuspid Valve
    See Tricuspid Valve
  Tumor
    Excision, 33120, 33130
  Ultrasound
    Myocardial Strain Imaging, 0399T
    Radiologic Guidance, 76932
  Unlisted Services and Procedures, 33999
  Ventriculography
    See Ventriculography
  Ventriculomyectomy, 33416
  Ventriculomyotomy, 33416
  Wound
    Repair, 33300, 33305
Heart Biopsy
  Ultrasound, Radiologic Guidance, 76932
Heartsbreath Test, 0085T
Heart Vessels
  Angiography, 93454-93461, 93563-93566
  Angioplasty, *[92920, 92921]*, *[92928, 92929]*, *[92937, 92938]*, *[92941]*, *[92943, 92944]*
  Injection, 93452-93461, 93563-93568
  Insertion
    Graft, 33330-33335
  Thrombolysis, *[92975, 92977]*
  Valvuloplasty
    See Valvuloplasty
    Percutaneous, 92986-92990
Heat Unstable Haemoglobin
  See Hemoglobin, Thermolabile
Heavy Lipoproteins
  See Lipoprotein
Heavy Metal, 83015, 83018
Heel
  See Calcaneus
  Collection of Blood, 36415, 36416
  X-ray, 73650
Heel Bone
  See Calcaneus
Heel Fracture
  See Calcaneus, Fracture
Heel Spur
  Excision, 28119
Heine–Medin Disease
  See Polio
Heine Operation
  See Cyclodialysis
Heinz Bodies, 85441, 85445
Helicobacter Pylori
  Antibody, 86677
  Antigen Detection
    Enzyme Immunoassay, 87338, 87339
  Breath Test, 78267, 78268, 83013
  Stool, 87338
  Urease Activity, 83009, 83013, 83014
Heller Procedure, 32665, 43279, 43330-43331
Helminth
  Antibody, 86682
Hemagglutination Inhibition Test, 86280

Hemangioma, 17106-17108
Hemapheresis, 36511-36516
Hematochezia, 82270, 82274
Hematologic Test
  See Blood Tests
Hematology
  Unlisted Services and Procedures, 85999
Hematoma
  Ankle, 27603
  Arm, Lower, 25028
  Arm, Upper
    Incision and Drainage, 23930
  Brain
    Drainage, 61154, 61156
    Evacuation, 61312-61315
    Incision and Drainage, 61312-61315
  Drain, 61108
  Ear, External
    Complicated, 69005
    Simple, 69000
  Elbow
    Incision and Drainage, 23930
  Epididymis
    Incision and Drainage, 54700
  Gums
    Incision and Drainage, 41800
  Hip, 26990
  Incision and Drainage
    Neck, 21501, 21502
    Skin, 10140
    Thorax, 21501, 21502
  Knee, 27301
  Leg, Lower, 27603
  Leg, Upper, 27301
  Mouth, 41005-41009, 41015-41018
    Incision and Drainage, 40800, 40801
  Nasal Septum
    Incision and Drainage, 30020
  Nose
    Incision and Drainage, 30000, 30020
  Pelvis, 26990
  Puncture Aspiration, 10160
  Scrotum
    Incision and Drainage, 54700
  Shoulder
    Drainage, 23030
  Skin
    Incision and Drainage, 10140
    Puncture Aspiration, 10160
  Subdural, 61108
  Subungual
    Evacuation, 11740
  Testis
    Incision and Drainage, 54700
  Tongue, 41000-41006, 41015
  Vagina
    Incision and Drainage, 57022, 57023
  Wrist, 25028
Hematopoietic Stem Cell Transplantation
  See Stem Cell, Transplantation
Hematopoietin
  See Erythropoietin
Hematuria
  See Blood, Urine
Hemic System
  Unlisted Procedure, 38999
Hemiephyseal Arrest
  Elbow, 24470
Hemifacial Microsomia
  Reconstruction Mandibular Condyle, 21247
Hemilaminectomy, 63020-63044
Hemilaryngectomy, 31370-31382
Hemipelvectomies
  See Amputation, Interperviabdominal
Hemiphalangectomy
  Toe, 28160
Hemispherectomy
  Partial, 61543
Hemochromatosis Gene Analysis, 81256
Hemocytoblast
  See Stem Cell
Hemodialysis, 90935, 90937, 99512
  Blood Flow Study, 90940
  Duplex Scan of Access, 93990
Hemofiltration, 90945, 90947
  Hemodialysis, 90935, 90937

Hemofiltration — *continued*
  Peritoneal Dialysis, 90945, 90947
Hemoglobin
  A1C, 83036
  Analysis
    O2 Affinity, 82820
  Antibody
    Fecal, 82274
  Carboxyhemoglobin, 82375-82376
  Chromatography, 83021
  Electrophoresis, 83020
  Fetal, 83030, 83033, 85460, 85461
  Fractionation and Quantitation, 83020
  Glycosylated (A1c), 83036-83037
  Methemoglobin, 83045, 83050
  Non–Automated, 83026
  Plasma, 83051
  Sulfhemoglobin, 83060
  Thermolabile, 83065, 83068
  Transcutaneous
    Carboxyhemoglobin, 88740
    Methemoglobin, 88741
  Urine, 83069
Hemoglobin F
  Fetal
    Chemical, 83030
    Qualitative, 83033
Hemoglobin, Glycosylated, 83036-83037
Hemoglobin (Hgb) quantitative
  Transcutaneous, 88738-88741
Hemogram
  Added Indices, 85025-85027
  Automated, 85025-85027
  Manual, 85014, 85018, 85032
Hemolysins, 85475
  with Agglutinins, 86940, 86941
Hemolytic Complement
  See Complement, Hemolytic
Hemolytic Complement, Total
  See Complement, Hemolytic, Total
Hemoperfusion, 90997
Hemophil
  See Clotting Factor
Hemophilus Influenza
  Antibody, 86684
  B Vaccine, 90647-90648, 90748
Hemorrhage
  Abdomen, 49002
  Anal
    Endoscopic Control, 46614
  Bladder
    Postoperative, 52214
  Chest Cavity
    Endoscopic Control, 32654
  Colon
    Endoscopic Control, 44391, 45382
  Colon–Sigmoid
    Endoscopic Control, 45334
  Esophagus
    Endoscopic Control, 43227
  Gastrointestinal, Upper
    Endoscopic Control, 43255
  Intestines, Small
    Endoscopic Control, 44366, 44378
  Liver
    Control, 47350
  Lung, 32110
  Nasal
    Cauterization, 30901-30906
    Endoscopic Control, 31238
  Nasopharynx, 42970-42972
  Nose
    Cauterization, 30901-30906
  Oropharynx, 42960-42962
  Rectum
    Endoscopic Control, 45317
  Throat, 42960-42962
  Uterus
    Postpartum, 59160
  Vagina, 57180
Hemorrhoidectomy
  External, 46250, *[46320]*
  Internal and External, 46255-46262
  Ligation, 46221 *[46945, 46946]*
  Whitehead, 46260
Hemorrhoidopexy, *[46947]*

Hemorrhoids
  Destruction, 46930
  Excision, 46250-46262, *[46320]*
  Incision, 46083
  Injection
    Sclerosing Solution, 46500
  Ligation, 45350, 46221 *[46945, 46946]*, *[45398]*
  Stapling, *[46947]*
Hemosiderin, 83070
Hemothorax
  Thoracostomy, 32551
Heparin, 85520
  Clotting Inhibitors, 85300-85305
  Neutralization, 85525
  Protamine Tolerance Test, 85530
Heparin Cofactor I
  See Antithrombin III
Hepatectomy
  Extensive, 47122
  Left Lobe, 47125
  Partial
    Donor, 47140-47142
    Lobe, 47120
  Right Lobe, 47130
  Total
    Donor, 47133
Hepatic Abscess
  See Abscess, Liver
Hepatic Arteries
  See Artery, Hepatic
Hepatic Artery Aneurysm
  See Artery, Hepatic, Aneurysm
Hepatic Duct
  Anastomosis
    with Intestines, 47765, 47802
  Exploration, 47400
  Incision and Drainage, 47400
  Nuclear Medicine
    Imaging, 78226-78227
  Removal
    Calculi (Stone), 47400
  Repair
    with Intestines, 47765, 47802
  Unlisted Services and Procedures, 47999
Hepatic Haemorrhage
  See Hemorrhage, Liver
Hepaticodochotomy
  See Hepaticostomy
Hepaticoenterostomy, 47802
Hepaticostomy, 47400
Hepaticotomy, 47400
Hepatic Portal Vein
  See Vein, Hepatic Portal
Hepatic Portoenterostomies
  See Hepaticoenterostomy
Hepatic Transplantation
  See Liver, Transplantation
Hepatitis A and Hepatitis B, 90636
Hepatitis Antibody
  A, 86708, 86709
  B core, 86704, 86705
  Be, 86707
  B Surface, 86706
  C, 86803, 86804
  Delta Agent, 86692
  IgG, 86704, 86708
  IgM, 86704, 86705, 86709
Hepatitis Antigen
  B, 87515-87517
  Be, 87350
  B Surface, 87340, 87341
  C, 87520-87522
  Delta Agent, 87380
  G, 87525-87527
Hepatitis A Vaccine
  Adolescent
    Pediatric
      Three Dose Schedule, 90634
      Two Dose Schedule, 90633
  Adult Dosage, 90632
Hepatitis B and Hib, 90748
Hepatitis B Immunization, 90739-90748
Hepatitis B Vaccine
  Dosage
    with Hemophilus Influenza Vaccine, 90748
    Adolescent, 90743-90744

Hepatitis B Vaccine — continued
  Dosage — continued
    Adult, 90739, 90746
    Dialysis Patient, 90747
    Immunosuppressed, 90740, 90747
    Pediatric, 90744
      Adolescent, 90743-90744
Hepatitis B Virus E Antibody
  See Antibody, Hepatitis
Hepatitis B Virus Surface ab
  See Antibody, Hepatitis B, Surface
Hepatobiliary System Imaging, 78226
  with Pharmacologic Intervention, 78227
Hepatorrhaphy
  See Liver, Repair
Hepatotomy
  Abscess, 47010
  Cyst, 47010
Hereditary Disorders
  Breast Cancer, 81432-81433
  Colon Cancer, 81435-81436
  Neuroendocrine Tumor, 81437-81438
  Retinal Disorders, 81434
Hernia
  Repair
    with Spermatic Cord, 55540
    Abdominal, 49560, 49565, 49590
      Incisional, 49560
      Recurrent, 49565
    Diaphragmatic, 39503-39541
      Chronic, 39541
      Neonatal, 39503
    Epigastric, 49570
      Incarcerated, 49572
    Femoral, 49550
      Incarcerated, 49553
      Recurrent, 49555
      Recurrent Incarcerated, 49557
      Reducible, 49550
    Incisional, 49561, 49566
      Incarcerated, 49561
    Inguinal, 49491, 49495-49500, 49505
      Incarcerated, 49492, 49496, 49501,
        49507, 49521
      Infant, Incarcerated
        Strangulated, 49496, 49501
      Infant, Reducible, 49495, 49500
      Laparoscopic, 49650, 49651
      Pediatric, Reducible, 49500, 49505
      Recurrent, Incarcerated
        Strangulated, 49521
      Recurrent, Reducible, 49520
      Sliding, 49525
      Strangulated, 49492
    Lumbar, 49540
    Lung, 32800
    Mayo, 49585
    Orchiopexy, 54640
    Recurrent Incisional
      Incarcerated, 49566
    Umbilicus, 49580, 49585
      Incarcerated, 49582, 49587
    Spigelian, 49590
Hernia, Cerebral
  See Encephalocele
Hernia, Rectovaginal
  See Rectocele
Hernia, Umbilical
  See Omphalocele
Heroin Test, [80305, 80306, 80307]
Herpes Simplex Virus
  Antibody, 86696
  Antigen Detection
    Immunofluorescence, 87273, 87274
    Nucleic Acid, 87528-87530
  Identification
    Smear and Stain, 87207
Herpes Smear, 87207
Herpesvirus 4 (Gamma), Human
  See Epstein–Barr Virus
Herpes Virus–6 Detection, 87531-87533
Herpetic Vesicle
  Destruction, 54050, 54065
Heteroantibodies
  See Antibody, Heterophile

Heterologous Transplant
  See Xenograft
Heterologous Transplantations
  See Heterograft
Heterophile Antibody, 86308-86310
Heterotropia
  See Strabismus
HEXA, 81255, 81406, 81412
Hexadecadrol
  See Dexamethasone
Hex B
  See b–Hexosaminidase
**Hexosaminidase A (Alpha Polypeptide) Gene
  Analysis**, 81255
Hexosephosphate Isomerase
  See Phosphohexose Isomerase
Heyman Procedure, 27179, 28264
HFE, 81256
H Flu
  See Hemophilus Influenza
Hgb, 83036, 83051, 83065, 83068, 85018
Hg Factor
  See Glucagon
HGH (Human Growth Hormone), 80418, 80428,
  80430, 83003, 86277
HHV–4
  See Epstein–Barr Virus
HIAA (Hydroxyindolacetic Acid, Urine), 83497
Hibb Operation, 22841
Hiberix, 90648
Hib Vaccine
  Four Dose Schedule
    Hib-MenCY, 90644
    PRP-T Four Dose Schedule, 90648
  Hib, 90647-90648
  PRP–OMP
    Three Dose Schedule, 90647
Hickmann Catheterization
  See Cannulization; Catheterization, Venous,
    Central Line; Venipuncture
Hicks–Pitney Test
  Thromboplastin, Partial Time, 85730, 85732
Hidradenitis
  See Sweat Gland
  Excision, 11450-11471
  Suppurative
    Incision and Drainage, 10060, 10061
High Altitude Simulation Test, 94452-94453
High Density Lipoprotein, 83718
Highly Selective Vagotomy
  See Vagotomy, Highly Selective
High Molecular Weight Kininogen
  See Fitzgerald Factor
Highmore Antrum
  See Sinus, Maxillary
Hill Procedure, 43842-43843
Hinton Positive
  See RPR
Hip
  See Femur; Pelvis
  Abscess
    Incision and Drainage, 26990
  Arthrocentesis, 20610-20611
  Arthrodesis, 27284, 27286
  Arthrography, 73525
  Arthroplasty, 27130, 27132
  Arthroscopy, 29860-29863 [29914, 29915,
    29916]
  Arthrotomy, 27030, 27033
  Biopsy, 27040, 27041
  Bone
    Drainage, 26992
  Bursa
    Incision and Drainage, 26991
  Capsulectomy
    with Release, Flexor Muscles, 27036
  Cast, 29305, 29325
  Craterization, 27070, 27071
  Cyst
    Excision, 27065-27067
  Denervation, 27035
  Echography
    Infant, 76885, 76886
  Endoprosthesis
    See Prosthesis, Hip
  Excision, 27070

Hip — continued
  Excision — continued
    Excess Skin, 15834
  Exploration, 27033
  Fasciotomy, 27025
  Fusion, 27284, 27286
  Hematoma
    Incision and Drainage, 26990
  Injection
    Radiologic, 27093, 27095, 27096
  Manipulation, 27275
  Reconstruction
    Total Replacement, 27130
  Removal
    Cast, 29710
    Foreign Body, 27033, 27086, 27087
      Arthroscopic, 29861
    Loose Body
      Arthroscopic, 29861
    Prosthesis, 27090, 27091
  Repair
    Muscle Transfer, 27100-27105, 27111
    Osteotomy, 27146-27156
    Tendon, 27097
  Saucerization, 27070
  Stem Prostheses
    See Arthroplasty, Hip
  Strapping, 29520
  Tenotomy
    Abductor Tendon, 27006
    Adductor Tendon, 27000-27003
    Iliopsoas Tendon, 27005
  Total Replacement, 27130, 27132
  Tumor
    Excision, 27047-27049 [27043, 27045,
      27059], 27065-27067, 27075-27078
  Ultrasound
    Infant, 76885, 76886
    X–ray, 73501-73503, 73521-73523
      with Contrast, 73525
Hip Joint
  Arthroplasty, 27132
    Revision, 27134-27138
  Arthrotomy, 27502
  Biopsy, 27502
  Capsulotomy
    with Release, Flexor Muscles, 27036
  Dislocation, 27250, 27252
    without Trauma, 27265, 27266
    Congenital, 27256-27259
    Open Treatment, 27253, 27254
  Manipulation, 27275
  Reconstruction
    Revision, 27134-27138
  Synovium
    Excision, 27054
    Arthroscopic, 29863
  Total Replacement, 27132
Hippocampus
  Excision, 61566
Hip Stem Prosthesis
  See Arthroplasty, Hip
Histamine, 83088
Histamine Release Test, 86343
Histochemistry, 88319
Histocompatibility Testing
  See Tissue Typing
Histoplasma
  Antibody, 86698
  Antigen, 87385
Histoplasma Capsulatum
  Antigen Detection
    Enzyme Immunoassay, 87385
Histoplasmin Test
  See Histoplasmosis, Skin Test
Histoplasmoses
  See Histoplasmosis
Histoplasmosis
  Skin Test, 86510
History and Physical
  See Evaluation and Management, Office and/or
    Other Outpatient Services
  Pelvic Exam under Anesthesia, 57410
  Preventive
    Established Patient, 99391-99397
    New Patient, 99381-99387

HIV, 86689, 86701-86703, 87389-87391, 87534-
  87539
  Antibody
    Confirmation Test, 86689
    Antigen HIV-1 with HIV-1 and HIV-2 Antibodies,
      87389
HIV–1
  Antigen Detection
    Enzyme Immunoassay, 87390
HIV–2
  Antigen Detection
    Enzyme Immunoassay, 87391
HIV Antibody, 86701-86703
HIV Detection
  Antibody, 86701-86703
  Antigen, 87390, 87391, 87534-87539
  Confirmation Test, 86689
HK3 Kallikrein
  See Antigen, Prostate Specific
HLA
  Antibody Detection, 86828-86835
  Crossmatch, 86825-86826
  Typing, 86812-86813, 86816-86817, 86821-
    86822
    Molecular Pathology Techniques, 81370-
      81383
HLCS, 81406
HMRK
  See Fitzgerald Factor
HNF1A, 81405
HNF1B, 81404-81405
HNF4A, 81406
Hoffman Apparatus, 20690
Hofmeister Operation, 43632
Holten Test, 82575
Holter Monitor, 93224-93227
Home Services
  Activities of Daily Living, 99509
  Catheter Care, 99507
  Enema Administration, 99511
  Established Patient, 99347-99350
  Hemodialysis, 99512
  Home Infusion Procedures, 99601, 99602
  Individual or Family Counseling, 99510
  Intramuscular Injections, 99506
  Mechanical Ventilation, 99504
  Newborn Care, 99502
  New Patient, 99341-99345
  Postnatal Assessment, 99501
  Prenatal Monitoring, 99500
  Respiratory Therapy, 99503
  Sleep Studies, 95805-95811 [95800, 95801]
  Stoma Care, 99505
  Unlisted Services and Procedures, 99600
Homocystine, 83090
  Urine, 82615
Homogenization, Tissue, 87176
Homologous Grafts
  See Graft, Skin
Homologous Transplantation
  See Homograft, Skin
Homovanillic Acid
  Urine, 83150
Horii Procedure (Carpal Bone), 25430
Hormone Adrenocorticotrophic
  See Adrenocorticotropic Hormone (ACTH)
Hormone Assay
  ACTH, 82024
  Aldosterone
    Blood or Urine, 82088
  Androstenedione
    Blood or Urine, 82157
  Androsterone
    Blood or Urine, 82160
  Angiotensin II, 82163
  Corticosterone, 82528
  Cortisol
    Total, 82533
  Dehydroepiandrosterone, 82626-82627
  Dihydrotestosterone, [80327, 80328]
  Epiandrosterone, [80327, 80328]
  Estradiol, 82670
  Estriol, 82677
  Estrogen, 82671, 82672
  Estrone, 82679
  Follicle Stimulating Hormone, 83001

Hormone Assay — *continued*
  Growth Hormone, 83003
    Suppression Panel, 80430
  Hydroxyprogesterone, 83498, 83499
  Luteinizing Hormone, 83002
  Somatotropin, 80430, 83003
  Testosterone, 84403
  Vasopressin, 84588
Hormone–Binding Globulin, Sex
  See Globulin, Sex Hormone Binding
Hormone, Corticotropin–Releasing
  See Corticotropic Releasing Hormone (CRH)
Hormone, Growth
  See Growth Hormone
Hormone, Human Growth
  See Growth Hormone, Human
Hormone, Interstitial Cell–Stimulation
  See Luteinizing Hormone (LH)
Hormone, Parathyroid
  See Parathormone
Hormone Pellet Implantation, 11980
Hormone, Pituitary Lactogenic
  See Prolactin
Hormone, Placental Lactogen
  See Lactogen, Human Placental
Hormones, Adrenal Cortex
  See Corticosteroids
Hormones, Antidiuretic
  See Antidiuretic Hormone
Hormone, Somatotropin Release–Inhibiting
  See Somatostatin
Hormone, Thyroid–Stimulating
  See Thyroid Stimulating Hormone (TSH)
Hospital Discharge Services
  See Discharge Services, Hospital
Hospital Services
  Inpatient Services
    Discharge Services, 99238, 99239
    Initial Care New or Established Patient,
      99221-99223
    Initial Hospital Care, 99221-99223
    Neonate, 99477
    Newborn, 99460-99465, 99466-99480
    Prolonged Services, 99356, 99357
    Subsequent Hospital Care, 99231-99233
  Normal Newborn, 99460-99463
  Observation
    Discharge Services, 99234-99236
    Initial Care, 99218-99220
      New or Established Patient, 99218-
        99220
    Intensive Neonatal, 99477
  Same Day Admission
    Discharge Services, 99234-99236
  Subsequent Newborn Care, 99462
Hot Pack Treatment, 97010
  See Physical Medicine and Rehabilitation
House Calls, 99341-99350
Howard Test
  Cystourethroscopy, Catheterization, Ureter,
    52005
HP, 83010, 83012
HPL, 83632
HRAS, 81403-81404
HSD11B2, 81404
HSD3B2, 81404
HSG, 58340, 74740
HSPB1, 81404
HTLV I
  Antibody
    Confirmatory Test, 86689
    Detection, 86687
HTLV–II
  Antibody, 86688
HTLV III
  See HIV
HTLV–IV
  See HIV–2
HTRA1, 81405
HTT, 81401
Hubbard Tank Therapy, 97036
  with Exercises, 97036, 97113
  See Physical Medicine/ Therapy/Occupational
    Therapy
Hue Test, 92283
Huggin Operation, 54520

Huhner Test, 89300-89320
Human
  Epididymis Protein 4 (HE4), 86305
  Growth Hormone, 80418, 80428, 80430
  Leukocyte Antigen, 86812-86826
  Papillomavirus Detection, [87623, 87624, 87625]
  Papillomavirus Vaccine, 90649-90651
Human Chorionic Gonadotropin
  See Chorionic Gonadotropin
Human Chorionic Somatomammotropin
  See Lactogen, HumanPlacental
Human Cytomegalovirus Group
  See Cytomegalovirus
Human Herpes Virus 4
  See Epstein–Barr Virus
Human Immunodeficiency Virus
  See HIV
Human Immunodeficiency Virus 1
  See HIV–1
Human Immunodeficiency Virus 2
  See HIV–2
Human Placental Lactogen, 83632
Human Platelet Antigen Genotyping, 81400
Human T Cell Leukemia Virus I
  See HTLV I
Human T Cell Leukemia Virus I Antibodies
  See Antibody, HTLV–I
Human T Cell Leukemia Virus II
  See HTLV II
Human T Cell Leukemia Virus II Antibodies
  See Antibody, HTLV–II
Humeral Epicondylitides, Lateral
  See Tennis Elbow
Humeral Fracture
  See Fracture, Humerus
Humerus
  See Arm, Upper; Shoulder
  Abscess
    Incision and Drainage, 23935
  Craterization, 23184, 24140
  Cyst
    Excision, 23150, 24110
      with Allograft, 23156, 24116
      with Autograft, 23155, 24115
  Diaphysectomy, 23184, 24140
  Excision, 23174, 23184, 23195, 23220, 24077-
    24079, 24110-24116, 24134, 24140,
    24150
  Fracture
    with Dislocation, 23665, 23670
    Closed Treatment, 24500, 24505
      with Manipulation, 23605
      without Manipulation, 23600
    Condyle
      Closed Treatment, 24576, 24577
      Open Treatment, 24579
      Percutaneous Fixation, 24582
    Epicondyle
      Closed Treatment, 24560, 24565
      Open Treatment, 24575
      Percutaneous Fixation, 24566
    Greater Tuberosity Fracture
      Closed Treatment with Manipulation,
        23625
      Closed Treatment without Manipula-
        tion, 23620
      Open Treatment, 23630
    Open Treatment, 23615, 23616
    Shaft
      Closed Treatment, 24500, 24505, 24516
      Open Treatment, 24515
    Supracondylar
      Closed Treatment, 24530, 24535
      Open Treatment, 24545, 24546
      Percutaneous Fixation, 24538
    Transcondylar
      Closed Treatment, 24530, 24535
      Open Treatment, 24545, 24546
      Percutaneous Fixation, 24538
  Osteomyelitis, 24134
  Pinning, Wiring, 23491, 24498
  Prophylactic Treatment, 23491, 24498
  Radical Resection, 23220, 24077-24079
  Repair, 24430
    with Graft, 24435
    Nonunion, Malunion, 24430, 24435

Humerus — *continued*
  Repair — *continued*
    Osteoplasty, 24420
    Osteotomy, 24400, 24410
  Resection Head, 23195
  Saucerization, 23184, 24140
  Sequestrectomy, 23174, 24134
  Tumor
    Excision, 23150-23156, 23220, 24075-24079
      [24071, 24073], 24110-24116
  X–ray, 73060
Hummelshein Operation, 67340
  Strabismus Repair
    Adjustable Sutures, 67335
    Extraocular Muscles, 67340
    One Horizontal Muscle, 67311
    One Vertical Muscle, 67314
    Posterior Fixation Suture Technique, 67335
    Previous Surgery not Involving Extraocular
      Muscles, 67331
    Release Extensive Scar Tissue, 67343
    Superior Oblique Muscle, 67318
    Transposition, 67320
    Two Horizontal Muscles, 67312
    Two or More Vertical Muscles, 67316
Humor Shunt, Aqueous
  See Aqueous Shunt
HVA (Homovanillic Acid), 83150
Hybridization Probes, DNA
  See Nucleic Acid Probe
Hydatid Disease
  See Echinococcosis
Hydatidiform Mole
  Evacuation and Curettage, 59870
  Excision, 59100
Hydatid Mole
  See Hydatidiform Mole
Hydration, 96360-96361
Hydrocarbons, Chlorinated
  See Chlorinated Hydrocarbons
Hydrocele
  Aspiration, 55000
  Excision
    Bilateral, Tunica Vaginalis, 55041
    Unilateral
      Spermatic Cord, 55500
      Tunica Vaginalis, 55040
  Repair, 55060
Hydrocelectomy, 49495-49501
Hydrocele, Tunica Vaginalis
  See Tunica Vaginalis, Hydrocele
Hydrochloric Acid, Gastric
  See Acid, Gastric
Hydrochloride, Vancomycin
  See Vancomycin
Hydrocodone
  See Dihydrocodeinone
Hydrogen Ion Concentration
  See pH
Hydrolase, Acetylcholine
  See Acetylcholinesterase
Hydrolases, Phosphoric Monoester
  See Phosphatase
Hydrolase, Triacylglycerol
  See Lipase
Hydrotherapy (Hubbard Tank), 97036
  with Exercises, 97036, 97113
  See Physical Medicine/Therapy/ Occupational
    Therapy
Hydrotubation, 58350
Hydroxyacetanilide
  See Acetaminophen
Hydroxycorticosteroid, 83491
Hydroxyindolacetic Acid, 83497
  Urine, 83497
Hydroxypregnenolone, 80406, 84143
Hydroxyprogesterone, 80402, 80406, 83498,
  83499
Hydroxyproline, 83500, 83505
Hydroxytyramine
  See Dopamine
Hygroma, Cystic
  Axillary or Cervical Excision, 38550, 38555
Hymen
  Excision, 56700
  Incision, 56442

Hymenal Ring
  Revision, 56700
Hymenectomy, 56700
Hymenotomy, 56442
Hyoid Bone
  Fracture
    Open Treatment, 31584
Hyperbaric Oxygen Pressurization, 99183
Hypercycloidal X–ray, 76101, 76102
Hyperdactylies
  See Supernumerary Digit
Hyperglycemic Glycogenolytic Factor
  See Glucagon
HyperRAB, 90375
HyperTED, 90389
Hypertelorism of Orbit
  See Orbital Hypertelorism
Hyperthermia Therapy
  See Thermotherapy
Hyperthermia Treatment, 77600-77620
Hypnotherapy, 90880
Hypodermis
  See Subcutaneous Tissue
Hypogastric Plexus
  Destruction, 64681
  Injection
    Anesthetic, 64517
    Neurolytic, 64681
Hypoglossal–Facial Anastomosis
  See Anastomosis, Nerve, Facial to Hypoglossal
Hypoglossal Nerve
  Anastomosis
    to Facial Nerve, 64868
Hypopharynges
  See Hypopharynx
Hypopharynx
  Diverticulectomy, 43130, 43180
Hypophysectomy, 61546, 61548, 62165
Hypophysis
  See Pituitary Gland
Hypopyrexia
  See Hypothermia
Hypospadias
  Repair, 54300, 54352
    Complications, 54340-54348
    First Stage, 54304
      Meatal Advancement, 54322
      Perineal, 54336
      Proximal Penile or Penoscrotal, 54332
    One Stage
      Meatal Advancement, 54322
      Perineal, 54336
    Urethroplasty by
      Local Skin Flaps, 54324
      Local Skin Flaps and Mobilization of
        Urethra, 54326
      Local Skin Flaps, Skin Graft Patch
        and/or Island Flap, 54328
      Urethroplasty for Second Stage, 54308-
        54316
      Free Skin Graft, 54316
      Urethroplasty for Third Stage, 54318
Hypotensive Anesthesia, 99135
Hypothermia, 99116, 99184
Hypothermic Anesthesia, 99116
Hypoxia
  Breathing Response, 94450
  High Altitude Simulation Test, 94452-94453
Hysterectomy
  Abdominal
    Radical, 58210
    Resection of Ovarian Malignancy, 58951,
      58953-58954, 58956
    Supracervical, 58180
    Total, 58150, 58200
      with Colpo–Urethrocystopexy, 58152
      with Omentectomy, 58956
      with Partial Vaginectomy, 58200
  Cesarean
    with Closure of Vesicouterine Fistula, 51925
    After Cesarean Section, 59525
  Laparoscopic, 58541-58544, 58548, 58570-
    58573
  Removal
    Lesion, 59100

Hysterectomy — *continued*
    Vaginal, 58260-58270, 58290-58294, 58550-58554
        with Colpectomy, 58275, 58280
        with Colpo–Urethrocystopexy, 58267, 58293
        See Lysis, Adhesions, Uterus
    Laparoscopic, 58550
    Radical, 58285
    Removal Tubes
        Ovaries, 52402, 58262, 58263, 58291-58292, 58552-58554
        Repair of Enterocele, 58263, 58292, 58294
    Wertheim, 58210
Hysterolysis, 58559
Hysteroplasty, 58540
Hysterorrhaphy, 58520, 59350
Hysterosalpingography, 74740
    Catheterization, 58345
        Introduction of Contrast, 58340
Hysterosalpingostomy
    See Implantation, Tubouterine
Hysteroscopy
    with Endometrial Ablation, 58563
    with Lysis of Adhesions, 58559
    Ablation
        Endometrial, 58563
    Diagnostic, 58555
    Lysis
        Adhesions, 58559
    Placement
        Fallopian Tube Implants, 58565
    Removal
        Impacted Foreign Body, 58562
        Leiomyomata, 58561
    Resection
        of Intrauterine Septum, 58560
    Surgical with Biopsy, 58558
    Unlisted Services and Procedures, 58579
Hysterosonography, 76831
    See Ultrasound
Hysterotomy, 59100
    See Ligation, Uterus
    Induced Abortion
        with Amniotic Injections, 59852
        with Vaginal Suppositories, 59857
Hysterotrachelectomy, 57530

I

IA, 36100-36140, 36260
IAB, 33970-33974
IABP, 33970-33974
IAC, 33970-33974
I Angiotensin, 84244
I Antibodies, HTLV, 86687, 86689
IBC, 83550
ICAM4, 81403
ICCE, 66920, 66930
Ichthyosis, Sex–Linked, 86592-86593
I Coagulation Factor, 85384-85385
ICSH, 80418, 80426, 83002
Identification
    Oocyte from Follicular Fluid, 89254
    Sentinel Node, 38792, 38900
    Sperm
        from Aspiration, 89257
        from Tissue, 89264
IDH (Isocitric Dehydrogenase, Blood), 83570
IDH1, 81403
IDH2, 81403
IDS, 81405
IDUA, 81406
IG, 82787, 84445, 86023
IgA, Gammaglobulin, 82784
IgD, Gammaglobulin, 82784
IgE
    Allergen Specific, 86003, 86005
    Gammaglobulin, 82785
IgG
    Allergen Specific, 86001
    Gammaglobulin, 82784
IGH@, 81261-81263
IGH@/BCL2 (t(14;18), 81401
IGK@, 81264
IgM, Gammaglobulin, 82784

I Heparin Co–Factor, 85300-85301
II, Coagulation Factor, 85610-85611
II, Cranial Nerve
    See Optic Nerve
IKBKAP, 81260, 81412
IL28B, 81400
IL2RG, 81405
Ileal Conduit
    Visualization, 50690
Ileocolostomy, 44160
Ileoproctostomy, 44150
Ileoscopy
    via Stoma, 44380-44384 *[44381]*
Ileostomy, 44310, 45136
    Continent (Kock Pouch), 44316
    Laparoscopic, 44186-44187
    Nontube, 44187
    Revision, 44312, 44314
Iliac Arteries
    See Artery, Iliac
Iliac Crest
    Free Osteocutaneous flap with Microvascular Anastomosis, 20970
Iliohypogastric Nerve
    Injection
        Anesthetic, 64425
Ilioinguinal Nerve
    Injection
        Anesthetic, 64425
Ilium
    Craterization, 27070, 27071
    Cyst, 27065-27067
    Excision, 27070-27071
    Fracture
        Open Treatment, 27215, 27218
    Saucerization, 27070, 27071
    Tumor, 27065-27067
Ilizarov Procedure
    Application, Bone Fixation Device, 20690, 20692
    Monticelli Type, 20692
Image-guided fluid collection drainage, percutaneous, 10030
Imaging
    See Vascular Studies
    Ophthalmic, 92132-92134, 92227-92228
    Tear film, 0330T
Imaging, Gamma Camera
    See Nuclear Medicine
Imaging, Magnetic Resonance
    See Magnetic Resonance Imaging (MRI)
Imaging, Ultrasonic
    See Echography
Imbrication
    Diaphragm, 39545
Imidobenzyle
    See Imipramine
IM Injection
    Chemotherapy/Complex Biological, 96401-96402
    Diagnostic, Prophylactic, Therapeutic, 96372
        Antineoplastic
            Hormonal, 96402
            Non-hormonal, 96401
Imipramine
    Assay, *[80335, 80336, 80337]*
Immune Complex Assay, 86332
Immune Globulin Administration, 96365-96368, 96372, 96374-96375
Immune Globulin E, 82785
Immune Globulins
    Antitoxin
        Botulinum, 90287
        Diphtheria, 90296
    Botulism, 90288
    Cytomegalovirus, 90291
    Hepatitis B, 90371
    Human, 90281, 90283-90284
    Rabies, 90375, 90376
    Rho (D), 90384-90386
    Tetanus, 90389
    Unlisted Immune Globulin, 90399
    Vaccinia, 90393
    Varicella–Zoster, 90396
Immune Serum Globulin
    Immunization, 90281, 90283

Immunization
    Active
        Acellular Pertussis, 90700, 90723
        BCG, 90585, 90586
        Cholera, *[90625]*
        Diphtheria, Tetanus Acellular
            Influenza B and Poliovirus Inactivated, Vaccine, 90698
        Diphtheria, Tetanus Toxoids, Acellular Pertussis, 90700, 90723
        Hemophilus Influenza B, 90647-90648, 90748
        Hepatitis A, 90632-90636
        Hepatitis B, 90740-90747, 90748
        Hepatitis B, Hemophilus Influenza B (HIB), 90748
        Influenza, 90655-90660
        Influenza B, 90647-90648
        Japanese Encephalitis, 90738
        Measles, Mumps, Rubella, 90707
        Measles, Mumps, Rubella, Varicella Vaccine, 90710
        Meningococcal Conjugate, 90734
        Meningococcal Polysaccharide, 90733
        Pneumococcal, 90732
        Poliomyelitis, 90713
        Rabies, 90675, 90676
        Rotavirus Vaccine, 90680-90681
        Tetanus Diphtheria and Acellular Pertussis, 90715
        Typhoid, 90690-90691
        Varicella (Chicken Pox), 90716
        Yellow Fever, 90717
    Administration
        with Counseling, 90460-90461
        without Counseling, 90471-90474
    Inactive
        Japanese Encephalitis Virus, 90738
    Passive
        Hyperimmune Serum Globulin, 90287-90399
        Immune Serum Globulin, 90281, 90283
    Unlisted Services and Procedures, 90749
Immunoassay
    Analyte, 83518-83520
    Calprotectin, Fecal, 83993
    Infectious Agent, 86317, 86318, 87449-87451, 87809
    Nonantibody, 83516-83519
    Tumor Antigen, 86294, 86316
        CA 125, 86304
        CA 15–3, 86300
        CA 19–9, 86301
Immunoblotting, Western
    HIV, 86689
    Protein, 84181-84182
    Tissue Analysis, 88371-88372
Immunochemical, Lysozyme (Muramidase), 85549
Immunocytochemistry, 88342-88344 *[88341]*
Immunodeficiency Virus, Human
    See HIV
Immunodeficiency Virus Type 1, Human, 87390
Immunodeficiency Virus Type 2, Human, 87391
Immunodiffusion, 86329, 86331
Immunoelectrophoresis, 86320-86327, 86334-86335
Immunofixation Electrophoresis, 86334-86335
Immunofluorescence, 88346, *[88350]*
Immunogen
    See Antigen
Immunoglobulin, 82787
    E, 86003-86005
    Heavy Chain Locus
        Gene Rearrangement Analysis, 81261-81262
        Variable Region Somatic Mutation Analysis, 81263
    Kappa Light Chain Locus Gene Rearrangement Analysis, 81264
    Platelet Associated, 86023
    Receptor Assay, 86243
    Thyroid Stimulating, 84445
Immunohistochemistry, 88342-88344 *[88341]*
Immunologic Skin Test
    See Skin, Tests

Immunology
    Unlisted Services and Procedures, 86849
Immunotherapies, Allergen
    See Allergen Immunotherapy
IMOVAX RABIES, 90675
Impedance Testing, 92567
    See Audiologic Function Tests
Imperfectly Descended Testis, 54550-54560
Implant
    Abdominal Wall
        Fascial Reinforcement, 0437T
    Artificial Heart, Intracorporeal, 0051T
    Biologic Implant Reinforcement
        for External Speech Processor/Cochlear Stimulator, 69714-69718
        Soft Tissue, 15777
    Brain
        Chemotherapy, 61517
        Thermal Perfusion Probe, 61107, 61210
    Breast
        Insertion, 19340-19342
        Preparation of Moulage, 19396
        Removal, 19328-19330
    Cardiac Event Recorder, 33282
    Carotid Sinus Baroreflex Activation Device, 0266T-0268T
    Cerebral Thermal Perfusion Probe, 61107, 61210
    Corneal Ring Segment
        Intrastomal, 65785
    Defibrillator System, 33240, *[33270, 33271]*
    Drug Delivery Device, 11981, 11983, 61517
    Electrode
        Brain, 61850-61870
        Gastric Implantation
            Laparoscopic
                Electrode, 43659
                Neurostimulator, 43647
            Open
                Electrode, 43999
                Neurostimulator, 43881
        Nerve, 64553-64581
        Spinal Cord, 63650, 63655
    External Speech Processor/Cochlear Stimulator, 69714-69718
    Eye
        Anterior Segment, 65920
        Aqueous Drainage Device, without Reservoir, 66183
        Aqueous Shunt
            into Subconjunctival Space, 0449T-0450T
            Revision, 66184-66185
            to Extraocular Reservoir, 66179-66180
        Corneal Ring Segments, 65785
        Placement or Replacement of Pegs, 65125
        Posterior Segment
            Extraocular, 67120
            Intraocular, 67121
        Replacement of Pegs, 65125
        Reservoir, 66180
        Vitreous
            Drug Delivery System, 67027
    Fallopian Tube, 58565
    Fascial Reinforcement
        Abdominal Wall, 0437T
    Glaucoma Drainage, 66180
    Hearing Aid
        Bone Conduction, 69710
    Hip Prosthesis
        See Arthroplasty, Hip
    Hormone Pellet, 11980
    Intraocular Lens
        See Insertion, Intraocular Lens
    Intraocular Retinal Electrode Array, 0100T
    Intrastomal Corneal Ring Segments, 65785
    Joint
        See Arthroplasty
    Mesh
        Closure of Necrotizing Soft Tissue Infection, 49568
        Hernia Repair, 49568, 49652-49657
        Vaginal Repair, 57267
    Nerve
        into Bone, 64787
        into Muscle, 64787

Implant — *continued*
  Neurostimulator
    Cranial, 61885-61886, 64568
    Gastric, 43647, 43881, 64590
    Spine, 64999
  Orbital, 67550
  Ovum, 58976
  Penile Prosthesis, 54400-54405
  Pulsatile Heart Assist System, 33999
  Pulse Generator
    Brain, 61885, 61886
    Spinal Cord, 63685
  Receiver
    Brain, 61885, 61886
    Nerve, 64590
    Spinal Cord, 63685
  Reinforcement Soft Tissue, 15777
  Removal, 20670, 20680
    Anesthesia, External Fixation, 20694
    Elbow, 24164
    Radius, 24164
    Wire, Pin, Rod, 20670
    Wire, Pin, Rod/Deep, 20680
  Reservoir Vascular Access Device
    Declotting, 36593
  Retinal Electrode Array, 0100T
  Subtalar Joint, Extra-osseous, 0335T
  Total Replacement Heart System, Intracorporeal, 0051T
  Tubouterine, 58752
  Ventricular Assist Device, 33976
    Intracorporeal, 0451T-0454T, 33979
Impression, Maxillofacial, 21076-21089
  Auricular Prosthesis, 21086
  Definitive Obturator Prosthesis, 21080
  Facial Prosthesis, 21088
  Interim Obturator, 21079
  Mandibular Resection Prosthesis, 21081
  Nasal Prosthesis, 21087
  Oral Surgical Splint, 21085
  Orbital Prosthesis, 21077
  Palatal Augmentation Prosthesis, 21082
  Palatal Lift Prosthesis, 21083
  Speech Aid Prosthesis, 21084
  Surgical Obturator, 21076
IMRT (Intensity Modulated Radiation Therapy)
  Plan, 77301
  Treatment
    Complex, [77386]
    Plan, 77301
    Simple, [77385]
IMT Testing, 0126T
Incision
  See Incision and Drainage
  Abdomen, 49000
    Exploration, 58960
  Abscess
    Soft Tissue, 20005
  Accessory Nerve, 63191
  Anal
    Fistula, 46270, 46280
    Septum, 46070
    Sphincter, 46080
  Ankle, 27607
    Tendon, 27605, 27606
  Anus
    See Anus, Incision
  Aortic Valve, 33390-33391
    for Stenosis, 33415
  Artery
    Nose, 30915, 30920
  Atrial Septum, 33735-33737
  Bile Duct
    Sphincter, 43262, 47460
  Bladder
    with Destruction, 51020, 51030
    with Radiotracer, 51020
    Catheterization, 51045
  Bladder Diverticulum, 52305
  Brachial Artery
    Exposure, 34834
  Brain
    Amygdalohippocampectomy, 61566
    Subpial, 61567
  Breast
    Capsules, 19370

Incision — *continued*
  Bronchus, 31899
  Burn Scab, 16035, 16036
  Cataract
    Secondary
      Laser Surgery, 66821
      Stab Incision Technique, 66820
  Colon
    Exploration, 44025
    Stoma
      Creation, 44320, 44322
      Revision, 44340-44346
  Cornea
    for Astigmatism, 65772
    for Keratoplasty, 0290T
  Corpus Callosum, 61541
  Cricothyroid Membrane, 31605
  Dentate Ligament, 63180, 63182
  Duodenum, 44010
  Ear, Inner
    Labyrinthectomy, 61596, 69801, 69905
      with Mastoidectomy, 69910
  Elbow, 24000
  Esophagus, 43020, 43045
    Esophageal Web, 43499
    Muscle, 43030
  Exploration
    Heart, 33310-33315
    Kidney, 50010
  Eye
    Adhesions, 65880
      Anterior Segment, 65860, 65865
      Anterior Synechiae, 65870
      Corneovitreal, 65880
      Posterior, 65875
    Anterior Chamber, 65820
    Trabecular, 65850
  Eyelid
    Canthus, 67715
    Sutures, 67710
  Femoral Artery
    Exposure, 34812, 34813
  Fibula, 27607
  Finger
    Decompression, 26035
    Tendon, 26060, 26455, 26460
    Tendon Sheath, 26055, 26060, 26455, 26460
  Foot
    Bone Cortex, 28005
    Capsule, 28260-28264
    Fascia, 28008
    for Infection, 28002, 28003
    Tendon, 28230, 28234
  for Implantation of Neurostimulator, 64568
  Gallbladder, 47490
  Hand Decompression, 26035, 26037
    Tendon, 26450, 26460
  Heart
    Exploration, 33310, 33315
    Incision, Not Specified, 33999
  Hemorrhoid
    External, 46083
  Hepatic Ducts
    See Hepaticostomy
  Hip
    Denervation, 27035
    Exploration, 27033
    Fasciotomy, 27025
    Joint Capsule for Flexor Release, 27036
    Tendon
      Abductor, 27006
      Adductor, 27000-27003
      Iliopsoas, 27005
  Hymen
    See Hymen, Incision
  Hymenotomy, 56442
  Hyoid, Muscle, 21685
  Iliac Artery
    Exposure, 34820, 34833
  Intercarpal Joint
    Dislocation, 25670
  Interphalangeal Joint
    Capsule, 26525
  Intestines (Except Rectum)
    See Enterotomy

Incision — *continued*
  Intestines, Small, 44010
    Biopsy, 44020
    Creation
      Pouch, 44316
      Stoma, 44300-44314
    Decompression, 44021
    Exploration, 44020
    Incision, 44020
    Removal
      Foreign Body, 44020
    Revision
      Stoma, 44312
  Intracranial Vessels, 37799
  Iris, 66500, 66505
  Kidney, 50010, 50045
    Calculus Removal, 50130
      Complicated, 50135
    Exploration, 50010
    Nephrotomy, with Exploration, 50045
    Pyelotomy, with Exploration, 50120
  Knee
    Capsule, 27435
    Exploration, 27310
    Fasciotomy, 27305
    Removal of Foreign Body, 27310
  Lacrimal Punctum, 68440
  Lacrimal Sac
    See Dacryocystotomy
  Larynx, 31300, 31320
  Leg, Lower
    Fasciotomy, 27600-27602
  Leg, Upper
    Fasciotomy, 27025, 27305
    Tenotomy, 27306, 27307, 27390-27392
  Lip
    Frenum, 40806
  Liver
    See Hepatotomy
  Lymphatic Channels, 38308
  Mastoid
    See Mastoidotomy
  Mesencephalic Tract, 61480
  Metacarpophalangeal Joint
    Capsule, 26520
  Mitral Valve, 33420, 33422
  Muscle
    See Myotomy
  Nerve, 64568, 64575-64580, 64585, 64595, 64702-64772
    Foot, 28035
    Root, 63185, 63190
    Sacral, 64581
    Vagus, 43640, 43641
  Nose
    See Rhinotomy
  Orbit
    See Orbitotomy
  Palm
    Fasciotomy, 26040, 26045
  Pancreas
    Sphincter, 43262
  Penis
    Prepuce, 54000, 54001
      Newborn, 54000
  Pericardium, 33030, 33031
    with Clot Removal, 33020
    with Foreign Body Removal, 33020
    with Tube Insertion, 33015
  Pharynx
    Stoma, 42955
  Pleural Cavity
    Empyema, 32035, 32036
    Pneumothorax, 32551
  Prostate
    Exposure
      Bilateral Pelvic Lymphadenectomy, 55865
      Insertion Radioactive Substance, 55860
      Lymph Node Biopsy, 55862
      Transurethral, 52450
  Pterygomaxillary Fossa, 31040
  Pulmonary Valve, 33470-33474
  Pyloric Sphincter, 43520
  Retina
    Encircling Material, 67115

Incision — *continued*
  Sclera
    Fistulization
      with Iridectomy, 66160
      Sclerectomy with Punch or Scissors with Iridectomy, 66160
      Thermocauterization with Iridectomy, 66155
      Trabeculectomy ab Externo in Absence Previous Surgery, 66170
    Trephination with Iridectomy, 66150
  Semicircular Canal Revision, 69840
    Fenestration, 69820
  Seminal Vesicle, 55600-55605
    Complicated, 55605
  Shoulder
    Bone, 23035
    Capsule Contracture Release, 23020
    Removal
      Calcareous Deposits, 23000
      Tenomyotomy, 23405-23406
  Shoulder Joint, 23040, 23044
  Sinus
    Frontal, 31070-31087
    Maxillary, 31020-31032
      Endoscopic, 31256, 31267
    Multiple, 31090
    Sphenoid
      Sinusotomy, 31050, 31051
  Skin, 10040-10180
  Skull, 61316, 62148
    Suture, 61550, 61552
  Spinal Cord, 63200
    Tract, 63170, 63194-63199
  Stomach
    Creation
      Stoma, 43830-43832
    Exploration, 43500
    Pyloric Sphincter, 43520
  Synovectomy, 26140
  Temporomandibular Joint, 21010-21070
  Tendon
    Arm, Upper, 24310
  Thigh
    Fasciotomy, 27025
  Thorax
    Empyema, 32035, 32036
    Pneumothorax, 32551
  Thyroid Gland
    See Thyrotomy
  Tibia, 27607
  Toe
    Capsule, 28270, 28272
    Fasciotomy, 28008
    Tendon, 28232, 28234
    Tenotomy, 28010, 28011
  Tongue
    Frenum, 41010
  Trachea
    with Flaps, 31610
    Emergency, 31603, 31605
    Planned, 31600
      Younger Than Two Years, 31601
  Tympanic Membrane, 69420
    with Anesthesia, 69421
  Ureter, 50600
  Ureterocele, 51535
  Urethra, 53000, 53010
    Meatus, 53020, 53025
  Uterus
    Remove Lesion, 59100
  Vagina
    Exploration, 57000
  Vas Deferens, 55200
    for X-ray, 55300
  Vestibule of Mouth
    See Mouth, Vestibule of, Incision
  Vitreous Strands
    Laser Surgery, 67031
    Pars Plana Approach, 67030
  Wrist, 25100-25105
    Capsule, 25085
    Decompression, 25020-25025
    Tendon Sheath, 25000, 25001
Incisional Hernia Repair
  See Hernia, Repair, Incisional

Incision and Drainage
See Drainage; Incision
Abdomen
  Fluid, 49082–49083
  Pancreatitis, 48000
Abscess
  Abdomen, Abdominal
    Open, 49040
    Pancreatitis, 48000
    Peritoneal, 49020
    Peritonitis, Localized, 49020
    Retroperitoneal, 49060
    Skin and Subcutaneous Tissue
      Complicated, 10061
        Multiple, 10061
        Simple, 10060
        Single, 10060
    Subdiaphragmatic, 49040
    Subphrenic, 49040
  Acne Surgery
    Comedomes, 10040
    Cysts, 10040
    Marsupialization, 10040
    Milia, Multiple, 10040
    Pustules, 10040
  Anal, 46045, 46050
  Ankle, 27603
  Appendix
    Open, 44900
  Arm, Lower, 25028, 25035
  Arm, Upper, 23930, 23931
  Auditory Canal, External, 69020
  Bartholin's Gland, 56420
  Bladder, 51080
  Brain, 61320, 61321
  Breast, 19020
  Ear, External
    Complicated, 69005
    Simple, 69000
  Elbow, 23930
  Epididymis, 54700
  Eyelid, 67700
  Finger, 26010, 26011
  Gums, 41800
  Hip, 26990
  Kidney
    Open, 50020
  Knee, 27301
  Leg, Lower, 27603
  Leg, Upper, 27301
  Liver
    Open, 47010
  Lung, 32200
  Lymph Node, 38300, 38305
  Mouth, 40800, 40801, 41005–41009, 41015–41018
  Nasal Septum, 30020
  Neck, 21501, 21502
  Nose, 30000, 30020
  Ovary, 58820, 58822
    Abdominal Approach, 58822
    Vaginal Approach, 58820
  Palate, 42000
  Paraurethral Gland, 53060
  Parotid Gland, 42300, 42305
  Pelvis, 26990, 45000
  Perineum, 56405
  Peritoneum
    Open, 49020
  Prostate, 55720, 55725
  Rectum, 45005, 45020, 46040, 46050, 46060
  Retroperitoneal
    Open, 49060
  Salivary Gland, 42300–42320
  Scrotum, 54700, 55100
  Shoulder, 23030
  Skene's Gland, 53060
  Skin, 10060, 10061
  Spine, 22010–22015
  Subdiaphragmatic
    Open, 49040
  Sublingual Gland, 42310, 42320
  Submaxillary Gland, 42310, 42320
  Subphrenic
    Open, 49040

Incision and Drainage — *continued*
Abscess — *continued*
  Testis, 54700
  Thorax, 21501, 21502
  Throat, 42700–42725
  Tongue, 41000–41006, 41015
  Tonsil, 42700
  Urethra, 53040
  Uvula, 42000
  Vagina, 57010, 57020
  Vulva, 56405
  Wrist, 25028, 25040
Ankle, 27610
Bile Duct, 47420, 47425
Bladder, 51040
Bulla
  Skin
    Puncture Aspiration, 10160
Bursa
  Ankle, 27604
  Arm, Lower, 25031
  Elbow, 23931
  Foot, 28001
  Hip, 26991
  Knee, 27301
  Leg, Lower, 27604
  Leg, Upper, 27301
  Palm, 26025, 26030
  Pelvis, 26991
  Wrist, 25031
Carbuncle
  Skin, 10060, 10061
Carpals, 25035, 26034
Comedones
  Skin, 10040
Cyst
  Conjunctiva, 68020
  Gums, 41800
  Liver
    Open, 47010
  Lung, 32200
  Mouth, 40800, 40801, 41005–41009, 41015–41018
  Ovarian, 58800, 58805
  Skin, 10040–10061
    Pilonidal, 10080, 10081
    Puncture Aspiration, 10160
  Spinal Cord, 63172, 63173
  Thyroid Gland, 60000
  Tongue, 41000–41006, 41015, 60000
Elbow
  Abscess, 23935
  Arthrotomy, 24000
Femur, 27303
Fluid Collection
  Skin, 10140
Foreign Body
  Skin, 10120, 10121
Furuncle, 10060, 10061
Gallbladder, 47480
Hematoma
  Ankle, 27603
  Arm, Lower, 25028
  Arm, Upper, 23930
  Brain, 61312–61315
  Ear, External
    Complicated, 69005
    Simple, 69000
  Elbow, 23930
  Epididymis, 54700
  Gums, 41800
  Hip, 26990
  Knee, 27301
  Leg, Lower, 27603
  Leg, Upper, 27301
  Mouth, 40800, 40801, 41005–41009, 41015–41018
  Nasal Septum, 30020
  Neck, 21501, 21502
  Nose, 30000, 30020
  Pelvis, 26990
  Scrotum, 54700
  Shoulder, 23030
  Skin, 10140
    Puncture Aspiration, 10160
  Skull, 61312–61315

Incision and Drainage — *continued*
Hematoma — *continued*
  Testis, 54700
  Thorax, 21501, 21502
  Tongue, 41000–41006, 41015
  Vagina, 57022, 57023
  Wrist, 25028
Hepatic Duct, 47400
Hip
  Bone, 26992, 27030
Humerus
  Abscess, 23935
Interphalangeal Joint
  Toe, 28024
Intertarsal Joint, 28020
Kidney, 50040, 50125
Knee, 27303, 27310
Lacrimal Gland, 68400
Lacrimal Sac, 68420
Liver
  Abscess or Cyst, 47010
Mediastinum, 39000, 39010
Metatarsophalangeal Joint, 28022
Milia, Multiple, 10040
Onychia, 10060, 10061
Orbit, 67405, 67440
Paronychia, 10060, 10061
Pelvic/Bone, 26992
Penis, 54015
Pericardium, 33025
Phalanges
  Finger, 26034
Pilonidal Cyst, 10080, 10081
Pustules
  Skin, 10040
Radius, 25035
Seroma
  Skin, 10140
Shoulder
  Abscess, 23030
  Arthrotomy
    Acromioclavicular Joint, 23044
    Glenohumeral Joint, 23040
    Sternoclavicular Joint, 23044
  Bursa, 23031
  Hematoma, 23030
Shoulder Joint
  Arthrotomy, Glenohumeral Joint, 23040
Tarsometatarsal Joint, 28020
Tendon Sheath
  Finger, 26020
  Palm, 26020
Thorax
  Deep, 21510
Toe, 28024
Ulna, 25035
Ureter, 50600
Vagina, 57020
Wound Infection
  Skin, 10180
Wrist, 25028, 25040
Inclusion Bodies
Fluid, 88106
Smear, 87207, 87210
Incomplete
Abortion, 59812
Indicator Dilution Studies, 93561, 93562
Induced
Abortion
  with Hysterotomy, 59100, 59852, 59857
  by Dilation and Curettage, 59840
  by Dilation and Evacuation, 59841
  by Saline, 59850, 59851
  by Vaginal Suppositories, 59855, 59856
Hyperthermia, 53850–53852
Induratio Penis Plastica
with Graft, 54110–54112
Injection, 54200
Surgical Exposure, 54205
INF2, 81406
Infantile Paralysis
See Polio
Infant, Newborn, Intensive Care
See Intensive Care, Neonatal
INFARIX, 90700

Infection
Actinomyces, 86602
Diagnosis
  Group A Strep Test, 3210F
Drainage
  Postoperative Wound, 10180
Filarioidea, 86280
Immunoassay, 86317, 86318
Rapid Test, 86403, 86406
Treatment
  Antibiotics Prescribed, 4045F
Infection, Bone
See Osteomyelitis
Infection, Wound
See Wound, Infection
Infectious Agent Detection
Antigen Detection
  Direct Fluorescence
    Bordetella, 87265
    Chlamydia Trachomatis, 87270
    Cryptosporidium, 87272
    Cytomegalovirus, 87271
    Enterovirus, 87267
    Giardia, 87269
    Influenza A, 87276
    Legionella Pneumophila, 87278
    Pertussis, 87265
    Respiratory Syncytial Virus, 87280
    Treponema Pallidum, 87285
    Varicella Zoster, 87290
  Direct Probe
    Vancomycin Resistance, 87500
  Enzyme Immunoassay
    Adenovirus, 87301
    Aspergillus, 87305
    Chlamydia Trachomatis, 87320
    Clostridium Difficile Toxin A, 87324
    Cryptococcus Neoformans, 87327
    Cryptosporidium, 87328
    Cytomegalovirus, 87332
    Entamoeba Histolytica Dispar Group, 87336
    Entamoeba Histolytica Group, 87337
    Escherichia coli 0157, 87335
    Giardia, 87329
    Helicobacter Pylori, 87338, 87339
    Hepatitis Be Antigen (HBeAg), 87350
    Hepatitis B Surface Antigen (HBsAg), 87340
    Hepatitis B Surface Antigen (HBsAg) Neutralization, 87341
    Hepatitis, Delta Agent, 87380
    Histoplasma Capsulatum, 87385
    HIV–1, 87390
    HIV–2, 87391
    Influenza A, 87400
    Influenza B, 87400
    Multiple Step Method, 87301–87449, 87451
      See specific agent
    Not Otherwise Specified, 87449–87451
    Respiratory Syncytial Virus, 87420
    Rotavirus, 87425
    Shiga–like Toxin, 87427
    Single Step Method, 87450
    Streptococcus, Group A, 87430
  Immunoassay
    Adenovirus, 87809
  Immunofluorescence, 87260, 87273–87275, 87277, 87279, 87281–87283, 87299–87300
    Adenovirus, 87260
    Herpes Simplex, 87273, 87274
    Influenza B, 87275
    Legionella Micdadei, 87277
    Not otherwise Specified, 87299
    Parainfluenza Virus, 87279
    Pneumocystis Carinii, 87281
    Polyvalent, 87300
    Rubeola, 87283
  Nucleic Acid
    Vancomycin Resistance, 87500
Concentration, 87015

Infectious Agent Detection — *continued*
  Detection
    by Immunoassay
      with Direct Optical Observation, 87802-87899
      Chlamydia Trachomatis, 87810
      Clostridium difficile, 87803
      HIV Antigen(s) with HIV-1 and HIV-2 Antibodies, [87806]
      Influenza, 87804
      Neisseria Gonorrhoeae, 87850
      Not Otherwise Specified, 87899
      Respiratory Syncytial Virus, 87807
      Streptococcus, Group A, 87880
      Streptococcus, Group B, 87802
      Trichomonas Vaginalis, 87808
    by Nucleic Acid
      Bartonella Henselae, 87470-87472
      Bartonella Quintana, 87470-87472
      Borrelia Burgdorferi, 87475-87477
      Candida Species, 87480-87482
      Central Nervous System Pathogen, 87483
      Chlamydia Pneumoniae, 87485-87487
      Chlamydia Trachomatis, 87490-87492
      Cytomegalovirus, 87495-87497
      Gardnerella Vaginalis, 87510-87512
      Hepatitis B Virus, 87515-87517
      Hepatitis C, 87520-87522
      Hepatitis G, 87525-87527
      Herpes Simplex Virus, 87528-87530
      Herpes Virus-6, 87531-87533
      HIV-1, 87534-87536
      HIV-2, 87537-87539
      Influenza, 87501-87503
      Intracellulare, 87560-87562
      Legionella Pneumophila, 87540-87542
      Multiple Organisms, 87800, 87801
      Mycobacteria Avium-Intracellularae, 87560-87562
      Mycobacteria Species, 87550-87552
      Mycobacteria Tuberculosis, 87555-87557
      Mycoplasma Pneumoniae, 87580-87582
      Neisseria Gonorrhoeae, 87590-87592
      Not Otherwise Specified, 87797-87799
      Papillomavirus, Human, [87623, 87624, 87625]
      Staphylococcus
        Aureus, 87640-87641
      Streptococcus
        Group A, 87650-87652
        Group B, 87653
      Trichomonas Vaginalis, 87660
  Enzymatic Activity, 87905
  Genotype Analysis
    by Nucleic Acid
      Hepatitis C Virus, 87902
      HIV-1 Protease/Reverse Transcriptase, 87901
  Phenotype Analysis
    by Nucleic Acid
      HIV-1 Drug Resistance, 87903, 87904
      HIV-1 Drug Resistance, 87900
  Phenotype Prediction
    by Genetic Database, 87900
  Vancomycin Resistance, 87500
Infectious Mononucleosis Virus
  See Epstein–Barr Virus
Inflammatory Process
  Localization
    Nuclear Medicine, 78805-78807
Inflation
  Eustachian Tube
    Myringotomy, 69420
      Anesthesia, 69424
Influenza A
  Antigen Detection
    Direct Fluorescent, 87276
    Enzyme Immunoassay, 87400
Influenza B
  Antigen Detection
    Enzyme Immunoassay, 87400
    Immunofluorescence, 87275
Influenza B Vaccine, 90647-90648, 90748

Influenza Vaccine, 90647-90648, 90653-90654, 90655-90660, 90661, 90662-90668, 90685-90688, 90697-90698, 90748, [90630], [90644], [90672], [90673], [90674]
Influenza Virus
  Antibody, 86710
  Vaccine, 90657-90660
  by Immunoassay
    with Direct Optical Observation, 87804
Infraorbital Nerve
  Avulsion, 64734
  Incision, 64734
  Transection, 64734
Infrared Light Treatment, 97026
  See Physical Medicine/Therapy/ Occupational Therapy
Infratentorial Craniotomy, 61520, 61521
Infusion
  Amnion, Transabdominal, 59072
  Cerebral
    Intravenous for Thrombolysis, 37195
  Chemotherapy, 96413-96417, 96423, 96425
  Continuous, by Catheter Paravertebral/Paraspinous Block
    Thoracic, [64463]
  Hydration, 96360-96361
  Intra-Arterial
    Chemotherapy or Complex Biological Agent, 96422-96425
    Diagnostic, Prophylactic, Diagnostic, 96373
    Unlisted, Intra-arterial, 96379
  Intracranial Administration
    Pharmacological Agent Other Than Thrombolysis, 61650-61651
  Intracranial for Thrombolysis, 61645
  Intraosseous, 36680
  IV
    Chemotherapy, Complex Biological Agent, 96413-96417
    Diagnostic, Prophylactic, Therapeutic, 96365-96368
    Hydration, 96360-96361
    Unlisted Intravenous Infusion, 96379
  Pump
    Electronic Analysis, 62367-62370, 95990-95991
    Insertion
      Intraarterial, 36260
    Intraarterial
      Removal, 36262
      Revision, 36261
    Intravenous
      Insertion, 36563
      Removal, 36590
      Revision, 36576, 36578
    Maintenance, 95990-95991, 96521-96522
      Chemotherapy, Pump Services, 96521-96522
    Refill, 62369-62370, 95990-95991
    Spinal Cord, 62361-62362, 62367-62370, 95990-95991
    Ventricular Catheter, 61215
  Radioelement, 77750
  Subcutaneous, 96369-96371
  Therapy, 62350, 62351, 62360-62362
    See Injection, Chemotherapy
    Arterial Catheterization, 36640
    Chemotherapy, 96401-96542, 96549
    Home Infusion Procedures, 99601-99602
    Intravenous, 96360-96361, 96365-96368
    Pain, 62360-62362, 62367-62368
  Transcatheter Therapy, 75894-75898, [37211, 37212, 37213, 37214]
Inguinal Hernia Repair
  See Hernia, Repair, Inguinal
INH
  See Drug Assay
Inhalation
  Pentamidine, 94642
Inhalation Provocation Tests
  See Bronchial Challenge Test
Inhalation Treatment, 94640-94645, 94664, 99503
  See Pulmonary, Therapeutic
Inhibin A, 86336
Inhibition, Fertilization
  See Contraception

Inhibition Test, Hemagglutination, 86280
Inhibitor
  Alpha 1-Protease, 82103-82104
  Alpha 2-Plasmin, 85410
  of Kappa Light Polypeptide Gene Enhancer in B-Cells, Kinase Complex-Associated Protein Gene Analysis, 81260
Inhibitory Concentration, Minimum
  See Minimum Inhibitory Concentration
Initial Inpatient Consultations
  See Consultation, Initial Inpatient
Injection
  Abdomen
    Air, 49400
    Contrast Material, 49400
  Allergen, 95115-95134
  Anesthetic
    Morton's Neuroma, 64455
    Paravertebral Facet, 64490-64495
    Paravertebral/Paraspinal Block, [64461, 64462, 64463]
    Plantar Common Digit, 64455
    Sympathetic Nerves, 64505-64530
    Transforaminal, 64479-64484
  Angiography
    Heart Vessels, 93454-93464, 93563-93568
    Pulmonary, 75746
  Ankle, 27648
  Antigen (Allergen), 95115-95125, 95145-95170
  Aponeurosis, 20550
  Application, on-body injector, 96377
  Bladder
    Radiologic, 51600-51610
  Bone Marrow, into, 38999
  Brain Canal, 61070
  Breast
    Radiologic, 19030
  Brisement, 20550-20551
  Bursa, 20600-20611
  Cardiac Catheterization, 93452-93461, 93563-93568
  Carpal Tunnel
    Therapeutic, 20526
  Chemotherapy, 96401-96549
  Cistern
    Medication or Other, 61055
  Contrast
    Central Venous Access Device, 36598
    Gastrostomy, Duodenostomy, Jejunostomy, Gastro-jejunostomy, or Cecostomy Tube, Percutaneous, 49465
    via Peritoneal Catheter, 49424
  Corpora Cavernosa, 54235
  Cyst
    Bone, 20615
    Kidney, 50390
    Pelvis, 50390
    Thyroid, 60300
  Dupuytren's Contracture, 20527
  Elbow
    Arthrography, Radiologic, 24220
  Enzyme
    Palmar Fascial Cord, 20527
  Epidural, 0228T-0231T, 62281-62282, 62320-62327, 64479-64484
  Esophageal Varices
    Endoscopy, 43243
  Esophagus
    Sclerosing Agent, 43204
    Submucosal, 43201
  Extremity
    Pseudoaneurysm, 36002
  Eye
    Air, 66020
    Medication, 66030
    Suprachoroidal, 0465T
  Eyelid
    Subconjunctival, 68200
  Ganglion
    Anesthetic, 64505, 64510
  Ganglion Cyst, 20612
  Gastric Secretion Stimulant, 43755
  Gastric Varices
    Endoscopy, 43243

Injection — *continued*
  Heart
    Therapeutic Substance into Pericardium, 33999
  Heart Vessels
    Cardiac Catheterization
      See Catheterization, Cardiac
  Hemorrhoids
    Sclerosing Solution, 46500
  Hip
    Radiologic, 27093, 27095
  Hydration, 96360-96361
  Insect Venom, 95130-95134
  Intervertebral Disc
    Chemonucleolysis Agent, 62292
    Radiological, 62290, 62291
  Intra–amniotic, 59850-59852
  Intra-arterial, 96373
    Chemotherapy, 96420-96425
  Intradermal, Tattooing, 11920-11922
  Intralesional, Skin, 11900, 11901
    Chemotherapy, 96405-96406
  Intramuscular, 96372, 99506
    Chemotherapy, 96401-96402
  Intravenous, 96365-96368
    Chemotherapy, 96409-96417
    Diagnostic, 96365-96368
    Thrombolytic, 37187-37188
    Vascular Flow Check, Graft, 15860
  Intravitreal
    Pharmacologic Agent, 67028
  Joint, 20600-20611
  Kidney
    Drugs, 50391
    Radiologic, [50430, 50431]
  Knee
    Radiologic, 27370
  Lacrimal Gland
    Radiologic, 68850
  Left Heart
    Radiologic, 93563-93566
  Lesion, Skin, 11900, 11901
    Chemotherapy, 96405-96411
  Ligament, 20550
  Liver, 47015
    Radiologic, 47531-47532
  Lymphangiography, 38790
  Mammary Ductogram
    Galactogram, 19030
  Muscle Endplate
    Cervical Spinal, 64616
    Extremity, 64642-64645
    Facial, 64612
    Trunk, 64646-64647
  Nephrostogram, Antegrade, [50430, 50431]
  Nerve
    Anesthetic, 01991-01992, 64400-64530
    Neurolytic Agent, 64600-64681 [64633, 64634, 64635, 64636]
  On-body Injector Application, 96377
  Orbit
    Retrobulbar
      Alcohol, 67505
      Medication, 67500
    Tenon's Capsule, 67515
  Palmar Fascial Cord, 20527
  Pancreatography, 48400
  Paravertebral
    Block, Thoracic, [64461, 64462, 64463]
    Facet Joint, 0213T-0218T, 64490-64495
  Penis
    for Erection, 54235
    Peyronie Disease, 54200
      with Surgical Exposure of Plaque, 54205
    Radiology, 54230
    Vasoactive Drugs, 54231
  Pericardium
    Injection of Therapeutic Substance, 33999
  Peritoneal Cavity Air
    See Pneumoperitoneum
  Platelet Rich Plasma, 0232T
  Radiologic
    Breast, 19030
    Radiopharmaceutical, 78808

[Resequenced]

Injection — continued
  Rectum
    Sclerosing Solution, 45520
  Right Heart
    Injection of Radiologic Substance, 93566
  Sacroiliac Joint
    for Arthrography, 27096
  Salivary Duct, 42660
  Salivary Gland
    Radiologic, 42550
  Sclerosing Agent
    Esophagus, 43204
    Intravenous, 36470, 36471
  Sentinel Node Identification Radioactive Tracer, 38792
  Shoulder
    Arthrography, Radiologic, 23350
  Shunt
    Peritoneal
      Venous, 49427
  Sinus Tract, 20500
    Diagnostic, 20501
  Spider Veins
    Telangiectasia, 36468
  Spinal Artery, 62294
  Spinal Cord
    Anesthetic, 62320-62327
    Blood, 62273
    Neurolytic Agent, 62280-62282
    Other, 62320-62327
    Radiologic, 62284
  Spleen
    Radiologic, 38200
  Steroids, 52283
    Morton's Neuroma, 64455
    Paravertebral
      Block (Paraspinous), Thoracic, [64461, 64462, 64463]
      Facet Joint, 0213T-0218T, 64490-64495
    Plantar Common Digital Nerve, 64455
    Stricture, 52283
    Sympathetic Nerves, 64505-64530
    Transforaminal, 64479-64484
  Subcutaneous, 96369-96371
    Chemotherapy, 96401-96402
  Suprachoroidal, 0465T
  Temporomandibular Joint
    Arthrography, 21116
  Tendon Origin, Insertion, 20551
  Tendon Sheath, 20550
  Therapeutic
    Extremity Pseudoaneurysm, 36002
    Lung, 32960
    Thyroid, 60300
    Turbinate, 30200
  Thoracic Cavity
    See Pleurodesis, Chemical
  Thrombolytic, 37184-37186
  Trachea
    Puncture, 31612
  Trigger Point(s)
    One or Two Muscle Groups, 20552
    Three or More Muscle Groups, 20553
  Turbinate, 30200
  Unlisted, 96379
  Ureter
    Drugs, 50391
    Radiologic, 50684, [50430, 50431]
  Ureteropyelography, 50690
  Venography, 36005
  Ventricular
    Dye, 61120
    Medication or Other, 61026
  Vitreous, 67028
    Fluid Substitute, 67025
  Vocal Cords
    Therapeutic, 31513, 31570, 31571
  Wrist
    Carpal Tunnel
      Therapeutic, 20526
    Radiologic, 25246
  Zygapophyseal, 0213T-0218T, 64490-64495
Inkblot Test, 96101-96103
Inner Ear
  See Ear, Inner

Innominate
  Tumor
    Excision, 27077
Innominate Arteries
  See Artery, Brachiocephalic
Inorganic Sulfates
  See Sulfate
Inpatient Consultations, 99251-99255
INR Test Review, 99363-99364
INS, 81404
Insemination
  Artificial, 58321, 58322, 89268
Insertion
  See Implantation; Intubation; Transplantation
  Aqueous Drainage Device, 0191T, 0449T-0450T, 66179-66185
  Balloon
    Intra–Aortic, 33967, 33973
  Breast
    Implants, 19340, 19342
  Cannula
    Arteriovenous, 36810, 36815
    Extracorporeal Circulation for Regional Chemotherapy of Extremity, 36823
    Thoracic Duct, 38794
    Vein to Vein, 36800
  Catheter
    Abdomen, 49324, 49419-49421, 49435
    Abdominal Artery, 36245-36248
    Aorta, 36200
    Bile Duct
      Percutaneous, 47533-47536
    Bladder, 51045, 51701-51703
    Brachiocephalic Artery, 36215-36218
    Brain, 61210, 61770, 64999
    Breast
      for Interstitial Radioelement Application, 19296-19298, 20555
    Bronchi, 31717
    Bronchus
      for Intracavitary Radioelement Application, 31643
    Cardiac
      See Catheterization, Cardiac
      Flow Directed, 93503
    Dialysis, 49421
    Flow Directed, 93503
    Gastrointestinal, Upper, 43241
    Head and/or Neck, 41019
    Intraperitoneal, 49418
    Jejunum, 44015
    Lower Extremity Artery, 36245-36248
    Nasotracheal, 31720
    Pelvic Artery, 36245-36248
    Pelvic Organs and/or Genitalia, 55920
    Pleural Cavity, 32550
    Portal Vein, 36481
    Prostate, 55875
    Pulmonary Artery, 36013-36015
    Renal Artery, 36251-36254
    Right Heart, 36013
    Skull, 61107
    Spinal Cord, 62350, 62351
    Suprapubic, 51102
    Thoracic Artery, 36215-36218
    Tracheobronchial, 31725
    Transthoracic, 33621
    Urethra, 51701-51703
    Vena Cava, 36010
    Venous, 36011, 36012, 36400-36425, 36500, 36510, 36555-36558, 36568-36569
  Cecostomy Tube, 49442
  Cervical Dilator, 59200
  Chest Wall Respiratory Sensor Electrode or Electrode Array, 0466T-0468T
  Cochlear Device, 69930
  Colonic Tube, 49442
  Defibrillator
    Heart, 33212, 33213
    Leads, 33216, 33217
    Pulse Generator Only, 33240
  Drug Delivery Implant, 11981, 11983
  Drug-Eluting Implant Lacrimal Canaliculus, 0356T

Insertion — continued
  Electrode
    Brain, 61531, 61533, 61760, 61850-61870
    Heart, 33202-33203, 33210-33217 [33221], 33224-33225, 93620-93622
    Nerve, 64553-64581
    Retina, 0100T
    Sphenoidal, 95830
    Spinal Cord, 63650, 63655
    Stomach
      Laparoscopic
        Gastric neurostimulator, 43647
      Open
        Gastric neurostimulator
          Antrum, 43881
          Lesser curvature, 43999
  Endotracheal Tube
    Emergency Intubation, 31500
  Filiform
    Urethra, 53620
  Gastrostomy Tube
    Laparoscopic, 43653
    Percutaneous, 43246, 49440
  Glucose Sensor, Interstitial, 0446T-0448T
  Graft
    Aorta, 33330-33335
    Heart Vessel, 33330-33335
  Guide
    Kidney, Pelvis, 50395
  Guide Wire
    Endoscopy, 43248
    Esophagoscopy, 43248
    with Dilation, 43226
  Hemodynamic Monitor, 0293T-0294T
  Heyman Capsule
    Uterus
      for Brachytherapy, 58346
  Iliac Artery
    Occlusion Device, 34808
  Implant
    Bone
      for External Speech Processor/Cochlear Stimulator, 69714-69718
  Implantable Defibrillator
    Leads, 33216-33220, 33224-33225
    Pulse Generator Only, 33240 [33230, 33231]
  Infusion Pump
    Intraarterial, 36260
    Intravenous, 36563
    Spinal Cord, 62361, 62362
  Interstitial Glucose Sensor, 0446T-0448T
  Intracardiac Ischemia Monitoring System, 0302T
    Device Only, 0304T
    Electrode Only, 0303T
  Intracatheter/Needle
    Aorta, 36160
    Arteriovenous Dialysis Circuit, 36901-36903
    Intraarterial, 36100-36140
    Intravenous, 36000
    Venous, 36000
  Intraocular Lens, 66983
    Manual or Mechanical Technique, 66982, 66984
    Not Associated with Concurrent Cataract Removal, 66985
  Intrauterine Device (IUD), 58300
  Ischemia Monitoring System, 0302T
  IVC Filter, 37191
  Jejunostomy Tube
    Endoscopy, 44372
    Percutaneous, 49441
  Keel
    Laryngoplasty, 31580
  Laminaria, 59200
  Mesh
    Pelvic Floor, 57267
  Needle
    Bone, 36680
    Head and/or Neck, 41019
    Intraosseous, 36680
    Pelvic Organs and/or Genitalia, 55920
    Prostate, 55875
  Needle Wire Dilator
    Stent
      Trachea, 31730
      Transtracheal for Oxygen, 31720

Insertion — continued
  Neurostimulator
    Pulse Generator, 64590
    Receiver, 64590
  Nose
    Septal Prosthesis, 30220
  Obturator/Larynx, 31527
  Ocular Implant
    with Foreign Material, 65155
    with or without Conjunctival Graft, 65150
    in Scleral Shell, 65130, 67550
    Muscles Attached, 65140
    Muscles Not Attached, 65135
    Telescope Prosthesis, 0308T
  Orbital Transplant, 67550
  Oviduct
    Chromotubation, 58350
    Hydrotubation, 58350
  Ovoid
    Vagina
      for Brachytherapy, 57155
  Pacemaker
    Heart, 33206-33208, 33212, 33213, [33221]
  Packing
    Vagina, 57180
  Penile Prosthesis Inflatable
    See Penile Prosthesis, Insertion, Inflatable
  Pessary
    Vagina, 57160
  PICC Line, 36568-36569
  Pin
    Skeletal Traction, 20650
  Port, 49419
  Posterior Spinous Process Distraction Devices, 22867-22870
  Probe
    Brain, 61770
  Prostaglandin, 59200
  Prostate
    Radioactive Substance, 55860
    Transprostatic Implant, 52441-52442
  Prosthesis
    Knee, 27438, 27445
    Nasal Septal, 30220
    Palate, 42281
    Pelvic Floor, 57267
    Penis
      Inflatable, 54401-54405
      Non–inflatable, 54400
    Speech, 31611
    Testis, 54660
    Urethral Sphincter, 53444-53445
  Pulse Generator
    Brain, 61885, 61886
    Heart, 33212, 33213
    Spinal Cord, 63685
  Radiation Afterloading Apparatus, 57156
  Radioactive Material
    Bladder, 51020
    Cystourethroscopy, 52250
    High Dose Electronic Brachytherapy, 0394T-0395T
    Interstitial Brachytherapy, 77770-77772
    Intracavitary Brachytherapy, 77761-77763, 77770-77772
    Intraocular, 0190T
    Prostate, 55860, 55875
    Remote Afterloading Brachytherapy, 77767-77768, 77770-77772
  Receiver
    Brain, 61885, 61886
    Spinal Cord, 63685
  Reservoir
    Brain, 61210, 61215
    Spinal Cord, 62360
  Shunt, 36835
    Abdomen
      Vein, 49425
      Venous, 49426
    Intrahepatic Portosystemic, 37182
  Spinal Instrument, 22849
    Spinous Process, 22841, 22867-22870
  Spinal Instrumentation
    Anterior, 22845-22847
    Internal Spinal Fixation, 22841, 22853-22854, 22867-22870, [22859]

Insertion — *continued*
  Spinal Instrumentation — *continued*
    Pelvic Fixation, 22848
    Posterior Non–segmental
      Harrington Rod Technique, 22840
    Posterior Segmental, 22842-22844
  Stent
    Bile Duct, 47801, *[43274]*
    Bladder, 51045
    Conjunctiva, 68750
    Esophagus, *[43212]*
    Gastrointestinal, Upper, *[43266]*
    Indwelling, 50605
    Lacrimal Canaliculus, Drug-Eluting, 0356T
    Lacrimal Duct, 68810-68815
    Pancreatic Duct, *[43274]*
    Small Intestines, 44370, 44379
    Ureteral, 50688, 50693-50695, 50947,
      52332
    Urethral, 52282, 53855
  Tamponade
    Esophagus, 43460
  Tandem
    Uterus
      for Brachytherapy, 57155
  Tendon Graft
    Finger, 26392
    Hand, 26392
  Testicular Prosthesis
    See Prosthesis, Testicular, Insertion
  Tissue Expanders, Skin, 11960-11971
  Tube
    Cecostomy, 49442
    Duodenostomy or Jejunostomy, 49441
    Esophagus, 43510
    Gastrointestinal, Upper, 43241
    Gastrostomy, 49440
    Small Intestines, 44379
    Trachea, 31730
    Ureter, 50688, 50693-50695
  Urethral
    Catheter, 51701-51703
    Guide Wire, 52344
    Implant Material, 51715
    Suppository, 53660-53661
  Vascular Pedicle
    Carpal Bone, 25430
  Venous Access Device
    Central, 36560-36566
    Peripheral, 36570, 36571
  Venous Shunt
    Abdomen, 49425
  Ventilating Tube, 69433
  Ventricular Assist Device, 33975
    Intracorporeal, 0451T-0454T
  Wire
    Skeletal Traction, 20650
In Situ Hybridization
  See Nucleic Acid Probe, Cytogenic Studies,
    Morphometric Analysis
Inspiratory Positive Pressure Breathing
  See Intermittent Positive Pressure Breathing
    (IPPB)
Instillation
  Agent for Pleurodesis, 32560-32562
  Drugs
    Bladder, 51720
    Kidney, 50391
    Ureter, 50391
Instillation, Bladder
  See Bladder, Instillation
Instrumentation
  See Application; Bone; Fixation; Spinal Instru-
    mentation
  Spinal
    Insertion, 22840-22848, 22853-22854,
      22867-22870, *[22859]*
    Reinsertion, 22849
    Removal, 22850, 22852, 22855
Insufflation, Eustachian Tube
  See Eustachian Tube, Inflation
Insulin, 80422, 80432-80435
  Antibody, 86337
  Blood, 83525
  Free, 83527

Insulin C–Peptide Measurement
  See C–Peptide
Insulin Like Growth Factors
  See Somatomedin
Insurance
  Basic Life and/or Disability Evaluation Services,
    99450
  Examination, 99450-99456
Integumentary System
  Ablation
    Breast, 19105
  Biopsy, 11100, 11101
  Breast
    Ablation, 19105
    Excision, 19100-19272
    Incision, 19000-19030
    Localization Device, 19281-19288
      with Biopsy, 19081-19086
    Reconstruction, 19316-19396
    Repair, 19316-19396
    Unlisted Services and Procedures, 19499
  Burns, 15002-15003, 15005, 16000-16036
  Debridement, 11000-11006, 11010-11044
    [11045, 11046]
  Destruction
    See Dermatology
    Actinotherapy, 96900
    Benign Lesion, 17000-17004
      by Photodynamic Therapy, 96567
    Chemical Exfoliation, 17360
    Cryotherapy, 17340
    Electrolysis Epilation, 17380
    Malignant Lesion, 17260-17286
      by Photodynamic Therapy, 96567
    Mohs Micrographic Surgery, 17311-17315
    Photodynamic Therapy, 96567, 96570,
      96571
    Premalignant Lesion, 17000-17004
    Unlisted Services and Procedures, 17999
  Drainage, 10040-10180
  Excision
    Benign Lesion, 11400-11471
    Debridement, 11000-11006, 11010-11044
      [11045, 11046]
    Malignant Lesion, 11600-11646
  Graft, 14000-14350, 15002-15278
    Autograft, 15040-15157
    Skin Substitute, 15271-15278
    Surgical Preparation, 15002-15005
    Tissue Transfer or Rearrangement, 14000-
      14350
  Implantation Biologic Implant, 15777
  Incision, 10040-10180
  Introduction
    Drug Delivery Implant, 11981, 11983
  Nails, 11719-11765
  Paring, 11055-11057
  Photography, 96904
  Pressure Ulcers, 15920-15999
  Removal
    Drug Delivery Implant, 11982, 11983
  Repair
    Adjacent Tissue Transfer
      Rearrangement, 14000-14350
    Complex, 13100-13160
    Flaps, 15740-15776
    Free Skin Grafts, 15002-15005, 15050-
      15136, 15200-15261
    Implantation Acellular Dermal Matrix,
      15777
    Intermediate, 12031-12057
    Other Procedures, 15780-15879
    Simple, 12001-12021
    Skin and/or Deep Tissue, 15570-15738
    Skin Substitute, 15271-15278
  Shaving of Epidermal or Dermal Lesion, 11300-
    11313
  Skin Tags
    Removal, 11200, 11201
Integumentum Commune
  See Integumentary System
Intelligence Test
  Computer-Assisted, 96103
  Psychiatric Diagnosis, Psychological Testing,
    96101-96103

Intensity Modulated Radiation Therapy (IMRT)
  Complex, *[77386]*
  Plan, 77301
  Simple, *[77385]*
Intensive Care
  Low Birth Weight Infant, 99478-99479
  Neonatal
    Initial Care, 99479
    Subsequent Care, 99478
Intercarpal Joint
  Arthrodesis, 25820, 25825
  Dislocation
    Closed Treatment, 25660
  Repair, 25447
Intercostal Nerve
  Destruction, 64620
  Injection
    Anesthetic, 64420, 64421
    Neurolytic Agent, 64620
Intercranial Arterial Perfusion
  Thrombolysis, 61624
Interdental Fixation
  without Fracture, 21497
  Device
    Application, 21110
  Mandibular Fracture
    Closed Treatment, 21453
    Open Treatment, 21462
Interdental Papilla
  See Gums
Interdental Wire Fixation
  Closed Treatment
    Craniofacial Separation, 21431
Interferometry
  Eye
    Biometry, 92136
Intermediate Care Facility (ICF) Visits, 99304-
  99318
Intermittent Positive Pressure Breathing (IPPB)
  See Continuous Negative Pressure Breathing
    (CNPB); Continuous Positive Airway
    Pressure (CPAP)
Internal Breast Prostheses
  See Breast, Implants
Internal Ear
  See Ear, Inner
Internal Rigid Fixation
  Reconstruction
    Mandibular Rami, 21196
International Normalized Ratio
  Test Review, 99363-99364
Internet E/M Service
  Nonphysician, 98969
  Physician, 99444
Interphalangeal Joint
  Arthrodesis, 26860-26863
  Arthroplasty, 26535, 26536
  Arthrotomy, 26080, 28054
  Biopsy
    Synovium, 26110
  Capsule
    Excision, 26525
    Incision, 26525
  Dislocation
    with Manipulation, 26340
    Closed Treatment, 26770
    Fingers/Hand
      with Manipulation, 26340
      Closed Treatment, 26770, 26775
      Open Treatment, 26785
      Percutaneous Fixation, 26776
    Open Treatment, 26785
    Percutaneous Fixation, 26776
    Toes/Foot
      Closed Treatment, 28660, 28665
      Open Treatment, 28675
      Percutaneous Fixation, 28666
  Excision, 28160
  Exploration, 26080, 28024
  Fracture
    with Manipulation, 26742
    Closed Treatment, 26740
    Open Treatment, 26746
  Fusion, 26860-26863
  Great Toe
    Arthrodesis, 28755

Interphalangeal Joint — *continued*
  Great Toe — *continued*
    Arthrodesis — *continued*
      with Tendon Transfer, 28760
    Fusion, 28755
      with Tendon Transfer, 28760
    Removal
      Foreign Body, 26080
      Loose Body, 28024
    Repair
      Collateral Ligament, 26545
      Volar Plate, 26548
    Synovectomy, 26140
    Synovial
      Biopsy, 28054
    Toe, 28272
      Arthrotomy, 28024
      Biopsy
        Synovial, 28054
      Dislocation, 28660-28665, 28675
        Percutaneous Fixation, 28666
      Excision, 28160
      Exploration, 28024
      Removal
        Foreign Body, 28024
        Loose Body, 28024
      Synovial
        Biopsy, 28054
Interrogation
  Cardio-Defibrillator, 93289, 93292, 93295
  Cardiovascular Monitoring System, 93290,
    93297, 93299
  Carotid Sinus Baroreflex Activation Device,
    0272T-0273T
  Intracardiac Ischemia Monitoring System, 0306T
  Loop Recorder, 93291, 93298-93299
  Pacemaker, 93288, 93294, 93296
  Ventricular Assist Device, 0463T, 93750
Interruption
  Vein
    Femoral, 37650
    Iliac, 37660
Intersex State
  Clitoroplasty, 56805
  Vaginoplasty, 57335
Intersex Surgery
  Female to Male, 55980
  Male to Female, 55970
Interstitial Cell Stimulating Hormone
  See Luteinizing Hormone (LH)
  Cystitides, Chronic
    See Cystitis, Interstitial
  Cystitis
    See Cystitis, Interstitial
  Fluid Pressure
    Monitoring, 20950
Interstitial Glucose Sensor
  Insertion, 0446T
  Removal, 0447T-0448T
Intertarsal Joint
  Arthrotomy, 28020, 28050
  Biopsy
    Synovial, 28050
  Exploration, 28020
  Removal
    Foreign Body, 28020
    Loose Body, 28020
  Synovial
    Biopsy, 28050
    Excision, 28070
Interthoracoscapular Amputation
  See Amputation, Interthoracoscapular
Intertrochanteric Femur Fracture
  See Femur, Fracture, Intertrochanteric
Intervertebral Chemonucleolysis
  See Chemonucleolysis
Intervertebral Disc
  Annuloplasty, 22526-22527
  Arthroplasty
    Cervical Interspace, 22856
    Each Additional Interspace, 0375T, *[22858]*
    Lumbar Interspace, 0163T, 22857-22865
    Removal, 0095T, 0164T
      Removal, 0095T
    Revision, 0098T, 0165T

Intervertebral Disc — *continued*
  Discography
    Cervical, 72285
    Lumbar, 72295
    Thoracic, 72285
  Excision
    Decompression, 62380, 63075-63078
    Herniated, 62380, 63020-63044, 63055-63066
  Injection
    Chemonucleolysis Agent, 62292
    X–ray, 62290, 62291
  X–ray with Contrast
    Cervical, 72285
    Lumbar, 72295
Intestinal Anastomosis
  See Anastomosis, Intestines
Intestinal Invagination
  See Intussusception
Intestinal Peptide, Vasoconstrictive
  See Vasoactive Intestinal Peptide
Intestine(s)
  Allotransplantation, 44135, 44136
    Removal, 44137
  Anastomosis, 44625, 44626
    Laparoscopic, 44227
  Biopsy, 44100
  Closure
    Enterostomy
      Large or Small, 44625, 44626
    Stoma, 44620, 44625
  Excision
    Donor, 44132, 44133
  Exclusion, 44700
  Laparoscopic Resection with Anastomosis, 44202, 44203, 44207, 44208
  Lesion
    Excision, 44110, 44111
  Lysis of Adhesions
    Laparoscopic, 44180
  Nuclear Medicine
    Imaging, 78290
  Reconstruction
    Bladder, 50820
    Colonic Reservoir, 45119
  Repair
    Diverticula, 44605
    Obstruction, 44615
    Ulcer, 44605
    Wound, 44605
  Resection, 44227
  Suture
    Diverticula, 44605
    Stoma, 44620, 44625
    Ulcer, 44605
    Wound, 44605
  Transplantation
    Allograft Preparation, 44715-44721
    Donor Enterectomy, 44132, 44133
    Removal of Allograft, 44137
  Unlisted Laparoscopic Procedure, 44238
Intestines, Large
  See Anus; Cecum; Colon; Rectum
Intestines, Small
  Anastomosis, 43845, 44130
  Biopsy, 44020, 44100
    Endoscopy, 44361
  Catheterization
    Jejunum, 44015
  Closure
    Stoma, 44620, 44625
  Decompression, 44021
  Destruction
    Lesion, 44369
    Tumor, 44369
  Endoscopy, 44360
    Biopsy, 44361, 44377
    Control of Bleeding, 44366, 44378
      via Stoma, 44382
    Destruction
      Lesion, 44369
      Tumor, 44369
    Diagnostic, 44376
    Exploration, 44360
    Hemorrhage, 44366

Intestines, Small — *continued*
  Endoscopy — *continued*
    Insertion
      Stent, 44370, 44379
      Tube, 44379
    Pelvic Pouch, 44385, 44386
    Place Tube, 44372
    Removal
      Foreign Body, 44363
      Lesion, 44365
      Polyp, 44364, 44365
      Tumor, 44364, 44365
    Tube Placement, 44372
    Tube Revision, 44373
    via Stoma, 44380-44384 *[44381]*
  Enterostomy, 44620-44626
    Tube Placement, 44300
  Excision, 44120-44128
    Partial with Anastomosis, 44140
  Exclusion, 44700
  Exploration, 44020
  Gastrostomy Tube, 44373
  Hemorrhage, 44378
  Hemorrhage Control, 44366
  Ileostomy, 44310-44314, 44316, 45136
    Continent, 44316
  Incision, 44010, 44020
    Creation
      Pouch, 44316
      Stoma, 44300-44310
    Decompression, 44021
    Exploration, 44020
    Revision
      Stoma, 44312
      Stoma Closure, 44620-44626
  Insertion
    Catheter, 44015
    Duodenostomy Tube, 49441
    Jejunostomy Tube, 44015, 44372
  Jejunostomy, 44310
    Laparoscopic, 44186
  Lesion
    Excision, 44110, 44111
  Lysis
    Adhesions, 44005
  Removal
    Foreign Body, 44020, 44363
  Repair
    Diverticula, 44602-44603
    Enterocele
      Abdominal Approach, 57270
      Vaginal Approach, 57268
    Fistula, 44640-44661
    Hernia, 44050
    Malrotation, 44055
    Obstruction, 44050, 44615
    Ulcer, 44602, 44603, 44605
    Volvulus, 44050
    Wound, 44602, 44603, 44605
  Revision
    Jejunostomy Tube, 44373, 49451-49452
  Specimen Collection, 43756-43757
  Suture
    Diverticula, 44602, 44603, 44605
    Fistula, 44640-44661
    Plication, 44680
    Stoma, 44620, 44625
    Ulcer, 44602, 44603, 44605
    Wound, 44602, 44603, 44605
  Unlisted Services and Procedures, 44799
  X–ray, 74245, 74249-74251
    Guide Intubation, 74355
Intestinovesical Fistula
  See Fistula, Enterovesical
Intima-Media Thickness Testing
  Artery
    Carotid, Common, 0126T
Intimectomy
  See Endarterectomy
Intra–Abdominal Manipulation
  Intestines, 44799
Intra–Abdominal Voiding Pressure Studies, *[51797]*
Intra-Aortic Balloon Pump Insertion, 33967-33974
Intra-Arterial Infusion Pump, 36260-36262

Intracapsular Extraction of Lens
  See Extraction, Lens, Intracapsular
Intracardiac Echocardiography, 93662
Intracranial
  Arterial Perfusion Thrombolysis, 61624
  Biopsy, 61140
  Microdissection, 69990
    with Surgical Microscope, 69990
  Percutaneous Thrombectomy/Thrombolysis, 61645
Intracranial Neoplasm, Acoustic Neuroma
  See Brain, Tumor, Excision
Intracranial Neoplasm, Craniopharyngioma
  See Craniopharyngioma
Intracranial Neoplasm, Meningioma
  See Meningioma
Intracranial Nerve
  Electrocoagulation
    Anesthesia, 00222
Intracranial Procedures
  Anesthesia, 00190, 00210-00222
Intradermal Influenza Virus Vaccine, 90654
Intradiscal Electrothermal Therapy (IDET), 22526-22527
Intrafallopian Transfer, Gamete
  See GIFT
Intra-Fraction Localization and Tracking
  Patient Motion During Radiation Therapy, *[77387]*
Intraluminal Angioplasty
  See Angioplasty
Intramuscular Autologous Bone Marrow Cell Therapy
  With Bone Marrow Harvest, 0263T
  Without Bone Marrow Harvest, 0264T
  Unilateral or Bilateral Bone Marrow Harvest Only, 0265T
Intramuscular Injection, 96372, 99506
Intraocular Lens
  Exchange, 66986
  Insertion, 66983
    Manual or Mechanical Technique, 66982, 66984
    Not Associated with Concurrent Cataract Removal, 66985
Intraoperative
  Manipulation of Stomach, 43659, 43999
  Neurophysiology Monitoring, *[95940, 95941]*
  Radiation Treatment Delivery, *[77424, 77425]*
  Radiation Treatment Management, 77469
Intraoral
  Skin Graft
    Pedicle Flap, 15576
Intra–Osseous Infusion
  See Infusion, Intraosseous
Intrathoracic Esophagoesophagostomy, 43499
Intrathoracic System
  Anesthesia, 00500-00580
Intratracheal Intubation
  See Insertion, Endotracheal Tube
Intrauterine
  Contraceptive Device (IUD)
    Insertion, 58300
    Removal, 58301
  Insemination, 58322
Intrauterine Synechiae
  Lysis, 58559
Intravascular Sensor
  Pressure
    Complete Study, 93982
Intravascular Stent
  See Transcatheter, Placement, Intravascular Stents
Intravascular Ultrasound
  Intraoperative Noncoronary Vessel, 37252-37253
Intravascular Vena Cava Filter (IVC), 37191
  Insertion, 37191
  Removal, 37193
  Reposition, 37192
Intravenous Pyelogram
  See Urography, Intravenous
Intravenous Therapy, 96360-96361, 96365-96368, 96374-96379
  See Injection, Chemotherapy

Intravesical Instillation
  See Bladder, Instillation
Intrinsic Factor, 83528
  Antibodies, 86340
Introduction
  Breast
    Localization Device, 19281-19288
    with Biopsy, 19081-19086
  Contraceptive Capsules
    Implantable, 11981
  Drug Delivery Implant, 11981, 11983
  Gastrointestinal Tube, 44500
    with Fluoroscopic Guidance, 74340
  Injections
    Intradermal, 11920-11922
    Intralesional, 11900, 11901
    Subcutaneous, 11950-11954
  Needle or Catheter
    Aorta, 36160, 36200
    Arterial System
      Brachiocephalic Branch, 36215-36218
      Lower Extremity, 36245-36248
      Pelvic Branch, 36245-36248
    AV Shunt
      Dialysis Circuit, 36901-36903
    Brachial Artery, 36120
    Carotid, 36100
    Extremity Artery, 36140
    Vertebral Artery, 36100
  Tissue Expanders, Skin, 11960-11971
Intubation
  Duodenal, 43756-43757
  Endotracheal Tube, 31500
  Eustachian Tube
    See Catheterization, Eustachian Tube
  Gastric, 43753-43755
Intubation Tube
  See Endotracheal Tube
Intussusception
  Barium Enema, 74283
  Reduction
    Laparotomy, 44050
Invagination, Intestinal
  See Intussusception
Inversion, Nipple, 19355
In Vitro Fertilization
  Biopsy Oocyte, 89290, 89291
  Culture Oocyte, 89250, 89251
    Extended, 89272
  Embryo Hatching, 89253
  Fertilize Oocyte, 89250
    Microtechnique, 89280, 89281
  Identify Oocyte, 89254
  Insemination of Oocyte, 89268
  Prepare Embryo, 89255, 89352
  Retrieve Oocyte, 58970
  Transfer Embryo, 58974, 58976
  Transfer Gamete, 58976
In Vivo NMR Spectroscopy
  See Magnetic Resonance Spectroscopy
Iodide Test
  Thyroid Uptake, 78012, 78014
IOL, 66825, 66983-66986
Ionization, Medical
  See Iontophoresis
Iontophoresis, 97033
  Sweat Collection, 89230
IP
  See Allergen Immunotherapy
Ipecac Administration, 99175
IPOL, 90713
IPV, 90713
Iridectomy
  with Corneoscleral or Corneal Section, 66600
  with Sclerectomy with Punch or Scissors, 66160
  with Thermocauterization, 66155
  with Transfixion as for Iris Bombe, 66605
  with Trephination, 66150
  by Laser Surgery, 66761
  Peripheral for Glaucoma, 66625
Iridocapsulectomy, 66830
Iridocapsulotomy, 66830
Iridodialysis, 66680
Iridoplasty, 66762
Iridotomy
  by Laser Surgery, 66761

Iridotomy — *continued*
  by Stab Incision, 66500
  Excision
    with Corneoscleral or Corneal Section,
      66600
    with Cyclectomy, 66605
    Optical, 66635
    Peripheral, 66625
  Incision
    with Transfixion as for Iris Bombe, 66505
    Stab, 66500
  Optical, 66635
  Peripheral, 66625
  Sector, 66630
Iris
  Cyst
    Destruction, 66770
  Excision
    Iridectomy
      with Corneoscleral or Corneal Section,
        66600
      with Cyclectomy, 66605
      Optical, 66635
      Peripheral, 66625
      Sector, 66630
  Incision
    Iridotomy
      with Transfixion as for Iris Bombe,
        66505
      Stab, 66500
  Lesion
    Destruction, 66770
  Repair, 66680
    Suture, 66682
  Revision
    Laser Surgery, 66761
    Photocoagulation, 66762
  Suture
    with Ciliary Body, 66682
Iron, 83540
Iron Binding Capacity, 83550
Iron Stain, 85536, 88313
Irradiation
  Blood Products, 86945
Irrigation
  Bladder, 51700
  Caloric Vestibular Test, 92533, 92537-92538
  Catheter
    Bladder, 51700
    Brain, 62194, 62225
    Venous Access Device, 96523
  Corpora Cavernosa
    Priapism, 54220
  Penis
    Priapism, 54220
  Peritoneal
    See Peritoneal Lavage
  Shunt
    Spinal Cord, 63744
  Sinus
    Maxillary, 31000
    Sphenoid, 31002
  Vagina, 57150
Irving Sterilization
  Ligation, Fallopian Tube, Oviduct, 58600-58611,
    58670
Ischemic Stroke
  Onset, 1065F-1066F
  Tissue Plasminogen Activator (tPA)
    Documentation that Administration was
      Considered, 4077F
Ischial
  Excision
    Bursa, 27060
    Tumor, 27078
Ischiectomy, 15941
Ischium
  Pressure Ulcer, 15940-15946
ISG Immunization, 90281, 90283
Island Pedicle Flaps, 15740
Islands of Langerhans
  See Islet Cell
Islet Cell
  Antibody, 86341
Isocitrate Dehydrogenase
  See Isocitric Dehydrogenase

Isocitric Dehydrogenase
  Blood, 83570
Isolation
  Sperm, 89260, 89261
Isomerase, Glucose 6 Phosphate
  See Phosphohexose Isomerase
Isopropanol
  See Isopropyl Alcohol
ISPD, 81405
Isthmusectomy
  Thyroid Gland, 60210-60225
ITPR1, 81408
IUD, 58300, 58301
  Insertion, 58300
  Removal, 58301
IUI (Intrauterine Insemination), 58322
IV, 96365-96368, 96374-96376
  Chemotherapy, 96413-96417
  Hydration, 96360-96361
IVC Filter
  Insertion, 37191
  Removal, 37193
  Reposition, 37192
IV, Coagulation Factor
  See Calcium
IVD, 81400, 81406
IVF (In Vitro Fertilization), 58970-58976, 89250-
  89255
IV Infusion Therapy, 96365-96368
  Chemotherapy, 96409, 96411, 96413-96417,
    96542
  Hydration, 96360-96361
IV Injection, 96374-96376
  Chemotherapy, 96409-96417
Ivor Lewis, 43117
IVP, 74400
Ivy Bleeding Time, 85002
IX Complex, Factor
  See Christmas Factor
IXIARO, 90738

J

Jaboulay Operation
  Gastroduodenostomy, 43810, 43850, 43855
JAG1, 81406-81407
JAK2, 81270, 81403
Janeway Procedure, 43832
Jannetta Procedure
  Decompression, Cranial Nerves, 61458
Janus Kinase 2 Gene Analysis, 81270
Japanese Encephalitis Virus Vaccine, 90738
Japanese, River Fever
  See Scrub Typhus
Jatene Procedure
  Repair, Great Arteries, 33770-33781
Jaw Joint
  See Facial Bones; Mandible; Maxilla
Jaws
  Muscle Reduction, 21295, 21296
  X–ray
    for Orthodontics, 70355
Jejunostomy
  with Pancreatic Drain, 48001
  Catheterization, 44015
  Insertion
    Catheter, 44015
    Laparoscopic, 44186
    Non–Tube, 44310
Jejunum
  Transfer with Microvascular Anastomosis, Free,
    43496
Johannsen Procedure, 53400
Johanson Operation
  See Reconstruction, Urethra
Joint
  See Specific Joint
  Acromioclavicular
    See Acromioclavicular Joint
  Arthrocentesis, 20600-20611
  Aspiration, 20600-20611
  Dislocation
    See Dislocation
  Drainage
    Acromioclavicular, 23044
    Ankle, 27610
    Carpometacarpal, 26070

Joint — *continued*
  Drainage — *continued*
    Glenohumeral, 23040
    Hip, 26990, 27030
    Interphalangeal, 26080, 28024
    Intertarsal, 28020
    Knee, 27301, 29871
    Metacarpophalangeal, 26075
    Metatarsophalangeal, 28022
    Midcarpal, 25040
    Pelvis, 26990
    Radiocarpal, 25040
    Sternoclavicular, 23044
    Thigh, 27301
    Wrist, 29843
  Finger
    See Intercarpal Joint
  Fixation (Surgical)
    See Arthrodesis
  Foot
    See Foot, Joint
  Hip
    See Hip, Joint
  Injection, 20600-20611
  Intertarsal
    See Intertarsal Joint
  Knee
    See Knee Joint
  Ligament
    See Ligament
  Metacarpophalangeal
    See Metacarpophalangeal Joint
  Metatarsophalangeal
    See Metatarsophalangeal Joint
  Mobilization, 97140
  Nuclear Medicine
    Imaging, 78300-78315
  Radiology
    Stress Views, 77071
  Sacroiliac
    See Sacroiliac Joint
  Shoulder
    See Glenohumeral Joint
  Sternoclavicular
    See Sternoclavicular Joint
  Survey, 77077
  Temporomandibular
    See Temporomandibular Joint (TMJ)
    Dislocation Temporomandibular
      See Dislocation, Temporomandibular
        Joint
    Implant
      See Prosthesis, Temporomandibular
        Joint
  Wrist
    See Radiocarpal Joint
Joint Syndrome, Temporomandibular
  See Temporomandibular Joint (TMJ)
Jones and Cantarow Test
  Clearance, Urea Nitrogen, 84545
Jones Procedure
  Arthrodesis, Interphalangeal Joint, Great Toe,
    28760
Jugal Bone
  See Cheekbone
Jugular Vein
  See Vein, Jugular
JUP, 81406

K

K+, 84132
Kader Operation
  Incision, Stomach, Creation of Stoma, 43830-
    43832
KAL1, 81406
Kala Azar Smear, 87207
Kallidin I/Kallidin 9
  See Bradykinin
Kallikrein HK3
  See Antigen, Prostate Specific
Kallikreinogen
  See Fletcher Factor
Kasai Procedure, 47701
KCNC3, 81403
KCNH2, 81406
KCNJ10, 81404

KCNJ1, 81404
KCNJ11, 81403
KCNJ2, 81403
KCNQ1, 81406
KCNQ1OT1/KCNQ1, 81401
KCNQ2, 81406
KDM5C, 81407
Kedani Fever, 86000
Keel Laryngoplasty, 31580
Keen Operation, 63198
  Laminectomy, 63600
Keitzer Test, 51727, 51729
Kelikian Procedure, 28280
Keller Procedure, 28292
Kelly Urethral Plication, 57220
Keratectomy
  Partial
    for Lesion, 65400
Keratomileusis, 65760
Keratophakia, 65765
Keratoplasty
  Lamellar, 65710
    in Aphakia, 65750
    in Pseudophakia, 65755
    Penetrating, 65730
Keratoprosthesis, 65770
Keratotomy
  Radial, 65771
Ketogenic Steroids, 83582
Ketone Body
  Acetone, 82009, 82010
Ketosteroids, 83586, 83593
KIAA0196, 81407
Kidner Procedure, 28238
Kidney
  Abscess
    Incision and Drainage
      Open, 50020
  Allograft Preparation, 50323-50329
    Donor Nephrectomy, 50300, 50320, 50547
    Implantation of Graft, 50360
    Recipient Nephrectomy, 50340, 50365
    Reimplantation Kidney, 50380
    Removal Transplant Renal Autograft, 50370
  Anesthesia
    Donor, 00862
    Recipient, 00868
  Biopsy, 50200, 50205
    Endoscopic, 50555-50557, 52354
    Renal Pelvis, 50606
  Catheterization
    Endoscopic, 50572
  Cyst
    Ablation, 50541
    Aspiration, 50390
    Excision, 50280, 50290
    Injection, 50390
    X–ray, 74470
  Destruction
    Calculus, 50590
    Endoscopic, 50557, 50576, 52354
  Dilation, 50395
  Endoscopy
    with Endopyelotomy, 50575
    Biopsy, 50555, 50574-50576, 52354
    Catheterization, 50553, 50572
    Destruction, 50557, 50576, 52354
    Dilation
      Intra–Renal Stricture, 52343, 52346
      Ureter, 50553
    Excision
      Tumor, 52355
    Exploration, 52351
    Lithotripsy, 52353
    Removal
      Calculus, 50561, 50580, 52352
      Foreign Body, 50561, 50580
    via Incision, 50570-50580
    via Stoma, 50551-50561
  Excision
    with Ureters, 50220-50236
    Donor, 50300, 50320, 50547
    Partial, 50240
    Recipient, 50340
    Transplantation, 50370
  Exploration, 50010, 50045, 50120

Kidney — *continued*
Incision, 50010, 50045, 50120, 50130, 50135
Incision and Drainage, 50040, 50125
Injection
Drugs, 50391
Insertion
Guide, 50395
Instillation
Drugs, 50391
Lithotripsy, 50590
Manometry
Pressure, 50396
Mass
Ablation, 50542
Cryosurgical, 50250
Radiofrequency, 50592
Mass Ablation, 50542
Needle Biopsy, 50200
Nuclear Medicine
Blood Flow, 78701-78709
Function Study, 78725
Imaging, 78700-78707, 78710
Unlisted Services and Procedures, 78799
Removal
Calculus, 50060-50081, 50130, 50561
Foreign Body, 50561, 50580
Tube
Nephrostomy, 50389
Renal Pelvis, 50405
Repair
Blood Vessels, 50100
Fistula, 50520-50526
Horseshoe Kidney, 50540
Renal Pelvis, 50400, 50405
Wound, 50500
Solitary, 50405
Suture
Fistula, 50520-50526
Horseshoe Kidney, 50540
Transplantation
Allograft Preparation, 50323-50329
Anesthesia
Donor, 00862
Recipient, 00868
Donor Nephrectomy, 50300-50320, 50547
Graft Implantation, 50360-50365
Implantation of Graft, 50360
Recipient Nephrectomy, 50340, 50365
Reimplantation Kidney, 50380
Removal Transplant Allograft, 50370
Tumor
Ablation
Cryotherapy, 50250, 50593
Ultrasound, 76770-76775, 76776
Kidney Stone
Removal, Calculi, 50060-50081, 50130, 50561, 50580
Killer Cell Immunoglobulin-like Receptor (KIR) Gene Family, 81403
Killian Operation, 31020
Sinusotomy, Frontal, 31070-31087
Kinase Creatine
Blood, 82550-82552
Kineplasty
Arm, Lower or Upper, 24940
Kinetic Therapy, 97530
Kininase A, 82164
Kininogen, 85293
Kininogen, High Molecular Weight, 85293
Kirsten Rat Sarcoma Viral Oncogene Homolog Gene Analysis, 81275
KIT, 81272
D816 Variant, 81273
Kleihauer–Betke Test, 85460
Kloramfenikol, 82415
Knee
See Femur; Fibula; Patella; Tibia
Abscess, 27301
Arthrocentesis, 20610-20611
Arthrodesis, 27580
Arthroplasty, 27440-27445, 27447
Intraoperative Balance Sensor, 0396T
Revision, 27486, 27487
Arthroscopy
Diagnostic, 29870
Surgical, 29866-29868, 29871-29889

Knee — *continued*
Arthrotomy, 27310, 27330-27335, 27403
Autograft, Osteochondral, Open, 27416
Biopsy, 27323, 27324, 27330, 27331
Synovium, 27330
Bone
Drainage, 27303
Bursa, 27301
Excision, 27340
Cyst
Excision, 27345, 27347
Disarticulation, 27598
Dislocation
Closed Treatment, 27550, 27552, 27560, 27562
Open Treatment, 27556-27558, 27566
Drainage, 27310
Excision
Cartilage, 27332, 27333
Ganglion, 27347
Lesion, 27347
Synovial Lining, 27334, 27335
Exploration, 27310, 27331
Fasciotomy, 27305, 27496-27499
Fracture, 27520, 27524
Arthroscopic Treatment, 29850, 29851
Fusion, 27580
Hematoma, 27301
Incision
Capsule, 27435
Injection
X–ray, 27370
Magnetic Resonance Imaging (MRI), 73721-73723
Manipulation, 27570
Meniscectomy, 27332, 27333
Osteochondral Graft, 27415-27416
Reconstruction, 27437, 27438
with Implantation, 27445
with Prosthesis, 27445
Ligament, 27427-27429
Removal
Foreign Body, 27310, 27331, 27372
Loose Body, 27331
Prosthesis, 27488
Repair
Ligament, 27405-27409
Collateral, 27405
Collateral and Cruciate, 27409
Cruciate, 27407, 27409
Meniscus, 27403
Tendon, 27380, 27381
Replacement, 27447
Retinacular
Release, 27425
Strapping, 29530
Suture
Tendon, 27380, 27381
Transplantation
Chondrocytes, 27412
Meniscus, 29868
Osteochondral
Allograft, 27415, 29867
Autograft, 27412, 29866
Tumor, 27327-27328 [27337, 27339], 27355-27358, 27364-27365 [27329]
Unlisted Services and Procedures, 27599
X–ray, 73560-73564
Arthrography, 73580
Bilateral, 73565
X–ray with Contrast
Angiography, 73706
Arthrography, 73580
Kneecap
Excision, 27350
Repair
Instability, 27420-27424
Knee Joint
Arthroplasty, 27446
Intraoperative Balance Sensor, 0396T
Knee Prosthesis
See Prosthesis, Knee
Knock–Knee Repair, 27455, 27457
Kocher Operation, 23650-23680
See Clavicle; Scapula; Shoulder, Dislocation, Closed Treatment

Kocher Pylorectomy
Gastrectomy, Partial, 43631
Kock Pouch, 44316
Formation, 50825
Kock Procedure, 44316
KOH
Hair, Nails, Tissue, Examination for Fungi, 87220
Konno Procedure, 33412
Koop Inguinal Orchiopexy, 54640
KRAS, 81275-81276, 81405
Kraske Procedure, 45116
Krause Operation
Gasserian Ganglion, Sensory Root, Decompression, 61450
Kroenlein Procedure, 67420
Krukenberg Procedure, 25915
Krupin-Denver Valve
Implant, 66180
Removal, 67120
Revision, 66185
KS, 83586, 83593
KUB, 74241, 74247, 74270, 74420
Kuhlmann Test, 96101-96103
Kuhnt–Szymanowski Procedure, 67917
K–Wire Fixation
Tongue, 41500
Kyphectomy
More than Two Segments, 22819
Up to Two Segments, 22818
Kyphoplasty, 22513-22515

L

L1CAM, 81407
Labial Adhesions
Lysis, 56441
Labyrinth
See Ear, Inner
Labyrinthectomy
with Mastoidectomy, 69910
with Skull Base Surgery, 61596
Transcanal, 69905
Labyrinthotomy
with Skull Base Surgery, 61596
Inner Ear, 69949
Transcanal, 69801
Laceration Repair
See Repair, Laceration, Skin
Lacrimal Duct
Balloon, 68816
Canaliculi
Incision, 68899
Repair, 68700
Dilation, 68816
Exploration, 68810
with Anesthesia, 68811
Canaliculi, 68840
Stent, 68815
Insertion
Stent, 68815
Nasolacrimal Duct Probing, 68816
Removal
Dacryolith, 68530
Foreign Body, 68530
X–ray with Contrast, 70170
Lacrimal Gland
Biopsy, 68510
Close Fistula, 68770
Excision
Partial, 68505
Total, 68500
Fistulization, 68720
Incision and Drainage, 68400
Injection
X–ray, 68850
Nuclear Medicine
Tear Flow, 78660
Removal
Dacryolith, 68530
Foreign Body, 68530
Repair
Fistula, 68770
Tumor
Excision
with Osteotomy, 68550
without Closure, 68540
X-Ray, 70170

Lacrimal Punctum
Closure
by Plug, 68761
by Thermocauterization, Ligation or Laser Surgery, 68760
Dilation, 68801
Incision, 68440
Repair, 68705
Lacrimal Sac
Biopsy, 68525
Excision, 68520
Incision and Drainage, 68420
Lacrimal System
Unlisted Services and Procedures, 68899
Lacryoaptography
Nuclear, 78660
Lactase Deficiency Breath Test, 91065
Lactate, 83605
Lactic Acid, 83605
Lactic Acid Measurement
See Lactate
Lactic Cytochrome Reductase
See Lactic Dehydrogenase
Lactic Dehydrogenase, 83615, 83625
Lactiferous Duct
Excision, 19112
Exploration, 19110
Lactoferrin
Fecal, 83630-83631
Lactogen, Human Placental, 83632
Lactogenic Hormone
See Prolactin
Lactose
Urine, 83633
Ladd Procedure, 44055
Lagophthalmos
Repair, 67912
Laki Lorand Factor
See Fibrin Stabilizing Factor
L–Alanine
See Aminolevulinic Acid (ALA)
LAMA2, 81408
LAMB2, 81407
Lamblia Intestinalis
See Giardia Lamblia
Lambrinudi Operation
Arthrodesis, Foot Joints, 28730, 28735, 28740
Lamellar Keratoplasties
See Keratoplasty, Lamellar
Laminaria
Insertion, 59200
Laminectomy, 62351, 63001-63003, 63005-63011, 63015-63044, 63180-63200, 63265-63290, 63600-63655
with Facetectomy, 63045-63048
Decompression
Cervical, 63001, 63015
with Facetectomy and Foraminotomy, 63045, 63048
Neural Elements, 0274T
Laminotomy
Initial
Cervical, 63020
Each Additional Space, 63035
Lumbar, 63030
Reexploration
Cervical, 63040
Each Additional Interspace, 63043
Lumbar, 63042
Each Additional Interspace, 63044
Lumbar, 63005, 63017
with Facetectomy and Foraminotomy, 63046, 63048
Neural Elements, 0275T
Sacral, 63011
Thoracic, 63003, 63016
with Facetectomy and Foraminotomy, 63047, 63048
Neural Elements, 0274T
Excision
Lesion, 63250-63273
Neoplasm, 63275-63290
Lumbar, 22630, 63012
Surgical, 63170-63200

Laminoplasty
Cervical, 63050-63051
Laminotomy
Cervical, One Interspace, 63020
Lumbar, 63042
One Interspace, 62380, 63030
Each Additional, 63035
Re–exploration, Cervical, 63040
Lamotrigine
Assay, 80175
LAMP2, 81405
Landboldt's Operation, 67971, 67973, 67975
Lane's Operation, 44150
Langerhans Islands
See Islet Cell
Language Evaluation, 92521-92524
Language Therapy, 92507, 92508
LAP, 83670
Laparoscopy
Abdominal, 49320-49329
Surgical, 49321-49326
Adrenalectomy, 60650
Adrenal Gland
Biopsy, 60650
Excision, 60650
Appendectomy, 44970
Aspiration, 49322
Biopsy, 49321
Lymph Nodes, 38570
Ovary, 49321
Bladder
Repair
Sling Procedure, 51992
Urethral Suspension, 51990
Unlisted, 51999
Cecostomy, 44188
Cholecystectomy, 47562-47564
Cholecystoenterostomy, 47570
Closure
Enterostomy, 44227
Colectomy
Partial, 44204-44208, 44213
Total, 44210-44212
Colostomy, 44188
Destruction
Lesion, 58662
Diagnostic, 49320
Drainage
Extraperitoneal Lymphocele, 49323
Ectopic Pregnancy, 59150
with Salpingectomy and/or Oophorectomy, 59151
Electrode
Implantation
Gastric
Antrum, 43647
Lesser Curvature, 43659
Removal
Gastric, 43648, 43659
Replacement
Gastric, 43647
Revision
Gastric, 43648, 43659
Enterectomy, 44202
Enterolysis, 44180
Enterostomy
Closure, 44227
Esophageal Lengthening, 43283
Esophagogastric Fundoplasty, 43280
Esophagomyotomy, 43279
Esophagus
Esophageal Lengthening, 43283
Esophageal Sphincter Augmentation, 43284
Removal, 43285
Esophagogastric Fundoplasty, 43280
Esophagomyotomy, 43279
Fimbrioplasty, 58672
Gastric Restrictive Procedures, 43644-43645, 43770-43774
Gastrostomy
Temporary, 43653
Graft Revision
Vaginal, 57426
Hernia Repair
Epigastric, 49652

Laparoscopy — *continued*
Hernia Repair — *continued*
Epigastric — *continued*
Incarcerated or Strangulated, 49653
Incisional, 49654
Incarcerated or Strangulated, 49655
Recurrent, 49656
Incarcerated or Strangulated, 49657
Initial, 49650
Recurrent, 49651
Spigelian, 49652
Incarcerated or Strangulated, 49653
Umbilical, 49652
Incarcerated or Strangulated, 49653
Ventral, 49652
Incarcerated or Strangulated, 49653
Hysterectomy, 58541-58554, 58570-58573
Radical, 58548
Total, 58570-58573
Ileostomy, 44187
Incontinence Repair, 51990, 51992
In Vitro Fertilization, 58976
Retrieve Oocyte, 58970
Transfer Embryo, 58974
Transfer Gamete, 58976
Jejunostomy, 44186-44187
Kidney
Ablation, 50541-50542
Ligation
Veins, Spermatic, 55500
Liver
Ablation
Tumor, 47370, 47371
Lymphadenectomy, 38571-38572
Lymphatic, 38570-38589
Lysis of Adhesions, 58660
Lysis of Intestinal Adhesions, 44180
Mobilization
Splenic Flexure, 44213
Nephrectomy, 50545-50548
Partial, 50543
Omentopexy, 49326
Orchiectomy, 54690
Orchiopexy, 54692
Ovary
Biopsy, 49321
Reimplantation, 59898
Suture, 59898
Oviduct Surgery, 58670, 58671, 58679
Pelvis, 49320
Placement Interstitial Device, 49327
Proctectomy, 45395, 45397
with Creation of Colonic Reservoir, 45397
Complete, 45395
Proctopexy, 45400, 45402
Prostatectomy, 55866
Pyloplasty, 50544
Rectum
Resection, 45395-45397
Unlisted, 45499
Removal
Fallopian Tubes, 58661
Leiomyomata, 58545-58546
Ovaries, 58661
Spleen, 38120
Testis, 54690
Resection
Intestines
with Anastomosis, 44202, 44203
Rectum, 45395-45397
Salpingostomy, 58673
Splenectomy, 38120, 38129
Splenic Flexure
Mobilization, 44213
Stomach, 43651-43659
Gastric Bypass, 43644-43645
Gastric Restrictive Procedures, 43770-43774, 43848, 43886-43888
Gastroenterostomy, 43644-43645
Roux–en–Y, 43644

Laparoscopy — *continued*
Surgical, 38570-38572, 43651-43653, 44180-44188, 44212, 44213, 44227, 44970, 45395-45402, 47370, 47371, 49321-49327, 49650, 49651, 50541, 50543, 50545, 50945-50948, 51992, 54690, 54692, 55550, 55866, 57425, 58545, 58546, 58552, 58554
Unlisted Services and Procedures, 38129, 38589, 43289, 43659, 44238, 44979, 45499, 47379, 47579, 49329, 49659, 50549, 50949, 51999, 54699, 55559, 58578, 58579, 58679, 59898
Ureterolithotomy, 50945
Ureteroneocystostomy, 50947-50948
Urethral Suspension, 51990
Uterus
Ablation
Fibroids, 58674
Vaginal Hysterectomy, 58550-58554
Vaginal Suspension, 57425
Vagus Nerve, 0312T-0314T
Vagus Nerves Transection, 43651, 43652
Laparotomy
with Biopsy, 49000
Electrode
Gastric
Implantation, 43881
Lesser Curvature, 43999
Removal, 43882
Replacement, 43881
Revision, 43882
Esophagogastric Fundoplasty, 43327
Exploration, 47015, 49000, 49002, 58960
for Staging, 49220
Hemorrhage Control, 49002
Hiatal Hernia, 43332-43333
Second Look, 58960
Staging, 58960
Surgical, 44050
Laparotomy, Exploratory, 47015, 49000-49002
Large Bowel
See Anus; Cecum; Rectum
Laroyenne Operation
Vagina, Abscess, Incision and Drainage, 57010
Laryngeal Function Study, 92520
Laryngeal Sensory Testing, 92614-92617
Laryngectomy, 31360-31382
Partial, 31367-31382
Subtotal, 31367, 31368
Total, 31360, 31365
Laryngocele
Removal, 31300
Laryngofissure, 31300
Laryngopharyngectomy
Excision, Larynx, with Pharynx, 31390, 31395
Laryngoplasty
Burns, 31599
Cricoid Split, 31587
Cricotracheal Resection, 31592
Laryngeal Stenosis, *[31551, 31552, 31553, 31554]*
Laryngeal Web, 31580
Medialization, 31591
Open Reduction of Fracture, 31584
Laryngoscopy
Diagnostic, 31505
Direct, 31515-31571
Exploration, 31505, 31520-31526, 31575
Indirect, 31505-31513
Newborn, 31520
Operative, 31530-31561
Telescopic, 31575-31579
with Stroboscopy, 31579
Laryngotomy
Diagnostic, 31320
Partial, 31370-31382
Removal
Tumor, 31300
Total, 31360-31368
Larynx
Aspiration
Endoscopy, 31515
Biopsy
Endoscopy, 31510, 31535, 31536, 31576
Dilation
Endoscopic, 31528, 31529

Larynx — *continued*
Electromyography
Needle, 95865
Endoscopy
Ablation, *[31572]*
Augmentation, *[31574]*
Destruction, *[31572]*
Direct, 31515-31571
Excision, 31545-31546
Exploration, 31505, 31520-31526, 31575
Indirect, 31505-31513
Injection, Therapeutic, *[31573]*
Operative, 31530-31561
Telescopic, 31575-31579
with Stroboscopy, 31579
Excision
with Pharynx, 31390, 31395
Lesion, Endoscopic, 31512, 31545-31546, 31578
Partial, 31367-31382
Total, 31360, 31365
Exploration
Endoscopic, 31505, 31520-31526, 31575
Fracture
Open Treatment, 31584
Insertion
Obturator, 31527
Nerve
Destruction, 31595
Pharynx
with Pharynx, 31390
Reconstruction
with Pharynx, 31395
Burns, 31599
Cricoid Split, 31587
Other, 31599
Stenosis, *[31551, 31552, 31553, 31554]*
Web, 31580
Removal
Foreign Body
Endoscopic, 31511, 31530, 31531, 31577
Lesion
Endoscopic, 31512, 31545-31546, 31578
Repair
Reinnervation Neuromuscular Pedicle, 31590
Stroboscopy, 31579
Tumor
Excision, 31300
Endoscopic, 31540, 31541
Unlisted Services and Procedures, 31599
Vocal Cord
Injection, 31513, 31570, 31571
X–ray, 70370
L Ascorbic Acid
See Ascorbic Acid
LASEK, 65760
Laser Surgery
Anal, 46917
Cautery
Esophagus, 43227
Eye
Anterior Segment Adhesions, 65860
Corneovitreal Adhesions, 66821
Iridectomy, 66761
Iridotomy, 66761
Lacrimal Punctum, 68760
Posterior Lens, 66821
Retinal Detachment, 67145
Secondary Cataract, 66821
Vitreous Strands/Adhesions, 67031
Lacrimal Punctum, 68760
Lens
Posterior, 66821
Lesion
Mouth, 40820
Nose, 30117, 30118
Penis, 54057
Skin, 17000-17111, 17260-17286
Prostate, 52647-52649
Spine
Diskectomy, 62287
Tumor
Urethra and Bladder, 52234-52240

Laser Surgery — *continued*
  Urethra and Bladder, 52214
Laser Treatment, 17000-17286, 96920-96922
  See Destruction
Lash Procedure
  Tracheoplasty, 31750-31760
LASIK, 65760
L Aspartate 2 Oxoglutarate Aminotransferase
  See Transaminase, Glutamic Oxaloacetic
Lateral Epicondylitis
  See Tennis Elbow
Latex Fixation, 86403, 86406
LATS, 80438, 80439
Latzko Procedure
  Colpocleisis, 57120
LAV
  See HIV
LAV-2, 86702-86703
Lavage
  Colon, 44701
  Gastric, 43753
  Lung
    Bronchial, 31624
    Total, 32997
  Peritoneal, 49084
LAV Antibodies, 86689, 86701-86703
LCM
  Antibody, 86727
LCT, 81400
LD (Lactic Dehydrogenase), 83615
LDB3, 81406
LDH, 83615, 83625
LDL, 83721
LDLR, 81405-81406
Lead, 83655
Leadbetter Procedure, 53431
Lecithin C
  See Tissue Typing
Lecithin–Sphingomyelin Ratio, 83661
Lee and White Test, 85345
LEEP Procedure, 57460
LeFort III Procedure
  Craniofacial Separation, 21431-21436
  Midface Reconstruction, 21154-21159
LeFort II Procedure
  Midface Reconstruction, 21150, 21151
  Nasomaxillary Complex Fracture, 21345-21348
LeFort I Procedure
  Midface Reconstruction, 21141-21147, 21155, 21160
  Palatal or Maxillary Fracture, 21421-21423
LeFort Procedure
  Vagina, 57120
Left Atrioventricular Valve
  See Mitral Valve
Left Heart Cardiac Catheterization
  See Cardiac Catheterization, Left Heart
Leg
  Cast
    Rigid Total Contact, 29445
  Excision
    Excess Skin, 15833
    Lipectomy, Suction Assisted, 15879
  Lower
    See Ankle; Fibula; Knee; Tibia
    Abscess
      Incision and Drainage, 27603
    Amputation, 27598, 27880-27882
      Revision, 27884, 27886
    Angiography, 73706
    Artery
      Ligation, 37618
    Biopsy, 27613, 27614
    Bursa
      Incision and Drainage, 27604
    Bypass Graft, 35903
    Cast, 29405-29435, 29450
    CT Scan, 73700-73706
    Decompression, 27600-27602
    Exploration
      Blood Vessel, 35860
    Fasciotomy, 27600-27602, 27892-27894
    Hematoma
      Incision and Drainage, 27603
    Lesion
      Excision, 27630

Leg — *continued*
  Lower — *continued*
    Magnetic Resonance Imaging, 73718-73720
    Repair
      Blood Vessel, 35226
        with Other Graft, 35286
        with Vein Graft, 35256
      Fascia, 27656
      Tendon, 27658-27692
    Skin Graft
      Delay of Flap, 15610
      Full Thickness, 15220, 15221
      Pedicle Flap, 15572
      Split, 15100, 15101
    Splint, 29515
    Strapping, 29580
    Tendon, 27658-27665
    Tissue Transfer, Adjacent, 14020, 14021
    Tumor, 27615-27619 [27632, 27634], 27635-27638, 27645-27647
    Ultrasound, 76881-76882
    Unlisted Services and Procedures, 27899
    Unna Boot, 29580
    X–ray, 73592
  Upper
    See Femur
    Abscess, 27301
    Amputation, 27590-27592
      at Hip, 27290, 27295
      Revision, 27594, 27596
    Angiography, 73706, 75635
    Artery
      Ligation, 37618
    Biopsy, 27323, 27324
    Bursa, 27301
    Bypass Graft, 35903
    Cast, 29345-29365, 29450
    Cast Brace, 29358
    CT Scan, 73700-73706, 75635
    Exploration
      Blood Vessel, 35860
    Fasciotomy, 27305, 27496-27499, 27892-27894
    Halo Application, 20663
    Hematoma, 27301
    Magnetic Resonance Imaging, 73718-73720
    Neurectomy, 27325, 27326
    Pressure Ulcer, 15950-15958
    Removal
      Cast, 29705
      Foreign Body, 27372
    Repair
      Blood Vessel
        with Other Graft, 35286
        with Vein Graft, 35256
      Muscle, 27385, 27386, 27400, 27430
      Tendon, 27393-27400
    Splint, 29505
    Strapping, 29580
    Suture
      Muscle, 27385, 27386
      Tendon, 27658-27665
    Tenotomy, 27306, 27307, 27390-27392
    Tumor
      Excision, 27327-27328 [27337, 27339], 27364-27365 [27329]
    Ultrasound, 76881-76882
    Unlisted Services and Procedures, 27599
    Unna Boot, 29580
    X–ray, 73592
  Wound Exploration
    Penetrating, 20103
Legionella
  Antibody, 86713
  Antigen, 87277, 87278, 87540-87542
Legionella Micdadei
  Immunofluorescence, 87277
Legionella Pneumophila
  Antigen Detection
    Direct Fluorescence, 87278
Leg Length Measurement X–Ray
  See Scanogram
Leiomyomata
  Embolization, 37243
  Removal, 58140, 58545-58546, 58561

Leishmania
  Antibody, 86717
Lempert's Fenestration, 69820
Lengthening
  Esophageal, 43338
  Radius and Ulna, 25391, 25393
  Tendons
    Lower Extremities, 27393-27395, 27685-27686
    Upper Extremities, 24305, 25280, 26476, 26478
  Tibia and Fibula, 27715
Lens
  Extracapsular, 66940
  Intracapsular, 66920
    Dislocated, 66930
  Intraocular
    Exchange, 66986
    Reposition, 66825
  Prosthesis
    Insertion, 66983
      Manual or Mechanical Technique, 66982, 66984
      not associated with Concurrent Cataract Removal, 66985
  Removal
    Lens Material
      Aspiration Technique, 66840
      Extracapsular, 66940
      Intracapsular, 66920, 66930
      Pars Plana Approach, 66852
      Phacofragmentation Technique, 66850
Lens Material
  Aspiration Technique, 66840
  Pars Plana Approach, 66852
  Phacofragmentation Technique, 66850
LEOPARD Syndrome, 81404, 81406, 81442
LEPR, 81406
Leptomeningioma
  See Meningioma
Leptospira
  Antibody, 86720
Leriche Operation
  Sympathectomy, Thoracolumbar, 64809
Lesion
  See Tumor
  Anal
    Destruction, 46900-46917, 46924
    Excision, 45108, 46922
  Ankle
    Tendon Sheath, 27630
  Arm, Lower
    Tendon Sheath Excision, 25110
  Auditory Canal, External
    Excision
      Exostosis, 69140
      Radical with Neck Dissection, 69155
      Radical without Neck Dissection, 69150
      Soft Tissue, 69145
  Bladder
    Destruction, 51030
  Brain
    Excision, 61534, 61536, 61600-61608, 61615, 61616
    Radiation Treatment, 77432
  Brainstem
    Excision, 61575, 61576
  Breast
    Excision, 19120-19126
  Carotid Body
    Excision, 60600, 60605
  Chemotherapy, 96405, 96406
    Destruction, 67220-67225
  Ciliary Body
    Destruction, 66770
  Colon
    Excision, 44110, 44111
  Conjunctiva
    Destruction, 68135
    Excision, 68110-68130
      with Adjacent Sclera, 68130
      over 1 cm, 68115
    Expression, 68040
  Cornea
    Destruction, 65450
    Excision, 65400

Lesion — *continued*
  Cornea — *continued*
    Excision — *continued*
      of Pterygium, 65420, 65426
  Cranium, 77432
  Destruction
    Ureter, 52341, 52342, 52344, 52345, 52354
  Ear, Middle
    Excision, 69540
  Epididymis
    Excision, 54830
  Esophagus
    Ablation, 43229
    Excision, 43100, 43101
    Removal, 43216
  Excision, 59100
    Bladder, 52224
    Urethra, 52224, 53265
  Eye
    Excision, 65900
  Eyelid
    Destruction, 67850
    Excision
      without Closure, 67840
      Multiple, Different Lids, 67805
      Multiple, Same Lid, 67801
      Single, 67800
      under Anesthesia, 67808
  Facial
    Destruction, 17000-17108, 17280-17286
  Femur
    Excision, 27062
  Finger
    Tendon Sheath, 26160
  Foot
    Excision, 28080, 28090
  Gums
    Destruction, 41850
    Excision, 41822-41828
  Hand
    Tendon Sheath, 26160
  Intestines
    Excision, 44110
  Intestines, Small
    Destruction, 44369
    Excision, 44111
  Iris
    Destruction, 66770
  Larynx
    Excision, 31545-31546
  Leg, Lower
    Tendon Sheath, 27630
  Lymph Node
    Incision and Drainage, 38300, 38305
  Mesentery
    Excision, 44820
  Mouth
    Destruction, 40820
    Excision, 40810-40816, 41116
    Vestibule
      Destruction, 40820
      Repair, 40830
  Nasopharynx
    Excision, 61586, 61600
  Nerve
    Excision, 64774-64792
  Nose
    Intranasal
      External Approach, 30118
      Internal Approach, 30117
  Orbit
    Excision, 61333, 67412
  Palate
    Destruction, 42160
    Excision, 42104-42120
  Pancreas
    Excision, 48120
  Pelvis
    Destruction, 58662
  Penis
    Destruction
      Any Method, 54065
      Cryosurgery, 54056
      Electrodesiccation, 54055
      Extensive, 54065
      Laser Surgery, 54057

Lesion — *continued*
  Penis — *continued*
    Destruction — *continued*
      Simple, 54050-54060
      Surgical Excision, 54060
    Excision, 54060
    Penile Plaque, 54110-54112
  Pharynx
    Destruction, 42808
    Excision, 42808
  Rectum
    Excision, 45108
  Removal
    Larynx, 31512, 31578
  Resection, 52354
  Retina
    Destruction
      Extensive, 67227, 67228
      Localized, 67208, 67210
    Radiation by Implantation of Source, 67218
  Sciatic Nerve
    Excision, 64786
  Sclera
    Excision, 66130
  Skin
    Abrasion, 15786, 15787
    Analysis, Multi-Spectral, 0400T-0401T
    Biopsy, 11100, 11101
    Destruction
      Benign, 17000-17250
      Malignant, 17260-17286
        by Photodynamic Therapy, 96567
      Premalignant, 17000-17004
    Excision
      Benign, 11400-11471
      Malignant, 11600-11646
    Injection, 11900, 11901
    Paring or Curettement, 11055-11057
      Benign Hyperkeratotic, 11055-11057
    Shaving, 11300-11313
  Skin Tags
    Removal, 11200, 11201
  Skull
    Excision, 61500, 61600-61608, 61615, 61616
  Spermatic Cord
    Excision, 55520
  Spinal Cord
    Destruction, 62280-62282
    Excision, 63265-63273
  Stomach
    Excision, 43611
  Testis
    Excision, 54512
  Toe
    Excision, 28092
  Tongue
    Excision, 41110-41114
  Uvula
    Destruction, 42145
    Excision, 42104-42107
  Vagina
    Destruction, 57061, 57065
  Vulva
    Destruction
      Extensive, 56515
      Simple, 56501
  Wrist Tendon
    Excision, 25110
Lesion of Sciatic Nerve
  See Sciatic Nerve, Lesion
Leu 2 Antigens
  See CD8
Leucine Aminopeptidase, 83670
Leukapheresis, 36511
Leukemia Lymphoma Virus I, Adult T Cell
  See HTLV–I
Leukemia Lymphoma Virus I Antibodies, Human T Cell
  See Antibody, HTLV–I
Leukemia Lymphoma Virus II Antibodies, Human T Cell
  See Antibody, HTLV–II
Leukemia Virus II, Hairy Cell Associated, Human T Cell
  See HTLV–II

Leukoagglutinins, 86021
Leukocyte
  See White Blood Cell
  Alkaline Phosphatase, 85540
  Antibody, 86021
  Histamine Release Test, 86343
  Phagocytosis, 86344
  Transfusion, 86950
Leukocyte Count, 85032, 85048, 89055
Leukocyte Histamine Release Test, 86343
Levarterenol
  See Noradrenalin
Levator Muscle Repair
  Blepharoptosis, Repair, 67901-67909
LeVeen Shunt
  Insertion, 49425
  Patency Test, 78291
  Revision, 49426
Levetiracetam
  Assay, 80177
Levulose
  See Fructose
L Glutamine
  See Glutamine
LGV
  Antibody, 86729
LH (Luteinizing Hormone), 80418, 80426, 83002
LHCGR, 81406
LHR (Leukocyte Histamine Release Test), 86343
Liberatory Maneuver, 69710
Lidocaine
  Assay, 80176
Lid Suture
  Blepharoptosis, Repair, 67901-67909
Life Support
  Organ Donor, 01990
Lift, Face
  See Face Lift
Ligament
  See Specific Site
  Collateral
    Repair, Knee with Cruciate Ligament, 27409
  Dentate
    Incision, 63180, 63182
    Section, 63180, 63182
  Injection, 20550
  Release
    Coracoacromial, 23415
    Transverse Carpal, 29848
  Repair
    Elbow, 24343-24346
    Knee Joint, 27405-27409
Ligation
  Appendage
    Dermal, 11200
  Artery
    Abdomen, 37617
    Carotid, 37600-37606
    Chest, 37616
    Coronary, 33502
    Coronary Artery, 33502
    Ethmoidal, 30915
    Extremity, 37618
    Fistula, 37607
    Maxillary, 30920
    Neck, 37615
    Temporal, 37609
  Bronchus, 31899
  Esophageal Varices, 43204, 43400
  Fallopian Tube
    Oviduct, 58600-58611, 58670
  Gastroesophageal, 43405
  Hemorrhoids, 0249T, 45350, 46221 *[46945, 46946]*, *[45398]*
  Inferior Vena Cava, 37619
  Oviducts, 59100
  Salivary Duct, 42665
  Shunt
    Aorta
      Pulmonary, 33924
    Peritoneal
      Venous, 49428
  Thoracic Duct, 38380
    Abdominal Approach, 38382
    Thoracic Approach, 38381
  Thyroid Vessels, 37615

Ligation — *continued*
  Ureter, 53899
  Vas Deferens, 55450
  Vein
    Clusters, 37785
    Esophagus, 43205, 43244, 43400
    Femoral, 37650
    Gastric, 43244
    Iliac, 37660
    Jugular, Internal, 37565
    Perforator, 37760-37761
    Saphenous, 37700-37735, 37780
    Vena Cava, 37619
Ligature Strangulation
  Skin Tags, 11200, 11201
Light Coagulation
  See Photocoagulation
Light Scattering Measurement
  See Nephelometry
Light Therapy, UV
  See Actinotherapy
Limb
  See Extremity
Limited Lymphadenectomy for Staging
  See Lymphadenectomy, Limited, for Staging
Limited Neck Dissection
  with Thyroidectomy, 60252
Limited Resection Mastectomies
  See Breast, Excision, Lesion
Lindholm Operation
  See Tenoplasty
Lingual Bone
  See Hyoid Bone
Lingual Frenectomy
  See Excision, Tongue, Frenum
Lingual Nerve
  Avulsion, 64740
  Incision, 64740
  Transection, 64740
Lingual Tonsil
  See Tonsils, Lingual
Linton Procedure, 37760
Lip
  Biopsy, 40490
  Excision, 40500-40530
    Frenum, 40819
  Incision
    Frenum, 40806
  Reconstruction, 40525, 40527
  Repair, 40650-40654
    Cleft Lip, 40700-40761
    Fistula, 42260
  Unlisted Services and Procedures, 40799
Lipase, 83690
Lip, Cleft
  See Cleft Lip
Lipectomies, Aspiration
  See Liposuction
Lipectomy
  Excision, 15830-15839
  Suction Assisted, 15876-15879
Lipids
  Feces, 82705, 82710
Lipo–Lutin
  See Progesterone
Lipolysis, Aspiration
  See Liposuction
Lipophosphodiesterase I
  See Tissue Typing
Lipoprotein
  (a), 83695
  Blood, 83695, 83700-83721
  LDL, 83700-83701, 83721
  Phospholipase A2, 0423T, 83698
Lipoprotein, Alpha
  See Lipoprotein
Lipoprotein, Pre–Beta
  See Lipoprotein, Blood
Liposuction, 15876-15879
Lips
  Skin Graft
    Delay of Flap, 15630
    Full Thickness, 15260, 15261
    Pedicle Flap, 15576
    Tissue Transfer, Adjacent, 14060, 14061

Lisfranc Operation
  Amputation, Foot, 28800, 28805
Listeria Monocytogenes
  Antibody, 86723
LITAF, 81404
Lithium
  Assay, 80178
Litholapaxy, 52317, 52318
Lithotripsy
  with Cystourethroscopy, 52353
  See Extracorporeal Shock Wave Therapy
  Bile Duct Calculi (Stone)
    Endoscopic, 43265
  Bladder, 52353
  Kidney, 50590, 52353
  Pancreatic Duct Calculi (Stone)
    Endoscopic, 43265
  Ureter, 52353
  Urethra, 52353
Lithotrity
  See Litholapaxy
Liver
  See Hepatic Duct
  Ablation
    Tumor, 47380-47383
      Laparoscopic, 47370-47371
  Abscess
    Aspiration, 47015
    Incision and Drainage
      Open, 47010
    Injection, 47015
  Aspiration, 47015
  Biopsy, 47100
    Anesthesia, 00702
  Cholangiography Injection
    Existing Access, 47531
    New Access, 47532
  Cyst
    Aspiration, 47015
    Incision and Drainage
      Open, 47010
  Excision
    Extensive, 47122
    Partial, 47120, 47125, 47130, 47140-47142
    Total, 47133
  Injection, 47015
    Cholangiography
      Existing Access, 47531
      New Access, 47532
  Lobectomy, 47125, 47130
    Partial, 47120
  Needle Biopsy, 47000, 47001
  Nuclear Medicine
    Imaging, 78201-78216
    Vascular Flow, 78206
  Repair
    Abscess, 47300
    Cyst, 47300
    Wound, 47350-47362
  Suture
    Wound, 47350-47362
  Transplantation, 47135
    Allograft preparation, 47143-47147
    Anesthesia, 00796, 01990
  Trisegmentectomy, 47122
  Ultrasound Scan (LUSS), 76705
  Unlisted Services and Procedures, 47379, 47399
Living Activities, Daily, 97535, 97537
LKP, 65710
L–Leucylnaphthylamidase, 83670
LMNA, 81406
Lobectomy
  Brain, 61323, 61537-61540
  Contralateral Subtotal
    Thyroid Gland, 60212, 60225
  Liver, 47120-47130
  Lung, 32480-32482
    Sleeve, 32486
  Parotid Gland, 42410, 42415
  Segmental, 32663
  Sleeve, 32486
  Temporal Lobe, 61537, 61538
  Thyroid Gland
    Partial, 60210, 60212
    Total, 60220, 60225
  Total, 32663

Local Excision Mastectomies
  See Breast, Excision, Lesion
Local Excision of Lesion or Tissue of Femur
  See Excision, Lesion, Femur
Localization
  Nodule Radiographic, Breast, 19281-19288
    with Biopsy, 19081-19086
  Patient Motion, [77387]
Log Hydrogen Ion Concentration
  See pH
Lombard Test, 92700
Long Acting Thyroid Stimulator
  See Thyrotropin Releasing Hormone (TRH)
Long Chain (C20–C22) Omega–3 Fatty Acids in RBC Membranes, 0111T
Longmire Operation, 47765
Long QT Syndrome Gene Analyses, 81413-81414
Long Term Care Facility Visits
  Annual Assessment, 99318
  Care Plan Oversight Services, 99379-99380
  Discharge Services, 99315-99316
  Initial, 99304-99306
  Subsequent, 99307-99310
Loopogram
  See Urography, Antegrade
Looposcopy, 53899
Loose Body
  Removal
    Ankle, 27620
    Carpometacarpal, 26070
    Elbow, 24101
    Interphalangeal Joint, 28020
      Toe, 28024
    Knee Joint, 27331
    Metatarsophalangeal Joint, 28022
    Tarsometatarsal Joint, 28020
    Toe, 28022
    Wrist, 25101
Lord Procedure
  Anal Sphincter, Dilation, 45905
Lorenz's Operation, 27258
Louis Bar Syndrome, 88248
Low Birth Weight Intensive Care Services, 99478-99480
Low Density Lipoprotein
  See Lipoprotein, LDL
Lower Extremities
  See Extremity, Lower
Lower GI Series
  See Barium Enema
Low Frequency Ultrasound, 97610
Lowsley's Operation, 54380
Low Vision Aids
  Fitting, 92354, 92355
LP, 62270
LRH (Luteinizing Releasing Hormone), 83727
LRP5, 81406
LRRK2, 81401, 81408
L/S, 83661
LSD (Lysergic Acid Diethylamide), 80299, [80305, 80306, 80307]
L/S Ratio
  Amniotic Fluid, 83661
LTH
  See Prolactin
Lucentis Injection, 67028
Lumbar
  See Spine
Lumbar Plexus
  Decompression, 64714
  Injection, Anesthetic, 64449
  Neuroplasty, 64714
  Release, 64714
  Repair
    Suture, 64862
Lumbar Puncture
  See Spinal Tap
Lumbar Spine Fracture
  See Fracture, Vertebra, Lumbar
Lumbar Sympathectomy
  See Sympathectomy, Lumbar
Lumbar Vertebra
  See Vertebra, Lumbar
Lumen Dilation, 74360
Lumpectomy, 19301-19302

Lunate
  Arthroplasty
    with Implant, 25444
  Dislocation
    Closed Treatment, 25690
    Open Treatment, 25695
Lung
  Ablation, 32998
  Abscess
    Incision and Drainage, 32200
  Angiography
    Injection, 93568
  Biopsy, 32096-32097, 32100
  Bullae
    Excision, 32141
      Endoscopic, 32655
  Cyst
    Incision and Drainage, 32200
    Removal, 32140
  Decortication
    with Parietal Pleurectomy, 32320
    Endoscopic, 32651, 32652
    Partial, 32225
    Total, 32220
  Empyema
    Excision, 32540
  Excision
    Bronchus Resection, 32486
    Completion, 32488
    Donor, 33930
      Heart Lung, 33930
      Lung, 32850
    Emphysematous, 32491
    Empyema, 32540
    Lobe, 32480, 32482
    Segment, 32484
    Total, 32440-32445
    Tumor, 32503-32504
    Wedge Resection, 32505-32507
      Endoscopic, 32666-32668
  Foreign Body
    Removal, 32151
  Hemorrhage, 32110
  Injection
    Radiologic, 93568
  Lavage
    Bronchial, 31624
    Total, 32997
  Lysis
    Adhesions, 32124
  Needle Biopsy, 32405
  Nuclear Medicine
    Imaging, Perfusion, 78580-78598
    Imaging, Ventilation, 78579, 78582, 78598
    Unlisted Services and Procedures, 78599
  Pneumolysis, 32940
  Pneumothorax, 32960
  Removal
    Bilobectomy, 32482
    Bronchoplasty, 32501
    Completion Pneumonectomy, 32488
    Extrapleural, 32445
    Single Lobe, 32480
    Single Segment, 32484
    Sleeve Lobectomy, 32486
    Sleeve Pneumonectomy, 32442
    Total Pneumonectomy, 32440-32445
    Two Lobes, 32482
    Volume Reduction, 32491
    Wedge Resection, 32505-32507
  Repair
    Hernia, 32800
  Segmentectomy, 32484
  Tear
    Repair, 32110
  Thoracotomy, 32110-32160
    with Excision–Plication of Bullae, 32141
    with Open Intrapleural Pneumonolysis, 32124
    Biopsy, 32096-32098
    Cardiac Massage, 32160
    for Post–Operative Complications, 32120
    Removal
      Bullae, 32141
      Cyst, 32140
      Intrapleural Foreign Body, 32150

Lung — *continued*
  Thoracotomy — *continued*
    Removal — *continued*
      Intrapulmonary Foreign Body, 32151
    Repair, 32110
  Transplantation, 32851-32854, 33935
    Allograft Preparation, 32855-32856, 33933
    Donor Pneumonectomy
      Heart–Lung, 33930
      Lung, 32850
  Tumor
    Removal, 32503-32504
  Unlisted Services and Procedures, 32999
  Volume Reduction
    Emphysematous, 32491
Lung Function Tests
  See Pulmonology, Diagnostic
Lupus Anticoagulant Assay, 85705
Lupus Band Test
  Immunofluorescence, 88346, [88350]
Luschke Procedure, 45120
LUSCS, 59514-59515, 59618, 59620, 59622
LUSS (Liver Ultrasound Scan), 76705
Luteinizing Hormone (LH), 80418, 80426, 83002
Luteinizing Release Factor, 83727
Luteotropic Hormone, 80418, 84146
Luteotropin, 80418, 84146
Luteotropin Placental, 83632
Lutrepulse Injection, 11980
LVRS, 32491
Lyme Disease, 86617, 86618
Lyme Disease ab, 86617
Lymphadenectomy
  Abdominal, 38747
  Bilateral Inguinofemoral, 54130, 56632, 56637
  Bilateral Pelvic, 51575, 51585, 51595, 54135, 55845, 55865
    Total, 38571, 38572, 57531, 58210
  Diaphragmatic Assessment, 58960
  Gastric, 38747
  Inguinofemoral, 38760, 38765
  Inguinofemoral, Iliac and Pelvic, 56640
  Injection
    Sentinel Node, 38792
  Limited, for Staging
    Para–Aortic, 38562
    Pelvic, 38562
    Retroperitoneal, 38564
  Limited Para–Aortic, Resection of Ovarian Malignancy, 58951
  Limited Pelvic, 55842, 55862, 58954
  Malignancy, 58951, 58954
  Mediastinal, 21632, 32674
  Para–Aortic, 58958
  Pelvic, 58958
  Peripancreatic, 38747
  Portal, 38747
  Radical
    Axillary, 38740, 38745
    Cervical, 38720, 38724
    Groin Area, 38760, 38765
    Pelvic, 54135, 55845, 58548
    Suprahyoid, 38700
  Retroperitoneal Transabdominal, 38780
  Thoracic, 38746
  Unilateral Inguinofemoral, 56631, 56634
Lymphadenitis
  Incision and Drainage, 38300, 38305
Lymphadenopathy Associated Antibodies
  See Antibody, HIV
Lymphadenopathy Associated Virus
  See HIV
Lymphangiogram, Abdominal
  See Lymphangiography, Abdomen
Lymphangiography
  Abdomen, 75805, 75807
  Arm, 75801, 75803
  Injection, 38790
  Leg, 75801, 75803
  Pelvis, 75805, 75807
Lymphangioma, Cystic
  See Hygroma
Lymphangiotomy, 38308
Lymphatic Channels
  Incision, 38308

Lymphatic Cyst
  Drainage
    Laparoscopic, 49323
    Open, 49062
Lymphatic System
  Anesthesia, 00320
  Unlisted Procedure, 38999
Lymph Duct
  Injection, 38790
Lymph Node(s)
  Abscess
    Incision and Drainage, 38300, 38305
  Biopsy, 38500, 38510-38530, 38570
    Needle, 38505
  Dissection, 38542
  Excision, 38500, 38510-38530
    Abdominal, 38747
    Inguinofemoral, 38760, 38765
    Laparoscopic, 38571, 38572
    Limited, for Staging
      Para–Aortic, 38562
      Pelvic, 38562
      Retroperitoneal, 38564
    Pelvic, 38770
    Radical
      Axillary, 38740, 38745
      Cervical, 38720, 38724
      Suprahyoid, 38720, 38724
    Retroperitoneal Transabdominal, 38780
    Thoracic, 38746
  Exploration, 38542
  Hygroma, Cystic
    Axillary
      Cervical
        Excision, 38550, 38555
  Nuclear Medicine
    Imaging, 78195
  Removal
    Abdominal, 38747
    Inguinofemoral, 38760, 38765
    Pelvic, 38747, 38770
    Retroperitoneal Transabdominal, 38780
    Thoracic, 38746
Lymphoblast Transformation
  See Blastogenesis
Lymphocele
  Drainage
    Laparoscopic, 49323
  Extraperitoneal
    Open Drainage, 49062
Lymphocyte
  Culture, 86821, 86822
  Toxicity Assay, 86805, 86806
  Transformation, 86353
Lymphocytes, CD4
  See CD4
Lymphocytes, CD8
  See CD8
Lymphocyte, Thymus–Dependent
  See T–Cells
Lymphocytic Choriomeningitis
  Antibody, 86727
Lymphocytotoxicity, 86805, 86806
Lymphogranuloma Venereum
  Antibody, 86729
Lymphoma Virus, Burkitt
  See Epstein–Barr Virus
Lymph Vessels
  Imaging
    Lymphangiography
      Abdomen, 75805-75807
      Arm, 75801-75803
      Leg, 75801-75803
      Pelvis, 75805-75807
    Nuclear Medicine, 78195
  Incision, 38308
Lynch Procedure, 31075
Lysergic Acid Diethylamide, 80299, [80305, 80306, 80307]
Lysergide, 80299, [80305, 80306, 80307]
Lysis
  Adhesions
    Bladder
      Intraluminal, 53899
    Corneovitreal, 65880
    Epidural, 62263, 62264

Lysis — continued
Adhesions — continued
Fallopian Tube, 58740
Foreskin, 54450
Intestinal, 44005
Labial, 56441
Lung, 32124
Nose, 30560
Ovary, 58740
Oviduct, 58740
Penile
Post–circumcision, 54162
Spermatic Cord, 54699, 55899
Tongue, 41599
Ureter, 50715-50725
Intraluminal, 53899
Urethra, 53500
Uterus, 58559
Euglobulin, 85360
Eye
Goniosynechiae, 65865
Synechiae
Anterior, 65870
Posterior, 65875
Labial
Adhesions, 56441
Nose
Intranasal Synechia, 30560
Transurethral
Adhesions, 53899
Lysozyme, 85549

M

MacEwen Operation
Hernia Repair, Inguinal, 49495-49500, 49505
Incarcerated, 49496, 49501, 49507, 49521
Laparoscopic, 49650, 49651
Recurrent, 49520
Sliding, 49525
Machado Test
Complement, Fixation Test, 86171
MacLean–De Wesselow Test
Clearance, Urea Nitrogen, 84540, 84545
Macrodactylia
Repair, 26590
Macroscopic Examination and Tissue Preparation, 88387
Intraoperative, 88388
Maculopathy, 67208-67218
Madlener Operation, 58600
Magnesium, 83735
Magnetic Resonance Angiography (MRA)
Abdomen, 74185
Arm, 73225
Chest, 71555
Fetal, 74712-74713
Head, 70544-70546
Leg, 73725
Neck, 70547-70549
Pelvis, 72198
Spine, 72159
Magnetic Resonance Spectroscopy, 76390
Magnetic Stimulation
Transcranial, 90867-90869
Magnetoencephalography (MEG), 95965-95967
Magnet Operation
Eye, Removal of Foreign Body
Conjunctival Embedded, 65210
Conjunctival Superficial, 65205
Corneal without Slit Lamp, 65220
Corneal with Slit Lamp, 65222
Intraocular, 65235-65265
Magnuson Procedure, 23450
MAGPI Operation, 54322
Magpi Procedure, 54322
Major Vestibular Gland
See Bartholin's Gland
Malar Area
Augmentation, 21270
Bone Graft, 21210
Fracture
with Bone Grafting, 21366
with Manipulation, 21355
Open Treatment, 21360-21366
Reconstruction, 21270

Malar Bone
See Cheekbone
Malaria Antibody, 86750
Malaria Smear, 87207
Malate Dehydrogenase, 83775
Maldescent, Testis
See Testis, Undescended
Male Circumcision
See Circumcision
Malformation, Arteriovenous
See Arteriovenous Malformation
Malic Dehydrogenase
See Malate Dehydrogenase
Malignant Hyperthermia Susceptibility
Caffeine Halothane Contracture Test (CHCT), 89049
Malleolus
See Ankle; Fibula; Leg, Lower; Tibia; Tibiofibular Joint
Metatarsophalangeal Joint, 27889
Mallet Finger Repair, 26432
Mallory–Weiss Procedure, 43502
Maltose
Tolerance Test, 82951, 82952
Malunion Repair
Femur
with Graft, 27472
without Graft, 27470
Metatarsal, 28322
Tarsal Joint, 28320
Mammalian Oviduct
See Fallopian Tube
Mammaplasties
See Breast, Reconstruction
Mammaplasty, 19318-19325
Mammary Abscess, 19020
Mammary Arteries
See Artery, Mammary
Mammary Duct
X–ray with Contrast, 77053, 77054
Mammary Ductogram
Injection, 19030
Radiologic Supervision and Interpretation, 77053-77054
Mammary Node
Dissection
Anesthesia, 00406
Mammary Stimulating Hormone, 80418, 84146
Mammilliplasty, 19350
Mammogram
with Computer-Aided Detection, 77065-77067
Diagnostic, 77065-77066
Guidance for Placement Localization Device, 19281-19282
Magnetic Resonance Imaging (MRI) with Computer-aided Detection, 0159T
Screening, 77067
Mammography
with Computer-Aided Detection, 77065-77067
Assessment, 3340F-3350F
Diagnostic, 77065-77066
Guidance for Placement Localization Device, 19281-19282
Magnetic Resonance Imaging (MRI) with Computer-Aided Detection, 0159T
Screening, 77067
Mammoplasty
Anesthesia, 00402
Augmentation, 19324, 19325
Reduction, 19318
Mammotomy
See Mastotomy
Mammotropic Hormone, Pituitary, 80418, 84146
Mammotropic Hormone, Placental, 83632
Mammotropin, 80418, 84146
Manchester Colporrhaphy, 58400
Mandated Services
Hospital, on call, 99026, 99027
Mandible
See Facial Bones; Maxilla; Temporomandibular Joint (TMJ)
Abscess
Excision, 21025
Bone Graft, 21215
Cyst
Excision, 21040, 21046, 21047

Mandible — continued
Dysostosis Repair, 21150-21151
Fracture
Closed Treatment
with Interdental Fixation, 21453
with Manipulation, 21451
without Manipulation, 21450
Open Treatment, 21454-21470
with Interdental Fixation, 21462
without Interdental Fixation, 21461
External Fixation, 21454
Percutaneous Treatment, 21452
Osteotomy, 21198, 21199
Reconstruction
with Implant, 21244-21246, 21248, 21249
Removal
Foreign Body, 41806
Torus Mandibularis
Excision, 21031
Tumor
Excision, 21040-21047
X–ray, 70100, 70110
Mandibular Body
Augmentation
with Bone Graft, 21127
with Prosthesis, 21125
Mandibular Condyle
Fracture
Open Treatment, 21465, 21470
Reconstruction, 21247
Mandibular Condylectomy
See Condylectomy
Mandibular Fracture
See Fracture, Mandible
Mandibular Rami
Reconstruction
with Bone Graft, 21194
with Internal Rigid Fixation, 21196
without Bone Graft, 21193
without Internal Rigid Fixation, 21195
Mandibular Resection Prosthesis, 21081
Mandibular Staple Bone Plate
Reconstruction
Mandible, 21244
Manganese, 83785
Manipulation
Chest Wall, 94667-94669
Chiropractic, 98940-98943
Dislocation and/or Fracture
Acetabulum, 27222
Acromioclavicular, 23545
Ankle, 27810, 27818, 27860
Carpometacarpal, 26670-26676
Clavicle, 23505
Elbow, 24300, 24640
Epicondyle, 24565
Femoral, 27232, 27502, 27510, 27517
Peritrochanteric, 27240
Fibula, 27781, 27788
Finger, 26725, 26727, 26742, 26755
Greater Tuberosity
Humeral, 23625
Hand, 26670-26676
Heel, 28405, 28406
Hip, 27257
Hip Socket, 27222
Humeral, 23605, 24505, 24535, 24577
Epicondyle, 24565
Intercarpal, 25660
Interphalangeal Joint, 26340, 26770-26776
Lunate, 25690
Malar Area, 21355
Mandibular, 21451
Metacarpal, 26605, 26607
Metacarpophalangeal, 26700-26706, 26742
Metacarpophalangeal Joint, 26340
Metatarsal Fracture, 28475, 28476
Nasal Bone, 21315, 21320
Orbit, 21401
Phalangeal Shaft, 26727
Distal, Finger or Thumb, 26755
Phalanges, Finger/Thumb, 26725
Phalanges
Finger, 26742, 26755, 26770-26776
Finger/Thumb, 26727
Great Toe, 28495, 28496

Manipulation — continued
Dislocation and/or Fracture — continued
Phalanges — continued
Toes, 28515
Radial, 24655, 25565
Radial Shaft, 25505
Radiocarpal, 25660
Radioulnar, 25675
Scapula, 23575
Shoulder, 23650, 23655
with Greater Tuberosity, 23665
with Surgical or Anatomical Neck, 23675
Sternoclavicular, 23525
with Surgical or Anatomical Neck, 23675
Talus, 28435, 28436
Tarsal, 28455, 28456
Thumb, 26641-26650
Tibial, 27532, 27752
Trans–Scaphoperilunar, 25680
Ulnar, 24675, 25535, 25565
Vertebral, 22315
Wrist, 25259, 25624, 25635, 25660, 25675, 25680, 25690
Foreskin, 54450
Globe, 92018, 92019
Hip, 27275
Interphalangeal Joint, Proximal, 26742
Knee, 27570
Osteopathic, 98925-98929
Palmar Fascial Cord, 26341
Physical Therapy, 97140
Shoulder
Application of Fixation Apparatus, 23700
Spine
Anesthesia, 22505
Stoma, 44799
Temporomandibular Joint (TMJ), 21073
Tibial, Distal, 27762
Manometric Studies
Kidney
Pressure, 50396
Rectum
Anus, 91122
Ureter
Pressure, 50686
Ureterostomy, 50686
Manometry
Esophageal, 43499
Esophagogastric, 91020
Rectum
Anus, 90911
Mantoux Test
Skin Test, 86580
Manual Therapy, 97140
MAP2K1, 81406
MAP2K2, 81406
Mapping
Brain, 96020
for Seizure Activity, 95961-95962
Sentinel Lymph Node, 38900
MAPT, 81406
Maquet Procedure, 27418
Marcellation Operation
Hysterectomy, Vaginal, 58260-58270, 58550
Marrow, Bone
Aspiration, 38220
Harvesting, 38230
Magnetic Resonance Imaging (MRI), 77084
Needle Biopsy, 38221
Nuclear Medicine Imaging, 78102-78104
Smear, 85097
T-Cell Transplantation, 38240-38242
Marshall–Marchetti–Krantz Procedure, 51840, 51841, 58152, 58267, 58293
Marsupialization
Bartholin's Gland Cyst, 56440
Cyst
Acne, 10040
Bartholin's Gland, 56440
Laryngeal, 31599
Splenic, 38999
Sublingual Salivary, 42409
Lesion
Kidney, 53899

Marsupialization — Metacarpal

Marsupialization — *continued*
  Liver
    Cyst or Abscess, 47300
  Pancreatic Cyst, 48500
  Skin, 10040
  Urethral Diverticulum, 53240
Mass
  Kidney
    Ablation, 50542
    Cryosurgery, 50250
Massage
  Cardiac, 32160
  Therapy, 97124
    See Physical Medicine/Therapy/Occupation-
      al Therapy
Masseter Muscle/Bone
  Reduction, 21295, 21296
Mass Spectrometry and Tandem Mass Spectrom-
  etry
  Analyte(s), 83789
Mastectomy
  Gynecomastia, 19300
  Modified Radical, 19307
  Partial, 19301-19302
  Radical, 19305-19306
  Simple, Complete, 19303
  Subcutaneous, 19304
Mastectomy, Halsted
  See Mastectomy, Radical
Masters' 2–Step Stress Test, 93799
Mastoid
  Excision
    Complete, 69502
    Radical, 69511
      Modified, 69505
      Petrous Apicectomy, 69530
      Simple, 69501
      Total, 69502
  Obliteration, 69670
  Repair
    with Apicectomy, 69605
    with Tympanoplasty, 69604
    by Excision, 69601-69603
    Fistula, 69700
Mastoid Cavity
  Debridement, 69220, 69222
Mastoidectomy
  with Apicectomy, 69605
  with Labyrinthectomy, 69910
  with Petrous Apicectomy, 69530
  with Skull Base Surgery, 61591, 61597
    Decompression, 61595
    Facial Nerve, 61595
  with Tympanoplasty, 69604, 69641-69646
    Ossicular Chain Reconstruction, 69642,
      69644, 69646
  Cochlear Device Implantation, 69930
  Complete, 69502
    Revision, 69601-69605
  Osseointegrated Implant
    for External Speech Processor/Cochlear
      Stimulator, 69715, 69718
  Ossicular Chain Reconstruction, 69605
  Radical, 69511
    Modified, 69505
    Revision, 69602, 69603
  Revision, 69601
  Simple, 69501
Mastoidotomy, 69635-69637
  with Tympanoplasty, 69635
    Ossicular Chain Reconstruction, 69636
      and Synthetic Prosthesis, 69637
Mastoids
  Polytomography, 76101, 76102
  X–ray, 70120, 70130
Mastopexy, 19316
Mastotomy, 19020
Maternity Care and Delivery, 0500F-0502F, 0503F,
  59400-59898
  See also Abortion, Cesarean Delivery, Ectopic
    Pregnancy, Vaginal Delivery
Maxilla
  See Facial Bones; Mandible
  Bone Graft, 21210
  CT Scan, 70486-70488
  Cyst, Excision, 21048, 21049

Maxilla — *continued*
  Excision, 21030, 21032-21034
  Fracture
    with Fixation, 21345-21347
    Closed Treatment, 21345, 21421
    Open Treatment, 21346-21348, 21422,
      21423
  Osteotomy, 21206
  Reconstruction
    with Implant, 21245, 21246, 21248, 21249
  Tumor
    Excision, 21048-21049
Maxillary Sinus
  Antrostomy, 31256-31267
  Dilation, 31295
  Excision, 31225-31230
  Exploration, 31020-31032
  Incision, 31020-31032, 31256-31267
  Irrigation, 31000
  Skull Base, 61581
Maxillary Torus Palatinus
  Tumor Excision, 21032
Maxillectomy, 31225, 31230
Maxillofacial Fixation
  Application
    Halo Type Appliance, 21100
Maxillofacial Impressions
  Auricular Prosthesis, 21086
  Definitive Obturator Prosthesis, 21080
  Facial Prosthesis, 21088
  Interim Obturator Prosthesis, 21079
  Mandibular Resection Prosthesis, 21081
  Nasal Prosthesis, 21087
  Oral Surgical Splint, 21085
  Orbital Prosthesis, 21077
  Palatal Augmentation Prosthesis, 21082
  Palatal Lift Prosthesis, 21083
  Speech Aid Prosthesis, 21084
  Surgical Obturator Prosthesis, 21076
Maxillofacial Procedures
  Unlisted Services and Procedures, 21299
Maxillofacial Prosthetics, 21076-21088
  Unlisted Services and Procedures, 21089
Maydl Operation, 45563, 50810
Mayo Hernia Repair, 49580-49587
Mayo Operation
  Varicose Vein Removal, 37700-37735, 37780,
    37785
Maze Procedure, 33254-33259, 33265-33266
MBC, 87181-87190
MC4R, 81403
McBurney Operation
  Hernia Repair, Inguinal, 49495-49500, 49505
    Incarcerated, 49496, 49501, 49507, 49521
    Recurrent, 49520
    Sliding, 49525
McCall Culdoplasty, 57283
McCannel Procedure, 66682
McCauley Procedure, 28240
MCCC1, 81406
MCCC2, 81406
McDonald Operation, 57700
McKissock Surgery, 19318
McIndoe Procedure, 57291
MCOLN1, 81290, 81412
McVay Operation
  Hernia Repair, Inguinal, 49495-49500, 49505
    Incarcerated, 49496, 49501, 49507, 49521
    Laparoscopic, 49650, 49651
    Recurrent, 49520
    Sliding, 49525
MEA (Microwave Endometrial Ablation), 58563
Measles, German
  Antibody, 86756
  Vaccine, 90707, 90710
Measles Immunization, 90707, 90710
Measles, Mumps, Rubella Vaccine, 90707
Measles Uncomplicated
  Antibody, 86765
  Antigen Detection, 87283
Measles Vaccine, 90707, 90710
Measurement
  Ocular Blood Flow, 0198T
  Spirometric Forced Expiratory Flow, 94011-
    94012

Meat Fibers
  Feces, 89160
Meatoplasty, 69310
Meatotomy, 53020-53025
  Contact Laser Vaporization with/without
    Transurethral Resection of Prostate,
    52648
    with Cystourethroscopy, 52281
  Infant, 53025
  Non–Contact Laser Coagulation Prostate, 52647
  Prostate
    Laser Coagulation, 52647
    Laser Vaporization, 52648
  Transurethral Electrosurgical Resection
    Prostate, 52601
  Ureter, 52290
  Urethral
    Cystourethroscopy, 52290-52305
Meckel's Diverticulum
  Excision, 44800
  Unlisted Services and Procedures, 44899
MECP2, 81302-81304
MED12, 81401
Median Nerve
  Decompression, 64721
  Neuroplasty, 64721
  Release, 64721
  Repair
    Suture
      Motor, 64835
  Transposition, 64721
Median Nerve Compression
  Decompression, 64721
    Endoscopy, 29848
    Injection, 20526
Mediastinoscopy
  with Biopsy, 39401-39402
  with Esophagogastric Fundoplasty, [43210]
Mediastinotomy
  Cervical Approach, 39000
  Transthoracic Approach, 39010
Mediastinum
  See Chest; Thorax
  Cyst
    Excision, 32662, 39200
  Endoscopy
    Biopsy, 39401-39402
    Esophagogastric Fundoplasty, [43210]
    Exploration, 39401
  Exploration, 39000, 39010
  Incision and Drainage, 39000, 39010
  Lymphadenectomy, 32674
  Needle Biopsy, 32405
  Removal
    Foreign Body, 39000, 39010
  Tumor
    Excision, 32662, 39200
  Unlisted Procedures, 39499
Medical Disability Evaluation Services, 99455,
  99456
Medical Genetics
  Counseling, 96040
Medical Nutrition Therapy, 97802-97804
Medical Team Conference, 99366-99368
Medical Testimony, 99075
Medication Therapy Management
  By a Pharmacist
    Initial Encounter, 99605-99606
    Subsequent Encounter, 99607
    Each Additional 15 Minutes, 99607
Medicine, Preventive
  See Preventive Medicine
Medicine, Pulmonary
  See Pulmonology
MEFV, 81402, 81404
MEG (Magnetoencephalography), 95965-95967
MEG3/DLK1, 81401
Meibomian Cyst
  Excision, 67805
    Multiple
      Different Lids, 67805
      Same Lid, 67801
    Single, 67800
    Under Anesthesia, 67808
Membrane, Mucous
  See Mucosa

Membrane, Tympanic
  See Ear, Drum
MEN1, 81404-81405
Menactra, 90734
Meninges
  Tumor
    Excision, 61512, 61519
Meningioma
  Excision, 61512, 61519
  Tumor
    Excision, 61512, 61519
Meningitis, Lymphocytic Benign
  Antibody, 86727
Meningocele Repair, 63700, 63702
Meningococcal Vaccine
  Conjugate, Serogroups A, C, Y, MCV4, Men-
    ACWY, W-135, 90734
  Conjugate, Serogroups C & Y and Hemophilus
    Influenza B, 90644
  Polysaccharide, Any Groups, 90733
  Recombinant, 90620-90621
Meningococcus, 86741
Meningomyelocele
  Repair, 63704-63706
Meniscal Temporal Lobectomy, 61566
Meniscectomy
  Knee Joint, 27332, 27333
  Temporomandibular Joint, 21060
Meniscus
  Knee
    Excision, 27332, 27333
    Repair, 27403
    Transplantation, 29868
Menomune, 90733
Mental Nerve
  Avulsion, 64736
  Incision, 64736
  Transection, 64736
Menveo, 90734
Meprobamate, [80369, 80370]
Mercury, 83015, 83825
Merskey Test
  Fibrin Degradation Products, 85362-85379
Mesencephalic Tract
  Incision, 61480
  Section, 61480
Mesencephalon
  Tractotomy, 61480
Mesenteric Arteries
  See Artery, Mesenteric
Mesentery
  Lesion
    Excision, 44820
  Repair, 44850
  Suture, 44850
  Unlisted Services and Procedures, 44899
Mesh
  Implantation
    Hernia, 49568
  Insertion
    Pelvic Floor, 57267
  Removal
    Abdominal Infected, 11008
Mesh Implantation
  Closure of Necrotizing Soft Tissue Infection,
    49568
  Incisional or Ventral Hernia, 49568
  Vagina, 57267
Metabisulfite Test
  Red Blood Cell, Sickling, 85660
Metabolic Panel
  Calcium Ionized, 80047
  Calcium Total, 80048
  Comprehensive, 80053
Metabolite
  Cocaine, [80353]
  Thromboxane, 84431
Metacarpal
  Amputation, 26910
  Craterization, 26230
  Cyst
    Excision, 26200, 26205
  Diaphysectomy, 26230
  Excision, 26230
    Radical for Tumor, 26250

Metacarpal — *continued*
Fracture
with Manipulation, 26605, 26607
without Manipulation, 26600
Closed Treatment, 26605
with Fixation, 26607
Open Treatment, 26615
Percutaneous Fixation, 26608
Ostectomy
Radical
for Tumor, 26250
Repair
Lengthening, 26568
Nonunion, 26546
Osteotomy, 26565
Saucerization, 26230
Tumor
Excision, 26200, 26205
Metacarpophalangeal Joint
Arthrodesis, 26850, 26852
Arthroplasty, 26530, 26531
Arthroscopy
Diagnostic, 29900
Surgical, 29901, 29902
Arthrotomy, 26075
Biopsy
Synovium, 26105
Capsule
Excision, 26520
Incision, 26520
Capsulodesis, 26516-26518
Dislocation
with Manipulation, 26340
Closed Treatment, 26700
Open Treatment, 26715
Percutaneous Fixation, 26705, 26706
Exploration, 26075
Fracture
with Manipulation, 26742
Closed Treatment, 26740
Open Treatment, 26746
Fusion, 26516-26518, 26850, 26852
Removal of Foreign Body, 26075
Repair
Collateral Ligament, 26540-26542
Synovectomy, 26135
Metadrenaline, 83835
Metals, Heavy, 83015, 83018
Metanephrine, 83835
Metatarsal
See Foot
Amputation, 28810
Condyle
Excision, 28288
Craterization, 28122
Cyst
Excision, 28104-28107
Diaphysectomy, 28122
Excision, 28110-28114, 28122, 28140
Fracture
Closed Treatment
with Manipulation, 28475, 28476
without Manipulation, 28470
Open Treatment, 28485
Percutaneous Fixation, 28476
Free Osteocutaneous Flap with Microvascular
Anastomosis, 20972
Repair, 28322
Lengthening, 28306, 28307
Osteotomy, 28306-28309
Saucerization, 28122
Tumor
Excision, 28104-28107, 28173
Metatarsectomy, 28140
Metatarsophalangeal Joint
Arthrotomy, 28022, 28052
Cheilectomy, 28289, 28291
Dislocation, 28630, 28635, 28645
Open Treatment, 28645
Percutaneous Fixation, 28636
Exploration, 28022
Great Toe
Arthrodesis, 28750
Fusion, 28750
Release, 28289, 28291

Metatarsophalangeal Joint — *continued*
Removal
of Foreign Body, 28022
of Loose Body, 28022
Repair
Hallux Rigidus, 28289, 28291
Synovial
Biopsy, 28052
Excision, 28072
Toe, 28270
Methadone, *[80358]*
Methaemoglobin, 83045-83050
Methamphetamine, *[80359]*
Methbipyranone, 80436
Methemalbumin, 83857
Methemoglobin, 83045, 83050, 88741
Methenamine Silver Stain, 88312
Methopyrapone, 80436
Methoxyhydroxymandelic Acid, 84585
Methsuximide, *[80339, 80340, 80341]*
Methyl Alcohol, *[80320]*
Methylamphetamine, *[80359]*
Methyl CpG Binding Protein 2 Gene Analysis,
81302-81304
Methylfluorprednisolone, 80420
Methylmorphine
See Codeine
Metroplasty, 58540
Metyrapone, 80436
MFN2, 81406
Mg, 83735
MGMT, *[81287]*
MIC (Minimum Inhibitory Concentration), 87186
MICA, 81403
Microalbumin
Urine, 82043, 82044
Microbiology, 87003-87999 *[87623, 87624, 87625,*
87806, 87906, 87910, 87912]
Microdissection, 88380-88381
Microfluorometries, Flow, 88182-88189
Diagnostic/Pretreatment, 3170F
Microglobulin, Beta 2
Blood, 82232
Urine, 82232
Micrographic Surgery
Mohs Technique, 17311-17315
Micro–Ophthalmia
Orbit Reconstruction, 21256
Micropigmentation
Correction, 11920-11922
Micro-Remodeling Female Bladder, 53860
Microsatellite Instability Analysis, 81301
Microscope, Surgical
See Operating Microscope
Microscopic Evaluation
Hair, 96902
Microscopies, Electron
See Electron Microscopy
Microscopy
Ear Exam, 92504
Microsomal Antibody, 86376
Microsomia, Hemifacial
See Hemifacial Microsomia
Microsurgery
Operating Microscope, 69990
Microvascular Anastomosis
Bone Graft
Fibula, 20955
Other, 20962
Facial Flap, Free, 15758
Muscle Flap, Free, 15756
Osteocutaneous Flap with, 20969-20973
Skin Flap, Free, 15757
Microvite A, 84590
Microvolt T-Wave Alternans, 93025
Microwave Therapy, 97024
See Physical Medicine/Therapy/Occupational
Therapy
Midbrain
See Brain; Brainstem; Mesencephalon; Skull Base
Surgery
Midcarpal Medioccipital Joint
Arthrotomy, 25040
Middle Cerebral Artery Velocimetry, 76821
Middle Ear
See Ear, Middle

Midface
Reconstruction
with Bone Graft, 21145-21159, 21188
without Bone Graft, 21141-21143
Forehead Advancement, 21159, 21160
MIF (Migration Inhibitory Factor), 86378
Migration Inhibitory Factor (MIF), 86378
Mile Operation, 44155, 44156
Milia, Multiple
Removal, 10040
Miller–Abbott Intubation, 44500, 74340
Miller Procedure, 28737
Millin-Read Operation, 57288
Minerva Cast, 29040
Removal, 29710
Minimum Inhibitory Concentration, 87186
Minimum Lethal Concentration, 87187
Minnesota Multiple Personality Inventory,
96101-96103
Miscarriage
Incomplete Abortion, 59812
Missed Abortion
First Trimester, 59820
Second Trimester, 59821
Septic Abortion, 59830
Missed Abortion
First Trimester, 59820
Second Trimester, 59821
Mitochondrial Antibody, 86255, 86256
Mitochondrial Genome Deletions, 81405
Mitogen Blastogenesis, 86353
Mitral Valve
Incision, 33420, 33422
Repair, 33420-33427
Incision, 33420, 33422
Transcatheter, 0345T, 33418-33419, 93590,
93592
Replacement, 33430
Mitrofanoff Operation, 50845
Miyagawanella
See Chlamydia
Antibody, 86631-86632
Antigen Detection
Direct Fluorescence, 87270
Enzyme Immunoassay, 87320
Culture, 87110
MLB Test, 92562
MLC, 86821
MLH1, 81292-81294, 81432-81433, 81435-81436,
[81288]
MLL/AFF1 (t(4;11)), 81401
MLL/MLLT3 (t(9;11)), 81401
MMAA, 81405
MMAB, 81405
MMACHC, 81404
MMK, 51841
MMPI, 96101-96103
Computer Assisted, 96103
MMRV, 90710
MMR Vaccine, 90707
Mobilization
Splenic Flexure, 44139
Laparoscopic, 44213
Stapes, 69650
Moderate Sedation, 99151-99157
Modified Radical Mastectomy, 19307
Modulation System, Cardiac, 0408T-0418T
Mohs Micrographic Surgery, 17311-17315
Molar Pregnancy
Evacuation and Curettage, 59870
Excision, 59100
Mold
Culture, 87107
Mole, Carneous
See Abortion
Molecular
Cytogenetics, 88271-88275
Interpretation and Report, 88291
MAAA, 81500-81599
Administrative, 0001M-0004M
Category I, 81500-81599
Oxygen Saturation, 82803-82810
Pathology
Tier 1 Procedures, 81200-81383, *[81161]*
Tier 2 Procedures, 81400-81408, 81479

Mole, Hydatid
Evacuation and Curettage, 59870
Excision, 59100
Molluscum Contagiosum Destruction
Penis, 54050-54060
Skin, 17110-17111
Vulva, 56501-56515
Molteno Procedure, 66180
Molteno Valve
Insertion, 66180
Removal, 67120
Revision, 66185
Monilia
Antibody, 86628
Skin Test, 86485
Monitoring
Blood Pressure, 24 hour, 93784-93790
Electrocardiogram
External, 93224-93272
Electroencephalogram, 95812, 95813, 95950-
95953, 95956
with Drug Activation, 95954
with Physical Activation, 95954
with WADA Activation, 95958
Fetal
During Labor, 59050, 59051, 99500
Interpretation Only, 59051
Glucose
Interstitial Fluid, 95250-95251
Interstitial Fluid Pressure, 20950
Intraocular Pressure, 0329T
Pediatric Apnea, 94774-94777
Prolonged, with Physician Attendance, 99354-
99360
Seizure, 61531, 61760
Monitoring, Sleep, 95808-95811
Monoethylene Glycol, 82693
Mononuclear Cell Antigen
Quantitative, 86356
Mononucleosis Virus, Infectious, 86663-86665
Monophosphate, Adenosine, 82030
Monophosphate, Adenosine Cyclic, 82030
Monospot Test, 86308
Monteggia Fracture, 24620, 24635
Monticelli Procedure, 20690, 20692
Morbilli
See Rubeola
Morphine Methyl Ether
See Codeine
Morphometric Analysis
Nerve, 88356
Skeletal Muscle, 88355
Tumor, 88358-88361
Morton's Neuroma
Excision, 28080
Mosaicplasty, 27416, 29866-29867
Moschcowitz Operation
Repair, Hernia, Femoral, 49550-49557
Mosenthal Test, 81002
Mother Cell
See Stem Cell
Motility Study
Colon, 91117
Duodenal, 91022
Esophagus, 91010, 91013
Imaging, 78258
Sperm, 89300
Motion Analysis
by Video and 3–D Kinematics, 96000, 96004
Computer–based, 96000, 96004
Motor Function Mapping Using nTMS, 0310T
Mousseaux–Barbin Procedure, 43510
Mouth
Abscess
Incision and Drainage, 40800, 40801,
41005-41009, 41015-41018
Biopsy, 40808, 41108
Cyst
Incision and Drainage, 40800, 40801,
41005-41009, 41015-41018
Excision
Frenum, 40819
Hematoma
Incision and Drainage, 40800, 40801,
41005-41009, 41015-41018

Mouth — *continued*
- Lesion
    - Destruction, 40820
    - Excision, 40810-40816, 41116
    - Vestibule of
        - Destruction, 40820
        - Repair, 40830
- Mucosa
    - Excision, 40818
- Reconstruction, 40840-40845
- Removal
    - Foreign Body, 40804, 40805
- Repair
    - Laceration, 40830, 40831
- Skin Graft
    - Full Thickness, 15240, 15241
    - Pedicle Flap, 15574
    - Split, 15120, 15121
- Tissue Transfer, Adjacent, 14040, 14041
- Unlisted Services and Procedures, 40899, 41599
- Vestibule
    - Excision
        - Destruction, 40808-40820
    - Incision, 40800-40806
    - Other Procedures, 40899
    - Removal
        - Foreign Body, 40804
    - Repair, 40830-40845

Move
- *See* Transfer
- Finger, 26555
- Toe Joint, 26556
- Toe to Hand, 26551-26554

Moynihan Test
- Gastrointestinal Tract, X–ray, with Contrast, 74246-74249

MPI, 81405
MPL, 81402-81403
MPO, 83876
MPR (Multifetal Pregnancy Reduction), 59866
MPV17, 81404-81405
MPZ, 81405
MRA (Magnetic Resonance Angiography), 71555, 72159, 72198, 73225, 73725, 74185
MRCP (Magnetic Resonance Cholangiopancreatography), 74181
MRI (Magnetic Resonance Imaging)
- 3D Rendering, 76376-76377
- Abdomen, 74181-74183
- Ankle, 73721-73723
- Arm, 73218-73220, 73223
- Bone Marrow Study, 77084
- Brain, 70551-70553
    - Functional, 70554-70555
    - Intraoperative, 0398T, 70557-70559
- Breast, 77058-77059
    - with Computer-Aided Detection, 0159T
- Chest, 71550-71552
- Elbow, 73221
- Face, 70540-70543
- Fetal, 74712-74713
- Finger Joint, 73221
- Foot, 73718, 73719
- Foot Joints, 73721-73723
- Guidance
    - Intracranial Stereotactic Ablation Lesion, 0398T
    - Needle Placement, 77021
    - Parenchymal Tissue Ablation, 77022
    - Tissue Ablation, 77022
- Hand, 73218-73220, 73223
- Heart, 75557-75563
    - Complete Study, 75557-75563, 75565
    - Flow Mapping, 75565
    - Morphology, 75557-75563
- Joint
    - Lower Extremity, 73721-73723
    - Upper Extremity, 73221-73223
- Knee, 73721-73723
- Leg, 73718-73720
- Neck, 70540-70543
- Orbit, 70540-70543
- Pelvis, 72195-72197
- Radiology
    - Unlisted Diagnostic Procedure, 76499
- Spectroscopy, 76390

MRI (Magnetic Resonance Imaging) — *continued*
- Spine
    - Cervical, 72141, 72142, 72156-72158
    - Lumbar, 72148-72158
    - Thoracic, 72146, 72147, 72156-72158
- Temporomandibular Joint (TMJ), 70336
- Toe, 73721-73723
- Unlisted, 76498
- Wrist, 73221

MRS (Magnetic Resonance Spectroscopy), 76390
MR Spectroscopy
- *See* Magnetic Resonance Spectroscopy
MSH2, 81295-81297, 81432-81433, 81435-81436
MSH6, 81298-81300, 81432-81433, 81435
MSLT, 95805
MT-ATP6, 81401
MTHFR, 81291
MTM1, 81405-81406
MT-ND4, 81401
MT-ND5, 81401
MT-ND6, 81401
MT-RNR1, 81401, 81403
MT-TK, 81401
MT-TL1, 81401
MT-TS1, 81401, 81403
MTWA (Microvolt T-Wave Alternans), 93025
Mucin
- Synovial Fluid, 83872
Mucocele
- Sinusotomy
    - Frontal, 31075
Mucolipin 1, 81290
Mucopolysaccharides, 83864
Mucormycoses
- *See* Mucormycosis
Mucormycosis
- Antibody, 86732
Mucosa
- Cautery, 30801-30802
- Destruction
    - Cautery, 30801-30802
    - Photodynamic Therapy, 96567
- Ectopic Gastric Imaging, 78290
- Excision of Lesion
    - Alveolar, Hyperplastic, 41828
    - Vestibule of Mouth, 40810-40818
    - via Esophagoscopy, 43229
    - via Small Intestinal Endoscopy, 44369
    - via Upper GI Endoscopy, [43270]
- Periodontal Grafting, 41870
- Urethra, Mucosal Advancement, 53450
- Vaginal Biopsy, 57100, 57105
Mucosa, Buccal
- *See* Mouth, Mucosa
Mucosectomy
- Rectal, 44799, 45113
Mucous Cyst
- Hand or finger, 26160
Mucous Membrane
- *See* Mouth, Mucosa
- Cutaneous
    - Biopsy, 11100, 11101
    - Excision
        - Benign Lesion, 11440-11446
        - Malignant, 11640-11646
    - Layer Closure, Wounds, 12051-12057
    - Simple Repair, Wounds, 12011-12018
- Excision
    - Sphenoid Sinus, 31288
- Lid Margin
    - Correction of Trichiasis, 67835
    - Nasal Test, 95065
    - Ophthalmic Test, 95060
- Rectum
    - Proctoplasty for Prolapse, 45505
Mucus Cyst
- *See* Mucous Cyst
MUGA (Multiple Gated Acquisition), 78453, 78454, 78472-78473, 78483
Muller Procedure
- Attended, 95806
- Unattended, 95807
Multianalyte Assays with Algorithmic Analyses, 0001M-0004M, 0006M-0009M, 81500, 81503-81504, 81506-81512, 81599

Multifetal Pregnancy Reduction, 59866
Multiple Sleep Latency Testing (MSLT), 95805
Multiple Valve Procedures
- *See* Valvuloplasty
Mumford Operation, 29824
Mumford Procedure, 23120, 29824
Mumps
- Antibody, 86735
- Immunization, 90707, 90710
- Vaccine
    - MMR, 90707
    - MMRV, 90710
Muramidase, 85549
Murine Typhus, 86000
Muscle(s)
- *See* Specific Muscle
- Abdomen
    - *See* Abdominal Wall
- Biofeedback Training, 90911
- Biopsy, 20200-20206
- Chemodenervation
    - Extremity, 64642-64645
    - Larynx, 64617
    - Neck, 64616
    - Trunk, 64646-64647
- Debridement
    - Infected, 11004-11006
- Heart
    - *See* Myocardium
- Neck
    - *See* Neck Muscle
- Removal
    - Foreign Body, 20520, 20525
- Repair
    - Extraocular, 65290
    - Forearm, 25260-25274
    - Wrist, 25260-25274
- Revision
    - Arm, Upper, 24330, 24331
    - Elbow, 24301
- Transfer
    - Arm, Upper, 24301, 24320
    - Elbow, 24301
    - Femur, 27110
    - Hip, 27100-27105, 27111
    - Shoulder, 23395, 23397, 24301, 24320
Muscle Compartment Syndrome
- Detection, 20950
Muscle Denervation
- *See* Chemodenervation
Muscle Division
- Scalenus Anticus, 21700, 21705
- Sternocleidomastoid, 21720, 21725
Muscle Flaps, 15731-15738
- Free, 15756
Muscle Grafts, 15841-15845
Muscle, Oculomotor
- *See* Eye Muscles
Muscle Testing
- Dynamometry, Eye, 92260
- Extraocular Multiple Muscles, 92265
- Manual, 95831-95834
Musculoplasty
- *See* Muscle, Repair
Musculoskeletal System
- Computer Assisted Surgical Navigational Procedure, 0054T-0055T, 20985
- Unlisted Services and Procedures, 20999, 21499, 24999, 25999, 26989, 27299, 27599, 27899
- Unlisted Services and Procedures, Head, 21499
Musculotendinous (Rotator) Cuff
- Repair, 23410, 23412
Mustard Procedure, 33774-33777
- *See* Repair, Great Arteries, Revision
MUT, 81406
MutL Homolog 1, Colon Cancer, Nonpolyposis Type 2 Gene Analysis, 81292-81294
MutS Homolog 2, Colon Cancer, Nonpolyposis Type 1 Gene Analysis, 81295-81297
MutS Homolog 6 (E. Coli) Gene Analysis, 81298-81300
MUTYH, 81401, 81406, 81435
MVD (Microvascular Decompression), 61450
MVR, 33430

Myasthenia Gravis
- Cholinesterase Inhibitor Challenge Test, 95857
Myasthenic, Gravis
- *See* Myasthenia Gravis
MYBPC3, 81407
Mycobacteria
- Culture, 87116
    - Identification, 87118
- Detection, 87550-87562
- Sensitivity Studies, 87190
Mycophenolate
- Assay, 80180
Mycoplasma
- Antibody, 86738
- Culture, 87109
- Detection, 87580-87582
Mycota
- *See* Fungus
Myectomy, Anorectal
- *See* Myomectomy, Anorectal
Myelencephalon
- *See* Medulla
Myelin Basic Protein
- Cerebrospinal Fluid, 83873
Myelography
- Brain, 70010
- Spine
    - Cervical, 62302, 72240
    - Lumbosacral, 62304, 72265
    - Thoracic, 62303, 72255
    - Two or More Regions, 62305, 72270
Myelomeningocele
- Repair, 63704, 63706
- Stereotaxis
    - Creation Lesion, 63600
Myeloperoxidase, 83876
Myelotomy, 63170
MYH11, 81408, 81410-81411
MYH6, 81407
MYH7, 81407
MYL2, 81405
MYL3, 81405
MYO15A, 81430
MYO7A, 81430
Myocardial
- Imaging, 0331T-0332T, 0399T, 78466, 78468, 78469
- Perfusion Imaging, 0439T, 78451-78454
    - *See* Nuclear Medicine
- Positron Emission Tomography (PET), 78459, 78491, 78492
- Repair
    - Postinfarction, 33542
Myocardium, 33140-33141
Myocutaneous Flaps, 15732-15738, 15756
Myofascial Pain Dysfunction Syndrome
- *See* Temporomandibular Joint (TMJ)
Myofascial Release, 97140
Myofibroma
- Embolization, 37243
- Removal, 58140, 58545-58546, 58561
Myoglobin, 83874
Myomectomy
- Anorectal, 45108
- Uterus, 58140-58146, 58545, 58546
Myoplasty
- Extraocular, 65290, 67346
MYOT, 81405
Myotomy
- Esophagus, 43030
- Hyoid, 21685
- Sigmoid Colon
    - Intestine, 44799
    - Rectum, 45999
Myringoplasty, 69620
Myringostomy, 69420-69421
Myringotomy, 69420, 69421
Myxoid Cyst
- Aspiration/Injection, 20612
- Drainage, 20612
- Wrist
    - Excision, 25111-25112

N

Na, 84295
Nabi-HIB, 90371

Naffziger Operation, 61330
Nagel Test, 92283
Nail Bed
  Reconstruction, 11762
  Repair, 11760
Nail Fold
  Excision
    Wedge, 11765
Nail Plate Separation
  See Onychia
Nails
  Avulsion, 11730, 11732
  Biopsy, 11755
  Debridement, 11720, 11721
  Drainage, 10060-10061
  Evacuation
    Hematoma, Subungual, 11740
  Excision, 11750
    Finger, 26236
    Toe, 28124, 28160
  KOH Examination, 87220
  Removal, 11730, 11732, 11750, 26236, 28124, 28160
  Trimming, 11719
Narcoanalysis, 90865
Narcosynthesis
  Diagnostic and Therapeutic, 90865
Nasal
  Abscess, 30000-30020
  Bleeding, 30901-30906, 31238
  Bone
    Fracture
      with Manipulation, 21315, 21320
      without Manipulation, 21310
      Closed Treatment, 21310-21320
      Open Treatment, 21325-21335
    X–ray, 70160
  Deformity Repair, 40700-40761
  Function Study, 92512
  Polyp
    Excision
      Extensive, 30115
      Simple, 30110
  Prosthesis
    Impression, 21087
  Septum
    Abscess
      Incision and Drainage, 30020
    Fracture
      Closed Treatment, 21337
      Open Treatment, 21336
    Hematoma
      Incision and Drainage, 30020
    Repair, 30630
    Submucous Resection, 30520
  Sinuses
    See Sinus; Sinuses
  Smear
    Eosinophils, 89190
  Turbinate
    Fracture
      Therapeutic, 30930
Nasoethmoid Complex
  Fracture
    Open Treatment, 21338, 21339
    Percutaneous Treatment, 21340
  Reconstruction, 21182-21184
Nasogastric Tube
  Placement, 43752
Nasolacrimal Duct
  Exploration, 68810
    with Anesthesia, 68811
  Insertion
    Stent, 68815
  Probing, 68816
  X–ray
    with Contrast, 70170
Nasomaxillary
  Fracture
    with Bone Grafting, 21348
    Closed Treatment, 21345
    Open Treatment, 21346-21348
Nasopharynges
  See Nasopharynx
Nasopharyngoscopy, 92511

Nasopharynx
  See Pharynx
  Biopsy, 42804, 42806
  Hemorrhage, 42970-42972
  Unlisted Services and Procedures, 42999
Natriuretic Peptide, 83880
Natural Killer Cells (NK)
  Total Count, 86357
Natural Ostium
  Sinus
    Maxillary, 31000
    Sphenoid, 31002
Navicular
  Arthroplasty
    with Implant, 25443
  Fracture
    with Manipulation, 25624
    Closed Treatment, 25622
    Open Treatment, 25628
  Repair, 25440
Navigation
  Computer Assisted, 20985, 61781-61783
NDP, 81403-81404
NDUFA1, 81404
NDUFAF2, 81404
NDUFS1, 81406
NDUFS4, 81404
NDUFS7, 81405
NDUFS8, 81405
NDUFV1, 81405
NEB, 81400, 81408
Neck
  Angiography, 70498, 70547-70549
  Artery
    Ligation, 37615
  Biopsy, 21550
  Bypass Graft, 35901
  CT Scan, 70490-70492, 70498
  Dissection, Radical
    See Radical Neck Dissection
  Exploration
    Blood Vessels, 35800
    Lymph Nodes, 38542
  Incision and Drainage
    Abscess, 21501, 21502
    Hematoma, 21501, 21502
  Lipectomy, Suction Assisted, 15876
  Magnetic Resonance Angiography (MRA), 70547-70549
  Magnetic Resonance Imaging (MRI), 70540-70543
  Nerve
    Graft, 64885, 64886
  Repair
    with Other Graft, 35261
    with Vein Graft, 35231
    Blood Vessel, 35201
  Rhytidectomy, 15825, 15828
  Skin
    Revision, 15819
  Skin Graft
    Delay of Flap, 15620
    Full Thickness, 15240, 15241
    Pedicle Flap, 15574
    Split, 15120, 15121
  Surgery, Unlisted, 21899
  Tissue Transfer, Adjacent, 14040, 14041
  Tumor, 21555-21558 *[21552, 21554]*
  Ultrasound Exam, 76536
  Unlisted Services and Procedures, 21899
  Urinary Bladder
    See Bladder, Neck
  Wound Exploration
    Penetrating, 20100
    X–ray, 70360
Neck, Humerus
  Fracture
    with Shoulder Dislocation
      Closed Treatment, 23680
      Open Treatment, 23675
Neck Muscle
  Division, Scalenus Anticus, 21700, 21705
    Sternocleidomastoid, 21720-21725
Necropsy
  Coroner Examination, 88045
  Forensic Examination, 88040

Necropsy — *continued*
  Gross and Microscopic Examination, 88020-88029
  Gross Examination, 88000-88016
  Organ, 88037
  Regional, 88036
  Unlisted Services and Procedures, 88099
Needle Biopsy
  See Biopsy
  Abdomen Mass, 49180
  Bone, 20220, 20225
  Bone Marrow, 38221
  Breast, 19100
  Colon
    Endoscopy, 45392
  Colon Sigmoid
    Endoscopy, 45342
  CT Scan Guidance, 77012
  Epididymis, 54800
  Esophagus
    Endoscopy, 43232, 43238
  Fluoroscopic Guidance, 77002
  Gastrointestinal, Upper
    Endoscopy, 43238, 43242
  Kidney, 50200
  Liver, 47000, 47001
  Lung, 32405
  Lymph Node, 38505
  Mediastinum, 32405
  Muscle, 20206
  Pancreas, 48102
  Pleura, 32400
  Prostate, 55700
    with Fluorescence Spectroscopy, 0443T
  Retroperitoneal Mass, 49180
  Salivary Gland, 42400
  Spinal Cord, 62269
  Testis, 54500
  Thyroid Gland, 60100
  Transbronchial, 31629, 31633
Needle Localization
  Breast
    with Biopsy, 19081-19086
    with Lesion Excision, 19125, 19126
    Placement, 19281-19288
  Magnetic Resonance Guidance, 77021
Needle Manometer Technique, 20950
Needle Wire
  Introduction
    Trachea, 31730
  Placement
    Breast, 19281-19288
Neer Procedure, 23470
NEFL, 81405
Negative Pressure Wound Therapy (NPWT), 97605-97608
Neisseria Gonorrhoeae, 87590-87592, 87850
Neisseria Meningitidis
  Antibody, 86741
Neobladder
  Construction, 51596
Neonatal Critical Care, 99468-99469
Neonatal Intensive Care
  See Newborn Care
  Initial, 99477-99480
  Subsequent, 99478-99480
Neoplasm
  See Tumor
Neoplastic Growth
  See Tumor
Nephelometry, 83883
Nephrectomy
  with Ureters, 50220-50236, 50546, 50548
  Donor, 50300, 50320, 50547
  Laparoscopic, 50545-50548
  Partial, 50240
    Laparoscopic, 50543
  Recipient, 50340
Nephrolith
  See Calculus, Removal, Kidney
Nephrolithotomy, 50060-50075
Nephropexy, 50400, 50405
Nephroplasty
  See Kidney, Repair
Nephropyeloplasty, 50400-50405, 50544
Nephrorrhaphy, 50500

Nephroscopy
  See Endoscopy, Kidney
Nephrostogram, *[50430, 50431]*
Nephrostolithotomy
  Percutaneous, 50080, 50081
Nephrostomy
  Change Tube, *[50435]*
    with Drainage, 50400
  Closure, 53899
  Endoscopic, 50562-50570
    with Exploration, 50045
  Percutaneous, 52334
  X–ray with Contrast
    to Guide Dilation, 74485
Nephrostomy Tract
  Establishment, 50395
Nephrotomogram
  See Nephrotomography
Nephrotomography, 74415
Nephrotomy, 50040, 50045
  with Exploration, 50045
Nerve
  Cranial
    See Cranial Nerve
  Facial
    See Facial Nerve
  Foot
    Incision, 28035
  Intercostal
    See Intercostal Nerve
  Median
    See Median Nerve
  Obturator
    See Obturator Nerve
  Peripheral
    See Peripheral Nerve
  Phrenic
    See Phrenic Nerve
  Sciatic
    See Sciatic Nerve
  Spinal
    See Spinal Nerve
  Tibial
    See Tibial Nerve
  Ulnar
    See Ulnar Nerve
  Vestibular
    See Vestibular Nerve
Nerve Conduction
  Motor and/or Sensory, 95905-95913
Nerve II, Cranial
  See Optic Nerve
Nerve Root
  See Cauda Equina; Spinal Cord
  Decompression, 62380, 63020-63048, 63055-63103
  Incision, 63185, 63190
  Section, 63185, 63190
Nerves
  Anastomosis
    Facial to Hypoglossal, 64868
    Facial to Spinal Accessory, 64866
  Avulsion, 64732-64772
  Biopsy, 64795
  Cryoablation, Percutaneous, 0440T-0442T
  Decompression, 62380, 64702-64727
  Destruction, 64600-64681 *[64633, 64634, 64635, 64636]*
  Laryngeal, Recurrent, 31595
  Paravertebral Facet Joint, *[64633, 64634, 64635, 64636]*
  Foot
    Excision, 28055
    Incision, 28035
  Graft, 64885-64907
  Implantation
    Electrode, 64553-64581
    to Bone, 64787
    to Muscle, 64787
  Incision, 43640, 43641, 64732-64772
  Injection
    Anesthetic, 01991-01992, 64400-64530
    Neurolytic Agent, 64600-64681 *[64633, 64634, 64635, 64636]*
  Insertion
    Electrode, 64553-64581

Nerves — *continued*
  Lesion
    Excision, 64774-64792
  Neurofibroma
    Excision, 64788-64792
  Neurolemmoma
    Excision, 64788-64792
  Neurolytic
    Internal, 64727
  Neuroma
    Excision, 64774-64786
  Neuroplasty, 64702-64721
  Nuclear Medicine
    Unlisted Services and Procedures, 78699
  Removal
    Electrode, 64585
  Repair
    Graft, 64885-64911
    Microdissection
      with Surgical Microscope, 69990
    Suture, 64831-64876
  Spinal Accessory
    Incision, 63191
    Section, 63191
  Suture, 64831-64876
  Sympathectomy
    Excision, 64802-64818
  Transection, 43640, 43641, 64732-64772
  Transposition, 64718-64721
  Unlisted Services and Procedures, 64999
Nerve Stimulation, Transcutaneous
  See Application, Neurostimulation
Nerve Teasing, 88362
Nerve V, Cranial
  See Trigeminal Nerve
Nerve VII, Cranial
  See Facial Nerve
Nerve X, Cranial
  See Vagus Nerve
Nerve XI, Cranial
  See Accessory Nerve
Nerve XII, Cranial
  See Hypoglossal Nerve
Nervous System
  Nuclear Medicine
    Unlisted Services and Procedures, 78699
Nesidioblast
  See Islet Cell
Neurectasis, 64999
Neurectomy
  Foot, 28055
  Gastrocnemius, 27326
  Hamstring Muscle, 27325
  Leg, Lower, 27326
  Leg, Upper, 27325
  Popliteal, 27326
  Tympanic, 69676
Neuroendoscopy
  Intracranial, 62160-62165
Neurofibroma
  Cutaneous Nerve
    Excision, 64788
  Extensive
    Destruction, 0419T-0420T
    Excision, 64792
  Peripheral Nerve
    Excision, 64790
Neurolemmoma
  Cutaneous Nerve
    Excision, 64788
  Extensive
    Excision, 64792
  Peripheral Nerve
    Excision, 64790
Neurologic System
  See Nervous System
Neurology
  Brain
    Cortex Magnetic Stimulation, 90867-90869
    Mapping, 96020
    Surface Electrode Stimulation, 95961-95962
  Central Motor
    Electrocorticogram
      Intraoperative, 95829
    Electroencephalogram (EEG)
      Brain Death, 95824

Neurology — *continued*
  Central Motor — *continued*
    Electroencephalogram — *continued*
      Electrode Placement, 95830
      Intraoperative, 95955
      Monitoring, 95812, 95813, 95950-95953, 95956
      Physical or Drug Activation, 95954
      Sleep, 95808, 95810, 95822, 95827
        Attended, 95806, 95807
        Standard, 95819
      WADA activation, 95958
    Electroencephalography (EEG)
      Digital Analysis, 95957
    Electromyography
      See Electromyography
      Fine Wire
        Dynamic, 96004
      Ischemic Limb Exercise Test, 95875
      Needle, 51785, 95860-95872
      Surface
        Dynamic, 96002-96004
    Higher Cerebral Function
      Aphasia Test, 96105
      Cognitive Function Tests, 96116
      Developmental Tests, 96110, 96111
    Magnetoencephalography (MEG), 95965-95967
    Motion Analysis
      by Video and 3–D Kinematics, 96000, 96004
      Computer–based, 96000, 96004
    Muscle Testing
      Manual, 95831-95834
    Nerve Conduction
      Motor and Sensory Nerve, 95905-95913
    Neuromuscular Junction Tests, 95937
    Neurophysiological Testing, 95921-95924
    Neuropsychological Testing, 96118-96120
    Plantar Pressure Measurements
      Dynamic, 96001, 96004
    Polysomnography, 95808-95811
    Range of Motion Test, 95851, 95852
    Reflex
      H–Reflex, 95907-95913
    Reflex Test
      Blink Reflex, 95933
    Sleep Study, 95808, 95810
      Attended, 95806
      Unattended, 95807
    Somatosensory Testing, 95925-95927 *[95938]*
    Transcranial Motor Stimulation, 95928-95929
    Unlisted Services and Procedures, 95999
    Urethral Sphincter, 51785
    Visual Evoked Potential, CNS, 95930
  Cognitive Performance, 96125
  Diagnostic
    Anal Sphincter, 51785
    Autonomic Nervous Function
      Heart Rate Response, 95921-95923
      Pseudomotor Response, 95921-95923
      Sympathetic Function, 95921-95923
    Brain Surface Electrode Stimulation, 95961, 95962
Neurolysis
  Nerve, 64704, 64708
  Internal, 64727
Neuroma
  Acoustic
    See Brain, Tumor, Excision
  Cutaneous Nerve
    Excision, 64774
  Digital Nerve
    Excision, 64776, 64778
  Excision, 64774
  Foot Nerve
    Excision, 28080, 64782, 64783
  Hand Nerve
    Excision, 64782, 64783
  Interdigital, 28080
  Peripheral Nerve
    Excision, 64784

Neuroma — *continued*
  Sciatic Nerve
    Excision, 64786
Neuromuscular Junction Tests, 95937
Neuromuscular Pedicle
  Reinnervation
    Larynx, 31590
Neuromuscular Reeducation, 97112
  See Physical Medicine/Therapy/Occupational Therapy
Neurophysiological Testing
  Autonomic Nervous Function
    Combined Parasympathetic and Sympathetic, 95924
    Heart Rate Response, 95921-95923
    Pseudomotor Response, 95921-95923
    Sympathetic Function, 95921-95923
Neuroplasty, 64712
  Cranial Nerve, 64716
  Digital Nerve, 64702, 64704
  Peripheral Nerve, 64708-64714, 64718-64721
Neuropsychological Testing, 96118-96120
  Computer Assisted, 96120
Neurorrhaphy, 64831-64876
  Peripheral Nerve
    with Graft, 64885-64907
    Conduit, 64910-64911
Neurostimulation
  Application, 64550
  Tibial, 64566
Neurostimulator
  Analysis, 95970-95982, 0317T
  Implantation
    Electrodes
      Incision, 64568, 64575-64581
      Laparoscopic, 0312T
      Percutaneous, 64553-64565
  Insertion
    Pulse Generator, 61885-61886, 64568, 64590
    Receiver, 61885-61886, 64590
  Removal
    Electrodes, 61880, 63661-63662, 64570, 64585, 0314T
    Pulse Generator, 61888, 64595, 0314T-0315T
    Receiver, 61888, 64595
  Replacement
    Electrodes, 43647, 43881, 63663-63664, 64569, 0313T
    Pulse Generator, 61885-61886, 63685, 64590, 0316T
    Receiver, 61885-61886, 63685, 64590
  Revision
    Electrode, 61880, 63663-63664, 64569, 64585, 0313T
    Pulse Generator, 61888, 63688, 64595
    Receiver, 61888, 63688, 64595
Neurotomy, Sympathetic
  See Gasserian Ganglion, Sensory Root, Decompression
Neurovascular Interventional Procedures
  Balloon Angioplasty, 61630
  Intracranial Balloon Dilatation, 61640-61642
  Occlusion
    Balloon, 61623
    Balloon Dilatation, 61640-61642
    Transcatheter, 61624
      Non-central nervous system, 61626
  Placement Intravascular Stent, 61635
  Vascular Catheterization, 61630, 61635
Neurovascular Pedicle Flaps, 15750
Neutralization Test
  Virus, 86382
Newborn Care, 99460-99465, 99502
  Attendance at Delivery, 99464
  Birthing Room, 99460-99463
  Blood Transfusion, 36450, 36456
    See Neonatal Intensive Care
  Circumcision
    Clamp or Other Device, 54150
    Surgical Excision, 54160
  Laryngoscopy, 31520
  Normal, 99460-99463
  Prepuce Slitting, 54000

Newborn Care — *continued*
  Preventive
    Office, 99461
  Resuscitation, 99465
  Standby for C–Section, 99360
  Subsequent Hospital Care, 99462
  Umbilical Artery Catheterization, 36660
New Patient
  Domiciliary or Rest Home Visit, 99324-99328
  Emergency Department Services, 99281-99288
  Home Services, 99341-99345
  Hospital Inpatient Services, 99221-99239
  Hospital Observation Services, 99217-99220
  Initial Inpatient Consultations, 99251-99255
  Initial Office Visit, 99201-99205
    See Evaluation and Management, Office and Other Outpatient
  Office and/or Other Outpatient Consultations, 99241-99245
  Outpatient Visit, 99211-99215
NF1, 81408
NF2, 81405-81406
NHLRC1, 81403
Nickel, 83885
Nicolas–Durand–Favre Disease
  See Lymphogranuloma Venerum
Nicotine, *[80323]*
Nidation
  See Implantation
Nikaidoh Procedure, 33782-33783
NIPA1, 81404
Nipples
  See Breast
  Inverted, 19355
  Reconstruction, 19350
Nissen Operation
  See Fundoplasty, Esophagogastric
Nitrate Reduction Test
  Urinalysis, 81000-81099
Nitric Oxide, 95012
Nitroblue Tetrazolium Dye Test, 86384
Nitrogen, Blood Urea
  See Blood Urea Nitrogen
NLGN3, 81405
NLGN4X, 81404-81405
N. Meningitidis, 86741
NMP22, 86386
NMR Imaging
  See Magnetic Resonance Spectroscopy
NMR Spectroscopies
  See Magnetic Resonance Spectroscopy
Noble Procedure, 44680
Nocardia
  Antibody, 86744
Nocturnal Penile Rigidity Test, 54250
Nocturnal Penile Tumescence Test, 54250
NOD2, 81401
Node Dissection, Lymph, 38542
Node, Lymph
  See Lymph Nodes
Nodes
  See Lymph Nodes
No Man's Land
  Tendon Repair, 26356-26358
Non-Invasive Arterial Pressure, 93050
Non–Invasive Vascular Imaging
  See Vascular Studies
Non–Office Medical Services, 99056
  Emergency Care, 99060
Non–Stress Test, Fetal, 59025
Nonunion Repair
  Femur
    with Graft, 27472
    without Graft, 27470
  Fibula, 27726
  Metatarsal, 28322
  Tarsal Joint, 28320
Noonan Spectrum Disorders (Noonan/Noonan-like Syndrome), 81442
Noradrenalin
  Blood, 82383, 82384
  Urine, 82382
Norchlorimipramine
  See Imipramine
Norepinephrine
  See Catecholamines

Norepinephrine — *continued*
Blood, 82383, 82384
Urine, 82382
Nortriptyline
Assay, [80335, 80336, 80337]
Norwood Procedure, 33619, 33622
Nose
Abscess
Incision and Drainage, 30000, 30020
Artery
Incision, 30915, 30920
Biopsy
Intranasal, 30100
Dermoid Cyst
Excision
Complex, 30125
Simple, 30124
Displacement Therapy, 30210
Endoscopy
Diagnostic, 31231-31235
Surgical, 31237-31294
Excision
Rhinectomy, 30150, 30160
Fracture
with Fixation, 21330, 21340, 21345-21347
Closed Treatment, 21345
Open Treatment, 21325-21336, 21338,
21339, 21346, 21347
Percutaneous Treatment, 21340
Hematoma
Hemorrhage
Cauterization, 30901-30906
Incision and Drainage, 30000, 30020
Insertion
Septal Prosthesis, 30220
Intranasal
Lesion
External Approach, 30118
Internal Approach, 30117
Lysis of Adhesions, 30560
Polyp
Excision
Extensive, 30115
Simple, 30110
Reconstruction
Cleft Lip
Cleft Palate, 30460, 30462
Dermatoplasty, 30620
Primary, 30400-30420
Secondary, 30430-30450
Septum, 30520
Removal
Foreign Body, 30300
with Anesthesia, 30310
by Lateral Rhinotomy, 30320
Repair
Adhesions, 30560
Cleft Lip, 40700-40761
Fistula, 30580, 30600, 42260
Rhinophyma, 30120
Septum, 30540, 30545, 30630
Synechia, 30560
Vestibular Stenosis, 30465
Skin
Excision, 30120
Surgical Planing, 30120
Skin Graft
Delay of Flap, 15630
Full Thickness, 15260, 15261
Pedicle Flap, 15576
Submucous Resection Turbinate
Excision, 30140
Tissue Transfer, Adjacent, 14060, 14061
Turbinate
Excision, 30130, 30140
Fracture, 30930
Injection, 30200
Turbinate Mucosa
Cauterization, 30801, 30802
Unlisted Services and Procedures, 30999
Nose Bleed, 30901-30906
See Hemorrhage, Nasal
NOTCH1, 81407
NOTCH3, 81406
NPC1, 81406
NPC2, 81404

NPHP1, 81405-81406
NPHS1, 81407
NPHS2, 81405
NPM1/ALK (t(2;5)), 81401
NPWT (Negative Pressure Wound Therapy),
97605-97608
NRAS, 81311
NROB1, 81404
NSD1, 81405-81406
NST, 59025
NSVD, 59400-59410, 59610-59614
NTD (Nitroblue Tetrazolium Dye Test), 86384
Nuclear Antigen
Antibody, 86235
Nuclear Imaging
See Nuclear Medicine
Nuclear Magnetic Resonance Imaging
See Magnetic Resonance Imaging (MRI)
Nuclear Magnetic Resonance Spectroscopy
See Magnetic Resonance Spectroscopy
Nuclear Matrix Protein 22 (NMP22), 86386
Nuclear Medicine
Abscess Localization, 78805, 78806, 78807
Adrenal Gland Imaging, 78075
Bladder
Residual Study, 78730
Blood
Flow Imaging, 78445
Iron
Plasma Volume, 78110, 78111
Platelet Survival, 78190, 78191
Red Cells, 78120, 78121, 78130-78140
Red Cell Survival, 78130, 78135
Unlisted Services and Procedures, 78199
Whole Blood Volume, 78122
Bone
Density Study, 78350, 78351
Imaging, 78300-78320
SPECT, 78320
Ultrasound, 76977
Unlisted Services and Procedures, 78399
Bone Marrow
Imaging, 78102-78104
Brain
Blood Flow, 78610
Cerebrospinal Fluid, 78630-78650
Imaging, 78600-78609
Vascular Flow, 78610
Endocrine Glands
Unlisted Services and Procedures, 78099
Esophagus
Imaging (Motility), 78258
Reflux Study, 78262
Gallbladder
Imaging, 78226-78227
Gastric Mucosa
Imaging, 78261
Gastrointestinal
Blood Loss Study, 78278
Protein Loss Study, 78282
Shunt Testing, 78291
Unlisted Services and Procedures, 78299
Genitourinary System
Unlisted Services and Procedures, 78799
Heart
Blood Flow, 78414
Blood Pool Imaging, 78472, 78473, 78481,
78483, 78494, 78496
Myocardial Imaging, 78459, 78466-78469
Myocardial Perfusion, 0439T, 78451-78454,
78491-78492
Shunt Detection, 78428
Unlisted Services and Procedures, 78499
Hepatobiliary System, 78226-78227
Inflammatory Process, 78805-78807
Intestines
Imaging, 78290
Kidney
Blood Flow, 78701-78709
Function Study, 78725
Imaging, 78700-78710
Lacrimal Gland
Tear Flow, 78660
Liver
Imaging, 78201-78216
Vascular Flow, 78206

Nuclear Medicine — *continued*
Lung
Imaging Perfusion, 78580-78598
Imaging Ventilation, 78579, 78582, 78598
Unlisted Services and Procedures, 78599
Lymphatics, 78195
Unlisted Services and Procedures, 78199
Lymph Nodes, 78195
Musculoskeletal System
Unlisted Services and Procedures, 78399
Nervous System
Unlisted Services and Procedures, 78699
Parathyroid Glands
Imaging, 78070
Pulmonary, 78579-78582, 78597-78598
Salivary Gland
Function Study, 78232
Imaging, 78230, 78231
Spleen
Imaging, 78185, 78215, 78216
Unlisted Services and Procedures, 78199
Stomach
Blood Loss Study, 78278
Emptying Study, 78264-78266
Protein Loss Study, 78282
Reflux Study, 78262
Vitamin B–12 Absorption, 78270-78272
Testes
Imaging, 78761
Therapeutic
Heart, 79440
Interstitial, 79300
Intra–arterial, 79445
Intra–articular, 79440
Intracavitary, 79200
Intravascular, 79101
Intravenous, 79101
Intravenous Infusion, 79101, 79403
Oral Administration, 79005
Radioactive Colloid Therapy, 79200, 79300
Thyroid, 79200, 79300
Unlisted Services and Procedures, 79999
Thyroid
Imaging, 78012-78014
for Metastases, 78015-78018
Metastases Uptake, 78020
Tumor Imaging
Positron Emission Tomography, 78811-
78816
with Computed Tomography, 78814-
78816
Tumor Localization, 78800-78804
Unlisted Services and Procedures, 78999
Urea Breath Test, 78267, 78268
Ureter
Reflux Study, 78740
Vein
Thrombosis Imaging, 78456-78458
Nucleases, DNA
Antibody, 86215
Nucleic Acid Probe
Amplified Probe Detection
Infectious Agent
Bartonella Henselae, 87471
Bartonella Quintana, 87471
Borrelia Burgdorferi, 87476
Candida Species, 87481
Central Nervous System Pathogen,
87483
Chlamydia Pneumoniae, 87486
Chlamydia Trachomatis, 87491
Enterovirus, 87498, 87500
Gardnerella Vaginalis, 87511
Hepatitis B Virus, 87516
Hepatitis C, 87521
Hepatitis G, 87526
Herpes Simplex Virus, 87529
HIV–1, 87535
HIV–2, 87538
Legionella Pneumophila, 87541
Multiple Organisms, 87801
Mycobacteria Avium-Intracellulare,
87561
Mycobacteria Species, 87551
Mycobacteria Tuberculosis, 87556
Mycoplasma Pneumoniae, 87581

Nucleic Acid Probe — *continued*
Amplified Probe Detection — *continued*
Infectious Agent — *continued*
Neisseria Gonorrhoeae, 87591
Not Otherwise Specified, 87798, 87801
Papillomavirus, Human, [87623, 87624,
87625]
Staphylococcus Aureus, 87640-87641
Streptococcus, Group A, 87651
Streptococcus, Group B, 87653
Direct Probe Detection
Infectious Agent
Bartonella Henselae, 87470
Bartonella Quintana, 87470
Borrelia Burgdorferi, 87475
Candida Species, 87480
Chlamydia Pneumoniae, 87485
Chlamydia Trachomatis, 87490
Cytomegalovirus, 87495
Gardnerella Vaginalis, 87510
Gastrointestinal Pathogens, 87505-
87507
Hepatitis B Virus, 87515
Hepatitis C, 87520
Hepatitis G, 87525
Herpes Simplex Virus, 87528
Herpes Virus-6, 87531
HIV–1, 87534
HIV–2, 87537
Legionella Pneumophila, 87540
Multiple Organisms, 87800
Mycobacteria Avium-Intracellulare,
87560
Mycobacteria Species, 87550
Mycobacteria Tuberculosis, 87555
Mycoplasma Pneumoniae, 87580
Neisseria Gonorrhoeae, 87590
Not Otherwise Specified, 87797
Papillomavirus, Human, [87623, 87624,
87625]
Streptococcus, Group A, 87650
Trichomonas Vaginalis, 87660
Genotype Analysis
Infectious Agent
Hepatitis C Virus, 87902
HIV–1, 87901
In Situ Hybridization, 88365-88369 [88364,
88373, 88374, 88377]
Nucleic Acid Microbial Identification, 87797-
87799
Phenotype Analysis
Infectious Agent
HIV–1 Drug Resistance, 87903, 87904
Quantification
Infectious Agent
Bartonella Henselae, 87472
Bartonella Quintana, 87472
Borrelia Burgdorferi, 87477
Candida Species, 87482
Chlamydia Pneumoniae, 87487
Chlamydia Trachomatis, 87492
Cytomegalovirus, 87497
Gardnerella Vaginalis, 87512
Hepatitis B Virus, 87517
Hepatitis C, 87522
Hepatitis G, 87527
Herpes Simplex Virus, 87530
Herpes Virus-6, 87533
HIV–1, 87536
HIV–2, 87539
Legionella Pneumophila, 87542
Mycobacteria Avium-Intracellulare,
87562
Mycobacteria Species, 87552
Mycobacteria Tuberculosis, 87557
Mycoplasma Pneumoniae, 87582
Neisseria Gonorrhoeae, 87592
Not Otherwise Specified, 87799
Papillomavirus, Human, [87623],
[87624, 87625]
Streptococcus, Group A, 87652
Nucleic Medicine
Vein
Thrombosis Imaging, 78456-78458
Nucleolysis, Intervertebral Disc
See Chemonucleolysis

[Resequenced]

Nucleophosmin Gene Analysis — Operation/Procedure

Nucleophosmin Gene Analysis, 81310
Nucleotidase, 83915
Nursemaid Elbow, 24640
Nursing Facility Services
  Annual Assessment, 99318
  Care Plan Oversight Services, 99379, 99380
  Discharge Services, 1110F-1111F, 99315-99316
  Initial, 99304-99306
  Subsequent Nursing Facility Care, 99307-99310
    New or Established Patient, 99307-99310
    See also Domiciliary Services
Nuss Procedure
  with Thoracoscopy, 21743
  without Thoracoscopy, 21742
Nutrition Therapy
  Group, 97804
  Home Infusion, 99601, 99602
  Initial Assessment, 97802
  Reassessment, 97803
Nystagmus Tests
  See Vestibular Function Tests
  Optokinetic, 92534, 92544
  Positional, 92532, 92542
  Spontaneous, 92531, 92541

O

O2 Saturation, 82805-82810, 94760-94762
OAE Test, 92587-92588
Ober–Yount Procedure, 27025
Obliteration
  Mastoid, 69670
  Vaginal
    Total, 57110-57112
    Vault, 57120
Obliteration, Total Excision of Vagina, 57110-57112
Obliteration, Vaginal Vault, 57120
Observation
  Discharge, 99217
  Initial, 99218-99220
  Same Date Admit/Discharge, 99234-99236
  Subsequent, *[99224, 99225, 99226]*
Obstetrical Care
  See Also Abortion; Cesarean Delivery; Ectopic Pregnancy
  Abortion
    Induced
      by Amniocentesis Injection, 59850-59852
      by Dilation and Curettage, 59840
      by Dilation and Evaluation, 59841
    Missed
      First Trimester, 59820
      Second Trimester, 59821
    Spontaneous, 59812
    Therapeutic, 59840-59852
  Antepartum Care, 59425-59426
  Cesarean Section
    with Hysterectomy, 59525
    with Postpartum Care, 59515
    for Failed VBAC
      with Postpartum Care, 59622
      Only, 59620
      Routine (Global), 59618
    Only, 59514
    Routine (Global), 59510
  Curettage
    Hydatidiform Mole, 59870
  Evacuation
    Hydatidiform Mole, 59870
  External Cephalic Version, 59412
  Miscarriage
    Surgical Completion, 59812-59821
  Placenta Delivery, 59414
  Postpartum Care
    Cesarean Delivery, 59510
    Following Vaginal Delivery After Prior Cesarean Section, 59610, 59614, 59618, 59622
    Postpartum care only, 59430
    Vaginal, 59400, 59410
  Septic Abortion, 59830
  Total (Global), 59400, 59510, 59610, 59618
  Unlisted Services and Procedures, 59898-59899
  Vaginal Delivery
    with Postpartum Care, 59410

Obstetrical Care — *continued*
  Vaginal Delivery — *continued*
    After C/S–VBAC (Global), 59610
      with Postpartum Care, 59614
    Delivery Only, 59612
    Only, 59409
    Routine (Global), 59400
Obstetric Tamponade
  Uterus, 59899
  Vagina, 59899
Obstruction
  Extracranial, 61623
  Fallopian Tube, 58565, 58615
  Head/Neck, 61623
  Intracranial, 61623
  Penis (Vein), 37790
  Umbilical Cord, 59072
Obstruction Clearance
  Venous Access Device, 36595-36596
Obstruction Colon, 44025-44050
Obstructive Material Removal
  Gastrostomy, Duodenostomy, Jejunostomy, Gastro-jejunostomy, or Cecostomy Tube, 49460
Obturator Nerve
  Avulsion, 64763-64766
  Incision, 64763-64766
  Transection, 64763-64766
Obturator Prosthesis
  Impression/Custom Preparation
    Definitive, 21080
    Interim, 21079
    Surgical, 21076
  Insertion
    Larynx, 31527
Occipital Nerve, Greater
  Avulsion, 64744
  Incision, 64744
  Injection
    Anesthetic, 64405
  Transection, 64744
Occlusion
  Extracranial/Intracranial, 61623
  Fallopian Tubes
    Oviduct, 58565, 58615
  Penis
    Vein, 37790
  Umbilical Cord, 59072
  Ureteral, 50705
Occlusive Disease of Artery, 35001, 35005-35021, 35045-35081, 35091, 35102, 35111, 35121, 35131, 35141, 35151
  See Also Repair, Artery; Revision
Occult Blood, 82270-82272
  by Hemoglobin Immunoassay, 82274
Occupational Therapy
  Evaluation, *[97165, 97166, 97167, 97168]*
OCT (Oxytocin Challenge), 59020
Ocular Implant
  See Also Orbital Implant
  Insertion
    in Scleral Shell, 65130
    Muscles Attached, 65140
    Muscles Not Attached, 65135
  Modification, 65125
  Reinsertion, 65150
    with Foreign Material, 65155
  Removal, 65175
Ocular Insert, Drug-eluting, 0444T-0445T
Ocular Muscle, 67311-67399
Ocular Orbit
  See Orbit
Ocular Photoscreening, 99174, *[99177]*
Ocular Prosthesis, 21077, 65770, 66982-66985, 92358
Oculomotor Muscle, 67311-67399
Oddi Sphincter
  Pressure Measurement, 43263
ODM, 92260
Odontoid Dislocation
  Open Treatment
    Reduction, 22318
      with Grafting, 22319
Odontoid Fracture
  Open Treatment
    Reduction, 22318

Odontoid Fracture — *continued*
  Open Treatment — *continued*
    Reduction — *continued*
      with Grafting, 22319
Odontoid Process
  Excisions, 22548
Oesophageal Neoplasm
  Endoscopic Removal
    Ablation, 43229
    Bipolar Cautery, 43216
    Hot Biopsy Forceps, 43216
    Snare, 43217
  Excision, Open, 43100-43101
Oesophageal Varices
  Injection Sclerosis, 43204, 43243
  Ligation, 43205, 43244, 43400
  Repair/Transection, 43401
Oesophagus
  See Esophagus
Oestradiol, 82670
  Response, 80415
Office and/or Other Outpatient Visits
  Consultation, 99241-99245
  Established Patient, 99211-99215
  New Patient, 99201-99205
  Normal Newborn, 99461
  Office Visit
    Established Patient, 99211-99215
    New Patient, 99201-99205
    Prolonged Service, 99354-99355
  Outpatient Visit
    Established Patient, 99211-99215
    New Patient, 99201-99205
    Prolonged Service, 99354-99355
Office Medical Services
  After Hours, 99050
  Emergency Care, 99058
  Extended Hours, 99051
Office or Other Outpatient Consultations, 99241-99245, 99354-99355
Olecranon
  See Also Elbow; Humerus; Radius; Ulna
  Bone Cyst
    Excision, 24120-24126
  Bursa
    Arthrocentesis, 20605-20606
    Excision, 24105
  Tumor, Benign, 25120-25126
    Cyst, 24120
    Excision, 24125, 24126
Olecranon Process
  Craterization, 24147
  Diaphysectomy, 24147
  Excision
    Cyst/Tumor, 24120-24126
    Partial, 24147
  Fracture
    Closed Treatment, 24670-24675
    Open Treatment, 24685
  Osteomyelitis, 24138, 24147
  Saucerization, 24147
  Sequestrectomy, 24138
Oligoclonal Immunoglobulin
  Cerebrospinal Fluid, 83916
Omentectomy, 49255, 58950-58958
  Laparotomy, 58960
  Oophorectomy, 58943
  Resection Ovarian Malignancy, 58950-58952
  Resection Peritoneal Malignancy, 58950-58958
  Resection Tubal Malignancy, 58950-58958
Omentum
  Excision, 49255, 58950-58958
  Flap, 49904-49905
    Free
      with Microvascular Anastomosis, 49906
  Unlisted Services and Procedures, 49999
Omphalectomy, 49250
Omphalocele
  Repair, 49600-49611
Omphalomesenteric Duct
  Excision, 44800
Omphalomesenteric Duct, Persistent
  Excision, 44800
OMT, 98925-98929
Oncology (Ovarian) Biochemical Assays, 81500, 81503-81504

Oncoprotein
  Des-Gamma-Carboxy Prothrombin (DCP), 83951
  HER–2/neu, 83950
One Stage Prothrombin Time, 85610-85611
On-Line Internet Assessment/Management
  Nonphysician, 98969
  Physician, 99444
On-Line Medical Evaluation
  Non-Physician, 98969
  Physician, 99444
ONSD, 67570
Onychectomy, 11750
Onychia
  Drainage, 10060-10061
Onychoplasty, 11760, 26236, 28124, 28160
Oocyte
  Assisted Fertilization, Microtechnique, 89280-89281
  Biopsy, 89290-89291
  Cryopreservation, 88240
  Culture
    with Co–Culture, 89251
    Extended, 89272
    Less than 4 days, 89250
  Identification, Follicular Fluid, 89254
  Insemination, 89268
  Retrieval
    for In Vitro Fertilization, 58970
  Storage, 89346
  Thawing, 89356
Oophorectomy, 58262-58263, 58291-58292, 58552, 58554, 58661, 58940-58943
  Ectopic Pregnancy
    Laparoscopic Treatment, 59151
    Surgical Treatment, 59120
Oophorectomy, Partial, 58920, 58940-58943
Oophorocystectomy, 58925
  Laparoscopic, 58662
OPA1, 81406-81407
Open Biopsy, Adrenal Gland, 60540-60545
Opening (Incision and Drainage)
  Acne
    Comedones, 10040
    Cysts, 10040
    Milia, Multiple, 10040
    Pustules, 10040
Operating Microscope, 69990
Operation/Procedure
  Blalock–Hanlon, 33735
  Blalock–Taussig Subclavian–Pulmonary Anastomosis, 33750
  Collis, 43283, 43338
  Damus-Kaye-Stansel, 33606
  Dana, 63185
  Dor, 33548
  Dunn, 28715
  Duvries, 27675-27676
  Estes, 58825
  Flip-flap, 54324
  Foley Pyeloplasty, 50400-50405
  Fontan, 33615-33617
  Fowler-Stephens, 54650
  Fox, 67923
  Fredet-Ramstedt, 43520
  Gardner, 63700-63702
  Green, 23400
  Harelip, 40700, 40761
  Heine, 66740
  Heller, 32665, 43330-43331
  Jaboulay Gastroduodenostomy, 43810, 43850-43855
  Johannsen, 53400
  Krause, 61450
  Kuhnt–Szymanowski, 67917
  Leadbetter Urethroplasty, 53431
  Maquet, 27418
  Mumford, 23120, 29824
  Nissen, 43280
  Norwood, 33611-33612, 33619
  Peet, 64802-64818
  Ramstedt, 43520
  Richardson Hysterectomy
    See Hysterectomy, Abdominal, Total
  Richardson Urethromeatoplasty, 53460
  Schanz, 27448
  Schlatter Total Gastrectomy, 43620-43622

Operation/Procedure — *continued*
   Smithwick, 64802-64818
   Stamm, 43830
      Laparoscopic, 43653
   SVR, SAVER, 33548
   Tenago, 53431
   Toupet, 43280
   Winiwarter Cholecystoenterostomy, 47720-47740
   Winter, 54435
Operculectomy, 41821
Operculum
   See Gums
Ophthalmic Biometry, 76516-76519, 92136
Ophthalmic Mucous Membrane Test, 95060
Ophthalmology
   Unlisted Services and Procedures, 92499
      See Also Ophthalmology, Diagnostic
Ophthalmology, Diagnostic
   Color Vision Exam, 92283
   Computerized Scanning, 92132-92134
   Computerized Screening, 99172, 99174, *[99177]*
   Dark Adaptation, 92284
   Electromyography, Needle, 92265
   Electro–oculography, 92270
   Electroretinography, 92275
   Endoscopy, 66990
   Eye Exam
      with Anesthesia, 92018-92019
      Established Patient, 92012-92014
      New Patient, 92002-92004
   Gonioscopy, 92020
   Ocular Photography
      External, 92285
      Internal, 92286-92287
   Ophthalmoscopy, 92225-92226
      with Angiography, 92235
      with Angioscopy, 92230
      with Dynamometry, 92260
      with Fluorescein Angiography, 92235
         and Indocyanine–Green, 92242
      with Fluorescein Angioscopy, 92230
      with Fundus Photography, 92250
      with Indocyanine–Green Angiography, 92240
         and Fluorescein, 92242
   Photoscreening, 99174, *[99177]*
   Refractive Determination, 92015
   Rotation Tests, 92499
   Sensorimotor Exam, 92060
   Tonometry
      Serial, 92100
   Ultrasound, 76510-76529
   Visual Acuity Screen, 99172-99173
   Visual Field Exam, 92081-92083
   Visual Function Screen, 99172, 99174, *[99177]*
Ophthalmoscopy, 92225-92226
   See Also Ophthalmology, Diagnostic
Opiates, *[80361, 80362, 80363, 80364]*
Opinion, Second
   See Confirmatory Consultations
Optical Coherence Tomography, Intraoperative
   Axillary Lymph Node, Each Specimen, Excised Tissue, 0351T-0352T
   Breast Tissue, Each Specimen, Excised Tissue, 0351T-0352T
   Surgical Cavity, 0353T-0354T
Optical Endomicroscopic Images, 88375
Optical Endomicroscopy, 0397T, 43206, 43252
Optic Nerve
   Decompression, 67570
      with Nasal/Sinus Endoscopy, 31294
   Head Evaluation, 2027F
OPTN, 81406
Optokinectic Nystagmus Test, 92534, 92544
Oral Lactose Tolerance Test, 82951-82952
Oral Mucosa
   Excision, 40818
Oral Surgical Splint, 21085
Orbit
   See Also Orbital Contents; Orbital Floor; Periorbital Region
   Biopsy, 61332
      Exploration, 67450
      Fine Needle Aspiration of Orbital Contents, 67415

Orbit — *continued*
   Biopsy — *continued*
      Orbitotomy without Bone Flap, 67400
   CT Scan, 70480-70482
   Decompression, 61330
      Bone Removal, 67414, 67445
   Exploration, 61332, 67400, 67450
      Lesion
         Excision, 61333
      Fracture
         Closed Treatment
            with Manipulation, 21401
            without Manipulation, 21400
         Open Treatment, 21406-21408
            Blowout Fracture, 21385-21395
      Incision and Drainage, 67405, 67440
      Injection
         Retrobulbar, 67500-67505
         Tenon's Capsule, 67515
      Insertion
         Implant, 67550
      Lesion
         Excision, 67412, 67420
      Magnetic Resonance Imaging (MRI), 70540-70543
      Removal
         Decompression, 67445
         Exploration, 61332-61333
         Foreign Body, 67413, 67430
         Implant, 67560
      Sella Turcica, 70482
      Unlisted Services and Procedures, 67599
      X–ray, 70190-70200
Orbital Contents
   Aspiration, 67415
Orbital Floor
   See Also Orbit; Periorbital Region
   Fracture
      Blow–Out, 21385-21395
Orbital Hypertelorism
   Osteotomy
      Periorbital, 21260-21263
Orbital Implant
   See Also Ocular Implant
   Insertion, 67550
   Removal, 67560
Orbital Prosthesis, 21077
Orbital Rim and Forehead
   Reconstruction, 21172-21180
Orbital Rims
   Reconstruction, 21182-21184
Orbital Transplant, 67560
Orbital Walls
   Reconstruction, 21182-21184
Orbit Area
   Reconstruction
      Secondary, 21275
Orbitocraniofacial Reconstruction
   Secondary, 21275
Orbitotomy
   with Bone Flap
      with Biopsy, 67450
      with Bone Removal for Decompression, 67445
      with Drainage, 67440
      with Foreign Body Removal, 67430
      with Lesion Removal, 67420
      for Exploration, 67450
   without Bone Flap
      with Biopsy, 67400
      with Bone Removal for Decompression, 67414
      with Drainage, 67405
      with Foreign Body Removal, 67413
      with Lesion Removal, 67412
      for Exploration, 67400
   Frontal Approach, 67400-67414
   Lateral Approach, 67420-67450
   Transconjunctival Approach, 67400-67414
Orbits
   Skin Graft
      Split, 15120-15121
Orbit Wall(s)
   Decompression
      with Nasal
         Sinus Endoscopy, 31292, 31293

Orbit Wall(s) — *continued*
   Reconstruction, 21182-21184
Orchidectomies
   Laparoscopic, 54690
   Partial, 54522
   Radical, 54530-54535
   Simple, 54520
   Tumor, 54530-54535
Orchidopexy, 54640-54650, 54692
Orchidoplasty
   Injury, 54670
   Suspension, 54620-54640
   Torsion, 54600
Orchiectomy
   Laparoscopic, 54690
   Partial, 54522
   Radical
      Abdominal Exploration, 54535
      Inguinal Approach, 54530
   Simple, 54520
Orchiopexy
   Abdominal Approach, 54650
   Inguinal Approach, 54640
   Intra–Abdominal Testis, 54692
   Koop Inguinal, 54640
Orchioplasty
   Injury, 54670
   Suspension, 54620-54640
   Torsion, 54600
Organ Donor
   Life Support, 01990
Organ Grafting
   See Transplantation
Organic Acids, 83918-83921
Organ or Disease Oriented Panel
   Electrolyte, 80051
   General Health Panel, 80050
   Hepatic Function Panel, 80076
   Hepatitis Panel, 80074
   Lipid Panel, 80061
   Metabolic
      Basic
         Calcium Ionized, 80047
         Calcium Total, 80048
      Comprehensive, 80053
   Obstetric Panel, 80055, *[80081]*
   Renal Function, 80069
Organ System, Neurologic
   See Nervous System
ORIF
   Dislocation
      Ankle, 27848
      Bennett, 26685-26686
      Bennett Thumb, 26665
      Carpometacarpal, 26685-26686
         Thumb, 26665
      Elbow, 24635
         Monteggia, 24635
      Galeazzi, 25525-25526
         with
            Repair
               Triangular Cartilage, 25526
      Hip
         Spontaneous, 27258
            with
               Femoral Shaft Shortening, 27259
         Traumatic, 27254
            with
               Fracture
                  Acetabular Wall, 27254
                  Femoral Head, 27254
      Interphalangeal
         Foot, 28675
         Hand, 26785
      Knee, 27556
         with
            Ligament, Ligamentous
               Augmentation, 27558
               Reconstruction, 27558
               Repair, 27557-27558
      Lunate, 25695
      Metacarpophalangeal, 26715
      Metatarsophalangeal Joint, 28645
      Monteggia, 24635
      Odontoid, 22318-22319

ORIF — *continued*
   Dislocation — *continued*
      Pelvic, Pelvis
         Ring
            Anterior
               Open, 27217
               Pubis Symphysis, 27217
               Rami, 27217
            Posterior
               Open, 27218
         Sacroiliac Joint
            Open, 27218
      Radioulnar
         Distal, 25676
      Sacroiliac Joint, 27218
      Sacrum, 27218
      Shoulder
         with
            Fracture
               Humeral, Humerus
                  Anatomical Neck, 23680
                  Surgical Neck, 23680
                  Tuberosity, 23670
      Talotarsal Joint, 28585
      Tarsal, 28555
      Tarsometatarsal Joint, 28615
      Temporomandibular, 21490
      Tibiofibular Joint, 27832
         with
            Excision
               Proximal
                  Fibula, 27832
      TMJ, 21490
      Trans–Scaphoperilunar, 25685
   Fracture
      Acetabulum, Acetabular
         Column
            Anterior, 27227-27228
            Posterior, 27227-27228
         T-Fracture, 27228
         Wall
            Anterior, 27226, 27228
            Posterior, 27226, 27228
            Traumatic, 27254
               with
                  Dislocation of Hip, 27254
      Alveolar Ridge, 21445
      Ankle
         Bimalleolar, 27814
         Trimalleolar, 27822
            with
               Fixation
                  Posterior Lip, 27823
               Malleolus Fracture
                  Lateral, 27822-27823
                  Medial, 27822-27823
      Calcaneal, Calcaneus, 28415
         with
            Bone Graft, 28420
      Capitate, 25645
      Carpal (Other), 25645
         Navicular, 25628
         Scaphoid, 25628
      Clavicle, 23515
      Clavicular, 23515
      Coccyx, Coccygeal, 27202
      Colles, 25607-25609
      Craniofacial, 21432-21436
      Cuboid, 28465
      Cuneiforms, 28465
      Elbow
         Monteggia, 24635
         Periarticular, 24586-24587
      Epiphysis, Epiphyseal, 27519
      Femur, Femoral
         Condyle
            Lateral, 27514
            Medial, 27514
         Distal, 27514
            Lateral Condyle, 27514
            Medial Condyle, 27514
         Epiphysis, Epiphyseal, 27519
         Head, 27254
            Traumatic, 27254
               with
                  Dislocation Hip, 27254

ORIF — continued
  Fracture — continued
    Femur, Femoral — continued
      Intertrochanteric, Intertrochanter, 27244-27245
        with/Intermedullary Implant, 27245
      Lateral condyle, 27514
      Medial condyle, 27514
      Peritrochanteric, Peritrochanter, 27244-27245
        with
          Intermedullary Implant, 27245
      Proximal End, 27236
        with
          Prosthetic Replacement, 27236
      Proximal Neck, 27236
        with
          Prosthetic Replacement, 27236
      Shaft, 27506-27507
        with
          Intermedullary Implant, 27245
      Subtrochanteric, Subtrochanter, 27244-27245
      Supracondylar, 27511-27513
        with
          Intercondylar Extension, 27513
      Transcondylar, 27511-27513
        with
          Intercondylar Extension, 27513
      Trochanteric, Trochanter
        Greater, 27248
        Intertrochanteric, Intertrochanter, 27244-27245
          with
            Intermedullary Implant, 27245
        Peritrochanteric, Peritrochanter, 27244-27245
          with
            Intermedullary implant, 27245
        Subtrochanteric, Subtrochanter, 27244-27245
          with
            Intermedullary Implant, 27245
    Fibula and Tibia, 27828
      Distal
        with
          Tibia Fracture, 27826
    Fibula, Fibular
      Distal, 27792
      Malleolus
        Lateral, 27792
      Proximal, 27784
      Shaft, 27784
    Foot
      Sesamoid, 28531
    Frontal Sinus, 21343-21344
    Galeazzi, 25525-25526
      with
        Fracture
          Radial Shaft, 25525-25526
        Repair
          Triangular Cartilage, 25526
    Great Toe, 28505
    Hamate, 25645
    Heel, 28415
      with
        Bone Graft, 28420
    Humeral, Humerus
      Anatomical Neck, 23615-23616
      Condylar
        Lateral, 24579
        Medial, 24579
      Epicondylar
        Lateral, 24575
        Medial, 24575
      Proximal, 23615-23616
      Shaft, 24515-24516
      Supracondylar, 24545-24546

ORIF — continued
  Fracture — continued
    Humeral, Humerus — continued
      Supracondylar — continued
        with
          Intercondylar Extension, 24546
      Surgical Neck, 23615-23616
      Transcondylar, 24545-24546
        with
          Intercondylar Extension, 24546
      Tuberosity, 23630
    Hyoid, 31584
    Interphalangeal, 26746
    Knee
      Intercondylar Spine, 27540
      Tuberosity, 27540
    Larynx, Laryngeal, 31584
    LeFort I, 21422-21423
    LeFort II, 21346-21348
    LeFort III, 21432-21436
    Lunate, 25645
    Malar (Area), 21365-21366
      with Malar Tripod, 21365-21366
      with Zygomatic Arch, 21365-21366
    Malleolus
      Lateral, 27792
        with
          Ankle Fracture
            Trimalleolar, 27822-27823
      Medial, 27766
        with
          Ankle Fracture
            Trimalleolar, 27822-27823
    Mandibular, Mandible, 21462, 21470
      Alveolar Ridge, 21445
      Condylar, Condyle, 21465
    Maxillary, Maxilla, 21422-21423
      Alveolar Ridge, 21445
    Metacarpal, 26615
    Metacarpophalangeal, 26715
    Metatarsal, 28485
    Monteggia, 24635
    Nasal Bone, 21330-21335
      with Nasal Septum, 21335
    Nasal Septum, 21335
    Nasoethmoid, 21339
    Nasomaxillary, 21346-21348
    Navicular
      Foot, 28465
      Hand, 25628
    Odontoid, 22318-22319
    Olecranon Process, 24685
    Orbit, 21406-21408
    Palate, Palatal, 21422-21423
    Patella, Patellar, 27524
      with
        Patellectomy
          Complete, 27524
          Partial, 27524
        Repair
          Soft Tissue, 27524
    Phalange, Phalangeal
      Foot, 28525
        Great Toe, 28505
      Hand, 26735
        Distal, 26765
    Pisiform, 25645
    Radial, Radius
      and
        Ulnar, Ulna, 25575
      Distal, 25606-25609
      Head, 24665-24666
      Neck, 24665-24666
      or
        Ulnar, Ulna, 25574
      Shaft, 25515, 25525-25526
        with Dislocation
          Distal
            Radio–Ulnar Joint, 25525-25526
        with Repair
          Triangular Cartilage, 25526
    Rib, 21811-21813
    Scaphoid, 25628

ORIF — continued
  Fracture — continued
    Scapula, Scapular, 23585
    Sesamoid, 28531
    Smith, 25607, 25608-25609
    Sternum, 21825
    Talar, Talus, 28445
    Tarsal
      Calcaneal, 28415
        with Bone Graft, 28420
      Cuboid, 28465
      Cuneiforms, 28465
      Navicular, 28465
      Talus, 28445
    T–Fracture, 27228
    Thigh
      Femur, Femoral
        Condyle
          Lateral, 27514
          Medial, 27514
        Distal, 27514
          Lateral Condyle, 27514
          Medial Condyle, 27514
          Epiphysis, Epiphyseal, 27519
        Head, 27254
          Traumatic, 27254
            with Dislocation Hip, 27254
        Intertrochanteric, Intertrochanter, 27244-27245
          with Intermedullary Implant, 27245
        Lateral Condyle, 27514
        Medial Condyle, 27514
        Peritrochanteric, Peritrochanter, 27244-27245
          with Intermedullary Implant, 27245
        Proximal End, 27236
          with Prosthetic Replacement, 27236
        Proximal Neck, 27236
          with Prosthetic Replacement, 27236
        Shaft, 27506-27507
          with Intermedullary Implant, 27245
        Subtrochanteric, Subtrochanter, 27244-27245
        Supracondylar, 27511-27513
          with Intercondylar Extension, 27513
        Transcondylar, 27511-27513
          with Intercondylar Extension, 27513
        Trochanteric, Trochanter
          Greater, 27248
          Intertrochanteric, Intertrochanter, 27244-27245
            with Intermedullary Implant, 27245
          Peritrochanteric, Peritrochanter, 27244-27245
            with Intermedullary Implant, 27245
          Subtrochanteric, Subtrochanter, 27244-27245
            with Intermedullary Implant, 27245
    Thumb, 26665
    Tibia and Fibula, 27828
    Tibia, Tibial
      Articular Surface, 27827
        with Fibula, Fibular
          Fracture, 27828
      Bicondylar, 27536
      Condylar
        Bicondylar, 27536
        Unicondylar, 27535
      Distal, 27826
      Pilon, 27827
        with Fibula, Fibular
          Fracture, 27828

ORIF — continued
  Fracture — continued
    Tibia, Tibial — continued
      Plafond, 27827
        with Fibula, Fibular
          Fracture, 27828
      Plateau, 27535-27536
      Proximal, 27535-27536
      Shaft, 27758-27759
        with Fibula, Fibular
          Fracture, 27758-27759
        with Intermedullary Implant, 27759
      Unicondylar, 27535
    Toe, 28525
      Great, 28505
    Trapezium, 25645
    Trapezoid, 25645
    Triquetral, 25645
    Ulna, Ulnar
      and Radial, Radius, 25575
      Monteggia, 24635
      Proximal, 24635, 24685
      Shaft, 25545
      or Radial, Radius, 25574
    Vertebral, 22325-22328
    Zygomatic Arch, 21365-21366
Ormond Disease
  Ureterolysis, 50715
Orogastric Tube
  Placement, 43752
Oropharynx
  Biopsy, 42800
Orthodontic Cephalogram, 70350
Orthomyxoviridae
  Antibody, 86710
  by Immunoassay with Direct Optical Observation, 87804
Orthomyxovirus, 86710, 87804
Orthopantogram, 70355
Orthopedic Cast
  See Cast
Orthopedic Surgery
  Computer Assisted Navigation, 20985
  Stereotaxis
    Computer Assisted, 20985
Orthoptic Training, 92065
Orthoroentgenogram, 77073
Orthosis/Orthotics
  Check–Out, 97762
  Management/Training, 97760
Os Calcis Fracture
  with Manipulation, 28405-28406
  without Manipulation, 28400
  Open Treatment, 28415-28420
  Percutaneous Fixation, 28406
Oscillometry, 94728
Osmolality
  Blood, 83930
  Urine, 83935
Osseous Survey, 77074-77076
Osseous Tissue
  See Bone
Ossicles
  Excision
    Stapes
      with Footplate Drill Out, 69661
      without Foreign Material, 69660-69661
  Reconstruction
    Ossicular Chain
      Tympanoplasty with Antrotomy or Mastoidotomy, 69636-69637
      Tympanoplasty with Mastoidectomy, 69642, 69644, 69646
      Tympanoplasty without Mastoidectomy, 69632-69633
  Release
    Stapes, 69650
  Replacement
    with Prosthesis, 69633, 69637
OST, 59020
Ostectomy
  Carpal, 25215
  Femur, 27365
  Humerus, 24999
  Metacarpal, 26250

Ostectomy — *continued*
  Metatarsal, 28288
  Phalanges
    Fingers, 26260-26262
  Pressure Ulcer
    Ischial, 15941, 15945
    Sacral, 15933, 15935, 15937
    Trochanteric, 15951, 15953, 15958
  Radius, 25999
  Scapula, 23190
  Sternum, 21620
  Ulna, 25999
Osteocalcin, 83937
Osteocartilaginous Exostosis
  Auditory Canal
    Excision, 69140
Osteochondroma
  Auditory Canal
    Excision, 69140
Osteoclasis
  Carpal, 26989
  Clavicle, 23929
  Femur, 27599
  Humerus, 24999
  Metacarpal, 26989
  Metatarsal, 28899
  Patella, 27599
  Radius, 26989
  Scapula, 23929
  Tarsal, 28899
  Thorax, 23929
  Ulna, 26989
Osteocutaneous Flap
  with Microvascular Anastomosis, 20969-20973
Osteoma
  Sinusotomy
    Frontal, 31075
Osteomyelitis
  Excision
    Clavicle, 23180
    Facial, 21026
    Femur, 27360
    Fibula
      Distal, 27641
      Proximal, 27360
    Humerus, 24140
      Proximal, 23184
    Mandible, 21025
    Metacarpal, 26230
    Olecranon Process, 24147
    Pelvis/Hip Joint
      Deep, 27071
      Superficial, 27070
    Phalanx (Toe), 28124
    Phalanx (Finger)
      Distal, 26236
      Proximal or Middle, 26235
    Radial Head/Neck, 24145
    Scapula, 23182
    Talus/Calcaneus, 28120
    Tarsal/Metatarsal, 28122
    Tibia
      Distal, 27640
      Proximal, 27360
    Ulna, 25150
  Incision
    Elbow, 23935
    Femur, 27303
    Foot, 28005
    Forearm, 25035
    Hand/Finger, 26034
    Hip Joint, 26992
    Humerus, 23935
    Knee, 27303
    Leg/Ankle, 27607
    Pelvis, 26992
    Shoulder, 23035
    Thorax, 21510
    Wrist, 25035
  Sequestrectomy
    Clavicle, 23170
    Forearm, 25145
    Humeral Head, 23174
    Humerus, Shaft or Distal, 24134
    Olecranon Process, 24138
    Radial Head/Neck, 24136

Osteomyelitis — *continued*
  Sequestrectomy — *continued*
    Scapula, 23172
    Skull, 61501
    Wrist, 25145
Osteopathic Manipulation, 98925-98929
Osteophytectomy, 63075-63078
Osteoplasty
  Carpal Bone, 25394
  Facial Bones
    Augmentation, 21208
    Reduction, 21209
  Femoral Neck, 27179
  Femur, 27179
    Lengthening, 27466-27468
    Shortening, 27465, 27468
  Fibula
    Lengthening, 27715
  Humerus, 24420
  Metacarpal, 26568
  Phalanges
    Finger, 26568
    Toe, 28299, 28310-28312
  Radius, 25390-25393
  Tibia
    Lengthening, 27715
  Ulna, 25390-25393
  Vertebra
    Cervicothoracic, 22510, 22512
    Lumbosacral, 22511-22512
Osteotomy
  with Graft
    Reconstruction
      Periorbital Region, 21267-21268
  Blount, 27455, 27475-27485
  Calcaneus, 28300
  Chin, 21121-21123
  Clavicle, 23480-23485
  Femur
    with Fixation, 27165
    with Open Reduction of Hip, 27156
    with Realignment, 27454
    without Fixation, 27448-27450
    Femoral Neck, 27161
    for Slipped Epiphysis, 27181
    Greater Trochanter, 27140
  Fibula, 27707-27712
  Hip, 27146-27156
    Femoral
      with Open Reduction, 27156
      Femur, 27151
  Humerus, 24400-24410
  Mandible, 21198-21199
    Extra–oral, 21047
    Intra–oral, 21046
  Maxilla, 21206
    Extra–oral, 21049
    Intra–oral, 21048
  Metacarpal, 26565
  Metatarsal, 28306-28309
  Orbit Reconstruction, 21256
  Patella
    Wedge, 27448
  Pelvis, 27158
  Pemberton, 27147
  Periorbital
    Orbital Hypertelorism, 21260-21263
    Osteotomy with Graft, 21267-21268
  Phalanges
    Finger, 26567
    Toe, 28299, 28310-28312
  Radius
    and Ulna, 25365, 25375
    Distal Third, 25350
    Middle or Proximal Third, 25355
    Multiple, 25370
  Salter, 27146
  Skull Base, 61582-61585, 61592
  Spine
    Anterior, 22220-22226
    Posterior/Posterolateral, 22210-22214
      Cervical, 22210
      Each Additional Vertebral Segment, 22208, 22216
      Lumbar, 22207, 22214
      Thoracic, 22206, 22212

Osteotomy — *continued*
  Spine — *continued*
    Posterior/Posterolateral — *continued*
      Three-Column, 22206-22208
  Talus, 28302
  Tarsal, 28304-28305
  Tibia, 27455-27457, 27705, 27709-27712
  Ulna, 25360
    and Radius, 25365, 25375
    Multiple, 25370
  Vertebra
    Additional Segment
      Anterior Approach, 22226
      Posterior/Posterolateral Approach, 22208, 22216
    Cervical
      Anterior Approach, 22220
      Posterior/Posterolateral Approach, 22210
    Lumbar
      Anterior Approach, 22224
      Posterior/Posterolateral Approach, 22214
    Thoracic
      Anterior Approach, 22222
      Posterior/Posterolateral Approach, 22212
OTC, 81405
Other Nonoperative Measurements and Examinations
  Acid Perfusion
    Esophagus, 91013, 91030
  Acid Reflux
    Esophagus, 91034-91035, 91037-91038
  Attenuation Measurements
    Ear Protector, 92596
  Bernstein Test, 91030
  Breath Hydrogen, 91065
  Bronchial Challenge Testing, 95070-95071
  Gastric Motility (Manometric) Studies, 91020
  Information
    Analysis of Data, 99090
  Iontophoresis, 97033
  Laryngeal Function Studies, 92520
  Manometry
    Anorectal, 91122
    Esophageal, 91010
  Photography
    Anterior Segment, 92286
    External Ocular, 92285
Otoacoustic Emission Evaluation, 92587-92588
Otolaryngology
  Diagnostic
    Exam under Anesthesia, 92502
Otomy
  See Incision
Otoplasty, 69300
Otorhinolaryngology
  Diagnostic
    Otolaryngology Exam, 92502
    Unlisted Services and Procedures, 92700
Ouchterlony Immunodiffusion, 86331
Outer Ear
  CT Scan, 70480-70482
Outpatient Visit, 99201-99215
Output, Cardiac
  by Indicator Dilution, 93561-93562
Ova
  Smear, 87177
Oval Window
  Repair Fistula, 69666
Oval Window Fistula
  Repair, 69666
Ovarian Cyst
  Excision, 58925
  Incision and Drainage, 58800-58805
Ovarian Vein Syndrome
  Ureterolysis, 50722
Ovariectomies, 58940-58943
  with Hysterectomy, 58262-58263, 58291-58292, 58542, 58544, 58552, 58554, 58571, 58573
  for Ectopic Pregnancy, 59120, 59151
Ovariolysis, 58740

Ovary
  Abscess
    Incision and Drainage, 58820-58822
      Abdominal Approach, 58822
      Vaginal Approach, 58820
  Biopsy, 58900
  Cryopreservation, 88240
  Cyst
    Incision and Drainage, 58800-58805
    Ovarian, 58805
  Excision, 58662, 58720
    Cyst, 58925
    Partial
      Oophorectomy, 58661, 58940
      Ovarian Malignancy, 58943
      Peritoneal Malignancy, 58943
      Tubal Malignancy, 58943
      Wedge Resection, 58920
    Total, 58940-58943
  Laparoscopy, 58660-58662, 58679
  Lysis
    Adhesions, 58660, 58740
  Radical Resection, 58950-58952
  Transposition, 58825
  Tumor
    Resection, 58950-58958
  Unlisted Services and Procedures, 58679, 58999
  Wedge Resection, 58920
Oviduct
  Anastomosis, 58750
  Chromotubation, 58350
  Ectopic Pregnancy, 59120-59121
  Excision, 58700-58720
  Fulguration
    Laparoscopic, 58670
  Hysterosalpingography, 74740
  Laparoscopy, 58679
  Ligation, 58600-58611
  Lysis
    Adhesions, 58740
  Occlusion, 58615
    Laparoscopic, 58671
  Repair, 58752
    Anastomosis, 58750
    Create Stoma, 58770
  Unlisted Services and Procedures, 58679, 58999
  X–ray with Contrast, 74740
Ovocyte
  See Oocyte
Ovulation Tests, 84830
Ovum Implantation, 58976
Ovum Transfer Surgery, 58976
Oxalate, 83945
Oxcarbazepine
  Assay, 80183
Oxidase, Ceruloplasmin, 82390
Oxidoreductase, Alcohol–Nad+, 84588
Oximetry (Noninvasive)
  See Also Pulmonology, Diagnostic
  Blood O2 Saturation
    Ear or Pulse, 94760-94762
Oxoisomerase, 84087
Oxosteroids, 83586-83593
Oxycodinone, *[80305, 80306, 80307], [80361, 80362, 80363, 80364]*
Oxygen Saturation, 82805-82810
  Ear Oximetry, 94760-94762
  Pulse Oximetry, 94760-94762
Oxyproline, 83500-83505
Oxytocin Stress Test, Fetal, 59020

P

PABPN1, 81401
Pacemaker, Heart
  See Also Cardiology, Defibrillator, Heart
  Conversion, 33214
  Electronic Analysis
    Antitachycardia System, 93724
  Electrophysiologic Evaluation, 93640-93642
  Evaluation, 93279-93281, 93286, 93288, 93293-93294, 93296
  Insertion, 33206-33208
    Electrode(s), 33202-33203, 33210-33211, 33216-33217, 33224-33225
    Pulse Generator, 33212-33213, 33240
  Interrogation, 93294, 93296

Pacemaker, Heart — *continued*
 Permanent Leadless, Ventricular
  Device Evaluation, 0389T-0391T
  Insertion, 0387T
  Removal, 0388T
  Replacement, 0387T
 Programming, 93279-93281
 Relocation
  Skin Pocket, 33222-33223
 Removal, 33236-33237
  Electrodes, 33234-33235, 33238, 33243-33244
  Pulse Generator
   Implantable Defibrillator, 33241
   Pacemaker, 33233
 Repair
  Electrode(s), 33218-33220
  Leads, 33218-33220
 Replacement, 33206-33208
  Catheter, 33210
  Electrode(s), 33210-33211
  Leads, 33210-33211
  Pulse Generator, 33212-33213
 Repositioning
  Electrodes, 33215, 33226, 33249
 Telephonic Analysis, 93293
 Upgrade, 33214
P-Acetamidophenol, *[80329, 80330, 80331]*
Pachymetry
 Eye, 76514
Packing
 Nasal Hemorrhage, 30901-30906
PAFAH1B1, 81405-81406
PAH, 81406
Pain Management
 Epidural, 62350-62351, 62360-62362, 99601-99602
 Intrathecal, 62350-62351, 62360-62362, 99601-99602
 Intravenous Therapy, 96360-96368, 96374-96376
Pain Therapy, 0278T, 62350-62365
Palatal Augmentation Prosthesis, 21082
Palatal Lift Prosthesis, 21083
Palate
 Abscess
  Incision and Drainage, 42000
 Biopsy, 42100
 Excision, 42120, 42145
 Fracture
  Closed Treatment, 21421
  Open Treatment, 21422-21423
 Lesion
  Destruction, 42160
  Excision, 42104-42120
 Prosthesis
  Augmentation, 21082
  Impression, 42280
  Insertion, 42281
  Lift, 21089
 Reconstruction
  Lengthening, 42226-42227
 Repair
  Cleft Palate, 42200-42225
  Laceration, 42180-42182
  Vomer Flap, 42235
 Unlisted Services and Procedures, 42299
Palate, Cleft
 Repair, 42200-42225
 Rhinoplasty, 30460-30462
Palatopharyngoplasty, 42145
Palatoplasty, 42200-42225
Palatoschisis, 42200-42225
PALB2, 81406, 81432
Palm
 Bursa
  Incision and Drainage, 26025-26030
 Fasciectomy, 26121-26125
 Fasciotomy, 26040-26045
 Tendon
  Excision, 26170
 Tendon Sheath
  Excision, 26145
  Incision and Drainage, 26020
Palsy, Seventh Nerve
 Graft/Repair, 15840-15845

PAMG-1, 84112
P&P, 85230
Pancoast Tumor Resection, 32503-32504
Pancreas
 Anastomosis
  with Intestines, 48520-48540, 48548
 Anesthesia, 00794
 Biopsy, 48100
  Needle Biopsy, 48102
 Cyst
  Anastomosis, 48520-48540
  Repair, 48500
 Debridement
  Peripancreatic Tissue, 48105
 Excision
  Ampulla of Vater, 48148
  Duct, 48148
  Partial, 48140-48146, 48150-48154, 48160
  Peripancreatic Tissue, 48105
  Total, 48155-48160
 Lesion
  Excision, 48120
 Needle Biopsy, 48102
 Placement
  Drains, 48000-48001
 Pseudocyst
  Drainage
   Open, 48510
 Removal
  Calculi (Stone), 48020
 Removal Transplanted Allograft, 48556
 Repair
  Cyst, 48500
 Resection, 48105
 Suture, 48545
 Transplantation, 48160, 48550, 48554-48556
  Allograft Preparation, 48550-48552
 Unlisted Services and Procedures, 48999
 X-ray with Contrast, 74300-74301
  Injection Procedure, 48400
Pancreas, Endocrine Only
 Islet Cell
  Antibody, 86341
  Transplantation, 48160
Pancreatectomy
 with Transplantation, 48160
 Donor, 48550
 Partial, 48140-48146, 48150-48154, 48160
 Total, 48155-48160
Pancreatic DNAse
 See DNAse
Pancreatic Duct
 Destruction
  Calculi (Stone), 43265
  Tumor, *[43278]*
 Dilation
  Endoscopy, *[43277]*
 Drainage
  of Cyst, 48999
 Endoscopy
  Collection
   Specimen, 43260
  Destruction
   Calculi (Stone), 43265
   Tumor, *[43278]*
  Dilation, *[43277]*
  Removal
   Calculi (Stone), 43264
   Foreign Body, *[43275]*
   Stent, *[43275, 43276]*
  Sphincterotomy, 43262
  Sphincter Pressure, 43263
 Incision
  Sphincter, 43262
 Placement
  Stent, *[43274]*
 Removal
  Calculi (Stone), 43264
  Foreign Body, *[43275]*
  Stent, *[43275, 43276]*
 Tumor
  Destruction, *[43278]*
 X-ray with Contrast
  Guide Catheter, 74329-74330
Pancreatic Elastase 1 (PE1), 82656
Pancreatic Islet Cell AB, 86341

Pancreaticojejunostomy, 48548
Pancreatitis
 Incision and Drainage, 48000
Pancreatography
 Injection Procedure, 48400
 Intraoperative, 74300-74301
Pancreatojejunostomies
 See Pancreaticojejunostomy
Pancreatorrhaphy, 48545
Pancreatotomy
 Sphincter, 43262
Pancreozymin–Secretin Test, 82938
Panel
 See Blood Tests; Organ or Disease Oriented panel
Panniculectomy, 15830
PAP, 88141-88167, 88174-88175
Papilla Excision, 46230 *[46220]*
Papilla, Interdental
 See Gums
Papilloma
 Destruction
  Anus, 46900-46924
  Penis, 54050-54065
Papillotomy, 43262
 Destruction
  Anus, 46900-46924
  Penis, 54050-54065
PAPP D, 83632
Pap Smears, 88141-88155, 88164-88167, 88174-88175
Paracentesis
 Abdomen, 49082-49083
 Eye
  Anterior Chamber
   with Diagnostic Aspiration of Aqueous, 65800
   with Removal of Blood, 65815
   with Removal Vitreous and
    or Discission of Anterior Hyaloid
    Membrane, 65810
Paracervical Nerve
 Injection
  Anesthetic, 64435
Paraffin Bath Therapy, 97018
Paraganglioma, Medullary, 80424
Parainfluenza Virus
 Antigen Detection
  Immunofluorescence, 87279
Paralysis, Facial Nerve
 Graft, 15840-15845
 Repair, 15840-15845
Paralysis, Infantile
 Polio
  Antibody, 86658
  Vaccine, 90713
Paranasal Sinuses
 See Sinus
Parasites
 Blood, 87206-87209
 Concentration, 87015
 Examination, 87169
 Smear, 87177
 Tissue, 87220
Parasitic Worms, 86682
Paraspinous Block, Thoracic, *[64461, 64462, 64463]*
Parathormone, 83970
Parathyrin, 83970
Parathyroid Autotransplantation, 60512
Parathyroidectomy, 60500-60505
Parathyroid Gland
 Autotransplant, 60512
 Biopsy, 60699
 Excision, 60500-60502
 Exploration, 60500-60505
 Nuclear Medicine
  Imaging, 78070-78072
Parathyroid Hormone, 83970
Parathyroid Hormone Measurement, 83970
Parathyroid Transplantation, 60512
Para-Tyrosine, 84510
Paraurethral Gland
 Abscess
  Incision and Drainage, 53060

Paravertebral Nerve
 Destruction, *[64633, 64634, 64635, 64636]*
 Injection
  Anesthetic, 64490-64495
  Neurolytic, *[64633, 64634, 64635, 64636]*
Parietal Cell Vagotomies, 43641
Parietal Craniotomy, 61556
Paring
 Skin Lesion
  Benign Hyperkeratotic
   More than Four Lesions, 11057
   Single Lesion, 11055
   Two to Four Lesions, 11056
PARK2, 81405-81406
Park Posterior Anal Repair, 46761
Paronychia
 Incision and Drainage, 10060-10061
Parotid Duct
 Diversion, 42507-42510
 Reconstruction, 42507-42510
Parotidectomy, 61590
Parotid Gland
 Abscess
  Incision and Drainage, 42300-42305
 Calculi (Stone)
  Excision, 42330, 42340
 Excision
  Partial, 42410-42415
  Total, 42420-42426
 Tumor
  Excision, 42410-42426
Parotitides, Epidemic
 See Mumps
Pars Abdominalis Aortae
 See Aorta, Abdominal
Partial Claviculectomy, 23120, 23180
Partial Colectomy, 44140-44147, 44160, 44204-44208, 44213
Partial Cystectomy, 51550-51565
Partial Esophagectomy, 43116-43124
Partial Gastrectomy, 43631-43635, 43845
Partial Glossectomy, 41120-41135
Partial Hepatectomy, 47120, 47125-47130, 47140-47142
Partial Mastectomies, 19301-19302
 See Also Breast, Excision, Lesion
Partial Nephrectomy, 50240, 50543
Partial Pancreatectomy, 48140-48146, 48150, 48153-48154, 48160
Partial Splenectomy, 38101, 38120
Partial Thromboplastin Time, 85730-85732
Partial Ureterectomy, 50220, 50546
Particle Agglutination, 86403-86406
Parvovirus
 Antibody, 86747
Patch
 Allergy Tests, 95044
Patella
 See Also Knee
 Dislocation, 27560-27566
 Excision, 27350
  with Reconstruction, 27424
 Fracture, 27520-27524
 Reconstruction, 27437-27438
 Repair
  Chondromalacia, 27418
  Instability, 27420-27424
Patellar Tendon Bearing (PTB) Cast, 29435
Patellectomy, 27350, 27524, 27566
 with Reconstruction, 27424
Patent Ductus Arteriosus
 Closure, 93582
Paternity Testing, 86910-86911
Patey's Operation
 Mastectomy, Modified Radical, 19307
Pathologic Dilatation
 See Dilation
Pathology
 Clinical
  Consultation, 80500-80502
   Intraoperative, 88329-88334
  Molecular, 81400-81408
  Report Includes pT Category, pN Category, Gleason Score, Statement of Margin Status, 3267F

Pathology — *continued*
Surgical
Consultation, 88321-88325
Intraoperative, 88329-88332
Decalcification Procedure, 88311
Electron Microscopy, 88348
Gross and Micro Exam
Level II, 88302
Level III, 88304
Level IV, 88305
Level V, 88307
Level VI, 88309
Gross Exam
Level I, 88300
Histochemistry, 88319
Immunocytochemistry, 88342, 88344, [88341]
Immunofluorescence, 88346, [88350]
In situ Hybridization, 88365, 88366, [88364]
Morphometry
Hybridization Techniques, 88367-88369 [88373, 88374], [88377]
Nerve, 88356
Skeletal Muscle, 88355
Tumor, 88358, 88361
Nerve Teasing, 88362
Special Stain, 88312-88314
Staining, 88312-88314
Unlisted Services and Procedures, 88399, 89240
Patient
Dialysis Training
Completed Course, 90989
Education
Heart Failure, 4003F
Patterson's Test
Blood Urea Nitrogen, 84520, 84525
Paul–Bunnell Test
See Antibody; Antibody Identification; Microsomal Antibody
PAX2, 81406
PAX8/PPARG (t(2;3)(q13;p25)), 81401
P B Antibodies, 86308-86310
PBG
Urine, 84106-84110
PBSCT (Peripheral Blood Stem Cell Transplant), 38240-38242
PC, 81406
PCCA, 81405-81406
PCCB, 81406
PCDH15, 81400, 81406-81407, 81430
PCDH19, 81405
PCL, 27407, 29889
PCP, 83992
PCSK9, 81406
PDE6A, 81434
PDE6B, 81434
PDGFRA, 81314
PDHA1, 81405-81406
PDHB, 81405
PDHX, 81406
PDX1, 81404
Peak Flow Rate, 94150
Pean's Operation
Amputation, Leg, Upper, at Hip, 27290
Pectoral Cavity
See Chest Cavity
Pectus Carinatum
Reconstructive Repair, 21740-21742
with Thoracoscopy, 21743
Pectus Excavatum Repair
Anesthesia, 00474
Reconstructive Repair, 21740-21742
with Thoracoscopy, 21743
PEDIARIX, 90723
Pediatric Critical Care
Initial, 99471
Subsequent, 99472
Pedicle Fixation, 22842-22844
Pedicle Flap
Formation, 15570-15576
Island, 15740
Neurovascular, 15750
Transfer, 15650
PedvaxHIB, 90647
PEEP, 94660

Peet Operation
See Nerves, Sympathectomy, Excision
PEG, 43246
Pelvic Adhesions, 58660, 58662, 58740
Pelvic Bone
Drainage, 26990
Pelvic Exam, 57410
Pelvic Exenteration, 51597
for Colorectal Malignancy, 45126
Pelvic Fixation
Insertion, 22848
Pelvic Lymphadenectomy, 38562, 38765
with Hysterectomy, 58210, 58548, 58951, 58954
with Prostatectomy, 55812-55815, 55842-55845
with Prostate Exposure, 55862-55865
with Trachelectomy, 57531
with Vaginectomy, 57112
with Vulvectomy, 56640
for Malignancy, 58951, 58958-58960
Laparoscopic, 38571-38572, 58548
Pelvimetry, 74710
Pelviolithotomy, 50130
Pelvis
See Also Hip
Abscess
Incision and Drainage, 26990, 45000
Angiography, 72191
Biopsy, 27040-27041
Bone
Drainage, 26992
Brace Application, 20662
Bursa
Incision and Drainage, 26991
CT Scan, 72191-72194
Cyst
Aspiration, 50390
Injection, 50390
Destruction
Lesion, 58662
Endoscopy
Destruction of Lesions, 58662
Lysis of Adhesions, 58660
Oviduct Surgery, 58670-58671
Exclusion
Small Intestine, 44700
Exenteration
for Colorectal Malignancy, 45126
for Gynecologic Malignancy, 58240
for Prostatic Malignancy, 51597
for Urethral Malignancy, 51597
for Vesical Malignancy, 51597
Fetal with Maternal Pelvic, 74712-74713
Halo, 20662
Hematoma
Incision and Drainage, 26990
Lysis
Adhesions, 58660
Magnetic Resonance Angiography, 72198
Magnetic Resonance Imaging (MRI), 72195-72197
Removal
Foreign Body, 27086-27087
Repair
Osteotomy, 27158
Tendon, 27098
Ring
Dislocation, 27197-27198, 27216-27218
Fracture, 27216-27218
Closed Treatment, 27197-27198
Tumor, 27047-27049 [27043, 27045], 27065, 27075-27078
Ultrasound, 76856-76857
Unlisted Services and Procedures, 27299
X–ray, 72170-72190
Manometry, 74710
Pelvi–Ureteroplasty, 50400-50405
Pemberton Osteotomy of Pelvis, 27158
Penectomy, 54120-54135
Penetrating Keratoplasties, 65730-65755
Penile Induration
Injection, 54200
with Surgical Exposure, 54205
Plaque Excision, 54110
with Graft, 54111-54112

Penile Prosthesis
Insertion
Inflatable, 54401-54405
Semi-Rigid, 54400
Removal Only
Inflatable, 54406, 54415
Semi–Rigid, 54415
Repair
Inflatable, 54408
Replacement
Inflatable, 54410-54411, 54416-54417
Semi–Rigid, 54416-54417
Penile Rigidity Test, 54250
Penile Tumescence Test, 54250
Penis
Amputation
Partial, 54120
Radical, 54130-54135
Total, 54125-54135
Biopsy, 54100-54105
Circumcision
with Clamp or Other Device, 54150
Newborn, 54150
Repair, 54163
Surgical Excision, 54161
Newborn, 54160
Excision
Partial, 54120
Prepuce, 54150-54161, 54163
Total, 54125-54135
Frenulum
Excision, 54164
Incision
and Drainage, 54015
Prepuce, 54000-54001
Injection
for Erection, 54235
Peyronie Disease, 54200
Surgical Exposure Plaque, 54205
Vasoactive Drugs, 54231
X-ray, 54230
Insertion
Prosthesis
Inflatable, 54401-54405
Noninflatable, 54400
Irrigation
Priapism, 54220
Lesion
Destruction
Any Method
Extensive, 54065
Cryosurgery, 54056
Electrodesiccation, 54055
Laser Surgery, 54057
Simple, 54050-54060
Surgical Excision, 54060
Excision, 54060
Penile Plaque, 54110-54112
Nocturnal Tumescence Test, 54250
Occlusion
Vein, 37790
Plaque
Excision, 54110-54112
Plethysmography, 54240
Prepuce
Stretch, 54450
Reconstruction
Angulation, 54360
Chordee, 54300-54304, 54328
Complications, 54340-54348
Epispadias, 54380-54390
Hypospadias, 54328-54352
Injury, 54440
Replantation, 54438
Removal
Foreign Body, 54115
Prosthesis
Inflatable, 54406, 54415
Semi–Rigid, 54415
Repair
Corporeal Tear, 54437
Fistulization, 54435
Priapism with Shunt, 54420-54430
Prosthesis
Inflatable, 54408

Penis — *continued*
Replacement
Prosthesis
Inflatable, 54410-54411, 54416-54417
Semi–Rigid, 54416-54417
Replantation, 54438
Revascularization, 37788
Rigidity Test, 54250
Test Erection, 54250
Unlisted Services and Procedures, 54699, 55899
Venous Studies, 93980-93981
Penis Adhesions
Lysis
Post–circumcision, 54162
Penis Prostheses
See Penile Prosthesis
Pentagastrin Test, 43755-43757
Pentamidine
Inhalation Treatment, 94640-94644
Peptidase P
Angiotensin Converting Enzyme (ACE), 82164
Peptidase S
Leucine Aminopeptidase, 83670
Peptide, Connecting, 80432, 84681
Peptide, Vasoactive Intestinal, 84586
Peptidyl Dipeptidase A
Angiotensin Converting Enzyme (ACE), 82164
Percutaneous
Access, Biliary, 47541
Aspiration
Bartholin's Gland, 58999
Gallbladder, 47999
Seminal Vesicle, 54699, 55899
Atherectomies, 0234T-0238T, 37225, 37227, 37229, 37231, 37233, 37235
Biopsy, Gallbladder/Bile Ducts, 47553
Cardiopulmonary Bypass, 33999
Cystostomy, 51100-51102, 53899
Discectomies, 62287
Electric Nerve Stimulation
Electrode Insertion, 64553-64565
Laminotomy/Laminectomy for Decompression
Neural Elements, 0274T-0275T
Lumbar Discectomy, 62287
Lysis of Adhesions
Epidural, 62263-62264
Nephrostomies, 50395, 52334
Transluminal Angioplasty
Aortic, [37246, 37247]
Brachiocephalic, [37246, 37247]
Coronary Artery, [92920, 92921]
with Atherectomy, [92924, 92925], [92933, 92934, 92937, 92938, 92941, 92943, 92944]
wtih Stent, [92928, 92929, 92933, 92934, 92937, 92938, 92941, 92943, 92944]
Femoral, Popliteal, 37224-37227
Iliac, 37220-37223
Pulmonary, 92997, 92998
Renal, [37246, 37247]
Tibioperoneal, 37228-37235
Vein, [37248, 37249]
Visceral, [37246, 37247]
Vertebral Augmentation, 22513-22515
Vertebroplasty, 22510-22512
Pereyra Procedure, 51845, 57289, 58267, 58293
Performance Measures
See Also Physician Quality Reporting System (PQRS)
ACE Inhibitor Therapy, 4010F
Acute Otitis
Examination
Membrane Mobility, 2035F
History
Auricular Pain, 1116F
Intervention
Antimicrobial Therapy, 4131F-4132F
Effusion Antihistamines, 4133F-4134F
Systemic Antimicrobials, 4131F-4132F
Systemic Steroids, 4135F-4136F
Topical Therapy, 4130F
Anginal Symptom Assessment, 1002F
Antiplatelet Therapy, 4011F
Aortic Aneurysm, 9001F-9004F
Beta–Blocker Therapy, 4008F

Performance Measures — *continued*
  Blood Pressure, 2000F
    Postpartum Care Visit, 0503F
    Prenatal Care Visit Initial, 0500F
    Prenatal Care Visit Subsequent, 0502F
    Prenatal Flow Sheet, 0501F
  Carotid Stenosis, 9005F-9007F
  Statin Therapy, 4013F
  Tobacco Use
    Assessment, 1000F, 1034F-1036F
    Counseling, 4000F
    Pharmacologic Therapy, 4001F
Performance Test
  See Also Physical Medicine/Therapy/Occupation-
    al Therapy
  Cognitive, 96125
  Performance Test Physical Therapy, 97750
  Psychological Test, 96101-96103
    Computer-Assisted, 96103
Perfusion
  Brain
    Imaging, 0042T
    Myocardial, 78451-78454
      Imaging, 0439T, 78466-78469
    Positron Emission Tomography (PET)
      Myocardial Imaging, 78491-78492
    Pulmonary, 78580, 78582, 78597-78598
Perfusion, Intracranial Arterial
  Percutaneous, 61645
  Thrombolysis, 61624
Perfusion Pump
  See Infusion Pump
Pericardectomies, 33030-33031
  Endoscopic, 32659
Pericardial Cyst
  See Cyst, Pericardial
  Excision, 33050
    Thoracoscopic, 32661
Pericardial Sac
  Drainage, 32659
Pericardial Window
  for Drainage, 33025
    Thoracoscopic, 32659
Pericardiectomy
  Complete, 33030-33031
  Subtotal, 33030-33031
Pericardiocentesis, 33010-33011
  Ultrasound Guidance, 76930
Pericardiostomy
  Tube, 33015
Pericardiotomy
  Removal
    Clot/Foreign Body, 33020
      via Thoracoscopy, 32658
Pericardium
  Cyst
    Excision, 32661, 33050
  Excision, 32659, 33030-33031
  Incision, 33030-33031
    with Tube, 33015
  Removal
    Clot, 33020
    Foreign Body, 33020
  Incision and Drainage, 33025
  Puncture Aspiration, 33010-33011
  Removal
    Clot
      Endoscopic, 32658
    Foreign Body
      Endoscopic, 32658
  Tumor
    Excision, 32661, 33050
Peridural Anesthesia
  See Anesthesia, Epidural
Peridural Injection, 62281-62282, 62320-62327,
    64479-64484
Perineal Prostatectomy
  Partial, 55801
  Radical, 55810-55815
Perineoplasty, 56810
Perineorrhaphy
  Repair
    Rectocele, 57250
Perineum
  Abscess
    Incision and Drainage, 56405

Perineum — *continued*
  Biopsy, 56605-56606
  Colposcopy, 99170
  Debridement
    Infected, 11004, 11006
  Removal
    Prosthesis, 53442
  Repair, 56810
  X–ray with Contrast, 74775
Perionychia, 10060-10061
Periorbital Region
  Reconstruction–Osteotomy
    with Graft, 21267-21268
  Repair–Osteotomy, 21260-21263
Peripheral Artery Disease (PAD) Rehabilitation,
    93668
Peripheral Blood Stem Cell Transplant, 38240-
    38242
Peripheral Nerve
  Repair/Suture
    Major, 64856, 64859
Periprostatic Placement Biodegradable Material
  Transperineal, 0438T
Periprosthetic Capsulotomy
  Breast, 19371
Peristaltic Pumps
  See Infusion Pump
Peritoneal Dialysis, 4055F, 90945-90947
  Kt/V Level, 3082F-3084F
  Training
    Counseling, 90989, 90993
Peritoneal Free Air, 49400
Peritoneal Lavage, 49084
Peritoneoscopy
  Biopsy, 49321
  Exploration, 49320
Peritoneum
  Abscess
    Incision and Drainage, 49020
  Chemotherapy Administration, 96446
  Endoscopy
    Drainage
      Lymphocele, 49323
  Exchange
    Drainage Catheter, 49423
  Injection
    Contrast
      Via Catheter, 49424
  Ligation
    Shunt, 49428
  Removal
    Cannula
      Catheter, 49422
    Foreign Body, 49402
    Shunt, 49429
  Tumor
    Resection, 58950-58954
  Unlisted Services and Procedures, 49999
  Venous Shunt, 49427
  X–ray, 74190
Persistent, Omphalomesenteric Duct
  Excision, 44800
Persistent Truncus Arteriosus
  See Truncus Arteriosus
  Repair, 33786
Personal Care
  See Self Care
Personality Test, 96101-96103
  Computer-Assisted, 96103
Pertussis Immunization, 90715, 90723
Pessary
  Insertion, 57160
Pesticides
  Chlorinated Hydrocarbons, 82441
PET
  with Computed Tomography (CT)
    Limited Area, 78814
    Skull Base to Mid-thigh, 78815
    Whole Body, 78816
  Brain, 78608-78609
  Heart, 78459
  Limited Area, 78811
  Myocardial Imaging Perfusion Study, 78491-
    78492
  Skull Base to Mid-thigh, 78812
  Whole Body, 78813

Petrous Temporal
  Excision
    Apex, 69530
Peyreva Procedure, 51845
Peyronie Disease
  with Graft, 54110-54112
  Injection, 54200
  Surgical Exposure, 54205
PFG (Percutaneous Fluoroscopic Gastrostomy),
    49440
PFT (Pulmonary Function Test), 94010-94799
PG, 84081, 84150
pH
  Blood Gases, 82800-82805
  Body Fluid, Not Otherwise Specified, 83986
  Exhaled Breath Condensate, 83987
Phacoemulsification
  Removal
    Extracapsular Cataract, 66982, 66984
    Secondary Membranous Cataract, 66850
Phagocytosis
  White Blood Cells, 86344
Phalangectomy
  Toe, 28150
    Partial, 28160
Phalanges (Hand)
  See Also Finger, Bone
  Incision, Bone Cortex, 26034
Phalanx, Finger
  Craterization, 26235, 26236
  Cyst
    Excision, 26210, 26215
  Diaphysectomy, 26235, 26236
  Excision, 26235, 26236
    Radical
      for Tumor, 26260-26262
  Fracture
    Articular
      with Manipulation, 26742
      Closed Treatment, 26740
      Open Treatment, 26746
    Distal, 26755, 26756
      Closed Treatment, 26750
      Open Treatment, 26765
      Percutaneous, 26756
    Open Treatment, 26735
      Distal, 26765
      Percutaneous Fixation, 26756
    Shaft, 26720-26727
      Open Treatment, 26735
  Incision and Drainage, 26034
  Ostectomy
    Radical
      for Tumor, 26260-26262
  Repair
    Lengthening, 26568
    Nonunion, 26546
    Osteotomy, 26567
  Saucerization, 26235, 26236
  Thumb
    Fracture
      Shaft, 26720-26727
  Tumor, 26115-26118 *[26111, 26113]*, 26210-
    26215, 26260-26262
Phalanx, Great Toe
  See Also Phalanx, Toe
  Fracture
    Closed Treatment, 28490
      with Manipulation, 28495
    Open Treatment, 28505
    Percutaneous Skeletal Fixation, 28496
Phalanx, Toe
  Condyle
    Excision, 28126
  Craterization, 28124
  Cyst
    Excision, 28108
  Diaphysectomy, 28124
  Excision, 28124, 28150-28160
  Fracture
    with Manipulation, 28515
    without Manipulation, 28510
    Open Treatment, 28525
  Repair
    Osteotomy, 28310, 28312
  Saucerization, 28124

Phalanx, Toe — *continued*
  Tumor
    Excision, 28108, 28175
Pharmaceutic Preparations
  See Drug
Pharmacotherapies
  See Chemotherapy
Pharyngeal Tonsil
  Excision, 42830-42836
    with Tonsils, 42820-42821
  Unlisted Services/Procedures, 42999
Pharyngectomy
  Partial, 42890
Pharyngolaryngectomy, 31390, 31395
Pharyngoplasty, 42950
Pharyngorrhaphy, 42900
Pharyngostomy, 42955
Pharyngotomy
  See Incision, Pharynx
Pharyngotympanic Tube
  Inflation
    with Myringotomy, 69420-69421
Pharynx
  See Also Nasopharynx; Throat
  Biopsy, 42800-42806
  Cineradiography, 70371, 74230
  Creation
    Stoma, 42955
  Excision, 42145
    with Larynx, 31390, 31395
    Partial, 42890
    Resection, 42892, 42894
  Hemorrhage, 42960-42962
  Lesion
    Destruction, 42808
    Excision, 42808
  Reconstruction, 42950
  Removal, Foreign Body, 42809
  Repair
    with Esophagus, 42953
  Unlisted Services and Procedures, 42999
  Video, 70371, 74230
  X–ray, 70370, 74210
Phencyclidine, 83992
Phenobarbital, *[80345]*
  Assay, 80184
Phenothiazine, *[80342, 80343, 80344]*
Phenotype Analysis
  by Nucleic Acid
    Infectious Agent
      HIV–1 Drug Resistance, 87903, 87904
Phenotype Prediction
  by Generic Database
    HIV–1
      Drug Susceptibility, 87900
    Using Regularly Updated Genotypic Bioinfor-
      matics, 87900
Phenylalanine, 84030
Phenylalanine–Tyrosine Ratio, 84030
Phenylketones, 84035
Phenylketonuria, 84030
Phenytoin
  Assay, 80185, 80186
Pheochromocytoma, 80424
Pheresis, 36511-36516
PHEX, 81406
Phlebectasia
  with Tissue Excision, 37735-37760
  Ablation, 36473-36479
  Removal, 37718-37735, 37765-37785
Phlebectomy
  Stab, 37765-37766
Phlebographies, 75820-75880, 75885, 75893,
    78445, 78457-78458
  Injection, 36005
Phleborrhaphy
  Femoral, 37650
  Iliac, 37660
Phlebotomy
  Therapeutic, 99195
Phonocardiogram
  Evaluation, 93799
  Intracardiac, 93799
  Tracing, 93799
Phoria
  See Strabismus

Phosphatase
Alkaline, 84075, 84080
Blood, 84078
Forensic Examination, 84061
Phosphatase, Acid, 84060
Blood, 84066
Phosphate, Pyridoxal, 84207
Phosphatidylcholine Cholinephosphohydrolase
See Tissue Typing
Phosphatidyl Glycerol, 84081
Phosphatidylglycerol, 84081
Phosphocreatine Phosphotransferase, ADP, 82550-82552
Phosphogluconate–6
Dehydrogenase, 84085
Phosphoglycerides, Glycerol, 84081
Phosphohexose Isomerase, 84087
Phosphohydrolases
Alkaline, 84075-84080
Forensic Examination, 84061
Phosphokinase, Creatine, 82550-82552
Phospholipase A2 (sPLA2-IIA), 0423T
Phospholipase C
See Tissue Typing
Phospholipid
Antibody, 86147-86148
Neutralization, 85598
Phosphomonoesterase, 84061, 84075-84080
Phosphoric Monoester Hydrolases, 84061, 84075-84080
Phosphorous, 84100
Urine, 84105
Phosphotransferase, ADP Phosphocreatine, 82550-82552
Photochemotherapies, Extracorporeal, 36522
Photochemotherapy, 96910-96913
See Also Dermatology
Endoscopic Light, 96570-96571
Photocoagulation
Endolaser Panretinal
Vitrectomy, 67040
Focal Endolaser
Vitrectomy, 67040
Iridoplasty, 66762
Lesion
Choroid, 67220
Cornea, 65450
Retina, 67210, 67228, 67229
Retinal Detachment
Prophylaxis, 67145
Repair, 67105, 67107, 67108, 67113
Retinopathy, 67228-67229
Photodynamic Therapy
Choroidal Lesions Eye, 67221, 67225
External, 96567
Photography
Ocular
Anterior Segment, 92286, 92287
External, 92285
Fundus, 92250
Skin, Diagnostic, 96904
Photo Patch
Allergy Test, 95052
See Also Allergy Tests
Photopheresis
Extracorporeal, 36522
Photophoresis
See Actinotherapy; Photochemotherapy
Photoradiation Therapies
See Actinotherapy
Photoscreen
Ocular, 99174
Photosensitivity Testing, 95056
See Also Allergy Tests
Phototherapies
See Actinotherapy
Phototherapy, Ultraviolet, 96900
PHOX2B, 81403-81404
Phrenic Nerve
Avulsion, 64746
Incision, 64746
Injection
Anesthetic, 64410
Transection, 64746

Physical Examination
Office and/or Other Outpatient Services, 99201-99205
Physical Medicine/Therapy/Occupational Therapy
See Also Neurology, Diagnostic
Activities of Daily Living, 97535, 99509
Aquatic Therapy
with Exercises, 97113
Athletic Training
Evaluation, [97169, 97170, 97171]
Re–evaluation, [97172]
Check–Out
Orthotics/Prosthetics
ADL, 97762
Cognitive Skills Development, 97532
Community/Work Reintegration, 97537
Evaluation, [97161, 97162, 97163, 97164, 97165, 97166, 97167, 97168, 97169, 97170, 97171, 97172]
Hydrotherapy
Hubbard Tank, 97036
Pool with Exercises, 97036, 97113
Joint Mobilization, 97140
Kinetic Therapy, 97530
Manipulation, 97140
Manual Therapy, 97140
Modalities
Contrast Baths, 97034
Diathermy Treatment, 97024
Electric Stimulation
Attended, Manual, 97032
Unattended, 97014
Hot or Cold Pack, 97010
Hydrotherapy (Hubbard Tank), 97036
Infrared Light Treatment, 97026
Iontophoresis, 97033
Microwave Therapy, 97024
Paraffin Bath, 97018
Traction, 97012
Ultrasound, 97035
Ultraviolet Light, 97028
Unlisted Services and Procedures, 97039
Vasopneumatic Device, 97016
Whirlpool Therapy, 97022
Orthotics Training, 97760
Osteopathic Manipulation, 98925-98929
Procedures
Aquatic Therapy, 97113
Direct, 97032
Gait Training, 97116
Group Therapeutic, 97150
Massage Therapy, 97124
Neuromuscular Reeducation, 97112
Physical Performance Test, 97750
Supervised, 97010-97028
Therapeutic Exercises, 4018F, 97110
Traction Therapy, 97140
Work Hardening, 97545, 97546
Prosthetic Training, 97761
Sensory Integration, 97533
Therapeutic Activities, 97530
Unlisted Services and Procedures, 97139, 97799
Wheelchair Management, 97542
Work Reintegration, 97537
Physical Therapy
See Physical Medicine/Therapy/Occupational Therapy
Physician Quality Reporting System (PQRS)
A1c, 3044F-3046F
ABO and RH Blood Typing, 3293F
Activity Level, 1003F, 3115F, 3119F
Advance Care Plan
Discussion, 1123F-1124F, 1158F
Document, 1157F
Age-Related Eye Disease Study (AREDS), 4177F
Alarm Symptoms, 1070F-1071F
Alcohol Use, 4320F
ALS See Amyotrophic Lateral Sclerosis
American Joint Committee on Cancer (AJCC)
Staging, 3300F, 3321F, 3370F-3390F
Amyotrophic Lateral Sclerosis (ALS)
Care Planning, 0580F
Cognitive/Behavior Screening, 3755F
Dysarthria Evaluation, 3762F-3763F

Physician Quality Reporting System (PQRS) — continued
Amyotrophic Lateral Sclerosis — continued
Noninvasive Respiratory Support Discussed, 4550F
Nutritional Support Offered, 4551F
Nutrition Evaluation, 3759F-3761F
Pharmacotherapy, 4540F-4541F
Planning for End-of-Life, 4553F
Pulmonary Function Tests, 3758F
Respiratory Insufficiency, 1503F-1505F
Speech Pathology Referral, 4552F
Symptom Evaluation, 3756F-3757F
Anesthesia
Duration, 4255F-4256F
Anesthesia Technique, 4560F
Angina, 0557F, 1002F, 1010F-1012F
Angiotensin Converting Enzyme (ACE), 4010F, 4480F-4481F
Antibiotic Therapy, 4120F, 4124F
Antidepressant Therapy, 4063F-4064F
Antihistamines or Decongestant, 4133F-4134F
Antimicrobial Therapy, 4131F-4132F
Antiretroviral Therapy, 4270F-4271F, 4276F
Anti -Tumor Necrosis Factor (TNF) Therapy, 6150F
Aortic Aneurysm, 9001F-9004F
Arterio-venous (AV) Fistula, 4051F
Aspirin Received 24 Hours Prior to Anesthesia, 4563F
Aspirin Therapy, 4084F, 4086F
Assessment
Alarm Symptoms, 1070F-1071F
Angina, 1002F, 1010F
Anti-Inflammatory/Analgesic Medications, 1007F
Asthma, 1005F, 1038F-1039F
Auricular or Periauricular Pain, 1116F
Back Pain and Function, 1130F
Cataract Surgery, 0014F
Chest X-ray, 3006F
Cognitive Impairment, 1494F, 3720F
Colonoscopy, 3018F
Colorectal Cancer Screening, 3017F
Community Acquired Bacterial Pneumonia, 0012F
Comorbid Conditions, 1026F
COPD, 1015F, 1018F-1019F
Dementia, 1175F
Depression, 1040F
DXA Results, 3095F-3096F
Dysphagia, 6010F, 6015F
Dyspnea, 1018F-1019F
Fall Risk, 1100F-1101F, 3288F
Functional Expiratory Volume, 3040F, 3042F
Functional Status, 1170F
Gastrointestinal and Renal Risk Factors, 1008F
GERD, 1118F
Heart Failure, 0001F
Hemoglobin A1c, 3044F-3046F
Hydration Status, 2018F, 2030F-2031F
Influenza Immunization, 1030F
LDL, 3048F-3050F
Left Ventricle, 3020F-3022F
Level of Activity, 1002F-1003F
Lipid Panel, 3011F
Mammogram, 3014F, 3340F-3350F
Melanoma, 0015F
Mental Status, 2014F, 2044F
Microalbuminuria, 3060F-3062F
Mobility
Tympanic Membrane, 2035F
Moles, 1050F
Neuropsychiatric Symptoms, 1181F
Optic Nerve Head, 2027F
Osteoarthritis, 0005F, 1006F-1008F, 2004F
Oxygen Saturation, 3028F, 3035F, 3037F
Pain, 1125F-1126F
Pneumococcus Immunization, 1022F
Pneumonia, 0012F
Preoperative, 3325F
Psychiatric Disorder, 3700F
Rehabilitation, 4079F
Retinopathy, 3072F

Physician Quality Reporting System (PQRS) — continued
Assessment — continued
Rh, 3290F-3291F
Rheumatoid Arthritis Prognosis, 3475F-3476F
Risk Factors
Thromboembolism, 1180F
Screen
Depression, 1220F, 3351F-3354F
Smoking, 1031F
Spirometry, 3023F, 3025F, 3027F
Suicide Risk, 3085F
Tissue Plasminogen Activator (t-PA), 4077F
Tobacco Use, 1000F, 1034F-1036F
Tympanic Membrane, 2035F
Type, Anatomic Location, and Activity, 1052F
Urinary Incontinence, 1090F-1091F
Visual Function, 1055F
Volume Overload, 1004F, 2002F
Asthma, 1005F, 1031F-1033F, 1038F-1039F, 2015F-2016F, 4000F, 4015F, 4140F, 4144F, 5250F
Barium Swallow, 3142F, 3200F
Barrett's Esophagus, 3140F
Beta Blocker, 4008F, 4115F, 4480F-4481F
Biopsy
Site Other Than Primary Tumor, 3250F
Biphosphonate Therapy, 4100F
Blood Pressure, 0513F, 2000F, 3074F-3080F
Body Mass Index (BMI), 3008F
Bone Scan, 3269F-3270F
Breast Imaging-Reporting and Data System (BI-RADS), 3340F-3345F
Information Entered into Internal Database, 7020F
Cancer
Adenoma, 3775F-3776F
American Joint Committee on Cancer (AJCC), 3300F, 3321F-3322F, 3370F-3390F
Breast, 3315F-3316F, 3370F-3380F, 3394F-3395F
Colon, 3382F-3390F
Melanoma, 0015F, 3319F-3322F
Metastatic, 3301F, 3323F
Pathology Report, 3317F-3318F
Stage, 3301F
Cardiac Rehab, 4500F, 4510F
Cardio Defibrillator, 4470F
Care Giver, 4322F
Care Plan, 0580F
Carotid, 3100F
Imaging Report, 3100F
Carotid Stenosis, 9005F-9007F
Cataract
Preoperative Assessment, 0014F
Presurgical Axial Length, 3073F
Visual Acuity, 4175F
CD4+, 3500F
Chemotherapy
Colon Cancer, 4180F
Planned Chemotherapy Regimen, 0519F
Chest X-ray, 3006F
Clostridium Difficile, 3520F
Cognition, 1494F
Cognitive and Behavioral Impairment Screening, 3755F
Colonoscopy
Detection of Adenoma, Other Neoplasm, 3775F-3776F
Follow-up (10 years), 0528F
Interval 3+ Years, 0529F
Communication
Diagnostic Mammogram, 5060F, 5062F
Risk
Fracture, 5100F
Treatment Plan, 5050F
Treatment Summary, 5020F
Composite Measure, 0001F-0015F
Compression Therapy, 4267F-4269F
Condition, 1127F
Coronary Artery Bypass Graft (CABG), 4110F

Physician Quality Reporting System (PQRS) — *continued*
Coronary Artery Disease, 1000F-1002F, 1034F, 3011F, 3021F-3022F, 4000F-4001F, 4004F, 4008F-4011F, 4013F, 4086F, 4145F, 4500F-4510F
Coronary Artery Stent, 4561F, 4562F
Corticosteroids, 3750F, 4003F, 4135F-4136F, 4140F-4142F
Counseling
    Against Bed Rest, 4248F
    Age-Related Eye Disease Study (AREDS), 4177F
    Alcohol, 4320F
        Risk with Hep-C, 4158F
    Contraceptive, 4159F
    Dementia, 6101F-6102F
    Driving Safety, 6110F
    Epilepsy, 4330F, 4340F, 6070F
    Exercise, 4242F
    Exercise and Calcium/Vitamin D, 4019F
    Glaucoma, 4174F
    Prostate Cancer, 4163F
    Resume Normal Activities, 4245F
    Safety Issues, 6090F
    Self Examination for Moles, 5005F
    Tobacco, 4004F
    Treatment Options
        Alcohol, 4320F
        Opioid, 4306F
    UV Protection, 4176F
CT or MRI
    Brain, 3111F-3112F
        Epilepsy, Ordered, Reviewed, or Requested, 3324F
        Hemorrhage , Mass Lesion, and Acute Infarction, 3110F
Culture
    Wound, 4260F-4261F
Cytogenic Testing
    Bone Marrow, 3155F
Deep Vein Thrombosis (DVT) Prophylaxis, 4070F
Dementia, 1175F, 1490F-1493F, 4350F, 6101F-6102F
Depression, 0545F, 1040F, 2060F, 3092F-3093F, 3351F-3354F, 3725F, 4060F-4067F
Diagnostic Imaging Studies
    Not Ordered, 3331F
    Ordered, 3319F-3320F, 3330F
Diagnostic Screening/Results, 3006F-3750F
Discharge
    Inpatient Facility, 1110F
    Instructions
        Heart Failure, 4014F
    Medications Reconciled, 1111F
    Within Last 60 Days, 1110F
Disease Activity
    Rheumatoid Arthritis (RA), 3470F-3472F
Disease Pharmacotherapy, 4540F
Dressing, 4265F-4266F
Dual-energy X-ray Absorptiometry (DXA), 3095F-3096F
Dysarthria, 3762F-3763F
Dysphagia, 3759F-3761F
ECG, 3120F
Education
    Alcohol Risk, 4158F
    Foot Care, 4305F
    Gastroenteritis, 4058F
    Heart Failure, 4003F
    Self-Care, 4450F
EEG, 3650F
Electroconvulsive Therapy (ECT), 4066F-4067F
Electrodiagnostic Studies, 3751F, 3752F
Elevation
    Head of Bed, 4167F
End of Life Services, 4553F
Endoscopy
    Upper, 3140F-3141F
Epilepsy, 1205F, 5200F, 6070F
Erythropoietin Therapy, 4090F, 4095F, 4171F-4172F
Esophageal Biopsy Report, 3126F
Esophagus, 3150F
Evaluation, 1501F

Physician Quality Reporting System (PQRS) — *continued*
Evaluation Hepatitis C
    Initial, 1119F
    Subsequent, 1121F
Exam
    Back, 0525F-0526F, 2040F
    Foot, 2028F
    Fundus, 2020F-2021F, 5010F
    Joints, 2004F
    Macular, 2019F, 2021F
    Retina, 2022F
    Skin, 2029F
Exercise
    Counseling, 4019F, 4242F
    Instruction, 4240F
    Therapeutic, 4018F
Falls, 3288F, 6080F
Fibrillation, 1060F-1061F
Follow-Up, 5005F-5250F
    Colonoscopy, 0528F-0529F
    Melanoma, 0015F
Functional Expiratory Volume, 3040F-3042F
GERD, 1118F, 3130F-3142F, 3150F
Glucocorticoid Therapy, 0540F, 4192F-4194F
Goals of care, 1152F-1153F
Hearing Test, 3230F
Heart Failure, 4014F
Hemodialysis, 0505F, 4052F-4054F
Hemoglobin Level, 3279F-3281F
Hepatitis, 1119F, 1121F, 3215F-3216F, 3218F, 3220F, 3265F-3266F, 3514F-3515F, 4148F-4159F
History, 1000F-1494F
    AIDS-Defining Condition, 3490F
    Moles, 1050F
HIV Status, 3292F, 3491F-3503F
Hypertension, 4050F, 4145F
ICU, 4168F-4169F
Influenza Immunization, 4035F, 4037F, 4274F
Inhalation Anesthesia, 4554F, 4555F
Insufficiency, 1503F, 1504F-1505F
International Normalization Ratio, 3555F
Interventions, 4000F-4526F
Intraocular Pressure (IOP), 3284F-3285F
Iron Stores, 3160F
Ischemic Stroke Symptoms, 1065F-1066F
Kt/V, 3082F-3084F
LDL-C, 3048F-3050F
Lipid
    Control, 0556F
    Panel, 3011F
Medications Documented and Reviewed, 1159F-1160F
Medication Therapy
    Alternative Long Term, 4144F
    Angiotensin Converting Enzyme (ACE) or Angiotensin Receptor Blockers (ARB), 4210F
    Anticonvulsant Medication, 4230F
    Digoxin, 4220F
    Diuretic Medication, 4221F
    Hypertension, 4145F
    Parkinson's Disease, 4324F
Melanoma
    Follow-Up, 0015F
    Greater than AJCC Stage 0 or 1A, 3321F-3322F
Microalbuminuria, 3060F-3062F
Nephropathy Treatment, 3066F
Neuropathy, 3753F
Neuropsychiatric, 1181F-1183F, 4526F
New York Hospital Association (NYHA), 3118F
Normothermia Maintained Intraoperatively, 4250F
Not Prescribed
    Antibiotic, 4124F
    Corticosteroids, 4192F
NPO Ordered, 6020F
Nutritional Support, 4551F
Oral Rehydration, 4056F
Ordered
    Calcium, Phosphorus, Parathyroid Hormone, Lipid Profile, 3278F
    Imaging Studies, 3319F, 3330F

Physician Quality Reporting System (PQRS) — *continued*
Osteoporosis
    Fracture, 5015F
    Pharmacologic Therapy, 4005F
Otitis Externa, 4130F
Oxygen Saturation, 3028F, 3035F, 3037F
Pain
    Auricular or Periauricular, 1116F
    Back, 1130F, 1134F-1137F, 2044F
    Query, 1502F
    Severity, 1125F-1126F
Parkinson's Disease, 1400F, 3700F-3720F, 4324F-4328F, 4400F, 6080F-6090F
Pathology, 3250F, 3260F, 3267F
Patient Information
    Entered into Internal Database, 7010F
    Entered into Reminder System, 7025F
Peginterferon and Ribavirin, 4153F
Performance Status Before Surgery, 3328F
Peritoneal Dialysis, 0507F, 4055F
Physical Exam, 2000F-2060F
Plan of Care
    Advance, 1123F-1124F
    Anemia, 0516F
    Blood Pressure, 0513F
    Chemotherapy, 0519F
    Depression, 0545F
    Dyspnea Management, 0535F
    Falls, 0518F
    Glaucoma, 0517F
    Glucorticoid Management, 0540F
    Hemodialysis, 0505F
    Hemoglobin Level, 0514F
    HIV RNA Control, 0575F
    Hypertension, 4050F
    Pain, 0521F
        Severity, 1125F-1126F
    Peritoneal dialysis, 0507F
    Urinary Incontinence, 0509F
Pneumatic Otoscopy, 2035F
Pneumococcal Vaccine Administration, 4040F
Polyneuropathy, 1500F
Post Operative Nausea and Vomiting, 4556F, 4557F
Postpartum Care, 0503F
Prenatal
    Rh, 3290F-3291F
Prenatal Care, 0500F-0502F
    Anti-D Immune Globulin, 4178F
Prescribed
    ACE Inhibitor or ARB Therapy, 4010F
    Adjuvant chemotherapy prescribed, 4180F
    Age Related Eye Disease Study (AREDS), 4177F
    Antibiotic, 4120F, 4124F
    Anticoagulant, 4075F
    Antidepressant, 4064F
    Anti-emetic Agent, 4558F
    Antihistamines or Decongestants, 4133F
    Anti-inflammatory Agent, 4016F
    Anti-inflammatory/Analgesic, 4016F
    Antimicrobial, 4131F-4132F
    Antiplatelet Therapy, 4011F, 4073F
    Antipsychotic, 4065F
    Antiviral, 4150F-4151F
    Asthma Treatment, 4015F
    Beta Blocker Therapy, 4008F
    Corticosteroids, 4135F
    Disease Modifying Anti-Rheumatic Drug Therapy Prescribed or Dispensed., 4187F
    Empiric Antibiotic, 4045F
    GI Prophylaxis for NSAIDS, 4017F
    Inhaled Bronchodilator, 4025F
    Osteoporosis Therapy, 4005F
    Otitis Externa Medication, 4130F
    Oxygen Therapy, 4030F
    Statin Therapy, 4013F
    Tamoxifen, 4179F
    Therapeutic Exercise, 4018F
    Warfarin Therapy, 4012F
Prophylaxis
    Antibiotic, 4041F-4043F, 4046F-4049F
    Cefazolin or Cefuroxime, 4041F
    for Deep Vein Thrombosis (DVT), 4070F

Physician Quality Reporting System (PQRS) — *continued*
Prophylaxis — *continued*
    for NSAID, 4017F
    Pneumocystis jiroveci pneumonia, 4279F-4280F
Prostate, 3268F-3274F
Prostate Specific Antigen (PSA), 3268F
Proton Pump Inhibitor (PPI) or Histamine H2 Receptor Antagonist (H2RA), 4185F-4186F
Psychotherapy, 4060F, 4062F
Pulmonary
    Function Test, 3038F
    Patient Referred for Pulmonary Function Testing or Peak Cough Expiratory Flow, 3758F
    Rehabilitation, 4033F
Radiation Therapy
    Conformal Radiation Therapy Not Received, 4182F
    Conformal Radiation Therapy Received, 4181F
    Dose Limits Established, 0520F
    Dose Reduction Device, 6040F
    Exposure Time, 6045F
    External Beam Radiotherapy, 4200F-4201F
    Prostate Cancer, 4164F-4165F
Rationale for Level of Care, 6005F
Recall System in Place, 7010F
Referral
    Arterio Venous (AV) Fistula, 4051F
    Electroconvulsive Therapy (ECT), 4066F
    Psychotherapy, 4062F
    Rehabilitative Therapy Options (Parkinsons), 4400F
Report
    Cytopathology, 0550F-0551F
Respiratory Support, 4550F
Results Reviewed
    Colorectal Cancer Screening, 3017F
    Malignancy, 3317F-3318F
    Mammography, 3014F
    Microalbuminuria Test Results, 3060F-3062F
    MRI or CT, 3324F
Retinopathy, 3072F
Rheumatoid Arthritis, 4192F-4196F
Risk
    Death within 1 year, 1150F-1151F
    Fracture, 3572F-3573F
    Prostate Cancer, 3272F-3274F
    Thromboembolism, 3550F-3552F
Safety, 6005F-6150F
Scintigraphy Study, 3570F
Screening
    Alcohol Use, 3016F
    Cervical Cancer, 3015F
    Colorectal Cancer, 3017F
    Depression, 1220F
    Diabetes, 3754F
    Drug Use, 4290F
    Dysarthria, 3763F
    Dysphagia, 3759F
    Dyspnea, 3450F-3452F
    Future Fall Risk, 1100F-1101F
    Group B Strep, 3294F
    Hepatitis B, 3513F
    Hepatitis C, 3514F
    High-Risk Behavior, 4290F, 4293F
    Mammography, 3014F
    STD, 3511F-3512F
    Suicide, 3085F
    TB, 3455F, 3510F
    Tobacco Use, 4004F
Seizure
    Type, 1200F
Self Care, 4450F
Signs and Symptoms Neuropathy, 3753F
Sleep Disturbance, 4328F
Smoking, 1031F-1036F, 4004F
Speech Language Pathology, 4552F
Spirometry, 3023F, 3025F-3027F
Statin Therapy, 4013F
Stereoscopic Photos, 2024F, 2026F
Sterile Barrier, 6030F

Physician Quality Reporting System (PQRS) —
continued
Strep Test
Group A, 3210F
Stroke, 1066F, 3110F-3112F
Structural Measures, 7010F-7025F
Symptom Management, 0555F, 1450F-1451F
Symptoms, ALS Related, 3756F-3757F
Temperature, 4559F
Therapeutic Monitoring
Angiotensin Converting Enzyme
(ACE)/Angiotensin Receptor Block-
ers (ARB), 4188F
Anticonvulsant, 4191F
Digoxin, 4189F
Diuretic, 4190F
Thromboembolism, 3550F
Timeout to Verify Correct Patient, Site, Proce-
dure, Documented, 6100F
Tobacco
Cessation, 4000F-4001F
Use, 1035F-1036F
Transfer, 0581F-0584F
Treatment
Options, 4325F
Plan, 5050F
Tuberculosis, 3455F, 3510F
Tympanometry, 2035F
Urinary Incontinence, 0509F, 1090F-1091F
Vaccine
Hepatitis
A, 4155F
B, 4149F, 4157F
Influenza, 4037F
Pneumococcal, 4040F
Vein Thromboembolism, 4069F
Ventricle, 3019F-3020F, 3055F-3056F
Verification, 6100F
Vital Signs Documented and Reviewed, 2010F
Volume Overload, 1004F, 2002F
Warfarin Therapy, 4012F, 4300F-4301F
Warming
Intraoperative, 4250F
Weight Recorded, 2001F
Wound, 2050F
Culture, 4260F-4261F
Dressings, 4265F-4266F
Physician Services
Care Plan Oversight Services, 99339-99340,
99374-99380
Domiciliary Facility, 99339-99340
Extracorporeal Liver Assist System, 0405T
Home Health Agency Care, 99374
Home/Rest Home Care, 99339-99340
Hospice, 99377, 99378
Nursing Facility, 99379, 99380
Case Management Services, 99366-99368
Direction, Advanced Life Support, 99288
Online, 99444
Prolonged
with Direct Patient Contact, 99354-99357
Outpatient Office, 99354, 99355
with Direct Patient Services
Inpatient, 99356, 99357
without Direct Patient Contact, 99358,
99359
Standby, 99360
Supervision, Care Plan Oversight Services,
0405T, 99339-99340, 99374-99380
Team Conference, 99367
Telephone, 99441-99443
Physiologic Recording of Tremor, 95999
PICC Line Insertion, 36568-36569
Pierce Ears, 69090
Piercing of Ear Lobe, 69090
PIK3CA, 81404
Piles
See Hemorrhoids
Pilon Fracture Treatment, 27824
Pilonidal Cyst
Excision, 11770-11772
Incision and Drainage, 10080, 10081
Pin
See Also Wire

Pin — *continued*
Insertion
Removal
Skeletal Traction, 20650
Prophylactic Treatment
Femur, 27187
Humerus, 24498
Shoulder, 23490, 23491
Pinch Graft, 15050
Pineal Gland
Excision
Partial, 60699
Total, 60699
Incision, 60699
PINK1, 81405
Pinna
See Ear, External
Pinworms
Examination, 87172
Pirogoff Procedure, 27888
Pituitary Epidermoid Tumor
See Craniopharyngioma
Pituitary Fossa
Exploration, 60699
Pituitary Gland
Excision, 61546, 61548
Incision, 60699
Tumor
Excision, 61546, 61548, 62165
Pituitary Growth Hormone
See Growth Hormone
Pituitary Lactogenic Hormone
See Prolactin
Pituitectomy
See Excision, Pituitary Gland
PKD1, 81407
PKD2, 81406
PKHD1, 81408
PKP, 65730-65755
PKP2, 81406
PKU, 84030
PL, 80418, 84146
Placement
Adjustable Gastric Restrictive Device, 43770
Amniotic Membrane
Ocular Surface, 65778-65779
Aqueous Drainage Device, 0191T, 0449T-0450T,
66179-66185, [0253T]
Breast Localization Device
with Guidance
Mammographic, 19281-19282
MRI, 19287-19288
Stereotactic, 19283-19284
Ultrasound, 19285-19286
Bronchial Stent, 31636-31637
Catheter
Aneurysm Sac Pressure Sensor, 34806
Complete Study, 93982
Bile Duct, 47533-47540
Brain for Chemotherapy, 64999
Bronchus
for Intracavitary Radioelement Applica-
tion, 31643
See Catheterization
for Interstitial Radioelement Application
Breast, 19296-19298
Genitalia, 55920
Head/Neck, 41019
Muscle, 20555
Pelvic Organs, 55920
Prostate, 55875
Soft Tissue, 20555
Pleural, 32550
Renal Artery, 36251-36254
Catheter, Cardiac, 93503
See Also Catheterization, Cardiac
Cecostomy Tube, 44300, 49442
Colonic Stent, 45327, 45347, 45389
Dosimeter
Prostate, 55876
Drainage
Pancreas, 48001
Drug-eluting Ocular Insert, 0444T-0445T
Duodenostomy Tube, 49441
Endovascular Prosthesis, Aorta, 33883-33886
Enterostomy Tube, 44300

Placement — *continued*
Fiducial Markers
Duodenum/Jejunum, 43253
Esophagus, 43253
Intra-abdominal, 49411
Intra-pelvic, 49411
Intrathoracic, 32553
Prostate, 55876
Retroperitoneum, 49411
Stomach, 43253
Gastrostomy Tube, 43246, 49440
Guidance Catheter
Abscess, 75989
Specimen, 75989
Interstitial Device
Bone, 0347T
Intra-abdominal, 49327, 49411-49412
Intra-pelvic, 49411
Intra-thoracic, 32553
Prostate, 55876
Retroperitoneum, 49411
Intrafacet Implant(s), 0219T-0222T
Intravascular Stent
Cervical Carotid Artery, 37215-37216
Innominate Artery, 37217-37218
Intracranial, 61635
Intrathoracic Common Carotid Artery,
37217-37218
IVC Filter, 37191
Jejunostomy Tube
Endoscopic, 44372
Percutaneous, 49441
Localization Device, Breast, 19281-19288
Nasogastric Tube, 43752
Needle
Bone, 36680
for Interstitial Radioelement Application
Genitalia, 55920
Head, 41019
Muscle, 20555
Neck, 41019
Pelvic Organs, 55920
Prostate, 55875
Soft Tissue, 20555
Head and/or Neck, 41019
Muscle or Soft Tissue
for Radioelement Application, 20555
Pelvic Organs and/or Genitalia, 55920
Prostate, 55875-55876
Needle Wire
Breast, 19281-19288
Orogastric Tube, 43752
Pharmacological Agent
Intravitreal Drug Delivery System, 67027
Pressure Sensor, 34806
Prosthesis, Thoracic Aorta, 75958-75959
Radiation Delivery Device
Intracoronary Artery, [92974]
Intraocular, 0190T
Sensor, Wireless
Endovascular Repair, 34806
Seton
Anal, 46020
Stereotactic Frame, 20660
Head Frame, 61800
Subconjunctival Retinal Prosthesis Receiver,
0100T
Tracheal Stent, 31631
Transcatheter
Extracranial, 0075T-0076T
Physiologic Sensor, 34806
Ureteral Stent, 50693-50695, 50947
Placenta
Delivery, 59414
Placental
Alpha Microglobulin-1, 84112
Lactogen, 83632
Placental Villi
See Chorionic Villus
Plafond Fracture Treatment
Tibial, 27824
Plagiocephaly, 21175
Planing
Nose
Skin, 30120

Plantar Digital Nerve
Decompression, 64726
Plantar Pressure Measurements
Dynamic, 96001, 96004
Plasma
Frozen Preparation, 86927
Injection, 0232T
Volume Determination, 78110, 78111
Plasma Prokallikrein
See Fletcher Factor
**Plasma Protein–A, Pregnancy Associated
(PAPP–A)**, 84163
Plasma Test
Volume Determination, 78110-78111
Plasma Thromboplastin
Antecedent, 85270
Component, 85250
Frozen Preparation, 86927
Plasmin, 85400
Plasmin Antiactivator
See Alpha–2 Antiplasmin
Plasminogen, 85420, 85421
Plasmodium
Antibody, 86750
Plastic Repair of Mouth
See Mouth, Repair
Plate, Bone
See Bone Plate
Platelet
See Also Blood Cell Count; Complete Blood
Count
Aggregation, 85576
Antibody, 86022, 86023
Assay, 85055
Blood, 85025
Count, 85032, 85049
Neutralization, 85597
Platelet Cofactor I
See Clotting Factor
Platelet Test
Survival Test, 78190, 78191
Platelet Thromboplastin Antecedent, 85270
Platysmal Flap, 15825
PLC, 86822
PLCE1, 81407
Pleoptic Training, 92065
Plethysmography
Extremities, 93922, 93923
Lung Volume, 94726
Penis, 54240
Pleura
Biopsy, 32098, 32400
Decortication, 32320
Empyema
Excision, 32540
Excision, 32310, 32320
Endoscopic, 32656
Foreign Body
Removal, 32150, 32151
Incision, 32320
Needle Biopsy, 32400
Removal
Foreign Body, 32150, 32653
Repair, 32215
Thoracotomy, 32096-32098, 32100-32160
Unlisted Services and Procedures, 32999
Pleural Cavity
Catheterization, 32550
Chemotherapy Administration, 96440, 96446
Fusion, 32560
Incision
Empyema, 32035, 32036
Pneumothorax, 32551
Puncture and Drainage, 32554-32557
Thoracostomy, 32035, 32036
Pleural Endoscopies
See Thoracoscopy
Pleural Scarification
for Repeat Pneumothorax, 32215
Pleural Tap
See Thoracentesis
Pleurectomy
Anesthesia, 00542
Parietal, 32310, 32320
Endoscopic, 32656
Pleuritis, Purulent, 21501-21502

Pleurodesis
Agent for Pleurodesis, 32560
Endoscopic, 32650
Pleurosclerosis
See Pleurodesis
Pleurosclerosis, Chemical
See Pleurodesis, Chemical
Plexectomy, Choroid
See Choroid Plexus, Excision
Plexus Brachialis
See Brachial Plexus
Plexus Cervicalis
See Cervical Plexus
Plexus, Choroid
See Choroid Plexus
Plexus Coeliacus
See Celiac Plexus
Plexus Lumbalis
See Lumbar Plexus
PLGN
See Plasminogen
Plication
Bullae, 32141
Diaphragm, 39599
Plication, Sphincter, Urinary Bladder
See Bladder, Repair, Neck
PLIF (Posterior Lumbar Interbody Fusion), 22630
PLN, 81403
PLP1, 81404-81405
PML/RARalpha, 81315-81316
PMP22, 81324-81326
PMS2, 81317-81319
Pneumocisternogram
See Cisternography
Pneumococcal Vaccine, 90670, 90732
Pneumocystis Carinii
Antigen Detection, 87281
Pneumoencephalogram, 78635
Pneumoencephalography
Anesthesia, 01935-01936
Pneumogastric Nerve
See Vagus Nerve
Pneumogram
Pediatric, 94772
Pneumolysis, 32940
Pneumonectomy, 32440-32445, 32671
Completion, 32488
Donor, 32850, 33930
Sleeve, 32442
Pneumonology
See Pulmonology
Pneumonolysis, 32940
Intrapleural, 32652
Open Intrapleural, 32124
Pneumonostomy, 32200
Pneumonotomy
See Incision, Lung
Pneumoperitoneum, 49400
Pneumothorax
Agent for Pleurodesis, 32560
Pleural Scarification for Repeat, 32215
Therapeutic
Injection Intrapleural Air, 32960
PNEUMOVAX 23, 90732
PNKD, 81406
POLG, 81406
Polio
Antibody, 86658
Vaccine, 90698, 90713
Poliovirus Vaccine, Inactivated
See Vaccines
Pollicization
Digit, 26550
Polya Anastomosis, 43632
Polya Gastrectomy, 43632
Polydactylism, 26587, 28344
Polydactylous Digit
Excision, Soft Tissue Only, 11200
Reconstruction, 26587
Repair, 26587
Polydactyly, Toes, 28344
Polyp
Antrochoanal
Removal, 31032
Esophagus
Ablation, 43229

Polyp — *continued*
Nose
Excision
Endoscopic, 31237-31240
Extensive, 30115
Simple, 30110
Removal
Sphenoid Sinus, 31051
Urethra
Excision, 53260
Polypectomy
Nose
Endoscopic, 0407T, 31237
Uterus, 58558
Polypeptide, Vasoactive Intestinal
See Vasoactive Intestinal Peptide
Polysomnography, 95808-95811
Pomeroy's Operation
Tubal Ligation, 58600
POMGNT1, 81406
POMT1, 81406
POMT2, 81406
Pooling
Blood Products, 86965
Pool Therapy with Exercises, 97036, 97113
Popliteal Arteries
See Artery, Popliteal
Popliteal Synovial Cyst
See Baker's Cyst
Poradenititstras
See Lymphogranuloma Venereum
PORP (Partial Ossicular Replacement Prosthesis),
69633, 69637
Porphobilinogen
Urine, 84106, 84110
Porphyrin Precursors, 82135
Porphyrins
Feces, 84126
Urine, 84119, 84120
Port
Peripheral
Insertion, 36569-36571
Removal, 36590
Replacement, 36578, 36585
Venous Access
Insertion, 36560-36561, 36566
Removal, 36590
Repair, 36576
Replacement, 36578, 36582-36583
Port-A-Cath
Insertion, 36560-36571
Removal, 36589-36590
Replacement, 36575-36585
Portal Vein
See Vein, Hepatic Portal
Porter–Silber Test
Corticosteroid, Blood, 82528
Port Film, 77417
Portoenterostomy, 47701
Portoenterostomy, Hepatic, 47802
Posadas–Wernicke Disease, 86490
Positional Nystagmus Test
See Nystagmus Test, Positional
Positive End Expiratory Pressure
See Pressure Breathing, Positive
Positive–Pressure Breathing, Inspiratory
See Intermittent Positive Pressure Breathing
(IPPB)
Positron Emission Tomography (PET)
with Computed Tomography (CT)
Limited, 78814
Skull Base to Mid-thigh, 78815
Whole Body, 78816
Brain, 78608, 78609
Heart, 78459
Limited, 78811
Myocardial Imaging Perfusion Study, 78491-78492
Perfusion Study, 78491, 78492
Skull Base to Mid-thigh, 78812
Whole Body, 78813
Postauricular Fistula
See Fistula, Postauricular
Postcaval Ureter
See Retrocaval Ureter

Postmeiotic Segregation Increased 2 (S. Cere-visiae) Gene Analysis, 81317-81319
Postmortem
See Autopsy
Postoperative Wound Infection
Incision and Drainage, 10180
Postop Vas Reconstruction
See Vasovasorrhaphy
Post–Op Visit, 99024
Postpartum Care
Cesarean Section, 59515
After Attempted Vaginal Delivery, 59622
Previous, 59610, 59614-59618, 59622
Postpartum Care Only, 59430
Vaginal Delivery, 59410, 59430
After Previous Cesarean Delivery, 59614
Potassium
Hydroxide Examination, 87220
Serum, 84132
Urine, 84133
Potential, Auditory Evoked
See Auditory Evoked Potentials
Potential, Evoked
See Evoked Potential
Potts-Smith Procedure, 33762
POU1F1, 81405
Pouch, Kock
See Kock Pouch
PPD, 86580
PPH, 59160
PPP, 85362-85379
PPP2R2B, 81401
PQBP1, 81404-81405
PRA, 86805-86808
Prealbumin, 84134
Prebeta Lipoproteins
See Lipoprotein, Blood
Pregl's Test
Cystourethroscopy, Catheterization, Urethral,
52005
Pregnancy
Abortion
Induced, 59855-59857
by Amniocentesis Injection, 59850-59852
by Dilation and Curettage, 59840
by Dilation and Evacuation, 59841
Septic, 59830
Therapeutic
by Dilation and Curettage, 59851
by Hysterotomy, 59852
by Saline, 59850
Antepartum Care, 0500F-0502F, 59425, 59426
Cesarean Section, 59618-59622
with Hysterectomy, 59525
Only, 59514
Postpartum Care, 0503F, 59514, 59515
Routine Care, 59510
Vaginal Birth After, 59610-59614
Ectopic
Abdominal, 59130
Cervix, 59140
Interstitial
Partial Resection Uterus, 59136
Total Hysterectomy, 59135
Laparoscopy
with Salpingectomy and/or
Oophorectomy, 59151
without Salpingectomy and/or
Oophorectomy, 59150
Miscarriage
Surgical Completion
Any Trimester, 59812
First Trimester, 59820
Second Trimester, 59821
Molar
See Hydatidiform Mole
Multifetal Reduction, 59866
Placenta Delivery, 59414
Tubal, 59121
with Salpingectomy and/or Oophorectomy,
59120
Vaginal Delivery, 59409, 59410
After Cesarean Section, 59610-59614
Antepartum Care, 59425-59426
Postpartum Care, 59430

Pregnancy — *continued*
Vaginal Delivery — *continued*
Total Obstetrical Care, 59400, 59610, 59618
Pregnancy Test
Blood, 84702-84703
Urine, 81025
Pregnanediol, 84135
Pregnanetriol, 84138
Pregnenolone, 84140
Prekallikrein
See Fletcher Factor
Prekallikrein Factor, 85292
Premature, Closure, Cranial Suture
See Craniosynostosis
Prenatal Procedure
Amnioinfusion
Transabdominal, 59070
Drainage
Fluid, 59074
Occlusion
Umbilical Cord, 59072
Shunt, 59076
Unlisted Procedure, 59897
Prenatal Testing
Amniocentesis, 59000
with Amniotic Fluid Reduction, 59001
Chorionic Villus Sampling, 59015
Cordocentesis, 59012
Fetal Blood Sample, 59030
Fetal Monitoring, 59050
Interpretation Only, 59051
Non–Stress Test, Fetal, 59025, 99500
Oxytocin Stress Test, 59020
Stress Test
Oxytocin, 59020
Ultrasound, 76801-76817
Fetal Biophysical Profile, 76818, 76819
Fetal Heart, 76825
Prentiss Operation
Orchiopexy, Inguinal Approach, 54640
Preparation
for Transfer
Embryo, 89255
for Transplantation
Heart, 33933, 33944
Heart/Lung, 33933
Intestines, 44715-44721
Kidney, 50323-50329
Liver, 47143-47147
Lung, 32855-32856, 33933
Pancreas, 48551-48552
Renal, 50323-50329
Thawing
Embryo
Cryopreserved, 89352
Oocytes
Cryopreserved, 89356
Reproductive Tissue
Cryopreserved, 89354
Sperm
Cryopreserved, 89353
Presacral Sympathectomy
See Sympathectomy, Presacral
Prescription
Contact Lens, 92310-92317
See Contact Lens Services
Pressure, Blood, 2000F, 2010F
24-Hour Monitoring, 93784-93790
Diastolic, 3078F-3080F
Systolic, 3074F-3075F
Venous, 93770
Pressure Breathing
See Pulmonology, Therapeutic
Negative
Continuous (CNP), 94662
Positive
Continuous (CPAP), 94660
Pressure Measurement of Sphincter of Oddi,
43263
Pressure Sensor, Aneurysm, 34806
Pressure Trousers
Application, 99199
Pressure Ulcer (Decubitus)
See Also Debridement; Skin Graft and Flap
Excision, 15920-15999
Coccygeal, 15920, 15922

[Resequenced]

Pressure Ulcer (Decubitus) — *continued*
  Excision — *continued*
    Ischial, 15940-15946
    Sacral, 15931-15937
    Trochanter, 15950-15958
    Unlisted Procedures and Services, 15999
Pressure, Venous, 93770
Pretreatment
  Red Blood Cell
    Antibody Identification, 86970-86972
  Serum
    Antibody Identification, 86975-86978
Prevention and Control
  See Prophylaxis/Prophylactic Treatment
Preventive Medicine, 99381-99387
  See Also Immunization; Newborn Care, Normal;
      Office and/or Other Outpatient Services;
      Prophylactic Treatment
  Administration and Interpretation of Health
    Risk Assessment, 96160-96161
  Counseling and/or Risk Factor Reduction Inter-
    vention, 99401-99429
  Established Patient, 99382-99397
  Established Patient Exam, 99391-99397
  Intervention, 99401-99429
    Behavior Change, 0403T, 99406-99408
    Calcium/Vitamin D Use, 4019F
    Exercise, 4019F
    Group Counseling, 99411-99412
    Individual Counseling, 99401-99404
    Self-Examination for Moles, 5005F
  Newborn Care, 99461
  New Patient Exam, 99381-99387
  Respiratory Pattern Recording, 94772
  Unlisted Services and Procedures, 99429
Prevnar 13, 90670
Priapism
  Repair
    with Shunt, 54420, 54430
    Fistulization, 54435
Primidone
  Assay, 80188
PRITS (Partial Resection Inferior Turbinates),
  30140
PRKAG2, 81406
PRKCG, 81406
PRL
  See Prolactin
PRNP, 81404
Proalbumin
  See Prealbumin
Probes, DNA
  See Nucleic Acid Probe
Probes, Nucleic Acid
  See Nucleic Acid Probe
Probing
  Nasolacrimal Duct, 68816
Procainamide
  Assay, 80190, 80192
Procalcitonin (PCT), 84145
Procedure, Fontan
  See Repair, Heart, Anomaly
Procedure, Maxillofacial
  See Maxillofacial Procedures
Process
  See Anatomic Term (e.g., coracoid, odontoid)
Process, Odontoid
  See Odontoid Process
Procidentia
  Rectal
    Excision, 45130, 45135
    Repair, 45900
Procoagulant Activity, Glomerular
  See Thromboplastin
Proconvertin, 85230
Proctectasis
  See Dilation, Rectum
Proctectomy
  Laparoscopic, 45395-45397
    with Colectomy/Ileostomy, 44211-44212
  Open Approach, 45110-45123
    with Colectomy, 45121
    with Colectomy/Ileostomy, 44155-44158
Proctocele
  See Rectocele
Proctopexy, 45400-45402, 45540-45550

Proctopexy — *continued*
  with Sigmoid Excision, 45550
Proctoplasty, 45500, 45505
Proctorrhaphy
  Fistula, 45800-45825
  Prolapse, 45540-45541
Proctoscopies
  See Anoscopy
Proctosigmoidoscopy
  Ablation
    Polyp or Lesion, 45320
  Biopsy, 45305
  Destruction
    Tumor, 45320
  Dilation, 45303
  Exploration, 45300
  Hemorrhage Control, 45317
  Placement
    Stent, 45327
  Removal
    Foreign Body, 45307
    Polyp, 45308-45315
    Tumor, 45315
  Stoma
    through Artificial, 45999
  Volvulus Repair, 45321
Proctostomy
  Closure, 45999
Proctotomy, 45160
Products, Gene
  See Protein
Proetz Therapy, 30210
Profibrinolysin, 85420-85421
Progenitor Cell
  See Stem Cell
Progesterone, 84144
Progesterone Receptors, 84234
Progestin Receptors, 84234
Programming
  Defibrillator System, 93282-93284, 93287
  Intracardiac Ischemia Monitoring System, 0305T
  Loop Recorder, 93285
  Pacemaker, 93279-93281, 93286
  Ventricular Assist Device, 0462T
Proinsulin, 84206
Pro–Insulin C Peptide
  See C–Peptide
Projective Test, 96101-96103
Prokallikrein, 85292
Prokallikrein, Plasma, 85292
Prokinogenase, 85292
Prolactin, 80418, 84146
Prolapse
  Anus, 46750-46751
  Proctopexy, 45400-45402, 45540-45541, 45550
  Proctoplasty, 45505, 45520
  Rectum, 45130-45135, 45900, 46753
  Urethra, 53275
Prolastin
  See Alpha–1 Antitrypsin
Prolonged Services
  with Direct Patient Contact, 99354-99355
  Before or After Direct Patient Contact, 99358,
    99359
  Inpatient or Observation, 99356-99357
  Physician Standby Services, 99360
PROM, 95851, 95852, 97110, 97530
Pronuclear Stage Tube Transfer (PROST), 58976
PROP1, 81404
Prophylactic Treatment
  See Also Preventive Medicine
  Antibiotic Documentation, 4042F-4043F, 4045F-
    4049F
  Antimicrobial Documentation, 4041F
  Clavicle, 23490
  Femoral Neck and Proximal Femur
    Nailing, 27187
    Pinning, 27187
    Wiring, 27187
  Femur, 27495
    Nailing, 27495
    Pinning, 27495
    Wiring, 27495
  Humerus, 23491
    Pinning, Wiring, 24498
  Radius, 25490, 25492

Prophylactic Treatment — *continued*
  Radius — *continued*
    Nailing, 25490, 25492
    Pinning, 25490, 25492
    Plating, 25490, 25492
    Wiring, 25490, 25492
  Shoulder
    Clavicle, 23490
    Humerus, 23491
  Tibia, 27745
  Ulna, 25491, 25492
    Nailing, 25491, 25492
    Pinning, 25491, 25492
    Plating, 25491, 25492
    Wiring, 25491, 25492
  Venous Thromboembolism (VTE), 4044F
Prophylaxis
  Anticoagulant Therapy, 4075F
  Deep Vein Thrombosis (DVT), 4070F
  Retinal Detachment
    Cryotherapy, 67141
      Cryotherapy, Diathermy, 67141
      Photocoagulation, 67145
    Diathermy, 67141
    Photocoagulation, 67145
ProQuad, 90710
PROST (Pronuclear Stage Tube Transfer), 58976
Prostaglandin, 84150
  Insertion, 59200
Prostanoids
  See Prostaglandin
Prostate
  Ablation
    Cryosurgery, 55873
    Transurethral Waterjet, 0419T
  Abscess
    Drainage, 52700
    Incision and Drainage, 55720, 55725
  Analysis, Fluorescence Spectroscopy, 0443T
  Biopsy, 55700, 55705, 55706
    with Fluorescence Spectroscopy, 0443T
  Brachytherapy
    Needle Insertion, 55875
  Coagulation
    Laser, 52647
  Destruction
    Cryosurgery, 55873
    Thermotherapy, 53850
      Microwave, 53850
      Radio Frequency, 53852
  Enucleation, Laser, 52649
  Excision
    Partial, 55801, 55821, 55831
    Perineal, 55801-55815
    Radical, 55810-55815, 55840-55845
    Retropubic, 55831-55845
    Suprapubic, 55821
    Transurethral, 52402, 52601
  Exploration
    with Nodes, 55862, 55865
    Exposure, 55860
  Incision
    Exposure, 55860-55865
    Transurethral, 52450
  Insertion
    Catheter, 55875
    Needle, 55875
    Radioactive Substance, 55860
  Needle Biopsy, 55700, 55706
    with Fluorescence Spectroscopy, 0443T
  Placement
    Catheter, 55875
    Dosimeter, 55876
    Fiducial Marker, 55876
    Interstitial Device, 55876
    Needle, 55875
  Thermotherapy
    Transurethral, 53850
  Ultrasound, 76872, 76873
  Unlisted Services and Procedures, 54699, 55899
    Urinary System, 53899
  Urethra
    Stent Insertion, 53855
  Vaporization
    Laser, 52648
Prostatectomy, 52601

Prostatectomy — *continued*
  Laparoscopic, 55866
  Perineal
    Partial, 55801
    Radical, 55810, 55815
  Retropubic
    Partial, 55831
    Radical, 55840-55845, 55866
  Suprapubic
    Partial, 55821
  Transurethral, 52601
  Walsh Modified Radical, 55810
Prostate Specific Antigen
  Complexed, 84152
  Free, 84154
  Total, 84153
Prostatic Abscess
  Incision and Drainage, 55720, 55725
    Prostatotomy, 55720, 55725
    Transurethral, 52700
Prostatotomy, 55720, 55725
Prosthesis
  Augmentation
    Mandibular Body, 21125
  Auricular, 21086
  Breast
    Insertion, 19340, 19342
    Removal, 19328, 19330
    Supply, 19396
  Check–Out, 97762
    See Physical Medicine/Therapy/ Occupation-
      al Therapy
  Cornea, 65770
  Elbow
    Removal, 24160-24164
  Endovascular
    Thoracic Aorta, 33883-33886
  Facial, 21088
  Hernia
    Mesh, 49568
  Hip
    Removal, 27090, 27091
  Impression and Custom Preparation (by Physi-
    cian)
    Auricular, 21086
    Facial, 21088
    Mandibular Resection, 21081
    Nasal, 21087
    Obturator
      Definitive, 21080
      Interim, 21079
      Surgical, 21076
    Oral Surgical Splint, 21085
    Orbital, 21077
    Palatal
      Augmentation, 21082
      Lift, 21083
    Speech Aid, 21084
  Intestines, 44700
  Knee
    Insertion, 27438, 27445
  Lens
    Insertion, 66982-66985
    Manual or Mechanical Technique, 66982-
      66984
    not Associated with Concurrent Cataract
      Removal, 66985
  Mandibular Resection, 21081
  Nasal, 21087
  Nasal Septum
    Insertion, 30220
  Obturator, 21076
    Definitive, 21080
    Interim, 21079
  Ocular, 21077, 65770, 66982-66985, 92358
    Fitting and Prescription, 92002-92014
    Loan, 92358
    Prescription, 92002-92014
  Orbital, 21077
  Orthotic
    Check-Out, 97762
    Training, 97761
  Ossicular Chain
    Partial or Total, 69633, 69637
  Palatal Augmentation, 21082
  Palatal Lift, 21083

Prosthesis — *continued*
Palate, 42280, 42281
Penile
  Fitting, 54699, 55899
  Insertion, 54400-54405
  Removal, 54406, 54410-54417
  Repair, 54408
  Replacement, 54410, 54411, 54416, 54417
Perineum
  Removal, 53442
Removal
  Elbow, 24160-24164
  Hip, 27090-27091
  Knee, 27488
  Shoulder, 23334-23335
  Wrist, 25250-25251
Shoulder
  Removal, 23334-23335
Skull Plate
  Removal, 62142
  Replacement, 62143
Spectacle
  Fitting, 92352, 92353
  Repair, 92371
Speech Aid, 21084
Spinal
  Insertion, 22853-22854, 22867-22870,
    [22859]
Synthetic, 69633, 69637
Temporomandibular Joint
  Arthroplasty, 21243
Testicular
  Insertion, 54660
Training, 97761
Urethral Sphincter
  Insertion, 53444, 53445
  Removal, 53446, 53447
  Repair, 53449
  Replacement, 53448
Vagina
  Insertion, 57267
Wrist
  Removal, 25250, 25251
Protease F, 85400
Protein
A, Plasma (PAPP-A), 84163
C–Reactive, 86140-86141
Electrophoresis, 84165-84166
Glycated, 82985
Myelin Basic, 83873
Osteocalcin, 83937
Other Fluids, 84166
Other Source, 84157
Prealbumin, 84134
Serum, 84155, 84165
Total, 84155-84160
Urine, 84156
  by Dipstick, 81000-81003
Western Blot, 84181, 84182, 88372
Protein Analysis, Tissue
Western Blot, 88371-88372
Protein Blotting, 84181-84182
Protein C Activator, 85337
Protein C Antigen, 85302
Protein C Assay, 85303
Protein C Resistance Assay, 85307
Protein S
Assay, 85306
Total, 85305
Prothrombase, 85260
Prothrombin, 85210
Coagulation Factor II Gene Analysis, 81240
Time, 85610, 85611
Prothrombinase
Inhibition, 85705
Inhibition Test, 85347
Partial Time, 85730, 85732
Prothrombokinase, 85230
Protime, 85610-85611
Proton Treatment Delivery
Complex, 77525
Intermediate, 77523
Simple, 77520, 77522
Protoporphyrin, 84202, 84203
Protozoa
Antibody, 86753

Provitamin A, 84590
Prower Factor, 85260
PRP, 67040
PRPF31, 81434
PRPH2, 81404, 81434
PRSS1, 81401, 81404
PRX, 81405
PSA, 84152
Free, 84154
Total, 84153
PSEN1, 81405
PSEN2, 81406
Pseudocyst, Pancreas
Drainage
  Open, 48510
PSG, 95808-95811
Psoriasis Treatment, 96910-96922
Psychiatric Diagnosis
Adaptive Behavior Assessments
  Behavioral Identification, 0359T
    Exposure Behavioral Followup, 0362T-
      0363T
    Observational Behavioral Followup, 0360T-
      0361T
Emotional/Behavioral Assessment, 96127
Evaluation, 90791-90792
Evaluation of Records, Reports, and Tests, 90885
Major Depressive Disorder (MDD), 3088F-3093F
  Diagnostic and Statistical Manual (DSM)
    Criteria Documented, 1040F
Narcosynthesis, 90865
Psychological Testing, 96101-96103
  Cognitive Performance, 96125
  Computer-Assisted, 96103
Suicide Risk Assessment, 3085F
Unlisted Services and Procedures, 90899
Psychiatric Treatment
Adaptive Behavior Treatment
  Family, 0370T
  Group, 0366T-0367T
  Individual Patient, 0364T-0365T, 0368T-
    0369T
  Multiple Family Group, 0371T
  Social Skills Group, 0372T
Biofeedback Training, 90875-90876
Consultation with Family, 90887
Electroconvulsive Therapy, 4066F, 90870
  Referral Documented, 4067F
Environmental Intervention, 90882
Exposure Adaptive Behavior Treatment, 0373T-
  0374T
Family, 90846-90849, 99510
Hypnotherapy, 90880
Individual Psychotherapy
  with Evaluation and Management Service,
    90833, 90836, 90838
  without Evaluation and Management Ser-
    vice, 90832, 90834, 90837
Narcosynthesis
  Analysis, 90865
Pharmacotherapy
  Antidepressant, 4064F
  Antipsychotic, 4065F
  Management, 90863
Psychoanalysis, 90845
Psychotherapy
  Family, 90846-90849
  Group, 90853
  Individual
    with Evaluation and Management Ser-
      vice, 90833, 90836, 90838
    without Evaluation and Management
      Service, 90832, 90834, 90837
  Interactive Complexity, 90785
Report Preparation, 90889
Suicide Risk Assessment, 3085F
Unlisted Services/Procedures, 90899
Psychoanalysis, 90845
Psychodrama, 90899
Psychophysiologic Feedback, 90875-90876
Psychotherapy
Behavior Identification Assessment, 0359T
Family, 90846-90849, 99510
Follow up Behavioral Assessment
  Exposure, 0362T-0363T
  Observational, 0360T-0361T

Psychotherapy — *continued*
Group, 90853
Home Visit by Nonphysician for Counseling,
  99510
Individual
  with Evaluation and Management Service,
    90833, 90836, 90838
  without Evaluation and Management Ser-
    vice, 90832, 90834, 90837
  for Crisis, 90839-90840
Interactive Complexity, 90785
Pharmacologic Management, 90863
Referral Documented, 4062F
Services Provided, 4060F
PT, 85610-85611
PTA (Factor XI), 85270
PTA, 36902-36903, 36905-36906, 37220-37235,
  92997-92998, [37246, 37247, 37248, 37249]
PTB, 29435
PTC, 85250
PTCA
Artery, Aortic, [37246, 37247]
PTC Factor, 85250
PTE (Prolonged Tissue Expansion), 11960, 19357
PTEN, 81321-81323
Pteroylglutamic Acid, 82746, 82747
Pterygium
Excision, 65420
  with Graft, 65426
Pterygomaxillary Fossa
Incision, 31040
Pterygopalatine Ganglion
Injection
  Anesthetic, 64505
PTH, 83970
PTK, 65400
Ptosis
See Blepharoptosis; Procidentia
PTPN11, 81406
PTT, 85730, 85732
Ptyalectasis, 42650-42660
Pubic Symphysis, 27282
Pubiotomy, 59899
Pubis
Craterization, 27070, 27071
Cyst
  Excision, 27065-27067
Excision, 27070
Saucerization, 27070, 27071
Tumor
  Excision, 27065-27067
PUBS (Percutaneous Umbilical Blood Sampling),
  59012
Pudendal Nerve
Destruction, 64630
Injection
  Anesthetic, 64430
  Neurolytic, 64630
Puestow Procedure, 48548
Pulled Elbow, 24640
Pulmonary, 78579-78582, 78597-78598
Pulmonary Artery, 33690
Angioplasty, 92997, 92998
Banding, 33690
Catheterization, 36013-36015
Embolism, 33910-33916
  Excision, 33910-33916
Percutaneous Transluminal Angioplasty, 92997,
  92998
Reimplantation, 33788
Repair, 33690, 33917-33920
  Reimplantation, 33788
Shunt
  from Aorta, 33755, 33762, 33924
  from Vena Cava, 33766, 33767
  Subclavian, 33750
Transection, 33922
Pulmonary Decortication, 32220, 32225, 32320,
  32651-32652
Pulmonary Hemorrhage, 32110
Pulmonary Valve
Incision, 33470-33474
Repair, 33470-33474
Replacement, 33475

Pulmonary Vein
Repair
  Complete, 33730
  Partial, 33724
  Stenosis, 33726
Stenosis
  Repair, 33726
Pulmonology
Diagnostic
  Airway Integrity, 94780-94781
  Airway Resistance, 94728
  Apnea Monitoring, Pediatric, 94774-94777
  Bronchodilation, 94664
  Bronchospasm Evaluation, 94060, 94070
  Carbon Dioxide Response
    Curve, 94400
  Diffusing Capacity, 94729
  Expired Gas Analysis
    Carbon Dioxide, 94770
    CO2, 94770
    NO, 95012
    O2 and CO2, 94681
    O2 Uptake, Direct, 94680
    O2 Uptake, Indirect, 94690
    Oxygen and Carbon Dioxide, 94681
    Oxygen Uptake, 94680
    Oxygen Uptake, Indirect, 94690
    Quantitative, 94250
  Flow–Volume Loop, 94375
  Hemoglobin Oxygen Affinity, 82820
  High Altitude Simulation Test (HAST),
    94452-94453
  Hypoxia Response Curve, 94450
  Inhalation Treatment, 94640, 94642, 94644-
    94645, 94664, 99503
  Lung Volume, 94726-94727
  Maximum Breathing Capacity, 94200
  Maximum Voluntary Ventilation, 94200
  Membrane Compliance, 94750
  Oximetry
    Ear or Pulse, 94760-94762
  Resistance to Airflow, 94728
  Spirometry, 94010-94070
    with Bronchospasm Evaluation, 94070
    Patient Initiated, 94014-94016
  Sputum Mobilization with Inhalants, 94664
  Stress Test, 94620-94621
  Unlisted Services and Procedures, 94799
  Vital Capacity, 94150
Therapeutic
  Expired Gas Analysis, 94250
  Inhalation Treatment, 94640, 94642, 94644-
    94645, 94664, 99503
  Intrapulmonary Surfactant Administration,
    94610
  Manipulation of Chest Wall, 94667-94669
  Pressure Ventilation
    Negative CNPB, 94662
    Positive CPAP, 94660
  Ventilation Assist, 94002-94005, 99504
Unlisted Noninvasive Vascular Diagnostic Study,
  93998
Unlisted Services and Procedures, 94799
Pulse Generator
Electronic Analysis, 95970-95979, 95980-95982
Heart
  Insertion/Replacement, 33212, 33213
Pulse Rate Increased
Heart
  Recording, 93609
Pump
See Chemotherapy, Pump Services; Infusion
  Pump
Pump, Infusion
See Infusion Pump
Pump Services
Oxygenator/Heat Exchange, 99190-99192
Pump Stomach for Poison, 43753
Punch Graft, 15775, 15776
Puncture
Artery, 36600
Chest
  with Imaging Guidance, 32555, 32557
  without Imaging Guidance, 32554, 32556
Cisternal, 61050-61055
Lumbar, 62270-62272

[Resequenced]

Puncture — continued
 Pericardium, 33010, 33011
 Pleural Cavity
  Drainage, 32556-32557
 Skull
  Drain Fluid, 61000-61020
   Cistern, 61050
  Inject Cistern, 61055
  Inject Ventricle, 61026
  Shunt
   Drainage of Fluid, 61070
   Injection, 61070
 Spinal Cord
  Diagnostic, 62270
  Drainage of Fluid, 62272
  Lumbar, 62270
 Spleen, 38999
 Tracheal
  Aspiration and/or Injection, 31612
Puncture Aspiration
 Abscess
  Skin, 10160
 Bulla, 10160
 Cyst
  Breast, 19000, 19001
  Skin, 10160
 Hematoma, 10160
Puncturing
 See Puncture
Pupillometry, Quantitative, 0341T
Pure–Tone Audiometry, 0208T-0209T, 92552, 92553
Pustules
 Removal, 10040
Putti–Platt Procedure, 23450
PUVA, 96912, 96913
PV, 90713
PVA (Percutaneous Vertebral Augmentation), 22513-22515
PVB (Paraspinous Vertebral Block), Thoracic, [64461, 64462, 64463]
Pyelogram
 See Urography, Intravenous; Urography, Retrograde
Pyelography, 74400, 74425
Pyelolithotomy, 50130
 Anatrophic, 50075
 Coagulum, 50130
Pyeloplasty, 50400, 50405, 50544
 Repair
  Horseshoe Kidney, 50540
 Secondary, 50405
Pyeloscopy
 with Cystourethroscopy, 52351
  Biopsy, 52354
  Destruction, 52354
  Lithotripsy, 52353
  Removal
   Calculus, 52352
  Tumor Excision, 52355
Pyelostolithotomy
 Percutaneous, 50080, 50081
Pyelostomy, 50125, 50400, 50405
 Closure, 53899
Pyelotomy
 with Drainage, 50125
 with Removal Calculus, 50130
 Complicated, 50135
 Endoscopic, 50570
 Exploration, 50120
Pyeloureteroplasty, 50400, 50405, 50544
PYGM, 81401, 81406
Pyloric Sphincter
 Incision, 43520
 Reconstruction, 43800
Pyloromyotomy, 43520
Pyloroplasty, 43800
 with Vagotomy, 43640
Pyothorax
 Incision and Drainage, 21501, 21502
Pyridoxal Phosphate, 84207
Pyrophosphate, Adenosine, 82030
Pyrophosphorylase, UDP Galactose, 82775-82776
Pyruvate, 84210, 84220

Q

Q Fever, 86000, 86638
Q Fever ab, 86638
QSART, 95923
QST (Quantitative Sensory Testing), 0106T-0110T
Quadrentectomy, 19301-19302
Quadriceps Repair, 27430
Qualifying Circumstances
 Anesthesia, 99100, 99116, 99135, 99140
Quantitative Carotid Atheroma Evaluation, 93895
Quantitative Carotid Intima Media Thickness Evaluation, 93895
Quantitative Pupillometry, 0341T
Quantitative Sensory Testing (QST)
 Using Cooling Stimuli, 0108T
 Using Heat–Pain Stimuli, 0109T
 Using Other Stimuli, 0110T
 Using Touch Pressure Stimuli, 0106T
 Using Vibration Stimuli, 0107T
Quick Test
 Prothrombin Time, 85610, 85611
Quinidine
 Assay, 80194
Quinine, 84228

R

RAB7A, 81405
RabAvert, 90675
Rabies
 Immune Globulin, 90375-90376
 Vaccine, 90675-90676
Rachicentesis, 62270-62272
Radial Arteries
 Aneurysm, 35045
 Embolectomy, 34111
 Sympathectomy, 64821
 Thrombectomy, 34111
Radial Head, Subluxation, 24640
Radial Keratotomy, 65771
Radiation
 Blood Products, 86945
Radiation Physics
 Consultation, 77336-77370
 Unlisted Services and Procedures, 77399
Radiation Therapy
 Consultation
  Radiation Physics, 77336-77370
 CT Scan Guidance, 77014
 Dose Plan, 77300, 77306-77331
  Brachytherapy, 77316-77318
  High-Dose Electronic Brachytherapy, 0394T-0395T
  Intensity Modulation, 77301
  Teletherapy, 77306-77321
 Field Set–Up, 77280-77290
 Guidance for Localization, [77387]
 Intraoperative, 77469, [77424, 77425]
 Localization of Patient Movement, [77387]
 Multi-leaf Collimator Device Design and Construction, 77338
 Planning, 77261-77290, 77293-77331 [77295]
 Special, 77470
 Stereotactic, 77371-77373, 77432
  Body, 77373
  Cranial Lesion, 77371-77372, 77432
 Treatment Delivery
  =>1MeV Complex, 77412
  =>1MeV Intermediate, 77407
  =>1MeV Simple, 77402
  Beam Modulation, [77385]
  Guidance for Localization, [77387]
  High Energy Neutron, 77422-77423
  Intensity Modulated Radiation (IMRT)
   Complex, [77386]
   Simple, [77385]
  Intraoperative, [77424, 77425]
  Proton Beam, 77520-77525
  Single, 77402
  Stereotactic
   Body, 77373
   Cranial Lesion(s), 77371-77372
  Superficial, 77401
  Three or More Areas, 77412
  Two Areas, 77407

Radiation Therapy — continued
 Treatment Delivery — continued
  Weekly, 77427
 Treatment Device, 77332-77334
 Treatment Management
  Intraoperative, 77469
  One or Two Fractions Only, 77431
  Stereotactic
   Body, 77435
   Cerebral, 77432
  Unlisted Services and Procedures, 77499
  Weekly, 77427
Radiation X
 See X–Ray
Radical Excision of Lymph Nodes
 Axillary, 38740-38745
 Cervical, 38720-38724
 Suprahyoid, 38700
Radical Mastectomies, Modified, 19307
Radical Neck Dissection
 with Auditory Canal Surgery, 69155
 with Thyroidectomy, 60254
 with Tongue Excision, 41135, 41145, 41153, 41155
 Laryngectomy, 31365-31368
 Pharyngolaryngectomy, 31390, 31395
Radical Vaginal Hysterectomy, 58285
Radical Vulvectomy, 56630-56640
Radioactive Colloid Therapy, 79300
Radioactive Substance
 Insertion
  Prostate, 55860
Radiocarpal Joint
 Arthrotomy, 25040
 Dislocation
  Closed Treatment, 25660
Radiocinematographies
 Esophagus, 74230
 Pharynx, 70371, 74230
 Speech Evaluation, 70371
 Swallowing Evaluation, 74230
 Unlisted Services and Procedures, 76120-76125
Radio–Cobalt B12 Schilling Test
 Vitamin B12 Absorption Study, 78270-78272
Radioelement
 Application, 77761-77772
  with Ultrasound, 76965
  Surface, 77789
 Handling, 77790
 Infusion, 77750
 Placement See Radioelement Substance
Radioelement Substance
 Catheterization, 55875
 Catheter Placement
  Breast, 19296-19298
  Bronchus, 31643
  Head and/or Neck, 41019
  Muscle and/or Soft Tissue, 20555
  Pelvic Organs or Genitalia, 55920
  Prostate, 55875
 Needle Placement
  Head and/or Neck, 41019
  Muscle and/or Soft Tissue, 20555
  Pelvic Organs and Genitalia, 55920
  Prostate, 55875
Radiography
 See Radiology, Diagnostic; X–Ray
Radioimmunosorbent Test
 Gammaglobulin, Blood, 82784-82785
Radioisotope Brachytherapy
 See Brachytherapy
Radioisotope Scan
 See Nuclear Medicine
Radiological Marker
 Preoperative Placement
  Excision of Breast Lesion, 19125, 19126
Radiology
 See Also Nuclear Medicine, Radiation Therapy, X–Ray, Ultrasound
 Diagnostic
  Unlisted Services and Procedures, 76499
 Examination, 70030
  Stress Views, 77071
 Joint Survey, 77077
 Therapeutic
  Field Set–Up, 77280-77290

Radiology — continued
 Therapeutic — continued
  Planning, 77261-77263, 77299
  Port Film, 77417
Radionuclide Therapy
 Heart, 79440
 Interstitial, 79300
 Intra–arterial, 79445
 Intra–articular, 79440
 Intracavitary, 79200
 Intravascular, 79101
 Intravenous, 79101, 79403
 Intravenous Infusion, 79101, 79403
 Oral, 79005
 Remote Afterloading, 77767-77768, 77770-77772
 Unlisted Services and Procedures, 79999
Radionuclide Tomography, Single–Photon Emission–Computed
 Abscess Localization, 78807
 Bone, 78320
 Brain, 78607
 Cerebrospinal Fluid, 78647
 Heart, 78451-78454
 Joint, 78320
 Kidney, 78710
 Liver, 78205
 Tumor Localization, 78803
Radiopharmaceutical Therapy
 Heart, 79440
 Interstitial, 79300
  Colloid Administration, 79300
 Intra-arterial Particulate, 79445
 Intra–articular, 79440
 Intracavitary, 79200
 Intravascular, 79101
 Intravenous, 78808, 79101, 79403
 Oral, 79005
 Unlisted Services and Procedures, 79999
Radiostereometic Analysis
 Lower Extremity, 0350T
 Placement Interstitial Device, 0347T
 Spine, 0348T
 Upper Extremity, 0349T
Radiosurgery
 Cranial Lesion, 61796-61799
 Spinal Lesion, 63620-63621
Radiotherapeutic
 See Radiation Therapy
Radiotherapies
 See Irradiation
Radiotherapy
 Afterloading, 77767-77768, 77770-77772
  Catheter Insertion, 19296-19298
  Planning, 77316-77318
Radiotherapy, Surface, 77789
Radioulnar Joint
 Arthrodesis
  with Ulnar Resection, 25830
 Dislocation
  Closed Treatment, 25525, 25675
  Open Treatment, 25676
  Percutaneous Fixation, 25671
Radius
 See Also Arm, Lower; Elbow; Ulna
 Arthroplasty, 24365
  with Implant, 24366, 25441
 Craterization, 24145, 25151
 Cyst
  Excision, 24125, 24126, 25120-25126
 Diaphysectomy, 24145, 25151
 Dislocation
  with Fracture
   Closed Treatment, 24620
   Open Treatment, 24635
  Partial, 24640
  Subluxate, 24640
 Excision, 24130, 24136, 24145, 24152
  Epiphyseal Bar, 20150
  Partial, 25145
  Styloid Process, 25230
 Fracture, 25605
  with Ulna, 25560, 25565
   Open Treatment, 25575
  Closed Treatment, 25500, 25505, 25520, 25600, 25605

Radius — *continued*
  Fracture — *continued*
    Closed Treatment — *continued*
      with Manipulation, 25605
      without Manipulation, 25600
    Colles, 25600, 25605
    Distal, 25600-25609
      Closed Treatment, 25600-25605
      Open Treatment, 25607-25609
    Head/Neck
      Closed Treatment, 24650, 24655
      Open Treatment, 24665, 24666
    Open Treatment, 25515, 25525, 25526, 25574
    Percutaneous Fixation, 25606
    Shaft, 25500-25526
      Open Treatment, 25515, 25574-25575
  Implant
    Removal, 24164
  Incision and Drainage, 25035
  Osteomyelitis, 24136, 24145
  Osteoplasty, 25390-25393
  Prophylactic Treatment, 25490, 25492
  Repair
    with Graft, 25405, 25420-25426
    Epiphyseal Arrest, 25450, 25455
    Epiphyseal Separation
      Closed, 25600
      Closed with Manipulation, 25605
      Open Treatment, 25607, 25608-25609
      Percutaneous Fixation, 25606
    Malunion or Nonunion, 25400, 25415
  Osteotomy, 25350, 25355, 25370, 25375
    and Ulna, 25365
  Saucerization, 24145, 25151
  Sequestrectomy, 24136, 25145
  Subluxation, 24640
  Tumor
    Cyst, 24120
    Excision, 24125, 24126, 25120-25126, 25170
RAF1, 81404, 81406
RA Factor
  Qualitative, 86430
  Quantitative, 86431
RAI1, 81405
Ramstedt Operation
  Pyloromyotomy, 43520
Ramus Anterior, Nervus Thoracicus
  Destruction, 64620
  Injection
    Anesthetic, 64420-64421
    Neurolytic, 64620
Range of Motion Test
  Extremities, 95851
  Eye, 92018, 92019
  Hand, 95852
  Rectum
    Biofeedback, 90911
  Trunk, 97530
Ranula
  Treatment of, 42408
Rapid Heart Rate
  Heart
    Recording, 93609
Rapid Plasma Reagin Test, 86592, 86593
Rapid Test for Infection, 86308, 86403, 86406
  Monospot Test, 86308
Rapoport Test, 52005
Raskind Procedure, 33735-33737
Rastelli Procedure, 33786
Rathke Pouch Tumor
  Excision, 61545
Rat Typhus, 86000
Rays, Roentgen
  See X–Ray
Raz Procedure, 51845
RBC, 78120, 78121, 78130-78140, 85007, 85014, 85041, 85547, 85555, 85557, 85651-85660, 86850-86870, 86970-86978
RBC ab, 86850-86870
RBL (Rubber Band Ligation)
  Hemorrhoids, 46221
  Skin Tags, 11200-11201
RCM, 96931-96936
RDH12,, 81434

Reaction
  Lip
    without Reconstruction, 40530
Realignment
  Femur, with Osteotomy, 27454
  Knee, Extensor, 27422
  Muscle, 20999
    Hand, 26989
  Tendon, Extensor, 26437
Reattachment
  Muscle, 20999
  Thigh, 27599
Receptor
  Antibody, 86243
  CD4, 86360
  Estrogen, 84233
  FC, 86243
  Progesterone, 84234
  Progestin, 84234
Receptor Assay
  Endocrine, 84235
  Estrogen, 84233
  Immunoglobulin, 86243
  Non–Hormone, 84238
  Progesterone, 84234
Recession
  Gastrocnemius
    Leg, Lower, 27687
  Tendon
    Hand, 26989
RECOMBIVAX HB, 90740, 90743-90744, 90746
Reconstruction
  See Also Revision
  Abdominal Wall
    Omental Flap, 49905
  Acetabulum, 27120, 27122
  Anal
    with Implant, 46762
    Congenital Absence, 46730-46740
    Fistula, 46742
    Graft, 46753
    Sphincter, 46750, 46751, 46760-46762
  Ankle, 27700-27703
  Apical–Aortic Conduit, 33404
  Atrial, 33254-33259
    Endoscopic, 33265-33266
    Open, 33254-33259
  Auditory Canal, External, 69310, 69320
  Bile Duct
    Anastomosis, 47800
  Bladder
    with Urethra, 51800, 51820
    from Colon, 50810
    from Intestines, 50820, 51960
  Breast
    with Free Flap, 19364
    with Latissimus Dorsi Flap, 19361
    with Other Techniques, 19366
    with Tissue Expander, 19357
    Augmentation, 19324, 19325
    Mammoplasty, 19318-19325
      Biesenberger, 19318
    Nipple, 19350, 19355
    Revision, 19380
    Transverse Rectus Abdominis Myocutaneous Flap, 19367-19369
  Bronchi
    with Lobectomy, 32501
    with Segmentectomy, 32501
    Graft Repair, 31770
    Stenosis, 31775
  Canthus, 67950
  Cardiac Anomaly, 33622
  Carpal, 25443
  Carpal Bone, 25394, 25430
  Cheekbone, 21270
  Chest Wall
    Omental Flap, 49905
    Trauma, 32820
  Cleft Palate, 42200-42225
  Conduit
    Apical–Aortic, 33404
  Conjunctiva, 68320-68335
    with Flap
      Bridge or Partial, 68360
      Total, 68362

Reconstruction — *continued*
  Cranial Bone
    Extracranial, 21181-21184
  Ear, Middle
    Tympanoplasty with Antrotomy or Mastoidectomy
      with Ossicular Chain Reconstruction, 69636, 69637
    Tympanoplasty with Mastoidectomy, 69641
      with Intact or Reconstructed Wall, 69643, 69644
      with Ossicular Chain Reconstruction, 69642
      Radical or Complete, 69644, 69645
    Tympanoplasty without Mastoidectomy, 69631
      with Ossicular Chain Reconstruction, 69632, 69633
  Elbow, 24360
    with Implant, 24361, 24362
    Total Replacement, 24363
  Esophagus, 43300, 43310, 43313
    Creation
      Stoma, 43351-43352
    Esophagostomy, 43351-43352
    Fistula, 43305, 43312, 43314
    Gastrointestinal, 43360-43361
  Eye
    Graft
      Conjunctiva, 65782
      Stem Cell, 65781
    Transplantation
      Amniotic Membrane, 65780
  Eyelid
    Canthus, 67950
    Second Stage, 67975
    Total, 67973-67975
    Total Eyelid
      Lower, One Stage, 67973
      Upper, One Stage, 67974
    Transfer Tarsoconjunctival Flap from Opposing Eyelid, 67971
  Facial Bones
    Secondary, 21275
  Fallopian Tube, 58673, 58750-58752, 58770
  Femur
    Knee, 27442, 27443
    Lengthening, 27466, 27468
    Shortening, 27465, 27468
  Fibula
    Lengthening, 27715
  Finger
    Polydactylous, 26587
  Foot
    Cleft, 28360
  Forehead, 21172-21180, 21182-21184
  Glenoid Fossa, 21255
  Gums
    Alveolus, 41874
    Gingiva, 41872
  Hand
    Tendon Pulley, 26500-26502
    Toe to Finger Transfer, 26551-26556
  Heart
    Atrial, 33254-33259
      Endoscopic, 33265-33266
      Open, 33254-33259
    Atrial Septum, 33735-33737
    Pulmonary Artery Shunt, 33924
    Vena Cava, 34502
  Hip
    Replacement, 27130, 27132
    Secondary, 27134-27138
  Hip Joint
    with Prosthesis, 27125
  Interphalangeal Joint, 26535, 26536
    Collateral Ligament, 26545
  Intestines, Small
    Anastomosis, 44130
  Knee, 27437, 27438
    with Implantation, 27445
    with Prosthesis, 27438, 27445
    Femur, 27442, 27443, 27446
    Instability, 27420, 27424
    Ligament, 27427-27429
    Replacement, 27447

Reconstruction — *continued*
  Knee — *continued*
    Revision, 27486, 27487
    Tibia
      Plateau, 27440-27443, 27446
  Kneecap
    Instability, 27420-27424
  Larynx
    Burns, 31599
    Cricoid Split, 31587
    Other, 31545-31546, 31599
    Stenosis, *[31551, 31552, 31553, 31554]*
    Web, 31580
  Lip, 40525, 40527, 40761
  Lunate, 25444
  Malar Augmentation
    with Bone Graft, 21210
    Prosthetic Material, 21270
  Mandible
    with Implant, 21244-21246, 21248, 21249
  Mandibular Condyle, 21247
  Mandibular Rami
    with Bone Graft, 21194
    with Internal Rigid Fixation, 21196
    without Bone Graft, 21193
    without Internal Rigid Fixation, 21195
  Maxilla
    with Implant, 21245, 21246, 21248, 21249
  Metacarpophalangeal Joint, 26530, 26531
  Midface, 21188
    with Bone Graft, 21145-21160, 21188
    with Internal Rigid Fixation, 21188
    without Bone Graft, 21141-21143
    without Internal Rigid Fixation, 21195
    Forehead Advancement, 21159, 21160
  Mouth, 40840-40845
  Nail Bed, 11762
  Nasoethmoid Complex, 21182-21184
  Navicular, 25443
  Nose
    Cleft Lip
      Cleft Palate, 30460, 30462
    Dermatoplasty, 30620
    Primary, 30400-30420
    Secondary, 30430-30462
    Septum, 30520
  Orbit, 21256
  Orbital Rim, 21172-21180
  Orbital Walls, 21182-21184
  Orbit Area
    Secondary, 21275
  Orbitocraniofacial
    Secondary Revision, 21275
  Orbit, with Bone Grafting, 21182-21184
  Oviduct
    Fimbrioplasty, 58760
  Palate
    Cleft Palate, 42200-42225
    Lengthening, 42226, 42227
  Parotid Duct
    Diversion, 42507-42510
  Patella, 27437, 27438
    Instability, 27420-27424
  Penis
    Angulation, 54360
    Chordee, 54300, 54304
    Complications, 54340-54348
    Epispadias, 54380-54390
    Hypospadias, 54332, 54352
      One Stage Distal with Urethroplasty, 54324-54328
      One Stage Perineal, 54336
  Periorbital Region
    Osteotomy with Graft, 21267, 21268
  Pharynx, 42950
  Pyloric Sphincter, 43800
  Radius, 24365, 25390-25393, 25441
    Arthroplasty
      with Implant, 24366
  Shoulder Joint
    with Implant, 23470, 23472
  Skull, 21172-21180
    Defect, 62140, 62141, 62145
  Sternum, 21740-21742
    with Thoracoscopy, 21743

Reconstruction — *continued*
- Stomach
  - with Duodenum, 43810, 43850, 43855, 43865
  - with Jejunum, 43820, 43825, 43860
  - for Obesity, 43644-43645, 43845-43848
  - Gastric Bypass, 43644-43846
  - Roux-en-Y, 43644, 43846
- Superior-Lateral Orbital Rim and Forehead, 21172, 21175
- Supraorbital Rim and Forehead, 21179, 21180
- Symblepharon, 68335
- Temporomandibular Joint
  - Arthroplasty, 21240-21243
- Throat, 42950
- Thumb
  - from Finger, 26550
  - Opponensplasty, 26490-26496
- Tibia
  - Lengthening, 27715
  - Tubercle, 27418
- Toe
  - Angle Deformity, 28313
  - Extra, 28344
  - Hammertoe, 28285, 28286
  - Macrodactyly, 28340, 28341
  - Polydactylous, 26587
  - Syndactyly, 28345
  - Webbed Toe, 28345
- Tongue
  - Frenum, 41520
- Trachea
  - Carina, 31766
  - Cervical, 31750
  - Fistula, 31755
  - Graft Repair, 31770
  - Intrathoracic, 31760
- Trapezium, 25445
- Tympanic Membrane, 69620
- Ulna, 25390-25393, 25442
  - Radioulnar, 25337
- Ureter, 50700
  - with Intestines, 50840
- Urethra, 53410-53440, 53445
  - Complications, 54340-54348
  - Hypospadias
    - Meatus, 53450, 53460
    - One Stage Distal with Meatal Advancement, 54322
    - One Stage Distal with Urethroplasty, 54324-54328
    - Suture to Bladder, 51840, 51841
    - Urethroplasty for Second Stage, 54308-54316
    - Urethroplasty for Third Stage, 54318
- Uterus, 58540
- Vas Deferens, 55400
- Vena Cava, 34502
  - with Resection, 37799
- Wound Repair, 13100-13160
- Wrist, 25332
  - Capsulectomy, 25320
  - Capsulorrhaphy, 25320
  - Realign, 25335
- Zygomatic Arch, 21255

Recording
- Tremor, 95999

Rectal Bleeding
- Endoscopic Control, 45317

Rectal Packing, 45999

Rectal Prolapse
- Excision, 45130-45135
- Repair, 45900

Rectal Sphincter
- Dilation, 45910

Rectocele
- Repair, 45560

Rectopexy
- Laparoscopic, 45400-45402
- Open, 45540-45550

Rectoplasty, 45500-45505

Rectorrhaphy, 45540-45541, 45800-45825

Rectovaginal Fistula
- *See* Fistula, Rectovaginal

Rectovaginal Hernia
- *See* Rectocele

Rectum
- *See Also* Anus
- Abscess
  - Incision and Drainage, 45005, 45020, 46040, 46060
- Biopsy, 45100
- Dilation
  - Endoscopy, 45303
- Endoscopy
  - Destruction
    - Tumor, 45320
  - Dilation, 45303
  - Exploration, 45300
  - Hemorrhage, 45317
  - Removal
    - Foreign Body, 45307
    - Polyp, 45308-45315
    - Tumor, 45308-45315
  - Volvulus, 45321
- Excision
  - with Colon, 45121
  - Partial, 45111, 45113-45116, 45123
  - Total, 45110, 45112, 45119, 45120
- Exploration
  - Endoscopic, 45300
  - Surgical, 45990
- Hemorrhage
  - Endoscopic, 45317
- Injection
  - Sclerosing Solution, 45520
- Laparoscopy, 45499
- Lesion
  - Excision, 45108
- Manometry, 91122
- Prolapse
  - Excision, 45130, 45135
- Removal
  - Fecal Impaction, 45915
  - Foreign Body, 45307, 45915
- Repair
  - with Sigmoid Excision, 45550
  - Fistula, 45800-45825, 46706-46707
  - Injury, 45562, 45563
  - Prolapse, 45505-45541, 45900
  - Rectocele, 45560
  - Stenosis, 45500
- Sensation, Tone, and Compliance Test, 91120
- Stricture
  - Excision, 45150
- Suture
  - Fistula, 45800-45825
  - Prolapse, 45540, 45541
- Tumor
  - Destruction, 45190, 45320
  - Excision, 45160, 45171-45172
- Unlisted Services and Procedures, 45999

Rectus Sheath Block
- Bilateral, 64488-64489
- Unilateral, 64486-64487

Red Blood Cell (RBC)
- Antibody, 86850-86870
  - Pretreatment, 86970-86972
- Count, 85032-85041
- Fragility
  - Mechanical, 85547
  - Osmotic, 85555, 85557
- Hematocrit, 85014
- Morphology, 85007
- Platelet Estimation, 85007
- Sedimentation Rate
  - Automated, 85652
  - Manual, 85651
- Sequestration, 78140
- Sickling, 85660
- Survival Test, 78130, 78135
- Volume Determination, 78120, 78121

Red Blood Cell ab, 86850-86870

Reductase, Glutathione, 82978

Reductase, Lactic Cytochrome, 83615, 83625

Reduction
- Blood Volume, 86960
- Dislocation
  - Acromioclavicular
    - Closed Treatment, 23545
    - Open Treatment, 23550, 23552

Reduction — *continued*
- Dislocation — *continued*
  - Ankle
    - Closed Treatment, 27840, 27842
    - Open Treatment, 27846, 27848
  - Bennet's
    - Closed Treatment, 26670, 26675
    - Open Treatment, 26665, 26685, 26686
    - Percutaneous Fixation, 26650, 26676
  - Carpometacarpal
    - Closed Treatment, 26641, 26645, 26670, 26675
    - Open Treatment, 26665, 26685, 26686
    - Percutaneous Fixation, 26650, 26676
  - Clavicle
    - Closed Treatment, 23540, 23545
    - Open Treatment, 23550, 23552
  - Elbow
    - Closed Treatment, 24600, 24605, 24620, 24640
    - Monteggia, 24620
    - Open Treatment
      - Acute, 24615
      - Chronic, 24615
      - Monteggia, 24635
      - Periarticular, 24586, 24587
  - Galeazzi
    - Closed Treatment, 25520
    - Open Treatment, 25525, 25526
      - with Fracture
        - Radial Shaft, 25525, 25526
      - with Repair
        - Triangular Cartilage, 25526
  - Hip
    - Post Arthroplasty
      - Closed Treatment, 27265, 27266
    - Spontaneous/Pathologic
      - Closed Treatment, 27257
      - Developmental/Congenital
        - Closed Treatment, 27257
        - Open Treatment, 27258
          - with Femoral Shaft Shortening, 27259
      - Open Treatment, 27258
        - with Femoral Shaft Shortening, 27259
    - Traumatic
      - Closed Treatment, 27250, 27252
      - Open Treatment, 27253, 27254
        - Acetabular Wall, 27254
        - Femoral Head, 27254
  - Intercarpal
    - Closed Treatment, 25660
    - Open Treatment, 25670
  - Interphalangeal Joint
    - Foot/Toe
      - Closed Treatment, 28660, 28665
      - Open Treatment, 28675
      - Percutaneous Fixation, 28666
    - Hand/Finger
      - Closed Treatment, 26770, 26775
      - Open Treatment, 26785
      - Percutaneous Fixation, 26776
  - Knee
    - Closed Treatment, 27550, 27552
    - Open Treatment, 27556-27558
  - Lunate
    - Closed Treatment, 25690
    - Open Treatment, 25695
  - Metacarpophalangeal Joint
    - Closed Treatment, 26700-26706
    - Open Treatment, 26715
  - Metatarsophalangeal Joint
    - Closed Treatment, 28630, 28635
    - Open Treatment, 28645
    - Percutaneous Fixation, 28636
  - Monteggia, 24635
  - Odontoid
    - Open Treatment, 22318, 22319
  - Patella, Patellar
    - Acute
      - Closed Treatment, 27560, 27562
      - Open Treatment, 27566
        - Partial, 27566
        - Total, 27566
      - Recurrent, 27420-27424

Reduction — *continued*
- Dislocation — *continued*
  - Patella, Patellar — *continued*
    - Recurrent — *continued*
      - with Patellectomy, 27424
  - Pelvic, Ring
    - Closed Treatment, 27197-27198
    - Open Treatment, 27217-27218
    - Percutaneous Fixation, 27216
  - Radiocarpal
    - Closed Treatment, 25660
    - Open Treatment, 25670
  - Radio-ulnar Joint
    - Closed Treatment, 25675
      - with Radial Fracture, 25520
    - Open Treatment, 25676
      - with Radial Fracture, 25525, 25526
  - Radius
    - with Fracture
      - Closed Treatment, 24620
      - Open Treatment, 24635
    - Closed Treatment, 24640
  - Sacrum, 27218
  - Shoulder
    - Closed Treatment with Manipulation, 23650, 23655
      - with Fracture of Greater Humeral Tuberosity, 23665
      - with Surgical or Anatomical Neck Fracture, 23675
    - Open Treatment, 23660
    - Recurrent, 23450-23466
  - Sternoclavicular
    - Closed Treatment, 23525
    - Open Treatment, 23530, 23532
  - Talotarsal joint
    - Closed Treatment, 28570, 28575
    - Open Treatment, 28585
    - Percutaneous Fixation, 28576
  - Tarsal
    - Closed Treatment, 28540, 28545
    - Open Treatment, 28555
    - Percutaneous Fixation, 28546
  - Tarsometatarsal joint
    - Closed Treatment, 28600
    - Open Treatment, 28615
    - Percutaneous Fixation, 28606
  - Temporomandibular
    - Closed Treatment, 21480, 21485
    - Open Treatment, 21490
  - Tibiofibular Joint
    - Closed Treatment, 27830, 27831
    - Open Treatment, 27832
  - TMJ
    - Closed Treatment, 21480, 21485
    - Open Treatment, 21490
  - Vertebral
    - Closed Treatment, 22315
    - Open Treatment, 22325, 22326-22328
- Forehead, 21137-21139
- Fracture
  - Acetabulum, Acetabular
    - Closed Treatment, 27222
    - Open Treatment, 27227, 27228
      - with Dislocation hip, 27254
  - Alveolar Ridge
    - Closed Treatment, 21440
    - Open Treatment, 21445
  - Ankle
    - Bimalleolar
      - Closed Treatment, 27810
      - Open Treatment, 27814
    - Trimalleolar
      - Closed Treatment, 27818
      - Open Treatment, 27822
        - with Fixation
          - Posterior Lip, 27823
        - with Malleolus Fracture
          - Lateral, 27822, 27823
          - Medial, 27822, 27823
  - Bennett
    - Closed Treatment, 26670, 26675
    - Open Treatment, 26665, 26685, 26686
    - Percutaneous Fixation, 26650, 26676
  - Blowout
    - Open Treatment, 21385-21395

Index

Reconstruction — Reduction

Reduction — *continued*
  Fracture — *continued*
    Bronchi, Bronchus
      Closed
        Endoscopic Treatment, 31630
    Calcaneal, Calcaneus
      Closed Treatment, 28405
      Open Treatment, 28415
        with
          Bone Graft, 28420
      Percutaneous Fixation, 28406
    Carpal Bone(s)
      Closed Treatment, 25624, 25635
        Capitate, 25635
        Hamate, 25635
        Lunate, 25635
        Navicular, 25624
        Pisiform, 25635
        Scaphoid, 25624
        Trapezium, 25635
        Trapezoid, 25635
        Triquetral, 25635
      Open Treatment, 25628, 25645
        Capitate, 25645
        Hamate, 25645
        Lunate, 25645
        Navicular, 25628
        Pisiform, 25645
        Scaphoid, 25628
        Trapezium, 25645
        Trapezoid, 25645
        Triquetral, 25645
    Carpometacarpal
      Closed Treatment, 26645
      Open Treatment, 26665
      Percutaneous Fixation, 26650
    Cheek
      Percutaneous, 21355
    Clavicle
      Closed Treatment, 23505
      Open Treatment, 23515
    Coccyx, Coccygeal
      Open Treatment, 27202
    Colles
      Closed Treatment, 25605
      Open Treatment, 25607-25609
      Percutaneous Fixation, 25606
    Craniofacial
      Open Treatment, 21432-21436
    Cuboid
      Closed Treatment, 28455
      Open Treatment, 28465
    Cuneiforms
      Closed Treatment, 28455
      Open Treatment, 28465
    Elbow
      Closed Treatment, 24620
      Open Treatment, 24586, 24587
    Epiphysis, Epiphyseal
      Closed Treatment, 27517
      Open Treatment, 27519
    Femur, Femoral
      Condyle
        Lateral
          Closed Treatment, 27510
          Open Treatment, 27514
        Medial
          Closed Treatment, 27510
          Open Treatment, 27514
      Distal
        Closed Treatment, 27510
          Lateral Condyle, 27510
          Medial Condyle, 27510
        Open Treatment, 27514
          Lateral Condyle, 27514
          Medial Condyle, 27514
      Epiphysis, Epiphyseal
        Closed Treatment, 27517
        Open Treatment, 27519
      Greater Trochanteric
        Open Treatment, 27248
      Head
        Traumatic, 27254
          with Dislocation Hip, 27254
          with Greater Trochanteric
            Open Treatment, 27248

Reduction — *continued*
  Fracture — *continued*
    Femur, Femoral — *continued*
      Intertrochanteric, Intertrochanter
        Closed Treatment, 27238, 27240
        Open Treatment, 27244, 27245
          with Intermedullary Implant,
            27245
      Peritrochanteric, Peritrochanter
        Closed Treatment, 27240
        Open Treatment, 27244, 27245
          with Intermedullary Implant,
            27245
      Proximal End
        Closed Treatment, 27232
        Open Treatment, 27236
          with Prosthetic Replacement,
            27236
      Proximal Neck
        Closed, 27232
        Open Treatment, 27236
          with Prosthetic Replacement,
            27236
      Shaft
        Closed Treatment, 27502
        Open Treatment, 27506, 27507
          with Intermedullary Implant,
            27245
      Subtrochanteric, Subtrochanter
        Closed Treatment, 27240
        Open Treatment, 27244, 27245
      Supracondylar
        Closed Treatment, 27503
          with Intercondylar Extension,
            27503
        Open Treatment, 27511, 27513
          with Intercondylar Extension,
            27513
      Transcondylar
        Closed Treatment, 27503
        Open Treatment, 27511, 27513
          with Intercondylar Extension,
            27513
    Fibula and Tibia, 27828
    Fibula, Fibular
      Distal
        Closed Treatment, 27788
        Open Treatment, 27792
          with Fracture
            Tibia, 27828
      Malleolus
        Lateral
          Closed Treatment, 27788
          Open Treatment, 27792
      Proximal
        Closed Treatment, 27781
        Open Treatment, 27784
      Shaft
        Closed Treatment, 27781
        Open Treatment, 27784
    Foot
      Sesamoid
        Open Treatment, 28531
    Frontal Sinus
      Open Treatment, 21343, 21344
    Great Toe
      Closed Treatment, 28495
      Open Treatment, 28505
      Percutaneous Fixation, 28496
    Heel
      Closed Treatment, 28405
      Open Treatment, 28415
        with Bone graft, 28420
    Humeral, Humerus
      Anatomical neck
        Closed Treatment, 23605
        Open Treatment, 23615, 23616
      Condylar
        Lateral
          Closed Treatment, 24577
          Open Treatment, 24579
          Percutaneous Fixation, 24582
        Medial
          Closed Treatment, 24577
          Open Treatment, 24579
          Percutaneous Fixation, 24566

Reduction — *continued*
  Fracture — *continued*
    Humeral, Humerus — *continued*
      Epicondylar
        Lateral
          Closed Treatment, 24565
          Open Treatment, 24575
          Percutaneous Fixation, 24566
        Medial
          Closed Treatment, 24565
          Open, 24575
          Percutaneous Fixation, 24566
      Proximal
        Closed Treatment, 23605
        Open Treatment, 23615, 23616
      Shaft
        Closed Treatment, 24505
        Open Treatment, 24515, 24516
      Supracondylar
        Closed Treatment, 24535
        Open Treatment, 24545, 24546
          with Intercondylar Extension,
            24546
      Surgical Neck
        Closed Treatment, 23605
        Open Treatment, 23615, 23616
      Transcondylar
        Closed Treatment, 24535
        Open Treatment, 24545, 24546
          with Intercondylar Extension,
            24546
      Tuberosity
        Closed Treatment, 23625
        Open Treatment, 23630
    Hyoid
      Open Treatment, 31584
    Iliac, Ilium
      Open Treatment
        Spine, 27215
        Tuberosity, 27215
        Wing, 27215
    Interphalangeal
      Closed Treatment
        Articular, 26742
      Open Treatment
        Articular, 26746
    Knee
      Intercondylar
        Spine
          Closed Treatment, 27538
          Open Treatment, 27540
        Tuberosity
          Open Treatment, 27540
    Larynx, Laryngeal
      Open Treatment, 31584
    LeFort I
      Open Treatment, 21422, 21423
    LeFort II
      Open Treatment, 21346-21348
    LeFort III
      Open Treatment, 21432-21436
    Lunate
      Closed Treatment, 25635
      Open Treatment, 25645
    Malar Area
      Open Treatment, 21360-21366
      Percutaneous Fixation, 21355
    Malar Tripod
      Open Treatment, 21360-21366
      Percutaneous Treatment, 21355
    Malleolus
      Lateral
        Closed Treatment, 27788
        Open Treatment, 27792
          with Fracture
            Ankle, Trimalleolar, 27822
      Medial
        Closed Treatment, 27762
        Open Treatment, 27766
          with Fracture
            Ankle, Trimalleolar, 27822
    Mandibular, Mandible
      Alveolar Ridge
        Closed Treatment, 21440
        Open Treatment, 21445
      Closed Treatment, 21451

Reduction — *continued*
  Fracture — *continued*
    Mandibular, Mandible — *continued*
      Condylar, Condyle
        Open Treatment, 21465
        Open Treatment, 21454-21462, 21470
      Metacarpal
        Closed Treatment, 26605, 26607
        Open Treatment, 26615
        Percutaneous Fixation, 26608
      Metacarpophalangeal
        Closed
          Articular, 26742
        Open
          Articular, 26746
      Metatarsal
        Closed Treatment, 28475
        Open Treatment, 28485
        Percutaneous Fixation, 28476
      Monteggia, 24635
      Nasal Bone
        Closed Treatment
          with Stabilization, 21320
          without Stabilization, 21315
        Open Treatment
          with External Fixation, 21330,
            21335
          with Fractured Septum, 21335
      Nasal, Nose
        Closed Treatment
          with Stabilization, 21320
          without Stabilization, 21315
        Open Treatment
          with External Fixation, 21330,
            21335
          with Fractured Septum, 21335
          with Internal Fixation, 21330,
            21335
      Nasal Septum
        Closed Treatment, 21337
          with Stabilization, 21337
          without Stabilization, 21337
        Open Treatment
          with Nasal Bone, 21335
          with Stabilization, 21336
          without Stabilization, 21336
      Nasoethmoid
        Open Treatment
          with External Fixation, 21339
          without External Fixation, 21338
      Nasomaxillary
        Closed Treatment
          LeFort II, 21345
        Open Treatment
          LeFort II, 21346-21348
      Navicular
        Foot
          Closed Treatment, 28455
          Open Treatment, 28465
          Percutaneous Fixation, 28456
        Hand
          Closed Treatment, 25624
          Open Treatment, 25628
      Odontoid
        Open Treatment, 22318, 22319
      Olecranon process
        Closed Treatment, 24675
        Open Treatment, 24685
      Orbit
        Closed Treatment, 21401
        Open Treatment, 21406-21408
      Orbital Floor
        Blowout, 21385-21395
        Open Treatment, 21385-21395
      Palate, Palatal
        Open Treatment, 21422, 21423
      Patella, Patellar
        Open Treatment, 27524
      Pelvic, Pelvis
        Iliac, Ilium
          Open Treatment
            Spine, 27215
            Tuberosity, 27215
            Wing, 27215
      Pelvic Ring
        Closed Treatment, 27197-27198

[Resequenced] © 2016 Optum360, LLC

Reduction — *continued*
  Fracture — *continued*
    Pelvic Ring — *continued*
      Open Treatment, 27217-27218
      Percutaneous Fixation, 27216
    Phalange, Phalanges, Phalangeal
      Foot
        Closed Treatment, 28515
          Great Toe, 28495, 28505
        Open Treatment, 28525
          Great Toe, 28505
        Percutaneous Fixation, 28496
          Great Toe, 28496
      Hand
        Closed Treatment, 26725
          Distal, 26755
        Open Treatment, 26735
          Distal, 26765
        Percutaneous Fixation, 26727,
          26756
    Pisiform
      Closed Treatment, 25635
      Open Treatment, 25645
    Radial, Radius
      Colles
        Closed Treatment, 25605
        Open Treatment, 25607-25609
        Percutaneous Fixation, 25606
      Distal
        Closed Treatment, 25605
          with Fracture
            Ulnar Styloid, 25600
        Open Treatment, 25607, 25608-
          25609
      Head
        Closed Treatment, 24655
        Open Treatment, 24665, 24666
      Neck
        Closed Treatment, 24655
        Open Treatment, 24665, 24666
      Shaft
        Closed Treatment, 25505
          with Dislocation
            Radio–Ulnar Joint, Distal,
              25520
        Open Treatment, 25515
          with Dislocation
            Radio–Ulnar Joint, Distal,
              25525, 25526
            Repair, Triangular Carti-
              lage, 25526
      Smith
        Closed Treatment, 25605
        Open Treatment, 25607, 25608-
          25609
        Percutaneous Fixation, 25606
    Rib
      Open Treatment, 21811-21813
    Sacroiliac Joint, 27218
    Sacrum, 27218
    Scaphoid
      Closed Treatment, 25624
      Open Treatment, 25628
    Scapula, Scapular
      Closed Treatment, 23575
      Open Treatment, 23585
    Sesamoid
      Open Treatment, 28531
    Sternum
      Open Treatment, 21825
    Talar, Talus
      Closed Treatment, 28435
      Open Treatment, 28445
      Percutaneous Fixation, 28436
    Tarsal
      Calcaneal
        Closed Treatment, 28405
        Open Treatment, 28415
          with Bone Graft, 28420
        Percutaneous Fixation, 28456
      Cuboid
        Closed Treatment, 28455
        Open Treatment, 28465
        Percutaneous Fixation, 28456
      Cuneiforms
        Closed Treatment, 28455

Reduction — *continued*
  Fracture — *continued*
    Tarsal — *continued*
      Cuneiforms — *continued*
        Open Treatment, 28465
        Percutaneous Fixation, 28456
      Navicular
        Closed Treatment, 28465
        Open Treatment, 28465
        Percutaneous Fixation, 28456
      Navicular Talus
        Closed Treatment, 28435
        Open Treatment, 28445
        Percutaneous Fixation, 28436
    T–Fracture, 27228
    Thigh
      Femur, Femoral
        Condyle
          Lateral
            Closed Treatment, 27510
            Open Treatment, 27514
          Medial
            Closed Treatment, 27510
            Open Treatment, 27514
        Distal
          Closed Treatment, 27510
            Lateral Condyle, 27510
            Medial Condyle, 27510
          Open, 27514
            Lateral Condyle, 27514
            Medial Condyle, 27514
        Epiphysis, Epiphyseal
          Closed, 27517
          Open, 27519
        Greater Trochanteric
          Open Treatment, 27248
        Head
          Traumatic, 27254
            with Dislocation Hip,
              27254
        Intertrochanter
          Closed Treatment, 27240
          Open Treatment, 27244,
           27245
            with Intermedullary Im-
             plant, 27245
        Peritrochanteric, Peritrochanter
          Closed Treatment, 27240
          Open Treatment, 27244,
           27245
            with Intermedullary Im-
             plant, 27245
        Proximal End
          Closed Treatment, 27232
          Open Treatment, 27236
            with Prosthetic Replace-
             ment, 27236
        Proximal Neck
          Closed Treatment, 27232
          Open Treatment, 27236
            with Prosthetic Replace-
             ment, 27236
        Shaft
          Closed Treatment, 27502
          Open Treatment, 27506,
           27507
            with Intermedullary Im-
             plant, 27245
        Subtrochanteric, Subtrochanter
          Closed Treatment, 27240
          Open Treatment, 27244,
           27245
        Supracondylar
          Closed Treatment, 27503
            with Intercondylar Exten-
             sion, 27503
        Transcondylar
          Closed Treatment, 27503
            with Intercondylar Exten-
             sion, 27503
          Open Treatment, 27511
            with Intercondylar Exten-
             sion, 27513
    Thumb
      Bennett, 26645
      Closed Treatment, 26645

Reduction — *continued*
  Fracture — *continued*
    Thumb — *continued*
      Open Treatment, 26665
      Percutaneous Fixation, 26650
    Tibia and Fibula, 27828
    Tibia, Tibial
      Articular Surface
        Closed Treatment, 27825
        Open Treatment, 27827
        with Fibula, Fibular
          Fracture, 27828
      Condylar
        Bicondylar, 27536
        Unicondylar, 27535
      Distal
        Closed Treatment, 27825
        Open Treatment, 27826
      Pilon
        Closed Treatment, 27825
        Open Treatment, 27827
        with Fibula, Fibular
          Fracture, 27828
      Plafond
        Closed Treatment, 27825
        Open Treatment, 27827
        with Fibula, Fibular
          Fracture, 27828
      Plateau
        Closed Treatment, 27532
        Open Treatment, 27535, 27536
      Proximal Plateau
        Closed Treatment, 27532
        Open Treatment, 27535, 27536
      Shaft
        Closed Treatment, 27752
        with Fibula, Fibular
          Fracture, 27752
        Open Treatment, 27758, 27759
        with Fibula, Fibular
          Fracture, 27758, 27759
        with Intermedullary Implant,
          27759
        Percutaneous Fixation, 27756
      Toe
        Closed Treatment, 28515
          Great, 28495
        Open Treatment, 28525
          Great, 28505
        Percutaneous Fixation, 28496
          Great, 28496
      Trachea, Tracheal
        Closed
          Endoscopic Treatment, 31630
      Trans–Scaphoperilunar
        Closed Treatment, 25680
        Open Treatment, 25685
      Trapezium
        Closed Treatment, 25635
        Open Treatment, 25645
      Trapezoid
        Closed Treatment, 25635
        Open Treatment, 25645
      Triquetral
        Closed Treatment, 25635
        Open Treatment, 25645
      Ulna, Ulnar
        Proximal
          Closed Treatment, 24675
          Open Treatment, 24685
          with Dislocation
            Radial Head, 24635
            Monteggia, 24635
        Shaft
          Closed Treatment, 25535
          And
           Radial, Radius, 25565
          Open Treatment, 25545
          and
           Radial, Radius, 25574,
           25575
        Styloid, 25650
      Vertebral
        Closed Treatment, 22315
        Open Treatment, 22325-22328, 63081-
          63091

Reduction — *continued*
  Fracture — *continued*
    Zygomatic Arch, 21356-21366
      Open Treatment, 21356-21366
        with Malar Area, 21360
        with Malar Tripod, 21360
      Percutaneous, 21355
  Lung Volume, 32491
  Mammoplasty, 19318
  Masseter Muscle/Bone, 21295, 21296
  Osteoplasty
    Facial Bones, 21209
  Pregnancy
    Multifetal, 59866
  Renal Pedicle
    Torsion, 53899
  Separation
    Craniofacial
      Open, 21432-21436
  Skull
    Craniomegalic, 62115-62117
  Subluxation
    Pelvic Ring
      Closed, 27197-27198
    Radial, 24640
      Head, 24640
      Neck, 24640
  Tongue Base
    Radiofrequency, 41530
  Ventricular Septum
    Non–surgical, 93799
REEP1, 81405
Refill
  Infusion Pump, 62369-62370, 95990-95991
Reflectance Confocal Microscopy, 96931-96936
Reflex Test
  Blink, Reflex, 95933
Reflux Study, 78262
  Gastroesophageal, 91034-91038
Refraction, 92015
Regnolli's Excision, 41140
Rehabilitation
  Artery
    Occlusive Disease, 93668
  Auditory
    Postlingual Hearing Loss, 92633
    Prelingual Hearing Loss, 92630
    Status Evaluation, 92626-92627
  Cardiac, 93797, 93798
  Services Considered Documentation, 4079F
Rehabilitation Facility
  Discharge Services, 1110F-1111F
Rehabilitative
  See Rehabilitation
Rehydration, 96360-96361
Reichstein's Substance S, 80436, 82634
Reimplantation
  Arteries
    Aorta Prosthesis, 35697
    Carotid, 35691, 35694, 35695
    Subclavian, 35693-35695
    Vertebral, 35691, 35693
    Visceral, 35697
  Coronary Ostia, 33783
  Kidney, 50380
  Ovary, 58825
  Pulmonary Artery, 33788
  Ureter
    to Bladder, 50780-50785
  Ureters, 51565
Reinnervation
  Larynx
    Neuromuscular Pedicle, 31590
Reinsch Test, 83015
Reinsertion
  Drug Delivery Implant, 11983
  Spinal Fixation Device, 22849
Relative Density
  Body Fluid, 84315
Release
  Carpal Tunnel, 64721
  Elbow Contracture
    with Radical Release of Capsule, 24149
  Flexor Muscles
    Hip, 27036

Release — *continued*
  Muscle
    Knee, 27422
    Thumb Contracture, 26508
  Nerve, 64702-64726
    Carpal Tunnel, 64721
    Neurolytic, 64727
  Retina
    Encircling Material, 67115
  Spinal Cord, 63200
  Stapes, 69650
  Tarsal Tunnel, 28035
  Tendon, 24332, 25295
  Thumb Contracture, 26508
Release–Inhibiting Hormone, Somatotropin, 84307
Relocation
  Defibrillator Site
    Chest, 33223
  Pacemaker Site
    Chest, 33222
Remodeling
  Bladder/Urethra, 53860
Remote Afterloading
  Brachytherapy, 77767-77768, 77770-77772
Remote Imaging
  Retinal Disease, 92227-92228
Removal
  Adjustable Gastric Restrictive Device, 43772-43774
  Adrenal Gland, 60650
  Allograft
    Intestinal, 44137
  Artificial Disc, 0095T, 0164T, 22864-22865
  Artificial Intervertebral Disc
    Cervical Interspace, 0095T, 22864
    Lumbar Interspace, 0164T, 22865
  Balloon
    Gastric, 43659, 43999
    Intra–Aortic, 33974
  Balloon Assist Device
    Intra–Aortic, 33968, 33971
  Bladder, 51597
    Electronic Stimulator, 53899
  Blood Clot
    Eye, 65930
  Blood Component
    Apheresis, 36511-36516
  Breast
    Capsules, 19371
    Implants, 19328, 19330
    Modified Radical, 19307
    Partial, 19301-19302
    Radical, 19305, 19306
    Simple, Complete, 19303
    Subcutaneous, 19304
  Calcaneous Deposits
    Subdeltoid, 23000
  Calculi (Stone)
    Bile Duct, 43264, 47420, 47425
      Percutaneous, 47554
    Bladder, 51050, 52310-52318, 52352
    Gallbladder, 47480
    Hepatic Duct, 47400
    Kidney, 50060-50081, 50130, 50561, 50580, 52352
    Pancreas, 48020
    Pancreatic Duct, 43264
    Salivary Gland, 42330-42340
    Ureter, 50610-50630, 50961, 50980, 51060, 51065, 52320-52330, 52352
    Urethra, 52310, 52315
  Cardiac Event Recorder, 33284
  Carotid Sinus Baroreflex Activation Device, 0269T-0270T
  Cast, 29700-29710
  Cataract
    with Replacement
      Extracapsular, 66982, 66984
      Intracapsular, 66983
      Not Associated with Concurrent, 66983
    Dilated Fundus Evaluation, 2021F
  Catheter
    Central Venous, 36589
    Peritoneum, 49422
    Pleural, 32552

Removal — *continued*
  Catheter — *continued*
    Spinal Cord, 62355
  Cerclage
    Cervix, 59871
  Cerumen
    Auditory Canal, External, 69209-69210
  Chest Wall Respiratory Sensor Electrode/Electrode Array, 0468T
  Clot
    Pericardium, 33020
    Endoscopic, 32658
  Comedones, 10040
  Contraceptive Capsules, 11976
  Cranial Tongs, 20665
  Cyst, 10040
  Dacryolith
    Lacrimal Duct, 68530
    Lacrimal Gland, 68530
  Defibrillator
    Heart, 33244
      Pulse Generator Only, 33241
      via Thoracotomy, 33243
    Subcutaneous Defibrillator Electrode Removal, *[33272]*
    Subcutaneous Pulse Generator, 33241, *[33262, 33263, 33264]*
  Drug Delivery Implant, 11982, 11983
  Ear Wax
    Auditory Canal, External, 69210
  Electrode
    Brain, 61535, 61880
    Cranial Nerve, 64570
    Heart, 33234-33238
    Nerve, 64585
    Neurostimulator, 64999
    Spinal Cord, 63661-63664
    Stomach, 43648, 43882
  Embolus, Artery
    Aortoiliac, 34151-34201
    Axillary, 34101
    Brachial, 34101
    Carotid, 34001
    Celiac, 34151
    Femoropopliteal, 34201
    Iliac, 34151, 34201
    Innominate, 34001-34101
    Mesentery, 34151
    Peroneal, 34203
    Popliteal, 34203
    Pulmonary, 33910-33916
    Radial, 34111
    Renal, 34151
    Subclavian, 34001-34101
    Tibial, 34203
    Ulnar, 34111
  External Fixation System, 20694, 20697
  Eye
    with Bone, 65112
    with Implant
      Muscles Attached, 65105
      Muscles not Attached, 65103
    with Muscle or Myocutaneous Flap, 65114
    without Implant, 65101
    Bone, 67414, 67445
    Ocular Contents
      with Implant, 65093
      without Implant, 65091
    Orbital Contents Only, 65110
  Fallopian Tube
    Laparoscopy, 58661
      with Hysterectomy, 58542, 58544, 58548
  Fat
    Lipectomy, 15876-15879
  Fecal Impaction
    Rectum, 45915
  Fibrin Deposit, 32150
  Fixation Device, 20670, 20680
  Foreign Bodies
    Adenoid, 42999
    Anal, 46608
    Ankle Joint, 27610, 27620
    Arm
      Lower, 25248
      Upper, 24200, 24201

Removal — *continued*
  Foreign Bodies — *continued*
    Auditory Canal, External, 69200
      with Anesthesia, 69205
    Bile Duct, *[43275]*
    Bladder, 52310, 52315
    Brain, 61570, 62163
    Bronchi, 31635
    Colon, 44025, 44390, 45379
    Colon–Sigmoid, 45332
    Conjunctival Embedded, 65210
    Cornea
      with Slit Lamp, 65222
      without Slit Lamp, 65220
    Duodenum, 44010
    Elbow, 24000, 24101, 24200, 24201
    Esophagus, 43020, 43045, 43194, 43215, 74235
    External Eye, 65205
    Eyelid, 67938
    Finger, 26075, 26080
    Foot, 28190-28193
    Gastrointestinal, Upper, 43247
    Gum, 41805
    Hand, 26070
    Hip, 27033, 27086, 27087
    Hysteroscopy, 58562
    Interphalangeal Joint
      Toe, 28024
    Intertarsal Joint, 28020
    Intestines, Small, 44020, 44363
    Intraocular, 65235
    Kidney, 50561, 50580
    Knee Joint, 27310, 27331, 27372
    Lacrimal Duct, 68530
    Lacrimal Gland, 68530
    Larynx, 31511, 31530, 31531, 31577
    Leg, Upper, 27372
    Lung, 32151
    Mandible, 41806
    Maxillary Sinus, 31299
    Mediastinum, 39000, 39010
    Metatarsophalangeal Joint, 28022
    Mouth, 40804, 40805
    Muscle, 20520, 20525
      Stimulator
        Skeletal, 20999
    Nose, 30300
      Anesthesia, Under, 30310
      Lateral Rhinotomy, 30320
    Orbit, 67413, 67430
      with Bone Flap, 67430
      without Bone Flap, 67413
    Pancreatic Duct, *[43275]*
    Patella
      See Patellectomy
    Pelvis, 27086, 27087
    Penile Tissue, 54115
    Penis, 54115
    Pericardium, 33020
      Endoscopic, 32658
    Peritoneum, 49402
    Pharynx, 42809
    Pleura, 32150, 32151
      Endoscopic, 32653
    Posterior Segment
      Magnetic Extraction, 65260
      Nonmagnetic Extraction, 65265
    Rectum, 45307, 45915
    Scrotum, 55120
    Shoulder, 23040, 23044
      Deep, 23333
      Subcutaneous, 23330
    Skin
      with Debridement, 11010-11012
    Stomach, 43500
    Subcutaneous, 10120, 10121
      with Debridement, 11010-11012
    Tarsometatarsal Joint, 28020
    Tendon Sheath, 20520, 20525
    Toe, 28022
    Ureter, 50961, 50980
    Urethra, 52310, 52315
    Uterus, 58562
    Vagina, 57415
    Wrist, 25040, 25101, 25248

Removal — *continued*
  Hair
    by Electrolysis, 17380
    Halo, 20665
    Harrington Rod, 22850
  Hearing Aid
    Bone Conduction, 69711
  Hematoma
    Brain, 61312-61315
  Implant, 20670, 20680
    Ankle, 27704
    Contraceptive Capsules, 11976
    Disc, 0164T, 22865
    Elbow, 24160
    Eye, 67120, 67121
    Finger, 26320
    Hand, 26320
    Pin, 20670, 20680
    Radius, 24164
    Rod, 20670, 20680
    Screw, 20670, 20680
    Wrist, 25449
  Implantable Defibrillator, 33241
  Infusion Pump
    Intra–Arterial, 36262
    Intravenous, 36590
    Spinal Cord, 62365
  Interstitial Glucose Sensor, 0447T-0448T
  Intra–Aortic Balloon, 33974
    Assist Device, 33968, 33971
  Intracardiac Ischemia Monitoring System, 0302T
    Device Only, 0304T, 0307T
    Electrode Only, 0303T
  Intrauterine Device (IUD), 58301
  Intravascular Vena Cava (IVC) Filter, 37193
  Keel
    Laryngoplasty, 31580
  Kidney
    Mechanical, 53899
  Lacrimal Gland
    Partial, 68505
    Total, 68500
  Lacrimal Sac
    Excision, 68520
  Laryngocele, 31300
  Leiomyomata, 58545, 58546, 58561
  Lens, 66920-66940
  Lens Material, 66840-66852
  Lesion
    Conjunctiva, 68040
    Larynx
      Endoscopic, 31512, 31545-31546, 31578
  Loose Body
    Ankle, 27620
    Carpometacarpal Joint, 26070
    Elbow, 24101
    Foot, 28020
    Interphalangeal Joint, Toe, 28024
    Intertarsal Joint, 28020
    Knee Joint, 27331
    Metatarsophalangeal Joint, 28022
    Tarsometatarsal Joint, 28020
    Toe, 28022
    Wrist, 25101
  Lung
    Apical Tumor, 32503-32504
    Bronchoplasty, 32501
    Completion Pneumonectomy, 32488
    Cyst, 32140
    Emphysematous, 32491
    Extrapleural, 32445
    Pneumonectomy, 32440-32445
    Single Lobe, 32480
    Single Segment, 32484
    Sleeve Lobectomy, 32486
    Sleeve Pneumonectomy, 32442
    Two Lobes, 32482
    Volume Reduction, 32491
  Lymph Nodes
    Abdominal, 38747
    Inguinofemoral, 38760, 38765
    Pelvic, 38770
    Retroperitoneal Transabdominal, 38780
    Thoracic, 38746
  Mammary Implant, 19328, 19330

Removal — *continued*
Mastoid
Air Cells, 69670
Mesh
Abdominal Wall, 11008
Milia, Multiple, 10040
Nail, 11730, 11732, 11750
Finger, 26236
Toe, 28124, 28160
Nephrostomy Tube, 50389
Neurostimulator
Electrode, 63661-63662, 64999
Pulse Generator, 64595, 64999
Receiver, 64595
Obstructive Material
Gastrostomy, Duodenostomy, Jejunostomy,
Gastro-jejunostomy, or Cecostomy
Tube, 49460
Ocular Implant, 65175, 65920
Orbital Implant, 67560
Ovaries
Laparoscopy, 58661
with Hysterectomy, 58542, 58544,
58548
Pacemaker
Heart, 33233-33237 *[33227, 33228, 33229]*
Patella, Complete, 27424
Plate
Skull, 62142
Polyp
Anal, 46610, 46612
Antrochoanal, 31032
Colon, 44392, 45385
Colon–Sigmoid, 45333
Endoscopy, 44364, 44365, 44394
Esophagus, 43217, 43250
Gastrointestinal, Upper, 43250, 43251
Rectum, 45315
Sphenoid Sinus, 31051
Prosthesis
Abdomen, 49606
Abdominal Wall, 11008
Elbow, 24160
Hip, 27090, 27091
Knee, 27488
Penis, 54406, 54410-54417
Perineum, 53442
Radius, 24164
Shoulder, 23334-23335
Skull, 62142
Urethral Sphincter, 53446, 53447
Wrist, 25250, 25251
Pulse Generator
Brain, 61888
Neurostimulator, 64999
Spinal Cord, 63688
Vagus Nerve Blocking Therapy, 0314T-
0315T
Pustules, 10040
Receiver
Brain, 61888
Spinal Cord, 63688
Reservoir, 62365
Seton
Anal, 46030
Shoulder Joint
Foreign or Loose Body, 23107
Shunt
Brain, 62256, 62258
Heart, 33924
Peritoneum, 49429
Spinal Cord, 63746
Skin Tags, 11200, 11201
Sling
Urethra, 53442
Vagina, 57287
Spinal Instrumentation
Anterior, 22855
Posterior Nonsegmental
Harrington Rod, 22850
Posterior Segmental, 22852
Stent
Bile Duct, *[43275, 43276]*
Pancreatic Duct, *[43275, 43276]*
Ureteral, 50382-50386

Removal — *continued*
Stone (Calculi)
Bile Duct, 43264, 47420, 47425
Percutaneous, 47554
Bladder, 51050, 52310-52318, 52352
Gallbladder, 47480
Hepatic Duct, 47400
Kidney, 50060-50081, 50130, 50561, 50580,
52352
Pancreas, 48020
Pancreatic Duct, 43264
Salivary Gland, 42330-42340
Ureter, 50610-50630, 50961, 50980, 51060,
51065, 52320-52330, 52352
Urethra, 52310, 52315
Subcutaneous Port for Gastric Restrictive Proce-
dure, 43887-43888
Suture
Anal, 46754
Anesthesia, 15850, 15851
Thrombus
See Thrombectomy
Tissue
Vaginal, Partial, 57107
Tissue Expanders, 11971
Transplant Intestines, 44137
Transplant Kidney, 50370
Tube
Ear, Middle, 69424
Finger, 26392, 26416
Hand, 26392, 26416
Nephrostomy, 50389
Tumor
Temporal Bone, 69970
Ureter
Ligature, 50940
Stent, 50382-50386
Urethral Stent
Bladder, 52310, 52315
Urethra, 52310, 52315
Vagina
Partial
with Nodes, 57109
Tissue, 57106
Wall, 57107, 57110, 57111
Vein
Clusters, 37785
Perforation, 37760
Saphenous, 37718-37735, 37780
Secondary, 37785
Varicose, 37765, 37766
Venous Access Device
Obstruction, 75901-75902
Ventilating Tube
Ear, Middle, 69424
Ventricular Assist Device, 33977, 33978
Intracorporeal, 0455T-0458T, 33980
Vitreous
Partial, 67005, 67010
Wire
Anal, 46754
Renal Abscess
Incision and Drainage, 50020
Renal Arteries
Aneurysm, 35121-35122
Angiography, 36251-36253
Angioplasty, *[37246, 37247]*
Atherectomy, 0234T
Bypass Graft, 35536, 35560, 35631-35636
Embolectomy, 34151
Thrombectomy, 34151
Thromboendarterectomy, 35341
Renal Autotransplantation, 50380
Renal Calculus
Removal, 50060-50081, 50130, 50561, 50580,
52352
Renal Cyst
Ablation, 50541
Aspiration, 50390
Excision, 50280, 50290
Injection, 50390
Xray, 74470
Renal Dialysis
Blood Flow Study, 90940
Documented Plan of Care, 0505F
Duplex Scan of Access, 93990

Renal Dialysis — *continued*
Kt/V Level, 3082F-3084F
via Catheter, 4054F
via Functioning Arteriovenous Fistula, 4052F
via Functioning Arteriovenous Graft, 4053F
Renal Disease Services
Arteriovenous Fistula
Revision, 36832, 36833
Thrombectomy, 36831
Arteriovenous Shunt
Revision, 36832, 36833
Thrombectomy, 36831
End Stage Renal Disease, 90951-90956, 90964,
90968
Hemodialysis, 90935, 90937
Blood Flow Study, 90940
Hemoperfusion, 90997
Patient Training, 90989, 90993
Peritoneal Dialysis, 90945-90947
Renal Pelvis Biopsy, 50606
Renal Transplantation
Allograft Preparation, 50323-50329
Anesthesia
Donor, 00862
Recipient, 00868
Donor Nephrectomy, 50300-50320, 50547
Graft Implantation, 50360-50365
Recipient Nephrectomy, 50340, 50365
Reimplantation Kidney, 50380
Removal Transplanted Allograft, 50370
Rendevous Procedure
Biliary Tree Access, 47541
Renin, 80408, 80416, 84244
Peripheral Vein, 80417
Renin–Converting Enzyme, 82164
Reoperation
Carotid
Thromboendarterectomy, 35390
Coronary Artery Bypass
Valve Procedure, 33530
Distal Vessel Bypass, 35700
Repair
See Also Revision
Abdomen, 49900
Hernia, 49491-49525, 49565, 49570, 49582-
49590
Omphalocele, 49600-49611
Suture, 49900
Abdominal Wall, 15830, 15847, 17999
Anal
Anomaly, 46744-46748
Fistula, 46288, 46706-46716
High Imperforate, 46730, 46735, 46740,
46742
Low Imperforate, 46715-46716
Park Posterior, 46761
Stricture, 46700, 46705
Aneurysm
Aorta
Abdominal, 34800-34805, 34825-
34832, 34841-34848, 35081-
35103, 75952-75953
Iliac Vessels, 35102-35103
Visceral Vessels, 35091-35092
Infrarenal, 34800-34805, 34825-34832
Imaging, 75952-75953
Thoracic, 33877-33886
Arteriovenous, 36832
Axillary-Brachial Artery, 35011, 35013
Carotid Artery, 35001-35002
Endovascular
Abdominal Aorta, 34800-34805
Iliac Artery, 34900
Thoracic Aorta, 33880-33891
Visceral Aorta, 34841-34848
Femoral, 35141-35142
Hepatic, Celiac, Renal, or Mesenteric Artery,
35121-35122
Iliac Artery, 34825-34826, 34900, 35131-
35132
Imaging, 75954
Innominate, Subclavian Artery, 35021-
35022
Intracranial Artery, 61697-61708
Popliteal Artery, 35151-35152
Radial or Ulnar Artery, 35045

Repair — *continued*
Aneurysm — *continued*
Sinus of Valsalva, 33720
Subclavian Artery, 35001-35002, 35021-
35022
Vertebral Artery, 35005
Ankle
Ligament, 27695-27698
Tendon, 27612, 27650-27654, 27680-27687
Anomaly
Artery Arborization, 33925-33926
Cardiac, 33608, 33610, 33615, 33617
Coronary Artery, 33502-33507
Pulmonary Venous Return, 33730
Aorta, 33320-33322, 33802, 33803
Coarctation, 33840-33851
Graft, 33860-33877
Sinus of Valsalva, 33702-33720
Thoracic
Endovascular, 33880-33891
Prosthesis Placement, 33886
Radiological Supervision and Interpre-
tation, 75956-75959
Visceral
Endovascular, 34841-34848
Aortic Arch
with Cardiopulmonary Bypass, 33853
without Cardiopulmonary Bypass, 33852
Aortic Valve, 93591-93592
Obstruction
Outflow Tract, 33414
Septal Hypertrophy, 33416
Stenosis, 33415
Valvuloplasty, 93591-93592
Arm
Lower, 25260, 25263, 25270
Fasciotomy, 24495
Secondary, 25265, 25272, 25274
Tendon, 25290
Tendon Sheath, 25275
Muscle, 24341
Tendon, 24332, 24341, 25280, 25295,
25310-25316
Upper
Muscle Revision, 24330, 24331
Muscle Transfer, 24301, 24320
Tendon Lengthening, 24305
Tendon Revision, 24320
Tendon Transfer, 24301
Tenotomy, 24310
Arteriovenous Aneurysm, 36832
Arteriovenous Fistula
Abdomen, 35182
Acquired or Traumatic, 35189
Extremities, 35184
Acquired or Traumatic, 35190
Head, 35180
Acquired or Traumatic, 35188
Neck, 35180
Acquired or Traumatic, 35188
Thorax, 35182
Acquired or Traumatic, 35189
Arteriovenous Malformation
Intracranial, 61680-61692
Intracranial Artery, 61705, 61708
Spinal Artery, 62294
Spinal Cord, 63250-63252
Arterioventricular Canal, 33665, 33670
Artery
Angioplasty
Aorta, *[37246, 37247]*
Axillary, *[37246, 37247]*
Brachiocephalic, *[37246, 37247]*
Bypass Graft, 35501-35571, 35601-35683,
35691-35700
Bypass In–Situ, 35583-35587
Bypass Venous Graft, 33510-33516, 35510-
35525
Coronary
Anomalous, 33502-33507
Dialysis Circuit, 36902-36903, 36905-36906,
36907
Iliac, 0254T-0255T, 34900, 37222-37223
Occlusive Disease, 35001, 35005-35021,
35045, 35081, 35091, 35102, 35111,
35121, 35131, 35141, 35151

Repair — continued

Artery — continued
Pulmonary, 33690, 33925-33926
Renal, [37246, 37247]
Renal or Visceral, [37246, 37247]
Subclavian, [37246, 37247]
Thromboendarterectomy, 35301-35321, 35341-35390
Venous Graft, 33510-33516, 35510-35525
Visceral, [37246, 37247]
Arytenoid Cartilage, 31400
Atria
Laparoscopic, 33265-33266
Open, 33254-33256
Atrial Fibrillation, 33254, 33255-33256
Bile Duct, 47701
with Intestines, 47760, 47780, 47785
Wound, 47900
Bladder
Exstrophy, 51940
Fistula, 44660, 44661, 45800, 45805, 51880-51925
Neck, 51845
Resection, 52500
Wound, 51860, 51865
Blepharoptosis
Conjunctivo-Tarso-Muller's Muscle Resection, 67908
Frontalis Muscle Technique
with Fascial Sling, 67902
Superior Rectus Technique with Fascial Sling, 67906
Tarso Levator Resection or Advancement, 67903-67904
Blood Vessel(s)
Abdomen, 35221, 35251, 35281
with Other Graft, 35281
with Vein Graft, 35251
Chest, 35211, 35216
with Other Graft, 35271, 35276
with Vein Graft, 35241, 35246
Finger, 35207
Graft Defect, 35870
Hand, 35207
Intrathoracic, 35211, 35216, 35241, 35246, 35271, 35276
Kidney, 50100
Lower Extremity, 35226, 35256, 35286
with Other Graft, 35286
with Vein Graft, 35256
Neck, 35201, 35231, 35261
with Other Graft, 35261
with Vein Graft, 35231
Upper Extremity, 35206, 35236, 35266
with Other Graft, 35266
with Vein Graft, 35236
Body Cast, 29720
Brain
Wound, 61571
Breast
Suspension, 19316
Bronchi, 31770, 32501
Fistula, 32815
Brow Ptosis, 67900
Bunion, 28289-28299 [28295]
Bypass Graft, 35901-35907
Fistula, 35870
Calcaneus
Osteotomy, 28300
Canaliculi, 68700
Cannula, 36860, 36861
Carpal, 25440
Carpal Bone, 25431
Cast
Spica, Body, or Jacket, 29720
Central Venous Catheter, 36575-36576
Cervix
Cerclage, 57700
Abdominal, 59320, 59325
Suture, 57720
Vaginal Approach, 57720
Chest Wall, 32905
Closure, 32810
Fistula, 32906
Pectus Excavatum, 21740

Repair — continued

Chin
Augmentation, 21120, 21123
Osteotomy, 21121-21123
Choanal Atresia, 30540, 30545
Chordee, 54304
Ciliary Body, 66680
Circumcision, 54163
Clavicle
Osteotomy, 23480, 23485
Cleft
Hand, 26580
Lip, 40525, 40527, 40700
Nasal Deformity, 40700, 40701, 40720, 40761
Cleft Palate, 42200-42225
See Cleft Palate Repair
Cloacal anomaly, 46744, 46746, 46748
Colon
Fistula, 44650-44661
Hernia, 44050
Malrotation, 44055
Obstruction, 44050
Conjunctiva, 65270, 65272
Cornea, 65275, 65280, 65285
Coronary Chamber Fistula, 33500, 33501
Cor Triatriatum or Supravalvular Mitral Ring, 33732
Cyst
Bartholin's Gland, 56440
Liver, 47300
Cystocele, 57240
Defect
Atrial Septal, 33647
Radius, 25425-25426
Septal, 33813-33814
Ulna, 25425-25426
Ventricular Septal, 33545
Defibrillator, Heart, 33218, 33220
Diaphragm
for Eventration, 39545
Hernia, 39503-39541
Lacerations, 39501
Dislocation
Ankle, 27846, 27848
Knee, 27556-27558
Ductus Arteriosus, 33820-33824
Dura, 61618-61619, 62010
Dura/Cerebrospinal Fluid Leak, 63707, 63709
Dysfunction
Prosthetic Valve, 33406
Ear, Middle
Oval Window Fistula, 69666
Round Window Fistula, 69667
Ectropion
Excision Tarsal Wedge, 67916, 67923
Extensive, 67917
Suture, 67914, 67921
Thermocauterization, 67915, 67922
Elbow
Fasciotomy, 24357-24359
Hemiepiphyseal Arrest, 24470
Ligament, 24343-24346
Muscle, 24341
Muscle Transfer, 24301
Tendon, 24340-24342
Each, 24341
Tendon Lengthening, 24305
Tendon Transfer, 24301
Tennis Elbow, 24357-24359
Electrode, 33218-33220
Electromagnetic Bone Conduction Hearing Device, 69711
Encephalocele, 62121
Enterocele
with Colporrhaphy, 57265
Hysterectomy, 58263, 58270, 58292, 58294
Vaginal Approach, 57268
Entropion, 67924
Epididymis, 54900, 54901
Episiotomy, 59300
Epispadias, 54380-54390
Esophageal Varices, 43401
Esophagus, 43300, 43310, 43312-43314
Esophagogastrostomy, 43320
Esophagojejunostomy, 43340, 43341

Repair — continued

Esophagus — continued
Fistula, 43305, 43312, 43314, 43420, 43425
Fundoplasty, 43325-43328
Hiatal Hernia, 43332-43337
Muscle, 43330, 43331
Preexisting Perforation, 43405
Varices, 43401
Wound, 43410, 43415
Extraocular muscle, 67340
Eye
Ciliary Body, 66680
Suture, 66682
Conjunctiva, 65270-65273
Wound, 65270-65273
Cornea, 65275
with Glue, 65286
Astigmatism, 65772, 65775
Wound, 65275-65285
Dehiscence, 66250
Fistula
Lacrimal Gland, 68770
Iris
with Ciliary Body, 66680
Suture, 66682
Lacrimal Duct
Canaliculi, 68700
Lacrimal Punctum, 68705
Retina
Detachment, 67101, 67113
Sclera
with Glue, 65286
with Graft, 66225
Reinforcement, 67250, 67255
Staphyloma, 66220, 66225
Wound, 65286, 66250
Strabismus
Chemodenervation, 67345
Symblepharon
with Graft, 68335
without Graft, 68330
Division, 68340
Trabeculae, 65855
Eyebrow
Ptosis, 67900
Eyelashes
Epilation
by Forceps, 67820
by Other than Forceps, 67825
Incision of Lid Margin, 67830
with Free Mucous Membrane Graft, 67835
Eyelid, 21280, 21282, 67961, 67966
Ectropion
Excision Tarsal Wedge, 67916
Suture, 67914
Tarsal Strip Operation, 67917
Thermocauterization, 67915
Entropion
Capsulopalpebral Fascia Repair, 67924
Excision Tarsal Wedge, 67923
Suture, 67921-67924
Tarsal Strip, 67924
Thermocauterization, 67922
Excisional, 67961, 67966
Lagophthalmos, 67912
Ptosis
Conjunctivo-Tarso-Muller's Muscle-Levator Resection, 67908
Frontalis Muscle Technique, 67901, 67902
Levator Resection, 67903, 67904
Reduction of Overcorrection, 67909
Superior Rectus Technique, 67906
Retraction, 67911
Wound
Extraocular Muscle, 65290
Suture, 67930, 67935
Eye Muscles
Strabismus
Adjustable Sutures, 67335
One Horizontal Muscle, 67311
One Vertical Muscle, 67314
Posterior Fixation Suture Technique, 67334, 67335

Repair — continued

Eye Muscles — continued
Strabismus — continued
Previous Surgery Not Involving Extraocular Muscles, 67331
Release Extensive Scar Tissue, 67343
Superior Oblique Muscle, 67318
Two Horizontal Muscles, 67312
Two or More Vertical Muscles, 67316
Wound
Extraocular Muscle, 65290
Facial Bones, 21208, 21209
Facial Nerve
Paralysis, 15840-15845
Suture
Intratemporal, Lateral to Geniculate Ganglion, 69740
Intratemporal, Medial to Geniculate Ganglion, 69745
Fallopian Tube, 58752
Anastomosis, 58750
Create Stoma, 58770
Fascial Defect, 50728
Leg, 27656
Femur, 27470, 27472
with Graft, 27170
Epiphysis, 27475-27485, 27742
Arrest, 27185
by Pinning, 27176
by Traction, 27175
Open Treatment, 27177, 27178
Osteoplasty, 27179
Osteotomy, 27181
Muscle Transfer, 27110
Osteotomy, 27140, 27151, 27450, 27454
with Fixation, 27165
with Open Reduction, 27156
Femoral Neck, 27161
Fibula
Epiphysis, 27477-27485, 27730-27742
Nonunion or Malunion, 27726
Osteotomy, 27707-27712
Finger
Claw Finger, 26499
Macrodactyly, 26590
Polydactylous, 26587
Syndactyly, 26560-26562
Tendon
Extensor, 26415-26434, 26445, 26449, 26455
Flexor, 26356-26358, 26440, 26442
Joint Stabilization, 26474
PIP Joint, 26471
Toe Transfer, 26551-26556
Trigger, 26055
Volar Plate, 26548
Web Finger, 26560
Fistula
Anal, 46706
Anoperineal, 46715-46716
Anorectal, 46707
Carotid–Cavernous, 61710
Coronary, 33500-33501
Graft-Enteric Fistula, 35870
Ileoanal Pouch, 46710-46712
Mastoid, 69700
Nasolabial, 42260
Neurovisceral, 50525-50526
Oromaxillary, 30580
Oronasal, 30600
Rectourethral, 46740-46742
Rectovaginal, 46740-46742, 57308
Sinus of Valsalva, 33702, 33710
Ureterovisceral, 50930
Foot
Fascia, 28250
Muscles, 28250
Tendon, 28200-28226, 28238
Fracture
Nasoethmoid, 21340
Patella, 27524
Radius, 25526
Talar Dome, 29892
Tibial Plafond, 29892
Gallbladder
with Gastroenterostomy, 47741

Repair — *continued*
Gallbladder — *continued*
with Intestines, 47720-47740
Laceration, 47999
Great Arteries, 33770-33781
Great Vessel, 33320-33322
Hallux Valgus, 28289-28299 *[28295]*
Hammertoe, 28285-28286
Hamstring, 27097
Hand
Cleft Hand, 26580
Muscles, 26591, 26593
Tendon
Extensor, 26410-26416, 26426, 26428, 26433-26437
Flexor, 26350-26358, 26440
Profundus, 26370-26373
Hearing Aid
Bone Conduction, 69711
Heart
Anomaly, 33600-33617
Aortic Sinus, 33702-33722
Artificial Heart
Intracorporeal, 0052T, 0053T
Atria
Laparoscopic, 33265-33266
Open, 33254-33256
Atrioventricular Canal, 33660, 33665
Complete, 33670
Atrioventricular Valve, 33660, 33665
Blood Vessel, 33320-33322
Cor Triatriatum, 33732
Fibrillation, 33254, 33255-33256
Infundibular, 33476, 33478
Mitral Valve, 33420-33427, 93590, 93592
Myocardium, 33542
Outflow Tract, 33476, 33478
Post–Infarction, 33542, 33545
Prosthetic Valve, 33670, 33852, 33853
Prosthetic Valve Dysfunction, 33496
Pulmonary Artery Shunt, 33924
Pulmonary Valve, 33470-33474
Septal Defect, 33545, 33608, 33610, 33681-33688, 33692-33697
Atrial and Ventricular, 33647
Atrium, 33641
Sinus of Valsalva, 33702-33722
Sinus Venosus, 33645
Tetralogy of Fallot, 33692
Total Replacement Heart System
Intracorporeal, 0052T, 0053T
Tricuspid Valve, 33465
Ventricle, 33611, 33612
Obstruction, 33619
Ventricular Tunnel, 33722
Wound, 33300, 33305
Hepatic Duct
with Intestines, 47765, 47802
Hernia
with Mesh, 49568
with Spermatic Cord, 54640
Abdomen, 49565, 49590
Incisional or Ventral, 49560
Diaphragmatic, 39503-39541
Epigastric
Incarcerated, 49572
Reducible, 49570
Femoral, 49550
Incarcerated, 49553
Initial
Incarcerated, 49553
Reducible, 49550
Recurrent, 49555
Recurrent Incarcerated, 49557
Reducible Recurrent, 49555
Hiatus, 43332-43337
Incisional
Initial
Incarcerated, 49566
Reducible, 49560
Recurrent
Reducible, 49565
Inguinal
Initial
by Laparoscopy, 49650
Incarcerated, 49496, 49501, 49507

Repair — *continued*
Hernia — *continued*
Inguinal — *continued*
Initial — *continued*
Reducible, 49491, 49495, 49500, 49505
Strangulated, 49492, 49496, 49501, 49507
Laparoscopy, 49650-49651
Older than 50 Weeks, Younger than 6 Months, 49496
Preterm Older than 50 weeks and younger than 6 months, full term infant younger than 6 months, 49495-49496
Preterm up to 50 Weeks, 49491-49492
Recurrent
by Laparoscopy, 49651
Incarcerated, 49521
Reducible, 49520
Strangulated, 49521
Sliding, 49525
Intestinal, 44025, 44050
Lumbar, 49540
Lung, 32800
Orchiopexy, 54640
Paracolostomy, 44346
Parasternal, 49999
Preterm Infant
Birth up to 50 Weeks, 49491-49492
Older than 50 weeks, 49495-49496
Reducible
Initial
Epigastric, 49570
Femoral, 49550
Incisional, 49560
Inguinal, 49495, 49500, 49505
Umbilical, 49580, 49585
Ventral, 49560
Recurrent
Femoral, 49555
Incisional, 49565
Inguinal, 49520
Ventral, 49560
Sliding, 49525
Spigelian, 49590
Umbilical, 49580, 49585
Incarcerated, 49582, 49587
Reducible, 49580, 49585
Ventral
Initial
Incarcerated, 49561
Reducible, 49565
Hip
Muscle Transfer, 27100-27105, 27111
Osteotomy, 27146-27156
Tendon, 27097
Humerus, 24420, 24430
with Graft, 24435
Osteotomy, 24400, 24410
Hypoplasia
Aortic Arch, 33619
Hypospadias, 54308, 54312, 54316, 54318, 54322, 54326, 54328, 54332, 54336, 54340, 54344, 54348, 54352
Ileoanal Pouch, 46710-46712
Ileostomy, 44310, 45136
Continent (Kock Pouch), 44316
Iliac Artery, 0254T-0255T, 34900, 37222-37223
Interphalangeal Joint
Volar Plate, 26548
Intestine
Large
Ulcer, 44605
Wound, 44605
Intestines
Enterocele
Abdominal Approach, 57270
Vaginal Approach, 57268
Large
Closure Enterostomy, 44620-44626
Diverticula, 44605
Obstruction, 44615
Intestines, Small
Closure Enterostomy, 44620-44626
Diverticula, 44602, 44603

Repair — *continued*
Intestines, Small — *continued*
Fistula, 44640-44661
Hernia, 44050
Malrotation, 44055
Obstruction, 44025, 44050
Ulcer, 44602, 44603
Wound, 44602, 44603
Introitus, Vagina, 56800
Iris, Ciliary Body, 66680
Jejunum
Free Transfer with Microvascular Anastomosis, 43496
Kidney
Fistula, 50520-50526
Horseshoe, 50540
Renal Pelvis, 50400, 50405
Wound, 50500
Knee
Cartilage, 27403
Instability, 27420
Ligament, 27405-27409
Collateral, 27405
Collateral and Cruciate, 27409
Cruciate, 27407, 27409
Meniscus, 27403
Tendons, 27380, 27381
Laceration, Skin
Abdomen
Complex, 13100-13102
Intermediate, 12031-12037
Layered, 12031-12037
Simple, 12001-12007
Superficial, 12001-12007
Arm, Arms
Complex, 13120-13122
Intermediate, 12031-12037
Layered, 12031-12037
Simple, 12001-12007
Superficial, 12001-12007
Axilla, Axillae
Complex, 13131-13133
Intermediate, 12031-12037
Layered, 12031-12037
Simple, 12001-12007
Superficial, 12001-12007
Back
Complex, 13100-13102
Intermediate, 12031-12037
Layered, 12031-12037
Simple, 12001-12007
Superficial, 12001-12007
Breast
Complex, 13100-13102
Intermediate, 12031-12037
Layered, 12031-12037
Simple, 12001-12007
Superficial, 12001-12007
Buttock
Complex, 13100-13102
Intermediate, 12031-12037
Layered, 12031-12037
Simple, 12001-12007
Superficial, 12001-12007
Cheek, Cheeks
Complex, 13131-13133
Intermediate, 12051-12057
Layered, 12051-12057
Simple, 12011-12018
Superficial, 12011-12018
Chest
Complex, 13100-13102
Intermediate, 12031-12037
Layered, 12031-12037
Simple, 12001-12007
Superficial, 12001-12007
Chin
Complex, 13131-13133
Intermediate, 12051-12057
Layered, 12051-12057
Simple, 12011-12018
Superficial, 12011-12018
Ear, Ears
Complex, 13151-13153
Intermediate, 12051-12057
Layered, 12051-12057

Repair — *continued*
Laceration, Skin — *continued*
Ear, Ears — *continued*
Layered — *continued*
2.5 cm or less, 12051
Simple, 12011-12018
Superficial, 12011-12018
External
Genitalia
Complex/Intermediate, 12041-12047
Layered, 12041-12047
Simple, 12001-12007
Superficial, 12041-12047
Extremity, Extremities
Complex, 13120-13122
Complex/Intermediate, 12031-12037
Intermediate, 12051-12057
Layered, 12031-12037
Simple, 12001-12007
Superficial, 12001-12007
Face
Complex/Intermediate, 12051-12057
Layered, 12051-12057
Simple, 12011-12018
Superficial, 12011-12018
Feet
Complex, 13131-13133
Intermediate, 12041-12047
Layered, 12041-12047
Simple, 12001-12007
Superficial, 12001-12007
Finger, Fingers
Complex, 13131-13133
Intermediate, 12041-12047
Layered, 12041-12047
Simple, 12001-12007
Superficial, 12001-12007
Foot
Complex, 13131-13133
Intermediate, 12041-12047
Layered, 12041-12047
Simple, 12001-12007
Superficial, 12001-12007
Forearm, Forearms
Complex, 13120-13122
Intermediate, 12031-12037
Layered, 12031-12037
Simple, 12001-12007
Superficial, 12001-12007
Forehead
Complex, 13131-13133
Intermediate, 12051-12057
Layered, 12051-12057
Simple, 12011-12018
Superficial, 12011-12018
Genitalia
Complex, 13131-13133
External
Complex/Intermediate, 12041-12047
Layered, 12041-12047
Simple, 12001-12007
Superficial, 12001-12007
Hand, Hands
Complex, 13131-13133
Intermediate, 12041-12047
Layered, 12041-12047
Simple, 12001-12007
Superficial, 12001-12007
Leg, Legs
Complex, 13120-13122
Intermediate, 12031-12037
Layered, 12031-12037
Simple, 12001-12007
Superficial, 12001-12007
Lip, Lips
Complex, 13151-13153
Intermediate, 12051-12057
Layered, 12051-12057
Simple, 12011-12018
Superficial, 12011-12018
Lower
Arm, Arms
Complex, 13120-13122
Intermediate, 12031-12037

Repair — continued
Laceration, Skin — continued
Lower — continued
Arm, Arms — continued
Layered, 12031-12037
Simple, 12001-12007
Superficial, 12001-12007
Extremity, Extremities
Complex, 13120-13122
Intermediate, 12031-12037
Layered, 12031-12037
Simple, 12001-12007
Superficial, 12001-12007
Leg, Legs
Complex, 13120-13122
Intermediate, 12031-12037
Layered, 12031-12037
Simple, 12001-12007
Superficial, 12001-12007
Mouth
Complex, 13131-13133
Mucous Membrane
Complex/Intermediate, 12051-12057
Layered, 12051-12057
Simple, 12011-12018
Superficial, 12011-12018
Neck
Complex, 13131-13133
Intermediate, 12041-12047
Layered, 12041-12047
Simple, 12001-12007
Superficial, 12001-12007
Nose
Complex, 13151-13153
Complex/Intermediate, 12051-12057
Layered, 12051-12057
Simple, 12011-12018
Superficial, 12011-12018
Palm, Palms
Complex, 13131-13133
Intermediate, 12041-12047
Layered, 12041-12047
Layered Simple, 12001-12007
Superficial, 12001-12007
Scalp
Complex, 13120-13122
Intermediate, 12031-12037
Layered, 12031-12037
Simple, 12001-12007
Superficial, 12001-12007
Toe, Toes
Complex, 13131-13133
Intermediate, 12041-12047
Layered, 12041-12047
Simple, 12001-12007
Superficial, 12001-12007
Trunk
Complex, 13100-13102
Intermediate, 12031-12037
Layered, 12031-12037
Simple, 12001-12007
Superficial, 12001-12007
Upper
Arm, Arms
Complex, 13120-13122
Intermediate, 12031-12037
Layered, 12031-12037
Simple, 12001-12007
Superficial, 12001-12007
Extremity
Complex, 13120-13122
Intermediate, 12031-12037
Layered, 12031-12037
Simple, 12001-12007
Superficial, 12001-12007
Leg, Legs
Complex, 13120-13122
Intermediate, 12031-12037
Layered, 12031-12037
Simple, 12001-12007
Superficial, 12001-12007
Larynx
Fracture, 31584
Reinnervation
Neuromuscular Pedicle, 31590

Repair — continued
Leak
Cerebrospinal Fluid, 31290-31291
Leg
Lower
Fascia, 27656
Tendon, 27658-27692
Upper
Muscles, 27385, 27386, 27400, 27430
Tendon, 27393-27400
Ligament
Ankle, 27695-27696, 27698
Anterior Cruciate, 29888
Collateral
Elbow, 24343, 24345
Metacarpophalangeal or Interpha-
langeal Joint, 26540
Knee, 27405, 27407, 27409
Posterior Cruciate Ligament, 29889
Lip, 40650-40654
Cleft Lip, 40700-40761
Fistula, 42260
Liver
Abscess, 47300
Cyst, 47300
Wound, 47350-47361
Lung
Hernia, 32800
Pneumolysis, 32940
Tear, 32110
Macrodactylia, 26590
Malunion
Femur, 27470, 27472
Fibula, 27726
Humerus, 24430
Metatarsal, 28322
Radius, 25400, 25405, 25415, 25420
Tarsal Bones, 28320
Tibia, 27720, 27722, 27724-27725
Ulna, 25400, 25405, 25415, 25420
Mastoidectomy
with Apicectomy, 69605
with Tympanoplasty, 69604
Complete, 69601
Modified Radical, 69602
Radical, 69603
Maxilla
Osteotomy, 21206
Meningocele, 63700, 63702
Meniscus
Knee, 27403, 29882-29883
Mesentery, 44850
Metacarpal
Lengthen, 26568
Nonunion, 26546
Osteotomy, 26565
Metacarpophalangeal Joint
Capsulodesis, 26516-26518
Collateral Ligament, 26540-26542
Fusion, 26516-26518
Metatarsal, 28322
Osteotomy, 28306-28309
Microsurgery, 69990
Mitral Valve, 33420-33427, 93590, 93592
Mouth
Floor, 41250
Laceration, 40830, 40831
Vestibule of, 40830-40845
Muscle
Hand, 26591
Upper Arm or Elbow, 24341
Musculotendinous Cuff, 23410, 23412
Myelomeningocele, 63704, 63706
Nail Bed, 11760
Nasal Deformity
Cleft Lip, 40700-40761
Nasal Septum, 30630
Navicular, 25440
Neck Muscles
Scalenus Anticus, 21700, 21705
Sternocleidomastoid, 21720, 21725
Nerve, 64876
Facial, 69955
Graft, 64885-64907
Microrepair
with Surgical Microscope, 69990

Repair — continued
Nerve — continued
Suture, 64831-64876
Nonunion
Carpal Bone, 25431
Femur, 27470, 27472
Fibula, 27726
Humerus, 24430
Metacarpal, 26546
Metatarsal, 28322
Navicular, 25440
Phalanx, 26546
Radius, 25400, 25405, 25415, 25420
Scaphoid, 25440
Tarsal Bones, 28320
Tibia, 27720, 27722, 27724-27725
Ulna, 25400, 25405, 25415, 25420
Nose
Adhesions, 30560
Fistula, 30580, 30600, 42260
Rhinophyma, 30120
Septum, 30540, 30545, 30630
Synechia, 30560
Vestibular Stenosis, 30465
Obstruction
Ventricular Outflow, 33414, 33619
Omentum, 49999
Omphalocele, 49600-49611
Osteochondritis Dissecans Lesion, 29892
Osteotomy
Femoral Neck, 27161
Radius and Ulna, 25365
Ulna and Radius, 25365
Vertebra
Additional Segment, 22216, 22226
Cervical, 22210, 22220
Lumbar, 22214, 22224
Thoracic, 22212, 22222
Oval Window
Fistula, 69666-69667
Oviduct, 58752
Create Stoma, 58770
Pacemaker
Heart
Electrode(s), 33218, 33220
Palate
Laceration, 42180, 42182
Vomer Flap, 42235
Pancreas
Cyst, 48500
Pseudocyst, 48510
Paravaginal Defect, 57284-57285, 57423
Pectus Carinatum, 21740-21742
with Thoracoscopy, 21743
Pectus Excavatum, 21740-21742
with Thoracoscopy, 21743
Pectus Excavatum or Carinatum, 21740, 21742-
21743
Pelvic Floor
with Prosthesis, 57267
Pelvis
Osteotomy, 27158
Tendon, 27098
Penis
Corporeal Tear, 54437
Fistulization, 54435
Injury, 54440
Priapism, 54420-54435
Prosthesis, 54408
Replantation, 54438
Shunt, 54420, 54430
Perforation
Septal, 30630
Perineum, 56810
Periorbital Region
Osteotomy, 21260-21263
Peritoneum, 49999
Phalanges
Finger
Lengthening, 26568
Osteotomy, 26567
Nonunion, 26546
Toe
Osteotomy, 28310, 28312
Pharynx
with Esophagus, 42953

Repair — continued
Pleura, 32215
Prosthesis
Penis, 54408
Pseudarthrosis
Tibia, 27727
Pulmonary Artery, 33917, 33920, 33925-33926
Reimplantation, 33788
Pulmonary Valve, 33470-33474
Pulmonary Venous
Anomaly, 33724
Stenosis, 33726
Quadriceps, 27430
Radius
with Graft, 25405, 25420-25426
Epiphyseal, 25450, 25455
Malunion or Nonunion, 25400-25420
Osteotomy, 25350, 25355, 25370, 25375
Rectocele, 45560, 57250
Rectovaginal Fistula, 57308
Rectum
with Sigmoid Excision, 45550
Fistula, 45800-45825, 46706-46707, 46715-
46716, 46740, 46742
Injury, 45562-45563
Prolapse, 45505-45541, 45900
Rectocele, 45560, 57250
Stenosis, 45500
Retinal Detachment, 67101-67113
Rotator Cuff, 23410-23412, 23420, 29827
Salivary Duct, 42500, 42505
Fistula, 42600
Scalenus Anticus, 21700, 21705
Scapula
Fixation, 23400
Scapulopexy, 23400
Sclera
with Glue, 65286
Reinforcement
with Graft, 67255
without Graft, 67250
Staphyloma
with Graft, 66225
without Graft, 66220
Wound
Operative, 66250
Tissue Glue, 65286
Scrotum, 55175, 55180
Septal Defect, 33813-33814
Septum, Nasal, 30420
Shoulder
Capsule, 23450-23466
Cuff, 23410, 23412
Ligament Release, 23415
Muscle Transfer, 23395, 23397
Musculotendinous (Rotator) Cuff, 23410,
23412
Rotator Cuff, 23415, 23420
Tendon, 23410, 23412, 23430, 23440
Tenomyotomy, 23405, 23406
Simple, Integumentary System, 12001-12021
Sinus
Ethmoid
Cerebrospinal Fluid Leak, 31290
Meningocele, 63700, 63702
Myelomeningocele, 63704, 63706
Sphenoid
Cerebrospinal Fluid Leak, 31291
Sinus of Valsalva, 33702-33722
Skin
See Also Repair, Laceration
Wound
Complex, 13100-13160
Intermediate, 12031-12057
Simple, 12020, 12021
Skull
Cerebrospinal Fluid Leak, 62100
Encephalocele, 62120
SLAP Lesion, 29807
Spectacles, 92370, 92371
Prosthesis, 92371
Sphincter, 53449
Spica Cast, 29720
Spinal Cord, 63700
Cerebrospinal Fluid Leak, 63707, 63709
Meningocele, 63700, 63702

Repair — *continued*
  Spinal Cord — *continued*
    Myelomeningocele, 63704, 63706
    Spinal Meningocele, 63700-63702
  Spine
    Cervical Vertebra, 22510, 22512
    Lumbar Vertebra, 22511-22512, 22514-22515
    Osteotomy, 22210-22226
    Sacral Vertebra, 22511-22512
    Thoracic Vertebra, 22510, 22512, 22513, 22515
  Spleen, 38115
  Stenosis
    Nasal Vestibular, 30465
    Pulmonary, 33782-33783
  Sternocleidomastoid, 21720, 21725
  Stomach
    Esophagogastrostomy, 43320
    Fistula, 43880
    Fundoplasty, 43325-43328
    Laceration, 43501, 43502
    Stoma, 43870
    Ulcer, 43501
  Symblepharon, 68330, 68335, 68340
  Syndactyly, 26560-26562
  Talus
    Osteotomy, 28302
  Tarsal, 28320
    Osteotomy, 28304, 28305
  Tear
    Lung, 32110
  Tendon
    Achilles, 27650, 27652, 27654
    Extensor, 26410, 26412, 26418, 26420, 26426, 26428, 26433-26434, 27664-27665
    Foot, 28208, 28210
    Flexor, 26350, 26352, 26356-26358, 27658-27659
    Leg, 28200, 28202
    Foot, 28200, 28202, 28208, 28210
    Leg, 27658-27659, 27664-27665
    Peroneal, 27675-27676
    Profundus, 26370, 26372-26373
    Upper Arm or Elbow, 24341
  Testis
    Injury, 54670
    Suspension, 54620, 54640
    Torsion, 54600
  Tetralogy of Fallot, 33692, 33694, 33697
  Throat
    Pharyngoesophageal, 42953
    Wound, 42900
  Thumb
    Muscle, 26508
    Tendon, 26510
  Tibia, 27720-27725
    Epiphysis, 27477-27485, 27730-27742
    Osteotomy, 27455, 27457, 27705, 27709, 27712
    Pseudoarthrosis, 27727
  Toe(s)
    Bunion, 28289-28299 *[28295]*
    Macrodactyly, 26590
    Muscle, 28240
    Polydactylous, 26587
    Ruiz–Mora Procedure, 28286
    Tendon, 28240
    Webbed Toe, 28280, 28345
  Tongue, 41250-41252
    Fixation, 41500
    Laceration, 41250-41252
    Mechanical, 41500
    Suture, 41510
  Trachea
    Fistula, 31755
      with Plastic Repair, 31825
      without Plastic Repair, 31820
    Stenosis, 31780, 31781
    Stoma, 31613, 31614
      with Plastic Repair, 31825
      without Plastic Repair, 31820
    Scar, 31830
    Wound
      Cervical, 31800

Repair — *continued*
  Trachea — *continued*
    Wound — *continued*
      Intrathoracic, 31805
  Transposition
    Great Arteries, 33770-33771, 33774-33781
  Triangular Fibrocartilage, 29846
  Tricuspid Valve, 33463-33465
  Trigger Finger, 26055
  Truncus Arteriosus
    Rastelli Type, 33786
  Tunica Vaginalis
    Hydrocele, 55060
  Tympanic Membrane, 69450, 69610, 69635-69637, 69641-69646
  Ulcer, 43501
  Ulna
    with Graft, 25405, 25420
    Epiphyseal, 25450, 25455
    Malunion or Nonunion, 25400-25415
    Osteotomy, 25360, 25370, 25375, 25425, 25426
  Umbilicus
    Omphalocele, 49600-49611
  Ureter
    Anastomosis, 50740-50825
    Continent Diversion, 50825
    Deligation, 50940
    Fistula, 50920, 50930
    Lysis Adhesions, 50715-50725
    Suture, 50900
    Urinary Undiversion, 50830
  Ureterocele, 51535
  Urethra
    with Replantation Penis, 54438
    Artificial Sphincter, 53449
    Diverticulum, 53240, 53400, 53405
    Fistula, 45820, 45825, 53400, 53405, 53520
    Prostatic or Membranous Urethra, 53415, 53420, 53425
    Stoma, 53520
    Stricture, 53400, 53405
    Urethrocele, 57230
    Wound, 53502-53515
  Urethral Sphincter, 57220
  Urinary Incontinence, 53431, 53440, 53445
  Uterus
    Anomaly, 58540
    Fistula, 51920, 51925
    Rupture, 58520, 59350
    Suspension, 58400, 58410
      Presacral Sympathectomy, 58410
  Vagina
    Anterior, 57240, 57289
      with Insertion of Mesh, 57267
      with Insertion of Prosthesis, 57267
    Cystocele, 57240, 57260
    Enterocele, 57265
    Episiotomy, 59300
    Fistula, 46715, 46716, 51900
      Rectovaginal, 57300-57307
      Transvesical and Vaginal Approach, 57330
      Urethrovaginal, 57310, 57311
      Vaginoenteric, 58999
      Vesicovaginal, 57320, 57330
    Hysterectomy, 58267, 58293
    Incontinence, 57288
    Pereyra Procedure, 57289
    Postpartum, 59300
    Prolapse, 57282, 57284
    Rectocele, 57250, 57260
    Suspension, 57280-57284
      Laparoscopic, 57425
    Wound, 57200, 57210
  Vaginal Wall Prolapse
    Anterior, 57240, 57267, 57289
    Anteroposterior, 57260-57267
    Nonobstetrical, 57200
    Posterior, 57250, 57267
  Vas Deferens
    Suture, 55400
  Vein
    Angioplasty, *[37248, 37249]*
    Femoral, 34501
    Graft, 34520

Repair — *continued*
  Vein — *continued*
    Pulmonary, 33730
    Transposition, 34510
    Ventricle, 33545, 33611-33612, 33782-33783
  Vulva
    Postpartum, 59300
  Wound
    Cardiac, 33300, 33305
    Complex, 13100-13160
    Extraocular Muscle, 65290
    Intermediate, 12031-12057
    Operative Wound Anterior Segment, 66250
    Simple, 12001-12021
  Wound Dehiscence
    Abdominal Wall, 49900
    Skin and Subcutaneous Tissue
      Complex, 13160
      Simple, 12020, 12021
  Wrist, 25260, 25263, 25270, 25447
    Bones, 25440
    Carpal Bone, 25431
    Cartilage, 25107
    Muscles, 25260-25274
    Removal
      Implant, 25449
    Secondary, 25265, 25272, 25274
    Tendon, 25280-25316
    Sheath, 25275
    Total Replacement, 25446

Repeat Surgeries
  Carotid
    Thromboendarterectomy, 35390
  Coronary Artery Bypass
    Valve Procedure, 33530
  Distal Vessel Bypass, 35700

Replacement
  Adjustable Gastric Restrictive Device, 43773
  Aortic Valve, 33405-33413
    Transcatheter, 33361-33369
  Arthroplasty
    Hip, 27125-27138
    Knee, 0396T, 27447
    Spine, 22856-22857, 22861-22862
  Artificial Heart
    Intracorporeal, 0052T-0053T
  Cardio-Defibrillator, 33249, *[33262, 33263, 33264]*
  Carotid Sinus Baroreflex Activation Device, 0266T-0268T
  Cecostomy Tube, 49450
  Cerebrospinal Fluid Shunt, 62160, 62194, 62225, 62230
  Chest Wall Respiratory Sensor Electrode or Electrode Array, 0467T
  Colonic Tube, 49450
  Contact Lens, 92326
    See Also Contact Lens Services
  Duodenostomy Tube, 49451
  Elbow
    Total, 24363
  Electrode
    Heart, 33210, 33211, 33216, 33217
    Stomach, 43647
  External Fixation, 20697
  Eye
    Drug Delivery System, 67121
  Gastro-jejunostomy Tube, 49452
  Gastrostomy Tube, 43760, 49450
  Hearing Aid
    Bone Conduction, 69710
  Heart
    Defibrillator
      Leads, 33249
  Hip, 27130, 27132
    Revision, 27134-27138
  Implant
    Bone
      for External Speech Processor/Cochlear Stimulator, 69717, 69718
  Intervertebral Disc
    Cervical Interspace, 0375T, 22856
    Lumbar Interspace, 0163T, 22862
  Intracardiac Ischemia Monitoring System, 0302T
    Device Only, 0304T
    Electrode Only, 0303T

Replacement — *continued*
  Jejunostomy Tube, 49451
  Knee
    Intraoperative Balance Sensor, 0396T
    Total, 27447
  Mitral Valve, 33430
  Nerve, 64726
  Neurostimulator
    Electrode, 63663-63664, 64569
    Pulse Generator/Receiver
      Intracranial, 61885
      Peripheral Nerve, 64590
      Spinal, 63685
  Ossicles
    with Prosthesis, 69633, 69637
  Ossicular Replacement, 69633, 69637
  Pacemaker, 33206-33208, *[33227, 33228, 33229]*
    Catheter, 33210
    Electrode, 33210, 33211, 33216, 33217
    Pulse Generator, 33212-33214 *[33221]*, 33224-33233 *[33227, 33228, 33229]*
  Pacing Cardioverter–Defibrillator
    Leads, 33243, 33244
    Pulse Generator Only, 33241
  Penile
    Prosthesis, 54410, 54411, 54416, 54417
  Prosthesis
    Skull, 62143
    Urethral Sphincter, 53448
  Pulmonary Valve, 33475
  Pulse Generator
    Brain, 61885
    Peripheral Nerve, 64590
    Spinal Cord, 63685
    Vagus Nerve Blocking Therapy, 0316T
  Receiver
    Brain, 61885
    Peripheral Nerve, 64590
    Spinal Cord, 63685
  Skin, 15002-15278
  Skull Plate, 62143
  Spinal Cord
    Reservoir, 62360
  Stent
    Ureteral, 50382, 50385
  Strut, 20697
  Subcutaneous Port for Gastric Restrictive Procedure, 43888
  Tissue Expanders
    Skin, 11970
  Total Replacement Heart System
    Intracorporeal, 0052T-0053T
  Total Replacement Hip, 27130-27132
  Tricuspid Valve, 33465
  Ureter
    with Intestines, 50840
    Electronic Stimulator, 53899
  Uterus
    Inverted, 59899
  Venous Access Device, 36582, 36583, 36585
    Catheter, 36578
  Venous Catheter
    Central, 36580, 36581, 36584
  Ventricular Assist Device, 0451T-0454T, 0459T, 33981-33983

Replantation, Reimplantation
  Adrenal Tissue, 60699
  Arm, Upper, 20802
  Digit, 20816, 20822
  Foot, 20838
  Forearm, 20805
  Hand, 20808
  Penis, 54438
  Scalp, 17999
  Thumb, 20824, 20827

Report Preparation
  Extended, Medical, 99080
  Psychiatric, 90889

Reposition
  Toe to Hand, 26551-26556

Repositioning
  Canalith, 95992
  Central Venous Catheter, Previously Placed, 36597
  Defibrillator, *[33273]*

Repositioning — *continued*
  Electrode
    Heart, 33215, 33226
  Gastrostomy Tube, 43761
  Intraocular Lens, 66825
  Intravascular Vena Cava Filter, 37192
  Tricuspid Valve, 33468
  Ventricular Assist Device, 0460T-0461T
Reproductive Tissue
  Preparation
    Thawing, 89354
  Storage, 89344
Reprogramming
  Infusion Pump, 62369-62370
  Peripheral Subcutaneous Field Stimulation
    Pulse Generator, 64999
  Shunt
    Brain, 62252
Reptilase
  Test, 85635
  Time, 85670-85675
Resection
  Abdomen, 51597
  Aortic Valve Stenosis, 33415
  Bladder Diverticulum, 52305
  Bladder Neck
    Transurethral, 52500
  Brain Lobe, 61323, 61537-61540
  Bullae, 32141
  Chest Wall, 19260-19272
  Cyst
    Mediastinal, 39200
  Diaphragm, 39560-39561
  Emphysematous Lung, 32672
  Endaural, 69905-69910
  Humeral Head, 23195
  Intestines, Small
    Laparoscopic, 44202-44203
  Lung, 32491, 32503-32504, 32672
  Mouth
    with Tongue Excision, 41153
  Myocardium
    Aneurysm, 33542
    Septal Defect, 33545
  Nasal Septum, Submucous, 30520
  Nose
    Septum, 30520
  Ovary, Wedge, 58920
  Palate, 42120
  Pancoast Tumor, 32503-32504
  Phalangeal Head
    Toe, 28153
  Prostate, Transurethral, 52601, 52630
  Radical
    Abdomen, 22904-22905, 51597
    Acetabulum, 27049 *[27059]*, 27076
    Ankle, 27615-27616, 27645-27647
    Arm, Lower, 24152, 25077-25078, 25170
    Arm, Upper, 23220, 24077-24079, 24150
    Back, 21935-21936
    Calcaneus, 27615-27616, 27647
    Elbow, 24077-24079, 24152
      Capsule Soft Tissue, 24149
    Face, 21015-21016
    Femur, 27364-27365 *[27329]*
    Fibula, 27615-27616, 27646
    Finger, 26117-26118, 26260-26262
    Flank, 21935-21936
    Foot, 28046-28047, 28171-28173
    Forearm, 25077-25078, 25170
    Hand, 26117-26118, 26250
    Hip, 27049 *[27059]*, 27075-27078
    Humerus, 23220, 24077-24079
    Innominate, 27049 *[27059]*, 27077
    Ischial, 27049 *[27059]*, 27078
    Knee, 27364-27365 *[27329]*
    Lymph Node(s)
      Abdomen, 38747
      Axillary, 38740, 38745
      Cervical, 38720, 38724
      Groin Area, 38760, 38765
      Pelvic, 38770
      Retroperitoneal, 38780
      Suprahyoid, 38700
      Thoracic, 38746
    Metacarpal, 26117-26118, 26250

Resection — *continued*
  Radical — *continued*
    Metatarsal, 28046-28047, 28173
    Mouth
      with Tongue Excision, 41150, 41155
    Neck, 21557-21558
    Ovarian Tumor
      with Radical Dissection for Debulking,
        58952-58954
      with Total Abdominal Hysterectomy,
        58951, 58953-58956
      Bilateral Salpingo–Oophorecto-
        my–Omentectomy, 58950-
        58954
      Omentectomy, 58950-58956
    Pelvis, 27049 *[27059]*, 27075-27078
    Peritoneal Tumor
      with Radical Dissection for Debulking,
        58952-58954
      Bilateral Salpingo–Oophorecto-
        my–Omentectomy, 58952-
        58954
    Phalanges
      Fingers, 26117-26118, 26260-26262
      Toes, 28046-28047, 28175
    Radius, 24152, 25077-25078, 25170
    Scalp, 21015-21016
    Scapula, 23077-23078, 23210
    Shoulder, 23077-23078, 23220
    Sternum, 21557-21558, 21630-21632
    Talus, 27615-27616, 27647
    Tarsal, 28046-28047, 28171
    Thigh, 27364-27365 *[27329]*
    Thorax, 21557-21558
    Tibia, 27615-27616, 27645
    Tonsil, 42842-42845
    Ulna, 25077-25078, 25170
    Wrist, 25077-25078, 25115-25116, 25170
  Rhinectomy
    Partial, 30150
    Total, 30160
  Ribs, 19260-19272, 32900
  Synovial Membrane
    See Synovectomy
  Temporal Bone, 69535
  Thoracotomy Wedge, 32505-32507
  Thymus, 32673
  Tumor
    Fallopian Tube, 58957-58958
    Lung, 32503-32504
    Mediastinal, 39220
    Ovary, 58957-58958
    Pericardial, 33050
    Peritoneum, 58957-58958
  Ulna
    Arthrodesis
      Radioulnar Joint, 25830
  Ureterocele
    Ectopic, 52301
    Orthotopic, 52300
  Vena Cava
    with Reconstruction, 37799
Residual Urine Collection, 51701
Resistance
  Airway, 94728
Resonance Spectroscopy, Magnetic, 76390
Respiration, Positive–Pressure, 94660
Respiratory Motion Management Simulation,
  77293
Respiratory Pattern Recording
  Preventive
    Infant, 94772
Respiratory Syncytial Virus
  Antibody, 86756
  Antigen Detection
    Direct Fluorescent Antibody, 87280
    Direct Optical Observation, 87807
    Enzyme Immunoassay, 87420
  Recombinant, 90378
Response, Auditory Evoked, 92585-92586
  See Also Audiologic Function Tests
Rest Home Visit
  Care Plan Oversight Services, 99339-99340
  Established Patient, 99334-99337
  New Patient, 99324-99328

Restoration
  Ventricular, 33548
Resuscitation
  Cardiac Massage via Thoracotomy, 32160
  Cardiopulmonary (CPR), 92950
  Newborn, 99460-99465
RET, 81404-81406
Reticulocyte
  Count, 85044-85045
Retina
  Computer-aided Animation and Analysis, 0380T
  Examination, Macula/Fundus, Dilated, 2019F-
    2021F
    Communication of Findings for Diabetes
      Management, 5010F
  Incision
    Encircling Material, 67115
  Lesion
    Extensive
      Destruction, 67227-67228
    Localized
      Destruction, 67208-67218
  Repair
    Detachment
      with Vitrectomy, 67108, 67113
      by Scleral Buckling, 67107-67108
      Cryotherapy, 67101
      Injection of Air, 67110
      Photocoagulation, 67105
      Scleral Dissection, 67107
    Prophylaxis
      Detachment, 67141, 67145
  Retinopathy
    Destruction
      Cryotherapy, Diathermy, 67227, 67229
      Photocoagulation, 67228-67229
      Preterm Infant, 67229
Retinacular
  Knee
    Release, 27425
Retinopathy
  Destruction/Treatment
    Cryotherapy, Diathermy, 67227, 67229
    Photocoagulation, 67228-67229
Retinopexy, Pneumatic, 67110
Retraction, Clot
  See Clot Retraction
Retrocaval Ureter
  Ureterolysis, 50725
**Retrograde Cholangiopancreatographies, Endo-
  scopic**
  See Cholangiopancreatography
Retrograde Cystourethrogram
  See Urethrocystography, Retrograde
Retrograde Pyelogram
  See Urography, Retrograde
Retroperitoneal Area
  Abscess
    Incision and Drainage
      Open, 49060
  Biopsy, 49010
  Cyst
    Destruction/Excision, 49203-49205
  Endometriomas
    Destruction/Excision, 49203-49205
  Exploration, 49010
  Needle Biopsy
    Mass, 49180
  Tumor
    Destruction
      Excision, 49203-49205
Retroperitoneal Fibrosis
  Ureterolysis, 50715
Retropubic Prostatectomies
  See Prostatectomy, Retropubic
Revascularization
  Distal Upper Extremity
    with Interval Ligation, 36838
  Femoral, Popliteal Artery, 37224-37227
  Heart
    Arterial Implant, 33999
    Myocardial Resection, 33542
    Other Tissue Grafts, 20926
  Iliac Artery, 37220-37223
  Interval Ligation
    Distal Upper Extremity, 36838

Revascularization — *continued*
  Penis, 37788
  Peroneal, Tibial, 37228-37235
  Popliteal, Femoral Artery, 37224-37227
  Tibial, Peroneal Artery, 37228-37235
  Transmyocardial, 33140-33141
Reversal, Vasectomy
  See Vasovasorrhaphy
Reverse T3, 84482
Reverse Triiodothyronine, 84482
Revision
  See Also Reconstruction
  Abdomen
    Intraperitoneal Catheter, 49325
    Peritoneal-Venous Shunt, 49426
  Adjustable Gastric Restrictive Device, 43771
  Aorta, 33404
  Arthroplasty
    Hip, 27125-27138
    Knee, 0396T, 27447
    Spine, 22861-22862
  Atrial, 33254-33256
  Blepharoplasty, 15820-15823
  Breast
    Implant, 19380
  Bronchial Stent, 31638
  Bronchus, 32501
  Bypass Graft
    Vein Patch, 35685
  Carotid Sinus Baroreflex Activation Device,
    0269T-0271T
  Cervicoplasty, 15819
  Chest Wall Respiratory Sensor Electrode/Elec-
    trode Array, 0467T
  Colostomy, 44340
    Paracolostomy Hernia, 44345-44346
  Cornea
    Prosthesis, 65770
    Reshaping
      Epikeratoplasty, 65767
      Keratomileusis, 65760
      Keratophakia, 65765
  Ear, Middle, 69662
  Electrode, 64999
    Stomach, 43648, 43882
  External Fixation System, 20693
  Eye
    Aqueous Shunt, 0449T-0450T, 66184-66185
  Gastric Restrictive Device, Adjustable, 43771
  Gastric Restrictive Procedure, 43848
    Adjustable Gastric Restrictive Device Com-
      ponent, 43771
    Subcutaneous Port Component, 43886
  Gastrostomy Tube, 44373
  Graft
    Vaginal, 57295-57296, 57426
  Hip Replacement
    See Replacement, Hip, Revision
  Hymenal Ring, 56700
  Ileostomy, 44312-44314
  Infusion Pump
    Intra–Arterial, 36261
    Intravenous, 36576-36578, 36582-36583
  Intracardiac Ischemia Monitoring System, 0302T
  Iris
    Iridoplasty, 66762
    Iridotomy, 66761
  Jejunostomy Tube, 44373
  Knee, 0396T, 27447
  Lower Extremity Arterial Bypass, 35879-35881
  Neurostimulator
    Chest Wall Respiratory Sensor, 0467T
    Electrode, 63663-63664, 64569, 64999
    Pulse Generator, 63688, 64999
    Receiver, 63688
  Rhytidectomy, 15824-15829
  Semicircular Canal
    Fenestration, 69840
  Shunt
    Intrahepatic Portosystemic, 37183
  Sling, 53442
  Stapedectomy, 69662
  Stomach
    for Obesity, 43848
  Subcutaneous Port for Gastric Restrictive Proce-
    dure, 43886

Revision — *continued*
　Tracheostomy
　　Scar, 31830
　Urinary–Cutaneous Anastomosis, 50727-50728
　Vagina
　　Graft, 57295-57296, 57426
　　Sling
　　　Stress Incontinence, 57287
　Venous Access Device, 36576-36578, 36582-
　　　36583, 36585
　Ventricle
　　Ventriculomyectomy, 33416
　　Ventriculomyotomy, 33416
　Vesicostomy, 51880
Rh (D), 86901
RHCE, 81403
RHD Deletion Analysis, 81403
Rheumatoid Factor, 86430-86431
Rh Immune Globulin, 90384-90386
Rhinectomy
　Partial, 30150
　Total, 30160
Rhinomanometry, 92512
Rhinopharynx
　Biopsy, 42804-42806
　Hemorrhage, 42970-42972
　Unlisted Services/Procedures, 42999
Rhinophyma
　Repair, 30120
Rhinoplasty
　Cleft Lip
　　Cleft Palate, 30460-30462
　　Primary, 30400-30420
　　Secondary, 30430-30450
Rhinoscopy
　Diagnostic, 31231-31235
　Surgical, 0406T-0407T, 31237-31294
　Unlisted Services/Procedures, 31299
Rhinotomy
　Lateral, 30118, 30320
Rhizotomy, 63185, 63190
RHO, 81404, 81434
Rho(D) Vaccine, 90384-90386
Rho Variant Du, 86905
Rh Type, 86901
Rhytidectomy, 15824-15829
　Cheek, 15828
　Chin, 15828
　Forehead, 15824
　Glabellar Frown Lines, 15826
　Neck, 15825, 15828
　Superficial Musculoaponeurotic System, 15829
Rhytidoplasties, 15824-15829
Rib
　Antibody, 86756
　Antigen Detection by Immunoassay with Direct
　　　Optical Observation
　　Direct Fluorescence, 87280
　　Enzyme Immunoassay, 87420
　Bone Graft
　　with Microvascular Anastomosis, 20962
　Excision, 21600-21616, 32900
　Fracture
　　Closed Treatment
　　　<i>See</i> E&M codes
　　External Fixation, 21899
　　Open Treatment, 21811-21813
　Free Osteocutaneous Flap with Microvascular
　　　Anastomosis, 20969
　Graft
　　to Face, 21230
　Resection, 19260-19272, 32900
　X-ray, 71100-71111
Riboflavin, 84252
Richardson Operation Hysterectomy, 58150
　See Also Hysterectomy, Abdominal, Total
Richardson Procedure, 53460
Rickettsia
　Antibody, 86757
Ridell Operation
　Sinusotomy, Frontal, 31075-31087
Ridge, Alveolar
　Fracture Treatment
　　Closed, 21440
　　Open, 21445
RIG (Rabies Immune Globulin), 90375-90376

Right Atrioventricular Valve, 33460-33468
Right Heart Cardiac Catheterization, 93456-
　　93457
　Congenital Cardiac Anomalies, 93530
Ripstein Operation
　Laparoscopic, 45400
　　with Sigmoid Resection, 45402
　Open, 45540-45541
　　with Sigmoid Excision, 45550
Risk Factor Reduction Intervention
　Behavior Change Interventions, 99406-99409
　Group Counseling, 0403T, 99411-99412
　Individual Counseling, 99401-99404
Risser Jacket, 29010-29015
　Removal, 29710
RK, 65771
Robotic Assistance
　Prostatectomy, 55866
Rocky Mountain Spotted Fever, 86000
Roentgenographic
　See X–Ray
Roentgenography
　See Radiology, Diagnostic
Roentgen Rays
　See X–Ray
ROM, 95851-95856, 97110, 97530
Ropes Test, 83872
Rorschach Test, 96101-96103
Ross Information Processing Assessment, 96125
Ross Procedure, 33413
Rotarix, 90681
RotaTeq, 90680
Rotation Flap, 14000-14350
Rotator Cuff
　Repair, 23410-23420
Rotavirus
　Antibody, 86759
　Antigen Detection
　　Enzyme Immunoassay, 87425
Rotavirus Vaccine, 90680-90681
Round Window
　Repair Fistula, 69667
Round Window Fistula, 69667
Roux–en–Y Procedures
　Biliary Tract, 47740-47741, 47780-47785
　Pancreas, 48540
　Stomach, 43621, 43633, 43644, 43846
　　Laparoscopic, 43644
RP1, 81404, 81434
RP2, 81434
RPE65, 81406, 81434
RPGR, 81434
RPP (Radical Perineal Prostatectomy), 55810-
　　55815
RPR, 86592-86593
RPS19, 81405
RRM2B, 81405
RRP (Radical Retropubic Prostatectomy), 55840-
　　55845
RSV
　Antibody, 86756
　Antigen Detection
　　Direct Fluorescent Antibody, 87280
　　Enzyme Immunoassay, 87420
　　Recombinant, 90378
RT3, 84482
Rubber Band Ligation
　Hemorrhoids, 46221
　Skin Tags, 11200-11201
Rubella
　Antibody, 86762
　Vaccine, 90707-90710
Rubella HI Test
　Hemagglutination Inhibition Test, 86280
Rubella Immunization
　MMR, 90707
　MMRV, 90710
Rubeola
　Antibody, 86765
　Antigen Detection
　　Immunofluorescence, 87283
Ruiz–Mora Procedure, 28286
RUNX1/RUNX1T1, 81401
Russell Viper Venom Time, 85612-85613
RYR1, 81406, 81408
RYR2, 81408

S

Saccomanno Technique, 88108
Sac, Endolymphatic
　Exploration, 69805-69806
Sacral Nerve
　Implantation
　　Electrode, 64561, 64581
　Insertion
　　Electrode, 64561, 64581
Sacroiliac Joint
　Arthrodesis, 27280
　Arthrotomy, 27050
　Biopsy, 27050
　Dislocation
　　Open Treatment, 27218
　Fusion, 27280
　Injection for Arthrography, 27096
　Stabilization for Arthrodesis, 27279
　X-ray, 72200-72202, 73525
Sacroplasty, 0200T-0201T
Sacrum
　Augmentation, 0200T-0201T
　Pressure Ulcer, 15931-15937
　Tumor
　　Excision, 49215
　X-ray, 72220
SAECG, 93278
SAH, 61566
Salabrasion, 15780-15787
Salicylate
　Assay, *[80329, 80330, 80331]*
Saline–Solution Abortion, 59850-59851
Salivary Duct
　Catheterization, 42660
　Dilation, 42650-42660
　Ligation, 42665
　Repair, 42500-42505
　　Fistula, 42600
Salivary Glands
　Abscess
　　Incision and Drainage, 42310-42320
　Biopsy, 42405
　Calculi (Stone)
　　Excision, 42330-42340
　Cyst
　　Drainage, 42409
　　Excision, 42408
　Injection
　　X-ray, 42550
　Needle Biopsy, 42400
　Nuclear Medicine
　　Function Study, 78232
　　Imaging, 78230-78231
　Parotid
　　Abscess, 42300-42305
　Unlisted Services and Procedures, 42699
　X-ray, 70380-70390
　　with Contrast, 70390
Salivary Gland Virus
　Antibody, 86644-86645
　Antigen Detection
　　Direct Fluorescence, 87271
　　Enzyme Immunoassay, 87332
　　Nucleic Acid, 87495-87497
Salmonella
　Antibody, 86768
Salpingectomy, 58262-58263, 58291-58292, 58552,
　　58554, 58661, 58700
　Ectopic Pregnancy
　　Laparoscopic Treatment, 59151
　　Surgical Treatment, 59120
　Oophorectomy, 58943
Salpingohysterostomy, 58752
Salpingolysis, 58740
Salpingoneostomy, 58673, 58770
Salpingo–Oophorectomy, 58720
　Resection Ovarian Malignancy, 58950-58956
　Resection Peritoneal Malignancy, 58950-58956
　Resection Tubal Malignancy, 58950-58956
Salpingostomy, 58673, 58770
　Laparoscopic, 58673
SALT, 84460
Salter Osteotomy of the Pelvis, 27146
Sampling
　See Biopsy; Brush Biopsy; Needle Biopsy

Sang–Park Procedure
　Septectomy, Atrial, 33735-33737
　　Balloon (Rashkind Type), 92992
　　Blade Method (Park), 92993
Sao Paulo Typhus, 86000
SAST, 84450
Saucerization
　Calcaneus, 28120
　Clavicle, 23180
　Femur, 27070, 27360
　Fibula, 27360, 27641
　Hip, 27070
　Humerus, 23184, 24140
　Ileum, 27070
　Metacarpal, 26230
　Metatarsal, 28122
　Olecranon Process, 24147
　Phalanges
　　Finger, 26235-26236
　　Toe, 28124
　Pubis, 27070
　Radius, 24145, 25151
　Scapula, 23182
　Talus, 28120
　Tarsal, 28122
　Tibia, 27360, 27640
　Ulna, 24147, 25150
Saundby Test, 82270, 82272
Sauve–Kapandji Procedure
　Arthrodesis, Distal Radioulnar Joint, 25830
SAVER (Surgical Anterior Ventricular Endocar-
　　dial Restoration), 33548
SBFT, 74249
SBRT (Stereotactic Body Radiation Therapy),
　　77373
Scabies, 87220
Scalenotomy, 21700-21705
Scalenus Anticus
　Division, 21700-21705
Scaling
　Chemical for Acne, 17360
Scalp
　Skin Graft
　　Delay of Flap, 15610
　　Full Thickness, 15220-15221
　　Pedicle Flap, 15572
　　Split, 15100-15101
　Tissue Transfer, Adjacent, 14020-14021
　Tumor Excision, 21011-21016
Scalp Blood Sampling, 59030
Scan
　See Also Specific Site; Nuclear Medicine
　Abdomen
　　Computed Tomography, 74150-74175,
　　　75635
　Computerized
　　Ophthalmic, 92132-92134
　CT
　　See CT Scan
　MRI
　　See Magnetic Resonance Imaging
　PET
　　With Computed Tomography (CT)
　　　Limited, 78814
　　　Skull Base to Mid-thigh, 78815
　　　Whole Body, 78816
　　Brain, 78608-78609
　　Heart, 78459
　　Limited Area, 78811
　　Myocardial Imaging Perfusion Study,
　　　78491-78492
　　Skull Base to Mid-Thigh, 78812
　　Whole Body, 78813
　Radionuclide, Brain, 78607
Scanning Radioisotope
　See Nuclear Medicine
Scanogram, 77073
Scaphoid
　Fracture
　　with Manipulation, 25624
　　Closed Treatment, 25622
　　Open Treatment, 25628
Scapula
　Craterization, 23182
　Cyst
　　Excision, 23140

Scapula — continued
  Cyst — continued
    Excision — continued
      with Allograft, 23146
      with Autograft, 23145
  Diaphysectomy, 23182
  Excision, 23172, 23190
    Partial, 23182
  Fracture
    Closed Treatment
      with Manipulation, 23575
      without Manipulation, 23570
    Open Treatment, 23585
  Ostectomy, 23190
  Repair
    Fixation, 23400
    Scapulopexy, 23400
  Saucerization, 23182
  Sequestrectomy, 23172
  Tumor
    Excision, 23140, 23210
      with Allograft, 23146
      with Autograft, 23145
      Radical Resection, 23210
  X–ray, 73010
Scapulopexy, 23400
Scarification
  Pleural, 32215
Scarification of Pleura
  Agent for Pleurodesis, 32560
  Endoscopic, 32650
SCBE (Single Contrast Barium Enema), 74270
Schanz Operation, 27448
Schauta Operation, 58285
Schede Procedure, 32905-32906
Scheie Procedure, 66155
Schilling Test, 78270-78272
Schlatter Operation, 43620
Schlemm's Canal Dilation, 66174-66175
Schlicter Test, 87197
Schocket Procedure, 66180
Schuchard Procedure
  Osteotomy
    Maxilla, 21206
Schwannoma, Acoustic
  See Brain, Tumor, Excision
Sciatic Nerve
  Decompression, 64712
  Injection
    Anesthetic, 64445-64446
  Lesion
    Excision, 64786
  Neuroma
    Excision, 64786
  Neuroplasty, 64712
  Release, 64712
  Repair
    Suture, 64858
Scintigraphy
  See Emission Computerized Tomography
  See Nuclear Medicine
Scissoring
  Skin Tags, 11200-11201
Sclera
  Excision, 66130
    Sclerectomy with Punch or Scissors, 66160
  Fistulization
    Sclerectomy with Punch or Scissors with Iridectomy, 66160
    Thermocauterization with Iridectomy, 66155
    Trabeculectomy ab Externo in Absence of Previous Surgery, 66170
    Trephination with Iridectomy, 66150
  Incision (Fistulization)
    Sclerectomy with Punch or Scissors with Iridectomy, 66160
    Thermocauterization with Iridectomy, 66155
    Trabeculectomy ab Externo in Absence of Previous Surgery, 66170
    Trephination with Iridectomy, 66150
  Lesion
    Excision, 66130
  Repair
    with Glue, 65286

Sclera — continued
  Repair — continued
    Reinforcement
      with Graft, 67255
      without Graft, 67250
    Staphyloma
      with Graft, 66225
      without Graft, 66220
    Wound (Operative), 66250
      Tissue Glue, 65286
Scleral Buckling Operation
  Retina, Repair, Detachment, 67107-67108, 67113
Scleral Ectasia
  Repair, 66220
    with Graft, 66225
Sclerectomy, 66160
Sclerotherapy
  Percutaneous (Cyst, Lymphocele, Seroma), 49185
  Venous, 36468-36471
Sclerotomy, 66150-66170
SCN1A, 81407
SCN1B, 81404
SCN4A, 81406
SCN5A, 81407
SCNN1A, 81406
SCNN1B, 81406
SCNN1G, 81406
SCO1, 81405
SCO2, 81404
Scoliosis Evaluation, Radiologic, 72081-72084
Scrambler Therapy, 0278T
Screening
  Abdominal Aortic Aneurysm (AAA), 76706
  Developmental, 96110
  Drug
    Alcohol and/or Substance Abuse, 99408-99409
  Evoked Otoacoustic Emissions, [92558]
  Mammography, 77067
Scribner Cannulization, 36810
Scrotal Varices
  Excision, 55530-55540
Scrotoplasty, 55175-55180
Scrotum
  Abscess
    Incision and Drainage, 54700, 55100
  Excision, 55150
  Exploration, 55110
  Hematoma
    Incision and Drainage, 54700
  Removal
    Foreign Body, 55120
  Repair, 55175-55180
  Ultrasound, 76870
  Unlisted Services and Procedures, 55899
Scrub Typhus, 86000
SDHA, 81406
SDHB, 81405, 81437-81438
SDHC, 81404-81405, 81437-81438
SDHD, 81404, 81437-81438
Second Look Surgery
  Carotid Thromboendarterectomy, 35390
  Coronary Artery Bypass, 33530
  Distal Vessel Bypass, 35700
  Valve Procedure, 33530
Secretory Type II Phospholipase A2 (sPLA2-IIA), 0423T
Section
  See Also Decompression
  Cesarean
    See Cesarean Delivery
  Cranial Nerve, 61460
    Spinal Access, 63191
  Dentate Ligament, 63180-63182
  Gasserian Ganglion
    Sensory Root, 61450
  Mesencephalic Tract, 61480
  Nerve Root, 63185-63190
  Spinal Accessory Nerve, 63191
  Spinal Cord Tract, 63194-63199
  Vestibular Nerve
    Transcranial Approach, 69950
    Translabyrinthine Approach, 69915

Sedation
  Moderate, 99155-99157
    with Independent Observation, 99151-99153
Seddon–Brookes Procedure, 24320
Sedimentation Rate
  Blood Cell
    Automated, 85652
    Manual, 85651
Segmentectomy
  Breast, 19301-19302
  Lung, 32484, 32669
Selective Cellular Enhancement Technique, 88112
Selenium, 84255
Self Care
  See Also Physical Medicine/ Therapy/Occupational Therapy
  Training, 97535, 98960-98962, 99509
Sella Turcica
  CT Scan, 70480-70482
  X–ray, 70240
Semen
  Cryopreservation
    Storage (per year), 89343
    Thawing, Each Aliquot, 89353
Semen Analysis, 89300-89322
  with Sperm Isolation, 89260-89261
  Sperm Analysis, 89329-89331
    Antibodies, 89325
Semenogelase, 84152-84154
Semicircular Canal
  Incision
    Fenestration, 69820
    Revised, 69840
Semilunar
  Bone
    See Lunate
Seminal Vesicle
  Cyst
    Excision, 55680
  Excision, 55650
  Incision, 55600, 55605
  Mullerian Duct
    Excision, 55680
  Unlisted Services and Procedures, 55899
Seminal Vesicles
  Vesiculography, 74440
  X–ray with Contrast, 74440
Seminin, 84152-84154
Semiquantitative, 81005
Semont Maneuver, 95992
Sengstaaken Tamponade
  Esophagus, 43460
Senning Procedure
  Repair, Great Arteries, 33774-33777
Senning Type, 33774-33777
Sensitivity Study
  Antibiotic
    Agar, 87181
    Disc, 87184
    Enzyme Detection, 87185
    Macrobroth, 87188
    MIC, 87186
    Microtiter, 87186
    MLC, 87187
    Mycobacteria, 87190
  Antiviral Drugs
    HIV–1
      Tissue Culture, 87904
Sensor, Chest Wall Respiratory Electrode or Electrode Array
  Insertion, 0466T
  Removal, 0468T
  Replacement, 0467T
  Revision, 0467T
Sensorimotor Exam, 92060
Sensor, Interstitial Glucose, 0446T-0448T
Sensor, Transcatheter Placement, 34806
Sensory Nerve
  Common
    Repair/Suture, 64834
Sensory Testing
  Quantitative (QST), Per Extremity
    Cooling Stimuli, 0108T
    Heat–Pain Stimuli, 0109T

Sensory Testing — continued
  Quantitative, Per Extremity — continued
    Touch Pressure Stimuli, 0106T
    Using Other Stimuli, 0110T
    Vibration Stimuli, 0107T
Sentinel Node
  Injection Procedure, 38792
SEP (Somatosensory Evoked Potentials), 95925-95927 [95938]
Separation
  Craniofacial
    Closed Treatment, 21431
    Open Treatment, 21432-21436
SEPT9, 81327
Septal Defect
  Repair, 33813-33814
  Ventricular
    Closure
      Open, 33675-33688
      Percutaneous, 93581
Septectomy
  Atrial, 33735-33737
    Balloon Type, 92992
    Blade Method, 92993
  Closed, 33735
  Submucous Nasal, 30520
Septic Abortion, 59830
Septoplasty, 30520
Septostomy
  Atrial, 33735-33737
    Balloon Type, 92992
    Blade Method, 92993
Septum, Nasal
  See Nasal Septum
Sequestrectomy
  with Alveolectomy, 41830
  Calcaneus, 28120
  Carpal, 25145
  Clavicle, 23170
  Forearm, 25145
  Humeral Head, 23174
  Humerus, 24134
  Olecranon Process, 24138
  Radius, 24136, 25145
  Scapula, 23172
  Skull, 61501
  Talus, 28120
  Ulna, 24138, 25145
  Wrist, 25145
Serialography
  Aorta, 75625
Serodiagnosis, Syphilis, 86592-86593
Serologic Test for Syphilis, 86592-86593
Seroma
  Incision and Drainage
    Skin, 10140
  Sclerotherapy, Percutaneous, 49185
Serotonin, 84260
SERPINA1, 81332
SERPINE1, 81400
Serpin Peptidase Inhibitor, Clade A, Alpha-1 Antiproteinase, Antitrypsin, Member 1 Gene Analysis, 81332
Serum
  Albumin, 82040
  Antibody Identification
    Pretreatment, 86975-86978
  CPK, 82550
  Serum Immune Globulin, 90281-90284
Serum Globulin Immunization, 90281-90284
Sesamoid Bone
  Excision, 28315
  Finger
    Excision, 26185
  Foot
    Fracture, 28530-28531
  Thumb
    Excision, 26185
Sesamoidectomy
  Toe, 28315
SETX, 81406
Severing of Blepharorrhaphy, 67710
Sever Procedure, 23020
Sex Change Operation
  Female to Male, 55980
  Male to Female, 55970

    [Resequenced]

Sex Chromatin, 88130
Sex Chromatin Identification, 88130-88140
Sex Hormone Binding Globulin, 84270
Sex–Linked Ichthyoses, 86592-86593
SG, 84315, 93503
SGCA, 81405
SGCB, 81405
SGCD, 81405
SGCE, 81405-81406
SGCG, 81404-81405
SGOT, 84450
SGPT, 84460
SH2D1A, 81403-81404
SH3TC2, 81406
Shaving
   Skin Lesion, 11300-11313
SHBG, 84270
Shelf Procedure
   Osteotomy, Hip, 27146-27151
      Femoral with Open Reduction, 27156
Shiga–Like Toxin
   Antigen Detection
      Enzyme Immunoassay, 87427
Shigella
   Antibody, 86771
Shirodkar Operation, 57700
SHOC2, 81400, 81405
Shock Wave Lithotripsy, 50590
Shock Wave (Extracorporeal) Therapy, 0101T-0102T, 28890
Shock Wave, Ultrasonic
   See Ultrasound
Shop Typhus of Malaya, 86000
Shoulder
   See Also Clavicle; Scapula
   Abscess
      Drainage, 23030
   Amputation, 23900-23921
   Arthrocentesis, 20610-20611
   Arthrodesis, 23800
      with Autogenous Graft, 23802
   Arthrography
      Injection
         Radiologic, 23350
   Arthroplasty
      with Implant, 23470-23472
   Arthroscopy
      Diagnostic, 29805
      Surgical, 29806-29828
   Arthrotomy
      with Removal Loose or Foreign Body, 23107
   Biopsy
      Deep, 23066
      Soft Tissue, 23065
   Blade
      See Scapula
   Bone
      Excision
         Acromion, 23130
         Clavicle, 23120-23125
         Clavicle Tumor, 23140-23146
      Incision, 23035
      Tumor
         Excision, 23140-23146
   Bursa
      Drainage, 23031
   Capsular Contracture Release, 23020
   Cast
      Figure Eight, 29049
      Removal, 29710
      Spica, 29055
      Velpeau, 29058
   Disarticulation, 23920-23921
   Dislocation
      with Greater Tuberosity Fracture
         Closed Treatment, 23665
         Open Treatment, 23670
      with Surgical or Anatomical Neck Fracture
         Closed Treatment with Manipulation, 23675
         Open Treatment, 23680
      Closed Treatment
         with Manipulation, 23650, 23655
      Open Treatment, 23660
   Excision
      Acromion, 23130

Shoulder — *continued*
   Excision — *continued*
      Torn Cartilage, 23101
   Exploration, 23107
   Hematoma
      Drainage, 23030
   Incision and Drainage, 23040-23044
      Superficial, 10060-10061
   Joint
      X–ray, 73050
   Manipulation
      Application of Fixation Apparatus, 23700
   Prophylactic Treatment, 23490-23491
   Prosthesis
      Removal, 23334-23335
   Radical Resection, 23077
   Removal
      Calcareous Deposits, 23000
      Cast, 29710
      Foreign Body, 23040-23044
         Deep, 23333
         Subcutaneous, 23330
      Foreign or Loose Body, 23107
      Prosthesis, 23334-23335
   Repair
      Capsule, 23450-23466
      Ligament Release, 23415
      Muscle Transfer, 23395-23397
      Rotator Cuff, 23410-23420
      Tendon, 23410-23412, 23430-23440
      Tenomyotomy, 23405-23406
   Strapping, 29240
   Surgery
      Unlisted Services and Procedures, 23929
   Tumor, 23075-23078 *[23071, 23073]*
   Unlisted Services and Procedures, 23929
   X–ray, 73020-73030
      with Contrast, 73040
Shoulder Bone
   Excision
      Acromion, 23130
      Clavicle, 23120-23125
   Tumor
      Excision, 23140-23146
Shoulder Joint
   See Also Clavicle; Scapula
   Arthroplasty
      with Implant, 23470-23472
   Arthrotomy
      with Biopsy, 23100-23101
      with Synovectomy, 23105-23106
   Dislocation
      with Greater Tuberosity Fracture
         Closed Treatment, 23665
         Open Treatment, 23670
      with Surgical or Anatomical Neck Fracture
         Closed Treatment with Manipulation, 23675
         Open Treatment, 23680
      Open Treatment, 23660
   Excision
      Torn Cartilage, 23101
   Exploration, 23040-23044, 23107
   Foreign Body Removal, 23040-23044
   Incision and Drainage, 23040-23044
   Removal
      Prosthesis, 23334-23335
   X–ray, 73050
SHOX, 81405
Shunt(s)
   Aqueous
      without Extraocular Reservoir, 0191T, 66183, *[0253T]*
      into Subconjunctival Space, 0449T-0450T
      Revision, 66184-66185
      to Extraocular Reservoir, 66179-66180
   Arteriovenous Shunt
      Dialysis Circuit, 36901-36909
   Brain
      Creation, 62180-62223
      Removal, 62256-62258
      Replacement, 62160, 62194, 62225-62230, 62258
      Reprogramming, 62252
   Cerebrospinal Fluid, 62180-62258, 63740-63746

Shunt(s) — *continued*
   Creation
      Arteriovenous
         with Bypass Graft, 35686
         with Graft, 36825-36830
         Direct, 36821
         ECMO
            Isolated with Chemotherapy Perfusion, 36823
         Thomas Shunt, 36835
         Transposition, 36818
      Fetal, 59076
      Great Vessel
         Aorta
            Pulmonary, 33924
         Aortic Pulmonary Artery
            Ascending, 33755
            Descending, 33762
            Central, 33764
            Subclavian–Pulmonary Artery, 33750
            Vena Cava to Pulmonary Artery, 33766-33768
      Intra–atrial, 33735-33737
      LeVeen
         Insertion, 49425
         Ligation, 49428
         Patency Test, 78291
         Removal, 49429
         Revision, 49426
      Nonvascular
         X–ray, 75809
      Peritoneal
         Venous
            Injection, 49427
            Ligation, 49428
            Removal, 49429
         X–ray, 75809
      Pulmonary Artery
         from Aorta, 33755-33762, 33924
         from Vena Cava, 33766-33767
         Subclavian, 33750
      Revision
         Arteriovenous, 36832
      Spinal Cord
         Creation, 63740-63741
         Irrigation, 63744
         Removal, 63746
         Replacement, 63744
      Superior Mesenteric–Cavel
         See Anastomosis, Caval to Mesenteric
      Transvenous Intrahepatic Portosystemic, 37182-37183
      Ureter to Colon, 50815
      Ventriculocisternal with Valve, 62180, 62200-62201
Shuntogram, 75809
Sialic Acid, 84275
Sialodochoplasty, 42500-42505
Sialogram, 70390
Sialography, 70390
Sialolithotomy, 42330-42340
Sickling
   Electrophoresis, 83020
Siderocytes, 85536
Siderophilin, 84466
Sigmoid
   See Colon–Sigmoid
Sigmoid Bladder
   Cystectomy, 51590
Sigmoidoscopy
   Ablation
      Polyp, *[45346]*
      Tumor, *[45346]*
   Biopsy, 45331
   Collection
      Specimen, 45331
   Exploration, 45330
   Hemorrhage Control, 45334
   Injection
      Submucosal, 45335
   Mucosal Resection, 45349
   Needle Biopsy, 45342
   Placement
      Stent, 45347
   Removal
      Foreign Body, 45332

Sigmoidoscopy — *continued*
   Removal — *continued*
      Polyp, 45333, 45338
      Tumor, 45333, 45338
   Repair
      Volvulus, 45337
   Ultrasound, 45341-45342
Signal–Averaged Electrocardiography, 93278
SIL1, 81405
Silica, 84285
Silicon Dioxide, 84285
Silicone
   Contouring Injections, 11950-11954
Simple Mastectomies
   See Mastectomy
Single Photon Absorptiometry
   Bone Density, 78350
Single Photon Emission Computed Tomography
   See SPECT
Sinogram, 76080
Sinus
   Ethmoidectomy
      Excision, 31254
   Pilonidal
      Excision, 11770-11772
      Incision and Drainage, 10080-10081
Sinusectomy, Ethmoid
   Endoscopic, 31254-31255
   Extranasal, 31205
   Intranasal, 31200-31201
Sinuses
   Ethmoid
      with Nasal
         Sinus Endoscopy, 0406T-0407T, 31254-31255
      Excision, 31200-31205
      Repair of Cerebrospinal Leak, 31290
   Frontal
      Destruction, 31080-31085
      Exploration, 31070-31075
      with Nasal
         Sinus Endoscopy, 31276
      Fracture
         Open Treatment, 21343-21344
      Incision, 31070-31087
   Injection, 20500
      Diagnostic, 20501
   Maxillary
      Antrostomy, 31256-31267
      Excision, 31225-31230
      Exploration, 31020-31032
         with Nasal/Sinus Endoscopy, 31233
      Incision, 31020-31032, 31256-31267
      Irrigation, 31000
      Skull Base Surgery, 61581
      Surgery, 61581
   Multiple
      Incision, 31090
      Paranasal Incision, 31090
   Repair of Cerebrospinal Leak, 31290
   Sphenoid
      Biopsy, 31050-31051
      Exploration, 31050-31051
      with Nasal
         Sinus Endoscopy, 31235
      Incision, 31050-31051
         with Nasal Sinus Endoscopy, 31287-31288
      Irrigation, 31002
      Repair of Cerebrospinal Leak, 31291
      Sinusotomy, 31050-31051
      Skull Base Surgery, 61580-61581
   Unlisted Services and Procedures, 31299
   X–ray, 70210-70220
Sinus of Valsalva
   Repair, 33702-33722
Sinusoidal Rotational Testing, 92546
Sinusoscopy
   Sinus
      Maxillary, 31233
      Sphenoid, 31235
Sinusotomy
   Combined, 31090
   Frontal Sinus
      Exploratory, 31070-31075
      Non–Obliterative, 31086-31087

[Resequenced]

Sinusotomy — *continued*
Frontal Sinus — *continued*
Obliterative, 31080-31085
Maxillary, 31020-31032
Multiple
Paranasal, 31090
Ridell, 31080
Sphenoid Sinus, 31050-31051
Sinu, Sphenoid
See Sinuses, Sphenoid
Sinus Venosus
Repair, 33645
Sirolimus Drug Assay, 80195
SISI Test, 92564
Sistrunk Operation
Cyst, Thyroid Gland, Excision, 60200
Six-Minute Walk Test, 94620
Size Reduction, Breast, 19318
Skeletal Fixation
Humeral Epicondyle
Percutaneous, 24566
Skeletal Traction
Insertion/Removal, 20650
Pin/Wire, 20650
Skene's Gland
Abscess
Incision and Drainage, 53060
Destruction, 53270
Excision, 53270
Skilled Nursing Facilities (SNFs)
Annual Assessment, 99318
Care Plan Oversight, 99379-99380
Discharge Services, 1110F-1111F, 99315-99316
Initial Care, 99304-99306
Subsequent Care, 99307-99310
Skin
Abrasion, 15786-15787
Chemical Peel, 15788-15793
Dermabrasion, 15780-15783
Abscess
Incision and Drainage, 10060-10061
Puncture Aspiration, 10160
Adjacent Tissue Transfer, 14000-14350
Autograft
Cultured, 15150-15152, 15155-15157
Dermal, 15130-15136
Biopsy, 11100-11101
Chemical Exfoliation, 17360
Cyst
Puncture Aspiration, 10160
Debridement, 11000-11006, 11010-11047
[11045, 11046]
with Open Fracture and/or Dislocation, 11010-11012
Eczematous, 11000-11001
Infected, 11000-11006
Subcutaneous Tissue, 11042-11047 *[11045, 11046]*
Infected, 11004-11006
Decubitus Ulcer(s)
Excision, 15920-15999
Desquamation, 17360
Destruction
Benign Lesion
Fifteen or More Lesions, 17111
One to Fourteen Lesions, 17110
Flat Warts, 17110-17111
Lesion(s), 17106-17108
Malignant Lesion, 17260-17286
by Photodynamic Therapy, 96567
Premalignant Lesions
by Photodynamic Therapy, 96567
Fifteen or More Lesions, 17004
First Lesion, 17000
Two to Fourteen Lesions, 17003
Excision
Debridement, 11000-11006, 11010-11044
[11045, 11046]
Excess Skin, 15830-15839, 15847
Hemangioma, 11400-11446
Lesion
Benign, 11400-11446
Malignant, 11600-11646
Fasciocutaneous Flaps, 15732-15738
Grafts
Free, 15200-15261

Skin — *continued*
Grafts — *continued*
Harvesting for Tissue Culture, 15040
Imaging, Microscopy, 96931-96936
Incision and Drainage, 10040-10180
See Also Incision, Skin
Lesion
See Lesion; Tumor
Analysis, Multi-Spectral, 0400T-0401T
Verrucous
Destruction, 17110-17111
Mole
History, 1050F
Patient Self-Examination Counseling, 5005F
Muscle Flaps, 15732-15738
Myocutaneous Flap, 15732-15738
Nevi
History, 1050F
Patient Self-Examination Counseling, 5005F
Nose
Surgical Planing, 30120
Paring, 11055-11057
Photography
Diagnostic, 96904
Removal
Skin Tag, 11200-11201
Revision
Blepharoplasty, 15820-15823
Cervicoplasty, 15819
Rhytidectomy, 15824-15829
Shaving, 11300-11313
Substitute Application, 15271-15278
Tags
Removal, 11200, 11201
Tests
See Also Allergy Tests
Candida, 86485
Coccidioidomycosis, 86490
Histoplasmosis, 86510
Other Antigen, 86356, 86486
Tuberculosis, 86580
Unlisted Antigen, 86486
Unlisted Services and Procedures, 17999
Wound Repair
Abdomen
Complex, 13100-13102
Intermediate, 12031-12037
Layered, 12031-12037
Simple, 12001-12007
Superficial, 12001-12007
Arm, Arms
Complex, 13120-13122
Intermediate, 12031-12037
Layered, 12031-12037
Simple, 12001-12007
Superficial, 12001-12007
Axilla, Axillae
Complex, 13131-13133
Intermediate, 12031-12037
Layered, 12031-12037
Simple, 12001-12007
Superficial, 12001-12007
Back
Complex, 13100-13102
Intermediate, 12031-12037
Layered, 12031-12037
Simple, 12001-12007
Superficial, 12001-12007
Breast
Complex, 13100-13102
Intermediate, 12031-12037
Layered, 12031-12037
Simple, 12001-12007
Superficial, 12001-12007
Buttock
Complex, 13100-13102
Intermediate, 12031-12037
Layered, 12031-12037
Simple, 12001-12007
Superficial, 12001-12007
Cheek, Cheeks
Complex, 13131-13133
Intermediate, 12051-12057
Layered, 12051-12057
Simple, 12011-12018
Superficial, 12011-12018

Skin — *continued*
Wound Repair — *continued*
Chest
Complex, 13100-13102
Intermediate, 12031-12037
Layered, 12031-12037
Simple, 12001-12007
Superficial, 12001-12007
Chin
Complex, 13131-13133
Intermediate, 12051-12057
Layered, 12051-12057
Simple, 12011-12018
Superficial, 12011-12018
Ear, Ears
Complex, 13151-13153
Intermediate, 12051-12057
Layered, 12051-12057
2.5 cm or less, 12051
Simple, 12011-12018
Superficial, 12011-12018
External
Genitalia
Complex/Intermediate, 12041-12047
Layered, 12041-12047
Simple, 12001-12007
Superficial, 12041-12047
Extremity, Extremities
Complex/Intermediate, 12031-12037
Layered, 12031-12037
Simple, 12001-12007
Superficial, 12001-12007
Eyelid, Eyelids
Complex, 13151-13153
Intermediate, 12051-12057
Layered, 12051-12057
Simple, 12011-12018
Superficial, 12011-12018
Face
Complex/Intermediate, 12051-12057
Layered, 12051-12057
Simple, 12011-12018
Superficial, 12011-12018
Feet
Complex, 13131-13133
Intermediate, 12041-12047
Layered, 12041-12047
Simple, 12001-12007
Superficial, 12001-12007
Finger, Fingers
Complex, 13131-13133
Intermediate, 12041-12047
Layered, 12041-12047
Simple, 12001-12007
Superficial, 12001-12007
Foot
Complex, 13131-13133
Intermediate, 12041-12047
Layered, 12041-12047
Simple, 12001-12007
Superficial, 12001-12007
Forearm, Forearms
Complex, 13120-13122
Intermediate, 12031-12037
Layered, 12031-12037
Simple, 12001-12007
Superficial, 12001-12007
Forehead
Complex, 13131-13133
Intermediate, 12051-12057
Layered, 12051-12057
Simple, 12011-12018
Superficial, 12011-12018
Genitalia
Complex, 13131-13133
External
Complex/Intermediate, 12041-12047
Layered, 12041-12047
Simple, 12001-12007
Superficial, 12001-12007
Hand, Hands
Complex, 13131-13133
Intermediate, 12041-12047
Layered, 12041-12047

Skin — *continued*
Wound Repair — *continued*
Hand, Hands — *continued*
Simple, 12001-12007
Superficial, 12001-12007
Leg, Legs
Complex, 13120-13122
Intermediate, 12031-12037
Layered, 12031-12037
Simple, 12001-12007
Superficial, 12001-12007
Lip, Lips
Complex, 13151-13153
Intermediate, 12051-12057
Layered, 12051-12057
Simple, 12011-12018
Superficial, 12011-12018
Lower
Arm, Arms
Complex, 13120-13122
Intermediate, 12031-12037
Layered, 12031-12037
Simple, 12001-12007
Superficial, 12001-12007
Extremity, Extremities
Complex, 13120-13122
Intermediate, 12031-12037
Layered, 12031-12037
Simple, 12001-12007
Superficial, 12001-12007
Leg, Legs
Complex, 13120-13122
Intermediate, 12031-12037
Layered, 12031-12037
Simple, 12001-12007
Superficial, 12001-12007
Mouth
Complex, 13131-13133
Mucous Membrane
Complex/Intermediate, 12051-12057
Layered, 12051-12057
Simple, 12011-12018
Superficial, 12011-12018
Neck
Complex, 13131-13133
Intermediate, 12041-12047
Layered, 12041-12047
Simple, 12001-12007
Superficial, 12001-12007
Nose
Complex, 13151-13153
Intermediate, 12051-12057
Layered, 12051-12057
Simple, 12011-12018
Superficial, 12011-12018
Palm, Palms
Complex, 13131-13133
Intermediate, 12041-12047
Layered, 12041-12047
Simple, 12001-12007
Superficial, 12001-12007
Scalp
Complex, 13120-13122
Intermediate, 12031-12057
Layered, 12031-12037
Simple, 12001-12007
Superficial, 12001-12007
Toe, Toes
Complex, 13131-13133
Intermediate, 12041-12047
Layered, 12041-12047
Simple, 12001-12007
Superficial, 12001-12007
Trunk
Complex, 13100-13102
Intermediate, 12031-12037
Layered, 12031-12037
Simple, 12001-12007
Superficial, 12001-12007
Upper
Arm, Arms
Complex, 13120-13122
Intermediate, 12031-12037
Layered, 12031-12037
Simple, 12001-12007
Superficial, 12001-12007

Skin — *continued*
  Wound Repair — *continued*
    Upper — *continued*
      Extremity
        Complex, 13120-13122
        Intermediate, 12031-12037
        Layered, 12031-12037
        Simple, 12001-12007
        Superficial, 12001-12007
      Leg, Legs
        Complex, 13120-13122
        Intermediate, 12031-12037
        Layered, 12031-12037
        Simple, 12001-12007
        Superficial, 12001-12007
Skin Graft and Flap
  Autograft
    Dermal, 15130-15136
    Epidermal, 15110-15116, 15150-15157
    Split-Thickness, 15100-15101, 15120-15121
  Composite Graft, 15760-15770
  Cross Finger Flap, 15574
  Delay of Flap, 15600-15630
  Derma–Fat–Fascia Graft, 15770
  Fascial
    Free, 15758
  Fasciocutaneous Flap, 15732-15738
  Formation, 15570-15576
  Free
    Full Thickness Skin Graft, 15200-15261
    Microvascular Anastomosis, 15756-15758
  Island Pedicle Flap, 15740
  Muscle, 15732-15738, 15842
    Free, 15756
  Myocutaneous, 15732-15738, 15756
  Pedicle Flap
    Formation, 15570-15576
    Island, 15740
    Neurovascular, 15750
    Transfer, 15650
  Pinch Graft, 15050
  Platysmal, 15825
  Punch Graft, 15775-15776
    for Hair Transplant, 15775-15776
  Recipient Site Preparation, 15002-15005
  Skin
    Free, 15757
  Split Graft, 15100-15101, 15120-15121
  Substitute Skin Application, 15271-15278
  Superficial Musculoaponeurotic System, 15829
  Tissue–Cultured, 15150-15157
  Tissue Transfer, 14000-14350
  Transfer, 15650
  Vascular Flow Check, 15860
Skull
  Burr Hole
    with Injection, 61120
    Biopsy Brain, 61140
    Drainage
      Abscess, 61150-61151
      Cyst, 61150-61151
      Hematoma, 61154-61156
    Exploration
      Infratentorial, 61253
      Supratentorial, 61250
    Insertion
      Catheter, 61210
      EEG Electrode, 61210
      Reservoir, 61210
    Intracranial Biopsy, 61140
  Decompression, 61322-61323, 61340-61345
    Orbit, 61330
  Drill Hole
    Catheter, 61107
    Drainage Hematoma, 61108
    Exploration, 61105
  Excision, 61501
  Exploration Drill Hole, 61105
  Fracture, 62000-62010
  Hematoma Drainage, 61108
  Incision
    Suture, 61550-61552
  Insertion
    Catheter, 61107
  Lesion
    Excision, 61500, 61600-61608, 61615-61616

Skull — *continued*
  Orbit
    Biopsy, 61332
    Excision
      Lesion, 61333
    Exploration, 61332-61333
  Puncture
    Cervical, 61050
    Cisternal, 61050
    Drain Fluid, 61070
    Injection, 61070
    Subdural, 61000-61001
    Ventricular Fluid, 61020
  Reconstruction, 21172-21180
    Defect, 62140-62141, 62145
  Reduction
    Craniomegalic, 62115-62117
  Removal
    Plate, 62142
    Prosthesis, 62142
  Repair
    Cerebrospinal Fluid Leak, 62100
    Encephalocele, 62120
  Replacement
    Plate, 62143
    Prosthesis, 62143
  Tumor
    Excision, 61500
  X–ray, 70250, 70260
Skull Base Surgery
  Anterior Cranial Fossa
    Bicoronal Approach, 61586
    Craniofacial Approach, 61580-61583
    Extradural, 61600, 61601
    LeFort I Osteotomy Approach, 61586
    Orbitocranial Approach, 61584, 61585
    Transzygomatic Approach, 61586
  Carotid Aneurysm, 61613
  Carotid Artery, 61610
    Transection
      Ligation, 61610-61612
  Craniotomy, 62121
  Dura
    Repair of Cerebrospinal Fluid Leak, 61618, 61619
  Middle Cranial Fossa
    Extradural, 61605, 61607
    Infratemporal Approach, 61590, 61591
    Intradural, 61606, 61608
    Orbitocranial Zygomatic Approach, 61592
  Posterior Cranial Fossa
    Extradural, 61615
    Intradural, 61616
    Transcondylar Approach, 61596, 61597
    Transpetrosal Approach, 61598
    Transtemporal Approach, 61595
SLC12A1, 81407
SLC12A3, 81407
SLC14A1, 81403
SLC16A2, 81404-81405
SLC22A5, 81405
SLC25A20, 81404-81405
SLC25A4, 81404
SLC26A4, 81406, 81430
SLC2A10, 81410
SLC2A1, 81405
SLC37A4, 81406
SLC4A1, 81403
SLC9A6, 81406
SLCO1B1, 81400
Sleep Apnea
  Central
    Neurostimulator System, 0424T-0436T
Sleep Study, 95803-95807 *[95800, 95801]*
  Polysomnography, 95808-95811 *[95782, 95783]*
  Unattended, *[95800, 95801]*
Sleeve Gastrectomy, 43775
Sliding Inlay Graft, Tibia
  Tibia, Repair, 27720-27725
Sling Operation
  Incontinence, 53440
    Removal, 53442
  Stress Incontinence, 51992, 57287
  Vagina, 57287, 57288
SMAD3, 81410
SMAD4, 81405-81406, 81436

Small Bowel
  See Also Intestines, Small
  Endoscopy, 44360-44386
    with Tumor Removal
      Ablation, 44369
      Bipolar Cautery, 44365
      Hot Biopsy Forceps, 44365
      Snare Technique, 44364
  Enterectomy, 44120-44128
    Laparoscopic, 44202-44203
  Enterotomy, 44020-44021
    for Lesion Removal, 44110-44111
Small Nuclear Ribonucleoprotein Polypeptide N and Ubiquitin Protein Ligase E3A Methylation Analysis, 81331
SMAS Flap, 15829
Smear
  Cervical, 88141-88143, 88155, 88164-88167, 88174-88175
  Papanicolaou, 88141-88155, 88164-88167, 88174-88175
Smear and Stain
  Cervical/Vaginal, 88141-88167, 88174-88175
  Cornea, 65430
  Fluorescent, 87206
  Gram or Giemsa, 87205
  Intracellular Parasites, 87207
  Ova
    Parasite, 87177, 87209
  Parasites, 87206-87209
  Wet Mount, 87210
Smith Fracture, 25600-25605, 25607, 25608-25609
Smith–Robinson Operation
  Arthrodesis, Vertebra, 22614
SMN1, 81400, 81403, 81405
SMN1/SMN2, 81401
Smoking and Tobacco Cessation, 99406-99407
Smooth Muscle Antibody, 86255
SMPD1, 81330, 81412
SNRPN/UBE3A, 81331
SO4
  Chondroitin Sulfate, 82485
  Dehydroepiandrosterone Sulfate, 82627
  Urine, 84392
Soave Procedure, 45120
Sodium, 84295, 84302
  Urine, 84300
Sodium Glycinate, Theophylline, 80198
Sofield Procedure, 24410
Soft Tissue
  Abscess, 20005
  Image-guided drainage with catheter, 10030
Solar Plexus
  Destruction, 64680
  Injection
    Anesthetic, 64530
    Neurolytic, 64680
Solitary Cyst, Bone
  Drainage, 20615
  Injection, 20615
Somatomammotropin, Chorionic, 83632
Somatomedin, 84305
Somatosensory Testing
  Lower Limbs, 95926
  Trunk or Head, 95927
  Upper Limbs, 95925
Somatostatin, 84307
Somatotropin, 83003
  Release Inhibiting Hormone, 84307
Somatropin, 80418, 80428-80430, 86277
Somnography, 95808-95811
Somophyllin T, 80198
Sonography
  See Echography
Sonohysterography, 76831
  Saline Infusion
    Injection Procedure, 58340
Sore, Bed
  Excision, 15920-15999
SOS1, 81406
Spasm, Eyelid
  Chemodenervation, 64612
SPAST, 81405-81406
SPC11, 81407
Special Services
  After Hours Medical Services, 99050

Special Services — *continued*
  Analysis
    Remote Physiologic Data, 99091
  Computer Data Analysis, 99090
  Device Handling, 99002
  Emergency Care in Office, 99058
    Out of Office, 99060
  Extended Hours, 99051-99053
  Group Education, 99078
    Self-Management, 98961-98962
  Hyperbaric Oxygen, 99183
  Hypothermia, 99116
  Individual Education
    Self-Management, 98960
  Medical Testimony, 99075
  Non–Office Medical Services, 99056
  On Call, Hospital Mandated, 99026, 99027
  Phlebotomy, 99199
  Postoperative Visit, 99024
  Prolonged Attendance, 99354-99360
  Psychiatric, 90889
  Pump Services, 99190-99192
  Reports and Forms
    Medical, 99080
    Psychiatric, 90889
  Specimen Handling, 99000, 99001
  Supply of Materials, 99070
    Educational, 99071
  Unlisted Services and Procedures, 99199
  Unusual Travel, 99082
Special Stain, 88312-88319
Specific Gravity
  with Urinalysis, 81000-81003
  Body Fluid, 84315
Specimen Collection
  Intestines, 43756-43757
  Stomach, 43754-43755
  Venous Catheter, 36591-36592
Specimen Concentration, 87015
Specimen Handling, 99000, 99001
Specimen X–ray Examination, 76098
SPECT
  See Also Emission Computerized Tomography
  Abscess Localization, 78807
  Bone, 78320
  Brain, 78607
  Cerebrospinal Fluid, 78647
  Heart, 78451-78452
  Kidney, 78710
  Liver, 78205-78206
  Localization
    Inflammatory Process, 78807
    Tumor, 78803
Spectacle Services
  Fitting
    Low Vision Aid, 92354, 92355
    Spectacle Prosthesis, 92352, 92353
    Spectacles, 92340-92342
  Repair, 92370, 92371
Spectometry
  Mass Analyte(s), 83789
Spectrophotometry, 84311
  Atomic Absorption, 82190
Spectroscopy
  Atomic Absorption, 82190
  Bioimpedance, 93702
  Coronary Vessel or Graft, 0205T
  Magnetic Resonance, 76390
  Prostate Tissue, 0443T
  Wound, 76499
Spectrum Analyses, 84311
Speech
  Audiometry Threshold, 0210T-0211T
  Evaluation, 92521-92524
    Cine, 70371
    for Prosthesis, 92597, 92607, 92608
    Video, 70371
  Prosthesis
    Creation, 31611
    Evaluation for Speech, 92567, 92607, 92608
    Insertion, 31611
    Preparation of, 21084
    Therapy, 92507, 92508
Speech Evaluation, 92521-92524
Sperm
  Antibodies, 89325

Sperm — *continued*
Cryopreservation, 89259
Evaluation, 89329-89331
Identification
from Aspiration, 89257
from Testis Tissue, 89264
Medicolegal, 88125
Isolation, 89260-89261
Storage (per year), 89343
Thawing, 89353
Sperm Analysis
Antibodies, 89325
Cervical Mucus Penetration Test, 89330
Cryopreservation, 89259
Hamster Penetration Test, 89329
Identification
from Aspiration, 89257
from Testis Tissue, 89264
Isolation and Preparation, 89260-89261
Spermatic Cord
Hydrocele
Excision, 55500
Laparoscopy, 55559
Lesion
Excision, 55520
Repair
Veins, 55530
with Hernia Repair, 55540
Abdominal Approach, 55535
Varicocele
Excision, 55530-55540
Spermatic Veins
Excision, 55530-55540
Ligation, 55500
Spermatocele
Excision, 54840
Spermatocystectomy, 54840
Sperm Evaluation, Cervical Mucus Penetration Test, 89330
Sperm Washing, 58323
SPG7, 81405-81406
Sphenoidotomy
with Nasal
Sinus Endoscopy, 31287, 31288
Sphenoid Sinus
See Sinuses, Sphenoid
Sphenopalatine Ganglion
Injection
Anesthetic, 64505
Sphenopalatine Ganglionectomy, 64999
Sphincter
See Also Specific Sphincter
Anal
Dilation, 45905
Incision, 46080
Artificial Genitourinary, 53444-53449
Esophageal Augmentation, 43284-43285
Pyloric
Incision, 43520
Reconstruction, 43800
Sphincter of Oddi
Pressure Measurement
Endoscopy, 43263
Sphincteroplasty
Anal, 46750-46751, 46760-46761
with Implant, 46762
Bile Duct, 47460, 47542
Bladder Neck, 51800, 51845
Pancreatic, 48999
Sphincterotomy
Anal, 46080
Bile Duct, 47460
Bladder, 52277
Sphingomyelin Phosphodiesterase 1, Acid Lysosomal Gene Analysis, 81330
Spica Cast
Hip, 29305, 29325
Repair, 29720
Shoulder, 29055
Spinal Accessory Nerve
Anastomosis
to Facial Nerve, 64866
Incision, 63191
Section, 63191
Spinal Column
See Spine

Spinal Cord
Biopsy, 63275-63290
Cyst
Aspiration, 62268
Incision and Drainage, 63172, 63173
Decompression, 62380, 63001-63103
with Cervical Laminoplasty, 63050-63051
Drain Fluid, 62272
Exploration, 63001-63044
Graft
Dura, 63710
Implantation
Electrode, 63650, 63655
Pulse Generator, 63685
Receiver, 63685
Incision, 63200
Dentate Ligament, 63180-63182
Nerve Root, 63185-63190
Tract, 63170, 63194-63199
Injection
Anesthesia, 62320-62327
Blood, 62273
CT Scan, 62284
Neurolytic Agent, 62280-62282
Other, 62320-62327
X-ray, 62284
Insertion
Electrode, 63650, 63655
Pulse Generator, 63685
Receiver, 63685
Lesion
Destruction, 62280-62282
Excision, 63265-63273, 63300-63308
Needle Biopsy, 62269
Neoplasm
Excision, 63275-63290
Puncture (Tap)
Diagnostic, 62270
Drainage of Fluid, 62272
Lumbar, 62270
Reconstruction
Dorsal Spine Elements, 63295
Release, 63200
Removal
Catheter, 62355
Electrode, 63661-63662
Pulse Generator, 63688
Pump, 62365
Receiver, 63688
Reservoir, 62365
Repair
Cerebrospinal Fluid Leak, 63707-63709
Meningocele, 63700-63702
Myelomeningocele, 63704-63706
Revision
Electrode, 63663-63664
Neurostimulator, 63688
Section
Dentate Ligament, 63180, 63182
Nerve Root, 63185-63190
Tract, 63194-63199
Shunt
Create, 63740, 63741
Irrigation, 63744
Removal, 63746
Replacement, 63744
Stereotaxis
Aspiration, 63615
Biopsy, 63615
Creation Lesion, 63600
Excision Lesion, 63615
Stimulation, 63610
Syrinx
Aspiration, 62268
Tumor
Excision, 63275-63290
Spinal Cord Neoplasms
Excision, 63275-63290
Spinal Fluid
Immunoelectrophoresis, 86325
Nuclear Imagine, 78630-78650
Spinal Fracture
See Fracture, Vertebra
Spinal Instrumentation
Anterior, 22845-22847
Removal, 22855

Spinal Instrumentation — *continued*
Internal Fixation, 22841
Pelvic Fixation, 22848
Posterior Nonsegmental
Harrington Rod Technique, 22840
Harrington Rod Technique Removal, 22850
Posterior Segmental, 22842-22844
Posterior Segmental Removal, 22852
Prosthetic Device, 22853-22854, 22867-22870, [22859]
Reinsertion of Spinal Fixation Device, 22849
Spinal Manipulation, 98940-98942
Spinal Nerve
Avulsion, 64772
Transection, 64772
Spinal Tap
Cervical Puncture, 61050-61055
Cisternal Puncture, 61050-61055
Drainage of Fluid, 62272
Lumbar, 62270
Subdural Tap, 61000-61001
Ventricular Puncture, 61020-61026, 61105-61120
Spine
See Also Intervertebral Disc; Spinal Cord; Vertebra; Vertebral Body; Vertebral Process
Allograft
Morselized, 20930
Structural, 20931
Arthroplasty
Cervical, 0098T, 22856, 22861, 22864, [22858]
Lumbar, 0163T-0165T, 22857, 22862, 22865
Augmentation
Lumbar Vertebra, 22514-22515
Thoracic Vertebra, 22513, 22515
Autograft
Local, 20936
Morselized, 20937
Structural, 20938
Biopsy, 20250, 20251
CT Scan
Cervical, 72125-72127
Lumbar, 72131-72133
Thoracic, 72128-72130
Fixation, 22842
Fusion
Anterior, 22808-22812
Anterior Approach, 22548-22585, 22812
Exploration, 22830
Lateral Extracavitary, 22532-22534
Posterior Approach, 22590-22802
Incision and Drainage
Abscess, 22010-22015
Insertion
Instrumentation, 22840-22848, 22853-22854, 22867-22870, [22859]
Kyphectomy, 22818, 22819
Magnetic Resonance Angiography, 72159
Magnetic Resonance Imaging
Cervical, 72141, 72142, 72156-72158
Lumbar, 72148-72158
Thoracic, 72146, 72147, 72156-72158
Manipulation
Anesthesia, 22505
Myelography
Cervical
with Radiological Supervision and Interpretation, 62302
Radiological Supervision and Interpretation Only, 72240
Lumbosacral
with Radiological Supervision and Interpretation, 62304
Radiological Supervision and Interpretation Only, 72265
Thoracic
with Radiological Supervision and Interpretation, 62303
Radiological Supervision and Interpretation Only, 72255
Two or More Regions
with Radiological Supervision and Interpretation, 62305
Radiological Supervision and Interpretation Only, 72270

Spine — *continued*
Percutaneous Vertebral Augmentation, 22513-22515
Percutaneous Vertebroplasty, 22510-22512
Reconstruction
Dorsal Spine Elements, 63295
Reinsertion Instrumentation, 22849
Removal Instrumentation, 22850, 22852-22855
Repair, Osteotomy
Anterior, 22220-22226
Posterior, 22210-22214
Cervical Laminoplasty, 63050-63051
Posterolateral, 22216
Surgery, NOS, 22899
Ultrasound, 76800
Unlisted Services and Procedures, 22899
X-Ray, 72020
with Contrast
Cervical, 72240
Lumbosacral, 72265
Thoracic, 72255
Total, 72270
Absorptiometry, 77080
Cervical, 72040-72052
Lumbosacral, 72100-72120
Thoracic, 72070-72074
Thoracolumbar, 72080, 72084
Thoracolumbar Junction, 72080
Spine Chemotherapy
Administration, 96450
See Also Chemotherapy
Spirometry, 94010-94070
Patient Initiated, 94014-94016
sPLA2-IIA, 0423T
Splanchnicectomy, 64802-64818
Spleen
Excision, 38100-38102
Laparoscopic, 38120
Injection
Radiologic, 38200
Nuclear Medicine
Imaging, 78185, 78215, 78216
Repair, 38115
Splenectomy
Laparoscopic, 38120
Partial, 38101
Partial with Repair, Ruptured Spleen, 38115
Total, 38100
En Bloc, 38102
Splenoplasty, 38115
Splenoportography, 75810
Injection Procedures, 38200
Splenorrhaphy, 38115
Splenotomy, 38999
Splint
See Also Casting; Strapping
Arm
Long, 29105
Short, 29125-29126
Finger, 29130-29131
Leg
Long, 29505
Short, 29515
Oral Surgical, 21085
Ureteral, 50400-50405
Split Grafts, 15100-15101, 15120-15121
Split Renal Function Test, 52005
Splitting
Blood Products, 86985
SPR (Selective Posterior Rhizotomy), 63185, 63190
SPRED1, 81405
Sprengel's Deformity, 23400
Spring Water Cyst, 33050
Excision, 33050
via Thoracoscopy, 32661
SPTBN2, 81407
Spur, Bone
See Also Exostosis
Calcaneal, 28119
External Auditory Canal, 69140
Sputum Analysis, 89220
SQ, 96369-96372
SRIH, 84307
SRS (Stereotactic Radiosurgery), 61796-61800, 63620-63621

SRT (Speech Reception Threshold), 92555
SRY, 81400
SS18/SSX1, 81401
SS18/SSX2 (t(X;18)), 81401
Ssabanejew–Frank Operation
   Incision, Stomach, Creation of Stoma, 43830-43832
Stabilizing Factor, Fibrin, 85290-85291
Stable Factor, 85230
Stain
   Special, 88312-88319
Stallard Procedure
   with Tube, 68750
   without Tube, 68745
Stamey Procedure, 51845
Standby Services, Physician, 99360
Standing X–ray, 73564, 73565
Stanford-Binet Test, 96101-96103
Stanftan, 96101-96103
Stapedectomy
   with Footplate Drill Out, 69661
   without Foreign Material, 69660
   Revision, 69662
Stapedotomy
   with Footplate Drill Out, 69661
   without Foreign Material, 69660
   Revision, 69662
Stapes
   Excision
      with Footplate Drill Out, 69661
      without Foreign Material, 69660
   Mobilization
      See Mobilization, Stapes
   Release, 69650
   Revision, 69662
Staphyloma
   Sclera
      Repair
         with Graft, 66225
         without Graft, 66220
STAT3, 81405
State Operation
   Proctectomy
      Partial, 45111, 45113-45116, 45123
      Total, 45110, 45112, 45120
         with Colon, 45121
Statin Therapy, 4013F
Statistics/Biometry, 76516-76519, 92136
Steindler Stripping, 28250
Steindler Type Advancement, 24330
Stellate Ganglion
   Injection
      Anesthetic, 64510
Stem, Brain
   Biopsy, 61575-61576
   Decompression, 61575-61576
   Evoked Potentials, 92585-92586
   Lesion Excision, 61575-61576
Stem Cell
   Cell Concentration, 38215
   Count, 86367
      Total Count, 86367
   Cryopreservation, 38207, 88240
   Donor Search, 38204
   Harvesting, 38205-38206
   Limbal
      Allograft, 65781
   Plasma Depletion, 38214
   Platelet Depletion, 38213
   Red Blood Cell Depletion, 38212
   T–cell Depletion, 38210
   Thawing, 38208, 38209, 88241
   Transplantation, 38240-38242
   Tumor Cell Depletion, 38211
   Washing, 38209
Stenger Test
   Pure Tone, 92565
   Speech, 92577
Stenosis
   Aortic
      Repair, 33415
         Supravalvular, 33417
   Bronchi, 31641
      Reconstruction, 31775
   Excision
      Trachea, 31780, 31781

Stenosis — *continued*
   Laryngoplasty, *[31551, 31552, 31553, 31554]*
   Reconstruction
      Auditory Canal, External, 69310
   Repair
      Trachea, 31780, 31781
   Tracheal, 31780-31781
   Urethral Stenosis, 52281
Stenson Duct, 42507-42510
Stent
   Exchange
      Bile Duct, *[43276]*
      Pancreatic Duct, *[43276]*
   Indwelling
      Insertion
         Ureter, 50605
   Intravascular, 0075T-0076T, 37215-37218, 37236-37239
   Placement
      Bronchoscopy, 31631, 31636-31637
      Colonoscopy, 44402, 45389
      Endoscopy
         Bile Duct, *[43274]*
         Esophagus, *[43212]*
         Gastrointestinal, Upper, *[43266]*
         Pancreatic Duct, *[43274]*
      Enteroscopy, 44370
      Percutaneous
         Bile Duct, 47538-47540
      Proctosigmoidoscopy, 45327
      Sigmoidoscopy, 45347
      Transcatheter
         Intravascular, 37215-37218, 37236-37239
         Extracranial, 0075T-0076T
      Ureteroneocystomy, 50947, 50948
      Urethral, 52282, 53855
   Removal
      Bile Duct, *[43275]*
      Pancreatic Duct, *[43275]*
   Revision
      Bronchoscopy, 31638
   Spanner, 53855
   Tracheal
      via Bronchoscopy, 31631
      Revision, 31638
   Ureteral
      Insertion, 50605, 52332
      Removal, 50384, 50386
      and Replacement, 50382, 50385
   Urethra, 52282
      Insertion, 52282, 53855
      Prostatic, 53855
Stereotactic Frame
   Application
      Removal, 20660
Stereotactic Radiosurgery
   Cranial Lesion, 61797-61799
   Spinal Lesion, 63620-63621
Stereotaxis
   Aspiration
      Brain Lesion, 61750
         with CT Scan and/or MRI, 61751
      Spinal Cord, 63615
   Biopsy
      Aspiration
         Brain Lesion, 61750
      Brain, 61750
      Brain with CT Scan and/or MRI, 61751
      Breast, 19081, 19283
      Prostate, 55706
      Spinal Cord, 63615
   Catheter Placement
      Brain
         Infusion, 64999
         Radiation Source, 61770
   Computer-Assisted
      Brain Surgery, 61781-61782
      Orthopedic Surgery, 20985
      Spinal Procedure, 61783
   Creation Lesion
      Brain
         Deep, 61720-61735
         Percutaneous, 61790
      Gasserian Ganglion, 61790
      Spinal Cord, 63600

Stereotaxis — *continued*
   Creation Lesion — *continued*
      Trigeminal Tract, 61791
   CT Scan
      Aspiration, 61751
      Biopsy, 61751
   Excision Lesion
      Brain, 61750-61751
      Spinal Cord, 63615
   Focus Beam
      Radiosurgery, 61796-61800, 63620-63621
   Guidance for Localization, *[77387]*
   Implantation Depth Electrodes, 61760
   Localization
      Brain, 61770
   MRI
      Brain
         Aspiration, 61751
         Biopsy, 61751
         Excision, 61751
   Stimulation
      Spinal Cord, 63610
   Treatment Delivery, 77371-77373, 77432, 77435
Sterile Coverings
   Burns, 16020-16030
   Change
      under Anesthesia, 15852
Sternal Fracture
   Closed Treatment, 21820
   Open Treatment, 21825
Sternoclavicular Joint
   Arthrotomy, 23044
      with Biopsy, 23101
      with Synovectomy, 23106
   Dislocation
      Closed Treatment
         with Manipulation, 23525
         without Manipulation, 23520
      Open Treatment, 23530-23532
         with Fascial Graft, 23532
Sternocleidomastoid
   Division, 21720-21725
Sternotomy
   Closure, 21750
Sternum
   Debridement, 21627
   Excision, 21620, 21630-21632
   Fracture
      Closed Treatment, 21820
      Open Treatment, 21825
   Ostectomy, 21620
   Radical Resection, 21630-21632
   Reconstruction, 21740-21742, 21750
      with Thoracoscopy, 21743
   X–Ray, 71120-71130
Steroid–Binding Protein, Sex, 84270
Steroids
   Anabolic
      See Androstenedione
   Injection
      Morton's Neuroma, 64455
      Paravertebral
         Facet Joint, 64490-64495
         Paraspinous Block, *[64461, 64462, 64463]*
      Plantar Common Digital Nerve, 64455
      Sympathetic Nerves, 64505-64530
      Transforaminal Epidural, 64479-64484
      Urethral Stricture, 52283
   Ketogenic
      Urine, 83582
STG, 15100-15121
STH, 83003
Stimson's Method Reduction, 23650, 23655
Stimulating Antibody, Thyroid, 84445
Stimulation
   Electric
      See Also Electrical Stimulation
      Brain Surface, 95961-95962
   Lymphocyte, 86353
   Spinal Cord
      Stereotaxis, 63610
   Transcutaneous Electric, 64550
Stimulator, Long–Acting Thyroid, 80438-80439
Stimulators, Cardiac, 33202-33213
   See Also Heart, Pacemaker

Stimulus Evoked Response, 51792
STK11, 81404-81405, 81432-81433, 81435-81436
Stoffel Operation
   Rhizotomy, 63185, 63190
Stoma
   Closure
      Intestines, 44620
   Creation
      Bladder, 51980
      Kidney, 50551-50561
      Stomach
         Neonatal, 43831
         Permanent, 43832
         Temporary, 43830, 43831
      Ureter, 50860
   Revision
      Colostomy, 44345
      Ileostomy
         Complicated, 44314
         Simple, 44312
   Ureter
      Endoscopy via, 50951-50961
Stomach
   Anastomosis
      with Duodenum, 43810, 43850-43855
      with Jejunum, 43820-43825, 43860-43865
   Biopsy, 43605
   Creation
      Stoma
         Permanent, 43832
         Temporary, 43830-43831
            Laparoscopic, 43653
   Electrode
      Implantation, 43647, 43881
      Removal/Revision, 43882
   Electrogastrography, 91132-91133
   Excision
      Partial, 43631-43635, 43845
      Total, 43620-43622
   Exploration, 43500
   Gastric Bypass, 43644-43645, 43846-43847
      Revision, 43848
   Gastric Restrictive Procedures, 43644-43645, 43770-43774, 43842-43848, 43886-43888
   Gastropexy, 43659, 43999
   Implantation
      Electrodes, 43647, 43881
   Incision, 43830-43832
      Exploration, 43500
      Pyloric Sphincter, 43520
      Removal
         Foreign Body, 43500
   Intubation, 43753-43756
   Laparoscopy, 43647-43648
   Nuclear Medicine
      Blood Loss Study, 78278
      Emptying Study, 78264-78266
      Imaging, 78261
      Protein Loss Study, 78282
      Reflux Study, 78262
      Vitamin B–12
         Absorption, 78270-78272
   Reconstruction
      for Obesity, 43644-43645, 43842-43847
      Roux–en–Y, 43644, 43846
   Removal
      Foreign Body, 43500
   Repair, 48547
      Fistula, 43880
      Fundoplasty, 43279-43282, 43325-43328
         Laparoscopic, 43280
      Laceration, 43501, 43502
      Stoma, 43870
      Ulcer, 43501
   Specimen Collection, 43754-43755
   Suture
      Fistula, 43880
      for Obesity, 43842, 43843
      Stoma, 43870
      Ulcer, 43840
      Wound, 43840
   Tumor
      Excision, 43610, 43611
   Ulcer
      Excision, 43610

Stomach — *continued*
Unlisted Services and Procedures, 43659, 43999
Stomatoplasty
Vestibule, 40840-40845
Stone
Calculi
Bile Duct, 43264, 47420, 47425
Percutaneous, 47554
Bladder, 51050, 52310-52318, 52352
Gallbladder, 47480
Hepatic Duct, 47400
Kidney, 50060-50081, 50130, 50561, 50580, 52352
Pancreas, 48020
Pancreatic Duct, 43264
Salivary Gland, 42330-42340
Ureter, 50610-50630, 50961, 50980, 51060, 51065, 52320-52330, 52352
Urethra, 52310, 52315, 52352
Stone, Kidney
Removal, 50060-50081, 50130, 50561, 50580, 52352
Stookey–Scarff Procedure
Ventriculocisternostomy, 62200
Stool Blood, 82270, 82272-82274
Storage
Embryo, 89342
Oocyte, 89346
Reproductive Tissue, 89344
Sperm, 89343
STR, 81265-81266
Strabismus
Chemodenervation, 67345
Repair
Adjustable Sutures, 67335
Extraocular Muscles, 67340
One Horizontal Muscle, 67311
One Vertical Muscle, 67314
Posterior Fixation Suture Technique, 67334, 67335
Previous Surgery not Involving Extraocular Muscles, 67331
Release Extensive Scar Tissue, 67343
Superior Oblique Muscle, 67318
Transposition, 67320
Two Horizontal Muscles, 67312
Two or More Vertical Muscles, 67316
Strapping
See Also Cast; Splint
Ankle, 29540
Chest, 29200
Elbow, 29260
Finger, 29280
Foot, 29540
Hand, 29280
Hip, 29520
Knee, 29530
Shoulder, 29240
Thorax, 29200
Toes, 29550
Unlisted Services and Procedures, 29799
Unna Boot, 29580
Wrist, 29260
Strassman Procedure, 58540
Strayer Procedure, 27687
Strep Quick Test, 86403
Streptococcus, Group A
Antigen Detection
Enzyme Immunoassay, 87430
Nucleic Acid, 87650-87652
Direct Optical Observation, 87880
Streptococcus, Group B
by Immunoassay
with Direct Optical Observation, 87802
Streptococcus Pneumoniae Vaccine
See Vaccines
Streptokinase, Antibody, 86590
Stress Tests
Cardiovascular, 93015-93024
Echocardiography, 93350-93351
with Contrast, 93352
Multiple Gated Acquisition (MUGA), 78472, 78473
Myocardial Perfusion Imaging, 0439T, 78451-78454
Pulmonary, 94620, 94621

Stress Tests — *continued*
Pulmonary — *continued*
See Pulmonology, Diagnostic
Stricture
Ureter, 50706
Urethra
Dilation, 52281
Repair, 53400
Strictureplasty
Intestines, 44615
Stroboscopy
Larynx, 31579
STS, 86592-86593
STSG, 15100-15121
Stuart–Prower Factor, 85260
Study
Color Vision, 92283
Common Carotid Intima–media Thickness (IMT), 0126T
Implanted Wireless Pressure Sensor, 93982
Sturmdorf Procedure, 57520
STXBP1, 81406
Styloidectomy
Radial, 25230
Styloid Process
Fracture, 25645, 25650
Radial
Excision, 25230
Stypven Time, 85612-85613
Subacromial Bursa
Arthrocentesis, 20610-20611
Subarachnoid Drug Administration, 0186T, 01996
Subclavian Arteries
Aneurysm, 35001-35002, 35021-35022
Angioplasty, [37246, 37247]
Bypass Graft, 35506, 35511-35516, 35526, 35606-35616, 35626, 35645
Embolectomy, 34001-34101
Thrombectomy, 34001-34101
Thromboendarterectomy, 35301, 35311
Transposition, 33889
Unlisted Services/Procedures, 37799
Subcutaneous
Chemotherapy, 96401-96402
Infusion, 96369-96371
Injection, 96372
Subcutaneous Implantable Defibrillator Device
Electrophysiologic Evaluation, [33270]
Insertion, [33270]
Defibrillator Electrode, [33271]
Implantable Defibrillator System and Electrode, [33270]
Pulse Generator with Existing Electrode, 33240
Interrogation Device Evaluation (In Person), [93261]
Programming Device Evaluation (In Person), [93260]
Removal
Electrode Only, [33272]
Pulse Generator Only, 33241
with Replacement, [33262, 33263, 33264]
Repositioning Electrode or Pulse Generator, [33273]
Subcutaneous Mastectomies, 19304
Subcutaneous Tissue
Excision, 15830-15839, 15847
Repair
Complex, 13100-13160
Intermediate, 12031-12057
Simple, 12020, 12021
Subdiaphragmatic Abscess, 49040
Subdural Electrode
Insertion, 61531-61533
Removal, 61535
Subdural Hematoma, 61108, 61154
Subdural Puncture, 61105-61108
Subdural Tap, 61000, 61001
Sublingual Gland
Abscess
Incision and Drainage, 42310-42320
Calculi (Stone)
Excision, 42330
Cyst
Drainage, 42409

Sublingual Gland — *continued*
Cyst — *continued*
Excision, 42408
Excision, 42450
Subluxation
Elbow, 24640
Submandibular Gland
Calculi (Stone)
Excision, 42330, 42335
Excision, 42440
Submaxillary Gland
Abscess
Incision and Drainage, 42310-42320
Submental Fat Pad
Excision
Excess Skin, 15838
Submucous Resection of Nasal Septum, 30520
Subperiosteal Implant
Reconstruction
Mandible, 21245, 21246
Maxilla, 21245, 21246
Subphrenic Abscess, 49040
Substance and/or Alcohol Abuse Screening and Intervention, 99408-99409
Substance S, Reichstein's, 80436, 82634
Substitute Skin Application, 15271-15278
Subtalar Joint Stabilization, 0335T
Subtrochanteric Fracture
with Implant, 27244-27245
Closed Treatment, 27238
with Manipulation, 27240
Sucrose Hemolysis Test, 85555-85557
Suction Lipectomies, 15876-15879
Sudiferous Gland
Excision
Axillary, 11450-11451
Inguinal, 11462-11463
Perianal, 11470-11471
Perineal, 11470-11471
Umbilical, 11470-11471
Sugars, 84375-84379
Sugar Water Test, 85555-85557
Sugiura Procedure
Esophagus, Repair, Varices, 43401
Sulfate
Chondroitin, 82485
DHA, 82627
Urine, 84392
Sulfation Factor, 84305
Sulphates
Chondroitin, 82485
DHA, 82627
Urine, 84392
Sumatran Mite Fever, 86000
Sunrise View X-Ray, 73560-73564
Superficial Musculoaponeurotic Systems (SMAS) Flap
Rhytidectomy, 15829
Supernumerary Digit
Reconstruction, 26587
Repair, 26587
Supervision
Home Health Agency Patient, 99374-99375
Supply
Chemotherapeutic Agent
See Chemotherapy
Educational Materials, 99071
Low Vision Aids
Fitting, 92354-92355
Repair, 92370
Materials, 99070
Prosthesis
Breast, 19396
Suppositories, Vaginal, 57160
for Induced Abortion, 59855-59857
Suppression, 80400-80408
Suppression/Testing, 80400-80439
Suppressor T Lymphocyte Marker, 86360
Suppurative Hidradenitis
Incision and Drainage, 10060-10061
Suprachoroidal Injection, 0465T
Suprahyoid
Lymphadenectomy, 38700
Supraorbital Nerve
Avulsion, 64732
Incision, 64732

Supraorbital Nerve — *continued*
Transection, 64732
Supraorbital Rim and Forehead
Reconstruction, 21179-21180
Suprapubic Prostatectomies, 55821
Suprarenal
Gland
Biopsy, 60540-60545, 60650
Excision, 60540-60545, 60650
Exploration, 60540-60545, 60650
Nuclear Medicine Imaging, 78075
Vein
Venography, 75840-75842
Suprascapular Nerve
Injection
Anesthetic, 64418
Suprasellar Cyst, 61545
SURF1, 81405
Surface CD4 Receptor, 86360
Surface Radiotherapy, 77789
Surgeries
Breast–Conserving, 19120-19126, 19301
Laser
Anus, 46614, 46917
Bladder/Urethra, 52214-52240
Esophagus, 43227
Lacrimal Punctum, 68760
Lens, Posterior, 66821
Lesion
Mouth, 40820
Nose, 30117-30118
Penis, 54057
Skin, 17000-17111, 17260-17286
Myocardium, 33140-33141
Prostate, 52647-52648
Spine, 62287
Mohs, 17311-17315
Repeat
Cardiac Valve Procedure, 33530
Carotid Thromboendarterectomy, 35390
Coronary Artery Bypass, 33530
Distal Vessel Bypass, 35700
Surgical
Avulsion
Nails, 11730-11732
Nerve, 64732-64772
Cartilage
Excision, 21060
Cataract Removal, 3073F, 66830, 66982-66984
Collapse Therapy, Thoracoplasty, 32905-32906
Diathermy
Ciliary Body, 66700
Lesions
Benign, 17000-17111
Malignant, 17260-17286
Premalignant, 17000-17111
Galvanism, 17380
Incision
See Incision
Meniscectomy, 21060
Microscopes, 69990
Pathology
See Pathology, Surgical
Planing
Nose
Skin, 30120
Pneumoperitoneum, 49400
Removal, Eye
with Implant, 65103-65105
without Implant, 65101
Revision
Cardiac Valve Procedure, 33530
Carotid Thromboendarterectomy, 35390
Coronary Artery Bypass, 33530
Distal Vessel Bypass, 35700
Services
Postoperative Visit, 99024
Ventricular Restoration, 33548
Surgical Correction
Uterus
Inverted, 59899
Surgical Services
Post–Operative Visit, 99024
Surveillance
See Monitoring

Suspension
Aorta, 33800
Hyoid, 21685
Kidney, 50400-50405
Tongue Base, 41512
Urethra, 51990, 57289
Uterine, 58400-58410
Vagina, 57280-57283, 57425
Vesical Neck, 51845
Suture
See Also Repair
Abdomen, 49900
Anus, 46999
Aorta, 33320, 33321
Bile Duct
Wound, 47900
Bladder
Fistulization, 44660-44661, 45800-45805,
51880-51925
Vesicouterine, 51920-51925
Vesicovaginal, 51900
Wound, 51860-51865
Cervix, 57720
Colon
Diverticula, 44604-44605
Fistula, 44650-44661
Plication, 44680
Stoma, 44620-44625
Ulcer, 44604-44605
Wound, 44604-44605
Esophagus
Wound, 43410, 43415
Eyelid, 67880
with Transposition of Tarsal Plate, 67882
Closure of, 67875
Wound
Full Thickness, 67935
Partial Thickness, 67930
Facial Nerve
Intratemporal
Lateral to Geniculate Ganglion, 69740
Medial to Geniculate Ganglion, 69745
Fallopian Tube
Simple, 58999
Foot
Tendon, 28200-28210
Gastroesophageal, 43405
Great Vessel, 33320-33322
Hemorrhoids, [46945], [46946]
Hepatic Duct, 47765, 47802
Intestines
Large, 44604-44605
Small, 44602-44603
Fistula, 44640-44661
Plication, 44680
Stoma, 44620-44625
Iris
with Ciliary Body, 66682
Kidney
Fistula, 50520-50526
Horseshoe, 50540
Wound, 50500
Leg, Lower
Tendon, 27658-27665
Leg, Upper
Muscles, 27385, 27386
Liver
Wound, 47350-47361
Mesentery, 44850
Nerve, 64831-64876
Pancreas, 48545
Pharynx
Wound, 42900
Rectum
Fistula, 45800-45825
Prolapse, 45540, 45541
Removal
Anesthesia, 15850, 15851
Spleen, 38115
Stomach
Fistula, 43880
Laceration, 43501, 43502
Stoma, 43870
Ulcer, 43501, 43840
Wound, 43840

Suture — *continued*
Tendon
Foot, 28200-28210
Knee, 27380, 27381
Testis
Injury, 54670
Suspension, 54620, 54640
Thoracic Duct
Abdominal Approach, 38382
Cervical Approach, 38380
Thoracic Approach, 38381
Throat
Wound, 42900
Tongue
to Lip, 41510
Trachea
Fistula, 31825
with Plastic Repair, 31825
without Plastic Repair, 31820
Stoma, 31825
with Plastic Repair, 31825
without Plastic Repair, 31820
Wound
Cervical, 31800
Intrathoracic, 31805
Ulcer, 44604-44605
Ureter, 50900, 50940
Deligation, 50940
Fistula, 50920-50930
Urethra
Fistula, 45820-45825, 53520
Stoma, 53520
to Bladder, 51840-51841
Wound, 53502-53515
Uterus
Fistula, 51920-51925
Rupture, 58520, 59350
Suspension, 58400-58410
Vagina
Cystocele, 57240, 57260
Enterocele, 57265
Fistula
Rectovaginal, 57300-57307
Transvesical and Vaginal Approach,
57330
Urethrovaginal, 57310-57311
Vesicovaginal, 51900, 57320-57330
Rectocele, 57250-57260
Suspension, 57280-57283
Wound, 57200-57210
Vas Deferens, 55400
Vein
Femoral, 37650
Iliac, 37660
Vena Cava, 37619
Wound, 44604-44605
Skin
Complex, 13100-13160
Intermediate, 12031-12057
Simple, 12020-12021
SUZI (Sub-Zonal Insemination), 89280
SVR (Surgical Ventricular Restoration), 33548
Swallowing
Cine, 74230
Evaluation, 92610-92613, 92616-92617
Therapy, 92526
Video, 74230
Swan-Ganz Catheter Insertion, 93503
Swanson Procedure
Repair, Metatarsal, 28322
Osteotomy, 28306-28309
Sweat Collection
Iontophoresis, 89230
Sweat Glands
Excision
Axillary, 11450, 11451
Inguinal, 11462, 11463
Perianal, 11470, 11471
Perineal, 11470, 11471
Umbilical, 11470, 11471
Sweat Test
Chloride, Blood, 82435
Swenson Procedure, 45120
Syme Procedure, 27888
Sympathectomy
with Rib Excision, 21616

Sympathectomy — *continued*
Artery
Digital, 64820
Radial, 64821
Superficial Palmar Arch, 64823
Ulnar, 64822
Cervical, 64802
Cervicothoracic, 64804
Digital Artery with Magnification, 64820
Lumbar, 64818
Presacral, 58410
Renal, 0338T-0339T
Thoracic, 32664
Thoracolumbar, 64809
Sympathetic Nerve
Excision, 64802-64818
Injection
Anesthetic, 64508, 64520-64530
Sympathins, 80424, 82382-82384
Symphysiotomy
Horseshoe Kidney, 50540
Symphysis, Pubic, 27282
Synagis, 90378
Syncytial Virus, Respiratory
Antibody, 86756
Antigen Detection
Direct Fluorescence, 87280
Direct Optical Observation, 87807
Enzyme Immunoassay, 87420
Syndactylism, Toes, 28280
Syndactyly
Repair, 26560-26562
Syndesmotomy
Coracoacromial
Arthroscopic, 29826
Open, 23130, 23415
Lateral Retinacular
Endoscopic, 29873
Open, 27425
Transverse Carpal, 29848
Syndrome
Adrenogenital, 56805, 57335
Ataxia–Telangiectasia
Chromosome Analysis, 88248
Bloom
Chromosome Analysis, 88245
Genomic Sequence Analysis, 81412
Carpal Tunnel
Decompression, 64721
Costen's
See Temporomandibular Joint (TMJ)
Erb–Goldflam, 95857
Ovarian Vein
Ureterolysis, 50722
Synechiae, Intrauterine
Lysis, 58559
Treacher Collins
Midface Reconstruction, 21150-21151
Urethral
Cystourethroscopy, 52285
Syngesterone, 84144
Synostosis (Cranial)
Bifrontal Craniotomy, 61557
Extensive Craniectomy, 61558-61559
Frontal Craniotomy, 61556
Parietal Craniotomy, 61556
Synovectomy
Arthrotomy with
Glenohumeral Joint, 23105
Sternoclavicular Joint, 23106
Elbow, 24102
Excision
Carpometacarpal Joint, 26130
Finger Joint, 26135-26140
Hip Joint, 27054
Interphalangeal Joint, 26140
Knee Joint, 27334-27335
Metacarpophalangeal Joint, 26135
Palm, 26145
Wrist, 25105, 25115-25119
Radical, 25115-25116
Synovial
Bursa
See Also Bursa
Joint Aspiration, 20600-20611

Synovial — *continued*
Cyst
See Also Ganglion
Aspiration, 20612
Membrane
See Synovium
Popliteal Space, 27345
Synovium
Biopsy
Carpometacarpal Joint, 26100
Interphalangeal Joint, 26110
Knee Joint, 27330
Metacarpophalangeal Joint
with Synovial Biopsy, 26105
Excision
Carpometacarpal Joint, 26130
Finger Joint, 26135-26140
Hip Joint, 27054
Interphalangeal Joint, 26140
Knee Joint, 27334-27335
Syphilis Nontreponemal Antibody, 86592-86593
Syphilis Test, 86592, 86593
Syrinx
Spinal Cord
Aspiration, 62268
System
Auditory, 69000-69979
Cardiac Contractility Modulation, 0408T-0418T
Cardiovascular, 33010-37799 [33221, 33227,
33228, 33229, 33230, 33231, 33262,
33263, 33264, 33270, 33271, 33272,
33273, 33962, 33963, 33964, 33965,
33966, 33969, 33984, 33985, 33986,
33987, 33988, 33989, 37211, 37212,
37213, 37214]
Digestive, 40490-49999 [43211, 43212, 43213,
43214, 43233, 43266, 43270, 43274,
43275, 43276, 43277, 43278, 44381,
44401, 45346, 45388, 45390, 45398,
45399, 46220, 46320, 46945, 46946,
46947]
Endocrine, 60000-60699
Eye/Ocular Adnexa, 65091-68899 [67810]
Genital
Female, 56405-58999
Male, 54000-55899
Hemic/Lymphatic, 38100-38999
Integumentary, 10040-19499 [11045, 11046]
Mediastinum/Diaphragm, 39000-39599
Musculoskeletal, 20005-29999 [21552, 21554,
22858, 23071, 23073, 24071, 24073,
25071, 25073, 26111, 26113, 27043,
27045, 27059, 27329, 27337, 27339,
27632, 27634, 28039, 28041, 29914,
29915, 29916]
Nervous, 61000-64999 [64633, 64634, 64635,
64636]
Neurostimulator
Central Sleep Apnea, 0424T-0436T
Respiratory, 30000-32999 [31651]
Urinary, 50010-53899 [51797, 52356]

T

T–3, 84480
T3 Free, 84481
T–4
T Cells, 86360-86361
Thyroxine, 84436-84439
T4 Molecule, 86360
T4 Total, 84436
T–7 Index
Thyroxine, Total, 84436
Triiodothyronine, 84480-84482
T–8, 86360
Taarnhoj Procedure
Decompression, Gasserian Ganglion, Sensory
Root, 61450
Tachycardia
Heart
Recording, 93609
TACO1, 81404
Tacrolimus
Assay, 80197
Tactile Breast Imaging, 0422T
Tag
Anus, 46230 [46220]

Tag — *continued*
  Skin Removal, 11200-11201
TAH, 51925, 58150, 58152, 58200-58240, 58951, 59525
TAHBSO, 58150, 58152, 58200-58240, 58951
Tail Bone
  Excision, 27080
  Fracture, 27200, 27202
Takeuchi Procedure, 33505
Talectomy, 28130
Talotarsal Joint
  Dislocation, 28570, 28575, 28585
  Percutaneous Fixation, 28576
Talus
  Arthrodesis
    Pantalar, 28705
    Subtalar, 28725
    Triple, 28715
  Arthroscopy
    Surgical, 29891, 29892
  Craterization, 28120
  Cyst
    Excision, 28100-28103
  Diaphysectomy, 28120
  Excision, 28120, 28130
  Fracture
    with Manipulation, 28435, 28436
    without Manipulation, 28430
    Open Treatment, 28445
    Percutaneous Fixation, 28436
  Osteochondral Graft, 28446
  Repair
    Osteochondritis Dissecans, 29892
    Osteotomy, 28302
  Saucerization, 28120
  Tumor
    Excision, 27647, 28100-28103
Tap
  Cisternal, 61050-61055
  Lumbar Diagnostic, 62270
TARDBP, 81405
Tarsal
  Fracture
    Percutaneous Fixation, 28456
Tarsal Bone
  See Ankle Bone
Tarsal Joint
  See Also Foot
  Arthrodesis, 28730, 28735, 28740
    with Advancement, 28737
    with Lengthening, 28737
  Craterization, 28122
  Cyst
    Excision, 28104-28107
  Diaphysectomy, 28122
  Dislocation, 28540, 28545, 28555
    Percutaneous Fixation, 28545, 28546
  Excision, 28116, 28122
  Fracture
    with Manipulation, 28455, 28456
    without Manipulation, 28450
    Open Treatment, 28465
  Fusion, 28730, 28735, 28740
    with Advancement, 28737
    with Lengthening, 28737
  Repair, 28320
    Osteotomy, 28304, 28305
  Saucerization, 28122
  Tumor
    Excision, 28104-28107, 28171
Tarsal Strip Procedure, 67917, 67924
Tarsal Tunnel Release, 28035
Tarsal Wedge Procedure, 67916, 67923
Tarsometatarsal Joint
  Arthrodesis, 28730, 28735, 28740
  Arthrotomy, 28020, 28050
  Biopsy
    Synovial, 28050, 28052
  Dislocation, 28600, 28605, 28615
    Percutaneous Fixation, 28606
  Exploration, 28020
  Fusion, 28730, 28735, 28740
  Removal
    Foreign Body, 28020
    Loose Body, 28020

Tarsometatarsal Joint — *continued*
  Synovial
    Biopsy, 28050
    Excision, 28070
Tarsorrhaphy, 67875
  Median, 67880
  Severing, 67710
    with Transposition of Tarsal Plate, 67882
Tattoo
  Cornea, 65600
  Skin, 11920-11922
Tay-Sachs Disease
  Genomic Sequence Analysis, 81412
TAZ, 81406
TB, 87015, 87116, 87190
TBG, 84442
TBNA (Transbronchial Needle Aspiration), 31629, 31633
TBP, 81401
TBS, 88164, 88166
TB Test
  Antigen Response, 86480
  Cell Mediated Immunity Measurement, 86480-86481
  Skin Test, 86580
TBX5, 81405
TCD (Transcranial Doppler), 93886-93893
TCD@, 81402
T Cell
  Antigen Receptor
    Beta Gene Rearrangement Analysis, 81340-81341
    Gamma Gene Rearrangement Analysis, 81342
  Leukemia Lymphoma Virus I, 86687, 86689
  Leukemia Lymphoma Virus II, 86688
T-Cell T8 Antigens, 86360
TCF4, 81405-81406
TCT, 85670
Tear Duct
  See Lacrimal Gland
Tear Film Imaging, 0330T
Tear Gland
  See Lacrimal Gland
Technique
  Pericardial Window, 33015
TEE, 93312-93318
Teeth
  X-ray, 70300-70320
Telangiectasia
  Chromosome Analysis, 88248
  Injection, 36468
Telangiectasia, Cerebello–Oculocutaneous
  Chromosome Analysis, 88248
Telephone
  Non-Face-to-Face
    Consult Physician, 99446-99449
    Nonphysician, 98966-98968
    Physician, 99441-99443
  Pacemaker Analysis, 93293
Teletherapy
  Dose Plan, 77306-77321
Temperature Gradient Studies, 93740
Temporal Arteries
  Biopsy, 37609
  Ligation, 37609
Temporal, Bone
  Electromagnetic Bone Conduction Hearing Device
    Implantation/Replacement, 69710
    Removal/Repair, 69711
  Excision, 69535
  Resection, 69535
  Tumor
    Removal, 69970
  Unlisted Services and Procedures, 69979
Temporal, Petrous
  Excision
    Apex, 69530
Temporomandibular Joint (TMJ)
  Arthrocentesis, 20605-20606
  Arthrography, 70328-70332
    Injection, 21116
  Arthroplasty, 21240-21243
  Arthroscopy
    Diagnostic, 29800

Temporomandibular Joint (TMJ) — *continued*
  Arthroscopy — *continued*
    Surgical, 29804
  Arthrotomy, 21010
  Cartilage
    Excision, 21060
  Condylectomy, 21050
  Coronoidectomy, 21070
  Dislocation
    Closed Treatment, 21480, 21485
    Open Treatment, 21490
  Injection
    Radiologic, 21116
  Magnetic Resonance Imaging, 70336
  Manipulation, 21073
  Meniscectomy, 21060
  Prostheses, 21243
  Reconstruction, 21240-21243
  X-ray with Contrast, 70328-70332
Tenago Procedure, 53431
Tendinosuture
  Foot, 28200-28210
  Knee, 27380-27381
Tendon
  Achilles
    Incision, 27605-27606
    Lengthening, 27612
    Repair, 27650-27654
  Arm, Upper
    Revision, 24320
  Finger
    Excision, 26180
  Forearm
    Repair, 25260-25274
  Graft
    Harvesting, 20924
  Insertion
    Biceps Tendon, 24342
  Lengthening
    Ankle, 27685, 27686
    Arm, Lower, 25280
    Arm, Upper, 24305
    Elbow, 24305
    Finger, 26476, 26478
    Forearm, 25280
    Hand, 26476, 26478
    Leg, Lower, 27685, 27686
    Leg, Upper, 27393-27395
    Toe, 28240
    Wrist, 25280
  Palm
    Excision, 26170
  Release
    Arm, Lower, 25295
    Arm, Upper, 24332
    Wrist, 25295
  Shortening
    Ankle, 27685, 27686
    Finger, 26477, 26479
    Hand, 26477, 26479
    Leg, Lower, 27685, 27686
  Transfer
    Arm, Lower, 25310, 25312, 25316
    Arm, Upper, 24301
    Elbow, 24301
    Finger, 26497, 26498
    Hand, 26480-26489
    Leg, Lower, 27690-27692
    Leg, Upper, 27400
    Pelvis, 27098
    Thumb, 26490, 26492, 26510
    Wrist, 25310, 25312, 25316, 25320
  Transplant
    Leg, Upper, 27396, 27397
  Wrist
    Repair, 25260-25274
Tendon Origin
  Insertion
    Injection, 20551
Tendon Pulley Reconstruction of Hand, 26500-26502
Tendon Sheath
  Arm
    Lower
      Repair, 25275

Tendon Sheath — *continued*
  Finger
    Incision, 26055
    Incision and Drainage, 26020
    Lesion, 26160
  Foot
    Excision, 28086, 28088
  Hand
    Lesion, 26160
  Injection, 20550
  Palm
    Incision and Drainage, 26020
  Removal
    Foreign Body, 20520, 20525
  Wrist
    Excision, 25115, 25116
    Incision, 25000, 25001
    Repair, 25275
Tendon Shortening
  Ankle, 27685, 27686
  Leg, Lower, 27685, 27686
Tenectomy, Tendon Sheath
  Foot, 28090
  Forearm/Wrist, 25110
  Hand/Finger, 26160
  Leg/Ankle, 27630
Tennis Elbow
  Repair, 24357-24359
Tenodesis
  Biceps Tendon
    at Elbow, 24340
    at Shoulder, 23430, 29828
  Finger, 26471, 26474
  Wrist, 25300, 25301
Tenolysis
  Ankle, 27680, 27681
  Arm, Lower, 25295
  Arm, Upper, 24332
  Finger
    Extensor, 26445, 26449
    Flexor, 26440, 26442
  Foot, 28220-28226
  Hand
    Extensor, 26445, 26449
    Flexor, 26440, 26442
  Leg, Lower, 27680, 27681
  Wrist, 25295
Tenomyotomy, 23405, 23406
Tenon's Capsule
  Injection, 67515
Tenoplasty
  Anesthesia, 01714
Tenorrhaphy
  Foot, 28200-28210, 28270
  Knee, 27380-27381
Tenosuspension
  at Wrist, 25300-25301
  Biceps, 29828
    at Elbow, 24340
    Long Tendon, 23430
  Interphalangeal Joint, 26471-26474
Tenosuture
  Foot, 28200-28210
  Knee, 27380-27381
Tenosynovectomy, 26145, 27626
Tenotomy
  Achilles Tendon, 27605, 27606
  Anesthesia, 01712
  Ankle, 27605, 27606
  Arm, Lower, 25290
  Arm, Upper, 24310
  Elbow, 24357
  Finger, 26060, 26455, 26460
  Foot, 28230, 28234
  Hand, 26450, 26460
  Hip
    Abductor, 27006
    Adductor, 27000-27003
    Iliopsoas Tendon, 27005
  Leg, Upper, 27306, 27307, 27390-27392
  Toe, 28010, 28011, 28232, 28234, 28240
  Wrist, 25290
TENS, 64550, 97014, 97032
Tensilon Test, 95857
TEP (Tracheoesophageal Puncture), 31611
Terman–Merrill Test, 96101-96103

Termination, Pregnancy
See Abortion
TEST (Tubal Embryo Stage Transfer), 58974
Tester, Color Vision, 92283
Testes
Cryopreservation, 89335
Nuclear Medicine
Imaging, 78761
Undescended
Exploration, 54550-54560
Testicular Vein
Excision, 55530-55540
Ligation, 55530-55540, 55550
Testimony, Medical, 99075
Testing
Acoustic Immittance, 92570
Actigraphy, 95803
Cognitive Performance, 96125
Developmental, 96111
Drug, Presumptive, [80305, 80306, 80307]
Neurobehavioral, 96116
Neuropsychological, 96118-96120
Psychological, 96101-96103
Range of Motion
Extremities, 95851
Eye, 92018-92019
Hand, 95852
Rectum
Biofeedback, 90911
Trunk, 97530
Testing, Histocompatibility, 86812-86817, 86821-86822
Testis
Abscess
Incision and Drainage, 54700
Biopsy, 54500, 54505
Cryopreservation, 89335
Excision
Laparoscopic, 54690
Partial, 54522
Radical, 54530, 54535
Simple, 54520
Hematoma
Incision and Drainage, 54700
Insertion
Prosthesis, 54660
Lesion
Excision, 54512
Needle Biopsy, 54500
Nuclear Medicine
Imaging, 78761
Repair
Injury, 54670
Suspension, 54620, 54640
Torsion, 54600
Suture
Injury, 54670
Suspension, 54620, 54640
Transplantation
to Thigh, 54680
Tumor
Excision, 54530, 54535
Undescended
Exploration, 54550, 54560
Unlisted Services and Procedures, 54699, 55899
Testosterone, 84402
Bioavailable, Direct, 84410
Response, 80414
Stimulation, 80414, 80415
Total, 84403
Testosterone Estradiol Binding Globulin, 84270
Test Tube Fertilization, 58321-58322
Tetanus, 86280
Antibody, 86774
Immunoglobulin, 90389
Tetanus Immunization, 90698-90702, 90714-90715, 90723
Tetralogy of Fallot, 33692-33697, 33924
TGFBR1, 81405, 81410-81411
TGFBR2, 81405, 81410-81411
TH, 81406
THA, 27130-27134
Thal–Nissen Procedure, 43325
THAP1, 81404

Thawing
Cryopreserved
Embryo, 89352
Oocytes, 89356
Reproductive Tissue, 89354
Sperm, 89353
Previously Frozen Cells, 38208, 38209
Thawing and Expansion
of Frozen Cell, 88241
THBR, 84479
Theleplasty, 19350
Theophylline
Assay, 80198
TheraCys, 90586
Therapeutic
Abortion, 59850-59852
Apheresis, 36511-36516
Drug Assay
See Drug Assay
Mobilization
See Mobilization
Photopheresis
See Photopheresis
Radiology
See Radiation Therapy
Therapeutic Activities
Music
Per 15 Minutes, 97530
Therapies
Actinotherapy, 96900
Cold
See Cryotherapy
Exercise, 97110-97113
Family, 99510
Psychotherapy, 90846-90849
Language, 92507-92508
Milieu, 90882
Occupational
Evaluation, [97165, 97166, 97167, 97168]
Photodynamic, 67221, 96567-96571
See Photochemotherapy
Physical
See Physical Medicine/ Therapy/ Occupational Therapy
Rhinophototherapy, 30999
Speech, 92507-92508
Tocolytic, 59412
Ultraviolet Light, 96900
Therapy
ACE Inhibitor Therapy, 4010F
Bone Marrow Cell, 0263T-0264T
Desensitization, 95180
Evaluation
Athletic Training, [97169, 97170, 97171, 97172]
Occupational, [97165, 97166, 97167, 97168]
Physical, [97161, 97162, 97163, 97164]
Hemodialysis
See Hemodialysis
Hot Pack, 97010
Pharmacologic, for Cessation of Tobacco Use, 4001F
Radiation
Blood Products, 86945
Speech, 92507-92508
Statin Therapy, Prescribed, 4013F
Vagus Nerve, 0312T-0317T
Warfarin, 4012F
Thermocauterization
Ectropion
Repair, 67922
Lesion
Cornea, 65450
Thermocoagulation, 17000-17286
Thermotherapy
Prostate, 53850-53852
Microwave, 53850
Radiofrequency, 53852
Thiamine, 84425
Thiersch Operation
Pinch Graft, 15050
Thiersch Procedure, 46753
Thigh
Excision
Excess Skin, 15832

Thigh — continued
Excision — continued
Tumor, 27327-27328 [27337, 27339], 27355-27358, 27364-27365 [27329]
Fasciotomy, 27025
ThinPrep, 88142
Thiocyanate, 84430
Thompson Procedure, 27430
Thompson Test
Smear and Stain, Routine, 87205
Urinalysis, Glass Test, 81020
Thoracectomy, 32905-32906
Thoracic
Anterior Ramus
Anesthetic Injection, 64400-64421
Destruction, 64620
Neurolytic Injection, 64620
Arteries
Catheterization, 36215-36218
Cavity
Bypass Graft Excision, 35905
Endoscopy
Exploration, 32601-32606
Surgical, 32650-32674
Duct
Cannulation, 38794
Ligation, 38380
Abdominal Approach, 38382
Thoracic Approach, 38381
Suture, 38380
Abdominal Approach, 38382
Cervical Approach, 38380
Thoracic Approach, 38381
Empyema
Incision and Drainage, 21501-21502
Surgery
Video–Assisted
See Thoracoscopy
Vertebra
See Also Vertebra, Thoracic
Corpectomy, 63085-63101, 63103
Intraspinal Lesion, 63300-63308
Decompression, 62380, 63055, 63057, 63064-63066
Discectomy, 63077-63078
Excision for Lesion, 22101, 22112
Injection Procedure
Diagnostic/Therapeutic, 62320-62327
for Discography, 62291
for Neurolysis, 62280-62282
Paravertebral, 64490-64495, [64461, 64462, 64463]
Laminectomy, 63003, 63016, 63046, 63048
Wall
See Chest Wall
Thoracoplasty, 32905
with Closure Bronchopleural Fistula, 32906
Thoracoscopy
Biopsy, 32604, 32607-32609
Diagnostic, 32601, 32604, 32606
Surgical, 32650-32674
Control Traumatic Hemorrhage, 32654
Creation Pericardial Window, 32659
Esophagomyotomy, 32665
Excision
Mediastinal Cyst, Tumor and/or Mass, 32662
Pericardial Cyst, Tumor and/or Mass, 32661
Lymphadenectomy, 32674
Parietal Pleurectomy, 32656
Partial Pulmonary Decortication, 32651
Pleurodesis, 32650
Removal
Clot, 32658
Foreign Body, 32653, 32658
Lung, 32671
Single Lobe, 32663
Single Lung Segment, 32669
Two Lobes, 32670
Resection
Thymus, 32673
Resection-Plication
Bullae, 32655
Emphysematous Lung, 32672
Sternum Reconstruction, 21743

Thoracoscopy — continued
Surgical — continued
Thoracic Sympathectomy, 32664
Total Pulmonary Decortication, 32652
Wedge Resection, 32666-32668
Thoracostomy
Empyema, 32035, 32036
Tube, 32551
Thoracotomy
Biopsy, 32096-32098
Cardiac Massage, 32160
Cyst Removal, 32140
Esophagogastric Fundoplasty, 43328
Exploration, 32100
for Postoperative Complications, 32120
Hemorrhage, 32110
Hiatal Hernia Repair, 43334-43335
Neonatal, 39503
Lung Repair, 32110
Open Intrapleural Pneumolysis, 32124
Removal
Bullae, 32141
Cyst, 32140
Defibrillator, 33243
Electrodes, 33238
Foreign Body
Intrapleural, 32150
Intrapulmonary, 32151
Pacemaker, 33236, 33237
Resection-Plication of Bullae, 32141
Transmyocardial Laser Revascularization, 33140, 33141
Wedge Resection, 32505-32507
Thorax
See Also Chest; Chest Cavity; Mediastinum
Angiography, 71275
Biopsy, 21550
CT Scan, 71250-71275
Incision
Empyema, 32035, 32036
Pneumothorax, 32551
Incision and Drainage
Abscess, 21501, 21502
Deep, 21510
Hematoma, 21501, 21502
Strapping, 29200
Tumor, 21555-21558 [21552, 21554]
Unlisted Services and Procedures, 21899
THRB, 81405
Three–Day Measles
Antibody, 86762
Vaccine, 90707-90710
Three Glass Test
Urinalysis, Glass Test, 81020
Throat
See Also Pharynx
Abscess
Incision and Drainage, 42700-42725
Biopsy, 42800-42806
Hemorrhage, 42960-42962
Reconstruction, 42950
Removal
Foreign Body, 42809
Repair
Pharyngoesophageal, 42953
Wound, 42900
Suture
Wound, 42900
Unlisted Services and Procedures, 42999
Thrombectomy
Aortoiliac Artery, 34151, 34201
Arterial, Mechanical, 37184-37185
Arteriovenous Fistula
Graft, 36904-36906
Axillary Artery, 34101
Axillary Vein, 34490
Brachial Artery, 34101
Bypass Graft, 35875, 35876
Noncoronary/Nonintracranial, 37184-37186
Carotid Artery, 34001
Celiac Artery, 34151
Dialysis Circuit, 36904-36906
Dialysis Graft
without Revision, 36831
Femoral, 34201
Femoropopliteal Vein, 34421, 34451

Thrombectomy — *continued*
Iliac Artery, 34151, 34201
Iliac Vein, 34401-34451
Innominate Artery, 34001-34101
Intracranial, Percutaneous, 61645
Mesenteric Artery, 34151
Percutaneous
Coronary Artery, [92973]
Noncoronary, Nonintracranial, 37184-37186
Vein, 37187-37188
Peroneal Artery, 34203
Popliteal Artery, 34203
Radial Artery, 34111
Renal Artery, 34151
Subclavian Artery, 34001-34101
Subclavian Vein, 34471, 34490
Tibial Artery, 34203
Ulnar Artery, 34111
Vena Cava, 34401-34451
Vena Caval, 50230
Venous, Mechanical, 37187-37188
Thrombin Inhibitor I, 85300-85301
Thrombin Time, 85670, 85675
Thrombocyte (Platelet)
Aggregation, 85576
Automated Count, 85049
Count, 85008
Manual Count, 85032
Thrombocyte ab, 86022-86023
Thromboendarterectomy
See Also Thrombectomy
Aorta, Abdominal, 35331
Aortoiliofemoral Artery, 35363
Axillary Artery, 35321
Brachial Artery, 35321
Carotid Artery, 35301, 35390
Celiac Artery, 35341
Femoral Artery, 35302, 35371-35372
Iliac Artery, 35351, 35361, 35363
Iliofemoral Artery, 35355, 35363
Innominate Artery, 35311
Mesenteric Artery, 35341
Peroneal Artery, 35305-35306
Popliteal Artery, 35303
Renal Artery, 35341
Subclavian Artery, 35301, 35311
Tibial Artery, 35305-35306
Vertebral Artery, 35301
Thrombokinase, 85260
Thrombolysin, 85400
Thrombolysis
Cerebral
Intravenous Infusion, 37195
Coronary Vessels, [92975, 92977]
Cranial Vessels, 37195
Intracranial, 61645
Other Than Coronary or Intracranial, [37211, 37212, 37213, 37214]
Thrombolysis Biopsy Intracranial
Arterial Perfusion, 61624
Thrombolysis Intracranial, 61645, 65205
See Also Ciliary Body; Cornea; Eye, Removal, Foreign Body; Iris; Lens; Retina; Sclera; Vitreous
Thrombomodulin, 85337
Thromboplastin
Inhibition, 85705
Inhibition Test, 85347
Partial Time, 85730, 85732
Thromboplastin Antecedent, Plasma, 85270
Thromboplastinogen, 85210-85293
Thromboplastinogen B, 85250
Thromboxane Metabolite(s), 84431
Thumb
Amputation, 26910-26952
Arthrodesis
Carpometacarpal Joint, 26841, 26842
Dislocation
with Fracture, 26645, 26650
Open Treatment, 26665
with Manipulation, 26641
Fracture
with Dislocation, 26645, 26650
Open Treatment, 26665

Thumb — *continued*
Fusion
in Opposition, 26820
Reconstruction
from Finger, 26550
Opponensplasty, 26490-26496
Repair
Muscle, 26508
Muscle Transfer, 26494
Tendon Transfer, 26510
Replantation, 20824, 20827
Sesamoidectomy, 26185
Unlisted Services and Procedures, 26989
Thymectomy, 60520, 60521
Sternal Split
Transthoracic Approach, 60521, 60522
Transcervical Approach, 60520
Thymotaxin, 82232
Thymus Gland, 60520
Excision, 60520, 60521
Exploration
Thymus Field, 60699
Incision, 60699
Other Operations, 60699
Repair, 60699
Transplantation, 60699
Thyrocalcitonin, 80410, 82308
Thyroglobulin, 84432
Antibody, 86800
Thyroglossal Duct
Cyst
Excision, 60280, 60281
Thyroidectomy
Partial, 60210-60225
Secondary, 60260
Total, 60240, 60271
Cervical Approach, 60271
for Malignancy
Limited Neck Dissection, 60252
Radical Neck Dissection, 60254
Removal All Thyroid Tissue, 60260
Sternal Split
Transthoracic Approach, 60270
Thyroid Gland
Biopsy
Open, 60699
Cyst
Aspiration, 60300
Excision, 60200
Incision and Drainage, 60000
Injection, 60300
Excision
for Malignancy
Limited Neck Dissection, 60252
Radical Neck Dissection, 60254
Partial, 60210-60225
Secondary, 60260
Total, 60240, 60271
Cervical Approach, 60271
Removal All Thyroid Tissue, 60260
Sternal Split
Transthoracic Approach, 60270
Transcervical Approach, 60520
Metastatic Cancer
Nuclear Imaging, 78015-78018
Needle Biopsy, 60100
Nuclear Medicine
Imaging for Metastases, 78015-78018
Metastases Uptake, 78020
Suture, 60699
Tissue
Reimplantation, 60699
Tumor
Excision, 60200
Thyroid Hormone Binding Ratio, 84479
Thyroid Hormone Uptake, 84479
Thyroid Isthmus
Transection, 60200
Thyroid Simulator, Long Acting, 80438-80439
Thyroid Stimulating Hormone (TSH), 80418, 80438, 84443
Thyroid Stimulating Hormone Receptor ab, 80438-80439
Thyroid Stimulating Immune Globulins (TSI), 84445

Thyroid Suppression Test
Nuclear Medicine Thyroid Uptake, 78012, 78014
Thyrolingual Cyst
Incision and Drainage, 60000
Thyrotomy, 31300
Thyrotropin Receptor ab, 80438-80439
Thyrotropin Releasing Hormone (TRH), 80438, 80439
Thyrotropin Stimulating Immunoglobulins, 84445
Thyroxine
Free, 84439
Neonatal, 84437
Total, 84436
True, 84436
Thyroxine Binding Globulin, 84442
Tiagabine
Assay, 80199
TIBC, 83550
Tibia
See Also Ankle
Arthroscopy Surgical, 29891, 29892
Craterization, 27360, 27640
Cyst
Excision, 27635-27638
Diaphysectomy, 27360, 27640
Excision, 27360, 27640
Epiphyseal Bar, 20150
Fracture
with Manipulation, 27825
without Manipulation, 27824
Incision, 27607
Arthroscopic Treatment, 29855, 29856
Plafond, 29892
Closed Treatment, 27824, 27825
with Manipulation, 27825
without Manipulation, 27824
Distal, 27824-27828
Intercondylar, 27538, 27540
Malleolus, 27760-27766, 27808-27814
Open Treatment, 27535, 27536, 27758, 27759, 27826-27828
Plateau, 29855, 29856
Closed Treatment, 27530, 27532
Shaft, 27752-27759
Osteoplasty
Lengthening, 27715
Prophylactic Treatment, 27745
Reconstruction, 27418
at Knee, 27440-27443, 27446
Repair, 27720-27725
Epiphysis, 27477-27485, 27730-27742
Osteochondritis Dissecans Arthroscopy, 29892
Osteotomy, 27455, 27457, 27705, 27709, 27712
Pseudoarthrosis, 27727
Saucerization, 27360, 27640
Tumor
Excision, 27635-27638, 27645
X-ray, 73590
Tibial
Arteries
Bypass Graft, 35566-35571, 35666-35671
Bypass In-Situ, 35585-35587
Embolectomy, 34203
Thrombectomy, 34203
Thromboendarterectomy, 35305-35306
Nerve
Repair/Suture
Posterior, 64840
Tibiofibular Joint
Arthrodesis, 27871
Dislocation, 27830-27832
Disruption
Open Treatment, 27829
Fusion, 27871
TIG, 90389
TIG (Tetanus Immune Globulin) Vaccine, 90389
Time
Bleeding, 85002
Prothrombin, 85610-85611
Reptilase, 85670-85675
Tinnitus
Assessment, 92625

TIPS (Transvenous Intrahepatic Portosystemic Shunt) Procedure, 37182-37183
Anesthesia, 01931
Tissue
Culture
Chromosome Analysis, 88230-88239
Homogenization, 87176
Non-neoplastic Disorder, 88230, 88237
Skin Grafts, 15040-15157
Solid tumor, 88239
Toxin/Antitoxin, 87230
Virus, 87252, 87253
Enzyme Activity, 82657
Examination for Ectoparasites, 87220
Examination for Fungi, 87220
Expander
Breast Reconstruction with, 19357
Insertion
Skin, 11960
Removal
Skin, 11971
Replacement
Skin, 11970
Grafts
Harvesting, 20926
Granulation
Cauterization, 17250
Homogenization, 87176
Hybridization In Situ, 88365-88369 [88364, 88373, 88374, 88377]
Mucosal
See Mucosa
Soft
Abscess, 20005
Transfer
Adjacent
Eyelids, 67961
Skin, 14000-14350
Facial Muscles, 15845
Finger Flap, 14350
Toe Flap, 14350
Typing
HLA Antibodies, 86812-86817
Lymphocyte Culture, 86821, 86822
Tissue Factor
Inhibition, 85705
Inhibition Test, 85347
Partial Time, 85730-85732
Tissue Transfer
Adjacent
Arms, 14020, 14021
Axillae, 14040, 14041
Cheeks, 14040, 14041
Chin, 14040, 14041
Ears, 14060, 14061
Eyelids, 67961
Face, 14040-14061
Feet, 14040, 14041
Finger, 14350
Forehead, 14040, 14041
Genitalia, 14040, 14041
Hand, 14040, 14041
Legs, 14020, 14021
Limbs, 14020, 14021
Lips, 14060, 14061
Mouth, 14040, 14041
Neck, 14040, 14041
Nose, 14060, 14061
Scalp, 14020, 14021
Skin, 14000-14350
Trunk, 14000, 14001
Facial Muscles, 15845
Finger Flap, 14350
Toe Flap, 14350
Tissue Typing
HLA Antibodies, 86812-86817
Lymphocyte Culture, 86821, 86822
TK2, 81405
TLC Screen, 84375
TMC1, 81430
TMEM43, 81406
TMEM67, 81407
TMJ
Arthrocentesis, 20605-20606
Arthrography, 70328-70332
Injection, 21116

TMJ — continued
Arthroplasty, 21240-21243
Arthroscopy
Diagnostic, 29800
TMPRSS3, 81430
TMR (Transmyocardial Revascularization), 33140-33141
TNA (Total Nail Avulsion), 11730, 11732
TNNC1, 81405
TNNI3, 81405
TNNT2, 81406
TNS, 64550
Tobacco Use
Assessment, 1000F, 1034F-1036F
Counseling, 4000F
Pharmacologic Therapy, 4001F
Tobramycin
Assay, 80200
Tocolysis, 59412
Tocopherol, 84446
Toe
See Also Interphalangeal Joint, Toe; Metatar-
sophalangeal Joint; Phalanx
Amputation, 28810-28825
Arthrocentesis, 20600-20604
Bunionectomy, 28289-28299 [28295]
Capsulotomy, 28270, 28272
Dislocation
See Specific Joint
Fasciotomy, 28008
Flap
Tissue Transfer, 14350
Lesion
Excision, 28092
Magnetic Resonance Imaging (MRI), 73721
Reconstruction
Angle Deformity, 28313
Extra Digit, 26587
Extra Toes, 28344
Hammer Toe, 28285, 28286
Macrodactyly, 28340, 28341
Syndactyly, 28345
Webbed Toe, 28345
Repair, 26590
Bunion, 28289-28299 [28295]
Extra Digit, 26587
Macrodactylia, 26590
Muscle, 28240
Tendon, 28232, 28234, 28240
Webbed, 28280, 28345
Webbed Toe, 28345
Reposition, 20973, 26551-26554
Reposition to Hand, 26551-26554, 26556
Strapping, 29550
Tenotomy, 28010, 28011, 28232, 28234
Tumor, 28043-28047 [28039, 28041], 28108, 28175
Unlisted Services and Procedures, 28899
X-Ray, 73660
Tolerance Test(s)
Glucagon, 82946
Glucose, 82951, 82952
Heparin–Protamine, 85530
Insulin, 80434, 80435
Maltose, 82951, 82952
Tomodensitometries
See CT Scan
Tomographic Scintigraphy, Computed, 78607, 78647
Tomographic SPECT
Myocardial Imaging, 78469
Tomographies, Computed X–Ray
See CT Scan
Tomography
Coherence
Optical
Axillary Node, Each Specimen, Excised Tissue, 0351T-0352T
Breast, Each Specimen, Excised Tissue, 0351T-0352T
Coronary Vessel or Graft, [92978, 92979]
Surgical Cavity, Breast, 0353T-0354T
Computed
Abdomen, 74150-74175, 75635
Head, 70450-70470, 70496

Tomography — continued
Computed — continued
Heart, 75571-75574
Tomosynthesis, Breast
Bilateral, 77062
Screening, 77063
Unilateral, 77061
Tompkins Metroplasty
Uterus Reconstruction, 58540
Tongue
Ablation, 41530
Abscess
Incision and Drainage, 41000-41006, 41015
Biopsy, 41100, 41105
Cyst
Incision and Drainage, 41000-41006, 41015, 60000
Excision
with Mouth Resection, 41150, 41153
with Radical Neck, 41135, 41145, 41153, 41155
Base
Radiofrequency, 41530
Complete, 41140-41155
Frenum, 41115
Partial, 41120-41135
Fixation, 41500
Hematoma
Incision and Drainage, 41000-41006, 41015
Incision
Frenum, 41010
Lesion
Excision, 41110-41114
Reconstruction
Frenum, 41520
Reduction for Sleep Apnea, 41530
Repair
Laceration, 41250-41252
Suture, 41510
Suspension, 41512
Unlisted Services and Procedures, 41599
Tonometry, Serial, 92100
Tonsillectomy, 42820-42826
with Adenoidectomy
Age 12 or Over, 42821
Younger Than Age 12, 42820
Primary
Age 12 or Over, 42826
Younger Than Age 12, 42825
Secondary
Age 12 or Over, 42826
Younger Than Age 12, 42825
Tonsil, Pharyngeal
Excision, 42830-42836
with Tonsillectomy, 42820-42821
Unlisted Services/Procedures, 42999
Tonsils
Abscess
Incision and Drainage, 42700
Excision, 42825, 42826
Excision with Adenoids, 42820, 42821
Lingual, 42870
Radical, 42842-42845
Tag, 42860
Lingual
Destruction, 42870
Removal
Foreign Body, 42999
Unlisted Services and Procedures, 42999
Topiramate
Assay, 80201
Topography
Corneal, 92025
TOR1A, 81400, 81404
Torek Procedure
Orchiopexy, 54650
Torkildsen Procedure, 62180
TORP (Total Ossicular Replacement Prosthesis), 69633, 69637
Torsion Swing Test, 92546
Torula, 86641, 87327
Torus Mandibularis
Tumor Excision, 21031
Total
Abdominal Hysterectomy, 58150
with Colpo-Urethrocystopexy, 58152

Total — continued
Abdominal Hysterectomy — continued
with Omentectomy, 58956
with Partial Vaginectomy, 58200
Bilirubin Level, 82247, 88720
Catecholamines, 82382
Cystectomy, 51570-51597
Dacryoadenectomy, 68500
Elbow Replacement, 24363
Esophagectomy, 43107-43113, 43124
Gastrectomy, 43620-43622
Hemolytic Complement, 86162
Hip Arthroplasty, 27130-27132
Knee Arthroplasty, 0396T, 27447
Mastectomies
See Mastectomy
Ostectomy of Patella, 27424
Splenectomy, 38100, 38102
Toupet Procedure, 43280
Touroff Operation/Ligation, Artery, Neck, 37615
Toxicology, [80305, 80306, 80307]
Toxin Assay, 87230
Tissue Culture, 87230
Toxin, Botulinum
Chemodenervation
Eccrine Glands, 64650-64653
Extraocular Muscle, 67345
Extremity Muscle, 64642-64645
for Blepharospasm, 64612
for Hemifacial Spasm, 64612
Internal Anal Sphincter, 46505
Neck Muscle, 64616
Trunk Muscle, 64646-64647
Toxoplasma
Antibody, 86777, 86778
TP53, 81404-81405, 81432
T–Phyl, 80198
TPM1, 81405
TPMT, 81401
TR3SVR, 33548
Trabeculectomy, 66170
Trabeculectomy Ab Externo
with Scarring Previous Surgery, 66172
in Absence of Previous Surgery, 66170
Trabeculoplasty
by Laser Surgery, 65855
Trabeculotomy Ab Externo
Eye, 65850
Trachea
Aspiration, 31720
Catheter, 31720, 31725
Dilation, 31630-31631, 31636-31638
Endoscopy
via Tracheostomy, 31615
Excision
Stenosis, 31780, 31781
Fistula
with Plastic Repair, 31825
without Plastic Repair, 31820
Repair, 31825
Fracture
Endoscopy, 31630
Incision
with Flaps, 31610
Emergency, 31603, 31605
Planned, 31600, 31601
Introduction
Needle Wire, 31730
Puncture
Aspiration and
or Injection, 31612
Reconstruction
Carina, 31766
Cervical, 31750
Fistula, 31755
Graft Repair, 31770
Intrathoracic, 31760
Repair
Cervical, 31750
Fistula, 31755
Intrathoracic, 31760
Stoma, 31613, 31614
Revision/Stoma/Scars, 31830
Scar
Revision, 31830

Trachea — continued
Stenosis
Excision, 31780, 31781
Repair, 31780, 31781
Stoma
Repair, 31825
with Plastic Repair, 31825
without Plastic Repair, 31820
Revision
Scars, 31830
Tumor
Excision
Cervical, 31785
Thoracic, 31786
Unlisted Services and Procedures, 31899
Bronchi, 31899
Wound
Suture
Cervical, 31800
Intrathoracic, 31805
Tracheal
Stent
Placement, 31631
Tube, 31500
Trachelectomy, 57530
Radical, 57531
Trachelorrhaphy, 57720
Tracheobronchoscopy
via Tracheostomy, 31615
Tracheoesophageal Fistula
Repair, 43305, 43312, 43314
Speech Prosthesis, 31611
Tracheoplasty
Cervical, 31750
Intrathoracic, 31760
Tracheopharyngeal Fistulization, 31755
Tracheoscopy, 31515-31529
Tracheostoma
Revision, 31613, 31614
Tracheostomy
with Flaps, 31610
Emergency, 31603, 31605
Planned, 31600, 31601
Revision
Scar, 31830
Surgical Closure
with Plastic Repair, 31825
without Plastic Repair, 31820
Tracheobronchoscopy through, 31615
Tracheotomy
Tube Change, 31502
Tracking Tests (Ocular), 92545
Traction Therapy
Manual, 97140
Mechanical, 97012
Skeletal, 20999
Tractotomy
Mesencephalon, 61480
Tract, Urinary
X-Ray with Contrast, 74400-74425
Training
Activities of Daily Living, 97535, 99509
Athletic, Evaluation, [97169, 97170, 97171, 97172]
Biofeedback, 90901, 90911
Cognitive Skills, 97532
Community
Work Reintegration, 97537
Home Management, 97535, 99509
Management
Propulsion, 97542
Orthoptic
Pleoptic, 92065
Orthotics, 97760
Prosthetics, 97761
Seeing Impaired, 97799
Braille, or Moon, 97799
Lead Dog, Use of, 97799
Self Care, 97535, 99509
Sensory Integration, 97533
Walking (Physical Therapy), 97116
Wheelchair Management
Propulsion, 97542
TRAM Flap
Breast Reconstruction, 19367-19369

Transabdominal Endoscopy
Intestine, Large, *[45399]*
Transaminase
Glutamic Oxaloacetic, 84450
Glutamic Pyruvic, 84460
Transbronchial Needle Aspiration (TBNA), 31629, 31633
Transcatheter
Biopsy, 37200
Closure
Left Atrial Appendage, 33340
Percutaneous, Heart, 93580-93582
Denervation
Renal Sympathetic, 0338T-0339T
Embolization
Cranial, 61624, 61626
Vascular, 37241-37244
Occlusion
Cranial, 61624, 61626
Vascular, 37241-37244
Placement
Intravascular Stent(s), 0075T-0076T, 37215-37217, 37236-37239
Wireless Physiologic Sensor, 34806
Removal, Foreign Body, 37197
Therapy
Embolization, 75894
Infusion, 75898, *[37211, 37212, 37213, 37214]*
Perfusion
Cranial, 61624, 61626
Septal Reduction, 93583
Transcortin, 84449
Transcranial
Doppler Study (TCP), 93886-93893
Stimulation, Motor, 95928-95929
Transcutaneous
Electrical Modulation Pain Reprocessing, 0278T
Electric Nerve Stimulation, 64550
Transdermal Electrostimulation, 64550
Transection
Artery
Carotid, 61610, 61612
Blood Vessel
Kidney, 50100
Brain
Subpial, 61597
Nerve, 64732-64772
Vagus, 43640, 43641
Pulmonary Artery, 33922
Transesophageal
Echocardiography, 93312-93318
Guidance for Intracardiac or Great Vessel Intervention, 93355
Transfer
Adjacent Tissue, 14000-14350
Blastocyst, 58974-58976
Cryopreserved, 89352
Finger Position, 26555
Gamete Intrafallopian, 58976
Jejunum
with Microvascular Anastomosis Preparation/Embryo, 89255
Free, 43496
Toe Joint, 26556
Toe to Hand, 26551-26554, 26556
Tubal Embryo Stage, 58974
Transferase
Aspartate Amino, 84450
Glutamic Oxaloacetic, 84450
Transferrin, 84466
Transformation
Lymphocyte, 86353
Transfusion
Blood, 36430
Exchange, 36450, 36455
Newborn, Partial, 36456
Fetal, 36460
Push
Infant, 36440
Unlisted Services and Procedures, 86999
White Blood Cells, 86950
Transfusion, Blood, Autologous, 86890-86891
Transillumination
Skull
Newborn, 95999

Transitional Care Management, 99495-99496
Translocation
Aortic Root, 33782-33783
Transluminal
Angioplasty
Arterial, 36902-36903, 36905-36906
Coronary, *[92920, 92921, 92924, 92925, 92928, 92929, 92933, 92934, 92937, 92938, 92941, 92943, 92944]*
Atherectomies, 0234T-0238T, 37227, 37229, 37231, 37233, 37235, *[92924, 92925], [92933, 92934], [92937, 92938], [92941], [92943, 92944], [92973]*
Transmyocardial Laser Revascularization, 33140, 33141
Transosteal Bone Plate
Reconstruction
Mandible, 21244
Transpeptidase, Gamma–Glutamyl, 82977
Transperineal Placement
Biodegradable Material
Periprostatic, 0438T
Transplant
See Also Graft
Bone
See Also Bone Graft
Allograft, Spine, 20930-20931
Autograft, Spine, 20936-20938
Hair, 15775-15776
See Hair, Transplant
Transplantation
See Also Graft
Amniotic Membrane, 65780
Backbench Preparation Prior to Transplantation
Intestine, 44715-44721
Kidney, 50323-50329
Liver, 47143-47147
Pancreas, 48551-48552
Bone Marrow, 38240, 38241
Harvesting, 38230
Cartilage
Knee, 27415, 29867
Allograft, 27415, 29867
Autograft, 27412, 29866
Chondrocytes
Knee, 27412
Conjunctiva, 65782
Cornea
Autograft/Homograft
Lamellar, 65710
Penetrating, 65730-65755
for Aphakia, 65750
Eye
Amniotic Membrane, 65780
Conjunctiva, 65782
Stem Cell, 65781
Hair
Punch Graft, 15775, 15776
Strip, 15220, 15221
Heart, 33945
Allograft Preparation, 33933, 33944
Heart–Lung, 33935
Intestines
Allograft Preparation, 44715-44721
Allotransplantation, 44135, 44136
Donor Enterectomy, 44132, 44133
Removal of Allograft, 44137
Liver, 47135
Allograft Preparation, 47143-47147
Lung
Allograft Preparation, 32855-32856, 33933
Donor Pneumonectomy, 32850
Double with Cardiopulmonary Bypass, 32854
Double, without Cardiopulmonary Bypass, 32853
Single, with Cardiopulmonary Bypass, 32852
Single, without Cardiopulmonary Bypass, 32851
Meniscus
Knee, 29868
Muscle, 15731-15738, 15756
Ovary, 58999
Pancreas, 48550, 48554-48556
Allograft Preparation, 48551-48552

Transplantation — *continued*
Pancreatic Islet Cell with Pancreatectomy, 48160
Parathyroid, 60512
Renal
Allograft Preparation, 50323-50329
Allotransplantation, 50360
with Recipient Nephrectomy, 50365
Autotransplantation, 50380
Donor Nephrectomy, 50300, 50320, 50547
Recipient Nephrectomy, 50340
Removal Transplanted Renal Allograft, 50370
Spleen, 38999
Stem Cells, 38240, 38241, 38242
Cell Concentration, 38215
Cryopreservation, 38207, 88240
Donor Search, 38204
Harvesting, 38205-38206
Plasma Depletion, 38214
Platelet Depletion, 38213
Red Blood Cell Depletion, 38212
T–cell Depletion, 38210
Thawing, 38208, 88241
Tumor Cell Depletion, 38211
Washing, 38209
Testis
to Thigh, 54680
Tissue, Harvesting, 20926
Transpleural Thoracoscopy
See Thoracoscopy
Transposition
Arteries
Carotid, 33889, 35691, 35694, 35695
Subclavian, 33889, 35693-35695
Vertebral, 35691, 35693
Cranial Nerve, 64716
Eye Muscles, 67320
Great Arteries
Repair, 33770-33781
Nerve, 64718-64721
Nipple, 19499
Ovary, 58825
Peripheral Nerve
Major, 64856
Vein Valve, 34510
Trans–Scaphoperilunar
Fracture
Dislocation, 25680, 25685
Closed Treatment, 25680
Open Treatment, 25685
Transthoracic Echocardiography, 0399T, 0439T, 93303-93350
Transthyretin, 84134
Transureteroureterostomy, 50770
Transurethral
See Also Specific Procedure
Fulguration
Postoperative Bleeding, 52214
Prostate
Ablation
Waterjet, 0421T
Incision, 52450
Resection, 52601, 52630-52640
Thermotherapy, 53850-53852
Microwave, 53850
Radiofrequency, 53852
Radiofrequency Micro-Remodeling
Female Bladder, 53860
Transversus Abdominis Plane (TAP) Block
Bilateral, 64488-64489
Unilateral, 64486-64487
Trapezium
Arthroplasty
with Implant, 25445
Travel, Unusual, 99082
TRB@, 81340-81341
TRD@, 81402
Treacher–Collins Syndrome
Midface Reconstruction, 21150, 21151
Treatment, Tocolytic, 59412
Trendelenburg Operation, 37785
Trephine Procedure
Sinusotomy
Frontal, 31070

Treponema Pallidum
Antibody, 86780
Antigen Detection
Direct Fluorescent Antibody, 87285
TRF (Thyrotropin Releasing Factor), 80439
TRG@, 81342
TRH, 80438, 80439
Triacylglycerol, 84478
Triacylglycerol Hydrolase, 83690
Triangular Cartilage
Repair with Fracture
Radial shaft, 25526
Triangular Fibrocartilage
Excision, 29846
Tributyrinase, 83690
Trichiasis
Repair, 67825
Epilation, by Forceps, 67820
Epilation, by Other than Forceps, 67825
Incision of Lid Margin, 67830
with Free Mucous Membrane Graft, 67835
Trichina, 86784, 96902
Trichinella
Antibody, 86784
Trichogram, 96902
Trichomonas Vaginalis
Antigen Detection
Nucleic Acid, 87660-87661
Trichrome Stain, 88313
Tricuspid Valve
Excision, 33460
Repair, 33463-33465
Replace, 33465
Repositioning, 33468
Tridymite, 84285
Trigeminal Ganglia, 61450, 61790
Trigeminal Nerve
Destruction, 64600-64610
Injection
Anesthetic, 64400
Neurolytic, 64600, 64605
Trigeminal Tract
Stereotactic
Create Lesion, 61791
Trigger Finger Repair, 26055
Trigger Point
Injection
One or Two Muscle Groups, 20552
Two or More Muscle Groups, 20553
Triglyceridase, 83690
Triglyceride Lipase, 83690
Triglycerides, 84478
Trigonocephaly, 21175
Triiodothyronine
Free, 84481
Resin Uptake, 84479
Reverse, 84482
Total, 84480
True, 84480
Triolean Hydrolase, 83690
Trioxopurine, 84550, 84560
Tripcellim
Duodenum, 84485
Feces, 84488-84490
Tripedia, 90700
Trisegmentectomy, 47122
Trocar Biopsy
Bone Marrow, 38221
Trochanter
Pressure Ulcer, 15950-15958
Trochanteric Femur Fracture, 27246-27248
Trophoblastic Tumor GTT, 59100, 59870
Troponin
Qualitative, 84512
Quantitative, 84484
TRPC6, 81406
Truncal Vagotomies, 43640
Truncus Arteriosus
Repair, 33786
Truncus Brachiocephalicus
Angioplasty, *[37246, 37247]*
Atherectomy, 0237T
Catheterization, 36215-36218
Trunk
Lipectomy, Suction Assisted, 15877

Trunk — *continued*
Skin Graft
Delay of Flap, 15600
Full Thickness, 15200
Muscle, Myocutaneous, or Fasciocutaneous
Flaps, 15734
Split, 15100, 15101
Tissue Transfer, Adjacent, 14000
TRUSP (Transrectal Ultrasound of Prostate),
76873
Trypanosomiases, 86171, 86280
Trypanosomiasis, 86171, 86280
Trypsin
Duodenum, 84485
Feces, 84488-84490
Trypsin Inhibitor, Alpha 1–Antitrypsin, 82103-
82104
Trypure
Duodenum, 84485
Feces, 84488-84490
TSA, 86316
Tsalicylate Intoxication, *[80329, 80330, 80331]*
TSC1, 81405-81406
TSC2, 81406-81407
TSH, 80418, 80438, 84443
TSI, 84445
Tsutsugamushi Disease, 86000
TT, 85670-85675
TT–3, 84480
TT–4, 84436
TTPA, 81404
TTR, 81404
T(15;17) Translocation Analysis, 81315-81316
T(9;22) Translocation Analysis, 81206-81208
Tuba, Auditoria (Auditiva)
Eustachian Tube Procedures, 69420-69421,
69799
Tubal Embryo Stage Transfer, 58976
Tubal Ligation, 58600
with Cesarean Section, 58611
Laparoscopic, 58670
Postpartum, 58605
Tubal Occlusion
with Cesarean Delivery
See Fallopian Tube, Occlusion; Occlusion
Create Lesion
See Fallopian Tube, Occlusion; Oc-
clusion, Fallopian Tube
See Fallopian Tube
Tubal Pregnancy, 59121
with Salpingectomy and/or Oophorectomy,
59120
Tube Change
Colonic, 49450
Duodenostomy, 49451
Gastro-Jejunostomy, 49452
Gastrostomy, 43760, 49446
Jejunostomy, 49451
Tracheotomy, 31502
Tube, Fallopian
See Fallopian Tube
Tubectomy, 58700, 58720
Tubed Pedicle Flap
Formation, 15570-15576
Walking Tube, 15650
Tube Placement
Cecostomy, 44300, 49442
Chest, 32551
Colonic, 49442
Duodenostomy, 49441
Enterostomy, 44300
Gastrostomy Tube, 43246, 49440
Jejunostomy, 49441
Nasogastric Tube, 43752
Orogastric Tube, 43752
Tubercle Bacilli
Culture, 87116
Tubercleplasty, Anterior Tibial, 27418
Tuberculin Test, 86580
Tuberculosis
Antigen Response Test, 86480
Cell Mediated Immunity Antigen, 86480-86481
Culture, 87116
Skin Test, 86580
Tuberculosis Vaccine (BCG), 90585, 90586

Tube Replacement
See Tube Change
Tubes
Chest, 32551
Endotracheal, 31500
Gastrostomy, 43246, 49440
See Also Gastrostomy Tube
Tudor "Rabbit Ear"
Urethra, Repair
Diverticulum, 53240, 53400, 53405
Fistula, 45820, 45825, 53400, 53405, 53520
Sphincter, 57220
Stricture, 53400, 53405
Urethrocele, 57230
Wound, 53502-53515
Tuffier Vaginal Hysterectomy
See Hysterectomy, Vaginal
TULIP, 52647-52648
Tumor
Abdomen
Destruction
Excision, 49203-49205
Abdominal Wall, 22900-22905
Acetabulum
Excision, 27076
Ankle, 27615-27619 *[27632]*
Arm, Lower, 24152, 25075-25078 *[25071, 25073]*
Arm, Upper, 23220, 24075-24079 *[24071,
24073]*, 24110-24126, 24150
Back, 21930-21936
Bile Duct
Ablation, *[43278]*
Extrahepatic, 47711
Intrahepatic, 47712
Bladder, 52234-52240
Excision, 51530, 52355
Brain, 61510
Excision, 61518, 61520, 61521, 61526,
61530, 61545, 62164
Breast
Excision, 19120-19126
Bronchi
Excision, 31640
Calcaneus, 28100-28103
Excision, 27647
Carpal, 25130-25136
Chest Wall
Excision, 19260-19272
Clavicle
Excision, 23140, 23200
with Allograft, 23146
with Autograft, 23145
Coccyx, 49215
Colon
Destruction, *[44401]*, *[45388]*
Removal, 44392, 44394, 45384-45385
Cranial Bone
Reconstruction, 21181, 21182
Destruction
Abdomen, 49203-49205
Chemosurgery, 17311-17315
Urethra, 53220
Ear, Middle
Extended, 69554
Transcanal, 69550
Transmastoid, 69552
Elbow, 24075-24079 *[24071, 24073]*, 24120-
24126, 24152
Esophagus
Ablation, 43229
Excision
Femur, 27355-27358
Face, 21011-21016
Facial Bones, 21029, 21030, 21034
Fallopian Tube
Resection, 58950, 58952-58956
Femoral, 27355-27358
Excision, 27365
Femur, 27065-27067
Excision, 27365
Fibula, 27635-27638
Excision, 27646
Finger
Excision, 26115-26117 *[26111, 26113]*
Foot, 28043, 28045, 28046
Flank, 21930-21936

Tumor — *continued*
Forearm
Radical Resection, 25077
Gums
Excision, 41825-41827
Hand, 26115-26117 *[26111, 26113]*
Heart
Excision, 33120, 33130
Hip, 27047-27049 *[27043, 27045]*, 27065-27067
Excision, 27075, 27076
Humerus, 23155-23156, 23220, 24115-24116,
24150
Ileum, 27065-27067
Immunoassay for Antigen, 86294, 86316
CA 125, 86304
CA 15–3, 86300
CA 19–9, 86301
Innominate
Excision, 27077
Intestines, Small
Destruction, 44369
Removal, 44364-44365
Ischial Tuberosity, 27078
Kidney
Excision, 52355
Knee
Excision, 27327-27328 *[27337, 27339]*,
27355-27358, 27364-27365 *[27329]*
Lacrimal Gland
Excision
with Osteotomy, 68550
Frontal Approach, 68540
Larynx, 31540, 31541
Excision, 31300
Endoscopic, 31540, 31541, 31578
Incision, 31300
Leg, Lower, 27615-27619 *[27632]*
Leg, Upper
Excision, 27327-27328 *[27337, 27339]*,
27355-27358, 27364-27365 *[27329]*
Liver
Ablation, 47380-47383
Localization
with Nuclear Medicine, 78800-78803
Mandible, 21040-21045
Maxillary Torus Palatinus, 21032
Mediastinal
Excision, 39220
Mediastinum, 32662
Meningioma
Excision, 61519
Metacarpal, 26200, 26205, 26250
Metatarsal, 28104-28107
Excision, 28173
Neck, 21555-21558 *[21552, 21554]*
Olecranon Process, 24075-24077 *[24071, 24073]*,
24120-24126
Ovary
Resection, 58950, 58952-58954
Pancreatic Duct
Ablation, *[43278]*
Parotid Gland
Excision, 42410-42426
Pelvis, 27047-27049 *[27043, 27045]*
Pericardial
Endoscopic, 32661
Excision, 33050
Peritoneum
Resection, 58950-58956
Phalanges
Finger, 26210, 26215, 26260-26262
Toe, 28108
Excision, 28175
Pituitary Gland
Excision, 61546, 61548
Pubis, 27065-27067
Radiation Therapy, *[77295]*
Radius, 25120-25126, 25170
with Allograft, 24126
with Autograft, 24125
Excision, 24120
Rectum, 0184T, 45160, 45171-45172, 45190
Resection
with Cystourethroscopy, 52355
Face, 21015
Scalp, 21015

Tumor — *continued*
Retroperitoneal
Destruction
Excision, 49203-49205
Sacrum, 49215
Scalp, 21011-21016
Scapula, 23140
Excision, 23140, 23210
with Allograft, 23146
with Autograft, 23145
Shoulder, 23075-23078 *[23071, 23073]*
Skull
Excision, 61500
Soft Tissue
Elbow
Excision, 24075
Finger
Excision, 26115
Forearm
Radical Resection, 25077
Hand
Excision, 26115
Spinal Cord
Excision, 63275-63290
Stomach
Excision, 43610, 43611
Talus, 28100-28103
Excision, 27647
Tarsal, 28104-28107
Excision, 28171
Temporal Bone
Removal, 69970
Testis
Excision, 54530, 54535
Thorax, 21555-21558 *[21552, 21554]*
Thyroid
Excision, 60200
Tibia, 27365, 27635-27638
Excision, 27645
Torus Mandibularis, 21031
Trachea
Excision
Cervical, 31785
Thoracic, 31786
Ulna, 25120-25126, 25170
with Allograft
Excision, 24126
with Autograft
Excision, 24125
Excision, 24120
Ureter
Excision, 52355
Urethra, 52234-52240, 53220
Excision, 52355
Uterus
Excision, 58140, 58145
Vagina
Excision, 57135
Vertebra
Additional Segment
Excision, 22103, 22116
Cervical
Excision, 22100
Lumbar, 22102
Thoracic
Excision, 22101
Wrist, 25075-25078 *[25071, 25073]*
**TUMT (Transurethral Microwave Thermothera-
py)**, 53850
TUNA, 53852
Tunica Vaginalis
Hydrocele
Aspiration, 55000
Excision, 55040, 55041
Repair, 55060
Turbinate
Excision, 30130, 30140
Fracture
Therapeutic, 30930
Injection, 30200
Submucous Resection
Nose
Excision, 30140
Turbinate Mucosa
Ablation, 30801, 30802
Turcica, Sella, 70240, 70480-70482

TURP, 52601, 52630
TVCB (Transvaginal Chorionic Villus Biopsy), 59015
TVH (Total Vaginal Hysterectomy), 58262-58263, 58285, 58291-58292
TVS (Transvaginal Sonography), 76817, 76830
TWINRIX, 90636
TWIST1, 81403-81404
Tylectomy, 19120-19126
Tylenol, [80329, 80330, 80331]
TYMP, 81405
Tympanic Membrane
   Create Stoma, 69433, 69436
   Incision, 69420, 69421
   Reconstruction, 69620
   Repair, 69450, 69610
Tympanic Nerve
   Excision, 69676
Tympanolysis, 69450
Tympanometry, 92550, 92567
Tympanoplasty
   with Antrotomy or Mastoidectomy, 69635
      with Ossicular Chain Reconstruction, 69636
        and Synthetic Prosthesis, 69637
   with Mastoidectomy, 69641
      with Intact or Reconstructed Wall
        without Ossicular Chain Reconstruction, 69643
        and Ossicular Chain Reconstruction, 69644
      and Ossicular Chain Reconstruction, 69644
      without Mastoidectomy, 69631
        with Ossicular Chain Reconstruction, 69632
        and Synthetic Prosthesis, 69633
   Myringoplasty, 69620
   Radical or Complete, 69645
      with Ossicular Chain Reconstruction, 69646
Tympanostomy, 69433, 69436
Tympanotomy, 69420-69421
TYMS, 81401
Typhin Vi, 90691
Typhoid Vaccine, 90690-90691
   Oral, 90690
   Polysaccharide, 90691
Typhus
   Endemic, 86000
   Mite–Bone, 86000
   Sao Paulo, 86000
   Tropical, 86000
Typing
   Blood, 86900-86906, 86910-86911, 86920-86923
   HLA, 81370-81383, 86812-86822
   Tissue, 81370-81383, 86812-86822
TYR, 81404
Tyrosine, 84510
Tzanck Smear, 88160-88161

U

UAC, 36660
UBA1, 81403
UBE3A, 81406
Uchida Procedure
   Tubal Ligation, 58600
UCX (Urine Culture), 87086-87088
UDP Galactose Pyrophosphorylase, 82775-82776
UDP Glucuronosyltransferase 1 Family, Polypeptide A1 Gene Analysis, 81350
UFR, 51736, 51741
UGT1A1, 81350
Ulcer
   Anal
      Destruction, 46940-46942
      Excision, 46200
   Decubitus
      See Debridement; Pressure Ulcer (Decubitus); Skin Graft and Flap
   Pinch Graft, 15050
   Pressure, 15920-15999
   Stomach
      Excision, 43610
Ulcerative, Cystitis, 52260-52265
Ulna
   See Also Arm, Lower; Elbow; Humerus; Radius

Ulna — *continued*
   Arthrodesis
      Radioulnar Joint
        with Resection, 25830
   Arthroplasty
      with Implant, 25442
   Centralization of Wrist, 25335
   Craterization, 24147, 25150
   Cyst
      Excision, 24125, 24126, 25120-25126
   Diaphysectomy, 24147, 25150, 25151
   Excision, 24147
      Abscess, 24138
      Complete, 25240
      Epiphyseal Bar, 20150
      Partial, 25145-25151, 25240
   Fracture, 25605
      with Dislocation
        Closed Treatment, 24620
        Open Treatment, 24635
      with Manipulation, 25535
      with Radius, 25560, 25565
        Open Treatment, 25575
      without Manipulation, 25530
      Closed Treatment, 25530, 25535
      Olecranon, 24670, 24675
        Open Treatment, 24685
      Open Treatment, 25545
      Shaft, 25530-25545
        Open Treatment, 25574
      Styloid Process
        Closed Treatment, 25650
        Open Treatment, 25652
        Percutaneous Fixation, 25651
   Incision and Drainage, 25035
   Osteoplasty, 25390-25393
   Prophylactic Treatment, 25491, 25492
   Reconstruction
      Radioulnar, 25337
   Repair, 25400, 25415
      with Graft, 25405, 25420-25426
        Malunion or Nonunion, 25400, 25415
      Epiphyseal Arrest, 25450, 25455
      Osteotomy, 25360, 25370, 25375
        and Radius, 25365
   Saucerization, 24147, 24150, 25151
   Sequestrectomy, 24138, 25145
   Tumor
      Cyst, 24120
      Excision, 24125, 24126, 25120-25126, 25170
Ulnar Arteries
   Aneurysm Repair, 35045
   Embolectomy, 34111
   Sympathectomy, 64822
   Thrombectomy, 34111
Ulnar Nerve
   Decompression, 64718
   Neuroplasty, 64718, 64719
   Reconstruction, 64718, 64719
   Release, 64718, 64719
   Repair
      Suture
        Motor, 64836
   Transposition, 64718, 64719
Ultrasonic Cardiography
   See Echocardiography
Ultrasonic Fragmentation Ureteral Calculus, 52325
Ultrasonography
   See Echography
Ultrasound
   3D Rendering, 76376-76377
   See Also Echocardiography; Echography
   Abdomen, 76700, 76705-76706
   Ablation
      Uterine Leiomyomata, 0071T-0072T, 0404T
   Arm, 76881-76882
   Artery
      Intracranial, 93886-93893
      Middle Cerebral, 76821
      Umbilical, 76820
   Bladder, 51798
   Bone Density Study, 76977
   Breast, 76641-76642
   Chest, 76604

Ultrasound — *continued*
   Colon
      Endoscopic, 45391-45392
   Colon–Sigmoid
      Endoscopic, 45341, 45342
   Computer Aided Surgical Navigation
      Intraoperative, 0054T-0055T
   Drainage
      Abscess, 75989
   Echoencephalography, 76506
   Esophagus
      Endoscopy, 43231, 43232
   Extremity, 76881-76882
   Eye, 76511-76513
      Biometry, 76514-76519
      Foreign Body, 76529
      Pachymetry, 76514
   Fetus, 76818, 76819
   Follow–Up, 76970
   for Physical Therapy, 97035
   Gastrointestinal, 76975
   Gastrointestinal, Upper
      Endoscopic, 43242, 43259
   Guidance
      Amniocentesis, 59001, 76946
      Amnioinfusion, 59070
      Arteriovenous Fistulae, 76936
      Chorionic Villus Sampling, 76945
      Cryosurgery, 55873
      Drainage
        Fetal Fluid, 59074
      Endometrial Ablation, 58356
      Esophagogastroduodenoscopy
        with Drainage Pseudocyst with Placement Catheters/Stents, 43240
        with Injection Diagnostic or Therapeutic Substance, 43253
        Examination, 43237, 43259
        Fine Needle Aspiration/Biopsy, 43238, 43242
      Fetal Cordocentesis, 76941
      Fetal Transfusion, 76941
      Heart Biopsy, 76932
      Injection Facet Joint, 0213T-0218T
      Needle Biopsy, 43232, 43242, 45342, 76942
      Occlusion
        Umbilical Cord, 59072
      Ova Retrieval, 76948
      Pericardiocentesis, 76930
      Pseudoaneurysm, 76936
      Radioelement, 76965
      Shunt Placement
        Fetal, 59076
      Thoracentesis, 76942
      Uterine Fibroid Ablation, 0404T, 58674
      Vascular Access, 76937
   Head, 76506, 76536
   Heart
      Fetal, 76825
   Hips
      Infant, 76885, 76886
   Hysterosonography, 76831
   Intraoperative, 76998
   Intravascular
      Intraoperative, 37252-37253
   Kidney, 76770-76776
   Leg, 76881-76882
   Neck, 76536
   Needle or Catheter Insertion, 20555
   Pelvis, 76856, 76857
   Physical Therapy, 97035
   Pregnant Uterus, 76801-76817
   Prostate, 76872, 76873
   Rectal, 76872, 76873
   Retroperitoneal, 76770, 76775
   Screening Study, Abdomen, 76706
   Scrotum, 76870
   Sonohysterography, 76831
   Stimulation to Aid Bone Healing, 20979
   Umbilical Artery, 76820
   Unlisted Services and Procedures, 76999
   Uterus
      Tumor Ablation, 0071T-0072T
   Vagina, 76830
   Wound Treatment, 97610
Ultraviolet A Therapy, 96912

Ultraviolet B Therapy, 96910
Ultraviolet Light Therapy
   Dermatology, 96900
      Ultraviolet A, 96912
      Ultraviolet B, 96910
   for Physical Medicine, 97028
Umbilectomy, 49250
Umbilical
   Artery Ultrasound, 76820
   Hernia
      Repair, 49580-49587
        Omphalocele, 49600-49611
   Vein Catheterization, 36510
Umbilical Cord
   Occlusion, 59072
Umbilicus
   Excision, 49250
   Repair
      Hernia, 49580-49587
      Omphalocele, 49600-49611
UMOD, 81406
Undescended Testicle
   Exploration, 54550-54560
Unguis
   See Nails
Unilateral Simple Mastectomy, 19303
Unlisted Services or Procedures, 99499
   Abdomen, 22999, 49329, 49999
   Allergy
      Immunology, 95199
   Anal, 46999
   Anesthesia, 01999
   Arm, Upper, 24999
   Arthroscopy, 29999
   Autopsy, 88099
   Bile Duct, 47999
   Bladder, 53899
   Brachytherapy, 77799
   Breast, 19499
   Bronchi, 31899
   Cardiac, 33999
   Cardiovascular Studies, 93799
   Casting, 29799
   Cervix, 58999
   Chemistry Procedure, 84999
   Chemotherapy, 96549
   Chest, 32999
   Coagulation, 85999
   Colon, [45399]
   Conjunctiva Surgery, 68399
   Craniofacial, 21299
   CT Scan, 76497
   Cytogenetic Study, 88299
   Cytopathology, 88199
   Dermatology, 96999
   Dialysis, 90999
   Diaphragm, 39599
   Ear
      External, 69399
      Inner, 69949
      Middle, 69799
   Endocrine System, 60699
   Epididymis, 55899
   Esophagus, 43289, 43499
   Evaluation and Management Services, 99499
   Eyelid, 67999
   Eye Muscle, 67399
   Eye Surgery
      Anterior Segment, 66999
      Posterior Segment, 67299
   Fluoroscopy, 76496
   Forearm, 25999
   Gallbladder Surgery, 47999
   Gastroenterology Test, 91299
   Gum Surgery, 41899
   Hand, 26989
   Hemic System, 38999
   Hepatic Duct, 47999
   Hip Joint, 27299
   Hysteroscopy, 58579
   Immunization, 90749
   Immunology, 86849
   Infusion, 96379
   Injection, 96379
   Injection of Medication, 96379
   Intestine, 44799

Unlisted Services or Procedures — *continued*
In Vivo, 88749
Kidney, 53899
Lacrimal System, 68899
Laparoscopy, 38129, 38589, 43289, 43659,
    44979, 47379, 47579, 49329, 49659,
    50549, 50949, 54699, 55559, 58578,
    58679, 59898, 60659
Larynx, 31599
Lip, 40799
Liver, 47379, 47399
Lungs, 32999
Lymphatic System, 38999
Magnetic Resonance, 76498
Maxillofacial, 21299
Maxillofacial Prosthetics, 21089
Meckel's Diverticulum, 44899
Mediastinum, 39499
Mesentery Surgery, 44899
Microbiology, 87999
Molecular Pathology, 81479
Mouth, 40899, 41599
Musculoskeletal, 25999, 26989
Musculoskeletal Surgery
    Abdominal Wall, 22999
    Neck, 21899
    Spine, 22899
    Thorax, 21899
Musculoskeletal System, 20999
    Ankle, 27899
    Arm, Upper, 24999
    Elbow, 24999
    Head, 21499
    Knee, 27599
    Leg, Lower, 27899
    Leg, Upper, 27599
Necropsy, 88099
Nervous System Surgery, 64999
Neurology
    Neuromuscular Testing, 95999
Noninvasive Vascular Diagnostic Study, 93998
Nose, 30999
Nuclear Medicine, 78999
    Blood, 78199
    Bone, 78399
    Endocrine Procedure, 78099
    Genitourinary System, 78799
    Heart, 78499
    Hematopoietic System, 78199
    Lymphatic System, 78199
    Musculoskeletal System, 78399
    Nervous System, 78699
    Therapeutic, 79999
Obstetric Care, 59898, 59899
Omentum, 49329, 49999
Ophthalmology, 92499
Orbit, 67599
Otorhinolaryngology, 92700
Ovary, 58679, 58999
Oviduct, 58679, 58999
Palate, 42299
Pancreas Surgery, 48999
Pathology, 89240
Pelvis, 27299
Penis, 55899
Peritoneum, 49329, 49999
Pharynx, 42999
Physical Therapy, 97039, 97139, 97799
Pleura, 32999
Pressure Ulcer, 15999
Preventive Medicine, 99429
Prostate, 55899
Psychiatric, 90899
Pulmonology, 94799
Radiation Physics, 77399
Radiation Therapy, 77499
    Planning, 77299
Radiology, Diagnostic, 76499
Radionuclide Therapy, 79999
Radiopharmaceutical Therapy, 79999
Rectum, 45999
Reproductive Medicine Lab, 89398
Salivary Gland, 42699
Scrotum, 55899
Seminal Vesicle, 54699, 55899
Shoulder, 23929

Unlisted Services or Procedures — *continued*
Sinuses, 31299
Skin, 17999
Small Intestine, 44799
Special Services and Reports, 99199
Spine, 22899
Stomach, 43659, 43999
Strapping, 29799
Surgical Pathology, 88399
Temporal Bone, 69979
Testis, 54699, 55899
Throat, 42999
Toe, 28899
Tongue, 41599
Tonsil
    Adenoid, 42999
Toxoid, 90749
Trachea, 31899
Transfusion, 86999
Ultrasound, 76999
Ureter, 50949
Urinary System, 53899
Uterus, 58578, 58579, 58999
Uvula, 42299
Vaccine, 90749
Vagina, 58999
Vascular, 37799
Vascular Endoscopy, 37501
Vascular Injection, 36299
Vascular Studies, 93799
Vas Deferens, 55899
Wrist, 25999
Unna Paste Boot, 29580
    Removal, 29700
UPD [uniparental disomy], 81402
UPP (Urethral Pressure Profile), 51727, 51729
Upper
    Digestive System Endoscopy
        See Endoscopy, Gastrointestinal, Upper
    Extremity
        See Arm, Upper; Elbow; Humerus
    Gastrointestinal Bleeding
        Endoscopic Control, 43255
    Gastrointestinal Endoscopy, Biopsy, 43239
    GI Tract
        See Gastrointestinal Tract, Upper
UPPP (Uvulopalatopharyngoplasty), 42145
Urachal Cyst
    Bladder
        Excision, 51500
Urea Breath Test, 78267, 78268, 83014
Urea Nitrogen, 84525
    Blood, 84520, 84525
    Clearance, 84545
    Quantitative, 84520
    Semiquantitative, 84525
    Urine, 84540
Urecholine Supersensitivity Test
    Cystometrogram, 51725, 51726
Ureter
    Anastomosis
        to Bladder, 50780-50785
        to Colon, 50810, 50815
        to Intestine, 50800, 50820, 50825
        to Kidney, 50740, 50750
        to Ureter, 50760, 50770
    Biopsy, 50606, 50955-50957, 50974-50976,
        52007
    Catheterization, 52005
    Continent Diversion, 50825
    Creation
        Stoma, 50860
    Destruction
        Endoscopic, 50957, 50976
    Dilation, 52341, 52342, 52344, 52345
        Endoscopic, 50553, 50572, 50953, 50972
    Endoscopy
        Biopsy, 50955-50957, 50974-50976, 52007,
            52354
        Catheterization, 50953, 50972, 52005
        Destruction, 50957, 50976, 52354
            Endoscopic, 50957, 50976
        Dilation, 52341, 52342, 52344, 52345
        Excision
            Tumor, 52355
        Exploration, 52351

Ureter — *continued*
    Endoscopy — *continued*
        Injection of Implant Material, 52327
        Insertion
            Stent, 50947, 52332, 52334
        Lithotripsy, 52353
            with Indwelling Stent, [52356]
        Manipulation of Ureteral Calculus, 52330
        Removal
            Calculus, 50961, 50980, 52320, 52325,
                52352
            Foreign Body, 50961, 50980
        Resection, 50970-50980, 52355
            via Incision, 50970-50980
            via Stoma, 50951-50961
    Exploration, 50600
    Incision and Drainage, 50600
    Injection
        Drugs, 50391
        Radiologic, 50684, 50690
    Insertion
        Stent, 50947, 52332, 52334
        Tube, 50688
    Instillation
        Drugs, 50391
    Lesion
        Destruction, 52354
    Lithotripsy, 52353
        with Indwelling Stent, [52356]
    Lysis
        Adhesions, 50715-50725
    Manometric Studies
        Pressure, 50686
    Meatotomy, 52290
    Nuclear Medicine
        Reflux Study, 78740
    Postcaval
        Ureterolysis, 50725
    Reconstruction, 50700
        with Intestines, 50840
    Reflux Study, 78740
    Reimplantation, 51565
    Removal
        Anastomosis, 50830
        Calculus, 50610-50630, 50961, 51060,
            51065, 52320, 52325
        Foreign Body, 50961
        Stent, 50382-50386
    Repair, 50900
        Anastomosis, 50740-50825
        Continent Diversion, 50825
        Deligation, 50940
        Fistula, 50920, 50930
        Lysis of Adhesions, 50715-50725
        Ureterocele, 51535
            Ectopic, 52301
            Orthotopic, 52300
        Urinary Undiversion, 50830
    Replacement
        with Intestines, 50840
        Stent, 50382
    Resection, 52355
    Revision
        Anastomosis, 50727, 50728
    Stent
        Change, 50382, 50688
        Insertion, 50688
        Removal, 50382-50387
        Replacement, 50382, 50688
    Suture, 50900
        Deligation, 50940
        Fistula, 50920, 50930
    Tube
        Change, 50688
        Insertion, 50688
    Tumor Resection, 50949
    Unlisted Services and Procedures, 53899
    Ureterocele
        Excision, 51535
        Incision, 51535
        Repair, 51535
    X-ray with Contrast
        Guide Dilation, 74485
Ureteral
    Biopsy, 50606, 52007

Ureteral — *continued*
    Catheterization
        Endoscopic, 50553, 50572, 50953, 50972,
            52005
        Injection, 50684
        Manometric Studies, 50396, 50686
    Endoscopy
        Biopsy, 52007
        Catheterization, 52005
        Guide Wire Insertion, 52334
        Meatotomy, 52290
            Splinting, 50400-50405
            Stent Insertion, 52332
Ureteral Splinting, 50400, 50405
Ureteral Stent
    Insertion, 52332
    Removal, 50384-50386
    Replacement, 50382, 50385
Ureteral Wire
    Insertion, 52334
Ureterectomy, 50650, 50660
    Partial, 50220
    Total, 50548
Ureterocalycostomy, 50750
    Excision, 51535
    Fulguration, 52300
        Ectopic, 52301
        Orthotopic, 52300
    Incision, 51535
    Repair, 51535
    Resection, 52300
        Ectopic, 52301
        Orthotopic, 52300
Ureterocolon Conduit, 50815
Ureteroenterostomy, 50800
    Revision, 50830
Ureterography
    Injection Procedure, 50684, [50430, 50431]
Ureteroileal Conduit, 50820
    Cystectomy, 51590
    Removal, 50830
Ureterolithotomy, 50610-50630
    Laparoscopy, 50945
    Transvesical, 51060
Ureterolysis
    for Ovarian Vein Syndrome, 50722
    for Retrocaval Ureter, 50725
    for Retroperitoneal Fibrosis, 50715
Ureteroneocystostomy, 50780-50785, 50830,
    51565
    Laparoscopic, 50947, 50948
Ureteropexy, 53899
Ureteroplasty, 50700
Ureteropyelography, 50951, 52005
    Injection Procedure, 50684, 50690
Ureteropyelostomy, 50740
Ureterorrhaphy, 50900
Ureteroscopy
    Dilation
        Intra-Renal Stricture, 52346
        Ureter, 52344, 52345
    Third Stage with Cystourethroscopy, 52351
        Biopsy, 52354
        Destruction, 52354
        Lithotripsy, 52353
    Removal
        Calculus, 52352
    Tumor Excision, 52355
Ureterosigmoidostomy, 50810
    Revision, 50830
Ureterostomy, 50860, 50951
    Injection Procedure, 50684
    Manometric Studies, 50686
    Stent
        Change, 50688
Ureterostomy Tube
    Change, 50688
Ureterotomy, 50600
    Insertion Indwelling Stent, 50605
Ureteroureterostomy, 50760, 50770, 50830
Urethra
    Abscess
        Incision and Drainage, 53040
    Adhesions
        Lysis, 53500

Urethra — *continued*
Artificial Sphincter
Repair, 53449
Biopsy, 52204, 52354, 53200
Destruction, 52214, 52224
Dilation, 52260, 52265, 53600, 53621
General, 53665
Suppository and/or Instillation, 53660, 53661
Diverticulum
Biopsy, 52204
Catheterization, 52010
Destruction, 52214, 52224
Endoscopy, 52000
Excision, 53230, 53235
Extravasation, 53080, 53085
Injection of Implant Material, 51715
Marsupialization, 53240
Repair, 53240
Drainage
Extravasation, 53080, 53085
Endoscopy, 52000
Biopsy, 52204, 52354
Catheterization, 52010
Destruction, 52354, 52400
Evacuation
Clot, 52001
Excision
Tumor, 52355
Exploration, 52351
Incision
Ejaculatory Duct, 52402
Injection of Implant Material, 51715
Lithotripsy, 52353
Removal
Calculus, 52352
Resection
Ejaculatory Duct, 52402
Vasectomy, 52402
Vasotomy, 52402
Excision
Diverticulum, 53230, 53235
Total
Female, 53210
Male, 53215
Incision, 53000, 53010
Meatus, 53020, 53025
Incision and Drainage, 53060
Insertion
Catheter, 51701-51703
Filiform, 53620, 53621
Stent, 52282, 53855
Lesion
Destruction, 53265
Excision, 53260
Lysis
Adhesions, 53500
Paraurethral Gland
Incision and Drainage, 53060
Polyp
Destruction, 53260
Excision, 53260
Pressure Profile Studies, 51727, 51729
Prolapse
Destruction, 53275
Excision, 53275
Repair, 53275
Radiotracer, 52250
Reconstruction, 53410-53440, 53445
Reconstruction and Bladder, 51800, 51820
Complications, 54340-54348
Hypospadias
First Stage, 54322-54328
Second Stage, 54308-54316
Third Stage, 54318
Meatus, 53450, 53460
Removal
Calculus, 52310, 52315
Foreign Body, 52310, 52315
Sling, 53442
Urethral Stent, 52315
Repair
with Replantation Penis, 54438
Diverticulum, 53240, 53400, 53405
Fistula, 45820, 45825, 53400, 53405, 53520
Sphincter, 57220

Urethra — *continued*
Repair — *continued*
Stricture, 53400, 53405
Urethrocele, 57230
Wound, 53502-53515
Skene's Gland
Incision and Drainage, 53060
Sphincter, 52277
Electromyography, 51784, 51785
Needle, 51785
Insertion
Prosthesis, 53444
Reconstruction, 53445
Removal
Prosthesis, 53446, 53447
Repair
Prosthesis, 53449
Replacement
Prosthesis, 53448
Suture
Fistula, 45820, 45825, 53520
to Bladder, 51840, 51841
Wound, 53502-53515
Thermotherapy, 53850-53852
Tumor
Destruction, 53220
Excision, 53220
Unlisted Services and Procedures, 53899
Urethrocystography, 74450, 74455
Urethrotomy, 52270-52276
X–ray with Contrast, 74450, 74455
Urethral
Diverticulum Marsupialization, 53240
Meatus, Dorsal
Reconstruction, 54385
Repair, 54380-54390
Pressure Profile, 51727, 51729
Sphincter
Biofeedback Training, 90911
Insertion
Prosthesis, 53444
Removal
Prosthesis, 53447
Replacement
Prosthesis, 53448
Stenosis
Dilation, 52281
Stent
Insertion, 52282, 53855
Removal
Bladder, 52310, 52315
Urethra, 52310, 52315
Stricture
Dilation, 52281, 53600-53621
Injection
Steroids, 52283
Syndrome
Cystourethroscopy, 52285
Urethral Calculus
Anesthesia, 00918
Urethral Diverticulum
Marsupialization, 53240
Urethral Guide Wire
Insertion, 52334
Urethral Pressure Profile, 51727, 51729
Urethral Sphincter
Biofeedback Training, 90911
Removal
Prosthesis, 53447
Urethral Stenosis
Dilation, 52281
Urethral Stent
Insertion, 52332
Removal
Bladder, 52310, 52315
Urethra, 52310, 52315
Urethral Stricture
Dilation, 52281, 53600, 53621
Injection
Steroids, 52283
Urethral Syndrome
Cystourethroscopy, 52285
Urethrectomy
Total
Female, 53210
Male, 53215

Urethrocele
Repair, 57230-57240
Urethrocystography, 74450, 74455
Contrast and/or Chain, 51605
Retrograde, 51610
Voiding, 51600
Urethrocystopexy, 51840-51841
Urethromeatoplasty, 53450, 53460
Urethropexy, 51840, 51841
Urethroplasty, 46744, 46746
First Stage, 53400
Hypospadias, 54322-54328
Reconstruction
Female Urethra, 53430
Male Anterior Urethra, 53410
Prostatic
Membranous Urethra
First Stage, 53420
One Stage, 53415
Second Stage, 53425
Second Stage, 53405
Hypospadias, 54308-54316
Third Stage
Hypospadias, 54318
Urethrorrhaphy, 53502-53515
Urethroscopy, 52000-52315, 52320-52402
Perineal, 53899
Urethrostomy, 53000, 53010
Urethrotomy, 53000, 53010
with Cystourethroscopy
Female, 52270
Male, 52275
Direct Vision
with Cystourethroscopy, 52276
Internal, 52601, 52647, 52648
Uric Acid
Blood, 84550
Other Source, 84560
Urine, 84560
Uridyltransferase, Galactose–1–Phosphate, 82775-82776
Uridylyltransferase, Galactosephophate, 82775-82776
Urinalysis, 81000-81099
without Microscopy, 81002
Automated, 81001, 81003
Glass Test, 81020
Microalbumin, 82043, 82044
Microscopic, 81015
Pregnancy Test, 81025
Qualitative, 81005
Routine, 81002
Screen, 81007
Semiquantitative, 81005
Unlisted Services and Procedures, 81099
Volume Measurement, 81050
Urinary Bladder
See Bladder
Urinary Catheter Irrigation, 51700
Urinary Sphincter, Artificial
Insertion, 53445
Removal, 53446
with Replacement, 53447-53448
Repair, 53449
Urinary Tract
X–ray with Contrast, 74400-74425
Urine
Albumin, 82042-82044
Blood, 81000-81005
Colony Count, 87086
Pregnancy Test, 81025
Tests, 81000-81099
Urine Sensitivity Test, 87181-87190
Urobilinogen
Feces, 84577
Urine, 84578-84583
Urodynamic Tests
Bladder Capacity
Ultrasound, 51798
Cystometrogram, 51725-51729
Electromyography Studies
Needle, 51785
Rectal, *[51797]*
Residual Urine
Ultrasound, 51798
Stimulus Evoked Response, 51792

Urodynamic Tests — *continued*
Urethra Pressure Profile, *[51797]*
Uroflowmetry, 51736, 51741
Voiding Pressure Studies
Bladder, 51728-51729
Intra–Abdominal, *[51797]*
Uroflowmetry, 51736, 51741
Urography
Antegrade, 74425
Infusion, 74410, 74415
Intravenous, 74400-74415
Retrograde, 74420
Uroporphyrin, 84120
Urostomy, 50727, 50728
Urothromboplastin
Inhibition, 85705
Inhibition Test, 85347
Partial Time, 85730-85732
USH1C, 81407, 81430
USH1G, 81404, 81430
USH2A, 81408, 81430, 81434
Uterine
Adhesion
Lysis, 58559
Cervix
See Cervix
Endoscopies
See Endoscopy, Uterus
Hemorrhage
Postpartum, 59160
Uterus
Ablation
Endometrium, 58353-58356
Tumor
Radiofrequency, 58674
Ultrasound Focused, 0071T-0072T
Uterine Fibroid
Transcervical, 0404T
Biopsy
Endometrium, 58100
Endoscopy, 58558
Catheterization
X–ray, 58340
Chromotubation, 58350
Curettage, 58356
Postpartum, 59160
Dilation and Curettage, 58120
Postpartum, 59160
Ectopic Pregnancy
Interstitial
Partial Resection Uterus, 59136
Total Hysterectomy, 59135
Endoscopy
Endometrial Ablation, 58563
Exploration, 58555
Surgery, 58558-58565
Treatment, 58558-58565
Excision
Laparoscopic, 58550
with Removal of Ovaries, 58552, 58554
Total, 58570-58573
Partial, 58180
Radical
Laparoscopic, 58548
Open, 58210, 58285
Removal of Tubes and/or Ovaries, 58262, 58263, 58291-58293, 58552, 58554
Sonohysterography, 76831
Total, 58150-58152, 58200, 58953-58956
Vaginal, 58260-58270, 58290-58294, 58550-58554
with Colpectomy, 58275, 58280
with Colpo–Urethrocystopexy, 58267
with Repair of Enterocele, 58270, 58294
Hemorrhage
Postpartum, 59160
Hydatidiform Mole
Excision, 59100
Hydrotubation, 58350
Hysterosalpingography, 74740
Hysterosonography, 76831
Incision
Removal of Lesion, 59100

Uterus — *continued*
Insertion
Heyman Capsule
for Brachytherapy, 58346
Intrauterine Device, 58300
Tandem
for Brachytherapy, 57155
Laparoscopy
Tumor Ablation, 58674
Unlisted, 58578
Lesion
Excision, 58545, 58546, 59100
Reconstruction, 58540
Removal
Intrauterine Device (IUD), 58301
Repair
Fistula, 51920, 51925
Rupture, 58520, 59350
Suspension, 58400
with Presacral Sympathectomy, 58410
Sonohysterography, 76831
Suture
Rupture, 59350
Tumor
Ablation
Radiofrequency, 58674
Ultrasound Focused, 0071T-0072T
Excision
Abdominal Approach, 58140, 58146
Vaginal Approach, 58145
Unlisted Services and Procedures, 58578, 58999
X-ray with Contrast, 74740
UTP Hexose 1 Phosphate Uridylyltransferase, 82775-82776
UVC, 36510
UV Light Therapy, 96900
Uvula
Abscess
Incision and Drainage, 42000
Biopsy, 42100
Excision, 42140, 42145
Lesion
Destruction, 42145
Excision, 42104-42107
Unlisted Services and Procedures, 42299
Uvulectomy, 42140
Uvulopalatopharyngoplasty, 42145
Uvulopharyngoplasty, 42145

V

Vaccines
Adenovirus, 90476, 90477
Anthrax, 90581
Chicken Pox, 90716
Cholera Injectable, [90625]
Diphtheria, Tetanus (DT), 90702
Diphtheria, Tetanus, Acellular Pertussis (DTaP), 90700
Diphtheria, Tetanus, Acellular Pertussis, and Poliovirus Inactivated (DTaP-IPV), 90696
Diphtheria, Tetanus, Acellular Pertussis, Hemophilus Influenza B, and Poliovirus Inactivated (DTaPp-IPV/Hib)), 90698
Diphtheria, Tetanus, Acellular Pertussis, Hemophilus Influenza B, Hepatitis B, and Poliovirus Inactivated (DTaP-IPV-Hib-HepB), 90697
Diphtheria, Tetanus, Acellular Pertussis, Hepatitis B, and Inactivated Poliovirus (DTaP-HepB-IPV), 90723
Diphtheria, Tetanus, and Acellular Pertussis, (Tdap), 90715
Encephalitis, Japanese, 90738
Hemophilus Influenza B, 90647-90648
Hepatitis A, 90632-90634
Hepatitis A and Hepatitis B, 90636
Hepatitis B, 90739-90747
Hepatitis B and Hemophilus Influenza B (HepB-Hib), 90748
Human Papilloma Virus, 90649-90651
Influenza, 90653-90668 [90630, 90672, 90673], 90685-90688, [90674]
Japanese Encephalitis, 90738
Measles, Mumps and Rubella (MMR), 90707
Measles, Mumps, Rubella and Varicella (MMRV), 90710

Vaccines — *continued*
Meningococcal, 90620-90621, 90644, 90733-90734
Pneumococcal, 90670, 90732
Poliovirus, Inactivated
Intramuscular, 90713
Subcutaneous, 90713
Rabies, 90675, 90676
Rotavirus, 90680-90681
Tetanus and Diphtheria, 90702, 90714
Tetanus, Diphtheria and Acellular Pertussis (Tdap), 90715
Tuberculosis (BCG), 90585
Typhoid, 90690-90691
Unlisted Vaccine
Toxoid, 90749
Varicella (Chicken Pox), 90716
Yellow Fever, 90717
Zoster, 90736
Vagina
Abscess
Incision and Drainage, 57010
Amines Test, 82120
Biopsy
Colposcopy, 57421
Endocervical, 57454
Extensive, 57105
Simple, 57100
Closure, 57120
Colposcopy, 57420-57421, 57455-57456, 57461
Construction
with Graft, 57292
without Graft, 57291
Cyst
Excision, 57135
Dilation, 57400
Endocervical
Biopsy, 57454
Exploration, 57452
Excision
Closure, 57120
Complete
with Removal of Paravaginal Tissue
with Lymphadenectomy, 57112
with Removal of Paravaginal Tissue, 57111
with Removal of Vaginal Wall, 57110
Partial
with Removal of Paravaginal Tissue
with Lymphadenectomy, 57109
with Removal of Paravaginal Tissue, 57107
with Removal of Vaginal Wall, 57106
Total, 57110
with Hysterectomy, 58275, 58280
with Repair of Enterocele, 58280
Exploration
Endocervical, 57452
Incision, 57000
Hematoma
Incision and Drainage, 57022, 57023
Hemorrhage, 57180
Hysterectomy, 58290, 58550, 58552-58554
Incision and Drainage, 57020
Insertion
Ovoid
for Brachytherapy, 57155
Packing for Bleeding, 57180
Pessary, 57160
Irrigation, 57150
Lesion
Destruction, 57061, 57065
Extensive, 57065
Simple, 57061
Prolapse
Sacrospinous Ligament Fixation, 57282
Removal
Foreign Body, 57415
Prosthetic Graft, 57295-57296
Sling
Stress Incontinence, 57287
Tissue, Partial, 57106
Wall, Partial, 57107
Repair, 56800

Vagina — *continued*
Repair — *continued*
Cystocele, 57240, 57260
Combined Anteroposterior, 57260, 57265
Posterior, 57240
Enterocele, 57265
Fistula, 51900
Rectovaginal, 57300-57308
Transvesical and Vaginal Approach, 57330
Urethrovaginal, 57310, 57311
Vesicovaginal, 51900, 57320, 57330
Hysterectomy, 58267, 58293
Incontinence, 57288
Obstetric, 59300
Paravaginal Defect, 57284
Pereyra Procedure, 57289
Prolapse, 57282, 57284
Prosthesis Insertion, 57267
Rectocele
Combined Anteroposterior, 57260, 57265
Posterior, 57250
Suspension, 57280-57283
Laparoscopic, 57425
Urethra Sphincter, 57220
Wound, 57200, 57210
Colpoperineorrhaphy, 57210
Colporrhaphy, 57200
Revision
Prosthetic Graft, 57295-57296, 57426
Sling
Stress Incontinence, 57287
Septum
Excision, 57130
Suspension, 57280-57283
Laparoscopic, 57425
Suture
Cystocele, 57240, 57260
Enterocele, 57265
Fistula, 51900, 57300-57330
Rectocele, 57250, 57260
Wound, 57200, 57210
Tumor
Excision, 57135
Ultrasound, 76830
Unlisted Services and Procedures, 58999
X-ray with Contrast, 74775
Vaginal Delivery, 59400, 59610-59614
After Previous Cesarean Section, 59610, 59612
Attempted, 59618-59622
Antepartum Care Only, 59425, 59426
Attempted, 59618-59622
Cesarean Delivery After Attempted
with Postpartum Care, 59622
Delivery Only, 59620
Delivery After Previous Vaginal Delivery Only
with Postpartum Care, 59614
Delivery Only, 59409
External Cephalic Version, 59412
Placenta, 59414
Postpartum Care only, 59410
Routine Care, 59400
Vaginal Smear, 88141-88155, 88164-88167, 88174-88175
Vaginal Suppositories
Induced Abortion, 59855
with Dilation and Curettage, 59856
with Hysterotomy, 59857
Vaginal Tissue
Removal, Partial, 57106
Vaginal Wall
Removal, Partial, 57107
Vaginectomy
Partial, 57109
with Nodes, 57109
Vaginoplasty
Intersex State, 57335
Vaginorrhaphy, 57200
See Also Colporrhaphy
Vaginoscopy
Biopsy, 57454
Exploration, 57452
Vaginotomy, 57000-57010

Vagotomy
With Gastroduodenostomy Revision/Reconstruction, 43855
With Gastrojejunostomy Revision/Reconstruction, 43865
With Partial Distal Gastrectomy, 43635
Abdominal, 64760
Highly Selective, 43641
Parietal Cell, 43641, 64755
Reconstruction, 43855
with Gastroduodenostomy Revision, 43855
with Gastrojejunostomy Revision, Reconstruction, 43865
Selective, 43640
Truncal, 43640
Vagus Nerve
Avulsion
Abdominal, 64760
Selective, 64755
Blocking Therapy
Laparoscopic Implantation Neurostimulator Electrode Array and Pulse Generator, 0312T
Laparoscopic Removal Neurostimulator Electrode Array and Pulse Generator, 0314T
Laparoscopic Revision or Replacement Electrode Array, Reconnect to Existing Pulse Generator, 0313T
Pulse Generator Electronic Analysis, 0317T
Removal Pulse Generator, 0315T
Replacement Pulse Generator, 0316T
Incision, 43640, 43641
Abdominal, 64760
Selective, 64755
Injection
Anesthetic, 64408
Transection, 43640, 43641
Abdominal, 64760
Selective, 43652, 64755
Truncal, 43651
Valentine's Test
Urinalysis, Glass Test, 81020
Valproic Acid, 80164
Valproic Acid Measurement, 80164
Valsalva Sinus
Repair, 33702-33720
Valva Atrioventricularis Sinistra (Valva Mitralis)
Incision, 33420, 33422
Repair, 33420-33427
Transcatheter, 33418-33419
Replacement, 33430
Valve
Aortic
Repair, Left Ventricle, 33414
Replacement, 33405-33413
Bicuspid
Incision, 33420, 33422
Repair, 33420-33427
Transcatheter, 33418-33419
Replacement, 33430
Mitral
Incision, 33420, 33422
Repair, 33420-33427
Transcatheter, 33418-33419
Replacement, 33430
Pulmonary
Incision, 33470-33474
Repair, 33470-33474
Replacement, 33475
Tricuspid
Excision, 33460
Repair, 33463-33465
Replace, 33465
Reposition, 33468
Valvectomy
Tricuspid Valve, 33460
Valve Stenosis, Aortic
Repair, 33415
Supravalvular, 33417
Valvotomy
Mitral Valve, 33420, 33422
Pulmonary Valve, 33470-33474
Reoperation, 33530
Valvuloplasty
Aortic Valve, 33390-33391

Valvuloplasty — *continued*
  Femoral Vein, 34501
  Mitral Valve, 33425-33427
  Percutaneous Balloon
    Aortic Valve, 92986
    Mitral Valve, 92987
    Pulmonary Valve, 92990
  Prosthetic Valve, 33496
  Reoperation, 33530
  Tricuspid Valve, 33460-33465
Vancomycin
  Assay, 80202
  Resistance, 87500
Van Den Bergh Test, 82247, 82248
Vanillymandelic Acid
  Urine, 84585
VAQTA, 90632-90633
VAR, 90716
Varicella (Chicken Pox)
  Immunization, 90710, 90716
Varicella–Zoster
  Antibody, 86787
  Antigen Detection
    Direct Fluorescent Antibody, 87290
Varices, Esophageal
  Injection Sclerosis, 43204
  Ligation, 43205, 43400
  Transection and Repair, 43401
Varicocele
  Spermatic Cord
    Excision, 55530-55540
Varicose Vein
  with Tissue Excision, 37735, 37760
  Ablation, 36473-36479
  Removal, 37718, 37722, 37735, 37765-37785
  Secondary Varicosity, 37785
VARIVAX, 90716
Vascular Flow Check, Graft, 15860
Vascular Injection
  Unlisted Services and Procedures, 36299
Vascular Lesion
  Cranial
    Excision, 61600-61608, 61615, 61616
  Cutaneous
    Destruction, 17106-17108
Vascular Malformation
  Cerebral
    Repair, 61710
  Finger
    Excision, 26115
  Hand
    Excision, 26115
Vascular Procedure(s)
  Angioscopy
    Noncoronary Vessels, 35400
  Brachytherapy
    Intracoronary Artery, *[92974]*
  Endoluminal Imaging
    Coronary Vessels, *[92978, 92979]*
  Endoscopy
    Surgical, 37500
  Harvest
    Lower Extremity Vein, 35572
  Thrombolysis
    Coronary Vessels, *[92975, 92977]*
    Cranial Vessels, 37195
    Intracranial Vessels, 61645
Vascular Rehabilitation, 93668
Vascular Studies
  See Also Doppler Scan, Duplex, Plethysmography
  Angioscopy
    Aorta, 93978, 93979
    Noncoronary Vessels, 35400
  Artery Studies
    Extracranial, 93880-93882
    Extremities, 93922-93924
    Intracranial, 93886, 93888
    Lower Extremity, 93922-93926
    Middle Cerebral Artery, Fetal, 76821
    Umbilical Artery, Fetal, 76820
    Upper Extremity, 93930, 93931
    Blood Pressure Monitoring, 24 Hour, 93784-93790
  Endothelial Function Assessment, 0337T
  Hemodialysis Access, 93990

Vascular Studies — *continued*
  Kidney
    Multiple Study with Pharmacological Intervention, 78709
    Single Study with Pharmacological Intervention, 78708
  Penile Vessels, 93980, 93981
  Temperature Gradient, 93740
  Unlisted Services and Procedures, 93799
  Venous Studies
    Extremities, 93970-93971
    Venous Pressure, 93770
  Visceral Studies, 93975-93979
Vascular Surgery
  Arm, Upper
    Anesthesia, 01770-01782
  Elbow
    Anesthesia, 01770-01782
  Endoscopy, 37500
  Unlisted Services and Procedures, 37799
Vas Deferens
  Anastomosis
    to Epididymis, 54900, 54901
  Excision, 55250
  Incision, 55200
    for X–Ray, 55300
  Ligation, 55450
  Repair
    Suture, 55400
  Unlisted Services and Procedures, 55899
  Vasography, 74440
  X–Ray with Contrast, 74440
Vasectomy, 55250
  Laser Coagulation of Prostate, 52647
  Laser Vaporization of Prostate, 52648
  Reversal, 55400
  Transurethral
    Cystourethroscopic, 52402
  Transurethral Electrosurgical Resection of Prostate, 52601
  Transurethral Resection of Prostate, 52648
Vasoactive Drugs
  Injection
    Penis, 54231
Vasoactive Intestinal Peptide, 84586
Vasogram, 74440
Vasography, 74440
Vasointestinal Peptide, 84586
Vasopneumatic Device Therapy, 97016
  See Also Physical Medicine/Therapy/ Occupational Therapy
Vasopressin, 84588
Vasotomy, 55200, 55300
  Transurethral
    Cystourethroscopic, 52402
Vasovasorrhaphy, 55400
Vasovasostomy, 55400
VATS
  See Thoracoscopy
VBAC, 59610-59614
VBG (Vertical Banding Gastroplasty), 43842
V, Cranial Nerve
  Destruction, 64600-64610
  Injection
    Neurolytic, 64600-64610
VCU (Voiding Cystourethrogram), 51600
VCUG (Voiding Cystourethrogram), 51600
VDRL, 86592-86593
Vectorcardiogram
  Evaluation, 93799
  Tracing, 93799
Vein
  Ablation
    Endovenous, 36473-36479
  Adrenal
    Venography, 75840, 75842
  Anastomosis
    Caval to Mesenteric, 37160
    Intrahepatic Portosystemic, 37182-37183
    Portocaval, 37140
    Reniportal, 37145
    Saphenopopliteal, 34530
    Splenorenal, 37180, 37181
    Vein, 34530, 37180, 37181
    to Vein, 37140-37160, 37182-37183

Vein — *continued*
  Angioplasty
    Transluminal, 36902, 36905, 36907, *[37246, 37247, 37248, 37249]*
  Arm
    Harvest of Vein for Bypass Graft, 35500
    Venography, 75820, 75822
  Axillary
    Thrombectomy, 34490
  Biopsy
    Transcatheter, 75970
  Cannulization
    to Artery, 36810, 36815
    to Vein, 36800
  Catheterization
    Central Insertion, 36555-36558
    Organ Blood, 36500
    Peripheral Insertion, 36568, 36569
    Removal, 36589
    Repair, 36575
    Replacement, 36578-36581, 36584
    Umbilical, 36510
  Endoscopic Harvest
    for Bypass Graft, 33508
  External Cannula Declotting, 36860, 36861
  Extremity
    Non–Invasive Studies, 93970-93971
  Femoral
    Repair, 34501
  Femoropopliteal
    Thrombectomy, 34421, 34451
  Guidance
    Fluoroscopic, 77001
    Ultrasound, 76937
  Hepatic Portal
    Splenoportography, 75810
    Venography, 75885, 75887
  Iliac
    Thrombectomy, 34401, 34421, 34451
  Injection
    Sclerosing Agent, 36468-36471
  Insertion
    IVC Filter, 37191
  Interrupt
    Femoral Vein, 37650
    Iliac, 37660
    Vena Cava, 37619
  Jugular
    Venography, 75860
  Leg
    Harvest for Vascular Reconstruction, 35572
    Venography, 75820, 75822
  Ligation
    Clusters, 37785
    Esophagus, 43205
    Jugular, 37565
    Perforation, 37760
    Saphenous, 37700-37735, 37780
    Secondary, 37785
  Liver
    Venography, 75860, 75889, 75891
  Neck
    Venography, 75860
  Nuclear Medicine
    Thrombosis Imaging, 78456-78458
  Orbit
    Venography, 75880
  Portal
    Catheterization, 36481
  Pulmonary
    Repair, 33730
  Removal
    Clusters, 37785
    Saphenous, 37700-37735, 37780
    Varicose, 37765, 37766
  Renal
    Venography, 75831, 75833
  Repair
    Angioplasty, *[37248, 37249]*
    Graft, 34520
  Sampling
    Venography, 75893
  Sinus
    Venography, 75870
  Skull
    Venography, 75870, 75872

Vein — *continued*
  Spermatic
    Excision, 55530-55540
    Ligation, 55500
  Splenic
    Splenoportography, 75810
  Stripping
    Saphenous, 37700-37735, 37780
  Subclavian
    Thrombectomy, 34471, 34490
  Thrombectomy
    Other than Hemodialysis Graft or Fistula, 35875, 35876
  Unlisted Services and Procedures, 37799
  Valve Transposition, 34510
  Varicose
    with Tissue Excision, 37735, 37760
    Ablation, 36473-36479
    Removal, 37700-37735, 37765-37785
    Secondary Varicosity, 37785
  Vena Cava
    Thrombectomy, 34401-34451
    Venography, 75825, 75827
Velpeau Cast, 29058
Vena Cava
  Catheterization, 36010
  Interruption, 37619
  Reconstruction, 34502
  Resection with Reconstruction, 37799
Vena Caval
  Thrombectomy, 50230
Venereal Disease Research Laboratory (VDRL), 86592-86593
Venesection
  Therapeutic, 99195
Venipuncture
  See Also Cannulation; Catheterization
  Child/Adult
    Cutdown, 36425
    Percutaneous, 36410
  Infant
    Cutdown, 36420
    Percutaneous, 36400-36406
  Routine, 36415
Venography
  Adrenal, 75840, 75842
  Arm, 75820, 75822
  Epidural, 75872
  Hepatic Portal, 75885, 75887
  Injection, 36005
  Jugular, 75860
  Leg, 75820, 75822
  Liver, 75889, 75891
  Neck, 75860
  Nuclear Medicine, 78445, 78457, 78458
  Orbit, 75880
  Renal, 75831, 75833
  Sagittal Sinus, 75870
  Vena Cava, 75825, 75827
  Venous Sampling, 75893
Venorrhaphy
  Femoral, 37650
  Iliac, 37660
  Vena Cava, 37619
Venotomy
  Therapeutic, 99195
Venous Access Device
  Blood Collection, 36591-36592
  Declotting, 36593
  Fluoroscopic Guidance, 77001
  Insertion
    Central, 36560-36566
    Peripheral, 36570, 36571
  Obstruction Clearance, 36595, 36596
    Guidance, 75901, 75902
  Removal, 36590
  Repair, 36576
  Replacement, 36582, 36583, 36585
    Catheter Only, 36578
Venous Blood Pressure, 93770
Venovenostomy
  Saphenopopliteal, 34530
Ventilating Tube
  Insertion, 69433
  Removal, 69424
Ventilation Assist, 94002-94005, 99504

Ventricular
Aneurysmectomy, 33542
Assist Device, 33975-33983, 33990-33993
Puncture, 61020, 61026, 61105-61120
Ventriculocisternostomy, 62180, 62200-62201
Ventriculography
Anesthesia
Brain, 00214
Cardia, 01920
Burr Holes, 01920
Cerebrospinal Fluid Flow, 78635
Nuclear Imaging, 78635
Ventriculomyectomy, 33416
Ventriculomyotomy, 33416
VEP, 95930
Vermiform Appendix
Abscess
Incision and Drainage, 44900
Excision, 44950-44960, 44970
Vermilionectomy, 40500
Verruca(e)
Destruction, 17110-17111
Verruca Plana
Destruction, 17110-17111
Version, Cephalic
External, of Fetus, 59412
Vertebra
See Also Spinal Cord; Spine; Vertebral Body;
Vertebral Process
Additional Segment
Excision, 22103, 22116
Arthrodesis
Anterior, 22548-22585
Exploration, 22830
Lateral Extracavitary, 22532-22534
Posterior, 22590-22802
Spinal Deformity
Anterior Approach, 22808-22812
Posterior Approach, 22800-22804
Arthroplasty, 0202T
Cervical
Artificial Disc, 22864
Excision for Tumor, 22100, 22110
Fracture, 23675, 23680
Fracture
Dislocation
Additional Segment
Open Treatment, 22328
Cervical
Open Treatment, 22326
Lumbar
Open Treatment, 22325
Thoracic
Open Treatment, 22327
Kyphectomy, 22818, 22819
Lumbar
Artificial Disc, 22865
Distraction Device, 22869-22870
Excision for Tumor, 22102, 22114
Osteoplasty
Cervicothoracic, 22510, 22512
Lumbosacral, 22511-22512
Osteotomy
Additional Segment
Anterior Approach, 22226
Posterior/Posterolateral Approach,
22216
Cervical
Anterior Approach, 22220
Posterior/Posterolateral Approach,
22210
Lumbar
Anterior Approach, 22224
Posterior/Posterolateral Approach,
22214
Thoracic
Anterior Approach, 22222
Posterior/Posterolateral Approach,
22212
Thoracic
Excision for Tumor, 22101, 22112
Vertebrae
See Also Vertebra
Arthrodesis
Anterior, 22548-22585
Lateral Extracavitary, 22532-22534

Vertebrae — *continued*
Arthrodesis — *continued*
Spinal Deformity, 22818, 22819
Vertebral
Arteries
Aneurysm, 35005, 61698, 61702
Bypass Graft, 35508, 35515, 35642-35645
Catheterization, 36100
Decompression, 61597
Thromboendarterectomy, 35301
Vertebral Body
Biopsy, 20250, 20251
Excision
with Skull Base Surgery, 61597
Decompression, 62380, 63081-63091
Lesion, 63300-63308
Fracture
Dislocation
Closed Treatment
without Manipulation, 22310
See also Evaluation and Manage-
ment Codes
Kyphectomy, 22818, 22819
Vertebral Column
See Spine
Vertebral Corpectomy, 63081-63308
Vertebral Fracture
Closed Treatment
with Manipulation, Casting, and/or Bracing,
22315
without Manipulation, 22310
Open Treatment
Additional Segment, 22328
Cervical, 22326
Lumbar, 22325
Posterior, 22325-22327
Thoracic, 22327
Vertebral Process
Fracture, Closed Treatment
See Evaluation and Management Codes
Vertebroplasty
Percutaneous
Cervicothoracic, 22510, 22512
Lumbosacral, 22511-22512
Vertical Banding Gastroplasty (VBG), 43842
Very Low Density Lipoprotein, 83719
Vesication
Puncture Aspiration, 10160
Vesicle, Seminal
Excision, 55650
Cyst, 55680
Mullerian Duct, 55680
Incision, 55600, 55605
Unlisted Services/Procedures, 55899
Vesiculography, 74440
X-Ray with Contrast, 74440
Vesico–Psoas Hitch, 50785
Vesicostomy
Cutaneous, 51980
Vesicourethropexy, 51840-51841
Vesicovaginal Fistula
Closure
Abdominal Approach, 51900
Transvesical/Vaginal Approach, 57330
Vaginal Approach, 57320
Vesiculectomy, 55650
Vesiculogram, Seminal, 55300, 74440
Vesiculography, 55300, 74440
Vesiculotomy, 55600, 55605
Complicated, 55605
Vessel, Blood
See Blood Vessels
Vessels Transposition, Great
Repair, 33770-33781
Vestibular Evaluation, 92540
Vestibular Function Tests
Additional Electrodes, 92547
Caloric Tests, 92533, 92537-92538
Nystagmus
Optokinetic, 92534, 92544
Positional, 92532, 92542
Spontaneous, 92531, 92541
Posturography, 92548
Sinusoidal Rotational Testing, 92546
Torsion Swing Test, 92546
Tracking Test, 92545

Vestibular Nerve
Section
Transcranial Approach, 69950
Translabyrinthine Approach, 69915
Vestibule of Mouth
Biopsy, 40808
Excision
Lesion, 40810-40816
Destruction, 40820
Mucosa for Graft, 40818
Vestibuloplasty, 40840-40845
VF, 92081-92083
V–Flap Procedure
One Stage Distal Hypospadias Repair, 54322
VHL, 81403-81404, 81437-81438
Vibration Perception Threshold (VPT), 0107T
ViCPs, 90691
Vicq D'Azyr Operation, 31600-31605
Vidal Procedure
Varicocele, Spermatic Cord, Excision, 55530-
55540
Video
Esophagus, 74230
Pharynx, 70371
Speech Evaluation, 70371
Swallowing Evaluation, 74230
Video–Assisted Thoracoscopic Surgery
See Thoracoscopy
Videoradiography
Unlisted Services and Procedures, 76120-76125
VII, Coagulation Factor, 85230
See Proconvertin
VII, Cranial Nerve
See Facial Nerve
VIII, Coagulation Factor, 85240-85247
Villus, Chorionic
Biopsy, 59015
Villusectomy
See Synovectomy
VIP, 84586
Viral
AIDS, 87390
Burkitt Lymphoma
Antibody, 86663-86665
Human Immunodeficiency
Antibody, 86701-86703
Antigen, 87389-87391, 87534-87539
Confirmation Test, 86689
Influenza
Antibody, 86710
Antigen Detection, 87804
Vaccine, 90653-90670 [*90672, 90673*],
90685-90688, [*90674*]
Respiratory Syncytial
Antibody, 86756
Antigen Detection, 87280, 87420, 87807
Recombinant, 90378
Salivary Gland
Cytomegalovirus
Antibody, 86644-86645
Antigen Detection, 87271, 87332,
87495-87497
Viral Antibodies, 86280
Viral Warts
Destruction, 17110-17111
Virtual Colonoscopy
Diagnostic, 74261-74262
Screening, 74263
Virus Identification
Immunofluorescence, 87254
Virus Isolation, 87250-87255
Visceral Aorta Repair, 34841-34848
Visceral Larva Migrans, 86280
Viscosities, Blood, 85810
Visit, Home, 99341-99350
Visual Acuity Screen, 0333T, 99172, 99173
Visual Evoked Potential, 0333T, 0464T
Visual Field Exam, 92081-92083
with Patient Initiated Data Transmission, 0378T-
0379T
Visual Function Screen, 1055F, 99172
Visualization
Ideal Conduit, 50690
Visual Reinforcement Audiometry, 92579
Vital Capacity Measurement, 94150

Vitamin
A, 84590
B–1, 84425
B–2, 84252
B–6, 84207
B–6 Measurement, 84207
B–12, 82607-82608
Absorption Study, 78270-78272
BC, 82746-82747
B Complex, 78270-78272
C, 82180
D, 82306 [*82652*]
E, 84446
K, 84597
Dependent Bone Protein, 83937
Dependent Protein S, 85305-85306
Epoxide Reductase Complex, Subunit 1
Gene Analysis, 81355
Not Otherwise Specified, 84591
Vitelline Duct
Excision, 44800
Vitrectomy
with Endolaser Panretinal Photocoagulation,
67040
with Epiretinal Membrane Stripping, 67041-
67043
with Focal Endolaser Photocoagulation, 67039
with Implantation of Intra–ocular Retinal Elec-
trode Array, 0100T
with Implantation or Replacement Drug Deliv-
ery System, 67027
with Placement of Subconjunctival Retinal
Prosthesis Receiver, 0100T
Anterior Approach
Partial, 67005
for Retinal Detachment, 67108, 67113
Pars Plana Approach, 67036, 67041-67043
Partial, 67005, 67010
Subtotal, 67010
Vitreous
Aspiration, 67015
Excision
with Epiretinal Membrane Stripping,
67041-67043
with Focal Endolaser Photocoagulation,
67039
Pars Plana Approach, 67036
Implantation
Drug Delivery System, 67027
Incision
Strands, 67030, 67031
Injection
Fluid Substitute, 67025
Pharmacologic Agent, 67028
Removal
Anterior Approach, 67005
Subtotal, 67010
Replacement
Drug Delivery System, 67027
Strands
Discission, 67030
Severing, 67031
Subtotal, 67010
Vitreous Humor
Anesthesia, 00145
Vivotif Berna, 90690
V-Ki-Ras2 Kirsten Rat Sarcoma Viral Oncogene
Gene Analysis, 81275
VKORC1, 81355
VLDL, 83719
VMA, 84585
Vocal Cords
Injection
Endoscopy, 31513
Therapeutic, 31570, 31571
Voice and Resonance Analysis, 92524
Voice Button
Speech Prosthesis, Creation, 31611
Voiding
EMG, 51784-51785
Pressure Studies
Abdominal, [*51797*]
Bladder, 51728-51729 [*51797*]
Rectum, [*51797*]
Volatiles, 84600
Volkman Contracture, 25315, 25316

Volume
  Lung, 94726-94727
  Reduction
    Blood Products, 86960
    Lung, 32491
Von Kraske Proctectomy
  Proctectomy, Partial, 45111-45123
VP, 51728-51729, *[51797]*
VPS13B, 81407-81408
VPT (Vibration Perception Threshold), 0107T
VRA, 92579
V-Raf Murine Sarcoma Viral Oncogene Homolog
  B1 Gene Analysis, 81210
Vulva
  Abscess
    Incision and Drainage, 56405
  Colposcopy., 56820
    Biopsy, 56821
  Excision
    Complete, 56625, 56633-56640
    Partial, 56620, 56630-56632
    Radical, 56630, 56631, 56633-56640
      Complete, 56633-56640
      Partial, 56630-56632
    Simple
      Complete, 56625
      Partial, 56620
  Lesion
    Destruction, 56501, 56515
  Perineum
    Biopsy, 56605, 56606
    Incision and Drainage, 56405
  Repair
    Obstetric, 59300
Vulvectomy
  Complete, 56625, 56633-56640
  Partial, 56620, 56630-56632
  Radical, 56630-56640
    Complete
      with Bilateral Inguinofemoral Lym-
        phadenectomy, 56637
      with Inguinofemoral, Iliac, and Pelvic
        Lymphadenectomy, 56640
      with Unilateral Inguinofemoral Lym-
        phadenectomy, 56634
    Partial, 56630-56632
    Simple
      Complete, 56625
      Partial, 56620
  Tricuspid Valve, 33460-33465
VWF, 81401, 81403-81406, 81408
V-Y Operation, Bladder, Neck, 51845
V-Y Plasty
  Skin, Adjacent Tissue Transfer, 14000-14350
VZIG, 90396

W

WADA Activation Test, 95958
WAIS, 96101-96103
  Psychiatric Diagnosis, Psychological Testing,
    96101-96103
Waldius Procedure, 27445
Wall, Abdominal
  See Abdominal Wall
Walsh Modified Radical Prostatectomy, 55810
Warfarin Therapy, 4012F
Warts
  Flat
    Destruction, 17110, 17111
WAS, 81406
Washing
  Sperm, 58323
Wasserman Test
  Syphilis Test, 86592-86593
Wassmund Procedure
  Osteotomy
    Maxilla, 21206
Waterjet Ablation
  Prostate, 0421T
Waterston Procedure, 33755
Water Wart
  Destruction
    Penis, 54050-54060
    Skin, 17110-17111
    Vulva, 56501-56515

Watson-Jones Procedure
  Repair, Ankle, Ligament, 27695-27698
Wave, Ultrasonic Shock
  See Ultrasound
WBC, 85007, 85009, 85025, 85048, 85540
WDR62, 81407
Webbed
  Toe
    Repair, 28280
Wechsler Memory Scales, 96118-96119
Wedge Excision
  Osteotomy, 21122
Wedge Resection
  Chest, 32505-32507, 32666-32668
  Ovary, 58920
Weight Recorded, 2001F
Well Child Care, 99381-99384, 99391-99394,
  99460-99463
Wellness Behavior
  Alcohol and/or Substance Abuse, 99408-99409
  Assessment, 96150
  Family Intervention, 96154-96155
  Group Intervention, 0403T, 96153
  Re-assessment, 96151
  Smoking and Tobacco Cessation Counseling,
    99406-99407
Wernicke-Posadas Disease, 86490
Wertheim Hysterectomy, 58210
Wertheim Operation, 58210
Westergren Test
  Sedimentation Rate, Blood Cell, 85651, 85652
Western Blot
  HIV, 86689
  Protein, 84181, 84182
  Tissue Analysis, 88371, 88372
West Nile Virus
  Antibody, 86788-86789
Wharton Ducts
  Ligation of, 42510
Wheelchair Management
  Propulsion
    Training, 97542
Wheeler Knife Procedure, 66820
Wheeler Procedure
  Blepharoplasty, 67924
  Discission Secondary Membranous Cataract,
    66820
Whipple Procedure, 48150
  without Pancreatojejunostomy, 48152
Whirlpool Therapy, 97022
White Blood Cell
  Alkaline Phosphatase, 85540
  Antibody, 86021
  Count, 85032, 85048, 89055
  Differential, 85004-85007, 85009
  Histamine Release Test, 86343
  Phagocytosis, 86344
  Transfusion, 86950
Whitehead Hemorrhoidectomy, 46260
Whitehead Operation, 46260
Whitman Astragalectomy, 28120, 28130
Whitman Procedure (Hip), 27120
Wick Catheter Technique, 20950
Widal Serum Test
  Agglutinin, Febrile, 86000
Wilke Type Procedure, 42507
Window
  Oval
    Fistula Repair, 69666
  Round
    Fistula Repair, 69667
Window Technic, Pericardial, 33015
Windpipe
  See Trachea
Winiwarter Operation, 47720-47740
Winter Procedure, 54435
Wintrobe Test
  Sedimentation Rate, Blood Cell, 85651, 85652
Wire
  Insertion
    Removal
      Skeletal Traction, 20650
  Intradental
    without Fracture, 21497

Wiring
  Prophylactic Treatment
    Humerus, 24498
Wirsung Duct
  See Pancreatic Duct
Wisconsin Card Sorting Test, 96118-96120
Witzel Operation, 43500, 43520, 43830-43832
Wolff-Parkinson-White Procedure, 33250
Womb
  See Uterus
Work Hardening, 97545-97546
Work Reintegration, 97545, 97546
Work Related Evaluation Services, 99455, 99456
Worm
  Helminth Antibody, 86682
Wound
  Abdominal wall, 49900
  Debridement
    Non-Selective, 97602
    Selective, 97597-97598
  Dehiscence
    Repair
      Abdominal wall, 49900
      Secondary
        Abdominal wall, 49900
        Skin and subcutaneous tissue
          Complex, 13160
          Complicated, 13160
          Extensive, 13160
        Skin and Subcutaneous Tissue
          Simple, 12020
            with Packing, 12021
          Superficial, 12020
            with Packing, 12021
    Suture
      Secondary
        Abdominal Wall, 49900
        Skin and Subcutaneous Tissue
          Complex, 13160
          Complicated, 13160
          Extensive, 13160
        Skin and Subcutaneous Tissue
          Simple, 12020
            with Packing, 12021
          Superficial, 12020
            with Packing, 12021
  Exploration
    Parathyroidectomy, 60502
    Penetrating
      Abdomen/Flank/Back, 20102
      Chest, 20101
      Extremity, 20103
      Neck, 20100
      Penetrating Trauma, 20100-20103
  Infection
    Incision and Drainage
      Postoperative, 10180
  Negative Pressure Therapy, 97605-97608
  Repair
    Skin
      Complex, 13100-13160
      Intermediate, 12031-12057
      Simple, 12001-12021
    Urethra, 53502-53515
  Secondary
    Abdominal Wall, 49900
    Skin and Subcutaneous Tissue
      Complex, 13160
      Complicated, 13160
      Extensive, 13160
      Simple, 12020
      Simple with Packing, 12021
      Superficial, 12020
        with Packing, 12021
  Suture
    Bladder, 51860, 51865
    Kidney, 50500
    Trachea
      Cervical, 31800
      Intrathoracic, 31805
    Urethra, 53502-53515
  Vagina
    Repair, 57200, 57210
W-Plasty
  Skin Surgery, Adjacent Tissue Transfer, 14000-
    14350

Wrist
  See Also Arm, Lower; Carpal Bone
  Abscess, 25028
  Arthrocentesis, 20605-20606
  Arthrodesis, 25800
    with Graft, 25810
    with Sliding Graft, 25805
  Arthrography, 73115
  Arthroplasty, 25332, 25443, 25447
    with Implant, 25441, 25442, 25444, 25445
    Revision, 25449
    Total Replacement, 25446
  Arthroscopy
    Diagnostic, 29840
    Surgical, 29843-29848
  Arthrotomy, 25040, 25100-25105
    for Repair, 25107
  Biopsy, 25065, 25066, 25100, 25101
  Bursa
    Excision, 25115, 25116
    Incision and Drainage, 25031
  Capsule
    Incision, 25085
  Cast, 29085
  Cyst, 25130-25136
  Decompression, 25020, 25023
  Disarticulation, 25920
    Reamputation, 25924
    Revision, 25922
  Dislocation
    with Fracture
      Closed Treatment, 25680
      Open Treatment, 25685
    with Manipulation, 25259, 25660, 25675
    Closed Treatment, 25660
    Intercarpal, 25660
      Open Treatment, 25670
    Open Treatment, 25660, 25670, 25676
    Percutaneous Fixation, 25671
    Radiocarpal, 25660
      Open Treatment, 25670
    Radioulnar
      Closed Treatment, 25675
      Percutaneous Fixation, 25671
  Excision
    Carpal, 25210, 25215
    Cartilage, 25107
    Tendon Sheath, 25115, 25116
    Tumor, 25075-25078 *[25071, 25073]*
  Exploration, 25040, 25101
  Fasciotomy, 25020-25025
  Fracture, 25645
    with Dislocation, 25680, 25685
    with Manipulation, 25259, 25624, 25635
    Closed Treatment, 25622, 25630
    Open Treatment, 25628
  Ganglion Cyst
    Excision, 25111, 25112
  Hematoma, 25028
  Incision, 25040, 25100-25105
    Tendon Sheath, 25000, 25001
  Injection
    Carpal Tunnel
      Therapeutic, 20526
    X-ray, 25246
  Joint
    See Radiocarpal Joint
  Lesion
    Excision, 25110
    Tendon Sheath, 25000
  Magnetic Resonance Imaging, 73221
  Reconstruction
    Capsulectomy, 25320
    Capsulorrhaphy, 25320
    Carpal Bone, 25394, 25430
    Realign, 25335
  Removal
    Foreign Body, 25040, 25101, 25248
    Implant, 25449
    Loose Body, 25101
    Prosthesis, 25250, 25251
  Repair, 25447
    Bone, 25440
    Carpal Bone, 25431
    Muscle, 25260, 25270
      Secondary, 25263, 25265, 25272, 25274

Wrist — *continued*
  Repair — *continued*
    Tendon, 25260, 25270, 25280-25316
      Secondary, 25263, 25265, 25272, 25274
    Tendon Sheath, 25275
  Strapping, 29260
  Synovium
    Excision, 25105, 25115-25119
  Tendon
    Excision, 25109
  Tendon Sheath
    Excision, 25115, 25116
  Tenodesis, 25300, 25301
  Tenotomy, 25290
  Unlisted Services and Procedures, 25999
  X-ray, 73100, 73110
    with Contrast, 73115
WT1, 81405

X

Xa, Coagulation Factor, 85260
X, Coagulation Factor, 85260
X, Cranial Nerve
  See Vagus Nerve
Xenoantibodies, 86308-86310
XI, Coagulation Factor, 85270
XI, Cranial Nerve
  See Accessory Nerve
XII, Coagulation Factor, 85280
XII, Cranial Nerve
  Hypoglossal Nerve
    Anastomosis to Facial Nerve, 64868
XIII, Coagulation Factor, 85290-85291
X-Linked Ichthyoses, 86592-86593
X-ray
  with Contrast
    Ankle, 73615
    Aorta, 75600-75630, 75952-75953
    Artery
      with Additional Vessels, 75774
      Abdominal, 75726
      Adrenal, 75731, 75733
      Arm, 75710, 75716
      Arteriovenous Shunt, 36901
      Brachial, 75658
      Leg, 75710, 75716
      Mammary, 75756
      Pelvic, 75736
      Pulmonary, 75741-75746
      Spine, 75705
      Transcatheter Therapy, 75894-75898
        Angiogram, 75898
        Embolization, 75894
    Bile Duct, 74301
      Guide Catheter, 74328, 74330
    Bladder, 74430, 74450, 74455
    Brain, 70010, 70015
    Central Venous Access Device, 36598
    Colon
      Barium Enema, 74270, 74280
    Corpora Cavernosa, 74445
    Elbow, 73085
    Epididymis, 74440
    Gallbladder, 74290
    Gastrointestinal Tract, 74246-74249
    Hip, 73525
    Iliac, 75953
    Iliofemoral Artery, 75630

X-ray — *continued*
  with Contrast — *continued*
    Intervertebral Disc
      Cervical, 72285
      Lumbar, 72295
      Thoracic, 72285
    Joint
      Stress Views, 77071
    Kidney
      Cyst, 74470
    Knee, 73560-73564, 73580
    Lacrimal Duct, 70170
    Lymph Vessel, 75805, 75807
      Abdomen, 75805, 75807
      Arm, 75801, 75803
      Leg, 75801, 75803
    Mammary Duct, 77053-77054
    Nasolacrimal Duct, 70170
      Guide Dilation, 74485
    Oviduct, 74740
    Pancreas, 74300, 74301
    Pancreatic Duct
      Guide Catheter, 74329, 74330
    Perineum, 74775
    Peritoneum, 74190
    Salivary Gland, 70390
    Seminal Vesicles, 74440
    Shoulder, 73040
    Spine
      Cervical, 72240
      Lumbosacral, 72265
      Thoracic, 72255
      Total, 72270
    Temporomandibular Joint (TMJ), 70328-70332
    Ureter
      Guide Dilation, 74485
    Urethra, 74450, 74455
    Urinary Tract, 74400-74425
    Uterus, 74740
    Vas Deferens, 74440
    Vein
      Adrenal, 75840, 75842
      Arm, 75820, 75822
        Hepatic Portal, 75810, 75885, 75887
      Jugular, 75860
      Leg, 75820, 75822
      Liver, 75889, 75891
      Neck, 75860
      Orbit, 75880
      Renal, 75831, 75833
      Sampling, 75893
      Sinus, 75870
      Skull, 75870, 75872
      Splenic, 75810
      Vena Cava, 75825, 75827
    Wrist, 73115
  Abdomen, 74000-74022
  Abscess, 76080
  Acromioclavicular Joint, 73050
  Ankle, 73600, 73610
  Arm, Lower, 73090
  Arm, Upper, 73092
  Auditory Meatus, 70134
  Barium Swallow Test, 3142F, 3200F
  Bile Duct
    Guide Dilation, 74360
  Body Section, 76100
    Motion, 76101, 76102

X-ray — *continued*
  Bone
    Age Study, 77072
    Dual Energy Absorptiometry, 77080-77081, [77086]
    Length Study, 77073
    Osseous Survey, 77074-77076
      Complete, 77075
      Infant, 77076
      Limited, 77074
    Ultrasound, 76977
  Breast, 77065-77067
    with Computer-aided Detection, 77065-77067
  Calcaneus, 73650
  Chest, 71010-71035
    with Computer-Aided Detection, 0174T-0175T
    with Fluoroscopy, 71023, 71034
    Complete (four views)
      with Fluoroscopy, 71034
    Partial (two views)
      with Fluoroscopy, 71023
    Stereo, 71015
  Clavicle, 73000
  Coccyx, 72220
  Consultation, 76140
  Duodenum, 74260
  Elbow, 73070, 73080
  Esophagus, 74220
  Eye, 70030
  Facial Bones, 70140, 70150
  Fallopian Tube, 74742
  Femur, 73551-73552
  Fibula, 73590
  Fingers, 73140
  Fistula, 76080
  Foot, 73620, 73630
  Gastrointestinal Tract, 74240-74245
    Guide Dilation, 74360
    Guide Intubation, 49440, 74340
    Upper, 3142F, 3200F
  Hand, 73120, 73130
  Head, 70350
  Heel, 73650
  Hip, 73501-73503, 73521-73523
  Humerus, 73060
  Intestines, Small, 74245, 74249-74251
    Guide Intubation, 74355
  Jaws, 70355
  Joint
    Stress Views, 77071
  Knee, 73560-73564, 73580
    Bilateral, 73565
  Larynx, 70370
  Leg, 73592
  Lumen Dilator, 74360
  Mandible, 70100, 70110
  Mastoids, 70120, 70130
  Nasal Bones, 70160
  Neck, 70360
  Nose to Rectum
    Foreign Body
      Child, 76010
  Orbit, 70190, 70200
  Pelvis, 72170, 72190
    Manometry, 74710
  Peritoneum, 74190
  Pharynx, 70370, 74210
  Ribs, 71100-71111

X-ray — *continued*
  Sacroiliac Joint, 72200, 72202
  Sacrum, 72220
  Salivary Gland, 70380
  Scapula, 73010
  Sella Turcica, 70240
  Shoulder, 73020, 73030, 73050
  Sinuses, 70210, 70220
  Sinus Tract, 76080
  Skull, 70250, 70260
  Specimen
    Surgical, 76098
  Spine, 72020
    Cervical, 72040-72052
    Lumbosacral, 72100-72120
    Thoracic, 72070-72074
    Thoracolumbar, 72080, 72084
    Thoracolumbar Junction, 72080
  Sternum, 71120, 71130
  Teeth, 70300-70320
  Tibia, 73590
  Toe, 73660
  Total Body
    Foreign Body, 76010
  Unlisted Services and Procedures, 76120, 76125
  Upper Gastrointestinal Series (Upper GI Series), 3142F, 3200F
  Wrist, 73100, 73110
X-Ray Tomography, Computed
  See CT Scan
Xylose Absorption Test
  Blood, 84620
  Urine, 84620

Y

Yacoub Procedure, 33864
YAG, 66821
Yeast
  Culture, 87106
Yellow Fever Vaccine, 90717
Yersinia
  Antibody, 86793
YF-VAX, 90717
Y-Plasty, 51800

Z

ZEB2, 81404-81405
Ziegler Procedure
  Discission Secondary Membranous Cataract, 66820
ZIFT, 58976
Zinc, 84630
Zinc Manganese Leucine Aminopeptidase, 83670
ZNF41, 81404
Zonisamide
  Assay, 80203
ZOSTAVAX, 90736
Z-Plasty, 26121-26125, 41520
Zygoma
  Fracture Treatment, 21355-21366
  Reconstruction, 21270
Zygomatic Arch
  Fracture
    with Manipulation, 21355
      Open Treatment, 21356-21366
  Reconstruction, 21255

00100-00126 Anesthesia for Cleft Lip, Ear, ECT, Eyelid, and Salivary Gland Procedures

CMS: 100-04,12,140.1 Qualified Nonphysician Anesthetists; 100-04,12,140.3 Payment for Qualified Nonphysician Anesthetists; 100-04,12,140.3.3 Billing Modifiers; 100-04,12,140.3.4 General Billing Instructions; 100-04,12,140.4.1 Anesthesiologist/Qualified Nonphysican Anesthetist; 100-04,12,140.4.2 Anesthetist and Anesthesiologist in a Single Procedure; 100-04,12,140.4.3 Payment for Medical /Surgical Services by CRNAs; 100-04,12,140.4.4 Conversion Factors for Anesthesia Services; 100-04,4,250.3.2 Anesthesia in a Hospital Outpatient Setting

00100 **Anesthesia for procedures on salivary glands, including biopsy**
0.00   0.00   **FUD** XXX   N
AMA: 2016,Jan,13; 2015,Jan,16; 2014,Aug,5; 2014,Jan,11; 2012,Jul,12-14; 2012,Jan,15-42; 2011,Oct,3-4; 2011,Jul,16-17; 2011,Jan,11

00102 **Anesthesia for procedures involving plastic repair of cleft lip**
0.00   0.00   **FUD** XXX   N
AMA: 2016,Jan,13; 2015,Jan,16; 2014,Aug,5; 2014,Jan,11; 2012,Jul,12-14; 2012,Jan,15-42; 2011,Oct,3-4; 2011,Jul,16-17; 2011,Jan,11

00103 **Anesthesia for reconstructive procedures of eyelid (eg, blepharoplasty, ptosis surgery)**
0.00   0.00   **FUD** XXX   N
AMA: 2016,Jan,13; 2015,Jan,16; 2014,Aug,5; 2014,Jan,11; 2012,Jul,12-14; 2012,Jan,15-42; 2011,Oct,3-4; 2011,Jul,16-17; 2011,Jan,11

00104 **Anesthesia for electroconvulsive therapy**
0.00   0.00   **FUD** XXX   N
AMA: 2016,Jan,13; 2015,Jan,16; 2014,Aug,5; 2014,Jan,11; 2012,Jul,12-14; 2012,Jan,15-42; 2011,Oct,3-4; 2011,Jul,16-17; 2011,Jan,11

00120 **Anesthesia for procedures on external, middle, and inner ear including biopsy; not otherwise specified**
0.00   0.00   **FUD** XXX   N
AMA: 2016,Jan,13; 2015,Jan,16; 2014,Aug,5; 2014,Jan,11; 2012,Jul,12-14; 2012,Jan,15-42; 2011,Oct,3-4; 2011,Jul,16-17; 2011,Jan,11

00124 **otoscopy**
0.00   0.00   **FUD** XXX   N
AMA: 2016,Jan,13; 2015,Jan,16; 2014,Aug,5; 2014,Jan,11; 2012,Jul,12-14; 2012,Jan,15-42; 2011,Oct,3-4; 2011,Jul,16-17; 2011,Jan,11

00126 **tympanotomy**
0.00   0.00   **FUD** XXX   N
AMA: 2016,Jan,13; 2015,Jan,16; 2014,Aug,5; 2014,Jan,11; 2012,Jul,12-14; 2012,Jan,15-42; 2011,Oct,3-4; 2011,Jul,16-17; 2011,Jan,11

00140-00148 Anesthesia for Eye Procedures

CMS: 100-04,12,140.1 Qualified Nonphysician Anesthetists; 100-04,12,140.3 Payment for Qualified Nonphysician Anesthetists; 100-04,12,140.3.3 Billing Modifiers; 100-04,12,140.3.4 General Billing Instructions; 100-04,12,140.4.1 Anesthesiologist/Qualified Nonphysican Anesthetist; 100-04,12,140.4.2 Anesthetist and Anesthesiologist in a Single Procedure; 100-04,12,140.4.3 Payment for Medical /Surgical Services by CRNAs; 100-04,12,140.4.4 Conversion Factors for Anesthesia Services; 100-04,4,250.3.2 Anesthesia in a Hospital Outpatient Setting

00140 **Anesthesia for procedures on eye; not otherwise specified**
0.00   0.00   **FUD** XXX   N
AMA: 2016,Jan,13; 2015,Jan,16; 2014,Aug,5; 2014,Jan,11; 2012,Jul,12-14; 2012,Jan,15-42; 2011,Oct,3-4; 2011,Jul,16-17; 2011,Jan,11

00142 **lens surgery**
0.00   0.00   **FUD** XXX   N
AMA: 2016,Jan,13; 2015,Jan,16; 2014,Aug,5; 2014,Jan,11; 2012,Jul,12-14; 2012,Jan,15-42; 2011,Oct,3-4; 2011,Jul,16-17; 2011,Jan,11

00144 **corneal transplant**
0.00   0.00   **FUD** XXX   N
AMA: 2016,Jan,13; 2015,Jan,16; 2014,Aug,5; 2014,Jan,11; 2012,Jul,12-14; 2012,Jan,15-42; 2011,Oct,3-4; 2011,Jul,16-17; 2011,Jan,11

00145 **vitreoretinal surgery**
0.00   0.00   **FUD** XXX   N
AMA: 2016,Jan,13; 2015,Jan,16; 2014,Aug,5; 2014,Jan,11; 2012,Jul,12-14; 2012,Jan,15-42; 2011,Oct,3-4; 2011,Jul,16-17; 2011,Jan,11

00147 **iridectomy**
0.00   0.00   **FUD** XXX   N
AMA: 2016,Jan,13; 2015,Jan,16; 2014,Aug,5; 2014,Jan,11; 2012,Jul,12-14; 2012,Jan,15-42; 2011,Oct,3-4; 2011,Jul,16-17; 2011,Jan,11

00148 **ophthalmoscopy**
0.00   0.00   **FUD** XXX   N
AMA: 2016,Jan,13; 2015,Jan,16; 2014,Aug,5; 2014,Jan,11; 2012,Jul,12-14; 2012,Jan,15-42; 2011,Oct,3-4; 2011,Jul,16-17; 2011,Jan,11

00160-00326 Anesthesia for Face and Head Procedures

CMS: 100-04,12,140.1 Qualified Nonphysician Anesthetists; 100-04,12,140.3 Payment for Qualified Nonphysician Anesthetists; 100-04,12,140.3.3 Billing Modifiers; 100-04,12,140.3.4 General Billing Instructions; 100-04,12,140.4.1 Anesthesiologist/Qualified Nonphysican Anesthetist; 100-04,12,140.4.2 Anesthetist and Anesthesiologist in a Single Procedure; 100-04,12,140.4.4 Conversion Factors for Anesthesia Services; 100-04,4,250.3.2 Anesthesia in a Hospital Outpatient Setting

00160 **Anesthesia for procedures on nose and accessory sinuses; not otherwise specified**
0.00   0.00   **FUD** XXX   N
AMA: 2016,Jan,13; 2015,Jan,16; 2014,Aug,5; 2014,Jan,11; 2012,Jul,12-14; 2012,Jan,15-42; 2011,Oct,3-4; 2011,Jul,16-17; 2011,Jan,11

00162 **radical surgery**
0.00   0.00   **FUD** XXX   N
AMA: 2016,Jan,13; 2015,Jan,16; 2014,Aug,5; 2014,Jan,11; 2012,Jul,12-14; 2012,Jan,15-42; 2011,Oct,3-4; 2011,Jul,16-17; 2011,Jan,11

00164 **biopsy, soft tissue**
0.00   0.00   **FUD** XXX   N
AMA: 2016,Jan,13; 2015,Jan,16; 2014,Aug,5; 2014,Jan,11; 2012,Jul,12-14; 2012,Jan,15-42; 2011,Oct,3-4; 2011,Jul,16-17; 2011,Jan,11

00170 **Anesthesia for intraoral procedures, including biopsy; not otherwise specified**
0.00   0.00   **FUD** XXX   N
AMA: 2016,Jan,13; 2015,Jan,16; 2014,Aug,5; 2014,Jan,11; 2012,Jul,12-14; 2012,Jan,15-42; 2011,Oct,3-4; 2011,Jul,16-17; 2011,Jan,11

00172 **repair of cleft palate**
0.00   0.00   **FUD** XXX   N
AMA: 2016,Jan,13; 2015,Jan,16; 2014,Aug,5; 2014,Jan,11; 2012,Jul,12-14; 2012,Jan,15-42; 2011,Oct,3-4; 2011,Jul,16-17; 2011,Jan,11

00174 **excision of retropharyngeal tumor**
0.00   0.00   **FUD** XXX   N
AMA: 2016,Jan,13; 2015,Jan,16; 2014,Aug,5; 2014,Jan,11; 2012,Jul,12-14; 2012,Jan,15-42; 2011,Oct,3-4; 2011,Jul,16-17; 2011,Jan,11

00176 **radical surgery**
0.00   0.00   **FUD** XXX   C
AMA: 2016,Jan,13; 2015,Jan,16; 2014,Aug,5; 2014,Jan,11; 2012,Jul,12-14; 2012,Jan,15-42; 2011,Oct,3-4; 2011,Jul,16-17; 2011,Jan,11

00190 **Anesthesia for procedures on facial bones or skull; not otherwise specified**
0.00   0.00   **FUD** XXX   N
AMA: 2016,Jan,13; 2015,Jan,16; 2014,Aug,5; 2014,Jan,11; 2012,Jul,12-14; 2012,Jan,15-42; 2011,Oct,3-4; 2011,Jul,16-17; 2011,Jan,11

Anesthesia

00192 — 00406

00192 radical surgery (including prognathism)
⚕ 0.00 ⚚ 0.00 **FUD** XXX [C][▢]
AMA: 2016,Jan,13; 2015,Jan,16; 2014,Aug,5; 2014,Jan,11; 2012,Jul,12-14; 2012,Jan,15-42; 2011,Oct,3-4; 2011,Jul,16-17; 2011,Jan,11

00210 Anesthesia for intracranial procedures; not otherwise specified
⚕ 0.00 ⚚ 0.00 **FUD** XXX [N][▢]
AMA: 2016,Jan,13; 2015,Jan,16; 2014,Aug,5; 2014,Jan,11; 2012,Jul,12-14; 2012,Jan,15-42; 2011,Oct,3-4; 2011,Jul,16-17; 2011,Jan,11

00211 craniotomy or craniectomy for evacuation of hematoma
⚕ 0.00 ⚚ 0.00 **FUD** XXX [C][▢]
AMA: 2016,Jan,13; 2015,Jan,16; 2014,Aug,5; 2014,Jan,11; 2012,Jul,12-14; 2012,Jan,15-42; 2011,Oct,3-4; 2011,Jul,16-17; 2011,Jan,11

00212 subdural taps
⚕ 0.00 ⚚ 0.00 **FUD** XXX [N][▢]
AMA: 2016,Jan,13; 2015,Jan,16; 2014,Aug,5; 2014,Jan,11; 2012,Jul,12-14; 2012,Jan,15-42; 2011,Oct,3-4; 2011,Jul,16-17; 2011,Jan,11

00214 burr holes, including ventriculography
⚕ 0.00 ⚚ 0.00 **FUD** XXX [C][▢]
AMA: 2016,Jan,13; 2015,Jan,16; 2014,Aug,5; 2014,Jan,11; 2012,Jul,12-14; 2012,Jan,15-42; 2011,Oct,3-4; 2011,Jul,16-17; 2011,Jan,11

00215 cranioplasty or elevation of depressed skull fracture, extradural (simple or compound)
⚕ 0.00 ⚚ 0.00 **FUD** XXX [C][▢]
AMA: 2016,Jan,13; 2015,Jan,16; 2014,Aug,5; 2014,Jan,11; 2012,Jul,12-14; 2012,Jan,15-42; 2011,Oct,3-4; 2011,Jul,16-17; 2011,Jan,11

00216 vascular procedures
⚕ 0.00 ⚚ 0.00 **FUD** XXX [N][▢]
AMA: 2016,Jan,13; 2015,Jan,16; 2014,Aug,5; 2014,Jan,11; 2012,Jul,12-14; 2012,Jan,15-42; 2011,Oct,3-4; 2011,Jul,16-17; 2011,Jan,11

00218 procedures in sitting position
⚕ 0.00 ⚚ 0.00 **FUD** XXX [N][▢]
AMA: 2016,Jan,13; 2015,Jan,16; 2014,Aug,5; 2014,Jan,11; 2012,Jul,12-14; 2012,Jan,15-42; 2011,Oct,3-4; 2011,Jul,16-17; 2011,Jan,11

00220 cerebrospinal fluid shunting procedures
⚕ 0.00 ⚚ 0.00 **FUD** XXX [N][▢]
AMA: 2016,Jan,13; 2015,Jan,16; 2014,Aug,5; 2014,Jan,11; 2012,Jul,12-14; 2012,Jan,15-42; 2011,Oct,3-4; 2011,Jul,16-17; 2011,Jan,11

00222 electrocoagulation of intracranial nerve
⚕ 0.00 ⚚ 0.00 **FUD** XXX [N][▢]
AMA: 2016,Jan,13; 2015,Jan,16; 2014,Aug,5; 2014,Jan,11; 2012,Jul,12-14; 2012,Jan,15-42; 2011,Oct,3-4; 2011,Jul,16-17; 2011,Jan,11

00300 Anesthesia for all procedures on the integumentary system, muscles and nerves of head, neck, and posterior trunk, not otherwise specified
⚕ 0.00 ⚚ 0.00 **FUD** XXX [N][▢]
AMA: 2016,Jan,13; 2015,Jan,16; 2014,Aug,5; 2014,Jan,11; 2012,Jul,12-14; 2012,Jan,15-42; 2011,Oct,3-4; 2011,Jul,16-17; 2011,Jan,11

00320 Anesthesia for all procedures on esophagus, thyroid, larynx, trachea and lymphatic system of neck; not otherwise specified, age 1 year or older
⚕ 0.00 ⚚ 0.00 **FUD** XXX [N][▢]
AMA: 2016,Jan,13; 2015,Jan,16; 2014,Aug,5; 2014,Jan,11; 2012,Jul,12-14; 2012,Jan,15-42; 2011,Oct,3-4; 2011,Jul,16-17; 2011,Jan,11

00322 needle biopsy of thyroid
EXCLUDES Cervical spine and spinal cord procedures (00600, 00604, 00670)
⚕ 0.00 ⚚ 0.00 **FUD** XXX [N][▢]
AMA: 2016,Jan,13; 2015,Jan,16; 2014,Aug,5; 2014,Jan,11; 2012,Jul,12-14; 2012,Jan,15-42; 2011,Oct,3-4; 2011,Jul,16-17; 2011,Jan,11

00326 Anesthesia for all procedures on the larynx and trachea in children younger than 1 year of age [A]
INCLUDES Anesthesia for patient of extreme age, younger than 1 year and older than 70 (99100)
⚕ 0.00 ⚚ 0.00 **FUD** XXX [N][▢]
AMA: 2016,Jan,13; 2015,Jan,16; 2014,Aug,5; 2014,Jan,11; 2012,Jul,12-14; 2012,Jan,15-42; 2011,Oct,3-4; 2011,Jul,16-17; 2011,Jan,11

00350-00352 Anesthesia for Neck Vessel Procedures

CMS: 100-04,12,140.1 Qualified Nonphysician Anesthetists; 100-04,12,140.3 Payment for Qualified Nonphysician Anesthetists; 100-04,12,140.3.3 Billing Modifiers; 100-04,12,140.3.4 General Billing Instructions; 100-04,12,140.4.1 Anesthesiologist/Qualified Nonphysican Anesthetist; 100-04,12,140.4.2 Anesthetist and Anesthesiologist in a Single Procedure; 100-04,12,140.4.3 Payment for Medical /Surgical Services by CRNAs; 100-04,12,140.4.4 Conversion Factors for Anesthesia Services; 100-04,4,250.3.2 Anesthesia in a Hospital Outpatient Setting
EXCLUDES Arteriography (01916)

00350 Anesthesia for procedures on major vessels of neck; not otherwise specified
⚕ 0.00 ⚚ 0.00 **FUD** XXX [N][▢]
AMA: 2016,Jan,13; 2015,Jan,16; 2014,Aug,5; 2014,Jan,11; 2012,Jul,12-14; 2012,Jan,15-42; 2011,Oct,3-4; 2011,Jul,16-17; 2011,Jan,11

00352 simple ligation
⚕ 0.00 ⚚ 0.00 **FUD** XXX [N][▢]
AMA: 2016,Jan,13; 2015,Jan,16; 2014,Aug,5; 2014,Jan,11; 2012,Jul,12-14; 2012,Jan,15-42; 2011,Oct,3-4; 2011,Jul,16-17; 2011,Jan,11

00400-00529 Anesthesia for Chest/Pectoral Girdle Procedures

CMS: 100-04,12,140.1 Qualified Nonphysician Anesthetists; 100-04,12,140.3 Payment for Qualified Nonphysician Anesthetists; 100-04,12,140.3.3 Billing Modifiers; 100-04,12,140.3.4 General Billing Instructions; 100-04,12,140.4.1 Anesthesiologist/Qualified Nonphysican Anesthetist; 100-04,12,140.4.2 Anesthetist and Anesthesiologist in a Single Procedure; 100-04,12,140.4.3 Payment for Medical /Surgical Services by CRNAs; 100-04,12,140.4.4 Conversion Factors for Anesthesia Services; 100-04,4,250.3.2 Anesthesia in a Hospital Outpatient Setting

00400 Anesthesia for procedures on the integumentary system on the extremities, anterior trunk and perineum; not otherwise specified
⚕ 0.00 ⚚ 0.00 **FUD** XXX [N][▢]
AMA: 2016,Jan,13; 2015,Jan,16; 2014,Aug,5; 2014,Jan,11; 2012,Jul,12-14; 2012,Jan,15-42; 2011,Oct,3-4; 2011,Jul,16-17; 2011,Jan,11

00402 reconstructive procedures on breast (eg, reduction or augmentation mammoplasty, muscle flaps)
⚕ 0.00 ⚚ 0.00 **FUD** XXX [N][▢]
AMA: 2016,Jan,13; 2015,Jan,16; 2014,Aug,5; 2014,Jan,11; 2012,Jul,12-14; 2012,Jan,15-42; 2011,Oct,3-4; 2011,Jul,16-17; 2011,Jan,11

00404 radical or modified radical procedures on breast
⚕ 0.00 ⚚ 0.00 **FUD** XXX [N][▢]
AMA: 2016,Jan,13; 2015,Jan,16; 2014,Aug,5; 2014,Jan,11; 2012,Jul,12-14; 2012,Jan,15-42; 2011,Oct,3-4; 2011,Jul,16-17; 2011,Jan,11

00406 radical or modified radical procedures on breast with internal mammary node dissection
⚕ 0.00 ⚚ 0.00 **FUD** XXX [N][▢]
AMA: 2016,Jan,13; 2015,Jan,16; 2014,Aug,5; 2014,Jan,11; 2012,Jul,12-14; 2012,Jan,15-42; 2011,Oct,3-4; 2011,Jul,16-17; 2011,Jan,11

00410 electrical conversion of arrhythmias

    0.00   0.00   **FUD** XXX   N

    AMA: 2016,Jan,13; 2015,Jan,16; 2014,Aug,5; 2014,Jan,11; 2012,Jul,12-14; 2012,Jan,15-42; 2011,Oct,3-4; 2011,Jul,16-17; 2011,Jan,11

00450 Anesthesia for procedures on clavicle and scapula; not otherwise specified

    0.00   0.00   **FUD** XXX   N

    AMA: 2016,Jan,13; 2015,Jan,16; 2014,Aug,5; 2014,Jan,11; 2012,Jul,12-14; 2012,Jan,15-42; 2011,Oct,3-4; 2011,Jul,16-17; 2011,Jan,11

00454 biopsy of clavicle

    0.00   0.00   **FUD** XXX   N

    AMA: 2016,Jan,13; 2015,Jan,16; 2014,Aug,5; 2014,Jan,11; 2012,Jul,12-14; 2012,Jan,15-42; 2011,Oct,3-4; 2011,Jul,16-17; 2011,Jan,11

00470 Anesthesia for partial rib resection; not otherwise specified

    0.00   0.00   **FUD** XXX   N

    AMA: 2016,Jan,13; 2015,Jan,16; 2014,Aug,5; 2014,Jan,11; 2012,Jul,12-14; 2012,Jan,15-42; 2011,Oct,3-4; 2011,Jul,16-17; 2011,Jan,11

00472 thoracoplasty (any type)

    0.00   0.00   **FUD** XXX   N

    AMA: 2016,Jan,13; 2015,Jan,16; 2014,Aug,5; 2014,Jan,11; 2012,Jul,12-14; 2012,Jan,15-42; 2011,Oct,3-4; 2011,Jul,16-17; 2011,Jan,11

00474 radical procedures (eg, pectus excavatum)

    0.00   0.00   **FUD** XXX   C

    AMA: 2016,Jan,13; 2015,Jan,16; 2014,Aug,5; 2014,Jan,11; 2012,Jul,12-14; 2012,Jan,15-42; 2011,Oct,3-4; 2011,Jul,16-17; 2011,Jan,11

00500 Anesthesia for all procedures on esophagus

    0.00   0.00   **FUD** XXX   N

    AMA: 2016,Jan,13; 2015,Jan,16; 2014,Aug,5; 2014,Jan,11; 2012,Jul,12-14; 2012,Jan,15-42; 2011,Oct,3-4; 2011,Jul,16-17; 2011,Jan,11

00520 Anesthesia for closed chest procedures; (including bronchoscopy) not otherwise specified

    0.00   0.00   **FUD** XXX   N

    AMA: 2016,Jan,13; 2015,Jan,16; 2014,Aug,5; 2014,Jan,11; 2012,Jul,12-14; 2012,Jan,15-42; 2011,Oct,3-4; 2011,Jul,16-17; 2011,Jan,11

00522 needle biopsy of pleura

    0.00   0.00   **FUD** XXX   N

    AMA: 2016,Jan,13; 2015,Jan,16; 2014,Aug,5; 2014,Jan,11; 2012,Jul,12-14; 2012,Jan,15-42; 2011,Oct,3-4; 2011,Jul,16-17; 2011,Jan,11

00524 pneumocentesis

    0.00   0.00   **FUD** XXX   C

    AMA: 2016,Jan,13; 2015,Jan,16; 2014,Aug,5; 2014,Jan,11; 2012,Jul,12-14; 2012,Jan,15-42; 2011,Oct,3-4; 2011,Jul,16-17; 2011,Jan,11

00528 mediastinoscopy and diagnostic thoracoscopy not utilizing 1 lung ventilation

    EXCLUDES   *Tracheobronchial reconstruction (00539)*

    0.00   0.00   **FUD** XXX   N

    AMA: 2016,Jan,13; 2015,Jan,16; 2014,Aug,5; 2014,Jan,11; 2012,Jul,12-14; 2012,Jan,15-42; 2011,Oct,3-4; 2011,Jul,16-17; 2011,Jan,11

00529 mediastinoscopy and diagnostic thoracoscopy utilizing 1 lung ventilation

    0.00   0.00   **FUD** XXX   N

    AMA: 2016,Jan,13; 2015,Jan,16; 2014,Aug,5; 2014,Jan,11; 2012,Jul,12-14; 2012,Jan,15-42; 2011,Oct,3-4; 2011,Jul,16-17; 2011,Jan,11

00530 Anesthesia for Cardiac Pacemaker Procedure

CMS: 100-03,10.6 Anesthesia in Cardiac Pacemaker Surgery; 100-04,12,140.1 Qualified Nonphysician Anesthetists; 100-04,12,140.3 Payment for Qualified Nonphysician Anesthetists; 100-04,12,140.3.3 Billing Modifiers; 100-04,12,140.3.4 General Billing Instructions; 100-04,12,140.4.1 Anesthesiologist/Qualified Nonphysican Anesthetist; 100-04,12,140.4.2 Anesthetist and Anesthesiologist in a Single Procedure; 100-04,12,140.4.3 Payment for Medical /Surgical Services by CRNAs; 100-04,12,140.4.4 Conversion Factors for Anesthesia Services; 100-04,4,250.3.2 Anesthesia in a Hospital Outpatient Setting

00530 Anesthesia for permanent transvenous pacemaker insertion

    0.00   0.00   **FUD** XXX   N

    AMA: 2016,Jan,13; 2015,Jan,16; 2014,Aug,5; 2014,Jan,11; 2012,Jul,12-14; 2012,Jan,15-42; 2011,Oct,3-4; 2011,Jul,16-17; 2011,Jan,11

00532-00550 Anesthesia for Heart and Lung Procedures

CMS: 100-04,12,140.1 Qualified Nonphysician Anesthetists; 100-04,12,140.3 Payment for Qualified Nonphysician Anesthetists; 100-04,12,140.3.3 Billing Modifiers; 100-04,12,140.3.4 General Billing Instructions; 100-04,12,140.4.1 Anesthesiologist/Qualified Nonphysican Anesthetist; 100-04,12,140.4.2 Anesthetist and Anesthesiologist in a Single Procedure; 100-04,12,140.4.3 Payment for Medical /Surgical Services by CRNAs; 100-04,12,140.4.4 Conversion Factors for Anesthesia Services; 100-04,4,250.3.2 Anesthesia in a Hospital Outpatient Setting

00532 Anesthesia for access to central venous circulation

    0.00   0.00   **FUD** XXX   N

    AMA: 2016,Jan,13; 2015,Jan,16; 2014,Aug,5; 2014,Jan,11; 2012,Jul,12-14; 2012,Jan,15-42; 2011,Oct,3-4; 2011,Jul,16-17; 2011,Jan,11

00534 Anesthesia for transvenous insertion or replacement of pacing cardioverter-defibrillator

    EXCLUDES   *Transthoracic approach (00560)*

    0.00   0.00   **FUD** XXX   N

    AMA: 2016,Jan,13; 2015,Jan,16; 2014,Aug,5; 2014,Jan,11; 2012,Jul,12-14; 2012,Jan,15-42; 2011,Oct,3-4; 2011,Jul,16-17; 2011,Jan,11

00537 Anesthesia for cardiac electrophysiologic procedures including radiofrequency ablation

    0.00   0.00   **FUD** XXX   N

    AMA: 2016,Jan,13; 2015,Jan,16; 2014,Aug,5; 2014,Jan,11; 2012,Jul,12-14; 2012,Jan,15-42; 2011,Oct,3-4; 2011,Jul,16-17; 2011,Jan,11

00539 Anesthesia for tracheobronchial reconstruction

    0.00   0.00   **FUD** XXX   N

    AMA: 2016,Jan,13; 2015,Jan,16; 2014,Aug,5; 2014,Jan,11; 2012,Jul,12-14; 2012,Jan,15-42; 2011,Oct,3-4; 2011,Jul,16-17; 2011,Jan,11

00540 Anesthesia for thoracotomy procedures involving lungs, pleura, diaphragm, and mediastinum (including surgical thoracoscopy); not otherwise specified

    EXCLUDES   *Thoracic spine and spinal cord procedures via anterior transthoracic approach (00625-00626)*

    0.00   0.00   **FUD** XXX   C

    AMA: 2016,Jan,13; 2015,Jan,16; 2014,Aug,5; 2014,Jan,11; 2012,Jul,12-14; 2012,Jan,15-42; 2011,Oct,3-4; 2011,Jul,16-17; 2011,Jan,11

00541 utilizing 1 lung ventilation

    EXCLUDES   *Thoracic spine and spinal cord procedures via anterior transthoracic approach (00625-00626)*

    0.00   0.00   **FUD** XXX   N

    AMA: 2016,Jan,13; 2015,Jan,16; 2014,Aug,5; 2014,Jan,11; 2012,Jul,12-14; 2012,Jan,15-42; 2011,Oct,3-4; 2011,Jul,16-17; 2011,Jan,11

00542 decortication

    0.00   0.00   **FUD** XXX   C

    AMA: 2016,Jan,13; 2015,Jan,16; 2014,Aug,5; 2014,Jan,11; 2012,Jul,12-14; 2012,Jan,15-42; 2011,Oct,3-4; 2011,Jul,16-17; 2011,Jan,11

Anesthesia

00546 — 00640

00546 **pulmonary resection with thoracoplasty**
  🚑 0.00   ⚕ 0.00   **FUD** XXX   C 🖵
  AMA: 2016,Jan,13; 2015,Jan,16; 2014,Aug,5; 2014,Jan,11;
  2012,Jul,12-14; 2012,Jan,15-42; 2011,Oct,3-4; 2011,Jul,16-17;
  2011,Jan,11

00548 **intrathoracic procedures on the trachea and bronchi**
  🚑 0.00   ⚕ 0.00   **FUD** XXX   N 🖵
  AMA: 2016,Jan,13; 2015,Jan,16; 2014,Aug,5; 2014,Jan,11;
  2012,Jul,12-14; 2012,Jan,15-42; 2011,Oct,3-4; 2011,Jul,16-17;
  2011,Jan,11

00550 **Anesthesia for sternal debridement**
  🚑 0.00   ⚕ 0.00   **FUD** XXX   N 🖵
  AMA: 2016,Jan,13; 2015,Jan,16; 2014,Aug,5; 2014,Jan,11;
  2012,Jul,12-14; 2012,Jan,15-42; 2011,Oct,3-4; 2011,Jul,16-17;
  2011,Jan,11

00560-00580 Anesthesia for Open Heart Procedures

CMS: 100-04,12,140.1 Qualified Nonphysician Anesthetists; 100-04,12,140.3 Payment for Qualified Nonphysician Anesthetists; 100-04,12,140.3.3 Billing Modifiers; 100-04,12,140.3.4 General Billing Instructions; 100-04,12,140.4.1 Anesthesiologist/Qualified Nonphysican Anesthetist; 100-04,12,140.4.2 Anesthetist and Anesthesiologist in a Single Procedure; 100-04,12,140.4.3 Payment for Medical /Surgical Services by CRNAs; 100-04,12,140.4.4 Conversion Factors for Anesthesia Services; 100-04,4,250.3.2 Anesthesia in a Hospital Outpatient Setting

00560 **Anesthesia for procedures on heart, pericardial sac, and great vessels of chest; without pump oxygenator**
  🚑 0.00   ⚕ 0.00   **FUD** XXX   C 🖵
  AMA: 2016,Jan,13; 2015,Jan,16; 2014,Aug,5; 2014,Jan,11;
  2012,Jul,12-14; 2012,Jan,15-42; 2011,Oct,3-4; 2011,Jul,16-17;
  2011,Jan,11

00561 **with pump oxygenator, younger than 1 year of age** A
  INCLUDES Anesthesia complicated by utilization of controlled hypotension (99135)
      Anesthesia complicated by utilization of total body hypothermia (99116)
      Anesthesia for patient of extreme age, younger than 1 year and older than 70 (99100)
  🚑 0.00   ⚕ 0.00   **FUD** XXX   C 🖵
  AMA: 2016,Jan,13; 2015,Jan,16; 2014,Aug,5; 2014,Jan,11;
  2012,Jul,12-14; 2012,Jan,15-42; 2011,Oct,3-4; 2011,Jul,16-17;
  2011,Jan,11

00562 **with pump oxygenator, age 1 year or older, for all noncoronary bypass procedures (eg, valve procedures) or for re-operation for coronary bypass more than 1 month after original operation** A
  🚑 0.00   ⚕ 0.00   **FUD** XXX   C 🖵
  AMA: 2016,Jan,13; 2015,Jan,16; 2014,Aug,5; 2014,Jan,11;
  2012,Jul,12-14; 2012,Jan,15-42; 2011,Oct,3-4; 2011,Jul,16-17;
  2011,Jan,11

00563 **with pump oxygenator with hypothermic circulatory arrest**
  🚑 0.00   ⚕ 0.00   **FUD** XXX   N 🖵
  AMA: 2016,Jan,13; 2015,Jan,16; 2014,Aug,5; 2014,Jan,11;
  2012,Jul,12-14; 2012,Jan,15-42; 2011,Oct,3-4; 2011,Jul,16-17;
  2011,Jan,11

00566 **Anesthesia for direct coronary artery bypass grafting; without pump oxygenator**
  🚑 0.00   ⚕ 0.00   **FUD** XXX   N 🖵
  AMA: 2016,Jan,13; 2015,Jan,16; 2014,Aug,5; 2014,Jan,11;
  2012,Jul,12-14; 2012,Jan,15-42; 2011,Oct,3-4; 2011,Jul,16-17;
  2011,Jan,11

00567 **with pump oxygenator**
  🚑 0.00   ⚕ 0.00   **FUD** XXX   C 🖵
  AMA: 2016,Jan,13; 2015,Jan,16; 2014,Aug,5; 2014,Jan,11;
  2012,Jul,12-14; 2012,Jan,15-42; 2011,Oct,3-4; 2011,Jul,16-17;
  2011,Jan,11

00580 **Anesthesia for heart transplant or heart/lung transplant**
  🚑 0.00   ⚕ 0.00   **FUD** XXX   C 🖵
  AMA: 2016,Jan,13; 2015,Jan,16; 2014,Aug,5; 2014,Jan,11;
  2012,Jul,12-14; 2012,Jan,15-42; 2011,Oct,3-4; 2011,Jul,16-17;
  2011,Jan,11

00600-00670 Anesthesia for Spinal Procedures

CMS: 100-04,12,140.1 Qualified Nonphysician Anesthetists; 100-04,12,140.3 Payment for Qualified Nonphysician Anesthetists; 100-04,12,140.3.3 Billing Modifiers; 100-04,12,140.3.4 General Billing Instructions; 100-04,12,140.4.1 Anesthesiologist/Qualified Nonphysican Anesthetist; 100-04,12,140.4.2 Anesthetist and Anesthesiologist in a Single Procedure; 100-04,12,140.4.3 Payment for Medical /Surgical Services by CRNAs; 100-04,12,140.4.4 Conversion Factors for Anesthesia Services; 100-04,4,250.3.2 Anesthesia in a Hospital Outpatient Setting

00600 **Anesthesia for procedures on cervical spine and cord; not otherwise specified**
  EXCLUDES Percutaneous image-guided spine and spinal cord anesthesia services (01935-01936)
  🚑 0.00   ⚕ 0.00   **FUD** XXX   N 🖵
  AMA: 2016,Jan,13; 2015,Jan,16; 2014,Aug,5; 2014,Jan,11;
  2012,Jul,12-14; 2012,Jan,15-42; 2011,Oct,3-4; 2011,Jul,16-17;
  2011,Jan,11

00604 **procedures with patient in the sitting position**
  🚑 0.00   ⚕ 0.00   **FUD** XXX   C 🖵
  AMA: 2016,Jan,13; 2015,Jan,16; 2014,Aug,5; 2014,Jan,11;
  2012,Jul,12-14; 2012,Jan,15-42; 2011,Oct,3-4; 2011,Jul,16-17;
  2011,Jan,11

00620 **Anesthesia for procedures on thoracic spine and cord, not otherwise specified**
  🚑 0.00   ⚕ 0.00   **FUD** XXX   N 🖵
  AMA: 2016,Jan,13; 2015,Jan,16; 2014,Aug,5; 2014,Jan,11;
  2012,Jul,12-14; 2012,Jan,15-42; 2011,Oct,3-4; 2011,Jul,16-17;
  2011,Jan,11

00625 **Anesthesia for procedures on the thoracic spine and cord, via an anterior transthoracic approach; not utilizing 1 lung ventilation**
  EXCLUDES Anesthesia services for thoracotomy procedures other than spine (00540-00541)
  🚑 0.00   ⚕ 0.00   **FUD** XXX   N 🖵
  AMA: 2016,Jan,13; 2015,Jan,16; 2014,Aug,5; 2014,Jan,11;
  2012,Jul,12-14; 2012,Jan,15-42; 2011,Oct,3-4; 2011,Jul,16-17;
  2011,Jan,11

00626 **utilizing 1 lung ventilation**
  EXCLUDES Anesthesia services for thoracotomy procedures other than spine (00540-00541)
  🚑 0.00   ⚕ 0.00   **FUD** XXX   N 🖵
  AMA: 2016,Jan,13; 2015,Jan,16; 2014,Aug,5; 2014,Jan,11;
  2012,Jul,12-14; 2012,Jan,15-42; 2011,Oct,3-4; 2011,Jul,16-17;
  2011,Jan,11

00630 **Anesthesia for procedures in lumbar region; not otherwise specified**
  🚑 0.00   ⚕ 0.00   **FUD** XXX   N 🖵
  AMA: 2016,Jan,13; 2015,Jan,16; 2014,Aug,5; 2014,Jan,11;
  2012,Jul,12-14; 2012,Jan,15-42; 2011,Oct,3-4; 2011,Jul,16-17;
  2011,Jan,11

00632 **lumbar sympathectomy**
  🚑 0.00   ⚕ 0.00   **FUD** XXX   C 🖵
  AMA: 2016,Jan,13; 2015,Jan,16; 2014,Aug,5; 2014,Jan,11;
  2012,Jul,12-14; 2012,Jan,15-42; 2011,Oct,3-4; 2011,Jul,16-17;
  2011,Jan,11

00635 **diagnostic or therapeutic lumbar puncture**
  🚑 0.00   ⚕ 0.00   **FUD** XXX   N 🖵
  AMA: 2016,Jan,13; 2015,Jan,16; 2014,Aug,5; 2014,Jan,11;
  2012,Jul,12-14; 2012,Jan,15-42; 2011,Oct,3-4; 2011,Jul,16-17;
  2011,Jan,11

00640 **Anesthesia for manipulation of the spine or for closed procedures on the cervical, thoracic or lumbar spine**
  🚑 0.00   ⚕ 0.00   **FUD** XXX   N 🖵
  AMA: 2016,Jan,13; 2015,Jan,16; 2014,Aug,5; 2014,Jan,11;
  2012,Jul,12-14; 2012,Jan,15-42; 2011,Oct,3-4; 2011,Jul,16-17;
  2011,Jan,11

26/TC **PC/TC Only**   AZ-Z3 **ASC Payment**   50 **Bilateral**   ♂ **Male Only**   ♀ **Female Only**   🚑 **Facility RVU**   ⚕ **Non-Facility RVU**   🖵 **CCI**
FUD Follow-up Days   **CMS:** IOM (Pub 100)   A-Y **OPPSI**   80/80 **Surg Assist Allowed / w/Doc**   **Lab Crosswalk**   **Radiology Crosswalk**   ☒ **CLIA**

4   CPT © 2016 American Medical Association. All Rights Reserved.   © 2016 Optum360, LLC

00670	Anesthesia for extensive spine and spinal cord procedures (eg, spinal instrumentation or vascular procedures)

    0.00   0.00   **FUD** XXX   C

AMA: 2016,Jan,13; 2015,Jan,16; 2014,Aug,5; 2014,Jan,11; 2012,Jul,12-14; 2012,Jan,15-42; 2011,Oct,3-4; 2011,Jul,16-17; 2011,Jan,11

00700-00882 Anesthesia for Abdominal Procedures

CMS: 100-04,12,140.1 Qualified Nonphysician Anesthetists; 100-04,12,140.3 Payment for Qualified Nonphysician Anesthetists; 100-04,12,140.3.3 Billing Modifiers; 100-04,12,140.3.4 General Billing Instructions; 100-04,12,140.4.1 Anesthesiologist/Qualified Nonphysican Anesthetist; 100-04,12,140.4.2 Anesthetist and Anesthesiologist in a Single Procedure; 100-04,12,140.4.3 Payment for Medical /Surgical Services by CRNAs; 100-04,12,140.4.4 Conversion Factors for Anesthesia Services; 100-04,4,250.3.2 Anesthesia in a Hospital Outpatient Setting

00700	Anesthesia for procedures on upper anterior abdominal wall; not otherwise specified

    0.00   0.00   **FUD** XXX   N

AMA: 2016,Jan,13; 2015,Jan,16; 2014,Aug,5; 2014,Jan,11; 2012,Jul,12-14; 2012,Jan,15-42; 2011,Oct,3-4; 2011,Jul,16-17; 2011,Jan,11

00702	percutaneous liver biopsy

    0.00   0.00   **FUD** XXX   N

AMA: 2016,Jan,13; 2015,Jan,16; 2014,Aug,5; 2014,Jan,11; 2012,Jul,12-14; 2012,Jan,15-42; 2011,Oct,3-4; 2011,Jul,16-17; 2011,Jan,11

00730	Anesthesia for procedures on upper posterior abdominal wall

    0.00   0.00   **FUD** XXX   N

AMA: 2016,Jan,13; 2015,Jan,16; 2014,Aug,5; 2014,Jan,11; 2012,Jul,12-14; 2012,Jan,15-42; 2011,Oct,3-4; 2011,Jul,16-17; 2011,Jan,11

00740	Anesthesia for upper gastrointestinal endoscopic procedures, endoscope introduced proximal to duodenum

    0.00   0.00   **FUD** XXX   N

AMA: 2016,Jan,13; 2015,Jan,16; 2014,Aug,5; 2014,Jan,11; 2012,Jul,12-14; 2012,Jan,15-42; 2011,Oct,3-4; 2011,Jul,16-17; 2011,Jan,11

00750	Anesthesia for hernia repairs in upper abdomen; not otherwise specified

    0.00   0.00   **FUD** XXX   N

AMA: 2016,Jan,13; 2015,Jan,16; 2014,Aug,5; 2014,Jan,11; 2012,Jul,12-14; 2012,Jan,15-42; 2011,Oct,3-4; 2011,Jul,16-17; 2011,Jan,11

00752	lumbar and ventral (incisional) hernias and/or wound dehiscence

    0.00   0.00   **FUD** XXX   N

AMA: 2016,Jan,13; 2015,Jan,16; 2014,Aug,5; 2014,Jan,11; 2012,Jul,12-14; 2012,Jan,15-42; 2011,Oct,3-4; 2011,Jul,16-17; 2011,Jan,11

00754	omphalocele

    0.00   0.00   **FUD** XXX   N

AMA: 2016,Jan,13; 2015,Jan,16; 2014,Aug,5; 2014,Jan,11; 2012,Jul,12-14; 2012,Jan,15-42; 2011,Oct,3-4; 2011,Jul,16-17; 2011,Jan,11

00756	transabdominal repair of diaphragmatic hernia

    0.00   0.00   **FUD** XXX   N

AMA: 2016,Jan,13; 2015,Jan,16; 2014,Aug,5; 2014,Jan,11; 2012,Jul,12-14; 2012,Jan,15-42; 2011,Oct,3-4; 2011,Jul,16-17; 2011,Jan,11

00770	Anesthesia for all procedures on major abdominal blood vessels

    0.00   0.00   **FUD** XXX   N

AMA: 2016,Jan,13; 2015,Jan,16; 2014,Aug,5; 2014,Jan,11; 2012,Jul,12-14; 2012,Jan,15-42; 2011,Oct,3-4; 2011,Jul,16-17; 2011,Jan,11

00790	Anesthesia for intraperitoneal procedures in upper abdomen including laparoscopy; not otherwise specified

    0.00   0.00   **FUD** XXX   N

AMA: 2016,Jan,13; 2015,Jan,16; 2014,Aug,5; 2014,Jan,11; 2012,Jul,12-14; 2012,Jan,15-42; 2011,Oct,3-4; 2011,Jul,16-17; 2011,Jan,11

00792	partial hepatectomy or management of liver hemorrhage (excluding liver biopsy)

    0.00   0.00   **FUD** XXX   C

AMA: 2016,Jan,13; 2015,Jan,16; 2014,Aug,5; 2014,Jan,11; 2012,Jul,12-14; 2012,Jan,15-42; 2011,Oct,3-4; 2011,Jul,16-17; 2011,Jan,11

00794	pancreatectomy, partial or total (eg, Whipple procedure)

    0.00   0.00   **FUD** XXX   C

AMA: 2016,Jan,13; 2015,Jan,16; 2014,Aug,5; 2014,Jan,11; 2012,Jul,12-14; 2012,Jan,15-42; 2011,Oct,3-4; 2011,Jul,16-17; 2011,Jan,11

00796	liver transplant (recipient)

EXCLUDES *Physiological support during liver harvest (01990)*

    0.00   0.00   **FUD** XXX   C

AMA: 2016,Jan,13; 2015,Jan,16; 2014,Aug,5; 2014,Jan,11; 2012,Jul,12-14; 2012,Jan,15-42; 2011,Oct,3-4; 2011,Jul,16-17; 2011,Jan,11

00797	gastric restrictive procedure for morbid obesity

    0.00   0.00   **FUD** XXX   N

AMA: 2016,Jan,13; 2015,Jan,16; 2014,Aug,5; 2014,Jan,11; 2012,Jul,12-14; 2012,Jan,15-42; 2011,Oct,3-4; 2011,Jul,16-17; 2011,Jan,11

00800	Anesthesia for procedures on lower anterior abdominal wall; not otherwise specified

    0.00   0.00   **FUD** XXX   N

AMA: 2016,Jan,13; 2015,Jan,16; 2014,Aug,5; 2014,Jan,11; 2012,Jul,12-14; 2012,Jan,15-42; 2011,Oct,3-4; 2011,Jul,16-17; 2011,Jan,11

00802	panniculectomy

    0.00   0.00   **FUD** XXX   C

AMA: 2016,Jan,13; 2015,Jan,16; 2014,Aug,5; 2014,Jan,11; 2012,Jul,12-14; 2012,Jan,15-42; 2011,Oct,3-4; 2011,Jul,16-17; 2011,Jan,11

00810	Anesthesia for lower intestinal endoscopic procedures, endoscope introduced distal to duodenum

    0.00   0.00   **FUD** XXX   N

AMA: 2016,Jan,13; 2015,Jan,16; 2014,Aug,5; 2014,Jan,11; 2012,Jul,12-14; 2012,Jan,15-42; 2011,Oct,3-4; 2011,Jul,16-17; 2011,Jan,11

00820	Anesthesia for procedures on lower posterior abdominal wall

    0.00   0.00   **FUD** XXX   N

AMA: 2016,Jan,13; 2015,Jan,16; 2014,Aug,5; 2014,Jan,11; 2012,Jul,12-14; 2012,Jan,15-42; 2011,Oct,3-4; 2011,Jul,16-17; 2011,Jan,11

00830	Anesthesia for hernia repairs in lower abdomen; not otherwise specified

EXCLUDES *Anesthesia for hernia repairs on infants one year old or less (00834, 00836)*

    0.00   0.00   **FUD** XXX   N

AMA: 2016,Jan,13; 2015,Jan,16; 2014,Aug,5; 2014,Jan,11; 2012,Jul,12-14; 2012,Jan,15-42; 2011,Oct,3-4; 2011,Jul,16-17; 2011,Jan,11

00832	ventral and incisional hernias

EXCLUDES *Anesthesia for hernia repairs on infants one year old or less (00834, 00836)*

    0.00   0.00   **FUD** XXX   N

AMA: 2016,Jan,13; 2015,Jan,16; 2014,Aug,5; 2014,Jan,11; 2012,Jul,12-14; 2012,Jan,15-42; 2011,Oct,3-4; 2011,Jul,16-17; 2011,Jan,11

● New Code   ▲ Revised Code   ○ Reinstated   ● New Web Release   ▲ Revised Web Release   Unlisted   Not Covered   # Resequenced
⊘ AMA Mod 51 Exempt   ⑤ Optum Mod 51 Exempt   ⑥ Mod 63 Exempt   ✗ Non-FDA Drug   ★ Telehealth   Ⓜ Maternity   Ⓐ Age Edit   + Add-on   **AMA:** CPT Asst

00834 Anesthesia for hernia repairs in the lower abdomen not otherwise specified, younger than 1 year of age ▲

INCLUDES Anesthesia for patient of extreme age, younger than 1 year and older than 70 (99100)

🚑 0.00 ⚕ 0.00 **FUD** XXX 🅽 ▢

AMA: 2016,Jan,13; 2015,Jan,16; 2014,Aug,5; 2014,Jan,11; 2012,Jul,12-14; 2012,Jan,15-42; 2011,Oct,3-4; 2011,Jul,16-17; 2011,Jan,11

00836 Anesthesia for hernia repairs in the lower abdomen not otherwise specified, infants younger than 37 weeks gestational age at birth and younger than 50 weeks gestational age at time of surgery ▲

INCLUDES Anesthesia for patient of extreme age, younger than 1 year and older than 70 (99100)

🚑 0.00 ⚕ 0.00 **FUD** XXX 🅽 ▢

AMA: 2016,Jan,13; 2015,Jan,16; 2014,Aug,5; 2014,Jan,11; 2012,Jul,12-14; 2012,Jan,15-42; 2011,Oct,3-4; 2011,Jul,16-17; 2011,Jan,11

00840 Anesthesia for intraperitoneal procedures in lower abdomen including laparoscopy; not otherwise specified

🚑 0.00 ⚕ 0.00 **FUD** XXX 🅽 ▢

AMA: 2016,Jan,13; 2015,Jan,16; 2014,Aug,5; 2014,Jan,11; 2012,Jul,12-14; 2012,Jan,15-42; 2011,Oct,3-4; 2011,Jul,16-17; 2011,Jan,11

00842 amniocentesis Ⓜ ♀

🚑 0.00 ⚕ 0.00 **FUD** XXX 🅽 ▢

AMA: 2016,Jan,13; 2015,Jan,16; 2014,Aug,5; 2014,Jan,11; 2012,Jul,12-14; 2012,Jan,15-42; 2011,Oct,3-4; 2011,Jul,16-17; 2011,Jan,11

00844 abdominoperineal resection Ⓒ ▢

🚑 0.00 ⚕ 0.00 **FUD** XXX

AMA: 2016,Jan,13; 2015,Jan,16; 2014,Aug,5; 2014,Jan,11; 2012,Jul,12-14; 2012,Jan,15-42; 2011,Oct,3-4; 2011,Jul,16-17; 2011,Jan,11

00846 radical hysterectomy ♀

🚑 0.00 ⚕ 0.00 **FUD** XXX Ⓒ ▢

AMA: 2016,Jan,13; 2015,Jan,16; 2014,Aug,5; 2014,Jan,11; 2012,Jul,12-14; 2012,Jan,15-42; 2011,Oct,3-4; 2011,Jul,16-17; 2011,Jan,11

00848 pelvic exenteration

🚑 0.00 ⚕ 0.00 **FUD** XXX Ⓒ ▢

AMA: 2016,Jan,13; 2015,Jan,16; 2014,Aug,5; 2014,Jan,11; 2012,Jul,12-14; 2012,Jan,15-42; 2011,Oct,3-4; 2011,Jul,16-17; 2011,Jan,11

00851 tubal ligation/transection ♀

🚑 0.00 ⚕ 0.00 **FUD** XXX 🅽 ▢

AMA: 2016,Jan,13; 2015,Jan,16; 2014,Oct,14; 2014,Aug,5; 2014,Jan,11; 2012,Jul,12-14; 2012,Jan,15-42; 2011,Oct,3-4; 2011,Jul,16-17; 2011,Jan,11

00860 Anesthesia for extraperitoneal procedures in lower abdomen, including urinary tract; not otherwise specified

🚑 0.00 ⚕ 0.00 **FUD** XXX 🅽 ▢

AMA: 2016,Jan,13; 2015,Jan,16; 2014,Aug,5; 2014,Jan,11; 2012,Jul,12-14; 2012,Jan,15-42; 2011,Oct,3-4; 2011,Jul,16-17; 2011,Jan,11

00862 renal procedures, including upper one-third of ureter, or donor nephrectomy

🚑 0.00 ⚕ 0.00 **FUD** XXX 🅽 ▢

AMA: 2016,Jan,13; 2015,Jan,16; 2014,Aug,5; 2014,Jan,11; 2012,Jul,12-14; 2012,Jan,15-42; 2011,Oct,3-4; 2011,Jul,16-17; 2011,Jan,11

00864 total cystectomy

🚑 0.00 ⚕ 0.00 **FUD** XXX Ⓒ ▢

AMA: 2016,Jan,13; 2015,Jan,16; 2014,Aug,5; 2014,Jan,11; 2012,Jul,12-14; 2012,Jan,15-42; 2011,Oct,3-4; 2011,Jul,16-17; 2011,Jan,11

00865 radical prostatectomy (suprapubic, retropubic) ♂

🚑 0.00 ⚕ 0.00 **FUD** XXX Ⓒ ▢

AMA: 2016,Jan,13; 2015,Jan,16; 2014,Aug,5; 2014,Jan,11; 2012,Jul,12-14; 2012,Jan,15-42; 2011,Oct,3-4; 2011,Jul,16-17; 2011,Jan,11

00866 adrenalectomy

🚑 0.00 ⚕ 0.00 **FUD** XXX Ⓒ ▢

AMA: 2016,Jan,13; 2015,Jan,16; 2014,Aug,5; 2014,Jan,11; 2012,Jul,12-14; 2012,Jan,15-42; 2011,Oct,3-4; 2011,Jul,16-17; 2011,Jan,11

00868 renal transplant (recipient)

EXCLUDES Anesthesia for donor nephrectomy (00862)
Physiological support during kidney harvest (01990)

🚑 0.00 ⚕ 0.00 **FUD** XXX Ⓒ ▢

AMA: 2016,Jan,13; 2015,Jan,16; 2014,Aug,5; 2014,Jan,11; 2012,Jul,12-14; 2012,Jan,15-42; 2011,Oct,3-4; 2011,Jul,16-17; 2011,Jan,11

00870 cystolithotomy

🚑 0.00 ⚕ 0.00 **FUD** XXX 🅽 ▢

AMA: 2016,Jan,13; 2015,Jan,16; 2014,Aug,5; 2014,Jan,11; 2012,Jul,12-14; 2012,Jan,15-42; 2011,Oct,3-4; 2011,Jul,16-17; 2011,Jan,11

00872 Anesthesia for lithotripsy, extracorporeal shock wave; with water bath

🚑 0.00 ⚕ 0.00 **FUD** XXX 🅽 ▢

AMA: 2016,Jan,13; 2015,Jan,16; 2014,Aug,5; 2014,Jan,11; 2012,Jul,12-14; 2012,Jan,15-42; 2011,Oct,3-4; 2011,Jul,16-17; 2011,Jan,11

00873 without water bath

🚑 0.00 ⚕ 0.00 **FUD** XXX 🅽 ▢

AMA: 2016,Jan,13; 2015,Jan,16; 2014,Aug,5; 2014,Jan,11; 2012,Jul,12-14; 2012,Jan,15-42; 2011,Oct,3-4; 2011,Jul,16-17; 2011,Jan,11

00880 Anesthesia for procedures on major lower abdominal vessels; not otherwise specified

🚑 0.00 ⚕ 0.00 **FUD** XXX 🅽 ▢

AMA: 2016,Jan,13; 2015,Jan,16; 2014,Aug,5; 2014,Jan,11; 2012,Jul,12-14; 2012,Jan,15-42; 2011,Oct,3-4; 2011,Jul,16-17; 2011,Jan,11

00882 inferior vena cava ligation

🚑 0.00 ⚕ 0.00 **FUD** XXX Ⓒ ▢

AMA: 2016,Jan,13; 2015,Jan,16; 2014,Aug,5; 2014,Jan,11; 2012,Jul,12-14; 2012,Jan,15-42; 2011,Oct,3-4; 2011,Jul,16-17; 2011,Jan,11

00902-00952 Anesthesia for Genitourinary Procedures

CMS: 100-04,12,140.1 Qualified Nonphysician Anesthetists; 100-04,12,140.3 Payment for Qualified Nonphysician Anesthetists; 100-04,12,140.3.3 Billing Modifiers; 100-04,12,140.3.4 General Billing Instructions; 100-04,12,140.4.1 Anesthesiologist/Qualified Nonphysican Anesthetist; 100-04,12,140.4.2 Anesthetist and Anesthesiologist in a Single Procedure; 100-04,12,140.4.3 Payment for Medical /Surgical Services by CRNAs; 100-04,12,140.4.4 Conversion Factors for Anesthesia Services; 100-04,4,250.3.2 Anesthesia in a Hospital Outpatient Setting

EXCLUDES Procedures on perineal skin, muscles, and nerves (00300, 00400)

00902 Anesthesia for; anorectal procedure

🚑 0.00 ⚕ 0.00 **FUD** XXX 🅽 ▢

AMA: 2016,Jan,13; 2015,Jan,16; 2014,Aug,5; 2014,Jan,11; 2012,Jul,12-14; 2012,Jan,15-42; 2011,Oct,3-4; 2011,Jul,16-17; 2011,Jan,11

00904 radical perineal procedure

🚑 0.00 ⚕ 0.00 **FUD** XXX Ⓒ ▢

AMA: 2016,Jan,13; 2015,Jan,16; 2014,Aug,5; 2014,Jan,11; 2012,Jul,12-14; 2012,Jan,15-42; 2011,Oct,3-4; 2011,Jul,16-17; 2011,Jan,11

00906 vulvectomy ♀

🚑 0.00 ⚕ 0.00 **FUD** XXX 🅽 ▢

AMA: 2016,Jan,13; 2015,Jan,16; 2014,Aug,5; 2014,Jan,11; 2012,Jul,12-14; 2012,Jan,15-42; 2011,Oct,3-4; 2011,Jul,16-17; 2011,Jan,11

26/TC PC/TC Only	A2-Z3 ASC Payment	50 Bilateral	♂ Male Only	🚑 Facility RVU	⚕ Non-Facility RVU	▢ CCI
FUD Follow-up Days	**CMS:** IOM (Pub 100)	A-Y OPPSI	80/80 Surg Assist Allowed / w/Doc	🔬 Lab Crosswalk	☢ Radiology Crosswalk	☒ CLIA
			♀ Female Only			

00908 perineal prostatectomy ♂
🔧 0.00 ⚕ 0.00 **FUD** XXX ⓒ🖵
AMA: 2016,Jan,13; 2015,Jan,16; 2014,Aug,5; 2014,Jan,11; 2012,Jul,12-14; 2012,Jan,15-42; 2011,Oct,3-4; 2011,Jul,16-17; 2011,Jan,11

00910 Anesthesia for transurethral procedures (including urethrocystoscopy); not otherwise specified
🔧 0.00 ⚕ 0.00 **FUD** XXX Ⓝ🖵
AMA: 2016,Jan,13; 2015,Jan,16; 2014,Aug,5; 2014,Jan,11; 2012,Jul,12-14; 2012,Jan,15-42; 2011,Oct,3-4; 2011,Jul,16-17; 2011,Jan,11

00912 transurethral resection of bladder tumor(s) Ⓝ🖵
🔧 0.00 ⚕ 0.00 **FUD** XXX
AMA: 2016,Jan,13; 2015,Jan,16; 2014,Aug,5; 2014,Jan,11; 2012,Jul,12-14; 2012,Jan,15-42; 2011,Oct,3-4; 2011,Jul,16-17; 2011,Jan,11

00914 transurethral resection of prostate ♂
🔧 0.00 ⚕ 0.00 **FUD** XXX Ⓝ🖵
AMA: 2016,Jan,13; 2015,Jan,16; 2014,Aug,5; 2014,Jan,11; 2012,Jul,12-14; 2012,Jan,15-42; 2011,Oct,3-4; 2011,Jul,16-17; 2011,Jan,11

00916 post-transurethral resection bleeding Ⓝ🖵
🔧 0.00 ⚕ 0.00 **FUD** XXX
AMA: 2016,Jan,13; 2015,Jan,16; 2014,Aug,5; 2014,Jan,11; 2012,Jul,12-14; 2012,Jan,15-42; 2011,Oct,3-4; 2011,Jul,16-17; 2011,Jan,11

00918 with fragmentation, manipulation and/or removal of ureteral calculus
🔧 0.00 ⚕ 0.00 **FUD** XXX Ⓝ🖵
AMA: 2016,Jan,13; 2015,Jan,16; 2014,Aug,5; 2014,Jan,11; 2012,Jul,12-14; 2012,Jan,15-42; 2011,Oct,3-4; 2011,Jul,16-17; 2011,Jan,11

00920 Anesthesia for procedures on male genitalia (including open urethral procedures); not otherwise specified ♂
🔧 0.00 ⚕ 0.00 **FUD** XXX Ⓝ🖵
AMA: 2016,Jan,13; 2015,Jan,16; 2014,Aug,5; 2014,Jan,11; 2012,Oct,14; 2012,Sep,16; 2012,Jul,12-14; 2012,Jan,15-42; 2011,Oct,3-4; 2011,Jul,16-17; 2011,Jan,11

00921 vasectomy, unilateral or bilateral ♂
🔧 0.00 ⚕ 0.00 **FUD** XXX Ⓝ🖵
AMA: 2016,Jan,13; 2015,Jan,16; 2014,Aug,5; 2014,Jan,11; 2012,Jul,12-14; 2012,Jan,15-42; 2011,Oct,3-4; 2011,Jul,16-17; 2011,Jan,11

00922 seminal vesicles ♂
🔧 0.00 ⚕ 0.00 **FUD** XXX Ⓝ🖵
AMA: 2016,Jan,13; 2015,Jan,16; 2014,Aug,5; 2014,Jan,11; 2012,Jul,12-14; 2012,Jan,15-42; 2011,Oct,3-4; 2011,Jul,16-17; 2011,Jan,11

00924 undescended testis, unilateral or bilateral ♂
🔧 0.00 ⚕ 0.00 **FUD** XXX Ⓝ🖵
AMA: 2016,Jan,13; 2015,Jan,16; 2014,Aug,5; 2014,Jan,11; 2012,Jul,12-14; 2012,Jan,15-42; 2011,Oct,3-4; 2011,Jul,16-17; 2011,Jan,11

00926 radical orchiectomy, inguinal ♂
🔧 0.00 ⚕ 0.00 **FUD** XXX Ⓝ🖵
AMA: 2016,Jan,13; 2015,Jan,16; 2014,Aug,5; 2014,Jan,11; 2012,Jul,12-14; 2012,Jan,15-42; 2011,Oct,3-4; 2011,Jul,16-17; 2011,Jan,11

00928 radical orchiectomy, abdominal ♂
🔧 0.00 ⚕ 0.00 **FUD** XXX Ⓝ🖵
AMA: 2016,Jan,13; 2015,Jan,16; 2014,Aug,5; 2014,Jan,11; 2012,Jul,12-14; 2012,Jan,15-42; 2011,Oct,3-4; 2011,Jul,16-17; 2011,Jan,11

00930 orchiopexy, unilateral or bilateral ♂
🔧 0.00 ⚕ 0.00 **FUD** XXX Ⓝ🖵
AMA: 2016,Jan,13; 2015,Jan,16; 2014,Aug,5; 2014,Jan,11; 2012,Jul,12-14; 2012,Jan,15-42; 2011,Oct,3-4; 2011,Jul,16-17; 2011,Jan,11

00932 complete amputation of penis ♂
🔧 0.00 ⚕ 0.00 **FUD** XXX ⓒ🖵
AMA: 2016,Jan,13; 2015,Jan,16; 2014,Aug,5; 2014,Jan,11; 2012,Jul,12-14; 2012,Jan,15-42; 2011,Oct,3-4; 2011,Jul,16-17; 2011,Jan,11

00934 radical amputation of penis with bilateral inguinal lymphadenectomy ♂
🔧 0.00 ⚕ 0.00 **FUD** XXX ⓒ🖵
AMA: 2016,Jan,13; 2015,Jan,16; 2014,Aug,5; 2014,Jan,11; 2012,Jul,12-14; 2012,Jan,15-42; 2011,Oct,3-4; 2011,Jul,16-17; 2011,Jan,11

00936 radical amputation of penis with bilateral inguinal and iliac lymphadenectomy ♂
🔧 0.00 ⚕ 0.00 **FUD** XXX ⓒ🖵
AMA: 2016,Jan,13; 2015,Jan,16; 2014,Aug,5; 2014,Jan,11; 2012,Jul,12-14; 2012,Jan,15-42; 2011,Oct,3-4; 2011,Jul,16-17; 2011,Jan,11

00938 insertion of penile prosthesis (perineal approach) ♂
🔧 0.00 ⚕ 0.00 **FUD** XXX Ⓝ🖵
AMA: 2016,Jan,13; 2015,Jan,16; 2014,Aug,5; 2014,Jan,11; 2012,Jul,12-14; 2012,Jan,15-42; 2011,Oct,3-4; 2011,Jul,16-17; 2011,Jan,11

00940 Anesthesia for vaginal procedures (including biopsy of labia, vagina, cervix or endometrium); not otherwise specified ♀
🔧 0.00 ⚕ 0.00 **FUD** XXX Ⓝ🖵
AMA: 2016,Jan,13; 2015,Jan,16; 2014,Aug,5; 2014,Jan,11; 2012,Jul,12-14; 2012,Jan,15-42; 2011,Oct,3-4; 2011,Jul,16-17; 2011,Jan,11

00942 colpotomy, vaginectomy, colporrhaphy, and open urethral procedures ♀
🔧 0.00 ⚕ 0.00 **FUD** XXX Ⓝ🖵
AMA: 2016,Jan,13; 2015,Jan,16; 2014,Aug,5; 2014,Jan,11; 2012,Jul,12-14; 2012,Jan,15-42; 2011,Oct,3-4; 2011,Jul,16-17; 2011,Jan,11

00944 vaginal hysterectomy ♀
🔧 0.00 ⚕ 0.00 **FUD** XXX ⓒ🖵
AMA: 2016,Jan,13; 2015,Jan,16; 2014,Aug,5; 2014,Jan,11; 2012,Jul,12-14; 2012,Jan,15-42; 2011,Oct,3-4; 2011,Jul,16-17; 2011,Jan,11

00948 cervical cerclage ♀
🔧 0.00 ⚕ 0.00 **FUD** XXX Ⓝ🖵
AMA: 2016,Jan,13; 2015,Jan,16; 2014,Aug,5; 2014,Jan,11; 2012,Jul,12-14; 2012,Jan,15-42; 2011,Oct,3-4; 2011,Jul,16-17; 2011,Jan,11

00950 culdoscopy ♀
🔧 0.00 ⚕ 0.00 **FUD** XXX Ⓝ🖵
AMA: 2016,Jan,13; 2015,Jan,16; 2014,Aug,5; 2014,Jan,11; 2012,Jul,12-14; 2012,Jan,15-42; 2011,Oct,3-4; 2011,Jul,16-17; 2011,Jan,11

00952 hysteroscopy and/or hysterosalpingography ♀
🔧 0.00 ⚕ 0.00 **FUD** XXX Ⓝ🖵
AMA: 2016,Jan,13; 2015,Jan,16; 2014,Aug,5; 2014,Jan,11; 2012,Jul,12-14; 2012,Jan,15-42; 2011,Oct,3-4; 2011,Jul,16-17; 2011,Jan,11

01112-01522 Anesthesia for Lower Extremity Procedures

CMS: 100-04,12,140.1 Qualified Nonphysician Anesthetists; 100-04,12,140.3 Payment for Qualified Nonphysician Anesthetists; 100-04,12,140.3.3 Billing Modifiers; 100-04,12,140.3.4 General Billing Instructions; 100-04,12,140.4.1 Anesthesiologist/Qualified Nonphysican Anesthetist; 100-04,12,140.4.2 Anesthetist and Anesthesiologist in a Single Procedure; 100-04,12,140.4.3 Payment for Medical /Surgical Services by CRNAs; 100-04,12,140.4.4 Conversion Factors for Anesthesia Services; 100-04,4,250.3.2 Anesthesia in a Hospital Outpatient Setting

01112 Anesthesia for bone marrow aspiration and/or biopsy, anterior or posterior iliac crest
🔧 0.00 ⚕ 0.00 **FUD** XXX Ⓝ🖵
AMA: 2016,Jan,13; 2015,Jan,16; 2014,Aug,5; 2014,Jan,11; 2012,Jul,12-14; 2012,Jan,15-42; 2011,Oct,3-4; 2011,Jul,16-17; 2011,Jan,11

● New Code ▲ Revised Code ○ Reinstated ● New Web Release ▲ Revised Web Release Unlisted Not Covered # Resequenced
⊘ AMA Mod 51 Exempt ⑤ Optum Mod 51 Exempt ⑥ Mod 63 Exempt ✗ Non-FDA Drug ★ Telehealth Ⓜ Maternity Ⓐ Age Edit ✚ Add-on **AMA:** CPT Asst

CPT © 2016 American Medical Association. All Rights Reserved.

01120 **Anesthesia for procedures on bony pelvis**
  0.00   0.00   **FUD** XXX   N
  AMA: 2016,Jan,13; 2015,Jan,16; 2014,Aug,5; 2014,Jan,11; 2012,Jul,12-14; 2012,Jan,15-42; 2011,Oct,3-4; 2011,Jul,16-17; 2011,Jan,11

01130 **Anesthesia for body cast application or revision**
  0.00   0.00   **FUD** XXX   N
  AMA: 2016,Jan,13; 2015,Jan,16; 2014,Aug,5; 2014,Jan,11; 2012,Jul,12-14; 2012,Jan,15-42; 2011,Oct,3-4; 2011,Jul,16-17; 2011,Jan,11

01140 **Anesthesia for interpelviabdominal (hindquarter) amputation**
  0.00   0.00   **FUD** XXX   C
  AMA: 2016,Jan,13; 2015,Jan,16; 2014,Aug,5; 2014,Jan,11; 2012,Jul,12-14; 2012,Jan,15-42; 2011,Oct,3-4; 2011,Jul,16-17; 2011,Jan,11

01150 **Anesthesia for radical procedures for tumor of pelvis, except hindquarter amputation**
  0.00   0.00   **FUD** XXX   C
  AMA: 2016,Jan,13; 2015,Jan,16; 2014,Aug,5; 2014,Jan,11; 2012,Jul,12-14; 2012,Jan,15-42; 2011,Oct,3-4; 2011,Jul,16-17; 2011,Jan,11

01160 **Anesthesia for closed procedures involving symphysis pubis or sacroiliac joint**
  0.00   0.00   **FUD** XXX   N
  AMA: 2016,Jan,13; 2015,Jan,16; 2014,Aug,5; 2014,Jan,11; 2012,Jul,12-14; 2012,Jan,15-42; 2011,Oct,3-4; 2011,Jul,16-17; 2011,Jan,11

01170 **Anesthesia for open procedures involving symphysis pubis or sacroiliac joint**
  0.00   0.00   **FUD** XXX   N
  AMA: 2016,Jan,13; 2015,Jan,16; 2014,Aug,5; 2014,Jan,11; 2012,Jul,12-14; 2012,Jan,15-42; 2011,Oct,3-4; 2011,Jul,16-17; 2011,Jan,11

01173 **Anesthesia for open repair of fracture disruption of pelvis or column fracture involving acetabulum**
  0.00   0.00   **FUD** XXX   N
  AMA: 2016,Jan,13; 2015,Jan,16; 2014,Aug,5; 2014,Jan,11; 2012,Jul,12-14; 2012,Jan,15-42; 2011,Oct,3-4; 2011,Jul,16-17; 2011,Jan,11

01180 **Anesthesia for obturator neurectomy; extrapelvic**
  0.00   0.00   **FUD** XXX   N
  AMA: 2016,Jan,13; 2015,Jan,16; 2014,Aug,5; 2014,Jan,11; 2012,Jul,12-14; 2012,Jan,15-42; 2011,Oct,3-4; 2011,Jul,16-17; 2011,Jan,11

01190   **intrapelvic**
  0.00   0.00   **FUD** XXX   N
  AMA: 2016,Jan,13; 2015,Jan,16; 2014,Aug,5; 2014,Jan,11; 2012,Jul,12-14; 2012,Jan,15-42; 2011,Oct,3-4; 2011,Jul,16-17; 2011,Jan,11

01200 **Anesthesia for all closed procedures involving hip joint**
  0.00   0.00   **FUD** XXX   N
  AMA: 2016,Jan,13; 2015,Jan,16; 2014,Aug,5; 2014,Jan,11; 2012,Jul,12-14; 2012,Jan,15-42; 2011,Oct,3-4; 2011,Jul,16-17; 2011,Jan,11

01202 **Anesthesia for arthroscopic procedures of hip joint**
  0.00   0.00   **FUD** XXX   N
  AMA: 2016,Jan,13; 2015,Jan,16; 2014,Aug,5; 2014,Jan,11; 2012,Jul,12-14; 2012,Jan,15-42; 2011,Oct,3-4; 2011,Jul,16-17; 2011,Jan,11

01210 **Anesthesia for open procedures involving hip joint; not otherwise specified**
  0.00   0.00   **FUD** XXX   N
  AMA: 2016,Jan,13; 2015,Jan,16; 2014,Aug,5; 2014,Jan,11; 2012,Jul,12-14; 2012,Jan,15-42; 2011,Oct,3-4; 2011,Jul,16-17; 2011,Jan,11

01212   **hip disarticulation**
  0.00   0.00   **FUD** XXX   C
  AMA: 2016,Jan,13; 2015,Jan,16; 2014,Aug,5; 2014,Jan,11; 2012,Jul,12-14; 2012,Jan,15-42; 2011,Oct,3-4; 2011,Jul,16-17; 2011,Jan,11

01214   **total hip arthroplasty**
  0.00   0.00   **FUD** XXX   C
  AMA: 2016,Jan,13; 2015,Jan,16; 2014,Aug,5; 2014,Jan,11; 2012,Jul,12-14; 2012,Jan,15-42; 2011,Oct,3-4; 2011,Jul,16-17; 2011,Jan,11

01215   **revision of total hip arthroplasty**
  0.00   0.00   **FUD** XXX   N
  AMA: 2016,Jan,13; 2015,Jan,16; 2014,Aug,5; 2014,Jan,11; 2012,Jul,12-14; 2012,Jan,15-42; 2011,Oct,3-4; 2011,Jul,16-17; 2011,Jan,11

01220 **Anesthesia for all closed procedures involving upper two-thirds of femur**
  0.00   0.00   **FUD** XXX   N
  AMA: 2016,Jan,13; 2015,Jan,16; 2014,Aug,5; 2014,Jan,11; 2012,Jul,12-14; 2012,Jan,15-42; 2011,Oct,3-4; 2011,Jul,16-17; 2011,Jan,11

01230 **Anesthesia for open procedures involving upper two-thirds of femur; not otherwise specified**
  0.00   0.00   **FUD** XXX   N
  AMA: 2016,Jan,13; 2015,Jan,16; 2014,Aug,5; 2014,Jan,11; 2012,Jul,12-14; 2012,Jan,15-42; 2011,Oct,3-4; 2011,Jul,16-17; 2011,Jan,11

01232   **amputation**
  0.00   0.00   **FUD** XXX   C
  AMA: 2016,Jan,13; 2015,Jan,16; 2014,Aug,5; 2014,Jan,11; 2012,Jul,12-14; 2012,Jan,15-42; 2011,Oct,3-4; 2011,Jul,16-17; 2011,Jan,11

01234   **radical resection**
  0.00   0.00   **FUD** XXX   C
  AMA: 2016,Jan,13; 2015,Jan,16; 2014,Aug,5; 2014,Jan,11; 2012,Jul,12-14; 2012,Jan,15-42; 2011,Oct,3-4; 2011,Jul,16-17; 2011,Jan,11

01250 **Anesthesia for all procedures on nerves, muscles, tendons, fascia, and bursae of upper leg**
  0.00   0.00   **FUD** XXX   N
  AMA: 2016,Jan,13; 2015,Jan,16; 2014,Aug,5; 2014,Jan,11; 2012,Jul,12-14; 2012,Jan,15-42; 2011,Oct,3-4; 2011,Jul,16-17; 2011,Jan,11

01260 **Anesthesia for all procedures involving veins of upper leg, including exploration**
  0.00   0.00   **FUD** XXX   N
  AMA: 2016,Jan,13; 2015,Jan,16; 2014,Aug,5; 2014,Jan,11; 2012,Jul,12-14; 2012,Jan,15-42; 2011,Oct,3-4; 2011,Jul,16-17; 2011,Jan,11

01270 **Anesthesia for procedures involving arteries of upper leg, including bypass graft; not otherwise specified**
  0.00   0.00   **FUD** XXX   N
  AMA: 2016,Jan,13; 2015,Jan,16; 2014,Aug,5; 2014,Jan,11; 2012,Jul,12-14; 2012,Jan,15-42; 2011,Oct,3-4; 2011,Jul,16-17; 2011,Jan,11

01272   **femoral artery ligation**
  0.00   0.00   **FUD** XXX   C
  AMA: 2016,Jan,13; 2015,Jan,16; 2014,Aug,5; 2014,Jan,11; 2012,Jul,12-14; 2012,Jan,15-42; 2011,Oct,3-4; 2011,Jul,16-17; 2011,Jan,11

01274   **femoral artery embolectomy**
  0.00   0.00   **FUD** XXX   C
  AMA: 2016,Jan,13; 2015,Jan,16; 2014,Aug,5; 2014,Jan,11; 2012,Jul,12-14; 2012,Jan,15-42; 2011,Oct,3-4; 2011,Jul,16-17; 2011,Jan,11

01320 Anesthesia for all procedures on nerves, muscles, tendons, fascia, and bursae of knee and/or popliteal area
⚕ 0.00   ⚗ 0.00   **FUD** XXX   Ⓝ ▯
AMA: 2016,Jan,13; 2015,Jan,16; 2014,Aug,5; 2014,Jan,11; 2012,Jul,12-14; 2012,Jan,15-42; 2011,Oct,3-4; 2011,Jul,16-17; 2011,Jan,11

01340 Anesthesia for all closed procedures on lower one-third of femur
⚕ 0.00   ⚗ 0.00   **FUD** XXX   Ⓝ ▯
AMA: 2016,Jan,13; 2015,Jan,16; 2014,Aug,5; 2014,Jan,11; 2012,Jul,12-14; 2012,Jan,15-42; 2011,Oct,3-4; 2011,Jul,16-17; 2011,Jan,11

01360 Anesthesia for all open procedures on lower one-third of femur
⚕ 0.00   ⚗ 0.00   **FUD** XXX   Ⓝ ▯
AMA: 2016,Jan,13; 2015,Jan,16; 2014,Aug,5; 2014,Jan,11; 2012,Jul,12-14; 2012,Jan,15-42; 2011,Oct,3-4; 2011,Jul,16-17; 2011,Jan,11

01380 Anesthesia for all closed procedures on knee joint
⚕ 0.00   ⚗ 0.00   **FUD** XXX   Ⓝ ▯
AMA: 2016,Jan,13; 2015,Jan,16; 2014,Aug,5; 2014,Jan,11; 2012,Jul,12-14; 2012,Jan,15-42; 2011,Oct,3-4; 2011,Jul,16-17; 2011,Jan,11

01382 Anesthesia for diagnostic arthroscopic procedures of knee joint
⚕ 0.00   ⚗ 0.00   **FUD** XXX   Ⓝ ▯
AMA: 2016,Jan,13; 2015,Jan,16; 2014,Aug,5; 2014,Jan,11; 2012,Jul,12-14; 2012,Jan,15-42; 2011,Oct,3-4; 2011,Jul,16-17; 2011,Jan,11

01390 Anesthesia for all closed procedures on upper ends of tibia, fibula, and/or patella
⚕ 0.00   ⚗ 0.00   **FUD** XXX   Ⓝ ▯
AMA: 2016,Jan,13; 2015,Jan,16; 2014,Aug,5; 2014,Jan,11; 2012,Jul,12-14; 2012,Jan,15-42; 2011,Oct,3-4; 2011,Jul,16-17; 2011,Jan,11

01392 Anesthesia for all open procedures on upper ends of tibia, fibula, and/or patella
⚕ 0.00   ⚗ 0.00   **FUD** XXX   Ⓝ ▯
AMA: 2016,Jan,13; 2015,Jan,16; 2014,Aug,5; 2014,Jan,11; 2012,Jul,12-14; 2012,Jan,15-42; 2011,Oct,3-4; 2011,Jul,16-17; 2011,Jan,11

01400 Anesthesia for open or surgical arthroscopic procedures on knee joint; not otherwise specified
⚕ 0.00   ⚗ 0.00   **FUD** XXX   Ⓝ ▯
AMA: 2016,Jan,13; 2015,Jan,16; 2014,Aug,5; 2014,Jan,11; 2012,Jul,12-14; 2012,Jan,15-42; 2011,Oct,3-4; 2011,Jul,16-17; 2011,Jan,11

01402 total knee arthroplasty
⚕ 0.00   ⚗ 0.00   **FUD** XXX   Ⓒ ▯
AMA: 2016,Jan,13; 2015,Jan,16; 2014,Aug,5; 2014,Jan,11; 2012,Jul,12-14; 2012,Jan,15-42; 2011,Oct,3-4; 2011,Jul,16-17; 2011,Jan,11

01404 disarticulation at knee
⚕ 0.00   ⚗ 0.00   **FUD** XXX   Ⓒ ▯
AMA: 2016,Jan,13; 2015,Jan,16; 2014,Aug,5; 2014,Jan,11; 2012,Jul,12-14; 2012,Jan,15-42; 2011,Oct,3-4; 2011,Jul,16-17; 2011,Jan,11

01420 Anesthesia for all cast applications, removal, or repair involving knee joint
⚕ 0.00   ⚗ 0.00   **FUD** XXX   Ⓝ ▯
AMA: 2016,Jan,13; 2015,Jan,16; 2014,Aug,5; 2014,Jan,11; 2012,Jul,12-14; 2012,Jan,15-42; 2011,Oct,3-4; 2011,Jul,16-17; 2011,Jan,11

01430 Anesthesia for procedures on veins of knee and popliteal area; not otherwise specified
⚕ 0.00   ⚗ 0.00   **FUD** XXX   Ⓝ ▯
AMA: 2016,Jan,13; 2015,Jan,16; 2014,Aug,5; 2014,Jan,11; 2012,Jul,12-14; 2012,Jan,15-42; 2011,Oct,3-4; 2011,Jul,16-17; 2011,Jan,11

01432 arteriovenous fistula
⚕ 0.00   ⚗ 0.00   **FUD** XXX   Ⓝ ▯
AMA: 2016,Jan,13; 2015,Jan,16; 2014,Aug,5; 2014,Jan,11; 2012,Jul,12-14; 2012,Jan,15-42; 2011,Oct,3-4; 2011,Jul,16-17; 2011,Jan,11

01440 Anesthesia for procedures on arteries of knee and popliteal area; not otherwise specified
⚕ 0.00   ⚗ 0.00   **FUD** XXX   Ⓝ ▯
AMA: 2016,Jan,13; 2015,Jan,16; 2014,Aug,5; 2014,Jan,11; 2012,Jul,12-14; 2012,Jan,15-42; 2011,Oct,3-4; 2011,Jul,16-17; 2011,Jan,11

01442 popliteal thromboendarterectomy, with or without patch graft
⚕ 0.00   ⚗ 0.00   **FUD** XXX   Ⓒ ▯
AMA: 2016,Jan,13; 2015,Jan,16; 2014,Aug,5; 2014,Jan,11; 2012,Jul,12-14; 2012,Jan,15-42; 2011,Oct,3-4; 2011,Jul,16-17; 2011,Jan,11

01444 popliteal excision and graft or repair for occlusion or aneurysm
⚕ 0.00   ⚗ 0.00   **FUD** XXX   Ⓒ ▯
AMA: 2016,Jan,13; 2015,Jan,16; 2014,Aug,5; 2014,Jan,11; 2012,Jul,12-14; 2012,Jan,15-42; 2011,Oct,3-4; 2011,Jul,16-17; 2011,Jan,11

01462 Anesthesia for all closed procedures on lower leg, ankle, and foot
⚕ 0.00   ⚗ 0.00   **FUD** XXX   Ⓝ ▯
AMA: 2016,Jan,13; 2015,Jan,16; 2014,Aug,5; 2014,Jan,11; 2012,Jul,12-14; 2012,Jan,15-42; 2011,Oct,3-4; 2011,Jul,16-17; 2011,Jan,11

01464 Anesthesia for arthroscopic procedures of ankle and/or foot
⚕ 0.00   ⚗ 0.00   **FUD** XXX   Ⓝ ▯
AMA: 2016,Jan,13; 2015,Jan,16; 2014,Aug,5; 2014,Jan,11; 2012,Jul,12-14; 2012,Jan,15-42; 2011,Oct,3-4; 2011,Jul,16-17; 2011,Jan,11

01470 Anesthesia for procedures on nerves, muscles, tendons, and fascia of lower leg, ankle, and foot; not otherwise specified
⚕ 0.00   ⚗ 0.00   **FUD** XXX   Ⓝ ▯
AMA: 2016,Jan,13; 2015,Jan,16; 2014,Aug,5; 2014,Jan,11; 2012,Jul,12-14; 2012,Jan,15-42; 2011,Oct,3-4; 2011,Jul,16-17; 2011,Jan,11

01472 repair of ruptured Achilles tendon, with or without graft
⚕ 0.00   ⚗ 0.00   **FUD** XXX   Ⓝ ▯
AMA: 2016,Jan,13; 2015,Jan,16; 2014,Aug,5; 2014,Jan,11; 2012,Jul,12-14; 2012,Jan,15-42; 2011,Oct,3-4; 2011,Jul,16-17; 2011,Jan,11

01474 gastrocnemius recession (eg, Strayer procedure)
⚕ 0.00   ⚗ 0.00   **FUD** XXX   Ⓝ ▯
AMA: 2016,Jan,13; 2015,Jan,16; 2014,Aug,5; 2014,Jan,11; 2012,Jul,12-14; 2012,Jan,15-42; 2011,Oct,3-4; 2011,Jul,16-17; 2011,Jan,11

01480 Anesthesia for open procedures on bones of lower leg, ankle, and foot; not otherwise specified
⚕ 0.00   ⚗ 0.00   **FUD** XXX   Ⓝ ▯
AMA: 2016,Jan,13; 2015,Jan,16; 2014,Aug,5; 2014,Jan,11; 2012,Jul,12-14; 2012,Jan,15-42; 2011,Oct,3-4; 2011,Jul,16-17; 2011,Jan,11

01482 radical resection (including below knee amputation)
⚕ 0.00   ⚗ 0.00   **FUD** XXX   Ⓝ ▯
AMA: 2016,Jan,13; 2015,Jan,16; 2014,Aug,5; 2014,Jan,11; 2012,Jul,12-14; 2012,Jan,15-42; 2011,Oct,3-4; 2011,Jul,16-17; 2011,Jan,11

01484 osteotomy or osteoplasty of tibia and/or fibula
⚕ 0.00   ⚗ 0.00   **FUD** XXX   Ⓝ ▯
AMA: 2016,Jan,13; 2015,Jan,16; 2014,Aug,5; 2014,Jan,11; 2012,Jul,12-14; 2012,Jan,15-42; 2011,Oct,3-4; 2011,Jul,16-17; 2011,Jan,11

01486 total ankle replacement
🚑 0.00   ⚕ 0.00   **FUD** XXX   C ▢
AMA: 2016,Jan,13; 2015,Jan,16; 2014,Aug,5; 2014,Jan,11; 2012,Jul,12-14; 2012,Jan,15-42; 2011,Oct,3-4; 2011,Jul,16-17; 2011,Jan,11

01490 Anesthesia for lower leg cast application, removal, or repair
🚑 0.00   ⚕ 0.00   **FUD** XXX   N ▢
AMA: 2016,Jan,13; 2015,Jan,16; 2014,Aug,5; 2014,Jan,11; 2012,Jul,12-14; 2012,Jan,15-42; 2011,Oct,3-4; 2011,Jul,16-17; 2011,Jan,11

01500 Anesthesia for procedures on arteries of lower leg, including bypass graft; not otherwise specified
🚑 0.00   ⚕ 0.00   **FUD** XXX   N ▢
AMA: 2016,Jan,13; 2015,Jan,16; 2014,Aug,5; 2014,Jan,11; 2012,Jul,12-14; 2012,Jan,15-42; 2011,Oct,3-4; 2011,Jul,16-17; 2011,Jan,11

01502 embolectomy, direct or with catheter
🚑 0.00   ⚕ 0.00   **FUD** XXX   C ▢
AMA: 2016,Jan,13; 2015,Jan,16; 2014,Aug,5; 2014,Jan,11; 2012,Jul,12-14; 2012,Jan,15-42; 2011,Oct,3-4; 2011,Jul,16-17; 2011,Jan,11

01520 Anesthesia for procedures on veins of lower leg; not otherwise specified
🚑 0.00   ⚕ 0.00   **FUD** XXX   N ▢
AMA: 2016,Jan,13; 2015,Jan,16; 2014,Aug,5; 2014,Jan,11; 2012,Jul,12-14; 2012,Jan,15-42; 2011,Oct,3-4; 2011,Jul,16-17; 2011,Jan,11

01522 venous thrombectomy, direct or with catheter
🚑 0.00   ⚕ 0.00   **FUD** XXX   N ▢
AMA: 2016,Jan,13; 2015,Jan,16; 2014,Aug,5; 2014,Jan,11; 2012,Jul,12-14; 2012,Jan,15-42; 2011,Oct,3-4; 2011,Jul,16-17; 2011,Jan,11

01610-01682 Anesthesia for Shoulder Procedures

CMS: 100-04,12,140.1 Qualified Nonphysician Anesthetists; 100-04,12,140.3 Payment for Qualified Nonphysician Anesthetists; 100-04,12,140.3.3 Billing Modifiers; 100-04,12,140.3.4 General Billing Instructions; 100-04,12,140.4.1 Anesthesiologist/Qualified Nonphysican Anesthetist; 100-04,12,140.4.2 Anesthetist and Anesthesiologist in a Single Procedure; 100-04,12,140.4.3 Payment for Medical /Surgical Services by CRNAs; 100-04,12,140.4.4 Conversion Factors for Anesthesia Services; 100-04,4,250.3.2 Anesthesia in a Hospital Outpatient Setting

INCLUDES   Acromioclavicular joint
Humeral head and neck
Shoulder joint
Sternoclavicular joint

01610 Anesthesia for all procedures on nerves, muscles, tendons, fascia, and bursae of shoulder and axilla
🚑 0.00   ⚕ 0.00   **FUD** XXX   N ▢
AMA: 2016,Jan,13; 2015,Jan,16; 2014,Aug,5; 2014,Jan,11; 2012,Jul,12-14; 2012,Jan,15-42; 2011,Oct,3-4; 2011,Jul,16-17; 2011,Jan,11

01620 Anesthesia for all closed procedures on humeral head and neck, sternoclavicular joint, acromioclavicular joint, and shoulder joint
🚑 0.00   ⚕ 0.00   **FUD** XXX   N ▢
AMA: 2016,Jan,13; 2015,Jan,16; 2014,Aug,5; 2014,Jan,11; 2012,Jul,12-14; 2012,Jan,15-42; 2011,Oct,3-4; 2011,Jul,16-17; 2011,Jan,11

01622 Anesthesia for diagnostic arthroscopic procedures of shoulder joint
🚑 0.00   ⚕ 0.00   **FUD** XXX   N ▢
AMA: 2016,Jan,13; 2015,Jan,16; 2014,Aug,5; 2014,Jan,11; 2012,Jul,12-14; 2012,Jan,15-42; 2011,Oct,3-4; 2011,Jul,16-17; 2011,Jan,11

01630 Anesthesia for open or surgical arthroscopic procedures on humeral head and neck, sternoclavicular joint, acromioclavicular joint, and shoulder joint; not otherwise specified
🚑 0.00   ⚕ 0.00   **FUD** XXX   N ▢
AMA: 2016,Jan,13; 2015,Jan,16; 2014,Aug,5; 2014,Jan,11; 2012,Jul,12-14; 2012,Jan,15-42; 2011,Oct,3-4; 2011,Jul,16-17; 2011,Jan,11

01634 shoulder disarticulation
🚑 0.00   ⚕ 0.00   **FUD** XXX   C ▢
AMA: 2016,Jan,13; 2015,Jan,16; 2014,Aug,5; 2014,Jan,11; 2012,Jul,12-14; 2012,Jan,15-42; 2011,Oct,3-4; 2011,Jul,16-17; 2011,Jan,11

01636 interthoracoscapular (forequarter) amputation
🚑 0.00   ⚕ 0.00   **FUD** XXX   C ▢
AMA: 2016,Jan,13; 2015,Jan,16; 2014,Aug,5; 2014,Jan,11; 2012,Jul,12-14; 2012,Jan,15-42; 2011,Oct,3-4; 2011,Jul,16-17; 2011,Jan,11

01638 total shoulder replacement
🚑 0.00   ⚕ 0.00   **FUD** XXX   C ▢
AMA: 2016,Jan,13; 2015,Jan,16; 2014,Aug,5; 2014,Jan,11; 2012,Jul,12-14; 2012,Jan,15-42; 2011,Oct,3-4; 2011,Jul,16-17; 2011,Jan,11

01650 Anesthesia for procedures on arteries of shoulder and axilla; not otherwise specified
🚑 0.00   ⚕ 0.00   **FUD** XXX   N ▢
AMA: 2016,Jan,13; 2015,Jan,16; 2014,Aug,5; 2014,Jan,11; 2012,Jul,12-14; 2012,Jan,15-42; 2011,Oct,3-4; 2011,Jul,16-17; 2011,Jan,11

01652 axillary-brachial aneurysm
🚑 0.00   ⚕ 0.00   **FUD** XXX   C ▢
AMA: 2016,Jan,13; 2015,Jan,16; 2014,Aug,5; 2014,Jan,11; 2012,Jul,12-14; 2012,Jan,15-42; 2011,Oct,3-4; 2011,Jul,16-17; 2011,Jan,11

01654 bypass graft
🚑 0.00   ⚕ 0.00   **FUD** XXX   C ▢
AMA: 2016,Jan,13; 2015,Jan,16; 2014,Aug,5; 2014,Jan,11; 2012,Jul,12-14; 2012,Jan,15-42; 2011,Oct,3-4; 2011,Jul,16-17; 2011,Jan,11

01656 axillary-femoral bypass graft
🚑 0.00   ⚕ 0.00   **FUD** XXX   C ▢
AMA: 2016,Jan,13; 2015,Jan,16; 2014,Aug,5; 2014,Jan,11; 2012,Jul,12-14; 2012,Jan,15-42; 2011,Oct,3-4; 2011,Jul,16-17; 2011,Jan,11

01670 Anesthesia for all procedures on veins of shoulder and axilla
🚑 0.00   ⚕ 0.00   **FUD** XXX   N ▢
AMA: 2016,Jan,13; 2015,Jan,16; 2014,Aug,5; 2014,Jan,11; 2012,Jul,12-14; 2012,Jan,15-42; 2011,Oct,3-4; 2011,Jul,16-17; 2011,Jan,11

01680 Anesthesia for shoulder cast application, removal or repair; not otherwise specified
🚑 0.00   ⚕ 0.00   **FUD** XXX   N ▢
AMA: 2016,Jan,13; 2015,Jan,16; 2014,Aug,5; 2014,Jan,11; 2012,Jul,12-14; 2012,Jan,15-42; 2011,Oct,3-4; 2011,Jul,16-17; 2011,Jan,11

01682 shoulder spica
🚑 0.00   ⚕ 0.00   **FUD** XXX   N ▢
AMA: 2016,Jan,13; 2015,Jan,16; 2014,Aug,5; 2014,Jan,11; 2012,Jul,12-14; 2012,Jan,15-42; 2011,Oct,3-4; 2011,Jul,16-17; 2011,Jan,11

01710-01860 Anesthesia for Upper Extremity Procedures

CMS: 100-04,12,140.1 Qualified Nonphysician Anesthetists; 100-04,12,140.3 Payment for Qualified Nonphysician Anesthetists; 100-04,12,140.3.3 Billing Modifiers; 100-04,12,140.3.4 General Billing Instructions; 100-04,12,140.4.1 Anesthesiologist/Qualified Nonphysican Anesthetist; 100-04,12,140.4.2 Anesthetist and Anesthesiologist in a Single Procedure; 100-04,12,140.4.3 Payment for Medical /Surgical Services by CRNAs; 100-04,12,140.4.4 Conversion Factors for Anesthesia Services; 100-04,4,250.3.2 Anesthesia in a Hospital Outpatient Setting

01710 Anesthesia for procedures on nerves, muscles, tendons, fascia, and bursae of upper arm and elbow; not otherwise specified

    🏷 0.00   ⚖ 0.00   **FUD** XXX   N ▣

    AMA: 2016,Jan,13; 2015,Jan,16; 2014,Aug,5; 2014,Jan,11; 2012,Jul,12-14; 2012,Jan,15-42; 2011,Oct,3-4; 2011,Jul,16-17; 2011,Jan,11

01712 tenotomy, elbow to shoulder, open

    🏷 0.00   ⚖ 0.00   **FUD** XXX   N ▣

    AMA: 2016,Jan,13; 2015,Jan,16; 2014,Aug,5; 2014,Jan,11; 2012,Jul,12-14; 2012,Jan,15-42; 2011,Oct,3-4; 2011,Jul,16-17; 2011,Jan,11

01714 tenoplasty, elbow to shoulder

    🏷 0.00   ⚖ 0.00   **FUD** XXX   N ▣

    AMA: 2016,Jan,13; 2015,Jan,16; 2014,Aug,5; 2014,Jan,11; 2012,Jul,12-14; 2012,Jan,15-42; 2011,Oct,3-4; 2011,Jul,16-17; 2011,Jan,11

01716 tenodesis, rupture of long tendon of biceps

    🏷 0.00   ⚖ 0.00   **FUD** XXX   N ▣

    AMA: 2016,Jan,13; 2015,Jan,16; 2014,Aug,5; 2014,Jan,11; 2012,Jul,12-14; 2012,Jan,15-42; 2011,Oct,3-4; 2011,Jul,16-17; 2011,Jan,11

01730 Anesthesia for all closed procedures on humerus and elbow

    🏷 0.00   ⚖ 0.00   **FUD** XXX   N ▣

    AMA: 2016,Jan,13; 2015,Jan,16; 2014,Aug,5; 2014,Jan,11; 2012,Jul,12-14; 2012,Jan,15-42; 2011,Oct,3-4; 2011,Jul,16-17; 2011,Jan,11

01732 Anesthesia for diagnostic arthroscopic procedures of elbow joint

    🏷 0.00   ⚖ 0.00   **FUD** XXX   N ▣

    AMA: 2016,Jan,13; 2015,Jan,16; 2014,Aug,5; 2014,Jan,11; 2012,Jul,12-14; 2012,Jan,15-42; 2011,Oct,3-4; 2011,Jul,16-17; 2011,Jan,11

01740 Anesthesia for open or surgical arthroscopic procedures of the elbow; not otherwise specified

    🏷 0.00   ⚖ 0.00   **FUD** XXX   N ▣

    AMA: 2016,Jan,13; 2015,Jan,16; 2014,Aug,5; 2014,Jan,11; 2012,Jul,12-14; 2012,Jan,15-42; 2011,Oct,3-4; 2011,Jul,16-17; 2011,Jan,11

01742 osteotomy of humerus

    🏷 0.00   ⚖ 0.00   **FUD** XXX   N ▣

    AMA: 2016,Jan,13; 2015,Jan,16; 2014,Aug,5; 2014,Jan,11; 2012,Jul,12-14; 2012,Jan,15-42; 2011,Oct,3-4; 2011,Jul,16-17; 2011,Jan,11

01744 repair of nonunion or malunion of humerus

    🏷 0.00   ⚖ 0.00   **FUD** XXX   N ▣

    AMA: 2016,Jan,13; 2015,Jan,16; 2014,Aug,5; 2014,Jan,11; 2012,Jul,12-14; 2012,Jan,15-42; 2011,Oct,3-4; 2011,Jul,16-17; 2011,Jan,11

01756 radical procedures

    🏷 0.00   ⚖ 0.00   **FUD** XXX   C ▣

    AMA: 2016,Jan,13; 2015,Jan,16; 2014,Aug,5; 2014,Jan,11; 2012,Jul,12-14; 2012,Jan,15-42; 2011,Oct,3-4; 2011,Jul,16-17; 2011,Jan,11

01758 excision of cyst or tumor of humerus

    🏷 0.00   ⚖ 0.00   **FUD** XXX   N ▣

    AMA: 2016,Jan,13; 2015,Jan,16; 2014,Aug,5; 2014,Jan,11; 2012,Jul,12-14; 2012,Jan,15-42; 2011,Oct,3-4; 2011,Jul,16-17; 2011,Jan,11

01760 total elbow replacement

    🏷 0.00   ⚖ 0.00   **FUD** XXX   N ▣

    AMA: 2016,Jan,13; 2015,Jan,16; 2014,Aug,5; 2014,Jan,11; 2012,Jul,12-14; 2012,Jan,15-42; 2011,Oct,3-4; 2011,Jul,16-17; 2011,Jan,11

01770 Anesthesia for procedures on arteries of upper arm and elbow; not otherwise specified

    🏷 0.00   ⚖ 0.00   **FUD** XXX   N ▣

    AMA: 2016,Jan,13; 2015,Jan,16; 2014,Aug,5; 2014,Jan,11; 2012,Jul,12-14; 2012,Jan,15-42; 2011,Oct,3-4; 2011,Jul,16-17; 2011,Jan,11

01772 embolectomy

    🏷 0.00   ⚖ 0.00   **FUD** XXX   N ▣

    AMA: 2016,Jan,13; 2015,Jan,16; 2014,Aug,5; 2014,Jan,11; 2012,Jul,12-14; 2012,Jan,15-42; 2011,Oct,3-4; 2011,Jul,16-17; 2011,Jan,11

01780 Anesthesia for procedures on veins of upper arm and elbow; not otherwise specified

    🏷 0.00   ⚖ 0.00   **FUD** XXX   N ▣

    AMA: 2016,Jan,13; 2015,Jan,16; 2014,Aug,5; 2014,Jan,11; 2012,Jul,12-14; 2012,Jan,15-42; 2011,Oct,3-4; 2011,Jul,16-17; 2011,Jan,11

01782 phleborrhaphy

    🏷 0.00   ⚖ 0.00   **FUD** XXX   N ▣

    AMA: 2016,Jan,13; 2015,Jan,16; 2014,Aug,5; 2014,Jan,11; 2012,Jul,12-14; 2012,Jan,15-42; 2011,Oct,3-4; 2011,Jul,16-17; 2011,Jan,11

01810 Anesthesia for all procedures on nerves, muscles, tendons, fascia, and bursae of forearm, wrist, and hand

    🏷 0.00   ⚖ 0.00   **FUD** XXX   N ▣

    AMA: 2016,Jan,13; 2015,Jan,16; 2014,Aug,5; 2014,Jan,11; 2012,Jul,12-14; 2012,Jan,15-42; 2011,Oct,3-4; 2011,Jul,16-17; 2011,Jan,11

01820 Anesthesia for all closed procedures on radius, ulna, wrist, or hand bones

    🏷 0.00   ⚖ 0.00   **FUD** XXX   N ▣

    AMA: 2016,Jan,13; 2015,Jan,16; 2014,Aug,5; 2014,Jan,11; 2012,Jul,12-14; 2012,Jan,15-42; 2011,Oct,3-4; 2011,Jul,16-17; 2011,Jan,11

01829 Anesthesia for diagnostic arthroscopic procedures on the wrist

    🏷 0.00   ⚖ 0.00   **FUD** XXX   N ▣

    AMA: 2016,Jan,13; 2015,Jan,16; 2014,Aug,5; 2014,Jan,11; 2012,Jul,12-14; 2012,Jan,15-42; 2011,Oct,3-4; 2011,Jul,16-17; 2011,Jan,11

01830 Anesthesia for open or surgical arthroscopic/endoscopic procedures on distal radius, distal ulna, wrist, or hand joints; not otherwise specified

    🏷 0.00   ⚖ 0.00   **FUD** XXX   N ▣

    AMA: 2016,Jan,13; 2015,Jan,16; 2014,Aug,5; 2014,Jan,11; 2012,Jul,12-14; 2012,Jan,15-42; 2011,Oct,3-4; 2011,Jul,16-17; 2011,Jan,11

01832 total wrist replacement

    🏷 0.00   ⚖ 0.00   **FUD** XXX   N ▣

    AMA: 2016,Jan,13; 2015,Jan,16; 2014,Aug,5; 2014,Jan,11; 2012,Jul,12-14; 2012,Jan,15-42; 2011,Oct,3-4; 2011,Jul,16-17; 2011,Jan,11

01840 Anesthesia for procedures on arteries of forearm, wrist, and hand; not otherwise specified

    🏷 0.00   ⚖ 0.00   **FUD** XXX   N ▣

    AMA: 2016,Jan,13; 2015,Jan,16; 2014,Aug,5; 2014,Jan,11; 2012,Jul,12-14; 2012,Jan,15-42; 2011,Oct,3-4; 2011,Jul,16-17; 2011,Jan,11

01842 embolectomy

    🏷 0.00   ⚖ 0.00   **FUD** XXX   N ▣

    AMA: 2016,Jan,13; 2015,Jan,16; 2014,Aug,5; 2014,Jan,11; 2012,Jul,12-14; 2012,Jan,15-42; 2011,Oct,3-4; 2011,Jul,16-17; 2011,Jan,11

01844 Anesthesia for vascular shunt, or shunt revision, any type (eg, dialysis)

    🏷 0.00   ⚖ 0.00   **FUD** XXX   N ▣

    AMA: 2016,Jan,13; 2015,Jan,16; 2014,Aug,5; 2014,Jan,11; 2012,Jul,12-14; 2012,Jan,15-42; 2011,Oct,3-4; 2011,Jul,16-17; 2011,Jan,11

● New Code   ▲ Revised Code   ○ Reinstated   ● New Web Release   ▲ Revised Web Release   Unlisted   Not Covered   # Resequenced
⊘ AMA Mod 51 Exempt   ⑪ Optum Mod 51 Exempt   ⑬ Mod 63 Exempt   ✗ Non-FDA Drug   ★ Telehealth   Ⓜ Maternity   Ⓐ Age Edit   + Add-on   **AMA:** CPT Asst

01850 **Anesthesia for procedures on veins of forearm, wrist, and hand; not otherwise specified**

    🔹 0.00   ⚬ 0.00   **FUD** XXX   N ▢

    AMA: 2016,Jan,13; 2015,Jan,16; 2014,Aug,5; 2014,Jan,11; 2012,Jul,12-14; 2012,Jan,15-42; 2011,Oct,3-4; 2011,Jul,16-17; 2011,Jan,11

01852 **phleborrhaphy**

    🔹 0.00   ⚬ 0.00   **FUD** XXX   N ▢

    AMA: 2016,Jan,13; 2015,Jan,16; 2014,Aug,5; 2014,Jan,11; 2012,Jul,12-14; 2012,Jan,15-42; 2011,Oct,3-4; 2011,Jul,16-17; 2011,Jan,11

01860 **Anesthesia for forearm, wrist, or hand cast application, removal, or repair**

    🔹 0.00   ⚬ 0.00   **FUD** XXX   N ▢

    AMA: 2016,Jan,13; 2015,Jan,16; 2014,Aug,5; 2014,Jan,11; 2012,Jul,12-14; 2012,Jan,15-42; 2011,Oct,3-4; 2011,Jul,16-17; 2011,Jan,11

01916-01936 Anesthesia for Interventional Radiology Procedures

CMS: 100-04,12,140.1 Qualified Nonphysician Anesthetists; 100-04,12,140.3 Payment for Qualified Nonphysician Anesthetists; 100-04,12,140.3.3 Billing Modifiers; 100-04,12,140.3.4 General Billing Instructions; 100-04,12,140.4.1 Anesthesiologist/Qualified Nonphysican Anesthetist; 100-04,12,140.4.2 Anesthetist and Anesthesiologist in a Single Procedure; 100-04,12,140.4.3 Payment for Medical /Surgical Services by CRNAs; 100-04,12,140.4.4 Conversion Factors for Anesthesia Services; 100-04,4,250.3.2 Anesthesia in a Hospital Outpatient Setting

01916 **Anesthesia for diagnostic arteriography/venography**

    EXCLUDES *Anesthesia for therapeutic interventional radiological procedures involving the arterial system (01924-01926)*

             Anesthesia for therapeutic interventional radiological procedures involving the venous/lymphatic system (01930-01933)

    🔹 0.00   ⚬ 0.00   **FUD** XXX   N ▢

    AMA: 2016,Jan,13; 2015,Jan,16; 2014,Aug,5; 2014,Jan,11; 2012,Jul,12-14; 2012,Jan,15-42; 2011,Oct,3-4; 2011,Jul,16-17; 2011,Jan,11

01920 **Anesthesia for cardiac catheterization including coronary angiography and ventriculography (not to include Swan-Ganz catheter)**

    🔹 0.00   ⚬ 0.00   **FUD** XXX   N ▢

    AMA: 2016,Jan,13; 2015,Jan,16; 2014,Aug,5; 2014,Jan,11; 2012,Jul,12-14; 2012,Jan,15-42; 2011,Oct,3-4; 2011,Jul,16-17; 2011,Jan,11

01922 **Anesthesia for non-invasive imaging or radiation therapy**

    🔹 0.00   ⚬ 0.00   **FUD** XXX   N ▢

    AMA: 2016,Jan,13; 2015,Jan,16; 2014,Aug,5; 2014,Jan,11; 2012,Jul,12-14; 2012,Jan,15-42; 2011,Oct,3-4; 2011,Jul,16-17; 2011,Jan,11

01924 **Anesthesia for therapeutic interventional radiological procedures involving the arterial system; not otherwise specified**

    🔹 0.00   ⚬ 0.00   **FUD** XXX   N ▢

    AMA: 2016,Jan,13; 2015,Jan,16; 2014,Aug,5; 2014,Jan,11; 2012,Jul,12-14; 2012,Jan,15-42; 2011,Oct,3-4; 2011,Jul,16-17; 2011,Jan,11

01925 **carotid or coronary**

    🔹 0.00   ⚬ 0.00   **FUD** XXX   N ▢

    AMA: 2016,Jan,13; 2015,Jan,16; 2014,Aug,5; 2014,Jan,11; 2012,Jul,12-14; 2012,Jan,15-42; 2011,Oct,3-4; 2011,Jul,16-17; 2011,Jan,11

01926 **intracranial, intracardiac, or aortic**

    🔹 0.00   ⚬ 0.00   **FUD** XXX   N ▢

    AMA: 2016,Jan,13; 2015,Jan,16; 2014,Aug,5; 2014,Jan,11; 2012,Jul,12-14; 2012,Jan,15-42; 2011,Oct,3-4; 2011,Jul,16-17; 2011,Jan,11

01930 **Anesthesia for therapeutic interventional radiological procedures involving the venous/lymphatic system (not to include access to the central circulation); not otherwise specified**

    🔹 0.00   ⚬ 0.00   **FUD** XXX   N ▢

    AMA: 2016,Jan,13; 2015,Jan,16; 2014,Aug,5; 2014,Jan,11; 2012,Jul,12-14; 2012,Jan,15-42; 2011,Oct,3-4; 2011,Jul,16-17; 2011,Jan,11

01931 **intrahepatic or portal circulation (eg, transvenous intrahepatic portosystemic shunt[s] [TIPS])**

    🔹 0.00   ⚬ 0.00   **FUD** XXX   N ▢

    AMA: 2016,Jan,13; 2015,Jan,16; 2014,Aug,5; 2014,Jan,11; 2012,Jul,12-14; 2012,Jan,15-42; 2011,Oct,3-4; 2011,Jul,16-17; 2011,Jan,11

01932 **intrathoracic or jugular**

    🔹 0.00   ⚬ 0.00   **FUD** XXX   N ▢

    AMA: 2016,Jan,13; 2015,Jan,16; 2014,Aug,5; 2014,Jan,11; 2012,Jul,12-14; 2012,Jan,15-42; 2011,Oct,3-4; 2011,Jul,16-17; 2011,Jan,11

01933 **intracranial**

    🔹 0.00   ⚬ 0.00   **FUD** XXX   N ▢

    AMA: 2016,Jan,13; 2015,Jan,16; 2014,Aug,5; 2014,Jan,11; 2012,Jul,12-14; 2012,Jan,15-42; 2011,Oct,3-4; 2011,Jul,16-17; 2011,Jan,11

01935 **Anesthesia for percutaneous image guided procedures on the spine and spinal cord; diagnostic**

    🔹 0.00   ⚬ 0.00   **FUD** XXX   N ▢

    AMA: 2016,Jan,13; 2015,Jan,16; 2014,Aug,5; 2014,Jan,11; 2012,Jul,12-14; 2012,Jan,15-42; 2011,Oct,3-4; 2011,Jul,16-17; 2011,Jan,11

01936 **therapeutic**

    🔹 0.00   ⚬ 0.00   **FUD** XXX   N ▢

    AMA: 2016,Jan,13; 2015,Jan,16; 2014,Aug,5; 2014,Jan,11; 2012,Jul,12-14; 2012,Jan,15-42; 2011,Oct,3-4; 2011,Jul,16-17; 2011,Jan,11

01951-01953 Anesthesia for Burn Procedures

CMS: 100-04,12,140.1 Qualified Nonphysician Anesthetists; 100-04,12,140.3 Payment for Qualified Nonphysician Anesthetists; 100-04,12,140.3.3 Billing Modifiers; 100-04,12,140.3.4 General Billing Instructions; 100-04,12,140.4.1 Anesthesiologist/Qualified Nonphysican Anesthetist; 100-04,12,140.4.2 Anesthetist and Anesthesiologist in a Single Procedure; 100-04,12,140.4.3 Payment for Medical /Surgical Services by CRNAs; 100-04,12,140.4.4 Conversion Factors for Anesthesia Services; 100-04,4,250.3.2 Anesthesia in a Hospital Outpatient Setting

01951 **Anesthesia for second- and third-degree burn excision or debridement with or without skin grafting, any site, for total body surface area (TBSA) treated during anesthesia and surgery; less than 4% total body surface area**

    🔹 0.00   ⚬ 0.00   **FUD** XXX   N ▢

    AMA: 2016,Jan,13; 2015,Jan,16; 2014,Aug,5; 2014,Jan,11; 2012,Jul,12-14; 2012,Jan,15-42; 2011,Oct,3-4; 2011,Jul,16-17; 2011,Jan,11

01952 **between 4% and 9% of total body surface area**

    🔹 0.00   ⚬ 0.00   **FUD** XXX   N ▢

    AMA: 2016,Jan,13; 2015,Jan,16; 2014,Aug,5; 2014,Jan,11; 2012,Jul,12-14; 2012,Jan,15-42; 2011,Oct,3-4; 2011,Jul,16-17; 2011,Jan,11

+ 01953 **each additional 9% total body surface area or part thereof (List separately in addition to code for primary procedure)**

    Code first (01952)

    🔹 0.00   ⚬ 0.00   **FUD** XXX   N ▢

    AMA: 2016,Jan,13; 2015,Jan,16; 2014,Aug,5; 2014,Jan,11; 2012,Jul,12-14; 2012,Jan,15-42; 2011,Oct,3-4; 2011,Jun,13; 2011,Jul,16-17; 2011,Jan,11

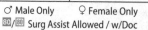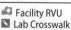

01958-01969 Anesthesia for Obstetric Procedures

CMS: 100-04,12,140.1 Qualified Nonphysician Anesthetists; 100-04,12,140.3 Payment for Qualified Nonphysician Anesthetists; 100-04,12,140.3.3 Billing Modifiers; 100-04,12,140.3.4 General Billing Instructions; 100-04,12,140.4.1 Anesthesiologist/Qualified Nonphysican Anesthetist; 100-04,12,140.4.2 Anesthetist and Anesthesiologist in a Single Procedure; 100-04,12,140.4.3 Payment for Medical /Surgical Services by CRNAs; 100-04,12,140.4.4 Conversion Factors for Anesthesia Services; 100-04,4,250.3.2 Anesthesia in a Hospital Outpatient Setting

01958 **Anesthesia for external cephalic version procedure** M

0.00   0.00   **FUD** XXX   N

AMA: 2016,Jan,13; 2015,Jan,16; 2014,Aug,5; 2014,Jan,11; 2012,Jul,12-14; 2012,Jan,15-42; 2011,Oct,3-4; 2011,Jul,16-17; 2011,Jan,11

01960 **Anesthesia for vaginal delivery only** M ♀

0.00   0.00   **FUD** XXX   N

AMA: 2016,Jan,13; 2015,Jan,16; 2014,Aug,5; 2014,Jan,11; 2012,Jul,12-14; 2012,Jan,15-42; 2011,Oct,3-4; 2011,Jul,16-17; 2011,Jan,11

01961 **Anesthesia for cesarean delivery only** M ♀

0.00   0.00   **FUD** XXX   N

AMA: 2016,Jan,13; 2015,Jan,16; 2014,Aug,5; 2014,Jan,11; 2012,Jul,12-14; 2012,Jan,15-42; 2011,Oct,3-4; 2011,Jul,16-17; 2011,Jan,11

01962 **Anesthesia for urgent hysterectomy following delivery** M ♀

0.00   0.00   **FUD** XXX   N

AMA: 2016,Jan,13; 2015,Jan,16; 2014,Aug,5; 2014,Jan,11; 2012,Jul,12-14; 2012,Jan,15-42; 2011,Oct,3-4; 2011,Jul,16-17; 2011,Jan,11

01963 **Anesthesia for cesarean hysterectomy without any labor analgesia/anesthesia care** M ♀

0.00   0.00   **FUD** XXX   N

AMA: 2016,Jan,13; 2015,Jan,16; 2014,Aug,5; 2014,Jan,11; 2012,Jul,12-14; 2012,Jan,15-42; 2011,Oct,3-4; 2011,Jul,16-17; 2011,Jan,11

01965 **Anesthesia for incomplete or missed abortion procedures** M ♀

0.00   0.00   **FUD** XXX   N

AMA: 2016,Jan,13; 2015,Jan,16; 2014,Aug,5; 2014,Jan,11; 2012,Jul,12-14; 2012,Jan,15-42; 2011,Oct,3-4; 2011,Jul,16-17; 2011,Jan,11

01966 **Anesthesia for induced abortion procedures** M ♀

0.00   0.00   **FUD** XXX   N

AMA: 2016,Jan,13; 2015,Jan,16; 2014,Aug,5; 2014,Jan,11; 2012,Jul,12-14; 2012,Jan,15-42; 2011,Oct,3-4; 2011,Jul,16-17; 2011,Jan,11

01967 **Neuraxial labor analgesia/anesthesia for planned vaginal delivery (this includes any repeat subarachnoid needle placement and drug injection and/or any necessary replacement of an epidural catheter during labor)** M ♀

0.00   0.00   **FUD** XXX   N

AMA: 2016,Jan,13; 2015,Jan,16; 2014,Oct,14; 2014,Aug,5; 2014,Jan,11; 2012,Jul,12-14; 2012,Jan,15-42; 2011,Oct,3-4; 2011,Jul,16-17; 2011,Jan,11

+ **01968** **Anesthesia for cesarean delivery following neuraxial labor analgesia/anesthesia (List separately in addition to code for primary procedure performed)** M ♀

Code first (01967)

0.00   0.00   **FUD** XXX   N

AMA: 2016,Jan,13; 2015,Jan,16; 2014,Oct,14; 2014,Aug,5; 2014,Jan,11; 2012,Jul,12-14; 2012,Jan,15-42; 2011,Oct,3-4; 2011,Jul,16-17; 2011,Jun,13; 2011,Jan,11

+ **01969** **Anesthesia for cesarean hysterectomy following neuraxial labor analgesia/anesthesia (List separately in addition to code for primary procedure performed)** M ♀

Code first (01967)

0.00   0.00   **FUD** XXX   N

AMA: 2016,Jan,13; 2015,Jan,16; 2014,Aug,5; 2014,Jan,11; 2012,Jul,12-14; 2012,Jan,15-42; 2011,Oct,3-4; 2011,Jun,13; 2011,Jul,16-17; 2011,Jan,11

01990-01999 Anesthesia Miscellaneous

CMS: 100-04,12,140.1 Qualified Nonphysician Anesthetists; 100-04,12,140.3 Payment for Qualified Nonphysician Anesthetists; 100-04,12,140.3.3 Billing Modifiers; 100-04,12,140.3.4 General Billing Instructions; 100-04,12,140.4.1 Anesthesiologist/Qualified Nonphysican Anesthetist; 100-04,12,140.4.2 Anesthetist and Anesthesiologist in a Single Procedure; 100-04,12,140.4.3 Payment for Medical /Surgical Services by CRNAs; 100-04,12,140.4.4 Conversion Factors for Anesthesia Services; 100-04,4,250.3.2 Anesthesia in a Hospital Outpatient Setting

01990 **Physiological support for harvesting of organ(s) from brain-dead patient**

0.00   0.00   **FUD** XXX   C

AMA: 2016,Jan,13; 2015,Jan,16; 2014,Aug,5; 2014,Jan,11; 2012,Jul,12-14; 2012,Jan,15-42; 2011,Oct,3-4; 2011,Jul,16-17; 2011,Jan,11

01991 **Anesthesia for diagnostic or therapeutic nerve blocks and injections (when block or injection is performed by a different physician or other qualified health care professional); other than the prone position**

EXCLUDES   Bier block for pain management (64999)
Moderate Sedation (99151-99157)
Pain management via intra-arterial or IV therapy (96373-96374)
Regional or local anesthesia of arms or legs for surgical procedure

0.00   0.00   **FUD** XXX   N

AMA: 2016,Jan,13; 2015,Jan,16; 2014,Aug,5; 2014,Jan,11; 2012,Jul,12-14; 2012,Jan,15-42; 2011,Oct,3-4; 2011,Jul,16-17; 2011,Jan,11

01992 **prone position**

EXCLUDES   Bier block for pain management (64999)
Moderate sedation (99151-99157)
Pain management via intra-arterial or IV therapy (96373-96374)
Regional or local anesthesia of arms or legs for surgical procedure

0.00   0.00   **FUD** XXX   N

AMA: 2016,Jan,13; 2015,Jan,16; 2014,Aug,5; 2014,Jan,11; 2012,Jul,12-14; 2012,Jan,15-42; 2011,Oct,3-4; 2011,Jul,16-17; 2011,Jan,11

01996 **Daily hospital management of epidural or subarachnoid continuous drug administration**

INCLUDES   Continuous epidural or subarachnoid drug services performed after insertion of an epidural or subarachnoid catheter

0.00   0.00   **FUD** XXX   N

AMA: 2016,Jan,13; 2015,May,10; 2015,Jan,16; 2014,Aug,5; 2014,Jan,11; 2012,Oct,14; 2012,Jul,3-6; 2012,Jul,12-14; 2012,Jan,15-42; 2011,Oct,3-4; 2011,Jul,16-17; 2011,Jan,11

01999 **Unlisted anesthesia procedure(s)**

0.00   0.00   **FUD** XXX   N

AMA: 2016,Jan,13; 2015,May,10; 2015,Jan,16; 2014,Aug,5; 2014,Aug,14; 2014,Jan,11; 2012,Jul,12-14; 2012,Jan,15-42; 2011,Oct,3-4; 2011,Jul,16-17; 2011,Jan,11

10021-10022 Fine Needle Aspiration

EXCLUDES *Percutaneous localization clip placement during breast biopsy (19081-19086)*
Percutaneous needle biopsy of:
Abdominal or retroperitoneal mass (49180)
Bone (20220, 20225)
Bone marrow (38220-38221)
Breast (19081-19086)
Epididymis (54800)
Kidney (50200)
Liver (47000)
Lung or mediastinum (32405)
Lymph node (38505)
Muscle (20206)
Nucleus pulposus, paravertebral tissue, intervertebral disc (62267)
Pancreas (48102)
Pleura (32400)
Prostate (55700, 55706)
Salivary gland (42400)
Spinal cord (62269)
Testis (54500)
Thyroid (60100)
Soft tissue percutaneous fluid drainage by catheter using image guidance (10030)

10021 **Fine needle aspiration; without imaging guidance**
(88172-88173)
2.00   3.49   **FUD** XXX   T P3 80
AMA: 2016,Jan,13; 2015,Jan,16; 2014,Jan,11; 2012,Jan,15-42; 2011,Jan,11

10022 **with imaging guidance**
(76942, 77002, 77012, 77021)
(88172-88173)
1.88   4.00   **FUD** XXX   T P3 80
AMA: 2016,Jan,13; 2015,Jan,16; 2014,Jan,11; 2012,Jan,15-42; 2011,Jan,11

10030-10180 Treatment of Lesions: Skin and Subcutaneous Tissues

EXCLUDES *Excision benign lesion (11400-11471)*

▲ **10030** **Image-guided fluid collection drainage by catheter (eg, abscess, hematoma, seroma, lymphocele, cyst), soft tissue (eg, extremity, abdominal wall, neck), percutaneous**
INCLUDES   Radiologic guidance (75989, 76942, 77002-77003, 77012, 77021)
EXCLUDES   *Percutaneous drainage with imaging guidance of:*
Peritoneal or retroperitoneal collections (49406)
Visceral collections (49405)
Transvaginal or transrectal drainage with imaging guidance of:
Peritoneal or retroperitoneal collections (49407)
Code also every instance of fluid collection drained using a separate catheter (10030)
4.87   22.1   **FUD** 000   T P2 80
AMA: 2016,Jan,13; 2015,Jan,16; 2014,May,9; 2014,May,3; 2013,Nov,9

10035 **Placement of soft tissue localization device(s) (eg, clip, metallic pellet, wire/needle, radioactive seeds), percutaneous, including imaging guidance; first lesion**
INCLUDES   Radiologic guidance (76942, 77002, 77012, 77021)
EXCLUDES   *Sites with a more specific code descriptor, such as the breast*
Use of code more than one time per site, regardless of the number of markers used
Code also each additional target on the same or opposite side (10036)
2.50   15.1   **FUD** 000   T N1 80 50
AMA: 2016,Jun,3

+ **10036** **each additional lesion (List separately in addition to code for primary procedure)**
INCLUDES   Radiologic guidance (76942, 77002, 77012, 77021)
EXCLUDES   *Sites with a more specific code descriptor, such as the breast*
Use of code more than one time per site, regardless of the number of markers used
Code first (10035)
1.26   13.2   **FUD** ZZZ   N N1 80
AMA: 2016,Jun,3

10040 **Acne surgery (eg, marsupialization, opening or removal of multiple milia, comedones, cysts, pustules)**
2.51   2.88   **FUD** 010   01 N1
AMA: 2016,Jan,13; 2015,Jan,16; 2014,Jan,11; 2012,Jan,15-42; 2011,Jan,11

10060 **Incision and drainage of abscess (eg, carbuncle, suppurative hidradenitis, cutaneous or subcutaneous abscess, cyst, furuncle, or paronychia); simple or single**
2.76   3.32   **FUD** 010   T P2
AMA: 2016,Jan,13; 2015,Jan,16; 2014,Jan,11; 2012,Oct,12; 2012,Sep,10; 2012,Jan,15-42; 2011,Jan,11

10061 **complicated or multiple**
5.12   5.85   **FUD** 010   T P3
AMA: 2016,Jan,13; 2015,Jan,16; 2014,Jan,11; 2012,Oct,12; 2012,Sep,10

10080 **Incision and drainage of pilonidal cyst; simple**
2.93   5.08   **FUD** 010   T P2
AMA: 2016,Jan,13; 2015,Jan,16; 2014,Jan,11

10081 **complicated**
EXCLUDES   *Excision of pilonidal cyst (11770-11772)*
4.85   7.61   **FUD** 010   T P3
AMA: 2016,Jan,13; 2015,Jan,16; 2014,Jan,11

10120 **Incision and removal of foreign body, subcutaneous tissues; simple**
2.95   4.30   **FUD** 010   T P3
AMA: 2016,Jan,13; 2015,Jan,16; 2014,Jan,11; 2013,Dec,16; 2013,Apr,10-11; 2012,Oct,12; 2012,Sep,10

10121 **complicated**
EXCLUDES   *Debridement associated with a fracture or dislocation (11010-11012)*
Exploration penetrating wound (20100-20103)
5.31   7.77   **FUD** 010   T A2
AMA: 2016,Jan,13; 2015,Jan,16; 2014,Jan,11; 2013,Dec,16; 2012,Oct,12; 2012,Sep,10

10140 **Incision and drainage of hematoma, seroma or fluid collection**
(76942, 77002, 77012, 77021)
3.38   4.62   **FUD** 010   T P3
AMA: 2016,Jan,13; 2015,Jan,16; 2014,Nov,5; 2014,Jan,11; 2012,Jan,15-42; 2011,Jan,11

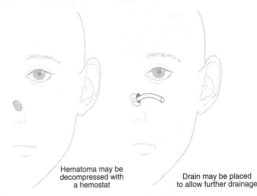

Hematoma may be decompressed with a hemostat

Drain may be placed to allow further drainage

10160 Puncture aspiration of abscess, hematoma, bulla, or cyst
☒ (76942, 77002, 77012, 77021)
🚗 2.74 ⚒ 3.69 **FUD** 010   T P3 ▢
AMA: 2016,Jan,13; 2015,Jan,16; 2014,Jan,11; 2012,Jan,15-42

10180 Incision and drainage, complex, postoperative wound
infection
EXCLUDES *Wound dehiscence (12020-12021, 13160)*
🚗 5.13 ⚒ 7.01 **FUD** 010   T A2 ▢
AMA: 2016,Jan,13; 2015,Jan,16; 2014,Nov,5; 2014,Jan,11;
2012,Jan,15-42; 2011,Jan,11

11000-11012 Removal of Foreign Substances and Infected/Devitalized Tissue

EXCLUDES *Debridement of:*
Burns (16000-16030)
Deeper tissue (11042-11047 [11045, 11046])
Nails (11720-11721)
Skin only (97597-97598)
Wounds (11042-11047 [11045, 11046])
Dermabrasions (15780-15783)
Pressure ulcer excision (15920-15999)

11000 Debridement of extensive eczematous or infected skin; up
to 10% of body surface
EXCLUDES *Necrotizing soft tissue infection of:*
Abdominal wall (11005-11006)
External genitalia and perineum (11004, 11006)
🚗 0.82 ⚒ 1.54 **FUD** 000   T P3 ▢
AMA: 2016,Jan,13; 2015,Jan,16; 2014,Jan,11; 2012,Oct,3-8;
2011,May,3-5

+ **11001** each additional 10% of the body surface, or part thereof
(List separately in addition to code for primary
procedure)
EXCLUDES *Necrotizing soft tissue infection of:*
Abdominal wall (11005-11006)
External genitalia and perineum (11004, 11006)
Code first (11000)
🚗 0.41 ⚒ 0.61 **FUD** ZZZ   N N1 ▢
AMA: 2016,Jan,13; 2015,Jan,16; 2014,Jan,11; 2012,Oct,3-8;
2011,May,3-5

11004 Debridement of skin, subcutaneous tissue, muscle and fascia
for necrotizing soft tissue infection; external genitalia and
perineum
EXCLUDES *Skin grafts or flaps (14000-14350, 15040-15770)*
🚗 16.7 ⚒ 16.7 **FUD** 000   C ▢
AMA: 2016,Jan,13; 2015,Jan,16; 2014,Jan,11; 2013,Oct,15;
2012,Oct,3-8; 2012,Jan,6-10; 2011,May,3-5

11005 abdominal wall, with or without fascial closure
EXCLUDES *Skin grafts or flaps (14000-14350, 15040-15770)*
🚗 22.6 ⚒ 22.6 **FUD** 000   C 80 ▢
AMA: 2016,Jan,13; 2015,Jan,16; 2014,Jan,11; 2013,Oct,15;
2012,Oct,3-8; 2012,Jan,6-10; 2011,May,3-5

11006 external genitalia, perineum and abdominal wall, with or
without fascial closure
EXCLUDES *Orchiectomy (54520)*
Skin grafts or flaps (14000-14350, 15040-15770)
Testicular transplant (54680)
🚗 20.3 ⚒ 20.3 **FUD** 000   C ▢
AMA: 2016,Jan,13; 2015,Jan,16; 2014,Jan,11; 2013,Oct,15;
2012,Oct,3-8; 2012,Jan,6-10; 2011,May,3-5

+ **11008** Removal of prosthetic material or mesh, abdominal wall for
infection (eg, for chronic or recurrent mesh infection or
necrotizing soft tissue infection) (List separately in addition
to code for primary procedure)
EXCLUDES *Debridement (11000-11001, 11010-11044 [11045,*
11046])
Insertion of mesh (49568)
Skin grafts or flaps (14000-14350, 15040-15770)
Code first (10180, 11004-11006)
🚗 7.98 ⚒ 7.98 **FUD** ZZZ   C 80 ▢
AMA: 2016,Jan,13; 2015,Jan,16; 2014,Jan,11; 2012,Oct,3-8;
2012,Jan,6-10; 2011,May,3-5

11010 Debridement including removal of foreign material at the
site of an open fracture and/or an open dislocation (eg,
excisional debridement); skin and subcutaneous tissues
🚗 8.04 ⚒ 13.9 **FUD** 010   T A2 ▢
AMA: 2016,Jan,13; 2015,Jan,16; 2014,Jan,11; 2012,Oct,3-8;
2012,Oct,13; 2012,Jan,15-42; 2011,May,3-5; 2011,Jan,11

11011 skin, subcutaneous tissue, muscle fascia, and muscle
🚗 8.62 ⚒ 15.2 **FUD** 000   T A2 ▢
AMA: 2016,Jan,13; 2015,Jan,16; 2014,Jan,11; 2012,Oct,3-8;
2012,Oct,13; 2011,May,3-5

11012 skin, subcutaneous tissue, muscle fascia, muscle, and
bone
🚗 12.3 ⚒ 20.3 **FUD** 000   T A2 ▢
AMA: 2016,Jan,13; 2015,Jan,16; 2014,Jan,11; 2012,Oct,3-8;
2012,Oct,13; 2012,Jan,15-42; 2011,May,3-5; 2011,Jan,11

11042-11047 [11045, 11046] Removal of Infected/Devitalized Tissue

INCLUDES Debridement reported by the size and depth
Debridement reported for multiple wounds by adding the total surface
area of wounds of the same depth
Injuries, wounds, chronic ulcers, infections
EXCLUDES *Debridement of:*
Burn (16020-16030)
Eczematous or infected skin (11000-11001)
Nails (11720-11721)
Necrotizing soft tissue infection of external genitalia, perineum, or
abdominal wall (11004-11006)
Non-elective debridement/active care management of same wound
(97597-97602)
Dermabrasions (15780-15783)
Excision of pressure ulcers (15920-15999)
Code also each additional single wound of different depths
Code also modifier 59 for additional wound debridement
Code also multiple wound groups of different depths

11042 Debridement, subcutaneous tissue (includes epidermis and
dermis, if performed); first 20 sq cm or less
🚗 1.77 ⚒ 3.30 **FUD** 000   T A2 ▢
AMA: 2016,Aug,9; 2016,Feb,13; 2016,Jan,13; 2015,Jan,16;
2014,Nov,5; 2014,Jan,11; 2013,Oct,15; 2013,Sep,17;
2013,Feb,16-17; 2012,Oct,3-8; 2012,Oct,13; 2012,Mar,3;
2012,Jan,15-42; 2012,Jan,6-10; 2011,Sep,11-12; 2011,May,3-5

+ # **11045** each additional 20 sq cm, or part thereof (List separately
in addition to code for primary procedure)
🚗 0.75 ⚒ 1.16 **FUD** ZZZ   N N1 80 ▢
AMA: 2016,Aug,9; 2016,Jan,13; 2015,Jan,16; 2014,Nov,5;
2014,Jan,11; 2013,Feb,16-17; 2012,Oct,13; 2012,Oct,3-8;
2012,Mar,3; 2012,Jan,6-10; 2011,Sep,11-12; 2011,May,3-5

11043 Debridement, muscle and/or fascia (includes epidermis,
dermis, and subcutaneous tissue, if performed); first 20 sq
cm or less
🚗 4.47 ⚒ 6.49 **FUD** 000   T A2 ▢
AMA: 2016,Aug,9; 2016,Jan,13; 2015,Jan,16; 2014,Nov,5;
2014,Jan,11; 2013,Feb,16-17; 2012,Oct,13; 2012,Oct,3-8;
2012,Mar,3; 2012,Jan,6-10; 2012,Jan,15-42; 2011,Sep,11-12;
2011,May,3-5; 2011,Jan,11

+ # **11046** each additional 20 sq cm, or part thereof (List separately in addition to code for primary procedure)
Code first (11043)
🔁 1.61 ⚕ 2.09 **FUD** ZZZ N M1 80 ▭
AMA: 2016,Aug,9; 2016,Jan,13; 2015,Jan,16; 2014,Nov,5; 2014,Jan,11; 2013,Feb,16-17; 2012,Oct,13; 2012,Oct,3-8; 2012,Mar,3; 2012,Jan,6-10; 2011,Sep,11-12; 2011,May,3-5

11044 Debridement, bone (includes epidermis, dermis, subcutaneous tissue, muscle and/or fascia, if performed); first 20 sq cm or less
🔁 6.66 ⚕ 8.96 **FUD** 000 T A2 ▭
AMA: 2016,Aug,9; 2016,Jan,13; 2015,Jan,16; 2014,Nov,5; 2014,Jan,11; 2013,Feb,16-17; 2012,Oct,3-8; 2012,Oct,13; 2012,Mar,3; 2012,Jan,6-10; 2012,Jan,15-42; 2011,Sep,11-12; 2011,May,3-5; 2011,Jan,11

11045 Resequenced code. See code following 11042.

11046 Resequenced code. See code following 11043.

+ **11047** each additional 20 sq cm, or part thereof (List separately in addition to code for primary procedure)
Code first (11044)
🔁 2.87 ⚕ 3.54 **FUD** ZZZ N M1 80 ▭
AMA: 2016,Aug,9; 2016,Jan,13; 2015,Jan,16; 2014,Nov,5; 2014,Jan,11; 2012,Oct,13; 2012,Oct,3-8; 2012,Mar,3; 2012,Jan,6-10; 2012,Jan,15-42; 2011,Sep,11-12; 2011,May,3-5

11055-11057 Excision Benign Hypertrophic Skin Lesions

CMS: 100-04,32,80.8 CSF Edits: Routine Foot Care
EXCLUDES *Destruction (17000-17004)*

11055 Paring or cutting of benign hyperkeratotic lesion (eg, corn or callus); single lesion
🔁 0.46 ⚕ 1.34 **FUD** 000 Q1 M1 ▭
AMA: 2016,Jan,13; 2015,Jan,16; 2014,Jan,11; 2012,Jan,15-42; 2011,Jan,11

11056 2 to 4 lesions
🔁 0.65 ⚕ 1.64 **FUD** 000 Q1 M1 ▭
AMA: 2016,Jan,13; 2015,Jan,16; 2014,Jan,11; 2012,Jan,15-42; 2011,Jan,11

11057 more than 4 lesions
🔁 0.85 ⚕ 1.85 **FUD** 000 T P3 ▭
AMA: 2016,Jan,13; 2015,Jan,16; 2014,Jan,11

11100-11101 Surgical Biopsy Skin and Mucous Membranes

INCLUDES Attaining tissue for pathologic exam
EXCLUDES *Biopsies performed during related procedures*
Biopsy of:
Conjunctiva (68100)
Eyelid ([67810])

11100 Biopsy of skin, subcutaneous tissue and/or mucous membrane (including simple closure), unless otherwise listed; single lesion
🔁 1.40 ⚕ 2.92 **FUD** 000 T P3 ▭
AMA: 2016,Jan,13; 2015,Jan,16; 2014,Jan,11; 2013,Mar,6-7; 2013,Feb,16-17

+ **11101** each separate/additional lesion (List separately in addition to code for primary procedure)
Code first (11100)
🔁 0.72 ⚕ 0.93 **FUD** ZZZ N M1 ▭
AMA: 2016,Jan,13; 2015,Jan,16; 2014,Jan,11; 2013,Mar,6-7; 2013,Feb,16-17

11200-11201 Skin Tag Removal - All Techniques

INCLUDES Chemical destruction
Electrocauterization
Electrosurgical destruction
Ligature strangulation
Removal with or without local anesthesia
Sharp excision or scissoring
EXCLUDES *Extensive or complicated secondary wound closure (13160)*

11200 Removal of skin tags, multiple fibrocutaneous tags, any area; up to and including 15 lesions
🔁 2.09 ⚕ 2.49 **FUD** 010 Q1 M1
AMA: 2016,Jan,13; 2015,Jan,16; 2014,Jan,11; 2012,Jan,15-42; 2011,Jun,13; 2011,Jan,11

+ **11201** each additional 10 lesions, or part thereof (List separately in addition to code for primary procedure)
Code first (11200)
🔁 0.48 ⚕ 0.54 **FUD** ZZZ N M1 ▭
AMA: 2016,Jan,13; 2015,Jan,16; 2014,Jan,11; 2012,Jan,15-42; 2011,Jun,13

11300-11313 Skin Lesion Removal: Shaving

INCLUDES Local anesthesia
Partial thickness excision by horizontal slicing
Wound cauterization

11300 Shaving of epidermal or dermal lesion, single lesion, trunk, arms or legs; lesion diameter 0.5 cm or less
🔁 1.01 ⚕ 2.74 **FUD** 000 Q1 M1 80 ▭
AMA: 2016,Jan,13; 2015,Jan,16; 2014,Jan,11; 2012,Jan,15-42; 2011,Jan,11

Shave excision of an elevated lesion; technique also used to biopsy

Elliptical excision is often used when tissue removal is larger than 4 mm or when deep pathology is suspected

A punch biopsy cuts a core of tissue as the tool is twisted downward

11301 lesion diameter 0.6 to 1.0 cm
🔁 1.54 ⚕ 3.38 **FUD** 000 Q1 M1 80 ▭
AMA: 2016,Jan,13; 2015,Jan,16; 2014,Jan,11; 2012,Jan,15-42; 2011,Jan,11

11302 lesion diameter 1.1 to 2.0 cm
🔁 1.81 ⚕ 3.98 **FUD** 000 Q1 M1 80 ▭
AMA: 2016,Jan,13; 2015,Jan,16; 2014,Jan,11; 2012,Jan,15-42; 2011,Jan,11

11303 lesion diameter over 2.0 cm
🔁 2.14 ⚕ 4.40 **FUD** 000 Q1 M1 80 ▭
AMA: 2016,Jan,13; 2015,Jan,16; 2014,Jan,11; 2012,Jan,15-42; 2011,Jan,11

11305 Shaving of epidermal or dermal lesion, single lesion, scalp, neck, hands, feet, genitalia; lesion diameter 0.5 cm or less
🔁 1.13 ⚕ 2.80 **FUD** 000 Q1 M1 80 ▭
AMA: 2016,Jan,13; 2015,Jan,16; 2014,Jan,11; 2012,Jan,15-42; 2011,Jan,11

11306 lesion diameter 0.6 to 1.0 cm
🔁 1.49 ⚕ 3.44 **FUD** 000 Q1 M1 80 ▭
AMA: 2016,Jan,13; 2015,Jan,16; 2014,Jan,11; 2012,Jan,15-42; 2011,Jan,11

11307 lesion diameter 1.1 to 2.0 cm
🔁 1.92 ⚕ 4.06 **FUD** 000 T P3 80 ▭
AMA: 2016,Jan,13; 2015,Jan,16; 2014,Jan,11; 2012,Jan,15-42; 2011,Jan,11

11308 lesion diameter over 2.0 cm
🔁 2.12 ⚕ 4.26 **FUD** 000 Q1 M1 80 ▭
AMA: 2016,Jan,13; 2015,Jan,16; 2014,Jan,11; 2012,Jan,15-42; 2011,Jan,11

11310 Shaving of epidermal or dermal lesion, single lesion, face, ears, eyelids, nose, lips, mucous membrane; lesion diameter 0.5 cm or less
🔁 1.36 ⚕ 3.20 **FUD** 000 T P3 80 ▭
AMA: 2016,Jan,13; 2015,Jan,16; 2014,Jan,11; 2013,Mar,6-7; 2013,Feb,16-17; 2012,Jan,15-42; 2011,Jan,11

11311   **lesion diameter 0.6 to 1.0 cm**
🚗 1.89   ⚕ 3.15   **FUD** 000   T P3 80 ▭
AMA: 2016,Jan,13; 2015,Jan,16; 2014,Jan,11; 2013,Mar,6-7; 2013,Feb,16-17; 2012,Jan,15-42; 2011,Jan,11

11312   **lesion diameter 1.1 to 2.0 cm**
🚗 2.25   ⚕ 4.53   **FUD** 000   T P3 80 ▭
AMA: 2016,Jan,13; 2015,Jan,16; 2014,Jan,11; 2013,Mar,6-7; 2013,Feb,16-17; 2012,Jan,15-42; 2011,Jan,11

11313   **lesion diameter over 2.0 cm**
🚗 2.89   ⚕ 5.25   **FUD** 000   T P3 80 ▭
AMA: 2016,Jan,13; 2015,Jan,16; 2014,Jan,11; 2013,Mar,6-7; 2013,Feb,16-17; 2012,Jan,15-42; 2011,Jan,11

11400-11446 Skin Lesion Removal: Benign

INCLUDES   Biopsy on same lesion
Full thickness removal including margins
Lesion measurement before excision at largest diameter plus margin
Local anesthesia
Simple, nonlayered closure
EXCLUDES   Adjacent tissue transfer. Report only adjacent tissue transfer (14000-14302)
Biopsy of eyelid ([67810])
Destruction of eyelid lesion (67850)
Excision and reconstruction of eyelid (67961-67975)
Excision of chalazion (67800-67808)
Eyelid procedures involving more than skin (67800 and subsequent codes)
Shave removal (11300-11313)
Code also complex closure (13100-13153)
Code also each separate lesion
Code also intermediate closure (12031-12057)
Code also modifier 22 if excision is complicated or unusual
Code also reconstruction (15002-15261, 15570-15770)

11400   **Excision, benign lesion including margins, except skin tag (unless listed elsewhere), trunk, arms or legs; excised diameter 0.5 cm or less**
🚗 2.29   ⚕ 3.50   **FUD** 010   T P3 ▭
AMA: 2016,Apr,3; 2016,Jan,13; 2015,Jan,16; 2014,Mar,4; 2014,Mar,12; 2014,Jan,11; 2012,May,13; 2012,Jan,15-42; 2011,Jan,9-10; 2011,Jan,11

11401   **excised diameter 0.6 to 1.0 cm**
🚗 2.96   ⚕ 4.21   **FUD** 010   T P3 ▭
AMA: 2016,Apr,3; 2016,Jan,13; 2015,Jan,16; 2014,Mar,4; 2014,Mar,12; 2014,Jan,11; 2012,May,13; 2012,Jan,15-42; 2011,Jan,9-10; 2011,Jan,11

11402   **excised diameter 1.1 to 2.0 cm**
🚗 3.26   ⚕ 4.68   **FUD** 010   T P3 ▭
AMA: 2016,Apr,3; 2016,Jan,13; 2015,Jan,16; 2014,Mar,4; 2014,Mar,12; 2014,Jan,11; 2012,May,13; 2012,Jan,15-42; 2011,Jan,11; 2011,Jan,9-10

11403   **excised diameter 2.1 to 3.0 cm**
🚗 4.22   ⚕ 5.43   **FUD** 010   T P3 ▭
AMA: 2016,Apr,3; 2016,Jan,13; 2015,Jan,16; 2014,Mar,4; 2014,Mar,12; 2014,Jan,11; 2012,May,13; 2011,Jan,9-10; 2011,Jan,11

11404   **excised diameter 3.1 to 4.0 cm**
🚗 4.65   ⚕ 6.17   **FUD** 010   T A2 ▭
AMA: 2016,Apr,3; 2016,Jan,13; 2015,Jan,16; 2014,Mar,4; 2014,Mar,12; 2014,Jan,11; 2012,May,13; 2012,Jan,15-42; 2011,Jan,11; 2011,Jan,9-10

11406   **excised diameter over 4.0 cm**
🚗 7.08   ⚕ 8.90   **FUD** 010   T A2 ▭
AMA: 2016,Apr,3; 2016,Jan,13; 2015,Jan,16; 2014,Mar,4; 2014,Mar,12; 2014,Jan,11; 2012,May,13; 2012,Jan,15-42; 2011,Jan,9-10; 2011,Jan,11

11420   **Excision, benign lesion including margins, except skin tag (unless listed elsewhere), scalp, neck, hands, feet, genitalia; excised diameter 0.5 cm or less**
🚗 2.33   ⚕ 3.46   **FUD** 010   T P3 ▭
AMA: 2016,Apr,3; 2016,Jan,13; 2015,Jan,16; 2014,Mar,4; 2014,Mar,12; 2014,Jan,11; 2013,Jan,15-16; 2012,May,13; 2012,Jan,15-42; 2011,Jan,11

11421   **excised diameter 0.6 to 1.0 cm**
🚗 3.14   ⚕ 4.43   **FUD** 010   T P3 ▭
AMA: 2016,Apr,3; 2016,Jan,13; 2015,Jan,16; 2014,Mar,4; 2014,Mar,12; 2014,Jan,11; 2013,Jan,15-16; 2012,May,13; 2011,Jan,11

11422   **excised diameter 1.1 to 2.0 cm**
🚗 3.87   ⚕ 4.96   **FUD** 010   T P3 ▭
AMA: 2016,Apr,3; 2016,Jan,13; 2015,Jan,16; 2014,Mar,4; 2014,Mar,12; 2014,Jan,11; 2013,Jan,15-16; 2012,May,13; 2012,Mar,4-7; 2011,Jan,11

11423   **excised diameter 2.1 to 3.0 cm**
🚗 4.50   ⚕ 5.72   **FUD** 010   T P3 ▭
AMA: 2016,Apr,3; 2016,Jan,13; 2015,Jan,16; 2014,Mar,4; 2014,Mar,12; 2014,Jan,11; 2013,Jan,15-16; 2012,May,13; 2011,Jan,11

11424   **excised diameter 3.1 to 4.0 cm**
🚗 5.15   ⚕ 6.62   **FUD** 010   T A2 ▭
AMA: 2016,Apr,3; 2016,Jan,13; 2015,Jan,16; 2014,Mar,4; 2014,Mar,12; 2014,Jan,11; 2013,Jan,15-16; 2012,May,13; 2011,Jan,11

11426   **excised diameter over 4.0 cm**
🚗 7.89   ⚕ 9.47   **FUD** 010   T A2 ▭
AMA: 2016,Apr,3; 2016,Jan,13; 2015,Jan,16; 2014,Mar,4; 2014,Mar,12; 2014,Jan,11; 2013,Jan,15-16; 2012,May,13; 2011,Jan,11

11440   **Excision, other benign lesion including margins, except skin tag (unless listed elsewhere), face, ears, eyelids, nose, lips, mucous membrane; excised diameter 0.5 cm or less**
🚗 2.94   ⚕ 3.81   **FUD** 010   T P3 ▭
AMA: 2016,Apr,3; 2016,Jan,13; 2015,Jan,16; 2014,Mar,4; 2014,Mar,12; 2014,Jan,11; 2012,May,13; 2012,Jan,15-42; 2011,Jan,11

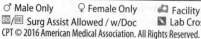

The physician removes a benign lesion from the external ear, nose, or mucous membranes

3.1 to 4.0 cm (11444)
Up to 0.5 cm (11440)
0.6 to 1.0 cm (11441)
Larger than 4.0 cm (11446)
1.1 to 2.0 cm (11442)
2.1 to 3.0 cm (11443)

11441   **excised diameter 0.6 to 1.0 cm**
🚗 3.76   ⚕ 4.75   **FUD** 010   T P3 ▭
AMA: 2016,Apr,3; 2016,Jan,13; 2015,Jan,16; 2014,Mar,4; 2014,Mar,12; 2014,Jan,11; 2012,May,13; 2012,Jan,15-42; 2011,Jan,11

11442   **excised diameter 1.1 to 2.0 cm**
🚗 4.16   ⚕ 5.32   **FUD** 010   T P3 ▭
AMA: 2016,Apr,3; 2016,Jan,13; 2015,Jan,16; 2014,Mar,4; 2014,Mar,12; 2014,Jan,11; 2012,May,13; 2012,Jan,15-42; 2011,Jan,11

11443   **excised diameter 2.1 to 3.0 cm**
🚗 5.11   ⚕ 6.35   **FUD** 010   T P3 ▭
AMA: 2016,Apr,3; 2016,Jan,13; 2015,Jan,16; 2014,Mar,4; 2014,Mar,12; 2014,Jan,11; 2012,May,13; 2011,Jan,11

11444   **excised diameter 3.1 to 4.0 cm**
🚗 6.51   ⚕ 7.98   **FUD** 010   T A2 ▭
AMA: 2016,Apr,3; 2016,Jan,13; 2015,Jan,16; 2014,Mar,4; 2014,Mar,12; 2014,Jan,11; 2012,May,13; 2011,Jan,11

11446   excised diameter over 4.0 cm
9.34   11.0   **FUD** 010   T A2

AMA: 2016,Apr,3; 2016,Jan,13; 2015,Jan,16; 2014,Mar,4; 2014,Mar,12; 2014,Jan,11; 2012,May,13; 2012,Jan,15-42; 2011,Jan,11

11450-11471 Treatment of Hidradenitis: Excision and Repair

Code also closure by skin graft or flap (14000-14350, 15040-15770)

11450   Excision of skin and subcutaneous tissue for hidradenitis, axillary; with simple or intermediate repair
7.23   10.8   **FUD** 090   T A2 50

AMA: 2016,Aug,9; 2016,Jan,13; 2015,Jan,16; 2014,Jan,11; 2012,May,13

Hidradenitis is a disease process stemming from clogged specialized sweat glands, principally of the axilla and groin areas

Hair shaft

Hair matrix

Sweat (eccrine gland)

Hidradenitis of the axilla

11451   with complex repair
9.32   13.7   **FUD** 090   T A2 80 50

AMA: 2016,Aug,9; 2016,Jan,13; 2015,Jan,16; 2014,Jan,11; 2012,May,13

11462   Excision of skin and subcutaneous tissue for hidradenitis, inguinal; with simple or intermediate repair
6.90   10.5   **FUD** 090   T A2 80 50

AMA: 2016,Aug,9; 2016,Jan,13; 2015,Jan,16; 2014,Jan,11; 2012,May,13

11463   with complex repair
9.35   13.9   **FUD** 090   T A2 80 50

AMA: 2016,Aug,9; 2016,Jan,13; 2015,Jan,16; 2014,Jan,11; 2012,May,13

11470   Excision of skin and subcutaneous tissue for hidradenitis, perianal, perineal, or umbilical; with simple or intermediate repair
8.07   11.7   **FUD** 090   T A2

AMA: 2016,Aug,9; 2016,Jan,13; 2015,Jan,16; 2014,Jan,11; 2012,May,13

11471   with complex repair
10.0   14.4   **FUD** 090   T A2 80

AMA: 2016,Aug,9; 2016,Jan,13; 2015,Jan,16; 2014,Jan,11; 2012,May,13

11600-11646 Skin Lesion Removal: Malignant

INCLUDES   Biopsy on same lesion
Excision of additional margin at same operative session
Full thickness removal including margins
Lesion measurement before excision at largest diameter plus margin
Local anesthesia
Simple, nonlayered closure

EXCLUDES   Adjacent tissue transfer. Report only adjacent tissue transfer (14000-14302)
Destruction (17260-17286)
Excision of additional margin at subsequent operative session (11600-11646)

Code also complex closure (13100-13153)
Code also each separate lesion
Code also intermediate closure (12031-12057)
Code also modifier 58 if re-excision is performed during postoperative period
Code also reconstruction (15002-15261, 15570-15770)

11600   Excision, malignant lesion including margins, trunk, arms, or legs; excised diameter 0.5 cm or less
3.41   5.44   **FUD** 010   T P3

AMA: 2016,Jan,13; 2015,Jan,16; 2014,Mar,4; 2014,Mar,12; 2014,Jan,11; 2012,Jul,12-14; 2012,May,13; 2012,Jan,15-42; 2011,Jan,11

11601   excised diameter 0.6 to 1.0 cm
4.27   6.47   **FUD** 010   T P3

AMA: 2016,Jan,13; 2015,Jan,16; 2014,Mar,4; 2014,Mar,12; 2014,Jan,11; 2012,Jul,12-14; 2012,May,13; 2012,Mar,4-7

11602   excised diameter 1.1 to 2.0 cm
4.69   7.02   **FUD** 010   T P3

AMA: 2016,Jan,13; 2015,Jan,16; 2014,Mar,4; 2014,Mar,12; 2014,Jan,11; 2012,May,13; 2012,Jul,12-14

11603   excised diameter 2.1 to 3.0 cm
5.62   8.03   **FUD** 010   T P3

AMA: 2016,Jan,13; 2015,Jan,16; 2014,Mar,4; 2014,Mar,12; 2014,Jan,11; 2012,May,13; 2012,Jul,12-14

11604   excised diameter 3.1 to 4.0 cm
6.19   8.93   **FUD** 010   T A2

AMA: 2016,Jan,13; 2015,Jan,16; 2014,Mar,4; 2014,Mar,12; 2014,Jan,11; 2012,May,13; 2012,Jul,12-14

11606   excised diameter over 4.0 cm
9.22   12.8   **FUD** 010   T A2

AMA: 2016,Jan,13; 2015,Jan,16; 2014,Mar,4; 2014,Mar,12; 2014,Jan,11; 2012,May,13; 2012,Jul,12-14

11620   Excision, malignant lesion including margins, scalp, neck, hands, feet, genitalia; excised diameter 0.5 cm or less
3.46   5.50   **FUD** 010   T P3

AMA: 2016,Jan,13; 2015,Jan,16; 2014,Mar,4; 2014,Mar,12; 2014,Jan,11; 2012,May,13; 2012,Jul,12-14

11621   excised diameter 0.6 to 1.0 cm
4.31   6.51   **FUD** 010   T P3

AMA: 2016,Jan,13; 2015,Jan,16; 2014,Mar,12; 2014,Mar,4; 2014,Jan,11; 2012,May,13

11622   excised diameter 1.1 to 2.0 cm
4.93   7.26   **FUD** 010   T P3

AMA: 2016,Jan,13; 2015,Jan,16; 2014,Mar,12; 2014,Mar,4; 2014,Jan,11; 2012,May,13

11623   excised diameter 2.1 to 3.0 cm
6.11   8.53   **FUD** 010   T P3

AMA: 2016,Jan,13; 2015,Jan,16; 2014,Mar,12; 2014,Mar,4; 2014,Jan,11; 2012,May,13

11624   excised diameter 3.1 to 4.0 cm
6.92   9.62   **FUD** 010   T A2

AMA: 2016,Jan,13; 2015,Jan,16; 2014,Mar,12; 2014,Mar,4; 2014,Jan,11; 2012,May,13

11626   excised diameter over 4.0 cm
8.49   11.6   **FUD** 010   T A2

AMA: 2016,Jan,13; 2015,Jan,16; 2014,Mar,12; 2014,Mar,4; 2014,Jan,11; 2012,May,13

11640   Excision, malignant lesion including margins, face, ears, eyelids, nose, lips; excised diameter 0.5 cm or less

EXCLUDES   Eyelid excision involving more than skin (67800-67808, 67840-67850, 67961-67966)
3.58   5.67   **FUD** 010   T P3

AMA: 2016,Jan,13; 2015,Jan,16; 2014,Mar,12; 2014,Mar,4; 2014,Jan,11; 2012,May,13

11641   excised diameter 0.6 to 1.0 cm

EXCLUDES   Eyelid excision involving more than skin (67800-67808, 67840-67850, 67961-67966)
4.49   6.74   **FUD** 010   T P3

AMA: 2016,Jan,13; 2015,Jan,16; 2014,Mar,12; 2014,Mar,4; 2014,Jan,11; 2012,May,13

11642   excised diameter 1.1 to 2.0 cm

EXCLUDES   Eyelid excision involving more than skin (67800-67808, 67840-67850, 67961-67966)
5.30   7.70   **FUD** 010   T P3

AMA: 2016,Jan,13; 2015,Jan,16; 2014,Mar,12; 2014,Mar,4; 2014,Jan,11; 2012,May,13

11643 **excised diameter 2.1 to 3.0 cm**
> EXCLUDES *Eyelid excision involving more than skin (67800-67808, 67840-67850, 67961-67966)*

🔧 6.63   ⚕ 9.08   **FUD** 010   T P3 ▢

AMA: 2016,Jan,13; 2015,Jan,16; 2014,Mar,12; 2014,Mar,4; 2014,Jan,11; 2012,May,13

11644 **excised diameter 3.1 to 4.0 cm**
> EXCLUDES *Eyelid excision involving more than skin (67800-67808, 67840-67850, 67961-67966)*

🔧 8.21   ⚕ 11.2   **FUD** 010   T A2 ▢

AMA: 2016,Jan,13; 2015,Jan,16; 2014,Mar,12; 2014,Mar,4; 2014,Jan,11; 2012,May,13

11646 **excised diameter over 4.0 cm**
> EXCLUDES *Eyelid excision involving more than skin (67800-67808, 67840-67850, 67961-67966)*

🔧 11.4   ⚕ 14.6   **FUD** 010   T A2 ▢

AMA: 2016,Jan,13; 2015,Jan,16; 2014,Mar,4; 2014,Mar,12; 2014,Jan,11; 2012,May,13; 2012,Jan,15-42; 2011,Jan,11

11719-11765 Nails and Supporting Structures

CMS: 100-02,15,290 Foot Care
> EXCLUDES *Drainage of paronychia or onychia (10060-10061)*

11719 **Trimming of nondystrophic nails, any number**

🔧 0.22   ⚕ 0.39   **FUD** 000   Q1 N1 ▢

AMA: 2016,Jan,13; 2015,Jan,16; 2014,Jan,11

11720 **Debridement of nail(s) by any method(s); 1 to 5**

🔧 0.42   ⚕ 0.91   **FUD** 000   Q1 N1 ▢

AMA: 2016,Jan,13; 2015,Jan,16; 2014,Jan,11

11721 **6 or more**

🔧 0.71   ⚕ 1.27   **FUD** 000   Q1 N1 ▢

AMA: 2016,Jan,13; 2015,Jan,16; 2014,Jan,11

11730 **Avulsion of nail plate, partial or complete, simple; single**

🔧 1.46   ⚕ 2.80   **FUD** 000   Q1 N1 ▢

AMA: 2016,Jan,13; 2015,Jan,16; 2014,Jan,11; 2012,Jan,15-42; 2011,Jan,11

+ 11732 **each additional nail plate (List separately in addition to code for primary procedure)**
Code first (11730)

🔧 0.58   ⚕ 1.01   **FUD** ZZZ   N N1 ▢

AMA: 2016,Jan,13; 2015,Jan,16; 2014,Jan,11

11740 **Evacuation of subungual hematoma**

🔧 0.93   ⚕ 1.40   **FUD** 000   Q1 N1 ▢

AMA: 2016,Jan,13; 2015,Jan,16; 2014,Jan,11

11750 **Excision of nail and nail matrix, partial or complete (eg, ingrown or deformed nail), for permanent removal;**
> EXCLUDES *Skin graft (15050)*

🔧 4.01   ⚕ 5.11   **FUD** 010   T P3 ▢

AMA: 2016,Jan,13; 2015,Jan,16; 2014,Jan,11

~~11752~~ **~~with amputation of tuft of distal phalanx~~**
To report, see ~15050, 26236, 28124, 28160

11755 **Biopsy of nail unit (eg, plate, bed, matrix, hyponychium, proximal and lateral nail folds) (separate procedure)**

🔧 2.23   ⚕ 3.78   **FUD** 000   T P3 80 ▢

AMA: 2016,Jan,13; 2015,Jan,16; 2014,Jan,11; 2012,Jan,15-42; 2011,Jan,11

11760 **Repair of nail bed**

🔧 3.34   ⚕ 5.50   **FUD** 010   T 62 ▢

AMA: 2016,Jan,13; 2015,Jan,16; 2014,Jan,11

11762 **Reconstruction of nail bed with graft**

🔧 5.26   ⚕ 7.94   **FUD** 010   T P3 ▢

AMA: 2016,Jan,13; 2015,Jan,16; 2014,Jan,11

11765 **Wedge excision of skin of nail fold (eg, for ingrown toenail)**
> INCLUDES *Cotting's operation*

🔧 2.68   ⚕ 4.73   **FUD** 010   Q1 N1 ▢

AMA: 2016,Jan,13; 2015,Jan,16; 2014,Jan,11

11770-11772 Treatment Pilonidal Cyst: Excision
> EXCLUDES *Incision of pilonidal cyst (10080-10081)*

11770 **Excision of pilonidal cyst or sinus; simple**

🔧 5.32   ⚕ 7.89   **FUD** 010   T A2 ▢

11771 **extensive**

🔧 12.4   ⚕ 16.3   **FUD** 090   T A2 ▢

11772 **complicated**

🔧 16.5   ⚕ 19.7   **FUD** 090   T A2 ▢

AMA: 2016,Jan,13; 2015,Sep,12

11900-11901 Treatment of Lesions: Injection
> EXCLUDES *Injection of local anesthesia performed preoperatively*
> *Injection of veins (36470-36471)*
> *Intralesional chemotherapy (96405-96406)*

11900 **Injection, intralesional; up to and including 7 lesions**

🔧 0.90   ⚕ 1.57   **FUD** 000   Q1 N1 ▢

AMA: 2016,Jan,13; 2015,Jan,16; 2014,Jan,11; 2013,Nov,14; 2012,Jan,15-42; 2011,Jan,11

11901 **more than 7 lesions**

🔧 1.39   ⚕ 1.98   **FUD** 000   Q1 N1 ▢

AMA: 2016,Jan,13; 2015,Jan,16; 2014,Jan,11; 2012,Jan,15-42; 2011,Jan,11

11920-11971 Tattoos, Tissue Expanders, and Dermal Fillers

CMS: 100-02,16,10 Exclusions from Coverage; 100-02,16,120 Cosmetic Procedures; 100-02,16,180 Services Related to Noncovered Procedures

11920 **Tattooing, intradermal introduction of insoluble opaque pigments to correct color defects of skin, including micropigmentation; 6.0 sq cm or less**

🔧 3.26   ⚕ 4.81   **FUD** 000   T P3 80 ▢

AMA: 2016,Aug,9

11921 **6.1 to 20.0 sq cm**

🔧 3.86   ⚕ 5.61   **FUD** 000   T P3 80 ▢

AMA: 2016,Aug,9

+ 11922 **each additional 20.0 sq cm, or part thereof (List separately in addition to code for primary procedure)**

🔧 0.85   ⚕ 1.74   **FUD** ZZZ   N N1 80 ▢

Code first (11921)

11950 **Subcutaneous injection of filling material (eg, collagen); 1 cc or less**

🔧 1.46   ⚕ 2.08   **FUD** 000   T P3 80 ▢

AMA: 2016,Jan,13; 2015,Jan,16; 2014,Jan,11; 2012,Jun,15-16

11951 **1.1 to 5.0 cc**

🔧 2.06   ⚕ 2.76   **FUD** 000   T P3 80 ▢

AMA: 2016,Jan,13; 2015,Jan,16; 2014,Jan,11; 2012,Jun,15-16

11952 **5.1 to 10.0 cc**

🔧 2.78   ⚕ 3.71   **FUD** 000   T P3 80 ▢

AMA: 2016,Jan,13; 2015,Jan,16; 2014,Jan,11; 2012,Jun,15-16

11954 **over 10.0 cc**

🔧 3.29   ⚕ 4.47   **FUD** 000   T P3 80 ▢

AMA: 2016,Jan,13; 2015,Jan,16; 2014,Jan,11; 2012,Jun,15-16

11960 **Insertion of tissue expander(s) for other than breast, including subsequent expansion**
> EXCLUDES *Breast reconstruction with tissue expander(s) (19357)*

🔧 27.0   ⚕ 27.0   **FUD** 090   T A2 ▢

AMA: 1991,Win,1

11970 **Replacement of tissue expander with permanent prosthesis**

🔧 17.4   ⚕ 17.4   **FUD** 090   J A2 50 ▢

AMA: 2016,Jan,13; 2015,Jan,16; 2014,Jan,11; 2013,Jan,15-16

11971 **Removal of tissue expander(s) without insertion of prosthesis**

🔧 9.11   ⚕ 13.3   **FUD** 090   Q2 A2 80 50 ▢

AMA: 2016,Jan,13; 2015,Jan,16; 2014,Jan,11; 2012,Jan,15-42; 2011,Jan,11

11976-11983 Drug Implantation

11976 Removal, implantable contraceptive capsules ♀
 ⊞ 2.69 ✂ 4.04 **FUD** 000 Q2 P3 80
 AMA: 1992,Win,1; 1991,Win,1

11980 Subcutaneous hormone pellet implantation (implantation of estradiol and/or testosterone pellets beneath the skin)
 ⊞ 1.61 ✂ 2.66 **FUD** 000 Q1 N1
 AMA: 2016,Jan,13; 2015,Jan,16; 2014,Jan,11

11981 Insertion, non-biodegradable drug delivery implant
 ⊞ 2.37 ✂ 3.98 **FUD** XXX Q1 N1 80
 AMA: 2016,Jan,13; 2015,Jan,16; 2014,Jan,11; 2012,Jan,15-42; 2011,Apr,12; 2011,Jan,11

11982 Removal, non-biodegradable drug delivery implant
 ⊞ 2.88 ✂ 4.52 **FUD** XXX Q1 N1 80
 AMA: 2016,Jan,13; 2015,Jan,16; 2014,Jan,11

11983 Removal with reinsertion, non-biodegradable drug delivery implant
 ⊞ 4.99 ✂ 6.31 **FUD** XXX Q1 N1 80

12001-12021 Suturing of Superficial Wounds

INCLUDES Administration of local anesthesia
Cauterization without closure
Simple:
 Exploration nerves, blood vessels, tendons
 Vessel ligation, in wound
Simple repair that involves:
 Routine debridement and decontamination
 Simple one layer closure
 Superficial tissues
 Sutures, staples, tissue adhesives
 Total length of several repairs in same code category

EXCLUDES *Adhesive strips only, see appropriate E&M service*
Complex repair nerves, blood vessels, tendons (see appropriate anatomical section)
Debridement:
 Performed separately, no closure (11042-11047 [11045, 11046])
 That requires:
  Comprehensive cleaning
  Removal of significant tissue
  Removal soft tissue and/or bone, no fracture/dislocation (11042-11047 [11045, 11046])
  Removal soft tissue and/or bone with open fracture/dislocation (11010-11012)
Deep tissue repair (12031-13153)
Major exploration (20100-20103)
Repair of nerves, blood vessels, tendons (See appropriate anatomical section. These repairs include simple and intermediate closure. Report complex closure with modifier 59.)
Secondary closure/dehiscence (13160)
Code also modifier 59 added to the less complicated procedure code if reporting more than one classification of wound repair

12001 Simple repair of superficial wounds of scalp, neck, axillae, external genitalia, trunk and/or extremities (including hands and feet); 2.5 cm or less
 ⊞ 1.27 ✂ 2.52 **FUD** 000 Q1 N1
 AMA: 2016,Jan,13; 2015,Jan,16; 2014,Jan,11; 2012,Mar,4-7; 2012,Jan,15-42; 2011,Jan,11

12002 2.6 cm to 7.5 cm
 ⊞ 1.67 ✂ 3.07 **FUD** 000 Q1 N1
 AMA: 2016,Jan,13; 2015,Jan,16; 2014,Oct,14; 2014,Jan,11; 2012,Jan,15-42; 2011,Jan,11

12004 7.6 cm to 12.5 cm
 ⊞ 2.09 ✂ 3.62 **FUD** 000 Q1 N1
 AMA: 2016,Jan,13; 2015,Jan,16; 2014,Jan,11; 2012,Jan,15-42; 2011,Jan,11

12005 12.6 cm to 20.0 cm
 ⊞ 2.72 ✂ 4.57 **FUD** 000 Q1 A2
 AMA: 2016,Jan,13; 2015,Jan,16; 2014,Jan,11; 2012,Jan,15-42; 2011,Jan,11

12006 20.1 cm to 30.0 cm
 ⊞ 3.34 ✂ 5.42 **FUD** 000 Q2 A2
 AMA: 2016,Jan,13; 2015,Jan,16; 2014,Jan,11; 2012,Jan,15-42; 2011,Jan,11

12007 over 30.0 cm
 ⊞ 4.22 ✂ 6.33 **FUD** 000 T A2
 AMA: 2016,Jan,13; 2015,Jan,16; 2014,Jan,11; 2012,Jan,15-42; 2011,Jan,11

12011 Simple repair of superficial wounds of face, ears, eyelids, nose, lips and/or mucous membranes; 2.5 cm or less
 ⊞ 1.58 ✂ 3.09 **FUD** 000 Q1 N1
 AMA: 2016,Jan,13; 2015,Jan,16; 2014,Jan,11; 2012,Jan,15-42; 2011,Jan,11

12013 2.6 cm to 5.0 cm
 ⊞ 1.66 ✂ 3.23 **FUD** 000 Q1 N1
 AMA: 2016,Jan,13; 2015,Jan,16; 2014,Jan,11; 2012,Jan,15-42; 2011,Jan,11

12014 5.1 cm to 7.5 cm
 ⊞ 2.14 ✂ 3.78 **FUD** 000 Q1 N1
 AMA: 2016,Jan,13; 2015,Jan,16; 2014,Jan,11; 2012,Jan,15-42; 2011,Jan,11

12015 7.6 cm to 12.5 cm
 ⊞ 2.69 ✂ 4.58 **FUD** 000 Q1 G2
 AMA: 2016,Jan,13; 2015,Jan,16; 2014,Jan,11; 2012,Jan,15-42; 2011,Jan,11

12016 12.6 cm to 20.0 cm
 ⊞ 3.68 ✂ 5.82 **FUD** 000 Q1 A2
 AMA: 2016,Jan,13; 2015,Jan,16; 2014,Jan,11; 2012,Jan,15-42; 2011,Jan,11

12017 20.1 cm to 30.0 cm
 ⊞ 4.41 ✂ 4.41 **FUD** 000 Q1 A2 80
 AMA: 2016,Jan,13; 2015,Jan,16; 2014,Jan,11; 2012,Jan,15-42; 2011,Jan,11

12018 over 30.0 cm
 ⊞ 5.00 ✂ 5.00 **FUD** 000 Q1 A2 80
 AMA: 2016,Jan,13; 2015,Jan,16; 2014,Jan,11; 2012,Jan,15-42; 2011,Jan,11

12020 Treatment of superficial wound dehiscence; simple closure
 EXCLUDES *Secondary closure major/complex wound or dehiscence (13160)*
 ⊞ 5.59 ✂ 8.23 **FUD** 010 T A2
 AMA: 2016,Jan,13; 2015,Jan,16; 2014,Jan,11; 2012,Jan,15-42; 2011,Jan,11

12021 with packing
 EXCLUDES *Secondary closure major/complex wound or dehiscence (13160)*
 ⊞ 4.05 ✂ 4.75 **FUD** 010 T A2
 AMA: 2016,Jan,13; 2015,Jan,16; 2014,Jan,11; 2012,Jan,15-42; 2011,Jan,11

12031-12057 Suturing of Intermediate Wounds

INCLUDES Administration of local anesthesia
Intermediate repair that involves:
 Closure of contaminated single layer wound
 Layer closure (e.g., subcutaneous tissue, superficial fascia)
 Removal foreign material (e.g. gravel, glass)
 Routine debridement and decontamination
Simple:
 Exploration nerves, blood vessels, tendons in wound
 Vessel ligation, in wound
Total length of several repairs in same code category

EXCLUDES *Debridement:*
 Performed separately, no closure (11042-11047 [11045, 11046])
 That requires:
  Removal soft tissue and/or bone, no fracture/dislocation (11042-11047 [11045, 11046])
  Removal soft tissue/bone due to open fracture/dislocation (11010-11012)
Major exploration (20100-20103)
Repair of nerves, blood vessels, tendons (See appropriate anatomical section. These repairs include simple and intermediate closure. Report complex closure with modifier 59.)
Secondary closure major/complex wound or dehiscence (13160)
Wound repair involving more than layer closure
Code also modifier 59 added to the less complicated procedure code if reporting more than one classification of wound repair

12031 Repair, intermediate, wounds of scalp, axillae, trunk and/or extremities (excluding hands and feet); 2.5 cm or less
 ⊞ 4.39 ✂ 6.70 **FUD** 010 T P2
 AMA: 2016,Jan,13; 2015,Jan,16; 2014,Jan,11; 2012,Jan,15-42; 2011,Jan,11

12032 | **2.6 cm to 7.5 cm**
🚑 5.60   ⚕ 8.58   **FUD** 010   T P2 ▢
AMA: 2016,Jan,13; 2015,Jan,16; 2014,Jan,11; 2012,Jan,15-42; 2011,Jan,11

12034 | **7.6 cm to 12.5 cm**
🚑 5.94   ⚕ 8.82   **FUD** 010   T A2 ▢
AMA: 2016,Jan,13; 2015,Jan,16; 2014,Jan,11; 2012,Jan,15-42; 2011,Jan,11

12035 | **12.6 cm to 20.0 cm**
🚑 6.91   ⚕ 10.8   **FUD** 010   T A2 ▢
AMA: 2016,Jan,13; 2015,Jan,16; 2014,Jan,11; 2012,Jan,15-42; 2011,Jan,11

12036 | **20.1 cm to 30.0 cm**
🚑 8.03   ⚕ 11.9   **FUD** 010   T A2 ▢
AMA: 2016,Jan,13; 2015,Jan,16; 2014,Jan,11; 2012,Jan,15-42; 2011,Jan,11

12037 | **over 30.0 cm**
🚑 9.40   ⚕ 13.5   **FUD** 010   T A2 80 ▢
AMA: 2016,Jan,13; 2015,Jan,16; 2014,Jan,11; 2012,Jan,15-42; 2011,Jan,11

12041 | **Repair, intermediate, wounds of neck, hands, feet and/or external genitalia; 2.5 cm or less**
🚑 4.32   ⚕ 6.70   **FUD** 010   02 P2 ▢
AMA: 2016,Jan,13; 2015,Jan,16; 2014,Jan,11; 2013,Jan,15-16; 2012,Jan,15-42; 2011,Jan,11

12042 | **2.6 cm to 7.5 cm**
🚑 5.76   ⚕ 8.18   **FUD** 010   T P2 ▢
AMA: 2016,Jan,13; 2015,Jan,16; 2014,Jan,11; 2013,Jan,15-16; 2012,Jan,15-42; 2011,Jan,11

12044 | **7.6 cm to 12.5 cm**
🚑 6.17   ⚕ 10.1   **FUD** 010   T A2 ▢
AMA: 2016,Jan,13; 2015,Jan,16; 2014,Jan,11; 2013,Jan,15-16; 2012,Jan,15-42; 2011,Jan,11

12045 | **12.6 cm to 20.0 cm**
🚑 7.77   ⚕ 11.4   **FUD** 010   T A2 ▢
AMA: 2016,Jan,13; 2015,Jan,16; 2014,Jan,11; 2013,Jan,15-16; 2012,Jan,15-42; 2011,Jan,11

12046 | **20.1 cm to 30.0 cm**
🚑 8.93   ⚕ 13.5   **FUD** 010   T A2 80 ▢
AMA: 2016,Jan,13; 2015,Jan,16; 2014,Jan,11; 2013,Jan,15-16; 2012,Jan,15-42; 2011,Jan,11

12047 | **over 30.0 cm**
🚑 9.93   ⚕ 14.7   **FUD** 010   T A2 80 ▢
AMA: 2016,Jan,13; 2015,Jan,16; 2014,Jan,11; 2013,Jan,15-16; 2012,Jan,15-42; 2011,Jan,11

12051 | **Repair, intermediate, wounds of face, ears, eyelids, nose, lips and/or mucous membranes; 2.5 cm or less**
🚑 4.93   ⚕ 7.31   **FUD** 010   T P2 ▢
AMA: 2016,Jan,13; 2015,Jan,16; 2014,Jan,11; 2012,Jan,15-42; 2011,Jan,11

12052 | **2.6 cm to 5.0 cm**
🚑 5.86   ⚕ 8.33   **FUD** 010   T P2 ▢
AMA: 2016,Jan,13; 2015,Jan,16; 2014,Jan,11; 2012,Jan,15-42; 2011,Jan,11

12053 | **5.1 cm to 7.5 cm**
🚑 6.26   ⚕ 9.77   **FUD** 010   T P2 ▢
AMA: 2016,Jan,13; 2015,Jan,16; 2014,Jan,11; 2012,Jan,15-42; 2011,Jan,11

12054 | **7.6 cm to 12.5 cm**
🚑 6.40   ⚕ 10.2   **FUD** 010   02 A2 ▢
AMA: 2016,Jan,13; 2015,Jan,16; 2014,Jan,11; 2012,Jan,15-42; 2011,Jan,11

12055 | **12.6 cm to 20.0 cm**
🚑 8.81   ⚕ 13.2   **FUD** 010   T A2 ▢
AMA: 2016,Jan,13; 2015,Jan,16; 2014,Jan,11; 2012,Jan,15-42; 2011,Jan,11

12056 | **20.1 cm to 30.0 cm**
🚑 10.8   ⚕ 15.4   **FUD** 010   02 A2 80 ▢
AMA: 2016,Jan,13; 2015,Jan,16; 2014,Jan,11; 2012,Jan,15-42; 2011,Jan,11

12057 | **over 30.0 cm**
🚑 11.7   ⚕ 15.9   **FUD** 010   T A2 80 ▢
AMA: 2016,Jan,13; 2015,Jan,16; 2014,Jan,11; 2012,Jan,15-42; 2011,Jan,11

13100-13160 Suturing of Complicated Wounds

INCLUDES
Creation of a limited defect for repair
Debridement complicated wounds/avulsions
More complicated than layered closure
Simple:
    Exploration nerves, vessels, tendons in wound
    Vessel ligation in wound
Total length of several repairs in same code category
Undermining, stents, retention sutures

EXCLUDES
Complex/secondary wound closure or dehiscence
Debridement of open fracture/dislocation (15002-15005)
Excision:
    Benign lesions (11400-11446)
    Malignant lesions (11600-11646)
Extensive exploration (20100-20103)
Repair of nerves, blood vessel, tendons (See appropriate anatomical section. These repairs include simple and intermediate closure. Report complex closure with modifier 59.)
Surgical preparation of a wound bed (15002-15005)
Code also modifier 59 added to the less complicated procedure code if reporting more than one classification of wound repair

13100 | **Repair, complex, trunk; 1.1 cm to 2.5 cm**
EXCLUDES Complex repair 1.0 cm or less (12001, 12031)
🚑 5.93   ⚕ 9.47   **FUD** 010   T A2 ▢
AMA: 2016,Jan,13; 2015,Jan,16; 2014,Jan,11; 2012,Dec,6-8; 2012,Jan,6-10; 2012,Jan,15-42; 2011,May,3-5; 2011,Jan,11

13101 | **2.6 cm to 7.5 cm**
🚑 7.30   ⚕ 11.2   **FUD** 010   T A2 ▢
AMA: 2016,Jan,13; 2015,Jan,16; 2014,Jan,11; 2012,Dec,6-8; 2012,Jan,6-10; 2012,Jan,15-42; 2011,May,3-5; 2011,May,6; 2011,Jan,11

+ **13102** | **each additional 5 cm or less (List separately in addition to code for primary procedure)**
Code first (13101)
🚑 2.15   ⚕ 3.45   **FUD** ZZZ   N N1 ▢
AMA: 2016,Jan,13; 2015,Jan,16; 2014,Jan,11; 2012,Dec,6-8; 2012,Jan,6-10; 2012,Jan,15-42; 2011,May,3-5; 2011,May,6; 2011,Jan,11

13120 | **Repair, complex, scalp, arms, and/or legs; 1.1 cm to 2.5 cm**
EXCLUDES Complex repair 1.0 cm or less (12001, 12031)
🚑 6.80   ⚕ 9.91   **FUD** 010   T A2 ▢
AMA: 2016,Jan,13; 2015,Jan,16; 2014,Jan,11; 2012,Dec,6-8; 2012,Jan,6-10; 2012,Jan,15-42; 2011,May,3-5; 2011,Jan,11

13121 | **2.6 cm to 7.5 cm**
🚑 7.71   ⚕ 12.1   **FUD** 010   T A2 ▢
AMA: 2016,Jan,13; 2015,Jan,16; 2014,Jan,11; 2012,Dec,6-8; 2012,Jan,6-10; 2012,Jan,15-42; 2011,May,6; 2011,May,3-5; 2011,Jan,11

+ **13122** | **each additional 5 cm or less (List separately in addition to code for primary procedure)**
Code first (13121)
🚑 2.47   ⚕ 3.78   **FUD** ZZZ   N N1 ▢
AMA: 2016,Jan,13; 2015,Jan,16; 2014,Jan,11; 2012,Dec,6-8; 2012,Jan,6-10; 2012,Jan,15-42; 2011,May,3-5; 2011,Jan,11

13131 | **Repair, complex, forehead, cheeks, chin, mouth, neck, axillae, genitalia, hands and/or feet; 1.1 cm to 2.5 cm**
EXCLUDES Complex repair 1.0 cm or less (12001, 12011, 12031, 12041, 12051)
🚑 7.20   ⚕ 10.9   **FUD** 010   T A2 ▢
AMA: 2016,Jan,13; 2015,Jan,16; 2014,Jan,11; 2013,Jan,15-16; 2012,Dec,6-8; 2012,Jan,6-10; 2012,Jan,15-42; 2011,May,3-5; 2011,May,6; 2011,Jan,11

26/TC PC/TC Only   A2-Z3 ASC Payment   50 Bilateral   ♂ Male Only   ♀ Female Only   🚑 Facility RVU   ⚕ Non-Facility RVU   ▢ CCI
FUD Follow-up Days   CMS: IOM (Pub 100)   A-Y OPPSI   80/80 Surg Assist Allowed / w/Doc   🔬 Lab Crosswalk   ☢ Radiology Crosswalk   ✖ CLIA

22

Integumentary System

12032 — 13131

13132	**2.6 cm to 7.5 cm**

🔧 9.08 ✂ 13.5 **FUD** 010 T A2 ▣

AMA: 2016,Jan,13; 2015,Jan,16; 2014,Oct,14; 2014,Jan,11; 2013,Jan,15-16; 2012,Dec,6-8; 2012,Jan,6-10; 2012,Jan,15-42; 2011,May,3-5; 2011,May,6; 2011,Jan,11

+ 13133 **each additional 5 cm or less (List separately in addition to code for primary procedure)**

Code first (13132)

🔧 3.79 ✂ 5.08 **FUD** ZZZ N N1 ▣

AMA: 2016,Jan,13; 2015,Jan,16; 2014,Jan,11; 2013,Jan,15-16; 2012,Dec,6-8; 2012,Jan,6-10; 2012,Jan,15-42; 2011,May,3-5; 2011,Jan,11

13151 **Repair, complex, eyelids, nose, ears and/or lips; 1.1 cm to 2.5 cm**

EXCLUDES Complex repair 1.0 cm or less (12011, 12051)

🔧 8.28 ✂ 11.9 **FUD** 010 T A2 ▣

AMA: 2016,Jan,13; 2015,Jan,16; 2014,May,3; 2014,Mar,12; 2014,Jan,11; 2012,Dec,6-8; 2012,Jan,6-10; 2012,Jan,15-42; 2011,May,3-5; 2011,Jan,11

13152 **2.6 cm to 7.5 cm**

🔧 10.0 ✂ 14.3 **FUD** 010 T A2 ▣

AMA: 2016,Jan,13; 2015,Jan,16; 2014,Oct,14; 2014,May,3; 2014,Mar,12; 2014,Jan,11; 2012,Dec,6-8; 2012,Jan,15-42; 2012,Jan,6-10; 2011,May,3-5; 2011,Jan,11

+ 13153 **each additional 5 cm or less (List separately in addition to code for primary procedure)**

Code first (13152)

🔧 4.09 ✂ 5.51 **FUD** ZZZ N N1 ▣

AMA: 2016,Jan,13; 2015,Jan,16; 2014,May,3; 2014,Mar,12; 2014,Jan,11; 2012,Dec,6-8; 2012,Jan,15-42; 2012,Jan,6-10; 2011,May,3-5; 2011,Jan,11

13160 **Secondary closure of surgical wound or dehiscence, extensive or complicated**

EXCLUDES Packing or simple secondary wound closure (12020-12021)

🔧 23.1 ✂ 23.1 **FUD** 090 T A2 ▣

AMA: 2016,Jan,13; 2015,Jan,16; 2014,Jan,11; 2012,Dec,6-8; 2012,Jan,15-42; 2011,May,3-5; 2011,Jan,11

14000-14350 Reposition Contiguous Tissue

INCLUDES Excision of lesion with repair by adjacent tissue transfer or tissue rearrangement
Size of defect includes primary (due to excision) and secondary (due to flap design)
Z-plasty, W-plasty, VY-plasty, rotation flap, advancement flap, double pedicle flap, random island flap

EXCLUDES Closure of wounds by undermining surrounding tissue without additional incisions (13100-13160)
Full thickness closure of:
Eyelid (67930-67935, 67961-67975)
Lip (40650-40654)
Code also skin graft necessary to repair secondary defect (15040-15731)

14000 **Adjacent tissue transfer or rearrangement, trunk; defect 10 sq cm or less**

INCLUDES Burrow's operation

EXCLUDES Excision of lesion with repair by adjacent tissue transfer or tissue rearrangement (11400-11446, 11600-11646)

🔧 14.4 ✂ 17.6 **FUD** 090 T A2 ▣

AMA: 2016,Jan,13; 2015,Sep,12; 2015,Feb,10; 2015,Jan,16; 2014,Apr,10; 2014,Jan,11; 2012,Dec,6-8; 2012,Nov,13-14; 2012,May,13; 2012,Jan,6-10; 2012,Jan,15-42; 2011,Jan,11

Example of common Z-plasty. Lesion is removed with oval-shaped incision

Two additional incisions (a. and b.) intersect the area

Skin of each incision is reflected back

The flaps are then transposed and the repair is closed

An adjacent flap, or other rearrangement flap, is performed to repair a defect of 10 sq cm or less (14000); a larger defect (up to 30 sq cm) is coded 14001

14001 **defect 10.1 sq cm to 30.0 sq cm**

EXCLUDES Excision of lesion with repair by adjacent tissue transfer or tissue rearrangement (11400-11446, 11600-11646)

🔧 18.8 ✂ 22.7 **FUD** 090 T A2 ▣

AMA: 2016,Jan,13; 2015,Feb,10; 2015,Jan,16; 2014,Apr,10; 2014,Jan,11; 2012,Dec,6-8; 2012,Nov,13-14; 2012,May,13; 2012,Jan,15-42; 2012,Jan,6-10; 2011,Jan,11

14020 **Adjacent tissue transfer or rearrangement, scalp, arms and/or legs; defect 10 sq cm or less**

EXCLUDES Excision of lesion with repair by adjacent tissue transfer or tissue rearrangement (11400-11446, 11600-11646)

🔧 16.3 ✂ 19.7 **FUD** 090 T A2 ▣

AMA: 2016,Jan,13; 2015,Jan,16; 2014,Jan,11; 2012,Dec,6-8; 2012,Nov,13-14; 2012,May,13; 2012,Jan,15-42; 2012,Jan,6-10; 2011,Jan,11

14021 **defect 10.1 sq cm to 30.0 sq cm**

EXCLUDES Excision of lesion with repair by adjacent tissue transfer or tissue rearrangement (11400-11446, 11600-11646)

🔧 20.6 ✂ 24.7 **FUD** 090 T A2 ▣

AMA: 2016,Jan,13; 2015,Jan,16; 2014,Jan,11; 2012,Dec,6-8; 2012,Nov,13-14; 2012,May,13; 2012,Jan,15-42; 2012,Jan,6-10; 2011,Jan,11

14040 **Adjacent tissue transfer or rearrangement, forehead, cheeks, chin, mouth, neck, axillae, genitalia, hands and/or feet; defect 10 sq cm or less**

INCLUDES Krimer's palatoplasty

EXCLUDES Excision of lesion with repair by adjacent tissue transfer or tissue rearrangement (11400-11446, 11600-11646)

🔧 18.1 ✂ 21.6 **FUD** 090 T A2 ▣

AMA: 2016,Jan,13; 2015,Jan,16; 2014,Jan,11; 2012,Dec,6-8; 2012,Nov,13-14; 2012,May,13; 2012,Jan,15-42; 2012,Jan,6-10; 2011,Jan,11

14041 **defect 10.1 sq cm to 30.0 sq cm**

EXCLUDES Excision of lesion with repair by adjacent tissue transfer or tissue rearrangement (11400-11446, 11600-11646)

🔧 22.3 ✂ 26.8 **FUD** 090 T A2 ▣

AMA: 2016,Jan,13; 2015,Jan,16; 2014,Jan,11; 2012,Dec,6-8; 2012,Nov,13-14; 2012,May,13; 2012,Jan,15-42; 2012,Jan,6-10; 2011,Jan,11

● New Code ▲ Revised Code ○ Reinstated ● New Web Release ▲ Revised Web Release **Unlisted** **Not Covered** # Resequenced
⊘ AMA Mod 51 Exempt ⑨ Optum Mod 51 Exempt ⑥⑨ Mod 63 Exempt ⁄ Non-FDA Drug ★ Telehealth M Maternity A Age Edit + Add-on **AMA:** CPT Asst

CPT © 2016 American Medical Association. All Rights Reserved. **23**

14060 Adjacent tissue transfer or rearrangement, eyelids, nose, ears and/or lips; defect 10 sq cm or less

INCLUDES Denonvillier's operation

EXCLUDES Excision of lesion with repair by adjacent tissue transfer or tissue rearrangement (11400-11446, 11600-11646)

Eyelid, full thickness (67961-67966)

�️ 19.3 ✂ 22.0 **FUD** 090   T A2 ▭

AMA: 2016,Jan,13; 2015,Jan,16; 2014,Jan,11; 2012,Dec,6-8; 2012,Nov,13-14; 2012,Aug,13-14; 2012,May,13; 2012,Jan,15-42; 2012,Jan,6-10; 2011,Jan,11

14061 defect 10.1 sq cm to 30.0 sq cm

EXCLUDES Excision of lesion with repair by adjacent tissue transfer or tissue rearrangement (11400-11446, 11600-11646)

Eyelid, full thickness (67961 and subsequent codes)

⏲ 23.9 ✂ 28.8 **FUD** 090   T A2 ▭

AMA: 2016,Jan,13; 2015,Jan,16; 2014,Jan,11; 2012,Dec,6-8; 2012,Nov,13-14; 2012,May,13; 2012,Jan,15-42; 2012,Jan,6-10; 2011,Jan,11

14301 Adjacent tissue transfer or rearrangement, any area; defect 30.1 sq cm to 60.0 sq cm

EXCLUDES Excision of lesion with repair by adjacent tissue transfer or tissue rearrangement (11400-11446, 11600-11646)

⏲ 25.4 ✂ 30.6 **FUD** 090   T G2 80 ▭

AMA: 2016,Jan,13; 2015,Jan,16; 2014,Jan,11; 2012,Dec,6-8; 2012,Nov,13-14; 2012,May,13

+ **14302** each additional 30.0 sq cm, or part thereof (List separately in addition to code for primary procedure)

EXCLUDES Excision of lesion with repair by adjacent tissue transfer or tissue rearrangement (11400-11446, 11600-11646)

Code first (14301)

⏲ 6.40 ✂ 6.40 **FUD** ZZZ   N N1 80 ▭

AMA: 2016,Jan,13; 2015,Jan,16; 2014,Jan,11; 2012,Dec,6-8; 2012,Nov,13-14; 2012,May,13

14350 Filleted finger or toe flap, including preparation of recipient site

⏲ 19.9 ✂ 19.9 **FUD** 090   T A2 80 ▭

AMA: 2016,Jan,13; 2015,Jan,16; 2014,Jan,11; 2012,Dec,6-8; 2012,May,13; 2012,Jan,15-42; 2011,Jan,11

15002-15005 Development of Base for Tissue Grafting

INCLUDES Add together the surface area of multiple wounds in the same anatomical locations as indicated in the code descriptor groups, such as face and scalp. Do not add together multiple wounds at different anatomical site groups such as trunk and face

Ankle or wrist if code description describes leg or arm

Cleaning and preparing a viable wound surface for grafting or negative pressure wound therapy used to heal the wound primarily

Code selection based on the defect size and location

Percentage applies to children younger than age 10

Removal of nonviable tissue in nonchronic wounds for primary healing

Square centimeters applies to children and adults age 10 or older

EXCLUDES Chronic wound management on wounds left to heal by secondary intention (11042-11047 [11045, 11046], 97597-97598)

Necrotizing soft tissue infections for specific anatomical locations (11004-11008)

15002 Surgical preparation or creation of recipient site by excision of open wounds, burn eschar, or scar (including subcutaneous tissues), or incisional release of scar contracture, trunk, arms, legs; first 100 sq cm or 1% of body area of infants and children

EXCLUDES Linear scar revision (13100-13153)

⏲ 6.54 ✂ 9.87 **FUD** 000   T A2 80 ▭

AMA: 2016,Jan,13; 2015,Jan,16; 2014,Mar,12; 2014,Jan,11; 2013,Feb,16-17; 2012,Dec,6-8; 2012,Oct,3-8; 2012,Oct,13; 2012,Jan,15-42; 2012,Jan,6-10; 2011,Jan,11

+ **15003** each additional 100 sq cm, or part thereof, or each additional 1% of body area of infants and children (List separately in addition to code for primary procedure)

Code first (15002)

⏲ 1.32 ✂ 2.15 **FUD** ZZZ   N N1 80 ▭

AMA: 2016,Jan,13; 2015,Jan,16; 2014,Mar,12; 2014,Jan,11; 2013,Feb,16-17; 2012,Oct,13; 2012,Oct,3-8; 2012,Jan,15-42; 2012,Jan,6-10; 2011,Jan,11

15004 Surgical preparation or creation of recipient site by excision of open wounds, burn eschar, or scar (including subcutaneous tissues), or incisional release of scar contracture, face, scalp, eyelids, mouth, neck, ears, orbits, genitalia, hands, feet and/or multiple digits; first 100 sq cm or 1% of body area of infants and children

⏲ 7.79 ✂ 11.4 **FUD** 000   T A2 80 ▭

AMA: 2016,Jan,13; 2015,Jan,16; 2014,Mar,12; 2014,Jan,11; 2013,Feb,16-17; 2012,Oct,3-8; 2012,Oct,13; 2012,Jan,15-42; 2012,Jan,6-10; 2011,Jan,11

+ **15005** each additional 100 sq cm, or part thereof, or each additional 1% of body area of infants and children (List separately in addition to code for primary procedure)

Code first (15004)

⏲ 2.63 ✂ 3.55 **FUD** ZZZ   N N1 80 ▭

AMA: 2016,Jan,13; 2015,Jan,16; 2014,Mar,12; 2014,Jan,11; 2013,Feb,16-17; 2012,Oct,13; 2012,Oct,3-8; 2012,Jan,15-42; 2012,Jan,6-10; 2011,Jan,11

15040 Obtain Autograft

INCLUDES Ankle or wrist if code description describes leg or arm

Percentage applies to children younger than age 10

Square centimeters applies to children and adults age 10 or older

15040 Harvest of skin for tissue cultured skin autograft, 100 sq cm or less

⏲ 3.69 ✂ 7.28 **FUD** 000   T A2 ▭

AMA: 2016,Jan,13; 2015,Jan,16; 2014,Jan,11; 2012,Jan,6-10; 2012,Jan,15-42; 2011,Jan,11

15050 Pinch Graft

INCLUDES Autologous skin graft harvest and application

Current graft removal

Fixation and anchoring skin graft

Simple cleaning

EXCLUDES Removal of devitalized tissue from wound(s), non-selective debridement, without anesthesia (97602)

Code also graft or flap necessary to repair donor site

15050 Pinch graft, single or multiple, to cover small ulcer, tip of digit, or other minimal open area (except on face), up to defect size 2 cm diameter

⏲ 12.7 ✂ 16.0 **FUD** 090   T A2 ▭

AMA: 2016,Jun,8; 2016,Jan,13; 2015,Jan,16; 2014,Jan,11; 2012,Jan,6-10; 2012,Jan,15-42; 2011,Mar,9; 2011,Jan,11

15100-15261 Skin Grafts and Replacements

INCLUDES Add together the surface area of multiple wounds in the same anatomical locations as indicated in the code description groups, such as face and scalp. Do not add together multiple wounds at different anatomical site groups such as trunk and face.
Ankle or wrist if code description describes leg or arm
Autologous skin graft harvest and application
Code selection based on recipient site location and size and type of graft
Current graft removal
Fixation and anchoring skin graft
Percentage applies to children younger than age 10
Simple cleaning
Simple tissue debridement
Square centimeters applies to children and adults age 10 or older

EXCLUDES *Debridement without immediate primary closure, when wound is grossly contaminated and extensive cleaning is needed, or when necrotic or contaminated tissue is removed (11042-11047 [11045, 11046], 97597-97598)*
Removal of devitalized tissue from wound(s), non-selective debridement, without anesthesia (97602)

Code also graft or flap necessary to repair donor site
Code also primary procedure requiring skin graft for definitive closure

15100 Split-thickness autograft, trunk, arms, legs; first 100 sq cm or less, or 1% of body area of infants and children (except 15050)
20.5 24.4 **FUD** 090 T A2
AMA: 2016,Jun,8; 2016,Jan,13; 2015,Jan,16; 2014,Jan,11; 2012,Oct,3-8; 2012,Jan,6-10; 2012,Jan,15-42; 2011,Mar,9; 2011,Jan,11

+ **15101** each additional 100 sq cm, or each additional 1% of body area of infants and children, or part thereof (List separately in addition to code for primary procedure)
Code first (15100)
3.21 5.29 **FUD** ZZZ N N1
AMA: 2016,Jun,8; 2016,Jan,13; 2015,Jan,16; 2014,Jan,11; 2012,Oct,3-8; 2012,Jan,6-10; 2012,Jan,15-42; 2011,Mar,9; 2011,Jan,11

15110 Epidermal autograft, trunk, arms, legs; first 100 sq cm or less, or 1% of body area of infants and children
20.0 22.8 **FUD** 090 T A2
AMA: 2016,Jan,13; 2015,Jan,16; 2014,Jan,11; 2012,Oct,3-8; 2012,Jan,6-10; 2012,Jan,15-42; 2011,Mar,9; 2011,Jan,11

+ **15111** each additional 100 sq cm, or each additional 1% of body area of infants and children, or part thereof (List separately in addition to code for primary procedure)
Code first (15110)
3.01 3.32 **FUD** ZZZ N N1
AMA: 2016,Jan,13; 2015,Jan,16; 2014,Jan,11; 2012,Oct,3-8; 2012,Jan,6-10; 2012,Jan,15-42; 2011,Mar,9; 2011,Jan,11

15115 Epidermal autograft, face, scalp, eyelids, mouth, neck, ears, orbits, genitalia, hands, feet, and/or multiple digits; first 100 sq cm or less, or 1% of body area of infants and children
20.5 23.4 **FUD** 090 T A2
AMA: 2016,Jan,13; 2015,Jan,16; 2014,Jan,11; 2012,Oct,3-8; 2012,Jan,6-10; 2012,Jan,15-42; 2011,Mar,9; 2011,Jan,11

+ **15116** each additional 100 sq cm, or each additional 1% of body area of infants and children, or part thereof (List separately in addition to code for primary procedure)
Code first (15115)
3.98 4.40 **FUD** ZZZ N N1
AMA: 2016,Jan,13; 2015,Jan,16; 2014,Jan,11; 2012,Oct,3-8; 2012,Jan,6-10; 2012,Jan,15-42; 2011,Mar,9; 2011,Jan,11

15120 Split-thickness autograft, face, scalp, eyelids, mouth, neck, ears, orbits, genitalia, hands, feet, and/or multiple digits; first 100 sq cm or less, or 1% of body area of infants and children (except 15050)
EXCLUDES *Other eyelid repair (67961-67975)*
20.0 24.2 **FUD** 090 T A2
AMA: 2016,Jun,8; 2016,Jan,13; 2015,Jan,16; 2014,Jan,11; 2012,Oct,3-8; 2012,Jan,6-10; 2012,Jan,15-42; 2011,Mar,9; 2011,Jan,11

+ **15121** each additional 100 sq cm, or each additional 1% of body area of infants and children, or part thereof (List separately in addition to code for primary procedure)
EXCLUDES *Other eyelid repair (67961-67975)*
Code first (15120)
3.83 5.93 **FUD** ZZZ N N1
AMA: 2016,Jun,8; 2016,Jan,13; 2015,Jan,16; 2014,Jan,11; 2012,Oct,3-8; 2012,Jan,6-10; 2012,Jan,15-42; 2011,Mar,9; 2011,Jan,11

15130 Dermal autograft, trunk, arms, legs; first 100 sq cm or less, or 1% of body area of infants and children
16.2 19.1 **FUD** 090 T A2
AMA: 2016,Jan,13; 2015,Jan,16; 2014,Jan,11; 2012,Oct,3-8; 2012,Jan,6-10; 2012,Jan,15-42; 2011,Mar,9; 2011,Jan,11

+ **15131** each additional 100 sq cm, or each additional 1% of body area of infants and children, or part thereof (List separately in addition to code for primary procedure)
Code first (15130)
2.62 2.85 **FUD** ZZZ N N1
AMA: 2016,Jan,13; 2015,Jan,16; 2014,Jan,11; 2012,Oct,3-8; 2012,Jan,6-10; 2012,Jan,15-42; 2011,Mar,9; 2011,Jan,11

15135 Dermal autograft, face, scalp, eyelids, mouth, neck, ears, orbits, genitalia, hands, feet, and/or multiple digits; first 100 sq cm or less, or 1% of body area of infants and children
21.1 24.0 **FUD** 090 T A2
AMA: 2016,Jan,13; 2015,Jan,16; 2014,Jan,11; 2012,Oct,3-8; 2012,Jan,6-10; 2012,Jan,15-42; 2011,Mar,9; 2011,Jan,11

+ **15136** each additional 100 sq cm, or each additional 1% of body area of infants and children, or part thereof (List separately in addition to code for primary procedure)
Code first (15135)
2.54 2.71 **FUD** ZZZ N N1
AMA: 2016,Jan,13; 2015,Jan,16; 2014,Jan,11; 2012,Oct,3-8; 2012,Jan,6-10; 2012,Jan,15-42; 2011,Mar,9; 2011,Jan,11

15150 Tissue cultured skin autograft, trunk, arms, legs; first 25 sq cm or less
18.2 19.9 **FUD** 090 T A2
AMA: 2016,Jan,13; 2015,Jan,16; 2014,Jan,11; 2012,Oct,3-8; 2012,Jan,6-10; 2012,Jan,15-42; 2011,Mar,9; 2011,Jan,11

+ **15151** additional 1 sq cm to 75 sq cm (List separately in addition to code for primary procedure)
EXCLUDES *Grafts over 75 sq cm (15152)*
Use of code more than one time per session
Code first (15150)
3.25 3.51 **FUD** ZZZ N N1
AMA: 2016,Jan,13; 2015,Jan,16; 2014,Jan,11; 2012,Oct,3-8; 2012,Jan,6-10; 2012,Jan,15-42; 2011,Mar,9; 2011,Jan,11

+ **15152** each additional 100 sq cm, or each additional 1% of body area of infants and children, or part thereof (List separately in addition to code for primary procedure)
Code first (15151)
4.04 4.31 **FUD** ZZZ N N1
AMA: 2016,Jan,13; 2015,Jan,16; 2014,Jan,11; 2012,Oct,3-8; 2012,Jan,6-10; 2012,Jan,15-42; 2011,Mar,9; 2011,Jan,11

15155 Tissue cultured skin autograft, face, scalp, eyelids, mouth, neck, ears, orbits, genitalia, hands, feet, and/or multiple digits; first 25 sq cm or less
19.1 20.6 **FUD** 090 T A2
AMA: 2016,Jan,13; 2015,Jan,16; 2014,Jan,11; 2012,Oct,3-8; 2012,Jan,6-10; 2012,Jan,15-42; 2011,Mar,9; 2011,Jan,11

+ **15156** **additional 1 sq cm to 75 sq cm (List separately in addition to code for primary procedure)**

> *EXCLUDES* *Grafts over 75 sq cm (15157)*
> *Use of code more than one time per session*
> Code first (15155)
> 4.31 4.54 **FUD** ZZZ N N1
>
> **AMA:** 2016,Jan,13; 2015,Jan,16; 2014,Jan,11; 2012,Oct,3-8; 2012,Jan,6-10; 2012,Jan,15-42; 2011,Mar,9; 2011,Jan,11

+ **15157** **each additional 100 sq cm, or each additional 1% of body area of infants and children, or part thereof (List separately in addition to code for primary procedure)**

> Code first (15156)
> 4.67 4.99 **FUD** ZZZ N N1
>
> **AMA:** 2016,Jan,13; 2015,Jan,16; 2014,Jan,11; 2012,Oct,3-8; 2012,Jan,6-10; 2012,Jan,15-42; 2011,Mar,9; 2011,Jan,11

15200 **Full thickness graft, free, including direct closure of donor site, trunk; 20 sq cm or less**

> 19.3 23.6 **FUD** 090 T A2
>
> **AMA:** 2016,Jun,8; 2016,Jan,13; 2015,Jan,16; 2014,Jan,11; 2012,Oct,3-8; 2012,Jan,6-10; 2012,Jan,15-42; 2011,Jan,11

+ **15201** **each additional 20 sq cm, or part thereof (List separately in addition to code for primary procedure)**

> Code first (15200)
> 2.27 4.20 **FUD** ZZZ N N1
>
> **AMA:** 2016,Jun,8; 2016,Jan,13; 2015,Jan,16; 2014,Jan,11; 2012,Oct,3-8; 2012,Jan,6-10; 2012,Jan,15-42; 2011,Jan,11

15220 **Full thickness graft, free, including direct closure of donor site, scalp, arms, and/or legs; 20 sq cm or less**

> 17.6 21.8 **FUD** 090 T A2
>
> **AMA:** 2016,Jun,8; 2016,Jan,13; 2015,Jan,16; 2014,Jan,11; 2012,Oct,3-8; 2012,Jan,6-10; 2012,Jan,15-42; 2011,Jan,11

+ **15221** **each additional 20 sq cm, or part thereof (List separately in addition to code for primary procedure)**

> Code first (15220)
> 2.06 3.88 **FUD** ZZZ N N1
>
> **AMA:** 2016,Jun,8; 2016,Jan,13; 2015,Jan,16; 2014,Jan,11; 2012,Oct,3-8; 2012,Jan,6-10; 2012,Jan,15-42; 2011,Jan,11

15240 **Full thickness graft, free, including direct closure of donor site, forehead, cheeks, chin, mouth, neck, axillae, genitalia, hands, and/or feet; 20 sq cm or less**

> *EXCLUDES* *Fingertip graft (15050)*
> *Syndactyly repair fingers (26560-26562)*
> 23.0 26.5 **FUD** 090 T A2
>
> **AMA:** 2016,Jun,8; 2016,Jan,13; 2015,Jan,16; 2014,Jan,11; 2012,Oct,3-8; 2012,Jan,6-10; 2012,Jan,15-42; 2011,Jan,11

+ **15241** **each additional 20 sq cm, or part thereof (List separately in addition to code for primary procedure)**

> Code first (15240)
> 3.22 5.25 **FUD** ZZZ N N1
>
> **AMA:** 2016,Jun,8; 2016,Jan,13; 2015,Jan,16; 2014,Jan,11; 2012,Oct,3-8; 2012,Jan,6-10; 2012,Jan,15-42; 2011,Jan,11

15260 **Full thickness graft, free, including direct closure of donor site, nose, ears, eyelids, and/or lips; 20 sq cm or less**

> *EXCLUDES* *Other eyelid repair (67961-67975)*
> 24.7 28.8 **FUD** 090 T A2
>
> **AMA:** 2016,Jun,8; 2016,Jan,13; 2015,Jan,16; 2014,Jan,11; 2012,Oct,3-8; 2012,Jan,6-10; 2012,Jan,15-42; 2011,Jan,11

+ **15261** **each additional 20 sq cm, or part thereof (List separately in addition to code for primary procedure)**

> *EXCLUDES* *Other eyelid repair (67961-67975)*
> Code first (15260)
> 4.05 6.14 **FUD** ZZZ N N1
>
> **AMA:** 2016,Jun,8; 2016,Jan,13; 2015,Jan,16; 2014,Jan,11; 2012,Oct,3-8; 2012,Jan,6-10; 2012,Jan,15-42; 2011,Jan,11

15271-15278 Skin Substitute Graft Application

INCLUDES Add together the surface area of multiple wounds in the same anatomical locations as indicated in the code description groups, such as face and scalp. Do not add together multiple wounds at different anatomical site groups such as trunk and face.
Ankle or wrist if code description describes leg or arm
Code selection based on defect site location and size
Fixation and anchoring skin graft
Graft types include:
  Biological material used for tissue engineering (e.g., scaffold) for growing skin
  Nonautologous human skin such as:
    Acellular
    Allograft
    Cellular
    Dermal
    Epidermal
    Homograft
  Nonhuman grafts
Percentage applies to children younger than age 10
Removing current graft
Simple cleaning
Simple tissue debridement
Square centimeters applies to children and adults age 10 or older

EXCLUDES *Application of nongraft dressing*
Injected skin substitutes
Removal of devitalized tissue from wound(s), non-selective debridement, without anesthesia (97602)
Skin application procedures, low cost (C5271-C5278)
Code also biologic implant for soft tissue reinforcement (15777)
Code also primary procedure requiring skin graft for definitive closure
Code also supply of high cost skin substitute product (C9349, C9363, Q4101, Q4103-Q4110, Q4116, Q4120-Q4123, Q4126-Q4128, Q4131-Q4133, Q4137-Q4138, Q4140-Q4141, Q4147-Q4148, Q4151-Q4154, Q4156, Q4159-Q4160)

15271 **Application of skin substitute graft to trunk, arms, legs, total wound surface area up to 100 sq cm; first 25 sq cm or less wound surface area**

> *EXCLUDES* *Total wound area greater than or equal to 100 sq cm (15273-15274)*
> 2.44 3.99 **FUD** 000 T G2
>
> **AMA:** 2016,Jan,13; 2015,Jan,16; 2014,Jun,14; 2014,Jan,11; 2013,Oct,15; 2012,Oct,3-8; 2012,Jan,6-10; 2012,Jan,15-42

+ **15272** **each additional 25 sq cm wound surface area, or part thereof (List separately in addition to code for primary procedure)**

> *EXCLUDES* *Total wound area greater than or equal to 100 sq cm (15273-15274)*
> Code first (15271)
> 0.50 0.77 **FUD** ZZZ N N1
>
> **AMA:** 2016,Jan,13; 2015,Jan,16; 2014,Jun,14; 2014,Jan,11; 2013,Oct,15; 2012,Oct,3-8; 2012,Jan,6-10; 2012,Jan,15-42

15273 **Application of skin substitute graft to trunk, arms, legs, total wound surface area greater than or equal to 100 sq cm; first 100 sq cm wound surface area, or 1% of body area of infants and children**

> *EXCLUDES* *Total wound surface area up to 100 cm (15271-15272)*
> 5.84 8.46 **FUD** 000 T G2
>
> **AMA:** 2016,Jan,13; 2015,Jan,16; 2014,Jun,14; 2014,Jan,11; 2013,Oct,15; 2013,Nov,14; 2012,Oct,3-8; 2012,Jan,6-10; 2012,Jan,15-42

+ **15274** **each additional 100 sq cm wound surface area, or part thereof, or each additional 1% of body area of infants and children, or part thereof (List separately in addition to code for primary procedure)**

> *EXCLUDES* *Total wound surface area up to 100 cm (15271-15272)*
> Code first (15273)
> 1.33 2.03 **FUD** ZZZ N N1
>
> **AMA:** 2016,Jan,13; 2015,Jan,16; 2014,Jun,14; 2014,Jan,11; 2013,Oct,15; 2013,Nov,14; 2012,Oct,3-8; 2012,Jan,6-10; 2012,Jan,15-42

15275 Application of skin substitute graft to face, scalp, eyelids, mouth, neck, ears, orbits, genitalia, hands, feet, and/or multiple digits, total wound surface area up to 100 sq cm; first 25 sq cm or less wound surface area

EXCLUDES Total wound area greater than or equal to 100 sq cm (15277-15278)

2.75 4.23 **FUD** 000 T G2

AMA: 2016,Jan,13; 2015,Jan,16; 2014,Jun,14; 2014,Jan,11; 2013,Oct,15; 2012,Oct,3-8; 2012,Jan,6-10; 2012,Jan,15-42

+ **15276** each additional 25 sq cm wound surface area, or part thereof (List separately in addition to code for primary procedure)

EXCLUDES Total wound area greater than or equal to 100 sq cm (15277-15278)

Code first (15275)

0.72 0.98 **FUD** ZZZ N N1

AMA: 2016,Jan,13; 2015,Jan,16; 2014,Jun,14; 2014,Jan,11; 2013,Oct,15; 2012,Oct,3-8; 2012,Jan,6-10; 2012,Jan,15-42

15277 Application of skin substitute graft to face, scalp, eyelids, mouth, neck, ears, orbits, genitalia, hands, feet, and/or multiple digits, total wound surface area greater than or equal to 100 sq cm; first 100 sq cm wound surface area, or 1% of body area of infants and children

EXCLUDES Total surface area up to 100 sq cm (15275-15276)

6.49 9.17 **FUD** 000 T G2

AMA: 2016,Jan,13; 2015,Jan,16; 2014,Jun,14; 2014,Jan,11; 2013,Oct,15; 2013,Nov,14; 2012,Oct,3-8; 2012,Jan,6-10; 2012,Jan,15-42

+ **15278** each additional 100 sq cm wound surface area, or part thereof, or each additional 1% of body area of infants and children, or part thereof (List separately in addition to code for primary procedure)

EXCLUDES Total surface area up to 100 sq cm (15275-15276)

Code first (15277)

1.65 2.42 **FUD** ZZZ N N1

AMA: 2016,Jan,13; 2015,Jan,16; 2014,Jun,14; 2014,Jan,11; 2013,Oct,15; 2013,Nov,14; 2012,Oct,3-8; 2012,Jan,6-10; 2012,Jan,15-42

15570-15731 Wound Reconstruction: Skin Flaps

INCLUDES Ankle or wrist if code description describes leg or arm
Code based on recipient site when the flap is attached in the transfer or to a final site and is based on donor site when a tube is created for transfer later or when the flap is delayed prior to transfer
Fixation and anchoring skin graft
Simple tissue debridement
Tube formation for later transfer

EXCLUDES Contiguous tissue transfer flaps (14000-14302)
Debridement without immediate primary closure (11042-11047 [11045, 11046], 97597-97598)
Excision of:
    Benign lesion (11400-11471)
    Burn eschar or scar (15002-15005)
    Malignant lesion (11600-11646)
Microvascular repair (15756-15758)
Primary procedure--see appropriate anatomical site

Code also application of extensive immobilization apparatus
Code also repair of donor site with skin grafts or flaps

15570 Formation of direct or tubed pedicle, with or without transfer; trunk

INCLUDES Flaps without a vascular pedicle

21.1 25.9 **FUD** 090 T A2

AMA: 2016,Jan,13; 2015,Jan,16; 2014,Jan,11; 2012,Dec,6-8; 2012,Jan,15-42; 2011,Jan,11

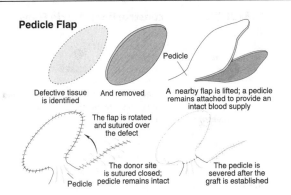

Pedicle Flap

Defective tissue is identified

And removed

A nearby flap is lifted; a pedicle remains attached to provide an intact blood supply

Pedicle

The flap is rotated and sutured over the defect

The donor site is sutured closed; pedicle remains intact

Pedicle

The pedicle is severed after the graft is established

15572 scalp, arms, or legs

INCLUDES Flaps without a vascular pedicle

21.4 25.2 **FUD** 090 T A2

AMA: 2016,Jan,13; 2015,Jan,16; 2014,Jan,11; 2012,Dec,6-8; 2012,Jan,15-42; 2011,Jan,11

15574 forehead, cheeks, chin, mouth, neck, axillae, genitalia, hands or feet

INCLUDES Flaps without a vascular pedicle

22.0 26.0 **FUD** 090 T A2

AMA: 2016,Jan,13; 2015,Jan,16; 2014,Jan,11; 2012,Dec,6-8; 2012,Jan,15-42; 2011,Jan,11

15576 eyelids, nose, ears, lips, or intraoral

INCLUDES Flaps without a vascular pedicle

19.2 22.9 **FUD** 090 T A2

AMA: 2016,Jan,13; 2015,Jan,16; 2014,Jan,11; 2012,Dec,6-8; 2012,Jan,15-42; 2011,Jan,11

15600 Delay of flap or sectioning of flap (division and inset); at trunk

5.92 9.13 **FUD** 090 T A2 80

AMA: 2016,Jan,13; 2015,Jan,16; 2014,Jan,11; 2012,Dec,6-8

15610 at scalp, arms, or legs

6.90 10.0 **FUD** 090 T A2 80

AMA: 2016,Jan,13; 2015,Jan,16; 2014,Jan,11; 2012,Dec,6-8

15620 at forehead, cheeks, chin, neck, axillae, genitalia, hands, or feet

9.35 12.4 **FUD** 090 T A2

AMA: 2016,Jan,13; 2015,Jan,16; 2014,Jan,11; 2012,Dec,6-8

15630 at eyelids, nose, ears, or lips

9.94 13.0 **FUD** 090 T A2

AMA: 2016,Jan,13; 2015,Jan,16; 2014,Jan,11; 2012,Dec,6-8

15650 Transfer, intermediate, of any pedicle flap (eg, abdomen to wrist, Walking tube), any location

EXCLUDES Defatting, revision, or rearranging of transferred pedicle flap or skin graft (13100-14302)
Eyelids, ears, lips, and nose - refer to anatomical area

10.9 14.2 **FUD** 090 T A2 80

AMA: 2016,Jan,13; 2015,Jan,16; 2014,Jan,11; 2012,Dec,6-8

15731 Forehead flap with preservation of vascular pedicle (eg, axial pattern flap, paramedian forehead flap)

EXCLUDES Muscle, myocutaneous, or fasciocutaneous flap of the head or neck (15732)

28.9 32.1 **FUD** 090 T A2 80

AMA: 2016,Jan,13; 2015,Jan,16; 2014,Jan,11; 2012,Dec,6-8

15732-15738 Wound Reconstruction: Muscle Flaps

INCLUDES Code based on donor site
EXCLUDES Contiguous tissue transfer flaps (14000-14302)
Microvascular repair (15756-15758)
Code also application of extensive immobilization apparatus
Code also repair of donor site with skin grafts or flaps

15732 Muscle, myocutaneous, or fasciocutaneous flap; head and neck (eg, temporalis, masseter muscle, sternocleidomastoid, levator scapulae)

EXCLUDES Forehead flap with preservation of vascular pedicle (15731)
🚗 32.0   ⚕ 36.6   **FUD** 090   T A2 ▢

AMA: 2016,Jan,13; 2015,Jan,16; 2014,Jan,11; 2012,Dec,6-8

15734 trunk
🚗 37.9   ⚕ 42.9   **FUD** 090   T A2 80 ▢

AMA: 2016,Jan,13; 2015,Jan,16; 2014,Apr,10; 2014,Jan,11; 2013,Oct,15; 2012,Dec,6-8

15736 upper extremity
🚗 32.7   ⚕ 37.7   **FUD** 090   T A2 ▢

AMA: 2016,Jan,13; 2015,Jan,16; 2014,Jan,11; 2013,Mar,13; 2012,Dec,6-8

15738 lower extremity
🚗 35.4   ⚕ 40.0   **FUD** 090   T A2 80 ▢

AMA: 2016,Jan,13; 2015,Jan,16; 2014,Jan,11; 2012,Dec,6-8; 2012,Jan,15-42; 2011,Jan,11

15740-15758 Wound Reconstruction: Other

INCLUDES Fixation and anchoring skin graft
Routine dressing
Simple tissue debridement
EXCLUDES Adjacent tissue transfer (14000-14302)
Excision of:
Benign lesion (11400-11471)
Burn eschar or scar (15002-15005)
Malignant lesion (11600-11646)
Flaps without addition of a vascular pedicle (15570-15576)
Primary procedure--see appropriate anatomical section
Skin graft for repair of donor site (15050-15278)
Code also repair of donor site with skin grafts or flaps (14000-14350, 15050-15278)

15740 Flap; island pedicle requiring identification and dissection of an anatomically named axial vessel

EXCLUDES V-Y subcutaneous flaps, random island flaps, and other flaps from adjacent areas (14000-14302)
🚗 24.5   ⚕ 29.0   **FUD** 090   T A2 ▢

AMA: 2016,Jan,13; 2015,Jan,16; 2014,Jan,11; 2012,Dec,6-8; 2012,Jan,15-42; 2011,Jan,11

15750 neurovascular pedicle

EXCLUDES V-Y subcutaneous flaps, random island flaps, and other flaps from adjacent areas (14000-14302)
🚗 26.3   ⚕ 26.3   **FUD** 090   T A2 80 ▢

AMA: 2010,Apr,3-4; 2002,Nov,5

15756 Free muscle or myocutaneous flap with microvascular anastomosis

INCLUDES Operating microscope (69990)
🚗 67.0   ⚕ 67.0   **FUD** 090   C 80 ▢

AMA: 2016,Feb,12; 2016,Jan,13; 2015,Jan,16; 2014,Jan,11

15757 Free skin flap with microvascular anastomosis

INCLUDES Operating microscope (69990)
🚗 66.2   ⚕ 66.2   **FUD** 090   C 80 ▢

AMA: 2016,Apr,8; 2016,Feb,12; 2016,Jan,13; 2015,Jan,16; 2014,Jan,11

15758 Free fascial flap with microvascular anastomosis

INCLUDES Operating microscope (69990)
🚗 66.3   ⚕ 66.3   **FUD** 090   C 80 ▢

AMA: 2016,Feb,12; 2016,Jan,13; 2015,Jan,16; 2014,Jan,11

15760-15770 Grafts Comprising Multiple Tissue Types

INCLUDES Fixation and anchoring skin graft
Routine dressing
Simple tissue debridement
EXCLUDES Adjacent tissue transfer (14000-14302)
Excision of:
Benign lesion (11400-11471)
Burn eschar or scar (15002-15005)
Malignant lesion (11600-11646)
Flaps without addition of vascular pedicle (15570-15576)
Microvascular repair (15756-15758)
Primary procedure (see appropriate anatomical site)
Repair of donor site with skin grafts or flaps (14000-14350, 15050-15278)

15760 Graft; composite (eg, full thickness of external ear or nasal ala), including primary closure, donor area
🚗 20.3   ⚕ 24.3   **FUD** 090   T A2 ▢

AMA: 2016,Jan,13; 2015,Jan,16; 2014,Jan,11

15770 derma-fat-fascia
🚗 19.2   ⚕ 19.2   **FUD** 090   T A2 80 ▢

AMA: 2016,Jan,13; 2015,Jan,16; 2014,Jan,11

15775-15839 Plastic, Reconstructive, and Aesthetic Surgery

CMS: 100-02,16,10 Exclusions from Coverage; 100-02,16,120 Cosmetic Procedures; 100-02,16,180 Services Related to Noncovered Procedures

15775 Punch graft for hair transplant; 1 to 15 punch grafts

EXCLUDES Strip transplant (15220)
🚗 6.42   ⚕ 8.56   **FUD** 000   T A2 80 ▢

AMA: 2016,Jan,13; 2015,Jan,16; 2014,Jan,11

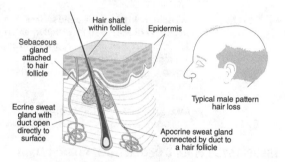

Hair shaft within follicle
Epidermis
Sebaceous gland attached to hair follicle
Ecrine sweat gland with duct open directly to surface
Apocrine sweat gland connected by duct to a hair follicle
Typical male pattern hair loss

15776 more than 15 punch grafts

EXCLUDES Strip transplant (15220)
🚗 10.2   ⚕ 14.1   **FUD** 000   T A2 80 ▢

AMA: 2016,Jan,13; 2015,Jan,16; 2014,Jan,11

+ **15777** Implantation of biologic implant (eg, acellular dermal matrix) for soft tissue reinforcement (ie, breast, trunk) (List separately in addition to code for primary procedure)

EXCLUDES Application of skin substitute (high cost) to an external wound (15271-15278)
Application of skin substitute (low cost) to an external wound (C5271-C5278)
Mesh implantation for:
Open repair of ventral or incisional hernia (49568)
Repair of devitalized soft tissue infection (49568)
Repair of pelvic floor (57267)
Repair anorectal fistula with plug (46707)
Soft tissue reinforcement with biologic implants other than in the breast or trunk (17999)
Code also synthetic or non-biological implant to reinforce abdominal wall (0437T)
Code also supply of biologic implant
Code first primary procedure
🚗 6.16   ⚕ 6.16   **FUD** ZZZ   N N1 50 ▢

AMA: 2016,Jan,13; 2015,Jan,16; 2014,Jan,11; 2013,Oct,15; 2012,Jan,6-10

15780 Dermabrasion; total face (eg, for acne scarring, fine wrinkling, rhytids, general keratosis)
🚗 18.1   ⚕ 23.9   **FUD** 090   T P3 80 ▢

AMA: 2016,Jan,13; 2015,Jan,16; 2014,Jan,11; 2012,Jan,15-42; 2011,Jan,11

15781 segmental, face
🚗 12.4 ✂ 15.7 **FUD** 090 T P2 ▢
AMA: 1997,Nov,1

15782 regional, other than face
🚗 12.7 ✂ 18.0 **FUD** 090 T P3 80 ▢
AMA: 1997,Nov,1

15783 superficial, any site (eg, tattoo removal)
🚗 10.3 ✂ 13.2 **FUD** 090 T P2 80 ▢
AMA: 2016,Jan,13; 2015,Jan,16; 2014,Jan,11

15786 Abrasion; single lesion (eg, keratosis, scar)
🚗 3.89 ✂ 6.93 **FUD** 010 Q1 N1 ▢
AMA: 1997,Nov,1

+ **15787** each additional 4 lesions or less (List separately in addition to code for primary procedure)
Code first (15786)
🚗 0.50 ✂ 1.39 **FUD** ZZZ N N1 ▢
AMA: 1997,Nov,1

15788 Chemical peel, facial; epidermal
🚗 7.07 ✂ 13.0 **FUD** 090 Q1 N1 ▢
AMA: 1997,Nov,1; 1993,Win,1

15789 dermal
🚗 11.8 ✂ 15.5 **FUD** 090 T P2 ▢
AMA: 1997,Nov,1; 1993,Win,1

15792 Chemical peel, nonfacial; epidermal
🚗 7.53 ✂ 12.5 **FUD** 090 Q1 N1 80 ▢
AMA: 1997,Nov,1; 1993,Win,1

15793 dermal
🚗 10.5 ✂ 13.9 **FUD** 090 Q1 N1 80 ▢
AMA: 1997,Nov,1; 1993,Win,1

15819 Cervicoplasty
🚗 21.1 ✂ 21.1 **FUD** 090 T G2 80 ▢
AMA: 1997,Nov,1

15820 Blepharoplasty, lower eyelid;
🚗 14.4 ✂ 15.9 **FUD** 090 T A2 80 50 ▢
AMA: 2016,Jan,13; 2015,Jan,16; 2014,Jan,11; 2012,Jan,15-42; 2011,Jan,11

15821 with extensive herniated fat pad
🚗 15.4 ✂ 17.1 **FUD** 090 T A2 80 50 ▢
AMA: 2016,Jan,13; 2015,Jan,16; 2014,Jan,11

15822 Blepharoplasty, upper eyelid;
🚗 11.1 ✂ 12.6 **FUD** 090 T A2 50 ▢
AMA: 2016,Jan,13; 2015,Jan,16; 2014,Jan,11

15823 with excessive skin weighting down lid
🚗 15.4 ✂ 17.1 **FUD** 090 T A2 50 ▢
AMA: 2016,Jan,13; 2015,Jan,16; 2014,Jan,11; 2011,Aug,8

15824 Rhytidectomy; forehead
EXCLUDES Repair of brow ptosis (67900)
🚗 0.00 ✂ 0.00 **FUD** 000 T A2 80 50 ▢
AMA: 1997,Nov,1

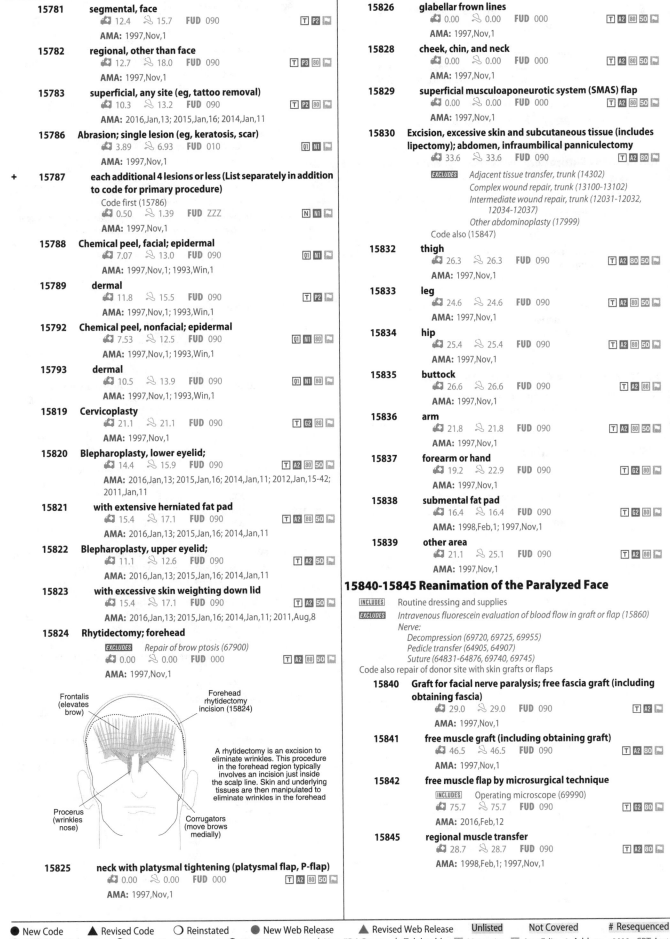

Frontalis (elevates brow)

Forehead rhytidectomy incision (15824)

A rhytidectomy is an excision to eliminate wrinkles. This procedure in the forehead region typically involves an incision just inside the scalp line. Skin and underlying tissues are then manipulated to eliminate wrinkles in the forehead

Procerus (wrinkles nose)

Corrugators (move brows medially)

15825 neck with platysmal tightening (platysmal flap, P-flap)
🚗 0.00 ✂ 0.00 **FUD** 000 T A2 80 50 ▢
AMA: 1997,Nov,1

15826 glabellar frown lines
🚗 0.00 ✂ 0.00 **FUD** 000 T A2 80 50 ▢
AMA: 1997,Nov,1

15828 cheek, chin, and neck
🚗 0.00 ✂ 0.00 **FUD** 000 T A2 80 50 ▢
AMA: 1997,Nov,1

15829 superficial musculoaponeurotic system (SMAS) flap
🚗 0.00 ✂ 0.00 **FUD** 000 T A2 80 50 ▢
AMA: 1997,Nov,1

15830 Excision, excessive skin and subcutaneous tissue (includes lipectomy); abdomen, infraumbilical panniculectomy
🚗 33.6 ✂ 33.6 **FUD** 090 T A2 80 ▢
EXCLUDES Adjacent tissue transfer, trunk (14302)
Complex wound repair, trunk (13100-13102)
Intermediate wound repair, trunk (12031-12032, 12034-12037)
Other abdominoplasty (17999)
Code also (15847)

15832 thigh
🚗 26.3 ✂ 26.3 **FUD** 090 T A2 80 50 ▢
AMA: 1997,Nov,1

15833 leg
🚗 24.6 ✂ 24.6 **FUD** 090 T A2 80 50 ▢
AMA: 1997,Nov,1

15834 hip
🚗 25.4 ✂ 25.4 **FUD** 090 T A2 80 50 ▢
AMA: 1997,Nov,1

15835 buttock
🚗 26.6 ✂ 26.6 **FUD** 090 T A2 80 ▢
AMA: 1997,Nov,1

15836 arm
🚗 21.8 ✂ 21.8 **FUD** 090 T A2 80 50 ▢
AMA: 1997,Nov,1

15837 forearm or hand
🚗 19.2 ✂ 22.9 **FUD** 090 T G2 80 ▢
AMA: 1997,Nov,1

15838 submental fat pad
🚗 16.4 ✂ 16.4 **FUD** 090 T G2 80 ▢
AMA: 1998,Feb,1; 1997,Nov,1

15839 other area
🚗 21.1 ✂ 25.1 **FUD** 090 T A2 80 ▢
AMA: 1997,Nov,1

15840-15845 Reanimation of the Paralyzed Face

INCLUDES Routine dressing and supplies
EXCLUDES Intravenous fluorescein evaluation of blood flow in graft or flap (15860)
Nerve:
Decompression (69720, 69725, 69955)
Pedicle transfer (64905, 64907)
Suture (64831-64876, 69740, 69745)
Code also repair of donor site with skin grafts or flaps

15840 Graft for facial nerve paralysis; free fascia graft (including obtaining fascia)
🚗 29.0 ✂ 29.0 **FUD** 090 T A2 ▢
AMA: 1997,Nov,1

15841 free muscle graft (including obtaining graft)
🚗 46.5 ✂ 46.5 **FUD** 090 T A2 80 ▢
AMA: 1997,Nov,1

15842 free muscle flap by microsurgical technique
INCLUDES Operating microscope (69990)
🚗 75.7 ✂ 75.7 **FUD** 090 T G2 80 ▢
AMA: 2016,Feb,12

15845 regional muscle transfer
🚗 28.7 ✂ 28.7 **FUD** 090 T A2 80 ▢
AMA: 1998,Feb,1; 1997,Nov,1

15847 Removal of Excess Abdominal Tissue Add-on

CMS: 100-02,16,10 Exclusions from Coverage; 100-02,16,120 Cosmetic Procedures; 100-02,16,180 Services Related to Noncovered Procedures

+ **15847** **Excision, excessive skin and subcutaneous tissue (includes lipectomy), abdomen (eg, abdominoplasty) (includes umbilical transposition and fascial plication) (List separately in addition to code for primary procedure)**

    🚑 0.00   ✂ 0.00   **FUD** YYY   N N1 80 ▢

    EXCLUDES Abdominal wall hernia repair (49491-49587)
         Other abdominoplasty (17999)
     Code first (15830)

15850-15852 Suture Removal/Dressing Change: Anesthesia Required

15850 **Removal of sutures under anesthesia (other than local), same surgeon**

    🚑 1.19   ✂ 2.52   **FUD** XXX   T G2 ▢

    AMA: 2016,Jan,13; 2015,Jan,16; 2014,Jan,11

15851 **Removal of sutures under anesthesia (other than local), other surgeon**

    🚑 1.31   ✂ 2.80   **FUD** 000   T P3 ▢

    AMA: 2016,Jan,13; 2015,Jan,16; 2014,Jan,11

15852 **Dressing change (for other than burns) under anesthesia (other than local)**

    EXCLUDES Dressing change for burns (16020-16030)

    🚑 1.35   ✂ 1.35   **FUD** 000   Q1 N1 ▢

    AMA: 1997,Nov,1

15860 Injection for Vascular Flow Determination

15860 **Intravenous injection of agent (eg, fluorescein) to test vascular flow in flap or graft**

    🚑 3.19   ✂ 3.19   **FUD** 000   Q1 N1 80 ▢

    AMA: 2002,May,7; 1997,Nov,1

15876-15879 Liposuction

CMS: 100-02,16,10 Exclusions from Coverage; 100-02,16,120 Cosmetic Procedures; 100-02,16,180 Services Related to Noncovered Procedures

15876 **Suction assisted lipectomy; head and neck**

    🚑 0.00   ✂ 0.00   **FUD** 000   T A2 80 ▢

    AMA: 1997,Nov,1

Cannula typically inserted through incision in front of ear

15877 **trunk**

    🚑 0.00   ✂ 0.00   **FUD** 000   T A2 80 ▢

    AMA: 2016,Jan,13; 2015,Jan,16; 2014,Jan,11; 2012,Jan,15-42; 2011,Jan,11

15878 **upper extremity**

    🚑 0.00   ✂ 0.00   **FUD** 000   T A2 80 50 ▢

    AMA: 1997,Nov,1

15879 **lower extremity**

    🚑 0.00   ✂ 0.00   **FUD** 000   T A2 80 50 ▢

    AMA: 1997,Nov,1

15920-15999 Treatment of Decubitus Ulcers

Code also free skin graft to repair ulcer or donor site

15920 **Excision, coccygeal pressure ulcer, with coccygectomy; with primary suture**

    🚑 17.3   ✂ 17.3   **FUD** 090   T A2 80 ▢

    AMA: 2011,May,3-5

15922 **with flap closure**

    🚑 22.3   ✂ 22.3   **FUD** 090   T A2 80 ▢

    AMA: 2011,May,3-5

15931 **Excision, sacral pressure ulcer, with primary suture;**

    🚑 19.7   ✂ 19.7   **FUD** 090   T A2 ▢

    AMA: 2011,May,3-5

15933 **with ostectomy**

    🚑 24.3   ✂ 24.3   **FUD** 090   T A2 80 ▢

    AMA: 2011,May,3-5

15934 **Excision, sacral pressure ulcer, with skin flap closure;**

    🚑 26.6   ✂ 26.6   **FUD** 090   T A2 ▢

    AMA: 2011,May,3-5

15935 **with ostectomy**

    🚑 31.3   ✂ 31.3   **FUD** 090   T A2 80 ▢

    AMA: 2011,May,3-5

15936 **Excision, sacral pressure ulcer, in preparation for muscle or myocutaneous flap or skin graft closure;**

    Code also any defect repair with:
       Muscle or myocutaneous flap (15734, 15738)
       Split skin graft (15100-15101)

    🚑 25.5   ✂ 25.5   **FUD** 090   T A2 ▢

    AMA: 2011,May,3-5

15937 **with ostectomy**

    Code also any defect repair with:
       Muscle or myocutaneous flap (15734, 15738)
       Split skin graft (15100-15101)

    🚑 29.6   ✂ 29.6   **FUD** 090   T A2 ▢

    AMA: 2011,May,3-5

15940 **Excision, ischial pressure ulcer, with primary suture;**

    🚑 20.1   ✂ 20.1   **FUD** 090   T A2 ▢

    AMA: 2011,May,3-5

15941 **with ostectomy (ischiectomy)**

    🚑 25.7   ✂ 25.7   **FUD** 090   T A2 80 ▢

    AMA: 2011,May,3-5

15944 **Excision, ischial pressure ulcer, with skin flap closure;**

    🚑 25.4   ✂ 25.4   **FUD** 090   T A2 80 ▢

    AMA: 2011,May,3-5

15945 **with ostectomy**

    🚑 27.9   ✂ 27.9   **FUD** 090   T A2 80 ▢

    AMA: 2011,May,3-5

15946 **Excision, ischial pressure ulcer, with ostectomy, in preparation for muscle or myocutaneous flap or skin graft closure**

    Code also any defect repair with:
       Muscle or myocutaneous flap (15734, 15738)
       Split skin graft (15100-15101)

    🚑 46.9   ✂ 46.9   **FUD** 090   T A2 ▢

    AMA: 2016,Jan,13; 2015,Jan,16; 2014,Jan,11; 2012,Jan,15-42; 2011,May,3-5; 2011,Jan,11

15950 **Excision, trochanteric pressure ulcer, with primary suture;**

    🚑 16.9   ✂ 16.9   **FUD** 090   T A2 ▢

    AMA: 2011,May,3-5

15951 **with ostectomy**

    🚑 25.1   ✂ 25.1   **FUD** 090   T A2 80 ▢

    AMA: 2011,May,3-5

15952 **Excision, trochanteric pressure ulcer, with skin flap closure;**

    🚑 25.6   ✂ 25.6   **FUD** 090   T A2 80 ▢

    AMA: 2011,May,3-5

15953 **with ostectomy**

    🚑 28.4   ✂ 28.4   **FUD** 090   T A2 ▢

    AMA: 2011,May,3-5

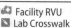

26/TC PC/TC Only   A2-Z3 ASC Payment   50 Bilateral   ♂ Male Only   ♀ Female Only   🚑 Facility RVU   ✂ Non-Facility RVU   ▢ CCI
FUD Follow-up Days   **CMS:** IOM (Pub 100)   A-Y OPPSI   80/80 Surg Assist Allowed / w/Doc   🔬 Lab Crosswalk   📷 Radiology Crosswalk   ✖ CLIA

15956 Excision, trochanteric pressure ulcer, in preparation for muscle or myocutaneous flap or skin graft closure;
  Code also any defect repair with:
    Muscle or myocutaneous flap (15734, 15738)
    Split skin graft (15100-15101)
  🔳 33.0 ⚖ 33.0 **FUD** 090   T A2 ▯
  AMA: 2011,May,3-5

15958 with ostectomy
  Code also any defect repair with:
    Muscle or myocutaneous flap (15734-15738)
    Split skin graft (15100-15101)
  🔳 33.6 ⚖ 33.6 **FUD** 090   T A2 ▯
  AMA: 2011,May,3-5

15999 Unlisted procedure, excision pressure ulcer
  🔳 0.00 ⚖ 0.00 **FUD** YYY   T 80 ▯
  AMA: 2011,May,3-5

16000-16036 Burn Care

INCLUDES Local care of burn surface only
EXCLUDES Application of skin grafts including all services described in the following codes (15100-15777)
E&M services
Flaps (15570-15650)

16000 Initial treatment, first degree burn, when no more than local treatment is required
  🔳 1.32 ⚖ 1.95 **FUD** 000   01 N1 ▯
  AMA: 2016,Jan,13; 2015,Jan,16; 2014,Jan,11; 2012,Oct,3-8

Head and neck 9%
Head and neck 9%
Each arm 9%
Posterior trunk 18%
Anterior trunk 18%
Genitalia 1%
Posterior leg 9%
Anterior leg 9%
9 9 9 9 9 9 9 9 9

16020 Dressings and/or debridement of partial-thickness burns, initial or subsequent; small (less than 5% total body surface area)
  INCLUDES Wound coverage other than skin graft
  🔳 1.55 ⚖ 2.31 **FUD** 000   01 N1 ▯
  AMA: 2016,Jan,13; 2015,Jan,16; 2014,Jan,11; 2012,Oct,3-8

16025 medium (eg, whole face or whole extremity, or 5% to 10% total body surface area)
  INCLUDES Wound coverage other than skin graft
  🔳 3.19 ⚖ 4.18 **FUD** 000   T A2 ▯
  AMA: 2016,Jan,13; 2015,Jan,16; 2014,Jan,11; 2012,Oct,3-8; 2012,Jan,15-42; 2011,Jan,11

16030 large (eg, more than 1 extremity, or greater than 10% total body surface area)
  INCLUDES Wound coverage other than skin graft
  🔳 3.84 ⚖ 5.27 **FUD** 000   T A2 ▯
  AMA: 2016,Jan,13; 2015,Jan,16; 2014,Jan,11; 2012,Oct,3-8; 2012,Jan,15-42; 2011,Jan,11

16035 Escharotomy; initial incision
  EXCLUDES Debridement or scraping of burn (16020-16030)
  🔳 5.61 ⚖ 5.61 **FUD** 000   T 62 ▯
  AMA: 2016,Jan,13; 2015,Jan,16; 2014,Jan,11; 2012,Oct,3-8

+ **16036** each additional incision (List separately in addition to code for primary procedure)
  EXCLUDES Debridement or scraping of burn (16020-16030)
  Code first (16035)
  🔳 2.33 ⚖ 2.33 **FUD** ZZZ   C ▯
  AMA: 2016,Jan,13; 2015,Jan,16; 2014,Jan,11; 2012,Oct,3-8

17000-17004 Destruction Any Method: Premalignant Lesion

CMS: 100-03,140.5 Laser Procedures
EXCLUDES Cryotherapy acne (17340)
Destruction of:
  Benign lesions other than cutaneous vascular proliferative lesions (17110-17111)
  Cutaneous vascular proliferative lesions (17106-17108)
  Malignant lesions (17260-17286)
  Plantar warts (17110-17111)
Destruction of lesion of:
  Anus (46900-46917, 46924)
  Conjunctiva (68135)
  Eyelid (67850)
  Penis (54050-54057, 54065)
  Vagina (57061, 57065)
  Vestibule of mouth (40820)
  Vulva (56501, 56515)
Destruction or excision of skin tags (11200-11201)
Localized chemotherapy treatment see appropriate office visit service code
Paring or excision of benign hyperkeratotic lesion (11055-11057)
Shaving skin lesions (11300-11313)
Treatment of inflammatory skin disease via laser (96920-96922)

17000 Destruction (eg, laser surgery, electrosurgery, cryosurgery, chemosurgery, surgical curettement), premalignant lesions (eg, actinic keratoses); first lesion
  🔳 1.52 ⚖ 1.89 **FUD** 010   01 N1 ▯
  AMA: 2016,Apr,3; 2016,Jan,13; 2015,Jan,16; 2014,Jan,11; 2012,May,13; 2012,Mar,4-7; 2012,Jan,15-42; 2011,Jan,11

+ **17003** second through 14 lesions, each (List separately in addition to code for first lesion)
  Code first (17000)
  🔳 0.07 ⚖ 0.16 **FUD** ZZZ   N N1 ▯
  AMA: 2016,Apr,3; 2016,Jan,13; 2015,Jan,16; 2014,Jan,11; 2012,May,13; 2012,Jan,15-42; 2011,Jan,11

17004 Destruction (eg, laser surgery, electrosurgery, cryosurgery, chemosurgery, surgical curettement), premalignant lesions (eg, actinic keratoses), 15 or more lesions
  EXCLUDES Use of code for destruction of less than 15 lesions (17000-17003)
  🔳 2.86 ⚖ 4.25 **FUD** 010   🚫 T P3 ▯
  AMA: 2016,Apr,3; 2016,Jan,13; 2015,Jan,16; 2014,Jan,11; 2012,May,13; 2012,Jan,15-42; 2011,Jan,11

17106-17250 Destruction Any Method: Vascular Proliferative Lesion

CMS: 100-02,16,10 Exclusions from Coverage; 100-02,16,120 Cosmetic Procedures
EXCLUDES Destruction of lesion of:
  Anus (46900-46917, 46924)
  Conjunctiva (68135)
  Eyelid (67850)
  Penis (54050-54057, 54065)
  Vagina (57061, 57065)
  Vestibule of mouth (40820)
  Vulva (56501, 56515)
Treatment of inflammatory skin disease via laser (96920-96922)

17106 Destruction of cutaneous vascular proliferative lesions (eg, laser technique); less than 10 sq cm
  🔳 7.90 ⚖ 9.68 **FUD** 090   T P3 ▯
  AMA: 2016,Apr,3; 2016,Jan,13; 2015,Jan,16; 2014,Jan,11; 2012,May,13; 2012,Jan,15-42; 2011,Jan,11

17107 10.0 to 50.0 sq cm
  🔳 9.94 ⚖ 12.3 **FUD** 090   T P2 ▯
  AMA: 2016,Apr,3; 2016,Jan,13; 2015,Jan,16; 2014,Jan,11; 2012,May,13; 2012,Jan,15-42; 2011,Jan,11

17108 over 50.0 sq cm
  🔳 15.0 ⚖ 18.1 **FUD** 090   T P3 80 ▯
  AMA: 2016,Apr,3; 2016,Jan,13; 2015,Jan,16; 2014,Jan,11; 2012,May,13; 2012,Jan,15-42; 2011,Jan,11

Integumentary System

17110 — 17312

17110 **Destruction (eg, laser surgery, electrosurgery, cryosurgery, chemosurgery, surgical curettement), of benign lesions other than skin tags or cutaneous vascular proliferative lesions; up to 14 lesions**
   1.99   3.13   **FUD** 010   [0] [M1] [▱]
   AMA: 2016,Apr,3; 2016,Jan,13; 2015,Jan,16; 2014,Jan,11; 2012,May,13; 2012,Jan,15-42; 2011,Jan,11

17111 **15 or more lesions**
   EXCLUDES   Destruction of neurofibromas, 50-100 lesions (0419T-0420T)
   2.45   3.71   **FUD** 010   [0] [M1] [▱]
   AMA: 2016,Apr,3; 2016,Jan,13; 2015,Jan,16; 2014,Jan,11; 2012,May,13; 2012,Jan,15-42; 2011,Jan,11

17250 **Chemical cauterization of granulation tissue (proud flesh, sinus or fistula)**
   EXCLUDES   Excision/removal codes for the same lesion
   1.06   2.24   **FUD** 000   [0] [M1] [▱]
   AMA: 2016,Jan,13; 2015,Jan,16; 2014,Jan,11; 2012,Dec,12; 2012,May,13; 2012,Jan,15-42; 2011,Jan,11

17260-17286 Destruction, Any Method: Malignant Lesion

CMS: 100-03,140.5 Laser Procedures

EXCLUDES   Destruction of lesion of:
   Anus (46900-46917, 46924)
   Conjunctiva (68135)
   Eyelid (67850)
   Penis (54050-54057, 54065)
   Vestibule of mouth (40820)
   Vulva (56501-56515)
   Localized chemotherapy treatment see appropriate office visit service code
   Shaving skin lesion (11300-11313)
   Treatment of inflammatory skin disease via laser (96920-96922)

17260 **Destruction, malignant lesion (eg, laser surgery, electrosurgery, cryosurgery, chemosurgery, surgical curettement), trunk, arms or legs; lesion diameter 0.5 cm or less**
   2.01   2.68   **FUD** 010   [0] [M1] [▱]
   AMA: 2016,Jan,13; 2015,Jan,16; 2014,Jan,11; 2012,May,13

17261 **lesion diameter 0.6 to 1.0 cm**
   2.62   4.06   **FUD** 010   [0] [M1] [▱]
   AMA: 2016,Jan,13; 2015,Jan,16; 2014,Jan,11; 2012,May,13

17262 **lesion diameter 1.1 to 2.0 cm**
   3.34   4.95   **FUD** 010   [0] [M1] [▱]
   AMA: 2016,Jan,13; 2015,Jan,16; 2014,Jan,11; 2012,May,13

17263 **lesion diameter 2.1 to 3.0 cm**
   3.71   5.41   **FUD** 010   [0] [M1] [▱]
   AMA: 2016,Jan,13; 2015,Jan,16; 2014,Jan,11; 2012,May,13

17264 **lesion diameter 3.1 to 4.0 cm**
   3.96   5.80   **FUD** 010   [T] [P2] [▱]
   AMA: 2016,Jan,13; 2015,Jan,16; 2014,Jan,11; 2012,May,13

17266 **lesion diameter over 4.0 cm**
   4.63   6.58   **FUD** 010   [T] [P3] [▱]
   AMA: 2016,Jan,13; 2015,Jan,16; 2014,Jan,11; 2012,May,13

17270 **Destruction, malignant lesion (eg, laser surgery, electrosurgery, cryosurgery, chemosurgery, surgical curettement), scalp, neck, hands, feet, genitalia; lesion diameter 0.5 cm or less**
   2.86   4.26   **FUD** 010   [T] [P3] [▱]
   AMA: 2016,Jan,13; 2015,Jan,16; 2014,Jan,11; 2012,May,13

17271 **lesion diameter 0.6 to 1.0 cm**
   3.18   4.61   **FUD** 010   [T] [P3] [▱]
   AMA: 2016,Jan,13; 2015,Jan,16; 2014,Jan,11; 2012,May,13

17272 **lesion diameter 1.1 to 2.0 cm**
   3.68   5.27   **FUD** 010   [0] [M1] [▱]
   AMA: 2016,Jan,13; 2015,Jan,16; 2014,Jan,11; 2012,May,13

17273 **lesion diameter 2.1 to 3.0 cm**
   4.15   5.88   **FUD** 010   [T] [P3] [▱]
   AMA: 2016,Jan,13; 2015,Jan,16; 2014,Jan,11; 2012,May,13

17274 **lesion diameter 3.1 to 4.0 cm**
   5.07   6.95   **FUD** 010   [T] [P3] [▱]
   AMA: 2016,Jan,13; 2015,Jan,16; 2014,Jan,11; 2012,May,13

17276 **lesion diameter over 4.0 cm**
   6.09   8.05   **FUD** 010   [T] [P3] [▱]
   AMA: 2016,Jan,13; 2015,Jan,16; 2014,Jan,11; 2012,May,13

17280 **Destruction, malignant lesion (eg, laser surgery, electrosurgery, cryosurgery, chemosurgery, surgical curettement), face, ears, eyelids, nose, lips, mucous membrane; lesion diameter 0.5 cm or less**
   2.60   3.98   **FUD** 010   [0] [M1] [▱]
   AMA: 2016,Jan,13; 2015,Jan,16; 2014,Jan,11; 2012,May,13

17281 **lesion diameter 0.6 to 1.0 cm**
   3.58   5.03   **FUD** 010   [T] [P3] [▱]
   AMA: 2016,Jan,13; 2015,Jan,16; 2014,Jan,11; 2012,May,13

17282 **lesion diameter 1.1 to 2.0 cm**
   4.14   5.79   **FUD** 010   [T] [P3] [▱]
   AMA: 2016,Jan,13; 2015,Jan,16; 2014,Jan,11; 2012,May,13

17283 **lesion diameter 2.1 to 3.0 cm**
   5.17   6.93   **FUD** 010   [T] [P2] [▱]
   AMA: 2016,Jan,13; 2015,Jan,16; 2014,Jan,11; 2012,May,13

17284 **lesion diameter 3.1 to 4.0 cm**
   6.03   7.92   **FUD** 010   [T] [P2] [▱]
   AMA: 2016,Jan,13; 2015,Jan,16; 2014,Jan,11; 2012,May,13

17286 **lesion diameter over 4.0 cm**
   8.09   10.1   **FUD** 010   [T] [P2] [▱]
   AMA: 2016,Jan,13; 2015,Jan,16; 2014,Jan,11; 2012,May,13

17311-17315 Mohs Surgery

INCLUDES   The following surgical/pathology services performed by the same physician or other qualified health care provider:
   Evaluation of skin margins by surgeon
   Pathology exam on Mohs surgery specimen (88302-88309)
   Routine frozen section stain (88314)
   Tumor removal, mapping, preparation, and examination of lesion

EXCLUDES   Frozen section if no prior diagnosis determination has been performed (88331)
Code also any special histochemical stain on a frozen section, nonroutine (with modifier 59) (88311-88314, 88342)
Code also biopsy (with modifier 59) if no prior diagnosis determination has been performed, if biopsy is indeterminate, or performed more than 90 days preoperatively (11100-11101)
Code also complex repair (13100-13160)
Code also flaps or grafts (14000-14350, 15050-15770)
Code also intermediate repair (12031-12057)
Code also simple repair (12001-12021)

17311 **Mohs micrographic technique, including removal of all gross tumor, surgical excision of tissue specimens, mapping, color coding of specimens, microscopic examination of specimens by the surgeon, and histopathologic preparation including routine stain(s) (eg, hematoxylin and eosin, toluidine blue), head, neck, hands, feet, genitalia, or any location with surgery directly involving muscle, cartilage, bone, tendon, major nerves, or vessels; first stage, up to 5 tissue blocks**
   10.9   18.7   **FUD** 000   [T] [P2] [▱]
   AMA: 2016,Jan,13; 2015,Jan,16; 2014,Oct,14; 2014,Feb,10; 2012,May,13

+ **17312** **each additional stage after the first stage, up to 5 tissue blocks (List separately in addition to code for primary procedure)**
   Code first (17311)
   5.80   11.0   **FUD** ZZZ   [N] [M1] [▱]
   AMA: 2016,Jan,13; 2015,Jan,16; 2014,Oct,14; 2014,Feb,10; 2012,May,13

[26]/[TC] PC/TC Only   [A2-Z3] ASC Payment   [50] Bilateral   ♂ Male Only   ♀ Female Only   ⌖ Facility RVU   ⌖ Non-Facility RVU   [▱] CCI
FUD Follow-up Days   **CMS:** IOM (Pub 100)   [A-Y] OPPSI   [80]/[80] Surg Assist Allowed / w/Doc   ⌖ Lab Crosswalk   ⌖ Radiology Crosswalk   [X] CLIA

32   CPT © 2016 American Medical Association. All Rights Reserved.   © 2016 Optum360, LLC

17313 Mohs micrographic technique, including removal of all gross tumor, surgical excision of tissue specimens, mapping, color coding of specimens, microscopic examination of specimens by the surgeon, and histopathologic preparation including routine stain(s) (eg, hematoxylin and eosin, toluidine blue), of the trunk, arms, or legs; first stage, up to 5 tissue blocks

📷 9.78   ⚕ 17.5   **FUD** 000   T P2 ▦

AMA: 2016,Jan,13; 2015,Jan,16; 2014,Oct,14; 2014,Feb,10; 2012,May,13

\+ **17314** each additional stage after the first stage, up to 5 tissue blocks (List separately in addition to code for primary procedure)

Code first (17313)

📷 5.38   ⚕ 10.5   **FUD** ZZZ   N N1 ▦

AMA: 2016,Jan,13; 2015,Jan,16; 2014,Oct,14; 2014,Feb,10; 2012,May,13

\+ **17315** Mohs micrographic technique, including removal of all gross tumor, surgical excision of tissue specimens, mapping, color coding of specimens, microscopic examination of specimens by the surgeon, and histopathologic preparation including routine stain(s) (eg, hematoxylin and eosin, toluidine blue), each additional block after the first 5 tissue blocks, any stage (List separately in addition to code for primary procedure)

Code first (17311-17314)

📷 1.53   ⚕ 2.26   **FUD** ZZZ   N N1 ▦

AMA: 2016,Jan,13; 2015,Jan,16; 2014,Oct,14; 2014,Feb,10; 2014,Jan,11; 2012,May,13

17340-17999 Treatment for Active Acne and Permanent Hair Removal

CMS: 100-02,16,10 Exclusions from Coverage; 100-02,16,120 Cosmetic Procedures

17340 Cryotherapy (CO2 slush, liquid N2) for acne

📷 1.40   ⚕ 1.46   **FUD** 010   Q1 N1 ▦

AMA: 2016,Jan,13; 2015,Jan,16; 2014,Jan,11; 2012,May,13

17360 Chemical exfoliation for acne (eg, acne paste, acid)

📷 2.82   ⚕ 3.65   **FUD** 010   Q1 N1 ▦

AMA: 2016,Jan,13; 2015,Jan,16; 2014,Jan,11; 2012,May,13

17380 Electrolysis epilation, each 30 minutes

EXCLUDES Actinotherapy (96900)

📷 0.00   ⚕ 0.00   **FUD** 000   T R2 80 ▦

AMA: 2016,Jan,13; 2015,Jan,16; 2014,Jan,11; 2012,May,13

17999 Unlisted procedure, skin, mucous membrane and subcutaneous tissue

📷 0.00   ⚕ 0.00   **FUD** YYY   Q1 80

AMA: 2016,May,13; 2016,Jan,13; 2015,Jan,16; 2014,Jan,11; 2013,Oct,15; 2012,May,13; 2012,Jan,15-42; 2011,Mar,9; 2011,Jan,11

19000-19030 Treatment of Breast Abscess and Cyst with Injection, Aspiration, Incision

19000 Puncture aspiration of cyst of breast;

⚕ (76942, 77021)

📷 1.26   ⚕ 3.21   **FUD** 000   T P3 ▦

AMA: 2016,Jan,13; 2015,Jan,16; 2014,Jan,11; 2013,Dec,16

\+ **19001** each additional cyst (List separately in addition to code for primary procedure)

Code first (19000)

⚕ (76942, 77021)

📷 0.63   ⚕ 0.77   **FUD** ZZZ   N N1 ▦

AMA: 2016,Jan,13; 2015,Jan,16; 2014,Jan,11; 2013,Dec,16

19020 Mastotomy with exploration or drainage of abscess, deep

📷 8.77   ⚕ 13.4   **FUD** 090   T A2 50 ▦

AMA: 2016,Jan,13; 2015,Jan,16; 2014,Dec,16; 2014,Dec,16; 2014,Jan,11

19030 Injection procedure only for mammary ductogram or galactogram

⚕ (77053-77054)

📷 2.24   ⚕ 4.69   **FUD** 000   N N1 50 ▦

AMA: 2016,Jan,13; 2015,Jan,16; 2014,Jan,11

19081-19086 Breast Biopsy with Imaging Guidance

CMS: 100-03,220.13 Percutaneous Image-guided Breast Biopsy; 100-04,12,40.7 Bilateral Procedures; 100-04,13,80.1 Physician Presence; 100-04,13,80.2 S&I Multiple Procedure Reduction

INCLUDES Breast biopsy with placement of localization devices
Fluoroscopic guidance for needle placement (77002)
Magnetic resonance guidance for needle placement (77021)
Radiological examination, surgical specimen (76098)
Ultrasonic guidance for needle placement (76942)

EXCLUDES Biopsy of breast without imaging guidance (19100-19101)
Lesion removal without concentration on surgical margins (19110-19126)
Open biopsy after placement of localization device (19101, 19281-19288)
Partial mastectomy (19301-19302)
Placement of localization devices only (19281-19288)
Total mastectomy (19303-19307)

Code also additional biopsies performed with different imaging modalities

19081 Biopsy, breast, with placement of breast localization device(s) (eg, clip, metallic pellet), when performed, and imaging of the biopsy specimen, when performed, percutaneous; first lesion, including stereotactic guidance

📷 4.90   ⚕ 19.7   **FUD** 000   T 62 80 50 ▦

AMA: 2016,Jun,3; 2016,Jan,13; 2015,May,8; 2015,Mar,5; 2015,Jan,16; 2014,Jun,14; 2014,May,3

\+ **19082** each additional lesion, including stereotactic guidance (List separately in addition to code for primary procedure)

Code first (19081)

📷 2.45   ⚕ 16.2   **FUD** ZZZ   N N1 80 ▦

AMA: 2016,Jun,3; 2016,Jan,13; 2015,May,8; 2015,Mar,5; 2015,Jan,16; 2014,Jun,14; 2014,May,3

19083 Biopsy, breast, with placement of breast localization device(s) (eg, clip, metallic pellet), when performed, and imaging of the biopsy specimen, when performed, percutaneous; first lesion, including ultrasound guidance

📷 4.59   ⚕ 19.0   **FUD** 000   T 62 80 50 ▦

AMA: 2016,Jun,3; 2016,Jan,13; 2015,May,8; 2015,Mar,5; 2015,Jan,16; 2014,Jun,14; 2014,May,3

\+ **19084** each additional lesion, including ultrasound guidance (List separately in addition to code for primary procedure)

Code first (19083)

📷 2.30   ⚕ 15.6   **FUD** ZZZ   N N1 80 ▦

AMA: 2016,Jun,3; 2016,Jan,13; 2015,May,8; 2015,Mar,5; 2015,Jan,16; 2014,Jun,14; 2014,May,3

19085 Biopsy, breast, with placement of breast localization device(s) (eg, clip, metallic pellet), when performed, and imaging of the biopsy specimen, when performed, percutaneous; first lesion, including magnetic resonance guidance

📷 5.39   ⚕ 29.2   **FUD** 000   T 62 80 50 ▦

AMA: 2016,Jun,3; 2016,Jan,13; 2015,May,8; 2015,Mar,5; 2015,Jan,16; 2014,Jun,14; 2014,May,3

\+ **19086** each additional lesion, including magnetic resonance guidance (List separately in addition to code for primary procedure)

Code first (19085)

📷 2.67   ⚕ 23.1   **FUD** ZZZ   N N1 80 ▦

AMA: 2016,Jun,3; 2016,Jan,13; 2015,May,8; 2015,Mar,5; 2015,Jan,16; 2014,Jun,14; 2014,May,3

19100-19101 Breast Biopsy Without Imaging Guidance

EXCLUDES Biopsy of breast with imaging guidance (19081-19086)
Lesion removal without concentration on surgical margins (19110-19126)
Partial mastectomy (19301-19302)
Total mastectomy (19303-19307)

19100 Biopsy of breast; percutaneous, needle core, not using imaging guidance (separate procedure)

EXCLUDES Fine needle aspiration:
With imaging guidance (10022)
Without imaging guidance (10021)

📷 2.02   ⚕ 4.28   **FUD** 000   T A2 50 ▦

AMA: 2016,Jan,13; 2015,Jan,16; 2014,May,3; 2014,Jan,11; 2012,Jan,15-42; 2011,Jan,11

● New Code   ▲ Revised Code   ○ Reinstated   ● New Web Release   ▲ Revised Web Release   Unlisted   Not Covered   # Resequenced
⊘ AMA Mod 51 Exempt   ⑨ Optum Mod 51 Exempt   ⑥③ Mod 63 Exempt   ✗ Non-FDA Drug   ★ Telehealth   M Maternity   A Age Edit   + Add-on   AMA: CPT Asst

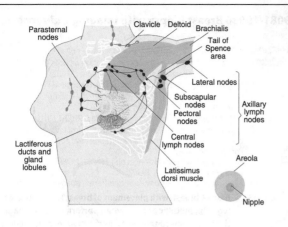

19101   open, incisional
Code also placement of localization device with imaging guidance (19281-19288)
📇 6.37   ⚕ 9.71   **FUD** 010   T A2 50 ▢
AMA: 2016,Jan,13; 2015,Jan,16; 2014,May,3; 2014,Jan,11; 2012,Jan,15-42; 2011,Jan,11

19105 Treatment of Fibroadenoma: Cryoablation

CMS: 100-04,13,80.1 Physician Presence; 100-04,13,80.2 S&I Multiple Procedure Reduction
INCLUDES Adjacent lesions treated with one cryoprobe
Ultrasound guidance (76940, 76942)

19105   Ablation, cryosurgical, of fibroadenoma, including ultrasound guidance, each fibroadenoma
📇 5.61   ⚕ 60.7   **FUD** 000   T P3 50 ▢
AMA: 2007,Mar,7-8

19110-19126 Excisional Procedures: Breast

INCLUDES Open removal of breast mass without concentration on surgical margins

19110   Nipple exploration, with or without excision of a solitary lactiferous duct or a papilloma lactiferous duct
📇 9.82   ⚕ 13.8   **FUD** 090   T A2 50 ▢
AMA: 2016,Jan,13; 2015,Jan,16; 2014,Jan,11

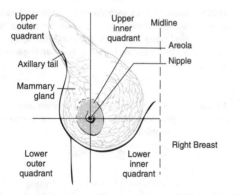

19112   Excision of lactiferous duct fistula
📇 8.92   ⚕ 12.9   **FUD** 090   T A2 80 50 ▢
AMA: 2016,Jan,13; 2015,Jan,16; 2014,Jan,11

19120   Excision of cyst, fibroadenoma, or other benign or malignant tumor, aberrant breast tissue, duct lesion, nipple or areolar lesion (except 19300), open, male or female, 1 or more lesions
📇 11.8   ⚕ 14.1   **FUD** 090   T A2 50 ▢
AMA: 2016,Jan,13; 2015,Mar,5; 2015,Jan,16; 2014,Mar,13; 2014,Jan,11; 2012,Jan,15-42; 2011,Jan,11

19125   Excision of breast lesion identified by preoperative placement of radiological marker, open; single lesion
📇 13.2   ⚕ 15.6   **FUD** 090   T A2 50 ▢
AMA: 2016,Jan,13; 2015,Mar,5; 2015,Jan,16; 2014,Jan,11; 2012,Jan,15-42; 2011,Jan,11

+ **19126   each additional lesion separately identified by a preoperative radiological marker (List separately in addition to code for primary procedure)**
Code first (19125)
📇 4.68   ⚕ 4.68   **FUD** ZZZ   N N1 ▢
AMA: 2016,Jan,13; 2015,Jan,16; 2014,Jan,11; 2012,Jan,15-42; 2011,Jan,11

19260-19272 Excisional Procedures: Chest Wall

EXCLUDES Resection of apical lung tumor (eg, Pancoast tumor), including chest wall resection, rib(s) resection(s), neurovascular dissection, when performed; without chest wall reconstruction(s) (32503-32504)
Thoracentesis, needle or catheter, aspiration of the pleural space; without imaging guidance (32554-32555)
Thoracotomy; with exploration (32100)
Tube thoracostomy, includes connection to drainage system (eg, water seal), when performed, open (separate procedure) (32551)

19260   Excision of chest wall tumor including ribs
📇 34.7   ⚕ 34.7   **FUD** 090   T 80 ▢
AMA: 2016,Jan,13; 2015,Jan,16; 2014,Jan,11; 2012,Oct,9-11; 2012,Sep,3-8

19271   Excision of chest wall tumor involving ribs, with plastic reconstruction; without mediastinal lymphadenectomy
📇 46.9   ⚕ 46.9   **FUD** 090   C 80 ▢
AMA: 2016,Jan,13; 2015,Jan,16; 2014,Jan,11; 2012,Oct,9-11; 2012,Sep,3-8

19272   with mediastinal lymphadenectomy
📇 51.3   ⚕ 51.3   **FUD** 090   C 80 ▢
AMA: 2016,Jan,13; 2015,Jan,16; 2014,Jan,11; 2012,Oct,9-11; 2012,Sep,3-8

19281-19288 Placement of Localization Markers

INCLUDES Placement of localization devices only
EXCLUDES Biopsy of breast without imaging guidance (19100-19101)
Fluoroscopic guidance for needle placement (77002)
Localization device placement with biopsy of breast (19081-19086)
Magnetic resonance guidance for needle placement (77021)
Ultrasonic guidance for needle placement (76942)
Code also open incisional breast biopsy when performed after localization device placement (19101)
Code also radiography of surgical specimen (76098)

19281   Placement of breast localization device(s) (eg, clip, metallic pellet, wire/needle, radioactive seeds), percutaneous; first lesion, including mammographic guidance
📇 2.93   ⚕ 6.80   **FUD** 000   Q1 N1 80 50 ▢
AMA: 2016,Jun,3; 2016,Jan,13; 2015,May,8; 2015,Jan,16; 2014,Jun,14; 2014,May,3

+ **19282   each additional lesion, including mammographic guidance (List separately in addition to code for primary procedure)**
Code first (19281)
📇 1.47   ⚕ 4.76   **FUD** ZZZ   N N1 80 ▢
AMA: 2016,Jun,3; 2016,Jan,13; 2015,May,8; 2015,Jan,16; 2014,Jun,14; 2014,May,3

19283   Placement of breast localization device(s) (eg, clip, metallic pellet, wire/needle, radioactive seeds), percutaneous; first lesion, including stereotactic guidance
📇 2.95   ⚕ 7.65   **FUD** 000   Q1 N1 80 50 ▢
AMA: 2016,Jun,3; 2016,May,13; 2016,Jan,13; 2015,May,8; 2015,Jan,16; 2014,May,3

+ **19284   each additional lesion, including stereotactic guidance (List separately in addition to code for primary procedure)**
Code first (19283)
📇 1.49   ⚕ 5.77   **FUD** ZZZ   N N1 80 ▢
AMA: 2016,Jun,3; 2016,May,13; 2016,Jan,13; 2015,May,8; 2015,Jan,16; 2014,May,3

Integumentary System

19285 Placement of breast localization device(s) (eg, clip, metallic pellet, wire/needle, radioactive seeds), percutaneous; first lesion, including ultrasound guidance
2.50   14.6   **FUD** 000   [01] [N1] [80] [50]
AMA: 2016,Jun,3; 2016,May,13; 2016,Jan,13; 2015,May,8; 2015,Jan,16; 2014,May,3

+ **19286** each additional lesion, including ultrasound guidance (List separately in addition to code for primary procedure)
Code first (19285)
1.26   12.8   **FUD** ZZZ   [N] [N1] [80]
AMA: 2016,Jun,3; 2016,May,13; 2016,Jan,13; 2015,May,8; 2015,Jan,16; 2014,May,3

19287 Placement of breast localization device(s) (eg clip, metallic pellet, wire/needle, radioactive seeds), percutaneous; first lesion, including magnetic resonance guidance
3.75   24.4   **FUD** 000   [01] [N1] [80] [50]
AMA: 2016,Jun,3; 2016,May,13; 2016,Jan,13; 2015,Jan,16; 2014,May,3

+ **19288** each additional lesion, including magnetic resonance guidance (List separately in addition to code for primary procedure)
Code first (19287)
1.87   19.7   **FUD** ZZZ   [N] [N1] [80]
AMA: 2016,Jun,3; 2016,May,13; 2016,Jan,13; 2015,Jan,16; 2014,May,3

19296-19298 Insertion Radiotherapy Afterloading Catheters
CMS: 100-04,12,40.7 Bilateral Procedures

19296 Placement of radiotherapy afterloading expandable catheter (single or multichannel) into the breast for interstitial radioelement application following partial mastectomy, includes imaging guidance; on date separate from partial mastectomy
6.10   112.   **FUD** 000   [J] [J8] [80] [50]
AMA: 2016,Jan,13; 2015,Jan,16; 2014,Jan,11; 2012,Jan,15-42; 2011,Jan,11

+ **19297** concurrent with partial mastectomy (List separately in addition to code for primary procedure)
Code first (19301-19302)
2.75   2.75   **FUD** ZZZ   [N] [N1] [80]
AMA: 2016,Jan,13; 2015,Jan,16; 2014,Jan,11; 2012,Jan,15-42

▲ **19298** Placement of radiotherapy after loading brachytherapy catheters (multiple tube and button type) into the breast for interstitial radioelement application following (at the time of or subsequent to) partial mastectomy, includes imaging guidance
9.43   29.8   **FUD** 000   [J] [J8] [80] [50]
AMA: 2016,Jan,13; 2015,Jan,16; 2014,Jan,11

19300-19307 Mastectomies: Partial, Simple, Radical
CMS: 100-04,12,40.7 Bilateral Procedures
EXCLUDES   Insertion of prosthesis (19340, 19342)

19300 Mastectomy for gynecomastia   ♂
11.8   14.9   **FUD** 090   [T] [A2] [50]
AMA: 2016,Jan,13; 2015,Jan,16; 2014,Mar,13; 2014,Jan,11

19301 Mastectomy, partial (eg, lumpectomy, tylectomy, quadrantectomy, segmentectomy);
EXCLUDES   Insertion of radiotherapy afterloading balloon or brachytherapy catheters (19296-19298)
18.8   18.8   **FUD** 090   [T] [A2] [80] [50]
AMA: 2016,Jan,13; 2015,Mar,5; 2015,Jan,16; 2014,Jan,11; 2013,Nov,14; 2012,Jan,15-42; 2011,Jan,11

19302 with axillary lymphadenectomy
EXCLUDES   Insertion of radiotherapy afterloading balloon or brachytherapy catheters (19296-19298)
25.9   25.9   **FUD** 090   [T] [A2] [80] [50]
AMA: 2016,Jan,13; 2015,Mar,5; 2015,Jan,16; 2014,Jan,11; 2012,Jan,15-42; 2011,Jan,11

19303 Mastectomy, simple, complete
EXCLUDES   Gynecomastia (19300)
29.1   29.1   **FUD** 090   [T] [A2] [80] [50]
AMA: 2016,Jan,13; 2015,Mar,5; 2015,Jan,16; 2014,Jan,11

19304 Mastectomy, subcutaneous
16.5   16.5   **FUD** 090   [T] [A2] [80] [50]
AMA: 2016,Jan,13; 2015,Jan,16; 2014,Jan,11; 2012,Jan,15-42; 2011,Jan,11

19305 Mastectomy, radical, including pectoral muscles, axillary lymph nodes
32.5   32.5   **FUD** 090   [C] [80] [50]
AMA: 2016,Jan,13; 2015,Jan,16; 2014,Jan,11

19306 Mastectomy, radical, including pectoral muscles, axillary and internal mammary lymph nodes (Urban type operation)
34.5   34.5   **FUD** 090   [C] [80] [50]
AMA: 2016,Jan,13; 2015,Jan,16; 2014,Jan,11

19307 Mastectomy, modified radical, including axillary lymph nodes, with or without pectoralis minor muscle, but excluding pectoralis major muscle
34.4   34.4   **FUD** 090   [T] [80] [50]
AMA: 2016,Jan,13; 2015,Mar,5; 2015,Jan,16; 2014,Jan,11

19316-19499 Plastic, Reconstructive, and Aesthetic Breast Procedures
CMS: 100-03,140.2 Breast Reconstruction Following Mastectomy; 100-04,12,40.7 Bilateral Procedures
Code also biologic implant for tissue reinforcement (15777)

19316 Mastopexy
22.0   22.0   **FUD** 090   [T] [A2] [80] [50]
AMA: 2016,Jan,13; 2015,Jan,16; 2014,Jan,11; 2012,Feb,11

19318 Reduction mammaplasty
INCLUDES   Aries-Pitanguy mammaplasty
Biesenberger mammaplasty
31.6   31.6   **FUD** 090   [T] [A2] [80] [50]
AMA: 2016,Jan,13; 2015,Jan,16; 2014,Apr,10; 2014,Jan,11; 2012,Jan,15-42; 2011,Jan,11

19324 Mammaplasty, augmentation; without prosthetic implant
14.0   14.0   **FUD** 090   [T] [A2] [80] [50]
AMA: 2016,Jan,13; 2015,Jan,16; 2014,Jan,11

19325 with prosthetic implant
EXCLUDES   Flap or graft (15100-15650)
18.3   18.3   **FUD** 090   [J] [J8] [80] [50]
AMA: 2016,Jan,13; 2015,Jan,16; 2014,Jan,11

19328 Removal of intact mammary implant
14.2   14.2   **FUD** 090   [02] [A2] [50]
AMA: 2016,Jan,13; 2015,Jan,16; 2014,Jan,11

19330 Removal of mammary implant material
18.1   18.1   **FUD** 090   [02] [A2] [50]
AMA: 2016,Jan,13; 2015,Jan,16; 2014,Jan,11; 2012,Jan,15-42; 2011,Jan,11

19340 Immediate insertion of breast prosthesis following mastopexy, mastectomy or in reconstruction
EXCLUDES   Supply of prosthetic implant (99070, L8030, L8039, L8600)
28.7   28.7   **FUD** 090   [T] [A2] [50]
AMA: 2016,Jan,13; 2015,Dec,18; 2015,Jan,16; 2014,Jan,11; 2012,Jan,15-42

19342 Delayed insertion of breast prosthesis following mastopexy, mastectomy or in reconstruction
EXCLUDES   Preparation of moulage for custom breast implant (19396)
26.4   26.4   **FUD** 090   [J] [J8] [80] [50]
AMA: 2016,Jan,13; 2015,Nov,10; 2015,Jan,16; 2014,Jan,11; 2013,Jan,15-16

19350 Nipple/areola reconstruction
19.3   23.4   **FUD** 090   [T] [A2] [50]
AMA: 2016,Aug,9; 2016,Jan,13; 2015,Jan,16; 2014,Jan,11; 2013,Jan,15-16; 2012,Jan,15-42; 2011,Jan,11

19355 **Correction of inverted nipples**
🚑 16.4 ✂ 20.1 **FUD** 090 T A2 80 50 ▢
AMA: 2016,Jan,13; 2015,Jan,16; 2014,Jan,11

19357 **Breast reconstruction, immediate or delayed, with tissue expander, including subsequent expansion**
🚑 43.1 ✂ 43.1 **FUD** 090 J J8 80 50 ▢
AMA: 2016,Jan,13; 2015,Feb,10; 2015,Jan,16; 2014,Jan,11; 2013,Oct,15; 2012,Jan,15-42

19361 **Breast reconstruction with latissimus dorsi flap, without prosthetic implant**
EXCLUDES *Implant of prosthesis (19340)*
🚑 45.2 ✂ 45.2 **FUD** 090 C 80 50 ▢
AMA: 2016,Jan,13; 2015,Feb,10; 2015,Jan,16; 2014,Jan,11

19364 **Breast reconstruction with free flap**
INCLUDES Closure of donor site
Harvesting of skin graft
Inset shaping of flap into breast
Microvascular repair
Operating microscope (69990)
🚑 79.2 ✂ 79.2 **FUD** 090 C 80 50 ▢
AMA: 2016,Feb,12; 2016,Jan,13; 2015,Feb,10; 2015,Jan,16; 2014,Apr,10; 2014,Jan,11; 2013,Mar,13; 2012,Jul,12-14; 2012,Jan,15-42; 2011,Dec,14-18; 2011,Jan,11

19366 **Breast reconstruction with other technique**
EXCLUDES *Operating microscope (69990)*
Code also implant of prosthesis if appropriate (19340, 19342)
🚑 40.4 ✂ 40.4 **FUD** 090 T A2 80 50 ▢
AMA: 2016,Jan,13; 2015,Feb,10; 2015,Jan,16; 2014,Apr,10; 2014,Jan,11; 2012,Jan,15-42; 2011,Dec,14-18

19367 **Breast reconstruction with transverse rectus abdominis myocutaneous flap (TRAM), single pedicle, including closure of donor site;**
🚑 51.4 ✂ 51.4 **FUD** 090 C 80 50 ▢
AMA: 2016,Jan,13; 2015,Feb,10; 2015,Jan,16; 2014,Jan,11

19368 **with microvascular anastomosis (supercharging)**
INCLUDES Operating microscope (69990)
🚑 63.3 ✂ 63.3 **FUD** 090 C 80 50 ▢
AMA: 2016,Feb,12; 2016,Jan,13; 2015,Feb,10; 2015,Jan,16; 2014,Jan,11

19369 **Breast reconstruction with transverse rectus abdominis myocutaneous flap (TRAM), double pedicle, including closure of donor site**
🚑 58.8 ✂ 58.8 **FUD** 090 C 80 50 ▢
AMA: 2016,Jan,13; 2015,Feb,10; 2015,Jan,16; 2014,Jan,11

19370 **Open periprosthetic capsulotomy, breast**
🚑 19.6 ✂ 19.6 **FUD** 090 T A2 50 ▢
AMA: 2016,Jan,13; 2015,Dec,18; 2015,Jan,16; 2014,Jan,11

19371 **Periprosthetic capsulectomy, breast**
🚑 22.4 ✂ 22.4 **FUD** 090 T A2 50 ▢
AMA: 2016,Jan,13; 2015,Jan,16; 2014,Jan,11; 2013,Jan,15-16; 2012,Jan,15-42; 2011,Jan,11

19380 **Revision of reconstructed breast**
🚑 22.1 ✂ 22.1 **FUD** 090 T A2 50 ▢
AMA: 2016,Jan,13; 2015,Dec,18; 2015,Jan,16; 2014,Jan,11

19396 **Preparation of moulage for custom breast implant**
🚑 4.03 ✂ 7.88 **FUD** 000 T G2 80 50 ▢
AMA: 2016,Jan,13; 2015,Jan,16; 2014,Jan,11

19499 **Unlisted procedure, breast**
🚑 0.00 ✂ 0.00 **FUD** YYY T 80 50
AMA: 2016,Jan,13; 2015,Mar,5; 2015,Jan,16; 2014,Dec,16; 2014,Dec,16; 2014,Jan,11; 2013,Nov,14; 2012,Jan,15-42; 2011,Jan,11

20005 Incisional Treatment Soft Tissue Abscess

EXCLUDES Superficial incision and drainage (10040-10160)

20005 **Incision and drainage of soft tissue abscess, subfascial (ie, involves the soft tissue below the deep fascia)**
🔧 6.72 ⚕ 8.83 **FUD** 010 T G2 🖵

20100-20103 Exploratory Surgery of Traumatic Wound

INCLUDES Debridement
Expanded dissection of wound for exploration
Extraction of foreign material
Open examination
Tying or coagulation of small vessels
EXCLUDES Cutaneous/subcutaneous incision and drainage procedures (10060-10061)
Laparotomy (49000-49010)
Repair of major vessels of:
Abdomen (35221, 35251, 35281)
Chest (35211, 35216, 35241, 35246, 35271, 35276)
Extremity (35206-35207, 35226, 35236, 35256, 35266, 35286)
Neck (35201, 35231, 35261)
Thoracotomy (32100-32160)

20100 **Exploration of penetrating wound (separate procedure); neck**
🔧 17.5 ⚕ 17.5 **FUD** 010 T 80 50 🖵
AMA: 2016,Jan,13; 2015,Jan,16; 2014,Jan,11; 2012,Jan,15-42; 2011,Jan,11

20101 **chest**
🔧 6.02 ⚕ 12.7 **FUD** 010 T 🖵
AMA: 2016,Jan,13; 2015,Jan,16; 2014,Jan,11; 2012,Jan,15-42; 2011,Jan,11

20102 **abdomen/flank/back**
🔧 7.39 ⚕ 14.0 **FUD** 010 T 🖵
AMA: 2016,Jan,13; 2015,Jan,16; 2014,Jan,11; 2012,Jan,15-42; 2011,Jan,11

20103 **extremity**
🔧 10.0 ⚕ 16.5 **FUD** 010 T G2 80 🖵
AMA: 2016,Jan,13; 2015,Jan,16; 2014,Jan,11; 2012,Jan,15-42; 2011,Jan,11

20150 Epiphyseal Bar Resection

EXCLUDES Bone marrow aspiration (38220)

20150 **Excision of epiphyseal bar, with or without autogenous soft tissue graft obtained through same fascial incision**
🔧 25.9 ⚕ 25.9 **FUD** 090 T G2 80 50 🖵
AMA: 1996,Nov,1

20200-20206 Muscle Biopsy

EXCLUDES Removal of muscle tumor (see appropriate anatomic section)

20200 **Biopsy, muscle; superficial**
🔧 2.76 ⚕ 5.90 **FUD** 000 T A2 🖵

20205 **deep**
🔧 4.51 ⚕ 8.25 **FUD** 000 T A2 🖵

20206 **Biopsy, muscle, percutaneous needle**
EXCLUDES Fine needle aspiration (10021-10022)
🔬 (76942, 77002, 77012, 77021)
🔍 (88172-88173)
🔧 1.71 ⚕ 6.72 **FUD** 000 T A2 🖵
AMA: 2001,Jan,8

20220-20225 Percutaneous Bone Biopsy

EXCLUDES Bone marrow biopsy (38221)

20220 **Biopsy, bone, trocar, or needle; superficial (eg, ilium, sternum, spinous process, ribs)**
🔬 (77002, 77012, 77021)
🔧 2.10 ⚕ 4.80 **FUD** 000 T A2 🖵
AMA: 2016,Jan,13; 2015,Jan,16; 2014,Jan,11

20225 **deep (eg, vertebral body, femur)**
EXCLUDES Percutaneous sacral augmentation (sacroplasty) (0200T-0201T)
Percutaneous vertebroplasty (22510-22515)
🔬 (77002, 77012, 77021)
🔧 3.14 ⚕ 14.9 **FUD** 000 T A2 🖵
AMA: 2016,Jan,13; 2015,Jan,8; 2015,Jan,16; 2014,Jan,11; 2012,Jun,10-11

20240-20251 Open Bone Biopsy

EXCLUDES Sequestrectomy or incision and drainage of bone abscess of:
Calcaneus (28120)
Carpal bone (25145)
Clavicle (23170)
Humeral head (23174)
Humerus (24134)
Olecranon process (24138)
Radius (24136, 25145)
Scapula (23172)
Skull (61501)
Talus (28120)
Ulna (24138, 24145)

▲ **20240** **Biopsy, bone, open; superficial (eg, sternum, spinous process, rib, patella, olecranon process, calcaneus, tarsal, metatarsal, carpal, metacarpal, phalanx)**
🔧 4.45 ⚕ 4.45 **FUD** 000 T A2 🖵
AMA: 2016,Jan,13; 2015,Jan,16; 2014,Jan,11; 2012,Jan,15-42; 2011,Jan,11

▲ **20245** **deep (eg, humeral shaft, ischium, femoral shaft)**
🔧 14.9 ⚕ 14.9 **FUD** 010 T A2 🖵
AMA: 2016,Jan,13; 2015,Jan,16; 2014,Jan,11

20250 **Biopsy, vertebral body, open; thoracic**
🔧 11.2 ⚕ 11.2 **FUD** 010 T A2 🖵
AMA: 2016,Jan,13; 2015,Jan,16; 2014,Jan,11

20251 **lumbar or cervical**
🔧 12.2 ⚕ 12.2 **FUD** 010 T A2 80 🖵
AMA: 2016,Jan,13; 2015,Jan,16; 2014,Jan,11

20500-20501 Injection Fistula/Sinus Tract

EXCLUDES Arthrography injection of:
Ankle (27648)
Elbow (24220)
Hip (27093, 27095)
Knee (27370)
Sacroiliac joint (27096)
Shoulder (23350)
Temporomandibular joint (TMJ) (21116)
Wrist (25246)

20500 **Injection of sinus tract; therapeutic (separate procedure)**
🔧 2.42 ⚕ 2.96 **FUD** 010 T P3 🖵
🔬 (76080)

20501 **diagnostic (sinogram)**
🔧 1.10 ⚕ 3.36 **FUD** 000 N N1 🖵
EXCLUDES Contrast injection or injections for radiological evaluation of existing gastrostomy, duodenostomy, jejunostomy, gastro-jejunostomy, or cecostomy (or other colonic) tube from percutaneous approach (49465)
🔬 (76080)

20520-20525 Foreign Body Removal

20520 **Removal of foreign body in muscle or tendon sheath; simple**
🔧 4.19 ⚕ 5.79 **FUD** 010 T P3 🖵

20525 **deep or complicated**
🔧 7.15 ⚕ 13.6 **FUD** 010 T A2 🖵

20526-20553 Therapeutic Injections: Tendons, Trigger Points

EXCLUDES Platelet rich plasma (PRP) injections (0232T)

20526 **Injection, therapeutic (eg, local anesthetic, corticosteroid), carpal tunnel**
🔧 1.65 ⚕ 2.19 **FUD** 000 T P3 50 🖵
AMA: 2016,Jan,13; 2015,Jan,16; 2014,Jan,11; 2012,Jan,15-42; 2011,Jan,11

● New Code ▲ Revised Code ○ Reinstated ● New Web Release ▲ Revised Web Release Unlisted Not Covered # Resequenced
⊘ AMA Mod 51 Exempt ⑤ Optum Mod 51 Exempt ⑥⑤ Mod 63 Exempt ✗ Non-FDA Drug ★ Telehealth M Maternity A Age Edit + Add-on AMA: CPT Asst

CPT © 2016 American Medical Association. All Rights Reserved.

20527 **Injection, enzyme (eg, collagenase), palmar fascial cord (ie, Dupuytren's contracture)**

EXCLUDES *Post injection palmar fascial cord manipulation (26341)*

1.91 2.39 FUD 000 T P3 50

AMA: 2016,Jan,13; 2015,Jan,16; 2014,Jan,11; 2012,Jul,8

20550 **Injection(s); single tendon sheath, or ligament, aponeurosis (eg, plantar "fascia")**

EXCLUDES *Morton's neuroma (64455, 64632)*

(76942, 77002, 77021)

1.20 1.67 FUD 000 T P3 50

AMA: 2016,Jan,13; 2015,Jan,16; 2014,Oct,9; 2014,Jan,11; 2012,Jul,8; 2012,Jan,15-42; 2011,Jan,11

20551 **single tendon origin/insertion**

(76942, 77002, 77021)

1.22 1.71 FUD 000 T P3

AMA: 2016,Jan,13; 2015,Jan,16; 2014,Oct,9; 2014,Jan,11; 2012,Jan,15-42; 2011,Jan,11

20552 **Injection(s); single or multiple trigger point(s), 1 or 2 muscle(s)**

(76942, 77002, 77021)

1.09 1.57 FUD 000 T P3

AMA: 2016,Jan,13; 2015,Jan,16; 2014,Oct,9; 2014,Jan,11; 2012,Apr,19; 2012,Jan,15-42; 2011,Jul,16-17; 2011,Feb,4-5; 2011,Jan,11

20553 **single or multiple trigger point(s), 3 or more muscles**

(76942, 77002, 77021)

1.24 1.81 FUD 000 T P3

AMA: 2016,Jan,13; 2015,Jan,16; 2014,Oct,9; 2014,Jan,11; 2012,Jan,15-42; 2011,Jul,16-17; 2011,Feb,4-5; 2011,Jan,11

20555 Placement of Catheters/Needles for Brachytherapy

CMS: 100-04,13,70.4 Clinical Brachytherapy

Code also interstitial radioelement application (77770-77772, 77778)

20555 **Placement of needles or catheters into muscle and/or soft tissue for subsequent interstitial radioelement application (at the time of or subsequent to the procedure)**

EXCLUDES *Interstitial radioelement:*

Devices placed into the breast (19296-19298)

Placement of needle, catheters, or devices into muscle or soft tissue of the head and neck (41019)

Placement of needles or catheters into pelvic organs or genitalia (55920)

Placement of needles or catheters into prostate (55875)

(76942, 77002, 77012, 77021)

9.43 9.43 FUD 000 T R2 80

AMA: 2016,Jan,13; 2015,Jan,16; 2014,Jan,11; 2012,Jan,15-42; 2011,Jan,11

20600-20611 Aspiration and/or Injection of Joint

CMS: 100-03,150.7 Prolotherapy, Joint Sclerotherapy, and Ligamentous Injections with Sclerosing Agents

EXCLUDES *Ultrasonic guidance for needle placement (76942)*

20600 **Arthrocentesis, aspiration and/or injection, small joint or bursa (eg, fingers, toes); without ultrasound guidance**

(77002, 77012, 77021)

1.02 1.35 FUD 000 T P3 50

AMA: 2016,Jan,13; 2015,Nov,10; 2015,Feb,6; 2015,Jan,16; 2014,Jan,11

20604 **with ultrasound guidance, with permanent recording and reporting**

(77002, 77012, 77021)

1.32 2.05 FUD 000 T P3 50

AMA: 2016,Jan,13; 2015,Jul,10; 2015,Feb,6

20605 **Arthrocentesis, aspiration and/or injection, intermediate joint or bursa (eg, temporomandibular, acromioclavicular, wrist, elbow or ankle, olecranon bursa); without ultrasound guidance**

(77002, 77012, 77021)

1.07 1.42 FUD 000 T P3 50

AMA: 2016,Jan,13; 2015,Nov,10; 2015,Feb,6; 2015,Jan,16; 2014,Jan,11

20606 **with ultrasound guidance, with permanent recording and reporting**

(77002, 77012, 77021)

1.51 2.27 FUD 000 T P3 50

AMA: 2016,Jan,13; 2015,Jul,10; 2015,Feb,6

20610 **Arthrocentesis, aspiration and/or injection, major joint or bursa (eg, shoulder, hip, knee, subacromial bursa); without ultrasound guidance**

EXCLUDES *Injection of contrast for knee arthrography (27370)*

(77002, 77012, 77021)

1.32 1.71 FUD 000 T P3 50

AMA: 2016,Jan,13; 2015,Nov,10; 2015,Aug,6; 2015,Feb,6; 2015,Jan,16; 2014,Dec,18; 2014,Jan,11; 2012,Jun,14; 2012,Mar,4-7; 2012,Jan,15-42; 2011,Jan,11

20611 **with ultrasound guidance, with permanent recording and reporting**

EXCLUDES *Injection of contrast for knee arthrography (27370)*

(77002, 77012, 77021)

1.77 2.60 FUD 000 T P3 50

AMA: 2016,Jan,13; 2015,Nov,10; 2015,Aug,6; 2015,Jul,10; 2015,Feb,6

20612-20615 Aspiration and/or Injection of Cyst

20612 **Aspiration and/or injection of ganglion cyst(s) any location**

1.20 1.72 FUD 000 T P3

Code also modifier 59 for multiple major joint aspirations or injections

20615 **Aspiration and injection for treatment of bone cyst**

4.69 6.96 FUD 010 T P3

20650-20697 Procedures Related to Bony Fixation

20650 **Insertion of wire or pin with application of skeletal traction, including removal (separate procedure)**

4.49 5.90 FUD 010 T A2

20660 **Application of cranial tongs, caliper, or stereotactic frame, including removal (separate procedure)**

7.13 7.13 FUD 000 Q2

AMA: 2016,Jan,13; 2015,Jan,16; 2014,Jan,11; 2012,Aug,14; 2012,Apr,13; 2012,Apr,11-13; 2012,Jan,15-42; 2011,Jan,11

20661 **Application of halo, including removal; cranial**

14.5 14.5 FUD 090 C

AMA: 2016,Jan,13; 2015,Jan,16; 2014,Jan,11; 2012,Aug,14

20662 **pelvic**

12.4 12.4 FUD 090 T R2 80

20663 **femoral**

13.4 13.4 FUD 090 T R2 80 50

20664 **Application of halo, including removal, cranial, 6 or more pins placed, for thin skull osteology (eg, pediatric patients, hydrocephalus, osteogenesis imperfecta)**

25.4 25.4 FUD 090 C

AMA: 2016,Jan,13; 2015,Jan,16; 2014,Jan,11; 2013,Aug,12; 2012,Aug,14

20665 **Removal of tongs or halo applied by another individual**

2.59 3.00 FUD 010 Q1 G2 80

AMA: 2016,Jan,13; 2015,Jan,16; 2014,Jan,11; 2012,Apr,11-13

20670 **Removal of implant; superficial (eg, buried wire, pin or rod) (separate procedure)**

4.22 10.7 FUD 010 Q2 A2

AMA: 2016,Jan,13; 2015,Jan,16; 2014,Jan,11; 2012,Apr,17-18; 2012,Jan,15-42; 2011,Jan,11

20680 deep (eg, buried wire, pin, screw, metal band, nail, rod or plate)
📷 12.1 🔧 17.6 **FUD** 090 [02] [A2] [80] 🖵
AMA: 2016,Jan,13; 2015,Nov,10; 2015,Jan,16; 2014,Mar,4; 2014,Jan,11; 2012,Oct,14; 2012,Sep,16; 2012,Jan,15-42; 2011,Jan,11

20690 Application of a uniplane (pins or wires in 1 plane), unilateral, external fixation system
📷 17.1 🔧 17.1 **FUD** 090 [J] [A2] 🖵
AMA: 2016,Jan,13; 2015,Jan,16; 2014,Jan,11; 2012,Jan,15-42; 2011,Jan,11

20692 Application of a multiplane (pins or wires in more than 1 plane), unilateral, external fixation system (eg, Ilizarov, Monticelli type)
📷 32.1 🔧 32.1 **FUD** 090 [J] [A2] [80] 🖵
AMA: 2016,Jan,13; 2015,Jan,16; 2014,Jan,11; 2012,Jan,15-42; 2011,Jan,11

20693 Adjustment or revision of external fixation system requiring anesthesia (eg, new pin[s] or wire[s] and/or new ring[s] or bar[s])
📷 12.8 🔧 12.8 **FUD** 090 [T] [A2] 🖵
AMA: 2016,Jan,13; 2015,Jan,16; 2014,Jan,11; 2012,Jan,15-42; 2011,Jan,11

20694 Removal, under anesthesia, of external fixation system
📷 9.72 🔧 12.1 **FUD** 090 [02] [A2] 🖵
AMA: 2016,Jan,13; 2015,Jan,16; 2014,Jan,11; 2012,Jan,15-42; 2011,Jan,11

20696 Application of multiplane (pins or wires in more than 1 plane), unilateral, external fixation with stereotactic computer-assisted adjustment (eg, spatial frame), including imaging; initial and subsequent alignment(s), assessment(s), and computation(s) of adjustment schedule(s)
EXCLUDES Application of multiplan external fixation system (20692)
Application of multiplan external fixation system, with stereotactic computer-assisted adjustment
📷 34.6 🔧 34.6 **FUD** 090 [J] [J8] [80] 🖵
AMA: 2016,Jan,13; 2015,Jan,16; 2014,Jan,11

20697 exchange (ie, removal and replacement) of strut, each
EXCLUDES Application of multiplane external fixation system (20692)
Exchange of strut for multiplane external fixation system
📷 56.2 🔧 56.2 **FUD** 000 ⊘ [T] [P2] [80] [TC]
AMA: 2016,Jan,13; 2015,Jan,16; 2014,Jan,11

20802-20838 Reimplantation Procedures

EXCLUDES Repair of incomplete amputation (see individual repair codes for bone(s), ligament(s), tendon(s), nerve(s), or blood vessel(s) and append modifier 52)

20802 Replantation, arm (includes surgical neck of humerus through elbow joint), complete amputation
📷 69.2 🔧 69.2 **FUD** 090 [C] [80] [50] 🖵
AMA: 1997,Apr,4

20805 Replantation, forearm (includes radius and ulna to radial carpal joint), complete amputation
📷 95.2 🔧 95.2 **FUD** 090 [C] [80] [50] 🖵
AMA: 1997,Apr,4

20808 Replantation, hand (includes hand through metacarpophalangeal joints), complete amputation
📷 115. 🔧 115. **FUD** 090 [C] [80] [50] 🖵
AMA: 1997,Apr,4

20816 Replantation, digit, excluding thumb (includes metacarpophalangeal joint to insertion of flexor sublimis tendon), complete amputation
📷 59.7 🔧 59.7 **FUD** 090 [C] [80] 🖵
AMA: 2016,Jan,13; 2015,Jan,16; 2014,Jan,11; 2012,Jan,15-42; 2011,Jan,11

20822 Replantation, digit, excluding thumb (includes distal tip to sublimis tendon insertion), complete amputation
📷 51.5 🔧 51.5 **FUD** 090 [T] [G2] [80] 🖵
AMA: 1997,Apr,4

20824 Replantation, thumb (includes carpometacarpal joint to MP joint), complete amputation
📷 58.6 🔧 58.6 **FUD** 090 [C] [80] [50] 🖵
AMA: 1997,Apr,4

20827 Replantation, thumb (includes distal tip to MP joint), complete amputation
📷 52.6 🔧 52.6 **FUD** 090 [C] [80] [50] 🖵
AMA: 1997,Apr,4

20838 Replantation, foot, complete amputation
📷 69.9 🔧 69.9 **FUD** 090 [C] [80] [50] 🖵
AMA: 1997,Apr,4

20900-20926 Bone and Tissue Autografts

EXCLUDES Acquisition of autogenous bone graft, cartilage, tendon, fascia lata through distinct incision unless included in the code description
Bone graft procedures on the spine (20930-20938)

20900 Bone graft, any donor area; minor or small (eg, dowel or button)
📷 5.48 🔧 11.9 **FUD** 000 [T] [A2] [80] 🖵
AMA: 2016,Jan,13; 2015,Jan,16; 2014,Jan,11; 2012,Jan,15-42; 2011,Jul,16-17; 2011,Jan,11

20902 major or large
📷 8.26 🔧 8.26 **FUD** 000 [J] [A2] [80] 🖵
AMA: 2016,Jan,13; 2015,Jan,16; 2014,Jan,11; 2012,Jan,15-42; 2011,Jul,16-17; 2011,Jan,11

20910 Cartilage graft; costochondral
EXCLUDES Graft with ear cartilage (21235)
📷 11.8 🔧 11.8 **FUD** 090 [T] [A2] [80] 🖵
AMA: 2016,Jan,13; 2015,Jan,16; 2014,Jan,11; 2013,Jan,15-16

20912 nasal septum
EXCLUDES Graft with ear cartilage (21235)
📷 13.8 🔧 13.8 **FUD** 090 [T] [A2] [80] 🖵
AMA: 2002,Apr,13; 1999,Aug,5

20920 Fascia lata graft; by stripper
📷 11.3 🔧 11.3 **FUD** 090 [T] [A2] 🖵
AMA: 2016,Jan,13; 2015,Jan,16; 2014,Jan,11

20922 by incision and area exposure, complex or sheet
📷 14.4 🔧 17.4 **FUD** 090 [T] [A2] [80] 🖵
AMA: 2016,Jan,13; 2015,Jan,16; 2014,Jan,11

20924 Tendon graft, from a distance (eg, palmaris, toe extensor, plantaris)
📷 14.5 🔧 14.5 **FUD** 090 [T] [A2] [80] 🖵
AMA: 2005,Jan,7-13; 2002,Apr,13

20926 Tissue grafts, other (eg, paratenon, fat, dermis)
EXCLUDES Platelet rich plasma injection (0232T)
📷 12.3 🔧 12.3 **FUD** 090 [T] [A2] 🖵
AMA: 2016,Jan,13; 2015,Jan,16; 2014,Jan,11; 2012,Jun,15-16; 2012,Apr,14-16; 2012,Jan,15-42; 2011,Jan,11

20930-20938 Bone Allograft and Autograft of Spine

EXCLUDES Bone marrow aspiration for bone grafting (38220)

+ **20930** Allograft, morselized, or placement of osteopromotive material, for spine surgery only (List separately in addition to code for primary procedure)
Code first (22319, 22532-22533, 22548-22558, 22590-22612, 22630, 22633-22634, 22800-22812)
📷 0.00 🔧 0.00 **FUD** XXX [N] [N1] 🖵
AMA: 2016,Jan,13; 2015,Jan,16; 2014,Jan,11; 2013,Jul,3-5; 2012,Jun,10-11; 2012,Apr,14-16; 2012,Jan,15-42; 2011,Dec,14-18; 2011,Jul,16-17; 2011,Jan,11

Musculoskeletal System

20931 — 21010

+ 20931 Allograft, structural, for spine surgery only (List separately in addition to code for primary procedure)
Code first (22319, 22532-22533, 22548-22558, 22590-22612, 22630, 22633-22634, 22800-22812)
🔧 3.29   🔧 3.29   **FUD** ZZZ   N N1
AMA: 2016,Jan,13; 2015,Jan,16; 2014,Jan,11; 2013,Jul,3-5; 2012,Jun,10-11; 2012,Apr,14-16; 2012,Jan,15-42; 2011,Dec,14-18; 2011,Sep,11-12; 2011,Jul,16-17; 2011,Jan,11

+ 20936 Autograft for spine surgery only (includes harvesting the graft); local (eg, ribs, spinous process, or laminar fragments) obtained from same incision (List separately in addition to code for primary procedure)
from person
Code first (22319, 22532-22533, 22548-22558, 22590-22612, 22630, 22633-22634, 22800-22812)
🔧 0.00   🔧 0.00   **FUD** XXX   N
AMA: 2016,Jan,13; 2015,Jan,16; 2014,Jan,11; 2013,Jul,3-5; 2012,Jun,10-11; 2012,Apr,14-16; 2012,Jan,15-42; 2011,Dec,14-18; 2011,Jan,11

+ 20937 morselized (through separate skin or fascial incision) (List separately in addition to code for primary procedure)
Code first (22319, 22532-22533, 22548-22558, 22590-22612, 22630, 22633-22634, 22800-22812)
🔧 4.89   🔧 4.89   **FUD** ZZZ   N 80
AMA: 2016,Jan,13; 2015,Jan,16; 2014,Jan,11; 2013,Jul,3-5; 2012,Jun,10-11; 2012,Apr,14-16; 2012,Jan,15-42; 2011,Dec,14-18; 2011,Jul,16-17; 2011,Jan,11

+ 20938 structural, bicortical or tricortical (through separate skin or fascial incision) (List separately in addition to code for primary procedure)
Code first (22319, 22532-22533, 22548-22558, 22590-22612, 22630, 22633-22634, 22800-22812)
🔧 5.40   🔧 5.40   **FUD** ZZZ   N 80
AMA: 2016,Jan,13; 2015,Jan,16; 2014,Jan,11; 2013,Jul,3-5; 2012,May,11-12; 2012,Jun,10-11; 2012,Apr,14-16; 2012,Apr,11-13; 2012,Jan,15-42; 2011,Dec,14-18; 2011,Jul,16-17; 2011,Jan,11

20950 Measurement of Intracompartmental Pressure

20950 Monitoring of interstitial fluid pressure (includes insertion of device, eg, wick catheter technique, needle manometer technique) in detection of muscle compartment syndrome
🔧 2.63   🔧 7.18   **FUD** 000   T 62 80
AMA: 2016,Jan,13; 2015,Jan,16; 2014,Jan,11; 2012,Jan,15-42; 2011,Jan,11

20955-20973 Bone and Osteocutaneous Grafts

INCLUDES   Operating microscope (69990)

20955 Bone graft with microvascular anastomosis; fibula
🔧 72.4   🔧 72.4   **FUD** 090   C 80
AMA: 2016,Feb,12; 2016,Jan,13; 2015,Jan,16; 2014,Jan,11

20956 iliac crest
🔧 76.6   🔧 76.6   **FUD** 090   C 80
AMA: 2016,Feb,12; 2016,Jan,13; 2015,Jan,16; 2014,Jan,11

20957 metatarsal
🔧 70.7   🔧 70.7   **FUD** 090   C 80
AMA: 2016,Feb,12; 2016,Jan,13; 2015,Jan,16; 2014,Jan,11

20962 other than fibula, iliac crest, or metatarsal
🔧 61.0   🔧 61.0   **FUD** 090   C 80
AMA: 2016,Feb,12

20969 Free osteocutaneous flap with microvascular anastomosis; other than iliac crest, metatarsal, or great toe
🔧 80.0   🔧 80.0   **FUD** 090   C 80
AMA: 2016,Feb,12; 2016,Jan,13; 2015,Jan,16; 2014,Jan,11

20970 iliac crest
🔧 84.5   🔧 84.5   **FUD** 090   C 80
AMA: 2016,Feb,12; 2016,Jan,13; 2015,Jan,16; 2014,Jan,11

20972 metatarsal
🔧 68.2   🔧 68.2   **FUD** 090   J 62 80
AMA: 2016,Feb,12; 2016,Jan,13; 2015,Jan,16; 2014,Jan,11

20973 great toe with web space
EXCLUDES   *Wrap-around repair (26551)*
🔧 76.1   🔧 76.1   **FUD** 090   J R2 80 50
AMA: 2016,Feb,12; 2016,Jan,13; 2015,Jan,16; 2014,Jan,11

20974-20979 Osteogenic Stimulation

CMS: 100-03,150.2 Osteogenic Stimulation

20974 Electrical stimulation to aid bone healing; noninvasive (nonoperative)
🔧 1.45   🔧 2.18   **FUD** 000   ⊘ A
AMA: 2016,Jan,13; 2015,Jan,16; 2014,Jan,11; 2012,Jan,15-42; 2011,Jan,11

20975 invasive (operative)
🔧 5.15   🔧 5.15   **FUD** 000   ⊘ N N1 80
AMA: 2002,Apr,13; 2000,Nov,8

20979 Low intensity ultrasound stimulation to aid bone healing, noninvasive (nonoperative)
🔧 0.93   🔧 1.49   **FUD** 000   01 N1
AMA: 2016,Jan,13; 2015,Jan,16; 2014,Jan,11; 2012,Jan,15-42; 2011,Jan,11

20982-20999 General Musculoskeletal Procedures

▲ **20982 Ablation therapy for reduction or eradication of 1 or more bone tumors (eg, metastasis) including adjacent soft tissue when involved by tumor extension, percutaneous, including imaging guidance when performed; radiofrequency**
EXCLUDES   *Radiologic guidance (76940, 77002, 77013, 77022)*
🔧 11.0   🔧 85.9   **FUD** 000   T 62 50
AMA: 2016,Jan,13; 2015,Sep,12; 2015,Jul,8

▲ **20983 cryoablation**
EXCLUDES   *Radiologic guidance (76940, 77002, 77013, 77022)*
🔧 11.7   🔧 206.   **FUD** 000   T 62 50
AMA: 2016,Jan,13; 2015,Jul,8

+ 20985 Computer-assisted surgical navigational procedure for musculoskeletal procedures, image-less (List separately in addition to code for primary procedure)
EXCLUDES   *Image guidance derived from intraoperative and preoperative obtained images (0054T-0055T)*
         Stereotactic computer-assisted navigational procedure; cranial or intradural (61781-61783)
Code first primary procedure
🔧 4.26   🔧 4.26   **FUD** ZZZ   N N1 80
AMA: 2016,Jan,13; 2015,Jan,16; 2014,Jan,11; 2011,Jul,12-13

20999 Unlisted procedure, musculoskeletal system, general
🔧 0.00   🔧 0.00   **FUD** YYY   T 80
AMA: 2016,Jan,13; 2015,Jul,8; 2015,Jan,16; 2014,Oct,9; 2014,Jan,11

21010 Temporomandibular Joint Arthrotomy

21010 Arthrotomy, temporomandibular joint
EXCLUDES   *Excision of foreign body from dentoalveolar site (41805-41806)*
         Soft tissue (subfascial) abscess drainage (20005)
         Superficial abscess and hematoma drainage (10060-10061)
🔧 21.4   🔧 21.4   **FUD** 090   J A2 80 50
AMA: 2002,Apr,13

21011-21016 Excision Soft Tissue Tumors Face and Scalp

INCLUDES Any necessary elevation of tissue planes or dissection
Measurement of tumor and necessary margin at greatest diameter prior to excision
Simple and intermediate repairs
Types of excision:
Fascial or subfascial soft tissue tumors: simple and marginal resection of tumors found either in or below the deep fascia, not including bone or excision of a substantial amount of normal tissue; primarily benign and intramuscular tumors
Radical resection soft tissue tumor: wide resection of tumor involving substantial margins of normal tissue and may include tissue removal from one or more layers; most often malignant or aggressive benign
Subcutaneous: simple and marginal resection of tumors in the subcutaneous tissue above the deep fascia; most often benign

EXCLUDES Complex repair
Excision of benign cutaneous lesions (eg, sebaceous cyst) (11420-11426)
Radical resection of cutaneous tumors (eg, melanoma) (11620-11646)
Significant exploration of vessels or neuroplasty

21011 Excision, tumor, soft tissue of face or scalp, subcutaneous; less than 2 cm
🖩 7.45 🔪 9.94 **FUD** 090 T P3 80 ▭
AMA: 2016,Jan,13; 2015,Jan,16; 2014,Jan,11

21012 2 cm or greater
🖩 9.75 🔪 9.75 **FUD** 090 T A2 80 ▭
AMA: 2016,Jan,13; 2015,Jan,16; 2014,Jan,11

21013 Excision, tumor, soft tissue of face and scalp, subfascial (eg, subgaleal, intramuscular); less than 2 cm
🖩 11.5 🔪 14.8 **FUD** 090 T P3 80 ▭
AMA: 2016,Jan,13; 2015,Jan,16; 2014,Jan,11

21014 2 cm or greater
🖩 15.0 🔪 15.0 **FUD** 090 T A2 80 ▭
AMA: 2016,Jan,13; 2015,Jan,16; 2014,Jan,11

21015 Radical resection of tumor (eg, sarcoma), soft tissue of face or scalp; less than 2 cm
EXCLUDES Removal of cranial tumor for osteomyelitis (61501)
🖩 20.4 🔪 20.4 **FUD** 090 T 62 ▭
AMA: 2016,Jan,13; 2015,Jan,16; 2014,Jan,11

21016 2 cm or greater
🖩 29.5 🔪 29.5 **FUD** 090 T 62 80 ▭
AMA: 2016,Jan,13; 2015,Jan,16; 2014,Jan,11

21025-21070 Procedures of Cranial and Facial Bones

INCLUDES Any necessary elevation of tissue planes or dissection
Measurement of tumor and necessary margins prior to excision
Radical resection of bone tumor involves resection of the tumor (may include entire bone) and wide margins of normal tissue primarily for malignant or aggressive benign tumors
Simple and intermediate repairs

EXCLUDES Complex repair
Excision of soft tissue tumors, face and scalp (21011-21016)
Radical resection of cutaneous tumors (e.g., melanoma) (11620-11646)
Significant exploration of vessels, neuroplasty, reconstruction, or complex bone repair

21025 Excision of bone (eg, for osteomyelitis or bone abscess); mandible
🖩 21.8 🔪 25.8 **FUD** 090 J A2 ▭
AMA: 2016,Jan,13; 2015,Jan,16; 2014,Jan,11; 2012,Jan,15-42; 2011,Oct,10

21026 facial bone(s)
🖩 14.4 🔪 17.8 **FUD** 090 T A2 ▭
AMA: 2002,Apr,13

21029 Removal by contouring of benign tumor of facial bone (eg, fibrous dysplasia)
🖩 18.4 🔪 22.0 **FUD** 090 T A2 80 ▭
AMA: 2002,Apr,13

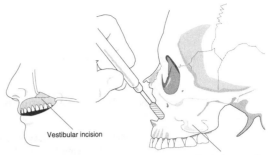

Vestibular incision

Burs, files, and osteotomes used to remove bone   Area of benign bone growth

21030 Excision of benign tumor or cyst of maxilla or zygoma by enucleation and curettage
🖩 12.1 🔪 15.0 **FUD** 090 T P3 50 ▭
AMA: 2016,Jan,13; 2015,Jan,16; 2014,Jan,11

21031 Excision of torus mandibularis
🖩 8.59 🔪 11.4 **FUD** 090 T P3 50 ▭
AMA: 2002,Apr,13

21032 Excision of maxillary torus palatinus
🖩 8.51 🔪 11.6 **FUD** 090 T P3 ▭
AMA: 2002,Apr,13

21034 Excision of malignant tumor of maxilla or zygoma
🖩 33.5 🔪 37.9 **FUD** 090 J A2 80 ▭
AMA: 2016,Jan,13; 2015,Jan,16; 2014,Jan,11

21040 Excision of benign tumor or cyst of mandible, by enucleation and/or curettage
INCLUDES Removal of benign tumor or cyst without osteotomy
EXCLUDES Removal of benign tumor or cyst with osteotomy (21046-21047)
🖩 12.1 🔪 15.1 **FUD** 090 T A2 ▭
AMA: 2016,Jan,13; 2015,Jan,16; 2014,Jan,11

21044 Excision of malignant tumor of mandible;
🖩 25.3 🔪 25.3 **FUD** 090 J A2 80 ▭
AMA: 2002,Apr,13

21045 radical resection
Code also bone graft procedure (21215)
🖩 35.5 🔪 35.5 **FUD** 090 C 80 ▭
AMA: 2002,Apr,13

21046 Excision of benign tumor or cyst of mandible; requiring intra-oral osteotomy (eg, locally aggressive or destructive lesion[s])
🖩 32.5 🔪 32.5 **FUD** 090 J A2 80 ▭
AMA: 2016,Jan,13; 2015,Jan,16; 2014,Jan,11

21047 requiring extra-oral osteotomy and partial mandibulectomy (eg, locally aggressive or destructive lesion[s])
🖩 38.3 🔪 38.3 **FUD** 090 J A2 80 ▭
AMA: 2016,Jan,13; 2015,Jan,16; 2014,Jan,11

21048 Excision of benign tumor or cyst of maxilla; requiring intra-oral osteotomy (eg, locally aggressive or destructive lesion[s])
🖩 33.3 🔪 33.3 **FUD** 090 J A2 80 ▭
AMA: 2016,Jan,13; 2015,Jan,16; 2014,Jan,11

21049 requiring extra-oral osteotomy and partial maxillectomy (eg, locally aggressive or destructive lesion[s])
🖩 35.1 🔪 35.1 **FUD** 090 J 80 ▭
AMA: 2016,Jan,13; 2015,Jan,16; 2014,Jan,11

21050 Condylectomy, temporomandibular joint (separate procedure)

🔧 24.3   ⚕ 24.3   **FUD** 090   J A2 80 50 ▭

AMA: 2002,Apr,13

21060 Meniscectomy, partial or complete, temporomandibular joint (separate procedure)

🔧 23.0   ⚕ 23.0   **FUD** 090   J A2 80 50 ▭

AMA: 2002,Apr,13

21070 Coronoidectomy (separate procedure)

🔧 17.6   ⚕ 17.6   **FUD** 090   J A2 80 50 ▭

AMA: 2002,Apr,13

21073 Temporomandibular Joint Manipulation with Anesthesia

21073 Manipulation of temporomandibular joint(s) (TMJ), therapeutic, requiring an anesthesia service (ie, general or monitored anesthesia care)

EXCLUDES   *Closed treatment of TMJ dislocation (21480, 21485)*
Manipulation of TMJ without general or MAC anesthesia (97140, 98925-98929, 98943)

🔧 7.35   ⚕ 11.1   **FUD** 090   T P3 80 50 ▭

AMA: 2016,Jan,13; 2015,Jan,16; 2014,Jan,11; 2012,Jan,15-42; 2011,Jan,11

21076-21089 Medical Impressions for Fabrication Maxillofacial Prosthesis

INCLUDES   Design, preparation, and professional services rendered by a physician or other qualified health care professional

EXCLUDES   *Application or removal of caliper or tongs (20660, 20665)*
Professional services rendered for outside laboratory designed and prepared prosthesis

21076 Impression and custom preparation; surgical obturator prosthesis

🔧 24.4   ⚕ 29.1   **FUD** 010   T P2 80 ▭

AMA: 2016,Jan,13; 2015,Jan,16; 2014,Jan,11; 2012,Jan,15-42; 2011,Jan,11

21077 orbital prosthesis

🔧 61.4   ⚕ 72.9   **FUD** 090   J P3 80 50 ▭

AMA: 2016,Jan,13; 2015,Jan,16; 2014,Jan,11

21079 interim obturator prosthesis

🔧 40.8   ⚕ 49.1   **FUD** 090   J P3 ▭

AMA: 2016,Jan,13; 2015,Jan,16; 2014,Jan,11

21080 definitive obturator prosthesis

🔧 45.5   ⚕ 55.1   **FUD** 090   J P3 ▭

AMA: 2016,Jan,13; 2015,Jan,16; 2014,Jan,11

21081 mandibular resection prosthesis

🔧 41.8   ⚕ 50.9   **FUD** 090   J P3 80 ▭

AMA: 2016,Jan,13; 2015,Jan,16; 2014,Jan,11

21082 palatal augmentation prosthesis

🔧 39.2   ⚕ 48.1   **FUD** 090   J P3 80 ▭

AMA: 2016,Jan,13; 2015,Jan,16; 2014,Jan,11

21083 palatal lift prosthesis

🔧 36.4   ⚕ 45.8   **FUD** 090   J P3 80 ▭

AMA: 2016,Jan,13; 2015,Jan,16; 2014,Jan,11

21084 speech aid prosthesis

🔧 42.2   ⚕ 52.7   **FUD** 090   J P3 80 ▭

AMA: 2016,Jan,13; 2015,Jan,16; 2014,Jan,11

21085 oral surgical splint

🔧 16.5   ⚕ 22.0   **FUD** 010   T P2 80 ▭

AMA: 2016,Jan,13; 2015,Jan,16; 2014,Jan,11

21086 auricular prosthesis

🔧 45.5   ⚕ 54.2   **FUD** 090   J P3 80 50 ▭

AMA: 2016,Jan,13; 2015,Jan,16; 2014,Jan,11

21087 nasal prosthesis

🔧 45.4   ⚕ 54.2   **FUD** 090   J P3 80 ▭

AMA: 2016,Jan,13; 2015,Jan,16; 2014,Jan,11

21088 facial prosthesis

🔧 0.00   ⚕ 0.00   **FUD** 090   J R2 80 ▭

AMA: 2016,Jan,13; 2015,Jan,16; 2014,Jan,11

21089 Unlisted maxillofacial prosthetic procedure

🔧 0.00   ⚕ 0.00   **FUD** YYY   T

AMA: 2016,Jan,13; 2015,Jan,16; 2014,Jan,11; 2012,Jan,15-42; 2011,Jan,11

21100-21110 Application Fixation Device

21100 Application of halo type appliance for maxillofacial fixation, includes removal (separate procedure)

🔧 14.4   ⚕ 29.5   **FUD** 090   J A2 80 ▭

AMA: 2002,Apr,13

21110 Application of interdental fixation device for conditions other than fracture or dislocation, includes removal

EXCLUDES   *Removal of interdental fixation by another individual (20670-20680)*

🔧 19.5   ⚕ 23.2   **FUD** 090   Q2 P2 ▭

AMA: 2016,Jan,13; 2015,Jan,16; 2014,Jan,11; 2013,Dec,16; 2012,Jan,15-42; 2011,Jan,11

21116 Injection for TMJ Arthrogram

CMS: 100-02,15,150.1 Treatment of Temporomandibular Joint (TMJ) Syndrome; 100-04,13,80.1 Physician Presence; 100-04,13,80.2 S&I Multiple Procedure Reduction

21116 Injection procedure for temporomandibular joint arthrography

⚕ (70332)

🔧 1.27   ⚕ 4.16   **FUD** 000   N N1 50 ▭

AMA: 2016,May,13; 2016,Jan,13; 2015,Aug,6

21120-21299 Repair/Reconstruction Craniofacial Bones

EXCLUDES   *Cranioplasty (21179-21180, 62120, 62140-62147)*

21120 Genioplasty; augmentation (autograft, allograft, prosthetic material)

🔧 15.0   ⚕ 18.9   **FUD** 090   J A2 ▭

AMA: 2002,Apr,13

Nasal bone — Frontal bone — Supraorbital margin — Frontonasal suture — Parietal bone — Frontomaxillary suture — Zygomatic process — Internasal suture — Zygomatic bone — Naso-maxillary suture — Zygomaxillary suture — Ramus — Nasal septum — Body of mandible — Alveolar process of maxilla — Mental foramen

21121 sliding osteotomy, single piece

🔧 19.5   ⚕ 23.4   **FUD** 090   T A2 80 ▭

AMA: 2002,Apr,13

21122 sliding osteotomies, 2 or more osteotomies (eg, wedge excision or bone wedge reversal for asymmetrical chin)

🔧 19.0   ⚕ 19.0   **FUD** 090   T A2 80 ▭

AMA: 2002,Apr,13

21123 sliding, augmentation with interpositional bone grafts (includes obtaining autografts)

🔧 27.0   ⚕ 27.0   **FUD** 090   T A2 80 ▭

AMA: 2002,Apr,13

21125 Augmentation, mandibular body or angle; prosthetic material

🔧 22.7   ⚕ 87.6   **FUD** 090   T A2 80 ▭

AMA: 2002,Apr,13

Musculoskeletal System

21050 — 21125

21127   with bone graft, onlay or interpositional (includes obtaining autograft)
  25.9   126.   **FUD** 090   J A2 80
  AMA: 2002,Apr,13

21137   Reduction forehead; contouring only
  21.8   21.8   **FUD** 090   T 62 80
  AMA: 2002,Apr,13

21138   contouring and application of prosthetic material or bone graft (includes obtaining autograft)
  25.6   25.6   **FUD** 090   J 62 80
  AMA: 2002,Apr,13

21139   contouring and setback of anterior frontal sinus wall
  27.4   27.4   **FUD** 090   J 62 80
  AMA: 2002,Apr,13

21141   Reconstruction midface, LeFort I; single piece, segment movement in any direction (eg, for Long Face Syndrome), without bone graft
  38.8   38.8   **FUD** 090   C 80
  AMA: 2002,Apr,13; 1995,Win,1

21142   2 pieces, segment movement in any direction, without bone graft
  40.7   40.7   **FUD** 090   C 80
  AMA: 2002,Apr,13; 1995,Win,1

21143   3 or more pieces, segment movement in any direction, without bone graft
  40.9   40.9   **FUD** 090   C 80
  AMA: 2002,Apr,13; 1995,Win,1

21145   single piece, segment movement in any direction, requiring bone grafts (includes obtaining autografts)
  45.7   45.7   **FUD** 090   C 80
  AMA: 2002,Apr,13; 1995,Win,1

21146   2 pieces, segment movement in any direction, requiring bone grafts (includes obtaining autografts) (eg, ungrafted unilateral alveolar cleft)
  44.7   44.7   **FUD** 090   C 80
  AMA: 2002,Apr,13; 1995,Win,1

21147   3 or more pieces, segment movement in any direction, requiring bone grafts (includes obtaining autografts) (eg, ungrafted bilateral alveolar cleft or multiple osteotomies)
  50.6   50.6   **FUD** 090   C 80
  AMA: 2002,Apr,13; 1995,Win,1

21150   Reconstruction midface, LeFort II; anterior intrusion (eg, Treacher-Collins Syndrome)
  48.6   48.6   **FUD** 090   J 62 80
  AMA: 2002,Apr,13

21151   any direction, requiring bone grafts (includes obtaining autografts)
  58.5   58.5   **FUD** 090   C 80
  AMA: 2002,Apr,13

21154   Reconstruction midface, LeFort III (extracranial), any type, requiring bone grafts (includes obtaining autografts); without LeFort I
  60.3   60.3   **FUD** 090   C 80
  AMA: 2002,Apr,13

21155   with LeFort I
  62.5   62.5   **FUD** 090   C 80
  AMA: 2002,Apr,13

Bicoronal scalp flap
Lower eyelid
Circum-vestibular
Typical transcutaneous and transoral incisions
LeFort III with LeFort I down-fracture

21159   Reconstruction midface, LeFort III (extra and intracranial) with forehead advancement (eg, mono bloc), requiring bone grafts (includes obtaining autografts); without LeFort I
  72.3   72.3   **FUD** 090   C 80
  AMA: 2002,Apr,13

21160   with LeFort I
  91.8   91.8   **FUD** 090   C 80
  AMA: 2002,Apr,13

21172   Reconstruction superior-lateral orbital rim and lower forehead, advancement or alteration, with or without grafts (includes obtaining autografts)
  EXCLUDES   Frontal or parietal craniotomy for craniosynostosis (61556)
  52.2   52.2   **FUD** 090   J 80
  AMA: 2002,Apr,13

21175   Reconstruction, bifrontal, superior-lateral orbital rims and lower forehead, advancement or alteration (eg, plagiocephaly, trigonocephaly, brachycephaly), with or without grafts (includes obtaining autografts)
  EXCLUDES   Bifrontal craniotomy for craniosynostosis (61557)
  62.0   62.0   **FUD** 090   J 80
  AMA: 2002,Apr,13

21179   Reconstruction, entire or majority of forehead and/or supraorbital rims; with grafts (allograft or prosthetic material)
  EXCLUDES   Extensive craniotomy for numerous suture craniosynostosis (61558-61559)
  41.8   41.8   **FUD** 090   C 80
  AMA: 2002,Apr,13

21180   with autograft (includes obtaining grafts)
  EXCLUDES   Extensive craniotomy for numerous suture craniosynostosis (61558-61559)
  44.6   44.6   **FUD** 090   C 80
  AMA: 2002,Apr,13

21181   Reconstruction by contouring of benign tumor of cranial bones (eg, fibrous dysplasia), extracranial
  21.2   21.2   **FUD** 090   J A2 80
  AMA: 2002,Apr,13

21182   Reconstruction of orbital walls, rims, forehead, nasoethmoid complex following intra- and extracranial excision of benign tumor of cranial bone (eg, fibrous dysplasia), with multiple autografts (includes obtaining grafts); total area of bone grafting less than 40 sq cm
  EXCLUDES   Removal of benign tumor of the skull (61563-61564)
  56.1   56.1   **FUD** 090   C 80
  AMA: 2002,May,7; 2002,Apr,13

21183 total area of bone grafting greater than 40 sq cm but less than 80 sq cm

> EXCLUDES *Removal of benign tumor of the skull (61563-61564)*
> 🚑 66.7 ⚖ 66.7 **FUD** 090   C 80 ▢
> AMA: 2002,Apr,13

21184 total area of bone grafting greater than 80 sq cm

> EXCLUDES *Removal of benign tumor of the skull (61563-61564)*
> 🚑 61.6 ⚖ 61.6 **FUD** 090   C 80 ▢
> AMA: 2002,Apr,13

21188 Reconstruction midface, osteotomies (other than LeFort type) and bone grafts (includes obtaining autografts)

> 🚑 46.7 ⚖ 46.7 **FUD** 090   C 80 ▢
> AMA: 2002,Apr,13

21193 Reconstruction of mandibular rami, horizontal, vertical, C, or L osteotomy; without bone graft

> 🚑 35.1 ⚖ 35.1 **FUD** 090   J 80 ▢
> AMA: 2016,Jan,13; 2015,Jan,16; 2014,Jan,11; 2012,Jan,15-42; 2011,Jan,11

21194 with bone graft (includes obtaining graft)

> 🚑 41.6 ⚖ 41.6 **FUD** 090   C 80 ▢
> AMA: 2016,Jan,13; 2015,Jan,16; 2014,Jan,11

21195 Reconstruction of mandibular rami and/or body, sagittal split; without internal rigid fixation

> 🚑 38.7 ⚖ 38.7 **FUD** 090   J 80 ▢
> AMA: 2016,Jan,13; 2015,Jan,16; 2014,Jan,11; 2012,Jan,15-42; 2011,Jan,11

21196 with internal rigid fixation

> 🚑 43.0 ⚖ 43.0 **FUD** 090   C 80 ▢
> AMA: 2016,Jan,13; 2015,Jan,16; 2014,Jan,11; 2012,Jan,15-42; 2011,Jan,11

21198 Osteotomy, mandible, segmental;

> EXCLUDES *Total maxillary osteotomy (21141-21160)*
> 🚑 33.9 ⚖ 33.9 **FUD** 090   T G2 80 ▢
> AMA: 2016,Jan,13; 2015,Jan,16; 2014,Jan,11; 2013,Dec,16

21199 with genioglossus advancement

> EXCLUDES *Total maxillary osteotomy (21141-21160)*
> 🚑 31.0 ⚖ 31.0 **FUD** 090   J G2 80 ▢
> AMA: 2016,Jan,13; 2015,Jan,16; 2014,Jan,11

21206 Osteotomy, maxilla, segmental (eg, Wassmund or Schuchard)

> 🚑 34.0 ⚖ 34.0 **FUD** 090   J A2 80 ▢
> AMA: 2002,Apr,13

21208 Osteoplasty, facial bones; augmentation (autograft, allograft, or prosthetic implant)

> 🚑 24.2 ⚖ 54.4 **FUD** 090   J A2 80 ▢
> AMA: 2002,Apr,13

21209 reduction

> 🚑 17.8 ⚖ 23.3 **FUD** 090   J A2 80 ▢
> AMA: 2002,Apr,13

21210 Graft, bone; nasal, maxillary or malar areas (includes obtaining graft)

> EXCLUDES *Cleft palate procedures (42200-42225)*
> 🚑 25.2 ⚖ 66.0 **FUD** 090   J A2 ▢
> AMA: 2002,Apr,13

21215 mandible (includes obtaining graft)

> 🚑 26.2 ⚖ 117. **FUD** 090   J A2 ▢
> AMA: 2002,Apr,13

21230 Graft; rib cartilage, autogenous, to face, chin, nose or ear (includes obtaining graft)

> EXCLUDES *Augmentation of facial bones (21208)*
> 🚑 20.5 ⚖ 20.5 **FUD** 090   J A2 80 ▢
> AMA: 2002,Apr,13

21235 ear cartilage, autogenous, to nose or ear (includes obtaining graft)

> EXCLUDES *Augmentation of facial bones (21208)*
> 🚑 16.3 ⚖ 20.8 **FUD** 090   T A2 ▢
> AMA: 2016,Jan,13; 2015,Jan,16; 2012,Jan,15-42; 2011,Jan,11

21240 Arthroplasty, temporomandibular joint, with or without autograft (includes obtaining graft)

> 🚑 32.5 ⚖ 32.5 **FUD** 090   J A2 80 50 ▢
> AMA: 2002,Apr,13; 1994,Win,1

Cutaway view of temporomandibular joint (TMJ)

TMJ syndrome is often related to stress and tooth-grinding; in other cases, arthritis, injury, poorly aligned teeth, or ill-fitting dentures may be the cause

Symptoms include facial pain and chewing problems; TMJ syndrome occurs more frequently in women

21242 Arthroplasty, temporomandibular joint, with allograft

> 🚑 29.8 ⚖ 29.8 **FUD** 090   J A2 80 50 ▢
> AMA: 2002,Apr,13

21243 Arthroplasty, temporomandibular joint, with prosthetic joint replacement

> 🚑 49.3 ⚖ 49.3 **FUD** 090   J J8 80 50 ▢
> AMA: 2002,Apr,13

21244 Reconstruction of mandible, extraoral, with transosteal bone plate (eg, mandibular staple bone plate)

> 🚑 30.9 ⚖ 30.9 **FUD** 090   J A2 80 ▢
> AMA: 2004,Mar,7; 2002,Apr,13

21245 Reconstruction of mandible or maxilla, subperiosteal implant; partial

> 🚑 25.6 ⚖ 32.0 **FUD** 090   J A2 80 ▢
> AMA: 2002,Apr,13

21246 complete

> 🚑 25.2 ⚖ 25.2 **FUD** 090   J A2 80 ▢
> AMA: 2002,Apr,13

21247 Reconstruction of mandibular condyle with bone and cartilage autografts (includes obtaining grafts) (eg, for hemifacial microsomia)

> 🚑 44.9 ⚖ 44.9 **FUD** 090   C 80 50 ▢
> AMA: 2002,Apr,13

21248 Reconstruction of mandible or maxilla, endosteal implant (eg, blade, cylinder); partial

> EXCLUDES *Midface reconstruction (21141-21160)*
> 🚑 26.3 ⚖ 32.2 **FUD** 090   J A2
> AMA: 2002,Apr,13

21249 complete

> EXCLUDES *Midface reconstruction (21141-21160)*
> 🚑 37.5 ⚖ 44.1 **FUD** 090   J A2 80 ▢
> AMA: 2002,Apr,13

21255 Reconstruction of zygomatic arch and glenoid fossa with bone and cartilage (includes obtaining autografts)

> 🚑 40.2 ⚖ 40.2 **FUD** 090   C 80 50 ▢
> AMA: 2002,Apr,13

21256 Reconstruction of orbit with osteotomies (extracranial) and with bone grafts (includes obtaining autografts) (eg, micro-ophthalmia)

> 🚑 34.6 ⚖ 34.6 **FUD** 090   J 80 50 ▢
> AMA: 2002,Apr,13

26/TC PC/TC Only A2-Z3 ASC Payment 50 Bilateral ♂ Male Only ♀ Female Only 🚑 Facility RVU ⚖ Non-Facility RVU ▢ CCI
FUD Follow-up Days CMS: IOM (Pub 100) A-Y OPPSI 80/80 Surg Assist Allowed / w/Doc ⚕ Lab Crosswalk ⚕ Radiology Crosswalk ✖ CLIA

21260	**Periorbital osteotomies for orbital hypertelorism, with bone grafts; extracranial approach**
	40.1 40.1 **FUD** 090 J G2 80
	AMA: 2002,Apr,13

21261	**combined intra- and extracranial approach**
	60.8 60.8 **FUD** 090 J 80
	AMA: 2002,Apr,13

21263	**with forehead advancement**
	56.1 56.1 **FUD** 090 J 80
	AMA: 2002,Apr,13

Grafts

In 21263, a frontal craniotomy is performed, the brain retracted, and the orbit approached from inside the skull; frontal bone is advanced and secured

Grafts are placed and the bony orbits realigned

Osteotomies are cut 360 degrees around the orbit; portions of nasal and ethmoid bones are removed

21267	**Orbital repositioning, periorbital osteotomies, unilateral, with bone grafts; extracranial approach**
	45.1 45.1 **FUD** 090 J A2 80 50
	AMA: 2002,Apr,13

21268	**combined intra- and extracranial approach**
	50.2 50.2 **FUD** 090 C 80 50
	AMA: 2002,Apr,13

21270	**Malar augmentation, prosthetic material**
	EXCLUDES *Bone graft (21210)*
	20.6 27.5 **FUD** 090 J A2 80 50
	AMA: 2002,Apr,13

21275	**Secondary revision of orbitocraniofacial reconstruction**
	24.0 24.0 **FUD** 090 J A2 80
	AMA: 2002,Apr,13

21280	**Medial canthopexy (separate procedure)**
	EXCLUDES *Reconstruction of canthus (67950)*
	16.2 16.2 **FUD** 090 J A2 80 50
	AMA: 2002,Apr,13

21282	**Lateral canthopexy**
	10.8 10.8 **FUD** 090 T A2 50
	AMA: 2002,Apr,13

21295	**Reduction of masseter muscle and bone (eg, for treatment of benign masseteric hypertrophy); extraoral approach**
	5.18 5.18 **FUD** 090 T A2 80 50
	AMA: 2002,Apr,13

21296	**intraoral approach**
	12.4 12.4 **FUD** 090 T A2 80 50
	AMA: 2002,Apr,13

21299	**Unlisted craniofacial and maxillofacial procedure**
	0.00 0.00 **FUD** YYY T 80
	AMA: 2002,Apr,13; 1995,Win,1

21310-21499 Care of Fractures/Dislocations of the Cranial and Facial Bones

EXCLUDES   *Closed treatment of skull fracture, report with appropriate E&M service*
Open treatment of skull fracture (62000-62010)

21310	**Closed treatment of nasal bone fracture without manipulation**
	0.78 3.76 **FUD** 000 T A2
	AMA: 2002,Apr,13

21315	**Closed treatment of nasal bone fracture; without stabilization**
	4.37 7.94 **FUD** 010 T A2
	AMA: 2002,Apr,13

21320	**with stabilization**
	3.90 7.36 **FUD** 010 T A2
	AMA: 2002,Apr,13

21325	**Open treatment of nasal fracture; uncomplicated**
	13.6 13.6 **FUD** 090 T A2 80
	AMA: 2002,Apr,13

21330	**complicated, with internal and/or external skeletal fixation**
	16.3 16.3 **FUD** 090 T A2 80
	AMA: 2002,Apr,13

21335	**with concomitant open treatment of fractured septum**
	20.9 20.9 **FUD** 090 T A2
	AMA: 2002,Apr,13

21336	**Open treatment of nasal septal fracture, with or without stabilization**
	18.5 18.5 **FUD** 090 T A2 80
	AMA: 2002,Apr,13

21337	**Closed treatment of nasal septal fracture, with or without stabilization**
	8.50 11.6 **FUD** 090 T A2 80
	AMA: 2002,Apr,13

21338	**Open treatment of nasoethmoid fracture; without external fixation**
	20.7 20.7 **FUD** 090 J A2 80
	AMA: 2002,Apr,13

21339	**with external fixation**
	22.1 22.1 **FUD** 090 T A2 80
	AMA: 2002,Apr,13

21340	**Percutaneous treatment of nasoethmoid complex fracture, with splint, wire or headcap fixation, including repair of canthal ligaments and/or the nasolacrimal apparatus**
	21.7 21.7 **FUD** 090 J A2 80
	AMA: 2002,Apr,13

21343	**Open treatment of depressed frontal sinus fracture**
	34.6 34.6 **FUD** 090 C 80
	AMA: 2002,Apr,13

21344	**Open treatment of complicated (eg, comminuted or involving posterior wall) frontal sinus fracture, via coronal or multiple approaches**
	40.2 40.2 **FUD** 090 C 80
	AMA: 2002,Apr,13

21345	**Closed treatment of nasomaxillary complex fracture (LeFort II type), with interdental wire fixation or fixation of denture or splint**
	18.8 23.3 **FUD** 090 T A2 80
	AMA: 2002,Apr,13

21346	**Open treatment of nasomaxillary complex fracture (LeFort II type); with wiring and/or local fixation**
	26.2 26.2 **FUD** 090 J
	AMA: 2002,Apr,13

21347	**requiring multiple open approaches**
	32.7 32.7 **FUD** 090 C 80
	AMA: 2002,Apr,13

21348	**with bone grafting (includes obtaining graft)**
	34.7 34.7 **FUD** 090 C 80
	AMA: 2002,Apr,13

21355	**Percutaneous treatment of fracture of malar area, including zygomatic arch and malar tripod, with manipulation**
	9.26 12.3 **FUD** 010 J A2 80 50
	AMA: 2002,Apr,13

21356 Open treatment of depressed zygomatic arch fracture (eg, Gillies approach)
🚑 10.9 ⚕ 14.4 **FUD** 010 T A2 80 50 ▭
AMA: 2002,Apr,13

21360 Open treatment of depressed malar fracture, including zygomatic arch and malar tripod
🚑 15.5 ⚕ 15.5 **FUD** 090 J G2 80 50 ▭
AMA: 2002,Apr,13

21365 Open treatment of complicated (eg, comminuted or involving cranial nerve foramina) fracture(s) of malar area, including zygomatic arch and malar tripod; with internal fixation and multiple surgical approaches
🚑 32.1 ⚕ 32.1 **FUD** 090 J 80 50 ▭
AMA: 2002,Apr,13

21366 with bone grafting (includes obtaining graft)
🚑 33.4 ⚕ 33.4 **FUD** 090 C 80 50 ▭
AMA: 2002,Apr,13

21385 Open treatment of orbital floor blowout fracture; transantral approach (Caldwell-Luc type operation)
🚑 19.6 ⚕ 19.6 **FUD** 090 J 80 50 ▭
AMA: 2002,Apr,13

21386 periorbital approach
🚑 19.9 ⚕ 19.9 **FUD** 090 J 80 50 ▭
AMA: 2002,Apr,13

21387 combined approach
🚑 20.5 ⚕ 20.5 **FUD** 090 J 80 50 ▭
AMA: 2002,Apr,13

21390 periorbital approach, with alloplastic or other implant
🚑 22.8 ⚕ 22.8 **FUD** 090 J G2 80 50 ▭
AMA: 2003,Jan,1; 2002,Apr,13

21395 periorbital approach with bone graft (includes obtaining graft)
🚑 28.8 ⚕ 28.8 **FUD** 090 J 80 50 ▭
AMA: 2002,Apr,13

21400 Closed treatment of fracture of orbit, except blowout; without manipulation
🚑 4.49 ⚕ 5.52 **FUD** 090 T A2 80 50 ▭
AMA: 2002,Apr,13

21401 with manipulation
🚑 8.25 ⚕ 12.6 **FUD** 090 T A2 80 50 ▭
AMA: 2002,Apr,13

21406 Open treatment of fracture of orbit, except blowout; without implant
🚑 14.9 ⚕ 14.9 **FUD** 090 J G2 80 50 ▭
AMA: 2002,Apr,13

21407 with implant
🚑 18.5 ⚕ 18.5 **FUD** 090 J G2 80 50 ▭
AMA: 2002,Apr,13

21408 with bone grafting (includes obtaining graft)
🚑 25.2 ⚕ 25.2 **FUD** 090 J 80 50 ▭
AMA: 2002,Apr,13

21421 Closed treatment of palatal or maxillary fracture (LeFort I type), with interdental wire fixation or fixation of denture or splint
🚑 18.4 ⚕ 21.8 **FUD** 090 J A2 80 ▭
AMA: 2002,Apr,13

21422 Open treatment of palatal or maxillary fracture (LeFort I type);
🚑 19.4 ⚕ 19.4 **FUD** 090 C 80 ▭
AMA: 2002,Apr,13

21423 complicated (comminuted or involving cranial nerve foramina), multiple approaches
🚑 23.6 ⚕ 23.6 **FUD** 090 C 80 ▭
AMA: 2002,Apr,13

21431 Closed treatment of craniofacial separation (LeFort III type) using interdental wire fixation of denture or splint
🚑 21.3 ⚕ 21.3 **FUD** 090 C 80 ▭
AMA: 2002,Apr,13

21432 Open treatment of craniofacial separation (LeFort III type); with wiring and/or internal fixation
🚑 18.9 ⚕ 18.9 **FUD** 090 C 80 ▭
AMA: 2002,Apr,13

21433 complicated (eg, comminuted or involving cranial nerve foramina), multiple surgical approaches
🚑 49.9 ⚕ 49.9 **FUD** 090 C 80 ▭
AMA: 2002,Apr,13

21435 complicated, utilizing internal and/or external fixation techniques (eg, head cap, halo device, and/or intermaxillary fixation)
EXCLUDES Removal of internal or external fixation (20670)
🚑 36.4 ⚕ 36.4 **FUD** 090 C 80 ▭
AMA: 2002,Apr,13

21436 complicated, multiple surgical approaches, internal fixation, with bone grafting (includes obtaining graft)
🚑 60.1 ⚕ 60.1 **FUD** 090 C 80 ▭
AMA: 2002,Apr,13

21440 Closed treatment of mandibular or maxillary alveolar ridge fracture (separate procedure)
🚑 13.5 ⚕ 16.7 **FUD** 090 T P3 80 ▭
AMA: 2002,Apr,13

21445 Open treatment of mandibular or maxillary alveolar ridge fracture (separate procedure)
🚑 18.1 ⚕ 22.3 **FUD** 090 J A2 80 ▭
AMA: 2002,Apr,13

21450 Closed treatment of mandibular fracture; without manipulation
🚑 14.3 ⚕ 17.9 **FUD** 090 T A2 80 ▭
AMA: 2002,Apr,13

21451 with manipulation
🚑 18.5 ⚕ 22.0 **FUD** 090 T A2 80 ▭
AMA: 2002,Apr,13

21452 Percutaneous treatment of mandibular fracture, with external fixation
🚑 10.1 ⚕ 17.2 **FUD** 090 T A2 80 ▭
AMA: 2002,Apr,13

In 21452, external fixation is necessary

Comminuted fractures

Metal or acrylic bar

Rods and pins placed in drilled holes

21453 Closed treatment of mandibular fracture with interdental fixation
🚑 22.6 ⚕ 26.4 **FUD** 090 J A2 80 ▭
AMA: 2016,Jan,13; 2015,Jan,16; 2014,Jan,11; 2012,Jan,15-42; 2011,Jan,11

21454 Open treatment of mandibular fracture with external fixation
🚑 17.1 ⚕ 17.1 **FUD** 090 J A2 80 ▭
AMA: 2002,Apr,13

26/TC PC/TC Only A2-Z3 ASC Payment 50 Bilateral ♂ Male Only ♀ Female Only 🚑 Facility RVU ⚕ Non-Facility RVU ▭ CCI
FUD Follow-up Days **CMS:** IOM (Pub 100) A-Y OPPSI 80/80 Surg Assist Allowed / w/Doc 🔬 Lab Crosswalk ☢ Radiology Crosswalk ✖ CLIA

46 CPT © 2016 American Medical Association. All Rights Reserved. © 2016 Optum360, LLC

21461	**Open treatment of mandibular fracture; without interdental fixation**
	🔧 27.2 ⚕ 61.8 **FUD** 090 J A2
	AMA: 2002,Apr,13
21462	**with interdental fixation**
	🔧 30.3 ⚕ 65.6 **FUD** 090 J A2 80
	AMA: 2002,Apr,13
21465	**Open treatment of mandibular condylar fracture**
	🔧 27.7 ⚕ 27.7 **FUD** 090 J A2 80 50
	AMA: 2002,Apr,13
21470	**Open treatment of complicated mandibular fracture by multiple surgical approaches including internal fixation, interdental fixation, and/or wiring of dentures or splints**
	🔧 34.9 ⚕ 34.9 **FUD** 090 J 80
	AMA: 2016,Jan,13; 2015,Jan,16; 2014,Jan,11; 2012,Jan,15-42; 2011,Jan,11
21480	**Closed treatment of temporomandibular dislocation; initial or subsequent**
	🔧 0.92 ⚕ 2.83 **FUD** 000 T A2 50
	AMA: 2002,Apr,13
21485	**complicated (eg, recurrent requiring intermaxillary fixation or splinting), initial or subsequent**
	🔧 17.0 ⚕ 20.3 **FUD** 090 T A2 80 50
	AMA: 2002,Apr,13
21490	**Open treatment of temporomandibular dislocation**
	EXCLUDES *Interdental wiring (21497)*
	🔧 26.5 ⚕ 26.5 **FUD** 090 J A2 80 50
	AMA: 2002,Apr,13
~~21495~~	~~Open treatment of hyoid fracture~~
	To report, see ~31584
21497	**Interdental wiring, for condition other than fracture**
	🔧 17.7 ⚕ 21.2 **FUD** 090 T A2 80
	AMA: 2016,Jan,13; 2015,Jan,16; 2014,Jan,11; 2012,Jan,15-42; 2011,Jan,11
21499	**Unlisted musculoskeletal procedure, head**
	EXCLUDES *Unlisted procedures of craniofacial or maxillofacial areas (21299)*
	🔧 0.00 ⚕ 0.00 **FUD** YYY T 80
	AMA: 2002,Apr,13; 1995,Win,1

21501-21510 Surgical Incision for Drainage: Chest and Soft Tissues of Neck

EXCLUDES *Biopsy of the flank or back (21920-21925)*
Simple incision and drainage of abscess or hematoma (10060, 10140)
Tumor removal of flank or back (21930-21936)

21501	**Incision and drainage, deep abscess or hematoma, soft tissues of neck or thorax;**
	EXCLUDES *Deep incision and drainage of posterior spine (22010-22015)*
	🔧 9.27 ⚕ 13.0 **FUD** 090 T A2
	AMA: 2016,Jan,13; 2015,Jan,16; 2014,Dec,16; 2014,Dec,16
21502	**with partial rib ostectomy**
	🔧 15.3 ⚕ 15.3 **FUD** 090 T A2 80
	AMA: 2002,Apr,13
21510	**Incision, deep, with opening of bone cortex (eg, for osteomyelitis or bone abscess), thorax**
	🔧 12.9 ⚕ 12.9 **FUD** 090 C 80
	AMA: 2002,Apr,13

21550 Soft Tissue Biopsy of Chest or Neck

EXCLUDES *Biopsy of bone (20220-20251)*
Soft tissue needle biopsy (20206)

21550	**Biopsy, soft tissue of neck or thorax**
	🔧 4.55 ⚕ 7.52 **FUD** 010 T G2
	AMA: 2002,Apr,13

21552-21558 [21552, 21554] Excision Soft Tissue Tumors Chest and Neck

INCLUDES Any necessary elevation of tissue planes or dissection
Measurement of tumor and necessary margin at greatest diameter prior to excision
Resection without removal of significant normal tissue
Simple and intermediate repairs
Types of excision:
  Fascial or subfascial soft tissue tumors: simple and marginal resection of tumors found either in or below the deep fascia, not involving bone or excision of a substantial amount of normal tissue; primarily benign and intramuscular tumors
  Radical resection soft tissue tumor: wide resection of tumor, involving substantial margins of normal tissue and may involve tissue removal from one or more layers; most often malignant or aggressive benign
  Subcutaneous: simple and marginal resection of tumors in the subcutaneous tissue above the deep fascia; most often benign

EXCLUDES *Complex repair*
Excision of benign cutaneous lesions (eg, sebaceous cyst) (11400-11426)
Radical resection of cutaneous tumors (eg, melanoma) (11600-11626)
Significant exploration of the vessels or neuroplasty

	21552	**Resequenced code. See code following 21555.**
	21554	**Resequenced code. See code following 21556.**
	21555	**Excision, tumor, soft tissue of neck or anterior thorax, subcutaneous; less than 3 cm**
		🔧 8.82 ⚕ 11.8 **FUD** 090 T G2
		AMA: 2016,Jan,13; 2015,Jan,16; 2014,Jan,11; 2012,Jan,15-42; 2011,Jan,11
#	21552	**3 cm or greater**
		🔧 12.8 ⚕ 12.8 **FUD** 090 T G2 80
	21556	**Excision, tumor, soft tissue of neck or anterior thorax, subfascial (eg, intramuscular); less than 5 cm**
		🔧 15.2 ⚕ 15.2 **FUD** 090 T G2
		AMA: 2002,Apr,13
#	21554	**5 cm or greater**
		🔧 21.1 ⚕ 21.1 **FUD** 090 T G2 80
	21557	**Radical resection of tumor (eg, sarcoma), soft tissue of neck or anterior thorax; less than 5 cm**
		🔧 27.6 ⚕ 27.6 **FUD** 090 T G2 80
		AMA: 2016,Jan,13; 2015,Jan,16; 2014,Jan,11
	21558	**5 cm or greater**
		🔧 38.9 ⚕ 38.9 **FUD** 090 T G2 80

21600-21632 Bony Resection Chest and Neck

21600	**Excision of rib, partial**
	EXCLUDES *Extensive debridement (11044, 11047)*
	Extensive tumor removal (19260)
	🔧 16.0 ⚕ 16.0 **FUD** 090 T A2 80
	AMA: 2016,Jan,13; 2015,Jan,16; 2014,Jan,11; 2013,Mar,13; 2012,Jul,12-14
21610	**Costotransversectomy (separate procedure)**
	🔧 34.7 ⚕ 34.7 **FUD** 090 T A2 80
	AMA: 2002,Apr,13
21615	**Excision first and/or cervical rib;**
	🔧 17.9 ⚕ 17.9 **FUD** 090 C 80 50
	AMA: 2016,Jan,13; 2015,Jan,16; 2014,Mar,13
21616	**with sympathectomy**
	🔧 21.7 ⚕ 21.7 **FUD** 090 C 80 50
	AMA: 2002,Apr,13
21620	**Ostectomy of sternum, partial**
	🔧 14.5 ⚕ 14.5 **FUD** 090 C 80
	AMA: 2002,Apr,13
21627	**Sternal debridement**
	EXCLUDES *Debridement with sternotomy closure (21750)*
	🔧 15.5 ⚕ 15.5 **FUD** 090 C 80
	AMA: 2016,Jan,13; 2015,Jan,16; 2014,Jan,11; 2011,May,3-5

21630 **Radical resection of sternum;**
    🔲 35.0   🔲 35.0   **FUD** 090   C 80 ▣
    AMA: 2002,Apr,13; 1994,Win,1

21632 **with mediastinal lymphadenectomy**
    🔲 35.0   🔲 35.0   **FUD** 090   C 80 ▣
    AMA: 2002,Apr,13

21685-21750 Repair/Reconstruction Chest and Soft Tissues Neck

EXCLUDES   *Biopsy of chest or neck (21550)*
       Repair of simple wounds (12001-12007)
       Tumor removal of chest or neck (21552-21558 [21552, 21554])

21685 **Hyoid myotomy and suspension**
    🔲 28.9   🔲 28.9   **FUD** 090   T G2 80 ▣
    AMA: 2016,Jan,13; 2015,Jan,16; 2014,Jan,11; 2012,Jan,15-42; 2011,Jan,11

21700 **Division of scalenus anticus; without resection of cervical rib**
    🔲 10.7   🔲 10.7   **FUD** 090   T A2 80 50 ▣
    AMA: 2002,Apr,13

21705 **with resection of cervical rib**
    🔲 16.0   🔲 16.0   **FUD** 090   C 80 50 ▣
    AMA: 2016,Jan,13; 2015,Jan,16; 2014,Mar,13

21720 **Division of sternocleidomastoid for torticollis, open operation; without cast application**
    EXCLUDES   *Transection of spinal accessory and cervical nerves (63191, 64722)*
    🔲 13.0   🔲 13.0   **FUD** 090   T A2 80 ▣
    AMA: 2002,Apr,13

21725 **with cast application**
    EXCLUDES   *Transection of spinal accessory and cervical nerves (63191, 64722)*
    🔲 15.2   🔲 15.2   **FUD** 090   T A2 80 ▣
    AMA: 2002,Apr,13

21740 **Reconstructive repair of pectus excavatum or carinatum; open**
    🔲 29.6   🔲 29.6   **FUD** 090   C 80 ▣
    AMA: 2002,Apr,13

21742 **minimally invasive approach (Nuss procedure), without thoracoscopy**
    🔲 0.00   🔲 0.00   **FUD** 090   T 80 ▣
    AMA: 2002,Apr,13

21743 **minimally invasive approach (Nuss procedure), with thoracoscopy**
    🔲 0.00   🔲 0.00   **FUD** 090   T 80 ▣
    AMA: 2002,Apr,13

21750 **Closure of median sternotomy separation with or without debridement (separate procedure)**
    🔲 19.8   🔲 19.8   **FUD** 090   C 80 ▣
    AMA: 2016,Jan,13; 2015,Jan,16; 2014,Jan,11; 2011,May,3-5

21811-21825 Fracture Care: Ribs and Sternum

EXCLUDES   *Closed treatment uncomplicated rib fractures*

21811 **Open treatment of rib fracture(s) with internal fixation, includes thoracoscopic visualization when performed, unilateral; 1-3 ribs**
    🔲 17.7   🔲 17.7   **FUD** 000   T 80 50 ▣
    AMA: 2016,Jan,13; 2015,Aug,3

21812 **4-6 ribs**
    🔲 21.2   🔲 21.2   **FUD** 000   T 80 50 ▣
    AMA: 2016,Jan,13; 2015,Aug,3

21813 **7 or more ribs**
    🔲 27.7   🔲 27.7   **FUD** 000   T 80 50 ▣
    AMA: 2016,Jan,13; 2015,Aug,3

21820 **Closed treatment of sternum fracture**
    🔲 4.12   🔲 4.02   **FUD** 090   T A2 ▣
    AMA: 2002,Apr,13

21825 **Open treatment of sternum fracture with or without skeletal fixation**
    EXCLUDES   *Treatment of sternoclavicular dislocation (23520-23532)*
    🔲 15.6   🔲 15.6   **FUD** 090   C 80 ▣
    AMA: 2002,Apr,13

21899 Unlisted Procedures of Chest or Neck

CMS: 100-04,4,180.3 Unlisted Service or Procedure

21899 **Unlisted procedure, neck or thorax**
    🔲 0.00   🔲 0.00   **FUD** YYY   T 80
    AMA: 2016,Jan,13; 2015,Aug,3

21920-21925 Biopsy Soft Tissue of Back and Flank

EXCLUDES   *Soft tissue needle biopsy (20206)*

21920 **Biopsy, soft tissue of back or flank; superficial**
    🔲 4.62   🔲 7.35   **FUD** 010   T P3 ▣
    AMA: 2002,Apr,13; 1993,Sum,25

21925 **deep**
    🔲 10.2   🔲 12.7   **FUD** 090   T A2 ▣
    AMA: 2002,Apr,13

21930-21936 Excision Soft Tissue Tumors Back or Flank

INCLUDES   Any necessary elevation of tissue planes or dissection
    Measurement of tumor and necessary margin at greatest diameter prior to excision
    Simple and intermediate repairs
    Types of excision:
       Fascial or subfascial soft tissue tumors: simple and marginal resection of tumors found either in or below the deep fascia, not involving bone or excision of a substantial amount of normal tissue; most often benign and intramuscular tumors
       Radical resection soft tissue tumor: wide resection of tumor, involving substantial margins of normal tissue and may include tissue removal from one or more layers; most often malignant or aggressive benign
       Subcutaneous: simple and marginal resection of tumors in the subcutaneous tissue above the deep fascia; most often benign

EXCLUDES   *Complex repair*
    Excision of benign cutaneous lesions (eg, sebaceous cyst) (11400-11406)
    Radical resection of cutaneous tumors (eg, melanoma) (11600-11606)
    Significant exploration of the vessels or neuroplasty

21930 **Excision, tumor, soft tissue of back or flank, subcutaneous; less than 3 cm**
    🔲 10.5   🔲 13.5   **FUD** 090   T G2 ▣
    AMA: 2016,Jan,13; 2015,Jan,16; 2014,Jan,11; 2012,Jan,15-42; 2011,Jan,11

21931 **3 cm or greater**
    🔲 13.5   🔲 13.5   **FUD** 090   T G2 80 ▣

21932 **Excision, tumor, soft tissue of back or flank, subfascial (eg, intramuscular); less than 5 cm**
    🔲 19.1   🔲 19.1   **FUD** 090   T G2 80 ▣

21933 **5 cm or greater**
    🔲 21.2   🔲 21.2   **FUD** 090   T G2 80 ▣

21935 **Radical resection of tumor (eg, sarcoma), soft tissue of back or flank; less than 5 cm**
    🔲 29.6   🔲 29.6   **FUD** 090   T G2 ▣
    AMA: 2002,Apr,13; 1990,Win,4

21936 **5 cm or greater**
    🔲 40.7   🔲 40.7   **FUD** 090   T G2 80 ▣

22010-22015 Incision for Drainage of Deep Spinal Abscess

EXCLUDES   *Incision and drainage of hematoma (10060, 10140)*
    Injection:
       Chemonucleolysis (62292)
       Discography (62290-62291)
       Facet joint (64490-64495, [64633, 64634, 64635, 64636])
       Myelography (62284)
    Needle/trocar biopsy (20220-20225)

22010 **Incision and drainage, open, of deep abscess (subfascial), posterior spine; cervical, thoracic, or cervicothoracic**
    🔲 27.5   🔲 27.5   **FUD** 090   C 80 ▣

26/TC PC/TC Only   A2-Z3 ASC Payment   50 Bilateral   ♂ Male Only   ♀ Female Only   🔲 Facility RVU   🔲 Non-Facility RVU   ▣ CCI
FUD Follow-up Days   CMS: IOM (Pub 100)   A-Y OPPSI   80/80 Surg Assist Allowed / w/Doc   🔲 Lab Crosswalk   🔲 Radiology Crosswalk   ❌ CLIA

48

22015	lumbar, sacral, or lumbosacral

🔪 26.6   🔨 26.6   **FUD** 090   C ▣

EXCLUDES   *Incision and drainage, complex, postoperative wound infection (10180)*
Incision and drainage, open, of deep abscess (subfascial), posterior spine; cervical, thoracic, or cervicothoracic (22010)
Removal of posterior nonsegmental instrumentation (eg, Harrington rod) (22850)
Removal of posterior segmental instrumentation (22852)

22100-22103 Partial Resection Vertebral Component

EXCLUDES   *Back or flank biopsy (21920-21925)*
Bone biopsy (20220-20251)
Injection:
Chemonucleolysis (62292)
Discography (62290-62291)
Facet joint (64490-64495, [64633, 64634, 64635, 64636])
Myelography (62284)
Removal of tumor flank or back (21930)
Soft tissue needle biopsy (20206)
Spinal reconstruction with vertebral body prosthesis:
Cervical (20931, 20938, 22554, 63081)
Thoracic (20931, 20938, 22556, 63085, 63087)

22100	Partial excision of posterior vertebral component (eg, spinous process, lamina or facet) for intrinsic bony lesion, single vertebral segment; cervical

🔪 25.2   🔨 25.2   **FUD** 090   T 80 ▣

AMA: 2016,Jan,13; 2015,Jan,16; 2013,Jul,3-5

22101	thoracic

🔪 24.6   🔨 24.6   **FUD** 090   T 80 ▣

AMA: 2016,Jan,13; 2015,Jan,16; 2013,Jul,3-5

22102	lumbar

Code also posterior spinous process distraction device insertion, if applicable (22867-22870)

🔪 22.8   🔨 22.8   **FUD** 090   T 62 80 ▣

AMA: 2016,Jan,13; 2015,Jan,16; 2013,Jul,3-5

+ 22103	each additional segment (List separately in addition to code for primary procedure)

Code first (22100-22102)

🔪 4.07   🔨 4.07   **FUD** ZZZ   N N1 80 ▣

AMA: 2003,Jan,1; 2002,Apr,13

22110-22116 Partial Resection Vertebral Component without Decompression

EXCLUDES   *Back or flank biopsy (21920-21925)*
Bone biopsy (20220-20251)
Bone grafting procedures (20930-20938)
Harvest bone graft (20931, 20938)
Injection:
Chemonucleolysis (62292)
Discography (62290-62291)
Facet joint (64490-64495, [64633, 64634, 64635, 64636])
Myelography (62284)
Osteotomy (22210-22226)
Removal of tumor flank or back (21930)
Restoration after vertebral body resection (22585, 63082, 63086, 63088, 63091)
Spinal restoration with graft:
Cervical (20931, 20938, 22554, 63081)
Lumbar (20931, 20938, 22558, 63087, 63090)
Thoracic (20931, 20938, 22556, 63085, 63087)
Spinal restoration with prosthesis:
Cervical (20931, 20938, 22554, 22853-22854 [22859], 63081)
Lumbar (20931, 20938, 22558, 22853-22854 [22859], 63087, 63090)
Thoracic (20931, 20938, 22556, 22853-22854 [22859], 63085, 63087)
Vertebral corpectomy (63081-63091)

22110	Partial excision of vertebral body, for intrinsic bony lesion, without decompression of spinal cord or nerve root(s), single vertebral segment; cervical

🔪 30.3   🔨 30.3   **FUD** 090   C 80 ▣

AMA: 2016,Jan,13; 2015,Jan,16; 2013,Jul,3-5

22112	thoracic

🔪 28.5   🔨 28.5   **FUD** 090   C 80 ▣

AMA: 2016,Jan,13; 2015,Jan,16; 2013,Jul,3-5

22114	lumbar

🔪 28.6   🔨 28.6   **FUD** 090   C 80 ▣

AMA: 2016,Jan,13; 2015,Jan,16; 2013,Jul,3-5

+ 22116	each additional vertebral segment (List separately in addition to code for primary procedure)

Code first (22110-22114)

🔪 4.14   🔨 4.14   **FUD** ZZZ   C 80 ▣

AMA: 2003,Feb,7; 2002,Apr,13

22206-22216 Spinal Osteotomy: Posterior/Posterolateral Approach

CMS: 100-04,12,40.8 Co-surgery and team surgery

EXCLUDES   *Decompression of the spinal cord and/or nerve roots (63001-63308)*
Injection:
Chemonucleolysis (62292)
Discography (62290-62292)
Facet joint (64490-64495, [64633, 64634, 64635, 64636])
Myelography (62284)
Procedures performed at same level (22210-22226, 22830, 63001-63048, 63055-63066, 63075-63091, 63101-63103)
Repair of vertebral fracture by the anterior approach, see appropriate arthrodesis, bone graft, instrumentation codes, and (63081-63091)
Code also arthrodesis (22590-22632)
Code also bone grafting procedures (20930-20938)
Code also spinal instrumentation (22840-22855 [22859])

22206	Osteotomy of spine, posterior or posterolateral approach, 3 columns, 1 vertebral segment (eg, pedicle/vertebral body subtraction); thoracic

EXCLUDES   *Osteotomy of spine, posterior or posterolateral approach, lumbar (22207)*
Procedures performed at same level (22210-22226, 22830, 63001-63048, 63055-63066, 63075-63091, 63101-63103)

🔪 70.9   🔨 70.9   **FUD** 090   C 80 ▣

AMA: 2016,Jan,13; 2015,Jan,16; 2014,Jan,11; 2013,Jul,3-5; 2012,Jan,15-42; 2011,Jan,11

22207	lumbar

EXCLUDES   *Osteotomy of spine, posterior or posterolateral approach, thoracic (22206)*
Procedures performed at the same level (22210-22226, 22830, 63001-63048, 63055-63066, 63075-63091, 63101-63103)

🔪 69.5   🔨 69.5   **FUD** 090   C 80 ▣

AMA: 2016,Jan,13; 2015,Jan,16; 2014,Jan,11; 2013,Jul,3-5; 2012,Jan,15-42; 2011,Jan,11

+ 22208	each additional vertebral segment (List separately in addition to code for primary procedure)

EXCLUDES   *Procedures performed at the same level (22210-22226, 22830, 63001-63048, 63055-63066, 63075-63091, 63101-63103)*

Code first (22206, 22207)

🔪 17.0   🔨 17.0   **FUD** ZZZ   C 80 ▣

AMA: 2016,Jan,13; 2015,Jan,16; 2014,Jan,11; 2012,Jan,15-42; 2011,Jan,11

22210	Osteotomy of spine, posterior or posterolateral approach, 1 vertebral segment; cervical

🔪 51.8   🔨 51.8   **FUD** 090   C 80 ▣

AMA: 2016,Jan,13; 2015,Jan,16; 2013,Jul,3-5

In 22210, patient is stabilized by halo and traction to correct cervical problem

C-6
C-7
T-1

Several sections may be removed

Report 22212 if thoracic; report 22214 if lumbar; report 22216 for each additional segment

Physician removes spinous processes, lamina

22212 thoracic
🔧 42.9 ✂ 42.9 **FUD** 090 C 80 📻
AMA: 2016,Jan,13; 2015,Jan,16; 2014,Jan,11; 2013,Jul,3-5

22214 lumbar
🔧 43.1 ✂ 43.1 **FUD** 090 C 80 📻
AMA: 2016,Jan,13; 2015,Jan,16; 2014,Dec,16; 2014,Dec,16; 2014,Jan,11; 2013,Jul,3-5

+ **22216** each additional vertebral segment (List separately in addition to primary procedure)
Code first (22210-22214)
🔧 10.6 ✂ 10.6 **FUD** ZZZ C 80 📻
AMA: 2016,Jan,13; 2015,Jan,16; 2014,Jan,11

22220-22226 Spinal Osteotomy: Anterior Approach

CMS: 100-04,12,40.8 Co-surgery and team surgery

EXCLUDES Corpectomy (63081-63091)
Decompression of the spinal cord and/or nerve roots (63001-63308)
Injection:
    Chemonucleolysis (62292)
    Discography (62290-62291)
    Facet joint (64490-64495, [64633], [64634], [64635], [64636])
    Myelography (62284)
    Needle/trocar biopsy (20220-20225)
    Repair of vertebral fracture by the anterior approach, see appropriate arthrodesis, bone graft, instrumentation codes, and (63081-63091)
Code also arthrodesis (22590-22632)
Code also bone grafting procedures (20930-20938)
Code also spinal instrumentation (22840-22855 [22859])

22220 Osteotomy of spine, including discectomy, anterior approach, single vertebral segment; cervical
🔧 46.3 ✂ 46.3 **FUD** 090 C 80 📻
AMA: 2016,Jan,13; 2015,Jan,16; 2013,Jul,3-5

22222 thoracic
🔧 44.9 ✂ 44.9 **FUD** 090 C 80 📻
AMA: 2016,Jan,13; 2015,Jan,16; 2014,Jan,11; 2013,Jul,3-5

22224 lumbar
🔧 45.8 ✂ 45.8 **FUD** 090 C 80 📻
AMA: 2016,Jan,13; 2015,Jan,16; 2013,Jul,3-5

+ **22226** each additional vertebral segment (List separately in addition to code for primary procedure)
Code first (22220-22224)
🔧 10.5 ✂ 10.5 **FUD** ZZZ C 80 📻
AMA: 2002,Feb,4; 2002,Apr,13

22305-22315 Closed Treatment Vertebral Fractures

EXCLUDES Injection:
    Chemonucleolysis (62292)
    Discography (62290-62291)
    Facet joint (64490-64495, [64633], [64634], [64635], [64636])
    Myelography (62284)
Code also arthrodesis (22590-22632)
Code also bone grafting procedures (20930-20938)
Code also spinal instrumentation (22840-22855 [22859])

~~**22305**~~ ~~Closed treatment of vertebral process fracture(s)~~
To report, see appropriate E&M codes

22310 Closed treatment of vertebral body fracture(s), without manipulation, requiring and including casting or bracing
EXCLUDES Percutaneous vertebroplasty performed at same level (22510-22515)
🔧 8.14 ✂ 8.82 **FUD** 090 T A2 📻
AMA: 2016,Jan,13; 2015,Jan,8; 2015,Jan,16; 2014,Jul,8; 2014,Jan,11; 2013,Jul,3-5; 2012,Jun,10-11; 2012,Jan,15-42; 2011,Jan,11

22315 Closed treatment of vertebral fracture(s) and/or dislocation(s) requiring casting or bracing, with and including casting and/or bracing by manipulation or traction
EXCLUDES Percutaneous vertebroplasty performed at same level (22510-22515)
Spinal manipulation (97140)
🔧 22.2 ✂ 25.4 **FUD** 090 T A2 📻
AMA: 2016,Jan,13; 2015,Jan,8; 2015,Jan,16; 2014,Jan,11; 2013,Jul,3-5; 2012,Jun,10-11; 2012,Apr,11-13

22318-22319 Open Treatment Odontoid Fracture: Anterior Approach

EXCLUDES Injection:
    Chemonucleolysis (62292)
    Discography (62290-62291)
    Facet joint (64490-64495, [64633, 64634, 64635, 64636])
    Myelography (62284)
    Needle/trocar biopsy (20220-20225)
Code also arthrodesis (22590-22632)
Code also bone grafting procedures (20930-20938)
Code also spinal instrumentation (22840-22855 [22859])

22318 Open treatment and/or reduction of odontoid fracture(s) and or dislocation(s) (including os odontoideum), anterior approach, including placement of internal fixation; without grafting
🔧 47.9 ✂ 47.9 **FUD** 090 C 80 📻
AMA: 2016,Jan,13; 2015,Jan,16; 2014,Jan,11; 2013,Jul,3-5; 2012,Apr,11-13

22319 with grafting
🔧 53.2 ✂ 53.2 **FUD** 090 C 80 📻
AMA: 2016,Jan,13; 2015,Jan,16; 2014,Jan,11; 2013,Jul,3-5; 2012,Apr,14-16

22325-22328 Open Treatment Vertebral Fractures: Posterior Approach

EXCLUDES Corpectomy (63081-63091)
Injection:
    Chemonucleolysis (62292)
    Discography (62290-62291)
    Facet joint (64490-64495, [64633], [64634], [64635], [64636])
    Myelography (62284)
Needle/trocar biopsy (20220-20225)
Spine decompression (63001-63091)
Vertebral fracture care by arthrodesis (22548-22632)
Vertebral fracture care frontal approach (63081-63091)
Code also arthrodesis (22548-22632)
Code also bone grafting procedures (20930-20938)
Code also spinal instrumentation (22840-22855 [22859])

22325 Open treatment and/or reduction of vertebral fracture(s) and/or dislocation(s), posterior approach, 1 fractured vertebra or dislocated segment; lumbar
EXCLUDES Percutaneous vertebral augmentation performed at same level (22514-22515)
Percutaneous vertebroplasty performed at same level (22511-22512)
🔧 41.7 ✂ 41.7 **FUD** 090 C 80 📻
AMA: 2016,Jan,13; 2015,Jan,16; 2015,Jan,8; 2014,Jan,11; 2013,Jul,3-5; 2012,Jun,10-11

22326 cervical
EXCLUDES Percutaneous vertebroplasty performed at same level (22510, 22512)
🔧 43.4 ✂ 43.4 **FUD** 090 C 80 📻
AMA: 2016,Jan,13; 2015,Jan,16; 2014,Jan,11; 2013,Jul,3-5

22327 thoracic
EXCLUDES Percutaneous vertebral augmentation performed at same level (22515)
Percutaneous vertebroplasty performed at same level (22510, 22512-22513)
🔧 43.6 ✂ 43.6 **FUD** 090 C 80 📻
AMA: 2016,Jan,13; 2015,Jan,16; 2015,Jan,8; 2014,Jan,11; 2013,Jul,3-5; 2012,Jun,10-11

+ **22328** each additional fractured vertebra or dislocated segment (List separately in addition to code for primary procedure)
Code first (22325-22327)
🔧 8.27 ✂ 8.27 **FUD** ZZZ C 80 📻
AMA: 2002,Apr,13; 1997,Nov,1

22505 Spinal Manipulation with Anesthesia

EXCLUDES *Manipulation not requiring anesthesia (97140)*

22505 **Manipulation of spine requiring anesthesia, any region**

⚙ 3.68 ⚖ 3.68 **FUD** 010 T A2 ▭

AMA: 2016,Jan,13; 2015,Jan,16; 2014,Jan,11; 2012,Jan,15-42; 2011,Jan,11

22510-22515 Percutaneous Vertebroplasty/Kyphoplasty

INCLUDES Bone biopsy when applicable (20225)
Radiological guidance

EXCLUDES *Closed treatment vertebral fractures (22310, 22315)*
Open treatment/reduction vertebral fractures (22325, 22327)
Sacroplasty/augmentation (0200T-0201T)

▲ **22510** **Percutaneous vertebroplasty (bone biopsy included when performed), 1 vertebral body, unilateral or bilateral injection, inclusive of all imaging guidance; cervicothoracic**

⚙ 13.0 ⚖ 50.3 **FUD** 010 T 62 ▭

AMA: 2016,Jan,13; 2015,Jan,8

▲ **22511** **lumbosacral**

⚙ 12.2 ⚖ 49.8 **FUD** 010 T 62 ▭

AMA: 2016,Jan,13; 2015,Apr,8; 2015,Jan,8

▲ + **22512** **each additional cervicothoracic or lumbosacral vertebral body (List separately in addition to code for primary procedure)**

Code first (22510-22511)

⚙ 6.09 ⚖ 27.9 **FUD** ZZZ N N1 ▭

AMA: 2016,Jan,13; 2015,Jan,8

▲ **22513** **Percutaneous vertebral augmentation, including cavity creation (fracture reduction and bone biopsy included when performed) using mechanical device (eg, kyphoplasty), 1 vertebral body, unilateral or bilateral cannulation, inclusive of all imaging guidance; thoracic**

⚙ 15.6 ⚖ 208. **FUD** 010 J 62 ▭

AMA: 2016,Jan,13; 2015,Jan,8

▲ **22514** **lumbar**

⚙ 14.5 ⚖ 208. **FUD** 010 J 62 ▭

AMA: 2016,Jan,13; 2015,Jan,8

▲ + **22515** **each additional thoracic or lumbar vertebral body (List separately in addition to code for primary procedure)**

Code first (22513-22514)

⚙ 6.59 ⚖ 126. **FUD** ZZZ N N1 ▭

AMA: 2016,Jan,13; 2015,Jan,8

22526-22527 Percutaneous Annuloplasty

CMS: 100-04,32,220.1 Thermal Intradiscal Procedures (TIPS)

INCLUDES Fluoroscopic guidance (77002, 77003)

EXCLUDES *Needle/trocar biopsy (20220-20225)*
Injection:
Chemonucleolysis (62292)
Discography (62290-62291)
Facet joint (64490-64495, [64633], [64634], [64635], [64636])
Myelography (62284)
Procedure performed by other methods (22899)

▲ **22526** **Percutaneous intradiscal electrothermal annuloplasty, unilateral or bilateral including fluoroscopic guidance; single level**

⚙ 10.1 ⚖ 67.8 **FUD** 010 E ▭

AMA: 2016,Jan,13; 2015,Jan,8; 2015,Jan,16; 2014,Jan,11; 2012,Jan,15-42; 2011,Jan,8; 2011,Jan,11

▲ + **22527** **1 or more additional levels (List separately in addition to code for primary procedure)**

Code first (22526)

⚙ 4.60 ⚖ 56.2 **FUD** ZZZ E ▭

AMA: 2016,Jan,13; 2015,Jan,8; 2015,Jan,16; 2014,Jan,11; 2011,Jan,8

22532-22534 Spinal Fusion: Lateral Extracavitary Approach

EXCLUDES *Corpectomy (63101-63103)*
Exploration of spinal fusion (22830)
Fracture care (22310-22328)
Injection:
Chemonucleolysis (62292)
Discography (62290-62291)
Facet joint (64490-64495, [64633], [64634], [64635], [64636])
Myelography (62284)
Laminectomy (63001-63017)
Needle/trocar biopsy (20220-20225)
Osteotomy (22206-22226)
Code also bone grafting procedures (20930-20938)
Code also spinal instrumentation (22840-22855 [22859])

22532 **Arthrodesis, lateral extracavitary technique, including minimal discectomy to prepare interspace (other than for decompression); thoracic**

⚙ 51.8 ⚖ 51.8 **FUD** 090 C 80 ▭

AMA: 2016,Jan,13; 2015,Jan,16; 2014,Jan,11; 2013,Jul,3-5; 2012,Apr,14-16

22533 **lumbar**

⚙ 47.9 ⚖ 47.9 **FUD** 090 C 80 ▭

AMA: 2016,Jan,13; 2015,Jan,16; 2014,Jan,11; 2013,Jul,3-5; 2012,Apr,14-16

+ **22534** **thoracic or lumbar, each additional vertebral segment (List separately in addition to code for primary procedure)**

Code first (22532-22533)

⚙ 10.5 ⚖ 10.5 **FUD** ZZZ C 80 ▭

AMA: 2002,Apr,13; 1993,Spr,36

22548-22634 Spinal Fusion: Anterior and Posterior Approach

EXCLUDES *Corpectomy (63081-63091)*
Exploration of spinal fusion (22830)
Fracture care (22310-22328)
Facet joint arthrodesis (0219T-0222T)
Injection:
Chemonucleolysis (62292)
Discography (62290-62291)
Facet joint (64490-64495, [64633], [64634], [64635], [64636])
Myelography (62284)
Laminectomy (63001-63017)
Needle/trocar biopsy (20220-20225)
Osteotomy (22206-22226)
Code also bone grafting procedures (20930-20938)
Code also spinal instrumentation (22840-22855 [22859])

22548 **Arthrodesis, anterior transoral or extraoral technique, clivus-C1-C2 (atlas-axis), with or without excision of odontoid process**

EXCLUDES *Laminectomy or laminotomy with disc removal (63020-63042)*

⚙ 57.8 ⚖ 57.8 **FUD** 090 C 80 ▭

AMA: 2016,Jan,13; 2015,Jan,16; 2014,Jan,11; 2013,Jul,3-5; 2012,Apr,14-16; 2012,Jan,15-42; 2011,Jan,11

● New Code ▲ Revised Code ○ Reinstated ● New Web Release ▲ Revised Web Release Unlisted Not Covered # Resequenced

⊘ AMA Mod 51 Exempt ⑤ Optum Mod 51 Exempt ⑥ Mod 63 Exempt ✗ Non-FDA Drug ★ Telehealth M Maternity A Age Edit + Add-on AMA: CPT Asst

© 2016 Optum360, LLC CPT © 2016 American Medical Association. All Rights Reserved. **51**

22551 **Arthrodesis, anterior interbody, including disc space preparation, discectomy, osteophytectomy and decompression of spinal cord and/or nerve roots; cervical below C2**

INCLUDES Operating microscope (69990)

🚑 50.0   ⚕ 50.0   **FUD** 090   [J] [J8] [80] 🔲

AMA: 2016,May,13; 2016,Feb,12; 2016,Jan,13; 2015,Jan,16; 2015,Jan,13; 2014,Jan,11; 2013,Jul,3-5; 2012,Apr,14-16; 2012,Jan,15-42; 2011,Jan,11

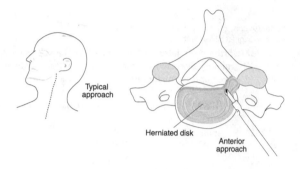

Typical approach

Herniated disk

Anterior approach

+ 22552 **cervical below C2, each additional interspace (List separately in addition to code for separate procedure)**

INCLUDES Operating microscope (69990)

Code first (22551)

🚑 11.7   ⚕ 11.7   **FUD** ZZZ   [N] [80] 🔲

AMA: 2016,Feb,12; 2016,Jan,13; 2015,Jan,16; 2014,Jan,11; 2013,Jul,3-5; 2012,Apr,14-16; 2012,Jan,15-42; 2011,Jan,11

22554 **Arthrodesis, anterior interbody technique, including minimal discectomy to prepare interspace (other than for decompression); cervical below C2**

EXCLUDES Anterior discectomy and interbody fusion during the same operative session (regardless if performed by multiple surgeons) (22551)

Discectomy, anterior, with decompression of spinal cord and/or nerve root(s), cervical (even by separate individual) (63075-63076)

🚑 36.5   ⚕ 36.5   **FUD** 090   [J] [J8] [80] 🔲

AMA: 2016,Jan,13; 2015,Apr,7; 2015,Jan,16; 2014,Jan,11; 2013,Jul,3-5; 2012,Apr,11-13; 2012,Apr,14-16; 2012,Jan,15-42; 2011,Jan,11

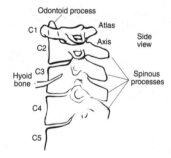

Odontoid process

C1   Atlas
C2   Axis   Side view

Hyoid bone   C3   Spinous processes

C4

C5

22556 **thoracic**

🚑 48.5   ⚕ 48.5   **FUD** 090   [C] [80] 🔲

AMA: 2016,Jan,13; 2015,Jan,16; 2014,Jan,11; 2013,Jul,3-5; 2012,Apr,14-16; 2012,Jan,15-42; 2011,Jan,11

22558 **lumbar**

EXCLUDES Arthrodesis using pre-sacral interbody technique (22586, 0195T)

🚑 44.7   ⚕ 44.7   **FUD** 090   [C] [80] 🔲

AMA: 2016,Jan,13; 2015,Mar,9; 2015,Jan,16; 2014,Jan,11; 2013,Jul,3-5; 2012,Apr,14-16; 2012,Jan,15-42; 2011,Jan,11

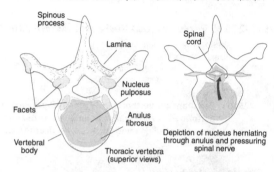

Spinous process

Lamina

Spinal cord

Nucleus pulposus

Facets

Anulus fibrosus

Vertebral body

Thoracic vertebra (superior views)

Depiction of nucleus herniating through anulus and pressuring spinal nerve

+ 22585 **each additional interspace (List separately in addition to code for primary procedure)**

EXCLUDES Anterior discectomy and interbody fusion during the same operative session (regardless if performed by multiple surgeons) (22552)

Discectomy, anterior, with decompression of spinal cord and/or nerve root(s), cervical (even by separate individual) (63075)

Code first (22554-22558)

🚑 9.64   ⚕ 9.64   **FUD** ZZZ   [C] [80] 🔲

AMA: 2016,Jan,13; 2015,Jan,16; 2014,Jan,11; 2012,Jan,15-42; 2011,Jan,11

22586 **Arthrodesis, pre-sacral interbody technique, including disc space preparation, discectomy, with posterior instrumentation, with image guidance, includes bone graft when performed, L5-S1 interspace**

🚑 52.7   ⚕ 52.7   **FUD** 090   [C] [80] 🔲

INCLUDES Radiologic guidance (77002-77003, 77011-77012)

EXCLUDES Allograft and autograft of spinal bone (20930-20938)

Epidurography, radiological supervision and interpretation (72275)

Pelvic fixation, other than sacrum (22848)

Posterior non-segmental instrumentation (22840)

22590 **Arthrodesis, posterior technique, craniocervical (occiput-C2)**

EXCLUDES Posterior intrafacet implant insertion (0219T-0222T)

🚑 46.1   ⚕ 46.1   **FUD** 090   [C] [80] 🔲

AMA: 2016,Jan,13; 2015,Jan,16; 2014,Jan,11; 2013,Jul,3-5; 2012,Apr,14-16

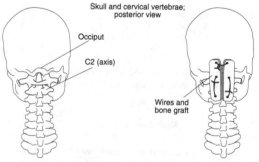

Skull and cervical vertebrae; posterior view

Occiput

C2 (axis)

Wires and bone graft

In 22590, the physician fuses skull to C2 (axis) to stabilize cervical vertebrae; anchor holes are drilled in the occiput of the skull

22595 **Arthrodesis, posterior technique, atlas-axis (C1-C2)**

EXCLUDES Posterior intrafacet implant insertion (0219T-0222T)

🚑 44.0   ⚕ 44.0   **FUD** 090   [C] [80] 🔲

AMA: 2016,Jan,13; 2015,Jan,16; 2014,Jan,11; 2013,Jul,3-5; 2012,Apr,14-16; 2012,Apr,11-13

22600 Arthrodesis, posterior or posterolateral technique, single level; cervical below C2 segment

> *EXCLUDES* *Posterior intrafacet implant insertion (0219T-0222T)*
> 🔧 37.5 ✄ 37.5 **FUD** 090 〔C〕〔80〕▢
> **AMA:** 2016,Jan,13; 2015,Jan,16; 2014,Jan,11; 2013,Jul,3-5; 2012,Jun,10-11; 2012,Apr,14-16

22610 thoracic (with lateral transverse technique, when performed)

> *EXCLUDES* *Posterior intrafacet implant insertion (0219T-0222T)*
> 🔧 36.7 ✄ 36.7 **FUD** 090 〔C〕〔80〕▢
> **AMA:** 2016,Jan,13; 2015,Jan,16; 2014,Jan,11; 2013,Jul,3-5; 2012,Jun,10-11; 2012,Apr,14-16

22612 lumbar (with lateral transverse technique, when performed)

> *EXCLUDES* *Arthrodesis performed at same interspace and segment (22630)*
> *Combined technique at the same interspace and segment (22633)*
> *Posterior intrafacet implant insertion (0219T-0222T)*
> 🔧 46.2 ✄ 46.2 **FUD** 090 〔J〕〔62〕〔80〕▢
> **AMA:** 2016,Jan,13; 2015,Jan,16; 2014,Jan,11; 2013,Dec,14; 2013,Jul,3-5; 2012,Jun,10-11; 2012,Apr,14-16; 2012,Jan,3-5; 2012,Jan,15-42; 2011,Dec,14-18; 2011,Jan,11

+ 22614 each additional vertebral segment (List separately in addition to code for primary procedure)

> *INCLUDES* Additional level fusion arthrodesis posterior or posterolateral interbody
> *EXCLUDES* *Additional level interbody arthrodesis combined posterolateral or posterior with posterior interbody arthrodesis (22634)*
> *Additional level posterior interbody arthrodesis (22632)*
> *Posterior intrafacet implant insertion (0219T-0222T)*
> Code first (22600, 22610, 22612, 22630, 22633)
> 🔧 11.4 ✄ 11.4 **FUD** ZZZ 〔N〕〔N1〕〔80〕▢
> **AMA:** 2016,Jan,13; 2015,Jan,16; 2014,Jan,11; 2013,Jul,3-5; 2012,Jun,10-11

22630 Arthrodesis, posterior interbody technique, including laminectomy and/or discectomy to prepare interspace (other than for decompression), single interspace; lumbar

> *EXCLUDES* *Arthrodesis performed at same interspace and segment (22612)*
> *Combined technique (22612 and 22630) for same interspace and segment (22633)*
> 🔧 45.7 ✄ 45.7 **FUD** 090 〔C〕〔80〕▢
> **AMA:** 2016,Jan,13; 2015,Jan,16; 2014,Jan,11; 2013,Jul,3-5; 2012,Jun,10-11; 2012,Apr,14-16; 2012,Jan,3-5; 2012,Jan,15-42; 2011,Dec,14-18; 2011,Jan,11

+ 22632 each additional interspace (List separately in addition to code for primary procedure)

> *INCLUDES* Includes posterior interbody fusion arthrodesis, additional level
> *EXCLUDES* *Additional level combined technique (22634)*
> *Additional level posterior or posterolateral fusion (22614)*
> Code first (22612, 22630, 22633)
> 🔧 9.42 ✄ 9.42 **FUD** ZZZ 〔C〕〔80〕▢
> **AMA:** 2016,Jan,13; 2015,Jan,16; 2014,Jan,11; 2013,Jul,3-5; 2012,Jun,10-11

22633 Arthrodesis, combined posterior or posterolateral technique with posterior interbody technique including laminectomy and/or discectomy sufficient to prepare interspace (other than for decompression), single interspace and segment; lumbar

> *EXCLUDES* *Arthrodesis performed at same interspace and segment (22612, 22630)*
> 🔧 53.9 ✄ 53.9 **FUD** 090 〔C〕〔80〕▢
> **AMA:** 2016,Jan,13; 2015,Jan,16; 2014,Jan,11; 2013,Jul,3-5; 2012,Jun,10-11; 2012,Jan,15-42; 2012,Jan,3-5; 2011,Dec,14-18

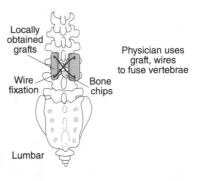

Locally obtained grafts

Physician uses graft, wires to fuse vertebrae

Wire fixation

Bone chips

Lumbar

Using a posterior or posterolateral technique the vertebral interbody is fused

+ 22634 each additional interspace and segment (List separately in addition to code for primary procedure)

> Code first (22633)
> 🔧 14.5 ✄ 14.5 **FUD** ZZZ 〔C〕〔80〕▢
> **AMA:** 2016,Jan,13; 2015,Jan,16; 2014,Jan,11; 2013,Jul,3-5; 2012,Jun,10-11; 2012,Jan,15-42; 2012,Jan,3-5; 2011,Dec,14-18

22800-22819 Procedures to Correct Anomalous Spinal Vertebrae

CMS: 100-03,150.2 Osteogenic Stimulation

> *EXCLUDES* *Facet injection (64490-64495, [64633, 64634, 64635, 64636])*
> Code also bone grafting procedures (20930-20938)
> Code also spinal instrumentation (22840-22855 [22859])

22800 Arthrodesis, posterior, for spinal deformity, with or without cast; up to 6 vertebral segments

> 🔧 39.2 ✄ 39.2 **FUD** 090 〔C〕〔80〕▢
> **AMA:** 2016,Jan,13; 2015,Jan,16; 2014,Jan,11; 2013,Jul,3-5; 2012,Apr,14-16

22802 7 to 12 vertebral segments

> 🔧 60.9 ✄ 60.9 **FUD** 090 〔C〕〔80〕▢
> **AMA:** 2016,Jan,13; 2015,Jan,16; 2014,Jan,11; 2013,Jul,3-5; 2012,Apr,14-16; 2012,Jan,15-42; 2011,Jan,11

22804 13 or more vertebral segments

> 🔧 70.4 ✄ 70.4 **FUD** 090 〔C〕〔80〕▢
> **AMA:** 2016,Jan,13; 2015,Jan,16; 2014,Jan,11; 2013,Jul,3-5; 2012,Apr,14-16

22808 Arthrodesis, anterior, for spinal deformity, with or without cast; 2 to 3 vertebral segments

> *INCLUDES* Smith-Robinson arthrodesis
> 🔧 53.4 ✄ 53.4 **FUD** 090 〔C〕〔80〕▢
> **AMA:** 2016,Jan,13; 2015,Jan,16; 2014,Jan,11; 2013,Jul,3-5; 2012,Apr,14-16

22810 4 to 7 vertebral segments

> 🔧 58.9 ✄ 58.9 **FUD** 090 〔C〕〔80〕▢
> **AMA:** 2016,Jan,13; 2015,Jan,16; 2014,Jan,11; 2013,Jul,3-5; 2012,Apr,14-16; 2012,Jan,15-42; 2011,Jan,11

22812 8 or more vertebral segments

> 🔧 70.0 ✄ 70.0 **FUD** 090 〔C〕〔80〕▢
> **AMA:** 2016,Jan,13; 2015,Jan,16; 2014,Jan,11; 2013,Jul,3-5; 2012,Apr,14-16

22818 Kyphectomy, circumferential exposure of spine and resection of vertebral segment(s) (including body and posterior elements); single or 2 segments

> EXCLUDES *Arthrodesis (22800-22804)*
>
> 🚑 62.9   ⚖ 62.9   **FUD** 090   C 80 ▭
>
> **AMA:** 2002,Apr,13; 1999,Dec,3

22819 3 or more segments

> EXCLUDES *Arthrodesis (22800-22804)*
>
> 🚑 81.0   ⚖ 81.0   **FUD** 090   C 80 ▭
>
> **AMA:** 2002,Apr,13; 1999,Dec,3

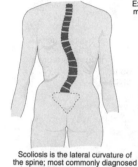
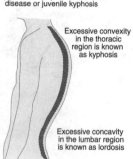

Excessively kyphotic thoracic spine may be caused by Scheuermann's disease or juvenile kyphosis

Excessive convexity in the thoracic region is known as kyphosis

Excessive concavity in the lumbar region is known as lordosis

Scoliosis is the lateral curvature of the spine; most commonly diagnosed during adolescence; occurrence is higher among females

22830 Surgical Exploration Previous Spinal Fusion

CMS: 100-03,150.2 Osteogenic Stimulation

> EXCLUDES *Arthrodesis (22532-22819)*
> *Bone grafting procedures (20930-20938)*
> *Facet injection (64490-64495, [64633, 64634, 64635, 64636])*
> *Instrumentation removal (22850, 22852, 22855)*
> *Spinal decompression (63001-63103)*
> Code also spinal instrumentation (22840-22855 [22859])

22830 Exploration of spinal fusion

> 🚑 23.5   ⚖ 23.5   **FUD** 090   C 80 ▭
>
> **AMA:** 2016,Jan,13; 2015,Jan,16; 2014,Jan,11; 2012,Jan,15-42; 2011,Jan,11

22840-22848 Posterior, Anterior, Pelvic Spinal Instrumentation

> INCLUDES Removal or revision of previously placed spinal instrumentation during same session as insertion of new instrumentation at levels including all or part of previously instrumented segments (22849, 22850, 22852, 22855)
>
> EXCLUDES *Arthrodesis (22532-22534, 22548-22812)*
> *Bone grafting procedures (20930-20938)*
> *Exploration of spinal fusion (22830)*
> *Fracture treatment (22325-22328)*

+ 22840 Posterior non-segmental instrumentation (eg, Harrington rod technique, pedicle fixation across 1 interspace, atlantoaxial transarticular screw fixation, sublaminar wiring at C1, facet screw fixation) (List separately in addition to code for primary procedure)

> Code first (22100-22102, 22110-22114, 22206-22207, 22210-22214, 22220-22224, 22310-22327, 22532-22533, 22548-22558, 22590-22612, 22630, 22633-22634, 22800-22812, 63001-63030, 63040-63042, 63045-63047, 63050-63056, 63064, 63075, 63077, 63081, 63085, 63087, 63090, 63101-63102, 63170-63290, 63300-63307)
>
> 🚑 22.2   ⚖ 22.2   **FUD** ZZZ   C 80 ▭
>
> **AMA:** 2016,Jan,13; 2015,Jan,16; 2014,Oct,14; 2014,Jan,11; 2013,Dec,16; 2013,Jul,3-5; 2012,Jun,10-11; 2012,Apr,11-13; 2012,Jan,15-42; 2011,Dec,14-18; 2011,Jan,11; 2011,Jan,9-10

+ 22841 Internal spinal fixation by wiring of spinous processes (List separately in addition to code for primary procedure)

> Code first (22100-22102, 22110-22114, 22206-22207, 22210-22214, 22220-22224, 22310-22327, 22532-22533, 22548-22558, 22590-22612, 22630, 22633-22634, 22800-22812, 63001-63030, 63040-63042, 63045-63047, 63050-63056, 63064, 63075, 63077, 63081, 63085, 63087, 63090, 63101-63102, 63170-63290, 63300-63307)
>
> 🚑 0.00   ⚖ 0.00   **FUD** XXX   C ▭
>
> **AMA:** 2016,Jan,13; 2015,Jan,16; 2014,Jan,11; 2013,Jul,3-5; 2012,Jun,10-11

+ 22842 Posterior segmental instrumentation (eg, pedicle fixation, dual rods with multiple hooks and sublaminar wires); 3 to 6 vertebral segments (List separately in addition to code for primary procedure)

> Code first (22100-22102, 22110-22114, 22206-22207, 22210-22214, 22220-22224, 22310-22327, 22532-22533, 22548-22558, 22590-22612, 22630, 22633-22634, 22800-22812, 63001-63030, 63040-63042, 63045-63047, 63050-63056, 63064, 63075, 63077, 63081, 63085, 63087, 63090, 63101-63102, 63170-63290, 63300-63307)
>
> 🚑 22.3   ⚖ 22.3   **FUD** ZZZ   C 80 ▭
>
> **AMA:** 2016,Jan,13; 2015,Jan,16; 2014,Jan,11; 2013,Jul,3-5; 2012,Jun,10-11; 2011,Dec,14-18

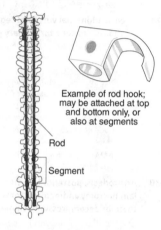

Example of rod hook; may be attached at top and bottom only, or also at segments

Rod

Segment

+ 22843 7 to 12 vertebral segments (List separately in addition to code for primary procedure)

> Code first (22100-22102, 22110-22114, 22206-22207, 22210-22214, 22220-22224, 22310-22327, 22532-22533, 22548-22558, 22590-22612, 22630, 22633-22634, 22800-22812, 63001-63030, 63040-63042, 63045-63047, 63050-63056, 63064, 63075, 63077, 63081, 63085, 63087, 63090, 63101-63102, 63170-63290, 63300-63307)
>
> 🚑 23.8   ⚖ 23.8   **FUD** ZZZ   C 80 ▭
>
> **AMA:** 2016,Jan,13; 2015,Jan,16; 2014,Jan,11; 2013,Jul,3-5; 2012,Jun,10-11; 2011,Dec,14-18

+ 22844 13 or more vertebral segments (List separately in addition to code for primary procedure)

> Code first (22100-22102, 22110-22114, 22206-22207, 22210-22214, 22220-22224, 22310-22327, 22532-22533, 22548-22558, 22590-22612, 22630, 22633-22634, 22800-22812, 63001-63030, 63040-63042, 63045-63047, 63050-63056, 63064, 63075, 63077, 63081, 63085, 63087, 63090, 63101-63102, 63170-63290, 63300-63307)
>
> 🚑 28.7   ⚖ 28.7   **FUD** ZZZ   C 80 ▭
>
> **AMA:** 2016,Jan,13; 2015,Jan,16; 2014,Jan,11; 2013,Jul,3-5; 2012,Jun,10-11; 2011,Dec,14-18

+ **22845** **Anterior instrumentation; 2 to 3 vertebral segments (List separately in addition to code for primary procedure)**

↗

INCLUDES Dwyer instrumentation technique

Code first (22100-22102, 22110-22114, 22206-22207, 22210-22214, 22220-22224, 22310-22327, 22532-22533, 22548-22558, 22590-22612, 22630, 22633-22634, 22800-22812, 63001-63030, 63040-63042, 63045-63047, 63050-63056, 63064, 63075, 63077, 63081, 63085, 63087, 63090, 63101-63102, 63170-63290, 63300-63307)

🔲 21.4   21.4   **FUD** ZZZ   C 80 ▢

AMA: 2016,May,13; 2016,Jan,13; 2015,Apr,7; 2015,Mar,9; 2015,Jan,16; 2015,Jan,13; 2014,Nov,14; 2014,Jan,11; 2013,Jul,3-5; 2012,Jun,10-11; 2012,Jan,15-42; 2011,Jan,11

+ **22846** **4 to 7 vertebral segments (List separately in addition to code for primary procedure)**

↗

INCLUDES Dwyer instrumentation technique

Code first (22100-22102, 22110-22114, 22206-22207, 22210-22214, 22220-22224, 22310-22327, 22532-22533, 22548-22558, 22590-22612, 22630, 22633-22634, 22800-22812, 63001-63030, 63040-63042, 63045-63047, 63050-63056, 63064, 63075, 63077, 63081, 63085, 63087, 63090, 63101-63102, 63170-63290, 63300-63307)

🔲 22.2   22.2   **FUD** ZZZ   C 80 ▢

AMA: 2016,May,13; 2016,Jan,13; 2015,Jan,16; 2014,Jan,11; 2013,Jul,3-5; 2012,Jun,10-11; 2012,Jan,15-42; 2011,Jan,11

+ **22847** **8 or more vertebral segments (List separately in addition to code for primary procedure)**

INCLUDES Dwyer instrumentation technique

Code first (22100-22102, 22110-22114, 22206-22207, 22210-22214, 22220-22224, 22310-22327, 22532-22533, 22548-22558, 22590-22612, 22630, 22633-22634, 22800-22812, 63001-63030, 63040-63042, 63045-63047, 63050-63056, 63064, 63075, 63077, 63081, 63085, 63087, 63090, 63101-63102, 63170-63290, 63300-63307)

🔲 24.2   24.2   **FUD** ZZZ   C 80 ▢

AMA: 2016,May,13; 2016,Jan,13; 2015,Jan,16; 2014,Jan,11; 2013,Jul,3-5; 2012,Jun,10-11; 2012,Jan,15-42; 2011,Jan,11

+ **22848** **Pelvic fixation (attachment of caudal end of instrumentation to pelvic bony structures) other than sacrum (List separately in addition to code for primary procedure)**

Code first (22100-22102, 22110-22114, 22206-22207, 22210-22214, 22220-22224, 22310-22327, 22532-22533, 22548-22558, 22590-22612, 22630, 22633-22634, 22800-22812, 63001-63030, 63040-63042, 63045-63047, 63050-63056, 63064, 63075, 63077, 63081, 63085, 63087, 63090, 63101-63102, 63170-63290, 63300-63307)

🔲 10.5   10.5   **FUD** ZZZ   C 80 ▢

AMA: 2016,Jan,13; 2015,Jan,16; 2014,Jan,11; 2013,Jul,3-5; 2012,Jun,10-11

22849-22855 [22859] Miscellaneous Spinal Instrumentation

EXCLUDES Arthrodesis (22532-22534, 22548-22812)
Bone grafting procedures (20930-20938)
Exploration of spinal fusion (22830)
Facet injection (64490-64495, [64633], [64634], [64635], [64636])
Fracture treatment (22325-22328)

22849 **Reinsertion of spinal fixation device**

INCLUDES Removal of instrumentation at the same level (22850, 22852, 22855)

🔲 37.8   37.8   **FUD** 090   C 80 ▢

AMA: 2016,May,13; 2016,Jan,13; 2015,Jan,16; 2014,Jan,11; 2013,Jul,3-5; 2012,Jun,10-11; 2012,Jan,15-42; 2011,Oct,10

22850 **Removal of posterior nonsegmental instrumentation (eg, Harrington rod)**

🔲 20.9   20.9   **FUD** 090   C 80 ▢

AMA: 2016,May,13; 2016,Jan,13; 2015,Jan,16; 2014,Jan,11; 2013,Jul,3-5; 2012,Jun,10-11

~~**22851** **Application of intervertebral biomechanical device(s) (eg, synthetic cage(s), methylmethacrylate) to vertebral defect or interspace (List separately in addition to code for primary procedure)**~~

To report, see ~22853-22854, [22859]

22852 **Removal of posterior segmental instrumentation**

🔲 20.1   20.1   **FUD** 090   C 80 ▢

AMA: 2016,Jan,13; 2015,Jan,16; 2014,Jan,11; 2012,Jun,10-11; 2012,Jan,15-42; 2011,Jan,11

● + **22853** **Insertion of interbody biomechanical device(s) (eg, synthetic cage, mesh) with integral anterior instrumentation for device anchoring (eg, screws, flanges), when performed, to intervertebral disc space in conjunction with interbody arthrodesis, each interspace (List separately in addition to code for primary procedure)**

Peek Cage

🔲 0.00   0.00   **FUD** 000

Code also interverterbral bone device/graft application (20930-20931, 20936-20938)
Code also subsequent disc spaces undergoing device insertion when disc spaces are not connected (22853-22854, [22859])
Code first (22100-22102, 22110-22114, 22206-22207, 22210-22214, 22220-22224, 22310-22327, 22532-22533, 22548-22558, 22590-22612, 22630, 22633-22634, 22800-22812, 63001-63030, 63040, 63042, 63045-63047, 63050-63056, 63064, 63075, 63077, 63081, 63085, 63087, 63090, 63101-63102, 63170-63290, 63300-63307)

● + **22854** **Insertion of intervertebral biomechanical device(s) (eg, synthetic cage, mesh) with integral anterior instrumentation for device anchoring (eg, screws, flanges), when performed, to vertebral corpectomy(ies) (vertebral body resection, partial or complete) defect, in conjunction with interbody arthrodesis, each contiguous defect (List separately in addition to code for primary procedure)**

Peek Cage

🔲 0.00   0.00   **FUD** 000

Code also interverterbral bone device/graft application (20930-20931, 20936-20938)
Code also subsequent disc spaces undergoing device insertion when disc spaces are not connected (22853-22854, [22859])
Code first (22100-22102, 22110-22114, 22206-22207, 22210-22214, 22220-22224, 22310-22327, 22532-22533, 22548-22558, 22590-22612, 22630, 22633-22634, 22800-22812, 63001-63030, 63040, 63042, 63045-63047, 63050-63056, 63064, 63075, 63077, 63081, 63085, 63087, 63090, 63101-63102, 63170-63290, 63300-63307)

● + # **22859** **Insertion of intervertebral biomechanical device(s) (eg, synthetic cage, mesh, methylmethacrylate) to intervertebral disc space or vertebral body defect without interbody arthrodesis, each contiguous defect (List separately in addition to code for primary procedure)**

🔲 0.00   0.00   **FUD** 000

Code also interverterbral bone device/graft application (20930-20931, 20936-20938)
Code also subsequent disc spaces undergoing device insertion when disc spaces are not connected (22853-22854, [22859])
Code first (22100-22102, 22110-22114, 22206-22207, 22210-22214, 22220-22224, 22310-22327, 22532-22533, 22548-22558, 22590-22612, 22630, 22633-22634, 22800-22812, 63001-63030, 63040-63042, 63045-63047, 63050-63056, 63064, 63075, 63077, 63081, 63085, 63087, 63090, 63101-63102, 63170-63290, 63300-63307)

22855 **Removal of anterior instrumentation**

🔲 32.2   32.2   **FUD** 090   C 80 ▢

AMA: 2016,Jan,13; 2015,Jan,16; 2014,Jan,11; 2012,Jun,10-11

22856-22865 [22858] Artificial Disc Replacement

EXCLUDES Fluoroscopy
Spinal decompression (63001-63048)

22856 Total disc arthroplasty (artificial disc), anterior approach, including discectomy with end plate preparation (includes osteophytectomy for nerve root or spinal cord decompression and microdissection); single interspace, cervical

INCLUDES Operating microscope (69990)

EXCLUDES Application of intervertebral biomechanical device(s) at the same level (22853-22854, [22859])
Arthrodesis at the same level (22554)
Cervical total disc arthroplasty, 3 or more levels (0375T)
Discectomy at the same level (63075)
Insertion of instrumentation at the same level (22845)

Code also ([22858])

🖪 47.2   ⚕ 47.2   **FUD** 090   J 80 🖵

AMA: 2016,Feb,12; 2016,Jan,13; 2015,Apr,7

+ # 22858 second level, cervical (List separately in addition to code for primary procedure)

EXCLUDES Cervical total disc arthroplasty, 3 or more levels (0375T)

Code first (22856)

🖪 14.7   ⚕ 14.7   **FUD** ZZZ   C 80 🖵

AMA: 2016,Feb,12; 2016,Jan,13; 2015,Apr,7

22857 Total disc arthroplasty (artificial disc), anterior approach, including discectomy to prepare interspace (other than for decompression), single interspace, lumbar

INCLUDES Operating microscope (69990)

EXCLUDES Application of intervertebral biomechanical device(s) at the same level (22853-22854, [22859])
Arthrodesis at the same level (22558)
Insertion of instrumentation at the same level (22845)
Retroperitoneal exploration (49010)

Code also arthroplasty more than one interspace, when performed (0163T)

🖪 57.1   ⚕ 57.1   **FUD** 090   C 80 🖵

AMA: 2016,Feb,12

22858 Resequenced code. See code following 22856.

22859 Resequenced code. See code following 22854.

22861 Revision including replacement of total disc arthroplasty (artificial disc), anterior approach, single interspace; cervical

INCLUDES Operating microscope (69990)

EXCLUDES Procedures performed at the same level (22845, 22853-22854, [22859], 22864, 63075)
Revision of additional cervical arthroplasty (0098T)

🖪 58.4   ⚕ 58.4   **FUD** 090   C 80 🖵

AMA: 2016,Feb,12

22862 lumbar

EXCLUDES Arthroplasty revision more than one interspace (0165T)
Procedures performed at the same level (22558, 22845, 22853-22854, [22859], 22865, 49010)

🖪 57.9   ⚕ 57.9   **FUD** 090   C 80 🖵

AMA: 2016,Jan,13; 2015,Jan,16; 2014,Jan,11

22864 Removal of total disc arthroplasty (artificial disc), anterior approach, single interspace; cervical

🖪 60.2   ⚕ 60.2   **FUD** 090   C 80 🖵

INCLUDES Operating microscope (69990)

EXCLUDES Cervical total disc arthroplasty with additional interspace removal (0095T)
Revision of total disc arthroplasty (22861)

22865 lumbar

EXCLUDES Arthroplasty more than one level (0164T)
Exploration, retroperitoneal area with or without biopsy(s) (49010)

🖪 59.3   ⚕ 59.3   **FUD** 090   C 80 🖵

AMA: 2016,Jan,13; 2015,Jan,16; 2014,Jan,11

22867-22899 Spinal Distraction/Stabilization Device

● **22867** Insertion of interlaminar/interspinous process stabilization/distraction device, without fusion, including image guidance when performed, with open decompression, lumbar; single level

EXCLUDES Interlaminar/interspinous stabilization/distraction device insertion (22869, 22870)
Procedures at the same level (22532-22534, 22558, 22612, 22614, 22630, 22632-22634, 22800, 22802, 22804, 22840-22842, 22869-22870, 63005, 63012, 63017, 63030, 63035, 63042, 63044, 63047-63048, 77003)

● + **22868** second level (List separately in addition to code for primary procedure)

🖪 0.00   ⚕ 0.00   **FUD** 000

EXCLUDES Interlaminar/interspinous stabilization/distraction device insertion (22869, 22870)
Procedures at the same level (22532-22534, 22558, 22612, 22614, 22630, 22632-22634, 22800, 22802, 22804, 22840-22842, 22869-22870, 63005, 63012, 63017, 63030, 63035, 63042, 63044, 63047-63048, 77003)

Code first (22867)

● **22869** Insertion of interlaminar/interspinous process stabilization/distraction device, without open decompression or fusion, including image guidance when performed, lumbar; single level

● + **22870** second level (List separately in addition to code for primary procedure)

🖪 0.00   ⚕ 0.00   **FUD** 000

EXCLUDES Procedures at the same level (22532-22534, 22558, 22612, 22614, 22630, 22632-22634, 22800, 22802, 22804, 22840-22842, 63005, 63012, 63017, 63030, 63035, 63042, 63044, 63047-63048, 77003)

Code first (22869)

22899 Unlisted procedure, spine

🖪 0.00   ⚕ 0.00   **FUD** YYY   T 80

AMA: 2016,Jan,13; 2015,Jan,16; 2015,Jan,8; 2014,Oct,14; 2014,Jan,11; 2013,Dec,14; 2013,Dec,16; 2012,Dec,12; 2012,Oct,14; 2012,Sep,16; 2012,Jan,15-42; 2012,Jan,13-14; 2011,Jan,11

22900-22999 Musculoskeletal Procedures of Abdomen

INCLUDES Any necessary elevation of tissue planes or dissection
Measurement of tumor and necessary margin at greatest diameter prior to excision
Simple and intermediate repairs
Types of excision:
Fascial or subfascial soft tissue tumors: simple and marginal resection of tumors found either in or below the deep fascia, not involving bone or excision of a substantial amount of normal tissue; primarily benign and intramuscular tumors
Radical resection soft tissue tumor: wide resection of tumor involving substantial margins of normal tissue and may include tissue removal from one or more layers; most often malignant or aggressive benign
Subcutaneous: simple and marginal resection of tumors in the subcutaneous tissue above the deep fascia; most often benign

EXCLUDES Complex repair
Excision of benign cutaneous lesions (eg, sebaceous cyst) (11400-11406)
Radical resection of cutaneous tumors (eg, melanoma) (11600-11606)
Significant exploration of the vessels or neuroplasty

22900 Excision, tumor, soft tissue of abdominal wall, subfascial (eg, intramuscular); less than 5 cm

🖪 16.2   ⚕ 16.2   **FUD** 090   T 62 80 🖵

AMA: 2002,Apr,13

22901 5 cm or greater

🖪 19.1   ⚕ 19.1   **FUD** 090   T 62 80 🖵

22902 Excision, tumor, soft tissue of abdominal wall, subcutaneous; less than 3 cm

🖪 9.54   ⚕ 12.5   **FUD** 090   T 62 80 🖵

22903 3 cm or greater

🖪 12.6   ⚕ 12.6   **FUD** 090   T 62 80 🖵

22904   Radical resection of tumor (eg, sarcoma), soft tissue of abdominal wall; less than 5 cm

    30.2   30.2   **FUD** 090   T G2 80

22905   5 cm or greater

    38.4   38.4   **FUD** 090   T G2 80

22999   Unlisted procedure, abdomen, musculoskeletal system

    0.00   0.00   **FUD** YYY   T 80

    AMA: 2002,Apr,13

23000-23044 Surgical Incision Shoulder: Drainage, Foreign Body Removal, Contracture Release

23000   Removal of subdeltoid calcareous deposits, open

    EXCLUDES   *Arthroscopic removal calcium deposits of bursa (29999)*

    10.6   16.6   **FUD** 090   T A2 80 50

    AMA: 2002,Apr,13

23020   Capsular contracture release (eg, Sever type procedure)

    EXCLUDES   *Simple incision and drainage (10040-10160)*

    19.7   19.7   **FUD** 090   T A2 80 50

    AMA: 2002,Apr,13; 1998,Nov,1

23030   Incision and drainage, shoulder area; deep abscess or hematoma

    7.36   12.5   **FUD** 010   T A2

    AMA: 2002,Apr,13

23031   infected bursa

    6.30   12.1   **FUD** 010   T A2 50

    AMA: 2002,Apr,13

Supraspinatus muscle and tendon
Acromion
Scapula
Bursa
Glenoid cavity
Head of humerus
Acromion
Clavicle
Deltoid muscle
Teres major muscle
Coracoid process
Humerus
Scapula
Triceps

The fibrous capsule enclosing the shoulder is thin and loose to allow freedom of movement; four rotator cuff muscles (supraspinatous, infraspinatous, teres minor, and scapularis) work together to hold the head of the humerus in the glenoid cavity

Section of left shoulder

23035   Incision, bone cortex (eg, osteomyelitis or bone abscess), shoulder area

    19.4   19.4   **FUD** 090   T A2 80 50

    AMA: 2003,Jan,1; 2002,Apr,13

23040   Arthrotomy, glenohumeral joint, including exploration, drainage, or removal of foreign body

    20.6   20.6   **FUD** 090   T A2 80 50

    AMA: 2002,Apr,13; 1998,Nov,1

23044   Arthrotomy, acromioclavicular, sternoclavicular joint, including exploration, drainage, or removal of foreign body

    16.3   16.3   **FUD** 090   T A2 50

    AMA: 2002,Apr,13; 1998,Nov,1

23065-23066 Shoulder Biopsy

EXCLUDES   *Soft tissue needle biopsy (20206)*

23065   Biopsy, soft tissue of shoulder area; superficial

    4.82   6.20   **FUD** 010   T P3 50

    AMA: 2002,Apr,13

23066   deep

    10.2   15.8   **FUD** 090   T A2 50

    AMA: 2002,Apr,13

23071-23078 [23071, 23073] Excision Soft Tissue Tumors of Shoulder

INCLUDES   Any necessary elevation of tissue planes or dissection

Measurement of tumor and necessary margin at greatest diameter prior to excision

Simple and intermediate repairs

Types of excision:

    Fascial or subfascial soft tissue tumors: simple and marginal resection of tumors found either in or below the deep fascia, not involving bone or excision of a substantial amount of normal tissue; primarily benign and intramuscular tumors

    Radical resection soft tissue tumor: wide resection of tumor, involving substantial margins of normal tissue and may involve tissue removal from one or more layers; most often malignant or aggressive benign

    Subcutaneous: simple and marginal resection of tumors in the subcutaneous tissue above the deep fascia; most often benign

EXCLUDES   *Complex repair*

Excision of benign cutaneous lesions (eg, sebaceous cyst) (11400-11406)

Radical resection of cutaneous tumors (eg, melanoma) (11600-11606)

Significant exploration of the vessels or neuroplasty

23071   **Resequenced code. See code following 23075.**

23073   **Resequenced code. See code following 23076.**

23075   Excision, tumor, soft tissue of shoulder area, subcutaneous; less than 3 cm

    9.39   13.3   **FUD** 090   T G2 50

    AMA: 2016,Jan,13; 2015,Jan,16; 2014,Jan,11

\#   **23071**   3 cm or greater

    12.1   12.1   **FUD** 090   T G2 80 50

    AMA: 2009,Oct,7,8&13

23076   Excision, tumor, soft tissue of shoulder area, subfascial (eg, intramuscular); less than 5 cm

    15.5   15.5   **FUD** 090   T G2 50

    AMA: 2016,Jan,13; 2015,Jan,16; 2014,Jan,11

\#   **23073**   5 cm or greater

    19.9   19.9   **FUD** 090   T G2 80 50

    AMA: 2009,Oct,7,8&13

23077   Radical resection of tumor (eg, sarcoma), soft tissue of shoulder area; less than 5 cm

    33.0   33.0   **FUD** 090   T G2 80 50

    AMA: 2002,Apr,13; 1990,Win,4

23078   5 cm or greater

    41.4   41.4   **FUD** 090   T G2 80 50

23100-23195 Bone and Joint Procedures of Shoulder

INCLUDES   Acromioclavicular joint

Clavicle

Head and neck of humerus

Scapula

Shoulder joint

Sternoclavicular joint

23100   Arthrotomy, glenohumeral joint, including biopsy

    14.2   14.2   **FUD** 090   T A2 80 50

    AMA: 2002,Apr,13; 1998,Nov,1

23101   Arthrotomy, acromioclavicular joint or sternoclavicular joint, including biopsy and/or excision of torn cartilage

    13.0   13.0   **FUD** 090   T A2 50

    AMA: 2002,Apr,13; 1998,Nov,1

23105   Arthrotomy; glenohumeral joint, with synovectomy, with or without biopsy

    18.3   18.3   **FUD** 090   T A2 80 50

    AMA: 2002,Apr,13; 1998,Nov,1

23106   sternoclavicular joint, with synovectomy, with or without biopsy

    14.1   14.1   **FUD** 090   T A2 50

    AMA: 2002,Apr,13; 1998,Nov,1

23107   Arthrotomy, glenohumeral joint, with joint exploration, with or without removal of loose or foreign body

    18.9   18.9   **FUD** 090   T A2 80 50

    AMA: 2002,Apr,13

● New Code   ▲ Revised Code   ○ Reinstated   ● New Web Release   ▲ Revised Web Release   Unlisted   Not Covered   # Resequenced

⊘ AMA Mod 51 Exempt   ⑪ Optum Mod 51 Exempt   ⊛ Mod 63 Exempt   ✗ Non-FDA Drug   ★ Telehealth   M Maternity   A Age Edit   + Add-on   AMA: CPT Asst

© 2016 Optum360, LLC   CPT © 2016 American Medical Association. All Rights Reserved.   **57**

23120 **Claviculectomy; partial**
INCLUDES Mumford operation
EXCLUDES *Arthroscopic claviculectomy (29824)*
🦴 16.7   ⚕ 16.7   **FUD** 090
  T A2 80 50 ▢
AMA: 2016,Jan,13; 2015,Jan,16; 2014,Jan,11; 2012,Oct,14; 2012,Sep,16

23125 **total**
🦴 20.3   ⚕ 20.3   **FUD** 090
  T A2 80 50 ▢
AMA: 2003,Jan,1; 2002,Apr,13

23130 **Acromioplasty or acromionectomy, partial, with or without coracoacromial ligament release**
🦴 17.5   ⚕ 17.5   **FUD** 090
  T A2 50 ▢
AMA: 2016,Jan,13; 2015,Mar,7; 2015,Feb,10; 2015,Jan,16; 2014,Jan,11; 2012,Jan,15-42; 2011,Jan,11

23140 **Excision or curettage of bone cyst or benign tumor of clavicle or scapula;**
🦴 15.3   ⚕ 15.3   **FUD** 090
  T A2 50 ▢
AMA: 2002,Apr,13

23145 **with autograft (includes obtaining graft)**
🦴 19.9   ⚕ 19.9   **FUD** 090
  T A2 80 50 ▢
AMA: 2002,Apr,13

23146 **with allograft**
🦴 17.8   ⚕ 17.8   **FUD** 090
  J A2 80 50 ▢
AMA: 2002,Apr,13

23150 **Excision or curettage of bone cyst or benign tumor of proximal humerus;**
🦴 18.8   ⚕ 18.8   **FUD** 090
  T A2 80 50 ▢
AMA: 2002,Apr,13

23155 **with autograft (includes obtaining graft)**
🦴 22.8   ⚕ 22.8   **FUD** 090
  T A2 80 50 ▢
AMA: 2002,Apr,13

23156 **with allograft**
🦴 19.4   ⚕ 19.4   **FUD** 090
  J A2 80 50 ▢
AMA: 2002,Apr,13

23170 **Sequestrectomy (eg, for osteomyelitis or bone abscess), clavicle**
🦴 15.9   ⚕ 15.9   **FUD** 090
  T A2 50 ▢
AMA: 2002,Apr,13

23172 **Sequestrectomy (eg, for osteomyelitis or bone abscess), scapula**
🦴 16.2   ⚕ 16.2   **FUD** 090
  T A2 80 50 ▢
AMA: 2002,Apr,13

23174 **Sequestrectomy (eg, for osteomyelitis or bone abscess), humeral head to surgical neck**
🦴 21.5   ⚕ 21.5   **FUD** 090
  T A2 80 50 ▢
AMA: 2002,Apr,13

23180 **Partial excision (craterization, saucerization, or diaphysectomy) bone (eg, osteomyelitis), clavicle**
🦴 19.1   ⚕ 19.1   **FUD** 090
  T A2 50 ▢
AMA: 2002,Apr,13; 1998,Nov,1

23182 **Partial excision (craterization, saucerization, or diaphysectomy) bone (eg, osteomyelitis), scapula**
🦴 18.7   ⚕ 18.7   **FUD** 090
  T A2 80 50 ▢
AMA: 2002,Apr,13; 1998,Nov,1

23184 **Partial excision (craterization, saucerization, or diaphysectomy) bone (eg, osteomyelitis), proximal humerus**
🦴 21.1   ⚕ 21.1   **FUD** 090
  T A2 80 50 ▢
AMA: 2002,Apr,13; 1998,Nov,1

23190 **Ostectomy of scapula, partial (eg, superior medial angle)**
🦴 16.3   ⚕ 16.3   **FUD** 090
  T A2 80 50 ▢
AMA: 2002,Apr,13

23195 **Resection, humeral head**
EXCLUDES *Arthroplasty with replacement with implant (23470)*
🦴 21.6   ⚕ 21.6   **FUD** 090
  J A2 80 50 ▢
AMA: 2003,Jan,1; 2002,Apr,13

23200-23220 Radical Resection of Bone Tumors of Shoulder

INCLUDES Any necessary elevation of tissue planes or dissection
Excision of adjacent soft tissue during bone tumor resection (23071-23078 [23071, 23073])
Measurement of tumor and necessary margin at greatest diameter prior to excision
Radical resection of cutaneous tumors (e.g., melanoma)
Resection of the tumor (may include entire bone) and wide margins of normal tissues primarily for malignant or aggressive benign tumors
Simple and intermediate repairs
EXCLUDES *Complex repair*
Significant exploration of vessels, neuroplasty, reconstruction, or complex bone repair

23200 **Radical resection of tumor; clavicle**
🦴 42.9   ⚕ 42.9   **FUD** 090
  C 80 50 ▢
AMA: 2002,Apr,13

23210 **scapula**
🦴 51.1   ⚕ 51.1   **FUD** 090
  C 80 50 ▢
AMA: 2002,Apr,13

23220 **Radical resection of tumor, proximal humerus**
🦴 55.9   ⚕ 55.9   **FUD** 090
  C 80 50 ▢
AMA: 2002,Apr,13; 1998,Nov,1

23330-23335 Removal Implant/Foreign Body from Shoulder

EXCLUDES *Bursal arthrocentesis or needling (20610)*
K-wire or pin insertion (20650)
K-wire or pin removal (20670, 20680)

23330 **Removal of foreign body, shoulder; subcutaneous**
🦴 4.32   ⚕ 6.80   **FUD** 010
  T A2 80 50 ▢
AMA: 2016,Jan,13; 2015,Jan,16; 2014,Mar,4; 2014,Jan,11

23333 **deep (subfascial or intramuscular)**
🦴 12.9   ⚕ 12.9   **FUD** 090
  T G2 80 50 ▢
AMA: 2016,Jan,13; 2015,Jan,16; 2014,Mar,4

23334 **Removal of prosthesis, includes debridement and synovectomy when performed; humeral or glenoid component**
EXCLUDES *Foreign body removal (23330, 23333)*
Prosthesis removal and replacement in same shoulder (eg, glenoid and/or humeral components) (23473-23474)
🦴 31.0   ⚕ 31.0   **FUD** 090
  T 62 50 ▢
AMA: 2016,Jan,13; 2015,Jan,16; 2014,Mar,4

23335 **humeral and glenoid components (eg, total shoulder)**
EXCLUDES *Foreign body removal (23330, 23333)*
Prosthesis removal and replacement in same shoulder (eg, glenoid and/or humeral components) (23473-23474)
🦴 36.8   ⚕ 36.8   **FUD** 090
  C 50 ▢
AMA: 2016,Jan,13; 2015,Jan,16; 2014,Mar,4

23350 Injection for Shoulder Arthrogram

23350 **Injection procedure for shoulder arthrography or enhanced CT/MRI shoulder arthrography**
EXCLUDES *Shoulder biopsy (29805-29826)*
📷 (73040, 73201-73202, 73222-73223, 77002)
🦴 1.47   ⚕ 3.71   **FUD** 000
  N N1 50 ▢
AMA: 2016,May,13; 2016,Jan,13; 2015,Aug,6; 2015,Jan,16; 2014,Jan,11

23395-23491 Repair/Reconstruction of Shoulder

23395 **Muscle transfer, any type, shoulder or upper arm; single**
🦴 37.0   ⚕ 37.0   **FUD** 090
  J A2 80 ▢
AMA: 2003,Jan,1; 2002,Apr,13

23397 **multiple**
🦴 32.8   ⚕ 32.8   **FUD** 090
  T A2 80 ▢
AMA: 2003,Jan,1; 2002,Apr,13

23400 **Scapulopexy (eg, Sprengels deformity or for paralysis)**
🦴 27.9   ⚕ 27.9   **FUD** 090
  J A2 80 50 ▢
AMA: 2003,Jan,1; 2002,Apr,13

23405   **Tenotomy, shoulder area; single tendon**
🔧 17.9   ⚖ 17.9   **FUD** 090   T A2 80 ▣
AMA: 2002,Apr,13; 1998,Nov,1

23406   **multiple tendons through same incision**
🔧 22.0   ⚖ 22.0   **FUD** 090   T A2 80 ▣
AMA: 2002,Apr,13; 1998,Nov,1

23410   **Repair of ruptured musculotendinous cuff (eg, rotator cuff) open; acute**
EXCLUDES   *Arthroscopic repair (29827)*
🔧 23.6   ⚖ 23.6   **FUD** 090   J A2 80 50 ▣
AMA: 2016,Jan,13; 2015,Jan,16; 2014,Jan,11; 2012,Jan,15-42; 2011,Jan,11

23412   **chronic**
EXCLUDES   *Arthroscopic repair (29827)*
🔧 24.5   ⚖ 24.5   **FUD** 090   J A2 80 50 ▣
AMA: 2016,Jan,13; 2015,Jun,10; 2015,Feb,10; 2015,Jan,16; 2014,Jan,11; 2012,Oct,14; 2012,Sep,16; 2012,Jan,15-42; 2011,Jan,11

23415   **Coracoacromial ligament release, with or without acromioplasty**
EXCLUDES   *Arthroscopic repair (29826)*
🔧 20.0   ⚖ 20.0   **FUD** 090   T A2 50 ▣
AMA: 2016,Jan,13; 2015,Mar,7

23420   **Reconstruction of complete shoulder (rotator) cuff avulsion, chronic (includes acromioplasty)**
🔧 27.8   ⚖ 27.8   **FUD** 090   J A2 80 50 ▣
AMA: 2016,Jan,13; 2015,Jan,16; 2014,Jan,11; 2012,Jan,15-42; 2011,Jan,11

23430   **Tenodesis of long tendon of biceps**
EXCLUDES   *Arthroscopic biceps tenodesis (29828)*
🔧 21.4   ⚖ 21.4   **FUD** 090   J A2 80 50 ▣
AMA: 2002,Apr,13; 1994,Win,1

23440   **Resection or transplantation of long tendon of biceps**
🔧 21.7   ⚖ 21.7   **FUD** 090   T A2 80 50 ▣
AMA: 2002,Apr,13; 1994,Win,1

23450   **Capsulorrhaphy, anterior; Putti-Platt procedure or Magnuson type operation**
EXCLUDES   *Arthroscopic thermal capsulorrhaphy (29999)*
🔧 27.1   ⚖ 27.1   **FUD** 090   T A2 80 50 ▣
AMA: 2002,Apr,13; 1998,Nov,1

23455   **with labral repair (eg, Bankart procedure)**
EXCLUDES   *Arthroscopic repair (29806)*
🔧 28.7   ⚖ 28.7   **FUD** 090   J A2 80 50 ▣
AMA: 2002,Apr,13; 1998,Nov,1

23460   **Capsulorrhaphy, anterior, any type; with bone block**
INCLUDES   Bristow procedure
🔧 31.4   ⚖ 31.4   **FUD** 090   T A2 80 50 ▣
AMA: 2002,Apr,13; 1994,Win,1

23462   **with coracoid process transfer**
EXCLUDES   *Open thermal capsulorrhaphy (23929)*
🔧 30.5   ⚖ 30.5   **FUD** 090   J A2 80 50 ▣
AMA: 2002,Apr,13

23465   **Capsulorrhaphy, glenohumeral joint, posterior, with or without bone block**
EXCLUDES   *Sternoclavicular and acromioclavicular joint repair (23530, 23550)*
🔧 32.0   ⚖ 32.0   **FUD** 090   J G2 80 50 ▣
AMA: 2002,Apr,13; 1998,Nov,1

23466   **Capsulorrhaphy, glenohumeral joint, any type multi-directional instability**
🔧 32.1   ⚖ 32.1   **FUD** 090   J A2 80 50 ▣
AMA: 2002,Apr,13; 1998,Nov,1

23470   **Arthroplasty, glenohumeral joint; hemiarthroplasty**
🔧 34.6   ⚖ 34.6   **FUD** 090   J 80 50 ▣
AMA: 2016,Jan,13; 2015,Jan,16; 2014,Mar,4

23472   **total shoulder (glenoid and proximal humeral replacement (eg, total shoulder))**
EXCLUDES   *Proximal humerus osteotomy (24400)*
           Removal of total shoulder components (23334-23335)
🔧 42.0   ⚖ 42.0   **FUD** 090   C 80 50 ▣
AMA: 2016,Jan,13; 2015,Jan,16; 2014,Mar,4; 2014,Jan,11; 2013,Mar,12; 2012,Jan,15-42; 2011,Jan,11

23473   **Revision of total shoulder arthroplasty, including allograft when performed; humeral or glenoid component**
EXCLUDES   *Removal of prosthesis only (glenoid and/or humeral component) (23334-23335)*
🔧 46.9   ⚖ 46.9   **FUD** 090   J 80 50 ▣
AMA: 2016,Jan,13; 2015,Jan,16; 2014,Mar,4; 2014,Jan,11; 2013,Mar,12; 2013,Feb,11-12

23474   **humeral and glenoid component**
EXCLUDES   *Removal of prosthesis only (glenoid and/or humeral component) (23334-23335)*
🔧 50.6   ⚖ 50.6   **FUD** 090   C 80 50 ▣
AMA: 2016,Jan,13; 2015,Jan,16; 2014,Mar,4; 2014,Jan,11; 2013,Mar,12; 2013,Feb,11-12

23480   **Osteotomy, clavicle, with or without internal fixation;**
🔧 23.6   ⚖ 23.6   **FUD** 090   T A2 50 ▣
AMA: 2002,Apr,13

23485   **with bone graft for nonunion or malunion (includes obtaining graft and/or necessary fixation)**
🔧 27.4   ⚖ 27.4   **FUD** 090   J G2 80 50 ▣
AMA: 2002,Apr,13

23490   **Prophylactic treatment (nailing, pinning, plating or wiring) with or without methylmethacrylate; clavicle**
🔧 24.2   ⚖ 24.2   **FUD** 090   J A2 80 50 ▣
AMA: 2002,Apr,13

23491   **proximal humerus**
🔧 29.1   ⚖ 29.1   **FUD** 090   J G2 80 50 ▣
AMA: 2002,Apr,13; 1998,Nov,1

23500-23680 Treatment of Shoulder Fracture/Dislocation

23500   **Closed treatment of clavicular fracture; without manipulation**
🔧 6.33   ⚖ 6.22   **FUD** 090   T A2 50 ▣
AMA: 2002,Apr,13

23505   **with manipulation**
🔧 9.52   ⚖ 10.0   **FUD** 090   T A2 50 ▣
AMA: 2002,Apr,13

23515   **Open treatment of clavicular fracture, includes internal fixation, when performed**
🔧 20.6   ⚖ 20.6   **FUD** 090   J A2 80 50 ▣
AMA: 2016,Jan,13; 2015,Jan,16; 2014,Jan,11

23520   **Closed treatment of sternoclavicular dislocation; without manipulation**
🔧 6.49   ⚖ 6.39   **FUD** 090   T A2 80 50 ▣
AMA: 2002,Apr,13

23525   **with manipulation**
🔧 9.92   ⚖ 10.7   **FUD** 090   T A2 80 50 ▣
AMA: 2002,Apr,13

23530   **Open treatment of sternoclavicular dislocation, acute or chronic;**
🔧 15.8   ⚖ 15.8   **FUD** 090   T A2 80 50 ▣
AMA: 2002,Apr,13

23532   **with fascial graft (includes obtaining graft)**
🔧 17.7   ⚖ 17.7   **FUD** 090   J A2 80 50 ▣
AMA: 2002,Apr,13

23540   **Closed treatment of acromioclavicular dislocation; without manipulation**
🔧 6.50   ⚖ 6.39   **FUD** 090   T A2 50 ▣
AMA: 2002,Apr,13

Musculoskeletal System

23545 — 24065

23545 **with manipulation**
8.80 | 9.67 | **FUD** 090 | T A2 80 50
AMA: 2002,Apr,13

23550 **Open treatment of acromioclavicular dislocation, acute or chronic;**
16.1 | 16.1 | **FUD** 090 | J A2 80 50
AMA: 2002,Apr,13

23552 **with fascial graft (includes obtaining graft)**
18.8 | 18.8 | **FUD** 090 | J 62 80 50
AMA: 2002,Apr,13

23570 **Closed treatment of scapular fracture; without manipulation**
6.81 | 6.61 | **FUD** 090 | T A2 50
AMA: 2002,Apr,13

23575 **with manipulation, with or without skeletal traction (with or without shoulder joint involvement)**
10.6 | 11.3 | **FUD** 090 | T A2 80 50
AMA: 2002,Apr,13

23585 **Open treatment of scapular fracture (body, glenoid or acromion) includes internal fixation, when performed**
28.2 | 28.2 | **FUD** 090 | J A2 80 50
AMA: 2016,Jan,13; 2015,Jan,16; 2014,Jan,11; 2012,Jan,15-42; 2011,Jan,11

23600 **Closed treatment of proximal humeral (surgical or anatomical neck) fracture; without manipulation**
8.76 | 9.29 | **FUD** 090 | T P2 50
AMA: 2002,Apr,13

23605 **with manipulation, with or without skeletal traction**
12.1 | 13.2 | **FUD** 090 | T A2 50
AMA: 2002,Apr,13

23615 **Open treatment of proximal humeral (surgical or anatomical neck) fracture, includes internal fixation, when performed, includes repair of tuberosity(s), when performed;**
25.4 | 25.4 | **FUD** 090 | J 62 80 50
AMA: 2016,Jan,13; 2015,Jan,16; 2014,Jan,11

23616 **with proximal humeral prosthetic replacement**
35.7 | 35.7 | **FUD** 090 | J J8 80 50
AMA: 2002,Apr,13

23620 **Closed treatment of greater humeral tuberosity fracture; without manipulation**
7.30 | 7.67 | **FUD** 090 | T P2 50
AMA: 2002,Apr,13; 1998,Nov,1

23625 **with manipulation**
10.0 | 10.8 | **FUD** 090 | T A2 50
AMA: 2002,Apr,13

23630 **Open treatment of greater humeral tuberosity fracture, includes internal fixation, when performed**
22.4 | 22.4 | **FUD** 090 | J A2 80 50
AMA: 2002,Apr,13; 1998,Nov,1

23650 **Closed treatment of shoulder dislocation, with manipulation; without anesthesia**
8.19 | 8.91 | **FUD** 090 | T A2 50
AMA: 2002,Apr,13

23655 **requiring anesthesia**
11.4 | 11.4 | **FUD** 090 | T A2 50
AMA: 2002,Apr,13

23660 **Open treatment of acute shoulder dislocation**
EXCLUDES *Chronic dislocation repair (23450-23466)*
16.6 | 16.6 | **FUD** 090 | T A2 80 50
AMA: 2016,Jan,13; 2015,Jan,16; 2014,Jan,11

23665 **Closed treatment of shoulder dislocation, with fracture of greater humeral tuberosity, with manipulation**
11.2 | 12.1 | **FUD** 090 | T A2 50
AMA: 2002,Apr,13; 1998,Nov,1

23670 **Open treatment of shoulder dislocation, with fracture of greater humeral tuberosity, includes internal fixation, when performed**
25.1 | 25.1 | **FUD** 090 | J A2 80 50
AMA: 2002,Apr,13; 1998,Nov,1

23675 **Closed treatment of shoulder dislocation, with surgical or anatomical neck fracture, with manipulation**
14.3 | 15.7 | **FUD** 090 | T A2 50
AMA: 2002,Apr,13

23680 **Open treatment of shoulder dislocation, with surgical or anatomical neck fracture, includes internal fixation, when performed**
26.6 | 26.6 | **FUD** 090 | J 62 80 50
AMA: 2002,Apr,13

23700-23929 Other/Unlisted Shoulder Procedures

23700 **Manipulation under anesthesia, shoulder joint, including application of fixation apparatus (dislocation excluded)**
5.64 | 5.64 | **FUD** 010 | T A2 50
AMA: 2016,Jan,13; 2015,Jun,10; 2015,Jan,16; 2014,Jan,11; 2012,Jan,15-42; 2011,Jan,11

23800 **Arthrodesis, glenohumeral joint;**
29.5 | 29.5 | **FUD** 090 | J 62 80 50
AMA: 2002,Apr,13; 1998,Nov,1

23802 **with autogenous graft (includes obtaining graft)**
36.3 | 36.3 | **FUD** 090 | J 62 80 50
AMA: 2002,Apr,13; 1998,Nov,1

23900 **Interthoracoscapular amputation (forequarter)**
40.0 | 40.0 | **FUD** 090 | C 80
AMA: 2002,Apr,13

23920 **Disarticulation of shoulder;**
32.3 | 32.3 | **FUD** 090 | C 80 50
AMA: 2002,Apr,13

23921 **secondary closure or scar revision**
13.4 | 13.4 | **FUD** 090 | T A2 50
AMA: 2002,Apr,13

23929 **Unlisted procedure, shoulder**
0.00 | 0.00 | **FUD** YYY | T 80
AMA: 2002,Apr,13

23930-24006 Surgical Incision Elbow/Upper Arm

EXCLUDES *Simple incision and drainage procedures (10040-10160)*

23930 **Incision and drainage, upper arm or elbow area; deep abscess or hematoma**
6.20 | 10.0 | **FUD** 010 | T A2 50
AMA: 2002,Apr,13

23931 **bursa**
4.58 | 8.18 | **FUD** 010 | T A2 50
AMA: 2002,Apr,13; 1998,Nov,1

23935 **Incision, deep, with opening of bone cortex (eg, for osteomyelitis or bone abscess), humerus or elbow**
14.5 | 14.5 | **FUD** 090 | T A2 80 50
AMA: 2002,Apr,13

24000 **Arthrotomy, elbow, including exploration, drainage, or removal of foreign body**
13.6 | 13.6 | **FUD** 090 | T A2 80 50
AMA: 2002,Apr,13; 1998,Nov,1

24006 **Arthrotomy of the elbow, with capsular excision for capsular release (separate procedure)**
20.2 | 20.2 | **FUD** 090 | T A2 80 50
AMA: 2002,Apr,13; 1996,Nov,1

24065-24066 Biopsy of Elbow/Upper Arm

EXCLUDES *Soft tissue needle biopsy (20206)*

24065 **Biopsy, soft tissue of upper arm or elbow area; superficial**
4.82 | 7.31 | **FUD** 010 | T P3 50
AMA: 2002,Apr,13

26/TC PC/TC Only | A2-Z3 ASC Payment | 50 Bilateral | ♂ Male Only | ♀ Female Only | Facility RVU | Non-Facility RVU | CCI
FUD Follow-up Days | CMS: IOM (Pub 100) | A-Y OPPSI | 80/80 Surg Assist Allowed / w/Doc | Lab Crosswalk | Radiology Crosswalk | CLIA
60

CPT © 2016 American Medical Association. All Rights Reserved.

© 2016 Optum360, LLC

24066 **deep (subfascial or intramuscular)**
📷 11.9　✂ 17.8　**FUD** 090　　　T A2 50 ▣
AMA: 2002,Apr,13; 1998,Nov,1

24071-24079 [24071, 24073] Excision Soft Tissue Tumors Elbow/Upper Arm

INCLUDES　Any necessary elevation of tissue planes or dissection
Measurement of tumor and necessary margin at greatest diameter prior to excision
Types of excision:
Fascial or subfascial soft tissue tumors: simple and marginal resection of tumors found either in or below the deep fascia, not involving bone or excision of a substantial amount of normal tissue; primarily benign and intramuscular tumors
Radical resection of soft tissue tumor: wide resection of tumor involving substantial margins of normal tissue and may involve tissue removal from one or more layers; most often malignant or aggressive benign
Subcutaneous: simple and marginal resection of tumors found in the subcutaneous tissue above the deep fascia; most often benign

EXCLUDES　Complex repair
Excision of benign cutaneous lesion (eg, sebaceous cyst) (11400-11406)
Radical resection of cutaneous tumors (eg, melanoma) (11600-11606)
Significant exploration of vessels or neuroplasty

24071 **Resequenced code. See code following 24075**

24073 **Resequenced code. See code following 24076.**

24075 **Excision, tumor, soft tissue of upper arm or elbow area, subcutaneous; less than 3 cm**
📷 9.49　✂ 14.0　**FUD** 090　　　T G2 50 ▣
AMA: 2002,Apr,13

\#　**24071** **3 cm or greater**
📷 11.7　✂ 11.7　**FUD** 090　　　T G2 80 50 ▣

24076 **Excision, tumor, soft tissue of upper arm or elbow area, subfascial (eg, intramuscular); less than 5 cm**
📷 15.6　✂ 15.6　**FUD** 090　　　T G2 50 ▣
AMA: 2002,Apr,13

\#　**24073** **5 cm or greater**
📷 19.9　✂ 19.9　**FUD** 090　　　T G2 80 50 ▣

24077 **Radical resection of tumor (eg, sarcoma), soft tissue of upper arm or elbow area; less than 5 cm**
📷 29.8　✂ 29.8　**FUD** 090　　　T G2 50 ▣
AMA: 2002,Apr,13; 1990,Win,4

24079 **5 cm or greater**
📷 38.1　✂ 38.1　**FUD** 090　　　T G2 80 50 ▣

24100-24149 Bone/Joint Procedures Upper Arm/Elbow

24100 **Arthrotomy, elbow; with synovial biopsy only**
📷 11.9　✂ 11.9　**FUD** 090　　　T A2 80 50 ▣
AMA: 2002,Apr,13; 1994,Win,1

24101 **with joint exploration, with or without biopsy, with or without removal of loose or foreign body**
📷 14.3　✂ 14.3　**FUD** 090　　　T A2 80 50 ▣
AMA: 2002,Apr,13

24102 **with synovectomy**
📷 17.6　✂ 17.6　**FUD** 090　　　T A2 80 50 ▣
AMA: 2002,Apr,13; 1994,Win,1

24105 **Excision, olecranon bursa**
📷 10.0　✂ 10.0　**FUD** 090　　　T A2 50 ▣
AMA: 2002,Apr,13

24110 **Excision or curettage of bone cyst or benign tumor, humerus;**
📷 16.6　✂ 16.6　**FUD** 090　　　T A2 50 ▣
AMA: 2002,Apr,13

24115 **with autograft (includes obtaining graft)**
📷 21.2　✂ 21.2　**FUD** 090　　　T A2 80 50 ▣
AMA: 2002,Apr,13

24116 **with allograft**
📷 24.8　✂ 24.8　**FUD** 090　　　T A2 80 50 ▣
AMA: 2002,Apr,13

24120 **Excision or curettage of bone cyst or benign tumor of head or neck of radius or olecranon process;**
📷 15.1　✂ 15.1　**FUD** 090　　　T A2 80 50 ▣
AMA: 2002,Apr,13

24125 **with autograft (includes obtaining graft)**
📷 17.6　✂ 17.6　**FUD** 090　　　T A2 80 50 ▣
AMA: 2002,Apr,13

24126 **with allograft**
📷 18.6　✂ 18.6　**FUD** 090　　　T A2 80 50 ▣
AMA: 2002,Apr,13

24130 **Excision, radial head**
EXCLUDES　Radial head arthroplasty with implant (24366)
📷 14.5　✂ 14.5　**FUD** 090　　　T A2 50 ▣
AMA: 2002,Apr,13

24134 **Sequestrectomy (eg, for osteomyelitis or bone abscess), shaft or distal humerus**
📷 21.4　✂ 21.4　**FUD** 090　　　J A2 80 50 ▣
AMA: 2002,Apr,13

24136 **Sequestrectomy (eg, for osteomyelitis or bone abscess), radial head or neck**
📷 17.9　✂ 17.9　**FUD** 090　　　T A2 50 ▣
AMA: 2002,Apr,13

24138 **Sequestrectomy (eg, for osteomyelitis or bone abscess), olecranon process**
📷 19.2　✂ 19.2　**FUD** 090　　　T A2 80 50 ▣
AMA: 2002,Apr,13

24140 **Partial excision (craterization, saucerization, or diaphysectomy) bone (eg, osteomyelitis), humerus**
📷 20.1　✂ 20.1　**FUD** 090　　　T A2 80 50 ▣
AMA: 2002,Apr,13; 1998,Nov,1

24145 **Partial excision (craterization, saucerization, or diaphysectomy) bone (eg, osteomyelitis), radial head or neck**
📷 17.0　✂ 17.0　**FUD** 090　　　T A2 50 ▣
AMA: 2002,Apr,13; 1998,Nov,1

24147 **Partial excision (craterization, saucerization, or diaphysectomy) bone (eg, osteomyelitis), olecranon process**
📷 17.8　✂ 17.8　**FUD** 090　　　T A2 50 ▣
AMA: 2002,Apr,13; 1998,Nov,1

24149 **Radical resection of capsule, soft tissue, and heterotopic bone, elbow, with contracture release (separate procedure)**
EXCLUDES　Capsular and soft tissue release (24006)
📷 33.7　✂ 33.7　**FUD** 090　　　T G2 80 50 ▣
AMA: 2002,Apr,13; 1996,Nov,1

24150-24152 Radical Resection Bone Tumor Upper Arm

INCLUDES　Any necessary elevation of tissue planes or dissection
Excision of adjacent soft tissue during bone tumor resection (24071-24079 [24071, 24073])
Measurement of tumor and necessary margin at greatest diameter prior to excision
Resection of the tumor (may include entire bone) and wide margins of normal tissue primarily for malignant or aggressive benign tumors
Simple and intermediate repairs

EXCLUDES　Complex repair
Significant exploration of vessels, neuroplasty, reconstruction, or complex bone repair

24150 **Radical resection of tumor, shaft or distal humerus**
📷 44.9　✂ 44.9　**FUD** 090　　　T 80 50 ▣
AMA: 2003,Jan,1; 2002,Apr,13

24152 **Radical resection of tumor, radial head or neck**
📷 38.1　✂ 38.1　**FUD** 090　　　T G2 80 50 ▣
AMA: 2003,Jan,1; 2002,Apr,13

24155 Elbow Arthrectomy

24155 **Resection of elbow joint (arthrectomy)**
📷 24.2　✂ 24.2　**FUD** 090　　　T A2 80 50 ▣
AMA: 2002,Apr,13; 1996,Nov,1

24160-24201 Removal Implant/Foreign Body from Elbow/Upper Arm

EXCLUDES   Bursal or joint arthrocentesis or needling (20605)
K-wire or pin insertion (20650)
K-wire or pin removal (20670, 20680)

24160   Removal of prosthesis, includes debridement and synovectomy when performed; humeral and ulnar components

INCLUDES   Prosthesis removal and replacement in same elbow (eg, humeral and/or ulnar component(s)) (24370-24371)

EXCLUDES   Foreign body removal (24200-24201)
Hardware removal other than prosthesis (20680)

🔪 36.4   ✂ 36.4   **FUD** 090   02 A2 50 ▢

AMA: 2016,Jan,13; 2015,Jan,16; 2014,Mar,4; 2014,Jan,11; 2013,Feb,11-12

24164   radial head

EXCLUDES   Foreign body removal (24200-24201)
Hardware removal other than prosthesis (20680)

🔪 21.0   ✂ 21.0   **FUD** 090   02 A2 50 ▢

AMA: 2016,Jan,13; 2015,Jan,16; 2014,Mar,4

24200   Removal of foreign body, upper arm or elbow area; subcutaneous

🔪 4.01   ✂ 5.90   **FUD** 010   T P3 80 50 ▢

AMA: 2016,Jan,13; 2015,Jan,16; 2014,Mar,4

24201   deep (subfascial or intramuscular)

🔪 10.3   ✂ 15.5   **FUD** 090   T A2 50 ▢

AMA: 2016,Jan,13; 2015,Jan,16; 2014,Mar,4

24220 Injection for Elbow Arthrogram

24220   Injection procedure for elbow arthrography

EXCLUDES   Injection tennis elbow (20550)

☢ (73085)

🔪 1.99   ✂ 4.56   **FUD** 000   N N1 80 50 ▢

AMA: 2016,May,13; 2016,Jan,13; 2015,Aug,6

24300-24498 Repair/Reconstruction of Elbow/Upper Arm

24300   Manipulation, elbow, under anesthesia

EXCLUDES   External fixation (20690, 20692)

🔪 11.9   ✂ 11.9   **FUD** 090   T G2 50 ▢

AMA: 2002,Apr,13

24301   Muscle or tendon transfer, any type, upper arm or elbow, single (excluding 24320-24331)

🔪 21.5   ✂ 21.5   **FUD** 090   T A2 80 ▢

AMA: 2002,Apr,13

24305   Tendon lengthening, upper arm or elbow, each tendon

🔪 16.5   ✂ 16.5   **FUD** 090   T A2 80 ▢

AMA: 2002,Apr,13; 1998,Nov,1

24310   Tenotomy, open, elbow to shoulder, each tendon

🔪 13.5   ✂ 13.5   **FUD** 090   T A2 80 ▢

AMA: 2002,Apr,13; 1998,Nov,1

24320   Tenoplasty, with muscle transfer, with or without free graft, elbow to shoulder, single (Seddon-Brookes type procedure)

🔪 22.4   ✂ 22.4   **FUD** 090   T A2 80 ▢

AMA: 2002,Apr,13

24330   Flexor-plasty, elbow (eg, Steindler type advancement);

🔪 20.6   ✂ 20.6   **FUD** 090   T A2 80 50 ▢

AMA: 2002,Apr,13

24331   with extensor advancement

🔪 22.6   ✂ 22.6   **FUD** 090   T A2 80 50 ▢

AMA: 2002,Apr,13

24332   Tenolysis, triceps

🔪 17.5   ✂ 17.5   **FUD** 090   T G2 50 ▢

AMA: 2002,Apr,13

24340   Tenodesis of biceps tendon at elbow (separate procedure)

🔪 17.5   ✂ 17.5   **FUD** 090   J A2 80 50 ▢

AMA: 2002,Apr,13; 1994,Win,1

24341   Repair, tendon or muscle, upper arm or elbow, each tendon or muscle, primary or secondary (excludes rotator cuff)

🔪 21.4   ✂ 21.4   **FUD** 090   T A2 80 50 ▢

AMA: 2002,Apr,13; 1996,Nov,1

24342   Reinsertion of ruptured biceps or triceps tendon, distal, with or without tendon graft

🔪 22.2   ✂ 22.2   **FUD** 090   T A2 80 50 ▢

AMA: 2002,Apr,13; 1996,Nov,1

24343   Repair lateral collateral ligament, elbow, with local tissue

🔪 20.2   ✂ 20.2   **FUD** 090   T G2 80 50 ▢

AMA: 2002,Apr,13

24344   Reconstruction lateral collateral ligament, elbow, with tendon graft (includes harvesting of graft)

🔪 31.5   ✂ 31.5   **FUD** 090   J G2 80 50 ▢

AMA: 2002,Apr,13

24345   Repair medial collateral ligament, elbow, with local tissue

🔪 20.1   ✂ 20.1   **FUD** 090   T A2 80 50 ▢

AMA: 2002,Apr,13

24346   Reconstruction medial collateral ligament, elbow, with tendon graft (includes harvesting of graft)

🔪 31.4   ✂ 31.4   **FUD** 090   J G2 80 50 ▢

AMA: 2002,Apr,13

24357   Tenotomy, elbow, lateral or medial (eg, epicondylitis, tennis elbow, golfer's elbow); percutaneous

EXCLUDES   Arthroscopy, elbow, surgical; debridement (29837-29838)

🔪 12.2   ✂ 12.2   **FUD** 090   T G2 80 50 ▢

AMA: 2016,Jan,13; 2015,Jan,16; 2014,Jan,11

24358   debridement, soft tissue and/or bone, open

EXCLUDES   Arthroscopy, elbow, surgical; debridement (29837-29838)

🔪 14.9   ✂ 14.9   **FUD** 090   T G2 80 50 ▢

AMA: 2016,Jan,13; 2015,Jan,16; 2014,Jan,11

24359   debridement, soft tissue and/or bone, open with tendon repair or reattachment

EXCLUDES   Arthroscopy, elbow, surgical; debridement (29837-29838)

🔪 18.9   ✂ 18.9   **FUD** 090   T G2 80 50 ▢

AMA: 2016,Jan,13; 2015,Jan,16; 2014,Jan,11

24360   Arthroplasty, elbow; with membrane (eg, fascial)

🔪 25.4   ✂ 25.4   **FUD** 090   J A2 80 50 ▢

AMA: 2002,Apr,13; 1998,Nov,1

24361   with distal humeral prosthetic replacement

🔪 28.7   ✂ 28.7   **FUD** 090   J J8 80 50 ▢

AMA: 2002,Apr,13

24362   with implant and fascia lata ligament reconstruction

🔪 30.5   ✂ 30.5   **FUD** 090   J J8 80 50 ▢

AMA: 2002,Apr,13

24363   with distal humerus and proximal ulnar prosthetic replacement (eg, total elbow)

EXCLUDES   Total elbow implant revision (24370-24371)

🔪 41.9   ✂ 41.9   **FUD** 090   J J8 80 50 ▢

AMA: 2016,Jan,13; 2015,Jan,16; 2014,Jan,11; 2013,Feb,11-12

24365   Arthroplasty, radial head;

🔪 18.2   ✂ 18.2   **FUD** 090   J G2 80 50 ▢

AMA: 2002,Apr,13

24366   with implant

🔪 19.5   ✂ 19.5   **FUD** 090   J J8 80 50 ▢

AMA: 2002,Apr,13

24370 Revision of total elbow arthroplasty, including allograft when performed; humeral or ulnar component

EXCLUDES *Prosthesis removal without replacement (eg, humeral and/or ulnar component/s) (24160)*

44.7   44.7   **FUD** 090   J J8 80 50

AMA: 2016,Jan,13; 2015,Jan,16; 2014,Mar,4; 2013,Feb,11-12

24371 humeral and ulnar component

EXCLUDES *Prosthesis removal without replacement (eg, humeral and/or ulnar component/s) (24160)*

51.3   51.3   **FUD** 090   J J8 80 50

AMA: 2016,Jan,13; 2015,Jan,16; 2014,Mar,4; 2013,Feb,11-12

24400 Osteotomy, humerus, with or without internal fixation

23.4   23.4   **FUD** 090   J A2 80 50

AMA: 2016,Jan,13; 2015,Jan,16; 2014,Mar,4

24410 Multiple osteotomies with realignment on intramedullary rod, humeral shaft (Sofield type procedure)

30.4   30.4   **FUD** 090   J J8 80 50

AMA: 2002,Apr,13

24420 Osteoplasty, humerus (eg, shortening or lengthening) (excluding 64876)

28.1   28.1   **FUD** 090   T A2 80 50

AMA: 2002,Apr,13

24430 Repair of nonunion or malunion, humerus; without graft (eg, compression technique)

30.3   30.3   **FUD** 090   J G2 80 50

AMA: 2002,Apr,13

24435 with iliac or other autograft (includes obtaining graft)

30.9   30.9   **FUD** 090   J J8 80 50

AMA: 2002,Apr,13

24470 Hemiepiphyseal arrest (eg, cubitus varus or valgus, distal humerus)

16.2   16.2   **FUD** 090   T A2 80 50

AMA: 2002,Apr,13; 1998,Nov,1

24495 Decompression fasciotomy, forearm, with brachial artery exploration

18.7   18.7   **FUD** 090   T A2 80 50

AMA: 2002,Apr,13

24498 Prophylactic treatment (nailing, pinning, plating or wiring), with or without methylmethacrylate, humeral shaft

24.9   24.9   **FUD** 090   J G2 80 50

AMA: 2002,Apr,13; 1998,Nov,1

24500-24685 Treatment of Fracture/Dislocation of Elbow/Upper Arm

INCLUDES Treatment for either closed or open fractures or dislocations

24500 Closed treatment of humeral shaft fracture; without manipulation

9.29   10.1   **FUD** 090   T A2 50

AMA: 2002,Apr,13

24505 with manipulation, with or without skeletal traction

12.8   14.2   **FUD** 090   T A2 50

AMA: 2002,Apr,13

24515 Open treatment of humeral shaft fracture with plate/screws, with or without cerclage

25.1   25.1   **FUD** 090   J G2 80 50

AMA: 2002,Apr,13

24516 Treatment of humeral shaft fracture, with insertion of intramedullary implant, with or without cerclage and/or locking screws

24.7   24.7   **FUD** 090   J G2 80 50

AMA: 2016,Jan,13; 2015,Jan,16; 2014,Jan,11

24530 Closed treatment of supracondylar or transcondylar humeral fracture, with or without intercondylar extension; without manipulation

9.82   10.8   **FUD** 090   T A2 50

AMA: 2002,Apr,13

24535 with manipulation, with or without skin or skeletal traction

16.2   17.5   **FUD** 090   T A2 50

AMA: 2002,Apr,13

24538 Percutaneous skeletal fixation of supracondylar or transcondylar humeral fracture, with or without intercondylar extension

21.3   21.3   **FUD** 090   T A2 50

AMA: 2016,Jan,13; 2015,Jan,16; 2014,Jan,11

24545 Open treatment of humeral supracondylar or transcondylar fracture, includes internal fixation, when performed; without intercondylar extension

26.7   26.7   **FUD** 090   J J8 80 50

AMA: 2002,Apr,13

24546 with intercondylar extension

29.8   29.8   **FUD** 090   J J8 80 50

AMA: 2002,Apr,13

24560 Closed treatment of humeral epicondylar fracture, medial or lateral; without manipulation

8.16   9.10   **FUD** 090   T A2 50

AMA: 2002,Apr,13

24565 with manipulation

13.9   15.1   **FUD** 090   T A2 50

AMA: 2002,Apr,13

24566 Percutaneous skeletal fixation of humeral epicondylar fracture, medial or lateral, with manipulation

20.5   20.5   **FUD** 090   T A2 50

AMA: 2002,Apr,13; 1993,Win,1

24575 Open treatment of humeral epicondylar fracture, medial or lateral, includes internal fixation, when performed

20.9   20.9   **FUD** 090   J G2 80 50

AMA: 2002,Apr,13

24576 Closed treatment of humeral condylar fracture, medial or lateral; without manipulation

8.69   9.66   **FUD** 090   T A2 50

AMA: 2002,Apr,13

24577 with manipulation

14.2   15.5   **FUD** 090   T A2 50

AMA: 2002,Apr,13

24579 Open treatment of humeral condylar fracture, medial or lateral, includes internal fixation, when performed

EXCLUDES *Closed treatment without manipulation (24530, 24560, 24576, 24650, 24670)*
Repair with manipulation (24535, 24565, 24577, 24675)

24.0   24.0   **FUD** 090   J G2 80 50

AMA: 2002,Apr,13

24582 Percutaneous skeletal fixation of humeral condylar fracture, medial or lateral, with manipulation

23.1   23.1   **FUD** 090   T A2 50

AMA: 2002,Apr,13; 1993,Win,1

24586 Open treatment of periarticular fracture and/or dislocation of the elbow (fracture distal humerus and proximal ulna and/or proximal radius);

31.1   31.1   **FUD** 090   J G2 80 50

AMA: 2002,Apr,13

24587 with implant arthroplasty

EXCLUDES *Distal humerus arthroplasty with implant (24361)*

31.0   31.0   **FUD** 090   J J8 80 50

AMA: 2002,Apr,13

24600 Treatment of closed elbow dislocation; without anesthesia

9.49   10.3   **FUD** 090   T A2 50

AMA: 2002,Apr,13

24605 requiring anesthesia

13.4   13.4   **FUD** 090   T A2 50

AMA: 2002,Apr,13

Musculoskeletal System

24615 — 25040

24615   **Open treatment of acute or chronic elbow dislocation**
    20.4   20.4   **FUD** 090   J A2 80 50
    AMA: 2002,Apr,13

24620   **Closed treatment of Monteggia type of fracture dislocation at elbow (fracture proximal end of ulna with dislocation of radial head), with manipulation**
    15.7   15.7   **FUD** 090   T A2 80 50
    AMA: 2002,Apr,13

24635   **Open treatment of Monteggia type of fracture dislocation at elbow (fracture proximal end of ulna with dislocation of radial head), includes internal fixation, when performed**
    19.3   19.3   **FUD** 090   J A2 80 50
    AMA: 2002,Apr,13

24640   **Closed treatment of radial head subluxation in child, nursemaid elbow, with manipulation**   A
    2.63   3.83   **FUD** 010   T P3 80 50
    AMA: 2002,Apr,13

24650   **Closed treatment of radial head or neck fracture; without manipulation**
    6.83   7.43   **FUD** 090   T P2 50
    AMA: 2002,Apr,13

24655   **with manipulation**
    11.2   12.3   **FUD** 090   T A2 50
    AMA: 2002,Apr,13

24665   **Open treatment of radial head or neck fracture, includes internal fixation or radial head excision, when performed;**
    18.6   18.6   **FUD** 090   J A2 80 50
    AMA: 2002,Apr,13

24666   **with radial head prosthetic replacement**
    21.0   21.0   **FUD** 090   J 62 80 50
    AMA: 2002,Apr,13

24670   **Closed treatment of ulnar fracture, proximal end (eg, olecranon or coronoid process[es]); without manipulation**
    7.48   8.27   **FUD** 090   T A2 50
    AMA: 2002,Apr,13

24675   **with manipulation**
    11.8   12.9   **FUD** 090   T A2 50
    AMA: 2002,Apr,13

24685   **Open treatment of ulnar fracture, proximal end (eg, olecranon or coronoid process[es]), includes internal fixation, when performed**
    EXCLUDES   *Arthrotomy, elbow (24100-24102)*
    18.7   18.7   **FUD** 090   J A2 80 50
    AMA: 2002,Apr,13

24800-24999 Other/Unlisted Elbow/Upper Arm Procedures

24800   **Arthrodesis, elbow joint; local**
    23.8   23.8   **FUD** 090   J A2 80 50
    AMA: 2002,Apr,13; 1998,Nov,1

24802   **with autogenous graft (includes obtaining graft)**
    28.1   28.1   **FUD** 090   J 62 80 50
    AMA: 2002,Apr,13; 1998,Nov,1

24900   **Amputation, arm through humerus; with primary closure**
    21.0   21.0   **FUD** 090   C 80 50
    AMA: 2002,Apr,13

24920   **open, circular (guillotine)**
    21.0   21.0   **FUD** 090   C 80 50
    AMA: 2002,Apr,13

24925   **secondary closure or scar revision**
    15.7   15.7   **FUD** 090   T A2 80 50
    AMA: 2002,Apr,13

24930   **re-amputation**
    22.1   22.1   **FUD** 090   C 80 50
    AMA: 2002,Apr,13

24931   **with implant**
    23.0   23.0   **FUD** 090   C 80 50
    AMA: 2002,Apr,13

24935   **Stump elongation, upper extremity**
    31.9   31.9   **FUD** 090   J 80 50
    AMA: 2002,Apr,13

24940   **Cineplasty, upper extremity, complete procedure**
    0.00   0.00   **FUD** 090   C 80 50
    AMA: 2002,Apr,13

24999   **Unlisted procedure, humerus or elbow**
    0.00   0.00   **FUD** YYY   T 80 50
    AMA: 2002,Apr,13

25000-25001 Incision Tendon Sheath of Wrist

25000   **Incision, extensor tendon sheath, wrist (eg, deQuervains disease)**
    EXCLUDES   *Carpal tunnel release (64721)*
    9.62   9.62   **FUD** 090   T A2 50
    AMA: 2002,Apr,13; 1998,Nov,1

25001   **Incision, flexor tendon sheath, wrist (eg, flexor carpi radialis)**
    9.77   9.77   **FUD** 090   T 62 50
    AMA: 2002,Apr,13

25020-25025 Decompression Fasciotomy Forearm/Wrist

25020   **Decompression fasciotomy, forearm and/or wrist, flexor OR extensor compartment; without debridement of nonviable muscle and/or nerve**
    EXCLUDES   *Brachial artery exploration (24495)*
                Superficial incision and drainage (10060-10160)
    16.4   16.4   **FUD** 090   T A2 50
    AMA: 2002,Apr,13

25023   **with debridement of nonviable muscle and/or nerve**
    EXCLUDES   *Debridement (11000-11044 [11045, 11046])*
                Decompression fasciotomy with exploration brachial artery exploration (24495)
                Superficial incision and drainage (10060-10160)
    31.5   31.5   **FUD** 090   T A2 80 50
    AMA: 2002,Apr,13

25024   **Decompression fasciotomy, forearm and/or wrist, flexor AND extensor compartment; without debridement of nonviable muscle and/or nerve**
    22.1   22.1   **FUD** 090   T A2 50
    AMA: 2002,Apr,13

25025   **with debridement of nonviable muscle and/or nerve**
    34.6   34.6   **FUD** 090   T A2 80 50
    AMA: 2002,Apr,13

25028-25040 Incision for Drainage/Foreign Body Removal

25028   **Incision and drainage, forearm and/or wrist; deep abscess or hematoma**
    14.9   14.9   **FUD** 090   T A2 50
    AMA: 2002,Apr,13

25031   **bursa**
    10.2   10.2   **FUD** 090   T A2 80 50
    AMA: 2002,Apr,13; 1998,Nov,1

25035   **Incision, deep, bone cortex, forearm and/or wrist (eg, osteomyelitis or bone abscess)**
    16.5   16.5   **FUD** 090   T A2 80 50
    AMA: 2002,Apr,13; 1998,Nov,1

25040   **Arthrotomy, radiocarpal or midcarpal joint, with exploration, drainage, or removal of foreign body**
    16.1   16.1   **FUD** 090   T A2 80 50
    AMA: 2002,Apr,13; 1994,Win,1

25065-25066 Biopsy Forearm/Wrist

EXCLUDES   *Soft tissue needle biopsy (20206)*

25065   **Biopsy, soft tissue of forearm and/or wrist; superficial**
📖 4.69   ⚖ 7.24   **FUD** 010   T P3 50 ▭
AMA: 2002,Apr,13

25066   **deep (subfascial or intramuscular)**
📖 10.2   ⚖ 10.2   **FUD** 090   T A2 50 ▭
AMA: 2002,Apr,13; 1998,Nov,1

25071-25078 [25071, 25073] Excision Soft Tissue Tumors Forearm/Wrist

INCLUDES   Any necessary elevation of tissue planes or dissection
Measurement of tumor and necessary margin at greatest diameter prior
to excision
Simple and intermediate repairs
Types of excision:
  Fascial or subfascial soft tissue tumors: simple and marginal resection
  of tumors found either in or below the deep fascia, not involving
  bone or excision of a substantial amount of normal tissue; primarily
  benign and intramuscular tumors
  Radical resection soft tissue tumor: wide resection of tumor involving
  substantial margins of normal tissue and may include tissue
  removal from one or more layers; most often malignant or
  aggressive benign
  Subcutaneous: simple and marginal resection of tumors in the
  subcutaneous tissue above the deep fascia; most often benign
EXCLUDES   *Complex repair*
Excision of benign cutaneous lesions (eg, sebaceous cyst) (11400-11406)
Radical resection of cutaneous tumors (eg, melanoma) (11600-11606)
Significant exploration of vessels or neuroplasty

25071   **Resequenced code. See code following 25075.**

25073   **Resequenced code. See code following 25076.**

25075   **Excision, tumor, soft tissue of forearm and/or wrist area,
subcutaneous; less than 3 cm**
📖 9.09   ⚖ 13.6   **FUD** 090   T 62 50 ▭
AMA: 2002,Apr,13

\#   **25071**   **3 cm or greater**
📖 12.2   ⚖ 12.2   **FUD** 090   T 62 80 50 ▭

25076   **Excision, tumor, soft tissue of forearm and/or wrist area,
subfascial (eg, intramuscular); less than 3 cm**
📖 14.8   ⚖ 14.8   **FUD** 090   T 62 50 ▭
AMA: 2002,Apr,13

\#   **25073**   **3 cm or greater**
📖 15.2   ⚖ 15.2   **FUD** 090   T 62 80 50 ▭

25077   **Radical resection of tumor (eg, sarcoma), soft tissue of
forearm and/or wrist area; less than 3 cm**
📖 25.4   ⚖ 25.4   **FUD** 090   T 62 50 ▭
AMA: 2002,Apr,13; 1990,Win,4

25078   **3 cm or greater**
📖 33.5   ⚖ 33.5   **FUD** 090   T 62 80 50 ▭

25085-25240 Procedures of Bones/Joints Lower Arm/Wrist

25085   **Capsulotomy, wrist (eg, contracture)**
📖 12.8   ⚖ 12.8   **FUD** 090   T A2 80 50 ▭
AMA: 2002,Apr,13; 1998,Nov,1

25100   **Arthrotomy, wrist joint; with biopsy**
📖 9.87   ⚖ 9.87   **FUD** 090   T A2 80 50 ▭
AMA: 2002,Apr,13; 2000,Dec,12

25101   **with joint exploration, with or without biopsy, with or
without removal of loose or foreign body**
📖 11.5   ⚖ 11.5   **FUD** 090   T A2 80 50 ▭
AMA: 2002,Apr,13

25105   **with synovectomy**
📖 13.7   ⚖ 13.7   **FUD** 090   T A2 80 50 ▭
AMA: 2002,Apr,13; 2000,Dec,12

25107   **Arthrotomy, distal radioulnar joint including repair of
triangular cartilage, complex**
📖 17.6   ⚖ 17.6   **FUD** 090   T A2 80 50 ▭
AMA: 2002,Apr,13; 1998,Nov,1

25109   **Excision of tendon, forearm and/or wrist, flexor or extensor,
each**
📖 15.3   ⚖ 15.3   **FUD** 090   T 62 50 ▭

25110   **Excision, lesion of tendon sheath, forearm and/or wrist**
📖 9.79   ⚖ 9.79   **FUD** 090   T A2 50 ▭
AMA: 2002,Apr,13

25111   **Excision of ganglion, wrist (dorsal or volar); primary**
EXCLUDES   *Excision of ganglion hand or finger (26160)*
📖 9.15   ⚖ 9.15   **FUD** 090   T A2 50 ▭
AMA: 2002,Apr,13

Synovial sheaths (blue) of the dorsum of right wrist, containing extensor tendons

Ganglion

Anatomical "snuffbox"

Anatomical "snuffbox"

Ganglions are round cystic swellings usually appearing on the dorsum of the wrist or hand; these swellings often communicate with the synovial sheath

Typical location of ganglion

25112   **recurrent**
EXCLUDES   *Excision of ganglion hand or finger (26160)*
📖 11.0   ⚖ 11.0   **FUD** 090   T A2 50 ▭
AMA: 2002,Apr,13

25115   **Radical excision of bursa, synovia of wrist, or forearm tendon
sheaths (eg, tenosynovitis, fungus, Tbc, or other granulomas,
rheumatoid arthritis); flexors**
EXCLUDES   *Finger synovectomy (26145)*
📖 21.7   ⚖ 21.7   **FUD** 090   T A2 50 ▭
AMA: 2016,Jan,13; 2015,Jan,16; 2012,Jun,15-16

25116   **extensors, with or without transposition of dorsal
retinaculum**
EXCLUDES   *Finger synovectomy (26145)*
📖 17.1   ⚖ 17.1   **FUD** 090   T A2 80 50 ▭
AMA: 2002,Apr,13

25118   **Synovectomy, extensor tendon sheath, wrist, single
compartment;**
EXCLUDES   *Finger synovectomy (26145)*
📖 10.9   ⚖ 10.9   **FUD** 090   T A2 50 ▭
AMA: 2016,Jan,13; 2015,Jun,10; 2015,Jan,16; 2014,Jan,11;
2012,Apr,17-18

25119   **with resection of distal ulna**
EXCLUDES   *Finger synovectomy (26145)*
📖 14.1   ⚖ 14.1   **FUD** 090   T A2 80 50 ▭
AMA: 2002,Apr,13

25120   **Excision or curettage of bone cyst or benign tumor of radius
or ulna (excluding head or neck of radius and olecranon
process);**
EXCLUDES   *Removal of bone cyst or tumor of radial head, neck, or
olecranon process (24120-24126)*
📖 14.2   ⚖ 14.2   **FUD** 090   T A2 80 50 ▭
AMA: 2002,Apr,13

25125   **with autograft (includes obtaining graft)**
📖 16.6   ⚖ 16.6   **FUD** 090   T A2 80 50 ▭
AMA: 2002,Apr,13

25126   **with allograft**
📖 17.0   ⚖ 17.0   **FUD** 090   T A2 80 50 ▭
AMA: 2002,Apr,13

25130   **Excision or curettage of bone cyst or benign tumor of carpal
bones;**
📖 12.7   ⚖ 12.7   **FUD** 090   T A2 80 50 ▭
AMA: 2002,Apr,13

25135 **with autograft (includes obtaining graft)**
📋 15.8   🔧 15.8   **FUD** 090   T A2 80 50 ▣
AMA: 2002,Apr,13

25136 **with allograft**
📋 14.0   🔧 14.0   **FUD** 090   T A2 80 50 ▣
AMA: 2002,Apr,13

25145 **Sequestrectomy (eg, for osteomyelitis or bone abscess), forearm and/or wrist**
📋 14.8   🔧 14.8   **FUD** 090   T A2 80 50 ▣
AMA: 2002,Apr,13

25150 **Partial excision (craterization, saucerization, or diaphysectomy) of bone (eg, for osteomyelitis); ulna**
📋 16.2   🔧 16.2   **FUD** 090   T A2 50 ▣
AMA: 2002,Apr,13

25151 **radius**
EXCLUDES   Partial removal of radial head, neck, or olecranon process (24145, 24147)
📋 16.7   🔧 16.7   **FUD** 090   T A2 80 50 ▣
AMA: 2002,Apr,13

25170 **Radical resection of tumor, radius or ulna**
INCLUDES   Any necessary elevation of tissue planes or dissection
Excision of adjacent soft tissue during bone tumor resection (25071-25078 [25071, 25073])
Measurement of tumor and necessary margin at greatest diameter prior to excision
Resection of the tumor (may include entire bone) and wide margins of normal tissue primarily for malignant or aggressive benign tumors
Resection without removal of significant normal tissue
Simple and intermediate repairs
EXCLUDES   Complex repair
Excision of adjacent soft tissue during bone tumor resection (25076-25078 [25073])
Radical resection of cutaneous tumors (e.g., melanoma) (11600-11646)
Significant exploration of vessels, neuroplasty, reconstruction, or complex bone repair
📋 42.6   🔧 42.6   **FUD** 090   T 80 50 ▣
AMA: 2003,Jan,1; 2002,Apr,13

25210 **Carpectomy; 1 bone**
EXCLUDES   Carpectomy with insertion of implant (25441-25445)
📋 13.9   🔧 13.9   **FUD** 090   T A2 80 ▣
AMA: 2002,Apr,13

25215 **all bones of proximal row**
📋 17.6   🔧 17.6   **FUD** 090   T A2 80 50 ▣
AMA: 2002,Apr,13

25230 **Radial styloidectomy (separate procedure)**
📋 12.3   🔧 12.3   **FUD** 090   T A2 50 ▣
AMA: 2002,Apr,13

25240 **Excision distal ulna partial or complete (eg, Darrach type or matched resection)**
EXCLUDES   Acquisition of fascia for interposition (20920, 20922)
Implant replacement (25442)
📋 12.2   🔧 12.2   **FUD** 090   T A2 80 50 ▣
AMA: 2002,Apr,13; 1994,Win,1

25246 Injection for Wrist Arthrogram

25246 **Injection procedure for wrist arthrography**
EXCLUDES   Excision of superficial foreign body (20520)
🔶 (73115)
📋 2.17   🔧 4.61   **FUD** 000   N N1 50 ▣
AMA: 2016,Jan,13; 2015,Aug,6

25248-25251 Removal Foreign Body of Wrist

EXCLUDES   Excision of superficial foreign body (20520)
K-wire, pin, or rod insertion (20650)
K-wire, pin, or rod removal (20670, 20680)

25248 **Exploration with removal of deep foreign body, forearm or wrist**
📋 11.9   🔧 11.9   **FUD** 090   T A2 50 ▣
AMA: 2002,Apr,13; 1994,Win,1

25250 **Removal of wrist prosthesis; (separate procedure)**
📋 14.9   🔧 14.9   **FUD** 090   Q2 A2 80 50 ▣
AMA: 2002,Apr,13

25251 **complicated, including total wrist**
📋 20.5   🔧 20.5   **FUD** 090   Q2 A2 80 50 ▣
AMA: 2002,Apr,13

25259 Manipulation of Wrist with Anesthesia

25259 **Manipulation, wrist, under anesthesia**
EXCLUDES   Application external fixation (20690, 20692)
📋 11.8   🔧 11.8   **FUD** 090   T G2 50 ▣
AMA: 2016,Jan,13; 2015,Jan,16; 2014,Jan,11; 2012,Jan,15-42; 2011,Jan,11

25260-25492 Repair/Reconstruction of Forearm/Wrist

25260 **Repair, tendon or muscle, flexor, forearm and/or wrist; primary, single, each tendon or muscle**
📋 18.0   🔧 18.0   **FUD** 090   T A2 ▣
AMA: 2002,Apr,13; 1996,Nov,1

25263 **secondary, single, each tendon or muscle**
📋 17.7   🔧 17.7   **FUD** 090   T A2 80 ▣
AMA: 2002,Apr,13; 1996,Nov,1

25265 **secondary, with free graft (includes obtaining graft), each tendon or muscle**
📋 21.4   🔧 21.4   **FUD** 090   T A2 80 ▣
AMA: 2002,Apr,13; 1996,Nov,1

25270 **Repair, tendon or muscle, extensor, forearm and/or wrist; primary, single, each tendon or muscle**
📋 13.9   🔧 13.9   **FUD** 090   T A2 80 ▣
AMA: 2002,Apr,13; 1996,Nov,1

25272 **secondary, single, each tendon or muscle**
📋 15.8   🔧 15.8   **FUD** 090   T A2 80 ▣
AMA: 2002,Apr,13; 1996,Nov,1

25274 **secondary, with free graft (includes obtaining graft), each tendon or muscle**
📋 19.0   🔧 19.0   **FUD** 090   T A2 80 ▣
AMA: 2002,Apr,13; 1996,Nov,1

25275 **Repair, tendon sheath, extensor, forearm and/or wrist, with free graft (includes obtaining graft) (eg, for extensor carpi ulnaris subluxation)**
📋 19.2   🔧 19.2   **FUD** 090   T A2 80 50 ▣
AMA: 2002,Apr,13

25280 **Lengthening or shortening of flexor or extensor tendon, forearm and/or wrist, single, each tendon**
📋 16.1   🔧 16.1   **FUD** 090   T A2 80 ▣
AMA: 2002,Apr,13

25290 **Tenotomy, open, flexor or extensor tendon, forearm and/or wrist, single, each tendon**
📋 12.4   🔧 12.4   **FUD** 090   T A2 ▣
AMA: 2002,Apr,13

25295 **Tenolysis, flexor or extensor tendon, forearm and/or wrist, single, each tendon**
📋 14.9   🔧 14.9   **FUD** 090   T A2 ▣
AMA: 2016,Jan,13; 2015,Jan,16; 2014,Jan,11; 2012,Jan,15-42; 2011,Jan,11

25300 **Tenodesis at wrist; flexors of fingers**
📋 19.5   🔧 19.5   **FUD** 090   T A2 80 50 ▣
AMA: 2002,Apr,13

25301 **extensors of fingers**
📋 18.4   🔧 18.4   **FUD** 090   T A2 80 50 ▣
AMA: 2002,Apr,13

25310 Tendon transplantation or transfer, flexor or extensor, forearm and/or wrist, single; each tendon
 🔧 17.7   ⚖ 17.7   **FUD** 090   T A2 80 ▣
AMA: 2016,Jan,13; 2015,Jan,16; 2014,Jan,11; 2012,Jan,15-42; 2011,Jan,11

25312 with tendon graft(s) (includes obtaining graft), each tendon
 🔧 20.4   ⚖ 20.4   **FUD** 090   T A2 80 ▣
AMA: 2002,Apr,13

25315 Flexor origin slide (eg, for cerebral palsy, Volkmann contracture), forearm and/or wrist;
 🔧 22.1   ⚖ 22.1   **FUD** 090   T A2 80 50 ▣
AMA: 2002,Apr,13; 1994,Win,1

25316 with tendon(s) transfer
 🔧 26.2   ⚖ 26.2   **FUD** 090   J A2 80 50 ▣
AMA: 2002,Apr,13; 1994,Win,1

25320 Capsulorrhaphy or reconstruction, wrist, open (eg, capsulodesis, ligament repair, tendon transfer or graft) (includes synovectomy, capsulotomy and open reduction) for carpal instability
 🔧 28.2   ⚖ 28.2   **FUD** 090   T A2 80 50 ▣
AMA: 2002,Apr,13; 1994,Win,1

25332 Arthroplasty, wrist, with or without interposition, with or without external or internal fixation
EXCLUDES   Acquiring fascia for interposition (20920, 20922)
Arthroplasty with prosthesis (25441-25446)
 🔧 24.1   ⚖ 24.1   **FUD** 090   T A2 80 50 ▣
AMA: 2016,Jan,13; 2015,Jan,16; 2014,Jan,11

25335 Centralization of wrist on ulna (eg, radial club hand)
 🔧 23.1   ⚖ 23.1   **FUD** 090   T A2 80 50 ▣
AMA: 2002,Apr,13

25337 Reconstruction for stabilization of unstable distal ulna or distal radioulnar joint, secondary by soft tissue stabilization (eg, tendon transfer, tendon graft or weave, or tenodesis) with or without open reduction of distal radioulnar joint
EXCLUDES   Acquiring fascia lata graft (20920, 20922)
 🔧 25.4   ⚖ 25.4   **FUD** 090   T A2 50 ▣
AMA: 2002,Apr,13; 1994,Win,1

25350 Osteotomy, radius; distal third
 🔧 19.3   ⚖ 19.3   **FUD** 090   J A2 80 50 ▣
AMA: 2002,Apr,13

25355 middle or proximal third
 🔧 21.5   ⚖ 21.5   **FUD** 090   T A2 80 50 ▣
AMA: 2002,Apr,13

25360 Osteotomy; ulna
 🔧 18.7   ⚖ 18.7   **FUD** 090   J A2 80 50 ▣
AMA: 2002,Apr,13

25365 radius AND ulna
 🔧 26.2   ⚖ 26.2   **FUD** 090   J A2 80 50 ▣
AMA: 2002,Apr,13

25370 Multiple osteotomies, with realignment on intramedullary rod (Sofield type procedure); radius OR ulna
 🔧 28.9   ⚖ 28.9   **FUD** 090   T A2 80 50 ▣
AMA: 2002,Apr,13

25375 radius AND ulna
 🔧 27.4   ⚖ 27.4   **FUD** 090   T A2 80 50 ▣
AMA: 2002,Apr,13

25390 Osteoplasty, radius OR ulna; shortening
 🔧 22.0   ⚖ 22.0   **FUD** 090   J A2 80 50 ▣
AMA: 2003,Jan,1; 2002,Apr,13

25391 lengthening with autograft
 🔧 28.6   ⚖ 28.6   **FUD** 090   J G2 80 50 ▣
AMA: 2003,Jan,1; 2002,Apr,13

25392 Osteoplasty, radius AND ulna; shortening (excluding 64876)
 🔧 24.9   ⚖ 24.9   **FUD** 090   T A2 80 50 ▣
AMA: 2003,Jan,1; 2002,Apr,13

25393 lengthening with autograft
 🔧 32.5   ⚖ 32.5   **FUD** 090   T A2 80 50 ▣
AMA: 2003,Jan,1; 2002,Apr,13

25394 Osteoplasty, carpal bone, shortening
 🔧 22.3   ⚖ 22.3   **FUD** 090   T G2 80 50 ▣
AMA: 2002,Apr,13

25400 Repair of nonunion or malunion, radius OR ulna; without graft (eg, compression technique)
 🔧 23.0   ⚖ 23.0   **FUD** 090   J A2 80 50 ▣
AMA: 2002,Apr,13

25405 with autograft (includes obtaining graft)
 🔧 29.7   ⚖ 29.7   **FUD** 090   J A2 80 50 ▣
AMA: 2002,Apr,13

25415 Repair of nonunion or malunion, radius AND ulna; without graft (eg, compression technique)
 🔧 27.6   ⚖ 27.6   **FUD** 090   J A2 80 50 ▣
AMA: 2002,Apr,13

25420 with autograft (includes obtaining graft)
 🔧 33.5   ⚖ 33.5   **FUD** 090   J G2 80 50 ▣
AMA: 2003,Jan,1; 2002,Apr,13

25425 Repair of defect with autograft; radius OR ulna
 🔧 27.7   ⚖ 27.7   **FUD** 090   T A2 80 50 ▣
AMA: 2002,Apr,13

25426 radius AND ulna
 🔧 32.3   ⚖ 32.3   **FUD** 090   T A2 80 50 ▣
AMA: 2002,Apr,13

25430 Insertion of vascular pedicle into carpal bone (eg, Hori procedure)
 🔧 21.0   ⚖ 21.0   **FUD** 090   T G2 50 ▣
AMA: 2002,Apr,13

25431 Repair of nonunion of carpal bone (excluding carpal scaphoid (navicular)) (includes obtaining graft and necessary fixation), each bone
 🔧 22.5   ⚖ 22.5   **FUD** 090   J G2 80 50 ▣
AMA: 2002,Apr,13

25440 Repair of nonunion, scaphoid carpal (navicular) bone, with or without radial styloidectomy (includes obtaining graft and necessary fixation)
 🔧 21.9   ⚖ 21.9   **FUD** 090   J A2 80 50 ▣
AMA: 2002,May,7; 2002,Apr,13

25441 Arthroplasty with prosthetic replacement; distal radius
 🔧 26.7   ⚖ 26.7   **FUD** 090   J J8 80 50 ▣
AMA: 2016,Jan,13; 2015,Jan,16; 2014,Jan,11

25442 distal ulna
 🔧 23.1   ⚖ 23.1   **FUD** 090   J J8 80 50 ▣
AMA: 2016,Jan,13; 2015,Jan,16; 2014,Jan,11

25443 scaphoid carpal (navicular)
 🔧 22.4   ⚖ 22.4   **FUD** 090   J A2 80 50 ▣
AMA: 2016,Jan,13; 2015,Jan,16; 2014,Jan,11

25444 lunate
 🔧 23.7   ⚖ 23.7   **FUD** 090   J J8 80 50 ▣
AMA: 2016,Jan,13; 2015,Jan,16; 2014,Jan,11

25445 trapezium
 🔧 20.7   ⚖ 20.7   **FUD** 090   J A2 50 ▣
AMA: 2016,Jan,13; 2015,Jan,16; 2014,Jan,11

25446 distal radius and partial or entire carpus (total wrist)
 🔧 33.6   ⚖ 33.6   **FUD** 090   J J8 80 50 ▣
AMA: 2016,Jan,13; 2015,Jan,16; 2014,Jan,11

25447 Arthroplasty, interposition, intercarpal or carpometacarpal joints

> EXCLUDES *Wrist arthroplasty (25332)*
> 🏥 23.7 ✂ 23.7 **FUD** 090   T A2 80 50 ▢
> **AMA:** 2016,Jan,13; 2015,Jan,16; 2014,Jan,11

25449 Revision of arthroplasty, including removal of implant, wrist joint

> 🏥 29.6 ✂ 29.6 **FUD** 090   J A2 80 50 ▢
> **AMA:** 2002,Apr,13

25450 Epiphyseal arrest by epiphysiodesis or stapling; distal radius OR ulna

> 🏥 14.8 ✂ 14.8 **FUD** 090   T A2 50 ▢
> **AMA:** 2002,Apr,13

25455 distal radius AND ulna

> 🏥 17.6 ✂ 17.6 **FUD** 090   T A2 50 ▢
> **AMA:** 2002,Apr,13

25490 Prophylactic treatment (nailing, pinning, plating or wiring) with or without methylmethacrylate; radius

> 🏥 20.6 ✂ 20.6 **FUD** 090   T A2 80 50 ▢
> **AMA:** 2002,Apr,13

25491 ulna

> 🏥 21.2 ✂ 21.2 **FUD** 090   J A2 80 50 ▢
> **AMA:** 2002,Apr,13

25492 radius AND ulna

> 🏥 26.0 ✂ 26.0 **FUD** 090   T A2 80 50 ▢
> **AMA:** 2002,Apr,13

25500-25695 Treatment of Fracture/Dislocation of Forearm/Wrist

Code also external fixation (20690)

25500 Closed treatment of radial shaft fracture; without manipulation

> 🏥 7.14 ✂ 7.77 **FUD** 090   T P2 50 ▢
> **AMA:** 2002,Apr,13

25505 with manipulation

> 🏥 13.1 ✂ 14.3 **FUD** 090   T A2 50 ▢
> **AMA:** 2003,May,7; 2002,Apr,13

25515 Open treatment of radial shaft fracture, includes internal fixation, when performed

> 🏥 19.1 ✂ 19.1 **FUD** 090   J A2 80 50 ▢
> **AMA:** 2002,Apr,13

25520 Closed treatment of radial shaft fracture and closed treatment of dislocation of distal radioulnar joint (Galeazzi fracture/dislocation)

> 🏥 15.1 ✂ 15.9 **FUD** 090   T A2 50 ▢
> **AMA:** 2002,Apr,13

25525 Open treatment of radial shaft fracture, includes internal fixation, when performed, and closed treatment of distal radioulnar joint dislocation (Galeazzi fracture/ dislocation), includes percutaneous skeletal fixation, when performed

> 🏥 22.5 ✂ 22.5 **FUD** 090   J A2 80 50 ▢
> **AMA:** 2002,Apr,13

25526 Open treatment of radial shaft fracture, includes internal fixation, when performed, and open treatment of distal radioulnar joint dislocation (Galeazzi fracture/ dislocation), includes internal fixation, when performed, includes repair of triangular fibrocartilage complex

> 🏥 27.3 ✂ 27.3 **FUD** 090   J A2 80 50 ▢
> **AMA:** 2002,Apr,13

25530 Closed treatment of ulnar shaft fracture; without manipulation

> 🏥 6.76 ✂ 7.45 **FUD** 090   T P2 50 ▢
> **AMA:** 2002,Apr,13

25535 with manipulation

> 🏥 12.9 ✂ 13.9 **FUD** 090   T A2 50 ▢
> **AMA:** 2010,Sep,6-7; 2002,Apr,13

25545 Open treatment of ulnar shaft fracture, includes internal fixation, when performed

> 🏥 17.8 ✂ 17.8 **FUD** 090   J A2 80 50 ▢
> **AMA:** 2016,Jan,13; 2015,Jan,16; 2014,Jan,11

25560 Closed treatment of radial and ulnar shaft fractures; without manipulation

> 🏥 7.14 ✂ 7.89 **FUD** 090   T P2 50 ▢
> **AMA:** 2002,Apr,13

25565 with manipulation

> 🏥 13.4 ✂ 14.8 **FUD** 090   T A2 50 ▢
> **AMA:** 2002,Apr,13

25574 Open treatment of radial AND ulnar shaft fractures, with internal fixation, when performed; of radius OR ulna

> 🏥 19.2 ✂ 19.2 **FUD** 090   J A2 80 50 ▢
> **AMA:** 2016,Jan,13; 2015,Jan,16; 2014,Jan,11

25575 of radius AND ulna

> 🏥 25.8 ✂ 25.8 **FUD** 090   J 62 80 50 ▢
> **AMA:** 2002,Apr,13

25600 Closed treatment of distal radial fracture (eg, Colles or Smith type) or epiphyseal separation, includes closed treatment of fracture of ulnar styloid, when performed; without manipulation

> INCLUDES *Closed treatment of ulnar styloid fracture (25650)*
> 🏥 8.82 ✂ 9.32 **FUD** 090   T P2 50 ▢
> **AMA:** 2016,Jan,13; 2015,Jan,16; 2014,Jan,11; 2013,Apr,10-11

25605 with manipulation

> INCLUDES *Closed treatment of ulnar styloid fracture (25650)*
> 🏥 14.6 ✂ 15.5 **FUD** 090   T A2 50 ▢
> **AMA:** 2016,Jan,13; 2015,Jan,16; 2014,Jan,11; 2013,Apr,10-11

25606 Percutaneous skeletal fixation of distal radial fracture or epiphyseal separation

> EXCLUDES *Closed treatment of ulnar styloid fracture (25650)*
>   *Open repair of ulnar styloid fracture (25652)*
>   *Percutaneous repair of ulnar styloid fracture (25651)*
> 🏥 19.0 ✂ 19.0 **FUD** 090   T A2 50 ▢
> **AMA:** 2007,Oct,7-10

25607 Open treatment of distal radial extra-articular fracture or epiphyseal separation, with internal fixation

> EXCLUDES *Closed treatment of ulnar styloid fracture (25650)*
>   *Open repair of ulnar styloid fracture (25652)*
>   *Percutaneous repair of ulnar styloid fracture (25651)*
> 🏥 21.0 ✂ 21.0 **FUD** 090   J A2 80 50 ▢
> **AMA:** 2016,Jan,13; 2015,Jan,16; 2014,Jan,11; 2012,Nov,13-14

25608 Open treatment of distal radial intra-articular fracture or epiphyseal separation; with internal fixation of 2 fragments

> EXCLUDES *Closed treatment of ulnar styloid fracture (25650)*
>   *Open repair of ulnar styloid fracture (25652)*
>   *Open treatment of distal radial intra-articular fracture or epiphyseal separation; with internal fixation of 3 or more fragments (25609, 25650)*
>   *Percutaneous repair of ulnar styloid fracture (25651)*
> 🏥 23.6 ✂ 23.6 **FUD** 090   J A2 80 50 ▢
> **AMA:** 2016,Jan,13; 2015,Jan,16; 2014,Jan,11

25609 with internal fixation of 3 or more fragments

> EXCLUDES *Closed treatment of ulnar styloid fracture (25650)*
>   *Open repair of ulnar styloid fracture (25652)*
>   *Percutaneous repair of ulnar styloid fracture (25651)*
> 🏥 30.0 ✂ 30.0 **FUD** 090   J A2 80 50 ▢
> **AMA:** 2016,Jan,13; 2015,Jan,16; 2014,Jan,11; 2013,Dec,14; 2013,Mar,13

25622 Closed treatment of carpal scaphoid (navicular) fracture; without manipulation

> 🏥 7.88 ✂ 8.64 **FUD** 090   T P2 50 ▢
> **AMA:** 2002,Apr,13

| 26/TC PC/TC Only | A2-Z6 ASC Payment | 50 Bilateral | ♂ Male Only | ♀ Female Only | 🏥 Facility RVU | ✂ Non-Facility RVU | ▢ CCI |
| FUD Follow-up Days | CMS: IOM (Pub 100) | A-Y OPPSI | 80/80 Surg Assist Allowed / w/Doc | | 🧪 Lab Crosswalk | ☢ Radiology Crosswalk | ✕ CLIA |

68   CPT © 2016 American Medical Association. All Rights Reserved.   © 2016 Optum360, LLC

25624   **with manipulation**
    12.3   13.5   **FUD** 090   T A2 80 50
    AMA: 2002,Apr,13

25628   **Open treatment of carpal scaphoid (navicular) fracture, includes internal fixation, when performed**
    20.6   20.6   **FUD** 090   T A2 80 50
    AMA: 2002,Apr,13

25630   **Closed treatment of carpal bone fracture (excluding carpal scaphoid [navicular]); without manipulation, each bone**
    7.98   8.67   **FUD** 090   T P2 50
    AMA: 2002,Apr,13

25635   **with manipulation, each bone**
    10.8   12.1   **FUD** 090   T A2 80 50
    AMA: 2002,Apr,13

25645   **Open treatment of carpal bone fracture (other than carpal scaphoid [navicular]), each bone**
    16.2   16.2   **FUD** 090   T A2 80 50
    AMA: 2002,Apr,13

25650   **Closed treatment of ulnar styloid fracture**
    EXCLUDES   *Closed treatment of distal radial fracture (25600, 25605)*
    Open treatment of distal radial extra-articular fracture or epiphyseal separation, with internal fixation (25607-25609)
    8.54   9.10   **FUD** 090   T P2 50
    AMA: 2016,Jan,13; 2015,Jan,16; 2014,Jan,11; 2013,Apr,10-11

25651   **Percutaneous skeletal fixation of ulnar styloid fracture**
    13.8   13.8   **FUD** 090   T G2 80 50
    AMA: 2007,Oct,7-10; 2002,Apr,13

25652   **Open treatment of ulnar styloid fracture**
    17.8   17.8   **FUD** 090   J G2 50
    AMA: 2016,Jan,13; 2015,Jan,16; 2014,Jan,11

25660   **Closed treatment of radiocarpal or intercarpal dislocation, 1 or more bones, with manipulation**
    11.6   11.6   **FUD** 090   T A2 80 50
    AMA: 2002,Apr,13

25670   **Open treatment of radiocarpal or intercarpal dislocation, 1 or more bones**
    17.3   17.3   **FUD** 090   T A2 80 50
    AMA: 2002,Apr,13

25671   **Percutaneous skeletal fixation of distal radioulnar dislocation**
    15.1   15.1   **FUD** 090   T A2 50
    AMA: 2002,Apr,13

25675   **Closed treatment of distal radioulnar dislocation with manipulation**
    11.2   12.3   **FUD** 090   T A2 80 50
    AMA: 2002,Apr,13

25676   **Open treatment of distal radioulnar dislocation, acute or chronic**
    17.9   17.9   **FUD** 090   J A2 80 50
    AMA: 2002,Apr,13

25680   **Closed treatment of trans-scaphoperilunar type of fracture dislocation, with manipulation**
    13.5   13.5   **FUD** 090   T A2 80 50
    AMA: 2002,Apr,13

25685   **Open treatment of trans-scaphoperilunar type of fracture dislocation**
    21.0   21.0   **FUD** 090   T A2 80 50
    AMA: 2002,Apr,13

25690   **Closed treatment of lunate dislocation, with manipulation**
    13.6   13.6   **FUD** 090   T A2 80 50
    AMA: 2002,Apr,13

25695   **Open treatment of lunate dislocation**
    18.1   18.1   **FUD** 090   T A2 80 50
    AMA: 2002,Apr,13

25800-25830 Wrist Fusion

25800   **Arthrodesis, wrist; complete, without bone graft (includes radiocarpal and/or intercarpal and/or carpometacarpal joints)**
    20.9   20.9   **FUD** 090   J G2 80 50
    AMA: 2002,Apr,13; 1998,Nov,1

25805   **with sliding graft**
    24.2   24.2   **FUD** 090   J A2 80 50
    AMA: 2002,Apr,13

25810   **with iliac or other autograft (includes obtaining graft)**
    24.8   24.8   **FUD** 090   J G2 80 50
    AMA: 2002,Apr,13

25820   **Arthrodesis, wrist; limited, without bone graft (eg, intercarpal or radiocarpal)**
    17.5   17.5   **FUD** 090   J A2 80 50
    AMA: 2002,Apr,13; 1998,Nov,1

25825   **with autograft (includes obtaining graft)**
    21.6   21.6   **FUD** 090   J A2 80 50
    AMA: 2016,Jan,13; 2015,Jan,16; 2014,Jan,11; 2012,Jul,12-14

25830   **Arthrodesis, distal radioulnar joint with segmental resection of ulna, with or without bone graft (eg, Sauve-Kapandji procedure)**
    27.0   27.0   **FUD** 090   J A2 80 50
    AMA: 2002,Apr,13; 1998,Nov,1

25900-25999 Amputation Through Forearm/Wrist

25900   **Amputation, forearm, through radius and ulna;**
    20.3   20.3   **FUD** 090   C 80 50
    AMA: 2002,Apr,13

25905   **open, circular (guillotine)**
    18.6   18.6   **FUD** 090   C 80 50
    AMA: 2002,Apr,13

25907   **secondary closure or scar revision**
    16.6   16.6   **FUD** 090   T A2 80 50
    AMA: 2002,Apr,13

25909   **re-amputation**
    19.6   19.6   **FUD** 090   T 80 50
    AMA: 2002,Apr,13

25915   **Krukenberg procedure**
    33.9   33.9   **FUD** 090   C 80 50
    AMA: 2002,Apr,13

25920   **Disarticulation through wrist;**
    19.9   19.9   **FUD** 090   C 80 50
    AMA: 2002,Apr,13

25922   **secondary closure or scar revision**
    16.4   16.4   **FUD** 090   T A2 80 50
    AMA: 2002,Apr,13

25924   **re-amputation**
    17.4   17.4   **FUD** 090   C 80 50
    AMA: 2002,Apr,13

25927   **Transmetacarpal amputation;**
    23.2   23.2   **FUD** 090   C 80 50
    AMA: 2002,Apr,13

25929   **secondary closure or scar revision**
    16.9   16.9   **FUD** 090   T A2 80 50
    AMA: 2002,Apr,13

25931   **re-amputation**
    19.0   19.0   **FUD** 090   T G2 50
    AMA: 2002,Apr,13

25999   **Unlisted procedure, forearm or wrist**
    0.00   0.00   **FUD** YYY   T 80 50
    AMA: 2002,Apr,13

26010-26037 Incision Hand/Fingers

26010 **Drainage of finger abscess; simple**
🔧 3.92 ✂ 7.48 **FUD** 010 `T` `P2` ▱
AMA: 2003,May,7; 2003,Sep,3

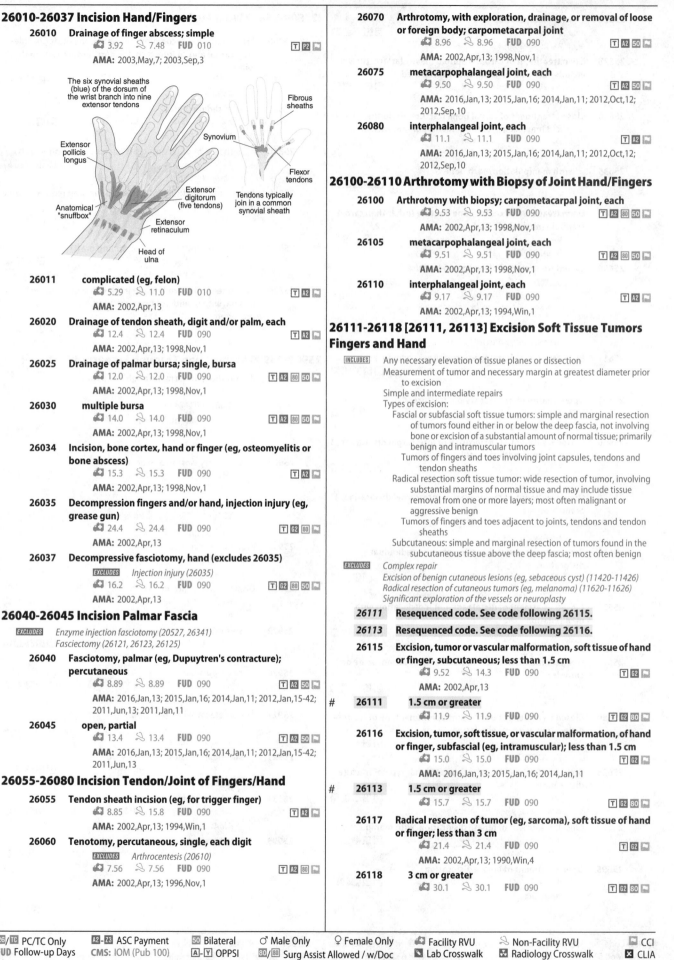

The six synovial sheaths (blue) of the dorsum of the wrist branch into nine extensor tendons

Extensor pollicis longus

Extensor digitorum (five tendons)

Anatomical "snuffbox"

Extensor retinaculum

Head of ulna

Fibrous sheaths

Synovium

Flexor tendons

Tendons typically join in a common synovial sheath

26011 **complicated (eg, felon)**
🔧 5.29 ✂ 11.0 **FUD** 010 `T` `A2` ▱
AMA: 2002,Apr,13

26020 **Drainage of tendon sheath, digit and/or palm, each**
🔧 12.4 ✂ 12.4 **FUD** 090 `T` `A2` ▱
AMA: 2002,Apr,13; 1998,Nov,1

26025 **Drainage of palmar bursa; single, bursa**
🔧 12.0 ✂ 12.0 **FUD** 090 `T` `A2` `80` `50` ▱
AMA: 2002,Apr,13; 1998,Nov,1

26030 **multiple bursa**
🔧 14.0 ✂ 14.0 **FUD** 090 `T` `A2` `80` `50` ▱
AMA: 2002,Apr,13; 1998,Nov,1

26034 **Incision, bone cortex, hand or finger (eg, osteomyelitis or bone abscess)**
🔧 15.3 ✂ 15.3 **FUD** 090 `T` `A2` ▱
AMA: 2002,Apr,13; 1998,Nov,1

26035 **Decompression fingers and/or hand, injection injury (eg, grease gun)**
🔧 24.4 ✂ 24.4 **FUD** 090 `T` `G2` `80` ▱
AMA: 2002,Apr,13

26037 **Decompressive fasciotomy, hand (excludes 26035)**
EXCLUDES Injection injury (26035)
🔧 16.2 ✂ 16.2 **FUD** 090 `T` `G2` `80` `50` ▱
AMA: 2002,Apr,13

26040-26045 Incision Palmar Fascia

EXCLUDES Enzyme injection fasciotomy (20527, 26341)
Fasciectomy (26121, 26123, 26125)

26040 **Fasciotomy, palmar (eg, Dupuytren's contracture); percutaneous**
🔧 8.89 ✂ 8.89 **FUD** 090 `T` `A2` `50` ▱
AMA: 2016,Jan,13; 2015,Jan,16; 2014,Jan,11; 2012,Jan,15-42; 2011,Jun,13; 2011,Jan,11

26045 **open, partial**
🔧 13.4 ✂ 13.4 **FUD** 090 `T` `A2` `50` ▱
AMA: 2016,Jan,13; 2015,Jan,16; 2014,Jan,11; 2012,Jan,15-42; 2011,Jun,13

26055-26080 Incision Tendon/Joint of Fingers/Hand

26055 **Tendon sheath incision (eg, for trigger finger)**
🔧 8.85 ✂ 15.8 **FUD** 090 `T` `A2` ▱
AMA: 2002,Apr,13; 1994,Win,1

26060 **Tenotomy, percutaneous, single, each digit**
EXCLUDES Arthrocentesis (20610)
🔧 7.56 ✂ 7.56 **FUD** 090 `T` `A2` `80` ▱
AMA: 2002,Apr,13; 1996,Nov,1

26070 **Arthrotomy, with exploration, drainage, or removal of loose or foreign body; carpometacarpal joint**
🔧 8.96 ✂ 8.96 **FUD** 090 `T` `A2` `50` ▱
AMA: 2002,Apr,13; 1998,Nov,1

26075 **metacarpophalangeal joint, each**
🔧 9.50 ✂ 9.50 **FUD** 090 `T` `A2` `50` ▱
AMA: 2016,Jan,13; 2015,Jan,16; 2014,Jan,11; 2012,Oct,12; 2012,Sep,10

26080 **interphalangeal joint, each**
🔧 11.1 ✂ 11.1 **FUD** 090 `T` `A2` ▱
AMA: 2016,Jan,13; 2015,Jan,16; 2014,Jan,11; 2012,Oct,12; 2012,Sep,10

26100-26110 Arthrotomy with Biopsy of Joint Hand/Fingers

26100 **Arthrotomy with biopsy; carpometacarpal joint, each**
🔧 9.53 ✂ 9.53 **FUD** 090 `T` `A2` `80` `50` ▱
AMA: 2002,Apr,13; 1998,Nov,1

26105 **metacarpophalangeal joint, each**
🔧 9.51 ✂ 9.51 **FUD** 090 `T` `A2` `80` `50` ▱
AMA: 2002,Apr,13; 1998,Nov,1

26110 **interphalangeal joint, each**
🔧 9.17 ✂ 9.17 **FUD** 090 `T` `A2` ▱
AMA: 2002,Apr,13; 1994,Win,1

26111-26118 [26111, 26113] Excision Soft Tissue Tumors Fingers and Hand

INCLUDES Any necessary elevation of tissue planes or dissection
Measurement of tumor and necessary margin at greatest diameter prior to excision
Simple and intermediate repairs
Types of excision:
  Fascial or subfascial soft tissue tumors: simple and marginal resection of tumors found either in or below the deep fascia, not involving bone or excision of a substantial amount of normal tissue; primarily benign and intramuscular tumors
  Tumors of fingers and toes involving joint capsules, tendons and tendon sheaths
  Radical resection soft tissue tumor: wide resection of tumor, involving substantial margins of normal tissue and may include tissue removal from one or more layers; most often malignant or aggressive benign
  Tumors of fingers and toes adjacent to joints, tendons and tendon sheaths
  Subcutaneous: simple and marginal resection of tumors found in the subcutaneous tissue above the deep fascia; most often benign

EXCLUDES Complex repair
Excision of benign cutaneous lesions (eg, sebaceous cyst) (11420-11426)
Radical resection of cutaneous tumors (eg, melanoma) (11620-11626)
Significant exploration of the vessels or neuroplasty

26111 **Resequenced code. See code following 26115.**

26113 **Resequenced code. See code following 26116.**

26115 **Excision, tumor or vascular malformation, soft tissue of hand or finger, subcutaneous; less than 1.5 cm**
🔧 9.52 ✂ 14.3 **FUD** 090 `T` `G2` ▱
AMA: 2002,Apr,13

\# **26111** **1.5 cm or greater**
🔧 11.9 ✂ 11.9 **FUD** 090 `T` `G2` `80` ▱

26116 **Excision, tumor, soft tissue, or vascular malformation, of hand or finger, subfascial (eg, intramuscular); less than 1.5 cm**
🔧 15.0 ✂ 15.0 **FUD** 090 `T` `G2` ▱
AMA: 2016,Jan,13; 2015,Jan,16; 2014,Jan,11

\# **26113** **1.5 cm or greater**
🔧 15.7 ✂ 15.7 **FUD** 090 `T` `G2` `80` ▱

26117 **Radical resection of tumor (eg, sarcoma), soft tissue of hand or finger; less than 3 cm**
🔧 21.4 ✂ 21.4 **FUD** 090 `T` `G2` ▱
AMA: 2002,Apr,13; 1990,Win,4

26118 **3 cm or greater**
🔧 30.1 ✂ 30.1 **FUD** 090 `T` `G2` `80` ▱

`26`/`TC` PC/TC Only   `A2`-`Z3` ASC Payment   `50` Bilateral   ♂ Male Only   ♀ Female Only   🔧 Facility RVU   ✂ Non-Facility RVU   ▱ CCI
FUD Follow-up Days   **CMS:** IOM (Pub 100)   `A`-`Y` OPPSI   `80`/`80` Surg Assist Allowed / w/Doc   🔲 Lab Crosswalk   🔧 Radiology Crosswalk   ☒ CLIA

70
CPT © 2016 American Medical Association. All Rights Reserved.
© 2016 Optum360, LLC

26121-26236 Procedures of Bones, Fascia, Joints and Tendons Hands and Fingers

26121   Fasciectomy, palm only, with or without Z-plasty, other local tissue rearrangement, or skin grafting (includes obtaining graft)

EXCLUDES   *Enzyme injection fasciotomy (20527, 26341)*
Fasciotomy (26040, 26045)

🔧 17.0   ⚕ 17.0   **FUD** 090   T A2 50 ▭

AMA: 2016,Jan,13; 2015,Jan,16; 2014,Jan,11; 2012,Jan,15-42; 2011,Jun,13

26123   Fasciectomy, partial palmar with release of single digit including proximal interphalangeal joint, with or without Z-plasty, other local tissue rearrangement, or skin grafting (includes obtaining graft);

EXCLUDES   *Enzyme injection fasciotomy (20527, 26341)*
Fasciotomy (26040, 26045)

🔧 23.8   ⚕ 23.8   **FUD** 090   T A2 50 ▭

AMA: 2016,Jan,13; 2015,Jan,16; 2014,Jan,11; 2012,Jan,15-42; 2011,Jun,13

+ 26125   each additional digit (List separately in addition to code for primary procedure)

EXCLUDES   *Enzyme injection fasciotomy (20527, 26341)*
Fasciotomy (26040, 26045)

Code first (26123)

🔧 7.91   ⚕ 7.91   **FUD** ZZZ   N N1 ▭

AMA: 2016,Jan,13; 2015,Jan,16; 2014,Jan,11; 2012,Jan,15-42; 2011,Jun,13

26130   Synovectomy, carpometacarpal joint

🔧 13.2   ⚕ 13.2   **FUD** 090   T A2 50 ▭

AMA: 2002,Apr,13

26135   Synovectomy, metacarpophalangeal joint including intrinsic release and extensor hood reconstruction, each digit

🔧 15.7   ⚕ 15.7   **FUD** 090   T A2 80 ▭

AMA: 2002,Apr,13

26140   Synovectomy, proximal interphalangeal joint, including extensor reconstruction, each interphalangeal joint

🔧 14.4   ⚕ 14.4   **FUD** 090   T A2 ▭

AMA: 2002,Apr,13

26145   Synovectomy, tendon sheath, radical (tenosynovectomy), flexor tendon, palm and/or finger, each tendon

EXCLUDES   *Wrist synovectomy (25115-25116)*

🔧 14.6   ⚕ 14.6   **FUD** 090   T A2 ▭

AMA: 2002,Apr,13; 1998,Nov,1

26160   Excision of lesion of tendon sheath or joint capsule (eg, cyst, mucous cyst, or ganglion), hand or finger

EXCLUDES   *Trigger finger (26055)*
Wrist ganglion removal (25111-25112)

🔧 9.53   ⚕ 16.2   **FUD** 090   T A2 ▭

AMA: 2002,Apr,13

26170   Excision of tendon, palm, flexor or extensor, single, each tendon

EXCLUDES   *Excision extensor tendon, with implantation of synthetic rod for delayed tendon graft, hand or finger, each rod (26415)*
Excision flexor tendon, with implantation of synthetic rod for delayed tendon graft, hand or finger, each rod (26390)

🔧 11.5   ⚕ 11.5   **FUD** 090   T A2 80 ▭

AMA: 2016,Jan,13; 2015,Jan,16; 2013,Jun,13

26180   Excision of tendon, finger, flexor or extensor, each tendon

EXCLUDES   *Excision extensor tendon, with implantation of synthetic rod for delayed tendon graft, hand or finger, each rod (26415)*
Excision flexor tendon, with implantation of synthetic rod for delayed tendon graft, hand or finger, each rod (26390)

🔧 12.6   ⚕ 12.6   **FUD** 090   T A2 80 ▭

AMA: 2002,Apr,13; 1998,Nov,1

26185   Sesamoidectomy, thumb or finger (separate procedure)

🔧 15.5   ⚕ 15.5   **FUD** 090   T A2 80 50 ▭

AMA: 2002,Apr,13; 1996,Nov,1

26200   Excision or curettage of bone cyst or benign tumor of metacarpal;

🔧 12.8   ⚕ 12.8   **FUD** 090   T A2 80 ▭

AMA: 2002,Apr,13

26205   with autograft (includes obtaining graft)

🔧 17.2   ⚕ 17.2   **FUD** 090   T A2 ▭

AMA: 2002,Apr,13

26210   Excision or curettage of bone cyst or benign tumor of proximal, middle, or distal phalanx of finger;

🔧 12.6   ⚕ 12.6   **FUD** 090   T A2 ▭

AMA: 2002,Apr,13

26215   with autograft (includes obtaining graft)

🔧 16.1   ⚕ 16.1   **FUD** 090   T A2 ▭

AMA: 2002,Apr,13

26230   Partial excision (craterization, saucerization, or diaphysectomy) bone (eg, osteomyelitis); metacarpal

🔧 14.2   ⚕ 14.2   **FUD** 090   T A2 80 ▭

AMA: 2002,Apr,13; 1998,Nov,1

26235   proximal or middle phalanx of finger

🔧 14.1   ⚕ 14.1   **FUD** 090   T A2 80 ▭

AMA: 2002,Apr,13

26236   distal phalanx of finger

🔧 12.6   ⚕ 12.6   **FUD** 090   T A2 ▭

AMA: 2002,Apr,13

26250-26262 Radical Resection Bone Tumor of Hand/Finger

INCLUDES   Any necessary elevation of tissue planes or dissection
Excision of adjacent soft tissue during bone tumor resection (26111-26118 [26111, 26113])
Measurement of tumor and necessary margin at greatest diameter prior to excision
Resection of the tumor (may include entire bone) and wide margins of normal tissue primarily for malignant or aggressive benign tumors
Simple and intermediate repairs

EXCLUDES   *Complex repair*
Significant exploration of vessels, neuroplasty, reconstruction, or complex bone repair

26250   Radical resection of tumor, metacarpal

🔧 30.9   ⚕ 30.9   **FUD** 090   T A2 80 ▭

AMA: 2002,Apr,13; 1998,Nov,1

26260   Radical resection of tumor, proximal or middle phalanx of finger

🔧 22.9   ⚕ 22.9   **FUD** 090   T A2 80 ▭

AMA: 2002,Apr,13; 1998,Nov,1

26262   Radical resection of tumor, distal phalanx of finger

🔧 17.9   ⚕ 17.9   **FUD** 090   T A2 80 ▭

AMA: 2002,Apr,13; 1998,Nov,1

26320 Implant Removal Hand/Finger

26320   Removal of implant from finger or hand

EXCLUDES   *Excision of foreign body (20520, 20525)*

🔧 9.91   ⚕ 9.91   **FUD** 090   Q2 A2 ▭

AMA: 2002,Apr,13

26340-26548 Repair/Reconstruction of Fingers and Hand

26340   Manipulation, finger joint, under anesthesia, each joint

EXCLUDES   *Application external fixation (20690, 20692)*

🔧 9.51   ⚕ 9.51   **FUD** 090   T G2 50 ▭

AMA: 2016,Jan,13; 2015,Jan,16; 2014,Jan,11; 2012,Jan,15-42; 2011,Jan,11

26341   Manipulation, palmar fascial cord (ie, Dupuytren's cord), post enzyme injection (eg, collagenase), single cord

EXCLUDES   *Enzyme injection fasciotomy (20527)*
Code also custom orthotic fabrication and/or fitting

🔧 2.14   ⚕ 2.81   **FUD** 010   T P3 50 ▭

AMA: 2016,Jan,13; 2015,Jan,16; 2014,Jan,11; 2012,Jul,8

26350 Repair or advancement, flexor tendon, not in zone 2 digital flexor tendon sheath (eg, no man's land); primary or secondary without free graft, each tendon
🔧 20.0 ⚕ 20.0 **FUD** 090 T A2 ▢
AMA: 2002,Apr,13; 1998,Nov,1

26352 secondary with free graft (includes obtaining graft), each tendon
🔧 23.1 ⚕ 23.1 **FUD** 090 T A2 80 ▢
AMA: 2002,Apr,13

26356 Repair or advancement, flexor tendon, in zone 2 digital flexor tendon sheath (eg, no man's land); primary, without free graft, each tendon
🔧 25.0 ⚕ 25.0 **FUD** 090 T A2 ▢
AMA: 2016,Jan,13; 2015,Jan,16; 2014,Sep,13; 2014,Jan,11; 2012,Jan,15-42; 2011,Jan,11

26357 secondary, without free graft, each tendon
🔧 24.6 ⚕ 24.6 **FUD** 090 T A2 80 ▢
AMA: 2002,Apr,13

26358 secondary, with free graft (includes obtaining graft), each tendon
🔧 27.3 ⚕ 27.3 **FUD** 090 T A2 80 ▢
AMA: 2002,Apr,13

26370 Repair or advancement of profundus tendon, with intact superficialis tendon; primary, each tendon
🔧 21.3 ⚕ 21.3 **FUD** 090 T A2 80 ▢
AMA: 2016,Jan,13; 2015,Jan,16; 2014,Jan,11; 2012,Jan,15-42

26372 secondary with free graft (includes obtaining graft), each tendon
🔧 24.8 ⚕ 24.8 **FUD** 090 T A2 80 ▢
AMA: 2002,Apr,13; 1998,Nov,1

26373 secondary without free graft, each tendon
🔧 23.8 ⚕ 23.8 **FUD** 090 T A2 80 ▢
AMA: 2002,Apr,13; 1998,Nov,1

26390 Excision flexor tendon, with implantation of synthetic rod for delayed tendon graft, hand or finger, each rod
🔧 23.6 ⚕ 23.6 **FUD** 090 J A2 80 ▢
AMA: 2002,Apr,13; 1998,Nov,1

26392 Removal of synthetic rod and insertion of flexor tendon graft, hand or finger (includes obtaining graft), each rod
🔧 27.3 ⚕ 27.3 **FUD** 090 J A2 80 ▢
AMA: 2002,Apr,13; 1998,Nov,1

26410 Repair, extensor tendon, hand, primary or secondary; without free graft, each tendon
🔧 15.9 ⚕ 15.9 **FUD** 090 T A2 ▢
AMA: 2002,Apr,13; 1998,Nov,1

26412 with free graft (includes obtaining graft), each tendon
🔧 19.1 ⚕ 19.1 **FUD** 090 T A2 80 ▢
AMA: 2002,Apr,13; 1998,Nov,1

26415 Excision of extensor tendon, with implantation of synthetic rod for delayed tendon graft, hand or finger, each rod
🔧 21.6 ⚕ 21.6 **FUD** 090 T A2 80 ▢
AMA: 2002,Apr,13; 1998,Nov,1

26416 Removal of synthetic rod and insertion of extensor tendon graft (includes obtaining graft), hand or finger, each rod
🔧 20.4 ⚕ 20.4 **FUD** 090 T A2 ▢
AMA: 2016,Jan,13; 2015,Jan,16; 2014,Jan,11

26418 Repair, extensor tendon, finger, primary or secondary; without free graft, each tendon
🔧 16.2 ⚕ 16.2 **FUD** 090 T A2 ▢
AMA: 2016,Jan,13; 2015,Jan,16; 2014,Jan,11; 2012,Jan,15-42; 2011,Jan,11

26420 with free graft (includes obtaining graft) each tendon
🔧 19.9 ⚕ 19.9 **FUD** 090 T A2 80 ▢
AMA: 2002,Apr,13

26426 Repair of extensor tendon, central slip, secondary (eg, boutonniere deformity); using local tissue(s), including lateral band(s), each finger
🔧 14.3 ⚕ 14.3 **FUD** 090 T A2 ▢
AMA: 2002,Apr,13; 1998,Nov,1

26428 with free graft (includes obtaining graft), each finger
🔧 21.2 ⚕ 21.2 **FUD** 090 T A2 80 ▢
AMA: 2002,Apr,13; 1998,Nov,1

26432 Closed treatment of distal extensor tendon insertion, with or without percutaneous pinning (eg, mallet finger)
🔧 14.0 ⚕ 14.0 **FUD** 090 T A2 ▢
AMA: 2002,Apr,13; 1998,Nov,1

26433 Repair of extensor tendon, distal insertion, primary or secondary; without graft (eg, mallet finger)
EXCLUDES *Trigger finger (26055)*
🔧 14.9 ⚕ 14.9 **FUD** 090 T A2 ▢
AMA: 2002,Apr,13; 1998,Nov,1

26434 with free graft (includes obtaining graft)
EXCLUDES *Trigger finger (26055)*
🔧 18.2 ⚕ 18.2 **FUD** 090 T A2 80 ▢
AMA: 2002,Apr,13

26437 Realignment of extensor tendon, hand, each tendon
🔧 17.5 ⚕ 17.5 **FUD** 090 T A2 ▢
AMA: 2002,Apr,13; 1998,Nov,1

26440 Tenolysis, flexor tendon; palm OR finger, each tendon
🔧 17.3 ⚕ 17.3 **FUD** 090 T A2 ▢
AMA: 2016,Jan,13; 2015,Jun,10; 2015,Jan,16; 2014,Jan,11; 2012,Jan,15-42; 2011,Jan,11

26442 palm AND finger, each tendon
🔧 27.1 ⚕ 27.1 **FUD** 090 T A2 ▢
AMA: 2002,Apr,13

26445 Tenolysis, extensor tendon, hand OR finger, each tendon
🔧 16.1 ⚕ 16.1 **FUD** 090 T A2 ▢
AMA: 2016,Jan,13; 2015,Jan,16; 2014,Jan,11; 2012,Jan,15-42; 2011,Jan,11

26449 Tenolysis, complex, extensor tendon, finger, including forearm, each tendon
🔧 19.8 ⚕ 19.8 **FUD** 090 T A2 80 ▢
AMA: 2002,Apr,13; 1998,Nov,1

26450 Tenotomy, flexor, palm, open, each tendon
🔧 11.4 ⚕ 11.4 **FUD** 090 T A2 80 ▢
AMA: 2002,Apr,13; 1998,Nov,1

26455 Tenotomy, flexor, finger, open, each tendon
🔧 11.3 ⚕ 11.3 **FUD** 090 T A2 80 ▢
AMA: 2002,Apr,13; 1998,Nov,1

26460 Tenotomy, extensor, hand or finger, open, each tendon
🔧 11.0 ⚕ 11.0 **FUD** 090 T A2 ▢
AMA: 2002,Apr,13; 1998,Nov,1

26471 Tenodesis; of proximal interphalangeal joint, each joint
🔧 17.2 ⚕ 17.2 **FUD** 090 T A2 80 ▢
AMA: 2002,Apr,13; 1998,Nov,1

26474 of distal joint, each joint
🔧 16.9 ⚕ 16.9 **FUD** 090 T A2 80 ▢
AMA: 2002,Apr,13; 1998,Nov,1

26476 Lengthening of tendon, extensor, hand or finger, each tendon
🔧 16.2 ⚕ 16.2 **FUD** 090 T A2 ▢
AMA: 2002,Apr,13; 1998,Nov,1

26477 Shortening of tendon, extensor, hand or finger, each tendon
🔧 16.3 ⚕ 16.3 **FUD** 090 T A2 ▢
AMA: 2002,Apr,13; 1998,Nov,1

26478 Lengthening of tendon, flexor, hand or finger, each tendon
🔧 17.4 ⚕ 17.4 **FUD** 090 T A2 80 ▢
AMA: 2016,Jan,13; 2015,Jan,16; 2014,Jan,11; 2013,Dec,16

26479 Shortening of tendon, flexor, hand or finger, each tendon
🔧 17.2 ⚕ 17.2 **FUD** 090   T A2 80 ▣
AMA: 2002,Apr,13; 1998,Nov,1

26480 Transfer or transplant of tendon, carpometacarpal area or dorsum of hand; without free graft, each tendon
🔧 21.1 ⚕ 21.1 **FUD** 090   T A2 80 ▣
AMA: 2016,Jan,13; 2015,Jan,16; 2014,Jan,11; 2013,Dec,16

26483 with free tendon graft (includes obtaining graft), each tendon
🔧 23.7 ⚕ 23.7 **FUD** 090   T A2 80 ▣
AMA: 2002,Apr,13

26485 Transfer or transplant of tendon, palmar; without free tendon graft, each tendon
🔧 22.7 ⚕ 22.7 **FUD** 090   T A2 80 ▣
AMA: 2002,Apr,13; 1998,Nov,1

26489 with free tendon graft (includes obtaining graft), each tendon
🔧 25.6 ⚕ 25.6 **FUD** 090   T A2 80 ▣
AMA: 2002,Apr,13

26490 Opponensplasty; superficialis tendon transfer type, each tendon
EXCLUDES Thumb fusion (26820)
🔧 22.1 ⚕ 22.1 **FUD** 090   T A2 80 ▣
AMA: 2002,Apr,13; 1998,Nov,1

26492 tendon transfer with graft (includes obtaining graft), each tendon
EXCLUDES Thumb fusion (26820)
🔧 24.5 ⚕ 24.5 **FUD** 090   T A2 80 ▣
AMA: 2002,Apr,13; 1998,Nov,1

26494 hypothenar muscle transfer
EXCLUDES Thumb fusion (26820)
🔧 22.2 ⚕ 22.2 **FUD** 090   T A2 80 ▣
AMA: 2002,Apr,13

26496 other methods
EXCLUDES Thumb fusion (26820)
🔧 24.1 ⚕ 24.1 **FUD** 090   T A2 80 ▣
AMA: 2002,Apr,13

26497 Transfer of tendon to restore intrinsic function; ring and small finger
🔧 24.5 ⚕ 24.5 **FUD** 090   T A2 80 ▣
AMA: 2002,Apr,13; 1998,Nov,1

26498 all 4 fingers
🔧 32.4 ⚕ 32.4 **FUD** 090   T A2 80 ▣
AMA: 2002,Apr,13

26499 Correction claw finger, other methods
🔧 23.4 ⚕ 23.4 **FUD** 090   T A2 80 ▣
AMA: 2002,Apr,13

26500 Reconstruction of tendon pulley, each tendon; with local tissues (separate procedure)
🔧 17.5 ⚕ 17.5 **FUD** 090   T A2 80 ▣
AMA: 2002,Apr,13; 1998,Nov,1

26502 with tendon or fascial graft (includes obtaining graft) (separate procedure)
🔧 19.6 ⚕ 19.6 **FUD** 090   T A2 80 ▣
AMA: 2002,Apr,13

26508 Release of thenar muscle(s) (eg, thumb contracture)
🔧 18.1 ⚕ 18.1 **FUD** 090   T A2 80 50 ▣
AMA: 2002,Apr,13; 1998,Nov,1

26510 Cross intrinsic transfer, each tendon
🔧 16.6 ⚕ 16.6 **FUD** 090   T A2 80 ▣
AMA: 2002,Apr,13

26516 Capsulodesis, metacarpophalangeal joint; single digit
🔧 19.6 ⚕ 19.6 **FUD** 090   T A2 80 50 ▣
AMA: 2002,Apr,13; 1998,Nov,1

26517 2 digits
🔧 23.2 ⚕ 23.2 **FUD** 090   T A2 80 50 ▣
AMA: 2002,Apr,13

26518 3 or 4 digits
🔧 23.2 ⚕ 23.2 **FUD** 090   T A2 80 50 ▣
AMA: 2002,Apr,13

26520 Capsulectomy or capsulotomy; metacarpophalangeal joint, each joint
EXCLUDES Carpometacarpal joint arthroplasty (25447)
🔧 18.2 ⚕ 18.2 **FUD** 090   T A2
AMA: 2002,Apr,13; 1998,Nov,1

26525 interphalangeal joint, each joint
EXCLUDES Carpometacarpal joint arthroplasty (25447)
🔧 18.3 ⚕ 18.3 **FUD** 090   T A2
AMA: 2016,Jan,13; 2015,Jun,10; 2015,Jan,16; 2014,Jan,11; 2012,Jan,15-42; 2011,Jan,11

26530 Arthroplasty, metacarpophalangeal joint; each joint
EXCLUDES Carpometacarpal joint arthroplasty (25447)
🔧 15.3 ⚕ 15.3 **FUD** 090   T A2 80 ▣
AMA: 2002,Apr,13; 1998,Nov,1

26531 with prosthetic implant, each joint
EXCLUDES Carpometacarpal joint arthroplasty (25447)
🔧 17.8 ⚕ 17.8 **FUD** 090   J A2 80 ▣
AMA: 2016,Jan,13; 2015,Jan,16; 2014,Jan,11; 2012,Jan,15-42; 2011,Sep,11-12

26535 Arthroplasty, interphalangeal joint; each joint
EXCLUDES Carpometacarpal joint arthroplasty (25447)
🔧 12.0 ⚕ 12.0 **FUD** 090   T A2
AMA: 2002,Apr,13; 1998,Nov,1

26536 with prosthetic implant, each joint
EXCLUDES Carpometacarpal joint arthroplasty (25447)
🔧 20.0 ⚕ 20.0 **FUD** 090   J A2 80 ▣
AMA: 2002,Apr,13; 1998,Nov,1

26540 Repair of collateral ligament, metacarpophalangeal or interphalangeal joint
🔧 18.4 ⚕ 18.4 **FUD** 090   T A2 80 ▣
AMA: 2002,Apr,13; 1996,Nov,1

26541 Reconstruction, collateral ligament, metacarpophalangeal joint, single; with tendon or fascial graft (includes obtaining graft)
🔧 22.5 ⚕ 22.5 **FUD** 090   T A2 80 ▣
AMA: 2016,Jan,13; 2015,Jan,16; 2014,Jan,11

26542 with local tissue (eg, adductor advancement)
🔧 19.0 ⚕ 19.0 **FUD** 090   T A2 80 ▣
AMA: 2016,Jan,13; 2015,Jan,16; 2014,Jan,11

26545 Reconstruction, collateral ligament, interphalangeal joint, single, including graft, each joint
🔧 19.4 ⚕ 19.4 **FUD** 090   T A2 80 ▣
AMA: 2002,Apr,13

26546 Repair non-union, metacarpal or phalanx (includes obtaining bone graft with or without external or internal fixation)
🔧 28.0 ⚕ 28.0 **FUD** 090   T A2 80 50 ▣
AMA: 2002,Apr,13; 1996,Nov,1

26548 Repair and reconstruction, finger, volar plate, interphalangeal joint
🔧 21.4 ⚕ 21.4 **FUD** 090   T A2 80 ▣
AMA: 2002,Apr,13

26550-26556 Reconstruction Procedures with Finger and Toe Transplants

26550 Pollicization of a digit
🔧 43.9 ⚕ 43.9 **FUD** 090   T A2 80 50 ▣
AMA: 2002,Apr,13

● New Code   ▲ Revised Code   ○ Reinstated   ● New Web Release   ▲ Revised Web Release   Unlisted   Not Covered   # Resequenced
⊘ AMA Mod 51 Exempt   ⑤ Optum Mod 51 Exempt   ⑥ Mod 63 Exempt   ⚕ Non-FDA Drug   ★ Telehealth   M Maternity   A Age Edit   + Add-on   AMA: CPT Asst

26551 Transfer, toe-to-hand with microvascular anastomosis; great toe wrap-around with bone graft

INCLUDES Operating microscope (69990)

EXCLUDES Big toe with web space (20973)

🚑 81.5 ⚕ 81.5 **FUD** 090 C 80 50 ▢

AMA: 2016,Feb,12; 2016,Jan,13; 2015,Jan,16; 2014,Jan,11

26553 other than great toe, single

INCLUDES Operating microscope (69990)

🚑 94.0 ⚕ 94.0 **FUD** 090 C 80 50 ▢

AMA: 2016,Feb,12; 2016,Jan,13; 2015,Jan,16; 2014,Jan,11

26554 other than great toe, double

INCLUDES Operating microscope (69990)

🚑 94.8 ⚕ 94.8 **FUD** 090 C 80 50 ▢

AMA: 2016,Feb,12; 2016,Jan,13; 2015,Jan,16; 2014,Jan,11

26555 Transfer, finger to another position without microvascular anastomosis

🚑 38.1 ⚕ 38.1 **FUD** 090 T A2 80 ▢

AMA: 2002,Apr,13; 1998,Nov,1

26556 Transfer, free toe joint, with microvascular anastomosis

INCLUDES Operating microscope (69990)

EXCLUDES Big toe to hand transfer (20973)

🚑 97.6 ⚕ 97.6 **FUD** 090 C 80 ▢

AMA: 2016,Feb,12; 2016,Jan,13; 2015,Jan,16; 2014,Jan,11

26560-26596 Repair of Other Deformities of the Fingers/Hand

26560 Repair of syndactyly (web finger) each web space; with skin flaps

🚑 15.7 ⚕ 15.7 **FUD** 090 T A2 80 ▢

AMA: 2002,Apr,13

26561 with skin flaps and grafts

🚑 26.2 ⚕ 26.2 **FUD** 090 T A2 80 ▢

AMA: 2002,Apr,13

26562 complex (eg, involving bone, nails)

🚑 38.1 ⚕ 38.1 **FUD** 090 T A2 80 ▢

AMA: 2002,Apr,13

26565 Osteotomy; metacarpal, each

🚑 19.0 ⚕ 19.0 **FUD** 090 T A2 80 ▢

AMA: 2002,Apr,13; 1998,Nov,1

26567 phalanx of finger, each

🚑 19.1 ⚕ 19.1 **FUD** 090 T A2 80 ▢

AMA: 2016,Jan,13; 2015,Jan,16; 2014,Jan,11; 2012,Apr,17-18

26568 Osteoplasty, lengthening, metacarpal or phalanx

🚑 25.4 ⚕ 25.4 **FUD** 090 T A2 80 ▢

AMA: 2002,Apr,13; 1998,Nov,1

26580 Repair cleft hand

INCLUDES Barsky's procedure

🚑 41.6 ⚕ 41.6 **FUD** 090 T A2 80 50 ▢

AMA: 2002,Apr,13

26587 Reconstruction of polydactylous digit, soft tissue and bone

EXCLUDES Soft tissue removal only (11200)

🚑 26.1 ⚕ 26.1 **FUD** 090 T A2 80 ▢

AMA: 2016,Jan,13; 2015,Jan,16; 2014,Jan,11; 2012,Jan,15-42; 2011,Jan,11

26590 Repair macrodactylia, each digit

🚑 38.4 ⚕ 38.4 **FUD** 090 T A2 80 ▢

AMA: 2016,Jan,13; 2015,Jan,16; 2014,Jan,11; 2012,Jan,15-42; 2011,Jan,11

26591 Repair, intrinsic muscles of hand, each muscle

🚑 12.2 ⚕ 12.2 **FUD** 090 T A2 80 ▢

AMA: 2016,Jan,13; 2015,Jan,16; 2014,Jan,11; 2012,Jan,15-42; 2011,Jan,11

26593 Release, intrinsic muscles of hand, each muscle

🚑 16.8 ⚕ 16.8 **FUD** 090 T A2 ▢

AMA: 2002,Apr,13; 1998,Nov,1

26596 Excision of constricting ring of finger, with multiple Z-plasties

EXCLUDES Graft repair or scar contracture release (11042, 14040-14041, 15120, 15240)

🚑 21.2 ⚕ 21.2 **FUD** 090 T A2 80 ▢

AMA: 2002,Apr,13

26600-26785 Treatment of Fracture/Dislocation of Fingers and Hand

INCLUDES Closed, percutaneous, and open treatment of fractures or dislocations

26600 Closed treatment of metacarpal fracture, single; without manipulation, each bone

🚑 7.87 ⚕ 8.35 **FUD** 090 T P2 ▢

AMA: 2002,Apr,13

26605 with manipulation, each bone

🚑 8.34 ⚕ 9.14 **FUD** 090 T A2 ▢

AMA: 2002,Apr,13

26607 Closed treatment of metacarpal fracture, with manipulation, with external fixation, each bone

🚑 12.9 ⚕ 12.9 **FUD** 090 T A2 80 ▢

AMA: 2002,Apr,13

26608 Percutaneous skeletal fixation of metacarpal fracture, each bone

🚑 13.6 ⚕ 13.6 **FUD** 090 T A2 80 ▢

AMA: 2002,Apr,13

26615 Open treatment of metacarpal fracture, single, includes internal fixation, when performed, each bone

🚑 16.4 ⚕ 16.4 **FUD** 090 T A2 ▢

AMA: 2002,Apr,13

26641 Closed treatment of carpometacarpal dislocation, thumb, with manipulation

🚑 9.55 ⚕ 10.4 **FUD** 090 T P2 80 50 ▢

AMA: 2002,Apr,13

26645 Closed treatment of carpometacarpal fracture dislocation, thumb (Bennett fracture), with manipulation

🚑 11.0 ⚕ 12.0 **FUD** 090 T A2 80 50 ▢

AMA: 2002,Apr,13

26650 Percutaneous skeletal fixation of carpometacarpal fracture dislocation, thumb (Bennett fracture), with manipulation

🚑 13.6 ⚕ 13.6 **FUD** 090 T A2 50 ▢

AMA: 2002,Apr,13

26665 Open treatment of carpometacarpal fracture dislocation, thumb (Bennett fracture), includes internal fixation, when performed

🚑 18.1 ⚕ 18.1 **FUD** 090 T A2 50 ▢

AMA: 2002,Apr,13

26670 Closed treatment of carpometacarpal dislocation, other than thumb, with manipulation, each joint; without anesthesia

🚑 8.75 ⚕ 9.63 **FUD** 090 T P2 80 ▢

AMA: 2002,Apr,13

26675 requiring anesthesia

🚑 11.8 ⚕ 12.8 **FUD** 090 T A2 80 ▢

AMA: 2002,Apr,13

26676 Percutaneous skeletal fixation of carpometacarpal dislocation, other than thumb, with manipulation, each joint

🚑 14.2 ⚕ 14.2 **FUD** 090 T A2 ▢

AMA: 2002,Apr,13

26685 Open treatment of carpometacarpal dislocation, other than thumb; includes internal fixation, when performed, each joint

🚑 16.4 ⚕ 16.4 **FUD** 090 T A2 ▢

AMA: 2002,Apr,13

26686 complex, multiple, or delayed reduction

🚑 17.8 ⚕ 17.8 **FUD** 090 T A2 80 ▢

AMA: 2002,Apr,13

26700   **Closed treatment of metacarpophalangeal dislocation, single, with manipulation; without anesthesia**
🚑 8.60   ⚕ 9.15   **FUD** 090   T P2 ▭
AMA: 2002,Apr,13

26705   **requiring anesthesia**
🚑 10.8   ⚕ 11.8   **FUD** 090   T A2 80 ▭
AMA: 2002,Apr,13

26706   **Percutaneous skeletal fixation of metacarpophalangeal dislocation, single, with manipulation**
🚑 12.5   ⚕ 12.5   **FUD** 090   T A2 ▭
AMA: 2002,Apr,13

26715   **Open treatment of metacarpophalangeal dislocation, single, includes internal fixation, when performed**
🚑 16.3   ⚕ 16.3   **FUD** 090   T A2 80 ▭
AMA: 2002,Apr,13

26720   **Closed treatment of phalangeal shaft fracture, proximal or middle phalanx, finger or thumb; without manipulation, each**
🚑 5.23   ⚕ 5.62   **FUD** 090   T P2 ▭
AMA: 2002,Apr,13

26725   **with manipulation, with or without skin or skeletal traction, each**
🚑 8.64   ⚕ 9.57   **FUD** 090   T P2 ▭
AMA: 2002,Apr,13

26727   **Percutaneous skeletal fixation of unstable phalangeal shaft fracture, proximal or middle phalanx, finger or thumb, with manipulation, each**
🚑 13.3   ⚕ 13.3   **FUD** 090   T A2 ▭
AMA: 2002,Apr,13

26735   **Open treatment of phalangeal shaft fracture, proximal or middle phalanx, finger or thumb, includes internal fixation, when performed, each**
🚑 17.0   ⚕ 17.0   **FUD** 090   T A2 ▭
AMA: 2002,Apr,13

26740   **Closed treatment of articular fracture, involving metacarpophalangeal or interphalangeal joint; without manipulation, each**
🚑 6.14   ⚕ 6.53   **FUD** 090   T P2 ▭
AMA: 2002,Apr,13

26742   **with manipulation, each**
🚑 9.52   ⚕ 10.4   **FUD** 090   T A2 ▭
AMA: 2002,Apr,13

26746   **Open treatment of articular fracture, involving metacarpophalangeal or interphalangeal joint, includes internal fixation, when performed, each**
🚑 21.2   ⚕ 21.2   **FUD** 090   T A2 ▭
AMA: 2002,Apr,13

26750   **Closed treatment of distal phalangeal fracture, finger or thumb; without manipulation, each**
🚑 5.23   ⚕ 5.22   **FUD** 090   T P2 ▭
AMA: 2002,Apr,13

26755   **with manipulation, each**
🚑 7.75   ⚕ 8.90   **FUD** 090   T G2 ▭
AMA: 2002,Apr,13

26756   **Percutaneous skeletal fixation of distal phalangeal fracture, finger or thumb, each**
🚑 11.9   ⚕ 11.9   **FUD** 090   T A2 80 ▭
AMA: 2002,Apr,13

26765   **Open treatment of distal phalangeal fracture, finger or thumb, includes internal fixation, when performed, each**
🚑 14.3   ⚕ 14.3   **FUD** 090   T A2 ▭
AMA: 2002,Apr,13

26770   **Closed treatment of interphalangeal joint dislocation, single, with manipulation; without anesthesia**
🚑 7.23   ⚕ 7.80   **FUD** 090   T G2 ▭
AMA: 2002,Apr,13

26775   **requiring anesthesia**
🚑 9.85   ⚕ 10.8   **FUD** 090   S P2 ▭
AMA: 2002,Apr,13

26776   **Percutaneous skeletal fixation of interphalangeal joint dislocation, single, with manipulation**
🚑 12.6   ⚕ 12.6   **FUD** 090   T A2 ▭
AMA: 2002,Apr,13

26785   **Open treatment of interphalangeal joint dislocation, includes internal fixation, when performed, single**
🚑 15.6   ⚕ 15.6   **FUD** 090   T A2 ▭
AMA: 2002,Apr,13

26820-26863 Fusion of Joint(s) of Fingers or Hand

26820   **Fusion in opposition, thumb, with autogenous graft (includes obtaining graft)**
🚑 22.2   ⚕ 22.2   **FUD** 090   T A2 80 50 ▭
AMA: 2002,Apr,13

26841   **Arthrodesis, carpometacarpal joint, thumb, with or without internal fixation;**
🚑 20.4   ⚕ 20.4   **FUD** 090   T A2 80 50 ▭
AMA: 2002,Apr,13

26842   **with autograft (includes obtaining graft)**
🚑 22.1   ⚕ 22.1   **FUD** 090   J A2 80 50 ▭
AMA: 2002,Apr,13

26843   **Arthrodesis, carpometacarpal joint, digit, other than thumb, each;**
🚑 20.8   ⚕ 20.8   **FUD** 090   J A2 80 ▭
AMA: 2016,Jan,13; 2015,Jan,16; 2014,Jan,11; 2012,Jan,15-42; 2011,Jan,11

26844   **with autograft (includes obtaining graft)**
🚑 22.8   ⚕ 22.8   **FUD** 090   J A2 80 ▭
AMA: 2002,Apr,13

26850   **Arthrodesis, metacarpophalangeal joint, with or without internal fixation;**
🚑 19.4   ⚕ 19.4   **FUD** 090   T A2 80 ▭
AMA: 2002,Apr,13

26852   **with autograft (includes obtaining graft)**
🚑 22.4   ⚕ 22.4   **FUD** 090   T A2 80 ▭
AMA: 2002,Apr,13

26860   **Arthrodesis, interphalangeal joint, with or without internal fixation;**
🚑 15.8   ⚕ 15.8   **FUD** 090   T A2 ▭
AMA: 2016,Jan,13; 2015,Jan,16; 2014,Jan,11; 2012,Jan,15-42; 2011,Jan,11

\+ 26861   **each additional interphalangeal joint (List separately in addition to code for primary procedure)**
Code first (26860)
🚑 2.98   ⚕ 2.98   **FUD** ZZZ   N N1 ▭
AMA: 2016,Jan,13; 2015,Jan,16; 2014,Jan,11; 2012,Jan,15-42; 2011,Jan,11

26862   **with autograft (includes obtaining graft)**
🚑 20.4   ⚕ 20.4   **FUD** 090   T A2 80 ▭
AMA: 2002,Apr,13

\+ 26863   **with autograft (includes obtaining graft), each additional joint (List separately in addition to code for primary procedure)**
Code first (26862)
🚑 6.65   ⚕ 6.65   **FUD** ZZZ   N N1 80 ▭
AMA: 2002,Apr,13

26910-26989 Amputations and Unlisted Procedures Finger/Hand

26910   **Amputation, metacarpal, with finger or thumb (ray amputation), single, with or without interosseous transfer**
EXCLUDES   *Repositioning (26550, 26555)*
         Transmetacarpal amputation of hand (25927)
🚑 20.3   ⚕ 20.3   **FUD** 090   T A2 ▭
AMA: 2002,Apr,13

26951 Amputation, finger or thumb, primary or secondary, any joint or phalanx, single, including neurectomies; with direct closure
> *EXCLUDES* *Repair necessitating flaps or grafts (15050-15758)*
> *Transmetacarpal amputation of hand (25927)*
> 🚗 18.4 ✂ 18.4 **FUD** 090   T A2 ▣
> AMA: 2002,Apr,13

26952 with local advancement flaps (V-Y, hood)
> *EXCLUDES* *Repair necessitating flaps or grafts (15050-15758)*
> *Transmetacarpal amputation of hand (25927)*
> 🚗 18.1 ✂ 18.1 **FUD** 090   T A2 ▣
> AMA: 2002,Apr,13

26989 Unlisted procedure, hands or fingers
> 🚗 0.00 ✂ 0.00 **FUD** YYY   T
> AMA: 2002,Apr,13

26990-26992 Incision for Drainage of Pelvis or Hip
> *EXCLUDES* *Simple incision and drainage procedures (10040-10160)*

26990 Incision and drainage, pelvis or hip joint area; deep abscess or hematoma
> 🚗 17.9 ✂ 17.9 **FUD** 090   T A2 ▣
> AMA: 2002,Apr,13

26991 infected bursa
> 🚗 14.9 ✂ 20.0 **FUD** 090   T A2 80 ▣
> AMA: 2002,Apr,13

26992 Incision, bone cortex, pelvis and/or hip joint (eg, osteomyelitis or bone abscess)
> 🚗 27.5 ✂ 27.5 **FUD** 090   C 80 ▣
> AMA: 2016,Jan,13; 2015,Jan,16; 2014,Jan,11; 2012,Oct,14; 2012,Jan,15-42; 2011,Jan,11

27000-27006 Tenotomy Procedures of Hip

27000 Tenotomy, adductor of hip, percutaneous (separate procedure)
> 🚗 11.9 ✂ 11.9 **FUD** 090   T A2 50 ▣
> AMA: 2002,Apr,13; 1998,Nov,1

27001 Tenotomy, adductor of hip, open
> 🚗 15.3 ✂ 15.3 **FUD** 090   T A2 80 50 ▣
> AMA: 2002,Apr,13; 1998,Nov,1

27003 Tenotomy, adductor, subcutaneous, open, with obturator neurectomy
> 🚗 17.0 ✂ 17.0 **FUD** 090   T A2 80 50 ▣
> AMA: 2002,Apr,13

27005 Tenotomy, hip flexor(s), open (separate procedure)
> 🚗 20.7 ✂ 20.7 **FUD** 090   C 80 50 ▣
> AMA: 2002,Apr,13; 1998,Nov,1

27006 Tenotomy, abductors and/or extensor(s) of hip, open (separate procedure)
> 🚗 21.1 ✂ 21.1 **FUD** 090   T 80 50 ▣
> AMA: 2002,Apr,13; 1998,Nov,1

27025-27036 Surgical Incision of Hip

27025 Fasciotomy, hip or thigh, any type
> 🚗 26.3 ✂ 26.3 **FUD** 090   C 80 50 ▣
> AMA: 2002,Apr,13

27027 Decompression fasciotomy(ies), pelvic (buttock) compartment(s) (eg, gluteus medius-minimus, gluteus maximus, iliopsoas, and/or tensor fascia lata muscle), unilateral
> 🚗 25.9 ✂ 25.9 **FUD** 090   T 80 50 ▣

27030 Arthrotomy, hip, with drainage (eg, infection)
> 🚗 26.9 ✂ 26.9 **FUD** 090   C 80 50 ▣
> AMA: 2002,Apr,13; 1998,Nov,1

27033 Arthrotomy, hip, including exploration or removal of loose or foreign body
> 🚗 27.9 ✂ 27.9 **FUD** 090   T A2 80 50 ▣
> AMA: 2016,Jan,13; 2015,Jan,16; 2014,Jan,11

27035 Denervation, hip joint, intrapelvic or extrapelvic intra-articular branches of sciatic, femoral, or obturator nerves
> *EXCLUDES* *Transection of obturator nerve (64763, 64766)*
> 🚗 33.0 ✂ 33.0 **FUD** 090   T A2 80 50 ▣
> AMA: 2016,Jan,13; 2015,Jan,16; 2014,Mar,13

27036 Capsulectomy or capsulotomy, hip, with or without excision of heterotopic bone, with release of hip flexor muscles (ie, gluteus medius, gluteus minimus, tensor fascia latae, rectus femoris, sartorius, iliopsoas)
> 🚗 29.0 ✂ 29.0 **FUD** 090   C 80 50 ▣
> AMA: 2002,Apr,13; 1996,Nov,1

27040-27041 Biopsy of Hip/Pelvis
> *EXCLUDES* *Soft tissue needle biopsy (20206)*

27040 Biopsy, soft tissue of pelvis and hip area; superficial
> 🚗 5.75 ✂ 9.81 **FUD** 010   T A2 50 ▣
> AMA: 2002,Apr,13

27041 deep, subfascial or intramuscular
> 🚗 19.8 ✂ 19.8 **FUD** 090   T A2 50 ▣
> AMA: 2002,Apr,13; 1998,Nov,1

27043-27049 [27043, 27045, 27059] Excision Soft Tissue Tumors Hip/ Pelvis
> *INCLUDES* Any necessary elevation of tissue planes or dissection
> Measurement of tumor and necessary margin at greatest diameter prior to excision
> Simple and intermediate repairs
> Types of excision:
>   Fascial or subfascial soft tissue tumors: simple and marginal resection of tumors found either in or below the deep fascia, not involving bone or excision of a substantial amount of normal tissue; primarily benign and intramuscular tumors
>   Radical resection of soft tissue tumor: wide resection of tumor involving substantial margins of normal tissue and may involve tissue removal from one or more layers; mostly malignant or aggressive benign,
>   Subcutaneous: simple and marginal resection of tumors found in the subcutaneous tissue above the deep fascia; most often benign
> *EXCLUDES* *Complex repair*
> *Excision of benign cutaneous lesions (eg, sebaceous cyst) (11400-11406)*
> *Radical resection of cutaneous tumors (eg, melanoma) (11600-11606)*
> *Significant exploration of vessels, neuroplasty, reconstruction, or complex bone repair*

27043 Resequenced code. See code following 27047.

27045 Resequenced code. See code following 27048.

27047 Excision, tumor, soft tissue of pelvis and hip area, subcutaneous; less than 3 cm
> 🚗 10.4 ✂ 13.3 **FUD** 090   T 62 50 ▣
> AMA: 2002,Apr,13; 1998,Nov,1

 # 27043 3 cm or greater
> 🚗 13.5 ✂ 13.5 **FUD** 090   T 62 50 ▣

27048 Excision, tumor, soft tissue of pelvis and hip area, subfascial (eg, intramuscular); less than 5 cm
> 🚗 17.6 ✂ 17.6 **FUD** 090   T 62 80 50 ▣
> AMA: 2002,Apr,13

 # 27045 5 cm or greater
> 🚗 21.6 ✂ 21.6 **FUD** 090   T 62 80 50 ▣

27049 Radical resection of tumor (eg, sarcoma), soft tissue of pelvis and hip area; less than 5 cm
> 🚗 38.9 ✂ 38.9 **FUD** 090   T 62 80 50 ▣
> AMA: 2002,Apr,13; 1998,Nov,1

 # 27059 5 cm or greater
> 🚗 52.5 ✂ 52.5 **FUD** 090   T 62 80 50 ▣

27050-27071 Procedures of Bones and Joints of Hip and Pelvis

27050 Arthrotomy, with biopsy; sacroiliac joint
> 🚗 11.0 ✂ 11.0 **FUD** 090   T A2 80 50 ▣
> AMA: 2002,Apr,13; 1994,Win,1

27052 **hip joint**
 16.5 16.5 **FUD** 090 T A2 80 50
AMA: 2002,Apr,13

27054 **Arthrotomy with synovectomy, hip joint**
 19.6 19.6 **FUD** 090 C 80 50
AMA: 2002,Apr,13; 1994,Win,1

27057 **Decompression fasciotomy(ies), pelvic (buttock) compartment(s) (eg, gluteus medius-minimus, gluteus maximus, iliopsoas, and/or tensor fascia lata muscle) with debridement of nonviable muscle, unilateral**
 29.2 29.2 **FUD** 090 T 80 50
AMA: 2002,Apr,13

27059 *Resequenced code. See code following 27049.*

27060 **Excision; ischial bursa**
 13.2 13.2 **FUD** 090 T A2 50
AMA: 2002,Apr,13

27062 **trochanteric bursa or calcification**
EXCLUDES *Arthrocentesis (20610)*
 13.1 13.1 **FUD** 090 T A2 50
AMA: 2002,Apr,13

27065 **Excision of bone cyst or benign tumor, wing of ilium, symphysis pubis, or greater trochanter of femur; superficial, includes autograft, when performed**
 14.6 14.6 **FUD** 090 T A2 80 50
AMA: 2002,Apr,13

27066 **deep (subfascial), includes autograft, when performed**
 23.2 23.2 **FUD** 090 T A2 80 50
AMA: 2002,Apr,13

27067 **with autograft requiring separate incision**
 29.4 29.4 **FUD** 090 T A2 80 50
AMA: 2002,Apr,13

27070 **Partial excision, wing of ilium, symphysis pubis, or greater trochanter of femur, (craterization, saucerization) (eg, osteomyelitis or bone abscess); superficial**
 24.3 24.3 **FUD** 090 C 80 50
AMA: 2002,Apr,13; 1998,Nov,1

27071 **deep (subfascial or intramuscular)**
 26.3 26.3 **FUD** 090 C 80 50
AMA: 2002,Apr,13

27075-27078 Radical Resection Bone Tumor of Hip/Pelvis

INCLUDES Any necessary elevation of tissue planes or dissection
Excision of adjacent soft tissue during bone tumor resection (27043-27049 [27043, 27045, 27059])
Measurement of tumor and necessary margin at greatest diameter prior to excision
Resection of the tumor (may include entire bone) and wide margins of normal tissue primarily for malignant or aggressive benign tumors
Simple and intermediate repairs
EXCLUDES *Complex repair*
Significant exploration of vessels, neuroplasty, reconstruction, or complex bone repair

27075 **Radical resection of tumor; wing of ilium, 1 pubic or ischial ramus or symphysis pubis**
 60.5 60.5 **FUD** 090 C 80
AMA: 2002,Apr,13; 1994,Win,1

27076 **ilium, including acetabulum, both pubic rami, or ischium and acetabulum**
 73.0 73.0 **FUD** 090 C 80
AMA: 2002,Apr,13

27077 **innominate bone, total**
 82.1 82.1 **FUD** 090 C 80
AMA: 2002,Apr,13

27078 **ischial tuberosity and greater trochanter of femur**
 59.6 59.6 **FUD** 090 C 80 50
AMA: 2002,Apr,13

27080 Excision of Coccyx

EXCLUDES *Surgical excision of decubitus ulcers (15920, 15922, 15931-15958)*

27080 **Coccygectomy, primary**
 14.7 14.7 **FUD** 090 T A2 80
AMA: 2002,Apr,13

27086-27091 Removal Foreign Body or Hip Prosthesis

27086 **Removal of foreign body, pelvis or hip; subcutaneous tissue**
 4.76 8.26 **FUD** 010 T A2 80 50
AMA: 2016,Jan,13; 2015,Jan,16; 2014,Jan,11

27087 **deep (subfascial or intramuscuiar)**
 18.0 18.0 **FUD** 090 T A2 80 50
AMA: 2002,Apr,13; 1998,Nov,1

Deep (27087)

A foreign body is removed from the pelvis or hip

27090 **Removal of hip prosthesis; (separate procedure)**
 23.8 23.8 **FUD** 090 C 80 50
AMA: 2002,Apr,13

27091 **complicated, including total hip prosthesis, methylmethacrylate with or without insertion of spacer**
 46.0 46.0 **FUD** 090 C 80 50
AMA: 2016,Jan,13; 2015,Jan,16; 2014,Jan,11

27093-27096 Injection for Arthrogram Hip/Sacroiliac Joint

27093 **Injection procedure for hip arthrography; without anesthesia**
 (73525)
 2.02 5.34 **FUD** 000 N N1 50
AMA: 2016,Jan,13; 2015,Aug,6; 2015,Jan,16; 2014,Jan,11; 2012,Jun,14

27095 **with anesthesia**
 (73525)
 2.38 6.87 **FUD** 000 N N1 50
AMA: 2016,Jan,11; 2016,Jan,13; 2015,Aug,6; 2015,Jan,16; 2014,Jan,11; 2012,Jun,14

27096 **Injection procedure for sacroiliac joint, anesthetic/steroid, with image guidance (fluoroscopy or CT) including arthrography when performed**
INCLUDES Confirmation of intra-articular needle placement with CT or fluoroscopy
Fluoroscopic guidance (77002-77003)
EXCLUDES *Procedure performed without fluoroscopy or CT guidance (20552)*
 2.43 4.59 **FUD** 000 B 50
AMA: 2016,Jan,13; 2015,Aug,6; 2015,Jan,16; 2014,Jan,11; 2012,Jan,3-5; 2012,Jan,15-42; 2011,Jan,11

27097-27187 Revision/Reconstruction Hip and Pelvis

INCLUDES Closed, open and percutaneous treatment of fractures and dislocations

27097 **Release or recession, hamstring, proximal**
 19.3 19.3 **FUD** 090 T A2 80 50
AMA: 2002,Apr,13; 1998,Nov,1

27098 **Transfer, adductor to ischium**
 19.2 19.2 **FUD** 090 T A2 80 50
AMA: 2002,Apr,13; 1998,Nov,1

● New Code ▲ Revised Code ○ Reinstated ● New Web Release ▲ Revised Web Release Unlisted Not Covered # Resequenced
Ⓝ AMA Mod 51 Exempt ⑨ Optum Mod 51 Exempt ⊛ Mod 63 Exempt ✗ Non-FDA Drug ★ Telehealth Ⓜ Maternity Ⓐ Age Edit + Add-on AMA: CPT Asst

27100 Transfer external oblique muscle to greater trochanter including fascial or tendon extension (graft)

INCLUDES   Eggers procedure

🚑 23.5   ℨ 23.5   **FUD** 090   J A2 80 50 ▢

AMA: 2002,Apr,13

27105 Transfer paraspinal muscle to hip (includes fascial or tendon extension graft)

🚑 24.9   ℨ 24.9   **FUD** 090   T A2 80 50 ▢

AMA: 2002,Apr,13

27110 Transfer iliopsoas; to greater trochanter of femur

🚑 27.8   ℨ 27.8   **FUD** 090   T A2 80 50 ▢

AMA: 2002,May,7; 2002,Apr,13

27111 to femoral neck

🚑 25.8   ℨ 25.8   **FUD** 090   T A2 80 50 ▢

AMA: 2002,Apr,13

27120 Acetabuloplasty; (eg, Whitman, Colonna, Haygroves, or cup type)

🚑 37.4   ℨ 37.4   **FUD** 090   C 80 50 ▢

AMA: 2002,Apr,13

27122 resection, femoral head (eg, Girdlestone procedure)

🚑 31.6   ℨ 31.6   **FUD** 090   C 80 50 ▢

AMA: 2002,Apr,13; 1998,Nov,1

27125 Hemiarthroplasty, hip, partial (eg, femoral stem prosthesis, bipolar arthroplasty)

EXCLUDES   Hip replacement following hip fracture (27236)

🚑 32.6   ℨ 32.6   **FUD** 090   C 80 50 ▢

AMA: 2016,Jan,13; 2015,Jan,16; 2014,Jan,11; 2012,Jan,15-42; 2011,Jan,11

Acetabulum remains intact

Prosthesis

27130 Arthroplasty, acetabular and proximal femoral prosthetic replacement (total hip arthroplasty), with or without autograft or allograft

🚑 39.1   ℨ 39.1   **FUD** 090   C 80 50 ▢

AMA: 2016,Jan,13; 2015,Jan,16; 2014,Jan,11; 2012,Jan,15-42; 2011,Dec,14-18

Damaged femur head ("ball") in degenerated socket (acetabulum)

Cuplike acetabular component of prosthesis fixed into hip bone

Prosthesis anchored into shaft of long bone

Damaged femur head replaced with prosthesis

27132 Conversion of previous hip surgery to total hip arthroplasty, with or without autograft or allograft

🚑 48.3   ℨ 48.3   **FUD** 090   C 80 50 ▢

AMA: 2016,Jan,13; 2015,Jan,16; 2014,Jan,11

27134 Revision of total hip arthroplasty; both components, with or without autograft or allograft

🚑 55.3   ℨ 55.3   **FUD** 090   C 80 50 ▢

AMA: 2016,Jan,13; 2015,Jan,16; 2014,Jan,11

27137 acetabular component only, with or without autograft or allograft

🚑 42.5   ℨ 42.5   **FUD** 090   C 80 50 ▢

AMA: 2016,Jan,13; 2015,Jan,16; 2014,Jan,11

27138 femoral component only, with or without allograft

🚑 44.1   ℨ 44.1   **FUD** 090   C 80 50 ▢

AMA: 2016,Jan,13; 2015,Jan,16; 2014,Jan,11

27140 Osteotomy and transfer of greater trochanter of femur (separate procedure)

🚑 25.7   ℨ 25.7   **FUD** 090   C 80 50 ▢

AMA: 2008,Dec,3-4; 2002,Apr,13

27146 Osteotomy, iliac, acetabular or innominate bone;

INCLUDES   Salter osteotomy

🚑 37.1   ℨ 37.1   **FUD** 090   C 80 50 ▢

AMA: 2016,Jan,13; 2015,Jan,16; 2014,Jan,11; 2012,Jan,15-42; 2011,Jan,11

Iliac crest   Sacrum   Ilium

Sacroiliac joint

Acetabulum

Head of femur

Ischium

Obturator foramen   Symphysis pubis   Neck of femur   Femur

27147 with open reduction of hip

INCLUDES   Pemberton osteotomy

🚑 42.4   ℨ 42.4   **FUD** 090   C 80 50 ▢

AMA: 2008,Dec,3-4; 2002,Apr,13

Ilium

Example of innominate osteotomy

Greater trochanter   Acetabu

Head of femur

Femoral head is reduced into the acetabulum

Kirschner wires are drilled through the ilium and into lower fragment

27151 with femoral osteotomy

🚑 45.8   ℨ 45.8   **FUD** 090   C 80 50 ▢

AMA: 2008,Dec,3-4; 2002,Apr,13

27156 with femoral osteotomy and with open reduction of hip

INCLUDES   Chiari osteotomy

🚑 49.5   ℨ 49.5   **FUD** 090   C 80 50 ▢

AMA: 2008,Dec,3-4; 2002,Apr,13

27158 Osteotomy, pelvis, bilateral (eg, congenital malformation)

🚑 41.1   ℨ 41.1   **FUD** 090   C 80 ▢

AMA: 2008,Dec,3-4; 2002,Apr,13

27161 Osteotomy, femoral neck (separate procedure)
35.0   35.0   **FUD** 090   C 80 50
AMA: 2008,Dec,3-4; 2002,Apr,13

27165 Osteotomy, intertrochanteric or subtrochanteric including internal or external fixation and/or cast
39.6   39.6   **FUD** 090   C 80 50
AMA: 2016,Jan,13; 2015,Jan,16; 2014,Jan,11

27170 Bone graft, femoral head, neck, intertrochanteric or subtrochanteric area (includes obtaining bone graft)
33.8   33.8   **FUD** 090   C 80 50
AMA: 2016,Jan,13; 2015,Jan,16; 2014,Jan,11

27175 Treatment of slipped femoral epiphysis; by traction, without reduction
19.2   19.2   **FUD** 090   C 80 50
AMA: 2008,Dec,3-4; 2002,Apr,13

27176 by single or multiple pinning, in situ
25.8   25.8   **FUD** 090   C 80 50
AMA: 2008,Dec,3-4; 2002,Apr,13

27177 Open treatment of slipped femoral epiphysis; single or multiple pinning or bone graft (includes obtaining graft)
32.1   32.1   **FUD** 090   C 80 50
AMA: 2008,Dec,3-4; 2002,Apr,13

27178 closed manipulation with single or multiple pinning
26.4   26.4   **FUD** 090   C 80 50
AMA: 2008,Dec,3-4; 2002,Apr,13

27179 osteoplasty of femoral neck (Heyman type procedure)
28.1   28.1   **FUD** 090   J 80 50
AMA: 2008,Dec,3-4; 2002,Apr,13

27181 osteotomy and internal fixation
27.7   27.7   **FUD** 090   C 80 50
AMA: 2008,Dec,3-4; 2002,Apr,13

27185 Epiphyseal arrest by epiphysiodesis or stapling, greater trochanter of femur
17.4   17.4   **FUD** 090   C 50
AMA: 2008,Dec,3-4; 2002,Apr,13

27187 Prophylactic treatment (nailing, pinning, plating or wiring) with or without methylmethacrylate, femoral neck and proximal femur
28.5   28.5   **FUD** 090   C 80 50
AMA: 2016,Jan,13; 2015,Jan,16; 2014,Jan,11

27193-27269 Treatment of Fracture/Dislocation Hip/Pelvis

27193 ~~Closed treatment of pelvic ring fracture, dislocation, diastasis or subluxation; without manipulation~~
To report, see ~27197

27194 ~~with manipulation, requiring more than local anesthesia~~
To report, see ~27198

● **27197** Closed treatment of posterior pelvic ring fracture(s), dislocation(s), diastasis or subluxation of the ilium, sacroiliac joint, and/or sacrum, with or without anterior pelvic ring fracture(s) and/or dislocation(s) of the pubic symphysis and/or superior/inferior rami, unilateral or bilateral; without manipulation

● **27198** with manipulation, requiring more than local anesthesia (ie, general anesthesia, moderate sedation, spinal/epidural)
EXCLUDES   Closed treatment anterior pelvic ring, pubic symphysis, inferior rami fracture/dislocation
See appropriate E&M codes

27200 Closed treatment of coccygeal fracture
5.37   5.15   **FUD** 090   T P2
AMA: 2008,Dec,3-4; 2002,Apr,13

27202 Open treatment of coccygeal fracture
15.2   15.2   **FUD** 090   T A2 80
AMA: 2008,Dec,3-4; 2002,Apr,13

27215 Open treatment of iliac spine(s), tuberosity avulsion, or iliac wing fracture(s), unilateral, for pelvic bone fracture patterns that do not disrupt the pelvic ring, includes internal fixation, when performed
17.9   17.9   **FUD** 090   E
AMA: 2008,Dec,3-4; 2002,Apr,13

27216 Percutaneous skeletal fixation of posterior pelvic bone fracture and/or dislocation, for fracture patterns that disrupt the pelvic ring, unilateral (includes ipsilateral ilium, sacroiliac joint and/or sacrum)
EXCLUDES   Sacroiliac joint arthrodesis without fracture and/or dislocation, percutaneous or minimally invasive (27279)
26.6   26.6   **FUD** 090   E
AMA: 2016,Jan,13; 2015,Jan,16; 2014,Mar,4; 2013,Sep,17

27217 Open treatment of anterior pelvic bone fracture and/or dislocation for fracture patterns that disrupt the pelvic ring, unilateral, includes internal fixation, when performed (includes pubic symphysis and/or ipsilateral superior/inferior rami)
24.9   24.9   **FUD** 090   E
AMA: 2008,Dec,3-4; 2002,Apr,13

27218 Open treatment of posterior pelvic bone fracture and/or dislocation, for fracture patterns that disrupt the pelvic ring, unilateral, includes internal fixation, when performed (includes ipsilateral ilium, sacroiliac joint and/or sacrum)
EXCLUDES   Sacroiliac joint arthrodesis without fracture and/or dislocation, percutaneous or minimally invasive (27279)
34.5   34.5   **FUD** 090   E
AMA: 2016,Jan,13; 2015,Jan,16; 2014,Mar,4

27220 Closed treatment of acetabulum (hip socket) fracture(s); without manipulation
15.0   15.2   **FUD** 090   T 62 50
AMA: 2008,Dec,3-4; 2002,Apr,13

27222 with manipulation, with or without skeletal traction
28.1   28.1   **FUD** 090   C 50
AMA: 2008,Dec,3-4; 2002,Apr,13

27226 Open treatment of posterior or anterior acetabular wall fracture, with internal fixation
30.4   30.4   **FUD** 090   C 80 50
AMA: 2008,Dec,3-4; 2002,Apr,13

27227 Open treatment of acetabular fracture(s) involving anterior or posterior (one) column, or a fracture running transversely across the acetabulum, with internal fixation
47.8   47.8   **FUD** 090   C 80 50
AMA: 2008,Dec,3-4; 2002,Apr,13

27228 Open treatment of acetabular fracture(s) involving anterior and posterior (two) columns, includes T-fracture and both column fracture with complete articular detachment, or single column or transverse fracture with associated acetabular wall fracture, with internal fixation
54.6   54.6   **FUD** 090   C 80 50
AMA: 2008,Dec,3-4; 2002,Apr,13

27230 Closed treatment of femoral fracture, proximal end, neck; without manipulation
13.5   13.5   **FUD** 090   T A2 50
AMA: 2008,Dec,3-4; 2002,Apr,13

27232 with manipulation, with or without skeletal traction
21.6   21.6   **FUD** 090   C 50
AMA: 2008,Dec,3-4; 2002,Apr,13

27235 Percutaneous skeletal fixation of femoral fracture, proximal end, neck
26.1   26.1   **FUD** 090   J 50
AMA: 2016,Jan,13; 2015,Jan,16; 2014,Jan,11

27236 Open treatment of femoral fracture, proximal end, neck, internal fixation or prosthetic replacement
🔲 34.4 　 34.4 　**FUD** 090 　　 C 80 50 ▢
AMA: 2016,Jan,13; 2015,Jan,16; 2014,Jan,11; 2012,Jan,15-42; 2011,Jan,11

27238 Closed treatment of intertrochanteric, peritrochanteric, or subtrochanteric femoral fracture; without manipulation
🔲 13.1 　 13.1 　**FUD** 090 　　 T A2 50 ▢
AMA: 2016,Jan,13; 2015,Jan,16; 2014,Jan,11

27240 with manipulation, with or without skin or skeletal traction
🔲 27.5 　 27.5 　**FUD** 090 　　 C 50 ▢
AMA: 2016,Jan,13; 2015,Jan,16; 2014,Jan,11

27244 Treatment of intertrochanteric, peritrochanteric, or subtrochanteric femoral fracture; with plate/screw type implant, with or without cerclage
🔲 35.5 　 35.5 　**FUD** 090 　　 C 80 50 ▢
AMA: 2016,Jan,13; 2015,Jan,16; 2014,Jan,11

27245 with intramedullary implant, with or without interlocking screws and/or cerclage
🔲 35.4 　 35.4 　**FUD** 090 　　 C 80 50 ▢
AMA: 2016,Jan,13; 2015,Jan,16; 2014,Jan,11; 2013,Sep,17

27246 Closed treatment of greater trochanteric fracture, without manipulation
🔲 11.0 　 11.0 　**FUD** 090 　　 T A2 50 ▢
AMA: 2008,Dec,3-4; 2002,Apr,13

27248 Open treatment of greater trochanteric fracture, includes internal fixation, when performed
🔲 21.3 　 21.3 　**FUD** 090 　　 C 80 50 ▢
AMA: 2008,Dec,3-4; 2002,Apr,13

27250 Closed treatment of hip dislocation, traumatic; without anesthesia
🔲 5.21 　 5.21 　**FUD** 000 　　 T A2 50 ▢
AMA: 2008,Dec,3-4; 2002,Apr,13

27252 requiring anesthesia
🔲 21.8 　 21.8 　**FUD** 090 　　 T A2 50 ▢
AMA: 2008,Dec,3-4; 2002,Apr,13

27253 Open treatment of hip dislocation, traumatic, without internal fixation
🔲 27.0 　 27.0 　**FUD** 090 　　 C 80 50 ▢
AMA: 2008,Dec,3-4; 2002,Apr,13

27254 Open treatment of hip dislocation, traumatic, with acetabular wall and femoral head fracture, with or without internal or external fixation
　EXCLUDES　 Acetabular fracture treatment (27226-27227)
🔲 36.5 　 36.5 　**FUD** 090 　　 C 80 50 ▢
AMA: 2008,Dec,3-4; 2002,Apr,13

27256 Treatment of spontaneous hip dislocation (developmental, including congenital or pathological), by abduction, splint or traction; without anesthesia, without manipulation
🔲 6.73 　 8.54 　**FUD** 010 　　 T G2 80 50 ▢
AMA: 2008,Dec,3-4; 2002,Apr,13

27257 with manipulation, requiring anesthesia
🔲 10.4 　 10.4 　**FUD** 010 　　 T A2 80 50 ▢
AMA: 2008,Dec,3-4; 2002,Apr,13

27258 Open treatment of spontaneous hip dislocation (developmental, including congenital or pathological), replacement of femoral head in acetabulum (including tenotomy, etc);
　INCLUDES　 Lorenz's operation
🔲 32.0 　 32.0 　**FUD** 090 　　 C 80 50 ▢
AMA: 2008,Dec,3-4; 2002,Apr,13

27259 with femoral shaft shortening
🔲 44.8 　 44.8 　**FUD** 090 　　 C 80 50 ▢
AMA: 2008,Dec,3-4; 2002,Apr,13

27265 Closed treatment of post hip arthroplasty dislocation; without anesthesia
🔲 11.3 　 11.3 　**FUD** 090 　　 T A2 50 ▢
AMA: 2008,Dec,3-4; 2002,Apr,13

27266 requiring regional or general anesthesia
🔲 16.7 　 16.7 　**FUD** 090 　　 T A2 50 ▢
AMA: 2008,Dec,3-4; 2002,Apr,13

27267 Closed treatment of femoral fracture, proximal end, head; without manipulation
🔲 12.4 　 12.4 　**FUD** 090 　　 T G2 80 50 ▢
AMA: 2016,Jan,13; 2015,Jan,16; 2014,Jan,11

27268 with manipulation
🔲 15.2 　 15.2 　**FUD** 090 　　 C 80 50 ▢
AMA: 2016,Jan,13; 2015,Jan,16; 2014,Jan,11

27269 Open treatment of femoral fracture, proximal end, head, includes internal fixation, when performed
　EXCLUDES　 Arthrotomy, hip (27033)
　　　　　Open treatment of hip dislocation, traumatic, without internal fixation (27253)
🔲 35.7 　 35.7 　**FUD** 090 　　 C 80 50 ▢
AMA: 2016,Jan,13; 2015,Jan,16; 2014,Jan,11

27275 Hip Manipulation with Anesthesia

27275 Manipulation, hip joint, requiring general anesthesia
🔲 5.21 　 5.21 　**FUD** 010 　　 T A2 ▢
AMA: 2016,May,13; 2016,Jan,13; 2016,Jan,11; 2015,Jan,16; 2014,Jan,11

27279-27286 Arthrodesis of Hip and Pelvis

27279 Arthrodesis, sacroiliac joint, percutaneous or minimally invasive (indirect visualization), with image guidance, includes obtaining bone graft when performed, and placement of transfixing device
🔲 20.0 　 20.0 　**FUD** 090 　　 J J8 80 50 ▢
27280 Arthrodesis, open, sacroiliac joint, including obtaining bone graft, including instrumentation, when performed
　EXCLUDES　 Sacroiliac joint arthrodesis without fracture and/or dislocation, percutaneous or minimally invasive (27279)
🔲 39.4 　 39.4 　**FUD** 090 　　 C 80 50 ▢
AMA: 2016,Jan,13; 2015,Jan,16; 2014,Mar,4; 2014,Jan,11; 2013,Sep,17

27282 Arthrodesis, symphysis pubis (including obtaining graft)
🔲 23.7 　 23.7 　**FUD** 090 　　 C 80 ▢
AMA: 2008,Dec,3-4; 2002,Apr,13

27284 Arthrodesis, hip joint (including obtaining graft);
🔲 44.9 　 44.9 　**FUD** 090 　　 C 80 50 ▢
AMA: 2008,Dec,3-4; 2002,Apr,13

27286 with subtrochanteric osteotomy
🔲 47.1 　 47.1 　**FUD** 090 　　 C 80 50 ▢
AMA: 2016,Jan,13; 2015,Jan,16; 2014,Jan,11

27290-27299 Amputations and Unlisted Procedures of Hip and Pelvis

27290 Interpelviabdominal amputation (hindquarter amputation)
　INCLUDES　 Pean's amputation
🔲 46.4 　 46.4 　**FUD** 090 　　 C 80 ▢
AMA: 2016,Jan,13; 2015,Jan,16; 2014,Jan,11

27295 Disarticulation of hip
🔲 36.3 　 36.3 　**FUD** 090 　　 C 80 50 ▢
AMA: 2016,Jan,13; 2015,Jan,16; 2014,Jan,11

27299 Unlisted procedure, pelvis or hip joint
🔲 0.00 　 0.00 　**FUD** YYY 　　 T 80 50
AMA: 2016,Jun,8; 2016,Jan,13; 2015,Jan,16; 2014,Mar,13; 2014,Jan,11; 2012,Nov,13-14; 2012,Oct,14; 2012,Jan,15-42; 2011,Jan,11

27301-27310 Incisional Procedures Femur or Knee

EXCLUDES Superficial incision and drainage (10040-10160)

27301 **Incision and drainage, deep abscess, bursa, or hematoma, thigh or knee region**
14.4 19.1 **FUD** 090 T A2 50
AMA: 2016,Jan,13; 2015,Jan,16; 2014,Jan,11

27303 **Incision, deep, with opening of bone cortex, femur or knee (eg, osteomyelitis or bone abscess)**
18.3 18.3 **FUD** 090 C 80
AMA: 2008,Dec,3-4; 2002,Apr,13

27305 **Fasciotomy, iliotibial (tenotomy), open**
EXCLUDES Ober-Yount (gluteal-iliotibial) fasciotomy (27025)
13.8 13.8 **FUD** 090 T A2 80 50
AMA: 2008,Dec,3-4; 2002,Apr,13

27306 **Tenotomy, percutaneous, adductor or hamstring; single tendon (separate procedure)**
10.1 10.1 **FUD** 090 T A2 80 50
AMA: 2008,Dec,3-4; 2002,Apr,13

27307 **multiple tendons**
13.2 13.2 **FUD** 090 T A2 80 50
AMA: 2008,Dec,3-4; 2002,Apr,13

27310 **Arthrotomy, knee, with exploration, drainage, or removal of foreign body (eg, infection)**
21.0 21.0 **FUD** 090 T A2 80 50
AMA: 2016,Jan,13; 2015,Jan,16; 2014,Jan,11

27323-27324 Biopsy Femur or Knee

EXCLUDES Soft tissue needle biopsy (20206)

27323 **Biopsy, soft tissue of thigh or knee area; superficial**
5.12 7.73 **FUD** 010 T A2 50
AMA: 2016,Jan,13; 2015,Jan,16; 2014,Jan,11

27324 **deep (subfascial or intramuscular)**
11.4 11.4 **FUD** 090 T A2 50
AMA: 2016,Jan,13; 2015,Jan,16; 2014,Jan,11

27325-27326 Neurectomy

27325 **Neurectomy, hamstring muscle**
15.6 15.6 **FUD** 090 T A2 80 50

27326 **Neurectomy, popliteal (gastrocnemius)**
14.8 14.8 **FUD** 090 T A2 80 50

27327-27329 [27337, 27339] Excision Soft Tissue Tumors Femur/ Knee

INCLUDES Any necessary elevation of tissue planes or dissection
Measurement of tumor and necessary margin at greatest diameter prior to excision
Simple and intermediate repairs
Types of excision:
Fascial or subfascial soft tissue tumors: simple and marginal resection of tumors found either in or below the deep fascia, not including bone or excision of a substantial amount of normal tissue; primarily benign and intramuscular tumors
Radical resection of soft tissue tumor: wide resection of tumor involving substantial margins of normal tissue and may involve tissue removal from one or more layers; most often malignant or aggressive benign
Subcutaneous: simple and marginal resection of tumors in the subcutaneous tissue above the deep fascia; most often benign
EXCLUDES Complex repair
Excision of benign cutaneous lesions (eg, sebaceous cyst) (11400-11406)
Radical resection of cutaneous tumors (eg, melanoma) (11600-11606)
Significant exploration of vessels or neuroplasty

27327 **Excision, tumor, soft tissue of thigh or knee area, subcutaneous; less than 3 cm**
9.03 13.1 **FUD** 090 T G2 50
AMA: 2002,Apr,13

\# **27337** **3 cm or greater**
12.0 12.0 **FUD** 090 T G2 80 50

27328 **Excision, tumor, soft tissue of thigh or knee area, subfascial (eg, intramuscular); less than 5 cm**
17.8 17.8 **FUD** 090 T G2 50
AMA: 2002,Apr,13

\# **27339** **5 cm or greater**
21.7 21.7 **FUD** 090 T G2 80 50

27329 Resequenced code. See code following 27360.

27330-27360 Resection Procedures Thigh/Knee

27330 **Arthrotomy, knee; with synovial biopsy only**
12.0 12.0 **FUD** 090 T A2 50
AMA: 2016,Jan,13; 2015,Jan,16; 2014,Jan,11; 2012,Mar,9-10

27331 **including joint exploration, biopsy, or removal of loose or foreign bodies**
13.6 13.6 **FUD** 090 T A2 80 50
AMA: 2016,Jan,13; 2015,Jan,16; 2014,Jan,11; 2012,Nov,13-14

27332 **Arthrotomy, with excision of semilunar cartilage (meniscectomy) knee; medial OR lateral**
18.3 18.3 **FUD** 090 T A2 80 50
AMA: 2002,Apr,13; 1998,Nov,1

Lateral meniscus
Posterior cruciate ligament
Medial meniscus
Bucket handle tear
Radial tear
Posterior horns
Anterior horns
Patellar ligament
Anterior cruciate ligament
Meniscus
Overhead view of right knee

27333 **medial AND lateral**
16.8 16.8 **FUD** 090 T A2 80 50
AMA: 2016,Jan,13; 2015,Jan,16; 2014,Jan,11; 2012,Mar,9-10

27334 **Arthrotomy, with synovectomy, knee; anterior OR posterior**
19.6 19.6 **FUD** 090 T A2 80 50
AMA: 2002,Apr,13; 1998,Nov,1

27335 **anterior AND posterior including popliteal area**
21.9 21.9 **FUD** 090 J A2 80 50
AMA: 2002,Apr,13

27337 Resequenced code. See code following 27327.

27339 Resequenced code. See code following 27328.

27340 **Excision, prepatellar bursa**
10.6 10.6 **FUD** 090 T A2 50
AMA: 2002,Apr,13

27345 **Excision of synovial cyst of popliteal space (eg, Baker's cyst)**
13.7 13.7 **FUD** 090 T A2 80 50
AMA: 2002,Apr,13; 1998,Nov,1

27347 **Excision of lesion of meniscus or capsule (eg, cyst, ganglion), knee**
15.2 15.2 **FUD** 090 T A2 80 50
AMA: 2002,Apr,13; 1998,Nov,1

27350 **Patellectomy or hemipatellectomy**
18.6 18.6 **FUD** 090 T A2 80 50
AMA: 2002,Apr,13

27355 **Excision or curettage of bone cyst or benign tumor of femur;**
17.2 17.2 **FUD** 090 T A2 80 50
AMA: 2002,Apr,13

27356 **with allograft**
🚑 21.1 ⚕ 21.1 **FUD** 090 [J] [J8] [80] [50] 🔲
AMA: 2002,Apr,13

27357 **with autograft (includes obtaining graft)**
🚑 23.3 ⚕ 23.3 **FUD** 090 [J] [A2] [80] [50] 🔲
AMA: 2016,Jan,13; 2015,Jan,16; 2014,Jan,11; 2012,Jan,15-42; 2011,Jan,11

+ 27358 **with internal fixation (List in addition to code for primary procedure)**
Code first (27355-27357)
🚑 8.04 ⚕ 8.04 **FUD** ZZZ [N] [N1] [80] 🔲
AMA: 2002,Apr,13

27360 **Partial excision (craterization, saucerization, or diaphysectomy) bone, femur, proximal tibia and/or fibula (eg, osteomyelitis or bone abscess)**
🚑 24.4 ⚕ 24.4 **FUD** 090 [T] [A2] [80] [50] 🔲
AMA: 2002,Apr,13; 1998,Nov,1

27364-27365 [27329] Radical Resection Tumor Knee/Thigh

INCLUDES Any necessary elevation of tissue planes or dissection
Excision of adjacent soft tissue during bone tumor resection
Measurement of tumor and necessary margin at greatest diameter prior to excision
Radical resection of bone tumor: resection of the tumor (may include entire bone) and wide margins of normal tissue primarily for malignant or aggressive benign tumors
Radical resection of soft tissue tumor: wide resection of tumor involving substantial margins of normal tissue that may include tissue removal from one or more layers; most often malignant or aggressive benign
Simple and intermediate repairs

EXCLUDES Complex repair
Radical resection of cutaneous tumors (eg, melanoma) (11600-11606)
Significant exploration of vessels, neuroplasty, reconstruction, or complex bone repair

 # 27329 **Radical resection of tumor (eg, sarcoma), soft tissue of thigh or knee area; less than 5 cm**
🚑 29.8 ⚕ 29.8 **FUD** 090 [T] [G2] [80] [50] 🔲
AMA: 2002,Apr,13; 1990,Win,4

27364 **5 cm or greater**
🚑 45.1 ⚕ 45.1 **FUD** 090 [T] [G2] [80] [50] 🔲

27365 **Radical resection of tumor, femur or knee**
EXCLUDES Soft tissue tumor excision thigh or knee area (27329, 27364)
🚑 59.7 ⚕ 59.7 **FUD** 090 [C] [80] [50] 🔲
AMA: 2002,Apr,13; 1994,Win,1

27370 Injection for Arthrogram of Knee

EXCLUDES Arthrocentesis, aspiration and/or injection, knee (20610-20611)
Arthroscopy, knee (29871)

27370 **Injection of contrast for knee arthrography**
📷 (73580)
🚑 1.46 ⚕ 4.41 **FUD** 000 [N] [N1] [50] 🔲
AMA: 2016,Jan,13; 2015,Aug,6; 2015,Feb,6

27372 Foreign Body Removal Femur or Knee

EXCLUDES Arthroscopic procedures (29870-29887)
Removal of knee prosthesis (27488)

27372 **Removal of foreign body, deep, thigh region or knee area**
🚑 11.5 ⚕ 17.3 **FUD** 090 [T] [A2] [80] [50] 🔲
AMA: 2002,Apr,13

27380-27499 Repair/Reconstruction of Femur or Knee

27380 **Suture of infrapatellar tendon; primary**
🚑 17.0 ⚕ 17.0 **FUD** 090 [T] [A2] [80] [50] 🔲
AMA: 2002,Apr,13

27381 **secondary reconstruction, including fascial or tendon graft**
🚑 22.8 ⚕ 22.8 **FUD** 090 [J] [A2] [80] [50] 🔲
AMA: 2002,Apr,13

27385 **Suture of quadriceps or hamstring muscle rupture; primary**
🚑 16.4 ⚕ 16.4 **FUD** 090 [T] [A2] [80] [50] 🔲
AMA: 2002,Apr,13

27386 **secondary reconstruction, including fascial or tendon graft**
🚑 23.8 ⚕ 23.8 **FUD** 090 [J] [A2] [80] [50] 🔲
AMA: 2002,Apr,13

27390 **Tenotomy, open, hamstring, knee to hip; single tendon**
🚑 12.8 ⚕ 12.8 **FUD** 090 [T] [A2] [80] [50] 🔲
AMA: 2002,Apr,13; 1998,Nov,1

27391 **multiple tendons, 1 leg**
🚑 16.5 ⚕ 16.5 **FUD** 090 [T] [A2] [80] 🔲
AMA: 2002,Apr,13; 1998,Nov,1

27392 **multiple tendons, bilateral**
🚑 20.3 ⚕ 20.3 **FUD** 090 [T] [A2] [80] 🔲
AMA: 2002,Apr,13; 1998,Nov,1

27393 **Lengthening of hamstring tendon; single tendon**
🚑 14.5 ⚕ 14.5 **FUD** 090 [T] [A2] [80] [50] 🔲
AMA: 2002,Apr,13; 1998,Nov,1

27394 **multiple tendons, 1 leg**
🚑 18.2 ⚕ 18.2 **FUD** 090 [T] [A2] [80] 🔲
AMA: 2002,Apr,13; 1998,Nov,1

27395 **multiple tendons, bilateral**
🚑 25.2 ⚕ 25.2 **FUD** 090 [T] [A2] [80] 🔲
AMA: 2002,Apr,13; 1998,Nov,1

27396 **Transplant or transfer (with muscle redirection or rerouting), thigh (eg, extensor to flexor); single tendon**
🚑 17.6 ⚕ 17.6 **FUD** 090 [T] [A2] [80] [50] 🔲
AMA: 2002,Apr,13; 1998,Nov,1

27397 **multiple tendons**
🚑 25.9 ⚕ 25.9 **FUD** 090 [T] [A2] [80] [50] 🔲
AMA: 2002,Apr,13; 1998,Nov,1

27400 **Transfer, tendon or muscle, hamstrings to femur (eg, Egger's type procedure)**
🚑 19.9 ⚕ 19.9 **FUD** 090 [T] [A2] [80] [50] 🔲
AMA: 2002,Apr,13; 1998,Nov,1

27403 **Arthrotomy with meniscus repair, knee**
EXCLUDES Arthroscopic treatment (29882)
🚑 18.3 ⚕ 18.3 **FUD** 090 [T] [A2] [80] [50] 🔲
AMA: 2002,Apr,13; 1998,Nov,1

27405 **Repair, primary, torn ligament and/or capsule, knee; collateral**
🚑 19.3 ⚕ 19.3 **FUD** 090 [T] [A2] [80] [50] 🔲
AMA: 2016,Jan,13; 2015,Jan,16; 2014,Jan,11; 2012,Dec,12

27407 **cruciate**
EXCLUDES Reconstruction (27427)
🚑 22.3 ⚕ 22.3 **FUD** 090 [J] [A2] [80] [50] 🔲
AMA: 2002,Apr,13; 1999,Nov,1

27409 **collateral and cruciate ligaments**
EXCLUDES Reconstruction (27427-27429)
🚑 27.4 ⚕ 27.4 **FUD** 090 [T] [A2] [80] [50] 🔲
AMA: 2002,Apr,13; 1999,Nov,1

27412 **Autologous chondrocyte implantation, knee**
EXCLUDES Arthrotomy, knee (27331)
Manipulation of knee joint under general anesthesia (27570)
Obtaining chondrocytes (29870)
Tissue grafts, other (eg, paratenon, fat, dermis) (20926)
🚑 47.7 ⚕ 47.7 **FUD** 090 [J] [80] [50] 🔲
AMA: 2002,Apr,13

27415   **Osteochondral allograft, knee, open**

EXCLUDES   *Arthroscopic procedure (29867)*
Osteochondral autograft knee (27416)

🚗 39.5   ⚕ 39.5   **FUD** 090   J G2 80 50 ▣

AMA: 2016,Jan,13; 2015,Jan,16; 2014,Jan,11; 2012,Jan,15-42;
2011,Jan,11

27416   **Osteochondral autograft(s), knee, open (eg, mosaicplasty)**
(includes harvesting of autograft[s])

EXCLUDES   *Procedures in the same compartment (29874, 29877,*
29879, 29885-29887)
Procedures performed at the same surgical session
(27415, 29870-29871, 29875, 29884)
Surgical arthroscopy of the knee with osteochondral
autograft(s) (29866)

🚗 28.1   ⚕ 28.1   **FUD** 090   J G2 80 50 ▣

AMA: 2016,Jan,13; 2015,Jan,16; 2014,Jan,11

27418   **Anterior tibial tubercleplasty (eg, Maquet type procedure)**

🚗 23.8   ⚕ 23.8   **FUD** 090   J A2 80 50 ▣

AMA: 2016,Jan,13; 2015,Jan,16; 2014,Jan,11; 2012,Jan,15-42;
2011,Jan,11

27420   **Reconstruction of dislocating patella; (eg, Hauser type**
procedure)

🚗 21.3   ⚕ 21.3   **FUD** 090   J A2 80 50 ▣

AMA: 2016,Jan,13; 2015,Jan,16; 2014,Jan,11; 2012,Nov,13-14

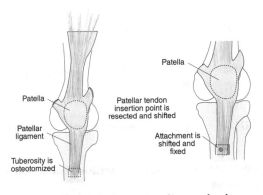

27422   **with extensor realignment and/or muscle advancement**
or release (eg, Campbell, Goldwaite type procedure)

🚗 21.3   ⚕ 21.3   **FUD** 090   T A2 80 50 ▣

AMA: 2016,Jan,13; 2015,Jan,16; 2014,Jan,11; 2012,Jan,15-42;
2011,Mar,9

27424   **with patellectomy**

🚗 21.5   ⚕ 21.5   **FUD** 090   T A2 80 50 ▣

AMA: 2002,Apr,13; 1998,Nov,1

27425   **Lateral retinacular release, open**

EXCLUDES   *Arthroscopic release (29873)*

🚗 12.8   ⚕ 12.8   **FUD** 090   T A2 50 ▣

AMA: 2016,Jan,13; 2015,Nov,7; 2015,Jan,16; 2014,Jan,11;
2012,Jan,15-42; 2011,Mar,9; 2011,Jan,11

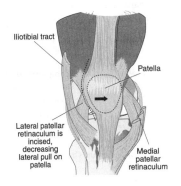

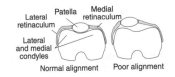

27427   **Ligamentous reconstruction (augmentation), knee;**
extra-articular

EXCLUDES   *Primary repair of ligament(s) (27405, 27407, 27409)*

🚗 20.4   ⚕ 20.4   **FUD** 090   J A2 80 50 ▣

AMA: 2016,Jan,13; 2015,Jan,16; 2014,Jan,11; 2012,Dec,12

27428   **intra-articular (open)**

EXCLUDES   *Primary repair of ligament(s) (27405, 27407, 27409)*

🚗 32.0   ⚕ 32.0   **FUD** 090   J G2 80 50 ▣

AMA: 2016,Jan,13; 2015,Jan,16; 2014,Jan,11; 2012,Jan,15-42;
2011,Jan,11

27429   **intra-articular (open) and extra-articular**

EXCLUDES   *Primary repair of ligament(s) (27405, 27407, 27409)*

🚗 35.8   ⚕ 35.8   **FUD** 090   J G2 80 50 ▣

AMA: 2016,Jan,13; 2015,Jan,16; 2014,Jan,11; 2012,Jan,15-42;
2011,Jan,11

27430   **Quadricepsplasty (eg, Bennett or Thompson type)**

🚗 21.2   ⚕ 21.2   **FUD** 090   T A2 80 50 ▣

AMA: 2002,Apr,13; 1998,Nov,1

27435   **Capsulotomy, posterior capsular release, knee**

🚗 23.1   ⚕ 23.1   **FUD** 090   T A2 80 50 ▣

AMA: 2002,Apr,13; 1998,Nov,1

27437   **Arthroplasty, patella; without prosthesis**

🚗 18.9   ⚕ 18.9   **FUD** 090   J A2 50 ▣

AMA: 2002,Apr,13

27438   **with prosthesis**

🚗 24.1   ⚕ 24.1   **FUD** 090   J J8 80 50 ▣

AMA: 2002,Apr,13

27440   **Arthroplasty, knee, tibial plateau;**

🚗 22.9   ⚕ 22.9   **FUD** 090   J J8 80 50 ▣

AMA: 2002,Apr,13

27441   **with debridement and partial synovectomy**

🚗 23.6   ⚕ 23.6   **FUD** 090   J J8 80 50 ▣

AMA: 2002,Apr,13

27442   **Arthroplasty, femoral condyles or tibial plateau(s), knee;**

🚗 25.0   ⚕ 25.0   **FUD** 090   J J8 80 50 ▣

AMA: 2016,Jun,8

27443   **with debridement and partial synovectomy**

🚗 23.2   ⚕ 23.2   **FUD** 090   J G2 80 50 ▣

AMA: 2002,Apr,13

27445 Arthroplasty, knee, hinge prosthesis (eg, Walldius type)
EXCLUDES Removal knee prosthesis (27488)
Revision knee arthroplasty (27487)
35.9   35.9   **FUD** 090   C 80 50
AMA: 2002,Apr,13; 1998,Nov,1

27446 Arthroplasty, knee, condyle and plateau; medial OR lateral compartment
EXCLUDES Removal knee prosthesis (27488)
Revision knee arthroplasty (27487)
33.4   33.4   **FUD** 090   J J8 80 50
AMA: 2002,Apr,13

27447 medial AND lateral compartments with or without patella resurfacing (total knee arthroplasty)
EXCLUDES Removal knee prosthesis (27488)
Revision knee arthroplasty (27487)
39.1   39.1   **FUD** 090   C 80 50
AMA: 2016,Jan,13; 2015,Jan,16; 2014,Jan,11

27448 Osteotomy, femur, shaft or supracondylar; without fixation
22.3   22.3   **FUD** 090   C 80 50
AMA: 2002,Apr,13

27450 with fixation
29.0   29.0   **FUD** 090   C 80 50
AMA: 2002,Apr,13

27454 Osteotomy, multiple, with realignment on intramedullary rod, femoral shaft (eg, Sofield type procedure)
37.5   37.5   **FUD** 090   C 80 50
AMA: 2002,Apr,13; 1998,Nov,1

27455 Osteotomy, proximal tibia, including fibular excision or osteotomy (includes correction of genu varus [bowleg] or genu valgus [knock-knee]); before epiphyseal closure
27.0   27.0   **FUD** 090   C 80 50
AMA: 2002,Apr,13

27457 after epiphyseal closure
27.2   27.2   **FUD** 090   C 80 50
AMA: 2002,Apr,13

27465 Osteoplasty, femur; shortening (excluding 64876)
35.6   35.6   **FUD** 090   C 80 50
AMA: 2002,Apr,13

27466 lengthening
33.9   33.9   **FUD** 090   C 80 50
AMA: 2002,Apr,13

27468 combined, lengthening and shortening with femoral segment transfer
35.4   35.4   **FUD** 090   C 80 50
AMA: 2002,Apr,13

27470 Repair, nonunion or malunion, femur, distal to head and neck; without graft (eg, compression technique)
33.8   33.8   **FUD** 090   C 80 50
AMA: 2002,Apr,13

27472 with iliac or other autogenous bone graft (includes obtaining graft)
36.3   36.3   **FUD** 090   C 80 50
AMA: 2002,Apr,13

27475 Arrest, epiphyseal, any method (eg, epiphysiodesis); distal femur
19.0   19.0   **FUD** 090   T 62 50
AMA: 2002,Apr,13; 2002,May,7

27477 tibia and fibula, proximal
21.0   21.0   **FUD** 090   T 50
AMA: 2002,May,7; 2002,Apr,13

27479 combined distal femur, proximal tibia and fibula
22.6   22.6   **FUD** 090   T 62 80 50
AMA: 2002,May,7; 2002,Apr,13

27485 Arrest, hemiepiphyseal, distal femur or proximal tibia or fibula (eg, genu varus or valgus)
19.2   19.2   **FUD** 090   T 50
AMA: 2002,Apr,13; 1998,Nov,1

27486 Revision of total knee arthroplasty, with or without allograft; 1 component
40.5   40.5   **FUD** 090   C 80 50
AMA: 2016,Jan,13; 2015,Jul,10; 2015,Jan,16; 2014,Jan,11; 2013,Dec,16

27487 femoral and entire tibial component
50.7   50.7   **FUD** 090   C 80 50
AMA: 2016,Jan,13; 2015,Jan,16; 2013,Jul,6

27488 Removal of prosthesis, including total knee prosthesis, methylmethacrylate with or without insertion of spacer, knee
34.6   34.6   **FUD** 090   C 80 50
AMA: 2016,Jan,13; 2015,Jan,16; 2013,Jul,6

27495 Prophylactic treatment (nailing, pinning, plating, or wiring) with or without methylmethacrylate, femur
32.4   32.4   **FUD** 090   C 80 50
AMA: 2002,Apr,13

27496 Decompression fasciotomy, thigh and/or knee, 1 compartment (flexor or extensor or adductor);
15.5   15.5   **FUD** 090   T A2 50
AMA: 2002,Apr,13

27497 with debridement of nonviable muscle and/or nerve
16.6   16.6   **FUD** 090   T A2 80 50
AMA: 2002,Apr,13

27498 Decompression fasciotomy, thigh and/or knee, multiple compartments;
18.5   18.5   **FUD** 090   T A2 80 50
AMA: 2002,Apr,13

27499 with debridement of nonviable muscle and/or nerve
20.0   20.0   **FUD** 090   T A2 80 50
AMA: 2002,Apr,13

27500-27566 Treatment of Fracture/Dislocation of Femur/Knee

INCLUDES Closed, percutaneous, and open treatment of fractures and dislocations

27500 Closed treatment of femoral shaft fracture, without manipulation
13.7   14.8   **FUD** 090   T A2 50
AMA: 2002,Apr,13

27501 Closed treatment of supracondylar or transcondylar femoral fracture with or without intercondylar extension, without manipulation
14.3   14.4   **FUD** 090   T A2 80 50
AMA: 2002,Apr,13

27502 Closed treatment of femoral shaft fracture, with manipulation, with or without skin or skeletal traction
21.9   21.9   **FUD** 090   T A2 50
AMA: 2016,Jan,13; 2015,Jan,16; 2014,Jan,11

27503 Closed treatment of supracondylar or transcondylar femoral fracture with or without intercondylar extension, with manipulation, with or without skin or skeletal traction
23.0   23.0   **FUD** 090   T A2 80 50
AMA: 2002,Apr,13

27506 Open treatment of femoral shaft fracture, with or without external fixation, with insertion of intramedullary implant, with or without cerclage and/or locking screws
38.5   38.5   **FUD** 090   C 80 50
AMA: 2016,Jan,13; 2015,Jan,16; 2014,Jan,11

27507 Open treatment of femoral shaft fracture with plate/screws, with or without cerclage
28.0   28.0   **FUD** 090   C 80 50
AMA: 2002,Apr,13

27508 Closed treatment of femoral fracture, distal end, medial or lateral condyle, without manipulation
🔧 14.1 ✂ 15.0 **FUD** 090 Ⓣ A2 50 ▣
AMA: 2002,Apr,13

27509 Percutaneous skeletal fixation of femoral fracture, distal end, medial or lateral condyle, or supracondylar or transcondylar, with or without intercondylar extension, or distal femoral epiphyseal separation
🔧 18.4 ✂ 18.4 **FUD** 090 Ⓙ A2 80 50 ▣
AMA: 2002,Apr,13; 1993,Win,1

Pins are placed percutaneously

27510 Closed treatment of femoral fracture, distal end, medial or lateral condyle, with manipulation
🔧 19.6 ✂ 19.6 **FUD** 090 Ⓣ A2 50 ▣
AMA: 2002,Apr,13

27511 Open treatment of femoral supracondylar or transcondylar fracture without intercondylar extension, includes internal fixation, when performed
🔧 28.7 ✂ 28.7 **FUD** 090 Ⓒ 80 50 ▣
AMA: 2002,Apr,13; 1996,May,6

27513 Open treatment of femoral supracondylar or transcondylar fracture with intercondylar extension, includes internal fixation, when performed
🔧 35.8 ✂ 35.8 **FUD** 090 Ⓒ 80 50 ▣
AMA: 2002,Apr,13

27514 Open treatment of femoral fracture, distal end, medial or lateral condyle, includes internal fixation, when performed
🔧 27.8 ✂ 27.8 **FUD** 090 Ⓒ 80 50 ▣
AMA: 2002,Apr,13

27516 Closed treatment of distal femoral epiphyseal separation; without manipulation
🔧 13.6 ✂ 14.5 **FUD** 090 Ⓣ A2 50 ▣
AMA: 2002,Apr,13

27517 with manipulation, with or without skin or skeletal traction
🔧 19.3 ✂ 19.3 **FUD** 090 Ⓣ A2 80 50 ▣
AMA: 2002,Apr,13

27519 Open treatment of distal femoral epiphyseal separation, includes internal fixation, when performed
🔧 25.7 ✂ 25.7 **FUD** 090 Ⓒ 80 50 ▣
AMA: 2002,Apr,13

27520 Closed treatment of patellar fracture, without manipulation
🔧 8.40 ✂ 9.20 **FUD** 090 Ⓣ A2 50 ▣
AMA: 2002,Apr,13

27524 Open treatment of patellar fracture, with internal fixation and/or partial or complete patellectomy and soft tissue repair
🔧 21.6 ✂ 21.6 **FUD** 090 Ⓣ 62 80 50 ▣
AMA: 2002,Apr,13

27530 Closed treatment of tibial fracture, proximal (plateau); without manipulation
EXCLUDES Arthroscopic repair (29855-29856)
🔧 8.00 ✂ 8.60 **FUD** 090 Ⓣ A2 50 ▣
AMA: 2002,Apr,13

27532 with or without manipulation, with skeletal traction
EXCLUDES Arthroscopic repair (29855-29856)
🔧 16.5 ✂ 17.6 **FUD** 090 Ⓣ A2 50 ▣
AMA: 2002,Apr,13

27535 Open treatment of tibial fracture, proximal (plateau); unicondylar, includes internal fixation, when performed
EXCLUDES Arthroscopic repair (29855-29856)
🔧 25.8 ✂ 25.8 **FUD** 090 Ⓒ 80 50 ▣
AMA: 2002,Apr,13

27536 bicondylar, with or without internal fixation
EXCLUDES Arthroscopic repair (29855-29856)
🔧 34.3 ✂ 34.3 **FUD** 090 Ⓒ 80 50 ▣
AMA: 2002,Apr,13

27538 Closed treatment of intercondylar spine(s) and/or tuberosity fracture(s) of knee, with or without manipulation
EXCLUDES Arthroscopic repair (29850-29851)
🔧 12.6 ✂ 13.4 **FUD** 090 Ⓣ A2 80 50 ▣
AMA: 2002,Apr,13

27540 Open treatment of intercondylar spine(s) and/or tuberosity fracture(s) of the knee, includes internal fixation, when performed
🔧 23.2 ✂ 23.2 **FUD** 090 Ⓒ 80 50 ▣
AMA: 2002,Apr,13

27550 Closed treatment of knee dislocation; without anesthesia
🔧 13.3 ✂ 14.4 **FUD** 090 Ⓣ A2 80 50 ▣
AMA: 2002,Apr,13

27552 requiring anesthesia
🔧 17.9 ✂ 17.9 **FUD** 090 Ⓣ A2 80 50 ▣
AMA: 2002,Apr,13

27556 Open treatment of knee dislocation, includes internal fixation, when performed; without primary ligamentous repair or augmentation/reconstruction
🔧 25.2 ✂ 25.2 **FUD** 090 Ⓒ 80 50 ▣
AMA: 2002,Apr,13

27557 with primary ligamentous repair
🔧 30.2 ✂ 30.2 **FUD** 090 Ⓒ 80 50 ▣
AMA: 2002,Apr,13

27558 with primary ligamentous repair, with augmentation/reconstruction
🔧 34.3 ✂ 34.3 **FUD** 090 Ⓒ 80 50 ▣
AMA: 2002,Apr,13

27560 Closed treatment of patellar dislocation; without anesthesia
EXCLUDES Recurrent dislocation (27420-27424)
🔧 9.51 ✂ 10.3 **FUD** 090 Ⓣ A2 50 ▣
AMA: 2002,Apr,13

27562 requiring anesthesia
EXCLUDES Recurrent dislocation (27420-27424)
🔧 13.4 ✂ 13.4 **FUD** 090 Ⓣ A2 80 50 ▣
AMA: 2002,Apr,13

27566 Open treatment of patellar dislocation, with or without partial or total patellectomy
EXCLUDES Recurrent dislocation (27420-27424)
🔧 25.6 ✂ 25.6 **FUD** 090 Ⓣ A2 80 50 ▣
AMA: 2002,Apr,13

● New Code ▲ Revised Code ○ Reinstated ● New Web Release ▲ Revised Web Release Unlisted Not Covered # Resequenced
⊘ AMA Mod 51 Exempt ⑨ Optum Mod 51 Exempt ⑥³ Mod 63 Exempt ⁄ Non-FDA Drug ★ Telehealth Ⓜ Maternity Ⓐ Age Edit + Add-on **AMA:** CPT Asst

27570 Knee Manipulation with Anesthesia

27570 Manipulation of knee joint under general anesthesia (includes application of traction or other fixation devices)
🚗 4.34　🔪 4.34　**FUD** 010　　T A2 50 ▢
AMA: 2016,Jan,13; 2015,Jan,16; 2014,Jan,11; 2012,Jan,15-42; 2011,Mar,9

27580 Knee Arthrodesis

27580 Arthrodesis, knee, any technique
INCLUDES　Albert's operation
🚗 41.4　🔪 41.4　**FUD** 090　　C 80 50 ▢
AMA: 2002,Apr,13

27590-27599 Amputations and Unlisted Procedures at Femur or Knee

27590 Amputation, thigh, through femur, any level;
🚗 23.4　🔪 23.4　**FUD** 090　　C 80 50 ▢
AMA: 2002,Apr,13

27591 immediate fitting technique including first cast
🚗 27.7　🔪 27.7　**FUD** 090　　C 80 50 ▢
AMA: 2002,Apr,13

27592 open, circular (guillotine)
🚗 19.8　🔪 19.8　**FUD** 090　　C 80 50 ▢
AMA: 2002,Apr,13

27594 secondary closure or scar revision
🚗 14.7　🔪 14.7　**FUD** 090　　T A2 50 ▢
AMA: 2002,Apr,13

27596 re-amputation
🚗 21.0　🔪 21.0　**FUD** 090　　C 50 ▢
AMA: 2002,Apr,13

27598 Disarticulation at knee
INCLUDES　Batch-Spittler-McFaddin operation
Callandar knee disarticulation
Gritti amputation
🚗 21.0　🔪 21.0　**FUD** 090　　C 80 50 ▢
AMA: 2002,Apr,13

27599 Unlisted procedure, femur or knee
🚗 0.00　🔪 0.00　**FUD** YYY　　T 80 50
AMA: 2016,Jun,8; 2016,Jan,13; 2015,Jan,16; 2015,Jan,13; 2014,Jan,9; 2014,Jan,11; 2012,Dec,12; 2012,Jan,15-42; 2011,Jan,11

27600-27602 Decompression Fasciotomy of Leg

EXCLUDES　Fasciotomy with debridement (27892-27894)
Simple incision and drainage (10140-10160)

27600 Decompression fasciotomy, leg; anterior and/or lateral compartments only
🚗 11.8　🔪 11.8　**FUD** 090　　T A2 50 ▢
AMA: 2002,Apr,13

27601 posterior compartment(s) only
🚗 12.7　🔪 12.7　**FUD** 090　　T A2 50 ▢
AMA: 2002,Apr,13

27602 anterior and/or lateral, and posterior compartment(s)
🚗 14.2　🔪 14.2　**FUD** 090　　T A2 80 50 ▢
AMA: 2002,Apr,13

27603-27612 Incisional Procedures Lower Leg and Ankle

27603 Incision and drainage, leg or ankle; deep abscess or hematoma
🚗 11.1　🔪 15.1　**FUD** 090　　T A2 50 ▢
AMA: 2002,Apr,13

27604 infected bursa
🚗 9.96　🔪 14.1　**FUD** 090　　T A2 80 50 ▢
AMA: 2002,Apr,13

27605 Tenotomy, percutaneous, Achilles tendon (separate procedure); local anesthesia
🚗 5.30　🔪 9.77　**FUD** 010　　T A2 80 50 ▢
AMA: 2002,Apr,13; 1998,Nov,1

27606 general anesthesia
🚗 8.15　🔪 8.15　**FUD** 010　　T A2 50 ▢
AMA: 2002,Apr,13

27607 Incision (eg, osteomyelitis or bone abscess), leg or ankle
🚗 17.4　🔪 17.4　**FUD** 090　　T A2 50 ▢
AMA: 2002,Apr,13; 1998,Nov,1

27610 Arthrotomy, ankle, including exploration, drainage, or removal of foreign body
🚗 18.7　🔪 18.7　**FUD** 090　　T A2 50 ▢
AMA: 2002,Apr,13; 1998,Nov,1

27612 Arthrotomy, posterior capsular release, ankle, with or without Achilles tendon lengthening
EXCLUDES　Lengthening or shortening tendon (27685)
🚗 16.0　🔪 16.0　**FUD** 090　　T A2 80 50 ▢
AMA: 2002,Apr,13; 1998,Nov,1

27613-27614 Biopsy Lower Leg and Ankle

EXCLUDES　Needle biopsy (20206)

27613 Biopsy, soft tissue of leg or ankle area; superficial
🚗 4.67　🔪 7.20　**FUD** 010　　T P3 50 ▢
AMA: 2002,Apr,13

27614 deep (subfascial or intramuscular)
🚗 11.6　🔪 16.5　**FUD** 090　　T A2 50 ▢
AMA: 2002,Apr,13; 1998,Nov,1

27615-27619 [27632, 27634] Excision Soft Tissue Tumors Lower Leg/Ankle

INCLUDES　Any necessary elevation of tissue planes or dissection
Measurement of tumor and necessary margin at greatest diameter prior to excision
Resection without removal of significant normal tissue
Simple and intermediate repairs
Types of excision:
　Fascial or subfascial soft tissue tumors: simple and marginal resection of most often benign and intramuscular tumors found either in or below the deep fascia, not involving bone
　Resection of the tumor (may include entire bone) and wide margins of normal tissue primarily for malignant or aggressive benign tumors
　Subcutaneous: simple and marginal resection of most often benign tumors found in the subcutaneous tissue above the deep fascia

EXCLUDES　Complex repair
Excision of benign cutaneous lesions (eg, sebaceous cyst) (11400-11406)
Radical resection of cutaneous tumors (eg, melanoma) (11600-11606)
Significant exploration of vessels or neuroplasty

27615 Radical resection of tumor (eg, sarcoma), soft tissue of leg or ankle area; less than 5 cm
🚗 29.5　🔪 29.5　**FUD** 090　　T G2 80 50 ▢
AMA: 2002,Apr,13; 1990,Win,4

27616 5 cm or greater
🚗 36.6　🔪 36.6　**FUD** 090　　T G2 80 50 ▢

27618 Excision, tumor, soft tissue of leg or ankle area, subcutaneous; less than 3 cm
🚗 8.83　🔪 12.8　**FUD** 090　　T G2 50 ▢
AMA: 2016,Jan,13; 2015,Jan,16; 2014,Jan,11

\# **27632** 3 cm or greater
🚗 11.9　🔪 11.9　**FUD** 090　　T G2 80 50 ▢

27619 Excision, tumor, soft tissue of leg or ankle area, subfascial (eg, intramuscular); less than 5 cm
🚗 13.4　🔪 13.4　**FUD** 090　　T G2 50 ▢
AMA: 2002,Apr,13

\# **27634** 5 cm or greater
🚗 19.7　🔪 19.7　**FUD** 090　　T G2 80 50 ▢

27620-27641 Bone and Joint Procedures Ankle/Leg

27620 Arthrotomy, ankle, with joint exploration, with or without biopsy, with or without removal of loose or foreign body
🚗 13.0　🔪 13.0　**FUD** 090　　T A2 80 50 ▢
AMA: 2002,Apr,13

27625 Arthrotomy, with synovectomy, ankle;
    16.8   16.8   **FUD** 090   T A2 80 50
    AMA: 2002,Apr,13; 1998,Nov,1

27626 including tenosynovectomy
    17.7   17.7   **FUD** 090   T A2 80 50
    AMA: 2002,Apr,13

27630 Excision of lesion of tendon sheath or capsule (eg, cyst or ganglion), leg and/or ankle
    10.5   16.0   **FUD** 090   T A2 50
    AMA: 2002,Apr,13

27632 Resequenced code. See code following 27618.

27634 Resequenced code. See code following 27619.

27635 Excision or curettage of bone cyst or benign tumor, tibia or fibula;
    16.8   16.8   **FUD** 090   T A2 50
    AMA: 2016,Jan,13; 2015,Jan,16; 2014,Jan,11; 2012,Apr,17-18

27637 with autograft (includes obtaining graft)
    21.5   21.5   **FUD** 090   J A2 80 50
    AMA: 2002,Apr,13

27638 with allograft
    21.9   21.9   **FUD** 090   J A2 80 50
    AMA: 2002,Apr,13

27640 Partial excision (craterization, saucerization, or diaphysectomy), bone (eg, osteomyelitis); tibia
    EXCLUDES *Excision of exostosis (27635)*
    24.0   24.0   **FUD** 090   T A2 50
    AMA: 2016,Jan,13; 2015,Jan,16; 2014,Jan,11; 2012,Apr,17-18

27641 fibula
    EXCLUDES *Excision of exostosis (27635)*
    19.2   19.2   **FUD** 090   T A2 50
    AMA: 2002,Apr,13

27645-27647 Radical Resection Bone Tumor Ankle/Leg

INCLUDES Any necessary elevation of tissue planes or dissection
Excision of adjacent soft tissue during bone tumor resection (27615-27619 [27632, 27634])
Measurement of tumor and necessary margin at greatest diameter prior to excision
Resection of the tumor (may include entire bone) and wide margins of normal tissue primarily for malignant or aggressive benign tumors
Simple and intermediate repairs

EXCLUDES *Complex repair*
Significant exploration of vessels, neuroplasty, reconstruction, or complex bone repair

27645 Radical resection of tumor; tibia
    51.2   51.2   **FUD** 090   C 80 50
    AMA: 2002,Apr,13; 1994,Win,1

27646 fibula
    44.3   44.3   **FUD** 090   C 80 50
    AMA: 2002,Apr,13; 1994,Win,1

27647 talus or calcaneus
    29.4   29.4   **FUD** 090   T A2 80 50
    AMA: 2002,Apr,13; 1994,Win,1

27648 Injection for Ankle Arthrogram

EXCLUDES *Arthroscopy (29894-29898)*

27648 Injection procedure for ankle arthrography
    (73615)
    1.52   4.67   **FUD** 000   N N1 80 50
    AMA: 2016,Jan,13; 2015,Aug,6

27650-27745 Repair/Reconstruction Lower Leg/Ankle

27650 Repair, primary, open or percutaneous, ruptured Achilles tendon;
    18.9   18.9   **FUD** 090   T A2 80 50
    AMA: 2016,Jan,13; 2015,Jan,16; 2014,Jul,5

27652 with graft (includes obtaining graft)
    19.6   19.6   **FUD** 090   J A2 50
    AMA: 2016,Jan,13; 2015,Jan,16; 2014,Jul,5

27654 Repair, secondary, Achilles tendon, with or without graft
    20.3   20.3   **FUD** 090   J A2 80 50
    AMA: 2016,Jan,13; 2015,Jan,16; 2014,Jul,5

27656 Repair, fascial defect of leg
    11.3   18.1   **FUD** 090   T A2 80 50
    AMA: 2002,Apr,13

27658 Repair, flexor tendon, leg; primary, without graft, each tendon
    10.7   10.7   **FUD** 090   T A2 80
    AMA: 2002,Apr,13; 1998,Nov,1

27659 secondary, with or without graft, each tendon
    13.8   13.8   **FUD** 090   T A2 80
    AMA: 2016,Jan,13; 2015,Jan,13

27664 Repair, extensor tendon, leg; primary, without graft, each tendon
    10.3   10.3   **FUD** 090   T A2 80
    AMA: 2016,Jan,13; 2015,Jan,13

27665 secondary, with or without graft, each tendon
    11.8   11.8   **FUD** 090   J A2 80
    AMA: 2002,Apr,13; 1998,Nov,1

27675 Repair, dislocating peroneal tendons; without fibular osteotomy
    13.9   13.9   **FUD** 090   T A2 80 50
    AMA: 2002,Apr,13; 1998,Nov,1

27676 with fibular osteotomy
    17.3   17.3   **FUD** 090   T A2 80 50
    AMA: 2002,Apr,13

27680 Tenolysis, flexor or extensor tendon, leg and/or ankle; single, each tendon
    12.3   12.3   **FUD** 090   T A2
    AMA: 2016,Jan,13; 2015,Jan,16; 2014,Jan,11

27681 multiple tendons (through separate incision[s])
    15.6   15.6   **FUD** 090   T A2 50
    AMA: 2002,Apr,13; 1998,Nov,1

27685 Lengthening or shortening of tendon, leg or ankle; single tendon (separate procedure)
    13.3   19.0   **FUD** 090   T A2 80 50
    AMA: 2016,Jan,13; 2015,Jan,16; 2014,Jan,11; 2012,Jan,15-42; 2011,Jan,11

27686 multiple tendons (through same incision), each
    16.0   16.0   **FUD** 090   T A2 50
    AMA: 2016,Jan,13; 2015,Jan,16; 2014,Jan,11; 2012,Jan,15-42; 2011,Jan,11

27687 Gastrocnemius recession (eg, Strayer procedure)
    13.0   13.0   **FUD** 090   T A2 80 50
    AMA: 2002,Apr,13

27690 Transfer or transplant of single tendon (with muscle redirection or rerouting); superficial (eg, anterior tibial extensors into midfoot)
    INCLUDES Toe extensors considered a single tendon with transplant into midfoot
    18.1   18.1   **FUD** 090   T A2 80 50
    AMA: 2002,Apr,13; 1995,Win,1

27691 deep (eg, anterior tibial or posterior tibial through interosseous space, flexor digitorum longus, flexor hallucis longus, or peroneal tendon to midfoot or hindfoot)
    INCLUDES Barr procedure
    Toe extensors considered a single tendon with transplant into midfoot
    21.5   21.5   **FUD** 090   T A2 80 50
    AMA: 2002,Apr,13; 1995,Win,1

Musculoskeletal System

27692 — 27759

+ **27692** **each additional tendon (List separately in addition to code for primary procedure)**
> INCLUDES Toe extensors considered a single tendon with transplant into midfoot
> Code first (27690-27691)
> 🦴 3.03 ⚖ 3.03 **FUD** ZZZ [N] [N1] [80] ▭
> **AMA:** 2003,Feb,7; 2002,Apr,13

27695 **Repair, primary, disrupted ligament, ankle; collateral**
> 🦴 13.6 ⚖ 13.6 **FUD** 090 [T] [A2] [50] ▭
> **AMA:** 2016,Jan,13; 2015,Jan,16; 2014,Mar,13; 2014,Jan,11

Lateral view of right ankle showing components of the collateral ligament

27696 **both collateral ligaments**
> 🦴 15.9 ⚖ 15.9 **FUD** 090 [T] [A2] [50] ▭
> **AMA:** 2016,Jan,13; 2015,Jan,16; 2014,Mar,13

27698 **Repair, secondary, disrupted ligament, ankle, collateral (eg, Watson-Jones procedure)**
> 🦴 18.4 ⚖ 18.4 **FUD** 090 [T] [A2] [80] [50] ▭
> **AMA:** 2016,Jan,13; 2015,Jan,16; 2014,Mar,13

27700 **Arthroplasty, ankle;**
> 🦴 17.1 ⚖ 17.1 **FUD** 090 [J] [A2] [80] [50] ▭
> **AMA:** 2002,Apr,13

27702 **with implant (total ankle)**
> 🦴 27.8 ⚖ 27.8 **FUD** 090 [C] [80] [50] ▭
> **AMA:** 2002,Apr,13

27703 **revision, total ankle**
> 🦴 31.9 ⚖ 31.9 **FUD** 090 [C] [80] [50] ▭
> **AMA:** 2002,Apr,13; 1998,Nov,1

27704 **Removal of ankle implant**
> 🦴 16.5 ⚖ 16.5 **FUD** 090 [02] [A2] [50] ▭
> **AMA:** 2002,Apr,13

27705 **Osteotomy; tibia**
> EXCLUDES Genu varus or genu valgus repair (27455-27457)
> 🦴 21.8 ⚖ 21.8 **FUD** 090 [T] [A2] [80] [50] ▭
> **AMA:** 2002,Apr,13

27707 **fibula**
> EXCLUDES Genu varus or genu valgus repair (27455-27457)
> 🦴 11.5 ⚖ 11.5 **FUD** 090 [T] [A2] [50] ▭
> **AMA:** 2002,Apr,13

27709 **tibia and fibula**
> EXCLUDES Genu varus or genu valgus repair (27455-27457)
> 🦴 33.6 ⚖ 33.6 **FUD** 090 [J] [A2] [80] [50] ▭
> **AMA:** 2002,Apr,13

27712 **multiple, with realignment on intramedullary rod (eg, Sofield type procedure)**
> EXCLUDES Genu varus or genu valgus repair (27455-27457)
> 🦴 31.7 ⚖ 31.7 **FUD** 090 [C] [80] [50] ▭
> **AMA:** 2002,Apr,13; 1998,Nov,1

27715 **Osteoplasty, tibia and fibula, lengthening or shortening**
> INCLUDES Anderson tibial lengthening
> 🦴 30.8 ⚖ 30.8 **FUD** 090 [C] [80] [50] ▭
> **AMA:** 2002,Apr,13; 1998,Nov,1

27720 **Repair of nonunion or malunion, tibia; without graft, (eg, compression technique)**
> 🦴 25.1 ⚖ 25.1 **FUD** 090 [J] [G2] [80] [50] ▭
> **AMA:** 2002,Apr,13

27722 **with sliding graft**
> 🦴 25.2 ⚖ 25.2 **FUD** 090 [J] [80] [50] ▭
> **AMA:** 2002,Apr,13

27724 **with iliac or other autograft (includes obtaining graft)**
> 🦴 36.4 ⚖ 36.4 **FUD** 090 [C] [80] [50] ▭
> **AMA:** 2016,Jan,13; 2015,Jan,16; 2014,Jan,11; 2012,May,11-12

27725 **by synostosis, with fibula, any method**
> 🦴 34.7 ⚖ 34.7 **FUD** 090 [C] [80] [50] ▭
> **AMA:** 2002,Apr,13

27726 **Repair of fibula nonunion and/or malunion with internal fixation**
> INCLUDES Osteotomy; fibula (27707)
> 🦴 27.8 ⚖ 27.8 **FUD** 090 [J] [G2] [50] ▭
> **AMA:** 2016,Jan,13; 2015,Jan,16; 2014,Jan,11; 2012,Jan,15-42; 2011,Jan,11

27727 **Repair of congenital pseudarthrosis, tibia**
> 🦴 29.8 ⚖ 29.8 **FUD** 090 [C] [80] [50] ▭
> **AMA:** 2002,Apr,13

27730 **Arrest, epiphyseal (epiphysiodesis), open; distal tibia**
> 🦴 16.3 ⚖ 16.3 **FUD** 090 [T] [A2] [50] ▭
> **AMA:** 2002,Apr,13; 1998,Nov,1

27732 **distal fibula**
> 🦴 11.6 ⚖ 11.6 **FUD** 090 [T] [A2] [50] ▭
> **AMA:** 2002,Apr,13

27734 **distal tibia and fibula**
> 🦴 18.8 ⚖ 18.8 **FUD** 090 [T] [A2] [50] ▭
> **AMA:** 2002,Apr,13

27740 **Arrest, epiphyseal (epiphysiodesis), any method, combined, proximal and distal tibia and fibula;**
> EXCLUDES Epiphyseal arrest of proximal tibia and fibula (27477)
> 🦴 20.3 ⚖ 20.3 **FUD** 090 [T] [A2] [80] [50] ▭
> **AMA:** 2002,Apr,13; 1998,Nov,1

27742 **and distal femur**
> EXCLUDES Epiphyseal arrest of proximal tibia and fibula (27477)
> 🦴 22.2 ⚖ 22.2 **FUD** 090 [T] [A2] [80] [50] ▭
> **AMA:** 2002,Apr,13

27745 **Prophylactic treatment (nailing, pinning, plating or wiring) with or without methylmethacrylate, tibia**
> 🦴 21.7 ⚖ 21.7 **FUD** 090 [J] [G2] [80] [50] ▭
> **AMA:** 2002,Apr,13

27750-27848 Treatment of Fracture/Dislocation Lower Leg/Ankle
INCLUDES Treatment of open or closed fracture or dislocation

27750 **Closed treatment of tibial shaft fracture (with or without fibular fracture); without manipulation**
> 🦴 9.07 ⚖ 9.87 **FUD** 090 [T] [A2] [50] ▭
> **AMA:** 2016,Jan,13; 2015,Jan,16; 2014,Jan,11; 2012,Jan,15-42; 2011,Jan,11

27752 **with manipulation, with or without skeletal traction**
> 🦴 14.2 ⚖ 15.3 **FUD** 090 [T] [A2] [50] ▭
> **AMA:** 2016,Jan,13; 2015,Jan,16; 2014,Jan,11

27756 **Percutaneous skeletal fixation of tibial shaft fracture (with or without fibular fracture) (eg, pins or screws)**
> 🦴 16.4 ⚖ 16.4 **FUD** 090 [J] [A2] [80] [50] ▭
> **AMA:** 2016,Jan,13; 2015,Jan,16; 2014,Jan,11

27758 **Open treatment of tibial shaft fracture (with or without fibular fracture), with plate/screws, with or without cerclage**
> 🦴 25.6 ⚖ 25.6 **FUD** 090 [J] [G2] [80] [50] ▭
> **AMA:** 2016,Jan,13; 2015,Jan,16; 2014,Jan,11; 2012,Jan,15-42; 2011,Jan,11

27759 **Treatment of tibial shaft fracture (with or without fibular fracture) by intramedullary implant, with or without interlocking screws and/or cerclage**
> 🦴 28.7 ⚖ 28.7 **FUD** 090 [J] [G2] [80] [50] ▭
> **AMA:** 2016,Jan,13; 2015,Jan,16; 2014,Jan,11

| 26/TC PC/TC Only | A2-Z3 ASC Payment | 50 Bilateral | ♂ Male Only | ♀ Female Only | 🦴 Facility RVU | ⚖ Non-Facility RVU | ▭ CCI |
| FUD Follow-up Days | CMS: IOM (Pub 100) | A-Y OPPSI | 80/80 Surg Assist Allowed / w/Doc | | 🧪 Lab Crosswalk | Radiology Crosswalk | ❌ CLIA |

88

CPT © 2016 American Medical Association. All Rights Reserved.

© 2016 Optum360, LLC

27760 Closed treatment of medial malleolus fracture; without manipulation
🦴 8.68 ⚕ 9.50 **FUD** 090   T A2 50 ▭
AMA: 2002,Apr,13; 1994,Sum,29

27762 with manipulation, with or without skin or skeletal traction
🦴 12.3 ⚕ 13.5 **FUD** 090   T A2 50 ▭
AMA: 2002,Apr,13; 1994,Sum,29

27766 Open treatment of medial malleolus fracture, includes internal fixation, when performed
🦴 17.5 ⚕ 17.5 **FUD** 090   T A2 50 ▭
AMA: 2002,Apr,13; 1994,Sum,29

27767 Closed treatment of posterior malleolus fracture; without manipulation
🦴 8.06 ⚕ 8.01 **FUD** 090   T P2 50 ▭
EXCLUDES *Treatment of bimalleolar ankle fracture (27808-27814)*
Treatment of trimalleolar ankle fracture (27816-27823)

27768 with manipulation
🦴 12.6 ⚕ 12.6 **FUD** 090   T G2 50 ▭
EXCLUDES *Treatment of bimalleolar ankle fracture (27808-27814)*
Treatment of trimalleolar ankle fracture (27816-27823)

27769 Open treatment of posterior malleolus fracture, includes internal fixation, when performed
🦴 21.0 ⚕ 21.0 **FUD** 090   J G2 50 ▭
EXCLUDES *Treatment of bimalleolar ankle fracture (27808-27814)*
Treatment of trimalleolar ankle fracture (27816-27823)

27780 Closed treatment of proximal fibula or shaft fracture; without manipulation
🦴 7.95 ⚕ 8.73 **FUD** 090   T A2 50 ▭
AMA: 2016,Jan,13; 2015,Jan,16; 2014,Jan,11

27781 with manipulation
🦴 11.1 ⚕ 12.0 **FUD** 090   T A2 50 ▭
AMA: 2002,Apr,13

27784 Open treatment of proximal fibula or shaft fracture, includes internal fixation, when performed
🦴 20.5 ⚕ 20.5 **FUD** 090   J A2 50 ▭
AMA: 2016,Jan,13; 2015,Jan,16; 2014,Jan,11; 2012,Jan,15-42; 2011,Jan,11

27786 Closed treatment of distal fibular fracture (lateral malleolus); without manipulation
🦴 8.16 ⚕ 9.01 **FUD** 090   T A2 50 ▭
AMA: 2002,Apr,13

27788 with manipulation
🦴 10.9 ⚕ 12.0 **FUD** 090   T A2 50 ▭
AMA: 2002,Apr,13

27792 Open treatment of distal fibular fracture (lateral malleolus), includes internal fixation, when performed
EXCLUDES *Repair of tibia and fibula shaft fracture (27750-27759)*
🦴 18.7 ⚕ 18.7 **FUD** 090   J A2 50 ▭
AMA: 2016,Jan,13; 2015,Jan,16; 2014,Jan,11

27808 Closed treatment of bimalleolar ankle fracture (eg, lateral and medial malleoli, or lateral and posterior malleoli or medial and posterior malleoli); without manipulation
🦴 8.56 ⚕ 9.52 **FUD** 090   T A2 50 ▭
AMA: 2002,Apr,13

27810 with manipulation
🦴 12.1 ⚕ 13.3 **FUD** 090   T A2 50 ▭
AMA: 2002,Apr,13

27814 Open treatment of bimalleolar ankle fracture (eg, lateral and medial malleoli, or lateral and posterior malleoli, or medial and posterior malleoli), includes internal fixation, when performed
🦴 22.2 ⚕ 22.2 **FUD** 090   J A2 80 50 ▭
AMA: 2016,Feb,13

27816 Closed treatment of trimalleolar ankle fracture; without manipulation
🦴 8.19 ⚕ 9.12 **FUD** 090   T A2 50 ▭
AMA: 2002,Apr,13

27818 with manipulation
🦴 12.4 ⚕ 13.8 **FUD** 090   T A2 50 ▭
AMA: 2002,Apr,13

27822 Open treatment of trimalleolar ankle fracture, includes internal fixation, when performed, medial and/or lateral malleolus; without fixation of posterior lip
🦴 24.1 ⚕ 24.1 **FUD** 090   J A2 80 50 ▭
AMA: 2002,Apr,13

27823 with fixation of posterior lip
🦴 27.4 ⚕ 27.4 **FUD** 090   J G2 80 50 ▭
AMA: 2002,Apr,13

27824 Closed treatment of fracture of weight bearing articular portion of distal tibia (eg, pilon or tibial plafond), with or without anesthesia; without manipulation
🦴 8.70 ⚕ 8.95 **FUD** 090   T A2 50 ▭
AMA: 2002,Apr,13

27825 with skeletal traction and/or requiring manipulation
🦴 14.1 ⚕ 15.5 **FUD** 090   T A2 80 50 ▭
AMA: 2002,Apr,13

27826 Open treatment of fracture of weight bearing articular surface/portion of distal tibia (eg, pilon or tibial plafond), with internal fixation, when performed; of fibula only
🦴 23.9 ⚕ 23.9 **FUD** 090   J A2 80 50 ▭
AMA: 2002,Apr,13

27827 of tibia only
🦴 31.0 ⚕ 31.0 **FUD** 090   J G2 80 50 ▭
AMA: 2002,Apr,13

27828 of both tibia and fibula
🦴 37.2 ⚕ 37.2 **FUD** 090   J G2 80 50 ▭
AMA: 2016,Jan,13; 2015,Jan,16; 2014,Apr,10

27829 Open treatment of distal tibiofibular joint (syndesmosis) disruption, includes internal fixation, when performed
🦴 19.6 ⚕ 19.6 **FUD** 090   T A2 80 50 ▭
AMA: 2016,Feb,13; 2016,Jan,13; 2015,Jan,16; 2014,Jan,11; 2012,Jan,15-42; 2011,Jan,11

27830 Closed treatment of proximal tibiofibular joint dislocation; without anesthesia
🦴 10.1 ⚕ 10.8 **FUD** 090   T A2 80 50 ▭
AMA: 2002,Apr,13

27831 requiring anesthesia
🦴 11.2 ⚕ 11.2 **FUD** 090   T A2 80 50 ▭
AMA: 2002,Apr,13

27832 Open treatment of proximal tibiofibular joint dislocation, includes internal fixation, when performed, or with excision of proximal fibula
🦴 21.7 ⚕ 21.7 **FUD** 090   J A2 80 50 ▭
AMA: 2002,Apr,13

27840 Closed treatment of ankle dislocation; without anesthesia
🦴 10.5 ⚕ 10.5 **FUD** 090   T A2 50 ▭
AMA: 2002,Apr,13

27842 requiring anesthesia, with or without percutaneous skeletal fixation
🦴 14.2 ⚕ 14.2 **FUD** 090   T A2 50 ▭
AMA: 2002,Apr,13

27846 Open treatment of ankle dislocation, with or without percutaneous skeletal fixation; without repair or internal fixation
EXCLUDES *Arthroscopy (29894-29898)*
🦴 20.8 ⚕ 20.8 **FUD** 090   T A2 80 50 ▭
AMA: 2002,Apr,13

27848 with repair or internal or external fixation

EXCLUDES *Arthroscopy (29894-29898)*

🔧 23.3   ⚕ 23.3   **FUD** 090   T A2 80 50 ▭

AMA: 2002,Apr,13

27860 Ankle Manipulation with Anesthesia

27860 Manipulation of ankle under general anesthesia (includes application of traction or other fixation apparatus)

🔧 5.03   ⚕ 5.03   **FUD** 010   T A2 80 50 ▭

AMA: 2002,Apr,13

27870-27871 Arthrodesis Lower Leg/Ankle

27870 Arthrodesis, ankle, open

EXCLUDES *Arthroscopic arthrodesis of ankle (29899)*

🔧 29.6   ⚕ 29.6   **FUD** 090   J J8 80 50 ▭

AMA: 2002,Apr,13; 2001,Dec,3

27871 Arthrodesis, tibiofibular joint, proximal or distal

🔧 19.6   ⚕ 19.6   **FUD** 090   J G2 80 50 ▭

AMA: 2002,Apr,13

27880-27889 Amputations of Lower Leg/Ankle

27880 Amputation, leg, through tibia and fibula;

INCLUDES Burgess amputation

🔧 26.7   ⚕ 26.7   **FUD** 090   C 80 50 ▭

AMA: 2002,Apr,13

27881 with immediate fitting technique including application of first cast

🔧 25.3   ⚕ 25.3   **FUD** 090   C 80 50 ▭

AMA: 2002,Apr,13

27882 open, circular (guillotine)

🔧 17.5   ⚕ 17.5   **FUD** 090   C 80 50 ▭

AMA: 2002,Apr,13

27884 secondary closure or scar revision

🔧 16.8   ⚕ 16.8   **FUD** 090   T A2 50 ▭

AMA: 2002,Apr,13

27886 re-amputation

🔧 19.2   ⚕ 19.2   **FUD** 090   C 50 ▭

AMA: 2002,Apr,13

27888 Amputation, ankle, through malleoli of tibia and fibula (eg, Syme, Pirogoff type procedures), with plastic closure and resection of nerves

🔧 19.8   ⚕ 19.8   **FUD** 090   C 80 50 ▭

AMA: 2002,Apr,13; 1998,Nov,1

27889 Ankle disarticulation

🔧 18.9   ⚕ 18.9   **FUD** 090   T A2 50 ▭

AMA: 2002,Apr,13

27892-27899 Decompression Fasciotomy Lower Leg

EXCLUDES *Decompression fasciotomy without debridement (27600-27602)*

27892 Decompression fasciotomy, leg; anterior and/or lateral compartments only, with debridement of nonviable muscle and/or nerve

🔧 15.9   ⚕ 15.9   **FUD** 090   T A2 80 50 ▭

AMA: 2002,Apr,13

27893 posterior compartment(s) only, with debridement of nonviable muscle and/or nerve

🔧 17.3   ⚕ 17.3   **FUD** 090   T A2 80 50 ▭

AMA: 2002,Apr,13

27894 anterior and/or lateral, and posterior compartment(s), with debridement of nonviable muscle and/or nerve

🔧 24.6   ⚕ 24.6   **FUD** 090   T A2 80 50 ▭

AMA: 2002,Apr,13

27899 Unlisted procedure, leg or ankle

🔧 0.00   ⚕ 0.00   **FUD** YYY   T 80 50

AMA: 2016,Jan,13; 2015,Jan,16; 2014,Jan,11; 2012,Jan,15-42; 2011,Jan,11

28001-28008 Surgical Incision Foot/Toe

EXCLUDES *Simple incision and drainage (10060-10160)*

28001 Incision and drainage, bursa, foot

🔧 4.87   ⚕ 7.96   **FUD** 010   T P3 ▭

AMA: 2002,Apr,13; 1998,Nov,1

28002 Incision and drainage below fascia, with or without tendon sheath involvement, foot; single bursal space

🔧 9.16   ⚕ 12.7   **FUD** 010   T A2 ▭

AMA: 2002,Apr,13; 1998,Nov,1

28003 multiple areas

🔧 16.3   ⚕ 20.4   **FUD** 090   T A2 ▭

AMA: 2002,Apr,13; 1998,Nov,1

28005 Incision, bone cortex (eg, osteomyelitis or bone abscess), foot

🔧 16.6   ⚕ 16.6   **FUD** 090   T A2 ▭

AMA: 2002,Apr,13; 1998,Nov,1

28008 Fasciotomy, foot and/or toe

EXCLUDES *Plantar fascia division (28250)*
Plantar fasciectomy (28060, 28062)

🔧 8.42   ⚕ 12.4   **FUD** 090   T A2 50 ▭

AMA: 2002,Apr,13

28010-28011 Tenotomy/Toe

EXCLUDES *Open tenotomy (28230-28234)*
Simple incision and drainage (10140-10160)

28010 Tenotomy, percutaneous, toe; single tendon

🔧 6.00   ⚕ 6.66   **FUD** 090   T P3 ▭

AMA: 2002,Apr,13; 1998,Nov,1

28011 multiple tendons

🔧 8.27   ⚕ 9.26   **FUD** 090   T A2 ▭

AMA: 2002,Apr,13; 1998,Nov,1

28020-28024 Arthrotomy Foot/Toe

EXCLUDES *Simple incision and drainage (10140-10160)*

28020 Arthrotomy, including exploration, drainage, or removal of loose or foreign body; intertarsal or tarsometatarsal joint

🔧 10.4   ⚕ 15.6   **FUD** 090   T A2 ▭

AMA: 2002,Apr,13; 1998,Nov,1

28022 metatarsophalangeal joint

🔧 9.36   ⚕ 14.0   **FUD** 090   T A2 ▭

AMA: 2002,Apr,13

28024 interphalangeal joint

🔧 8.77   ⚕ 13.3   **FUD** 090   T A2 ▭

AMA: 2002,Apr,13

28035 Tarsal Tunnel Release

EXCLUDES *Other nerve decompression (64722)*
Other neuroplasty (64704)

28035 Release, tarsal tunnel (posterior tibial nerve decompression)

🔧 10.2   ⚕ 15.1   **FUD** 090   T A2 50 ▭

AMA: 2002,Apr,13; 1998,Nov,1

26/TC PC/TC Only	A2-Z3 ASC Payment	50 Bilateral	♂ Male Only	♀ Female Only	🔧 Facility RVU	⚕ Non-Facility RVU	▭ CCI
FUD Follow-up Days	**CMS:** IOM (Pub 100)	A-Y OPPSI			🧪 Lab Crosswalk	📊 Radiology Crosswalk	❌ CLIA

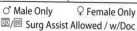 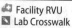

80/80 Surg Assist Allowed / w/Doc

90

CPT © 2016 American Medical Association. All Rights Reserved.

© 2016 Optum360, LLC

28039-28047 [28039, 28041] Excision Soft Tissue Tumors Foot/Toe

INCLUDES Any necessary elevation of tissue planes or dissection
Measurement of tumor and necessary margin at greatest diameter prior to excision
Simple and intermediate repairs
Types of excision:
Fascial or subfascial soft tissue tumors: simple and marginal resection of tumors found either in or below the deep fascia, not involving bone or excision of a substantial amount of normal tissue; primarily benign and intramuscular tumors
Tumors of fingers and toes involving joint capsules, tendons and tendon sheaths
Radical resection soft tissue tumor: wide resection of tumor, involving substantial margins of normal tissue and may involve tissue removal from one or more layers; most often malignant or aggressive benign
Tumors of fingers and toes adjacent to joints, tendons and tendon sheaths
Subcutaneous: simple and marginal resection of tumors in the subcutaneous tissue above the deep fascia; most often benign

EXCLUDES Complex repair
Excision of benign cutaneous lesions (eg, sebaceous cyst) (11420-11426)
Radical resection of cutaneous tumors (eg, melanoma) (11620-11626)
Significant exploration of vessels, neuroplasty, or reconstruction

28039 Resequenced code. See code following 28043.

28041 Resequenced code. See code following 28045.

28043 Excision, tumor, soft tissue of foot or toe, subcutaneous; less than 1.5 cm
🔧 7.55 👤 11.5 **FUD** 090 T G2 50 ▣
AMA: 2002,Apr,13; 1998,Nov,1

 # 28039 1.5 cm or greater
🔧 10.1 👤 14.7 **FUD** 090 T G2 80 50 ▣

28045 Excision, tumor, soft tissue of foot or toe, subfascial (eg, intramuscular); less than 1.5 cm
🔧 10.0 👤 14.2 **FUD** 090 T G2 80 50 ▣
AMA: 2002,Apr,13

 # 28041 1.5 cm or greater
🔧 13.2 👤 13.2 **FUD** 090 T G2 80 50 ▣

28046 Radical resection of tumor (eg, sarcoma), soft tissue of foot or toe; less than 3 cm
🔧 21.0 👤 21.0 **FUD** 090 T G2 50 ▣
AMA: 2002,Apr,13; 1990,Win,4

28047 3 cm or greater
🔧 30.8 👤 30.8 **FUD** 090 T G2 80 50 ▣

28050-28160 Resection Procedures Foot/Toes

28050 Arthrotomy with biopsy; intertarsal or tarsometatarsal joint
🔧 8.04 👤 12.2 **FUD** 090 T A2 50 ▣
AMA: 2002,Apr,13; 1998,Nov,1

28052 metatarsophalangeal joint
🔧 8.22 👤 12.9 **FUD** 090 T A2 50 ▣
AMA: 2002,Apr,13

28054 interphalangeal joint
🔧 7.03 👤 11.3 **FUD** 090 T A2 80 50 ▣
AMA: 2002,Apr,13

28055 Neurectomy, intrinsic musculature of foot
🔧 10.7 👤 10.7 **FUD** 090 T A2 80 50 ▣

28060 Fasciectomy, plantar fascia; partial (separate procedure)
EXCLUDES Plantar fasciotomy (28008, 28250)
🔧 10.2 👤 14.9 **FUD** 090 T A2 50 ▣
AMA: 2016,Jan,13; 2015,Jan,16; 2014,Jan,11; 2012,Jan,15-42; 2011,Jan,11

28062 radical (separate procedure)
EXCLUDES Plantar fasciotomy (28008, 28250)
🔧 11.7 👤 16.9 **FUD** 090 T A2 50 ▣
AMA: 2002,Apr,13

28070 Synovectomy; intertarsal or tarsometatarsal joint, each
🔧 10.2 👤 15.3 **FUD** 090 T A2 ▣
AMA: 2002,Apr,13

28072 metatarsophalangeal joint, each
🔧 9.55 👤 14.6 **FUD** 090 T A2 ▣
AMA: 2002,Apr,13

28080 Excision, interdigital (Morton) neuroma, single, each
🔧 10.5 👤 15.1 **FUD** 090 T A2 80 ▣
AMA: 2016,Jan,13; 2015,Jan,16; 2014,Jan,11

Plantar view of right foot showing common location of Morton neuroma

Morton neuroma is a chronic inflammation or irritation of the nerves in the web space between the heads of the metatarsals and phalanges

28086 Synovectomy, tendon sheath, foot; flexor
🔧 10.4 👤 15.8 **FUD** 090 T A2 80 50 ▣
AMA: 2002,Apr,13

28088 extensor
🔧 8.13 👤 12.9 **FUD** 090 T A2 80 50 ▣
AMA: 2002,Apr,13

28090 Excision of lesion, tendon, tendon sheath, or capsule (including synovectomy) (eg, cyst or ganglion); foot
🔧 8.87 👤 13.5 **FUD** 090 T A2 50 ▣
AMA: 2002,Apr,13; 1998,Nov,1

28092 toe(s), each
🔧 7.73 👤 12.2 **FUD** 090 T A2 ▣
AMA: 2002,Apr,13; 1998,Nov,1

28100 Excision or curettage of bone cyst or benign tumor, talus or calcaneus;
🔧 11.8 👤 17.5 **FUD** 090 T A2 80 50 ▣
AMA: 2002,Apr,13

28102 with iliac or other autograft (includes obtaining graft)
🔧 17.3 👤 17.3 **FUD** 090 J A2 80 50 ▣
AMA: 2002,Apr,13

28103 with allograft
🔧 11.2 👤 11.2 **FUD** 090 J A2 80 50 ▣
AMA: 2002,Apr,13

28104 Excision or curettage of bone cyst or benign tumor, tarsal or metatarsal, except talus or calcaneus;
🔧 10.1 👤 15.2 **FUD** 090 T A2 80 ▣
AMA: 2002,May,7; 2002,Apr,13

28106 with iliac or other autograft (includes obtaining graft)
🔧 13.3 👤 13.3 **FUD** 090 T A2 80 ▣
AMA: 2002,May,7; 2002,Apr,13

28107 with allograft
🔧 10.7 👤 16.1 **FUD** 090 J A2 80 ▣
AMA: 2002,May,7; 2002,Apr,13

28108 Excision or curettage of bone cyst or benign tumor, phalanges of foot
EXCLUDES Partial excision bone, toe (28124)
🔧 8.29 👤 12.7 **FUD** 090 T A2
AMA: 2002,Apr,13

28110 Ostectomy, partial excision, fifth metatarsal head (bunionette) (separate procedure)
🔧 8.33 👤 13.3 **FUD** 090 T A2 50 ▣
AMA: 2016,Jan,13; 2015,Jan,16; 2014,Jan,11; 2012,Jan,15-42; 2011,Jan,11

28111 Ostectomy, complete excision; first metatarsal head
🦵 9.40   ⚕ 14.2   **FUD** 090   T A2 50 ▣
AMA: 2002,Apr,13

28112 other metatarsal head (second, third or fourth)
🦵 9.02   ⚕ 14.1   **FUD** 090   T A2 50 ▣
AMA: 2002,Apr,13

28113 fifth metatarsal head
🦵 12.2   ⚕ 17.0   **FUD** 090   T A2 80 50 ▣
AMA: 2002,Apr,13

28114 all metatarsal heads, with partial proximal phalangectomy, excluding first metatarsal (eg, Clayton type procedure)
🦵 24.1   ⚕ 30.9   **FUD** 090   T A2 80 50 ▣
AMA: 2002,Apr,13; 1998,Nov,1

28116 Ostectomy, excision of tarsal coalition
🦵 16.4   ⚕ 21.7   **FUD** 090   T A2 50 ▣
AMA: 2002,Apr,13

28118 Ostectomy, calcaneus;
🦵 11.8   ⚕ 17.1   **FUD** 090   T A2 80 50 ▣
AMA: 2016,Jan,13; 2015,Jan,16; 2015,Jan,13; 2014,Jan,11; 2012,Jan,15-42; 2011,May,9

28119 for spur, with or without plantar fascial release
🦵 10.3   ⚕ 15.1   **FUD** 090   T A2 50 ▣
AMA: 2016,Jan,13; 2015,Jan,16; 2014,Jan,11; 2012,Jan,15-42; 2011,May,9

28120 Partial excision (craterization, saucerization, sequestrectomy, or diaphysectomy) bone (eg, osteomyelitis or bossing); talus or calcaneus
INCLUDES   Barker operation
🦵 14.3   ⚕ 19.5   **FUD** 090   T A2 50 ▣
AMA: 2016,Jan,13; 2015,Jan,16; 2014,Jan,11; 2012,Jan,15-42; 2011,May,9

28122 tarsal or metatarsal bone, except talus or calcaneus
EXCLUDES   Hallux rigidus cheilectomy (28289)
     Partial removal of talus or calcaneus (28120)
🦵 12.6   ⚕ 17.2   **FUD** 090   T A2 80 50 ▣
AMA: 2002,Apr,13; 1998,Nov,1

28124 phalanx of toe
🦵 9.49   ⚕ 13.7   **FUD** 090   T P3 50 ▣
AMA: 2002,Apr,13

28126 Resection, partial or complete, phalangeal base, each toe
🦵 7.15   ⚕ 11.4   **FUD** 090   T A2 ▣
AMA: 2016,Jan,13; 2015,Mar,9

28130 Talectomy (astragalectomy)
INCLUDES   Whitman astragalectomy
EXCLUDES   Calcanectomy (28118)
🦵 18.4   ⚕ 18.4   **FUD** 090   T A2 80 50 ▣
AMA: 2002,Apr,13

28140 Metatarsectomy
🦵 12.7   ⚕ 17.2   **FUD** 090   T A2 ▣
AMA: 2002,Apr,13

28150 Phalangectomy, toe, each toe
🦵 8.09   ⚕ 12.3   **FUD** 090   T A2 ▣
AMA: 2002,Apr,13; 1998,Nov,1

28153 Resection, condyle(s), distal end of phalanx, each toe
🦵 7.58   ⚕ 11.8   **FUD** 090   T A2 ▣
AMA: 2016,Jan,13; 2015,Jan,16; 2014,Jan,11; 2012,Jan,15-42; 2011,Dec,14-18

28160 Hemiphalangectomy or interphalangeal joint excision, toe, proximal end of phalanx, each
🦵 7.77   ⚕ 12.1   **FUD** 090   T A2 ▣
AMA: 2002,Apr,13; 1998,Nov,1

28171-28175 Radical Resection Bone Tumor Foot/Toes

INCLUDES   Any necessary elevation of tissue planes or dissection
Excision of adjacent soft tissue during bone tumor resection (28039-28047 [28039, 28041])
Measurement of tumor and necessary margin at greatest diameter prior to excision
Resection of the tumor (may include entire bone) and wide margins of normal tissue primarily for malignant or aggressive benign tumors
Simple and intermediate repairs
EXCLUDES   Complex repair
Radical tumor resection calcaneus or talus (27647)
Significant exploration of vessels, neuroplasty, reconstruction, or complex bone repair

28171 Radical resection of tumor; tarsal (except talus or calcaneus)
🦵 24.3   ⚕ 24.3   **FUD** 090   T A2 80 ▣
AMA: 2002,Apr,13; 1994,Win,1

28173 metatarsal
🦵 21.9   ⚕ 21.9   **FUD** 090   T A2 ▣
AMA: 2002,Apr,13; 1994,Win,1

28175 phalanx of toe
🦵 14.0   ⚕ 14.0   **FUD** 090   T A2 ▣
AMA: 2002,Apr,13

28190-28193 Foreign Body Removal: Foot

28190 Removal of foreign body, foot; subcutaneous
🦵 3.85   ⚕ 7.40   **FUD** 010   T P3 50 ▣
AMA: 2016,Jan,13; 2015,Jan,16; 2014,Jan,11; 2013,Dec,16

28192 deep
🦵 9.05   ⚕ 13.6   **FUD** 090   T A2 50 ▣
AMA: 2016,Jan,13; 2015,Jan,16; 2014,Jan,11; 2013,Dec,16

28193 complicated
🦵 10.6   ⚕ 15.3   **FUD** 090   T A2 50 ▣
AMA: 2002,Apr,13

28200-28360 [28295] Repair/Reconstruction of Foot/Toe

INCLUDES   Closed, open, and percutaneous treatment of fractures and dislocations

28200 Repair, tendon, flexor, foot; primary or secondary, without free graft, each tendon
🦵 9.25   ⚕ 14.1   **FUD** 090   T A2 ▣
AMA: 2016,Feb,15; 2016,Jan,13; 2015,Jan,16; 2014,Jul,5; 2014,Jan,11; 2012,Jan,15-42; 2011,May,9

28202 secondary with free graft, each tendon (includes obtaining graft)
🦵 12.2   ⚕ 17.2   **FUD** 090   J A2 80 ▣
AMA: 2002,Apr,13

28208 Repair, tendon, extensor, foot; primary or secondary, each tendon
🦵 8.96   ⚕ 13.6   **FUD** 090   T A2 ▣
AMA: 2002,Apr,13; 1998,Nov,1

28210 secondary with free graft, each tendon (includes obtaining graft)
🦵 11.7   ⚕ 16.5   **FUD** 090   J A2 80 ▣
AMA: 2002,Apr,13

28220 Tenolysis, flexor, foot; single tendon
🦵 8.67   ⚕ 12.9   **FUD** 090   T P3 50 ▣
AMA: 2002,Apr,13; 1998,Nov,1

28222 multiple tendons
🦵 10.0   ⚕ 14.6   **FUD** 090   T A2 50 ▣
AMA: 2002,Apr,13; 1998,Nov,1

28225 Tenolysis, extensor, foot; single tendon
🦵 7.46   ⚕ 11.8   **FUD** 090   T A2 50 ▣
AMA: 2002,Apr,13; 1998,Nov,1

28226 multiple tendons
🦵 11.2   ⚕ 17.5   **FUD** 090   T A2 50 ▣
AMA: 2002,Apr,13; 1998,Nov,1

28230 Tenotomy, open, tendon flexor; foot, single or multiple tendon(s) (separate procedure)
🖩 8.14　🔪 12.5　**FUD** 090　　　T P3 50 ▣
AMA: 2002,Apr,13; 1998,Nov,1

28232 toe, single tendon (separate procedure)
🖩 6.99　🔪 11.1　**FUD** 090　　　T P3 ▣
AMA: 2016,Jan,13; 2015,Mar,9

28234 Tenotomy, open, extensor, foot or toe, each tendon
EXCLUDES　Tendon transfer (27690-27691)
🖩 7.58　🔪 11.8　**FUD** 090　　　T A2 ▣
AMA: 2016,Jan,13; 2015,Jan,16; 2014,Jan,11; 2011,Jan,11

28238 Reconstruction (advancement), posterior tibial tendon with excision of accessory tarsal navicular bone (eg, Kidner type procedure)
EXCLUDES　Extensor hallucis longus transfer with big toe fusion (28760)
　　　　　Jones procedure (28760)
　　　　　Subcutaneous tenotomy (28010-28011)
　　　　　Transfer or transplant of tendon with muscle redirection or rerouting (27690-27692)
🖩 14.0　🔪 19.3　**FUD** 090　　　T A2 80 50 ▣
AMA: 2002,Apr,13; 2002,May,7

28240 Tenotomy, lengthening, or release, abductor hallucis muscle
🖩 8.35　🔪 12.7　**FUD** 090　　　T A2 50 ▣
AMA: 2002,Apr,13

28250 Division of plantar fascia and muscle (eg, Steindler stripping) (separate procedure)
🖩 11.6　🔪 16.8　**FUD** 090　　　T A2 80 50 ▣
AMA: 2002,Apr,13; 1998,Nov,1

28260 Capsulotomy, midfoot; medial release only (separate procedure)
🖩 14.6　🔪 19.8　**FUD** 090　　　T A2 80 50 ▣
AMA: 2002,Apr,13

28261 with tendon lengthening
🖩 22.3　🔪 28.2　**FUD** 090　　　T A2 80 50 ▣
AMA: 2002,Apr,13

28262 extensive, including posterior talotibial capsulotomy and tendon(s) lengthening (eg, resistant clubfoot deformity)
🖩 34.1　🔪 42.4　**FUD** 090　　　J A2 80 50 ▣
AMA: 2002,Apr,13; 1998,Nov,1

28264 Capsulotomy, midtarsal (eg, Heyman type procedure)
🖩 21.9　🔪 28.8　**FUD** 090　　　T A2 80 50 ▣
AMA: 2002,Apr,13; 1998,Nov,1

28270 Capsulotomy; metatarsophalangeal joint, with or without tenorrhaphy, each joint (separate procedure)
🖩 9.60　🔪 14.1　**FUD** 090　　　T A2 50 ▣
AMA: 2016,Jan,13; 2015,Jan,16; 2014,Sep,13; 2014,Jan,11; 2012,Jan,15-42; 2011,Sep,11-12; 2011,Jan,11

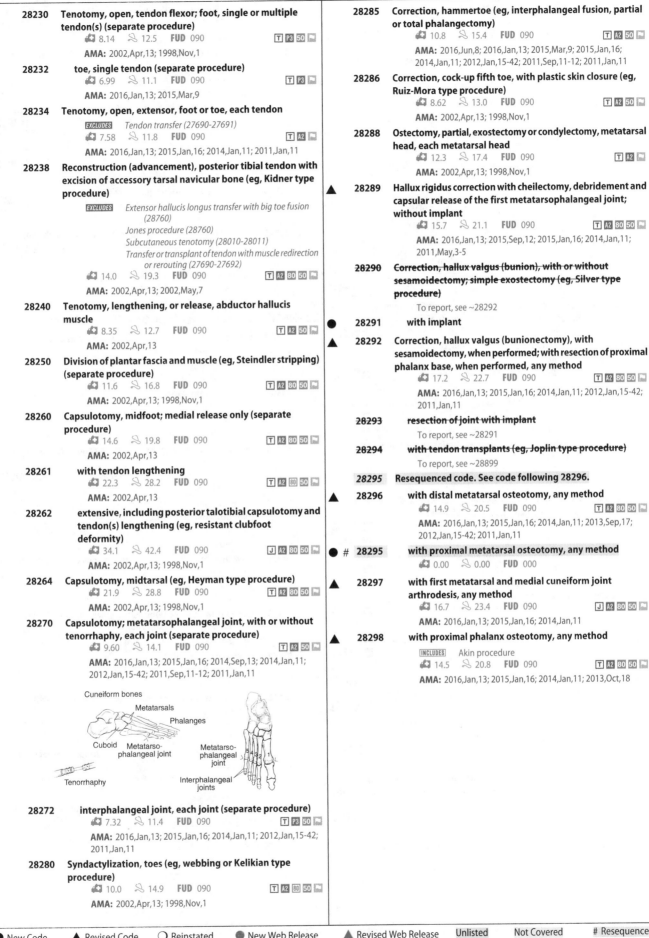

Cuneiform bones
Metatarsals
Phalanges
Cuboid
Metatarso-phalangeal joint
Metatarso-phalangeal joint
Interphalangeal joints
Tenorrhaphy

28272 interphalangeal joint, each joint (separate procedure)
🖩 7.32　🔪 11.4　**FUD** 090　　　T P3 50 ▣
AMA: 2016,Jan,13; 2015,Jan,16; 2014,Jan,11; 2012,Jan,15-42; 2011,Jan,11

28280 Syndactylization, toes (eg, webbing or Kelikian type procedure)
🖩 10.0　🔪 14.9　**FUD** 090　　　T A2 80 50 ▣
AMA: 2002,Apr,13; 1998,Nov,1

28285 Correction, hammertoe (eg, interphalangeal fusion, partial or total phalangectomy)
🖩 10.8　🔪 15.4　**FUD** 090　　　T A2 50 ▣
AMA: 2016,Jun,8; 2016,Jan,13; 2015,Mar,9; 2015,Jan,16; 2014,Jan,11; 2012,Jan,15-42; 2011,Sep,11-12; 2011,Jan,11

28286 Correction, cock-up fifth toe, with plastic skin closure (eg, Ruiz-Mora type procedure)
🖩 8.62　🔪 13.0　**FUD** 090　　　T A2 50 ▣
AMA: 2002,Apr,13; 1998,Nov,1

28288 Ostectomy, partial, exostectomy or condylectomy, metatarsal head, each metatarsal head
🖩 12.3　🔪 17.4　**FUD** 090　　　T A2 ▣
AMA: 2002,Apr,13; 1998,Nov,1

▲ **28289** Hallux rigidus correction with cheilectomy, debridement and capsular release of the first metatarsophalangeal joint; without implant
🖩 15.7　🔪 21.1　**FUD** 090　　　T A2 80 50 ▣
AMA: 2016,Jan,13; 2015,Sep,12; 2015,Jan,16; 2014,Jan,11; 2011,May,3-5

~~**28290**~~ ~~Correction, hallux valgus (bunion), with or without sesamoidectomy; simple exostectomy (eg, Silver type procedure)~~
To report, see ~28292

● **28291** with implant

▲ **28292** Correction, hallux valgus (bunionectomy), with sesamoidectomy, when performed; with resection of proximal phalanx base, when performed, any method
🖩 17.2　🔪 22.7　**FUD** 090　　　T A2 80 50 ▣
AMA: 2016,Jan,13; 2015,Jan,16; 2014,Jan,11; 2012,Jan,15-42; 2011,Jan,11

~~**28293**~~ ~~resection of joint with implant~~
To report, see ~28291

~~**28294**~~ ~~with tendon transplants (eg, Joplin type procedure)~~
To report, see ~28899

28295 Resequenced code. See code following 28296.

▲ **28296** with distal metatarsal osteotomy, any method
🖩 14.9　🔪 20.5　**FUD** 090　　　T A2 80 50 ▣
AMA: 2016,Jan,13; 2015,Jan,16; 2014,Jan,11; 2013,Sep,17; 2012,Jan,15-42; 2011,Jan,11

● # **28295** with proximal metatarsal osteotomy, any method
🖩 0.00　🔪 0.00　**FUD** 000

▲ **28297** with first metatarsal and medial cuneiform joint arthrodesis, any method
🖩 16.7　🔪 23.4　**FUD** 090　　　J A2 80 50 ▣
AMA: 2016,Jan,13; 2015,Jan,16; 2014,Jan,11

▲ **28298** with proximal phalanx osteotomy, any method
INCLUDES　Akin procedure
🖩 14.5　🔪 20.8　**FUD** 090　　　T A2 80 50 ▣
AMA: 2016,Jan,13; 2015,Jan,16; 2014,Jan,11; 2013,Oct,18

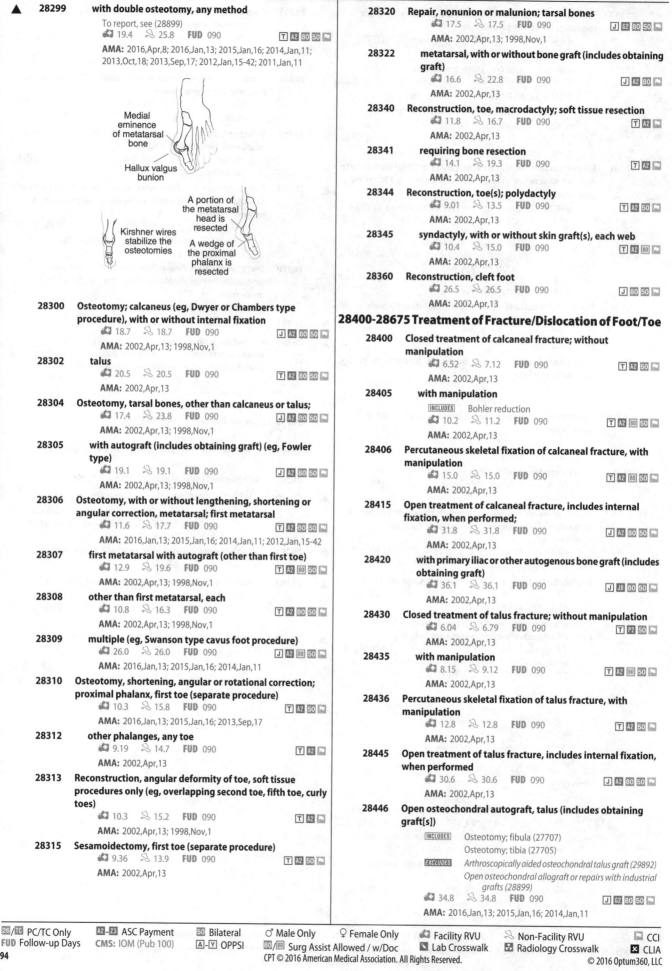

▲ **28299** **with double osteotomy, any method**
To report, see (28899)
🖩 19.4   ⚕ 25.8   **FUD** 090   ⬚ T A2 80 50
AMA: 2016,Apr,8; 2016,Jan,13; 2015,Jan,16; 2014,Jan,11; 2013,Oct,18; 2013,Sep,17; 2012,Jan,15-42; 2011,Jan,11

Medial eminence of metatarsal bone

Hallux valgus bunion

Kirshner wires stabilize the osteotomies

A portion of the metatarsal head is resected

A wedge of the proximal phalanx is resected

28300 **Osteotomy; calcaneus (eg, Dwyer or Chambers type procedure), with or without internal fixation**
🖩 18.7   ⚕ 18.7   **FUD** 090   ⬚ J A2 80 50
AMA: 2002,Apr,13; 1998,Nov,1

28302 **talus**
🖩 20.5   ⚕ 20.5   **FUD** 090   ⬚ T A2 80 50
AMA: 2002,Apr,13

28304 **Osteotomy, tarsal bones, other than calcaneus or talus;**
🖩 17.4   ⚕ 23.8   **FUD** 090   ⬚ J A2 80 50
AMA: 2002,Apr,13; 1998,Nov,1

28305 **with autograft (includes obtaining graft) (eg, Fowler type)**
🖩 19.1   ⚕ 19.1   **FUD** 090   ⬚ J A2 80 50
AMA: 2002,Apr,13; 1998,Nov,1

28306 **Osteotomy, with or without lengthening, shortening or angular correction, metatarsal; first metatarsal**
🖩 11.6   ⚕ 17.7   **FUD** 090   ⬚ T A2 80 50
AMA: 2016,Jan,13; 2015,Jan,16; 2014,Jan,11; 2012,Jan,15-42

28307 **first metatarsal with autograft (other than first toe)**
🖩 12.9   ⚕ 19.6   **FUD** 090   ⬚ T A2 80 50
AMA: 2002,Apr,13; 1998,Nov,1

28308 **other than first metatarsal, each**
🖩 10.8   ⚕ 16.3   **FUD** 090   ⬚ T A2 80 50
AMA: 2002,Apr,13; 1998,Nov,1

28309 **multiple (eg, Swanson type cavus foot procedure)**
🖩 26.0   ⚕ 26.0   **FUD** 090   ⬚ J A2 80 50
AMA: 2016,Jan,13; 2015,Jan,16; 2014,Jan,11

28310 **Osteotomy, shortening, angular or rotational correction; proximal phalanx, first toe (separate procedure)**
🖩 10.3   ⚕ 15.8   **FUD** 090   ⬚ T A2 50
AMA: 2016,Jan,13; 2015,Jan,16; 2013,Sep,17

28312 **other phalanges, any toe**
🖩 9.19   ⚕ 14.7   **FUD** 090   ⬚ T A2
AMA: 2002,Apr,13

28313 **Reconstruction, angular deformity of toe, soft tissue procedures only (eg, overlapping second toe, fifth toe, curly toes)**
🖩 10.3   ⚕ 15.2   **FUD** 090   ⬚ T A2
AMA: 2002,Apr,13; 1998,Nov,1

28315 **Sesamoidectomy, first toe (separate procedure)**
🖩 9.36   ⚕ 13.9   **FUD** 090   ⬚ T A2 50
AMA: 2002,Apr,13

28320 **Repair, nonunion or malunion; tarsal bones**
🖩 17.5   ⚕ 17.5   **FUD** 090   ⬚ J 62 80 50
AMA: 2002,Apr,13; 1998,Nov,1

28322 **metatarsal, with or without bone graft (includes obtaining graft)**
🖩 16.6   ⚕ 22.8   **FUD** 090   ⬚ J A2 80
AMA: 2002,Apr,13

28340 **Reconstruction, toe, macrodactyly; soft tissue resection**
🖩 11.8   ⚕ 16.7   **FUD** 090   ⬚ T A2
AMA: 2002,Apr,13

28341 **requiring bone resection**
🖩 14.1   ⚕ 19.3   **FUD** 090   ⬚ T A2
AMA: 2002,Apr,13

28344 **Reconstruction, toe(s); polydactyly**
🖩 9.01   ⚕ 13.5   **FUD** 090   ⬚ T A2 50
AMA: 2002,Apr,13

28345 **syndactyly, with or without skin graft(s), each web**
🖩 10.4   ⚕ 15.0   **FUD** 090   ⬚ T A2 80
AMA: 2002,Apr,13

28360 **Reconstruction, cleft foot**
🖩 26.5   ⚕ 26.5   **FUD** 090   ⬚ J 80 50
AMA: 2002,Apr,13

28400-28675 Treatment of Fracture/Dislocation of Foot/Toe

28400 **Closed treatment of calcaneal fracture; without manipulation**
🖩 6.52   ⚕ 7.12   **FUD** 090   ⬚ T A2 50
AMA: 2002,Apr,13

28405 **with manipulation**
INCLUDES   Bohler reduction
🖩 10.2   ⚕ 11.2   **FUD** 090   ⬚ T A2 80 50
AMA: 2002,Apr,13

28406 **Percutaneous skeletal fixation of calcaneal fracture, with manipulation**
🖩 15.0   ⚕ 15.0   **FUD** 090   ⬚ T A2 80 50
AMA: 2002,Apr,13

28415 **Open treatment of calcaneal fracture, includes internal fixation, when performed;**
🖩 31.8   ⚕ 31.8   **FUD** 090   ⬚ J A2 80 50
AMA: 2002,Apr,13

28420 **with primary iliac or other autogenous bone graft (includes obtaining graft)**
🖩 36.1   ⚕ 36.1   **FUD** 090   ⬚ J J8 80 50
AMA: 2002,Apr,13

28430 **Closed treatment of talus fracture; without manipulation**
🖩 6.04   ⚕ 6.79   **FUD** 090   ⬚ T P2 50
AMA: 2002,Apr,13

28435 **with manipulation**
🖩 8.15   ⚕ 9.12   **FUD** 090   ⬚ T A2 80 50
AMA: 2002,Apr,13

28436 **Percutaneous skeletal fixation of talus fracture, with manipulation**
🖩 12.8   ⚕ 12.8   **FUD** 090   ⬚ T A2 50
AMA: 2002,Apr,13

28445 **Open treatment of talus fracture, includes internal fixation, when performed**
🖩 30.6   ⚕ 30.6   **FUD** 090   ⬚ J A2 80 50
AMA: 2002,Apr,13

28446 **Open osteochondral autograft, talus (includes obtaining graft[s])**
INCLUDES   Osteotomy; fibula (27707)
Osteotomy; tibia (27705)
EXCLUDES   *Arthroscopically aided osteochondral talus graft (29892)*
Open osteochondral allograft or repairs with industrial grafts (28899)
🖩 34.8   ⚕ 34.8   **FUD** 090   ⬚ J 62 80 50
AMA: 2016,Jan,13; 2015,Jan,16; 2014,Jan,11

28450 Treatment of tarsal bone fracture (except talus and calcaneus); without manipulation, each
🔧 5.52   🔨 6.19   **FUD** 090   T P2 ▢
AMA: 2016,Jan,13; 2015,Jan,16; 2014,Jan,11; 2012,Jan,15-42; 2011,Jan,11

28455 with manipulation, each
🔧 7.47   🔨 8.30   **FUD** 090   T P3 80 ▢
AMA: 2002,Apr,13

28456 Percutaneous skeletal fixation of tarsal bone fracture (except talus and calcaneus), with manipulation, each
🔧 9.16   🔨 9.16   **FUD** 090   J A2 ▢
AMA: 2002,Apr,13

28465 Open treatment of tarsal bone fracture (except talus and calcaneus), includes internal fixation, when performed, each
🔧 17.9   🔨 17.9   **FUD** 090   J A2 ▢
AMA: 2002,Apr,13

28470 Closed treatment of metatarsal fracture; without manipulation, each
🔧 5.87   🔨 6.28   **FUD** 090   T P2 ▢
AMA: 2002,Apr,13

28475 with manipulation, each
🔧 6.54   🔨 7.37   **FUD** 090   T P2 ▢
AMA: 2002,Apr,13

28476 Percutaneous skeletal fixation of metatarsal fracture, with manipulation, each
🔧 10.1   🔨 10.1   **FUD** 090   T A2 80 ▢
AMA: 2002,Apr,13

28485 Open treatment of metatarsal fracture, includes internal fixation, when performed, each
🔧 15.1   🔨 15.1   **FUD** 090   T A2 ▢
AMA: 2002,Apr,13

28490 Closed treatment of fracture great toe, phalanx or phalanges; without manipulation
🔧 3.59   🔨 4.17   **FUD** 090   T P2 50 ▢
AMA: 2002,Apr,13

28495 with manipulation
🔧 4.29   🔨 5.10   **FUD** 090   T P2 50 ▢
AMA: 2002,Apr,13

28496 Percutaneous skeletal fixation of fracture great toe, phalanx or phalanges, with manipulation
🔧 6.72   🔨 12.6   **FUD** 090   T A2 50 ▢
AMA: 2002,Apr,13

28505 Open treatment of fracture, great toe, phalanx or phalanges, includes internal fixation, when performed
🔧 14.3   🔨 19.2   **FUD** 090   T A2 50 ▢
AMA: 2002,Apr,13

28510 Closed treatment of fracture, phalanx or phalanges, other than great toe; without manipulation, each
🔧 3.46   🔨 3.55   **FUD** 090   T P3 ▢
AMA: 2002,Apr,13

28515 with manipulation, each
🔧 4.09   🔨 4.63   **FUD** 090   T P3 ▢
AMA: 2002,Apr,13

28525 Open treatment of fracture, phalanx or phalanges, other than great toe, includes internal fixation, when performed, each
🔧 11.4   🔨 16.3   **FUD** 090   T A2 80 ▢
AMA: 2002,Apr,13

28530 Closed treatment of sesamoid fracture
🔧 2.94   🔨 3.31   **FUD** 090   T P3 80 50 ▢
AMA: 2002,Apr,13

28531 Open treatment of sesamoid fracture, with or without internal fixation
🔧 5.29   🔨 9.98   **FUD** 090   T A2 50 ▢
AMA: 2002,Apr,13

28540 Closed treatment of tarsal bone dislocation, other than talotarsal; without anesthesia
🔧 5.36   🔨 5.94   **FUD** 090   T P2 80 50 ▢
AMA: 2002,Apr,13

28545 requiring anesthesia
🔧 7.43   🔨 8.37   **FUD** 090   T A2 80 50 ▢
AMA: 2002,Apr,13

28546 Percutaneous skeletal fixation of tarsal bone dislocation, other than talotarsal, with manipulation
🔧 9.46   🔨 16.0   **FUD** 090   T A2 80 50 ▢
AMA: 2002,Apr,13

28555 Open treatment of tarsal bone dislocation, includes internal fixation, when performed
🔧 19.2   🔨 25.4   **FUD** 090   J A2 80 50 ▢
AMA: 2002,Apr,13

28570 Closed treatment of talotarsal joint dislocation; without anesthesia
🔧 5.41   🔨 6.38   **FUD** 090   T P2 80 50 ▢
AMA: 2002,Apr,13

28575 requiring anesthesia
🔧 9.48   🔨 10.4   **FUD** 090   T A2 80 50 ▢
AMA: 2002,Apr,13

28576 Percutaneous skeletal fixation of talotarsal joint dislocation, with manipulation
🔧 11.2   🔨 11.2   **FUD** 090   T A2 80 50 ▢
AMA: 2002,Apr,13

28585 Open treatment of talotarsal joint dislocation, includes internal fixation, when performed
🔧 19.2   🔨 24.6   **FUD** 090   T A2 80 50 ▢
AMA: 2016,Jan,13; 2015,Jan,16; 2014,Jan,11; 2012,Jan,15-42; 2011,Sep,11-12

28600 Closed treatment of tarsometatarsal joint dislocation; without anesthesia
🔧 5.39   🔨 6.26   **FUD** 090   T P2 80 ▢
AMA: 2002,Apr,13

28605 requiring anesthesia
🔧 8.41   🔨 9.34   **FUD** 090   T A2 80 ▢
AMA: 2002,Apr,13

28606 Percutaneous skeletal fixation of tarsometatarsal joint dislocation, with manipulation
🔧 11.3   🔨 11.3   **FUD** 090   T A2 ▢
AMA: 2002,Apr,13

28615 Open treatment of tarsometatarsal joint dislocation, includes internal fixation, when performed
🔧 22.7   🔨 22.7   **FUD** 090   J A2 80 ▢
AMA: 2002,Apr,13

28630 Closed treatment of metatarsophalangeal joint dislocation; without anesthesia
🔧 3.15   🔨 4.50   **FUD** 010   T P3 80 ▢
AMA: 2002,Apr,13

28635 requiring anesthesia
🔧 3.77   🔨 5.01   **FUD** 010   T A2 80 ▢
AMA: 2002,Apr,13

28636 Percutaneous skeletal fixation of metatarsophalangeal joint dislocation, with manipulation
🔧 5.24   🔨 8.18   **FUD** 010   T A2 ▢
AMA: 2002,Apr,13

28645 Open treatment of metatarsophalangeal joint dislocation, includes internal fixation, when performed
🔧 13.9   🔨 18.9   **FUD** 010   T A2 ▢
AMA: 2016,Jan,13; 2015,Jan,16; 2014,Sep,13

28660 Closed treatment of interphalangeal joint dislocation; without anesthesia
🔧 2.55   🔨 3.34   **FUD** 010   T P3 ▢
AMA: 2002,Apr,13

28665 **requiring anesthesia**
🚑 3.76   ⚕ 4.41   **FUD** 010   S A2 80 ▭
AMA: 2002,Apr,13

28666 **Percutaneous skeletal fixation of interphalangeal joint dislocation, with manipulation**
🚑 5.39   ⚕ 5.39   **FUD** 010   T A2 ▭
AMA: 2002,Apr,13

28675 **Open treatment of interphalangeal joint dislocation, includes internal fixation, when performed**
🚑 11.8   ⚕ 16.8   **FUD** 090   T A2 ▭
AMA: 2002,Apr,13

28705-28760 Arthrodesis of Foot/Toe

28705 **Arthrodesis; pantalar**
🚑 36.1   ⚕ 36.1   **FUD** 090   J J8 80 50 ▭
AMA: 2002,Apr,13

28715 **triple**
🚑 27.0   ⚕ 27.0   **FUD** 090   J J8 80 50 ▭
AMA: 2002,Apr,13; 1998,Nov,1

28725 **subtalar**
INCLUDES   Dunn arthrodesis
       Grice arthrosis
🚑 22.4   ⚕ 22.4   **FUD** 090   J G2 80 50 ▭
AMA: 2016,Jan,13; 2015,Jan,16; 2014,Jan,11; 2012,Jan,15-42; 2011,Sep,11-12

28730 **Arthrodesis, midtarsal or tarsometatarsal, multiple or transverse;**
INCLUDES   Lambrinudi arthrodesis
🚑 21.1   ⚕ 21.1   **FUD** 090   J G2 80 50 ▭
AMA: 2002,Apr,13

28735 **with osteotomy (eg, flatfoot correction)**
🚑 22.5   ⚕ 22.5   **FUD** 090   J J8 80 50 ▭
AMA: 2002,Apr,13; 1998,Nov,1

28737 **Arthrodesis, with tendon lengthening and advancement, midtarsal, tarsal navicular-cuneiform (eg, Miller type procedure)**
🚑 19.8   ⚕ 19.8   **FUD** 090   J G2 80 50 ▭
AMA: 2002,Apr,13; 2002,May,7

28740 **Arthrodesis, midtarsal or tarsometatarsal, single joint**
🚑 17.9   ⚕ 24.4   **FUD** 090   J G2 80 ▭
AMA: 2016,Jan,13; 2015,Jan,16; 2014,Jan,11; 2012,Jan,15-42; 2011,Jan,11

28750 **Arthrodesis, great toe; metatarsophalangeal joint**
🚑 17.0   ⚕ 23.4   **FUD** 090   J A2 80 50 ▭
AMA: 2016,Jan,13; 2015,Jan,16; 2014,Jan,11

28755 **interphalangeal joint**
🚑 9.52   ⚕ 14.6   **FUD** 090   T A2 50 ▭
AMA: 2002,Apr,13

28760 **Arthrodesis, with extensor hallucis longus transfer to first metatarsal neck, great toe, interphalangeal joint (eg, Jones type procedure)**
EXCLUDES   *Hammer toe repair or interphalangeal fusion (28285)*
🚑 16.6   ⚕ 22.7   **FUD** 090   J A2 80 50 ▭
AMA: 2002,Apr,13; 1998,Nov,1

28800-28825 Amputation Foot/Toe

28800 **Amputation, foot; midtarsal (eg, Chopart type procedure)**
🚑 15.6   ⚕ 15.6   **FUD** 090   C 80 50 ▭
AMA: 2002,Apr,13; 1998,Nov,1

28805 **transmetatarsal**
🚑 21.2   ⚕ 21.2   **FUD** 090   T 80 50 ▭
AMA: 2002,Apr,13; 1997,May,4

28810 **Amputation, metatarsal, with toe, single**
🚑 12.5   ⚕ 12.5   **FUD** 090   T A2 80 ▭
AMA: 2002,Apr,13

28820 **Amputation, toe; metatarsophalangeal joint**
🚑 11.4   ⚕ 16.3   **FUD** 090   T A2 ▭
AMA: 2002,Apr,13; 1997,May,4

28825 **interphalangeal joint**
🚑 10.7   ⚕ 15.6   **FUD** 090   T A2 ▭
AMA: 2002,Apr,13

28890-28899 Other/Unlisted Procedures Foot/Toe

28890 **Extracorporeal shock wave, high energy, performed by a physician or other qualified health care professional, requiring anesthesia other than local, including ultrasound guidance, involving the plantar fascia**
EXCLUDES   *Extracorporeal shock wave therapy of integumentary system not otherwise specified (0299T-0300T)*
      Extracorporeal shock wave therapy of musculoskeletal system not otherwise specified (0101T-0102T)
🚑 6.44   ⚕ 9.28   **FUD** 090   T P3 50 ▭
AMA: 2016,Jan,13; 2015,Jan,16; 2014,Jan,11; 2012,Jan,15-42; 2011,Jan,11

28899 **Unlisted procedure, foot or toes**
🚑 0.00   ⚕ 0.00   **FUD** YYY   T 60
AMA: 2016,Jun,8; 2016,Jan,13; 2015,Nov,10; 2015,Jan,16; 2014,Jan,11; 2012,Jan,15-42; 2011,Sep,11-12; 2011,Jan,11

29000-29086 Casting: Arm/Shoulder/Torso

INCLUDES   Application of cast or strapping when provided as:
     An initial service to stabilize the fracture or injury without restorative treatment
     A replacement procedure
     Removal of cast
EXCLUDES   *Cast or splint material*
     E&M services provided as part of the initial service when restorative treatment is not provided
     Orthotic supervision and training (97760-97762)

29000 **Application of halo type body cast (see 20661-20663 for insertion)**
🚑 5.04   ⚕ 8.25   **FUD** 000   S G2 80 ▭
AMA: 2016,Jan,13; 2015,Jan,16; 2014,Jan,11

29010 **Application of Risser jacket, localizer, body; only**
🚑 4.24   ⚕ 6.80   **FUD** 000   S P2 80 ▭
AMA: 2016,Jan,13; 2015,Jan,16; 2014,Jan,11

29015 **including head**
🚑 5.14   ⚕ 8.15   **FUD** 000   S P2 80 ▭
AMA: 2016,Jan,13; 2015,Jan,16; 2014,Jan,11

29035 **Application of body cast, shoulder to hips;**
🚑 3.45   ⚕ 5.57   **FUD** 000   S P2 80 ▭
AMA: 2016,Jan,13; 2015,Jan,16; 2014,Jan,11

29040 **including head, Minerva type**
🚑 4.19   ⚕ 6.46   **FUD** 000   S G2 80 ▭
AMA: 2016,Jan,13; 2015,Jan,16; 2014,Jan,11

29044 **including 1 thigh**
🚑 4.35   ⚕ 8.09   **FUD** 000   S P2 80 ▭
AMA: 2016,Jan,13; 2015,Jan,16; 2014,Jan,11

29046 **including both thighs**
🚑 4.55   ⚕ 6.95   **FUD** 000   S G2 80 ▭
AMA: 2016,Jan,13; 2015,Jan,16; 2014,Jan,11

29049 **Application, cast; figure-of-eight**
🚑 1.79   ⚕ 2.40   **FUD** 000   S P3 80 ▭
AMA: 2016,Jan,13; 2015,Jan,16; 2014,Jan,11

29055 **shoulder spica**
🚑 4.00   ⚕ 6.38   **FUD** 000   S P2 80 ▭
AMA: 2016,Jan,13; 2015,Jan,16; 2014,Jan,11

29058 **plaster Velpeau**
🚑 2.67   ⚕ 3.50   **FUD** 000   S P3 80 ▭
AMA: 2016,Jan,13; 2015,Jan,16; 2014,Jan,11

29065 **shoulder to hand (long arm)**
🚑 1.97   ⚕ 2.75   **FUD** 000   S P3 50 ▭
AMA: 2016,Jan,13; 2015,Jan,16; 2014,Jan,11

29075	elbow to finger (short arm)
	1.79 2.48 **FUD** 000 S P3 50
	AMA: 2016,Jan,13; 2015,Jan,16; 2014,Jan,11

29085	hand and lower forearm (gauntlet)
	1.94 2.73 **FUD** 000 S P3 50
	AMA: 2016,Jan,13; 2015,Jan,16; 2014,Jan,11; 2012,Jan,15-42; 2011,Jan,11

29086	finger (eg, contracture)
	1.47 2.24 **FUD** 000 S P3 50
	AMA: 2016,Jan,13; 2015,Jan,16; 2014,Jan,11

29105-29280 Splinting and Strapping: Torso/Upper Extremities

INCLUDES   Application of splint or strapping when provided as:
        An initial service to stabilize the fracture or dislocation
        A replacement procedure
EXCLUDES   E&M services provided as part of the initial service when restorative treatment is not provided
        Orthotic supervision and training (97760-97762)
        Splinting and strapping material

29105	**Application of long arm splint (shoulder to hand)**
	1.70 2.51 **FUD** 000 S P3 50
	AMA: 2016,Jan,13; 2015,Jan,16; 2014,Jan,11; 2012,Jan,15-42; 2011,Jan,11

29125	**Application of short arm splint (forearm to hand); static**
	1.13 1.84 **FUD** 000 01 N1 50
	AMA: 2016,Jan,13; 2015,Jan,16; 2014,Jan,11

29126	**dynamic**
	1.39 2.19 **FUD** 000 01 N1 50
	AMA: 2016,Jan,13; 2015,Jan,16; 2014,Jan,11

29130	**Application of finger splint; static**
	0.82 1.17 **FUD** 000 01 N1 50
	AMA: 2016,Jan,13; 2015,Jan,16; 2014,Jan,11

29131	**dynamic**
	0.94 1.45 **FUD** 000 01 N1 50
	AMA: 2016,Jan,13; 2015,Jan,16; 2014,Jan,11

29200	**Strapping; thorax**
	EXCLUDES Strapping of low back (29799)
	0.52 0.84 **FUD** 000 S P3
	AMA: 2016,Jan,13; 2015,Jan,16; 2014,Jan,11

29240	**shoulder (eg, Velpeau)**
	0.53 0.82 **FUD** 000 01 N1 50
	AMA: 2016,Jan,13; 2015,Jan,16; 2014,Jan,11; 2011,Jan,11

29260	**elbow or wrist**
	0.56 0.83 **FUD** 000 01 N1 50
	AMA: 2016,Jan,13; 2015,Jan,16; 2014,Jan,11

29280	**hand or finger**
	0.58 0.84 **FUD** 000 01 N1 50
	AMA: 2016,Jan,13; 2015,Jan,16; 2014,Jan,11

29305-29450 Casting: Legs

INCLUDES   Application of cast when provided as:
        An initial service to stabilize the fracture or injury without restorative treatment
        A replacement procedure
        Removal of cast
EXCLUDES   Cast or splint materials
        E&M services provided as part of the initial service when restorative treatment is not provided
        Orthotic supervision and training (97760-97762)

29305	**Application of hip spica cast; 1 leg**
	EXCLUDES Hip spica cast thighs only (29046)
	4.59 7.08 **FUD** 000 S P2 80
	AMA: 2016,Jan,13; 2015,Jan,16; 2014,Jan,11

29325	**1 and one-half spica or both legs**
	EXCLUDES Hip spica cast thighs only (29046)
	5.13 7.79 **FUD** 000 S P2 80
	AMA: 2016,Jan,13; 2015,Jan,16; 2014,Jan,11

29345	**Application of long leg cast (thigh to toes);**
	2.90 3.90 **FUD** 000 S P3 50
	AMA: 2016,Jan,13; 2015,Jan,16; 2014,Jan,11; 2011,Sep,11-12

29355	**walker or ambulatory type**
	3.06 4.03 **FUD** 000 S P3 50
	AMA: 2016,Jan,13; 2015,Jan,16; 2014,Jan,11; 2011,Sep,11-12

29358	**Application of long leg cast brace**
	3.00 4.60 **FUD** 000 S P3 50
	AMA: 2016,Jan,13; 2015,Jan,16; 2014,Jan,11; 2011,Sep,11-12

29365	**Application of cylinder cast (thigh to ankle)**
	2.52 3.51 **FUD** 000 S P3 50
	AMA: 2016,Jan,13; 2015,Jan,16; 2014,Jan,11; 2011,Sep,11-12

29405	**Application of short leg cast (below knee to toes);**
	1.72 2.34 **FUD** 000 S P3 50
	AMA: 2016,Jan,13; 2015,Jan,16; 2014,Jan,11; 2011,Sep,11-12

29425	**walking or ambulatory type**
	1.63 2.25 **FUD** 000 S P3 50
	AMA: 2016,Jan,13; 2015,Jan,16; 2014,Jan,11; 2011,Sep,11-12

29435	**Application of patellar tendon bearing (PTB) cast**
	2.38 3.33 **FUD** 000 S P3 50
	AMA: 2016,Jan,13; 2015,Jan,16; 2014,Jan,11; 2011,Sep,11-12

29440	**Adding walker to previously applied cast**
	0.83 1.25 **FUD** 000 S P3 50
	AMA: 2016,Jan,13; 2015,Jan,16; 2014,Jan,11

29445	**Application of rigid total contact leg cast**
	2.99 3.85 **FUD** 000 S P3 50
	AMA: 2016,Jan,13; 2015,Jan,16; 2014,Jan,11; 2012,Jan,15-42; 2011,Sep,11-12

29450	**Application of clubfoot cast with molding or manipulation, long or short leg**
	3.23 4.10 **FUD** 000 S P3 50
	AMA: 2016,Jan,13; 2015,Jan,16; 2014,Jan,11

29505-29584 Splinting and Strapping Ankle/Foot/Leg/Toes

INCLUDES   Application of splinting and strapping when provided as:
        An initial service to stabilize the fracture or injury without restorative treatment
        A replacement procedure
EXCLUDES   E&M services provided as part of the initial service when restorative treatment is not provided
        Orthotic supervision and training (97760-97762)

29505	**Application of long leg splint (thigh to ankle or toes)**
	1.43 2.38 **FUD** 000 S P3 50
	AMA: 2016,Jan,13; 2015,Jan,16; 2014,Jan,11; 2012,Jan,15-42; 2011,Jan,11

29515	**Application of short leg splint (calf to foot)**
	1.42 2.05 **FUD** 000 S P3 50
	AMA: 2016,Jan,13; 2015,Jan,16; 2014,Jan,11

29520	**Strapping; hip**
	0.53 0.89 **FUD** 000 01 N1 80 50
	AMA: 2016,Jan,13; 2015,Jan,16; 2014,Jan,11

29530	**knee**
	0.53 0.82 **FUD** 000 01 N1 50
	AMA: 2016,Jan,13; 2015,Jan,16; 2014,Jan,11

29540	**ankle and/or foot**
	EXCLUDES Application of multi-layer compression system (29581-29582)
	0.52 0.74 **FUD** 000 S P3 50
	AMA: 2016,Aug,3; 2016,Jan,13; 2015,Jan,16; 2014,Mar,4; 2014,Jan,11; 2012,Oct,14; 2012,Sep,16; 2012,Jan,15-42; 2011,Jan,11

29550	**toes**
	0.33 0.54 **FUD** 000 01 N1 50
	AMA: 2016,Jan,13; 2015,Jan,16; 2014,Jan,11

29580   **Unna boot**
> EXCLUDES   *Application of multi-layer compression system (29581-29582)*
> 🛠 1.02   🔧 1.50   **FUD** 000   S P3 50 📧
> **AMA:** 2016,Aug,3; 2016,Jan,13; 2015,Jan,16; 2014,Mar,4; 2014,Jan,11; 2012,Oct,14; 2012,Sep,16; 2012,Jan,15-42; 2011,Jan,11

29581   **Application of multi-layer compression system; leg (below knee), including ankle and foot**
> EXCLUDES   *Application of multi-layer compression system (29582)*
> *Endovenous ablation therapy of incompetent vein (36475-36476, 36478-36479)*
> *Strapping (29540, 29580)*
> 🛠 0.36   🔧 1.75   **FUD** 000   S P3 80 50 📧
> **AMA:** 2016,Aug,3; 2016,Jan,13; 2015,Mar,9; 2015,Jan,16; 2014,Oct,6; 2014,Mar,4; 2014,Jan,11; 2013,Sep,17; 2012,Oct,14; 2012,Sep,16; 2011,May,3-5

29582   **thigh and leg, including ankle and foot, when performed**
> EXCLUDES   *Endovenous ablation therapy of incompetent vein (36475-36476, 36478-36479)*
> *Strapping (29540, 29580-29581)*
> 🛠 0.45   🔧 1.99   **FUD** 000   S P3 80 50 📧
> **AMA:** 2016,Aug,3; 2016,Jan,13; 2015,Mar,9; 2015,Jan,16; 2014,Oct,6; 2014,Mar,4

29583   **upper arm and forearm**
> EXCLUDES   *Application of multi-layer compression system (29584)*
> 🛠 0.32   🔧 1.24   **FUD** 000   S P3 80 50 📧
> **AMA:** 2016,Aug,3; 2016,Jan,13; 2015,Mar,9

29584   **upper arm, forearm, hand, and fingers**
> EXCLUDES   *Application of multi-layer compression system (29583)*
> 🛠 0.45   🔧 1.99   **FUD** 000   S P3 80 50 📧
> **AMA:** 2016,Aug,3; 2016,Jan,13; 2015,Mar,9

29700-29799 Casting Services Other Than Application

INCLUDES   Casts applied by treating individual
Removal of casts applied by treating individual

29700   **Removal or bivalving; gauntlet, boot or body cast**
> 🛠 0.96   🔧 1.79   **FUD** 000   S P3 📧
> **AMA:** 2016,Jan,13; 2015,Jan,16; 2014,Jan,11

29705   **full arm or full leg cast**
> 🛠 1.36   🔧 1.91   **FUD** 000   S P3 50 📧
> **AMA:** 2016,Jan,13; 2015,Jan,16; 2014,Jan,11

29710   **shoulder or hip spica, Minerva, or Risser jacket, etc.**
> 🛠 2.39   🔧 3.49   **FUD** 000   S P3 80 50 📧
> **AMA:** 2016,Jan,13; 2015,Jan,16; 2014,Jan,11

29720   **Repair of spica, body cast or jacket**
> 🛠 1.28   🔧 2.43   **FUD** 000   S P3 📧
> **AMA:** 2016,Jan,13; 2015,Jan,16; 2014,Jan,11

29730   **Windowing of cast**
> 🛠 1.30   🔧 1.85   **FUD** 000   S P3 📧
> **AMA:** 2016,Jan,13; 2015,Jan,16; 2014,Jan,11

29740   **Wedging of cast (except clubfoot casts)**
> 🛠 2.03   🔧 2.85   **FUD** 000   S P3 📧
> **AMA:** 2016,Jan,13; 2015,Jan,16; 2014,Jan,11

29750   **Wedging of clubfoot cast**
> 🛠 1.93   🔧 2.55   **FUD** 000   S P3 80 50 📧
> **AMA:** 2016,Jan,13; 2015,Jan,16; 2014,Jan,11

29799   **Unlisted procedure, casting or strapping**
> 🛠 0.00   🔧 0.00   **FUD** YYY   S 80
> **AMA:** 2016,Aug,3; 2016,Jan,13; 2015,Jan,16; 2014,Jan,11; 2012,Oct,14; 2012,Sep,16

29800-29999 [29914, 29915, 29916] Arthroscopic Procedures

INCLUDES   Diagnostic arthroscopy with surgical arthroscopy
Code also modifier 51 if arthroscopy is performed with arthrotomy

29800   **Arthroscopy, temporomandibular joint, diagnostic, with or without synovial biopsy (separate procedure)**
> 🛠 14.6   🔧 14.6   **FUD** 090   T A2 80 50 📧
> **AMA:** 2016,Jan,13; 2015,Jan,16; 2013,May,12

29804   **Arthroscopy, temporomandibular joint, surgical**
> EXCLUDES   *Open surgery (21010)*
> 🛠 18.6   🔧 18.6   **FUD** 090   T A2 80 50 📧
> **AMA:** 2016,Jan,13; 2015,Jan,16; 2013,May,12

29805   **Arthroscopy, shoulder, diagnostic, with or without synovial biopsy (separate procedure)**
> EXCLUDES   *Open surgery (23065-23066, 23100-23101)*
> 🛠 13.5   🔧 13.5   **FUD** 090   T A2 50 📧
> **AMA:** 2016,Jan,13; 2015,Jun,10; 2015,Jan,16; 2013,May,12

29806   **Arthroscopy, shoulder, surgical; capsulorrhaphy**
> EXCLUDES   *Open surgery (23450-23466)*
> *Thermal capsulorrhaphy (29999)*
> 🛠 30.5   🔧 30.5   **FUD** 090   J A2 50 📧
> **AMA:** 2016,Jan,13; 2015,Jul,10; 2015,Mar,7; 2015,Jan,16; 2013,May,12

29807   **repair of SLAP lesion**
> 🛠 29.8   🔧 29.8   **FUD** 090   J A2 50 📧
> **AMA:** 2016,Jan,13; 2015,Mar,7; 2015,Jan,16; 2013,May,12

29819   **with removal of loose body or foreign body**
> EXCLUDES   *Open surgery (23040-23044, 23107)*
> 🛠 16.8   🔧 16.8   **FUD** 090   T A2 50 📧
> **AMA:** 2016,Jan,13; 2015,Mar,7; 2015,Jan,16; 2013,May,12

29820   **synovectomy, partial**
> EXCLUDES   *Open surgery (23105)*
> 🛠 15.3   🔧 15.3   **FUD** 090   T A2 80 50 📧
> **AMA:** 2016,Jan,13; 2015,Mar,7; 2015,Jan,16; 2013,Jun,13; 2013,May,12

29821   **synovectomy, complete**
> EXCLUDES   *Open surgery (23105)*
> 🛠 16.7   🔧 16.7   **FUD** 090   T A2 80 50 📧
> **AMA:** 2016,Jan,13; 2015,Mar,7; 2015,Jan,16; 2013,Jun,13; 2013,May,12

29822   **debridement, limited**
> EXCLUDES   *Open surgery (see specific shoulder section)*
> 🛠 16.3   🔧 16.3   **FUD** 090   T A2 80 50 📧
> **AMA:** 2016,Jan,13; 2015,Mar,7; 2015,Jan,16; 2014,Jan,11; 2013,May,12; 2012,Oct,14; 2012,Sep,16; 2012,Apr,17-18

29823   **debridement, extensive**
> EXCLUDES   *Open surgery (see specific shoulder section)*
> 🛠 17.7   🔧 17.7   **FUD** 090   T A2 80 50 📧
> **AMA:** 2016,Jan,13; 2015,Mar,7; 2015,Jan,16; 2014,Jan,11; 2013,May,12; 2012,Oct,14; 2012,Sep,16; 2012,Apr,17-18

29824   **distal claviculectomy including distal articular surface (Mumford procedure)**
> INCLUDES   Mumford procedure
> EXCLUDES   *Open surgery (23120)*
> 🛠 19.1   🔧 19.1   **FUD** 090   T A2 80 50 📧
> **AMA:** 2016,Jan,13; 2015,Mar,7; 2015,Jan,16; 2013,May,12

29825   **with lysis and resection of adhesions, with or without manipulation**
> EXCLUDES   *Open surgery (see specific shoulder section)*
> 🛠 16.6   🔧 16.6   **FUD** 090   T A2 80 50 📧
> **AMA:** 2016,Jan,13; 2015,Mar,7; 2015,Jan,16; 2013,May,12

+ **29826**   **decompression of subacromial space with partial acromioplasty, with coracoacromial ligament (ie, arch) release, when performed (List separately in addition to code for primary procedure)**
> EXCLUDES   *Open surgery (23130, 23415)*
> Code first (29806-29825, 29827-29828)
> 🛠 5.09   🔧 5.09   **FUD** ZZZ   N N1 80 50 📧
> **AMA:** 2016,Jan,13; 2015,Mar,7; 2015,Jan,16; 2014,Jan,11; 2013,May,12; 2012,Oct,14; 2012,Sep,16

| 26/TC PC/TC Only | A2-Z3 ASC Payment | 50 Bilateral | ♂ Male Only | ♀ Female Only | 🛠 Facility RVU | 🔧 Non-Facility RVU | 📧 CCI |
| **FUD** Follow-up Days | **CMS:** IOM (Pub 100) | A-Y OPPSI | 80/80 Surg Assist Allowed / w/Doc | | 🔬 Lab Crosswalk | ☢ Radiology Crosswalk | ✖ CLIA |

98   CPT © 2016 American Medical Association. All Rights Reserved.   © 2016 Optum360, LLC

29827 **with rotator cuff repair**

EXCLUDES Distal clavicle excision (29824)
Open surgery or mini open repair (23412)
Subacromial decompression (29826)

🔧 30.4 ✂ 30.4 **FUD** 090 J A2 80 50 ▢

AMA: 2016,Jul,8; 2016,Jan,13; 2015,Mar,7; 2015,Jan,16; 2014,Jan,11; 2013,May,12; 2012,Jan,15-42; 2011,Jan,11

29828 **biceps tenodesis**

EXCLUDES Arthroscopy, shoulder, diagnostic, with or without synovial biopsy (29805)
Arthroscopy, shoulder, surgical; debridement, limited (29822)
Arthroscopy, shoulder, surgical; synovectomy, partial (29820)
Tenodesis of long tendon of biceps (23430)

🔧 26.2 ✂ 26.2 **FUD** 090 J G2 80 50 ▢

AMA: 2016,Jul,8; 2016,Jan,13; 2015,Mar,7; 2015,Jan,16; 2014,Jan,11; 2013,May,12; 2012,Jan,15-42; 2011,Jan,11

29830 **Arthroscopy, elbow, diagnostic, with or without synovial biopsy (separate procedure)**

🔧 13.0 ✂ 13.0 **FUD** 090 T A2 50 ▢

AMA: 2016,Jan,13; 2015,Jan,16; 2013,May,12

29834 **Arthroscopy, elbow, surgical; with removal of loose body or foreign body**

🔧 13.9 ✂ 13.9 **FUD** 090 T A2 80 50 ▢

AMA: 2016,Jan,13; 2015,Jan,16; 2013,May,12

29835 **synovectomy, partial**

🔧 14.5 ✂ 14.5 **FUD** 090 T A2 80 50 ▢

AMA: 2016,Jan,13; 2015,Jan,16; 2013,May,12

29836 **synovectomy, complete**

🔧 16.3 ✂ 16.3 **FUD** 090 T A2 80 50 ▢

AMA: 2016,Jan,13; 2015,Jan,16; 2013,May,12

29837 **debridement, limited**

🔧 15.0 ✂ 15.0 **FUD** 090 T A2 80 50 ▢

AMA: 2016,Jan,13; 2015,Jan,16; 2013,May,12

29838 **debridement, extensive**

🔧 16.8 ✂ 16.8 **FUD** 090 T A2 80 50 ▢

AMA: 2016,Jan,13; 2015,Jan,16; 2013,May,12

29840 **Arthroscopy, wrist, diagnostic, with or without synovial biopsy (separate procedure)**

🔧 13.0 ✂ 13.0 **FUD** 090 T A2 80 50 ▢

AMA: 2016,Jan,13; 2015,Jan,16; 2013,May,12

29843 **Arthroscopy, wrist, surgical; for infection, lavage and drainage**

🔧 13.9 ✂ 13.9 **FUD** 090 T A2 80 50 ▢

AMA: 2016,Jan,13; 2015,Jan,16; 2013,May,12

29844 **synovectomy, partial**

🔧 14.2 ✂ 14.2 **FUD** 090 T A2 80 50 ▢

AMA: 2016,Jan,13; 2015,Jan,16; 2013,May,12

29845 **synovectomy, complete**

🔧 16.5 ✂ 16.5 **FUD** 090 T A2 80 50 ▢

AMA: 2016,Jan,13; 2015,Jan,16; 2014,Jan,11; 2013,May,12; 2012,Jan,15-42; 2011,Jan,11

29846 **excision and/or repair of triangular fibrocartilage and/or joint debridement**

🔧 14.9 ✂ 14.9 **FUD** 090 T A2 80 50 ▢

AMA: 2016,Jan,13; 2015,Jan,16; 2014,Jan,11; 2013,May,12; 2012,Jan,15-42; 2011,Jan,11

29847 **internal fixation for fracture or instability**

🔧 15.3 ✂ 15.3 **FUD** 090 T A2 80 50 ▢

AMA: 2016,Jan,13; 2015,Jan,16; 2013,May,12

29848 **Endoscopy, wrist, surgical, with release of transverse carpal ligament**

EXCLUDES Open surgery (64721)

🔧 14.6 ✂ 14.6 **FUD** 090 T A2 50 ▢

AMA: 2016,Jan,13; 2015,Jul,10; 2015,Jan,16; 2014,Jan,11; 2013,May,12

29850 **Arthroscopically aided treatment of intercondylar spine(s) and/or tuberosity fracture(s) of the knee, with or without manipulation; without internal or external fixation (includes arthroscopy)**

🔧 17.7 ✂ 17.7 **FUD** 090 T A2 80 50 ▢

AMA: 2016,Jan,13; 2015,Jan,16; 2013,May,12

29851 **with internal or external fixation (includes arthroscopy)**

EXCLUDES Bone graft (20900, 20902)

🔧 25.4 ✂ 25.4 **FUD** 090 T A2 80 50 ▢

AMA: 2016,Jan,13; 2015,Jan,16; 2013,May,12

29855 **Arthroscopically aided treatment of tibial fracture, proximal (plateau); unicondylar, includes internal fixation, when performed (includes arthroscopy)**

EXCLUDES Bone graft (20900, 20902)

🔧 22.5 ✂ 22.5 **FUD** 090 J A2 80 50 ▢

AMA: 2016,Jan,13; 2015,Jan,16; 2013,May,12

29856 **bicondylar, includes internal fixation, when performed (includes arthroscopy)**

EXCLUDES Bone graft (20900, 20902)

🔧 28.7 ✂ 28.7 **FUD** 090 J A2 80 50 ▢

AMA: 2016,Jan,13; 2015,Jan,16; 2013,May,12

29860 **Arthroscopy, hip, diagnostic with or without synovial biopsy (separate procedure)**

🔧 19.0 ✂ 19.0 **FUD** 090 T A2 80 50 ▢

AMA: 2016,Jan,13; 2015,Jan,16; 2014,Jan,11; 2013,May,12; 2011,Sep,5-7

29861 **Arthroscopy, hip, surgical; with removal of loose body or foreign body**

🔧 20.7 ✂ 20.7 **FUD** 090 T A2 80 50 ▢

AMA: 2016,Jan,13; 2015,Jan,16; 2014,Jan,11; 2013,May,12; 2011,Sep,5-7

29862 **with debridement/shaving of articular cartilage (chondroplasty), abrasion arthroplasty, and/or resection of labrum**

🔧 23.2 ✂ 23.2 **FUD** 090 J A2 80 50 ▢

AMA: 2016,Jan,13; 2015,Jan,16; 2014,Jan,11; 2013,May,12; 2011,Sep,5-7

29863 **with synovectomy**

🔧 23.2 ✂ 23.2 **FUD** 090 T A2 80 50 ▢

AMA: 2016,Jan,13; 2015,Jan,16; 2014,Jan,11; 2013,May,12; 2011,Sep,5-7

29914 **with femoroplasty (ie, treatment of cam lesion)**

EXCLUDES Arthroscopy, hip, surgical; with debridement/shaving of articular cartilage (chondroplasty), abrasion arthroplasty, and/or resection of labrum (29862)
Arthroscopy, hip, surgical; with synovectomy (29863)

🔧 28.6 ✂ 28.6 **FUD** 090 J G2 80 50 ▢

AMA: 2016,Jan,13; 2015,Jan,16; 2014,Jan,11; 2012,Jan,15-42; 2011,Sep,5-7

29915 **with acetabuloplasty (ie, treatment of pincer lesion)**

EXCLUDES Arthroscopy, hip, surgical; with debridement/shaving of articular cartilage (chondroplasty), abrasion arthroplasty, and/or resection of labrum (29862)
Arthroscopy, hip, surgical; with synovectomy (29863)

🔧 29.1 ✂ 29.1 **FUD** 090 J G2 80 50 ▢

AMA: 2016,Jan,13; 2015,Jan,16; 2014,Jan,11; 2012,Jan,15-42; 2011,Sep,5-7

29916 **with labral repair**

EXCLUDES Arthroscopy, hip, surgical; with acetabuloplasty ([29915])
Arthroscopy, hip, surgical; with synovectomy (29863)
Labral repair secondary to acetabuloplasty (29862)

🔧 29.1 ✂ 29.1 **FUD** 090 J G2 80 50 ▢

AMA: 2016,Jan,13; 2015,Jan,16; 2014,Jan,11; 2012,Jan,15-42; 2011,Sep,5-7

29866 **Arthroscopy, knee, surgical; osteochondral autograft(s) (eg, mosaicplasty) (includes harvesting of the autograft[s])**

> EXCLUDES *Open osteochondral autograft of the knee (27416)*
> *Procedures performed at the same surgical session (29870-29871, 29875, 29884)*
> *Procedures performed in the same compartment (29874, 29877, 29879, 29885-29887)*

🚑 30.0 🔧 30.0 **FUD** 090 J 62 80 50 ▣

AMA: 2016,Jan,13; 2015,Jan,16; 2013,May,12

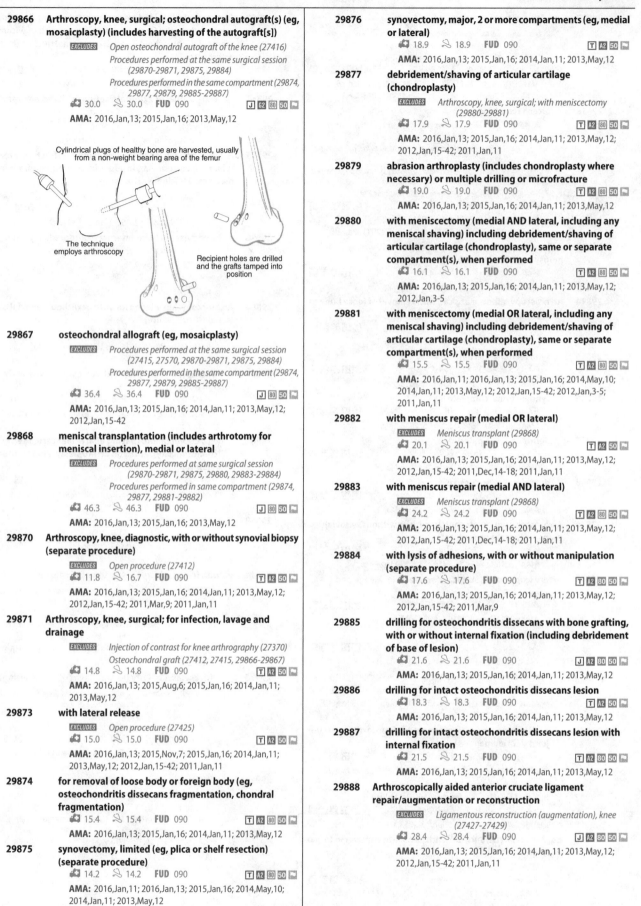

Cylindrical plugs of healthy bone are harvested, usually from a non-weight bearing area of the femur

The technique employs arthroscopy

Recipient holes are drilled and the grafts tamped into position

29867 **osteochondral allograft (eg, mosaicplasty)**

> EXCLUDES *Procedures performed at the same surgical session (27415, 27570, 29870-29871, 29875, 29884)*
> *Procedures performed in the same compartment (29874, 29877, 29879, 29885-29887)*

🚑 36.4 🔧 36.4 **FUD** 090 J 80 50 ▣

AMA: 2016,Jan,13; 2015,Jan,16; 2014,Jan,11; 2013,May,12; 2012,Jan,15-42

29868 **meniscal transplantation (includes arthrotomy for meniscal insertion), medial or lateral**

> EXCLUDES *Procedures performed at same surgical session (29870-29871, 29875, 29880, 29883-29884)*
> *Procedures performed in same compartment (29874, 29877, 29881-29882)*

🚑 46.3 🔧 46.3 **FUD** 090 J 80 50 ▣

AMA: 2016,Jan,13; 2015,Jan,16; 2013,May,12

29870 **Arthroscopy, knee, diagnostic, with or without synovial biopsy (separate procedure)**

> EXCLUDES *Open procedure (27412)*

🚑 11.8 🔧 16.7 **FUD** 090 T A2 50 ▣

AMA: 2016,Jan,13; 2015,Jan,16; 2014,Jan,11; 2013,May,12; 2012,Jan,15-42; 2011,Mar,9; 2011,Jan,11

29871 **Arthroscopy, knee, surgical; for infection, lavage and drainage**

> EXCLUDES *Injection of contrast for knee arthrography (27370)*
> *Osteochondral graft (27412, 27415, 29866-29867)*

🚑 14.8 🔧 14.8 **FUD** 090 T A2 50 ▣

AMA: 2016,Jan,13; 2015,Aug,6; 2015,Jan,16; 2014,Jan,11; 2013,May,12

29873 **with lateral release**

> EXCLUDES *Open procedure (27425)*

🚑 15.0 🔧 15.0 **FUD** 090 T A2 50 ▣

AMA: 2016,Jan,13; 2015,Nov,7; 2015,Jan,16; 2014,Jan,11; 2013,May,12; 2012,Jan,15-42; 2011,Jan,11

29874 **for removal of loose body or foreign body (eg, osteochondritis dissecans fragmentation, chondral fragmentation)**

🚑 15.4 🔧 15.4 **FUD** 090 T A2 80 50 ▣

AMA: 2016,Jan,13; 2015,Jan,16; 2014,Jan,11; 2013,May,12

29875 **synovectomy, limited (eg, plica or shelf resection) (separate procedure)**

🚑 14.2 🔧 14.2 **FUD** 090 T A2 80 50 ▣

AMA: 2016,Jan,11; 2016,Jan,13; 2015,Jan,16; 2014,May,10; 2014,Jan,11; 2013,May,12

29876 **synovectomy, major, 2 or more compartments (eg, medial or lateral)**

🚑 18.9 🔧 18.9 **FUD** 090 T A2 50 ▣

AMA: 2016,Jan,13; 2015,Jan,16; 2014,Jan,11; 2013,May,12

29877 **debridement/shaving of articular cartilage (chondroplasty)**

> EXCLUDES *Arthroscopy, knee, surgical; with meniscectomy (29880-29881)*

🚑 17.9 🔧 17.9 **FUD** 090 T A2 80 50 ▣

AMA: 2016,Jan,13; 2015,Jan,16; 2014,Jan,11; 2013,May,12; 2012,Jan,15-42; 2011,Jan,11

29879 **abrasion arthroplasty (includes chondroplasty where necessary) or multiple drilling or microfracture**

🚑 19.0 🔧 19.0 **FUD** 090 T A2 80 50 ▣

AMA: 2016,Jan,13; 2015,Jan,16; 2014,Jan,11; 2013,May,12

29880 **with meniscectomy (medial AND lateral, including any meniscal shaving) including debridement/shaving of articular cartilage (chondroplasty), same or separate compartment(s), when performed**

🚑 16.1 🔧 16.1 **FUD** 090 T A2 80 50 ▣

AMA: 2016,Jan,13; 2015,Jan,16; 2014,Jan,11; 2013,May,12; 2012,Jan,3-5

29881 **with meniscectomy (medial OR lateral, including any meniscal shaving) including debridement/shaving of articular cartilage (chondroplasty), same or separate compartment(s), when performed**

🚑 15.5 🔧 15.5 **FUD** 090 T A2 80 50 ▣

AMA: 2016,Jan,11; 2016,Jan,13; 2015,Jan,16; 2014,May,10; 2014,Jan,11; 2013,May,12; 2012,Jan,15-42; 2012,Jan,3-5; 2011,Jan,11

29882 **with meniscus repair (medial OR lateral)**

> EXCLUDES *Meniscus transplant (29868)*

🚑 20.1 🔧 20.1 **FUD** 090 T A2 50 ▣

AMA: 2016,Jan,13; 2015,Jan,16; 2014,Jan,11; 2013,May,12; 2012,Jan,15-42; 2011,Dec,14-18; 2011,Jan,11

29883 **with meniscus repair (medial AND lateral)**

> EXCLUDES *Meniscus transplant (29868)*

🚑 24.2 🔧 24.2 **FUD** 090 T A2 80 50 ▣

AMA: 2016,Jan,13; 2015,Jan,16; 2014,Jan,11; 2013,May,12; 2012,Jan,15-42; 2011,Dec,14-18; 2011,Jan,11

29884 **with lysis of adhesions, with or without manipulation (separate procedure)**

🚑 17.6 🔧 17.6 **FUD** 090 T A2 80 50 ▣

AMA: 2016,Jan,13; 2015,Jan,16; 2014,Jan,11; 2013,May,12; 2012,Jan,15-42; 2011,Mar,9

29885 **drilling for osteochondritis dissecans with bone grafting, with or without internal fixation (including debridement of base of lesion)**

🚑 21.6 🔧 21.6 **FUD** 090 J A2 80 50 ▣

AMA: 2016,Jan,13; 2015,Jan,16; 2014,Jan,11; 2013,May,12

29886 **drilling for intact osteochondritis dissecans lesion**

🚑 18.3 🔧 18.3 **FUD** 090 T A2 50 ▣

AMA: 2016,Jan,13; 2015,Jan,16; 2014,Jan,11; 2013,May,12

29887 **drilling for intact osteochondritis dissecans lesion with internal fixation**

🚑 21.5 🔧 21.5 **FUD** 090 T A2 80 50 ▣

AMA: 2016,Jan,13; 2015,Jan,16; 2014,Jan,11; 2013,May,12

29888 **Arthroscopically aided anterior cruciate ligament repair/augmentation or reconstruction**

> EXCLUDES *Ligamentous reconstruction (augmentation), knee (27427-27429)*

🚑 28.4 🔧 28.4 **FUD** 090 J A2 80 50 ▣

AMA: 2016,Jan,13; 2015,Jan,16; 2014,Jan,11; 2013,May,12; 2012,Jan,15-42; 2011,Jan,11

29889	**Arthroscopically aided posterior cruciate ligament repair/augmentation or reconstruction**
	EXCLUDES *Ligamentous reconstruction (augmentation), knee (27427-27429)*
	🚗 35.2 ⚕ 35.2 **FUD** 090 [J] [J8] [80] [50] [▣]
	AMA: 2016,Jan,13; 2015,Jan,16; 2014,Jan,11; 2013,May,12; 2012,Jan,15-42; 2011,Jan,11

29891	**Arthroscopy, ankle, surgical, excision of osteochondral defect of talus and/or tibia, including drilling of the defect**
	🚗 19.4 ⚕ 19.4 **FUD** 090 [T] [A2] [80] [50] [▣]
	AMA: 2016,Jan,13; 2015,Jan,16; 2013,May,12

29892	**Arthroscopically aided repair of large osteochondritis dissecans lesion, talar dome fracture, or tibial plafond fracture, with or without internal fixation (includes arthroscopy)**
	🚗 16.7 ⚕ 16.7 **FUD** 090 [T] [A2] [80] [50] [▣]
	AMA: 2016,Jan,13; 2015,Jan,16; 2014,Jan,11; 2013,May,12

29893	**Endoscopic plantar fasciotomy**
	🚗 12.2 ⚕ 17.6 **FUD** 090 [T] [A2] [50] [▣]
	AMA: 2016,Jan,13; 2015,Jan,16; 2013,May,12

29894	**Arthroscopy, ankle (tibiotalar and fibulotalar joints), surgical; with removal of loose body or foreign body**
	🚗 14.4 ⚕ 14.4 **FUD** 090 [T] [A2] [80] [50] [▣]
	AMA: 2016,Jan,13; 2015,Jan,16; 2013,May,12

29895	**synovectomy, partial**
	🚗 13.7 ⚕ 13.7 **FUD** 090 [T] [A2] [80] [50] [▣]
	AMA: 2016,Jan,13; 2015,Jan,16; 2014,Jan,11; 2013,May,12; 2012,Jan,15-42

29897	**debridement, limited**
	🚗 14.5 ⚕ 14.5 **FUD** 090 [T] [A2] [80] [50] [▣]
	AMA: 2016,Jan,13; 2015,Jan,16; 2013,May,12

29898	**debridement, extensive**
	🚗 16.2 ⚕ 16.2 **FUD** 090 [T] [A2] [80] [50] [▣]
	AMA: 2016,Jan,13; 2015,Jan,16; 2013,May,12

29899	**with ankle arthrodesis**
	EXCLUDES *Open procedure (27870)*
	🚗 29.8 ⚕ 29.8 **FUD** 090 [J] [G2] [80] [50] [▣]
	AMA: 2016,Jan,13; 2015,Jan,16; 2013,May,12

29900	**Arthroscopy, metacarpophalangeal joint, diagnostic, includes synovial biopsy**
	EXCLUDES *Arthroscopy, metacarpophalangeal joint, surgical (29901-29902)*
	🚗 13.0 ⚕ 13.0 **FUD** 090 [T] [A2] [80] [50] [▣]
	AMA: 2016,Jan,13; 2015,Jan,16; 2013,May,12

29901	**Arthroscopy, metacarpophalangeal joint, surgical; with debridement**
	🚗 15.3 ⚕ 15.3 **FUD** 090 [T] [A2] [80] [50] [▣]
	AMA: 2016,Jan,13; 2015,Jan,16; 2013,May,12

29902	**with reduction of displaced ulnar collateral ligament (eg, Stenar lesion)**
	🚗 16.1 ⚕ 16.1 **FUD** 090 [T] [A2] [80] [50] [▣]
	AMA: 2016,Jan,13; 2015,Jan,16; 2013,May,12

29904	**Arthroscopy, subtalar joint, surgical; with removal of loose body or foreign body**
	🚗 18.3 ⚕ 18.3 **FUD** 090 [T] [G2] [80] [50] [▣]
	AMA: 2016,Jan,13; 2015,Jan,16; 2013,May,12

29905	**with synovectomy**
	🚗 19.7 ⚕ 19.7 **FUD** 090 [T] [G2] [80] [50] [▣]
	AMA: 2016,Jan,13; 2015,Jan,16; 2013,May,12

29906	**with debridement**
	🚗 20.7 ⚕ 20.7 **FUD** 090 [T] [G2] [80] [50] [▣]
	AMA: 2016,Jan,13; 2015,Jan,16; 2013,May,12

29907	**with subtalar arthrodesis**
	🚗 25.2 ⚕ 25.2 **FUD** 090 [J] [G2] [80] [50] [▣]
	AMA: 2016,Jan,13; 2015,Jan,16; 2013,May,12

29914	**Resequenced code. See code following 29863.**

29915	**Resequenced code. See code following 29863.**
29916	**Resequenced code. See code before 29866.**
29999	**Unlisted procedure, arthroscopy**
	🚗 0.00 ⚕ 0.00 **FUD** YYY [T] [80] [50] [▣]
	AMA: 2016,Jan,13; 2015,Dec,16; 2015,Jan,16; 2014,Jan,11; 2013,May,12; 2012,Apr,17-18; 2012,Jan,15-42; 2011,Dec,14-18; 2011,Jan,11

30000-30115 I&D, Biopsy, Excision Procedures of the Nose

30000 Drainage abscess or hematoma, nasal, internal approach

EXCLUDES *Incision and drainage (10060, 10140)*

🔧 3.39 ⚕ 6.58 **FUD** 010 [T] [P2] [80] ▣

AMA: 2005,May,13-14; 1994,Spr,24

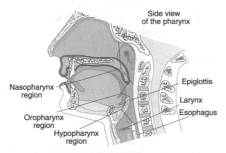

Side view of the pharynx

Nasopharynx region
Oropharynx region
Hypopharynx region
Epiglottis
Larynx
Esophagus

The nasopharynx is the membranous passage above the level of the soft palate; the oropharynx is the region between the soft palate and the upper edge of the epiglottis; the hypopharynx is the region of the epiglottis to the juncture of the larynx and esophagus; the three regions are collectively known as the pharynx

30020 Drainage abscess or hematoma, nasal septum

🔧 3.42 ⚕ 6.67 **FUD** 010 [T] [P2] ▣

EXCLUDES *Lateral rhinotomy incision (30118, 30320)*

30100 Biopsy, intranasal

🔧 1.98 ⚕ 4.04 **FUD** 000 [T] [P3] ▣

EXCLUDES *Superficial biopsy of nose (11100-11101)*

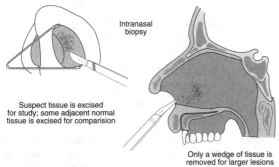

Intranasal biopsy

Suspect tissue is excised for study; some adjacent normal tissue is excised for comparision

Only a wedge of tissue is removed for larger lesions

30110 Excision, nasal polyp(s), simple

🔧 3.74 ⚕ 6.60 **FUD** 010 [T] [P3] [50] ▣

30115 Excision, nasal polyp(s), extensive

🔧 12.3 ⚕ 12.3 **FUD** 090 [T] [A2] [50] ▣

30117-30118 Destruction Procedures Nose

CMS: 100-03,140.5 Laser Procedures

30117 Excision or destruction (eg, laser), intranasal lesion; internal approach

🔧 9.77 ⚕ 25.1 **FUD** 090 [T] [A2] ▣

AMA: 1990,Win,4

30118 external approach (lateral rhinotomy)

🔧 22.0 ⚕ 22.0 **FUD** 090 [T] [A2] ▣

30120-30140 Excision Procedures Nose, Turbinate

30120 Excision or surgical planing of skin of nose for rhinophyma

🔧 12.5 ⚕ 14.8 **FUD** 090 [T] [A2] ▣

AMA: 2016,Jan,13; 2015,Jan,16; 2014,Jan,11; 2012,Jan,15-42; 2011,Jan,11

30124 Excision dermoid cyst, nose; simple, skin, subcutaneous

🔧 8.19 ⚕ 8.19 **FUD** 090 [T] [R2] ▣

30125 complex, under bone or cartilage

🔧 17.4 ⚕ 17.4 **FUD** 090 [J] [A2] [80] ▣

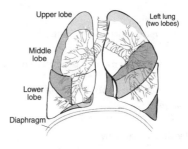

Upper lobe
Middle lobe
Lower lobe
Diaphragm
Left lung (two lobes)

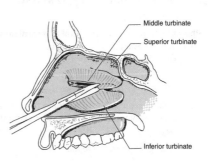

Middle turbinate
Superior turbinate
Inferior turbinate

30130 Excision inferior turbinate, partial or complete, any method

EXCLUDES *Ablation, soft tissue of inferior turbinates, unilateral or bilateral, any method (30801-30802)*
Excision middle/superior turbinate(s) (30999)
Fracture nasal inferior turbinate(s), therapeutic (30930)

🔧 10.9 ⚕ 10.9 **FUD** 090 [T] [A2] [50] ▣

AMA: 2016,Jan,13; 2015,Jan,16; 2014,Jan,11; 2012,Jan,15-42; 2011,Jan,11

30140 Submucous resection inferior turbinate, partial or complete, any method

EXCLUDES *Ablation, soft tissue of inferior turbinates, unilateral or bilateral, any method (30801-30802)*
Endoscopic resection of concha bullosa of middle turbinate (31240)
Fracture nasal inferior turbinate(s), therapeutic (30930)
Submucous resection:
Nasal septum (30520)
Superior or middle turbinate (30999)

🔧 12.6 ⚕ 12.6 **FUD** 090 [T] [A2] [50] ▣

AMA: 2016,Jan,13; 2015,Jan,16; 2014,Jan,11; 2012,Jan,15-42; 2011,Jan,11

30150-30160 Surgical Removal: Nose

EXCLUDES *Reconstruction and/or closure (primary or delayed primary intention) (13151-13160, 14060-14302, 15120-15121, 15260-15261, 15760, 20900-20912)*

30150 Rhinectomy; partial

🔧 22.0 ⚕ 22.0 **FUD** 090 [J] [A2] ▣

30160 total

🔧 22.1 ⚕ 22.1 **FUD** 090 [J] [A2] [80] ▣

30200-30320 Turbinate Injection, Removal Foreign Substance in the Nose

30200 Injection into turbinate(s), therapeutic

🔧 1.71 ⚕ 3.26 **FUD** 000 [T] [P3] ▣

AMA: 2016,Jan,13; 2015,Jan,16; 2014,Jan,11; 2012,Jan,15-42; 2011,Jan,11

30210 **Displacement therapy (Proetz type)**
🚗 2.85   ⚕ 4.29   **FUD** 010   [T] [P3] ▭
AMA: 2016,Jan,13; 2015,Jan,16; 2014,Jan,11; 2012,Jan,15-42; 2011,Jan,11

30220 **Insertion, nasal septal prosthesis (button)**
🚗 3.59   ⚕ 8.68   **FUD** 010   [T] [A2] ▭

30300 **Removal foreign body, intranasal; office type procedure**
🚗 3.03   ⚕ 5.32   **FUD** 010   [01] [N1] ▭
AMA: 2016,Jan,13; 2015,Jan,16; 2014,Jan,11; 2012,Jan,13-14

30310 **requiring general anesthesia**
🚗 5.91   ⚕ 5.91   **FUD** 010   [T] [A2] [80] ▭

30320 **by lateral rhinotomy**
🚗 12.7   ⚕ 12.7   **FUD** 090   [T] [A2] [80] ▭

30400-30630 Reconstruction or Repair of Nose

EXCLUDES   Bone/tissue grafts (20900-20926, 21210)

30400 **Rhinoplasty, primary; lateral and alar cartilages and/or elevation of nasal tip**
🚗 28.9   ⚕ 28.9   **FUD** 090   [T] [A2] [80] ▭

     INCLUDES   Carpue's operation
     EXCLUDES   Reconstruction of columella (13151-13153)

30410 **complete, external parts including bony pyramid, lateral and alar cartilages, and/or elevation of nasal tip**
🚗 33.8   ⚕ 33.8   **FUD** 090   [J] [A2] [80] ▭

30420 **including major septal repair**
🚗 39.2   ⚕ 39.2   **FUD** 090   [J] [A2] ▭
AMA: 2016,Jul,8

30430 **Rhinoplasty, secondary; minor revision (small amount of nasal tip work)**
🚗 27.5   ⚕ 27.5   **FUD** 090   [T] [A2] [80] ▭

30435 **intermediate revision (bony work with osteotomies)**
🚗 31.7   ⚕ 31.7   **FUD** 090   [J] [A2] [80] ▭

30450 **major revision (nasal tip work and osteotomies)**
🚗 42.8   ⚕ 42.8   **FUD** 090   [J] [A2] [80] ▭

30460 **Rhinoplasty for nasal deformity secondary to congenital cleft lip and/or palate, including columellar lengthening; tip only**
🚗 20.4   ⚕ 20.4   **FUD** 090   [J] [A2] [80] ▭
AMA: 2016,Jan,13; 2015,Jan,16; 2014,Dec,18

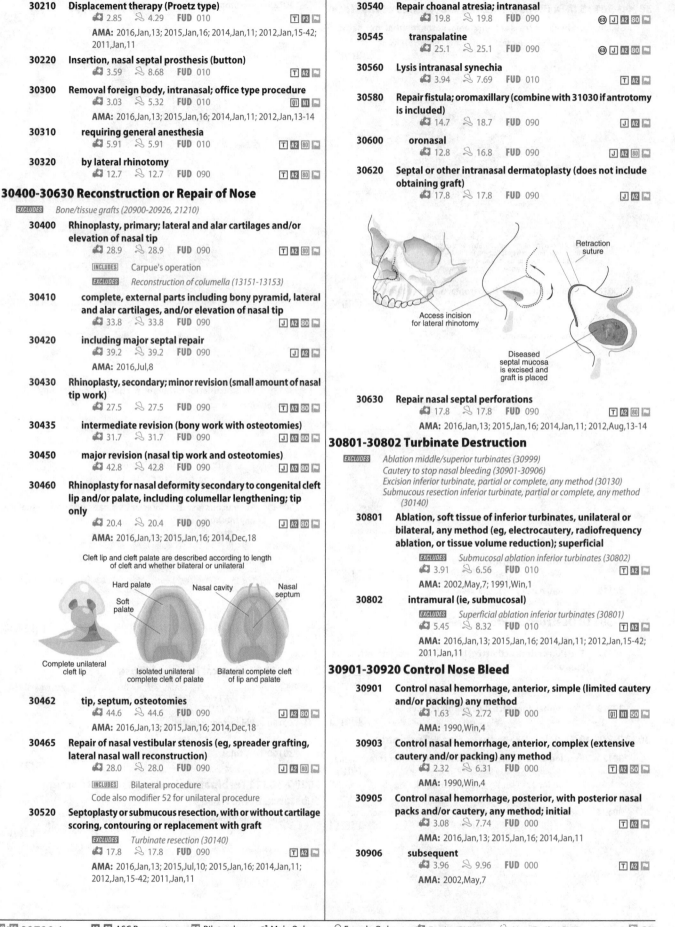

Cleft lip and cleft palate are described according to length of cleft and whether bilateral or unilateral

Hard palate   Nasal cavity   Nasal septum
Soft palate

Complete unilateral cleft lip   Isolated unilateral complete cleft of palate   Bilateral complete cleft of lip and palate

30462 **tip, septum, osteotomies**
🚗 44.6   ⚕ 44.6   **FUD** 090   [J] [A2] [80] ▭
AMA: 2016,Jan,13; 2015,Jan,16; 2014,Dec,18

30465 **Repair of nasal vestibular stenosis (eg, spreader grafting, lateral nasal wall reconstruction)**
🚗 28.0   ⚕ 28.0   **FUD** 090   [J] [A2] [80] ▭

     INCLUDES   Bilateral procedure
     Code also modifier 52 for unilateral procedure

30520 **Septoplasty or submucous resection, with or without cartilage scoring, contouring or replacement with graft**
     EXCLUDES   Turbinate resection (30140)
🚗 17.8   ⚕ 17.8   **FUD** 090   [T] [A2] ▭
AMA: 2016,Jan,13; 2015,Jul,10; 2015,Jan,16; 2014,Jan,11; 2012,Jan,15-42; 2011,Jan,11

30540 **Repair choanal atresia; intranasal**
🚗 19.8   ⚕ 19.8   **FUD** 090   [63] [J] [A2] [80] ▭

30545 **transpalatine**
🚗 25.1   ⚕ 25.1   **FUD** 090   [63] [J] [A2] [80] ▭

30560 **Lysis intranasal synechia**
🚗 3.94   ⚕ 7.69   **FUD** 010   [T] [A2] ▭

30580 **Repair fistula; oromaxillary (combine with 31030 if antrotomy is included)**
🚗 14.7   ⚕ 18.7   **FUD** 090   [J] [A2] ▭

30600 **oronasal**
🚗 12.8   ⚕ 16.8   **FUD** 090   [J] [A2] [80] ▭

30620 **Septal or other intranasal dermatoplasty (does not include obtaining graft)**
🚗 17.8   ⚕ 17.8   **FUD** 090   [J] [A2] ▭

Retraction suture

Access incision for lateral rhinotomy

Diseased septal mucosa is excised and graft is placed

30630 **Repair nasal septal perforations**
🚗 17.8   ⚕ 17.8   **FUD** 090   [T] [A2] [80] ▭
AMA: 2016,Jan,13; 2015,Jan,16; 2014,Jan,11; 2012,Aug,13-14

30801-30802 Turbinate Destruction

EXCLUDES   Ablation middle/superior turbinates (30999)
     Cautery to stop nasal bleeding (30901-30906)
     Excision inferior turbinate, partial or complete, any method (30130)
     Submucous resection inferior turbinate, partial or complete, any method (30140)

30801 **Ablation, soft tissue of inferior turbinates, unilateral or bilateral, any method (eg, electrocautery, radiofrequency ablation, or tissue volume reduction); superficial**
     EXCLUDES   Submucosal ablation inferior turbinates (30802)
🚗 3.91   ⚕ 6.56   **FUD** 010   [T] [A2] ▭
AMA: 2002,May,7; 1991,Win,1

30802 **intramural (ie, submucosal)**
     EXCLUDES   Superficial ablation inferior turbinates (30801)
🚗 5.45   ⚕ 8.32   **FUD** 010   [T] [A2] ▭
AMA: 2016,Jan,13; 2015,Jan,16; 2014,Jan,11; 2012,Jan,15-42; 2011,Jan,11

30901-30920 Control Nose Bleed

30901 **Control nasal hemorrhage, anterior, simple (limited cautery and/or packing) any method**
🚗 1.63   ⚕ 2.72   **FUD** 000   [01] [N1] [50] ▭
AMA: 1990,Win,4

30903 **Control nasal hemorrhage, anterior, complex (extensive cautery and/or packing) any method**
🚗 2.32   ⚕ 6.31   **FUD** 000   [T] [A2] [50] ▭
AMA: 1990,Win,4

30905 **Control nasal hemorrhage, posterior, with posterior nasal packs and/or cautery, any method; initial**
🚗 3.08   ⚕ 7.74   **FUD** 000   [T] [A2] ▭
AMA: 2016,Jan,13; 2015,Jan,16; 2014,Jan,11

30906 **subsequent**
🚗 3.96   ⚕ 9.96   **FUD** 000   [T] [A2] ▭
AMA: 2002,May,7

| 26/TC PC/TC Only | A2-Z3 ASC Payment | 50 Bilateral | ♂ Male Only | ♀ Female Only | 🚗 Facility RVU | ⚕ Non-Facility RVU | ▭ CCI |
| **FUD** Follow-up Days | **CMS:** IOM (Pub 100) | A-Y OPPSI | 80/80 Surg Assist Allowed / w/Doc | | 🔬 Lab Crosswalk | 📊 Radiology Crosswalk | ❌ CLIA |

104   CPT © 2016 American Medical Association. All Rights Reserved.   © 2016 Optum360, LLC

30915 Ligation arteries; ethmoidal
🔧 16.5　⚬ 16.5　**FUD** 090　　T A2 🖥

EXCLUDES　*External carotid artery (37600)*

30920 internal maxillary artery, transantral
🔧 23.9　⚬ 23.9　**FUD** 090　　T A2 🖥

EXCLUDES　*External carotid artery (37600)*

30930-30999 Other and Unlisted Procedures of Nose

30930 Fracture nasal inferior turbinate(s), therapeutic

EXCLUDES　*Excision inferior turbinate, partial or complete, any method (30130)*
Fracture of superior or middle turbinate(s) (30999)
Submucous resection inferior turbinate, partial or complete, any method (30140)

🔧 3.53　⚬ 3.53　**FUD** 010　　T A2 50 🖥

AMA: 2016,Jul,8; 2016,Jan,13; 2015,Jan,16; 2014,Jan,11; 2012,Jan,15-42; 2011,Jan,11

30999 Unlisted procedure, nose
🔧 0.00　⚬ 0.00　**FUD** YYY　　T 80

AMA: 2016,Jan,13; 2015,Jan,16; 2013,Feb,13

31000-31230 Opening Sinuses

31000 Lavage by cannulation; maxillary sinus (antrum puncture or natural ostium)
🔧 3.04　⚬ 5.26　**FUD** 010　　T P3 50 🖥

AMA: 2016,Jan,13; 2015,Jan,16; 2014,Apr,10

Schematic showing lateral wall of the nasal cavity (above) and coronal section showing nasal and paranasal sinuses (left)

31002 sphenoid sinus
🔧 5.54　⚬ 5.54　**FUD** 010　　T R2 80 50 🖥

31020 Sinusotomy, maxillary (antrotomy); intranasal
🔧 10.3　⚬ 13.8　**FUD** 090　　T A2 50 🖥

31030 radical (Caldwell-Luc) without removal of antrochoanal polyps
🔧 15.1　⚬ 19.8　**FUD** 090　　J A2 50 🖥

31032 radical (Caldwell-Luc) with removal of antrochoanal polyps
🔧 16.4　⚬ 16.4　**FUD** 090　　J A2 50 🖥

31040 Pterygomaxillary fossa surgery, any approach
🔧 21.8　⚬ 21.8　**FUD** 090　　T R2 50 🖥

EXCLUDES　*Transantral ligation internal maxillary artery (30920)*

31050 Sinusotomy, sphenoid, with or without biopsy;
🔧 13.9　⚬ 13.9　**FUD** 090　　J A2 50 🖥

31051 with mucosal stripping or removal of polyp(s)
🔧 18.4　⚬ 18.4　**FUD** 090　　J A2 50 🖥

31070 Sinusotomy frontal; external, simple (trephine operation)
🔧 12.5　⚬ 12.5　**FUD** 090　　J A2 50 🖥

INCLUDES　Killian operation

EXCLUDES　*Intranasal frontal sinusotomy (31276)*

31075 transorbital, unilateral (for mucocele or osteoma, Lynch type)
🔧 22.5　⚬ 22.5　**FUD** 090　　J A2 80 50 🖥

31080 obliterative without osteoplastic flap, brow incision (includes ablation)
🔧 29.6　⚬ 29.6　**FUD** 090　　J A2 80 50 🖥

INCLUDES　Ridell sinusotomy

31081 obliterative, without osteoplastic flap, coronal incision (includes ablation)
🔧 42.3　⚬ 42.3　**FUD** 090　　J A2 80 50 🖥

31084 obliterative, with osteoplastic flap, brow incision
🔧 33.1　⚬ 33.1　**FUD** 090　　J A2 80 50 🖥

31085 obliterative, with osteoplastic flap, coronal incision
🔧 45.1　⚬ 45.1　**FUD** 090　　J A2 80 50 🖥

31086 nonobliterative, with osteoplastic flap, brow incision
🔧 32.3　⚬ 32.3　**FUD** 090　　J A2 80 50 🖥

31087 nonobliterative, with osteoplastic flap, coronal incision
🔧 31.0　⚬ 31.0　**FUD** 090　　J A2 80 50 🖥

31090 Sinusotomy, unilateral, 3 or more paranasal sinuses (frontal, maxillary, ethmoid, sphenoid)
🔧 29.3　⚬ 29.3　**FUD** 090　　J A2 50 🖥

AMA: 1998,Nov,1; 1997,Nov,1

31200 Ethmoidectomy; intranasal, anterior
🔧 16.2　⚬ 16.2　**FUD** 090　　J A2 50 🖥

AMA: 2016,Feb,10

31201 intranasal, total
🔧 21.1　⚬ 21.1　**FUD** 090　　T A2 50 🖥

AMA: 2016,Feb,10

31205 extranasal, total
🔧 25.5　⚬ 25.5　**FUD** 090　　T A2 80 50 🖥

AMA: 2016,Feb,10

31225 Maxillectomy; without orbital exenteration
🔧 53.8　⚬ 53.8　**FUD** 090　　C 80 50 🖥

31230 with orbital exenteration (en bloc)
🔧 59.7　⚬ 59.7　**FUD** 090　　C 80 50 🖥

EXCLUDES　*Orbital exenteration without maxillectomy (65110-65114)*
Skin grafts (15120-15121)

31231-31235 Nasal Endoscopy, Diagnostic

INCLUDES　Complete sinus exam (e.g., nasal cavity, turbinates, sphenoethmoidal recess)

31231 Nasal endoscopy, diagnostic, unilateral or bilateral (separate procedure)
🔧 1.87　⚬ 6.00　**FUD** 000　　T P2 🖥

AMA: 2016,Feb,10; 2016,Jan,13; 2015,Jan,16; 2014,Jan,11

31233 Nasal/sinus endoscopy, diagnostic with maxillary sinusoscopy (via inferior meatus or canine fossa puncture)

EXCLUDES　*Nasal/sinus endoscopy, surgical; with dilation of maxillary sinus ostium (31295)*

🔧 3.94　⚬ 7.52　**FUD** 000　　T A2 80 50 🖥

AMA: 2016,Jan,13; 2015,Jan,16; 2014,Jan,11; 2011,Jun,11-12

31235 Nasal/sinus endoscopy, diagnostic with sphenoid sinusoscopy (via puncture of sphenoidal face or cannulation of ostium)

EXCLUDES　*Nasal/sinus endoscopy, surgical; with dilation of sphenoid sinus ostium (31297)*

🔧 4.67　⚬ 8.57　**FUD** 000　　T A2 80 50 🖥

AMA: 2016,Jan,13; 2015,Jan,16; 2014,Jan,11; 2011,Jun,11-12

Respiratory System

31237 — 31287

31237-31240 Nasal Endoscopy, Surgical

INCLUDES Diagnostic nasal/sinus endoscopy
Unilateral procedure

EXCLUDES *Frontal sinus exploration (31276)*
Maxillary antrostomy (31256)
*Osteomeatal complex (OMC) resection and/or partial (anterior)
ethmoidectomy (31254)*
Removal of maxillary sinus tissue (31267)
Total (anterior and posterior) ethmoidectomy (31255)

31237 **Nasal/sinus endoscopy, surgical; with biopsy, polypectomy
or debridement (separate procedure)**

🗁 4.66   ⚕ 7.41   **FUD** 000   T A2 50 ▱

AMA: 2016,Feb,10; 2016,Jan,13; 2015,Jan,16; 2015,Jan,13;
2014,Jan,11; 2012,Jan,15-42; 2011,Dec,13; 2011,Jun,11-12;
2011,Jan,11

31238 **with control of nasal hemorrhage**

🗁 4.88   ⚕ 7.40   **FUD** 000   T A2 80 50 ▱

AMA: 2016,Jan,13; 2015,Jan,16; 2014,Jan,11; 2011,Jun,11-12

31239 **with dacryocystorhinostomy**

🗁 17.6   ⚕ 17.6   **FUD** 010   T A2 80 50 ▱

AMA: 2016,Jan,13; 2015,Jan,16; 2014,Jan,11; 2011,Jun,11-12

31240 **with concha bullosa resection**

🗁 4.65   ⚕ 4.65   **FUD** 000   T A2 80 50 ▱

AMA: 2016,Feb,10; 2016,Jan,13; 2015,Jan,16; 2014,Jan,11;
2011,Jun,11-12

31254-31255 Nasal Endoscopy with Ethmoid Removal

INCLUDES Diagnostic nasal/sinus endoscopy
Sinusotomy, when applicable

31254 **Nasal/sinus endoscopy, surgical; with ethmoidectomy, partial
(anterior)**

Code also any combination of the following endoscopic
procedures when performed in conjunction with partial
(anterior) ethmoidectomy and/or osteomeatal complex
(OMC) resection, regardless of whether polyps are removed:
Antrostomy, with or without removal of maxillary
sinus tissue; either (31256, 31267)
Frontal sinus exploration (31276)

🗁 7.88   ⚕ 7.88   **FUD** 000   T A2 50 ▱

AMA: 2016,Feb,10; 2016,Jan,13; 2015,Jan,16; 2014,Jan,11;
2012,Jan,15-42; 2011,Jun,11-12; 2011,Jan,11

31255 **with ethmoidectomy, total (anterior and posterior)**

Code also any combination of the following endoscopic
procedures when performed in conjunction with total
(anterior and posterior) ethmoidectomy, regardless of
whether polyps are removed:
Antrostomy, with or without removal of maxillary
sinus tissue; either (31256, 31267)
Frontal sinus exploration (31276)
Sphenoidotomy, with or without removal of tissue;
either (31287, 31288)

🗁 11.5   ⚕ 11.5   **FUD** 000   T A2 50 ▱

AMA: 2016,Feb,10; 2016,Jan,13; 2015,Jan,16; 2014,Jan,11;
2012,Jan,15-42; 2011,Jun,11-12; 2011,Jan,11

31256-31267 Nasal Endoscopy with Maxillary Procedures

INCLUDES Diagnostic nasal/sinus endoscopy
Nasal/sinus endoscopy, surgical; with dilation of maxillary sinus ostium
(31295)
Sinusotomy, when applicable

31256 **Nasal/sinus endoscopy, surgical, with maxillary
antrostomy;**

Code also any combination of the following endoscopic
procedures when performed in conjunction with maxillary
antrostomy, regardless if polyps are removed:
Frontal sinus exploration (31276)
Sphenoidotomy, with or without removal of tissue;
either (31287, 31288)
Total (anterior and posterior) ethmoidectomy (31255)

🗁 5.71   ⚕ 5.71   **FUD** 000   T A2 50 ▱

AMA: 2016,Jan,13; 2015,Jan,16; 2014,Jan,11; 2013,Jun,13;
2011,Jun,11-12

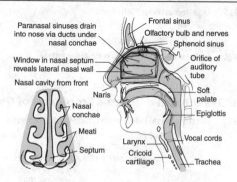

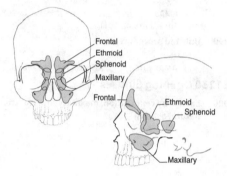

31267 **with removal of tissue from maxillary sinus**

Code also any combination of the following endoscopic
procedures when performed in conjunction with maxillary
antrostomy with removal of maxillary sinus tissue,
regardless of whether polyps are removed:
Frontal sinus exploration (31276)
Sphenoidotomy, with or without removal of tissue;
either (31287, 31288)
Total (anterior and posterior) ethmoidectomy (31255)

🗁 9.17   ⚕ 9.17   **FUD** 000   T A2 50 ▱

AMA: 2016,Jan,13; 2015,Jan,16; 2014,Jan,11; 2012,Jan,15-42;
2011,Jun,11-12; 2011,Jan,11

31276 Nasal Endoscopy with Frontal Sinus Examination

INCLUDES Diagnostic nasal/sinus endoscopy
Sinusotomy, when applicable
Unilateral procedure

EXCLUDES *Unilateral endoscopy two or more sinuses (31231-31235)*

Code also any combination of the following endoscopic procedures when performed
in conjunction with frontal sinus exploration, regardless of whether polyps are
removed:
Antrostomy, with or without removal of maxillary sinus tissue; either
(31256, 31267)
Nasal/sinus endoscopy, surgical; with dilation of frontal sinus ostium
(different sinus) (31296)
Sphenoidotomy, with or without removal of tissue; either (31287, 31288)
Total (anterior and posterior) ethmoidectomy (31255)

31276 **Nasal/sinus endoscopy, surgical with frontal sinus exploration,
with or without removal of tissue from frontal sinus**

🗁 14.5   ⚕ 14.5   **FUD** 000   T A2 50 ▱

AMA: 2016,Jan,13; 2015,Jan,16; 2014,Jan,11; 2012,Jan,15-42;
2011,Jun,11-12; 2011,Jan,11

31287-31288 Nasal Endoscopy with Sphenoid Procedures

INCLUDES Diagnostic nasal/sinus endoscopy
Sinusotomy, when applicable

Code also nasal/sinus endoscopy, surgical; with dilation of sphenoid sinus ostium
(different sinus) (31297)

31287 **Nasal/sinus endoscopy, surgical, with sphenoidotomy;**

🗁 6.70   ⚕ 6.70   **FUD** 000   T A2 80 50 ▱

AMA: 2016,Jan,13; 2015,Jan,16; 2014,Jan,11; 2011,Jun,11-12

31288   **with removal of tissue from the sphenoid sinus**
     7.76   7.76   **FUD** 000   T A2 80 50
     AMA: 2016,Feb,10; 2016,Jan,13; 2015,Jan,16; 2014,Jan,11; 2011,Jun,11-12

31290-31294 Nasal Endoscopy with Repair and Decompression

INCLUDES   Diagnostic nasal/sinus endoscopy
     Sinusotomy, when applicable

31290   **Nasal/sinus endoscopy, surgical, with repair of cerebrospinal fluid leak; ethmoid region**
     33.3   33.3   **FUD** 010   C 80 50
     AMA: 2016,Feb,10; 2016,Jan,13; 2015,Jan,16; 2014,Jan,11; 2011,Jun,11-12

31291   **sphenoid region**
     35.5   35.5   **FUD** 010   C 80 50
     AMA: 2016,Jan,13; 2015,Jan,16; 2014,Jan,11; 2011,Jun,11-12

31292   **Nasal/sinus endoscopy, surgical; with medial or inferior orbital wall decompression**
     28.8   28.8   **FUD** 010   T 80 50
     AMA: 2016,Jan,13; 2015,Jan,16; 2014,Jan,11; 2011,Jun,11-12

31293   **with medial orbital wall and inferior orbital wall decompression**
     31.2   31.2   **FUD** 010   T 80 50
     AMA: 2016,Jan,13; 2015,Jan,16; 2014,Jan,11; 2011,Jun,11-12

31294   **with optic nerve decompression**
     35.7   35.7   **FUD** 010   T 80 50
     AMA: 2016,Jan,13; 2015,Jan,16; 2014,Jan,11; 2011,Jun,11-12

31295-31297 Nasal Endoscopy with Sinus Ostia Dilation

INCLUDES   Any method of tissue displacement
     Fluoroscopy, when performed

31295   **Nasal/sinus endoscopy, surgical; with dilation of maxillary sinus ostium (eg, balloon dilation), transnasal or via canine fossa**
     EXCLUDES   *When performed in the same sinus:*
       Nasal/sinus endoscopy, diagnostic with maxillary sinusoscopy (31233)
       Nasal/sinus endoscopy, surgical, with maxillary antrostomy (31256-31267)
     4.74   58.3   **FUD** 000   T P2 80 50
     AMA: 2016,Jan,13; 2015,Jan,16; 2014,Jan,11; 2011,Jun,11-12

31296   **with dilation of frontal sinus ostium (eg, balloon dilation)**
     EXCLUDES   *When performed in the same sinus:*
       Nasal/sinus endoscopy, surgical with frontal sinus exploration (31276)
     5.68   59.5   **FUD** 000   T P2 80 50
     AMA: 2016,Jan,13; 2015,Jan,16; 2014,Jan,11; 2011,Jun,11-12

31297   **with dilation of sphenoid sinus ostium (eg, balloon dilation)**
     EXCLUDES   *When performed in the same sinus:*
       Nasal/sinus endoscopy, diagnostic with sphenoid sinusoscopy (31235)
       Nasal/sinus endoscopy, surgical, with sphenoidotomy (31287-31288)
     4.64   58.4   **FUD** 000   T P2 80 50
     AMA: 2016,Jan,13; 2015,Jan,16; 2014,Jan,11; 2011,Jun,11-12

31299 Unlisted Procedures of Accessory Sinuses

CMS: 100-04,4,180.3 Unlisted Service or Procedure
EXCLUDES   *Hypophysectomy (61546, 61548)*

31299   **Unlisted procedure, accessory sinuses**
     0.00   0.00   **FUD** YYY   T 80
     AMA: 2016,Feb,10; 2016,Jan,13; 2015,Jul,10; 2015,Jan,16; 2014,Jan,11; 2013,Jun,13; 2012,Jan,15-42; 2011,Jun,11-12

31300-31502 Procedures of the Larynx

31300   **Laryngotomy (thyrotomy, laryngofissure); with removal of tumor or laryngocele, cordectomy**
     37.6   37.6   **FUD** 090   T A2 80

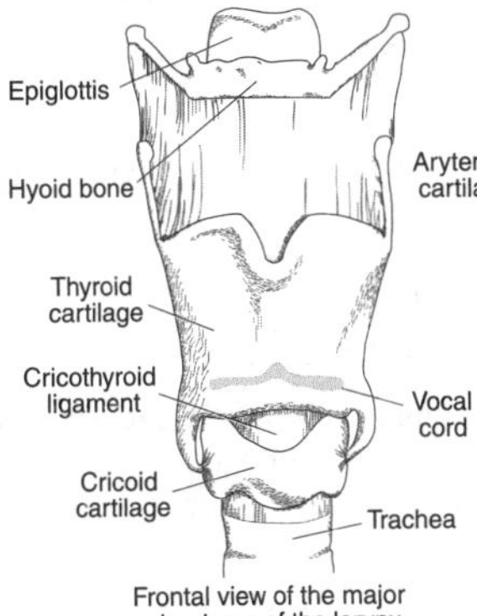

Frontal view of the major structures of the larynx

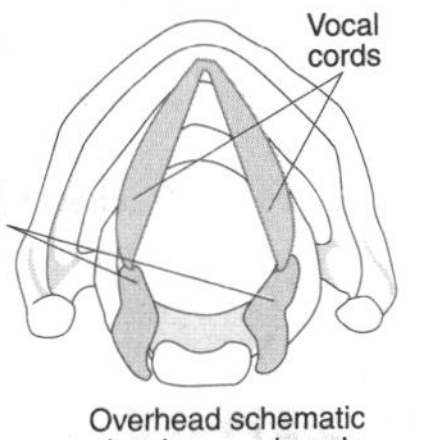

The larynx is the air passage of the neck area, serving as the voice mechanism as well as the valve to prevent food and other particles from entering the respiratory tract

Overhead schematic showing vocal cords

31320   **diagnostic**
     19.8   19.8   **FUD** 090   J A2 80

31360   **Laryngectomy; total, without radical neck dissection**
     61.0   61.0   **FUD** 090   C 80
     AMA: 2016,Jan,13; 2015,Jan,16; 2014,Jan,11

31365   **total, with radical neck dissection**
     75.3   75.3   **FUD** 090   C 80
     AMA: 2016,Jan,13; 2015,Jan,16; 2014,Jan,11; 2012,Jan,15-42; 2011,Jan,11

31367   **subtotal supraglottic, without radical neck dissection**
     64.6   64.6   **FUD** 090   C 80
     AMA: 2016,Jan,13; 2015,Jan,16; 2014,Jan,11

31368   **subtotal supraglottic, with radical neck dissection**
     72.1   72.1   **FUD** 090   C 80

31370   **Partial laryngectomy (hemilaryngectomy); horizontal**
     60.9   60.9   **FUD** 090   C 80

31375   **laterovertical**
     57.5   57.5   **FUD** 090   C 80

31380   **anterovertical**
     56.9   56.9   **FUD** 090   C 80

31382   **antero-latero-vertical**
     62.6   62.6   **FUD** 090   C 80

31390   **Pharyngolaryngectomy, with radical neck dissection; without reconstruction**
     83.9   83.9   **FUD** 090   C 80

31395   **with reconstruction**
     88.7   88.7   **FUD** 090   C 80

31400   **Arytenoidectomy or arytenoidopexy, external approach**
     28.2   28.2   **FUD** 090   J A2 80
     EXCLUDES   *Endoscopic arytenoidectomy (31560)*

31420   **Epiglottidectomy**
     23.9   23.9   **FUD** 090   J A2 80

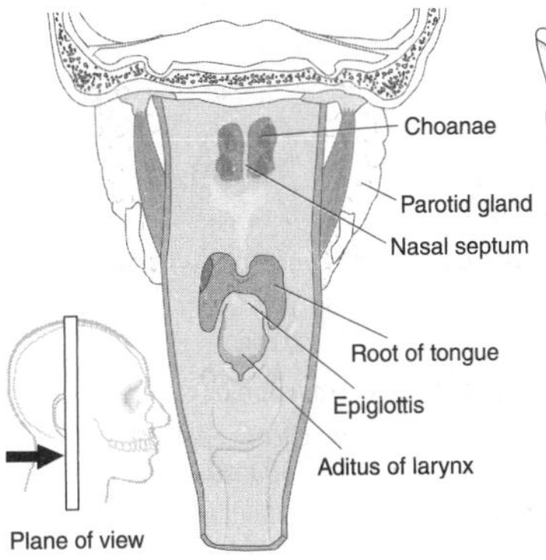

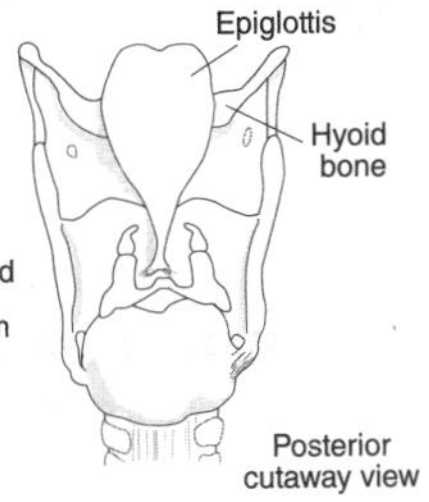

Plane of view

Posterior cutaway view

● New Code   ▲ Revised Code   ○ Reinstated   ● New Web Release   ▲ Revised Web Release   Unlisted   Not Covered   # Resequenced
Ⓢ AMA Mod 51 Exempt   ⑤ Optum Mod 51 Exempt   ⑥ Mod 63 Exempt   ✗ Non-FDA Drug   ★ Telehealth   M Maternity   A Age Edit   + Add-on   AMA: CPT Asst

Respiratory System *(side tab)*

31500 — 31574 *(side tab)*

31500   **Intubation, endotracheal, emergency procedure**
    🚑 3.16   3.16   **FUD** 000   ⊘ Ⓣ G2 ▭
    AMA: 2016,May,3; 2016,Jan,13; 2015,Jan,16; 2014,Jan,11;
    2012,Jan,15-42; 2011,Jan,11

31502   **Tracheotomy tube change prior to establishment of fistula tract**
    🚑 1.01   1.01   **FUD** 000   Ⓣ G2 ▭
    AMA: 1990,Win,4

31505-31541 Endoscopy of the Larynx

31505   **Laryngoscopy, indirect; diagnostic (separate procedure)**
    🚑 1.42   2.38   **FUD** 000   Ⓣ P3 ▭
    AMA: 2016,Jan,13; 2015,Jan,16; 2014,Jan,11

31510   **with biopsy**
    🚑 3.51   6.04   **FUD** 000   Ⓣ A2 80 ▭
    AMA: 2016,Jan,13; 2015,Jan,16; 2014,Jan,11

31511   **with removal of foreign body**
    🚑 3.76   6.07   **FUD** 000   Ⓣ A2 ▭
    AMA: 2016,Jan,13; 2015,Jan,16; 2014,Jan,11

31512   **with removal of lesion**
    🚑 3.74   5.87   **FUD** 000   Ⓣ A2 80 ▭
    AMA: 2016,Jan,13; 2015,Jan,16; 2014,Jan,11

31513   **with vocal cord injection**
    🚑 3.82   3.82   **FUD** 000   Ⓣ A2 80 ▭
    AMA: 2016,Jan,13; 2015,Jan,16; 2014,Jan,11

31515   **Laryngoscopy direct, with or without tracheoscopy; for aspiration**
    🚑 3.03   5.30   **FUD** 000   Ⓣ A2 ▭
    AMA: 1998,Nov,1; 1997,Nov,1

31520   **diagnostic, newborn**
    🚑 4.53   4.53   **FUD** 000   A
    🚑 4.53   4.53   63 Ⓣ G2 80 ▭
    AMA: 1998,Nov,1; 1997,Nov,1

31525   **diagnostic, except newborn**
    🚑 4.65   7.27   **FUD** 000   Ⓣ A2 ▭
    AMA: 2016,Jan,13; 2015,Jan,16; 2014,Jan,11

31526   **diagnostic, with operating microscope or telescope**
    INCLUDES   Operating microscope (69990)
    🚑 4.57   4.57   **FUD** 000   Ⓣ A2 ▭
    AMA: 2016,Feb,12

31527   **with insertion of obturator**
    🚑 5.64   5.64   **FUD** 000   Ⓣ A2 80 ▭
    AMA: 1998,Nov,1; 1997,Nov,1

31528   **with dilation, initial**
    🚑 4.20   4.20   **FUD** 000   Ⓣ A2 80 ▭
    AMA: 2002,May,7; 1998,Nov,1

31529   **with dilation, subsequent**
    🚑 4.70   4.70   **FUD** 000   Ⓣ A2 80 ▭
    AMA: 2002,May,7; 1998,Nov,1

31530   **Laryngoscopy, direct, operative, with foreign body removal;**
    🚑 5.75   5.75   **FUD** 000   Ⓣ A2 ▭
    AMA: 1998,Nov,1; 1997,Nov,1

31531   **with operating microscope or telescope**
    INCLUDES   Operating microscope (69990)
    🚑 6.18   6.18   **FUD** 000   Ⓣ A2 80 ▭
    AMA: 2016,Feb,12

31535   **Laryngoscopy, direct, operative, with biopsy;**
    🚑 5.51   5.51   **FUD** 000   Ⓣ A2 ▭
    AMA: 1998,Nov,1; 1997,Nov,1

31536   **with operating microscope or telescope**
    INCLUDES   Operating microscope (69990)
    🚑 6.13   6.13   **FUD** 000   Ⓣ A2 ▭
    AMA: 2016,Feb,12

31540   **Laryngoscopy, direct, operative, with excision of tumor and/or stripping of vocal cords or epiglottis;**
    🚑 7.03   7.03   **FUD** 000   Ⓣ A2 ▭
    AMA: 1998,Nov,1; 1997,Nov,1

31541   **with operating microscope or telescope**
    INCLUDES   Operating microscope (69990)
    🚑 7.68   7.68   **FUD** 000   Ⓣ A2 ▭
    AMA: 2016,Feb,12

31545-31554 Endoscopy of Larynx with Reconstruction

INCLUDES   Operating microscope (69990)
EXCLUDES   *Laryngoscopy, direct, operative, with excision of tumor and/or stripping of vocal cords or epiglottis (31540-31541)*
    Vocal cord reconstruction with allograft (31599)

31545   **Laryngoscopy, direct, operative, with operating microscope or telescope, with submucosal removal of non-neoplastic lesion(s) of vocal cord; reconstruction with local tissue flap(s)**
    🚑 10.5   10.5   **FUD** 000   Ⓣ A2 50 ▭
    AMA: 2016,Feb,12

31546   **reconstruction with graft(s) (includes obtaining autograft)**
    EXCLUDES   *Tissue grafts, other (eg, paratenon, fat, dermis) (20926)*
    🚑 16.0   16.0   **FUD** 000   Ⓣ A2 50 ▭
    AMA: 2016,Feb,12; 2016,Jan,13; 2015,Jan,16; 2014,Jan,11;
    2012,Jan,15-42; 2011,Jan,11

31551   **Resequenced code. See code following 31580.**

31552   **Resequenced code. See code following 31580.**

31553   **Resequenced code. See code following 31580.**

31554   **Resequenced code. See code following 31580.**

31560-31571 Endoscopy of Larynx with Arytenoid Removal, Vocal Cord Injection

31560   **Laryngoscopy, direct, operative, with arytenoidectomy;**
    🚑 9.11   9.11   **FUD** 000   Ⓣ A2 80 ▭
    AMA: 1998,Nov,1; 1997,Nov,1

31561   **with operating microscope or telescope**
    INCLUDES   Operating microscope (69990)
    🚑 9.98   9.98   **FUD** 000   Ⓣ A2 80 ▭
    AMA: 2016,Feb,12

31570   **Laryngoscopy, direct, with injection into vocal cord(s), therapeutic;**
    🚑 6.68   9.76   **FUD** 000   Ⓣ A2 ▭
    AMA: 2016,Jan,13; 2015,Jan,16; 2014,Jan,6

31571   **with operating microscope or telescope**
    INCLUDES   Operating microscope (69990)
    🚑 7.27   7.27   **FUD** 000   Ⓣ A2 ▭
    AMA: 2016,Feb,12; 2016,Jan,13; 2015,Jan,16; 2014,Jan,6;
    2014,Jan,11; 2012,Nov,13-14

31572-31579 [31572, 31573, 31574] Endoscopy of Larynx, Flexible Fiberoptic

EXCLUDES   *Evaluation by flexible fiberoptic endoscope:*
    Sensory assessment (92614-92615)
    Swallowing (92612-92613)
    Swallowing and sensory assessment (92616-92617)
    Flexible fiberoptic endoscopic examination/testing by cine or video recording (92612-92617)

31572   **Resequenced code. See code following 31578.**

31573   **Resequenced code. See code following 31578.**

31574   **Resequenced code. See code following 31578.**

▲ **31575** **Laryngoscopy, flexible; diagnostic**

EXCLUDES *Diagnostic nasal endoscopy not through additional endoscope (31231)*

Procedures during same session (31572-31574, 31576-31578, 43197-43198, 92511, 92612, 92614, 92616)

🚑 2.21 ⚕ 3.27 **FUD** 000 〔T〕〔P3〕🖥

AMA: 1999,Nov,1; 1997,Nov,1

▲ **31576** **with biopsy(ies)**

EXCLUDES *Destruction or excision of lesion (31572, 31578)*

🚑 3.58 ⚕ 6.43 **FUD** 000 〔T〕〔A2〕🖥

AMA: 1997,Nov,1

▲ **31577** **with removal of foreign body(s)**

🚑 4.34 ⚕ 6.94 **FUD** 000 〔T〕〔A2〕〔80〕🖥

AMA: 1997,Nov,1

▲ **31578** **with removal of lesion(s), non-laser**

🚑 4.99 ⚕ 8.01 **FUD** 000 〔T〕〔A2〕〔80〕🖥

AMA: 1997,Nov,1

● # **31572** **with ablation or destruction of lesion(s) with laser, unilateral**

🚑 0.00 ⚕ 0.00 **FUD** 000

EXCLUDES *Biopsy or excision of lesion (31576, 31578)*

Swallowing evaluation or sensory testing (92612-92617)

● # **31573** **with therapeutic injection(s) (eg, chemodenervation agent or corticosteroid, injected percutaneous, transoral, or via endoscope channel), unilateral**

🚑 0.00 ⚕ 0.00 **FUD** 000

● # **31574** **with injection(s) for augmentation (eg, percutaneous, transoral), unilateral**

🚑 0.00 ⚕ 0.00 **FUD** 000

▲ **31579** **Laryngoscopy, flexible or rigid telescopic, with stroboscopy**

🚑 4.08 ⚕ 6.04 **FUD** 000 〔T〕〔P3〕🖥

AMA: 1997,Nov,1; 1995,Win,1

31580-31599 [31551, 31552, 31553, 31554] Larynx Reconstruction

▲ **31580** **Laryngoplasty; for laryngeal web, with indwelling keel or stent insertion**

🚑 35.1 ⚕ 35.1 **FUD** 090 〔J〕〔A2〕〔80〕🖥

EXCLUDES *Keel or stent removal (31599)*

Tracheostomy (31600-31601, 31603, 31605, 31610)

Treatment of laryngeal stenosis (31551-31554)

● # **31551** **for laryngeal stenosis, with graft, without indwelling stent placement, younger than 12 years of age**

🚑 0.00 ⚕ 0.00 **FUD** 000

EXCLUDES *Cartilage graft obtained through same incision*

Procedure during same session (31552-31554, 31580)

Tracheostomy (31600-31601, 31603, 31605, 31610)

● # **31552** **for laryngeal stenosis, with graft, without indwelling stent placement, age 12 years or older**

🚑 0.00 ⚕ 0.00 **FUD** 000

EXCLUDES *Cartilage graft obtained through same incision*

Procedure during same session (31551, 31553-31554, 31580)

Tracheostomy (31600-31601, 31603, 31605, 31610)

● # **31553** **for laryngeal stenosis, with graft, with indwelling stent placement, younger than 12 years of age**

🚑 0.00 ⚕ 0.00 **FUD** 000

EXCLUDES *Cartilage graft obtained through same incision*

Procedure during same session (31551-31552, 31554, 31580)

Stent removal (31599)

Tracheostomy (31600-31601, 31603, 31605, 31610)

● # **31554** **for laryngeal stenosis, with graft, with indwelling stent placement, age 12 years or older**

🚑 0.00 ⚕ 0.00 **FUD** 000

EXCLUDES *Cartilage graft obtained through same incision*

Procedure during same session (31551-31553, 31580)

Stent removal (31599)

Tracheostomy (31600-31601, 31603, 31605, 31610)

~~**31582** **for laryngeal stenosis, with graft or core mold, including tracheotomy**~~

To report, see ~[31551, 31552, 31553, 31554]

▲ **31584** **with open reduction and fixation of (eg, plating) fracture, includes tracheostomy, if performed**

🚑 43.5 ⚕ 43.5 **FUD** 090 〔C〕〔80〕🖥

EXCLUDES *Cartilage graft obtained through same incision*

▲ **31587** **Laryngoplasty, cricoid split, without graft placement**

🚑 28.8 ⚕ 28.8 **FUD** 090 〔C〕〔80〕🖥

EXCLUDES *Tracheostomy (31600-31601, 31603, 31605, 31610)*

~~**31588** **Laryngoplasty, not otherwise specified (eg, for burns, reconstruction after partial laryngectomy)**~~

To report, see ~31599

31590 **Laryngeal reinnervation by neuromuscular pedicle**

🚑 25.7 ⚕ 25.7 **FUD** 090 〔J〕〔A2〕〔80〕🖥

● **31591** **Laryngoplasty, medialization, unilateral**

● **31592** **Cricotracheal resection**

EXCLUDES *Advancement or rotational flaps performed not requiring additional incision*

Cartilage graft obtained through same incision

Tracheal stenosis excision/anastomosis (31780-31781)

Tracheostomy (31600-31601, 31603, 31605, 31610)

31595 **Section recurrent laryngeal nerve, therapeutic (separate procedure), unilateral**

🚑 21.9 ⚕ 21.9 **FUD** 090 〔J〕〔A2〕〔80〕〔50〕🖥

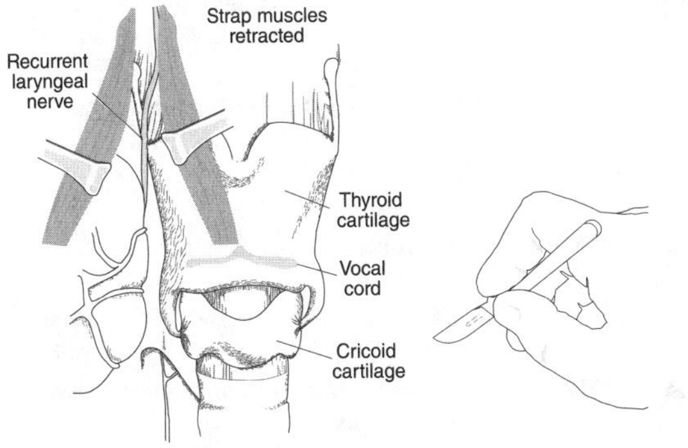

31599 **Unlisted procedure, larynx**

🚑 0.00 ⚕ 0.00 **FUD** YYY 〔T〕〔80〕

AMA: 2016,Jan,13; 2015,Jan,16; 2014,Jan,11; 2012,Nov,13-14

31600-31610 Stoma Creation: Trachea

EXCLUDES *Aspiration of trachea, direct vision (31515)*

Endotracheal intubation (31500)

31600 **Tracheostomy, planned (separate procedure);**

🚑 11.5 ⚕ 11.5 **FUD** 000 〔T〕🖥

AMA: 2010,Aug,3-7; 2010,Aug,3-7

31601 **younger than 2 years** 〔A〕

🚑 7.31 ⚕ 7.31 **FUD** 000 〔T〕〔80〕🖥

31603 **Tracheostomy, emergency procedure; transtracheal**

🚑 6.48 ⚕ 6.48 **FUD** 000 〔T〕〔A2〕🖥

31605 **cricothyroid membrane**

🚑 5.32 ⚕ 5.32 **FUD** 000 〔T〕〔G2〕🖥

31610 **Tracheostomy, fenestration procedure with skin flaps**

🚑 20.5 ⚕ 20.5 **FUD** 090 〔J〕🖥

● New Code ▲ Revised Code ○ Reinstated ● New Web Release ▲ Revised Web Release Unlisted Not Covered # Resequenced

⊘ AMA Mod 51 Exempt ⑤ Optum Mod 51 Exempt ⑥₃ Mod 63 Exempt ⊮ Non-FDA Drug ★ Telehealth 〔M〕 Maternity 〔A〕 Age Edit + Add-on **AMA:** CPT Asst

© 2016 Optum360, LLC CPT © 2016 American Medical Association. All Rights Reserved. **109**

31611-31614 Procedures of the Trachea

31611 Construction of tracheoesophageal fistula and subsequent insertion of an alaryngeal speech prosthesis (eg, voice button, Blom-Singer prosthesis)
  🔧 15.5 🔧 15.5 **FUD** 090 T A2 80 ▢

31612 Tracheal puncture, percutaneous with transtracheal aspiration and/or injection
  EXCLUDES *Tracheal aspiration under direct vision (31515)*
  🔧 1.41 🔧 2.41 **FUD** 000 J A2 80 ▢
  AMA: 1994,Win,1

31613 Tracheostoma revision; simple, without flap rotation
  🔧 13.0 🔧 13.0 **FUD** 090 T A2 ▢

31614   complex, with flap rotation
  🔧 21.7 🔧 21.7 **FUD** 090 J A2 ▢

31615 Endoscopy Through Tracheostomy

INCLUDES Diagnostic bronchoscopy
EXCLUDES *Endobronchial ultrasound [EBUS] guided biopsies of mediastinal or hilar lymph nodes (31652-31653)*
  Tracheoscopy (31515-31578)
Code also endobronchial ultrasound [EBUS] during diagnostic/therapeutic peripheral lesion intervention (31654)

▲ **31615** Tracheobronchoscopy through established tracheostomy incision
  🔧 3.71 🔧 5.22 **FUD** 000 T A2 ▢
  AMA: 2016,Jan,13; 2015,Jan,16; 2014,Jan,11; 2013,Mar,8-9; 2012,Nov,13-14

31622-31654 [31651] Endoscopy of Lung

INCLUDES Diagnostic bronchoscopy with surgical bronchoscopy procedures
  Fluoroscopic imaging guidance, when performed

▲ **31622** Bronchoscopy, rigid or flexible, including fluoroscopic guidance, when performed; diagnostic, with cell washing, when performed (separate procedure)
  🔧 4.16 🔧 8.67 **FUD** 000 T A2 ▢
  AMA: 2016,Apr,5; 2016,Jan,13; 2015,Jan,16; 2014,Jan,11; 2013,Mar,8-9; 2012,Jan,15-42; 2011,Feb,8-9; 2011,Jan,6-7; 2011,Jan,11

▲ **31623**   with brushing or protected brushings
  🔧 4.22 🔧 9.43 **FUD** 000 T A2 ▢
  AMA: 2016,Apr,5; 2016,Jan,13; 2015,Jan,16; 2014,Jan,11; 2013,Mar,8-9; 2012,Jan,15-42; 2011,Jan,6-7; 2011,Jan,11

▲ **31624**   with bronchial alveolar lavage
  🔧 4.26 🔧 8.93 **FUD** 000 T A2 ▢
  AMA: 2016,Apr,5; 2016,Jan,13; 2015,Jan,16; 2014,Jan,11; 2013,Mar,8-9; 2012,Jan,15-42; 2011,Jan,6-7; 2011,Jan,11

▲ **31625**   with bronchial or endobronchial biopsy(s), single or multiple sites
  🔧 4.88 🔧 11.2 **FUD** 000 T A2 ▢
  AMA: 2016,Apr,5; 2016,Jan,13; 2015,Jan,16; 2014,Jan,11; 2013,Mar,8-9; 2012,Jan,15-42; 2011,Jan,6-7; 2011,Jan,11

▲ **31626**   with placement of fiducial markers, single or multiple
  Code also device
  🔧 6.10 🔧 25.8 **FUD** 000 T G2 80 ▢
  AMA: 2016,Apr,5; 2016,Jan,13; 2015,Jun,6; 2015,Jan,16; 2014,Jan,11; 2013,Mar,8-9; 2011,Jan,6-7

▲ + **31627**   with computer-assisted, image-guided navigation (List separately in addition to code for primary procedure[s])
  INCLUDES 3D reconstruction (76376-76377)
  Code first (31615, 31622-31626, 31628-31631, 31635-31636, 31638-31643)
  🔧 2.81 🔧 40.1 **FUD** ZZZ N N1 80 ▢
  AMA: 2016,Jan,13; 2015,Jan,16; 2014,Jan,11; 2013,Mar,8-9; 2011,Jan,6-7

▲ **31628**   with transbronchial lung biopsy(s), single lobe
  INCLUDES All biopsies taken from lobe
  EXCLUDES *Transbronchial biopsies by needle aspiration (31629, 31633)*
  Code also transbronchial biopsies of additional lobe(s) (31632)
  🔧 5.43 🔧 11.8 **FUD** 000 T A2 ▢
  AMA: 2016,Apr,5; 2016,Jan,13; 2015,Jan,16; 2014,Jan,11; 2013,Mar,8-9; 2012,Jan,15-42; 2011,Jan,6-7; 2011,Jan,11

▲ **31629**   with transbronchial needle aspiration biopsy(s), trachea, main stem and/or lobar bronchus(i)
  INCLUDES All biopsies from same lobe or upper airway
  EXCLUDES *Transbronchial biopsies of lung (31628, 31632)*
  Code also transbronchial needle biopsies of additional lobe(s) (31633)
  🔧 5.75 🔧 14.1 **FUD** 000 T A2 ▢
  AMA: 2016,Apr,5; 2016,Jan,13; 2015,Jan,16; 2014,Jan,11; 2013,Mar,8-9; 2012,Jan,15-42; 2011,Apr,12; 2011,Jan,6-7; 2011,Jan,11

31630   with tracheal/bronchial dilation or closed reduction of fracture
  🔧 5.78 🔧 5.78 **FUD** 000 T A2 ▢
  AMA: 2016,Jan,13; 2015,Jan,16; 2014,Jan,11; 2013,Mar,8-9; 2011,Jan,6-7

31631   with placement of tracheal stent(s) (includes tracheal/bronchial dilation as required)
  EXCLUDES *Bronchial stent placement (31636-31637)*
  Revision bronchial or tracheal stent (31638)
  🔧 6.65 🔧 6.65 **FUD** 000 T A2 ▢
  AMA: 2016,Jan,13; 2015,Jan,16; 2014,Jan,11; 2013,Mar,8-9; 2011,Jan,6-7

▲ + **31632**   with transbronchial lung biopsy(s), each additional lobe (List separately in addition to code for primary procedure)
  INCLUDES All biopsies of additional lobe of lung
  Code first (31628)
  🔧 1.42 🔧 2.13 **FUD** ZZZ N N1 ▢
  AMA: 2016,Jan,13; 2015,Jan,16; 2014,Jan,11; 2013,Mar,8-9

▲ + **31633**   with transbronchial needle aspiration biopsy(s), each additional lobe (List separately in addition to code for primary procedure)
  INCLUDES All needle biopsies from another lobe or from trachea
  Code first (31629)
  🔧 1.83 🔧 2.63 **FUD** ZZZ N N1 ▢
  AMA: 2016,Jan,13; 2015,Jan,16; 2014,Jan,11; 2013,Mar,8-9; 2012,Jan,15-42; 2011,Apr,12; 2011,Jan,11

▲ **31634**   with balloon occlusion, with assessment of air leak, with administration of occlusive substance (eg, fibrin glue), if performed
  EXCLUDES *Bronchoscopy, rigid or flexible, including fluoroscopic guidance, when performed; with balloon occlusion, when performed, assessment of air leak, airway sizing, and insertion of bronchial valve(s), initial lobe (31647, [31651])*
  🔧 5.96 🔧 52.9 **FUD** 000 T G2 80 ▢
  AMA: 2016,Jan,13; 2015,Jan,16; 2014,Jan,11; 2013,Mar,8-9; 2011,Jan,6-7

▲ **31635**   with removal of foreign body
  EXCLUDES *Removal implanted bronchial valves (31648-31649)*
  🔧 5.44 🔧 9.94 **FUD** 000 T A2 ▢
  AMA: 2016,Jan,13; 2015,Jan,16; 2014,Jan,11; 2013,Mar,8-9; 2012,Jan,15-42; 2011,Jan,6-7; 2011,Jan,11

31636   with placement of bronchial stent(s) (includes tracheal/bronchial dilation as required), initial bronchus
  🔧 6.40 🔧 6.40 **FUD** 000 T A2 ▢
  AMA: 2016,Jan,13; 2015,Jan,16; 2014,Jan,11; 2013,Mar,8-9; 2011,Jan,6-7

+ 31637 each additional major bronchus stented (List separately in addition to code for primary procedure)
Code first (31636)
🔧 2.14 ⚖ 2.14 **FUD** ZZZ N N1 ▭
AMA: 2016,Jan,13; 2015,Jan,16; 2014,Jan,11; 2013,Mar,8-9

31638 with revision of tracheal or bronchial stent inserted at previous session (includes tracheal/bronchial dilation as required)
🔧 7.31 ⚖ 7.31 **FUD** 000 T A2 ▭
AMA: 2016,Jan,13; 2015,Jan,16; 2014,Jan,11; 2013,Mar,8-9; 2011,Jan,6-7

31640 with excision of tumor
🔧 7.35 ⚖ 7.35 **FUD** 000 T A2 ▭
AMA: 2016,Apr,5; 2016,Jan,13; 2015,Jan,16; 2014,Jan,11; 2013,Mar,8-9; 2011,Jan,6-7

31641 with destruction of tumor or relief of stenosis by any method other than excision (eg, laser therapy, cryotherapy)
Code also any photodynamic therapy via bronchoscopy (96570-96571)
🔧 7.45 ⚖ 7.45 **FUD** 000 T A2 ▭
AMA: 2016,Jan,13; 2015,Jan,16; 2014,Jan,11; 2013,Apr,8-9; 2013,Mar,8-9; 2011,Oct,3-4; 2011,Jan,6-7

31643 with placement of catheter(s) for intracavitary radioelement application
Code also if appropriate (77761-77763, 77770-77772)
🔧 5.10 ⚖ 5.10 **FUD** 000 T A2 ▭
AMA: 2016,Apr,5; 2016,Jan,13; 2015,Jan,16; 2014,Jan,11; 2013,Mar,8-9; 2011,Jan,6-7

▲ **31645** with therapeutic aspiration of tracheobronchial tree, initial (eg, drainage of lung abscess)
EXCLUDES Bedside aspiration of trachea, bronchi (31725)
🔧 4.65 ⚖ 9.22 **FUD** 000 T A2 ▭
AMA: 2016,Apr,5; 2016,Jan,13; 2015,Jan,16; 2014,Jan,11; 2013,Mar,8-9; 2011,Jan,6-7

▲ **31646** with therapeutic aspiration of tracheobronchial tree, subsequent
EXCLUDES Bedside aspiration of trachea, bronchi (31725)
🔧 4.02 ⚖ 8.27 **FUD** 000 T A2 ▭
AMA: 2016,Apr,5; 2016,Jan,13; 2015,Jan,16; 2014,Jan,11; 2013,Mar,8-9; 2011,Jan,6-7

▲ **31647** with balloon occlusion, when performed, assessment of air leak, airway sizing, and insertion of bronchial valve(s), initial lobe
🔧 6.39 ⚖ 6.39 **FUD** 000 T G2 ▭
AMA: 2016,Jan,13; 2015,Jan,16; 2014,Jan,11; 2013,Mar,8-9

▲ + # **31651** with balloon occlusion, when performed, assessment of air leak, airway sizing, and insertion of bronchial valve(s), each additional lobe (List separately in addition to code for primary procedure[s])
Code first (31647)
🔧 2.29 ⚖ 2.29 **FUD** ZZZ N N1 ▭
AMA: 2016,Jan,13; 2015,Jan,16; 2014,Jan,11; 2013,Mar,8-9

▲ **31648** with removal of bronchial valve(s), initial lobe
EXCLUDES Removal with reinsertion bronchial valve during same session (31647 and 31648) and ([31651])
🔧 5.91 ⚖ 5.91 **FUD** 000 T G2 ▭
AMA: 2016,Jan,13; 2015,Jan,16; 2014,Jan,11; 2013,Mar,8-9

▲ + **31649** with removal of bronchial valve(s), each additional lobe (List separately in addition to code for primary procedure)
Code first (31648)
🔧 2.01 ⚖ 2.01 **FUD** ZZZ 02 G2 ▭
AMA: 2016,Jan,13; 2015,Jan,16; 2014,Jan,11; 2013,Mar,8-9

31651 Resequenced code. See code following 31647.

▲ **31652** with endobronchial ultrasound (EBUS) guided transtracheal and/or transbronchial sampling (eg, aspiration[s]/biopsy[ies]), one or two mediastinal and/or hilar lymph node stations or structures
EXCLUDES Procedures performed more than one time per session
🔧 6.75 ⚖ 25.7 **FUD** 000 T G2 ▭
AMA: 2016,Apr,5

▲ **31653** with endobronchial ultrasound (EBUS) guided transtracheal and/or transbronchial sampling (eg, aspiration[s]/biopsy[ies]), 3 or more mediastinal and/or hilar lymph node stations or structures
EXCLUDES Procedures performed more than one time per session
🔧 7.45 ⚖ 27.3 **FUD** 000 T G2 ▭
AMA: 2016,Apr,5

▲ + **31654** with transendoscopic endobronchial ultrasound (EBUS) during bronchoscopic diagnostic or therapeutic intervention(s) for peripheral lesion(s) (List separately in addition to code for primary procedure[s])
EXCLUDES Endobronchial ultrasound [EBUS] for mediastinal/hilar lymph node station/adjacent structure access (31652-31653)
Procedures performed more than one time per session
Code first (31622-31626, 31628-31629, 31640, 31643-31646)
🔧 1.95 ⚖ 4.10 **FUD** ZZZ N N1 ▭
AMA: 2016,Apr,5

31660-31661 Bronchial Thermoplasty

INCLUDES Fluoroscopic imaging guidance, when performed

▲ **31660** Bronchoscopy, rigid or flexible, including fluoroscopic guidance, when performed; with bronchial thermoplasty, 1 lobe
🔧 6.05 ⚖ 6.05 **FUD** 000 T ▭
AMA: 2016,Jan,13; 2015,Jan,16; 2014,Jan,11; 2013,Mar,8-9

▲ **31661** with bronchial thermoplasty, 2 or more lobes
🔧 6.35 ⚖ 6.35 **FUD** 000 T ▭
AMA: 2016,Jan,13; 2015,Jan,16; 2014,Jan,11; 2013,Mar,8-9

31717-31899 Respiratory Procedures

EXCLUDES Endotracheal intubation (31500)
Tracheal aspiration under direct vision (31515)

31717 Catheterization with bronchial brush biopsy
🔧 3.12 ⚖ 7.42 **FUD** 000 T A2 ▭
AMA: 2016,Jan,13; 2015,Jan,16; 2014,Jan,11; 2012,Jan,15-42; 2011,Jan,11

31720 Catheter aspiration (separate procedure); nasotracheal
🔧 1.48 ⚖ 1.48 **FUD** 000 01 N1 ▭
AMA: 1994,Win,1

▲ **31725** tracheobronchial with fiberscope, bedside
🔧 2.58 ⚖ 2.58 **FUD** 000 C ▭

31730 Transtracheal (percutaneous) introduction of needle wire dilator/stent or indwelling tube for oxygen therapy
🔧 4.29 ⚖ 35.0 **FUD** 000 T A2 ▭
AMA: 1992,Win,1

31750 Tracheoplasty; cervical
🔧 40.6 ⚖ 40.6 **FUD** 090 J A2 80 ▭

31755 tracheopharyngeal fistulization, each stage
🔧 50.9 ⚖ 50.9 **FUD** 090 J A2 80 ▭

31760 intrathoracic
🔧 40.4 ⚖ 40.4 **FUD** 090 C 80 ▭

31766 Carinal reconstruction
🔧 51.8 ⚖ 51.8 **FUD** 090 C 80 ▭

31770 Bronchoplasty; graft repair
🔧 38.9 ⚖ 38.9 **FUD** 090 C 80 ▭
EXCLUDES Bronchoplasty done with lobectomy (32501)

31775 excision stenosis and anastomosis
🔧 37.5 ⚖ 37.5 **FUD** 090 C 80 ▭
EXCLUDES Bronchoplasty done with lobectomy (32501)

● New Code   ▲ Revised Code   ○ Reinstated   ● New Web Release   ▲ Revised Web Release   Unlisted   Not Covered   # Resequenced
⊘ AMA Mod 51 Exempt   51 Optum Mod 51 Exempt   63 Mod 63 Exempt   ✗ Non-FDA Drug   ★ Telehealth   M Maternity   ▲ Age Edit   + Add-on   AMA: CPT Asst

31780 Excision tracheal stenosis and anastomosis; cervical
🖢 34.1 ⚕ 34.1 **FUD** 090
C 80 📭

31781 cervicothoracic
🖢 41.8 ⚕ 41.8 **FUD** 090
C 80 📭

31785 Excision of tracheal tumor or carcinoma; cervical
🖢 31.4 ⚕ 31.4 **FUD** 090
T 80 📭
AMA: 2003,Jan,1

31786 thoracic
🖢 41.7 ⚕ 41.7 **FUD** 090
C 80 📭

31800 Suture of tracheal wound or injury; cervical
🖢 21.2 ⚕ 21.2 **FUD** 090
C 80 📭
AMA: 1994,Win,1

31805 intrathoracic
🖢 23.9 ⚕ 23.9 **FUD** 090
C 80 📭

31820 Surgical closure tracheostomy or fistula; without plastic repair
🖢 9.47 ⚕ 12.4 **FUD** 090
T A2 80 📭
EXCLUDES   Tracheoesophageal fistula repair (43305, 43312)

31825 with plastic repair
🖢 13.8 ⚕ 17.2 **FUD** 090
T A2 80 📭
EXCLUDES   Tracheoesophageal fistula repair (43305, 43312)

31830 Revision of tracheostomy scar
🖢 9.91 ⚕ 12.7 **FUD** 090
T A2 80 📭

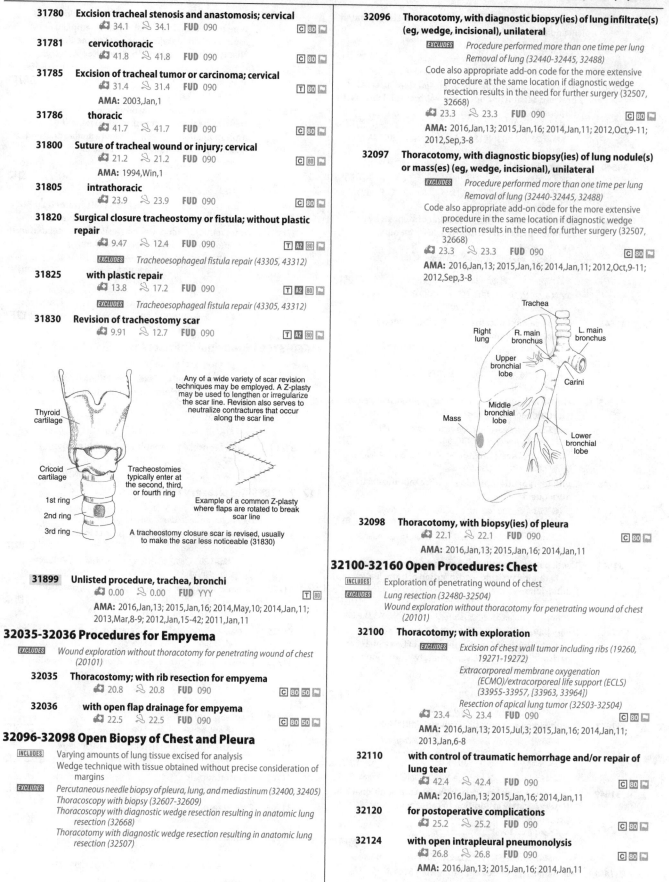

Thyroid cartilage

Cricoid cartilage

Tracheostomies typically enter at the second, third, or fourth ring

1st ring
2nd ring
3rd ring

Any of a wide variety of scar revision techniques may be employed. A Z-plasty may be used to lengthen or irregularize the scar line. Revision also serves to neutralize contractures that occur along the scar line

Example of a common Z-plasty where flaps are rotated to break scar line

A tracheostomy closure scar is revised, usually to make the scar less noticeable (31830)

31899 Unlisted procedure, trachea, bronchi
🖢 0.00 ⚕ 0.00 **FUD** YYY
T 80
AMA: 2016,Jan,13; 2015,Jan,16; 2014,May,10; 2014,Jan,11; 2013,Mar,8-9; 2012,Jan,15-42; 2011,Jan,11

32035-32036 Procedures for Empyema
EXCLUDES   Wound exploration without thoracotomy for penetrating wound of chest (20101)

32035 Thoracostomy; with rib resection for empyema
🖢 20.8 ⚕ 20.8 **FUD** 090
C 80 50 📭

32036 with open flap drainage for empyema
🖢 22.5 ⚕ 22.5 **FUD** 090
C 80 50 📭

32096-32098 Open Biopsy of Chest and Pleura
INCLUDES   Varying amounts of lung tissue excised for analysis
Wedge technique with tissue obtained without precise consideration of margins
EXCLUDES   Percutaneous needle biopsy of pleura, lung, and mediastinum (32400, 32405)
Thoracoscopy with biopsy (32607-32609)
Thoracoscopy with diagnostic wedge resection resulting in anatomic lung resection (32668)
Thoracotomy with diagnostic wedge resection resulting in anatomic lung resection (32507)

32096 Thoracotomy, with diagnostic biopsy(ies) of lung infiltrate(s) (eg, wedge, incisional), unilateral
EXCLUDES   Procedure performed more than one time per lung
Removal of lung (32440-32445, 32488)
Code also appropriate add-on code for the more extensive procedure at the same location if diagnostic wedge resection results in the need for further surgery (32507, 32668)
🖢 23.3 ⚕ 23.3 **FUD** 090
C 80 📭
AMA: 2016,Jan,13; 2015,Jan,16; 2014,Jan,11; 2012,Oct,9-11; 2012,Sep,3-8

32097 Thoracotomy, with diagnostic biopsy(ies) of lung nodule(s) or mass(es) (eg, wedge, incisional), unilateral
EXCLUDES   Procedure performed more than one time per lung
Removal of lung (32440-32445, 32488)
Code also appropriate add-on code for the more extensive procedure in the same location if diagnostic wedge resection results in the need for further surgery (32507, 32668)
🖢 23.3 ⚕ 23.3 **FUD** 090
C 80 📭
AMA: 2016,Jan,13; 2015,Jan,16; 2014,Jan,11; 2012,Oct,9-11; 2012,Sep,3-8

Trachea

Right lung

R. main bronchus

L. main bronchus

Upper bronchial lobe

Carini

Middle bronchial lobe

Mass

Lower bronchial lobe

32098 Thoracotomy, with biopsy(ies) of pleura
🖢 22.1 ⚕ 22.1 **FUD** 090
C 80 📭
AMA: 2016,Jan,13; 2015,Jan,16; 2014,Jan,11

32100-32160 Open Procedures: Chest
INCLUDES   Exploration of penetrating wound of chest
EXCLUDES   Lung resection (32480-32504)
Wound exploration without thoracotomy for penetrating wound of chest (20101)

32100 Thoracotomy; with exploration
EXCLUDES   Excision of chest wall tumor including ribs (19260, 19271-19272)
Extracorporeal membrane oxygenation (ECMO)/extracorporeal life support (ECLS) (33955-33957, [33963, 33964])
Resection of apical lung tumor (32503-32504)
🖢 23.4 ⚕ 23.4 **FUD** 090
C 80 📭
AMA: 2016,Jan,13; 2015,Jul,3; 2015,Jan,16; 2014,Jan,11; 2013,Jan,6-8

32110 with control of traumatic hemorrhage and/or repair of lung tear
🖢 42.4 ⚕ 42.4 **FUD** 090
C 80 📭
AMA: 2016,Jan,13; 2015,Jan,16; 2014,Jan,11

32120 for postoperative complications
🖢 25.2 ⚕ 25.2 **FUD** 090
C 80 📭

32124 with open intrapleural pneumonolysis
🖢 26.8 ⚕ 26.8 **FUD** 090
C 80 📭
AMA: 2016,Jan,13; 2015,Jan,16; 2014,Jan,11

32140 with cyst(s) removal, includes pleural procedure when performed

🔧 28.9   ✂ 28.9   **FUD** 090   C 80 ▭

AMA: 2016,Jan,13; 2015,Jan,16; 2014,Jan,11

32141 with resection-plication of bullae, includes any pleural procedure when performed

EXCLUDES   *Lung volume reduction (32491)*

🔧 44.3   ✂ 44.3   **FUD** 090   C 80 ▭

AMA: 2016,Jan,13; 2015,Jan,16; 2014,Jan,11

32150 with removal of intrapleural foreign body or fibrin deposit

🔧 29.1   ✂ 29.1   **FUD** 090   C 80 ▭

AMA: 2016,Jan,13; 2015,Jan,16; 2014,Jan,11

32151 with removal of intrapulmonary foreign body

🔧 29.1   ✂ 29.1   **FUD** 090   C 80 ▭

32160 with cardiac massage

🔧 22.8   ✂ 22.8   **FUD** 090   C 80 ▭

32200-32320 Open Procedures: Lung

32200 Pneumonostomy, with open drainage of abscess or cyst

EXCLUDES   *Image-guided, percutaneous drainage (eg, abscess, cyst) of lungs/mediastinum via catheter (49405)*

🔧 (75989)

🔧 32.9   ✂ 32.9   **FUD** 090   C 80 ▭

AMA: 2013,Nov,9

32215 Pleural scarification for repeat pneumothorax

🔧 23.1   ✂ 23.1   **FUD** 090   C 80 50 ▭

32220 Decortication, pulmonary (separate procedure); total

🔧 45.9   ✂ 45.9   **FUD** 090   C 80 50 ▭

32225 partial

🔧 28.8   ✂ 28.8   **FUD** 090   C 80 50 ▭

32310 Pleurectomy, parietal (separate procedure)

🔧 26.4   ✂ 26.4   **FUD** 090   C 80 ▭

AMA: 1994,Win,1

32320 Decortication and parietal pleurectomy

🔧 46.3   ✂ 46.3   **FUD** 090   C 80 ▭

AMA: 1994,Fall,1

32400-32405 Lung Biopsy

EXCLUDES   *Open lung biopsy (32096-32097)*
Open mediastinal biopsy (39000-39010)
Thoracoscopic (VATS) biopsy of lung, pericardium, pleural or mediastinal space (32604-32609)

32400 Biopsy, pleura, percutaneous needle

EXCLUDES   *Fine needle aspiration (10021-10022)*

🔧 (76942, 77002, 77012, 77021)

🔧 2.52   ✂ 4.32   **FUD** 000   T A2 ▭

AMA: 2016,Jan,13; 2015,Jan,16; 2014,Jan,11

▲ **32405** Biopsy, lung or mediastinum, percutaneous needle

EXCLUDES   *Fine needle aspiration (10022)*

🔧 (76942, 77002, 77012, 77021)

🔧 3.00   ✂ 12.8   **FUD** 000   T A2 ▭

AMA: 2016,Jan,13; 2015,Jan,16; 2014,Jan,11; 2012,Jan,15-42; 2011,Jan,11

32440-32501 Lung Resection

32440 Removal of lung, pneumonectomy;

Code also excision of chest wall tumor (19260-19272)

🔧 45.4   ✂ 45.4   **FUD** 090   C 80 ▭

AMA: 2016,Jan,13; 2015,Jan,16; 2014,Jan,11; 2012,Oct,9-11; 2012,Sep,3-8

32442 with resection of segment of trachea followed by broncho-tracheal anastomosis (sleeve pneumonectomy)

Code also excision of chest wall tumor (19260-19272)

🔧 93.1   ✂ 93.1   **FUD** 090   C 80 ▭

AMA: 2016,Jan,13; 2015,Jan,16; 2014,Jan,11; 2012,Oct,9-11; 2012,Sep,3-8

32445 extrapleural

Code also empyemectomy with extrapleural pneumonectomy (32540)

Code also excision of chest wall tumor (19260-19272)

🔧 103.   ✂ 103.   **FUD** 090   C 80 ▭

AMA: 2016,Jan,13; 2015,Jan,16; 2014,Jan,11; 2012,Oct,9-11; 2012,Sep,3-8

32480 Removal of lung, other than pneumonectomy; single lobe (lobectomy)

EXCLUDES   *Lung removal with bronchoplasty (32501)*

Code also decortication (32320)

Code also excision of chest wall tumor (19260-19272)

🔧 42.9   ✂ 42.9   **FUD** 090   C 80 ▭

AMA: 2016,Jan,13; 2015,Jan,16; 2014,Jan,11; 2012,Oct,9-11; 2012,Sep,3-8

32482 2 lobes (bilobectomy)

EXCLUDES   *Lung removal with bronchoplasty (32501)*

Code also decortication (32320)

Code also excision of chest wall tumor (19260-19272)

🔧 45.9   ✂ 45.9   **FUD** 090   C 80 ▭

AMA: 2016,Jan,13; 2015,Jan,16; 2014,Jan,11; 2012,Oct,9-11; 2012,Sep,3-8; 2012,Jan,15-42; 2011,Jan,11

32484 single segment (segmentectomy)

EXCLUDES   *Lung removal with bronchoplasty (32501)*

Code also decortication (32320)

Code also excision of chest wall tumor (19260-19272)

🔧 41.7   ✂ 41.7   **FUD** 090   C 80 ▭

AMA: 2016,Jan,13; 2015,Jan,16; 2014,Jan,11; 2012,Oct,9-11; 2012,Sep,3-8

32486 with circumferential resection of segment of bronchus followed by broncho-bronchial anastomosis (sleeve lobectomy)

Code also decortication (32320)

Code also excision of chest wall tumor (19260-19272)

🔧 68.4   ✂ 68.4   **FUD** 090   C 80 ▭

AMA: 2016,Jan,13; 2015,Jan,16; 2014,Jan,11; 2012,Oct,9-11; 2012,Sep,3-8

32488 **with all remaining lung following previous removal of a portion of lung (completion pneumonectomy)**
Code also decortication (32320)
Code also excision of chest wall tumor (19260-19272)
🔪 69.5   ✂ 69.5   **FUD** 090   C 80 ▢
AMA: 2016,Jan,13; 2015,Jan,16; 2014,Jan,11; 2012,Oct,9-11; 2012,Sep,3-8

32491 **with resection-plication of emphysematous lung(s) (bullous or non-bullous) for lung volume reduction, sternal split or transthoracic approach, includes any pleural procedure, when performed**
🔪 42.8   ✂ 42.8   **FUD** 090   C 80 50 ▢
AMA: 2016,Jan,13; 2015,Jan,16; 2014,Jan,11

+ **32501** **Resection and repair of portion of bronchus (bronchoplasty) when performed at time of lobectomy or segmentectomy (List separately in addition to code for primary procedure)**
INCLUDES   Plastic closure of bronchus, not closure of a resected end of bronchus
Code first (32480-32484)
🔪 7.14   ✂ 7.14   **FUD** ZZZ   C 80 ▢
AMA: 1995,Win,1

32503-32504 Excision of Lung Neoplasm

EXCLUDES   *Excision of chest wall tumor involving ribs (19260, 19271-19272)*
Lung resection performed in conjunction with chest wall resection
Thoracentesis, needle or catheter, aspiration of the pleural space (32554-32555)
Thoracotomy; with exploration (32100)
Tube thoracostomy (32551)

32503 **Resection of apical lung tumor (eg, Pancoast tumor), including chest wall resection, rib(s) resection(s), neurovascular dissection, when performed; without chest wall reconstruction(s)**
🔪 52.5   ✂ 52.5   **FUD** 090   C 80 ▢
AMA: 2012,Oct,9-11; 2012,Sep,3-8

32504 **with chest wall reconstruction**
🔪 59.9   ✂ 59.9   **FUD** 090   C 80 ▢
AMA: 2012,Oct,9-11; 2012,Sep,3-8

32505-32507 Thoracotomy with Wedge Resection

INCLUDES   Wedge technique with tissue obtained with precise consideration of margins and complete resection
Code also resection of chest wall tumor with lung resection when performed (19260-19272)

32505 **Thoracotomy; with therapeutic wedge resection (eg, mass, nodule), initial**
EXCLUDES   *Removal of lung (32440, 32442, 32445, 32488)*
Code also a more extensive procedure of the lung when performed on the contralateral lung or different lobe with modifier 59 regardless of intraoperative pathology consultation
🔪 27.0   ✂ 27.0   **FUD** 090   C 80 ▢
AMA: 2016,Jan,13; 2015,Jan,16; 2014,Jan,11; 2012,Oct,9-11; 2012,Sep,3-8

+ **32506** **with therapeutic wedge resection (eg, mass or nodule), each additional resection, ipsilateral (List separately in addition to code for primary procedure)**
Code also a more extensive procedure of the lung when performed on the contralateral lung or different lobe with modifier 59
Code first (32505)
🔪 4.57   ✂ 4.57   **FUD** ZZZ   C 80 ▢
AMA: 2016,Jan,13; 2015,Jan,16; 2014,Jan,11; 2012,Oct,9-11; 2012,Sep,3-8

+ **32507** **with diagnostic wedge resection followed by anatomic lung resection (List separately in addition to code for primary procedure)**
INCLUDES   Classification as a diagnostic wedge resection if intraoperative pathology consultation dictates more extensive resection in the same anatomical area
EXCLUDES   *Diagnostic wedge resection by thoracoscopy (32668)*
Therapeutic wedge resection (32505-32506, 32666-32667)
Code first (32440, 32442, 32445, 32480-32488, 32503-32504)
🔪 4.56   ✂ 4.56   **FUD** ZZZ   C 80 ▢
AMA: 2016,Jan,13; 2015,Jan,16; 2014,Jan,11; 2012,Oct,9-11; 2012,Sep,3-8

32540 Removal of Empyema

32540 **Extrapleural enucleation of empyema (empyemectomy)**
EXCLUDES   *Lung removal code when empyemectomy is performed with lobectomy (see appropriate lung removal code)*
Code also appropriate removal of lung code when done with lobectomy (32480-32488)
🔪 50.4   ✂ 50.4   **FUD** 090   C 80 ▢
AMA: 1994,Fall,1

32550-32552 Chest Tube/Catheter

▲ **32550** **Insertion of indwelling tunneled pleural catheter with cuff**
EXCLUDES   *Procedures performed on same side of chest with (32554-32557)*
🔲 (75989)
🔪 6.43   ✂ 22.2   **FUD** 000   T 62 ▢
AMA: 2016,Jan,13; 2015,Jan,16; 2014,May,3; 2014,Mar,13; 2014,Jan,11; 2012,Nov,3-5; 2012,Jan,15-42; 2011,Jan,11

▲ **32551** **Tube thoracostomy, includes connection to drainage system (eg, water seal), when performed, open (separate procedure)**
🔪 4.92   ✂ 4.92   **FUD** 000   T 50 ▢
AMA: 2016,Jan,13; 2015,Jan,16; 2014,May,3; 2014,Jan,11; 2012,Nov,3-5; 2011,Aug,3-5

32552 **Removal of indwelling tunneled pleural catheter with cuff**
🔪 4.61   ✂ 5.32   **FUD** 010   02 62 80 ▢
AMA: 2016,Jan,13; 2015,Jan,16; 2014,Jan,11; 2012,Nov,3-5; 2012,Jan,15-42; 2011,Jan,11

32553 Intrathoracic Placement Radiation Therapy Devices

EXCLUDES   *Percutaneous placement of interstitial device(s) for radiation therapy guidance: intra-abdominal, intrapelvic, and/or retroperitoneal (49411)*
Code also device

▲ **32553** **Placement of interstitial device(s) for radiation therapy guidance (eg, fiducial markers, dosimeter), percutaneous, intra-thoracic, single or multiple**
🔲 (76942, 77002, 77012, 77021)
🔪 5.62   ✂ 16.8   **FUD** 000   S 62 80 ▢
AMA: 2016,Jun,3; 2016,Jan,13; 2015,Jun,6; 2015,Jan,16; 2014,Jan,11

32554-32557 Pleural Aspiration and Drainage

EXCLUDES   *Open tube thoracostomy (32551)*
Placement of indwelling tunneled pleural drainage catheter (cuffed) (32550)
Procedures performed on same side of chest with (32550-32551)
Radiologic guidance (75989, 76942, 77002, 77012, 77021)

32554 **Thoracentesis, needle or catheter, aspiration of the pleural space; without imaging guidance**
🔪 2.59   ✂ 5.70   **FUD** 000   T 62 50 ▢
AMA: 2016,Jan,13; 2015,Jan,16; 2014,Jan,11; 2013,Nov,9; 2012,Nov,3-5

32555 **with imaging guidance**
🔪 3.25   ✂ 8.25   **FUD** 000   T 62 50 ▢
AMA: 2016,Jan,13; 2015,Jan,16; 2014,Jan,11; 2013,Nov,9; 2012,Nov,3-5

32556	**Pleural drainage, percutaneous, with insertion of indwelling catheter; without imaging guidance**

🔧 3.57　✂ 15.3　**FUD** 000　　T 62 50 ▢

AMA: 2016,Jan,13; 2015,Jan,16; 2014,Jan,11; 2013,Nov,9; 2012,Nov,3-5

32557	**with imaging guidance**

🔧 4.45　✂ 14.6　**FUD** 000　　T 62 50 ▢

AMA: 2016,Jan,13; 2015,Jan,16; 2014,May,3; 2014,Jan,11; 2013,Nov,9; 2012,Nov,3-5

32560-32562 Instillation Drug/Chemical by Chest Tube

EXCLUDES　*Insertion of chest tube (32551)*

32560	**Instillation, via chest tube/catheter, agent for pleurodesis (eg, talc for recurrent or persistent pneumothorax)**

🔧 2.26　✂ 6.96　**FUD** 000　　T ▢

AMA: 2016,Jan,13; 2015,Jan,16; 2014,Jan,11

32561	**Instillation(s), via chest tube/catheter, agent for fibrinolysis (eg, fibrinolytic agent for break up of multiloculated effusion); initial day**

EXCLUDES　*Procedure reported more than one time on the date of initial treatment*

🔧 1.98　✂ 2.65　**FUD** 000　　T 80 ▢

AMA: 2016,Jan,13; 2015,Jan,16; 2014,Jan,11

32562	**subsequent day**

Procedure reported more than one time on each day of initial treatment

🔧 1.79　✂ 2.39　**FUD** 000　　T 80 ▢

AMA: 2016,Jan,13; 2015,Jan,16; 2014,Jan,11

32601-32674 Thoracic Surgery: Video-Assisted (VATS)

INCLUDES　Diagnostic thoracoscopy in surgical thoracoscopy

32601	**Thoracoscopy, diagnostic (separate procedure); lungs, pericardial sac, mediastinal or pleural space, without biopsy**

🔧 8.97　✂ 8.97　**FUD** 000　　T 80 ▢

AMA: 2016,Jan,13; 2015,Jan,16; 2014,Jan,11; 2013,Aug,13; 2012,Oct,9-11; 2012,Sep,3-8

32604	**pericardial sac, with biopsy**

EXCLUDES　*Open biopsy of pericardium (39010)*

🔧 14.0　✂ 14.0　**FUD** 000　　T 80 ▢

AMA: 2016,Jan,13; 2015,Jan,16; 2014,Jan,11; 2013,Aug,13; 2012,Oct,9-11; 2012,Sep,3-8

32606	**mediastinal space, with biopsy**

🔧 13.4　✂ 13.4　**FUD** 000　　T 80 ▢

AMA: 2016,Jan,13; 2015,Jan,16; 2014,Jan,11; 2013,Aug,13; 2012,Oct,9-11; 2012,Sep,3-8

32607	**Thoracoscopy; with diagnostic biopsy(ies) of lung infiltrate(s) (eg, wedge, incisional), unilateral**

EXCLUDES　*Procedure reported more than one time per lung*
Removal of lung (32440-32445, 32488)
Thoracoscopy, surgical; with removal of lung (32671)

🔧 8.98　✂ 8.98　**FUD** 000　　T 80 ▢

AMA: 2016,Jan,13; 2015,Jan,16; 2014,Jan,11; 2013,Aug,13; 2012,Oct,9-11; 2012,Sep,3-8

32608	**with diagnostic biopsy(ies) of lung nodule(s) or mass(es) (eg, wedge, incisional), unilateral**

EXCLUDES　*Procedure reported more than one time per lung*
Removal of lung (32440-32445, 32488)
Thoracoscopy, surgical; with removal of lung (32671)

🔧 11.0　✂ 11.0　**FUD** 000　　T 80 ▢

AMA: 2016,Jan,13; 2015,Jan,16; 2014,Jan,11; 2013,Aug,13; 2012,Oct,9-11; 2012,Sep,3-8

32609	**with biopsy(ies) of pleura**

🔧 7.53　✂ 7.53　**FUD** 000　　T 80 ▢

AMA: 2016,Jan,13; 2015,Jan,16; 2014,Jan,11; 2013,Aug,13; 2012,Oct,9-11; 2012,Sep,3-8

32650	**Thoracoscopy, surgical; with pleurodesis (eg, mechanical or chemical)**

🔧 19.3　✂ 19.3　**FUD** 090　　C 80 50 ▢

AMA: 2016,Jan,13; 2015,Jan,16; 2014,Jan,11; 2013,Aug,13

32651	**with partial pulmonary decortication**

🔧 31.8　✂ 31.8　**FUD** 090　　C 80 50 ▢

AMA: 2016,Jan,13; 2015,Jan,16; 2014,Jan,11; 2013,Aug,13

32652	**with total pulmonary decortication, including intrapleural pneumonolysis**

🔧 48.3　✂ 48.3　**FUD** 090　　C 80 50 ▢

AMA: 2016,Jan,13; 2015,Jan,16; 2014,Jan,11; 2013,Aug,13

32653	**with removal of intrapleural foreign body or fibrin deposit**

🔧 30.7　✂ 30.7　**FUD** 090　　C 80 ▢

AMA: 2016,Jan,13; 2015,Jan,16; 2014,Jan,11; 2013,Aug,13

32654	**with control of traumatic hemorrhage**

🔧 34.4　✂ 34.4　**FUD** 090　　C 80 50 ▢

AMA: 2016,Jan,13; 2015,Jan,16; 2014,Jan,11; 2013,Aug,13

32655	**with resection-plication of bullae, includes any pleural procedure when performed**

EXCLUDES　*Thoracoscopic lung volume reduction surgery (32672)*

🔧 27.7　✂ 27.7　**FUD** 090　　C 80 50 ▢

AMA: 2016,Jan,13; 2015,Jan,16; 2014,Jan,11; 2013,Aug,13; 2012,Jan,15-42; 2011,Jan,11

32656	**with parietal pleurectomy**

🔧 23.3　✂ 23.3　**FUD** 090　　C 80 50 ▢

AMA: 2016,Jan,13; 2015,Jan,16; 2014,Jan,11; 2013,Aug,13

32658	**with removal of clot or foreign body from pericardial sac**

🔧 20.7　✂ 20.7　**FUD** 090　　C 80 ▢

AMA: 2016,Jan,13; 2015,Jan,16; 2014,Jan,11; 2013,Aug,13

32659	**with creation of pericardial window or partial resection of pericardial sac for drainage**

🔧 21.2　✂ 21.2　**FUD** 090　　C 80 ▢

AMA: 2016,Jan,13; 2015,Jan,16; 2014,Jan,11; 2013,Aug,13

32661	**with excision of pericardial cyst, tumor, or mass**

🔧 23.2　✂ 23.2　**FUD** 090　　C 80 ▢

AMA: 2016,Jan,13; 2015,Jan,16; 2014,Jan,11; 2013,Aug,13

32662	**with excision of mediastinal cyst, tumor, or mass**

🔧 25.9　✂ 25.9　**FUD** 090　　C 80 ▢

AMA: 2016,Jan,13; 2015,Jan,16; 2014,Jan,11; 2013,Aug,13; 2012,Jan,15-42; 2011,Jan,11

32663	**with lobectomy (single lobe)**

EXCLUDES　*Thoracoscopic segmentectomy (32669)*

🔧 40.7　✂ 40.7　**FUD** 090　　C 80 ▢

AMA: 2016,Jan,13; 2015,Jan,16; 2014,Jan,11; 2013,Aug,13; 2012,Oct,9-11; 2012,Sep,3-8

32664	**with thoracic sympathectomy**

🔧 24.7　✂ 24.7　**FUD** 090　　C 80 50 ▢

AMA: 2016,Jan,13; 2015,Dec,16; 2015,Jan,16; 2014,Jan,11; 2013,Aug,13; 2012,Jan,15-42; 2011,Jan,11

32665	**with esophagomyotomy (Heller type)**

EXCLUDES　*Exploratory thoracoscopy with and without biopsy (32601-32609)*

🔧 35.5　✂ 35.5　**FUD** 090　　C 80 ▢

AMA: 2016,Jan,13; 2015,Jan,16; 2014,Jan,11; 2013,Aug,13

32666	**with therapeutic wedge resection (eg, mass, nodule), initial unilateral**

EXCLUDES　*Removal of lung (32440-32445, 32488)*
Thoracoscopy, surgical; with removal of lung (32671)

Code also a more extensive procedure of the lung when performed on the contralateral lung or different lobe with modifier 59 regardless of pathology consultation

🔧 25.3　✂ 25.3　**FUD** 090　　C 80 50 ▢

AMA: 2016,Jan,13; 2015,Jan,16; 2014,Jan,11; 2013,Aug,13; 2012,Oct,9-11; 2012,Sep,3-8

+ 32667 **with therapeutic wedge resection (eg, mass or nodule), each additional resection, ipsilateral (List separately in addition to code for primary procedure)**

> EXCLUDES *Removal of lung (32440-32445, 32488)*
> *Thoracoscopy, surgical; with removal of lung (32671)*

Code also a more extensive procedure of the lung when performed on the contralateral lung or different lobe with modifier 59 regardless of intraoperative pathology consultation

Code first (32666)

🚗 4.58 ✂ 4.58 **FUD** ZZZ

C 80 ▣

AMA: 2016,Jan,13; 2015,Jan,16; 2014,Jan,11; 2013,Aug,13; 2012,Oct,9-11; 2012,Sep,3-8

+ 32668 **with diagnostic wedge resection followed by anatomic lung resection (List separately in addition to code for primary procedure)**

> INCLUDES Classification as a diagnostic wedge resection if intraoperative pathology consultation dictates more extensive resection in the same anatomical area

Code first (32440-32488, 32503-32504, 32663, 32669-32671)

🚗 4.57 ✂ 4.57 **FUD** ZZZ

C 80 ▣

AMA: 2016,Jan,13; 2015,Jan,16; 2014,Jan,11; 2013,Aug,13; 2012,Oct,9-11; 2012,Sep,3-8

32669 **with removal of a single lung segment (segmentectomy)**

🚗 39.1 ✂ 39.1 **FUD** 090

C 80 ▣

AMA: 2016,Jan,13; 2015,Jan,16; 2014,Jan,11; 2013,Aug,13; 2012,Oct,9-11; 2012,Sep,3-8

32670 **with removal of two lobes (bilobectomy)**

🚗 46.5 ✂ 46.5 **FUD** 090

C 80 ▣

AMA: 2016,Jan,13; 2015,Jan,16; 2014,Jan,11; 2013,Aug,13; 2012,Oct,9-11; 2012,Sep,3-8

32671 **with removal of lung (pneumonectomy)**

🚗 51.5 ✂ 51.5 **FUD** 090

C 80 ▣

AMA: 2016,Jan,13; 2015,Jan,16; 2014,Jan,11; 2013,Aug,13; 2012,Oct,9-11; 2012,Sep,3-8

32672 **with resection-plication for emphysematous lung (bullous or non-bullous) for lung volume reduction (LVRS), unilateral includes any pleural procedure, when performed**

🚗 44.2 ✂ 44.2 **FUD** 090

C 80 ▣

AMA: 2016,Jan,13; 2015,Jan,16; 2014,Jan,11; 2013,Aug,13; 2012,Oct,9-11; 2012,Sep,3-8

32673 **with resection of thymus, unilateral or bilateral**

> EXCLUDES *Exploratory thoracoscopy with and without biopsy (32601-32609)*
> *Open excision mediastinal cyst (39200)*
> *Open excision mediastinal tumor (39220)*
> *Open thymectomy (60520-60522)*

🚗 35.4 ✂ 35.4 **FUD** 090

C 80 ▣

AMA: 2016,Jan,13; 2015,Jan,16; 2014,Jan,11; 2013,Aug,13; 2012,Oct,9-11; 2012,Sep,3-8

+ 32674 **with mediastinal and regional lymphadenectomy (List separately in addition to code for primary procedure)**

> INCLUDES Mediastinal lymph nodes:
> Left side:
> Aortopulmonary window
> Inferior pulmonary ligament
> Paraesophageal
> Subcarinal
> Right side:
> Inferior pulmonary ligament
> Paraesophageal
> Paratracheal
> Subcarinal

> EXCLUDES *Mediastinal and regional lymphadenectomy by thoracotomy (38746)*

Code first (19260, 31760, 31766, 31786, 32096-32200, 32220-32320, 32440-32491, 32503-32505, 32601-32663, 32666, 32669-32673, 32815, 33025, 33030, 33050-33130, 39200-39220, 39560-39561, 43101, 43112, 43117-43118, 43122-43123, 43351, 60270, 60505)

🚗 6.29 ✂ 6.29 **FUD** ZZZ

C 80 ▣

AMA: 2016,Jan,13; 2015,Jan,16; 2014,May,3; 2014,Jan,11; 2013,Aug,13; 2012,Oct,9-11; 2012,Sep,3-8

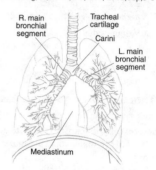

R. main bronchial segment — Tracheal cartilage — Carini — L. main bronchial segment — Mediastinum

32701 Target Delineation for Stereotactic Radiation Therapy

> INCLUDES Collaboration between the radiation oncologist and surgeon
> Correlation of tumor and contiguous body structures
> Determination of borders and volume of tumor
> Identification of fiducial markers
> Verification of target when fiducial markers are not used

> EXCLUDES *Fiducial marker insertion (31626, 32553)*
> *Procedure performed by same physician as radiation treatment management (77427-77499)*
> *Radiation oncology services (77295, 77331, 77370, 77373, 77435)*
> *Therapeutic radiology (77261-77799 [77295, 77385, 77386, 77387, 77424, 77425])*

32701 **Thoracic target(s) delineation for stereotactic body radiation therapy (SRS/SBRT), (photon or particle beam), entire course of treatment**

🚗 6.32 ✂ 6.32 **FUD** XXX

B 80 26 ▣

AMA: 2016,Jan,13; 2015,Jun,6

32800-32820 Chest Repair and Reconstruction Procedures

32800 **Repair lung hernia through chest wall**

🚗 27.4 ✂ 27.4 **FUD** 090

C 80 ▣

32810 **Closure of chest wall following open flap drainage for empyema (Clagett type procedure)**

🚗 26.1 ✂ 26.1 **FUD** 090

C 80 ▣

32815 **Open closure of major bronchial fistula**

🚗 81.3 ✂ 81.3 **FUD** 090

C 80 ▣

32820 **Major reconstruction, chest wall (posttraumatic)**

🚗 38.7 ✂ 38.7 **FUD** 090

C 80 ▣

26/TC PC/TC Only   A2-Z3 ASC Payment   50 Bilateral   ♂ Male Only   ♀ Female Only   🚗 Facility RVU   ✂ Non-Facility RVU   ▣ CCI
FUD Follow-up Days   **CMS:** IOM (Pub 100)   A-Y OPPSI   80/80 Surg Assist Allowed / w/Doc   ▨ Lab Crosswalk   ▨ Radiology Crosswalk   ☒ CLIA

116

32850-32856 Lung Transplant Procedures

INCLUDES Harvesting donor lung(s), cold preservation, preparation of donor lung(s), transplantation into recipient

EXCLUDES Repairs or resection of donor lung(s) (32491, 32505-32507, 35216, 35276)

32850 **Donor pneumonectomy(s) (including cold preservation), from cadaver donor**
   0.00   0.00 **FUD** XXX   C ▢
   AMA: 1993,Win,1

32851 **Lung transplant, single; without cardiopulmonary bypass**
   95.9   95.9 **FUD** 090   C 80 ▢
   AMA: 1993,Win,1

32852 **with cardiopulmonary bypass**
   104.   104. **FUD** 090   C 80 ▢
   AMA: 1993,Win,1

32853 **Lung transplant, double (bilateral sequential or en bloc); without cardiopulmonary bypass**
   133.   133. **FUD** 090   C 80 ▢
   AMA: 1993,Win,1

32854 **with cardiopulmonary bypass**
   142.   142. **FUD** 090   C 80 ▢
   AMA: 1993,Win,1

32855 **Backbench standard preparation of cadaver donor lung allograft prior to transplantation, including dissection of allograft from surrounding soft tissues to prepare pulmonary venous/atrial cuff, pulmonary artery, and bronchus; unilateral**
   0.00   0.00 **FUD** XXX   C 80 ▢

32856 **bilateral**
   0.00   0.00 **FUD** XXX   C 80 ▢

32900-32997 Chest and Respiratory Procedures

32900 **Resection of ribs, extrapleural, all stages**
   40.7   40.7 **FUD** 090   C 80 ▢

32905 **Thoracoplasty, Schede type or extrapleural (all stages);**
   38.9   38.9 **FUD** 090   C 80 ▢

32906 **with closure of bronchopleural fistula**
   48.1   48.1 **FUD** 090   C 80 ▢

EXCLUDES Open closure of bronchial fistula (32815)
     Resection first rib for thoracic compression (21615-21616)

32940 **Pneumonolysis, extraperiosteal, including filling or packing procedures**
   35.8   35.8 **FUD** 090   C 80 ▢

32960 **Pneumothorax, therapeutic, intrapleural injection of air**
   2.89   4.05 **FUD** 000   T 02 ▢

32997 **Total lung lavage (unilateral)**
EXCLUDES Broncho-alveolar lavage by bronchoscopy (31624)
   9.91   9.91 **FUD** 000   C 50 ▢
   AMA: 2016,Jan,13; 2015,Jan,16; 2014,Jan,11

32998-32999 Destruction of Lung Neoplasm

32998 **Ablation therapy for reduction or eradication of 1 or more pulmonary tumor(s) including pleura or chest wall when involved by tumor extension, percutaneous, radiofrequency, unilateral**
   8.24   68.0 **FUD** 000   T 02 80 50 ▢
   (76940, 77013, 77022)

32999 **Unlisted procedure, lungs and pleura**
   0.00   0.00 **FUD** YYY   T
   AMA: 2016,Jan,13; 2015,Dec,16; 2015,Jun,6; 2015,Jan,16; 2014,Jan,11; 2012,Jan,15-42; 2011,Aug,9-10; 2011,Jan,11

33010-33050 Procedures of the Pericardial Sac

EXCLUDES *Surgical thoracoscopy (video-assisted thoracic surgery [VATS]) procedures of pericardium (32601, 32604, 32658-32659, 32661)*

▲ **33010** **Pericardiocentesis; initial**

✴ (76930)

🔳 3.49 ⚕ 3.49 **FUD** 000 　　　　　T A2 ▭

AMA: 2016,Sep,9; 2016,Jan,13; 2015,Feb,10

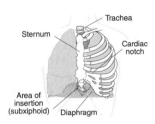

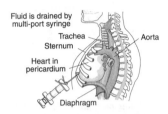

A centesis syringe is inserted into the pericardial sac, either under fluoroscopic guidance or by use of anatomical landmarks, and excess fluid is removed

▲ **33011** **subsequent**

✴ (76930)

🔳 3.51 ⚕ 3.51 **FUD** 000 　　　　T A2 80 ▭

AMA: 2016,Sep,9; 2016,Jan,13; 2015,Feb,10; 2015,Jan,16; 2014,Jan,11

33015 **Tube pericardiostomy**

🔳 14.7 ⚕ 14.7 **FUD** 090 　　　　C ▭

AMA: 2016,Jan,13; 2015,Jan,16; 2014,Aug,14

33020 **Pericardiotomy for removal of clot or foreign body (primary procedure)**

🔳 25.5 ⚕ 25.5 **FUD** 090 　　　　C 80 ▭

AMA: 1997,Nov,1

33025 **Creation of pericardial window or partial resection for drainage**

EXCLUDES *Surgical thoracoscopy (video-assisted thoracic surgery [VATS]) creation of pericardial window (32659)*

🔳 23.1 ⚕ 23.1 **FUD** 090 　　　　C 80 ▭

AMA: 1997,Nov,1

33030 **Pericardiectomy, subtotal or complete; without cardiopulmonary bypass**

INCLUDES Delorme pericardiectomy

🔳 58.2 ⚕ 58.2 **FUD** 090 　　　　C 80 ▭

AMA: 1997,Nov,1; 1994,Win,1

33031 **with cardiopulmonary bypass**

🔳 71.9 ⚕ 71.9 **FUD** 090 　　　　C 80 ▭

AMA: 1997,Nov,1; 1994,Win,1

33050 **Resection of pericardial cyst or tumor**

EXCLUDES *Open biopsy of pericardium (39010)*
Surgical thoracoscopy (video-assisted thoracic surgery [VATS]) resection of cyst, mass, or tumor of pericardium (32661)

🔳 29.0 ⚕ 29.0 **FUD** 090 　　　　C 80 ▭

AMA: 1997,Nov,1

33120-33130 Neoplasms of Heart

Code also removal of thrombus through a separate heart incision, when performed (33310-33315); append modifier 59 to (33315)

33120 **Excision of intracardiac tumor, resection with cardiopulmonary bypass**

🔳 61.0 ⚕ 61.0 **FUD** 090 　　　　C 80 ▭

AMA: 2016,Jan,13; 2015,Jan,16; 2014,Jan,11

33130 **Resection of external cardiac tumor**

🔳 40.1 ⚕ 40.1 **FUD** 090 　　　　C 80 ▭

AMA: 2016,Jan,13; 2015,Jan,16; 2014,Jan,11

33140-33141 Transmyocardial Revascularization

33140 **Transmyocardial laser revascularization, by thoracotomy; (separate procedure)**

🔳 45.7 ⚕ 45.7 **FUD** 090 　　　　C 80 ▭

AMA: 2016,Jan,13; 2015,Jan,16; 2014,Jan,11; 2012,Jan,15-42; 2011,Jan,11

+ **33141** **performed at the time of other open cardiac procedure(s) (List separately in addition to code for primary procedure)**

Code first (33390-33391, 33400-33496, 33510-33536, 33542)

🔳 3.84 ⚕ 3.84 **FUD** ZZZ 　　　　C 80 ▭

AMA: 2016,Jan,13; 2015,Jan,16; 2014,Jan,11

33202-33203 Placement Epicardial Leads

Code also insertion of pulse generator when performed by same physician/same surgical session (33212-33213, [33221], 33230-33231, 33240)

33202 **Insertion of epicardial electrode(s); open incision (eg, thoracotomy, median sternotomy, subxiphoid approach)**

🔳 22.5 ⚕ 22.5 **FUD** 090 　　　　C ▭

AMA: 2016,Aug,5; 2016,May,5; 2016,Jan,13; 2015,May,3; 2015,Jan,16; 2014,Nov,5; 2014,Jan,11; 2012,Jun,3-9

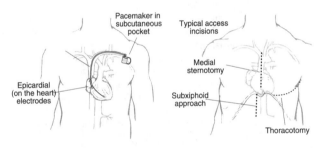

Epicardial electrodes are placed on the outside of the heart in an open procedure

33203 **endoscopic approach (eg, thoracoscopy, pericardioscopy)**

🔳 23.4 ⚕ 23.4 **FUD** 090 　　　　C ▭

AMA: 2016,Aug,5; 2016,May,5; 2016,Jan,13; 2015,May,3; 2015,Jan,16; 2014,Nov,5; 2014,Jan,11; 2012,Jun,3-9

33206-33214 [33221] Pacemakers

INCLUDES Device evaluation (93279-93299 [93260, 93261])
Dual lead: device that paces and senses in two heart chambers
Multiple lead: device that paces and senses in three or more heart chambers
Radiological supervision and interpretation for pacemaker procedure
Single lead: device that paces and senses in one heart chamber
Skin pocket revision, when performed
If revision includes incision/drainage of a wound infection or hematoma code also (10140, 10180, 11042-11047 [11045, 11046])

EXCLUDES *Electrode repositioning:*
Left ventricle (33226)
Pacemaker (33215)
Insertion of lead for left ventricular (biventricular) pacing (33224-33225)
Leadless pacemaker systems (0387T-0391T)

▲ **33206** **Insertion of new or replacement of permanent pacemaker with transvenous electrode(s); atrial**

INCLUDES Pulse generator insertion/transvenous electrode placement

EXCLUDES *Insertion of transvenous electrode (33216-33217)*
Removal and replacement of pacemaker pulse generator (33227-33229)

Code also removal of pacemaker pulse generator and electrodes when removal and replacement of pulse generator and electrodes is performed (33233, 33234, 33235)

🚑 13.3 ⚕ 13.3 **FUD** 090 J J8 ▢

AMA: 2016,Aug,5; 2016,May,5; 2016,Jan,13; 2015,May,3; 2015,Jan,16; 2014,Nov,5; 2014,Jan,11; 2013,Apr,10-11; 2012,Jun,3-9; 2012,Jan,15-42; 2011,Jan,11

▲ **33207** **ventricular**

EXCLUDES *Insertion of transvenous electrode (33216-33217)*
Removal and replacement of pacemaker pulse generator (33227-33229)

Code also removal of pacemaker pulse generator and electrodes when removal and replacement of pulse generator and electrodes is performed (33224, 33225, 33233)

🚑 14.2 ⚕ 14.2 **FUD** 090 J J8 ▢

AMA: 2016,Aug,5; 2016,May,5; 2016,Jan,13; 2015,May,3; 2015,Jan,16; 2014,Nov,5; 2014,Jan,11; 2013,Apr,10-11; 2012,Jun,3-9; 2012,Jan,15-42; 2011,Jan,11

▲ **33208** **atrial and ventricular**

INCLUDES Pulse generator insertion/transvenous electrode placement

EXCLUDES *Insertion of transvenous electrode (33216-33217)*
Removal and replacement of pacemaker pulse generator (33227-33229)

Code also removal of pacemaker pulse generator and electrodes when removal and replacement of pulse generator and electrodes is performed (33233, 33234, 33235)

🚑 15.4 ⚕ 15.4 **FUD** 090 J J8 ▢

AMA: 2016,Aug,5; 2016,May,5; 2016,Jan,13; 2015,May,3; 2015,Jan,16; 2014,Nov,5; 2014,Jan,11; 2013,Apr,10-11; 2012,Jun,3-9; 2012,Jan,15-42; 2011,Jan,11

▲ **33210** **Insertion or replacement of temporary transvenous single chamber cardiac electrode or pacemaker catheter (separate procedure)**

🚑 5.20 ⚕ 5.20 **FUD** 000 J J8 ▢

AMA: 2016,Aug,5; 2016,May,5; 2016,Jan,13; 2015,May,3; 2015,Jan,16; 2014,Nov,5; 2014,Jan,11; 2013,Jan,6-8; 2012,Jun,3-9; 2011,Aug,3-5

▲ **33211** **Insertion or replacement of temporary transvenous dual chamber pacing electrodes (separate procedure)**

🚑 5.32 ⚕ 5.32 **FUD** 000 J J8 ▢

AMA: 2016,Aug,5; 2016,May,5; 2016,Jan,13; 2015,May,3; 2015,Jan,16; 2014,Nov,5; 2014,Jan,11; 2012,Jun,3-9; 2011,Aug,3-5

▲ **33212** **Insertion of pacemaker pulse generator only; with existing single lead**

EXCLUDES *Insertion of a single transvenous electrode (33216-33217, 33233)*
Removal and replacement of pacemaker pulse generator (33227-33229)
Removal of permanent pacemaker pulse generator only (33233)

Code also placement of epicardial leads by same physician/same surgical session (33202-33203)

🚑 9.67 ⚕ 9.67 **FUD** 090 J J8 ▢

AMA: 2016,Aug,5; 2016,May,5; 2016,Jan,13; 2015,May,3; 2015,Jan,16; 2014,Nov,5; 2014,Jan,11; 2012,Jun,3-9; 2012,Jan,15-42; 2011,Jan,11

▲ **33213** **with existing dual leads**

EXCLUDES *Insertion of a single transvenous electrode (33216-33217)*
Removal and replacement of pacemaker pulse generator (33227-33229)
Removal of permanent pacemaker pulse generator only (33233)

Code also placement of epicardial leads by same physician/same surgical session (33202-33203)

🚑 10.0 ⚕ 10.0 **FUD** 090 J J8 ▢

AMA: 2016,Aug,5; 2016,May,5; 2016,Jan,13; 2015,May,3; 2015,Jan,16; 2014,Nov,5; 2014,Jan,11; 2012,Jun,3-9; 2012,Jan,15-42; 2011,Jan,11

▲ # **33221** **with existing multiple leads**

EXCLUDES *Insertion of a single transvenous electrode (33216-33217)*
Removal and replacement of pacemaker pulse generator (33227-33229)
Removal of permanent pacemaker pulse generator only (33233)

Code also placement of epicardial leads by same physician/same surgical session (33202-33203)

🚑 10.8 ⚕ 10.8 **FUD** 090 J J8 ▢

AMA: 2016,Aug,5; 2016,May,5; 2016,Jan,13; 2015,May,3; 2015,Jan,16; 2014,Nov,5; 2014,Jan,11; 2012,Jun,3-9

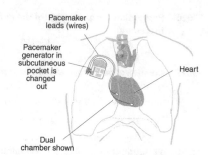

Pacemaker leads (wires)

Pacemaker generator in subcutaneous pocket is changed out

Heart

Dual chamber shown

▲ **33214** **Upgrade of implanted pacemaker system, conversion of single chamber system to dual chamber system (includes removal of previously placed pulse generator, testing of existing lead, insertion of new lead, insertion of new pulse generator)**

EXCLUDES *Insertion of a single transvenous electrode (33216-33217)*
Removal and replacement of pacemaker pulse generator (33227-33229)

🚑 14.1 ⚕ 14.1 **FUD** 090 J J8 80 ▢

AMA: 2016,Aug,5; 2016,May,5; 2016,Jan,13; 2015,May,3; 2015,Jan,16; 2014,Nov,5; 2014,Jan,11; 2012,Jun,3-9

26/TC PC/TC Only   A2-Z3 ASC Payment   50 Bilateral   ♂ Male Only   ♀ Female Only   🚑 Facility RVU   ⚕ Non-Facility RVU   ▢ CCI
FUD Follow-up Days   CMS: IOM (Pub 100)   A-Y OPPSI   80/80 Surg Assist Allowed / w/Doc   ▣ Lab Crosswalk   ✚ Radiology Crosswalk   ✖ CLIA
120

CPT © 2016 American Medical Association. All Rights Reserved.   © 2016 Optum360, LLC

33215-33249 [33227, 33228, 33229, 33230, 33231, 33262, 33263, 33264] Pacemakers/Implantable Defibrillator/Electrode Insertion/Replacement/Revision/Repair

INCLUDES Device evaluation (93279-93299 [93260, 93261])
Dual lead: device that paces and senses in two heart chambers
Multiple lead: device that paces and senses in three or more heart chambers
Radiological supervision and interpretation for pacemaker or pacing cardioverter-defibrillator procedure
Single lead: device that paces and senses in one heart chamber
Skin pocket revision, when performed
If revision includes incision/drainage of a wound infection or hematoma code also (10140, 10180, 11042-11047 [11045, 11046])

EXCLUDES Electrode repositioning:
Left ventricle (33226)
Pacemaker or implantable defibrillator (33215)
Fluoroscopic guidance for lead evaluation without lead change, insertion, or revision (76000)
Insertion of lead for left ventricular (biventricular) pacing (33224-33225)
Removal of leadless pacemaker system (0388T)
Removal of subcutaneous implantable defibrillator electrode ([33272])
Testing of defibrillator threshold (DFT) during follow-up evaluation (93642-93644)
Testing of defibrillator threshold (DFT) during insertion/replacement (93640-93641)

33215 Repositioning of previously implanted transvenous pacemaker or implantable defibrillator (right atrial or right ventricular) electrode
⏱ 8.98 ⚖ 8.98 **FUD** 090 T G2 ▭
AMA: 2016,Aug,5; 2016,May,5; 2016,Jan,13; 2015,May,3; 2015,Jan,16; 2014,Nov,5; 2014,Jan,11; 2012,Jun,3-9

▲ **33216** Insertion of a single transvenous electrode, permanent pacemaker or implantable defibrillator
EXCLUDES Insertion or replacement of a lead for a cardiac venous system (33224-33225)
Insertion or replacement of permanent implantable defibrillator generator or system (33249)
Removal and replacement of permanent pacemaker or implantable defibrillator (33206-33208, 33212-33213, [33221], 33227-33229, 33230-33231, 33240, [33262, 33263, 33264])
⏱ 11.0 ⚖ 11.0 **FUD** 090 J J8 ▭
AMA: 2016,Aug,5; 2016,May,5; 2016,Jan,13; 2015,May,3; 2015,Jan,16; 2014,Nov,5; 2014,Jan,11; 2012,Jun,3-9; 2012,Jan,15-42; 2011,Jan,11

▲ **33217** Insertion of 2 transvenous electrodes, permanent pacemaker or implantable defibrillator
EXCLUDES Insertion or replacement of a lead for a cardiac venous system (33224-33225)
Insertion or replacement of permanent implantable defibrillator generator or system (33249)
Removal and replacement of permanent pacemaker or implantable defibrillator (33206-33208, 33212-33213, [33221], 33227-33229, 33230-33231, 33240, [33262, 33263, 33264])
⏱ 10.8 ⚖ 10.8 **FUD** 090 J J8 ▭
AMA: 2016,Aug,5; 2016,May,5; 2016,Jan,13; 2015,May,3; 2015,Jan,16; 2014,Nov,5; 2014,Jan,11; 2012,Jun,3-9; 2012,Jan,15-42; 2011,Jan,11

▲ **33218** Repair of single transvenous electrode, permanent pacemaker or implantable defibrillator
Code also replacement of implantable defibrillator pulse generator, when performed ([33262, 33263, 33264])
Code also replacement of pacemaker pulse generator, when performed (33227-33229)
⏱ 11.6 ⚖ 11.6 **FUD** 090 T G2 ▭
AMA: 2016,Aug,5; 2016,May,5; 2016,Jan,13; 2015,May,3; 2015,Jan,16; 2014,Nov,5; 2014,Jan,11; 2012,Jun,3-9; 2012,Jan,15-42; 2011,Jan,11

▲ **33220** Repair of 2 transvenous electrodes for permanent pacemaker or implantable defibrillator
Code also modifier 52 Reduced services, when one electrode of a two-chamber system is repaired
Code also replacement of implantable defibrillator pulse generator, when performed ([33263, 33264])
Code also replacement of pacemaker pulse generator, when performed (33228-33229)
⏱ 11.6 ⚖ 11.6 **FUD** 090 T G2 ▭
AMA: 2016,Aug,5; 2016,May,5; 2016,Jan,13; 2015,May,3; 2015,Jan,16; 2014,Nov,5; 2014,Jan,11; 2012,Jun,3-9; 2012,Jan,15-42; 2011,Jan,11

33221 Resequenced code. See code following 33213.

▲ **33222** Relocation of skin pocket for pacemaker
INCLUDES Formation of the new pocket
Procedures related to the existing pocket:
Accessing the pocket
Incision/drainage of any abscess or hematoma (10140, 10180)
Pocket closure (13100-13102)
EXCLUDES Debridement, subcutaneous tissue (11042-11047 [11045, 11046])
Code also removal and replacement of an existing generator
⏱ 10.1 ⚖ 10.1 **FUD** 090 T A2 ▭
AMA: 2016,Aug,5; 2016,May,5; 2016,Jan,13; 2015,May,3; 2015,Jan,16; 2014,Nov,5; 2014,Jan,11; 2012,Jun,3-9

▲ **33223** Relocation of skin pocket for implantable defibrillator
INCLUDES Formation of the new pocket
Procedures related to the existing pocket:
Accessing the pocket
Incision/drainage of any abscess or hematoma (10140, 10180)
Pocket closure (11042-11047 [11045, 11046])
EXCLUDES Debridement, subcutaneous tissue (11042-11047 [11045, 11046])
Code also removal and replacement of an existing generator
⏱ 12.1 ⚖ 12.1 **FUD** 090 T A2 80 ▭
AMA: 2016,Aug,5; 2016,Jan,13; 2015,Jan,16; 2014,Nov,5; 2014,Jan,11; 2012,Jun,3-9

33224 Insertion of pacing electrode, cardiac venous system, for left ventricular pacing, with attachment to previously placed pacemaker or implantable defibrillator pulse generator (including revision of pocket, removal, insertion, and/or replacement of existing generator)
Code also placement of epicardial electrode when appropriate (33202-33203)
⏱ 14.9 ⚖ 14.9 **FUD** 000 J J8 ▭
AMA: 2016,Aug,5; 2016,May,5; 2016,Jan,13; 2015,May,3; 2015,Jan,16; 2014,Nov,5; 2014,Jan,11; 2012,Jun,3-9; 2012,Jan,15-42; 2011,Jan,11

+ **33225** Insertion of pacing electrode, cardiac venous system, for left ventricular pacing, at time of insertion of implantable defibrillator or pacemaker pulse generator (eg, for upgrade to dual chamber system) (List separately in addition to code for primary procedure)
Code first (33206-33208, 33212-33213, [33221], 33214, 33216-33217, 33223, 33228-33229, 33230-33231, 33233, 33234-33235, 33240, [33263, 33264], 33249)
Code first (33223) for relocation of pocket for implantable defibrillator
Code first (33222) for relocation of pocket for pacemaker pulse generator
⏱ 13.5 ⚖ 13.5 **FUD** ZZZ N N1 ▭
AMA: 2016,Aug,5; 2016,May,5; 2016,Jan,13; 2015,May,3; 2015,Jan,16; 2014,Nov,5; 2014,Jan,11; 2012,Jun,3-9; 2012,Jan,15-42; 2011,Jan,11

33226 Repositioning of previously implanted cardiac venous system (left ventricular) electrode (including removal, insertion and/or replacement of existing generator)
⏱ 14.3 ⚖ 14.3 **FUD** 000 T G2 ▭
AMA: 2016,Aug,5; 2016,May,5; 2016,Jan,13; 2015,May,3; 2015,Jan,16; 2014,Nov,5; 2014,Jan,11; 2012,Jun,3-9

33227 Resequenced code. See code following 33233.

33228 Resequenced code. See code following 33233.

33229 Resequenced code. See code before 33234.

33230 Resequenced code. See code following 33240.

33231 Resequenced code. See code before 33241.

▲ **33233** Removal of permanent pacemaker pulse generator only

> EXCLUDES Removal and replacement of pacemaker pulse
> generator and transvenous electrode(s): code
> 33233 with (33206, 33207, 33208, 33234, 33235)
> Removal of permanent pacemaker pulse generator with
> replacement of pacemaker pulse generator; single
> lead system (33227-33229)

🖛 7.02 ✎ 7.02 **FUD** 090 [02] [J8] 🖵

AMA: 2016,Aug,5; 2016,May,5; 2016,Jan,13; 2015,Jan,16;
2014,Nov,5; 2014,Jan,11; 2012,Jun,3-9; 2012,Jan,15-42;
2011,Jan,11

▲ # **33227** Removal of permanent pacemaker pulse generator with
replacement of pacemaker pulse generator; single lead
system

🖛 10.1 ✎ 10.1 **FUD** 090 [J] [J8] 🖵

AMA: 2016,Aug,5; 2016,May,5; 2016,Jan,13; 2015,Jan,16;
2014,Nov,5; 2014,Jan,11; 2013,Apr,10-11; 2012,Jun,3-9

▲ # **33228** dual lead system

🖛 10.6 ✎ 10.6 **FUD** 090 [J] [J8] 🖵

AMA: 2016,Aug,5; 2016,May,5; 2016,Jan,13; 2015,Jan,16;
2014,Nov,5; 2014,Jan,11; 2013,Apr,10-11; 2012,Jun,3-9

▲ # **33229** multiple lead system

🖛 11.1 ✎ 11.1 **FUD** 090 [J] [J8] 🖵

AMA: 2016,Aug,5; 2016,May,5; 2016,Jan,13; 2015,Jan,16;
2014,Nov,5; 2014,Jan,11; 2013,Apr,10-11; 2012,Jun,3-9

▲ **33234** Removal of transvenous pacemaker electrode(s); single lead
system, atrial or ventricular

> EXCLUDES Removal and replacement of pacemaker pulse
> generator and transvenous electrode 33234 and
> 33233 and (33206, 33207, 33208)
> Thoracotomy to remove electrodes (33238, 33243)
> Code also pacing electrode insertion in cardiac venous system
> for pacing of left ventricle during insertion of pulse
> generator (pacemaker or implantable defibrillator) when
> performed (33225)

🖛 14.3 ✎ 14.3 **FUD** 090 [02] [G2] 🖵

AMA: 2016,Aug,5; 2016,May,5; 2016,Jan,13; 2015,Jan,16;
2014,Nov,5; 2014,Jan,11; 2012,Oct,14; 2012,Jun,3-9

▲ **33235** dual lead system

> EXCLUDES Removal and replacement of pacemaker pulse
> generator and transvenous electrode(s) 33235 and
> 33233 and (33206, 33207, 33208, 33233, 33235)
> Thoracotomy to remove electrode(s) (33238, 33243)
> Code also pacing electrode insertion in cardiac venous system
> for pacing of left ventricle during insertion of pulse
> generator (pacemaker or implantable defibrillator) when
> performed (33225)

🖛 18.7 ✎ 18.7 **FUD** 090 [02] [G2] 🖵

AMA: 2016,Aug,5; 2016,May,5; 2016,Jan,13; 2015,Jan,16;
2014,Nov,5; 2014,Jan,11; 2013,Dec,14; 2012,Oct,14; 2012,Jun,3-9

33236 Removal of permanent epicardial pacemaker and electrodes
by thoracotomy; single lead system, atrial or ventricular

> EXCLUDES Removal of implantable defibrillator electrode(s) by
> thoracotomy (33243)
> Removal of transvenous electrodes by thoracotomy
> (33238)
> Removal of transvenous pacemaker electrodes, single
> or dual lead system; without thoracotomy (33234,
> 33235)

🖛 22.7 ✎ 22.7 **FUD** 090 [C] [80] 🖵

AMA: 2016,Aug,5; 2016,May,5; 2016,Jan,13; 2015,Jan,16;
2014,Nov,5; 2014,Jan,11; 2012,Jun,3-9

33237 dual lead system

> EXCLUDES Removal of implantable defibrillator electrode(s) by
> thoracotomy (33243)
> Removal of transvenous electrodes by thoracotomy
> (33238)
> Removal of transvenous pacemaker electrodes, single
> or dual lead system; without thoracotomy (33234,
> 33235)

🖛 24.4 ✎ 24.4 **FUD** 090 [C] [80] 🖵

AMA: 2016,Aug,5; 2016,May,5; 2016,Jan,13; 2015,Jan,16;
2014,Nov,5; 2014,Jan,11; 2012,Jun,3-9

33238 Removal of permanent transvenous electrode(s) by
thoracotomy

> EXCLUDES Removal of implantable defibrillator electrode(s) by
> thoracotomy (33243)
> Removal of transvenous pacemaker electrodes, single
> or dual lead system; without thoracotomy (33234,
> 33235)

🖛 27.0 ✎ 27.0 **FUD** 090 [C] [80] 🖵

AMA: 2016,Aug,5; 2016,May,5; 2016,Jan,13; 2015,Jan,16;
2014,Nov,5; 2014,Jan,11; 2012,Jun,3-9

▲ **33240** Insertion of implantable defibrillator pulse generator only;
with existing single lead

> EXCLUDES Insertion of electrode (33216-33217, [33271])
> Programming and interrogation of device
> (93260-93261)
> Removal and replacement of implantable defibrillator
> pulse generator ([33262, 33263, 33264])
> Code also placement of epicardial leads by same physician/same
> surgical session as generator insertion (33202-33203)

🖛 10.9 ✎ 10.9 **FUD** 090 [J] [J8] 🖵

AMA: 2016,Aug,5; 2016,Jan,13; 2015,Jan,16; 2014,Nov,5;
2014,Jan,11; 2012,Jun,3-9; 2012,Jan,15-42; 2011,Jan,11

▲ # **33230** with existing dual leads

> EXCLUDES Insertion of a single transvenous electrode, permanent
> pacemaker or implantable defibrillator
> (33216-33217)
> Removal and replacement of implantable defibrillator
> pulse generator ([33262, 33263, 33264])
> Code also placement of epicardial leads by same physician/same
> surgical session as generator insertion (33202-33203)

🖛 11.5 ✎ 11.5 **FUD** 090 [J] [J8]

AMA: 2016,Aug,5; 2016,Jan,13; 2015,Jan,16; 2014,Nov,5;
2014,Jan,11; 2012,Jun,3-9

▲ # **33231** with existing multiple leads

> EXCLUDES Insertion of a single transvenous electrode, permanent
> pacemaker or implantable defibrillator
> (33216-33217)
> Removal and replacement of implantable defibrillator
> pulse generator ([33262, 33263, 33264])
> Code also placement of epicardial leads by same physician/same
> surgical session as generator placement (33202-33203)

🖛 11.9 ✎ 11.9 **FUD** 090 [J] [J8]

AMA: 2016,Aug,5; 2016,Jan,13; 2015,Jan,16; 2014,Nov,5;
2014,Jan,11; 2012,Jun,3-9

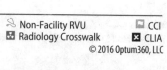

R. atrium — Aorta — L. coronary artery — Right coronary artery — Subclavian vein — Pulse generator (pacemaker) in subcutaneous pocket — Extravascular or vascular electrode leads — Thoracotomy incision — Electrodes on surface of heart

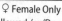 PC/TC Only   [A2-Z3] ASC Payment   [50] Bilateral   ♂ Male Only   ♀ Female Only   🖛 Facility RVU   ✎ Non-Facility RVU   🖵 CCI
FUD Follow-up Days   **CMS:** IOM (Pub 100)   [A]-[Y] OPPSI   [80]/[80] Surg Assist Allowed / w/Doc   🧪 Lab Crosswalk   ☢ Radiology Crosswalk   [X] CLIA

122

CPT © 2016 American Medical Association. All Rights Reserved.

© 2016 Optum360, LLC

▲ **33241** **Removal of implantable defibrillator pulse generator only**

> EXCLUDES *Insertion of implantable defibrillator pulse generator only*
> *Programming and interrogation of device (93260-93261)*
> *Removal and replacement of implantable defibrillator pulse generator ([33262, 33263, 33264])*

Code also electrode removal by thoracotomy (33243)
Code also insertion of subcutaneous defibrillator system and removal of subcutaneous defibrillator lead, when performed ([33270], [33272])
Code also removal of defibrillator leads and insertion of defibrillator system, when performed (33243, 33244, 33249)
Code also transvenous removal of electrode(s) (33244)

🚗 6.61 ⚖ 6.61 **FUD** 090 [Q2] [G2] ▣

AMA: 2016,Aug,5; 2016,Jan,13; 2015,Jan,16; 2014,Nov,5; 2014,Jan,11; 2012,Jun,3-9

▲ # **33262** **Removal of implantable defibrillator pulse generator with replacement of implantable defibrillator pulse generator; single lead system**

> EXCLUDES *Insertion of electrode (33216-33217, [33271])*
> *Programming and interrogation of device (93260-93261)*
> *Removal of implantable defibrillator pulse generator only (33241)*
> *Repair of implantable defibrillator pulse generator and/or leads (33218, 33220)*

Code also electrode(s) removal by thoracotomy (33243)
Code also subcutaneous electrode removal ([33272])
Code also transvenous removal of electrode(s) (33244)

🚗 11.1 ⚖ 11.1 **FUD** 090 [J] [J8] ▣

AMA: 2016,Aug,5; 2016,Jan,13; 2015,Jan,16; 2014,Nov,5; 2014,Jan,11; 2012,Jun,3-9

▲ # **33263** **dual lead system**

> EXCLUDES *Insertion of a single transvenous electrode, permanent pacemaker or implantable defibrillator (33216-33217)*
> *Removal of implantable defibrillator pulse generator only (33241)*
> *Repair of implantable defibrillator pulse generator and/or leads (33218, 33220)*

Code also removal of electrodes by thoracotomy (33243)
Code also subcutaneous electrode removal ([33272])
Code also transvenous removal of electrodes (33244)

🚗 11.6 ⚖ 11.6 **FUD** 090 [J] [J8] ▣

AMA: 2016,Aug,5; 2016,Jan,13; 2015,Jan,16; 2014,Nov,5; 2014,Jan,11; 2013,Dec,16; 2012,Jun,3-9

▲ # **33264** **multiple lead system**

> EXCLUDES *Insertion of a single transvenous electrode, permanent pacemaker or implantable defibrillator (33216-33217)*
> *Removal of implantable defibrillator pulse generator only (33241)*
> *Repair of implantable defibrillator pulse generator and/or leads (33218, 33220)*

Code also removal of electrodes by thoracotomy (33243)
Code also subcutaneous electrode removal ([33272])
Code also transvenous removal of electrodes (33244)

🚗 12.0 ⚖ 12.0 **FUD** 090 [J] [J8] ▣

AMA: 2016,Aug,5; 2016,Jan,13; 2015,Jan,16; 2014,Nov,5; 2014,Jan,11; 2013,Dec,16; 2012,Jun,3-9

33243 **Removal of single or dual chamber implantable defibrillator electrode(s); by thoracotomy**

> EXCLUDES *Transvenous removal of defibrillator electrode(s) (33244)*

Code also removal of defibrillator generator and insertion/replacement of defibrillator system (generator and leads), when performed (33241, 33249)

🚗 39.7 ⚖ 39.7 **FUD** 090 [C] [80] ▣

AMA: 2016,Aug,5; 2016,Jan,13; 2015,Jan,16; 2014,Nov,5; 2014,Jan,11; 2012,Jun,3-9

▲ **33244** **by transvenous extraction**

> EXCLUDES *Thoracotomy to remove electrodes (33238, 33243)*

Code also removal of defibrillator generator and insertion/replacement of defibrillator system (generator and leads), when performed (33241, 33249)

🚗 25.2 ⚖ 25.2 **FUD** 090 [Q2] ▣

AMA: 2016,Aug,5; 2016,Jan,13; 2015,Jan,16; 2014,Nov,5; 2014,Jan,11; 2012,Jun,3-9

▲ **33249** **Insertion or replacement of permanent implantable defibrillator system, with transvenous lead(s), single or dual chamber**

> EXCLUDES *Insertion of a single transvenous electrode, permanent pacemaker or implantable defibrillator (33216-33217)*

Code also removal of defibrillator generator and removal of leads (by thoracotomy or transvenous), when performed (33241, 33243, 33244)
Code also removal of defibrillator generator when upgrading from single to dual-chamber system (33241)

🚗 26.8 ⚖ 26.8 **FUD** 090 [J] [J8] ▣

AMA: 2016,Aug,5; 2016,Jan,13; 2015,Jan,16; 2014,Nov,5; 2014,Jan,11; 2012,Jun,3-9

[33270, 33271, 33272, 33273] Subcutaneous Implantable Defibrillator

> INCLUDES Defibrillation threshold testing (DFT) during subcutaneous defibrillator implant (93640-93641)
> Programming and interrogation of device (93260-93261)

33270 **Insertion or replacement of permanent subcutaneous implantable defibrillator system, with subcutaneous electrode, including defibrillation threshold evaluation, induction of arrhythmia, evaluation of sensing for arrhythmia termination, and programming or reprogramming of sensing or therapeutic parameters, when performed**

> EXCLUDES *Electrophysiologic evaluation of subcutaneous implantable defibrillator (93644)*
> *Insertion of subcutaneous implantable defibrillator electrode ([33271])*

Code also removal of defibrillator generator and subcutaneous electrode, when performed (33241, [33272])

🚗 17.1 ⚖ 17.1 **FUD** 090 [J] [J8] ▣

AMA: 2016,Aug,5; 2016,Jan,13; 2015,Jan,16; 2014,Nov,5

33271 **Insertion of subcutaneous implantable defibrillator electrode**

> EXCLUDES *Insertion of implantable defibrillator pulse generator only (33240)*
> *Insertion or replacement of permanent subcutaneous implantable defibrillator system ([33270])*
> *Removal and replacement of implantable defibrillator pulse generator ([33262])*

🚗 14.4 ⚖ 14.4 **FUD** 090 [J] [J8] ▣

AMA: 2016,Aug,5; 2016,Jan,13; 2015,Jan,16; 2014,Nov,5

33272 **Removal of subcutaneous implantable defibrillator electrode**

Code also removal defibrillator generator and insertion/replacement subcutaneous defibrillator system (generator and leads), when performed (33241, [33270])
Code also removal of defibrillator generator with replacement, when performed ([33262])
Code also removal of defibrillator generator (without replacement), when performed (33241)

🚗 10.1 ⚖ 10.1 **FUD** 090 [Q2] ▣

AMA: 2016,Aug,5; 2016,Jan,13; 2015,Jan,16; 2014,Nov,5

33273 **Repositioning of previously implanted subcutaneous implantable defibrillator electrode**

🚗 11.6 ⚖ 11.6 **FUD** 090 [T] [G2] ▣

AMA: 2016,Aug,5; 2016,Jan,13; 2015,Jan,16; 2014,Nov,5

33250-33251 Surgical Ablation Arrhythmogenic Foci, Supraventricular

INCLUDES Procedures using cryotherapy, laser, microwave, radiofrequency, and ultrasound

33250 Operative ablation of supraventricular arrhythmogenic focus or pathway (eg, Wolff-Parkinson-White, atrioventricular node re-entry), tract(s) and/or focus (foci); without cardiopulmonary bypass

EXCLUDES *Pacing and mapping during surgery by other provider (93631)*

🚑 42.6 ⚕ 42.6 **FUD** 090 C 80 ▢

AMA: 2016,Jan,13; 2015,Jan,16; 2014,Jan,11

33251 with cardiopulmonary bypass

🚑 47.2 ⚕ 47.2 **FUD** 090 C 80 ▢

AMA: 2016,Jan,13; 2015,Jan,16; 2014,Jan,11

33254-33256 Surgical Ablation Arrhythmogenic Foci, Atrial (e.g., Maze)

INCLUDES Excision or isolation of the left atrial appendage
Procedures using cryotherapy, laser, microwave, radiofrequency, and ultrasound

EXCLUDES *Any procedure involving median sternotomy or cardiopulmonary bypass*
Aortic valve procedures (33390-33391, 33404-33415)
Aortoplasty (33417)
Ascending aorta graft, with cardiopulmonary bypass (33860-33864)
Coronary artery bypass (33510-33516, 33517-33523, 33533-33536)
Excision of intracardiac tumor, resection with cardiopulmonary bypass (33120)
Insertion or replacement of temporary transvenous single chamber cardiac electrode or pacemaker catheter (separate procedure) (33210-33211)
Mitral valve procedures (33418-33430)
Outflow tract augmentation (33478)
Prosthetic valve repair (33496)
Pulmonary artery embolectomy; with cardiopulmonary bypass (33910-33920)
Pulmonary valve procedures (33470-33476)
Repair aberrant coronary artery anatomy (33500-33507)
Repair aberrant heart anatomy (33600-33853)
Resection of external cardiac tumor (33130)
Temporary pacemaker (33210-33211)
Thoracotomy; with exploration (32100)
Transcatheter pulmonary valve implantation (33477)
Tricuspid valve procedures (33460-33468)
Tube thoracostomy, includes connection to drainage system (32551)
Ventricular reconstruction (33542-33548)
Ventriculomyotomy (33416)

33254 Operative tissue ablation and reconstruction of atria, limited (eg, modified maze procedure)

🚑 39.8 ⚕ 39.8 **FUD** 090 C 80 ▢

AMA: 2016,Jan,13; 2015,Jan,16; 2014,Jan,11

33255 Operative tissue ablation and reconstruction of atria, extensive (eg, maze procedure); without cardiopulmonary bypass

🚑 47.0 ⚕ 47.0 **FUD** 090 C 80 ▢

AMA: 2016,Jan,13; 2015,Jan,16; 2014,Jan,11

33256 with cardiopulmonary bypass

🚑 56.8 ⚕ 56.8 **FUD** 090 C 80 ▢

AMA: 2016,Jan,13; 2015,Jan,16; 2014,Jan,11

33257-33259 Surgical Ablation Arrhythmogenic Foci, Atrial, with Other Heart Procedure(s)

EXCLUDES *Endoscopy, surgical; operative tissue ablation and reconstruction of atria, limited (33265-33266)*
Operative tissue ablation and reconstruction of atria, limited (33254-33256)
Temporary pacemaker (33210-33211)
Tube thoracostomy, includes connection to drainage system (32551)

+ 33257 Operative tissue ablation and reconstruction of atria, performed at the time of other cardiac procedure(s), limited (eg, modified maze procedure) (List separately in addition to code for primary procedure)

🚑 16.9 ⚕ 16.9 **FUD** ZZZ C 80 ▢

Code first (33120-33130, 33250-33251, 33261, 33300-33335, 33390-33391, 33404-33496, 33500-33507, 33510-33516, 33533-33548, 33600-33619, 33641-33697, 33702-33732, 33735-33767, 33770-33814, 33840-33877, 33910-33922, 33925-33926, 33935, 33945, 33975-33980)

+ 33258 Operative tissue ablation and reconstruction of atria, performed at the time of other cardiac procedure(s), extensive (eg, maze procedure), without cardiopulmonary bypass (List separately in addition to code for primary procedure)

🚑 18.9 ⚕ 18.9 **FUD** ZZZ C 80 ▢

Code first, if performed without cardiopulmonary bypass (33130, 33250, 33300, 33310, 33320-33321, 33330, 33390-33391, 33414-33417, 33420, 33470-33471, 33501-33503, 33510-33516, 33533-33536, 33690, 33735, 33737, 33800-33813, 33840-33852, 33915, 33925)

+ 33259 Operative tissue ablation and reconstruction of atria, performed at the time of other cardiac procedure(s), extensive (eg, maze procedure), with cardiopulmonary bypass (List separately in addition to code for primary procedure)

🚑 24.5 ⚕ 24.5 **FUD** ZZZ C 80 ▢

Code first, if performed with cardiopulmonary bypass (33120, 33251, 33261, 33305, 33315, 33322, 33335, 33390-33391, 33404-33413, 33422-33468, 33474-33478, 33496, 33500, 33504-33507, 33510-33516, 33533-33548, 33600-33688, 33692-33722, 33730, 33732, 33736, 33750-33767, 33770-33781, 33786-33788, 33814, 33853, 33860-33877, 33910, 33916-33922, 33926, 33935, 33945, 33975-33980)

33261-33264 Surgical Ablation Arrhythmogenic Foci, Ventricular

33261 Operative ablation of ventricular arrhythmogenic focus with cardiopulmonary bypass

🚑 47.6 ⚕ 47.6 **FUD** 090 C 80 ▢

AMA: 2016,Jan,13; 2015,Jan,16; 2014,Jan,11

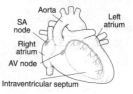

Impulse centers that are causing arrhythmia are treated with ablation

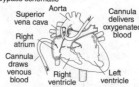

33262 Resequenced code. See code following 33241.

33263 Resequenced code. See code following 33241.

33264 Resequenced code. See code before 33243.

33265-33273 Surgical Ablation Arrhythmogenic Foci, Endoscopic

EXCLUDES *Insertion or replacement of temporary transvenous single chamber cardiac electrode or pacemaker catheter (separate procedure) (33210-33211)*
Tube thoracostomy, includes connection to drainage system (32551)

33265 Endoscopy, surgical; operative tissue ablation and reconstruction of atria, limited (eg, modified maze procedure), without cardiopulmonary bypass

🚑 39.5 ⚕ 39.5 **FUD** 090 C 80 ▢

AMA: 2016,Jan,13; 2015,Jan,16; 2014,Jan,11

33266 operative tissue ablation and reconstruction of atria, extensive (eg, maze procedure), without cardiopulmonary bypass

🚑 53.7 ⚕ 53.7 **FUD** 090 C 80 ▢

AMA: 2016,Jan,13; 2015,Jan,16; 2014,Jan,11

33270 Resequenced code. See code following 33249.

33271 Resequenced code. See code following 33249.

33272 Resequenced code. See code following 33249.

33273 Resequenced code. See code following 33249.

33282-33284 Implantable Loop Recorder

▲ **33282** **Implantation of patient-activated cardiac event recorder**

INCLUDES Initial programming of device

EXCLUDES *Subsequent electronic analysis and/or reprogramming of device (93285, 93291, 93298-93299)*

🚑 6.91 ⚖ 6.91 **FUD** 090 [J] [J8] 🔲

AMA: 2016,Jan,13; 2015,Jan,16; 2014,Jan,11; 2012,Jan,15-42; 2011,Jan,11

▲ **33284** **Removal of an implantable, patient-activated cardiac event recorder**

🚑 6.11 ⚖ 6.11 **FUD** 090 [02] [62] 🔲

AMA: 2016,Jan,13; 2015,Jan,16; 2014,Jan,11

33300-33315 Procedures for Injury of the Heart

INCLUDES Procedures with and without cardiopulmonary bypass

EXCLUDES *Cardiac assist services (33946-33949, 33967-33983, 33990-33993)*

33300 **Repair of cardiac wound; without bypass**

🚑 71.3 ⚖ 71.3 **FUD** 090 [C] [80] 🔲

AMA: 1997,Nov,1

33305 **with cardiopulmonary bypass**

🚑 119. ⚖ 119. **FUD** 090 [C] [80] 🔲

AMA: 1997,Nov,1

33310 **Cardiotomy, exploratory (includes removal of foreign body, atrial or ventricular thrombus); without bypass**

EXCLUDES *Other cardiac procedures unless separate incision into heart is necessary in order to remove thrombus*

🚑 34.1 ⚖ 34.1 **FUD** 090 [C] [80] 🔲

AMA: 1997,Nov,1

33315 **with cardiopulmonary bypass**

EXCLUDES *Other cardiac procedures unless separate incision into heart is necessary in order to remove thrombus*

Code also excision of thrombus with cardiopulmonary bypass and append modifier 59 if separate incision is required with (33120, 33130, 33420-33430, 33460-33468, 33496, 33542, 33545, 33641-33647, 33670, 33681, 33975-33980)

🚑 55.6 ⚖ 55.6 **FUD** 090 [C] [80] 🔲

AMA: 2016,Jan,13; 2015,Jan,16; 2014,Jan,11; 2012,Jan,15-42; 2011,Jan,11

33320-33335 Procedures for Injury of the Aorta/Great Vessels

33320 **Suture repair of aorta or great vessels; without shunt or cardiopulmonary bypass**

🚑 30.9 ⚖ 30.9 **FUD** 090 [C] [80] 🔲

AMA: 2016,Jan,13; 2015,Jan,16; 2014,Jan,11

33321 **with shunt bypass**

🚑 35.7 ⚖ 35.7 **FUD** 090 [C] [80] 🔲

AMA: 1997,Nov,1; 1994,Win,1

33322 **with cardiopulmonary bypass**

🚑 40.4 ⚖ 40.4 **FUD** 090 [C] [80] 🔲

AMA: 2016,Jan,13; 2015,Jan,16; 2014,Jan,11

33330 **Insertion of graft, aorta or great vessels; without shunt, or cardiopulmonary bypass**

🚑 41.4 ⚖ 41.4 **FUD** 090 [C] [80] 🔲

AMA: 1997,Nov,1; 1994,Win,1

33335 **with cardiopulmonary bypass**

🚑 54.4 ⚖ 54.4 **FUD** 090 [C] [80] 🔲

AMA: 1997,Nov,1

33340 Closure Left Atrial Appendage

EXCLUDES *Cardiac catheterization except for reasons other than closure left atrial appendage (93451-93453, 93456, 93458-93461, 93462, 93530-93533)*

● **33340** **Percutaneous transcatheter closure of the left atrial appendage with endocardial implant, including fluoroscopy, transseptal puncture, catheter placement(s), left atrial angiography, left atrial appendage angiography, when performed, and radiological supervision and interpretation**

33361-33369 Transcatheter Aortic Valve Replacement

CMS: 100-03,20.32 Transcatheter Aortic Valve Replacement (TAVR); 100-04,32,290.1.1 Coding Requirements for TAVR Services; 100-04,32,290.2 Claims Processing for TAVR/ Professional Claims; 100-04,32,290.3 Claims Processing TAVR Inpatient; 100-04,32,290.4 Payment of TAVR for MA Plan Participants

INCLUDES Access and implantation of the aortic valve (33361-33366)
Access sheath placement
Advancement of valve delivery system
Arteriotomy closure
Balloon aortic valvuloplasty
Cardiac or open arterial approach
Deployment of valve
Percutaneous access
Temporary pacemaker
Valve repositioning when necessary
Radiology procedures:
Angiography during and after procedure
Assessment of access site for closure
Documentation of completion of the intervention
Guidance for valve placement
Supervision and interpretation

EXCLUDES *Cardiac catheterization procedures included in the TAVR/TAVI service (93452-93453, 93458-93461, 93567)*
Percutaneous coronary interventional procedures
Transvascular ventricular support (33967, 33970, 33973, 33975-33976, 33990-33993, 33999)

Code also cardiac catheterization services for purposes other than TAVR/TAVI

Code also diagnostic coronary angiography at a different session from the interventional procedure

Code also diagnostic coronary angiography at the same time as TAVR/TAVI when:
A previous study is available, but documentation states the patient's condition has changed since the previous study, visualization of the anatomy/pathology is inadequate, or a change occurs during the procedure warranting additional evaluation of an area outside the current target area
No previous catheter-based coronary angiography study is available, and a full diagnostic study is performed, with the decision to perform the intervention based on that study

Code also modifier 59 when diagnostic coronary angiography procedures are performed as separate and distinct procedural services on the same day or session as TAVR/TAVI

Code also modifier 62 as all TAVI/TAVR procedures require the work of two physicians

33361 **Transcatheter aortic valve replacement (TAVR/TAVI) with prosthetic valve; percutaneous femoral artery approach**

Code also cardiopulmonary bypass when performed (33367-33369)

🚑 39.5 ⚖ 39.5 **FUD** 000 [C] [80] 🔲

AMA: 2016,Jan,13; 2015,Mar,9; 2015,Jan,16; 2014,Jul,8; 2014,Jan,11; 2014,Jan,5; 2013,Jan,6-8

33362 **open femoral artery approach**

Code also cardiopulmonary bypass when performed (33367-33369)

🚑 43.2 ⚖ 43.2 **FUD** 000 [C] [80] 🔲

AMA: 2016,Jan,13; 2015,Mar,9; 2015,Jan,16; 2014,Jul,8; 2014,Jan,11; 2014,Jan,5; 2013,Jan,6-8

33363 **open axillary artery approach**

Code also cardiopulmonary bypass when performed (33367-33369)

🚑 44.9 ⚖ 44.9 **FUD** 000 [C] [80] 🔲

AMA: 2016,Jan,13; 2015,Mar,9; 2015,Jan,16; 2014,Jul,8; 2014,Jan,11; 2014,Jan,5; 2013,Jan,6-8

33364 **open iliac artery approach**

Code also cardiopulmonary bypass when performed (33367-33369)

🚑 47.0 ⚖ 47.0 **FUD** 000 [C] [80] 🔲

AMA: 2016,Jan,13; 2015,Mar,9; 2015,Jan,16; 2014,Jul,8; 2014,Jan,11; 2014,Jan,5; 2013,Jan,6-8

33365 **transaortic approach (eg, median sternotomy, mediastinotomy)**

Code also cardiopulmonary bypass when performed (33367-33369)

🚑 51.8 ⚖ 51.8 **FUD** 000 [C] [80] 🔲

AMA: 2016,Jan,13; 2015,Mar,9; 2015,Jan,16; 2014,Jul,8; 2014,Jan,11; 2014,Jan,5; 2013,Jan,6-8

33366 transapical exposure (eg, left thoracotomy)

Code also cardiopulmonary bypass when performed (33367-33369)

⏢ 56.1 ⚕ 56.1 **FUD** 000 [C] [80] [⬜]

AMA: 2016,Jan,13; 2015,Mar,9; 2015,Jan,16; 2014,Jul,8; 2014,Jan,5

+ 33367 cardiopulmonary bypass support with percutaneous peripheral arterial and venous cannulation (eg, femoral vessels) (List separately in addition to code for primary procedure)

EXCLUDES *Cardiopulmonary bypass support with open or central arterial and venous cannulation (33368-33369)*

Code first (33361-33366, 33418, 33477)

⏢ 18.2 ⚕ 18.2 **FUD** ZZZ [C] [80] [⬜]

AMA: 2016,Mar,5; 2016,Jan,13; 2015,Sep,3; 2015,Jan,16; 2013,Jan,6-8

+ 33368 cardiopulmonary bypass support with open peripheral arterial and venous cannulation (eg, femoral, iliac, axillary vessels) (List separately in addition to code for primary procedure)

EXCLUDES *Cardiopulmonary bypass support with percutaneous or central arterial and venous cannulation (33367, 33369)*

Code first (33361-33366, 33418, 33477)

⏢ 21.7 ⚕ 21.7 **FUD** ZZZ [C] [80] [⬜]

AMA: 2016,Mar,5; 2016,Jan,13; 2015,Sep,3; 2015,Jan,16; 2013,Jan,6-8

+ 33369 cardiopulmonary bypass support with central arterial and venous cannulation (eg, aorta, right atrium, pulmonary artery) (List separately in addition to code for primary procedure)

EXCLUDES *Cardiopulmonary bypass support with percutaneous or open arterial and venous cannulation (33367-33368)*

Code first (33361-33366, 33418, 33477)

⏢ 28.8 ⚕ 28.8 **FUD** ZZZ [C] [80] [⬜]

AMA: 2016,Mar,5; 2016,Jan,13; 2015,Sep,3; 2015,Jan,16; 2013,Jan,6-8

33390-33415 Aortic Valve Procedures

● **33390** Valvuloplasty, aortic valve, open, with cardiopulmonary bypass; simple (ie, valvotomy, debridement, debulking, and/or simple commissural resuspension)

● **33391** complex (eg, leaflet extension, leaflet resection, leaflet reconstruction, or annuloplasty)

INCLUDES Simple aortic valvuloplasty (33390)

~~33400~~ ~~Valvuloplasty, aortic valve; open, with cardiopulmonary bypass~~

To report, see ~33990-33991

~~33401~~ ~~open, with inflow occlusion~~

To report, see ~33390-33391

~~33403~~ ~~using transventricular dilation, with cardiopulmonary bypass~~

To report, see ~33390-33391

33404 Construction of apical-aortic conduit

⏢ 51.2 ⚕ 51.2 **FUD** 090 [C] [80] [⬜]

AMA: 2016,Jan,13; 2015,Jan,16; 2014,Jan,11; 2012,Jan,15-42; 2011,Jan,11

▲ **33405** Replacement, aortic valve, open, with cardiopulmonary bypass; with prosthetic valve other than homograft or stentless valve

⏢ 66.0 ⚕ 66.0 **FUD** 090 [C] [80] [⬜]

AMA: 2016,Jan,13; 2015,Jan,16; 2014,Jan,11; 2013,Jan,6-8; 2011,Aug,3-5

▲ **33406** with allograft valve (freehand)

⏢ 83.7 ⚕ 83.7 **FUD** 090 [C] [80] [⬜]

AMA: 2016,Jan,13; 2015,Jan,16; 2014,Jan,11; 2011,Aug,3-5

▲ **33410** with stentless tissue valve

⏢ 73.7 ⚕ 73.7 **FUD** 090 [C] [80] [⬜]

AMA: 2016,Jan,13; 2015,Jan,16; 2014,Jan,11; 2011,Aug,3-5

33411 Replacement, aortic valve; with aortic annulus enlargement, noncoronary sinus

⏢ 97.7 ⚕ 97.7 **FUD** 090 [C] [80] [⬜]

AMA: 2016,Jan,13; 2015,Jan,16; 2014,Jan,11; 2012,Jan,15-42; 2011,Aug,3-5

Replacement valve ⟶ 19 mm

The aortic valve is replaced

Tricuspid valve · Noncoronary leaflet · Mitral valve · Incision line to widen annulus · R. coronary artery · Incision · Valve annulus · Aortic valve (replaced) · Pulmonary valve · L. coronary artery

Overhead schematic of major heart valves

33412 with transventricular aortic annulus enlargement (Konno procedure)

⏢ 92.4 ⚕ 92.4 **FUD** 090 [C] [80] [⬜]

AMA: 2016,Jan,13; 2015,Jan,16; 2014,Jan,11; 2011,Aug,3-5

33413 by translocation of autologous pulmonary valve with allograft replacement of pulmonary valve (Ross procedure)

⏢ 94.7 ⚕ 94.7 **FUD** 090 [C] [80] [⬜]

AMA: 2016,Jan,13; 2015,Jan,16; 2014,Jan,11; 2011,Aug,3-5

33414 Repair of left ventricular outflow tract obstruction by patch enlargement of the outflow tract

⏢ 62.9 ⚕ 62.9 **FUD** 090 [C] [80] [⬜]

AMA: 2016,Jan,13; 2015,Jan,16; 2014,Jan,11

33415 Resection or incision of subvalvular tissue for discrete subvalvular aortic stenosis

⏢ 58.9 ⚕ 58.9 **FUD** 090 [C] [80] [⬜]

AMA: 2016,Jan,13; 2015,Jan,16; 2014,Jan,11

33416 Ventriculectomy

CMS: 100-03,20.26 Partial Ventriculectomy

EXCLUDES *Percutaneous transcatheter septal reduction therapy (93583)*

33416 Ventriculomyotomy (-myectomy) for idiopathic hypertrophic subaortic stenosis (eg, asymmetric septal hypertrophy)

⏢ 59.1 ⚕ 59.1 **FUD** 090 [C] [80] [⬜]

AMA: 2016,Jan,13; 2015,Jan,16; 2014,Jan,11

33417 Repair of Supravalvular Stenosis by Aortoplasty

33417 Aortoplasty (gusset) for supravalvular stenosis

⏢ 48.7 ⚕ 48.7 **FUD** 090 [C] [80] [⬜]

AMA: 2016,Jan,13; 2015,Jan,16; 2014,Jan,11

33418-33419 Transcatheter Mitral Valve Procedures

INCLUDES Access sheath placement
Advancement of valve delivery system
Deployment of valve
Radiology procedures:
  Angiography during and after procedure
  Documentation of completion of the intervention
  Guidance for valve placement
  Supervision and interpretation
Valve repositioning when necessary

EXCLUDES *Cardiac catheterization services for purposes other than TMVR*
Diagnostic angiography at different session from interventional procedure
Percutaneous coronary interventional procedures

Code also cardiopulmonary bypass:
  Central (33369)
  Open peripheral (33368)
  Percutaneous peripheral (33367)
Code also diagnostic coronary angiography and cardiac catheterization procedures
  when:
  No previous study available and full diagnostic study performed
  Previous study inadequate or patient's clinical indication for the study changed
    prior to or during the procedure
  Use modifier 59 with cardiac catheterization procedures when on same day or
    same session as TMVR
Code also transvascular ventricular support:
  Balloon pump (33967, 33970, 33973)
  Ventricular assist device (33990-33993)

33418 **Transcatheter mitral valve repair, percutaneous approach, including transseptal puncture when performed; initial prosthesis**

Code also left heart catheterization when performed by
  transapical puncture (93462)
🚗 52.2   ⚕ 52.2   **FUD** 090   C 80 ▭

AMA: 2016,Jan,13; 2015,Sep,3

+ **33419** **additional prosthesis(es) during same session (List separately in addition to code for primary procedure)**

EXCLUDES *Percutaneous approach through the coronary sinus for TMVR (0345T)*
Procedures performed more than one time per session

Code first (33418)
🚗 12.3   ⚕ 12.3   **FUD** ZZZ   N N1 80 ▭

AMA: 2016,Jan,13; 2015,Sep,3

33420-33430 Mitral Valve Procedures

Code also removal of thrombus through a separate heart incision, when performed
  (33310-33315); append modifier 59 to (33315)

33420 **Valvotomy, mitral valve; closed heart**
🚗 42.4   ⚕ 42.4   **FUD** 090   C ▭
AMA: 2016,Jan,13; 2015,Sep,3; 2015,Jan,16; 2014,Jan,11

33422 **open heart, with cardiopulmonary bypass**
🚗 48.6   ⚕ 48.6   **FUD** 090   C 80 ▭
AMA: 2016,Jan,13; 2015,Sep,3; 2015,Jan,16; 2014,Jan,11

33425 **Valvuloplasty, mitral valve, with cardiopulmonary bypass;**
🚗 79.5   ⚕ 79.5   **FUD** 090   C 80 ▭
AMA: 2016,Jan,13; 2015,Sep,3; 2015,Jan,16; 2014,Jan,11;
2012,Jan,15-42; 2011,Jan,11

33426 **with prosthetic ring**
🚗 69.3   ⚕ 69.3   **FUD** 090   C 80 ▭
AMA: 2016,Jan,13; 2015,Sep,3; 2015,Jan,16; 2014,Jan,11

33427 **radical reconstruction, with or without ring**
🚗 71.1   ⚕ 71.1   **FUD** 090   C 80 ▭
AMA: 2016,Jan,13; 2015,Sep,3; 2015,Jan,16; 2014,Jan,11

33430 **Replacement, mitral valve, with cardiopulmonary bypass**
🚗 81.4   ⚕ 81.4   **FUD** 090   C 80 ▭
AMA: 2016,Jan,13; 2015,Sep,3; 2015,Jan,16; 2014,Jan,11

33460-33468 Tricuspid Valve Procedures

Code also removal of thrombus through a separate heart incision, when performed
  (33310-33315); append modifier 59 to (33315)

33460 **Valvectomy, tricuspid valve, with cardiopulmonary bypass**
🚗 71.0   ⚕ 71.0   **FUD** 090   C 80 ▭
AMA: 2016,Jan,13; 2015,Jan,16; 2014,Jan,11

33463 **Valvuloplasty, tricuspid valve; without ring insertion**
🚗 89.9   ⚕ 89.9   **FUD** 090   C 80 ▭
AMA: 2016,Jan,13; 2015,Jan,16; 2014,Jan,11

33464 **with ring insertion**
🚗 71.0   ⚕ 71.0   **FUD** 090   C 80 ▭
AMA: 2016,Jan,13; 2015,Jan,16; 2014,Jan,11

33465 **Replacement, tricuspid valve, with cardiopulmonary bypass**
🚗 80.2   ⚕ 80.2   **FUD** 090   C 80 ▭
AMA: 2016,Jan,13; 2015,Jan,16; 2014,Jan,11

33468 **Tricuspid valve repositioning and plication for Ebstein anomaly**
🚗 71.8   ⚕ 71.8   **FUD** 090   C 80 ▭
AMA: 2016,Jan,13; 2015,Jan,16; 2014,Jan,11

33470-33474 Pulmonary Valvotomy

INCLUDES Brock's operation
Code also the concurrent ligation/takedown of a systemic-to-pulmonary artery shunt
  (33924)

33470 **Valvotomy, pulmonary valve, closed heart; transventricular**
🚗 37.7   ⚕ 37.7   **FUD** 090   63 C 80 ▭
AMA: 2016,Jan,13; 2015,Jan,16; 2014,Jan,11

33471 **via pulmonary artery**
EXCLUDES *Percutaneous valvuloplasty of pulmonary valve (92990)*
🚗 40.3   ⚕ 40.3   **FUD** 090   C 80 ▭
AMA: 2016,Jan,13; 2015,Jan,16; 2014,Jan,11

33474 **Valvotomy, pulmonary valve, open heart, with cardiopulmonary bypass**
🚗 63.7   ⚕ 63.7   **FUD** 090   C 80 ▭
AMA: 2007,Mar,1-3; 2005,Feb,13-16

33475-33476 Other Procedures Pulmonary Valve

Code also the concurrent ligation/takedown of a systemic-to-pulmonary artery shunt
  (33924)

33475 **Replacement, pulmonary valve**
🚗 67.8   ⚕ 67.8   **FUD** 090   C 80 ▭
AMA: 2016,Jan,13; 2015,Jan,16; 2014,Jan,11

33476 **Right ventricular resection for infundibular stenosis, with or without commissurotomy**
INCLUDES Brock's operation
🚗 44.5   ⚕ 44.5   **FUD** 090   C 80 ▭
AMA: 2016,Jan,13; 2015,Jan,16; 2014,Jan,11

33477 Transcatheter Pulmonary Valve Implantation

INCLUDES Cardiac catheterization, contrast injection, angiography, fluoroscopic
  guidance and the supervision and interpretation for device placement
Percutaneous balloon angioplasty within the treatment area
Valvulopasty or stent insertion in pulmonary valve conduit (37236-37237,
  92997-92998)
Pre-, intra-, and post-operative hemodynamic measurements

EXCLUDES *Balloon pump insertion (33967, 33970, 33973)*
Cardiopulmonary bypass performed in the same session (33367-33369)
Extracorporeal membrane oxygenation (ECMO) (33946-33959 [33962, 33963,
  33964, 33965, 33966, 33969, 33984, 33985, 33986, 33987, 33988, 33989])
Fluoroscopy (76000-76001)
Injection procedure during cardiac catheterization (93563, 93566-93568)
Percutaneous cardiac intervention procedures, when performed
Procedures performed more than one time per session
Right heart catheterization (93451, 93453-93461, 93530-93533)
Ventricular assist device (VAD) (33990-33993)

Code also the concurrent ligation/takedown of a systemic-to-pulmonary artery shunt
  (33924)

33477 **Transcatheter pulmonary valve implantation, percutaneous approach, including pre-stenting of the valve delivery site, when performed**
🚗 37.5   ⚕ 37.5   **FUD** 000   C 80 ▭
AMA: 2016,Aug,9; 2016,Mar,5

33478 Outflow Tract Augmentation

Code also for cavopulmonary anastamosis to a second superior vena cava (33768)
Code also the concurrent ligation/takedown of a systemic-to-pulmonary artery shunt
  (33924)

33478 **Outflow tract augmentation (gusset), with or without commissurotomy or infundibular resection**
🚗 46.0   ⚕ 46.0   **FUD** 090   C 80 ▭
AMA: 2016,Jan,13; 2015,Jan,16; 2014,Jan,11

33496 Prosthetic Valve Repair

Code also removal of thrombus through a separate heart incision, when performed (33310-33315); append modifier 59 to (33315)
Code also reoperation if performed (33530)

33496 **Repair of non-structural prosthetic valve dysfunction with cardiopulmonary bypass (separate procedure)**
⚙ 48.6 ⚖ 48.6 **FUD** 090 C 80 ▣
AMA: 2016,Jan,13; 2015,Jan,16; 2014,Jan,11

33500-33507 Repair Aberrant Coronary Artery Anatomy

INCLUDES Angioplasty and/or endarterectomy

33500 **Repair of coronary arteriovenous or arteriocardiac chamber fistula; with cardiopulmonary bypass**
⚙ 45.5 ⚖ 45.5 **FUD** 090 C 80 ▣
AMA: 2007,Mar,1-3; 1997,Nov,1

33501 **without cardiopulmonary bypass**
⚙ 32.9 ⚖ 32.9 **FUD** 090 C 80 ▣
AMA: 2007,Mar,1-3; 1997,Nov,1

33502 **Repair of anomalous coronary artery from pulmonary artery origin; by ligation**
⚙ 37.3 ⚖ 37.3 **FUD** 090 63 C 80 ▣
AMA: 2007,Mar,1-3; 1997,Nov,1

33503 **by graft, without cardiopulmonary bypass**
⚙ 38.8 ⚖ 38.8 **FUD** 090 63 C 80 ▣
AMA: 2007,Mar,1-3; 1997,Nov,1

33504 **by graft, with cardiopulmonary bypass**
⚙ 42.8 ⚖ 42.8 **FUD** 090 C 80 ▣
AMA: 2007,Mar,1-3; 1997,Nov,1

33505 **with construction of intrapulmonary artery tunnel (Takeuchi procedure)**
⚙ 60.4 ⚖ 60.4 **FUD** 090 63 C 80 ▣
AMA: 2007,Mar,1-3; 1997,Nov,1

33506 **by translocation from pulmonary artery to aorta**
⚙ 60.2 ⚖ 60.2 **FUD** 090 63 C 80 ▣
AMA: 2007,Mar,1-3; 1997,Nov,1

33507 **Repair of anomalous (eg, intramural) aortic origin of coronary artery by unroofing or translocation**
⚙ 50.5 ⚖ 50.5 **FUD** 090 C 80 ▣
AMA: 2016,Jan,13; 2015,Jan,16; 2014,Jan,11

33508 Endoscopic Harvesting of Venous Graft

INCLUDES Diagnostic endoscopy
EXCLUDES Harvesting of vein of upper extremity (35500)
Code first (33510-33523)

+ **33508** **Endoscopy, surgical, including video-assisted harvest of vein(s) for coronary artery bypass procedure (List separately in addition to code for primary procedure)**
⚙ 0.47 ⚖ 0.47 **FUD** ZZZ N N1 80 ▣
AMA: 1997,Nov,1

33510-33516 Coronary Artery Bypass: Venous Grafts

INCLUDES Obtaining saphenous vein grafts
Venous bypass grafting only
EXCLUDES Arterial bypass (33533-33536)
Combined arterial-venous bypass (33517-33523, 33533-33536)
Obtaining vein graft:
Femoropopliteal vein (35572)
Upper extremity vein (35500)
Percutaneous ventricular assist devices (33990-33993)
Code also modifier 80 when assistant at surgery obtains grafts

33510 **Coronary artery bypass, vein only; single coronary venous graft**
⚙ 56.2 ⚖ 56.2 **FUD** 090 C 80 ▣
AMA: 2016,Jan,13; 2015,Jan,16; 2014,Aug,14; 2014,Jan,11; 2012,Apr,3-9; 2012,Jan,15-42; 2011,Jan,11

33511 **2 coronary venous grafts**
⚙ 61.8 ⚖ 61.8 **FUD** 090 C 80 ▣
AMA: 2016,Jan,13; 2015,Jan,16; 2014,Aug,14; 2014,Jan,11; 2012,Apr,3-9

33512 **3 coronary venous grafts**
⚙ 70.2 ⚖ 70.2 **FUD** 090 C 80 ▣
AMA: 2016,Jan,13; 2015,Jan,16; 2014,Aug,14; 2014,Jan,11; 2012,Apr,3-9

33513 **4 coronary venous grafts**
⚙ 72.2 ⚖ 72.2 **FUD** 090 C 80 ▣
AMA: 2016,Jan,13; 2015,Jan,16; 2014,Aug,14; 2014,Jan,11; 2012,Apr,3-9

33514 **5 coronary venous grafts**
⚙ 76.0 ⚖ 76.0 **FUD** 090 C 80 ▣
AMA: 2016,Jan,13; 2015,Jan,16; 2014,Aug,14; 2014,Jan,11; 2012,Apr,3-9

33516 **6 or more coronary venous grafts**
⚙ 79.4 ⚖ 79.4 **FUD** 090 C 80 ▣
AMA: 2016,Jan,13; 2015,Jan,16; 2014,Aug,14; 2014,Jan,11; 2012,Apr,3-9

33517-33523 Coronary Artery Bypass: Venous AND Arterial Grafts

INCLUDES Obtaining saphenous vein grafts
EXCLUDES Obtaining arterial graft:
Upper extremity (35600)
Obtaining vein graft:
Femoropopliteal vein graft (35572)
Upper extremity (35500)
Percutaneous ventricular assist devices (33990-33993)
Code also modifier 80 when assistant at surgery obtains grafts
Code first (33533-33536)

+ **33517** **Coronary artery bypass, using venous graft(s) and arterial graft(s); single vein graft (List separately in addition to code for primary procedure)**
⚙ 5.46 ⚖ 5.46 **FUD** ZZZ C 80 ▣
AMA: 2016,Jan,13; 2015,Jan,16; 2014,Jan,11; 2012,Apr,3-9

+ **33518** **2 venous grafts (List separately in addition to code for primary procedure)**
⚙ 12.0 ⚖ 12.0 **FUD** ZZZ C 80 ▣
AMA: 2016,Jan,13; 2015,Jan,16; 2014,Jan,11; 2012,Apr,3-9

+ **33519** **3 venous grafts (List separately in addition to code for primary procedure)**
⚙ 15.8 ⚖ 15.8 **FUD** ZZZ C 80 ▣
AMA: 2016,Jan,13; 2015,Jan,16; 2014,Jan,11; 2012,Apr,3-9

+ **33521** **4 venous grafts (List separately in addition to code for primary procedure)**
⚙ 19.0 ⚖ 19.0 **FUD** ZZZ C 80 ▣
AMA: 2016,Jan,13; 2015,Jan,16; 2014,Jan,11; 2012,Apr,3-9

+ **33522** **5 venous grafts (List separately in addition to code for primary procedure)**
⚙ 21.3 ⚖ 21.3 **FUD** ZZZ C 80 ▣
AMA: 2016,Jan,13; 2015,Jan,16; 2014,Jan,11; 2012,Apr,3-9

+ **33523** **6 or more venous grafts (List separately in addition to code for primary procedure)**
⚙ 24.2 ⚖ 24.2 **FUD** ZZZ C 80 ▣
AMA: 2016,Jan,13; 2015,Jan,16; 2014,Jan,11; 2012,Apr,3-9

33530 Reoperative Coronary Artery Bypass Graft or Valve Procedure

EXCLUDES *Percutaneous ventricular assist devices (33990-33993)*
Code first (33390-33391, 33400-33496, 33510-33536, 33863)

+ **33530** **Reoperation, coronary artery bypass procedure or valve procedure, more than 1 month after original operation (List separately in addition to code for primary procedure)**
15.3   15.3   **FUD** ZZZ   C 80
AMA: 2016,Jan,13; 2015,Jan,16; 2014,Jan,11; 2012,Apr,3-9; 2012,Jan,15-42; 2011,Feb,8-9; 2011,Jan,11

33533-33536 Coronary Artery Bypass: Arterial Grafts

INCLUDES Obtaining arterial graft (eg, epigastric, internal mammary, gastroepiploic and others)
EXCLUDES *Obtaining arterial graft:*
Upper extremity (35600)
Obtaining venous graft:
Femoropopliteal vein (35572)
Upper extremity (35500)
Percutaneous ventricular assist devices (33990-33993)
Venous bypass (33510-33516)
Code also (33517-33523)
Code also modifier 80 when assistant at surgery obtains grafts

33533 **Coronary artery bypass, using arterial graft(s); single arterial graft**
54.3   54.3   **FUD** 090   C 80
AMA: 2016,Jan,13; 2015,Jan,16; 2014,Nov,14; 2014,Jan,11; 2012,Apr,3-9

33534 **2 coronary arterial grafts**
63.9   63.9   **FUD** 090   C 80
AMA: 2016,Jan,13; 2015,Jan,16; 2014,Jan,11; 2012,Apr,3-9

33535 **3 coronary arterial grafts**
71.3   71.3   **FUD** 090   C 80
AMA: 2016,Jan,13; 2015,Jan,16; 2014,Jan,11; 2012,Apr,3-9

33536 **4 or more coronary arterial grafts**
76.9   76.9   **FUD** 090   C 80
AMA: 2016,Jan,13; 2015,Jan,16; 2014,Nov,14; 2014,Jan,11; 2012,Apr,3-9

33542-33548 Ventricular Reconstruction

33542 **Myocardial resection (eg, ventricular aneurysmectomy)**
Code also removal of thrombus through a separate heart incision, when performed (33310-33315); append modifier 59 to (33315)
76.4   76.4   **FUD** 090   C 80
AMA: 2016,Jan,13; 2015,Jan,16; 2014,Jan,11

33545 **Repair of postinfarction ventricular septal defect, with or without myocardial resection**
Code also removal of thrombus through a separate heart incision, when performed (33310-33315); append modifier 59 to (33315)
90.2   90.2   **FUD** 090   C 80
AMA: 2016,Jan,13; 2015,Jan,16; 2014,Jan,11

33548 **Surgical ventricular restoration procedure, includes prosthetic patch, when performed (eg, ventricular remodeling, SVR, SAVER, Dor procedures)**
EXCLUDES *Batista procedure or pachopexy (33999)*
Cardiotomy, exploratory (33310, 33315)
Temporary pacemaker (33210-33211)
Tube thoracostomy (32551)
86.2   86.2   **FUD** 090   C 80
AMA: 2016,Jan,13; 2015,Jan,16; 2014,Jan,11; 2012,Jan,15-42; 2011,Jan,11

33572 Endarterectomy with CABG (LAD, RCA, Cx)

Code first (33510-33516, 33533-33536)

+ **33572** **Coronary endarterectomy, open, any method, of left anterior descending, circumflex, or right coronary artery performed in conjunction with coronary artery bypass graft procedure, each vessel (List separately in addition to primary procedure)**
6.72   6.72   **FUD** ZZZ   C 80
AMA: 1997,Nov,1; 1994,Win,1

33600-33622 Repair Aberrant Heart Anatomy

33600 **Closure of atrioventricular valve (mitral or tricuspid) by suture or patch**
50.3   50.3   **FUD** 090   C 80
AMA: 2016,Jan,13; 2015,Jan,16; 2014,Jan,11

33602 **Closure of semilunar valve (aortic or pulmonary) by suture or patch**
Code also the concurrent ligation/takedown of a systemic-to-pulmonary artery shunt (33924)
48.8   48.8   **FUD** 090   C 80
AMA: 2007,Mar,1-3; 1997,Nov,1

33606 **Anastomosis of pulmonary artery to aorta (Damus-Kaye-Stansel procedure)**
Code also the concurrent ligation/takedown of a systemic-to-pulmonary artery shunt (33924)
54.4   54.4   **FUD** 090   C 80
AMA: 2007,Mar,1-3; 1997,Nov,1

33608 **Repair of complex cardiac anomaly other than pulmonary atresia with ventricular septal defect by construction or replacement of conduit from right or left ventricle to pulmonary artery**
EXCLUDES *Unifocalization of arborization anomalies of pulmonary artery (33925, 33926)*
Code also the concurrent ligation/takedown of a systemic-to-pulmonary artery shunt (33924)
52.7   52.7   **FUD** 090   C 80
AMA: 2007,Mar,1-3; 1997,Nov,1

33610 **Repair of complex cardiac anomalies (eg, single ventricle with subaortic obstruction) by surgical enlargement of ventricular septal defect**
Code also the concurrent ligation/takedown of a systemic-to-pulmonary artery shunt (33924)
51.9   51.9   **FUD** 090   63 C 80
AMA: 2007,Mar,1-3; 2002,May,7

33611 **Repair of double outlet right ventricle with intraventricular tunnel repair;**
Code also the concurrent ligation/takedown of a systemic-to-pulmonary artery shunt (33924)
60.1   60.1   **FUD** 090   63 C 80
AMA: 2007,Mar,1-3; 1997,Nov,1

33612 **with repair of right ventricular outflow tract obstruction**
Code also the concurrent ligation/takedown of a systemic-to-pulmonary artery shunt (33924)
58.7   58.7   **FUD** 090   C 80
AMA: 2007,Mar,1-3; 1997,Nov,1

33615 **Repair of complex cardiac anomalies (eg, tricuspid atresia) by closure of atrial septal defect and anastomosis of atria or vena cava to pulmonary artery (simple Fontan procedure)**
Code also the concurrent ligation/takedown of a systemic-to-pulmonary artery shunt (33924)
58.4   58.4   **FUD** 090   C 80
AMA: 2007,Mar,1-3; 1997,Nov,1

33617 **Repair of complex cardiac anomalies (eg, single ventricle) by modified Fontan procedure**
Code also cavopulmonary anastomosis to a second superior vena cava (33768)
Code also the concurrent ligation/takedown of a systemic-to-pulmonary artery shunt (33924)
63.3   63.3   **FUD** 090   C 80
AMA: 2007,Mar,1-3; 1997,Nov,1

33619 **Repair of single ventricle with aortic outflow obstruction and aortic arch hypoplasia (hypoplastic left heart syndrome) (eg, Norwood procedure)**
79.8   79.8   **FUD** 090   63 C 80
AMA: 2016,Jul,3; 2016,Jan,13; 2015,Jan,16; 2014,Jan,11; 2012,May,14-15; 2011,Apr,3-8

Cardiovascular, Hemic, and Lymphatic

33620 — 33692

33620 **Application of right and left pulmonary artery bands (eg, hybrid approach stage 1)**

> EXCLUDES *Banding of main pulmonary artery related to septal defect (33690)*
>
> Code also transthoracic insertion of catheter for stent placement with removal of catheter and closure when performed during same session
>
> 🚗 48.3 ⚕ 48.3 **FUD** 090 〔C〕〔80〕🖥
>
> **AMA:** 2016,Jul,3; 2016,Jan,13; 2015,Jan,16; 2014,Jan,11; 2012,May,14-15; 2011,Apr,3-8

33621 **Transthoracic insertion of catheter for stent placement with catheter removal and closure (eg, hybrid approach stage 1)**

> Code also application of right and left pulmonary artery bands when performed during same session (33620)
>
> Code also stent placement (37236)
>
> 🚗 27.2 ⚕ 27.2 **FUD** 090 〔C〕〔80〕🖥
>
> **AMA:** 2016,Jul,3; 2016,Jan,13; 2015,Jan,16; 2014,Jan,11; 2012,May,14-15; 2011,Apr,3-8

33622 **Reconstruction of complex cardiac anomaly (eg, single ventricle or hypoplastic left heart) with palliation of single ventricle with aortic outflow obstruction and aortic arch hypoplasia, creation of cavopulmonary anastomosis, and removal of right and left pulmonary bands (eg, hybrid approach stage 2, Norwood, bidirectional Glenn, pulmonary artery debanding)**

> EXCLUDES *Excision of coarctation of aorta (33840, 33845, 33851)*
>
> *Repair of hypoplastic or interrupted aortic arch (33853)*
>
> *Repair of patent ductus arteriosus (33822)*
>
> *Repair of pulmonary artery stenosis by reconstruction with patch or graft (33917)*
>
> *Repair of single ventricle with aortic outflow obstruction and aortic arch hypoplasia (33619)*
>
> *Shunt; superior vena cava to pulmonary artery for flow to both lungs (33767)*
>
> Code also anastomosis, cavopulmonary, second superior vena cava for bilateral bidirectional Glenn procedure (33768)
>
> Code also the concurrent ligation/takedown of a systemic-to-pulmonary artery shunt (33924)
>
> 🚗 106. ⚕ 106. **FUD** 090 〔C〕〔80〕🖥
>
> **AMA:** 2016,Jul,3; 2016,Jan,13; 2015,Jan,16; 2014,Jan,11; 2012,May,14-15; 2011,Apr,3-8

33641-33645 Closure of Defect: Atrium

Code also removal of thrombus through a separate heart incision, when performed (33310-33315); append modifier 59 to (33315)

33641 **Repair atrial septal defect, secundum, with cardiopulmonary bypass, with or without patch**

> 🚗 48.0 ⚕ 48.0 **FUD** 090 〔C〕〔80〕🖥
>
> **AMA:** 2016,Jan,13; 2015,Jan,16; 2014,Jan,11; 2012,Jan,15-42

33645 **Direct or patch closure, sinus venosus, with or without anomalous pulmonary venous drainage**

> EXCLUDES *Repair of isolated partial anomalous pulmonary venous return (33724)*
>
> *Repair of pulmonary venous stenosis (33726)*
>
> 🚗 50.6 ⚕ 50.6 **FUD** 090 〔C〕〔80〕🖥
>
> **AMA:** 2007,Mar,1-3; 1997,Nov,1

33647 Closure of Septal Defect: Atrium AND Ventricle

EXCLUDES *Tricuspid atresia repair procedures (33615)*

Code also removal of thrombus through a separate heart incision, when performed (33310-33315); append modifier 59 to (33315)

33647 **Repair of atrial septal defect and ventricular septal defect, with direct or patch closure**

> 🚗 53.2 ⚕ 53.2 **FUD** 090 〔63〕〔C〕〔80〕🖥
>
> **AMA:** 2007,Mar,1-3; 1997,Nov,1

33660-33670 Closure of Defect: Atrioventricular Canal

33660 **Repair of incomplete or partial atrioventricular canal (ostium primum atrial septal defect), with or without atrioventricular valve repair**

> 🚗 51.4 ⚕ 51.4 **FUD** 090 〔C〕〔80〕🖥
>
> **AMA:** 2007,Mar,1-3; 1997,Nov,1

33665 **Repair of intermediate or transitional atrioventricular canal, with or without atrioventricular valve repair**

> 🚗 56.0 ⚕ 56.0 **FUD** 090 〔C〕〔80〕🖥
>
> **AMA:** 2007,Mar,1-3; 1997,Nov,1

33670 **Repair of complete atrioventricular canal, with or without prosthetic valve**

> Code also removal of thrombus through a separate heart incision, when performed (33310-33315); append modifier 59 to (33315)
>
> 🚗 57.8 ⚕ 57.8 **FUD** 090 〔63〕〔C〕〔80〕🖥
>
> **AMA:** 2007,Mar,1-3; 1997,Nov,1

33675-33677 Closure of Multiple Septal Defects: Ventricle

EXCLUDES *Closure of single ventricular septal defect (33681, 33684, 33688)*

Insertion or replacement of temporary transvenous single chamber cardiac electrode or pacemaker catheter (33210)

Percutaneous closure (93581)

Thoracentesis (32554-32555)

Thoracotomy (32100)

Tube thoracostomy (32551)

33675 **Closure of multiple ventricular septal defects;**

> 🚗 57.8 ⚕ 57.8 **FUD** 090 〔C〕〔80〕🖥
>
> **AMA:** 2016,Jan,13; 2015,Jan,16; 2014,Jan,11

33676 **with pulmonary valvotomy or infundibular resection (acyanotic)**

> 🚗 62.3 ⚕ 62.3 **FUD** 090 〔C〕〔80〕🖥
>
> **AMA:** 2016,Jan,13; 2015,Jan,16; 2014,Jan,11

33677 **with removal of pulmonary artery band, with or without gusset**

> 🚗 64.8 ⚕ 64.8 **FUD** 090 〔C〕〔80〕🖥
>
> **AMA:** 2016,Jan,13; 2015,Jan,16; 2014,Jan,11

33681-33688 Closure of Septal Defect: Ventricle

EXCLUDES *Repair of pulmonary vein that requires creating an atrial septal defect (33724)*

33681 **Closure of single ventricular septal defect, with or without patch;**

> Code also removal of thrombus through a separate heart incision, when performed (33310-33315); append modifier 59 to (33315)
>
> 🚗 53.8 ⚕ 53.8 **FUD** 090 〔C〕〔80〕🖥
>
> **AMA:** 2016,Jan,13; 2015,Jan,16; 2014,Jan,11

33684 **with pulmonary valvotomy or infundibular resection (acyanotic)**

> Code also concurrent ligation/takedown of a systemic-to-pulmonary artery shunt if performed (33924)
>
> 🚗 58.1 ⚕ 58.1 **FUD** 090 〔C〕〔80〕🖥
>
> **AMA:** 2007,Mar,1-3; 1997,Nov,1

33688 **with removal of pulmonary artery band, with or without gusset**

> Code also the concurrent ligation/takedown of a systemic-to-pulmonary artery shunt if performed (33924)
>
> 🚗 55.2 ⚕ 55.2 **FUD** 090 〔C〕〔80〕🖥
>
> **AMA:** 2007,Mar,1-3; 1997,Nov,1

33690 Reduce Pulmonary Overcirculation in Septal Defects

EXCLUDES *Left and right pulmonary artery banding in a single ventricle (33620)*

33690 **Banding of pulmonary artery**

> 🚗 35.1 ⚕ 35.1 **FUD** 090 〔63〕〔C〕〔80〕🖥
>
> **AMA:** 2016,Jan,13; 2015,Jan,16; 2014,Jan,11; 2012,May,14-15; 2011,Apr,3-8

33692-33697 Repair of Defects of Tetralogy of Fallot

Code also the concurrent ligation/takedown of a systemic-to-pulmonary artery shunt (33924)

33692 **Complete repair tetralogy of Fallot without pulmonary atresia;**

> 🚗 60.4 ⚕ 60.4 **FUD** 090 〔C〕〔80〕🖥
>
> **AMA:** 2007,Mar,1-3; 1997,Nov,1

26/TC PC/TC Only	A2-Z3 ASC Payment	50 Bilateral	♂ Male Only	♀ Female Only	🚗 Facility RVU	⚕ Non-Facility RVU	🖥 CCI
FUD Follow-up Days	**CMS:** IOM (Pub 100)	A-Y OPPSI	80/80 Surg Assist Allowed / w/Doc		🗊 Lab Crosswalk	🔀 Radiology Crosswalk	✖ CLIA

130   CPT © 2016 American Medical Association. All Rights Reserved.   © 2016 Optum360, LLC

33694   **with transannular patch**
  📷 60.1   ⚒ 60.1   **FUD** 090   ⑥③ ⓒ 80 ▢
  AMA: 2007,Mar,1-3; 1997,Nov,1

33697   **Complete repair tetralogy of Fallot with pulmonary atresia including construction of conduit from right ventricle to pulmonary artery and closure of ventricular septal defect**
  📷 60.2   ⚒ 60.2   **FUD** 090   ⓒ 80 ▢
  AMA: 2016,Jan,13; 2015,Jan,16; 2014,Jan,11

33702-33722 Repair Anomalies Sinus of Valsalva

33702   **Repair sinus of Valsalva fistula, with cardiopulmonary bypass;**
  📷 45.2   ⚒ 45.2   **FUD** 090   ⓒ 80 ▢
  AMA: 2016,Jan,13; 2015,Jan,16; 2014,Jan,11

33710   **with repair of ventricular septal defect**
  📷 63.2   ⚒ 63.2   **FUD** 090   ⓒ 80 ▢
  AMA: 2007,Mar,1-3; 1997,Nov,1

33720   **Repair sinus of Valsalva aneurysm, with cardiopulmonary bypass**
  📷 45.2   ⚒ 45.2   **FUD** 090   ⓒ 80 ▢
  AMA: 2007,Mar,1-3; 1997,Nov,1

33722   **Closure of aortico-left ventricular tunnel**
  📷 47.6   ⚒ 47.6   **FUD** 090   ⓒ 80 ▢
  AMA: 2016,Jan,13; 2015,Jan,16; 2014,Jan,11

33724-33732 Repair Aberrant Pulmonary Venous Connection

33724   **Repair of isolated partial anomalous pulmonary venous return (eg, Scimitar Syndrome)**
  EXCLUDES   *Temporary pacemaker (33210-33211)*
               Tube thoracostomy (32551)
  📷 45.0   ⚒ 45.0   **FUD** 090   ⓒ 80 ▢
  AMA: 2016,Jan,13; 2015,Jan,16; 2014,Jan,11

33726   **Repair of pulmonary venous stenosis**
  EXCLUDES   *Temporary pacemaker (33210-33211)*
               Tube thoracostomy (32551)
  📷 59.5   ⚒ 59.5   **FUD** 090   ⓒ 80 ▢
  AMA: 2016,Jan,13; 2015,Jan,16; 2014,Jan,11

33730   **Complete repair of anomalous pulmonary venous return (supracardiac, intracardiac, or infracardiac types)**
  EXCLUDES   *Partial anomalous pulmonary venous return (33724)*
               Repair of pulmonary venous stenosis (33726)
  📷 58.7   ⚒ 58.7   **FUD** 090   ⑥③ ⓒ 80 ▢
  AMA: 2016,Jan,13; 2015,Jan,16; 2014,Jan,11

33732   **Repair of cor triatriatum or supravalvular mitral ring by resection of left atrial membrane**
  📷 48.2   ⚒ 48.2   **FUD** 090   ⑥③ ⓒ 80 ▢
  AMA: 2016,Jan,13; 2015,Jan,16; 2014,Jan,11

33735-33737 Creation of Atrial Septal Defect

Code also the concurrent ligation/takedown of a systemic-to-pulmonary artery shunt (33924)

33735   **Atrial septectomy or septostomy; closed heart (Blalock-Hanlon type operation)**
  📷 37.9   ⚒ 37.9   **FUD** 090   ⑥③ ⓒ 80 ▢
  AMA: 2016,Jan,13; 2015,Jan,16; 2014,Jan,11

33736   **open heart with cardiopulmonary bypass**
  📷 41.1   ⚒ 41.1   **FUD** 090   ⑥③ ⓒ 80 ▢
  AMA: 2007,Mar,1-3; 1997,Nov,1

33737   **open heart, with inflow occlusion**
  EXCLUDES   *Atrial septectomy/septostomy:*
               Blade method (92993)
               Transvenous balloon method (92992)
  📷 39.5   ⚒ 39.5   **FUD** 090   ⓒ 80 ▢
  AMA: 2007,Mar,1-3; 1997,Nov,1

33750-33767 Systemic Vessel to Pulmonary Artery Shunts

Code also the concurrent ligation/takedown of a systemic-to-pulmonary artery shunt (33924)

33750   **Shunt; subclavian to pulmonary artery (Blalock-Taussig type operation)**
  📷 36.9   ⚒ 36.9   **FUD** 090   ⑥③ ⓒ 80 ▢
  AMA: 2007,Mar,1-3; 1997,Nov,1

33755   **ascending aorta to pulmonary artery (Waterston type operation)**
  📷 38.5   ⚒ 38.5   **FUD** 090   ⑥③ ⓒ 80 ▢
  AMA: 2007,Mar,1-3; 1997,Nov,1

33762   **descending aorta to pulmonary artery (Potts-Smith type operation)**
  📷 39.1   ⚒ 39.1   **FUD** 090   ⑥③ ⓒ 80 ▢
  AMA: 2007,Mar,1-3; 1997,Nov,1

33764   **central, with prosthetic graft**
  📷 38.5   ⚒ 38.5   **FUD** 090   ⓒ 80 ▢
  AMA: 2007,Mar,1-3; 1997,Nov,1

33766   **superior vena cava to pulmonary artery for flow to 1 lung (classical Glenn procedure)**
  📷 38.9   ⚒ 38.9   **FUD** 090   ⓒ 80 ▢
  AMA: 2007,Mar,1-3; 1997,Nov,1

33767   **superior vena cava to pulmonary artery for flow to both lungs (bidirectional Glenn procedure)**
  📷 41.6   ⚒ 41.6   **FUD** 090   ⓒ 80 ▢
  AMA: 2016,Jul,3; 2011,Apr,3-8

33768 Cavopulmonary Anastomosis to Decrease Volume Load

EXCLUDES   *Temporary pacemaker (33210-33211)*
             Tube thoracostomy (32551)
Code first (33478, 33617, 33622, 33767)

+   **33768**   **Anastomosis, cavopulmonary, second superior vena cava (List separately in addition to primary procedure)**
  📷 12.2   ⚒ 12.2   **FUD** ZZZ   ⓒ 80 ▢
  AMA: 2016,Jul,3; 2016,Jan,13; 2015,Jan,16; 2014,Jan,11; 2011,Apr,3-8

33770-33783 Repair Aberrant Anatomy: Transposition Great Vessels

Code also the concurrent ligation/takedown of a systemic-to-pulmonary artery shunt (33924)

33770   **Repair of transposition of the great arteries with ventricular septal defect and subpulmonary stenosis; without surgical enlargement of ventricular septal defect**
  📷 65.3   ⚒ 65.3   **FUD** 090   ⓒ 80 ▢
  AMA: 2016,Jan,13; 2015,Jan,16; 2014,Jan,11

33771   **with surgical enlargement of ventricular septal defect**
  📷 67.4   ⚒ 67.4   **FUD** 090   ⓒ 80 ▢
  AMA: 2007,Mar,1-3; 1997,Nov,1

33774   **Repair of transposition of the great arteries, atrial baffle procedure (eg, Mustard or Senning type) with cardiopulmonary bypass;**
  📷 52.6   ⚒ 52.6   **FUD** 090   ⓒ 80 ▢
  AMA: 2007,Mar,1-3; 1997,Nov,1

33775   **with removal of pulmonary band**
  📷 56.7   ⚒ 56.7   **FUD** 090   ⓒ 80 ▢
  AMA: 2007,Mar,1-3; 1997,Nov,1

33776   **with closure of ventricular septal defect**
  📷 60.0   ⚒ 60.0   **FUD** 090   ⓒ 80 ▢
  AMA: 2007,Mar,1-3; 1997,Nov,1

33777   **with repair of subpulmonic obstruction**
  📷 58.1   ⚒ 58.1   **FUD** 090   ⓒ 80 ▢
  AMA: 2007,Mar,1-3; 1997,Nov,1

Cardiovascular, Hemic, and Lymphatic

33778 — 33870

33778 **Repair of transposition of the great arteries, aortic pulmonary artery reconstruction (eg, Jatene type);**
72.3   72.3   **FUD** 090   63 C 80
AMA: 2007,Mar,1-3; 1997,Nov,1

33779 **with removal of pulmonary band**
71.9   71.9   **FUD** 090   C 80
AMA: 2007,Mar,1-3; 1997,Nov,1

33780 **with closure of ventricular septal defect**
69.4   69.4   **FUD** 090   C 80
AMA: 2007,Mar,1-3; 1997,Nov,1

33781 **with repair of subpulmonic obstruction**
71.5   71.5   **FUD** 090   C 80
AMA: 2016,Jan,13; 2015,Jan,16; 2014,Jan,11

33782 **Aortic root translocation with ventricular septal defect and pulmonary stenosis repair (ie, Nikaidoh procedure); without coronary ostium reimplantation**
94.6   94.6   **FUD** 090   C 80
EXCLUDES   Closure of single ventricular septal defect (33681)
           Repair of complex cardiac anomaly other than pulmonary atresia (33608)
           Repair of pulmonary atresia with ventricular septal defect (33920)
           Repair of transposition of the great arteries (33770-33771, 33778, 33780)
           Replacement, aortic valve (33412-33413)

33783 **with reimplantation of 1 or both coronary ostia**
107.   107.   **FUD** 090   C 80

33786-33788 Repair Aberrant Anatomy: Truncus Arteriosus

33786 **Total repair, truncus arteriosus (Rastelli type operation)**
Code also the concurrent ligation/takedown of a systemic-to-pulmonary artery shunt (33924)
66.6   66.6   **FUD** 090   63 C 80
AMA: 2016,Jan,13; 2015,Jan,16; 2014,Jan,11

33788 **Reimplantation of an anomalous pulmonary artery**
EXCLUDES   Pulmonary artery banding (33690)
47.0   47.0   **FUD** 090   C 80
AMA: 2016,Jan,13; 2015,Jan,16; 2014,Jan,11

33800-33853 Repair Aberrant Anatomy: Aorta

33800 **Aortic suspension (aortopexy) for tracheal decompression (eg, for tracheomalacia) (separate procedure)**
28.9   28.9   **FUD** 090   C 80
AMA: 2016,Jan,13; 2015,Jan,16; 2014,Jan,11

33802 **Division of aberrant vessel (vascular ring);**
31.7   31.7   **FUD** 090   C 80
AMA: 2007,Mar,1-3; 1997,Nov,1

33803 **with reanastomosis**
33.6   33.6   **FUD** 090   C 80
AMA: 2007,Mar,1-3; 1997,Nov,1

33813 **Obliteration of aortopulmonary septal defect; without cardiopulmonary bypass**
37.7   37.7   **FUD** 090   C 80
AMA: 2007,Mar,1-3; 1997,Nov,1

33814 **with cardiopulmonary bypass**
44.5   44.5   **FUD** 090   C 80
AMA: 2007,Mar,1-3; 1997,Nov,1

33820 **Repair of patent ductus arteriosus; by ligation**
EXCLUDES   Percutaneous transcatheter closure patent ductus arteriosus (93582)
28.3   28.3   **FUD** 090   C 80
AMA: 2016,Jan,13; 2015,Jan,16; 2014,Jan,11

33822 **by division, younger than 18 years**   A
EXCLUDES   Percutaneous transcatheter closure patent ductus arteriosus (93582)
31.1   31.1   **FUD** 090   C 80
AMA: 2016,Jul,3; 2016,Jan,13; 2015,Jan,16; 2014,Jan,11; 2011,Apr,3-8

33824 **by division, 18 years and older**
EXCLUDES   Percutaneous closure patent ductus arteriosus (93582)
34.5   34.5   **FUD** 090   C 80
AMA: 2007,Mar,1-3; 1997,Nov,1

33840 **Excision of coarctation of aorta, with or without associated patent ductus arteriosus; with direct anastomosis**
36.2   36.2   **FUD** 090   C 80
AMA: 2016,Jul,3; 2011,Apr,3-8

33845 **with graft**
39.0   39.0   **FUD** 090   C 80
AMA: 2016,Jul,3; 2011,Apr,3-8

33851 **repair using either left subclavian artery or prosthetic material as gusset for enlargement**
37.2   37.2   **FUD** 090   C 80
AMA: 2016,Jul,3; 2011,Apr,3-8

33852 **Repair of hypoplastic or interrupted aortic arch using autogenous or prosthetic material; without cardiopulmonary bypass**
EXCLUDES   Hypoplastic left heart syndrome repair by excision of coarctation of aorta (33619)
40.9   40.9   **FUD** 090   C 80
AMA: 2007,Mar,1-3; 1997,Nov,1

33853 **with cardiopulmonary bypass**
EXCLUDES   Hypoplastic left heart syndrome repair by excision of coarctation of aorta (33619)
53.6   53.6   **FUD** 090   C 80
AMA: 2016,Jul,3; 2016,Jan,13; 2015,Jan,16; 2014,Jan,11; 2011,Apr,3-8

33860-33877 Aortic Graft Procedures

33860 **Ascending aorta graft, with cardiopulmonary bypass, includes valve suspension, when performed**
93.5   93.5   **FUD** 090   C 80
AMA: 2016,Jan,13; 2015,Jan,16; 2014,Jan,11; 2011,Aug,3-5

33863 **Ascending aorta graft, with cardiopulmonary bypass, with aortic root replacement using valved conduit and coronary reconstruction (eg, Bentall)**
INCLUDES   Ascending aorta graft, with cardiopulmonary bypass, includes valve suspension, when performed (33860)
EXCLUDES   Replacement, aortic valve, with cardiopulmonary bypass (33405-33406, 33410-33413)
91.7   91.7   **FUD** 090   C 80
AMA: 2016,Jan,13; 2015,Jan,16; 2014,Jan,11; 2012,Jan,15-42; 2011,Aug,3-5

33864 **Ascending aorta graft, with cardiopulmonary bypass with valve suspension, with coronary reconstruction and valve-sparing aortic root remodeling (eg, David Procedure, Yacoub Procedure)**
INCLUDES   Ascending aorta graft with cardiopulmonary bypass (33860-33863)
93.8   93.8   **FUD** 090   C 80
AMA: 2016,Jan,13; 2015,Jan,16; 2014,Jan,11; 2012,Jan,15-42; 2011,Aug,3-5

33870 **Transverse arch graft, with cardiopulmonary bypass**
73.3   73.3   **FUD** 090   C 80
AMA: 1997,Nov,1

| 26/TC | PC/TC Only | A2-Z3 | ASC Payment | 50 | Bilateral | ♂ | Male Only | ♀ | Female Only | Facility RVU | Non-Facility RVU | CCI |
| FUD | Follow-up Days | CMS: | IOM (Pub 100) | A-Y | OPPSI | 80/80 | Surg Assist Allowed / w/Doc | | | Lab Crosswalk | Radiology Crosswalk | CLIA |

132   CPT © 2016 American Medical Association. All Rights Reserved.   © 2016 Optum360, LLC

33875 Descending thoracic aorta graft, with or without bypass

🔧 80.1 ⚕ 80.1 **FUD** 090 C 80 ▣

AMA: 1997,Nov,1

33877 Repair of thoracoabdominal aortic aneurysm with graft, with or without cardiopulmonary bypass

🔧 106. ⚕ 106. **FUD** 090 C 80 ▣

AMA: 1997,Nov,1

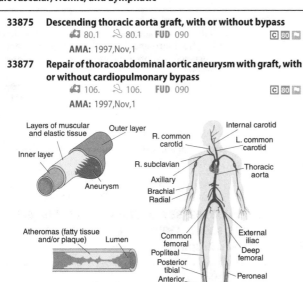

33880-33891 Endovascular Repair Aortic Aneurysm: Thoracic

INCLUDES Balloon angioplasty
Deployment of stent
Introduction, manipulation, placement, and deployment of the device

EXCLUDES *Additional interventional procedures provided during the endovascular repair*
Carotid-carotid bypass (33891)
Guidewire and catheter insertion (36140, 36200-36218)
Open exposure of artery/subsequent closure (34812, 34820, 34833-34834)
Study, interpretation, and report of implanted wireless pressure sensor in an aneurysmal sac (93982)
Subclavian to carotid artery transposition (33889)
Substantial artery repair/replacement (35226, 35286)
Transcatheter insertion of wireless physiologic sensor in an aneurysmal sac (34806)

33880 Endovascular repair of descending thoracic aorta (eg, aneurysm, pseudoaneurysm, dissection, penetrating ulcer, intramural hematoma, or traumatic disruption); involving coverage of left subclavian artery origin, initial endoprosthesis plus descending thoracic aortic extension(s), if required, to level of celiac artery origin

INCLUDES Placement of distal extensions in distal thoracic aorta

EXCLUDES *Proximal extensions*

🔧 (75956)

🔧 52.9 ⚕ 52.9 **FUD** 090 C 80 ▣

AMA: 2016,Jan,13; 2015,Jan,16; 2014,Jan,11

33881 not involving coverage of left subclavian artery origin, initial endoprosthesis plus descending thoracic aortic extension(s), if required, to level of celiac artery origin

INCLUDES Placement of distal extensions in distal thoracic aorta

EXCLUDES *Procedure where the placement of extension includes coverage of left subclavian artery origin (33880)*
Proximal extensions

🔧 (75957)

🔧 45.4 ⚕ 45.4 **FUD** 090 C 80 ▣

AMA: 2016,Jan,13; 2015,Jan,16; 2014,Jan,11

33883 Placement of proximal extension prosthesis for endovascular repair of descending thoracic aorta (eg, aneurysm, pseudoaneurysm, dissection, penetrating ulcer, intramural hematoma, or traumatic disruption); initial extension

EXCLUDES *Procedure where the placement of extension includes coverage of left subclavian artery origin (33880)*

🔧 (75958)

🔧 32.9 ⚕ 32.9 **FUD** 090 C 80 ▣

AMA: 2016,Jan,13; 2015,Jan,16; 2014,Jan,11

+ 33884 each additional proximal extension (List separately in addition to code for primary procedure)

Code first (33883)

🔧 (75958)

🔧 12.0 ⚕ 12.0 **FUD** ZZZ C 80 ▣

AMA: 2016,Jan,13; 2015,Jan,16; 2014,Jan,11

33886 Placement of distal extension prosthesis(s) delayed after endovascular repair of descending thoracic aorta

INCLUDES All modules deployed

EXCLUDES *Endovascular repair of descending thoracic aorta (33880, 33881)*

🔧 (75959)

🔧 28.4 ⚕ 28.4 **FUD** 090 C 80 ▣

AMA: 2016,Jan,13; 2015,Jan,16; 2014,Jan,11

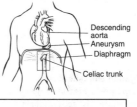

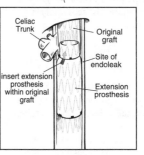

Repair of endoleak in descending thoracic aorta

33889 Open subclavian to carotid artery transposition performed in conjunction with endovascular repair of descending thoracic aorta, by neck incision, unilateral

EXCLUDES *Transposition and/or reimplantation; subclavian to carotid artery (35694)*

🔧 23.2 ⚕ 23.2 **FUD** 000 C 80 50 ▣

AMA: 2016,Jan,13; 2015,Jan,16; 2014,Jan,11

33891 Bypass graft, with other than vein, transcervical retropharyngeal carotid-carotid, performed in conjunction with endovascular repair of descending thoracic aorta, by neck incision

EXCLUDES *Bypass graft (35509, 35601)*

🔧 28.5 ⚕ 28.5 **FUD** 000 C 80 50 ▣

AMA: 2016,Jan,13; 2015,Jan,16; 2014,Jan,11

33910-33926 Surgical Procedures of Pulmonary Artery

33910 Pulmonary artery embolectomy; with cardiopulmonary bypass

🔧 76.5 ⚕ 76.5 **FUD** 090 C 80 ▣

AMA: 2016,Jan,13; 2015,Jan,16; 2014,Jan,11

33915 without cardiopulmonary bypass

🔧 37.1 ⚕ 37.1 **FUD** 090 C 80 ▣

AMA: 2016,Jan,13; 2015,Jan,16; 2014,Jan,11

33916 Pulmonary endarterectomy, with or without embolectomy, with cardiopulmonary bypass

🔧 122. ⚕ 122. **FUD** 090 C 80 ▣

AMA: 2016,Jan,13; 2015,Jan,16; 2014,Jan,11

33917 **Repair of pulmonary artery stenosis by reconstruction with patch or graft**

> Code also the concurrent ligation/takedown of a systemic-to-pulmonary artery shunt (33924)
>
> 🚑 42.6   ⚕ 42.6   **FUD** 090   C 80 ▭
>
> **AMA:** 2016,Jul,3; 2016,Jan,13; 2015,Jan,16; 2014,Jan,11; 2011,Apr,3-8

33920 **Repair of pulmonary atresia with ventricular septal defect, by construction or replacement of conduit from right or left ventricle to pulmonary artery**

> *EXCLUDES*   *Repair of complicated cardiac anomalies by creating/replacing conduit from ventricle to pulmonary artery (33608)*
>
> Code also the concurrent ligation/takedown of a systemic-to-pulmonary artery shunt (33924)
>
> 🚑 55.6   ⚕ 55.6   **FUD** 090   C 80 ▭
>
> **AMA:** 2016,Jan,13; 2015,Jan,16; 2014,Jan,11

33922 **Transection of pulmonary artery with cardiopulmonary bypass**

> Code also the concurrent ligation/takedown of a systemic-to-pulmonary artery shunt (33924)
>
> 🚑 40.6   ⚕ 40.6   **FUD** 090   63 C 80 ▭
>
> **AMA:** 1997,Nov,1; 1995,Win,1

+ 33924 **Ligation and takedown of a systemic-to-pulmonary artery shunt, performed in conjunction with a congenital heart procedure (List separately in addition to code for primary procedure)**

> Code first (33470-33478, 33600-33617, 33622, 33684-33688, 33692-33697, 33735-33767, 33770-33783, 33786, 33917, 33920-33922, 33925-33926, 33935, 33945)
>
> 🚑 8.38   ⚕ 8.38   **FUD** ZZZ   C 80 ▭
>
> **AMA:** 1997,Nov,1; 1995,Win,1

33925 **Repair of pulmonary artery arborization anomalies by unifocalization; without cardiopulmonary bypass**

> 🚑 50.3   ⚕ 50.3   **FUD** 090   C 80 ▭
>
> Code also the concurrent ligation/takedown of a systemic-to-pulmonary artery shunt (33924)

33926 **with cardiopulmonary bypass**

> 🚑 74.6   ⚕ 74.6   **FUD** 090   C 80 ▭
>
> Code also the concurrent ligation/takedown of a systemic-to-pulmonary artery shunt (33924)

33930-33945 Heart and Heart-Lung Transplants

CMS: 100-03,260.9 Heart Transplants; 100-04,3,90.2 Heart Transplants

> *INCLUDES*   Backbench work to prepare the donor heart and/or lungs for transplantation (33933, 33944)
> Harvesting of donor organs with cold preservation (33930, 33940)
> Transplantation of heart and/or lungs into recipient (33935, 33945)
>
> *EXCLUDES*   *Implantation/repair/replacement of artificial heart or components (0051T-0053T)*

33930 **Donor cardiectomy-pneumonectomy (including cold preservation)**

> 🚑 0.00   ⚕ 0.00   **FUD** XXX   C ▭
>
> **AMA:** 1997,Nov,1

33933 **Backbench standard preparation of cadaver donor heart/lung allograft prior to transplantation, including dissection of allograft from surrounding soft tissues to prepare aorta, superior vena cava, inferior vena cava, and trachea for implantation**

> 🚑 0.00   ⚕ 0.00   **FUD** XXX   C 80 ▭
>
> **AMA:** 1997,Nov,1

33935 **Heart-lung transplant with recipient cardiectomy-pneumonectomy**

> Code also the concurrent ligation/takedown of a systemic-to-pulmonary artery shunt (33924)
>
> 🚑 145.   ⚕ 145.   **FUD** 090   C 80 ▭
>
> **AMA:** 1997,Nov,1

33940 **Donor cardiectomy (including cold preservation)**

> 🚑 0.00   ⚕ 0.00   **FUD** XXX   C ▭
>
> **AMA:** 2016,Jan,13; 2015,Jan,16; 2014,Jan,11

33944 **Backbench standard preparation of cadaver donor heart allograft prior to transplantation, including dissection of allograft from surrounding soft tissues to prepare aorta, superior vena cava, inferior vena cava, pulmonary artery, and left atrium for implantation**

> *EXCLUDES*   *Procedures performed on donor heart (33300, 33310, 33320, 33390, 33463-33464, 33510, 33641, 35216, 35276, 35685)*
>
> 🚑 0.00   ⚕ 0.00   **FUD** XXX   C 80 ▭
>
> **AMA:** 1997,Nov,1

33945 **Heart transplant, with or without recipient cardiectomy**

> Code also the concurrent ligation/takedown of a systemic-to-pulmonary artery shunt (33924)
>
> 🚑 141.   ⚕ 141.   **FUD** 090   C 80 ▭
>
> **AMA:** 1997,May,4; 1997,Nov,1

33946-33959 [33962, 33963, 33964, 33965, 33966, 33969, 33984, 33985, 33986, 33987, 33988, 33989] Extracorporeal Circulatory and Respiratory Support

> *INCLUDES*   Cannula repositioning and cannula insertion performed during same session
> Cannula repositioning and initiation of ECMO/ECLS on the same day
> Multiple physician and nonphysician team collaboration
> Veno-arterial ECMO/ECLS for heart and lung support
> Veno-venous ECMO/ECLS for lung support
>
> *EXCLUDES*   *Overall daily management services needed to manage a patient; report the appropriate observation, hospital inpatient, or critical care E/M codes*
> Code also extensive arterial repair/replacement (35266, 35286, 35371, 35665)

33946 **Extracorporeal membrane oxygenation (ECMO)/extracorporeal life support (ECLS) provided by physician; initiation, veno-venous**

> *EXCLUDES*   *Daily ECMO/ECLS veno-venous management on day of initial service (33948)*
> *Repositioning of ECMO/ECLS cannula on day of initial service (33957-33959 [33962, 33963, 33964])*
> Code also cannula insertion (33951-33956)
>
> 🚑 8.91   ⚕ 8.91   **FUD** XXX   63 C ▭
>
> **AMA:** 2016,Mar,5; 2016,Jan,13; 2015,Jul,3

33947 **initiation, veno-arterial**

> *EXCLUDES*   *Daily ECMO/ECLS veno-arterial management on day of initial service (33949)*
> *Repositioning of ECMO/ECLS cannula on day of initial service (33957-33959 [33962, 33963, 33964])*
> Code also cannula insertion (33951-33956)
>
> 🚑 9.85   ⚕ 9.85   **FUD** XXX   63 C ▭
>
> **AMA:** 2016,Mar,5; 2016,Jan,13; 2015,Jul,3

33948 **daily management, each day, veno-venous**

> *EXCLUDES*   *ECMO/ECLS initiation, veno-venous (33946)*
>
> 🚑 7.03   ⚕ 7.03   **FUD** XXX   63 C ▭
>
> **AMA:** 2016,Mar,5; 2016,Jan,13; 2015,Jul,3

33949 **daily management, each day, veno-arterial**

> *EXCLUDES*   *ECMO/ECLS initiation, veno-arterial (33947)*
>
> 🚑 6.84   ⚕ 6.84   **FUD** XXX   63 C ▭
>
> **AMA:** 2016,Mar,5; 2016,Jan,13; 2015,Jul,3

33951 **insertion of peripheral (arterial and/or venous) cannula(e), percutaneous, birth through 5 years of age (includes fluoroscopic guidance, when performed)**   A

> *INCLUDES*   Cannula replacement in same vessel
> Cannula repositioning during same episode of care
> Code also cannula removal if new cannula inserted in different vessel with ([33965, 33966, 33969, 33984, 33985, 33986])
> Code also ECMO/ECLS initiation or daily management (33946-33947, 33948-33949)
>
> 🚑 12.1   ⚕ 12.1   **FUD** 000   C 80 ▭
>
> **AMA:** 2016,Mar,5; 2016,Jan,13; 2015,Jul,3

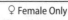 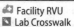

33952 insertion of peripheral (arterial and/or venous) cannula(e), percutaneous, 6 years and older (includes fluoroscopic guidance, when performed) Ⓐ

INCLUDES Cannula replacement in same vessel
Cannula repositioning during same episode of care
Code also cannula removal if new cannula inserted in different vessel with ([33965, 33966, 33969, 33984, 33985, 33986])
Code also ECMO/ECLS initiation or daily management (33946-33947, 33948-33949)

🔧 12.5　 ⚬ 12.5　**FUD** 000　Ⓒ 80 ▣

AMA: 2016,Mar,5; 2016,Jan,13; 2015,Jul,3

33953 insertion of peripheral (arterial and/or venous) cannula(e), open, birth through 5 years of age Ⓐ

INCLUDES Cannula replacement in same vessel
Cannula repositioning during same episode of care
EXCLUDES *Open artery exposure for delivery/deployment of endovascular prosthesis (34812, 34820, 34834)*
Code also cannula removal if new cannula inserted in different vessel with ([33965, 33966, 33969, 33984, 33985, 33986])
Code also ECMO/ECLS initiation or daily management (33496-33947, 33948-33949)

🔧 13.5　 ⚬ 13.5　**FUD** 000　Ⓒ 80 ▣

AMA: 2016,Mar,5; 2016,Jan,13; 2015,Jul,3

33954 insertion of peripheral (arterial and/or venous) cannula(e), open, 6 years and older Ⓐ

INCLUDES Cannula replacement in same vessel
Cannula repositioning during same episode of care
EXCLUDES *Open artery exposure for delivery/deployment of endovascular prosthesis (34812, 34820, 34834)*
Code also cannula removal if new cannula inserted in different vessel with ([33965, 33966, 33969, 33984, 33985, 33986])
Code also ECMO/ECLS initiation or daily management (33946-33947, 33948-33949)

🔧 14.0　 ⚬ 14.0　**FUD** 000　Ⓒ 80 ▣

AMA: 2016,Mar,5; 2016,Jan,13; 2015,Jul,3

33955 insertion of central cannula(e) by sternotomy or thoracotomy, birth through 5 years of age Ⓐ

INCLUDES Cannula replacement in same vessel
Cannula repositioning during same episode of care
EXCLUDES *Mediastinotomy (39010)*
Thoracotomy (32100)
Code also cannula removal if new cannula inserted in different vessel with ([33965, 33966, 33969, 33984, 33985, 33986])
Code also ECMO/ECLS initiation or daily management (33946-33947, 33948-33949)

🔧 24.3　 ⚬ 24.3　**FUD** 000　Ⓒ 80 ▣

AMA: 2016,Mar,5; 2016,Jan,13; 2015,Jul,3

33956 insertion of central cannula(e) by sternotomy or thoracotomy, 6 years and older Ⓐ

INCLUDES Cannula replacement in same vessel
Cannula repositioning during same episode of care
EXCLUDES *Mediastinotomy (39010)*
Thoracotomy (32100)
Code also cannula removal if new cannula inserted in different vessel with ([33965, 33966, 33969, 33984, 33985, 33986])
Code also ECMO/ECLS initiation or daily management (33946-33947, 33948-33949)

🔧 24.4　 ⚬ 24.4　**FUD** 000　Ⓒ 80 ▣

AMA: 2016,Mar,5; 2016,Jan,13; 2015,Jul,3

33957 reposition peripheral (arterial and/or venous) cannula(e), percutaneous, birth through 5 years of age (includes fluoroscopic guidance, when performed) Ⓐ

INCLUDES Fluoroscopic guidance
EXCLUDES *ECMO/ECLS initiation, veno-arterial (33947)*
ECMO/ECLS initiation, veno-venous (33946)
ECMO/ECLS insertion of cannula (33951-33956)
Open artery exposure for delivery/deployment of endovascular prosthesis (34812, 34820, 34834)

🔧 5.42　 ⚬ 5.42　**FUD** 000　Ⓒ 80 ▣

AMA: 2016,Mar,5; 2016,Jan,13; 2015,Jul,3

33958 reposition peripheral (arterial and/or venous) cannula(e), percutaneous, 6 years and older (includes fluoroscopic guidance, when performed) Ⓐ

INCLUDES Fluoroscopic guidance
EXCLUDES *ECMO/ECLS initiation, veno-arterial (33947)*
ECMO/ECLS initiation, veno-venous (33946)
ECMO/ECLS insertion of cannula (33951-33956)
Open artery exposure for delivery/deployment of endovascular prosthesis (34812, 34820, 34834)

🔧 5.34　 ⚬ 5.34　**FUD** 000　Ⓒ 80 ▣

AMA: 2016,Mar,5; 2016,Jan,13; 2015,Jul,3

33959 reposition peripheral (arterial and/or venous) cannula(e), open, birth through 5 years of age (includes fluoroscopic guidance, when performed) Ⓐ

INCLUDES Fluoroscopic guidance
EXCLUDES *ECMO/ECLS initiation, veno-arterial (33947)*
ECMO/ECLS initiation, veno-venous (33946)
ECMO/ECLS insertion of cannula (33951-33956)
Open artery exposure for delivery/deployment of endovascular prosthesis (34812, 34820, 34834)

🔧 6.88　 ⚬ 6.88　**FUD** 000　Ⓒ 80 ▣

AMA: 2016,Mar,5; 2016,Jan,13; 2015,Jul,3

#　33962 reposition peripheral (arterial and/or venous) cannula(e), open, 6 years and older (includes fluoroscopic guidance, when performed) Ⓐ

INCLUDES Fluoroscopic guidance
EXCLUDES *ECMO/ECLS initiation, veno-arterial (33947)*
ECMO/ECLS initiation, veno-venous (33946)
ECMO/ECLS insertion of cannula (33951-33956)
Open artery exposure for delivery/deployment of endovascular prosthesis (34812, 34820, 34834)

🔧 6.96　 ⚬ 6.96　**FUD** 000　Ⓒ 80 ▣

AMA: 2016,Mar,5; 2016,Jan,13; 2015,Jul,3

#　33963 reposition of central cannula(e) by sternotomy or thoracotomy, birth through 5 years of age (includes fluoroscopic guidance, when performed) Ⓐ

INCLUDES Fluoroscopic guidance
EXCLUDES *ECMO/ECLS initiation, veno-atrial (33947)*
ECMO/ECLS initiation, veno-venous (33946)
ECMO/ECLS insertion of cannula (33951-33956)
Mediastinotomy (39010)
Open artery exposure for delivery/deployment of endovascular prosthesis (34812, 34820, 34834)
Thoracotomy (32100)

🔧 13.7　 ⚬ 13.7　**FUD** 000　Ⓒ 80 ▣

AMA: 2016,Mar,5; 2016,Jan,13; 2015,Jul,3

#　33964 reposition central cannula(e) by sternotomy or thoracotomy, 6 years and older (includes fluoroscopic guidance, when performed) Ⓐ

INCLUDES Fluoroscopic guidance
EXCLUDES *ECMO/ECLS initiation, veno-atrial (33947)*
ECMO/ECLS initiation, veno-venous (33946)
ECMO/ECLS insertion of cannula (33951-33956)
Mediastinotomy (39010)
Thoracotomy (32100)

🔧 14.3　 ⚬ 14.3　**FUD** 000　Ⓒ 80 ▣

AMA: 2016,Mar,5; 2016,Jan,13; 2015,Jul,3

#　33965 removal of peripheral (arterial and/or venous) cannula(e), percutaneous, birth through 5 years of age Ⓐ

Code also extensive arterial repair/replacement, when performed (35266, 35286, 35371, 35665)
Code also new cannula insertion into different vessel (33951-33956)

🔧 5.42　 ⚬ 5.42　**FUD** 000　Ⓒ 80 ▣

AMA: 2016,Mar,5; 2016,Jan,13; 2015,Jul,3

Cardiovascular, Hemic, and Lymphatic

33966 — 33975

removal of peripheral (arterial and/or venous) cannula(e), percutaneous, 6 years and older Ⓐ

\# **33966**

Code also new cannula insertion into different vessel (33951-33956)

Code also extensive arterial repair/replacement, when performed (35266, 35286, 35371, 35665)

🔧 6.87   ⚕ 6.87   **FUD** 000   Ⓒ 80 ▢

AMA: 2016,Mar,5; 2016,Jan,13; 2015,Jul,3

\# **33969** **removal of peripheral (arterial and/or venous) cannula(e), open, birth through 5 years of age** Ⓐ

EXCLUDES   Repair blood vessel (35201, 35206, 35211, 35216, 35226)

Open artery exposure for delivery/deployment of endovascular prosthesis (34812, 34820, 34834)

Code also extensive arterial repair/replacement, when performed (35266, 35286, 35371, 35665)

Code also new cannula insertion into different vessel (33951-33956)

🔧 8.01   ⚕ 8.01   **FUD** 000   Ⓒ 80 ▢

AMA: 2016,Mar,5; 2016,Jan,13; 2015,Jul,3

\# **33984** **removal of peripheral (arterial and/or venous) cannula(e), open, 6 years and older** Ⓐ

EXCLUDES   Repair blood vessel (35201, 35206, 35211, 35216, 35226)

Open artery exposure for delivery/deployment of endovascular prosthesis (34812, 34820, 34834)

Code also extensive arterial repair/replacement, when performed (35266, 35286, 35371, 35665)

Code also new cannula insertion into different vessel (33951-33956)

🔧 8.33   ⚕ 8.33   **FUD** 000   Ⓒ 80 ▢

AMA: 2016,Mar,5; 2016,Jan,13; 2015,Jul,3

\# **33985** **removal of central cannula(e) by sternotomy or thoracotomy, birth through 5 years of age** Ⓐ

EXCLUDES   Repair blood vessel (35201, 35206, 35211, 35216, 35226)

Code also extensive arterial repair/replacement, when performed (35266, 35286, 35371, 35665)

Code also new cannula insertion into different vessel (33951-33956)

🔧 15.1   ⚕ 15.1   **FUD** 000   Ⓒ 80 ▢

AMA: 2016,Mar,5; 2016,Jan,13; 2015,Jul,3

\# **33986** **removal of central cannula(e) by sternotomy or thoracotomy, 6 years and older** Ⓐ

EXCLUDES   Repair blood vessel (35201, 35206, 35211, 35216, 35226)

Code also extensive arterial repair/replacement, when performed (35266, 35286, 35371, 35665)

Code also new cannula insertion into different vessel (33951-33956)

🔧 15.4   ⚕ 15.4   **FUD** 000   Ⓒ 80 ▢

AMA: 2016,Mar,5; 2016,Jan,13; 2015,Jul,3

+ \# **33987** **Arterial exposure with creation of graft conduit (eg, chimney graft) to facilitate arterial perfusion for ECMO/ECLS (List separately in addition to code for primary procedure)**

EXCLUDES   Open artery exposure for delivery of endovascular prosthesis (34833)

Code first (33953-33956)

🔧 6.08   ⚕ 6.08   **FUD** ZZZ   Ⓒ 80 ▢

AMA: 2016,Mar,5; 2016,Jan,13; 2015,Jul,3

\# **33988** **Insertion of left heart vent by thoracic incision (eg, sternotomy, thoracotomy) for ECMO/ECLS**

🔧 22.6   ⚕ 22.6   **FUD** 000   Ⓒ 80 ▢

AMA: 2016,Mar,5; 2016,Jan,13; 2015,Jul,3

\# **33989** **Removal of left heart vent by thoracic incision (eg, sternotomy, thoracotomy) for ECMO/ECLS**

🔧 14.6   ⚕ 14.6   **FUD** 000   Ⓒ 80 ▢

AMA: 2016,Mar,5; 2016,Jan,13; 2015,Jul,3

33962-33999 Mechanical Circulatory Support

33962 **Resequenced code. See code following 33959.**

33963 **Resequenced code. See code following 33959.**

33964 **Resequenced code. See code following 33959.**

33965 **Resequenced code. See code following 33959.**

33966 **Resequenced code. See code following 33959.**

33967 **Insertion of intra-aortic balloon assist device, percutaneous**

🔧 7.56   ⚕ 7.56   **FUD** 000   Ⓒ 80 ▢

AMA: 2016,Mar,5; 2016,Jan,13; 2015,Sep,3; 2015,Jul,3; 2015,Jan,16; 2014,Jan,11; 2013,Mar,10-11; 2012,Jan,15-42

33968 **Removal of intra-aortic balloon assist device, percutaneous**

EXCLUDES   Removal of implantable aortic couterpulsation ventricular assist system (0455T-0458T)

🔧 0.98   ⚕ 0.98   **FUD** 000   Ⓒ ▢

AMA: 2016,Mar,5; 2016,Jan,13; 2015,Jul,3; 2015,Jan,16; 2014,Jan,11; 2012,Jan,15-42; 2011,Jan,11

33969 **Resequenced code. See code following 33959.**

33970 **Insertion of intra-aortic balloon assist device through the femoral artery, open approach**

EXCLUDES   Insertion/replacement implantable aortic counterpulsation ventricular assist system (0451T-0454T)

Percutaneous insertion of intra-aortic balloon assist device (33967)

🔧 10.3   ⚕ 10.3   **FUD** 000   Ⓒ 80 ▢

AMA: 2016,Mar,5; 2016,Jan,13; 2015,Sep,3; 2015,Jul,3; 2015,Jan,16; 2014,Jan,11; 2013,Mar,10-11

33971 **Removal of intra-aortic balloon assist device including repair of femoral artery, with or without graft**

EXCLUDES   Removal of implantable aortic counterpulsation ventricular assist system (0455T-0458T)

🔧 20.6   ⚕ 20.6   **FUD** 090   Ⓒ

AMA: 2016,Mar,5; 2016,Jan,13; 2015,Jul,3; 2015,Jan,16; 2014,Jan,11

33973 **Insertion of intra-aortic balloon assist device through the ascending aorta**

EXCLUDES   Insertion/replacement of implantable aortic counterpulsation ventricular assist system (0451T-0454T)

🔧 15.0   ⚕ 15.0   **FUD** 000   Ⓒ 80 ▢

AMA: 2016,Mar,5; 2016,Jan,13; 2015,Sep,3; 2015,Jul,3; 2015,Jan,16; 2014,Jan,11; 2013,Mar,10-11

33974 **Removal of intra-aortic balloon assist device from the ascending aorta, including repair of the ascending aorta, with or without graft**

EXCLUDES   Removal of implantable aortic counterpulsation ventricular assist system (0455T-0458T)

🔧 25.8   ⚕ 25.8   **FUD** 090   Ⓒ ▢

AMA: 2016,Mar,5; 2016,Jan,13; 2015,Jul,3; 2015,Jan,16; 2014,Jan,11

33975 **Insertion of ventricular assist device; extracorporeal, single ventricle**

INCLUDES   Insertion of the new pump with de-airing, connection, and initiation

Removal of the old pump with replacement of the entire ventricular assist device system, including pump(s) and cannulas

Transthoracic approach

EXCLUDES   Percutaneous approach (33990-33991)

Replacement percutaneous transseptal approach (33999)

Code also removal of thrombus through a separate heart incision, when performed (33310-33315); append modifier 59 to (33315)

🔧 38.4   ⚕ 38.4   **FUD** XXX   Ⓒ 80 ▢

AMA: 2016,Mar,5; 2016,Jan,13; 2015,Jul,3; 2015,Jan,16; 2014,Jan,11; 2013,Mar,10-11; 2012,Jan,15-42; 2011,Jan,11

33976 **extracorporeal, biventricular**

 INCLUDES Insertion of the new pump with de-airing, connection, and initiation

  Removal with replacement of the entire ventricular assist device system, including pump(s) and cannulas

  Transthoracic approach

 EXCLUDES *Percutaneous approach (33990-33991)*

  Replacement percutaneous transseptal approach (33999)

  Code also removal of thrombus through a separate heart incision, when performed (33310-33315); append modifier 59 to (33315)

 🚑 46.8 ⚒ 46.8 **FUD** XXX C 80 📁

 AMA: 2016,Mar,5; 2016,Jan,13; 2015,Jul,3; 2015,Jan,16; 2014,Jan,11; 2013,Mar,10-11; 2012,Jan,15-42

33977 **Removal of ventricular assist device; extracorporeal, single ventricle**

 INCLUDES Removal of the entire device and the cannulas

 EXCLUDES *Removal of ventricular assist device when performed at the same time of insertion of a new device*

  Replacement percutaneous transseptal approach (33999)

  Code also removal of thrombus through a separate heart incision, when performed (33310-33315); append modifier 59 to (33315)

 🚑 32.9 ⚒ 32.9 **FUD** XXX C 80 📁

 AMA: 2016,Mar,5; 2016,Jan,13; 2015,Jul,3; 2015,Jan,16; 2014,Jan,11; 2013,Mar,10-11; 2012,Jan,15-42

33978 **extracorporeal, biventricular**

 INCLUDES Removal of the entire device and the cannulas

 EXCLUDES *Removal of ventricular assist device when performed at the same time of insertion of a new device*

  Replacement percutaneous transseptal approach (33999)

  Code also removal of thrombus through a separate heart incision, when performed (33310-33315); append modifier 59 to (33315)

 🚑 39.0 ⚒ 39.0 **FUD** XXX C 80 📁

 AMA: 2016,Mar,5; 2016,Jan,13; 2015,Jul,3; 2015,Jan,16; 2014,Jan,11; 2013,Mar,10-11; 2012,Jan,15-42

33979 **Insertion of ventricular assist device, implantable intracorporeal, single ventricle**

 INCLUDES New pump insertion with connection, de-airing, and initiation

  Removal with replacement of the entire ventricular assist device system, including pump(s) and cannulas

  Transthoracic approach

 EXCLUDES *Insertion/replacement of implantable aortic counterpulsation ventricular assist system (0451T-0454T)*

  Percutaneous approach (33990-33991)

  Replacement percutaneous transseptal approach (33999)

  Code also removal of thrombus through a separate heart incision, when performed (33310-33315); append modifier 59 to (33315)

 🚑 57.0 ⚒ 57.0 **FUD** XXX C 80 📁

 AMA: 2016,Mar,5; 2016,Jan,13; 2015,Jul,3; 2015,Jan,16; 2014,Jan,11; 2013,Mar,10-11; 2012,Jan,15-42

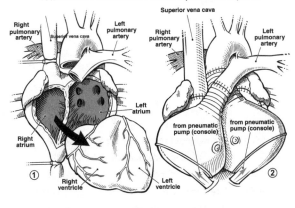

Total Internal Biventricular Heart Replacement System

33980 **Removal of ventricular assist device, implantable intracorporeal, single ventricle**

 INCLUDES Removal of the entire device and the cannulas

 EXCLUDES *Removal of implantable aortic counterpulsation ventricular assist system (0455T-0458T)*

  Removal of ventricular assist device when performed at the same time of insertion of a new device

  Percutaneous transseptal approach (33999)

  Code also removal of thrombus through a separate heart incision, when performed (33310-33315); append modifier 59 to (33315)

 🚑 52.1 ⚒ 52.1 **FUD** XXX C 80 📁

 AMA: 2016,Mar,5; 2016,Jan,13; 2015,Jul,3; 2015,Jan,16; 2014,Jan,11; 2013,Mar,10-11

33981 **Replacement of extracorporeal ventricular assist device, single or biventricular, pump(s), single or each pump**

 INCLUDES Insertion of the new pump with de-airing, connection, and initiation

  Removal of the old pump

 EXCLUDES *Percutaneous transseptal approach (33999)*

 🚑 24.4 ⚒ 24.4 **FUD** XXX C 80 📁

 AMA: 2016,Mar,5; 2016,Jan,13; 2015,Jul,3; 2015,Jan,16; 2014,Jan,11

33982 **Replacement of ventricular assist device pump(s); implantable intracorporeal, single ventricle, without cardiopulmonary bypass**

 INCLUDES New pump insertion with connection, de-airing, and initiation

  Removal of the old pump

 EXCLUDES *Percutaneous transseptal approach (33999)*

 🚑 57.8 ⚒ 57.8 **FUD** XXX C 80 📁

 AMA: 2016,Mar,5; 2016,Jan,13; 2015,Jul,3; 2015,Jan,16; 2014,Jan,11

● New Code ▲ Revised Code ○ Reinstated ● New Web Release ▲ Revised Web Release Unlisted Not Covered # Resequenced

⊘ AMA Mod 51 Exempt ⑤ Optum Mod 51 Exempt ⑥ Mod 63 Exempt ⁄ Non-FDA Drug ★ Telehealth M Maternity A Age Edit + Add-on **AMA:** CPT Asst

© 2016 Optum360, LLC CPT © 2016 American Medical Association. All Rights Reserved. **137**

33983   **implantable intracorporeal, single ventricle, with cardiopulmonary bypass**

INCLUDES   Insertion of the new pump with de-airing, connection, and initiation
Removal of the old pump

EXCLUDES   *Insertion/replacement of implantable aortic counterpulsation ventricular assist system (0451T-0454T)*
Percutaneous transseptal approach (33999)

🚑 67.6   🔧 67.6   **FUD** XXX   C 80 ▣

AMA: 2016,Mar,5; 2016,Jan,13; 2015,Jul,3; 2015,Jan,16; 2014,Jan,11

33984   Resequenced code. See code following 33959.

33985   Resequenced code. See code following 33959.

33986   Resequenced code. See code following 33959.

33987   Resequenced code. See code following 33959.

33988   Resequenced code. See code following 33959.

33989   Resequenced code. See code following 33959.

▲ **33990**   **Insertion of ventricular assist device, percutaneous including radiological supervision and interpretation; arterial access only**

INCLUDES   Initial insertion and replacement of percutaneous ventricular assist device

EXCLUDES   *Extensive artery repair/replacement (35226, 35286)*
Open arterial approach to aid insertion of percutaneous ventricular assist device, when used (34812)
Removal of percutaneous ventricular assist device at time of replacement of the entire system (33992)
Transthoracic approach (33975-33976)

🚑 12.8   🔧 12.8   **FUD** XXX   C 80 ▣

AMA: 2016,Mar,5; 2016,Jan,13; 2015,Sep,3; 2015,Jan,16; 2014,Oct,14; 2014,Jan,11; 2013,Mar,10-11

▲ **33991**   **both arterial and venous access, with transseptal puncture**

INCLUDES   Initial insertion as well as replacement of percutaneous ventricular assist device

EXCLUDES   *Extensive artery repair/replacement (35226, 35286)*
Insertion/replacement of implantable aortic counterpulsation ventricular assist system (0451T-0454T)
Open arterial approach to aid with insertion of percutaneous ventricular assist device, when performed (34812)
Removal of percutaneous ventricular assist device at time of replacement of the entire system (33992)
Transthoracic approach (33975-33976)

🚑 18.6   🔧 18.6   **FUD** XXX   C 80 ▣

AMA: 2016,Mar,5; 2016,Jan,13; 2015,Sep,3; 2015,Jan,16; 2014,Jan,11; 2013,Mar,10-11

▲ **33992**   **Removal of percutaneous ventricular assist device at separate and distinct session from insertion**

INCLUDES   Removal of device and cannulas

EXCLUDES   *Removal of implantable aortic counterpulsation ventricular assist system (0455T-0458T)*

Code also modifier 59 when percutaneous ventricular assist device is removed on the same day as the insertion, but at a different session

🚑 6.05   🔧 6.05   **FUD** XXX   C 80 ▣

AMA: 2016,Mar,5; 2016,Jan,13; 2015,Sep,3; 2015,Jan,16; 2014,Jan,11; 2013,Mar,10-11

▲ **33993**   **Repositioning of percutaneous ventricular assist device with imaging guidance at separate and distinct session from insertion**

EXCLUDES   *Repositioning of a percutaneous ventricular assist device without image guidance*
Repositioning of device/electrode (0460T-0461T)
Repositioning of the percutaneous ventricular assist device at the same session as the insertion (33990-33991)
Skin pocket relocation with replacement implantable aortic counterpulsation ventricular assist device and electrodes (0459T)

Code also modifier 59 when percutaneous ventricular assist device is repositioned using imaging guidance on the same day as the insertion, but at a different session

🚑 5.31   🔧 5.31   **FUD** XXX   C 80 ▣

AMA: 2016,Mar,5; 2016,Jan,13; 2015,Sep,3; 2015,Jan,16; 2014,Jan,11; 2013,Mar,10-11

33999   **Unlisted procedure, cardiac surgery**

🚑 0.00   🔧 0.00   **FUD** YYY   T 80

AMA: 2016,May,5; 2016,Jan,13; 2015,Jan,16; 2014,Dec,16; 2014,Dec,16; 2014,Jan,11; 2013,Dec,14; 2013,Mar,10-11; 2013,Feb,13; 2012,Jan,15-42; 2011,Jan,11

34001-34530 Surgical Revascularization: Veins and Arteries

INCLUDES   Repair of blood vessel
Surgeon's component of operative arteriogram

34001   **Embolectomy or thrombectomy, with or without catheter; carotid, subclavian or innominate artery, by neck incision**

🚑 28.7   🔧 28.7   **FUD** 090   C 80 50 ▣

AMA: 1997,Nov,1

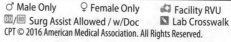

Subclavian artery · Axillary artery · Major arteries of the arm · Brachial artery · Superior ulnar collateral · Posterior ulnar recurrent · Radial artery · Ulnar artery · Common interosseous · Aorto-femoral artery · Femoral and deep femoral branches · Popliteal artery · Peroneal artery · Major arteries of the leg · Anterior tibial artery · Posterior tibial artery · Arteries (red) are usually accompanied by at least one vein (blue)

34051   **innominate, subclavian artery, by thoracic incision**

🚑 28.9   🔧 28.9   **FUD** 090   C 80 50 ▣

AMA: 1997,Nov,1

34101   **axillary, brachial, innominate, subclavian artery, by arm incision**

🚑 17.7   🔧 17.7   **FUD** 090   T 80 50 ▣

AMA: 1997,Nov,1

34111   **radial or ulnar artery, by arm incision**

🚑 17.7   🔧 17.7   **FUD** 090   T 80 50 ▣

AMA: 1997,Nov,1

34151   **renal, celiac, mesentery, aortoiliac artery, by abdominal incision**

🚑 41.3   🔧 41.3   **FUD** 090   C 80 50 ▣

AMA: 1997,Nov,1

34201   **femoropopliteal, aortoiliac artery, by leg incision**

🚑 30.5   🔧 30.5   **FUD** 090   T 80 50 ▣

AMA: 2016,Jan,13; 2015,Jan,16; 2014,Jan,11; 2012,Jan,15-42; 2011,Aug,9-10

34203   **popliteal-tibio-peroneal artery, by leg incision**

🚑 28.2   🔧 28.2   **FUD** 090   T 80 50 ▣

AMA: 1997,Nov,1

34401 Thrombectomy, direct or with catheter; vena cava, iliac vein, by abdominal incision
🔧 42.6 ✂ 42.6 **FUD** 090 C 80 50 ▣
AMA: 1997,Nov,1

34421 vena cava, iliac, femoropopliteal vein, by leg incision
🔧 21.5 ✂ 21.5 **FUD** 090 T 80 50 ▣
AMA: 2016,Jan,13; 2015,Jan,16; 2014,Jan,11

34451 vena cava, iliac, femoropopliteal vein, by abdominal and leg incision
🔧 42.6 ✂ 42.6 **FUD** 090 C 80 50 ▣
AMA: 1997,Nov,1

34471 subclavian vein, by neck incision
🔧 31.9 ✂ 31.9 **FUD** 090 T 50 ▣
AMA: 1997,Nov,1

34490 axillary and subclavian vein, by arm incision
🔧 17.9 ✂ 17.9 **FUD** 090 T 62 50 ▣
AMA: 1997,Nov,1

34501 Valvuloplasty, femoral vein
🔧 28.7 ✂ 28.7 **FUD** 090 T 80 50 ▣
AMA: 1997,Nov,1

34502 Reconstruction of vena cava, any method
🔧 45.0 ✂ 45.0 **FUD** 090 C 80 ▣
AMA: 1997,Nov,1

34510 Venous valve transposition, any vein donor
🔧 34.9 ✂ 34.9 **FUD** 090 T 80 50 ▣
AMA: 1997,Nov,1

34520 Cross-over vein graft to venous system
🔧 29.6 ✂ 29.6 **FUD** 090 T 80 50 ▣
AMA: 1997,Nov,1

34530 Saphenopopliteal vein anastomosis
🔧 32.1 ✂ 32.1 **FUD** 090 T 80 50 ▣
AMA: 1997,Nov,1

34800-34834 Endovascular Stent Grafting for Abdominal Aneurysms

INCLUDES Balloon angioplasty/stent deployment within the target treatment zone
Introduction, manipulation, placement, and deployment of the device
Open exposure of femoral or iliac artery/subsequent closure
Thromboendarterectomy at site of aneurysm

EXCLUDES Additional interventional procedures outside of target treatment zone
Guidewire and catheter insertion (36140, 36200, 36245-36248)
Study, interpretation, and report of implanted wireless pressure sensor in an aneurysmal sac (93982)
Substantial artery repair/replacement (35226, 35286)
Transcatheter insertion of wireless physiologic sensor in an aneurysmal sac (34806)

34800 Endovascular repair of infrarenal abdominal aortic aneurysm or dissection; using aorto-aortic tube prosthesis
🔧 33.4 ✂ 33.4 **FUD** 090 C 80 ▣
AMA: 2016,Jan,13; 2015,Jan,16; 2014,Jan,11; 2013,Dec,8; 2012,Apr,3-9; 2012,Jan,15-42; 2011,Jan,11

Abdominal aorta — Renal arteries
Tube prosthesis
Infrarenal aneurysm — Iliac arteries
Unibody bifurcated device
Main aortic prosthesis
Single limb modular device

34802 using modular bifurcated prosthesis (1 docking limb)
🔧 36.8 ✂ 36.8 **FUD** 090 C 80 ▣
AMA: 2016,Jan,13; 2015,Jan,16; 2014,Jan,11; 2013,Dec,8; 2012,Apr,3-9; 2012,Jan,15-42; 2011,Jan,11

34803 using modular bifurcated prosthesis (2 docking limbs)
EXCLUDES Endovascular repair of visceral aorta (34841-34848)
Code also open arterial exposure as appropriate (34812, 34820, 34833, 34834)
🔄 (75952)
🔧 38.0 ✂ 38.0 **FUD** 090 C 80 ▣
AMA: 2016,Jan,13; 2015,Jan,16; 2014,Jan,11; 2013,Dec,8; 2012,Apr,3-9

34804 using unibody bifurcated prosthesis
EXCLUDES Endovascular repair of visceral aorta (34841-34848)
Code also open arterial exposure as appropriate (34812, 34820, 34833, 34834)
🔄 (75952)
🔧 36.8 ✂ 36.8 **FUD** 090 C 80 ▣
AMA: 2016,Jan,13; 2015,Jan,16; 2014,Jan,11; 2013,Dec,8; 2012,Apr,3-9

34805 using aorto-uniiliac or aorto-unifemoral prosthesis
EXCLUDES Endovascular repair of visceral aorta (34841-34848)
Code also open arterial exposure as appropriate (34812, 34820, 34833, 34834)
🔄 (75952)
🔧 35.2 ✂ 35.2 **FUD** 090 C 80 ▣
AMA: 2016,Jan,13; 2015,Jan,16; 2014,Jan,11; 2013,Dec,8; 2012,Apr,3-9; 2012,Jan,15-42; 2011,Jan,11

+ **34806** Transcatheter placement of wireless physiologic sensor in aneurysmal sac during endovascular repair, including radiological supervision and interpretation, instrument calibration, and collection of pressure data (List separately in addition to code for primary procedure)
EXCLUDES Noninvasive physiologic study of implanted wireless pressure sensor in aneurysmal sac following endovascular repair (93982)
Code also open arterial exposure as appropriate (34812, 34820, 34833-34834)
Code first (33880-33881, 33886, 34800-34805, 34825, 34900)
🔧 2.96 ✂ 2.96 **FUD** ZZZ C 80 ▣
AMA: 2016,Jan,13; 2015,Jan,16; 2014,Jan,11; 2012,Apr,3-9

+ **34808** Endovascular placement of iliac artery occlusion device (List separately in addition to code for primary procedure)
Code also open arterial exposure as appropriate (34812, 34820, 34833-34834)
Code first (34800, 34805, 34813, 34825-34826)
🔧 6.12 ✂ 6.12 **FUD** ZZZ C 80 ▣
AMA: 2016,Jan,13; 2015,Jan,16; 2014,Jan,11; 2012,Apr,3-9

34812 Open femoral artery exposure for delivery of endovascular prosthesis, by groin incision, unilateral
EXCLUDES ECMO/ECLS insertion, removal or repositioning (33953-33954, 33959, [33962], [33969], [33984])
Code also as appropriate (34800-34808)
🔧 9.97 ✂ 9.97 **FUD** 000 C 80 50 ▣
AMA: 2016,Jan,13; 2015,Jul,3; 2015,Jan,16; 2014,Jan,11; 2013,Dec,8; 2013,Mar,10-11; 2012,Apr,3-9; 2012,Jan,15-42; 2011,Jan,11

+ **34813** Placement of femoral-femoral prosthetic graft during endovascular aortic aneurysm repair (List separately in addition to code for primary procedure)
EXCLUDES Grafting of femoral artery (35521, 35533, 35539, 35540, 35556, 35558, 35566, 35621, 35646, 35654-35661, 35666, 35700)
Code first (34812)
🔧 7.00 ✂ 7.00 **FUD** ZZZ C 80 ▣
AMA: 2016,Jan,13; 2015,Jan,16; 2014,Jan,11; 2012,Apr,3-9

34820 Open iliac artery exposure for delivery of endovascular prosthesis or iliac occlusion during endovascular therapy, by abdominal or retroperitoneal incision, unilateral
EXCLUDES ECMO/ECLS insertion, removal or repositioning (33953-33954, 33959, [33962], [33969], [33984])
Code also as appropriate (34800-34808)
🔧 14.5 ✂ 14.5 **FUD** 000 C 80 50 ▣
AMA: 2016,Jan,13; 2015,Jul,3; 2015,Jan,16; 2014,Jan,11; 2012,Apr,3-9; 2012,Jan,15-42; 2011,Jan,11

34825 Placement of proximal or distal extension prosthesis for endovascular repair of infrarenal abdominal aortic or iliac aneurysm, false aneurysm, or dissection; initial vessel

Code also as appropriate (34800-34805, 34900)
☒ (75953)
⚕ 20.5 ✄ 20.5 **FUD** 090   C 80 ▭

AMA: 2016,Jan,13; 2015,Jan,16; 2014,Jan,11; 2013,Dec,8; 2012,Apr,3-9

+ 34826 each additional vessel (List separately in addition to code for primary procedure)

Code also as appropriate (34800-34805, 34900)
Code first (34825)
☒ (75953)
⚕ 6.07 ✄ 6.07 **FUD** ZZZ   C 80 ▭

AMA: 2016,Jan,13; 2015,Jan,16; 2014,Jan,11; 2013,Dec,8; 2012,Apr,3-9

34830 Open repair of infrarenal aortic aneurysm or dissection, plus repair of associated arterial trauma, following unsuccessful endovascular repair; tube prosthesis

⚕ 52.1 ✄ 52.1 **FUD** 090   C 80 ▭

AMA: 2016,Jan,13; 2015,Jan,16; 2014,Jan,11; 2012,Jan,15-42; 2011,Jan,11

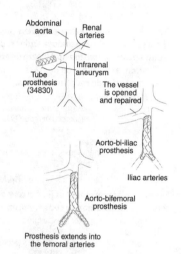

Abdominal aorta
Renal arteries
Tube prosthesis (34830)
Infrarenal aneurysm
The vessel is opened and repaired
Aorto-bi-iliac prosthesis
Iliac arteries
Aorto-bifemoral prosthesis
Prosthesis extends into the femoral arteries

An infrarenal aortic aneurysm or dissection is treated in an open surgical session following an unsuccessful endovascular treatment attempt. A tube prosthesis is placed and any associated arterial trauma is repaired

34831 aorto-bi-iliac prosthesis
⚕ 56.2 ✄ 56.2 **FUD** 090   C 80 ▭

AMA: 2016,Jan,13; 2015,Jan,16; 2014,Jan,11; 2012,Jan,15-42; 2011,Jan,11

34832 aorto-bifemoral prosthesis
⚕ 55.8 ✄ 55.8 **FUD** 090   C 80 ▭

AMA: 2016,Jan,13; 2015,Jan,16; 2014,Jan,11; 2012,Jan,15-42; 2011,Jan,11

34833 Open iliac artery exposure with creation of conduit for delivery of aortic or iliac endovascular prosthesis, by abdominal or retroperitoneal incision, unilateral

EXCLUDES *Arterial exposure with creation of graft conduit (eg, chimney graft) to facilitate arterial perfusion for ECMO/ECLS ([33987])*
Open iliac artery exposure for delivery of endovascular prosthesis or iliac occlusion during endovascular therapy (34820)
Code also as appropriate (34800-34805)
⚕ 17.9 ✄ 17.9 **FUD** 000   C 80 50 ▭

AMA: 2016,Jan,13; 2015,Jul,3; 2015,Jan,16; 2014,Jan,11; 2012,Jan,15-42; 2011,Jan,11

34834 Open brachial artery exposure to assist in the deployment of aortic or iliac endovascular prosthesis by arm incision, unilateral

EXCLUDES *ECMO/ECLS insertion, removal or repositioning (33953-33954, 33959, [33962], [33969], [33984])*
Code also as appropriate (34800-34805)
⚕ 8.06 ✄ 8.06 **FUD** 000   C 80 50 ▭

AMA: 2016,Jan,13; 2015,Jul,3; 2015,Jan,16; 2014,Jan,11

34839-34848 Repair Visceral Aorta with Fenestrated Endovascular Grafts

INCLUDES
Angiography
Balloon angioplasty before and after deployment of graft
Fluoroscopic guidance
Guidewire and catheter insertion of vessels in the target treatment zone
Radiologic supervision and interpretation
Visceral aorta (34841-34844)
Visceral aorta and associated infrarenal abdominal aorta (34845-34848)

EXCLUDES *Catheterization of:*
Arterial families outside treatment zone
Hypogastric arteries
Distal extension prosthesis terminating in the common femoral, external iliac, or internal iliac artery (34825-34826, 75953, 0254T-0255T)
Insertion of bare metal or covered intravascular stents in visceral branches in the target treatment zone (37236-37237)
Interventional procedures outside treatment zone
Open exposure of access vessels (34812)
Repair of abdominal aortic aneurysm without a fenestrated graft (34800-34805)
Substantial artery repair (35226, 35286)
Code also associated endovascular repair of descending thoracic aorta (33880-33886, 75956-75959)

34839 Physician planning of a patient-specific fenestrated visceral aortic endograft requiring a minimum of 90 minutes of physician time

⚕ 0.00 ✄ 0.00 **FUD** YYY   B 80 ▭

EXCLUDES *3D rendering with interpretation and reporting of imaging (76376-76377)*
Endovascular repair procedure on day of or day after planning (34841-34848)
Planning on day of or day before endovascular repair procedure
Total planning time of less than 90 minutes

34841 Endovascular repair of visceral aorta (eg, aneurysm, pseudoaneurysm, dissection, penetrating ulcer, intramural hematoma, or traumatic disruption) by deployment of a fenestrated visceral aortic endograft and all associated radiological supervision and interpretation, including target zone angioplasty, when performed; including one visceral artery endoprosthesis (superior mesenteric, celiac or renal artery)

INCLUDES *Repairs extending from the visceral aorta to one or more of the four visceral artery origins to the level of the infrarenal aorta*
EXCLUDES *Endovascular repair of aorta (34800, 34802-34805, 34845-34848)*
Physician planning of a patient-specific fenestrated visceral aortic endograft (34839)
Radiological supervision and interpretation, endovascular repair, aorta (75952)
⚕ 0.00 ✄ 0.00 **FUD** YYY   C 80 ▭

AMA: 2016,Jan,13; 2015,Jan,16; 2014,Jan,11; 2013,Dec,8

34842 including two visceral artery endoprostheses (superior mesenteric, celiac and/or renal artery[s])

INCLUDES *Repairs extending from the visceral aorta to one or more of the four visceral artery origins to the level of the infrarenal aorta*
EXCLUDES *Endovascular repair of aorta (34800, 34802-34805, 34845-34848)*
Physician planning of a patient-specific fenestrated visceral aortic endograft (34839)
Radiological supervision and interpretation, endovascular repair, aorta (75952)
⚕ 0.00 ✄ 0.00 **FUD** YYY   C 80 ▭

AMA: 2016,Jan,13; 2015,Jan,16; 2014,Jan,11; 2013,Dec,8

26/TC PC/TC Only   A2-Z3 ASC Payment   50 Bilateral   ♂ Male Only   ♀ Female Only   ⚕ Facility RVU   ✄ Non-Facility RVU   ▭ CCI
FUD Follow-up Days   CMS: IOM (Pub 100)   A-Y OPPSI   80/80 Surg Assist Allowed / w/Doc   ☒ Lab Crosswalk   ☒ Radiology Crosswalk   ☒ CLIA

140

34843 including three visceral artery endoprostheses (superior mesenteric, celiac and/or renal artery[s])

> INCLUDES   Repairs extending from the visceral aorta to one or more of the four visceral artery origins to the level of the infrarenal aorta
>
> EXCLUDES   *Endovascular repair of aorta (34800, 34802-34805, 34845-34848)*
> *Physician planning of a patient-specific fenestrated visceral aortic endograft (34839)*
> *Radiological supervision and interpretation, endovascular repair, aorta (75952)*

🚑 0.00   🔧 0.00   **FUD** YYY   C 80 🖥

AMA: 2016,Jan,13; 2015,Jan,16; 2014,Jan,11; 2013,Dec,8

34844 including four or more visceral artery endoprostheses (superior mesenteric, celiac and/or renal artery[s])

> INCLUDES   Repairs extending from the visceral aorta to one or more of the four visceral artery origins to the level of the infrarenal aorta
>
> EXCLUDES   *Endovascular repair of aorta (34800, 34802-34805, 34845-34848)*
> *Physician planning of a patient-specific fenestrated visceral aortic endograft (34839)*
> *Radiological supervision and interpretation, endovascular repair, aorta (75952)*

🚑 0.00   🔧 0.00   **FUD** YYY   C 80 🖥

AMA: 2016,Jan,13; 2015,Jan,16; 2014,Jan,11; 2013,Dec,8

34845 Endovascular repair of visceral aorta and infrarenal abdominal aorta (eg, aneurysm, pseudoaneurysm, dissection, penetrating ulcer, intramural hematoma, or traumatic disruption) with a fenestrated visceral aortic endograft and concomitant unibody or modular infrarenal aortic endograft and all associated radiological supervision and interpretation, including target zone angioplasty, when performed; including one visceral artery endoprosthesis (superior mesenteric, celiac or renal artery)

> INCLUDES   Placement of device and extensions into the common iliac arteries
> Repairs extending from the visceral aorta into the common iliac arteries
>
> EXCLUDES   *Direct repair aneurysm (35081, 35102)*
> *Endovascular repair of aorta (34800, 34802-34805, 34841-34844)*
> *Physician planning of a patient-specific fenestrated visceral aortic endograft (34839)*
> *Radiological supervision and interpretation, endovascular repair, aorta (75952)*

Code also iliac artery revascularization when performed outside zone of target treatment (37220-37223)

🚑 0.00   🔧 0.00   **FUD** YYY   C 80 🖥

AMA: 2016,Jan,13; 2015,Jan,16; 2014,Jan,11; 2013,Dec,8

34846 including two visceral artery endoprostheses (superior mesenteric, celiac and/or renal artery[s])

> INCLUDES   Placement of device and extensions into the common iliac arteries
> Repairs extending from the visceral aorta into the common iliac arteries
>
> EXCLUDES   *Direct repair aneurysm (35081, 35102)*
> *Endovascular repair of aorta (34800, 34802-34805, 34841-34844)*
> *Physician planning of a patient-specific fenestrated visceral aortic endograft (34839)*
> *Radiological supervision and interpretation, endovascular repair, aorta (75952)*

Code also iliac artery revascularization when performed outside zone of target treatment (37220-37223)

🚑 0.00   🔧 0.00   **FUD** YYY   C 80 🖥

AMA: 2016,Jan,13; 2015,Jan,16; 2014,Jan,11; 2013,Dec,8

34847 including three visceral artery endoprostheses (superior mesenteric, celiac and/or renal artery[s])

> INCLUDES   Placement of device and extensions into the common iliac arteries
> Repairs extending from the visceral aorta into the common iliac arteries
>
> EXCLUDES   *Direct repair aneurysm (35081, 35102)*
> *Endovascular repair of aorta (34800, 34802-34805, 34841-34844)*
> *Physician planning of a patient-specific fenestrated visceral aortic endograft (34839)*
> *Radiological supervision and interpretation, endovascular repair, aorta (75952)*

Code also iliac artery revascularization when performed outside zone of target treatment (37220-37223)

🚑 0.00   🔧 0.00   **FUD** YYY   C 80 🖥

AMA: 2016,Jan,13; 2015,Jan,16; 2014,Jan,11; 2013,Dec,8

34848 including four or more visceral artery endoprostheses (superior mesenteric, celiac and/or renal artery[s])

> INCLUDES   Placement of device and extensions into the common iliac arteries
> Repairs extending from the visceral aorta into the common iliac arteries
>
> EXCLUDES   *Direct repair aneurysm (35081, 35102)*
> *Endovascular repair of aorta (34800, 34802-34805, 34841-34844)*
> *Physician planning of a patient-specific fenestrated visceral aortic endograft (34839)*
> *Radiological supervision and interpretation, endovascular repair, aorta (75952)*

Code also iliac artery revascularization when performed outside zone of target treatment (37220-37223)

🚑 0.00   🔧 0.00   **FUD** YYY   C 80 🖥

AMA: 2016,Jul,6; 2016,Jan,13; 2015,Jan,16; 2014,Jan,11; 2013,Dec,8

34900 Endovascular Stent Grafting Iliac Artery

> INCLUDES   Balloon angioplasty/stent deployment within the target treatment zone
> Introduction, manipulation, placement, and deployment
>
> EXCLUDES   *Endovascular repair of iliac artery bifurcation (e.g., aneurysm, arteriovenous malformation, pseudoaneurysm, trauma) using bifurcated endoprosthesis (0254T)*
> *Insertion guidewires, catheters (36200, 36245-36248)*
> *Open exposure femoral or iliac artery (34812, 34820)*
> *Other concurrent interventional procedures outside of target zone*
> *Placement extension prosthesis (34825-34826)*
> *Substantial artery repair/replacement (35206-35286)*
> *Supervision and interpretation for placement distal extension prosthesis (75953)*

34900 Endovascular repair of iliac artery (eg, aneurysm, pseudoaneurysm, arteriovenous malformation, trauma) using ilio-iliac tube endoprosthesis

> 📷 (75954)

🚑 26.4   🔧 26.4   **FUD** 090   C 80 50 🖥

AMA: 2016,Jan,13; 2015,Jan,16; 2014,Jan,11; 2012,Apr,3-9

35001-35152 Repair Aneurysm, False Aneurysm, Related Arterial Disease

> INCLUDES   Endarterectomy procedures
>
> EXCLUDES   *Endovascular repairs of:*
> *Abdominal aortic aneurysm (34800-34826)*
> *Aneurysm of iliac artery (34900)*
> *Thoracic aortic aneurysm (33880-33891)*
> *Intracranial aneurysms (61697-61710)*
> *Open repairs thoracic aortic aneurysm (33860-33875)*
> *Repairs related to occlusive disease only (35201-35286)*

35001 Direct repair of aneurysm, pseudoaneurysm, or excision (partial or total) and graft insertion, with or without patch graft; for aneurysm and associated occlusive disease, carotid, subclavian artery, by neck incision

🚑 33.1   🔧 33.1   **FUD** 090   C 80 50 🖥

AMA: 2002,May,7; 2000,Dec,1

35002 for ruptured aneurysm, carotid, subclavian artery, by neck incision

🚗 33.6   ⚕ 33.6   **FUD** 090   C 80 50 ▱

AMA: 2002,May,7; 1997,Nov,1

35005 for aneurysm, pseudoaneurysm, and associated occlusive disease, vertebral artery

🚗 31.9   ⚕ 31.9   **FUD** 090   C 80 50 ▱

AMA: 2002,May,7; 1997,Nov,1

An incision is made in the back of the neck to directly approach an aneurysm or false aneurysm of the vertebral artery. The artery is either repaired directly or excised with a graft

Graft repair

Vertebral artery

Subclavian artery

35011 for aneurysm and associated occlusive disease, axillary-brachial artery, by arm incision

🚗 29.6   ⚕ 29.6   **FUD** 090   T 80 50 ▱

AMA: 2002,May,7; 1997,Nov,1

35013 for ruptured aneurysm, axillary-brachial artery, by arm incision

🚗 37.0   ⚕ 37.0   **FUD** 090   C 80 50 ▱

AMA: 2002,May,7; 1997,Nov,1

35021 for aneurysm, pseudoaneurysm, and associated occlusive disease, innominate, subclavian artery, by thoracic incision

🚗 36.7   ⚕ 36.7   **FUD** 090   C 80 50 ▱

AMA: 2002,May,7; 1997,Nov,1

35022 for ruptured aneurysm, innominate, subclavian artery, by thoracic incision

🚗 40.9   ⚕ 40.9   **FUD** 090   C 80 50 ▱

AMA: 2002,May,7; 1997,Nov,1

35045 for aneurysm, pseudoaneurysm, and associated occlusive disease, radial or ulnar artery

🚗 29.3   ⚕ 29.3   **FUD** 090   T 80 50 ▱

AMA: 2002,May,7; 1997,Nov,1

35081 for aneurysm, pseudoaneurysm, and associated occlusive disease, abdominal aorta

🚗 51.7   ⚕ 51.7   **FUD** 090   C 80 ▱

AMA: 2016,Jan,13; 2015,Jan,16; 2014,Jan,11; 2013,Dec,8; 2012,Jan,15-42; 2011,Jan,11

35082 for ruptured aneurysm, abdominal aorta

🚗 64.9   ⚕ 64.9   **FUD** 090   C 80 ▱

AMA: 2002,May,7; 1997,Nov,1

35091 for aneurysm, pseudoaneurysm, and associated occlusive disease, abdominal aorta involving visceral vessels (mesenteric, celiac, renal)

🚗 53.0   ⚕ 53.0   **FUD** 090   C 80 50 ▱

AMA: 2016,Jan,13; 2015,Jan,16; 2014,Jan,11

35092 for ruptured aneurysm, abdominal aorta involving visceral vessels (mesenteric, celiac, renal)

🚗 76.9   ⚕ 76.9   **FUD** 090   C 80 50 ▱

AMA: 2002,May,7; 1997,Nov,1

35102 for aneurysm, pseudoaneurysm, and associated occlusive disease, abdominal aorta involving iliac vessels (common, hypogastric, external)

🚗 55.9   ⚕ 55.9   **FUD** 090   C 80 50 ▱

AMA: 2016,Jan,13; 2015,Jan,16; 2014,Jan,11; 2013,Dec,8

35103 for ruptured aneurysm, abdominal aorta involving iliac vessels (common, hypogastric, external)

🚗 66.4   ⚕ 66.4   **FUD** 090   C 80 50 ▱

AMA: 2002,May,7; 1997,Nov,1

35111 for aneurysm, pseudoaneurysm, and associated occlusive disease, splenic artery

🚗 44.9   ⚕ 44.9   **FUD** 090   C 80 50 ▱

AMA: 2002,May,7; 1997,Nov,1

35112 for ruptured aneurysm, splenic artery

🚗 54.1   ⚕ 54.1   **FUD** 090   C 80 50 ▱

AMA: 2002,May,7; 1997,Nov,1

35121 for aneurysm, pseudoaneurysm, and associated occlusive disease, hepatic, celiac, renal, or mesenteric artery

🚗 48.6   ⚕ 48.6   **FUD** 090   C 80 50 ▱

AMA: 2002,May,7; 1997,Nov,1

35122 for ruptured aneurysm, hepatic, celiac, renal, or mesenteric artery

🚗 63.1   ⚕ 63.1   **FUD** 090   C 80 50 ▱

AMA: 2002,May,7; 1997,Nov,1

35131 for aneurysm, pseudoaneurysm, and associated occlusive disease, iliac artery (common, hypogastric, external)

🚗 41.0   ⚕ 41.0   **FUD** 090   C 80 50 ▱

AMA: 2016,Jan,13; 2015,Jan,16; 2014,Jan,11

35132 for ruptured aneurysm, iliac artery (common, hypogastric, external)

🚗 48.2   ⚕ 48.2   **FUD** 090   C 80 50 ▱

AMA: 2002,May,7; 1997,Nov,1

35141 for aneurysm, pseudoaneurysm, and associated occlusive disease, common femoral artery (profunda femoris, superficial femoral)

🚗 32.7   ⚕ 32.7   **FUD** 090   C 80 50 ▱

AMA: 2002,May,7; 1997,Nov,1

35142 for ruptured aneurysm, common femoral artery (profunda femoris, superficial femoral)

🚗 39.1   ⚕ 39.1   **FUD** 090   C 80 50 ▱

AMA: 2002,May,7; 1997,Nov,1

35151 for aneurysm, pseudoaneurysm, and associated occlusive disease, popliteal artery

🚗 36.7   ⚕ 36.7   **FUD** 090   C 80 50 ▱

AMA: 2002,May,7; 1997,Nov,1

35152 for ruptured aneurysm, popliteal artery

🚗 41.4   ⚕ 41.4   **FUD** 090   C 80 50 ▱

AMA: 2002,May,7; 1997,Nov,1

35180-35190 Surgical Repair Arteriovenous Fistula

35180 Repair, congenital arteriovenous fistula; head and neck

🚗 27.3   ⚕ 27.3   **FUD** 090   T 80 ▱

AMA: 2016,Jan,13; 2015,Jan,16; 2014,Jan,11; 2012,Jan,15-42; 2011,Aug,9-10

35182 thorax and abdomen

🚗 52.3   ⚕ 52.3   **FUD** 090   C 80 ▱

AMA: 2016,Jan,13; 2015,Jan,16; 2014,Jan,11; 2012,Jan,15-42; 2011,Aug,9-10

35184 extremities

🚗 30.7   ⚕ 30.7   **FUD** 090   T 80 ▱

AMA: 2016,Jan,13; 2015,Jan,16; 2014,Jan,11; 2012,Jan,15-42; 2011,Aug,9-10

35188 Repair, acquired or traumatic arteriovenous fistula; head and neck

🚗 33.8   ⚕ 33.8   **FUD** 090   T A2 80 ▱

AMA: 2016,Jan,13; 2015,Jan,16; 2014,Jan,11; 2012,Jan,15-42; 2011,Aug,9-10

35189 thorax and abdomen

🚗 45.3   ⚕ 45.3   **FUD** 090   C 80 ▱

AMA: 2016,Jan,13; 2015,Jan,16; 2014,Jan,11; 2012,Jan,15-42; 2011,Aug,9-10

35190	**extremities**						T 80 🔲
	🔧 22.4	⚒ 22.4	**FUD** 090				

AMA: 2016,Jan,13; 2015,Jan,16; 2014,Jan,11; 2012,Jan,15-42; 2011,Aug,9-10

35201-35286 Surgical Repair Artery or Vein

EXCLUDES Arteriovenous fistula repair (35180-35190)
Primary open vascular procedures

35201	**Repair blood vessel, direct; neck**					T 80 50 🔲
	EXCLUDES Removal ECMO/ECLS of cannula ([33969, 33984, 33985, 33986])					
	🔧 27.9	⚒ 27.9	**FUD** 090			

AMA: 2016,Jan,13; 2015,Jul,3; 2015,Jan,16; 2014,Mar,8

35206	**upper extremity**					T 80 50 🔲
	EXCLUDES Removal ECMO/ECLS of cannula ([33969, 33984, 33985, 33986])					
	🔧 22.8	⚒ 22.8	**FUD** 090			

AMA: 2016,Jan,13; 2015,Jul,3; 2015,Jan,16; 2014,Apr,10; 2014,Jan,11; 2012,Apr,3-9

35207	**hand, finger**					T A2 50 🔲
	🔧 21.8	⚒ 21.8	**FUD** 090			

AMA: 2012,Apr,3-9

35211	**intrathoracic, with bypass**					C 80 50 🔲
	EXCLUDES Removal ECMO/ECLS of cannula ([33969, 33984, 33985, 33986])					
	🔧 40.2	⚒ 40.2	**FUD** 090			

AMA: 2015,Jul,3; 2012,Apr,3-9

35216	**intrathoracic, without bypass**					C 80 50 🔲
	EXCLUDES Removal ECMO/ECLS of cannula ([33969, 33984, 33985, 33986])					
	🔧 59.9	⚒ 59.9	**FUD** 090			

AMA: 2016,Jan,13; 2015,Jan,16; 2014,Jan,11; 2012,Apr,3-9

35221	**intra-abdominal**					C 80 50 🔲
	🔧 42.7	⚒ 42.7	**FUD** 090			

AMA: 2012,Apr,3-9

35226	**lower extremity**					T 80 50 🔲
	EXCLUDES Removal ECMO/ECLS of cannula ([33969, 33984, 33985, 33986])					
	🔧 24.5	⚒ 24.5	**FUD** 090			

AMA: 2016,Jul,6; 2016,Jan,13; 2015,Jul,3; 2015,Jan,16; 2014,Jan,11; 2013,Dec,8; 2013,Mar,10-11; 2012,Apr,3-9

35231	**Repair blood vessel with vein graft; neck**					T 80 50 🔲
	🔧 35.7	⚒ 35.7	**FUD** 090			

AMA: 2012,Apr,3-9

35236	**upper extremity**					T 80 50 🔲
	🔧 28.9	⚒ 28.9	**FUD** 090			

AMA: 2016,Jan,13; 2015,Jan,16; 2014,Jan,11; 2012,Apr,3-9

35241	**intrathoracic, with bypass**					C 80 50 🔲
	🔧 40.3	⚒ 40.3	**FUD** 090			

AMA: 2012,Apr,3-9

35246	**intrathoracic, without bypass**					C 80 50 🔲
	🔧 46.0	⚒ 46.0	**FUD** 090			

AMA: 2012,Apr,3-9

35251	**intra-abdominal**					C 80 50 🔲
	🔧 50.0	⚒ 50.0	**FUD** 090			

AMA: 2012,Apr,3-9

35256	**lower extremity**					T 80 50 🔲
	🔧 30.1	⚒ 30.1	**FUD** 090			

AMA: 2012,Apr,3-9

35261	**Repair blood vessel with graft other than vein; neck**					T 80 50 🔲
	🔧 31.2	⚒ 31.2	**FUD** 090			

AMA: 2012,Apr,3-9

35266	**upper extremity**					T 80 50 🔲
	🔧 25.7	⚒ 25.7	**FUD** 090			

AMA: 2016,Jan,13; 2015,Jan,16; 2014,Jan,11; 2012,Apr,3-9

35271	**intrathoracic, with bypass**					C 80 50 🔲
	🔧 40.1	⚒ 40.1	**FUD** 090			

AMA: 2012,Apr,3-9

35276	**intrathoracic, without bypass**					C 80 50 🔲
	🔧 42.5	⚒ 42.5	**FUD** 090			

AMA: 2012,Apr,3-9

35281	**intra-abdominal**					C 80 50 🔲
	🔧 47.7	⚒ 47.7	**FUD** 090			

AMA: 2012,Apr,3-9

35286	**lower extremity**					T 80 50 🔲
	🔧 27.6	⚒ 27.6	**FUD** 090			

AMA: 2016,Jul,6; 2016,Jan,13; 2015,Jan,16; 2014,Jan,11; 2013,Dec,8; 2013,Mar,10-11; 2012,Apr,3-9

35301-35372 Surgical Thromboendarterectomy Peripheral and Visceral Arteries

INCLUDES Obtaining saphenous or arm vein for graft
Thrombectomy/embolectomy

EXCLUDES Coronary artery bypass procedures (33510-33536, 33572)
Thromboendarterectomy for vascular occlusion on a different vessel during the same session

35301	**Thromboendarterectomy, including patch graft, if performed; carotid, vertebral, subclavian, by neck incision**					C 80 50 🔲
	🔧 33.5	⚒ 33.5	**FUD** 090			

AMA: 2016,Jan,13; 2015,Jan,16; 2014,Jan,11

Vertebral
Thrombus (blood clot)
External carotid
Carotid artery
Internal carotid
Subclavian artery
Aorta
Plaque
Tool to remove clot and/or plaque

35302	**superficial femoral artery**					C 80 50 🔲
	EXCLUDES Harvest of upper extremity vein, 1 segment, for lower extremity or coronary artery bypass procedure (35500)					
	Revascularization, endovascular, open or percutaneous, femoral, popliteal artery(s) (37225, 37227)					
	🔧 33.3	⚒ 33.3	**FUD** 090			

AMA: 2016,Jan,13; 2015,Jan,16; 2014,Jan,11

35303	**popliteal artery**					C 80 50 🔲
	EXCLUDES Harvest of upper extremity vein, 1 segment, for lower extremity or coronary artery bypass procedure (35500)					
	Revascularization, endovascular, open or percutaneous, femoral, popliteal artery(s) (37225, 37227)					
	🔧 36.8	⚒ 36.8	**FUD** 090			

AMA: 2016,Jan,13; 2015,Jan,16; 2014,Jan,11

35304	**tibioperoneal trunk artery**					C 80 50 🔲
	EXCLUDES Harvest of upper extremity vein, 1 segment, for lower extremity or coronary artery bypass procedure (35500)					
	Revascularization, endovascular, open or percutaneous, tibial/peroneal artery (37229, 37231, 37233, 37235)					
	🔧 38.0	⚒ 38.0	**FUD** 090			

AMA: 2016,Jan,13; 2015,Jan,16; 2014,Jan,11

35305	**tibial or peroneal artery, initial vessel**					C 80 50 🔲
	EXCLUDES Harvest of upper extremity vein, 1 segment, for lower extremity or coronary artery bypass procedure (35500)					
	Revascularization, endovascular, open or percutaneous, tibial/peroneal artery (37229, 37231, 37233, 37235)					
	🔧 36.4	⚒ 36.4	**FUD** 090			

AMA: 2016,Jan,13; 2015,Jan,16; 2014,Jan,11; 2012,Jan,15-42; 2011,Jan,11

+ 35306 each additional tibial or peroneal artery (List separately in addition to code for primary procedure)

> EXCLUDES *Harvest of upper extremity vein, 1 segment, for lower extremity or coronary artery bypass procedure (35500)*
> *Revascularization, endovascular, open or percutaneous, tibial/peroneal artery (37229, 37231, 37233, 37235)*
> Code first (35305)
> 📷 13.5 📎 13.5 **FUD** ZZZ 🅒 80 📄
> **AMA:** 2016,Jan,13; 2015,Jan,16; 2014,Jan,11

35311 subclavian, innominate, by thoracic incision
> 📷 43.0 📎 43.0 **FUD** 090 🅒 80 50 📄
> **AMA:** 1997,Nov,1

35321 axillary-brachial
> 📷 26.3 📎 26.3 **FUD** 090 🆃 80 50 📄
> **AMA:** 1997,Nov,1

35331 abdominal aorta
> 📷 42.9 📎 42.9 **FUD** 090 🅒 80 50 📄
> **AMA:** 1997,Nov,1

35341 mesenteric, celiac, or renal
> 📷 40.4 📎 40.4 **FUD** 090 🅒 80 50 📄
> **AMA:** 1997,Nov,1

35351 iliac
> 📷 37.9 📎 37.9 **FUD** 090 🅒 80 50 📄
> **AMA:** 1997,Nov,1

35355 iliofemoral
> 📷 30.6 📎 30.6 **FUD** 090 🅒 80 50 📄
> **AMA:** 1997,Nov,1

35361 combined aortoiliac
> 📷 45.5 📎 45.5 **FUD** 090 🅒 80 50 📄
> **AMA:** 1997,Nov,1

35363 combined aortoiliofemoral
> 📷 51.7 📎 51.7 **FUD** 090 🅒 80 50 📄
> **AMA:** 1997,Nov,1

35371 common femoral
> 📷 24.2 📎 24.2 **FUD** 090 🅒 80 50 📄
> **AMA:** 2016,Jan,13; 2015,Jan,16; 2014,Jan,11; 2012,Apr,3-9

35372 deep (profunda) femoral
> 📷 29.0 📎 29.0 **FUD** 090 🅒 80 50 📄
> **AMA:** 2016,Jan,13; 2015,Jan,16; 2014,Jan,11

35390 Surgical Thromboendarterectomy: Carotid Reoperation

Code first (35301)

+ 35390 Reoperation, carotid, thromboendarterectomy, more than 1 month after original operation (List separately in addition to code for primary procedure)
> 📷 4.71 📎 4.71 **FUD** ZZZ 🅒 80 📄
> **AMA:** 1997,Nov,1; 1993,Win,1

35400 Endoscopic Visualization of Vessels

Code first the therapeutic intervention

+ 35400 Angioscopy (noncoronary vessels or grafts) during therapeutic intervention (List separately in addition to code for primary procedure)
> 📷 4.41 📎 4.41 **FUD** ZZZ 🅒 80 📄
> **AMA:** 1997,Dec,1; 1997,Nov,1

35450-35460 Transluminal Angioplasty: Open

35450 ~~Transluminal balloon angioplasty, open; renal or other visceral artery~~
> To report, see ~36902, 36905, 36907, [37246, 37247, 37248, 37249]

35452 ~~aortic~~
> To report, see ~36902, 36905, 36907, [37246, 37247, 37248, 37249]

35458 ~~brachiocephalic trunk or branches, each vessel~~
> To report, see ~36902, 36905, 36907, [37246, 37247, 37248, 37249]

35460 ~~venous~~
> To report, see ~36902, 36905, 36907, [37246, 37247, 37248, 37249]

35471-35476 Transluminal Angioplasty: Percutaneous

35471 ~~Transluminal balloon angioplasty, percutaneous; renal or visceral artery~~
> To report, see ~36902, 36905, 36907, [37246, 37247, 37248, 37249]

35472 ~~aortic~~
> To report, see ~36902, 36905, 36907, [37246, 37247, 37248, 37249]

35475 ~~brachiocephalic trunk or branches, each vessel~~
> To report, see ~36902, 36905, 36907, [37246, 37247, 37248, 37249]

35476 ~~venous~~
> To report, see ~36902, 36905, 36907, [37246, 37247, 37248, 37249]

35500 Obtain Arm Vein for Graft

> EXCLUDES *Endoscopic harvest (33508)*
> *Harvesting of multiple vein segments (35682, 35683)*
> Code first (33510-33536, 35556, 35566, 35570-35571, 35583-35587)

+ 35500 Harvest of upper extremity vein, 1 segment, for lower extremity or coronary artery bypass procedure (List separately in addition to code for primary procedure)
> 📷 9.43 📎 9.43 **FUD** ZZZ 🅝 80 📄
> **AMA:** 2016,Jan,13; 2015,Jan,16; 2014,Jan,11; 2012,Apr,3-9

35501-35571 Arterial Bypass Using Vein Grafts

> INCLUDES Obtaining saphenous vein grafts
> EXCLUDES *Obtaining multiple vein segments (35682, 35683)*
> *Obtaining vein grafts, upper extremity or femoropopliteal (35500, 35572)*
> *Treatment of different sites with different bypass procedures during the same operative session*

35501 Bypass graft, with vein; common carotid-ipsilateral internal carotid
> 📷 44.2 📎 44.2 **FUD** 090 🅒 80 50 📄
> **AMA:** 2016,Jan,13; 2015,Jan,16; 2014,Jan,11; 2012,Apr,3-9

35506 carotid-subclavian or subclavian-carotid
> 📷 37.7 📎 37.7 **FUD** 090 🅒 80 50 📄
> **AMA:** 2016,Jan,13; 2015,Jan,16; 2014,Jan,11

35508 carotid-vertebral
> INCLUDES Endoscopic procedure
> 📷 40.1 📎 40.1 **FUD** 090 🅒 80 50 📄
> **AMA:** 1999,Mar,6; 1999,Apr,11

35509 carotid-contralateral carotid
> 📷 41.7 📎 41.7 **FUD** 090 🅒 80 50 📄
> **AMA:** 2016,Jan,13; 2015,Jan,16; 2014,Jan,11; 2012,Jan,15-42; 2011,Jan,11

35510 carotid-brachial
> 📷 36.4 📎 36.4 **FUD** 090 🅒 80 50 📄
> **AMA:** 2016,Jan,13; 2015,Jan,16; 2014,Jan,11; 2012,Jan,15-42; 2011,Jan,11

35511 subclavian-subclavian
> 📷 33.2 📎 33.2 **FUD** 090 🅒 80 50 📄
> **AMA:** 2016,Jan,13; 2015,Jan,16; 2014,Jan,11

35512 subclavian-brachial
> 📷 36.1 📎 36.1 **FUD** 090 🅒 80 50 📄
> **AMA:** 2016,Jan,13; 2015,Jan,16; 2014,Jan,11

35515 subclavian-vertebral
> 📷 42.4 📎 42.4 **FUD** 090 🅒 80 50 📄
> **AMA:** 1999,Mar,6; 1999,Apr,11

35516 subclavian-axillary
> 📷 36.1 📎 36.1 **FUD** 090 🅒 80 50 📄
> **AMA:** 1999,Mar,6; 1999,Apr,11

26/TC PC/TC Only A2-Z3 ASC Payment 50 Bilateral ♂ Male Only ♀ Female Only 📷 Facility RVU 📎 Non-Facility RVU 📄 CCI
FUD Follow-up Days CMS: IOM (Pub 100) A-Y OPPSI 80/80 Surg Assist Allowed / w/Doc 🅽 Lab Crosswalk 📻 Radiology Crosswalk ❌ CLIA

144
CPT © 2016 American Medical Association. All Rights Reserved.
© 2016 Optum360, LLC

35518 axillary-axillary
  🚑 34.3 ⚕ 34.3 **FUD** 090 C 80 50 ▭
  AMA: 2016,Jan,13; 2015,Jan,16; 2014,Jan,11

35521 axillary-femoral
  EXCLUDES Synthetic graft (35621)
  🚑 36.6 ⚕ 36.6 **FUD** 090 C 80 50 ▭
  AMA: 2016,Jan,13; 2015,Jan,16; 2014,Jan,11; 2012,Apr,3-9

35522 axillary-brachial
  🚑 35.7 ⚕ 35.7 **FUD** 090 C 80 50 ▭
  AMA: 2016,Jan,13; 2015,Jan,16; 2014,Jan,11

35523 brachial-ulnar or -radial
  🚑 37.9 ⚕ 37.9 **FUD** 090 C 80 50 ▭

  EXCLUDES Bypass graft using synthetic conduit (37799)
    Bypass graft, with vein; brachial-brachial (35525)
    Distal revascularization and interval ligation (DRIL),
      upper extremity hemodialysis access (steal
      syndrome) (36838)
    Harvest of upper extremity vein, 1 segment, for lower
      extremity or coronary artery bypass procedure
      (35500)
    Repair blood vessel, direct; upper extremity (35206)

35525 brachial-brachial
  🚑 33.8 ⚕ 33.8 **FUD** 090 C 80 50 ▭
  AMA: 2016,Jan,13; 2015,Jan,16; 2014,Jan,11

35526 aortosubclavian, aortoinnominate, or aortocarotid
  EXCLUDES Synthetic graft (35626)
  🚑 50.1 ⚕ 50.1 **FUD** 090 C 80 50 ▭
  AMA: 1999,Mar,6; 1999,Apr,11

35531 aortoceliac or aortomesenteric
  🚑 59.8 ⚕ 59.8 **FUD** 090 C 80 50 ▭
  AMA: 1999,Mar,6; 1999,Apr,11

35533 axillary-femoral-femoral
  EXCLUDES Synthetic graft (35654)
  🚑 44.3 ⚕ 44.3 **FUD** 090 C 80 50 ▭
  AMA: 2012,Apr,3-9

35535 hepatorenal
  🚑 56.7 ⚕ 56.7 **FUD** 090 C 80 50 ▭

  EXCLUDES Bypass graft (35536, 35560, 35631, 35636)
    Harvest of upper extremity vein, 1 segment, for lower
      extremity or coronary artery bypass procedure
      (35500)
    Repair blood vessel (35221, 35251, 35281)

35536 splenorenal
  🚑 50.0 ⚕ 50.0 **FUD** 090 C 80 50 ▭
  AMA: 2016,Jan,13; 2015,Jan,16; 2014,Jan,11; 2012,Jan,15-42;
    2011,Jan,11

35537 aortoiliac
  EXCLUDES Bypass graft, with vein; aortobi-iliac (35538)
    Synthetic graft (35637)
  🚑 64.8 ⚕ 64.8 **FUD** 090 C 80 ▭
  AMA: 2016,Jan,13; 2015,Jan,16; 2014,Jan,11; 2012,Apr,3-9

35538 aortobi-iliac
  EXCLUDES Bypass graft, with vein; aortoiliac (35537)
    Synthetic graft (35638)
  🚑 69.5 ⚕ 69.5 **FUD** 090 C 80 ▭
  AMA: 2016,Jan,13; 2015,Jan,16; 2014,Jan,11; 2012,Apr,3-9

Report 35539 for aortofemoral
or 35540 for grafts aortobifemoral

Aorta
Common iliac
Femoral

Blockage in lower aorta

Femoral arteries
(bilateral graft shown)

35539 aortofemoral
  EXCLUDES Bypass graft, with vein; aortobifemoral (35540)
    Synthetic graft (35647)
  🚑 65.0 ⚕ 65.0 **FUD** 090 C 80 50 ▭
  AMA: 2016,Jan,13; 2015,Jan,16; 2014,Jan,11; 2012,Apr,3-9

35540 aortobifemoral
  EXCLUDES Bypass graft, with vein; aortofemoral (35539)
    Synthetic graft (35646)
  🚑 72.6 ⚕ 72.6 **FUD** 090 C 50 ▭
  AMA: 2016,Jan,13; 2015,Jan,16; 2014,Jan,11; 2012,Apr,3-9

35556 femoral-popliteal
  🚑 41.5 ⚕ 41.5 **FUD** 090 C 80 50 ▭
  AMA: 2016,Jan,13; 2015,Jan,16; 2014,Jan,11; 2012,Apr,3-9

35558 femoral-femoral
  🚑 36.5 ⚕ 36.5 **FUD** 090 C 80 50 ▭
  AMA: 2012,Apr,3-9

35560 aortorenal
  🚑 50.8 ⚕ 50.8 **FUD** 090 C 80 50 ▭
  AMA: 2016,Jan,13; 2015,Jan,16; 2014,Jan,11; 2012,Jan,15-42;
    2011,Jan,11

35563 ilioiliac
  🚑 39.4 ⚕ 39.4 **FUD** 090 C 80 50 ▭
  AMA: 1999,Mar,6; 1999,Apr,11

35565 iliofemoral
  🚑 39.2 ⚕ 39.2 **FUD** 090 C 80 50 ▭
  AMA: 2012,Apr,3-9

35566 femoral-anterior tibial, posterior tibial, peroneal artery
  or other distal vessels
  🚑 49.5 ⚕ 49.5 **FUD** 090 C 80 50 ▭
  AMA: 2016,Jan,13; 2015,Jan,16; 2014,Jan,11; 2012,Apr,3-9

35570 tibial-tibial, peroneal-tibial, or tibial/peroneal
  trunk-tibial
  EXCLUDES Repair of blood vessel with graft (35256, 35286)
  🚑 45.0 ⚕ 45.0 **FUD** 090 C 80 50 ▭
  AMA: 2016,Jan,13; 2015,Jan,16; 2014,Jan,11; 2012,Apr,3-9

35571 popliteal-tibial, -peroneal artery or other distal vessels
  🚑 39.4 ⚕ 39.4 **FUD** 090 C 80 50 ▭
  AMA: 2016,Jan,13; 2015,Jan,16; 2014,Jan,11; 2012,Apr,3-9

35572 Obtain Femoropopliteal Vein for Graft

Code first (33510-33523, 33533-33536, 34502, 34520, 35001-35002, 35011-35022,
  35102-35103, 35121-35152, 35231-35256, 35501-35587, 35879-35907)

35572 Harvest of femoropopliteal vein, 1 segment, for vascular
  reconstruction procedure (eg, aortic, vena caval, coronary,
  peripheral artery) (List separately in addition to code for
  primary procedure)
+ 🚑 10.2 ⚕ 10.2 **FUD** ZZZ N N1 80
  AMA: 2016,Jan,13; 2015,Jan,16; 2014,Jan,11; 2012,Jan,15-42;
    2011,Jan,11

35583-35587 Lower Extremity Revascularization: In-situ Vein Bypass

INCLUDES Obtaining saphenous vein grafts
EXCLUDES Obtaining multiple vein segments (35682, 35683)
  Obtaining vein graft, upper extremity or femoropopliteal (35500, 35572)

35583 In-situ vein bypass; femoral-popliteal
  Code also aortobifemoral bypass graft other than vein for
    aortobifemoral bypass using synthetic conduit and
    femoral-popliteal bypass with vein conduit in situ (35646)
  Code also concurrent aortofemoral bypass for aortofemoral
    bypass graft with synthetic conduit and femoral-popliteal
    bypass with vein conduit in-situ (35647)
  Code also concurrent aortofemoral bypass (vein) for an
    aortofemoral bypass using a vein conduit or a
    femoral-popliteal bypass with vein conduit in-situ (35539)
  🚑 42.9 ⚕ 42.9 **FUD** 090 C 80 50 ▭
  AMA: 2016,Jan,13; 2015,Jan,16; 2014,Jan,11; 2012,Apr,3-9

Cardiovascular, Hemic, and Lymphatic

35585 — 35647

35585   **femoral-anterior tibial, posterior tibial, or peroneal artery**
    🔹 49.8   🔸 49.8   **FUD** 090   [C] [80] [50] [▣]
    AMA: 2016,Jan,13; 2015,Jan,16; 2014,Jan,11; 2012,Apr,3-9

35587   **popliteal-tibial, peroneal**
    🔹 40.5   🔸 40.5   **FUD** 090   [C] [80] [50] [▣]
    AMA: 2016,Jan,13; 2015,Jan,16; 2014,Jan,11; 2012,Apr,3-9

35600 Obtain Arm Artery for Coronary Bypass

EXCLUDES   *Transposition and/or reimplantation of arteries (35691-35695)*
Code first (33533-33536)

+   **35600**   **Harvest of upper extremity artery, 1 segment, for coronary artery bypass procedure (List separately in addition to code for primary procedure)**
    🔹 7.45   🔸 7.45   **FUD** ZZZ   [C] [80] [▣]
    AMA: 2016,Jan,13; 2015,Jan,16; 2014,Jan,11; 2012,Jan,15-42; 2011,Jan,11

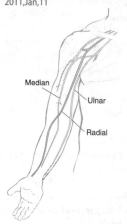

Median
Ulnar
Radial

An upper extremity artery or segment is harvested for a coronary artery bypass procedure

35601-35671 Arterial Bypass: Grafts Other Than Veins

EXCLUDES   *Transposition and/or reimplantation of arteries (35691-35695)*

35601   **Bypass graft, with other than vein; common carotid-ipsilateral internal carotid**
    EXCLUDES   *Open transcervical common carotid-common carotid bypass with endovascular repair of descending thoracic aorta (33891)*
    🔹 41.5   🔸 41.5   **FUD** 090   [C] [80] [50] [▣]
    AMA: 2016,Jan,13; 2015,Jan,16; 2014,Jan,11

35606   **carotid-subclavian**
    EXCLUDES   *Open subclavian to carotid artery transposition performed with endovascular thoracic aneurysm repair via neck incision (33889)*
    🔹 34.8   🔸 34.8   **FUD** 090   [C] [80] [50] [▣]
    AMA: 1997,Nov,1

35612   **subclavian-subclavian**
    🔹 31.8   🔸 31.8   **FUD** 090   [C] [80] [50] [▣]
    AMA: 1997,Nov,1

35616   **subclavian-axillary**
    🔹 32.6   🔸 32.6   **FUD** 090   [C] [80] [50] [▣]
    AMA: 1997,Nov,1

35621   **axillary-femoral**
    🔹 32.5   🔸 32.5   **FUD** 090   [C] [80] [50] [▣]
    AMA: 2016,Jan,13; 2015,Jan,16; 2014,Jan,11; 2012,Apr,3-9

35623   **axillary-popliteal or -tibial**
    🔹 38.9   🔸 38.9   **FUD** 090   [C] [80] [50] [▣]
    AMA: 2012,Apr,3-9

35626   **aortosubclavian, aortoinnominate, or aortocarotid**
    🔹 46.4   🔸 46.4   **FUD** 090   [C] [80] [50] [▣]
    AMA: 1997,Nov,1

35631   **aortoceliac, aortomesenteric, aortorenal**
    🔹 54.8   🔸 54.8   **FUD** 090   [C] [80] [50] [▣]
    AMA: 1997,Nov,1

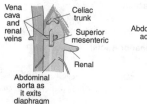
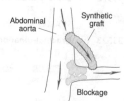

Vena cava and renal veins
Celiac trunk
Superior mesenteric
Renal
Abdominal aorta as it exits diaphragm
Abdominal aorta
Synthetic graft
Blockage

35632   **ilio-celiac**
    🔹 53.4   🔸 53.4   **FUD** 090   [C] [80] [50] [▣]
    EXCLUDES   *Bypass graft (35531, 35631)*
          Repair of blood vessel (35221, 35251, 35281)

35633   **ilio-mesenteric**
    🔹 59.4   🔸 59.4   **FUD** 090   [C] [80] [50] [▣]
    EXCLUDES   *Bypass graft (35531, 35631)*
          Repair of blood vessel (35221, 35251, 35281)

35634   **iliorenal**
    🔹 52.3   🔸 52.3   **FUD** 090   [C] [80] [50] [▣]
    EXCLUDES   *Bypass graft (35536, 35560, 35631)*
          Repair of blood vessel (35221, 35251, 35281)

35636   **splenorenal (splenic to renal arterial anastomosis)**
    🔹 47.4   🔸 47.4   **FUD** 090   [C] [80] [50] [▣]
    AMA: 1997,Nov,1; 1994,Win,1

35637   **aortoiliac**
    EXCLUDES   *Bypass graft (35638, 35646)*
    🔹 51.1   🔸 51.1   **FUD** 090   [C] [80] [▣]
    AMA: 2016,Jan,13; 2015,Jan,16; 2014,Jan,11; 2012,Jan,15-42; 2011,Jan,11

35638   **aortobi-iliac**
    EXCLUDES   *Bypass graft (35637, 35646)*
          Open placement of aorto-bi-iliac prosthesis after a failed endovascular repair (34831)
    🔹 52.2   🔸 52.2   **FUD** 090   [C] [80] [▣]
    AMA: 2016,Jan,13; 2015,Jan,16; 2014,Jan,11; 2012,Jan,15-42; 2011,Jan,11

35642   **carotid-vertebral**
    🔹 29.2   🔸 29.2   **FUD** 090   [C] [80] [50] [▣]
    AMA: 1997,Nov,1

35645   **subclavian-vertebral**
    🔹 30.1   🔸 30.1   **FUD** 090   [C] [80] [50] [▣]
    AMA: 1997,Nov,1

35646   **aortobifemoral**
    EXCLUDES   *Bypass graft using vein graft (35540)*
          Open placement of aortobifemoral prosthesis after a failed endovascular repair (34832)
    🔹 50.9   🔸 50.9   **FUD** 090   [C] [80] [▣]
    AMA: 2016,Jan,13; 2015,Jan,16; 2014,Jan,11; 2012,Apr,3-9

35647   **aortofemoral**
    EXCLUDES   *Bypass graft using vein graft (35539)*
    🔹 46.1   🔸 46.1   **FUD** 090   [C] [80] [50] [▣]
    AMA: 2016,Jan,13; 2015,Jan,16; 2014,Jan,11

35650	**axillary-axillary**
	🛠 32.0　⚕ 32.0　**FUD** 090　　C 80 50 ▣
	AMA: 1997,Nov,1

35654	**axillary-femoral-femoral**
	🛠 40.6　⚕ 40.6　**FUD** 090　　C 80 ▣
	AMA: 2016,Jan,13; 2015,Jan,16; 2014,Jan,11; 2012,Apr,3-9

35656	**femoral-popliteal**
	🛠 32.1　⚕ 32.1　**FUD** 090　　C 80 50 ▣
	AMA: 2016,Jan,13; 2015,Jan,16; 2014,Jan,11; 2012,Apr,3-9

35661	**femoral-femoral**
	🛠 32.1　⚕ 32.1　**FUD** 090　　C 80 50 ▣
	AMA: 2016,Jan,13; 2015,Jan,16; 2014,Jan,11; 2012,Apr,3-9

35663	**ilioiliac**
	🛠 37.2　⚕ 37.2　**FUD** 090　　C 80 50 ▣
	AMA: 1997,Nov,1

35665	**iliofemoral**
	🛠 34.8　⚕ 34.8　**FUD** 090　　C 80 50 ▣
	AMA: 2016,Jan,13; 2015,Jan,16; 2014,Jan,11

35666	**femoral-anterior tibial, posterior tibial, or peroneal artery**
	🛠 37.6　⚕ 37.6　**FUD** 090　　C 80 50 ▣
	AMA: 2016,Jan,13; 2015,Jan,16; 2014,Jan,11; 2012,Apr,3-9

35671	**popliteal-tibial or -peroneal artery**
	🛠 33.1　⚕ 33.1　**FUD** 090　　C 80 50 ▣
	AMA: 2012,Apr,3-9

35681-35683 Arterial Bypass Using Combination Synthetic and Donor Graft

INCLUDES　Acquiring multiple segments of vein from sites other than the extremity for which the arterial bypass is performed
Anastomosis of vein segments to creat bypass graft conduits

+	35681	**Bypass graft; composite, prosthetic and vein (List separately in addition to code for primary procedure)**
		EXCLUDES　Bypass graft (35682, 35683)
		Code first primary procedure
		🛠 2.37　⚕ 2.37　**FUD** ZZZ　　C 80 ▣
		AMA: 2016,Jan,13; 2015,Jan,16; 2014,Jan,11; 2012,Jan,15-42; 2011,Jan,11

+	35682	**autogenous composite, 2 segments of veins from 2 locations (List separately in addition to code for primary procedure)**
		EXCLUDES　Bypass graft (35681, 35683)
		Code first (35556, 35566, 35570-35571, 35583-35587)
		🛠 10.4　⚕ 10.4　**FUD** ZZZ　　C 80 ▣
		AMA: 2016,Jan,13; 2015,Jan,16; 2014,Jan,11; 2012,Jan,15-42

+	35683	**autogenous composite, 3 or more segments of vein from 2 or more locations (List separately in addition to code for primary procedure)**
		EXCLUDES　Bypass graft (35681-35682)
		Code first (35556, 35566, 35570-35571, 35583-35587)
		🛠 12.2　⚕ 12.2　**FUD** ZZZ　　C 80 ▣
		AMA: 2016,Jan,13; 2015,Jan,16; 2014,Jan,11; 2012,Jan,15-42; 2011,Jan,11

35685-35686 Supplemental Procedures

INCLUDES　Additional procedures that may be needed with a bypass graft to increase the patency of the graft
EXCLUDES　Composite grafts (35681-35683)

+	35685	**Placement of vein patch or cuff at distal anastomosis of bypass graft, synthetic conduit (List separately in addition to code for primary procedure)**
		INCLUDES　Connection of a segment of vein (cuff or patch) between the distal portion of the synthetic graft and the native artery
		Code first (35656, 35666, 35671)
		🛠 5.89　⚕ 5.89　**FUD** ZZZ　　N 80 ▣
		AMA: 2016,Jan,13; 2015,Jan,16; 2014,Jan,11

+	35686	**Creation of distal arteriovenous fistula during lower extremity bypass surgery (non-hemodialysis) (List separately in addition to code for primary procedure)**
		INCLUDES　Creation of a fistula between the peroneal or tibial artery and vein at or past the site of the distal anastomosis
		Code first (35556, 35566, 35570-35571, 35583-35587, 35623, 35656, 35666, 35671)
		🛠 4.78　⚕ 4.78　**FUD** ZZZ　　N 80 ▣
		AMA: 2016,Jan,13; 2015,Jan,16; 2014,Jan,11; 2012,Apr,3-9

35691-35697 Arterial Translocation

CMS: 100-03,160.8 Electroencephalographic Monitoring During Cerebral Vasculature Surgery

35691	**Transposition and/or reimplantation; vertebral to carotid artery**
	🛠 28.4　⚕ 28.4　**FUD** 090　　C 80 50 ▣
	AMA: 1997,Nov,1; 1993,Win,1

35693	**vertebral to subclavian artery**
	🛠 24.1　⚕ 24.1　**FUD** 090　　C 80 50 ▣
	AMA: 1997,Nov,1; 1994,Sum,29

35694	**subclavian to carotid artery**
	EXCLUDES　Subclavian to carotid artery transposition procedure (open) with concurrent repair of descending thoracic aorta (endovascular) (33889)
	🛠 29.3　⚕ 29.3　**FUD** 090　　C 80 50 ▣
	AMA: 1997,Nov,1; 1993,Win,1

35695	**carotid to subclavian artery**
	🛠 31.1　⚕ 31.1　**FUD** 090　　C 80 50 ▣
	AMA: 1997,Nov,1; 1993,Win,1

+	35697	**Reimplantation, visceral artery to infrarenal aortic prothesis, each artery (List separately in addition to code for primary procedure)**
		EXCLUDES　Repair of thoracoabdominal aortic aneurysm with graft (33877)
		Code first primary procedure
		🛠 4.37　⚕ 4.37　**FUD** ZZZ　　C 80 ▣
		AMA: 1997,Nov,1

35700 Reoperative Bypass Lower Extremities

Code first (35556, 35566, 35570-35571, 35583, 35585, 35587, 35656, 35666, 35671)

+	35700	**Reoperation, femoral-popliteal or femoral (popliteal)-anterior tibial, posterior tibial, peroneal artery, or other distal vessels, more than 1 month after original operation (List separately in addition to code for primary procedure)**
		🛠 4.53　⚕ 4.53　**FUD** ZZZ　　C 80 ▣
		AMA: 2016,Jan,13; 2015,Jan,16; 2014,Jan,11; 2012,Apr,3-9

35701-35761 Arterial Exploration without Repair

35701	**Exploration (not followed by surgical repair), with or without lysis of artery; carotid artery**
	🛠 16.6　⚕ 16.6　**FUD** 090　　C 80 50 ▣
	AMA: 1997,Nov,1

35721	**femoral artery**
	🛠 13.4　⚕ 13.4　**FUD** 090　　C 80 50 ▣
	AMA: 2016,Jan,13; 2015,Jan,16; 2014,Jan,11

35741	**popliteal artery**
	🛠 15.2　⚕ 15.2　**FUD** 090　　C 80 50 ▣
	AMA: 1997,Nov,1

35761	**other vessels**
	🛠 11.4　⚕ 11.4　**FUD** 090　　T 62 80 50 ▣
	AMA: 1997,Nov,1

35800-35860 Arterial Exploration for Postoperative Complication

INCLUDES　Return to the operating room for postoperative hemorrhage

35800	**Exploration for postoperative hemorrhage, thrombosis or infection; neck**
	🛠 20.9　⚕ 20.9　**FUD** 090　　C 80 ▣
	AMA: 1997,Nov,1

35820　**chest**
　　🔄 58.6　⅋ 58.6　**FUD** 090　　　　C 80 ▢
　　AMA: 1997,Nov,1

35840　**abdomen**
　　🔄 34.7　⅋ 34.7　**FUD** 090　　　　C 80 ▢
　　AMA: 1997,May,4; 1997,Nov,1

35860　**extremity**
　　🔄 24.8　⅋ 24.8　**FUD** 090　　　　T 80 ▢
　　AMA: 2016,Jan,13; 2015,Jan,16; 2014,Apr,10

35870 Repair Secondary Aortoenteric Fistula

35870　**Repair of graft-enteric fistula**
　　🔄 36.8　⅋ 36.8　**FUD** 090　　　　C 80 ▢
　　AMA: 1997,Nov,1

35875-35876 Removal of Thrombus from Graft

EXCLUDES　Thrombectomy dialysis fistula or graft (36831, 36833)
Thrombectomy with blood vessel repair, lower extremity, vein graft (35256)
Thrombectomy with blood vessel repair, lower extremity, with/without patch angioplasty (35226)

35875　**Thrombectomy of arterial or venous graft (other than hemodialysis graft or fistula);**
　　🔄 17.6　⅋ 17.6　**FUD** 090　　　　T A2 ▢
　　AMA: 2016,Jan,13; 2015,Jan,16; 2014,Jan,11; 2012,Jan,15-42; 2011,Jan,11

35876　**with revision of arterial or venous graft**
　　🔄 28.0　⅋ 28.0　**FUD** 090　　　　T A2 80 ▢
　　AMA: 1999,Mar,6; 1999,Nov,1

35879-35884 Revision Lower Extremity Bypass Graft

EXCLUDES　Removal of infected graft (35901-35907)
Revascularization following removal of infected graft(s)
Thrombectomy dialysis fistula or graft (36831, 36833)
Thrombectomy with blood vessel repair, lower extremity, vein graft (35256)
Thrombectomy with blood vessel repair, lower extremity, with/without patch angioplasty (35226)
Thrombectomy with graft revision (35876)

35879　**Revision, lower extremity arterial bypass, without thrombectomy, open; with vein patch angioplasty**
　　🔄 27.3　⅋ 27.3　**FUD** 090　　　　T 80 50 ▢
　　AMA: 2016,Jan,13; 2015,Jan,16; 2014,Jan,11

35881　**with segmental vein interposition**
　　EXCLUDES　Revision of femoral anastomosis of synthetic arterial bypass graft (35883-35884)
　　🔄 30.2　⅋ 30.2　**FUD** 090　　　　T 80 50 ▢
　　AMA: 2016,Jan,13; 2015,Jan,16; 2014,Jan,11

35883　**Revision, femoral anastomosis of synthetic arterial bypass graft in groin, open; with nonautogenous patch graft (eg, Dacron, ePTFE, bovine pericardium)**
　　EXCLUDES　Reoperation, femoral-popliteal or femoral (popliteal)-anterior tibial, posterior tibial, peroneal artery, or other distal vessels (35700)
　　Revision, femoral anastomosis of synthetic arterial bypass graft in groin, open; with autogenous vein patch graft (35884)
　　Thrombectomy of arterial or venous graft (35875)
　　🔄 35.8　⅋ 35.8　**FUD** 090　　　　T 80 50 ▢
　　AMA: 2016,Jan,13; 2015,Jan,16; 2014,Jan,11; 2012,Jan,15-42; 2011,Jan,11

35884　**with autogenous vein patch graft**
　　EXCLUDES　Reoperation, femoral-popliteal or femoral (popliteal)-anterior tibial, posterior tibial, peroneal artery, or other distal vessels (35700)
　　Revision, femoral anastomosis of synthetic arterial bypass graft in groin, open; with autogenous vein patch graft (35883)
　　Thrombectomy of arterial or venous graft (35875-35876)
　　🔄 36.7　⅋ 36.7　**FUD** 090　　　　T 80 50 ▢
　　AMA: 2016,Jan,13; 2015,Jan,16; 2014,Jan,11; 2012,Jan,15-42; 2011,Jan,11

35901-35907 Removal of Infected Graft

35901　**Excision of infected graft; neck**
　　🔄 13.9　⅋ 13.9　**FUD** 090　　　　C 80 ▢
　　AMA: 1997,Nov,1; 1993,Win,1

Infected graft is removed

In 35901, the physician removes an infected graft from the neck and repairs the blood vessel. If a new graft is placed, report the appropriate revascularization code

35903　**extremity**
　　🔄 16.7　⅋ 16.7　**FUD** 090　　　　T 80 ▢
　　AMA: 1997,Nov,1; 1993,Win,1

35905　**thorax**
　　🔄 49.8　⅋ 49.8　**FUD** 090　　　　C 80 ▢
　　AMA: 1997,Nov,1; 1993,Win,1

35907　**abdomen**
　　🔄 56.6　⅋ 56.6　**FUD** 090　　　　C 80 ▢
　　AMA: 1997,Nov,1; 1993,Win,1

36000 Intravenous Access Established

INCLUDES　Venous access for phlebotomy, prophylactic intravenous access, infusion therapy, chemotherapy, hydration, transfusion, drug administration, etc. which is included in the work value of the primary procedure

36000　**Introduction of needle or intracatheter, vein**
　　🔄 0.27　⅋ 0.73　**FUD** XXX　　　　N N1 ▢
　　AMA: 2016,Jan,13; 2015,Jan,16; 2014,Oct,6; 2014,Sep,13; 2014,May,4; 2014,Jan,11; 2012,Jan,15-42; 2011,Jan,11

36002 Injection Treatment of Pseudoaneurysm

INCLUDES　Insertion of needle or catheter, local anesthesia, injection of contrast, power injections, and all pre- and postinjection care provided
EXCLUDES　Arteriotomy site sealant
Compression repair pseudoaneurysm, ultrasound guided (76936)
Medications, contrast material, catheters

36002　**Injection procedures (eg, thrombin) for percutaneous treatment of extremity pseudoaneurysm**
　　🔅 (76942, 77002, 77012, 77021)
　　🔄 3.10　⅋ 4.64　**FUD** 000　　　　S 62 50 ▢
　　AMA: 2016,Jan,13; 2015,Jan,16; 2014,Oct,6; 2014,Jan,11; 2013,Nov,6

36005-36015 Insertion Needle or Intracatheter: Venous

INCLUDES　Insertion of needle/catheter, local anesthesia, injection of contrast, power injections, all pre- and postinjection care
EXCLUDES　Medications, contrast materials, catheters
Code also catheterization of second order vessels (or higher) supplied by the same first order branch, same vascular family (36012)
Code also each vascular family (e.g., bilateral procedures are separate vascular families)

36005　**Injection procedure for extremity venography (including introduction of needle or intracatheter)**
　　🔅 (75820, 75822)
　　🔄 1.41　⅋ 9.23　**FUD** 000　　　　N N1 80 50 ▢
　　AMA: 2016,Jul,6; 2016,Jan,13; 2015,Jan,16; 2014,Oct,6

▲ **36010**　**Introduction of catheter, superior or inferior vena cava**
　　🔄 3.57　⅋ 14.3　**FUD** XXX　　　　N N1 50 ▢
　　AMA: 2016,Jul,6; 2016,Jan,13; 2015,Jan,16; 2014,Jan,11; 2012,Apr,3-9; 2012,Jan,15-42; 2011,Jan,11

36011　**Selective catheter placement, venous system; first order branch (eg, renal vein, jugular vein)**
　　🔄 4.58　⅋ 23.7　**FUD** XXX　　　　N N1 50 ▢
　　AMA: 2016,Jul,6; 2016,Jan,13; 2015,Jan,16; 2014,Jan,11; 2012,Apr,3-9

26/TC PC/TC Only　　A2-Z3 ASC Payment　　50 Bilateral　　♂ Male Only　　♀ Female Only　　🔄 Facility RVU　　⅋ Non-Facility RVU　　▢ CCI
FUD Follow-up Days　　CMS: IOM (Pub 100)　　A-Y OPPSI　　80/80 Surg Assist Allowed / w/Doc　　🔅 Lab Crosswalk　　🔅 Radiology Crosswalk　　❌ CLIA

148　　CPT © 2016 American Medical Association. All Rights Reserved.　　© 2016 Optum360, LLC

36012 second order, or more selective, branch (eg, left adrenal vein, petrosal sinus)

🔧 5.08 ⚕ 24.5 **FUD** XXX [N] [N1] [50] 🖵

AMA: 2016,Jul,6; 2016,Jan,13; 2015,Jan,16; 2014,Jan,11; 2012,Apr,3-9

36013 Introduction of catheter, right heart or main pulmonary artery

🔧 3.65 ⚕ 22.3 **FUD** XXX [N] [N1] 🖵

AMA: 2016,Jul,6; 2016,Jan,13; 2015,Jan,16; 2014,Jan,11; 2012,Jan,15-42; 2011,Jan,11

36014 Selective catheter placement, left or right pulmonary artery

🔧 4.37 ⚕ 23.1 **FUD** XXX [N] [N1] [50] 🖵

AMA: 2016,Jul,6; 2016,Jan,13; 2015,Jan,16; 2014,Jan,11

36015 Selective catheter placement, segmental or subsegmental pulmonary artery

EXCLUDES *Placement of Swan Ganz/other flow directed catheter for monitoring (93503)*
Selective blood sampling, specific organs (36500)

🔧 5.00 ⚕ 24.7 **FUD** XXX [N] [N1] [50] 🖵

AMA: 2016,Jul,6; 2016,Jan,13; 2015,Jan,16; 2014,Jan,11; 2012,Mar,9-10

36100-36218 Insertion Needle or Intracatheter: Arterial

INCLUDES Introduction of the catheter and catheterization of all lesser order vessels used for the approach
Local anesthesia, placement of catheter/needle, injection of contrast, power injections, all pre- and postinjection care

EXCLUDES *Angiography (36222-36228, 75600-75774)*
Angioplasty ([37246, 37247])
Chemotherapy injections (96401-96549)
Injection procedures for cardiac catheterizations (93455, 93457, 93459, 93461, 93530-93533, 93564)
Internal mammary artery angiography without left heart catheterization (36216, 36217)
Medications, contrast, catheters
Transcatheter interventions (37200, [37211], [37213, 37214], 37236-37239, 37241-37244, 61624, 61626)

Code also additional first order or higher catheterization for vascular families if the vascular family is supplied by a first order vessel that is different from one already coded
Code also catheterization of second and third order vessels supplied by the same first order branch, same vascular family (36218, 36248)

36100 Introduction of needle or intracatheter, carotid or vertebral artery

🔧 4.53 ⚕ 14.2 **FUD** XXX [N] [N1] [50] 🖵

AMA: 2000,Oct,4; 1998,Apr,1

36120 Introduction of needle or intracatheter; retrograde brachial artery

EXCLUDES *Arteriovenous cannula insertion (36810-36821)*

🔧 2.93 ⚕ 12.0 **FUD** XXX [N] [N1] 🖵

AMA: 2016,Jan,13; 2015,Jan,16; 2014,Jan,11; 2012,Jan,15-42; 2011,Jan,11

▲ **36140** extremity artery

EXCLUDES *Arteriovenous cannula insertion (36810-36821)*

🔧 3.01 ⚕ 12.4 **FUD** XXX [N] [N1] 🖵

AMA: 2016,Jan,13; 2015,Jan,16; 2014,Jan,11; 2012,Jan,15-42; 2011,Jul,3-11; 2011,Jan,11

~~**36147** Introduction of needle and/or catheter, arteriovenous shunt created for dialysis (graft/fistula); initial access with complete radiological evaluation of dialysis access, including fluoroscopy, image documentation and report (includes access of shunt, injection[s] of contrast, and all necessary imaging from the arterial anastomosis and adjacent artery through entire venous outflow including the inferior or superior vena cava)~~
To report, see ~36901-36906

~~**36148** additional access for therapeutic intervention (List separately in addition to code for primary procedure)~~
To report, see ~36901-36906

36160 Introduction of needle or intracatheter, aortic, translumbar

🔧 3.60 ⚕ 14.0 **FUD** XXX [N] [N1] 🖵

AMA: 2016,Jan,13; 2015,Jan,16; 2014,Jan,11

▲ **36200** Introduction of catheter, aorta

EXCLUDES *Nonselective angiography of the extracranial carotid and/or cerebral vessels and cervicocerebral arch (36221)*

🔧 4.48 ⚕ 17.7 **FUD** 000 [N] [N1] [50] 🖵

AMA: 2016,Jul,6; 2016,Jan,13; 2015,Jan,16; 2014,Jan,11; 2013,Feb,16-17; 2012,Apr,3-9; 2012,Jan,15-42; 2011,Oct,9; 2011,Jul,3-11; 2011,Jan,11

36215 Selective catheter placement, arterial system; each first order thoracic or brachiocephalic branch, within a vascular family

INCLUDES Introduction of catheter into the aorta (36200)
EXCLUDES *Placement of catheter for coronary angiography (93454-93461)*

🔧 6.85 ⚕ 32.0 **FUD** XXX [N] [N1] 🖵

AMA: 2016,Jul,6; 2016,Jan,13; 2015,Jan,16; 2014,Jan,11; 2012,Apr,3-9; 2012,Jan,15-42; 2011,Jan,11

36216 initial second order thoracic or brachiocephalic branch, within a vascular family

🔧 8.04 ⚕ 33.9 **FUD** XXX [N] [N1] 🖵

AMA: 2016,Jul,6; 2016,Jan,13; 2015,Jan,16; 2014,Jan,11; 2013,Nov,14; 2012,Apr,3-9; 2011,Dec,9-12

36217 initial third order or more selective thoracic or brachiocephalic branch, within a vascular family

🔧 9.56 ⚕ 55.9 **FUD** XXX [N] [N1] 🖵

AMA: 2016,Jul,6; 2016,Jan,13; 2015,Jan,16; 2014,Jan,11; 2012,Apr,3-9; 2011,Dec,9-12

+ **36218** additional second order, third order, and beyond, thoracic or brachiocephalic branch, within a vascular family (List in addition to code for initial second or third order vessel as appropriate)

Code also transcatheter therapy procedures (37200, [37211], [37213, 37214], 37236-37239, 37241-37244, 61624, 61626)
Code first (36216-36217, 36225-36226)

🔧 1.55 ⚕ 5.49 **FUD** ZZZ [N] [N1] 🖵

AMA: 2016,Jul,6; 2016,Jan,13; 2015,Jan,16; 2014,Jan,11; 2013,May,3-5; 2012,Apr,3-9

36221-36228 Diagnostic Studies: Aortic Arch/Carotid/Vertebral Arteries

INCLUDES Accessing the vessel
Arterial contrast injection that includes arterial, capillary, and venous phase imaging, when performed
Arteriotomy closure (pressure or closure device)
Catheter placement
Radiologic supervision and interpretation
Reporting of selective catheter placement based on intensity of services in the following hierarchy:
36226>36225
36224>36223>36222

EXCLUDES *3D rendering when performed (76376-76377)*
Interventional procedures
Transcatheter intravascular stent placement of common carotid or innominate artery on the same side (37217)
Ultrasound guidance (76937)

Code also diagnostic angiography of upper extremities/other vascular beds during the same session, if performed (75774)

▲ **36221** Non-selective catheter placement, thoracic aorta, with angiography of the extracranial carotid, vertebral, and/or intracranial vessels, unilateral or bilateral, and all associated radiological supervision and interpretation, includes angiography of the cervicocerebral arch, when performed

EXCLUDES *Selective catheter placement, common carotid or innominate artery (36222-36226)*
Transcatheter intravascular stent placement of common carotid or innominate artery on the same side (37217)

🔧 6.29 ⚕ 31.2 **FUD** 000 [02] [N1] 🖵

AMA: 2016,Mar,3; 2016,Jan,13; 2015,Nov,3; 2015,May,7; 2015,Jan,16; 2014,Mar,8; 2014,Jan,11; 2013,Oct,18; 2013,Jun,12; 2013,May,3-5; 2013,Feb,16-17

● New Code ▲ Revised Code ○ Reinstated ● New Web Release ▲ Revised Web Release Unlisted Not Covered # Resequenced
⊘ AMA Mod 51 Exempt ⑪ Optum Mod 51 Exempt ⑬ Mod 63 Exempt ✎ Non-FDA Drug ★ Telehealth [M] Maternity [A] Age Edit + Add-on AMA: CPT Asst

Cardiovascular, Hemic, and Lymphatic

36222 — 36246

▲ **36222** Selective catheter placement, common carotid or innominate artery, unilateral, any approach, with angiography of the ipsilateral extracranial carotid circulation and all associated radiological supervision and interpretation, includes angiography of the cervicocerebral arch, when performed

> INCLUDES Unilateral catheterization of artery
> EXCLUDES *Transcatheter placement of intravascular stent(s) (37215-37218)*
> Code also modifier 59 when different territories on both sides of the body are being studied
> 🚗 8.62 ⚖ 37.5 **FUD** 000 02 N1 50 🖵

> **AMA:** 2016,Mar,3; 2016,Jan,13; 2015,Nov,3; 2015,Nov,10; 2015,May,7; 2015,Jan,16; 2014,Mar,8; 2014,Jan,11; 2013,Oct,18; 2013,Nov,14; 2013,Jun,12; 2013,May,3-5; 2013,Feb,16-17

▲ **36223** Selective catheter placement, common carotid or innominate artery, unilateral, any approach, with angiography of the ipsilateral intracranial carotid circulation and all associated radiological supervision and interpretation, includes angiography of the extracranial carotid and cervicocerebral arch, when performed

> INCLUDES Unilateral catheterization of artery
> EXCLUDES *Transcatheter placement of intravascular stent(s) (37215-37218)*
> Code also modifier 59 when different territories on both sides of the body are being studied
> 🚗 9.42 ⚖ 43.8 **FUD** 000 02 N1 50 🖵

> **AMA:** 2016,Mar,3; 2016,Jan,13; 2015,Nov,3; 2015,Jan,16; 2014,Mar,8; 2014,Jan,11; 2013,Oct,18; 2013,Jun,12; 2013,May,3-5; 2013,Feb,16-17

▲ **36224** Selective catheter placement, internal carotid artery, unilateral, with angiography of the ipsilateral intracranial carotid circulation and all associated radiological supervision and interpretation, includes angiography of the extracranial carotid and cervicocerebral arch, when performed

> INCLUDES Unilateral catheterization of artery
> EXCLUDES *Transcatheter placement of intravascular stent(s) (37215-37218)*
> Code also modifier 59 when different territories on both sides of the body are being studied
> 🚗 10.4 ⚖ 51.6 **FUD** 000 02 N1 50 🖵

> **AMA:** 2016,Mar,3; 2016,Jan,13; 2015,Nov,3; 2015,Jan,16; 2014,Mar,8; 2014,Jan,11; 2013,Oct,18; 2013,Jun,12; 2013,May,3-5; 2013,Feb,16-17

▲ **36225** Selective catheter placement, subclavian or innominate artery, unilateral, with angiography of the ipsilateral vertebral circulation and all associated radiological supervision and interpretation, includes angiography of the cervicocerebral arch, when performed

> EXCLUDES *Transcatheter placement of intravascular stent(s) (37217)*
> 🚗 9.28 ⚖ 42.8 **FUD** 000 02 N1 50 🖵

> **AMA:** 2016,Mar,3; 2016,Jan,13; 2015,Nov,3; 2015,Jan,16; 2014,Mar,8; 2014,Jan,11; 2013,Oct,18; 2013,Nov,14; 2013,Jun,12; 2013,May,3-5

▲ **36226** Selective catheter placement, vertebral artery, unilateral, with angiography of the ipsilateral vertebral circulation and all associated radiological supervision and interpretation, includes angiography of the cervicocerebral arch, when performed

> EXCLUDES *Transcatheter placement of intravascular stent(s)*
> 🚗 10.5 ⚖ 52.4 **FUD** 000 02 N1 50 🖵

> **AMA:** 2016,Mar,3; 2016,Jan,13; 2015,Nov,3; 2015,Jan,16; 2014,Mar,8; 2013,Oct,18; 2013,Jun,12; 2013,May,3-5

▲ + **36227** Selective catheter placement, external carotid artery, unilateral, with angiography of the ipsilateral external carotid circulation and all associated radiological supervision and interpretation (List separately in addition to code for primary procedure)

> INCLUDES Unilateral catheter placement/diagnostic imaging of ipsilateral external carotid circulation
> EXCLUDES *Transcatheter placement of intravascular stent(s)*
> Code first (36222-36224)
> 🚗 3.32 ⚖ 7.19 **FUD** ZZZ N N1 50 🖵

> **AMA:** 2016,Jan,13; 2015,Nov,10; 2015,Jan,16; 2014,Mar,8; 2014,Jan,11; 2013,Oct,18; 2013,Jun,12; 2013,May,3-5; 2013,Feb,16-17

▲ + **36228** Selective catheter placement, each intracranial branch of the internal carotid or vertebral arteries, unilateral, with angiography of the selected vessel circulation and all associated radiological supervision and interpretation (eg, middle cerebral artery, posterior inferior cerebellar artery) (List separately in addition to code for primary procedure)

> INCLUDES Unilateral catheter placement/imaging of initial and each additional intracranial branch of internal carotid or vertebral arteries
> EXCLUDES *Procedure performed more than 2 times per side*
> *Transcatheter placement of intravascular stent(s)*
> Code first (36223-36226)
> 🚗 6.79 ⚖ 34.6 **FUD** ZZZ N N1 50 🖵

> **AMA:** 2016,Jan,13; 2015,Nov,3; 2015,Jan,16; 2014,Jan,11; 2013,Oct,18; 2013,Jun,12; 2013,May,3-5; 2013,Feb,16-17

36245-36254 Catheter Placement: Arteries of the Lower Body

> INCLUDES Introduction of the catheter and catheterization of all lesser order vessels used for the approach
> Local anesthesia, placement of catheter/needle, injection of contrast, power injections
> EXCLUDES *Angiography (36222-36228, 75600-75774)*
> *Chemotherapy injections (96401-96549)*
> *Injection procedures for cardiac catheterizations (93455, 93457, 93459, 93461, 93530-93533, 93564)*
> *Internal mammary artery angiography without left heart catheterization (36216-36217)*
> *Medications, contrast, catheters*
> *Transcatheter procedures (37200, [37211], [37213, 37214], 37236-37239, 37241-37244, 61624, 61626)*
> Code also additional first order or higher catheterization for vascular families if the vascular family is supplied by a first order vessel that is different from one already coded
> Code also catheterization of second and third order vessels supplied by the same first order branch, same vascular family (36218, 36248)
> 🖸 (75600-75774)

▲ **36245** Selective catheter placement, arterial system; each first order abdominal, pelvic, or lower extremity artery branch, within a vascular family

> 🚗 7.38 ⚖ 39.0 **FUD** XXX N N1 50 🖵

> **AMA:** 2016,Jul,6; 2016,Jan,13; 2015,Jan,16; 2014,Jan,11; 2013,Nov,14; 2012,Apr,3-9; 2012,Jan,15-42; 2011,Oct,9; 2011,Jul,3-11; 2011,Jan,11

▲ **36246** initial second order abdominal, pelvic, or lower extremity artery branch, within a vascular family

> 🚗 7.86 ⚖ 25.4 **FUD** 000 N N1 50 🖵

> **AMA:** 2016,Jul,6; 2016,Jan,13; 2015,Jan,16; 2014,Jan,11; 2013,Nov,14; 2012,Apr,3-9; 2012,Jan,15-42; 2011,Oct,9; 2011,Jul,3-11; 2011,Jan,11

2G/TG PC/TC Only	A2-Z3 ASC Payment	50 Bilateral	♂ Male Only	♀ Female Only	🚗 Facility RVU	⚖ Non-Facility RVU	🖵 CCI
FUD Follow-up Days	CMS: IOM (Pub 100)	A-Y OPPSI	80/80 Surg Assist Allowed / w/Doc		🖵 Lab Crosswalk	🖸 Radiology Crosswalk	✖ CLIA

150

CPT © 2016 American Medical Association. All Rights Reserved.

© 2016 Optum360, LLC

▲ **36247** **initial third order or more selective abdominal, pelvic, or lower extremity artery branch, within a vascular family**
📷 9.29   ⚕ 45.0   **FUD** 000   N N1 50
AMA: 2016,Jul,6; 2016,Jan,13; 2015,Jan,16; 2014,Jan,11; 2013,Nov,14; 2012,Apr,3-9; 2012,Jan,15-42; 2011,Jul,3-11; 2011,Jan,11

▲ + **36248** **additional second order, third order, and beyond, abdominal, pelvic, or lower extremity artery branch, within a vascular family (List in addition to code for initial second or third order vessel as appropriate)**
Code first (36246, 36247)
📷 1.45   ⚕ 4.37   **FUD** ZZZ   N N1 ▱
AMA: 2016,Jul,6; 2016,Jan,13; 2015,Jan,16; 2014,Jan,11; 2012,Apr,3-9; 2012,Jan,15-42; 2011,Jul,3-11; 2011,Jan,11

▲ **36251** **Selective catheter placement (first-order), main renal artery and any accessory renal artery(s) for renal angiography, including arterial puncture and catheter placement(s), fluoroscopy, contrast injection(s), image postprocessing, permanent recording of images, and radiological supervision and interpretation, including pressure gradient measurements when performed, and flush aortogram when performed; unilateral**
INCLUDES   Closure device placement at vascular access site
EXCLUDES   *Transcatheter renal sympathetic denervation, percutaneous approach (0338T-0339T)*
📷 8.22   ⚕ 40.6   **FUD** 000   Q2 N1 ▱
AMA: 2016,Jan,13; 2015,Jan,16; 2014,Jan,11; 2013,Nov,14; 2012,Aug,13-14; 2012,Apr,3-9; 2012,Jan,15-42

▲ **36252** **bilateral**
INCLUDES   Closure device placement at vascular access site
EXCLUDES   *Transcatheter renal sympathetic denervation, percutaneous approach (0338T-0339T)*
📷 10.9   ⚕ 44.0   **FUD** 000   Q2 N1 ▱
AMA: 2016,Jan,13; 2015,Jan,16; 2014,Jan,11; 2012,Apr,3-9; 2012,Jan,15-42

▲ **36253** **Superselective catheter placement (one or more second order or higher renal artery branches) renal artery and any accessory renal artery(s) for renal angiography, including arterial puncture, catheterization, fluoroscopy, contrast injection(s), image postprocessing, permanent recording of images, and radiological supervision and interpretation, including pressure gradient measurements when performed, and flush aortogram when performed; unilateral**
INCLUDES   Closure device placement at vascular access site
EXCLUDES   *Procedure performed on same kidney with (36251)*
Transcatheter renal sympathetic denervation, percutaneous approach (0338T-0339T)
📷 11.0   ⚕ 64.6   **FUD** 000   Q2 N1 ▱
AMA: 2016,Jan,13; 2015,Jan,16; 2014,Jan,11; 2013,Nov,14; 2012,Aug,13-14; 2012,Apr,3-9; 2012,Jan,15-42

▲ **36254** **bilateral**
INCLUDES   Closure device placement at vascular access site
EXCLUDES   *Selective catheter placement (first-order), main renal artery and any accessory renal artery(s) for renal angiography (36252)*
Transcatheter renal sympathetic denervation, percutaneous approach (0338T-0339T)
📷 12.7   ⚕ 62.8   **FUD** 000   Q2 N1 ▱
AMA: 2016,Jan,13; 2015,Jan,16; 2014,Jan,11; 2012,Aug,13-14; 2012,Apr,3-9; 2012,Jan,15-42

36260-36299 Implanted Infusion Pumps: Intra-arterial

36260 **Insertion of implantable intra-arterial infusion pump (eg, for chemotherapy of liver)**
📷 18.2   ⚕ 18.2   **FUD** 090   T A2 ▱
AMA: 2016,Jan,13; 2015,Jan,16; 2014,Jan,11

36261 **Revision of implanted intra-arterial infusion pump**
📷 11.6   ⚕ 11.6   **FUD** 090   T G2 80 ▱
AMA: 2000,Oct,4; 1997,Nov,1

36262 **Removal of implanted intra-arterial infusion pump**
📷 8.86   ⚕ 8.86   **FUD** 090   Q2 G2
AMA: 2000,Oct,4; 1997,Nov,1

36299 **Unlisted procedure, vascular injection**
📷 0.00   ⚕ 0.00   **FUD** YYY   N 80
AMA: 2000,Oct,4; 1997,Nov,1

36400-36425 Specimen Collection: Phlebotomy

EXCLUDES   *Collection of specimen from:*
A completely implantable device (36591)
An established catheter (36592)

36400 **Venipuncture, younger than age 3 years, necessitating the skill of a physician or other qualified health care professional, not to be used for routine venipuncture; femoral or jugular vein**   A
📷 0.58   ⚕ 0.85   **FUD** XXX   N N1 ▱
AMA: 2016,Jan,13; 2015,Jan,16; 2014,May,4; 2014,Jan,11

36405 **scalp vein**   A
📷 0.47   ⚕ 0.75   **FUD** XXX   N N1 ▱
AMA: 2016,Jan,13; 2015,Jan,16; 2014,May,4; 2014,Jan,11

36406 **other vein**   A
📷 0.24   ⚕ 0.47   **FUD** XXX   N N1 ▱
AMA: 2016,Jan,13; 2015,Jan,16; 2014,May,4; 2014,Jan,11

36410 **Venipuncture, age 3 years or older, necessitating the skill of a physician or other qualified health care professional (separate procedure), for diagnostic or therapeutic purposes (not to be used for routine venipuncture)**   A
📷 0.27   ⚕ 0.48   **FUD** XXX   N N1 ▱
AMA: 2016,Jan,13; 2015,Jan,16; 2014,Oct,6; 2014,Jan,11; 2013,Sep,17; 2012,Jan,15-42; 2011,Jan,11

36415 **Collection of venous blood by venipuncture**
📷 0.00   ⚕ 0.00   **FUD** XXX   63 Q N1 ▱
AMA: 2016,Jan,13; 2015,Jan,16; 2014,May,4; 2014,Jan,11; 2012,Jan,15-42; 2011,Jan,11

36416 **Collection of capillary blood specimen (eg, finger, heel, ear stick)**
📷 0.00   ⚕ 0.00   **FUD** XXX   N N1 ▱
AMA: 2008,Apr,-9; 2003,Feb,7

36420 **Venipuncture, cutdown; younger than age 1 year** A
📷 1.51   ⚕ 1.51   **FUD** XXX   63 Q1 N1 80 ▱
AMA: 2016,Jan,13; 2015,Jan,16; 2014,Jan,11

36425 **age 1 or over**   A
EXCLUDES   *Endovenous ablation therapy of incompetent vein, extremity (36475-36476, 36478-36479)*
📷 1.15   ⚕ 1.15   **FUD** XXX   Q1 N1 ▱
AMA: 2016,Jan,13; 2015,Jan,16; 2014,Oct,6

36430-36460 Transfusions

CMS: 100-01,3,20.5 Blood Deductibles; 100-03,110.16 Transfusion in Kidney Transplants; 100-03,110.7 Blood Transfusions; 100-03,110.8 Blood Platelet Transfusions

36430 **Transfusion, blood or blood components**
EXCLUDES   *Infant partial exchange transfusion (36456)*
📷 0.98   ⚕ 0.98   **FUD** XXX   S P3
AMA: 2016,Jan,13; 2015,Jan,16; 2014,Jan,11; 2012,Jan,15-42; 2011,Jan,11

36440 **Push transfusion, blood, 2 years or younger**   A
EXCLUDES   *Infant partial exchange transfusion (36456)*
📷 1.65   ⚕ 1.65   **FUD** XXX   S R2 80 ▱
AMA: 2016,Jan,13; 2015,Jan,16; 2014,Jan,11

36450 **Exchange transfusion, blood; newborn**   A
EXCLUDES   *Infant partial exchange transfusion (36456)*
📷 3.37   ⚕ 3.37   **FUD** XXX   63 S R2 80 ▱
AMA: 2003,Apr,7; 1997,Nov,1

36455 **other than newborn**   A
📷 3.65   ⚕ 3.65   **FUD** XXX   S G2 ▱
AMA: 2003,Apr,7; 1997,Nov,1

● New Code   ▲ Revised Code   ○ Reinstated   ● New Web Release   ▲ Revised Web Release   Unlisted   Not Covered   # Resequenced
⊘ AMA Mod 51 Exempt   ⑤ Optum Mod 51 Exempt   63 Mod 63 Exempt   ✗ Non-FDA Drug   ★ Telehealth   M Maternity   A Age Edit   + Add-on   AMA: CPT Asst

● **36456** **Partial exchange transfusion, blood, plasma or crystalloid necessitating the skill of a physician or other qualified health care professional, newborn**

> EXCLUDES   *Transfusions of other types (36430-36450)*

36460 **Transfusion, intrauterine, fetal**   A ♀
> ✚ (76941)
> 🚑 9.95   ⚖ 9.95   **FUD** XXX   ⑥③ Ⓢ 80 ▭
> **AMA:** 2003,Apr,7; 1997,Nov,1

36468-36471 Destruction Spider Veins

> EXCLUDES   *Embolization or occlusion services in the same operative field (37241-37244)*
> *Imaging guidance with ultrasound*

36468 **Single or multiple injections of sclerosing solutions, spider veins (telangiectasia), limb or trunk**
> 🚑 0.00   ⚖ 0.00   **FUD** 000   ⓪① N1 80 ▭
> **AMA:** 2016,Jan,13; 2015,Apr,10; 2015,Jan,16; 2014,Oct,6; 2014,Aug,14; 2013,Nov,6

36470 **Injection of sclerosing solution; single vein**
> 🚑 2.42   ⚖ 4.27   **FUD** 010   T P3 50 ▭
> **AMA:** 2016,Jan,13; 2015,Nov,10; 2015,Apr,10; 2015,Jan,16; 2014,Oct,6; 2014,Aug,14; 2013,Nov,6

36471 **multiple veins, same leg**
> 🚑 2.91   ⚖ 4.99   **FUD** 010   T P3 50 ▭
> **AMA:** 2016,Jan,13; 2015,Nov,10; 2015,Aug,8; 2015,Apr,10; 2015,Jan,16; 2014,Oct,6; 2014,Aug,14; 2013,Nov,6

36473-36479 Vein Ablation

> INCLUDES   In same operative field:
> Compression system of lower extremities (29581-29582)
> Venous access/injections (36000-36410, 36425)
> Infiltration with tumescent fluid (36475-36476, 36478-36479)
> Local anesthesia (36473-36474)
> Patient monitoring
> Radiological guidance (76000-76001, 76937, 76942, 76998, 77002)
> EXCLUDES   *Transcatheter embolization (75894)*

● **36473** **Endovenous ablation therapy of incompetent vein, extremity, inclusive of all imaging guidance and monitoring, percutaneous, mechanochemical; first vein treated**
> EXCLUDES   *Laser ablation incompetent vein (36478-36479)*
> *Radiofrequency ablation incompetent vein (36475-36476)*
> *Vascular embolization or occlusion (37241)*

● + **36474** **subsequent vein(s) treated in a single extremity, each through separate access sites (List separately in addition to code for primary procedure)**
> 🚑 0.00   ⚖ 0.00   **FUD** 000
> EXCLUDES   *Laser ablation incompetent vein (36478-36479)*
> *Radiofrequency ablation incompetent vein (36475-36476)*
> *Use of code more than one time per extremity treated*
> *Vascular embolization or occlusion (37241)*
> Code first (36473)

36475 **Endovenous ablation therapy of incompetent vein, extremity, inclusive of all imaging guidance and monitoring, percutaneous, radiofrequency; first vein treated**
> EXCLUDES   *Endovenous ablation therapy of incompetent vein (36478-36479)*
> *Vascular embolization or occlusion (37241-37244)*
> 🚑 8.21   ⚖ 43.8   **FUD** 000   T A2 50 ▭
> **AMA:** 2016,Aug,3; 2016,Jan,13; 2015,Apr,10; 2015,Jan,16; 2014,Oct,6; 2014,Aug,14; 2014,Mar,4; 2014,Jan,11; 2013,Nov,6; 2012,Jan,15-42

▲ + **36476** **subsequent vein(s) treated in a single extremity, each through separate access sites (List separately in addition to code for primary procedure)**
> EXCLUDES   *Endovenous ablation therapy of incompetent vein (36478-36479)*
> *Use of code more than one time per extremity treated*
> *Vascular embolization or occlusion (37241-37244)*
> Code first (36475)
> 🚑 3.98   ⚖ 8.51   **FUD** ZZZ   N N1 50 ▭
> **AMA:** 2016,Aug,3; 2016,Jan,13; 2015,Apr,10; 2015,Jan,16; 2014,Oct,6; 2014,Aug,14; 2014,Mar,4; 2014,Jan,11; 2013,Nov,6; 2012,Jan,15-42

36478 **Endovenous ablation therapy of incompetent vein, extremity, inclusive of all imaging guidance and monitoring, percutaneous, laser; first vein treated**
> EXCLUDES   *Endovenous ablation therapy of incompetent vein (36475-36476)*
> *Vascular embolization or occlusion (37241)*
> 🚑 8.16   ⚖ 34.3   **FUD** 000   T A2 50 ▭
> **AMA:** 2016,Aug,3; 2016,Jan,13; 2015,Apr,10; 2015,Jan,16; 2014,Oct,6; 2014,Aug,14; 2014,Mar,4; 2014,Jan,11; 2013,Nov,6; 2012,Jul,12-14

▲ + **36479** **subsequent vein(s) treated in a single extremity, each through separate access sites (List separately in addition to code for primary procedure)**
> EXCLUDES   *Endovenous ablation therapy of incompetent vein (36475-36476)*
> *Use of code more than one time per extremity treated*
> *Vascular embolization or occlusion (37241)*
> Code first (36478)
> 🚑 3.98   ⚖ 8.83   **FUD** ZZZ   N N1 50 ▭
> **AMA:** 2016,Aug,3; 2016,Jan,13; 2015,Apr,10; 2015,Jan,16; 2014,Oct,6; 2014,Aug,14; 2014,Mar,4; 2014,Jan,11; 2013,Nov,6; 2012,Jul,12-14; 2012,Jan,15-42

36481-36510 Other Venous Catheterization Procedures

> EXCLUDES   *Collection of a specimen from:*
> *A completely implantable device (36591)*
> *An established catheter (36592)*

▲ **36481** **Percutaneous portal vein catheterization by any method**
> ✚ (75885, 75887)
> 🚑 10.1   ⚖ 58.0   **FUD** 000   N N1
> **AMA:** 2016,Jan,13; 2015,Jan,16; 2014,Jan,11; 2012,Jan,15-42; 2011,Jan,11

36500 **Venous catheterization for selective organ blood sampling**
> EXCLUDES   *Inferior or superior vena cava catheterization (36010)*
> ✚ (75893)
> 🚑 5.30   ⚖ 5.30   **FUD** 000   N N1 ▭
> **AMA:** 2014,Jan,11

36510 **Catheterization of umbilical vein for diagnosis or therapy, newborn**   A
> EXCLUDES   *Collection of a specimen from:*
> *Capillary blood (36416)*
> *Venipuncture (36415)*
> 🚑 1.60   ⚖ 2.58   **FUD** 000   ⑥③ N N1 80 ▭
> **AMA:** 2016,May,3; 2016,Jan,13; 2015,Jan,16; 2014,Jan,11

36511-36516 Apheresis

> **CMS:** 100-03,110.14 Apheresis (Therapeutic Pheresis); 100-04,4,231.9 Billing for Pheresis and Apheresis Services
> EXCLUDES   *Collection of a specimen from:*
> *A completely implantable device (36591)*
> *An established catheter (36592)*
> Code also modifier 26 for a professional evaluation

36511 **Therapeutic apheresis; for white blood cells**
> 🚑 2.69   ⚖ 2.69   **FUD** 000   Ⓢ 62 ▭
> **AMA:** 2016,Jan,13; 2015,Jan,16; 2014,Jan,11; 2013,Oct,3; 2011,Jan,11

 PC/TC Only   ASC Payment   50 Bilateral   ♂ Male Only   ♀ Female Only    Facility RVU   ⚖ Non-Facility RVU   ▭ CCI

FUD Follow-up Days   **CMS:** IOM (Pub 100)   OPPSI   80/80 Surg Assist Allowed / w/Doc   Lab Crosswalk   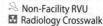 Radiology Crosswalk   ✖ CLIA

152   CPT © 2016 American Medical Association. All Rights Reserved.   © 2016 Optum360, LLC

36512	**for red blood cells**		

🚑 2.71   🔪 2.71   **FUD** 000   S G2 ▭

AMA: 2016,Jan,13; 2015,Jan,16; 2014,Jan,11; 2013,Oct,3; 2011,Jan,11

36513	**for platelets**		

🚑 2.80   🔪 2.80   **FUD** 000   S G2 ▭

AMA: 2016,Jan,13; 2015,Jan,16; 2014,Jan,11; 2013,Oct,3; 2012,Jan,15-42; 2011,Jan,11

36514	**for plasma pheresis**		

🚑 2.68   🔪 15.3   **FUD** 000   S G2 ▭

AMA: 2016,Jan,13; 2015,Jan,16; 2014,Jan,11; 2013,Oct,3; 2011,Jan,11

36515	**with extracorporeal immunoadsorption and plasma reinfusion**		

🚑 2.53   🔪 58.7   **FUD** 000   S P2 ▭

AMA: 2016,Jan,13; 2015,Jan,16; 2014,Jan,11; 2013,Oct,3; 2011,Jan,11

36516	**with extracorporeal selective adsorption or selective filtration and plasma reinfusion**		

🚑 2.01   🔪 59.1   **FUD** 000   S P2 ▭

AMA: 2016,Jan,13; 2015,Jan,16; 2014,Jan,11; 2013,Oct,3; 2011,Jan,11

36522 Extracorporeal Photopheresis

CMS: 100-03,110.4 Extracorporeal Photopheresis; 100-04,32,190 Billing for Extracorporeal Photopheresis; 100-04,32,190.2 Extracorporeal Photopheresis; 100-04,32,190.3 Medicare Denial Codes; 100-04,4,231.9 Billing for Pheresis and Apheresis Services

36522	**Photopheresis, extracorporeal**		

🚑 2.93   🔪 39.7   **FUD** 000   S G2 ▭

AMA: 2016,Jan,13; 2015,Jan,16; 2014,Jan,11; 2013,Oct,3; 2012,Jan,15-42; 2011,Jan,11

36555-36571 Placement of Implantable Venous Access Device

INCLUDES Devices accessed by an exposed catheter, or a subcutaneous port or pump
Devices inserted via cutdown or percutaneous access:
   Centrally (eg, femoral, jugular, subclavian veins, or inferior vena cava)
   Peripherally (eg, basilic or cephalic)
Devices terminating in the brachiocephalic (innominate), iliac, or subclavian veins, vena cava, or right atrium
Venous access obtained by cutdown or percutaneously with any size catheter
EXCLUDES Maintenance/refilling of implantable pump/reservoir (96522)
Code also removal of central venous access device (if code available) when a new device is placed through a separate venous access

▲ 36555   **Insertion of non-tunneled centrally inserted central venous catheter; younger than 5 years of age**   A

EXCLUDES Peripheral insertion (36568)

🚑 3.41   🔪 7.33   **FUD** 000   T A2 ▭

AMA: 2016,Jan,13; 2015,Jan,16; 2014,Jan,11

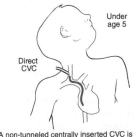

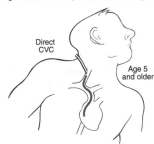

A non-tunneled centrally inserted CVC is inserted. Report 36555 for a patient under age 5 and 36556 for patients older than age 5

36556	**age 5 years or older**		A

EXCLUDES Peripheral insertion (36569)

🚑 3.49   🔪 6.66   **FUD** 000   T A2 ▭

AMA: 2016,Jan,13; 2015,Jan,16; 2014,Jan,11

▲ 36557   **Insertion of tunneled centrally inserted central venous catheter, without subcutaneous port or pump; younger than 5 years of age**   A

🚑 9.55   🔪 28.7   **FUD** 010   T A2 80 50 ▭

AMA: 2016,Jan,13; 2015,Jan,16; 2014,Jan,11

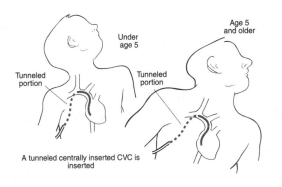

A tunneled centrally inserted CVC is inserted

▲ 36558   **age 5 years or older**   A

EXCLUDES Peripheral insertion (36571)

🚑 8.04   🔪 22.3   **FUD** 010   T A2 80 50 ▭

AMA: 2016,Jan,13; 2015,Jan,16; 2015,Jan,13; 2014,Jan,11

▲ 36560   **Insertion of tunneled centrally inserted central venous access device, with subcutaneous port; younger than 5 years of age**   A

EXCLUDES Peripheral insertion (36570)

🚑 11.3   🔪 38.3   **FUD** 010   T A2 80 50 ▭

AMA: 2016,Jan,13; 2015,Jan,16; 2014,Jan,11; 2012,Jan,15-42; 2011,Jan,11

▲ **36561**　　**age 5 years or older**　　　　　　　　　　　A
> EXCLUDES　*Peripheral insertion (36571)*
> 🚗 10.2　　⚕ 33.5　　**FUD** 010　　T A2 80 50 ▣
>
> **AMA:** 2016,Jan,13; 2015,Jan,16; 2014,Jan,11; 2012,Jan,15-42; 2011,Jan,11

▲ **36563**　**Insertion of tunneled centrally inserted central venous access device with subcutaneous pump**
> 🚗 11.1　　⚕ 37.9　　**FUD** 010　　T A2 80 ▣
>
> **AMA:** 2016,Jan,13; 2015,Jan,16; 2014,Jan,11

▲ **36565**　**Insertion of tunneled centrally inserted central venous access device, requiring 2 catheters via 2 separate venous access sites; without subcutaneous port or pump (eg, Tesio type catheter)**
> 🚗 10.1　　⚕ 27.7　　**FUD** 010　　T A2 80 50 ▣
>
> **AMA:** 2016,Jan,13; 2015,Jan,16; 2014,Jan,11

▲ **36566**　　**with subcutaneous port(s)**
> 🚗 11.2　　⚕ 155.　　**FUD** 010　　T A2 80 50 ▣
>
> **AMA:** 2016,Jan,13; 2015,Jan,16; 2014,Jan,11

▲ **36568**　**Insertion of peripherally inserted central venous catheter (PICC), without subcutaneous port or pump; younger than 5 years of age**　　　　　　　　A
> EXCLUDES　*Centrally inserted placement (36555)*
> 　　　　*PICC line removal with codes for removal of tunneled central venous catheters; report appropriate E&M code*
> 🚗 2.81　　⚕ 8.58　　**FUD** 000　　T A2 ▣
>
> **AMA:** 2016,Jan,13; 2015,Jan,16; 2014,Jan,11; 2012,Nov,13-14; 2012,Jan,15-42; 2011,Jan,11

　　36569　　**age 5 years or older**　　　　　　　　　A
> EXCLUDES　*Centrally inserted placement (36556)*
> 　　　　*PICC line removal with codes for removal of tunneled central venous catheters; report appropriate E&M code*
> 🚗 2.65　　⚕ 7.13　　**FUD** 000　　T A2 ▣
>
> **AMA:** 2016,Jan,13; 2015,Jan,16; 2014,Sep,13; 2014,Jan,11; 2013,Sep,17; 2012,Nov,13-14; 2012,Jan,15-42; 2011,Jan,11

▲ **36570**　**Insertion of peripherally inserted central venous access device, with subcutaneous port; younger than 5 years of age**　　　　　　　　A
> EXCLUDES　*Centrally inserted placement (36560)*
> 🚗 9.02　　⚕ 33.0　　**FUD** 010　　T A2 80 50 ▣
>
> **AMA:** 2016,Jan,13; 2015,Jan,16; 2014,Jan,11; 2012,Jan,15-42

▲ **36571**　　**age 5 years or older**　　　　　　　　　A
> EXCLUDES　*Centrally inserted placement (36561)*
> 🚗 9.39　　⚕ 37.1　　**FUD** 010　　T A2 80 50 ▣
>
> **AMA:** 2016,Jan,13; 2015,Jan,16; 2014,Jan,11; 2012,Jan,15-42

36575-36590 Repair, Removal, and Replacement Implantable Venous Access Device

> EXCLUDES　*Mechanical removal obstructive material, pericatheter/intraluminal (36595, 36596)*
>
> Code also a frequency of two for procedures involving both catheters from a multicatheter device

　　36575　**Repair of tunneled or non-tunneled central venous access catheter, without subcutaneous port or pump, central or peripheral insertion site**
> INCLUDES　Repair of the device without replacing any parts
> 🚗 1.02　　⚕ 4.75　　**FUD** 000　　T A2 80 ▣
>
> **AMA:** 2016,Jan,13; 2015,Jan,16; 2014,Jan,11

▲ **36576**　**Repair of central venous access device, with subcutaneous port or pump, central or peripheral insertion site**
> INCLUDES　Repair of the device without replacing any parts
> 🚗 5.75　　⚕ 11.1　　**FUD** 010　　T A2 80 ▣
>
> **AMA:** 2016,Jan,13; 2015,Jan,16; 2014,Jan,11

▲ **36578**　**Replacement, catheter only, of central venous access device, with subcutaneous port or pump, central or peripheral insertion site**
> INCLUDES　Partial replacement (catheter only)
> EXCLUDES　*Total replacement of the entire device using the same venous access sites (36582-36583)*
> 🚗 6.28　　⚕ 14.8　　**FUD** 010　　T A2 80 ▣
>
> **AMA:** 2016,Jan,13; 2015,Jan,16; 2014,Jan,11

　　36580　**Replacement, complete, of a non-tunneled centrally inserted central venous catheter, without subcutaneous port or pump, through same venous access**
> INCLUDES　Complete replacement (replace all components/same access site)
> 🚗 1.94　　⚕ 6.13　　**FUD** 000　　T A2 ▣
>
> **AMA:** 2016,Jan,13; 2015,Jan,16; 2014,Jan,11

▲ **36581**　**Replacement, complete, of a tunneled centrally inserted central venous catheter, without subcutaneous port or pump, through same venous access**
> INCLUDES　Complete replacement (replace all components/same access site)
> EXCLUDES　*Removal of old device and insertion of new device using a separate venous access site*
> 🚗 5.70　　⚕ 21.9　　**FUD** 010　　T A2 80 ▣
>
> **AMA:** 2016,Jan,13; 2015,Jan,16; 2014,Jan,11

▲ **36582**　**Replacement, complete, of a tunneled centrally inserted central venous access device, with subcutaneous port, through same venous access**
> INCLUDES　Complete replacement (replace all components/same access site)
> EXCLUDES　*Removal of old device and insertion of new device using a separate venous access site*
> 🚗 8.90　　⚕ 31.4　　**FUD** 010　　T A2 80 ▣
>
> **AMA:** 2016,Jan,13; 2015,Jan,16; 2014,Jan,11

▲ **36583**　**Replacement, complete, of a tunneled centrally inserted central venous access device, with subcutaneous pump, through same venous access**
> INCLUDES　Complete replacement (replace all components/same access site)
> EXCLUDES　*Removal of old device and insertion of new device using a separate venous access site*
> 🚗 9.85　　⚕ 38.9　　**FUD** 010　　T A2 80 ▣
>
> **AMA:** 2016,Jan,13; 2015,Jan,16; 2014,Jan,11

　　36584　**Replacement, complete, of a peripherally inserted central venous catheter (PICC), without subcutaneous port or pump, through same venous access**
> INCLUDES　Complete replacement (replace all components/same access site)
> 🚗 1.93　　⚕ 5.84　　**FUD** 000　　T A2 ▣
>
> **AMA:** 2016,Jan,13; 2015,Jan,16; 2014,Jan,11

▲ **36585**　**Replacement, complete, of a peripherally inserted central venous access device, with subcutaneous port, through same venous access**
> INCLUDES　Complete replacement (replace all components/same access site)
> 🚗 8.26　　⚕ 32.8　　**FUD** 010　　T A2 80 ▣
>
> **AMA:** 2016,Jan,13; 2015,Jan,16; 2014,Jan,11

　　36589　**Removal of tunneled central venous catheter, without subcutaneous port or pump**
> INCLUDES　Complete removal/all components
> EXCLUDES　*Non-tunneled central venous catheter removal; report appropriate E&M code*
> 🚗 3.99　　⚕ 4.73　　**FUD** 010　　02 A2 80 ▣
>
> **AMA:** 2016,Jan,13; 2015,Nov,10; 2015,Jan,16; 2014,Jan,11

26/TC PC/TC Only　　A2-Z3 ASC Payment　　50 Bilateral　　♂ Male Only　　♀ Female Only　　🚗 Facility RVU　　⚕ Non-Facility RVU　　▣ CCI
FUD Follow-up Days　　CMS: IOM (Pub 100)　　A-Y OPPSI　　80/80 Surg Assist Allowed / w/Doc　　🔬 Lab Crosswalk　　☢ Radiology Crosswalk　　CLIA

154　　　　　　　　　　　　　　　　CPT © 2016 American Medical Association. All Rights Reserved.　　　　　　　　　　　© 2016 Optum360, LLC

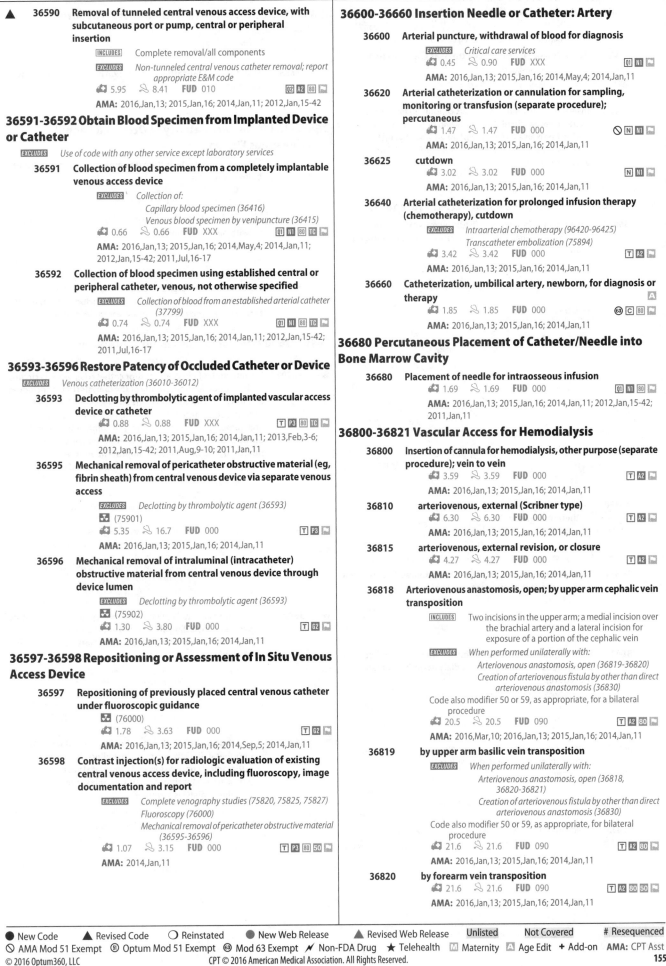

▲ 36590 **Removal of tunneled central venous access device, with subcutaneous port or pump, central or peripheral insertion**
INCLUDES Complete removal/all components
EXCLUDES *Non-tunneled central venous catheter removal; report appropriate E&M code*
🔧 5.95 ⚕ 8.41 **FUD** 010 [02][A2][80][▣]
AMA: 2016,Jan,13; 2015,Jan,16; 2014,Jan,11; 2012,Jan,15-42

36591-36592 Obtain Blood Specimen from Implanted Device or Catheter
EXCLUDES *Use of code with any other service except laboratory services*

36591 **Collection of blood specimen from a completely implantable venous access device**
EXCLUDES *Collection of:*
Capillary blood specimen (36416)
Venous blood specimen by venipuncture (36415)
🔧 0.66 ⚕ 0.66 **FUD** XXX [01][N1][80][TC][▣]
AMA: 2016,Jan,13; 2015,Jan,16; 2014,May,4; 2014,Jan,11; 2012,Jan,15-42; 2011,Jul,16-17

36592 **Collection of blood specimen using established central or peripheral catheter, venous, not otherwise specified**
EXCLUDES *Collection of blood from an established arterial catheter (37799)*
🔧 0.74 ⚕ 0.74 **FUD** XXX [01][N1][80][TC][▣]
AMA: 2016,Jan,13; 2015,Jan,16; 2014,Jan,11; 2012,Jan,15-42; 2011,Jul,16-17

36593-36596 Restore Patency of Occluded Catheter or Device
EXCLUDES *Venous catheterization (36010-36012)*

36593 **Declotting by thrombolytic agent of implanted vascular access device or catheter**
🔧 0.88 ⚕ 0.88 **FUD** XXX [T][P3][80][TC][▣]
AMA: 2016,Jan,13; 2015,Jan,16; 2014,Jan,11; 2013,Feb,3-6; 2012,Jan,15-42; 2011,Aug,9-10; 2011,Jan,11

36595 **Mechanical removal of pericatheter obstructive material (eg, fibrin sheath) from central venous device via separate venous access**
EXCLUDES *Declotting by thrombolytic agent (36593)*
🔧 (75901)
🔧 5.35 ⚕ 16.7 **FUD** 000 [T][P3][▣]
AMA: 2016,Jan,13; 2015,Jan,16; 2014,Jan,11

36596 **Mechanical removal of intraluminal (intracatheter) obstructive material from central venous device through device lumen**
EXCLUDES *Declotting by thrombolytic agent (36593)*
🔧 (75902)
🔧 1.30 ⚕ 3.80 **FUD** 000 [T][G2][▣]
AMA: 2016,Jan,13; 2015,Jan,16; 2014,Jan,11

36597-36598 Repositioning or Assessment of In Situ Venous Access Device

36597 **Repositioning of previously placed central venous catheter under fluoroscopic guidance**
🔧 (76000)
🔧 1.78 ⚕ 3.63 **FUD** 000 [T][G2][▣]
AMA: 2016,Jan,13; 2015,Jan,16; 2014,Sep,5; 2014,Jan,11

36598 **Contrast injection(s) for radiologic evaluation of existing central venous access device, including fluoroscopy, image documentation and report**
EXCLUDES *Complete venography studies (75820, 75825, 75827)*
Fluoroscopy (76000)
Mechanical removal of pericatheter obstructive material (36595-36596)
🔧 1.07 ⚕ 3.15 **FUD** 000 [T][P3][80][50][▣]
AMA: 2014,Jan,11

36600-36660 Insertion Needle or Catheter: Artery

36600 **Arterial puncture, withdrawal of blood for diagnosis**
EXCLUDES *Critical care services*
🔧 0.45 ⚕ 0.90 **FUD** XXX [01][N1][▣]
AMA: 2016,Jan,13; 2015,Jan,16; 2014,May,4; 2014,Jan,11

36620 **Arterial catheterization or cannulation for sampling, monitoring or transfusion (separate procedure); percutaneous**
🔧 1.47 ⚕ 1.47 **FUD** 000 [🚫][N][N1][▣]
AMA: 2016,Jan,13; 2015,Jan,16; 2014,Jan,11

36625 **cutdown**
🔧 3.02 ⚕ 3.02 **FUD** 000 [N][N1][▣]
AMA: 2016,Jan,13; 2015,Jan,16; 2014,Jan,11

36640 **Arterial catheterization for prolonged infusion therapy (chemotherapy), cutdown**
EXCLUDES *Intraarterial chemotherapy (96420-96425)*
Transcatheter embolization (75894)
🔧 3.42 ⚕ 3.42 **FUD** 000 [T][A2][▣]
AMA: 2016,Jan,13; 2015,Jan,16; 2014,Jan,11

36660 **Catheterization, umbilical artery, newborn, for diagnosis or therapy** [A]
🔧 1.85 ⚕ 1.85 **FUD** 000 [63][C][80][▣]
AMA: 2016,Jan,13; 2015,Jan,16; 2014,Jan,11

36680 Percutaneous Placement of Catheter/Needle into Bone Marrow Cavity

36680 **Placement of needle for intraosseous infusion**
🔧 1.69 ⚕ 1.69 **FUD** 000 [01][N1][80][▣]
AMA: 2016,Jan,13; 2015,Jan,16; 2014,Jan,11; 2012,Jan,15-42; 2011,Jan,11

36800-36821 Vascular Access for Hemodialysis

36800 **Insertion of cannula for hemodialysis, other purpose (separate procedure); vein to vein**
🔧 3.59 ⚕ 3.59 **FUD** 000 [T][A2][▣]
AMA: 2016,Jan,13; 2015,Jan,16; 2014,Jan,11

36810 **arteriovenous, external (Scribner type)**
🔧 6.30 ⚕ 6.30 **FUD** 000 [T][A2][▣]
AMA: 2016,Jan,13; 2015,Jan,16; 2014,Jan,11

36815 **arteriovenous, external revision, or closure**
🔧 4.27 ⚕ 4.27 **FUD** 000 [T][A2][▣]
AMA: 2016,Jan,13; 2015,Jan,16; 2014,Jan,11

36818 **Arteriovenous anastomosis, open; by upper arm cephalic vein transposition**
INCLUDES Two incisions in the upper arm; a medial incision over the brachial artery and a lateral incision for exposure of a portion of the cephalic vein
EXCLUDES *When performed unilaterally with:*
Arteriovenous anastomosis, open (36819-36820)
Creation of arteriovenous fistula by other than direct arteriovenous anastomosis (36830)
Code also modifier 50 or 59, as appropriate, for a bilateral procedure
🔧 20.5 ⚕ 20.5 **FUD** 090 [T][A2][80][▣]
AMA: 2016,Mar,10; 2016,Jan,13; 2015,Jan,16; 2014,Jan,11

36819 **by upper arm basilic vein transposition**
EXCLUDES *When performed unilaterally with:*
Arteriovenous anastomosis, open (36818, 36820-36821)
Creation of arteriovenous fistula by other than direct arteriovenous anastomosis (36830)
Code also modifier 50 or 59, as appropriate, for bilateral procedure
🔧 21.6 ⚕ 21.6 **FUD** 090 [T][A2][80][▣]
AMA: 2016,Jan,13; 2015,Jan,16; 2014,Jan,11

36820 **by forearm vein transposition**
🔧 21.6 ⚕ 21.6 **FUD** 090 [T][A2][80][50][▣]
AMA: 2016,Jan,13; 2015,Jan,16; 2014,Jan,11

36821 direct, any site (eg, Cimino type) (separate procedure)

🚑 19.6   ⚖ 19.6   **FUD** 090   [T] [A2] [80] [□]

AMA: 2016,Jan,13; 2015,Aug,8; 2015,Jan,16; 2014,Jan,11

36823 Vascular Access for Extracorporeal Circulation

INCLUDES   Chemotherapy perfusion

EXCLUDES   *Chemotherapy administration (96409-96425)*
Maintenance for extracorporeal circulation (33946-33949)

36823 Insertion of arterial and venous cannula(s) for isolated extracorporeal circulation including regional chemotherapy perfusion to an extremity, with or without hyperthermia, with removal of cannula(s) and repair of arteriotomy and venotomy sites

🚑 39.2   ⚖ 39.2   **FUD** 090   [C] [□]

AMA: 2014,Jan,11

36825-36835 Permanent Vascular Access Procedures

36825 Creation of arteriovenous fistula by other than direct arteriovenous anastomosis (separate procedure); autogenous graft

EXCLUDES   *Direct arteriovenous (AV) anastomosis (36821)*

🚑 23.6   ⚖ 23.6   **FUD** 090   [T] [A2] [80] [□]

AMA: 2016,Jan,13; 2015,Jan,16; 2014,Jan,11

In 36825, the artery and vein are connected by a vein graft in an end-to-side manner, creating an arteriovenous fistula

Radial artery

Radial artery

Graft

Basilic vein

Basilic vein

In 36830, the artery and vein are connected by a synthetic graft

36830 nonautogenous graft (eg, biological collagen, thermoplastic graft)

EXCLUDES   *Direct arteriovenous (AV) anastomosis (36821)*

🚑 19.7   ⚖ 19.7   **FUD** 090   [T] [A2] [80] [□]

AMA: 2016,Jan,13; 2015,Jan,16; 2015,Jan,13; 2014,Jan,11

36831 Thrombectomy, open, arteriovenous fistula without revision, autogenous or nonautogenous dialysis graft (separate procedure)

🚑 18.2   ⚖ 18.2   **FUD** 090   [T] [A2] [80] [□]

AMA: 2016,Jan,13; 2015,Jan,16; 2014,Jan,11; 2012,Jan,15-42; 2011,Jan,11

36832 Revision, open, arteriovenous fistula; without thrombectomy, autogenous or nonautogenous dialysis graft (separate procedure)

INCLUDES   Revision of an arteriovenous access fistula or graft

🚑 22.4   ⚖ 22.4   **FUD** 090   [T] [A2] [80] [□]

AMA: 2016,Jan,13; 2015,Jan,16; 2014,Jan,11; 2012,Jan,15-42; 2011,Jan,11

36833 with thrombectomy, autogenous or nonautogenous dialysis graft (separate procedure)

EXCLUDES   *Hemodialysis circuit procedures (36901-36906)*

🚑 24.0   ⚖ 24.0   **FUD** 090   [T] [A2] [80] [□]

AMA: 2016,Jan,13; 2015,Jan,16; 2014,Jan,11; 2012,Jan,15-42; 2011,Jan,11

36835 Insertion of Thomas shunt (separate procedure)

🚑 14.4   ⚖ 14.4   **FUD** 090   [T] [A2] [□]

AMA: 2014,Jan,11

36838 DRIL Procedure for Ischemic Steal Syndrome

EXCLUDES   *Bypass graft, with vein (35512, 35522-35523)*
Ligation (37607, 37618)
Revision, open, arteriovenous fistula (36832)

36838 Distal revascularization and interval ligation (DRIL), upper extremity hemodialysis access (steal syndrome)

🚑 33.8   ⚖ 33.8   **FUD** 090   [T] [80] [50] [□]

AMA: 2014,Jan,11

36860-36870 Restore Patency of Occluded Cannula or Arteriovenous Fistula

36860 External cannula declotting (separate procedure); without balloon catheter

☒ (76000)

🚑 3.19   ⚖ 5.94   **FUD** 000   [T] [A2]

AMA: 2016,Jan,13; 2015,Jan,16; 2014,Jan,11

36861 with balloon catheter

☒ (76000)

🚑 3.85   ⚖ 3.85   **FUD** 000   [T] [A2] [□]

AMA: 2016,Jan,13; 2015,Jan,16; 2014,Jan,11

36870 ~~Thrombectomy, percutaneous, arteriovenous fistula, autogenous or nonautogenous graft (includes mechanical thrombus extraction and intra-graft thrombolysis)~~

To report, see ~36904-36906

36901-36909 Hemodialysis Circuit Procedures

EXCLUDES   *Arteriography to assess inflow to hemodialysis circuit when performed*

● **36901** Introduction of needle(s) and/or catheter(s), dialysis circuit, with diagnostic angiography of the dialysis circuit, including all direct puncture(s) and catheter placement(s), injection(s) of contrast, all necessary imaging from the arterial anastomosis and adjacent artery through entire venous outflow including the inferior or superior vena cava, fluoroscopic guidance, radiological supervision and interpretation and image documentation and report;

INCLUDES   Access
Catheter advancement (e.g., imaging of accessory veins, assess all sections of circuit)
Contrast injection

EXCLUDES   *Balloon angioplasty of peripheral segment (36902)*
Open revision with thrombectomy of arteriovenous fistula (36833)
Percutaneous transluminal procedures of peripheral segment (36904-36906)
Stent placement in peripheral segment (36903)
Use of code more than one time per procedure

● **36902** with transluminal balloon angioplasty, peripheral dialysis segment, including all imaging and radiological supervision and interpretation necessary to perform the angioplasty

EXCLUDES   *Open revision with thrombectomy of arteriovenous fistula (36833)*
Percutaneous transluminal procedures of peripheral segment (36904-36906)
Stent placement in peripheral segment (36903)
Use of code more than one time per procedure

● **36903** with transcatheter placement of intravascular stent(s), peripheral dialysis segment, including all imaging and radiological supervision and interpretation necessary to perform the stenting, and all angioplasty within the peripheral dialysis segment

INCLUDES   Balloon angioplasty of peripheral segment (36902)

EXCLUDES   *Central hemodialysis circuit procedures (36907-36908)*
Open revision with thrombectomy of arteriovenous fistula (36833)
Percutaneous transluminal procedures of peripheral segment (36904-36906)
Use of code more than one time per procedure

● **36904** Percutaneous transluminal mechanical thrombectomy and/or infusion for thrombolysis, dialysis circuit, any method, including all imaging and radiological supervision and interpretation, diagnostic angiography, fluoroscopic guidance, catheter placement(s), and intraprocedural pharmacological thrombolytic injection(s);

> EXCLUDES *Open thrombectomy of arteriovenous fistula with/without revision (36831, 36833)*
> *Use of code more than one time per procedure*

● **36905** with transluminal balloon angioplasty, peripheral dialysis segment, including all imaging and radiological supervision and interpretation necessary to perform the angioplasty

> INCLUDES Percutaneous mechanical thrombectomy (36904)
> EXCLUDES *Use of code more than one time per procedure*

● **36906** with transcatheter placement of intravascular stent(s), peripheral dialysis segment, including all imaging and radiological supervision and interpretation necessary to perform the stenting, and all angioplasty within the peripheral dialysis circuit

> INCLUDES Percutaneous transluminal balloon angioplasty (36905)
> Percutaneous transluminal thrombectomy (36904)
> EXCLUDES *Hemodialysis circuit procedures provided by catheter or needle access (36901-36903)*
> *Use of code more than one time per procedure*
> Code also balloon angioplasty of central veins, when performed (36907)
> Code also stent placement in central veins, when performed (36908)

● + **36907** Transluminal balloon angioplasty, central dialysis segment, performed through dialysis circuit, including all imaging and radiological supervision and interpretation required to perform the angioplasty (List separately in addition to code for primary procedure)

> 📇 0.00 ⌀ 0.00 **FUD** 000
> INCLUDES All central hemodialysis segment angiography
> EXCLUDES *Angiography with stent placement (36908)*
> Code first (36818-36833, 36901-36906)

● + **36908** Transcatheter placement of intravascular stent(s), central dialysis segment, performed through dialysis circuit, including all imaging radiological supervision and interpretation required to perform the stenting, and all angioplasty in the central dialysis segment (List separately in addition to code for primary procedure)

> 📇 0.00 ⌀ 0.00 **FUD** 000
> INCLUDES All central hemodialysis segment stent(s) placed
> Ballooon angioplasty central dialysis segment (36907)
> Code first when performed (36818-36833, 36901-36906)

● + **36909** Dialysis circuit permanent vascular embolization or occlusion (including main circuit or any accessory veins), endovascular, including all imaging and radiological supervision and interpretation necessary to complete the intervention (List separately in addition to code for primary procedure)

> 📇 0.00 ⌀ 0.00 **FUD** 000
> INCLUDES All embolization/occlusion procedures performed in the hemodialysis circuit
> EXCLUDES *Banding/ligation of arteriovenous fistula (37607)*
> *Use of code more than one time per day*
> Code first (36901-36906)

37140-37181 Open Decompression of Portal Circulation

> EXCLUDES *Peritoneal-venous shunt (49425)*

37140 Venous anastomosis, open; portocaval

> 📇 66.7 ⌀ 66.7 **FUD** 090   C 🖵
> **AMA:** 2014,Jan,11

37145 renoportal

> 📇 62.5 ⌀ 62.5 **FUD** 090   C 80 🖵
> **AMA:** 2014,Jan,11

37160 caval-mesenteric

> 📇 64.2 ⌀ 64.2 **FUD** 090   C 80 🖵
> **AMA:** 2014,Jan,11

37180 splenorenal, proximal

> 📇 59.2 ⌀ 59.2 **FUD** 090   C 80 🖵
> **AMA:** 2014,Jan,11

37181 splenorenal, distal (selective decompression of esophagogastric varices, any technique)

> EXCLUDES *Percutaneous procedure (37182)*
> 📇 67.6 ⌀ 67.6 **FUD** 090   C 80 🖵
> **AMA:** 2014,Jan,11

37182-37183 Transvenous Decompression of Portal Circulation

> INCLUDES Percutaneous transhepatic portography (75885, 75887)

37182 Insertion of transvenous intrahepatic portosystemic shunt(s) (TIPS) (includes venous access, hepatic and portal vein catheterization, portography with hemodynamic evaluation, intrahepatic tract formation/dilatation, stent placement and all associated imaging guidance and documentation)

> EXCLUDES *Open procedure (37140)*
> 📇 24.2 ⌀ 24.2 **FUD** 000   C 80 🖵
> **AMA:** 2016,Jan,13; 2015,Jan,16; 2014,Jan,11; 2013,Sep,17; 2012,Jan,15-42; 2011,Jan,11

▲ **37183** Revision of transvenous intrahepatic portosystemic shunt(s) (TIPS) (includes venous access, hepatic and portal vein catheterization, portography with hemodynamic evaluation, intrahepatic tract recanulization/dilatation, stent placement and all associated imaging guidance and documentation)

> EXCLUDES *Arteriovenous (AV) aneurysm repair (36832)*
> 📇 11.4 ⌀ 168. **FUD** 000   J 80 🖵
> **AMA:** 2016,Jan,13; 2015,Jan,16; 2014,Jan,11; 2012,Jan,15-42; 2011,Jan,11

37184-37188 Removal of Thrombus from Vessel: Percutaneous

> INCLUDES Fluoroscopic guidance (76000-76001)
> Injection(s) of thrombolytics during the procedure
> Postprocedure evaluation
> Pretreatment planning
> EXCLUDES *Continuous infusion of thrombolytics prior to and after the procedure ([37211, 37212, 37213, 37214])*
> *Diagnostic studies*
> *Intracranial arterial mechanical thrombectomy or infusion (61645)*
> *Mechanical thrombectomy, coronary (92973)*
> *Other interventions performed percutaneously (e.g., balloon angioplasty)*
> *Placement of catheters*
> *Radiological supervision/interpretation*

▲ **37184** Primary percutaneous transluminal mechanical thrombectomy, noncoronary, non-intracranial, arterial or arterial bypass graft, including fluoroscopic guidance and intraprocedural pharmacological thrombolytic injection(s); initial vessel

> EXCLUDES *Intracranial arterial mechanical thrombectomy (61645)*
> *Mechanical thrombectomy for embolus/thrombus complicating another percutaneous interventional procedure (37186)*
> *Mechanical thrombectomy of another vascular family/separate access site, append modifier 51 to code, as appropriate*
> *Moderate sedation services (99151-99157)*
> *Therapeutic, prophylactic, or diagnostic injection (96374)*
> 📇 13.4 ⌀ 64.9 **FUD** 000   T 62 50 🖵
> **AMA:** 2016,Jul,6; 2016,Mar,3; 2016,Jan,13; 2015,Nov,3; 2015,Apr,10; 2015,Jan,16; 2014,Jan,11; 2013,Feb,3-6

▲ + **37185** **second and all subsequent vessel(s) within the same vascular family (List separately in addition to code for primary mechanical thrombectomy procedure)**

INCLUDES Treatment of second and all succeeding vessel(s) in same vascular family

EXCLUDES *Intravenous drug injections administered subsequent to an initial service*

Mechanical thrombectomy for treating of embolus/thrombus complicating another percutaneous interventional procedure (37186)

Mechanical thrombectomy of another vascular family/separate access site, append modifier 51 to code as appropriate

Therapeutic, prophylactic, or diagnostic injection (96375)

Code first (37184)

🚗 4.92   ⚕ 20.6   **FUD** ZZZ   N N1 ▣

AMA: 2016,Jul,6; 2016,Jan,13; 2015,Nov,3; 2015,Apr,10; 2015,Jan,16; 2014,Jan,11; 2013,Feb,3-6

▲ + **37186** **Secondary percutaneous transluminal thrombectomy (eg, nonprimary mechanical, snare basket, suction technique), noncoronary, non-intracranial, arterial or arterial bypass graft, including fluoroscopic guidance and intraprocedural pharmacological thrombolytic injections, provided in conjunction with another percutaneous intervention other than primary mechanical thrombectomy (List separately in addition to code for primary procedure)**

INCLUDES Removal of small emboli/thrombi prior to or after another percutaneous procedure

Primary percutaneous transluminal mechanical thrombectomy, noncoronary, non-intracranial (37184-37185)

Therapeutic, prophylactic, or diagnostic injection (96375)

Code first primary procedure

🚗 7.31   ⚕ 39.3   **FUD** ZZZ   N N1 ▣

AMA: 2016,Jul,6; 2016,Jan,13; 2015,Nov,3; 2015,Jan,16; 2014,Jan,11; 2013,Feb,3-6; 2012,Jan,15-42; 2011,Jul,3-11; 2011,Jan,11

▲ **37187** **Percutaneous transluminal mechanical thrombectomy, vein(s), including intraprocedural pharmacological thrombolytic injections and fluoroscopic guidance**

INCLUDES Secondary or subsequent intravenous injection after another initial service

EXCLUDES *Therapeutic, prophylactic, or diagnostic injection (96375)*

🚗 11.9   ⚕ 58.8   **FUD** 000   T G2 50 ▣

AMA: 2016,Jul,6; 2016,Mar,3; 2016,Jan,13; 2015,Nov,3; 2015,Jan,16; 2014,Jan,11; 2013,Feb,3-6

▲ **37188** **Percutaneous transluminal mechanical thrombectomy, vein(s), including intraprocedural pharmacological thrombolytic injections and fluoroscopic guidance, repeat treatment on subsequent day during course of thrombolytic therapy**

EXCLUDES *Therapeutic, prophylactic, or diagnostic injection (96375)*

🚗 8.57   ⚕ 50.7   **FUD** 000   T G2 50 ▣

AMA: 2016,Jul,6; 2016,Mar,3; 2016,Jan,13; 2015,Nov,3; 2015,Jan,16; 2014,Jan,11; 2013,Feb,3-6

37191-37193 Vena Cava Filters

▲ **37191** **Insertion of intravascular vena cava filter, endovascular approach including vascular access, vessel selection, and radiological supervision and interpretation, intraprocedural roadmapping, and imaging guidance (ultrasound and fluoroscopy), when performed**

EXCLUDES *Open ligation of inferior vena cava via laparotomy or retroperitoneal approach (37619)*

🚗 6.97   ⚕ 75.0   **FUD** 000   T ▣

AMA: 2016,May,11; 2016,Jan,13; 2015,Jan,16; 2014,Jan,11; 2013,Feb,3-6; 2012,Apr,3-9

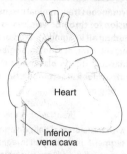

Heart

Inferior vena cava

The inverior vena cava (or IVC) is the major return vessel of the lower body. It extends from the right atrium of the heart down to the bifurcation of the iliac veins

An intravascular "umbrella" device in the IVC. Such devices are intended to entrap clots and prevent clot passage into the pulmonary arteries

▲ **37192** **Repositioning of intravascular vena cava filter, endovascular approach including vascular access, vessel selection, and radiological supervision and interpretation, intraprocedural roadmapping, and imaging guidance (ultrasound and fluoroscopy), when performed**

EXCLUDES *Insertion of intravascular vena cava filter (37191)*

🚗 10.7   ⚕ 44.2   **FUD** 000   T ▣

AMA: 2016,May,11; 2016,Jan,13; 2015,Jan,16; 2014,Jan,11; 2013,Feb,3-6; 2012,Apr,3-9

▲ **37193** **Retrieval (removal) of intravascular vena cava filter, endovascular approach including vascular access, vessel selection, and radiological supervision and interpretation, intraprocedural roadmapping, and imaging guidance (ultrasound and fluoroscopy), when performed**

EXCLUDES *Transcatheter retrieval, percutaneous, of intravascular foreign body (37197)*

🚗 10.6   ⚕ 45.6   **FUD** 000   T ▣

AMA: 2016,May,11; 2016,Jan,13; 2015,Jan,16; 2014,Jan,11; 2013,Feb,3-6; 2012,Apr,3-9

37195 Intravenous Cerebral Thrombolysis

37195 **Thrombolysis, cerebral, by intravenous infusion**

🚗 0.00   ⚕ 0.00   **FUD** XXX   T 80 ▣

AMA: 2014,Jan,11

37197-37214 [37211, 37212, 37213, 37214] Transcatheter Procedures: Infusions, Biopsy, Foreign Body Removal

▲ **37197** **Transcatheter retrieval, percutaneous, of intravascular foreign body (eg, fractured venous or arterial catheter), includes radiological supervision and interpretation, and imaging guidance (ultrasound or fluoroscopy), when performed**

EXCLUDES *Percutaneous vena cava filter retrieval (37193)*
Removal leadless pacemaker system (0388T)

🚗 9.24   ⚕ 43.3   **FUD** 000   T G2 ▣

AMA: 2016,May,11; 2016,Jan,13; 2015,Jan,16; 2014,Jan,11; 2013,Feb,3-6

37200 **Transcatheter biopsy**

📷 (75970)

🚗 6.40   ⚕ 6.40   **FUD** 000   T G2 ▣

AMA: 2014,Jan,11

▲ # **37211** **Transcatheter therapy, arterial infusion for thrombolysis other than coronary or intracranial, any method, including radiological supervision and interpretation, initial treatment day**

INCLUDES
Catheter exchange or position change
E&M services on the day of and related to thrombolysis
First day of transcatheter thrombolytic infusion
Fluoroscopic guidance
Follow-up arteriography or venography
Radiologic supervision and interpretation

EXCLUDES
Angiography through existing catheter for follow-up study for transcatheter therapy, embolization or infusion, other than for thrombolysis (75898)
Catheter placement
Declotting of implanted catheter or vascular access device by thrombolytic agent (36593)
Diagnostic studies
Intracranial arterial mechanical thrombectomy or infusion (61645)
Percutaneous interventions
Procedure performed more than one time per date of service
Ultrasound guidance (76937)

Code also significant, separately identifiable E&M service on the day of thrombolysis using modifier 25

🚑 11.6   ⚕ 11.6   **FUD** 000   [T] [62] [50] 🔲

AMA: 2016,Jul,6; 2016,Mar,3; 2016,Jan,13; 2015,Nov,3; 2015,Jan,16; 2014,Jan,11; 2013,Feb,3-6

▲ # **37212** **Transcatheter therapy, venous infusion for thrombolysis, any method, including radiological supervision and interpretation, initial treatment day**

INCLUDES
Catheter position change or exchange
E&M services on the day of and related to thrombolysis
First day of transcatheter thrombolytic infusion
Fluoroscopic guidance
Follow-up arteriography or venography
Initiation and completion of thrombolysis on same date of service
Radiologic supervision and interpretation

EXCLUDES
Angiography through existing catheter for follow-up study for transcatheter therapy, embolization or infusion, other than for thrombolysis (75898)
Catheter placement
Declotting of implanted catheter or vascular access device by thrombolytic agent (36593)
Diagnostic studies
Percutaneous interventions
Procedure performed more than one time per date of service
Ultrasound guidance (76937)

Code also significant, separately identifiable E&M service on the same day as thrombolysis using modifier 25

🚑 10.2   ⚕ 10.2   **FUD** 000   [T] [62] [50] 🔲

AMA: 2016,Jul,6; 2016,Mar,3; 2016,Jan,13; 2015,Nov,3; 2015,Jan,16; 2014,Jan,11; 2013,Feb,3-6

▲ # **37213** **Transcatheter therapy, arterial or venous infusion for thrombolysis other than coronary, any method, including radiological supervision and interpretation, continued treatment on subsequent day during course of thrombolytic therapy, including follow-up catheter contrast injection, position change, or exchange, when performed;**

INCLUDES
Continued thrombolytic infusions on subsequent days besides the initial and last days of treatment
E&M services on the day of and related to the thrombolysis
Fluoroscopic guidance
Radiologic supervision and interpretation

EXCLUDES
Angiography through existing catheter for follow-up study for transcatheter therapy, embolization or infusion, other than for thrombolysis (75898)
Catheter placement
Declotting of implanted catheter or vascular access device by thrombolytic agent (36593)
Diagnostic studies
Percutaneous interventions
Procedure performed more than one time per date of service
Ultrasound guidance (76937)

Code also significant, separately identifiable E&M services not related to the thrombolysis using modifier 25

🚑 7.22   ⚕ 7.22   **FUD** 000   [T] 🔲

AMA: 2016,Jul,6; 2016,Mar,3; 2016,Jan,13; 2015,Nov,3; 2015,Jan,16; 2014,Jan,11; 2013,Feb,3-6

▲ # **37214** **cessation of thrombolysis including removal of catheter and vessel closure by any method**

INCLUDES
E&M services on the day of and related to the thrombolysis
Fluoroscopic guidance
Last day of transcatheter thrombolytic infusions
Radiologic supervision and interpretation

EXCLUDES
Angiography through existing catheter for follow-up study for transcatheter therapy, embolization or infusion, other than for thrombolysis (75898)
Catheter placement
Declotting of implanted catheter or vascular access device by thrombolytic agent (36593)
Diagnostic studies
Percutaneous interventions
Procedure performed more than one time per date of service
Ultrasound guidance (76937)

Code also significant, separately identifiable E&M service not related to thrombolysis using modifier 25

🚑 3.96   ⚕ 3.96   **FUD** 000   [T] 🔲

AMA: 2016,Jul,6; 2016,Mar,3; 2016,Jan,13; 2015,Nov,3; 2015,Jan,16; 2014,Jan,11; 2013,Feb,3-6

37211	Resequenced code. See code following 37200.
37212	Resequenced code. See code following 37200.
37213	Resequenced code. See code following 37200.
37214	Resequenced code. See code following 37200.

37215-37216 Stenting of Cervical Carotid Artery with/without Insertion Distal Embolic Protection Device

INCLUDES
Carotid stenting, if required
Ipsilateral cerebral and cervical carotid diagnostic imaging/supervision and interpretation
Ipsilateral selective carotid catheterization

EXCLUDES
Carotid catheterization and imaging, if carotid stenting not required
Selective catheter placement, common carotid or innominate artery (36222-36224)
Transcatheter placement extracranial vertebral artery stents, open or percutaneous (0075T, 0076T)

▲ **37215** **Transcatheter placement of intravascular stent(s), cervical carotid artery, open or percutaneous, including angioplasty, when performed, and radiological supervision and interpretation; with distal embolic protection**

🚑 29.4   ⚕ 29.4   **FUD** 090   [C] [80] [50] 🔲

AMA: 2016,Jan,13; 2015,Jan,16; 2014,Mar,8; 2014,Jan,11; 2013,Feb,3-6

● New Code   ▲ Revised Code   ○ Reinstated   ● New Web Release   ▲ Revised Web Release   Unlisted   Not Covered   # Resequenced
⊗ AMA Mod 51 Exempt   ⑤ Optum Mod 51 Exempt   ⊛ Mod 63 Exempt   ⊘ Non-FDA Drug   ★ Telehealth   Ⓜ Maternity   Ⓐ Age Edit   + Add-on   **AMA:** CPT Asst
© 2016 Optum360, LLC   CPT © 2016 American Medical Association. All Rights Reserved.   **159**

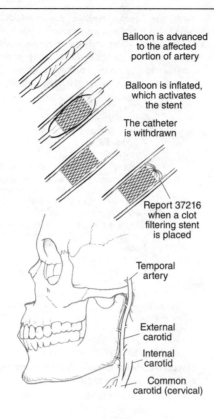

Balloon is advanced to the affected portion of artery

Balloon is inflated, which activates the stent

The catheter is withdrawn

Report 37216 when a clot filtering stent is placed

Temporal artery

External carotid

Internal carotid

Common carotid (cervical)

▲ **37216** **without distal embolic protection**

🔧 0.00   ⚕ 0.00   **FUD** 090   E 🔲

AMA: 2016,Jan,13; 2015,Jan,16; 2014,Mar,8; 2014,Jan,11; 2013,Feb,3-6

37217-37218 Stenting of Intrathoracic Carotid Artery/Innominate Artery

INCLUDES Access to vessel (open)
Arteriotomy closure by suture
Catheterization of the vessel (selective)
Imaging during and after the procedure
Radiological supervision and interpretation

EXCLUDES *Transcatheter insertion extracranial vertebral artery stents, open or percutaneous (0075T-0076T)*
Transcatheter insertion intracranial stents (61635)
Transcatheter insertion intravascular cervical carotid artery stents, open or percutaneous (37215-37216)

37217 **Transcatheter placement of intravascular stent(s), intrathoracic common carotid artery or innominate artery by retrograde treatment, open ipsilateral cervical carotid artery exposure, including angioplasty, when performed, and radiological supervision and interpretation**

EXCLUDES *Services performed on the same side:*
Non-selective catheter placement, thoracic aorta (36221-36227)
Repair blood vessel, direct; neck (35201)
Transluminal balloon angioplasty ([37246, 37247])
Code also revascularization of carotid artery, when performed (33891, 35301, 35509-35510, 35601, 35606)

🔧 32.2   ⚕ 32.2   **FUD** 090   C 80 50 🔲

AMA: 2016,Jan,13; 2015,May,7; 2015,Jan,16; 2014,Mar,8; 2014,Jan,11

▲ **37218** **Transcatheter placement of intravascular stent(s), intrathoracic common carotid artery or innominate artery, open or percutaneous antegrade approach, including angioplasty, when performed, and radiological supervision and interpretation**

EXCLUDES *Selective catheter placement, common carotid or innominate artery (36222-36224)*

🔧 24.0   ⚕ 24.0   **FUD** 090   C 80 50 🔲

AMA: 2016,Jan,13; 2015,May,7

37220-37235 Endovascular Revascularization Lower Extremities

INCLUDES Percutaneous and open interventional and associated procedures for lower extremity occlusive disease; unilateral
Accessing the vessel
Arteriotomy closure by suturing of puncture or pressure with application of arterial closure device
Atherectomy (e.g., directional, laser, rotational)
Balloon angioplasty (e.g., cryoplasty, cutting balloon, low-profile)
Catheterization of the vessel (selective)
Embolic protection
Imaging once procedure is complete
Radiological supervision and interpretation of intervention(s)
Stenting (e.g., bare metal, balloon-expandable, covered, drug-eluting, self-expanding)
Transversing of the lesion
Reporting the most comprehensive treatment in a given vessel according to the following hierarchy:
1. Stent and atherectomy
2. Atherectomy
3. Stent
4. PTA
Revascularization procedures for three arterial vascular territories:
Femoral/popliteal vascular territory including the common, deep, and superficial femoral arteries, and the popliteal artery (one extremity = a single vessel) (37224-37227)
Iliac vascular territory: common iliac, external iliac, internal iliac (37220-37223)
Tibial/peroneal territory: includes anterior tibial, peroneal artery, posterior tibial (37228-37235)

EXCLUDES *Assignment of more than one code from this family for each lower extremity vessel treated*
Assignment of more than one code when multiple vessels are treated in the femoral/popliteal territory (report the most complex service for more than one lesion in the territory); when a contiguous lesion that spans from one territory to another can be opened with a single procedure; or when more than one stent is deployed in the same vessel
Extensive repair or replacement of artery (35226, 35286)
Mechanical thrombectomy and/or thrombolysis
Code also add-on codes for different vessels, but not different lesions in the same vessel; and for multiple territories in the same leg
Code also modifier 59 for a bilateral procedure
Code first one primary code for the initial service in each leg

▲ **37220** **Revascularization, endovascular, open or percutaneous, iliac artery, unilateral, initial vessel; with transluminal angioplasty**

Code also only when transluminal angioplasty is performed outside the treatment target zone of (34802-34805, 34825-34826, 34845-34848, 34900, 0254T)

🔧 12.2   ⚕ 90.1   **FUD** 000   J 62 50 🔲

AMA: 2016,Jul,8; 2016,Jan,13; 2015,Jan,16; 2014,Jan,11; 2013,Dec,8; 2011,Oct,9; 2011,Jul,3-11

▲ **37221** **with transluminal stent placement(s), includes angioplasty within the same vessel, when performed**

Code also only when transluminal angioplasty is performed outside the treatment target zone of (34802-34805, 34825-34826, 34845-34848, 34900, 0254T)

🔧 15.0   ⚕ 132.   **FUD** 000   J J8 80 50 🔲

AMA: 2016,Jul,6; 2016,Jul,8; 2016,Jan,13; 2015,Jan,16; 2015,Jan,13; 2014,Jan,11; 2013,Dec,8; 2012,Apr,3-9; 2012,Jan,15-42; 2011,Oct,9; 2011,Jul,16-17; 2011,Jul,3-11

▲ + **37222** **Revascularization, endovascular, open or percutaneous, iliac artery, each additional ipsilateral iliac vessel; with transluminal angioplasty (List separately in addition to code for primary procedure)**
> Code also only when transluminal angioplasty is performed outside the treatment target zone of (34802-34805, 34825-34826, 34845-34848, 34900, 0254T)
> Code first (37220-37221)
> 🚑 5.51   ⚕ 25.3   **FUD** ZZZ   N N1 80 50 ▣
>
> **AMA:** 2016,Jul,8; 2016,Jan,13; 2015,Jan,16; 2014,Jan,11; 2013,Dec,8; 2011,Oct,9; 2011,Jul,3-11

▲ + **37223** **with transluminal stent placement(s), includes angioplasty within the same vessel, when performed (List separately in addition to code for primary procedure)**
> Code also only when transluminal angioplasty is performed outside the treatment target zone of (34802-34805, 34825-34826, 34845-34848, 34900, 0254T)
> Code first (37221)
> 🚑 6.32   ⚕ 73.8   **FUD** ZZZ   N N1 80 50 ▣
>
> **AMA:** 2016,Jul,6; 2016,Jul,8; 2016,Jan,13; 2015,Jan,16; 2014,Jan,11; 2013,Dec,8; 2012,Apr,3-9; 2011,Oct,9; 2011,Jul,3-11

▲ **37224** **Revascularization, endovascular, open or percutaneous, femoral, popliteal artery(s), unilateral; with transluminal angioplasty**
> 🚑 13.4   ⚕ 109.   **FUD** 000   J G2 80 50 ▣
>
> **AMA:** 2016,Jul,8; 2016,Jan,13; 2015,Jan,16; 2014,Jan,11; 2012,Jan,15-42; 2011,Dec,14-18; 2011,Oct,9; 2011,Jul,3-11

▲ **37225** **with atherectomy, includes angioplasty within the same vessel, when performed**
> 🚑 18.2   ⚕ 314.   **FUD** 000   J J8 80 50 ▣
>
> **AMA:** 2016,Jul,8; 2016,Jan,13; 2015,Jan,16; 2014,Jan,11; 2011,Oct,9; 2011,Jul,3-11

▲ **37226** **with transluminal stent placement(s), includes angioplasty within the same vessel, when performed**
> 🚑 15.8   ⚕ 258.   **FUD** 000   J J8 80 50 ▣
>
> **AMA:** 2016,Jul,6; 2016,Jul,8; 2016,Jan,13; 2015,Jan,16; 2014,Jan,11; 2012,Jan,15-42; 2011,Dec,14-18; 2011,Oct,9; 2011,Jul,3-11

▲ **37227** **with transluminal stent placement(s) and atherectomy, includes angioplasty within the same vessel, when performed**
> 🚑 21.9   ⚕ 424.   **FUD** 000   J J8 80 50 ▣
>
> **AMA:** 2016,Jul,6; 2016,Jul,8; 2016,Jan,13; 2015,Jan,16; 2014,Jan,11; 2011,Oct,9; 2011,Jul,3-11

▲ **37228** **Revascularization, endovascular, open or percutaneous, tibial, peroneal artery, unilateral, initial vessel; with transluminal angioplasty**
> 🚑 16.4   ⚕ 155.   **FUD** 000   J J8 80 50 ▣
>
> **AMA:** 2016,Jul,8; 2016,Jan,13; 2015,Jan,16; 2014,Jan,11; 2011,Oct,9; 2011,Jul,3-11

▲ **37229** **with atherectomy, includes angioplasty within the same vessel, when performed**
> 🚑 21.2   ⚕ 309.   **FUD** 000   J J8 80 50 ▣
>
> **AMA:** 2016,Jul,8; 2016,Jan,13; 2015,Jan,16; 2014,Jan,11; 2012,Apr,3-9; 2011,Oct,9; 2011,Jul,3-11

▲ **37230** **with transluminal stent placement(s), includes angioplasty within the same vessel, when performed**
> 🚑 20.9   ⚕ 236.   **FUD** 000   J J8 80 50 ▣
>
> **AMA:** 2016,Jul,6; 2016,Jul,8; 2016,Jan,13; 2015,Jan,16; 2014,Jan,11; 2012,Apr,3-9; 2011,Oct,9; 2011,Jul,3-11

▲ **37231** **with transluminal stent placement(s) and atherectomy, includes angioplasty within the same vessel, when performed**
> 🚑 22.7   ⚕ 380.   **FUD** 000   J J8 80 50 ▣
>
> **AMA:** 2016,Jul,6; 2016,Jul,8; 2016,Jan,13; 2015,Jan,16; 2014,Jan,11; 2012,Apr,3-9; 2011,Oct,9; 2011,Jul,3-11

▲ + **37232** **Revascularization, endovascular, open or percutaneous, tibial/peroneal artery, unilateral, each additional vessel; with transluminal angioplasty (List separately in addition to code for primary procedure)**
> Code first (37228-37231)
> 🚑 5.97   ⚕ 34.5   **FUD** ZZZ   N N1 80 50 ▣
>
> **AMA:** 2016,Jul,8; 2016,Jan,13; 2015,Jan,16; 2014,Jan,11; 2012,Apr,3-9; 2011,Oct,9; 2011,Jul,3-11

▲ + **37233** **with atherectomy, includes angioplasty within the same vessel, when performed (List separately in addition to code for primary procedure)**
> Code first (37229, 37231)
> 🚑 9.72   ⚕ 41.7   **FUD** ZZZ   N N1 80 50 ▣
>
> **AMA:** 2016,Jul,8; 2016,Jan,13; 2015,Jan,16; 2014,Jan,11; 2012,Apr,3-9; 2011,Oct,9; 2011,Jul,3-11

▲ + **37234** **with transluminal stent placement(s), includes angioplasty within the same vessel, when performed (List separately in addition to code for primary procedure)**
> Code first (37229-37231)
> 🚑 8.37   ⚕ 110.   **FUD** ZZZ   N N1 80 50 ▣
>
> **AMA:** 2016,Jul,6; 2016,Jul,8; 2016,Jan,13; 2015,Jan,16; 2014,Jan,11; 2012,Apr,3-9; 2011,Oct,9; 2011,Jul,3-11

▲ + **37235** **with transluminal stent placement(s) and atherectomy, includes angioplasty within the same vessel, when performed (List separately in addition to code for primary procedure)**
> Code first (37231)
> 🚑 11.9   ⚕ 116.   **FUD** ZZZ   N N1 80 50 ▣
>
> **AMA:** 2016,Jul,6; 2016,Jul,8; 2016,Jan,13; 2015,Jan,16; 2014,Jan,11; 2011,Oct,9; 2011,Jul,3-11

[37246, 37247, 37248, 37249] Transluminal Balloon Angioplasty

| INCLUDES | Open and percutaneous balloon angioplasty
| | Radiological supervision and interpretation |
| EXCLUDES | *Angioplasty of other vessels:* |

> EXCLUDES *Angioplasty of other vessels:*
> *Aortic/visceral arteries (with endovascular repair) (34841-34848)*
> *Coronary artery (92920-92944)*
> *Intracranial artery (61630, 61635)*
> *Performed in a hemodialysis circuit (36901-36909)*
> *Revascularization lower extremities (37220-37235)*
> *Percutaneous removal of thrombus/infusion of thrombolytics (37184-37188, [37211, 37212, 37213, 37214])*
> *Pulmonary artery (92997-92998)*
> *Use of codes more than one time for all services performed in a single vessel or treatable with one angioplasty procedure*

Code also angioplasty of different vessel, when performed ([37247], [37249])
Code also extensive repair or replacement of artery, when performed (35226, 35286)
Code also intravascular ultrasound, when performed (37252-37253)

● # **37246** **Transluminal balloon angioplasty (except lower extremity artery(ies) for occlusive disease, intracranial, coronary, pulmonary, or dialysis circuit), open or percutaneous, including all imaging and radiological supervision and interpretation necessary to perform the angioplasty within the same artery; initial artery**
> 🚑 0.00   ⚕ 0.00   **FUD** 000
>
> EXCLUDES *Intravascular stent placement except lower extremities (37236-37237)*
> *Stent placement:*
> *Cervical carotid artery (37215-37216)*
> *Intrathoracic carotid or innominate artery (37217-37218)*

● + # **37247** **each additional artery (List separately in addition to code for primary procedure)**
> 🚑 0.00   ⚕ 0.00   **FUD** 000
>
> EXCLUDES *Intravascular stent placement except lower extremities (37236-37237)*
> *Stent placement:*
> *Cervical carotid artery (37215-37216)*
> *Intrathoracic carotid or innominate artery (37217-37218)*
>
> Code first ([37246])

● # **37248** **Transluminal balloon angioplasty (except dialysis circuit), open or percutaneous, including all imaging and radiological supervision and interpretation necessary to perform the angioplasty within the same vein; initial vein**

🚑 0.00   ⚕ 0.00   **FUD** 000

> *EXCLUDES* *Placement of intravascular (venous) stent in same vein, same session as (37238-37239)*

● + # **37249** **each additional vein (List separately in addition to code for primary procedure)**

🚑 0.00   ⚕ 0.00   **FUD** 000

> *EXCLUDES* *Placement of intravascular (venous) stent in same vein, same session as (37238-37239)*

Code first (37239)

37236-37239 Endovascular Revascularization Excluding Lower Extremities

INCLUDES Arteriotomy closure by suturing of a puncture, pressure or application of arterial closure device
Balloon angioplasty
   Post-dilation after stent deployment
   Predilation performed as primary or secondary angioplasty
   Treatment of lesion inside same vessel but outside of stented portion
   Treatment using different-sized balloons to accomplish the procedure
Endovascular revascularization of arteries and veins other than carotid, coronary, extracranial, intracranial, lower extremities
Imaging once procedure is complete
Radiological supervision and interpretation
Stent placement provided as the only treatment

EXCLUDES *Angioplasty in an unrelated vessel*
Extensive repair or replacement of an artery (35226, 35286)
Insertion of multiple stents in a single vessel using more than one code
Intravascular ultrasound (37252-37253)
Mechanical thrombectomy (37184-37188)
Selective and nonselective catheterization (36005, 36010-36015, 36200, 36215-36218, 36245-36248)
Stent placement in:
   Arteries of the lower extremities for occlusive disease (37221, 37223, 37226-37227, 37230-37231, 37234-37235)
   Cervical carotid artery (37215-37216)
   Extracranial vertebral (0075T-0076T)
   Intracoronary (92928-92929, 92933-92934, 92937-92938, 92941, 92943-92944)
   Intracranial (61635)
   Intrathoracic common carotid or innominate artery, retrograde or antegrade approach (37218)
   Visceral arteries with fenestrated aortic repair (34841-34848)
Hemodialysis circuit (36903, 36905, 36908)
Thrombolytic therapy ([37211, 37212, 37213, 37214])
Ultrasound guidance (76937)
Code also add-on codes for different vessels treated during the same operative session

▲ **37236** **Transcatheter placement of an intravascular stent(s) (except lower extremity artery(s) for occlusive disease, cervical carotid, extracranial vertebral or intrathoracic carotid, intracranial, or coronary), open or percutaneous, including radiological supervision and interpretation and including all angioplasty within the same vessel, when performed; initial artery**

> *EXCLUDES* *Procedures in the same target treatment zone with (34841-34848)*

🚑 13.3   ⚕ 117.   **FUD** 000

AMA: 2016,Jul,6; 2016,Jul,3; 2016,Mar,5; 2016,Jan,13; 2015,May,7; 2015,Jan,16; 2014,Jan,11; 2013,Dec,8

▲ + **37237** **each additional artery (List separately in addition to code for primary procedure)**

> *EXCLUDES* *Procedures in the same target treatment zone with (34841-34848)*

Code first (37236)

🚑 6.27   ⚕ 70.1   **FUD** ZZZ

AMA: 2016,Jul,6; 2016,Mar,5; 2016,Jan,13; 2015,Jan,16; 2014,Jan,11; 2013,Dec,8

▲ **37238** **Transcatheter placement of an intravascular stent(s), open or percutaneous, including radiological supervision and interpretation and including angioplasty within the same vessel, when performed; initial vein**

🚑 9.21   ⚕ 119.   **FUD** 000

AMA: 2016,Jul,6; 2016,Jun,8; 2014,Jan,11

▲ + **37239** **each additional vein (List separately in addition to code for primary procedure)**

Code first (37238)

🚑 4.39   ⚕ 57.9   **FUD** ZZZ

AMA: 2016,Jul,6; 2014,Jan,11

37241-37249 Therapeutic Vascular Embolization/Occlusion

INCLUDES Embolization or occlusion of arteries, lymphatics, and veins except for head/neck and central nervous system
Imaging once procedure is complete
Intraprocedural guidance
Radiological supervision and interpretation
Roadmapping
Stent placement provided as support for embolization

EXCLUDES *Embolization code assigned more than once per operative field*
Head, neck, or central nervous system embolization (61624, 61626, 61710)
Multiple codes for indications that overlap, code only the indication needing the most immediate attention
Stent deployment as primary management of aneurysm, pseudoaneurysm, or vascular extravasation
Vein destruction with sclerosing solution (36468-36471)
Code also additional embolization procedure(s) and the appropriate modifiers (eg, modifier 59) when embolization procedures are performed in multiple operative fields
Code also diagnostic angiography and catheter placement using modifier 59 when appropriate

▲ **37241** **Vascular embolization or occlusion, inclusive of all radiological supervision and interpretation, intraprocedural roadmapping, and imaging guidance necessary to complete the intervention; venous, other than hemorrhage (eg, congenital or acquired venous malformations, venous and capillary hemangiomas, varices, varicoceles)**

> *EXCLUDES* *Embolization of side branch(s) of an outflow vein from a hemodialysis access (36909)*
> *Procedure in same operative field with:*
>   *Endovenous ablation therapy of incompetent vein (36475-36479)*
>   *Injection of sclerosing solution; single vein (36470-36471)*
>   *Transcatheter embolization procedures (75894, 75898)*
>   *Vein destruction (36468-36479)*

🚑 13.2   ⚕ 136.   **FUD** 000

AMA: 2016,Jan,13; 2015,Nov,3; 2015,Aug,8; 2015,Apr,10; 2015,Jan,16; 2014,Oct,6; 2014,Aug,14; 2014,Jan,11; 2013,Nov,6; 2013,Nov,14

▲ **37242** **arterial, other than hemorrhage or tumor (eg, congenital or acquired arterial malformations, arteriovenous malformations, arteriovenous fistulas, aneurysms, pseudoaneurysms)**

> *EXCLUDES* *Percutaneous treatment of pseudoaneurysm of an extremity (36002)*

🚑 14.4   ⚕ 218.   **FUD** 000

AMA: 2016,Jan,13; 2015,Nov,3; 2015,Jan,16; 2014,Oct,6; 2014,Jan,11; 2013,Nov,6; 2013,Nov,14

▲ **37243** **for tumors, organ ischemia, or infarction**

> *INCLUDES* Embolization of uterine fibroids (37244)
> *EXCLUDES* *Procedure in same operative field:*
>   *Angiography (75898)*
>   *Transcatheter embolization in same operative field (75894)*
> Code also chemotherapy when provided with embolization procedure (96420-96425)
> Code also injection of radioisotopes when provided with embolization procedure (79445)

🚑 17.0   ⚕ 277.   **FUD** 000

AMA: 2016,Jan,13; 2015,Nov,3; 2015,Jan,16; 2014,Oct,6; 2014,Jan,11; 2013,Nov,6; 2013,Nov,14

▲ **37244** **for arterial or venous hemorrhage or lymphatic extravasation**

> *INCLUDES* Embolization of uterine arteries for hemorrhage

🚑 19.9   ⚕ 193.   **FUD** 000

AMA: 2016,Jan,13; 2015,Nov,3; 2015,Jan,16; 2014,Oct,6; 2014,Aug,14; 2014,Jan,11; 2013,Nov,6; 2013,Nov,14

26/TC PC/TC Only	A2-Z3 ASC Payment	50 Bilateral	♂ Male Only	♀ Female Only	🚑 Facility RVU	⚕ Non-Facility RVU	CCI
FUD Follow-up Days	**CMS:** IOM (Pub 100)	A-Y OPPSI	80/80 Surg Assist Allowed / w/Doc		Lab Crosswalk	Radiology Crosswalk	CLIA

162   CPT © 2016 American Medical Association. All Rights Reserved.   © 2016 Optum360, LLC

37246	Resequenced code. See code following 37235.
37247	Resequenced code. See code following 37235.
37248	Resequenced code. See code following 37235.
37249	Resequenced code. See code following 37235.

37252-37253 Intravascular Ultrasound: Noncoronary

INCLUDES Manipulation and repositioning of the transducer prior to and after therapeutic interventional procedures

EXCLUDES Selective or non-selective catheter placement for access (36005-36248)
Transcatheter procedures (37200, 37236-37239, 37241-37244, 61624, 61626)
Vena cava filter procedures (37191-37193, 37197)

▲ + **37252** Intravascular ultrasound (noncoronary vessel) during diagnostic evaluation and/or therapeutic intervention, including radiological supervision and interpretation; initial noncoronary vessel (List separately in addition to code for primary procedure)

Code first primary procedure
🔲 2.70 🔨 39.8 **FUD** ZZZ   N N1 80 ▣

AMA: 2016,Jul,6; 2016,May,11

▲ + **37253** each additional noncoronary vessel (List separately in addition to code for primary procedure)

Code first (37252)
🔲 2.16 🔨 6.19 **FUD** ZZZ   N N1 80 ▣

AMA: 2016,Jul,6; 2016,May,11

37500-37501 Vascular Endoscopic Procedures

INCLUDES Diagnostic endoscopy

EXCLUDES Open procedure (37760)

37500 Vascular endoscopy, surgical, with ligation of perforator veins, subfascial (SEPS)
🔲 22.2 🔨 22.2 **FUD** 090   T A2 50 ▣

AMA: 2016,Jan,13; 2015,Jan,16; 2014,Jan,11

37501 Unlisted vascular endoscopy procedure
🔲 0.00 🔨 0.00 **FUD** YYY   T 50

AMA: 2014,Jan,11

37565-37606 Ligation Procedures: Jugular Vein, Carotid Arteries

CMS: 100-03,160.8 Electroencephalographic Monitoring During Cerebral Vasculature Surgery

EXCLUDES Arterial balloon occlusion, endovascular, temporary (61623)
Suture of arteries and veins (35201-35286)
Transcatheter arterial embolization/occlusion, permanent (61624-61626)
Treatment of intracranial aneurysm (61703)

37565 Ligation, internal jugular vein
🔲 21.1 🔨 21.1 **FUD** 090   T 80 50 ▣

AMA: 2014,Jan,11

37600 Ligation; external carotid artery
🔲 20.7 🔨 20.7 **FUD** 090   T 80 ▣

AMA: 2014,Jan,11

External carotid artery is ligated

External carotid artery
Internal carotid artery

Sternocleidomastoid muscle

Carotid artery

37605 internal or common carotid artery
🔲 23.4 🔨 23.4 **FUD** 090   T 80 ▣

AMA: 2014,Jan,11

37606 internal or common carotid artery, with gradual occlusion, as with Selverstone or Crutchfield clamp
🔲 16.9 🔨 16.9 **FUD** 090   T 80 ▣

AMA: 2014,Jan,11

37607-37609 Ligation Hemodialysis Angioaccess or Temporal Artery

EXCLUDES Suture of arteries and veins (35201-35286)

37607 Ligation or banding of angioaccess arteriovenous fistula
🔲 11.0 🔨 11.0 **FUD** 090   T A2 ▣

AMA: 2014,Jan,11

37609 Ligation or biopsy, temporal artery
🔲 6.03 🔨 8.92 **FUD** 010   T A2 50 ▣

AMA: 2014,Jan,11

37615-37618 Arterial Ligation, Major Vessel, for Injury/Rupture

EXCLUDES Suture of arteries and veins (35201-35286)

37615 Ligation, major artery (eg, post-traumatic, rupture); neck
INCLUDES Touroff ligation
🔲 14.8 🔨 14.8 **FUD** 090   T 80 ▣

AMA: 2014,Jan,11

37616 chest
INCLUDES Bardenheuer operation
🔲 32.1 🔨 32.1 **FUD** 090   C 80 ▣

AMA: 2014,Jan,11

37617 abdomen
🔲 39.0 🔨 39.0 **FUD** 090   C 80 ▣

AMA: 2016,Jan,13; 2015,Jan,16; 2014,Jan,11; 2013,Aug,13

37618 extremity
🔲 11.2 🔨 11.2 **FUD** 090   C 80 ▣

AMA: 2014,Jan,11

37619 Ligation Inferior Vena Cava

EXCLUDES Suture of arteries and veins (35201-35286)
Endovascular delivery of inferior vena cava filter (37191)

37619 Ligation of inferior vena cava
🔲 47.9 🔨 47.9 **FUD** 090   T 80 ▣

AMA: 2016,Jan,13; 2015,Jan,16; 2014,Jan,11; 2012,Apr,3-9

37650-37660 Venous Ligation, Femoral and Common Iliac

EXCLUDES Suture of arteries and veins (35201-35286)

37650 Ligation of femoral vein
🔲 14.9 🔨 14.9 **FUD** 090   T A2 50 ▣

AMA: 2014,Jan,11

37660 Ligation of common iliac vein
🔲 34.0 🔨 34.0 **FUD** 090   C 80 50 ▣

AMA: 2014,Jan,11

37700-37785 Treatment of Varicose Veins of Legs

EXCLUDES Suture of arteries and veins (35201-35286)

37700 Ligation and division of long saphenous vein at saphenofemoral junction, or distal interruptions
INCLUDES Babcock operation
EXCLUDES Ligation, division, and stripping of vein (37718, 37722)
🔲 7.33 🔨 7.33 **FUD** 090   T A2 50 ▣

AMA: 2016,Jan,13; 2015,Jan,16; 2014,Jan,11; 2012,Jan,15-42; 2011,Jan,11

37718 Ligation, division, and stripping, short saphenous vein
EXCLUDES Ligation, division, and stripping of vein (37700, 37735, 37780)
🔲 12.8 🔨 12.8 **FUD** 090   T A2 50 ▣

AMA: 2014,Jan,11

37722 Ligation, division, and stripping, long (greater) saphenous veins from saphenofemoral junction to knee or below
EXCLUDES Ligation, division, and stripping of vein (37700, 37718, 37735)
🔲 14.1 🔨 14.1 **FUD** 090   T A2 50 ▣

AMA: 2014,Jan,11; 2011,Jul,3-11

37735 Ligation and division and complete stripping of long or short saphenous veins with radical excision of ulcer and skin graft and/or interruption of communicating veins of lower leg, with excision of deep fascia

EXCLUDES Ligation, division, and stripping of vein (37700, 37718, 37722, 37780)

⚙ 20.1 ⚲ 20.1 **FUD** 090 T A2 50 ▭

AMA: 2016,Jan,13; 2015,Jan,16; 2014,Jan,11; 2011,Jul,3-11

37760 Ligation of perforator veins, subfascial, radical (Linton type), including skin graft, when performed, open, 1 leg

EXCLUDES Duplex scan of extremity veins (93971)
Ligation of subfascial perforator veins, endoscopic (37500)
Ultrasonic guidance (76937, 76942, 76998)

⚙ 18.1 ⚲ 18.1 **FUD** 090 T A2 50 ▭

AMA: 2016,Jan,13; 2015,Jan,16; 2014,Jan,11

37761 Ligation of perforator vein(s), subfascial, open, including ultrasound guidance, when performed, 1 leg

EXCLUDES Duplex scan of extremity veins (93971)
Ligation of subfascial perforator veins, endoscopic (37500)
Ultrasonic guidance (76937, 76942, 76998)

⚙ 16.2 ⚲ 16.2 **FUD** 090 T R2 80 50 ▭

AMA: 2016,Jan,13; 2015,Jan,16; 2014,Jan,11

37765 Stab phlebectomy of varicose veins, 1 extremity; 10-20 stab incisions

EXCLUDES Fewer than 10 incisions (37799)
More than 20 incisions (37766)

⚙ 13.2 ⚲ 18.8 **FUD** 090 T P3 50 ▭

AMA: 2016,Jan,13; 2015,Jan,16; 2014,Oct,6; 2014,Jan,11

37766 more than 20 incisions

EXCLUDES Fewer than 10 incisions (37799)
10-20 incisions (37765)

⚙ 16.1 ⚲ 22.4 **FUD** 090 T P3 50 ▭

AMA: 2016,Jan,13; 2015,Jan,16; 2014,Oct,6; 2014,Jan,11; 2013,Sep,17

37780 Ligation and division of short saphenous vein at saphenopopliteal junction (separate procedure)

⚙ 7.47 ⚲ 7.47 **FUD** 090 T A2 50 ▭

AMA: 2016,Jan,13; 2015,Jan,16; 2014,Jan,11; 2012,Jan,15-42; 2011,Jan,11

37785 Ligation, division, and/or excision of varicose vein cluster(s), 1 leg

⚙ 7.69 ⚲ 10.3 **FUD** 090 T A2 50 ▭

AMA: 2016,Jan,13; 2015,Jan,16; 2014,Jan,11; 2012,Jan,15-42; 2011,Jan,11

37788-37790 Treatment of Vascular Disease of the Penis

37788 Penile revascularization, artery, with or without vein graft ♂

⚙ 37.2 ⚲ 37.2 **FUD** 090 C 80 ▭

AMA: 2014,Jan,11

37790 Penile venous occlusive procedure

⚙ 14.5 ⚲ 14.5 **FUD** 090 T A2 80 ▭

AMA: 2014,Jan,11

37799 Unlisted Vascular Surgery Procedures

CMS: 100-04,32,161 Intracranial Percutaneous Transluminal Angioplasty (PTA) With Stenting; 100-04,4,180.3 Unlisted Service or Procedure

37799 Unlisted procedure, vascular surgery

⚙ 0.00 ⚲ 0.00 **FUD** YYY T 80

AMA: 2016,Jan,13; 2015,Apr,10; 2015,Jan,16; 2014,Oct,6; 2014,Aug,14; 2014,Mar,8; 2014,Jan,11; 2013,Nov,14; 2012,Jan,15-42; 2011,Aug,9-10; 2011,Jan,11

38100-38200 Splenic Procedures

38100 Splenectomy; total (separate procedure)

⚙ 33.4 ⚲ 33.4 **FUD** 090 C 80 ▭

AMA: 2016,Jan,13; 2015,Jan,16; 2014,Jan,11; 2012,Oct,3-8; 2012,Sep,11-13

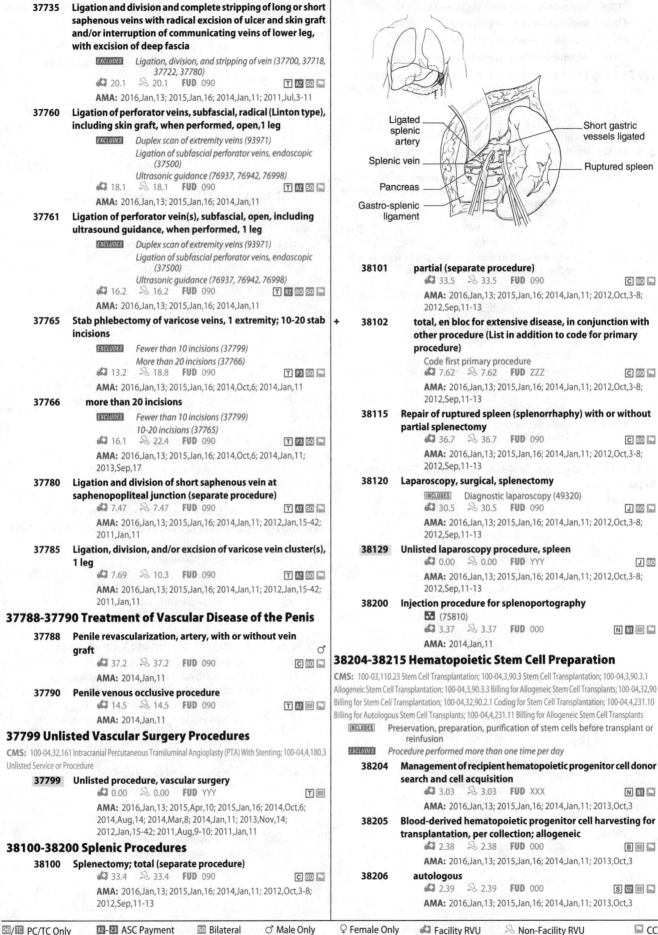

Ligated splenic artery

Splenic vein

Pancreas

Gastro-splenic ligament

Short gastric vessels ligated

Ruptured spleen

38101 partial (separate procedure)

⚙ 33.5 ⚲ 33.5 **FUD** 090 C 80 ▭

AMA: 2016,Jan,13; 2015,Jan,16; 2014,Jan,11; 2012,Oct,3-8; 2012,Sep,11-13

+ **38102** total, en bloc for extensive disease, in conjunction with other procedure (List in addition to code for primary procedure)

Code first primary procedure

⚙ 7.62 ⚲ 7.62 **FUD** ZZZ C 80 ▭

AMA: 2016,Jan,13; 2015,Jan,16; 2014,Jan,11; 2012,Oct,3-8; 2012,Sep,11-13

38115 Repair of ruptured spleen (splenorrhaphy) with or without partial splenectomy

⚙ 36.7 ⚲ 36.7 **FUD** 090 C 80 ▭

AMA: 2016,Jan,13; 2015,Jan,16; 2014,Jan,11; 2012,Oct,3-8; 2012,Sep,11-13

38120 Laparoscopy, surgical, splenectomy

INCLUDES Diagnostic laparoscopy (49320)

⚙ 30.5 ⚲ 30.5 **FUD** 090 J 80 ▭

AMA: 2016,Jan,13; 2015,Jan,16; 2014,Jan,11; 2012,Oct,3-8; 2012,Sep,11-13

38129 Unlisted laparoscopy procedure, spleen

⚙ 0.00 ⚲ 0.00 **FUD** YYY J 80

AMA: 2016,Jan,13; 2015,Jan,16; 2014,Jan,11; 2012,Oct,3-8; 2012,Sep,11-13

38200 Injection procedure for splenoportography

⚡ (75810)

⚙ 3.37 ⚲ 3.37 **FUD** 000 N N1 80 ▭

AMA: 2014,Jan,11

38204-38215 Hematopoietic Stem Cell Preparation

CMS: 100-03,110.23 Stem Cell Transplantation; 100-04,3,90.3 Stem Cell Transplantation; 100-04,3,90.3.1 Allogeneic Stem Cell Transplantation; 100-04,3,90.3.3 Billing for Allogeneic Stem Cell Transplants; 100-04,32,90 Billing for Stem Cell Transplantation; 100-04,32,90.2.1 Coding for Stem Cell Transplantation; 100-04,4,231.10 Billing for Autologous Stem Cell Transplants; 100-04,4,231.11 Billing for Allogeneic Stem Cell Transplants

INCLUDES Preservation, preparation, purification of stem cells before transplant or reinfusion

EXCLUDES Procedure performed more than one time per day

38204 Management of recipient hematopoietic progenitor cell donor search and cell acquisition

⚙ 3.03 ⚲ 3.03 **FUD** XXX N N1 ▭

AMA: 2016,Jan,13; 2015,Jan,16; 2014,Jan,11; 2013,Oct,3

38205 Blood-derived hematopoietic progenitor cell harvesting for transplantation, per collection; allogeneic

⚙ 2.38 ⚲ 2.38 **FUD** 000 B 80 ▭

AMA: 2016,Jan,13; 2015,Jan,16; 2014,Jan,11; 2013,Oct,3

38206 autologous

⚙ 2.39 ⚲ 2.39 **FUD** 000 S G2 80 ▭

AMA: 2016,Jan,13; 2015,Jan,16; 2014,Jan,11; 2013,Oct,3

38207 Transplant preparation of hematopoietic progenitor cells; cryopreservation and storage

EXCLUDES *Flow cytometry (88182, 88184-88189)*

(88240)

1.35 ⚕ 1.35 **FUD** XXX [S][▢]

AMA: 2016,Jan,13; 2015,Jan,16; 2014,Jan,11; 2013,Oct,3

38208 thawing of previously frozen harvest, without washing, per donor

EXCLUDES *Flow cytometry (88182, 88184-88189)*

(88241)

0.85 ⚕ 0.85 **FUD** XXX [S][▢]

AMA: 2016,Jan,13; 2015,Jan,16; 2014,Jan,11; 2013,Oct,3

38209 thawing of previously frozen harvest, with washing, per donor

EXCLUDES *Flow cytometry (88182, 88184-88189)*

0.36 ⚕ 0.36 **FUD** XXX [S][▢]

AMA: 2016,Jan,13; 2015,Jan,16; 2014,Jan,11; 2013,Oct,3

38210 specific cell depletion within harvest, T-cell depletion

EXCLUDES *Flow cytometry (88182, 88184-88189)*

2.38 ⚕ 2.38 **FUD** XXX [S][▢]

AMA: 2016,Jan,13; 2015,Jan,16; 2014,Jan,11; 2013,Oct,3

38211 tumor cell depletion

EXCLUDES *Flow cytometry (88182, 88184-88189)*

2.15 ⚕ 2.15 **FUD** XXX [S][▢]

AMA: 2016,Jan,13; 2015,Jan,16; 2014,Jan,11; 2013,Oct,3

38212 red blood cell removal

EXCLUDES *Flow cytometry (88182, 88184-88189)*

1.43 ⚕ 1.43 **FUD** XXX [S][▢]

AMA: 2016,Jan,13; 2015,Jan,16; 2014,Jan,11; 2013,Oct,3

38213 platelet depletion

EXCLUDES *Flow cytometry (88182, 88184-88189)*

0.36 ⚕ 0.36 **FUD** XXX [S][▢]

AMA: 2016,Jan,13; 2015,Jan,16; 2014,Jan,11; 2013,Oct,3

38214 plasma (volume) depletion

EXCLUDES *Flow cytometry (88182, 88184-88189)*

1.23 ⚕ 1.23 **FUD** XXX [S][▢]

AMA: 2016,Jan,13; 2015,Jan,16; 2014,Jan,11; 2013,Oct,3

38215 cell concentration in plasma, mononuclear, or buffy coat layer

EXCLUDES *Flow cytometry (88182, 88184-88189)*

1.43 ⚕ 1.43 **FUD** XXX [S][▢]

AMA: 2016,Jan,13; 2015,Jan,16; 2014,Jan,11; 2013,Oct,3

38220-38232 Bone Marrow Procedures

CMS: 100-03,110.23 Stem Cell Transplantation; 100-04,3,90.3 Stem Cell Transplantation; 100-04,32,90 Billing for Stem Cell Transplantation; 100-04,4,231.11 Billing for Allogeneic Stem Cell Transplants

38220 Bone marrow; aspiration only

INCLUDES Bone marrow aspiration for bone graft

EXCLUDES *Bone marrow aspiration for platelet rich stem cell injection (0232T)*

1.77 ⚕ 4.68 **FUD** XXX [T][P3][80][50][▢]

AMA: 2016,Jan,13; 2015,Mar,9; 2015,Jan,16; 2014,Jan,11; 2013,Oct,3; 2012,May,11-12; 2012,Apr,14-16; 2012,Jan,15-42; 2011,Jan,11

38221 biopsy, needle or trocar

EXCLUDES *Bone marrow aspiration for platelet rich stem cell injection (0232T)*

(88305)

2.15 ⚕ 4.76 **FUD** XXX [T][P3][80][50][▢]

AMA: 2016,Jan,13; 2015,Mar,9; 2014,Jan,11; 2012,May,11-12

38230 Bone marrow harvesting for transplantation; allogeneic

EXCLUDES *Bone marrow aspiration for platelet rich stem cell injection (0232T)*

Harvesting of blood-derived hematopoietic progenitor cells for transplant (allogeneic) (38205)

5.72 ⚕ 5.72 **FUD** 000 [S][G2][80][▢]

AMA: 2016,Jan,13; 2015,Jan,16; 2014,Jan,11; 2013,Oct,3; 2012,May,11-12

38232 autologous

EXCLUDES *Aspiration of bone marrow (38220)*

Harvesting of blood-derived peripheral stem cells for transplant (autologous) (38206)

5.70 ⚕ 5.70 **FUD** 000 [S][G2][80][▢]

AMA: 2016,Jan,13; 2015,Jan,16; 2014,Jan,11; 2013,Oct,3; 2012,May,11-12

38240-38243 [38243] Hematopoietic Progenitor Cell Transplantation

CMS: 100-03,110.23 Stem Cell Transplantation; 100-04,3,90.3 Stem Cell Transplantation; 100-04,3,90.3.1 Allogeneic Stem Cell Transplantation; 100-04,3,90.3.2 Autologous Stem Cell Transplantation (AuSCT); 100-04,3,90.3.3 Billing for Allogeneic Stem Cell Transplants; 100-04,32,90 Billing for Stem Cell Transplantation; 100-04,32,90.2 Allogeneic Stem Cell Transplantation; 100-04,32,90.2.1 Coding for Stem Cell Transplantation; 100-04,32,90.3 Autologous Stem Cell Transplantation; 100-04,32,90.4 Edits Stem Cell Transplant; 100-04,32,90.6 Clinical Trials for Stem Cell Transplant for Myelodysplastic Syndrome (; 100-04,4,231.10 Billing for Autologous Stem Cell Transplants; 100-04,4,231.11 Billing for Allogeneic Stem Cell Transplants

INCLUDES Evaluation of patient prior to, during, and after the infusion
Management of uncomplicated adverse reactions such as hives or nausea
Monitoring of physiological parameters
Physician presence during the infusion
Supervision of clinical staff

EXCLUDES *Administration of fluids for the transplant or for incidental hydration separately*
Concurrent administration of medications with the infusion for the transplant
Cryopreservation, freezing, and storage of hematopoietic progenitor cells for transplant (38207)
Human leukocyte antigen (HLA) testing (81370-81383, 86812-86822)
Modification, treatment, processing of hematopoietic progenitor cell specimens for transplant (38210-38215)
Thawing and expansion of hematopoietic progenitor cells for transplant (38208-38209)

Code also administration of medications and/or fluids not related to the transplant with modifier 59

Code also E&M service for the treatment of more complicated adverse reactions after the infusion, as appropriate

Code also separately identifiable E&M service on the same date, using modifier 25 as appropriate (99211-99215, 99217-99220, [99224, 99225, 99226], 99221-99223, 99231-99239, 99471-99472, 99475-99476)

38240 Hematopoietic progenitor cell (HPC); allogeneic transplantation per donor

EXCLUDES *Allogeneic lymphocyte infusions on same date of service with (38242)*
Hematopoietic progenitor cell (HPC); HPC boost on same date of service with ([38243])

6.43 ⚕ 6.43 **FUD** XXX [S][80][▢]

AMA: 2016,Jan,13; 2015,Jan,16; 2014,Jan,11; 2013,Oct,3

38241 autologous transplantation

4.82 ⚕ 4.82 **FUD** XXX [S][G2][80][▢]

AMA: 2016,Jan,13; 2015,Jan,16; 2014,Jan,11; 2013,Oct,3

\# **38243** HPC boost

EXCLUDES *Allogeneic lymphocyte infusions on same date of service with (38242)*
Hematopoietic progenitor cell (HPC); allogeneic transplantation per donor on same date of service with

3.37 ⚕ 3.37 **FUD** 000 [S][R2][80][▢]

AMA: 2016,Jan,13; 2015,Feb,10; 2015,Jan,16; 2014,Jan,11; 2013,Oct,3; 2013,Jun,13

38242 **Allogeneic lymphocyte infusions**

EXCLUDES *Aspiration of bone marrow (38220)*

Hematopoietic progenitor cell (HPC); allogeneic transplantation per donor on same date of service with (38240)

Hematopoietic progenitor cell (HPC); HPC boost on same date of service with ([38243])

⌧ (81379-81383, 86812-86822)

🏥 3.38 ⚕ 3.38 **FUD** 000 　　　　　S R2 80 ▣

AMA: 2016,Jan,13; 2015,Jan,16; 2014,Jan,11; 2013,Oct,3; 2013,Jun,13

38243 **Resequenced code. See code following 38241.**

38300-38382 Incision Lymphatic Vessels

38300 **Drainage of lymph node abscess or lymphadenitis; simple**

🏥 5.33 ⚕ 7.91 **FUD** 010 　　　　　T A2 ▣

AMA: 2014,Jan,11

38305 **extensive**

🏥 13.7 ⚕ 13.7 **FUD** 090 　　　　　T A2 ▣

AMA: 2014,Jan,11

38308 **Lymphangiotomy or other operations on lymphatic channels**

🏥 12.9 ⚕ 12.9 **FUD** 090 　　　　　T A2 80 ▣

AMA: 2014,Jan,11

Cervical lymph nodes
Intercostal lymph nodes
Entrance of thoracic duct into subclavian vein
Cisterna chyli
Spleen
Axillary nodes
Lumbar nodes
Thymus
Thoracic duct
Retosacral nodes
Mesenteric nodes
Iliac nodes
Intestinal nodes
Inguinal nodes
Mesocolic nodes

38380 **Suture and/or ligation of thoracic duct; cervical approach**

🏥 16.4 ⚕ 16.4 **FUD** 090 　　　　　C 80 ▣

AMA: 2014,Jan,11

38381 **thoracic approach**

🏥 23.2 ⚕ 23.2 **FUD** 090 　　　　　C 80 ▣

AMA: 2014,Jan,11

38382 **abdominal approach**

🏥 17.8 ⚕ 17.8 **FUD** 090 　　　　　C 80 ▣

AMA: 2014,Jan,11

38500-38555 Biopsy/Excision Lymphatic Vessels

EXCLUDES *Injection for sentinel node identification (38792)*
Percutaneous needle biopsy retroperitoneal mass (49180)

38500 **Biopsy or excision of lymph node(s); open, superficial**

EXCLUDES *Lymphadenectomy (38700-38780)*

🏥 7.35 ⚕ 9.52 **FUD** 010 　　　　　T A2 50 ▣

AMA: 2016,Jan,13; 2015,Jan,16; 2014,Jan,11; 2012,Jun,15-16; 2012,Jan,15-42; 2011,Jan,11

38505 **by needle, superficial (eg, cervical, inguinal, axillary)**

EXCLUDES *Fine needle aspiration (10021-10022)*

⌧ (76942, 77002, 77012, 77021)

🏥 2.06 ⚕ 3.62 **FUD** 000 　　　　　T A2 50 ▣

AMA: 2016,Jan,13; 2015,Jan,16; 2014,Jan,11; 2012,Jan,15-42; 2011,Jan,11

38510 **open, deep cervical node(s)**

🏥 12.1 ⚕ 14.9 **FUD** 010 　　　　　T A2 50 ▣

AMA: 2016,Jan,13; 2015,Jan,16; 2014,Jan,11; 2012,Jun,15-16; 2012,Jan,15-42; 2011,Jan,11

38520 **open, deep cervical node(s) with excision scalene fat pad**

🏥 13.4 ⚕ 13.4 **FUD** 090 　　　　　T A2 50 ▣

AMA: 2016,Jan,13; 2015,Jan,16; 2014,Jan,11; 2012,Jan,15-42; 2011,Jan,11

38525 **open, deep axillary node(s)**

🏥 12.6 ⚕ 12.6 **FUD** 090 　　　　　T A2 50 ▣

AMA: 2016,Jan,13; 2015,Mar,5; 2015,Jan,16; 2014,Apr,10; 2014,Jan,11; 2012,Jan,15-42; 2011,Jan,11

38530 **open, internal mammary node(s)**

EXCLUDES *Fine needle aspiration (10022)*
Lymphadenectomy (38720-38746)

🏥 15.8 ⚕ 15.8 **FUD** 090 　　　　T A2 80 50 ▣

AMA: 2016,Jan,13; 2015,Jan,16; 2014,Apr,10; 2014,Jan,11

38542 **Dissection, deep jugular node(s)**

EXCLUDES *Complete cervical lymphadenectomy (38720)*

🏥 15.0 ⚕ 15.0 **FUD** 090 　　　　J A2 80 50 ▣

AMA: 2016,Jan,13; 2015,Jan,16; 2014,Jan,11

38550 **Excision of cystic hygroma, axillary or cervical; without deep neurovascular dissection**

🏥 14.6 ⚕ 14.6 **FUD** 090 　　　　T A2 80 ▣

AMA: 2014,Jan,11

38555 **with deep neurovascular dissection**

🏥 29.0 ⚕ 29.0 **FUD** 090 　　　　T A2 80 ▣

AMA: 2014,Jan,11

38562-38564 Limited Lymphadenectomy: Staging

38562 **Limited lymphadenectomy for staging (separate procedure); pelvic and para-aortic**

EXCLUDES *Prostatectomy (55812, 55842)*
Radioactive substance inserted into prostate (55862)

🏥 20.2 ⚕ 20.2 **FUD** 090 　　　　　C 80 ▣

AMA: 2016,Jan,13; 2015,Jan,16; 2014,Jan,11; 2012,Jan,15-42; 2011,Jan,11

38564 **retroperitoneal (aortic and/or splenic)**

🏥 20.3 ⚕ 20.3 **FUD** 090 　　　　　C 80 ▣

AMA: 2014,Jan,11

38570-38589 Laparoscopic Lymph Node Procedures

INCLUDES Diagnostic laparoscopy (49320)

EXCLUDES *Laparoscopy with draining of lymphocele to peritoneal cavity (49323)*
Limited lymphadenectomy:
Pelvic (38562)
Retroperitoneal (38564)

38570 **Laparoscopy, surgical; with retroperitoneal lymph node sampling (biopsy), single or multiple**

🏥 14.5 ⚕ 14.5 **FUD** 010 　　　　J A2 80 ▣

AMA: 2016,Jan,13; 2015,Jan,16; 2014,Jan,11

38571 **with bilateral total pelvic lymphadenectomy**

🏥 19.2 ⚕ 19.2 **FUD** 010 　　　　J A2 80 ▣

AMA: 2016,Jan,13; 2015,Jan,16; 2014,Jan,11

38572 **with bilateral total pelvic lymphadenectomy and peri-aortic lymph node sampling (biopsy), single or multiple**

🏥 26.8 ⚕ 26.8 **FUD** 010 　　　　J A2 80 ▣

AMA: 2016,Jan,13; 2015,Jan,16; 2015,Jan,13; 2014,Jan,11

38589 **Unlisted laparoscopy procedure, lymphatic system**

🏥 0.00 ⚕ 0.00 **FUD** YYY 　　　　J 80 50

AMA: 2016,Jan,13; 2015,Jan,16; 2014,Jan,11

38700-38780 Lymphadenectomy Procedures

INCLUDES Lymph node biopsy/excision (38500)

EXCLUDES *Excision of lymphedematous skin and subcutaneous tissue (15004-15005)*
Limited lymphadenectomy
Pelvic (38562)
Retroperitoneal (38564)
Repair of lymphademiatous skin and tissue (15570-15650)

38700 **Suprahyoid lymphadenectomy**

🏥 23.3 ⚕ 23.3 **FUD** 090 　　　　T 62 80 50 ▣

AMA: 2016,Jan,13; 2015,Jan,16; 2014,Jan,11

26/TC PC/TC Only	A2-Z3 ASC Payment	50 Bilateral	♂ Male Only	♀ Female Only	🏥 Facility RVU	⚕ Non-Facility RVU	▣ CCI
FUD Follow-up Days	CMS: IOM (Pub 100)	A-Y OPPSI	80/80 Surg Assist Allowed / w/Doc		⌧ Lab Crosswalk	Radiology Crosswalk	CLIA

38720 Cervical lymphadenectomy (complete)
  38.9 ⚕ 38.9 **FUD** 090   T 80 50 ▣
  AMA: 2016,Jan,13; 2015,Jan,16; 2014,Jan,11; 2012,Jan,15-42; 2011,Jan,11

38724 Cervical lymphadenectomy (modified radical neck dissection)
  42.1 ⚕ 42.1 **FUD** 090   C 80 50 ▣
  AMA: 2016,Jan,13; 2015,Jan,16; 2014,Jan,11; 2012,Dec,3-5; 2012,Jan,15-42; 2011,Jan,11

38740 Axillary lymphadenectomy; superficial
  20.0 ⚕ 20.0 **FUD** 090   J A2 80 50 ▣
  AMA: 2016,Jan,13; 2015,Jan,16; 2014,Apr,10; 2014,Jan,11

38745 complete
  25.3 ⚕ 25.3 **FUD** 090   J A2 80 50 ▣
  AMA: 2014,Jan,11

+ **38746** Thoracic lymphadenectomy by thoracotomy, mediastinal and regional lymphadenectomy (List separately in addition to code for primary procedure)
  INCLUDES   Left side
       Aortopulmonary window
       Inferior pulmonary ligament
       Paraesophageal
       Subcarinal
     Right side
       Inferior pulmonary ligament
       Paraesophageal
       Paratracheal
       Subcarinal
  EXCLUDES   *Thoracoscopic mediastinal and regional lymphadenectomy (32674)*
  Code first primary procedure (19260, 31760, 31766, 31786, 32096-32200, 32220-32320, 32440-32491, 32503-32505, 33025, 33030, 33050-33130, 39200-39220, 39560-39561, 43101, 43112, 43117-43118, 43122-43123, 43351, 60270, 60505)
  6.27 ⚕ 6.27 **FUD** ZZZ   C 80 ▣
  AMA: 2016,Jan,13; 2015,Jan,16; 2014,May,3; 2014,Jan,11; 2012,Oct,9-11; 2012,Sep,3-8

Parasternal nodes

Central nodes

+ **38747** Abdominal lymphadenectomy, regional, including celiac, gastric, portal, peripancreatic, with or without para-aortic and vena caval nodes (List separately in addition to code for primary procedure)
  Code first primary procedure
  7.76 ⚕ 7.76 **FUD** ZZZ   C 80 ▣
  AMA: 2014,Jan,11

38760 Inguinofemoral lymphadenectomy, superficial, including Cloquet's node (separate procedure)
  24.3 ⚕ 24.3 **FUD** 090   T A2 80 50 ▣
  AMA: 2016,Jan,13; 2015,Jan,16; 2014,Jan,11; 2012,Jan,15-42; 2011,Jan,11

38765 Inguinofemoral lymphadenectomy, superficial, in continuity with pelvic lymphadenectomy, including external iliac, hypogastric, and obturator nodes (separate procedure)
  37.3 ⚕ 37.3 **FUD** 090   C 80 50 ▣
  AMA: 2016,Jan,13; 2015,Jan,16; 2014,Jan,11; 2012,Jan,15-42; 2011,Jan,11

38770 Pelvic lymphadenectomy, including external iliac, hypogastric, and obturator nodes (separate procedure)
  23.2 ⚕ 23.2 **FUD** 090   C 80 50 ▣
  AMA: 2014,Jan,11

38780 Retroperitoneal transabdominal lymphadenectomy, extensive, including pelvic, aortic, and renal nodes (separate procedure)
  29.5 ⚕ 29.5 **FUD** 090   C 80 ▣
  AMA: 2014,Jan,11

38790-38999 Cannulation/Injection/Other Procedures

38790 Injection procedure; lymphangiography
  ⬛ (75801-75807)
  2.40 ⚕ 2.40 **FUD** 000   N N1 50 ▣
  AMA: 2014,Jan,11

38792   radioactive tracer for identification of sentinel node
  EXCLUDES   *Sentinel node excision (38500-38542)*
       Sentinel node(s) identification (mapping) intraoperative with nonradioactive dye injection (38900)
  ⬛ (78195)
  1.15 ⚕ 1.15 **FUD** 000   01 N1 50 ▣
  AMA: 2016,Jan,13; 2015,Mar,5; 2015,Jan,16; 2014,Jan,11

38794 Cannulation, thoracic duct
  8.64 ⚕ 8.64 **FUD** 090   N N1 80 ▣
  AMA: 2014,Jan,11

+ **38900** Intraoperative identification (eg, mapping) of sentinel lymph node(s) includes injection of non-radioactive dye, when performed (List separately in addition to code for primary procedure)
  EXCLUDES   *Injection of tracer for sentinel node identification (38792)*
  Code first (19302, 19307, 38500, 38510, 38520, 38525, 38530, 38542, 38740, 38745)
  4.01 ⚕ 4.01 **FUD** ZZZ   N N1 80 50 ▣
  AMA: 2016,Jan,13; 2015,Mar,5; 2014,Jan,11

38999 Unlisted procedure, hemic or lymphatic system
  0.00 ⚕ 0.00 **FUD** YYY   S 80
  AMA: 2016,Jan,13; 2015,Jan,16; 2014,Jan,11; 2012,Jan,15-42; 2011,Jan,11

39000-39499 Surgical Procedures: Mediastinum

39000 Mediastinotomy with exploration, drainage, removal of foreign body, or biopsy; cervical approach
  14.4 ⚕ 14.4 **FUD** 090   C 80 ▣
  AMA: 2014,Jan,11

39010   transthoracic approach, including either transthoracic or median sternotomy
  EXCLUDES   *ECMO/ECLS insertion or reposition of cannula (33955-33956, [33963, 33964])*
       Video-assisted thoracic surgery (VATS) pericardial biopsy (32604)
  22.8 ⚕ 22.8 **FUD** 090   C 80 ▣
  AMA: 2016,Jan,13; 2015,Jul,3; 2015,Jan,16; 2014,Jan,11; 2014,Jan,5; 2013,Jan,6-8

39200 Resection of mediastinal cyst
  25.6 ⚕ 25.6 **FUD** 090   C 80 ▣
  AMA: 2014,Jan,11; 2012,Oct,9-11; 2012,Sep,3-8

39220 Resection of mediastinal tumor
  EXCLUDES   *Thymectomy (60520)*
       Thyroidectomy, substernal (60270)
       Video-assisted thoracic surgery (VATS) resection cyst, mass, or tumor of mediastinum (32662)
  33.0 ⚕ 33.0 **FUD** 090   C 80 ▣
  AMA: 2014,Jan,11; 2012,Oct,9-11; 2012,Sep,3-8

39401 Mediastinoscopy; includes biopsy(ies) of mediastinal mass (eg, lymphoma), when performed
  9.05 ⚕ 9.05 **FUD** 000   T
  AMA: 2016,Jun,4

● New Code ▲ Revised Code ○ Reinstated ● New Web Release ▲ Revised Web Release Unlisted Not Covered # Resequenced
⊘ AMA Mod 51 Exempt ⑨ Optum Mod 51 Exempt ⑥ Mod 63 Exempt ✗ Non-FDA Drug ★ Telehealth Ⓜ Maternity Ⓐ Age Edit + Add-on **AMA:** CPT Asst

39402 **with lymph node biopsy(ies) (eg, lung cancer staging)**
⏣ 11.8   ⬦ 11.8   **FUD** 000   🅣 ▭
AMA: 2016,Jun,4

39499 **Unlisted procedure, mediastinum**
⏣ 0.00   ⬦ 0.00   **FUD** YYY   🅒 80
AMA: 2014,Jan,11

39501-39599 Surgical Procedures: Diaphragm

EXCLUDES *Esophagogastric fundoplasty, with fundic patch (43325)*
Repair of diaphragmatic (esophageal) hernias:
  Laparoscopic with fundoplication (43280-43282)
  Laparotomy (43332-43333)
  Thoracoabdominal (43336-43337)
  Thoracotomy (43334-43335)

39501 **Repair, laceration of diaphragm, any approach**
⏣ 24.5   ⬦ 24.5   **FUD** 090   🅒 80 ▭
AMA: 2016,Jan,13; 2015,Jan,16; 2014,Dec,16; 2014,Dec,16;
2014,Jan,11

39503 **Repair, neonatal diaphragmatic hernia, with or without chest tube insertion and with or without creation of ventral hernia** 🅐
⏣ 178.   ⬦ 178.   **FUD** 090   ㉖ 🅒 80 ▭
AMA: 2016,Jan,13; 2015,Jan,16; 2014,Jan,11; 2012,Feb,3-7

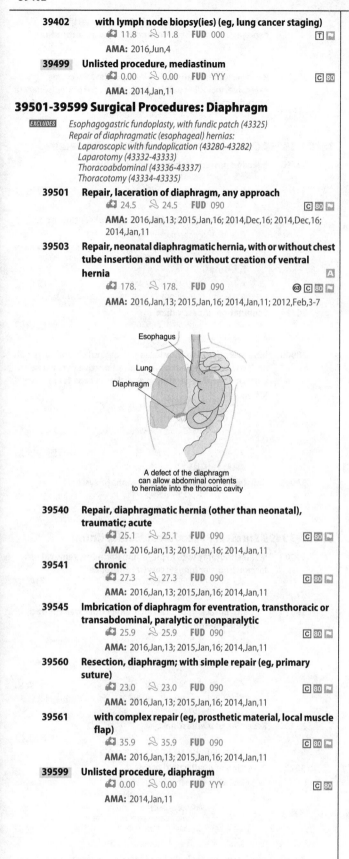

A defect of the diaphragm
can allow abdominal contents
to herniate into the thoracic cavity

39540 **Repair, diaphragmatic hernia (other than neonatal), traumatic; acute**
⏣ 25.1   ⬦ 25.1   **FUD** 090   🅒 80 ▭
AMA: 2016,Jan,13; 2015,Jan,16; 2014,Jan,11

39541 **chronic**
⏣ 27.3   ⬦ 27.3   **FUD** 090   🅒 80 ▭
AMA: 2016,Jan,13; 2015,Jan,16; 2014,Jan,11

39545 **Imbrication of diaphragm for eventration, transthoracic or transabdominal, paralytic or nonparalytic**
⏣ 25.9   ⬦ 25.9   **FUD** 090   🅒 80 ▭
AMA: 2016,Jan,13; 2015,Jan,16; 2014,Jan,11

39560 **Resection, diaphragm; with simple repair (eg, primary suture)**
⏣ 23.0   ⬦ 23.0   **FUD** 090   🅒 80 ▭
AMA: 2016,Jan,13; 2015,Jan,16; 2014,Jan,11

39561 **with complex repair (eg, prosthetic material, local muscle flap)**
⏣ 35.9   ⬦ 35.9   **FUD** 090   🅒 80 ▭
AMA: 2016,Jan,13; 2015,Jan,16; 2014,Jan,11

39599 **Unlisted procedure, diaphragm**
⏣ 0.00   ⬦ 0.00   **FUD** YYY   🅒 80
AMA: 2014,Jan,11

40490-40799 Resection and Repair Procedures of the Lips

EXCLUDES *Procedures on the skin of lips-see integumenary section codes*

40490 **Biopsy of lip**
🔧 2.12 ⚕ 3.68 **FUD** 000 T P3 ▭
AMA: 2014,Jan,11

40500 **Vermilionectomy (lip shave), with mucosal advancement**
🔧 10.5 ⚕ 14.5 **FUD** 090 T A2 ▭
AMA: 2014,Jan,11

40510 **Excision of lip; transverse wedge excision with primary closure**
EXCLUDES *Excision of mucous lesions (40810-40816)*
🔧 10.3 ⚕ 13.9 **FUD** 090 T A2 ▭
AMA: 2014,Jan,11

40520 **V-excision with primary direct linear closure**
EXCLUDES *Excision of mucous lesions (40810-40816)*
🔧 10.4 ⚕ 14.1 **FUD** 090 T A2 ▭
AMA: 2014,Jan,11

40525 **full thickness, reconstruction with local flap (eg, Estlander or fan)**
🔧 16.0 ⚕ 16.0 **FUD** 090 T A2 ▭
AMA: 2014,Jan,11

40527 **full thickness, reconstruction with cross lip flap (Abbe-Estlander)**
INCLUDES *Cleft lip repair with cross lip pedicle flap (Abbe-Estlander type), without pedicle sectioning and insertion*
EXCLUDES *Cleft lip repair with cross lip pedicle flap (Abbe-Estlander type), with pedicle sectioning and insertion (40761)*
🔧 17.9 ⚕ 17.9 **FUD** 090 J A2 80 ▭
AMA: 2014,Jan,11

40530 **Resection of lip, more than one-fourth, without reconstruction**
EXCLUDES *Reconstruction (13131-13153)*
🔧 11.7 ⚕ 15.5 **FUD** 090 T A2 ▭
AMA: 2014,Jan,11

40650 **Repair lip, full thickness; vermilion only**
🔧 8.68 ⚕ 12.7 **FUD** 090 T A2 80 ▭
AMA: 2016,Jan,13; 2015,Jan,16; 2014,Jan,11; 2012,Jan,15-42; 2011,Jan,11

40652 **up to half vertical height**
🔧 10.1 ⚕ 14.0 **FUD** 090 T A2 80 ▭
AMA: 2016,Jan,13; 2015,Jan,16; 2014,Jan,11; 2012,Jan,15-42; 2011,Jan,11

40654 **over one-half vertical height, or complex**
🔧 12.3 ⚕ 16.4 **FUD** 090 T A2 ▭
AMA: 2014,Jan,11

40700 **Plastic repair of cleft lip/nasal deformity; primary, partial or complete, unilateral**
EXCLUDES *Cleft lip repair with cross lip pedicle flap (Abbe-Estlander type):*
With pedicle sectioning and insertion (40761)
Without pedicle sectioning and insertion (40527)
Rhinoplasty for nasal deformity secondary to congenital cleft lip (30460, 30462)
🔧 26.2 ⚕ 26.2 **FUD** 090 J A2 80 ▭
AMA: 2016,Jan,13; 2015,Jan,16; 2014,Dec,18; 2014,Jan,11

40701 **primary bilateral, 1-stage procedure**
EXCLUDES *Cleft lip repair with cross lip pedicle flap (Abbe-Estlander type):*
With pedicle sectioning and insertion (40761)
Without pedicle sectioning and insertion (40527)
Rhinoplasty for nasal deformity secondary to congenital cleft lip (30460, 30462)
🔧 29.4 ⚕ 29.4 **FUD** 090 J A2 80 ▭
AMA: 2016,Jan,13; 2015,Jan,16; 2014,Dec,18; 2014,Jan,11

Bilateral cleft lip

Cleft margins on both sides are incised

Margins are closed, correcting cleft

40702 **primary bilateral, 1 of 2 stages**
EXCLUDES *Cleft lip repair with cross lip pedicle flap (Abbe-Estlander type):*
With pedicle sectioning and insertion (40761)
Without pedicle sectioning and insertion (40527)
Rhinoplasty for nasal deformity secondary to congenital cleft lip (30460, 30462)
🔧 24.7 ⚕ 24.7 **FUD** 090 J R2 80 ▭
AMA: 2016,Jan,13; 2015,Jan,16; 2014,Dec,18; 2014,Jan,11

40720 **secondary, by recreation of defect and reclosure**
EXCLUDES *Cleft lip repair with cross lip pedicle flap (Abbe-Estlander type):*
With pedicle sectioning and insertion (40761)
Without pedicle sectioning and insertion (40527)
Rhinoplasty for nasal deformity secondary to congenital cleft lip (30460, 30462)
🔧 29.5 ⚕ 29.5 **FUD** 090 J A2 80 50 ▭
AMA: 2016,Jan,13; 2015,Jan,16; 2014,Dec,18; 2014,Jan,11

40761 **with cross lip pedicle flap (Abbe-Estlander type), including sectioning and inserting of pedicle**
EXCLUDES *Cleft lip repair with cross lip pedicle flap (Abbe-Estlander type) without sectioning and insertion of pedicle (40527)*
Cleft palate repair (42200-42225)
Other reconstructive procedures (14060-14061, 15120-15261, 15574, 15576, 15630)
🔧 31.2 ⚕ 31.2 **FUD** 090 J A2 ▭
AMA: 2014,Jan,11

40799 **Unlisted procedure, lips**
🔧 0.00 ⚕ 0.00 **FUD** YYY T 80
AMA: 2014,Jan,11

40800-40819 Incision and Resection of Buccal Cavity

INCLUDES Mucosal/submucosal tissue of lips/cheeks
Oral cavity outside the dentoalveolar structures

40800 **Drainage of abscess, cyst, hematoma, vestibule of mouth; simple**
🔧 3.87 ⚕ 6.20 **FUD** 010 T P2 ▭
AMA: 2014,Jan,11

40801 **complicated**
🔧 6.54 ⚕ 9.22 **FUD** 010 T A2 ▭
AMA: 2014,Jan,11

40804 **Removal of embedded foreign body, vestibule of mouth; simple**
🔧 3.43 ⚕ 5.55 **FUD** 010 Q1 N1 80 ▭
AMA: 2014,Jan,11

40805　**complicated**
🏥 6.52　⚕ 10.7　**FUD** 010　T P3 ▢
AMA: 2014,Jan,11

40806　**Incision of labial frenum (frenotomy)**
🏥 0.94　⚕ 3.29　**FUD** 000　T P3 80 ▢
AMA: 2014,Jan,11

40808　**Biopsy, vestibule of mouth**
🏥 3.19　⚕ 5.45　**FUD** 010　T P3 ▢
AMA: 2014,Jan,11

40810　**Excision of lesion of mucosa and submucosa, vestibule of mouth; without repair**
🏥 3.75　⚕ 6.03　**FUD** 010　T P3 ▢
AMA: 2014,Jan,11

40812　**with simple repair**
🏥 5.82　⚕ 8.44　**FUD** 010　T P3 ▢
AMA: 2014,Jan,11

40814　**with complex repair**
🏥 8.99　⚕ 11.2　**FUD** 090　T A2 ▢
AMA: 2014,Jan,11

40816　**complex, with excision of underlying muscle**
🏥 9.33　⚕ 11.7　**FUD** 090　T A2 ▢
AMA: 2014,Jan,11

40818　**Excision of mucosa of vestibule of mouth as donor graft**
🏥 7.98　⚕ 10.4　**FUD** 090　T A2 80 ▢
AMA: 2014,Jan,11

40819　**Excision of frenum, labial or buccal (frenumectomy, frenulectomy, frenectomy)**
🏥 7.08　⚕ 9.26　**FUD** 090　T A2 80 ▢
AMA: 2014,Jan,11

40820 Destruction of Lesion of Buccal Cavity

CMS: 100-03,140.5 Laser Procedures
INCLUDES　Mucosal/submucosal tissue of lips/cheeks
　　　　　Oral cavity outside the dentoalveolar structures

40820　**Destruction of lesion or scar of vestibule of mouth by physical methods (eg, laser, thermal, cryo, chemical)**
🏥 5.06　⚕ 7.75　**FUD** 010　T P3 ▢
AMA: 2014,Jan,11

40830-40899 Repair Procedures of the Buccal Cavity

INCLUDES　Mucosal/submucosal tissue of lips/cheeks
　　　　　Oral cavity outside the dentoalveolar structures
EXCLUDES　Skin grafts (15002-15630)

40830　**Closure of laceration, vestibule of mouth; 2.5 cm or less**
🏥 4.84　⚕ 7.74　**FUD** 010　T C2 80 ▢
AMA: 2014,Jan,11

40831　**over 2.5 cm or complex**
🏥 6.59　⚕ 9.83　**FUD** 010　T A2 80 ▢
AMA: 2014,Jan,11

40840　**Vestibuloplasty; anterior**
🏥 18.3　⚕ 23.6　**FUD** 090　T A2 80 ▢
AMA: 2014,Jan,11

40842　**posterior, unilateral**
🏥 17.6　⚕ 22.7　**FUD** 090　J A2 80 ▢
AMA: 2014,Jan,11

40843　**posterior, bilateral**
🏥 24.8　⚕ 31.5　**FUD** 090　T A2 80 ▢
AMA: 2014,Jan,11

40844　**entire arch**
🏥 30.6　⚕ 37.7　**FUD** 090　J A2 80 ▢
AMA: 2014,Jan,11

40845　**complex (including ridge extension, muscle repositioning)**
🏥 35.7　⚕ 42.4　**FUD** 090　J A2 80 ▢
AMA: 2014,Jan,11

40899　**Unlisted procedure, vestibule of mouth**
🏥 0.00　⚕ 0.00　**FUD** YYY　T 80
AMA: 2014,Jan,11

41000-41018 Surgical Incision of Floor of Mouth or Tongue

EXCLUDES　Frenoplasty (41520)

41000　**Intraoral incision and drainage of abscess, cyst, or hematoma of tongue or floor of mouth; lingual**
🏥 3.30　⚕ 4.74　**FUD** 010　T P3 ▢
AMA: 2014,Jan,11

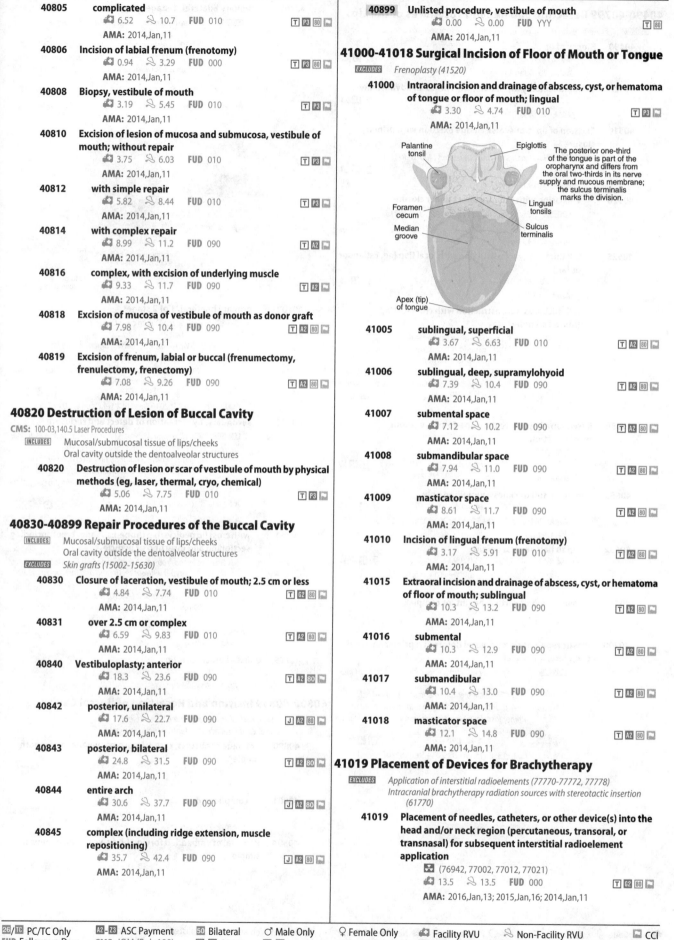

Palatine tonsil
Epiglottis
The posterior one-third of the tongue is part of the oropharynx and differs from the oral two-thirds in its nerve supply and mucous membrane; the sulcus terminalis marks the division.
Foramen cecum
Lingual tonsils
Median groove
Sulcus terminalis
Apex (tip) of tongue

41005　**sublingual, superficial**
🏥 3.67　⚕ 6.63　**FUD** 010　T A2 80 ▢
AMA: 2014,Jan,11

41006　**sublingual, deep, supramylohyoid**
🏥 7.39　⚕ 10.4　**FUD** 090　T A2 80 ▢
AMA: 2014,Jan,11

41007　**submental space**
🏥 7.12　⚕ 10.2　**FUD** 090　T A2 80 ▢
AMA: 2014,Jan,11

41008　**submandibular space**
🏥 7.94　⚕ 11.0　**FUD** 090　T A2 80 ▢
AMA: 2014,Jan,11

41009　**masticator space**
🏥 8.61　⚕ 11.7　**FUD** 090　T A2 80 ▢
AMA: 2014,Jan,11

41010　**Incision of lingual frenum (frenotomy)**
🏥 3.17　⚕ 5.91　**FUD** 010　T A2 80 ▢
AMA: 2014,Jan,11

41015　**Extraoral incision and drainage of abscess, cyst, or hematoma of floor of mouth; sublingual**
🏥 10.3　⚕ 13.2　**FUD** 090　T A2 80 ▢
AMA: 2014,Jan,11

41016　**submental**
🏥 10.3　⚕ 12.9　**FUD** 090　T A2 80 ▢
AMA: 2014,Jan,11

41017　**submandibular**
🏥 10.4　⚕ 13.0　**FUD** 090　T A2 80 ▢
AMA: 2014,Jan,11

41018　**masticator space**
🏥 12.1　⚕ 14.8　**FUD** 090　T A2 80 ▢
AMA: 2014,Jan,11

41019 Placement of Devices for Brachytherapy

EXCLUDES　Application of interstitial radioelements (77770-77772, 77778)
　　　　　Intracranial brachytherapy radiation sources with stereotactic insertion (61770)

41019　**Placement of needles, catheters, or other device(s) into the head and/or neck region (percutaneous, transoral, or transnasal) for subsequent interstitial radioelement application**
☢ (76942, 77002, 77012, 77021)
🏥 13.5　⚕ 13.5　**FUD** 000　T C2 80 ▢
AMA: 2016,Jan,13; 2015,Jan,16; 2014,Jan,11

41100-41599 Resection and Repair of the Tongue

41100 **Biopsy of tongue; anterior two-thirds**
3.16　4.90　**FUD** 010　　T P3 ▭
AMA: 2014,Jan,11

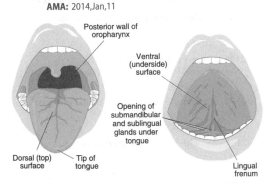

Posterior wall of oropharynx

Ventral (underside) surface

Opening of submandibular and sublingual glands under tongue

Dorsal (top) surface

Tip of tongue

Lingual frenum

Anterior (front) two-thirds of tongue comprises most of easily visible portions; the base, or root, comprises the remainder of tongue

41105 **posterior one-third**
3.27　4.98　**FUD** 010　　T P3 ▭
AMA: 2014,Jan,11

41108 **Biopsy of floor of mouth**
2.66　4.32　**FUD** 010　　T P3 ▭
AMA: 2014,Jan,11

41110 **Excision of lesion of tongue without closure**
3.86　6.19　**FUD** 010　　T P3 ▭
AMA: 2014,Jan,11

41112 **Excision of lesion of tongue with closure; anterior two-thirds**
7.45　9.79　**FUD** 090　　T A2 ▭
AMA: 2014,Jan,11

41113 **posterior one-third**
8.25　10.7　**FUD** 090　　T A2 ▭
AMA: 2014,Jan,11

41114 **with local tongue flap**
INCLUDES　Excision lesion of tongue with closure anterior/posterior two-thirds (41112-41113)
18.6　18.6　**FUD** 090　　T A2 80 ▭
AMA: 2014,Jan,11

41115 **Excision of lingual frenum (frenectomy)**
4.49　7.23　**FUD** 010　　T P3 80 ▭
AMA: 2014,Jan,11

41116 **Excision, lesion of floor of mouth**
6.48　9.69　**FUD** 090　　T A2 ▭
AMA: 2014,Jan,11

41120 **Glossectomy; less than one-half tongue**
31.7　31.7　**FUD** 090　　J A2 80 ▭
AMA: 2016,Jan,13; 2015,Jan,16; 2014,Jan,11

41130 **hemiglossectomy**
39.0　39.0　**FUD** 090　　C 80 ▭
AMA: 2016,Jan,13; 2015,Jan,16; 2014,Jan,11

41135 **partial, with unilateral radical neck dissection**
64.0　64.0　**FUD** 090　　C 80 ▭
AMA: 2016,Jan,13; 2015,Jan,16; 2014,Jan,11

41140 **complete or total, with or without tracheostomy, without radical neck dissection**
INCLUDES　Regnoli's excision
64.6　64.6　**FUD** 090　　C 80 ▭
AMA: 2016,Jan,13; 2015,Jan,16; 2014,Jan,11

41145 **complete or total, with or without tracheostomy, with unilateral radical neck dissection**
82.0　82.0　**FUD** 090　　C 80 ▭
AMA: 2016,Jan,13; 2015,Jan,16; 2014,Jan,11

41150 **composite procedure with resection floor of mouth and mandibular resection, without radical neck dissection**
65.0　65.0　**FUD** 090　　C 80 ▭
AMA: 2016,Jan,13; 2015,Jan,16; 2014,Jan,11

41153 **composite procedure with resection floor of mouth, with suprahyoid neck dissection**
70.7　70.7　**FUD** 090　　C 80 ▭
AMA: 2016,Jan,13; 2015,Jan,16; 2014,Jan,11

41155 **composite procedure with resection floor of mouth, mandibular resection, and radical neck dissection (Commando type)**
88.7　88.7　**FUD** 090　　C 80 ▭
AMA: 2016,Jan,13; 2015,Jan,16; 2014,Jan,11; 2012,Jan,15-42; 2011,Jan,11

41250 **Repair of laceration 2.5 cm or less; floor of mouth and/or anterior two-thirds of tongue**
4.48　7.78　**FUD** 010　　Q1 N1 80 ▭
AMA: 2014,Jan,11

41251 **posterior one-third of tongue**
5.34　8.48　**FUD** 010　　T A2 80 ▭
AMA: 2014,Jan,11

41252 **Repair of laceration of tongue, floor of mouth, over 2.6 cm or complex**
6.15　9.16　**FUD** 010　　T A2 80 ▭
AMA: 2014,Jan,11

41500 **Fixation of tongue, mechanical, other than suture (eg, K-wire)**
12.1　12.1　**FUD** 090　　T A2 80 ▭
AMA: 2016,Jan,13; 2015,Jan,16; 2014,Jan,11

41510 **Suture of tongue to lip for micrognathia (Douglas type procedure)**
12.3　12.3　**FUD** 090　　T A2 80 ▭
AMA: 2016,Jan,13; 2015,Jan,16; 2014,Jan,11

41512 **Tongue base suspension, permanent suture technique**
EXCLUDES　Mechanical fixation of tongue, other than suture (41500)
Suture tongue to lip for micrognathia (41510)
19.4　19.4　**FUD** 090　　J 62 80 ▭
AMA: 2016,Jan,13; 2015,Jan,16; 2014,Jan,11; 2012,Aug,13-14

41520 **Frenoplasty (surgical revision of frenum, eg, with Z-plasty)**
EXCLUDES　Frenotomy (40806, 41010)
7.61　10.3　**FUD** 090　　J A2 80 ▭
AMA: 2014,Jan,11

41530 **Submucosal ablation of the tongue base, radiofrequency, 1 or more sites, per session**
11.0　28.6　**FUD** 000　　T R2 80 ▭
AMA: 2016,Jan,13; 2015,Jan,16; 2014,Jan,11

41599 **Unlisted procedure, tongue, floor of mouth**
0.00　0.00　**FUD** YYY　　T 80
AMA: 2016,Jan,13; 2015,Jan,16; 2014,Jan,11; 2012,Jan,15-42; 2011,Jan,11

41800-41899 Procedures of the Teeth and Supporting Structures

41800 **Drainage of abscess, cyst, hematoma from dentoalveolar structures**
4.30　7.90　**FUD** 010　　Q1 N1 ▭
AMA: 2014,Jan,11

41805 **Removal of embedded foreign body from dentoalveolar structures; soft tissues**
5.14　7.54　**FUD** 010　　T P3 80 ▭
AMA: 2014,Jan,11

41806 **bone**
7.68　10.3　**FUD** 010　　T P3 80 ▭
AMA: 2014,Jan,11

41820 **Gingivectomy, excision gingiva, each quadrant**
🦷 0.00 ⚕ 0.00 **FUD** 000 [T] [R2] [80] [▢]
AMA: 2014,Jan,11

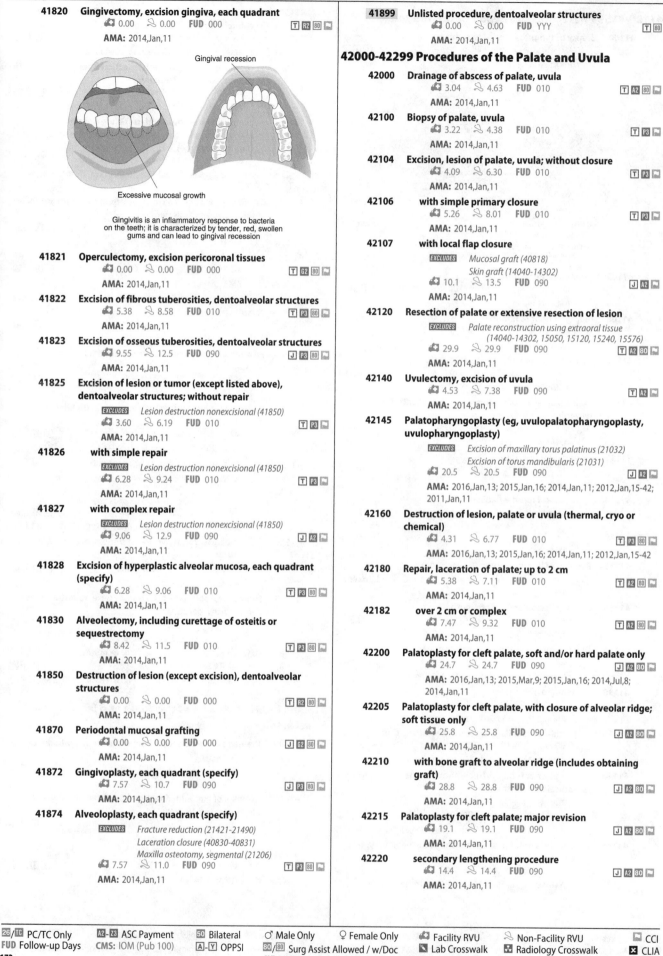

Gingival recession

Excessive mucosal growth

Gingivitis is an inflammatory response to bacteria on the teeth; it is characterized by tender, red, swollen gums and can lead to gingival recession

41821 **Operculectomy, excision pericoronal tissues**
🦷 0.00 ⚕ 0.00 **FUD** 000 [T] [G2] [80] [▢]
AMA: 2014,Jan,11

41822 **Excision of fibrous tuberosities, dentoalveolar structures**
🦷 5.38 ⚕ 8.58 **FUD** 010 [T] [P3] [80] [▢]
AMA: 2014,Jan,11

41823 **Excision of osseous tuberosities, dentoalveolar structures**
🦷 9.55 ⚕ 12.5 **FUD** 090 [J] [P3] [80] [▢]
AMA: 2014,Jan,11

41825 **Excision of lesion or tumor (except listed above), dentoalveolar structures; without repair**
EXCLUDES *Lesion destruction nonexcisional (41850)*
🦷 3.60 ⚕ 6.19 **FUD** 010 [T] [P3] [▢]
AMA: 2014,Jan,11

41826 **with simple repair**
EXCLUDES *Lesion destruction nonexcisional (41850)*
🦷 6.28 ⚕ 9.24 **FUD** 010 [T] [P3] [▢]
AMA: 2014,Jan,11

41827 **with complex repair**
EXCLUDES *Lesion destruction nonexcisional (41850)*
🦷 9.06 ⚕ 12.9 **FUD** 090 [J] [A2] [▢]
AMA: 2014,Jan,11

41828 **Excision of hyperplastic alveolar mucosa, each quadrant (specify)**
🦷 6.28 ⚕ 9.06 **FUD** 010 [T] [P3] [80] [▢]
AMA: 2014,Jan,11

41830 **Alveolectomy, including curettage of osteitis or sequestrectomy**
🦷 8.42 ⚕ 11.5 **FUD** 010 [T] [P3] [80] [▢]
AMA: 2014,Jan,11

41850 **Destruction of lesion (except excision), dentoalveolar structures**
🦷 0.00 ⚕ 0.00 **FUD** 000 [T] [R2] [80] [▢]
AMA: 2014,Jan,11

41870 **Periodontal mucosal grafting**
🦷 0.00 ⚕ 0.00 **FUD** 000 [J] [G2] [80] [▢]
AMA: 2014,Jan,11

41872 **Gingivoplasty, each quadrant (specify)**
🦷 7.57 ⚕ 10.7 **FUD** 090 [J] [P3] [80] [▢]
AMA: 2014,Jan,11

41874 **Alveoloplasty, each quadrant (specify)**
EXCLUDES *Fracture reduction (21421-21490)*
Laceration closure (40830-40831)
Maxilla osteotomy, segmental (21206)
🦷 7.57 ⚕ 11.0 **FUD** 090 [T] [P3] [80] [▢]
AMA: 2014,Jan,11

41899 **Unlisted procedure, dentoalveolar structures**
🦷 0.00 ⚕ 0.00 **FUD** YYY [T] [80]
AMA: 2014,Jan,11

42000-42299 Procedures of the Palate and Uvula

42000 **Drainage of abscess of palate, uvula**
🦷 3.04 ⚕ 4.63 **FUD** 010 [T] [A2] [80] [▢]
AMA: 2014,Jan,11

42100 **Biopsy of palate, uvula**
🦷 3.22 ⚕ 4.38 **FUD** 010 [T] [P3] [▢]
AMA: 2014,Jan,11

42104 **Excision, lesion of palate, uvula; without closure**
🦷 4.09 ⚕ 6.30 **FUD** 010 [T] [P3] [▢]
AMA: 2014,Jan,11

42106 **with simple primary closure**
🦷 5.26 ⚕ 8.01 **FUD** 010 [T] [P3] [▢]
AMA: 2014,Jan,11

42107 **with local flap closure**
EXCLUDES *Mucosal graft (40818)*
Skin graft (14040-14302)
🦷 10.1 ⚕ 13.5 **FUD** 090 [J] [A2] [▢]
AMA: 2014,Jan,11

42120 **Resection of palate or extensive resection of lesion**
EXCLUDES *Palate reconstruction using extraoral tissue (14040-14302, 15050, 15120, 15240, 15576)*
🦷 29.9 ⚕ 29.9 **FUD** 090 [T] [A2] [80] [▢]
AMA: 2014,Jan,11

42140 **Uvulectomy, excision of uvula**
🦷 4.53 ⚕ 7.38 **FUD** 090 [T] [A2] [▢]
AMA: 2014,Jan,11

42145 **Palatopharyngoplasty (eg, uvulopalatopharyngoplasty, uvulopharyngoplasty)**
EXCLUDES *Excision of maxillary torus palatinus (21032)*
Excision of torus mandibularis (21031)
🦷 20.5 ⚕ 20.5 **FUD** 090 [J] [A2] [▢]
AMA: 2016,Jan,13; 2015,Jan,16; 2014,Jan,11; 2012,Jan,15-42; 2011,Jan,11

42160 **Destruction of lesion, palate or uvula (thermal, cryo or chemical)**
🦷 4.31 ⚕ 6.77 **FUD** 010 [T] [P3] [80] [▢]
AMA: 2016,Jan,13; 2015,Jan,16; 2014,Jan,11; 2012,Jan,15-42

42180 **Repair, laceration of palate; up to 2 cm**
🦷 5.38 ⚕ 7.11 **FUD** 010 [T] [A2] [80] [▢]
AMA: 2014,Jan,11

42182 **over 2 cm or complex**
🦷 7.47 ⚕ 9.32 **FUD** 010 [T] [A2] [80] [▢]
AMA: 2014,Jan,11

42200 **Palatoplasty for cleft palate, soft and/or hard palate only**
🦷 24.7 ⚕ 24.7 **FUD** 090 [J] [A2] [80] [▢]
AMA: 2016,Jan,13; 2015,Mar,9; 2015,Jan,16; 2014,Jul,8; 2014,Jan,11

42205 **Palatoplasty for cleft palate, with closure of alveolar ridge; soft tissue only**
🦷 25.8 ⚕ 25.8 **FUD** 090 [J] [A2] [80] [▢]
AMA: 2014,Jan,11

42210 **with bone graft to alveolar ridge (includes obtaining graft)**
🦷 28.8 ⚕ 28.8 **FUD** 090 [J] [A2] [80] [▢]
AMA: 2014,Jan,11

42215 **Palatoplasty for cleft palate; major revision**
🦷 19.1 ⚕ 19.1 **FUD** 090 [J] [A2] [80] [▢]
AMA: 2014,Jan,11

42220 **secondary lengthening procedure**
🦷 14.4 ⚕ 14.4 **FUD** 090 [J] [A2] [80] [▢]
AMA: 2014,Jan,11

42225	attachment pharyngeal flap

⚷ 25.6   ⚸ 25.6   **FUD** 090   J G2 80 ▭

AMA: 2016,Jan,13; 2015,Jan,16; 2014,Jan,11; 2012,Jan,15-42; 2011,Jan,11

42226	Lengthening of palate, and pharyngeal flap

⚷ 26.1   ⚸ 26.1   **FUD** 090   J A2 80 ▭

AMA: 2014,Jan,11

42227	Lengthening of palate, with island flap

⚷ 24.8   ⚸ 24.8   **FUD** 090   J G2 80 ▭

AMA: 2014,Jan,11

42235	Repair of anterior palate, including vomer flap

EXCLUDES   *Oronasal fistula repair (30600)*

⚷ 21.4   ⚸ 21.4   **FUD** 090   J A2 80 ▭

AMA: 2016,Jan,13; 2015,Mar,9; 2015,Jan,16; 2014,Jul,8; 2014,Jan,11

42260	Repair of nasolabial fistula

EXCLUDES   *Cleft lip repair (40700-40761)*

⚷ 19.3   ⚸ 23.6   **FUD** 090   T A2 80 ▭

AMA: 2014,Jan,11

42280	Maxillary impression for palatal prosthesis

⚷ 3.23   ⚸ 4.83   **FUD** 010   T P3 80 ▭

AMA: 2014,Jan,11

42281	Insertion of pin-retained palatal prosthesis

⚷ 4.41   ⚸ 5.97   **FUD** 010   T G2 80 ▭

AMA: 2014,Jan,11

42299	Unlisted procedure, palate, uvula

⚷ 0.00   ⚸ 0.00   **FUD** YYY   T 80

AMA: 2016,Jan,13; 2015,Jan,16; 2014,Jul,8; 2014,Jan,11; 2012,Jan,15-42; 2011,Jan,11

42300-42699 Procedures of the Salivary Ducts and Glands

42300	Drainage of abscess; parotid, simple

⚷ 4.46   ⚸ 6.10   **FUD** 010   T A2 ▭

AMA: 2014,Jan,11

42305	parotid, complicated

⚷ 12.5   ⚸ 12.5   **FUD** 090   T A2 80 ▭

AMA: 2014,Jan,11

42310	Drainage of abscess; submaxillary or sublingual, intraoral

⚷ 3.61   ⚸ 4.68   **FUD** 010   T A2 80 ▭

AMA: 2014,Jan,11

42320	submaxillary, external

⚷ 5.12   ⚸ 7.27   **FUD** 010   T A2 80 ▭

AMA: 2014,Jan,11

42330	Sialolithotomy; submandibular (submaxillary), sublingual or parotid, uncomplicated, intraoral

⚷ 4.82   ⚸ 6.76   **FUD** 010   T P3 ▭

AMA: 2014,Jan,11

42335	submandibular (submaxillary), complicated, intraoral

⚷ 7.54   ⚸ 10.9   **FUD** 090   T P3 ▭

AMA: 2014,Jan,11

42340	parotid, extraoral or complicated intraoral

⚷ 9.79   ⚸ 13.5   **FUD** 090   T A2 80 50 ▭

AMA: 2014,Jan,11

42400	Biopsy of salivary gland; needle

EXCLUDES   *Fine needle aspiration (10021-10022)*

⚙ (76942, 77002, 77012, 77021)

◧ (88172-88173)

⚷ 1.60   ⚸ 3.07   **FUD** 000   T P3 ▭

AMA: 2014,Jan,11

42405	incisional

⚙ (76942, 77002, 77012, 77021)

⚷ 6.59   ⚸ 8.67   **FUD** 010   T A2 ▭

AMA: 2014,Jan,11

42408	Excision of sublingual salivary cyst (ranula)

⚷ 9.50   ⚸ 13.1   **FUD** 090   T A2 80 ▭

AMA: 2014,Jan,11

42409	Marsupialization of sublingual salivary cyst (ranula)

⚷ 6.46   ⚸ 9.67   **FUD** 090   T A2 80 ▭

AMA: 2014,Jan,11

42410	Excision of parotid tumor or parotid gland; lateral lobe, without nerve dissection

EXCLUDES   *Facial nerve suture or graft (64864, 64865, 69740, 69745)*

⚷ 18.0   ⚸ 18.0   **FUD** 090   J A2 80 50 ▭

AMA: 2014,Jan,11

Hard palate
Soft palate
Sublingual gland and ducts
Wharton duct
Parotid gland and duct
Submandibular gland
Vestibule
Tonsils

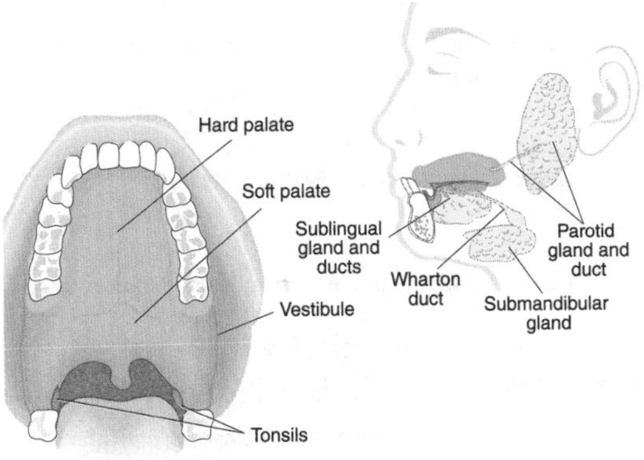

42415	lateral lobe, with dissection and preservation of facial nerve

EXCLUDES   *Facial nerve suture or graft (64864, 64865, 69740, 69745)*

⚷ 30.6   ⚸ 30.6   **FUD** 090   J A2 80 50 ▭

AMA: 2014,Jan,11

42420	total, with dissection and preservation of facial nerve

EXCLUDES   *Facial nerve suture or graft (64864, 64865, 69740, 69745)*

⚷ 34.4   ⚸ 34.4   **FUD** 090   J A2 80 50 ▭

AMA: 2014,Jan,11

42425	total, en bloc removal with sacrifice of facial nerve

EXCLUDES   *Facial nerve suture or graft (64864, 64865, 69740, 69745)*

⚷ 24.2   ⚸ 24.2   **FUD** 090   J A2 80 50 ▭

AMA: 2014,Jan,11

42426	total, with unilateral radical neck dissection

EXCLUDES   *Facial nerve suture or graft (64864, 64865, 69740, 69745)*

⚷ 39.1   ⚸ 39.1   **FUD** 090   C 80 50 ▭

AMA: 2016,Jan,13; 2015,Jan,16; 2014,Jan,11

42440	Excision of submandibular (submaxillary) gland

⚷ 11.9   ⚸ 11.9   **FUD** 090   J A2 80 50 ▭

AMA: 2014,Jan,11

42450	Excision of sublingual gland

⚷ 10.4   ⚸ 13.1   **FUD** 090   J A2 80 ▭

AMA: 2014,Jan,11

42500	Plastic repair of salivary duct, sialodochoplasty; primary or simple

⚷ 10.0   ⚸ 12.6   **FUD** 090   T A2 80 ▭

AMA: 2014,Jan,11

42505	secondary or complicated

⚷ 13.2   ⚸ 16.1   **FUD** 090   J A2

AMA: 2014,Jan,11

42507	Parotid duct diversion, bilateral (Wilke type procedure);

⚷ 15.0   ⚸ 15.0   **FUD** 090   J A2 80 ▭

AMA: 2014,Jan,11

42509	with excision of both submandibular glands

⚷ 24.5   ⚸ 24.5   **FUD** 090   J A2 80 ▭

AMA: 2014,Jan,11

42510	with ligation of both submandibular (Wharton's) ducts

⚷ 18.7   ⚸ 18.7   **FUD** 090   J A2 80 ▭

AMA: 2014,Jan,11

● New Code   ▲ Revised Code   ○ Reinstated   ● New Web Release   ▲ Revised Web Release   Unlisted   Not Covered   # Resequenced
⊘ AMA Mod 51 Exempt   ⑤⑩ Optum Mod 51 Exempt   ⑥③ Mod 63 Exempt   ⤴ Non-FDA Drug   ★ Telehealth   M Maternity   A Age Edit   + Add-on   AMA: CPT Asst

42550	Injection procedure for sialography
	(70390)
	1.83 3.87 **FUD** 000 N M1
	AMA: 2014,Jan,11

42600	Closure salivary fistula
	10.1 13.9 **FUD** 090 T A2 80
	AMA: 2014,Jan,11

42650	Dilation salivary duct
	1.71 2.43 **FUD** 000 T P3
	AMA: 2014,Jan,11

42660	Dilation and catheterization of salivary duct, with or without injection
	2.61 3.72 **FUD** 000 T P3 80
	AMA: 2014,Jan,11

42665	Ligation salivary duct, intraoral
	5.97 8.98 **FUD** 090 J A2 80
	AMA: 2014,Jan,11

42699	Unlisted procedure, salivary glands or ducts
	0.00 0.00 **FUD** YYY T 80
	AMA: 2014,Jan,11

42700-42999 Procedures of the Adenoids/Throat/Tonsils

42700	Incision and drainage abscess; peritonsillar
	3.95 5.51 **FUD** 010 T A2
	AMA: 2014,Jan,11

42720	retropharyngeal or parapharyngeal, intraoral approach
	11.4 13.2 **FUD** 010 T A2 80
	AMA: 2014,Jan,11

42725	retropharyngeal or parapharyngeal, external approach
	23.8 23.8 **FUD** 090 J A2 80
	AMA: 2014,Jan,11

42800	Biopsy; oropharynx
	EXCLUDES *Laryngoscopy with biopsy (31510, 31535-31536, 31576)*
	3.26 4.61 **FUD** 010 T P3
	AMA: 2014,Jan,11

The nasal cavities and paranasal sinuses are lined with a continuous mucous membrane

Nasal cavity

Auditory tube

Epiglottis

Orbit

Nasopharynx region

Ethmoidal cells

Oropharynx region

Hypopharynx region

Maxillary sinus

Vocal cord and larynx

Trachea

Middle and inferior meatus

Frontal coronal section of left side of skull showing sinuses

The pharynx is a transitional zone between the oral cavity and the rest of the digestive canal. It is the common route for both air and food

42804	nasopharynx, visible lesion, simple
	EXCLUDES *Laryngoscopy with biopsy (31510, 31535-31536)*
	3.30 5.68 **FUD** 010 T A2
	AMA: 2014,Jan,11

42806	nasopharynx, survey for unknown primary lesion
	EXCLUDES *Laryngoscopy with biopsy (31510, 31535-31536)*
	3.85 6.38 **FUD** 010 T A2
	AMA: 2014,Jan,11

42808	Excision or destruction of lesion of pharynx, any method
	4.73 6.60 **FUD** 010 T A2
	AMA: 2014,Jan,11

42809	Removal of foreign body from pharynx
	3.56 5.87 **FUD** 010 Q1 N1
	AMA: 2014,Jan,11

42810	Excision branchial cleft cyst or vestige, confined to skin and subcutaneous tissues
	8.42 11.2 **FUD** 090 T A2 80 50
	AMA: 2014,Jan,11

42815	Excision branchial cleft cyst, vestige, or fistula, extending beneath subcutaneous tissues and/or into pharynx
	16.2 16.2 **FUD** 090 J A2 80 50
	AMA: 2014,Jan,11

42820	Tonsillectomy and adenoidectomy; younger than age 12 A
	8.45 8.45 **FUD** 090 T A2 80
	AMA: 2016,Jan,13; 2015,Jan,16; 2014,Jan,11; 2012,Jan,15-42; 2011,Jan,11

42821	age 12 or over A
	8.77 8.77 **FUD** 090 T A2 80
	AMA: 2016,Jan,13; 2015,Jan,16; 2014,Jan,11; 2012,Jan,15-42; 2011,Jan,11

42825	Tonsillectomy, primary or secondary; younger than age 12 A
	7.63 7.63 **FUD** 090 J A2 80
	AMA: 2016,Jan,13; 2015,Jan,16; 2014,Jan,11; 2012,Jan,15-42; 2011,Jan,11

42826	age 12 or over A
	7.32 7.32 **FUD** 090 T A2
	AMA: 2016,Jan,13; 2015,Jan,16; 2014,Jan,11; 2012,Jan,15-42; 2011,Jan,11

42830	Adenoidectomy, primary; younger than age 12 A
	6.03 6.03 **FUD** 090 J A2 80
	AMA: 2016,Jan,13; 2015,Jan,16; 2014,Jan,11

42831	age 12 or over A
	6.52 6.52 **FUD** 090 T A2 80
	AMA: 2016,Jan,13; 2015,Jan,16; 2014,Jan,11

42835	Adenoidectomy, secondary; younger than age 12 A
	5.60 5.60 **FUD** 090 T A2 80
	AMA: 2016,Jan,13; 2015,Jan,16; 2014,Jan,11

42836	age 12 or over A
	7.01 7.01 **FUD** 090 T A2 80
	AMA: 2016,Jan,13; 2015,Jan,16; 2014,Jan,11; 2012,Jan,15-42; 2011,Jan,11

42842	Radical resection of tonsil, tonsillar pillars, and/or retromolar trigone; without closure
	29.8 29.8 **FUD** 090 J 80
	AMA: 2016,Jan,13; 2015,Jan,16; 2014,Jan,11

42844	closure with local flap (eg, tongue, buccal)
	40.9 40.9 **FUD** 090 J 80
	AMA: 2016,Jan,13; 2015,Jan,16; 2014,Jan,11

42845	closure with other flap
	Code also closure with other flap(s)
	Code also radical neck dissection when combined (38720)
	65.9 65.9 **FUD** 090 C 80
	AMA: 2016,Jan,13; 2015,Jan,16; 2014,Jan,11

© 2016 Optum360, LLC

42860 **Excision of tonsil tags**
🚑 5.48 ⚕ 5.48 **FUD** 090   J A2 80 ▭
AMA: 2014,Jan,11

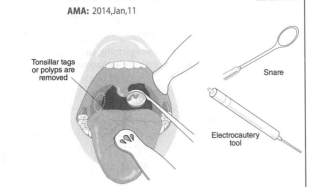

Tonsillar tags or polyps are removed

Snare

Electrocautery tool

42870 **Excision or destruction lingual tonsil, any method (separate procedure)**
EXCLUDES *Nasopharynx resection (juvenile angiofibroma) by transzygomatic/bicoronal approach (61586, 61600)*
🚑 17.6 ⚕ 17.6 **FUD** 090   T A2 80 ▭
AMA: 2014,Jan,11

42890 **Limited pharyngectomy**
Code also radical neck dissection when combined (38720)
🚑 42.2 ⚕ 42.2 **FUD** 090   J A2 80 ▭
AMA: 2014,Jan,11

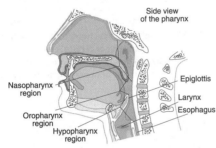

Side view of the pharynx

Nasopharynx region

Oropharynx region

Hypopharynx region

Epiglottis

Larynx

Esophagus

The nasopharynx is the membranous passage above the level of the soft palate; the oropharynx is the region between the soft palate and the upper edge of the epiglottis; the hypopharynx is the region of the epiglottis to the juncture of the larynx and esophagus; the three regions are collectively known as the pharynx

42892 **Resection of lateral pharyngeal wall or pyriform sinus, direct closure by advancement of lateral and posterior pharyngeal walls**
Code also radical neck dissection when combined (38720)
🚑 55.7 ⚕ 55.7 **FUD** 090   J A2 80 ▭
AMA: 2016,Jan,13; 2015,Jan,16; 2014,Jan,11

42894 **Resection of pharyngeal wall requiring closure with myocutaneous or fasciocutaneous flap or free muscle, skin, or fascial flap with microvascular anastomosis**
EXCLUDES *Flap used for reconstruction (15732, 15734, 15756-15758)*
Code also radical neck dissection when combined (38720)
🚑 70.0 ⚕ 70.0 **FUD** 090   C 80 ▭
AMA: 2016,Jan,13; 2015,Jan,16; 2014,Jan,11; 2012,Jan,15-42; 2011,Jan,11

42900 **Suture pharynx for wound or injury**
🚑 9.82 ⚕ 9.82 **FUD** 010   T A2 80 ▭
AMA: 2014,Jan,11

42950 **Pharyngoplasty (plastic or reconstructive operation on pharynx)**
EXCLUDES *Pharyngeal flap (42225)*
🚑 24.0 ⚕ 24.0 **FUD** 090   J A2 80 ▭
AMA: 2016,Apr,8; 2014,Jan,11

42953 **Pharyngoesophageal repair**
Code also closure using myocutaneous or other flap
🚑 28.9 ⚕ 28.9 **FUD** 090   C 80 ▭
AMA: 2014,Jan,11

42955 **Pharyngostomy (fistulization of pharynx, external for feeding)**
🚑 22.7 ⚕ 22.7 **FUD** 090   T A2 80 ▭
AMA: 2014,Jan,11

42960 **Control oropharyngeal hemorrhage, primary or secondary (eg, post-tonsillectomy); simple**
🚑 4.95 ⚕ 4.95 **FUD** 010   T A2 80 ▭
AMA: 2014,Jan,11

42961 **complicated, requiring hospitalization**
🚑 12.3 ⚕ 12.3 **FUD** 090   C 80 ▭
AMA: 2014,Jan,11

42962 **with secondary surgical intervention**
🚑 15.0 ⚕ 15.0 **FUD** 090   T A2 ▭
AMA: 2014,Jan,11

42970 **Control of nasopharyngeal hemorrhage, primary or secondary (eg, postadenoidectomy); simple, with posterior nasal packs, with or without anterior packs and/or cautery**
🚑 11.7 ⚕ 11.7 **FUD** 090   T R2 ▭
AMA: 2014,Jan,11

42971 **complicated, requiring hospitalization**
🚑 13.2 ⚕ 13.2 **FUD** 090   C 80 ▭
AMA: 2014,Jan,11

42972 **with secondary surgical intervention**
🚑 14.8 ⚕ 14.8 **FUD** 090   T A2 80 ▭
AMA: 2014,Jan,11

42999 **Unlisted procedure, pharynx, adenoids, or tonsils**
🚑 0.00 ⚕ 0.00 **FUD** YYY   T 80
AMA: 2016,Jan,13; 2015,Jan,16; 2014,Feb,11; 2014,Jan,11

43020-43135 Incision/Resection of Esophagus

EXCLUDES *Gastrointestinal reconstruction for previous esophagectomy (43360-43361)*
Gastrotomy with intraluminal tube insertion (43510)

43020 **Esophagotomy, cervical approach, with removal of foreign body**
EXCLUDES *Laparotomy with esophageal intubation (43510)*
🚑 15.3 ⚕ 15.3 **FUD** 090   T 80 ▭
AMA: 2014,Jan,11

43030 **Cricopharyngeal myotomy**
EXCLUDES *Laparotomy with esophageal intubation (43510)*
🚑 15.0 ⚕ 15.0 **FUD** 090   J G2 80 ▭
AMA: 2014,Jan,11

43045 **Esophagotomy, thoracic approach, with removal of foreign body**
EXCLUDES *Laparotomy with esophageal intubation (43510)*
🚑 37.9 ⚕ 37.9 **FUD** 090   C 80 ▭
AMA: 2014,Jan,11

43100 **Excision of lesion, esophagus, with primary repair; cervical approach**
EXCLUDES *Wide excision of malignant lesion of cervical esophagus, with total laryngectomy:*
With radical neck dissection (31365, 43107, 43116, 43124)
Without radical neck dissection (31360, 43107, 43116, 43124)
🚑 18.1 ⚕ 18.1 **FUD** 090   C 80 ▭
AMA: 2014,Jan,11

43101   **thoracic or abdominal approach**

> EXCLUDES   *Wide excision of malignant lesion of cervical esophagus with total laryngectomy:*
> *With radical neck dissection (31365, 43107, 43116, 43124)*
> *Without radical neck dissection (31360, 43107, 43116, 43124)*

🚗 29.5   ⚖ 29.5   **FUD** 090   C 80 ▭

AMA: 2016,Jan,13; 2015,Jan,16; 2014,Jan,11

43107   **Total or near total esophagectomy, without thoracotomy; with pharyngogastrostomy or cervical esophagogastrostomy, with or without pyloroplasty (transhiatal)**

🚗 74.3   ⚖ 74.3   **FUD** 090   C 80 ▭

AMA: 2014,Jan,11

43108   **with colon interposition or small intestine reconstruction, including intestine mobilization, preparation and anastomosis(es)**

🚗 133.   ⚖ 133.   **FUD** 090   C 80 ▭

AMA: 2014,Jan,11

43112   **Total or near total esophagectomy, with thoracotomy; with pharyngogastrostomy or cervical esophagogastrostomy, with or without pyloroplasty**

🚗 78.5   ⚖ 78.5   **FUD** 090   C 80 ▭

AMA: 2016,Jan,13; 2015,Jan,16; 2014,Jan,11; 2013,Aug,13

43113   **with colon interposition or small intestine reconstruction, including intestine mobilization, preparation, and anastomosis(es)**

🚗 132.   ⚖ 132.   **FUD** 090   C 80 ▭

AMA: 2014,Jan,11

43116   **Partial esophagectomy, cervical, with free intestinal graft, including microvascular anastomosis, obtaining the graft and intestinal reconstruction**

> INCLUDES   Operating microscope (69990)
>
> EXCLUDES   *Free jejunal graft with microvascular anastomosis done by a different physician (43496)*
>
> Code also modifier 52 if intestinal or free jejunal graft with microvascular anastomosis is done by another physician

🚗 146.   ⚖ 146.   **FUD** 090   C 80 ▭

AMA: 2016,Feb,12; 2014,Jan,11

43117   **Partial esophagectomy, distal two-thirds, with thoracotomy and separate abdominal incision, with or without proximal gastrectomy; with thoracic esophagogastrostomy, with or without pyloroplasty (Ivor Lewis)**

> EXCLUDES   *Esophagogastrectomy (lower third) and vagotomy (43122)*
> *Total esophagectomy with gastropharyngostomy (43107, 43124)*

🚗 71.9   ⚖ 71.9   **FUD** 090   C 80 ▭

AMA: 2014,Jan,11

43118   **with colon interposition or small intestine reconstruction, including intestine mobilization, preparation, and anastomosis(es)**

> EXCLUDES   *Esophagogastrectomy (lower third) and vagotomy (43122)*
> *Total esophagectomy with gastropharyngostomy (43107, 43124)*

🚗 107.   ⚖ 107.   **FUD** 090   C 80 ▭

AMA: 2014,Jan,11

43121   **Partial esophagectomy, distal two-thirds, with thoracotomy only, with or without proximal gastrectomy, with thoracic esophagogastrostomy, with or without pyloroplasty**

🚗 83.7   ⚖ 83.7   **FUD** 090   C 80 ▭

AMA: 2014,Jan,11

43122   **Partial esophagectomy, thoracoabdominal or abdominal approach, with or without proximal gastrectomy; with esophagogastrostomy, with or without pyloroplasty**

🚗 74.7   ⚖ 74.7   **FUD** 090   C 80 ▭

AMA: 2014,Jan,11

43123   **with colon interposition or small intestine reconstruction, including intestine mobilization, preparation, and anastomosis(es)**

🚗 137.   ⚖ 137.   **FUD** 090   C 80 ▭

AMA: 2014,Jan,11

43124   **Total or partial esophagectomy, without reconstruction (any approach), with cervical esophagostomy**

🚗 111.   ⚖ 111.   **FUD** 090   C 80 ▭

AMA: 2016,Jan,13; 2015,Jan,16; 2014,Jan,11

43130   **Diverticulectomy of hypopharynx or esophagus, with or without myotomy; cervical approach**

> EXCLUDES   *Diverticulectomy hypopharynx or cervical esophagus, endoscopic (43180)*

🚗 22.8   ⚖ 22.8   **FUD** 090   J 62 80 ▭

AMA: 2016,Jan,13; 2015,Jan,16; 2014,Jan,11; 2012,Jan,15-42; 2011,Jan,11

43135   **thoracic approach**

> EXCLUDES   *Diverticulectomy hypopharynx or cervical esophagus, endoscopic (43180)*

🚗 43.2   ⚖ 43.2   **FUD** 090   C 80 ▭

AMA: 2016,Jan,13; 2015,Jan,16; 2014,Jan,11; 2012,Jan,15-42; 2011,Jan,11

43180-43233 [43211, 43212, 43213, 43214] Endoscopic Procedures: Esophagus

> INCLUDES   Control of bleeding as result of the endoscopic procedure during same operative session
> Diagnostic endoscopy with surgical endoscopy
> Examination of upper esophageal sphincter (cricopharyngeus muscle) to/including the gastroesophageal junction
> Retroflexion examination of proximal region of stomach

43180   **Esophagoscopy, rigid, transoral with diverticulectomy of hypopharynx or cervical esophagus (eg, Zenker's diverticulum), with cricopharyngeal myotomy, includes use of telescope or operating microscope and repair, when performed**

> INCLUDES   Operating microscope (69990)
>
> EXCLUDES   *Esophagogastroduodenoscopy, flexible, transoral; with esophagogastric fundoplasty (43210)*
> *Open diverticulectomy hypopharynx or esophagus (43130-43135)*

🚗 15.9   ⚖ 15.9   **FUD** 090   T 62 ▭

AMA: 2016,Feb,12; 2016,Jan,13; 2015,Nov,8

43191   **Esophagoscopy, rigid, transoral; diagnostic, including collection of specimen(s) by brushing or washing when performed (separate procedure)**

> EXCLUDES   *Flexible, transnasal (43197-43198)*
>
> EXCLUDES   *Esophagogastroduodenoscopy, flexible, transoral; with esophagogastric fundoplasty (43210)*
> *Esophagoscopy, rigid, transoral (43192-43198)*
> *Flexible, transoral (43200)*

🚗 4.48   ⚖ 4.48   **FUD** 000   T 62 ▭

AMA: 2016,Jan,13; 2015,Nov,8; 2015,Jan,16; 2014,Feb,9; 2014,Jan,11; 2013,Dec,3

43192   **with directed submucosal injection(s), any substance**

> EXCLUDES   *Esophagoscopy, flexible, transnasal; with biopsy, single or multiple (43198)*
> *Esophagoscopy, rigid or flexible, diagnostic (43191, 43197)*
> *Flexible, transoral (43201)*
> *Injection sclerosis of esophageal varices:*
> *Flexible, transoral (43204)*
> *Rigid, transoral (43499)*

🚗 4.95   ⚖ 4.95   **FUD** 000   T 62 ▭

AMA: 2016,Jan,13; 2015,Jan,16; 2014,Feb,9; 2014,Jan,11; 2013,Dec,3

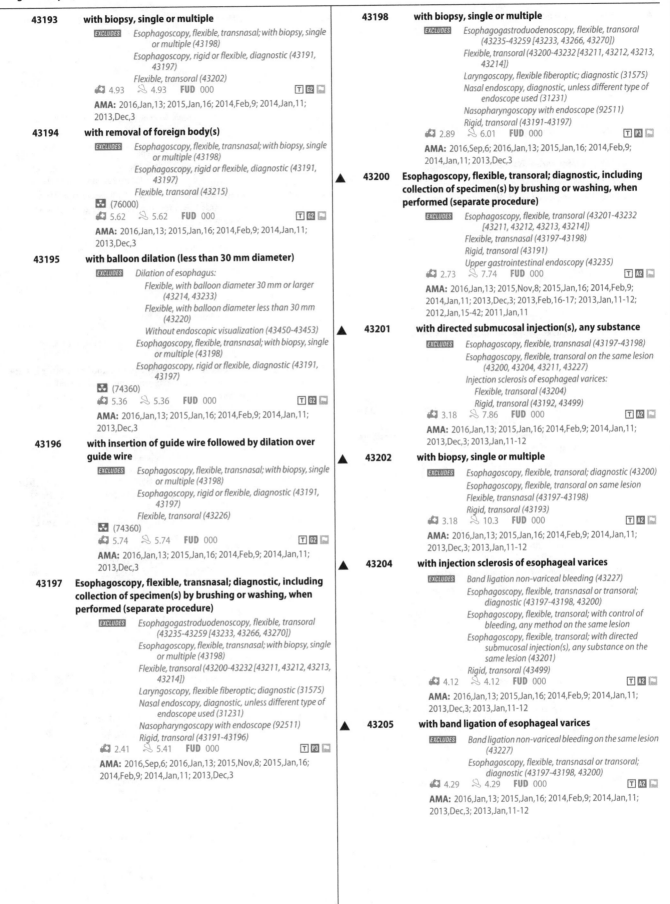

43193 **with biopsy, single or multiple**

EXCLUDES Esophagoscopy, flexible, transnasal; with biopsy, single or multiple (43198)

Esophagoscopy, rigid or flexible, diagnostic (43191, 43197)

Flexible, transoral (43202)

4.93 ⚕ 4.93 **FUD** 000 T G2 ▭

AMA: 2016,Jan,13; 2015,Jan,16; 2014,Feb,9; 2014,Jan,11; 2013,Dec,3

43194 **with removal of foreign body(s)**

EXCLUDES Esophagoscopy, flexible, transnasal; with biopsy, single or multiple (43198)

Esophagoscopy, rigid or flexible, diagnostic (43191, 43197)

Flexible, transoral (43215)

(76000)

5.62 ⚕ 5.62 **FUD** 000 T G2 ▭

AMA: 2016,Jan,13; 2015,Jan,16; 2014,Feb,9; 2014,Jan,11; 2013,Dec,3

43195 **with balloon dilation (less than 30 mm diameter)**

EXCLUDES Dilation of esophagus:

Flexible, with balloon diameter 30 mm or larger (43214, 43233)

Flexible, with balloon diameter less than 30 mm (43220)

Without endoscopic visualization (43450-43453)

Esophagoscopy, flexible, transnasal; with biopsy, single or multiple (43198)

Esophagoscopy, rigid or flexible, diagnostic (43191, 43197)

(74360)

5.36 ⚕ 5.36 **FUD** 000 T G2 ▭

AMA: 2016,Jan,13; 2015,Jan,16; 2014,Feb,9; 2014,Jan,11; 2013,Dec,3

43196 **with insertion of guide wire followed by dilation over guide wire**

EXCLUDES Esophagoscopy, flexible, transnasal; with biopsy, single or multiple (43198)

Esophagoscopy, rigid or flexible, diagnostic (43191, 43197)

Flexible, transoral (43226)

(74360)

5.74 ⚕ 5.74 **FUD** 000 T G2 ▭

AMA: 2016,Jan,13; 2015,Jan,16; 2014,Feb,9; 2014,Jan,11; 2013,Dec,3

43197 **Esophagoscopy, flexible, transnasal; diagnostic, including collection of specimen(s) by brushing or washing, when performed (separate procedure)**

EXCLUDES Esophagogastroduodenoscopy, flexible, transoral (43235-43259 [43233, 43266, 43270])

Esophagoscopy, flexible, transnasal; with biopsy, single or multiple (43198)

Flexible, transoral (43200-43232 [43211, 43212, 43213, 43214])

Laryngoscopy, flexible fiberoptic; diagnostic (31575)

Nasal endoscopy, diagnostic, unless different type of endoscope used (31231)

Nasopharyngoscopy with endoscope (92511)

Rigid, transoral (43191-43196)

2.41 ⚕ 5.41 **FUD** 000 T P3 ▭

AMA: 2016,Sep,6; 2016,Jan,13; 2015,Nov,8; 2015,Jan,16; 2014,Feb,9; 2014,Jan,11; 2013,Dec,3

43198 **with biopsy, single or multiple**

EXCLUDES Esophagogastroduodenoscopy, flexible, transoral (43235-43259 [43233, 43266, 43270])

Flexible, transoral (43200-43232 [43211, 43212, 43213, 43214])

Laryngoscopy, flexible fiberoptic; diagnostic (31575)

Nasal endoscopy, diagnostic, unless different type of endoscope used (31231)

Nasopharyngoscopy with endoscope (92511)

Rigid, transoral (43191-43197)

2.89 ⚕ 6.01 **FUD** 000 T P3 ▭

AMA: 2016,Sep,6; 2016,Jan,13; 2015,Jan,16; 2014,Feb,9; 2014,Jan,11; 2013,Dec,3

▲ **43200** **Esophagoscopy, flexible, transoral; diagnostic, including collection of specimen(s) by brushing or washing, when performed (separate procedure)**

EXCLUDES Esophagoscopy, flexible, transoral (43201-43232 [43211, 43212, 43213, 43214])

Flexible, transnasal (43197-43198)

Rigid, transoral (43191)

Upper gastrointestinal endoscopy (43235)

2.73 ⚕ 7.74 **FUD** 000 T A2 ▭

AMA: 2016,Jan,13; 2015,Nov,8; 2015,Jan,16; 2014,Feb,9; 2014,Jan,11; 2013,Dec,3; 2013,Feb,16-17; 2013,Jan,11-12; 2012,Jan,15-42; 2011,Jan,11

▲ **43201** **with directed submucosal injection(s), any substance**

EXCLUDES Esophagoscopy, flexible, transnasal (43197-43198)

Esophagoscopy, flexible, transoral on the same lesion (43200, 43204, 43211, 43227)

Injection sclerosis of esophageal varices:

Flexible, transoral (43204)

Rigid, transoral (43192, 43499)

3.18 ⚕ 7.86 **FUD** 000 T A2 ▭

AMA: 2016,Jan,13; 2015,Jan,16; 2014,Feb,9; 2014,Jan,11; 2013,Dec,3; 2013,Jan,11-12

▲ **43202** **with biopsy, single or multiple**

EXCLUDES Esophagoscopy, flexible, transoral; diagnostic (43200)

Esophagoscopy, flexible, transoral on same lesion

Flexible, transnasal (43197-43198)

Rigid, transoral (43193)

3.18 ⚕ 10.3 **FUD** 000 T A2 ▭

AMA: 2016,Jan,13; 2015,Jan,16; 2014,Feb,9; 2014,Jan,11; 2013,Dec,3; 2013,Jan,11-12

▲ **43204** **with injection sclerosis of esophageal varices**

EXCLUDES Band ligation non-variceal bleeding (43227)

Esophagoscopy, flexible, transnasal or transoral; diagnostic (43197-43198, 43200)

Esophagoscopy, flexible, transoral; with control of bleeding, any method on the same lesion

Esophagoscopy, flexible, transoral; with directed submucosal injection(s), any substance on the same lesion (43201)

Rigid, transoral (43499)

4.12 ⚕ 4.12 **FUD** 000 T A2 ▭

AMA: 2016,Jan,13; 2015,Jan,16; 2014,Feb,9; 2014,Jan,11; 2013,Dec,3; 2013,Jan,11-12

▲ **43205** **with band ligation of esophageal varices**

EXCLUDES Band ligation non-variceal bleeding on the same lesion (43227)

Esophagoscopy, flexible, transnasal or transoral; diagnostic (43197-43198, 43200)

4.29 ⚕ 4.29 **FUD** 000 T A2 ▭

AMA: 2016,Jan,13; 2015,Jan,16; 2014,Feb,9; 2014,Jan,11; 2013,Dec,3; 2013,Jan,11-12

▲ **43206** **with optical endomicroscopy**

EXCLUDES *Esophagoscopy, flexible, transnasal or transoral; diagnostic (43197-43198, 43200)*

Optical endomicroscopic image(s), interpretation and report (88375)

Code also contrast agent

4.11 ⚕ 9.40 **FUD** 000 T G2 ▣

AMA: 2016,Jan,13; 2015,Jan,16; 2014,Feb,9; 2014,Jan,11; 2013,Dec,3; 2013,Aug,5; 2013,Jan,11-12

43210 Resequenced code. See code following 43259.

43211 Resequenced code. See code following 43217.

43212 Resequenced code. See code following 43217.

43213 Resequenced code. See code following 43220.

43214 Resequenced code. See code following 43220.

▲ **43215** **with removal of foreign body(s)**

EXCLUDES *Esophagoscopy, flexible, transnasal or transoral; diagnostic (43197-43198, 43200)*

Rigid, transoral (43194)

Upper gastrointestinal endoscopy (43247)

(76000)

4.32 ⚕ 11.9 **FUD** 000 T A2 ▣

AMA: 2016,Jan,13; 2015,Jan,16; 2014,Feb,9; 2014,Jan,11; 2013,Dec,3; 2013,Jan,11-12

▲ **43216** **with removal of tumor(s), polyp(s), or other lesion(s) by hot biopsy forceps**

EXCLUDES *Esophagoscopy, flexible, transnasal or transoral; diagnostic (43197-43198, 43200)*

Removal by snare technique (43217)

4.08 ⚕ 11.7 **FUD** 000 T A2 ▣

AMA: 2016,Jan,13; 2015,Jan,16; 2014,Feb,9; 2014,Jan,11; 2013,Dec,3; 2013,Jan,11-12

▲ **43217** **with removal of tumor(s), polyp(s), or other lesion(s) by snare technique**

EXCLUDES *Esophagoscopy, flexible, transnasal or transoral; diagnostic (43197-43198, 43200)*

Esophagoscopy, flexible, transoral; with endoscopic mucosal resection on the same lesion (43211)

Upper gastrointestinal endoscopy with snare technique (43251)

4.87 ⚕ 12.7 **FUD** 000 T A2 ▣

AMA: 2016,Jan,13; 2015,Jan,16; 2014,Feb,9; 2014,Jan,11; 2013,Dec,3; 2013,Jan,11-12

▲ # **43211** **with endoscopic mucosal resection**

EXCLUDES *Esophagoscopy, flexible, transnasal or transoral; diagnostic (43197-43198, 43200)*

Esophagoscopy, flexible, transoral; with directed submucosal injection(s) (43201-43202)

Esophagoscopy, flexible, transoral; with removal of tumor(s), polyp(s), or other lesion(s) by snare technique (43217)

7.07 ⚕ 7.07 **FUD** 000 T G2 ▣

AMA: 2016,Jan,13; 2015,Jan,16; 2014,Feb,9; 2014,Jan,11; 2013,Dec,3

▲ # **43212** **with placement of endoscopic stent (includes pre- and post-dilation and guide wire passage, when performed)**

EXCLUDES *Esophagogastroduodenoscopy, flexible, transoral; with insertion of intraluminal tube or catheter (43241)*

Esophagoscopy, flexible, transnasal or transoral; diagnostic (43197-43198, 43200)

Esophagoscopy, flexible, transoral; with insertion of guide wire followed by passage of dilator(s) over guide wire (43226)

Esophagoscopy, flexible, transoral; with transendoscopic balloon dilation (43220)

(74360)

5.73 ⚕ 5.73 **FUD** 000 J G2 ▣

AMA: 2016,Jan,13; 2015,Jan,16; 2014,Feb,9; 2014,Jan,11; 2013,Dec,3

▲ **43220** **with transendoscopic balloon dilation (less than 30 mm diameter)**

EXCLUDES *Dilation of esophagus:*

Rigid, with balloon diameter 30 mm or larger (43214)

Rigid, with balloon diameter less than 30mm (43195)

Without endoscopic visualization (43450, 43453)

Esophagoscopy, flexible, transnasal; diagnostic (43197-43198)

Esophagoscopy, flexible, transoral (43200, 43212, 43226, 43229)

(74360)

3.62 ⚕ 32.1 **FUD** 000 T A2 ▣

AMA: 2016,Jan,13; 2015,Jan,16; 2014,Feb,9; 2014,Jan,11; 2013,Dec,3; 2013,Jan,11-12; 2012,Jan,15-42; 2011,Jan,11

▲ # **43213** **with dilation of esophagus, by balloon or dilator, retrograde (includes fluoroscopic guidance, when performed)**

INCLUDES Fluoroscopy (76000-76001)

EXCLUDES *Esophagoscopy, flexible, transnasal or transoral; diagnostic (43197-43198, 43200)*

Intraluminal dilation of strictures and/or obstructions (eg, esophagus), radiological supervision and interpretation (74360)

Code also each additional stricture treated in same operative session with modifier 59 and (43213)

7.73 ⚕ 34.7 **FUD** 000 T G2 ▣

AMA: 2016,Jan,13; 2015,Jan,16; 2014,Feb,9; 2014,Jan,11; 2013,Dec,3

▲ # **43214** **with dilation of esophagus with balloon (30 mm diameter or larger) (includes fluoroscopic guidance, when performed)**

INCLUDES Fluoroscopy (76000-76001)

EXCLUDES *Esophagoscopy, flexible, transnasal or transoral; diagnostic (43197-43198, 43200)*

Intraluminal dilation of strictures and/or obstructions (eg, esophagus), radiological supervision and interpretation (74360)

5.78 ⚕ 5.78 **FUD** 000 T G2 ▣

AMA: 2016,Jan,13; 2015,Jan,16; 2014,Feb,9; 2014,Jan,11; 2013,Dec,3

▲ **43226** **with insertion of guide wire followed by passage of dilator(s) over guide wire**

EXCLUDES *Esophagoscopy, flexible, transnasal or transoral; diagnostic (43197-43198, 43200)*

Esophagoscopy, flexible, transoral; with ablation of tumor(s), polyp(s), or other lesion(s) on the same lesion (43229)

Esophagoscopy, flexible, transoral; with placement of endoscopic stent (43212)

Esophagoscopy, flexible, transoral; with transendoscopic balloon dilation (43220)

Rigid, transoral (43196)

(74360)

3.99 ⚕ 10.8 **FUD** 000 T A2 ▣

AMA: 2016,Jan,13; 2015,Jan,16; 2014,Feb,9; 2014,Jan,11; 2013,Dec,3; 2013,Jan,11-12

▲ **43227** **with control of bleeding, any method**

EXCLUDES *Esophagoscopy, flexible, transnasal or transoral; diagnostic (43197-43198, 43200)*

Esophagoscopy, flexible, transoral; with directed submucosal injection(s) on the same lesion (43201)

Esophagoscopy, flexible, transoral; with injection sclerosis of esophageal varices on the same lesion (43204-43205)

5.01 ⚕ 19.7 **FUD** 000 T A2 ▣

AMA: 2016,Jan,13; 2015,Jan,16; 2014,Feb,9; 2014,Feb,11; 2014,Jan,11; 2013,Dec,3; 2013,Jan,11-12

26/TC PC/TC Only   A2-Z3 ASC Payment   50 Bilateral   ♂ Male Only   ♀ Female Only   Facility RVU   ⚕ Non-Facility RVU   ▣ CCI

FUD Follow-up Days   **CMS:** IOM (Pub 100)   A-Y OPPSI   80/80 Surg Assist Allowed / w/Doc   Lab Crosswalk   Radiology Crosswalk   CLIA

178   CPT © 2016 American Medical Association. All Rights Reserved.   © 2016 Optum360, LLC

▲ **43229** **with ablation of tumor(s), polyp(s), or other lesion(s) (includes pre- and post-dilation and guide wire passage, when performed)**

> EXCLUDES *Esophagoscopy, flexible, transnasal or transoral; diagnostic (43197-43198, 43200)*
> *Esophagoscopy, flexible, transoral; with insertion of guide wire followed by passage of dilator(s) over guide wire on the same lesion (43226)*
> *Esophagoscopy, flexible, transoral; with transendoscopic balloon dilation on the same lesion (43220)*
> Code also esophagoscopic photodynamic therapy, when performed (96570-96571)

🔲 5.95 ⚕ 20.5 **FUD** 000 Ⓣ G2 ▭

AMA: 2016,Jan,13; 2015,Jan,16; 2014,Feb,9; 2014,Jan,11; 2013,Dec,3

▲ **43231** **with endoscopic ultrasound examination**

> INCLUDES Gastrointestinal endoscopic ultrasound, supervision and interpretation (76975)
> EXCLUDES *Esophagoscopy, flexible, transnasal or transoral; diagnostic (43197-43198, 43200)*
> *Esophagoscopy, flexible, transoral; with transendoscopic ultrasound-guided intramural or transmural fine needle aspiration/biopsy(s) (43232)*
> *Procedure performed more than one time per operative session*

🔲 4.86 ⚕ 11.3 **FUD** 000 Ⓣ A2 ▭

AMA: 2016,Jan,13; 2015,Jan,16; 2014,Feb,9; 2014,Jan,11; 2013,Dec,3; 2013,Jan,11-12

▲ **43232** **with transendoscopic ultrasound-guided intramural or transmural fine needle aspiration/biopsy(s)**

> EXCLUDES *Esophagoscopy, flexible, transnasal or transoral; diagnostic (43197-43198, 43200)*
> *Esophagoscopy, flexible, transoral; with endoscopic ultrasound examination (43231)*
> *Gastrointestinal endoscopic ultrasound, supervision and interpretation (76975)*
> *Procedure performed more than one time per operative session*
> *Ultrasonic guidance (76942)*

🔲 5.97 ⚕ 13.5 **FUD** 000 Ⓣ A2 ▭

AMA: 2016,Jan,13; 2015,Jan,16; 2014,Feb,9; 2014,Jan,11; 2013,Dec,3; 2013,Jan,11-12; 2012,Jan,15-42; 2011,Jan,11

43233 **Resequenced code. See code following 43249.**

43235-43259 [43210, 43233, 43266, 43270] Endoscopic Procedures: Esophagogastroduodenoscopy (EGD)

> INCLUDES Control of bleeding as result of the endoscopic procedure during same operative session
> Diagnostic endoscopy with surgical endoscopy
> EXCLUDES *Exam of jejunum distal to the anastomosis in surgically altered stomach, including post-gastroenterostomy (Billroth II) and gastric bypass (43235-43259 [43233, 43266, 43270])*
> *Exam of upper esophageal sphincter (cricopharyngeus muscle) to/including gastroesophageal junction and/or retroflexion exam of proximal region of stomach (43197-43232 [43211, 43212, 43213, 43214])*
> Code also modifier 52 when duodenum is not examined either deliberately or due to significant issues and repeat procedure will not be performed
> Code also modifier 53 when duodenum is not examined either deliberately or due to significant issues and repeat procedure is planned

▲ **43235** **Esophagogastroduodenoscopy, flexible, transoral; diagnostic, including collection of specimen(s) by brushing or washing, when performed (separate procedure)**

> EXCLUDES *Endoscopy of small intestine (44360-44379)*
> *Esophagogastroduodenoscopy, flexible, transoral; with esophagogastric fundoplasty (43210)*
> *Esophagoscopy, flexible, transnasal; diagnostic (43197-43198)*
> *Procedure performed with surgical endoscopy (43236-43259 [43233, 43266, 43270])*

🔲 3.75 ⚕ 8.84 **FUD** 000 Ⓣ A2 ▭

AMA: 2016,Jan,13; 2015,Nov,8; 2015,Jan,16; 2014,Jan,11; 2013,Dec,3; 2013,Jan,11-12; 2012,Jan,15-42; 2011,Jan,11

▲ **43236** **with directed submucosal injection(s), any substance**

> EXCLUDES *Endoscopy of small intestine (44360-44379)*
> *Esophagogastroduodenoscopy, flexible, transoral; with control of bleeding, any method (43255)*
> *Esophagogastroduodenoscopy, flexible, transoral; with endoscopic mucosal resection on the same lesion (43254)*
> *Esophagogastroduodenoscopy, flexible, transoral; with injection sclerosis of esophageal/gastric varices on the same lesion (43243)*
> *Esophagoscopy, flexible, transnasal or transoral; diagnostic (43197-43198, 43235)*
> *Injection sclerosis of varices, esophageal/gastric (43243)*

🔲 4.23 ⚕ 11.0 **FUD** 000 Ⓣ A2 ▭

AMA: 2016,Jan,13; 2015,Jan,16; 2014,Jan,11; 2013,Dec,3; 2013,Jan,11-12

▲ **43237** **with endoscopic ultrasound examination limited to the esophagus, stomach or duodenum, and adjacent structures**

> INCLUDES Gastrointestinal endoscopic ultrasound, supervision and interpretation (76975)
> EXCLUDES *Endoscopy of small intestine (44360-44379)*
> *Esophagogastroduodenoscopy, flexible, transoral (43235, 43238, 43242, 43253, 43259)*
> *Esophagoscopy, flexible, transnasal; diagnostic (43197-43198)*
> *Procedure performed more than one time per operative session*

🔲 5.90 ⚕ 5.90 **FUD** 000 Ⓣ A2 ▭

AMA: 2016,Jan,11; 2016,Jan,13; 2015,Jan,16; 2014,Jan,11; 2013,Dec,3; 2013,Jan,11-12

▲ **43238** **with transendoscopic ultrasound-guided intramural or transmural fine needle aspiration/biopsy(s), (includes endoscopic ultrasound examination limited to the esophagus, stomach or duodenum, and adjacent structures)**

> INCLUDES Gastrointestinal endoscopic ultrasound, supervision and interpretation (76975)
> Ultrasonic guidance (76942)
> EXCLUDES *Endoscopy of small intestine (44360-44379)*
> *Esophagogastroduodenoscopy, flexible, transoral (43235, 43237, 43242)*
> *Esophagoscopy, flexible, transnasal (43197-43198)*
> *Procedure performed more than one time per operative session*

🔲 6.99 ⚕ 6.99 **FUD** 000 Ⓣ A2 ▭

AMA: 2016,Jan,13; 2015,Jan,16; 2014,Jan,11; 2013,Dec,3; 2013,Jan,11-12

▲ **43239** **with biopsy, single or multiple**

> EXCLUDES *Endoscopy of small intestine (44360-44379)*
> *Esophagogastroduodenoscopy, flexible, transoral; diagnostic (43235)*
> *Esophagogastroduodenoscopy, flexible, transoral; with endoscopic mucosal resection on the same lesion (43254)*
> *Esophagoscopy, flexible, transnasal (43197-43198)*

🔲 4.23 ⚕ 11.2 **FUD** 000 Ⓣ A2 ▭

AMA: 2016,Jan,13; 2015,Jan,16; 2014,Jan,11; 2013,Dec,3; 2013,Jan,11-12; 2012,Jan,15-42; 2011,Jan,11

Digestive System

43240 — 43233

▲ **43240** **with transmural drainage of pseudocyst (includes placement of transmural drainage catheter[s]/stent[s], when performed, and endoscopic ultrasound, when performed)**

EXCLUDES *Endoscopic pancreatic necrosectomy (48999)*
Endoscopy of small intestine (44360-44379)
Esophagogastroduodenoscopy, flexible, transoral (43235, 43242, [43266], 43259)
Esophagogastroduodenoscopy, flexible, transoral; with transendoscopic ultrasound-guided transmural injection of diagnostic or therapeutic substance(s) on the same lesion (43253)
Esophagoscopy, flexible, transnasal (43197-43198)
Procedure performed more than one time per operative session

⚕ 11.6   ⚕ 11.6   **FUD** 000   T A2 ▢

AMA: 2016,Jan,13; 2015,Jan,16; 2014,Jan,11; 2013,Dec,3; 2013,Jan,11-12

▲ **43241** **with insertion of intraluminal tube or catheter**

EXCLUDES *Endoscopy of small intestine (44360-44379)*
Esophagogastroduodenoscopy, flexible, transoral (43235, [43266])
Esophagoscopy, flexible, transnasal or transoral (43197-43198, 43212)
Tube placement:
Enteric, non-endoscopic (44500, 74340)
Naso or oro-gastric requiring professional skill and fluoroscopic guidance (43752)

⚕ 4.34   ⚕ 4.34   **FUD** 000   T A2 ▢

AMA: 2016,Jan,13; 2015,Jan,16; 2014,Jan,11; 2013,Dec,3; 2013,Jan,11-12

▲ **43242** **with transendoscopic ultrasound-guided intramural or transmural fine needle aspiration/biopsy(s) (includes endoscopic ultrasound examination of the esophagus, stomach, and either the duodenum or a surgically altered stomach where the jejunum is examined distal to the anastomosis)**

INCLUDES *Gastrointestinal endoscopic ultrasound, supervision and interpretation (76975)*
Ultrasonic guidance (76942)
EXCLUDES *Endoscopy of small intestine (44360-44379)*
Esophagogastroduodenoscopy, flexible, transoral (43235, 43237-43238, 43240, 43259)
Esophagoscopy, flexible, transnasal (43197-43198)
Procedure performed more than one time per operative session
Transmural fine needle biopsy/aspiration with ultrasound guidance, transendoscopic, esophagus/stomach/duodenum/neighboring structure (43238)

⊠ 88172-88173

⚕ 7.89   ⚕ 7.89   **FUD** 000   T A2 ▢

AMA: 2016,Jan,13; 2015,Jan,16; 2014,Jan,11; 2013,Dec,3; 2013,Jan,11-12

▲ **43243** **with injection sclerosis of esophageal/gastric varices**

EXCLUDES *Endoscopy of small intestine (44360-44379)*
Esophagogastroduodenoscopy, flexible, transoral; diagnostic (43235)
Esophagogastroduodenoscopy, flexible, transoral with on the same lesion (43236, 43255)
Esophagoscopy, flexible, transnasal (43197-43198)

⚕ 7.12   ⚕ 7.12   **FUD** 000   T A2 ▢

AMA: 2016,Jan,13; 2015,Jan,16; 2014,Jan,11; 2013,Dec,3; 2013,Jan,11-12

▲ **43244** **with band ligation of esophageal/gastric varices**

EXCLUDES *Band ligation, non-variceal bleeding (43255)*
Endoscopy of small intestine (44360-44379)
Esophagogastroduodenoscopy, flexible, transoral (43235, 43255)
Esophagoscopy, flexible, transnasal (43197-43198)

⚕ 7.37   ⚕ 7.37   **FUD** 000   T A2 ▢

AMA: 2016,Jan,13; 2015,Jan,16; 2014,Jan,11; 2013,Dec,3; 2013,Jan,11-12; 2012,Jan,15-42; 2011,Jun,13

▲ **43245** **with dilation of gastric/duodenal stricture(s) (eg, balloon, bougie)**

EXCLUDES *Endoscopy of small intestine (44360-44379)*
Esophagogastroduodenoscopy, flexible, transoral (43235, [43266])
Esophagoscopy, flexible, transnasal (43197-43198)
🔆 (74360)

⚕ 5.32   ⚕ 17.4   **FUD** 000   T A2 ▢

AMA: 2016,Jan,13; 2015,Jan,16; 2014,Jan,11; 2013,Dec,3; 2013,Jan,11-12; 2012,Jan,15-42; 2011,Jan,11

▲ **43246** **with directed placement of percutaneous gastrostomy tube**

EXCLUDES *Endoscopy of small intestine (44360-44372, 44376-44379)*
Esophagogastroduodenoscopy, flexible, transoral; diagnostic (43235)
Esophagoscopy, flexible, transnasal (43197-43198)
Gastrostomy tube replacement without endoscopy or imaging (43760)
Percutaneous insertion of gastrostomy tube, nonendoscopic (49440)

⚕ 6.03   ⚕ 6.03   **FUD** 000   T A2 80 ▢

AMA: 2016,Jan,13; 2015,Jan,16; 2014,Jan,11; 2013,Dec,3; 2013,May,12; 2013,Jan,11-12; 2012,Jan,15-42; 2011,Jan,11

▲ **43247** **with removal of foreign body(s)**

EXCLUDES *Endoscopy of small intestine (44360-44379)*
Esophagogastroduodenoscopy, flexible, transoral; diagnostic (43235)
Esophagoscopy, flexible, transnasal (43197-43198)
🔆 (76000)

⚕ 5.36   ⚕ 11.8   **FUD** 000   T A2 ▢

AMA: 2016,Jan,13; 2015,Jan,16; 2014,Jan,11; 2013,Dec,3; 2013,Jan,11-12; 2012,Jan,15-42; 2011,Jan,11

▲ **43248** **with insertion of guide wire followed by passage of dilator(s) through esophagus over guide wire**

EXCLUDES *Endoscopy of small intestine (44360-44379)*
Esophagogastroduodenoscopy, flexible, transoral (43235, [43266], [43270])
Esophagoscopy, flexible, transnasal (43197-43198)
🔆 (74360)

⚕ 5.04   ⚕ 11.6   **FUD** 000   T A2 ▢

AMA: 2016,Jan,13; 2015,Jan,16; 2014,Jan,11; 2013,Dec,3; 2013,Jan,11-12; 2012,Jan,15-42; 2011,Jan,11

▲ **43249** **with transendoscopic balloon dilation of esophagus (less than 30 mm diameter)**

EXCLUDES *Endoscopy of small intestine (44360-44379)*
Esophagogastroduodenoscopy, flexible, transoral (43235, [43266], [43270])
Esophagoscopy, flexible, transnasal (43197-43198)
🔆 (74360)

⚕ 4.66   ⚕ 30.4   **FUD** 000   T A2 ▢

AMA: 2016,Jan,13; 2015,Jan,16; 2014,Jan,11; 2013,Dec,3; 2013,Jan,11-12

▲ # **43233** **with dilation of esophagus with balloon (30 mm diameter or larger) (includes fluoroscopic guidance, when performed)**

INCLUDES *Fluoroscopy (76000-76001)*
Intraluminal dilation of strictures and/or obstructions (74360)
EXCLUDES *Endoscopy of small intestine (44360-44379)*
Esophagogastroduodenoscopy, flexible, transoral; diagnostic (43235)
Esophagoscopy, flexible, transnasal (43197-43198)

⚕ 6.84   ⚕ 6.84   **FUD** 000   T G2 ▢

AMA: 2016,Jan,13; 2015,Jan,16; 2014,Jan,11; 2013,Dec,3

26/TC PC/TC Only	A2-Z3 ASC Payment	50 Bilateral	♂ Male Only	♀ Female Only	⚕ Facility RVU	⚕ Non-Facility RVU	▢ CCI
FUD Follow-up Days	CMS: IOM (Pub 100)	A-Y OPPSI	80/80 Surg Assist Allowed / w/Doc		⊠ Lab Crosswalk	🔆 Radiology Crosswalk	⊠ CLIA

180

CPT © 2016 American Medical Association. All Rights Reserved.

© 2016 Optum360, LLC

▲ **43250** **with removal of tumor(s), polyp(s), or other lesion(s) by hot biopsy forceps**

EXCLUDES Endoscopy of small intestine (44360-44379)
Esophagogastroduodenoscopy, flexible, transoral (43235)
Esophagoscopy, flexible, transnasal (43197-43198)

🔧 5.15 ⚕ 12.9 **FUD** 000 T A2 💻

AMA: 2016,Jan,13; 2015,Jan,16; 2014,Jan,11; 2013,Dec,3; 2013,Jan,11-12; 2012,Jan,15-42; 2011,Jan,11

▲ **43251** **with removal of tumor(s), polyp(s), or other lesion(s) by snare technique**

EXCLUDES Endoscopic mucosal resection when performed on same lesion (43254)
Endoscopy of small intestine (44360-44379)
Esophagogastroduodenoscopy, flexible, transoral (43235)
Esophagoscopy, flexible, transnasal (43197-43198)

🔧 5.92 ⚕ 14.1 **FUD** 000 T A2 💻

AMA: 2016,Jan,13; 2015,Jan,16; 2014,Jan,11; 2013,Dec,3; 2013,Jan,11-12; 2012,Jan,15-42; 2011,Jun,13

▲ **43252** **with optical endomicroscopy**

EXCLUDES Endoscopy of small intestine (44360-44379)
Esophagogastroduodenoscopy, flexible, transoral (43235)
Esophagoscopy, flexible, transnasal (43197-43198)
Optical endomicroscopic image(s), interpretation and report (88375)

Code also contrast agent

🔧 5.09 ⚕ 10.4 **FUD** 000 T G2 💻

AMA: 2016,Jan,13; 2015,Jan,16; 2014,Jan,11; 2013,Dec,3; 2013,Aug,5; 2013,Jan,11-12

▲ **43253** **with transendoscopic ultrasound-guided transmural injection of diagnostic or therapeutic substance(s) (eg, anesthetic, neurolytic agent) or fiducial marker(s) (includes endoscopic ultrasound examination of the esophagus, stomach, and either the duodenum or a surgically altered stomach where the jejunum is examined distal to the anastomosis)**

INCLUDES Gastrointestinal endoscopic ultrasound, supervision and interpretation (76975)
Ultrasonic guidance (76942)

EXCLUDES Endoscopy of small intestine (44360-44379)
Esophagogastroduodenoscopy, flexible, transoral (43235, 43237, 43259)
Esophagogastroduodenoscopy, flexible, transoral; with transmural drainage of pseudocyst on the same lesion with (43240)
Esophagoscopy, flexible, transnasal (43197-43198)
Procedure performed more than one time per operative session
Transmural fine needle biopsy/aspiration with ultrasound guidance, transendoscopic, esophagus/stomach/duodenum/neighboring structures (43238, 43242)

🔧 7.87 ⚕ 7.87 **FUD** 000 T G2 💻

AMA: 2016,Jan,13; 2015,Jan,16; 2014,Jan,11; 2013,Dec,3

▲ **43254** **with endoscopic mucosal resection**

EXCLUDES Endoscopy of small intestine (44360-44379)
Esophagogastroduodenoscopy, flexible, transoral; diagnostic (43235)
Esophagogastroduodenoscopy, flexible, transoral on the same lesion (43236, 43239, 43251)
Esophagoscopy, flexible, transnasal (43197-43198)

🔧 8.11 ⚕ 8.11 **FUD** 000 T G2 💻

AMA: 2016,Jan,13; 2015,Jan,16; 2014,Jan,11; 2013,Dec,3

▲ **43255** **with control of bleeding, any method**

EXCLUDES Endoscopy of small intestine (44360-44379)
Esophagogastroduodenoscopy, flexible, transoral (43235)
Esophagogastroduodenoscopy, flexible, transoral on the same lesion (43236, 43243-43244)
Esophagoscopy, flexible, transnasal (43197-43198)

🔧 6.05 ⚕ 20.7 **FUD** 000 T A2 💻

AMA: 2016,Jan,13; 2015,Jan,16; 2014,Jan,11; 2013,Dec,3; 2013,Jan,11-12

▲ # **43266** **with placement of endoscopic stent (includes pre- and post-dilation and guide wire passage, when performed)**

EXCLUDES Endoscopy of small intestine (44360-44379)
Esophagogastroduodenoscopy, flexible, transoral (43235, 43240-43241, 43245, 43248-43249)
Esophagoscopy, flexible, transnasal (43197-43198)

🔧 (74360)

🔧 6.80 ⚕ 6.80 **FUD** 000 J G2 💻

AMA: 2016,Jan,13; 2015,Jan,16; 2014,Jan,11; 2013,Dec,3

▲ **43257** **with delivery of thermal energy to the muscle of lower esophageal sphincter and/or gastric cardia, for treatment of gastroesophageal reflux disease**

EXCLUDES Endoscopy small intestine (44360-44379)
Esophageal lesion ablation (43229, [43270])
Esophagogastroduodenoscopy, flexible, transoral; diagnostic (43235)
Esophagoscopy, flexible, transnasal (43197-43198)

🔧 7.00 ⚕ 7.00 **FUD** 000 T A2 💻

AMA: 2016,Jan,13; 2015,Jan,16; 2014,Jan,11; 2013,Dec,3; 2013,Jan,11-12

▲ # **43270** **with ablation of tumor(s), polyp(s), or other lesion(s) (includes pre- and post-dilation and guide wire passage, when performed)**

EXCLUDES Endoscopy of small intestine (44360-44379)
Esophagogastroduodenoscopy, flexible, transoral (43235, 43248-43249)
Esophagoscopy, flexible, transnasal (43197-43198)

Code also esophagoscopic photodynamic therapy, when performed (96570-96571)

🔧 6.99 ⚕ 21.3 **FUD** 000 T G2 💻

AMA: 2016,Jan,13; 2015,Jan,16; 2014,Jan,11; 2013,Dec,3

▲ **43259** **with endoscopic ultrasound examination, including the esophagus, stomach, and either the duodenum or a surgically altered stomach where the jejunum is examined distal to the anastomosis**

INCLUDES Gastrointestinal endoscopic ultrasound, supervision and interpretation (76975)

EXCLUDES Endoscopy of small intestine (44360-44379)
Esophagogastroduodenoscopy, flexible, transoral (43235, 43237, 43240, 43242, 43253)
Esophagoscopy, flexible, transnasal (43197-43198)
Procedure performed more than one time per operative session

🔧 6.80 ⚕ 6.80 **FUD** 000 T A2 💻

AMA: 2016,Jan,11; 2016,Jan,13; 2015,Jan,16; 2014,Jan,11; 2013,Dec,3; 2013,Jan,11-12

43210 **with esophagogastric fundoplasty, partial or complete, includes duodenoscopy when performed**

EXCLUDES Esophagogastroduodenoscopy, flexible, transoral (43235)
Esophagoscopy, flexible, transnasal or transoral; diagnostic (43197, 43200)
Esophagoscopy, rigid, transoral (43180, 43191)

🔧 12.4 ⚕ 12.4 **FUD** 000 J G2 💻

AMA: 2016,Jan,13; 2015,Nov,8

● New Code ▲ Revised Code ○ Reinstated ● New Web Release ▲ Revised Web Release Unlisted Not Covered # Resequenced
⊘ AMA Mod 51 Exempt ⑤ Optum Mod 51 Exempt ⑥ Mod 63 Exempt ✔ Non-FDA Drug ★ Telehealth Ⓜ Maternity Ⓐ Age Edit ✚ Add-on AMA: CPT Asst

CPT © 2016 American Medical Association. All Rights Reserved.

Digestive System

43260 — 43275

43260-43278 [43274, 43275, 43276, 43277, 43278]
Endoscopic Procedures: ERCP

INCLUDES Diagnostic endoscopy with surgical endoscopy
Pancreaticobiliary system:
Biliary tree (right and left hepatic ducts, cystic duct/gallbladder, and common bile ducts)
Pancreas (major and minor ducts)

EXCLUDES ERCP via Roux-en-Y anatomy (for instance post-gastric or bariatric bypass or post total gastrectomy) or via gastrostomy (open or laparoscopic) (47999, 48999)
Optical endomicroscopy of biliary tract and pancreas, report one time per session (0397T)
Percutaneous biliary catheter procedures (47490-47544)

Code also appropriate endoscopy of each anatomic site examined
Code also sphincteroplasty or ductal stricture dilation, when performed prior to the debris/stone removal from the duct ([43277])
Code also the appropriate ERCP procedure when performed on altered postoperative anatomy (i.e. Billroth II gastroenterostomy)
📷 (74328-74330)

▲ **43260** **Endoscopic retrograde cholangiopancreatography (ERCP); diagnostic, including collection of specimen(s) by brushing or washing, when performed (separate procedure)**

EXCLUDES Endoscopic retrograde cholangiopancreatography (ERCP) (43261-43270 [43274, 43275, 43276, 43277, 43278])

📷 9.63   ⬚ 9.63   **FUD** 000   T A2 ▣

AMA: 2016,Jan,13; 2015,Dec,3; 2015,Jan,16; 2014,Jan,11; 2013,Dec,3; 2013,Jan,11-12; 2012,Jan,15-42; 2012,Jan,11-12; 2011,Jan,11

▲ **43261** **with biopsy, single or multiple**

EXCLUDES Endoscopic retrograde cholangiopancreatography (ERCP); diagnostic (43260)
Percutaneous endoluminal biopsy of biliary tree (47543)

📷 10.1   ⬚ 10.1   **FUD** 000   T A2 ▣

AMA: 2016,Jan,13; 2015,Dec,3; 2015,Jan,16; 2014,Jan,11; 2013,Dec,3; 2013,Jan,11-12; 2012,Jan,15-42; 2011,Jun,13

▲ **43262** **with sphincterotomy/papillotomy**

EXCLUDES Endoscopic retrograde cholangiopancreatography (ERCP) (43260, [43277])
Endoscopic retrograde cholangiopancreatography (ERCP) with placement or exchange of stent in the same location ([43274])
Endoscopic retrograde cholangiopancreatography (ERCP) with removal foreign body in the same location ([43276])
Esophagogastroduodenoscopy, flexible, transoral with ablation of tumor(s), polyp(s), or other lesion(s) in the same location ([43270])
Percutaneous balloon dilation biliary duct or ampulla (47542)

Code also procedure performed with sphincterotomy (43261, 43263-43265, [43275], [43278])

📷 10.6   ⬚ 10.6   **FUD** 000   T A2 ▣

AMA: 2016,Jan,13; 2015,Dec,3; 2015,Jan,16; 2014,Jan,11; 2013,Dec,3; 2013,Jan,11-12; 2012,Jan,15-42; 2011,Jan,11

Diaphragm
Endoscope entering the sphincter of Oddi
Stomach
Pancreas
Pancreatic duct
Common bile duct
Proximal duodenum
Report 43263 when a pressure measurement is made of the sphincter

An endoscope is fed through the stomach and into the duodenum. Usually a smaller sub-scope is fed up the sphincter of Oddi and into the ducts that drain the pancreas and the gallbladder (common bile).

▲ **43263** **with pressure measurement of sphincter of Oddi**

EXCLUDES Endoscopic retrograde cholangiopancreatography (ERCP); diagnostic (43260)
Procedure performed more than one time per session

📷 10.6   ⬚ 10.6   **FUD** 000   T A2 ▣

AMA: 2016,Jan,13; 2015,Jan,16; 2014,Jan,11; 2013,Dec,3; 2013,Jan,11-12

▲ **43264** **with removal of calculi/debris from biliary/pancreatic duct(s)**

INCLUDES Incidental dilation due to passage of instrument

EXCLUDES Endoscopic retrograde cholangiopancreatography (ERCP) (43260, 43265)
Findings without debris or calculi, even if balloon was used
Percutaneous calculus/debris removal (47544)

Code also sphincteroplasty when dilation is necessary in order to access the area of debris/stones ([43277])

📷 10.8   ⬚ 10.8   **FUD** 000   T A2 ▣

AMA: 2016,Jan,13; 2015,Dec,3; 2015,Jan,16; 2014,Jan,11; 2013,Dec,3; 2013,Jan,11-12; 2012,Jan,15-42; 2011,Jan,11

▲ **43265** **with destruction of calculi, any method (eg, mechanical, electrohydraulic, lithotripsy)**

INCLUDES Incidental dilation due to passage of instrument
Stone removal when in the same ductal system

EXCLUDES Endoscopic retrograde cholangiopancreatography (ERCP) (43260, 43264)
Findings without debris or calculi, even if balloon was used
Percutaneous calculus/debris removal (47544)

Code also sphincteroplasty when dilation is necessary in order to access the area of debris/stones ([43277])

📷 12.8   ⬚ 12.8   **FUD** 000   T A2 ▣

AMA: 2016,Jan,13; 2015,Dec,3; 2015,Jan,16; 2014,Jan,11; 2013,Dec,3; 2013,Jan,11-12

43266 Resequenced code. See code following 43255.

43270 Resequenced code. See code following 43257.

▲ # **43274** **with placement of endoscopic stent into biliary or pancreatic duct, including pre- and post-dilation and guide wire passage, when performed, including sphincterotomy, when performed, each stent**

INCLUDES Balloon dilation when in the same duct
Tube placement for naso-pancreatic or naso-biliary drainage

EXCLUDES Percutaneous placement biliary stent (47538-47540)
Procedures for stent placement or exchange in the same duct (43262, 43270 [43275, 43276, 43277])

Code also for each additional stent placement in different ducts or side by side in same duct in same session/day, using modifier 59 with ([43274])

📷 13.7   ⬚ 13.7   **FUD** 000   J G2 ▣

AMA: 2016,Jan,13; 2015,Jan,16; 2014,Jan,11; 2013,Dec,3

▲ # **43275** **with removal of foreign body(s) or stent(s) from biliary/pancreatic duct(s)**

EXCLUDES Endoscopic retrograde cholangiopancreatography (ERCP) (43260, [43274], [43276])
Pancreatic or biliary duct stent removal without ERCP (43247)
Percutaneous calculus/debris removal (47544)
Procedure performed more than one time per session

📷 11.2   ⬚ 11.2   **FUD** 000   T G2 ▣

AMA: 2016,Jan,13; 2015,Jan,16; 2014,Jan,11; 2013,Dec,3

▲ # 43276 **with removal and exchange of stent(s), biliary or pancreatic duct, including pre- and post-dilation and guide wire passage, when performed, including sphincterotomy, when performed, each stent exchanged**

INCLUDES Balloon dilation when in the same duct
Stent placement or exchange of one stent

EXCLUDES Endoscopic retrograde cholangiopancreatography (ERCP) (43260, [43275])
Procedures for stent insertion or exchange of stent in same duct (43262, [43274])

Code also each additional stent exchanged in same session/day, using modifier 59 with ([43276])

📷 14.3   ⚕ 14.3   **FUD** 000   J 62 ▣

AMA: 2016,Jan,13; 2015,Jan,16; 2014,Jan,11; 2013,Dec,3

▲ # 43277 **with trans-endoscopic balloon dilation of biliary/pancreatic duct(s) or of ampulla (sphincteroplasty), including sphincterotomy, when performed, each duct**

EXCLUDES Endoscopic retrograde cholangiopancreatography (ERCP) (43260, 43262, [43274], [43276])
Endoscopic retrograde cholangiopancreatography (ERCP); with ablation of tumor(s), polyp(s), or other lesion(s) for the same lesion ([43278])
Percutaneous dilation biliary duct/ampulla (47542)
Removal of stone/debris, dilation incidental to instrument passage (43264-43265)

Code also both right and left hepatic duct (bilateral) balloon dilation, using ([43277]) and append modifier 59 to second procedure

Code also each additional balloon dilation in different ducts or side by side in same duct in same session/day, using modifier 59 with ([43277])

Code also same session sphincterotomy without sphincteroplasty in different duct, using modifier 59 with (43262)

📷 11.2   ⚕ 11.2   **FUD** 000   T 62 ▣

AMA: 2016,Jan,13; 2015,Dec,3; 2015,Jan,16; 2014,Jan,11; 2013,Dec,3

▲ # 43278 **with ablation of tumor(s), polyp(s), or other lesion(s), including pre- and post-dilation and guide wire passage, when performed**

EXCLUDES Ampullectomy (43254)
Endoscopic retrograde cholangiopancreatography (ERCP); diagnostic (43260)
Endoscopic retrograde cholangiopancreatography (ERCP); with trans-endoscopic balloon dilation of biliary/pancreatic duct(s) or of ampulla (sphincteroplasty) on the same lesion with ([43277])

📷 12.8   ⚕ 12.8   **FUD** 000   T 62 ▣

AMA: 2016,Jan,13; 2015,Jan,16; 2014,Jan,11; 2013,Dec,3

▲ + 43273 **Endoscopic cannulation of papilla with direct visualization of pancreatic/common bile duct(s) (List separately in addition to code(s) for primary procedure)**

EXCLUDES Procedure performed more than one time per session

Code first (43260-43270 [43274, 43275, 43276, 43277, 43278])

📷 3.51   ⚕ 3.51   **FUD** ZZZ   N N1 80 ▣

AMA: 2016,Jan,13; 2015,Jan,16; 2014,Jan,11; 2013,Dec,3; 2013,Jan,11-12; 2012,Jan,15-42; 2011,Jan,11

43274   Resequenced code. See code following 43265.

43275   Resequenced code. See code following 43265.

43276   Resequenced code. See code following 43265.

43277   Resequenced code. See code before 43273.

43278   Resequenced code. See code before 43273.

43279-43289 Laparoscopic Procedures of Esophagus

INCLUDES Diagnostic laparoscopy with surgical laparoscopy (49320)

43279 **Laparoscopy, surgical, esophagomyotomy (Heller type), with fundoplasty, when performed**

EXCLUDES Esophagomyotomy, open method (43330-43331)
Laparoscopy, surgical, esophagogastric fundoplasty (43280)

📷 37.5   ⚕ 37.5   **FUD** 090   C 80 ▣

AMA: 2016,Jan,13; 2015,Jan,16; 2014,Jan,11; 2013,Jan,11-12; 2012,Feb,3-7; 2011,Jun,8-10

43280 **Laparoscopy, surgical, esophagogastric fundoplasty (eg, Nissen, Toupet procedures)**

EXCLUDES Esophagogastric fundoplasty, open method (43327-43328)
Esophagogastroduodenoscopy fundoplasty, transoral (43210)
Laparoscopy, surgical, esophageal sphincter augmentation (43284-43285)
Laparoscopy, surgical, esophagomyotomy (43279)

📷 31.4   ⚕ 31.4   **FUD** 090   J 80 ▣

AMA: 2016,Jan,13; 2015,Nov,8; 2015,Jan,16; 2014,Dec,16; 2014,Dec,16; 2014,Jan,11; 2013,Jan,11-12; 2012,Feb,3-7; 2011,Jun,8-10

43281 **Laparoscopy, surgical, repair of paraesophageal hernia, includes fundoplasty, when performed; without implantation of mesh**

EXCLUDES Dilation of esophagus (43450, 43453)
Implantation of mesh or other prosthesis (49568)
Laparoscopy, surgical, esophagogastric fundoplasty (43280)
Transabdominal repair of paraesophageal hiatal hernia (43332-43333)
Transthoracic repair of diaphragmatic hernia (43334-43335)

📷 44.8   ⚕ 44.8   **FUD** 090   J 80 ▣

AMA: 2016,Jan,13; 2015,Jan,16; 2014,Dec,16; 2014,Dec,16; 2014,Jan,11; 2013,Jan,11-12; 2012,Feb,3-7; 2011,Jun,8-10

43282 **with implantation of mesh**

EXCLUDES Dilation of esophagus (43450, 43453)
Implantation of mesh or other prosthesis (49568)
Laparoscopy, surgical, esophagogastric fundoplasty (43280)
Transabdominal paraesophageal hernia repair (43332-43333)
Transthoracic paraesophageal hernia repair (43334-43335)

📷 50.4   ⚕ 50.4   **FUD** 090   C 80 ▣

AMA: 2016,Aug,9; 2016,Jan,13; 2015,Jan,16; 2014,Dec,16; 2014,Dec,16; 2014,Jan,11; 2013,Jan,11-12; 2012,Feb,3-7; 2011,Jun,8-10

+ 43283 **Laparoscopy, surgical, esophageal lengthening procedure (eg, Collis gastroplasty or wedge gastroplasty) (List separately in addition to code for primary procedure)**

Code first (43280-43282)

📷 4.62   ⚕ 4.62   **FUD** ZZZ   C 80 ▣

AMA: 2016,Jan,13; 2015,Jan,16; 2014,Jan,11; 2013,Jan,11-12; 2012,Feb,3-7; 2011,Jun,8-10

● 43284 **Laparoscopy, surgical, esophageal sphincter augmentation procedure, placement of sphincter augmentation device (ie, magnetic band), including cruroplasty when performed**

EXCLUDES Performed during the same session (43279-43282)

● 43285 **Removal of esophageal sphincter augmentation device**

43289 **Unlisted laparoscopy procedure, esophagus**

📷 0.00   ⚕ 0.00   **FUD** YYY   J 80 50

AMA: 2016,Jan,13; 2015,Jan,16; 2014,Dec,16; 2014,Dec,16; 2014,Jan,11; 2013,Jan,11-12

43300-43425 Open Esophageal Repair Procedures

43300 Esophagoplasty (plastic repair or reconstruction), cervical approach; without repair of tracheoesophageal fistula
🔧 17.9 ⚕ 17.9 **FUD** 090 ☐ C 80 ▣
AMA: 2014,Jan,11; 2013,Jan,11-12

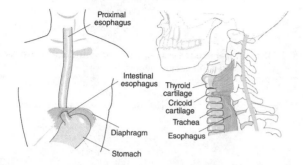

Proximal esophagus
Intestinal esophagus
Thyroid cartilage
Cricoid cartilage
Trachea
Esophagus
Diaphragm
Stomach

43305 with repair of tracheoesophageal fistula
🔧 31.9 ⚕ 31.9 **FUD** 090 ☐ C 80 ▣
AMA: 2014,Jan,11; 2013,Jan,11-12

43310 Esophagoplasty (plastic repair or reconstruction), thoracic approach; without repair of tracheoesophageal fistula
🔧 43.3 ⚕ 43.3 **FUD** 090 ☐ C 80 ▣
AMA: 2014,Jan,11; 2013,Jan,11-12

43312 with repair of tracheoesophageal fistula
🔧 47.0 ⚕ 47.0 **FUD** 090 ☐ C 80 ▣
AMA: 2014,Jan,11; 2013,Jan,11-12

43313 Esophagoplasty for congenital defect (plastic repair or reconstruction), thoracic approach; without repair of congenital tracheoesophageal fistula
🔧 78.6 ⚕ 78.6 **FUD** 090 63 C 80 ▣
AMA: 2014,Jan,11; 2013,Jan,11-12

43314 with repair of congenital tracheoesophageal fistula
🔧 89.8 ⚕ 89.8 **FUD** 090 63 C 80 ▣
AMA: 2014,Jan,11; 2013,Jan,11-12

43320 Esophagogastrostomy (cardioplasty), with or without vagotomy and pyloroplasty, transabdominal or transthoracic approach
EXCLUDES Laparoscopic approach (43280)
🔧 40.4 ⚕ 40.4 **FUD** 090 ☐ C 80 ▣
AMA: 2014,Jan,11; 2013,Jan,11-12

43325 Esophagogastric fundoplasty, with fundic patch (Thal-Nissen procedure)
EXCLUDES Myotomy, cricopharyngeal (43030)
🔧 38.9 ⚕ 38.9 **FUD** 090 ☐ C 80 ▣
AMA: 2014,Jan,11; 2013,Jan,11-12

43327 Esophagogastric fundoplasty partial or complete; laparotomy
🔧 23.8 ⚕ 23.8 **FUD** 090 ☐ C 80 ▣
AMA: 2016,Jan,13; 2015,Nov,8; 2015,Jan,16; 2014,Jan,11; 2013,Jan,11-12; 2012,Feb,3-7; 2011,Jun,8-10

43328 thoracotomy
EXCLUDES Esophagogastroduodenoscopy fundoplasty, transoral (43210)
🔧 33.0 ⚕ 33.0 **FUD** 090 ☐ C 80 ▣
AMA: 2016,Jan,13; 2015,Nov,8; 2015,Jan,16; 2014,Jan,11; 2013,Jan,11-12; 2012,Feb,3-7; 2011,Jun,8-10

43330 Esophagomyotomy (Heller type); abdominal approach
EXCLUDES Esophagomyotomy, laparoscopic method (43279)
🔧 38.5 ⚕ 38.5 **FUD** 090 ☐ C 80 ▣
AMA: 2016,Jan,13; 2015,Jan,16; 2014,Jan,11; 2013,Jan,11-12; 2012,Feb,3-7; 2011,Jun,8-10

43331 thoracic approach
EXCLUDES Thoracoscopy with esophagomyotomy (32665)
🔧 39.1 ⚕ 39.1 **FUD** 090 ☐ C 80 ▣
AMA: 2016,Jan,13; 2015,Jan,16; 2014,Jan,11; 2013,Jan,11-12; 2012,Feb,3-7; 2011,Jun,8-10

43332 Repair, paraesophageal hiatal hernia (including fundoplication), via laparotomy, except neonatal; without implantation of mesh or other prosthesis
EXCLUDES Neonatal diaphragmatic hernia repair (39503)
🔧 33.7 ⚕ 33.7 **FUD** 090 ☐ C 80 ▣
AMA: 2016,Jan,13; 2015,Jan,16; 2014,Jan,11; 2013,Jan,11-12; 2012,Feb,3-7; 2011,Jun,8-10

43333 with implantation of mesh or other prosthesis
EXCLUDES Neonatal diaphragmatic hernia repair (39503)
🔧 36.7 ⚕ 36.7 **FUD** 090 ☐ C 80 ▣
AMA: 2016,Jan,13; 2015,Jan,16; 2014,Jan,11; 2013,Jan,11-12; 2012,Feb,3-7; 2011,Jun,8-10

43334 Repair, paraesophageal hiatal hernia (including fundoplication), via thoracotomy, except neonatal; without implantation of mesh or other prosthesis
EXCLUDES Neonatal diaphragmatic hernia repair (39503)
🔧 36.4 ⚕ 36.4 **FUD** 090 ☐ C 80 ▣
AMA: 2016,Jan,13; 2015,Jan,16; 2014,Jan,11; 2013,Jan,11-12; 2012,Feb,3-7; 2011,Jun,8-10

43335 with implantation of mesh or other prosthesis
EXCLUDES Neonatal diaphragmatic hernia repair (39503)
🔧 39.0 ⚕ 39.0 **FUD** 090 ☐ C 80 ▣
AMA: 2016,Jan,13; 2015,Jan,16; 2014,Jan,11; 2013,Jan,11-12; 2012,Feb,3-7; 2011,Jun,8-10

43336 Repair, paraesophageal hiatal hernia, (including fundoplication), via thoracoabdominal incision, except neonatal; without implantation of mesh or other prosthesis
EXCLUDES Neonatal diaphragmatic hernia repair (39503)
🔧 43.9 ⚕ 43.9 **FUD** 090 ☐ C 80 ▣
AMA: 2016,Jan,13; 2015,Jan,16; 2014,Jan,11; 2013,Jan,11-12; 2012,Feb,3-7; 2011,Jun,8-10

+ 43337 with implantation of mesh or other prosthesis
EXCLUDES Neonatal diaphragmatic hernia repair (39503)
🔧 47.4 ⚕ 47.4 **FUD** 090 ☐ C 80 ▣
AMA: 2016,Jan,13; 2015,Jan,16; 2014,Jan,11; 2013,Jan,11-12; 2012,Feb,3-7; 2011,Jun,8-10

43338 Esophageal lengthening procedure (eg, Collis gastroplasty or wedge gastroplasty) (List separately in addition to code for primary procedure)
Code first (43280, 43327-43337)
🔧 3.39 ⚕ 3.39 **FUD** ZZZ ☐ C 80 ▣
AMA: 2016,Jan,13; 2015,Jan,16; 2014,Jan,11; 2013,Jan,11-12; 2012,Feb,3-7; 2011,Jun,8-10

43340 Esophagojejunostomy (without total gastrectomy); abdominal approach
🔧 39.6 ⚕ 39.6 **FUD** 090 ☐ C 80 ▣
AMA: 2014,Jan,11; 2013,Jan,11-12

43341 thoracic approach
🔧 40.9 ⚕ 40.9 **FUD** 090 ☐ C 80 ▣
AMA: 2014,Jan,11; 2013,Jan,11-12

43351 Esophagostomy, fistulization of esophagus, external; thoracic approach
🔧 37.4 ⚕ 37.4 **FUD** 090 ☐ C 80 ▣
AMA: 2014,Jan,11; 2013,Jan,11-12

43352 cervical approach
🔧 31.1 ⚕ 31.1 **FUD** 090 ☐ C 80 ▣
AMA: 2014,Jan,11; 2013,Jan,11-12

Digestive System

43300 — 43352

43360	Gastrointestinal reconstruction for previous esophagectomy, for obstructing esophageal lesion or fistula, or for previous esophageal exclusion; with stomach, with or without pyloroplasty

🔧 68.8 ⚕ 68.8 **FUD** 090   C 80 ▢

AMA: 2014,Jan,11; 2013,Jan,11-12

43361	with colon interposition or small intestine reconstruction, including intestine mobilization, preparation, and anastomosis(es)

🔧 74.3 ⚕ 74.3 **FUD** 090   C 80 ▢

AMA: 2014,Jan,11; 2013,Jan,11-12

43400	Ligation, direct, esophageal varices

🔧 43.1 ⚕ 43.1 **FUD** 090   C 80 ▢

AMA: 2014,Jan,11; 2013,Jan,11-12

43401	Transection of esophagus with repair, for esophageal varices

🔧 45.2 ⚕ 45.2 **FUD** 090   C 80 ▢

AMA: 2014,Jan,11; 2013,Jan,11-12

43405	Ligation or stapling at gastroesophageal junction for pre-existing esophageal perforation

🔧 42.5 ⚕ 42.5 **FUD** 090   C 80 ▢

AMA: 2014,Jan,11; 2013,Jan,11-12

43410	Suture of esophageal wound or injury; cervical approach

🔧 30.5 ⚕ 30.5 **FUD** 090   C 80 ▢

AMA: 2016,Jan,13; 2015,Jan,16; 2014,Jan,11; 2013,Jan,11-12

43415	transthoracic or transabdominal approach

🔧 74.9 ⚕ 74.9 **FUD** 090   C 80 ▢

AMA: 2014,Jan,11; 2013,Jan,11-12

43420	Closure of esophagostomy or fistula; cervical approach

EXCLUDES   Paraesophageal hiatal hernia repair:
Transabdominal (43332-43333)
Transthoracic (43334-43335)

🔧 29.5 ⚕ 29.5 **FUD** 090   T 80 ▢

AMA: 2014,Jan,11; 2013,Jan,11-12

43425	transthoracic or transabdominal approach

EXCLUDES   Paraesophageal hiatal hernia repair:
Transabdominal (43332-43333)
Transthoracic (43334-43335)

🔧 41.9 ⚕ 41.9 **FUD** 090   C 80 ▢

AMA: 2014,Jan,11; 2013,Jan,11-12

43450-43453 Esophageal Dilation

43450	Dilation of esophagus, by unguided sound or bougie, single or multiple passes

✂ (74220, 74360)

🔧 2.48 ⚕ 6.01 **FUD** 000   T A2 ▢

AMA: 2016,Jan,13; 2015,Jan,16; 2014,Jan,11; 2013,Dec,3; 2013,Jan,11-12; 2012,Jan,15-42; 2011,Jan,11

▲ | 43453 | Dilation of esophagus, over guide wire |
|---|---|

EXCLUDES   Dilation performed with direct visualization (43195, 43226)
Endoscopic dilation by dilator or balloon:
Balloon diameter 30 mm or larger (43214, 43233)
Balloon diameter less than 30 mm (43195, 43220, 43249)

✂ (74220, 74360)

🔧 2.67 ⚕ 27.4 **FUD** 000   T A2 ▢

AMA: 2016,Jan,13; 2015,Jan,16; 2014,Jan,11; 2013,Dec,3; 2013,Jan,11-12; 2012,Jan,15-42; 2011,Jan,11

43460-43499 Other/Unlisted Esophageal Procedures

43460	Esophagogastric tamponade, with balloon (Sengstaken type)

EXCLUDES   Removal of foreign body of the esophagus with balloon catheter (43499, 74235)

✂ (74220)

🔧 6.25 ⚕ 6.25 **FUD** 000   C ▢

AMA: 2014,Jan,11; 2013,Jan,11-12

In 43460, laryngoscope guides tube through vocal cords

Endotracheal tube — Inflated cuff — Esophageal balloon — Esophagus — Gastric aspiration tube — Tube to gastric balloon — Tube to esophageal balloon — Diaphragm — Fundus of stomach — Inferior esophageal sphincter — Gastric balloon and aspiration tube — Cutaway view of Sengstaken-type esophagogastric tamponade with balloons inflated

Side view schematic (above) of inflated endotracheal cuff generally used to provide air passage and prevent tracheal collapse

43496	Free jejunum transfer with microvascular anastomosis

INCLUDES   Operating microscope (69990)

🔧 0.00 ⚕ 0.00 **FUD** 090   C 80 ▢

AMA: 2016,Feb,12; 2016,Jan,13; 2015,Jan,16; 2014,Jan,11; 2013,Jan,11-12

43499	Unlisted procedure, esophagus

🔧 0.00 ⚕ 0.00 **FUD** YYY   T

AMA: 2016,Jan,13; 2015,Nov,10; 2015,Nov,8; 2015,Jan,16; 2014,Jan,11; 2013,Dec,3; 2013,Mar,13; 2013,Jan,11-12; 2012,Jan,15-42; 2011,Dec,19; 2011,May,9; 2011,Jan,11

43500-43641 Open Gastric Incisional and Resection Procedures

43500	Gastrotomy; with exploration or foreign body removal

🔧 22.7 ⚕ 22.7 **FUD** 090   C 80 ▢

AMA: 2014,Jan,11; 2013,Jan,11-12

Esophagus — Mucosal and muscle layers — Rugae (folds lining the stomach) — Pyloric sphincter — Duodenum — Inner stomach — Fundus — Esophagus — Cardiac notch — Diaphragm

43501	with suture repair of bleeding ulcer

🔧 39.0 ⚕ 39.0 **FUD** 090   C 80 ▢

AMA: 2014,Jan,11; 2013,Jan,11-12

43502	with suture repair of pre-existing esophagogastric laceration (eg, Mallory-Weiss)

🔧 44.1 ⚕ 44.1 **FUD** 090   C 80 ▢

AMA: 2014,Jan,11; 2013,Jan,11-12

43510	with esophageal dilation and insertion of permanent intraluminal tube (eg, Celestin or Mousseaux-Barbin)

🔧 27.3 ⚕ 27.3 **FUD** 090   T 80 ▢

AMA: 2014,Jan,11; 2013,Jan,11-12

43520	Pyloromyotomy, cutting of pyloric muscle (Fredet-Ramstedt type operation)

🔧 19.9 ⚕ 19.9 **FUD** 090   63 C 80 ▢

AMA: 2014,Jan,11; 2013,Jan,11-12

43605 **Biopsy of stomach, by laparotomy**
🚑 24.2   ⚖ 24.2   **FUD** 090   C 80 ▣
AMA: 2014,Jan,11; 2013,Jan,11-12

43610 **Excision, local; ulcer or benign tumor of stomach**
🚑 28.4   ⚖ 28.4   **FUD** 090   C 80 ▣
AMA: 2014,Jan,11; 2013,Jan,11-12

43611 **malignant tumor of stomach**
🚑 35.4   ⚖ 35.4   **FUD** 090   C 80 ▣
AMA: 2014,Jan,11; 2013,Jan,11-12

43620 **Gastrectomy, total; with esophagoenterostomy**
🚑 56.7   ⚖ 56.7   **FUD** 090   C 80 ▣
AMA: 2014,Jan,11; 2013,Jan,11-12

43621 **with Roux-en-Y reconstruction**
🚑 65.9   ⚖ 65.9   **FUD** 090   C 80 ▣
AMA: 2014,Jan,11; 2013,Jan,11-12

43622 **with formation of intestinal pouch, any type**
🚑 67.2   ⚖ 67.2   **FUD** 090   C 80 ▣
AMA: 2014,Jan,11; 2013,Jan,11-12

43631 **Gastrectomy, partial, distal; with gastroduodenostomy**
INCLUDES   Billroth operation
🚑 42.0   ⚖ 42.0   **FUD** 090   C 80 ▣
AMA: 2014,Jan,11; 2013,Jan,11-12

43632 **with gastrojejunostomy**
INCLUDES   Polya anastomosis
🚑 59.0   ⚖ 59.0   **FUD** 090   C 80 ▣
AMA: 2014,Jan,11; 2013,Jan,11-12

43633 **with Roux-en-Y reconstruction**
🚑 55.7   ⚖ 55.7   **FUD** 090   C 80 ▣
AMA: 2014,Jan,11; 2013,Jan,11-12

43634 **with formation of intestinal pouch**
🚑 61.4   ⚖ 61.4   **FUD** 090   C 80 ▣
AMA: 2014,Jan,11; 2013,Jan,11-12

+ 43635 **Vagotomy when performed with partial distal gastrectomy (List separately in addition to code[s] for primary procedure)**
Code first as appropriate (43631-43634)
🚑 3.27   ⚖ 3.27   **FUD** ZZZ   C 80 ▣
AMA: 2014,Jan,11; 2013,Jan,11-12

43640 **Vagotomy including pyloroplasty, with or without gastrostomy; truncal or selective**
EXCLUDES   Pyloroplasty (43800)
            Vagotomy (64755, 64760)
🚑 34.2   ⚖ 34.2   **FUD** 090   C 80 ▣
AMA: 2014,Jan,11; 2013,Jan,11-12

43641 **parietal cell (highly selective)**
EXCLUDES   Upper gastrointestinal endoscopy (43235-43259 [43233, 43266, 43270])
🚑 34.4   ⚖ 34.4   **FUD** 090   C 80 ▣
AMA: 2014,Jan,11; 2013,Jan,11-12

43644-43645 Laparoscopic Gastric Bypass with Small Bowel Resection

CMS: 100-03,100.1 Bariatric Surgery for Treatment Co-morbid Conditions Due to Morbid Obesity; 100-04,32,150.1 Bariatric Surgery: Treatment of Co-Morbid Conditions Due to Morbid Obesity; 100-04,32,150.2 HCPCS Procedure Codes for Bariatric Surgery; 100-04,32,150.5 ICD Diagnosis Codes for BMI ≥35; 100-04,32,150.6 Bariatric Surgery Claims Guidance

INCLUDES   Diagnostic laparoscopy (49320)
EXCLUDES   Endoscopy, upper gastrointestinal, (esophagus/stomach/duodenum/jejunum) (43235-43259 [43233, 43266, 43270])

43644 **Laparoscopy, surgical, gastric restrictive procedure; with gastric bypass and Roux-en-Y gastroenterostomy (roux limb 150 cm or less)**
EXCLUDES   Roux limb less than 150 cm (43846)
            Roux limb greater than 150 cm (43645)
🚑 50.3   ⚖ 50.3   **FUD** 090   C 80 ▣
AMA: 2014,Jan,11; 2013,Jan,11-12

43645 **with gastric bypass and small intestine reconstruction to limit absorption**
EXCLUDES   Roux limb less than 150 cm (43847)
🚑 53.7   ⚖ 53.7   **FUD** 090   C 80 ▣
AMA: 2016,Jan,13; 2015,Jan,16; 2014,Jan,11; 2013,Jan,11-12

43647-43659 Other and Unlisted Laparoscopic Gastric Procedures

INCLUDES   Diagnostic laparoscopy (49320)
EXCLUDES   Endoscopy, upper gastrointestinal, (esophagus/stomach/duodenum/jejunum) (43235-43259 [43233, 43266, 43270])

43647 **Laparoscopy, surgical; implantation or replacement of gastric neurostimulator electrodes, antrum**
EXCLUDES   Electronic analysis/programming gastric neurostimulator (95980-95982)
            Insertion gastric neurostimulator pulse generator (64590)
            Laparoscopy with implantation, removal, or revision of gastric neurostimulator electrodes on the lesser curvature of the stomach (43659)
            Open method (43881)
            Vagus nerve blocking pulse generator and/or neurostimulator electrode array implantation, reprogramming, replacement, revision, or removal at the esophagogastric junction performed laparoscopically (0312T-0317T)
🚑 0.00   ⚖ 0.00   **FUD** YYY   J 80 ▣
AMA: 2016,Jan,13; 2015,Jan,16; 2014,Jan,11; 2013,Jan,11-12; 2012,Jan,15-42; 2011,Jan,11

43648 **revision or removal of gastric neurostimulator electrodes, antrum**
EXCLUDES   Electronic analysis/programming gastric neurostimulator (95980-95982)
            Laparoscopy with implantation, removal, or revision of gastric neurostimulator electrodes on the lesser curvature of the stomach (43659)
            Open method (43882)
            Revision/removal gastric neurostimulator pulse generator (64595)
            Vagus nerve blocking pulse generator and/or neurostimulator electrode array implantation, reprogramming, replacement, revision, or removal at the esophagogastric junction performed laparoscopically (0312T-0317T)
🚑 0.00   ⚖ 0.00   **FUD** YYY   J 80 ▣
AMA: 2016,Jan,13; 2015,Jan,16; 2014,Jan,11; 2013,Jan,11-12

43651 **Laparoscopy, surgical; transection of vagus nerves, truncal**
🚑 18.9   ⚖ 18.9   **FUD** 090   J 80 ▣
AMA: 2016,Jan,13; 2015,Jan,16; 2014,Jan,11; 2013,Jan,11-12

43652 **transection of vagus nerves, selective or highly selective**
🚑 22.2   ⚖ 22.2   **FUD** 090   J 80 ▣
AMA: 2016,Jan,13; 2015,Jan,16; 2014,Jan,11; 2013,Jan,11-12

43653 **gastrostomy, without construction of gastric tube (eg, Stamm procedure) (separate procedure)**
🚑 16.5   ⚖ 16.5   **FUD** 090   J A2 80 ▣
AMA: 2016,Jan,13; 2015,Jan,16; 2014,Jan,11; 2013,Jan,11-12

43659 **Unlisted laparoscopy procedure, stomach**
🚑 0.00   ⚖ 0.00   **FUD** YYY   J 80 50
AMA: 2016,Jan,13; 2015,Jan,16; 2014,Jan,11; 2013,Jun,13; 2013,Feb,13; 2013,Jan,11-12; 2012,Jan,15-42; 2011,Dec,19; 2011,Jun,8-10; 2011,Jan,11

43752-43761 Nonsurgical Gastric Tube Procedures

43752 Naso- or oro-gastric tube placement, requiring physician's skill and fluoroscopic guidance (includes fluoroscopy, image documentation and report)

EXCLUDES *Critical care services (99291-99292)*

Initial inpatient neonatal/pediatric critical care, per day (99468-99469, 99471-99472)

Percutaneous insertion of gastrostomy tube (43246, 49440)

Placement of enteric tube (44500, 74340)

Subsequent intensive care, per day, for low birth weight infant (99478-99479)

1.18　　1.18　**FUD** 000　　　03 G2

AMA: 2016,Jan,13; 2015,Jan,16; 2014,May,4; 2014,Jan,11; 2013,Jan,11-12; 2012,Jan,15-42; 2011,Sep,3-4; 2011,Jan,11

43753 Gastric intubation and aspiration(s) therapeutic, necessitating physician's skill (eg, for gastrointestinal hemorrhage), including lavage if performed

0.63　　0.63　**FUD** 000　　　Q1 N1 80

AMA: 2016,Jan,13; 2015,Jan,16; 2014,May,4; 2014,Jan,11; 2013,Jan,11-12; 2011,Sep,3-4

43754 Gastric intubation and aspiration, diagnostic; single specimen (eg, acid analysis)

EXCLUDES *Analysis of gastic acid (82930)*

Naso- or oro-gastric tube placement using fluoroscopic guidance (43752)

0.95　　3.02　**FUD** 000　　　Q1 N1 80

AMA: 2016,Jan,13; 2015,Jan,16; 2014,Jan,11; 2013,Jan,11-12; 2011,Sep,3-4

43755 collection of multiple fractional specimens with gastric stimulation, single or double lumen tube (gastric secretory study) (eg, histamine, insulin, pentagastrin, calcium, secretin), includes drug administration

EXCLUDES *Analysis of gastic acid (82930)*

Naso- or oro-gastric tube placement using fluoroscopic guidance (43752)

Code also drugs or substances administered

1.78　　4.00　**FUD** 000　　　S G2 80

AMA: 2016,Jan,13; 2015,Jan,16; 2014,Jan,11; 2013,Jan,11-12; 2011,Sep,3-4

43756 Duodenal intubation and aspiration, diagnostic, includes image guidance; single specimen (eg, bile study for crystals or afferent loop culture)

Code also drugs or substances administered

(89049-89240)

1.48　　5.84　**FUD** 000　　　Q1 G2 80

AMA: 2016,Jan,13; 2015,Jan,16; 2014,Jan,11; 2013,Jan,11-12; 2011,Sep,3-4

43757 collection of multiple fractional specimens with pancreatic or gallbladder stimulation, single or double lumen tube, includes drug administration

Code also drugs or substances administered

(89049-89240)

2.25　　8.25　**FUD** 000　　　T G2 80

AMA: 2016,Jan,13; 2015,Jan,16; 2014,Jan,11; 2013,Jan,11-12; 2011,Sep,3-4

43760 Change of gastrostomy tube, percutaneous, without imaging or endoscopic guidance

EXCLUDES *Endoscopic placement of gastrostomy tube (43246)*

Gastrostomy tube replacement using fluoroscopy (49450)

1.36　　13.8　**FUD** 000　　　T A2

AMA: 2016,Jan,13; 2015,Jan,16; 2014,Jan,11; 2013,Jan,11-12; 2012,Jan,15-42; 2011,Jan,11

43761 Repositioning of a naso- or oro-gastric feeding tube, through the duodenum for enteric nutrition

EXCLUDES *Conversion of gastrostomy tube to gastro-jejunostomy tube, percutaneous (49446)*

Gastrostomy tube converted endoscopically to jejunostomy tube (44373)

Introduction of long gastrointestinal tube into the duodenum (44500)

(76000)

2.97　　3.35　**FUD** 000　　　T A2

AMA: 2016,Jan,13; 2015,Jan,16; 2014,Jan,11; 2013,Jan,11-12

43770-43775 Laparoscopic Bariatric Procedures

CMS: 100-03,100.1 Bariatric Surgery for Treatment Co-morbid Conditions Due to Morbid Obesity; 100-04,32,150.1 Bariatric Surgery: Treatment of Co-Morbid Conditions Due to Morbid Obesity; 100-04,32,150.2 HCPCS Procedure Codes for Bariatric Surgery; 100-04,32,150.5 ICD Diagnosis Codes for BMI ≥35; 100-04,32,150.6 Bariatric Surgery Claims Guidance

INCLUDES Diagnostic laparoscopy (49320)

Stomach/duodenum/jejunum/ileum

Subsequent band adjustments (change of the gastric band component diameter by injection/aspiration of fluid through the subcutaneous port component) during the postoperative period

43770 Laparoscopy, surgical, gastric restrictive procedure; placement of adjustable gastric restrictive device (eg, gastric band and subcutaneous port components)

Code also modifier 52 for placement of individual component

32.4　　32.4　**FUD** 090　　　J 80

AMA: 2016,Jan,13; 2015,Jan,16; 2014,Jan,11; 2013,Jan,11-12; 2012,Jan,15-42; 2011,Jan,11

43771 revision of adjustable gastric restrictive device component only

36.9　　36.9　**FUD** 090　　　C 80

AMA: 2016,Jan,13; 2015,Jan,16; 2014,Jan,11; 2013,Jan,11-12

43772 removal of adjustable gastric restrictive device component only

27.5　　27.5　**FUD** 090　　　C 80

AMA: 2016,Jan,13; 2015,Jan,16; 2014,Jan,11; 2013,Jan,11-12

43773 removal and replacement of adjustable gastric restrictive device component only

EXCLUDES *Laparoscopy, surgical, gastric restrictive procedure; removal of adjustable gastric restrictive device component only (43772)*

36.8　　36.8　**FUD** 090　　　C 80

AMA: 2016,Jan,13; 2015,Jan,16; 2014,Jan,11; 2013,Jan,11-12

43774 removal of adjustable gastric restrictive device and subcutaneous port components

EXCLUDES *Removal/replacement of subcutaneous port components and gastric band (43659)*

27.8　　27.8　**FUD** 090　　　C 80

AMA: 2016,Jan,13; 2015,Jan,16; 2014,Jan,11; 2013,Jan,11-12; 2012,Jan,15-42; 2011,Jan,11

43775 longitudinal gastrectomy (ie, sleeve gastrectomy)

EXCLUDES *Open gastric restrictive procedure for morbid obesity, without gastric bypass, other than vertical-banded gastroplasty (43843)*

Vagus nerve blocking pulse generator and/or neurostimulator electrode array implantation, reprogramming, replacement, revision, or removal at the esophagogastric junction performed laparoscopically (0312T-0317T)

32.0　　32.0　**FUD** 090　　　C 80

AMA: 2014,Jan,11; 2013,Jan,11-12

43800-43840 Open Gastric Incisional/Repair/Resection Procedures

43800 Pyloroplasty

EXCLUDES *Vagotomy with pyloroplasty (43640)*

26.9　　26.9　**FUD** 090　　　C 80

AMA: 2014,Jan,11; 2013,Jan,11-12

43810 Gastroduodenostomy

29.5　　29.5　**FUD** 090　　　C 80

AMA: 2014,Jan,11; 2013,Jan,11-12

43820 Gastrojejunostomy; without vagotomy
🔪 38.9 ⚕ 38.9 **FUD** 090 C 80 ▣
AMA: 2014,Jan,11; 2013,Jan,11-12

43825 with vagotomy, any type
🔪 37.8 ⚕ 37.8 **FUD** 090 C 80 ▣
AMA: 2014,Jan,11; 2013,Jan,11-12

43830 Gastrostomy, open; without construction of gastric tube (eg, Stamm procedure) (separate procedure)
🔪 20.2 ⚕ 20.2 **FUD** 090 T 80 ▣
AMA: 2016,Jan,13; 2015,Jan,16; 2014,Jan,11; 2013,Jan,11-12

43831 neonatal, for feeding A
EXCLUDES Change of gastrostomy tube (43760)
🔪 16.8 ⚕ 16.8 **FUD** 090 63 T 80 ▣
AMA: 2016,Jan,13; 2015,Jan,16; 2014,Jan,11; 2013,Jan,11-12

43832 with construction of gastric tube (eg, Janeway procedure)
EXCLUDES Endoscopic placement of percutaneous gastrostomy tube (43246)
🔪 30.1 ⚕ 30.1 **FUD** 090 C 80 ▣
AMA: 2016,Jan,13; 2015,Jan,16; 2014,Jan,11; 2013,Jan,11-12

43840 Gastrorrhaphy, suture of perforated duodenal or gastric ulcer, wound, or injury
🔪 39.4 ⚕ 39.4 **FUD** 090 C 80 ▣
AMA: 2014,Jan,11; 2013,Jan,11-12

43842-43848 Open Bariatric Procedures for Morbid Obesity

CMS: 100-03,100.1 Bariatric Surgery for Treatment Co-morbid Conditions Due to Morbid Obesity; 100-04,32,150.1 Bariatric Surgery: Treatment of Co-Morbid Conditions Due to Morbid Obesity; 100-04,32,150.2 HCPCS Procedure Codes for Bariatric Surgery; 100-04,32,150.5 ICD Diagnosis Codes for BMI ≥35; 100-04,32,150.6 Bariatric Surgery Claims Guidance

43842 Gastric restrictive procedure, without gastric bypass, for morbid obesity; vertical-banded gastroplasty
🔪 34.4 ⚕ 34.4 **FUD** 090 E ▣
AMA: 2016,Jan,13; 2015,Jan,16; 2014,Jan,11; 2013,Jan,11-12

43843 other than vertical-banded gastroplasty
EXCLUDES Laparoscopic longitudinal gastrectomy (e.g., sleeve gastrectomy) (43775)
🔪 37.0 ⚕ 37.0 **FUD** 090 C 80 ▣
AMA: 2016,Jan,13; 2015,Jan,16; 2014,Jan,11; 2013,Jan,11-12

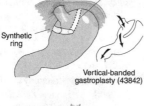

Surgical staples partition off a portion of stomach
Synthetic ring
Vertical-banded gastroplasty (43842)

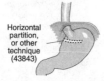

Horizontal partition, or other technique (43843)

The stomach is surgically restricted to treat morbid obesity. A vertical-banded technique is coded 43842 and any other gastroplasty technique that does not employ gastric bypass is coded 43843. These partitioning techniques give the patient a sensation of fullness, thus decreasing daily caloric intake

43845 Gastric restrictive procedure with partial gastrectomy, pylorus-preserving duodenoileostomy and ileoileostomy (50 to 100 cm common channel) to limit absorption (biliopancreatic diversion with duodenal switch)
EXCLUDES Enteroenterostomy, anastomosis of intestine (44130)
Exploratory laparotomy, exploratory celiotomy (49000)
Gastrectomy, partial, distal; with Roux-en-Y reconstruction (43633)
Gastric restrictive procedure, with gastric bypass for morbid obesity; with small intestine reconstruction (43847)
🔪 57.0 ⚕ 57.0 **FUD** 090 C 80 ▣
AMA: 2016,Jan,13; 2015,Jan,16; 2014,Jan,11; 2013,Jan,11-12

43846 Gastric restrictive procedure, with gastric bypass for morbid obesity; with short limb (150 cm or less) Roux-en-Y gastroenterostomy
EXCLUDES Performed laparoscopically (43644)
Roux limb more than 150 cm (43847)
🔪 46.8 ⚕ 46.8 **FUD** 090 C 80 ▣
AMA: 2016,Jan,13; 2015,Jan,16; 2014,Jan,11; 2013,Jan,11-12

43847 with small intestine reconstruction to limit absorption
EXCLUDES Performed laparoscopically (43645)
🔪 51.5 ⚕ 51.5 **FUD** 090 C 80 ▣
AMA: 2016,Jan,13; 2015,Jan,16; 2014,Jan,11; 2013,Jan,11-12

43848 Revision, open, of gastric restrictive procedure for morbid obesity, other than adjustable gastric restrictive device (separate procedure)
EXCLUDES Gastric restrictive port procedures (43886-43888)
Procedures for adjustable gastric restrictive devices (43770-43774)
🔪 55.8 ⚕ 55.8 **FUD** 090 C 80 ▣
AMA: 2016,Jan,13; 2015,Jan,16; 2014,Jan,11; 2013,Jan,11-12

43850-43882 Open Gastric Procedures: Closure/Implantation/Replacement/Revision

43850 Revision of gastroduodenal anastomosis (gastroduodenostomy) with reconstruction; without vagotomy
🔪 47.0 ⚕ 47.0 **FUD** 090 C 80 ▣
AMA: 2014,Jan,11; 2013,Jan,11-12

43855 with vagotomy
🔪 47.7 ⚕ 47.7 **FUD** 090 C 80 ▣
AMA: 2014,Jan,11; 2013,Jan,11-12

43860 Revision of gastrojejunal anastomosis (gastrojejunostomy) with reconstruction, with or without partial gastrectomy or intestine resection; without vagotomy
🔪 47.4 ⚕ 47.4 **FUD** 090 C 80 ▣
AMA: 2014,Jan,11; 2013,Jan,11-12

43865 with vagotomy
🔪 49.4 ⚕ 49.4 **FUD** 090 C 80 ▣
AMA: 2014,Jan,11; 2013,Jan,11-12

43870 Closure of gastrostomy, surgical
🔪 20.6 ⚕ 20.6 **FUD** 090 T A2 80 ▣
AMA: 2014,Jan,11; 2013,Jan,11-12

43880 Closure of gastrocolic fistula
🔪 46.3 ⚕ 46.3 **FUD** 090 C 80 ▣
AMA: 2014,Jan,11; 2013,Jan,11-12

43881 Implantation or replacement of gastric neurostimulator electrodes, antrum, open

> EXCLUDES Electronic analysis and programming (95980-95982)
> Implantation/removal/revision gastric neurostimulator electrodes, lesser curvature or vagal trunk (EGJ):
> Laparoscopically (43659)
> Open, lesser curvature (43999)
> Implantation/replacement performed laparoscopically (43647)
> Insertion of gastric neurostimulator pulse generator (64590)
> Vagus nerve blocking pulse generator and/or neurostimulator electrode array implantation, reprogramming, replacement, revision, or removal at the esophagogastric junction performed laparoscopically (0312T-0317T)

🔧 0.00   ⚕ 0.00   **FUD** YYY   C 80 ▭

AMA: 2016,Jan,13; 2015,Jan,16; 2014,Jan,11; 2013,Jan,11-12

43882 Revision or removal of gastric neurostimulator electrodes, antrum, open

> EXCLUDES Electronic analysis and programming (95980-95982)
> Implantation/removal/revision gastric neurostimulator electrodes, lesser curvature or vagal trunk (EGJ):
> Laparoscopic (43659)
> Open, lesser curvature (43999)
> Revision/removal gastric neurostimulator electrodes, antrum, performed laparoscopically (43648)
> Revision/removal gastric neurostimulator pulse generator (64595)
> Vagus nerve blocking pulse generator and/or neurostimulator electrode array implantation, reprogramming, replacement, revision, or removal at the esophagogastric junction performed laparoscopically (0312T-0317T)

🔧 0.00   ⚕ 0.00   **FUD** YYY   C 80 ▭

AMA: 2016,Jan,13; 2015,Jan,16; 2014,Jan,11; 2013,Jan,11-12

43886-43999 Bariatric Procedures: Removal/Replacement/Revision Port Components

CMS: 100-04,32,150.1 Bariatric Surgery: Treatment of Co-Morbid Conditions Due to Morbid Obesity; 100-04,32,150.2 HCPCS Procedure Codes for Bariatric Surgery; 100-04,32,150.5 ICD Diagnosis Codes for BMI ≥35; 100-04,32,150.6 Bariatric Surgery Claims Guidance

43886 Gastric restrictive procedure, open; revision of subcutaneous port component only

🔧 10.4   ⚕ 10.4   **FUD** 090   T 62 80 ▭

AMA: 2016,Jan,13; 2015,Jan,16; 2014,Jan,11; 2013,Jan,11-12

43887 removal of subcutaneous port component only

> EXCLUDES Gastric band and subcutaneous port components:
> Removal and replacement performed laparoscopically (43659)
> Removal performed laparoscopically (43774)

🔧 9.36   ⚕ 9.36   **FUD** 090   02 62 80 ▭

AMA: 2016,Jan,13; 2015,Jan,16; 2014,Jan,11; 2013,Jan,11-12

43888 removal and replacement of subcutaneous port component only

> EXCLUDES Gastric band and subcutaneous port components:
> Removal and replacement performed laparoscopically (43659)
> Removal performed laparoscopically (43774)
> Gastric restrictive procedure, open; removal of subcutaneous port component only (43887)

🔧 13.2   ⚕ 13.2   **FUD** 090   T 62 80 ▭

AMA: 2016,Jan,13; 2015,Jan,16; 2014,Jan,11; 2013,Jan,11-12

43999 Unlisted procedure, stomach

🔧 0.00   ⚕ 0.00   **FUD** YYY   T 80

AMA: 2016,Jan,13; 2015,Jan,16; 2014,Jan,11; 2013,Feb,13; 2013,Jan,11-12; 2012,Jan,15-42; 2011,Jun,13; 2011,Jan,11

44005-44130 Incisional and Resection Procedures of Bowel

44005 Enterolysis (freeing of intestinal adhesion) (separate procedure)

> EXCLUDES Enterolysis performed laparoscopically (44180)
> Excision of ileoanal reservoir with ileostomy (45136)

🔧 31.7   ⚕ 31.7   **FUD** 090   C 80 ▭

AMA: 2016,Jan,13; 2015,Jan,16; 2014,Jan,11; 2013,Jan,11-12; 2012,Jan,15-42; 2011,Jan,11

44010 Duodenotomy, for exploration, biopsy(s), or foreign body removal

🔧 25.0   ⚕ 25.0   **FUD** 090   C 80 ▭

AMA: 2014,Jan,11; 2013,Jan,11-12

+ **44015** Tube or needle catheter jejunostomy for enteral alimentation, intraoperative, any method (List separately in addition to primary procedure)

Code first the primary procedure

🔧 4.14   ⚕ 4.14   **FUD** ZZZ   C 80 ▭

AMA: 2016,Jan,13; 2015,Jan,16; 2014,Jan,11; 2013,Jan,11-12; 2012,Jan,15-42; 2011,Jan,11

44020 Enterotomy, small intestine, other than duodenum; for exploration, biopsy(s), or foreign body removal

🔧 28.2   ⚕ 28.2   **FUD** 090   C 80 ▭

AMA: 2014,Jan,11; 2013,Jan,11-12

44021 for decompression (eg, Baker tube)

🔧 28.2   ⚕ 28.2   **FUD** 090   C 80 ▭

AMA: 2014,Jan,11; 2013,Jan,11-12

Anterior abdominal skin. Baker-type tube. Depicted at left is a tube threaded through intestine for decompression. Peritoneum. Bowel lumen. Note that the bowel is sutured to the abdominal wall

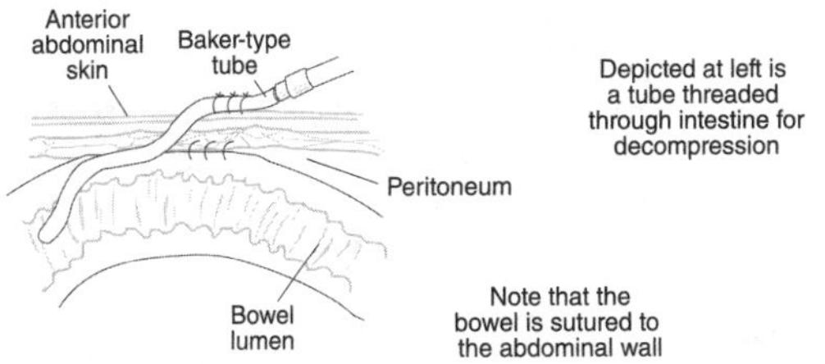

44025 Colotomy, for exploration, biopsy(s), or foreign body removal

> INCLUDES Amussat's operation
> EXCLUDES Intestine exteriorization (Mikulicz resection with crushing of spur) (44602-44605)

🔧 28.5   ⚕ 28.5   **FUD** 090   C 80 ▭

AMA: 2014,Jan,11; 2013,Jan,11-12

44050 Reduction of volvulus, intussusception, internal hernia, by laparotomy

🔧 27.1   ⚕ 27.1   **FUD** 090   C 80 ▭

AMA: 2014,Jan,11; 2013,Jan,11-12

44055 Correction of malrotation by lysis of duodenal bands and/or reduction of midgut volvulus (eg, Ladd procedure)

🔧 43.2   ⚕ 43.2   **FUD** 090   63 C 80 ▭

AMA: 2014,Jan,11; 2013,Jan,11-12

44100 Biopsy of intestine by capsule, tube, peroral (1 or more specimens)

🔧 3.16   ⚕ 3.16   **FUD** 000   T A2 ▭

AMA: 2014,Jan,11; 2013,Jan,11-12

44110 Excision of 1 or more lesions of small or large intestine not requiring anastomosis, exteriorization, or fistulization; single enterotomy

🔧 24.7   ⚕ 24.7   **FUD** 090   C 80 ▭

AMA: 2014,Jan,11; 2013,Jan,11-12

44111 multiple enterotomies

🔧 28.5   ⚕ 28.5   **FUD** 090   C 80 ▭

AMA: 2014,Jan,11; 2013,Jan,11-12

44120 Enterectomy, resection of small intestine; single resection and anastomosis

> EXCLUDES Excision of ileoanal reservoir with ileostomy (45136)

🔧 35.5   ⚕ 35.5   **FUD** 090   C 80 ▭

AMA: 2016,Jan,13; 2015,Jan,16; 2014,Jan,11; 2013,Jan,11-12

● New Code   ▲ Revised Code   ○ Reinstated   ● New Web Release   ▲ Revised Web Release   Unlisted   Not Covered   # Resequenced

⊘ AMA Mod 51 Exempt   ⑤ Optum Mod 51 Exempt   ⑥ Mod 63 Exempt   ✗ Non-FDA Drug   ★ Telehealth   M Maternity   A Age Edit   + Add-on   **AMA:** CPT Asst

© 2016 Optum360, LLC   CPT © 2016 American Medical Association. All Rights Reserved.   **189**

Digestive System

44121 — 44158

+ **44121** **each additional resection and anastomosis (List separately in addition to code for primary procedure)**
Code first (44120)
🔧 7.05   ✂ 7.05   **FUD** ZZZ   C 80 ▭
AMA: 2014,Jan,11; 2013,Jan,11-12

44125 **with enterostomy**
🔧 34.2   ✂ 34.2   **FUD** 090   C 80 ▭
AMA: 2014,Jan,11; 2013,Jan,11-12

44126 **Enterectomy, resection of small intestine for congenital atresia, single resection and anastomosis of proximal segment of intestine; without tapering**
🔧 71.6   ✂ 71.6   **FUD** 090   63 C 80 ▭
AMA: 2014,Jan,11; 2013,Jan,11-12

44127 **with tapering**
🔧 82.2   ✂ 82.2   **FUD** 090   63 C 80 ▭
AMA: 2014,Jan,11; 2013,Jan,11-12

+ **44128** **each additional resection and anastomosis (List separately in addition to code for primary procedure)**
Code first single resection of small intestine (44126, 44127)
🔧 7.12   ✂ 7.12   **FUD** ZZZ   63 C 80 ▭
AMA: 2014,Jan,11; 2013,Jan,11-12

44130 **Enteroenterostomy, anastomosis of intestine, with or without cutaneous enterostomy (separate procedure)**
🔧 38.0   ✂ 38.0   **FUD** 090   C 80 ▭
AMA: 2014,Jan,11; 2013,Jan,11-12

44132-44137 Intestine Transplant Procedures

CMS: 100-03,260.5 Intestinal and Multi-Visceral Transplantation; 100-04,3,90.6 Intestinal and Multi-Visceral Transplants

44132 **Donor enterectomy (including cold preservation), open; from cadaver donor**
INCLUDES   Graft:
Cold preservation
Harvest
EXCLUDES   Preparation/reconstruction of backbench intestinal graft (44715, 44720-44721)
🔧 0.00   ✂ 0.00   **FUD** XXX   C 80 ▭
AMA: 2014,Jan,11; 2013,Jan,11-12

44133 **partial, from living donor**
INCLUDES   Donor care
Graft:
Cold preservation
Harvest
EXCLUDES   Preparation/reconstruction of backbench intestinal graft (44715, 44720-44721)
🔧 0.00   ✂ 0.00   **FUD** XXX   C 80 ▭
AMA: 2014,Jan,11; 2013,Jan,11-12

44135 **Intestinal allotransplantation; from cadaver donor**
INCLUDES   Allograft transplantation
Recipient care
🔧 0.00   ✂ 0.00   **FUD** XXX   C 80 ▭
AMA: 2014,Jan,11; 2013,Jan,11-12

44136 **from living donor**
INCLUDES   Allograft transplantation
Recipient care
🔧 0.00   ✂ 0.00   **FUD** XXX   C 80 ▭
AMA: 2014,Jan,11; 2013,Jan,11-12

44137 **Removal of transplanted intestinal allograft, complete**
EXCLUDES   Partial removal of transplant allograft (44120-44121, 44140)
🔧 0.00   ✂ 0.00   **FUD** XXX   C 80 ▭
AMA: 2014,Jan,11; 2013,Jan,11-12

44139-44160 Colon Resection Procedures

+ **44139** **Mobilization (take-down) of splenic flexure performed in conjunction with partial colectomy (List separately in addition to primary procedure)**
Code first partial colectomy (44140-44147)
🔧 3.53   ✂ 3.53   **FUD** ZZZ   C 80 ▭
AMA: 2014,Jan,11; 2013,Jan,11-12

44140 **Colectomy, partial; with anastomosis**
EXCLUDES   Laparoscopic method (44204)
🔧 38.9   ✂ 38.9   **FUD** 090   C 80 ▭
AMA: 2016,Jan,13; 2015,Jan,16; 2014,Jan,11; 2013,Jan,11-12

44141 **with skin level cecostomy or colostomy**
🔧 52.9   ✂ 52.9   **FUD** 090   C 80 ▭
AMA: 2016,Jan,13; 2015,Jan,16; 2014,Jan,11; 2013,Jan,11-12

44143 **with end colostomy and closure of distal segment (Hartmann type procedure)**
EXCLUDES   Laparoscopic method (44206)
🔧 48.3   ✂ 48.3   **FUD** 090   C 80 ▭
AMA: 2016,Jan,13; 2015,Jan,16; 2014,Jan,11; 2013,Jan,11-12

44144 **with resection, with colostomy or ileostomy and creation of mucofistula**
🔧 51.4   ✂ 51.4   **FUD** 090   C 80 ▭
AMA: 2016,Jan,13; 2015,Jan,16; 2014,Jan,11; 2013,Jan,11-12

44145 **with coloproctostomy (low pelvic anastomosis)**
EXCLUDES   Laparoscopic method (44207)
🔧 48.1   ✂ 48.1   **FUD** 090   C 80 ▭
AMA: 2014,Jan,11; 2013,Jan,11-12

44146 **with coloproctostomy (low pelvic anastomosis), with colostomy**
EXCLUDES   Laparoscopic method (44208)
🔧 61.4   ✂ 61.4   **FUD** 090   C 80 ▭
AMA: 2016,Jan,13; 2015,Jan,16; 2014,Jan,11; 2013,Jan,11-12

44147 **abdominal and transanal approach**
🔧 56.4   ✂ 56.4   **FUD** 090   C 80 ▭
AMA: 2016,Jan,13; 2015,Jan,16; 2014,Jan,11; 2013,Jan,11-12

44150 **Colectomy, total, abdominal, without proctectomy; with ileostomy or ileoproctostomy**
INCLUDES   Lane's operation
EXCLUDES   Laparoscopic method (44210)
🔧 54.2   ✂ 54.2   **FUD** 090   C 80 ▭
AMA: 2014,Jan,11; 2013,Jan,11-12

44151 **with continent ileostomy**
🔧 62.0   ✂ 62.0   **FUD** 090   C 80 ▭
AMA: 2014,Jan,11; 2013,Jan,11-12

44155 **Colectomy, total, abdominal, with proctectomy; with ileostomy**
INCLUDES   Miles' colectomy
EXCLUDES   Laparoscopic method (44212)
🔧 60.4   ✂ 60.4   **FUD** 090   C 80 ▭
AMA: 2014,Jan,11; 2013,Jan,11-12

44156 **with continent ileostomy**
🔧 66.6   ✂ 66.6   **FUD** 090   C 80 ▭
AMA: 2014,Jan,11; 2013,Jan,11-12

44157 **with ileoanal anastomosis, includes loop ileostomy, and rectal mucosectomy, when performed**
🔧 62.4   ✂ 62.4   **FUD** 090   C 80 ▭
AMA: 2014,Jan,11; 2013,Jan,11-12

44158 **with ileoanal anastomosis, creation of ileal reservoir (S or J), includes loop ileostomy, and rectal mucosectomy, when performed**
EXCLUDES   Laparoscopic method (44211)
🔧 61.7   ✂ 61.7   **FUD** 090   C 80 ▭
AMA: 2014,Jan,11; 2013,Jan,11-12

44160 Colectomy, partial, with removal of terminal ileum with ileocolostomy

EXCLUDES *Laparoscopic method (44205)*

36.0 ⚕ 36.0 **FUD** 090 C 80

AMA: 2016,Jan,13; 2015,Jan,16; 2014,Jan,11; 2013,Jan,11-12

44180 Laparoscopic Enterolysis

INCLUDES Diagnostic laparoscopy (49320)

EXCLUDES *Laparoscopic salpingolysis/ovariolysis (58660)*

44180 Laparoscopy, surgical, enterolysis (freeing of intestinal adhesion) (separate procedure)

26.6 ⚕ 26.6 **FUD** 090 J 80

AMA: 2016,Jan,13; 2015,Jan,16; 2014,Jan,11; 2013,Jan,11-12

44186-44238 Laparoscopic Enterostomy Procedures

INCLUDES Diagnostic laparoscopy (49320)

44186 Laparoscopy, surgical; jejunostomy (eg, for decompression or feeding)

18.9 ⚕ 18.9 **FUD** 090 J 80

AMA: 2016,Jan,13; 2015,Jan,16; 2014,Jan,11; 2013,Jan,11-12

44187 ileostomy or jejunostomy, non-tube

EXCLUDES *Open method (44310)*

32.0 ⚕ 32.0 **FUD** 090 C 80

AMA: 2016,Jan,13; 2015,Jan,16; 2014,Jan,11; 2013,Jan,11-12

44188 Laparoscopy, surgical, colostomy or skin level cecostomy

EXCLUDES *Laparoscopy, surgical, appendectomy (44970)*
Open method (44320)

35.5 ⚕ 35.5 **FUD** 090 C 80

AMA: 2016,Jan,13; 2015,Jan,16; 2014,Jan,11; 2013,Jan,11-12; 2012,Jan,15-42; 2011,Jan,11

44202 Laparoscopy, surgical; enterectomy, resection of small intestine, single resection and anastomosis

EXCLUDES *Open method (44120)*

40.2 ⚕ 40.2 **FUD** 090 C 80

AMA: 2016,Jan,13; 2015,Jan,16; 2014,Jan,11; 2013,Jan,11-12

+ 44203 each additional small intestine resection and anastomosis (List separately in addition to code for primary procedure)

EXCLUDES *Open method (44121)*
Code first single resection of small intestine (44202)

7.02 ⚕ 7.02 **FUD** ZZZ C 80

AMA: 2016,Jan,13; 2015,Jan,16; 2014,Jan,11; 2013,Jan,11-12

44204 colectomy, partial, with anastomosis

EXCLUDES *Open method (44140)*

44.6 ⚕ 44.6 **FUD** 090 C 80

AMA: 2016,Jan,13; 2015,Jan,16; 2014,Jan,11; 2013,Jan,11-12; 2012,Jan,15-42; 2011,Jan,11

44205 colectomy, partial, with removal of terminal ileum with ileocolostomy

EXCLUDES *Open method (44160)*

38.8 ⚕ 38.8 **FUD** 090 C 80

AMA: 2016,Jan,13; 2015,Jan,16; 2014,Jan,11; 2013,Jan,11-12

44206 colectomy, partial, with end colostomy and closure of distal segment (Hartmann type procedure)

EXCLUDES *Open method (44143)*

50.9 ⚕ 50.9 **FUD** 090 C 80

AMA: 2016,Jan,13; 2015,Jan,16; 2014,Jan,11; 2013,Jan,11-12

44207 colectomy, partial, with anastomosis, with coloproctostomy (low pelvic anastomosis)

EXCLUDES *Open method (44145)*

52.8 ⚕ 52.8 **FUD** 090 C 80

AMA: 2016,Jan,13; 2015,Jan,16; 2014,Jan,11; 2013,Jan,11-12

44208 colectomy, partial, with anastomosis, with coloproctostomy (low pelvic anastomosis) with colostomy

EXCLUDES *Open method (44146)*

57.6 ⚕ 57.6 **FUD** 090 C 80

AMA: 2016,Jan,13; 2015,Jan,16; 2014,Jan,11; 2013,Jan,11-12

44210 colectomy, total, abdominal, without proctectomy, with ileostomy or ileoproctostomy

EXCLUDES *Open method (44150)*

51.6 ⚕ 51.6 **FUD** 090 C 80

AMA: 2016,Jan,13; 2015,Jan,16; 2014,Jan,11; 2013,Jan,11-12

44211 colectomy, total, abdominal, with proctectomy, with ileoanal anastomosis, creation of ileal reservoir (S or J), with loop ileostomy, includes rectal mucosectomy, when performed

EXCLUDES *Open method (44157-44158)*

63.2 ⚕ 63.2 **FUD** 090 C 80

AMA: 2016,Jan,13; 2015,Jan,16; 2014,Jan,11; 2013,Jan,11-12

44212 colectomy, total, abdominal, with proctectomy, with ileostomy

EXCLUDES *Open method (44155)*

59.3 ⚕ 59.3 **FUD** 090 C 80

AMA: 2016,Jan,13; 2015,Jan,16; 2014,Jan,11; 2013,Jan,11-12

+ 44213 Laparoscopy, surgical, mobilization (take-down) of splenic flexure performed in conjunction with partial colectomy (List separately in addition to primary procedure)

EXCLUDES *Open method (44139)*
Code first partial colectomy (44204-44208)

5.47 ⚕ 5.47 **FUD** ZZZ C 80

AMA: 2016,Jan,13; 2015,Jan,16; 2014,Jan,11; 2013,Jan,11-12; 2012,Jan,15-42; 2011,Jan,11

44227 Laparoscopy, surgical, closure of enterostomy, large or small intestine, with resection and anastomosis

EXCLUDES *Open method (44625-44626)*

48.4 ⚕ 48.4 **FUD** 090 C 80

AMA: 2016,Jan,13; 2015,Jan,16; 2014,Jan,11; 2013,Jan,11-12

44238 Unlisted laparoscopy procedure, intestine (except rectum)

0.00 ⚕ 0.00 **FUD** YYY J 80 50

AMA: 2016,Jan,13; 2015,Jan,16; 2014,Jan,11; 2013,Jan,11-12

44300-44346 Open Enterostomy Procedures

44300 Placement, enterostomy or cecostomy, tube open (eg, for feeding or decompression) (separate procedure)

EXCLUDES *Other gastrointestinal tube(s) placed percutaneously with fluoroscopic imaging guidance (49441-49442)*

24.4 ⚕ 24.4 **FUD** 090 C 80

AMA: 2016,Jan,13; 2015,Jan,16; 2014,Jan,11; 2013,Jan,11-12; 2012,Jan,15-42; 2011,Jan,11

44310 Ileostomy or jejunostomy, non-tube

EXCLUDES *Colectomy, partial; with resection, with colostomy or ileostomy and creation of mucofistula (44144)*
Colectomy, total, abdominal (44150-44151, 44155-44156)
Excision of ileoanal reservoir with ileostomy (45136)
Laparoscopic method (44187)
Proctectomy (45113, 45119)

30.2 ⚕ 30.2 **FUD** 090 C 80

AMA: 2016,Jan,13; 2015,Jan,16; 2014,Jan,11; 2013,Jan,11-12; 2012,Jan,15-42; 2011,Jan,11

44312 Revision of ileostomy; simple (release of superficial scar) (separate procedure)

17.0 ⚕ 17.0 **FUD** 090 T A2 80

AMA: 2014,Jan,11; 2013,Jan,11-12

44314 complicated (reconstruction in-depth) (separate procedure)

29.0 ⚕ 29.0 **FUD** 090 C 80

AMA: 2014,Jan,11; 2013,Jan,11-12

44316 **Continent ileostomy (Kock procedure) (separate procedure)**
> *EXCLUDES* Fiberoptic evaluation (44385)
> 🚗 41.1 ⚕ 41.1 **FUD** 090   C 80 ▣
> **AMA:** 2014,Jan,11; 2013,Jan,11-12

44320 **Colostomy or skin level cecostomy;**
> *EXCLUDES* Closure of fistula (45805, 45825, 57307)
> Colectomy, partial (44141, 44144, 44146)
> Exploration, repair, and presacral drainage (45563)
> Laparoscopic method (44188)
> Pelvic exenteration (45126, 51597, 58240)
> Proctectomy (45110, 45119)
> Suture of large intestine (44605)
> Ureterosigmoidostomy (50810)
> 🚗 34.8 ⚕ 34.8 **FUD** 090   C 80 ▣
> **AMA:** 2016,Jan,13; 2015,Jan,16; 2014,Jan,11; 2013,Jan,11-12

44322 **with multiple biopsies (eg, for congenital megacolon) (separate procedure)**
> 🚗 28.9 ⚕ 28.9 **FUD** 090   C 80 ▣
> **AMA:** 2014,Jan,11; 2013,Jan,11-12

44340 **Revision of colostomy; simple (release of superficial scar) (separate procedure)**
> 🚗 18.1 ⚕ 18.1 **FUD** 090   T A2 ▣
> **AMA:** 2014,Jan,11; 2013,Jan,11-12

44345 **complicated (reconstruction in-depth) (separate procedure)**
> 🚗 30.4 ⚕ 30.4 **FUD** 090   C 80 ▣
> **AMA:** 2014,Jan,11; 2013,Jan,11-12

44346 **with repair of paracolostomy hernia (separate procedure)**
> 🚗 34.3 ⚕ 34.3 **FUD** 090   C 80 ▣
> **AMA:** 2016,Jan,13; 2015,Jan,16; 2014,Jan,11; 2013,Jan,11-12; 2012,Jan,15-42; 2011,Jan,11

Herniations that have formed around the site of a colostomy are repaired

Skin

The colon is mobilized, trimmed if necessary, and a new stoma is often created

44360-44379 Endoscopy of Small Intestine

INCLUDES Control of bleeding as result of endoscopic procedure during same operative session
EXCLUDES Esophagogastroduodenoscopy, flexible, transoral (43235-43259 [43233, 43266, 43270])
Retrograde exam through anus/colon stoma (44799)

▲ **44360** **Small intestinal endoscopy, enteroscopy beyond second portion of duodenum, not including ileum; diagnostic, including collection of specimen(s) by brushing or washing, when performed (separate procedure)**
> *EXCLUDES* Small intestinal endoscopy, enteroscopy (44376-44379)
> 🚗 4.37 ⚕ 4.37 **FUD** 000   T A2 ▣
> **AMA:** 2016,Jan,13; 2015,Jan,16; 2014,Nov,3; 2014,Jan,11; 2013,Dec,3; 2013,Jan,11-12; 2012,Jan,15-42; 2011,Mar,9

▲ **44361** **with biopsy, single or multiple**
> *EXCLUDES* Small intestinal endoscopy, enteroscopy (44376-44379)
> 🚗 4.82 ⚕ 4.82 **FUD** 000   T A2 ▣
> **AMA:** 2014,Nov,3; 2014,Jan,11; 2013,Dec,3; 2013,Jan,11-12

▲ **44363** **with removal of foreign body(s)**
> *EXCLUDES* Small intestinal endoscopy, enteroscopy (44376-44379)
> 🚗 5.78 ⚕ 5.78 **FUD** 000   T A2 80 ▣
> **AMA:** 2014,Nov,3; 2014,Jan,11; 2013,Dec,3; 2013,Jan,11-12

▲ **44364** **with removal of tumor(s), polyp(s), or other lesion(s) by snare technique**
> *EXCLUDES* Small intestinal endoscopy, enteroscopy (44376-44379)
> 🚗 6.15 ⚕ 6.15 **FUD** 000   T A2 80 ▣
> **AMA:** 2014,Nov,3; 2014,Jan,11; 2013,Dec,3; 2013,Jan,11-12

▲ **44365** **with removal of tumor(s), polyp(s), or other lesion(s) by hot biopsy forceps or bipolar cautery**
> *EXCLUDES* Small intestinal endoscopy, enteroscopy (44376-44379)
> 🚗 5.41 ⚕ 5.41 **FUD** 000   T A2 80 ▣
> **AMA:** 2014,Nov,3; 2014,Jan,11; 2013,Dec,3; 2013,Jan,11-12

▲ **44366** **with control of bleeding (eg, injection, bipolar cautery, unipolar cautery, laser, heater probe, stapler, plasma coagulator)**
> *EXCLUDES* Small intestinal endoscopy, enteroscopy (44376-44379)
> 🚗 7.22 ⚕ 7.22 **FUD** 000   T A2 ▣
> **AMA:** 2016,Jan,13; 2015,Jan,16; 2014,Nov,3; 2014,Jan,11; 2013,Dec,3; 2013,Jan,11-12

▲ **44369** **with ablation of tumor(s), polyp(s), or other lesion(s) not amenable to removal by hot biopsy forceps, bipolar cautery or snare technique**
> *EXCLUDES* Small intestinal endoscopy, enteroscopy (44376-44379)
> 🚗 7.38 ⚕ 7.38 **FUD** 000   T A2 80 ▣
> **AMA:** 2014,Nov,3; 2014,Jan,11; 2013,Dec,3; 2013,Jan,11-12

▲ **44370** **with transendoscopic stent placement (includes predilation)**
> *EXCLUDES* Small intestinal endoscopy, enteroscopy (44376-44379)
> 🚗 8.00 ⚕ 8.00 **FUD** 000   J A2 80 ▣
> **AMA:** 2016,Jan,13; 2015,Jan,16; 2014,Nov,3; 2014,Jan,11; 2013,Dec,3; 2013,Jan,11-12

▲ **44372** **with placement of percutaneous jejunostomy tube**
> *EXCLUDES* Small intestinal endoscopy, enteroscopy (44376-44379)
> 🚗 7.21 ⚕ 7.21 **FUD** 000   T A2 ▣
> **AMA:** 2016,Jan,13; 2015,Jan,16; 2014,Nov,3; 2014,Jan,11; 2013,Dec,3; 2013,Jan,11-12

▲ **44373** **with conversion of percutaneous gastrostomy tube to percutaneous jejunostomy tube**
> *EXCLUDES* Jejunostomy, fiberoptic, through stoma (43235)
> Small intestinal endoscopy, enteroscopy (44376-44379)
> 🚗 5.80 ⚕ 5.80 **FUD** 000   T A2 ▣
> **AMA:** 2016,Jan,13; 2015,Jan,16; 2014,Nov,3; 2014,Jan,11; 2013,Dec,3; 2013,Jan,11-12

▲ **44376** **Small intestinal endoscopy, enteroscopy beyond second portion of duodenum, including ileum; diagnostic, with or without collection of specimen(s) by brushing or washing (separate procedure)**
> *EXCLUDES* Small intestinal endoscopy, enteroscopy (44360-44373)
> 🚗 8.50 ⚕ 8.50 **FUD** 000   T A2 80 ▣
> **AMA:** 2016,Jan,13; 2015,Jan,16; 2014,Nov,3; 2014,Jan,11; 2013,Dec,3; 2013,Jan,11-12; 2011,Mar,9

▲ **44377** **with biopsy, single or multiple**
> *EXCLUDES* Small intestinal endoscopy, enteroscopy (44360-44373)
> 🚗 8.97 ⚕ 8.97 **FUD** 000   T A2 80 ▣
> **AMA:** 2016,Jan,13; 2015,Jan,16; 2014,Nov,3; 2014,Jan,11; 2013,Dec,3; 2013,Jan,11-12

▲ **44378** **with control of bleeding (eg, injection, bipolar cautery, unipolar cautery, laser, heater probe, stapler, plasma coagulator)**
> *EXCLUDES* Small intestinal endoscopy, enteroscopy (44360-44373)
> 🚗 11.4 ⚕ 11.4 **FUD** 000   T A2 80 ▣
> **AMA:** 2016,Jan,13; 2015,Jan,16; 2014,Nov,3; 2014,Jan,11; 2013,Dec,3; 2013,Jan,11-12; 2012,Apr,17-18

▲ **44379** **with transendoscopic stent placement (includes predilation)**
> *EXCLUDES* Small intestinal endoscopy, enteroscopy (44360-44373)
> 🚗 12.2 ⚕ 12.2 **FUD** 000   J A2 80 ▣
> **AMA:** 2016,Jan,13; 2015,Jan,16; 2014,Nov,3; 2014,Jan,11; 2013,Dec,3; 2013,Jan,11-12

44380-44384 [44381] Ileoscopy Via Stoma

INCLUDES Control of bleeding as result of endoscopic procedure during same operative session

EXCLUDES *Computed tomographic colonography (74261-74263)*

Code also exam of nonfunctional distal colon/rectum, when performed, with:
Anoscopy (46600, 46604-46606, 46608-46615)
Proctosigmoidoscopy (45300-45327)
Sigmoidoscopy (45330-45347 [45346])

▲ **44380** **Ileoscopy, through stoma; diagnostic, including collection of specimen(s) by brushing or washing, when performed (separate procedure)**

EXCLUDES *Ileoscopy, through stoma (44382-44384 [44381])*

🚑 1.81 ⚕ 6.26 **FUD** 000 T A2 ▭

AMA: 2016,Jan,13; 2015,Jan,16; 2014,Dec,3; 2014,Nov,3; 2014,Jan,11; 2013,Dec,3; 2013,Jan,11-12

44381 **Resequenced code. See code following 44382.**

▲ **44382** **with biopsy, single or multiple**

EXCLUDES *Ileoscopy, through stoma; diagnostic (44380)*

🚑 2.30 ⚕ 9.07 **FUD** 000 T A2 ▭

AMA: 2016,Jan,13; 2015,Jan,16; 2014,Dec,3; 2014,Nov,3; 2014,Jan,11; 2013,Dec,3; 2013,Jan,11-12

▲ # **44381** **with transendoscopic balloon dilation**

EXCLUDES *Ileoscopy, through stoma (44380, 44384)*

Code also each additional stricture dilated in same session, using modifier 59 with (44381)

🔀 (74360)

🚑 2.64 ⚕ 28.3 **FUD** 000 T G2 ▭

AMA: 2016,Jan,13; 2015,Jan,16; 2014,Dec,3; 2014,Nov,3

▲ **44384** **with placement of endoscopic stent (includes pre- and post-dilation and guide wire passage, when performed)**

EXCLUDES *Ileoscopy, through stoma (44380-44381)*

🔀 (74360)

🚑 4.59 ⚕ 4.59 **FUD** 000 J G2 ▭

AMA: 2016,Jan,13; 2015,Jan,16; 2014,Dec,3; 2014,Nov,3

44385-44386 Endoscopy of Small Intestinal Pouch

INCLUDES Control of bleeding as result of the endoscopic procedure during same operative session

EXCLUDES *Computed tomographic colonography (74261-74263)*

▲ **44385** **Endoscopic evaluation of small intestinal pouch (eg, Kock pouch, ileal reservoir [S or J]); diagnostic, including collection of specimen(s) by brushing or washing, when performed (separate procedure)**

EXCLUDES *Endoscopic evaluation of small intestinal pouch (44386)*

🚑 2.24 ⚕ 6.90 **FUD** 000 T A2 ▭

AMA: 2016,Jan,13; 2015,Jan,16; 2014,Dec,3; 2014,Nov,3; 2014,Jan,11; 2013,Dec,3; 2013,Jan,11-12

▲ **44386** **with biopsy, single or multiple**

EXCLUDES *Endoscopic evaluation of small intestinal pouch (44385)*

🚑 2.75 ⚕ 9.71 **FUD** 000 T A2 ▭

AMA: 2016,Jan,13; 2015,Jan,16; 2014,Dec,3; 2014,Nov,3; 2014,Jan,11; 2013,Dec,3; 2013,Jan,11-12

44388-44408 [44401] Colonoscopy Via Stoma

INCLUDES Control of bleeding as result of endoscopic procedure during same operative session

EXCLUDES *Colonoscopy via rectum (45378, 45392-45393 [45390, 45398])*
Computed tomographic colonography (74261-74263)

Code also exam of nonfunctional distal colon/rectum, when performed, with:
Anoscopy (46600, 46604-46606, 46608-46615)
Proctosigmoidoscopy (45300-45327)
Sigmoidoscopy (45330-45347 [45346])

▲ **44388** **Colonoscopy through stoma; diagnostic, including collection of specimen(s) by brushing or washing, when performed (separate procedure)**

EXCLUDES *Colonoscopy through stoma (44389-44408 [44401])*

Code also modifier 53 when planned total colonoscopy cannot be completed

🚑 4.74 ⚕ 10.0 **FUD** 000 T A2 ▭

AMA: 2016,Jan,13; 2015,Jan,16; 2014,Dec,3; 2014,Nov,3; 2014,Jan,11; 2013,Dec,3; 2013,Jan,11-12; 2012,Jan,15-42; 2011,Jan,11

▲ **44389** **with biopsy, single or multiple**

EXCLUDES *Colonoscopy through stoma; diagnostic (44388)*
Colonoscopy through stoma; with endoscopic mucosal resection on the same lesion (44403)

Code also modifier 52 when colonoscope fails to reach the junction of the small intestine

🚑 5.20 ⚕ 12.6 **FUD** 000 T A2 ▭

AMA: 2016,Jan,13; 2015,Jan,16; 2014,Dec,3; 2014,Nov,3; 2014,Jan,11; 2013,Dec,3; 2013,Jan,11-12

▲ **44390** **with removal of foreign body(s)**

EXCLUDES *Colonoscopy through stoma; diagnostic (44388)*

Code also modifier 52 when colonoscope fails to reach the junction of the small intestine

🔀 (76000)

🚑 6.34 ⚕ 12.6 **FUD** 000 T A2 ▭

AMA: 2016,Jan,13; 2015,Jan,16; 2014,Dec,3; 2014,Nov,3; 2014,Jan,11; 2013,Dec,3; 2013,Jan,11-12

▲ **44391** **with control of bleeding, any method**

EXCLUDES *Colonoscopy through stoma; diagnostic (44388)*
Colonoscopy through stoma; with directed submucosal injection(s) on the same lesion (44404)

Code also modifier 52 when colonoscope fails to reach the junction of the small intestine

🚑 6.93 ⚕ 21.7 **FUD** 000 T A2 ▭

AMA: 2016,Jan,13; 2015,Jan,16; 2014,Dec,3; 2014,Nov,3; 2014,Jan,11; 2013,Dec,3; 2013,Jan,11-12

▲ **44392** **with removal of tumor(s), polyp(s), or other lesion(s) by hot biopsy forceps**

EXCLUDES *Colonoscopy through stoma; diagnostic (44388)*

Code also modifier 52 when colonoscope fails to reach the junction of the small intestine

🚑 5.98 ⚕ 11.8 **FUD** 000 T A2 ▭

AMA: 2016,Jan,13; 2015,Jan,16; 2014,Dec,3; 2014,Nov,3; 2014,Jan,11; 2013,Dec,3; 2013,Jan,11-12

▲ # **44401** **with ablation of tumor(s), polyp(s), or other lesion(s) (includes pre-and post-dilation and guide wire passage, when performed)**

EXCLUDES *Colonoscopy through stoma; diagnostic (44388)*
Colonoscopy through stoma; with transendoscopic balloon dilation on the same lesion (44405)

Code also modifier 52 when colonoscope fails to reach the junction of the small intestine

🚑 7.27 ⚕ 92.4 **FUD** 000 T G2 ▭

AMA: 2016,Jan,13; 2015,Jan,16; 2014,Dec,3; 2014,Nov,3

▲ **44394** **with removal of tumor(s), polyp(s), or other lesion(s) by snare technique**

EXCLUDES *Colonoscopy through stoma; diagnostic (44388)*
Colonoscopy through stoma; with endoscopic mucosal resection on the same lesion (44403)

Code also modifier 52 when colonoscope fails to reach the junction of the small intestine

🚑 6.79 ⚕ 13.3 **FUD** 000 T A2 ▭

AMA: 2016,Jan,13; 2015,Jan,16; 2014,Dec,3; 2014,Nov,3; 2014,Jan,11; 2013,Dec,3; 2013,Jan,11-12

44401 **Resequenced code. See code following 44392.**

▲ **44402** **with endoscopic stent placement (including pre- and post-dilation and guide wire passage, when performed)**

> EXCLUDES *Colonoscopy through stoma (44388, 44405)*
> Code also modifier 52 when colonoscope fails to reach the junction of the small intestine
> ⚡ (74360)
> 💰 7.87 ⚖ 7.87 **FUD** 000 [J] [62] [🖵]
> **AMA:** 2016,Jan,13; 2015,Jan,16; 2014,Dec,3; 2014,Nov,3

▲ **44403** **with endoscopic mucosal resection**

> EXCLUDES *Colonoscopy through stoma; diagnostic (44388)*
> *Colonoscopy through stoma on the same lesion (44389, 44394, 44404)*
> Code also modifier 52 when colonoscope fails to reach the junction of the small intestine
> 💰 9.04 ⚖ 9.04 **FUD** 000 [T] [62] [🖵]
> **AMA:** 2016,Jan,13; 2015,Jan,16; 2014,Dec,3; 2014,Nov,3

▲ **44404** **with directed submucosal injection(s), any substance**

> EXCLUDES *Colonoscopy through stoma; diagnostic (44388)*
> *Colonoscopy through stoma on the same lesion (44391, 44403)*
> Code also modifier 52 when colonoscope fails to reach the junction of the small intestine
> 💰 5.21 ⚖ 12.1 **FUD** 000 [T] [62] [🖵]
> **AMA:** 2016,Jan,13; 2015,Jan,16; 2014,Dec,3; 2014,Nov,3

▲ **44405** **with transendoscopic balloon dilation**

> EXCLUDES *Colonoscopy through stoma (44388, [44401], 44402)*
> Code also each additional stricture dilated in same session, using modifier 59 with (44405)
> Code also modifier 52 when colonoscope fails to reach the junction of the small intestine
> ⚡ (74360)
> 💰 5.54 ⚖ 17.3 **FUD** 000 [T] [62] [🖵]
> **AMA:** 2016,Jan,13; 2015,Jan,16; 2014,Dec,3; 2014,Nov,3

▲ **44406** **with endoscopic ultrasound examination, limited to the sigmoid, descending, transverse, or ascending colon and cecum and adjacent structures**

> INCLUDES *Gastrointestinal endoscopic ultrasound, supervision and interpretation (76975)*
> EXCLUDES *Colonoscopy through stoma (44388, 44407)*
> *Procedure performed more than one time per operative session*
> Code also modifier 52 when colonoscope fails to reach the junction of the small intestine
> 💰 6.90 ⚖ 6.90 **FUD** 000 [T] [62] [🖵]
> **AMA:** 2016,Jan,13; 2015,Jan,16; 2014,Dec,3; 2014,Nov,3

▲ **44407** **with transendoscopic ultrasound guided intramural or transmural fine needle aspiration/biopsy(s), includes endoscopic ultrasound examination limited to the sigmoid, descending, transverse, or ascending colon and cecum and adjacent structures**

> INCLUDES *Gastrointestinal endoscopic ultrasound, supervision and interpretation (76975)*
> *Ultrasonic guidance (76942)*
> EXCLUDES *Colonoscopy through stoma (44388, 44406)*
> *Procedure performed more than one time per operative session*
> Code also modifier 52 when colonoscope fails to reach the junction of the small intestine
> 💰 8.26 ⚖ 8.26 **FUD** 000 [T] [62] [🖵]
> **AMA:** 2016,Jan,13; 2015,Jan,16; 2014,Dec,3; 2014,Nov,3

▲ **44408** **with decompression (for pathologic distention) (eg, volvulus, megacolon), including placement of decompression tube, when performed**

> EXCLUDES *Colonoscopy through stoma; diagnostic (44388)*
> *Procedure performed more than one time per operative session*
> 💰 6.97 ⚖ 6.97 **FUD** 000 [T] [62] [🖵]
> **AMA:** 2016,Jan,13; 2015,Jan,16; 2014,Dec,3; 2014,Nov,3

44500 Gastrointestinal Intubation

▲ **44500** **Introduction of long gastrointestinal tube (eg, Miller-Abbott) (separate procedure)**

> EXCLUDES *Placement of oro- or naso-gastric tube (43752)*
> ⚡ (74340)
> 💰 0.71 ⚖ 0.71 **FUD** 000 [⊘] [T] [62] [80] [🖵]
> **AMA:** 2016,Sep,9; 2016,Jan,13; 2015,Jan,16; 2014,Jan,11; 2013,Dec,3; 2013,Jan,11-12

44602-44680 Open Repair Procedures of Intestines

44602 **Suture of small intestine (enterorrhaphy) for perforated ulcer, diverticulum, wound, injury or rupture; single perforation**

> 💰 41.0 ⚖ 41.0 **FUD** 090 [C] [80] [🖵]
> **AMA:** 2014,Jan,11; 2013,Dec,3; 2013,Jan,11-12

44603 **multiple perforations**

> 💰 47.0 ⚖ 47.0 **FUD** 090 [C] [80] [🖵]
> **AMA:** 2014,Jan,11; 2013,Dec,3; 2013,Jan,11-12

44604 **Suture of large intestine (colorrhaphy) for perforated ulcer, diverticulum, wound, injury or rupture (single or multiple perforations); without colostomy**

> 💰 30.6 ⚖ 30.6 **FUD** 090 [C] [80] [🖵]
> **AMA:** 2014,Jan,11; 2013,Dec,3; 2013,Jan,11-12

44605 **with colostomy**

> 💰 37.8 ⚖ 37.8 **FUD** 090 [C] [80] [🖵]
> **AMA:** 2014,Jan,11; 2013,Dec,3; 2013,Jan,11-12

44615 **Intestinal stricturoplasty (enterotomy and enterorrhaphy) with or without dilation, for intestinal obstruction**

> 💰 31.2 ⚖ 31.2 **FUD** 090 [C] [80] [🖵]
> **AMA:** 2014,Jan,11; 2013,Dec,3; 2013,Jan,11-12

44620 **Closure of enterostomy, large or small intestine;**

> EXCLUDES *Laparoscopic method (44227)*
> 💰 25.1 ⚖ 25.1 **FUD** 090 [C] [80] [🖵]
> **AMA:** 2014,Jan,11; 2013,Dec,3; 2013,Jan,11-12

44625 **with resection and anastomosis other than colorectal**

> EXCLUDES *Laparoscopic method (44227)*
> 💰 29.4 ⚖ 29.4 **FUD** 090 [C] [80] [🖵]
> **AMA:** 2014,Jan,11; 2013,Dec,3; 2013,Jan,11-12

44626 **with resection and colorectal anastomosis (eg, closure of Hartmann type procedure)**

> EXCLUDES *Laparoscopic method (44227)*
> 💰 46.5 ⚖ 46.5 **FUD** 090 [C] [80] [🖵]
> **AMA:** 2014,Jan,11; 2013,Dec,3; 2013,Jan,11-12

44640 **Closure of intestinal cutaneous fistula**

> 💰 40.7 ⚖ 40.7 **FUD** 090 [C] [80] [🖵]
> **AMA:** 2014,Jan,11; 2013,Dec,3; 2013,Jan,11-12

44650 **Closure of enteroenteric or enterocolic fistula**

> 💰 42.0 ⚖ 42.0 **FUD** 090 [C] [80] [🖵]
> **AMA:** 2014,Jan,11; 2013,Dec,3; 2013,Jan,11-12

44660 **Closure of enterovesical fistula; without intestinal or bladder resection**

> EXCLUDES *Closure of fistula:*
> *Gastrocolic (43880)*
> *Rectovesical (45800, 45805)*
> *Renocolic (50525-50526)*
> 💰 38.5 ⚖ 38.5 **FUD** 090 [C] [80] [🖵]
> **AMA:** 2014,Jan,11; 2013,Dec,3; 2013,Jan,11-12

44661 **with intestine and/or bladder resection**

> EXCLUDES *Closure of fistula:*
> *Gastrocolic (43880)*
> *Rectovesical (45800, 45805)*
> *Renocolic (50525-50526)*
> 💰 45.0 ⚖ 45.0 **FUD** 090 [C] [80] [🖵]
> **AMA:** 2014,Jan,11; 2013,Dec,3; 2013,Jan,11-12

44680 **Intestinal plication (separate procedure)**

> INCLUDES *Noble intestinal plication*
> 💰 30.9 ⚖ 30.9 **FUD** 090 [C] [80] [🖵]
> **AMA:** 2014,Jan,11; 2013,Dec,3; 2013,Jan,11-12

26/TC PC/TC Only	A2-Z3 ASC Payment	50 Bilateral	♂ Male Only	♀ Female Only	💰 Facility RVU	⚖ Non-Facility RVU	🖵 CCI
FUD Follow-up Days	**CMS:** IOM (Pub 100)	A-Y OPPSI	80/80 Surg Assist Allowed / w/Doc		⚡ Lab Crosswalk	⚡ Radiology Crosswalk	⚡ CLIA

194

44700-44705 Other Intestinal Procedures

44700 Exclusion of small intestine from pelvis by mesh or other prosthesis, or native tissue (eg, bladder or omentum)

EXCLUDES *Therapeutic radiation clinical treatment (77261-77799 [77295, 77385, 77386, 77387, 77424, 77425])*

🔧 29.5   ✂ 29.5   **FUD** 090   C 80 ▣

AMA: 2014,Jan,11; 2013,Dec,3; 2013,Jan,11-12

+ 44701 Intraoperative colonic lavage (List separately in addition to code for primary procedure)

EXCLUDES *Appendectomy (44950-44960)*

Placement, enterostomy or cecostomy, tube open (44300)

Code first as appropriate (44140, 44145, 44150, 44604)

🔧 4.90   ✂ 4.90   **FUD** ZZZ   N N1 80 ▣

AMA: 2014,Jan,11; 2013,Dec,3; 2013,Jan,11-12

44705 Preparation of fecal microbiota for instillation, including assessment of donor specimen

EXCLUDES *Fecal instillation by enema or oro-nasogastric tube (44799)*

Therapeutic enema (74283)

🔧 0.00   ✂ 0.00   **FUD** XXX   B ▣

AMA: 2016,Jan,13; 2015,Jan,16; 2014,Jan,11; 2013,Dec,3; 2013,May,12; 2013,Jan,11-12

44715-44799 Backbench Transplant Procedures

CMS: 100-04,3,90.6 Intestinal and Multi-Visceral Transplants

44715 Backbench standard preparation of cadaver or living donor intestine allograft prior to transplantation, including mobilization and fashioning of the superior mesenteric artery and vein

INCLUDES Mobilization/fashioning of superior mesenteric vein/artery

🔧 0.00   ✂ 0.00   **FUD** XXX   C 80 ▣

AMA: 2014,Jan,11; 2013,Dec,3; 2013,Jan,11-12

44720 Backbench reconstruction of cadaver or living donor intestine allograft prior to transplantation; venous anastomosis, each

🔧 8.01   ✂ 8.01   **FUD** XXX   C 80 ▣

AMA: 2014,Jan,11; 2013,Dec,3; 2013,Jan,11-12

44721 arterial anastomosis, each

🔧 11.2   ✂ 11.2   **FUD** XXX   C 80 ▣

AMA: 2016,Jan,13; 2015,Jan,16; 2014,Jan,11; 2013,Dec,3; 2013,Jan,11-12

44799 Unlisted procedure, small intestine

EXCLUDES *Unlisted colon procedure (45399)*

Unlisted intestinal procedure performed laparoscopically (44238)

Unlisted rectal procedure (45499, 45999)

🔧 0.00   ✂ 0.00   **FUD** YYY   T

AMA: 2016,Jan,13; 2015,Jan,16; 2014,Nov,3; 2014,Jan,11; 2013,Dec,3; 2013,May,12; 2013,Jan,11-12; 2012,Jan,15-42; 2011,May,9; 2011,Mar,9; 2011,Jan,11

44800-44899 Meckel's Diverticulum and Mesentery Procedures

44800 Excision of Meckel's diverticulum (diverticulectomy) or omphalomesenteric duct

🔧 22.1   ✂ 22.1   **FUD** 090   C 80 ▣

AMA: 2014,Jan,11; 2013,Dec,3; 2013,Jan,11-12

44820 Excision of lesion of mesentery (separate procedure)

EXCLUDES *Resection of intestine (44120-44128, 44140-44160)*

🔧 24.3   ✂ 24.3   **FUD** 090   C 80 ▣

AMA: 2014,Jan,11; 2013,Dec,3; 2013,Jan,11-12

44850 Suture of mesentery (separate procedure)

EXCLUDES *Internal hernia repair/reduction (44050)*

🔧 21.7   ✂ 21.7   **FUD** 090   C 80 ▣

AMA: 2014,Jan,11; 2013,Dec,3; 2013,Jan,11-12

44899 Unlisted procedure, Meckel's diverticulum and the mesentery

🔧 0.00   ✂ 0.00   **FUD** YYY   C 80

AMA: 2014,Jan,11; 2013,Dec,3; 2013,Jan,11-12

44900-44979 Open and Endoscopic Appendix Procedures

44900 Incision and drainage of appendiceal abscess, open

EXCLUDES *Image guided percutaneous catheter drainage (49406)*

🔧 22.3   ✂ 22.3   **FUD** 090   C 80 ▣

AMA: 2014,Jan,11; 2013,Nov,9; 2013,Dec,3; 2013,Jan,11-12

44950 Appendectomy;

INCLUDES Battle's operation

EXCLUDES *Procedure performed with other intra-abdominal procedure(s) when appendectomy is incidental*

🔧 18.6   ✂ 18.6   **FUD** 090   T 80 ▣

AMA: 2016,Jan,13; 2015,Jan,16; 2014,Jan,11; 2013,Dec,3; 2013,Jan,11-12

Failure to treat appendicitis can lead to peritonitis

Ascending colon

Ileum

Cecum

Free tenia

Appendix and appendicular artery

Mesoappendix

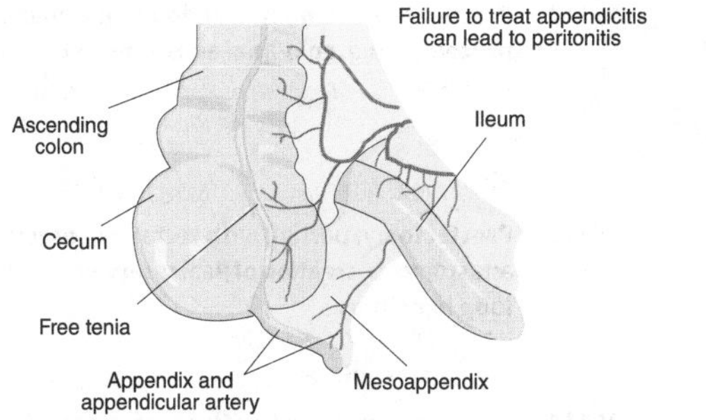

+ 44955 when done for indicated purpose at time of other major procedure (not as separate procedure) (List separately in addition to code for primary procedure)

Code first primary procedure

🔧 2.44   ✂ 2.44   **FUD** ZZZ   N 80 ▣

AMA: 2016,Jan,13; 2015,Jan,16; 2014,Jan,11; 2013,Dec,3; 2013,Jan,11-12; 2012,Jan,13-14

44960 for ruptured appendix with abscess or generalized peritonitis

INCLUDES Battle's operation

🔧 25.3   ✂ 25.3   **FUD** 090   C 80 ▣

AMA: 2016,Jan,13; 2015,Jan,16; 2014,Jan,11; 2013,Dec,3; 2013,Jan,11-12

44970 Laparoscopy, surgical, appendectomy

INCLUDES Diagnostic laparoscopy

🔧 17.4   ✂ 17.4   **FUD** 090   J 80 ▣

AMA: 2016,Jan,13; 2015,Mar,3; 2015,Jan,16; 2014,Jan,11; 2013,Dec,3; 2013,Jan,11-12; 2012,Jan,15-42; 2011,Jan,11

44979 Unlisted laparoscopy procedure, appendix

🔧 0.00   ✂ 0.00   **FUD** YYY   J 80 50

AMA: 2016,Jan,13; 2015,Jan,16; 2014,Jan,11; 2013,Dec,3; 2013,Jan,11-12; 2012,Jan,13-14

45000-45190 Open and Transrectal Procedures of Rectum

45000 Transrectal drainage of pelvic abscess

EXCLUDES *Image guided transrectal catheter drainage (49407)*

🔧 12.2   ✂ 12.2   **FUD** 090   T A2 ▣

AMA: 2014,Jan,11; 2013,Nov,9; 2013,Dec,3; 2013,Jan,11-12

45005 Incision and drainage of submucosal abscess, rectum

🔧 4.66   ✂ 7.85   **FUD** 010   T A2 ▣

AMA: 2014,Jan,11; 2013,Dec,3; 2013,Jan,11-12

45020 Incision and drainage of deep supralevator, pelvirectal, or retrorectal abscess

EXCLUDES *Incision and drainage of perianal, ischiorectal, intramural abscess (46050, 46060)*

🔧 16.5   ✂ 16.5   **FUD** 090   T A2 ▣

AMA: 2014,Jan,11; 2013,Dec,3; 2013,Jan,11-12

● New Code　▲ Revised Code　○ Reinstated　● New Web Release　▲ Revised Web Release　Unlisted　Not Covered　# Resequenced
⊘ AMA Mod 51 Exempt　⑤ Optum Mod 51 Exempt　㊿ Mod 63 Exempt　✐ Non-FDA Drug　★ Telehealth　M Maternity　A Age Edit　+ Add-on　AMA: CPT Asst

　CPT © 2016 American Medical Association. All Rights Reserved.

Digestive System

45100 — 45300

45100 **Biopsy of anorectal wall, anal approach (eg, congenital megacolon)**
EXCLUDES　Biopsy performed endoscopically (45305)
📷 8.64　　🔧 8.64　　**FUD** 090　　　　　T A2 ⬜
AMA: 2014,Jan,11; 2013,Dec,3; 2013,Jan,11-12

45108 **Anorectal myomectomy**
📷 10.5　　🔧 10.5　　**FUD** 090　　　　　T A2 ⬜
AMA: 2014,Jan,11; 2013,Dec,3; 2013,Jan,11-12

45110 **Proctectomy; complete, combined abdominoperineal, with colostomy**
EXCLUDES　Laparoscopic method (45395)
📷 53.5　　🔧 53.5　　**FUD** 090　　　　　C 80 ⬜
AMA: 2014,Jan,11; 2013,Dec,3; 2013,Jan,11-12

45111 **partial resection of rectum, transabdominal approach**
INCLUDES　Luschka proctectomy
📷 31.4　　🔧 31.4　　**FUD** 090　　　　　C 80 ⬜
AMA: 2014,Jan,11; 2013,Dec,3; 2013,Jan,11-12

45112 **Proctectomy, combined abdominoperineal, pull-through procedure (eg, colo-anal anastomosis)**
EXCLUDES　Proctectomy for colo-anal anastomosis with creation of colonic pouch or reservoir (45119)
📷 54.4　　🔧 54.4　　**FUD** 090　　　　　C 80 ⬜
AMA: 2014,Jan,11; 2013,Dec,3; 2013,Jan,11-12

45113 **Proctectomy, partial, with rectal mucosectomy, ileoanal anastomosis, creation of ileal reservoir (S or J), with or without loop ileostomy**
📷 54.8　　🔧 54.8　　**FUD** 090　　　　　C 80 ⬜
AMA: 2014,Jan,11; 2013,Dec,3; 2013,Jan,11-12

45114 **Proctectomy, partial, with anastomosis; abdominal and transsacral approach**
📷 52.7　　🔧 52.7　　**FUD** 090　　　　　C 80 ⬜
AMA: 2014,Jan,11; 2013,Dec,3; 2013,Jan,11-12

45116 **transsacral approach only (Kraske type)**
📷 47.7　　🔧 47.7　　**FUD** 090　　　　　C 80 ⬜
AMA: 2014,Jan,11; 2013,Dec,3; 2013,Jan,11-12

45119 **Proctectomy, combined abdominoperineal pull-through procedure (eg, colo-anal anastomosis), with creation of colonic reservoir (eg, J-pouch), with diverting enterostomy when performed**
EXCLUDES　Laparoscopic method (45397)
📷 56.4　　🔧 56.4　　**FUD** 090　　　　　C 80 ⬜
AMA: 2016,Jan,13; 2015,Jan,16; 2014,Jan,11; 2013,Dec,3; 2013,Jan,11-12

45120 **Proctectomy, complete (for congenital megacolon), abdominal and perineal approach; with pull-through procedure and anastomosis (eg, Swenson, Duhamel, or Soave type operation)**
📷 43.5　　🔧 43.5　　**FUD** 090　　　　　C 80 ⬜
AMA: 2014,Jan,11; 2013,Dec,3; 2013,Jan,11-12

45121 **with subtotal or total colectomy, with multiple biopsies**
📷 50.4　　🔧 50.4　　**FUD** 090　　　　　C 80 ⬜
AMA: 2014,Jan,11; 2013,Dec,3; 2013,Jan,11-12

45123 **Proctectomy, partial, without anastomosis, perineal approach**
📷 32.4　　🔧 32.4　　**FUD** 090　　　　　C 80 ⬜
AMA: 2014,Jan,11; 2013,Dec,3; 2013,Jan,11-12

45126 **Pelvic exenteration for colorectal malignancy, with proctectomy (with or without colostomy), with removal of bladder and ureteral transplantations, and/or hysterectomy, or cervicectomy, with or without removal of tube(s), with or without removal of ovary(s), or any combination thereof**
📷 80.9　　🔧 80.9　　**FUD** 090　　　　　C 80 ⬜
AMA: 2014,Jan,11; 2013,Dec,3; 2013,Jan,11-12

45130 **Excision of rectal procidentia, with anastomosis; perineal approach**
INCLUDES　Altemeier procedure
📷 31.4　　🔧 31.4　　**FUD** 090　　　　　C 80 ⬜
AMA: 2014,Jan,11; 2013,Dec,3; 2013,Jan,11-12

45135 **abdominal and perineal approach**
INCLUDES　Altemeier procedure
📷 39.7　　🔧 39.7　　**FUD** 090　　　　　C 80 ⬜
AMA: 2014,Jan,11; 2013,Dec,3; 2013,Jan,11-12

45136 **Excision of ileoanal reservoir with ileostomy**
EXCLUDES　Enterectomy (44120)
Enterolysis (44005)
Ileostomy or jejunostomy, non-tube (44310)
📷 52.4　　🔧 52.4　　**FUD** 090　　　　　C 80 ⬜
AMA: 2014,Jan,11; 2013,Dec,3; 2013,Jan,11-12

45150 **Division of stricture of rectum**
📷 11.2　　🔧 11.2　　**FUD** 090　　　　　T A2 80 ⬜
AMA: 2014,Jan,11; 2013,Dec,3; 2013,Jan,11-12

45160 **Excision of rectal tumor by proctotomy, transsacral or transcoccygeal approach**
📷 29.6　　🔧 29.6　　**FUD** 090　　　　　T A2 80 ⬜
AMA: 2014,Jan,11; 2013,Dec,3; 2013,Jan,11-12

45171 **Excision of rectal tumor, transanal approach; not including muscularis propria (ie, partial thickness)**
EXCLUDES　Transanal destruction of rectal tumor (45190)
Transanal endoscopic microsurgical tumor excision (TEMS) (0184T)
📷 17.3　　🔧 17.3　　**FUD** 090　　　　　T 62 80 ⬜
AMA: 2016,Jan,13; 2015,Jan,16; 2014,Jan,11; 2013,Dec,3; 2013,Jan,11-12

45172 **including muscularis propria (ie, full thickness)**
EXCLUDES　Transanal destruction of rectal tumor (45190)
Transanal endoscopic microsurgical tumor excision (TEMS) (0184T)
📷 23.3　　🔧 23.3　　**FUD** 090　　　　　T 62 80 ⬜
AMA: 2016,Jan,13; 2015,Jan,16; 2014,Jan,11; 2013,Dec,3; 2013,Jan,11-12

45190 **Destruction of rectal tumor (eg, electrodesiccation, electrosurgery, laser ablation, laser resection, cryosurgery) transanal approach**
EXCLUDES　Transanal endoscopic microsurgical tumor excision (TEMS) (0184T)
Transanal excision of rectal tumor (45171-45172)
📷 20.0　　🔧 20.0　　**FUD** 090　　　　　T A2 ⬜
AMA: 2016,Jan,13; 2015,Jan,16; 2014,Jan,11; 2013,Dec,3; 2013,Jan,11-12

45300-45327 Rigid Proctosigmoidoscopy Procedures

INCLUDES　Control of bleeding as result of the endoscopic procedure during same operative session
Exam of:
Entire rectum
Portion of sigmoid colon
EXCLUDES　Computed tomographic colonography (74261-74263)
Code also examination of colon through stoma:
Colonoscopy via stoma (44388-44408 [44401])
Ileoscopy via stoma (44380-44384 [44381])

45300 **Proctosigmoidoscopy, rigid; diagnostic, with or without collection of specimen(s) by brushing or washing (separate procedure)**
📷 1.56　　🔧 3.50　　**FUD** 000　　　　　T P3 ⬜
AMA: 2016,Jan,13; 2015,Jan,16; 2014,Jan,11; 2013,Dec,3; 2013,Jan,11-12

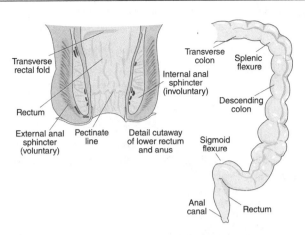

▲ 45303 **with dilation (eg, balloon, guide wire, bougie)**
🔗 (74360)
🚑 2.67 ⚕ 27.2 **FUD** 000 　 T P2 ▢
AMA: 2016,Jan,13; 2015,Jan,16; 2014,Jan,11; 2013,Dec,3; 2013,Jan,11-12

▲ 45305 **with biopsy, single or multiple**
🚑 2.28 ⚕ 5.56 **FUD** 000 　 T A2 ▢
AMA: 2016,Jan,13; 2015,Jan,16; 2014,Jan,11; 2013,Dec,3; 2013,Jan,11-12

▲ 45307 **with removal of foreign body**
🚑 3.08 ⚕ 6.66 **FUD** 000 　 T A2 80 ▢
AMA: 2016,Jan,13; 2015,Jan,16; 2014,Jan,11; 2013,Dec,3; 2013,Jan,11-12

▲ 45308 **with removal of single tumor, polyp, or other lesion by hot biopsy forceps or bipolar cautery**
🚑 2.58 ⚕ 6.15 **FUD** 000 　 T A2 ▢
AMA: 2016,Jan,13; 2015,Jan,16; 2014,Jan,11; 2013,Dec,3; 2013,Jan,11-12

▲ 45309 **with removal of single tumor, polyp, or other lesion by snare technique**
🚑 2.75 ⚕ 6.44 **FUD** 000 　 T A2 ▢
AMA: 2016,Jan,13; 2015,Jan,16; 2014,Jan,11; 2013,Dec,3; 2013,Jan,11-12

▲ 45315 **with removal of multiple tumors, polyps, or other lesions by hot biopsy forceps, bipolar cautery or snare technique**
🚑 3.03 ⚕ 6.44 **FUD** 000 　 T A2 ▢
AMA: 2016,Jan,13; 2015,Jan,16; 2014,Jan,11; 2013,Dec,3; 2013,Jan,11-12

▲ 45317 **with control of bleeding (eg, injection, bipolar cautery, unipolar cautery, laser, heater probe, stapler, plasma coagulator)**
🚑 3.40 ⚕ 6.93 **FUD** 000 　 T A2 ▢
AMA: 2016,Jan,13; 2015,Jan,16; 2014,Jan,11; 2013,Dec,3; 2013,Jan,11-12

▲ 45320 **with ablation of tumor(s), polyp(s), or other lesion(s) not amenable to removal by hot biopsy forceps, bipolar cautery or snare technique (eg, laser)**
🚑 3.20 ⚕ 6.94 **FUD** 000 　 T A2 ▢
AMA: 2016,Jan,13; 2015,Jan,16; 2014,Jan,11; 2013,Dec,3; 2013,Jan,11-12

▲ 45321 **with decompression of volvulus**
🚑 3.11 ⚕ 3.11 **FUD** 000 　 T A2 ▢
AMA: 2016,Jan,13; 2015,Jan,16; 2014,Jan,11; 2013,Dec,3; 2013,Jan,11-12

▲ 45327 **with transendoscopic stent placement (includes predilation)**
🚑 3.54 ⚕ 3.54 **FUD** 000 　 J A2 ▢
AMA: 2016,Jan,13; 2015,Jan,16; 2014,Jan,11; 2013,Dec,3; 2013,Jan,11-12

45330-45350 [45346] Flexible Sigmoidoscopy Procedures

INCLUDES Control of bleeding as result of the endoscopic procedure during same operative session
Exam of:
Entire rectum
Entire sigmoid colon
Portion of descending colon (when performed)
EXCLUDES *Computed tomographic colonography (74261-74263)*
Code also examination of colon through stoma when appropriate:
Colonoscopy (44388-44408 [44401])
Ileoscopy (44380-44384 [44381])

45330 **Sigmoidoscopy, flexible; diagnostic, including collection of specimen(s) by brushing or washing, when performed (separate procedure)**
EXCLUDES *Sigmoidoscopy, flexible (45331-45350 [45346])*
🚑 1.63 ⚕ 4.74 **FUD** 000 　 T P3 ▢
AMA: 2016,Feb,13; 2016,Jan,13; 2015,Sep,12; 2015,Jan,16; 2014,Dec,3; 2014,Dec,18; 2014,Jan,11; 2013,Dec,3; 2013,Jan,11-12; 2012,Jan,15-42; 2011,Jan,11

45331 **with biopsy, single or multiple**
EXCLUDES *Sigmoidoscopy, flexible; with endoscopic mucosal resection on the same lesion (45349)*
🚑 2.10 ⚕ 7.27 **FUD** 000 　 T A2 ▢
AMA: 2016,Feb,13; 2016,Jan,13; 2015,Jan,16; 2014,Dec,3; 2014,Dec,18; 2014,Jan,11; 2013,Dec,3; 2013,Jan,11-12; 2012,Jan,15-42; 2011,Jan,11

▲ 45332 **with removal of foreign body(s)**
EXCLUDES *Sigmoidoscopy, flexible; diagnostic (45330)*
🔗 (76000)
🚑 3.24 ⚕ 8.82 **FUD** 000 　 T A2 ▢
AMA: 2016,Feb,13; 2016,Jan,13; 2015,Jan,16; 2014,Dec,3; 2014,Dec,18; 2014,Jan,11; 2013,Dec,3; 2013,Jan,11-12

▲ 45333 **with removal of tumor(s), polyp(s), or other lesion(s) by hot biopsy forceps**
EXCLUDES *Sigmoidoscopy, flexible; diagnostic (45330)*
🚑 2.90 ⚕ 9.90 **FUD** 000 　 T A2 ▢
AMA: 2016,Feb,13; 2016,Jan,13; 2015,Jan,16; 2014,Dec,3; 2014,Dec,18; 2014,Jan,11; 2013,Dec,3; 2013,Jan,11-12

▲ 45334 **with control of bleeding, any method**
EXCLUDES *Sigmoidoscopy, flexible; diagnostic (45330)*
Sigmoidoscopy, flexible; with band ligation on the same lesion (45350)
Sigmoidoscopy, flexible; with directed submucosal injection on the same lesion (45335)
🚑 3.61 ⚕ 17.2 **FUD** 000 　 T A2 ▢
AMA: 2016,Feb,13; 2016,Jan,13; 2015,Jan,16; 2014,Dec,3; 2014,Dec,18; 2014,Jan,11; 2013,Dec,3; 2013,Jan,11-12; 2012,Jan,15-42; 2011,Jan,11

▲ 45335 **with directed submucosal injection(s), any substance**
EXCLUDES *Sigmoidoscopy, flexible; diagnostic (45330)*
Sigmoidoscopy, flexible; with control of bleeding on the same lesion (45334)
Sigmoidoscopy, flexible; with endoscopic mucosal resection on the same lesion (45349)
🚑 2.10 ⚕ 8.20 **FUD** 000 　 T A2 ▢
AMA: 2016,Feb,13; 2016,Jan,13; 2015,Jan,16; 2014,Dec,3; 2014,Dec,18; 2014,Jan,11; 2013,Dec,3; 2013,Jan,11-12; 2012,Jan,15-42; 2011,Jan,11

Digestive System

45337 — 45382

▲ **45337** **with decompression (for pathologic distention) (eg, volvulus, megacolon), including placement of decompression tube, when performed**

EXCLUDES *Procedure performed more than one time per operative session*

Sigmoidoscopy, flexible; diagnostic (45330)

🔲 3.53   🔲 3.53   **FUD** 000   T A2 🔲

AMA: 2016,Feb,13; 2016,Jan,13; 2015,Jan,16; 2014,Dec,3; 2014,Dec,18; 2014,Jan,11; 2013,Dec,3; 2013,Jan,11-12

▲ **45338** **with removal of tumor(s), polyp(s), or other lesion(s) by snare technique**

EXCLUDES *Sigmoidoscopy, flexible; diagnostic (45330)*

Sigmoidoscopy, flexible; with endoscopic mucosal resection on the same lesion (45349)

🔲 3.68   🔲 9.21   **FUD** 000   T A2 🔲

AMA: 2016,Feb,13; 2016,Jan,13; 2015,Jan,16; 2014,Dec,3; 2014,Dec,18; 2014,Jan,11; 2013,Dec,3; 2013,Jan,11-12

▲ # **45346** **with ablation of tumor(s), polyp(s), or other lesion(s) (includes pre- and post-dilation and guide wire passage, when performed)**

EXCLUDES *Sigmoidoscopy, flexible; diagnostic (45330)*

Sigmoidoscopy, flexible; with transendoscopic balloon dilation on same lesion (45340)

🔲 4.86   🔲 88.4   **FUD** 000   T G2 🔲

AMA: 2016,Feb,13; 2016,Jan,13; 2015,Jan,16; 2014,Dec,3

▲ **45340** **with transendoscopic balloon dilation**

EXCLUDES *Sigmoidoscopy, flexible (45330, [45346], 45347)*

Code also each additional stricture dilated in same session, using modifier 59 with (45340)

🔲 (74360)

🔲 2.43   🔲 13.9   **FUD** 000   T A2 🔲

AMA: 2016,Feb,13; 2016,Jan,13; 2015,Jan,16; 2014,Dec,3; 2014,Dec,18; 2014,Jan,11; 2013,Dec,3; 2013,Jan,11-12

▲ **45341** **with endoscopic ultrasound examination**

INCLUDES Ultrasound, transrectal (76872)

EXCLUDES *Gastrointestinal endoscopic ultrasound, supervision and interpretation (76975)*

Procedure performed more than one time per operative session

Sigmoidoscopy, flexible (45330, 45342)

🔲 3.79   🔲 3.79   **FUD** 000   T A2 🔲

AMA: 2016,Feb,13; 2016,Jan,13; 2015,Jan,16; 2014,Dec,3; 2014,Dec,18; 2014,Jan,11; 2013,Dec,3; 2013,Jan,11-12

▲ **45342** **with transendoscopic ultrasound guided intramural or transmural fine needle aspiration/biopsy(s)**

INCLUDES Gastrointestinal endoscopic ultrasound, supervision and interpretation (76975)

Ultrasonic guidance (76942)

Ultrasound, transrectal (76872)

EXCLUDES *Sigmoidoscopy, flexible (45330, 45341)*

Procedure performed more than one time per operative session

🔲 5.14   🔲 5.14   **FUD** 000   T A2 🔲

AMA: 2016,Feb,13; 2016,Jan,13; 2015,Jan,16; 2014,Dec,3; 2014,Dec,18; 2014,Jan,11; 2013,Dec,3; 2013,Jan,11-12

45346 **Resequenced code. See code following 45338.**

▲ **45347** **with placement of endoscopic stent (includes pre- and post-dilation and guide wire passage, when performed)**

EXCLUDES *Sigmoidoscopy, flexible (45330, 45340)*

🔲 (74360)

🔲 4.69   🔲 4.69   **FUD** 000   J G2 🔲

AMA: 2016,Feb,13; 2016,Jan,13; 2015,Jan,16; 2014,Dec,3

▲ **45349** **with endoscopic mucosal resection**

EXCLUDES *Procedure performed on the same lesion with (45331, 45335, 45338, 45350)*

Sigmoidoscopy, flexible; diagnostic (45330)

🔲 5.97   🔲 5.97   **FUD** 000   T G2 🔲

AMA: 2016,Jan,13; 2015,Jan,16; 2014,Dec,3

▲ **45350** **with band ligation(s) (eg, hemorrhoids)**

EXCLUDES *Hemorrhoidectomy, internal, by rubber band ligation (46221)*

Procedure performed more than one time per operative session

Sigmoidoscopy, flexible; diagnostic (45330)

Sigmoidoscopy, flexible; with control of bleeding, same lesion (45334)

Sigmoidoscopy, flexible; with endoscopic mucosal resection (45349)

🔲 3.10   🔲 16.5   **FUD** 000   T G2 🔲

AMA: 2016,Jan,13; 2015,Jan,16; 2014,Dec,3

45378-45393 [45388, 45390, 45398] Flexible and Rigid Colonoscopy Procedures

INCLUDES Control of bleeding as result of the endoscopic procedure during same operative session

Exam of:
Entire colon (rectum to cecum)
Terminal ileum (when performed)

EXCLUDES *Computed tomographic colonography (74261-74263)*

Code also modifier 53 (physician), or 73, 74 (facility) for an incomplete colonoscopy

▲ **45378** **Colonoscopy, flexible; diagnostic, including collection of specimen(s) by brushing or washing, when performed (separate procedure)**

EXCLUDES *Colonoscopy, flexible (45379-45393 [45388, 45390, 45398])*

Decompression for pathological distention (45393)

Code also modifier 53 (physician), or 73, 74 (facility) for an incomplete colonoscopy

🔲 5.58   🔲 10.7   **FUD** 000   T A2 🔲

AMA: 2016,Jan,13; 2015,Sep,12; 2015,Jan,16; 2014,Dec,3; 2014,Nov,3; 2014,Jan,11; 2013,Dec,3; 2013,Jan,11-12; 2012,Jan,15-42; 2011,Apr,12

▲ **45379** **with removal of foreign body(s)**

EXCLUDES *Colonoscopy, flexible; diagnostic (45378)*

Code also modifier 52 when colonoscope fails to reach the junction of the small intestine

🔲 (76000)

🔲 7.18   🔲 13.5   **FUD** 000   T A2 🔲

AMA: 2016,Jan,13; 2015,Jan,16; 2014,Dec,3; 2014,Jan,11; 2013,Dec,3; 2013,Jan,11-12

▲ **45380** **with biopsy, single or multiple**

EXCLUDES *Colonoscopy, flexible; diagnostic (45378)*

Colonoscopy, flexible; with endoscopic mucosal resection on the same lesion (45390)

Code also modifier 52 when colonoscope fails to reach the junction of the small intestine

🔲 6.05   🔲 13.3   **FUD** 000   T A2 🔲

AMA: 2016,Jan,13; 2015,Jan,16; 2014,Dec,3; 2014,Jan,11; 2013,Dec,3; 2013,Jan,11-12; 2012,Jan,15-42; 2011,Jan,11

▲ **45381** **with directed submucosal injection(s), any substance**

EXCLUDES *Colonoscopy, flexible; diagnostic (45378)*

Colonoscopy, flexible; with control of bleeding on the same lesion (45382)

Colonoscopy, flexible; with endoscopic mucosal resection on the same lesion (45390)

Code also modifier 52 when colonoscope fails to reach the junction of the small intestine

🔲 6.05   🔲 12.8   **FUD** 000   T A2 🔲

AMA: 2016,Jan,13; 2015,Jan,16; 2014,Dec,3; 2014,Jan,11; 2013,Dec,3; 2013,Jan,11-12; 2012,Jan,15-42; 2011,Jan,11

▲ **45382** **with control of bleeding, any method**

EXCLUDES *Colonoscopy, flexible; diagnostic (45378)*

Colonoscopy, flexible; with band ligation on the same lesion ([45398])

Colonoscopy, flexible; with directed submucosal injection on the same lesion (45381)

Code also modifier 52 when colonoscope fails to reach the junction of the small intestine

🔲 7.78   🔲 22.5   **FUD** 000   T A2 🔲

AMA: 2016,Jan,13; 2015,Jan,16; 2014,Dec,3; 2014,Jan,11; 2013,Dec,3; 2013,Jan,11-12

▲ # **45388** **with ablation of tumor(s), polyp(s), or other lesion(s) (includes pre- and post-dilation and guide wire passage, when performed)**

EXCLUDES Colonoscopy, flexible (45378, 45386)

Code also modifier 53 (physician), or 73, 74 (facility) for an incomplete colonoscopy

🔧 8.11 ⚕ 92.9 **FUD** 000 T G2 ▢

AMA: 2016,Jan,13; 2015,Jan,16; 2014,Dec,3

▲ **45384** **with removal of tumor(s), polyp(s), or other lesion(s) by hot biopsy forceps**

EXCLUDES Colonoscopy, flexible; diagnostic (45378)

Code also modifier 52 when colonoscope fails to reach the junction of the small intestine

🔧 6.86 ⚕ 14.6 **FUD** 000 T A2 ▢

AMA: 2016,Jan,13; 2015,Jun,10; 2015,Jan,16; 2014,Dec,3; 2014,Jan,11; 2013,Dec,3; 2013,Jan,11-12; 2012,Jan,15-42; 2011,Apr,12; 2011,Jan,11

▲ **45385** **with removal of tumor(s), polyp(s), or other lesion(s) by snare technique**

EXCLUDES Colonoscopy, flexible; diagnostic (45378)
Colonoscopy, flexible; with endoscopic mucosal resection on the same lesion (45390)

🔧 7.64 ⚕ 13.9 **FUD** 000 T A2 ▢

AMA: 2016,Jan,13; 2015,Jan,16; 2014,Dec,3; 2014,Jan,11; 2013,Dec,3; 2013,Jan,11-12; 2012,Jan,15-42; 2011,Jan,11

▲ **45386** **with transendoscopic balloon dilation**

EXCLUDES Colonoscopy, flexible (45378, [45388], 45389)

Code also each additional stricture dilated in same operative session, using modifier 59 with (45386)

➕ (74360)

🔧 6.38 ⚕ 18.6 **FUD** 000 T A2 ▢

AMA: 2016,Jan,13; 2015,Jan,16; 2014,Dec,3; 2014,Jan,11; 2013,Dec,3; 2013,Jan,11-12

45388 **Resequenced code. See code following 45382.**

▲ **45389** **with endoscopic stent placement (includes pre- and post-dilation and guide wire passage, when performed)**

EXCLUDES Colonoscopy, flexible (45378, 45386)

➕ (74360)

🔧 8.68 ⚕ 8.68 **FUD** 000 J G2 ▢

AMA: 2016,Jan,13; 2015,Jan,16; 2014,Dec,3

45390 **Resequenced code. See code following 45392.**

▲ **45391** **with endoscopic ultrasound examination limited to the rectum, sigmoid, descending, transverse, or ascending colon and cecum, and adjacent structures**

INCLUDES Gastrointestinal endoscopic ultrasound, supervision and interpretation (76975)
Ultrasound, transrectal (76872)

EXCLUDES Colonoscopy, flexible (45378, 45392)
Procedure performed more than one time per operative session

🔧 7.73 ⚕ 7.73 **FUD** 000 T A2 ▢

AMA: 2016,Jan,13; 2015,Jan,16; 2014,Dec,3; 2014,Jan,11; 2013,Dec,3; 2013,Jan,11-12

▲ **45392** **with transendoscopic ultrasound guided intramural or transmural fine needle aspiration/biopsy(s), includes endoscopic ultrasound examination limited to the rectum, sigmoid, descending, transverse, or ascending colon and cecum, and adjacent structures**

INCLUDES Gastrointestinal endoscopic ultrasound, supervision and interpretation (76975)
Ultrasonic guidance (76942)
Ultrasound, transrectal (76872)

EXCLUDES Colonoscopy, flexible (45378, 45391)
Procedure performed more than one time per operative session

🔧 9.10 ⚕ 9.10 **FUD** 000 T A2 ▢

AMA: 2016,Jan,13; 2015,Jan,16; 2014,Dec,3; 2014,Jan,11; 2013,Dec,3; 2013,Jan,11-12

▲ # **45390** **with endoscopic mucosal resection**

EXCLUDES Colonoscopy, flexible; diagnostic (45378)
Colonoscopy, flexible; with band ligation on the same lesion ([45398])
Colonoscopy, flexible; with biopsy on the same lesion (45380-45381)
Colonoscopy, flexible; with removal of tumor(s), polyp(s), or other lesion(s) by snare technique on the same lesion (45385)

🔧 9.91 ⚕ 9.91 **FUD** 000 T G2 ▢

AMA: 2016,Jan,13; 2015,Jan,16; 2014,Dec,3

▲ **45393** **with decompression (for pathologic distention) (eg, volvulus, megacolon), including placement of decompression tube, when performed**

EXCLUDES Colonoscopy, flexible; diagnostic (45378)
Procedure performed more than one time per operative session

🔧 7.58 ⚕ 7.58 **FUD** 000 T G2 ▢

AMA: 2016,Jan,13; 2015,Jan,16; 2014,Dec,3

▲ # **45398** **with band ligation(s) (eg, hemorrhoids)**

EXCLUDES Bleeding control by band ligation (45382)
Colonoscopy, flexible (45378, 45390)
Hemorrhoidectomy, internal, by rubber band ligation (46221)
Procedure performed more than one time per operative session

Code also modifier 52 when colonoscope fails to reach the junction of the small intestine

🔧 7.06 ⚕ 20.7 **FUD** 000 T G2 ▢

AMA: 2016,Jan,13; 2015,Jan,16; 2014,Dec,3

45395-45499 Laparoscopic Procedures of Rectum

INCLUDES Diagnostic laparoscopy

45395 **Laparoscopy, surgical; proctectomy, complete, combined abdominoperineal, with colostomy**

EXCLUDES Open method (45110)

🔧 57.3 ⚕ 57.3 **FUD** 090 C 80 ▢

AMA: 2016,Jan,13; 2015,Jan,16; 2014,Jan,11; 2013,Jan,11-12

45397 **proctectomy, combined abdominoperineal pull-through procedure (eg, colo-anal anastomosis), with creation of colonic reservoir (eg, J-pouch), with diverting enterostomy, when performed**

EXCLUDES Open method (45119)

🔧 62.4 ⚕ 62.4 **FUD** 090 C 80 ▢

AMA: 2016,Jan,13; 2015,Jan,16; 2014,Jan,11; 2013,Jan,11-12; 2012,Jan,15-42; 2011,Jan,11

45398 **Resequenced code. See code following 45393.**

45399 **Resequenced code. See code before 45990.**

45400 **Laparoscopy, surgical; proctopexy (for prolapse)**

EXCLUDES Open method (45540-45541)

🔧 33.0 ⚕ 33.0 **FUD** 090 C 80 ▢

AMA: 2016,Jan,13; 2015,Jan,16; 2014,Jan,11; 2013,Jan,11-12

45402 **proctopexy (for prolapse), with sigmoid resection**

EXCLUDES Open method (45550)

🔧 44.0 ⚕ 44.0 **FUD** 090 C 80 ▢

AMA: 2016,Jan,13; 2015,Jan,16; 2014,Jan,11; 2013,Jan,11-12

45499 **Unlisted laparoscopy procedure, rectum**

EXCLUDES Unlisted rectal procedure performed via open technique (45999)

🔧 0.00 ⚕ 0.00 **FUD** YYY J 80

AMA: 2014,Jan,11; 2013,Jan,11-12

45500-45825 Open Repairs of Rectum

45500 **Proctoplasty; for stenosis**

🔧 15.0 ⚕ 15.0 **FUD** 090 T A2 80 ▢

AMA: 2014,Jan,11; 2013,Jan,11-12

Digestive System

45505 — 46045

45505   for prolapse of mucous membrane
🔲 17.1   ⚖ 17.1   **FUD** 090   T A2 🔲
AMA: 2016,Jan,13; 2015,Mar,9; 2015,Jan,16; 2014,Jan,11;
2013,Oct,18; 2013,Jan,11-12

45520   Perirectal injection of sclerosing solution for prolapse
🔲 1.16   ⚖ 4.47   **FUD** 000   Q1 N1 🔲
AMA: 2016,Jan,13; 2015,Jan,16; 2014,Jan,11; 2013,Jan,11-12;
2012,Jan,15-42; 2011,Jan,11

45540   Proctopexy (eg, for prolapse); abdominal approach
EXCLUDES   *Laparoscopic method (45400)*
🔲 30.6   ⚖ 30.6   **FUD** 090   C 80 🔲
AMA: 2014,Jan,11; 2013,Jan,11-12

45541   perineal approach
🔲 27.3   ⚖ 27.3   **FUD** 090   T 62 80 🔲
AMA: 2014,Jan,11; 2013,Jan,11-12

45550   with sigmoid resection, abdominal approach
INCLUDES   Frickman proctopexy
EXCLUDES   *Laparoscopic method (45402)*
🔲 42.2   ⚖ 42.2   **FUD** 090   C 80 🔲
AMA: 2014,Jan,11; 2013,Jan,11-12

45560   Repair of rectocele (separate procedure)
EXCLUDES   *Posterior colporrhaphy with rectocele repair (57250)*
🔲 19.8   ⚖ 19.8   **FUD** 090   T A2 80 🔲
AMA: 2014,Jan,11; 2013,Jan,11-12

45562   Exploration, repair, and presacral drainage for rectal injury;
🔲 32.4   ⚖ 32.4   **FUD** 090   C 80 🔲
AMA: 2014,Jan,11; 2013,Jan,11-12

45563   with colostomy
INCLUDES   Maydl colostomy
🔲 47.8   ⚖ 47.8   **FUD** 090   C 80 🔲
AMA: 2014,Jan,11; 2013,Jan,11-12

45800   Closure of rectovesical fistula;
🔲 34.8   ⚖ 34.8   **FUD** 090   C 80 🔲
AMA: 2014,Jan,11; 2013,Jan,11-12

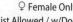

Bladder — Pubic symphysis — Urethra — Pubic symphysis — An anal fistula leading from the rectum to the skin near the anus contains a continual discharge that irritates the skin and causes discomfort or pain — Rectoperineal fistula — Rectum

45805   with colostomy
🔲 42.4   ⚖ 42.4   **FUD** 090   C 80 🔲
AMA: 2014,Jan,11; 2013,Jan,11-12

45820   Closure of rectourethral fistula;
EXCLUDES   *Closure of fistula, rectovaginal (57300-57308)*
🔲 34.4   ⚖ 34.4   **FUD** 090   C 80 🔲
AMA: 2014,Jan,11; 2013,Jan,11-12

45825   with colostomy
EXCLUDES   *Closure of fistula, rectovaginal (57300-57308)*
🔲 40.0   ⚖ 40.0   **FUD** 090   C 80 🔲
AMA: 2014,Jan,11; 2013,Jan,11-12

45900-45999 [45399] Closed Procedures of Rectum With Anesthesia

45900   Reduction of procidentia (separate procedure) under anesthesia
🔲 5.86   ⚖ 5.86   **FUD** 010   T A2 80 🔲
AMA: 2014,Jan,11; 2013,Jan,11-12

45905   Dilation of anal sphincter (separate procedure) under anesthesia other than local
🔲 4.89   ⚖ 4.89   **FUD** 010   T A2 🔲
AMA: 2014,Jan,11; 2013,Jan,11-12

45910   Dilation of rectal stricture (separate procedure) under anesthesia other than local
🔲 5.61   ⚖ 5.61   **FUD** 010   T A2 🔲
AMA: 2014,Jan,11; 2013,Jan,11-12

45915   Removal of fecal impaction or foreign body (separate procedure) under anesthesia
🔲 6.53   ⚖ 9.48   **FUD** 010   T A2 🔲
AMA: 2016,Jan,13; 2015,Jan,16; 2014,Jan,11; 2013,Jan,11-12;
2012,Jan,15-42; 2011,Jan,11

\#   **45399   Unlisted procedure, colon**
🔲 0.00   ⚖ 0.00   **FUD** XXX   T 🔲
AMA: 2016,Jan,13; 2015,Jan,16; 2014,Dec,3; 2014,Nov,3

45990   Anorectal exam, surgical, requiring anesthesia (general, spinal, or epidural), diagnostic
INCLUDES   Diagnostic:
Anoscopy
Proctoscopy, rigid
Exam:
Pelvic (when performed)
Perineal, external
Rectal, digital
EXCLUDES   *Anogenital examination (99170)*
Anoscopy; diagnostic (46600)
Pelvic examination under anesthesia (57410)
Proctosigmoidoscopy, rigid (45300-45327)
🔲 3.11   ⚖ 3.11   **FUD** 000   T A2 80 🔲
AMA: 2016,Jan,13; 2015,Jan,16; 2014,Jan,11; 2013,Jan,11-12;
2012,Jan,15-42; 2011,Jan,11

45999   Unlisted procedure, rectum
EXCLUDES   *Unlisted rectal procedure performed laparoscopically (45499)*
🔲 0.00   ⚖ 0.00   **FUD** YYY   T 80
AMA: 2016,Jan,13; 2015,Jan,16; 2014,Jan,11; 2013,Jan,11-12

46020-46083 Surgical Incision of Anus

EXCLUDES   *Cryosurgical destruction of hemorrhoid(s) (46999)*
Fistulotomy, subcutaneous (46270)
Hemorrhoidopexy ([46947])
Injection of hemorrhoid(s) (46500)
Thermal energy destruction of internal hemorrhoid(s) (46930)

46020   Placement of seton
EXCLUDES   *Anoscopy; diagnostic (46600)*
Incision and drainage of ischiorectal or intramural abscess (46060)
Ligation, hemorrhoidal vascular bundle (0249T)
Ligation, hemorrhoidal vascular bundle (46280)
🔲 6.76   ⚖ 7.92   **FUD** 010   T A2 🔲
AMA: 2014,Jan,11; 2013,Jan,11-12

46030   Removal of anal seton, other marker
🔲 2.60   ⚖ 3.98   **FUD** 010   T A2 80 🔲
AMA: 2014,Jan,11; 2013,Jan,11-12

46040   Incision and drainage of ischiorectal and/or perirectal abscess (separate procedure)
🔲 11.9   ⚖ 15.3   **FUD** 090   T A2 🔲
AMA: 2014,Jan,11; 2013,Jan,11-12

46045   Incision and drainage of intramural, intramuscular, or submucosal abscess, transanal, under anesthesia
🔲 12.5   ⚖ 12.5   **FUD** 090   T A2 🔲
AMA: 2014,Jan,11; 2013,Jan,11-12

46050 Incision and drainage, perianal abscess, superficial
> *EXCLUDES* *Incision and drainage abscess:*
> *Ischiorectal/intramural (46060)*
> *Supralevator/pelvirectal/retrorectal (45020)*
> 2.80 ☐ 5.74 **FUD** 010 ☐T☐A2☐
> **AMA:** 2014,Jan,11; 2013,Jan,11-12

46060 Incision and drainage of ischiorectal or intramural abscess, with fistulectomy or fistulotomy, submuscular, with or without placement of seton
> *EXCLUDES* *Incision and drainage abscess:*
> *Supralevator/pelvirectal/retrorectal (45020)*
> *Placement of seton (46020)*
> 13.7 ☐ 13.7 **FUD** 090 ☐T☐A2☐
> **AMA:** 2014,Jan,11; 2013,Jan,11-12

46070 Incision, anal septum (infant) ☐A
> *EXCLUDES* *Anoplasty (46700-46705)*
> 6.53 ☐ 6.53 **FUD** 090 ☐63☐T☐63☐80☐
> **AMA:** 2014,Jan,11; 2013,Jan,11-12

46080 Sphincterotomy, anal, division of sphincter (separate procedure)
> 4.60 ☐ 7.09 **FUD** 010 ☐T☐A2☐
> **AMA:** 2014,Jan,11; 2013,Jan,11-12

46083 Incision of thrombosed hemorrhoid, external
> 3.06 ☐ 5.02 **FUD** 010 ☐T☐P2☐
> **AMA:** 2016,Jan,13; 2015,Jan,16; 2014,Jan,11; 2013,Jan,11-12; 2012,Jan,15-42; 2011,Jan,11

46200-46262 [46220, 46320, 46945, 46946] Anal Resection and Hemorrhoidectomies

> *EXCLUDES* *Cryosurgical destruction of hemorrhoid(s) (46999)*
> *Hemorrhoidopexy ([46947])*
> *Injection of hemorrhoid(s) (46500)*
> *Thermal energy destruction of internal hemorrhoid(s) (46930)*

46200 Fissurectomy, including sphincterotomy, when performed
> 9.36 ☐ 12.7 **FUD** 090 ☐T☐A2☐
> **AMA:** 2014,Jan,11; 2013,Jan,11-12

46220 Resequenced code. See code before 46230.

46221 Hemorrhoidectomy, internal, by rubber band ligation(s)
> *EXCLUDES* *Colonoscopy or sigmoidoscopy, flexible; with band ligation (45350, [45398])*
> *Ligation of hemorrhoidal vascular bundles including ultrasound guidance (0249T)*
> 5.47 ☐ 7.65 **FUD** 010 ☐T☐P3☐
> **AMA:** 2016,Jan,13; 2015,Apr,10; 2015,Jan,16; 2014,Dec,3; 2014,Jan,11; 2013,Jan,11-12

\# **46945** Hemorrhoidectomy, internal, by ligation other than rubber band; single hemorrhoid column/group
> *EXCLUDES* *Other hemorrhoid procedures:*
> *Destruction (46930)*
> *Excision (46250-46262)*
> *Injection sclerosing solution (46500)*
> *Ligation, hemorrhoidal vascular bundle (0249T)*
> 6.49 ☐ 8.82 **FUD** 090 ☐T☐P3☐
> **AMA:** 2016,Jan,13; 2015,Apr,10; 2014,Jan,11; 2013,Jan,11-12

\# **46946** 2 or more hemorrhoid columns/groups
> *EXCLUDES* *Ligation, hemorrhoidal vascular bundle (0249T)*
> 6.48 ☐ 8.96 **FUD** 090 ☐T☐A2☐
> **AMA:** 2016,Jan,13; 2015,Apr,10; 2014,Jan,11; 2013,Jan,11-12

\# **46220** Excision of single external papilla or tag, anus
> 3.42 ☐ 5.88 **FUD** 010 ☐T☐A2☐
> **AMA:** 2014,Jan,11; 2013,Jan,11-12

46230 Excision of multiple external papillae or tags, anus
> 4.97 ☐ 7.80 **FUD** 010 ☐T☐A2☐
> **AMA:** 2014,Jan,11; 2013,Jan,11-12

\# **46320** Excision of thrombosed hemorrhoid, external
> 3.19 ☐ 5.24 **FUD** 010 ☐T☐P3☐
> **AMA:** 2014,Jan,11; 2013,Jan,11-12

46250 Hemorrhoidectomy, external, 2 or more columns/groups
> *EXCLUDES* *Hemorrhoidectomy, external, single column/group (46999)*
> *Ligation, hemorrhoidal vascular bundle (0249T)*
> 9.10 ☐ 13.2 **FUD** 090 ☐T☐A2☐
> **AMA:** 2014,Jan,11; 2013,Jan,11-12

46255 Hemorrhoidectomy, internal and external, single column/group;
> *EXCLUDES* *Ligation, hemorrhoidal vascular bundle (0249T)*
> 10.2 ☐ 14.5 **FUD** 090 ☐T☐A2☐
> **AMA:** 2016,Jan,13; 2015,Jan,16; 2014,Oct,14; 2014,Jan,11; 2013,Jan,11-12

46257 with fissurectomy
> *EXCLUDES* *Ligation, hemorrhoidal vascular bundle (0249T)*
> 12.1 ☐ 12.1 **FUD** 090 ☐T☐A2☐
> **AMA:** 2014,Jan,11; 2013,Jan,11-12

46258 with fistulectomy, including fissurectomy, when performed
> *EXCLUDES* *Ligation, hemorrhoidal vascular bundle (0249T)*
> 13.4 ☐ 13.4 **FUD** 090 ☐T☐A2☐80☐
> **AMA:** 2014,Jan,11; 2013,Jan,11-12

46260 Hemorrhoidectomy, internal and external, 2 or more columns/groups;
> *INCLUDES* *Whitehead hemorrhoidectomy*
> *EXCLUDES* *Ligation, hemorrhoidal vascular bundle (0249T)*
> 13.7 ☐ 13.7 **FUD** 090 ☐T☐A2☐
> **AMA:** 2014,Jan,11; 2013,Jan,11-12

46261 with fissurectomy
> *EXCLUDES* *Ligation, hemorrhoidal vascular bundle (0249T)*
> 15.0 ☐ 15.0 **FUD** 090 ☐T☐A2☐
> **AMA:** 2014,Jan,11; 2013,Jan,11-12

46262 with fistulectomy, including fissurectomy, when performed
> *EXCLUDES* *Ligation, hemorrhoidal vascular bundle (0249T)*
> 15.9 ☐ 15.9 **FUD** 090 ☐T☐A2☐
> **AMA:** 2016,Jan,13; 2015,Jan,16; 2014,Jan,11; 2013,Jan,11-12

46270-46320 Resection of Anal Fistula

46270 Surgical treatment of anal fistula (fistulectomy/fistulotomy); subcutaneous
> 11.3 ☐ 14.5 **FUD** 090 ☐T☐A2☐
> **AMA:** 2014,Jan,11; 2013,Jan,11-12

46275 intersphincteric
> 11.9 ☐ 15.3 **FUD** 090 ☐T☐A2☐
> **AMA:** 2014,Jan,11; 2013,Jan,11-12

46280 transsphincteric, suprasphincteric, extrasphincteric or multiple, including placement of seton, when performed
> *EXCLUDES* *Placement of seton (46020)*
> 13.5 ☐ 13.5 **FUD** 090 ☐T☐A2☐
> **AMA:** 2014,Jan,11; 2013,Jan,11-12

46285 second stage
> 11.8 ☐ 15.2 **FUD** 090 ☐T☐A2☐
> **AMA:** 2014,Jan,11; 2013,Jan,11-12

46288 Closure of anal fistula with rectal advancement flap
> 15.8 ☐ 15.8 **FUD** 090 ☐T☐A2☐
> **AMA:** 2014,Jan,11; 2013,Jan,11-12

46320 Resequenced code. See code following 46230.

Digestive System

46500 — 46730

46500 Other Hemorrhoid Procedures

EXCLUDES *Anoscopic injection of bulking agent, submucosal, for fecal incontinence (0377T)*

46500 **Injection of sclerosing solution, hemorrhoids**

🔧 3.54 ⚖ 5.55 **FUD** 010 T P3 ▢

AMA: 2016,Jan,13; 2015,Jan,16; 2014,Jan,11; 2013,Jan,11-12

Rectum

Valve cusps become incompetent in the varicose vein causing blood to pool

Anal sphincter

Internal hemorrhoid

External hemorrhoid

Thrombus (blood clot)

46505 Chemodenervation Anal Sphincter

EXCLUDES *Chemodenervation of:*
Extremity muscles (64642-64645)
Muscles/facial nerve (64612)
Neck muscles (64616)
Other peripheral nerve/branch (64640)
Pudendal nerve (64630)
Trunk muscles (64646-64647)
Code also drug(s)/substance(s) given

46505 **Chemodenervation of internal anal sphincter**

🔧 6.88 ⚖ 8.17 **FUD** 010 T G2 50 ▢

AMA: 2016,Jan,13; 2015,Jan,16; 2014,Jan,11; 2013,Jan,11-12

46600-46615 Anoscopic Procedures

INCLUDES Diagnostic endoscopy (49320)
EXCLUDES *Delivery of thermal energy via anoscope to the muscle of the anal canal (46999)*
Injection of bulking agent, submucosal, for fecal incontinence (0377T)

46600 **Anoscopy; diagnostic, including collection of specimen(s) by brushing or washing, when performed (separate procedure)**

EXCLUDES *Excision of rectal tumor, transanal endoscopic microsurgical approach (ie, TEMS) (0184T)*
High-resolution anoscopy (HRA), diagnostic (46601)
Ligation, hemorrhoidal vascular bundle (0249T)
Surgical incision of anus (46020-46762 [46220, 46320, 46945, 46946, 46947])

🔧 1.18 ⚖ 2.52 **FUD** 000 01 N1 ▢

AMA: 2016,Jan,13; 2015,Jan,16; 2014,Jan,11; 2013,Jan,11-12; 2012,Jan,15-42; 2011,Aug,9-10

46601 **diagnostic, with high-resolution magnification (HRA) (eg, colposcope, operating microscope) and chemical agent enhancement, including collection of specimen(s) by brushing or washing, when performed**

INCLUDES Operating microscope (69990)

🔧 2.70 ⚖ 3.90 **FUD** 000 01 N1 ▢

AMA: 2016,Feb,12

46604 **with dilation (eg, balloon, guide wire, bougie)**

🔧 1.92 ⚖ 17.5 **FUD** 000 T P3 ▢

AMA: 2016,Jan,13; 2015,Jan,16; 2014,Jan,11; 2013,Jan,11-12

46606 **with biopsy, single or multiple**

EXCLUDES *High resolution anoscopy (HRA) with biopsy (46607)*

🔧 2.20 ⚖ 6.43 **FUD** 000 T P3 ▢

AMA: 2016,Jan,13; 2015,Jan,16; 2014,Jan,11; 2013,Jan,11-12

46607 **with high-resolution magnification (HRA) (eg, colposcope, operating microscope) and chemical agent enhancement, with biopsy, single or multiple**

INCLUDES Operating microscope (69990)

🔧 3.64 ⚖ 5.46 **FUD** 000 T G2 ▢

AMA: 2016,Feb,12

46608 **with removal of foreign body**

🔧 2.34 ⚖ 6.61 **FUD** 000 T A2 ▢

AMA: 2016,Jan,13; 2015,Jan,16; 2014,Jan,11; 2013,Jan,11-12

46610 **with removal of single tumor, polyp, or other lesion by hot biopsy forceps or bipolar cautery**

🔧 2.34 ⚖ 6.44 **FUD** 000 T A2 ▢

AMA: 2016,Jan,13; 2015,Jan,16; 2014,Jan,11; 2013,Jan,11-12

46611 **with removal of single tumor, polyp, or other lesion by snare technique**

🔧 2.35 ⚖ 5.01 **FUD** 000 T A2 ▢

AMA: 2016,Jan,13; 2015,Jan,16; 2014,Jan,11; 2013,Jan,11-12

46612 **with removal of multiple tumors, polyps, or other lesions by hot biopsy forceps, bipolar cautery or snare technique**

🔧 2.70 ⚖ 7.34 **FUD** 000 T A2 ▢

AMA: 2016,Jan,13; 2015,Jan,16; 2014,Jan,11; 2013,Jan,11-12

46614 **with control of bleeding (eg, injection, bipolar cautery, unipolar cautery, laser, heater probe, stapler, plasma coagulator)**

🔧 1.87 ⚖ 3.66 **FUD** 000 T P3 ▢

AMA: 2016,Jan,13; 2015,Jan,16; 2014,Jan,11; 2013,Jan,11-12

46615 **with ablation of tumor(s), polyp(s), or other lesion(s) not amenable to removal by hot biopsy forceps, bipolar cautery or snare technique**

🔧 2.68 ⚖ 4.11 **FUD** 000 T A2 ▢

AMA: 2016,Jan,13; 2015,Jan,16; 2014,Jan,11; 2013,Jan,11-12

46700-46762 [46947] Anal Repairs and Stapled Hemorrhoidopexy

46700 **Anoplasty, plastic operation for stricture; adult**

🔧 18.8 ⚖ 18.8 **FUD** 090 T A2 ▢

AMA: 2014,Jan,11; 2013,Jan,11-12

46705 **infant**

EXCLUDES *Anal septum incision (46070)*

🔧 14.4 ⚖ 14.4 **FUD** 090 63 C 80 ▢

AMA: 2014,Jan,11; 2013,Jan,11-12

46706 **Repair of anal fistula with fibrin glue**

🔧 4.78 ⚖ 4.78 **FUD** 010 T A2 ▢

AMA: 2014,Jan,11; 2013,Jan,11-12

46707 **Repair of anorectal fistula with plug (eg, porcine small intestine submucosa [SIS])**

🔧 13.7 ⚖ 13.7 **FUD** 090 T G2 80 ▢

AMA: 2016,Jan,13; 2015,Jan,16; 2014,Jan,11; 2013,Oct,15; 2013,Jan,11-12; 2012,Jan,6-10

46710 **Repair of ileoanal pouch fistula/sinus (eg, perineal or vaginal), pouch advancement; transperineal approach**

🔧 30.3 ⚖ 30.3 **FUD** 090 C 80 ▢

AMA: 2016,Jan,13; 2015,Jan,16; 2014,Jan,11; 2013,Jan,11-12

46712 **combined transperineal and transabdominal approach**

🔧 61.8 ⚖ 61.8 **FUD** 090 C 80 ▢

AMA: 2016,Jan,13; 2015,Jan,16; 2014,Jan,11; 2013,Jan,11-12

46715 **Repair of low imperforate anus; with anoperineal fistula (cut-back procedure)**

🔧 15.6 ⚖ 15.6 **FUD** 090 63 C 80 ▢

AMA: 2014,Jan,11; 2013,Jan,11-12

46716 **with transposition of anoperineal or anovestibular fistula**

🔧 31.9 ⚖ 31.9 **FUD** 090 63 C 80 ▢

AMA: 2014,Jan,11; 2013,Jan,11-12

46730 **Repair of high imperforate anus without fistula; perineal or sacroperineal approach**

🔧 52.6 ⚖ 52.6 **FUD** 090 63 C 80 ▢

AMA: 2014,Jan,11; 2013,Jan,11-12

46735 combined transabdominal and sacroperineal approaches
🚗 60.9   ⚕ 60.9   **FUD** 090   ⑥³ Ⓒ 80 ▣
AMA: 2014,Jan,11; 2013,Jan,11-12

46740 Repair of high imperforate anus with rectourethral or rectovaginal fistula; perineal or sacroperineal approach
🚗 62.2   ⚕ 62.2   **FUD** 090   ⑥³ Ⓒ 80 ▣
AMA: 2014,Jan,11; 2013,Jan,11-12

46742 combined transabdominal and sacroperineal approaches
🚗 70.3   ⚕ 70.3   **FUD** 090   ⑥³ Ⓒ 80 ▣
AMA: 2014,Jan,11; 2013,Jan,11-12

46744 Repair of cloacal anomaly by anorectovaginoplasty and urethroplasty, sacroperineal approach   ♀
🚗 102.   ⚕ 102.   **FUD** 090   ⑥³ Ⓒ 80 ▣
AMA: 2014,Jan,11; 2013,Jan,11-12

46746 Repair of cloacal anomaly by anorectovaginoplasty and urethroplasty, combined abdominal and sacroperineal approach;   ♀
🚗 105.   ⚕ 105.   **FUD** 090   Ⓒ 80 ▣
AMA: 2014,Jan,11; 2013,Jan,11-12

46748 with vaginal lengthening by intestinal graft or pedicle flaps   ♀
🚗 114.   ⚕ 114.   **FUD** 090   Ⓒ 80 ▣
AMA: 2014,Jan,11; 2013,Jan,11-12

46750 Sphincteroplasty, anal, for incontinence or prolapse; adult
🚗 21.7   ⚕ 21.7   **FUD** 090   T A2 80 ▣
AMA: 2014,Jan,11; 2013,Jan,11-12

46751 child   Ⓐ
🚗 17.2   ⚕ 17.2   **FUD** 090   Ⓒ 80 ▣
AMA: 2014,Jan,11; 2013,Jan,11-12

46753 Graft (Thiersch operation) for rectal incontinence and/or prolapse
🚗 17.6   ⚕ 17.6   **FUD** 090   T A2 ▣
AMA: 2014,Jan,11; 2013,Jan,11-12

46754 Removal of Thiersch wire or suture, anal canal
🚗 6.55   ⚕ 8.36   **FUD** 010   T A2 80 ▣
AMA: 2014,Jan,11; 2013,Jan,11-12

46760 Sphincteroplasty, anal, for incontinence, adult; muscle transplant
🚗 31.4   ⚕ 31.4   **FUD** 090   T A2 80 ▣
AMA: 2014,Jan,11; 2013,Jan,11-12

46761 levator muscle imbrication (Park posterior anal repair)
🚗 26.6   ⚕ 26.6   **FUD** 090   T A2 80 ▣
AMA: 2014,Jan,11; 2013,Jan,11-12

46762 implantation artificial sphincter
EXCLUDES   *Anoscopic injection of bulking agent, submucosal, for fecal incontinence (0377T)*
🚗 26.7   ⚕ 26.7   **FUD** 090   J A2 80 ▣
AMA: 2014,Jan,11; 2013,Jan,11-12

\#   **46947** Hemorrhoidopexy (eg, for prolapsing internal hemorrhoids) by stapling
🚗 11.0   ⚕ 11.0   **FUD** 090   T A2 ▣
AMA: 2016,Jan,13; 2015,Jan,16; 2014,Jan,11; 2013,Jan,11-12; 2012,Jan,15-42; 2011,Jan,11

46900-46999 Destruction Procedures: Anus

46900 Destruction of lesion(s), anus (eg, condyloma, papilloma, molluscum contagiosum, herpetic vesicle), simple; chemical
🚗 3.95   ⚕ 6.91   **FUD** 010   T P2 ▣
AMA: 2014,Jan,11; 2013,Jan,11-12

46910 electrodesiccation
🚗 3.86   ⚕ 7.32   **FUD** 010   T P3 ▣
AMA: 2014,Jan,11; 2013,Jan,11-12

46916 cryosurgery
🚗 4.12   ⚕ 6.54   **FUD** 010   T P2 ▣
AMA: 2014,Jan,11; 2013,Jan,11-12

46917 laser surgery
🚗 3.79   ⚕ 12.8   **FUD** 010   T A2 ▣
AMA: 2014,Jan,11; 2013,Jan,11-12

46922 surgical excision
🚗 3.90   ⚕ 7.61   **FUD** 010   T A2 ▣
AMA: 2014,Jan,11; 2013,Jan,11-12

46924 Destruction of lesion(s), anus (eg, condyloma, papilloma, molluscum contagiosum, herpetic vesicle), extensive (eg, laser surgery, electrosurgery, cryosurgery, chemosurgery)
🚗 5.29   ⚕ 15.1   **FUD** 010   T A2 ▣
AMA: 2014,Jan,11; 2013,Jan,11-12

46930 Destruction of internal hemorrhoid(s) by thermal energy (eg, infrared coagulation, cautery, radiofrequency)
EXCLUDES   *Other hemorrhoid procedures:*
Cryosurgery destruction (46999)
Excision ([46320], 46250-46262)
Hemorrhoidopexy ([46947])
Incision (46083)
Injection sclerosing solution (46500)
Ligation (46221, [46945, 46946])
🚗 4.22   ⚕ 5.86   **FUD** 090   T P3 80 ▣
AMA: 2016,Jul,8; 2016,Jan,13; 2015,Apr,10; 2014,Jan,11; 2013,Jan,11-12

46940 Curettage or cautery of anal fissure, including dilation of anal sphincter (separate procedure); initial
🚗 4.22   ⚕ 6.52   **FUD** 010   T P3 ▣
AMA: 2014,Jan,11; 2013,Jan,11-12

46942 subsequent
🚗 3.78   ⚕ 6.16   **FUD** 010   T P3 80 ▣
AMA: 2014,Jan,11; 2013,Jan,11-12

46945 Resequenced code. See code following 46221.

46946 Resequenced code, See code following 46221.

46947 Resequenced code, See code following 46762.

46999 Unlisted procedure, anus
🚗 0.00   ⚕ 0.00   **FUD** YYY   T 80
AMA: 2016,Jan,13; 2015,Apr,10; 2015,Jan,16; 2014,Jan,11; 2013,Jan,11-12

47000-47001 Needle Biopsy of Liver

EXCLUDES   *Fine needle aspiration (10021, 10022)*

▲   **47000** Biopsy of liver, needle; percutaneous
▣ (76942, 77002, 77012, 77021)
◣ (88172-88173)
🚗 2.98   ⚕ 10.3   **FUD** 000   T A2 ▣
AMA: 2016,Jan,13; 2015,Jan,16; 2014,Jan,11; 2013,Jan,11-12; 2012,Jan,15-42; 2011,Jan,11

+   **47001** when done for indicated purpose at time of other major procedure (List separately in addition to code for primary procedure)
Code first primary procedure
▣ (76942, 77002)
◣ (88172-88173)
🚗 3.02   ⚕ 3.02   **FUD** ZZZ   N N1 ▣
AMA: 2016,Jan,13; 2015,Jan,16; 2014,Jan,11; 2013,Jan,11-12; 2012,Jan,15-42; 2011,Jan,11

47010-47130 Open Incisional and Resection Procedures of Liver

47010 Hepatotomy, for open drainage of abscess or cyst, 1 or 2 stages
EXCLUDES   *Image guided percutaneous catheter drainage (49505)*
🚗 34.9   ⚕ 34.9   **FUD** 090   Ⓒ 80 ▣
AMA: 2014,Jan,11; 2013,Nov,9; 2013,Jan,11-12

● New Code   ▲ Revised Code   ○ Reinstated   ● New Web Release   ▲ Revised Web Release   Unlisted   Not Covered   \# Resequenced
⊘ AMA Mod 51 Exempt   ⑤⓪ Optum Mod 51 Exempt   ⑥³ Mod 63 Exempt   ✎ Non-FDA Drug   ★ Telehealth   Ⓜ Maternity   Ⓐ Age Edit   ✛ Add-on   **AMA:** CPT Asst
© 2016 Optum360, LLC   CPT © 2016 American Medical Association. All Rights Reserved.   **203**

47015 Laparotomy, with aspiration and/or injection of hepatic parasitic (eg, amoebic or echinococcal) cyst(s) or abscess(es)

   33.1   33.1   **FUD** 090   C 80

   AMA: 2014,Jan,11; 2013,Jan,11-12

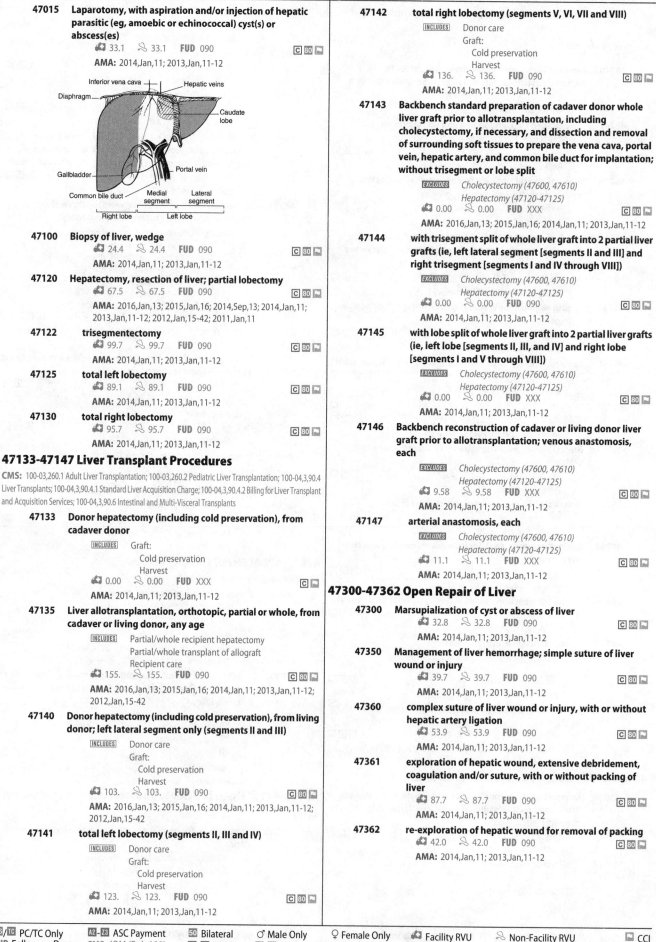

47100 Biopsy of liver, wedge

   24.4   24.4   **FUD** 090   C 80

   AMA: 2014,Jan,11; 2013,Jan,11-12

47120 Hepatectomy, resection of liver; partial lobectomy

   67.5   67.5   **FUD** 090   C 80

   AMA: 2016,Jan,13; 2015,Jan,16; 2014,Sep,13; 2014,Jan,11; 2013,Jan,11-12; 2012,Jan,15-42; 2011,Jan,11

47122 trisegmentectomy

   99.7   99.7   **FUD** 090   C 80

   AMA: 2014,Jan,11; 2013,Jan,11-12

47125 total left lobectomy

   89.1   89.1   **FUD** 090   C 80

   AMA: 2014,Jan,11; 2013,Jan,11-12

47130 total right lobectomy

   95.7   95.7   **FUD** 090   C 80

   AMA: 2014,Jan,11; 2013,Jan,11-12

47133-47147 Liver Transplant Procedures

CMS: 100-03,260.1 Adult Liver Transplantation; 100-03,260.2 Pediatric Liver Transplantation; 100-04,3,90.4 Liver Transplants; 100-04,3,90.4.1 Standard Liver Acquisition Charge; 100-04,3,90.4.2 Billing for Liver Transplant and Acquisition Services; 100-04,3,90.6 Intestinal and Multi-Visceral Transplants

47133 Donor hepatectomy (including cold preservation), from cadaver donor

   INCLUDES   Graft:
          Cold preservation
          Harvest

   0.00   0.00   **FUD** XXX   C

   AMA: 2014,Jan,11; 2013,Jan,11-12

47135 Liver allotransplantation, orthotopic, partial or whole, from cadaver or living donor, any age

   INCLUDES   Partial/whole recipient hepatectomy
          Partial/whole transplant of allograft
          Recipient care

   155.   155.   **FUD** 090   C 80

   AMA: 2016,Jan,13; 2015,Jan,16; 2014,Jan,11; 2013,Jan,11-12; 2012,Jan,15-42

47140 Donor hepatectomy (including cold preservation), from living donor; left lateral segment only (segments II and III)

   INCLUDES   Donor care
          Graft:
             Cold preservation
             Harvest

   103.   103.   **FUD** 090   C 80

   AMA: 2016,Jan,13; 2015,Jan,16; 2014,Jan,11; 2013,Jan,11-12; 2012,Jan,15-42

47141 total left lobectomy (segments II, III and IV)

   INCLUDES   Donor care
          Graft:
             Cold preservation
             Harvest

   123.   123.   **FUD** 090   C 80

   AMA: 2014,Jan,11; 2013,Jan,11-12

47142 total right lobectomy (segments V, VI, VII and VIII)

   INCLUDES   Donor care
          Graft:
             Cold preservation
             Harvest

   136.   136.   **FUD** 090   C 80

   AMA: 2014,Jan,11; 2013,Jan,11-12

47143 Backbench standard preparation of cadaver donor whole liver graft prior to allotransplantation, including cholecystectomy, if necessary, and dissection and removal of surrounding soft tissues to prepare the vena cava, portal vein, hepatic artery, and common bile duct for implantation; without trisegment or lobe split

   EXCLUDES   Cholecystectomy (47600, 47610)
          Hepatectomy (47120-47125)

   0.00   0.00   **FUD** XXX   C 80

   AMA: 2016,Jan,13; 2015,Jan,16; 2014,Jan,11; 2013,Jan,11-12

47144 with trisegment split of whole liver graft into 2 partial liver grafts (ie, left lateral segment [segments II and III] and right trisegment [segments I and IV through VIII])

   EXCLUDES   Cholecystectomy (47600, 47610)
          Hepatectomy (47120-47125)

   0.00   0.00   **FUD** 090   C 80

   AMA: 2014,Jan,11; 2013,Jan,11-12

47145 with lobe split of whole liver graft into 2 partial liver grafts (ie, left lobe [segments II, III, and IV] and right lobe [segments I and V through VIII])

   EXCLUDES   Cholecystectomy (47600, 47610)
          Hepatectomy (47120-47125)

   0.00   0.00   **FUD** XXX   C 80

   AMA: 2014,Jan,11; 2013,Jan,11-12

47146 Backbench reconstruction of cadaver or living donor liver graft prior to allotransplantation; venous anastomosis, each

   EXCLUDES   Cholecystectomy (47600, 47610)
          Hepatectomy (47120-47125)

   9.58   9.58   **FUD** XXX   C 80

   AMA: 2014,Jan,11; 2013,Jan,11-12

47147 arterial anastomosis, each

   EXCLUDES   Cholecystectomy (47600, 47610)
          Hepatectomy (47120-47125)

   11.1   11.1   **FUD** XXX   C 80

   AMA: 2014,Jan,11; 2013,Jan,11-12

47300-47362 Open Repair of Liver

47300 Marsupialization of cyst or abscess of liver

   32.8   32.8   **FUD** 090   C 80

   AMA: 2014,Jan,11; 2013,Jan,11-12

47350 Management of liver hemorrhage; simple suture of liver wound or injury

   39.7   39.7   **FUD** 090   C 80

   AMA: 2014,Jan,11; 2013,Jan,11-12

47360 complex suture of liver wound or injury, with or without hepatic artery ligation

   53.9   53.9   **FUD** 090   C 80

   AMA: 2014,Jan,11; 2013,Jan,11-12

47361 exploration of hepatic wound, extensive debridement, coagulation and/or suture, with or without packing of liver

   87.7   87.7   **FUD** 090   C 80

   AMA: 2014,Jan,11; 2013,Jan,11-12

47362 re-exploration of hepatic wound for removal of packing

   42.0   42.0   **FUD** 090   C 80

   AMA: 2014,Jan,11; 2013,Jan,11-12

26/TC PC/TC Only   A2-Z3 ASC Payment   50 Bilateral   ♂ Male Only   ♀ Female Only   Facility RVU   Non-Facility RVU   CCI
FUD Follow-up Days   **CMS:** IOM (Pub 100)   A-Y OPPSI   80/80 Surg Assist Allowed / w/Doc   Lab Crosswalk   Radiology Crosswalk   CLIA

204

CPT © 2016 American Medical Association. All Rights Reserved.

© 2016 Optum360, LLC

47370-47379 Laparoscopic Ablation Liver Tumors

INCLUDES Diagnostic laparoscopy (49320)

47370 Laparoscopy, surgical, ablation of 1 or more liver tumor(s); radiofrequency
(76940)
36.1 36.1 **FUD** 090 J 80
AMA: 2016,Jan,13; 2015,Jan,16; 2014,Jan,11; 2013,Jan,11-12

47371 cryosurgical
(76940)
32.7 32.7 **FUD** 090 J 80
AMA: 2014,Jan,11; 2013,Jan,11-12

47379 Unlisted laparoscopic procedure, liver
0.00 0.00 **FUD** YYY J 80
AMA: 2016,Jan,13; 2015,Jan,16; 2014,Dec,18; 2014,Jan,11; 2013,Jan,11-12; 2012,Jan,15-42; 2011,Jan,11

47380-47399 Open/Percutaneous Ablation Liver Tumors

47380 Ablation, open, of 1 or more liver tumor(s); radiofrequency
(76940)
41.8 41.8 **FUD** 090 C 80
AMA: 2016,Jan,13; 2015,Jan,16; 2014,Jan,11; 2013,Jan,11-12

47381 cryosurgical
(76940)
38.6 38.6 **FUD** 090 C 80
AMA: 2014,Jan,11; 2013,Jan,11-12

▲ **47382** Ablation, 1 or more liver tumor(s), percutaneous, radiofrequency
(76940, 77013, 77022)
22.3 142. **FUD** 010 T 62
AMA: 2016,Jan,13; 2015,Jan,16; 2014,Jan,11; 2013,Jan,11-12

▲ **47383** Ablation, 1 or more liver tumor(s), percutaneous, cryoablation
(76940, 77013, 77022)
14.2 214. **FUD** 010 T 62
AMA: 2016,Jan,13; 2015,Jan,16; 2014,Dec,18

47399 Unlisted procedure, liver
0.00 0.00 **FUD** YYY T
AMA: 2016,Jan,13; 2015,Jan,16; 2014,Dec,18; 2014,Jan,11; 2013,Jan,11-12

47400-47490 Biliary Tract Procedures

47400 Hepaticotomy or hepaticostomy with exploration, drainage, or removal of calculus
62.4 62.4 **FUD** 090 C 80
AMA: 2014,Jan,11; 2013,Jan,11-12

47420 Choledochotomy or choledochostomy with exploration, drainage, or removal of calculus, with or without cholecystotomy; without transduodenal sphincterotomy or sphincteroplasty
38.9 38.9 **FUD** 090 C 80
AMA: 2014,Jan,11; 2013,Jan,11-12

47425 with transduodenal sphincterotomy or sphincteroplasty
39.2 39.2 **FUD** 090 C 80
AMA: 2014,Jan,11; 2013,Jan,11-12

47460 Transduodenal sphincterotomy or sphincteroplasty, with or without transduodenal extraction of calculus (separate procedure)
36.3 36.3 **FUD** 090 C 80
AMA: 2014,Jan,11; 2013,Jan,11-12

47480 Cholecystotomy or cholecystostomy, open, with exploration, drainage, or removal of calculus (separate procedure)
EXCLUDES Percutaneous cholecystostomy (47490)
25.3 25.3 **FUD** 090 C 80
AMA: 2016,Jan,13; 2015,Jan,16; 2014,Jan,11; 2013,Jan,11-12; 2012,Jan,15-42; 2011,Apr,12

R. hepatic duct
Gallbladder
L. hepatic duct
Common hepatic duct
Drainage tube
Cystic duct
Common bile duct (choledochus)
Calculi (stones) are removed if present

47490 Cholecystostomy, percutaneous, complete procedure, including imaging guidance, catheter placement, cholecystogram when performed, and radiological supervision and interpretation
INCLUDES Radiological guidance (75989, 76942, 77002, 77012, 77021)
EXCLUDES Injection procedure for cholangiography (47531-47532)
Open cholecystostomy (47480)
9.60 9.60 **FUD** 010 T
AMA: 2016,Jan,13; 2015,Dec,3; 2015,Jan,16; 2014,Jan,11; 2013,Nov,9; 2013,Jan,11-12; 2012,Jan,15-42; 2011,Apr,12

47531-47532 Injection/Insertion Procedures of Biliary Tract

INCLUDES Contrast material injection
Radiologic supervision and interpretation
EXCLUDES Intraoperative cholangiography (74300-74301)
Procedures performed via the same access (47490, 47533-47541)

47531 Injection procedure for cholangiography, percutaneous, complete diagnostic procedure including imaging guidance (eg, ultrasound and/or fluoroscopy) and all associated radiological supervision and interpretation; existing access
2.78 10.5 **FUD** 000 02 N1
AMA: 2015,Dec,3

▲ **47532** new access (eg, percutaneous transhepatic cholangiogram)
6.27 23.3 **FUD** 000 02 N1
AMA: 2015,Dec,3

47533-47544 Percutaneous Procedures of the Biliary Tract

▲ **47533** Placement of biliary drainage catheter, percutaneous, including diagnostic cholangiography when performed, imaging guidance (eg, ultrasound and/or fluoroscopy), and all associated radiological supervision and interpretation; external
EXCLUDES Conversion to internal-external drainage catheter (47535)
Percutaneous placement stent in bile duct (47538)
Placement stent into bile duct, new access (47540)
Replacement existing internal drainage catheter (47536)
8.88 38.0 **FUD** 000 T 62
AMA: 2015,Dec,3

▲ **47534** internal-external
EXCLUDES Conversion to external only drainage catheter (47536)
Percutaneous placement stent in bile duct (47538)
Placement stent into bile duct, new access (47540)
11.7 46.8 **FUD** 000 T 62
AMA: 2015,Dec,3

▲ **47535** **Conversion of external biliary drainage catheter to internal-external biliary drainage catheter, percutaneous, including diagnostic cholangiography when performed, imaging guidance (eg, fluoroscopy), and all associated radiological supervision and interpretation**
🚑 6.78   ⚖ 31.4   **FUD** 000   T 62 ▢
AMA: 2015,Dec,3

▲ **47536** **Exchange of biliary drainage catheter (eg, external, internal-external, or conversion of internal-external to external only), percutaneous, including diagnostic cholangiography when performed, imaging guidance (eg, fluoroscopy), and all associated radiological supervision and interpretation**
INCLUDES   Exchange of one drainage catheter
EXCLUDES   Placement of stent(s) into a bile duct, percutaneous (47538)
Code also exchange of additional catheters in same session with modifier 59 (47536)
🚑 4.28   ⚖ 23.2   **FUD** 000   T 62 ▢
AMA: 2015,Dec,3

47537 **Removal of biliary drainage catheter, percutaneous, requiring fluoroscopic guidance (eg, with concurrent indwelling biliary stents), including diagnostic cholangiography when performed, imaging guidance (eg, fluoroscopy), and all associated radiological supervision and interpretation**
EXCLUDES   Placement of stent(s) into a bile duct via the same access (47538)
Removal without use of fluoroscopic guidance; report with appropriate E&M service code
🚑 2.89   ⚖ 11.4   **FUD** 000   02 62 ▢
AMA: 2015,Dec,3

▲ **47538** **Placement of stent(s) into a bile duct, percutaneous, including diagnostic cholangiography, imaging guidance (eg, fluoroscopy and/or ultrasound), balloon dilation, catheter exchange(s) and catheter removal(s) when performed, and all associated radiological supervision and interpretation; existing access**
EXCLUDES   Drainage catheter inserted following stent placement (47536)
Procedures performed via the same access (47536-47537)
Treatment of same lesion in same operative session ([43277], 47542, 47555-47556)
Code also multiple stents placed during same session when: (47538-47540)
Serial stents placed within the same bile duct;
Stent placement via two or more percutaneous access sites or the space between two other stents
Two or more stents inserted through the same percutaneous access
🚑 9.55   ⚖ 128.   **FUD** 000   T 62 ▢
AMA: 2016,Mar,10; 2015,Dec,3

▲ **47539** **new access, without placement of separate biliary drainage catheter**
EXCLUDES   Treatment of same lesion in same session ([43277], 47542, 47555-47556)
Code also multiple stents placed during same session when: (47538-47540)
Serial stents placed within the same bile duct
Stent placement via two or more percutaneous access sites or the space between two other stents
Two or more stents inserted through the same percutaneous access
🚑 12.9   ⚖ 139.   **FUD** 000   T 62 ▢
AMA: 2016,Mar,10; 2015,Dec,3

▲ **47540** **new access, with placement of separate biliary drainage catheter (eg, external or internal-external)**
EXCLUDES   Procedure performed via the same access (47533-47534)
Treatment of same lesion in same session ([43277], 47542, 47555-47556)
Code also multiple stents placed during same session when: (47538-47540)
Serial stents placed within the same bile duct;
Stent placement via two or more percutaneous access sites or the space between two other stents;
Two or more stents inserted through the same percutaneous access
🚑 15.4   ⚖ 145.   **FUD** 000   T 62 ▢
AMA: 2016,Mar,10; 2015,Dec,3

▲ **47541** **Placement of access through the biliary tree and into small bowel to assist with an endoscopic biliary procedure (eg, rendezvous procedure), percutaneous, including diagnostic cholangiography when performed, imaging guidance (eg, ultrasound and/or fluoroscopy), and all associated radiological supervision and interpretation, new access**
EXCLUDES   Access through biliary tree into small bowel for endoscopic biliary procedure (47535-47537)
Conversion, exchange, or removal of external biliary drainage catheter (47535-47537)
Injection procedure for cholangiography (47531-47532)
Placement of biliary drainage catheter (47533-47534)
Placement of stent(s) into a bile duct (47538-47540)
Procedure performed when previous catheter access exists
🚑 8.21   ⚖ 33.5   **FUD** 000   T 62 ▢
AMA: 2015,Dec,3

▲ + **47542** **Balloon dilation of biliary duct(s) or of ampulla (sphincteroplasty), percutaneous, including imaging guidance (eg, fluoroscopy), and all associated radiological supervision and interpretation, each duct (List separately in addition to code for primary procedure)**
EXCLUDES   Biliary endoscopy, with dilation of biliary duct stricture (47555-47556)
Endoscopic balloon dilation ([43277], 47555-47556)
Endoscopic retrograde cholangiopancreatography (ERCP) (43262, [43277])
Placement of stent(s) into a bile duct (47538-47540)
Procedure performed with balloon used to remove calculi, debris, sludge without dilation (47544)
Code also one additional dilation code when more than one dilation performed in same session, using modifier 59 with (47542)
Code first (47531-47537, 47541)
🚑 3.88   ⚖ 14.7   **FUD** ZZZ   N N1 ▢
AMA: 2015,Dec,3

▲ + **47543** **Endoluminal biopsy(ies) of biliary tree, percutaneous, any method(s) (eg, brush, forceps, and/or needle), including imaging guidance (eg, fluoroscopy), and all associated radiological supervision and interpretation, single or multiple (List separately in addition to code for primary procedure)**
EXCLUDES   Endoscopic biopsy (46261, 47553)
Endoscopic brushings (43260, 47552)
Procedure performed more than one time per session
Code first (47531-47540)
🚑 4.88   ⚖ 37.7   **FUD** ZZZ   N N1 ▢
AMA: 2015,Dec,3

▲ + **47544** Removal of calculi/debris from biliary duct(s) and/or gallbladder, percutaneous, including destruction of calculi by any method (eg, mechanical, electrohydraulic, lithotripsy) when performed, imaging guidance (eg, fluoroscopy), and all associated radiological supervision and interpretation (List separately in addition to code for primary procedure)

EXCLUDES *Device deployment without findings of calculi/debris*
Endoscopic calculi removal/destruction (43264-43265, 47554)
Endoscopic retrograde cholangiopancreatography (ERCP); with removal of calculi/debris from biliary/pancreatic duct(s) (43264)
Procedures with removal of incidental debris (47531-47543)

Code first when debris removal not incidental, as appropriate (47531-47540)

⚙ 6.25   ⚕ 23.2   **FUD** ZZZ   Ⓝ N1 ⌷

AMA: 2015,Dec,3

47550-47556 Endoscopic Procedures of the Biliary Tract

INCLUDES Diagnostic endoscopy (49320)
EXCLUDES *Endoscopic retrograde cholangiopancreatography (ERCP) (43260-43265, [43274], [43275], [43276], [43277], [43278], 74328-74330, 74363)*

+ **47550** Biliary endoscopy, intraoperative (choledochoscopy) (List separately in addition to code for primary procedure)
Code first primary procedure
⚙ 4.82   ⚕ 4.82   **FUD** ZZZ   Ⓒ 80 ⌷
AMA: 2014,Jan,11; 2013,Jan,11-12

47552 Biliary endoscopy, percutaneous via T-tube or other tract; diagnostic, with collection of specimen(s) by brushing and/or washing, when performed (separate procedure)
⚙ 9.04   ⚕ 9.04   **FUD** 000   Ⓣ A2 ⌷
AMA: 2016,Jan,13; 2015,Dec,3; 2015,Jan,16; 2014,Jan,11; 2013,Jan,11-12; 2012,Jan,15-42; 2011,Jan,11

47553 with biopsy, single or multiple
⚙ 8.92   ⚕ 8.92   **FUD** 000   Ⓣ A2 ⌷
AMA: 2016,Jan,13; 2015,Dec,3; 2015,Jan,16; 2014,Jan,11; 2013,Jan,11-12; 2012,Jan,15-42; 2011,Jan,11

47554 with removal of calculus/calculi
⚙ 13.8   ⚕ 13.8   **FUD** 000   Ⓣ A2 ⌷
AMA: 2016,Jan,13; 2015,Dec,3; 2015,Jan,16; 2014,Jan,11; 2013,Jan,11-12; 2012,Jan,15-42; 2011,Jan,11

47555 with dilation of biliary duct stricture(s) without stent
🔧 (74363)
⚙ 10.6   ⚕ 10.6   **FUD** 000   Ⓣ A2 ⌷
AMA: 2016,Jan,13; 2015,Dec,3; 2015,Jan,16; 2014,Jan,11; 2013,Jan,11-12; 2012,Jan,15-42; 2011,Jan,11

47556 with dilation of biliary duct stricture(s) with stent
🔧 (74363)
⚙ 12.1   ⚕ 12.1   **FUD** 000   Ⓣ A2 ⌷
AMA: 2016,Jan,13; 2015,Dec,3; 2015,Jan,16; 2014,Jan,11; 2013,Jan,11-12; 2012,Jan,15-42; 2011,Jan,11

47562-47579 Laparoscopic Gallbladder Procedures

INCLUDES Diagnostic laparoscopy (49320)

47562 Laparoscopy, surgical; cholecystectomy
⚙ 19.0   ⚕ 19.0   **FUD** 090   Ⓙ 62 80 ⌷
AMA: 2016,Jan,13; 2015,Jan,16; 2014,Jan,11; 2013,Jan,11-12; 2012,Jan,15-42; 2011,Jan,11

47563 cholecystectomy with cholangiography
EXCLUDES *Percutaneous cholangiography (47531-47532)*
Code also intraoperative radiology supervision and interpretation (74300-74301)
⚙ 20.7   ⚕ 20.7   **FUD** 090   Ⓙ 62 80 ⌷
AMA: 2016,Jan,13; 2015,Jan,16; 2014,Jan,11; 2013,Jan,11-12; 2012,Jan,15-42; 2011,Jan,11

47564 cholecystectomy with exploration of common duct
⚙ 32.2   ⚕ 32.2   **FUD** 090   Ⓙ 62 80 ⌷
AMA: 2016,Jan,13; 2015,Jan,16; 2014,Jan,11; 2013,Jan,11-12; 2012,Jan,15-42; 2011,Jan,11

47570 cholecystoenterostomy
⚙ 22.1   ⚕ 22.1   **FUD** 090   Ⓒ 80 ⌷
AMA: 2016,Jan,13; 2015,Jan,16; 2014,Jan,11; 2013,Jan,11-12

47579 Unlisted laparoscopy procedure, biliary tract
⚙ 0.00   ⚕ 0.00   **FUD** YYY   Ⓙ 80 50
AMA: 2016,Jan,13; 2015,Jan,16; 2014,Jan,11; 2013,Jan,11-12

47600-47620 Open Gallbladder Procedures

47600 Cholecystectomy;
EXCLUDES *Laparoscopic method (47562-47564)*
⚙ 30.9   ⚕ 30.9   **FUD** 090   Ⓒ 80 ⌷
AMA: 2016,Jan,13; 2015,Jan,16; 2014,Jan,11; 2013,Jan,11-12

47605 with cholangiography
EXCLUDES *Laparoscopic method (47563-47564)*
⚙ 32.5   ⚕ 32.5   **FUD** 090   Ⓒ 80 ⌷
AMA: 2016,Jan,13; 2015,Jan,16; 2014,Jan,11; 2013,Jan,11-12; 2012,Jan,15-42; 2011,Jan,11

47610 Cholecystectomy with exploration of common duct;
EXCLUDES *Laparoscopic method (47564)*
Code also biliary endoscopy when performed in conjunction with cholecystectomy with exploration of common duct (47550)
⚙ 36.3   ⚕ 36.3   **FUD** 090   Ⓒ 80 ⌷
AMA: 2016,Jan,13; 2015,Jan,16; 2014,Jan,11; 2013,Jan,11-12; 2012,Jan,15-42; 2011,Jan,11

47612 with choledochoenterostomy
⚙ 36.8   ⚕ 36.8   **FUD** 090   Ⓒ 80 ⌷
AMA: 2014,Jan,11; 2013,Jan,11-12

47620 with transduodenal sphincterotomy or sphincteroplasty, with or without cholangiography
⚙ 39.9   ⚕ 39.9   **FUD** 090   Ⓒ 80 ⌷
AMA: 2014,Jan,11; 2013,Jan,11-12

47700-47999 Open Resection and Repair of Biliary Tract

47700 Exploration for congenital atresia of bile ducts, without repair, with or without liver biopsy, with or without cholangiography
⚙ 30.1   ⚕ 30.1   **FUD** 090   63 Ⓒ 80 ⌷
AMA: 2014,Jan,11; 2013,Jan,11-12

47701 Portoenterostomy (eg, Kasai procedure)
⚙ 49.2   ⚕ 49.2   **FUD** 090   63 Ⓒ 80 ⌷
AMA: 2014,Jan,11; 2013,Jan,11-12

47711 Excision of bile duct tumor, with or without primary repair of bile duct; extrahepatic
EXCLUDES *Anastomosis (47760-47800)*
⚙ 45.1   ⚕ 45.1   **FUD** 090   Ⓒ 80 ⌷
AMA: 2014,Jan,11; 2013,Jan,11-12

47712 intrahepatic
EXCLUDES *Anastomosis (47760-47800)*
⚙ 57.7   ⚕ 57.7   **FUD** 090   Ⓒ 80 ⌷
AMA: 2014,Jan,11; 2013,Jan,11-12

47715 **Excision of choledochal cyst**
🔧 38.6 ✂ 38.6 **FUD** 090 Ⓒ 80 ▢

AMA: 2016,Jan,13; 2015,Jan,16; 2014,Jan,11; 2013,Jan,11-12; 2012,Jan,15-42; 2011,Jan,11

47720 **Cholecystoenterostomy; direct**
EXCLUDES Laparoscopic method (47570)
🔧 33.3 ✂ 33.3 **FUD** 090 Ⓒ 80 ▢

AMA: 2016,Jan,13; 2015,Jan,16; 2014,Jan,11; 2013,Jan,11-12

47721 **with gastroenterostomy**
🔧 39.3 ✂ 39.3 **FUD** 090 Ⓒ 80 ▢

AMA: 2014,Jan,11; 2013,Jan,11-12

47740 **Roux-en-Y**
🔧 37.7 ✂ 37.7 **FUD** 090 Ⓒ 80 ▢

AMA: 2014,Jan,11; 2013,Jan,11-12

47741 **Roux-en-Y with gastroenterostomy**
🔧 42.6 ✂ 42.6 **FUD** 090 Ⓒ 80 ▢

AMA: 2014,Jan,11; 2013,Jan,11-12

47760 **Anastomosis, of extrahepatic biliary ducts and gastrointestinal tract**
🔧 65.5 ✂ 65.5 **FUD** 090 Ⓒ 80 ▢

AMA: 2014,Jan,11; 2013,Jan,11-12

47765 **Anastomosis, of intrahepatic ducts and gastrointestinal tract**
INCLUDES Longmire anastomosis
🔧 88.0 ✂ 88.0 **FUD** 090 Ⓒ 80 ▢

AMA: 2014,Jan,11; 2013,Jan,11-12

47780 **Anastomosis, Roux-en-Y, of extrahepatic biliary ducts and gastrointestinal tract**
🔧 71.7 ✂ 71.7 **FUD** 090 Ⓒ 80 ▢

AMA: 2014,Jan,11; 2013,Jan,11-12

47785 **Anastomosis, Roux-en-Y, of intrahepatic biliary ducts and gastrointestinal tract**
🔧 94.2 ✂ 94.2 **FUD** 090 Ⓒ 80 ▢

AMA: 2014,Jan,11; 2013,Jan,11-12

47800 **Reconstruction, plastic, of extrahepatic biliary ducts with end-to-end anastomosis**
🔧 45.6 ✂ 45.6 **FUD** 090 Ⓒ 80 ▢

AMA: 2014,Jan,11; 2013,Jan,11-12

47801 **Placement of choledochal stent**
🔧 28.9 ✂ 28.9 **FUD** 090 Ⓒ 80 ▢

AMA: 2016,Jan,13; 2015,Jan,16; 2014,Jan,11; 2013,Jan,11-12; 2012,Jan,15-42

47802 **U-tube hepaticoenterostomy**
🔧 43.8 ✂ 43.8 **FUD** 090 Ⓒ 80 ▢

AMA: 2014,Jan,11; 2013,Jan,11-12

47900 **Suture of extrahepatic biliary duct for pre-existing injury (separate procedure)**
🔧 39.7 ✂ 39.7 **FUD** 090 Ⓒ 80 ▢

AMA: 2014,Jan,11; 2013,Jan,11-12

47999 **Unlisted procedure, biliary tract**
🔧 0.00 ✂ 0.00 **FUD** YYY Ⓣ

AMA: 2016,Jan,13; 2015,Jan,16; 2014,Jan,11; 2013,Jan,11-12; 2012,Jan,15-42; 2011,May,9

48000-48548 Open Procedures of the Pancreas

EXCLUDES Peroral pancreatic procedures performed endoscopically (43260-43265, 43270 [43274, 43275, 43276, 43277, 43278])

48000 **Placement of drains, peripancreatic, for acute pancreatitis;**
🔧 54.2 ✂ 54.2 **FUD** 090 Ⓒ 80 ▢

AMA: 2014,Jan,11; 2013,Jan,11-12

Pancreas

48001 **with cholecystostomy, gastrostomy, and jejunostomy**
🔧 66.4 ✂ 66.4 **FUD** 090 Ⓒ 80 ▢

AMA: 2014,Jan,11; 2013,Jan,11-12

48020 **Removal of pancreatic calculus**
🔧 33.9 ✂ 33.9 **FUD** 090 Ⓒ 80 ▢

AMA: 2014,Jan,11; 2013,Jan,11-12

48100 **Biopsy of pancreas, open (eg, fine needle aspiration, needle core biopsy, wedge biopsy)**
🔧 25.7 ✂ 25.7 **FUD** 090 Ⓒ 80 ▢

AMA: 2014,Jan,11; 2013,Jan,11-12

48102 **Biopsy of pancreas, percutaneous needle**
EXCLUDES Aspiration, fine needle (10022)
📷 (76942, 77002, 77012, 77021)
🔬 (88172-88173)
🔧 7.03 ✂ 15.2 **FUD** 010 Ⓣ A2 ▢

AMA: 2014,Jan,11; 2013,Jan,11-12

48105 **Resection or debridement of pancreas and peripancreatic tissue for acute necrotizing pancreatitis**
🔧 82.7 ✂ 82.7 **FUD** 090 Ⓒ 80 ▢

AMA: 2014,Jan,11; 2013,Jan,11-12

48120 **Excision of lesion of pancreas (eg, cyst, adenoma)**
🔧 32.1 ✂ 32.1 **FUD** 090 Ⓒ 80 ▢

AMA: 2014,Jan,11; 2013,Jan,11-12

48140 **Pancreatectomy, distal subtotal, with or without splenectomy; without pancreaticojejunostomy**
🔧 45.3 ✂ 45.3 **FUD** 090 Ⓒ 80 ▢

AMA: 2014,Jan,11; 2013,Jan,11-12

48145 **with pancreaticojejunostomy**
🔧 47.1 ✂ 47.1 **FUD** 090 Ⓒ 80 ▢

AMA: 2014,Jan,11; 2013,Jan,11-12

26/TC PC/TC Only A2-Z3 ASC Payment 50 Bilateral ♂ Male Only ♀ Female Only 🔧 Facility RVU ✂ Non-Facility RVU ▢ CCI
FUD Follow-up Days CMS: IOM (Pub 100) A-Y OPPSI 80/80 Surg Assist Allowed / w/Doc 🔬 Lab Crosswalk 📷 Radiology Crosswalk ✖ CLIA

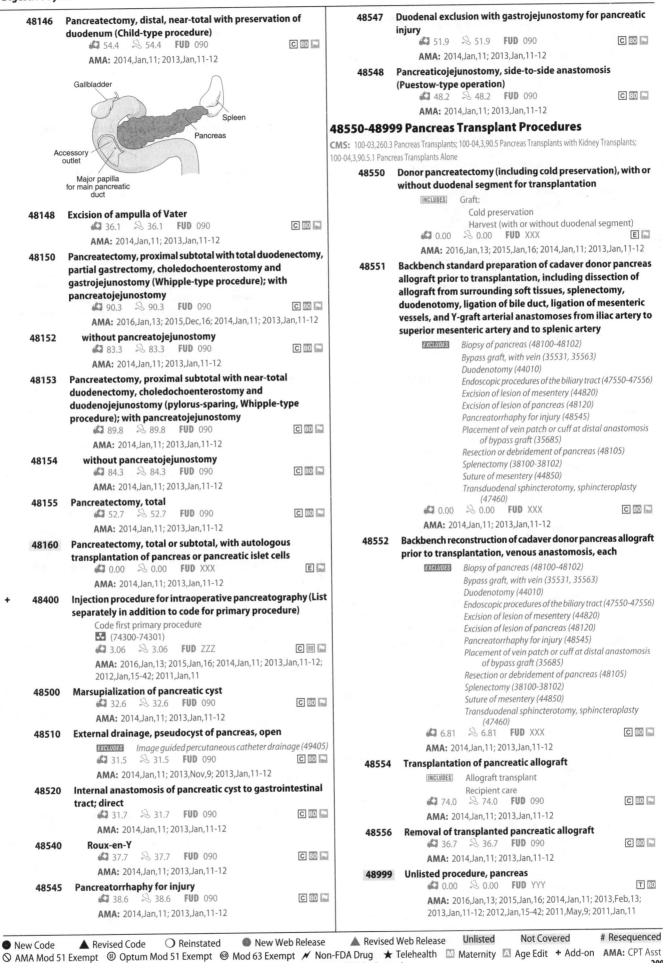

48146 Pancreatectomy, distal, near-total with preservation of duodenum (Child-type procedure)
54.4   54.4   **FUD** 090   C 80
AMA: 2014,Jan,11; 2013,Jan,11-12

Diagram labels: Gallbladder, Spleen, Pancreas, Accessory outlet, Major papilla for main pancreatic duct

48148 Excision of ampulla of Vater
36.1   36.1   **FUD** 090   C 80
AMA: 2014,Jan,11; 2013,Jan,11-12

48150 Pancreatectomy, proximal subtotal with total duodenectomy, partial gastrectomy, choledochoenterostomy and gastrojejunostomy (Whipple-type procedure); with pancreatojejunostomy
90.3   90.3   **FUD** 090   C 80
AMA: 2016,Jan,13; 2015,Dec,16; 2014,Jan,11; 2013,Jan,11-12

48152 without pancreatojejunostomy
83.3   83.3   **FUD** 090   C 80
AMA: 2014,Jan,11; 2013,Jan,11-12

48153 Pancreatectomy, proximal subtotal with near-total duodenectomy, choledochoenterostomy and duodenojejunostomy (pylorus-sparing, Whipple-type procedure); with pancreatojejunostomy
89.8   89.8   **FUD** 090   C 80
AMA: 2014,Jan,11; 2013,Jan,11-12

48154 without pancreatojejunostomy
84.3   84.3   **FUD** 090   C 80
AMA: 2014,Jan,11; 2013,Jan,11-12

48155 Pancreatectomy, total
52.7   52.7   **FUD** 090   C 80
AMA: 2014,Jan,11; 2013,Jan,11-12

48160 Pancreatectomy, total or subtotal, with autologous transplantation of pancreas or pancreatic islet cells
0.00   0.00   **FUD** XXX   E
AMA: 2014,Jan,11; 2013,Jan,11-12

+ **48400** Injection procedure for intraoperative pancreatography (List separately in addition to code for primary procedure)
Code first primary procedure
(74300-74301)
3.06   3.06   **FUD** ZZZ   C 80
AMA: 2016,Jan,13; 2015,Jan,16; 2014,Jan,11; 2013,Jan,11-12; 2012,Jan,15-42; 2011,Jan,11

48500 Marsupialization of pancreatic cyst
32.6   32.6   **FUD** 090   C 80
AMA: 2014,Jan,11; 2013,Jan,11-12

48510 External drainage, pseudocyst of pancreas, open
EXCLUDES Image guided percutaneous catheter drainage (49405)
31.5   31.5   **FUD** 090   C 80
AMA: 2014,Jan,11; 2013,Nov,9; 2013,Jan,11-12

48520 Internal anastomosis of pancreatic cyst to gastrointestinal tract; direct
31.7   31.7   **FUD** 090   C 80
AMA: 2014,Jan,11; 2013,Jan,11-12

48540 Roux-en-Y
37.7   37.7   **FUD** 090   C 80
AMA: 2014,Jan,11; 2013,Jan,11-12

48545 Pancreatorrhaphy for injury
38.6   38.6   **FUD** 090   C 80
AMA: 2014,Jan,11; 2013,Jan,11-12

48547 Duodenal exclusion with gastrojejunostomy for pancreatic injury
51.9   51.9   **FUD** 090   C 80
AMA: 2014,Jan,11; 2013,Jan,11-12

48548 Pancreaticojejunostomy, side-to-side anastomosis (Puestow-type operation)
48.2   48.2   **FUD** 090   C 80
AMA: 2014,Jan,11; 2013,Jan,11-12

48550-48999 Pancreas Transplant Procedures

CMS: 100-03,260.3 Pancreas Transplants; 100-04,3,90.5 Pancreas Transplants with Kidney Transplants; 100-04,3,90.5.1 Pancreas Transplants Alone

48550 Donor pancreatectomy (including cold preservation), with or without duodenal segment for transplantation
INCLUDES Graft:
    Cold preservation
    Harvest (with or without duodenal segment)
0.00   **FUD** XXX   E
AMA: 2016,Jan,13; 2015,Jan,16; 2014,Jan,11; 2013,Jan,11-12

48551 Backbench standard preparation of cadaver donor pancreas allograft prior to transplantation, including dissection of allograft from surrounding soft tissues, splenectomy, duodenotomy, ligation of bile duct, ligation of mesenteric vessels, and Y-graft arterial anastomoses from iliac artery to superior mesenteric artery and to splenic artery
EXCLUDES Biopsy of pancreas (48100-48102)
    Bypass graft, with vein (35531, 35563)
    Duodenotomy (44010)
    Endoscopic procedures of the biliary tract (47550-47556)
    Excision of lesion of mesentery (44820)
    Excision of lesion of pancreas (48120)
    Pancreatorrhaphy for injury (48545)
    Placement of vein patch or cuff at distal anastomosis of bypass graft (35685)
    Resection or debridement of pancreas (48105)
    Splenectomy (38100-38102)
    Suture of mesentery (44850)
    Transduodenal sphincterotomy, sphincteroplasty (47460)
0.00   0.00   **FUD** XXX   C 80
AMA: 2014,Jan,11; 2013,Jan,11-12

48552 Backbench reconstruction of cadaver donor pancreas allograft prior to transplantation, venous anastomosis, each
EXCLUDES Biopsy of pancreas (48100-48102)
    Bypass graft, with vein (35531, 35563)
    Duodenotomy (44010)
    Endoscopic procedures of the biliary tract (47550-47556)
    Excision of lesion of mesentery (44820)
    Excision of lesion of pancreas (48120)
    Pancreatorrhaphy for injury (48545)
    Placement of vein patch or cuff at distal anastomosis of bypass graft (35685)
    Resection or debridement of pancreas (48105)
    Splenectomy (38100-38102)
    Suture of mesentery (44850)
    Transduodenal sphincterotomy, sphincteroplasty (47460)
6.81   6.81   **FUD** XXX   C 80
AMA: 2014,Jan,11; 2013,Jan,11-12

48554 Transplantation of pancreatic allograft
INCLUDES Allograft transplant
    Recipient care
74.0   74.0   **FUD** 090   C 80
AMA: 2014,Jan,11; 2013,Jan,11-12

48556 Removal of transplanted pancreatic allograft
36.7   36.7   **FUD** 090   C 80
AMA: 2014,Jan,11; 2013,Jan,11-12

48999 Unlisted procedure, pancreas
0.00   0.00   **FUD** YYY   T 80
AMA: 2016,Jan,13; 2015,Jan,16; 2014,Jan,11; 2013,Feb,13; 2013,Jan,11-12; 2012,Jan,15-42; 2011,May,9; 2011,Jan,11

Digestive System

49000 — 49203

49000-49084 Exploratory and Drainage Procedures: Abdomen/Peritoneum

49000 Exploratory laparotomy, exploratory celiotomy with or without biopsy(s) (separate procedure)

> EXCLUDES Exploration of penetrating wound without laparotomy (20102)
> Percutaneous image-guided drainage of peritoneal abscess/peritonitis via catheter (49406)
> Transrectal/transvaginal image-guided drainage of peritoneal abscess via catheter (49407)

🚗 22.3   ⚕ 22.3   **FUD** 090   C 80 ▣

AMA: 2016,Jan,13; 2015,Jan,16; 2014,Jan,11; 2013,Jan,11-12; 2012,Oct,3-8; 2012,Sep,11-13; 2012,Jan,15-42; 2011,Jan,11

49002 Reopening of recent laparotomy

> EXCLUDES Hepatic wound re-exploration for packing removal (47362)

🚗 30.3   ⚕ 30.3   **FUD** 090   C 80 ▣

AMA: 2016,Jan,13; 2015,Jan,16; 2014,Jan,11; 2013,Jan,11-12

49010 Exploration, retroperitoneal area with or without biopsy(s) (separate procedure)

> EXCLUDES Exploration of penetrating wound without laparotomy (20102)

🚗 27.0   ⚕ 27.0   **FUD** 090   C 80 ▣

AMA: 2014,Jan,11; 2013,Jan,11-12

49020 Drainage of peritoneal abscess or localized peritonitis, exclusive of appendiceal abscess, open

> EXCLUDES Appendiceal abscess (44900)
> Image guided percutaneous catheter drainage of abscess/peritonitis via catheter (49406)
> Image-guided transrectal/transvaginal drainage of peritoneal abscess via catheter (49407)

🚗 46.1   ⚕ 46.1   **FUD** 090   C 80 ▣

AMA: 2014,Jan,11; 2013,Nov,9; 2013,Jan,11-12

49040 Drainage of subdiaphragmatic or subphrenic abscess, open

> EXCLUDES Image-guided percutaneous drainage of subdiaphragmatic/subphrenic abscess via catheter (49406)

🚗 28.9   ⚕ 28.9   **FUD** 090   C 80 ▣

AMA: 2014,Jan,11; 2013,Nov,9; 2013,Jan,11-12

49060 Drainage of retroperitoneal abscess, open

> EXCLUDES Image-guided percutaneous drainage of retroperitoneal abscess via catheter (49406)
> Transrectal/transvaginal image-guided drainage of retroperitoneal abscess via catheter (49407)

🚗 31.8   ⚕ 31.8   **FUD** 090   C ▣

AMA: 2016,Jan,13; 2015,Jan,16; 2014,Jan,11; 2013,Nov,9; 2013,Jan,11-12; 2012,Jan,15-42; 2011,Jan,11

49062 Drainage of extraperitoneal lymphocele to peritoneal cavity, open

> EXCLUDES Drainage of lymphocele to peritoneal cavity, laparoscopic (49323)
> Image-guided percutaneous drainage of retroperitoneal lymphocele via catheter (49406)

🚗 21.3   ⚕ 21.3   **FUD** 090   C 80 ▣

AMA: 2016,Jan,13; 2015,Jan,16; 2014,Jan,11; 2013,Jan,11-12; 2012,Jan,15-42; 2011,Jan,11

49082 Abdominal paracentesis (diagnostic or therapeutic); without imaging guidance

🚗 2.15   ⚕ 5.46   **FUD** 000   T 62 ▣

AMA: 2016,Jan,13; 2015,Jan,16; 2014,Jan,11; 2013,Nov,9; 2013,Jan,11-12; 2012,Dec,9-10

49083 with imaging guidance

> INCLUDES Radiological guidance (76942, 77002, 77012, 77021)
> EXCLUDES Image-guided percutaneous drainage of retroperitoneal abscess via catheter (49406)

🚗 3.15   ⚕ 8.36   **FUD** 000   T 62 ▣

AMA: 2016,Jan,13; 2015,Jan,16; 2014,Mar,13; 2014,Jan,11; 2013,Nov,9; 2013,Jan,11-12; 2012,Dec,9-10

49084 Peritoneal lavage, including imaging guidance, when performed

> INCLUDES Radiological guidance (76942, 77002, 77012, 77021)
> EXCLUDES Image-guided percutaneous drainage of retroperitoneal abscess via catheter (49406)

🚗 3.15   ⚕ 3.15   **FUD** 000   T 62 ▣

AMA: 2016,Jan,13; 2015,Jan,16; 2014,Jan,11; 2013,Nov,9; 2013,Jan,11-12; 2012,Dec,9-10

49180 Biopsy of Mass: Abdomen/Retroperitoneum

> EXCLUDES Aspiration, fine needle (10021, 10022)
> Lysis of intestinal adhesions (44005)

49180 Biopsy, abdominal or retroperitoneal mass, percutaneous needle

> 🔘 (76942, 77002, 77012, 77021)
> 🔳 (88172-88173)

🚗 2.48   ⚕ 4.66   **FUD** 000   T A2 ▣

AMA: 2016,Jan,13; 2015,Jan,16; 2014,Jan,11; 2013,Jan,11-12

49185 Sclerotherapy of a Fluid Collection

49185 Sclerotherapy of a fluid collection (eg, lymphocele, cyst, or seroma), percutaneous, including contrast injection(s), sclerosant injection(s), diagnostic study, imaging guidance (eg, ultrasound, fluoroscopy) and radiological supervision and interpretation when performed

> INCLUDES Multiple lesions treated via same access
> EXCLUDES Contrast injection for assessment of abscess or cyst (49424)
> Pleurodesis (32560)
> Radiologic examination, abscess, fistula or sinus tract stud (76080)
> Sclerosis of veins/endovenous ablation of incompetent veins of extremity (36468, 36470-36471, 36475-36476, 36478-36479)
> Sclerotherapy of lymphatic/vascular malformation (37241)

Code also access or drainage via needle or catheter (10030, 10160, 49405-49407, 50390)

Code also existing catheter exchange pre- or post-sclerosant injection (49423, 75984)

Code also modifier 59 for treatment of multiple lesions in same session via separate access

🚗 3.57   ⚕ 28.2   **FUD** 000   T ▣

AMA: 2016,Mar,10

49203-49205 Open Destruction or Excision: Abdominal Tumors

> EXCLUDES Ablation, open, 1 or more renal mass lesion(s), cryosurgical
> Biopsy of kidney or ovary (50205, 58900)
> Cryoablation of renal tumor (50250, 50593)
> Excision of perinephric cyst (50290)
> Excision of presacral or sacrococcygeal tumor (49215)
> Exploration, renal or retroperitoneal area (49010, 50010)
> Exploratory laparotomy (49000)
> Laparotomy, for staging or restaging of ovarian, tubal, or primary peritoneal malignancy (58960)
> Lysis of intestinal adhesions (44005)
> Nephrectomy (50225, 50236)
> Oophorectomy (58940-58958)
> Ovarian cystectomy (58925)
> Pelvic or retroperitoneal lymphadenectomy (38770, 38780)
> Primary, recurrent ovarian, uterine, or tubal resection (58957-58958)
> Wedge resection or bisection of ovary (58920)

Code also colectomy (44140)
Code also nephrectomy (50220, 50240)
Code also vena caval resection with reconstruction (37799)
Code also small bowel resection (44120)

49203 Excision or destruction, open, intra-abdominal tumors, cysts or endometriomas, 1 or more peritoneal, mesenteric, or retroperitoneal primary or secondary tumors; largest tumor 5 cm diameter or less

🚗 34.6   ⚕ 34.6   **FUD** 090   C 80 ▣

AMA: 2016,Jan,13; 2015,Jan,16; 2014,Jan,11; 2013,Jan,11-12

49204 largest tumor 5.1-10.0 cm diameter
🚑 44.3 ⚕ 44.3 **FUD** 090 C 80 ▢
AMA: 2016,Jan,13; 2015,Jan,16; 2014,Jan,11; 2013,Jan,11-12

49205 largest tumor greater than 10.0 cm diameter
🚑 50.9 ⚕ 50.9 **FUD** 090 C 80 ▢
AMA: 2016,Jan,13; 2015,Jan,16; 2014,Jan,11; 2013,Jan,11-12

49215 Resection Presacral/Sacrococcygeal Tumor

49215 Excision of presacral or sacrococcygeal tumor
🚑 64.3 ⚕ 64.3 **FUD** 090 ⑥③ C 80 ▢
AMA: 2014,Jan,11; 2013,Jan,11-12

49220-49255 Other Open Abdominal Procedures

EXCLUDES *Lysis of intestinal adhesions (44005)*

49220 Staging laparotomy for Hodgkins disease or lymphoma (includes splenectomy, needle or open biopsies of both liver lobes, possibly also removal of abdominal nodes, abdominal node and/or bone marrow biopsies, ovarian repositioning)
🚑 25.7 ⚕ 25.7 **FUD** 090 C 80 ▢
AMA: 2014,Jan,11; 2013,Jan,11-12

49250 Umbilectomy, omphalectomy, excision of umbilicus (separate procedure)
🚑 16.9 ⚕ 16.9 **FUD** 090 T A2 ▢
AMA: 2014,Jan,11; 2013,Jan,11-12

49255 Omentectomy, epiploectomy, resection of omentum (separate procedure)
🚑 22.9 ⚕ 22.9 **FUD** 090 C 80 ▢
AMA: 2016,Jan,13; 2015,Jan,16; 2014,Jan,11; 2013,Jan,11-12

49320-49329 Laparoscopic Procedures of the Abdomen/Peritoneum/Omentum

INCLUDES Diagnostic laparoscopy (49320)
EXCLUDES *Fulguration/excision of lesions of ovary/pelvic viscera/peritoneal surface, performed laparoscopically (58662)*

49320 Laparoscopy, abdomen, peritoneum, and omentum, diagnostic, with or without collection of specimen(s) by brushing or washing (separate procedure)
🚑 9.41 ⚕ 9.41 **FUD** 010 J A2 80 ▢
AMA: 2016,Jan,13; 2015,Dec,16; 2015,Jan,16; 2014,Jan,11; 2013,Jan,11-12; 2012,Jan,15-42; 2011,Jan,11

49321 Laparoscopy, surgical; with biopsy (single or multiple)
🚑 9.99 ⚕ 9.99 **FUD** 010 J A2 80 ▢
AMA: 2016,Jan,13; 2015,Jan,16; 2014,Jan,11; 2013,Jan,11-12

49322 with aspiration of cavity or cyst (eg, ovarian cyst) (single or multiple)
🚑 10.6 ⚕ 10.6 **FUD** 010 J A2 80 ▢
AMA: 2016,Jan,13; 2015,Jan,16; 2014,Jan,11; 2013,Jan,11-12

49323 with drainage of lymphocele to peritoneal cavity
EXCLUDES *Open drainage of lymphocele to peritoneal cavity (49062)*
🚑 18.4 ⚕ 18.4 **FUD** 090 J 80 ▢
AMA: 2016,Jan,13; 2015,Jan,16; 2014,Jan,11; 2013,Jan,11-12; 2012,Jan,15-42; 2011,Jan,11

49324 with insertion of tunneled intraperitoneal catheter
EXCLUDES *Open approach (49421)*
Code also insertion of subcutaneous extension to intraperitoneal cannula with remote chest exit site, when appropriate (49435)
🚑 11.3 ⚕ 11.3 **FUD** 010 J G2 80 ▢
AMA: 2014,Jan,11; 2013,Jan,11-12

49325 with revision of previously placed intraperitoneal cannula or catheter, with removal of intraluminal obstructive material if performed
🚑 12.0 ⚕ 12.0 **FUD** 010 J G2 80 ▢
AMA: 2014,Jan,11; 2013,Jan,11-12

+ **49326** with omentopexy (omental tacking procedure) (List separately in addition to code for primary procedure)
Code first laparoscopy with permanent intraperitoneal cannula or catheter insertion or revision of previously placed catheter/cannula (49324, 49325)
🚑 5.51 ⚕ 5.51 **FUD** ZZZ N N1 80 ▢
AMA: 2014,Jan,11; 2013,Jan,11-12

+ **49327** with placement of interstitial device(s) for radiation therapy guidance (eg, fiducial markers, dosimeter), intra-abdominal, intrapelvic, and/or retroperitoneum, including imaging guidance, if performed, single or multiple (List separately in addition to code for primary procedure)
EXCLUDES *Open approach (49412)*
Percutaneous approach (49411)
Code first laparoscopic abdominal, pelvic or retroperitoneal procedures
🚑 3.81 ⚕ 3.81 **FUD** ZZZ N N1 80 ▢
AMA: 2014,Jan,11; 2013,Jan,11-12

49329 Unlisted laparoscopy procedure, abdomen, peritoneum and omentum
🚑 0.00 ⚕ 0.00 **FUD** YYY J 80 50
AMA: 2016,Jan,13; 2015,Jan,16; 2014,Jan,11; 2013,Oct,18; 2013,Jan,11-12; 2012,Jan,15-42; 2011,Dec,14-18; 2011,Jan,11

49400-49436 Peritoneal and Visceral Procedures: Drainage/Insertion/Modifications/Removal

49400 Injection of air or contrast into peritoneal cavity (separate procedure)
📷 (74190)
🚑 2.72 ⚕ 3.89 **FUD** 000 N N1 ▢
AMA: 2016,Jan,13; 2015,Jan,16; 2014,Jan,11; 2013,Jan,11-12; 2012,Jan,15-42; 2011,Jan,11

49402 Removal of peritoneal foreign body from peritoneal cavity
EXCLUDES *Enterolysis (44005)*
Percutaneous or open drainage or lavage (49020, 49040, 49082-49084, 49406)
Percutaneous tunneled intraperitoneal catheter insertion without subcutaneous port (49418)
🚑 24.8 ⚕ 24.8 **FUD** 090 T A2 ▢
AMA: 2014,Jan,11; 2013,Jan,11-12

▲ **49405** Image-guided fluid collection drainage by catheter (eg, abscess, hematoma, seroma, lymphocele, cyst); visceral (eg, kidney, liver, spleen, lung/mediastinum), percutaneous
INCLUDES Radiological guidance (75989, 76942, 77002-77003, 77012, 77021)
EXCLUDES *Open drainage (32200, 47010, 48510, 50020)*
Percutaneous cholecystostomy (47490)
Percutaneous pleural drainage (32556-32557)
Pneumonostomy (32200)
Thoracentesis (32554-32555)
Code also each individual collection drained per separate catheter
🚑 6.14 ⚕ 24.9 **FUD** 000 T ▢
AMA: 2016,Jan,13; 2015,Jan,16; 2014,May,9; 2014,Jan,11; 2013,Nov,9

Digestive System

49406 — 49440

▲ **49406** **peritoneal or retroperitoneal, percutaneous**

> INCLUDES Radiological guidance (75989, 76942, 77002-77003, 77012, 77021)
>
> EXCLUDES *Diagnostic or therapeutic percutaneous abdominal paracentesis (49082-49083)*
> *Open peritoneal/retroperitoneal drainage (44900, 49020-49062, 49084, 50020, 58805, 58822)*
> *Open transrectal drainage pelvic abscess (45000)*
> *Percutaneous tunneled intraperitoneal catheter insertion without subcutaneous port (49418)*
> *Transrectal/transvaginal image-guided peritoneal/retroperitoneal drainage via catheter (49407)*
>
> Code also each individual collection drained per separate catheter
>
> 🚑 6.14   🔧 24.9   **FUD** 000   T 62 📵
>
> **AMA:** 2016,Jan,13; 2015,Jan,16; 2014,May,9; 2014,Jan,11; 2013,Nov,9

▲ **49407** **peritoneal or retroperitoneal, transvaginal or transrectal**

> INCLUDES Radiological guidance (75989, 76942, 77002-77003, 77012, 77021)
>
> EXCLUDES *Image guided percutaneous catheter drainage of soft tissue (eg, abdominal wall, neck, extremity) (10030)*
> *Open transrectal/transvaginal drainage (45000, 58800, 58820)*
> *Percutaneous pleural drainage (32556-32557)*
> *Peritoneal drainage or lavage, open or percutaneous (49020, 49040, 49060)*
> *Thoracentesis (32554-32555)*
>
> Code also each individual collection drained per separate catheter
>
> 🚑 6.59   🔧 20.8   **FUD** 000   T 62 📵
>
> **AMA:** 2016,Jan,13; 2015,Jan,16; 2014,May,9; 2014,Jan,11; 2013,Nov,9

▲ **49411** **Placement of interstitial device(s) for radiation therapy guidance (eg, fiducial markers, dosimeter), percutaneous, intra-abdominal, intra-pelvic (except prostate), and/or retroperitoneum, single or multiple**

> EXCLUDES *Placement (percutaneous) of interstitial device(s) for intrathoracic radiation therapy guidance (32553)*
>
> Code also supply of device
> ✚ (76942, 77002, 77012, 77021)
>
> 🚑 5.73   🔧 15.6   **FUD** 000   S P3 80 📵
>
> **AMA:** 2016,Jun,3; 2016,Jan,13; 2015,Jan,16; 2014,Jan,11; 2013,Jan,11-12

+ **49412** **Placement of interstitial device(s) for radiation therapy guidance (eg, fiducial markers, dosimeter), open, intra-abdominal, intrapelvic, and/or retroperitoneum, including image guidance, if performed, single or multiple (List separately in addition to code for primary procedure)**

> EXCLUDES *Laparoscopic approach (49327)*
> *Percutaneous approach (49411)*
>
> Code first open abdominal, pelvic or retroperitoneal procedure(s)
>
> 🚑 2.41   🔧 2.41   **FUD** ZZZ   C 80 📵
>
> **AMA:** 2014,Jan,11; 2013,Jan,11-12

▲ **49418** **Insertion of tunneled intraperitoneal catheter (eg, dialysis, intraperitoneal chemotherapy instillation, management of ascites), complete procedure, including imaging guidance, catheter placement, contrast injection when performed, and radiological supervision and interpretation, percutaneous**

> 🚑 6.34   🔧 40.9   **FUD** 000   T 62 80 📵
>
> **AMA:** 2014,Jan,11; 2013,Nov,9; 2013,Jan,11-12

49419 **Insertion of tunneled intraperitoneal catheter, with subcutaneous port (ie, totally implantable)**

> EXCLUDES *Removal of catheter/cannula (49422)*
>
> 🚑 12.8   🔧 12.8   **FUD** 090   T A2 📵
>
> **AMA:** 2014,Jan,11; 2013,Jan,11-12

49421 **Insertion of tunneled intraperitoneal catheter for dialysis, open**

> EXCLUDES *Laparoscopic approach (49324)*
>
> Code also insertion of subcutaneous extension to intraperitoneal cannula with remote chest exit site, when appropriate (49435)
>
> 🚑 6.70   🔧 6.70   **FUD** 000   T 62 📵
>
> **AMA:** 2016,Jan,13; 2015,Jan,16; 2014,Jan,11; 2013,Jan,11-12; 2012,Jan,15-42; 2011,Jan,11

49422 **Removal of tunneled intraperitoneal catheter**

> EXCLUDES *Removal temporary catheter or cannula (Use appropriate E&M code)*
>
> 🚑 11.0   🔧 11.0   **FUD** 010   02 A2 📵
>
> **AMA:** 2014,Jan,11; 2013,Jan,11-12

49423 **Exchange of previously placed abscess or cyst drainage catheter under radiological guidance (separate procedure)**

> ✚ (75984)
>
> 🚑 2.09   🔧 15.6   **FUD** 000   T 62 80 📵
>
> **AMA:** 2016,Jan,13; 2015,Jan,16; 2014,Jan,11; 2013,Jan,11-12

49424 **Contrast injection for assessment of abscess or cyst via previously placed drainage catheter or tube (separate procedure)**

> ✚ (76080)
>
> 🚑 1.11   🔧 4.17   **FUD** 000   N N1 80 📵
>
> **AMA:** 2016,Jan,13; 2015,Jan,16; 2014,Jan,11; 2013,Jan,11-12; 2012,Jan,15-42; 2011,Jan,11

49425 **Insertion of peritoneal-venous shunt**

> 🚑 21.2   🔧 21.2   **FUD** 090   C 80 📵
>
> **AMA:** 2014,Jan,11; 2013,Jan,11-12

49426 **Revision of peritoneal-venous shunt**

> EXCLUDES *Shunt patency test (78291)*
>
> 🚑 17.7   🔧 17.7   **FUD** 090   T A2 📵
>
> **AMA:** 2014,Jan,11; 2013,Jan,11-12

49427 **Injection procedure (eg, contrast media) for evaluation of previously placed peritoneal-venous shunt**

> ✚ (75809, 78291)
>
> 🚑 1.34   🔧 1.34   **FUD** 000   N N1 80 📵
>
> **AMA:** 2014,Jan,11; 2013,Jan,11-12

49428 **Ligation of peritoneal-venous shunt**

> 🚑 12.5   🔧 12.5   **FUD** 010   C 📵
>
> **AMA:** 2014,Jan,11; 2013,Jan,11-12

49429 **Removal of peritoneal-venous shunt**

> 🚑 13.2   🔧 13.2   **FUD** 010   02 62 📵
>
> **AMA:** 2014,Jan,11; 2013,Jan,11-12

+ **49435** **Insertion of subcutaneous extension to intraperitoneal cannula or catheter with remote chest exit site (List separately in addition to code for primary procedure)**

> Code first permanent insertion of intraperitoneal catheter/cannula (49324, 49421)
>
> 🚑 3.50   🔧 3.50   **FUD** ZZZ   N N1 80 📵
>
> **AMA:** 2014,Jan,11; 2013,Jan,11-12

49436 **Delayed creation of exit site from embedded subcutaneous segment of intraperitoneal cannula or catheter**

> 🚑 5.41   🔧 5.41   **FUD** 010   T 62 80 📵
>
> **AMA:** 2014,Jan,11; 2013,Jan,11-12

49440-49442 Insertion of Percutaneous Gastrointestinal Tube

> EXCLUDES *Naso- or oro-gastric tube placement (43752)*

▲ **49440** **Insertion of gastrostomy tube, percutaneous, under fluoroscopic guidance including contrast injection(s), image documentation and report**

> INCLUDES Needle placement with fluoroscopic guidance (77002)
>
> Code also gastrostomy to gastro-jejunostomy tube conversion with initial gastrostomy tube insertion, when performed (49446)
>
> 🚑 6.43   🔧 29.6   **FUD** 010   T 62 80 📵
>
> **AMA:** 2016,Jan,13; 2015,Jan,16; 2014,Dec,18; 2014,Sep,5; 2014,Jan,11; 2013,Jan,11-12; 2012,Jan,15-42; 2011,Jan,11

▲ **49441** Insertion of duodenostomy or jejunostomy tube, percutaneous, under fluoroscopic guidance including contrast injection(s), image documentation and report

> EXCLUDES *Gastrostomy tube to gastrojejunostomy tube conversion (49446)*

> 📖 7.45 ⚖ 33.4 **FUD** 010 T G2 80 ▣

> **AMA:** 2016,Jan,13; 2015,Jan,16; 2014,Dec,18; 2014,Sep,5; 2014,Jan,11; 2013,Jan,11-12; 2012,Jan,15-42; 2011,Jan,11

▲ **49442** Insertion of cecostomy or other colonic tube, percutaneous, under fluoroscopic guidance including contrast injection(s), image documentation and report

> 📖 6.43 ⚖ 27.5 **FUD** 010 T G2 80 ▣

> **AMA:** 2016,Jan,13; 2015,Jan,16; 2014,Dec,18; 2014,Sep,5; 2014,Jan,11; 2013,Jan,11-12; 2012,Jan,15-42; 2011,Jan,11

49446 Percutaneous Conversion: Gastrostomy to Gastro-jejunostomy Tube

> EXCLUDES *Code also initial gastrostomy tube insertion (49440) when conversion is performed at the same time*

▲ **49446** Conversion of gastrostomy tube to gastro-jejunostomy tube, percutaneous, under fluoroscopic guidance including contrast injection(s), image documentation and report

> 📖 4.72 ⚖ 28.5 **FUD** 000 T G2 80 ▣

> **AMA:** 2016,Jan,13; 2015,Jan,16; 2014,Sep,5; 2014,Jan,11; 2013,Jan,11-12; 2012,Jan,15-42; 2011,Jan,11

49450-49452 Replacement Gastrointestinal Tube

> EXCLUDES *Placement of new tube whether gastrostomy, jejunostomy, duodenostomy, gastro-jejunostomy, or cecostomy at different percutaneous site (49440-49442)*

49450 Replacement of gastrostomy or cecostomy (or other colonic) tube, percutaneous, under fluoroscopic guidance including contrast injection(s), image documentation and report

> EXCLUDES *Change of gastrostomy tube, percutaneous, without imaging or endoscopic guidance (43760)*

> 📖 1.95 ⚖ 19.0 **FUD** 000 T G2 80 ▣

> **AMA:** 2016,Jan,13; 2015,Jan,16; 2014,Sep,5; 2014,Jan,11; 2013,Dec,16; 2013,Jan,11-12; 2012,Jan,15-42; 2011,Jan,11

49451 Replacement of duodenostomy or jejunostomy tube, percutaneous, under fluoroscopic guidance including contrast injection(s), image documentation and report

> 📖 2.64 ⚖ 20.7 **FUD** 000 T G2 80 ▣

> **AMA:** 2016,Jan,13; 2015,Jan,16; 2014,Dec,18; 2014,Sep,5; 2014,Jan,11; 2013,Jan,11-12; 2012,Jan,15-42; 2011,Jan,11

49452 Replacement of gastro-jejunostomy tube, percutaneous, under fluoroscopic guidance including contrast injection(s), image documentation and report

> 📖 4.06 ⚖ 25.6 **FUD** 000 T G2 80 ▣

> **AMA:** 2016,Jan,13; 2015,Jan,16; 2014,Sep,5; 2014,Jan,11; 2013,Jan,11-12; 2012,Jan,15-42; 2011,Jan,11

49460-49465 Removal of Obstruction/Injection for Contrast Through Gastrointestinal Tube

49460 Mechanical removal of obstructive material from gastrostomy, duodenostomy, jejunostomy, gastro-jejunostomy, or cecostomy (or other colonic) tube, any method, under fluoroscopic guidance including contrast injection(s), if performed, image documentation and report

> INCLUDES Contrast injection (49465)

> EXCLUDES *Replacement of gastrointestinal tube (49450-49452)*

> 📖 1.40 ⚖ 20.9 **FUD** 000 T G2 80 ▣

> **AMA:** 2016,Jan,13; 2015,Jan,16; 2014,Sep,5; 2014,Jan,11; 2013,Jan,11-12

49465 Contrast injection(s) for radiological evaluation of existing gastrostomy, duodenostomy, jejunostomy, gastro-jejunostomy, or cecostomy (or other colonic) tube, from a percutaneous approach including image documentation and report

> EXCLUDES *Mechanical removal of obstructive material from gastrointestinal tube (49460)*
> *Replacement of gastrointestinal tube (49450-49452)*

> 📖 0.90 ⚖ 4.64 **FUD** 000 01 G2 80 ▣

> **AMA:** 2016,Jan,13; 2015,Jan,16; 2014,Sep,5; 2014,Jan,11; 2013,Jan,11-12

49491-49492 Inguinal Hernia Repair on Premature Infant

> INCLUDES Hernia repairs done on preterm infants younger than or equal to 50 weeks postconception age but younger than 6 months of age since birth
> Initial repair: no previous repair required
> Mesh or other prosthesis

> EXCLUDES *Abdominal wall debridement (11042, 11043)*
> *Intra-abdominal hernia repair/reduction (44050)*

> Code also repair or excision of testicle(s), intestine, ovaries if performed (44120, 54520, 58940)

49491 Repair, initial inguinal hernia, preterm infant (younger than 37 weeks gestation at birth), performed from birth up to 50 weeks postconception age, with or without hydrocelectomy; reducible A

> 📖 23.0 ⚖ 23.0 **FUD** 090 63 T 80 50 ▣

> **AMA:** 2016,Jan,13; 2015,Jan,16; 2014,Jan,11; 2013,Jan,11-12; 2012,Jan,15-42; 2011,Jan,11

49492 incarcerated or strangulated A

> 📖 27.7 ⚖ 27.7 **FUD** 090 63 T 80 50 ▣

> **AMA:** 2016,Jan,13; 2015,Jan,16; 2014,Jan,11; 2013,Jan,11-12

49495-49557 Hernia Repair: Femoral/Inguinal /Lumbar

> INCLUDES Initial repair: no previous repair required
> Mesh or other prosthesis
> Recurrent repair: required previous repair(s)

> EXCLUDES *Abdominal wall debridement (11042, 11043)*
> *Intra-abdominal hernia repair/reduction (44050)*

> Code also repair or excision of testicle(s), intestine, ovaries if performed (44120, 54520, 58940)

49495 Repair, initial inguinal hernia, full term infant younger than age 6 months, or preterm infant older than 50 weeks postconception age and younger than age 6 months at the time of surgery, with or without hydrocelectomy; reducible A

> INCLUDES Hernia repairs done on preterm infants older than 50 weeks postconception age and younger than 6 months

> 📖 11.0 ⚖ 11.0 **FUD** 090 63 T A2 80 50 ▣

> **AMA:** 2016,Jan,13; 2015,Jan,16; 2014,Jan,11; 2013,Jan,11-12; 2012,Jan,15-42; 2011,Jan,11

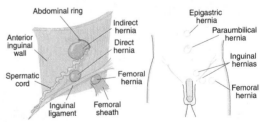

A hernia is a protrusion, usually through an abdominal wall containment

49496 incarcerated or strangulated A

> INCLUDES Hernia repairs done on preterm infants older than 50 weeks postconception age and younger than 6 months

> 📖 17.8 ⚖ 17.8 **FUD** 090 63 T A2 80 50 ▣

> **AMA:** 2016,Jan,13; 2015,Jan,16; 2014,Jan,11; 2013,Jan,11-12; 2012,Jan,15-42; 2011,Jan,11

49500 Repair initial inguinal hernia, age 6 months to younger than 5 years, with or without hydrocelectomy; reducible [A]

INCLUDES Repairs performed on patients 6 months to younger than 5 years old

🔢 10.3 ✂ 10.3 **FUD** 090 [T] [A2] [80] [50] [⌐]

AMA: 2016,Jan,13; 2015,Jan,16; 2014,Nov,14; 2014,Jan,11; 2013,Jan,11-12; 2012,Jan,15-42; 2011,Jan,11

49501 incarcerated or strangulated [A]

INCLUDES Repairs performed on patients 6 months to younger than 5 years old

🔢 16.8 ✂ 16.8 **FUD** 090 [T] [A2] [80] [50] [⌐]

AMA: 2016,Jan,13; 2015,Jan,16; 2014,Jan,11; 2013,Jan,11-12; 2012,Jan,15-42; 2011,Jan,11

49505 Repair initial inguinal hernia, age 5 years or older; reducible [A]

INCLUDES MacEwen hernia repair
Code also when performed:
Excision of hydrocele (55040)
Excision of spermatocele (54840)
Simple orchiectomy (54520)

🔢 15.0 ✂ 15.0 **FUD** 090 [T] [A2] [80] [50] [⌐]

AMA: 2016,Jan,13; 2015,Jan,16; 2014,Jan,11; 2013,Jan,11-12; 2012,Jan,15-42; 2011,Jan,11

49507 incarcerated or strangulated [A]

Code also when performed:
Excision of hydrocele (55040)
Excision of spermatocele (54840)
Simple orchiectomy (54520)

🔢 16.9 ✂ 16.9 **FUD** 090 [T] [A2] [80] [50] [⌐]

AMA: 2016,Jan,13; 2015,Jan,16; 2014,Jan,11; 2013,Jan,11-12; 2012,Jan,15-42; 2011,Jan,11

49520 Repair recurrent inguinal hernia, any age; reducible

🔢 18.3 ✂ 18.3 **FUD** 090 [T] [A2] [80] [50] [⌐]

AMA: 2016,Jan,13; 2015,Jan,16; 2014,Jan,11; 2013,Jan,11-12; 2012,Jan,15-42; 2011,Jan,11

49521 incarcerated or strangulated

🔢 20.7 ✂ 20.7 **FUD** 090 [T] [A2] [80] [50] [⌐]

AMA: 2016,Jan,13; 2015,Jan,16; 2014,Jan,11; 2013,Jan,11-12; 2012,Jan,15-42; 2011,Jan,11

49525 Repair inguinal hernia, sliding, any age

EXCLUDES Inguinal hernia repair, incarcerated/strangulated (49496, 49501, 49507, 49521)

🔢 16.5 ✂ 16.5 **FUD** 090 [T] [A2] [80] [50] [⌐]

AMA: 2016,Jan,13; 2015,Jan,16; 2014,Jan,11; 2013,Jan,11-12; 2012,Jan,15-42; 2011,Jan,11

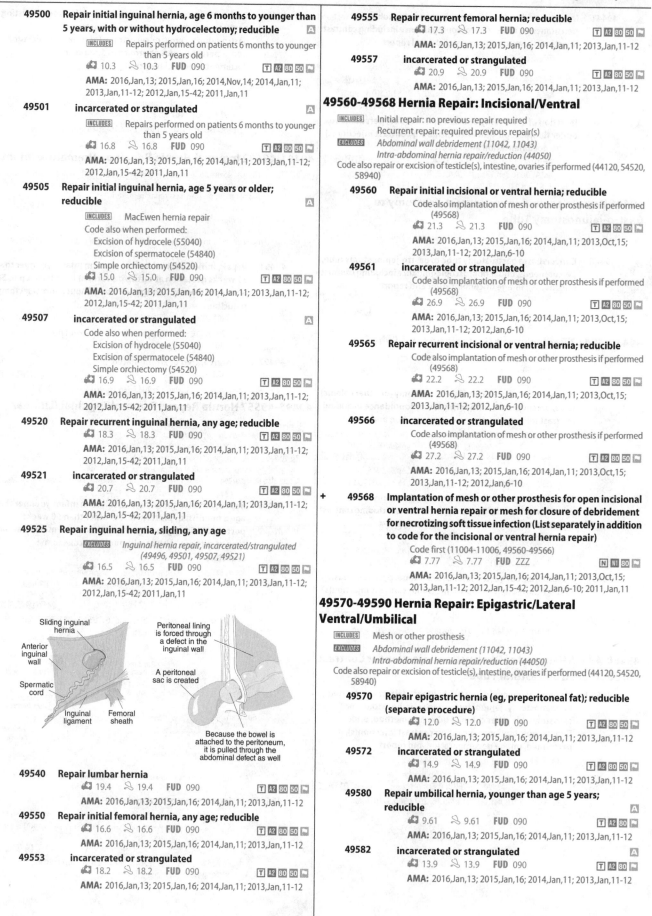

49540 Repair lumbar hernia

🔢 19.4 ✂ 19.4 **FUD** 090 [T] [A2] [80] [50] [⌐]

AMA: 2016,Jan,13; 2015,Jan,16; 2014,Jan,11; 2013,Jan,11-12

49550 Repair initial femoral hernia, any age; reducible

🔢 16.6 ✂ 16.6 **FUD** 090 [T] [A2] [80] [50] [⌐]

AMA: 2016,Jan,13; 2015,Jan,16; 2014,Jan,11; 2013,Jan,11-12

49553 incarcerated or strangulated

🔢 18.2 ✂ 18.2 **FUD** 090 [T] [A2] [80] [50] [⌐]

AMA: 2016,Jan,13; 2015,Jan,16; 2014,Jan,11; 2013,Jan,11-12

49555 Repair recurrent femoral hernia; reducible

🔢 17.3 ✂ 17.3 **FUD** 090 [T] [A2] [80] [50] [⌐]

AMA: 2016,Jan,13; 2015,Jan,16; 2014,Jan,11; 2013,Jan,11-12

49557 incarcerated or strangulated

🔢 20.9 ✂ 20.9 **FUD** 090 [T] [A2] [80] [50] [⌐]

AMA: 2016,Jan,13; 2015,Jan,16; 2014,Jan,11; 2013,Jan,11-12

49560-49568 Hernia Repair: Incisional/Ventral

INCLUDES Initial repair: no previous repair required
Recurrent repair: required previous repair(s)
EXCLUDES Abdominal wall debridement (11042, 11043)
Intra-abdominal hernia repair/reduction (44050)
Code also repair or excision of testicle(s), intestine, ovaries if performed (44120, 54520, 58940)

49560 Repair initial incisional or ventral hernia; reducible

Code also implantation of mesh or other prosthesis if performed (49568)

🔢 21.3 ✂ 21.3 **FUD** 090 [T] [A2] [80] [50] [⌐]

AMA: 2016,Jan,13; 2015,Jan,16; 2014,Jan,11; 2013,Oct,15; 2013,Jan,11-12; 2012,Jan,6-10

49561 incarcerated or strangulated

Code also implantation of mesh or other prosthesis if performed (49568)

🔢 26.9 ✂ 26.9 **FUD** 090 [T] [A2] [80] [50] [⌐]

AMA: 2016,Jan,13; 2015,Jan,16; 2014,Jan,11; 2013,Oct,15; 2013,Jan,11-12; 2012,Jan,6-10

49565 Repair recurrent incisional or ventral hernia; reducible

Code also implantation of mesh or other prosthesis if performed (49568)

🔢 22.2 ✂ 22.2 **FUD** 090 [T] [A2] [80] [50] [⌐]

AMA: 2016,Jan,13; 2015,Jan,16; 2014,Jan,11; 2013,Oct,15; 2013,Jan,11-12; 2012,Jan,6-10

49566 incarcerated or strangulated

Code also implantation of mesh or other prosthesis if performed (49568)

🔢 27.2 ✂ 27.2 **FUD** 090 [T] [A2] [80] [50] [⌐]

AMA: 2016,Jan,13; 2015,Jan,16; 2014,Jan,11; 2013,Oct,15; 2013,Jan,11-12; 2012,Jan,6-10

+ 49568 Implantation of mesh or other prosthesis for open incisional or ventral hernia repair or mesh for closure of debridement for necrotizing soft tissue infection (List separately in addition to code for the incisional or ventral hernia repair)

Code first (11004-11006, 49560-49566)

🔢 7.77 ✂ 7.77 **FUD** ZZZ [N] [N1] [80] [⌐]

AMA: 2016,Jan,13; 2015,Jan,16; 2014,Jan,11; 2013,Oct,15; 2013,Jan,11-12; 2012,Jan,15-42; 2012,Jan,6-10; 2011,Jan,11

49570-49590 Hernia Repair: Epigastric/Lateral Ventral/Umbilical

INCLUDES Mesh or other prosthesis
EXCLUDES Abdominal wall debridement (11042, 11043)
Intra-abdominal hernia repair/reduction (44050)
Code also repair or excision of testicle(s), intestine, ovaries if performed (44120, 54520, 58940)

49570 Repair epigastric hernia (eg, preperitoneal fat); reducible (separate procedure)

🔢 12.0 ✂ 12.0 **FUD** 090 [T] [A2] [80] [50] [⌐]

AMA: 2016,Jan,13; 2015,Jan,16; 2014,Jan,11; 2013,Jan,11-12

49572 incarcerated or strangulated

🔢 14.9 ✂ 14.9 **FUD** 090 [T] [A2] [80] [50] [⌐]

AMA: 2016,Jan,13; 2015,Jan,16; 2014,Jan,11; 2013,Jan,11-12

49580 Repair umbilical hernia, younger than age 5 years; reducible [A]

🔢 9.61 ✂ 9.61 **FUD** 090 [T] [A2] [80] [⌐]

AMA: 2016,Jan,13; 2015,Jan,16; 2014,Jan,11; 2013,Jan,11-12

49582 incarcerated or strangulated [A]

🔢 13.9 ✂ 13.9 **FUD** 090 [T] [A2] [80] [⌐]

AMA: 2016,Jan,13; 2015,Jan,16; 2014,Jan,11; 2013,Jan,11-12

| 26/TC PC/TC Only | A2-Z3 ASC Payment | 50 Bilateral | ♂ Male Only | ♀ Female Only | 🔢 Facility RVU | ✂ Non-Facility RVU | ⌐ CCI |
| **FUD** Follow-up Days | **CMS:** IOM (Pub 100) | A-Y OPPSI | 80/80 Surg Assist Allowed / w/Doc | | Lab Crosswalk | Radiology Crosswalk | CLIA |

214

CPT © 2016 American Medical Association. All Rights Reserved.

© 2016 Optum360, LLC

49500 — 49582

Digestive System

49585 Repair umbilical hernia, age 5 years or older; reducible ⒜
    INCLUDES Mayo hernia repair
    🚗 12.8   ✂ 12.8   **FUD** 090   T A2 80 ▣
    AMA: 2016,Jan,13; 2015,Jan,16; 2014,Jan,11; 2013,Jan,11-12

49587 incarcerated or strangulated ⒜
    🚗 13.7   ✂ 13.7   **FUD** 090   T A2 80 ▣
    AMA: 2016,Jan,13; 2015,Jan,16; 2014,Jan,11; 2013,Jan,11-12

49590 Repair spigelian hernia
    🚗 16.5   ✂ 16.5   **FUD** 090   T A2 80 50 ▣
    AMA: 2016,Jan,13; 2015,Jan,16; 2014,Jan,11; 2013,Jan,11-12

49600-49611 Repair Birth Defect Abdominal Wall: Omphalocele/Gastroschisis

INCLUDES Mesh or other prosthesis
EXCLUDES *Abdominal wall debridement (11042, 11043)*
    Intra-abdominal hernia repair/reduction (44050)
    Repair of:
      Diaphragmatic or hiatal hernia (39503, 43332-43337)
      Omentum (49999)

49600 Repair of small omphalocele, with primary closure
    🚗 20.3   ✂ 20.3   **FUD** 090   63 T A2 80 ▣
    AMA: 2016,Jan,13; 2015,Jan,16; 2014,Jan,11; 2013,Jan,11-12

49605 Repair of large omphalocele or gastroschisis; with or without prosthesis
    🚗 143.   ✂ 143.   **FUD** 090   63 C 80 ▣
    AMA: 2016,Jan,13; 2015,Jan,16; 2014,Jan,11; 2013,Jan,11-12

49606 with removal of prosthesis, final reduction and closure, in operating room
    🚗 32.3   ✂ 32.3   **FUD** 090   63 C 80 ▣
    AMA: 2016,Jan,13; 2015,Jan,16; 2014,Jan,11; 2013,Jan,11-12

49610 Repair of omphalocele (Gross type operation); first stage
    🚗 19.9   ✂ 19.9   **FUD** 090   63 C 80 ▣
    AMA: 2016,Jan,13; 2015,Jan,16; 2014,Jan,11; 2013,Jan,11-12

49611 second stage
    🚗 17.5   ✂ 17.5   **FUD** 090   63 C 80 ▣
    AMA: 2016,Jan,13; 2015,Jan,16; 2014,Jan,11; 2013,Jan,11-12; 2012,Jan,15-42; 2011,Jan,11

49650-49659 Laparoscopic Hernia Repair

INCLUDES Diagnostic laparoscopy (49320)

49650 Laparoscopy, surgical; repair initial inguinal hernia
    🚗 12.3   ✂ 12.3   **FUD** 090   J A2 80 50 ▣
    AMA: 2016,Jan,13; 2015,Jan,16; 2014,Jul,5; 2014,Jan,11; 2013,Jan,11-12

49651 repair recurrent inguinal hernia
    🚗 16.1   ✂ 16.1   **FUD** 090   J A2 80 50 ▣
    AMA: 2016,Jan,13; 2015,Jan,16; 2014,Jan,11; 2013,Jan,11-12

49652 Laparoscopy, surgical, repair, ventral, umbilical, spigelian or epigastric hernia (includes mesh insertion, when performed); reducible
    INCLUDES Laparoscopy, surgical, enterolysis (44180)
    EXCLUDES *Implantation of mesh or other prosthesis (49568)*
    🚗 21.5   ✂ 21.5   **FUD** 090   J G2 80 50 ▣
    AMA: 2014,Jan,11; 2013,Jan,11-12

49653 incarcerated or strangulated
    INCLUDES Laparoscopy, surgical, enterolysis (44180)
    EXCLUDES *Implantation of mesh or other prosthesis (49568)*
    🚗 26.8   ✂ 26.8   **FUD** 090   J G2 80 50 ▣
    AMA: 2014,Jan,11; 2013,Jan,11-12

49654 Laparoscopy, surgical, repair, incisional hernia (includes mesh insertion, when performed); reducible
    INCLUDES Laparoscopy, surgical, enterolysis (44180)
    EXCLUDES *Implantation of mesh or other prosthesis (49568)*
    🚗 24.5   ✂ 24.5   **FUD** 090   J G2 80 50 ▣
    AMA: 2014,Jan,11; 2013,Jan,11-12

49655 incarcerated or strangulated
    INCLUDES Laparoscopy, surgical, enterolysis (44180)
    EXCLUDES *Implantation of mesh or other prosthesis (49568)*
    🚗 29.9   ✂ 29.9   **FUD** 090   J G2 80 50 ▣
    AMA: 2014,Jan,11; 2013,Jan,11-12

49656 Laparoscopy, surgical, repair, recurrent incisional hernia (includes mesh insertion, when performed); reducible
    INCLUDES Laparoscopy, surgical, enterolysis (44180)
    EXCLUDES *Implantation of mesh or other prosthesis (49568)*
    🚗 26.6   ✂ 26.6   **FUD** 090   J G2 80 50 ▣
    AMA: 2014,Jan,11; 2013,Jan,11-12

49657 incarcerated or strangulated
    INCLUDES Laparoscopy, surgical, enterolysis (44180)
    EXCLUDES *Implantation of mesh or other prosthesis (49568)*
    🚗 38.2   ✂ 38.2   **FUD** 090   J G2 80 50 ▣
    AMA: 2014,Jan,11; 2013,Jan,11-12

49659 Unlisted laparoscopy procedure, hernioplasty, herniorrhaphy, herniotomy
    🚗 0.00   ✂ 0.00   **FUD** YYY   J 80 50 ▣
    AMA: 2016,Jan,13; 2015,Jan,16; 2014,Dec,16; 2014,Dec,16; 2014,Jul,5; 2014,Jan,11; 2013,Jan,11-12; 2012,Jan,15-42; 2011,Jan,11

49900 Surgical Repair Abdominal Wall

EXCLUDES *Abdominal wall debridement (11042, 11043)*
    Suture of ruptured diaphragm (39540-39541)

49900 Suture, secondary, of abdominal wall for evisceration or dehiscence
    🚗 23.5   ✂ 23.5   **FUD** 090   C 80 ▣
    AMA: 2016,Jan,13; 2015,Jan,16; 2014,Jan,11; 2013,Jan,11-12

49904-49999 Harvesting of Omental Flap

49904 Omental flap, extra-abdominal (eg, for reconstruction of sternal and chest wall defects)
    INCLUDES Harvest and transfer
    EXCLUDES *Omental flap harvest by second surgeon: both surgeons code 49904 with modifier 62 (49904)*
    🚗 41.2   ✂ 41.2   **FUD** 090   C ▣
    AMA: 2014,Jan,11; 2013,Jan,11-12

+ 49905 Omental flap, intra-abdominal (List separately in addition to code for primary procedure)
    EXCLUDES *Exclusion of small intestine from pelvis by mesh or other prosthesis, or native tissue (44700)*
    Code first primary procedure
    🚗 10.2   ✂ 10.2   **FUD** ZZZ   C 80 ▣
    AMA: 2016,Jan,13; 2015,Jan,16; 2014,Jan,11; 2013,Jan,11-12; 2012,Jan,15-42; 2011,Jan,11

49906 Free omental flap with microvascular anastomosis
    INCLUDES Operating microscope (69990)
    🚗 0.00   ✂ 0.00   **FUD** 090   C ▣
    AMA: 2016,Feb,12; 2016,Jan,13; 2015,Jan,16; 2014,Jan,11; 2013,Jan,11-12

49999 Unlisted procedure, abdomen, peritoneum and omentum
    🚗 0.00   ✂ 0.00   **FUD** YYY   T
    AMA: 2016,Jan,13; 2015,Jan,16; 2014,Jan,9; 2014,Jan,11; 2013,Jan,11-12; 2012,Jan,15-42; 2011,Jun,13; 2011,Jan,11

50010-50045 Kidney Procedures for Exploration or Drainage

EXCLUDES Donor nephrectomy performed laparoscopically (50547)
Retroperitoneal
  Abscess drainage (49060)
  Exploration (49010)
  Tumor/cyst excision (49203-49205)

50010 Renal exploration, not necessitating other specific procedures

EXCLUDES Laparoscopic ablation of mass lesions of kidney (50542)

⚕ 21.2   ⚒ 21.2   FUD 090   C 80 50 ▣

AMA: 2014,Jan,11

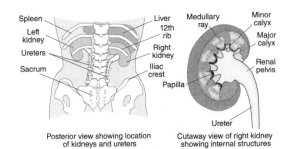

Spleen
Left kidney
Ureters
Sacrum
Liver
12th rib
Right kidney
Iliac crest
Medullary ray
Minor calyx
Major calyx
Renal pelvis
Papilla
Ureter

Posterior view showing location of kidneys and ureters

Cutaway view of right kidney showing internal structures

50020 Drainage of perirenal or renal abscess, open

EXCLUDES Image-guided percutaneous of perirenal or renal abscess (49405)

⚕ 29.2   ⚒ 29.2   FUD 090   T ▣

AMA: 2016,Jan,13; 2015,Jan,16; 2014,May,9; 2014,Jan,11; 2013,Nov,9

50040 Nephrostomy, nephrotomy with drainage

⚕ 26.6   ⚒ 26.6   FUD 090   C 50 ▣

AMA: 2016,Jan,13; 2015,Jan,16; 2014,Jan,11

50045 Nephrotomy, with exploration

EXCLUDES Renal endoscopy through nephrotomy (50570-50580)

⚕ 27.6   ⚒ 27.6   FUD 090   C 80 50 ▣

AMA: 2016,Jan,13; 2015,Jan,16; 2014,Jan,11

50060-50081 Treatment of Kidney Stones

CMS: 100-03,230.1 NCD for Treatment of Kidney Stones

EXCLUDES Retroperitoneal:
  Abscess drainage (49060)
  Exploration (49010)
  Tumor/cyst excision (49203-49205)

50060 Nephrolithotomy; removal of calculus

⚕ 32.8   ⚒ 32.8   FUD 090   C 80 50 ▣

AMA: 2016,Jan,13; 2015,Jan,16; 2014,Jan,11

50065 secondary surgical operation for calculus

⚕ 34.7   ⚒ 34.7   FUD 090   C 80 50 ▣

AMA: 2016,Jan,13; 2015,Jan,16; 2014,Jan,11

50070 complicated by congenital kidney abnormality

⚕ 34.0   ⚒ 34.0   FUD 090   C 80 50 ▣

AMA: 2016,Jan,13; 2015,Jan,16; 2014,Jan,11

50075 removal of large staghorn calculus filling renal pelvis and calyces (including anatrophic pyelolithotomy)

⚕ 41.9   ⚒ 41.9   FUD 090   C 80 50 ▣

AMA: 2016,Jan,13; 2015,Jan,16; 2014,Jan,11

50080 Percutaneous nephrostolithotomy or pyelostolithotomy, with or without dilation, endoscopy, lithotripsy, stenting, or basket extraction; up to 2 cm

EXCLUDES Nephrostomy without nephrostolithotomy (50040, 50395, 52334)

▣ (76000, 76001)

⚕ 25.0   ⚒ 25.0   FUD 090   J J8 50 ▣

AMA: 2016,Jan,13; 2015,Jan,16; 2014,Jan,11; 2012,Jan,15-42; 2011,Jan,11

50081 over 2 cm

EXCLUDES Nephrostomy without nephrostolithotomy (50040, 50395, 52334)

▣ (76000, 76001)

⚕ 36.7   ⚒ 36.7   FUD 090   J J8 80 50 ▣

AMA: 2016,Jan,13; 2015,Jan,16; 2014,Jan,11; 2012,Jan,15-42; 2011,Jan,11

50100 Repair of Anomalous Vessels of the Kidney

EXCLUDES Retroperitoneal:
  Abscess drainage (49060)
  Exploration (49010)
  Tumor/cyst excision (49203-49205)

50100 Transection or repositioning of aberrant renal vessels (separate procedure)

⚕ 30.5   ⚒ 30.5   FUD 090   C 80 50 ▣

AMA: 2016,Jan,13; 2015,Jan,16; 2014,Jan,11

50120-50135 Procedures of Renal Pelvis

EXCLUDES Retroperitoneal:
  Abscess drainage (49060)
  Exploration (49010)
  Tumor/cyst excision (49203-49205)

50120 Pyelotomy; with exploration

INCLUDES Gol-Vernet pyelotomy

EXCLUDES Renal endoscopy through pyelotomy (50570-50580)

⚕ 27.2   ⚒ 27.2   FUD 090   C 80 50 ▣

AMA: 2016,Jan,13; 2015,Jan,16; 2014,Jan,11

50125 with drainage, pyelostomy

⚕ 29.6   ⚒ 29.6   FUD 090   C 80 50 ▣

AMA: 2016,Jan,13; 2015,Jan,16; 2014,Jan,11

50130 with removal of calculus (pyelolithotomy, pelviolithotomy, including coagulum pyelolithotomy)

⚕ 29.6   ⚒ 29.6   FUD 090   C 80 50 ▣

AMA: 2016,Jan,13; 2015,Jan,16; 2014,Jan,11

50135 complicated (eg, secondary operation, congenital kidney abnormality)

⚕ 32.7   ⚒ 32.7   FUD 090   C 80 50 ▣

AMA: 2016,Jan,13; 2015,Jan,16; 2014,Jan,11

50200-50205 Biopsy of Kidney

EXCLUDES Laparoscopic renal mass lesion ablation (50542)
Retroperitoneal tumor/cyst excision (49203-49205)

▲ **50200** Renal biopsy; percutaneous, by trocar or needle

EXCLUDES Fine needle aspiration (10022)

▣ (76942, 77002, 77012, 77021)

▣ (88172-88173)

⚕ 4.11   ⚒ 17.4   FUD 000   T A2 50 ▣

AMA: 2016,Jan,13; 2015,Jan,16; 2014,Jan,11

50205 by surgical exposure of kidney

⚕ 21.8   ⚒ 21.8   FUD 090   C 80 50 ▣

AMA: 2016,Jan,13; 2015,Jan,16; 2014,Jan,11

50220-50240 Nephrectomy Procedures

EXCLUDES Laparoscopic renal mass lesion ablation (50542)
Retroperitoneal tumor/cyst excision (49203-49205)

50220 Nephrectomy, including partial ureterectomy, any open approach including rib resection;

⚕ 30.1   ⚒ 30.1   FUD 090   C 80 50 ▣

AMA: 2016,Jan,13; 2015,Jan,16; 2014,Jan,11

50225 complicated because of previous surgery on same kidney

⚕ 34.6   ⚒ 34.6   FUD 090   C 80 50 ▣

AMA: 2016,Jan,13; 2015,Jan,16; 2014,Jan,11

50230 radical, with regional lymphadenectomy and/or vena caval thrombectomy

EXCLUDES Vena caval resection with reconstruction (37799)

⚕ 36.8   ⚒ 36.8   FUD 090   C 80 50 ▣

AMA: 2016,Jan,13; 2015,Jan,16; 2014,Jan,11

50234 **Nephrectomy with total ureterectomy and bladder cuff; through same incision**
📷 37.4 ⚖ 37.4 **FUD** 090 C 80 50 ▣
AMA: 2016,Jan,13; 2015,Jan,16; 2014,Jan,11

50236 **through separate incision**
📷 42.2 ⚖ 42.2 **FUD** 090 C 80 50 ▣
AMA: 2016,Jan,13; 2015,Jan,16; 2014,Jan,11

50240 **Nephrectomy, partial**
EXCLUDES *Laparoscopic partial nephrectomy (50543)*
📷 38.0 ⚖ 38.0 **FUD** 090 C 80 50 ▣
AMA: 2016,Jan,13; 2015,Jan,16; 2014,Jan,11

50250-50290 Open Removal Kidney Lesions

EXCLUDES *Open destruction or excision intra-abdominal tumors (49203-49205)*

50250 **Ablation, open, 1 or more renal mass lesion(s), cryosurgical, including intraoperative ultrasound guidance and monitoring, if performed**
EXCLUDES *Laparoscopic renal mass lesion ablation (50542)*
Percutaneous renal tumor ablation (50592-50593)
📷 34.9 ⚖ 34.9 **FUD** 090 C 80 ▣
AMA: 2016,Jan,13; 2015,Jan,16; 2014,Jan,11; 2012,Jan,15-42; 2011,Jan,11

50280 **Excision or unroofing of cyst(s) of kidney**
EXCLUDES *Renal cyst laparoscopic ablation (50541)*
📷 27.4 ⚖ 27.4 **FUD** 090 C 80 50 ▣
AMA: 2016,Jan,13; 2015,Jan,16; 2014,Jan,11

50290 **Excision of perinephric cyst**
📷 25.8 ⚖ 25.8 **FUD** 090 C 80 ▣
AMA: 2016,Jan,13; 2015,Jan,16; 2014,Jan,11

50300-50380 Kidney Transplant Procedures

CMS: 100-04,3,90.1 Kidney Transplant - General; 100-04,3,90.1.1 Standard Kidney Acquisition Charge; 100-04,3,90.1.2 Billing for Kidney Transplant and Acquisition Services; 100-04,3,90.5 Pancreas Transplants with Kidney Transplants

EXCLUDES *Dialysis procedures (90935-90999)*
Lymphocele drainage to peritoneal cavity performed laparoscopically (49323)

50300 **Donor nephrectomy (including cold preservation); from cadaver donor, unilateral or bilateral**
INCLUDES Graft:
Cold preservation
Harvesting
EXCLUDES *Donor nephrectomy performed laparoscopically (50547)*
📷 0.00 ⚖ 0.00 **FUD** XXX C
AMA: 2016,Jan,13; 2015,Jan,16; 2014,Jan,11

50320 **open, from living donor**
INCLUDES Donor care
Graft:
Cold preservation
Harvesting
EXCLUDES *Donor nephrectomy performed laparoscopically (50547)*
📷 41.9 ⚖ 41.9 **FUD** 090 C 80 50 ▣
AMA: 2016,Jan,13; 2015,Jan,16; 2014,Jan,11

50323 **Backbench standard preparation of cadaver donor renal allograft prior to transplantation, including dissection and removal of perinephric fat, diaphragmatic and retroperitoneal attachments, excision of adrenal gland, and preparation of ureter(s), renal vein(s), and renal artery(s), ligating branches, as necessary**
EXCLUDES *Adrenalectomy (60540, 60545)*
📷 0.00 ⚖ 0.00 **FUD** XXX C 80 ▣
AMA: 2016,Jan,13; 2015,Jan,16; 2014,Jan,11

50325 **Backbench standard preparation of living donor renal allograft (open or laparoscopic) prior to transplantation, including dissection and removal of perinephric fat and preparation of ureter(s), renal vein(s), and renal artery(s), ligating branches, as necessary**
📷 0.00 ⚖ 0.00 **FUD** XXX C 80 ▣
AMA: 2014,Jan,11

50327 **Backbench reconstruction of cadaver or living donor renal allograft prior to transplantation; venous anastomosis, each**
📷 6.30 ⚖ 6.30 **FUD** XXX C 80 ▣
AMA: 2014,Jan,11

50328 **arterial anastomosis, each**
📷 5.53 ⚖ 5.53 **FUD** XXX C 80 ▣
AMA: 2014,Jan,11

50329 **ureteral anastomosis, each**
📷 5.17 ⚖ 5.17 **FUD** XXX C 80 ▣
AMA: 2014,Jan,11

50340 **Recipient nephrectomy (separate procedure)**
📷 27.0 ⚖ 27.0 **FUD** 090 C 80 50 ▣
AMA: 2014,Jan,11

50360 **Renal allotransplantation, implantation of graft; without recipient nephrectomy**
INCLUDES Allograft transplantation
Recipient care
Code also backbench work (50323, 50325, 50327-50329)
Code also donor nephrectomy (cadaver or living donor) (50300, 50320, 50547)
📷 70.1 ⚖ 70.1 **FUD** 090 C 80 ▣
AMA: 2014,Jan,11

50365 **with recipient nephrectomy**
INCLUDES Allograft transplantation
Recipient care
📷 81.9 ⚖ 81.9 **FUD** 090 C 80 50 ▣
AMA: 2016,Jan,13; 2015,Jan,16; 2014,Jan,11

50370 **Removal of transplanted renal allograft**
📷 34.7 ⚖ 34.7 **FUD** 090 C 80 ▣
AMA: 2014,Jan,11

50380 **Renal autotransplantation, reimplantation of kidney**
INCLUDES Reimplantation of autograft
EXCLUDES *Secondary procedures:*
Nephrolithotomy (50060-50075)
Partial nephrectomy (50240, 50543)
📷 57.5 ⚖ 57.5 **FUD** 090 C 80 ▣
AMA: 2016,Jan,13; 2015,Jan,16; 2014,Jan,11

50382-50386 Removal With/Without Replacement Internal Ureteral Stent

INCLUDES Radiological supervision and interpretation

▲ **50382** **Removal (via snare/capture) and replacement of internally dwelling ureteral stent via percutaneous approach, including radiological supervision and interpretation**
EXCLUDES *Introduction of guide into renal pelvis and/or ureter with dilation (50395)*
Removal and replacement of an internally dwelling ureteral stent using a transurethral approach (50385)
📷 7.84 ⚖ 33.8 **FUD** 000 T 62 50 ▣
AMA: 2016,Jan,3; 2016,Jan,13; 2015,Jan,16; 2014,Jan,11

▲ **50384** **Removal (via snare/capture) of internally dwelling ureteral stent via percutaneous approach, including radiological supervision and interpretation**
EXCLUDES *Introduction of guide into renal pelvis and/or ureter with dilation (50395)*
Removal of an internally dwelling ureteral stent using a transurethral approach (50386)
📷 7.12 ⚖ 26.9 **FUD** 000 02 62 50 ▣
AMA: 2016,Jan,3; 2016,Jan,13; 2015,Jan,16; 2014,Jan,11

▲ **50385** **Removal (via snare/capture) and replacement of internally dwelling ureteral stent via transurethral approach, without use of cystoscopy, including radiological supervision and interpretation**
📷 6.71 ⚖ 32.5 **FUD** 000 T 62 80 50 ▣
AMA: 2016,Jan,3; 2016,Jan,13; 2015,Jan,16; 2014,Jan,11

▲ **50386** Removal (via snare/capture) of internally dwelling ureteral stent via transurethral approach, without use of cystoscopy, including radiological supervision and interpretation

🔧 5.10 ⚕ 21.1 **FUD** 000 [02] [P3] [80] [50] 🖵

AMA: 2016,Jan,3; 2016,Jan,13; 2015,Jan,16; 2014,Jan,11

50387 Remove/Replace Accessible Ureteral Stent

EXCLUDES *Removal and replacement of ureteral stent through ureterostomy tube or ileal conduit (50688)*
Removal without replacement of externally accessible ureteral stent without fluoroscopic guidance, report with appropriate E&M code

▲ **50387** Removal and replacement of externally accessible nephroureteral catheter (eg, external/internal stent) requiring fluoroscopic guidance, including radiological supervision and interpretation

🔧 2.82 ⚕ 15.5 **FUD** 000 [T] [62] [80] [50] 🖵

AMA: 2016,Mar,10; 2016,Jan,13; 2016,Jan,3; 2015,Oct,5; 2015,Jan,16; 2014,Jan,11; 2012,Mar,9-10

50389-50396 [50430, 50431, 50432, 50433, 50434, 50435] Percutaneous and Injection Procedures With/Without Indwelling Tube/Catheter Access

50389 Removal of nephrostomy tube, requiring fluoroscopic guidance (eg, with concurrent indwelling ureteral stent)

EXCLUDES *Nephrostomy tube removal without fluoroscopic guidance, report with appropriate E&M code*

🔧 1.57 ⚕ 8.45 **FUD** 000 [02] [62] [50] 🖵

AMA: 2016,Jan,3; 2016,Jan,13; 2015,Oct,5; 2015,Jan,16; 2014,Jan,11

50390 Aspiration and/or injection of renal cyst or pelvis by needle, percutaneous

EXCLUDES *Antegrade nephrostogram/pyelogram ([50430, 50431])*
📷 (74425, 74470, 76942, 77002, 77012, 77021)

🔧 2.80 ⚕ 2.80 **FUD** 000 [T] [A2] [50] 🖵

AMA: 2016,Jan,13; 2015,Oct,5; 2015,Jan,16; 2014,Jan,11

50391 Instillation(s) of therapeutic agent into renal pelvis and/or ureter through established nephrostomy, pyelostomy or ureterostomy tube (eg, anticarcinogenic or antifungal agent)

Code also therapeutic agent

🔧 2.82 ⚕ 3.48 **FUD** 000 [T] [P3] [50] 🖵

AMA: 2016,Jan,13; 2015,Oct,5; 2015,Jan,16; 2014,Jan,11

50395 Introduction of guide into renal pelvis and/or ureter with dilation to establish nephrostomy tract, percutaneous

EXCLUDES *Percutaneous nephrostolithotomy (50080-50081)*
Placement of nephrostomy catheter ([50432, 50433])
Removal, replacement internally dwelling ureteral stent (50382, 50384)
Renal endoscopy (50551-50561)
Retrograde percutaneous nephrostomy (52334)
📷 (74485)

🔧 5.17 ⚕ 5.17 **FUD** 000 [T] [A2] [50] 🖵

AMA: 2016,Jan,13; 2015,Oct,5; 2015,Jan,16; 2014,Jan,11; 2012,Jan,15-42; 2011,Jan,11

50396 Manometric studies through nephrostomy or pyelostomy tube, or indwelling ureteral catheter

📷 (74425)

🔧 3.41 ⚕ 3.41 **FUD** 000 [T] [A2] [80] [50] 🖵

AMA: 2016,Jan,13; 2015,Jan,16; 2014,Jan,11

▲ # **50430** Injection procedure for antegrade nephrostogram and/or ureterogram, complete diagnostic procedure including imaging guidance (eg, ultrasound and fluoroscopy) and all associated radiological supervision and interpretation; new access

INCLUDES Renal pelvis and associated ureter as a single element
EXCLUDES *Procedure performed with for same renal collecting system/ureter ([50432, 50433, 50434, 50435], 50693-50695, 74425)*

🔧 4.84 ⚕ 14.8 **FUD** 000 [02] [N1] [80] [50] 🖵

AMA: 2016,Jan,3; 2016,Jan,13; 2015,Oct,5

50431 existing access

INCLUDES Renal pelvis and associated ureter as a single element
EXCLUDES *Procedure performed with for same renal collecting system/ureter ([50432, 50433, 50434, 50435], 50693-50695, 74425)*

🔧 1.92 ⚕ 4.61 **FUD** 000 [02] [N1] [50] 🖵

AMA: 2016,Jan,3; 2016,Jan,13; 2015,Oct,5

▲ # **50432** Placement of nephrostomy catheter, percutaneous, including diagnostic nephrostogram and/or ureterogram when performed, imaging guidance (eg, ultrasound and/or fluoroscopy) and all associated radiological supervision and interpretation

INCLUDES Renal pelvis and associated ureter as a single element
EXCLUDES *Procedure performed with dilation of nephrostomy tube tract (50395)*
Procedure performed with for same renal collecting system/ureter ([50432, 50433, 50434, 50435], 50693-50695, 74425)

🔧 6.40 ⚕ 24.0 **FUD** 000 [T] [62] [50] 🖵

AMA: 2016,Jan,3; 2016,Jan,13; 2015,Oct,5

▲ # **50433** Placement of nephroureteral catheter, percutaneous, including diagnostic nephrostogram and/or ureterogram when performed, imaging guidance (eg, ultrasound and/or fluoroscopy) and all associated radiological supervision and interpretation, new access

INCLUDES Renal pelvis and associated ureter as a single element
EXCLUDES *Dilation of nephroureteral catheter tract (50395)*
Nephroureteral catheter removal/replacement (50387)
Procedures performed for same renal collecting system/ureter ([50430, 50431, 50432], 50693-50695, 74425)

🔧 7.89 ⚕ 32.3 **FUD** 000 [T] [62] [50] 🖵

AMA: 2016,Jan,3; 2016,Jan,13; 2015,Oct,5

▲ # **50434** Convert nephrostomy catheter to nephroureteral catheter, percutaneous, including diagnostic nephrostogram and/or ureterogram when performed, imaging guidance (eg, ultrasound and/or fluoroscopy) and all associated radiological supervision and interpretation, via pre-existing nephrostomy tract

INCLUDES Renal pelvis and associated ureter as a single element
EXCLUDES *Procedure performed for same renal collecting system/ureter ([50430, 50431], [50435], 50684, 50693, 74425)*

🔧 6.05 ⚕ 25.5 **FUD** 000 [T] [62] [50] 🖵

AMA: 2016,Jan,3; 2016,Jan,13; 2015,Oct,5

50435 Exchange nephrostomy catheter, percutaneous, including diagnostic nephrostogram and/or ureterogram when performed, imaging guidance (eg, ultrasound and/or fluoroscopy) and all associated radiological supervision and interpretation

INCLUDES Renal pelvis and associated ureter as a single element
EXCLUDES *Procedure performed for same renal collecting system/ureter ([50430, 50431], [50434], 50693, 74425)*
Removal nephrostomy catheter that requires fluoroscopic guidance (50389)

🔧 2.94 ⚕ 13.4 **FUD** 000 [T] [62] [50] 🖵

AMA: 2016,Jan,3; 2016,Jan,13; 2015,Oct,5

50400-50540 Open Surgical Procedures of Kidney

50400 Pyeloplasty (Foley Y-pyeloplasty), plastic operation on renal pelvis, with or without plastic operation on ureter, nephropexy, nephrostomy, pyelostomy, or ureteral splinting; simple

EXCLUDES *Laparoscopic pyeloplasty (50544)*

🔧 33.3 ⚕ 33.3 **FUD** 090 [C] [80] [50] 🖵

AMA: 2016,Jan,13; 2015,Jan,16; 2014,Jan,11

● New Code ▲ Revised Code ○ Reinstated ● New Web Release ▲ Revised Web Release Unlisted Not Covered # Resequenced
⊘ AMA Mod 51 Exempt ⑤ Optum Mod 51 Exempt ⑥ Mod 63 Exempt ✗ Non-FDA Drug ★ Telehealth [M] Maternity [A] Age Edit + Add-on **AMA:** CPT Asst

Urinary System *(side tab)*

50405 — 50570 *(side tab)*

50405 **complicated (congenital kidney abnormality, secondary pyeloplasty, solitary kidney, calycoplasty)**
EXCLUDES *Laparoscopic pyeloplasty (50544)*
🚗 40.1 ✂ 40.1 **FUD** 090 [C] [80] [50] 🔲
AMA: 2016,Jan,13; 2015,Jan,16; 2014,Jan,11

50430 Resequenced code. See code following 50396.

50431 Resequenced code. See code following 50396.

50432 Resequenced code. See code following 50396.

50433 Resequenced code. See code following 50396.

50434 Resequenced code. See code following 50396.

50435 Resequenced code. See code following 50396.

50500 **Nephrorrhaphy, suture of kidney wound or injury**
🚗 36.8 ✂ 36.8 **FUD** 090 [C] [80] 🔲
AMA: 2014,Jan,11

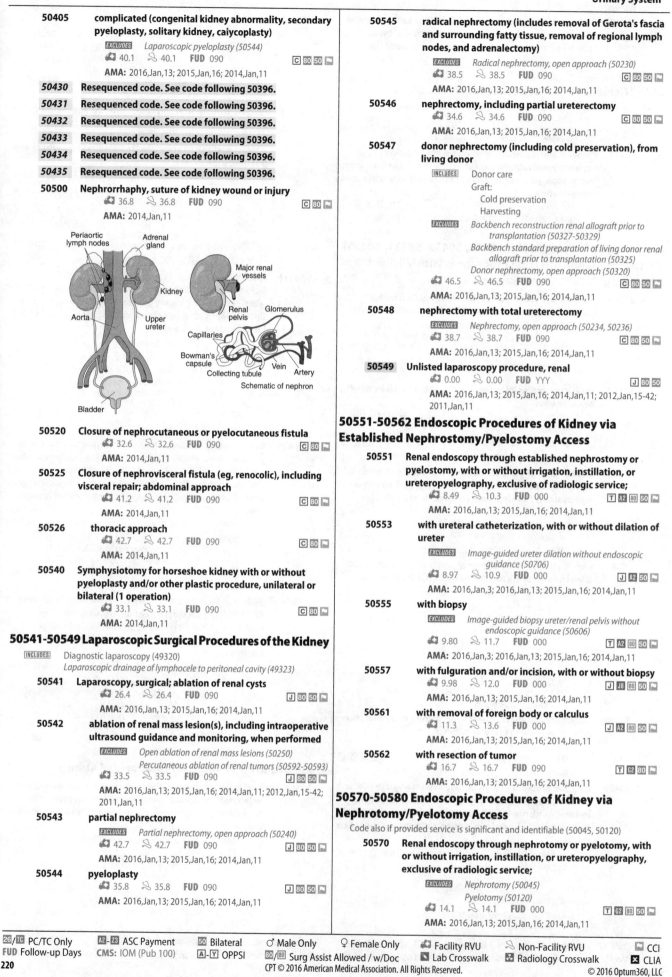

Schematic of nephron (labels: Periaortic lymph nodes, Adrenal gland, Major renal vessels, Kidney, Renal pelvis, Glomerulus, Aorta, Upper ureter, Capillaries, Bowman's capsule, Vein, Artery, Collecting tubule, Bladder)

50520 **Closure of nephrocutaneous or pyelocutaneous fistula**
🚗 32.6 ✂ 32.6 **FUD** 090 [C] [80] 🔲
AMA: 2014,Jan,11

50525 **Closure of nephrovisceral fistula (eg, renocolic), including visceral repair; abdominal approach**
🚗 41.2 ✂ 41.2 **FUD** 090 [C] [80] 🔲
AMA: 2014,Jan,11

50526 **thoracic approach**
🚗 42.7 ✂ 42.7 **FUD** 090 [C] [80] 🔲
AMA: 2014,Jan,11

50540 **Symphysiotomy for horseshoe kidney with or without pyeloplasty and/or other plastic procedure, unilateral or bilateral (1 operation)**
🚗 33.1 ✂ 33.1 **FUD** 090 [C] [80] 🔲
AMA: 2014,Jan,11

50541-50549 Laparoscopic Surgical Procedures of the Kidney
INCLUDES Diagnostic laparoscopy (49320)
Laparoscopic drainage of lymphocele to peritoneal cavity (49323)

50541 **Laparoscopy, surgical; ablation of renal cysts**
🚗 26.4 ✂ 26.4 **FUD** 090 [J] [80] [50] 🔲
AMA: 2016,Jan,13; 2015,Jan,16; 2014,Jan,11

50542 **ablation of renal mass lesion(s), including intraoperative ultrasound guidance and monitoring, when performed**
EXCLUDES *Open ablation of renal mass lesions (50250)*
Percutaneous ablation of renal tumors (50592-50593)
🚗 33.5 ✂ 33.5 **FUD** 090 [J] [80] [50] 🔲
AMA: 2016,Jan,13; 2015,Jan,16; 2014,Jan,11; 2012,Jan,15-42; 2011,Jan,11

50543 **partial nephrectomy**
EXCLUDES *Partial nephrectomy, open approach (50240)*
🚗 42.7 ✂ 42.7 **FUD** 090 [J] [80] [50] 🔲
AMA: 2016,Jan,13; 2015,Jan,16; 2014,Jan,11

50544 **pyeloplasty**
🚗 35.8 ✂ 35.8 **FUD** 090 [J] [80] [50] 🔲
AMA: 2016,Jan,13; 2015,Jan,16; 2014,Jan,11

50545 **radical nephrectomy (includes removal of Gerota's fascia and surrounding fatty tissue, removal of regional lymph nodes, and adrenalectomy)**
EXCLUDES *Radical nephrectomy, open approach (50230)*
🚗 38.5 ✂ 38.5 **FUD** 090 [C] [80] [50] 🔲
AMA: 2016,Jan,13; 2015,Jan,16; 2014,Jan,11

50546 **nephrectomy, including partial ureterectomy**
🚗 34.6 ✂ 34.6 **FUD** 090 [C] [80] [50] 🔲
AMA: 2016,Jan,13; 2015,Jan,16; 2014,Jan,11

50547 **donor nephrectomy (including cold preservation), from living donor**
INCLUDES Donor care
Graft:
    Cold preservation
    Harvesting
EXCLUDES *Backbench reconstruction renal allograft prior to transplantation (50327-50329)*
Backbench standard preparation of living donor renal allograft prior to transplantation (50325)
Donor nephrectomy, open approach (50320)
🚗 46.5 ✂ 46.5 **FUD** 090 [C] [80] [50] 🔲
AMA: 2016,Jan,13; 2015,Jan,16; 2014,Jan,11

50548 **nephrectomy with total ureterectomy**
EXCLUDES *Nephrectomy, open approach (50234, 50236)*
🚗 38.7 ✂ 38.7 **FUD** 090 [C] [80] [50] 🔲
AMA: 2016,Jan,13; 2015,Jan,16; 2014,Jan,11

50549 **Unlisted laparoscopy procedure, renal**
🚗 0.00 ✂ 0.00 **FUD** YYY [J] [80] [50]
AMA: 2016,Jan,13; 2015,Jan,16; 2014,Jan,11; 2012,Jan,15-42; 2011,Jan,11

50551-50562 Endoscopic Procedures of Kidney via Established Nephrostomy/Pyelostomy Access

50551 **Renal endoscopy through established nephrostomy or pyelostomy, with or without irrigation, instillation, or ureteropyelography, exclusive of radiologic service;**
🚗 8.49 ✂ 10.3 **FUD** 000 [T] [A2] [80] [50] 🔲
AMA: 2016,Jan,13; 2015,Jan,16; 2014,Jan,11

50553 **with ureteral catheterization, with or without dilation of ureter**
EXCLUDES *Image-guided ureter dilation without endoscopic guidance (50706)*
🚗 8.97 ✂ 10.9 **FUD** 000 [J] [A2] [50] 🔲
AMA: 2016,Jan,3; 2016,Jan,13; 2015,Jan,16; 2014,Jan,11

50555 **with biopsy**
EXCLUDES *Image-guided biopsy ureter/renal pelvis without endoscopic guidance (50606)*
🚗 9.80 ✂ 11.7 **FUD** 000 [T] [A2] [80] [50] 🔲
AMA: 2016,Jan,3; 2016,Jan,13; 2015,Jan,16; 2014,Jan,11

50557 **with fulguration and/or incision, with or without biopsy**
🚗 9.98 ✂ 12.0 **FUD** 000 [J] [J8] [80] [50] 🔲
AMA: 2016,Jan,13; 2015,Jan,16; 2014,Jan,11

50561 **with removal of foreign body or calculus**
🚗 11.3 ✂ 13.6 **FUD** 000 [J] [A2] [80] [50] 🔲
AMA: 2016,Jan,13; 2015,Jan,16; 2014,Jan,11

50562 **with resection of tumor**
🚗 16.7 ✂ 16.7 **FUD** 090 [T] [G2] [80] 🔲
AMA: 2016,Jan,13; 2015,Jan,16; 2014,Jan,11

50570-50580 Endoscopic Procedures of Kidney via Nephrotomy/Pyelotomy Access
Code also if provided service is significant and identifiable (50045, 50120)

50570 **Renal endoscopy through nephrotomy or pyelotomy, with or without irrigation, instillation, or ureteropyelography, exclusive of radiologic service;**
EXCLUDES *Nephrotomy (50045)*
Pyelotomy (50120)
🚗 14.1 ✂ 14.1 **FUD** 000 [T] [G2] [80] [50] 🔲
AMA: 2016,Jan,13; 2015,Jan,16; 2014,Jan,11

50572	with ureteral catheterization, with or without dilation of ureter

EXCLUDES *Image-guided ureter dilation without endoscopic guidance (50706)*

🔲 15.3   🔾 15.3   **FUD** 000   T 62 80 50 🔲

AMA: 2016,Jan,3; 2016,Jan,13; 2015,Jan,16; 2014,Jan,11

50574	with biopsy

EXCLUDES *Image-guide ureter/renal pelvis biopsy without endoscopic guidance (50606)*

🔲 16.3   🔾 16.3   **FUD** 000   T 62 80 50 🔲

AMA: 2016,Jan,3; 2016,Jan,13; 2015,Jan,16; 2014,Jan,11

50575	with endopyelotomy (includes cystoscopy, ureteroscopy, dilation of ureter and ureteral pelvic junction, incision of ureteral pelvic junction and insertion of endopyelotomy stent)

🔲 20.5   🔾 20.5   **FUD** 000   J 62 50 🔲

AMA: 2016,Jan,13; 2015,Jan,16; 2014,Jan,11; 2012,Jan,15-42; 2011,Jan,11

50576	with fulguration and/or incision, with or without biopsy

🔲 16.2   🔾 16.2   **FUD** 000   T 62 80 50 🔲

AMA: 2016,Jan,13; 2015,Jan,16; 2014,Jan,11

50580	with removal of foreign body or calculus

🔲 17.5   🔾 17.5   **FUD** 000   T 62 80 50 🔲

AMA: 2016,Jan,13; 2015,Jan,16; 2014,Jan,11

50590-50593 Noninvasive and Minimally Invasive Procedures of the Kidney

50590	Lithotripsy, extracorporeal shock wave

🔲 16.3   🔾 20.5   **FUD** 090   J 62 50 🔲

AMA: 2016,Jan,13; 2015,Jan,16; 2014,Jan,11; 2012,Jan,15-42; 2011,Jan,11

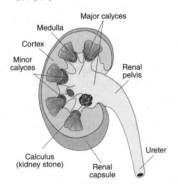

▲	50592	Ablation, 1 or more renal tumor(s), percutaneous, unilateral, radiofrequency

🔲 (76940, 77013, 77022)

🔲 10.4   🔾 72.3   **FUD** 010   T 62 50 🔲

AMA: 2014,Jan,11

▲	50593	Ablation, renal tumor(s), unilateral, percutaneous, cryotherapy

🔲 (76940, 77013, 77022)

🔲 13.8   🔾 131.   **FUD** 010   T 62 80 50 🔲

AMA: 2014,Jan,11

50600-50940 Open and Injection Procedures of Ureter

50600	Ureterotomy with exploration or drainage (separate procedure)

Code also ureteral endoscopy through ureterotomy when procedures constitute a significant identifiable service (50970-50980)

🔲 27.1   🔾 27.1   **FUD** 090   C 80 50 🔲

AMA: 2014,Jan,11

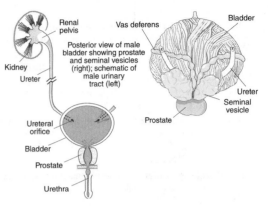

Posterior view of male bladder showing prostate and seminal vesicles (right); schematic of male urinary tract (left)

50605	Ureterotomy for insertion of indwelling stent, all types

🔲 28.4   🔾 28.4   **FUD** 090   C 80 50 🔲

AMA: 2016,Jan,13; 2015,Jan,16; 2014,Jan,11; 2012,Apr,17-18; 2012,Jan,15-42; 2011,Jan,11

▲ +	50606	Endoluminal biopsy of ureter and/or renal pelvis, non-endoscopic, including imaging guidance (eg, ultrasound and/or fluoroscopy) and all associated radiological supervision and interpretation (List separately in addition to code for primary procedure)

INCLUDES Renal pelvis and associated ureter as a single element

EXCLUDES *Procedure performed for same renal collecting system/associated ureter with (50555, 50574, 50955, 50974, 52007, 74425)*

Code first (50382-50389, [50430, 50431, 50432, 50433, 50434, 50435], 50684, 50688, 50690, 50693-50695, 51610)

🔲 4.56   🔾 15.0   **FUD** ZZZ   N M 50 🔲

AMA: 2016,Jan,3

50610	Ureterolithotomy; upper one-third of ureter

EXCLUDES *Cystotomy with calculus basket extraction of ureteral calculus (51065)*
Transvesical ureterolithotomy (51060)
Ureteral calculus manipulation/extraction performed endoscopically (50080-50081, 50561, 50961, 50980, 52320-52330, 52352-52353, [52356])
Ureterolithotomy performed laparoscopically (50945)

🔲 28.1   🔾 28.1   **FUD** 090   C 80 50 🔲

AMA: 2016,Jan,13; 2015,Jan,16; 2014,Jan,11

50620	middle one-third of ureter

EXCLUDES *Cystotomy with calculus basket extraction of ureteral calculus (51065)*
Transvesical ureterolithotomy (51060)
Ureteral calculus manipulation/extraction performed endoscopically (50080-50081, 50561, 50961, 50980, 52320-52330, 52352-52353, [52356])
Ureterolithotomy performed laparoscopically (50945)

🔲 26.0   🔾 26.0   **FUD** 090   C 80 50 🔲

AMA: 2016,Jan,13; 2015,Jan,16; 2014,Jan,11

50630	lower one-third of ureter

EXCLUDES *Cystotomy with calculus basket extraction of ureteral calculus (51065)*
Transvesical ureterolithotomy (51060)
Ureteral calculus manipulation/extraction performed endoscopically (50080-50081, 50561, 50961, 50980, 52320-52330, 52352-52353, [52356])
Ureterolithotomy performed laparoscopically (50945)

🔲 25.6   🔾 25.6   **FUD** 090   C 80 50 🔲

AMA: 2016,Jan,13; 2015,Jan,16; 2014,May,3; 2014,Jan,11

Urinary System

50650   **Ureterectomy, with bladder cuff (separate procedure)**
- *EXCLUDES*   *Ureterocele (51535, 52300)*
- 🚜 29.7   ⚖ 29.7   **FUD** 090   C 80 50 ▣
- **AMA:** 2014,Jan,11

50660   **Ureterectomy, total, ectopic ureter, combination abdominal, vaginal and/or perineal approach**
- *EXCLUDES*   *Ureterocele (51535, 52300)*
- 🚜 33.0   ⚖ 33.0   **FUD** 090   C 80 ▣
- **AMA:** 2014,Jan,11

50684   **Injection procedure for ureterography or ureteropyelography through ureterostomy or indwelling ureteral catheter**
- *EXCLUDES*   *Placement of nephroureteral catheter ([50433, 50434])*
  - *Placement of ureteral stent (50693-50695)*
- ✪ (74425)
- 🚜 1.45   ⚖ 3.02   **FUD** 000   N N1 50 ▣
- **AMA:** 2016,Jan,3; 2015,Oct,5; 2014,Jan,11

50686   **Manometric studies through ureterostomy or indwelling ureteral catheter**
- 🚜 2.54   ⚖ 4.08   **FUD** 000   S P2 80 ▣
- **AMA:** 2014,Jan,11

50688   **Change of ureterostomy tube or externally accessible ureteral stent via ileal conduit**
- ✪ (75984)
- 🚜 2.30   ⚖ 2.30   **FUD** 010   T A2 ▣
- **AMA:** 2016,Jan,3; 2014,Jan,11

50690   **Injection procedure for visualization of ileal conduit and/or ureteropyelography, exclusive of radiologic service**
- ✪ (74425)
- 🚜 2.03   ⚖ 2.81   **FUD** 000   N N1 ▣
- **AMA:** 2016,Jan,3; 2014,Jan,11

▲ **50693**   **Placement of ureteral stent, percutaneous, including diagnostic nephrostogram and/or ureterogram when performed, imaging guidance (eg, ultrasound and/or fluoroscopy), and all associated radiological supervision and interpretation; pre-existing nephrostomy tract**
- *INCLUDES*   Renal pelvis and associated ureter as a single element
- *EXCLUDES*   *Procedure performed for the same renal collecting system/ureter ([50430, 50431, 50432, 50433, 50434, 50435], 50684, 74425)*
- 🚜 6.33   ⚖ 30.1   **FUD** 000   T G2 50 ▣
- **AMA:** 2016,Jan,3; 2016,Jan,13; 2015,Oct,5

▲ **50694**   **new access, without separate nephrostomy catheter**
- *INCLUDES*   Renal pelvis and associated ureter as a single element
- *EXCLUDES*   *Procedure performed for the same renal collecting system/ureter ([50430, 50431, 50432, 50433, 50434, 50435], 50684, 74425)*
- 🚜 8.18   ⚖ 33.1   **FUD** 000   T G2 50 ▣
- **AMA:** 2016,Jan,3; 2016,Jan,13; 2015,Oct,5

▲ **50695**   **new access, with separate nephrostomy catheter**
- *INCLUDES*   Placement of separate ureteral stent and nephrostomy catheter into a ureter/associated renal pelvis through a new access
  - Renal pelvis and associated ureter as a single element
- *EXCLUDES*   *Procedure performed for the same renal collecting system/ureter ([50430, 50431, 50432, 50433, 50434, 50435], 50684, 74425)*
- 🚜 10.3   ⚖ 40.4   **FUD** 000   T G2 50 ▣
- **AMA:** 2016,Jan,3; 2016,Jan,13; 2015,Oct,5

50700   **Ureteroplasty, plastic operation on ureter (eg, stricture)**
- 🚜 26.7   ⚖ 26.7   **FUD** 090   C 80 50 ▣
- **AMA:** 2014,Jan,11

▲ + **50705**   **Ureteral embolization or occlusion, including imaging guidance (eg, ultrasound and/or fluoroscopy) and all associated radiological supervision and interpretation (List separately in addition to code for primary procedure)**
- *INCLUDES*   Renal pelvis and associated ureter as a single element
- *EXCLUDES*   *Percutaneous nephrostomy/nephroureteral catheter/ureteral catheter placement (50385, 50387, [50432, 50433, 50434, 50435], 50693-50695)*
- Code also when performed:
  - additional catheter insertions
  - diagnostic pyelography/ureterography
  - other interventions
- Code first (50382-50389, [50430, 50431, 50432, 50433, 50434, 50435], 50684, 50688, 50690, 50693-50695, 51610)
- 🚜 5.84   ⚖ 48.4   **FUD** ZZZ   N N1 50 ▣
- **AMA:** 2016,Jan,3

▲ + **50706**   **Balloon dilation, ureteral stricture, including imaging guidance (eg, ultrasound and/or fluoroscopy) and all associated radiological supervision and interpretation (List separately in addition to code for primary procedure)**
- *INCLUDES*   Dilation of nephrostomy, ureters, or urethra (74485)
  - Renal pelvis and associated ureter as a single element
- *EXCLUDES*   *Cystourethroscopy (52341, 52344-52345)*
  - *Percutaneous nephrostomy/nephroureteral catheter/ureteral catheter placement (50385, 50387, [50432, 50433, 50434, 50435], 50693-50695)*
  - *Renal endoscopy (50553, 50572)*
  - *Ureteral endoscopy (50953, 50972)*
- Code also when performed:
  - additional catheter insertions
  - diagnostic pyelography/ureterography
  - other interventions
- Code first (50382-50389, [50430, 50431, 50432, 50433, 50434, 50435], 50684, 50688, 50690, 50693-50695, 51610)
- 🚜 5.43   ⚖ 21.7   **FUD** ZZZ   N N1 50 ▣
- **AMA:** 2016,Jan,3

50715   **Ureterolysis, with or without repositioning of ureter for retroperitoneal fibrosis**
- 🚜 35.1   ⚖ 35.1   **FUD** 090   C 80 50 ▣
- **AMA:** 2014,Jan,11

50722   **Ureterolysis for ovarian vein syndrome**   ♀
- 🚜 29.3   ⚖ 29.3   **FUD** 090   C 80 ▣
- **AMA:** 2014,Jan,11

50725   **Ureterolysis for retrocaval ureter, with reanastomosis of upper urinary tract or vena cava**
- 🚜 32.4   ⚖ 32.4   **FUD** 090   C 80 ▣
- **AMA:** 2014,Jan,11

50727   **Revision of urinary-cutaneous anastomosis (any type urostomy);**
- 🚜 14.5   ⚖ 14.5   **FUD** 090   T G2 80 ▣
- **AMA:** 2014,Jan,11

50728   **with repair of fascial defect and hernia**
- 🚜 20.1   ⚖ 20.1   **FUD** 090   C 80 ▣
- **AMA:** 2014,Jan,11

50740   **Ureteropyelostomy, anastomosis of ureter and renal pelvis**
- 🚜 35.4   ⚖ 35.4   **FUD** 090   C 80 50 ▣
- **AMA:** 2016,Jan,13; 2015,Jan,16; 2014,Jan,11

50750   **Ureterocalycostomy, anastomosis of ureter to renal calyx**
- 🚜 33.1   ⚖ 33.1   **FUD** 090   C 80 50 ▣
- **AMA:** 2016,Jan,13; 2015,Jan,16; 2014,Jan,11

50760   **Ureteroureterostomy**
- 🚜 32.5   ⚖ 32.5   **FUD** 090   C 80 50 ▣
- **AMA:** 2016,Jan,13; 2015,Jan,16; 2014,Jan,11

50770   **Transureteroureterostomy, anastomosis of ureter to contralateral ureter**
- 🚜 33.1   ⚖ 33.1   **FUD** 090   C 80 ▣
- **AMA:** 2014,Jan,11

50780   Ureteroneocystostomy; anastomosis of single ureter to bladder
    INCLUDES   Minor procedures to prevent vesicoureteral reflux
    EXCLUDES   Cystourethroplasty with ureteroneocystostomy (51820)
    🔲 31.8   ⚖ 31.8   FUD 090   C 80 50 ▣
    AMA: 2016,Jan,13; 2015,Jan,16; 2014,Jan,11

50782   anastomosis of duplicated ureter to bladder
    INCLUDES   Minor procedures to prevent vesicoureteral reflux
    🔲 30.3   ⚖ 30.3   FUD 090   C 80 50 ▣
    AMA: 2016,Jan,13; 2015,Jan,16; 2014,Jan,11

50783   with extensive ureteral tailoring
    INCLUDES   Minor procedures to prevent vesicoureteral reflux
    🔲 32.5   ⚖ 32.5   FUD 090   C 80 50 ▣
    AMA: 2016,Jan,13; 2015,Jan,16; 2014,Jan,11

50785   with vesico-psoas hitch or bladder flap
    INCLUDES   Minor procedures to prevent vesicoureteral reflux
    🔲 34.9   ⚖ 34.9   FUD 090   C 80 50 ▣
    AMA: 2016,Jan,13; 2015,Jan,16; 2014,Jan,11

50800   Ureteroenterostomy, direct anastomosis of ureter to intestine
    EXCLUDES   Cystectomy with ureterosigmoidostomy/ureteroileal conduit (51580-51595)
    🔲 26.5   ⚖ 26.5   FUD 090   C 80 50 ▣
    AMA: 2016,Jan,13; 2015,Jan,16; 2014,Jan,11

50810   Ureterosigmoidostomy, with creation of sigmoid bladder and establishment of abdominal or perineal colostomy, including intestine anastomosis
    EXCLUDES   Cystectomy with ureterosigmoidostomy/ureteroileal conduit (51580-51595)
    🔲 36.2   ⚖ 36.2   FUD 090   C 80 ▣
    AMA: 2016,Jan,13; 2015,Jan,16; 2014,Jan,11

50815   Ureterocolon conduit, including intestine anastomosis
    EXCLUDES   Cystectomy with ureterosigmoidostomy/ureteroileal conduit (51580-51595)
    🔲 35.2   ⚖ 35.2   FUD 090   C 80 50 ▣
    AMA: 2016,Jan,13; 2015,Jan,16; 2014,Jan,11

50820   Ureteroileal conduit (ileal bladder), including intestine anastomosis (Bricker operation)
    EXCLUDES   Cystectomy with ureterosigmoidostomy/ureteroileal conduit (51580-51595)
    🔲 37.8   ⚖ 37.8   FUD 090   C 80 50 ▣
    AMA: 2016,Jan,13; 2015,Jan,16; 2014,Jan,11

50825   Continent diversion, including intestine anastomosis using any segment of small and/or large intestine (Kock pouch or Camey enterocystoplasty)
    🔲 47.6   ⚖ 47.6   FUD 090   C 80 ▣
    AMA: 2016,Jan,13; 2015,Jan,16; 2014,Jan,11

50830   Urinary undiversion (eg, taking down of ureteroileal conduit, ureterosigmoidostomy or ureteroenterostomy with ureteroureterostomy or ureteroneocystostomy)
    🔲 52.1   ⚖ 52.1   FUD 090   C 80 ▣
    AMA: 2016,Jan,13; 2015,Jan,16; 2014,Jan,11

50840   Replacement of all or part of ureter by intestine segment, including intestine anastomosis
    🔲 35.4   ⚖ 35.4   FUD 090   C 80 50 ▣
    AMA: 2016,Jan,13; 2015,Jan,16; 2014,Jan,11

50845   Cutaneous appendico-vesicostomy
    INCLUDES   Mitrofanoff operation
    🔲 35.9   ⚖ 35.9   FUD 090   C 80 ▣
    AMA: 2014,Jan,11

50860   Ureterostomy, transplantation of ureter to skin
    🔲 27.1   ⚖ 27.1   FUD 090   C 80 50 ▣
    AMA: 2014,Jan,11

50900   Ureterorrhaphy, suture of ureter (separate procedure)
    🔲 24.7   ⚖ 24.7   FUD 090   C 80 50 ▣
    AMA: 2014,Jan,11

50920   Closure of ureterocutaneous fistula
    🔲 25.3   ⚖ 25.3   FUD 090   C 80 ▣
    AMA: 2014,Jan,11

50930   Closure of ureterovisceral fistula (including visceral repair)
    🔲 33.9   ⚖ 33.9   FUD 090   C 80 ▣
    AMA: 2014,Jan,11

50940   Deligation of ureter
    EXCLUDES   Ureteroplasty/ureterolysis (50700-50860)
    🔲 25.4   ⚖ 25.4   FUD 090   C 80 50 ▣
    AMA: 2014,Jan,11

50945-50949 Laparoscopic Procedures of Ureter

    INCLUDES   Diagnostic laparoscopy (49320)
                Ureteroneocystostomy, open approach (50780-50785)

50945   Laparoscopy, surgical; ureterolithotomy
    🔲 27.9   ⚖ 27.9   FUD 090   J 80 50 ▣
    AMA: 2016,Jan,13; 2015,Jan,16; 2014,Jan,11; 2012,Jan,15-42; 2011,Jan,11

50947   ureteroneocystostomy with cystoscopy and ureteral stent placement
    🔲 39.9   ⚖ 39.9   FUD 090   J A2 80 50 ▣
    AMA: 2016,Jan,13; 2015,Jan,16; 2014,Jan,11

50948   ureteroneocystostomy without cystoscopy and ureteral stent placement
    🔲 36.7   ⚖ 36.7   FUD 090   J A2 80 50 ▣
    AMA: 2016,Jan,13; 2015,Jan,16; 2014,Jan,11

50949   Unlisted laparoscopy procedure, ureter
    🔲 0.00   ⚖ 0.00   FUD YYY   J 80 50
    AMA: 2016,Jan,13; 2015,Jan,16; 2014,Jan,11

50951-50961 Endoscopic Procedures of Ureter via Established Ureterostomy Access

50951   Ureteral endoscopy through established ureterostomy, with or without irrigation, instillation, or ureteropyelography, exclusive of radiologic service;
    🔲 8.84   ⚖ 10.7   FUD 000   T A2 80 50 ▣
    AMA: 2016,Jan,13; 2015,Jan,16; 2014,Jan,11; 2012,Jan,15-42; 2011,Jan,11

50953   with ureteral catheterization, with or without dilation of ureter
    EXCLUDES   Image-guided ureter dilation without endoscopic guidance (50706)
    🔲 9.37   ⚖ 11.3   FUD 000   T A2 80 50 ▣
    AMA: 2016,Jan,3; 2016,Jan,13; 2015,Jan,16; 2014,Jan,11

50955   with biopsy
    EXCLUDES   Image-guided biopsy of ureter and/or renal pelvis without endoscopic guidance (50606)
    🔲 10.1   ⚖ 12.1   FUD 000   T A2 80 50 ▣
    AMA: 2016,Jan,3; 2016,Jan,13; 2015,Jan,16; 2014,Jan,11

50957   with fulguration and/or incision, with or without biopsy
    🔲 10.2   ⚖ 12.2   FUD 000   J A2 80 50 ▣
    AMA: 2016,Jan,13; 2015,Jan,16; 2014,Jan,11

50961   with removal of foreign body or calculus
    🔲 9.15   ⚖ 11.0   FUD 000   T A2 80 50 ▣
    AMA: 2016,Jan,13; 2015,Jan,16; 2014,Jan,11; 2012,Jan,15-42; 2011,Jan,11

50970-50980 Endoscopic Procedures of Ureter via Ureterotomy

    EXCLUDES   Ureterotomy (50600)

50970   Ureteral endoscopy through ureterotomy, with or without irrigation, instillation, or ureteropyelography, exclusive of radiologic service;
    🔲 10.7   ⚖ 10.7   FUD 000   T A2 80 50 ▣
    AMA: 2016,Jan,13; 2015,Jan,16; 2014,Jan,11

Urinary System

50972 — 51595

50972   with ureteral catheterization, with or without dilation of ureter

> EXCLUDES   *Image-guided ureter dilation without endoscopic guidance (50706)*

> 10.4   10.4   **FUD** 000   T A2 80 50

AMA: 2016,Jan,3; 2016,Jan,13; 2015,Jan,16; 2014,Jan,11

50974   with biopsy

> EXCLUDES   *Image-guided biopsy of ureter and/or renal pelvis without endoscopic guidance (50606)*

> 13.6   13.6   **FUD** 000   J A2 80 50

AMA: 2016,Jan,3; 2016,Jan,13; 2015,Jan,16; 2014,Jan,11

50976   with fulguration and/or incision, with or without biopsy

> 13.4   13.4   **FUD** 000   J A2 80 50

AMA: 2016,Jan,13; 2015,Jan,16; 2014,Jan,11

50980   with removal of foreign body or calculus

> 10.2   10.2   **FUD** 000   T A2 80 50

AMA: 2016,Jan,13; 2015,Jan,16; 2014,Jan,11

51020-51080 Open Incisional Procedures of Bladder

51020   Cystotomy or cystostomy; with fulguration and/or insertion of radioactive material

> 13.4   13.4   **FUD** 090   T A2 80

AMA: 2014,Jan,11

51030   with cryosurgical destruction of intravesical lesion

> 13.6   13.6   **FUD** 090   T A2 80

AMA: 2014,Jan,11

51040   Cystostomy, cystotomy with drainage

> 8.30   8.30   **FUD** 090   T A2 80

AMA: 2014,Jan,11

51045   Cystotomy, with insertion of ureteral catheter or stent (separate procedure)

> 14.1   14.1   **FUD** 090   T A2 80

AMA: 2014,Jan,11

51050   Cystolithotomy, cystotomy with removal of calculus, without vesical neck resection

> 13.5   13.5   **FUD** 090   J A2 80

AMA: 2014,Jan,11

51060   Transvesical ureterolithotomy

> 16.7   16.7   **FUD** 090   T 80

AMA: 2014,Jan,11

51065   Cystotomy, with calculus basket extraction and/or ultrasonic or electrohydraulic fragmentation of ureteral calculus

> 16.6   16.6   **FUD** 090   J A2 80

AMA: 2014,Jan,11

51080   Drainage of perivesical or prevesical space abscess

> EXCLUDES   *Image-guided percutaneous catheter drainage (49406)*

> 11.7   11.7   **FUD** 090   T A2 80

AMA: 2014,Jan,11

51100-51102 Bladder Aspiration Procedures

51100   Aspiration of bladder; by needle

> (76942, 77002, 77012)

> 1.13   1.74   **FUD** 000   T P3

AMA: 2016,Jan,13; 2015,Jan,16; 2014,Jan,11

51101   by trocar or intracatheter

> (76942, 77002, 77012)

> 1.50   3.53   **FUD** 000   S P3

AMA: 2016,Jan,13; 2015,Jan,16; 2014,Jan,11

51102   with insertion of suprapubic catheter

> (76942, 77002, 77012)

> 4.17   6.46   **FUD** 000   T A2

AMA: 2016,Jan,13; 2015,Jan,16; 2014,Jan,11

51500-51597 Open Excisional Procedures of Bladder

51500   Excision of urachal cyst or sinus, with or without umbilical hernia repair

> 18.3   18.3   **FUD** 090   T A2 80

AMA: 2014,Jan,11

51520   Cystotomy; for simple excision of vesical neck (separate procedure)

> 17.1   17.1   **FUD** 090   T A2 80

AMA: 2014,Jan,11

51525   for excision of bladder diverticulum, single or multiple (separate procedure)

> EXCLUDES   *Transurethral resection (52305)*

> 24.7   24.7   **FUD** 090   C 80

AMA: 2014,Jan,11

51530   for excision of bladder tumor

> EXCLUDES   *Transurethral resection (52234-52240, 52305)*

> 22.9   22.9   **FUD** 090   C 80

AMA: 2014,Jan,11

51535   Cystotomy for excision, incision, or repair of ureterocele

> EXCLUDES   *Transurethral excision (52300)*

> 22.4   22.4   **FUD** 090   T 62 80 50

AMA: 2014,Jan,11

51550   Cystectomy, partial; simple

> 27.7   27.7   **FUD** 090   C 80

AMA: 2014,Jan,11

51555   complicated (eg, postradiation, previous surgery, difficult location)

> 36.4   36.4   **FUD** 090   C 80

AMA: 2014,Jan,11

51565   Cystectomy, partial, with reimplantation of ureter(s) into bladder (ureteroneocystostomy)

> 37.4   37.4   **FUD** 090   C 80

AMA: 2014,Jan,11

51570   Cystectomy, complete; (separate procedure)

> 42.5   42.5   **FUD** 090   C 80

AMA: 2014,Jan,11

51575   with bilateral pelvic lymphadenectomy, including external iliac, hypogastric, and obturator nodes

> 52.4   52.4   **FUD** 090   C 80

AMA: 2014,Jan,11

51580   Cystectomy, complete, with ureterosigmoidostomy or ureterocutaneous transplantations;

> 54.5   54.5   **FUD** 090   C 80

AMA: 2014,Jan,11

51585   with bilateral pelvic lymphadenectomy, including external iliac, hypogastric, and obturator nodes

> 60.6   60.6   **FUD** 090   C 80

AMA: 2014,Jan,11

51590   Cystectomy, complete, with ureteroileal conduit or sigmoid bladder, including intestine anastomosis;

> 55.6   55.6   **FUD** 090   C 80

AMA: 2014,Jan,11

51595   with bilateral pelvic lymphadenectomy, including external iliac, hypogastric, and obturator nodes

> 62.9   62.9   **FUD** 090   C 80

AMA: 2014,Jan,11

Diaphragm
Umbilicus
Access is from above the pubic bone
Pubic bone
Hip and pubic bone
Urethral orifice
Labia majora
Vaginal canal
Ovary
Uterus
Rectouterine pouch
Bladder
Cervix
Rectum
Anus

51596 Cystectomy, complete, with continent diversion, any open technique, using any segment of small and/or large intestine to construct neobladder
⏴ 67.6 ⏵ 67.6 **FUD** 090 `C` `80` ▯
AMA: 2014,Jan,11

51597 Pelvic exenteration, complete, for vesical, prostatic or urethral malignancy, with removal of bladder and ureteral transplantations, with or without hysterectomy and/or abdominoperineal resection of rectum and colon and colostomy, or any combination thereof
EXCLUDES *Pelvic exenteration for gynecologic malignancy (58240)*
⏴ 66.1 ⏵ 66.1 **FUD** 090 `C` `80` ▯
AMA: 2014,Jan,11

51600-51720 Injection/Insertion/Instillation Procedures of Bladder

51600 Injection procedure for cystography or voiding urethrocystography
⊠ (74430, 74455)
⏴ 1.28 ⏵ 5.21 **FUD** 000 `N` `N1` ▯
AMA: 2014,Jan,11

51605 Injection procedure and placement of chain for contrast and/or chain urethrocystography
⊠ (74430)
⏴ 1.10 ⏵ 1.10 **FUD** 000 `N` `N1` ▯
AMA: 2014,Jan,11

51610 Injection procedure for retrograde urethrocystography
⊠ (74450)
⏴ 1.85 ⏵ 3.03 **FUD** 000 `N` `N1` ▯
AMA: 2016,Jan,3; 2014,Jan,11

51700 Bladder irrigation, simple, lavage and/or instillation
⏴ 1.29 ⏵ 2.36 **FUD** 000 `T` `P3` ▯
AMA: 2014,Jan,11

51701 Insertion of non-indwelling bladder catheter (eg, straight catheterization for residual urine)
EXCLUDES *Catheterization for specimen collection (P9612)*
Insertion of catheter as an inclusive component of another procedure
⏴ 0.80 ⏵ 1.55 **FUD** 000 `Q1` `N1` ▯
AMA: 2016,Jan,13; 2015,Jan,16; 2014,Jan,11; 2012,Jan,15-42; 2011,Jan,11

51702 Insertion of temporary indwelling bladder catheter; simple (eg, Foley)
EXCLUDES *Focused ultrasound ablation of uterine leiomyomata (0071T-0072T)*
Insertion of catheter as an inclusive component of another procedure
⏴ 0.87 ⏵ 1.99 **FUD** 000 `Q1` `N1` ▯
AMA: 2016,Jan,13; 2015,Jan,16; 2014,May,3; 2014,Jan,11; 2012,Jan,15-42; 2011,Jan,11

51703 complicated (eg, altered anatomy, fractured catheter/balloon)
⏴ 2.34 ⏵ 3.68 **FUD** 000 `S` `P2` ▯
AMA: 2016,Jan,13; 2015,Jan,16; 2014,Jan,11

51705 Change of cystostomy tube; simple
⏴ 1.49 ⏵ 2.58 **FUD** 000 `T` `P3` ▯
AMA: 2016,Jan,13; 2015,Jan,16; 2014,Jan,11; 2012,Jan,15-42; 2011,Jan,11

51710 complicated
⊠ (75984)
⏴ 2.30 ⏵ 3.65 **FUD** 000 `T` `A2` ▯
AMA: 2016,Jan,13; 2015,Jan,16; 2014,Jan,11

51715 Endoscopic injection of implant material into the submucosal tissues of the urethra and/or bladder neck
EXCLUDES *Injection of bulking agent (submucosal) for fecal incontinence, via anoscope (0377T)*
⏴ 5.75 ⏵ 8.27 **FUD** 000 `T` `A2` `80` ▯
AMA: 2014,Jan,11

51720 Bladder instillation of anticarcinogenic agent (including retention time)
Code also bacillus Calmette-Guerin vaccine (BCG) (90586)
⏴ 2.30 ⏵ 3.10 **FUD** 000 `T` `P3` ▯
AMA: 2016,Jan,13; 2015,Jan,16; 2014,Jan,11; 2012,Jan,15-42; 2011,Jan,11

51725-51798 [51797] Uroflowmetric Evaluations

INCLUDES Equipment
Fees for services of technician
Medications
Supplies
Code also modifier 26 if physician/other qualified health care professional provides only interpretation of results and/or operates the equipment

51725 Simple cystometrogram (CMG) (eg, spinal manometer)
⏴ 5.30 ⏵ 5.30 **FUD** 000 `T` `P3` `80` ▯
AMA: 2016,Jan,13; 2015,Jan,16; 2014,Jan,11

51726 Complex cystometrogram (ie, calibrated electronic equipment);
⏴ 7.44 ⏵ 7.44 **FUD** 000 `T` `A2` ▯
AMA: 2016,Jan,13; 2015,Jan,16; 2014,Jan,11

51727 with urethral pressure profile studies (ie, urethral closure pressure profile), any technique
⏴ 8.81 ⏵ 8.81 **FUD** 000 `T` `P3` `80` ▯
AMA: 2016,Jan,13; 2015,Jan,16; 2014,Jan,11

51728 with voiding pressure studies (ie, bladder voiding pressure), any technique
⏴ 8.89 ⏵ 8.89 **FUD** 000 `T` `P3` `80` ▯
AMA: 2016,Jan,13; 2015,Jan,16; 2014,Jan,11

51729 with voiding pressure studies (ie, bladder voiding pressure) and urethral pressure profile studies (ie, urethral closure pressure profile), any technique
⏴ 9.61 ⏵ 9.61 **FUD** 000 `T` `P3` `80` ▯
AMA: 2016,Jan,13; 2015,Jan,16; 2014,Jan,11

+ # 51797 Voiding pressure studies, intra-abdominal (ie, rectal, gastric, intraperitoneal) (List separately in addition to code for primary procedure)
Code first (51728-51729)
⏴ 3.16 ⏵ 3.16 **FUD** ZZZ `N` `N1` `80` ▯
AMA: 2016,Jan,13; 2015,Jan,16; 2014,Jan,11; 2012,Jan,15-42; 2011,Jan,11

51736 Simple uroflowmetry (UFR) (eg, stop-watch flow rate, mechanical uroflowmeter)
⏴ 0.44 ⏵ 0.44 **FUD** XXX `Q1` `N1` `80` ▯
AMA: 2016,Jan,13; 2015,Jan,16; 2014,Jan,11

51741 Complex uroflowmetry (eg, calibrated electronic equipment)
⏴ 0.45 ⏵ 0.45 **FUD** XXX `Q1` `N1` ▯
AMA: 2016,Jan,13; 2015,Jan,16; 2014,Sep,13; 2014,Jan,11

51784 Electromyography studies (EMG) of anal or urethral sphincter, other than needle, any technique
EXCLUDES *Stimulus evoked response (51792)*
⏴ 5.44 ⏵ 5.44 **FUD** 000 `S` `P2` ▯
AMA: 2016,Jan,13; 2015,Jan,16; 2014,Sep,13; 2014,Feb,11; 2014,Jan,11

51785 Needle electromyography studies (EMG) of anal or urethral sphincter, any technique
⏴ 7.48 ⏵ 7.48 **FUD** 000 `T` `A2` `80` ▯
AMA: 2016,Jan,13; 2015,Jan,16; 2014,Jan,11; 2012,Jan,15-42; 2011,Jan,11

51792 Stimulus evoked response (eg, measurement of bulbocavernosus reflex latency time)
EXCLUDES *Electromyography studies (EMG) of anal or urethral sphincter (51784)*
⏴ 5.98 ⏵ 5.98 **FUD** 000 `Q1` `N1` `80` ▯
AMA: 2016,Jan,13; 2015,Jan,16; 2014,Feb,11; 2014,Jan,11

51797 Resequenced code, See code following 51729.

Urinary System

51798 Measurement of post-voiding residual urine and/or bladder capacity by ultrasound, non-imaging
🔧 0.54 ⚕ 0.54 **FUD** XXX   01 N1 80 TC
AMA: 2016,Jan,13; 2015,Jan,16; 2014,Jan,11

51800-51980 Open Repairs Urinary System

51800 Cystoplasty or cystourethroplasty, plastic operation on bladder and/or vesical neck (anterior Y-plasty, vesical fundus resection), any procedure, with or without wedge resection of posterior vesical neck
🔧 29.9 ⚕ 29.9 **FUD** 090   C 80
AMA: 2014,Jan,11

51820 Cystourethroplasty with unilateral or bilateral ureteroneocystostomy
🔧 31.9 ⚕ 31.9 **FUD** 090   C 80
AMA: 2014,Jan,11

51840 Anterior vesicourethropexy, or urethropexy (eg, Marshall-Marchetti-Krantz, Burch); simple
EXCLUDES Pereyra type urethropexy (57289)
🔧 18.8 ⚕ 18.8 **FUD** 090   C 80
AMA: 2016,Jan,13; 2015,Jan,16; 2014,Jan,11; 2012,Aug,13-14; 2012,Jan,15-42; 2011,Jan,11

51841 complicated (eg, secondary repair)
EXCLUDES Pereyra type urethropexy (57289)
🔧 22.3 ⚕ 22.3 **FUD** 090   C 80
AMA: 2016,Jan,13; 2015,Jan,16; 2014,Jan,11; 2012,Aug,13-14

51845 Abdomino-vaginal vesical neck suspension, with or without endoscopic control (eg, Stamey, Raz, modified Pereyra) ♀
🔧 16.8 ⚕ 16.8 **FUD** 090   J 80
AMA: 2016,Jan,13; 2015,Jan,16; 2014,Jan,11

51860 Cystorrhaphy, suture of bladder wound, injury or rupture; simple
🔧 21.4 ⚕ 21.4 **FUD** 090   J 80
AMA: 2014,Jan,11

51865 complicated
🔧 25.7 ⚕ 25.7 **FUD** 090   C 80
AMA: 2014,Jan,11

51880 Closure of cystostomy (separate procedure)
🔧 13.4 ⚕ 13.4 **FUD** 090   T A2 80
AMA: 2014,Jan,11

51900 Closure of vesicovaginal fistula, abdominal approach ♀
EXCLUDES Vesicovaginal fistula closure, vaginal approach (57320-57330)
🔧 24.0 ⚕ 24.0 **FUD** 090   C 80
AMA: 2014,Jan,11

51920 Closure of vesicouterine fistula; ♀
EXCLUDES Enterovesical fistula closure (44660-44661)
Rectovesical fistula closure (45800-45805)
🔧 24.9 ⚕ 24.9 **FUD** 090   C 80
AMA: 2014,Jan,11

51925 with hysterectomy ♀
EXCLUDES Enterovesical fistula closure (44660-44661)
Rectovesical fistula closure (45800-45805)
🔧 31.4 ⚕ 31.4 **FUD** 090   C 80
AMA: 2014,Jan,11

51940 Closure, exstrophy of bladder
EXCLUDES Epispadias reconstruction with exstrophy of bladder (54390)
🔧 47.5 ⚕ 47.5 **FUD** 090   C 80
AMA: 2014,Jan,11

51960 Enterocystoplasty, including intestinal anastomosis
🔧 40.0 ⚕ 40.0 **FUD** 090   C 80
AMA: 2014,Jan,11

51980 Cutaneous vesicostomy
🔧 20.4 ⚕ 20.4 **FUD** 090   C 80
AMA: 2014,Jan,11

51990-51999 Laparoscopic Procedures of Urinary System

CMS: 100-03,230.10 Incontinence Control Devices
INCLUDES Diagnostic laparoscopy (49320)

51990 Laparoscopy, surgical; urethral suspension for stress incontinence
🔧 21.5 ⚕ 21.5 **FUD** 090   J 80
AMA: 2016,Jan,13; 2015,Jan,16; 2014,Jan,11; 2012,Aug,13-14; 2012,Mar,9-10

51992 sling operation for stress incontinence (eg, fascia or synthetic)
EXCLUDES Removal/revision of sling for stress incontinence (57287)
Sling operation for stress incontinence, open approach (57288)
🔧 24.1 ⚕ 24.1 **FUD** 090   J A2 80
AMA: 2016,Jan,13; 2015,Jan,16; 2014,Jan,11; 2012,Aug,13-14; 2012,Mar,9-10

51999 Unlisted laparoscopy procedure, bladder
🔧 0.00 ⚕ 0.00 **FUD** YYY   J 80
AMA: 2014,Jan,11

52000-52318 Endoscopic Procedures via Urethra: Bladder and Urethra

INCLUDES Diagnostic and therapeutic endoscopy of bowel segments utilized as replacements for native bladder

52000 Cystourethroscopy (separate procedure)
EXCLUDES Cystourethroscopy (52001, 52320, 52325, 52327, 52330, 52332, 52334, 52341-52343, [52356])
🔧 3.63 ⚕ 5.80 **FUD** 000   T A2
AMA: 2016,Jan,13; 2015,Jan,16; 2014,May,3; 2014,Jan,11; 2013,Mar,13; 2012,Jan,15-42; 2011,Jan,11

52001 Cystourethroscopy with irrigation and evacuation of multiple obstructing clots
INCLUDES Cystourethroscopy (separate procedure) (52000)
🔧 8.28 ⚕ 10.5 **FUD** 000   T A2
AMA: 2014,Jan,11

52005 Cystourethroscopy, with ureteral catheterization, with or without irrigation, instillation, or ureteropyelography, exclusive of radiologic service;
INCLUDES Howard test
🔧 3.83 ⚕ 7.53 **FUD** 000   T A2
AMA: 2016,Jan,13; 2015,Jan,16; 2014,Jan,11; 2012,Jan,15-42; 2011,Jan,11

52007 with brush biopsy of ureter and/or renal pelvis
EXCLUDES Image-guided ureter/renal pelvis biopsy without endoscopic guidance (50606)
🔧 4.77 ⚕ 12.5 **FUD** 000   T A2 50
AMA: 2016,Jan,3; 2016,Jan,13; 2015,Jan,16; 2014,Jan,11

52010 Cystourethroscopy, with ejaculatory duct catheterization, with or without irrigation, instillation, or duct radiography, exclusive of radiologic service ♂
🔧 (74440)
🔧 4.81 ⚕ 10.5 **FUD** 000   T A2
AMA: 2016,Jan,13; 2015,Jan,16; 2014,Jan,11

52204 Cystourethroscopy, with biopsy(s)
🔧 4.08 ⚕ 10.4 **FUD** 000   T A2
AMA: 2016,May,12; 2016,Jan,13; 2015,Jan,16; 2014,Jan,11; 2012,Jan,15-42; 2011,Jan,11

52214 Cystourethroscopy, with fulguration (including cryosurgery or laser surgery) of trigone, bladder neck, prostatic fossa, urethra, or periurethral glands
Code also modifier 78 when performed by same physician:
During postoperative period (52601, 52630)
During the postoperative period of a related surgical procedure
For postoperative bleeding
🔧 5.08 ⚕ 18.6 **FUD** 000   T A2
AMA: 2016,May,12; 2016,Jan,13; 2015,Jan,16; 2014,Jan,11

 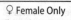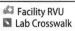

52224 Cystourethroscopy, with fulguration (including cryosurgery or laser surgery) or treatment of MINOR (less than 0.5 cm) lesion(s) with or without biopsy
🚑 5.87 ✄ 19.5 **FUD** 000 T A2 ▣
AMA: 2016,May,12; 2016,Jan,13; 2015,Jan,16; 2014,Jan,11; 2012,Jan,15-42; 2011,Jan,11

52234 Cystourethroscopy, with fulguration (including cryosurgery or laser surgery) and/or resection of; SMALL bladder tumor(s) (0.5 up to 2.0 cm)
EXCLUDES Bladder tumor excision through cystotomy (51530)
🚑 7.09 ✄ 7.09 **FUD** 000 T A2 ▣
AMA: 2016,May,12; 2016,Jan,13; 2015,Jan,16; 2014,Jan,11; 2012,Jan,15-42; 2011,Jan,11

52235 MEDIUM bladder tumor(s) (2.0 to 5.0 cm)
EXCLUDES Bladder tumor excision through cystotomy (51530)
🚑 8.32 ✄ 8.32 **FUD** 000 T A2 ▣
AMA: 2016,May,12; 2016,Jan,13; 2015,Jan,16; 2014,Jan,11

52240 LARGE bladder tumor(s)
EXCLUDES Bladder tumor excision through cystotomy (51530)
🚑 11.3 ✄ 11.3 **FUD** 000 T A2 ▣
AMA: 2016,May,12; 2016,Jan,13; 2015,Jan,16; 2014,Jan,11

52250 Cystourethroscopy with insertion of radioactive substance, with or without biopsy or fulguration
🚑 6.91 ✄ 6.91 **FUD** 000 T A2 ▣
AMA: 2016,Jan,13; 2015,Jan,16; 2014,Jan,11

52260 Cystourethroscopy, with dilation of bladder for interstitial cystitis; general or conduction (spinal) anesthesia
🚑 6.06 ✄ 6.06 **FUD** 000 T A2 ▣
AMA: 2016,Jan,13; 2015,Jan,16; 2014,Jan,11; 2012,Jan,15-42; 2011,Jan,11

52265 local anesthesia
🚑 4.69 ✄ 10.3 **FUD** 000 T P3 ▣
AMA: 2016,Jan,13; 2015,Jan,16; 2014,Jan,11

52270 Cystourethroscopy, with internal urethrotomy; female ♀
🚑 5.23 ✄ 10.0 **FUD** 000 T A2 ▣
AMA: 2016,Jan,13; 2015,Jan,16; 2014,Jan,11

52275 male ♂
🚑 7.16 ✄ 13.5 **FUD** 000 T A2 ▣
AMA: 2016,Jan,13; 2015,Jan,16; 2014,Jan,11

52276 Cystourethroscopy with direct vision internal urethrotomy
🚑 7.63 ✄ 7.63 **FUD** 000 T A2 ▣
AMA: 2016,Jan,13; 2015,Jan,16; 2014,Jan,11; 2012,Jan,15-42; 2011,Jan,11

52277 Cystourethroscopy, with resection of external sphincter (sphincterotomy)
🚑 9.32 ✄ 9.32 **FUD** 000 T A2 80 ▣
AMA: 2016,Jan,13; 2015,Jan,16; 2014,Jan,11

52281 Cystourethroscopy, with calibration and/or dilation of urethral stricture or stenosis, with or without meatotomy, with or without injection procedure for cystography, male or female
🚑 4.38 ✄ 7.72 **FUD** 000 T A2 ▣
AMA: 2016,Jan,13; 2015,Jan,16; 2014,Jan,11; 2012,Jan,15-42; 2011,Jan,11

52282 Cystourethroscopy, with insertion of permanent urethral stent
EXCLUDES Placement of temporary prostatic urethral stent (53855)
🚑 9.70 ✄ 9.70 **FUD** 000 T A2 ▣
AMA: 2016,Jan,13; 2015,Jun,5; 2015,Jan,16; 2014,Jan,11

52283 Cystourethroscopy, with steroid injection into stricture
🚑 5.80 ✄ 7.87 **FUD** 000 T A2 ▣
AMA: 2016,Jan,13; 2015,Mar,9; 2015,Jan,16; 2014,Jan,11

52285 Cystourethroscopy for treatment of the female urethral syndrome with any or all of the following: urethral meatotomy, urethral dilation, internal urethrotomy, lysis of urethrovaginal septal fibrosis, lateral incisions of the bladder neck, and fulguration of polyp(s) of urethra, bladder neck, and/or trigone ♀
🚑 5.64 ✄ 7.94 **FUD** 000 T A2 ▣
AMA: 2016,Jan,13; 2015,Jan,16; 2014,Jan,11

52287 Cystourethroscopy, with injection(s) for chemodenervation of the bladder
Code also supply of chemodenervation agent
🚑 4.87 ✄ 8.83 **FUD** 000 T G2 ▣
AMA: 2014,Jan,11

52290 Cystourethroscopy; with ureteral meatotomy, unilateral or bilateral
🚑 7.03 ✄ 7.03 **FUD** 000 T A2 ▣
AMA: 2016,Jan,13; 2015,Jan,16; 2014,Jan,11

52300 with resection or fulguration of orthotopic ureterocele(s), unilateral or bilateral
🚑 8.09 ✄ 8.09 **FUD** 000 T A2 80 ▣
AMA: 2016,Jan,13; 2015,Jan,16; 2014,Jan,11

52301 with resection or fulguration of ectopic ureterocele(s), unilateral or bilateral
🚑 8.36 ✄ 8.36 **FUD** 000 T A2 80 ▣
AMA: 2016,Jan,13; 2015,Jan,16; 2014,Jan,11

52305 with incision or resection of orifice of bladder diverticulum, single or multiple
🚑 8.04 ✄ 8.04 **FUD** 000 J A2 ▣
AMA: 2016,Jan,13; 2015,Jan,16; 2014,Jan,11

Diverticulum of bladder
Bladder
Pubic bone
Rectum
Urethra

52310 Cystourethroscopy, with removal of foreign body, calculus, or ureteral stent from urethra or bladder (separate procedure); simple
Code also modifier 58 for removal of a self-retaining, indwelling ureteral stent
🚑 4.37 ✄ 6.91 **FUD** 000 T A2 ▣
AMA: 2016,Jan,13; 2015,Jun,5; 2015,Jan,16; 2014,Jan,11

52315 complicated
Code also modifier 58 for removal of a self-retaining, indwelling ureteral stent
🚑 7.91 ✄ 11.7 **FUD** 000 T A2 ▣
AMA: 2016,Jan,13; 2015,Jan,16; 2014,Jan,11

52317 Litholapaxy: crushing or fragmentation of calculus by any means in bladder and removal of fragments; simple or small (less than 2.5 cm)
🚑 10.0 ✄ 22.7 **FUD** 000 T A2 ▣
AMA: 2016,Jan,13; 2015,Jan,16; 2014,Jan,11; 2012,Feb,11

52318 complicated or large (over 2.5 cm)
🚑 13.6 ✄ 13.6 **FUD** 000 J A2 ▣
AMA: 2016,Jan,13; 2015,Jan,16; 2014,Jan,11; 2012,Feb,11

52320-52356 [52356] Endoscopic Procedures via Urethra: Renal Pelvis and Ureter

INCLUDES   Diagnostic cystourethroscopy when performed with therapeutic cystourethroscopy
Insertion/removal of temporary ureteral catheter (52005)

EXCLUDES   Diagnostic cystourethroscopy only (52000)
Self-retaining/indwelling ureteral stent removal by cystourethroscope, with modifier 58 if appropriate (52310, 52315)
Code also the insertion of an indwelling stent performed in addition to other procedures within this section (52332)

52320   **Cystourethroscopy (including ureteral catheterization); with removal of ureteral calculus**

INCLUDES   Cystourethroscopy (separate procedure) (52000)
🚑 7.11   ⚕ 7.11   **FUD** 000   T A2 50 ▢
AMA: 2016,Jan,13; 2015,Jan,16; 2014,Jan,11; 2012,Jan,15-42; 2011,Jan,11

52325   **with fragmentation of ureteral calculus (eg, ultrasonic or electro-hydraulic technique)**

INCLUDES   Cystourethroscopy (separate procedure) (52000)
🚑 9.26   ⚕ 9.26   **FUD** 000   T A2 50 ▢
AMA: 2016,Jan,13; 2015,Jan,16; 2014,Jan,11; 2012,Jan,15-42; 2011,Jan,11

52327   **with subureteric injection of implant material**

INCLUDES   Cystourethroscopy (separate procedure) (52000)
🚑 7.55   ⚕ 7.55   **FUD** 000   T A2 50 ▢
AMA: 2016,Jan,13; 2015,Jan,16; 2014,Jan,11

52330   **with manipulation, without removal of ureteral calculus**

INCLUDES   Cystourethroscopy (separate procedure) (52000)
🚑 7.60   ⚕ 13.9   **FUD** 000   T A2 50 ▢
AMA: 2016,Jan,13; 2015,Jan,16; 2014,May,3; 2014,Jan,11; 2012,Jan,15-42; 2011,Jan,11

52332   **Cystourethroscopy, with insertion of indwelling ureteral stent (eg, Gibbons or double-J type)**

INCLUDES   Cystourethroscopy (separate procedure) (52000)
EXCLUDES   Cystourethroscopy, with ureteroscopy and/or pyeloscopy; with lithotripsy when performed on the same side with (52353, [52356])
🚑 4.48   ⚕ 13.8   **FUD** 000   T A2 50 ▢
AMA: 2016,Jan,13; 2015,Jan,16; 2014,May,3; 2014,Jan,11; 2012,Jan,15-42; 2011,Jan,11

52334   **Cystourethroscopy with insertion of ureteral guide wire through kidney to establish a percutaneous nephrostomy, retrograde**

INCLUDES   Cystourethroscopy (separate procedure) (52000)
EXCLUDES   Cystourethroscopy with incision/fulguration/resection of congenital posterior urethral valves/obstructive hypertrophic mucosal folds (52400)
Cystourethroscopy with pyeloscopy and/or ureteroscopy (52351-52353 [52356])
Nephrostomy tract establishment only (50395)
Percutaneous nephrostolithotomy (50080, 50081)
🚑 7.39   ⚕ 7.39   **FUD** 000   T A2 50 ▢
AMA: 2016,Jan,13; 2015,Jan,16; 2014,May,3; 2014,Jan,11

52341   **Cystourethroscopy; with treatment of ureteral stricture (eg, balloon dilation, laser, electrocautery, and incision)**

Cystourethroscopy (52000, 52351)
EXCLUDES   Balloon dilation, ureteral stricture (50706)
🚑 8.19   ⚕ 8.19   **FUD** 000   T A2 50 ▢
AMA: 2016,Jan,3; 2016,Jan,13; 2015,Jan,16; 2014,Jan,11

52342   **with treatment of ureteropelvic junction stricture (eg, balloon dilation, laser, electrocautery, and incision)**

INCLUDES   Cystourethroscopy (separate procedure)
EXCLUDES   Balloon dilation with imaging guidance (50706)
Diagnostic cystourethroscopy (52351)
🚑 8.91   ⚕ 8.91   **FUD** 000   T A2 50 ▢
AMA: 2016,Jan,13; 2015,Jan,16; 2014,Jan,11; 2012,Jan,15-42; 2011,Jan,11

52343   **with treatment of intra-renal stricture (eg, balloon dilation, laser, electrocautery, and incision)**

INCLUDES   Diagnostic cystourethroscopy (52351)
EXCLUDES   Balloon dilation with imaging guidance (50706)
Cystourethroscopy (separate procedure) (52000)
🚑 9.92   ⚕ 9.92   **FUD** 000   T A2 50 ▢
AMA: 2016,Jan,13; 2015,Jan,16; 2014,May,3; 2014,Jan,11

52344   **Cystourethroscopy with ureteroscopy; with treatment of ureteral stricture (eg, balloon dilation, laser, electrocautery, and incision)**

INCLUDES   Diagnostic cystourethroscopy (52351)
EXCLUDES   Balloon dilation, ureteral stricture (50706)
Cystourethroscopy with transurethral resection or incision of ejaculatory ducts (52402)
🚑 10.6   ⚕ 10.6   **FUD** 000   T A2 50 ▢
AMA: 2016,Jan,3; 2016,Jan,13; 2015,Jan,16; 2014,Jan,11

52345   **with treatment of ureteropelvic junction stricture (eg, balloon dilation, laser, electrocautery, and incision)**

INCLUDES   Diagnostic cystourethroscopy (52351)
EXCLUDES   Balloon dilation, ureteral stricture (50706)
Cystourethroscopy with transurethral resection or incision of ejaculatory ducts (52402)
🚑 11.3   ⚕ 11.3   **FUD** 000   T A2 80 50 ▢
AMA: 2016,Jan,3; 2016,Jan,13; 2015,Jan,16; 2014,Jan,11

52346   **with treatment of intra-renal stricture (eg, balloon dilation, laser, electrocautery, and incision)**

INCLUDES   Diagnostic cystourethroscopy (52351)
EXCLUDES   Balloon dilation with imaging guidance (50706)
Cystourethroscopy with transurethral resection or incision of ejaculatory ducts (52402)
🚑 12.8   ⚕ 12.8   **FUD** 000   J A2 80 50 ▢
AMA: 2016,Jan,13; 2015,Jan,16; 2014,May,3; 2014,Jan,11

52351   **Cystourethroscopy, with ureteroscopy and/or pyeloscopy; diagnostic**

EXCLUDES   Cystourethroscopy (52341-52346, 52352-52353 [52356])
📷 (74485)
🚑 8.73   ⚕ 8.73   **FUD** 000   T A2 ▢
AMA: 2016,Jan,13; 2015,Jan,16; 2014,May,3; 2014,Jan,11

52352   **with removal or manipulation of calculus (ureteral catheterization is included)**

INCLUDES   Diagnostic cystourethroscopy (52351)
🚑 10.2   ⚕ 10.2   **FUD** 000   T A2 50 ▢
AMA: 2016,Jan,13; 2015,Jan,16; 2014,Jan,11; 2012,Jan,15-42; 2011,Jan,11

52353   **with lithotripsy (ureteral catheterization is included)**

INCLUDES   Diagnostic cystourethroscopy (52351)
EXCLUDES   Cystourethroscopy when performed on the same side (52332, [52356])
🚑 11.3   ⚕ 11.3   **FUD** 000   J A2 50 ▢
AMA: 2016,Jan,13; 2015,Jan,16; 2014,May,3; 2014,Jan,11; 2012,Jan,15-42; 2011,Jan,11

\# **52356**   **with lithotripsy including insertion of indwelling ureteral stent (eg, Gibbons or double-J type)**

INCLUDES   Diagnostic cystourethroscopy (52000, 52351)
EXCLUDES   Cystourethroscopy when performed on the same side with (52332, 52353)
🚑 11.9   ⚕ 11.9   **FUD** 000   J 62 50 ▢
AMA: 2016,Jan,13; 2015,Jan,16; 2014,May,3; 2014,Jan,11

52354   **with biopsy and/or fulguration of ureteral or renal pelvic lesion**

INCLUDES   Diagnostic cystourethroscopy (52351)
EXCLUDES   Image guided biopsy without endoscopic guidance (50606)
🚑 12.0   ⚕ 12.0   **FUD** 000   T A2 50 ▢
AMA: 2016,Jan,13; 2015,Jan,16; 2014,May,3; 2014,Jan,11

52355 with resection of ureteral or renal pelvic tumor
INCLUDES Diagnostic cystourethroscopy (52351)
⚙ 13.4 ⚕ 13.4 **FUD** 000 J A2 50 ▭
AMA: 2016,Jan,13; 2015,Jan,16; 2014,May,3; 2014,Jan,11

52356 Resequenced code. See code following 52353.

52400-52700 Endoscopic Procedures via Urethra: Prostate and Vesical Neck

52400 Cystourethroscopy with incision, fulguration, or resection of congenital posterior urethral valves, or congenital obstructive hypertrophic mucosal folds
⚙ 13.7 ⚕ 13.7 **FUD** 090 T A2 ▭
AMA: 2016,Jan,13; 2015,Jan,16; 2014,Jan,11

52402 Cystourethroscopy with transurethral resection or incision of ejaculatory ducts ♂
⚙ 7.69 ⚕ 7.69 **FUD** 000 T A2 ▭
AMA: 2014,Jan,11

52441 Cystourethroscopy, with insertion of permanent adjustable transprostatic implant; single implant
⚙ 6.58 ⚕ 35.1 **FUD** 000 B ▭
AMA: 2016,Jan,13; 2015,Jun,5

+ **52442** each additional permanent adjustable transprostatic implant (List separately in addition to code for primary procedure)
EXCLUDES Permanent urethral stent insertion (52282)
Removal of stent, calculus or foreign body (implant) (52310)
Temporary prostatic urethral stent insertion (53855)
Code first (52441)
⚙ 1.75 ⚕ 26.8 **FUD** ZZZ B ▭
AMA: 2016,Jan,13; 2015,Jun,5

52450 Transurethral incision of prostate ♂
⚙ 13.5 ⚕ 13.5 **FUD** 090 T A2 ▭
AMA: 2016,Jan,13; 2015,Jun,5; 2015,Jan,16; 2014,Jan,11; 2012,Jan,15-42; 2011,Jan,11

52500 Transurethral resection of bladder neck (separate procedure)
⚙ 14.0 ⚕ 14.0 **FUD** 090 T A2 ▭
AMA: 2016,Jan,13; 2015,Jan,16; 2014,Jan,11; 2012,Jan,15-42; 2011,Jan,11

52601 Transurethral electrosurgical resection of prostate, including control of postoperative bleeding, complete (vasectomy, meatotomy, cystourethroscopy, urethral calibration and/or dilation, and internal urethrotomy are included) ♂
INCLUDES Stage 1 of partial transurethral resection of prostate
EXCLUDES Ablation by waterjet (0421T)
Excision of prostate (55801-55845)
Transurethral fulguration of prostate (52214)
Code also modifier 58 for stage 2 partial transurethral resection of prostate
⚙ 24.3 ⚕ 24.3 **FUD** 090 J A2 ▭
AMA: 2016,Jan,13; 2015,Jun,5; 2015,Jan,16; 2014,Jan,11; 2012,Jan,15-42; 2011,Oct,10

52630 Transurethral resection; residual or regrowth of obstructive prostate tissue including control of postoperative bleeding, complete (vasectomy, meatotomy, cystourethroscopy, urethral calibration and/or dilation, and internal urethrotomy are included) ♂
EXCLUDES Ablation by waterjet (0421T)
Excision of prostate (55801-55845)
Code also modifier 78 when performed by same physician within the postoperative period of a related procedure
⚙ 11.4 ⚕ 11.4 **FUD** 090 J A2 ▭
AMA: 2016,Jan,13; 2015,Jan,16; 2014,Jan,11

52640 of postoperative bladder neck contracture
EXCLUDES Excision of prostate (55801-55845)
⚙ 9.04 ⚕ 9.04 **FUD** 090 T A2 ▭
AMA: 2016,Jan,13; 2015,Jan,16; 2014,Jan,11

52647 Laser coagulation of prostate, including control of postoperative bleeding, complete (vasectomy, meatotomy, cystourethroscopy, urethral calibration and/or dilation, and internal urethrotomy are included if performed) ♂
⚙ 18.6 ⚕ 50.3 **FUD** 090 J A2 ▭
AMA: 2016,Jan,13; 2015,Jan,16; 2014,Jan,11; 2012,Jan,15-42; 2011,Jan,11

52648 Laser vaporization of prostate, including control of postoperative bleeding, complete (vasectomy, meatotomy, cystourethroscopy, urethral calibration and/or dilation, internal urethrotomy and transurethral resection of prostate are included if performed) ♂
⚙ 19.8 ⚕ 51.8 **FUD** 090 J A2 ▭
AMA: 2016,Jan,13; 2015,Jun,5; 2015,Jan,16; 2014,Jan,11; 2012,Jan,15-42; 2011,Jan,11

52649 Laser enucleation of the prostate with morcellation, including control of postoperative bleeding, complete (vasectomy, meatotomy, cystourethroscopy, urethral calibration and/or dilation, internal urethrotomy and transurethral resection of prostate are included if performed) ♂
INCLUDES Cystourethroscopy (52000, 52276, 52281)
Laser coagulation of prostate (52647-52648)
Meatotomy (53020)
Transurethral resection of prostate (52601)
Vasectomy (55250)
⚙ 23.6 ⚕ 23.6 **FUD** 090 J G2 80 ▭
AMA: 2016,Jan,13; 2015,Jun,5; 2014,Jan,11

52700 Transurethral drainage of prostatic abscess ♂
EXCLUDES Litholapaxy (52317, 52318)
⚙ 12.6 ⚕ 12.6 **FUD** 090 T A2 80 ▭
AMA: 2016,Jan,13; 2015,Jan,16; 2014,Jan,11

Bladder Prostate Urethra

53000-53520 Open Surgical Procedures of Urethra

EXCLUDES Endoscopic procedures; cystoscopy, urethroscopy, cystourethroscopy (52000-52700 [52356])
Urethrocystography injection procedure (51600-51610)

53000 Urethrotomy or urethrostomy, external (separate procedure); pendulous urethra
⚙ 4.25 ⚕ 4.25 **FUD** 010 T A2 ▭
AMA: 2014,Jan,11

53010 perineal urethra, external
⚙ 8.48 ⚕ 8.48 **FUD** 090 J A2 ▭
AMA: 2014,Jan,11

53020 Meatotomy, cutting of meatus (separate procedure); except infant
⚙ 2.79 ⚕ 2.79 **FUD** 000 T A2 ▭
AMA: 2014,Jan,11

53025 infant A
⚙ 2.07 ⚕ 2.07 **FUD** 000 63 T R2 80 ▭
AMA: 2014,Jan,11

● New Code ▲ Revised Code ○ Reinstated ● New Web Release ▲ Revised Web Release Unlisted Not Covered # Resequenced
◯ AMA Mod 51 Exempt ⑪ Optum Mod 51 Exempt ⑥ Mod 63 Exempt ✗ Non-FDA Drug ★ Telehealth ▣ Maternity ▲ Age Edit + Add-on **AMA:** CPT Asst

Urinary System

53040 **Drainage of deep periurethral abscess**
EXCLUDES *Incision and drainage of subcutaneous abscess (10060-10061)*
⚙ 11.2 ⚕ 11.2 **FUD** 090 T A2 80 ▭
AMA: 2014,Jan,11

53060 **Drainage of Skene's gland abscess or cyst**
⚙ 4.71 ⚕ 5.23 **FUD** 010 T P3 ▭
AMA: 2014,Jan,11

53080 **Drainage of perineal urinary extravasation; uncomplicated (separate procedure)**
⚙ 12.0 ⚕ 12.0 **FUD** 090 T A2 ▭
AMA: 2014,Jan,11

53085 **complicated**
⚙ 19.2 ⚕ 19.2 **FUD** 090 T G2 80 ▭
AMA: 2014,Jan,11

53200 **Biopsy of urethra**
⚙ 4.09 ⚕ 4.47 **FUD** 000 T A2 ▭
AMA: 2014,Jan,11

53210 **Urethrectomy, total, including cystostomy; female** ♀
⚙ 22.1 ⚕ 22.1 **FUD** 090 J A2 80 ▭
AMA: 2014,Jan,11

53215 **male** ♂
⚙ 26.7 ⚕ 26.7 **FUD** 090 J A2 80 ▭
AMA: 2014,Jan,11

53220 **Excision or fulguration of carcinoma of urethra**
⚙ 13.0 ⚕ 13.0 **FUD** 090 T A2 80 ▭
AMA: 2014,Jan,11

53230 **Excision of urethral diverticulum (separate procedure); female** ♀
⚙ 17.3 ⚕ 17.3 **FUD** 090 T A2 80 ▭
AMA: 2014,Jan,11

53235 **male** ♂
⚙ 18.1 ⚕ 18.1 **FUD** 090 J A2 80 ▭
AMA: 2014,Jan,11

53240 **Marsupialization of urethral diverticulum, male or female**
⚙ 12.2 ⚕ 12.2 **FUD** 090 J A2 ▭
AMA: 2014,Jan,11

53250 **Excision of bulbourethral gland (Cowper's gland)**
⚙ 11.8 ⚕ 11.8 **FUD** 090 T A2 ▭
AMA: 2014,Jan,11

53260 **Excision or fulguration; urethral polyp(s), distal urethra**
EXCLUDES *Endoscopic method (52214, 52224)*
⚙ 5.18 ⚕ 5.76 **FUD** 010 T A2 ▭
AMA: 2014,Jan,11

53265 **urethral caruncle**
EXCLUDES *Endoscopic method (52214, 52224)*
⚙ 5.34 ⚕ 6.22 **FUD** 010 T A2 ▭
AMA: 2014,Jan,11

53270 **Skene's glands**
EXCLUDES *Endoscopic method (52214, 52224)*
⚙ 5.34 ⚕ 5.95 **FUD** 010 T A2 ▭
AMA: 2014,Jan,11

53275 **urethral prolapse**
EXCLUDES *Endoscopic method (52214, 52224)*
⚙ 7.54 ⚕ 7.54 **FUD** 010 T A2 ▭
AMA: 2014,Jan,11

53400 **Urethroplasty; first stage, for fistula, diverticulum, or stricture (eg, Johannsen type)**
EXCLUDES *Hypospadias repair (54300-54352)*
⚙ 23.0 ⚕ 23.0 **FUD** 090 J A2 80 ▭
AMA: 2014,Jan,11

53405 **second stage (formation of urethra), including urinary diversion**
EXCLUDES *Hypospadias repair (54300-54352)*
⚙ 25.1 ⚕ 25.1 **FUD** 090 J A2 80 ▭
AMA: 2014,Jan,11

53410 **Urethroplasty, 1-stage reconstruction of male anterior urethra** ♂
EXCLUDES *Hypospadias repair (54300-54352)*
⚙ 28.1 ⚕ 28.1 **FUD** 090 J A2 80 ▭
AMA: 2014,Jan,11

53415 **Urethroplasty, transpubic or perineal, 1-stage, for reconstruction or repair of prostatic or membranous urethra** ♂
⚙ 32.4 ⚕ 32.4 **FUD** 090 C 80 ▭
AMA: 2014,Jan,11

53420 **Urethroplasty, 2-stage reconstruction or repair of prostatic or membranous urethra; first stage** ♂
⚙ 24.5 ⚕ 24.5 **FUD** 090 J A2 ▭
AMA: 2014,Jan,11

53425 **second stage** ♂
⚙ 26.9 ⚕ 26.9 **FUD** 090 J A2 80 ▭
AMA: 2014,Jan,11

53430 **Urethroplasty, reconstruction of female urethra** ♀
⚙ 27.6 ⚕ 27.6 **FUD** 090 T A2 80 ▭
AMA: 2014,Jan,11

53431 **Urethroplasty with tubularization of posterior urethra and/or lower bladder for incontinence (eg, Tenago, Leadbetter procedure)**
⚙ 33.2 ⚕ 33.2 **FUD** 090 J A2 80 ▭
AMA: 2014,Jan,11

53440 **Sling operation for correction of male urinary incontinence (eg, fascia or synthetic)** ♂
⚙ 21.6 ⚕ 21.6 **FUD** 090 J J8 80 ▭
AMA: 2014,Jan,11

53442 **Removal or revision of sling for male urinary incontinence (eg, fascia or synthetic)** ♂
⚙ 22.4 ⚕ 22.4 **FUD** 090 J A2 80 ▭
AMA: 2014,Jan,11

53444 **Insertion of tandem cuff (dual cuff)**
⚙ 22.7 ⚕ 22.7 **FUD** 090 J J8 80 ▭
AMA: 2014,Jan,11

53445 **Insertion of inflatable urethral/bladder neck sphincter, including placement of pump, reservoir, and cuff**
⚙ 21.6 ⚕ 21.6 **FUD** 090 J J8 80 ▭
AMA: 2014,Jan,11

53446 **Removal of inflatable urethral/bladder neck sphincter, including pump, reservoir, and cuff**
⚙ 18.4 ⚕ 18.4 **FUD** 090 02 A2 80 ▭
AMA: 2014,Jan,11

53447 **Removal and replacement of inflatable urethral/bladder neck sphincter including pump, reservoir, and cuff at the same operative session**
⚙ 23.2 ⚕ 23.2 **FUD** 090 J J8 80 ▭
AMA: 2014,Jan,11

53448 **Removal and replacement of inflatable urethral/bladder neck sphincter including pump, reservoir, and cuff through an infected field at the same operative session including irrigation and debridement of infected tissue**
INCLUDES *Debridement (11042, 11043)*
⚙ 36.9 ⚕ 36.9 **FUD** 090 C 80 ▭
AMA: 2014,Jan,11

53449 **Repair of inflatable urethral/bladder neck sphincter, including pump, reservoir, and cuff**
⚙ 17.5 ⚕ 17.5 **FUD** 090 J A2 80 ▭
AMA: 2014,Jan,11

53450	Urethromeatoplasty, with mucosal advancement

EXCLUDES Meatotomy (53020, 53025)

🔧 11.7 ✂ 11.7 **FUD** 090 T A2 📵

AMA: 2016,Jan,13; 2015,Jan,16; 2014,Jan,11; 2012,Oct,14; 2012,Sep,16

53460	Urethromeatoplasty, with partial excision of distal urethral segment (Richardson type procedure)

🔧 13.1 ✂ 13.1 **FUD** 090 T A2 80 📵

AMA: 2014,Jan,11

53500	Urethrolysis, transvaginal, secondary, open, including cystourethroscopy (eg, postsurgical obstruction, scarring)

INCLUDES Cystourethroscopy (separate procedure) (52000)

EXCLUDES Retropubic approach (53899)

🔧 21.4 ✂ 21.4 **FUD** 090 T 80 📵

AMA: 2016,Jan,13; 2015,Jan,16; 2014,Jan,11

53502	Urethrorrhaphy, suture of urethral wound or injury, female ♀

🔧 13.9 ✂ 13.9 **FUD** 090 T A2 📵

AMA: 2014,Jan,11

53505	Urethrorrhaphy, suture of urethral wound or injury; penile ♂

🔧 14.0 ✂ 14.0 **FUD** 090 J A2 80 📵

AMA: 2014,Jan,11

53510	perineal ♂

🔧 18.1 ✂ 18.1 **FUD** 090 J A2 80 📵

AMA: 2014,Jan,11

53515	prostatomembranous ♂

🔧 22.8 ✂ 22.8 **FUD** 090 J A2 80 📵

AMA: 2014,Jan,11

53520	Closure of urethrostomy or urethrocutaneous fistula, male (separate procedure) ♂

EXCLUDES Closure of fistula:
    Urethrorectal (45820, 45825)
    Urethrovaginal (57310)

🔧 15.9 ✂ 15.9 **FUD** 090 J A2 📵

AMA: 2014,Jan,11

53600-53665 Urethral Dilation

EXCLUDES Endoscopic procedures; cystoscopy, urethroscopy, cystourethroscopy
(52000-52700 [52356])
Urethral catheterization (51701-51703)
Urethrocystography injection procedure (51600-51610)
📷 (74485)

53600	Dilation of urethral stricture by passage of sound or urethral dilator, male; initial ♂

🔧 1.83 ✂ 2.37 **FUD** 000 T P3 📵

AMA: 2014,Jan,11

53601	subsequent ♂

🔧 1.54 ✂ 2.30 **FUD** 000 01 N1 📵

AMA: 2014,Jan,11

53605	Dilation of urethral stricture or vesical neck by passage of sound or urethral dilator, male, general or conduction (spinal) anesthesia ♂

EXCLUDES Procedure performed under local anesthesia
(53600-53601, 53620-53621)

🔧 1.86 ✂ 1.86 **FUD** 000 T A2 📵

AMA: 2014,Jan,11

53620	Dilation of urethral stricture by passage of filiform and follower, male; initial ♂

🔧 2.51 ✂ 3.30 **FUD** 000 T P3 📵

AMA: 2014,Jan,11

53621	subsequent ♂

🔧 2.08 ✂ 3.11 **FUD** 000 T P3 📵

AMA: 2014,Jan,11

53660	Dilation of female urethra including suppository and/or instillation; initial ♀

🔧 1.20 ✂ 2.00 **FUD** 000 S P3 📵

AMA: 2014,Jan,11

53661	subsequent ♀

🔧 1.16 ✂ 1.96 **FUD** 000 01 N1 📵

AMA: 2014,Jan,11

53665	Dilation of female urethra, general or conduction (spinal) anesthesia ♀

EXCLUDES Procedure performed under local anesthesia
(53660-53661)

🔧 1.11 ✂ 1.11 **FUD** 000 T A2 📵

AMA: 2014,Jan,11

53850-53899 Transurethral Procedures

EXCLUDES Endoscopic procedures; cystoscopy, urethroscopy, cystourethroscopy
(52000-52700 [52356])

53850	Transurethral destruction of prostate tissue; by microwave thermotherapy ♂

📷 (81020)

🔧 17.4 ✂ 58.5 **FUD** 090 T P2 📵

AMA: 2016,Jan,13; 2015,Jun,5; 2015,Jan,16; 2014,Jan,11

53852	by radiofrequency thermotherapy ♂

📷 (81020)

🔧 17.8 ✂ 53.9 **FUD** 090 J P3 📵

AMA: 2016,Jan,13; 2015,Jun,5; 2015,Jan,16; 2014,Jan,11

53855	Insertion of a temporary prostatic urethral stent, including urethral measurement

EXCLUDES Permanent urethral stent insertion (52282)

🔧 2.38 ✂ 21.8 **FUD** 000 T P2 80 📵

AMA: 2016,Jan,13; 2015,Jun,5; 2015,Jan,16; 2014,Jan,11

53860	Transurethral radiofrequency micro-remodeling of the female bladder neck and proximal urethra for stress urinary incontinence ♀

🔧 6.51 ✂ 43.6 **FUD** 090 T P2 80 📵

AMA: 2014,Jan,11

53899	Unlisted procedure, urinary system

🔧 0.00 ✂ 0.00 **FUD** YYY T 80

AMA: 2016,Jan,13; 2015,Jun,5; 2015,Mar,9; 2015,Jan,16; 2014,Jan,11; 2012,Jan,15-42; 2011,Jan,11

CPT © 2016 American Medical Association. All Rights Reserved.

54000-54015 Procedures of Penis: Incisional

EXCLUDES *Debridement of abdominal perineal gangrene (11004-11006)*

54000 **Slitting of prepuce, dorsal or lateral (separate procedure); newborn** A ♂
🔪 3.10 ⚖ 4.21 **FUD** 010 ⑥③ T A2 80 ▣
AMA: 2014,Jan,11

Prostate · Dorsal surface · Reservoir · Ventral surface · Corpus spongiosum · An implanted, inflatable penile prosthesis (left); schematic of the main features of the penis (far left) · Corpus cavernosum · Prepuce · Glans · Pump in scrotum · External urethral orifice

54001 **except newborn** ♂
🔪 3.97 ⚖ 5.25 **FUD** 010 T A2 ▣
AMA: 2014,Jan,11

54015 **Incision and drainage of penis, deep** ♂
EXCLUDES *Abscess, skin/subcutaneous (10060-10160)*
🔪 8.91 ⚖ 8.91 **FUD** 010 T A2 80 ▣
AMA: 2014,Jan,11

54050-54065 Destruction of Penis Lesions: Multiple Methods

EXCLUDES *Excision/destruction other lesions (11420-11426, 11620-11626, 17000-17250, 17270-17276)*

54050 **Destruction of lesion(s), penis (eg, condyloma, papilloma, molluscum contagiosum, herpetic vesicle), simple; chemical** ♂
🔪 3.01 ⚖ 3.75 **FUD** 010 01 N1 ▣
AMA: 2014,Jan,11

54055 **electrodesiccation** ♂
🔪 2.65 ⚖ 3.37 **FUD** 010 T P3 ▣
AMA: 2014,Jan,11

54056 **cryosurgery** ♂
🔪 3.18 ⚖ 4.04 **FUD** 010 01 N1 ▣
AMA: 2014,Jan,11

54057 **laser surgery** ♂
🔪 2.72 ⚖ 3.85 **FUD** 010 T A2 ▣
AMA: 2014,Jan,11

54060 **surgical excision** ♂
🔪 3.74 ⚖ 5.10 **FUD** 010 T A2 ▣
AMA: 2014,Jan,11

54065 **Destruction of lesion(s), penis (eg, condyloma, papilloma, molluscum contagiosum, herpetic vesicle), extensive (eg, laser surgery, electrosurgery, cryosurgery, chemosurgery)** ♂
🔪 4.97 ⚖ 6.23 **FUD** 010 T A2 ▣
AMA: 2014,Jan,11

54100-54115 Procedures of Penis: Excisional

54100 **Biopsy of penis; (separate procedure)** ♂
🔪 3.62 ⚖ 5.64 **FUD** 000 T A2 ▣
AMA: 2016,Jan,13; 2015,Jan,16; 2014,Jan,11

54105 **deep structures** ♂
🔪 6.12 ⚖ 7.53 **FUD** 010 T A2 ▣
AMA: 2014,Jan,11

54110 **Excision of penile plaque (Peyronie disease);** ♂
🔪 18.1 ⚖ 18.1 **FUD** 090 T A2 80 ▣
AMA: 2014,Jan,11

54111 **with graft to 5 cm in length** ♂
🔪 23.0 ⚖ 23.0 **FUD** 090 J A2 80 ▣
AMA: 2016,Jan,13; 2015,Jan,16; 2014,Jan,11; 2012,Jan,15-42; 2011,Jan,11

54112 **with graft greater than 5 cm in length** ♂
🔪 27.0 ⚖ 27.0 **FUD** 090 J J8 80 ▣
AMA: 2014,Jan,11

54115 **Removal foreign body from deep penile tissue (eg, plastic implant)** ♂
🔪 12.2 ⚖ 12.9 **FUD** 090 T A2 80 ▣
AMA: 2014,Jan,11

54120-54135 Amputation of Penis

EXCLUDES *Lymphadenectomy (separate procedure) (38760-38770)*

54120 **Amputation of penis; partial** ♂
🔪 18.1 ⚖ 18.1 **FUD** 090 T A2 80 ▣
AMA: 2014,Jan,11

54125 **complete** ♂
🔪 23.3 ⚖ 23.3 **FUD** 090 C 80 ▣
AMA: 2014,Jan,11

54130 **Amputation of penis, radical; with bilateral inguinofemoral lymphadenectomy** ♂
🔪 34.2 ⚖ 34.2 **FUD** 090 C 80 ▣
AMA: 2014,Jan,11

54135 **in continuity with bilateral pelvic lymphadenectomy, including external iliac, hypogastric and obturator nodes** ♂
🔪 43.1 ⚖ 43.1 **FUD** 090 C 80 ▣
AMA: 2014,Jan,11

54150-54164 Circumcision Procedures

54150 **Circumcision, using clamp or other device with regional dorsal penile or ring block** ♂
Code also modifier 52 when performed without dorsal penile or ring block
🔪 2.81 ⚖ 4.38 **FUD** 000 ⑥③ T A2 80 ▣
AMA: 2016,Jan,13; 2015,Jan,16; 2014,Jan,11; 2012,Jan,15-42; 2011,Jan,11

54160 **Circumcision, surgical excision other than clamp, device, or dorsal slit; neonate (28 days of age or less)** A ♂
🔪 4.19 ⚖ 6.34 **FUD** 010 ⑥③ T A2
AMA: 2016,Jan,13; 2015,Jan,16; 2014,Jan,11; 2012,Jan,15-42; 2011,Jan,11

54161 **older than 28 days of age** A ♂
🔪 5.65 ⚖ 5.65 **FUD** 010 T A2
AMA: 2016,Jan,13; 2015,Jan,16; 2014,Jan,11; 2012,Jan,15-42; 2011,Jan,11

54162 **Lysis or excision of penile post-circumcision adhesions** ♂
🔪 5.72 ⚖ 7.33 **FUD** 010 T A2 ▣
AMA: 2014,Jan,11

54163 **Repair incomplete circumcision** ♂
🔪 6.28 ⚖ 6.28 **FUD** 010 T A2 ▣
AMA: 2014,Jan,11

54164 **Frenulotomy of penis** ♂
EXCLUDES *Circumcision (54150-54163)*
🔪 5.54 ⚖ 5.54 **FUD** 010 T A2 ▣
AMA: 2014,Jan,11

54200-54250 Evaluation and Treatment of Erectile Abnormalities

54200 **Injection procedure for Peyronie disease;** ♂
🔪 2.40 ⚖ 3.04 **FUD** 010 T P3 ▣
AMA: 2014,Jan,11

54205 with surgical exposure of plaque ♂
🏥 15.2 ✂ 15.2 **FUD** 090 [J] [A2] [80] ⚑
AMA: 2014,Jan,11

54220 Irrigation of corpora cavernosa for priapism ♂
🏥 3.86 ✂ 5.81 **FUD** 000 [T] [A2] ⚑
AMA: 2014,Jan,11

54230 Injection procedure for corpora cavernosography ♂
☢ (74445)
🏥 2.29 ✂ 2.76 **FUD** 000 [N] [N1] ⚑
AMA: 2014,Jan,11

54231 Dynamic cavernosometry, including intracavernosal injection of vasoactive drugs (eg, papaverine, phentolamine) ♂
🏥 3.34 ✂ 4.00 **FUD** 000 [T] [P3] ⚑
AMA: 2014,Jan,11

54235 Injection of corpora cavernosa with pharmacologic agent(s) (eg, papaverine, phentolamine) ♂
🏥 2.11 ✂ 2.57 **FUD** 000 [T] [P3] ⚑
AMA: 2016,Jan,13; 2015,Jan,16; 2014,Jan,11; 2012,Jan,15-42; 2011,Jan,11

54240 Penile plethysmography ♂
🏥 2.91 ✂ 2.91 **FUD** 000 [S] [P3] [80] ⚑
AMA: 2014,Jan,11

54250 Nocturnal penile tumescence and/or rigidity test ♂
🏥 3.46 ✂ 3.46 **FUD** 000 [T] [P3] [80] ⚑
AMA: 2014,Jan,11

54300-54390 Hypospadias Repair and Related Procedures

[EXCLUDES] *Other urethroplasties (53400-53430)*
Revascularization of penis (37788)

54300 Plastic operation of penis for straightening of chordee (eg, hypospadias), with or without mobilization of urethra ♂
🏥 18.4 ✂ 18.4 **FUD** 090 [T] [A2] [80] ⚑
AMA: 2016,Jan,13; 2015,Jan,16; 2014,Dec,16; 2014,Dec,16; 2014,Jan,11

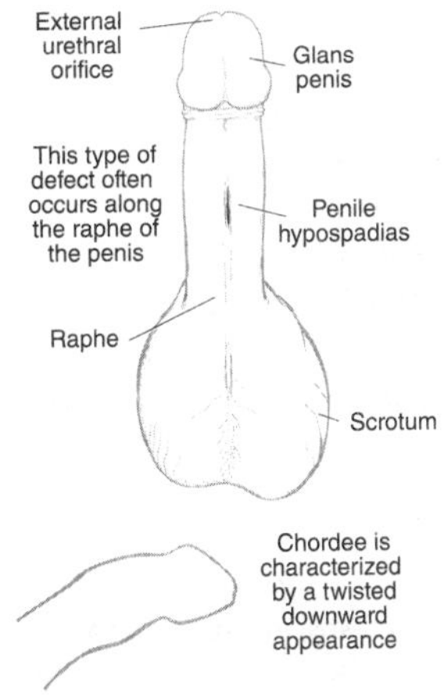
External urethral orifice
Glans penis
This type of defect often occurs along the raphe of the penis
Penile hypospadias
Raphe
Scrotum
Chordee is characterized by a twisted downward appearance

54304 Plastic operation on penis for correction of chordee or for first stage hypospadias repair with or without transplantation of prepuce and/or skin flaps ♂
🏥 21.5 ✂ 21.5 **FUD** 090 [T] [A2] [80] ⚑
AMA: 2014,Jan,11

54308 Urethroplasty for second stage hypospadias repair (including urinary diversion); less than 3 cm ♂
🏥 20.5 ✂ 20.5 **FUD** 090 [J] [A2] [80] ⚑
AMA: 2014,Jan,11

54312 greater than 3 cm ♂
🏥 24.7 ✂ 24.7 **FUD** 090 [T] [A2] [80] ⚑
AMA: 2014,Jan,11

54316 Urethroplasty for second stage hypospadias repair (including urinary diversion) with free skin graft obtained from site other than genitalia ♂
🏥 30.1 ✂ 30.1 **FUD** 090 [J] [A2] [80] ⚑
AMA: 2014,Jan,11

54318 Urethroplasty for third stage hypospadias repair to release penis from scrotum (eg, third stage Cecil repair) ♂
🏥 21.4 ✂ 21.4 **FUD** 090 [T] [A2] [80] ⚑
AMA: 2014,Jan,11

54322 1-stage distal hypospadias repair (with or without chordee or circumcision); with simple meatal advancement (eg, Magpi, V-flap) ♂
🏥 22.0 ✂ 22.0 **FUD** 090 [T] [A2] [80] ⚑
AMA: 2014,Jan,11

54324 with urethroplasty by local skin flaps (eg, flip-flap, prepucial flap) ♂
[INCLUDES] Browne's operation
🏥 28.6 ✂ 28.6 **FUD** 090 [T] [A2] [80] ⚑
AMA: 2014,Jan,11

54326 with urethroplasty by local skin flaps and mobilization of urethra ♂
🏥 27.1 ✂ 27.1 **FUD** 090 [J] [A2] [80] ⚑
AMA: 2014,Jan,11

54328 with extensive dissection to correct chordee and urethroplasty with local skin flaps, skin graft patch, and/or island flap ♂
[EXCLUDES] *Urethroplasty/straightening of chordee (54308)*
🏥 27.0 ✂ 27.0 **FUD** 090 [T] [A2] [80] ⚑
AMA: 2016,Jan,13; 2015,Jan,16; 2014,Jan,11; 2012,Jan,15-42; 2011,Jan,11

54332 1-stage proximal penile or penoscrotal hypospadias repair requiring extensive dissection to correct chordee and urethroplasty by use of skin graft tube and/or island flap ♂
🏥 30.7 ✂ 30.7 **FUD** 090 [T] [80] ⚑
AMA: 2016,Jan,13; 2015,Jan,16; 2014,Jan,11; 2012,Jan,15-42; 2011,Jan,11

54336 1-stage perineal hypospadias repair requiring extensive dissection to correct chordee and urethroplasty by use of skin graft tube and/or island flap ♂
🏥 35.9 ✂ 35.9 **FUD** 090 [T] [80] ⚑
AMA: 2016,Jan,13; 2015,Jan,16; 2014,Jan,11; 2012,Jan,15-42; 2011,Jan,11

54340 Repair of hypospadias complications (ie, fistula, stricture, diverticula); by closure, incision, or excision, simple ♂
🏥 16.3 ✂ 16.3 **FUD** 090 [T] [A2] [80] ⚑
AMA: 2014,Jan,11

54344 requiring mobilization of skin flaps and urethroplasty with flap or patch graft ♂
🏥 29.9 ✂ 29.9 **FUD** 090 [J] [A2] [80] ⚑
AMA: 2014,Jan,11

54348 requiring extensive dissection and urethroplasty with flap, patch or tubed graft (includes urinary diversion) ♂
🏥 29.1 ✂ 29.1 **FUD** 090 [T] [A2] [80] ⚑
AMA: 2014,Jan,11

54352 Repair of hypospadias cripple requiring extensive dissection and excision of previously constructed structures including re-release of chordee and reconstruction of urethra and penis by use of local skin as grafts and island flaps and skin brought in as flaps or grafts ♂
🏥 40.7 ✂ 40.7 **FUD** 090 [J] [A2] [80] ⚑
AMA: 2014,Jan,11

54360 Plastic operation on penis to correct angulation ♂
🏥 20.7 ✂ 20.7 **FUD** 090 [T] [A2] [80] ⚑
AMA: 2014,Jan,11

54380 Plastic operation on penis for epispadias distal to external sphincter; ♂

    INCLUDES Lowsley's operation

    🚜 22.9   ⚕ 22.9   **FUD** 090   T A2 80 ▣

    AMA: 2014,Jan,11

54385 with incontinence ♂

    🚜 28.0   ⚕ 28.0   **FUD** 090   T A2 80 ▣

    AMA: 2014,Jan,11

54390 with exstrophy of bladder ♂

    🚜 37.4   ⚕ 37.4   **FUD** 090   C 80 ▣

    AMA: 2014,Jan,11

54400-54417 Procedures to Treat Impotence

CMS: 100-03,230.4 Diagnosis and Treatment of Impotence

    EXCLUDES Other urethroplasties (53400-53430)

    Revascularization of penis (37788)

54400 Insertion of penile prosthesis; non-inflatable (semi-rigid) ♂

    EXCLUDES Replacement/removal penile prosthesis (54415, 54416)

    🚜 15.2   ⚕ 15.2   **FUD** 090   J J8 ▣

    AMA: 2014,Jan,11

54401 inflatable (self-contained) ♂

    EXCLUDES Replacement/removal penile prosthesis (54415, 54416)

    🚜 18.8   ⚕ 18.8   **FUD** 090   J J8 ▣

    AMA: 2014,Jan,11

54405 Insertion of multi-component, inflatable penile prosthesis, including placement of pump, cylinders, and reservoir ♂

    Code also modifier 52 for reduced services

    🚜 23.2   ⚕ 23.2   **FUD** 090   J J8 80 ▣

    AMA: 2014,Jan,11

54406 Removal of all components of a multi-component, inflatable penile prosthesis without replacement of prosthesis ♂

    Code also modifier 52 for reduced services

    🚜 20.9   ⚕ 20.9   **FUD** 090   02 A2 80 ▣

    AMA: 2014,Jan,11

54408 Repair of component(s) of a multi-component, inflatable penile prosthesis ♂

    🚜 22.7   ⚕ 22.7   **FUD** 090   J A2 80 ▣

    AMA: 2014,Jan,11

54410 Removal and replacement of all component(s) of a multi-component, inflatable penile prosthesis at the same operative session ♂

    🚜 24.6   ⚕ 24.6   **FUD** 090   J J8 80 ▣

    AMA: 2014,Jan,11

54411 Removal and replacement of all components of a multi-component inflatable penile prosthesis through an infected field at the same operative session, including irrigation and debridement of infected tissue ♂

    INCLUDES Debridement (11042, 11043)

    Code also modifier 52 for reduced services

    🚜 29.4   ⚕ 29.4   **FUD** 090   J 80 ▣

    AMA: 2014,Jan,11

54415 Removal of non-inflatable (semi-rigid) or inflatable (self-contained) penile prosthesis, without replacement of prosthesis ♂

    🚜 15.1   ⚕ 15.1   **FUD** 090   02 A2 80 ▣

    AMA: 2014,Jan,11

54416 Removal and replacement of non-inflatable (semi-rigid) or inflatable (self-contained) penile prosthesis at the same operative session ♂

    🚜 20.3   ⚕ 20.3   **FUD** 090   J J8 80 ▣

    AMA: 2014,Jan,11

54417 Removal and replacement of non-inflatable (semi-rigid) or inflatable (self-contained) penile prosthesis through an infected field at the same operative session, including irrigation and debridement of infected tissue ♂

    INCLUDES Debridement (11042, 11043)

    🚜 25.8   ⚕ 25.8   **FUD** 090   J 80 ▣

    AMA: 2014,Jan,11

54420-54450 Other Procedures of the Penis

    EXCLUDES Other urethroplasties (53400-53430)

    Revascularization of penis (37788)

54420 Corpora cavernosa-saphenous vein shunt (priapism operation), unilateral or bilateral ♂

    🚜 20.2   ⚕ 20.2   **FUD** 090   T A2 80 ▣

    AMA: 2014,Jan,11

54430 Corpora cavernosa-corpus spongiosum shunt (priapism operation), unilateral or bilateral ♂

    🚜 18.3   ⚕ 18.3   **FUD** 090   C 80 ▣

    AMA: 2014,Jan,11

54435 Corpora cavernosa-glans penis fistulization (eg, biopsy needle, Winter procedure, rongeur, or punch) for priapism ♂

    🚜 11.9   ⚕ 11.9   **FUD** 090   T A2 ▣

    AMA: 2014,Jan,11

54437 Repair of traumatic corporeal tear(s) ♂

    🚜 19.5   ⚕ 19.5   **FUD** 090   T G2 80 ▣

    EXCLUDES Urethral repair (53410, 53415)

54438 Replantation, penis, complete amputation including urethral repair ♂

    🚜 39.4   ⚕ 39.4   **FUD** 090   C 80 ▣

    EXCLUDES Replantation/repair of corporeal tear in incomplete amputation penis (54437)

    Replantation/urethral repair in incomplete amputation penis (53410-53415)

54440 Plastic operation of penis for injury ♂

    🚜 0.00   ⚕ 0.00   **FUD** 090   T A2 80 ▣

    AMA: 2014,Jan,11

54450 Foreskin manipulation including lysis of preputial adhesions and stretching ♂

    🚜 1.66   ⚕ 2.00   **FUD** 000   T A2 ▣

    AMA: 2014,Jan,11

54500-54560 Testicular Procedures: Incisional

    EXCLUDES Debridement of abdominal perineal gangrene (11004-11006)

54500 Biopsy of testis, needle (separate procedure) ♂

    EXCLUDES Fine needle aspiration (10021, 10022)

    🔬 (88172-88173)

    🚜 2.14   ⚕ 2.14   **FUD** 000   T A2 80 50 ▣

    AMA: 2014,Jan,11

54505 Biopsy of testis, incisional (separate procedure) ♂

    Code also when combined with epididymogram, seminal vesiculogram or vasogram (55300)

    🚜 6.04   ⚕ 6.04   **FUD** 010   T A2 80 50 ▣

    AMA: 2016,Jan,13; 2015,Jan,16; 2014,Jan,11

54512 Excision of extraparenchymal lesion of testis ♂

    🚜 15.5   ⚕ 15.5   **FUD** 090   T A2 50 ▣

    AMA: 2016,Jan,13; 2015,Jan,16; 2014,Jan,11; 2012,Jan,15-42; 2011,Jan,11

54520 Orchiectomy, simple (including subcapsular), with or without testicular prosthesis, scrotal or inguinal approach ♂

    INCLUDES Huggins' orchiectomy

    EXCLUDES Lymphadenectomy, radical retroperitoneal (38780)

    Code also hernia repair if performed (49505, 49507)

    🚜 9.37   ⚕ 9.37   **FUD** 090   T A2 50 ▣

    AMA: 2016,Jan,13; 2015,Jan,16; 2014,Jan,11

54522 **Orchiectomy, partial** ♂

EXCLUDES *Lymphadenectomy, radical retroperitoneal (38780)*

17.8   17.8   **FUD** 090   T A2 80 50 ▢

AMA: 2016,Jan,13; 2015,Jan,16; 2014,Jan,11

54530 **Orchiectomy, radical, for tumor; inguinal approach** ♂

EXCLUDES *Lymphadenectomy, radical retroperitoneal (38780)*

14.5   14.5   **FUD** 090   T A2 80 50 ▢

AMA: 2016,Jan,13; 2015,Jan,16; 2014,Jan,11

54535 **with abdominal exploration** ♂

EXCLUDES *Lymphadenectomy, radical retroperitoneal (38780)*

21.3   21.3   **FUD** 090   T 80 50 ▢

AMA: 2016,Jan,13; 2015,Jan,16; 2014,Jan,11

54550 **Exploration for undescended testis (inguinal or scrotal area)** ♂

14.1   14.1   **FUD** 090   T A2 80 50 ▢

AMA: 2016,Jan,13; 2015,Jan,16; 2014,Jan,11

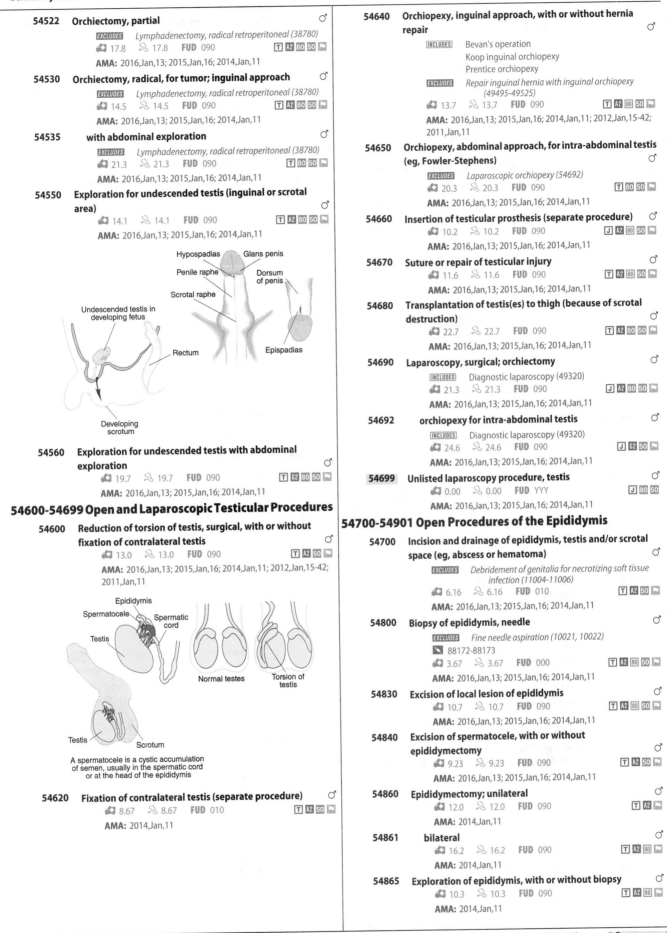

54560 **Exploration for undescended testis with abdominal exploration** ♂

19.7   19.7   **FUD** 090   T G2 80 50 ▢

AMA: 2016,Jan,13; 2015,Jan,16; 2014,Jan,11

54600-54699 Open and Laparoscopic Testicular Procedures

54600 **Reduction of torsion of testis, surgical, with or without fixation of contralateral testis** ♂

13.0   13.0   **FUD** 090   T A2 50 ▢

AMA: 2016,Jan,13; 2015,Jan,16; 2014,Jan,11; 2012,Jan,15-42; 2011,Jan,11

54620 **Fixation of contralateral testis (separate procedure)** ♂

8.67   8.67   **FUD** 010   T A2 50 ▢

AMA: 2014,Jan,11

54640 **Orchiopexy, inguinal approach, with or without hernia repair** ♂

INCLUDES Bevan's operation
Koop inguinal orchiopexy
Prentice orchiopexy

EXCLUDES *Repair inguinal hernia with inguinal orchiopexy (49495-49525)*

13.7   13.7   **FUD** 090   T A2 80 50 ▢

AMA: 2016,Jan,13; 2015,Jan,16; 2014,Jan,11; 2012,Jan,15-42; 2011,Jan,11

54650 **Orchiopexy, abdominal approach, for intra-abdominal testis (eg, Fowler-Stephens)** ♂

EXCLUDES *Laparoscopic orchiopexy (54692)*

20.3   20.3   **FUD** 090   T 80 50 ▢

AMA: 2016,Jan,13; 2015,Jan,16; 2014,Jan,11

54660 **Insertion of testicular prosthesis (separate procedure)** ♂

10.2   10.2   **FUD** 090   J A2 80 50 ▢

AMA: 2016,Jan,13; 2015,Jan,16; 2014,Jan,11

54670 **Suture or repair of testicular injury** ♂

11.6   11.6   **FUD** 090   T A2 80 50 ▢

AMA: 2016,Jan,13; 2015,Jan,16; 2014,Jan,11

54680 **Transplantation of testis(es) to thigh (because of scrotal destruction)** ♂

22.7   22.7   **FUD** 090   T A2 80 50 ▢

AMA: 2016,Jan,13; 2015,Jan,16; 2014,Jan,11

54690 **Laparoscopy, surgical; orchiectomy** ♂

INCLUDES Diagnostic laparoscopy (49320)

21.3   21.3   **FUD** 090   J A2 80 50 ▢

AMA: 2016,Jan,13; 2015,Jan,16; 2014,Jan,11

54692 **orchiopexy for intra-abdominal testis** ♂

INCLUDES Diagnostic laparoscopy (49320)

24.6   24.6   **FUD** 090   J G2 50 ▢

AMA: 2016,Jan,13; 2015,Jan,16; 2014,Jan,11

54699 **Unlisted laparoscopy procedure, testis** ♂

0.00   0.00   **FUD** YYY   J 80 50

AMA: 2016,Jan,13; 2015,Jan,16; 2014,Jan,11

54700-54901 Open Procedures of the Epididymis

54700 **Incision and drainage of epididymis, testis and/or scrotal space (eg, abscess or hematoma)** ♂

EXCLUDES *Debridement of genitalia for necrotizing soft tissue infection (11004-11006)*

6.16   6.16   **FUD** 010   T A2 50 ▢

AMA: 2016,Jan,13; 2015,Jan,16; 2014,Jan,11

54800 **Biopsy of epididymis, needle** ♂

EXCLUDES *Fine needle aspiration (10021, 10022)*

88172-88173

3.67   3.67   **FUD** 000   T A2 80 50 ▢

AMA: 2016,Jan,13; 2015,Jan,16; 2014,Jan,11

54830 **Excision of local lesion of epididymis** ♂

10.7   10.7   **FUD** 090   T A2 80 50 ▢

AMA: 2016,Jan,13; 2015,Jan,16; 2014,Jan,11

54840 **Excision of spermatocele, with or without epididymectomy** ♂

9.23   9.23   **FUD** 090   T A2 50 ▢

AMA: 2016,Jan,13; 2015,Jan,16; 2014,Jan,11

54860 **Epididymectomy; unilateral** ♂

12.0   12.0   **FUD** 090   T A2 ▢

AMA: 2014,Jan,11

54861 **bilateral** ♂

16.2   16.2   **FUD** 090   T A2 80 ▢

AMA: 2014,Jan,11

54865 **Exploration of epididymis, with or without biopsy** ♂

10.3   10.3   **FUD** 090   T A2 80 ▢

AMA: 2014,Jan,11

54900 Epididymovasostomy, anastomosis of epididymis to vas deferens; unilateral ♂

EXCLUDES Operating microscope (69990)

🚗 24.1 ✂ 24.1 **FUD** 090 [T] [A2] [80] [📋]

AMA: 2016,Jan,13; 2015,Jan,16; 2014,Jan,11; 2012,Jan,15-42; 2011,Jan,11

54901 bilateral ♂

EXCLUDES Operating microscope (69990)

🚗 31.9 ✂ 31.9 **FUD** 090 [T] [A2] [80] [📋]

AMA: 2016,Jan,13; 2015,Jan,16; 2014,Jan,11; 2012,Jan,15-42; 2011,Jan,11

55000-55180 Procedures of the Tunica Vaginalis and Scrotum

55000 Puncture aspiration of hydrocele, tunica vaginalis, with or without injection of medication ♂

🚗 2.45 ✂ 3.34 **FUD** 000 [T] [P3] [50] [📋]

AMA: 2014,Jan,11

Schematic showing a communicating hydrocele flowing through unclosed processus vaginalis

55040 Excision of hydrocele; unilateral ♂

EXCLUDES Repair of hernia with hydrocelectomy (49495-49501)

🚗 9.72 ✂ 9.72 **FUD** 090 [T] [A2] [📋]

AMA: 2016,Jan,13; 2015,Jan,16; 2014,Jan,11

55041 bilateral ♂

EXCLUDES Repair of hernia with hydrocelectomy (49495-49501)

🚗 14.6 ✂ 14.6 **FUD** 090 [T] [A2] [📋]

AMA: 2014,Jan,11

55060 Repair of tunica vaginalis hydrocele (Bottle type) ♂

🚗 10.9 ✂ 10.9 **FUD** 090 [T] [A2] [80] [50] [📋]

AMA: 2016,Jan,13; 2015,Jan,16; 2014,Nov,14; 2014,Jan,11

55100 Drainage of scrotal wall abscess ♂

EXCLUDES Debridement of genitalia for necrotizing soft tissue infection (11004-11006)
Incision and drainage of scrotal space (54700)

🚗 4.78 ✂ 6.16 **FUD** 010 [T] [A2] [📋]

AMA: 2014,Jan,11

55110 Scrotal exploration ♂

🚗 11.1 ✂ 11.1 **FUD** 090 [T] [A2] [📋]

AMA: 2014,Jan,11

55120 Removal of foreign body in scrotum ♂

🚗 10.2 ✂ 10.2 **FUD** 090 [T] [A2] [80] [📋]

AMA: 2014,Jan,11

55150 Resection of scrotum ♂

EXCLUDES Lesion excision of skin of scrotum (11420-11426, 11620-11626)

🚗 14.1 ✂ 14.1 **FUD** 090 [T] [A2] [80] [📋]

AMA: 2014,Jan,11

55175 Scrotoplasty; simple ♂

🚗 10.4 ✂ 10.4 **FUD** 090 [T] [A2] [80] [📋]

AMA: 2016,Jan,13; 2015,Jan,16; 2014,Dec,16; 2014,Dec,16; 2014,Jan,11

55180 complicated ♂

🚗 19.9 ✂ 19.9 **FUD** 090 [J] [A2] [80] [📋]

AMA: 2014,Jan,11

55200-55680 Procedures of Other Male Genital Ducts and Glands

55200 Vasotomy, cannulization with or without incision of vas, unilateral or bilateral (separate procedure) ♂

🚗 8.00 ✂ 12.3 **FUD** 090 [T] [A2] [80] [📋]

AMA: 2014,Jan,11

55250 Vasectomy, unilateral or bilateral (separate procedure), including postoperative semen examination(s) ♂

🚗 6.52 ✂ 10.9 **FUD** 090 [T] [A2] [📋]

AMA: 2016,Jan,13; 2015,Jan,16; 2014,Jan,11; 2012,Jan,15-42; 2011,Jan,11

55300 Vasotomy for vasograms, seminal vesiculograms, or epididymograms, unilateral or bilateral ♂

Code also biopsy of testis and modifier 51 when combined (54505)

❌ (74440)

🚗 5.39 ✂ 5.39 **FUD** 000 [N] [N1] [80] [📋]

AMA: 2014,Jan,11

55400 Vasovasostomy, vasovasorrhaphy ♂

EXCLUDES Operating microscope (69990)

🚗 14.6 ✂ 14.6 **FUD** 090 [T] [A2] [80] [50] [📋]

AMA: 2016,Jan,13; 2015,Jan,16; 2014,Jan,11; 2012,Jan,15-42; 2011,Jan,11

55450 Ligation (percutaneous) of vas deferens, unilateral or bilateral (separate procedure) ♂

🚗 7.39 ✂ 10.2 **FUD** 010 [T] [P3] [80] [📋]

AMA: 2014,Jan,11

55500 Excision of hydrocele of spermatic cord, unilateral (separate procedure) ♂

🚗 11.4 ✂ 11.4 **FUD** 090 [T] [A2] [80] [50] [📋]

AMA: 2016,Jan,13; 2015,Jan,16; 2014,Jan,11

55520 Excision of lesion of spermatic cord (separate procedure) ♂

🚗 13.0 ✂ 13.0 **FUD** 090 [T] [A2] [80] [50] [📋]

AMA: 2016,Jan,13; 2015,Jan,16; 2014,Jan,11; 2012,Jan,15-42; 2011,Jan,11

55530 Excision of varicocele or ligation of spermatic veins for varicocele; (separate procedure) ♂

🚗 10.1 ✂ 10.1 **FUD** 090 [T] [A2] [50] [📋]

AMA: 2016,Jan,13; 2015,Jan,16; 2014,Jan,11

55535 abdominal approach ♂

🚗 12.3 ✂ 12.3 **FUD** 090 [T] [A2] [80] [50] [📋]

AMA: 2016,Jan,13; 2015,Jan,16; 2014,Jan,11

55540 with hernia repair ♂

🚗 15.6 ✂ 15.6 **FUD** 090 [T] [A2] [50] [📋]

AMA: 2016,Jan,13; 2015,Jan,16; 2014,Jan,11

55550 Laparoscopy, surgical, with ligation of spermatic veins for varicocele ♂

INCLUDES Diagnostic laparoscopy (49320)

🚗 12.3 ✂ 12.3 **FUD** 090 [J] [A2] [80] [50] [📋]

AMA: 2016,Jan,13; 2015,Jan,16; 2014,Jan,11

55559 Unlisted laparoscopy procedure, spermatic cord ♂

🚗 0.00 ✂ 0.00 **FUD** YYY [J] [80] [50]

AMA: 2016,Jan,13; 2015,Jan,16; 2014,Jan,11

55600 Vesiculotomy; ♂

🚗 12.1 ✂ 12.1 **FUD** 090 [T] [R2] [80] [50] [📋]

AMA: 2014,Jan,11

55605 complicated ♂

🚗 15.7 ✂ 15.7 **FUD** 090 [C] [80] [50] [📋]

AMA: 2014,Jan,11

55650 Vesiculectomy, any approach ♂

🚗 20.6 ✂ 20.6 **FUD** 090 [C] [80] [50] [📋]

AMA: 2014,Jan,11

26/TC PC/TC Only A2-Z3 ASC Payment 50 Bilateral ♂ Male Only ♀ Female Only 🚗 Facility RVU ✂ Non-Facility RVU 📋 CCI
FUD Follow-up Days CMS: IOM (Pub 100) A-Y OPPSI 80/80 Surg Assist Allowed / w/Doc 🔬 Lab Crosswalk ❌ Radiology Crosswalk ❌ CLIA

55680 Excision of Mullerian duct cyst ♂
    EXCLUDES *Injection procedure (52010, 55300)*
    🔷 10.2   10.2   **FUD** 090   T A2 80 50
    AMA: 2014,Jan,11

55700-55725 Procedures of Prostate: Incisional

55700 Biopsy, prostate; needle or punch, single or multiple, any approach ♂
    EXCLUDES *Fine needle aspiration (10021, 10022)*
    Needle biopsy of prostate, saturation sampling for prostate mapping (55706)
    🔳 (76942, 77002, 77012, 77021)
    🔲 (88172-88173)
    🔷 4.01   6.19   **FUD** 000   T A2
    AMA: 2016,Jan,13; 2015,Jan,16; 2014,Jan,11

Bladder
Pubic bone
Suprapubic approach
Pubic bone
Ischial tuberosity
Rectum
Vesicle
Urethra
Prostate
Perineal approach (retropubic) to prostate (above) and side view schematic of suprapubic approach

55705 incisional, any approach ♂
    🔷 7.65   7.65   **FUD** 010   T A2
    AMA: 2014,Jan,11

55706 Biopsies, prostate, needle, transperineal, stereotactic template guided saturation sampling, including imaging guidance ♂
    EXCLUDES *Biopsy, prostate; needle or punch (55700)*
    🔷 10.7   10.7   **FUD** 010   T G2 80
    AMA: 2016,Jan,13; 2015,Jan,16; 2014,Jan,11; 2012,Jan,15-42; 2011,Jan,11

55720 Prostatotomy, external drainage of prostatic abscess, any approach; simple ♂
    EXCLUDES *Drainage of prostatic abscess, transurethral (52700)*
    🔷 13.0   13.0   **FUD** 090   T A2 80
    AMA: 2014,Jan,11

55725 complicated ♂
    EXCLUDES *Drainage of prostatic abscess, transurethral (52700)*
    🔷 17.0   17.0   **FUD** 090   T A2 80
    AMA: 2014,Jan,11

55801-55845 Open Prostatectomy

EXCLUDES *Limited pelvic lymphadenectomy for staging (separate procedure) (38562)*
Node dissection, independent (38770-38780)
Transurethral prostate
Destruction (53850-53852)
Resection (52601-52640)

55801 Prostatectomy, perineal, subtotal (including control of postoperative bleeding, vasectomy, meatotomy, urethral calibration and/or dilation, and internal urethrotomy) ♂
    🔷 31.6   31.6   **FUD** 090   C 80
    AMA: 2014,Jan,11

55810 Prostatectomy, perineal radical; ♂
    INCLUDES Walsh modified radical prostatectomy
    🔷 37.9   37.9   **FUD** 090   C 80
    AMA: 2014,Jan,11

55812 with lymph node biopsy(s) (limited pelvic lymphadenectomy) ♂
    🔷 46.2   46.2   **FUD** 090   C 80
    AMA: 2014,Jan,11

55815 with bilateral pelvic lymphadenectomy, including external iliac, hypogastric and obturator nodes ♂
    EXCLUDES *When performed on separate days, report: (38770, 55810)*
    Pelvic lymphadenectomy, bilateral, and append modifier 50 (38770)
    Perineal radical prostatectomy (55810)
    🔷 50.9   50.9   **FUD** 090   C 80
    AMA: 2014,Jan,11

55821 Prostatectomy (including control of postoperative bleeding, vasectomy, meatotomy, urethral calibration and/or dilation, and internal urethrotomy); suprapubic, subtotal, 1 or 2 stages ♂
    🔷 25.1   25.1   **FUD** 090   C 80
    AMA: 2014,Jan,11

55831 retropubic, subtotal ♂
    🔷 27.1   27.1   **FUD** 090   C 80
    AMA: 2014,Jan,11

55840 Prostatectomy, retropubic radical, with or without nerve sparing; ♂
    EXCLUDES *Prostatectomy, radical retropubic, performed laparoscopically (55866)*
    🔷 33.7   33.7   **FUD** 090   C 80
    AMA: 2014,Jan,11

55842 with lymph node biopsy(s) (limited pelvic lymphadenectomy) ♂
    EXCLUDES *Prostatectomy, retropubic radical, performed laparoscopically (55866)*
    🔷 33.6   33.6   **FUD** 090   C 80
    AMA: 2014,Jan,11

55845 with bilateral pelvic lymphadenectomy, including external iliac, hypogastric, and obturator nodes ♂
    EXCLUDES *Prostatectomy, retropubic radical, performed laparoscopically (55866)*
    When performed on separate days, report: (38770, 55840)
    Pelvic lymphadenectomy, bilateral, and append modifier 50 (38770)
    Radical prostatectomy, retropubic, with or without nerve sparing (55840)
    🔷 39.2   39.2   **FUD** 090   C 80
    AMA: 2014,Jan,11

55860-55865 Prostate Exposure for Radiation Source Application

55860 Exposure of prostate, any approach, for insertion of radioactive substance; ♂
    EXCLUDES *Interstitial radioelement application (77770-77772, 77778)*
    🔷 25.1   25.1   **FUD** 090   T G2
    AMA: 2014,Jan,11

55862 with lymph node biopsy(s) (limited pelvic lymphadenectomy) ♂
    🔷 33.1   33.1   **FUD** 090   C 80
    AMA: 2014,Jan,11

55865 with bilateral pelvic lymphadenectomy, including external iliac, hypogastric and obturator nodes ♂
    🔷 38.3   38.3   **FUD** 090   C 80
    AMA: 2014,Jan,11

55866 Laparoscopic Prostatectomy

55866 Laparoscopy, surgical prostatectomy, retropubic radical, including nerve sparing, includes robotic assistance, when performed ♂
    INCLUDES Diagnostic laparoscopy (49320)
    EXCLUDES *Open method (55840)*
    🔷 40.3   40.3   **FUD** 090   C 80
    AMA: 2016,Jan,13; 2015,Jan,16; 2014,Jan,11; 2012,Mar,9-10

55870-55899 Miscellaneous Prostate Procedures

55870 **Electroejaculation** ♂

> EXCLUDES *Artificial insemination (58321-58322)*

🔧 4.10 🔪 5.01 **FUD** 000   T P3 ▢

AMA: 2014,Jan,11

55873 **Cryosurgical ablation of the prostate (includes ultrasonic guidance and monitoring)** ♂

🔧 22.0 🔪 200. **FUD** 090   J J8 ▢

AMA: 2016,Jan,13; 2015,Sep,12; 2015,Jan,16; 2014,Jan,11

55875 **Transperineal placement of needles or catheters into prostate for interstitial radioelement application, with or without cystoscopy** ♂

> Code also interstitial radioelement application (77770-77772, 77778)
> 🔧 (76965)

🔧 21.9 🔪 21.9 **FUD** 090   Q3 A2 80 ▢

AMA: 2016,Jan,13; 2015,Jan,16; 2014,Jan,11

55876 **Placement of interstitial device(s) for radiation therapy guidance (eg, fiducial markers, dosimeter), prostate (via needle, any approach), single or multiple** ♂

> Code also supply of device
> 🔧 (76942, 77002, 77012, 77021)

🔧 2.89 🔪 3.86 **FUD** 000   S P3 ▢

AMA: 2016,Jun,3; 2016,Jan,13; 2015,Jan,16; 2014,Jan,11; 2012,Jan,15-42; 2011,Jan,11

55899 **Unlisted procedure, male genital system** ♂

🔧 0.00 🔪 0.00 **FUD** YYY   T 80

AMA: 2016,Jan,13; 2015,Jun,5; 2015,Jan,16; 2014,Jan,11

55920 Insertion Brachytherapy Catheters/Needles Pelvis/Genitalia, Male/Female

55920 **Placement of needles or catheters into pelvic organs and/or genitalia (except prostate) for subsequent interstitial radioelement application**

> EXCLUDES *Insertion of Heyman capsules for purposes of brachytherapy (58346)*
> *Insertion of vaginal ovoids and/or uterine tandems for purposes of brachytherapy (57155)*
> *Placement of catheters or needles, prostate (55875)*

🔧 12.8 🔪 12.8 **FUD** 000   T G2 80 ▢

AMA: 2016,Jan,13; 2015,Jan,16; 2014,Jan,11

55970-55980 Transsexual Surgery

CMS: 100-02,16,10 Exclusions from Coverage; 100-02,16,180 Services Related to Noncovered Procedures

55970 **Intersex surgery; male to female** ♂

🔧 0.00 🔪 0.00 **FUD** YYY   T ▢

AMA: 2014,Jan,11

55980 **female to male** ♀

🔧 0.00 🔪 0.00 **FUD** YYY   T ▢

AMA: 2014,Jan,11

56405-56420 Incision and Drainage of Abscess

> EXCLUDES *Incision and drainage Skene's gland cyst/abscess (53060)*
> *Incision and drainage subcutaneous abscess/cyst/furuncle (10040, 10060, 10061)*

56405 **Incision and drainage of vulva or perineal abscess** ♀

🔧 3.07 🔪 3.09 **FUD** 010   T P3 ▢

AMA: 2014,Jan,11

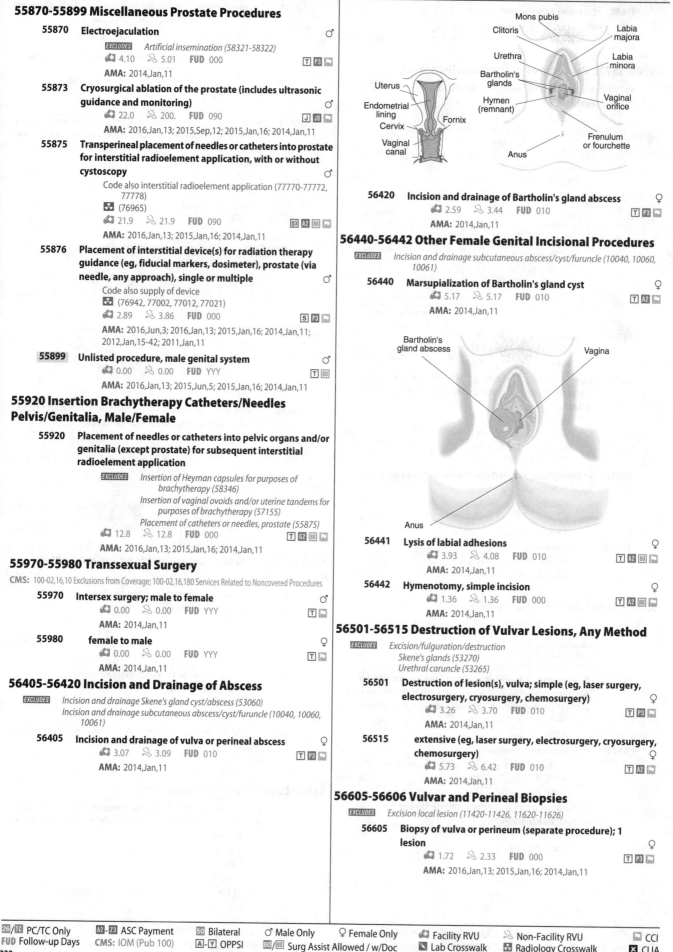

56420 **Incision and drainage of Bartholin's gland abscess** ♀

🔧 2.59 🔪 3.44 **FUD** 010   T P3 ▢

AMA: 2014,Jan,11

56440-56442 Other Female Genital Incisional Procedures

> EXCLUDES *Incision and drainage subcutaneous abscess/cyst/furuncle (10040, 10060, 10061)*

56440 **Marsupialization of Bartholin's gland cyst** ♀

🔧 5.17 🔪 5.17 **FUD** 010   T A2 ▢

AMA: 2014,Jan,11

56441 **Lysis of labial adhesions** ♀

🔧 3.93 🔪 4.08 **FUD** 010   T A2 80 ▢

AMA: 2014,Jan,11

56442 **Hymenotomy, simple incision** ♀

🔧 1.36 🔪 1.36 **FUD** 000   T A2 80 ▢

AMA: 2014,Jan,11

56501-56515 Destruction of Vulvar Lesions, Any Method

> EXCLUDES *Excision/fulguration/destruction*
> *Skene's glands (53270)*
> *Urethral caruncle (53265)*

56501 **Destruction of lesion(s), vulva; simple (eg, laser surgery, electrosurgery, cryosurgery, chemosurgery)** ♀

🔧 3.26 🔪 3.70 **FUD** 010   T P3 ▢

AMA: 2014,Jan,11

56515 **extensive (eg, laser surgery, electrosurgery, cryosurgery, chemosurgery)** ♀

🔧 5.73 🔪 6.42 **FUD** 010   T A2 ▢

AMA: 2014,Jan,11

56605-56606 Vulvar and Perineal Biopsies

> EXCLUDES *Excision local lesion (11420-11426, 11620-11626)*

56605 **Biopsy of vulva or perineum (separate procedure); 1 lesion** ♀

🔧 1.72 🔪 2.33 **FUD** 000   T P3 ▢

AMA: 2016,Jan,13; 2015,Jan,16; 2014,Jan,11

26/TC PC/TC Only   A2-Z3 ASC Payment   50 Bilateral   ♂ Male Only   ♀ Female Only   🔧 Facility RVU   🔪 Non-Facility RVU   ▢ CCI

FUD Follow-up Days   **CMS:** IOM (Pub 100)   A-Y OPPSI   80/80 Surg Assist Allowed / w/Doc   📋 Lab Crosswalk   🔧 Radiology Crosswalk   ❌ CLIA

238

+ **56606** each separate additional lesion (List separately in addition to code for primary procedure) ♀
Code first (56605)
⚐ 0.85 ⚗ 1.07 **FUD** ZZZ N N1 ▣
AMA: 2014,Jan,11

56620-56640 Vulvectomy Procedures

INCLUDES Removal of:
Greater than 80% of the vulvar area - complete procedure
Less than 80% of the vulvar area - partial procedure
Skin and deep subcutaneous tissue - radical procedure
Skin and superficial subcutaneous tissues - simple procedure
EXCLUDES Skin graft (15004-15005, 15120-15121, 15240-15241)

56620 Vulvectomy simple; partial ♀
⚐ 14.8 ⚗ 14.8 **FUD** 090 T A2 80 ▣
AMA: 2016,Jan,13; 2015,Jan,16; 2014,Jan,11; 2013,Dec,14

56625 complete ♀
⚐ 18.0 ⚗ 18.0 **FUD** 090 T A2 80 ▣
AMA: 2014,Jan,11

56630 Vulvectomy, radical, partial; ♀
⚐ 26.6 ⚗ 26.6 **FUD** 090 C 80 ▣
AMA: 2014,Jan,11

56631 with unilateral inguinofemoral lymphadenectomy ♀
INCLUDES Bassett's operation
⚐ 34.0 ⚗ 34.0 **FUD** 090 C 80 ▣
AMA: 2014,Jan,11

56632 with bilateral inguinofemoral lymphadenectomy ♀
INCLUDES Bassett's operation
⚐ 39.4 ⚗ 39.4 **FUD** 090 C 80 ▣
AMA: 2014,Jan,11

56633 Vulvectomy, radical, complete; ♀
INCLUDES Bassett's operation
⚐ 34.8 ⚗ 34.8 **FUD** 090 C 80 ▣
AMA: 2014,Jan,11

56634 with unilateral inguinofemoral lymphadenectomy ♀
INCLUDES Bassett's operation
⚐ 37.6 ⚗ 37.6 **FUD** 090 C 80 ▣
AMA: 2014,Jan,11

56637 with bilateral inguinofemoral lymphadenectomy ♀
INCLUDES Bassett's operation
⚐ 43.3 ⚗ 43.3 **FUD** 090 C 80 ▣
AMA: 2014,Jan,11

56640 Vulvectomy, radical, complete, with inguinofemoral, iliac, and pelvic lymphadenectomy ♀
INCLUDES Bassett's operation
EXCLUDES Lymphadenectomy (38760-38780)
⚐ 43.6 ⚗ 43.6 **FUD** 090 C 80 50 ▣
AMA: 2014,Jan,11

56700-56740 Other Excisional Procedures: External Female Genitalia

56700 Partial hymenectomy or revision of hymenal ring ♀
⚐ 5.28 ⚗ 5.28 **FUD** 010 T A2 80 ▣
AMA: 2014,Jan,11

56740 Excision of Bartholin's gland or cyst ♀
EXCLUDES Excision/fulguration/marsupialization:
Skene's glands (53270)
Urethral carcinoma (53220)
Urethral caruncle (53265)
Urethral diverticulum (53230, 53240)
⚐ 8.56 ⚗ 8.56 **FUD** 010 T A2 50 ▣
AMA: 2014,Jan,11

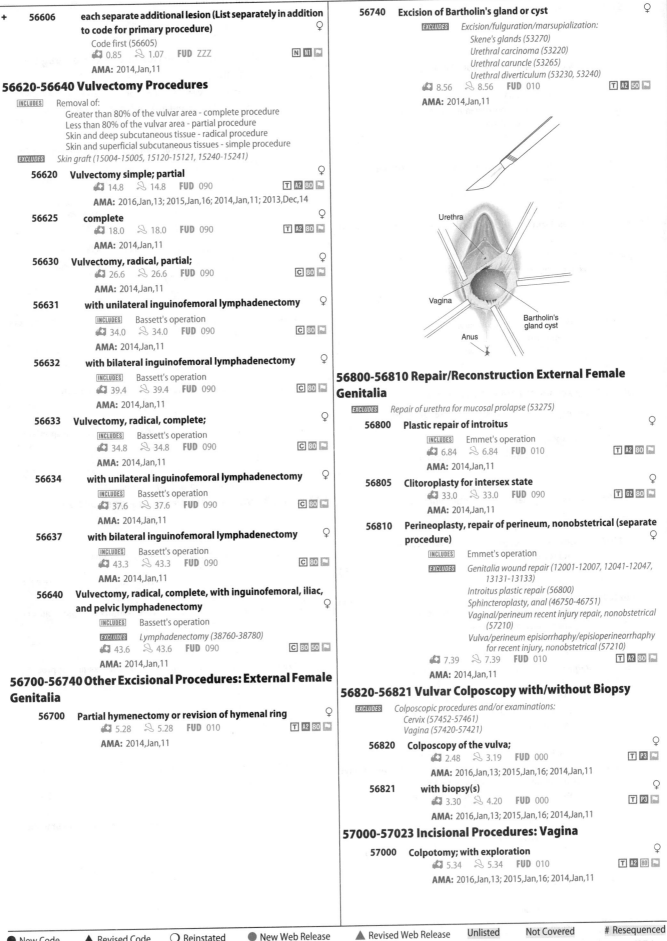

56800-56810 Repair/Reconstruction External Female Genitalia

EXCLUDES Repair of urethra for mucosal prolapse (53275)

56800 Plastic repair of introitus ♀
INCLUDES Emmet's operation
⚐ 6.84 ⚗ 6.84 **FUD** 010 T A2 80 ▣
AMA: 2014,Jan,11

56805 Clitoroplasty for intersex state ♀
⚐ 33.0 ⚗ 33.0 **FUD** 090 T G2 80 ▣
AMA: 2014,Jan,11

56810 Perineoplasty, repair of perineum, nonobstetrical (separate procedure) ♀
INCLUDES Emmet's operation
EXCLUDES Genitalia wound repair (12001-12007, 12041-12047, 13131-13133)
Introitus plastic repair (56800)
Sphincteroplasty, anal (46750-46751)
Vaginal/perineum recent injury repair, nonobstetrical (57210)
Vulva/perineum episiorrhaphy/episioperineorrhaphy for recent injury, nonobstetrical (57210)
⚐ 7.39 ⚗ 7.39 **FUD** 010 T A2 80 ▣
AMA: 2014,Jan,11

56820-56821 Vulvar Colposcopy with/without Biopsy

EXCLUDES Colposcopic procedures and/or examinations:
Cervix (57452-57461)
Vagina (57420-57421)

56820 Colposcopy of the vulva; ♀
⚐ 2.48 ⚗ 3.19 **FUD** 000 T P3 ▣
AMA: 2016,Jan,13; 2015,Jan,16; 2014,Jan,11

56821 with biopsy(s) ♀
⚐ 3.30 ⚗ 4.20 **FUD** 000 T P3 ▣
AMA: 2016,Jan,13; 2015,Jan,16; 2014,Jan,11

57000-57023 Incisional Procedures: Vagina

57000 Colpotomy; with exploration ♀
⚐ 5.34 ⚗ 5.34 **FUD** 010 T A2 80 ▣
AMA: 2016,Jan,13; 2015,Jan,16; 2014,Jan,11

● New Code ▲ Revised Code ○ Reinstated ● New Web Release ▲ Revised Web Release Unlisted Not Covered # Resequenced
⊘ AMA Mod 51 Exempt ⑤ Optum Mod 51 Exempt ⑥③ Mod 63 Exempt ✗ Non-FDA Drug ★ Telehealth M Maternity A Age Edit + Add-on **AMA:** CPT Asst
© 2016 Optum360, LLC CPT © 2016 American Medical Association. All Rights Reserved. **239**

Genital System

57010 — 57250

57010 with drainage of pelvic abscess ♀
INCLUDES Laroyenne operation
🚜 12.2 ⚕ 12.2 **FUD** 090
T A2 80
AMA: 2014,Jan,11

57020 Colpocentesis (separate procedure) ♀
🚜 2.30 ⚕ 2.63 **FUD** 000
T A2 80
AMA: 2014,Jan,11

57022 Incision and drainage of vaginal hematoma; obstetrical/postpartum ♀
🚜 4.82 ⚕ 4.82 **FUD** 010
T R2 80
AMA: 2014,Jan,11

57023 non-obstetrical (eg, post-trauma, spontaneous bleeding) ♀
🚜 8.79 ⚕ 8.79 **FUD** 010
T A2 80
AMA: 2014,Jan,11

57061-57065 Destruction of Vaginal Lesions, Any Method

CMS: 100-03,140.5 Laser Procedures

57061 Destruction of vaginal lesion(s); simple (eg, laser surgery, electrosurgery, cryosurgery, chemosurgery) ♀
🚜 2.79 ⚕ 3.22 **FUD** 010
T P3
AMA: 2016,Jan,13; 2015,Jan,16; 2014,Jan,11; 2012,Jan,15-42; 2011,Jan,11

57065 extensive (eg, laser surgery, electrosurgery, cryosurgery, chemosurgery) ♀
🚜 4.97 ⚕ 5.53 **FUD** 010
T A2
AMA: 2016,Jan,13; 2015,Jan,16; 2014,Jan,11; 2012,Jan,15-42; 2011,Jan,11

57100-57135 Excisional Procedures: Vagina

57100 Biopsy of vaginal mucosa; simple (separate procedure) ♀
🚜 1.91 ⚕ 2.53 **FUD** 000
T P3
AMA: 2014,Jan,11

57105 extensive, requiring suture (including cysts) ♀
🚜 3.59 ⚕ 3.87 **FUD** 010
T A2
AMA: 2014,Jan,11

57106 Vaginectomy, partial removal of vaginal wall; ♀
🚜 14.1 ⚕ 14.1 **FUD** 090
T 80
AMA: 2016,Jan,13; 2015,Jan,16; 2014,Jan,11

57107 with removal of paravaginal tissue (radical vaginectomy) ♀
🚜 41.6 ⚕ 41.6 **FUD** 090
T 80
AMA: 2016,Jan,13; 2015,Jan,16; 2014,Jan,11

57109 with removal of paravaginal tissue (radical vaginectomy) with bilateral total pelvic lymphadenectomy and para-aortic lymph node sampling (biopsy) ♀
🚜 49.8 ⚕ 49.8 **FUD** 090
T 80
AMA: 2016,Jan,13; 2015,Jan,16; 2014,Jan,11

57110 Vaginectomy, complete removal of vaginal wall; ♀
🚜 25.3 ⚕ 25.3 **FUD** 090
C 80
AMA: 2016,Jan,13; 2015,Jan,16; 2014,Jan,11

57111 with removal of paravaginal tissue (radical vaginectomy) ♀
🚜 45.7 ⚕ 45.7 **FUD** 090
C 80
AMA: 2016,Jan,13; 2015,Jan,16; 2014,Jan,11

57112 with removal of paravaginal tissue (radical vaginectomy) with bilateral total pelvic lymphadenectomy and para-aortic lymph node sampling (biopsy) ♀
🚜 53.2 ⚕ 53.2 **FUD** 090
C 80
AMA: 2016,Jan,13; 2015,Jan,16; 2014,Jan,11

57120 Colpocleisis (Le Fort type) ♀
🚜 14.4 ⚕ 14.4 **FUD** 090
J G2 80
AMA: 2014,Jan,11

57130 Excision of vaginal septum ♀
🚜 4.50 ⚕ 5.00 **FUD** 010
T A2 80
AMA: 2014,Jan,11

57135 Excision of vaginal cyst or tumor ♀
🚜 4.92 ⚕ 5.44 **FUD** 010
T A2
AMA: 2014,Jan,11

57150-57180 Irrigation/Insertion/Introduction Vaginal Medication or Supply

57150 Irrigation of vagina and/or application of medicament for treatment of bacterial, parasitic, or fungoid disease ♀
🚜 0.82 ⚕ 1.27 **FUD** 000
Q1 N1
AMA: 2014,Jan,11

▲ **57155** Insertion of uterine tandem and/or vaginal ovoids for clinical brachytherapy ♀
EXCLUDES Insertion of radioelement sources or ribbons (77761-77763, 77770-77772)
The placement of needles or catheters into the pelvic organs and/or genitalia (except for the prostate) for interstitial radioelement application (55920)
🚜 8.32 ⚕ 12.2 **FUD** 000
T A2
AMA: 2016,Jan,13; 2015,Jan,16; 2014,Jan,11

57156 Insertion of a vaginal radiation afterloading apparatus for clinical brachytherapy ♀
🚜 4.19 ⚕ 5.62 **FUD** 000
T G2 80
AMA: 2014,Jan,11

57160 Fitting and insertion of pessary or other intravaginal support device ♀
🚜 1.33 ⚕ 2.15 **FUD** 000
T P3
AMA: 2016,Jan,13; 2015,Jan,16; 2014,Jan,11; 2012,Jan,15-42; 2011,Jan,11

57170 Diaphragm or cervical cap fitting with instructions ♀
🚜 1.38 ⚕ 1.72 **FUD** 000
T P3 80
AMA: 2014,Jan,11

57180 Introduction of any hemostatic agent or pack for spontaneous or traumatic nonobstetrical vaginal hemorrhage (separate procedure) ♀
🚜 2.99 ⚕ 3.97 **FUD** 010
T A2
AMA: 2016,Jan,13; 2015,Jan,16; 2014,Jan,11

57200-57335 Vaginal Repair and Reconstruction

EXCLUDES Marshall-Marchetti-Kranz type urethral suspension, abdominal approach (51840-51841)
Urethral suspension performed laparoscopically (51990)

57200 Colporrhaphy, suture of injury of vagina (nonobstetrical) ♀
🚜 8.59 ⚕ 8.59 **FUD** 090
T A2 80
AMA: 2014,Jan,11

57210 Colpoperineorrhaphy, suture of injury of vagina and/or perineum (nonobstetrical) ♀
🚜 10.4 ⚕ 10.4 **FUD** 090
T A2 80
AMA: 2014,Jan,11

57220 Plastic operation on urethral sphincter, vaginal approach (eg, Kelly urethral plication) ♀
🚜 9.04 ⚕ 9.04 **FUD** 090
J A2 80
AMA: 2014,Jan,11

57230 Plastic repair of urethrocele ♀
🚜 11.1 ⚕ 11.1 **FUD** 090
T A2 80
AMA: 2014,Jan,11

57240 Anterior colporrhaphy, repair of cystocele with or without repair of urethrocele ♀
🚜 19.0 ⚕ 19.0 **FUD** 090
J A2 80
AMA: 2016,Jan,13; 2015,Jan,16; 2014,Jan,11

57250 Posterior colporrhaphy, repair of rectocele with or without perineorrhaphy ♀
EXCLUDES Rectocele repair (separate procedure) without posterior colporrhaphy (45560)
🚜 19.1 ⚕ 19.1 **FUD** 090
J A2 80
AMA: 2016,Jan,13; 2015,Jan,16; 2014,Jan,11; 2012,Jan,15-42; 2011,May,9

57260 **Combined anteroposterior colporrhaphy;** ♀
🚗 23.6 ⚕ 23.6 **FUD** 090 [J] [A2] [80] [▣]
AMA: 2016,Jan,13; 2015,Jan,16; 2014,Jan,11

57265 **with enterocele repair** ♀
🚗 25.8 ⚕ 25.8 **FUD** 090 [J] [A2] [80] [▣]
AMA: 2016,Jan,13; 2015,Jan,16; 2014,Jan,11

+ **57267** **Insertion of mesh or other prosthesis for repair of pelvic floor defect, each site (anterior, posterior compartment), vaginal approach (List separately in addition to code for primary procedure)** ♀
Code first (45560, 57240-57265, 57285)
🚗 7.29 ⚕ 7.29 **FUD** ZZZ [N] [N1] [80] [▣]
AMA: 2016,Jan,13; 2015,Jan,16; 2014,Jan,11; 2013,Oct,15; 2012,Jan,6-10; 2012,Jan,15-42; 2011,May,9; 2011,Jan,11

57268 **Repair of enterocele, vaginal approach (separate procedure)** ♀
🚗 13.7 ⚕ 13.7 **FUD** 090 [T] [A2] [80] [▣]
AMA: 2016,Jan,13; 2015,Jan,16; 2014,Jan,11

57270 **Repair of enterocele, abdominal approach (separate procedure)** ♀
🚗 22.7 ⚕ 22.7 **FUD** 090 [C] [80] [▣]
AMA: 2016,Jan,13; 2015,Jan,16; 2014,Jan,11

57280 **Colpopexy, abdominal approach** ♀
🚗 27.0 ⚕ 27.0 **FUD** 090 [C] [80] [▣]
AMA: 2016,Jan,13; 2015,Jan,16; 2014,Jan,11

57282 **Colpopexy, vaginal; extra-peritoneal approach (sacrospinous, iliococcygeus)** ♀
🚗 14.2 ⚕ 14.2 **FUD** 090 [J] [80] [▣]
AMA: 2016,Jan,13; 2015,Jan,16; 2014,Jan,11

57283 **intra-peritoneal approach (uterosacral, levator myorrhaphy)** ♀
EXCLUDES Excision of cervical stump (57556)
Vaginal hysterectomy (58263, 58270, 58280, 58292, 58294)
🚗 19.5 ⚕ 19.5 **FUD** 090 [J] [80] [▣]
AMA: 2016,Jan,13; 2015,Jan,16; 2014,Jan,11; 2012,Jan,15-42; 2011,May,9

57284 **Paravaginal defect repair (including repair of cystocele, if performed); open abdominal approach** ♀
EXCLUDES Anterior colporrhaphy (57240)
Anterior vesicourethropexy (51840-51841)
Combined anteroposterior colporrhaphy (57260-57265)
Hysterectomy (58152, 58267)
Laparoscopy, surgical; urethral suspension for stress incontinence (51990)
🚗 23.1 ⚕ 23.1 **FUD** 090 [J] [80] [▣]
AMA: 2016,Jan,13; 2015,Jan,16; 2014,Jan,11; 2012,Jan,15-42; 2011,Jan,11

57285 **vaginal approach** ♀
EXCLUDES Anterior colporrhaphy (57240)
Combined anteroposterior colporrhaphy (57260-57265)
Laparoscopy, surgical; urethral suspension for stress incontinence (51990)
Vaginal hysterectomy (58267)
🚗 19.0 ⚕ 19.0 **FUD** 090 [J] [80] [▣]
AMA: 2016,Jan,13; 2015,Jan,16; 2014,Jan,11

57287 **Removal or revision of sling for stress incontinence (eg, fascia or synthetic)** ♀
🚗 19.3 ⚕ 19.3 **FUD** 090 [G2] [G2] [80] [▣]
AMA: 2016,Jan,13; 2015,Jan,16; 2014,Jan,11; 2012,Jan,15-42; 2011,Jan,11

57288 **Sling operation for stress incontinence (eg, fascia or synthetic)** ♀
INCLUDES Millin-Read operation
EXCLUDES Sling operation for stress incontinence performed laparoscopically (51992)
🚗 20.3 ⚕ 20.3 **FUD** 090 [J] [A2] [80] [▣]
AMA: 2016,Jan,13; 2015,Jan,16; 2014,Jan,11; 2012,Jan,15-42; 2011,Jan,11

57289 **Pereyra procedure, including anterior colporrhaphy** ♀
🚗 20.9 ⚕ 20.9 **FUD** 090 [J] [A2] [80] [▣]
AMA: 2016,Jan,13; 2015,Jan,16; 2014,Jan,11

57291 **Construction of artificial vagina; without graft** ♀
INCLUDES McIndoe vaginal construction
🚗 17.4 ⚕ 17.4 **FUD** 090 [T] [A2] [80] [▣]
AMA: 2014,Jan,11

57292 **with graft** ♀
🚗 23.3 ⚕ 23.3 **FUD** 090 [J] [80] [▣]
AMA: 2014,Jan,11

57295 **Revision (including removal) of prosthetic vaginal graft; vaginal approach** ♀
EXCLUDES Laparoscopic approach (57426)
🚗 13.5 ⚕ 13.5 **FUD** 090 [T] [G2] [80] [▣]
AMA: 2014,Jan,11

57296 **open abdominal approach** ♀
EXCLUDES Laparoscopic approach (57426)
🚗 26.8 ⚕ 26.8 **FUD** 090 [C] [80] [▣]
AMA: 2014,Jan,11

57300 **Closure of rectovaginal fistula; vaginal or transanal approach** ♀
🚗 16.0 ⚕ 16.0 **FUD** 090 [T] [A2] [80] [▣]
AMA: 2014,Jan,11

57305 **abdominal approach** ♀
🚗 26.7 ⚕ 26.7 **FUD** 090 [C] [80] [▣]
AMA: 2014,Jan,11

57307 **abdominal approach, with concomitant colostomy** ♀
🚗 31.0 ⚕ 31.0 **FUD** 090 [C] [80] [▣]
AMA: 2014,Jan,11

57308 **transperineal approach, with perineal body reconstruction, with or without levator plication** ♀
🚗 18.7 ⚕ 18.7 **FUD** 090 [C] [80] [▣]
AMA: 2014,Jan,11

57310 **Closure of urethrovaginal fistula;** ♀
🚗 13.2 ⚕ 13.2 **FUD** 090 [J] [G2] [80] [▣]
AMA: 2014,Jan,11

57311 **with bulbocavernosus transplant** ♀
🚗 15.1 ⚕ 15.1 **FUD** 090 [C] [80] [▣]
AMA: 2014,Jan,11

57320 **Closure of vesicovaginal fistula; vaginal approach** ♀
EXCLUDES Cystostomy, concomitant (51020-51040, 51101-51102)
🚗 15.2 ⚕ 15.2 **FUD** 090 [J] [G2] [80] [▣]
AMA: 2014,Jan,11

57330 **transvesical and vaginal approach** ♀
EXCLUDES Vesicovaginal fistula closure, abdominal approach (51900)
🚗 21.2 ⚕ 21.2 **FUD** 090 [J] [80] [▣]
AMA: 2014,Jan,11

57335 **Vaginoplasty for intersex state** ♀
🚗 32.3 ⚕ 32.3 **FUD** 090 [T] [80] [▣]
AMA: 2014,Jan,11

57400-57415 Treatment of Vaginal Disorders Under Anesthesia

57400 Dilation of vagina under anesthesia (other than local) ♀
🚑 3.84 ✄ 3.84 **FUD** 000 [T] [A2] [80] ▭
AMA: 2014,Jan,11

57410 Pelvic examination under anesthesia (other than local) ♀
🚑 3.07 ✄ 3.07 **FUD** 000 [T] [A2] ▭
AMA: 2016,Jan,13; 2015,Jan,16; 2014,Jan,11

57415 Removal of impacted vaginal foreign body (separate procedure) under anesthesia (other than local) ♀
EXCLUDES *Removal of impacted vaginal foreign body without anesthesia, report with appropriate E&M code*
🚑 4.55 ✄ 4.55 **FUD** 010 [T] [A2] [80] ▭
AMA: 2014,Jan,11

57420-57426 Endoscopic Vaginal Procedures

57420 Colposcopy of the entire vagina, with cervix if present; ♀
EXCLUDES *Colposcopic procedures and/or examinations:*
Cervix (57452-57461)
Vulva (56820-56821)
Code also endometrial sampling (biopsy) performed at the same time as colposcopy (58110)
Code also modifier 51 for colposcopic procedures of different sites, as appropriate
🚑 2.62 ✄ 3.34 **FUD** 000 [T] [P3] ▭
AMA: 2016,Jan,13; 2015,Jan,16; 2014,Jan,11

57421 with biopsy(s) of vagina/cervix ♀
EXCLUDES *Colposcopic procedures and/or examinations:*
Cervix (57452-57461)
Vulva (56820-56821)
Code also endometrial sampling (biopsy) performed at the same time as colposcopy (58110)
Code also modifier 51 for colposcopic procedures of multiple sites, as appropriate
🚑 3.56 ✄ 4.48 **FUD** 000 [T] [P3] ▭
AMA: 2016,Jan,13; 2015,Jan,16; 2014,Jan,11; 2012,Jan,15-42; 2011,Jan,11

57423 Paravaginal defect repair (including repair of cystocele, if performed), laparoscopic approach ♀
EXCLUDES *Anterior colporrhaphy (57240)*
Anterior vesicourethropexy (51840-51841)
Combined anteroposterior colporrhaphy (57260)
Diagnostic laparoscopy (49320)
Hysterectomy (58152, 58267)
Laparoscopy, surgical; urethral suspension for stress incontinence (51990)
🚑 25.8 ✄ 25.8 **FUD** 090 [J] [80] ▭
AMA: 2016,Jan,13; 2015,Jan,16; 2014,Jan,11

57425 Laparoscopy, surgical, colpopexy (suspension of vaginal apex) ♀
🚑 27.5 ✄ 27.5 **FUD** 090 [J] [80] ▭
AMA: 2014,Jan,11

57426 Revision (including removal) of prosthetic vaginal graft, laparoscopic approach ♀
EXCLUDES *Open abdominal approach (57296)*
Vaginal approach (57295)
🚑 23.9 ✄ 23.9 **FUD** 090 [J] [G2] [80] ▭
AMA: 2014,Jan,11

57452-57461 Endoscopic Cervical Procedures

EXCLUDES *Colposcopic procedures and/or examinations:*
Vagina (57420-57421)
Vulva (56820-56821)
Code also endometrial sampling (biopsy) performed at the same time as colposcopy (58110)

57452 Colposcopy of the cervix including upper/adjacent vagina; ♀
🚑 2.63 ✄ 3.09 **FUD** 000 [T] [P3] ▭
AMA: 2016,Jan,13; 2015,Jan,16; 2014,Jan,11

57454 with biopsy(s) of the cervix and endocervical curettage ♀
INCLUDES Colposcopy of the cervix (57452)
🚑 3.86 ✄ 4.33 **FUD** 000 [T] [P3] ▭
AMA: 2016,Jan,13; 2015,Jan,16; 2014,Jan,11; 2012,Jan,15-42; 2011,Aug,9-10

57455 with biopsy(s) of the cervix ♀
INCLUDES Colposcopy of the cervix (57452)
🚑 3.15 ✄ 4.04 **FUD** 000 [T] [P3] ▭
AMA: 2016,Jan,13; 2015,Jan,16; 2014,Jan,11

57456 with endocervical curettage ♀
INCLUDES Colposcopy of the cervix (57452)
EXCLUDES *Colposcopy of the cervix including upper/adjacent vagina; with loop electrode conization of the cervix (57461)*
🚑 2.93 ✄ 3.81 **FUD** 000 [T] [P3] ▭
AMA: 2016,Jan,13; 2015,Jan,16; 2014,Jan,11; 2012,Jan,15-42; 2011,Jan,11

57460 with loop electrode biopsy(s) of the cervix ♀
INCLUDES Colposcopy of the cervix (57452)
🚑 4.63 ✄ 7.99 **FUD** 000 [T] [P3] ▭
AMA: 2016,Jan,13; 2015,Jan,16; 2014,Jan,11; 2012,Jan,15-42; 2011,Jan,11

57461 with loop electrode conization of the cervix ♀
INCLUDES Colposcopy of the cervix (57452)
EXCLUDES *Colposcopy of the cervix including upper/adjacent vagina; with endocervical curettage (57456)*
🚑 5.34 ✄ 9.03 **FUD** 000 [T] [P3] ▭
AMA: 2016,Jan,13; 2015,Jan,16; 2014,Jan,11; 2012,Jan,15-42; 2011,Jan,11

57500-57556 Cervical Procedures: Multiple Techniques

EXCLUDES *Radical surgical procedures (58200-58240)*

57500 Biopsy of cervix, single or multiple, or local excision of lesion, with or without fulguration (separate procedure) ♀
🚑 2.16 ✄ 3.61 **FUD** 000 [T] [P3] ▭
AMA: 2014,Jan,11

57505 Endocervical curettage (not done as part of a dilation and curettage) ♀
🚑 2.62 ✄ 2.89 **FUD** 010 [T] [P3] ▭
AMA: 2016,Jan,13; 2015,Jan,16; 2014,Jan,11; 2012,Jan,15-42; 2011,Jan,11

57510 Cautery of cervix; electro or thermal ♀
🚑 3.28 ✄ 3.71 **FUD** 010 [T] [P3] ▭
AMA: 2014,Jan,11

57511 cryocautery, initial or repeat ♀
🚑 3.74 ✄ 4.10 **FUD** 010 [T] [P3] ▭
AMA: 2014,Jan,11

57513 laser ablation ♀
🚑 3.81 ✄ 4.11 **FUD** 010 [T] [A2] ▭
AMA: 2014,Jan,11

57520 Conization of cervix, with or without fulguration, with or without dilation and curettage, with or without repair; cold knife or laser ♀
EXCLUDES *Dilation and curettage, diagnostic/therapeutic, nonobstetrical (58120)*
🚑 7.83 ✄ 8.71 **FUD** 090 [T] [A2] ▭
AMA: 2016,Jan,13; 2015,Jan,16; 2014,Jan,11

57522 loop electrode excision ♀
🚑 6.91 ✄ 7.45 **FUD** 090 [T] [A2] ▭
AMA: 2016,Jan,13; 2015,Jan,16; 2014,Jan,11; 2012,Jan,15-42; 2011,Jan,11

57530 Trachelectomy (cervicectomy), amputation of cervix (separate procedure) ♀
🚑 9.87 ✄ 9.87 **FUD** 090 [T] [A2] [80] ▭
AMA: 2014,Jan,11

Genital System

57400 — 57530

57531 Radical trachelectomy, with bilateral total pelvic lymphadenectomy and para-aortic lymph node sampling biopsy, with or without removal of tube(s), with or without removal of ovary(s) ♀

    📅 52.5   ✂ 52.5   **FUD** 090   C 80 🖵

    AMA: 2014,Jan,11

57540 Excision of cervical stump, abdominal approach; ♀

    📅 22.2   ✂ 22.2   **FUD** 090   C 80 🖵

    AMA: 2014,Jan,11

57545 with pelvic floor repair ♀

    📅 24.0   ✂ 24.0   **FUD** 090   C 80 🖵

    AMA: 2014,Jan,11

57550 Excision of cervical stump, vaginal approach; ♀

    📅 11.5   ✂ 11.5   **FUD** 090   T A2 80 🖵

    AMA: 2014,Jan,11

57555 with anterior and/or posterior repair ♀

    📅 16.9   ✂ 16.9   **FUD** 090   J 80 🖵

    AMA: 2014,Jan,11

57556 with repair of enterocele ♀

    EXCLUDES   *Insertion of hemostatic agent/pack for spontaneous/traumatic nonobstetrical vaginal hemorrhage (57180)*

                 Intrauterine device insertion (58300)

    📅 16.0   ✂ 16.0   **FUD** 090   J A2 80 🖵

    AMA: 2014,Jan,11

57558-57800 Cervical Procedures: Dilation, Suturing, or Instrumentation

57558 Dilation and curettage of cervical stump ♀

    EXCLUDES   *Radical surgical procedures (58200-58240)*

    📅 3.21   ✂ 3.52   **FUD** 010   T A2 🖵

    AMA: 2014,Jan,11

57700 Cerclage of uterine cervix, nonobstetrical ♀

    INCLUDES   McDonald cerclage

                 Shirodker operation

    📅 9.02   ✂ 9.02   **FUD** 090   T A2 80 🖵

    AMA: 2014,Jan,11

57720 Trachelorrhaphy, plastic repair of uterine cervix, vaginal approach ♀

    INCLUDES   Emmet operation

    📅 8.69   ✂ 8.69   **FUD** 090   T A2 80 🖵

    AMA: 2014,Jan,11

57800 Dilation of cervical canal, instrumental (separate procedure) ♀

    📅 1.38   ✂ 1.71   **FUD** 000   T P3 🖵

    AMA: 2014,Jan,11

58100-58120 Procedures Involving the Endometrium

58100 Endometrial sampling (biopsy) with or without endocervical sampling (biopsy), without cervical dilation, any method (separate procedure) ♀

    EXCLUDES   *Endocervical curettage only (57505)*

                 Endometrial sampling (biopsy) performed in conjunction with colposcopy (58110)

    📅 2.49   ✂ 3.09   **FUD** 000   T P3 🖵

    AMA: 2014,Jan,11

+ **58110** Endometrial sampling (biopsy) performed in conjunction with colposcopy (List separately in addition to code for primary procedure) ♀

    Code first colposcopy (57420-57421, 57452-57461)

    📅 1.16   ✂ 1.36   **FUD** ZZZ   N N1 80 🖵

    AMA: 2016,Jan,13; 2015,Jan,16; 2014,Jan,11

58120 Dilation and curettage, diagnostic and/or therapeutic (nonobstetrical) ♀

    EXCLUDES   *Postpartum hemorrhage (59160)*

    📅 6.22   ✂ 7.32   **FUD** 010   T A2 🖵

    AMA: 2016,Jan,13; 2015,Jan,16; 2014,Jan,11; 2012,Jan,15-42; 2011,Jan,11

58140-58146 Myomectomy Procedures

58140 Myomectomy, excision of fibroid tumor(s) of uterus, 1 to 4 intramural myoma(s) with total weight of 250 g or less and/or removal of surface myomas; abdominal approach ♀

    📅 26.2   ✂ 26.2   **FUD** 090   C 80 🖵

    AMA: 2016,Jan,13; 2015,Jan,16; 2014,Jan,11; 2012,Jan,15-42; 2011,Jan,11

58145 vaginal approach ♀

    📅 15.5   ✂ 15.5   **FUD** 090   T A2 80 🖵

    AMA: 2014,Jan,11

58146 Myomectomy, excision of fibroid tumor(s) of uterus, 5 or more intramural myomas and/or intramural myomas with total weight greater than 250 g, abdominal approach ♀

    EXCLUDES   *Hysterectomy (58150-58240)*

                 Myomectomy procedures (58140-58145)

    📅 32.5   ✂ 32.5   **FUD** 090   C 80 🖵

    AMA: 2016,Jan,13; 2015,Jan,16; 2014,Jan,11; 2012,Jan,15-42; 2011,Jan,11

58150-58294 Abdominal and Vaginal Hysterectomies

CMS: 100-03,230.3 Sterilization

    EXCLUDES   *Destruction/excision of endometriomas, open method (49203-49205, 58957-58958)*

                 Paracentesis (49082-49084)

                 Pelvic laparotomy (49000)

                 Secondary closure disruption or evisceration of abdominal wall (49900)

58150 Total abdominal hysterectomy (corpus and cervix), with or without removal of tube(s), with or without removal of ovary(s); ♀

    📅 28.8   ✂ 28.8   **FUD** 090   C 80 🖵

    AMA: 2016,Jan,13; 2015,Jan,16; 2014,Jan,11; 2012,Jan,15-42; 2011,Jan,11

58152 with colpo-urethrocystopexy (eg, Marshall-Marchetti-Krantz, Burch) ♀

    EXCLUDES   *Urethrocystopexy without hysterectomy (51840-51841)*

    📅 35.4   ✂ 35.4   **FUD** 090   C 80 🖵

    AMA: 2016,Jan,13; 2015,Jan,16; 2014,Jan,11

58180 Supracervical abdominal hysterectomy (subtotal hysterectomy), with or without removal of tube(s), with or without removal of ovary(s) ♀

    📅 27.3   ✂ 27.3   **FUD** 090   C 80 🖵

    AMA: 2014,Jan,11

58200 Total abdominal hysterectomy, including partial vaginectomy, with para-aortic and pelvic lymph node sampling, with or without removal of tube(s), with or without removal of ovary(s) ♀

    📅 39.2   ✂ 39.2   **FUD** 090   C 80 🖵

    AMA: 2014,Jan,11

58210 Radical abdominal hysterectomy, with bilateral total pelvic lymphadenectomy and para-aortic lymph node sampling (biopsy), with or without removal of tube(s), with or without removal of ovary(s) ♀

    INCLUDES   Wertheim hysterectomy

    EXCLUDES   *Chemotherapy (96401-96549)*

                 Hysterectomy, radical, with transposition of ovary(s) (58825)

    📅 52.9   ✂ 52.9   **FUD** 090   C 80 🖵

    AMA: 2016,Jan,13; 2015,Jan,16; 2014,Jan,11; 2012,May,14-15

58240 Pelvic exenteration for gynecologic malignancy, with total abdominal hysterectomy or cervicectomy, with or without removal of tube(s), with or without removal of ovary(s), with removal of bladder and ureteral transplantations, and/or abdominoperineal resection of rectum and colon and colostomy, or any combination thereof ♀

EXCLUDES Chemotherapy (96401-96549)
Pelvic exenteration for male genital malignancy or lower urinary tract (51597)

83.5 ⚕ 83.5 **FUD** 090 C 80 ▢

AMA: 2014,Jan,11

58260 Vaginal hysterectomy, for uterus 250 g or less; ♀

23.3 ⚕ 23.3 **FUD** 090 J 62 80 ▢

AMA: 2016,Jan,13; 2015,Jan,16; 2014,Jan,11; 2011,May,9

58262 with removal of tube(s), and/or ovary(s) ♀

26.1 ⚕ 26.1 **FUD** 090 J 62 80 ▢

AMA: 2014,Jan,11

58263 with removal of tube(s), and/or ovary(s), with repair of enterocele ♀

28.0 ⚕ 28.0 **FUD** 090 J 80 ▢

AMA: 2014,Jan,11

58267 with colpo-urethrocystopexy (Marshall-Marchetti-Krantz type, Pereyra type) with or without endoscopic control ♀

29.8 ⚕ 29.8 **FUD** 090 C 80 ▢

AMA: 2016,Jan,13; 2015,Jan,16; 2014,Jan,11

58270 with repair of enterocele ♀

EXCLUDES Vaginal hysterectomy with repair of enterocele and removal of tubes and/or ovaries (58263)

24.9 ⚕ 24.9 **FUD** 090 J 80 ▢

AMA: 2014,Jan,11

58275 Vaginal hysterectomy, with total or partial vaginectomy; ♀

27.8 ⚕ 27.8 **FUD** 090 C 80 ▢

AMA: 2014,Jan,11

58280 with repair of enterocele ♀

29.6 ⚕ 29.6 **FUD** 090 C 80 ▢

AMA: 2014,Jan,11

58285 Vaginal hysterectomy, radical (Schauta type operation) ♀

38.0 ⚕ 38.0 **FUD** 090 C 80 ▢

AMA: 2016,Jan,13; 2015,Jan,16; 2014,Jan,11

58290 Vaginal hysterectomy, for uterus greater than 250 g; ♀

32.5 ⚕ 32.5 **FUD** 090 J 80 ▢

AMA: 2014,Jan,11

58291 with removal of tube(s) and/or ovary(s) ♀

35.1 ⚕ 35.1 **FUD** 090 J 80 ▢

AMA: 2014,Jan,11

58292 with removal of tube(s) and/or ovary(s), with repair of enterocele ♀

37.1 ⚕ 37.1 **FUD** 090 J 80 ▢

AMA: 2014,Jan,11

58293 with colpo-urethrocystopexy (Marshall-Marchetti-Krantz type, Pereyra type) with or without endoscopic control ♀

38.5 ⚕ 38.5 **FUD** 090 C 80 ▢

AMA: 2014,Jan,11

58294 with repair of enterocele ♀

34.5 ⚕ 34.5 **FUD** 090 J 80 ▢

AMA: 2014,Jan,11

58300-58323 Contraception and Reproduction Procedures

58300 Insertion of intrauterine device (IUD) ♀

EXCLUDES Insertion and/or removal of implantable contraceptive capsules (11976, 11981-11983)

1.54 ⚕ 2.06 **FUD** XXX E ▢

AMA: 2016,Jan,13; 2015,Jan,16; 2014,Jan,11; 2012,Jan,15-42; 2011,Jan,11

58301 Removal of intrauterine device (IUD) ♀

EXCLUDES Insertion and/or removal of implantable contraceptive capsules (11976, 11981-11983)

1.92 ⚕ 2.68 **FUD** 000 02 P3 80 ▢

AMA: 2016,Jan,13; 2015,Jan,16; 2014,Jan,11; 2012,Jan,15-42; 2011,Jan,11

58321 Artificial insemination; intra-cervical ♀

1.39 ⚕ 2.17 **FUD** 000 T P3 80 ▢

AMA: 2014,Jan,11

58322 intra-uterine ♀

1.66 ⚕ 2.42 **FUD** 000 T P3 80 ▢

AMA: 2014,Jan,11

58323 Sperm washing for artificial insemination ♀

0.34 ⚕ 0.43 **FUD** 000 T P3 80 ▢

AMA: 2014,Jan,11

58340-58350 Fallopian Tube Patency and Brachytherapy Procedures

58340 Catheterization and introduction of saline or contrast material for saline infusion sonohysterography (SIS) or hysterosalpingography ♀

▨ (74740, 76831)

1.66 ⚕ 3.36 **FUD** 000 N N1 ▢

AMA: 2016,Jan,13; 2015,Jan,16; 2014,Jan,11; 2012,Jan,15-42; 2011,Jan,11

58345 Transcervical introduction of fallopian tube catheter for diagnosis and/or re-establishing patency (any method), with or without hysterosalpingography ♀

▨ (74742)

7.71 ⚕ 7.71 **FUD** 010 T R2 80 50 ▢

AMA: 2016,Jan,13; 2015,Jan,16; 2014,Jan,11; 2012,Jan,15-42; 2011,Jan,11

58346 Insertion of Heyman capsules for clinical brachytherapy ♀

EXCLUDES Insertion of radioelement sources or ribbons (77761-77763, 77770-77772)
The placement of needles or catheters into the pelvic organs and/or genitalia (except for the prostate) for interstitial radioelement application (55920)

12.7 ⚕ 12.7 **FUD** 090 T A2 ▢

AMA: 2016,Jan,13; 2015,Jan,16; 2014,Jan,11

58350 Chromotubation of oviduct, including materials ♀

2.22 ⚕ 2.71 **FUD** 010 J A2 50 ▢

AMA: 2016,Jan,13; 2015,Jan,16; 2014,Jan,11; 2012,Jan,15-42; 2011,Jan,11

Mild pressure drives solution into tubes

Uterus

Ovary

Cervix

Delivery apparatus

Saline or medicated solution is injected into uterus

26/TC PC/TC Only	A2-Z3 ASC Payment	50 Bilateral	♂ Male Only	♀ Female Only	Facility RVU	⚕ Non-Facility RVU	▢ CCI
FUD Follow-up Days	**CMS:** IOM (Pub 100)	A-Y OPPSI	80/80 Surg Assist Allowed / w/Doc		▨ Lab Crosswalk	▨ Radiology Crosswalk	✕ CLIA

244

58353-58356 Ablation of Endometrium

EXCLUDES *Destruction/excision of endometriomas, open method (49203-49205)*

58353 **Endometrial ablation, thermal, without hysteroscopic guidance** ♀

EXCLUDES *Endometrial ablation performed hysteroscopically (58563)*

🚗 6.20 ⚕ 28.3 **FUD** 010 J A2 🖵

AMA: 2016,Jan,13; 2015,Jan,16; 2014,Jan,11; 2012,Jan,15-42; 2011,Jan,11

58356 **Endometrial cryoablation with ultrasonic guidance, including endometrial curettage, when performed** ♀

EXCLUDES *Dilation and curettage (58120)*
Endometrial biopsy (58100)
Hysterosalpingography (58340)
Ultrasound (76700, 76856)

🚗 9.80 ⚕ 53.0 **FUD** 010 J P3 80 🖵

AMA: 2014,Jan,11

58400-58540 Uterine Repairs: Vaginal and Abdominal

58400 **Uterine suspension, with or without shortening of round ligaments, with or without shortening of sacrouterine ligaments; (separate procedure)** ♀

INCLUDES Alexander's operation
Baldy-Webster operation
Manchester colporrhaphy

EXCLUDES *Anastomosis of tubes to uterus (58752)*

🚗 12.4 ⚕ 12.4 **FUD** 090 C 80 🖵

AMA: 2014,Jan,11

58410 **with presacral sympathectomy** ♀

INCLUDES Alexander's operation

EXCLUDES *Anastomosis of tubes to uterus (58752)*

🚗 23.2 ⚕ 23.2 **FUD** 090 C 80 🖵

AMA: 2016,Jan,13; 2015,Jan,16; 2014,Jan,11; 2012,Jan,15-42; 2011,Jan,11

58520 **Hysterorrhaphy, repair of ruptured uterus (nonobstetrical)** ♀

🚗 24.2 ⚕ 24.2 **FUD** 090 C 80 🖵

AMA: 2014,Jan,11

58540 **Hysteroplasty, repair of uterine anomaly (Strassman type)** ♀

INCLUDES Strassman type

EXCLUDES *Vesicouterine fistula closure (51920)*

🚗 25.6 ⚕ 25.6 **FUD** 090 C 80 🖵

AMA: 2014,Jan,11

58541-58554 Laparoscopic Procedures of the Uterus

CMS: 100-03,230.3 Sterilization

INCLUDES Diagnostic laparoscopy

EXCLUDES *Hysteroscopy (58555-58565)*

58541 **Laparoscopy, surgical, supracervical hysterectomy, for uterus 250 g or less;** ♀

EXCLUDES *Colpotomy (57000)*
Hysteroscopy (58561)
Laparoscopy (49320, 58545-58546, 58661, 58670-58671)
Myomectomy procedures (58140-58146)
Pelvic examination under anesthesia (57410)
Treatment of nonobstetrical vaginal hemorrhage (57180)

🚗 20.3 ⚕ 20.3 **FUD** 090 J G2 80 🖵

AMA: 2016,Jan,13; 2015,Jan,16; 2014,Jan,11

58542 **with removal of tube(s) and/or ovary(s)** ♀

EXCLUDES *Colpotomy (57000)*
Hysteroscopy (58561)
Laparoscopy (49320, 58545-58546, 58661, 58670-58671)
Myomectomy procedures (58140-58146)
Pelvic examination under anesthesia (57410)
Treatment of nonobstetrical vaginal hemorrhage (57180)

🚗 23.2 ⚕ 23.2 **FUD** 090 J G2 80 🖵

AMA: 2016,Jan,13; 2015,Jan,16; 2014,Jan,11

58543 **Laparoscopy, surgical, supracervical hysterectomy, for uterus greater than 250 g;** ♀

EXCLUDES *Colpotomy (57000)*
Hysteroscopy (58561)
Laparoscopy (49320, 58545-58546, 58661, 58670-58671)
Myomectomy procedures (58140-58146)
Pelvic examination under anesthesia (57410)
Treatment of nonobstetrical vaginal hemorrhage (57180)

🚗 23.4 ⚕ 23.4 **FUD** 090 J G2 80 🖵

AMA: 2016,Jan,13; 2015,Jan,16; 2014,Jan,11

58544 **with removal of tube(s) and/or ovary(s)** ♀

EXCLUDES *Colpotomy (57000)*
Hysteroscopy (58561)
Laparoscopy (49320, 58545-58546, 58661, 58670-58671)
Myomectomy procedures (58140-58146)
Pelvic examination under anesthesia (57410)
Treatment of nonobstetrical vaginal hemorrhage (57180)

🚗 25.6 ⚕ 25.6 **FUD** 090 J G2 80 🖵

AMA: 2016,Jan,13; 2015,Jan,16; 2014,Jan,11

58545 **Laparoscopy, surgical, myomectomy, excision; 1 to 4 intramural myomas with total weight of 250 g or less and/or removal of surface myomas** ♀

🚗 25.6 ⚕ 25.6 **FUD** 090 J A2 80 🖵

AMA: 2014,Jan,11

58546 **5 or more intramural myomas and/or intramural myomas with total weight greater than 250 g** ♀

🚗 31.7 ⚕ 31.7 **FUD** 090 J A2 80 🖵

AMA: 2016,Jan,13; 2015,Jan,16; 2014,Jan,11; 2012,Jan,15-42; 2011,Jan,11

58548 **Laparoscopy, surgical, with radical hysterectomy, with bilateral total pelvic lymphadenectomy and para-aortic lymph node sampling (biopsy), with removal of tube(s) and ovary(s), if performed** ♀

EXCLUDES *Laparoscopy (38570-38572, 58550-58554)*
Radical hysterectomy (58210, 58285)

🚗 54.5 ⚕ 54.5 **FUD** 090 C 80 🖵

AMA: 2016,Jan,13; 2015,Sep,12; 2015,Jan,16; 2014,Jan,11

58550 **Laparoscopy, surgical, with vaginal hysterectomy, for uterus 250 g or less;** ♀

EXCLUDES *Colpotomy (57000)*
Hysteroscopy (58561)
Laparoscopy (49320, 58545-58546, 58661, 58670-58671)
Myomectomy procedures (58140-58146)
Pelvic examination under anesthesia (57410)
Treatment of nonobstetrical vaginal hemorrhage (57180)

🚗 24.9 ⚕ 24.9 **FUD** 090 J A2 80 🖵

AMA: 2016,Jan,13; 2015,Jan,16; 2014,Jan,11

58552 **with removal of tube(s) and/or ovary(s)** ♀

EXCLUDES Colpotomy (57000)
Hysteroscopy (58561)
Laparoscopy (49320, 58545-58546, 58661, 58670-58671)
Myomectomy procedures (58140-58146)
Pelvic examination under anesthesia (57410)
Treatment of nonobstetrical vaginal hemorrhage (57180)

⚙ 28.0 ✂ 28.0 **FUD** 090 J G2 80 ▭

AMA: 2016,Jan,13; 2015,Jan,16; 2014,Jan,11

58553 **Laparoscopy, surgical, with vaginal hysterectomy, for uterus greater than 250 g;** ♀

EXCLUDES Colpotomy (57000)
Hysteroscopy (58561)
Laparoscopy (49320, 58545-58546, 58661, 58670-58671)
Myomectomy procedures (58140-58146)
Pelvic examination under anesthesia (57410)
Treatment of nonobstetrical vaginal hemorrhage (57180)

⚙ 32.2 ✂ 32.2 **FUD** 090 J G2 80 ▭

AMA: 2014,Jan,11

58554 **with removal of tube(s) and/or ovary(s)** ♀

EXCLUDES Colpotomy (57000)
Hysteroscopy (58561)
Laparoscopy (49320, 58545-58546, 58661, 58670-58671)
Myomectomy procedures (58140-58146)
Pelvic examination under anesthesia (57410)
Treatment of nonobstetrical vaginal hemorrhage (57180)

⚙ 37.7 ✂ 37.7 **FUD** 090 J G2 80 ▭

AMA: 2014,Jan,11

58555-58565 Hysteroscopy

INCLUDES Diagnostic hysteroscopy (58555)
EXCLUDES Laparoscopy (58541-58554, 58570-58578)

58555 **Hysteroscopy, diagnostic (separate procedure)** ♀

⚙ 5.37 ✂ 8.80 **FUD** 000 T A2 80 ▭

AMA: 2016,Jan,13; 2015,Jan,16; 2014,Jan,11

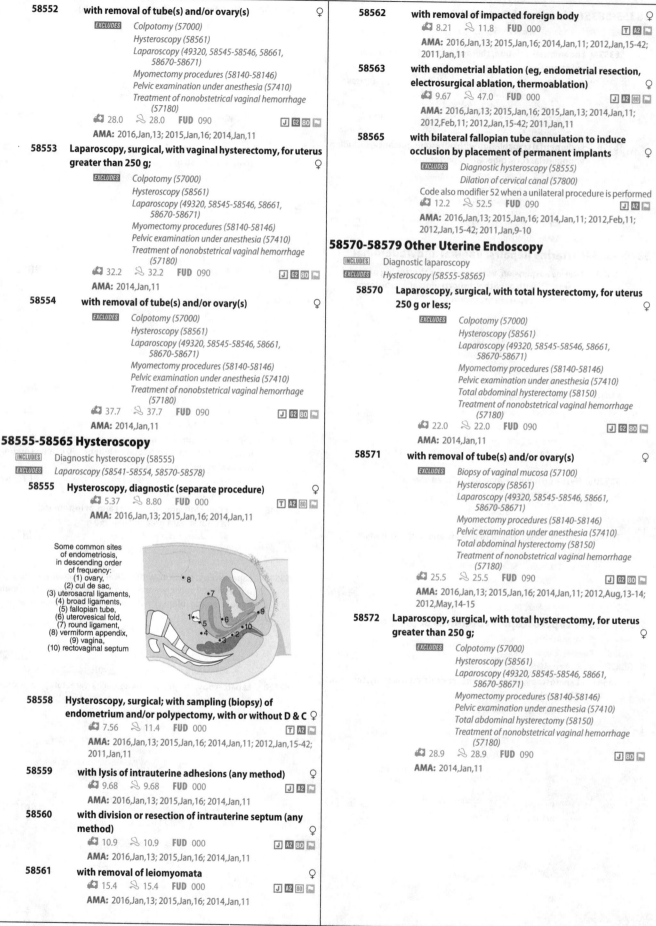

Some common sites of endometriosis, in descending order of frequency:
(1) ovary,
(2) cul de sac,
(3) uterosacral ligaments,
(4) broad ligaments,
(5) fallopian tube,
(6) uterovesical fold,
(7) round ligament,
(8) vermiform appendix,
(9) vagina,
(10) rectovaginal septum

58558 **Hysteroscopy, surgical; with sampling (biopsy) of endometrium and/or polypectomy, with or without D & C** ♀

⚙ 7.56 ✂ 11.4 **FUD** 000 T A2 ▭

AMA: 2016,Jan,13; 2015,Jan,16; 2014,Jan,11; 2012,Jan,15-42; 2011,Jan,11

58559 **with lysis of intrauterine adhesions (any method)** ♀

⚙ 9.68 ✂ 9.68 **FUD** 000 J A2 ▭

AMA: 2016,Jan,13; 2015,Jan,16; 2014,Jan,11

58560 **with division or resection of intrauterine septum (any method)** ♀

⚙ 10.9 ✂ 10.9 **FUD** 000 J A2 80 ▭

AMA: 2016,Jan,13; 2015,Jan,16; 2014,Jan,11

58561 **with removal of leiomyomata** ♀

⚙ 15.4 ✂ 15.4 **FUD** 000 J A2 80 ▭

AMA: 2016,Jan,13; 2015,Jan,16; 2014,Jan,11

58562 **with removal of impacted foreign body** ♀

⚙ 8.21 ✂ 11.8 **FUD** 000 T A2 ▭

AMA: 2016,Jan,13; 2015,Jan,16; 2014,Jan,11; 2012,Jan,15-42; 2011,Jan,11

58563 **with endometrial ablation (eg, endometrial resection, electrosurgical ablation, thermoablation)** ♀

⚙ 9.67 ✂ 47.0 **FUD** 000 J A2 80 ▭

AMA: 2016,Jan,13; 2015,Jan,16; 2015,Jan,13; 2014,Jan,11; 2012,Feb,11; 2012,Jan,15-42; 2011,Jan,11

58565 **with bilateral fallopian tube cannulation to induce occlusion by placement of permanent implants** ♀

EXCLUDES Diagnostic hysteroscopy (58555)
Dilation of cervical canal (57800)
Code also modifier 52 when a unilateral procedure is performed

⚙ 12.2 ✂ 52.5 **FUD** 090 J A2 ▭

AMA: 2016,Jan,13; 2015,Jan,16; 2014,Jan,11; 2012,Feb,11; 2012,Jan,15-42; 2011,Jan,9-10

58570-58579 Other Uterine Endoscopy

INCLUDES Diagnostic laparoscopy
EXCLUDES Hysteroscopy (58555-58565)

58570 **Laparoscopy, surgical, with total hysterectomy, for uterus 250 g or less;** ♀

EXCLUDES Colpotomy (57000)
Hysteroscopy (58561)
Laparoscopy (49320, 58545-58546, 58661, 58670-58671)
Myomectomy procedures (58140-58146)
Pelvic examination under anesthesia (57410)
Total abdominal hysterectomy (58150)
Treatment of nonobstetrical vaginal hemorrhage (57180)

⚙ 22.0 ✂ 22.0 **FUD** 090 J G2 80 ▭

AMA: 2014,Jan,11

58571 **with removal of tube(s) and/or ovary(s)** ♀

EXCLUDES Biopsy of vaginal mucosa (57100)
Hysteroscopy (58561)
Laparoscopy (49320, 58545-58546, 58661, 58670-58671)
Myomectomy procedures (58140-58146)
Pelvic examination under anesthesia (57410)
Total abdominal hysterectomy (58150)
Treatment of nonobstetrical vaginal hemorrhage (57180)

⚙ 25.5 ✂ 25.5 **FUD** 090 J G2 80 ▭

AMA: 2016,Jan,13; 2015,Jan,16; 2014,Jan,11; 2012,Aug,13-14; 2012,May,14-15

58572 **Laparoscopy, surgical, with total hysterectomy, for uterus greater than 250 g;** ♀

EXCLUDES Colpotomy (57000)
Hysteroscopy (58561)
Laparoscopy (49320, 58545-58546, 58661, 58670-58671)
Myomectomy procedures (58140-58146)
Pelvic examination under anesthesia (57410)
Total abdominal hysterectomy (58150)
Treatment of nonobstetrical vaginal hemorrhage (57180)

⚙ 28.9 ✂ 28.9 **FUD** 090 J 80 ▭

AMA: 2014,Jan,11

58573 with removal of tube(s) and/or ovary(s) ♀

EXCLUDES Colpotomy (57000)
Hysteroscopy (58561)
Laparoscopy (49320, 58545-58546, 58661, 58670-58671)
Myomectomy procedures (58140-58146)
Pelvic examination under anesthesia (57410)
Total abdominal hysterectomy (58150)
Treatment of nonobstetrical vaginal hemorrhage (57180)

⏱ 34.6 ⚕ 34.6 **FUD** 090 J G2 80 ▣

AMA: 2016,Jan,13; 2015,Jan,16; 2014,Jan,11; 2012,Aug,13-14; 2012,May,14-15

58578 Unlisted laparoscopy procedure, uterus ♀

⏱ 0.00 ⚕ 0.00 **FUD** YYY J 80 50

AMA: 2016,Jan,13; 2015,Jan,16; 2014,Jan,11; 2012,Jan,15-42; 2011,Jan,11

58579 Unlisted hysteroscopy procedure, uterus ♀

⏱ 0.00 ⚕ 0.00 **FUD** YYY T 80 50

AMA: 2016,Jan,13; 2015,Jan,16; 2014,Jan,11

58600-58615 Sterilization by Tubal Interruption

CMS: 100-03,230.3 Sterilization

EXCLUDES Destruction/excision of endometriomas, open method (49203-49205)

58600 Ligation or transection of fallopian tube(s), abdominal or vaginal approach, unilateral or bilateral ♀

INCLUDES Madlener operation

⏱ 10.2 ⚕ 10.2 **FUD** 090 T G2 80 ▣

AMA: 2016,Jan,13; 2015,Jan,16; 2014,Jan,11

58605 Ligation or transection of fallopian tube(s), abdominal or vaginal approach, postpartum, unilateral or bilateral, during same hospitalization (separate procedure) ♀

EXCLUDES Laparoscopic methods (58670-58671)

⏱ 9.32 ⚕ 9.32 **FUD** 090 C 80 ▣

AMA: 2016,Jan,13; 2015,Jan,16; 2014,Jan,11

+ **58611** Ligation or transection of fallopian tube(s) when done at the time of cesarean delivery or intra-abdominal surgery (not a separate procedure) (List separately in addition to code for primary procedure) ♀

Code first primary procedure

⏱ 2.19 ⚕ 2.19 **FUD** ZZZ C 80 ▣

AMA: 2014,Jan,11

58615 Occlusion of fallopian tube(s) by device (eg, band, clip, Falope ring) vaginal or suprapubic approach ♀

EXCLUDES Laparoscopic method (58671)
Lysis of adnexal adhesions (58740)

⏱ 6.88 ⚕ 6.88 **FUD** 010 T G2 80 ▣

AMA: 2016,Jan,13; 2015,Jan,16; 2014,Jan,11

58660-58679 Endoscopic Procedures Fallopian Tubes and/or Ovaries

CMS: 100-03,230.3 Sterilization

INCLUDES Diagnostic laparoscopy (49320)
Laparoscopy with biopsy of fallopian tube or ovary (49321)
Laparoscopy with ovarian cyst aspiration (49322)

58660 Laparoscopy, surgical; with lysis of adhesions (salpingolysis, ovariolysis) (separate procedure) ♀

⏱ 19.1 ⚕ 19.1 **FUD** 090 J A2 80 ▣

AMA: 2016,Jan,13; 2015,Jan,16; 2014,Jan,11; 2012,Jan,15-42; 2011,Dec,14-18; 2011,Jan,11

58661 with removal of adnexal structures (partial or total oophorectomy and/or salpingectomy) ♀

⏱ 18.4 ⚕ 18.4 **FUD** 010 J A2 80 50 ▣

AMA: 2016,Jan,13; 2015,Jan,16; 2014,Jan,11; 2012,Jan,15-42; 2011,Jan,11

58662 with fulguration or excision of lesions of the ovary, pelvic viscera, or peritoneal surface by any method ♀

⏱ 20.1 ⚕ 20.1 **FUD** 090 J A2 80 ▣

AMA: 2016,Jan,13; 2015,Jan,16; 2014,Jan,11

58670 with fulguration of oviducts (with or without transection) ♀

⏱ 10.3 ⚕ 10.3 **FUD** 090 J A2 ▣

AMA: 2016,Jan,13; 2015,Jan,16; 2014,Jan,11

58671 with occlusion of oviducts by device (eg, band, clip, or Falope ring) ♀

⏱ 10.3 ⚕ 10.3 **FUD** 090 J A2 ▣

AMA: 2016,Jan,13; 2015,Jan,16; 2014,Jan,11

58672 with fimbrioplasty ♀

⏱ 20.7 ⚕ 20.7 **FUD** 090 J A2 80 50 ▣

AMA: 2016,Jan,13; 2015,Jan,16; 2014,Jan,11

58673 with salpingostomy (salpingoneostomy) ♀

⏱ 22.5 ⚕ 22.5 **FUD** 090 J A2 80 50 ▣

AMA: 2016,Jan,13; 2015,Jan,16; 2014,Jan,11; 2012,Jan,15-42; 2011,Jan,11

● **58674** Laparoscopy, surgical, ablation of uterine fibroid(s) including intraoperative ultrasound guidance and monitoring, radiofrequency

EXCLUDES Hysterectomy (58541-58554, 58570-58573)
Ultrasonic guidance (76998)

58679 Unlisted laparoscopy procedure, oviduct, ovary ♀

⏱ 0.00 ⚕ 0.00 **FUD** YYY J 80 50

AMA: 2016,Jan,13; 2015,Jan,16; 2014,Jan,11

58700-58770 Open Procedures Fallopian Tubes, with/without Ovaries

EXCLUDES Destruction/excision of endometriomas, open method (49203-49205, 58957-58958)

58700 Salpingectomy, complete or partial, unilateral or bilateral (separate procedure) ♀

⏱ 22.2 ⚕ 22.2 **FUD** 090 C 80 ▣

AMA: 2014,Jan,11

58720 Salpingo-oophorectomy, complete or partial, unilateral or bilateral (separate procedure) ♀

⏱ 20.9 ⚕ 20.9 **FUD** 090 C 80 ▣

AMA: 2016,Jan,13; 2015,Jan,16; 2014,Jan,11; 2012,Jan,15-42; 2011,Jan,11

58740 Lysis of adhesions (salpingolysis, ovariolysis) ♀

EXCLUDES Excision/fulguration of lesions performed laparoscopically (58662)
Laparoscopic method (58660)

⏱ 25.1 ⚕ 25.1 **FUD** 090 C 80 ▣

AMA: 2016,Jan,13; 2015,Jan,16; 2014,Jan,11

58750 Tubotubal anastomosis ♀

⏱ 27.7 ⚕ 27.7 **FUD** 090 C 80 50 ▣

AMA: 2014,Jan,11

Occluded section of tube is excised

Ovary

Tube ends are sutured

58752 Tubouterine implantation ♀

⏱ 26.3 ⚕ 26.3 **FUD** 090 C 80 50 ▣

AMA: 2014,Jan,11

58760 **Fimbrioplasty** ♀

EXCLUDES *Laparoscopic method (58672)*

🏥 23.3   ✋ 23.3   **FUD** 090

C 80 50 ▭

AMA: 2016,Jan,13; 2015,Jan,16; 2014,Jan,11

58770 **Salpingostomy (salpingoneostomy)** ♀

EXCLUDES *Laparoscopic method (58673)*

🏥 26.3   ✋ 26.3   **FUD** 090

T 80 50 ▭

AMA: 2016,Jan,13; 2015,Jan,16; 2014,Jan,11

58800-58925 Open Procedures: Ovary

CMS: 100-03,230.3 Sterilization

EXCLUDES *Destruction/excision of endometriomas, open method (49203-49205, 58957-58958)*

58800 **Drainage of ovarian cyst(s), unilateral or bilateral (separate procedure); vaginal approach** ♀

🏥 8.43   ✋ 8.97   **FUD** 090

T A2 ▭

AMA: 2014,Jan,11; 2013,Nov,9

58805 **abdominal approach** ♀

🏥 11.4   ✋ 11.4   **FUD** 090

T 62 80 ▭

AMA: 2014,Jan,11; 2013,Nov,9

58820 **Drainage of ovarian abscess; vaginal approach, open** ♀

EXCLUDES *Transrectal fluid drainage using catheter, image guided (49407)*

🏥 8.82   ✋ 8.82   **FUD** 090

T A2 80 50 ▭

AMA: 2014,Jan,11; 2013,Nov,9

58822 **abdominal approach** ♀

EXCLUDES *Transrectal fluid drainage using catheter, image guided (49407)*

🏥 21.4   ✋ 21.4   **FUD** 090

C 80 50 ▭

AMA: 2014,Jan,11; 2013,Nov,9

58825 **Transposition, ovary(s)** ♀

🏥 19.7   ✋ 19.7   **FUD** 090

C 80 ▭

AMA: 2014,Jan,11

58900 **Biopsy of ovary, unilateral or bilateral (separate procedure)** ♀

EXCLUDES *Laparoscopy with biopsy of fallopian tube or ovary (49321)*

🏥 13.0   ✋ 13.0   **FUD** 090

T A2 80 ▭

AMA: 2016,Jan,13; 2015,Jan,16; 2014,Jan,11

58920 **Wedge resection or bisection of ovary, unilateral or bilateral** ♀

🏥 21.8   ✋ 21.8   **FUD** 090

J 80 ▭

AMA: 2014,Jan,11

58925 **Ovarian cystectomy, unilateral or bilateral** ♀

🏥 21.2   ✋ 21.2   **FUD** 090

J 80 ▭

AMA: 2014,Jan,11

58940-58960 Removal Ovary(s) with/without Multiple Procedures for Malignancy

CMS: 100-03,230.3 Sterilization

EXCLUDES *Chemotherapy (96401-96549)*
Destruction/excision of tumors, cysts, or endometriomas, open method (49203-49205)

58940 **Oophorectomy, partial or total, unilateral or bilateral;** ♀

EXCLUDES *Oophorectomy with tumor debulking for ovarian malignancy (58952)*

🏥 15.0   ✋ 15.0   **FUD** 090

C 80 ▭

AMA: 2016,Jan,13; 2015,Jan,16; 2014,Jan,11

58943 **for ovarian, tubal or primary peritoneal malignancy, with para-aortic and pelvic lymph node biopsies, peritoneal washings, peritoneal biopsies, diaphragmatic assessments, with or without salpingectomy(s), with or without omentectomy** ♀

🏥 33.7   ✋ 33.7   **FUD** 090

C 80 ▭

AMA: 2014,Jan,11; 2011,Jan,11

58950 **Resection (initial) of ovarian, tubal or primary peritoneal malignancy with bilateral salpingo-oophorectomy and omentectomy;** ♀

EXCLUDES *Resection/tumor debulking of recurrent ovarian/tubal/primary peritoneal/uterine malignancy (58957-58958)*

🏥 32.3   ✋ 32.3   **FUD** 090

C 80 ▭

AMA: 2014,Jan,11; 2011,Jan,11

58951 **with total abdominal hysterectomy, pelvic and limited para-aortic lymphadenectomy** ♀

EXCLUDES *Resection/tumor debulking of recurrent ovarian/tubal/primary peritoneal/uterine malignancy (58957-58958)*

🏥 41.6   ✋ 41.6   **FUD** 090

C 80 ▭

AMA: 2016,Jan,13; 2015,Jan,16; 2014,Jan,11; 2012,Jan,15-42; 2011,Jan,11

58952 **with radical dissection for debulking (ie, radical excision or destruction, intra-abdominal or retroperitoneal tumors)** ♀

EXCLUDES *Resection/tumor debulking of recurrent ovarian/tubal/primary peritoneal/uterine malignancy (58957-58958)*

🏥 47.1   ✋ 47.1   **FUD** 090

C 80 ▭

AMA: 2016,Jan,13; 2015,Jan,16; 2014,Jan,11; 2012,Jan,15-42; 2011,Jan,11

58953 **Bilateral salpingo-oophorectomy with omentectomy, total abdominal hysterectomy and radical dissection for debulking;** ♀

🏥 58.3   ✋ 58.3   **FUD** 090

C 80 ▭

AMA: 2016,Jan,13; 2015,Jan,16; 2014,May,10; 2014,Jan,11; 2011,Jan,11

58954 **with pelvic lymphadenectomy and limited para-aortic lymphadenectomy** ♀

🏥 63.4   ✋ 63.4   **FUD** 090

C 80 ▭

AMA: 2016,Jan,13; 2015,Jan,16; 2014,Jan,11; 2011,Jan,11

58956 **Bilateral salpingo-oophorectomy with total omentectomy, total abdominal hysterectomy for malignancy** ♀

EXCLUDES *Biopsy of ovary (58900)*
Hysterectomy (58150, 58262-58263)
Laparoscopy (58550, 58661)
Omentectomy (49255)
Oophorectomy (58940)
Ovarian cystectomy (58925)
Resection of malignancy (58957-58958)
Salpingectomy salpingo-oophorectomy, (58700, 58720)

🏥 39.5   ✋ 39.5   **FUD** 090

C 80 ▭

AMA: 2016,Jan,13; 2015,Jan,16; 2014,May,10; 2014,Jan,11

58957 **Resection (tumor debulking) of recurrent ovarian, tubal, primary peritoneal, uterine malignancy (intra-abdominal, retroperitoneal tumors), with omentectomy, if performed;** ♀

EXCLUDES *Biopsy of ovary (58900-58960)*
Destruction, excision cysts, endometriomas, or tumors (49203-49215)
Enterolysis (44005)
Exploratory laparotomy (49000)
Lymphadenectomy (38770, 38780)
Omentectomy (49255)

🏥 45.5   ✋ 45.5   **FUD** 090

C 80 ▭

AMA: 2014,Jan,11

58958 with pelvic lymphadenectomy and limited para-aortic lymphadenectomy ♀

EXCLUDES *Biopsy of ovary (58900-58960)*
Destruction, excision cysts, endometriomas, or tumors (49203-49215)
Enterolysis (44005)
Exploratory laparotomy (49000)
Lymphadenectomy (38770, 38780)
Omentectomy (49255)

🔧 50.0 ⚕ 50.0 **FUD** 090 C 80 💻

AMA: 2014,Jan,11

58960 Laparotomy, for staging or restaging of ovarian, tubal, or primary peritoneal malignancy (second look), with or without omentectomy, peritoneal washing, biopsy of abdominal and pelvic peritoneum, diaphragmatic assessment with pelvic and limited para-aortic lymphadenectomy ♀

EXCLUDES *Resection of malignancy (58957-58958)*

🔧 27.9 ⚕ 27.9 **FUD** 090 C 80 💻

AMA: 2014,Jan,11

58970-58999 Procedural Components: In Vitro Fertilization

58970 Follicle puncture for oocyte retrieval, any method M ♀

📟 (76948)

🔧 5.68 ⚕ 6.30 **FUD** 000 T A2 80 💻

AMA: 2014,Jan,11

58974 Embryo transfer, intrauterine M ♀

🔧 0.00 ⚕ 0.00 **FUD** 000 T A2 80 💻

AMA: 2014,Jan,11

58976 Gamete, zygote, or embryo intrafallopian transfer, any method M ♀

EXCLUDES *Adnexal procedures performed laparoscopically (58660-58673)*

🔧 6.22 ⚕ 7.19 **FUD** 000 T A2 80 💻

AMA: 2016,Jan,13; 2015,Jan,16; 2014,Jan,11

58999 Unlisted procedure, female genital system (nonobstetrical) ♀

🔧 0.00 ⚕ 0.00 **FUD** YYY T

AMA: 2016,Jan,13; 2015,Jan,16; 2014,Jan,11; 2012,Jan,15-42; 2011,Jan,11

59000-59001 Aspiration of Amniotic Fluid

EXCLUDES *Intrauterine fetal transfusion (36460)*
Unlisted fetal invasive procedure (59897)

59000 Amniocentesis; diagnostic M ♀

📟 (76946)

🔧 2.34 ⚕ 3.60 **FUD** 000 T P3 💻

AMA: 2016,Jan,13; 2015,Jan,16; 2014,Jan,11

59001 therapeutic amniotic fluid reduction (includes ultrasound guidance) M ♀

🔧 5.21 ⚕ 5.21 **FUD** 000 T R2 💻

AMA: 2016,Jan,13; 2015,Jan,16; 2014,Jan,11

59012-59076 Fetal Testing and Treatment

EXCLUDES *Intrauterine fetal transfusion (36460)*
Unlisted fetal invasive procedures (59897)

59012 Cordocentesis (intrauterine), any method M ♀

📟 (76941)

🔧 5.88 ⚕ 5.88 **FUD** 000 T 62 80 💻

AMA: 2014,Jan,11

59015 Chorionic villus sampling, any method M ♀

📟 (76945)

🔧 3.82 ⚕ 4.48 **FUD** 000 T P3 80 💻

AMA: 2016,Jan,13; 2015,Jan,16; 2014,Jan,11

59020 Fetal contraction stress test M ♀

🔧 2.03 ⚕ 2.03 **FUD** 000 T P3 80 💻

AMA: 2016,Jan,13; 2015,Jan,16; 2014,Jan,11

59025 Fetal non-stress test M ♀

🔧 1.38 ⚕ 1.38 **FUD** 000 T P3 80 💻

AMA: 2016,Jan,13; 2015,Jan,16; 2014,Jan,11; 2012,Jan,15-42; 2011,Jan,11

59030 Fetal scalp blood sampling M ♀

Code also modifier 76 or 77, as appropriate, for repeat fetal scalp blood sampling

🔧 2.90 ⚕ 2.90 **FUD** 000 T 80 💻

AMA: 2014,Jan,11

59050 Fetal monitoring during labor by consulting physician (ie, non-attending physician) with written report; supervision and interpretation M ♀

🔧 1.47 ⚕ 1.47 **FUD** XXX M 80 💻

AMA: 2014,Jan,11

59051 interpretation only M ♀

🔧 1.22 ⚕ 1.22 **FUD** XXX B 80 💻

AMA: 2014,Jan,11

59070 Transabdominal amnioinfusion, including ultrasound guidance M ♀

🔧 8.74 ⚕ 11.4 **FUD** 000 T 62 80 💻

AMA: 2016,Jan,13; 2015,Jan,16; 2014,Jan,11; 2012,Jan,15-42; 2011,Jan,11

59072 Fetal umbilical cord occlusion, including ultrasound guidance M ♀

🔧 13.5 ⚕ 13.5 **FUD** 000 T 62 💻

AMA: 2016,Jan,13; 2015,Jan,16; 2014,Jan,11; 2012,Jan,15-42; 2011,Jan,11

59074 Fetal fluid drainage (eg, vesicocentesis, thoracocentesis, paracentesis), including ultrasound guidance M ♀

🔧 8.66 ⚕ 10.9 **FUD** 000 T 62 80 💻

AMA: 2016,Jan,13; 2015,Jan,16; 2014,Jan,11; 2012,Jan,15-42; 2011,Jan,11

59076 Fetal shunt placement, including ultrasound guidance M ♀

🔧 13.5 ⚕ 13.5 **FUD** 000 T 62 80 💻

AMA: 2016,Jan,13; 2015,Jan,16; 2014,Jan,11; 2012,Jan,15-42; 2011,Jan,11

59100-59151 Tubal Pregnancy/Hysterotomy Procedures

CMS: 100-03,230.3 Sterilization

59100 Hysterotomy, abdominal (eg, for hydatidiform mole, abortion) M ♀

Code also ligation of fallopian tubes when performed at the same time as hysterotomy (58611)

🔧 22.8 ⚕ 22.8 **FUD** 090 T R2 80 💻

AMA: 2014,Jan,11

59120 Surgical treatment of ectopic pregnancy; tubal or ovarian, requiring salpingectomy and/or oophorectomy, abdominal or vaginal approach M ♀

🔧 22.9 ⚕ 22.9 **FUD** 090 C 80 💻

AMA: 2014,Jan,11

59121 tubal or ovarian, without salpingectomy and/or oophorectomy M ♀

🔧 22.9 ⚕ 22.9 **FUD** 090 C 80 💻

AMA: 2014,Jan,11

59130 abdominal pregnancy M ♀

🔧 26.8 ⚕ 26.8 **FUD** 090 C 80 💻

AMA: 2014,Jan,11

59135 interstitial, uterine pregnancy requiring total hysterectomy M ♀

🔧 23.8 ⚕ 23.8 **FUD** 090 C 80 💻

AMA: 2014,Jan,11

59136 interstitial, uterine pregnancy with partial resection of uterus M ♀

🔧 24.4 ⚕ 24.4 **FUD** 090 C 80 💻

AMA: 2014,Jan,11

59140 **cervical, with evacuation** Ⓜ ♀
🔪 11.5 ⚕ 11.5 **FUD** 090 Ⓒ 80 ▢
AMA: 2014,Jan,11

59150 **Laparoscopic treatment of ectopic pregnancy; without salpingectomy and/or oophorectomy** Ⓜ ♀
🔪 22.2 ⚕ 22.2 **FUD** 090 Ⓙ 62 80 ▢
AMA: 2016,Jan,13; 2015,Jan,16; 2014,Jan,11

59151 **with salpingectomy and/or oophorectomy** Ⓜ ♀
🔪 21.5 ⚕ 21.5 **FUD** 090 Ⓙ 62 80 ▢
AMA: 2014,Jan,11

[Anatomical illustration showing: Abdominal pregnancy, Site of interstitial pregnancy, Ectopic pregnancy in tube, Ovarian pregnancy, Cervix and cervical canal, Uterus, Ectopic pregnancy in cervix, Broad ligament (mesometric)]

59160-59200 Procedures of Uterus Prior To/After Delivery

59160 **Curettage, postpartum** Ⓜ ♀
🔪 5.00 ⚕ 5.86 **FUD** 010 Ⓣ A2 80 ▢
AMA: 2016,Jan,13; 2015,Jan,16; 2014,Jan,11; 2012,Jan,15-42; 2011,Jan,11

59200 **Insertion of cervical dilator (eg, laminaria, prostaglandin) (separate procedure)** Ⓜ ♀
EXCLUDES *Fetal transfusion, intrauterine (36460)*
Hypertonic solution/prostaglandin introduction for labor initiation (59850-59857)
🔪 1.29 ⚕ 2.05 **FUD** 000 Ⓣ P3 ▢
AMA: 2016,Jan,13; 2015,Jan,16; 2014,Jan,11

59300-59350 Postpartum Vaginal/Cervical/Uterine Repairs

EXCLUDES *Nonpregnancy-related cerclage (57700)*

59300 **Episiotomy or vaginal repair, by other than attending** Ⓜ ♀
🔪 4.30 ⚕ 5.55 **FUD** 000 Ⓣ P3 80 ▢
AMA: 2014,Jan,11

59320 **Cerclage of cervix, during pregnancy; vaginal** Ⓜ ♀
🔪 4.41 ⚕ 4.41 **FUD** 000 Ⓣ A2 80 ▢
AMA: 2016,Jan,13; 2015,Jan,16; 2014,Jan,11; 2012,Jan,15-42; 2011,Jan,11

59325 **abdominal** Ⓜ ♀
🔪 7.03 ⚕ 7.03 **FUD** 000 Ⓒ 80 ▢
AMA: 2016,Jan,13; 2015,Jan,16; 2014,Jan,11; 2012,Jan,15-42; 2011,Jan,11

59350 **Hysterorrhaphy of ruptured uterus** Ⓜ ♀
🔪 7.67 ⚕ 7.67 **FUD** 000 Ⓒ 80 ▢
AMA: 2014,Jan,11

59400-59410 Vaginal Delivery: Comprehensive and Component Services

CMS: 100-02,15,180 Nurse-Midwife (CNM) Services; 100-02,15,20.1 Physician Expense for Surgery, Childbirth, and Treatment for Infertility

INCLUDES Care provided for an uncomplicated pregnancy including delivery as well as antepartum and postpartum care:
Admission history
Admission to hospital
Artificial rupture of membranes
Management of uncomplicated labor
Physical exam
Vaginal delivery with or without episiotomy or forceps

EXCLUDES *Medical complications of pregnancy, labor, and delivery:*
Cardiac problems
Diabetes
Hyperemesis
Hypertension
Neurological problems
Premature rupture of membranes
Pre-term labor
Toxemia
Trauma
Newborn circumcision (54150, 54160)
Services incidental to or unrelated to the pregnancy

59400 **Routine obstetric care including antepartum care, vaginal delivery (with or without episiotomy, and/or forceps) and postpartum care** Ⓜ ♀
INCLUDES Fetal heart tones
Hospital/office visits following cesarean section or vaginal delivery
Initial/subsequent history
Physical exams
Recording of weight/blood pressures
Routine chemical urinalysis
Routine prenatal visits:
Each month up to 28 weeks gestation
Every other week from 29 to 36 weeks gestation
Weekly from 36 weeks until delivery
🔪 60.1 ⚕ 60.1 **FUD** MMM Ⓑ ▢
AMA: 2016,Jan,13; 2015,Jan,16; 2014,Jan,11; 2012,Jan,15-42; 2011,Jan,11

[Illustration showing breech presentation (left) and Simpson forceps delivery of aftercoming head (right); Vacuum extractor attached to posterior fontanelle to flex head downward (below left)]

59409 **Vaginal delivery only (with or without episiotomy and/or forceps);** Ⓜ ♀
EXCLUDES *Inpatient management after delivery/discharge services (99217-99239 [99224, 99225, 99226])*
🔪 23.5 ⚕ 23.5 **FUD** MMM Ⓣ 80 ▢
AMA: 2016,Jan,13; 2015,Jan,16; 2014,Jan,11; 2012,Jan,15-42; 2011,Jan,11

59410 **including postpartum care** Ⓜ ♀
INCLUDES Hospital/office visits following cesarean section or vaginal delivery
🔪 30.0 ⚕ 30.0 **FUD** MMM Ⓑ ▢
AMA: 2014,Jan,11

59412-59414 Other Maternity Services

CMS: 100-02,15,180 Nurse-Midwife (CNM) Services; 100-02,15,20.1 Physician Expense for Surgery, Childbirth, and Treatment for Infertility

59412 External cephalic version, with or without tocolysis [M] ♀

Code also delivery code(s)
🗐 3.00 ✂ 3.00 **FUD** MMM [T][G2][80][▦]

AMA: 2014,Jan,11

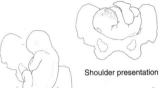
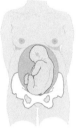
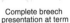

Complete breech presentation at term

"Footling"

Shoulder presentation

Brow presentation

59414 Delivery of placenta (separate procedure) [M] ♀

🗐 2.66 ✂ 2.66 **FUD** MMM [T][G2][80][▦]

AMA: 2016,Jan,13; 2015,Jan,16; 2014,Jan,11; 2012,Jan,15-42; 2011,Jan,11

59425-59430 Prenatal and Postpartum Visits

CMS: 100-02,15,180 Nurse-Midwife (CNM) Services; 100-02,15,20.1 Physician Expense for Surgery, Childbirth, and Treatment for Infertility

INCLUDES Physician/other qualified health care professional providing all or a portion of antepartum/postpartum care, but no delivery due to:
Referral to another physician for delivery
Termination of pregnancy by abortion

EXCLUDES *Antepartum care, 1-3 visits, report with appropriate evaluation and management service code*
Medical complications of pregnancy, labor, and delivery:
Cardiac problems
Diabetes
Hyperemesis
Hypertension
Neurological problems
Premature rupture of membranes
Pre-term labor
Toxemia
Trauma
Newborn circumcision (54150, 54160)
Services incidental to or unrelated to the pregnancy

59425 Antepartum care only; 4-6 visits [M] ♀

INCLUDES Fetal heart tones
Initial/subsequent history
Physical exams
Recording of weight/blood pressures
Routine chemical urinalysis
Routine prenatal visits:
Each month up to 28 weeks gestation
Every other week from 29 to 36 weeks gestation
Weekly from 36 weeks until delivery

🗐 10.2 ✂ 13.0 **FUD** MMM [B][80][▦]

AMA: 2016,Jan,13; 2015,Jan,16; 2014,Jan,11; 2012,Jan,15-42; 2011,Jan,11

59426 7 or more visits [M] ♀

INCLUDES Biweekly visits to 36 weeks gestation
Fetal heart tones
Initial/subsequent history
Monthly visits up to 28 weeks gestation
Physical exams
Recording of weight/blood pressures
Routine chemical urinalysis
Weekly visits until delivery

🗐 18.1 ✂ 23.3 **FUD** MMM [B][80][▦]

AMA: 2016,Jan,13; 2015,Jan,16; 2014,Jan,11; 2012,Jan,15-42; 2011,Jan,11

59430 Postpartum care only (separate procedure) [M] ♀

INCLUDES Office/other outpatient visits following cesarean section or vaginal delivery

🗐 4.02 ✂ 5.29 **FUD** MMM [B][▦]

AMA: 2016,Jan,13; 2015,Jan,16; 2014,Jan,11; 2012,Jan,15-42; 2011,Jan,11

59510-59525 Cesarean Section Delivery: Comprehensive and Components of Care

CMS: 100-02,15,20.1 Physician Expense for Surgery, Childbirth, and Treatment for Infertility

INCLUDES Classic cesarean section
Low cervical cesarean section

EXCLUDES *Infant standby attendance (99360)*
Medical complications of pregnancy, labor, and delivery:
Cardiac problems
Diabetes
Hyperemesis
Hypertension
Neurological problems
Premature rupture of membranes
Pre-term labor
Toxemia
Trauma
Newborn circumcision (54150, 54160)
Services incidental to or unrelated to the pregnancy
Vaginal delivery after prior cesarean section (59610-59614)

59510 Routine obstetric care including antepartum care, cesarean delivery, and postpartum care [M] ♀

INCLUDES Admission history
Admission to hospital
Cesarean delivery
Fetal heart tones
Hospital/office visits following cesarean section
Initial/subsequent history
Management of uncomplicated labor
Physical exam
Recording of weight/blood pressures
Routine chemical urinalysis
Routine prenatal visits:
Each month up to 28 weeks gestation
Every other week 29 to 36 weeks gestation
Weekly from 36 weeks until delivery

EXCLUDES *Medical problems complicating labor and delivery*

🗐 66.7 ✂ 66.7 **FUD** MMM [B][▦]

AMA: 2016,Jan,13; 2015,Jan,16; 2014,Jan,11; 2013,Mar,13; 2012,Jan,15-42; 2011,Jan,11

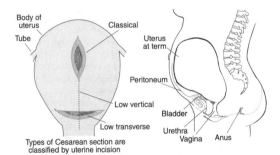

Body of uterus
Tube
Classical
Uterus at term
Peritoneum
Low vertical
Bladder
Low transverse
Urethra
Vagina
Anus
Types of Cesarean section are classified by uterine incision

59514 Cesarean delivery only; [M] ♀

INCLUDES Admission history
Admission to hospital
Cesarean delivery
Management of uncomplicated labor
Physical exam

EXCLUDES *Inpatient management after delivery/discharge services (99217-99239 [99224, 99225, 99226])*
Medical problems complicating labor and delivery

🗐 26.5 ✂ 26.5 **FUD** MMM [C][80][▦]

AMA: 2016,Jan,13; 2015,Jan,16; 2014,Jan,11; 2013,Mar,13; 2012,Jan,15-42; 2011,Jan,11

Genital System

59515 — 59830

59515 including postpartum care   M ♀

    INCLUDES Admission history
Admission to hospital
Cesarean delivery
Hospital/office visits following cesarean section or
      vaginal delivery
Management of uncomplicated labor
Physical exam

    EXCLUDES *Medical problems complicating labor and delivery*

    ⏱ 36.5   ✂ 36.5   **FUD** MMM   B ▯

    AMA: 2016,Jan,13; 2015,Jan,16; 2014,Jan,11; 2013,Mar,13

+ 59525 **Subtotal or total hysterectomy after cesarean delivery (List separately in addition to code for primary procedure)** M ♀

    Code first cesarean delivery (59510, 59514, 59515, 59618, 59620, 59622)

    ⏱ 13.9   ✂ 13.9   **FUD** ZZZ   C 80 ▯

    AMA: 2014,Jan,11

59610-59614 Vaginal Delivery After Prior Cesarean Section: Comprehensive and Components of Care

CMS: 100-02,15,180 Nurse-Midwife (CNM) Services; 100-02,15,20.1 Physician Expense for Surgery, Childbirth, and Treatment for Infertility

    INCLUDES Admission history
Admission to hospital
Management of uncomplicated labor
Patients with previous cesarean delivery who present with the expectation
      of a vaginal delivery
Physical exam
Successful vaginal delivery after previous cesarean delivery (VBAC)
Vaginal delivery with or without episiotomy or forceps

    EXCLUDES *Elective cesarean delivery (59510, 59514, 59515)*
Medical complications of pregnancy, labor, and delivery:
    Cardiac problems
    Diabetes
    Hyperemesis
    Hypertension
    Neurological problems
    Premature rupture of membranes
    Pre-term labor
    Toxemia
    Trauma
Newborn circumcision (54150, 54160)
Services incidental to or unrelated to the pregnancy

59610 **Routine obstetric care including antepartum care, vaginal delivery (with or without episiotomy, and/or forceps) and postpartum care, after previous cesarean delivery** M ♀

    INCLUDES Fetal heart tones
Hospital/office visits following cesarean section or
      vaginal delivery
Initial/subsequent history
Physical exams
Recording of weight/blood pressures
Routine chemical urinalysis
Routine prenatal visits:
    Each month up to 28 weeks gestation
    Every other week 29 to 36 weeks gestation
    Weekly from 36 weeks until delivery

    ⏱ 63.3   ✂ 63.3   **FUD** MMM   B 80 ▯

    AMA: 2016,Jan,13; 2015,Jan,16; 2014,Jan,11

59612 **Vaginal delivery only, after previous cesarean delivery (with or without episiotomy and/or forceps);** M ♀

    EXCLUDES *Inpatient management after delivery/discharge services (99217-99239 [99224, 99225, 99226])*

    ⏱ 26.5   ✂ 26.5   **FUD** MMM   T 80 ▯

    AMA: 2016,Jan,13; 2015,Jan,16; 2014,Jan,11

59614 including postpartum care   M ♀

    INCLUDES Hospital/office visits following cesarean section or
      vaginal delivery

    ⏱ 33.0   ✂ 33.0   **FUD** MMM   B 80 ▯

    AMA: 2016,Jan,13; 2015,Jan,16; 2014,Jan,11

59618-59622 Cesarean Section After Attempted Vaginal Birth/Prior C-Section

CMS: 100-02,15,20.1 Physician Expense for Surgery, Childbirth, and Treatment for Infertility

    INCLUDES Admission history
Admission to hospital
Cesarean delivery
Cesarean delivery following an unsuccessful vaginal delivery attempt after
      previous cesarean delivery
Management of uncomplicated labor
Patients with previous cesarean delivery who present with the expectation
      of a vaginal delivery
Physical exam

    EXCLUDES *Elective cesarean delivery (59510, 59514, 59515)*
Medical complications of pregnancy, labor, and delivery:
    Cardiac problems
    Diabetes
    Hyperemesis
    Hypertension
    Neurological problems
    Premature rupture of membranes
    Pre-term labor
    Toxemia
    Trauma
Newborn circumcision (54150, 54160)
Services incidental to or unrelated to the pregnancy

59618 **Routine obstetric care including antepartum care, cesarean delivery, and postpartum care, following attempted vaginal delivery after previous cesarean delivery** M ♀

    INCLUDES Fetal heart tones
Hospital/office visits following cesarean section or
      vaginal delivery
Initial/subsequent history
Physical exams
Recording of weight/blood pressures
Routine chemical urinalysis
Routine prenatal visits:
    Each month up to 28 weeks gestation
    Every two weeks 29 to 36 weeks gestation
    Weekly from 36 weeks until delivery

    ⏱ 67.7   ✂ 67.7   **FUD** MMM   B 80 ▯

    AMA: 2016,Jan,13; 2015,Jan,16; 2014,Jan,11

59620 **Cesarean delivery only, following attempted vaginal delivery after previous cesarean delivery;** M ♀

    EXCLUDES *Inpatient management after delivery/discharge services (99217-99239 [99224, 99225, 99226])*

    ⏱ 27.2   ✂ 27.2   **FUD** MMM   C 80 ▯

    AMA: 2016,Jan,13; 2015,Jan,16; 2014,Jan,11

59622 including postpartum care   M ♀

    INCLUDES Hospital/office visits following cesarean section or
      vaginal delivery

    ⏱ 37.5   ✂ 37.5   **FUD** MMM   B 80 ▯

    AMA: 2016,Jan,13; 2015,Jan,16; 2014,Jan,11

59812-59830 Treatment of Miscarriage

CMS: 100-02,15,20.1 Physician Expense for Surgery, Childbirth, and Treatment for Infertility

    EXCLUDES *Medical treatment of spontaneous complete abortion, any trimester (99201-99233 [99224, 99225, 99226])*

59812 **Treatment of incomplete abortion, any trimester, completed surgically** M ♀

    INCLUDES Surgical treatment of spontaneous abortion

    ⏱ 8.52   ✂ 9.15   **FUD** 090   T A2 ▯

    AMA: 2016,Jan,13; 2015,Jan,16; 2014,Jan,11

59820 **Treatment of missed abortion, completed surgically; first trimester** M ♀

    ⏱ 10.2   ✂ 10.8   **FUD** 090   T A2 ▯

    AMA: 2016,Jan,13; 2015,Jan,16; 2014,Jan,11

59821 second trimester   M ♀

    ⏱ 10.2   ✂ 10.9   **FUD** 090   T A2 80 ▯

    AMA: 2016,Jan,13; 2015,Jan,16; 2014,Jan,11

59830 **Treatment of septic abortion, completed surgically** M ♀

    ⏱ 12.5   ✂ 12.5   **FUD** 090   C 80 ▯

    AMA: 2016,Jan,13; 2015,Jan,16; 2014,Jan,11

59840-59866 Elective Abortions

CMS: 100-02,1,90 Termination of Pregnancy; 100-02,15,20.1 Physician Expense for Surgery, Childbirth, and Treatment for Infertility; 100-03,140.1 Abortion; 100-04,3,100.1 Billing for Abortion Services

59840 **Induced abortion, by dilation and curettage** M ♀
6.00 ≈ 6.25 **FUD** 010 T A2 80 ▭
AMA: 2016,Jan,13; 2015,Jan,16; 2014,Jan,11; 2012,Jan,15-42; 2011,Jan,11

59841 **Induced abortion, by dilation and evacuation** M ♀
10.4 ≈ 11.0 **FUD** 010 T A2 80 ▭
AMA: 2016,Jan,13; 2015,Jan,16; 2014,Jan,11

59850 **Induced abortion, by 1 or more intra-amniotic injections (amniocentesis-injections), including hospital admission and visits, delivery of fetus and secundines;** M ♀
EXCLUDES *Cervical dilator insertion (59200)*
10.0 ≈ 10.0 **FUD** 090 C 80 ▭
AMA: 2016,Jan,13; 2015,Jan,16; 2014,Jan,11

59851 **with dilation and curettage and/or evacuation** M ♀
EXCLUDES *Cervical dilator insertion (59200)*
10.6 ≈ 10.6 **FUD** 090 C 80 ▭
AMA: 2016,Jan,13; 2015,Jan,16; 2014,Jan,11

59852 **with hysterotomy (failed intra-amniotic injection)** M ♀
EXCLUDES *Cervical dilator insertion (59200)*
14.4 ≈ 14.4 **FUD** 090 C 80 ▭
AMA: 2016,Jan,13; 2015,Jan,16; 2014,Jan,11

59855 **Induced abortion, by 1 or more vaginal suppositories (eg, prostaglandin) with or without cervical dilation (eg, laminaria), including hospital admission and visits, delivery of fetus and secundines;** M ♀
11.9 ≈ 11.9 **FUD** 090 C 80 ▭
AMA: 2014,Jan,11

59856 **with dilation and curettage and/or evacuation** M ♀
14.0 ≈ 14.0 **FUD** 090 C 80 ▭
AMA: 2014,Jan,11

59857 **with hysterotomy (failed medical evacuation)** M ♀
14.8 ≈ 14.8 **FUD** 090 C 80 ▭
AMA: 2014,Jan,11

59866 **Multifetal pregnancy reduction(s) (MPR)** M ♀
6.23 ≈ 6.23 **FUD** 000 T 92 80 ▭
AMA: 2014,Jan,11

59870-59899 Miscellaneous Obstetrical Procedures

CMS: 100-02,15,20.1 Physician Expense for Surgery, Childbirth, and Treatment for Infertility

59870 **Uterine evacuation and curettage for hydatidiform mole** M ♀
13.6 ≈ 13.6 **FUD** 090 T A2 80 ▭
AMA: 2016,Jan,13; 2015,Jan,16; 2014,Jan,11; 2012,Jan,15-42; 2011,Jan,11

59871 **Removal of cerclage suture under anesthesia (other than local)** M ♀
3.86 ≈ 3.86 **FUD** 000 92 A2 80 ▭
AMA: 2016,Jan,13; 2015,Jan,16; 2014,Jan,11

59897 **Unlisted fetal invasive procedure, including ultrasound guidance, when performed** ♀
0.00 ≈ 0.00 **FUD** YYY T ▭
AMA: 2014,Jan,11

59898 **Unlisted laparoscopy procedure, maternity care and delivery** M ♀
0.00 ≈ 0.00 **FUD** YYY J 80 50
AMA: 2016,Jan,13; 2015,Jan,16; 2014,Jan,11

59899 **Unlisted procedure, maternity care and delivery** M ♀
0.00 ≈ 0.00 **FUD** YYY T 80
AMA: 2016,Jan,13; 2015,Jan,16; 2014,Jan,11; 2013,Oct,3; 2012,Jan,15-42; 2011,Jan,11

60000 I&D of Infected Thyroglossal Cyst

60000 Incision and drainage of thyroglossal duct cyst, infected

📷 4.42   🔪 4.91   **FUD** 010   T A2 80 ▣

AMA: 2014,Jan,11

60100 Core Needle Biopsy: Thyroid

EXCLUDES Fine needle aspiration (10021-10022)

60100 Biopsy thyroid, percutaneous core needle

🔲 (76942, 77002, 77012, 77021)

🔲 (88172-88173)

📷 2.28   🔪 3.22   **FUD** 000   T P3 ▣

AMA: 2016,Jan,13; 2015,Jan,16; 2014,Jan,11; 2012,Jan,15-42; 2011,Jan,11

60200 Surgical Removal Thyroid Cyst or Mass; Division of Isthmus

60200 Excision of cyst or adenoma of thyroid, or transection of isthmus

📷 19.0   🔪 19.0   **FUD** 090   J A2 80 ▣

AMA: 2016,Jan,13; 2015,Jan,16; 2014,Jan,11; 2012,Dec,3-5; 2011,Aug,9-10

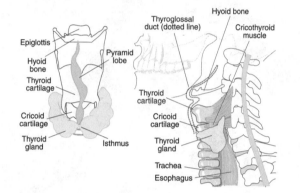

60210-60225 Subtotal Thyroidectomy

60210 Partial thyroid lobectomy, unilateral; with or without isthmusectomy

📷 20.4   🔪 20.4   **FUD** 090   J G2 80 ▣

AMA: 2016,Jan,13; 2015,Jan,16; 2014,Jan,11; 2012,Dec,3-5; 2012,Jan,15-42; 2011,Aug,9-10

60212 with contralateral subtotal lobectomy, including isthmusectomy

📷 29.1   🔪 29.1   **FUD** 090   J G2 80 ▣

AMA: 2016,Jan,13; 2015,Jan,16; 2014,Jan,11; 2012,Dec,3-5

60220 Total thyroid lobectomy, unilateral; with or without isthmusectomy

📷 20.4   🔪 20.4   **FUD** 090   J G2 80 ▣

AMA: 2016,Jan,13; 2015,Jan,16; 2014,Jan,11; 2012,Dec,3-5; 2012,Jan,15-42; 2011,Aug,9-10; 2011,Jan,11

60225 with contralateral subtotal lobectomy, including isthmusectomy

📷 26.9   🔪 26.9   **FUD** 090   J G2 80 ▣

AMA: 2016,Jan,13; 2015,Jan,16; 2014,Jan,11; 2012,Dec,3-5

60240-60271 Complete Thyroidectomy Procedures

60240 Thyroidectomy, total or complete

EXCLUDES Subtotal or partial thyroidectomy (60271)

📷 26.6   🔪 26.6   **FUD** 090   J G2 80 ▣

AMA: 2016,Jan,13; 2015,Jan,16; 2014,Jan,11; 2012,Dec,3-5

60252 Thyroidectomy, total or subtotal for malignancy; with limited neck dissection

📷 38.2   🔪 38.2   **FUD** 090   J 80 ▣

AMA: 2016,Jan,13; 2015,Jan,16; 2014,Jan,11; 2012,Dec,3-5; 2012,Jan,15-42; 2011,Jan,11

60254 with radical neck dissection

📷 48.4   🔪 48.4   **FUD** 090   C 80 ▣

AMA: 2016,Jan,13; 2015,Jan,16; 2014,Jan,11; 2012,Dec,3-5; 2012,Jan,15-42; 2011,Jan,11

60260 Thyroidectomy, removal of all remaining thyroid tissue following previous removal of a portion of thyroid

📷 31.6   🔪 31.6   **FUD** 090   J 80 50 ▣

AMA: 2016,Jan,13; 2015,Jan,16; 2014,Jan,11; 2012,Dec,3-5; 2012,Jan,15-42; 2011,Jan,11

60270 Thyroidectomy, including substernal thyroid; sternal split or transthoracic approach

📷 39.5   🔪 39.5   **FUD** 090   C 80 ▣

AMA: 2016,Jan,13; 2015,Jan,16; 2014,Jan,11; 2012,Dec,3-5

60271 cervical approach

📷 30.6   🔪 30.6   **FUD** 090   J 80 ▣

AMA: 2016,Jan,13; 2015,Jan,16; 2014,Jan,11; 2012,Dec,3-5

60280-60300 Treatment of Cyst/Sinus of Thyroid

60280 Excision of thyroglossal duct cyst or sinus;

EXCLUDES Thyroid ultrasound (76536)

📷 12.8   🔪 12.8   **FUD** 090   J A2 80 ▣

AMA: 2014,Jan,11

60281 recurrent

EXCLUDES Thyroid ultrasound (76536)

📷 16.9   🔪 16.9   **FUD** 090   J A2 80 ▣

AMA: 2014,Jan,11

60300 Aspiration and/or injection, thyroid cyst

EXCLUDES Fine needle aspiration (10021-10022)

🔲 (76942, 77012)

📷 1.44   🔪 3.38   **FUD** 000   T P3 ▣

AMA: 2014,Jan,11

60500-60512 Parathyroid Procedures

60500 Parathyroidectomy or exploration of parathyroid(s);

📷 27.9   🔪 27.9   **FUD** 090   J G2 80 ▣

AMA: 2016,Jan,13; 2015,Jan,16; 2014,Jan,11; 2012,Dec,3-5

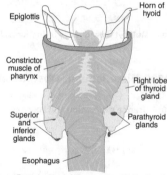

Posterior view of pharynx, thyroid glands, and parathyroid glands

60502 re-exploration

📷 37.2   🔪 37.2   **FUD** 090   J 80 ▣

AMA: 2016,Jan,13; 2015,Jan,16; 2014,Jan,11; 2012,Dec,3-5

60505 with mediastinal exploration, sternal split or transthoracic approach

📷 40.0   🔪 40.0   **FUD** 090   C 80 ▣

AMA: 2016,Jan,13; 2015,Jan,16; 2014,Jan,11; 2012,Dec,3-5

+ **60512** Parathyroid autotransplantation (List separately in addition to code for primary procedure)

Code first (60212, 60225, 60240, 60252, 60254, 60260, 60270-60271, 60500, 60502, 60505)

📷 7.07   🔪 7.07   **FUD** ZZZ   N 80 ▣

AMA: 2016,Jan,13; 2015,Jan,16; 2014,Jan,11; 2012,Dec,3-5; 2012,Jan,15-42; 2011,Aug,9-10

26/TC PC/TC Only   A2-Z3 ASC Payment   50 Bilateral   ♂ Male Only   ♀ Female Only   📷 Facility RVU   🔪 Non-Facility RVU   ▣ CCI

FUD Follow-up Days   **CMS:** IOM (Pub 100)   A-Y OPPSI   80/80 Surg Assist Allowed / w/Doc   🔲 Lab Crosswalk   🔲 Radiology Crosswalk   ✖ CLIA

254   CPT © 2016 American Medical Association. All Rights Reserved.   © 2016 Optum360, LLC

60520-60522 Thymus Procedures

EXCLUDES Surgical thoracoscopy (video-assisted thoracic surgery (VATS) thymectomy (32673)

60520 Thymectomy, partial or total; transcervical approach (separate procedure)
30.2   30.2   **FUD** 090   J 80
AMA: 2014,Jan,11; 2012,Oct,9-11; 2012,Sep,3-8

60521 sternal split or transthoracic approach, without radical mediastinal dissection (separate procedure)
32.5   32.5   **FUD** 090   C 80
AMA: 2016,Jan,13; 2015,Jan,16; 2014,Jan,11; 2012,Oct,9-11; 2012,Sep,3-8; 2012,Jan,15-42; 2011,Jan,11

60522 sternal split or transthoracic approach, with radical mediastinal dissection (separate procedure)
39.4   39.4   **FUD** 090   C 80
AMA: 2014,Jan,11; 2012,Oct,9-11; 2012,Sep,3-8

60540-60545 Adrenal Gland Procedures

EXCLUDES Laparoscopic approach (60650)
Removal of remote or disseminated pheochromocytoma (49203-49205)
Standard backbench preparation of cadaver donor (50323)

60540 Adrenalectomy, partial or complete, or exploration of adrenal gland with or without biopsy, transabdominal, lumbar or dorsal (separate procedure);
30.6   30.6   **FUD** 090   C 80 50
AMA: 2014,Jan,11

60545 with excision of adjacent retroperitoneal tumor
35.1   35.1   **FUD** 090   C 80 50
AMA: 2014,Jan,11

60600-60605 Carotid Body Procedures

60600 Excision of carotid body tumor; without excision of carotid artery
40.4   40.4   **FUD** 090   C 80
AMA: 2014,Jan,11

60605 with excision of carotid artery
50.0   50.0   **FUD** 090   C 80
AMA: 2016,Sep,8; 2016,Jul,10; 2014,Jan,11

60650-60699 Laparoscopic and Unlisted Procedures

INCLUDES Diagnostic laparoscopy (49320)

60650 Laparoscopy, surgical, with adrenalectomy, partial or complete, or exploration of adrenal gland with or without biopsy, transabdominal, lumbar or dorsal
EXCLUDES Peritoneoscopy performed as separate procedure (49320)
34.5   34.5   **FUD** 090   C 80 50
AMA: 2016,Jan,13; 2015,Jan,16; 2014,Jan,11

60659 Unlisted laparoscopy procedure, endocrine system
0.00   0.00   **FUD** YYY   J 80 50
AMA: 2016,Jan,13; 2015,Jan,16; 2014,Jan,11

60699 Unlisted procedure, endocrine system
0.00   0.00   **FUD** YYY   J 80
AMA: 2016,Jan,13; 2015,Jan,16; 2014,Jan,11; 2012,Jan,15-42; 2011,Jan,11

61000-61253 Transcranial Access via Puncture, Burr Hole, Twist Hole, or Trephine

EXCLUDES Injection for:
Cerebral angiography (36100-36218)

61000 Subdural tap through fontanelle, or suture, infant, unilateral or bilateral; initial ⒶA

EXCLUDES Injection for:
Pneumoencephalography (61055)
Ventriculography (61026, 61120)

🔧 3.37   ⚕ 3.37   **FUD** 000   T R2 ▢

AMA: 2014,Jan,11

Overhead view of newborn skull

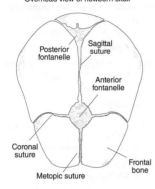

Posterior fontanelle
Sagittal suture
Anterior fontanelle
Coronal suture
Frontal bone
Metopic suture

An initial tap through to the subdural
level is performed on an infant via a
fontanelle or suture, either unilateral
or bilateral.

61001 subsequent taps ⒶA

🔧 2.45   ⚕ 2.45   **FUD** 000   T R2 ▢

AMA: 2014,Jan,11

61020 Ventricular puncture through previous burr hole, fontanelle, suture, or implanted ventricular catheter/reservoir; without injection

🔧 2.94   ⚕ 2.94   **FUD** 000   T A2 ▢

AMA: 2014,Jan,11

61026 with injection of medication or other substance for diagnosis or treatment

INCLUDES Injection for ventriculography

🔧 2.98   ⚕ 2.98   **FUD** 000   T A2 ▢

AMA: 2014,Jan,11

61050 Cisternal or lateral cervical (C1-C2) puncture; without injection (separate procedure)

🔧 2.47   ⚕ 2.47   **FUD** 000   T A2 80 ▢

AMA: 2014,Jan,11

61055 with injection of medication or other substance for diagnosis or treatment

INCLUDES Injection for pneumoencephalography

EXCLUDES Myelography via lumbar injection (62302-62305)
Radiology procedures except when furnished by a different provider

🔧 3.49   ⚕ 3.49   **FUD** 000   T A2 ▢

AMA: 2014,Sep,3; 2014,Jan,11

61070 Puncture of shunt tubing or reservoir for aspiration or injection procedure

🔀 (75809)

🔧 1.67   ⚕ 1.67   **FUD** 000   T A2 ▢

AMA: 2016,Jan,13; 2015,Jan,16; 2014,Jan,11; 2012,Jan,15-42; 2011,Jan,11

61105 Twist drill hole for subdural or ventricular puncture

🔧 13.3   ⚕ 13.3   **FUD** 090   C 80 ▢

AMA: 2014,Jan,11

61107 Twist drill hole(s) for subdural, intracerebral, or ventricular puncture; for implanting ventricular catheter, pressure recording device, or other intracerebral monitoring device

Code also intracranial neuroendoscopic ventricular catheter insertion or reinsertion, when performed (62160)

🔧 9.32   ⚕ 9.32   **FUD** 000   ⊘ C ▢

AMA: 2014,Jan,11

61108 for evacuation and/or drainage of subdural hematoma

🔧 26.5   ⚕ 26.5   **FUD** 090   C ▢

AMA: 2014,Jan,11

61120 Burr hole(s) for ventricular puncture (including injection of gas, contrast media, dye, or radioactive material)

INCLUDES Includes: Injection for ventriculography

🔧 21.8   ⚕ 21.8   **FUD** 090   C 80 ▢

AMA: 2014,Jan,11

61140 Burr hole(s) or trephine; with biopsy of brain or intracranial lesion

🔧 37.1   ⚕ 37.1   **FUD** 090   C 80 ▢

AMA: 2014,Jan,11

61150 with drainage of brain abscess or cyst

🔧 39.3   ⚕ 39.3   **FUD** 090   C ▢

AMA: 2014,Jan,11

61151 with subsequent tapping (aspiration) of intracranial abscess or cyst

🔧 29.3   ⚕ 29.3   **FUD** 090   C ▢

AMA: 2014,Jan,11

61154 Burr hole(s) with evacuation and/or drainage of hematoma, extradural or subdural

🔧 37.2   ⚕ 37.2   **FUD** 090   C 80 50 ▢

AMA: 2014,Jan,11

61156 Burr hole(s); with aspiration of hematoma or cyst, intracerebral

🔧 36.5   ⚕ 36.5   **FUD** 090   C 80 ▢

AMA: 2014,Jan,11

61210 for implanting ventricular catheter, reservoir, EEG electrode(s), pressure recording device, or other cerebral monitoring device (separate procedure)

Code also intracranial neuroendoscopic ventricular catheter insertion or reinsertion, when performed (62160)

🔧 10.9   ⚕ 10.9   **FUD** 000   C ▢

AMA: 2016,Jan,13; 2015,Jan,16; 2014,Jan,11; 2012,Jan,15-42; 2011,Jan,11

61215 Insertion of subcutaneous reservoir, pump or continuous infusion system for connection to ventricular catheter

EXCLUDES Chemotherapy (96450)
Refilling and maintenance of implantable infusion pump (95990)

🔧 14.8   ⚕ 14.8   **FUD** 090   T A2 ▢

AMA: 2016,Jan,13; 2015,Jan,16; 2014,Jan,11

61250 Burr hole(s) or trephine, supratentorial, exploratory, not followed by other surgery

EXCLUDES Burr hole or trephine followed by craniotomy at same operative session (61304-61321)

🔧 23.6   ⚕ 23.6   **FUD** 090   C 80 50 ▢

AMA: 2014,Jan,11

61253 Burr hole(s) or trephine, infratentorial, unilateral or bilateral

EXCLUDES Burr hole or trephine followed by craniotomy at same operative session (61304-61321)

🔧 23.6   ⚕ 23.6   **FUD** 090   C 80 ▢

AMA: 2016,Jan,13; 2015,Jan,16; 2014,Jan,11; 2012,Jan,15-42; 2011,Jan,11

Nervous System

61304 — 61458

61304-61323 Craniectomy/Craniotomy: By Indication/Specific Area of Brain

EXCLUDES Injection for:
Cerebral angiography (36100-36218)
Pneumoencephalography (61055)
Ventriculography (61026, 61120)

61304 Craniectomy or craniotomy, exploratory; supratentorial

EXCLUDES *Other craniectomy/craniotomy procedures when performed at the same anatomical site and during the same surgical encounter*

🚑 48.3 ⚕ 48.3 **FUD** 090 C 80 ▢

AMA: 2014,Jan,11

61305 infratentorial (posterior fossa)

EXCLUDES *Other craniectomy/craniotomy procedures when performed at the same anatomical site and during the same surgical encounter*

🚑 58.9 ⚕ 58.9 **FUD** 090 C 80 ▢

AMA: 2014,Jan,11

61312 Craniectomy or craniotomy for evacuation of hematoma, supratentorial; extradural or subdural

🚑 61.2 ⚕ 61.2 **FUD** 090 C 80 ▢

AMA: 2016,Jan,13; 2015,Jan,16; 2014,Jan,11

61313 intracerebral

🚑 58.3 ⚕ 58.3 **FUD** 090 C 80 ▢

AMA: 2014,Jan,11

61314 Craniectomy or craniotomy for evacuation of hematoma, infratentorial; extradural or subdural

🚑 53.5 ⚕ 53.5 **FUD** 090 C 80 ▢

AMA: 2014,Jan,11

61315 intracerebellar

🚑 60.8 ⚕ 60.8 **FUD** 090 C 80 ▢

AMA: 2014,Jan,11

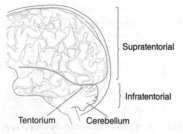

Supratentorial

Infratentorial

Tentorium   Cerebellum

The tentorium is a dural
septum that separates the cerebellum from
the occipital lobes

+ 61316 Incision and subcutaneous placement of cranial bone graft (List separately in addition to code for primary procedure)

Code first (61304, 61312-61313, 61322-61323, 61340, 61570-61571, 61680-61705)

🚑 2.60 ⚕ 2.60 **FUD** ZZZ C ▢

AMA: 2014,Jan,11

61320 Craniectomy or craniotomy, drainage of intracranial abscess; supratentorial

🚑 55.9 ⚕ 55.9 **FUD** 090 C 80 ▢

AMA: 2014,Jan,11

61321 infratentorial

🚑 61.7 ⚕ 61.7 **FUD** 090 C 80 ▢

AMA: 2014,Jan,11

61322 Craniectomy or craniotomy, decompressive, with or without duraplasty, for treatment of intracranial hypertension, without evacuation of associated intraparenchymal hematoma; without lobectomy

EXCLUDES *Craniectomy or craniotomy for evacuation of hematoma (61313)*
Subtemporal decompression (61340)

🚑 69.9 ⚕ 69.9 **FUD** 090 C 80 ▢

AMA: 2014,Jan,11

61323 with lobectomy

EXCLUDES *Craniectomy or craniotomy for evacuation of hematoma (61313)*
Subtemporal decompression (61340)

🚑 70.8 ⚕ 70.8 **FUD** 090 C ▢

AMA: 2014,Jan,11

61330-61530 Craniectomy/Craniotomy/Decompression Brain By Surgical Approach/Specific Area of Brain

EXCLUDES Injection for:
Cerebral angiography (36100-36218)
Pneumoencephalography (61055)
Ventriculography (61026, 61120)

61330 Decompression of orbit only, transcranial approach

INCLUDES Naffziger operation

🚑 46.7 ⚕ 46.7 **FUD** 090 J 62 80 50 ▢

AMA: 2014,Jan,11

61332 Exploration of orbit (transcranial approach); with biopsy

🚑 51.3 ⚕ 51.3 **FUD** 090 C 80 50 ▢

AMA: 2014,Jan,11

61333 with removal of lesion

🚑 53.0 ⚕ 53.0 **FUD** 090 C 80 50 ▢

AMA: 2014,Jan,11

61340 Subtemporal cranial decompression (pseudotumor cerebri, slit ventricle syndrome)

EXCLUDES *Decompression craniotomy or craniectomy for intracranial hypertension, without hematoma removal (61322-61323)*

🚑 41.8 ⚕ 41.8 **FUD** 090 C 80 50 ▢

AMA: 2014,Jan,11

61343 Craniectomy, suboccipital with cervical laminectomy for decompression of medulla and spinal cord, with or without dural graft (eg, Arnold-Chiari malformation)

🚑 64.5 ⚕ 64.5 **FUD** 090 C 80 ▢

AMA: 2014,Jan,11

61345 Other cranial decompression, posterior fossa

EXCLUDES *Kroenlein procedure (67445)*
Orbital decompression using a lateral wall approach (67445)

🚑 59.8 ⚕ 59.8 **FUD** 090 C 80 ▢

AMA: 2014,Jan,11

61450 Craniectomy, subtemporal, for section, compression, or decompression of sensory root of gasserian ganglion

INCLUDES Frazier-Spiller procedure
Hartley-Krause
Krause decompression
Taarnhoj procedure

🚑 56.5 ⚕ 56.5 **FUD** 090 C 80 ▢

AMA: 2014,Jan,11

61458 Craniectomy, suboccipital; for exploration or decompression of cranial nerves

INCLUDES Jannetta decompression

🚑 59.0 ⚕ 59.0 **FUD** 090 C 80 ▢

AMA: 2014,Jan,11

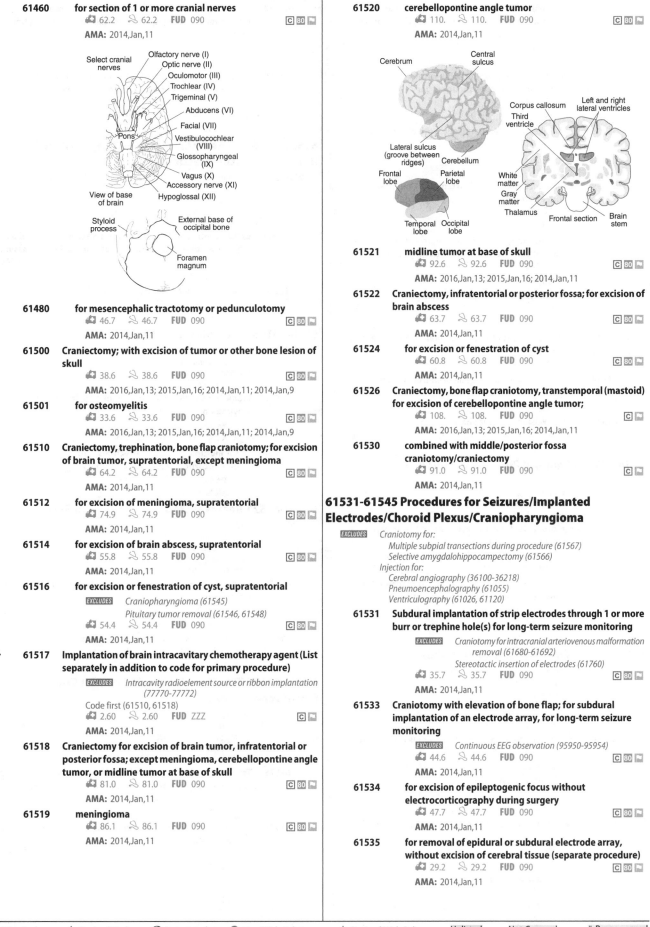

61460   for section of 1 or more cranial nerves
    62.2 62.2 **FUD** 090   C 80
    AMA: 2014,Jan,11

Select cranial nerves
Olfactory nerve (I)
Optic nerve (II)
Oculomotor (III)
Trochlear (IV)
Trigeminal (V)
Abducens (VI)
Facial (VII)
Pons
Vestibulocochlear (VIII)
Glossopharyngeal (IX)
Vagus (X)
Accessory nerve (XI)
View of base of brain
Hypoglossal (XII)

Styloid process
External base of occipital bone
Foramen magnum

61480   for mesencephalic tractotomy or pedunculotomy
    46.7 46.7 **FUD** 090   C 80
    AMA: 2014,Jan,11

61500   Craniectomy; with excision of tumor or other bone lesion of skull
    38.6 38.6 **FUD** 090   C 80
    AMA: 2016,Jan,13; 2015,Jan,16; 2014,Jan,11; 2014,Jan,9

61501   for osteomyelitis
    33.6 33.6 **FUD** 090   C 80
    AMA: 2016,Jan,13; 2015,Jan,16; 2014,Jan,11; 2014,Jan,9

61510   Craniectomy, trephination, bone flap craniotomy; for excision of brain tumor, supratentorial, except meningioma
    64.2 64.2 **FUD** 090   C 80
    AMA: 2014,Jan,11

61512   for excision of meningioma, supratentorial
    74.9 74.9 **FUD** 090   C 80
    AMA: 2014,Jan,11

61514   for excision of brain abscess, supratentorial
    55.8 55.8 **FUD** 090   C 80
    AMA: 2014,Jan,11

61516   for excision or fenestration of cyst, supratentorial
    EXCLUDES *Craniopharyngioma (61545)*
    Pituitary tumor removal (61546, 61548)
    54.4 54.4 **FUD** 090   C 80
    AMA: 2014,Jan,11

\+ **61517   Implantation of brain intracavitary chemotherapy agent (List separately in addition to code for primary procedure)**
    EXCLUDES *Intracavity radioelement source or ribbon implantation (77770-77772)*
    Code first (61510, 61518)
    2.60 2.60 **FUD** ZZZ   C
    AMA: 2014,Jan,11

61518   Craniectomy for excision of brain tumor, infratentorial or posterior fossa; except meningioma, cerebellopontine angle tumor, or midline tumor at base of skull
    81.0 81.0 **FUD** 090   C 80
    AMA: 2014,Jan,11

61519   meningioma
    86.1 86.1 **FUD** 090   C 80
    AMA: 2014,Jan,11

61520   cerebellopontine angle tumor
    110. 110. **FUD** 090   C 80
    AMA: 2014,Jan,11

Cerebrum
Central sulcus
Corpus callosum
Left and right lateral ventricles
Third ventricle
Lateral sulcus (groove between ridges)
Cerebellum
Frontal lobe
Parietal lobe
White matter
Gray matter
Thalamus
Frontal section
Brain stem
Temporal lobe
Occipital lobe

61521   midline tumor at base of skull
    92.6 92.6 **FUD** 090   C 80
    AMA: 2016,Jan,13; 2015,Jan,16; 2014,Jan,11

61522   Craniectomy, infratentorial or posterior fossa; for excision of brain abscess
    63.7 63.7 **FUD** 090   C 80
    AMA: 2014,Jan,11

61524   for excision or fenestration of cyst
    60.8 60.8 **FUD** 090   C 80
    AMA: 2014,Jan,11

61526   Craniectomy, bone flap craniotomy, transtemporal (mastoid) for excision of cerebellopontine angle tumor;
    108. 108. **FUD** 090   C
    AMA: 2016,Jan,13; 2015,Jan,16; 2014,Jan,11

61530   combined with middle/posterior fossa craniotomy/craniectomy
    91.0 91.0 **FUD** 090   C
    AMA: 2014,Jan,11

61531-61545 Procedures for Seizures/Implanted Electrodes/Choroid Plexus/Craniopharyngioma

EXCLUDES *Craniotomy for:*
    Multiple subpial transections during procedure (61567)
    Selective amygdalohippocampectomy (61566)
    Injection for:
    Cerebral angiography (36100-36218)
    Pneumoencephalography (61055)
    Ventriculography (61026, 61120)

61531   Subdural implantation of strip electrodes through 1 or more burr or trephine hole(s) for long-term seizure monitoring
    EXCLUDES *Craniotomy for intracranial arteriovenous malformation removal (61680-61692)*
    Stereotactic insertion of electrodes (61760)
    35.7 35.7 **FUD** 090   C 80
    AMA: 2014,Jan,11

61533   Craniotomy with elevation of bone flap; for subdural implantation of an electrode array, for long-term seizure monitoring
    EXCLUDES *Continuous EEG observation (95950-95954)*
    44.6 44.6 **FUD** 090   C 80
    AMA: 2014,Jan,11

61534   for excision of epileptogenic focus without electrocorticography during surgery
    47.7 47.7 **FUD** 090   C 80
    AMA: 2014,Jan,11

61535   for removal of epidural or subdural electrode array, without excision of cerebral tissue (separate procedure)
    29.2 29.2 **FUD** 090   C 80
    AMA: 2014,Jan,11

61536 for excision of cerebral epileptogenic focus, with electrocorticography during surgery (includes removal of electrode array)
🔧 76.3   ⚕ 76.3   **FUD** 090   C 80 ▣
AMA: 2014,Jan,11

61537 for lobectomy, temporal lobe, without electrocorticography during surgery
🔧 72.4   ⚕ 72.4   **FUD** 090   C 80 ▣
AMA: 2014,Jan,11

61538 for lobectomy, temporal lobe, with electrocorticography during surgery
🔧 78.8   ⚕ 78.8   **FUD** 090   C 80 ▣
AMA: 2014,Jan,11

61539 for lobectomy, other than temporal lobe, partial or total, with electrocorticography during surgery
🔧 69.0   ⚕ 69.0   **FUD** 090   C 80 ▣
AMA: 2014,Jan,11

61540 for lobectomy, other than temporal lobe, partial or total, without electrocorticography during surgery
🔧 64.5   ⚕ 64.5   **FUD** 090   C 80 ▣
AMA: 2014,Jan,11

61541 for transection of corpus callosum
🔧 63.5   ⚕ 63.5   **FUD** 090   C 80 ▣
AMA: 2014,Jan,11

61543 for partial or subtotal (functional) hemispherectomy
🔧 62.1   ⚕ 62.1   **FUD** 090   C 80 ▣
AMA: 2014,Jan,11

61544 for excision or coagulation of choroid plexus
🔧 56.2   ⚕ 56.2   **FUD** 090   C 80 ▣
AMA: 2014,Jan,11

61545 for excision of craniopharyngioma
🔧 94.2   ⚕ 94.2   **FUD** 090   C 80 ▣
AMA: 2014,Jan,11

61546-61548 Removal Pituitary Gland/Tumor

EXCLUDES Injection for:
Cerebral angiography (36100-36218)
Pneumoencephalography (61055)
Ventriculography (61026, 61120)

61546 Craniotomy for hypophysectomy or excision of pituitary tumor, intracranial approach
🔧 68.2   ⚕ 68.2   **FUD** 090   C 80 ▣
AMA: 2014,Jan,11

61548 Hypophysectomy or excision of pituitary tumor, transnasal or transseptal approach, nonstereotactic
INCLUDES Operating microscope (69990)
🔧 46.0   ⚕ 46.0   **FUD** 090   C 80 ▣
AMA: 2016,Feb,12; 2014,Jan,11

61550-61559 Craniosynostosis Procedures

EXCLUDES Injection for:
Cerebral angiography (36100-36218)
Pneumoencephalography (61055)
Ventriculography (61026, 61120)
Orbital hypertelorism reconstruction (21260-21263)
Reconstruction (21172-21180)

61550 Craniectomy for craniosynostosis; single cranial suture
🔧 27.9   ⚕ 27.9   **FUD** 090   C 80 ▣
AMA: 2016,Jan,13; 2015,Jan,16; 2014,Jan,11; 2012,Feb,11

61552 multiple cranial sutures
🔧 33.5   ⚕ 33.5   **FUD** 090   C 80 ▣
AMA: 2016,Jan,13; 2015,Jan,16; 2014,Jan,11; 2012,Feb,11

61556 Craniotomy for craniosynostosis; frontal or parietal bone flap
🔧 46.1   ⚕ 46.1   **FUD** 090   C 80 ▣
AMA: 2016,Jan,13; 2015,Jan,16; 2014,Jan,11; 2012,Feb,11

61557 bifrontal bone flap
🔧 46.9   ⚕ 46.9   **FUD** 090   C 80 ▣
AMA: 2016,Jan,13; 2015,Jan,16; 2014,Jan,11; 2012,Feb,11

61558 Extensive craniectomy for multiple cranial suture craniosynostosis (eg, cloverleaf skull); not requiring bone grafts
🔧 55.4   ⚕ 55.4   **FUD** 090   C 80 ▣
AMA: 2016,Jan,13; 2015,Jan,16; 2014,Jan,11; 2012,Feb,11

61559 recontouring with multiple osteotomies and bone autografts (eg, barrel-stave procedure) (includes obtaining grafts)
🔧 61.3   ⚕ 61.3   **FUD** 090   C 80 ▣
AMA: 2016,Jan,13; 2015,Jan,16; 2014,Jan,11; 2012,Feb,11

61563-61564 Removal Cranial Bone Tumor With/Without Optic Nerve Decompression

EXCLUDES Injection for:
Cerebral angiography (36100-36218)
Pneumoencephalography (61055)
Ventriculography (61026, 61120)
Reconstruction (21181-21183)

61563 Excision, intra and extracranial, benign tumor of cranial bone (eg, fibrous dysplasia); without optic nerve decompression
🔧 56.0   ⚕ 56.0   **FUD** 090   C 80 ▣
AMA: 2014,Jan,11

61564 with optic nerve decompression
🔧 67.6   ⚕ 67.6   **FUD** 090   C 80 50 ▣
AMA: 2014,Jan,11

61566-61567 Craniotomy for Seizures

EXCLUDES Injection for:
Cerebral angiography (36100-36218)
Pneumoencephalography (61055)
Ventriculography (61026, 61120)

61566 Craniotomy with elevation of bone flap; for selective amygdalohippocampectomy
🔧 66.1   ⚕ 66.1   **FUD** 090   C 80 ▣
AMA: 2014,Jan,11

61567 for multiple subpial transections, with electrocorticography during surgery
🔧 75.7   ⚕ 75.7   **FUD** 090   C 80 ▣
AMA: 2014,Jan,11

61570-61571 Removal of Foreign Body from Brain

EXCLUDES Injection for:
Cerebral angiography (36100-36218)
Pneumoencephalography (61055)
Ventriculography (61026, 61120)
Sequestrectomy for osteomyelitis (61501)

61570 Craniectomy or craniotomy; with excision of foreign body from brain
🔧 54.8   ⚕ 54.8   **FUD** 090   C 80 ▣
AMA: 2014,Jan,11

61571 with treatment of penetrating wound of brain
🔧 58.4   ⚕ 58.4   **FUD** 090   C 80 ▣
AMA: 2014,Jan,11

61575-61576 Transoral Approach Posterior Cranial Fossa/Upper Cervical Cord

EXCLUDES Arthrodesis (22548)
Injection for:
Cerebral angiography (36100-36218)
Pneumoencephalography (61055)
Ventriculography (61026, 61120)

61575 Transoral approach to skull base, brain stem or upper spinal cord for biopsy, decompression or excision of lesion;
🔧 62.3   ⚕ 62.3   **FUD** 090   C 80 ▣
AMA: 2014,Jan,11

61576 requiring splitting of tongue and/or mandible (including tracheostomy)
🔧 105.   ⚕ 105.   **FUD** 090   C 80 ▣
AMA: 2014,Jan,11

26/TC	PC/TC Only	A2-Z3 ASC Payment	50 Bilateral	♂ Male Only	🔧 Facility RVU	⚕ Non-Facility RVU	▣ CCI
FUD	Follow-up Days	CMS: IOM (Pub 100)	A-Y OPPSI	80/80 Surg Assist Allowed / w/Doc	🔬 Lab Crosswalk	🔧 Radiology Crosswalk	✖ CLIA

260
CPT © 2016 American Medical Association. All Rights Reserved.
© 2016 Optum360, LLC

Nervous System

61580 — 61611

61580-61598 Surgical Approach: Cranial Fossae

EXCLUDES Definitive surgery (61600-61616)
Dural repair and/or reconstruction (61618-61619)
Injection for:
Cerebral angiography (36100-36218)
Pneumoencephalography (61055)
Ventriculography (61026, 61120)
Primary closure (15732, 15756-15758)

61580 Craniofacial approach to anterior cranial fossa; extradural, including lateral rhinotomy, ethmoidectomy, sphenoidectomy, without maxillectomy or orbital exenteration
72.8 72.8 **FUD** 090 C 50
AMA: 2016,Jan,13; 2015,Jan,16; 2014,Jan,11

61581 extradural, including lateral rhinotomy, orbital exenteration, ethmoidectomy, sphenoidectomy and/or maxillectomy
77.0 77.0 **FUD** 090 C 50
AMA: 2016,Jan,13; 2015,Jan,16; 2014,Jan,11

61582 extradural, including unilateral or bifrontal craniotomy, elevation of frontal lobe(s), osteotomy of base of anterior cranial fossa
84.6 84.6 **FUD** 090 C 80
AMA: 2016,Jan,13; 2015,Jan,16; 2014,Jan,11

61583 intradural, including unilateral or bifrontal craniotomy, elevation or resection of frontal lobe, osteotomy of base of anterior cranial fossa
84.7 84.7 **FUD** 090 C 80
AMA: 2016,Jan,13; 2015,Jan,16; 2014,Jan,11

61584 Orbitocranial approach to anterior cranial fossa, extradural, including supraorbital ridge osteotomy and elevation of frontal and/or temporal lobe(s); without orbital exenteration
83.6 83.6 **FUD** 090 C 80 50
AMA: 2016,Jan,13; 2015,Jan,16; 2014,Jan,11

61585 with orbital exenteration
94.7 94.7 **FUD** 090 C 80 50
AMA: 2016,Jan,13; 2015,Jan,16; 2014,Jan,11

61586 Bicoronal, transzygomatic and/or LeFort I osteotomy approach to anterior cranial fossa with or without internal fixation, without bone graft
70.4 70.4 **FUD** 090 C 80
AMA: 2014,Jan,11

61590 Infratemporal pre-auricular approach to middle cranial fossa (parapharyngeal space, infratemporal and midline skull base, nasopharynx), with or without disarticulation of the mandible, including parotidectomy, craniotomy, decompression and/or mobilization of the facial nerve and/or petrous carotid artery
88.4 88.4 **FUD** 090 C 80 50
AMA: 2016,Jan,13; 2015,Jan,16; 2014,Jan,11

61591 Infratemporal post-auricular approach to middle cranial fossa (internal auditory meatus, petrous apex, tentorium, cavernous sinus, parasellar area, infratemporal fossa) including mastoidectomy, resection of sigmoid sinus, with or without decompression and/or mobilization of contents of auditory canal or petrous carotid artery
90.2 90.2 **FUD** 090 C 80 50
AMA: 2016,Jan,13; 2015,Jan,16; 2014,Jan,11

61592 Orbitocranial zygomatic approach to middle cranial fossa (cavernous sinus and carotid artery, clivus, basilar artery or petrous apex) including osteotomy of zygoma, craniotomy, extra- or intradural elevation of temporal lobe
93.0 93.0 **FUD** 090 C 80 50
AMA: 2016,Jan,13; 2015,Jan,16; 2014,Jan,11

61595 Transtemporal approach to posterior cranial fossa, jugular foramen or midline skull base, including mastoidectomy, decompression of sigmoid sinus and/or facial nerve, with or without mobilization
68.7 68.7 **FUD** 090 C 50
AMA: 2016,Jan,13; 2015,Jan,16; 2014,Jan,11

61596 Transcochlear approach to posterior cranial fossa, jugular foramen or midline skull base, including labyrinthectomy, decompression, with or without mobilization of facial nerve and/or petrous carotid artery
70.6 70.6 **FUD** 090 C 80 50
AMA: 2016,Jan,13; 2015,Jan,16; 2014,Jan,11

61597 Transcondylar (far lateral) approach to posterior cranial fossa, jugular foramen or midline skull base, including occipital condylectomy, mastoidectomy, resection of C1-C3 vertebral body(s), decompression of vertebral artery, with or without mobilization
82.4 82.4 **FUD** 090 C 80 50
AMA: 2016,Jan,13; 2015,Jan,16; 2014,Jan,11

61598 Transpetrosal approach to posterior cranial fossa, clivus or foramen magnum, including ligation of superior petrosal sinus and/or sigmoid sinus
83.2 83.2 **FUD** 090 C 80
AMA: 2016,Jan,13; 2015,Jan,16; 2014,Jan,11

61600-61616 Definitive Procedures: Cranial Fossae

EXCLUDES Dural repair and/or reconstruction (61618-61619)
Injection for:
Cerebral angiography (36100-36218)
Pneumoencephalography (61055)
Ventriculography (61026, 61120)
Primary closure (15732, 15756-15758)
Surgical approach (61580-61598)

61600 Resection or excision of neoplastic, vascular or infectious lesion of base of anterior cranial fossa; extradural
62.1 62.1 **FUD** 090 C 80
AMA: 2016,Jan,13; 2015,Jan,16; 2014,Jan,11

61601 intradural, including dural repair, with or without graft
70.8 70.8 **FUD** 090 C 80
AMA: 2016,Jan,13; 2015,Jan,16; 2014,Jan,11

61605 Resection or excision of neoplastic, vascular or infectious lesion of infratemporal fossa, parapharyngeal space, petrous apex; extradural
63.0 63.0 **FUD** 090 C 80
AMA: 2016,Jan,13; 2015,Jan,16; 2014,Jan,11

61606 intradural, including dural repair, with or without graft
87.3 87.3 **FUD** 090 C 80
AMA: 2016,Jan,13; 2015,Jan,16; 2014,Jan,11

61607 Resection or excision of neoplastic, vascular or infectious lesion of parasellar area, cavernous sinus, clivus or midline skull base; extradural
79.2 79.2 **FUD** 090 C 80
AMA: 2016,Jan,13; 2015,Jan,16; 2014,Jan,11

61608 intradural, including dural repair, with or without graft
95.3 95.3 **FUD** 090 C 80
AMA: 2016,Jan,13; 2015,Jan,16; 2014,Jan,11

+ **61610** Transection or ligation, carotid artery in cavernous sinus, with repair by anastomosis or graft (List separately in addition to code for primary procedure)
Code first (61605-61608)
44.9 44.9 **FUD** ZZZ C 80
AMA: 2016,Jan,13; 2015,Jan,16; 2014,Jan,11

+ **61611** Transection or ligation, carotid artery in petrous canal; without repair (List separately in addition to code for primary procedure)
Code first (61605-61608)
11.2 11.2 **FUD** ZZZ C 80
AMA: 2016,Jan,13; 2015,Jan,16; 2014,Jan,11

+ 61612 with repair by anastomosis or graft (List separately in addition to code for primary procedure)
Code first (61605-61608)
🔲 42.2 🔲 42.2 **FUD** ZZZ C 80 🔲
AMA: 2016,Jan,13; 2015,Jan,16; 2014,Jan,11

61613 Obliteration of carotid aneurysm, arteriovenous malformation, or carotid-cavernous fistula by dissection within cavernous sinus
🔲 94.5 🔲 94.5 **FUD** 090 C 80 50 🔲
AMA: 2016,Jan,13; 2015,Jan,16; 2014,Jan,11

61615 Resection or excision of neoplastic, vascular or infectious lesion of base of posterior cranial fossa, jugular foramen, foramen magnum, or C1-C3 vertebral bodies; extradural
🔲 66.0 🔲 66.0 **FUD** 090 C 80 🔲
AMA: 2016,Jan,13; 2015,Jan,16; 2014,Jan,11

61616 intradural, including dural repair, with or without graft
🔲 97.6 🔲 97.6 **FUD** 090 C 80 🔲
AMA: 2016,Jan,13; 2015,Jan,16; 2014,Jan,11

61618-61619 Reconstruction Post-Surgical Cranial Fossae Defects

EXCLUDES Definitive surgery (61600-61616)
Injection for:
Cerebral angiography (36100-36218)
Pneumoencephalography (61055)
Ventriculography (61026, 61120)
Primary closure (15732, 15756-15758)
Surgical approach (61580-61598)

61618 Secondary repair of dura for cerebrospinal fluid leak, anterior, middle or posterior cranial fossa following surgery of the skull base; by free tissue graft (eg, pericranium, fascia, tensor fascia lata, adipose tissue, homologous or synthetic grafts)
🔲 37.9 🔲 37.9 **FUD** 090 C 80 🔲
AMA: 2016,Jan,13; 2015,Jan,16; 2014,Jan,11; 2012,Jan,15-42; 2011,Jan,11

61619 by local or regionalized vascularized pedicle flap or myocutaneous flap (including galea, temporalis, frontalis or occipitalis muscle)
🔲 42.1 🔲 42.1 **FUD** 090 C 80 🔲
AMA: 2016,Jan,13; 2015,Jan,16; 2014,Jan,11; 2012,Jan,15-42; 2011,Jan,11

61623-61651 Neurovascular Interventional Procedures

61623 Endovascular temporary balloon arterial occlusion, head or neck (extracranial/intracranial) including selective catheterization of vessel to be occluded, positioning and inflation of occlusion balloon, concomitant neurological monitoring, and radiologic supervision and interpretation of all angiography required for balloon occlusion and to exclude vascular injury post occlusion

EXCLUDES Diagnostic angiography of target artery just before temporary occlusion; report only radiological supervision and interpretation
Selective catheterization and angiography of artery besides the target artery; report catheterization and radiological supervision and interpretation codes as appropriate
🔲 16.5 🔲 16.5 **FUD** 000 J 🔲
AMA: 2016,Jan,13; 2015,Jan,16; 2014,Jan,11

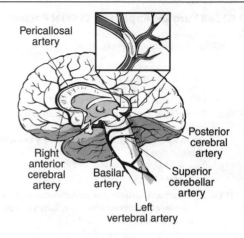

Pericallosal artery

Posterior cerebral artery

Right anterior cerebral artery

Basilar artery

Superior cerebellar artery

Left vertebral artery

61624 Transcatheter permanent occlusion or embolization (eg, for tumor destruction, to achieve hemostasis, to occlude a vascular malformation), percutaneous, any method; central nervous system (intracranial, spinal cord)

EXCLUDES Non-central nervous system transcatheter occlusion or embolization other than head or neck (37241-37244)
🔲 (75894)
🔲 33.2 🔲 33.2 **FUD** 000 C 🔲
AMA: 2016,Jan,13; 2015,Jan,16; 2014,Jan,11; 2013,Nov,6; 2012,Jan,15-42; 2011,Jan,11

61626 non-central nervous system, head or neck (extracranial, brachiocephalic branch)

EXCLUDES Non-central nervous system transcatheter occlusion or embolization other than head or neck (37241-37244)
🔲 (75894)
🔲 25.0 🔲 25.0 **FUD** 000 J 🔲
AMA: 2016,Jan,13; 2015,Jan,16; 2014,Jan,11; 2013,Nov,6

61630 Balloon angioplasty, intracranial (eg, atherosclerotic stenosis), percutaneous

INCLUDES Diagnostic arteriogram if stent or angioplasty is necessary
Radiology services for arteriography of target vascular family
Selective catheterization of the target vascular family

EXCLUDES Diagnostic arteriogram if stent or angioplasty is not necessary (use applicable code for selective catheterization and radiology services)
Percutaneous arterial transluminal mechanical thrombectomy and/or infusion for thrombolysis performed in the same vascular territory (61645)
🔲 38.7 🔲 38.7 **FUD** XXX C 80 🔲
AMA: 2016,Mar,3; 2016,Jan,13; 2015,Nov,3; 2015,Jan,16; 2014,Jan,11

61635 **Transcatheter placement of intravascular stent(s), intracranial (eg, atherosclerotic stenosis), including balloon angioplasty, if performed**

INCLUDES   Diagnostic arteriogram if stent or angioplasty is necessary
Radiology services for arteriography of target vascular family
Selective catheterization of the target vascular family

EXCLUDES   *Craniotomy with elevation of bone flap performed in the same vascular territory (61545)*
Diagnostic arteriogram if stent or angioplasty is not necessary (use applicable code for selective catheterization and radiology services)

🚑 41.5   ⚕ 41.5   **FUD** XXX   C 80 📠

AMA: 2016,Mar,3; 2016,Jan,13; 2015,Nov,3; 2015,Jan,16; 2014,Mar,8; 2014,Jan,11

61640 **Balloon dilatation of intracranial vasospasm, percutaneous; initial vessel**

INCLUDES   Angiography after dilation of vessel
Fluoroscopic guidance
Injection of contrast material
Roadmapping
Selective catheterization of target vessel
Vessel analysis

EXCLUDES   *Endovascular intracranial prolonged administration of pharmacologic agent performed in the same vascular territory (61650-61651)*

🚑 18.7   ⚕ 18.7   **FUD** 000   E 📠

AMA: 2016,Mar,3; 2016,Jan,13; 2015,Nov,3; 2015,Jan,16; 2014,May,10; 2014,Jan,11

+ 61641 **each additional vessel in same vascular family (List separately in addition to code for primary procedure)**

INCLUDES   Angiography after dilation of vessel
Fluoroscopic guidance
Injection of contrast material
Roadmapping
Selective catheterization of target vessel
Vessel analysis

Code first (61640)

🚑 6.57   ⚕ 6.57   **FUD** ZZZ   E 📠

AMA: 2016,Mar,3; 2016,Jan,13; 2015,Nov,3; 2015,Jan,16; 2014,May,10; 2014,Jan,11

+ 61642 **each additional vessel in different vascular family (List separately in addition to code for primary procedure)**

INCLUDES   Angiography after dilation of vessel
Fluoroscopic guidance
Injection of contrast material
Roadmapping
Selective catheterization of target vessel
Vessel analysis

EXCLUDES   *Endovascular intracranial prolonged administration of pharmacologic agent performed in the same vascular territory (61650-61651)*

Code first (61640)

🚑 13.1   ⚕ 13.1   **FUD** ZZZ   E 📠

AMA: 2016,Mar,3; 2016,Jan,13; 2015,Nov,3; 2015,Jan,16; 2014,May,10; 2014,Jan,11

61645 **Percutaneous arterial transluminal mechanical thrombectomy and/or infusion for thrombolysis, intracranial, any method, including diagnostic angiography, fluoroscopic guidance, catheter placement, and intraprocedural pharmacological thrombolytic injection(s)**

INCLUDES   Interventions performed in an intracranial artery including:
Angiography with radiologic supervision and interpretation (diagnostic and subsequent)
Closure of arteriotomy by any method
Fluoroscopy
Patient monitoring
Procedures performed in vascular territories:
Left carotid
Right carotid
Vertebro-basilar

EXCLUDES   *Procedure performed in the same vascular target area:*
Balloon angioplasty, intracranial (61630)
Diagnostic studies: aortic arch, carotid, and vertebral arteries (36221-36228)
Endovascular intracranial prolonged administration of pharmacologic agent (61650-61651)
Transcatheter placement of intravascular stent (61635)
Transluminal thrombectomy (37184, 37186)
Venous thrombectomy or thrombolysis (37187-37188, [37212], [37214])

🚑 22.5   ⚕ 22.5   **FUD** 000   E 80 50 📠

AMA: 2016,Mar,3; 2016,Jan,13; 2015,Dec,18; 2015,Nov,3

61650 **Endovascular intracranial prolonged administration of pharmacologic agent(s) other than for thrombolysis, arterial, including catheter placement, diagnostic angiography, and imaging guidance; initial vascular territory**

INCLUDES   Interventions performed in an intracranial artery, including:
Angiography with radiologic supervision and interpretation (diagnostic and subsequent)
Closure of arteriotomy by any method
Fluoroscopy
Patient monitoring
Procedures performed in vascular territories:
Left carotid
Right carotid
Vertebro-basilar
Prolonged (at least 10 minutes) arterial administration of non-thrombolytic agents

EXCLUDES   *Procedure performed in the same vascular target area:*
Balloon dilatation of intracranial vasospasm (61640-61642)
Chemotherapy administration (96420-96425)
Diagnostic studies: aortic arch, carotid, and vertebral arteries (36221-36228)
Transluminal thrombectomy (37184, 37186, 61645)
Treatment of an iatrogenic condition
Venous thrombectomy or thrombolysis

🚑 15.0   ⚕ 15.0   **FUD** 000   C 📠

AMA: 2016,Mar,3; 2016,Jan,13; 2015,Nov,3

Nervous System

61651 — 61711

+ **61651** **each additional vascular territory (List separately in addition to code for primary procedure)**

INCLUDES   Interventions performed in an intracranial artery including:

  Angiography with radiologic supervision and interpretation (diagnostic and subsequent)
  Closure of arteriotomy by any method
  Fluoroscopy
  Patient monitoring
  Procedures performed in vascular territories:
    Left carotid
    Right carotid
    Vertebro-basilar
  Prolonged (at least 10 minutes) arterial administration of non-thrombolytic agents

EXCLUDES   *Procedure performed in the same vascular target area:*
  Balloon dilatation of intracranial vasospasm (61640-61642)
  Chemotherapy administration (96420-96425)
  Diagnostic studies: aortic arch, carotid, and vertebral arteries (36221-36228)
  Transluminal thrombectomy (37184, 37186, 61645)
  Treatment of an iatrogenic condition
  Venous thrombectomy or thrombolysis

Code first (61650)

🚗 6.40   ✂ 6.40   **FUD** ZZZ   C 🖵

AMA: 2016,Mar,3; 2016,Jan,13; 2015,Nov,3

61680-61692 Surgical Treatment of Arteriovenous Malformation of the Brain

INCLUDES   Craniotomy

61680 **Surgery of intracranial arteriovenous malformation; supratentorial, simple**

🚗 65.9   ✂ 65.9   **FUD** 090   C 80 🖵

AMA: 2014,Jan,11

61682 **supratentorial, complex**

🚗 122.   ✂ 122.   **FUD** 090   C 80 🖵

AMA: 2016,Jan,13; 2015,Jan,16; 2014,Jan,11; 2013,Jun,13

61684 **infratentorial, simple**

🚗 84.1   ✂ 84.1   **FUD** 090   C 80 🖵

AMA: 2014,Jan,11

61686 **infratentorial, complex**

🚗 132.   ✂ 132.   **FUD** 090   C 80 🖵

AMA: 2016,Jan,13; 2015,Jan,16; 2014,Jan,11; 2013,Jun,13

61690 **dural, simple**

🚗 63.7   ✂ 63.7   **FUD** 090   C 80 🖵

AMA: 2014,Jan,11

61692 **dural, complex**

🚗 107.   ✂ 107.   **FUD** 090   C 80 🖵

AMA: 2016,Jan,13; 2015,Jan,16; 2014,Jan,11; 2013,Jun,13

61697-61703 Surgical Treatment Brain Aneurysm

INCLUDES   Craniotomy

61697 **Surgery of complex intracranial aneurysm, intracranial approach; carotid circulation**

INCLUDES   Aneurysms bigger than 15 mm
  Calcification of the aneurysm neck
  Inclusion of normal vessels in aneurysm neck
  Surgery needing temporary vessel occlusion, trapping, or cardiopulmonary bypass to treat aneurysm

🚗 124.   ✂ 124.   **FUD** 090   C 🖵

AMA: 2014,Jan,11

61698 **vertebrobasilar circulation**

INCLUDES   Aneurysm bigger than 15 mm
  Calcification of aneurysm neck
  Inclusion of normal vessels into aneurysm neck
  Surgery needing temporary vessel occlusion, trapping, or cardiopulmonary bypass to treat aneurysm

🚗 136.   ✂ 136.   **FUD** 090   C 80 🖵

AMA: 2014,Jan,11

61700 **Surgery of simple intracranial aneurysm, intracranial approach; carotid circulation**

🚗 100.   ✂ 100.   **FUD** 090   C 80 🖵

AMA: 2016,Jan,13; 2015,Jan,16; 2014,Jan,11; 2012,Jan,15-42; 2011,Jan,11

61702 **vertebrobasilar circulation**

🚗 118.   ✂ 118.   **FUD** 090   C 80 🖵

AMA: 2014,Jan,11

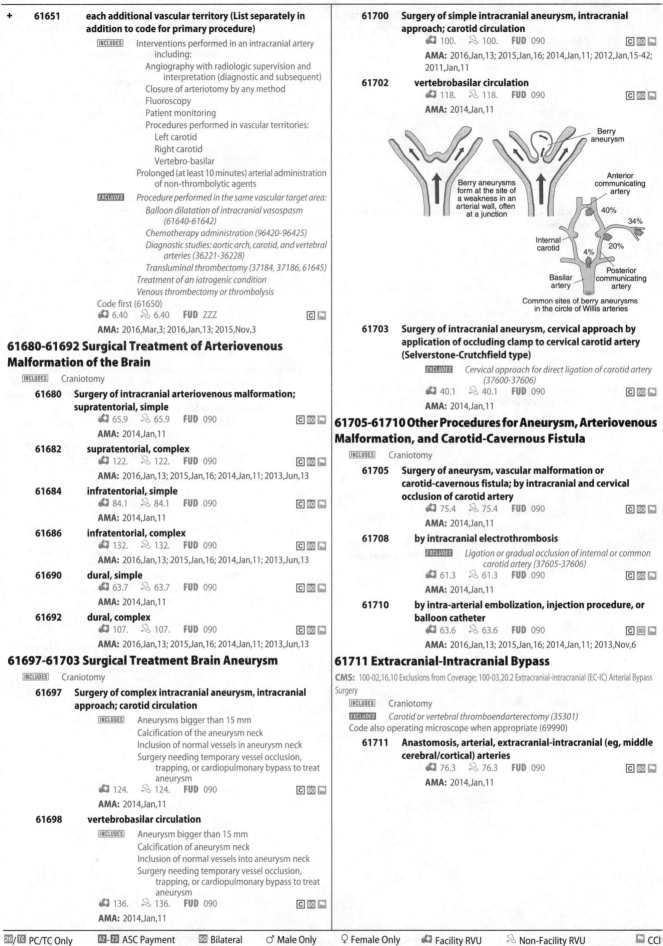

Berry aneurysm

Berry aneurysms form at the site of a weakness in an arterial wall, often at a junction

Anterior communicating artery

Internal carotid

40%
34%
4%   20%

Basilar artery
Posterior communicating artery

Common sites of berry aneurysms in the circle of Willis arteries

61703 **Surgery of intracranial aneurysm, cervical approach by application of occluding clamp to cervical carotid artery (Selverstone-Crutchfield type)**

EXCLUDES   *Cervical approach for direct ligation of carotid artery (37600-37606)*

🚗 40.1   ✂ 40.1   **FUD** 090   C 80 🖵

AMA: 2014,Jan,11

61705-61710 Other Procedures for Aneurysm, Arteriovenous Malformation, and Carotid-Cavernous Fistula

INCLUDES   Craniotomy

61705 **Surgery of aneurysm, vascular malformation or carotid-cavernous fistula; by intracranial and cervical occlusion of carotid artery**

🚗 75.4   ✂ 75.4   **FUD** 090   C 80 🖵

AMA: 2014,Jan,11

61708 **by intracranial electrothrombosis**

EXCLUDES   *Ligation or gradual occlusion of internal or common carotid artery (37605-37606)*

🚗 61.3   ✂ 61.3   **FUD** 090   C 80 🖵

AMA: 2014,Jan,11

61710 **by intra-arterial embolization, injection procedure, or balloon catheter**

🚗 63.6   ✂ 63.6   **FUD** 090   C 80 🖵

AMA: 2016,Jan,13; 2015,Jan,16; 2014,Jan,11; 2013,Nov,6

61711 Extracranial-Intracranial Bypass

CMS: 100-02,16,10 Exclusions from Coverage; 100-03,20.2 Extracranial-intracranial (EC-IC) Arterial Bypass Surgery

INCLUDES   Craniotomy

EXCLUDES   *Carotid or vertebral thromboendarterectomy (35301)*

Code also operating microscope when appropriate (69990)

61711 **Anastomosis, arterial, extracranial-intracranial (eg, middle cerebral/cortical) arteries**

🚗 76.3   ✂ 76.3   **FUD** 090   C 80 🖵

AMA: 2014,Jan,11

26/TC PC/TC Only   A2-Z3 ASC Payment   50 Bilateral   ♂ Male Only   ♀ Female Only   🚗 Facility RVU   ✂ Non-Facility RVU   🖵 CCI
FUD Follow-up Days   CMS: IOM (Pub 100)   A-Y OPPSI   80/80 Surg Assist Allowed / w/Doc   🔬 Lab Crosswalk   🏥 Radiology Crosswalk   ❌ CLIA

264   CPT © 2016 American Medical Association. All Rights Reserved.   © 2016 Optum360, LLC

61720-61791 Stereotactic Procedures of the Brain

61720 Creation of lesion by stereotactic method, including burr hole(s) and localizing and recording techniques, single or multiple stages; globus pallidus or thalamus

⏢ 37.5 ⚖ 37.5 **FUD** 090 T 🖳

AMA: 2016,Jan,13; 2015,Jan,16; 2014,Jul,8; 2014,Jan,11; 2011,Jul,12-13

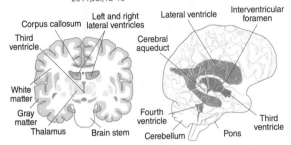

Frontal secion of the brain (left) and lateral view schematic showing the ventricular system in blue (right)

61735 subcortical structure(s) other than globus pallidus or thalamus

⏢ 46.3 ⚖ 46.3 **FUD** 090 C 🖳

AMA: 2014,Jul,8; 2014,Jan,11; 2011,Jul,12-13

61750 Stereotactic biopsy, aspiration, or excision, including burr hole(s), for intracranial lesion;

⏢ 41.3 ⚖ 41.3 **FUD** 090 C 🖳

AMA: 2016,Jan,13; 2015,Jan,16; 2014,Jul,8; 2014,Jan,11; 2011,Jul,12-13

61751 with computed tomography and/or magnetic resonance guidance

🔢 (70450, 70460, 70470, 70551-70553)

⏢ 40.6 ⚖ 40.6 **FUD** 090 C 🖳

AMA: 2016,Jan,13; 2015,Jan,16; 2014,Jul,8; 2014,Jan,11; 2012,Jan,15-42; 2011,Jul,12-13; 2011,Jan,11

61760 Stereotactic implantation of depth electrodes into the cerebrum for long-term seizure monitoring

⏢ 46.7 ⚖ 46.7 **FUD** 090 C 🖳

AMA: 2014,Jul,8; 2014,Jan,11; 2011,Jul,12-13

61770 Stereotactic localization, including burr hole(s), with insertion of catheter(s) or probe(s) for placement of radiation source

⏢ 47.6 ⚖ 47.6 **FUD** 090 T 63 🖳

AMA: 2016,Jan,13; 2015,Jan,16; 2014,Jul,8; 2014,Jan,11; 2011,Jul,12-13

+ **61781** Stereotactic computer-assisted (navigational) procedure; cranial, intradural (List separately in addition to code for primary procedure)

> *EXCLUDES* Creation of lesion by stereotactic method (61720-61791)
> Extradural sterotactic computer-assisted procedure for same surgical session by same individual (61782)
> Radiation treatment delivery, stereotactic radiosurgery (SRS) (77371-77373)
> Stereotactic implantation of neurostimulator electrode array (61863-61868)
> Stereotactic radiation treatment management (77432)
> Stereotactic radiosurgery (61796-61799)
> Ventriculocisternostomy (62201)

Code first primary procedure

⏢ 6.96 ⚖ 6.96 **FUD** ZZZ N N1 80 🖳

AMA: 2016,Jan,13; 2015,Jan,16; 2014,Sep,13; 2014,Jul,8; 2014,Jan,11; 2011,Jul,12-13

+ **61782** cranial, extradural (List separately in addition to code for primary procedure)

> *EXCLUDES* Intradural stereotactic computer-assisted procedure for same surgical session by same individual (61781)
> Stereotactic radiosurgery (61796-61799)

Code first primary procedure

⏢ 5.11 ⚖ 5.11 **FUD** ZZZ N N1 80 🖳

AMA: 2016,Jan,13; 2015,Jan,16; 2014,Jul,8; 2014,Jan,11; 2011,Jul,12-13

+ **61783** spinal (List separately in addition to code for primary procedure)

> *EXCLUDES* Stereotactic radiosurgery (61796-61799, 63620-63621)

Code first primary procedure

⏢ 6.85 ⚖ 6.85 **FUD** ZZZ N N1 80 🖳

AMA: 2016,Jan,13; 2015,Jan,16; 2014,Jul,8; 2014,Jan,11; 2011,Jul,12-13

61790 Creation of lesion by stereotactic method, percutaneous, by neurolytic agent (eg, alcohol, thermal, electrical, radiofrequency); gasserian ganglion

⏢ 25.9 ⚖ 25.9 **FUD** 090 T A2 50 🖳

AMA: 2014,Jul,8; 2014,Jan,11; 2011,Jul,12-13

61791 trigeminal medullary tract

⏢ 31.3 ⚖ 31.3 **FUD** 090 T A2 80 50 🖳

AMA: 2016,Jan,13; 2015,Jan,16; 2014,Jul,8; 2014,Jan,11; 2011,Jul,12-13

61796-61800 Stereotactic Radiosurgery (SRS): Brain

> *INCLUDES* Planning, dosimetry, targeting, positioning or blocking performed by the neurosurgeon
> *EXCLUDES* Application of cranial tongs, caliper, or stereotactic frame (20660)
> Intensity modulated beam delivery plan and treatment (77301, 77385-77386)
> Radiation treatment management and radiosurgery by the same provider (77427-77435)
> Treatment planning, physics and dosimetry, and treatment delivery performed by the radiation oncologist
> Stereotactic body radiation therapy (77373, 77435)
> Sterotactic radiosurgery more than once per lesion per treatment course

61796 Stereotactic radiosurgery (particle beam, gamma ray, or linear accelerator); 1 simple cranial lesion

> *INCLUDES* Lesions < 3.5 cm
> *EXCLUDES* Stereotactic computer-assisted proceudres (61781-61783)
> Stereotactic radiosurgery (61798)
> Treatment of complex lesions: (61798-61799)
> Arteriovenous malformations (AVM)
> Brainstem lesions
> Cavernous sinus/parasellar/petroclival tumors, glomus tumors, pituitary tumors, and tumors of pineal region
> Lesions located <= 5 mm from the optic nerve, chasm, or tract
> Schwannomas

Code also stereotactic headframe application, when performed (61800)

⏢ 29.8 ⚖ 29.8 **FUD** 090 B 80 🖳

AMA: 2016,Jan,13; 2015,Jun,6; 2015,Jan,16; 2014,Jul,8; 2014,Jan,11; 2012,Apr,11-13; 2011,Jul,12-13

+ **61797** each additional cranial lesion, simple (List separately in addition to code for primary procedure)

> *INCLUDES* Lesions < 3.5 cm
> *EXCLUDES* Stereotactic computer-assisted procedures (61781-61783)
> Treatment of complex lesions: (61798-61799)
> Arteriovenous malformations (AVM)
> Brainstem lesion
> Cavernous sinus/parasellar/petroclival tumors, glomus tumors, pituitary tumor, tumors of pineal region
> Lesions located <= 5 mm from the optic nerve, chasm, or tract
> Schwannomas
> Use of code for additional stereotactic radiosurgery more than four times in total per treatment course when used alone or in combination with (61799)

Code first (61796, 61798)

⏢ 6.54 ⚖ 6.54 **FUD** ZZZ B 80 🖳

AMA: 2016,Jan,13; 2015,Jun,6; 2015,Jan,16; 2014,Jul,8; 2014,Jan,11; 2012,Apr,11-13; 2011,Jul,12-13

61720 — 61797

61798 **1 complex cranial lesion**

INCLUDES All therapeutic lesion creation procedures
Treatment of complex lesions:
Arteriovenous malformations (AVM)
Brainstem lesions
Cavernous sinus, parasellar, petroclival, glomus, pineal region, and pituitary tumors
Lesions located <= 5 mm from the optic nerve, chasm, or tract
Lesions >= 3.5 cm
Schwannomas
Treatment of multiple lesions as long as one is complex

EXCLUDES Stereotactic computer-assisted procedures (61781-61783)
Stereotactic radiosurgery (61796)
Code also stereotactic headframe application, when performed (61800)

🖾 40.7 ⚕ 40.7 **FUD** 090 B 80 ▢

AMA: 2016,Jan,13; 2015,Jun,6; 2015,Jan,16; 2014,Jul,8; 2014,Jan,11; 2012,Apr,11-13; 2011,Jul,12-13

+ 61799 **each additional cranial lesion, complex (List separately in addition to code for primary procedure)**

INCLUDES All therapeutic lesion creation procedures
Treatment of complex lesions:
Arteriovenous malformations (AVM)
Brainstem lesions
Cavernous sinus, parasellar, petroclival, glomus, pineal region, and pituitary tumors
Lesions located <= 5 mm from the optic nerve, chasm, or tract
Lesions >= 3.5 cm
Schwannomas

EXCLUDES Stereotactic computer-assisted procedures (61781-61783)
Use of code for additional stereotactic radiosurgery more than four times in total per treatment course when used alone or in combination with (61797)
Code first (61798)

🖾 9.01 ⚕ 9.01 **FUD** ZZZ B 80 ▢

AMA: 2016,Jan,13; 2015,Jun,6; 2015,Jan,16; 2014,Jul,8; 2014,Jan,11; 2012,Apr,11-13; 2011,Jul,12-13

+ 61800 **Application of stereotactic headframe for stereotactic radiosurgery (List separately in addition to code for primary procedure)**

Code first (61796, 61798)

🖾 4.56 ⚕ 4.56 **FUD** ZZZ B 80 ▢

AMA: 2016,Jan,13; 2015,Jun,6; 2015,Jan,16; 2014,Jan,11; 2012,Apr,11-13

61850-61888 Intracranial Neurostimulation

INCLUDES Microelectrode recording by operating surgeon
EXCLUDES Electronic analysis and reprogramming of neurostimulator pulse generator (95970-95975)
Neurophysiological mapping by another physician/qualified health care professional (95961-95962)

61850 **Twist drill or burr hole(s) for implantation of neurostimulator electrodes, cortical**

🖾 28.9 ⚕ 28.9 **FUD** 090 C 80 ▢

AMA: 2016,Jan,13; 2015,Jan,16; 2014,Jan,11

61860 **Craniectomy or craniotomy for implantation of neurostimulator electrodes, cerebral, cortical**

🖾 46.2 ⚕ 46.2 **FUD** 090 C 80 ▢

AMA: 2016,Jan,13; 2015,Jan,16; 2014,Jan,11

61863 **Twist drill, burr hole, craniotomy, or craniectomy with stereotactic implantation of neurostimulator electrode array in subcortical site (eg, thalamus, globus pallidus, subthalamic nucleus, periventricular, periaqueductal gray), without use of intraoperative microelectrode recording; first array**

🖾 44.1 ⚕ 44.1 **FUD** 090 C 80 50 ▢

AMA: 2016,Jan,13; 2015,Jan,16; 2014,Jul,8; 2014,Jan,11; 2012,Jan,15-42; 2011,Jul,12-13; 2011,Jan,11

+ 61864 **each additional array (List separately in addition to primary procedure)**

Code first (61863)

🖾 8.43 ⚕ 8.43 **FUD** ZZZ C 80 ▢

AMA: 2014,Jul,8; 2014,Jan,11; 2011,Jul,12-13

61867 **Twist drill, burr hole, craniotomy, or craniectomy with stereotactic implantation of neurostimulator electrode array in subcortical site (eg, thalamus, globus pallidus, subthalamic nucleus, periventricular, periaqueductal gray), with use of intraoperative microelectrode recording; first array**

🖾 67.0 ⚕ 67.0 **FUD** 090 C 80 50 ▢

AMA: 2014,Jul,8; 2014,Jan,11; 2011,Jul,12-13

+ 61868 **each additional array (List separately in addition to primary procedure)**

Code first (61867)

🖾 14.7 ⚕ 14.7 **FUD** ZZZ C 80 ▢

AMA: 2016,Jan,13; 2015,Jan,16; 2014,Jul,8; 2014,Jan,11; 2011,Jul,12-13

61870 **Craniectomy for implantation of neurostimulator electrodes, cerebellar, cortical**

🖾 33.6 ⚕ 33.6 **FUD** 090 C 80 ▢

AMA: 2014,Jan,11

61880 **Revision or removal of intracranial neurostimulator electrodes**

🖾 16.7 ⚕ 16.7 **FUD** 090 02 62 80 50 ▢

AMA: 2014,Jan,11

61885 **Insertion or replacement of cranial neurostimulator pulse generator or receiver, direct or inductive coupling; with connection to a single electrode array**

EXCLUDES Percutaneous procedure to place cranial nerve neurostimulator electrode(s) (64553)
Revision or replacement cranial nerve neurostimulator electrode array (64569)

🖾 15.0 ⚕ 15.0 **FUD** 090 J J8 80 50 ▢

AMA: 2016,Jan,13; 2015,Jan,16; 2014,Jan,11; 2012,Jan,15-42; 2011,Sep,9-10; 2011,Sep,8; 2011,Feb,4-5

61886 **with connection to 2 or more electrode arrays**

EXCLUDES Percutaneous procedure to place cranial nerve neurostimulator electrode(s) (64553)
Revision or replacement cranial nerve neurostimulator electrode array (64569)

🖾 24.7 ⚕ 24.7 **FUD** 090 J J8 80 ▢

AMA: 2016,Jan,13; 2015,Jan,16; 2014,Jan,11; 2012,Jan,15-42; 2011,Sep,9-10; 2011,Sep,8; 2011,Feb,4-5

61888 **Revision or removal of cranial neurostimulator pulse generator or receiver**

EXCLUDES Insertion or replacement of cranial neurostimulator pulse generator or receiver (61885-61886)

🖾 11.6 ⚕ 11.6 **FUD** 010 J J8 50 ▢

AMA: 2016,Jan,13; 2015,Jan,16; 2014,Jan,11; 2012,Jan,15-42; 2011,Sep,8; 2011,Sep,9-10; 2011,Feb,4-5

62000-62148 Repair of Skull and/or Cerebrospinal Fluid Leaks

62000 **Elevation of depressed skull fracture; simple, extradural**

🖾 30.3 ⚕ 30.3 **FUD** 090 J ▢

AMA: 2014,Jan,11

62005 **compound or comminuted, extradural**

🖾 36.4 ⚕ 36.4 **FUD** 090 C 80 ▢

AMA: 2014,Jan,11

62010 **with repair of dura and/or debridement of brain**

🖾 44.9 ⚕ 44.9 **FUD** 090 C 80 ▢

AMA: 2014,Jan,11

62100 **Craniotomy for repair of dural/cerebrospinal fluid leak, including surgery for rhinorrhea/otorrhea**

EXCLUDES Repair of spinal fluid leak (63707, 63709)

🖾 46.7 ⚕ 46.7 **FUD** 090 C 80 ▢

AMA: 2014,Jan,11

62115 Reduction of craniomegalic skull (eg, treated hydrocephalus); not requiring bone grafts or cranioplasty
🚑 37.8   ⚕ 37.8   **FUD** 090   C 80 ▢
AMA: 2014,Jan,11

62117 requiring craniotomy and reconstruction with or without bone graft (includes obtaining grafts)
🚑 47.2   ⚕ 47.2   **FUD** 090   C 80 ▢
AMA: 2014,Jan,11

62120 Repair of encephalocele, skull vault, including cranioplasty
🚑 48.3   ⚕ 48.3   **FUD** 090   C 80 ▢
AMA: 2014,Jan,11

62121 Craniotomy for repair of encephalocele, skull base
🚑 46.5   ⚕ 46.5   **FUD** 090   C 80 ▢
AMA: 2014,Jan,11

62140 Cranioplasty for skull defect; up to 5 cm diameter
🚑 30.2   ⚕ 30.2   **FUD** 090   C 80 ▢
AMA: 2016,Jan,13; 2015,Jan,16; 2014,Jan,11; 2014,Jan,9

62141 larger than 5 cm diameter
🚑 33.3   ⚕ 33.3   **FUD** 090   C 80 ▢
AMA: 2016,Jan,13; 2015,Jan,16; 2014,Jan,11; 2014,Jan,9

62142 Removal of bone flap or prosthetic plate of skull
🚑 25.9   ⚕ 25.9   **FUD** 090   C 80 ▢
AMA: 2016,Jan,13; 2015,Jan,16; 2014,Jan,11; 2014,Jan,9

62143 Replacement of bone flap or prosthetic plate of skull
🚑 30.4   ⚕ 30.4   **FUD** 090   C 80 ▢
AMA: 2016,Jan,13; 2015,Jan,16; 2014,Jan,11; 2014,Jan,9

62145 Cranioplasty for skull defect with reparative brain surgery
🚑 41.4   ⚕ 41.4   **FUD** 090   C 80 ▢
AMA: 2016,Jan,13; 2015,Jan,16; 2014,Jan,11; 2014,Jan,9

62146 Cranioplasty with autograft (includes obtaining bone grafts); up to 5 cm diameter
🚑 36.5   ⚕ 36.5   **FUD** 090   C 80 ▢
AMA: 2016,Jan,13; 2015,Jan,16; 2014,Jan,11; 2014,Jan,9

62147 larger than 5 cm diameter
🚑 41.5   ⚕ 41.5   **FUD** 090   C 80 ▢
AMA: 2016,Jan,13; 2015,Jan,16; 2014,Jan,11; 2014,Jan,9

+ 62148 Incision and retrieval of subcutaneous cranial bone graft for cranioplasty (List separately in addition to code for primary procedure)
Code first (62140-62147)
🚑 3.77   ⚕ 3.77   **FUD** ZZZ   C ▢
AMA: 2014,Jan,11

62160-62165 Neuroendoscopic Brain Procedures

INCLUDES   Diagnostic endoscopy

+ 62160 Neuroendoscopy, intracranial, for placement or replacement of ventricular catheter and attachment to shunt system or external drainage (List separately in addition to code for primary procedure)
Code first (61107, 61210, 62220-62230, 62258)
🚑 5.64   ⚕ 5.64   **FUD** ZZZ   N N1 ▢
AMA: 2016,Jan,13; 2015,Jan,16; 2014,Jan,11; 2012,Dec,12; 2012,Jan,15-42; 2011,Jan,11

62161 Neuroendoscopy, intracranial; with dissection of adhesions, fenestration of septum pellucidum or intraventricular cysts (including placement, replacement, or removal of ventricular catheter)
🚑 44.7   ⚕ 44.7   **FUD** 090   C 80 ▢
AMA: 2014,Jan,11

62162 with fenestration or excision of colloid cyst, including placement of external ventricular catheter for drainage
🚑 55.5   ⚕ 55.5   **FUD** 090   C 80 ▢
AMA: 2014,Jan,11

62163 with retrieval of foreign body
🚑 32.5   ⚕ 32.5   **FUD** 090   C 80 ▢
AMA: 2014,Jan,11

62164 with excision of brain tumor, including placement of external ventricular catheter for drainage
🚑 61.1   ⚕ 61.1   **FUD** 090   C 80 ▢
AMA: 2014,Jan,11

62165 with excision of pituitary tumor, transnasal or trans-sphenoidal approach
🚑 45.2   ⚕ 45.2   **FUD** 090   C 80 ▢
AMA: 2014,Jan,11

62180-62258 Cerebrospinal Fluid Diversion Procedures

62180 Ventriculocisternostomy (Torkildsen type operation)
🚑 46.9   ⚕ 46.9   **FUD** 090   C 80 ▢
AMA: 2014,Jan,11

62190 Creation of shunt; subarachnoid/subdural-atrial, -jugular, -auricular
🚑 25.8   ⚕ 25.8   **FUD** 090   C ▢
AMA: 2014,Jan,11

Origin of shunt is subarachnoid/subdural

Shunt to pleura, peritoneum, or other site (62192)

Shunt to jugular, atria, or auricle (62190)

62192 subarachnoid/subdural-peritoneal, -pleural, other terminus
🚑 28.6   ⚕ 28.6   **FUD** 090   C 80 ▢
AMA: 2014,Jan,11

62194 Replacement or irrigation, subarachnoid/subdural catheter
🚑 13.5   ⚕ 13.5   **FUD** 010   T A2 80 ▢
AMA: 2016,Jan,13; 2015,Jan,16; 2014,Jan,11; 2011,Dec,6-7

62200 Ventriculocisternostomy, third ventricle;
INCLUDES   Dandy ventriculocisternostomy
🚑 40.5   ⚕ 40.5   **FUD** 090   C 80 ▢
AMA: 2014,Jan,11

62201 stereotactic, neuroendoscopic method
EXCLUDES   Intracranial neuroendoscopic surgery (62161-62165)
🚑 35.4   ⚕ 35.4   **FUD** 090   C ▢
AMA: 2016,Jan,13; 2015,Jan,16; 2014,Jul,8; 2014,Jan,11; 2012,Jan,15-42; 2011,Jul,12-13; 2011,Jan,11

62220 Creation of shunt; ventriculo-atrial, -jugular, -auricular
Code also intracranial neuroendoscopic ventricular catheter insertion, when performed (62160)
🚑 30.2   ⚕ 30.2   **FUD** 090   C 80 ▢
AMA: 2014,Jan,11

62223 ventriculo-peritoneal, -pleural, other terminus

Code also intracranial neuroendoscopic ventricular catheter insertion, when performed (62160)

⚕ 30.7 ⚗ 30.7 **FUD** 090 C 80 ▭

AMA: 2014,Jan,11

62225 Replacement or irrigation, ventricular catheter

Code also intracranial neuroendoscopic ventricular catheter insertion, when performed (62160)

⚕ 15.3 ⚗ 15.3 **FUD** 090 T A2 ▭

AMA: 2016,Jan,13; 2015,Jan,16; 2014,Jan,11; 2012,Jan,15-42; 2011,Dec,6-7

62230 Replacement or revision of cerebrospinal fluid shunt, obstructed valve, or distal catheter in shunt system

Code also intracranial neuroendoscopic ventricular catheter insertion, when performed (62160)

Code also when proximal catheter and valve are replaced (62225)

⚕ 24.7 ⚗ 24.7 **FUD** 090 T A2 80 ▭

AMA: 2016,Jan,13; 2015,Jan,16; 2014,Jan,11; 2012,Dec,12; 2012,Jan,15-42; 2011,Dec,6-7

62252 Reprogramming of programmable cerebrospinal shunt

⚕ 2.47 ⚗ 2.47 **FUD** XXX S P3 80 ▭

AMA: 2014,Jan,11

62256 Removal of complete cerebrospinal fluid shunt system; without replacement

EXCLUDES Reprogramming cerebrospinal fluid (CSF) shunt (62252)

⚕ 17.5 ⚗ 17.5 **FUD** 090 C 80 ▭

AMA: 2014,Jan,11

62258 with replacement by similar or other shunt at same operation

EXCLUDES Reprogramming of a cerebrospinal fluid (CSF) shunt (62252)

Code also intracranial neuroendoscopic ventricular catheter insertion, when performed (62160)

⚕ 33.0 ⚗ 33.0 **FUD** 090 C 80 ▭

AMA: 2016,Jan,13; 2015,Jan,16; 2014,Jan,11; 2012,Jan,15-42; 2011,Dec,6-7

62263-62264 Lysis of Epidural Lesions with Injection of Solution/Mechanical Methods

INCLUDES Epidurography (72275)
Fluoroscopic guidance (77003)
Percutaneous mechanical lysis

62263 Percutaneous lysis of epidural adhesions using solution injection (eg, hypertonic saline, enzyme) or mechanical means (eg, catheter) including radiologic localization (includes contrast when administered), multiple adhesiolysis sessions; 2 or more days

INCLUDES All adhesiolysis treatments, injections, and infusions during course of treatment
Percutaneous epidural catheter insertion and removal for neurolytic agent injections during a series of treatment sessions

EXCLUDES Procedure performed more than one time for the complete series spanning two or more treatment days

⚕ 9.78 ⚗ 18.6 **FUD** 010 T A2 ▭

AMA: 2016,Jan,13; 2015,Jan,16; 2014,Jan,11; 2012,Jun,12-13; 2012,Jan,15-42; 2011,Jan,11; 2011,Jan,8

62264 1 day

INCLUDES Multiple treatment sessions performed on the same day

EXCLUDES Percutaneous lysis of epidural adhesions using solution injection, 2 or more days (62263)

⚕ 6.88 ⚗ 12.0 **FUD** 010 T A2 ▭

AMA: 2016,Jan,13; 2015,Jan,16; 2014,Jan,11; 2012,Jun,12-13; 2012,Jan,15-42; 2011,Jan,11; 2011,Jan,8

62267-62269 Percutaneous Procedures of Spinal Cord

62267 Percutaneous aspiration within the nucleus pulposus, intervertebral disc, or paravertebral tissue for diagnostic purposes

EXCLUDES Bone biopsy (20225)
Decompression of intervertebral disc (62287)
Fine needle aspiration (10022)
Injection for discography (62290-62291)

Code also fluoroscopic guidance (77003)

⚕ 4.61 ⚗ 7.11 **FUD** 000 T 62 80 ▭

AMA: 2016,Jan,13; 2015,Jan,16; 2014,Jan,11; 2012,Jul,3-6; 2011,Jan,8

62268 Percutaneous aspiration, spinal cord cyst or syrinx

📷 (76942, 77002, 77012)

⚕ 7.48 ⚗ 7.48 **FUD** 000 T A2 ▭

AMA: 2014,Jan,11

62269 Biopsy of spinal cord, percutaneous needle

EXCLUDES Fine needle aspiration (10021-10022)

📷 (76942, 77002, 77012)

🔬 (88172-88173)

⚕ 7.82 ⚗ 7.82 **FUD** 000 T A2 80 ▭

AMA: 2014,Jan,11

62270-62272 Spinal Puncture, Subarachnoid Space, Diagnostic/Therapeutic

INCLUDES Fluoroscopic guidance (77003)

62270 Spinal puncture, lumbar, diagnostic

⚕ 2.25 ⚗ 4.54 **FUD** 000 T A2 ▭

AMA: 2016,Jan,13; 2015,Jan,16; 2014,Sep,3; 2014,Jan,11; 2012,Mar,4-7; 2011,Jan,8

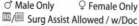

Meninges

62272 Spinal puncture, therapeutic, for drainage of cerebrospinal fluid (by needle or catheter)

⚕ 2.42 ⚗ 5.76 **FUD** 000 T A2 ▭

AMA: 2016,Jan,13; 2015,Jan,16; 2014,Jan,11; 2013,Dec,14; 2011,Jan,8

62273 Epidural Blood Patch

CMS: 100-03,10.5 NCD for Autogenous Epidural Blood Graft (10.5)

EXCLUDES Injection of diagnostic or therapeutic material (62320-62327)

Code also fluoroscopic guidance (77003)

62273 Injection, epidural, of blood or clot patch

⚕ 3.28 ⚗ 4.95 **FUD** 000 T A2 ▭

AMA: 2016,Jan,13; 2015,Jan,16; 2014,Jan,11; 2011,Jan,8

62280-62282 Neurolysis

INCLUDES Contrast injection during fluoroscopic guidance/localization

EXCLUDES Injection of diagnostic or therapeutic material only (62320-62327)

Code also fluoroscopic guidance and localization unless a formal contrast study is performed (77003)

62280 Injection/infusion of neurolytic substance (eg, alcohol, phenol, iced saline solutions), with or without other therapeutic substance; subarachnoid

⚕ 4.65 ⚗ 8.73 **FUD** 010 T A2 ▭

AMA: 2016,Jan,13; 2015,Jan,16; 2014,Jan,11; 2012,Jun,12-13; 2011,Jan,8

62281   **epidural, cervical or thoracic**
    4.53   6.88 **FUD** 010   T A2
    AMA: 2016,Jan,13; 2015,Jan,16; 2014,Jan,11; 2012,Jun,12-13; 2011,Jan,8

62282   **epidural, lumbar, sacral (caudal)**
    4.19   8.36 **FUD** 010   T A2
    AMA: 2016,Jan,13; 2015,Jan,16; 2014,Jan,11; 2012,Jun,12-13; 2012,Jan,15-42; 2011,Jan,11; 2011,Jan,8

62284-62294 Injection/Aspiration of Spine, Diagnostic/Therapeutic

62284   **Injection procedure for myelography and/or computed tomography, lumbar**
    EXCLUDES Injection at C1-C2 (61055)
           Myelography (62302-62305, 72240, 72255, 72265, 72270)
    2.48   5.20 **FUD** 000   N N1
    AMA: 2016,Jan,13; 2015,Jan,16; 2014,Sep,3; 2014,Jan,11; 2012,Jan,15-42; 2011,Jan,11

▲ 62287   **Decompression procedure, percutaneous, of nucleus pulposus of intervertebral disc, any method utilizing needle based technique to remove disc material under fluoroscopic imaging or other form of indirect visualization, with discography and/or epidural injection(s) at the treated level(s), when performed, single or multiple levels, lumbar**
    INCLUDES Endoscopic approach
    EXCLUDES Injection for discography (62290)
           Injection of diagnostic or therapeutic substance(s) (62322)
           Lumbar discography (72295)
           Percutaneous aspiration, diagnostic (62267)
           Percutaneous decompression of nucleus pulposus of an intervertebral disc, non-needle based technique (0274T-0275T)
           Radiological guidance (77003, 77012)
    16.3   16.3 **FUD** 090   T A2
    AMA: 2016,Jan,13; 2015,Mar,9; 2015,Jan,16; 2014,Apr,10; 2014,Jan,11; 2012,Oct,14; 2012,Jul,3-6; 2012,Jan,15-42; 2011,Jan,11

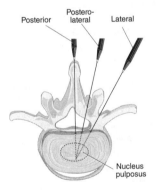

Posterior   Postero-lateral   Lateral

Nucleus pulposus

62290   **Injection procedure for discography, each level; lumbar**
    (72295)
    4.98   9.53 **FUD** 000   N N1
    AMA: 2016,Jan,13; 2015,Jan,16; 2014,Jan,11; 2012,Jul,3-6; 2012,Jan,15-42; 2011,Mar,7; 2011,Jan,11

62291   **cervical or thoracic**
    (72285)
    4.93   9.44 **FUD** 000   N N1
    AMA: 2016,Jan,13; 2015,Jan,16; 2014,Jan,11; 2011,Mar,7

62292   **Injection procedure for chemonucleolysis, including discography, intervertebral disc, single or multiple levels, lumbar**
    16.7   16.7 **FUD** 090   T R2 80
    AMA: 2016,Jan,13; 2015,Jan,16; 2014,Jan,11; 2012,Jan,15-42; 2011,Jan,11

62294   **Injection procedure, arterial, for occlusion of arteriovenous malformation, spinal**
    22.6   22.6 **FUD** 090   T A2
    AMA: 2014,Jan,11

62302-62305 Myelography

    EXCLUDES C1-C2 injection (61055)
           Lumbar myelogram furnished by other providers (62284, 72240, 72255, 72265, 72270)

62302   **Myelography via lumbar injection, including radiological supervision and interpretation; cervical**
    3.54   6.88 **FUD** 000   Q2 N1
    EXCLUDES Myelography (62303-62305)

62303   **thoracic**
    3.60   7.15 **FUD** 000   Q2 N1
    EXCLUDES Myelography (62302, 62304-62305)

62304   **lumbosacral**
    3.49   6.81 **FUD** 000   Q2 N1
    EXCLUDES Myelography (62302-62303, 62305)

62305   **2 or more regions (eg, lumbar/thoracic, cervical/thoracic, lumbar/cervical, lumbar/thoracic/cervical)**
    3.64   7.42 **FUD** 000   Q2 N1
    EXCLUDES Myelography (62302-62305)

62310-62327 Injection/Infusion Diagnostic/Therapeutic Material

    EXCLUDES Epidurography (72275)
           Transforaminal epidural injection (64479-64484)
           Use of code more than one time even when catheter tip or injected drug travels into a different area of the spine

~~62310~~   ~~Injection(s), of diagnostic or therapeutic substance(s) (including anesthetic, antispasmodic, opioid, steroid, other solution), not including neurolytic substances, including needle or catheter placement, includes contrast for localization when performed, epidural or subarachnoid; cervical or thoracic~~
    To report, see ~62320-62321

~~62311~~   ~~lumbar or sacral (caudal)~~
    To report, see ~62322-62323

~~62318~~   ~~Injection(s), including indwelling catheter placement, continuous infusion or intermittent bolus, of diagnostic or therapeutic substance(s) (including anesthetic, antispasmodic, opioid, steroid, other solution), not including neurolytic substances, includes contrast for localization when performed, epidural or subarachnoid; cervical or thoracic~~
    To report, see ~62324-62325

~~62319~~   ~~lumbar or sacral (caudal)~~
    To report, see ~62326-62327

● 62320   **Injection(s), of diagnostic or therapeutic substance(s) (eg, anesthetic, antispasmodic, opioid, steroid, other solution), not including neurolytic substances, including needle or catheter placement, interlaminar epidural or subarachnoid, cervical or thoracic; without imaging guidance**

● 62321   **with imaging guidance (ie, fluoroscopy or CT)**
    INCLUDES Radiologic guidance (76942, 77003, 77012)

● 62322   **Injection(s), of diagnostic or therapeutic substance(s) (eg, anesthetic, antispasmodic, opioid, steroid, other solution), not including neurolytic substances, including needle or catheter placement, interlaminar epidural or subarachnoid, lumbar or sacral (caudal); without imaging guidance**

Nervous System

62323 — 63012

● **62323** **with imaging guidance (ie, fluoroscopy or CT)**

> INCLUDES Radiologic guidance (76942, 77003, 77012)

● **62324** **Injection(s), including indwelling catheter placement, continuous infusion or intermittent bolus, of diagnostic or therapeutic substance(s) (eg, anesthetic, antispasmodic, opioid, steroid, other solution), not including neurolytic substances, interlaminar epidural or subarachnoid, cervical or thoracic; without imaging guidance**

> Code also hospital management of continuous infusion of drug, epidural or subarachnoid (01996)

● **62325** **with imaging guidance (ie, fluoroscopy or CT)**

> INCLUDES Radiologic guidance (76942, 77003, 77012)
>
> Code also hospital management of continuous infusion of drug, epidural or subarachnoid (01996)

● **62326** **Injection(s), including indwelling catheter placement, continuous infusion or intermittent bolus, of diagnostic or therapeutic substance(s) (eg, anesthetic, antispasmodic, opioid, steroid, other solution), not including neurolytic substances, interlaminar epidural or subarachnoid, lumbar or sacral (caudal); without imaging guidance**

> Code also hospital management of continuous infusion of drug, epidural or subarachnoid (01996)

● **62327** **with imaging guidance (ie, fluoroscopy or CT)**

> INCLUDES Radiologic guidance (76942, 77003, 77012)
>
> Code also hospital management of continuous infusion of drug, epidural or subarachnoid (01996)

62350-62370 Procedures Related to Epidural and Intrathecal Catheters

> EXCLUDES Epidural blood patch (62273)
> Injection epidural/subarachnoid diagnostic/therapeutic drugs (62320-62327)
> Injection for lumbar computed tomography/myelography (62284)
> Injection/infusion neurolytic substances (62280-62282)
> Spinal puncture (62270-62272)

62350 **Implantation, revision or repositioning of tunneled intrathecal or epidural catheter, for long-term medication administration via an external pump or implantable reservoir/infusion pump; without laminectomy**

> 11.6 ⚖ 11.6 **FUD** 010   T A2
>
> **AMA:** 2016,Jan,13; 2015,Jan,16; 2014,Jan,11

62351 **with laminectomy**

> 25.3 ⚖ 25.3 **FUD** 090   J 80
>
> **AMA:** 2016,Jan,13; 2015,Jan,16; 2014,Jan,11

62355 **Removal of previously implanted intrathecal or epidural catheter**

> 7.80 ⚖ 7.80 **FUD** 010   Q2 A2 80
>
> **AMA:** 2014,Jan,11

62360 **Implantation or replacement of device for intrathecal or epidural drug infusion; subcutaneous reservoir**

> 9.04 ⚖ 9.04 **FUD** 010   J J8 80
>
> **AMA:** 2014,Jan,11

62361 **nonprogrammable pump**

> 10.4 ⚖ 10.4 **FUD** 010   J J8 80
>
> **AMA:** 2014,Jan,11

62362 **programmable pump, including preparation of pump, with or without programming**

> 11.2 ⚖ 11.2 **FUD** 010   J J8 80
>
> **AMA:** 2016,Jan,13; 2015,Jan,16; 2014,Jan,11; 2012,Jan,15-42; 2011,Jan,11

62365 **Removal of subcutaneous reservoir or pump, previously implanted for intrathecal or epidural infusion**

> 8.61 ⚖ 8.61 **FUD** 010   Q2 A2 80
>
> **AMA:** 2014,Jan,11

62367 **Electronic analysis of programmable, implanted pump for intrathecal or epidural drug infusion (includes evaluation of reservoir status, alarm status, drug prescription status); without reprogramming or refill**

> 0.73 ⚖ 1.18 **FUD** XXX   S P3
>
> **AMA:** 2016,Jan,13; 2015,Jan,16; 2014,Jan,11; 2012,Aug,10-12; 2012,Jul,3-6

62368 **with reprogramming**

> 1.02 ⚖ 1.62 **FUD** XXX   S P3
>
> **AMA:** 2016,Jan,13; 2015,Jan,16; 2014,Jan,11; 2012,Aug,10-12; 2012,Jul,3-6; 2012,Jan,15-42; 2011,Jan,11

62369 **with reprogramming and refill**

> 1.03 ⚖ 3.43 **FUD** XXX   S P3
>
> **AMA:** 2016,Jan,13; 2015,Jan,16; 2014,Jan,11; 2012,Aug,10-12; 2012,Jul,3-6

62370 **with reprogramming and refill (requiring skill of a physician or other qualified health care professional)**

> 1.35 ⚖ 3.61 **FUD** XXX   S P3
>
> **AMA:** 2016,Jan,13; 2015,Jan,16; 2014,Jan,11; 2012,Aug,10-12; 2012,Jul,3-6

62380 Endoscopic Decompression/Laminectomy/Laminotomy

> EXCLUDES Open decompression (63030, 63056)
> Percutaneous decompression (62267, 0274T-0275T)
> Code also operating microscope, when applicable (69990)

● **62380** **Endoscopic decompression of spinal cord, nerve root(s), including laminotomy, partial facetectomy, foraminotomy, discectomy and/or excision of herniated intervertebral disc, 1 interspace, lumbar**

63001-63048 Posterior Midline Approach: Laminectomy/Laminotomy/Decompression

> INCLUDES Endoscopic assistance through open and direct visualization
> EXCLUDES Arthrodesis (22590-22614)
> Percutaneous decompression (62287, 0274T, 0275T)
> Code also operating microscope, when applicable (69990)

63001 **Laminectomy with exploration and/or decompression of spinal cord and/or cauda equina, without facetectomy, foraminotomy or discectomy (eg, spinal stenosis), 1 or 2 vertebral segments; cervical**

> 36.3 ⚖ 36.3 **FUD** 090   J G2 80
>
> **AMA:** 2016,Jan,13; 2015,Jan,16; 2014,Jan,11; 2013,Jul,3-5; 2012,Jul,3-6; 2012,Jan,15-42; 2011,Jul,12-13; 2011,Jan,11

63003 **thoracic**

> 36.1 ⚖ 36.1 **FUD** 090   J G2 80
>
> **AMA:** 2016,Jan,13; 2015,Jan,16; 2014,Jan,11; 2013,Jul,3-5; 2012,Jul,3-6; 2012,Jan,15-42; 2011,Jul,12-13; 2011,Jan,11

63005 **lumbar, except for spondylolisthesis**

> 34.4 ⚖ 34.4 **FUD** 090   J G2 80
>
> **AMA:** 2016,Jan,13; 2015,Jan,16; 2014,Jan,11; 2013,Dec,16; 2013,Jul,3-5; 2012,Jul,3-6; 2012,Jan,15-42; 2011,Jul,12-13; 2011,Jan,11

63011 **sacral**

> 31.8 ⚖ 31.8 **FUD** 090   J 80
>
> **AMA:** 2016,Jan,13; 2015,Jan,16; 2014,Jan,11; 2013,Jul,3-5; 2012,Jan,15-42; 2011,Jul,12-13; 2011,Jan,11

63012 **Laminectomy with removal of abnormal facets and/or pars inter-articularis with decompression of cauda equina and nerve roots for spondylolisthesis, lumbar (Gill type procedure)**

> 34.7 ⚖ 34.7 **FUD** 090   J 80
>
> **AMA:** 2016,Jan,13; 2015,Jan,16; 2014,Jan,11; 2013,Jul,3-5; 2012,Jan,15-42; 2011,Jul,12-13; 2011,Jan,11

63015 Laminectomy with exploration and/or decompression of spinal cord and/or cauda equina, without facetectomy, foraminotomy or discectomy (eg, spinal stenosis), more than 2 vertebral segments; cervical
43.4 ⚕ 43.4 **FUD** 090 J 80 🏴
AMA: 2016,Jan,13; 2015,Jan,16; 2014,Jan,11; 2013,Jul,3-5; 2012,Jan,15-42; 2011,Jul,12-13; 2011,Jan,11

63016 thoracic
44.4 ⚕ 44.4 **FUD** 090 J 80 🏴
AMA: 2016,Jan,13; 2015,Jan,16; 2014,Jan,11; 2013,Jul,3-5; 2012,Jan,15-42; 2011,Jul,12-13; 2011,Jan,11

63017 lumbar
36.6 ⚕ 36.6 **FUD** 090 J 80 🏴
AMA: 2016,Jan,13; 2015,Jan,16; 2014,Jan,11; 2013,Jul,3-5; 2012,Jan,15-42; 2011,Jul,12-13; 2011,Jan,11

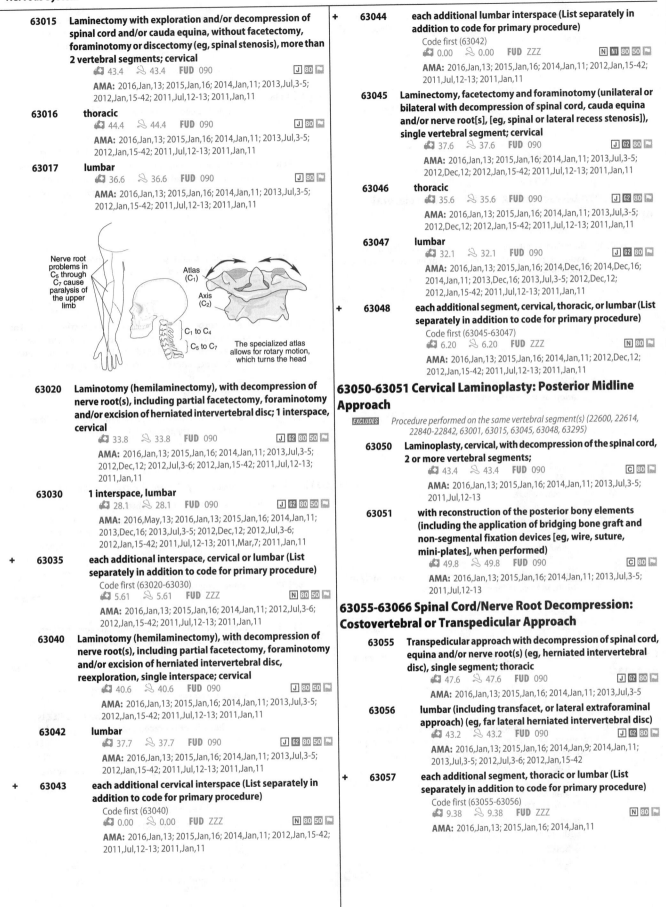

Nerve root problems in C_5 through C_7 cause paralysis of the upper limb

Atlas (C_1)

Axis (C_2)

C_1 to C_4

C_5 to C_7

The specialized atlas allows for rotary motion, which turns the head

63020 Laminotomy (hemilaminectomy), with decompression of nerve root(s), including partial facetectomy, foraminotomy and/or excision of herniated intervertebral disc; 1 interspace, cervical
33.8 ⚕ 33.8 **FUD** 090 J 62 80 50 🏴
AMA: 2016,Jan,13; 2015,Jan,16; 2014,Jan,11; 2013,Jul,3-5; 2012,Dec,12; 2012,Jul,3-6; 2012,Jan,15-42; 2011,Jul,12-13; 2011,Jan,11

63030 1 interspace, lumbar
28.1 ⚕ 28.1 **FUD** 090 J 62 80 50 🏴
AMA: 2016,May,13; 2016,Jan,13; 2015,Jan,16; 2014,Jan,11; 2013,Dec,16; 2013,Jul,3-5; 2012,Dec,12; 2012,Jul,3-6; 2012,Jan,15-42; 2011,Jul,12-13; 2011,Mar,7; 2011,Jan,11

+ 63035 each additional interspace, cervical or lumbar (List separately in addition to code for primary procedure)
Code first (63020-63030)
5.61 ⚕ 5.61 **FUD** ZZZ N 80 50 🏴
AMA: 2016,Jan,13; 2015,Jan,16; 2014,Jan,11; 2012,Jul,3-6; 2012,Jan,15-42; 2011,Jul,12-13; 2011,Jan,11

63040 Laminotomy (hemilaminectomy), with decompression of nerve root(s), including partial facetectomy, foraminotomy and/or excision of herniated intervertebral disc, reexploration, single interspace; cervical
40.6 ⚕ 40.6 **FUD** 090 J 80 50 🏴
AMA: 2016,Jan,13; 2015,Jan,16; 2014,Jan,11; 2013,Jul,3-5; 2012,Jan,15-42; 2011,Jul,12-13; 2011,Jan,11

63042 lumbar
37.7 ⚕ 37.7 **FUD** 090 J 62 80 50 🏴
AMA: 2016,Jan,13; 2015,Jan,16; 2014,Jan,11; 2013,Jul,3-5; 2012,Jan,15-42; 2011,Jul,12-13; 2011,Jan,11

+ 63043 each additional cervical interspace (List separately in addition to code for primary procedure)
Code first (63040)
0.00 ⚕ 0.00 **FUD** ZZZ N 80 50 🏴
AMA: 2016,Jan,13; 2015,Jan,16; 2014,Jan,11; 2012,Jan,15-42; 2011,Jul,12-13; 2011,Jan,11

+ 63044 each additional lumbar interspace (List separately in addition to code for primary procedure)
Code first (63042)
0.00 ⚕ 0.00 **FUD** ZZZ N N1 80 50 🏴
AMA: 2016,Jan,13; 2015,Jan,16; 2014,Jan,11; 2012,Jan,15-42; 2011,Jul,12-13; 2011,Jan,11

63045 Laminectomy, facetectomy and foraminotomy (unilateral or bilateral with decompression of spinal cord, cauda equina and/or nerve root[s], [eg, spinal or lateral recess stenosis]), single vertebral segment; cervical
37.6 ⚕ 37.6 **FUD** 090 J 62 80 🏴
AMA: 2016,Jan,13; 2015,Jan,16; 2014,Jan,11; 2013,Jul,3-5; 2012,Dec,12; 2012,Jan,15-42; 2011,Jul,12-13; 2011,Jan,11

63046 thoracic
35.6 ⚕ 35.6 **FUD** 090 J 62 80 🏴
AMA: 2016,Jan,13; 2015,Jan,16; 2014,Jan,11; 2013,Jul,3-5; 2012,Dec,12; 2012,Jan,15-42; 2011,Jul,12-13; 2011,Jan,11

63047 lumbar
32.1 ⚕ 32.1 **FUD** 090 J 62 80 🏴
AMA: 2016,Jan,13; 2015,Jan,16; 2014,Dec,16; 2014,Dec,16; 2014,Jan,11; 2013,Dec,16; 2013,Jul,3-5; 2012,Dec,12; 2012,Jan,15-42; 2011,Jul,12-13; 2011,Jan,11

+ 63048 each additional segment, cervical, thoracic, or lumbar (List separately in addition to code for primary procedure)
Code first (63045-63047)
6.20 ⚕ 6.20 **FUD** ZZZ N 80 🏴
AMA: 2016,Jan,13; 2015,Jan,16; 2014,Jan,11; 2012,Dec,12; 2012,Jan,15-42; 2011,Jul,12-13; 2011,Jan,11

63050-63051 Cervical Laminoplasty: Posterior Midline Approach

EXCLUDES Procedure performed on the same vertebral segment(s) (22600, 22614, 22840-22842, 63001, 63015, 63045, 63048, 63295)

63050 Laminoplasty, cervical, with decompression of the spinal cord, 2 or more vertebral segments;
43.4 ⚕ 43.4 **FUD** 090 C 80 🏴
AMA: 2016,Jan,13; 2015,Jan,16; 2014,Jan,11; 2013,Jul,3-5; 2011,Jul,12-13

63051 with reconstruction of the posterior bony elements (including the application of bridging bone graft and non-segmental fixation devices [eg, wire, suture, mini-plates], when performed)
49.8 ⚕ 49.8 **FUD** 090 C 80 🏴
AMA: 2016,Jan,13; 2015,Jan,16; 2014,Jan,11; 2013,Jul,3-5; 2011,Jul,12-13

63055-63066 Spinal Cord/Nerve Root Decompression: Costovertebral or Transpedicular Approach

63055 Transpedicular approach with decompression of spinal cord, equina and/or nerve root(s) (eg, herniated intervertebral disc), single segment; thoracic
47.6 ⚕ 47.6 **FUD** 090 J 62 80 🏴
AMA: 2016,Jan,13; 2015,Jan,16; 2014,Jan,11; 2013,Jul,3-5

63056 lumbar (including transfacet, or lateral extraforaminal approach) (eg, far lateral herniated intervertebral disc)
43.2 ⚕ 43.2 **FUD** 090 J 62 80 🏴
AMA: 2016,Jan,13; 2015,Jan,16; 2014,Jan,9; 2014,Jan,11; 2013,Jul,3-5; 2012,Jul,3-6; 2012,Jan,15-42

+ 63057 each additional segment, thoracic or lumbar (List separately in addition to code for primary procedure)
Code first (63055-63056)
9.38 ⚕ 9.38 **FUD** ZZZ N 80 🏴
AMA: 2016,Jan,13; 2015,Jan,16; 2014,Jan,11

63064 Costovertebral approach with decompression of spinal cord or nerve root(s) (eg, herniated intervertebral disc), thoracic; single segment

> EXCLUDES Laminectomy with intraspinal thoracic lesion removal (63266, 63271, 63276, 63281, 63286)

🔲 51.6 ⚕ 51.6 **FUD** 090 　J 80 🔲

AMA: 2016,Jan,13; 2015,Jan,16; 2014,Jan,11; 2013,Jul,3-5

+ **63066** each additional segment (List separately in addition to code for primary procedure)

> EXCLUDES Laminectomy with intraspinal thoracic lesion removal (63266, 63271, 63276, 63281, 63286)

Code first (63064)
🔲 6.14 ⚕ 6.14 **FUD** ZZZ 　N 80 🔲

AMA: 2014,Jan,11

63075-63078 Discectomy: Anterior or Anterolateral Approach

INCLUDES Operating microscope (69990)

63075 Discectomy, anterior, with decompression of spinal cord and/or nerve root(s), including osteophytectomy; cervical, single interspace

> EXCLUDES Anterior cervical discectomy and anterior interbody fusion at same level during same operative session (22551)
>
> Anterior interbody arthrodesis (even by another provider) (22554)

🔲 39.5 ⚕ 39.5 **FUD** 090 　J 80 🔲

AMA: 2016,Feb,12; 2016,Jan,13; 2015,Apr,7; 2015,Jan,16; 2014,Jan,11; 2013,Jul,3-5; 2012,Jan,15-42; 2011,Jan,11

+ **63076** cervical, each additional interspace (List separately in addition to code for primary procedure)

> EXCLUDES Anterior cervical discectomy and anterior interbody fusion at same level during same operative session (22552)
>
> Anterior interbody arthrodesis (even by another provider) (22554)

Code first (63075)
🔲 7.24 ⚕ 7.24 **FUD** ZZZ 　N 80 🔲

AMA: 2016,Feb,12; 2016,Jan,13; 2015,Jan,16; 2014,Jan,11; 2012,Jan,15-42; 2011,Jan,11

63077 thoracic, single interspace
🔲 43.7 ⚕ 43.7 **FUD** 090 　C 80 🔲

AMA: 2016,Feb,12; 2016,Jan,13; 2015,Jan,16; 2014,Jan,11; 2013,Jul,3-5; 2012,Jan,15-42; 2011,Jan,11

+ **63078** thoracic, each additional interspace (List separately in addition to code for primary procedure)
Code first (63077)
🔲 5.66 ⚕ 5.66 **FUD** ZZZ 　C 80 🔲

AMA: 2016,Feb,12; 2016,Jan,13; 2015,Jan,16; 2014,Jan,11; 2012,Jan,15-42; 2011,Jan,11

63081-63091 Vertebral Corpectomy, All Levels, Anterior Approach

INCLUDES Disc removal at the level below and/or above vertebral segment
EXCLUDES Arthrodesis (22548-22812)
Code also reconstruction (20930-20938, 22548-22812, 22840-22855 [22859])

63081 Vertebral corpectomy (vertebral body resection), partial or complete, anterior approach with decompression of spinal cord and/or nerve root(s); cervical, single segment

> EXCLUDES Transoral approach (61575-61576)

🔲 51.3 ⚕ 51.3 **FUD** 090 　C 80 🔲

AMA: 2016,Apr,8; 2016,Jan,13; 2015,Jun,10; 2015,Jan,16; 2014,Jan,11; 2013,Jul,3-5

+ **63082** cervical, each additional segment (List separately in addition to code for primary procedure)

> EXCLUDES Transoral approach (61575-61576)

Code first (63081)
🔲 7.81 ⚕ 7.81 **FUD** ZZZ 　C 80 🔲

AMA: 2016,Apr,8; 2016,Jan,13; 2015,Jan,16; 2014,Jan,11

63085 Vertebral corpectomy (vertebral body resection), partial or complete, transthoracic approach with decompression of spinal cord and/or nerve root(s); thoracic, single segment
🔲 55.7 ⚕ 55.7 **FUD** 090 　C 80 🔲

AMA: 2016,Apr,8; 2016,Jan,13; 2015,Jan,16; 2014,Jan,11; 2013,Jul,3-5

+ **63086** thoracic, each additional segment (List separately in addition to code for primary procedure)
Code first (63085)
🔲 5.57 ⚕ 5.57 **FUD** ZZZ 　C 80 🔲

AMA: 2016,Apr,8; 2016,Jan,13; 2015,Jan,16; 2014,Jan,11

63087 Vertebral corpectomy (vertebral body resection), partial or complete, combined thoracolumbar approach with decompression of spinal cord, cauda equina or nerve root(s), lower thoracic or lumbar; single segment
🔲 70.1 ⚕ 70.1 **FUD** 090 　C 80 🔲

AMA: 2016,Apr,8; 2016,Jan,13; 2015,Jan,16; 2014,Jan,11; 2013,Jul,3-5

+ **63088** each additional segment (List separately in addition to code for primary procedure)
Code first (63087)
🔲 7.59 ⚕ 7.59 **FUD** ZZZ 　C 80 🔲

AMA: 2016,Apr,8; 2016,Jan,13; 2015,Jan,16; 2014,Jan,11

63090 Vertebral corpectomy (vertebral body resection), partial or complete, transperitoneal or retroperitoneal approach with decompression of spinal cord, cauda equina or nerve root(s), lower thoracic, lumbar, or sacral; single segment
🔲 56.8 ⚕ 56.8 **FUD** 090 　C 80 🔲

AMA: 2016,Apr,8; 2016,Jan,13; 2015,Jan,16; 2014,Jan,11; 2013,Jul,3-5

+ **63091** each additional segment (List separately in addition to code for primary procedure)
Code first (63090)
🔲 5.16 ⚕ 5.16 **FUD** ZZZ 　C 80 🔲

AMA: 2016,Apr,8; 2016,Jan,13; 2015,Jan,16; 2014,Jan,11

63101-63103 Corpectomy: Lateral Extracavitary Approach

63101 Vertebral corpectomy (vertebral body resection), partial or complete, lateral extracavitary approach with decompression of spinal cord and/or nerve root(s) (eg, for tumor or retropulsed bone fragments); thoracic, single segment
🔲 67.6 ⚕ 67.6 **FUD** 090 　C 80 🔲

AMA: 2016,Jan,13; 2015,Jan,16; 2014,Jan,11; 2013,Jul,3-5

63102 lumbar, single segment
🔲 66.2 ⚕ 66.2 **FUD** 090 　C 80 🔲

AMA: 2016,Jan,13; 2015,Jan,16; 2014,Jan,11; 2013,Jul,3-5

+ **63103** thoracic or lumbar, each additional segment (List separately in addition to code for primary procedure)
Code first (63101-63102)
🔲 8.59 ⚕ 8.59 **FUD** ZZZ 　C 80 🔲

AMA: 2014,Jan,11

63170-63295 Laminectomies

63170 Laminectomy with myelotomy (eg, Bischof or DREZ type), cervical, thoracic, or thoracolumbar
🔲 47.0 ⚕ 47.0 **FUD** 090 　C 80 🔲

AMA: 2016,Jan,13; 2015,Jan,16; 2014,Jan,11; 2013,Jul,3-5

63172 Laminectomy with drainage of intramedullary cyst/syrinx; to subarachnoid space
🔲 40.6 ⚕ 40.6 **FUD** 090 　C 80 🔲

AMA: 2016,Jan,13; 2015,Jan,16; 2014,Jan,11; 2013,Jul,3-5

63173 to peritoneal or pleural space
🔲 50.3 ⚕ 50.3 **FUD** 090 　C 80 🔲

AMA: 2016,Jan,13; 2015,Jan,16; 2014,Jan,11; 2013,Jul,3-5

63180 Laminectomy and section of dentate ligaments, with or without dural graft, cervical; 1 or 2 segments
🔲 43.8 ⚕ 43.8 **FUD** 090 　C 80 🔲

AMA: 2016,Jan,13; 2015,Jan,16; 2014,Jan,11; 2013,Jul,3-5

26/TC PC/TC Only　　A2-Z6 ASC Payment　　50 Bilateral　　♂ Male Only　　♀ Female Only　　⚡ Facility RVU　　⚕ Non-Facility RVU　　🔲 CCI
FUD Follow-up Days　　CMS: IOM (Pub 100)　　A-Y OPPSI　　80/80 Surg Assist Allowed / w/Doc　　🔲 Lab Crosswalk　　⚡ Radiology Crosswalk　　☒ CLIA

272　　CPT © 2016 American Medical Association. All Rights Reserved.　　© 2016 Optum360, LLC

63182 **more than 2 segments**
40.5 40.5 **FUD** 090 C 80
AMA: 2016,Jan,13; 2015,Jan,16; 2014,Jan,11; 2013,Jul,3-5

63185 **Laminectomy with rhizotomy; 1 or 2 segments**
INCLUDES Dana rhizotomy
Stoffel rhizotomy
33.0 33.0 **FUD** 090 C 80
AMA: 2016,Jan,13; 2015,Jan,16; 2014,Jan,11; 2013,Jul,3-5

63190 **more than 2 segments**
36.6 36.6 **FUD** 090 C 80
AMA: 2016,Jan,13; 2015,Jan,16; 2014,Jan,11; 2013,Jul,3-5

63191 **Laminectomy with section of spinal accessory nerve**
EXCLUDES *Division of sternocleidomastoid muscle for torticollis (21720)*
39.7 39.7 **FUD** 090 C 80 50
AMA: 2016,Jan,13; 2015,Jan,16; 2014,Jan,11; 2013,Jul,3-5

63194 **Laminectomy with cordotomy, with section of 1 spinothalamic tract, 1 stage; cervical**
47.1 47.1 **FUD** 090 C 80
AMA: 2016,Jan,13; 2015,Jan,16; 2014,Jan,11; 2013,Jul,3-5

63195 **thoracic**
45.4 45.4 **FUD** 090 C 80
AMA: 2016,Jan,13; 2015,Jan,16; 2014,Jan,11; 2013,Jul,3-5

63196 **Laminectomy with cordotomy, with section of both spinothalamic tracts, 1 stage; cervical**
40.8 40.8 **FUD** 090 C 80
AMA: 2016,Jan,13; 2015,Jan,16; 2014,Jan,11; 2013,Jul,3-5

63197 **thoracic**
50.5 50.5 **FUD** 090 C 80
AMA: 2016,Jan,13; 2015,Jan,16; 2014,Jan,11; 2013,Jul,3-5

63198 **Laminectomy with cordotomy with section of both spinothalamic tracts, 2 stages within 14 days; cervical**
INCLUDES Keen laminectomy
48.1 48.1 **FUD** 090 C 80
AMA: 2016,Jan,13; 2015,Jan,16; 2014,Jan,11; 2013,Jul,3-5

63199 **thoracic**
50.5 50.5 **FUD** 090 C 80
AMA: 2016,Jan,13; 2015,Jan,16; 2014,Jan,11; 2013,Jul,3-5

63200 **Laminectomy, with release of tethered spinal cord, lumbar**
45.0 45.0 **FUD** 090 C 80
AMA: 2016,Jan,13; 2015,Jan,16; 2014,Jan,11; 2013,Jul,3-5

63250 **Laminectomy for excision or occlusion of arteriovenous malformation of spinal cord; cervical**
82.3 82.3 **FUD** 090 C 80
AMA: 2016,Jan,13; 2015,Jan,16; 2014,Jan,11; 2013,Jul,3-5

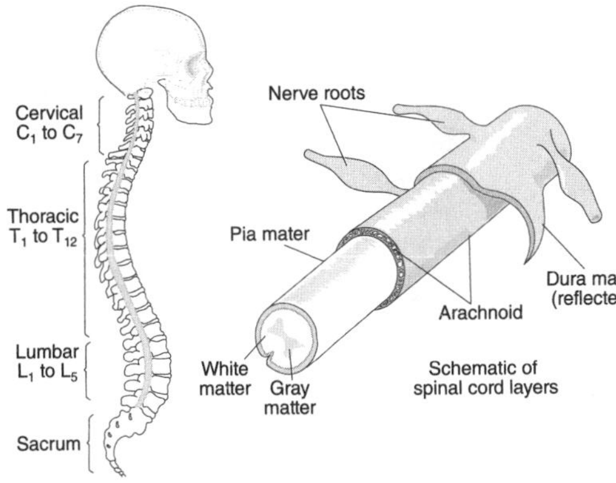
Cervical C1 to C7
Thoracic T1 to T12
Lumbar L1 to L5
Sacrum
Nerve roots
Pia mater
Arachnoid
Dura mater (reflected)
White matter
Gray matter
Schematic of spinal cord layers

63251 **thoracic**
89.5 89.5 **FUD** 090 C 80
AMA: 2016,Jan,13; 2015,Jan,16; 2014,Jan,11; 2013,Jul,3-5

63252 **thoracolumbar**
89.4 89.4 **FUD** 090 C 80
AMA: 2016,Jan,13; 2015,Jan,16; 2014,Jan,11; 2013,Jul,3-5

63265 **Laminectomy for excision or evacuation of intraspinal lesion other than neoplasm, extradural; cervical**
48.9 48.9 **FUD** 090 C 80
AMA: 2016,Jan,13; 2015,Jan,16; 2014,Jan,11; 2013,Jul,3-5

63266 **thoracic**
50.3 50.3 **FUD** 090 C 80
AMA: 2014,Jan,11; 2013,Jul,3-5

63267 **lumbar**
40.0 40.0 **FUD** 090 C 80
AMA: 2016,Jan,13; 2015,Jan,16; 2014,Jan,11; 2013,Jul,3-5

63268 **sacral**
42.0 42.0 **FUD** 090 C 80
AMA: 2016,Jan,13; 2015,Jan,16; 2014,Jan,11; 2013,Jul,3-5

63270 **Laminectomy for excision of intraspinal lesion other than neoplasm, intradural; cervical**
61.2 61.2 **FUD** 090 C 80
AMA: 2016,Jan,13; 2015,Jan,16; 2014,Jan,11; 2013,Jul,3-5

63271 **thoracic**
60.6 60.6 **FUD** 090 C 80
AMA: 2016,Jan,13; 2015,Jan,16; 2014,Jan,11; 2013,Jul,3-5

63272 **lumbar**
55.3 55.3 **FUD** 090 C 80
AMA: 2016,Jan,13; 2015,Jan,16; 2014,Jan,11; 2013,Jul,3-5

63273 **sacral**
54.8 54.8 **FUD** 090 C 80
AMA: 2016,Jan,13; 2015,Jan,16; 2014,Jan,11; 2013,Jul,3-5

63275 **Laminectomy for biopsy/excision of intraspinal neoplasm; extradural, cervical**
52.7 52.7 **FUD** 090 C 80
AMA: 2016,Jan,13; 2015,Jan,16; 2014,Jan,11; 2013,Jul,3-5

63276 **extradural, thoracic**
52.3 52.3 **FUD** 090 C 80
AMA: 2016,Jan,13; 2015,Jan,16; 2014,Jan,11; 2013,Jul,3-5

63277 **extradural, lumbar**
45.3 45.3 **FUD** 090 C 80
AMA: 2016,Jan,13; 2015,Jan,16; 2014,Jan,11; 2013,Jul,3-5

63278 **extradural, sacral**
46.9 46.9 **FUD** 090 C 80
AMA: 2016,Jan,13; 2015,Jan,16; 2014,Jan,11; 2013,Jul,3-5

63280 **intradural, extramedullary, cervical**
62.0 62.0 **FUD** 090 C 80
AMA: 2016,Jan,13; 2015,Jan,16; 2014,Jan,11; 2013,Jul,3-5

63281 **intradural, extramedullary, thoracic**
61.2 61.2 **FUD** 090 C 80
AMA: 2016,Jan,13; 2015,Jan,16; 2014,Jan,11; 2013,Jul,3-5

63282 **intradural, extramedullary, lumbar**
57.6 57.6 **FUD** 090 C 80
AMA: 2016,Jan,13; 2015,Jan,16; 2014,Jan,11; 2013,Jul,3-5

63283 **intradural, sacral**
55.4 55.4 **FUD** 090 C 80
AMA: 2016,Jan,13; 2015,Jan,16; 2014,Jan,11; 2013,Jul,3-5

63285 **intradural, intramedullary, cervical**
77.1 77.1 **FUD** 090 C 80
AMA: 2016,Jan,13; 2015,Jan,16; 2014,Jan,11; 2013,Jul,3-5

63286 **intradural, intramedullary, thoracic**
75.9 75.9 **FUD** 090 C 80
AMA: 2016,Jan,13; 2015,Jan,16; 2014,Jan,11; 2013,Jul,3-5

63287 **intradural, intramedullary, thoracolumbar**
81.2 81.2 **FUD** 090 C 80
AMA: 2016,Jan,13; 2015,Jan,16; 2014,Jan,11; 2013,Jul,3-5

63290 **combined extradural-intradural lesion, any level**
EXCLUDES *Drainage intramedullary cyst or syrinx (63172-63173)*
81.0 81.0 **FUD** 090 C 80
AMA: 2016,Jan,13; 2015,Jan,16; 2014,Jan,11; 2013,Jul,3-5

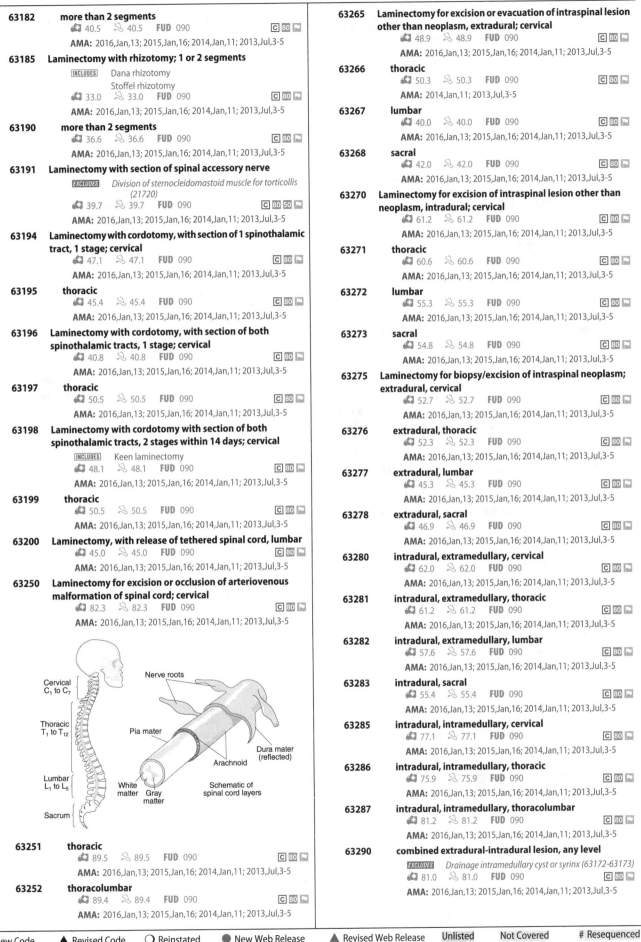

63295 — **63655**

Nervous System

+ **63295** Osteoplastic reconstruction of dorsal spinal elements, following primary intraspinal procedure (List separately in addition to code for primary procedure)

> *EXCLUDES* Procedure performed at the same vertebral segment(s) (22590-22614, 22840-22844, 63050-63051)
> Code first (63172-63173, 63185, 63190, 63200-63290)
> 🔩 9.85 🔪 9.85 **FUD** ZZZ C 80
> **AMA:** 2014,Jan,11

63300-63308 Vertebral Corpectomy for Intraspinal Lesion: Anterior/Anterolateral Approach

> *EXCLUDES* Arthrodesis (22548-22585)
> Spinal reconstruction (20930-20938)

63300 Vertebral corpectomy (vertebral body resection), partial or complete, for excision of intraspinal lesion, single segment; extradural, cervical
> 🔩 53.8 🔪 53.8 **FUD** 090 C 80
> **AMA:** 2016,Jan,13; 2015,Jan,16; 2014,Jan,11; 2013,Jul,3-5

63301 extradural, thoracic by transthoracic approach
> 🔩 64.8 🔪 64.8 **FUD** 090 C 80
> **AMA:** 2016,Jan,13; 2015,Jan,16; 2014,Jan,11; 2013,Jul,3-5

63302 extradural, thoracic by thoracolumbar approach
> 🔩 63.8 🔪 63.8 **FUD** 090 C 80
> **AMA:** 2016,Jan,13; 2015,Jan,16; 2014,Jan,11; 2013,Jul,3-5

63303 extradural, lumbar or sacral by transperitoneal or retroperitoneal approach
> 🔩 67.9 🔪 67.9 **FUD** 090 C 80
> **AMA:** 2016,Jan,13; 2015,Jan,16; 2014,Jan,11; 2013,Jul,3-5

63304 intradural, cervical
> 🔩 68.5 🔪 68.5 **FUD** 090 C 80
> **AMA:** 2016,Jan,13; 2015,Jan,16; 2014,Jan,11; 2013,Jul,3-5

63305 intradural, thoracic by transthoracic approach
> 🔩 71.2 🔪 71.2 **FUD** 090 C 80
> **AMA:** 2016,Jan,13; 2015,Jan,16; 2014,Jan,11; 2013,Jul,3-5

63306 intradural, thoracic by thoracolumbar approach
> 🔩 67.4 🔪 67.4 **FUD** 090 C 80
> **AMA:** 2016,Jan,13; 2015,Jan,16; 2014,Jan,11; 2013,Jul,3-5

63307 intradural, lumbar or sacral by transperitoneal or retroperitoneal approach
> 🔩 67.5 🔪 67.5 **FUD** 090 C 80
> **AMA:** 2016,Jan,13; 2015,Jan,16; 2014,Jan,11; 2013,Jul,3-5

+ **63308** each additional segment (List separately in addition to codes for single segment)
> Code first (63300-63307)
> 🔩 9.53 🔪 9.53 **FUD** ZZZ C 80
> **AMA:** 2014,Jan,11

63600-63615 Stereotactic Procedures of the Spinal Cord

63600 Creation of lesion of spinal cord by stereotactic method, percutaneous, any modality (including stimulation and/or recording)
> 🔩 26.1 🔪 26.1 **FUD** 090 T A2 80
> **AMA:** 2014,Jan,11

63610 Stereotactic stimulation of spinal cord, percutaneous, separate procedure not followed by other surgery
> 🔩 12.3 🔪 12.3 **FUD** 000 T A2 80
> **AMA:** 2014,Jan,11

63615 Stereotactic biopsy, aspiration, or excision of lesion, spinal cord
> 🔩 28.2 🔪 28.2 **FUD** 090 T R2
> **AMA:** 2014,Jan,11

63620-63621 Stereotactic Radiosurgery (SRS): Spine

> *INCLUDES* Computer assisted planning
> Planning dosimetry, targeting, positioning, or blocking by neurosurgeon
> *EXCLUDES* Arteriovenous malformations (see Radiation Oncology Section)
> Intensity modulated beam delivery plan and treatment (77301, 77385-77386)
> Radiation treatment management by the same provider (77427-77432)
> Stereotactic body radiation therapy (77373, 77435)
> Stereotactic computer-assisted procedures (61781-61783)
> Treatment planning, physics, dosimetry, treatment delivery and management provided by the radiation oncologist (77261-77790 [77295, 77385, 77386, 77387, 77424, 77425])

63620 Stereotactic radiosurgery (particle beam, gamma ray, or linear accelerator); 1 spinal lesion
> *EXCLUDES* Use of code more than one time per treatment course
> 🔩 32.8 🔪 32.8 **FUD** 090 B 80
> **AMA:** 2016,Jan,13; 2015,Jun,6; 2015,Jan,16; 2014,Jan,11; 2011,Jul,12-13

+ **63621** each additional spinal lesion (List separately in addition to code for primary procedure)
> *EXCLUDES* Use of code more than one time per lesion
> Use of code more than two times per entire treatment course
> Code first (63620)
> 🔩 7.52 🔪 7.52 **FUD** ZZZ B 80
> **AMA:** 2016,Jan,13; 2015,Jun,6; 2015,Jan,16; 2014,Jan,11; 2011,Jul,12-13

63650-63688 Spinal Neurostimulation

> *INCLUDES* Complex and simple neurostimulators
> *EXCLUDES* Analysis and programming of neurostimulator pulse generator (95970-95975)

63650 Percutaneous implantation of neurostimulator electrode array, epidural
> *INCLUDES* The following are components of a neurostimulator system:
> Collection of contacts of which four or more provide the electrical stimulation in the epidural space
> Contacts on a catheter-type lead (array)
> Extension
> External controller
> Implanted neurostimulator
> 🔩 11.9 🔪 37.8 **FUD** 010 J J8
> **AMA:** 2016,Jan,11; 2016,Jan,13; 2015,Dec,18; 2015,Jan,16; 2014,Jan,11; 2013,Oct,18; 2012,Jan,15-42; 2011,Apr,9; 2011,Apr,10-11; 2011,Jan,11

63655 Laminectomy for implantation of neurostimulator electrodes, plate/paddle, epidural
> *INCLUDES* The following are components of a neurostimulator system:
> Collection of contacts of which four or more provide the electrical stimulation in the epidural space
> Contacts on a plate or paddle-shaped surface for systems placed by open exposure
> Extension
> External controller
> Implanted neurostimulator
> 🔩 24.0 🔪 24.0 **FUD** 090 J J8 80
> **AMA:** 2016,Jan,13; 2015,Jan,16; 2014,Jan,11; 2012,Jan,15-42; 2011,Apr,10-11; 2011,Apr,9

63661 Removal of spinal neurostimulator electrode percutaneous array(s), including fluoroscopy, when performed

INCLUDES The following are components of a neurostimulator system:
Collection of contacts of which four or more provide the electrical stimulation in the epidural space
Contacts on a catheter-type lead (array)
Extension
External controller
Implanted neurostimulator

EXCLUDES Use of code when removing or replacing a temporary array placed percutaneously for an external generator

9.29   16.5   **FUD** 010   Q2 G2 80

AMA: 2016,Jan,13; 2015,Jan,16; 2014,Jan,11; 2011,Apr,10-11; 2011,Apr,9; 2011,Jan,8

63662 Removal of spinal neurostimulator electrode plate/paddle(s) placed via laminotomy or laminectomy, including fluoroscopy, when performed

INCLUDES The following are components of a neurostimulator system:
Collection of contacts of which four or more provide the electrical stimulation in the epidural space
Contacts on a plate or paddle-shaped surface for systems placed by open exposure
Extension
External controller
Implanted neurostimulator

24.2   24.2   **FUD** 090   Q2 G2 80

AMA: 2016,Jan,13; 2015,Jan,16; 2014,Jan,11; 2011,Apr,10-11; 2011,Apr,9; 2011,Jan,8

63663 Revision including replacement, when performed, of spinal neurostimulator electrode percutaneous array(s), including fluoroscopy, when performed

INCLUDES The following are components of a neurostimulator system:
Collection of contacts of which four or more provide the electrical stimulation in the epidural space
Contacts on a catheter-type lead (array)
Extension
External controller
Implanted neurostimulator

EXCLUDES Removal of spinal neurostimulator electrode percutaneous array(s), plate/paddle(s) (63661-63662)
Use of code when removing or replacing a temporary array placed percutaneously for an external generator

13.0   22.6   **FUD** 010   J J8 80

AMA: 2016,Jan,13; 2015,Jan,16; 2014,Jan,11; 2011,Apr,10-11; 2011,Apr,9; 2011,Jan,8

63664 Revision including replacement, when performed, of spinal neurostimulator electrode plate/paddle(s) placed via laminotomy or laminectomy, including fluoroscopy, when performed

INCLUDES The following are components of a neurostimulator system:
Collection of contacts of which four or more provide the electrical stimulation in the epidural space
Contacts on a plate or paddle-shaped surface for systems placed by open exposure
Extension
External controller
Implanted neurostimulator

EXCLUDES Removal of spinal neurostimulator electrode percutaneous array(s), plate/paddle(s) (63661-63662)

25.0   25.0   **FUD** 090   J J8 80

AMA: 2016,Jan,13; 2015,Jan,16; 2014,Jan,11; 2011,Apr,10-11; 2011,Apr,9; 2011,Jan,8

63685 Insertion or replacement of spinal neurostimulator pulse generator or receiver, direct or inductive coupling

EXCLUDES Revision/removal neurostimulator pulse generator/receiver (63688)
Use of code for insertion/replacement with code for revision/removal (63688)

10.6   10.6   **FUD** 010   J J8 80

AMA: 2016,Jan,13; 2015,Jan,16; 2014,Jan,11; 2012,Jan,15-42; 2011,Apr,10-11; 2011,Jan,11

63688 Revision or removal of implanted spinal neurostimulator pulse generator or receiver

EXCLUDES Use of code for revision/removal with code for insertion/replacement (63685)

10.7   10.7   **FUD** 010   Q2 A2

AMA: 2016,Jan,13; 2015,Jan,16; 2014,Jan,11; 2011,Apr,10-11

63700-63706 Repair Congenital Neural Tube Defects

EXCLUDES Complex skin repair (see appropriate integumentary closure code)

63700 Repair of meningocele; less than 5 cm diameter

33.8   33.8   **FUD** 090   63 C 80

AMA: 2014,Jan,11

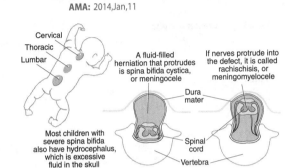

Cervical
Thoracic
Lumbar

A fluid-filled herniation that protrudes is spina bifida cystica, or meningocele

If nerves protrude into the defect, it is called rachischisis, or meningomyelocele

Dura mater

Most children with severe spina bifida also have hydrocephalus, which is excessive fluid in the skull

Spinal cord

Vertebra

63702 larger than 5 cm diameter

36.8   36.8   **FUD** 090   63 C 80

AMA: 2014,Jan,11

63704 Repair of myelomeningocele; less than 5 cm diameter

48.6   48.6   **FUD** 090   63 C 80

AMA: 2014,Jan,11

63706 larger than 5 cm diameter

49.3   49.3   **FUD** 090   63 C 80

AMA: 2014,Jan,11

63707-63710 Repair Dural Cerebrospinal Fluid Leak

63707 Repair of dural/cerebrospinal fluid leak, not requiring laminectomy

26.7   26.7   **FUD** 090   C 80

AMA: 2014,Jan,11

63709 Repair of dural/cerebrospinal fluid leak or pseudomeningocele, with laminectomy

32.0   32.0   **FUD** 090   C 80

AMA: 2014,Jan,11

63710 Dural graft, spinal

EXCLUDES Laminectomy and section of dentate ligament (63180, 63182)

31.5   31.5   **FUD** 090   C 80

AMA: 2014,Jan,11

63740-63746 Cerebrospinal Fluid (CSF) Shunt: Lumbar

EXCLUDES Placement of subarachnoid catheter with reservoir and/or pump:
Not requiring laminectomy (62350, 62360-62362)
With laminectomy (62351, 62360-62362)

63740 Creation of shunt, lumbar, subarachnoid-peritoneal, -pleural, or other; including laminectomy

27.5   27.5   **FUD** 090   C 80

AMA: 2014,Jan,11

63741 percutaneous, not requiring laminectomy

19.7   19.7   **FUD** 090   T 80

AMA: 2014,Jan,11

Nervous System

63744 — 64463

63744	**Replacement, irrigation or revision of lumbosubarachnoid shunt**

⚙ 19.6   ⚕ 19.6   **FUD** 090   T A2 80 ▭

AMA: 2014,Jan,11

63746	**Removal of entire lumbosubarachnoid shunt system without replacement**

⚙ 17.6   ⚕ 17.6   **FUD** 090   Q2 A2 80 ▭

AMA: 2014,Jan,11

64400-64463 Nerve Blocks

EXCLUDES   Epidural or subarachnoid injection (62320-62327)
Nerve destruction (62280-62282, 64600-64681 [64633, 64634, 64635, 64636])

64400	**Injection, anesthetic agent; trigeminal nerve, any division or branch**

⚙ 2.04   ⚕ 3.63   **FUD** 000   T P3 50 ▭

AMA: 2016,Jan,13; 2015,Jan,16; 2014,Jan,11; 2013,Jan,13-14; 2012,Jan,15-42; 2011,Feb,4-5; 2011,Jan,11

64402	**facial nerve**

⚙ 2.26   ⚕ 3.71   **FUD** 000   Q1 N1 50 ▭

AMA: 2016,Jan,13; 2015,Jan,16; 2014,Jan,11; 2013,Jan,13-14; 2012,Jan,15-42; 2011,Feb,4-5; 2011,Jan,11

64405	**greater occipital nerve**

⚙ 1.82   ⚕ 2.88   **FUD** 000   T P3 50 ▭

AMA: 2016,Jan,13; 2015,Jan,16; 2014,Jan,11; 2013,Jan,13-14; 2012,Jan,15-42; 2011,Feb,4-5; 2011,Jan,11

64408	**vagus nerve**

⚙ 2.14   ⚕ 2.91   **FUD** 000   T P3 80 50 ▭

AMA: 2016,Jan,13; 2015,Jan,16; 2014,Jan,11; 2013,Jan,13-14; 2012,Jan,15-42; 2011,Feb,4-5; 2011,Jan,11

64410	**phrenic nerve**

⚙ 2.00   ⚕ 3.48   **FUD** 000   T A2 80 50 ▭

AMA: 2016,Jan,13; 2015,Jan,16; 2014,Jan,11; 2013,Jan,13-14; 2012,Jan,15-42; 2011,Feb,4-5; 2011,Jan,11

64413	**cervical plexus**

⚙ 2.33   ⚕ 3.61   **FUD** 000   T P3 50 ▭

AMA: 2016,Jan,13; 2015,Jan,16; 2014,Jan,11; 2013,Jan,13-14; 2012,Jan,15-42; 2011,Feb,4-5; 2011,Jan,11

64415	**brachial plexus, single**

⚙ 1.87   ⚕ 3.36   **FUD** 000   T A2 50 ▭

AMA: 2016,Jan,13; 2015,Jan,16; 2014,Jan,11; 2013,Jan,13-14; 2012,Jan,15-42; 2011,Feb,4-5; 2011,Jan,11

64416	**brachial plexus, continuous infusion by catheter (including catheter placement)**

EXCLUDES   Management of epidural or subarachnoid continuous drug administration (01996)

⚙ 2.26   ⚕ 2.26   **FUD** 000   T 62 50 ▭

AMA: 2016,Jan,13; 2015,Jan,16; 2014,Jan,11; 2013,Jan,13-14; 2012,Jan,15-42; 2011,Feb,4-5; 2011,Jan,11

64417	**axillary nerve**

⚙ 2.04   ⚕ 3.68   **FUD** 000   T A2 50 ▭

AMA: 2016,Jan,13; 2015,Jan,16; 2014,Jan,11; 2013,Jan,13-14; 2012,Jan,15-42; 2011,Feb,4-5; 2011,Jan,11

64418	**suprascapular nerve**

⚙ 2.19   ⚕ 4.14   **FUD** 000   T P3 50 ▭

AMA: 2016,Jan,13; 2015,Jan,16; 2014,Jan,11; 2013,Jan,13-14; 2012,Jan,15-42; 2011,Feb,4-5; 2011,Jan,11

64420	**intercostal nerve, single**

⚙ 1.96   ⚕ 3.20   **FUD** 000   T A2 ▭

AMA: 2016,Jan,13; 2016,Jan,9; 2015,Jun,3; 2015,Jan,16; 2014,Jan,11; 2013,Jan,13-14; 2012,Jan,15-42; 2011,Feb,4-5; 2011,Jan,11

64421	**intercostal nerves, multiple, regional block**

⚙ 2.64   ⚕ 4.29   **FUD** 000   T A2 50 ▭

AMA: 2016,Jan,13; 2016,Jan,9; 2015,Jun,3; 2015,Jan,16; 2014,Jan,11; 2013,Jan,13-14; 2012,Jan,15-42; 2011,Feb,4-5; 2011,Jan,11

64425	**ilioinguinal, iliohypogastric nerves**

⚙ 2.68   ⚕ 3.76   **FUD** 000   T P3 50 ▭

AMA: 2016,Jan,13; 2015,Jun,3; 2015,Jan,16; 2014,Jan,11; 2013,Jan,13-14; 2012,Jan,15-42; 2011,Feb,4-5; 2011,Jan,11

64430	**pudendal nerve**

⚙ 2.36   ⚕ 3.94   **FUD** 000   T A2 50 ▭

AMA: 2016,Jan,13; 2015,Jan,16; 2014,Jan,11; 2013,Jan,13-14; 2012,Jan,15-42; 2011,Feb,4-5; 2011,Jan,11

64435	**paracervical (uterine) nerve** ♀

⚙ 2.39   ⚕ 3.87   **FUD** 000   T P3 50 ▭

AMA: 2016,Jan,13; 2015,Jan,16; 2014,Jan,11; 2013,Jan,13-14; 2012,Feb,11; 2012,Jan,15-42; 2011,Feb,4-5; 2011,Jan,11

64445	**sciatic nerve, single**

⚙ 2.08   ⚕ 3.87   **FUD** 000   T P3 50 ▭

AMA: 2016,Jan,13; 2015,Jan,16; 2014,Jan,11; 2013,Jan,13-14; 2012,Apr,19; 2011,Dec,8-9; 2011,Feb,4-5

64446	**sciatic nerve, continuous infusion by catheter (including catheter placement)**

EXCLUDES   Management of epidural or subarachnoid continuous drug administration (01996)

⚙ 2.27   ⚕ 2.27   **FUD** 000   T 62 50 ▭

AMA: 2016,Jan,13; 2015,Jan,16; 2014,Jan,11; 2013,Jan,13-14; 2011,Feb,4-5

64447	**femoral nerve, single**

EXCLUDES   Management of epidural or subarachnoid continuous drug administration (01996)

⚙ 1.90   ⚕ 3.41   **FUD** 000   T P3 50 ▭

AMA: 2016,Jan,13; 2015,Sep,12; 2015,Jan,16; 2014,Dec,16; 2014,Dec,16; 2014,Nov,14; 2014,Jan,11; 2013,Jan,13-14; 2011,Feb,4-5

64448	**femoral nerve, continuous infusion by catheter (including catheter placement)**

EXCLUDES   Management of epidural or subarachnoid continuous drug administration (01996)

⚙ 2.04   ⚕ 2.04   **FUD** 000   T 62 50 ▭

AMA: 2016,Jan,13; 2015,Sep,12; 2015,Jan,16; 2014,Dec,16; 2014,Dec,16; 2014,Nov,14; 2014,Jan,11; 2013,Jan,13-14; 2011,Feb,4-5

64449	**lumbar plexus, posterior approach, continuous infusion by catheter (including catheter placement)**

EXCLUDES   Management of epidural or subarachnoid continuous drug administration (01996)

⚙ 2.41   ⚕ 2.41   **FUD** 000   T 62 50 ▭

AMA: 2016,Jan,13; 2015,Jan,16; 2014,Jan,11; 2013,Jan,13-14; 2011,Feb,4-5

64450	**other peripheral nerve or branch**

EXCLUDES   Morton's neuroma (64455, 64632)

⚙ 1.31   ⚕ 2.27   **FUD** 000   T P3 50 ▭

AMA: 2016,Jan,13; 2015,Nov,10; 2015,Sep,12; 2015,Jun,3; 2015,Jan,16; 2014,Jan,11; 2013,Jan,13-14; 2012,Jan,15-42; 2011,Feb,4-5; 2011,Jan,11

64455	**Injection(s), anesthetic agent and/or steroid, plantar common digital nerve(s) (eg, Morton's neuroma)**

EXCLUDES   Destruction by neurolytic agent; plantar common digital nerve (64632)

⚙ 1.00   ⚕ 1.36   **FUD** 000   T P3 80 50 ▭

AMA: 2016,Jan,13; 2015,Jan,16; 2014,Jan,11; 2013,Nov,14; 2013,Jan,13-14; 2012,Sep,14-15; 2012,Sep,14-15; 2011,Feb,4-5

64461	**Resequenced code. See code following 64484.**
64462	**Resequenced code. See code following 64484.**
64463	**Resequenced code. See code following 64484.**

64479-64484 Transforaminal Injection

INCLUDES Imaging guidance (fluoroscopy or CT) and contrast injection
EXCLUDES Epidural or subarachnoid injection (62320-62327)
Nerve destruction (62280-62282, 64600-64681 [64633, 64634, 64635, 64636])

64479 Injection(s), anesthetic agent and/or steroid, transforaminal epidural, with imaging guidance (fluoroscopy or CT); cervical or thoracic, single level

> **EXCLUDES** Transforaminal epidural injection using ultrasonic guidance (0228T)

> 🚗 3.81 ⚕ 6.72 **FUD** 000 T A2 50 ▫

> **AMA:** 2016,Jan,13; 2016,Jan,9; 2015,Jan,16; 2014,Jan,11; 2012,Jul,3-6; 2012,Jan,15-42; 2011,Jul,16-17; 2011,Feb,4-5; 2011,Jan,8

Thoracic vertebra (superior view) — Spinous process, Transverse costal facet, Lamina, Superior articular facets, Pedicle, Superior articular facets, Superior costal facet, Vertebral body. Superior view of C7 — Spinous process, Superior articular facets, Vertebral body

+ 64480 cervical or thoracic, each additional level (List separately in addition to code for primary procedure)

> **EXCLUDES** Transforaminal epidural injection at T12-L1 level (64479)
> Transforaminal epidural injection using ultrasonic guidance (0229T)

> Code first (64479)

> 🚗 1.82 ⚕ 3.22 **FUD** ZZZ N N1 50 ▫

> **AMA:** 2016,Jan,13; 2016,Jan,9; 2015,Jan,16; 2014,Jan,11; 2012,Jul,3-6; 2012,Jan,15-42; 2011,Jul,16-17; 2011,Feb,4-5; 2011,Jan,11; 2011,Jan,8

64483 lumbar or sacral, single level

> **EXCLUDES** Transforaminal epidural injection using ultrasonic guidance (0230T)

> 🚗 3.25 ⚕ 6.26 **FUD** 000 T A2 50 ▫

> **AMA:** 2016,Jan,9; 2016,Jan,13; 2015,Jan,16; 2014,Jan,11; 2012,Jul,3-6; 2012,May,14-15; 2011,Jul,16-17; 2011,Feb,4-5; 2011,Jan,8

+ 64484 lumbar or sacral, each additional level (List separately in addition to code for primary procedure)

> **EXCLUDES** Transforaminal epidural injection using ultrasonic guidance (0231T)

> Code first (64483)

> 🚗 1.50 ⚕ 2.50 **FUD** ZZZ N N1 50 ▫

> **AMA:** 2016,Jan,13; 2016,Jan,9; 2015,Jan,16; 2014,Jan,11; 2012,Jul,3-6; 2012,Jan,15-42; 2011,Jul,16-17; 2011,Feb,4-5; 2011,Jan,11

[64461, 64462, 64463] Paravertebral Blocks

INCLUDES Radiological guidance (76942, 77002-77003)
EXCLUDES Injection of:
Anesthetic agent (64420-64421, 64479-64480)
Diagnostic or therapeutic substance (62320, 62324, 64490-64492)

 # 64461 Paravertebral block (PVB) (paraspinous block), thoracic; single injection site (includes imaging guidance, when performed)

> 🚗 2.49 ⚕ 4.22 **FUD** 000 T P3 50 ▫

> **AMA:** 2016,Jan,9

+ # 64462 second and any additional injection site(s) (includes imaging guidance, when performed) (List separately in addition to code for primary procedure)

> **EXCLUDES** Procedure performed more than one time per day

> Code first (64461)

> 🚗 1.57 ⚕ 2.39 **FUD** ZZZ N N1 50 ▫

> **AMA:** 2016,Jan,9

 # 64463 continuous infusion by catheter (includes imaging guidance, when performed)

> 🚗 2.41 ⚕ 4.59 **FUD** 000 T P3 50 ▫

> **AMA:** 2016,Jan,9

64486-64489 Transversus Abdominis Plane (TAP) Block

64486 Transversus abdominis plane (TAP) block (abdominal plane block, rectus sheath block) unilateral; by injection(s) (includes imaging guidance, when performed)

> 🚗 1.82 ⚕ 3.54 **FUD** 000 N N1 50 ▫

> **AMA:** 2016,Jan,13; 2015,Jun,3

64487 by continuous infusion(s) (includes imaging guidance, when performed)

> 🚗 2.13 ⚕ 4.36 **FUD** 000 N N1 50 ▫

> **AMA:** 2016,Jan,13; 2015,Jun,3

64488 Transversus abdominis plane (TAP) block (abdominal plane block, rectus sheath block) bilateral; by injections (includes imaging guidance, when performed)

> 🚗 2.30 ⚕ 4.37 **FUD** 000 N N1 ▫

> **AMA:** 2016,Jan,13; 2015,Jun,3

64489 by continuous infusions (includes imaging guidance, when performed)

> 🚗 2.59 ⚕ 6.08 **FUD** 000 N N1 ▫

> **AMA:** 2016,Jan,13; 2015,Jun,3

64490-64495 Paraspinal Nerve Injections

INCLUDES Image guidance (CT or fluoroscopy) and any contrast injection
EXCLUDES Injection without imaging (20552-20553)
Ultrasonic guidance (0213T-0218T)

64490 Injection(s), diagnostic or therapeutic agent, paravertebral facet (zygapophyseal) joint (or nerves innervating that joint) with image guidance (fluoroscopy or CT), cervical or thoracic; single level

> **INCLUDES** Injection of T12-L1 joint and nerves that innervate that joint

> 🚗 3.07 ⚕ 5.43 **FUD** 000 T 62 80 50 ▫

> **AMA:** 2016,Jan,13; 2016,Jan,9; 2015,Jan,16; 2014,Jan,11; 2012,Oct,14; 2012,Jun,10-11; 2012,Jan,15-42; 2011,Feb,4-5; 2011,Jan,11; 2011,Jan,8

+ 64491 second level (List separately in addition to code for primary procedure)

> Code first (64490)

> 🚗 1.74 ⚕ 2.68 **FUD** ZZZ N N1 80 50 ▫

> **AMA:** 2016,Jan,13; 2016,Jan,9; 2015,Jan,16; 2014,Jan,11; 2012,Oct,14; 2012,Jun,10-11; 2012,Jan,15-42; 2011,Feb,4-5; 2011,Jan,11; 2011,Jan,8

+ 64492 third and any additional level(s) (List separately in addition to code for primary procedure)

> **EXCLUDES** Procedure performed more than one time per day

> Code also when appropriate (64491)

> Code first (64490)

> 🚗 1.76 ⚕ 2.69 **FUD** ZZZ N N1 80 50 ▫

> **AMA:** 2016,Jan,13; 2016,Jan,9; 2015,Jan,16; 2014,Jan,11; 2012,Oct,14; 2012,Jun,10-11; 2012,Jan,15-42; 2011,Feb,4-5; 2011,Jan,8

64493 Injection(s), diagnostic or therapeutic agent, paravertebral facet (zygapophyseal) joint (or nerves innervating that joint) with image guidance (fluoroscopy or CT), lumbar or sacral; single level

> 🚗 2.63 ⚕ 4.93 **FUD** 000 T 62 80 50 ▫

> **AMA:** 2016,Jan,13; 2015,Jan,16; 2014,Jan,11; 2012,Oct,14; 2012,Jun,10-11; 2012,Jan,15-42; 2011,Feb,4-5; 2011,Feb,8-9; 2011,Jan,8

+ 64494 second level (List separately in addition to code for primary procedure)

> Code first (64493)

> 🚗 1.50 ⚕ 2.47 **FUD** ZZZ N N1 80 50 ▫

> **AMA:** 2016,Jan,13; 2015,Jan,16; 2014,Jan,11; 2012,Oct,14; 2012,Jun,10-11; 2011,Feb,4-5; 2011,Jan,8

Nervous System

64495 — 64590

+ **64495** third and any additional level(s) (List separately in addition to code for primary procedure)

EXCLUDES Procedure performed more than one time per day
Code also when appropriate (64494)
Code first (64493)

📋 1.52 ⚕ 2.48 **FUD** ZZZ N N1 80 50 ▣

AMA: 2016,Jan,13; 2015,Jan,16; 2014,Jan,11; 2012,Oct,14; 2012,Jun,10-11; 2011,Feb,4-5; 2011,Jan,8

64505-64530 Sympathetic Nerve Blocks

64505 Injection, anesthetic agent; sphenopalatine ganglion

📋 2.50 ⚕ 2.98 **FUD** 000 T P3 50 ▣

AMA: 2016,Jan,13; 2015,Jan,16; 2014,Jul,8; 2014,Jan,11; 2013,Jan,13-14; 2012,Jan,15-42; 2011,Feb,4-5; 2011,Jan,11

64508 carotid sinus (separate procedure)

📋 2.11 ⚕ 1.78 **FUD** 000 T P3 80 50 ▣

AMA: 2016,Jan,13; 2015,Jan,16; 2014,Jan,11; 2013,Jan,13-14; 2011,Feb,4-5

64510 stellate ganglion (cervical sympathetic)

📋 2.12 ⚕ 3.62 **FUD** 000 T A2 50 ▣

AMA: 2016,Jan,13; 2015,Jan,16; 2014,Jan,11; 2013,Jan,13-14; 2011,Feb,4-5

64517 superior hypogastric plexus

📋 3.52 ⚕ 5.19 **FUD** 000 T A2 ▣

AMA: 2016,Jan,13; 2015,Jan,16; 2014,Jan,11; 2013,Jan,13-14; 2012,Jan,15-42; 2011,Feb,4-5; 2011,Jan,11

64520 lumbar or thoracic (paravertebral sympathetic)

📋 2.33 ⚕ 5.30 **FUD** 000 T A2 50 ▣

AMA: 2016,Jan,13; 2015,Jan,16; 2014,Jan,11; 2013,Jan,13-14; 2012,Jan,15-42; 2011,Feb,4-5; 2011,Jan,11

64530 celiac plexus, with or without radiologic monitoring

EXCLUDES Transmural anesthetic injection with transendoscopic ultrasound-guidance (43253)

📋 2.65 ⚕ 5.43 **FUD** 000 T A2 ▣

AMA: 2016,Jan,13; 2015,Jan,16; 2014,Jan,11; 2013,Jan,13-14; 2012,Jan,15-42; 2011,Feb,4-5; 2011,Jan,11

64550 Transcutaneous Electrical Nerve Stimulation

CMS: 100-03,10.2 Transcutaneous Electrical Nerve Stimulation (TENS) for Acute Postoperative Pain

EXCLUDES Analysis and programming neurostimulator pulse generator (95970-95975)
Implantation of electrode array(s), either trial or permanent, with pulse generator for peripheral subcutaneous field stimulation (64999)

64550 Application of surface (transcutaneous) neurostimulator

📋 0.25 ⚕ 0.45 **FUD** 000 A ▣

AMA: 2016,Jan,13; 2015,Jan,16; 2014,Jan,11; 2012,Jan,15-42; 2011,Feb,4-5; 2011,Jan,11

64553-64570 Electrical Nerve Stimulation: Insertion/Replacement/Removal/Revision

INCLUDES Simple and complex neurostimulators
EXCLUDES Analysis and programming of neurostimulator pulse generator (95970-95975)

64553 Percutaneous implantation of neurostimulator electrode array; cranial nerve

EXCLUDES Open procedure (61885-61886)

📋 4.48 ⚕ 5.95 **FUD** 010 J J8 80 ▣

AMA: 2016,Jan,13; 2015,Jan,16; 2014,Jan,11; 2011,Feb,4-5

64555 peripheral nerve (excludes sacral nerve)

EXCLUDES Posterior tibial neurostimulation (64566)

📋 4.40 ⚕ 6.01 **FUD** 010 J J8 ▣

AMA: 2016,Feb,13; 2016,Jan,13; 2015,Jan,16; 2015,Jan,13; 2014,Jan,11; 2012,Jan,15-42; 2011,Feb,4-5

64561 sacral nerve (transforaminal placement) including image guidance, if performed

📋 8.69 ⚕ 23.2 **FUD** 010 J J8 50 ▣

AMA: 2016,Jan,13; 2015,Jan,16; 2014,Sep,5; 2014,Jan,11; 2012,Dec,12; 2011,Feb,4-5

64565 neuromuscular

📋 3.78 ⚕ 5.39 **FUD** 010 J J8 ▣

AMA: 2016,Jan,13; 2015,Jan,16; 2014,Jan,11; 2012,Jan,15-42; 2011,Feb,4-5; 2011,Jan,11

64566 Posterior tibial neurostimulation, percutaneous needle electrode, single treatment, includes programming

EXCLUDES Electronic analysis of implanted neurostimulator pulse generator system (95970-95972)
Percutaneous implantation of neurostimulator electrode array; peripheral nerve (64555)

📋 0.88 ⚕ 3.60 **FUD** 000 T P3 80 ▣

AMA: 2016,Jan,13; 2015,Jan,16; 2014,Jan,11; 2011,Sep,8; 2011,Feb,4-5

64568 Incision for implantation of cranial nerve (eg, vagus nerve) neurostimulator electrode array and pulse generator

EXCLUDES Insertion, replacement of cranial neurostimulator pulse generator or receiver (61885-61886)
Removal of neurostimulator electrode array and pulse generator (64570)

📋 19.1 ⚕ 19.1 **FUD** 090 J J8 80 50 ▣

AMA: 2016,Jan,13; 2015,Jan,16; 2014,Jan,11; 2012,Jan,15-42; 2011,Sep,8; 2011,Sep,11-12; 2011,Sep,9-10; 2011,Feb,4-5

64569 Revision or replacement of cranial nerve (eg, vagus nerve) neurostimulator electrode array, including connection to existing pulse generator

EXCLUDES Removal of neurostimulator electrode array and pulse generator (64570)
Replacement of pulse generator (61885)
Revision, removal pulse generator (61888)

📋 22.8 ⚕ 22.8 **FUD** 090 J J8 80 50 ▣

AMA: 2016,Jan,13; 2015,Jan,16; 2014,Jan,11; 2011,Sep,8; 2011,Sep,9-10; 2011,Feb,4-5

64570 Removal of cranial nerve (eg, vagus nerve) neurostimulator electrode array and pulse generator

EXCLUDES Laparoscopic revision, replacement, removal, or implantation of vagus nerve blocking neurostimulator pulse generator and/or electrode array at the esophagogastric junction (0312T-0317T)
Revision, removal pulse generator (61888)

📋 18.9 ⚕ 18.9 **FUD** 090 02 G2 80 50 ▣

AMA: 2016,Jan,13; 2015,Jan,16; 2014,Jan,11; 2011,Sep,8; 2011,Sep,9-10; 2011,Feb,4-5

64575-64595 Implantation/Revision/Removal Neurostimulators: Incisional

INCLUDES Simple and complex neurostimulators
EXCLUDES Analysis and programming neurostimulator pulse generator (95970-95975)

64575 Incision for implantation of neurostimulator electrode array; peripheral nerve (excludes sacral nerve)

📋 9.19 ⚕ 9.19 **FUD** 090 J J8 ▣

AMA: 2014,Jan,11; 2011,Feb,4-5

64580 neuromuscular

📋 8.72 ⚕ 8.72 **FUD** 090 J J8 80 ▣

AMA: 2014,Jan,11; 2011,Feb,4-5

64581 sacral nerve (transforaminal placement)

📋 19.0 ⚕ 19.0 **FUD** 090 J J8 ▣

AMA: 2016,Jan,13; 2015,Jan,16; 2014,Sep,5; 2014,Jan,11; 2012,Dec,12; 2011,Feb,4-5

64585 Revision or removal of peripheral neurostimulator electrode array

📋 4.11 ⚕ 6.96 **FUD** 010 02 A2 ▣

AMA: 2014,Jan,11; 2011,Feb,4-5

64590 Insertion or replacement of peripheral or gastric neurostimulator pulse generator or receiver, direct or inductive coupling

EXCLUDES Revision, removal of neurostimulator pulse generator (64595)

📋 4.61 ⚕ 7.53 **FUD** 010 J J8 ▣

AMA: 2016,Jan,13; 2015,Jan,16; 2015,Jan,13; 2014,Jan,11; 2012,Dec,12; 2012,Jan,15-42; 2011,Sep,9-10; 2011,Feb,4-5

64595 Revision or removal of peripheral or gastric neurostimulator pulse generator or receiver

> EXCLUDES Revision, removal of neurostimulator pulse generator (64595)

> 🚑 3.63   ⚕ 6.98   **FUD** 010   Q2 A2 ▢

> **AMA:** 2016,Jan,13; 2015,Jan,16; 2014,Jan,11; 2012,Jan,15-42; 2011,Feb,4-5; 2011,Jan,11

64600-64610 Chemical Denervation Trigeminal Nerve

INCLUDES   Injection of therapeutic medication
EXCLUDES   *The following chemodenervation procedures:*
  Anal sphincter (46505)
  Bladder (52287)
  Muscle electrical stimulation or EMG with needle guidance (95873, 95874)
  Strabismus that involves the extraocular muscles (67345)
  Treatments that do not destroy the target nerve (64999)
Code also chemodenervation agent

64600 Destruction by neurolytic agent, trigeminal nerve; supraorbital, infraorbital, mental, or inferior alveolar branch

> 🚑 6.32   ⚕ 11.1   **FUD** 010   T A2 ▢

> **AMA:** 2016,Jan,13; 2015,Jan,16; 2014,Jan,11; 2012,Sep,14-15; 2012,Sep,14-15; 2011,Feb,4-5

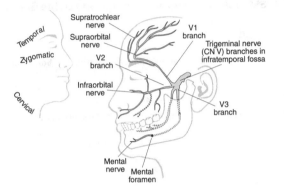

64605 second and third division branches at foramen ovale

> 🚑 11.9   ⚕ 21.4   **FUD** 010   T A2 80 50 ▢

> **AMA:** 2016,Jan,13; 2015,Jan,16; 2014,Jan,11; 2012,Sep,14-15; 2012,Sep,14-15; 2011,Feb,4-5

64610 second and third division branches at foramen ovale under radiologic monitoring

> 🚑 14.2   ⚕ 21.3   **FUD** 010   T A2 50 ▢

> **AMA:** 2016,Jan,13; 2015,Jan,16; 2014,Jan,11; 2012,Sep,14-15; 2012,Sep,14-15; 2011,Feb,4-5

64611-64617 Chemical Denervation Procedures Head and Neck

INCLUDES   Injection of therapeutic medication
EXCLUDES   *Electromyography or muscle electric stimulation guidance (95873-95874)*
  Nerve destruction of:
   Anal sphincter (46505)
   Bladder (52287)
   Extraocular muscles to treat strabismus (67345)
  Treatments that do not destroy the target nerve (64999)

64611 Chemodenervation of parotid and submandibular salivary glands, bilateral

> Code also modifier 52 for injection of fewer than four salivary glands

> 🚑 2.94   ⚕ 3.35   **FUD** 010   T P3 80 ▢

> **AMA:** 2016,Jan,13; 2015,Jan,16; 2014,Jan,11; 2012,Sep,14-15; 2012,Sep,14-15; 2011,Feb,4-5

64612 Chemodenervation of muscle(s); muscle(s) innervated by facial nerve, unilateral (eg, for blepharospasm, hemifacial spasm)

> 🚑 3.37   ⚕ 3.77   **FUD** 010   T P3 50 ▢

> **AMA:** 2016,Jan,13; 2015,Jan,16; 2014,May,5; 2014,Jan,6; 2014,Jan,11; 2013,Dec,10; 2013,Apr,5-6; 2012,Sep,14-15; 2012,Sep,14-15; 2012,Jan,15-42; 2011,Dec,19; 2011,Feb,4-5; 2011,Jan,11

64615 muscle(s) innervated by facial, trigeminal, cervical spinal and accessory nerves, bilateral (eg, for chronic migraine)

> EXCLUDES Chemodenervation (64612, 64616-64617, 64642-64647)
>   *Procedure performed more than one time per session*
> Code also any guidance performed but report only once (95873-95874)

> 🚑 3.60   ⚕ 4.14   **FUD** 010   T P3 ▢

> **AMA:** 2016,Jan,13; 2015,Jan,16; 2014,Jan,11; 2014,Jan,6; 2013,Apr,5-6

64616 neck muscle(s), excluding muscles of the larynx, unilateral (eg, for cervical dystonia, spasmodic torticollis)

> Code also guidance by muscle electrical stimulation or needle electromyography, but report only once (95873-95874)

> 🚑 3.15   ⚕ 3.62   **FUD** 010   T P3 50 ▢

> **AMA:** 2016,Jan,13; 2015,Jan,16; 2014,May,5; 2014,Jan,11; 2014,Jan,6

64617 larynx, unilateral, percutaneous (eg, for spasmodic dysphonia), includes guidance by needle electromyography, when performed

> EXCLUDES Chemodenervation of larynx via direct laryngoscopy (31570-31571)
>   *Diagnostic needle electromyography of larynx (95865)*
>   *Electrical stimulation guidance for chemodenervation (95873-95874)*

> 🚑 3.59   ⚕ 5.61   **FUD** 010   T P3 50 ▢

> **AMA:** 2016,Jan,13; 2015,Jan,16; 2014,Jan,11; 2014,Jan,6

64620-64640 [64633, 64634, 64635, 64636] Chemical Denervation Intercostal, Facet Joint, Plantar, and Pudendal Nerve(s)

INCLUDES   Injection of therapeutic medication

64620 Destruction by neurolytic agent, intercostal nerve

> 🚑 4.93   ⚕ 5.82   **FUD** 010   T A2 ▢

> **AMA:** 2016,Jan,13; 2015,Jan,16; 2014,Jan,6; 2014,Jan,11; 2012,Sep,14-15; 2012,Sep,14-15; 2011,Feb,4-5

\# **64633** Destruction by neurolytic agent, paravertebral facet joint nerve(s), with imaging guidance (fluoroscopy or CT); cervical or thoracic, single facet joint

> INCLUDES Paravertebral facet destruction of T12-L1 joint or nerve(s) that innervate that joint
>   Radiological guidance (77003, 77012)
> EXCLUDES *Denervation performed using chemical, low grade thermal, or pulsed radiofrequency methods (64999)*
>   *Destruction of paravertebral facet joint nerve(s) without imaging guidance (64999)*

> 🚑 6.54   ⚕ 12.0   **FUD** 010   T 62 50 ▢

> **AMA:** 2016,Jan,13; 2015,Feb,9; 2015,Jan,16; 2014,Jan,11; 2013,Apr,10-11; 2012,Sep,14-15; 2012,Sep,14-15; 2012,Jul,3-6; 2012,Jun,10-11

+ \# **64634** cervical or thoracic, each additional facet joint (List separately in addition to code for primary procedure)

> INCLUDES Radiological guidance (77003, 77012)
> EXCLUDES *Denervation performed using chemical, low grade thermal, or pulsed radiofrequency methods (64999)*
>   *Destruction of paravertebral facet joint nerve(s) without imaging guidance (64999)*
> Code first ([64633])

> 🚑 1.98   ⚕ 5.42   **FUD** ZZZ   N N1 50 ▢

> **AMA:** 2016,Jan,13; 2015,Feb,9; 2015,Jan,16; 2014,Jan,11; 2013,Apr,10-11; 2012,Sep,14-15; 2012,Sep,14-15; 2012,Jul,3-6; 2012,Jun,10-11

Nervous System

64635 — 64704

lumbar or sacral, single facet joint

 # 64635   lumbar or sacral, single facet joint

INCLUDES   Radiological guidance (77003, 77012)

EXCLUDES   Denervation performed using chemical, low grade thermal, or pulsed radiofrequency methods (64999)
Destruction of individual nerves, sacroiliac joint, by neurolytic agent (64640)
Destruction of paravertebral facet joint nerve(s) without imaging guidance (64999)

6.45   11.9   **FUD** 010   T 62 50

AMA: 2016,Jan,13; 2015,Feb,9; 2015,Jan,16; 2014,Jan,11; 2013,Apr,10-11; 2012,Sep,14-15; 2012,Sep,14-15; 2012,Jul,3-6; 2012,Jun,10-11

+ # 64636   lumbar or sacral, each additional facet joint (List separately in addition to code for primary procedure)

INCLUDES   Radiological guidance (77003, 77012)

EXCLUDES   Denervation performed using chemical, low grade thermal, or pulsed radiofrequency methods (64999)
Destruction of individual nerves, sacroiliac joint, by neurolytic agent (64640)
Destruction of paravertebral facet joint nerve(s) without imaging guidance (64999)

Code first ([64635])

1.73   4.93   **FUD** ZZZ   N N1 50

AMA: 2016,Jan,13; 2015,Feb,9; 2015,Jan,16; 2014,Jan,11; 2013,Apr,10-11; 2012,Sep,14-15; 2012,Sep,14-15; 2012,Jul,3-6; 2012,Jun,10-11

64630   Destruction by neurolytic agent; pudendal nerve

5.55   6.64   **FUD** 010   T A2 80

AMA: 2016,Jan,13; 2015,Jan,16; 2014,Jan,11; 2012,Sep,14-15; 2012,Sep,14-15; 2011,Feb,4-5

64632   plantar common digital nerve

EXCLUDES   Injection(s), anesthetic agent and/or steroid (64455)

1.97   2.43   **FUD** 010   T P3 80 50

AMA: 2016,Jan,13; 2015,Jul,10; 2015,Jan,16; 2014,Jan,11; 2013,Nov,14; 2013,Jan,13-14; 2012,Sep,14-15; 2012,Sep,14-15; 2011,Feb,4-5

64633   Resequenced code. See code following 64620.

64634   Resequenced code. See code following 64620.

64635   Resequenced code. See code following 64620.

64636   Resequenced code. See code before 64630.

64640   other peripheral nerve or branch

INCLUDES   Neurolytic destruction of nerves of sacroiliac joint

2.67   3.79   **FUD** 010   T P3 50

AMA: 2016,Jan,13; 2015,Jan,16; 2014,Jan,11; 2012,Sep,14-15; 2012,Sep,14-15; 2012,Jun,15-16; 2012,Jan,15-42; 2011,Feb,4-5; 2011,Jan,11

64642-64645 Chemical Denervation Extremity Muscles

INCLUDES   Trunk muscles include erector spine, obliques, paraspinal and rectus abdominus. The rest of the muscles are considered neck, head or extremity muscles.

EXCLUDES   Chemodenervation with needle-guided electromyography or with guidance provided by muscle electrical stimulation (95873-95874)
Procedure performed more than once per extremity

Code also other extremities when appropriate, up to a total of 4 units per patient (if all extremities are injected) (64642-64645)

64642   Chemodenervation of one extremity; 1-4 muscle(s)

EXCLUDES   Use of more than one base code per session (64642)

3.13   4.05   **FUD** 000   T P3

AMA: 2016,Jan,13; 2015,Jan,16; 2014,Oct,14; 2014,Jan,11; 2014,Jan,6

+ 64643   each additional extremity, 1-4 muscle(s) (List separately in addition to code for primary procedure)

Code first (64642, 64644)

2.10   2.66   **FUD** ZZZ   N N1

AMA: 2016,Jan,13; 2015,Jan,16; 2014,Oct,14; 2014,Jan,11; 2014,Jan,6

♀ 64644   Chemodenervation of one extremity; 5 or more muscles

3.43   4.65   **FUD** 000   T P3

AMA: 2016,Jan,13; 2015,Jan,16; 2014,Oct,14; 2014,Jan,11; 2014,Jan,6

+ 64645   each additional extremity, 5 or more muscles (List separately in addition to code for primary procedure)

Code first (64644)

2.41   3.27   **FUD** ZZZ   N N1

AMA: 2016,Jan,13; 2015,Jan,16; 2014,Oct,14; 2014,Jan,11; 2014,Jan,6

64646-64647 Chemical Denervation Trunk Muscles

EXCLUDES   Procedure performed more than once per extremity

64646   Chemodenervation of trunk muscle(s); 1-5 muscle(s)

EXCLUDES   Use of more than once per session (64646-64647)

3.38   4.30   **FUD** 000   T P3

AMA: 2016,Jan,13; 2015,Jan,16; 2014,Jan,11; 2014,Jan,6

64647   6 or more muscles

EXCLUDES   Use of more than once per session (64646-64647)

3.95   5.08   **FUD** 000   T P3

AMA: 2016,Jan,13; 2015,Jan,16; 2014,Jan,11; 2014,Jan,6

64650-64653 Chemical Denervation Eccrine Glands

INCLUDES   Injection of therapeutic medication

EXCLUDES   Chemodenervation of extremities (64999)

Code also drugs or other substances used

64650   Chemodenervation of eccrine glands; both axillae

1.21   2.20   **FUD** 000   T P3 80

AMA: 2016,Jan,13; 2015,Jan,16; 2014,Jan,11; 2012,Sep,14-15; 2012,Sep,14-15; 2011,Feb,4-5

64653   other area(s) (eg, scalp, face, neck), per day

EXCLUDES   Bladder chemodenervation (52287)
Hands or feet (64999)

1.57   2.76   **FUD** 000   T P3 80

AMA: 2016,Jan,13; 2015,Jan,16; 2014,Jan,11; 2012,Sep,14-15; 2012,Sep,14-15; 2011,Feb,4-5

64680-64681 Neurolysis: Celiac Plexus, Superior Hypogastric Plexus

INCLUDES   Injection of therapeutic medication
Only for lesions that abut the dura matter or that affect the spinal neural tissue

64680   Destruction by neurolytic agent, with or without radiologic monitoring; celiac plexus

EXCLUDES   Transmural neurolytic agent injection with transendoscopic ultrasound guidance (43253)

4.78   8.82   **FUD** 010   T A2

AMA: 2016,Jan,13; 2015,Jan,16; 2014,Jan,11; 2012,Sep,14-15; 2012,Sep,14-15; 2012,Jan,15-42; 2011,Feb,4-5; 2011,Jan,11

64681   superior hypogastric plexus

5.47   9.76   **FUD** 010   T A2

AMA: 2016,Jan,13; 2015,Jan,16; 2014,Jan,11; 2012,Sep,14-15; 2012,Sep,14-15; 2012,Jan,15-42; 2011,Feb,4-5; 2011,Jan,11

64702-64727 Decompression and/or Transposition of Nerve

INCLUDES   External neurolysis and/or transposition to repair or restore a nerve
Neuroplasty with nerve wrapping
Surgical decompression/freeing of nerve from scar tissue

EXCLUDES   Facial nerve decompression (69720)
Percutaneous neurolysis (62263-62264, 62280-62282)

64702   Neuroplasty; digital, 1 or both, same digit

14.3   14.3   **FUD** 090   T A2

AMA: 2016,Jan,13; 2015,Jan,16; 2014,Jan,11; 2012,Jan,15-42; 2011,Jan,11

64704   nerve of hand or foot

9.12   9.12   **FUD** 090   T A2 80

AMA: 2016,Jan,13; 2015,Jan,16; 2014,Jan,11; 2012,Jan,15-42; 2011,Jan,11

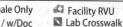 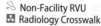

26/TC PC/TC Only   A2-B3 ASC Payment   50 Bilateral   ♂ Male Only   ♀ Female Only   Facility RVU   Non-Facility RVU   CCI
FUD Follow-up Days   **CMS:** IOM (Pub 100)   A-Y OPPSI   80/80 Surg Assist Allowed / w/Doc   Lab Crosswalk   Radiology Crosswalk   CLIA

64708 Neuroplasty, major peripheral nerve, arm or leg, open; other than specified
- 14.2   14.2 **FUD** 090   T G2 80
AMA: 2016,Jan,13; 2015,Jan,16; 2014,Jan,11; 2012,Jun,12-13; 2012,Jan,15-42; 2011,Jan,11

64712 sciatic nerve
- 16.5   16.5 **FUD** 090   T G2 80 50
AMA: 2016,Jan,13; 2015,Jan,16; 2014,Jan,11; 2012,Jun,12-13; 2012,Jan,15-42; 2011,Jan,11

64713 brachial plexus
- 20.8   20.8 **FUD** 090   T G2 80 50
AMA: 2016,Jan,13; 2015,Jan,16; 2014,Jan,11; 2013,May,12; 2012,Jun,12-13; 2012,Jan,15-42; 2011,Jan,11

64714 lumbar plexus
- 18.4   18.4 **FUD** 090   T G2 80 50
AMA: 2016,Jan,13; 2015,Jan,16; 2014,Jan,11; 2013,Dec,16; 2012,Jun,12-13; 2012,Jan,15-42; 2011,Jan,11

64716 Neuroplasty and/or transposition; cranial nerve (specify)
- 15.4   15.4 **FUD** 090   T A2 80
AMA: 2016,Jan,13; 2015,Jan,16; 2014,Jan,11; 2012,Jan,15-42; 2011,Jan,11

64718 ulnar nerve at elbow
- 16.9   16.9 **FUD** 090   T A2 80 50
AMA: 2016,Jan,13; 2015,Jan,16; 2014,Jan,11; 2012,Jan,15-42; 2011,Jan,11

64719 ulnar nerve at wrist
- 11.4   11.4 **FUD** 090   T A2 50
AMA: 2016,Jan,13; 2015,Jan,16; 2014,Jan,11; 2012,Jan,15-42; 2011,Jan,11

64721 median nerve at carpal tunnel
EXCLUDES Arthroscopic procedure (29848)
- 12.2   12.3 **FUD** 090   T A2 50
AMA: 2016,Jan,13; 2015,Jul,10; 2015,Jan,16; 2014,Jan,11; 2013,Dec,14; 2012,Oct,14; 2012,Sep,16; 2012,Jun,15-16; 2012,Jan,15-42; 2011,Jan,11

64722 Decompression; unspecified nerve(s) (specify)
- 10.6   10.6 **FUD** 090   T A2 80
AMA: 2016,Jan,13; 2015,Jan,16; 2014,Jan,11; 2012,Jan,15-42; 2011,Jan,11

64726 plantar digital nerve
- 7.87   7.87 **FUD** 090   T A2
AMA: 2016,Jan,13; 2015,Jan,16; 2014,Jan,11; 2012,Jan,15-42; 2011,Jan,11

+ **64727** Internal neurolysis, requiring use of operating microscope (List separately in addition to code for neuroplasty) (Neuroplasty includes external neurolysis)
INCLUDES Operating microscope (69990)
Code first neuroplasty (64702-64721)
- 5.33   5.33 **FUD** ZZZ   N N1
AMA: 2016,Feb,12; 2016,Jan,13; 2015,Jan,16; 2014,Jan,11; 2012,Jun,12-13; 2012,Jan,15-42; 2011,Jan,11

64732-64772 Surgical Avulsion/Transection of Nerve
EXCLUDES Stereotactic lesion of gasserian ganglion (61790)

64732 Transection or avulsion of; supraorbital nerve
- 10.7   10.7 **FUD** 090   T A2 80 50
AMA: 2016,Jan,13; 2015,Jan,16; 2014,Jan,11

64734 infraorbital nerve
- 11.8   11.8 **FUD** 090   T A2 80 50
AMA: 2014,Jan,11

64736 mental nerve
- 11.4   11.4 **FUD** 090   T A2 80 50
AMA: 2014,Jan,11

64738 inferior alveolar nerve by osteotomy
- 12.1   12.1 **FUD** 090   T A2 80 50
AMA: 2014,Jan,11

64740 lingual nerve
- 13.1   13.1 **FUD** 090   T A2 80 50
AMA: 2014,Jan,11

64742 facial nerve, differential or complete
- 13.9   13.9 **FUD** 090   T A2 80 50
AMA: 2014,Jan,11

64744 greater occipital nerve
- 14.2   14.2 **FUD** 090   T A2 80 50
AMA: 2014,Jan,11

64746 phrenic nerve
EXCLUDES Section of recurrent unilateral laryngeal nerve (31595)
- 12.9   12.9 **FUD** 090   T A2 80 50
AMA: 2014,Jan,11

64755 vagus nerves limited to proximal stomach (selective proximal vagotomy, proximal gastric vagotomy, parietal cell vagotomy, supra- or highly selective vagotomy)
EXCLUDES Laparoscopic procedure (43652)
- 26.6   26.6 **FUD** 090   C 80
AMA: 2016,Jan,13; 2015,Jan,16; 2014,Jan,11

64760 vagus nerve (vagotomy), abdominal
EXCLUDES Laparoscopic procedure (43651)
- 14.5   14.5 **FUD** 090   C 80
AMA: 2016,Jan,13; 2015,Jan,16; 2014,Jan,11

64763 Transection or avulsion of obturator nerve, extrapelvic, with or without adductor tenotomy
- 14.6   14.6 **FUD** 090   T G2 80 50
AMA: 2014,Jan,11

64766 Transection or avulsion of obturator nerve, intrapelvic, with or without adductor tenotomy
- 17.3   17.3 **FUD** 090   T G2 80 50
AMA: 2014,Jan,11

64771 Transection or avulsion of other cranial nerve, extradural
- 17.2   17.2 **FUD** 090   T A2 80
AMA: 2014,Jan,11

64772 Transection or avulsion of other spinal nerve, extradural
EXCLUDES Removal of tender scar and soft tissue including neuroma if necessary (11400-11446, 13100-13153)
- 16.1   16.1 **FUD** 090   T A2 80
AMA: 2016,Jan,13; 2015,Apr,10; 2014,Jan,11

64774-64823 Excisional Nerve Procedures
EXCLUDES Morton neuroma excision (28080)

64774 Excision of neuroma; cutaneous nerve, surgically identifiable
- 11.9   11.9 **FUD** 090   T A2
AMA: 2014,Jan,11

64776 digital nerve, 1 or both, same digit
- 11.2   11.2 **FUD** 090   T A2 80
AMA: 2014,Jan,11

+ **64778** digital nerve, each additional digit (List separately in addition to code for primary procedure)
Code first (64776)
- 4.13   4.13 **FUD** ZZZ   N N1
AMA: 2014,Jan,11

64782 hand or foot, except digital nerve
- 13.0   13.0 **FUD** 090   T A2
AMA: 2014,Jan,11

+ **64783** hand or foot, each additional nerve, except same digit (List separately in addition to code for primary procedure)
Code first (64782)
- 6.38   6.38 **FUD** ZZZ   N N1
AMA: 2014,Jan,11

64784 major peripheral nerve, except sciatic
- 21.0   21.0 **FUD** 090   T A2 80
AMA: 2014,Jan,11

64786 sciatic nerve
⚙ 30.9 ✂ 30.9 **FUD** 090 T A2 80 50 ▢
AMA: 2014,Jan,11

+ **64787** Implantation of nerve end into bone or muscle (List separately in addition to neuroma excision)
Code also, when appropriate (64774-64786)
⚙ 7.02 ✂ 7.02 **FUD** ZZZ N N1 80 ▢
AMA: 2014,Jan,11

64788 Excision of neurofibroma or neurolemmoma; cutaneous nerve
⚙ 11.4 ✂ 11.4 **FUD** 090 T A2 ▢
AMA: 2016,Apr,3; 2014,Jan,11

64790 major peripheral nerve
⚙ 24.2 ✂ 24.2 **FUD** 090 T A2 80 ▢
AMA: 2016,Apr,3; 2014,Jan,11

64792 extensive (including malignant type)
EXCLUDES Destruction neurofibroma of skin (0419T-0420T)
⚙ 34.9 ✂ 34.9 **FUD** 090 T A2 80 ▢
AMA: 2016,Apr,3; 2014,Jan,11

64795 Biopsy of nerve
⚙ 5.58 ✂ 5.58 **FUD** 000 T A2 ▢
AMA: 2014,Jan,11

64802 Sympathectomy, cervical
⚙ 19.1 ✂ 19.1 **FUD** 090 T A2 80 50 ▢
AMA: 2014,Jan,11

64804 Sympathectomy, cervicothoracic
⚙ 28.9 ✂ 28.9 **FUD** 090 T 80 50 ▢
AMA: 2014,Jan,11

64809 Sympathectomy, thoracolumbar
INCLUDES Leriche sympathectomy
⚙ 29.5 ✂ 29.5 **FUD** 090 C 80 50 ▢
AMA: 2014,Jan,11

64818 Sympathectomy, lumbar
⚙ 17.7 ✂ 17.7 **FUD** 090 C 80 50 ▢
AMA: 2014,Jan,11

64820 Sympathectomy; digital arteries, each digit
INCLUDES Operating microscope (69990)
⚙ 20.8 ✂ 20.8 **FUD** 090 T G2 ▢
AMA: 2016,Feb,12; 2016,Jan,13; 2015,Jan,16; 2014,Jan,11; 2012,Jan,15-42; 2011,Jan,11

64821 radial artery
INCLUDES Operating microscope (69990)
⚙ 19.7 ✂ 19.7 **FUD** 090 T A2 50 ▢
AMA: 2016,Feb,12; 2014,Jan,11

64822 ulnar artery
INCLUDES Operating microscope (69990)
⚙ 19.7 ✂ 19.7 **FUD** 090 T G2 50 ▢
AMA: 2016,Feb,12; 2014,Jan,11

64823 superficial palmar arch
INCLUDES Operating microscope (69990)
⚙ 22.4 ✂ 22.4 **FUD** 090 T G2 50 ▢
AMA: 2016,Feb,12; 2014,Jan,11

64831-64907 Nerve Repair: Suture and Nerve Grafts

64831 Suture of digital nerve, hand or foot; 1 nerve
⚙ 19.6 ✂ 19.6 **FUD** 090 T A2 50 ▢
AMA: 2016,Jan,13; 2015,Jan,16; 2014,Sep,13; 2014,Jan,11

+ **64832** each additional digital nerve (List separately in addition to code for primary procedure)
Code first (64831)
⚙ 9.76 ✂ 9.76 **FUD** ZZZ N N1 80 ▢
AMA: 2016,Jan,13; 2015,Jan,16; 2014,Jan,11

64834 Suture of 1 nerve; hand or foot, common sensory nerve
⚙ 21.3 ✂ 21.3 **FUD** 090 T A2 80 50 ▢
AMA: 2014,Jan,11

64835 median motor thenar
⚙ 23.2 ✂ 23.2 **FUD** 090 T A2 80 50 ▢
AMA: 2014,Jan,11

64836 ulnar motor
⚙ 23.3 ✂ 23.3 **FUD** 090 T A2 80 50 ▢
AMA: 2014,Jan,11

+ **64837** Suture of each additional nerve, hand or foot (List separately in addition to code for primary procedure)
Code first (64834-64836)
⚙ 10.7 ✂ 10.7 **FUD** ZZZ N N1 80 ▢
AMA: 2014,Jan,11

64840 Suture of posterior tibial nerve
⚙ 29.3 ✂ 29.3 **FUD** 090 T A2 80 50 ▢
AMA: 2014,Jan,11

64856 Suture of major peripheral nerve, arm or leg, except sciatic; including transposition
⚙ 29.2 ✂ 29.2 **FUD** 090 T A2 ▢
AMA: 2014,Jan,11

64857 without transposition
⚙ 30.3 ✂ 30.3 **FUD** 090 T A2 80 ▢
AMA: 2014,Jan,11

64858 Suture of sciatic nerve
⚙ 32.6 ✂ 32.6 **FUD** 090 T A2 80 50 ▢
AMA: 2014,Jan,11

+ **64859** Suture of each additional major peripheral nerve (List separately in addition to code for primary procedure)
Code first (64856-64857)
⚙ 7.31 ✂ 7.31 **FUD** ZZZ N N1 80 ▢
AMA: 2014,Jan,11

64861 Suture of; brachial plexus
⚙ 38.2 ✂ 38.2 **FUD** 090 T A2 80 50 ▢
AMA: 2014,Jan,11

64862 lumbar plexus
⚙ 44.9 ✂ 44.9 **FUD** 090 T A2 80 50 ▢
AMA: 2014,Jan,11

64864 Suture of facial nerve; extracranial
⚙ 25.3 ✂ 25.3 **FUD** 090 T A2 80 ▢
AMA: 2014,Jan,11

64865 infratemporal, with or without grafting
⚙ 32.5 ✂ 32.5 **FUD** 090 T A2 80 ▢
AMA: 2014,Jan,11

64866 Anastomosis; facial-spinal accessory
⚙ 33.2 ✂ 33.2 **FUD** 090 C 80 ▢
AMA: 2014,Jan,11

64868 facial-hypoglossal
INCLUDES Korte-Ballance anastomosis
⚙ 29.3 ✂ 29.3 **FUD** 090 C 80 ▢
AMA: 2014,Jan,11

+ **64872** Suture of nerve; requiring secondary or delayed suture (List separately in addition to code for primary neurorrhaphy)
Code first (64831-64865)
⚙ 3.50 ✂ 3.50 **FUD** ZZZ N N1 80 ▢
AMA: 2014,Jan,11

+ **64874** requiring extensive mobilization, or transposition of nerve (List separately in addition to code for nerve suture)
Code first (64831-64865)
⚙ 4.97 ✂ 4.97 **FUD** ZZZ N N1 80 ▢
AMA: 2014,Jan,11

+ **64876** requiring shortening of bone of extremity (List separately in addition to code for nerve suture)
Code first (64831-64865)
⚙ 5.12 ✂ 5.12 **FUD** ZZZ N N1 80 ▢
AMA: 2014,Jan,11

64885 Nerve graft (includes obtaining graft), head or neck; up to 4 cm in length

🚗 33.2   ⚓ 33.2   **FUD** 090   T A2 80 ▣

AMA: 2016,Jan,13; 2015,Jan,16; 2014,Jan,11; 2012,Jan,15-42; 2011,Jan,11

64886 more than 4 cm length

🚗 37.6   ⚓ 37.6   **FUD** 090   T A2 80 ▣

AMA: 2016,Jan,13; 2015,Jan,16; 2014,Jan,11; 2012,Jan,15-42; 2011,Jan,11

64890 Nerve graft (includes obtaining graft), single strand, hand or foot; up to 4 cm length

🚗 31.4   ⚓ 31.4   **FUD** 090   T A2 80 ▣

AMA: 2016,Jan,13; 2015,Aug,8; 2015,Apr,10; 2014,Jan,11

64891 more than 4 cm length

🚗 33.6   ⚓ 33.6   **FUD** 090   T A2 80 ▣

AMA: 2014,Jan,11

64892 Nerve graft (includes obtaining graft), single strand, arm or leg; up to 4 cm length

🚗 30.0   ⚓ 30.0   **FUD** 090   T A2 80 ▣

AMA: 2014,Jan,11

64893 more than 4 cm length

🚗 32.7   ⚓ 32.7   **FUD** 090   T A2 80 ▣

AMA: 2014,Jan,11

64895 Nerve graft (includes obtaining graft), multiple strands (cable), hand or foot; up to 4 cm length

🚗 38.5   ⚓ 38.5   **FUD** 090   T A2 80 ▣

AMA: 2016,Jan,13; 2015,Jan,16; 2014,Jan,11

64896 more than 4 cm length

🚗 41.4   ⚓ 41.4   **FUD** 090   T A2 80 ▣

AMA: 2016,Jan,13; 2015,Jan,16; 2014,Jan,11

64897 Nerve graft (includes obtaining graft), multiple strands (cable), arm or leg; up to 4 cm length

🚗 35.8   ⚓ 35.8   **FUD** 090   T A2 80 ▣

AMA: 2016,Jan,13; 2015,Jan,16; 2014,Jan,11

64898 more than 4 cm length

🚗 39.4   ⚓ 39.4   **FUD** 090   T A2 80 ▣

AMA: 2016,Jan,13; 2015,Jan,16; 2014,Jan,11

+ 64901 Nerve graft, each additional nerve; single strand (List separately in addition to code for primary procedure)

Code first (64885-64893)

🚗 16.1   ⚓ 16.1   **FUD** ZZZ   N N1 80 ▣

AMA: 2016,Jan,13; 2015,Jan,16; 2014,Jan,11

+ 64902 multiple strands (cable) (List separately in addition to code for primary procedure)

Code first (64885-64886, 64895-64898)

🚗 19.0   ⚓ 19.0   **FUD** ZZZ   N N1 80 ▣

AMA: 2016,Jan,13; 2015,Jan,16; 2014,Jan,11

64905 Nerve pedicle transfer; first stage

🚗 29.6   ⚓ 29.6   **FUD** 090   T A2 80 ▣

AMA: 2014,Jan,11

64907 second stage

🚗 39.8   ⚓ 39.8   **FUD** 090   T A2 80 ▣

AMA: 2014,Jan,11

64910-64999 Nerve Repair: Synthetic and Vein Grafts

64910 Nerve repair; with synthetic conduit or vein allograft (eg, nerve tube), each nerve

INCLUDES   Operating microscope (69990)

🚗 23.7   ⚓ 23.7   **FUD** 090   T G2 80 ▣

AMA: 2016,Jan,13; 2015,Aug,8; 2015,Apr,10; 2015,Jan,16; 2014,Jan,11

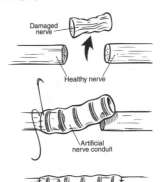

Damaged nerve

Healthy nerve

Artificial nerve conduit

A synthetic "bridge" is affixed to each end of a severed nerve with sutures
This procedure is performed using an operating microscope

64911 with autogenous vein graft (includes harvest of vein graft), each nerve

INCLUDES   Operating microscope (69990)

🚗 29.1   ⚓ 29.1   **FUD** 090   T 80 ▣

AMA: 2016,Jan,13; 2015,Jan,16; 2014,Jan,11

64999 Unlisted procedure, nervous system

🚗 0.00   ⚓ 0.00   **FUD** YYY   T 80

AMA: 2016,Feb,13; 2016,Jan,13; 2015,Oct,9; 2015,Aug,8; 2015,Jul,10; 2015,Apr,10; 2015,Feb,9; 2015,Jan,16; 2014,Jul,8; 2014,Feb,11; 2014,Jan,8; 2014,Jan,9; 2014,Jan,11; 2013,Dec,14; 2013,Nov,14; 2013,Jun,13; 2013,Apr,5-6; 2013,Apr,10-11; 2012,Dec,12; 2012,Sep,14-15; 2012,Oct,14; 2012,Sep,14-15; 2012,Sep,16; 2012,May,14-15; 2012,Feb,11; 2012,Jan,15-42; 2012,Jan,13-14; 2011,Sep,11-12; 2011,Jul,12-13; 2011,Jul,16-17; 2011,Apr,12; 2011,Jan,11

65091-65093 Surgical Removal of Eyeball Contents

INCLUDES Operating microscope (69990)

65091   Evisceration of ocular contents; without implant
🔧 17.9 ⚖ 17.9 **FUD** 090   T A2 80 50 ▣
AMA: 2016,Feb,12; 2014,Jan,11

Conjunctiva
Sclera
Muscles are severed at their attachment to the eyeball

Evisceration involves removal of the contents of the eyeball: the vitreous; retina; choroid; lens; iris; and ciliary muscle. Only the scleral shell remains. A temporary or permanent implant is usually inserted

Enucleation involves severing the extraorbital muscles and optic nerve with removal of the eyeball. An implant is usually inserted and, if permanent, may involve attachment to the severed extraorbital muscles

65093   with implant
🔧 17.7 ⚖ 17.7 **FUD** 090   T A2 50 ▣
AMA: 2016,Feb,12; 2014,Jan,11

65101-65105 Surgical Removal of Eyeball

INCLUDES Operating microscope (69990)
EXCLUDES Conjunctivoplasty following enucleation (68320-68328)

65101   Enucleation of eye; without implant
🔧 20.8 ⚖ 20.8 **FUD** 090   T A2 50 ▣
AMA: 2016,Feb,12; 2014,Jan,11

65103   with implant, muscles not attached to implant
🔧 21.7 ⚖ 21.7 **FUD** 090   T A2 50 ▣
AMA: 2016,Feb,12; 2014,Jan,11

65105   with implant, muscles attached to implant
🔧 24.0 ⚖ 24.0 **FUD** 090   T A2 80 50 ▣
AMA: 2016,Feb,12; 2014,Jan,11

65110-65114 Surgical Removal of Orbital Contents

INCLUDES Operating microscope (69990)
EXCLUDES Free full thickness graft (15260-15261)
Repair more extensive than skin (67930-67975)
Skin graft (15120-15121)

65110   Exenteration of orbit (does not include skin graft), removal of orbital contents; only
🔧 34.6 ⚖ 34.6 **FUD** 090   T A2 80 50 ▣
AMA: 2016,Feb,12; 2014,Jan,11

65112   with therapeutic removal of bone
🔧 40.2 ⚖ 40.2 **FUD** 090   T A2 80 50 ▣
AMA: 2016,Feb,12; 2014,Jan,11

65114   with muscle or myocutaneous flap
🔧 42.2 ⚖ 42.2 **FUD** 090   T A2 80 50 ▣
AMA: 2016,Feb,12; 2014,Jan,11

65125-65175 Implant Procedures: Insertion, Removal, and Revision

INCLUDES Operating microscope (69990)
EXCLUDES Orbital implant insertion outside muscle cone (67550)
Orbital implant removal or revision outside muscle cone (67560)

65125   Modification of ocular implant with placement or replacement of pegs (eg, drilling receptacle for prosthesis appendage) (separate procedure)
🔧 8.28 ⚖ 12.9 **FUD** 090   T 82 50 ▣
AMA: 2016,Feb,12; 2014,Jan,11

65130   Insertion of ocular implant secondary; after evisceration, in scleral shell
🔧 20.6 ⚖ 20.6 **FUD** 090   T A2 50 ▣
AMA: 2016,Feb,12; 2014,Jan,11

65135   after enucleation, muscles not attached to implant
🔧 20.9 ⚖ 20.9 **FUD** 090   T A2 50 ▣
AMA: 2016,Feb,12; 2014,Jan,11

65140   after enucleation, muscles attached to implant
🔧 22.8 ⚖ 22.8 **FUD** 090   T A2 50 ▣
AMA: 2016,Feb,12; 2014,Jan,11

65150   Reinsertion of ocular implant; with or without conjunctival graft
🔧 16.1 ⚖ 16.1 **FUD** 090   T A2 80 50 ▣
AMA: 2016,Feb,12; 2014,Jan,11

65155   with use of foreign material for reinforcement and/or attachment of muscles to implant
🔧 23.9 ⚖ 23.9 **FUD** 090   T A2 50 ▣
AMA: 2016,Feb,12; 2014,Jan,11

65175   Removal of ocular implant
🔧 18.5 ⚖ 18.5 **FUD** 090   T A2 50 ▣
AMA: 2016,Feb,12; 2014,Jan,11

65205-65265 Foreign Body Removal By Area of Eye

INCLUDES Operating microscope (69990)
EXCLUDES Removal:
Anterior segment implant (65920)
Ocular implant (65175)
Orbital implant outside muscle cone (67560)
Posterior segment implant (67120)
Removal of foreign body:
Eyelid (67938)
Lacrimal system (68530)
Orbit:
Lateral approach (67430)
Frontal approach (67413)

65205   Removal of foreign body, external eye; conjunctival superficial
🔬 (70030, 76529)
🔧 1.25 ⚖ 1.58 **FUD** 000   Q1 N1 50 ▣
AMA: 2016,Feb,12; 2016,Jan,13; 2015,Jan,16; 2014,Jan,11; 2013,Oct,18; 2012,Jan,15-42; 2011,Jan,11

65210   conjunctival embedded (includes concretions), subconjunctival, or scleral nonperforating
🔬 (70030, 76529)
🔧 1.51 ⚖ 1.94 **FUD** 000   Q1 N1 50 ▣
AMA: 2016,Feb,12; 2014,Jan,11

65220   corneal, without slit lamp
EXCLUDES Repair of corneal wound with foreign body (65275)
🔬 (70030, 76529)
🔧 1.20 ⚖ 1.64 **FUD** 000   Q1 N1 50 ▣
AMA: 2016,Feb,12; 2016,Jan,13; 2015,Jan,16; 2014,Jan,11; 2012,Jan,15-42; 2011,Jan,11

65222   corneal, with slit lamp
EXCLUDES Repair of corneal wound with foreign body (65275)
🔬 (70030, 76529)
🔧 1.48 ⚖ 1.88 **FUD** 000   Q1 N1 50 ▣
AMA: 2016,Feb,12; 2016,Jan,13; 2015,Jan,16; 2014,Jan,11; 2012,Jan,15-42; 2011,Jan,11

65235   Removal of foreign body, intraocular; from anterior chamber of eye or lens
🔬 (70030, 76529)
🔧 20.1 ⚖ 20.1 **FUD** 090   T A2 80 50 ▣
AMA: 2016,Feb,12; 2016,Jan,13; 2015,Jan,16; 2014,Jan,11

65260   from posterior segment, magnetic extraction, anterior or posterior route
🔬 (70030, 76529)
🔧 27.1 ⚖ 27.1 **FUD** 090   T A2 80 50 ▣
AMA: 2016,Feb,12; 2014,Jan,11

65265   from posterior segment, nonmagnetic extraction
🔬 (70030, 76529)
🔧 30.6 ⚖ 30.6 **FUD** 090   T A2 80 50 ▣
AMA: 2016,Feb,12; 2014,Jan,11

65270-65290 Laceration Repair External Eye

INCLUDES Conjunctival flap
Operating microscope (69990)
Restoration of anterior chamber with air or saline injection

EXCLUDES Repair:
Ciliary body or iris (66680)
Eyelid laceration (12011-12018, 12051-12057, 13151-13160, 67930, 67935)
Lacrimal system injury (68700)
Surgical wound (66250)
Treatment of orbit fracture (21385-21408)

65270 **Repair of laceration; conjunctiva, with or without nonperforating laceration sclera, direct closure**
🔲 3.98 🔲 7.53 **FUD** 010 T A2 80 50 ▣
AMA: 2016,Feb,12; 2016,Jan,13; 2015,Jan,16; 2014,Jan,11; 2012,Aug,9

65272 **conjunctiva, by mobilization and rearrangement, without hospitalization**
🔲 9.95 🔲 14.1 **FUD** 090 T A2 50 ▣
AMA: 2016,Feb,12; 2014,Jan,11

65273 **conjunctiva, by mobilization and rearrangement, with hospitalization**
🔲 10.8 🔲 10.8 **FUD** 090 C 50 ▣
AMA: 2016,Feb,12; 2014,Jan,11

65275 **cornea, nonperforating, with or without removal foreign body**
🔲 13.1 🔲 16.3 **FUD** 090 T A2 80 50 ▣
AMA: 2016,Feb,12; 2014,Jan,11

65280 **cornea and/or sclera, perforating, not involving uveal tissue**
EXCLUDES Procedure performed for surgical wound repair
🔲 19.0 🔲 19.0 **FUD** 090 J A2 80 50 ▣
AMA: 2016,Feb,12; 2016,Jan,13; 2015,Jan,16; 2014,Jan,11; 2012,Aug,9

65285 **cornea and/or sclera, perforating, with reposition or resection of uveal tissue**
EXCLUDES Procedure performed for surgical wound repair
🔲 31.4 🔲 31.4 **FUD** 090 J A2 50 ▣
AMA: 2016,Feb,12; 2016,Jan,13; 2015,Jan,16; 2014,Jan,11; 2012,Aug,9

65286 **application of tissue glue, wounds of cornea and/or sclera**
🔲 14.0 🔲 19.8 **FUD** 090 T P3 50 ▣
AMA: 2016,Feb,12; 2016,Jan,13; 2015,Jan,16; 2014,Jan,11

65290 **Repair of wound, extraocular muscle, tendon and/or Tenon's capsule**
🔲 13.8 🔲 13.8 **FUD** 090 T A2 50 ▣
AMA: 2016,Feb,12; 2014,Jan,11

65400-65600 Removal Corneal Lesions

INCLUDES Operating microscope (69990)

65400 **Excision of lesion, cornea (keratectomy, lamellar, partial), except pterygium**
🔲 17.0 🔲 19.2 **FUD** 090 T A2 50 ▣
AMA: 2016,Feb,12; 2016,Jan,13; 2015,Jan,16; 2014,Jan,11

65410 **Biopsy of cornea**
🔲 2.96 🔲 4.04 **FUD** 000 T A2 80 50 ▣
AMA: 2016,Feb,12; 2016,Jan,13; 2015,Jan,16; 2014,Jan,11

65420 **Excision or transposition of pterygium; without graft**
🔲 10.7 🔲 14.5 **FUD** 090 T A2 50 ▣
AMA: 2016,Feb,12; 2016,Jan,13; 2015,Jan,16; 2014,Jan,11; 2012,Jan,15-42; 2011,Jan,11

The conjunctiva is subject to numerous acute and chronic irritations and disorders

65426 **with graft**
🔲 13.5 🔲 18.4 **FUD** 090 T A2 50 ▣
AMA: 2016,Feb,12; 2016,Jan,13; 2015,Jan,16; 2014,Jan,11

65430 **Scraping of cornea, diagnostic, for smear and/or culture**
🔲 2.93 🔲 3.23 **FUD** 000 Q1 N1 50 ▣
AMA: 2016,Feb,12; 2014,Jan,11

65435 **Removal of corneal epithelium; with or without chemocauterization (abrasion, curettage)**
EXCLUDES Collagen cross-linking of cornea (0402T)
🔲 1.97 🔲 2.25 **FUD** 000 T P3 50 ▣
AMA: 2016,Feb,12; 2016,Jan,13; 2015,Jan,16; 2014,Jan,11; 2012,Jan,15-42; 2011,Jan,11

65436 **with application of chelating agent (eg, EDTA)**
🔲 10.5 🔲 10.9 **FUD** 090 T P3 50 ▣
AMA: 2016,Feb,12; 2014,Jan,11

65450 **Destruction of lesion of cornea by cryotherapy, photocoagulation or thermocauterization**
🔲 9.11 🔲 9.19 **FUD** 090 T G2 50 ▣
AMA: 2016,Feb,12; 2014,Jan,11

65600 **Multiple punctures of anterior cornea (eg, for corneal erosion, tattoo)**
🔲 9.75 🔲 11.1 **FUD** 090 T P3 50 ▣
AMA: 2016,Feb,12; 2014,Jan,11

65710-65757 Corneal Transplants

CMS: 100-03,80.7 Refractive Keratoplasty

INCLUDES Operating microscope (69990)
EXCLUDES Computerized corneal topography (92025)
Processing, preserving, and transporting corneal tissue (V2785)

65710 **Keratoplasty (corneal transplant); anterior lamellar**
INCLUDES Use and preparation of fresh or preserved graft
EXCLUDES Refractive keratoplasty surgery (65760-65767)
🔲 31.3 🔲 31.3 **FUD** 090 J A2 80 50 ▣
AMA: 2016,Feb,12; 2016,Jan,13; 2015,Jan,16; 2014,Jan,11; 2012,Aug,9

65730 **penetrating (except in aphakia or pseudophakia)**
INCLUDES Use and preparation of fresh or preserved graft
EXCLUDES Refractive keratoplasty surgery (65760-65767)
🔲 34.7 🔲 34.7 **FUD** 090 J A2 80 50 ▣
AMA: 2016,Feb,12; 2016,Jan,13; 2015,Jan,16; 2014,Jan,11; 2012,Aug,9; 2012,Jan,15-42; 2011,Jan,11

65750 **penetrating (in aphakia)**
INCLUDES Use and preparation of fresh or preserved graft
EXCLUDES Refractive keratoplasty surgery (65760-65767)
🔲 34.9 🔲 34.9 **FUD** 090 J A2 80 50 ▣
AMA: 2016,Feb,12; 2016,Jan,13; 2015,Jan,16; 2014,Jan,11; 2012,Aug,9; 2011,Jan,11

65755 **penetrating (in pseudophakia)**
INCLUDES Use and preparation of fresh or preserved graft
EXCLUDES *Refractive keratoplasty surgery (65760-65767)*
⚙ 34.7 ⚕ 34.7 **FUD** 090 [J] [A2] [80] [50] 🔲
AMA: 2016,Feb,12; 2016,Jan,13; 2015,Jan,16; 2014,Jan,11;
2012,Aug,9

65756 **endothelial**
EXCLUDES *Refractive keratoplasty surgery (65760-65767)*
Code also donor material
Code also if appropriate (65757)
⚙ 33.5 ⚕ 33.5 **FUD** 090 [J] [G2] [80] [50] 🔲
AMA: 2016,Feb,12; 2016,Jan,13; 2015,Jan,16; 2014,Jan,11;
2012,Jan,15-42; 2011,Jan,11

\+ **65757** **Backbench preparation of corneal endothelial allograft prior to transplantation (List separately in addition to code for primary procedure)**
Code first (65756)
⚙ 0.00 ⚕ 0.00 **FUD** ZZZ [N] [N1] [80] 🔲
AMA: 2016,Feb,12; 2016,Jan,13; 2015,Jan,16; 2014,Aug,14;
2014,Jan,11; 2012,Jan,15-42; 2011,Jan,11

65760-65785 Corneal Refractive Procedures

CMS: 100-03,80.7 Refractive Keratoplasty
INCLUDES Operating microscope (69990)
EXCLUDES *Unlisted corneal procedures (66999)*

65760 **Keratomileusis**
EXCLUDES *Computerized corneal topography (92025)*
⚙ 0.00 ⚕ 0.00 **FUD** XXX [E] 🔲
AMA: 2016,Feb,12; 2014,Jan,11

65765 **Keratophakia**
EXCLUDES *Computerized corneal topography (92025)*
⚙ 0.00 ⚕ 0.00 **FUD** XXX [E] 🔲
AMA: 2016,Feb,12; 2014,Jan,11

65767 **Epikeratoplasty**
EXCLUDES *Computerized corneal topography (92025)*
⚙ 0.00 ⚕ 0.00 **FUD** XXX [E] 🔲
AMA: 2016,Feb,12; 2014,Jan,11

65770 **Keratoprosthesis**
EXCLUDES *Computerized corneal topography (92025)*
⚙ 39.7 ⚕ 39.7 **FUD** 090 [J] [G2] [80] [50] 🔲
AMA: 2016,Feb,12; 2014,Jan,11

65771 **Radial keratotomy**
EXCLUDES *Computerized corneal topography (92025)*
⚙ 0.00 ⚕ 0.00 **FUD** XXX [E] 🔲
AMA: 2016,Feb,12; 2014,Jan,11

65772 **Corneal relaxing incision for correction of surgically induced astigmatism**
⚙ 11.5 ⚕ 12.7 **FUD** 090 [T] [A2] [50] 🔲
AMA: 2016,Feb,12; 2014,Jan,11

65775 **Corneal wedge resection for correction of surgically induced astigmatism**
EXCLUDES *Fitting of contact lens to treat disease (92071-92072)*
⚙ 15.6 ⚕ 15.6 **FUD** 090 [T] [A2] [50] 🔲
AMA: 2016,Feb,12; 2016,Jan,13; 2015,Jan,16; 2014,Jan,11;
2012,Aug,9

65778 **Placement of amniotic membrane on the ocular surface; without sutures**
EXCLUDES *Ocular surface reconstruction (65780)*
Removal of corneal epithelium (65435)
Scraping of cornea, diagnostic (65430)
Use of tissue glue to place amniotic membrane (66999)
⚙ 1.66 ⚕ 40.5 **FUD** 000 [Q2] [N1] [80] [50] 🔲
AMA: 2016,Feb,12; 2016,Jan,13; 2015,Jan,16; 2014,May,5;
2014,Jan,11

65779 **single layer, sutured**
EXCLUDES *Ocular surface reconstruction (65780)*
Removal of corneal epithelium (65435)
Scraping of cornea, diagnostic (65430)
Use of tissue glue to place amniotic membrane (66999)
⚙ 4.32 ⚕ 33.9 **FUD** 000 [Q2] [N1] [80] [50] 🔲
AMA: 2016,Feb,12; 2016,Jan,13; 2015,Jan,16; 2014,May,5;
2014,Jan,11

65780 **Ocular surface reconstruction; amniotic membrane transplantation, multiple layers**
⚙ 20.3 ⚕ 20.3 **FUD** 090 [T] [A2] [50] 🔲
AMA: 2016,Feb,12; 2016,Jan,13; 2015,Jan,16; 2014,May,5;
2014,Jan,11; 2012,Jan,15-42; 2011,Jan,11

65781 **limbal stem cell allograft (eg, cadaveric or living donor)**
⚙ 37.7 ⚕ 37.7 **FUD** 090 [J] [A2] [80] [50] 🔲
AMA: 2016,Feb,12; 2016,Jan,13; 2015,Jan,16; 2014,Jan,11

65782 **limbal conjunctival autograft (includes obtaining graft)**
EXCLUDES *Conjunctival allograft harvest from a living donor (68371)*
⚙ 32.5 ⚕ 32.5 **FUD** 090 [T] [A2] [50] 🔲
AMA: 2016,Feb,12; 2016,Jan,13; 2015,Jan,16; 2014,Jan,11;
2012,Jan,15-42; 2011,Jan,11

65785 **Implantation of intrastromal corneal ring segments**
⚙ 11.0 ⚕ 59.8 **FUD** 090 [J] [R2] [50] 🔲
AMA: 2016,Feb,12

65800-66030 Anterior Segment Procedures

INCLUDES Operating microscope (69990)
EXCLUDES *Unlisted procedures of anterior segment (66999)*

65800 **Paracentesis of anterior chamber of eye (separate procedure); with removal of aqueous**
EXCLUDES *Insertion of ocular telescope prosthesis (0308T)*
⚙ 2.60 ⚕ 3.37 **FUD** 000 [T] [A2] [50] 🔲
AMA: 2016,Feb,12; 2016,Jan,13; 2015,Jan,16; 2014,Jan,11;
2013,Mar,6-7; 2012,Nov,10

65810 **with removal of vitreous and/or discission of anterior hyaloid membrane, with or without air injection**
EXCLUDES *Insertion of ocular telescope prosthesis (0308T)*
⚙ 13.1 ⚕ 13.1 **FUD** 090 [T] [A2] [50] 🔲
AMA: 2016,Feb,12; 2016,Jan,13; 2015,Jan,16; 2014,Jan,11;
2012,Nov,10

65815 **with removal of blood, with or without irrigation and/or air injection**
EXCLUDES *Injection only (66020-66030)*
Insertion of ocular telescope prosthesis (0308T)
Removal of blood clot only (65930)
⚙ 13.5 ⚕ 18.0 **FUD** 090 [T] [A2] [50] 🔲
AMA: 2016,Feb,12; 2016,Jan,13; 2015,Jan,16; 2014,Jan,11;
2012,Nov,10

65820 **Goniotomy**
INCLUDES Barkan's operation
Code also ophthalmic endoscope if used (69990)
⚙ 21.2 ⚕ 21.2 **FUD** 090 [63] [J] [A2] [80] [50] 🔲
AMA: 2016,Feb,12; 2016,Jan,13; 2015,Jan,16; 2014,Jan,11

65850 **Trabeculotomy ab externo**
⚙ 23.7 ⚕ 23.7 **FUD** 090 [T] [A2] [50] 🔲
AMA: 2016,Feb,12; 2014,Jan,11

65855 **Trabeculoplasty by laser surgery**
EXCLUDES *Severing adhesions of anterior segment (65860-65880)*
Trabeculectomy ab externo (66170)
Code also modifier 22 Increased procedural services, or 52 Reduced services, as appropriate, for re-treatment after several months for advancing disease
⚙ 6.81 ⚕ 7.73 **FUD** 010 [T] [P3] [50] 🔲
AMA: 2016,Feb,12; 2016,Jan,13; 2015,Jan,16; 2014,Jan,11;
2012,Jan,15-42; 2011,Jan,11

65860 Severing adhesions of anterior segment, laser technique (separate procedure)

🚑 7.18 ⚕ 8.73 **FUD** 090   T P3 80 50 ▣

AMA: 2016,Feb,12; 2014,Jan,11

65865 Severing adhesions of anterior segment of eye, incisional technique (with or without injection of air or liquid) (separate procedure); goniosynechiae

EXCLUDES   *Laser trabeculectomy (65855)*

🚑 13.3 ⚕ 13.3 **FUD** 090   T A2 50 ▣

AMA: 2016,Feb,12; 2014,Jan,11

65870 anterior synechiae, except goniosynechiae

🚑 16.7 ⚕ 16.7 **FUD** 090   T A2 50 ▣

AMA: 2016,Feb,12; 2014,Jan,11

65875 posterior synechiae

Code also ophthalmic endoscope if used (66990)

🚑 17.8 ⚕ 17.8 **FUD** 090   T A2 50 ▣

AMA: 2016,Feb,12; 2016,Jan,13; 2015,Jan,16; 2014,Jan,11

65880 corneovitreal adhesions

EXCLUDES   *Laser procedure (66821)*

🚑 18.7 ⚕ 18.7 **FUD** 090   T A2 50 ▣

AMA: 2016,Feb,12; 2014,Jan,11

65900 Removal of epithelial downgrowth, anterior chamber of eye

🚑 27.1 ⚕ 27.1 **FUD** 090   T A2 80 50 ▣

AMA: 2016,Feb,12; 2014,Jan,11

65920 Removal of implanted material, anterior segment of eye

Code also ophthalmic endoscope if used (66990)

🚑 22.3 ⚕ 22.3 **FUD** 090   T A2 50 ▣

AMA: 2016,Feb,12; 2016,Jan,13; 2015,Jan,16; 2014,Jan,11

65930 Removal of blood clot, anterior segment of eye

🚑 18.0 ⚕ 18.0 **FUD** 090   T A2 50 ▣

AMA: 2016,Feb,12; 2014,Jan,11

66020 Injection, anterior chamber of eye (separate procedure); air or liquid

EXCLUDES   *Insertion of ocular telescope prosthesis (0308T)*

🚑 3.73 ⚕ 5.27 **FUD** 010   T A2 50 ▣

AMA: 2016,Feb,12; 2016,Jan,13; 2015,Jan,16; 2014,Jan,11; 2012,Nov,10

66030 medication

EXCLUDES   *Insertion of ocular telescope prosthesis (0308T)*

🚑 3.14 ⚕ 4.68 **FUD** 010   T A2 50 ▣

AMA: 2016,Feb,12; 2014,Jan,11; 2012,Nov,10

66130 Excision Scleral Lesion

INCLUDES   Operating microscope (69990)

EXCLUDES   *Intraocular foreign body removal (65235)*
Surgery on posterior sclera (67250, 67255)

66130 Excision of lesion, sclera

🚑 16.1 ⚕ 19.6 **FUD** 090   T A2 80 50 ▣

AMA: 2016,Feb,12; 2014,Jan,11

66150-66185 Procedures for Glaucoma

INCLUDES   Operating microscope (69990)

EXCLUDES   *Intraocular foreign body removal (65235)*
Surgery on posterior sclera (67250, 67255)

66150 Fistulization of sclera for glaucoma; trephination with iridectomy

🚑 24.8 ⚕ 24.8 **FUD** 090   J A2 50 ▣

AMA: 2016,Feb,12; 2014,Jan,11

66155 thermocauterization with iridectomy

🚑 24.7 ⚕ 24.7 **FUD** 090   T A2 50 ▣

AMA: 2016,Feb,12; 2014,Jan,11

66160 sclerectomy with punch or scissors, with iridectomy

INCLUDES   Knapp's operation

🚑 27.9 ⚕ 27.9 **FUD** 090   T A2 50 ▣

AMA: 2016,Feb,12; 2014,Jan,11

66170 trabeculectomy ab externo in absence of previous surgery

EXCLUDES   *Repair of surgical wound (66250)*
Trabeculectomy ab externo (65850)

🚑 27.4 ⚕ 27.4 **FUD** 090   T A2 80 50 ▣

AMA: 2016,Feb,12; 2016,Jan,13; 2015,Jan,16; 2014,Jan,11; 2012,Dec,12

66172 trabeculectomy ab externo with scarring from previous ocular surgery or trauma (includes injection of antifibrotic agents)

🚑 34.6 ⚕ 34.6 **FUD** 090   T A2 80 50 ▣

AMA: 2016,Feb,12; 2016,Jan,13; 2015,Jan,16; 2014,Jan,11; 2012,Dec,12

66174 Transluminal dilation of aqueous outflow canal; without retention of device or stent

🚑 26.8 ⚕ 26.8 **FUD** 090   T A2 80 50 ▣

AMA: 2016,Feb,12; 2014,Jan,11

66175 with retention of device or stent

🚑 28.1 ⚕ 28.1 **FUD** 090   J A2 80 50 ▣

AMA: 2016,Feb,12; 2014,Jan,11

66179 Aqueous shunt to extraocular equatorial plate reservoir, external approach; without graft

🚑 30.5 ⚕ 30.5 **FUD** 090   J 62 80 50 ▣

AMA: 2016,Feb,12; 2016,Jan,13; 2015,Jan,10

66180 with graft

EXCLUDES   *Scleral reinforcement (67255)*

🚑 32.2 ⚕ 32.2 **FUD** 090   J A2 80 50 ▣

AMA: 2016,Feb,12; 2016,Jan,13; 2015,Jan,10; 2015,Jan,16; 2014,Jan,11; 2012,Jun,15-16

66183 Insertion of anterior segment aqueous drainage device, without extraocular reservoir, external approach

🚑 29.1 ⚕ 29.1 **FUD** 090   J 62 80 50 ▣

AMA: 2016,Feb,12; 2016,Jan,13; 2015,Jan,16; 2014,May,5; 2014,Jan,11

66184 Revision of aqueous shunt to extraocular equatorial plate reservoir; without graft

🚑 22.2 ⚕ 22.2 **FUD** 090   T 62 80 50 ▣

AMA: 2016,Feb,12; 2016,Jan,13; 2015,Jan,10

66185 with graft

EXCLUDES   *Implanted shunt removal (67120)*
Scleral reinforcement (67255)

🚑 23.9 ⚕ 23.9 **FUD** 090   T A2 80 50 ▣

AMA: 2016,Feb,12; 2016,Jan,13; 2015,Jan,10; 2014,Jan,11

66220-66225 Staphyloma Repair

INCLUDES   Operating microscope (69990)

EXCLUDES   *Scleral procedures with retinal procedures (67101-67228)*
Scleral reinforcement (67250, 67255)

66220 Repair of scleral staphyloma; without graft

🚑 21.1 ⚕ 21.1 **FUD** 090   T A2 80 50 ▣

AMA: 2016,Feb,12; 2014,Jan,11

66225 with graft

🚑 26.3 ⚕ 26.3 **FUD** 090   T A2 50 ▣

AMA: 2016,Feb,12; 2014,Jan,11

66250 Anterior Segment Operative Wound Revision or Repair

INCLUDES   Operating microscope (69990)

EXCLUDES   *Unlisted procedures of anterior sclera (66999)*

66250 Revision or repair of operative wound of anterior segment, any type, early or late, major or minor procedure

🚑 15.7 ⚕ 21.1 **FUD** 090   T A2 50 ▣

AMA: 2016,Feb,12; 2016,Jan,13; 2015,Jan,16; 2014,Jan,11; 2012,Jan,15-42; 2011,Jan,11

66500-66505 Iridotomy With/Without Transfixion

INCLUDES   Operating microscope (69990)

EXCLUDES   *Photocoagulation iridotomy (66761)*

26/TC PC/TC Only   A2-Z3 ASC Payment   50 Bilateral   ♂ Male Only   ♀ Female Only   🚑 Facility RVU   ⚕ Non-Facility RVU   ▣ CCI
FUD Follow-up Days   CMS: IOM (Pub 100)   A-Y OPPSI   80/80 Surg Assist Allowed / w/Doc   ▨ Lab crosswalk   ▧ Radiology crosswalk   ☒ CLIA

288   CPT © 2016 American Medical Association. All Rights Reserved.   © 2016 Optum360, LLC

66500 Iridotomy by stab incision (separate procedure); except transfixion
📷 10.0 ⚖ 10.0 **FUD** 090 [T] [A2] [50] 📷
AMA: 2016,Feb,12; 2014,Jan,11

66505 with transfixion as for iris bombe
📷 10.9 ⚖ 10.9 **FUD** 090 [T] [A2] [50] 📷
AMA: 2016,Feb,12; 2014,Jan,11

66600-66635 Iridectomy Procedures

INCLUDES Operating microscope (69990)
EXCLUDES Insertion of ocular telescope prosthesis (0308T)
Photocoagulation coreoplasty (66762)

66600 Iridectomy, with corneoscleral or corneal section; for removal of lesion
📷 23.5 ⚖ 23.5 **FUD** 090 [T] [A2] [50] 📷
AMA: 2016,Feb,12; 2014,Jan,11

66605 with cyclectomy
📷 29.9 ⚖ 29.9 **FUD** 090 [T] [A2] [50] 📷
AMA: 2016,Feb,12; 2014,Jan,11

66625 peripheral for glaucoma (separate procedure)
📷 12.1 ⚖ 12.1 **FUD** 090 [T] [A2] [50] 📷
AMA: 2016,Feb,12; 2014,Jan,11

66630 sector for glaucoma (separate procedure)
📷 16.1 ⚖ 16.1 **FUD** 090 [T] [A2] [50] 📷
AMA: 2016,Feb,12; 2014,Jan,11

66635 optical (separate procedure)
📷 16.2 ⚖ 16.2 **FUD** 090 [T] [A2] [50] 📷
AMA: 2016,Feb,12; 2014,Jan,11

66680-66770 Other Procedures of the Uveal Tract

INCLUDES Operating microscope (69990)
EXCLUDES Unlisted procedures of ciliary body or iris (66999)

66680 Repair of iris, ciliary body (as for iridodialysis)
EXCLUDES Resection or repositioning of uveal tissue for perforating laceration of cornea and/or sclera (65285)
📷 14.6 ⚖ 14.6 **FUD** 090 [T] [A2] [50] 📷
AMA: 2016,Feb,12; 2014,Jan,11

66682 Suture of iris, ciliary body (separate procedure) with retrieval of suture through small incision (eg, McCannel suture)
📷 18.0 ⚖ 18.0 **FUD** 090 [T] [A2] [50] 📷
AMA: 2016,Feb,12; 2014,Jan,11

66700 Ciliary body destruction; diathermy
INCLUDES Heine's operation
📷 11.1 ⚖ 12.7 **FUD** 090 [T] [A2] [80] [50] 📷
AMA: 2016,Feb,12; 2014,Jan,11

66710 cyclophotocoagulation, transscleral
📷 11.1 ⚖ 12.4 **FUD** 090 [T] [A2] [50] 📷
AMA: 2016,Feb,12; 2016,Jan,13; 2015,Jan,16; 2014,Jan,11; 2012,Jan,15-42; 2011,Jan,11

66711 cyclophotocoagulation, endoscopic
📷 18.1 ⚖ 18.1 **FUD** 090 [T] [A2] [50] 📷
AMA: 2016,Feb,12; 2016,Jan,13; 2015,Jan,16; 2014,Jan,11; 2012,Jan,15-42; 2011,Jan,11

▲ **66720** cryotherapy
📷 12.0 ⚖ 13.4 **FUD** 090 [T] [A2] [50] 📷
AMA: 2016,Feb,12; 2014,Jan,11

66740 cyclodialysis
📷 11.1 ⚖ 12.3 **FUD** 090 [T] [A2] [50] 📷
AMA: 2016,Feb,12; 2014,Jan,11

66761 Iridotomy/iridectomy by laser surgery (eg, for glaucoma) (per session)
EXCLUDES Insertion of ocular telescope prosthesis (0308T)
📷 6.69 ⚖ 8.38 **FUD** 010 [T] [P3] [50] 📷
AMA: 2016,Feb,12; 2016,Jan,13; 2015,Jan,16; 2014,Jan,11

66762 Iridoplasty by photocoagulation (1 or more sessions) (eg, for improvement of vision, for widening of anterior chamber angle)
📷 12.0 ⚖ 13.4 **FUD** 090 [T] [P2] [50] 📷
AMA: 2016,Feb,12; 2016,Jan,13; 2015,Jan,16; 2014,Jan,11

66770 Destruction of cyst or lesion iris or ciliary body (nonexcisional procedure)
EXCLUDES Excision:
Epithelial downgrowth (65900)
Iris, ciliary body lesion (66600-66605)
📷 13.7 ⚖ 14.9 **FUD** 090 [T] [P2] [50] 📷
AMA: 2016,Feb,12; 2014,Jan,11

66820-66825 Post-Cataract Surgery Procedures

INCLUDES Operating microscope (69990)

66820 Discission of secondary membranous cataract (opacified posterior lens capsule and/or anterior hyaloid); stab incision technique (Ziegler or Wheeler knife)
📷 11.1 ⚖ 11.1 **FUD** 090 [T] [62] [50] 📷
AMA: 2016,Feb,12; 2014,Jan,11

Cataract / Iris / Lens / Artificial lens / Cornea / Opaque lens capsule / Iris

An after-cataract is a cataract that develops in a lens tissue that remains after most of the lens has already been removed

66821 laser surgery (eg, YAG laser) (1 or more stages)
📷 8.81 ⚖ 9.33 **FUD** 090 [T] [A2] [50] 📷
AMA: 2016,Feb,12; 2014,Jan,11

66825 Repositioning of intraocular lens prosthesis, requiring an incision (separate procedure)
EXCLUDES Insertion of ocular telescope prosthesis (0308T)
📷 21.5 ⚖ 21.5 **FUD** 090 [T] [A2] [80] [50] 📷
AMA: 2016,Feb,12; 2014,Jan,11

66830-66940 Cataract Extraction; Without Insertion Intraocular Lens

CMS: 100-03,80.10 Phacoemulsification Procedure--Cataract Extraction
INCLUDES Anterior and/or posterior capsulotomy
Enzymatic zonulysis
Iridectomy/iridotomy
Lateral canthotomy
Medications
Operating microscope (69990)
Subconjunctival injection
Subtenon injection
Use of viscoelastic material
EXCLUDES Removal of intralenticular foreign body without lens excision (65235)
Repair of surgical laceration (66250)

66830 Removal of secondary membranous cataract (opacified posterior lens capsule and/or anterior hyaloid) with corneo-scleral section, with or without iridectomy (iridocapsulotomy, iridocapsulectomy)
INCLUDES Graefe's operation
📷 20.1 ⚖ 20.1 **FUD** 090 [T] [A2] [50] 📷
AMA: 2016,Feb,12; 2014,Jan,11

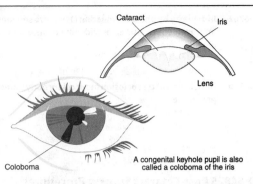

Cataract

Iris

Lens

Coloboma

A congenital keyhole pupil is also called a coloboma of the iris

66840 **Removal of lens material; aspiration technique, 1 or more stages**

INCLUDES Fukala's operation

19.7   19.7   **FUD** 090   T A2 50

AMA: 2016,Sep,9; 2016,Jun,6; 2016,Apr,8; 2016,Feb,12; 2016,Jan,13; 2015,Jan,16; 2014,Jan,11; 2012,Jan,15-42; 2011,Jan,11

66850 **phacofragmentation technique (mechanical or ultrasonic) (eg, phacoemulsification), with aspiration**

22.4   22.4   **FUD** 090   T A2 50

AMA: 2016,Jun,6; 2016,Feb,12; 2016,Jan,13; 2015,Jan,16; 2014,Jan,11; 2012,Jan,15-42; 2011,Jan,11

66852 **pars plana approach, with or without vitrectomy**

23.9   23.9   **FUD** 090   J A2 80 50

AMA: 2016,Jun,6; 2016,Feb,12; 2016,Jan,13; 2015,Jan,16; 2014,Jan,11; 2012,Jan,15-42; 2011,Jan,11

66920 **intracapsular**

21.3   21.3   **FUD** 090   T A2 80 50

AMA: 2016,Feb,12; 2016,Jan,13; 2015,Jan,16; 2014,Jan,11; 2012,Jan,15-42; 2011,Jan,11

66930 **intracapsular, for dislocated lens**

24.2   24.2   **FUD** 090   J A2 80 50

AMA: 2016,Feb,12; 2016,Jan,13; 2015,Jan,16; 2014,Jan,11; 2012,Jan,15-42; 2011,Jan,11

66940 **extracapsular (other than 66840, 66850, 66852)**

22.1   22.1   **FUD** 090   T A2 80 50

AMA: 2016,Jun,6; 2016,Feb,12; 2016,Jan,13; 2015,Jan,16; 2014,Jan,11; 2012,Jan,15-42; 2011,Jan,11

66982-66984 Cataract Extraction: With Insertion Intraocular Lens

CMS: 100-03,80.10 Phacoemulsification Procedure--Cataract Extraction; 100-04,32,120.2 PC-IOL and A-C IOL Billing

INCLUDES   Anterior or posterior capsulotomy
Enzymatic zonulysis
Iridectomy/iridotomy
Lateral canthotomy
Medications
Operating microscope (69990)
Subconjunctival injection
Subtenon injection
Use of viscoelastic material

EXCLUDES   *Implanted material removal from the anterior segment (65920)*
Insertion of ocular telescope prosthesis
Ocular telescope prosthesis insertion with lens removal (0308T)
Secondary fixation (66682)
Supply of intraocular lens

66982 **Extracapsular cataract removal with insertion of intraocular lens prosthesis (1-stage procedure), manual or mechanical technique (eg, irrigation and aspiration or phacoemulsification), complex, requiring devices or techniques not generally used in routine cataract surgery (eg, iris expansion device, suture support for intraocular lens, or primary posterior capsulorrhexis) or performed on patients in the amblyogenic developmental stage**

(76519)

22.5   22.5   **FUD** 090   T A2 50

AMA: 2016,Mar,10; 2016,Feb,12; 2016,Jan,13; 2015,Jan,16; 2014,Jan,11; 2013,Mar,6-7; 2012,Jan,15-42; 2011,Jan,11

66983 **Intracapsular cataract extraction with insertion of intraocular lens prosthesis (1 stage procedure)**

(76519)

20.9   20.9   **FUD** 090   T A2 50

AMA: 2016,Feb,12; 2016,Jan,13; 2015,Jan,16; 2014,Jan,11; 2013,Mar,6-7; 2012,Jan,15-42; 2011,Jan,11

66984 **Extracapsular cataract removal with insertion of intraocular lens prosthesis (1 stage procedure), manual or mechanical technique (eg, irrigation and aspiration or phacoemulsification)**

EXCLUDES   *Complex extracapsular cataract removal (66982)*

(76519)

18.1   18.1   **FUD** 090   T A2 50

AMA: 2016,Feb,12; 2016,Jan,13; 2015,Jan,16; 2014,Jan,11; 2013,Mar,6-7; 2012,Jan,15-42; 2011,Jan,11

66985-66986 Secondary Insertion or Replacement of Intraocular Lens

CMS: 100-03,80.10 Phacoemulsification Procedure--Cataract Extraction; 100-03,80.12 Intraocular Lenses (IOLs); 100-04,32,120.2 PC-IOL and A-C IOL Billing

INCLUDES   Operating microscope (69990)

EXCLUDES   *Implanted material removal from the anterior segment (65920)*
Insertion of ocular telescope prosthesis (0308T)
Secondary fixation (66682)
Supply of intraocular lens
Code also ophthalmic endoscope if used (66990)

66985 **Insertion of intraocular lens prosthesis (secondary implant), not associated with concurrent cataract removal**

EXCLUDES   *Insertion of lens at the time of cataract procedure (66982-66984)*

(76519)

21.8   21.8   **FUD** 090   T A2 50

AMA: 2016,Feb,12; 2016,Jan,13; 2015,Jan,16; 2014,Jan,11; 2013,Mar,6-7; 2012,Jan,15-42; 2011,Dec,14-18; 2011,Jan,11

66986 **Exchange of intraocular lens**

(76519)

25.7   25.7   **FUD** 090   T A2 50

AMA: 2016,Feb,12; 2016,Jan,13; 2015,Jan,16; 2014,Jan,11

66990-66999 Ophthalmic Endoscopy

INCLUDES   Operating microscope (69990)

+ **66990** **Use of ophthalmic endoscope (List separately in addition to code for primary procedure)**

Code first (65820, 65875, 65920, 66985-66986, 67036, 67039-67043, 67113)

2.57   2.57   **FUD** ZZZ   N N1

AMA: 2016,Sep,5; 2016,Feb,12; 2016,Jan,13; 2015,Jan,16; 2014,Jan,11; 2012,Jan,15-42; 2011,Jan,11

66999 **Unlisted procedure, anterior segment of eye**

0.00   0.00   **FUD** YYY   T 80 50

AMA: 2016,Apr,8; 2016,Feb,12; 2016,Jan,13; 2015,Jan,16; 2014,Jan,11

67005-67015 Vitrectomy: Partial and Subtotal

INCLUDES   Operating microscope (69990)

67005   **Removal of vitreous, anterior approach (open sky technique or limbal incision); partial removal**

EXCLUDES   *Anterior chamber vitrectomy by paracentesis (65810)*
Severing of corneovitreal adhesions (65880)

⏱ 13.3   ⚕ 13.3   **FUD** 090   T A2 50 ▣

AMA: 2016,Feb,12; 2016,Jan,13; 2015,Jan,16; 2014,Jan,11

67010   **subtotal removal with mechanical vitrectomy**

EXCLUDES   *Anterior chamber vitrectomy by paracentesis (65810)*
Severing of corneovitreal adhesions (65880)

⏱ 15.3   ⚕ 15.3   **FUD** 090   T A2 50 ▣

AMA: 2016,Feb,12; 2016,Jan,13; 2015,Jan,16; 2014,Jan,11

67015   **Aspiration or release of vitreous, subretinal or choroidal fluid, pars plana approach (posterior sclerotomy)**

⏱ 16.4   ⚕ 16.4   **FUD** 090   T A2 50 ▣

AMA: 2016,Sep,5; 2016,Jun,6; 2016,Feb,12; 2014,Jan,11

67025-67028 Intravitreal Injection/Implantation

INCLUDES   Operating microscope (69990)

67025   **Injection of vitreous substitute, pars plana or limbal approach (fluid-gas exchange), with or without aspiration (separate procedure)**

⏱ 17.9   ⚕ 20.5   **FUD** 090   T A2 50 ▣

AMA: 2016,Feb,12; 2014,Jan,11

67027   **Implantation of intravitreal drug delivery system (eg, ganciclovir implant), includes concomitant removal of vitreous**

EXCLUDES   *Removal of drug delivery system (67121)*

⏱ 24.1   ⚕ 24.1   **FUD** 090   J A2 80 50 ▣

AMA: 2016,Feb,12; 2016,Jan,13; 2015,Jan,16; 2014,Jan,11; 2012,Jan,15-42; 2011,Jan,11

67028   **Intravitreal injection of a pharmacologic agent (separate procedure)**

⏱ 2.84   ⚕ 2.89   **FUD** 000   S P3 50 ▣

AMA: 2016,Feb,12; 2016,Jan,13; 2015,Jan,16; 2014,Jan,11; 2012,Oct,14

67030-67031 Incision of Vitreous Strands/Membranes

INCLUDES   Operating microscope (69990)

67030   **Discission of vitreous strands (without removal), pars plana approach**

⏱ 15.0   ⚕ 15.0   **FUD** 090   T A2 50 ▣

AMA: 2016,Feb,12; 2014,Jan,11

67031   **Severing of vitreous strands, vitreous face adhesions, sheets, membranes or opacities, laser surgery (1 or more stages)**

⏱ 10.1   ⚕ 10.9   **FUD** 090   T A2 50 ▣

AMA: 2016,Feb,12; 2014,Jan,11

67036-67043 Pars Plana Mechanical Vitrectomy

INCLUDES   Operating microscope (69990)
EXCLUDES   *Foreign body removal (65260, 65265)*
Lens removal (66850)
Unlisted vitreal procedures (67299)
Vitrectomy in retinal detachment (67108, 67113)
Code also ophthalmic endoscope if used (66990)

67036   **Vitrectomy, mechanical, pars plana approach;**

Code also placement of intraocular radiation source applicator (0190T)

⏱ 25.5   ⚕ 25.5   **FUD** 090   T A2 80 50 ▣

AMA: 2016,Sep,5; 2016,Feb,12; 2016,Jan,13; 2015,Jan,16; 2014,Jan,11

67039   **with focal endolaser photocoagulation**

⏱ 27.3   ⚕ 27.3   **FUD** 090   J A2 80 50 ▣

AMA: 2016,Sep,5; 2016,Feb,12; 2016,Jan,13; 2015,Jan,16; 2014,Jan,11; 2012,Jan,15-42; 2011,Jan,11

67040   **with endolaser panretinal photocoagulation**

⏱ 29.5   ⚕ 29.5   **FUD** 090   J A2 80 50 ▣

AMA: 2016,Sep,5; 2016,Feb,12; 2016,Jan,13; 2015,Jan,16; 2014,Jan,11; 2012,Jan,15-42; 2011,Jan,11

67041   **with removal of preretinal cellular membrane (eg, macular pucker)**

⏱ 32.6   ⚕ 32.6   **FUD** 090   T 62 80 50 ▣

AMA: 2016,Sep,5; 2016,Feb,12; 2016,Jan,13; 2015,Jan,16; 2014,Jan,11

67042   **with removal of internal limiting membrane of retina (eg, for repair of macular hole, diabetic macular edema), includes, if performed, intraocular tamponade (ie, air, gas or silicone oil)**

⏱ 32.6   ⚕ 32.6   **FUD** 090   J 62 80 50 ▣

AMA: 2016,Sep,5; 2016,Feb,12; 2016,Jan,13; 2015,Jan,16; 2014,Jan,11

67043   **with removal of subretinal membrane (eg, choroidal neovascularization), includes, if performed, intraocular tamponade (ie, air, gas or silicone oil) and laser photocoagulation**

⏱ 34.4   ⚕ 34.4   **FUD** 090   J 62 80 50 ▣

AMA: 2016,Sep,5; 2016,Feb,12; 2016,Jan,13; 2015,Jan,16; 2014,Jan,11

67101-67115 Detached Retina Repair

INCLUDES   Operating microscope (69990)
Primary technique when cryotherapy and/or diathermy and/or photocoagulation are used in combination

▲ **67101**   **Repair of retinal detachment, including drainage of subretinal fluid when performed; cryotherapy**

⏱ 19.0   ⚕ 22.1   **FUD** 090   T P3 50 ▣

AMA: 2016,Sep,5; 2016,Jun,6; 2016,Feb,12; 2016,Jan,13; 2015,Jan,16; 2014,Jan,11

Vitreous
Optic nerve
Optic disc
Choroid
Sclera
Retina
Pars plana
Posterior chamber

▲ **67105**   **photocoagulation**

⏱ 18.2   ⚕ 20.3   **FUD** 090   T P2 50 ▣

AMA: 2016,Sep,5; 2016,Jun,6; 2016,Feb,12; 2016,Jan,13; 2015,Jan,16; 2014,Jan,11

67107   **Repair of retinal detachment; scleral buckling (such as lamellar scleral dissection, imbrication or encircling procedure), including, when performed, implant, cryotherapy, photocoagulation, and drainage of subretinal fluid**

INCLUDES   Gonin's operation

⏱ 28.8   ⚕ 28.8   **FUD** 090   J 62 80 50 ▣

AMA: 2016,Sep,5; 2016,Jun,6; 2016,Feb,12; 2014,Jan,11

67108   **with vitrectomy, any method, including, when performed, air or gas tamponade, focal endolaser photocoagulation, cryotherapy, drainage of subretinal fluid, scleral buckling, and/or removal of lens by same technique**

⏱ 36.7   ⚕ 36.7   **FUD** 090   J 62 80 50 ▣

AMA: 2016,Sep,5; 2016,Jun,6; 2016,Feb,12; 2016,Jan,13; 2015,Jan,16; 2014,Jan,11; 2012,Mar,9-10; 2012,Jan,15-42; 2011,Jan,11

67110   **by injection of air or other gas (eg, pneumatic retinopexy)**

⏱ 19.7   ⚕ 21.5   **FUD** 090   T P3 50 ▣

AMA: 2016,Sep,5; 2016,Jun,6; 2016,Feb,12; 2014,Jan,11

67113 Repair of complex retinal detachment (eg, proliferative vitreoretinopathy, stage C-1 or greater, diabetic traction retinal detachment, retinopathy of prematurity, retinal tear of greater than 90 degrees), with vitrectomy and membrane peeling, including, when performed, air, gas, or silicone oil tamponade, cryotherapy, endolaser photocoagulation, drainage of subretinal fluid, scleral buckling, and/or removal of lens

EXCLUDES *Vitrectomy for other than retinal detachment, pars plana approach (67036-67043)*
Code also ophthalmic endoscope if used (66990)

🔧 39.9 ⚖ 39.9 **FUD** 090 Ⓙ G2 80 50 🖵

AMA: 2016,Sep,5; 2016,Jun,6; 2016,Feb,12; 2016,Jan,13; 2015,Jan,16; 2014,Jan,11

67115 Release of encircling material (posterior segment)

🔧 14.1 ⚖ 14.1 **FUD** 090 T A2 50 🖵

AMA: 2016,Feb,12; 2014,Jan,11

67120-67121 Removal of Previously Implanted Prosthetic Device

INCLUDES Operating microscope (69990)
EXCLUDES *Foreign body removal (65260, 65265)*
Removal of implanted material anterior segment (65920)

67120 Removal of implanted material, posterior segment; extraocular

🔧 15.8 ⚖ 18.5 **FUD** 090 T A2 50 🖵

AMA: 2016,Feb,12; 2014,Jan,11

67121 intraocular

🔧 25.7 ⚖ 25.7 **FUD** 090 T A2 80 50 🖵

AMA: 2016,Feb,12; 2014,Jan,11

67141-67145 Retinal Detachment: Preventative Procedures

INCLUDES Operating microscope (69990)
Treatment at one or more sessions that may occur at different encounters
EXCLUDES *Procedure performed more than one time during a defined period of treatment*

67141 Prophylaxis of retinal detachment (eg, retinal break, lattice degeneration) without drainage, 1 or more sessions; cryotherapy, diathermy

🔧 13.8 ⚖ 14.8 **FUD** 090 T A2 50 🖵

AMA: 2016,Sep,5; 2016,Feb,12; 2016,Jan,13; 2015,Jan,16; 2014,Jan,11

67145 photocoagulation (laser or xenon arc)

🔧 14.1 ⚖ 14.9 **FUD** 090 T P2 50 🖵

AMA: 2016,Sep,5; 2016,Feb,12; 2016,Jan,13; 2015,Jan,16; 2014,Jan,11

67208-67218 Destruction of Retinal Lesions

INCLUDES Operating microscope (69990)
Treatment at one or more sessions that may occur at different encounters
EXCLUDES *Procedure performed more than one time during a defined period of treatment*
Unlisted retinal procedures (67299)

67208 Destruction of localized lesion of retina (eg, macular edema, tumors), 1 or more sessions; cryotherapy, diathermy

🔧 16.3 ⚖ 16.9 **FUD** 090 T P2 50 🖵

AMA: 2016,Feb,12; 2016,Jan,13; 2015,Jan,16; 2014,Jan,11

67210 photocoagulation

🔧 14.1 ⚖ 14.6 **FUD** 090 T P2 50 🖵

AMA: 2016,Feb,12; 2016,Jan,13; 2015,Jan,16; 2014,Jan,11; 2012,Jan,3-5

67218 radiation by implantation of source (includes removal of source)

🔧 39.2 ⚖ 39.2 **FUD** 090 T A2 50 🖵

AMA: 2016,Feb,12; 2016,Jan,13; 2015,Jan,16; 2014,Jan,11

67220-67225 Destruction of Choroidal Lesions

INCLUDES Operating microscope (69990)

67220 Destruction of localized lesion of choroid (eg, choroidal neovascularization); photocoagulation (eg, laser), 1 or more sessions

INCLUDES Treatment at one or more sessions that may occur at different encounters
EXCLUDES *Procedure performed more than one time during a defined period of treatment*

🔧 14.1 ⚖ 15.1 **FUD** 090 T P2 50 🖵

AMA: 2016,Feb,12; 2016,Jan,13; 2015,Jan,16; 2014,Jan,11; 2012,Jan,3-5; 2012,Jan,15-42; 2011,Jan,11

67221 photodynamic therapy (includes intravenous infusion)

🔧 6.06 ⚖ 8.11 **FUD** 000 T P3 🖵

AMA: 2016,Feb,12; 2016,Jan,13; 2015,Jan,16; 2014,Jan,11; 2012,Jan,15-42; 2011,Jan,11

+ **67225** photodynamic therapy, second eye, at single session (List separately in addition to code for primary eye treatment)

Code first (67221)

🔧 0.79 ⚖ 0.84 **FUD** ZZZ N N1 🖵

AMA: 2016,Feb,12; 2016,Jan,13; 2015,Jan,16; 2014,Jan,11; 2012,Jan,15-42; 2011,Jan,11

67227-67229 Destruction Retinopathy

INCLUDES Operating microscope (69990)
EXCLUDES *Unlisted retinal procedures (67299)*

67227 Destruction of extensive or progressive retinopathy (eg, diabetic retinopathy), cryotherapy, diathermy

🔧 7.28 ⚖ 8.19 **FUD** 010 T G2 50 🖵

AMA: 2016,Feb,12; 2016,Jan,13; 2015,Jan,16; 2014,Jan,11; 2012,Jan,15-42; 2011,Jan,11

67228 Treatment of extensive or progressive retinopathy (eg, diabetic retinopathy), photocoagulation

🔧 8.71 ⚖ 9.64 **FUD** 010 T P3 50 🖵

AMA: 2016,Feb,12; 2016,Jan,13; 2015,Jan,16; 2014,Jan,11

67229 Treatment of extensive or progressive retinopathy, 1 or more sessions, preterm infant (less than 37 weeks gestation at birth), performed from birth up to 1 year of age (eg, retinopathy of prematurity), photocoagulation or cryotherapy

EXCLUDES *Procedure performed more than one time during a defined period of treatment*

🔧 31.6 ⚖ 31.6 **FUD** 090 T A2 50 🖵

AMA: 2016,Feb,12; 2016,Jan,13; 2015,Jan,16; 2014,Jan,11

67250-67255 Reinforcement of Posterior Sclera

INCLUDES Operating microscope (69990)
EXCLUDES *Removal of lesion of sclera (66130)*
Repair scleral staphyloma (66220, 66225)

67250 Scleral reinforcement (separate procedure); without graft

🔧 22.1 ⚖ 22.1 **FUD** 090 T A2 50 🖵

AMA: 2016,Feb,12; 2014,Jan,11

67255 with graft

EXCLUDES *Aqueous shunt to extraocular equatorial plate reservoir (66180)*
Revision of aqueous shunt to extraocular equatorial plate reservoir; with graft (66185)

🔧 19.3 ⚖ 19.3 **FUD** 090 T A2 80 50 🖵

AMA: 2016,Feb,12; 2016,Jan,13; 2015,Jan,16; 2015,Jan,10; 2014,Jan,11; 2012,Jun,15-16

67299 Unlisted Posterior Segment Procedure

CMS: 100-04,4,180.3 Unlisted Service or Procedure
INCLUDES Operating microscope (69990)

67299 Unlisted procedure, posterior segment

🔧 0.00 ⚖ 0.00 **FUD** YYY T 80 50

AMA: 2016,Feb,12; 2016,Jan,13; 2015,Jan,16; 2014,Jan,11; 2012,Jan,15-42; 2011,Jan,11

26/TC PC/TC Only   A2-Z3 ASC Payment   50 Bilateral   ♂ Male Only   ♀ Female Only   🔧 Facility RVU   ⚖ Non-Facility RVU   🖵 CCI
FUD Follow-up Days   CMS: IOM (Pub 100)   A-Y OPPSI   80/80 Surg Assist Allowed / w/Doc   🔬 Lab crosswalk   📊 Radiology crosswalk   ❌ CLIA

CPT © 2016 American Medical Association. All Rights Reserved.   © 2016 Optum360, LLC

Eye, Ocular Adnexa, and Ear

67113 — 67299

67311-67334 Strabismus Procedures on Extraocular Muscles

INCLUDES Operating microscope (69990)
Code also adjustable sutures (67335)

67311 Strabismus surgery, recession or resection procedure; 1 horizontal muscle

🔧 16.9 ✂ 16.9 **FUD** 090 T A2 50

AMA: 2016,Feb,12; 2016,Jan,13; 2015,Jan,16; 2014,Jan,11; 2012,Jan,15-42; 2011,Jan,11

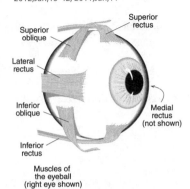

Superior rectus
Superior oblique
Lateral rectus
Inferior oblique
Inferior rectus
Medial rectus (not shown)
Muscles of the eyeball (right eye shown)

67312 2 horizontal muscles

🔧 20.1 ✂ 20.1 **FUD** 090 T A2 50

AMA: 2016,Feb,12; 2016,Jan,13; 2015,Jan,16; 2014,Jan,11; 2012,Jan,15-42; 2011,Jan,11

67314 1 vertical muscle (excluding superior oblique)

🔧 19.0 ✂ 19.0 **FUD** 090 T A2 50

AMA: 2016,Feb,12; 2016,Jan,13; 2015,Jan,16; 2014,Jan,11

67316 2 or more vertical muscles (excluding superior oblique)

🔧 22.7 ✂ 22.7 **FUD** 090 T A2 80 50

AMA: 2016,Feb,12; 2016,Jan,13; 2015,Jan,16; 2014,Jan,11

67318 Strabismus surgery, any procedure, superior oblique muscle

🔧 19.9 ✂ 19.9 **FUD** 090 T A2 50

AMA: 2016,Feb,12; 2016,Jan,13; 2015,Jan,16; 2014,Jan,11

+ 67320 Transposition procedure (eg, for paretic extraocular muscle), any extraocular muscle (specify) (List separately in addition to code for primary procedure)

Code first (67311-67318)

🔧 9.17 ✂ 9.17 **FUD** ZZZ N N1

AMA: 2016,Feb,12; 2016,Jan,13; 2015,Jan,16; 2014,Jan,11

+ 67331 Strabismus surgery on patient with previous eye surgery or injury that did not involve the extraocular muscles (List separately in addition to code for primary procedure)

Code first (67311-67318)

🔧 8.70 ✂ 8.70 **FUD** ZZZ N N1 50

AMA: 2016,Feb,12; 2016,Jan,13; 2015,Jan,16; 2014,Jan,11

+ 67332 Strabismus surgery on patient with scarring of extraocular muscles (eg, prior ocular injury, strabismus or retinal detachment surgery) or restrictive myopathy (eg, dysthyroid ophthalmopathy) (List separately in addition to code for primary procedure)

Code first (67311-67318)

🔧 9.44 ✂ 9.44 **FUD** ZZZ N N1 50

AMA: 2016,Feb,12; 2016,Jan,13; 2015,Jan,16; 2014,Jan,11

+ 67334 Strabismus surgery by posterior fixation suture technique, with or without muscle recession (List separately in addition to code for primary procedure)

Code first (67311-67318)

🔧 8.58 ✂ 8.58 **FUD** ZZZ N N1 50

AMA: 2016,Feb,12; 2016,Jan,13; 2015,Jan,16; 2014,Jan,11

67335-67399 Other Procedures of Extraocular Muscles

INCLUDES Operating microscope (69990)

+ 67335 Placement of adjustable suture(s) during strabismus surgery, including postoperative adjustment(s) of suture(s) (List separately in addition to code for specific strabismus surgery)

Code first (67311-67334)

🔧 4.22 ✂ 4.22 **FUD** ZZZ N N1 50

AMA: 2016,Feb,12; 2016,Jan,13; 2015,Jan,16; 2014,Jan,11

+ 67340 Strabismus surgery involving exploration and/or repair of detached extraocular muscle(s) (List separately in addition to code for primary procedure)

INCLUDES Hummelsheim operation
Code first (67311-67334)

🔧 10.2 ✂ 10.2 **FUD** ZZZ N N1 80

AMA: 2016,Feb,12; 2016,Jan,13; 2015,Jan,16; 2014,Jan,11

67343 Release of extensive scar tissue without detaching extraocular muscle (separate procedure)

Code also if these procedures are performed on other than the affected muscle (67311-67340)

🔧 18.5 ✂ 18.5 **FUD** 090 T A2 50

AMA: 2016,Feb,12; 2016,Jan,13; 2015,Jan,16; 2014,Jan,11

67345 Chemodenervation of extraocular muscle

EXCLUDES Nerve destruction for blepharospasm and other neurological disorders (64612, 64616)

🔧 6.21 ✂ 6.89 **FUD** 010 T P3 50

AMA: 2016,Feb,12; 2016,Jan,13; 2015,Jan,16; 2014,May,5; 2014,Jan,11; 2013,Dec,10; 2012,Jan,15-42; 2011,Jan,11

67346 Biopsy of extraocular muscle

EXCLUDES Repair laceration extraocular muscle, tendon, or Tenon's capsule (65290)

🔧 5.50 ✂ 5.50 **FUD** 000 T A2 80 50

AMA: 2016,Feb,12; 2014,Jan,11

67399 Unlisted procedure, extraocular muscle

🔧 0.00 ✂ 0.00 **FUD** YYY T 80 50

AMA: 2016,Feb,12; 2014,Jan,11

67400-67415 Frontal Orbitotomy

INCLUDES Operating microscope (69990)

67400 Orbitotomy without bone flap (frontal or transconjunctival approach); for exploration, with or without biopsy

🔧 26.3 ✂ 26.3 **FUD** 090 T A2 50

AMA: 2016,Feb,12; 2014,Jan,11

67405 with drainage only

🔧 22.4 ✂ 22.4 **FUD** 090 T A2 50

AMA: 2016,Feb,12; 2016,Jan,13; 2015,Jan,16; 2014,Jan,11; 2012,Jan,15-42; 2011,Jan,11

67412 with removal of lesion

🔧 24.0 ✂ 24.0 **FUD** 090 T A2 50

AMA: 2016,Feb,12; 2014,Jan,11

67413 with removal of foreign body

🔧 24.2 ✂ 24.2 **FUD** 090 T A2 80 50

AMA: 2016,Feb,12; 2014,Jan,11

67414 with removal of bone for decompression

🔧 37.5 ✂ 37.5 **FUD** 090 T G2 80 50

AMA: 2016,Feb,12; 2016,Jan,13; 2015,Jan,16; 2014,Jan,11; 2012,Jan,15-42; 2011,Jan,11

67415 Fine needle aspiration of orbital contents

EXCLUDES Decompression optic nerve (67570)
Exenteration, enucleation, and repair (65101-65175)

🔧 2.97 ✂ 2.97 **FUD** 000 T A2 80 50

AMA: 2016,Feb,12; 2014,Jan,11

67420-67450 Lateral Orbitotomy

INCLUDES Operating microscope (69990)
EXCLUDES Orbital implant (67550, 67560)
Surgical removal of all or some of the orbital contents or repair after removal (65091-65175)
Transcranial approach orbitotomy (61330-61333)

67420 Orbitotomy with bone flap or window, lateral approach (eg, Kroenlein); with removal of lesion
🚗 45.8 ⚖ 45.8 **FUD** 090 T A2 80 50 ▢
AMA: 2016,Feb,12; 2014,Jan,11

67430 with removal of foreign body
🚗 35.0 ⚖ 35.0 **FUD** 090 T A2 80 50 ▢
AMA: 2016,Feb,12; 2014,Jan,11

67440 with drainage
🚗 34.0 ⚖ 34.0 **FUD** 090 T A2 80 50 ▢
AMA: 2016,Feb,12; 2014,Jan,11

67445 with removal of bone for decompression
EXCLUDES Decompression optic nerve sheath (67570)
🚗 39.7 ⚖ 39.7 **FUD** 090 T A2 80 50 ▢
AMA: 2016,Feb,12; 2014,Jan,11

67450 for exploration, with or without biopsy
🚗 35.5 ⚖ 35.5 **FUD** 090 T A2 80 50 ▢
AMA: 2016,Feb,12; 2014,Jan,11

67500-67515 Eye Injections

INCLUDES Operating microscope (69990)

67500 Retrobulbar injection; medication (separate procedure, does not include supply of medication)
🚗 2.05 ⚖ 2.22 **FUD** 000 T G2 50 ▢
AMA: 2016,Feb,12; 2016,Jan,13; 2015,Jan,16; 2014,Jan,11; 2012,Nov,10

67505 alcohol
🚗 2.31 ⚖ 2.52 **FUD** 000 T P3 50 ▢
AMA: 2016,Feb,12; 2014,Jan,11

67515 Injection of medication or other substance into Tenon's capsule
EXCLUDES Subconjunctival injection (68200)
🚗 2.53 ⚖ 2.74 **FUD** 000 T P3 50 ▢
AMA: 2016,Feb,12; 2016,Jan,13; 2015,Jan,16; 2014,Jan,11; 2012,Nov,10

67550-67560 Orbital Implant

INCLUDES Operating microscope (69990)
EXCLUDES Fracture repair malar area, orbit (21355-21408)
Ocular implant inside muscle cone (65093-65105, 65130-65175)

67550 Orbital implant (implant outside muscle cone); insertion
🚗 27.2 ⚖ 27.2 **FUD** 090 T A2 50 ▢
AMA: 2016,Feb,12; 2014,Jan,11

67560 removal or revision
🚗 27.9 ⚖ 27.9 **FUD** 090 T A2 80 50 ▢
AMA: 2016,Feb,12; 2014,Jan,11

67570-67599 Other and Unlisted Orbital Procedures

INCLUDES Operating microscope (69990)

67570 Optic nerve decompression (eg, incision or fenestration of optic nerve sheath)
🚗 32.9 ⚖ 32.9 **FUD** 090 T A2 80 50 ▢
AMA: 2016,Feb,12; 2014,Jan,11

67599 Unlisted procedure, orbit
🚗 0.00 ⚖ 0.00 **FUD** YYY T 80 50
AMA: 2016,Feb,12; 2014,Jan,11

67700-67715 [67810] Incisional Procedures of Eyelids

INCLUDES Operating microscope (69990)

67700 Blepharotomy, drainage of abscess, eyelid
🚗 3.30 ⚖ 7.56 **FUD** 010 T P2 50 ▢
AMA: 2016,Feb,12; 2016,Jan,13; 2015,Jan,16; 2014,Jan,11; 2013,Mar,6-7

67710 Severing of tarsorrhaphy
🚗 2.76 ⚖ 6.30 **FUD** 010 T P3 50 ▢
AMA: 2016,Feb,12; 2016,Jan,13; 2015,Jan,16; 2014,Jan,11; 2013,Mar,6-7

67715 Canthotomy (separate procedure)
EXCLUDES Canthoplasty (67950)
Symblepharon division (68340)
🚗 3.08 ⚖ 6.72 **FUD** 010 T A2 50 ▢
AMA: 2016,Feb,12; 2016,Jan,13; 2015,Jan,16; 2014,Jan,11; 2013,Mar,6-7

\# **67810** Incisional biopsy of eyelid skin including lid margin
EXCLUDES Biopsy of eyelid skin (11100-11101, 11310-11313)
🚗 2.05 ⚖ 4.86 **FUD** 000 T P3 50 ▢
AMA: 2016,Feb,12; 2016,Jan,13; 2015,Jan,16; 2014,Jan,11; 2013,Mar,6-7; 2013,Feb,16-17; 2012,Jan,15-42; 2011,Jan,11

67800-67808 Excision of Chalazion (Meibomian Cyst)

INCLUDES Lesion removal requiring more than skin:
Lid margin
Palpebral conjunctiva
Tarsus
Operating microscope (69990)
EXCLUDES Blepharoplasty, graft, or reconstructive procedures (67930-67975)
Excision/destruction skin lesion of eyelid (11310-11313, 11440-11446, 11640-11646, 17000-17004)

67800 Excision of chalazion; single
🚗 2.93 ⚖ 3.59 **FUD** 010 T P3
AMA: 2016,Feb,12; 2016,Jan,13; 2015,Jan,16; 2014,Jan,11; 2013,Mar,6-7; 2012,Jan,15-42; 2011,Jan,11

67801 multiple, same lid
🚗 3.79 ⚖ 4.58 **FUD** 010 T P3 ▢
AMA: 2016,Feb,12; 2014,Jan,11; 2013,Mar,6-7

67805 multiple, different lids
🚗 4.67 ⚖ 5.70 **FUD** 010 T P3 ▢
AMA: 2016,Feb,12; 2016,Jan,13; 2015,Jan,16; 2014,Jan,11; 2013,Mar,6-7; 2012,Jan,15-42; 2011,Jan,11

67808 under general anesthesia and/or requiring hospitalization, single or multiple
🚗 10.4 ⚖ 10.4 **FUD** 090 T A2 ▢
AMA: 2016,Feb,12; 2014,Jan,11; 2013,Mar,6-7

67810-67850 Other Eyelid Procedures

INCLUDES Operating microscope (69990)

67810 Resequenced code. See code following 67715.

67820 Correction of trichiasis; epilation, by forceps only
🚗 1.51 ⚖ 1.41 **FUD** 000 01 N1 50 ▢
AMA: 2016,Feb,12; 2016,Jan,13; 2015,Jan,16; 2014,Jan,11; 2012,Jan,15-42; 2011,Jan,11

67825 epilation by other than forceps (eg, by electrosurgery, cryotherapy, laser surgery)
🚗 3.44 ⚖ 3.63 **FUD** 010 T P3 50 ▢
AMA: 2016,Feb,12; 2016,Jan,13; 2015,Jan,16; 2014,Jan,11; 2012,Jan,15-42; 2011,Jan,11

67830 incision of lid margin
🚗 3.92 ⚖ 7.51 **FUD** 010 T A2 50 ▢
AMA: 2016,Feb,12; 2014,Jan,11

67835 incision of lid margin, with free mucous membrane graft
🚗 12.4 ⚖ 12.4 **FUD** 090 T A2 80 50 ▢
AMA: 2016,Feb,12; 2014,Jan,11

67840 Excision of lesion of eyelid (except chalazion) without closure or with simple direct closure
EXCLUDES Eyelid resection and reconstruction (67961, 67966)
🚗 4.49 ⚖ 7.76 **FUD** 010 T P3 50 ▢
AMA: 2016,Feb,12; 2014,Jan,11

67850 Destruction of lesion of lid margin (up to 1 cm)
EXCLUDES Mohs micro procedures (17311-17315)
Topical chemotherapy (99201-99215)
🚗 3.87 ⚖ 6.06 **FUD** 010 T P3 50 ▢
AMA: 2016,Feb,12; 2014,Jan,11

67875-67882 Suturing of the Eyelids

INCLUDES Operating microscope (69990)
EXCLUDES Canthoplasty (67950)
Canthotomy (67715)
Severing of tarsorrhaphy (67710)

67875 **Temporary closure of eyelids by suture (eg, Frost suture)**
2.76 4.84 **FUD** 000 T G2 50
AMA: 2016,Feb,12; 2014,Jan,11

67880 **Construction of intermarginal adhesions, median tarsorrhaphy, or canthorrhaphy;**
10.4 12.9 **FUD** 090 T A2 50
AMA: 2016,Feb,12; 2014,Jan,11

67882 **with transposition of tarsal plate**
13.3 15.9 **FUD** 090 T A2 50
AMA: 2016,Feb,12; 2014,Jan,11

67900-67912 Repair of Ptosis/Retraction Eyelids, Eyebrows

INCLUDES Operating microscope (69990)

67900 **Repair of brow ptosis (supraciliary, mid-forehead or coronal approach)**
EXCLUDES Forehead rhytidectomy (15824)
14.4 18.0 **FUD** 090 T A2 50
AMA: 2016,Feb,12; 2016,Jan,13; 2015,Jan,16; 2014,Jan,11; 2012,Jan,15-42; 2011,Jan,11

67901 **Repair of blepharoptosis; frontalis muscle technique with suture or other material (eg, banked fascia)**
16.3 21.3 **FUD** 090 T A2 50
AMA: 2016,Feb,12; 2016,Jan,13; 2015,Jan,16; 2014,Jan,11

67902 **frontalis muscle technique with autologous fascial sling (includes obtaining fascia)**
20.5 20.5 **FUD** 090 T A2 50
AMA: 2016,Feb,12; 2016,Jan,13; 2015,Jan,16; 2014,Jan,11

67903 **(tarso) levator resection or advancement, internal approach**
13.7 16.7 **FUD** 090 T A2 50
AMA: 2016,Feb,12; 2016,Jan,13; 2015,Jan,16; 2014,Jan,11

67904 **(tarso) levator resection or advancement, external approach**
INCLUDES Everbusch's operation
16.9 20.6 **FUD** 090 T A2 50
AMA: 2016,Feb,12; 2016,Jan,13; 2015,Jan,16; 2014,Jan,11; 2011,Aug,8

67906 **superior rectus technique with fascial sling (includes obtaining fascia)**
14.3 14.3 **FUD** 090 T A2 50
AMA: 2016,Feb,12; 2016,Jan,13; 2015,Jan,16; 2014,Jan,11

67908 **conjunctivo-tarso-Muller's muscle-levator resection (eg, Fasanella-Servat type)**
12.0 13.9 **FUD** 090 T A2 50
AMA: 2016,Feb,12; 2016,Jan,13; 2015,Jan,16; 2014,Jan,11

67909 **Reduction of overcorrection of ptosis**
12.4 15.1 **FUD** 090 T A2 50
AMA: 2016,Feb,12; 2016,Jan,13; 2015,Jan,16; 2014,Jan,11

67911 **Correction of lid retraction**
EXCLUDES Graft harvest (20920, 20922, 20926)
Mucous membrane graft repair of trichiasis (67835)
15.9 15.9 **FUD** 090 T A2 50
AMA: 2016,Feb,12; 2016,Jan,13; 2015,Jan,16; 2014,Jan,11

67912 **Correction of lagophthalmos, with implantation of upper eyelid lid load (eg, gold weight)**
13.9 24.9 **FUD** 090 T A2 50
AMA: 2016,Feb,12; 2016,Jan,13; 2015,Jan,16; 2014,Jan,11; 2012,Jan,15-42; 2011,Jan,11

67914-67924 Repair Ectropion/Entropion

INCLUDES Operating microscope (69990)
EXCLUDES Cicatricial ectropion or entropion with scar excision or graft (67961-67966)

67914 **Repair of ectropion; suture**
9.28 13.2 **FUD** 090 T A2 50
AMA: 2016,Feb,12; 2016,Jan,13; 2015,Jan,16; 2014,Jan,11

67915 **thermocauterization**
5.61 8.25 **FUD** 090 T P3 50
AMA: 2016,Feb,12; 2016,Jan,13; 2015,Jan,16; 2014,Jan,11

67916 **excision tarsal wedge**
12.2 16.7 **FUD** 090 T A2 50
AMA: 2016,Feb,12; 2016,Jan,13; 2015,Jan,16; 2014,Jan,11; 2012,Jan,15-42; 2011,Jan,11

67917 **extensive (eg, tarsal strip operations)**
EXCLUDES Repair of everted punctum (68705)
12.9 17.0 **FUD** 090 T A2 50
AMA: 2016,Feb,12; 2016,Jan,13; 2015,Jan,16; 2014,Jan,11; 2012,Jan,15-42; 2011,Jan,11

67921 **Repair of entropion; suture**
8.80 12.9 **FUD** 090 T A2 50
AMA: 2016,Feb,12; 2016,Jan,13; 2015,Jan,16; 2014,Jan,11

67922 **thermocauterization**
5.60 8.18 **FUD** 090 T P3 50
AMA: 2016,Feb,12; 2016,Jan,13; 2015,Jan,16; 2014,Jan,11

67923 **excision tarsal wedge**
12.2 16.6 **FUD** 090 T A2 50
AMA: 2016,Feb,12; 2016,Jan,13; 2015,Jan,16; 2014,Jan,11

67924 **extensive (eg, tarsal strip or capsulopalpebral fascia repairs operation)**
12.9 17.7 **FUD** 090 T A2 50
AMA: 2016,Feb,12; 2016,Jan,13; 2015,Jan,16; 2014,Jan,11

67930-67935 Repair Eyelid Wound

INCLUDES Operating microscope (69990)
Repairs involving more than skin:
Lid margin
Palpebral conjunctiva
Tarsus
EXCLUDES Blepharoplasty for entropion or ectropion (67916-67917, 67923-67924)
Correction of lid retraction and blepharoptosis (67901-67911)
Free graft (15120-15121, 15260-15261)
Graft preparation (15004)
Plastic repair of lacrimal canaliculi (68700)
Removal of eyelid lesion (67800 [67810], 67840-67850)
Repair involving skin of eyelid (12011-12018, 12051-12057, 13151-13153)
Repair of blepharochalasis (15820-15823)
Skin adjacent tissue transfer (14060-14061)
Tarsorrhaphy, canthorrhaphy (67880, 67882)

67930 **Suture of recent wound, eyelid, involving lid margin, tarsus, and/or palpebral conjunctiva direct closure; partial thickness**
6.81 10.2 **FUD** 010 T P3 50
AMA: 2016,Feb,12; 2014,Jan,11

67935 **full thickness**
12.5 16.7 **FUD** 090 T A2 50
AMA: 2016,Feb,12; 2014,Jan,11

67938-67999 Eyelid Reconstruction/Repair/Removal Deep Foreign Body

INCLUDES Operating microscope (69990)

EXCLUDES *Blepharoplasty for entropion or ectropion (67916-67917, 67923-67924)*
Correction of lid retraction and blepharoptosis (67901-67911)
Free graft (15120-15121, 15260-15261)
Graft preparation (15004)
Plastic repair of lacrimal canaliculi (68700)
Removal of eyelid lesion (67800-67808, 67840-67850)
Repair involving skin of eyelid (12011-12018, 12051-12057, 13151-13153)
Repair of blepharochalasis (15820-15823)
Skin adjacent tissue transfer (14060-14061)
Tarsorrhaphy, canthorrhaphy (67880, 67882)

67938 **Removal of embedded foreign body, eyelid**
🚗 3.28   🔪 6.82   **FUD** 010   T P2 50 ▢
AMA: 2016,Feb,12; 2016,Jan,13; 2015,Jan,16; 2014,May,5; 2014,Jan,11

67950 **Canthoplasty (reconstruction of canthus)**
🚗 13.1   🔪 16.1   **FUD** 090   T A2 50 ▢
AMA: 2016,Feb,12; 2014,Jan,11

67961 **Excision and repair of eyelid, involving lid margin, tarsus, conjunctiva, canthus, or full thickness, may include preparation for skin graft or pedicle flap with adjacent tissue transfer or rearrangement; up to one-fourth of lid margin**
EXCLUDES *Canthoplasty (67950)*
Delay flap (15630)
Flap attachment (15650)
Free skin grafts (15120-15121, 15260-15261)
Tubed pedicle flap preparation (15576)
🚗 12.8   🔪 16.2   **FUD** 090   T A2 80 50 ▢
AMA: 2016,Feb,12; 2016,Jan,13; 2015,Jan,16; 2014,Jan,11

67966 **over one-fourth of lid margin**
EXCLUDES *Canthoplasty (67950)*
Delay flap (15630)
Flap attachment (15650)
Free skin grafts (15120-15121, 15260-15261)
Tubed pedicle flap preparation (15576)
🚗 18.6   🔪 21.7   **FUD** 090   T A2 50 ▢
AMA: 2016,Feb,12; 2016,Jan,13; 2015,Jan,16; 2014,Jan,11; 2012,Nov,13-14

67971 **Reconstruction of eyelid, full thickness by transfer of tarsoconjunctival flap from opposing eyelid; up to two-thirds of eyelid, 1 stage or first stage**
INCLUDES Dupuy-Dutemp reconstruction
Landboldt's operation
🚗 20.5   🔪 20.5   **FUD** 090   T A2 50 ▢
AMA: 2016,Feb,12; 2014,Jan,11

67973 **total eyelid, lower, 1 stage or first stage**
INCLUDES Landboldt's operation
🚗 26.3   🔪 26.3   **FUD** 090   T A2 80 50 ▢
AMA: 2016,Feb,12; 2014,Jan,11

67974 **total eyelid, upper, 1 stage or first stage**
INCLUDES Landboldt's operation
🚗 26.3   🔪 26.3   **FUD** 090   T A2 80 50 ▢
AMA: 2016,Feb,12; 2014,Jan,11

67975 **second stage**
INCLUDES Landboldt's operation
🚗 19.4   🔪 19.4   **FUD** 090   T A2 50 ▢
AMA: 2016,Feb,12; 2014,Jan,11

67999 **Unlisted procedure, eyelids**
🚗 0.00   🔪 0.00   **FUD** YYY   T 80 50
AMA: 2016,Feb,12; 2016,Jan,13; 2015,Jan,16; 2014,Jan,11; 2012,Jan,15-42; 2011,Jan,11

68020-68200 Conjunctival Biopsy/Injection/Treatment of Lesions

INCLUDES Operating microscope (69990)

EXCLUDES *Foreign body removal (65205-65265)*

68020 **Incision of conjunctiva, drainage of cyst**
🚗 3.13   🔪 3.38   **FUD** 010   T P3 50 ▢
AMA: 2016,Feb,12; 2014,Jan,11

68040 **Expression of conjunctival follicles (eg, for trachoma)**
EXCLUDES *Automated evacuation meibomian glands with heat/pressure (0207T)*
🚗 1.44   🔪 1.77   **FUD** 0207T   T P3 50 ▢
AMA: 2016,Feb,12; 2016,Jan,13; 2015,Jan,16; 2014,May,5; 2014,Jan,11

68100 **Biopsy of conjunctiva**
🚗 2.76   🔪 4.79   **FUD** 000   T P3 50 ▢
AMA: 2016,Feb,12; 2014,Jan,11

68110 **Excision of lesion, conjunctiva; up to 1 cm**
🚗 4.21   🔪 6.36   **FUD** 010   T P3 50 ▢
AMA: 2016,Feb,12; 2014,Jan,11

68115 **over 1 cm**
🚗 5.22   🔪 8.79   **FUD** 010   T A2 50 ▢
AMA: 2016,Feb,12; 2014,Jan,11

68130 **with adjacent sclera**
🚗 11.6   🔪 15.2   **FUD** 090   T A2 50 ▢
AMA: 2016,Feb,12; 2014,Jan,11

68135 **Destruction of lesion, conjunctiva**
🚗 4.28   🔪 4.43   **FUD** 010   T P3 50 ▢
AMA: 2016,Feb,12; 2014,Jan,11

68200 **Subconjunctival injection**
EXCLUDES *Retrobulbar or Tenon's capsule injection (67500-67515)*
🚗 0.99   🔪 1.17   **FUD** 000   01 N1 50 ▢
AMA: 2016,Feb,12; 2016,Jan,13; 2015,Jan,16; 2014,Jan,11; 2012,Nov,10; 2012,Jan,15-42; 2011,Jan,11

68320-68340 Conjunctivoplasty Procedures

INCLUDES Operating microscope (69990)

EXCLUDES *Conjunctival foreign body removal (65205, 65210)*
Laceration repair (65270-65273)

68320 **Conjunctivoplasty; with conjunctival graft or extensive rearrangement**
🚗 15.2   🔪 20.4   **FUD** 090   T A2 50 ▢
AMA: 2016,Feb,12; 2016,Jan,13; 2015,Jan,16; 2014,Jan,11; 2012,Jan,15-42; 2011,Jan,11

68325 **with buccal mucous membrane graft (includes obtaining graft)**
🚗 18.6   🔪 18.6   **FUD** 090   T A2 50 ▢
AMA: 2016,Feb,12; 2014,Jan,11

68326 **Conjunctivoplasty, reconstruction cul-de-sac; with conjunctival graft or extensive rearrangement**
🚗 18.3   🔪 18.3   **FUD** 090   T A2 50 ▢
AMA: 2016,Feb,12; 2014,Jan,11

68328 **with buccal mucous membrane graft (includes obtaining graft)**
🚗 20.0   🔪 20.0   **FUD** 090   T A2 80 50 ▢
AMA: 2016,Feb,12; 2014,Jan,11

68330 **Repair of symblepharon; conjunctivoplasty, without graft**
🚗 13.0   🔪 17.0   **FUD** 090   T A2 80 50 ▢
AMA: 2016,Feb,12; 2014,Jan,11

68335 **with free graft conjunctiva or buccal mucous membrane (includes obtaining graft)**
🚗 18.3   🔪 18.3   **FUD** 090   T A2 50 ▢
AMA: 2016,Feb,12; 2014,Jan,11

68340 **division of symblepharon, with or without insertion of conformer or contact lens**
🚗 11.3   🔪 15.3   **FUD** 090   T A2 80 50 ▢
AMA: 2016,Feb,12; 2014,Jan,11

68360-68399 Conjunctival Flaps and Unlisted Procedures

INCLUDES Operating microscope (69990)

68360 Conjunctival flap; bridge or partial (separate procedure)

EXCLUDES *Conjunctival flap for injury (65280, 65285)*
Conjunctival foreign body removal (65205, 65210)
Surgical wound repair (66250)

11.6   15.0   **FUD** 090   T A2 50

AMA: 2016,Feb,12; 2014,Jan,11

68362 total (such as Gunderson thin flap or purse string flap)

EXCLUDES *Conjunctival flap for injury (65280, 65285)*
Conjunctival foreign body removal (65205, 65210)
Surgical wound repair (66250)

18.6   18.6   **FUD** 090   T A2 50

AMA: 2016,Feb,12; 2016,Jan,13; 2015,Jan,16; 2014,Jan,11

68371 Harvesting conjunctival allograft, living donor

11.7   11.7   **FUD** 010   T A2 50

AMA: 2016,Feb,12; 2016,Jan,13; 2015,Jan,16; 2014,Jan,11

68399 Unlisted procedure, conjunctiva

0.00   0.00   **FUD** YYY   T 80 50

AMA: 2016,Feb,12; 2016,Jan,13; 2015,Jan,16; 2014,Jan,11

68400-68899 Nasolacrimal System Procedures

INCLUDES Operating microscope (69990)

68400 Incision, drainage of lacrimal gland

3.74   8.00   **FUD** 010   T P3 50

AMA: 2016,Feb,12; 2014,Jan,11

Left eye

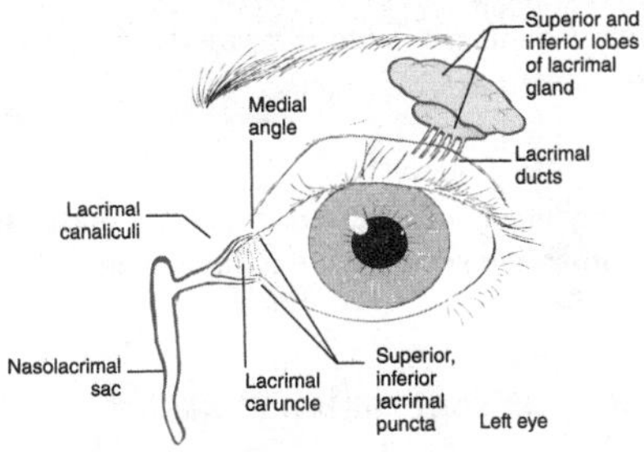

68420 Incision, drainage of lacrimal sac (dacryocystotomy or dacryocystostomy)

4.78   9.07   **FUD** 010   T P3 50

AMA: 2016,Feb,12; 2014,Jan,11

68440 Snip incision of lacrimal punctum

2.81   2.89   **FUD** 010   T P3 50

AMA: 2016,Feb,12; 2014,Jan,11

68500 Excision of lacrimal gland (dacryoadenectomy), except for tumor; total

27.6   27.6   **FUD** 090   T A2 50

AMA: 2016,Feb,12; 2014,Jan,11

68505 partial

27.4   27.4   **FUD** 090   T A2 50

AMA: 2016,Feb,12; 2014,Jan,11

68510 Biopsy of lacrimal gland

8.30   12.5   **FUD** 000   T A2 80 50

AMA: 2016,Feb,12; 2014,Jan,11

68520 Excision of lacrimal sac (dacryocystectomy)

19.4   19.4   **FUD** 090   T A2 80 50

AMA: 2016,Feb,12; 2014,Jan,11

68525 Biopsy of lacrimal sac

7.49   7.49   **FUD** 000   T A2 50

AMA: 2016,Feb,12; 2014,Jan,11

68530 Removal of foreign body or dacryolith, lacrimal passages

INCLUDES Meller's excision

7.31   12.0   **FUD** 010   T P2 50

AMA: 2016,Feb,12; 2014,Jan,11

68540 Excision of lacrimal gland tumor; frontal approach

26.3   26.3   **FUD** 090   T A2 50

AMA: 2016,Feb,12; 2014,Jan,11

68550 involving osteotomy

31.3   31.3   **FUD** 090   T A2 50

AMA: 2016,Feb,12; 2014,Jan,11

68700 Plastic repair of canaliculi

17.1   17.1   **FUD** 090   T A2 50

AMA: 2016,Feb,12; 2014,Jan,11

68705 Correction of everted punctum, cautery

4.72   6.67   **FUD** 010   T P2 50

AMA: 2016,Feb,12; 2016,Jan,13; 2015,Jan,16; 2014,Jan,11

68720 Dacryocystorhinostomy (fistulization of lacrimal sac to nasal cavity)

21.4   21.4   **FUD** 090   T A2 80 50

AMA: 2016,Feb,12; 2016,Jan,13; 2015,Jan,16; 2014,Jan,11; 2012,Jan,15-42; 2011,Jan,11

68745 Conjunctivorhinostomy (fistulization of conjunctiva to nasal cavity); without tube

21.5   21.5   **FUD** 090   T A2 80 50

AMA: 2016,Feb,12; 2014,Jan,11

68750 with insertion of tube or stent

22.2   22.2   **FUD** 090   T A2 80 50

AMA: 2016,Feb,12; 2016,Jan,13; 2015,Jan,16; 2014,Jan,11; 2012,Jan,15-42; 2011,Jan,11

68760 Closure of the lacrimal punctum; by thermocauterization, ligation, or laser surgery

4.14   5.68   **FUD** 010   T P3 50

AMA: 2016,Feb,12; 2014,Jan,11

68761 by plug, each

EXCLUDES *Drug-eluting lacrimal implant (0356T)*
Drug-eluting ocular insert (0444T-0445T)

3.37   4.17   **FUD** 010   T P3 80 50

AMA: 2016,Feb,12; 2016,Jan,13; 2015,Jan,16; 2014,Jan,11; 2012,Jan,15-42; 2011,Jan,11

68770 Closure of lacrimal fistula (separate procedure)

17.8   17.8   **FUD** 090   T A2 80 50

AMA: 2016,Feb,12; 2014,Jan,11

68801 Dilation of lacrimal punctum, with or without irrigation

2.46   2.84   **FUD** 010   Q1 N1 50

AMA: 2016,Feb,12; 2014,Jan,11

68810 Probing of nasolacrimal duct, with or without irrigation;

EXCLUDES *Ophthalmological exam under anesthesia (92018)*

4.30   5.51   **FUD** 010   T A2 50

AMA: 2016,Feb,12; 2016,Jan,13; 2015,Jan,16; 2014,Jan,11

68811 requiring general anesthesia

EXCLUDES *Ophthalmological exam under anesthesia (92018)*

4.72   4.72   **FUD** 010   T A2 50

AMA: 2016,Feb,12; 2016,Jan,13; 2015,Jan,16; 2014,Jan,11; 2012,Jan,15-42; 2011,Jan,11

68815 with insertion of tube or stent

EXCLUDES *Drug eluting ocular insert (0444T-0445T)*
Ophthalmological exam under anesthesia (92018)

6.29   11.2   **FUD** 010   T A2 50

AMA: 2016,Feb,12; 2016,Jan,13; 2015,Jan,16; 2014,Jan,11; 2012,Jan,15-42; 2011,Jan,11

68816 with transluminal balloon catheter dilation

EXCLUDES *Probing of nasolacrimal duct (68810-68811, 68815)*

5.73   18.1   **FUD** 010   T G2 50

AMA: 2016,Feb,12; 2016,Jan,13; 2015,Jan,16; 2014,Jan,11

68840 Probing of lacrimal canaliculi, with or without irrigation

3.31   3.61   **FUD** 010   T P3 50

AMA: 2016,Feb,12; 2014,Jan,11

68850 Injection of contrast medium for dacryocystography

(70170, 78660)

1.59   1.73   **FUD** 000   N N1 50

AMA: 2016,Feb,12; 2016,Jan,13; 2015,Jan,16; 2014,Jan,11; 2012,Jan,15-42; 2011,Jan,11

● New Code   ▲ Revised Code   ○ Reinstated   ● New Web Release   ▲ Revised Web Release   Unlisted   Not Covered   # Resequenced
⊘ AMA Mod 51 Exempt   ⑤① Optum Mod 51 Exempt   ⑥③ Mod 63 Exempt   ✎ Non-FDA Drug   ★ Telehealth   Ⓜ Maternity   ⚠ Age Edit   + Add-on   **AMA:** CPT Asst

Eye, Ocular Adnexa, and Ear

68899 — 69420

68899   Unlisted procedure, lacrimal system
🔧 0.00   ✂ 0.00   **FUD** YYY   T 80 50
AMA: 2014,Jan,11

69000-69020 Treatment External Abscess/Hematoma

69000   Drainage external ear, abscess or hematoma; simple
🔧 3.42   ✂ 5.35   **FUD** 010   T P2 50 ▭
AMA: 2016,Jan,13; 2015,Jan,16; 2014,Jan,11; 2012,Jan,15-42;
2011,Jan,11

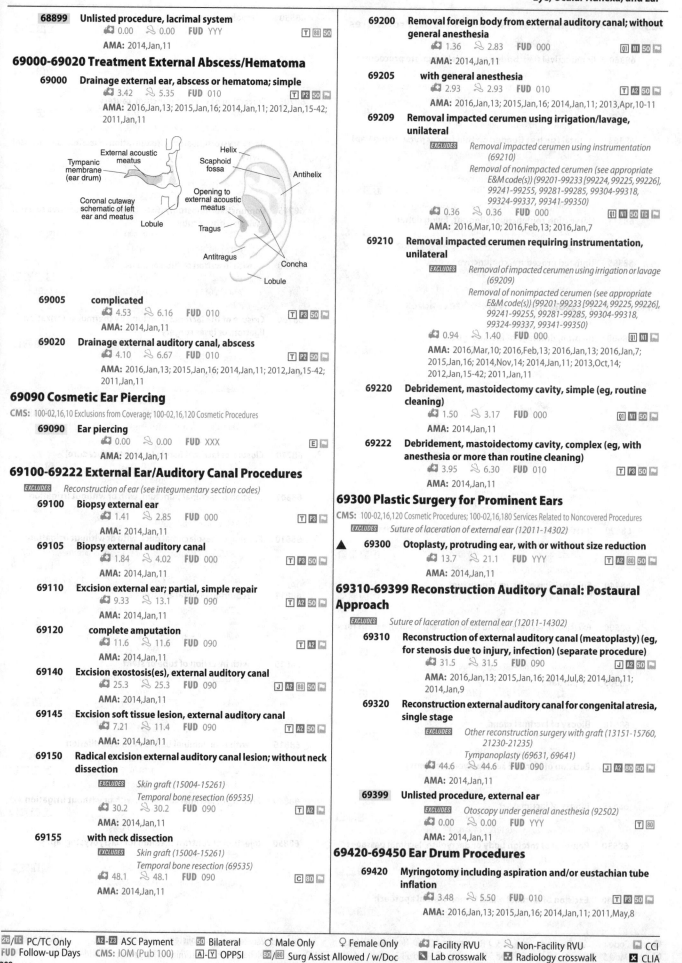

69005   complicated
🔧 4.53   ✂ 6.16   **FUD** 010   T P3 50 ▭
AMA: 2014,Jan,11

69020   Drainage external auditory canal, abscess
🔧 4.10   ✂ 6.67   **FUD** 010   T P2 50 ▭
AMA: 2016,Jan,13; 2015,Jan,16; 2014,Jan,11; 2012,Jan,15-42;
2011,Jan,11

69090 Cosmetic Ear Piercing

CMS: 100-02,16,10 Exclusions from Coverage; 100-02,16,120 Cosmetic Procedures

69090   Ear piercing
🔧 0.00   ✂ 0.00   **FUD** XXX   E ▭
AMA: 2014,Jan,11

69100-69222 External Ear/Auditory Canal Procedures

EXCLUDES   *Reconstruction of ear (see integumentary section codes)*

69100   Biopsy external ear
🔧 1.41   ✂ 2.85   **FUD** 000   T P3
AMA: 2014,Jan,11

69105   Biopsy external auditory canal
🔧 1.84   ✂ 4.02   **FUD** 000   T P3 50 ▭
AMA: 2014,Jan,11

69110   Excision external ear; partial, simple repair
🔧 9.33   ✂ 13.1   **FUD** 090   T A2 50 ▭
AMA: 2014,Jan,11

69120   complete amputation
🔧 11.6   ✂ 11.6   **FUD** 090   T A2 ▭
AMA: 2014,Jan,11

69140   Excision exostosis(es), external auditory canal
🔧 25.3   ✂ 25.3   **FUD** 090   J A2 80 50 ▭
AMA: 2014,Jan,11

69145   Excision soft tissue lesion, external auditory canal
🔧 7.21   ✂ 11.4   **FUD** 090   T A2 50 ▭
AMA: 2014,Jan,11

69150   Radical excision external auditory canal lesion; without neck
dissection
EXCLUDES   *Skin graft (15004-15261)*
Temporal bone resection (69535)
🔧 30.2   ✂ 30.2   **FUD** 090   T A2 ▭
AMA: 2014,Jan,11

69155   with neck dissection
EXCLUDES   *Skin graft (15004-15261)*
Temporal bone resection (69535)
🔧 48.1   ✂ 48.1   **FUD** 090   C 80 ▭
AMA: 2014,Jan,11

69200   Removal foreign body from external auditory canal; without
general anesthesia
🔧 1.36   ✂ 2.83   **FUD** 000   Q1 N1 50 ▭
AMA: 2014,Jan,11

69205   with general anesthesia
🔧 2.93   ✂ 2.93   **FUD** 010   T A2 50 ▭
AMA: 2016,Jan,13; 2015,Jan,16; 2014,Jan,11; 2013,Apr,10-11

69209   Removal impacted cerumen using irrigation/lavage,
unilateral
EXCLUDES   *Removal impacted cerumen using instrumentation
(69210)*
*Removal of nonimpacted cerumen (see appropriate
E&M code(s)) (99201-99233 [99224, 99225, 99226],
99241-99255, 99281-99285, 99304-99318,
99324-99337, 99341-99350)*
🔧 0.36   ✂ 0.36   **FUD** 000   Q1 N1 50 TC ▭
AMA: 2016,Mar,10; 2016,Feb,13; 2016,Jan,7

69210   Removal impacted cerumen requiring instrumentation,
unilateral
EXCLUDES   *Removal of impacted cerumen using irrigation or lavage
(69209)*
*Removal of nonimpacted cerumen (see appropriate
E&M code(s)) (99201-99233 [99224, 99225, 99226],
99241-99255, 99281-99285, 99304-99318,
99324-99337, 99341-99350)*
🔧 0.94   ✂ 1.40   **FUD** 000   Q1 N1 ▭
AMA: 2016,Mar,10; 2016,Feb,13; 2016,Jan,13; 2016,Jan,7;
2015,Jan,16; 2014,Nov,14; 2014,Jan,11; 2013,Oct,14;
2012,Jan,15-42; 2011,Jan,11

69220   Debridement, mastoidectomy cavity, simple (eg, routine
cleaning)
🔧 1.50   ✂ 3.17   **FUD** 000   Q1 N1 50 ▭
AMA: 2014,Jan,11

69222   Debridement, mastoidectomy cavity, complex (eg, with
anesthesia or more than routine cleaning)
🔧 3.95   ✂ 6.30   **FUD** 010   T P3 50 ▭
AMA: 2014,Jan,11

69300 Plastic Surgery for Prominent Ears

CMS: 100-02,16,120 Cosmetic Procedures; 100-02,16,180 Services Related to Noncovered Procedures
EXCLUDES   *Suture of laceration of external ear (12011-14302)*

▲ **69300**   Otoplasty, protruding ear, with or without size reduction
🔧 13.7   ✂ 21.1   **FUD** YYY   T A2 80 50 ▭
AMA: 2014,Jan,11

69310-69399 Reconstruction Auditory Canal: Postaural Approach

EXCLUDES   *Suture of laceration of external ear (12011-14302)*

69310   Reconstruction of external auditory canal (meatoplasty) (eg,
for stenosis due to injury, infection) (separate procedure)
🔧 31.5   ✂ 31.5   **FUD** 090   J A2 50 ▭
AMA: 2016,Jan,13; 2015,Jan,16; 2014,Jul,8; 2014,Jan,11;
2014,Jan,9

69320   Reconstruction external auditory canal for congenital atresia,
single stage
EXCLUDES   *Other reconstruction surgery with graft (13151-15760,
21230-21235)*
Tympanoplasty (69631, 69641)
🔧 44.6   ✂ 44.6   **FUD** 090   J A2 80 50 ▭
AMA: 2014,Jan,11

69399   Unlisted procedure, external ear
EXCLUDES   *Otoscopy under general anesthesia (92502)*
🔧 0.00   ✂ 0.00   **FUD** YYY   T 80
AMA: 2014,Jan,11

69420-69450 Ear Drum Procedures

69420   Myringotomy including aspiration and/or eustachian tube
inflation
🔧 3.48   ✂ 5.50   **FUD** 010   T P3 50 ▭
AMA: 2016,Jan,13; 2015,Jan,16; 2014,Jan,11; 2011,May,8

| 26/TC PC/TC Only | A2-Z3 ASC Payment | 50 Bilateral | ♂ Male Only | ♀ Female Only | 🔧 Facility RVU | ✂ Non-Facility RVU | ▭ CCI |
| FUD Follow-up Days | CMS: IOM (Pub 100) | A-Y OPPSI | 80/80 Surg Assist Allowed / w/Doc | | 🔳 Lab crosswalk | 🔳 Radiology crosswalk | ✖ CLIA |

298   CPT © 2016 American Medical Association. All Rights Reserved.   © 2016 Optum360, LLC

69421 Myringotomy including aspiration and/or eustachian tube inflation requiring general anesthesia
🔧 4.30 🔪 4.30 **FUD** 010 Ⓣ A2 50 ▢
AMA: 2016,Jan,13; 2015,Jan,16; 2014,Jan,11; 2011,May,8

69424 Ventilating tube removal requiring general anesthesia
EXCLUDES Cochlear device implantation (69930)
Eardrum repair (69610-69646)
Foreign body removal (69205)
Implantation, replacement of electromagnetic bone conduction hearing device in temporal bone (69710-69745)
Labyrinth procedures (69801-69915)
Mastoid obliteration (69670)
Myringotomy (69420-69421)
Polyp, glomus tumor removal (69535-69554)
Removal impacted cerumen requiring instrumentation (69210)
Repair of window (69666-69667)
Revised mastoidectomy (69601-69605)
Stapes procedures (69650-69662)
Transmastoid excision (69501-69530)
Tympanic neurectomy (69676)
Tympanostomy, tympanolysis (69433-69450)
🔧 1.80 🔪 3.66 **FUD** 000 02 P3 50 ▢
AMA: 2016,Jan,13; 2015,Jan,16; 2014,Jan,11; 2012,Jan,15-42; 2011,Jan,11

69433 Tympanostomy (requiring insertion of ventilating tube), local or topical anesthesia
🔧 3.83 🔪 5.81 **FUD** 010 Ⓣ P3 50 ▢
AMA: 2016,Jan,13; 2015,Jan,16; 2014,Jan,11; 2011,May,8

69436 Tympanostomy (requiring insertion of ventilating tube), general anesthesia
🔧 4.63 🔪 4.63 **FUD** 010 Ⓣ A2 50 ▢
AMA: 2016,Jan,13; 2015,Jan,16; 2014,Jan,11; 2012,May,14-15; 2011,May,8

69440 Middle ear exploration through postauricular or ear canal incision
EXCLUDES Atticotomy (69601-69605)
🔧 19.9 🔪 19.9 **FUD** 090 Ⓙ A2 50 ▢
AMA: 2014,Jan,11

69450 Tympanolysis, transcanal
🔧 15.7 🔪 15.7 **FUD** 090 Ⓙ A2 80 50 ▢
AMA: 2014,Jan,11

69501-69530 Transmastoid Excision
EXCLUDES Mastoidectomy cavity debridement (69220, 69222)
Skin graft (15004-15770)

69501 Transmastoid antrotomy (simple mastoidectomy)
🔧 21.2 🔪 21.2 **FUD** 090 Ⓙ A2 50 ▢
AMA: 2016,Jan,13; 2015,Jan,16; 2014,Jan,11

69502 Mastoidectomy; complete
🔧 28.1 🔪 28.1 **FUD** 090 Ⓙ A2 80 50 ▢
AMA: 2016,Jan,13; 2015,Jan,16; 2014,Jan,11

69505 modified radical
🔧 34.7 🔪 34.7 **FUD** 090 Ⓙ A2 80 50 ▢
AMA: 2016,Jan,13; 2015,Jan,16; 2014,Jan,11

69511 radical
🔧 35.5 🔪 35.5 **FUD** 090 Ⓙ A2 80 50 ▢
AMA: 2016,Jan,13; 2015,Jan,16; 2014,Jan,11

69530 Petrous apicectomy including radical mastoidectomy
🔧 47.8 🔪 47.8 **FUD** 090 Ⓙ A2 80 50 ▢
AMA: 2014,Jan,11

69535-69554 Polyp and Glomus Tumor Removal

69535 Resection temporal bone, external approach
EXCLUDES Middle fossa approach (69950-69970)
🔧 77.6 🔪 77.6 **FUD** 090 Ⓒ 50 ▢
AMA: 2014,Jan,11

69540 Excision aural polyp
🔧 3.67 🔪 6.00 **FUD** 010 Ⓣ P3 50 ▢
AMA: 2014,Jan,11

69550 Excision aural glomus tumor; transcanal
🔧 30.0 🔪 30.0 **FUD** 090 Ⓙ A2 80 50 ▢
AMA: 2014,Jan,11

69552 transmastoid
🔧 45.1 🔪 45.1 **FUD** 090 Ⓙ A2 80 50 ▢
AMA: 2014,Jan,11

69554 extended (extratemporal)
🔧 70.3 🔪 70.3 **FUD** 090 Ⓒ 80 50 ▢
AMA: 2014,Jan,11

69601-69605 Revised Mastoidectomy
EXCLUDES Skin graft (15120-15121, 15260-15261)

69601 Revision mastoidectomy; resulting in complete mastoidectomy
🔧 30.2 🔪 30.2 **FUD** 090 Ⓙ A2 80 50 ▢
AMA: 2016,Jan,13; 2015,Jan,16; 2014,Jan,11

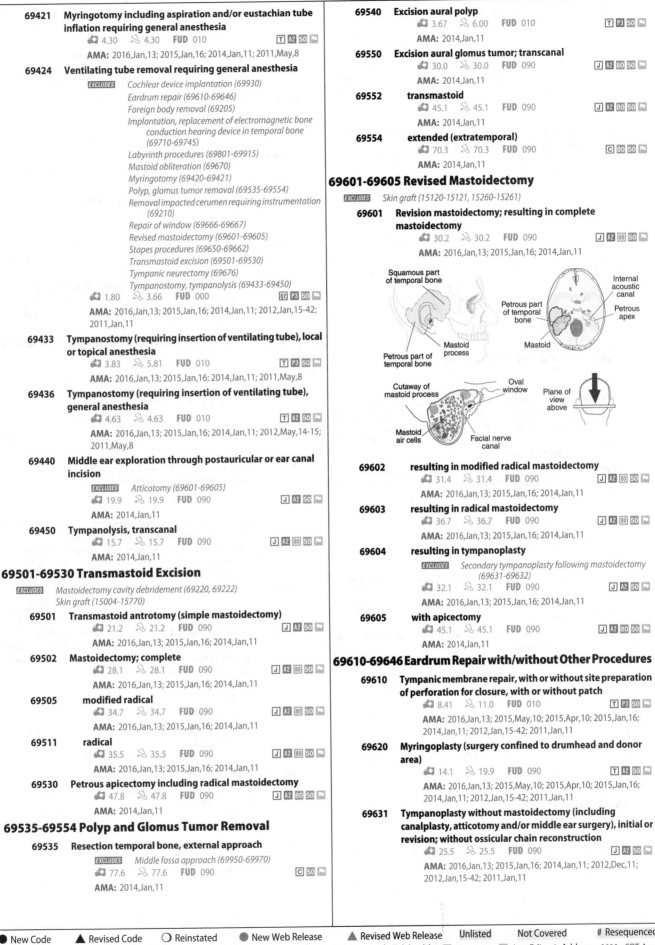

69602 resulting in modified radical mastoidectomy
🔧 31.4 🔪 31.4 **FUD** 090 Ⓙ A2 80 50 ▢
AMA: 2016,Jan,13; 2015,Jan,16; 2014,Jan,11

69603 resulting in radical mastoidectomy
🔧 36.7 🔪 36.7 **FUD** 090 Ⓙ A2 80 50 ▢
AMA: 2016,Jan,13; 2015,Jan,16; 2014,Jan,11

69604 resulting in tympanoplasty
EXCLUDES Secondary tympanoplasty following mastoidectomy (69631-69632)
🔧 32.1 🔪 32.1 **FUD** 090 Ⓙ A2 50 ▢
AMA: 2016,Jan,13; 2015,Jan,16; 2014,Jan,11

69605 with apicectomy
🔧 45.1 🔪 45.1 **FUD** 090 Ⓙ A2 80 50 ▢
AMA: 2014,Jan,11

69610-69646 Eardrum Repair with/without Other Procedures

69610 Tympanic membrane repair, with or without site preparation of perforation for closure, with or without patch
🔧 8.41 🔪 11.0 **FUD** 010 Ⓣ P3 50 ▢
AMA: 2016,Jan,13; 2015,May,10; 2015,Apr,10; 2015,Jan,16; 2014,Jan,11; 2012,Jan,15-42; 2011,Jan,11

69620 Myringoplasty (surgery confined to drumhead and donor area)
🔧 14.1 🔪 19.9 **FUD** 090 Ⓣ A2 50 ▢
AMA: 2016,Jan,13; 2015,May,10; 2015,Apr,10; 2015,Jan,16; 2014,Jan,11; 2012,Jan,15-42; 2011,Jan,11

69631 Tympanoplasty without mastoidectomy (including canalplasty, atticotomy and/or middle ear surgery), initial or revision; without ossicular chain reconstruction
🔧 25.5 🔪 25.5 **FUD** 090 Ⓙ A2 50 ▢
AMA: 2016,Jan,13; 2015,Jan,16; 2014,Jan,11; 2012,Dec,11; 2012,Jan,15-42; 2011,Jan,11

69632 with ossicular chain reconstruction (eg, postfenestration)
🔧 31.1   ✂ 31.1   **FUD** 090   J A2 50 ▱
AMA: 2016,Jan,13; 2015,Jan,16; 2014,Jan,11

69633 with ossicular chain reconstruction and synthetic prosthesis (eg, partial ossicular replacement prosthesis [PORP], total ossicular replacement prosthesis [TORP])
🔧 30.2   ✂ 30.2   **FUD** 090   J A2 50 ▱
AMA: 2016,Jan,13; 2015,Jan,16; 2014,Jan,11

69635 Tympanoplasty with antrotomy or mastoidotomy (including canalplasty, atticotomy, middle ear surgery, and/or tympanic membrane repair); without ossicular chain reconstruction
🔧 35.7   ✂ 35.7   **FUD** 090   J A2 50 ▱
AMA: 2016,Jan,13; 2015,Jan,16; 2014,Jan,11

Helix, Scaphoid fossa, Semicircular canals, Ossicular chain, Cochlear nerve, Malleus, External acoustic canal, Incus, Stapes, Tympanic membrane (eardrum), Cochlea, Concha, Lobule, Detail of ossicular chain

69636 with ossicular chain reconstruction
🔧 39.9   ✂ 39.9   **FUD** 090   J A2 80 50 ▱
AMA: 2016,Jan,13; 2015,Jan,16; 2014,Jan,11

69637 with ossicular chain reconstruction and synthetic prosthesis (eg, partial ossicular replacement prosthesis [PORP], total ossicular replacement prosthesis [TORP])
🔧 39.7   ✂ 39.7   **FUD** 090   J A2 80 50 ▱
AMA: 2016,Jan,13; 2015,Jan,16; 2014,Jan,11

69641 Tympanoplasty with mastoidectomy (including canalplasty, middle ear surgery, tympanic membrane repair); without ossicular chain reconstruction
🔧 30.1   ✂ 30.1   **FUD** 090   J A2 50 ▱
AMA: 2016,Jan,13; 2015,Jan,16; 2014,Jan,11

69642 with ossicular chain reconstruction
🔧 38.6   ✂ 38.6   **FUD** 090   J A2 50 ▱
AMA: 2016,Jan,13; 2015,Jan,16; 2014,Jan,11

69643 with intact or reconstructed wall, without ossicular chain reconstruction
🔧 35.3   ✂ 35.3   **FUD** 090   J A2 50 ▱
AMA: 2016,Jan,13; 2015,Jan,16; 2014,Jan,11

69644 with intact or reconstructed canal wall, with ossicular chain reconstruction
🔧 42.7   ✂ 42.7   **FUD** 090   J A2 50 ▱
AMA: 2016,Jan,13; 2015,Jan,16; 2014,Jan,11

69645 radical or complete, without ossicular chain reconstruction
🔧 42.0   ✂ 42.0   **FUD** 090   J A2 50 ▱
AMA: 2016,Jan,13; 2015,Jan,16; 2014,Jan,11

69646 radical or complete, with ossicular chain reconstruction
🔧 44.6   ✂ 44.6   **FUD** 090   J A2 80 50 ▱
AMA: 2016,Jan,13; 2015,Jan,16; 2014,Jan,11

69650-69662 Stapes Procedures

69650 Stapes mobilization
🔧 23.2   ✂ 23.2   **FUD** 090   J A2 50 ▱
AMA: 2014,Jan,11

69660 Stapedectomy or stapedotomy with reestablishment of ossicular continuity, with or without use of foreign material;
🔧 26.8   ✂ 26.8   **FUD** 090   J A2 50 ▱
AMA: 2014,Jan,11

69661 with footplate drill out
🔧 34.9   ✂ 34.9   **FUD** 090   J A2 80 50 ▱
AMA: 2014,Jan,11

69662 Revision of stapedectomy or stapedotomy
🔧 33.5   ✂ 33.5   **FUD** 090   J A2 50 ▱
AMA: 2014,Jan,11

69666-69700 Other Inner Ear Procedures

69666 Repair oval window fistula
🔧 23.3   ✂ 23.3   **FUD** 090   T A2 80 50 ▱
AMA: 2014,Jan,11

69667 Repair round window fistula
🔧 23.3   ✂ 23.3   **FUD** 090   T A2 80 50 ▱
AMA: 2014,Jan,11

69670 Mastoid obliteration (separate procedure)
🔧 27.3   ✂ 27.3   **FUD** 090   J A2 80 50 ▱
AMA: 2014,Jan,11

69676 Tympanic neurectomy
🔧 24.0   ✂ 24.0   **FUD** 090   T A2 50 ▱
AMA: 2014,Jan,11

69700 Closure postauricular fistula, mastoid (separate procedure)
🔧 19.8   ✂ 19.8   **FUD** 090   T A2 50 ▱
AMA: 2014,Jan,11

69710-69718 Procedures Related to Hearing Aids/Auditory Implants

CMS: 100-02,16,100 Hearing Devices

69710 Implantation or replacement of electromagnetic bone conduction hearing device in temporal bone
INCLUDES   Removal of existing device when performing replacement procedure
🔧 0.00   ✂ 0.00   **FUD** XXX   E ▱
AMA: 2014,Jan,11

69711 Removal or repair of electromagnetic bone conduction hearing device in temporal bone
🔧 24.9   ✂ 24.9   **FUD** 090   J A2 80 50 ▱
AMA: 2014,Jan,11

69714 Implantation, osseointegrated implant, temporal bone, with percutaneous attachment to external speech processor/cochlear stimulator; without mastoidectomy
🔧 31.1   ✂ 31.1   **FUD** 090   J J8 50 ▱
AMA: 2016,Jan,13; 2015,Jan,16; 2014,Jan,11; 2013,Oct,18

69715 with mastoidectomy
🔧 38.4   ✂ 38.4   **FUD** 090   J J8 50 ▱
AMA: 2014,Jan,11

69717 Replacement (including removal of existing device), osseointegrated implant, temporal bone, with percutaneous attachment to external speech processor/cochlear stimulator; without mastoidectomy
🔧 32.7   ✂ 32.7   **FUD** 090   J G2 50 ▱
AMA: 2014,Jan,11

69718 with mastoidectomy
🔧 38.8   ✂ 38.8   **FUD** 090   J G2 50 ▱
AMA: 2014,Jan,11

69720-69799 Procedures of the Facial Nerve

EXCLUDES   *Extracranial suture of facial nerve (64864)*

69720 Decompression facial nerve, intratemporal; lateral to geniculate ganglion
🔧 35.2   ✂ 35.2   **FUD** 090   J A2 80 50 ▱
AMA: 2014,Jan,11

69725 including medial to geniculate ganglion
🔧 54.4   ✂ 54.4   **FUD** 090   J 80 50 ▱
AMA: 2014,Jan,11

26/TC PC/TC Only   A2-Z3 ASC Payment   50 Bilateral   ♂ Male Only   ♀ Female Only   🔧 Facility RVU   ✂ Non-Facility RVU   ▱ CCI
FUD Follow-up Days   CMS: IOM (Pub 100)   A-Y OPPSI   80/80 Surg Assist Allowed / w/Doc   🔲 Lab crosswalk   ✚ Radiology crosswalk   ✗ CLIA

300

CPT © 2016 American Medical Association. All Rights Reserved.   © 2016 Optum360, LLC

69740	**Suture facial nerve, intratemporal, with or without graft or decompression; lateral to geniculate ganglion**	
	33.7 33.7 **FUD** 090	J A2 80 50 ▭
	AMA: 2014,Jan,11	
69745	**including medial to geniculate ganglion**	
	40.3 40.3 **FUD** 090	J A2 80 50 ▭
	AMA: 2014,Jan,11	
69799	**Unlisted procedure, middle ear**	
	0.00 0.00 **FUD** YYY	T 80 50
	AMA: 2016,Jan,13; 2015,Jan,16; 2014,Jan,11	

69801-69915 Procedures of the Labyrinth

69801	**Labyrinthotomy, with perfusion of vestibuloactive drug(s), transcanal**	
	EXCLUDES *Myringotomy, tympanostomy on the same ear (69420-69421, 69433, 69436)*	
	Procedure performed more than one time per day	
	3.64 5.63 **FUD** 000	T P3 80 50 ▭
	AMA: 2016,Jan,13; 2015,Jan,16; 2014,Jan,11; 2012,Jan,15-42; 2011,May,8; 2011,May,7; 2011,Jan,11	

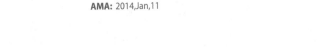

Anterior semicircular canal
Lateral semicircular canal
Window
Posterior semicircular canal
Cochlea

Side view schematic of semicircular canals (left). Sound (below) as registered in the cochlea
- Low tone
- Mid range
- High tones

Petrous apex
Internal acoustic canal
Mastoid

69805	**Endolymphatic sac operation; without shunt**	
	30.4 30.4 **FUD** 090	J A2 80 50 ▭
	AMA: 2014,Jan,11	
69806	**with shunt**	
	27.3 27.3 **FUD** 090	J A2 50 ▭
	AMA: 2014,Jan,11	
69820	**Fenestration semicircular canal**	
	INCLUDES Lempert's fenestration	
	24.7 24.7 **FUD** 090	J A2 80 50 ▭
	AMA: 2014,Jan,11	
69840	**Revision fenestration operation**	
	26.0 26.0 **FUD** 090	J A2 80 50 ▭
	AMA: 2014,Jan,11	
69905	**Labyrinthectomy; transcanal**	
	26.5 26.5 **FUD** 090	J A2 50 ▭
	AMA: 2014,Jan,11	
69910	**with mastoidectomy**	
	29.4 29.4 **FUD** 090	J A2 80 50 ▭
	AMA: 2014,Jan,11	
69915	**Vestibular nerve section, translabyrinthine approach**	
	EXCLUDES *Transcranial approach (69950)*	
	44.5 44.5 **FUD** 090	J A2 80 50 ▭
	AMA: 2014,Jan,11	

69930-69949 Cochlear Implantation

CMS: 100-02,16,100 Hearing Devices

69930	**Cochlear device implantation, with or without mastoidectomy**	
	35.4 35.4 **FUD** 090	J J8 80 50 ▭
	AMA: 2014,Jan,11	

69949	**Unlisted procedure, inner ear**	
	0.00 0.00 **FUD** YYY	T 80 50
	AMA: 2014,Jan,11	

69950-69979 Inner Ear Procedures via Craniotomy

EXCLUDES   *External approach (69535)*

69950	**Vestibular nerve section, transcranial approach**	
	51.5 51.5 **FUD** 090	C 80 50 ▭
	AMA: 2014,Jan,11	
69955	**Total facial nerve decompression and/or repair (may include graft)**	
	57.7 57.7 **FUD** 090	J 80 50 ▭
	AMA: 2014,Jan,11	
69960	**Decompression internal auditory canal**	
	55.5 55.5 **FUD** 090	J 80 50 ▭
	AMA: 2014,Jan,11	
69970	**Removal of tumor, temporal bone**	
	62.0 62.0 **FUD** 090	J 80 50 ▭
	AMA: 2014,Jan,11	
69979	**Unlisted procedure, temporal bone, middle fossa approach**	
	0.00 0.00 **FUD** YYY	T 80 50
	AMA: 2016,Jan,13; 2015,Jan,16; 2014,Sep,13; 2014,Jan,11	

69990 Operating Microscope

EXCLUDES   *Magnifying loupes*

+ **69990**	**Microsurgical techniques, requiring use of operating microscope (List separately in addition to code for primary procedure)**	
	Code first primary procedure	
	6.45 6.45 **FUD** ZZZ	N N1 80 ▭
	AMA: 2016,Feb,12; 2016,Jan,13; 2015,Jan,16; 2014,Sep,13; 2014,Apr,10; 2014,Jan,11; 2014,Jan,8; 2013,Oct,14; 2012,Dec,12; 2012,Jun,12-13; 2012,Mar,9-10; 2012,Jan,15-42; 2011,Jan,11	

70010-70015 Radiography: Neurodiagnostic

70010 Myelography, posterior fossa, radiological supervision and interpretation

🔲 1.75   🔲 1.75   **FUD** XXX   02 N1 80 ▢

AMA: 2016,Jan,13; 2015,Jan,16; 2014,Jan,11; 2012,Feb,9-10

70015 Cisternography, positive contrast, radiological supervision and interpretation

🔲 4.32   🔲 4.32   **FUD** XXX   02 N1 80 ▢

AMA: 2014,Jan,11; 2012,Feb,9-10

70030-70390 Radiography: Head, Neck, Orofacial Structures

INCLUDES Minimum number of views or more views when needed to adequately complete the study

Radiographs that have to be repeated during the encounter due to substandard quality; only one unit of service is reported

EXCLUDES Obtaining more films after review of initial films, based on the discretion of the radiologist, an order for the test, and a change in the patient's condition

70030 Radiologic examination, eye, for detection of foreign body

🔲 0.78   🔲 0.78   **FUD** XXX   01 N1 80 ▢

AMA: 2014,Jan,11; 2012,Feb,9-10

70100 Radiologic examination, mandible; partial, less than 4 views

🔲 0.92   🔲 0.92   **FUD** XXX   01 N1 80 ▢

AMA: 2014,Jan,11; 2012,Feb,9-10

70110 complete, minimum of 4 views

🔲 1.06   🔲 1.06   **FUD** XXX   01 N1 80 ▢

AMA: 2014,Jan,11; 2012,Feb,9-10

70120 Radiologic examination, mastoids; less than 3 views per side

🔲 0.95   🔲 0.95   **FUD** XXX   01 N1 80 ▢

AMA: 2014,Jan,11; 2012,Feb,9-10

70130 complete, minimum of 3 views per side

🔲 1.53   🔲 1.53   **FUD** XXX   01 N1 80 ▢

AMA: 2014,Jan,11; 2012,Feb,9-10

70134 Radiologic examination, internal auditory meati, complete

🔲 1.44   🔲 1.44   **FUD** XXX   01 N1 80 ▢

AMA: 2014,Jan,11; 2012,Feb,9-10

The internal auditory meatus is radiologically imaged

70140 Radiologic examination, facial bones; less than 3 views

🔲 0.83   🔲 0.83   **FUD** XXX   01 N1 80 ▢

AMA: 2014,Jan,11; 2012,Feb,9-10

An x-ray of the facial bones is performed

70150 complete, minimum of 3 views

🔲 1.16   🔲 1.16   **FUD** XXX   01 N1 80 ▢

AMA: 2014,Jan,11; 2012,Feb,9-10

70160 Radiologic examination, nasal bones, complete, minimum of 3 views

🔲 0.91   🔲 0.91   **FUD** XXX   01 N1 80 ▢

AMA: 2014,Jan,11; 2012,Feb,9-10

70170 Dacryocystography, nasolacrimal duct, radiological supervision and interpretation

EXCLUDES Injection of contrast (68850)

🔲 0.00   🔲 0.00   **FUD** XXX   02 N1 80 ▢

AMA: 2014,Jan,11; 2012,Feb,9-10

70190 Radiologic examination; optic foramina

🔲 1.00   🔲 1.00   **FUD** XXX   01 N1 80 ▢

AMA: 2014,Jan,11; 2012,Feb,9-10

70200 orbits, complete, minimum of 4 views

🔲 1.18   🔲 1.18   **FUD** XXX   01 N1 80 ▢

AMA: 2014,Jan,11; 2012,Feb,9-10

An x-ray of the orbits is performed

70210 Radiologic examination, sinuses, paranasal, less than 3 views

🔲 0.83   🔲 0.83   **FUD** XXX   01 N1 80 ▢

AMA: 2014,Jan,11; 2012,Feb,9-10

70220 Radiologic examination, sinuses, paranasal, complete, minimum of 3 views

🔲 1.05   🔲 1.05   **FUD** XXX   01 N1 80 ▢

AMA: 2014,Jan,11; 2012,Feb,9-10

70240 Radiologic examination, sella turcica

🔲 0.84   🔲 0.84   **FUD** XXX   01 N1 80 ▢

AMA: 2014,Jan,11; 2012,Feb,9-10

70250 Radiologic examination, skull; less than 4 views

🔲 1.01   🔲 1.01   **FUD** XXX   01 N1 80 ▢

AMA: 2014,Jan,11; 2012,Feb,9-10

70260 complete, minimum of 4 views

🔲 1.28   🔲 1.28   **FUD** XXX   01 N1 80 ▢

AMA: 2014,Jan,11; 2012,Feb,9-10

Radiology

70300 — 70492

70300 **Radiologic examination, teeth; single view**
🎞 0.42 ⚕ 0.42 **FUD** XXX `Q1` `N1` `80` `▢`
AMA: 2014,Jan,11; 2012,Feb,9-10

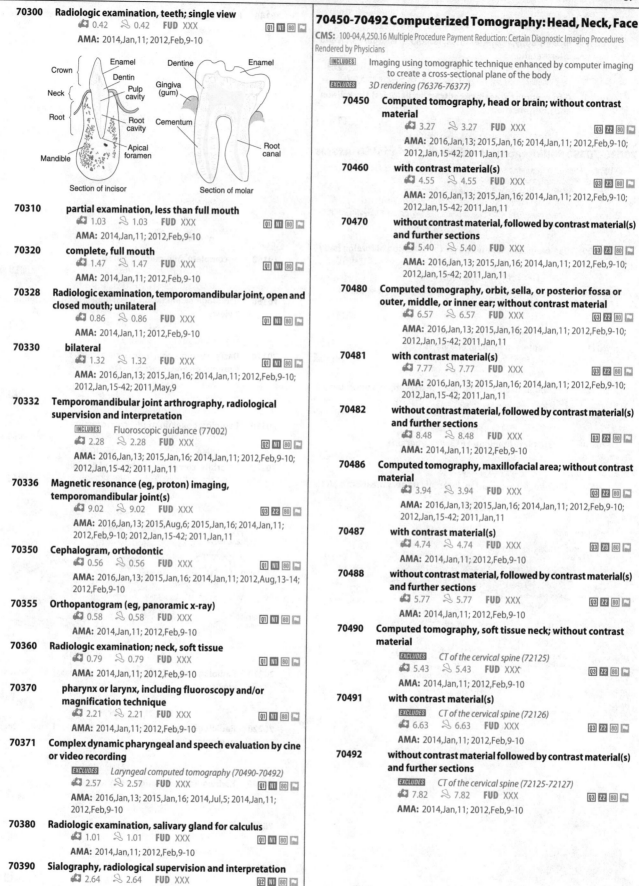

Section of incisor — Section of molar

Labels: Crown, Enamel, Dentin, Neck, Dentine, Enamel, Pulp cavity, Gingiva (gum), Root, Root cavity, Cementum, Apical foramen, Mandible, Root canal

70310 **partial examination, less than full mouth**
🎞 1.03 ⚕ 1.03 **FUD** XXX `Q1` `N1` `80` `▢`
AMA: 2014,Jan,11; 2012,Feb,9-10

70320 **complete, full mouth**
🎞 1.47 ⚕ 1.47 **FUD** XXX `Q1` `N1` `80` `▢`
AMA: 2014,Jan,11; 2012,Feb,9-10

70328 **Radiologic examination, temporomandibular joint, open and closed mouth; unilateral**
🎞 0.86 ⚕ 0.86 **FUD** XXX `Q1` `N1` `80` `▢`
AMA: 2014,Jan,11; 2012,Feb,9-10

70330 **bilateral**
🎞 1.32 ⚕ 1.32 **FUD** XXX `Q1` `N1` `80` `▢`
AMA: 2016,Jan,13; 2015,Jan,16; 2014,Jan,11; 2012,Feb,9-10; 2012,Jan,15-42; 2011,May,9

70332 **Temporomandibular joint arthrography, radiological supervision and interpretation**
INCLUDES Fluoroscopic guidance (77002)
🎞 2.28 ⚕ 2.28 **FUD** XXX `Q2` `N1` `80` `▢`
AMA: 2016,Jan,13; 2015,Jan,16; 2014,Jan,11; 2012,Feb,9-10; 2012,Jan,15-42; 2011,Jan,11

70336 **Magnetic resonance (eg, proton) imaging, temporomandibular joint(s)**
🎞 9.02 ⚕ 9.02 **FUD** XXX `Q3` `Z2` `80` `▢`
AMA: 2016,Jan,13; 2015,Aug,6; 2015,Jan,16; 2014,Jan,11; 2012,Feb,9-10; 2012,Jan,15-42; 2011,Jan,11

70350 **Cephalogram, orthodontic**
🎞 0.56 ⚕ 0.56 **FUD** XXX `Q1` `N1` `80` `▢`
AMA: 2016,Jan,13; 2015,Jan,16; 2014,Jan,11; 2012,Aug,13-14; 2012,Feb,9-10

70355 **Orthopantogram (eg, panoramic x-ray)**
🎞 0.58 ⚕ 0.58 **FUD** XXX `Q1` `N1` `80` `▢`
AMA: 2014,Jan,11; 2012,Feb,9-10

70360 **Radiologic examination; neck, soft tissue**
🎞 0.79 ⚕ 0.79 **FUD** XXX `Q1` `N1` `80` `▢`
AMA: 2014,Jan,11; 2012,Feb,9-10

70370 **pharynx or larynx, including fluoroscopy and/or magnification technique**
🎞 2.21 ⚕ 2.21 **FUD** XXX `Q1` `N1` `80` `▢`
AMA: 2014,Jan,11; 2012,Feb,9-10

70371 **Complex dynamic pharyngeal and speech evaluation by cine or video recording**
EXCLUDES Laryngeal computed tomography (70490-70492)
🎞 2.57 ⚕ 2.57 **FUD** XXX `Q1` `N1` `80` `▢`
AMA: 2016,Jan,13; 2015,Jan,16; 2014,Jul,5; 2014,Jan,11; 2012,Feb,9-10

70380 **Radiologic examination, salivary gland for calculus**
🎞 1.01 ⚕ 1.01 **FUD** XXX `Q1` `N1` `80` `▢`
AMA: 2014,Jan,11; 2012,Feb,9-10

70390 **Sialography, radiological supervision and interpretation**
🎞 2.64 ⚕ 2.64 **FUD** XXX `Q2` `N1` `80` `▢`
AMA: 2014,Jan,11; 2012,Feb,9-10

70450-70492 Computerized Tomography: Head, Neck, Face

CMS: 100-04,4,250.16 Multiple Procedure Payment Reduction: Certain Diagnostic Imaging Procedures Rendered by Physicians
INCLUDES Imaging using tomographic technique enhanced by computer imaging to create a cross-sectional plane of the body
EXCLUDES 3D rendering (76376-76377)

70450 **Computed tomography, head or brain; without contrast material**
🎞 3.27 ⚕ 3.27 **FUD** XXX `Q3` `Z2` `80` `▢`
AMA: 2016,Jan,13; 2015,Jan,16; 2014,Jan,11; 2012,Feb,9-10; 2012,Jan,15-42; 2011,Jan,11

70460 **with contrast material(s)**
🎞 4.55 ⚕ 4.55 **FUD** XXX `Q3` `Z3` `80` `▢`
AMA: 2016,Jan,13; 2015,Jan,16; 2014,Jan,11; 2012,Feb,9-10; 2012,Jan,15-42; 2011,Jan,11

70470 **without contrast material, followed by contrast material(s) and further sections**
🎞 5.40 ⚕ 5.40 **FUD** XXX `Q3` `Z3` `80` `▢`
AMA: 2016,Jan,13; 2015,Jan,16; 2014,Jan,11; 2012,Feb,9-10; 2012,Jan,15-42; 2011,Jan,11

70480 **Computed tomography, orbit, sella, or posterior fossa or outer, middle, or inner ear; without contrast material**
🎞 6.57 ⚕ 6.57 **FUD** XXX `Q3` `Z2` `80` `▢`
AMA: 2016,Jan,13; 2015,Jan,16; 2014,Jan,11; 2012,Feb,9-10; 2012,Jan,15-42; 2011,Jan,11

70481 **with contrast material(s)**
🎞 7.77 ⚕ 7.77 **FUD** XXX `Q3` `Z2` `80` `▢`
AMA: 2016,Jan,13; 2015,Jan,16; 2014,Jan,11; 2012,Feb,9-10; 2012,Jan,15-42; 2011,Jan,11

70482 **without contrast material, followed by contrast material(s) and further sections**
🎞 8.48 ⚕ 8.48 **FUD** XXX `Q3` `Z2` `80` `▢`
AMA: 2014,Jan,11; 2012,Feb,9-10

70486 **Computed tomography, maxillofacial area; without contrast material**
🎞 3.94 ⚕ 3.94 **FUD** XXX `Q3` `Z2` `80` `▢`
AMA: 2016,Jan,13; 2015,Jan,16; 2014,Jan,11; 2012,Feb,9-10; 2012,Jan,15-42; 2011,Jan,11

70487 **with contrast material(s)**
🎞 4.74 ⚕ 4.74 **FUD** XXX `Q3` `Z3` `80` `▢`
AMA: 2014,Jan,11; 2012,Feb,9-10

70488 **without contrast material, followed by contrast material(s) and further sections**
🎞 5.77 ⚕ 5.77 **FUD** XXX `Q3` `Z2` `80` `▢`
AMA: 2014,Jan,11; 2012,Feb,9-10

70490 **Computed tomography, soft tissue neck; without contrast material**
EXCLUDES CT of the cervical spine (72125)
🎞 5.43 ⚕ 5.43 **FUD** XXX `Q3` `Z2` `80` `▢`
AMA: 2014,Jan,11; 2012,Feb,9-10

70491 **with contrast material(s)**
EXCLUDES CT of the cervical spine (72126)
🎞 6.63 ⚕ 6.63 **FUD** XXX `Q3` `Z2` `80` `▢`
AMA: 2014,Jan,11; 2012,Feb,9-10

70492 **without contrast material followed by contrast material(s) and further sections**
EXCLUDES CT of the cervical spine (72125-72127)
🎞 7.82 ⚕ 7.82 **FUD** XXX `Q3` `Z2` `80` `▢`
AMA: 2014,Jan,11; 2012,Feb,9-10

70496-70498 Computerized Tomographic Angiography: Head and Neck

CMS: 100-04,4,250.16 Multiple Procedure Payment Reduction: Certain Diagnostic Imaging Procedures Rendered by Physicians

INCLUDES Multiple rapid thin section CT scans to create cross-sectional images of bones, organs and tissues

70496 **Computed tomographic angiography, head, with contrast material(s), including noncontrast images, if performed, and image postprocessing**
8.28   8.28   **FUD** XXX   03 Z2 80
AMA: 2016,Jan,13; 2015,Jan,16; 2014,Jan,11; 2012,Feb,9-10

70498 **Computed tomographic angiography, neck, with contrast material(s), including noncontrast images, if performed, and image postprocessing**
8.25   8.25   **FUD** XXX   03 Z2 80
AMA: 2016,Jan,13; 2015,Jan,16; 2014,Jan,11; 2012,Feb,9-10

70540-70543 Magnetic Resonance Imaging: Face, Neck, Orbits

CMS: 100-04,4,250.16 Multiple Procedure Payment Reduction: Certain Diagnostic Imaging Procedures Rendered by Physicians

INCLUDES Application of an external magnetic field that forces alignment of hydrogen atom nuclei in soft tissues which converts to sets of tomographic images that can be displayed as three-dimensional images

EXCLUDES *Magnetic resonance angiography head/neck (70544-70549)*
Procedure performed more than one time per session

70540 **Magnetic resonance (eg, proton) imaging, orbit, face, and/or neck; without contrast material(s)**
10.1   10.1   **FUD** XXX   03 Z2 80
AMA: 2016,Jan,13; 2015,Jan,16; 2014,Jan,11; 2012,Feb,9-10; 2012,Jan,15-42

70542 **with contrast material(s)**
11.3   11.3   **FUD** XXX   03 Z2 80
AMA: 2016,Jan,13; 2015,Jan,16; 2014,Jan,11; 2012,Feb,9-10; 2012,Jan,15-42

70543 **without contrast material(s), followed by contrast material(s) and further sequences**
13.8   13.8   **FUD** XXX   03 Z2 80
AMA: 2016,Jan,13; 2015,Jan,16; 2014,Jan,11; 2012,Feb,9-10; 2012,Jan,15-42

70544-70549 Magnetic Resonance Angiography: Head and Neck

CMS: 100-04,13,40.1.1 Magnetic Resonance Angiography; 100-04,13,40.1.2 HCPCS Coding Requirements; 100-04,4,250.16 Multiple Procedure Payment Reduction: Certain Diagnostic Imaging Procedures Rendered by Physicians

INCLUDES Use of magnetic fields and radio waves to produce detailed cross-sectional images of internal body structures

EXCLUDES *Use of code with the following unless a separate diagnostic MRI is performed (70551-70553)*

70544 **Magnetic resonance angiography, head; without contrast material(s)**
11.0   11.0   **FUD** XXX   03 Z2 80
AMA: 2016,Jan,13; 2015,Jan,16; 2014,Jan,11; 2012,Feb,9-10

70545 **with contrast material(s)**
10.8   10.8   **FUD** XXX   03 Z2 80
AMA: 2016,Jan,13; 2015,Jan,16; 2014,Jan,11; 2012,Feb,9-10

70546 **without contrast material(s), followed by contrast material(s) and further sequences**
16.8   16.8   **FUD** XXX   03 Z2 80
AMA: 2016,Jan,13; 2015,Jan,16; 2014,Jan,11; 2012,Feb,9-10

70547 **Magnetic resonance angiography, neck; without contrast material(s)**
11.0   11.0   **FUD** XXX   03 Z2 80
AMA: 2016,Jan,13; 2015,Jan,16; 2014,Jan,11; 2012,Feb,9-10

70548 **with contrast material(s)**
11.6   11.6   **FUD** XXX   03 Z2 80
AMA: 2016,Jan,13; 2015,Jan,16; 2014,Jan,11; 2012,Feb,9-10

70549 **without contrast material(s), followed by contrast material(s) and further sequences**
16.9   16.9   **FUD** XXX   03 Z2 80
AMA: 2016,Jan,13; 2015,Jan,16; 2014,Jan,11; 2012,Feb,9-10

70551-70553 Magnetic Resonance Imaging: Brain and Brain Stem

CMS: 100-04,4,200.3.2 Multi-Source Photon Stereotactic RadiosurgeryPlanning and Delivery; 100-04,4,250.16 Multiple Procedure Payment Reduction: Certain Diagnostic Imaging Procedures Rendered by Physicians

INCLUDES Application of an external magnetic field that forces alignment of hydrogen atom nuclei in soft tissues which converts to sets of tomographic images that can be displayed as three-dimensional images

EXCLUDES *Magnetic spectroscopy (76390)*

70551 **Magnetic resonance (eg, proton) imaging, brain (including brain stem); without contrast material**
6.48   6.48   **FUD** XXX   03 Z2 80
AMA: 2016,Jan,13; 2015,Jan,16; 2014,Jan,11; 2012,Feb,9-10; 2012,Jan,15-42; 2011,Jan,11

70552 **with contrast material(s)**
8.99   8.99   **FUD** XXX   03 Z3 80
AMA: 2016,Jan,13; 2015,Jan,16; 2014,Jan,11; 2012,Feb,9-10; 2012,Jan,15-42; 2011,Jan,11

70553 **without contrast material, followed by contrast material(s) and further sequences**
10.6   10.6   **FUD** XXX   03 Z2 80
AMA: 2016,Jan,13; 2015,Jan,16; 2014,Jan,11; 2012,Feb,9-10; 2012,Jan,15-42; 2011,Jan,11

70554-70555 Magnetic Resonance Imaging: Brain Mapping

INCLUDES Neuroimaging technique using MRI to identify and map signals related to brain activity

EXCLUDES *Use of code with the following unless a separate diagnostic MRI is performed (70551-70553)*

70554 **Magnetic resonance imaging, brain, functional MRI; including test selection and administration of repetitive body part movement and/or visual stimulation, not requiring physician or psychologist administration**
EXCLUDES *Functional brain mapping (96020)*
Testing performed by a physician or psychologist (70555)
12.6   12.6   **FUD** XXX   03 Z2 80
AMA: 2016,Jan,13; 2015,Jan,16; 2014,Jan,11; 2012,Feb,9-10; 2012,Jan,15-42; 2011,Jan,11

70555 **requiring physician or psychologist administration of entire neurofunctional testing**
EXCLUDES *Testing performed by a technologist, nonphysician, or nonpsychologist (70554)*
Code also (96020)
0.00   0.00   **FUD** XXX   S Z2 80
AMA: 2016,Jan,13; 2015,Jan,16; 2014,Jan,11; 2012,Feb,9-10

70557-70559 Magnetic Resonance Imaging: Intraoperative

EXCLUDES *Intracranial lesion stereotaxic biopsy with magnetic resonance guidance (61751)*
Procedures performed more than one time per surgical encounter
Magnetic resonance guidance (77021-77022)
Stereotactic biopsy, aspiration, or excision (61751)
Use of codes unless a separate report is generated

70557 **Magnetic resonance (eg, proton) imaging, brain (including brain stem and skull base), during open intracranial procedure (eg, to assess for residual tumor or residual vascular malformation); without contrast material**
0.00   0.00   **FUD** XXX   S Z2 80
AMA: 2014,Jan,11; 2012,Feb,9-10

70558 **with contrast material(s)**
0.00   0.00   **FUD** XXX   S Z2 80
AMA: 2014,Jan,11; 2012,Feb,9-10

70559 **without contrast material(s), followed by contrast material(s) and further sequences**
0.00   0.00   **FUD** XXX   S Z2 80
AMA: 2014,Jan,11; 2012,Feb,9-10

71010-71130 Radiography: Thorax

EXCLUDES *Needle placement guidance (76942, 77002)*

71010   Radiologic examination, chest; single view, frontal

EXCLUDES *Concurrent computer-aided detection (0174T)*
Critical care, evaluation and management (99291-99292)
Remotely performed CAD (0175T)

🚑 0.63   ⚕ 0.63   **FUD** XXX   [03] [Z3] [80] [▭]

AMA: 2016,Jan,13; 2015,Jan,16; 2014,May,4; 2014,Jan,11; 2013,Sep,17; 2012,Feb,9-10; 2012,Jan,15-42; 2011,Jan,11

71015   stereo, frontal

EXCLUDES *Critical care, evaluation and management (99291-99292)*

🚑 0.78   ⚕ 0.78   **FUD** XXX   [03] [Z3] [80] [▭]

AMA: 2016,Jan,13; 2015,Jan,16; 2014,May,4; 2014,Jan,11; 2012,Feb,9-10

71020   Radiologic examination, chest, 2 views, frontal and lateral;

EXCLUDES *Concurrent computer-aided detection (0174T)*
Critical care, evaluation and management (99291-99292)
Remotely performed CAD (0175T)

🚑 0.78   ⚕ 0.78   **FUD** XXX   [03] [Z3] [80] [▭]

AMA: 2016,Jan,13; 2015,Jan,16; 2014,Jun,14; 2014,May,4; 2014,Jan,11; 2013,Sep,17; 2012,Feb,9-10; 2012,Jan,15-42; 2011,Jan,11

71021   with apical lordotic procedure

EXCLUDES *Concurrent computer-aided detection (0174T)*
Remotely performed CAD (0175T)

🚑 0.95   ⚕ 0.95   **FUD** XXX   [01] [N1] [80] [▭]

AMA: 2014,Jan,11; 2012,Feb,9-10

71022   with oblique projections

EXCLUDES *Concurrent computer-aided detection (0174T)*
Remotely performed CAD (0175T)

🚑 1.17   ⚕ 1.17   **FUD** XXX   [01] [N1] [80] [▭]

AMA: 2016,Jan,13; 2015,Jan,16; 2014,Jan,11; 2012,Feb,9-10

71023   with fluoroscopy

🚑 1.78   ⚕ 1.78   **FUD** XXX   [01] [N1] [80] [▭]

AMA: 2016,Aug,5; 2016,Jan,13; 2015,Jan,16; 2014,Sep,5; 2014,Jan,11; 2013,Sep,17; 2013,Mar,10-11; 2013,Feb,3-6; 2012,Feb,9-10; 2012,Jan,15-42; 2011,Jul,3-11; 2011,Jan,11

71030   Radiologic examination, chest, complete, minimum of 4 views;

EXCLUDES *Concurrent computer-aided detection (0174T)*
Remotely performed CAD (0175T)

🚑 1.17   ⚕ 1.17   **FUD** XXX   [01] [N1] [80] [▭]

AMA: 2016,Jan,13; 2015,Jan,16; 2014,Jan,11; 2012,Feb,9-10; 2011,Jan,11

71034   with fluoroscopy

EXCLUDES *Separate fluoroscopy of chest (76000)*

🚑 2.34   ⚕ 2.34   **FUD** XXX   [01] [N1] [80] [▭]

AMA: 2016,Aug,5; 2016,Jan,13; 2015,Jan,16; 2014,Sep,5; 2014,Jan,11; 2013,Sep,17; 2013,Mar,10-11; 2013,Feb,3-6; 2012,Feb,9-10; 2012,Jan,15-42; 2011,Jul,3-11; 2011,Jan,11

71035   Radiologic examination, chest, special views (eg, lateral decubitus, Bucky studies)

🚑 0.92   ⚕ 0.92   **FUD** XXX   [01] [N1] [80] [▭]

AMA: 2016,Jan,13; 2015,Jan,16; 2014,Jan,11; 2013,Sep,17; 2012,Feb,9-10; 2012,Jan,15-42; 2011,Jan,11

71100   Radiologic examination, ribs, unilateral; 2 views

🚑 0.92   ⚕ 0.92   **FUD** XXX   [01] [N1] [80] [▭]

AMA: 2014,Jan,11; 2012,Feb,9-10

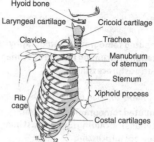

71101   including posteroanterior chest, minimum of 3 views

🚑 1.02   ⚕ 1.02   **FUD** XXX   [01] [N1] [80] [▭]

AMA: 2014,Jan,11; 2012,Feb,9-10

71110   Radiologic examination, ribs, bilateral; 3 views

🚑 1.05   ⚕ 1.05   **FUD** XXX   [01] [N1] [80] [▭]

AMA: 2014,Jan,11; 2012,Feb,9-10

71111   including posteroanterior chest, minimum of 4 views

🚑 1.34   ⚕ 1.34   **FUD** XXX   [01] [N1] [80] [▭]

AMA: 2014,Jan,11; 2012,Feb,9-10

71120   Radiologic examination; sternum, minimum of 2 views

🚑 0.83   ⚕ 0.83   **FUD** XXX   [01] [N1] [80] [▭]

AMA: 2014,Jan,11; 2012,Feb,9-10

71130   sternoclavicular joint or joints, minimum of 3 views

🚑 1.01   ⚕ 1.01   **FUD** XXX   [01] [N1] [80] [▭]

AMA: 2014,Jan,11; 2012,Feb,9-10

71250-71270 Computerized Tomography: Thorax

CMS: 100-04,4,250.16 Multiple Procedure Payment Reduction: Certain Diagnostic Imaging Procedures Rendered by Physicians

INCLUDES Imaging using tomographic technique enhanced by computer imaging to create a cross-sectional plane of the body

EXCLUDES *3D rendering (76376-76377)*
CT of the heart (75571-75574)

71250   Computed tomography, thorax; without contrast material

🚑 5.08   ⚕ 5.08   **FUD** XXX   [03] [Z2] [80] [▭]

AMA: 2016,Jan,13; 2015,Jan,16; 2014,Jan,11; 2012,Feb,9-10; 2012,Jan,15-42; 2011,Aug,9-10; 2011,Jan,11

71260   with contrast material(s)

🚑 6.45   ⚕ 6.45   **FUD** XXX   [03] [Z2] [80] [▭]

AMA: 2016,Jan,13; 2015,Jan,16; 2014,Jan,11; 2012,Feb,9-10; 2012,Jan,15-42; 2011,Jan,11

71270   without contrast material, followed by contrast material(s) and further sections

🚑 7.74   ⚕ 7.74   **FUD** XXX   [03] [Z2] [80] [▭]

AMA: 2016,Jan,13; 2015,Jan,16; 2014,Jan,11; 2012,Feb,9-10; 2012,Jan,15-42; 2011,Jan,11

71275 Computerized Tomographic Angiography: Thorax

CMS: 100-04,4,250.16 Multiple Procedure Payment Reduction: Certain Diagnostic Imaging Procedures Rendered by Physicians

INCLUDES Multiple rapid thin section CT scans to create cross-sectional images of bones, organs and tissues

EXCLUDES *CT angiography of coronary arteries that includes calcification score and/or cardiac morphology (75574)*

71275   Computed tomographic angiography, chest (noncoronary), with contrast material(s), including noncontrast images, if performed, and image postprocessing

🚑 8.43   ⚕ 8.43   **FUD** XXX   [03] [Z2] [80] [▭]

AMA: 2016,Jan,13; 2015,Jan,16; 2014,Jan,11; 2012,Feb,9-10; 2012,Jan,15-42; 2011,Aug,9-10; 2011,Jan,11

[26]/[TC] PC/TC Only   [A2]-[Z3] ASC Payment   [50] Bilateral   ♂ Male Only   ♀ Female Only   🚑 Facility RVU   ⚕ Non-Facility RVU   [▭] CCI
FUD Follow-up Days   **CMS:** IOM (Pub 100)   [A]-[Y] OPPSI   [80]/[80] Surg Assist Allowed / w/Doc   [◨] Lab Crosswalk   [◨] Radiology Crosswalk   [✕] CLIA

306   CPT © 2016 American Medical Association. All Rights Reserved.   © 2016 Optum360, LLC

71550-71552 Magnetic Resonance Imaging: Thorax

CMS: 100-04,4,250.16 Multiple Procedure Payment Reduction: Certain Diagnostic Imaging Procedures Rendered by Physicians

INCLUDES Application of an external magnetic field that forces alignment of hydrogen atom nuclei in soft tissues which converts to sets of tomographic images that can be displayed as three-dimensional images

EXCLUDES *MRI of the breast (77058-77059)*

71550 **Magnetic resonance (eg, proton) imaging, chest (eg, for evaluation of hilar and mediastinal lymphadenopathy); without contrast material(s)**
11.6   11.6   **FUD** XXX   Q3 Z2 80 ▭
AMA: 2016,Jan,13; 2015,Jan,16; 2014,Jan,11; 2012,Feb,9-10; 2012,Jan,15-42; 2011,Jan,11

71551 **with contrast material(s)**
12.8   12.8   **FUD** XXX   Q3 Z2 80 ▭
AMA: 2016,Jan,13; 2015,Jan,16; 2014,Jan,11; 2012,Feb,9-10; 2012,Jan,15-42; 2011,Jan,11

71552 **without contrast material(s), followed by contrast material(s) and further sequences**
16.3   16.3   **FUD** XXX   Q3 Z2 80 ▭
AMA: 2016,Jan,13; 2015,Jan,16; 2014,Jan,11; 2012,Feb,9-10; 2012,Jan,15-42; 2011,Jan,11

71555 Magnetic Resonance Angiography: Thorax

CMS: 100-04,13,40.1.1 Magnetic Resonance Angiography; 100-04,13,40.1.2 HCPCS Coding Requirements; 100-04,4,250.16 Multiple Procedure Payment Reduction: Certain Diagnostic Imaging Procedures Rendered by Physicians

71555 **Magnetic resonance angiography, chest (excluding myocardium), with or without contrast material(s)**
11.1   11.1   **FUD** XXX   B 80 ▭
AMA: 2016,Jan,13; 2015,Jan,16; 2014,Jan,11; 2012,Feb,9-10

72020-72120 Radiography: Spine

INCLUDES Minimum number of views or more views when needed to adequately complete the study
Radiographs that have to be repeated during the encounter due to substandard quality; only one unit of service is reported

EXCLUDES *Obtaining more films after review of initial films, based on the discretion of the radiologist, an order for the test, and a change in the patient's condition*

72020 **Radiologic examination, spine, single view, specify level**
EXCLUDES *Single view of entire thoracic and lumbar spine (72081)*
0.62   0.62   **FUD** XXX   Q1 N1 80 ▭
AMA: 2016,Sep,4; 2016,Jan,13; 2015,Oct,9; 2015,Jan,16; 2014,Jan,11; 2013,Jul,10; 2012,Feb,9-10

72040 **Radiologic examination, spine, cervical; 2 or 3 views**
0.93   0.93   **FUD** XXX   Q1 N1 80 ▭
AMA: 2016,Jan,13; 2015,Jan,16; 2014,Jan,11; 2013,Jul,10; 2012,Feb,9-10

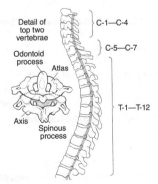

An x-ray of the cervical spine is performed

72050 **4 or 5 views**
1.26   1.26   **FUD** XXX   Q1 N1 80 ▭
AMA: 2014,Jan,11; 2012,Feb,9-10

72052 **6 or more views**
1.58   1.58   **FUD** XXX   Q1 N1 80 ▭
AMA: 2014,Jan,11; 2012,Feb,9-10

72070 **Radiologic examination, spine; thoracic, 2 views**
0.95   0.95   **FUD** XXX   Q1 N1 80 ▭
AMA: 2016,Jan,13; 2015,Jan,16; 2014,Jan,11; 2012,Feb,9-10

72072 **thoracic, 3 views**
0.97   0.97   **FUD** XXX   Q1 N1 80 ▭
AMA: 2016,Jan,13; 2015,Jan,16; 2014,Jan,11; 2012,Feb,9-10

72074 **thoracic, minimum of 4 views**
1.10   1.10   **FUD** XXX   Q1 N1 80 ▭
AMA: 2016,Jan,13; 2015,Jan,16; 2014,Jan,11; 2012,Feb,9-10

72080 **thoracolumbar junction, minimum of 2 views**
EXCLUDES *Single view of thoracolumbar junction (72020)*
0.86   0.86   **FUD** XXX   Q1 N1 80 ▭
AMA: 2016,Sep,4; 2016,Jan,13; 2015,Oct,9; 2015,Jan,16; 2014,Jan,11; 2012,Feb,9-10

72081 **Radiologic examination, spine, entire thoracic and lumbar, including skull, cervical and sacral spine if performed (eg, scoliosis evaluation); one view**
1.09   1.09   **FUD** XXX   Q1 80 ▭
AMA: 2016,Sep,4

72082 **2 or 3 views**
1.75   1.75   **FUD** XXX   Q1 80 ▭
AMA: 2016,Sep,4

72083 **4 or 5 views**
1.90   1.90   **FUD** XXX   S Z2 80 ▭
AMA: 2016,Sep,4

72084 **minimum of 6 views**
2.27   2.27   **FUD** XXX   S Z2 80 ▭
AMA: 2016,Sep,4

72100 **Radiologic examination, spine, lumbosacral; 2 or 3 views**
0.98   0.98   **FUD** XXX   Q1 N1 80 ▭
AMA: 2016,Jan,13; 2015,Jan,16; 2014,Jan,11; 2012,Feb,9-10

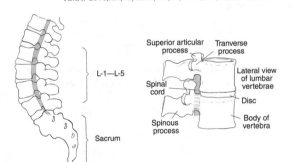

72110 **minimum of 4 views**
1.37   1.37   **FUD** XXX   Q1 N1 80 ▭
AMA: 2016,Jan,13; 2015,Jan,16; 2014,Jan,11; 2012,Feb,9-10

72114 **complete, including bending views, minimum of 6 views**
1.75   1.75   **FUD** XXX   Q1 N1 80 ▭
AMA: 2014,Jan,11; 2012,Feb,9-10

72120 **bending views only, 2 or 3 views**
1.13   1.13   **FUD** XXX   Q1 N1 80 ▭
AMA: 2016,Aug,7; 2014,Jan,11; 2012,Feb,9-10

72125-72133 Computerized Tomography: Spine

CMS: 100-04,12,20.4.7 Services Not Meeting National Electrical Manufacturers Association (NEMA) Standard; 100-04,4,20.6.12 Use of HCPCS Modifier – CT; 100-04,4,250.16 Multiple Procedure Payment Reduction: Certain Diagnostic Imaging Procedures Rendered by Physicians

INCLUDES Imaging using tomographic technique enhanced by computer imaging to create a cross-sectional plane of the body

EXCLUDES *3D rendering (76376-76377)*
Code also intrathecal injection procedure when performed (61055, 62284)

72125 **Computed tomography, cervical spine; without contrast material**
5.19   5.19   **FUD** XXX   Q3 Z2 80 ▭
AMA: 2014,Jan,11; 2012,Feb,9-10

72126 **with contrast material**
🚑 6.44 ☁ 6.44 **FUD** XXX   [Q3] [Z3] [80] [▢]
AMA: 2016,Jan,13; 2015,Jan,16; 2014,Jan,11; 2012,Feb,9-10

72127 **without contrast material, followed by contrast material(s) and further sections**
🚑 7.62 ☁ 7.62 **FUD** XXX   [Q3] [Z2] [80] [▢]
AMA: 2014,Jan,11; 2012,Feb,9-10

72128 **Computed tomography, thoracic spine; without contrast material**
🚑 5.07 ☁ 5.07 **FUD** XXX   [Q3] [Z2] [80] [▢]
AMA: 2014,Jan,11; 2012,Feb,9-10

72129 **with contrast material**
🚑 6.45 ☁ 6.45 **FUD** XXX   [Q3] [Z2] [80] [▢]
AMA: 2016,Jan,13; 2015,Jan,16; 2014,Jan,11; 2012,Feb,9-10

72130 **without contrast material, followed by contrast material(s) and further sections**
🚑 7.67 ☁ 7.67 **FUD** XXX   [Q3] [Z2] [80] [▢]
AMA: 2014,Jan,11; 2012,Feb,9-10

72131 **Computed tomography, lumbar spine; without contrast material**
🚑 5.05 ☁ 5.05 **FUD** XXX   [Q3] [Z2] [80] [▢]
AMA: 2014,Jan,11; 2012,Feb,9-10

72132 **with contrast material**
🚑 6.43 ☁ 6.43 **FUD** XXX   [Q3] [Z3] [80] [▢]
AMA: 2016,Jan,13; 2015,Jan,16; 2014,Jan,11; 2012,Feb,9-10

72133 **without contrast material, followed by contrast material(s) and further sections**
🚑 7.61 ☁ 7.61 **FUD** XXX   [Q3] [Z2] [80] [▢]
AMA: 2014,Jan,11; 2012,Feb,9-10

72141-72158 Magnetic Resonance Imaging: Spine

CMS: 100-04,4,250.16 Multiple Procedure Payment Reduction: Certain Diagnostic Imaging Procedures Rendered by Physicians

[INCLUDES] Application of an external magnetic field that forces alignment of hydrogen atom nuclei in soft tissues which converts to sets of tomographic images that can be displayed as three-dimensional images
Code also intrathecal injection procedure when performed (61055, 62284)

72141 **Magnetic resonance (eg, proton) imaging, spinal canal and contents, cervical; without contrast material**
🚑 6.30 ☁ 6.30 **FUD** XXX   [Q3] [Z3] [80] [▢]
AMA: 2016,Jan,13; 2015,Jan,16; 2014,Jun,14; 2014,Jan,11; 2012,Feb,9-10

72142 **with contrast material(s)**
[EXCLUDES] MRI of cervical spinal canal performed without contrast followed by repeating the study with contrast (72156)
🚑 9.14 ☁ 9.14 **FUD** XXX   [Q3] [Z3] [80] [▢]
AMA: 2016,Jan,13; 2015,Jan,16; 2014,Jan,11; 2012,Feb,9-10

72146 **Magnetic resonance (eg, proton) imaging, spinal canal and contents, thoracic; without contrast material**
🚑 6.30 ☁ 6.30 **FUD** XXX   [Q3] [Z3] [80] [▢]
AMA: 2016,Jan,13; 2015,Jan,16; 2014,Jun,14; 2014,Jan,11; 2012,Feb,9-10

72147 **with contrast material(s)**
[EXCLUDES] MRI of thoracic spinal canal performed without contrast followed by repeating the study with contrast (72157)
🚑 9.04 ☁ 9.04 **FUD** XXX   [Q3] [Z3] [80] [▢]
AMA: 2016,Jan,13; 2015,Jan,16; 2014,Jan,11; 2012,Feb,9-10; 2012,Jan,15-42; 2011,Jan,11

72148 **Magnetic resonance (eg, proton) imaging, spinal canal and contents, lumbar; without contrast material**
🚑 6.27 ☁ 6.27 **FUD** XXX   [Q3] [Z3] [80] [▢]
AMA: 2016,Jan,13; 2015,Jan,16; 2014,Jun,14; 2014,Jan,11; 2012,Feb,9-10; 2012,Jan,15-42; 2011,Jan,11

72149 **with contrast material(s)**
[EXCLUDES] MRI of lumbar spinal canal performed without contrast followed by repeating the study with contrast (72158)
🚑 9.03 ☁ 9.03 **FUD** XXX   [Q3] [Z3] [80] [▢]
AMA: 2014,Jan,11; 2012,Feb,9-10

72156 **Magnetic resonance (eg, proton) imaging, spinal canal and contents, without contrast material, followed by contrast material(s) and further sequences; cervical**
🚑 10.6 ☁ 10.6 **FUD** XXX   [Q3] [Z2] [80] [▢]
AMA: 2014,Jan,11; 2012,Feb,9-10

72157 **thoracic**
🚑 10.6 ☁ 10.6 **FUD** XXX   [Q3] [Z2] [80] [▢]
AMA: 2014,Jan,11; 2012,Feb,9-10

72158 **lumbar**
🚑 10.6 ☁ 10.6 **FUD** XXX   [Q3] [Z2] [80] [▢]
AMA: 2014,Jan,11; 2012,Feb,9-10

Superior view of thoracic spine and surrounding paraspinal muscles

72159 Magnetic Resonance Angiography: Spine

CMS: 100-04,13,40.1.1 Magnetic Resonance Angiography; 100-04,13,40.1.2 HCPCS Coding Requirements; 100-04,4,250.16 Multiple Procedure Payment Reduction: Certain Diagnostic Imaging Procedures Rendered by Physicians

72159 **Magnetic resonance angiography, spinal canal and contents, with or without contrast material(s)**
🚑 11.7 ☁ 11.7 **FUD** XXX   [B] [80] [▢]
AMA: 2016,Jan,13; 2015,Jan,16; 2014,Jan,11; 2012,Feb,9-10

72170-72190 Radiography: Pelvis

[INCLUDES] Minimum number of views or more views when needed to adequately complete the study
Radiographs that have to be repeated during the encounter due to substandard quality; only one unit of service is reported

[EXCLUDES] A second interpretation by the requesting physician (included in E&M service)
Combined CT or CT angiography of abdomen and pelvis (74174, 74176-74178)
Obtaining more films after review of initial films, based on the discretion of the radiologist, an order for the test, and a change in the patient's condition
Pelvimetry (74710)

72170 **Radiologic examination, pelvis; 1 or 2 views**
🚑 0.89 ☁ 0.89 **FUD** XXX   [01] [N1] [80] [▢]
AMA: 2016,Aug,7; 2016,Jun,5; 2016,Jan,13; 2015,Jan,16; 2014,Jan,11; 2012,Feb,9-10; 2012,Jan,15-42; 2011,Jan,11

72190 **complete, minimum of 3 views**
🚑 1.07 ☁ 1.07 **FUD** XXX   [01] [N1] [80] [▢]
AMA: 2016,Jun,5; 2014,Jan,11; 2012,Feb,9-10

72191 Computerized Tomographic Angiography: Pelvis

CMS: 100-04,4,250.16 Multiple Procedure Payment Reduction: Certain Diagnostic Imaging Procedures Rendered by Physicians

[EXCLUDES] Computed tomographic angiography (73706, 74174-74175, 75635)

72191 **Computed tomographic angiography, pelvis, with contrast material(s), including noncontrast images, if performed, and image postprocessing**
🚑 8.59 ☁ 8.59 **FUD** XXX   [Q3] [Z2] [80] [▢]
AMA: 2016,Jan,13; 2015,Jan,16; 2014,Jan,11; 2012,Feb,9-10

72192-72194 Computerized Tomography: Pelvis

CMS: 100-04,4,250.16 Multiple Procedure Payment Reduction: Certain Diagnostic Imaging Procedures Rendered by Physicians

> EXCLUDES 3D rendering (76376-76377)
> Combined CT of abdomen and pelvis (74176-74178)
> CT colonography, diagnostic (74261-74262)
> CT colonography, screening (74263)

72192 **Computed tomography, pelvis; without contrast material**
> 4.11   4.11 **FUD** XXX   Q3 Z2 80
>
> **AMA:** 2016,Jan,13; 2015,Jan,16; 2014,Jan,11; 2012,Oct,12; 2012,Feb,9-10; 2012,Jan,15-42; 2011,Jan,11

72193 **with contrast material(s)**
> 6.36   6.36 **FUD** XXX   Q3 Z2 80
>
> **AMA:** 2016,Jan,13; 2015,Jan,16; 2014,Jan,11; 2012,Oct,12; 2012,Feb,9-10

72194 **without contrast material, followed by contrast material(s) and further sections**
> 7.33   7.33 **FUD** XXX   Q3 Z2 80
>
> **AMA:** 2016,Jan,13; 2015,Jan,16; 2014,Jan,11; 2012,Oct,12; 2012,Feb,9-10; 2012,Jan,15-42; 2011,Jan,11

72195-72197 Magnetic Resonance Imaging: Pelvis

CMS: 100-04,4,250.16 Multiple Procedure Payment Reduction: Certain Diagnostic Imaging Procedures Rendered by Physicians

> INCLUDES Application of an external magnetic field that forces alignment of hydrogen atom nuclei in soft tissues which converts to sets of tomographic images that can be displayed as three-dimensional images
> EXCLUDES Magnetic resonance imaging of fetus(es) (74712-74713)

72195 **Magnetic resonance (eg, proton) imaging, pelvis; without contrast material(s)**
> 10.5   10.5 **FUD** XXX   Q3 Z2 80
>
> **AMA:** 2016,Jun,5; 2016,Jan,13; 2015,Jan,16; 2014,Jun,14; 2014,Jan,11; 2012,Feb,9-10; 2012,Jan,15-42; 2011,Jan,11

72196 **with contrast material(s)**
> 11.5   11.5 **FUD** XXX   Q3 Z2 80
>
> **AMA:** 2016,Jun,5; 2016,Jan,13; 2015,Jan,16; 2014,Jan,11; 2012,Feb,9-10; 2012,Jan,15-42; 2011,Jan,11

72197 **without contrast material(s), followed by contrast material(s) and further sequences**
> 14.2   14.2 **FUD** XXX   Q3 Z2 80
>
> **AMA:** 2016,Jun,5; 2016,Jan,13; 2015,Jan,16; 2014,Jan,11; 2012,Feb,9-10

72198 Magnetic Resonance Angiography: Pelvis

CMS: 100-04,13,40.1.1 Magnetic Resonance Angiography; 100-04,13,40.1.2 HCPCS Coding Requirements; 100-04,4,250.16 Multiple Procedure Payment Reduction: Certain Diagnostic Imaging Procedures Rendered by Physicians

> INCLUDES Use of magnetic fields and radio waves to produce detailed cross-sectional images of internal body structures

72198 **Magnetic resonance angiography, pelvis, with or without contrast material(s)**
> 11.2   11.2 **FUD** XXX   B 80
>
> **AMA:** 2016,Jan,13; 2015,Jan,16; 2014,Jan,11; 2012,Feb,9-10

72200-72220 Radiography: Pelvisacral

> INCLUDES Minimum number of views or more views when needed to adequately complete the study
> Radiographs that have to be repeated during the encounter due to substandard quality; only one unit of service is reported
> EXCLUDES Injection procedure for myelography
> Myelography
> Obtaining more films after review of initial films, based on the discretion of the radiologist, an order for the test, and a change in the patient's condition
> Second interpretation by the requesting physician (included in E&M service)

72200 **Radiologic examination, sacroiliac joints; less than 3 views**
> 0.80   0.80 **FUD** XXX   Q1 N1 80
>
> **AMA:** 2014,Jan,11; 2012,Feb,9-10

72202 **3 or more views**
> 0.92   0.92 **FUD** XXX   Q1 N1 80
>
> **AMA:** 2014,Jan,11; 2012,Feb,9-10

72220 **Radiologic examination, sacrum and coccyx, minimum of 2 views**
> 0.79   0.79 **FUD** XXX   Q1 N1 80
>
> **AMA:** 2014,Jan,11; 2012,Feb,9-10

72240-72270 Myelography with Contrast: Spinal Cord

CMS: 100-04,13,40.1.3.1 Payment for Low Osmolar Contrast Material

> INCLUDES Fluoroscopic guidance for subarachnoid puncture for diagnostic radiographic myelography (77003)
> EXCLUDES Arthrodesis (22586, 0195T-0196T, 0309T)
> Injection procedure for myelography (62284)
> Myelography (62302-62305)

72240 **Myelography, cervical, radiological supervision and interpretation**
> Code also injection for myelogram at C1-C2 when appropriate (61055)
> 2.75   2.75 **FUD** XXX   Q2 N1 80
>
> **AMA:** 2016,Jan,13; 2015,Jan,16; 2014,Sep,3; 2014,Jan,11; 2012,Feb,9-10

72255 **Myelography, thoracic, radiological supervision and interpretation**
> 2.74   2.74 **FUD** XXX   Q2 N1 80
>
> **AMA:** 2016,Jan,13; 2015,Jan,16; 2014,Sep,3; 2014,Jan,11; 2012,Feb,9-10

72265 **Myelography, lumbosacral, radiological supervision and interpretation**
> 2.59   2.59 **FUD** XXX   Q2 N1 80
>
> **AMA:** 2016,Jan,13; 2015,Jan,16; 2014,Sep,3; 2014,Jan,11; 2012,Feb,9-10

72270 **Myelography, 2 or more regions (eg, lumbar/thoracic, cervical/thoracic, lumbar/cervical, lumbar/thoracic/cervical), radiological supervision and interpretation**
> 3.58   3.58 **FUD** XXX   Q2 N1 80
>
> **AMA:** 2016,Jan,13; 2015,Jan,16; 2014,Sep,3; 2014,Jan,11; 2012,Feb,9-10

72275 Radiography: Epidural Space

> INCLUDES Epidurogram, documentation of images, formal written report
> Fluoroscopic guidance (77003)
> EXCLUDES Arthrodesis (22586, 0195T-0196T, 0309T)
> Second interpretation by the requesting physician (included in E&M service)
> Code also injection procedure as appropriate (62280-62282, 62320-62327, 64479-64484)

72275 **Epidurography, radiological supervision and interpretation**
> 3.25   3.25 **FUD** XXX   N N1
>
> **AMA:** 2016,Jan,13; 2015,Jan,16; 2014,Jan,11; 2012,Jul,3-6; 2012,Jun,12-13; 2012,Feb,9-10; 2012,Jan,15-42; 2011,Jan,11

72285 Radiography: Intervertebral Disc (Cervical/Thoracic)

CMS: 100-04,13,30.1.3.1 Payment for Low Osmolar Contrast Material
Code also discography injection procedure (62291)

72285 **Discography, cervical or thoracic, radiological supervision and interpretation**
> 3.21   3.21 **FUD** XXX   Q2 N1 80
>
> **AMA:** 2016,Jan,13; 2015,Jan,16; 2014,Jan,11; 2012,Feb,9-10; 2011,Mar,7

72295 Radiography: Intervertebral Disc (Lumbar)

CMS: 100-04,13,30.1.3.1 Payment for Low Osmolar Contrast Material
Code also discography injection procedure (62290)

72295 **Discography, lumbar, radiological supervision and interpretation**
> 2.78   2.78 **FUD** XXX   Q2 N1 80
>
> **AMA:** 2016,Jan,13; 2015,Jan,16; 2014,Jan,11; 2012,Jul,3-6; 2012,Feb,9-10; 2012,Jan,15-42; 2011,Mar,7; 2011,Jan,11

73000-73085 Radiography: Shoulder and Upper Arm

INCLUDES Minimum number of views or more views when needed to adequately complete the study
Radiographs that have to be repeated during the encounter due to substandard quality; only one unit of service is reported

EXCLUDES *Fluoroscopic guidance*
Obtaining more films after review of initial films, based on the discretion of the radiologist, an order for the test, and a change in the patient's condition
Second interpretation by the requesting physician (included in E&M service)
Stress views of upper body joint(s), when performed (77071)

73000 **Radiologic examination; clavicle, complete**
🏥 0.77 ⚕ 0.77 **FUD** XXX
AMA: 2014,Jan,11; 2012,Feb,9-10

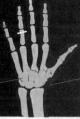

Gold wedding band absorbs all x-rays (white)

Air allows all rays to reach film (black)

Calcium in bone absorbs most of rays and is nearly white

Radiograph (left)

Film

X-ray beam

Soft tissues absorb part of rays and will vary in gray intensity

Posterioranterior (PA) chest study; lateral views also common

73010 **scapula, complete**
🏥 0.84 ⚕ 0.84 **FUD** XXX
AMA: 2014,Jan,11; 2012,Feb,9-10

73020 **Radiologic examination, shoulder; 1 view**
🏥 0.64 ⚕ 0.64 **FUD** XXX
AMA: 2014,Jan,11; 2012,Feb,9-10

73030 **complete, minimum of 2 views**
🏥 0.81 ⚕ 0.81 **FUD** XXX
AMA: 2014,Jan,11; 2012,Feb,9-10

73040 **Radiologic examination, shoulder, arthrography, radiological supervision and interpretation**
INCLUDES Fluoroscopic guidance (77002)
Code also arthrography injection procedure (23350)
🏥 2.81 ⚕ 2.81 **FUD** XXX
AMA: 2016,Jan,13; 2015,Jan,16; 2014,Jan,11; 2012,Feb,9-10; 2012,Jan,15-42; 2011,Jan,11

73050 **Radiologic examination; acromioclavicular joints, bilateral, with or without weighted distraction**
🏥 0.99 ⚕ 0.99 **FUD** XXX
AMA: 2014,Jan,11; 2012,Feb,9-10

73060 **humerus, minimum of 2 views**
🏥 0.81 ⚕ 0.81 **FUD** XXX
AMA: 2014,Jan,11; 2012,Feb,9-10

73070 **Radiologic examination, elbow; 2 views**
🏥 0.76 ⚕ 0.76 **FUD** XXX
AMA: 2016,Jan,13; 2015,Jan,16; 2014,Jan,11; 2012,Feb,9-10

73080 **complete, minimum of 3 views**
🏥 0.87 ⚕ 0.87 **FUD** XXX
AMA: 2014,Jan,11; 2012,Feb,9-10

73085 **Radiologic examination, elbow, arthrography, radiological supervision and interpretation**
INCLUDES Fluoroscopic guidance (77002)
Code also arthrography injection procedure (24220)
🏥 2.73 ⚕ 2.73 **FUD** XXX
AMA: 2016,Jan,13; 2015,Jan,16; 2014,Jan,11; 2012,Feb,9-10

73090-73140 Radiography: Forearm and Hand

INCLUDES Minimum number of views or more views when needed to adequately complete the study
Radiographs that have to be repeated during the encounter due to substandard quality; only one unit of service is reported

EXCLUDES *Obtaining more films after review of initial films, based on the discretion of the radiologist, an order for the test, and a change in the patient's condition*
Second interpretation by the requesting physician (included in E&M service)
Stress views of upper body joint(s), when performed (77071)

73090 **Radiologic examination; forearm, 2 views**
🏥 0.72 ⚕ 0.72 **FUD** XXX
AMA: 2016,Jan,13; 2015,Jan,16; 2014,Jan,11; 2012,Feb,9-10

73092 **upper extremity, infant, minimum of 2 views**
🏥 0.76 ⚕ 0.76 **FUD** XXX
AMA: 2014,Jan,11; 2012,Feb,9-10

73100 **Radiologic examination, wrist; 2 views**
🏥 0.81 ⚕ 0.81 **FUD** XXX
AMA: 2016,Jan,13; 2015,Jan,16; 2014,Jan,11; 2012,Feb,9-10

73110 **complete, minimum of 3 views**
🏥 0.99 ⚕ 0.99 **FUD** XXX
AMA: 2016,Jan,13; 2015,Jan,16; 2014,Jan,11; 2012,Feb,9-10; 2012,Jan,15-42; 2011,Jan,11

73115 **Radiologic examination, wrist, arthrography, radiological supervision and interpretation**
INCLUDES Fluoroscopic guidance (77002)
Code also arthrography injection procedure (25246)
🏥 3.00 ⚕ 3.00 **FUD** XXX
AMA: 2016,Jan,13; 2015,Jan,16; 2014,Jan,11; 2012,Feb,9-10

73120 **Radiologic examination, hand; 2 views**
🏥 0.73 ⚕ 0.73 **FUD** XXX
AMA: 2014,Jan,11; 2012,Feb,9-10

73130 **minimum of 3 views**
🏥 0.86 ⚕ 0.86 **FUD** XXX
AMA: 2014,Jan,11; 2012,Feb,9-10

73140 **Radiologic examination, finger(s), minimum of 2 views**
🏥 0.88 ⚕ 0.88 **FUD** XXX
AMA: 2016,Jan,13; 2015,Jan,16; 2014,Jan,11; 2012,Feb,9-10

73200-73202 Computerized Tomography: Shoulder, Arm, Hand

CMS: 100-04,4,250.16 Multiple Procedure Payment Reduction: Certain Diagnostic Imaging Procedures Rendered by Physicians

INCLUDES Imaging using tomographic technique enhanced by computer imaging to create a cross-sectional plane of the body
Intravascular, intrathecal, or intra-articular contrast materials when noted in code descriptor

EXCLUDES *3D rendering (76376-76377)*

73200 **Computed tomography, upper extremity; without contrast material**
🏥 5.04 ⚕ 5.04 **FUD** XXX
AMA: 2016,Jan,13; 2015,Jan,16; 2014,Jan,11; 2012,Feb,9-10; 2012,Jan,15-42; 2011,Jul,16-17; 2011,Feb,8-9

73201 **with contrast material(s)**
🏥 6.27 ⚕ 6.27 **FUD** XXX
AMA: 2016,Jan,13; 2015,Aug,6; 2015,Jan,16; 2014,Jan,11; 2012,Feb,9-10; 2012,Jan,15-42; 2011,Jul,16-17

73202 **without contrast material, followed by contrast material(s) and further sections**
🏥 7.81 ⚕ 7.81 **FUD** XXX
AMA: 2014,Jan,11; 2012,Feb,9-10; 2011,Jul,16-17

73206 Computerized Tomographic Angiography: Shoulder, Arm, and Hand

CMS: 100-04,4,250.16 Multiple Procedure Payment Reduction: Certain Diagnostic Imaging Procedures Rendered by Physicians

INCLUDES Intravascular, intrathecal, or intra-articular contrast materials when noted in code descriptor
Multiple rapid thin section CT scans to create cross-sectional images of bones, organs and tissues

73206 Computed tomographic angiography, upper extremity, with contrast material(s), including noncontrast images, if performed, and image postprocessing
9.21   9.21   **FUD** XXX   Q3 Z2 80
AMA: 2016,Jan,13; 2015,Jan,16; 2014,Jan,11; 2012,Feb,9-10

73218-73223 Magnetic Resonance Imaging: Shoulder, Arm, Hand

CMS: 100-04,4,250.16 Multiple Procedure Payment Reduction: Certain Diagnostic Imaging Procedures Rendered by Physicians

INCLUDES Application of an external magnetic field that forces alignment of hydrogen atom nuclei in soft tissues which converts to sets of tomographic images that can be displayed as three-dimensional images
Intravascular, intrathecal, or intra-articular contrast materials when noted in code descriptor

73218 Magnetic resonance (eg, proton) imaging, upper extremity, other than joint; without contrast material(s)
10.2   10.2   **FUD** XXX   Q3 Z2 80
AMA: 2016,Jan,13; 2015,Jan,16; 2014,Jan,11; 2012,Feb,9-10; 2012,Jan,15-42; 2011,Feb,8-9

73219 with contrast material(s)
11.3   11.3   **FUD** XXX   Q3 Z2 80
AMA: 2016,Jan,13; 2015,Jan,16; 2014,Jan,11; 2012,Feb,9-10; 2012,Jan,15-42

73220 without contrast material(s), followed by contrast material(s) and further sequences
14.0   14.0   **FUD** XXX   Q3 Z2 80
AMA: 2016,Jan,13; 2015,Jan,16; 2014,Jan,11; 2012,Feb,9-10

73221 Magnetic resonance (eg, proton) imaging, any joint of upper extremity; without contrast material(s)
6.64   6.64   **FUD** XXX   Q3 Z2 80
AMA: 2016,Jan,13; 2015,Jan,16; 2014,Jan,11; 2012,Feb,9-10; 2012,Jan,15-42; 2011,Feb,8-9

73222 with contrast material(s)
10.6   10.6   **FUD** XXX   Q3 Z2 80
AMA: 2016,Jan,13; 2015,Aug,6; 2015,Jan,16; 2014,Jan,11; 2012,Feb,9-10

73223 without contrast material(s), followed by contrast material(s) and further sequences
13.1   13.1   **FUD** XXX   Q3 Z2 80
AMA: 2016,Jan,13; 2015,Jan,16; 2014,Jan,11; 2012,Feb,9-10

73225 Magnetic Resonance Angiography: Shoulder, Arm, Hand

CMS: 100-04,13,40.1.1 Magnetic Resonance Angiography; 100-04,4,250.16 Multiple Procedure Payment Reduction: Certain Diagnostic Imaging Procedures Rendered by Physicians

INCLUDES Intravascular, intrathecal, or intra-articular contrast materials when noted in code descriptor
Use of magnetic fields and radio waves to produce detailed cross-sectional images of internal body structures

73225 Magnetic resonance angiography, upper extremity, with or without contrast material(s)
11.3   11.3   **FUD** XXX   B 80
AMA: 2016,Jan,13; 2015,Jan,16; 2014,Jan,11; 2012,Feb,9-10

73501-73552 Radiography: Pelvic Region and Thigh

EXCLUDES Stress views of lower body joint(s), when performed (77071)

73501 Radiologic examination, hip, unilateral, with pelvis when performed; 1 view
0.83   0.83   **FUD** XXX   01 80
AMA: 2016,Aug,7; 2016,Jun,8; 2016,Jan,13; 2015,Oct,9

73502 2-3 views
1.16   1.16   **FUD** XXX   01 80
AMA: 2016,Aug,7; 2016,Jun,8; 2016,Jan,13; 2015,Oct,9

73503 minimum of 4 views
1.45   1.45   **FUD** XXX   01 80
AMA: 2016,Aug,7; 2016,Jun,8; 2016,Jan,13; 2015,Oct,9

73521 Radiologic examination, hips, bilateral, with pelvis when performed; 2 views
1.11   1.11   **FUD** XXX   01 80
AMA: 2016,Aug,7; 2016,Jun,8; 2016,Jan,13; 2015,Oct,9

73522 3-4 views
1.37   1.37   **FUD** XXX   01 80
AMA: 2016,Aug,7; 2016,Jun,8; 2016,Jan,13; 2015,Oct,9

73523 minimum of 5 views
1.59   1.59   **FUD** XXX   S 80
AMA: 2016,Aug,7; 2016,Jun,8; 2016,Jan,13; 2015,Oct,9

73525 Radiologic examination, hip, arthrography, radiological supervision and interpretation
INCLUDES Fluoroscopic guidance (77002)
2.85   2.85   **FUD** XXX   Q2 N1 80
AMA: 2016,Aug,7; 2016,Jan,13; 2015,Jan,16; 2014,Jan,11; 2012,Jun,14; 2012,Feb,9-10

73551 Radiologic examination, femur; 1 view
0.78   0.78   **FUD** XXX   01 80
AMA: 2016,Aug,7

73552 minimum 2 views
0.91   0.91   **FUD** XXX   01 80
AMA: 2016,Aug,7

73560-73660 Radiography: Lower Leg, Ankle, and Foot

EXCLUDES Stress views of lower body joint(s), when performed (77071)

73560 Radiologic examination, knee; 1 or 2 views
0.87   0.87   **FUD** XXX   01 N1 80
AMA: 2016,Jan,13; 2015,May,10; 2015,Feb,10; 2014,Jan,11; 2012,Feb,9-10

73562 3 views
1.00   1.00   **FUD** XXX   01 N1 80
AMA: 2014,Jan,11; 2012,Feb,9-10

73564 complete, 4 or more views
1.10   1.10   **FUD** XXX   01 N1 80
AMA: 2016,Jan,13; 2015,May,10; 2015,Feb,10; 2015,Jan,16; 2014,Jan,11; 2012,Feb,9-10; 2012,Jan,15-42; 2011,Jan,11

73565 both knees, standing, anteroposterior
1.00   1.00   **FUD** XXX   01 N1 80
AMA: 2016,Jan,13; 2015,May,10; 2015,Feb,10; 2014,Jan,11; 2012,Feb,9-10

73580 Radiologic examination, knee, arthrography, radiological supervision and interpretation
INCLUDES Fluoroscopic guidance (77002)
3.24   3.24   **FUD** XXX   Q2 N1 80
AMA: 2016,Jan,13; 2015,Aug,6; 2015,Jan,16; 2014,Jan,11; 2012,Feb,9-10

73590 Radiologic examination; tibia and fibula, 2 views
0.80   0.80   **FUD** XXX   01 N1 80
AMA: 2016,Jan,13; 2015,Jan,16; 2014,Jan,11; 2012,Feb,9-10

73592 lower extremity, infant, minimum of 2 views
0.78   0.78   **FUD** XXX   01 N1 80
AMA: 2014,Jan,11; 2012,Feb,9-10

73600 Radiologic examination, ankle; 2 views
0.84   0.84   **FUD** XXX   01 N1 80
AMA: 2016,Jan,13; 2015,Jan,16; 2014,Jan,11; 2012,Feb,9-10

73610 complete, minimum of 3 views
0.87   0.87   **FUD** XXX   01 N1 80
AMA: 2016,Jan,13; 2015,Jan,16; 2014,Jan,11; 2012,Feb,9-10

Radiology

73615 Radiologic examination, ankle, arthrography, radiological supervision and interpretation
INCLUDES Fluoroscopic guidance (77002)
🚑 2.94 📊 2.94 **FUD** XXX [02] [N1] [80] [▣]
AMA: 2016,Jan,13; 2015,Jan,16; 2014,Jan,11; 2012,Feb,9-10

73620 Radiologic examination, foot; 2 views
🚑 0.73 📊 0.73 **FUD** XXX [01] [N1] [80] [▣]
AMA: 2016,Jan,13; 2015,Jan,16; 2014,Jan,11; 2012,Feb,9-10

73630 complete, minimum of 3 views
🚑 0.81 📊 0.81 **FUD** XXX [01] [N1] [80] [▣]
AMA: 2014,Jan,11; 2012,Feb,9-10

73650 Radiologic examination; calcaneus, minimum of 2 views
🚑 0.76 📊 0.76 **FUD** XXX [01] [N1] [80] [▣]
AMA: 2014,Jan,11; 2012,Feb,9-10

73660 toe(s), minimum of 2 views
🚑 0.79 📊 0.79 **FUD** XXX [01] [N1] [80] [▣]
AMA: 2014,Jan,11; 2012,Feb,9-10

73700-73702 Computerized Tomography: Leg, Ankle, and Foot

CMS: 100-04,4,250.16 Multiple Procedure Payment Reduction: Certain Diagnostic Imaging Procedures Rendered by Physicians
EXCLUDES 3D rendering (76376-76377)

73700 Computed tomography, lower extremity; without contrast material
🚑 5.04 📊 5.04 **FUD** XXX [03] [Z2] [80] [▣]
AMA: 2016,Jan,13; 2015,Jan,16; 2014,Jan,11; 2012,Feb,9-10; 2012,Jan,15-42; 2011,Jul,16-17

73701 with contrast material(s)
🚑 6.36 📊 6.36 **FUD** XXX [03] [Z2] [80] [▣]
AMA: 2016,Jan,13; 2015,Jan,16; 2014,Jan,11; 2012,Feb,9-10; 2011,Jul,16-17

73702 without contrast material, followed by contrast material(s) and further sections
🚑 7.72 📊 7.72 **FUD** XXX [03] [Z2] [80] [▣]
AMA: 2016,Jan,13; 2015,Jan,16; 2014,Jan,11; 2012,Feb,9-10; 2011,Jul,16-17

73706 Computerized Tomographic Angiography: Leg, Ankle, and Foot

CMS: 100-04,4,250.16 Multiple Procedure Payment Reduction: Certain Diagnostic Imaging Procedures Rendered by Physicians
EXCLUDES CT angiography for aorto-iliofemoral runoff (75635)

73706 Computed tomographic angiography, lower extremity, with contrast material(s), including noncontrast images, if performed, and image postprocessing
🚑 9.91 📊 9.91 **FUD** XXX [03] [Z2] [80] [▣]
AMA: 2016,Jan,13; 2015,Jan,16; 2014,Jan,11; 2012,Feb,9-10; 2012,Jan,15-42; 2011,Apr,12; 2011,Jan,11

73718-73723 Magnetic Resonance Imaging: Leg, Ankle, and Foot

CMS: 100-04,4,250.16 Multiple Procedure Payment Reduction: Certain Diagnostic Imaging Procedures Rendered by Physicians

73718 Magnetic resonance (eg, proton) imaging, lower extremity other than joint; without contrast material(s)
🚑 10.2 📊 10.2 **FUD** XXX [03] [Z2] [80] [▣]
AMA: 2016,Jan,13; 2015,Jan,16; 2014,Jan,11; 2012,Feb,9-10

73719 with contrast material(s)
🚑 11.3 📊 11.3 **FUD** XXX [03] [Z2] [80] [▣]
AMA: 2016,Jan,13; 2015,Jan,16; 2014,Jan,11; 2012,Feb,9-10

73720 without contrast material(s), followed by contrast material(s) and further sequences
🚑 14.1 📊 14.1 **FUD** XXX [03] [Z2] [80] [▣]
AMA: 2016,Jan,13; 2015,Jan,16; 2014,Jan,11; 2012,Feb,9-10

73721 Magnetic resonance (eg, proton) imaging, any joint of lower extremity; without contrast material
🚑 6.65 📊 6.65 **FUD** XXX [03] [Z2] [80] [▣]
AMA: 2016,Jan,13; 2015,Jan,16; 2014,Jan,11; 2012,Feb,9-10; 2012,Jan,15-42; 2011,Jan,11

73722 with contrast material(s)
🚑 10.7 📊 10.7 **FUD** XXX [03] [Z2] [80] [▣]
AMA: 2016,Jan,13; 2015,Aug,6; 2015,Jan,16; 2014,Jan,11; 2012,Feb,9-10

73723 without contrast material(s), followed by contrast material(s) and further sequences
🚑 13.2 📊 13.2 **FUD** XXX [03] [Z2] [80] [▣]
AMA: 2016,Jan,13; 2015,Jan,16; 2014,Jan,11; 2012,Feb,9-10

73725 Magnetic Resonance Angiography: Leg, Ankle, and Foot

CMS: 100-04,13,40.1.2 HCPCS Coding Requirements; 100-04,4,250.16 Multiple Procedure Payment Reduction: Certain Diagnostic Imaging Procedures Rendered by Physicians

73725 Magnetic resonance angiography, lower extremity, with or without contrast material(s)
🚑 11.2 📊 11.2 **FUD** XXX [B] [80] [▣]
AMA: 2016,Jan,13; 2015,Jan,16; 2014,Jan,11; 2012,Feb,9-10

74000-74022 Radiography: Abdomen--General

74000 Radiologic examination, abdomen; single anteroposterior view
🚑 0.66 📊 0.66 **FUD** XXX [01] [N1] [80] [▣]
AMA: 2016,Jun,5; 2014,Jan,11; 2012,Feb,9-10

74010 anteroposterior and additional oblique and cone views
🚑 0.99 📊 0.99 **FUD** XXX [01] [N1] [80] [▣]
AMA: 2016,Jun,5; 2016,Jan,13; 2015,Jan,16; 2014,Jun,14; 2014,Jan,11; 2012,Feb,9-10

74020 complete, including decubitus and/or erect views
🚑 1.05 📊 1.05 **FUD** XXX [01] [N1] [80] [▣]
AMA: 2016,Jun,5; 2014,Jan,11; 2012,Feb,9-10

74022 complete acute abdomen series, including supine, erect, and/or decubitus views, single view chest
🚑 1.25 📊 1.25 **FUD** XXX [01] [N1] [80] [▣]
AMA: 2016,Jun,5; 2014,Jan,11; 2012,Feb,9-10

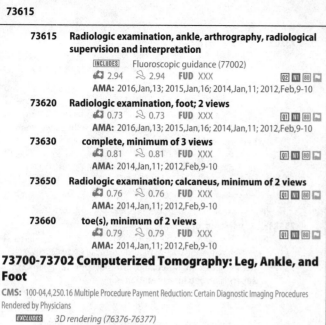

Esophagus
Diaphragm
Liver
Abdomen
Pelvis area

74150-74170 Computerized Tomography: Abdomen--General

CMS: 100-04,4,250.16 Multiple Procedure Payment Reduction: Certain Diagnostic Imaging Procedures Rendered by Physicians
EXCLUDES 3D rendering (76376-76377)
Combined CT of abdomen and pelvis (74176-74178)
CT colonography, diagnostic (74261-74262)
CT colonography, screening (74263)

74150 Computed tomography, abdomen; without contrast material
🚑 4.21 📊 4.21 **FUD** XXX [03] [Z2] [80] [▣]
AMA: 2016,Jun,5; 2016,Jan,13; 2015,Jan,16; 2014,Jan,11; 2012,Oct,12; 2012,Feb,9-10; 2012,Jan,15-42; 2011,Jan,11

74160 with contrast material(s)
🚑 6.49 📊 6.49 **FUD** XXX [03] [Z2] [80] [▣]
AMA: 2016,Jun,5; 2016,Jan,13; 2015,Jan,16; 2014,Jan,11; 2012,Oct,12; 2012,Feb,9-10

74170 without contrast material, followed by contrast material(s) and further sections
🚑 7.38 📊 7.38 **FUD** XXX [03] [Z2] [80] [▣]
AMA: 2016,Jun,5; 2016,Jan,13; 2015,Jan,16; 2014,Jan,11; 2012,Oct,12; 2012,Feb,9-10

© 2016 Optum360, LLC

74174-74175 Computerized Tomographic Angiography: Abdomen and Pelvis

CMS: 100-04,4,250.16 Multiple Procedure Payment Reduction: Certain Diagnostic Imaging Procedures Rendered by Physicians

> EXCLUDES CT angiography for aorto-iliofemoral runoff (75635)
> CT angiography, lower extremity (73706)
> CT angiography, pelvis (72191)

74174 Computed tomographic angiography, abdomen and pelvis, with contrast material(s), including noncontrast images, if performed, and image postprocessing

> EXCLUDES 3D rendering (76376-76377)
> Computed tomographic angiography abdomen (74175)

🔧 10.9　⚕ 10.9　**FUD** XXX　[S][Z2][80][📺]

AMA: 2014,Jan,11; 2012,Feb,9-10

74175 Computed tomographic angiography, abdomen, with contrast material(s), including noncontrast images, if performed, and image postprocessing

🔧 8.63　⚕ 8.63　**FUD** XXX　[Q3][Z2][80][📺]

AMA: 2016,Jan,13; 2015,Jan,16; 2014,Jan,11; 2012,Feb,9-10; 2012,Jan,15-42; 2011,Apr,12

74176-74178 Computerized Tomography: Abdomen and Pelvis

CMS: 100-04,4,250.16 Multiple Procedure Payment Reduction: Certain Diagnostic Imaging Procedures Rendered by Physicians

> EXCLUDES Computed tomography of abdomen or pelvis alone (72192-72194, 74150-74170)
> Procedure performed more than one time for each combined examination of the abdomen and pelvis

74176 Computed tomography, abdomen and pelvis; without contrast material

🔧 5.64　⚕ 5.64　**FUD** XXX　[Q3][Z2][📺]

AMA: 2016,Jan,13; 2015,Jan,16; 2014,Jan,11; 2012,Feb,9-10

74177 with contrast material(s)

🔧 8.75　⚕ 8.75　**FUD** XXX　[Q3][Z2][📺]

AMA: 2016,Jan,13; 2015,Jan,16; 2014,Jan,11; 2012,Feb,9-10

74178 without contrast material in one or both body regions, followed by contrast material(s) and further sections in one or both body regions

🔧 9.93　⚕ 9.93　**FUD** XXX　[Q3][Z2][📺]

AMA: 2016,Jan,13; 2015,Jan,16; 2014,Jan,11; 2012,Feb,9-10

74181-74183 Magnetic Resonance Imaging: Abdomen–General

CMS: 100-04,4,250.16 Multiple Procedure Payment Reduction: Certain Diagnostic Imaging Procedures Rendered by Physicians

74181 Magnetic resonance (eg, proton) imaging, abdomen; without contrast material(s)

🔧 9.37　⚕ 9.37　**FUD** XXX　[Q3][Z2][80][📺]

AMA: 2016,Jan,13; 2015,Jan,16; 2014,Jan,11; 2012,Feb,9-10; 2012,Jan,15-42; 2011,Jan,11

74182 with contrast material(s)

🔧 12.7　⚕ 12.7　**FUD** XXX　[Q3][Z2][80][📺]

AMA: 2016,Jan,13; 2015,Jan,16; 2014,Jan,11; 2012,Feb,9-10; 2012,Jan,15-42; 2011,Jan,11

74183 without contrast material(s), followed by with contrast material(s) and further sequences

🔧 14.2　⚕ 14.2　**FUD** XXX　[Q3][Z2][80][📺]

AMA: 2016,Jan,13; 2015,Jan,16; 2014,Jan,11; 2012,Feb,9-10

74185 Magnetic Resonance Angiography: Abdomen–General

CMS: 100-04,13,40.1.1 Magnetic Resonance Angiography; 100-04,13,40.1.2 HCPCS Coding Requirements; 100-04,4,250.16 Multiple Procedure Payment Reduction: Certain Diagnostic Imaging Procedures Rendered by Physicians

74185 Magnetic resonance angiography, abdomen, with or without contrast material(s)

🔧 11.3　⚕ 11.3　**FUD** XXX　[B][80][📺]

AMA: 2016,Jan,13; 2015,Jan,16; 2014,Jan,11; 2012,Feb,9-10

74190 Peritoneography

74190 Peritoneogram (eg, after injection of air or contrast), radiological supervision and interpretation

> EXCLUDES Computed tomography, pelvis or abdomen (72192, 74150)

Code also injection procedure (49400)

🔧 0.00　⚕ 0.00　**FUD** XXX　[Q2][N1][80][📺]

AMA: 2016,Jan,13; 2015,Jan,16; 2014,Jan,11; 2012,Feb,9-10; 2012,Jan,15-42; 2011,Jan,11

74210-74235 Radiography: Throat and Esophagus

> EXCLUDES Percutaneous placement of gastrostomy tube, endoscopic (43246)
> Percutaneous placement of gastrostomy tube, fluoroscopic guidance (49440)

74210 Radiologic examination; pharynx and/or cervical esophagus

🔧 2.18　⚕ 2.18　**FUD** XXX　[Q1][N1][80][📺]

AMA: 2014,Jan,11; 2012,Feb,9-10

74220 esophagus

🔧 2.49　⚕ 2.49　**FUD** XXX　[Q1][N1][80][📺]

AMA: 2014,Jan,11; 2012,Feb,9-10

74230 Swallowing function, with cineradiography/videoradiography

🔧 3.60　⚕ 3.60　**FUD** XXX　[Q1][N1][80][📺]

AMA: 2016,Jan,13; 2015,Jan,16; 2014,Jul,5; 2014,Jan,11; 2012,Feb,9-10

74235 Removal of foreign body(s), esophageal, with use of balloon catheter, radiological supervision and interpretation

Code also procedure (43499)

🔧 0.00　⚕ 0.00　**FUD** XXX　[N][N1][80][📺]

AMA: 2014,Jan,11; 2012,Feb,9-10

74240-74283 Radiography: Intestines

> EXCLUDES Percutaneous placement of gastrostomy tube, endoscopic (43246)
> Percutaneous placement of gastrostomy tube, fluoroscopic guidance (49440)

74240 Radiologic examination, gastrointestinal tract, upper; with or without delayed images, without KUB

🔧 3.18　⚕ 3.18　**FUD** XXX　[Q1][Z2][80][📺]

AMA: 2016,Sep,7; 2014,Jan,11; 2012,Feb,9-10

74241 with or without delayed images, with KUB

🔧 3.31　⚕ 3.31　**FUD** XXX　[Q1][Z2][80][📺]

AMA: 2016,Sep,7; 2014,Jan,11; 2012,Feb,9-10

74245 with small intestine, includes multiple serial images

🔧 4.82　⚕ 4.82　**FUD** XXX　[S][Z2][80][📺]

AMA: 2016,Sep,7; 2014,Jan,11; 2012,Feb,9-10

74246 Radiological examination, gastrointestinal tract, upper, air contrast, with specific high density barium, effervescent agent, with or without glucagon; with or without delayed images, without KUB

> INCLUDES Moynihan test

🔧 3.58　⚕ 3.58　**FUD** XXX　[Q1][Z2][80][📺]

AMA: 2016,Sep,7; 2014,Jan,11; 2012,Feb,9-10

74247 with or without delayed images, with KUB

🔧 3.96　⚕ 3.96　**FUD** XXX　[Q1][Z2][80][📺]

AMA: 2016,Sep,7; 2014,Jan,11; 2012,Feb,9-10

74249 with small intestine follow-through

🔧 5.17　⚕ 5.17　**FUD** XXX　[S][Z2][80][📺]

AMA: 2014,Jan,11; 2012,Feb,9-10

74250 Radiologic examination, small intestine, includes multiple serial images;

🔧 2.92　⚕ 2.92　**FUD** XXX　[Q1][Z2][80][📺]

AMA: 2016,Sep,7; 2014,Jan,11; 2012,Feb,9-10

74251 via enteroclysis tube

🔧 11.7　⚕ 11.7　**FUD** XXX　[S][Z2][80][📺]

AMA: 2016,Sep,7; 2014,Jan,11; 2012,Feb,9-10

74260 Duodenography, hypotonic

🔧 9.92　⚕ 9.92　**FUD** XXX　[Q1][N1][80][📺]

AMA: 2014,Jan,11; 2012,Feb,9-10

● New Code　▲ Revised Code　○ Reinstated　● New Web Release　▲ Revised Web Release　Unlisted　Not Covered　# Resequenced
⊘ AMA Mod 51 Exempt　⑤ Optum Mod 51 Exempt　⑥ Mod 63 Exempt　⊁ Non-FDA Drug　★ Telehealth　Ⓜ Maternity　Ⓐ Age Edit　+ Add-on　**AMA:** CPT Asst

Radiology

74261 Computed tomographic (CT) colonography, diagnostic, including image postprocessing; without contrast material

EXCLUDES 3D rendering (76376-76377)
Computed tomography of abdomen or pelvis alone (72192-72194, 74150-74170)
Screening computed tomographic (CT) colonography (74263)

🚑 13.6   ⚕ 13.6   **FUD** XXX   03 Z2 80 ▯

AMA: 2016,Jan,13; 2015,Jan,16; 2014,Jan,11; 2012,Feb,9-10

74262 with contrast material(s) including non-contrast images, if performed

EXCLUDES 3D rendering (76376-76377)
Computed tomography of abdomen or pelvis alone (72192-72194, 74150-74170)
Screening computed tomographic (CT) colonography (74263)

🚑 15.1   ⚕ 15.1   **FUD** XXX   03 Z2 80 ▯

AMA: 2016,Jan,13; 2015,Jan,16; 2014,Jan,11; 2012,Feb,9-10

74263 Computed tomographic (CT) colonography, screening, including image postprocessing

EXCLUDES 3D rendering (76376-76377)
Computed tomography of abdomen or pelvis alone (72192-72194, 74150-74170)
Computed tomographic (CT) colonography (74261)

🚑 21.2   ⚕ 21.2   **FUD** XXX   E ▯

AMA: 2016,Jan,13; 2015,Jan,16; 2014,Jan,11; 2012,Feb,9-10

74270 Radiologic examination, colon; contrast (eg, barium) enema, with or without KUB

🚑 4.23   ⚕ 4.23   **FUD** XXX   01 N1 80 ▯

AMA: 2016,Jan,13; 2015,Jan,16; 2014,Jan,11; 2012,Feb,9-10; 2012,Jan,15-42; 2011,Jan,11

74280 air contrast with specific high density barium, with or without glucagon

🚑 5.98   ⚕ 5.98   **FUD** XXX   S Z2 80 ▯

AMA: 2014,Jan,11; 2012,Feb,9-10

74283 Therapeutic enema, contrast or air, for reduction of intussusception or other intraluminal obstruction (eg, meconium ileus)

🚑 5.78   ⚕ 5.78   **FUD** XXX   S Z2 80 ▯

AMA: 2014,Jan,11; 2012,Feb,9-10

74290-74330 Radiography: Biliary Tract

74290 Cholecystography, oral contrast

🚑 1.97   ⚕ 1.97   **FUD** XXX   01 N1 80 ▯

AMA: 2014,Jan,11; 2012,Feb,9-10

74300 Cholangiography and/or pancreatography; intraoperative, radiological supervision and interpretation

🚑 0.00   ⚕ 0.00   **FUD** XXX   N N1 80 ▯

AMA: 2016,Jan,13; 2015,Dec,3; 2015,Jan,16; 2014,Jan,11; 2012,Feb,9-10; 2012,Jan,15-42; 2011,Jan,11

+ **74301** additional set intraoperative, radiological supervision and interpretation (List separately in addition to code for primary procedure)

Code first (74300)

🚑 0.00   ⚕ 0.00   **FUD** ZZZ   N N1 80 ▯

AMA: 2015,Dec,3; 2014,Jan,11; 2012,Feb,9-10

74328 Endoscopic catheterization of the biliary ductal system, radiological supervision and interpretation

Code also ERCP (43260-43270 [43274, 43275, 43276, 43277, 43278])

🚑 0.00   ⚕ 0.00   **FUD** XXX   N N1 80 ▯

AMA: 2016,Jan,13; 2015,Jan,16; 2014,Jan,11; 2012,Feb,9-10; 2012,Jan,15-42; 2011,Jan,11

74329 Endoscopic catheterization of the pancreatic ductal system, radiological supervision and interpretation

Code also ERCP (43260-43270 [43274, 43275, 43276, 43277, 43278])

🚑 0.00   ⚕ 0.00   **FUD** XXX   N N1 80 ▯

AMA: 2014,Jan,11; 2012,Feb,9-10

74330 Combined endoscopic catheterization of the biliary and pancreatic ductal systems, radiological supervision and interpretation

Code also ERCP (43260-43270 [43274, 43275, 43276, 43277, 43278])

🚑 0.00   ⚕ 0.00   **FUD** XXX   N N1 80 ▯

AMA: 2014,Jan,11; 2012,Feb,9-10

74340-74363 Radiography: Bilidigestive Intubation

EXCLUDES Percutaneous insertion of gastrostomy tube, endoscopic (43246)
Percutaneous placement of gastrostomy tube, fluoroscopic guidance (49440)

74340 Introduction of long gastrointestinal tube (eg, Miller-Abbott), including multiple fluoroscopies and images, radiological supervision and interpretation

Code also placement of tube (44500)

🚑 0.00   ⚕ 0.00   **FUD** XXX   N N1 80 ▯

AMA: 2016,Sep,9; 2014,Jan,11; 2012,Feb,9-10

74355 Percutaneous placement of enteroclysis tube, radiological supervision and interpretation

INCLUDES Fluoroscopic guidance (77002)

🚑 0.00   ⚕ 0.00   **FUD** XXX   N N1 80 ▯

AMA: 2016,Jan,13; 2015,Jan,16; 2014,Jan,11; 2012,Feb,9-10; 2011,Jan,8

74360 Intraluminal dilation of strictures and/or obstructions (eg, esophagus), radiological supervision and interpretation

EXCLUDES Esophagoscopy, flexible, transoral; with dilation of esophagus (43213-43214)
Esophagogastroduodenoscopy, flexible, transoral; with dilation of esophagus (43233)

🚑 0.00   ⚕ 0.00   **FUD** XXX   N N1 80 ▯

AMA: 2016,Jan,13; 2015,Jan,16; 2014,Jan,11; 2012,Feb,9-10

74363 Percutaneous transhepatic dilation of biliary duct stricture with or without placement of stent, radiological supervision and interpretation

EXCLUDES Surgical procedure (47555-47556)

🚑 0.00   ⚕ 0.00   **FUD** XXX   N N1 80 ▯

AMA: 2014,Jan,11; 2012,Feb,9-10

74400-74775 Radiography: Urogenital

74400 Urography (pyelography), intravenous, with or without KUB, with or without tomography

🚑 3.09   ⚕ 3.09   **FUD** XXX   S Z2 80 ▯

AMA: 2014,Jan,11; 2012,Feb,9-10

74410 Urography, infusion, drip technique and/or bolus technique;

🚑 3.04   ⚕ 3.04   **FUD** XXX   S Z2 80 ▯

AMA: 2014,Jan,11; 2012,Feb,9-10

74415 with nephrotomography

🚑 3.84   ⚕ 3.84   **FUD** XXX   S Z2 80 ▯

AMA: 2014,Jan,11; 2012,Feb,9-10

74420 Urography, retrograde, with or without KUB

🚑 0.00   ⚕ 0.00   **FUD** XXX   S Z2 80 ▯

AMA: 2016,Jan,13; 2015,Jan,16; 2014,Jan,11; 2012,Feb,9-10; 2012,Jan,15-42; 2011,Jan,11

74425 Urography, antegrade (pyelostogram, nephrostogram, loopogram), radiological supervision and interpretation

EXCLUDES Injection for antegrade nephrostogram and/or ureterogram ([50430, 50431, 50432, 50433, 50434, 50435])
Ureteral stent placement (50693-50695)

🚑 0.00   ⚕ 0.00   **FUD** XXX   02 N1 80 ▯

AMA: 2016,Jan,3; 2016,Jan,13; 2015,Oct,5; 2015,Jan,16; 2014,Jan,11; 2012,Feb,9-10

74430 Cystography, minimum of 3 views, radiological supervision and interpretation

🚑 1.06   ⚕ 1.06   **FUD** XXX   02 N1 80 ▯

AMA: 2014,Jan,11; 2012,Feb,9-10

74440 Vasography, vesiculography, or epididymography, radiological supervision and interpretation ♂
🚑 2.28 ⚕ 2.28 **FUD** XXX Q2 N1 80 ▭
AMA: 2014,Jan,11; 2012,Feb,9-10

74445 Corpora cavernosography, radiological supervision and interpretation ♂
INCLUDES Needle placement with fluoroscopic guidance (77002)
🚑 0.00 ⚕ 0.00 **FUD** XXX Q2 N1 80 ▭
AMA: 2016,Jan,13; 2015,Jan,16; 2014,Jan,11; 2012,Feb,9-10; 2011,Jan,8

74450 Urethrocystography, retrograde, radiological supervision and interpretation
🚑 0.00 ⚕ 0.00 **FUD** XXX Q2 N1 80 ▭
AMA: 2014,Jan,11; 2012,Feb,9-10

74455 Urethrocystography, voiding, radiological supervision and interpretation
🚑 2.29 ⚕ 2.29 **FUD** XXX Q2 N1 80 ▭
AMA: 2014,Jan,11; 2012,Feb,9-10

74470 Radiologic examination, renal cyst study, translumbar, contrast visualization, radiological supervision and interpretation
INCLUDES Needle placement with fluoroscopic guidance (77002)
🚑 0.00 ⚕ 0.00 **FUD** XXX Q2 N1 80 ▭
AMA: 2016,Jan,13; 2015,Jan,16; 2014,Jan,11; 2012,Feb,9-10; 2011,Jan,8

74485 Dilation of nephrostomy, ureters, or urethra, radiological supervision and interpretation
EXCLUDES Change of pyelostomy/nephrostomy tube ([50435])
Ureter dilation without radiologic guidance (52341, 52344)
🚑 2.59 ⚕ 2.59 **FUD** XXX Q2 N1 80 ▭
AMA: 2016,Jan,3; 2016,Jan,13; 2015,Oct,5; 2015,Jan,16; 2014,Jan,11; 2012,Feb,9-10; 2012,Jan,15-42; 2011,Jan,11

74710 Pelvimetry, with or without placental localization ♀
EXCLUDES Imaging procedures on abdomen and pelvis (72170-72190, 74000-74170)
🚑 1.03 ⚕ 1.03 **FUD** XXX Q1 N1 80 ▭
AMA: 2014,Jan,11; 2012,Feb,9-10

74712 Magnetic resonance (eg, proton) imaging, fetal, including placental and maternal pelvic imaging when performed; single or first gestation ♀
EXCLUDES Imaging of maternal pelvis or placenta without fetal imaging (72195-72197)
🚑 13.5 ⚕ 13.5 **FUD** XXX S Z2 80 ▭
AMA: 2016,Jun,5

+ **74713** each additional gestation (List separately in addition to code for primary procedure) ♀
EXCLUDES Imaging of maternal pelvis or placenta without fetal imaging (72195-72197)
Code first (74712)
🚑 6.52 ⚕ 6.52 **FUD** ZZZ N 80 ▭
AMA: 2016,Jun,5

74740 Hysterosalpingography, radiological supervision and interpretation ♀
EXCLUDES Imaging procedures on abdomen and pelvis (72170-72190, 74000-74170)
Code also injection of saline/contrast (58340)
🚑 2.10 ⚕ 2.10 **FUD** XXX Q2 N1 80 ▭
AMA: 2016,Jan,13; 2015,Jan,16; 2014,Jan,11; 2012,Feb,9-10; 2012,Jan,15-42; 2011,Jan,11

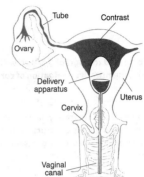

Hysterosalpingography (imaging of the uterus and tubes) is performed. Report for radiological supervision and interpretation

74742 Transcervical catheterization of fallopian tube, radiological supervision and interpretation ♀
EXCLUDES Imaging procedures on abdomen and pelvis (72170-72190, 74000-74170)
Code also (58345)
🚑 0.00 ⚕ 0.00 **FUD** XXX N N1 80 ▭
AMA: 2016,Jan,13; 2015,Jan,16; 2014,Jan,11; 2012,Feb,9-10

74775 Perineogram (eg, vaginogram, for sex determination or extent of anomalies) M ♀
EXCLUDES Imaging procedures on abdomen and pelvis (72170-72190, 74000-74170)
🚑 0.00 ⚕ 0.00 **FUD** XXX S Z2 80 ▭
AMA: 2014,Jan,11; 2012,Feb,9-10

75557-75565 Magnetic Resonance Imaging: Heart Structure and Physiology

INCLUDES Physiologic evaluation of cardiac function
EXCLUDES 3D rendering (76376-76377)
Cardiac catheterization procedures (93451-93572)
Use of more than one code in this group per session
Code also separate vascular injection (36000-36299)

75557 Cardiac magnetic resonance imaging for morphology and function without contrast material;
🚑 8.95 ⚕ 8.95 **FUD** XXX Q3 Z2 80 ▭
AMA: 2016,Jan,13; 2015,Jan,16; 2014,Jan,11; 2012,Feb,9-10

75559 with stress imaging
INCLUDES Pharmacologic wall motion stress evaluation without contrast
Code also stress testing when performed (93015-93018)
🚑 12.2 ⚕ 12.2 **FUD** XXX Q3 Z2 80 ▭
AMA: 2016,Jan,13; 2015,Jan,16; 2014,Jan,11; 2012,Feb,9-10

75561 Cardiac magnetic resonance imaging for morphology and function without contrast material(s), followed by contrast material(s) and further sequences;
🚑 11.9 ⚕ 11.9 **FUD** XXX Q3 Z2 80 ▭
AMA: 2016,Jan,13; 2015,Jan,16; 2014,Jan,11; 2012,Feb,9-10

75563 with stress imaging
INCLUDES Pharmacologic perfusion stress evaluation with contrast
Code also stress testing when performed (93015-93018)
🚑 14.1 ⚕ 14.1 **FUD** XXX Q3 Z3 80 ▭
AMA: 2016,Jan,13; 2015,Jan,16; 2014,Jan,11; 2012,Feb,9-10

+ **75565** Cardiac magnetic resonance imaging for velocity flow mapping (List separately in addition to code for primary procedure)

Code first (75557, 75559, 75561, 75563)
🚑 1.54 ⚖ 1.54 **FUD** ZZZ   Ⓝ N1 80 ▭
AMA: 2016,Jan,13; 2015,Jan,16; 2014,Jan,11; 2012,Feb,9-10

75571-75574 Computed Tomographic Imaging: Heart

CMS: 100-04,12,20.4.7 Services Not Meeting National Electrical Manufacturers Association (NEMA) Standard; 100-04,4,20.6.12 Use of HCPCS Modifier – CT; 100-04,4,250.16 Multiple Procedure Payment Reduction: Certain Diagnostic Imaging Procedures Rendered by Physicians

EXCLUDES   3D rendering (76376-76377)
Use of more than one code in this group per session

75571 Computed tomography, heart, without contrast material, with quantitative evaluation of coronary calcium
🚑 2.82 ⚖ 2.82 **FUD** XXX   Q1 N1 80 ▭
AMA: 2016,Jan,13; 2015,Jan,16; 2014,Jan,11; 2012,Feb,9-10

75572 Computed tomography, heart, with contrast material, for evaluation of cardiac structure and morphology (including 3D image postprocessing, assessment of cardiac function, and evaluation of venous structures, if performed)
🚑 7.99 ⚖ 7.99 **FUD** XXX   Ⓢ Z2 80 ▭
AMA: 2016,Jan,13; 2015,Jan,16; 2014,Jan,11; 2012,Feb,9-10

75573 Computed tomography, heart, with contrast material, for evaluation of cardiac structure and morphology in the setting of congenital heart disease (including 3D image postprocessing, assessment of LV cardiac function, RV structure and function and evaluation of venous structures, if performed)
🚑 11.0 ⚖ 11.0 **FUD** XXX   Ⓢ Z2 80 ▭
AMA: 2016,Jan,13; 2015,Jan,16; 2014,Jan,11; 2012,Feb,9-10

75574 Computed tomographic angiography, heart, coronary arteries and bypass grafts (when present), with contrast material, including 3D image postprocessing (including evaluation of cardiac structure and morphology, assessment of cardiac function, and evaluation of venous structures, if performed)
🚑 11.7 ⚖ 11.7 **FUD** XXX   Ⓢ Z2 80 ▭
AMA: 2016,Jan,13; 2015,Jan,16; 2014,Jan,11; 2012,Feb,9-10

75600-75791 Radiography: Arterial

INCLUDES   Diagnostic angiography specifically included in the interventional code description
The following diagnostic procedures with interventional supervision and interpretation:
Angiography
Contrast injection
Fluoroscopic guidance for intervention
Post-angioplasty/atherectomy/stent angiography
Roadmapping
Vessel measurement

EXCLUDES   Catheterization codes for diagnostic angiography of lower extremity when an access site other than the site used for the therapy is required
Diagnostic angiogram during a separate encounter from the interventional procedure
Diagnostic angiography with interventional procedure if:
1. No previous catheter-based angiogram is accessible and a complete diagnostic procedure is performed and the decision to proceed with an interventional procedure is based on the diagnostic service, OR
2. The previous diagnostic angiogram is accessible but the documentation in the medical record specifies that:
A. the patient's condition has changed
B. there is insufficient imaging of the patient's anatomy and/or disease, OR
C. there is a clinical change during the procedure that necessitates a new examination away from the site of the intervention
3. Modifier 59 is appended to the code(s) for the diagnostic radiological supervision and interpretation service to indicate the guidelines were met
Intra-arterial procedures (36100-36248)
Intravenous procedures (36000, 36005-36015)

75600 Aortography, thoracic, without serialography, radiological supervision and interpretation
EXCLUDES   Supravalvular aortography (93567)
🚑 5.57 ⚖ 5.57 **FUD** XXX   02 N1 80 ▭
AMA: 2014,Jan,11; 2012,Feb,9-10

75605 Aortography, thoracic, by serialography, radiological supervision and interpretation
EXCLUDES   Supravalvular aortography (93567)
🚑 3.92 ⚖ 3.92 **FUD** XXX   02 N1 80 ▭
AMA: 2016,Jan,13; 2015,Jan,16; 2014,Jan,11; 2013,Jan,6-8; 2012,Feb,9-10; 2012,Jan,15-42; 2011,Jan,11

75625 Aortography, abdominal, by serialography, radiological supervision and interpretation
EXCLUDES   Supravalvular aortography (93567)
🚑 3.91 ⚖ 3.91 **FUD** XXX   02 N1 80 ▭
AMA: 2016,Jan,13; 2015,Jan,16; 2014,Jan,11; 2013,Feb,16-17; 2013,Jan,6-8; 2012,Feb,9-10; 2012,Jan,15-42; 2011,Jul,3-11; 2011,Jan,11

75630 Aortography, abdominal plus bilateral iliofemoral lower extremity, catheter, by serialography, radiological supervision and interpretation
EXCLUDES   Supravalvular aortography (93567)
🚑 4.83 ⚖ 4.83 **FUD** XXX   02 N1 80 ▭
AMA: 2016,Jan,13; 2015,Jan,16; 2014,Jan,11; 2012,Feb,9-10; 2012,Jan,15-42; 2011,Jul,3-11; 2011,Jan,11

75635 Computed tomographic angiography, abdominal aorta and bilateral iliofemoral lower extremity runoff, with contrast material(s), including noncontrast images, if performed, and image postprocessing
EXCLUDES   3D rendering (76376-76377)
Computed tomographic angiography, abdomen, lower extremity, pelvis (72191, 73706, 74174-74175)
🚑 10.7 ⚖ 10.7 **FUD** XXX   02 N1 80 ▭
AMA: 2016,Jan,13; 2015,Jan,16; 2014,Jan,11; 2012,Feb,9-10; 2012,Jan,15-42; 2011,Apr,12

75658 Angiography, brachial, retrograde, radiological supervision and interpretation
🚑 4.73 ⚖ 4.73 **FUD** XXX   02 N1 80 ▭
AMA: 2014,Jan,11; 2012,Feb,9-10

75705 Angiography, spinal, selective, radiological supervision and interpretation
🚑 6.90 ⚖ 6.90 **FUD** XXX   02 N1 80 ▭
AMA: 2014,Jan,11; 2012,Feb,9-10

Angiography of a specific area of the spine is performed

75710 Angiography, extremity, unilateral, radiological supervision and interpretation
🚑 4.63 ⚖ 4.63 **FUD** XXX   02 N1 80 ▭
AMA: 2016,Jan,13; 2015,Jan,16; 2014,Jan,11; 2012,Feb,9-10; 2012,Jan,15-42; 2011,Jan,11

75716 Angiography, extremity, bilateral, radiological supervision and interpretation
🚑 5.31 ⚖ 5.31 **FUD** XXX   02 N1 80 ▭
AMA: 2016,Jan,13; 2015,Jan,16; 2014,Jan,11; 2012,Feb,9-10; 2012,Jan,15-42; 2011,Jan,11

| 26/TC PC/TC Only | A2-Z3 ASC Payment | 50 Bilateral | ♂ Male Only | ♀ Female Only | 🚑 Facility RVU | ⚖ Non-Facility RVU | ▭ CCI |
| FUD Follow-up Days | CMS: IOM (Pub 100) | A-Y OPPSI | 80/80 Surg Assist Allowed / w/Doc | | 🔲 Lab Crosswalk | 🔳 Radiology Crosswalk | ☒ CLIA |

316   CPT © 2016 American Medical Association. All Rights Reserved.   © 2016 Optum360, LLC

75726 Angiography, visceral, selective or supraselective (with or without flush aortogram), radiological supervision and interpretation

> *EXCLUDES* *Selective angiography, each additional visceral vessel examined after basic examination (75774)*
>
> 4.23   4.23   **FUD** XXX   02 N1 80
>
> **AMA:** 2014,Jan,11; 2012,Feb,9-10

75731 Angiography, adrenal, unilateral, selective, radiological supervision and interpretation

> 4.87   4.87   **FUD** XXX   02 N1 80
>
> **AMA:** 2014,Jan,11; 2012,Feb,9-10

75733 Angiography, adrenal, bilateral, selective, radiological supervision and interpretation

> 5.20   5.20   **FUD** XXX   02 N1 80
>
> **AMA:** 2014,Jan,11; 2012,Feb,9-10

75736 Angiography, pelvic, selective or supraselective, radiological supervision and interpretation

> 4.55   4.55   **FUD** XXX   02 N1 80
>
> **AMA:** 2014,Jan,11; 2012,Feb,9-10

75741 Angiography, pulmonary, unilateral, selective, radiological supervision and interpretation

> 4.28   4.28   **FUD** XXX   02 N1 80
>
> **AMA:** 2016,Jan,13; 2015,Jan,16; 2014,Jan,11; 2013,Jan,6-8; 2012,Feb,9-10; 2012,Mar,9-10

75743 Angiography, pulmonary, bilateral, selective, radiological supervision and interpretation

> 4.80   4.80   **FUD** XXX   02 N1 80
>
> **AMA:** 2016,Jan,13; 2015,Jan,16; 2014,Jan,11; 2013,Jan,6-8; 2012,Feb,9-10

75746 Angiography, pulmonary, by nonselective catheter or venous injection, radiological supervision and interpretation

> *EXCLUDES* *Nonselective injection procedure or catheter introduction with cardiac cath (93568)*
>
> 4.30   4.30   **FUD** XXX   02 N1 80
>
> **AMA:** 2014,Jan,11; 2012,Feb,9-10

75756 Angiography, internal mammary, radiological supervision and interpretation

> *EXCLUDES* *Internal mammary angiography with cardiac cath (93455, 93457, 93459, 93461, 93564)*
>
> 4.73   4.73   **FUD** XXX   02 N1 80
>
> **AMA:** 2016,Jan,13; 2015,Jan,16; 2014,Jan,11; 2012,Feb,9-10; 2011,Dec,9-12

+ 75774 Angiography, selective, each additional vessel studied after basic examination, radiological supervision and interpretation (List separately in addition to code for primary procedure)

> *EXCLUDES* *Angiography (75600-75756)*
> *Cardiac cath procedures (93452-93462, 93531-93533, 93563-93568)*
> *Catheterizations (36215-36248)*
> *Dialysis circuit angiography (current access), use modifier 52 with (36901)*
> *Nonselective catheter placement, thoracic aorta (36221-36228)*
>
> Code first initial vessel
> Code first diagnostic angiography of upper extremities and other vascular beds (except cervicocerebral vessels)
>
> 2.48   2.48   **FUD** ZZZ   N N1 80
>
> **AMA:** 2016,Jan,13; 2015,Jan,16; 2014,Jan,11; 2013,Oct,18; 2013,Jun,12; 2013,May,3-5; 2013,Feb,16-17; 2012,Feb,9-10; 2012,Jan,15-42; 2011,Apr,12; 2011,Jan,11

75791 ~~Angiography, arteriovenous shunt (eg, dialysis patient fistula/graft), complete evaluation of dialysis access, including fluoroscopy, image documentation and report (includes injections of contrast and all necessary imaging from the arterial anastomosis and adjacent artery through entire venous outflow including the inferior or superior vena cava), radiological supervision and interpretation~~

> To report, see ~36901-36906

75801-75893 Radiography: Lymphatic and Venous

> *INCLUDES* Diagnostic venography specifically included in the interventional code description
> The following diagnostic procedures with interventional supervision and interpretation:
> Contrast injection
> Fluoroscopic guidance for intervention
> Post-angioplasty/venography
> Roadmapping
> Venography
> Vessel measurement
>
> *EXCLUDES* Diagnostic venogram during a separate encounter from the interventional procedure
> Diagnostic venography with interventional procedure if:
> 1. No previous catheter-based venogram is accessible and a complete diagnostic procedure is performed and the decision to proceed with an interventional procedure is based on the diagnostic service, OR
> 2. The previous diagnostic venogram is accessible but the documentation in the medical record specifies that:
>   A. The patient's condition has changed
>   B. There is insufficient imaging of the patient's anatomy and/or disease, OR
>   C. There is a clinical change during the procedure that necessitates a new examination away from the site of the intervention
> Intravenous procedures (36000-36015, 36400-36510)
> Lymphatic injection procedures (38790)

75801 Lymphangiography, extremity only, unilateral, radiological supervision and interpretation

> 0.00   0.00   **FUD** XXX   02 N1 80
>
> **AMA:** 2014,Jan,11; 2012,Feb,9-10

75803 Lymphangiography, extremity only, bilateral, radiological supervision and interpretation

> 0.00   0.00   **FUD** XXX   02 N1 80
>
> **AMA:** 2014,Jan,11; 2012,Feb,9-10

75805 Lymphangiography, pelvic/abdominal, unilateral, radiological supervision and interpretation

> 0.00   0.00   **FUD** XXX   02 N1 80
>
> **AMA:** 2014,Jan,11; 2012,Feb,9-10

75807 Lymphangiography, pelvic/abdominal, bilateral, radiological supervision and interpretation

> 0.00   0.00   **FUD** XXX   02 N1 80
>
> **AMA:** 2014,Jan,11; 2012,Feb,9-10

75809 Shuntogram for investigation of previously placed indwelling nonvascular shunt (eg, LeVeen shunt, ventriculoperitoneal shunt, indwelling infusion pump), radiological supervision and interpretation

> *INCLUDES* Needle placement with fluoroscopic guidance (77002)
> Code also surgical procedure (49427, 61070)
>
> 2.80   2.80   **FUD** XXX   02 N1 80
>
> **AMA:** 2016,Jan,13; 2015,Jan,16; 2014,Jan,11; 2012,Feb,9-10; 2012,Jan,15-42; 2011,Jan,11; 2011,Jan,8

75810 Splenoportography, radiological supervision and interpretation

> *INCLUDES* Needle placement with fluoroscopic guidance (77002)
>
> 0.00   0.00   **FUD** XXX   02 N1 80
>
> **AMA:** 2016,Jan,13; 2015,Jan,16; 2014,Jan,11; 2012,Feb,9-10; 2011,Jan,8

75820 Venography, extremity, unilateral, radiological supervision and interpretation

> 3.26   3.26   **FUD** XXX   02 N1 80
>
> **AMA:** 2016,May,5; 2016,Jan,13; 2015,May,3; 2015,Jan,16; 2014,Jan,11; 2012,Feb,9-10; 2012,Jan,15-42; 2011,Jan,11

75822 Venography, extremity, bilateral, radiological supervision and interpretation

> 3.89   3.89   **FUD** XXX   02 N1 80
>
> **AMA:** 2014,Jan,11; 2012,Feb,9-10

75825 Venography, caval, inferior, with serialography, radiological supervision and interpretation

> 3.86   3.86   **FUD** XXX   02 N1 80
>
> **AMA:** 2016,Jan,13; 2015,Jan,16; 2014,Jan,11; 2012,Feb,9-10; 2012,Jan,15-42; 2011,Jan,11

Radiology (sidebar, vertical)

75827 — 75901 (sidebar, vertical)

75827 Venography, caval, superior, with serialography, radiological supervision and interpretation
　3.93　3.93　**FUD** XXX　02 N1 80
AMA: 2016,Jan,13; 2015,Jan,16; 2014,Jan,11; 2012,Feb,9-10

75831 Venography, renal, unilateral, selective, radiological supervision and interpretation
　3.99　3.99　**FUD** XXX　02 N1 80
AMA: 2014,Jan,11; 2012,Feb,9-10

75833 Venography, renal, bilateral, selective, radiological supervision and interpretation
　4.66　4.66　**FUD** XXX　02 N1 80
AMA: 2014,Jan,11; 2012,Feb,9-10

75840 Venography, adrenal, unilateral, selective, radiological supervision and interpretation
　4.20　4.20　**FUD** XXX　02 N1 80
AMA: 2014,Jan,11; 2012,Feb,9-10

75842 Venography, adrenal, bilateral, selective, radiological supervision and interpretation
　5.10　5.10　**FUD** XXX　02 N1 80
AMA: 2014,Jan,11; 2012,Feb,9-10

75860 Venography, venous sinus (eg, petrosal and inferior sagittal) or jugular, catheter, radiological supervision and interpretation
　4.05　4.05　**FUD** XXX　02 N1 80
AMA: 2014,Jan,11; 2012,Feb,9-10

75870 Venography, superior sagittal sinus, radiological supervision and interpretation
　4.18　4.18　**FUD** XXX　02 N1 80
AMA: 2014,Jan,11; 2012,Feb,9-10

75872 Venography, epidural, radiological supervision and interpretation
　3.97　3.97　**FUD** XXX　02 N1 80
AMA: 2014,Jan,11; 2012,Feb,9-10

75880 Venography, orbital, radiological supervision and interpretation
　4.03　4.03　**FUD** XXX　02 N1 80
AMA: 2014,Jan,11; 2012,Feb,9-10

75885 Percutaneous transhepatic portography with hemodynamic evaluation, radiological supervision and interpretation
INCLUDES　Needle placement with fluoroscopic guidance (77002)
　4.48　4.48　**FUD** XXX　02 N1 80
AMA: 2016,Jan,13; 2015,Jan,16; 2014,Jan,11; 2012,Feb,9-10; 2012,Jan,15-42; 2011,Jan,11; 2011,Jan,8

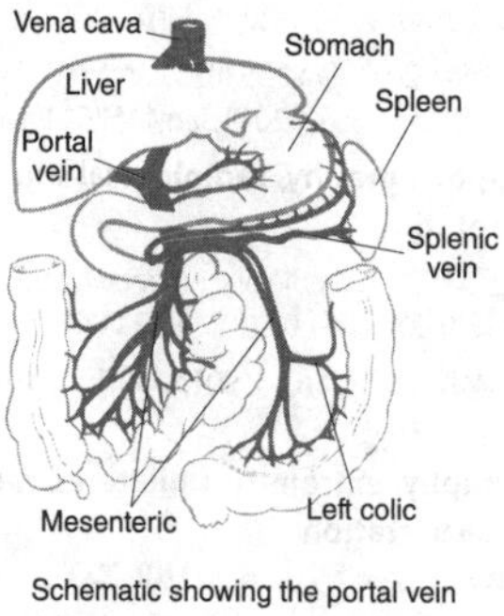

Schematic showing the portal vein

75887 Percutaneous transhepatic portography without hemodynamic evaluation, radiological supervision and interpretation
INCLUDES　Needle placement with fluoroscopic guidance (77002)
　4.51　4.51　**FUD** XXX　02 N1 80
AMA: 2016,Jan,13; 2015,Jan,16; 2014,Jan,11; 2012,Feb,9-10; 2012,Jan,15-42; 2011,Jan,11; 2011,Jan,8

75889 Hepatic venography, wedged or free, with hemodynamic evaluation, radiological supervision and interpretation
　4.08　4.08　**FUD** XXX　02 N1 80
AMA: 2014,Jan,11; 2012,Feb,9-10

75891 Hepatic venography, wedged or free, without hemodynamic evaluation, radiological supervision and interpretation
　4.11　4.11　**FUD** XXX　02 N1 80
AMA: 2014,Jan,11; 2012,Feb,9-10

75893 Venous sampling through catheter, with or without angiography (eg, for parathyroid hormone, renin), radiological supervision and interpretation
Code also surgical procedure (36500)
　3.35　3.35　**FUD** XXX　02 N1 80
AMA: 2014,Jan,11; 2012,Feb,9-10

75894-75902 Transcatheter Procedures

INCLUDES　The following diagnostic procedures with interventional supervision and interpretation:
Angiography/venography
Completion angiography/venography except for those services allowed by (75898)
Contrast injection
Fluoroscopic guidance for intervention
Roadmapping
Vessel measurement

EXCLUDES　Diagnostic angiography/venography performed at the same session as transcatheter therapy unless it is specifically included in the code descriptor or is excluded in the venography/angiography notes (75600-75893)

75894 Transcatheter therapy, embolization, any method, radiological supervision and interpretation
EXCLUDES　Endovenous ablation therapy of incompetent vein (36478-36479)
Transluminal balloon angioplasty (36475-36476)
Vascular embolization or occlusion (37241-37244)
　0.00　0.00　**FUD** XXX　N N1 80
AMA: 2016,Jan,13; 2015,Jan,16; 2014,Oct,6; 2014,Jan,11; 2013,Nov,6; 2013,Nov,14; 2012,Feb,9-10; 2012,Apr,3-9

75898 Angiography through existing catheter for follow-up study for transcatheter therapy, embolization or infusion, other than for thrombolysis
EXCLUDES　Noncoronary thrombolysis infusion ([37211, 37212, 37213, 37214], 61645)
Non-thrombolysis infusion other than coronary (61650-61651)
Percutaneous arterial transluminal mechanical thrombectomy (61645)
Prolonged endovascular intracranial administration of pharmacologic agent(s) (61650-61651)
Transcatheter therapy, arterial infusion for thrombolysis ([37211, 37212, 37213, 37214])
Vascular embolization or occlusion (37241-37244)
　0.00　0.00　**FUD** XXX　02 N1 80
AMA: 2016,Jan,13; 2015,Nov,3; 2015,Jan,16; 2014,Oct,6; 2014,Jan,11; 2013,Nov,6; 2013,Nov,14; 2012,Feb,9-10; 2012,Jan,15-42; 2011,Jan,11

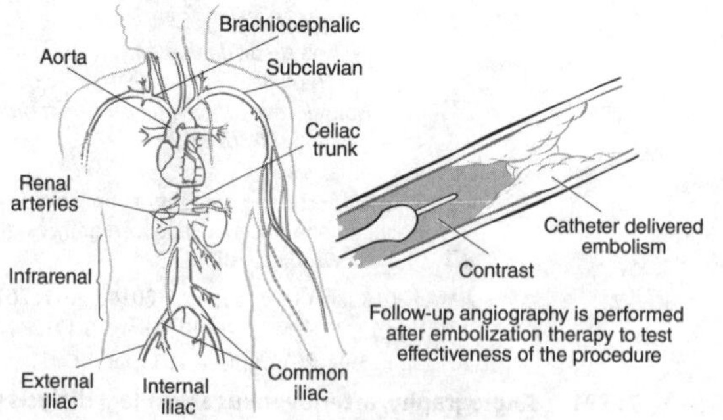

Follow-up angiography is performed after embolization therapy to test effectiveness of the procedure

75901 Mechanical removal of pericatheter obstructive material (eg, fibrin sheath) from central venous device via separate venous access, radiologic supervision and interpretation
EXCLUDES　Venous catheterization (36010-36012)
Code also surgical procedure (36595)
　5.00　5.00　**FUD** XXX　N N1 80
AMA: 2016,Jan,13; 2015,Jan,16; 2014,Jan,11; 2012,Feb,9-10

75902 Mechanical removal of intraluminal (intracatheter) obstructive material from central venous device through device lumen, radiologic supervision and interpretation

> EXCLUDES *Venous catheterization (36010-36012)*
> Code also surgical procedure (36596)
> 🔲 2.03 　 2.03 　 **FUD** XXX 　　 N N1 80 🖳
> **AMA:** 2016,Jan,13; 2015,Jan,16; 2014,Jan,11; 2012,Feb,9-10

75952-75959 Endovascular Aneurysm Repair

INCLUDES The following diagnostic procedures with interventional supervision and interpretation:
Angiography/venography
Completion angiography/venography except for those services allowed by (75898)
Contrast injection
Fluoroscopic guidance for intervention
Roadmapping
Vessel measurement

EXCLUDES *Diagnostic angiography/venography performed at the same session as transcatheter therapy unless it is specifically included in the code descriptor (75600-75893)*

75952 Endovascular repair of infrarenal abdominal aortic aneurysm or dissection, radiological supervision and interpretation

> EXCLUDES *Endovascular repair of visceral aorta with or without infrarenal abdominal aorta repair, radiologic supervision and interpretation (34841-34848)*
> *Implantation endovascular grafts (34800-34805)*
> 🔲 0.00 　 0.00 　 **FUD** XXX 　　 C 80 🖳
> **AMA:** 2016,Jan,13; 2015,Jan,16; 2014,Jan,11; 2013,Dec,8; 2012,Feb,9-10; 2012,Apr,3-9

75953 Placement of proximal or distal extension prosthesis for endovascular repair of infrarenal aortic or iliac artery aneurysm, pseudoaneurysm, or dissection, radiological supervision and interpretation

> EXCLUDES *Placement of endovascular extension prostheses (34825-34826)*
> 🔲 0.00 　 0.00 　 **FUD** XXX 　　 C 80 🖳
> **AMA:** 2016,Jan,13; 2015,Jan,16; 2014,Jan,11; 2013,Dec,8; 2012,Feb,9-10

75954 Endovascular repair of iliac artery aneurysm, pseudoaneurysm, arteriovenous malformation, or trauma, using ilio-iliac tube endoprosthesis, radiological supervision and interpretation

> EXCLUDES *Endovascular repair of iliac artery aneurysm, arteriovenous malformation, pseudoaneurysm, or trauma with bifurcated endoprosthesis, radiological supervision and interpretation (0255T)*
> *Placement of endovascular graft (34900)*
> 🔲 0.00 　 0.00 　 **FUD** XXX 　　 C 80 🖳
> **AMA:** 2016,Jan,13; 2015,Jan,16; 2014,Jan,11; 2012,Feb,9-10

75956 Endovascular repair of descending thoracic aorta (eg, aneurysm, pseudoaneurysm, dissection, penetrating ulcer, intramural hematoma, or traumatic disruption); involving coverage of left subclavian artery origin, initial endoprosthesis plus descending thoracic aortic extension(s), if required, to level of celiac artery origin, radiological supervision and interpretation

> INCLUDES All angiography
> Fluoroscopy for component delivery
> Code also endovascular graft implantation (33880)
> 🔲 0.00 　 0.00 　 **FUD** XXX 　　 C 80 🖳
> **AMA:** 2016,Jan,13; 2015,Jan,16; 2014,Jan,11; 2012,Feb,9-10

75957 not involving coverage of left subclavian artery origin, initial endoprosthesis plus descending thoracic aortic extension(s), if required, to level of celiac artery origin, radiological supervision and interpretation

> INCLUDES All angiography
> Fluoroscopy for component delivery
> Code also endovascular graft implantation (33881)
> 🔲 0.00 　 0.00 　 **FUD** XXX 　　 C 80 🖳
> **AMA:** 2016,Jan,13; 2015,Jan,16; 2014,Jan,11; 2012,Feb,9-10

75958 Placement of proximal extension prosthesis for endovascular repair of descending thoracic aorta (eg, aneurysm, pseudoaneurysm, dissection, penetrating ulcer, intramural hematoma, or traumatic disruption), radiological supervision and interpretation

> Code also placement of each additional proximal extension(s) (75958)
> Code also proximal endovascular extension implantation (33883-33884)
> 🔲 0.00 　 0.00 　 **FUD** XXX 　　 C 80 🖳
> **AMA:** 2016,Jan,13; 2015,Jan,16; 2014,Jan,11; 2012,Feb,9-10

75959 Placement of distal extension prosthesis(s) (delayed) after endovascular repair of descending thoracic aorta, as needed, to level of celiac origin, radiological supervision and interpretation

> INCLUDES Corresponding services for placement of distal thoracic endovascular extension(s) placed during procedure following the principal procedure
> Code also placement of distal endovascular extension (33886)
> EXCLUDES *Endovascular repair of descending thoracic aorta (75956-75957)*
> *Use of code more than one time no matter how many modules are deployed*
> 🔲 0.00 　 0.00 　 **FUD** XXX 　　 C 80 🖳
> **AMA:** 2016,Jan,13; 2015,Jan,16; 2014,Jan,11; 2012,Feb,9-10

75962-75978 Percutaneous Transluminal Angioplasty

INCLUDES The following diagnostic procedures with interventional supervision and interpretation:
Angiography/venography
Completion angiography/venography except for those services allowed by (75898)
Contrast injection
Fluoroscopic guidance for intervention
Roadmapping
Vessel measurement

EXCLUDES *Diagnostic angiography/venography performed at the same session as transcatheter therapy unless it is specifically included in the code descriptor (75600-75893)*
Radiological supervision and interpretation for transluminal balloon angioplasty in:
Femoral/popliteal arteries (37224-37227)
Iliac artery (37220-37223)
Tibial/peroneal artery (37228-37235)

75962 ~~Transluminal balloon angioplasty, peripheral artery other than renal, or other visceral artery, iliac or lower extremity, radiological supervision and interpretation~~

> To report, see ~36902, 36905, [37246, 37247]

75964 ~~Transluminal balloon angioplasty, each additional peripheral artery other than renal or other visceral artery, iliac or lower extremity, radiological supervision and interpretation (List separately in addition to code for primary procedure)~~

> To report, see ~36902, 36905, [37246, 37247]

75966 ~~Transluminal balloon angioplasty, renal or other visceral artery, radiological supervision and interpretation~~

> To report, see ~36902, 36905, [37246, 37247]

75968 ~~Transluminal balloon angioplasty, each additional visceral artery, radiological supervision and interpretation (List separately in addition to code for primary procedure)~~

> To report, see ~36902, 36905, [37246, 37247]

75970 Transcatheter biopsy, radiological supervision and interpretation

> EXCLUDES *Injection procedure only for transcatheter therapy or biopsy (36100-36299)*
> *Percutaneous needle biopsy*
> *Pancreas (48102)*
> *Retroperitoneal lymph node/mass (49180)*
> *Transcatheter renal/ureteral biopsy (52007)*
> 🔲 0.00 　 0.00 　 **FUD** XXX 　　 N N1 80 🖳
> **AMA:** 2014,Jan,11; 2012,Feb,9-10

75978 ~~Transluminal balloon angioplasty, venous (eg, subclavian stenosis), radiological supervision and interpretation~~

> To report, see ~36902, 36905, 36907, [37248], [37249]

75984-75989 Percutaneous Drainage

INCLUDES The following diagnostic procedures with interventional supervision and interpretation:
Angiography/venography
Completion angiography/venography except for those services allowed by (75898)
Contrast injection
Fluoroscopic guidance for intervention
Roadmapping
Vessel measurement

EXCLUDES Diagnostic angiography/venography performed at the same session as transcatheter therapy unless it is specifically included in the code descriptor (75600-75893)

75984 **Change of percutaneous tube or drainage catheter with contrast monitoring (eg, genitourinary system, abscess), radiological supervision and interpretation**

EXCLUDES Change only of nephrostomy/pyelostomy tube ([50435])
Cholecystostomy, percutaneous (47490)
Introduction procedure only for percutaneous biliary drainage (47531-47544)
Nephrostolithotomy/pyelostolithotomy, percutaneous (50080-50081)
Percutaneous replacement of gastrointestinal tube using fluoroscopic guidance (49450-49452)
Removal and/or replacement of internal ureteral stent using transurethral approach (50385-50386)

🚑 3.00 ⚖ 3.00 **FUD** XXX [N] [N1] [80] ▭

AMA: 2014,Jan,11; 2012,Feb,9-10

75989 **Radiological guidance (ie, fluoroscopy, ultrasound, or computed tomography), for percutaneous drainage (eg, abscess, specimen collection), with placement of catheter, radiological supervision and interpretation**

INCLUDES Needle placement with fluoroscopic guidance (77002)

EXCLUDES Cholecystostomy (47490)
Image-guided fluid collection drainage by catheter (10030, 49405-49407)
Thoracentesis (32554-32557)

🚑 3.41 ⚖ 3.41 **FUD** XXX [N] [N1] [80] ▭

AMA: 2016,Jan,13; 2015,Dec,3; 2015,Jan,16; 2014,May,9; 2014,Jan,11; 2013,Nov,9; 2012,Nov,3-5; 2012,Feb,9-10; 2012,Jan,15-42; 2011,Apr,12; 2011,Jan,8

76000-76140 Miscellaneous Techniques

EXCLUDES Arthrography:
Ankle (73615)
Elbow (73085)
Hip (73525)
Knee (73580)
Shoulder (73040)
Wrist (73115)
CT cerebral perfusion test (0042T)

76000 **Fluoroscopy (separate procedure), up to 1 hour physician or other qualified health care professional time, other than 71023 or 71034 (eg, cardiac fluoroscopy)**

EXCLUDES Extracorporeal membrane oxygenation (ECMO)/extracorporeal life support (ECLS) (33957-33959, [33962, 33963, 33964])

🚑 1.33 ⚖ 1.33 **FUD** XXX [S] [Z3] [80] ▭

AMA: 2016,Aug,5; 2016,May,5; 2016,May,13; 2016,Mar,5; 2016,Jan,13; 2016,Jan,11; 2015,Nov,3; 2015,Sep,3; 2015,May,3; 2015,Jan,16; 2014,Dec,3; 2014,Nov,5; 2014,Oct,6; 2014,Sep,5; 2014,Jan,11; 2013,Sep,17; 2013,Mar,10-11; 2013,Feb,3-6; 2012,Feb,9-10; 2012,Jan,15-42; 2011,Jul,3-11; 2011,Jan,8; 2011,Jan,11

76001 **Fluoroscopy, physician or other qualified health care professional time more than 1 hour, assisting a nonradiologic physician or other qualified health care professional (eg, nephrostolithotomy, ERCP, bronchoscopy, transbronchial biopsy)**

EXCLUDES Extracorporeal membrane oxygenation (ECMO)/extracorporeal life support (ECLS) (33957-33959, [33962, 33963, 33964])

🚑 0.00 ⚖ 0.00 **FUD** XXX [N] [N1] [80] ▭

AMA: 2016,Mar,5; 2016,Jan,13; 2015,Nov,3; 2015,Sep,3; 2015,Jan,16; 2014,Oct,6; 2014,Sep,5; 2014,Jan,11; 2013,Mar,10-11; 2013,Feb,3-6; 2012,Feb,9-10; 2012,Jan,15-42; 2011,Jan,11; 2011,Jan,8

76010 **Radiologic examination from nose to rectum for foreign body, single view, child** [A]

🚑 0.73 ⚖ 0.73 **FUD** XXX [Q1] [N1] [80] ▭

AMA: 2016,Jan,13; 2015,Jan,16; 2014,Jan,11; 2012,Feb,9-10; 2012,Jan,15-42; 2011,Jan,11

76080 **Radiologic examination, abscess, fistula or sinus tract study, radiological supervision and interpretation**

EXCLUDES Contrast injections, radiology evaluation, and guidance via fluoroscopy of gastrostomy, duodenostomy, jejunostomy, gastro-jejunostomy, or cecostomy tube (49465)

🚑 1.56 ⚖ 1.56 **FUD** XXX [Q2] [N1] [80] ▭

AMA: 2016,Jan,13; 2015,Jan,16; 2014,Jan,11; 2012,Feb,9-10; 2012,Jan,15-42; 2011,Jan,11

76098 **Radiological examination, surgical specimen**

EXCLUDES Breast biopsy with placement of breast localization device(s) (19081-19086)

🚑 0.47 ⚖ 0.47 **FUD** XXX [Q2] [N1] [80] ▭

AMA: 2012,Feb,9-10

76100 **Radiologic examination, single plane body section (eg, tomography), other than with urography**

🚑 2.60 ⚖ 2.60 **FUD** XXX [Q1] [N1] [80] ▭

AMA: 2012,Feb,9-10

76101 **Radiologic examination, complex motion (ie, hypercycloidal) body section (eg, mastoid polytomography), other than with urography; unilateral**

EXCLUDES Nephrotomography (74415)
Panoramic x-ray (70355)
Procedure performed more than one time per day

🚑 3.70 ⚖ 3.70 **FUD** XXX [Q1] [Z2] [80] ▭

AMA: 2012,Feb,9-10

76102 **bilateral**

EXCLUDES Nephrotomography (74415)
Panoramic x-ray (70355)
Procedure performed more than one time per day

🚑 4.90 ⚖ 4.90 **FUD** XXX [S] [Z2] [80] ▭

AMA: 2012,Feb,9-10

76120 **Cineradiography/videoradiography, except where specifically included**

🚑 2.35 ⚖ 2.35 **FUD** XXX [Q1] [N1] [80] ▭

AMA: 2016,Jan,13; 2015,Jan,16; 2014,Jan,11; 2012,Feb,9-10; 2011,Apr,13

+ **76125** **Cineradiography/videoradiography to complement routine examination (List separately in addition to code for primary procedure)**

Code first primary procedure

🚑 0.00 ⚖ 0.00 **FUD** ZZZ [N] [N1] [80] ▭

AMA: 2016,Jan,13; 2015,Jan,16; 2014,Jan,11; 2012,Feb,9-10

76140 **Consultation on X-ray examination made elsewhere, written report**

🚑 0.00 ⚖ 0.00 **FUD** XXX [E] ▭

AMA: 2016,Jan,13; 2015,Jan,16; 2014,Jan,11; 2012,Feb,9-10; 2012,Jan,15-42; 2011,Jan,11

76376-76377 Three-dimensional Manipulation

INCLUDES Concurrent physician supervision of image postprocessing
3D manipulation of volumetric data set
Rendering of image

EXCLUDES Arthrography:
Ankle (73615)
Elbow (73085)
Hip (73525)
Knee (73580)
Shoulder (73040)
Wrist (73115)
Computer-aided detection of MRI data for lesion, breast MRI (0159T)
CT cerebral perfusion test (0042T)
Code also base imaging procedure(s)

76376 **3D rendering with interpretation and reporting of computed tomography, magnetic resonance imaging, ultrasound, or other tomographic modality with image postprocessing under concurrent supervision; not requiring image postprocessing on an independent workstation**

EXCLUDES 3D rendering (76377)
Bronchoscopy, with computer-assisted, image-guided navigation (31627)
Cardiac magnetic resonance imaging (75557, 75559, 75561, 75563, 75565)
Computer-aided detection (0159T)
Computed tomographic angiography (70496, 70498, 71275, 72191, 73206, 73706, 74174-74175, 74261-74263, 75571-75574, 75635)
Digital breast tomosynthesis (77061-77063)
Echocardiography, transesophageal (TEE) for guidance (93355)
Magnetic resonance angiography (70544-70549, 71555, 72159, 72198, 73225, 73725, 74185)
Nuclear radiology procedures (78012-78999)
Physician planning of a patient-specific fenestrated visceral aortic endograft (34839)

🔲 0.65 🔲 0.65 **FUD** XXX N NI 80 ▢

AMA: 2016,Apr,8; 2016,Jan,13; 2015,Jan,16; 2014,Jan,11; 2013,Jun,12; 2013,May,3-5; 2012,Feb,9-10; 2012,Jan,15-42; 2011,Jan,11

76377 **requiring image postprocessing on an independent workstation**

EXCLUDES 3D rendering (76376)
Cardiac magnetic resonance imaging (75557, 75559, 75561, 75563, 75565)
Computer-aided detection (0159T)
Computed tomographic angiography (70496, 70498, 71275, 72191, 73206, 73706, 74174-74175, 74261-74263, 75571-75574, 75635)
Digital breast tomosynthesis (77061)
Echocardiography, transesophageal (TEE) for guidance (93355)
Magnetic resonance angiography (70544-70549, 71555, 72159, 72198, 73225, 73725, 74185)
Nuclear radiology procedures (78012-78999)
Physician planning of a patient-specific fenestrated visceral aortic endograft (34839)

🔲 2.01 🔲 2.01 **FUD** XXX N NI 80 ▢

AMA: 2016,Apr,8; 2016,Jan,13; 2015,Jan,16; 2014,Jan,11; 2013,Jun,12; 2013,May,3-5; 2012,Feb,9-10; 2012,Jan,15-42; 2011,Jan,11

76380 Computerized Tomography: Delimited

EXCLUDES Arthrography:
Ankle (73615)
Elbow (73085)
Hip (73525)
Knee (73580)
Shoulder (73040)
Wrist (73115)
CT cerebral perfusion test (0042T)

76380 **Computed tomography, limited or localized follow-up study**

🔲 4.12 🔲 4.12 **FUD** XXX 01 NI 80 ▢

AMA: 2016,Jan,13; 2015,Jan,16; 2014,Jan,11; 2012,Feb,9-10

76390 Magnetic Resonance Spectroscopy

CMS: 100-03,220.2.1 Magnetic Resonance Spectroscopy

EXCLUDES Arthrography:
Ankle (73615)
Elbow (73085)
Hip (73525)
Knee (73580)
Shoulder (73040)
Wrist (73115)
CT cerebral perfusion test (0042T)

76390 **Magnetic resonance spectroscopy**

EXCLUDES MRI
🔲 12.4 🔲 12.4 **FUD** XXX E ▢

AMA: 2012,Feb,9-10

76496-76499 Unlisted Radiology Procedures

76496 **Unlisted fluoroscopic procedure (eg, diagnostic, interventional)**

🔲 0.00 🔲 0.00 **FUD** XXX 01 NI 80 ▢

AMA: 2012,Feb,9-10

76497 **Unlisted computed tomography procedure (eg, diagnostic, interventional)**

🔲 0.00 🔲 0.00 **FUD** XXX 01 NI 80 ▢

AMA: 2016,Jan,13; 2015,Jan,16; 2014,Jan,11; 2012,Feb,9-10; 2012,Jan,15-42; 2011,Jan,11

76498 **Unlisted magnetic resonance procedure (eg, diagnostic, interventional)**

🔲 0.00 🔲 0.00 **FUD** XXX S 72 80 ▢

AMA: 2016,Jan,13; 2015,Jan,16; 2014,Jan,11; 2012,Feb,9-10; 2012,Jan,15-42; 2011,Dec,14-18; 2011,Jan,11

76499 **Unlisted diagnostic radiographic procedure**

🔲 0.00 🔲 0.00 **FUD** XXX 01 NI 80

AMA: 2016,Jul,8; 2016,Jan,13; 2015,Jan,16; 2014,Jan,11; 2013,Dec,16; 2012,Feb,9-10; 2012,Jan,15-42; 2011,Dec,14-18; 2011,Jan,11

76506 Ultrasound: Brain

INCLUDES Required permanent documentation of ultrasound images except when diagnostic purpose is biometric measurement
Written documentation

EXCLUDES Noninvasive vascular studies, diagnostic (93880-93990)
Ultrasound exam that does not include thorough assessment of organ or site, recorded image, and written report

76506 **Echoencephalography, real time with image documentation (gray scale) (for determination of ventricular size, delineation of cerebral contents, and detection of fluid masses or other intracranial abnormalities), including A-mode encephalography as secondary component where indicated**

🔲 3.36 🔲 3.36 **FUD** XXX 01 NI 80 ▢

AMA: 2016,Jan,13; 2015,Jan,16; 2014,Jan,11; 2012,Feb,9-10

76510-76529 Ultrasound: Eyes

INCLUDES Required permanent documentation of ultrasound images except when diagnostic purpose is biometric measurement
Written documentation

76510 **Ophthalmic ultrasound, diagnostic; B-scan and quantitative A-scan performed during the same patient encounter**

🔲 4.81 🔲 4.81 **FUD** XXX 01 NI 80 ▢

AMA: 2016,Jan,13; 2015,Jan,16; 2014,Jan,11; 2012,Feb,9-10

76511 **quantitative A-scan only**

🔲 2.86 🔲 2.86 **FUD** XXX 01 NI 80 ▢

AMA: 2016,Jan,13; 2015,Jan,16; 2014,Jan,11; 2012,Feb,9-10

76512 **B-scan (with or without superimposed non-quantitative A-scan)**

🔲 2.62 🔲 2.62 **FUD** XXX 01 NI 80 ▢

AMA: 2016,Jan,13; 2015,Jan,16; 2014,Jan,11; 2012,Feb,9-10

76513 **anterior segment ultrasound, immersion (water bath) B-scan or high resolution biomicroscopy**

EXCLUDES *Computerized ophthalmic testing other than by ultrasound (92132-92134)*

📖 2.69 ⅄ 2.69 **FUD** XXX Q1 N1 80 ▣

AMA: 2016,Jan,13; 2015,Jan,16; 2014,Jan,11; 2013,Apr,7; 2012,Feb,9-10; 2012,Jan,15-42; 2011,Jan,11

76514 **corneal pachymetry, unilateral or bilateral (determination of corneal thickness)**

INCLUDES Biometric measurement for which permanent documentation of images is not required

EXCLUDES *Collagen cross-linking of cornea (0402T)*

📖 0.43 ⅄ 0.43 **FUD** XXX Q1 N1 80 ▣

AMA: 2016,Feb,12; 2016,Jan,13; 2015,Jan,16; 2014,Jan,11; 2012,Feb,9-10; 2012,Jan,15-42; 2011,Jan,11

76516 **Ophthalmic biometry by ultrasound echography, A-scan;**

INCLUDES Biometric measurement for which permanent documentation of images is not required

📖 2.22 ⅄ 2.22 **FUD** XXX Q1 N1 80 ▣

AMA: 2016,Jan,13; 2015,Jan,16; 2014,Jan,11; 2012,Feb,9-10; 2012,Jan,15-42; 2011,Jan,11

76519 **with intraocular lens power calculation**

INCLUDES Biometric measurement for which permanent documentation of images is not required
Written prescription that satisfies requirement for written report

EXCLUDES *Partial coherence interferometry (92136)*

📖 2.37 ⅄ 2.37 **FUD** XXX Q1 N1 80 ▣

AMA: 2016,Jan,13; 2015,Jan,16; 2014,Jan,11; 2012,Feb,9-10; 2012,Jan,15-42; 2011,Jan,11

76529 **Ophthalmic ultrasonic foreign body localization**

📖 2.24 ⅄ 2.24 **FUD** XXX Q1 N1 80 ▣

AMA: 2016,Jan,13; 2015,Jan,16; 2014,Jan,11; 2012,Feb,9-10

76536-76800 Ultrasound: Neck, Thorax, Abdomen, and Spine

INCLUDES Required permanent documentation of ultrasound images except when diagnostic purpose is biometric measurement
Written documentation

EXCLUDES *Focused ultrasound ablation of uterine leiomyomata (0071T-0072T)*
Ultrasound exam that does not include thorough assessment of organ or site, recorded image, and written report

76536 **Ultrasound, soft tissues of head and neck (eg, thyroid, parathyroid, parotid), real time with image documentation**

📖 3.29 ⅄ 3.29 **FUD** XXX Q1 N1 80 ▣

AMA: 2016,Jan,13; 2015,Jan,16; 2014,Jan,11; 2012,Feb,9-10

76604 **Ultrasound, chest (includes mediastinum), real time with image documentation**

📖 2.49 ⅄ 2.49 **FUD** XXX Q1 N1 80 ▣

AMA: 2016,Jan,13; 2015,Jan,16; 2014,Jan,11; 2012,Nov,3-5; 2012,Feb,9-10

76641 **Ultrasound, breast, unilateral, real time with image documentation, including axilla when performed; complete**

INCLUDES Complete examination of all four quadrants, retroareolar region, and axilla when performed

EXCLUDES *Procedure performed more than one time per breast per session*

📖 3.04 ⅄ 3.04 **FUD** XXX Q1 N1 80 50 ▣

AMA: 2016,Jan,13; 2015,Aug,8

76642 **limited**

📖 2.50 ⅄ 2.50 **FUD** XXX Q1 N1 80 50 ▣

INCLUDES Examination not including all of the elements in complete examination

EXCLUDES *Procedure performed more than one time per breast per session*

76700 **Ultrasound, abdominal, real time with image documentation; complete**

INCLUDES Real time scans of:
Common bile duct
Gall bladder
Inferior vena cava
Kidneys
Liver
Pancreas
Spleen
Upper abdominal aorta

📖 3.47 ⅄ 3.47 **FUD** XXX Q3 Z3 80 ▣

AMA: 2016,Jan,13; 2015,Jan,16; 2014,Jan,11; 2012,Feb,9-10

76705 **limited (eg, single organ, quadrant, follow-up)**

📖 2.59 ⅄ 2.59 **FUD** XXX Q3 Z3 80 ▣

AMA: 2016,Jan,13; 2015,Jan,16; 2014,Jan,11; 2012,Dec,9-10; 2012,Mar,9-10; 2012,Feb,9-10; 2012,Jan,15-42; 2011,Jan,11

● **76706** **Ultrasound, abdominal aorta, real time with image documentation, screening study for abdominal aortic aneurysm (AAA)**

EXCLUDES *Diagnostic ultrasound of aorta (76770-76775)*
Duplex scan of aorta (93978-93979)

76770 **Ultrasound, retroperitoneal (eg, renal, aorta, nodes), real time with image documentation; complete**

INCLUDES Complete assessment of kidneys and bladder if history indicates urinary pathology
Real time scans of:
Abdominal aorta
Common iliac artery origins
Inferior vena cava
Kidneys

📖 3.21 ⅄ 3.21 **FUD** XXX Q3 Z3 80 ▣

AMA: 2016,Jan,13; 2015,Jan,16; 2014,Jan,11; 2012,Feb,9-10

76775 **limited**

📖 1.64 ⅄ 1.64 **FUD** XXX Q1 N1 80 ▣

AMA: 2016,Jan,13; 2015,Jan,16; 2014,Jan,11; 2012,Feb,9-10; 2012,Jan,15-42; 2011,Jan,11

76776 **Ultrasound, transplanted kidney, real time and duplex Doppler with image documentation**

EXCLUDES *Abdominal/pelvic/scrotal contents/retroperitoneal duplex scan (93975, 93976)*
Transplanted kidney ultrasound without duplex doppler (76775)

📖 4.44 ⅄ 4.44 **FUD** XXX Q3 Z2 80 ▣

AMA: 2016,Jan,13; 2015,Jan,16; 2014,Jan,11; 2012,Feb,9-10

76800 **Ultrasound, spinal canal and contents**

📖 4.00 ⅄ 4.00 **FUD** XXX Q1 N1 80 ▣

AMA: 2016,Jan,13; 2015,Jan,16; 2014,Jan,11; 2012,Feb,9-10; 2012,Jan,15-42; 2011,Jan,11

76801-76802 Ultrasound: Pregnancy Less Than 14 Weeks

INCLUDES Determination of the number of gestational sacs and fetuses
Gestational sac/fetal measurement appropriate for gestational age (younger than 14 weeks 0 days)
Inspection of the maternal uterus and adnexa
Quality analysis of amniotic fluid volume/gestational sac shape
Visualization of fetal and placental anatomic formation
Written documentation of each component of exam

EXCLUDES *Focused ultrasound ablation of uterine leiomyomata (0071T-0072T)*
Ultrasound exam that does not include thorough assessment of organ or site, recorded image, and written report

76801 **Ultrasound, pregnant uterus, real time with image documentation, fetal and maternal evaluation, first trimester (< 14 weeks 0 days), transabdominal approach; single or first gestation** M ♀

EXCLUDES *Fetal nuchal translucency measurement, first trimester (76813)*

📖 3.49 ⅄ 3.49 **FUD** XXX S Z3 80 ▣

AMA: 2016,Jan,13; 2015,Jan,16; 2014,Jan,11; 2012,Feb,9-10; 2012,Jan,15-42; 2011,Jan,11

+ 76802 each additional gestation (List separately in addition to code for primary procedure) Ⓜ ♀

> EXCLUDES *Fetal nuchal translucency measurement, first trimester (76814)*
> Code first (76801)
> 🚑 1.84 ⚕ 1.84 **FUD** ZZZ Ⓝ N1 80 ▢
> **AMA:** 2016,Jan,13; 2015,Jan,16; 2014,Jan,11; 2012,Feb,9-10; 2012,Jan,15-42; 2011,Jan,11

76805-76810 Ultrasound: Pregnancy of 14 Weeks or More

> INCLUDES Determination of the number of gestational/chorionic sacs and fetuses
> Evaluation of:
>   Amniotic fluid
>   Four chambered heart
>   Intracranial, spinal, abdominal anatomy
>   Placenta location
>   Umbilical cord insertion site
> Examination of maternal adnexa if visible
> Gestational sac/fetal measurement appropriate for gestational age (older than or equal to 14 weeks 0 days)
> Written documentation of each component of exam
> EXCLUDES *Focused ultrasound ablation of uterine leiomyomata (0071T-0072T)*
> *Ultrasound exam that does not include thorough assessment of organ or site, recorded image, and written report*

76805 Ultrasound, pregnant uterus, real time with image documentation, fetal and maternal evaluation, after first trimester (> or = 14 weeks 0 days), transabdominal approach; single or first gestation Ⓜ ♀

> 🚑 4.03 ⚕ 4.03 **FUD** XXX S Z2 80 ▢
> **AMA:** 2016,Jan,13; 2015,Jan,16; 2014,Jan,11; 2012,Feb,9-10

+ 76810 each additional gestation (List separately in addition to code for primary procedure) Ⓜ ♀

> Code first (76805)
> 🚑 2.65 ⚕ 2.65 **FUD** ZZZ Ⓝ N1 80 ▢
> **AMA:** 2016,Jan,13; 2015,Jan,16; 2014,Jan,11; 2012,Feb,9-10

76811-76812 Ultrasound: Pregnancy, with Additional Studies of Fetus

> INCLUDES Determination of the number of gestational/chorionic sacs and fetuses
> Evaluation of:
>   Abdominal organ specific anatomy
>   Amniotic fluid
>   Chest anatomy
>   Face
>   Fetal brain/ventricles
>   Four chambered heart
>   Heart/outflow tracts and chest anatomy
>   Intracranial, spinal, abdominal anatomy
>   Limbs including number, length, and architecture
>   Other fetal anatomy as indicated
>   Placenta location
>   Umbilical cord insertion site
> Examination of maternal adnexa if visible
> Gestational sac/fetal measurement appropriate for gestational age (older than or equal to 14 weeks 0 days)
> Written documentation of each component of exam, including reason for nonvisualization, when applicable
> EXCLUDES *Focused ultrasound ablation of uterine leiomyomata (0071T-0072T)*
> *Ultrasound exam that does not include thorough assessment organ or site, recorded image, and written report*

76811 Ultrasound, pregnant uterus, real time with image documentation, fetal and maternal evaluation plus detailed fetal anatomic examination, transabdominal approach; single or first gestation Ⓜ ♀

> 🚑 5.17 ⚕ 5.17 **FUD** XXX S Z3 80 ▢
> **AMA:** 2016,Jan,13; 2015,Jan,16; 2014,Jan,11; 2012,Feb,9-10

+ 76812 each additional gestation (List separately in addition to code for primary procedure) Ⓜ ♀

> Code first (76811)
> 🚑 5.87 ⚕ 5.87 **FUD** ZZZ Ⓝ N1 80 ▢
> **AMA:** 2016,Jan,13; 2015,Jan,16; 2014,Jan,11; 2012,Feb,9-10

76813-76828 Ultrasound: Other Fetal Evaluations

> INCLUDES Required permanent documentation of ultrasound images except when diagnostic purpose is biometric measurement
> Written documentation
> EXCLUDES *Focused ultrasound ablation of uterine leiomyomata (0071T-0072T)*
> *Ultrasound exam that does not include thorough assessment of organ or site, recorded image, and written report*

76813 Ultrasound, pregnant uterus, real time with image documentation, first trimester fetal nuchal translucency measurement, transabdominal or transvaginal approach; single or first gestation Ⓜ ♀

> 🚑 3.44 ⚕ 3.44 **FUD** XXX 01 N1 80 ▢
> **AMA:** 2016,Jan,13; 2015,Jan,16; 2014,Jan,11; 2012,Feb,9-10

+ 76814 each additional gestation (List separately in addition to code for primary procedure) Ⓜ ♀

> Code first (76813)
> 🚑 2.31 ⚕ 2.31 **FUD** XXX Ⓝ N1 80 ▢
> **AMA:** 2016,Jan,13; 2015,Jan,16; 2014,Jan,11; 2012,Feb,9-10

76815 Ultrasound, pregnant uterus, real time with image documentation, limited (eg, fetal heart beat, placental location, fetal position and/or qualitative amniotic fluid volume), 1 or more fetuses Ⓜ ♀

> INCLUDES Exam concentrating on one or more elements
> Reporting only one time per exam, instead of per element
> EXCLUDES *Fetal nuchal translucency measurement, first trimester (76813-76814)*
> 🚑 2.39 ⚕ 2.39 **FUD** XXX 01 N1 80 ▢
> **AMA:** 2016,Jan,13; 2015,Jan,16; 2014,Jan,11; 2012,Feb,9-10; 2012,Jan,15-42; 2011,Jan,11

76816 Ultrasound, pregnant uterus, real time with image documentation, follow-up (eg, re-evaluation of fetal size by measuring standard growth parameters and amniotic fluid volume, re-evaluation of organ system(s) suspected or confirmed to be abnormal on a previous scan), transabdominal approach, per fetus Ⓜ ♀

> INCLUDES Re-evaluation of fetal size, interval growth, or aberrancies noted on a prior ultrasound
> Code also modifier 59 for examination of each additional fetus in a multiple pregnancy
> 🚑 3.27 ⚕ 3.27 **FUD** XXX 01 N1 80 ▢
> **AMA:** 2016,Jan,13; 2015,Jan,16; 2014,Jan,11; 2012,Feb,9-10; 2012,Jan,15-42; 2011,Jan,11

76817 Ultrasound, pregnant uterus, real time with image documentation, transvaginal Ⓜ ♀

> EXCLUDES *Transvaginal ultrasound, non-obstetrical (76830)*
> Code also transabdominal obstetrical ultrasound, if performed
> 🚑 2.76 ⚕ 2.76 **FUD** XXX 01 N1 80 ▢
> **AMA:** 2016,Jan,13; 2015,Jan,16; 2014,Jan,11; 2012,Feb,9-10; 2012,Jan,15-42

76818 Fetal biophysical profile; with non-stress testing Ⓜ ♀

> Code also modifier 59 for each additional fetus
> 🚑 3.46 ⚕ 3.46 **FUD** XXX S Z3 80 ▢
> **AMA:** 2016,Jan,13; 2015,Jan,16; 2014,Jan,11; 2012,Feb,9-10; 2012,Jan,15-42; 2011,Jan,11

76819 without non-stress testing Ⓜ ♀

> EXCLUDES *Amniotic fluid index without non-stress test (76815)*
> Code also modifier 59 for each additional fetus
> 🚑 2.52 ⚕ 2.52 **FUD** XXX S Z3 80 ▢
> **AMA:** 2016,Jan,13; 2015,Jan,16; 2014,Jan,11; 2012,Feb,9-10; 2012,Jan,15-42; 2011,Jan,11

76820 Doppler velocimetry, fetal; umbilical artery Ⓜ

> 🚑 1.34 ⚕ 1.34 **FUD** XXX 01 N1 80 ▢
> **AMA:** 2016,Jul,8; 2016,Jan,13; 2015,Jan,16; 2014,Jan,11; 2012,Feb,9-10

76821 middle cerebral artery Ⓜ

> 🚑 2.64 ⚕ 2.64 **FUD** XXX 01 N1 80 ▢
> **AMA:** 2016,Jan,13; 2015,Jan,16; 2014,Jan,11; 2012,Feb,9-10

Radiology (vertical, left margin)

76825 — 76886 (vertical, left margin)

76825 **Echocardiography, fetal, cardiovascular system, real time with image documentation (2D), with or without M-mode recording;** Ⓜ ♀
🚑 7.84   ☇ 7.84   **FUD** XXX   Ⓢ Ⓩ3 80 🖵
AMA: 2016,Jan,13; 2015,Jan,16; 2014,Jan,11; 2012,Feb,9-10

76826 **follow-up or repeat study** Ⓜ ♀
🚑 4.63   ☇ 4.63   **FUD** XXX   Ⓢ Ⓩ3 80 🖵
AMA: 2012,Feb,9-10

76827 **Doppler echocardiography, fetal, pulsed wave and/or continuous wave with spectral display; complete** Ⓜ ♀
🚑 2.15   ☇ 2.15   **FUD** XXX   01 N1 80 🖵
AMA: 2016,Jan,13; 2015,Jan,16; 2014,Jan,11; 2012,Feb,9-10

76828 **follow-up or repeat study** Ⓜ ♀
EXCLUDES   *Color mapping (93325)*
🚑 1.52   ☇ 1.52   **FUD** XXX   01 N1 80 🖵
AMA: 2016,Jan,13; 2015,Jan,16; 2014,Jan,11; 2012,Feb,9-10

76830-76873 Ultrasound: Male and Female Genitalia

INCLUDES   Required permanent documentation of ultrasound images except when diagnostic purpose is biometric measurement
  Written documentation
EXCLUDES   *Focused ultrasound ablation of uterine leiomyomata (0071T-0072T)*
  Ultrasound exam that does not include thorough assessment of organ or site, recorded image, and written report

76830 **Ultrasound, transvaginal** ♀
EXCLUDES   *Transvaginal ultrasound, obstetric (76817)*
Code also transabdominal non-obstetrical ultrasound, if performed
🚑 3.46   ☇ 3.46   **FUD** XXX   Ⓢ Ⓩ2 80 🖵
AMA: 2016,Jan,13; 2015,Jan,16; 2014,Jan,11; 2012,Feb,9-10; 2012,Jan,15-42; 2011,Jan,11

Nonpregnant uterus
Ovary
Pubic bone
Bladder
Rectum
Ultrasonic lead in vaginal canal

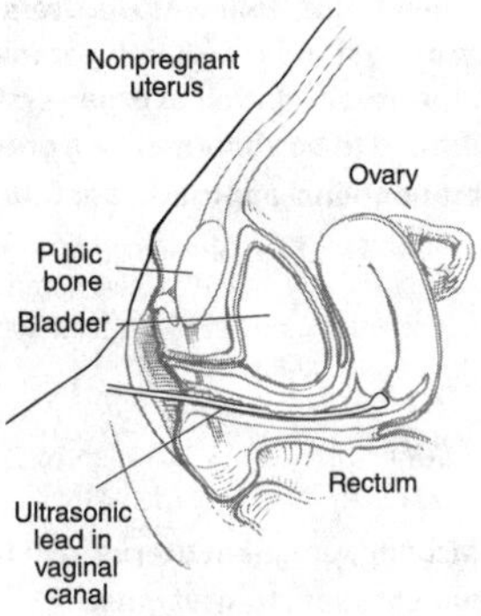

Ultrasound is performed in real time with image documentation by a transvaginal approach

76831 **Saline infusion sonohysterography (SIS), including color flow Doppler, when performed** ♀
Code also saline introduction for saline infusion sonohysterography (58340)
🚑 3.36   ☇ 3.36   **FUD** XXX   03 Ⓩ3 80 🖵
AMA: 2016,Jan,13; 2015,Jan,16; 2014,Jan,11; 2012,Feb,9-10; 2012,Jan,15-42; 2011,Jan,11

76856 **Ultrasound, pelvic (nonobstetric), real time with image documentation; complete**
INCLUDES   Total examination of the female pelvic anatomy which includes:
  Bladder measurement
  Description and measurement of the uterus and adnexa
  Description of any pelvic pathology
  Measurement of the endometrium
  Total examination of the male pelvis which includes:
  Bladder measurement
  Description of any pelvic pathology
  Evaluation of prostate and seminal vesicles
🚑 3.11   ☇ 3.11   **FUD** XXX   03 Ⓩ3 80 🖵
AMA: 2016,Aug,9; 2016,Jan,13; 2015,Jan,16; 2014,Jan,11; 2012,Feb,9-10; 2012,Jan,15-42; 2011,Jan,11

76857 **limited or follow-up (eg, for follicles)**
INCLUDES   Focused evaluation limited to:
  Evaluation of one or more elements listed in 76856 and/or
  Reevaluation of one or more pelvic aberrancies noted on a prior ultrasound
  Urinary bladder alone
EXCLUDES   *Bladder volume or post-voided residual measurement without imaging the bladder (51798)*
  Urinary bladder and kidneys (76770)
🚑 1.35   ☇ 1.35   **FUD** XXX   03 Ⓩ3 80 🖵
AMA: 2016,Jan,13; 2015,Jan,16; 2014,Jan,11; 2012,Feb,9-10; 2012,Jan,15-42; 2011,Jan,11

76870 **Ultrasound, scrotum and contents** ♂
🚑 1.91   ☇ 1.91   **FUD** XXX   01 N1 80 🖵
AMA: 2012,Feb,9-10

76872 **Ultrasound, transrectal;**
EXCLUDES   *Colonoscopy (45391-45392)*
  Ligation, hemorrhoidal vascular bundle(s) (0249T)
  Sigmoidoscopy (45341-45342)
  Transurethral prostate ablation (0421T)
🚑 2.66   ☇ 2.66   **FUD** XXX   Ⓢ Ⓩ3 80 🖵
AMA: 2016,Jan,13; 2015,Jan,16; 2014,Jan,11; 2012,Feb,9-10

76873 **prostate volume study for brachytherapy treatment planning (separate procedure)** ♂
🚑 4.75   ☇ 4.75   **FUD** XXX   Ⓢ Ⓩ2 🖵
AMA: 2016,Jan,13; 2015,Jan,16; 2014,Jan,11; 2012,Feb,9-10

76881-76886 Ultrasound: Extremities

EXCLUDES   *Doppler studies of the extremities (93925-93926, 93930-93931, 93970-93971)*

76881 **Ultrasound, extremity, nonvascular, real-time with image documentation; complete**
INCLUDES   Real time scans of a specific joint including assessment of:
  Joint
  Muscles
  Other soft tissue
  Tendons
🚑 3.24   ☇ 3.24   **FUD** XXX   Ⓢ Ⓩ3 🖵
AMA: 2016,Sep,9; 2012,Feb,9-10

76882 **limited, anatomic specific**
INCLUDES   Limited examination of a certain anatomical structure (e.g. muscle or tendon) or for evaluation of a soft-tissue mass
🚑 1.02   ☇ 1.02   **FUD** XXX   01 N1 🖵
AMA: 2016,Sep,9; 2012,Feb,9-10

76885 **Ultrasound, infant hips, real time with imaging documentation; dynamic (requiring physician or other qualified health care professional manipulation)** Ⓐ
🚑 4.13   ☇ 4.13   **FUD** XXX   01 N1 80 🖵
AMA: 2012,Feb,9-10

76886 **limited, static (not requiring physician or other qualified health care professional manipulation)** Ⓐ
🚑 3.00   ☇ 3.00   **FUD** XXX   01 N1 80 🖵
AMA: 2012,Feb,9-10

26/TC PC/TC Only   A2-Z3 ASC Payment   50 Bilateral   ♂ Male Only   ♀ Female Only   🚑 Facility RVU   ☇ Non-Facility RVU   🖵 CCI
FUD Follow-up Days   CMS: IOM (Pub 100)   A-Y OPPSI   80/80 Surg Assist Allowed / w/Doc   ☒ Lab Crosswalk   ☒ Radiology Crosswalk   ☒ CLIA

324
CPT © 2016 American Medical Association. All Rights Reserved.   © 2016 Optum360, LLC

76930-76970 Imaging Guidance: Ultrasound

INCLUDES Required permanent documentation of ultrasound images except when diagnostic purpose is biometric measurement
Written documentation

EXCLUDES *Focused ultrasound ablation of uterine leiomyomata (0071T-0072T)*
Ultrasound exam that does not include thorough assessment of organ or site, recorded image, and written report

76930 **Ultrasonic guidance for pericardiocentesis, imaging supervision and interpretation**

🔧 0.00   ✂ 0.00   **FUD** XXX   N N1 80 📷

AMA: 2016,Sep,9; 2012,Feb,9-10

76932 **Ultrasonic guidance for endomyocardial biopsy, imaging supervision and interpretation**

🔧 0.00   ✂ 0.00   **FUD** YYY   N N1 80 📷

AMA: 2012,Feb,9-10

76936 **Ultrasound guided compression repair of arterial pseudoaneurysm or arteriovenous fistulae (includes diagnostic ultrasound evaluation, compression of lesion and imaging)**

🔧 7.71   ✂ 7.71   **FUD** XXX   S Z2 80 📷

AMA: 2012,Feb,9-10

+ **76937** **Ultrasound guidance for vascular access requiring ultrasound evaluation of potential access sites, documentation of selected vessel patency, concurrent realtime ultrasound visualization of vascular needle entry, with permanent recording and reporting (List separately in addition to code for primary procedure)**

INCLUDES Ultrasonic guidance (76942)

EXCLUDES *Extremity venous noninvasive vascular diagnostic study performed separately from venous access guidance (93970-93971)*
Insertion of intravascular vena cava filter (37191-37193)
Ligation perforator veins (37760-37761)

Code first primary procedure

🔧 0.89   ✂ 0.89   **FUD** ZZZ   N N1 80 📷

AMA: 2016,Jul,6; 2016,Jan,13; 2015,Jul,10; 2015,Jan,16; 2014,Oct,6; 2014,Jan,11; 2013,Sep,17; 2013,Jun,12; 2013,May,3-5; 2013,Feb,3-6; 2012,Feb,9-10; 2012,Apr,3-9; 2011,Jan,8

76940 **Ultrasound guidance for, and monitoring of, parenchymal tissue ablation**

INCLUDES Ultrasonic guidance (76998)

EXCLUDES *Ablation (20982-20983, 32998, 47370-47383, 50250, 50542, 50592-50593, 0340T)*

🔧 0.00   ✂ 0.00   **FUD** YYY   N N1 80 📷

AMA: 2016,Jan,13; 2015,Jul,8; 2015,Jan,16; 2014,Jan,11; 2012,Feb,9-10

76941 **Ultrasonic guidance for intrauterine fetal transfusion or cordocentesis, imaging supervision and interpretation**   M ♀

Code also surgical procedure (36460, 59012)

🔧 0.00   ✂ 0.00   **FUD** XXX   N N1 80 📷

AMA: 2012,Feb,9-10

76942 **Ultrasonic guidance for needle placement (eg, biopsy, aspiration, injection, localization device), imaging supervision and interpretation**

EXCLUDES *Arthrocentesis (20604, 20606, 20611)*
Breast biopsy with placement of localization device(s) (19083)
Destruction/reduction of malignant breast tumor (0301T)
Esophagogastroduodenoscopy (43237, 43242)
Esophagoscopy (43232)
Gastrointestinal endoscopic ultrasound (76975)
Image-guided fluid collection drainage by catheter (10030)
Injection procedures (27096, 64479-64484, 0228T, 0231T-0232T)
Ligation (37760-37761, 0249T)
Placement of breast localization device(s) (19285)
Sigmoidoscopy (45341-45342)
Thoracentesis (32554-32557)

🔧 1.72   ✂ 1.72   **FUD** XXX   N N1 80 📷

AMA: 2016,Jun,3; 2016,Jan,13; 2016,Jan,9; 2015,Dec,3; 2015,Nov,10; 2015,Aug,8; 2015,Feb,6; 2015,Jan,16; 2014,Oct,6; 2014,Jan,11; 2013,Dec,3; 2013,Nov,9; 2012,Dec,9-10; 2012,Nov,3-5; 2012,Feb,9-10; 2012,Jan,15-42; 2011,Apr,12; 2011,Mar,9; 2011,Feb,4-5; 2011,Jan,11

76945 **Ultrasonic guidance for chorionic villus sampling, imaging supervision and interpretation**   M ♀

Code also surgical procedure (59015)

🔧 0.00   ✂ 0.00   **FUD** XXX   N N1 80 📷

AMA: 2012,Feb,9-10

76946 **Ultrasonic guidance for amniocentesis, imaging supervision and interpretation**   M ♀

🔧 0.93   ✂ 0.93   **FUD** XXX   N N1 80 📷

AMA: 2012,Feb,9-10

76948 **Ultrasonic guidance for aspiration of ova, imaging supervision and interpretation**   M ♀

🔧 1.97   ✂ 1.97   **FUD** XXX   N N1 80 📷

AMA: 2012,Feb,9-10

76965 **Ultrasonic guidance for interstitial radioelement application**

🔧 2.55   ✂ 2.55   **FUD** XXX   N N1 80 📷

AMA: 2012,Feb,9-10

76970 **Ultrasound study follow-up (specify)**

🔧 2.63   ✂ 2.63   **FUD** XXX   Q1 N1 80 📷

AMA: 2012,Feb,9-10

76975 Endoscopic Ultrasound

CMS: 100-04,12,30.1 Upper Gastrointestinal Endoscopy Including Endoscopic Ultrasound (EUS)

INCLUDES Required permanent documentation of ultrasound images except when diagnostic purpose is biometric measurement
Written documentation

EXCLUDES *Focused ultrasound ablation of uterine leiomyomata (0071T-0072T)*
Ultrasound exam that does not include thorough assessment of organ or site, recorded image, and written report

76975 **Gastrointestinal endoscopic ultrasound, supervision and interpretation**

INCLUDES Ultrasonic guidance (76942)

EXCLUDES *Colonoscopy (44406-44407, 45391-45392)*
Esophagogastroduodenoscopy (43237-43238, 43240, 43242, 43259)
Esophagoscopy (43231-43232)
Sigmoidoscopy (45341-45342)

🔧 0.00   ✂ 0.00   **FUD** XXX   Q2 N1 80 📷

AMA: 2016,Jan,13; 2015,Jan,16; 2014,Jan,11; 2013,Dec,3; 2012,Feb,9-10

Radiology

76977 — 77011

76977 Bone Density Measurements: Ultrasound

CMS: 100-02,15,80.5.5 Frequency Standards; 100-04,13,30.1.3.1 Payment for Low Osmolar Contrast Material

INCLUDES Required permanent documentation of ultrasound images except when diagnostic purpose is biometric measurement
Written documentation

EXCLUDES Ultrasound exam that does not include thorough assessment of organ or site, recorded image, and written report

76977 **Ultrasound bone density measurement and interpretation, peripheral site(s), any method**

🔌 0.20   🔗 0.20   **FUD** XXX   S Z3 80 🖵

AMA: 2012,Feb,9-10

76998-76999 Imaging Guidance During Surgery: Ultrasound

INCLUDES Required permanent documentation of ultrasound images except when diagnostic purpose is biometric measurement
Written documentation

EXCLUDES Focused ultrasound ablation of uterine leiomyomata (0071T-0072T)
Ultrasound exam that does not include thorough assessment of organ or site, recorded image, and written report

76998 **Ultrasonic guidance, intraoperative**

EXCLUDES Ablation (47370-47382, 76940)
Destruction/reduction of malignant breast tumor (0301T)
Endovenous ablation therapy of incompetent vein (36475, 36479)
Ligation (37760-37761, 0249T)

🔌 0.00   🔗 0.00   **FUD** XXX   N N1 80 🖵

AMA: 2016,Jan,13; 2015,Aug,8; 2015,Jan,16; 2014,Oct,6; 2014,Jan,11; 2014,Jan,5; 2013,Jan,6-8; 2012,Feb,9-10

76999 **Unlisted ultrasound procedure (eg, diagnostic, interventional)**

🔌 0.00   🔗 0.00   **FUD** XXX   01 N1 80

AMA: 2016,Jan,13; 2015,Jan,16; 2014,Jan,11; 2012,Feb,9-10

77001-77022 Imaging Guidance Techniques

+ 77001 **Fluoroscopic guidance for central venous access device placement, replacement (catheter only or complete), or removal (includes fluoroscopic guidance for vascular access and catheter manipulation, any necessary contrast injections through access site or catheter with related venography radiologic supervision and interpretation, and radiographic documentation of final catheter position) (List separately in addition to code for primary procedure)**

INCLUDES Fluoroscopic guidance for needle placement (77002)

EXCLUDES Any procedure codes that include fluoroscopic guidance in the code descriptor
Extracorporeal membrane oxygenation (ECMO)/extracorporeal life support (ECLS) (33957-33959, [33962, 33963, 33964])
Formal extremity venography performed separately from venous access and interpreted separately (36005, 75820, 75822, 75825, 75827)
Code first primary procedure

🔌 1.98   🔗 1.98   **FUD** ZZZ   N N1 🖵

AMA: 2016,Jan,13; 2015,Jan,16; 2014,Jan,11; 2012,Feb,9-10; 2012,Jan,15-42; 2011,Jan,8; 2011,Jan,11

▲ + 77002 **Fluoroscopic guidance for needle placement (eg, biopsy, aspiration, injection, localization device) (List separately in addition to code for primary procedure)**

EXCLUDES Ablation therapy (20982-20983)
Any procedure codes that include fluoroscopic guidance in the code descriptor:
Corpora cavernosography (74445)
Insertion of gastrostomy tube (49440)
Placement of enteroclysis tube (74355)
Radiological guidance for percutaneous drainage by catheter (75989)
Renal cyst study (74470)
Shuntogram (75809-75810)
Transhepatic portography (75885, 75887)
Arthrography procedure(s) (70332, 73040, 73085, 73115, 73525, 73580, 73615, 74470)
Biopsy, breast, with placement of breast localization device(s) (19081-19086)
Image-guided fluid collection drainage by catheter (10030)
Placement of breast localization device(s) (19281-19288)
Platelet rich plasma injection(s) (0232T)
Thoracentesis (32554-32557)
Code first surgical procedure (10022, 10160, 20206, 20220, 20225, 20525-20526, 20550-20555, 20600, 20605, 20610, 20612, 20615, 21116, 21550, 23350, 24220, 25246, 27093-27095, 27370, 27648, 32400-32405, 32553, 36002, 38220-38221, 38505, 38794, 41019, 42400-42405, 47000-47001, 48102, 49180, 49411, 50200, 50390, 51100-51102, 55700, 55876, 60100, 62268-62269, 64505-64508, 64600-64605)

🔌 2.62   🔗 2.62   **FUD** XXX   N N1 🖵

AMA: 2016,Sep,9; 2016,Aug,7; 2016,Jun,3; 2016,Jan,9; 2016,Jan,13; 2015,Dec,3; 2015,Aug,6; 2015,Jul,8; 2015,Feb,6; 2015,Feb,10; 2015,Jan,16; 2014,Jan,11; 2013,Nov,9; 2012,Dec,9-10; 2012,Nov,3-5; 2012,Jun,14; 2012,Feb,11; 2012,Apr,19; 2012,Feb,9-10; 2012,Jan,15-42; 2011,Apr,12; 2011,Jan,11; 2011,Jan,8

▲ + 77003 **Fluoroscopic guidance and localization of needle or catheter tip for spine or paraspinous diagnostic or therapeutic injection procedures (epidural or subarachnoid) (List separately in addition to code for primary procedure)**

EXCLUDES Any procedure codes that include fluoroscopic guidance in the code descriptor
Arthrodesis (22586, 0195T-0196T, 0309T)
Image-guided fluid collection drainage by catheter (10030)
Injection of medication (subarachnoid/interlaminar epidural) (62320-62327)
Code first primary procedure (61050-61055, 62267, 62270-62273, 62280-62284, 64510, 64517, 64520, 64610)

🔌 2.41   🔗 2.41   **FUD** XXX   N N1 🖵

AMA: 2016,Jan,13; 2016,Jan,11; 2016,Jan,9; 2015,Jan,16; 2014,Jan,11; 2013,Dec,14; 2013,Nov,9; 2012,Sep,14-15; 2012,Sep,14-15; 2012,Jul,3-6; 2012,Jun,12-13; 2012,Feb,9-10; 2012,Jan,15-42; 2011,Jul,16-17; 2011,Mar,7; 2011,Feb,4-5; 2011,Jan,11; 2011,Jan,8

77011 **Computed tomography guidance for stereotactic localization**

EXCLUDES Arthrodesis (22586, 0195T-0196T, 0309T)

🔌 6.28   🔗 6.28   **FUD** XXX   N N1 🖵

AMA: 2016,Jan,13; 2015,Jan,16; 2014,Jan,11; 2012,Feb,9-10

77012 **Computed tomography guidance for needle placement (eg, biopsy, aspiration, injection, localization device), radiological supervision and interpretation**

EXCLUDES *Arthrodesis (22586, 0195T-0196T, 0309T)*
Destruction of paravertebral facet joint nerve by neurolysis ([64633, 64634, 64635, 64636])
Image-guided fluid collection drainage by catheter (10030)
Injection, paravertebral facet joint (64490-64495)
Platelet rich plasma injection(s) (0232T)
Sacroiliac joint arthrography (27096)
Thoracentesis (32554-32557)
Transforaminal epidural needle placement/injection (64479-64484)

🚑 3.52   ⚖ 3.52   **FUD** XXX   N N1 ▣

AMA: 2016,Jun,3; 2016,Jan,13; 2015,Dec,3; 2015,Feb,6; 2015,Jan,16; 2014,Jan,11; 2013,Nov,9; 2012,Dec,9-10; 2012,Nov,3-5; 2012,Sep,14-15; 2012,Sep,14-15; 2012,Jul,3-6; 2012,Feb,9-10; 2012,Jan,15-42; 2011,Apr,12; 2011,Feb,4-5

77013 **Computed tomography guidance for, and monitoring of, parenchymal tissue ablation**

EXCLUDES *Ablation therapy (20982-20983, 32998, 47382-47383, 50592-50593, 0340T)*

🚑 0.00   ⚖ 0.00   **FUD** XXX   N N1 80 ▣

AMA: 2016,Jan,13; 2015,Jul,8; 2015,Jan,16; 2014,Jan,11; 2012,Feb,9-10

77014 **Computed tomography guidance for placement of radiation therapy fields**

Code also placement of interstitial device(s) for radiation therapy guidance (31627, 32553, 49411, 55876)

🚑 3.32   ⚖ 3.32   **FUD** XXX   N N1 ▣

AMA: 2016,Feb,3; 2016,Jan,13; 2015,Apr,10; 2015,Jan,16; 2014,Jan,11; 2012,Feb,9-10

77021 **Magnetic resonance guidance for needle placement (eg, for biopsy, needle aspiration, injection, or placement of localization device) radiological supervision and interpretation**

EXCLUDES *Biopsy, breast, with placement of breast localization device(s) (19085)*
Image-guided fluid collection drainage by catheter (10030)
Placement of breast localization device(s) (19287)
Platelet rich plasma injection(s) (0232T)
Surgical procedure
Thoracentesis (32554-32557)

🚑 11.3   ⚖ 11.3   **FUD** XXX   N N1 ▣

AMA: 2016,Jun,3; 2016,Jan,13; 2015,Dec,3; 2015,Feb,6; 2015,Jan,16; 2014,Jan,11; 2013,Nov,9; 2012,Dec,9-10; 2012,Nov,3-5; 2012,Feb,9-10; 2011,Apr,12

77022 **Magnetic resonance guidance for, and monitoring of, parenchymal tissue ablation**

EXCLUDES *Ablation:*
Percutaneous radiofrequency (32998, 47382-47383, 50592-50593)
Pulmonary tumor (0340T)
Reduction or eradication of 1 or more bone tumors (20982-20983)
Uterine leiomyomata by focused ablation (0071T-0072T)

🚑 0.00   ⚖ 0.00   **FUD** XXX   N N1 80 ▣

AMA: 2016,Jan,13; 2015,Jul,8; 2015,Jan,16; 2014,Oct,6; 2014,Jan,11; 2012,Feb,9-10

77051-77067 Radiography: Breast

77051 ~~Computer-aided detection (computer algorithm analysis of digital image data for lesion detection) with further review for interpretation, with or without digitization of film radiographic images; diagnostic mammography (List separately in addition to code for primary procedure)~~

To report, see ~77065-77066

77052 ~~screening mammography (List separately in addition to code for primary procedure)~~

To report, see ~77067

77053 **Mammary ductogram or galactogram, single duct, radiological supervision and interpretation**

Code also injection procedure (19030)

🚑 1.64   ⚖ 1.64   **FUD** XXX   02 N1 ▣

AMA: 2016,Jan,13; 2015,Jan,16; 2014,Jan,11; 2012,Feb,9-10

77054 **Mammary ductogram or galactogram, multiple ducts, radiological supervision and interpretation**

🚑 2.16   ⚖ 2.16   **FUD** XXX   02 N1 ▣

AMA: 2016,Jan,13; 2015,Jan,16; 2014,Jan,11; 2012,Feb,9-10

77055 ~~Mammography; unilateral~~

To report, see ~77065

77056 ~~bilateral~~

To report, see ~77066

77057 ~~Screening mammography, bilateral (2-view study of each breast)~~

To report, see ~77067

77058 **Magnetic resonance imaging, breast, without and/or with contrast material(s); unilateral**

🚑 15.1   ⚖ 15.1   **FUD** XXX   B ▣

AMA: 2016,Jan,13; 2015,Jan,16; 2014,Jan,11; 2012,Feb,9-10

77059 **bilateral**

🚑 15.0   ⚖ 15.0   **FUD** XXX   B ▣

AMA: 2016,Jan,13; 2015,Jan,16; 2014,Jan,11; 2012,Feb,9-10

77061 **Digital breast tomosynthesis; unilateral**

🚑 0.00   ⚖ 0.00   **FUD** XXX   E ▣

EXCLUDES *3D rendering (76376-76377)*
Screening mammography (77067)

77062 **bilateral**

🚑 0.00   ⚖ 0.00   **FUD** XXX   E ▣

EXCLUDES *3D rendering (76376-76377)*
Screening mammography (77067)

+ 77063 **Screening digital breast tomosynthesis, bilateral (List separately in addition to code for primary procedure)**

🚑 1.56   ⚖ 1.56   **FUD** ZZZ   A ▣

EXCLUDES *3D rendering (76376-76377)*
Diagnostic mammography (77065-77066)
Code first (77067)

● **77065** **Diagnostic mammography, including computer-aided detection (CAD) when performed; unilateral**

● **77066** **bilateral**

● **77067** **Screening mammography, bilateral (2-view study of each breast), including computer-aided detection (CAD) when performed**

EXCLUDES *Breast scan, electrical impedance (76499)*

77071-77086 [77085, 77086] Additional Evaluations of Bones and Joints

77071 **Manual application of stress performed by physician or other qualified health care professional for joint radiography, including contralateral joint if indicated**

Code also interpretation of stressed images according to anatomical site and number of views

🚑 1.36   ⚖ 1.36   **FUD** XXX   01 N1 80 26 ▣

AMA: 2016,Jan,13; 2015,Jan,16; 2014,Jan,11; 2012,Feb,9-10

77072 **Bone age studies**

🚑 0.65   ⚖ 0.65   **FUD** XXX   01 N1 80 ▣

AMA: 2016,Jan,13; 2015,Jan,16; 2014,Jan,11; 2012,Feb,9-10

77073 **Bone length studies (orthoroentgenogram, scanogram)**

🚑 1.01   ⚖ 1.01   **FUD** XXX   01 N1 80 ▣

AMA: 2016,Jan,13; 2015,Jan,16; 2014,Jan,11; 2012,Feb,9-10

77074 Radiologic examination, osseous survey; limited (eg, for metastases)
1.81   1.81   **FUD** XXX   01 N1 80
AMA: 2016,Jan,13; 2015,Jan,16; 2014,Jan,11; 2012,Feb,9-10

77075 complete (axial and appendicular skeleton)
2.46   2.46   **FUD** XXX   01 N1 80
AMA: 2016,Jan,13; 2015,Jan,16; 2014,Jan,11; 2012,Feb,9-10

77076 Radiologic examination, osseous survey, infant
2.70   2.70   **FUD** XXX   01 N1 80
AMA: 2016,Jan,13; 2015,Jan,16; 2014,Jan,11; 2012,Feb,9-10

77077 Joint survey, single view, 2 or more joints (specify)
1.05   1.05   **FUD** XXX   01 N1 80
AMA: 2016,Jan,13; 2015,Jan,16; 2014,Jan,11; 2012,Feb,9-10

77078 Computed tomography, bone mineral density study, 1 or more sites, axial skeleton (eg, hips, pelvis, spine)
3.20   3.20   **FUD** XXX   S Z2 80
AMA: 2016,Jan,13; 2015,Jan,16; 2014,Jan,11; 2012,Feb,9-10

77080 Dual-energy X-ray absorptiometry (DXA), bone density study, 1 or more sites; axial skeleton (eg, hips, pelvis, spine)
EXCLUDES   *Dual-energy x-ray absorptiometry (DXA), bone density study ([77085])*
Vertebral fracture assessment via dual-energy x-ray absorptiometry (DXA) ([77086])
1.16   1.16   **FUD** XXX   S Z3 80
AMA: 2016,Jan,13; 2015,Jan,16; 2014,Jan,11; 2012,Feb,9-10

77081 appendicular skeleton (peripheral) (eg, radius, wrist, heel)
0.79   0.79   **FUD** XXX   S Z3 80
AMA: 2016,Jan,13; 2015,Jan,16; 2014,Jan,11; 2012,Feb,9-10

\#   **77085** axial skeleton (eg, hips, pelvis, spine), including vertebral fracture assessment
1.59   1.59   **FUD** XXX   01 N1 80
EXCLUDES   *Dual-energy x-ray absorptiometry (DXA), bone density study (77080)*
Vertebral fracture assessment via dual-energy x-ray absorptiometry (DXA) ([77086])

\#   **77086** Vertebral fracture assessment via dual-energy X-ray absorptiometry (DXA)
1.00   1.00   **FUD** XXX   01 N1 80
EXCLUDES   *Dual-energy x-ray absorptiometry (DXA), bone density study (77080)*
Therapy performed more than one time for treatment to a specific area
Vertebral fracture assessment via dual-energy X-ray absorptiometry (DXA) ([77085])

77084 Magnetic resonance (eg, proton) imaging, bone marrow blood supply
10.9   10.9   **FUD** XXX   S Z2 80
AMA: 2016,Jan,13; 2015,Jan,16; 2014,Jan,11; 2012,Feb,9-10

77085 Resequenced code. See code following 77081.

77086 Resequenced code. See code before 77084.

77261-77263 Therapeutic Radiology: Treatment Planning

INCLUDES   Determination of:
Appropriate treatment devices
Number and size of treatment ports
Treatment method
Treatment time/dosage
Treatment volume
Interpretation of special testing
Tumor localization
EXCLUDES   *Brachytherapy (0394T-0395T)*
Radiation treatment delivery, superficial (77401)

77261 Therapeutic radiology treatment planning; simple
INCLUDES   Planning for single treatment area included in a single port or simple parallel opposed ports with simple or no blocking
2.14   2.14   **FUD** XXX   B 80 26
AMA: 2016,Feb,3; 2016,Jan,13; 2015,Jan,16; 2014,Jan,11; 2012,Feb,9-10

77262 intermediate
INCLUDES   Planning for three or more converging ports, two separate treatment sites, multiple blocks, or special time dose constraints
3.20   3.20   **FUD** XXX   B 80 26
AMA: 2016,Feb,3; 2016,Jan,13; 2015,Jan,16; 2014,Jan,11; 2012,Feb,9-10

77263 complex
INCLUDES   Planning for very complex blocking, custom shielding blocks, tangential ports, special wedges or compensators, three or more separate treatment areas, rotational or special beam considerations, combination of treatment modalities
4.68   4.68   **FUD** XXX   B 80 26
AMA: 2016,Feb,3; 2016,Jan,13; 2015,Jan,16; 2014,Jan,11; 2012,Feb,9-10

77280-77299 Radiation Therapy Simulation

CMS: 100-04,4,200.3.1 Billing for IMRT Planning and Delivery

77280 Therapeutic radiology simulation-aided field setting; simple
INCLUDES   Simulation of a single treatment site
7.71   7.71   **FUD** XXX   S Z2 80
AMA: 2016,Jan,13; 2015,Apr,10; 2015,Jan,16; 2014,Jan,11; 2013,Nov,11; 2012,Feb,9-10; 2012,Jan,15-42; 2011,Jan,11

77285 intermediate
INCLUDES   Two different treatment sites
12.1   12.1   **FUD** XXX   S Z2 80
AMA: 2016,Jan,13; 2015,Apr,10; 2015,Jan,16; 2014,Jan,11; 2013,Nov,11; 2012,Feb,9-10

77290 complex
INCLUDES   Brachytherapy
Complex blocking
Contrast material
Custom shielding blocks
Hyperthermia probe verification
Rotation, arc or particle therapy
Simulation to ≥ 3 treatment sites
14.5   14.5   **FUD** XXX   S Z2 80
AMA: 2016,Sep,9; 2016,Jan,13; 2015,Apr,10; 2015,Jan,16; 2014,Jan,11; 2013,Nov,11; 2012,Feb,9-10; 2012,Jan,15-42; 2011,Jan,11

\+   **77293** Respiratory motion management simulation (List separately in addition to code for primary procedure)
Code first (77295, 77301)
13.1   13.1   **FUD** ZZZ   N 80
AMA: 2016,Jan,13; 2015,Dec,16; 2013,Nov,11

77295 Resequenced code. See code before 77300.

77299 Unlisted procedure, therapeutic radiology clinical treatment planning
0.00   0.00   **FUD** XXX   S Z2 80
AMA: 2016,Jan,13; 2015,Jan,16; 2014,Jan,11; 2013,Nov,11; 2012,Feb,9-10; 2012,Jan,15-42; 2011,Jan,11

77300-77370 [77295] Radiation Physics Services

CMS: 100-04,13,70.5 Radiation Physics Services

\#   **77295** 3-dimensional radiotherapy plan, including dose-volume histograms
13.8   13.8   **FUD** XXX   S Z3 80
AMA: 2016,Jan,13; 2015,Dec,16; 2015,Jun,6; 2015,Jan,16; 2014,Jan,11; 2013,Nov,11; 2012,Feb,9-10

| 26/TC PC/TC Only | A2-Z3 ASC Payment | 50 Bilateral | ♂ Male Only | ♀ Female Only | 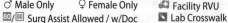 Facility RVU | Non-Facility RVU | CCI |
| FUD Follow-up Days | CMS: IOM (Pub 100) | A-Y OPPSI | 80/80 Surg Assist Allowed / w/Doc | | Lab Crosswalk | Radiology Crosswalk | CLIA |

328   CPT © 2016 American Medical Association. All Rights Reserved.   © 2016 Optum360, LLC

77300 Basic radiation dosimetry calculation, central axis depth dose calculation, TDF, NSD, gap calculation, off axis factor, tissue inhomogeneity factors, calculation of non-ionizing radiation surface and depth dose, as required during course of treatment, only when prescribed by the treating physician

> EXCLUDES *Brachytherapy (77316-77318, 77767-77772, 0394T-0395T)*
> *Teletherapy plan (77306-77307, 77321)*

🗇 1.88   ⚕ 1.88   **FUD** XXX   ⓢ Z3 80 ▣

AMA: 2016,Jan,13; 2015,Jan,16; 2014,Jan,11; 2013,Nov,11; 2012,Feb,9-10; 2012,Jan,15-42; 2011,Jan,11

77301 Intensity modulated radiotherapy plan, including dose-volume histograms for target and critical structure partial tolerance specifications

🗇 55.1   ⚕ 55.1   **FUD** XXX   ⓢ Z2 80 ▣

AMA: 2016,Jan,13; 2015,Jan,16; 2014,Jan,11; 2013,Nov,11; 2012,Feb,9-10; 2012,Jan,15-42; 2011,Jan,11

77306 Teletherapy isodose plan; simple (1 or 2 unmodified ports directed to a single area of interest), includes basic dosimetry calculation(s)

> EXCLUDES *Brachytherapy (0394T-0395T)*
> *Radiation dosimetry calculation (77300)*
> *Radiation treatment delivery (77401)*
> *Therapy performed more than one time for treatment to a specific area*

🗇 4.22   ⚕ 4.22   **FUD** XXX   ⓢ Z3 80 ▣

AMA: 2016,Feb,3

77307 complex (multiple treatment areas, tangential ports, the use of wedges, blocking, rotational beam, or special beam considerations), includes basic dosimetry calculation(s)

> EXCLUDES *Brachytherapy (0394T-0395T)*
> *Radiation dosimetry calculation (77300)*
> *Radiation treatment delivery (77401)*
> *Therapy performed more than one time for treatment to a specific area*

🗇 8.15   ⚕ 8.15   **FUD** XXX   ⓢ Z3 80 ▣

AMA: 2016,Feb,3

77316 Brachytherapy isodose plan; simple (calculation[s] made from 1 to 4 sources, or remote afterloading brachytherapy, 1 channel), includes basic dosimetry calculation(s)

> EXCLUDES *Brachytherapy (0394T-0395T)*
> *Radiation dosimetry calculation (77300)*
> *Radiation treatment delivery (77401)*

🗇 5.33   ⚕ 5.33   **FUD** XXX   ⓢ Z2 80 ▣

AMA: 2016,Feb,3

77317 intermediate (calculation[s] made from 5 to 10 sources, or remote afterloading brachytherapy, 2-12 channels), includes basic dosimetry calculation(s)

🗇 6.94   ⚕ 6.94   **FUD** XXX   ⓢ Z3 80 ▣

> EXCLUDES *Brachytherapy (0394T-0395T)*
> *Radiation dosimetry calculation (77300)*
> *Radiation treatment delivery (77401)*

77318 complex (calculation[s] made from over 10 sources, or remote afterloading brachytherapy, over 12 channels), includes basic dosimetry calculation(s)

> EXCLUDES *Brachytherapy (0394T-0395T)*
> *Radiation dosimetry calculation (77300)*
> *Radiation treatment delivery (77401)*

🗇 10.0   ⚕ 10.0   **FUD** XXX   ⓢ Z2 80 ▣

AMA: 2016,Feb,3

77321 Special teletherapy port plan, particles, hemibody, total body

🗇 2.62   ⚕ 2.62   **FUD** XXX   ⓢ Z3 80 ▣

AMA: 2016,Jan,13; 2015,Jan,16; 2014,Jan,11; 2013,Nov,11; 2012,Feb,9-10

77331 Special dosimetry (eg, TLD, microdosimetry) (specify), only when prescribed by the treating physician

🗇 1.80   ⚕ 1.80   **FUD** XXX   ⓢ Z3 80 ▣

AMA: 2016,Jan,13; 2015,Jun,6; 2015,Jan,16; 2014,Jan,11; 2013,Nov,11; 2012,Feb,9-10

77332 Treatment devices, design and construction; simple (simple block, simple bolus)

> EXCLUDES *Brachytherapy (0394T-0395T)*
> *Radiation treatment delivery (77401)*

🗇 2.34   ⚕ 2.34   **FUD** XXX   ⓢ Z3 80 ▣

AMA: 2016,Feb,3; 2016,Jan,13; 2015,Jan,16; 2014,Jan,11; 2013,Nov,11; 2012,Feb,9-10; 2012,Jan,15-42

77333 intermediate (multiple blocks, stents, bite blocks, special bolus)

> EXCLUDES *Brachytherapy (0394T-0395T)*
> *Radiation treatment delivery (77401)*

🗇 1.50   ⚕ 1.50   **FUD** XXX   ⓢ Z3 80 ▣

AMA: 2016,Feb,3; 2016,Jan,13; 2015,Jan,16; 2014,Jan,11; 2013,Nov,11; 2012,Feb,9-10

77334 complex (irregular blocks, special shields, compensators, wedges, molds or casts)

> EXCLUDES *Brachytherapy (0394T-0395T)*
> *Radiation treatment delivery (77401)*

🗇 4.31   ⚕ 4.31   **FUD** XXX   ⓢ Z3 80 ▣

AMA: 2016,Sep,9; 2016,Feb,3; 2016,Jan,13; 2015,Dec,16; 2015,Jan,16; 2014,Jan,11; 2013,Nov,11; 2012,Feb,9-10; 2012,Jan,15-42

77336 Continuing medical physics consultation, including assessment of treatment parameters, quality assurance of dose delivery, and review of patient treatment documentation in support of the radiation oncologist, reported per week of therapy

> EXCLUDES *Brachytherapy (0394T-0395T)*
> *Radiation treatment delivery (77401)*

🗇 2.24   ⚕ 2.24   **FUD** XXX   ⓢ Z2 80 TC ▣

AMA: 2016,Feb,3; 2016,Jan,13; 2015,Jan,16; 2014,Jan,11; 2013,Nov,11; 2012,Feb,9-10

77338 Multi-leaf collimator (MLC) device(s) for intensity modulated radiation therapy (IMRT), design and construction per IMRT plan

> EXCLUDES *Immobilization in IMRT treatment (77332-77334)*
> *Intensity modulated radiation treatment delivery (IMRT) (77385)*
> *Use of code more than one time per IMRT plan*

🗇 14.3   ⚕ 14.3   **FUD** XXX   ⓢ Z2 80 ▣

AMA: 2016,Jan,13; 2015,Jan,16; 2014,Jan,11; 2013,Nov,11; 2012,Feb,9-10; 2012,Jan,15-42; 2011,Jan,11

77370 Special medical radiation physics consultation

🗇 3.44   ⚕ 3.44   **FUD** XXX   ⓢ Z2 80 TC ▣

AMA: 2016,Feb,3; 2016,Jan,13; 2015,Jun,6; 2015,Jan,16; 2014,Jan,11; 2013,Nov,11; 2012,Feb,9-10; 2012,Jan,15-42; 2011,Jan,11

77371-77399 Stereotactic Radiosurgery (SRS) Planning and Delivery

CMS: 100-04,13,70.5 Radiation Physics Services

▲ **77371** Radiation treatment delivery, stereotactic radiosurgery (SRS), complete course of treatment of cranial lesion(s) consisting of 1 session; multi-source Cobalt 60 based

> EXCLUDES *Guidance with computed tomography for radiation therapy field placement (77014)*

🗇 0.00   ⚕ 0.00   **FUD** XXX   ⓙ 80 TC ▣

AMA: 2016,Jan,13; 2015,Jan,16; 2014,Jul,8; 2014,Jan,11; 2012,Feb,9-10; 2011,Jul,12-13

77372 **linear accelerator based**

    EXCLUDES   *Guidance with computed tomography for radiation therapy field placement (77014)*

        Radiation treatment supervision (77432)

    🚑 30.2   ⚕ 30.2   **FUD** XXX   J 80 TC 🔲

    AMA: 2016,Jan,13; 2015,Jan,16; 2014,Jul,8; 2014,Jan,11; 2012,Feb,9-10; 2011,Jul,12-13

77373 **Stereotactic body radiation therapy, treatment delivery, per fraction to 1 or more lesions, including image guidance, entire course not to exceed 5 fractions**

    EXCLUDES   *Guidance with computed tomography for radiation therapy field placement (77014)*

        Intensity modulated radiation treatment delivery (IMRT) (77385-77386)

        Radiation treatment delivery (77401-77402, 77407, 77412)

        Single fraction cranial lesion(s) (77371-77372)

    🚑 38.4   ⚕ 38.4   **FUD** XXX   S 80 TC 🔲

    AMA: 2016,Jan,13; 2015,Jun,6; 2015,Jan,16; 2014,Jul,8; 2014,Jan,11; 2012,Feb,9-10; 2011,Jul,12-13

77385 **Resequenced code. See code following 77417.**

77386 **Resequenced code. See code following 77417.**

77387 **Resequenced code. See code following 77417.**

77399 **Unlisted procedure, medical radiation physics, dosimetry and treatment devices, and special services**

    🚑 0.00   ⚕ 0.00   **FUD** XXX   S Z2 80 🔲

    AMA: 2016,Jan,13; 2015,Jan,16; 2014,Jan,11; 2012,Feb,9-10

77401-77417 [77385, 77386, 77387, 77424, 77425] Radiation Treatment

    INCLUDES   Technical component and assorted energy levels

77401 **Radiation treatment delivery, superficial and/or ortho voltage, per day**

    EXCLUDES   *Continuing medical physics consultation (77336)*

        Isodose plan:

            Brachytherapy (77316-77318)

            Teletherapy (77306-77307)

        Management of:

            Intraoperative radiation treatment (77469-77470)

            Radiation therapy (77431-77432)

            Radiation treatment (77427)

            Stereotactic body radiation therapy (77435)

        Stereotactic body radiation therapy, treatment delivery (77373)

        Therapeutic radiology treatment planning (77261-77263)

        Treatment devices, design and construction (77332-77334)

        Unlisted procedure, therapeutic radiology treatment management (77499)

    Code also E&M services when performed alone, as appropriate

    🚑 0.68   ⚕ 0.68   **FUD** XXX   S Z3 80 TC 🔲

    AMA: 2016,Feb,3; 2016,Jan,13; 2015,Dec,14; 2015,Jan,16; 2014,Jan,11; 2012,Feb,9-10

77402 **Radiation treatment delivery, ≥1 MeV; simple1 MeV; simple**

    EXCLUDES   *Stereotactic body radiation therapy, treatment delivery (77373)*

    🚑 0.00   ⚕ 0.00   **FUD** XXX   S Z2 80 TC 🔲

    AMA: 2016,Jun,9; 2016,Mar,7; 2016,Feb,3; 2016,Jan,13; 2015,Dec,14; 2015,Jan,16; 2014,Jan,11; 2012,Feb,9-10

77407 **intermediate**

    EXCLUDES   *Stereotactic body radiation therapy, treatment delivery (77373)*

    🚑 0.00   ⚕ 0.00   **FUD** XXX   S Z2 80 TC 🔲

    AMA: 2016,Jun,9; 2016,Mar,7; 2016,Feb,3; 2016,Jan,13; 2015,Dec,14; 2015,Jan,16; 2014,Jan,11; 2012,Feb,9-10

77412 **complex**

    EXCLUDES   *Stereotactic body radiation therapy, treatment delivery (77373)*

    🚑 0.00   ⚕ 0.00   **FUD** XXX   S Z2 80 TC 🔲

    AMA: 2016,Jun,9; 2016,Mar,7; 2016,Feb,3; 2016,Jan,13; 2015,Dec,14; 2015,Jan,16; 2014,Jan,11; 2012,Feb,9-10

77417 **Therapeutic radiology port image(s)**

    EXCLUDES   *Intensity modulated treatment planning (77301)*

    🚑 0.31   ⚕ 0.31   **FUD** XXX   N N1 80 TC 🔲

    AMA: 2016,Jan,13; 2015,Dec,14; 2015,Jan,16; 2014,Jan,11; 2012,Feb,9-10; 2012,Jan,15-42; 2011,Jan,11

\# **77385** **Intensity modulated radiation treatment delivery (IMRT), includes guidance and tracking, when performed; simple**

    EXCLUDES   *Radiation treatment delivery, stereotactic radiosurgery (SRS) (77371-77373)*

    Code also modifier 26 for professional component tracking and guidance with (77387)

    🚑 0.00   ⚕ 0.00   **FUD** XXX   S Z2 80 TC

    AMA: 2016,Feb,3

\# **77386** **complex**

    EXCLUDES   *Radiation treatment delivery, stereotactic radiosurgery (SRS) (77371-77373)*

    Code also modifier 26 for professional component tracking and guidance with (77387)

    🚑 0.00   ⚕ 0.00   **FUD** XXX   S Z2 80 TC

    AMA: 2016,Feb,3

\# **77387** **Guidance for localization of target volume for delivery of radiation treatment delivery, includes intrafraction tracking, when performed**

    EXCLUDES   *Guidance with computed tomography for radiation therapy field placement (77014)*

        Intensity modulated radiation treatment delivery (IMRT) (77385)

        Radiation treatment delivery, stereotactic radiosurgery (SRS) (77371-77373)

    🚑 0.00   ⚕ 0.00   **FUD** XXX   N N1 80

    AMA: 2016,Feb,3; 2016,Jan,13; 2015,Dec,16; 2015,Dec,14

\# **77424** **Intraoperative radiation treatment delivery, x-ray, single treatment session**

    🚑 0.00   ⚕ 0.00   **FUD** XXX   J Z2 🔲

    AMA: 2016,Jan,13; 2015,Dec,14; 2012,Feb,9-10

\# **77425** **Intraoperative radiation treatment delivery, electrons, single treatment session**

    🚑 0.00   ⚕ 0.00   **FUD** XXX   J Z2 🔲

    AMA: 2016,Jan,13; 2015,Dec,14; 2015,Jan,16; 2014,Jan,11; 2012,Feb,9-10

77422-77425 Neutron Therapy

77422 **High energy neutron radiation treatment delivery; single treatment area using a single port or parallel-opposed ports with no blocks or simple blocking**

    🚑 0.00   ⚕ 0.00   **FUD** XXX   S Z3 80 TC 🔲

    AMA: 2016,Jan,13; 2015,Dec,14; 2015,Jan,16; 2014,Jan,11; 2012,Feb,9-10

77423 **1 or more isocenter(s) with coplanar or non-coplanar geometry with blocking and/or wedge, and/or compensator(s)**

    🚑 0.00   ⚕ 0.00   **FUD** XXX   S Z3 80 TC 🔲

    AMA: 2016,Jan,13; 2015,Dec,14; 2015,Jan,16; 2014,Jan,11; 2012,Feb,9-10

77424 **Resequenced code. See code before 77422.**

77425 **Resequenced code. See code before 77422.**

77427-77499 Radiation Therapy Management

INCLUDES Assessment of patient for medical evaluation and management (at least one per treatment management service) that includes:
Coordination of care/treatment
Evaluation of patient's response to treatment
Review of:
Dose delivery
Dosimetry
Lab tests
Patient treatment set-up
Port film
Treatment parameters
X-rays
Units of five fractions or treatment sessions regardless of time. Two or more fractions performed on the same day can be counted separately provided there is a distinct break in service between sessions and the fractions are of the character usually furnished on different days.

EXCLUDES High dose rate electronic brachytherapy (0394T-0395T)
Radiation treatment delivery (77401)

77427   Radiation treatment management, 5 treatments

INCLUDES 3 or 4 fractions beyond a multiple of five at the end of a treatment period

EXCLUDES Use of code separately when one or two more fractions are provided beyond a multiple of five at the end of a course of treatment

🚗 5.24   ⚲ 5.24   **FUD** XXX   Ⓑ 26 🖩

AMA: 2016,Feb,3; 2016,Jan,13; 2015,Jun,6; 2015,Jan,16; 2014,Jan,11; 2012,Feb,9-10

77431   Radiation therapy management with complete course of therapy consisting of 1 or 2 fractions only

EXCLUDES Use of code when used to fill in the last week of a protracted therapy course

🚗 2.88   ⚲ 2.88   **FUD** XXX   Ⓑ 80 26 🖩

AMA: 2016,Feb,3; 2016,Jan,13; 2015,Jun,6; 2015,Jan,16; 2014,Jan,11; 2012,Feb,9-10

77432   Stereotactic radiation treatment management of cranial lesion(s) (complete course of treatment consisting of 1 session)

INCLUDES Guidance for localization of target volume for radiation delivery (professional component)

EXCLUDES Stereotactic body radiation therapy treatment (77432, 77435)
Stereotactic radiosurgery by same physician (61796-61800)

Code also technical component of guidance for localization of target volume by appending modifier TC to (77387)

🚗 11.8   ⚲ 11.8   **FUD** XXX   Ⓑ 80 26 🖩

AMA: 2016,Feb,3; 2016,Jan,13; 2015,Dec,14; 2015,Dec,16; 2015,Jun,6; 2015,Jan,16; 2014,Jul,8; 2014,Jan,11; 2012,Feb,9-10; 2012,Jan,15-42; 2011,Jul,12-13; 2011,Jan,11

77435   Stereotactic body radiation therapy, treatment management, per treatment course, to 1 or more lesions, including image guidance, entire course not to exceed 5 fractions

INCLUDES Guidance for localization of target volume for radiation delivery (professional component)

EXCLUDES Radiation treatment management (77435)
Stereotactic radiosurgery by same physician (32701, 63620-63621)

Code also technical component of guidance for localization of target volume by appending modifier TC to (77387)

🚗 17.8   ⚲ 17.8   **FUD** XXX   Ⓝ N1 80 26 🖩

AMA: 2016,Feb,3; 2016,Jan,13; 2015,Dec,14; 2015,Jun,6; 2015,Jan,16; 2014,Jan,11; 2012,Feb,9-10; 2012,Jan,15-42

77469   Intraoperative radiation treatment management

EXCLUDES Medical E&M services provided outside of the intraoperative treatment management

🚗 9.10   ⚲ 9.10   **FUD** XXX   Ⓑ 80 🖩

AMA: 2016,Feb,3; 2015,Jun,6; 2012,Feb,9-10

77470   Special treatment procedure (eg, total body irradiation, hemibody radiation, per oral or endocavitary irradiation)

EXCLUDES Daily or weekly patient management
Intraoperative radiation treatment delivery and management ([77424, 77425], 77469)
Procedure performed more than one time per course of therapy

🚗 4.41   ⚲ 4.41   **FUD** XXX   Ⓢ Z3 80 🖩

AMA: 2016,Feb,3; 2016,Jan,13; 2015,Jun,6; 2015,Jan,16; 2014,Jan,11; 2012,Feb,9-10

77499   Unlisted procedure, therapeutic radiology treatment management

🚗 0.00   ⚲ 0.00   **FUD** XXX   Ⓑ 80 🖩

AMA: 2016,Feb,3; 2016,Jan,13; 2015,Jun,6; 2015,Jan,16; 2014,Jan,11; 2012,Feb,9-10

77520-77525 Proton Therapy

EXCLUDES High dose rate electronic brachytherapy, per fraction (0394T-0395T)

77520   Proton treatment delivery; simple, without compensation

INCLUDES Single treatment site using:
Single nontangential/oblique port

🚗 0.00   ⚲ 0.00   **FUD** XXX   Ⓢ Z2 80 TC 🖩

AMA: 2016,Jan,13; 2015,Jan,16; 2014,Jan,11; 2012,Feb,9-10

77522   simple, with compensation

INCLUDES Single treatment site using:
Custom block with compensation
Single nontangential/oblique port

🚗 0.00   ⚲ 0.00   **FUD** XXX   Ⓢ Z2 80 TC 🖩

AMA: 2012,Feb,9-10

77523   intermediate

INCLUDES One or more treatment sites using:
One or more tangential/oblique ports with custom blocks and compensators OR
Two or more ports with custom blocks and compensators

🚗 0.00   ⚲ 0.00   **FUD** XXX   Ⓢ Z2 80 TC 🖩

AMA: 2016,Jan,13; 2015,Jan,16; 2014,Jan,11; 2012,Feb,9-10

77525   complex

INCLUDES One or more treatment sites using:
Two or more ports with matching or patching fields and custom blocks and compensators

🚗 0.00   ⚲ 0.00   **FUD** XXX   Ⓢ Z2 80 TC 🖩

AMA: 2012,Feb,9-10

77600-77620 Hyperthermia Treatment

CMS: 100-03,110.1 Hyperthermia for Treatment of Cancer

INCLUDES Interstitial insertion of temperature sensors
Management during the course of therapy
Normal follow-up care for three months after completion
Physics planning
Use of heat generating devices

EXCLUDES Initial E&M service
Radiation therapy treatment (77371-77373, 77401-77412, 77422-77423)

▲ **77600   Hyperthermia, externally generated; superficial (ie, heating to a depth of 4 cm or less)**

🚗 11.8   ⚲ 11.8   **FUD** XXX   Ⓢ Z2 80 🖩

AMA: 2016,Jan,13; 2015,Jan,16; 2014,Jan,11; 2013,Dec,16; 2012,Feb,9-10

▲ **77605   deep (ie, heating to depths greater than 4 cm)**

EXCLUDES Microwave thermotherapy of the breast (0301T)

🚗 22.5   ⚲ 22.5   **FUD** XXX   Ⓢ Z2 80 🖩

AMA: 2016,Jan,13; 2015,Jan,16; 2014,Jan,11; 2013,Dec,16; 2012,Feb,9-10

▲ **77610   Hyperthermia generated by interstitial probe(s); 5 or fewer interstitial applicators**

🚗 28.0   ⚲ 28.0   **FUD** XXX   Ⓢ Z2 80 🖩

AMA: 2016,Jan,13; 2015,Jan,16; 2014,Jan,11; 2013,Dec,16; 2012,Feb,9-10

▲ **77615**   **more than 5 interstitial applicators**
🔲 30.0   ⚖ 30.0   **FUD** XXX   Ⓢ Z2 80 🔲
AMA: 2016,Jan,13; 2015,Jan,16; 2014,Jan,11; 2013,Dec,16; 2012,Feb,9-10

77620   **Hyperthermia generated by intracavitary probe(s)**
🔲 10.8   ⚖ 10.8   **FUD** XXX   Ⓢ Z2 80 🔲
AMA: 2016,Jan,13; 2015,Jan,16; 2014,Jan,11; 2013,Dec,16; 2012,Feb,9-10

77750-77799 Brachytherapy

CMS: 100-04,13,70.4 Clinical Brachytherapy; 100-04,4,61.4.4 Billing for Brachytherapy Source Supervision, Handling and Loading Costs

INCLUDES Hospital admission and daily visits
EXCLUDES Placement of:
Heyman capsules (58346)
Ovoids and tandems (57155)

77750   **Infusion or instillation of radioelement solution (includes 3-month follow-up care)**
EXCLUDES Monoclonal antibody infusion (79403)
Nonantibody radiopharmaceutical therapy infusion without follow-up care (79101)
🔲 10.4   ⚖ 10.4   **FUD** 090   Ⓢ Z2 80 🔲
AMA: 2016,Jan,13; 2015,Jan,16; 2014,Jan,11; 2012,Feb,9-10

77761   **Intracavitary radiation source application; simple**
INCLUDES One to four sources/ribbons
EXCLUDES High dose rate electronic brachytherapy (0394T-0395T)
🔲 11.0   ⚖ 11.0   **FUD** 090   Ⓢ Z3 80 🔲
AMA: 2016,Jan,13; 2015,Jan,16; 2014,Jan,11; 2012,Feb,9-10; 2012,Jan,15-42; 2011,Jan,11

77762   **intermediate**
INCLUDES Five to ten sources/ribbons
EXCLUDES High dose rate electronic brachytherapy (0394T-0395T)
🔲 14.6   ⚖ 14.6   **FUD** 090   Ⓢ Z3 80 🔲
AMA: 2016,Jan,13; 2015,Jan,16; 2014,Jan,11; 2012,Feb,9-10

77763   **complex**
INCLUDES More than ten sources/ribbons
EXCLUDES High dose rate electronic brachytherapy (0394T-0395T)
🔲 20.7   ⚖ 20.7   **FUD** 090   Ⓢ Z3 80 🔲
AMA: 2016,Jan,13; 2015,Jan,16; 2014,Jan,11; 2012,Feb,9-10

77767   **Remote afterloading high dose rate radionuclide skin surface brachytherapy, includes basic dosimetry, when performed; lesion diameter up to 2.0 cm or 1 channel**
🔲 6.35   ⚖ 6.35   **FUD** XXX   Ⓢ Z2 80 🔲
EXCLUDES Basic radiation dosimetry calculation (77300)
High dose rate electronic brachytherapy (0394T-0395T)
Superficial non-brachytherapy superficial treatment delivery (77401)

77768   **lesion diameter over 2.0 cm and 2 or more channels, or multiple lesions**
🔲 9.95   ⚖ 9.95   **FUD** XXX   Ⓢ Z2 80 🔲
EXCLUDES Basic radiation dosimetry calculation (77300)
High dose rate electronic brachytherapy (0394T-0395T)
Superficial non-brachytherapy superficial treatment delivery (77401)

77770   **Remote afterloading high dose rate radionuclide interstitial or intracavitary brachytherapy, includes basic dosimetry, when performed; 1 channel**
🔲 9.06   ⚖ 9.06   **FUD** XXX   Ⓢ Z2 80 🔲
EXCLUDES Basic radiation dosimetry calculation (77300)
High dose rate electronic brachytherapy (0394T-0395T)
Superficial non-brachytherapy superficial treatment delivery (77401)

77771   **2-12 channels**
🔲 16.8   ⚖ 16.8   **FUD** XXX   Ⓢ Z2 80 🔲
EXCLUDES Basic radiation dosimetry calculation (77300)
High dose rate electronic brachytherapy (0394T-0395T)
Superficial non-brachytherapy superficial treatment delivery (77401)

77772   **over 12 channels**
🔲 25.7   ⚖ 25.7   **FUD** XXX   Ⓢ Z2 80 🔲
EXCLUDES Basic radiation dosimetry calculation (77300)
High dose rate electronic brachytherapy (0394T-0395T)
Superficial non-brachytherapy superficial treatment delivery (77401)

77778   **Interstitial radiation source application, complex, includes supervision, handling, loading of radiation source, when performed**
INCLUDES More than ten sources/ribbons
EXCLUDES High dose rate electronic brachytherapy (0394T-0395T)
Supervision, handling, loading of radiation source (77790)
🔲 22.0   ⚖ 22.0   **FUD** 000   Q3 Z3 80 🔲
AMA: 2016,Jan,13; 2015,Jan,16; 2014,Jan,11; 2012,Feb,9-10

77789   **Surface application of low dose rate radionuclide source**
EXCLUDES High dose rate electronic brachytherapy (0394T-0395T)
Radiation treatment delivery, superficial and/or ortho voltage (77401)
Remote afterloading high dose rate radionuclide skin surface brachytherapy (77767-77768)
🔲 3.38   ⚖ 3.38   **FUD** 000   Ⓢ Z3 80 🔲
AMA: 2016,Jan,13; 2015,Jan,16; 2014,Jan,11; 2012,Feb,9-10

77790   **Supervision, handling, loading of radiation source**
EXCLUDES Interstitial radiation source application, complex (77778)
🔲 0.42   ⚖ 0.42   **FUD** XXX   Ⓝ N1 80 TC 🔲
AMA: 2016,Jan,13; 2015,Jan,16; 2014,Jan,11; 2012,Feb,9-10

77799   **Unlisted procedure, clinical brachytherapy**
🔲 0.00   ⚖ 0.00   **FUD** XXX   Ⓢ Z2 80
AMA: 2016,Jan,13; 2015,Jan,16; 2014,Jan,11; 2012,Feb,9-10

78012-78099 Nuclear Radiology: Thyroid, Parathyroid, Adrenal

EXCLUDES Diagnostic services (see appropriate sections)
Follow-up care (see appropriate section)
Radioimmunoassays (82009-84999 [82652])
Code also radiopharmaceutical(s) and/or drug(s) supplied

78012   **Thyroid uptake, single or multiple quantitative measurement(s) (including stimulation, suppression, or discharge, when performed)**
🔲 2.30   ⚖ 2.30   **FUD** XXX   Ⓢ Z2 80 🔲
AMA: 2016,Jan,13; 2015,Jan,16; 2013,Jun,9-11

78013   **Thyroid imaging (including vascular flow, when performed);**
🔲 5.56   ⚖ 5.56   **FUD** XXX   Ⓢ Z2 80 🔲
AMA: 2016,Jan,13; 2015,Jan,16; 2013,Jun,9-11

78014   **with single or multiple uptake(s) quantitative measurement(s) (including stimulation, suppression, or discharge, when performed)**
🔲 7.04   ⚖ 7.04   **FUD** XXX   Ⓢ Z2 80 🔲
AMA: 2016,Jan,13; 2015,Jan,16; 2013,Jun,9-11

78015   **Thyroid carcinoma metastases imaging; limited area (eg, neck and chest only)**
🔲 6.41   ⚖ 6.41   **FUD** XXX   Ⓢ Z2 80 🔲
AMA: 2016,Jan,13; 2015,Jan,16; 2014,Jan,11; 2012,Feb,9-10

78016   **with additional studies (eg, urinary recovery)**
🔲 8.13   ⚖ 8.13   **FUD** XXX   Ⓢ Z2 80 🔲
AMA: 2016,Jan,13; 2015,Jan,16; 2014,Jan,11; 2012,Feb,9-10

78018   **whole body**
🔲 9.11   ⚖ 9.11   **FUD** XXX   Ⓢ Z2 80 🔲
AMA: 2016,Jan,13; 2015,Jan,16; 2014,Jan,11; 2012,Feb,9-10

+ **78020**   **Thyroid carcinoma metastases uptake (List separately in addition to code for primary procedure)**
Code first (78018)
🔲 2.43   ⚖ 2.43   **FUD** ZZZ   Ⓝ N1 80 🔲
AMA: 2016,Jan,13; 2015,Jan,16; 2014,Jan,11; 2012,Feb,9-10; 2012,Jan,15-42; 2011,Jan,11

78070 Parathyroid planar imaging (including subtraction, when performed);
🚗 8.73　⚕ 8.73　**FUD** XXX　Ⓢ Z2 80 🖥
AMA: 2016,Jan,13; 2015,Jan,16; 2014,Jan,11; 2012,Feb,9-10

78071 with tomographic (SPECT)
🚗 10.4　⚕ 10.4　**FUD** XXX　Ⓢ Z2 80 🖥

78072 with tomographic (SPECT), and concurrently acquired computed tomography (CT) for anatomical localization
🚗 12.0　⚕ 12.0　**FUD** XXX　Ⓢ Z2 80 🖥

78075 Adrenal imaging, cortex and/or medulla
🚗 12.4　⚕ 12.4　**FUD** XXX　Ⓢ Z2 80 🖥
AMA: 2016,Jan,13; 2015,Jan,16; 2014,Jan,11; 2012,Feb,9-10

78099 Unlisted endocrine procedure, diagnostic nuclear medicine
🚗 0.00　⚕ 0.00　**FUD** XXX　Ⓢ Z2 80
AMA: 2016,Jan,13; 2015,Jan,16; 2014,Jan,11; 2012,Feb,9-10

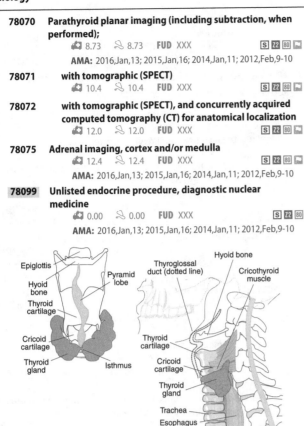

78102-78199 Nuclear Radiology: Blood Forming Organs

EXCLUDES　Diagnostic services (see appropriate sections)
Follow-up care (see appropriate section)
Radioimmunoassays (82009-84999 [82652])
Code also radiopharmaceutical(s) and/or drug(s) supplied

78102 Bone marrow imaging; limited area
🚗 4.94　⚕ 4.94　**FUD** XXX　Ⓢ Z2 80 🖥
AMA: 2016,Jan,13; 2015,Jan,16; 2014,Jan,11; 2012,Feb,9-10

78103 multiple areas
🚗 6.48　⚕ 6.48　**FUD** XXX　Ⓢ Z2 80 🖥
AMA: 2012,Feb,9-10

78104 whole body
🚗 7.14　⚕ 7.14　**FUD** XXX　Ⓢ Z2 80 🖥
AMA: 2012,Feb,9-10

78110 Plasma volume, radiopharmaceutical volume-dilution technique (separate procedure); single sampling
🚗 2.73　⚕ 2.73　**FUD** XXX　Ⓢ Z2 80 🖥
AMA: 2012,Feb,9-10

78111 multiple samplings
🚗 2.80　⚕ 2.80　**FUD** XXX　Ⓢ Z2 80 🖥
AMA: 2012,Feb,9-10

78120 Red cell volume determination (separate procedure); single sampling
🚗 2.73　⚕ 2.73　**FUD** XXX　Ⓢ Z2 80 🖥
AMA: 2012,Feb,9-10

78121 multiple samplings
🚗 2.97　⚕ 2.97　**FUD** XXX　Ⓢ Z2 80 🖥
AMA: 2012,Feb,9-10

78122 Whole blood volume determination, including separate measurement of plasma volume and red cell volume (radiopharmaceutical volume-dilution technique)
🚗 2.84　⚕ 2.84　**FUD** XXX　Ⓢ Z2 80 🖥
AMA: 2012,Feb,9-10

78130 Red cell survival study;
🚗 4.89　⚕ 4.89　**FUD** XXX　Ⓢ Z2 80 🖥
AMA: 2012,Feb,9-10

78135 differential organ/tissue kinetics (eg, splenic and/or hepatic sequestration)
🚗 10.2　⚕ 10.2　**FUD** XXX　Ⓢ Z2 80 🖥
AMA: 2012,Feb,9-10

78140 Labeled red cell sequestration, differential organ/tissue (eg, splenic and/or hepatic)
🚗 3.97　⚕ 3.97　**FUD** XXX　Ⓢ Z2 80 🖥
AMA: 2012,Feb,9-10

78185 Spleen imaging only, with or without vascular flow
EXCLUDES　Liver imaging (78215-78216)
🚗 6.17　⚕ 6.17　**FUD** XXX　Ⓢ Z2 80 🖥
AMA: 2012,Feb,9-10

78190 Kinetics, study of platelet survival, with or without differential organ/tissue localization
🚗 11.4　⚕ 11.4　**FUD** XXX　Ⓢ Z2 80 🖥
AMA: 2012,Feb,9-10

78191 Platelet survival study
🚗 4.89　⚕ 4.89　**FUD** XXX　Ⓢ Z2 80 🖥
AMA: 2012,Feb,9-10

78195 Lymphatics and lymph nodes imaging
EXCLUDES　Sentinel node identification without scintigraphy (38792)
Sentinel node removal (38500-38542)
🚗 10.3　⚕ 10.3　**FUD** XXX　Ⓢ Z2 80 🖥
AMA: 2016,Jan,13; 2015,Jan,16; 2014,Jan,11; 2012,Feb,9-10

78199 Unlisted hematopoietic, reticuloendothelial and lymphatic procedure, diagnostic nuclear medicine
🚗 0.00　⚕ 0.00　**FUD** XXX　Ⓢ Z2 80
AMA: 2016,Jan,13; 2015,Jan,16; 2014,Jan,11; 2012,Feb,9-10

78201-78299 Nuclear Radiology: Digestive System

EXCLUDES　Diagnostic services (see appropriate sections)
Follow-up care (see appropriate section)
Radioimmunoassays (82009-84999 [82652])
Code also radiopharmaceutical(s) and/or drug(s) supplied

78201 Liver imaging; static only
EXCLUDES　Spleen imaging only (78185)
🚗 5.47　⚕ 5.47　**FUD** XXX　Ⓢ Z2 80 🖥
AMA: 2016,Jan,13; 2015,Jan,16; 2014,Jan,11; 2012,Feb,9-10

78202 with vascular flow
EXCLUDES　Spleen imaging only (78185)
🚗 5.88　⚕ 5.88　**FUD** XXX　Ⓢ Z2 80 🖥
AMA: 2012,Feb,9-10

78205 Liver imaging (SPECT);
🚗 6.16　⚕ 6.16　**FUD** XXX　Ⓢ Z2 80 🖥
AMA: 2012,Feb,9-10

78206 with vascular flow
🚗 9.98　⚕ 9.98　**FUD** XXX　Ⓢ Z2 80 🖥
AMA: 2012,Feb,9-10

78215 Liver and spleen imaging; static only
🚗 5.67　⚕ 5.67　**FUD** XXX　Ⓢ Z2 80 🖥
AMA: 2012,Feb,9-10

78216 with vascular flow
🚗 3.66　⚕ 3.66　**FUD** XXX　Ⓢ Z2 80 🖥
AMA: 2012,Feb,9-10

78226 Hepatobiliary system imaging, including gallbladder when present;
🚗 9.67　⚕ 9.67　**FUD** XXX　Ⓢ Z2 80 🖥
AMA: 2012,Feb,9-10

78227 with pharmacologic intervention, including quantitative measurement(s) when performed
🚗 13.1　⚕ 13.1　**FUD** XXX　Ⓢ Z2 80 🖥
AMA: 2012,Feb,9-10

78230 **Salivary gland imaging;**
🚑 4.11 ⚕ 4.11 **FUD** XXX
⬜S ⬜Z2 ⬜80 ⬜
AMA: 2012,Feb,9-10

78231 **with serial images**
🚑 3.79 ⚕ 3.79 **FUD** XXX
⬜S ⬜Z2 ⬜80 ⬜
AMA: 2012,Feb,9-10

78232 **Salivary gland function study**
🚑 2.87 ⚕ 2.87 **FUD** XXX
⬜S ⬜Z2 ⬜80 ⬜
AMA: 2012,Feb,9-10

78258 **Esophageal motility**
🚑 6.46 ⚕ 6.46 **FUD** XXX
⬜S ⬜Z2 ⬜80 ⬜
AMA: 2012,Feb,9-10

78261 **Gastric mucosa imaging**
🚑 7.24 ⚕ 7.24 **FUD** XXX
⬜S ⬜Z2 ⬜80 ⬜
AMA: 2012,Feb,9-10

78262 **Gastroesophageal reflux study**
🚑 7.12 ⚕ 7.12 **FUD** XXX
⬜S ⬜Z2 ⬜80 ⬜
AMA: 2016,Jan,13; 2015,Dec,11; 2012,Feb,9-10

78264 **Gastric emptying imaging study (eg, solid, liquid, or both);**
EXCLUDES Procedure performed more than one time per study
🚑 9.75 ⚕ 9.75 **FUD** XXX
⬜S ⬜Z2 ⬜80 ⬜
AMA: 2016,Jan,13; 2015,Dec,11; 2012,Feb,9-10

78265 **with small bowel transit**
EXCLUDES Procedure performed more than one time per study
🚑 11.6 ⚕ 11.6 **FUD** XXX
⬜S ⬜Z2 ⬜80 ⬜
AMA: 2015,Dec,11;

78266 **with small bowel and colon transit, multiple days**
EXCLUDES Procedure performed more than one time per study
🚑 13.8 ⚕ 13.8 **FUD** XXX
⬜S ⬜Z2 ⬜80 ⬜
AMA: 2015,Dec,11

78267 **Urea breath test, C-14 (isotopic); acquisition for analysis**
EXCLUDES Breath hydrogen/methane test (91065)
🚑 0.00 ⚕ 0.00 **FUD** XXX
⬜A ⬜
AMA: 2016,Jan,13; 2015,Jan,16; 2014,Jan,11; 2012,Feb,9-10

78268 **analysis**
EXCLUDES Breath hydrogen/methane test (91065)
🚑 0.00 ⚕ 0.00 **FUD** XXX
⬜A ⬜
AMA: 2016,Jan,13; 2015,Jan,16; 2014,Jan,11; 2012,Feb,9-10

78270 **Vitamin B-12 absorption study (eg, Schilling test); without intrinsic factor**
🚑 2.94 ⚕ 2.94 **FUD** XXX
⬜S ⬜Z2 ⬜80 ⬜
AMA: 2012,Feb,9-10

78271 **with intrinsic factor**
🚑 2.62 ⚕ 2.62 **FUD** XXX
⬜S ⬜Z2 ⬜80 ⬜
AMA: 2012,Feb,9-10

78272 **Vitamin B-12 absorption studies combined, with and without intrinsic factor**
🚑 2.81 ⚕ 2.81 **FUD** XXX
⬜S ⬜Z2 ⬜80 ⬜
AMA: 2012,Feb,9-10

78278 **Acute gastrointestinal blood loss imaging**
🚑 10.1 ⚕ 10.1 **FUD** XXX
⬜S ⬜Z2 ⬜80 ⬜
AMA: 2012,Feb,9-10

78282 **Gastrointestinal protein loss**
🚑 0.00 ⚕ 0.00 **FUD** XXX
⬜S ⬜Z2 ⬜80 ⬜
AMA: 2012,Feb,9-10

78290 **Intestine imaging (eg, ectopic gastric mucosa, Meckel's localization, volvulus)**
🚑 9.73 ⚕ 9.73 **FUD** XXX
⬜S ⬜Z2 ⬜80 ⬜
AMA: 2012,Feb,9-10

78291 **Peritoneal-venous shunt patency test (eg, for LeVeen, Denver shunt)**
Code also (49427)
🚑 7.34 ⚕ 7.34 **FUD** XXX
⬜S ⬜Z2 ⬜80 ⬜
AMA: 2012,Feb,9-10

78299 **Unlisted gastrointestinal procedure, diagnostic nuclear medicine**
🚑 0.00 ⚕ 0.00 **FUD** XXX
⬜S ⬜Z2 ⬜80
AMA: 2016,Jan,13; 2015,Jan,16; 2014,Jan,11; 2012,Feb,9-10

78300-78399 Nuclear Radiology: Bones and Joints

EXCLUDES Diagnostic services (see appropriate sections)
Follow-up care (see appropriate section)
Radioimmunoassays (82009-84999 [82652])
Code also radiopharmaceutical(s) and/or drug(s) supplied

78300 **Bone and/or joint imaging; limited area**
🚑 5.27 ⚕ 5.27 **FUD** XXX
⬜S ⬜Z2 ⬜80 ⬜
AMA: 2016,Jan,13; 2015,Jan,16; 2014,Jan,11; 2012,Feb,9-10; 2012,Jan,15-42; 2011,Jan,11

78305 **multiple areas**
🚑 6.73 ⚕ 6.73 **FUD** XXX
⬜S ⬜Z2 ⬜80 ⬜
AMA: 2016,Jan,13; 2015,Jan,16; 2014,Jan,11; 2012,Feb,9-10

78306 **whole body**
🚑 7.35 ⚕ 7.35 **FUD** XXX
⬜S ⬜Z2 ⬜80 ⬜
AMA: 2016,Jan,13; 2015,Jan,16; 2014,Jan,11; 2012,Feb,9-10; 2012,Jan,15-42; 2011,Jan,11

78315 **3 phase study**
🚑 10.1 ⚕ 10.1 **FUD** XXX
⬜S ⬜Z2 ⬜80 ⬜
AMA: 2016,Jan,13; 2015,Jan,16; 2014,Jan,11; 2012,Feb,9-10; 2012,Jan,15-42; 2011,Jan,11

78320 **tomographic (SPECT)**
🚑 6.64 ⚕ 6.64 **FUD** XXX
⬜S ⬜Z2 ⬜80 ⬜
AMA: 2016,Jan,13; 2015,Jan,16; 2014,Jan,11; 2012,Feb,9-10; 2012,Jan,15-42; 2011,Jan,11

78350 **Bone density (bone mineral content) study, 1 or more sites; single photon absorptiometry**
🚑 0.93 ⚕ 0.93 **FUD** XXX
⬜E ⬜
AMA: 2012,Feb,9-10

78351 **dual photon absorptiometry, 1 or more sites**
🚑 0.43 ⚕ 0.43 **FUD** XXX
⬜E ⬜
AMA: 2012,Feb,9-10

78399 **Unlisted musculoskeletal procedure, diagnostic nuclear medicine**
🚑 0.00 ⚕ 0.00 **FUD** XXX
⬜S ⬜Z2 ⬜80
AMA: 2016,Jan,13; 2015,Jan,16; 2014,Jan,11; 2012,Feb,9-10

78414-78499 Nuclear Radiology: Heart and Vascular

EXCLUDES Diagnostic services (see appropriate sections)
Follow-up care (see appropriate section)
Radioimmunoassays (82009-84999 [82652])
Code also radiopharmaceutical(s) and/or drug(s) supplied

78414 **Determination of central c-v hemodynamics (non-imaging) (eg, ejection fraction with probe technique) with or without pharmacologic intervention or exercise, single or multiple determinations**
🚑 0.00 ⚕ 0.00 **FUD** XXX
⬜S ⬜Z2 ⬜80 ⬜
AMA: 2016,Jan,13; 2015,Jan,16; 2014,Jan,11; 2012,Feb,9-10

78428 **Cardiac shunt detection**
🚑 5.25 ⚕ 5.25 **FUD** XXX
⬜S ⬜Z2 ⬜80 ⬜
AMA: 2016,Jan,13; 2015,Jan,16; 2014,Jan,11; 2012,Feb,9-10

78445 **Non-cardiac vascular flow imaging (ie, angiography, venography)**
🚑 5.10 ⚕ 5.10 **FUD** XXX
⬜S ⬜Z2 ⬜80 ⬜
AMA: 2016,Jan,13; 2015,Jan,16; 2014,Jan,11; 2012,Feb,9-10

78451 **Myocardial perfusion imaging, tomographic (SPECT) (including attenuation correction, qualitative or quantitative wall motion, ejection fraction by first pass or gated technique, additional quantification, when performed); single study, at rest or stress (exercise or pharmacologic)**
Code also stress testing when performed (93015-93018)
🚑 9.94 ⚕ 9.94 **FUD** XXX
⬜S ⬜Z2 ⬜80 ⬜
AMA: 2016,Jan,13; 2015,Jan,16; 2014,Jan,11; 2012,Feb,9-10; 2012,Jan,15-42; 2011,Feb,8-9

26/TC PC/TC Only
FUD Follow-up Days
A2-Z3 ASC Payment
CMS: IOM (Pub 100)
50 Bilateral
A-Y OPPSI
♂ Male Only
80/80 Surg Assist Allowed / w/Doc
♀ Female Only
🚑 Facility RVU
⚕ Lab Crosswalk
Non-Facility RVU
Radiology Crosswalk
⬜ CCI
❌ CLIA
334
CPT © 2016 American Medical Association. All Rights Reserved.
© 2016 Optum360, LLC

78452 multiple studies, at rest and/or stress (exercise or pharmacologic) and/or redistribution and/or rest reinjection
Code also stress testing when performed (93015-93018)
🖼 13.7   ⚕ 13.7   **FUD** XXX   S Z2 80 ▢
AMA: 2016,Jan,13; 2015,Jan,16; 2014,Jan,11; 2012,Feb,9-10; 2012,Jan,15-42; 2011,Feb,8-9

78453 Myocardial perfusion imaging, planar (including qualitative or quantitative wall motion, ejection fraction by first pass or gated technique, additional quantification, when performed); single study, at rest or stress (exercise or pharmacologic)
Code also stress testing when performed (93015-93018)
🖼 8.86   ⚕ 8.86   **FUD** XXX   S Z2 80 ▢
AMA: 2016,Jan,13; 2015,Jan,16; 2014,Jan,11; 2012,Feb,9-10

78454 multiple studies, at rest and/or stress (exercise or pharmacologic) and/or redistribution and/or rest reinjection
Code also stress testing when performed (93015-93018)
🖼 12.7   ⚕ 12.7   **FUD** XXX   S Z2 80 ▢
AMA: 2016,Jan,13; 2015,Jan,16; 2014,Jan,11; 2012,Feb,9-10

78456 Acute venous thrombosis imaging, peptide
🖼 9.20   ⚕ 9.20   **FUD** XXX
AMA: 2016,Jan,13; 2015,Jan,16; 2014,Jan,11; 2012,Feb,9-10

78457 Venous thrombosis imaging, venogram; unilateral
🖼 5.48   ⚕ 5.48   **FUD** XXX
AMA: 2016,Jan,13; 2015,Jan,16; 2014,Jan,11; 2012,Feb,9-10

78458 bilateral
🖼 4.87   ⚕ 4.87   **FUD** XXX   S Z2 80 ▢
AMA: 2016,Jan,13; 2015,Jan,16; 2014,Jan,11; 2012,Feb,9-10

78459 Myocardial imaging, positron emission tomography (PET), metabolic evaluation
EXCLUDES   Myocardial perfusion studies (78491-78492)
🖼 0.00   ⚕ 0.00   **FUD** XXX   S Z2 80 ▢
AMA: 2016,Jan,13; 2015,Jan,16; 2014,Jan,11; 2012,Feb,9-10

78466 Myocardial imaging, infarct avid, planar; qualitative or quantitative
🖼 5.55   ⚕ 5.55   **FUD** XXX   S Z2 80 ▢
AMA: 2012,Feb,9-10

78468 with ejection fraction by first pass technique
🖼 5.76   ⚕ 5.76   **FUD** XXX   S Z2 80 ▢
AMA: 2016,Jan,13; 2015,Jan,16; 2014,Jan,11; 2012,Feb,9-10

78469 tomographic SPECT with or without quantification
EXCLUDES   Myocardial sympathetic innervation imaging (0331T-0332T)
🖼 6.59   ⚕ 6.59   **FUD** XXX   S Z2 80 ▢
AMA: 2016,Jan,13; 2015,Jan,16; 2014,Jan,11; 2012,Feb,9-10

78472 Cardiac blood pool imaging, gated equilibrium; planar, single study at rest or stress (exercise and/or pharmacologic), wall motion study plus ejection fraction, with or without additional quantitative processing
EXCLUDES   Cardiac blood pool imaging (78481, 78483, 78494)
   Myocardial perfusion imaging (78451-78454)
   Right ventricular ejection fraction by first pass technique (78496)
Code also stress testing when performed (93015-93018)
🖼 6.68   ⚕ 6.68   **FUD** XXX   S Z2 80 ▢
AMA: 2016,Jan,13; 2015,Jan,16; 2014,Jan,11; 2012,Feb,9-10

78473 multiple studies, wall motion study plus ejection fraction, at rest and stress (exercise and/or pharmacologic), with or without additional quantification
EXCLUDES   Cardiac blood pool imaging (78481, 78483, 78494)
   Myocardial perfusion imaging (78451-78454)
Code also stress testing when performed (93015-93018)
🖼 8.41   ⚕ 8.41   **FUD** XXX   S Z2 80 ▢
AMA: 2016,Jan,13; 2015,Jan,16; 2014,Jan,11; 2012,Feb,9-10

78481 Cardiac blood pool imaging (planar), first pass technique; single study, at rest or with stress (exercise and/or pharmacologic), wall motion study plus ejection fraction, with or without quantification
EXCLUDES   Myocardial perfusion imaging (78451-78454)
Code also stress testing when performed (93015-93018)
🖼 5.07   ⚕ 5.07   **FUD** XXX   S Z2 80 ▢
AMA: 2016,Jan,13; 2015,Jan,16; 2014,Jan,11; 2012,Feb,9-10

78483 multiple studies, at rest and with stress (exercise and/or pharmacologic), wall motion study plus ejection fraction, with or without quantification
EXCLUDES   Blood flow studies of the brain (78610)
   Myocardial perfusion imaging (78451-78454)
Code also stress testing when performed (93015-93018)
🖼 7.02   ⚕ 7.02   **FUD** XXX   S Z2 80 ▢
AMA: 2016,Jan,13; 2015,Jan,16; 2014,Jan,11; 2012,Feb,9-10

78491 Myocardial imaging, positron emission tomography (PET), perfusion; single study at rest or stress
Code also stress testing when performed (93015-93018)
🖼 0.00   ⚕ 0.00   **FUD** XXX   S Z2 80 ▢
AMA: 2016,Jan,13; 2015,Jan,16; 2014,Jan,11; 2012,Feb,9-10

78492 multiple studies at rest and/or stress
Code also stress testing when performed (93015-93018)
🖼 0.00   ⚕ 0.00   **FUD** XXX   S Z2 80 ▢
AMA: 2016,Jan,13; 2015,Jan,16; 2014,Jan,11; 2012,Feb,9-10

78494 Cardiac blood pool imaging, gated equilibrium, SPECT, at rest, wall motion study plus ejection fraction, with or without quantitative processing
🖼 6.54   ⚕ 6.54   **FUD** XXX   S Z2 80 ▢
AMA: 2016,Jan,13; 2015,Jan,16; 2014,Jan,11; 2012,Feb,9-10

+ **78496** Cardiac blood pool imaging, gated equilibrium, single study, at rest, with right ventricular ejection fraction by first pass technique (List separately in addition to code for primary procedure)
Code first (78472)
🖼 1.28   ⚕ 1.28   **FUD** ZZZ   N 51 80 ▢
AMA: 2016,Jan,13; 2015,Jan,16; 2014,Jan,11; 2012,Feb,9-10; 2012,Jan,15-42; 2011,Jan,11

78499 Unlisted cardiovascular procedure, diagnostic nuclear medicine
🖼 0.00   ⚕ 0.00   **FUD** XXX   S Z2 80
AMA: 2016,Jan,13; 2015,Jan,16; 2014,Jan,11; 2012,Feb,9-10

78579-78599 Nuclear Radiology: Lungs

EXCLUDES   Diagnostic services (see appropriate sections)
   Follow-up care (see appropriate sections)
   Radioimmunoassays (82009-84999 [82652])
Code also radiopharmaceutical(s) and/or drug(s) supplied

78579 Pulmonary ventilation imaging (eg, aerosol or gas)
EXCLUDES   Procedure performed more than one time per imaging session
🖼 5.44   ⚕ 5.44   **FUD** XXX   S Z2 80 ▢
AMA: 2012,Feb,9-10

78580 Pulmonary perfusion imaging (eg, particulate)
EXCLUDES   Myocardial perfusion imaging (78451-78454)
   Procedure performed more than one time per imaging session
🖼 6.98   ⚕ 6.98   **FUD** XXX   S Z2 80 ▢
AMA: 2016,Jan,13; 2015,Jan,16; 2014,Jan,11; 2012,Feb,9-10

78582 Pulmonary ventilation (eg, aerosol or gas) and perfusion imaging
EXCLUDES   Myocardial perfusion imaging (78451-78454)
   Procedure performed more than one time per imaging session
🖼 9.77   ⚕ 9.77   **FUD** XXX   S Z2 80 ▢
AMA: 2012,Feb,9-10

● New Code   ▲ Revised Code   ○ Reinstated   ● New Web Release   ▲ Revised Web Release   Unlisted   Not Covered   # Resequenced
Ⓢ AMA Mod 51 Exempt   ⑤ Optum Mod 51 Exempt   ⑥ Mod 63 Exempt   ✗ Non-FDA Drug   ★ Telehealth   M Maternity   A Age Edit   + Add-on   **AMA:** CPT Asst

78597 Quantitative differential pulmonary perfusion, including imaging when performed

> EXCLUDES Myocardial perfusion imaging (78451-78454)
> Procedure performed more than one time per imaging session

🚑 5.89   ⚖ 5.89   **FUD** XXX   [S] [Z2] [80] [📠]

AMA: 2012,Feb,9-10

78598 Quantitative differential pulmonary perfusion and ventilation (eg, aerosol or gas), including imaging when performed

> EXCLUDES Myocardial perfusion imaging (78451-78454)
> Procedure performed more than one time per imaging session

🚑 8.95   ⚖ 8.95   **FUD** XXX   [S] [Z2] [80] [📠]

AMA: 2012,Feb,9-10

78599 Unlisted respiratory procedure, diagnostic nuclear medicine

🚑 0.00   ⚖ 0.00   **FUD** XXX   [S] [Z2] [80]

AMA: 2016,Jan,13; 2015,Jan,16; 2014,Jan,11; 2012,Feb,9-10

78600-78650 Nuclear Radiology: Brain/Cerebrospinal Fluid

EXCLUDES Diagnostic services (see appropriate sections)
Follow-up care (see appropriate section)
Radioimmunoassays (82009-84999 [82652])
Code also radiopharmaceutical(s) and/or drug(s) supplied

78600 Brain imaging, less than 4 static views;

🚑 5.40   ⚖ 5.40   **FUD** XXX   [S] [Z2] [80] [📠]

AMA: 2016,Jan,13; 2015,Jan,16; 2014,Jan,11; 2012,Feb,9-10

Diagram of tomography principal (left)

X-ray beam
Plane of study
Focal point
Detection plate

Schematic of frontal coronal CT section of skull

78601 with vascular flow

🚑 6.23   ⚖ 6.23   **FUD** XXX   [S] [Z2] [80] [📠]

AMA: 2012,Feb,9-10

78605 Brain imaging, minimum 4 static views;

🚑 5.80   ⚖ 5.80   **FUD** XXX   [S] [Z2] [80] [📠]

AMA: 2012,Feb,9-10

78606 with vascular flow

🚑 9.65   ⚖ 9.65   **FUD** XXX   [S] [Z2] [80] [📠]

AMA: 2012,Feb,9-10

78607 Brain imaging, tomographic (SPECT)

🚑 10.2   ⚖ 10.2   **FUD** XXX   [S] [Z2] [80] [📠]

AMA: 2012,Feb,9-10

78608 Brain imaging, positron emission tomography (PET); metabolic evaluation

🚑 0.00   ⚖ 0.00   **FUD** XXX   [S] [Z2] [80] [📠]

AMA: 2012,Feb,9-10

78609 perfusion evaluation

🚑 2.11   ⚖ 2.11   **FUD** XXX   [E] [📠]

AMA: 2012,Feb,9-10

78610 Brain imaging, vascular flow only

🚑 5.10   ⚖ 5.10   **FUD** XXX   [S] [Z2] [80] [📠]

AMA: 2012,Feb,9-10

78630 Cerebrospinal fluid flow, imaging (not including introduction of material); cisternography

Code also injection procedure (61000-61070, 62270-62327)

🚑 9.87   ⚖ 9.87   **FUD** XXX   [S] [Z2] [80] [📠]

AMA: 2012,Feb,9-10

78635 ventriculography

Code also injection procedure (61000-61070, 62270-62294)

🚑 9.88   ⚖ 9.88   **FUD** XXX   [S] [Z2] [60] [📠]

AMA: 2012,Feb,9-10

78645 shunt evaluation

Code also injection procedure (61000-61070, 62270-62294)

🚑 9.41   ⚖ 9.41   **FUD** XXX   [S] [Z2] [80] [📠]

AMA: 2012,Feb,9-10

78647 tomographic (SPECT)

🚑 10.2   ⚖ 10.2   **FUD** XXX   [S] [Z2] [80] [📠]

AMA: 2012,Feb,9-10

78650 Cerebrospinal fluid leakage detection and localization

Code also injection procedure (61000-61070, 62270-62294)

🚑 9.60   ⚖ 9.60   **FUD** XXX   [S] [Z2] [80] [📠]

AMA: 2012,Feb,9-10

78660-78699 Nuclear Radiology: Lacrimal Duct System

Code also radiopharmaceutical(s) and/or drug(s) supplied

78660 Radiopharmaceutical dacryocystography

🚑 5.25   ⚖ 5.25   **FUD** XXX   [S] [Z2] [80] [📠]

AMA: 2012,Feb,9-10

78699 Unlisted nervous system procedure, diagnostic nuclear medicine

🚑 0.00   ⚖ 0.00   **FUD** XXX   [S] [Z2] [80]

AMA: 2016,Jan,13; 2015,Jan,16; 2014,Jan,11; 2012,Feb,9-10

78700-78725 Nuclear Radiology: Renal Anatomy and Function

EXCLUDES Diagnostic services (see appropriate sections)
Follow-up care (see appropriate section)
Radioimmunoassays (82009-84999 [82652])
Renal endoscopy with insertion of radioactive substances (77778)
Code also radiopharmaceutical(s) and/or drug(s) supplied

78700 Kidney imaging morphology;

🚑 5.01   ⚖ 5.01   **FUD** XXX   [S] [Z2] [80] [📠]

AMA: 2016,Jan,13; 2015,Jan,16; 2014,Jan,11; 2012,Feb,9-10

78701 with vascular flow

🚑 6.14   ⚖ 6.14   **FUD** XXX   [S] [Z2] [80] [📠]

AMA: 2012,Feb,9-10

78707 with vascular flow and function, single study without pharmacological intervention

🚑 6.77   ⚖ 6.77   **FUD** XXX   [S] [Z2] [80] [📠]

AMA: 2016,Jan,13; 2015,Jan,16; 2014,Jan,11; 2012,Feb,9-10

78708 with vascular flow and function, single study, with pharmacological intervention (eg, angiotensin converting enzyme inhibitor and/or diuretic)

🚑 5.06   ⚖ 5.06   **FUD** XXX   [S] [Z2] [80] [📠]

AMA: 2016,Jan,13; 2015,Jan,16; 2014,Jan,11; 2012,Feb,9-10

78709 with vascular flow and function, multiple studies, with and without pharmacological intervention (eg, angiotensin converting enzyme inhibitor and/or diuretic)

🚑 10.5   ⚖ 10.5   **FUD** XXX   [S] [Z2] [80] [📠]

AMA: 2016,Jan,13; 2015,Jan,16; 2014,Jan,11; 2012,Feb,9-10

78710 tomographic (SPECT)

🚑 5.83   ⚖ 5.83   **FUD** XXX   [S] [Z2] [80] [📠]

AMA: 2016,Jan,13; 2015,Jan,16; 2014,Jan,11; 2012,Feb,9-10

78725 Kidney function study, non-imaging radioisotopic study

🚑 3.16   ⚖ 3.16   **FUD** XXX   [S] [Z2] [80] [📠]

AMA: 2012,Feb,9-10

78730-78799 Nuclear Radiology: Urogenital

EXCLUDES Diagnostic services (see appropriate sections)
Follow-up care (see appropriate section)
Radioimmunoassays (82009-84999 [82652])
Code also radiopharmaceutical(s) and/or drug(s) supplied

+ **78730** Urinary bladder residual study (List separately in addition to code for primary procedure)

> EXCLUDES Measurement of postvoid residual urine and/or bladder capacity using ultrasound (51798)
> Ultrasound imaging of the bladder only with measurement of postvoid residual urine (76857)

Code first (78740)

🚑 2.22   ⚖ 2.22   **FUD** ZZZ   [N] [N1] [80] [📠]

AMA: 2016,Jan,13; 2015,Jan,16; 2014,Jan,11; 2012,Feb,9-10

78740 Ureteral reflux study (radiopharmaceutical voiding cystogram)

> EXCLUDES *Catheterization (51701-51703)*

Code also urinary bladder residual study (78730)

🔲 6.35   🔲 6.35   FUD XXX   [S] [Z2] [80]

AMA: 2012,Feb,9-10

78761 Testicular imaging with vascular flow ♂

🔲 6.08   🔲 6.08   FUD XXX   [S] [Z2] [80]

AMA: 2016,Jan,13; 2015,Jan,16; 2014,Jan,11; 2012,Feb,9-10

78799 Unlisted genitourinary procedure, diagnostic nuclear medicine

🔲 0.00   🔲 0.00   FUD XXX   [S] [Z2] [80]

AMA: 2016,Jan,13; 2015,Jan,16; 2014,Jan,11; 2012,Feb,9-10

78800-78804 Nuclear Radiology: Tumor Localization

Code also radiopharmaceutical(s) and/or drug(s) supplied

78800 Radiopharmaceutical localization of tumor or distribution of radiopharmaceutical agent(s); limited area

> INCLUDES Ocular radiophosphorus tumor identification

> EXCLUDES *Specific organ (see appropriate site)*

🔲 5.57   🔲 5.57   FUD XXX   [S] [Z2] [80] [▢]

AMA: 2016,Jan,13; 2015,Jan,16; 2014,Jan,11; 2012,Feb,9-10; 2012,Jan,15-42; 2011,Dec,14-18

78801 multiple areas

🔲 7.60   🔲 7.60   FUD XXX   [S] [Z2] [80] [▢]

AMA: 2016,Jan,13; 2015,Jan,16; 2014,Jan,11; 2012,Feb,9-10; 2012,Jan,15-42; 2011,Dec,14-18

78802 whole body, single day imaging

🔲 9.47   🔲 9.47   FUD XXX   [S] [Z2] [80] [▢]

AMA: 2012,Feb,9-10

78803 tomographic (SPECT)

🔲 9.91   🔲 9.91   FUD XXX   [S] [Z2] [80] [▢]

AMA: 2016,Jan,13; 2015,Oct,9; 2012,Feb,9-10

78804 whole body, requiring 2 or more days imaging

🔲 16.5   🔲 16.5   FUD XXX   [S] [Z2] [80] [▢]

AMA: 2012,Feb,9-10

78805-78807 Nuclear Radiology: Inflammation and Infection

> EXCLUDES *Imaging bone infectious or inflammatory disease with bone imaging radiopharmaceutical (78300, 78305-78306)*

Code also radiopharmaceutical(s) and/or drug(s) supplied

78805 Radiopharmaceutical localization of inflammatory process; limited area

🔲 5.31   🔲 5.31   FUD XXX   [S] [Z2] [80] [▢]

AMA: 2016,Jan,13; 2015,Jan,16; 2014,Jan,11; 2012,Feb,9-10

78806 whole body

🔲 9.71   🔲 9.71   FUD XXX   [S] [Z2] [80] [▢]

AMA: 2016,Jan,13; 2015,Jan,16; 2014,Jan,11; 2012,Feb,9-10

78807 tomographic (SPECT)

🔲 9.91   🔲 9.91   FUD XXX   [S] [Z2] [80] [▢]

AMA: 2012,Feb,9-10

78808 Intravenous Injection for Radiopharmaceutical Localization

Code also radiopharmaceutical(s) and/or drug(s) supplied

78808 Injection procedure for radiopharmaceutical localization by non-imaging probe study, intravenous (eg, parathyroid adenoma)

> EXCLUDES *Identification of sentinel node (38792)*

🔲 1.31   🔲 1.31   FUD XXX   [Q1] [N1] [80] [▢]

AMA: 2012,Feb,9-10

78811-78999 Nuclear Radiology: Diagnosis, Staging, Restaging or Monitoring Cancer

CMS: 100-03,220.6.17 Positron Emission Tomography (FDG) for Oncologic Conditions; 100-03,220.6.19 NaF-18 PET to Identify Bone Metastasis of Cancer; 100-03,220.6.9 FDG PET for Refractory Seizures; 100-04,13,60 Positron Emission Tomography (PET) Scans - General Information; 100-04,13,60.13 Billing for PET Scans for Specific Indications of Cervical Cancer; 100-04,13,60.15 Billing for CMS-Approved Clinical Trials for PET Scans; 100-04,13,60.16 Billing and Coverage for PET Scans; 100-04,13,60.17 Billing and Coverage Changes for PET Scans for Cervical Cancer; 100-04,13,60.18 Billing and Coverage for PET (NaF-18) Scans to Identify Bone Metastasis; 100-04,13,60.2 Use of Gamma Cameras, Full and Partial Ring PET Scanners; 100-04,13,60.3 PET Scan Qualifying Conditions; 100-04,13,60.3.1 Appropriate Codes for PET Scans; 100-04,13,60.3.2 Tracer Codes Required for PET Scans

> EXCLUDES *CT scan performed for other than attenuation correction and anatomical localization (report with the appropriate site-specific CT code and modifier 59)*
> *Ocular radiophosphorus tumor identification (78800)*
> *PET brain scan (78608-78609)*
> *PET myocardial imaging (78459, 78491-78492)*
> *Procedure performed more than one time per imaging session*

Code also radiopharmaceutical(s) and/or drug(s) supplied

78811 Positron emission tomography (PET) imaging; limited area (eg, chest, head/neck)

🔲 0.00   🔲 0.00   FUD XXX   [S] [Z2] [80] [▢]

AMA: 2016,Jan,13; 2015,Jan,16; 2014,Jan,11; 2012,Feb,9-10

78812 skull base to mid-thigh

🔲 0.00   🔲 0.00   FUD XXX   [S] [Z2] [80] [▢]

AMA: 2016,Jan,13; 2015,Jan,16; 2014,Jan,11; 2013,Feb,16-17; 2012,Feb,9-10

78813 whole body

🔲 0.00   🔲 0.00   FUD XXX   [S] [Z2] [80] [▢]

AMA: 2016,Jan,13; 2015,Jan,16; 2014,Jan,11; 2013,Feb,16-17; 2012,Feb,9-10

78814 Positron emission tomography (PET) with concurrently acquired computed tomography (CT) for attenuation correction and anatomical localization imaging; limited area (eg, chest, head/neck)

🔲 0.00   🔲 0.00   FUD XXX   [S] [Z2] [80] [▢]

AMA: 2016,Jan,13; 2015,Jan,16; 2014,Jan,11; 2013,Feb,16-17; 2012,Feb,9-10; 2012,Jan,15-42; 2011,Jan,11

78815 skull base to mid-thigh

🔲 0.00   🔲 0.00   FUD XXX   [S] [Z2] [80] [▢]

AMA: 2016,Jan,13; 2015,Jan,16; 2014,Jan,11; 2013,Feb,16-17; 2012,Feb,9-10; 2012,Jan,15-42; 2011,Jan,11

78816 whole body

🔲 0.00   🔲 0.00   FUD XXX   [S] [Z2] [80] [▢]

AMA: 2016,Jan,13; 2015,Jan,16; 2014,Jan,11; 2013,Feb,16-17; 2012,Feb,9-10; 2012,Jan,15-42; 2011,Jan,11

78999 Unlisted miscellaneous procedure, diagnostic nuclear medicine

🔲 0.00   🔲 0.00   FUD XXX   [S] [Z2] [80]

AMA: 2016,Jan,13; 2015,Oct,9; 2015,Jan,16; 2014,Jan,11; 2012,Feb,9-10

79005-79999 Systemic Radiopharmaceutical Therapy

> EXCLUDES *Imaging guidance*
> *Injection into artery, body cavity, or joint (see appropriate injection codes)*
> *Radiological supervision and interpretation*

79005 Radiopharmaceutical therapy, by oral administration

> EXCLUDES *Monoclonal antibody treatment (79403)*

🔲 3.89   🔲 3.89   FUD XXX   [S] [Z3] [80] [▢]

AMA: 2016,Jan,13; 2015,Jan,16; 2014,Jan,11; 2012,Feb,9-10

79101 Radiopharmaceutical therapy, by intravenous administration

> EXCLUDES *Administration of nonantibody radioelement solution including follow-up care (77750)*
> *Hydration infusion (96360)*
> *Intravenous injection, IV push (96374-96375, 96409)*
> *Radiolabeled monoclonal antibody IV infusion (79403)*
> *Venipuncture (36400, 36410)*

🔲 4.06   🔲 4.06   FUD XXX   [S] [Z3] [80] [▢]

AMA: 2016,Jan,13; 2015,Jan,16; 2014,Jan,11; 2012,Feb,9-10

● New Code   ▲ Revised Code   ○ Reinstated   ● New Web Release   ▲ Revised Web Release   Unlisted   Not Covered   # Resequenced
⊘ AMA Mod 51 Exempt   ⑨ Optum Mod 51 Exempt   ⑥⑨ Mod 63 Exempt   ⁄ Non-FDA Drug   ★ Telehealth   [M] Maternity   [A] Age Edit   + Add-on   AMA: CPT Asst

79200 **Radiopharmaceutical therapy, by intracavitary administration**
    📷 4.54   🔬 4.54 **FUD** XXX   S Z3 80 ▣
    AMA: 2016,Jan,13; 2015,Jan,16; 2014,Jan,11; 2012,Feb,9-10

79300 **Radiopharmaceutical therapy, by interstitial radioactive colloid administration**
    📷 0.00   🔬 0.00 **FUD** XXX   S Z2 80 ▣
    AMA: 2016,Jan,13; 2015,Jan,16; 2014,Jan,11; 2012,Feb,9-10

79403 **Radiopharmaceutical therapy, radiolabeled monoclonal antibody by intravenous infusion**
    EXCLUDES *Intravenous radiopharmaceutical therapy (79101)*
    📷 5.48   🔬 5.48 **FUD** XXX   S Z3 80 ▣
    AMA: 2016,Jan,13; 2015,Jan,16; 2014,Jan,11; 2012,Feb,9-10

79440 **Radiopharmaceutical therapy, by intra-articular administration**
    📷 4.12   🔬 4.12 **FUD** XXX   S Z3 80 ▣
    AMA: 2016,Jan,13; 2015,Jan,16; 2014,Jan,11; 2012,Feb,9-10

79445 **Radiopharmaceutical therapy, by intra-arterial particulate administration**
    EXCLUDES *Intra-arterial injections (96373, 96420)*
              Procedural and radiological supervision and interpretation for angiographic and interventional procedures before intra-arterial radiopharmaceutical therapy
    📷 0.00   🔬 0.00 **FUD** XXX   S Z2 80 ▣
    AMA: 2016,Jan,13; 2015,Jan,16; 2014,Jan,11; 2013,Nov,6; 2012,Feb,9-10

79999 **Radiopharmaceutical therapy, unlisted procedure**
    📷 0.00   🔬 0.00 **FUD** XXX   S Z2 80
    AMA: 2016,Jan,13; 2015,Jan,16; 2014,Jan,11; 2012,Feb,9-10

80047-80081 [80081] Multi-test Laboratory Panels

INCLUDES Groups of specified tests that may be reported as a panel

EXCLUDES *Reporting two or more panel codes that include the same tests; report the panel with the highest number of tests in common to meet the definition of the panel code*

Code also individual tests that are not part of the panel, when appropriate

80047 Basic metabolic panel (Calcium, ionized)

INCLUDES Calcium, ionized (82330)
Carbon dioxide (bicarbonate) (82374)
Chloride (82435)
Creatinine (82565)
Glucose (82947)
Potassium (84132)
Sodium (84295)
Urea nitrogen (BUN) (84520)

⚏ 0.00   ⚕ 0.00   **FUD** XXX   ☒ ◘ ▭

AMA: 2016,Jan,13; 2015,Jan,16; 2014,Jan,11; 2013,Apr,10-11

80048 Basic metabolic panel (Calcium, total)

INCLUDES Calcium, total (82310)
Carbon dioxide (bicarbonate) (82374)
Chloride (82435)
Creatinine (82565)
Glucose (82947)
Potassium (84132)
Sodium (84295)
Urea nitrogen (BUN) (84520)

⚏ 0.00   ⚕ 0.00   **FUD** XXX   ☒ ◘ ▭

AMA: 2016,Jan,13; 2015,Jan,16; 2014,Jan,11

80050 General health panel

INCLUDES Complete blood count (CBC), automated, with:
Manual differential WBC count
Blood smear with manual differential AND complete (CBC), automated (85007, 85027)
Manual differential WBC count, buffy coat AND complete (CBC), automated (85009, 85027)
OR
Automated differential WBC count
Automated differential WBC count AND complete (CBC), automated/automated differential WBC count (85004, 85025)
Automated differential WBC count AND complete (CBC), automated (85004, 85027)
Comprehensive metabolic profile (80053)
Thyroid stimulating hormone (84443)

⚏ 0.00   ⚕ 0.00   **FUD** XXX   ☒

AMA: 2016,Jan,13; 2015,Jan,16; 2014,Jan,11; 2012,Jan,15-42; 2011,Jan,11

80051 Electrolyte panel

INCLUDES Carbon dioxide (bicarbonate) (82374)
Chloride (82435)
Potassium (84132)
Sodium (84295)

⚏ 0.00   ⚕ 0.00   **FUD** XXX   ☒ ◘ ▭

AMA: 2016,Jan,13; 2015,Jan,16; 2014,Jan,11; 2012,Jan,15-42; 2011,Jan,11

80053 Comprehensive metabolic panel

INCLUDES Albumin (82040)
Bilirubin, total (82247)
Calcium, total (82310)
Carbon dioxide (bicarbonate) (82374)
Chloride (82435)
Creatinine (82565)
Glucose (82947)
Phosphatase, alkaline (84075)
Potassium (84132)
Protein, total (84155)
Sodium (84295)
Transferase, alanine amino (ALT) (SGPT) (84460)
Transferase, aspartate amino (AST) (SGOT) (84450)
Urea nitrogen (BUN) (84520)

⚏ 0.00   ⚕ 0.00   **FUD** XXX   ☒ ◘ ▭

AMA: 2016,Jan,13; 2015,Jan,16; 2014,Jan,11; 2013,Apr,10-11; 2012,Jan,15-42; 2011,Jan,11

80055 Obstetric panel   Ⓜ ♀

INCLUDES Complete blood count (CBC), automated, with:
Manual differential WBC count
Blood smear with manual differential AND complete (CBC), automated (85007, 85027)
Manual differential WBC count, buffy coat AND complete (CBC), automated (85009, 85027)
OR
Automated differential WBC count
Automated differential WBC count AND complete (CBC), automated/automated differential WBC count (85004, 85025)
Automated differential WBC count AND complete (CBC), automated (85004, 85027)
Blood typing, ABO and Rh (86900-86901)
Hepatitis B surface antigen (HBsAg) (87340)
RBC antibody screen, each serum technique (86850)
Rubella antibody (86762)
Syphilis test, non-treponemal antibody qualitative (86592)

EXCLUDES *Use of code when syphilis screening is provided using a treponemal antibody approach. Instead, assign individual codes for tests performed in the OB panel (86780)*

⚏ 0.00   ⚕ 0.00   **FUD** XXX   ▣

AMA: 2016,Jan,13; 2015,Jan,16; 2014,Jan,11; 2012,Jan,15-42; 2011,Jan,11

80081 Obstetric panel (includes HIV testing)   ♀

INCLUDES Complete blood count (CBC), automated, with:
Manual differential WBC count
Blood smear with manual differential AND complete (CBC), automated (85007, 85027)
Manual differential WBC count, buffy count AND complete (CBC), automated (85009, 85027)
OR
Automated differential WBC count
Automated differential WBC count AND complete (CBC), automated/automated differential WBC count (85004, 85025)
Automated differential WBC count AND complete (CBC), automated (85004, 85027)
Blood typing, ABO and Rh (86900-86901)
Hepatitis B surface antigen (HBsAg) (87340)
HIV-1 antigens, with HIV-1 and HIV-2 antibodies, single result (87389)
RBC antibody screen, each serum technique (86850)
Rubella antibody (86762)
Syphilis test, non-treponemal antibody qualitative (86592)

EXCLUDES *Use of code when syphilis screening is provided using a treponemal antibody approach. Instead, assign individual codes for tests performed in the OB panel (86780)*

⚏ 0.00   ⚕ 0.00   **FUD** XXX   ◘ ▭

AMA: 2016,Jan,13

80061 **Lipid panel**

INCLUDES Cholesterol, serum, total (82465)
Lipoprotein, direct measurement, high density cholesterol (HDL cholesterol) (83718)
Triglycerides (84478)

📋 0.00 ⚗ 0.00 **FUD** XXX ☒ Ⓐ 🖿

AMA: 2016,Jan,13; 2015,Jan,16; 2014,Jan,11; 2012,Jan,15-42; 2011,Jan,11

80069 **Renal function panel**

INCLUDES Albumin (82040)
Calcium, total (82310)
Carbon dioxide (bicarbonate) (82374)
Chloride (82435)
Creatinine (82565)
Glucose (82947)
Phosphorus inorganic (phosphate) (84100)
Potassium (84132)
Sodium (84295)
Urea nitrogen (BUN) (84520)

📋 0.00 ⚗ 0.00 **FUD** XXX ☒ Ⓠ 🖿

AMA: 2016,Jan,13; 2015,Jan,16; 2014,Jan,11; 2012,Jan,15-42; 2011,Jan,11

80074 **Acute hepatitis panel**

INCLUDES Hepatitis A antibody (HAAb) IgM (86709)
Hepatitis B core antibody (HBcAb), IgM (86705)
Hepatitis B surface antigen (HBsAg) (87340)
Hepatitis C antibody (86803)

📋 0.00 ⚗ 0.00 **FUD** XXX Ⓠ 🖿

AMA: 2016,Jan,13; 2015,Jan,16; 2014,Jan,11; 2012,Jan,15-42; 2011,Jan,11

80076 **Hepatic function panel**

INCLUDES Albumin (82040)
Bilirubin, direct (82248)
Bilirubin, total (82247)
Phosphatase, alkaline (84075)
Protein, total (84155)
Transferase, alanine amino (ALT) (SGPT) (84460)
Transferase, aspartate amino (AST) (SGOT) (84450)

📋 0.00 ⚗ 0.00 **FUD** XXX Ⓠ 🖿

AMA: 2016,Jan,13; 2015,Jan,16; 2014,Jan,11; 2012,Jan,15-42; 2011,Jan,11

80081 **Resequenced code. See code following 80055.**

[80300, 80301, 80302, 80303, 80304, 80305, 80306, 80307] Nonspecific Drug Screening

INCLUDES All testing procedures provided despite the number of tests performed per modality

EXCLUDES *Confirmatory drug testing ([80320, 80321, 80322, 80323, 80324, 80325, 80326, 80327, 80328, 80329, 80330, 80331, 80332, 80333, 80334, 80335, 80336, 80337, 80338, 80339, 80340, 80341, 80342, 80343, 80344, 80345, 80346, 80347, 80348, 80349, 80350, 80351, 80352, 80353, 80354, 80355, 80356, 80357, 80358, 80359, 80360, 80361, 80362, 80363, 80364, 80365, 80366, 80367, 80368, 80369, 80370, 80371, 80372, 80373, 80374, 80375, 80376, 80377, 83992], [83992])*
Validation testing

~~**80300** Drug screen, any number of drug classes from Drug Class List A; any number of non-TLC devices or procedures, (eg, immunoassay) capable of being read by direct optical observation, including instrumented-assisted when performed (eg, dipsticks, cups, cards, cartridges), per date of service~~

To report, see ~[80305, 80306]

~~**80301** single drug class method, by instrumented test systems (eg, discrete multichannel chemistry analyzers utilizing immunoassay or enzyme assay), per date of service~~

To report, see ~[80307]

~~**80302** Drug screen, presumptive, single drug class from Drug Class List B, by immunoassay (eg, ELISA) or non-TLC chromatography without mass spectrometry (eg, GC, HPLC), each procedure~~

To report, see ~[80307]

~~**80303** Drug screen, any number of drug classes, presumptive, single or multiple drug class method; thin layer chromatography procedure(s) (TLC) (eg, acid, neutral, alkaloid plate), per date of service~~

To report, see ~[80307]

~~**80304** not otherwise specified presumptive procedure (eg, TOF, MALDI, LDTD, DESI, DART), each procedure~~

To report, see ~[80307]

● # **80305** **Drug test(s), presumptive, any number of drug classes, any number of devices or procedures (eg, immunoassay); capable of being read by direct optical observation only (eg, dipsticks, cups, cards, cartridges) includes sample validation when performed, per date of service**

📋 0.00 ⚗ 0.00 **FUD** 000

● # **80306** **read by instrument assisted direct optical observation (eg, dipsticks, cups, cards, cartridges), includes sample validation when performed, per date of service**

📋 0.00 ⚗ 0.00 **FUD** 000

● # **80307** **Drug test(s), presumptive, any number of drug classes, any number of devices or procedures, by instrument chemistry analyzers (eg, utilizing immunoassay [eg, EIA, ELISA, EMIT, FPIA, IA, KIMS, RIA]), chromatography (eg, GC, HPLC), and mass spectrometry either with or without chromatography, (eg, DART, DESI, GC-MS, GC-MS/MS, LC-MS, LC-MS/MS, LDTD, MALDI, TOF) includes sample validation when performed, per date of service**

📋 0.00 ⚗ 0.00 **FUD** 000

[80320, 80321, 80322, 80323, 80324, 80325, 80326, 80327, 80328, 80329, 80330, 80331, 80332, 80333, 80334, 80335, 80336, 80337, 80338, 80339, 80340, 80341, 80342, 80343, 80344, 80345, 80346, 80347, 80348, 80349, 80350, 80351, 80352, 80353, 80354, 80355, 80356, 80357, 80358, 80359, 80360, 80361, 80362, 80363, 80364, 80365, 80366, 80367, 80368, 80369, 80370, 80371, 80372, 80373, 80374, 80375, 80376, 80377, 83992] Confirmatory Drug Testing

INCLUDES Antihistamine drug tests ([80375, 80376, 80377])
Detection of specific drugs using methods other than immunoassay or enzymatic technique

EXCLUDES *Metabolites separate from the code for the drug except when a distinct code is available*

80320 **Alcohols**

📋 0.00 ⚗ 0.00 **FUD** XXX Ⓑ

AMA: 2016,Jan,13; 2015,Apr,3

80321 **Alcohol biomarkers; 1 or 2**

📋 0.00 ⚗ 0.00 **FUD** XXX Ⓑ

AMA: 2015,Apr,3

80322 **3 or more**

📋 0.00 ⚗ 0.00 **FUD** XXX Ⓑ

AMA: 2015,Apr,3

80323 **Alkaloids, not otherwise specified**

📋 0.00 ⚗ 0.00 **FUD** XXX Ⓑ

AMA: 2015,Apr,3

80324 **Amphetamines; 1 or 2**

📋 0.00 ⚗ 0.00 **FUD** XXX Ⓑ

AMA: 2015,Apr,3

80325 **3 or 4**

📋 0.00 ⚗ 0.00 **FUD** XXX Ⓑ

AMA: 2015,Apr,3

80326 **5 or more**

📋 0.00 ⚗ 0.00 **FUD** XXX Ⓑ

AMA: 2015,Apr,3

80327 **Anabolic steroids; 1 or 2**

📋 0.00 ⚗ 0.00 **FUD** XXX Ⓑ

AMA: 2015,Apr,3

#	80328	**3 or more**

🔧 0.00   ⚕ 0.00   **FUD** XXX   Ⓑ
AMA: 2015,Apr,3

#	80329	**Analgesics, non-opioid; 1 or 2**

🔧 0.00   ⚕ 0.00   **FUD** XXX   Ⓑ
AMA: 2015,Apr,3

#	80330	**3-5**

🔧 0.00   ⚕ 0.00   **FUD** XXX   Ⓑ
AMA: 2015,Apr,3

#	80331	**6 or more**

🔧 0.00   ⚕ 0.00   **FUD** XXX   Ⓑ
AMA: 2015,Apr,3

#	80332	**Antidepressants, serotonergic class; 1 or 2**

🔧 0.00   ⚕ 0.00   **FUD** XXX   Ⓑ
AMA: 2015,Apr,3

#	80333	**3-5**

🔧 0.00   ⚕ 0.00   **FUD** XXX   Ⓑ
AMA: 2015,Apr,3

#	80334	**6 or more**

🔧 0.00   ⚕ 0.00   **FUD** XXX   Ⓑ
AMA: 2015,Apr,3

#	80335	**Antidepressants, tricyclic and other cyclicals; 1 or 2**

🔧 0.00   ⚕ 0.00   **FUD** XXX   Ⓑ
AMA: 2015,Apr,3

#	80336	**3-5**

🔧 0.00   ⚕ 0.00   **FUD** XXX   Ⓑ
AMA: 2015,Apr,3

#	80337	**6 or more**

🔧 0.00   ⚕ 0.00   **FUD** XXX   Ⓑ
AMA: 2015,Apr,3

#	80338	**Antidepressants, not otherwise specified**

🔧 0.00   ⚕ 0.00   **FUD** XXX   Ⓑ
AMA: 2015,Apr,3

#	80339	**Antiepileptics, not otherwise specified; 1-3**

🔧 0.00   ⚕ 0.00   **FUD** XXX   Ⓑ
AMA: 2015,Apr,3

#	80340	**4-6**

🔧 0.00   ⚕ 0.00   **FUD** XXX   Ⓑ
AMA: 2015,Apr,3

#	80341	**7 or more**

🔧 0.00   ⚕ 0.00   **FUD** XXX   Ⓑ
AMA: 2015,Apr,3

#	80342	**Antipsychotics, not otherwise specified; 1-3**

🔧 0.00   ⚕ 0.00   **FUD** XXX   Ⓑ
AMA: 2015,Apr,3

#	80343	**4-6**

🔧 0.00   ⚕ 0.00   **FUD** XXX   Ⓑ
AMA: 2015,Apr,3

#	80344	**7 or more**

🔧 0.00   ⚕ 0.00   **FUD** XXX   Ⓑ
AMA: 2015,Apr,3

#	80345	**Barbiturates**

🔧 0.00   ⚕ 0.00   **FUD** XXX   Ⓑ
AMA: 2015,Apr,3

#	80346	**Benzodiazepines; 1-12**

🔧 0.00   ⚕ 0.00   **FUD** XXX   Ⓑ
AMA: 2015,Apr,3

#	80347	**13 or more**

🔧 0.00   ⚕ 0.00   **FUD** XXX   Ⓑ
AMA: 2015,Apr,3

#	80348	**Buprenorphine**

🔧 0.00   ⚕ 0.00   **FUD** XXX   Ⓑ
AMA: 2015,Apr,3

#	80349	**Cannabinoids, natural**

🔧 0.00   ⚕ 0.00   **FUD** XXX   Ⓑ
AMA: 2015,Apr,3

#	80350	**Cannabinoids, synthetic; 1-3**

🔧 0.00   ⚕ 0.00   **FUD** XXX   Ⓑ
AMA: 2015,Apr,3

#	80351	**4-6**

🔧 0.00   ⚕ 0.00   **FUD** XXX   Ⓑ
AMA: 2015,Apr,3

#	80352	**7 or more**

🔧 0.00   ⚕ 0.00   **FUD** XXX   Ⓑ
AMA: 2015,Apr,3

#	80353	**Cocaine**

🔧 0.00   ⚕ 0.00   **FUD** XXX   Ⓑ
AMA: 2015,Apr,3

#	80354	**Fentanyl**

🔧 0.00   ⚕ 0.00   **FUD** XXX   Ⓑ
AMA: 2015,Apr,3

#	80355	**Gabapentin, non-blood**

🔧 0.00   ⚕ 0.00   **FUD** XXX   Ⓑ
AMA: 2016,Jan,13; 2015,Apr,3

#	80356	**Heroin metabolite**

🔧 0.00   ⚕ 0.00   **FUD** XXX   Ⓑ
AMA: 2015,Apr,3

#	80357	**Ketamine and norketamine**

🔧 0.00   ⚕ 0.00   **FUD** XXX   Ⓑ
AMA: 2015,Apr,3

#	80358	**Methadone**

🔧 0.00   ⚕ 0.00   **FUD** XXX   Ⓑ
AMA: 2015,Apr,3

#	80359	**Methylenedioxyamphetamines (MDA, MDEA, MDMA)**

🔧 0.00   ⚕ 0.00   **FUD** XXX   Ⓑ
AMA: 2015,Apr,3

#	80360	**Methylphenidate**

🔧 0.00   ⚕ 0.00   **FUD** XXX   Ⓑ
AMA: 2015,Apr,3

#	80361	**Opiates, 1 or more**

🔧 0.00   ⚕ 0.00   **FUD** XXX   Ⓑ
AMA: 2015,Apr,3

#	80362	**Opioids and opiate analogs; 1 or 2**

🔧 0.00   ⚕ 0.00   **FUD** XXX   Ⓑ
AMA: 2015,Apr,3

#	80363	**3 or 4**

🔧 0.00   ⚕ 0.00   **FUD** XXX   Ⓑ
AMA: 2015,Apr,3

#	80364	**5 or more**

🔧 0.00   ⚕ 0.00   **FUD** XXX   Ⓑ
AMA: 2015,Apr,3

#	80365	**Oxycodone**

🔧 0.00   ⚕ 0.00   **FUD** XXX   Ⓑ
AMA: 2015,Apr,3

#	83992	**Phencyclidine (PCP)**

🔧 0.00   ⚕ 0.00   **FUD** XXX   Ⓑ
AMA: 2016,Jan,13; 2015,Jun,10; 2015,Apr,3

#	80366	**Pregabalin**

🔧 0.00   ⚕ 0.00   **FUD** XXX   Ⓑ
AMA: 2015,Apr,3

#	80367	**Propoxyphene**

🔧 0.00   ⚕ 0.00   **FUD** XXX   Ⓑ
AMA: 2015,Apr,3

#	80368	**Sedative hypnotics (non-benzodiazepines)**

🔧 0.00   ⚕ 0.00   **FUD** XXX   Ⓑ
AMA: 2015,Apr,3

Pathology and Laboratory

80369 — 80192

80369 Skeletal muscle relaxants; 1 or 2
🚑 0.00   ⚕ 0.00   **FUD** XXX   B
AMA: 2015,Apr,3

80370 3 or more
🚑 0.00   ⚕ 0.00   **FUD** XXX   B
AMA: 2015,Apr,3

80371 Stimulants, synthetic
🚑 0.00   ⚕ 0.00   **FUD** XXX   B
AMA: 2015,Apr,3

80372 Tapentadol
🚑 0.00   ⚕ 0.00   **FUD** XXX   B
AMA: 2015,Apr,3

80373 Tramadol
🚑 0.00   ⚕ 0.00   **FUD** XXX   B
AMA: 2015,Apr,3

80374 Stereoisomer (enantiomer) analysis, single drug class
Code also index drug analysis if appropriate
🚑 0.00   ⚕ 0.00   **FUD** XXX   B
AMA: 2015,Apr,3

80375 Drug(s) or substance(s), definitive, qualitative or quantitative, not otherwise specified; 1-3
🚑 0.00   ⚕ 0.00   **FUD** XXX   B
AMA: 2016,Jan,13; 2015,Apr,3

80376 4-6
🚑 0.00   ⚕ 0.00   **FUD** XXX   B
AMA: 2016,Jan,13; 2015,Apr,3

80377 7 or more
🚑 0.00   ⚕ 0.00   **FUD** XXX   B
AMA: 2016,Jan,13; 2015,Apr,3

80150-80377 [80164, 80165, 80171] Therapeutic Drug Levels

INCLUDES   Testing of drug and metabolite(s) in primary code
Tests on specimens from blood and blood components, and spinal fluid

80150 **Amikacin**
🚑 0.00   ⚕ 0.00   **FUD** XXX   Q
AMA: 2016,Jan,13; 2015,Apr,3; 2015,Jan,16; 2014,Jan,11; 2012,Jan,15-42; 2011,Mar,9

80155 **Caffeine**
🚑 0.00   ⚕ 0.00   **FUD** XXX   Q
AMA: 2015,Apr,3; 2014,Jan,11

80156 **Carbamazepine; total**
🚑 0.00   ⚕ 0.00   **FUD** XXX   Q
AMA: 2016,Jan,13; 2015,Apr,3; 2015,Jan,16; 2014,Jan,11; 2011,Mar,9

80157 **free**
🚑 0.00   ⚕ 0.00   **FUD** XXX   Q
AMA: 2016,Jan,13; 2015,Apr,3; 2015,Jan,16; 2014,Jan,11; 2011,Mar,9

80158 **Cyclosporine**
🚑 0.00   ⚕ 0.00   **FUD** XXX   Q
AMA: 2016,Jan,13; 2015,Apr,3; 2015,Jan,16; 2014,Jan,11; 2011,Mar,9

80159 **Clozapine**
🚑 0.00   ⚕ 0.00   **FUD** XXX   Q
AMA: 2015,Apr,3; 2014,Jan,11

80162 **Digoxin; total**
🚑 0.00   ⚕ 0.00   **FUD** XXX   Q
AMA: 2016,Jan,13; 2015,Apr,3; 2015,Jan,16; 2014,Jan,11; 2011,Mar,9

80163 **free**
🚑 0.00   ⚕ 0.00   **FUD** XXX   Q
AMA: 2016,Jan,13; 2015,Apr,3

80164 Resequenced code. See code following 80201.

80165 Resequenced code. See code following 80201.

80168 **Ethosuximide**
🚑 0.00   ⚕ 0.00   **FUD** XXX   Q
AMA: 2016,Jan,13; 2015,Apr,3; 2015,Jan,16; 2014,Jan,11; 2011,Mar,9

80169 **Everolimus**
🚑 0.00   ⚕ 0.00   **FUD** XXX   Q
AMA: 2015,Apr,3; 2014,Jan,11

80171 Gabapentin, whole blood, serum, or plasma
🚑 0.00   ⚕ 0.00   **FUD** XXX   Q
AMA: 2016,Jan,13; 2015,Apr,3; 2014,Jan,11

80170 **Gentamicin**
🚑 0.00   ⚕ 0.00   **FUD** XXX   Q
AMA: 2016,Jan,13; 2015,Apr,3; 2015,Jan,16; 2014,Jan,11; 2011,Mar,9

80171 Resequenced code. See code following 80169.

80173 **Haloperidol**
🚑 0.00   ⚕ 0.00   **FUD** XXX   Q
AMA: 2016,Jan,13; 2015,Apr,3; 2015,Jan,16; 2014,Jan,11; 2011,Mar,9

80175 **Lamotrigine**
🚑 0.00   ⚕ 0.00   **FUD** XXX   Q
AMA: 2015,Apr,3; 2014,Jan,11

80176 **Lidocaine**
🚑 0.00   ⚕ 0.00   **FUD** XXX   Q
AMA: 2016,Jan,13; 2015,Apr,3; 2015,Jan,16; 2014,Jan,11; 2011,Mar,9

80177 **Levetiracetam**
🚑 0.00   ⚕ 0.00   **FUD** XXX   Q
AMA: 2015,Apr,3; 2014,Jan,11

80178 **Lithium**
🚑 0.00   ⚕ 0.00   **FUD** XXX   X Q
AMA: 2016,Jan,13; 2015,Apr,3; 2015,Jan,16; 2014,Jan,11; 2011,Mar,9

80180 **Mycophenolate (mycophenolic acid)**
🚑 0.00   ⚕ 0.00   **FUD** XXX   Q
AMA: 2015,Apr,3; 2014,Jan,11

80183 **Oxcarbazepine**
🚑 0.00   ⚕ 0.00   **FUD** XXX   Q
AMA: 2015,Apr,3; 2014,Jan,11

80184 **Phenobarbital**
🚑 0.00   ⚕ 0.00   **FUD** XXX   Q
AMA: 2016,Jan,13; 2015,Apr,3; 2015,Jan,16; 2014,Jan,11; 2011,Mar,9

80185 **Phenytoin; total**
🚑 0.00   ⚕ 0.00   **FUD** XXX   Q
AMA: 2016,Jan,13; 2015,Apr,3; 2015,Jan,16; 2014,Jan,11; 2011,Mar,9

80186 **free**
🚑 0.00   ⚕ 0.00   **FUD** XXX   Q
AMA: 2016,Jan,13; 2015,Apr,3; 2015,Jan,16; 2014,Jan,11; 2011,Mar,9

80188 **Primidone**
🚑 0.00   ⚕ 0.00   **FUD** XXX   Q
AMA: 2016,Jan,13; 2015,Apr,3; 2015,Jan,16; 2014,Jan,11; 2011,Mar,9

80190 **Procainamide;**
🚑 0.00   ⚕ 0.00   **FUD** XXX   Q
AMA: 2016,Jan,13; 2015,Apr,3; 2015,Jan,16; 2014,Jan,11; 2011,Mar,9

80192 **with metabolites (eg, n-acetyl procainamide)**
🚑 0.00   ⚕ 0.00   **FUD** XXX   Q ▢
AMA: 2016,Jan,13; 2015,Apr,3; 2015,Jan,16; 2014,Jan,11; 2011,Mar,9

	80194	**Quinidine**	
		🔧 0.00 ⚖ 0.00 **FUD** XXX	Q
		AMA: 2016,Jan,13; 2015,Apr,3; 2015,Jan,16; 2014,Jan,11; 2011,Mar,9	

	80195	**Sirolimus**	
		🔧 0.00 ⚖ 0.00 **FUD** XXX	Q
		AMA: 2016,Jan,13; 2015,Apr,3; 2015,Jan,16; 2014,Jan,11; 2011,Mar,9	

	80197	**Tacrolimus**	
		🔧 0.00 ⚖ 0.00 **FUD** XXX	Q
		AMA: 2016,Jan,13; 2015,Apr,3; 2015,Jan,16; 2014,Jan,11; 2011,Mar,9	

	80198	**Theophylline**	
		🔧 0.00 ⚖ 0.00 **FUD** XXX	Q
		AMA: 2016,Jan,13; 2015,Apr,3; 2015,Jan,16; 2014,Jan,11; 2011,Mar,9	

	80199	**Tiagabine**	
		🔧 0.00 ⚖ 0.00 **FUD** XXX	Q
		AMA: 2015,Apr,3; 2014,Jan,11	

	80200	**Tobramycin**	
		🔧 0.00 ⚖ 0.00 **FUD** XXX	Q
		AMA: 2016,Jan,13; 2015,Apr,3; 2015,Jan,16; 2014,Jan,11; 2011,Mar,9	

	80201	**Topiramate**	
		🔧 0.00 ⚖ 0.00 **FUD** XXX	Q
		AMA: 2016,Jan,13; 2015,Apr,3; 2015,Jan,16; 2014,Jan,11; 2011,Mar,9	

#	80164	**Valproic acid (dipropylacetic acid); total**	
		🔧 0.00 ⚖ 0.00 **FUD** XXX	Q
		AMA: 2016,Jan,13; 2015,Apr,3; 2015,Jan,16; 2014,Jan,11; 2011,Mar,9	

#	80165	**free**	
		🔧 0.00 ⚖ 0.00 **FUD** XXX	Q
		AMA: 2016,Jan,13; 2015,Apr,3	

	80202	**Vancomycin**	
		🔧 0.00 ⚖ 0.00 **FUD** XXX	Q
		AMA: 2016,Jan,13; 2015,Apr,3; 2015,Jan,16; 2014,Jan,11; 2012,Jan,15-42; 2011,Mar,9	

	80203	**Zonisamide**	
		🔧 0.00 ⚖ 0.00 **FUD** XXX	Q
		AMA: 2015,Apr,3; 2014,Jan,11	

	80299	**Quantitation of therapeutic drug, not elsewhere specified**	
		🔧 0.00 ⚖ 0.00 **FUD** XXX	Q
		AMA: 2016,Jan,13; 2015,Apr,3; 2015,Jan,16; 2014,Jan,11; 2012,Jan,15-42; 2011,Mar,9; 2011,Jan,11	

	80300	Resequenced code. See code before 80150.
	80301	Resequenced code. See code before 80150.
	80302	Resequenced code. See code before 80150.
	80303	Resequenced code. See code before 80150.
	80304	Resequenced code. See code before 80150.
	80305	Resequenced code. See code before 80150.
	80306	Resequenced code. See code before 80150.
	80307	Resequenced code. See code before 80150.
	80320	Resequenced code. See code before 80150.
	80321	Resequenced code. See code before 80150.
	80322	Resequenced code. See code before 80150.
	80323	Resequenced code. See code before 80150.
	80324	Resequenced code. See code before 80150.
	80325	Resequenced code. See code before 80150.
	80326	Resequenced code. See code before 80150.
	80327	Resequenced code. See code before 80150.
	80328	Resequenced code. See code before 80150.

80329	Resequenced code. See code before 80150.
80330	Resequenced code. See code before 80150.
80331	Resequenced code. See code before 80150.
80332	Resequenced code. See code before 80150.
80333	Resequenced code. See code before 80150.
80334	Resequenced code. See code before 80150.
80335	Resequenced code. See code before 80150.
80336	Resequenced code. See code before 80150.
80337	Resequenced code. See code before 80150.
80338	Resequenced code. See code before 80150.
80339	Resequenced code. See code before 80150.
80340	Resequenced code. See code before 80150.
80341	Resequenced code. See code before 80150.
80342	Resequenced code. See code before 80150.
80343	Resequenced code. See code before 80150.
80344	Resequenced code. See code before 80150.
80345	Resequenced code. See code before 80150.
80346	Resequenced code. See code before 80150.
80347	Resequenced code. See code before 80150.
80348	Resequenced code. See code before 80150.
80349	Resequenced code. See code before 80150.
80350	Resequenced code. See code before 80150.
80351	Resequenced code. See code before 80150.
80352	Resequenced code. See code before 80150.
80353	Resequenced code. See code before 80150.
80354	Resequenced code. See code before 80150.
80355	Resequenced code. See code before 80150.
80356	Resequenced code. See code before 80150.
80357	Resequenced code. See code before 80150.
80358	Resequenced code. See code before 80150.
80359	Resequenced code. See code before 80150.
80360	Resequenced code. See code before 80150.
80361	Resequenced code. See code before 80150.
80362	Resequenced code. See code before 80150.
80363	Resequenced code. See code before 80150.
80364	Resequenced code. See code before 80150.
80365	Resequenced code. See code following 80364.
80366	Resequenced code. See code following 83992.
80367	Resequenced code. See code following 80366.
80368	Resequenced code. See code following 80367.
80369	Resequenced code. See code following 80368.
80370	Resequenced code. See code following 80369.
80371	Resequenced code. See code following 80370.
80372	Resequenced code. See code following 80371.
80373	Resequenced code. See code following 80372.
80374	Resequenced code. See code following 80373.
80375	Resequenced code. See code following 80374.
80376	Resequenced code. See code following 80375.
80377	Resequenced code. See code following 80376.

80400-80439 Stimulation and Suppression Test Panels

EXCLUDES Administration of evocative or suppressive material (96365-96368, 96372, 96374-96376, C8957)
Evocative or suppression test substances, as applicable
Physician monitoring and attendance during test (see E&M services)

80400   ACTH stimulation panel; for adrenal insufficiency
INCLUDES   Cortisol x 2 (82533)
🚑 0.00   🔪 0.00   FUD XXX   Q 🖬
AMA: 2016,Jan,13; 2015,Jan,16; 2014,Jan,11

80402   for 21 hydroxylase deficiency
INCLUDES   17 hydroxyprogesterone X 2 (83498)
Cortisol x 2 (82533)
🚑 0.00   🔪 0.00   FUD XXX   Q 🖬
AMA: 2014,Jan,11

80406   for 3 beta-hydroxydehydrogenase deficiency
INCLUDES   17 hydroxypregnenolone x 2 (84143)
Cortisol x 2 (82533)
🚑 0.00   🔪 0.00   FUD XXX   Q 🖬
AMA: 2014,Jan,11

80408   Aldosterone suppression evaluation panel (eg, saline infusion)
INCLUDES   Aldosterone x 2 (82088)
Renin x 2 (84244)
🚑 0.00   🔪 0.00   FUD XXX   Q 🖬
AMA: 2014,Jan,11

80410   Calcitonin stimulation panel (eg, calcium, pentagastrin)
INCLUDES   Calcitonin x 3 (82308)
🚑 0.00   🔪 0.00   FUD XXX   Q 🖬
AMA: 2014,Jan,11

80412   Corticotropic releasing hormone (CRH) stimulation panel
INCLUDES   Adrenocorticotropic hormone (ACTH) x 6 (82024)
Cortisol x 6 (82533)
🚑 0.00   🔪 0.00   FUD XXX   Q 🖬
AMA: 2014,Jan,11

80414   Chorionic gonadotropin stimulation panel; testosterone response
INCLUDES   Testosterone x 2 on three pooled blood samples (84403)
🚑 0.00   🔪 0.00   FUD XXX   Q 🖬
AMA: 2014,Jan,11

80415   estradiol response
INCLUDES   Estradiol x 2 on three pooled blood samples (82670)
🚑 0.00   🔪 0.00   FUD XXX   Q 🖬
AMA: 2014,Jan,11

80416   Renal vein renin stimulation panel (eg, captopril)
INCLUDES   Renin x 6 (84244)
🚑 0.00   🔪 0.00   FUD XXX   Q 🖬
AMA: 2014,Jan,11

80417   Peripheral vein renin stimulation panel (eg, captopril)
INCLUDES   Renin x 2 (84244)
🚑 0.00   🔪 0.00   FUD XXX   Q 🖬
AMA: 2014,Jan,11

80418   Combined rapid anterior pituitary evaluation panel
INCLUDES   Adrenocorticotropic hormone (ACTH) x 4 (82024)
Cortisol x 4 (82533)
Follicle stimulating hormone (FSH) x 4 (83001)
Human growth hormone x 4 (83003)
Luteinizing hormone (LH) x 4 (83002)
Prolactin x 4 (84146)
Thyroid stimulating hormone (TSH) x 4 (84443)
🚑 0.00   🔪 0.00   FUD XXX   Q 🖬
AMA: 2014,Jan,11

80420   Dexamethasone suppression panel, 48 hour
INCLUDES   Cortisol x 2 (82533)
Free cortisol, urine x 2 (82530)
Volume measurement for timed collection x 2 (81050)
EXCLUDES   Single dose dexamethasone (82533)
🚑 0.00   🔪 0.00   FUD XXX   Q 🖬
AMA: 2014,Jan,11

80422   Glucagon tolerance panel; for insulinoma
INCLUDES   Glucose x 3 (82947)
Insulin x 3 (83525)
🚑 0.00   🔪 0.00   FUD XXX   Q 🖬
AMA: 2014,Jan,11

80424   for pheochromocytoma
INCLUDES   Catecholamines, fractionated x 2 (82384)
🚑 0.00   🔪 0.00   FUD XXX   Q 🖬
AMA: 2014,Jan,11

80426   Gonadotropin releasing hormone stimulation panel
INCLUDES   Follicle stimulating hormone (FSH) x 4 (83001)
Luteinizing hormone (LH) x 4 (83002)
🚑 0.00   🔪 0.00   FUD XXX   Q 🖬
AMA: 2014,Jan,11

80428   Growth hormone stimulation panel (eg, arginine infusion, l-dopa administration)
INCLUDES   Human growth hormone (HGH) x 4 (83003)
🚑 0.00   🔪 0.00   FUD XXX   Q 🖬
AMA: 2014,Jan,11

80430   Growth hormone suppression panel (glucose administration)
INCLUDES   Glucose x 3 (82947)
Human growth hormone (HGH) x 4 (83003)
🚑 0.00   🔪 0.00   FUD XXX   Q 🖬
AMA: 2014,Jan,11

80432   Insulin-induced C-peptide suppression panel
INCLUDES   C-peptide x 5 (84681)
Glucose x 5 (82947)
Insulin (83525)
🚑 0.00   🔪 0.00   FUD XXX   Q 🖬
AMA: 2014,Jan,11

80434   Insulin tolerance panel; for ACTH insufficiency
INCLUDES   Cortisol x 5 (82533)
Glucose x 5 (82947)
🚑 0.00   🔪 0.00   FUD XXX   Q 🖬
AMA: 2014,Jan,11

80435   for growth hormone deficiency
INCLUDES   Glucose x 5 (82947)
Human growth hormone (HGH) x 5 (83003)
🚑 0.00   🔪 0.00   FUD XXX   Q 🖬
AMA: 2014,Jan,11

80436   Metyrapone panel
INCLUDES   11 deoxycortisol x 2 (82634)
Cortisol x 2 (82533)
🚑 0.00   🔪 0.00   FUD XXX   Q 🖬
AMA: 2014,Jan,11

80438   Thyrotropin releasing hormone (TRH) stimulation panel; 1 hour
INCLUDES   Thyroid stimulating hormone (TSH) x 3 (84443)
🚑 0.00   🔪 0.00   FUD XXX   Q 🖬
AMA: 2014,Jan,11

80439   2 hour
INCLUDES   Thyroid stimulating hormone (TSH) x 4 (84443)
🚑 0.00   🔪 0.00   FUD XXX   Q 🖬
AMA: 2014,Jan,11

80500-80502 Consultation By Clinical Pathologist

INCLUDES   Pharmacokinetic consultations
Written report by pathologist for tests requiring additional medical judgment and requested by a physician or other qualified health care professional
EXCLUDES   Consultations that include patient examination
Use of code when a medical interpretive assessment is not provided

80500   Clinical pathology consultation; limited, without review of patient's history and medical records
🚑 0.55   🔪 0.62   FUD XXX   Q 80 🖬
AMA: 2016,Jan,13; 2015,Jan,16; 2014,Jan,11

80502 comprehensive, for a complex diagnostic problem, with review of patient's history and medical records
🚑 1.95 🔎 2.02 **FUD** XXX 01 80 📟
AMA: 2016,Jan,13; 2015,Jan,16; 2014,Jan,11

81000-81099 Urine Tests

81000 Urinalysis, by dip stick or tablet reagent for bilirubin, glucose, hemoglobin, ketones, leukocytes, nitrite, pH, protein, specific gravity, urobilinogen, any number of these constituents; non-automated, with microscopy
🚑 0.00 🔎 0.00 **FUD** XXX Q 📟
AMA: 2016,Jan,13; 2015,Jan,16; 2014,Jan,11

81001 automated, with microscopy
🚑 0.00 🔎 0.00 **FUD** XXX Q 📟
AMA: 2014,Jan,11

81002 non-automated, without microscopy
[INCLUDES] Mosenthal test
🚑 0.00 🔎 0.00 **FUD** XXX X Q 📟
AMA: 2016,Jan,13; 2015,Jan,16; 2014,Jan,11

81003 automated, without microscopy
🚑 0.00 🔎 0.00 **FUD** XXX X Q 📟
AMA: 2016,Jan,13; 2015,Jan,16; 2014,Jan,11

81005 Urinalysis; qualitative or semiquantitative, except immunoassays
[INCLUDES] Benedict test for dextrose
[EXCLUDES] *Immunoassay, qualitative or semiquantitative (83518)*
Microalbumin (82043-82044)
Nonimmunoassay reagent strip analysis (81000, 81002)
🚑 0.00 🔎 0.00 **FUD** XXX Q 📟
AMA: 2016,Jan,13; 2015,Jan,16; 2014,Jan,11

81007 bacteriuria screen, except by culture or dipstick
[EXCLUDES] *Culture (87086-87088)*
Dipstick (81000, 81002)
🚑 0.00 🔎 0.00 **FUD** XXX X Q 📟
AMA: 2014,Jan,11

81015 microscopic only
[EXCLUDES] *Sperm evaluation for retrograde ejaculation (89331)*
🚑 0.00 🔎 0.00 **FUD** XXX Q
AMA: 2014,Jan,11

81020 2 or 3 glass test
[INCLUDES] Valentine's test
🚑 0.00 🔎 0.00 **FUD** XXX Q 📟
AMA: 2014,Jan,11

81025 Urine pregnancy test, by visual color comparison methods
🚑 0.00 🔎 0.00 **FUD** XXX X Q
AMA: 2016,Jan,13; 2015,Jan,16; 2014,Jan,11

81050 Volume measurement for timed collection, each
🚑 0.00 🔎 0.00 **FUD** XXX Q
AMA: 2014,Jan,11

81099 Unlisted urinalysis procedure
🚑 0.00 🔎 0.00 **FUD** XXX Q
AMA: 2016,Jan,13; 2015,Jan,16; 2014,Jan,11

81161-81355 [81161, 81162, 81287, 81288] Gene Analysis: Tier 1 Procedures

[INCLUDES] All analytical procedures in the evaluation such as:
Amplification
Cell lysis
Detection
Digestion
Extraction
Nucleic acid stabilization
Code selection based on specific gene being reviewed
Evaluation of constitutional or somatic gene variations
Evaluation of the presence of gene variants using the common gene variant name
Examples of proteins or diseases in the code description that are not all inclusive
Generally all the listed gene variants in the code description would be tested but lists are not all inclusive
Gene specific and genomic testing
Genes described using Human Genome Organization (HUGO) approved names
Qualitative results unless otherwise stated
Tier 1 molecular pathology codes (81200-81355 [81161, 81162, 81287, 81288])

[EXCLUDES] *Full gene sequencing using separate gene variant assessment codes unless it is specifically stated in the code description*
In situ hybridization analyses (88271-88275, 88365-88368 [88364, 88373, 88374])
Microbial identification (87149-87153, 87470-87801 [87623, 87624, 87625], 87900-87904 [87906, 87910, 87912])
Other related gene variants not listed in code
Tier 1 molecular pathology codes (81370-81383)
Tier 2 codes (81400-81408)
Unlisted molecular pathology procedures ([81479])
Code also modifier 26 when only interpretation and report are performed
Code also services required before cell lysis

81161 Resequenced code. See code following 81229.

81162 Resequenced code. See code following 81211.

81170 *ABL1 (ABL proto-oncogene 1, non-receptor tyrosine kinase)* (eg, acquired imatinib tyrosine kinase inhibitor resistance), gene analysis, variants in the kinase domain
🚑 0.00 🔎 0.00 **FUD** XXX A 📟
AMA: 2016,Aug,9

81200 *ASPA (aspartoacylase)* (eg, Canavan disease) gene analysis, common variants (eg, E285A, Y231X)
🚑 0.00 🔎 0.00 **FUD** XXX A 📟
AMA: 2016,Aug,9; 2016,Jan,13; 2015,Jan,16; 2014,Jan,11; 2013,Sep,3-12; 2012,May,3-10

81201 *APC (adenomatous polyposis coli)* (eg, familial adenomatosis polyposis [FAP], attenuated FAP) gene analysis; full gene sequence
🚑 0.00 🔎 0.00 **FUD** XXX A 📟
AMA: 2016,Aug,9; 2016,Jan,13; 2015,Jan,16; 2014,Jan,11; 2013,Sep,3-12

81202 known familial variants
🚑 0.00 🔎 0.00 **FUD** XXX A 📟
AMA: 2016,Aug,9; 2016,Jan,13; 2015,Jan,16; 2014,Jan,11; 2013,Sep,3-12

81203 duplication/deletion variants
🚑 0.00 🔎 0.00 **FUD** XXX A 📟
AMA: 2016,Aug,9; 2016,Jan,13; 2015,Jan,16; 2014,Jan,11; 2013,Sep,3-12

81205 *BCKDHB (branched-chain keto acid dehydrogenase E1, beta polypeptide)* (eg, maple syrup urine disease) gene analysis, common variants (eg, R183P, G278S, E422X)
🚑 0.00 🔎 0.00 **FUD** XXX A 📟
AMA: 2016,Aug,9; 2016,Jan,13; 2015,Jan,16; 2014,Jan,11; 2013,Sep,3-12; 2012,May,3-10

81206 *BCR/ABL1 (t(9;22))* (eg, chronic myelogenous leukemia) translocation analysis; major breakpoint, qualitative or quantitative
🚑 0.00 🔎 0.00 **FUD** XXX A 📟
AMA: 2016,Aug,9; 2016,Jan,13; 2015,Jan,16; 2014,Jan,11; 2013,Sep,3-12; 2012,May,3-10

Pathology and Laboratory

80502 — 81206

81207 **minor breakpoint, qualitative or quantitative**
🚑 0.00 ⚕ 0.00 **FUD** XXX [A][📠]
AMA: 2016,Aug,9; 2016,Jan,13; 2015,Jan,16; 2014,Jan,11; 2013,Sep,3-12; 2012,May,3-10

81208 **other breakpoint, qualitative or quantitative**
🚑 0.00 ⚕ 0.00 **FUD** XXX [A][📠]
AMA: 2016,Aug,9; 2016,Jan,13; 2015,Jan,16; 2014,Jan,11; 2013,Sep,3-12; 2012,May,3-10

81209 *BLM (Bloom syndrome, RecQ helicase-like) (eg, Bloom syndrome) gene analysis, 2281del6ins7 variant*
🚑 0.00 ⚕ 0.00 **FUD** XXX [A][📠]
AMA: 2016,Aug,9; 2016,Jan,13; 2015,Jan,16; 2014,Jan,11; 2013,Sep,3-12; 2012,May,3-10

81210 *BRAF (B-Raf proto-oncogene, serine/threonine kinase) (eg, colon cancer, melanoma), gene analysis, V600 variant(s)*
🚑 0.00 ⚕ 0.00 **FUD** XXX [A][📠]
AMA: 2016,Aug,9; 2016,Jan,13; 2015,Jan,16; 2014,Jan,11; 2013,Sep,3-12; 2012,May,3-10

81211 *BRCA1, BRCA2 (breast cancer 1 and 2) (eg, hereditary breast and ovarian cancer) gene analysis; full sequence analysis and common duplication/deletion variants in BRCA1 (ie, exon 13 del 3.835kb, exon 13 dup 6kb, exon 14-20 del 26kb, exon 22 del 510bp, exon 8-9 del 7.1kb)*
> **EXCLUDES** *BRCA1, BRCA2 (breast cancer 1 and 2) (81162)*
🚑 0.00 ⚕ 0.00 **FUD** XXX [A][📠]
AMA: 2016,Aug,9; 2016,Jan,13; 2015,Jan,16; 2014,Jan,11; 2013,Sep,3-12; 2012,May,3-10

\# **81162** **full sequence analysis and full duplication/deletion analysis**
> **EXCLUDES** *BRCA1, BRCA2 (breast cancer 1 and 2) (81211, 81213-81214)*
> *BRCA2 (breast cancer 2) (81216)*
🚑 0.00 ⚕ 0.00 **FUD** XXX [A][📠]
AMA: 2016,Aug,9

81212 **185delAG, 5385insC, 6174delT variants**
🚑 0.00 ⚕ 0.00 **FUD** XXX [A][📠]
AMA: 2016,Aug,9; 2016,Jan,13; 2015,Jan,16; 2014,Jan,11; 2013,Sep,3-12; 2012,May,3-10

81213 **uncommon duplication/deletion variants**
> **EXCLUDES** *BRCA1, BRCA2 (breast cancer 1 and 2) (81162)*
🚑 0.00 ⚕ 0.00 **FUD** XXX [A][📠]
AMA: 2016,Aug,9; 2016,Jan,13; 2015,Jan,16; 2014,Jan,11; 2013,Sep,3-12; 2012,May,3-10

81214 *BRCA1 (breast cancer 1) (eg, hereditary breast and ovarian cancer) gene analysis; full sequence analysis and common duplication/deletion variants (ie, exon 13 del 3.835kb, exon 13 dup 6kb, exon 14-20 del 26kb, exon 22 del 510bp, exon 8-9 del 7.1kb)*
> **EXCLUDES** *BRCA1 with BRCA2 full sequence testing (81162, 81211)*
🚑 0.00 ⚕ 0.00 **FUD** XXX [A][📠]
AMA: 2016,Aug,9; 2016,Jan,13; 2015,Jan,16; 2014,Jan,11; 2013,Sep,3-12; 2012,May,3-10

81215 **known familial variant**
🚑 0.00 ⚕ 0.00 **FUD** XXX [A][📠]
AMA: 2016,Aug,9; 2016,Jan,13; 2015,Jan,16; 2014,Jan,11; 2013,Sep,3-12; 2012,May,3-10

81216 *BRCA2 (breast cancer 2) (eg, hereditary breast and ovarian cancer) gene analysis; full sequence analysis*
> **EXCLUDES** *BRCA1 with BRCA2 full sequence testing (81162, 81211)*
🚑 0.00 ⚕ 0.00 **FUD** XXX [A][📠]
AMA: 2016,Aug,9; 2016,Jan,13; 2015,Jan,16; 2014,Jan,11; 2013,Sep,3-12; 2012,May,3-10

81217 **known familial variant**
🚑 0.00 ⚕ 0.00 **FUD** XXX [A][📠]
AMA: 2016,Aug,9; 2016,Jan,13; 2015,Jan,16; 2014,Jan,11; 2013,Sep,3-12; 2012,May,3-10

81218 *CEBPA (CCAAT/enhancer binding protein [C/EBP], alpha) (eg, acute myeloid leukemia), gene analysis, full gene sequence*
🚑 0.00 ⚕ 0.00 **FUD** XXX [A][📠]
AMA: 2016,Aug,9

81219 *CALR (calreticulin) (eg, myeloproliferative disorders), gene analysis, common variants in exon 9*
🚑 0.00 ⚕ 0.00 **FUD** XXX [A][📠]
AMA: 2016,Aug,9

81220 *CFTR (cystic fibrosis transmembrane conductance regulator) (eg, cystic fibrosis) gene analysis; common variants (eg, ACMG/ACOG guidelines)*
> **EXCLUDES** *CFTR (cystic fibrosis transmembrane conductance regulator) (81224)*
🚑 0.00 ⚕ 0.00 **FUD** XXX [A][📠]
AMA: 2016,Aug,9; 2016,Jan,13; 2015,Jan,16; 2014,Jan,11; 2013,Sep,3-12; 2012,May,3-10

81221 **known familial variants**
🚑 0.00 ⚕ 0.00 **FUD** XXX [A][📠]
AMA: 2016,Aug,9; 2016,Jan,13; 2015,Jan,16; 2014,Jan,11; 2013,Sep,3-12; 2012,May,3-10

81222 **duplication/deletion variants**
🚑 0.00 ⚕ 0.00 **FUD** XXX [A][📠]
AMA: 2016,Aug,9; 2016,Jan,13; 2015,Jan,16; 2014,Jan,11; 2013,Sep,3-12; 2012,May,3-10

81223 **full gene sequence**
🚑 0.00 ⚕ 0.00 **FUD** XXX [A][📠]
AMA: 2016,Aug,9; 2016,Jan,13; 2015,Jan,16; 2014,Jan,11; 2013,Sep,3-12; 2012,May,3-10

81224 **intron 8 poly-T analysis (eg, male infertility)**
🚑 0.00 ⚕ 0.00 **FUD** XXX [A][📠]
AMA: 2016,Aug,9; 2016,Jan,13; 2015,Jan,16; 2014,Jan,11; 2013,Sep,3-12; 2012,May,3-10

81225 *CYP2C19 (cytochrome P450, family 2, subfamily C, polypeptide 19) (eg, drug metabolism), gene analysis, common variants (eg, *2, *3, *4, *8, *17)*
🚑 0.00 ⚕ 0.00 **FUD** XXX [A][📠]
AMA: 2016,Aug,9; 2016,Jan,13; 2015,Jan,16; 2014,Jan,11; 2013,Sep,3-12; 2012,May,3-10

81226 *CYP2D6 (cytochrome P450, family 2, subfamily D, polypeptide 6) (eg, drug metabolism), gene analysis, common variants (eg, *2, *3, *4, *5, *6, *9, *10, *17, *19, *29, *35, *41, *1XN, *2XN, *4XN)*
🚑 0.00 ⚕ 0.00 **FUD** XXX [A][📠]
AMA: 2016,Aug,9; 2016,Jan,13; 2015,Jan,16; 2014,Jan,11; 2013,Sep,3-12; 2012,May,3-10

81227 *CYP2C9 (cytochrome P450, family 2, subfamily C, polypeptide 9) (eg, drug metabolism), gene analysis, common variants (eg, *2, *3, *5, *6)*
🚑 0.00 ⚕ 0.00 **FUD** XXX [A][📠]
AMA: 2016,Aug,9; 2016,Jan,13; 2015,Jan,16; 2014,Jan,11; 2013,Sep,3-12; 2012,May,3-10

81228 **Cytogenomic constitutional (genome-wide) microarray analysis; interrogation of genomic regions for copy number variants (eg, bacterial artificial chromosome [BAC] or oligo-based comparative genomic hybridization [CGH] microarray analysis)**
> **EXCLUDES** *Cytogenomic constitutional microarray analysis (genome-wide) (81229)*
> *Cytogenomic constitutional microarray analysis (not genome-wide), report code for targeted analysis or unlisted molecular pathology (81405, [81479])*
> *Molecular cytogenetics (88271)*
> *Use of code with analyte-specific procedures when the analytes are included in the microarray analysis*
🚑 0.00 ⚕ 0.00 **FUD** XXX [A][📠]
AMA: 2016,Aug,9; 2016,Jan,13; 2015,Jan,16; 2014,Jan,11; 2013,Sep,3-12; 2012,May,3-10

26/TC PC/TC Only   **A2-Z3** ASC Payment   **50** Bilateral   ♂ Male Only   ♀ Female Only   🚑 Facility RVU   ⚕ Non-Facility RVU   📠 CCI
FUD Follow-up Days   **CMS:** IOM (Pub 100)   [A]-[Y] OPPSI   **80/80** Surg Assist Allowed / w/Doc   📠 Lab Crosswalk   📠 Radiology Crosswalk   ☒ CLIA

346   CPT © 2016 American Medical Association. All Rights Reserved.   © 2016 Optum360, LLC

81229 interrogation of genomic regions for copy number and single nucleotide polymorphism (SNP) variants for chromosomal abnormalities

> EXCLUDES *Cytogenomic constitutional microarray analysis (genome-wide) (81228)*
> *Cytogenomic constitutional microarray analysis (not genome-wide), report code for targeted analysis or unlisted molecular pathology (81405, [81479])*
> *Fetal chromosome analysis using maternal blood ([81479], 81420-81422)*
> *Molecular cytogenetics (88271)*
> *Use of code with analyte-specific procedures when the analytes are included in the microarray analysis*

🔷 0.00　🔶 0.00　**FUD** XXX　Ⓐ ▯

AMA: 2016,Aug,9; 2016,Jan,13; 2015,Jan,16; 2014,Jan,11; 2013,Sep,3-12; 2012,May,3-10

\# **81161** *DMD (dystrophin) (eg, Duchenne/Becker muscular dystrophy) deletion analysis, and duplication analysis, if performed*

🔷 0.00　🔶 0.00　**FUD** XXX　Ⓐ ▯

AMA: 2016,Aug,9; 2014,Jan,11

81235 *EGFR (epidermal growth factor receptor) (eg, non-small cell lung cancer) gene analysis, common variants (eg, exon 19 LREA deletion, L858R, T790M, G719A, G719S, L861Q)*

🔷 0.00　🔶 0.00　Ⓐ ▯

AMA: 2016,Aug,9; 2016,Jan,13; 2015,Jan,16; 2014,Jan,11; 2013,Sep,3-12

81240 *F2 (prothrombin, coagulation factor II) (eg, hereditary hypercoagulability) gene analysis, 20210G>A variant*

🔷 0.00　🔶 0.00　**FUD** XXX　Ⓐ ▯

AMA: 2016,Aug,9; 2016,Jan,13; 2015,Jan,16; 2014,Jan,11; 2013,Sep,3-12; 2012,May,3-10

81241 *F5 (coagulation factor V) (eg, hereditary hypercoagulability) gene analysis, Leiden variant*

🔷 0.00　🔶 0.00　**FUD** XXX　Ⓐ ▯

AMA: 2016,Aug,9; 2016,Jan,13; 2015,Jan,16; 2014,Jan,11; 2013,Sep,3-12; 2012,May,3-10

81242 *FANCC (Fanconi anemia, complementation group C) (eg, Fanconi anemia, type C) gene analysis, common variant (eg, IVS4+4A>T)*

🔷 0.00　🔶 0.00　**FUD** XXX　Ⓐ ▯

AMA: 2016,Aug,9; 2016,Jan,13; 2015,Jan,16; 2014,Jan,11; 2013,Sep,3-12; 2012,May,3-10

81243 *FMR1 (fragile X mental retardation 1) (eg, fragile X mental retardation) gene analysis; evaluation to detect abnormal (eg, expanded) alleles*

> INCLUDES *Testing for detection and characterization of abnormal alleles using a single assay such as PCR*

🔷 0.00　🔶 0.00　**FUD** XXX　Ⓐ ▯

AMA: 2016,Aug,9; 2016,Jan,13; 2015,Jan,16; 2014,Jan,11; 2013,Sep,3-12; 2012,May,3-10

81244 characterization of alleles (eg, expanded size and methylation status)

> EXCLUDES *Testing for detection and characterization of abnormal alleles using a single assay such as PCR (81243)*

🔷 0.00　🔶 0.00　**FUD** XXX　Ⓐ ▯

AMA: 2016,Aug,9; 2016,Jan,13; 2015,Jan,16; 2014,Jan,11; 2013,Sep,3-12; 2012,May,3-10

81245 *FLT3 (fms-related tyrosine kinase 3) (eg, acute myeloid leukemia), gene analysis; internal tandem duplication (ITD) variants (ie, exons 14, 15)*

🔷 0.00　🔶 0.00　**FUD** XXX　Ⓐ ▯

AMA: 2016,Aug,9; 2016,Jan,13; 2015,Jan,16; 2015,Jan,3; 2014,Jan,11; 2013,Sep,3-12; 2012,May,3-10

81246 tyrosine kinase domain (TKD) variants (eg, D835, I836)

🔷 0.00　🔶 0.00　**FUD** XXX　Ⓐ ▯

AMA: 2016,Aug,9; 2016,Jan,13; 2015,Jan,3

81250 *G6PC (glucose-6-phosphatase, catalytic subunit) (eg, Glycogen storage disease, type 1a, von Gierke disease) gene analysis, common variants (eg, R83C, Q347X)*

🔷 0.00　🔶 0.00　**FUD** XXX　Ⓐ ▯

AMA: 2016,Aug,9; 2016,Jan,13; 2015,Jan,16; 2014,Jan,11; 2013,Sep,3-12; 2012,May,3-10

81251 *GBA (glucosidase, beta, acid) (eg, Gaucher disease) gene analysis, common variants (eg, N370S, 84GG, L444P, IVS2+1G>A)*

🔷 0.00　🔶 0.00　**FUD** XXX　Ⓐ ▯

AMA: 2016,Aug,9; 2016,Jan,13; 2015,Jan,16; 2014,Jan,11; 2013,Sep,3-12; 2012,May,3-10

81252 *GJB2 (gap junction protein, beta 2, 26kDa, connexin 26) (eg, nonsyndromic hearing loss) gene analysis; full gene sequence*

🔷 0.00　🔶 0.00　**FUD** XXX　Ⓐ ▯

AMA: 2016,Aug,9; 2016,Jan,13; 2015,Jan,16; 2014,Jan,11; 2013,Sep,3-12

81253 known familial variants

🔷 0.00　🔶 0.00　**FUD** XXX　Ⓐ ▯

AMA: 2016,Aug,9; 2016,Jan,13; 2015,Jan,16; 2014,Jan,11; 2013,Sep,3-12

81254 *GJB6 (gap junction protein, beta 6, 30kDa, connexin 30) (eg, nonsyndromic hearing loss) gene analysis, common variants (eg, 309kb [del(GJB6-D13S1830)] and 232kb [del(GJB6-D13S1854)])*

🔷 0.00　🔶 0.00　**FUD** XXX　Ⓐ ▯

AMA: 2016,Aug,9; 2016,Jan,13; 2015,Jan,16; 2014,Jan,11; 2013,Sep,3-12

81255 *HEXA (hexosaminidase A [alpha polypeptide]) (eg, Tay-Sachs disease) gene analysis, common variants (eg, 1278insTATC, 1421+1G>C, G269S)*

🔷 0.00　🔶 0.00　**FUD** XXX　Ⓐ ▯

AMA: 2016,Aug,9; 2016,Jan,13; 2015,Jan,16; 2014,Jan,11; 2013,Sep,3-12; 2012,May,3-10

81256 *HFE (hemochromatosis) (eg, hereditary hemochromatosis) gene analysis, common variants (eg, C282Y, H63D)*

🔷 0.00　🔶 0.00　**FUD** XXX　Ⓐ ▯

AMA: 2016,Aug,9; 2016,Jan,13; 2015,Jan,16; 2014,Jan,11; 2013,Sep,3-12; 2012,May,3-10

81257 *HBA1/HBA2 (alpha globin 1 and alpha globin 2) (eg, alpha thalassemia, Hb Bart hydrops fetalis syndrome, HbH disease), gene analysis, for common deletions or variant (eg, Southeast Asian, Thai, Filipino, Mediterranean, alpha3.7, alpha4.2, alpha20.5, and Constant Spring)*

🔷 0.00　🔶 0.00　**FUD** XXX　Ⓐ ▯

AMA: 2016,Aug,9; 2016,Jan,13; 2015,Jan,16; 2014,Jan,11; 2013,Sep,3-12; 2012,May,3-10

81260 *IKBKAP (inhibitor of kappa light polypeptide gene enhancer in B-cells, kinase complex-associated protein) (eg, familial dysautonomia) gene analysis, common variants (eg, 2507+6T>C, R696P)*

🔷 0.00　🔶 0.00　**FUD** XXX　Ⓐ ▯

AMA: 2016,Aug,9; 2016,Jan,13; 2015,Jan,16; 2014,Jan,11; 2013,Sep,3-12; 2012,May,3-10

81261 *IGH@ (Immunoglobulin heavy chain locus) (eg, leukemias and lymphomas, B-cell), gene rearrangement analysis to detect abnormal clonal population(s); amplified methodology (eg, polymerase chain reaction)*

🔷 0.00　🔶 0.00　**FUD** XXX　Ⓐ ▯

AMA: 2016,Aug,9; 2016,Jan,13; 2015,Jan,16; 2014,Jan,11; 2013,Sep,3-12; 2012,May,3-10

81262 direct probe methodology (eg, Southern blot)

🔷 0.00　🔶 0.00　**FUD** XXX　Ⓐ ▯

AMA: 2016,Aug,9; 2016,Jan,13; 2015,Jan,16; 2014,Jan,11; 2013,Sep,3-12; 2012,May,3-10

81263 **IGH@ (Immunoglobulin heavy chain locus)** *(eg, leukemia and lymphoma, B-cell), variable region somatic mutation analysis*

    0.00   0.00   **FUD** XXX   A

    AMA: 2016,Aug,9; 2016,Jan,13; 2015,Jan,16; 2014,Jan,11; 2013,Sep,3-12; 2012,May,3-10

81264 **IGK@ (Immunoglobulin kappa light chain locus)** *(eg, leukemia and lymphoma, B-cell), gene rearrangement analysis, evaluation to detect abnormal clonal population(s)*

    EXCLUDES   *Immunoglobulin kappa deleting element (IGKDEL) analysis ([81479])*

                Immunoglobulin lambda gene (IGL@) rearrangement ([81479])

    0.00   0.00   **FUD** XXX   A

    AMA: 2016,Aug,9; 2016,Jan,13; 2015,Jan,16; 2014,Jan,11; 2013,Sep,3-12; 2012,May,3-10

81265 **Comparative analysis using Short Tandem Repeat (STR) markers; patient and comparative specimen (eg, pre-transplant recipient and donor germline testing, post-transplant non-hematopoietic recipient germline [eg, buccal swab or other germline tissue sample] and donor testing, twin zygosity testing, or maternal cell contamination of fetal cells)**

    Code also the following codes for chimerism testing if comparative short tandem repeat (STR) analysis of recipient (using buccal swab or other germline tissue sample) and donor are performed after hematopoietic stem cell transplantation (81266-81268)

    0.00   0.00   **FUD** XXX   A

    AMA: 2016,Aug,9; 2016,Jan,13; 2015,Jan,16; 2014,Jan,11; 2013,Sep,3-12; 2012,May,3-10

+ 81266 **each additional specimen (eg, additional cord blood donor, additional fetal samples from different cultures, or additional zygosity in multiple birth pregnancies) (List separately in addition to code for primary procedure)**

    Code also the following codes for chimerism testing if comparative short tandem repeat (STR) analysis of recipient (using buccal swab or other germline tissue sample) and donor are performed after hematopoietic stem cell transplantation (81267-81268)

    Code first (81265)

    0.00   0.00   **FUD** XXX   A

    AMA: 2016,Aug,9; 2016,Jan,13; 2015,Jan,16; 2014,Jan,11; 2013,Sep,3-12; 2012,May,3-10

81267 **Chimerism (engraftment) analysis, post transplantation specimen (eg, hematopoietic stem cell), includes comparison to previously performed baseline analyses; without cell selection**

    Code also the following codes for chimerism testing if comparative short tandem repeat (STR) analysis of recipient (using buccal swab or other germline tissue sample) and donor are performed after hematopoietic stem cell transplantation (81265-81266, 81268)

    0.00   0.00   **FUD** XXX   A

    AMA: 2016,Aug,9; 2016,Jan,13; 2015,Jan,16; 2014,Jan,11; 2013,Sep,3-12; 2012,May,3-10

81268 **with cell selection (eg, CD3, CD33), each cell type**

    Code also the following codes for chimerism testing if comparative short tandem repeat (STR) analysis of recipient (using buccal swab or other germline tissue sample) and donor are performed after hematopoietic stem cell transplantation (81265-81267)

    0.00   0.00   **FUD** XXX   A

    AMA: 2016,Aug,9; 2016,Jan,13; 2015,Jan,16; 2014,Jan,11; 2013,Sep,3-12; 2012,May,3-10

81270 **JAK2 (Janus kinase 2)** *(eg, myeloproliferative disorder) gene analysis, p.Val617Phe (V617F) variant*

    0.00   0.00   **FUD** XXX   A

    AMA: 2016,Aug,9; 2016,Jan,13; 2015,Jan,16; 2014,Jan,11; 2013,Sep,3-12; 2012,May,3-10

81272 **KIT (v-kit Hardy-Zuckerman 4 feline sarcoma viral oncogene homolog)** *(eg, gastrointestinal stromal tumor [GIST], acute myeloid leukemia, melanoma), gene analysis, targeted sequence analysis (eg, exons 8, 11, 13, 17, 18)*

    0.00   0.00   **FUD** XXX   A

    AMA: 2016,Aug,9

81273 **KIT (v-kit Hardy-Zuckerman 4 feline sarcoma viral oncogene homolog)** *(eg, mastocytosis), gene analysis, D816 variant*

    0.00   0.00   **FUD** XXX   A

    AMA: 2016,Aug,9

81275 **KRAS (Kirsten rat sarcoma viral oncogene homolog)** *(eg, carcinoma) gene analysis; variants in exon 2 (eg, codons 12 and 13)*

    0.00   0.00   **FUD** XXX   A

    AMA: 2016,Aug,9; 2016,Jan,13; 2015,Jan,16; 2014,Jan,11; 2013,Sep,3-12; 2012,May,3-10

81276 **additional variant(s) (eg, codon 61, codon 146)**

    0.00   0.00   **FUD** XXX   A

    AMA: 2016,Aug,9

81280 ~~Long QT syndrome gene analyses (eg, *KCNQ1, KCNH2, SCN5A, KCNE1, KCNE2, KCNJ2, CACNA1C, CAV3, SCN4B, AKAP, SNTA1,* and *ANK2*); full sequence analysis~~

81281 ~~known familial sequence variant~~

81282 ~~duplication/deletion variants~~

81287 **Resequenced code. See code following 81290.**

81288 **Resequenced code. See code following 81292.**

81290 **MCOLN1 (mucolipin 1)** *(eg, Mucolipidosis, type IV) gene analysis, common variants (eg, IVS3-2A>G, del6.4kb)*

    0.00   0.00   **FUD** XXX   A

    AMA: 2016,Aug,9; 2016,Jan,13; 2015,Jan,16; 2014,Jan,11; 2013,Sep,3-12; 2012,May,3-10

 # 81287 **MGMT (O-6-methylguanine-DNA methyltransferase)** *(eg, glioblastoma multiforme), methylation analysis*

    0.00   0.00   **FUD** XXX   A

    AMA: 2016,Aug,9; 2014,Jan,11

81291 **MTHFR (5,10-methylenetetrahydrofolate reductase)** *(eg, hereditary hypercoagulability) gene analysis, common variants (eg, 677T, 1298C)*

    0.00   0.00   **FUD** XXX   A

    AMA: 2016,Aug,9; 2016,Jan,13; 2015,Jan,16; 2014,Jan,11; 2013,Sep,3-12; 2012,May,3-10

81292 **MLH1 (mutL homolog 1, colon cancer, nonpolyposis type 2)** *(eg, hereditary non-polyposis colorectal cancer, Lynch syndrome) gene analysis; full sequence analysis*

    0.00   0.00   **FUD** XXX   A

    AMA: 2016,Aug,9; 2016,Jan,13; 2015,Jan,16; 2015,Jan,3; 2014,Jan,11; 2013,Sep,3-12; 2012,May,3-10

 # 81288 **promoter methylation analysis**

    0.00   0.00   **FUD** XXX   A

    AMA: 2016,Aug,9; 2016,Jan,13; 2015,Jan,3

81293 **known familial variants**

    0.00   0.00   **FUD** XXX   A

    AMA: 2016,Aug,9; 2016,Jan,13; 2015,Jan,16; 2014,Jan,11; 2013,Sep,3-12; 2012,May,3-10

81294 **duplication/deletion variants**

    0.00   0.00   **FUD** XXX   A

    AMA: 2016,Aug,9; 2016,Jan,13; 2015,Jan,16; 2014,Jan,11; 2013,Sep,3-12; 2012,May,3-10

81295 **MSH2 (mutS homolog 2, colon cancer, nonpolyposis type 1)** *(eg, hereditary non-polyposis colorectal cancer, Lynch syndrome) gene analysis; full sequence analysis*

    0.00   0.00   **FUD** XXX   A

    AMA: 2016,Aug,9; 2016,Jan,13; 2015,Jan,16; 2014,Jan,11; 2013,Sep,3-12; 2012,May,3-10

26/TC PC/TC Only   **A2-Z3** ASC Payment   **50** Bilateral   ♂ Male Only   ♀ Female Only   Facility RVU   Non-Facility RVU   CCI
FUD Follow-up Days   **CMS:** IOM (Pub 100)   **A-Y** OPPSI   **80/80** Surg Assist Allowed / w/Doc   Lab Crosswalk   Radiology Crosswalk   **X** CLIA

348   CPT © 2016 American Medical Association. All Rights Reserved.   © 2016 Optum360, LLC

81296   **known familial variants**
    🔲 0.00   ⚕ 0.00   **FUD** XXX   Ⓐ 🔲
    AMA: 2016,Aug,9; 2016,Jan,13; 2015,Jan,16; 2014,Jan,11;
    2013,Sep,3-12; 2012,May,3-10

81297   **duplication/deletion variants**
    🔲 0.00   ⚕ 0.00   **FUD** XXX   Ⓐ 🔲
    AMA: 2016,Aug,9; 2016,Jan,13; 2015,Jan,16; 2014,Jan,11;
    2013,Sep,3-12; 2012,May,3-10

81298   *MSH6 (mutS homolog 6 [E. coli]) (eg, hereditary non-polyposis
    colorectal cancer, Lynch syndrome) gene analysis; full
    sequence analysis*
    🔲 0.00   ⚕ 0.00   **FUD** XXX   Ⓐ 🔲
    AMA: 2016,Aug,9; 2016,Jan,13; 2015,Jan,16; 2014,Jan,11;
    2013,Sep,3-12; 2012,May,3-10

81299   **known familial variants**
    🔲 0.00   ⚕ 0.00   **FUD** XXX   Ⓐ 🔲
    AMA: 2016,Aug,9; 2016,Jan,13; 2015,Jan,16; 2014,Jan,11;
    2013,Sep,3-12; 2012,May,3-10

81300   **duplication/deletion variants**
    🔲 0.00   ⚕ 0.00   **FUD** XXX   Ⓐ 🔲
    AMA: 2016,Aug,9; 2016,Jan,13; 2015,Jan,16; 2014,Jan,11;
    2013,Sep,3-12; 2012,May,3-10

81301   **Microsatellite instability analysis (eg, hereditary
    non-polyposis colorectal cancer, Lynch syndrome) of markers
    for mismatch repair deficiency (eg, BAT25, BAT26), includes
    comparison of neoplastic and normal tissue, if performed**
    🔲 0.00   ⚕ 0.00   **FUD** XXX   Ⓐ 🔲
    AMA: 2016,Aug,9; 2016,Jan,13; 2015,Jan,16; 2014,Jan,11;
    2013,Sep,3-12; 2012,May,3-10

81302   *MECP2 (methyl CpG binding protein 2) (eg, Rett syndrome)
    gene analysis; full sequence analysis*
    🔲 0.00   ⚕ 0.00   **FUD** XXX   Ⓐ 🔲
    AMA: 2016,Aug,9; 2016,Jan,13; 2015,Jan,16; 2014,Jan,11;
    2013,Sep,3-12; 2012,May,3-10

81303   **known familial variant**
    🔲 0.00   ⚕ 0.00   **FUD** XXX   Ⓐ 🔲
    AMA: 2016,Aug,9; 2016,Jan,13; 2015,Jan,16; 2014,Jan,11;
    2013,Sep,3-12; 2012,May,3-10

81304   **duplication/deletion variants**
    🔲 0.00   ⚕ 0.00   **FUD** XXX   Ⓐ 🔲
    AMA: 2016,Aug,9; 2016,Jan,13; 2015,Jan,16; 2014,Jan,11;
    2013,Sep,3-12; 2012,May,3-10

81310   *NPM1 (nucleophosmin) (eg, acute myeloid leukemia) gene
    analysis, exon 12 variants*
    🔲 0.00   ⚕ 0.00   **FUD** XXX   Ⓐ 🔲
    AMA: 2016,Aug,9; 2016,Jan,13; 2015,Jan,16; 2014,Jan,11;
    2013,Sep,3-12; 2012,May,3-10

81311   *NRAS (neuroblastoma RAS viral [v-ras] oncogene homolog) (eg,
    colorectal carcinoma), gene analysis, variants in exon 2 (eg,
    codons 12 and 13) and exon 3 (eg, codon 61)*
    🔲 0.00   ⚕ 0.00   **FUD** XXX   Ⓐ 🔲
    AMA: 2016,Aug,9

81313   *PCA3/KLK3 (prostate cancer antigen 3 [non-protein
    coding]/kallikrein-related peptidase 3 [prostate specific
    antigen]) ratio (eg, prostate cancer)*
    🔲 0.00   ⚕ 0.00   **FUD** XXX   Ⓐ 🔲
    AMA: 2016,Aug,9; 2016,Jan,13; 2015,Jan,3

81314   *PDGFRA (platelet-derived growth factor receptor, alpha
    polypeptide) (eg, gastrointestinal stromal tumor [GIST]), gene
    analysis, targeted sequence analysis (eg, exons 12, 18)*
    🔲 0.00   ⚕ 0.00   **FUD** XXX   Ⓐ 🔲
    AMA: 2016,Aug,9

81315   *PML/RARalpha, (t(15;17)), (promyelocytic leukemia/retinoic
    acid receptor alpha) (eg, promyelocytic leukemia)
    translocation analysis; common breakpoints (eg, intron 3 and
    intron 6), qualitative or quantitative*
    INCLUDES   Intron 3 and 6 (and exon 6 if performed) testing
    🔲 0.00   ⚕ 0.00   **FUD** XXX   Ⓐ 🔲
    AMA: 2016,Aug,9; 2016,Jan,13; 2015,Jan,16; 2014,Jan,11;
    2013,Sep,3-12; 2012,May,3-10

81316   **single breakpoint (eg, intron 3, intron 6 or exon 6),
    qualitative or quantitative**
    EXCLUDES   Intron 3 and 6 (and exon 6 if performed) testing (81315)
            Use of more than one unit of this code for testing intron
            6 and exon 6 without intron 3 (81316)
    🔲 0.00   ⚕ 0.00   **FUD** XXX   Ⓐ 🔲
    AMA: 2016,Aug,9; 2016,Jan,13; 2015,Jan,16; 2014,Jan,11;
    2013,Sep,3-12; 2012,May,3-10

81317   *PMS2 (postmeiotic segregation increased 2 [S. cerevisiae]) (eg,
    hereditary non-polyposis colorectal cancer, Lynch syndrome)
    gene analysis; full sequence analysis*
    🔲 0.00   ⚕ 0.00   **FUD** XXX   Ⓐ 🔲
    AMA: 2016,Aug,9; 2016,Jan,13; 2015,Jan,16; 2014,Jan,11;
    2013,Sep,3-12; 2012,May,3-10

81318   **known familial variants**
    🔲 0.00   ⚕ 0.00   **FUD** XXX   Ⓐ 🔲
    AMA: 2016,Aug,9; 2016,Jan,13; 2015,Jan,16; 2014,Jan,11;
    2013,Sep,3-12; 2012,May,3-10

81319   **duplication/deletion variants**
    🔲 0.00   ⚕ 0.00   **FUD** XXX   Ⓐ 🔲
    AMA: 2016,Aug,9; 2016,Jan,13; 2015,Jan,16; 2014,Jan,11;
    2013,Sep,3-12; 2012,May,3-10

81321   *PTEN (phosphatase and tensin homolog) (eg, Cowden
    syndrome, PTEN hamartoma tumor syndrome) gene analysis;
    full sequence analysis*
    🔲 0.00   ⚕ 0.00   **FUD** XXX   Ⓐ 🔲
    AMA: 2016,Aug,9; 2016,Jan,13; 2015,Jan,16; 2014,Jan,11;
    2013,Sep,3-12

81322   **known familial variant**
    🔲 0.00   ⚕ 0.00   **FUD** XXX   Ⓐ 🔲
    AMA: 2016,Aug,9; 2016,Jan,13; 2015,Jan,16; 2014,Jan,11;
    2013,Sep,3-12

81323   **duplication/deletion variant**
    🔲 0.00   ⚕ 0.00   **FUD** XXX   Ⓐ 🔲
    AMA: 2016,Aug,9; 2016,Jan,13; 2015,Jan,16; 2014,Jan,11;
    2013,Sep,3-12

81324   *PMP22 (peripheral myelin protein 22) (eg,
    Charcot-Marie-Tooth, hereditary neuropathy with liability to
    pressure palsies) gene analysis; duplication/deletion
    analysis*
    🔲 0.00   ⚕ 0.00   **FUD** XXX   Ⓐ 🔲
    AMA: 2016,Aug,9; 2016,Jan,13; 2015,Jan,16; 2014,Jan,11;
    2013,Sep,3-12

81325   **full sequence analysis**
    🔲 0.00   ⚕ 0.00   **FUD** XXX   Ⓐ 🔲
    AMA: 2016,Aug,9; 2016,Jan,13; 2015,Jan,16; 2014,Jan,11;
    2013,Sep,3-12

81326   **known familial variant**
    🔲 0.00   ⚕ 0.00   **FUD** XXX   Ⓐ 🔲
    AMA: 2016,Aug,9; 2016,Jan,13; 2015,Jan,16; 2014,Jan,11;
    2013,Sep,3-12

● **81327**   *SEPT9 (Septin9) (eg, colorectal cancer) methylation analysis*

81330   *SMPD1(sphingomyelin phosphodiesterase 1, acid lysosomal)
    (eg, Niemann-Pick disease, Type A) gene analysis, common
    variants (eg, R496L, L302P, fsP330)*
    🔲 0.00   ⚕ 0.00   **FUD** XXX   Ⓐ 🔲
    AMA: 2016,Aug,9; 2016,Jan,13; 2015,Jan,16; 2014,Jan,11;
    2013,Sep,3-12; 2012,May,3-10

● New Code   ▲ Revised Code   ○ Reinstated   ● New Web Release   ▲ Revised Web Release   Unlisted   Not Covered   # Resequenced
⊘ AMA Mod 51 Exempt   ⑩ Optum Mod 51 Exempt   ⑥③ Mod 63 Exempt   ✎ Non-FDA Drug   ★ Telehealth   Ⓜ Maternity   Ⓐ Age Edit   + Add-on   **AMA:** CPT Asst

81331 *SNRPN/UBE3A (small nuclear ribonucleoprotein polypeptide N and ubiquitin protein ligase E3A) (eg, Prader-Willi syndrome and/or Angelman syndrome), methylation analysis*
⏣ 0.00 ⚷ 0.00 **FUD** XXX 🅐 🖳
AMA: 2016,Aug,9; 2016,Jan,13; 2015,Jan,16; 2014,Jan,11; 2013,Sep,3-12; 2012,May,3-10

81332 *SERPINA1 (serpin peptidase inhibitor, clade A, alpha-1 antiproteinase, antitrypsin, member 1) (eg, alpha-1-antitrypsin deficiency), gene analysis, common variants (eg, *S and *Z)*
⏣ 0.00 ⚷ 0.00 **FUD** XXX 🅐 🖳
AMA: 2016,Aug,9; 2016,Jan,13; 2015,Jan,16; 2014,Jan,11; 2013,Sep,3-12; 2012,May,3-10

81340 *TRB@ (T cell antigen receptor, beta) (eg, leukemia and lymphoma), gene rearrangement analysis to detect abnormal clonal population(s); using amplification methodology (eg, polymerase chain reaction)*
⏣ 0.00 ⚷ 0.00 **FUD** XXX 🅐 🖳
AMA: 2016,Aug,9; 2016,Jan,13; 2015,Jan,16; 2014,Jan,11; 2013,Sep,3-12; 2012,May,3-10

81341 *using direct probe methodology (eg, Southern blot)*
⏣ 0.00 ⚷ 0.00 **FUD** XXX 🅐 🖳
AMA: 2016,Aug,9; 2016,Jan,13; 2015,Jan,16; 2014,Jan,11; 2013,Sep,3-12; 2012,May,3-10

81342 *TRG@ (T cell antigen receptor, gamma) (eg, leukemia and lymphoma), gene rearrangement analysis, evaluation to detect abnormal clonal population(s)*
EXCLUDES *T cell antigen alpha [TRA@] gene arrangement testing ([81479])*
T cell antigen delta [TRD@] gene arrangement testing (81402)
⏣ 0.00 ⚷ 0.00 **FUD** XXX 🅐 🖳
AMA: 2016,Aug,9; 2016,Jan,13; 2015,Jan,16; 2014,Jan,11; 2013,Sep,3-12; 2012,May,3-10

81350 *UGT1A1 (UDP glucuronosyltransferase 1 family, polypeptide A1) (eg, irinotecan metabolism), gene analysis, common variants (eg, *28, *36, *37)*
⏣ 0.00 ⚷ 0.00 **FUD** XXX 🅐 🖳
AMA: 2016,Aug,9; 2016,Jan,13; 2015,Jan,16; 2014,Jan,11; 2013,Sep,3-12; 2012,May,3-10

81355 *VKORC1 (vitamin K epoxide reductase complex, subunit 1) (eg, warfarin metabolism), gene analysis, common variant(s) (eg, -1639G>A, c.173+1000C>T)*
⏣ 0.00 ⚷ 0.00 **FUD** XXX 🅐 🖳
AMA: 2016,Aug,9; 2016,Jan,13; 2015,Jan,16; 2014,Jan,11; 2013,Sep,3-12; 2012,May,3-10

81370-81383 Human Leukocyte Antigen (HLA) Testing

INCLUDES Additional testing that must be performed to resolve ambiguous allele combinations for high-resolution typing
All analytical procedures in the evaluation such as:
Amplification
Cell lysis
Detection
Digestion
Extraction
Nucleic acid stabilization
Analysis to identify human leukocyte antigen (HLA) alleles and allele groups connected to specific diseases and individual response to drug therapy in addition to other clinical uses
Code selection based on specific gene being reviewed
Evaluation of the presence of gene variants using the common gene variant name
Examples of proteins or diseases in the code description that are not all inclusive
Generally all the listed gene variants in the code description would be tested but lists are not all inclusive
Genes described using Human Genome Organization (HUGO) approved names
High-resolution typing resolves the common well-defined (CWD) alleles and is usually identified by at least four-digits. There are some instances when high-resolution typing may include some ambiguities for rare alleles, and those may be reported as a string of alleles or an NMDP code
Histocompatibility antigen testing
Intermediate resolution HLA testing is identified by a string of alleles or a National Marrow Donor Program (NMDP) code
Low and intermediate resolution are considered low resolution for code assignment
Low-resolution HLA type reporting is identified by two-digit HLA name
Multiple variant alleles or allele groups that can be identified by typing
One or more HLA genes in specific clinical circumstances
Qualitative results unless otherwise stated
Typing performed to determine the compatibility of recipients and potential donors undergoing solid organ or hematopoietic stem cell pretransplantation testing
EXCLUDES Full gene sequencing using separate gene variant assessment codes unless it is specifically stated in the code description
HLA antigen typing by nonmolecular pathology methods (86812-86822)
Microbial identification (87149-87153, 87470-87801 [87623, 87624, 87625], 87900-87904 [87906, 87910, 87912])
Other related gene variants not listed in code
Tier 1 molecular pathology codes (81200-81355 [81161, 81162, 81287, 81288])
Tier 2 and unlisted mocular pathology procedures (81400-81408, [81479])
Code also modifier 26 when only interpretation and report are performed
Code also services required before cell lysis

81370 HLA Class I and II typing, low resolution (eg, antigen equivalents); HLA-A, -B, -C, -DRB1/3/4/5, and -DQB1
⏣ 0.00 ⚷ 0.00 **FUD** XXX 🅐 🖳
AMA: 2016,Aug,9; 2016,Jan,13; 2015,Jan,16; 2014,Jan,11; 2013,Sep,3-12; 2012,May,3-10; 2012,Jun,15-16

81371 *HLA-A, -B, and -DRB1(eg, verification typing)*
⏣ 0.00 ⚷ 0.00 **FUD** XXX 🅐 🖳
AMA: 2016,Aug,9; 2016,Jan,13; 2015,Jan,16; 2014,Jan,11; 2013,Sep,3-12; 2012,May,3-10; 2012,Jun,15-16

81372 HLA Class I typing, low resolution (eg, antigen equivalents); complete (ie, HLA-A, -B, and -C)
EXCLUDES *Class I and II low-resolution HLA typing for HLA-A, -B, -C, -DRB1/3/4/5, and -DQB1 (81370)*
⏣ 0.00 ⚷ 0.00 **FUD** XXX 🅐 🖳
AMA: 2016,Aug,9; 2016,Jan,13; 2015,Jan,16; 2014,Jan,11; 2013,Sep,3-12; 2012,May,3-10; 2012,Jun,15-16

81373 one locus (eg, HLA-A, -B, or -C), each
EXCLUDES *A complete Class 1 (HLA-A, -B, and -C) low-resolution typing (81372)*
Reporting the presence or absence of a single antigen equivalent using low-resolution methodology (81374)
⏣ 0.00 ⚷ 0.00 **FUD** XXX 🅐 🖳
AMA: 2016,Aug,9; 2016,Jan,13; 2015,Jan,16; 2014,Jan,11; 2013,Sep,3-12; 2012,May,3-10; 2012,Jun,15-16

81374   one antigen equivalent (eg, B*27), each

EXCLUDES   *Testing for the presence or absence of more than 2 antigen equivalents at a locus, use the following code for each locus test (81373)*

💰 0.00   ⚕ 0.00   **FUD** XXX   🅰 ▱

AMA: 2016,Aug,9; 2016,Jan,13; 2015,Jan,16; 2014,Jan,11; 2013,Sep,3-12; 2012,May,3-10; 2012,Jun,15-16

81375   HLA Class II typing, low resolution (eg, antigen equivalents); *HLA-DRB1/3/4/5 and -DQB1*

EXCLUDES   *Class I and II low-resolution HLA typing for HLA-A, -B, -C, -DRB 1/3/4/5, and DQB1 (81370)*

💰 0.00   ⚕ 0.00   **FUD** XXX   🅰 ▱

AMA: 2016,Aug,9; 2016,Jan,13; 2015,Jan,16; 2014,Jan,11; 2013,Sep,3-12; 2012,May,3-10; 2012,Jun,15-16

81376   one locus (eg, *HLA-DRB1, -DRB3/4/5, -DQB1, -DQA1, -DPB1, or -DPA1*), each

INCLUDES   Low-resolution typing, HLA-DRB1/3/4/5 reported as a single locus

EXCLUDES   *Low-resolution typing for HLA-DRB1/3/4/5 and -DQB1 (81375)*

💰 0.00   ⚕ 0.00   **FUD** XXX   🅰 ▱

AMA: 2016,Aug,9; 2016,Jan,13; 2015,Jan,16; 2014,Jan,11; 2013,Sep,3-12; 2012,May,3-10; 2012,Jun,15-16

81377   one antigen equivalent, each

EXCLUDES   *Testing for presence or absence of more than two antigen equivalents at a locus (81376)*

💰 0.00   ⚕ 0.00   **FUD** XXX   🅰 ▱

AMA: 2016,Aug,9; 2016,Jan,13; 2015,Jan,16; 2014,Jan,11; 2013,Sep,3-12; 2012,May,3-10; 2012,Jun,15-16

81378   HLA Class I and II typing, high resolution (ie, alleles or allele groups), *HLA-A, -B, -C, and -DRB1*

💰 0.00   ⚕ 0.00   **FUD** XXX   🅰 ▱

AMA: 2016,Aug,9; 2016,Jan,13; 2015,Jan,16; 2014,Jan,11; 2013,Sep,3-12; 2012,May,3-10; 2012,Jun,15-16

81379   HLA Class I typing, high resolution (ie, alleles or allele groups); complete (ie, *HLA-A, -B, and -C*)

💰 0.00   ⚕ 0.00   **FUD** XXX   🅰 ▱

AMA: 2016,Aug,9; 2016,Jan,13; 2015,Jan,16; 2014,Jan,11; 2013,Sep,3-12; 2012,May,3-10; 2012,Jun,15-16

81380   one locus (eg, *HLA-A, -B, or -C*), each

EXCLUDES   *Complete Class I high-resolution typing for HLA-A, -B, and -C (81379)*

Testing for presence or absence of a single allele or allele group using high-resolution methodology (81381)

💰 0.00   ⚕ 0.00   **FUD** XXX   🅰 ▱

AMA: 2016,Aug,9; 2016,Jan,13; 2015,Jan,16; 2014,Jan,11; 2013,Sep,3-12; 2012,May,3-10; 2012,Jun,15-16

81381   one allele or allele group (eg, *B*57:01P*), each

EXCLUDES   *Testing for the presence or absence of more than two alleles or allele groups of locus, report the following code for each locus (81380)*

💰 0.00   ⚕ 0.00   **FUD** XXX   🅰 ▱

AMA: 2016,Aug,9; 2016,Jan,13; 2015,Jan,16; 2014,Jan,11; 2013,Sep,3-12; 2012,May,3-10; 2012,Jun,15-16

81382   HLA Class II typing, high resolution (ie, alleles or allele groups); one locus (eg, *HLA-DRB1, -DRB3/4/5, -DQB1, -DQA1, -DPB1, or -DPA1*), each

INCLUDES   Typing of one or all of the DRB3/4/5 genes is regarded as one locus

EXCLUDES   *Testing for just the presence or absence of a single allele or allele group using high-resolution methodology (81383)*

💰 0.00   ⚕ 0.00   **FUD** XXX   🅰 ▱

AMA: 2016,Jan,13; 2015,Jan,16; 2014,Jan,11; 2013,Sep,3-12; 2012,May,3-10; 2012,Jun,15-16

81383   one allele or allele group (eg, *HLA-DQB1*06:02P*), each

EXCLUDES   *For testing for the presence or absence of more than two alleles or allele groups at a locus, report the following code for each locus (81382)*

💰 0.00   ⚕ 0.00   **FUD** XXX   🅰 ▱

AMA: 2016,Jan,13; 2015,Jan,16; 2014,Jan,11; 2013,Sep,3-12; 2012,May,3-10; 2012,Jun,15-16

81400-81408 [81479] Molecular Pathology Tier 2 Procedures

INCLUDES   All analytical procedures in the evaluation such as:
Amplification
Cell lysis
Detection
Digestion
Extraction
Nucleic acid stabilization
Code selection based on specific gene being reviewed
Codes that are arranged by level of technical resources and work involved
Evaluation of the presence of a gene variant using the common gene variant name
Examples of proteins or diseases in the code description (not all inclusive)
Generally all the listed gene variants in the code description would be tested but lists are not all inclusive
Genes described using the Human Genome Organization (HUGO) approved names
Histocompatibility testing
Qualitative results unless otherwise stated
Specific analytes listed after the code description to use for selecting the appropriate molecular pathology procedure
Targeted genomic testing (81410-81471)
Testing for diseases that are more rare

EXCLUDES   *Full gene sequencing using separate gene variant assessment codes unless it is specifically stated in the code description*
Microbial identification (87149-87153, 87470-87801 [87623, 87624, 87625], 87900-87904 [87906, 87910, 87912])
Other related gene variants not listed in code
Tier 1 molecular pathology (81200-81383 [81161, 81162, 81287, 81288])
Tier 2 codes (Error)
Unlisted molecular pathology procedures ([81479])

Code also modifier 26 when only interpretation and report are performed
Code also services required before cell lysis

81400   Molecular pathology procedure, Level 1(eg, identification of single germline variant [eg, SNP] by techniques such as restriction enzyme digestion or melt curve analysis)

ACADM (acyl-CoA dehydrogenase, C-4 to C-12 straight chain, MCAD) (eg, medium chain acyl dehydrogenase deficiency), K304E variant

ACE (angiotensin converting enzyme) (eg, hereditary blood pressure regulation), insertion/deletion variant

AGTR1 (angiotensin II receptor, type 1) (eg, essential hypertension), 1166A>C variant

BCKDHA (branched chain keto acid dehydrogenase E1, alpha polypeptide) (eg, maple syrup urine disease, type 1A), Y438N variant

CCR5 (chemokine C-C motif receptor 5) (eg, HIV resistance), 32-bp deletion mutation/794 825del32 deletion

CLRN1 (clarin 1) (eg, Usher syndrome, type 3), N48K variant

DPYD (dihydropyrimidine dehydrogenase) (eg, 5-fluorouracil/5-FU and capecitabine drug metabolism), IVS14+1G>A variant

F2 (coagulation factor 2) (eg, hereditary hypercoagulability), 1199G>A variant

F5 (coagulation factor V) (eg, hereditary hypercoagulability), HR2 variant

F7 (coagulation factor VII [serum prothrombin conversion accelerator]) (eg, hereditary hypercoagulability), R353Q variant

F13B (coagulation factor XIII, B polypeptide) (eg, hereditary hypercoagulability), V34L variant

FGB (fibrinogen beta chain) (eg, hereditary ischemic heart disease), -455G>A variant

FGFR1 (fibroblast growth factor receptor 1) (eg, Pfeiffer syndrome type 1, craniosynostosis), P252R variant

FGFR3 (fibroblast growth factor receptor 3) (eg, Muenke syndrome), P250R variant

FKTN (fukutin) (eg, Fukuyama congenital muscular dystrophy), retrotransposon insertion variant

GNE (glucosamine [UDP-N-acetyl]-2 -epimerase/N-acetylmannosamine kinase) (eg, inclusion body myopathy 2 [IBM2], Nonaka myopathy), M712T variant

Human platelet antigen 1 genotyping (HPA-1), ITGB3 (integrin, beta 3 [platelet glycoprotein IIIa], antigen CD61 [GPIIIa]) (eg, neonatal alloimmune thrombocytopenia [NAIT], post-transfusion purpura), HPA-1a/b (L33P)

Human platelet antigen 2 genotyping (HPA-2), GP1BA (glycoprotein Ib [platelet], alpha polypeptide [GPIba]) (eg, neonatal alloimmune thrombocytopenia [NAIT], post-transfusion purpura), HPA-2a/b (T145M)

Human platelet antigen 3 genotyping (HPA-3), ITGA2B (integrin, alpha 2b [platelet glycoprotein IIb of IIb/IIIa complex], antigen CD41 [GPIIb]) (eg, neonatal alloimmune thrombocytopenia [NAIT], post-transfusion purpura), HPA-3a/b (I843S)

Human platelet antigen 4 genotyping (HPA-4), ITGB3 (integrin, beta 3 [platelet glycoprotein IIIa], antigen CD61 [GPIIIa]) (eg, neonatal alloimmune thrombocytopenia [NAIT], post-transfusion purpura), HPA-4a/b (R143Q)

Human platelet antigen 5 genotyping (HPA-5), ITGA2 (integrin, alpha 2 [CD49B, alpha 2 subunit of VLA-2 receptor] [GPIa]) (eg, neonatal alloimmune thrombocytopenia [NAIT], post-transfusion purpura), HPA-5a/b (K505E)

Human platelet antigen 6 genotyping (HPA-6w), ITGB3 (integrin, beta 3 [platelet glycoprotein IIIa, antigen CD61] [GPIIIa]) (eg, neonatal alloimmune thrombocytopenia [NAIT], post-transfusion purpura), HPA-6a/b (R489Q)

Human platelet antigen 9 genotyping (HPA-9w), ITGA2B (integrin, alpha 2b [platelet glycoprotein IIb of IIb/IIIa complex, antigen CD41] [GPIIb]) (eg, neonatal alloimmune thrombocytopenia [NAIT], post-transfusion purpura), HPA-9a/b (V837M)

Human platelet antigen 15 genotyping (HPA-15), CD109 (CD109 molecule) (eg, neonatal alloimmune thrombocytopenia [NAIT], post-transfusion purpura), HPA-15a/b (S682Y)

IL28B (interleukin 28B [interferon, lambda 3]) (eg, drug response), rs12979860 variant

IVD (isovaleryl-CoA dehydrogenase) (eg, isovaleric acidemia), A282V variant

LCT (lactase-phlorizin hydrolase) (eg, lactose intolerance), 13910 C>T variant

NEB (nebulin) (eg, nemaline myopathy 2), exon 55 deletion variant

PCDH15 (protocadherin-related 15) (eg, Usher syndrome type 1F), R245X variant

SERPINE1 (serpine peptidase inhibitor clade E, member 1, plasminogen activator inhibitor -1, PAI-1) (eg, thrombophilia), 4G variant

SHOC2 (soc-2 suppressor of clear homolog) (eg, Noonan-like syndrome with loose anagen hair), S2G variant

SLCO1B1 (solute carrier organic anion transporter family, member 1B1) (eg, adverse drug reaction), V174A variant

SMN1 (survival of motor neuron 1, telomeric) (eg, spinal muscular atrophy), exon 7 deletion

SRY (sex determining region Y) (eg, 46,XX testicular disorder of sex development, gonadal dysgenesis), gene analysis

TOR1A (torsin family 1, member A [torsin A]) (eg, early-onset primary dystonia [DYT1]), 907_909delGAG (904_906delGAG) variant

    📋 0.00 ✂ 0.00 **FUD** XXX   Ⓐ▯

AMA: 2016,Aug,9; 2016,Jan,13; 2015,Jan,3; 2015,Jan,16; 2014,Jan,11; 2013,Sep,3-12; 2013,Jul,11-12; 2012,May,3-10

▲ **81401** **Molecular pathology procedure, Level 2 (eg, 2-10 SNPs, 1 methylated variant, or 1 somatic variant [typically using nonsequencing target variant analysis], or detection of a dynamic mutation disorder/triplet repeat)**

ABCC8 (ATP-binding cassette, sub-family C [CFTR/MRP], member 8) (eg, familial hyperinsulinism), common variants (eg, c.3898-9G>A [c.3992-9G>A], F1388del)

ABL1 (ABL proto oncogene 1, non-receptor tyrosine kinase) (eg, acquired imatinib resistance), T315I variant

ACADM (acyl-CoA dehydrogenase, C-4 to C-12 straight chain, MCAD) (eg, medium chain acyl dehydrogenase deficiency), common variants (eg, K304E, Y42H)

ADRB2 (adrenergic beta-2 receptor surface) (eg, drug metabolism), common variants (eg, G16R, Q27E)

AFF2 (AF4/FMR2 family, member 2 [FMR2]) (eg, fragile X mental retardation 2 [FRAXE]), evaluation to detect abnormal (eg, expanded) alleles

APOB (apolipoprotein B) (eg, familial hypercholesterolemia type B), common variants (eg, R3500Q, R3500W)

APOE (apolipoprotein E) (eg, hyperlipoproteinemia type III, cardiovascular disease, Alzheimer disease), common variants (eg, *2, *3, *4)

AR (androgen receptor) (eg, spinal and bulbar muscular atrophy, Kennedy disease, X chromosome inactivation), characterization of alleles (eg, expanded size or methylation status)

ATN1 (atrophin 1) (eg, dentatorubral-pallidoluysian atrophy), evaluation to detect abnormal (eg, expanded) alleles

ATXN1 (ataxin 1) (eg, spinocerebellar ataxia), evaluation to detect abnormal (eg, expanded) alleles

ATXN2 (ataxin 2) (eg, spinocerebellar ataxia), evaluation to detect abnormal (eg, expanded) alleles

ATXN3 (ataxin 3) (eg, spinocerebellar ataxia, Machado-Joseph disease), evaluation to detect abnormal (eg, expanded) alleles

ATXN7 (ataxin 7) (eg, spinocerebellar ataxia), evaluation to detect abnormal (eg, expanded) alleles

ATXN8OS (ATXN8 opposite strand [non-protein coding]) (eg, spinocerebellar ataxia), evaluation to detect abnormal (eg, expanded) alleles

ATXN10 (ataxin 10) (eg, spinocerebellar ataxia), evaluation to detect abnormal (eg, expanded) alleles

CACNA1A (calcium channel, voltage-dependent, P/Q type, alpha 1A subunit) (eg, spinocerebellar ataxia), evaluation to detect abnormal (eg, expanded) alleles

CBFB/MYH11 (inv(16)) (eg, acute myeloid leukemia), qualitative, and quantitative, if performed

CBS (cystathionine-beta-synthase) (eg, homocystinuria, cystathionine beta-synthase deficiency), common variants (eg, I278T, G307S)

CCND1/IGH (BCL1/IgH, t(11;14)) (eg, mantle cell lymphoma) translocation analysis, major breakpoint, qualitative and quantitative, if performed

CFH/ARMS2 (complement factor H/age-related maculopathy susceptibility 2) (eg, macular degeneration), common variants (eg, Y402H [CFH], A69S [ARMS2])

CNBP (CCHC-type zinc finger, nucleic acid binding protein) (eg, myotonic dystrophy type 2), evaluation to detect abnormal (eg, expanded) alleles

CSTB (cystatin B [stefin B]) (eg, Unverricht-Lundborg disease), evaluation to detect abnormal (eg, expanded) alleles

CYP3A4 (cytochrome P450, family 3, subfamily A, polypeptide 4) (eg, drug metabolism), common variants (eg, *2, *3, *4, *5, *6)

CYP3A5 (cytochrome P450, family 3, subfamily A, polypeptide 5) (eg, drug metabolism), common variants (eg, *2, *3, *4, *5, *6)

DEK/NUP214 (t(6;9)) (eg, acute myeloid leukemia), translocation analysis, qualitative, and quantitative, if performed

DMPK (dystrophia myotonica-protein kinase) (eg, myotonic dystrophy, type 1), evaluation to detect abnormal (eg, expanded) alleles

| 26/TC PC/TC Only | A2-Z3 ASC Payment | 50 Bilateral | ♂ Male Only | ♀ Female Only | 📋 Facility RVU | ✎ Non-Facility RVU | ▢ CCI |
| **FUD** Follow-up Days | **CMS:** IOM (Pub 100) | A-Y OPPSI | 80/80 Surg Assist Allowed / w/Doc | | ▣ Lab Crosswalk | ▣ Radiology Crosswalk | ✖ CLIA |

352

CPT © 2016 American Medical Association. All Rights Reserved.   © 2016 Optum360, LLC

E2A/PBX1 (t(1;19)) (eg, acute lymphocytic leukemia), translocation analysis, qualitative, and quantitative, if performed

EML4/ALK (inv(2)) (eg, non-small cell lung cancer), translocation or inversion analysis

ETV6/NTRK3 (t(12;15)) (eg, congenital/infantile fibrosarcoma), translocation analysis, qualitative, and quantitative, if performed

ETV6/RUNX1 (t(12;21)) (eg, acute lymphocytic leukemia), translocation analysis, qualitative and quantitative, if performed

EWSR1/ATF1 (t(12;22)) (eg, clear cell sarcoma), translocation analysis, qualitative, and quantitative, if performed

EWSR1/ERG (t(21;22)) (eg, Ewing sarcoma/peripheral neuroectodermal tumor), translocation analysis, qualitative and quantitative, if performed

EWSR1/FLI1 (t(11;22)) (eg, Ewing sarcoma/peripheral neuroectodermal tumor), translocation analysis, qualitative and quantitative, if performed

EWSR1/WT1 (t(11;22)) (eg, desmoplastic small round cell tumor), translocation analysis, qualitative and quantitative, if performed

F11 (coagulation factor XI) (eg, coagulation disorder), common variants (eg, E117X [Type II], F283L [Type III], IVS14del14, and IVS14+1G>A [Type I])

FGFR3 (fibroblast growth factor receptor 3) (eg, achondroplasia, hypochondroplasia), common variants (eg, 1138G>A, 1138G>C, 1620C>A, 1620C>G)

FIP1L1/PDGFRA (del[4q12]) (eg, imatinib-sensitive chronic eosinophilic leukemia), qualitative and quantitative, if performed

FLG (filaggrin) (eg, ichthyosis vulgaris), common variants (eg, R501X, 2282del4, R2447X, S3247X, 3702delG)

FOXO1/PAX3 (t(2;13)) (eg, alveolar rhabdomyosarcoma), translocation analysis, qualitative and quantitative, if performed

FOXO1/PAX7 (t(1;13)) (eg, alveolar rhabdomyosarcoma), translocation analysis, qualitative and quantitative, if performed

FUS/DDIT3 (t(12;16)) (eg, myxoid liposarcoma), translocation analysis, qualitative, and quantitative, if performed

FXN (frataxin) (eg, Friedreich ataxia), evaluation to detect abnormal (expanded) alleles

GALC (galactosylceramidase) (eg, Krabbe disease), common variants (eg, c.857G>A, 30-kb deletion)

GALT (galactose-1-phosphate uridylyltransferase) (eg, galactosemia), common variants (eg, Q188R, S135L, K285N, T138M, L195P, Y209C, IVS2-2A>G, P171S, del5kb, N314D, L218L/N314D)

H19 (imprinted maternally expressed transcript [non-protein coding]) (eg, Beckwith-Wiedemann syndrome), methylation analysis

HBB (hemoglobin, beta) (eg, sickle cell anemia, hemoglobin C, hemoglobin E), common variants (eg, HbS, HbC, HbE)

HTT (huntingtin) (eg, Huntington disease), evaluation to detect abnormal (eg, expanded) alleles

IGH@/BCL2 (t(14;18)) (eg, follicular lymphoma), translocation and analysis; single breakpoint (eg) major breakpoint region [MBR] or minor cluster region [mcr]), qualitative or quantitative(When both MBR and mcr breakpoints are performed, use 81402)

KCNQ10T1 (KCNQ1 overlapping transcript 1 [non-protein coding]) (e.g, Beckwith-Wiedemann syndrome), methylation analysis

LRRK2 (leucine-rich repeat kinase 2) (eg, Parkinson disease), common variants (eg, R1441G, G2019S, I2020T)

MED12 (mediator complex subunit 12) (eg, FG syndrome type 1, Lujan syndrome), common variants (eg, R961W, N1007S)

MEG3/DLK1 (maternally expressed 3 [non-protein coding]/delta-like 1 homolog [Drosophila]) (eg, intrauterine growth retardation), methylation analysis

MLL/AFF1 (t(4;11)) (eg acute lymphoblastic leukemia), translocation analysis, qualitative and quantitative, if performed

MLL/MLLT3 (t(9;11)) (eg, acute myeloid leukemia) translocation analysis, qualitative and quantitative, if performed

MT-RNR1 (mitochondrially encoded 12S RNA) (eg, nonsyndromic hearing loss), common variants (eg, m.1555G>G, m1494C>T)

MUTYH (mutY homolog [E.coli]) (eg, MYH-associated polyposis), common variants (eg, Y165C, G382D)

MT-ATP6 (mitochondrially encoded ATP synthase 6) (eg, neuropathy with ataxia and retinitis pigmentosa [NARP], Leigh syndrome), common variants (eg, m.8993T>G, m.8993T>C)

MT-ND4, MT-ND6 (mitochondrially encoded NADH dehydrogenase 4, mitochondrially encoded NADH dehydrogenase 6) (eg, Leber hereditary optic neuropathy [LHON]), common variants (eg m.11778G>A, m3460G>A, m14484T>C)

MT-ND5 (mitochondrially encoded tRNA leucine 1 [UUA/G], mitochondrially encoded NADH dehydrogenase 5) (eg, mitochondrial encephalopathy with lactic acidosis and stroke-like episodes [MELAS]), common variants (eg, m.3243A>G, m.3271T>C, m.3252A>G, m.13513G>A)

MT-TK (mitochondrially encoded tRNA lysine) (eg, myoclonic epilepsy with ragged-red fibers [MERRF]), common variants (eg, m8344A>G, m.8356T>C)

MT-TL1 (mitochondrially encoded tRNA leucine 1[UUA/G]) (eg, diabetes and hearing loss), common variants (eg, m.3243A>G, m.14709 T>C) MT-TL1

MT-TS1, MT-RNR1 (mitochondrially encoded tRNA serine 1 [UCN], mitochondrially encoded 12S RNA) (eg, nonsyndromic sensorineural deafness [including aminoglycoside-induced nonsyndromic deafness]) common variants (eg, m.7445A>G, m.1555A>G)

NOD2 (nucleotide-binding oligomerization domain containing 2) (eg, Crohn's disease, Blau syndrome), common variants (eg, SNP 8, SNP 12, SNP 13)

NPM/ALK (t(2;5)) (eg, anaplastic large cell lymphoma), translocation analysis

PABPN1 (poly[A] binding protein, nuclear 1) (eg, oculopharyngeal muscular dystrophy), evaluation to detect abnormal (eg, expanded) alleles

PAX8/PPARG (t(2;3) (q13;p25)) (eg, follicular thyroid carcinoma), translocation analysis

PPP2R2B (protein phosphatase 2, regulatory subunit B, beta) (eg, spinocerebellar ataxia), evaluation to detect abnormal (eg, expanded) alleles

PRSS1 (protease, serine, 1 [trypsin 1]) (eg, hereditary pancreatitis), common variants (eg, N29I, A16V, R122H)

PYGM (phosphorylase, glycogen, muscle) (eg, glycogen storage disease type V, McArdle disease), common variants (eg, R50X, G205S)

RUNX1/RUNX1T1 (t(8;21)) (eg, acute myeloid leukemia) translocation analysis, qualitative and quantitative, if performed

SMN1/SMN2 (survival of motor neuron 1, telomeric/survival of motor neuron 2, centromeric) (eg, spinal muscular atrophy), dosage analysis (eg, carrier testing)

SMN1/SMN2 duplication/deletion analysis

SS18/SSX1 (t(X;18)) (eg, synovial sarcoma), translocation analysis, qualitative and quantitative, if performed

SS18/SSX2 (t(X;18)) (eg, synovial sarcoma), translocation analysis, qualitative and quantitative, if performed

TBP (TATA box binding protein) (eg, spinocerebellar ataxia), evaluation to detect abnormal (eg, expanded) alleles

TPMT (thiopurine S-methyltransferase) (eg, drug metabolism), common variants (eg, *2, *3)

TYMS (thymidylate synthetase) (eg, 5-fluorouracil/5-FU drug metabolism), tandem repeat variant

VWF (von Willebrand factor) (eg, von Willebrand disease type 2N), common variants (eg, T791M, R816W, R854Q)

🔧 0.00   ⚕ 0.00   **FUD** XXX   🅰 ▢

AMA: 2016,Aug,9; 2016,Jan,13; 2015,Jan,3; 2015,Jan,16; 2014,Jan,11; 2013,Sep,3-12; 2013,Jul,11-12; 2012,May,3-10

81402 **Molecular pathology procedure, Level 3 (eg, >10 SNPs, 2-10 methylated variants, or 2-10 somatic variants [typically using non-sequencing target variant analysis], immunoglobulin and T-cell receptor gene rearrangements, duplication/deletion variants of 1 exon, loss of heterozygosity [LOH], uniparental disomy [UPD])**

Chromosome 1p-/19q- (eg, glial tumors), deletion analysis

Chromosome 18q- (eg, D18S55, D18S58, D18S61, D18S64, and D18S69) (eg, colon cancer), allelic imbalance assessment (ie, loss of heterozygosity)

COL1A1/PDGFB (t(17;22)) (eg, dermatofibrosarcoma protuberans), translocation analysis, multiple breakpoints, qualitative, and quantitative, if performed

CYP21A2 (cytochrome P450, family 21, subfamily A, polypeptide 2) (eg, congenital adrenal hyperplasia, 21-hydroxylase deficiency), common variants (eg, IVS2-13G, P30L, I172N, exon 6 mutation cluster [I235N, V236E, M238K], V281L, L307FfsX6, Q318X, R356W, P453S, G110VfsX21, 30-kb deletion variant)

ESR1/PGR (receptor 1/progesterone receptor) ratio (eg, breast cancer)

IGH@/BCL2 (t(14;18)) (eg, follicular lymphoma), translocation analysis; major breakpoint region (MBR) and minor cluster region (mcr) breakpoints, qualitative or quantitative

MEFV (Mediterranean fever) (eg, familial Mediterranean fever), common variants (eg, E148Q, P369S, F479L, M680I, I692del, M694V, M694I, K695R, V726A, A744S, R761H)

MPL (myeloproliferative leukemia virus oncogene, thrombopoietin receptor, TPOR) (eg, myeloproliferative disorder), common variants (eg, W515A, W515K, W515L, W515R)

TRD@ (T cell antigen receptor, delta) (eg, leukemia and lymphoma), gene rearrangement analysis, evaluation to detect abnormal clonal population

Uniparental disomy (UPD) (eg, Russell-Silver syndrome, Prader-Willi/Angelman syndrome), short tandem repeat (STR) analysis

🔁 0.00   ⚖ 0.00   **FUD** XXX   Ⓐ 🖵

AMA: 2016,Aug,9; 2016,Jan,13; 2015,Jan,3; 2015,Jan,16; 2014,Jan,11; 2013,Sep,3-12; 2013,Jul,11-12; 2012,May,3-10

▲ **81403** **Molecular pathology procedure, Level 4 (eg, analysis of single exon by DNA sequence analysis, analysis of >10 amplicons using multiplex PCR in 2 or more independent reactions, mutation scanning or duplication/deletion variants of 2-5 exons)**

ANG (angiogenin, ribonuclease, RNase A family, 5) (eg, amyotrophic lateral sclerosis), full gene sequence

ARX (aristaless-related homeobox) (eg, X-linked lissencephaly with ambiguous genitalia, X-linked mental retardation), duplication/deletion analysis

CEL (carboxyl ester lipase [bile salt-stimulated lipase]) (eg, maturity-onset diabetes of the young [MODY]), targeted sequence analysis of exon 11 (eg, c.1785delC, c.1686delT)

CTNNB1 (catenin [cadherin-associated protein], beta 1, 88kDa) (eg, desmoid tumors), targeted sequence analysis (eg, exon 3)

DAZ/SRY (deleted in azoospermia and sex determining region Y) (eg, male infertility), common deletions (eg, AZFa, AZFb, AZFc, AZFd)

DNMT3A (DNA [cytosine-5-]-methyltransferase 3 alpha) (eg, acute myeloid leukemia), targeted sequence analysis (eg, exon 23)

EPCAM (epithelial cell adhesion molecule) (eg, Lynch syndrome), duplication/deletion analysis

F8 (coagulation factor VIII) (eg, hemophilia A), inversion analysis, intron 1 and intron 22A

F12 (coagulation factor XII [Hageman factor]) (eg, angioedema, hereditary, type III; factor XII deficiency), targeted sequence analysis of exon 9

FGFR3 (fibroblast growth factor receptor 3) (eg, isolated craniosynostosis), targeted sequence analysis (eg, exon 7)

(For targeted sequence analysis of multiple FGFR3 exons, use 81404)

GJB1 (gap junction protein, beta 1) (eg, Charcot-Marie-Tooth X-linked), full gene sequence

GNAQ (guanine nucleotide-binding protein G[q] subunit alpha) (eg, uveal melanoma), common variants (eg, R183, Q209)

HBB (hemoglobin, beta, beta-globin) (eg, beta thalassemia), duplication/deletion analysis

Human erythrocyte antigen gene analyses (eg, SLC14A1 [Kidd blood group], BCAM [Lutheran blood group], ICAM4 [Landsteiner-Wiener blood group], SLC4A1 [Diego blood group], AQP1 [Colton blood group], ERMAP [Scianna blood group], RHCE [Rh blood group, CcEe antigens], KEL [Kell blood group], DARC [Duffy blood group], GYPA, GYPB, GYPE [MNS blood group], ART4 [Dombrock blood group]) (eg, sickle-cell disease, thalassemia, hemolytic transfusion reactions, hemolytic disease of the fetus or newborn), common variants

HRAS (v-Ha-ras Harvey rat sarcoma viral oncogene homolog) (eg, Costello syndrome), exon 2 sequence

IDH1 (isocitrate dehydrogenase 1 [NADP+], soluble) (eg, glioma), common exon 4 variants (eg, R132H, R132C)

IDH2 (isocitrate dehydrogenase 2 [NADP+], mitochondrial) (eg, glioma), common exon 4 variants (eg, R140W, R172M)

JAK2 (Janus kinase 2) (eg, myeloproliferative disorder), exon 12 sequence and exon 13 sequence, if performed

KCNC3 (potassium voltage-gated channel, Shaw-related subfamily, member 3) (eg, spinocerebellar ataxia), targeted sequence analysis (eg, exon 2)

KCNJ2 (potassium inwardly-rectifying channel, subfamily J, member 2) (eg, Andersen-Tawil syndrome), full gene sequence

KCNJ11 (potassium inwardly-rectifying channel, subfamily J, member 11) (eg, familial hyperinsulinism), full gene sequence

Killer cell immunoglobulin-like receptor (KIR) gene family (eg, hematopoietic stem cell transplantation), genotyping of KIR family genes

Known familial variant, not otherwise specified, for gene listed in Tier 1 or Tier 2, or identified during a genomic sequencing procedure, DNA sequence analysis, each variant exon

(For a known familial variant that is considered a common variant, use specific common variant Tier 1 or Tier 2 code)

MC4R (melanocortin 4 receptor) (eg, obesity), full gene sequence

*MICA (MHC class I polypeptide-related sequence A) (eg, solid organ transplantation), common variants (eg, *001, *002)*

MPL (myeloproliferative leukemia virus oncogene, thrombopoietin receptor, TPOR) (eg, myeloproliferative disorder), exon 10 sequence

MT-RNR1 (mitochondrially encoded 12S RNA) (eg, nonsyndromic hearing loss), full gene sequence

MT-TS1 (mitochondrially encoded tRNA serine 1) (eg, nonsyndromic hearing loss), full gene sequence

NDP (Norrie disease [pseudoglioma]) (eg, Norrie disease), duplication/deletion analysis

NHLRC1 (NHL repeat containing 1) (eg, progressive myoclonus epilepsy), full gene sequence

PHOX2B (paired-like homeobox 2b) (eg, congenital central hypoventilation syndrome), duplication/deletion analysis

PLN (phospholamban) (eg, dilated cardiomyopathy, hypertrophic cardiomyopathy), full gene sequence

RHD (Rh blood group, D antigen) (eg, hemolytic disease of the fetus and newborn, Rh maternal/fetal compatibility), deletion analysis (eg, exons 4, 5, and 7, pseudogene)

RHD (Rh blood group, D antigen) (eg, hemolytic disease of the fetus and newborn, Rh maternal/fetal compatibility), deletion analysis (eg,

| 26/TC PC/TC Only | A2-Z3 ASC Payment | 50 Bilateral | ♂ Male Only | ♀ Female Only | ⬥ Facility RVU | ⬥ Non-Facility RVU | 🖵 CCI |
| FUD Follow-up Days | CMS: IOM (Pub 100) | A-Y OPPSI | 80/80 Surg Assist Allowed / w/Doc | | ⬥ Lab Crosswalk | ⬥ Radiology Crosswalk | ❌ CLIA |

354

exons 4, 5, and 7, pseudogene), performed on cell-free fetal DNA in maternal blood

(For human erythrocyte gene analysis of RHD, use a separate unit of 81403)

SH2D1A (SH2 domain containing 1A) (eg, X-linked lymphoproliferative syndrome), duplication/deletion analysis

SMN1 (survival of motor neuron 1, telomeric) (eg, spinal muscular atrophy), known familial sequence variant(s)

TWIST1 (twist homolog 1 [Drosophila]) (eg, Saethre-Chotzen syndrome), duplication/deletion analysis

UBA1 (ubiquitin-like modifier activating enzyme 1) (eg, spinal muscular atrophy, X-linked), targeted sequence analysis (eg, exon 15)

VHL (von Hippel-Lindau tumor suppressor) (eg, von Hippel-Lindau familial cancer syndrome), deletion/duplication analysis

VWF (von Willebrand factor) (eg, von Willebrand disease types 2A, 2B, 2M), targeted sequence analysis (eg, exon 28)

📖 0.00   ⚒ 0.00   **FUD** XXX   🅰 🖵

AMA: 2016,Aug,9; 2016,Jan,13; 2015,Jan,3; 2015,Jan,16; 2014,Jan,11; 2013,Sep,3-12; 2013,Jul,11-12; 2012,May,3-10

81404 **Molecular pathology procedure, Level 5 (eg, analysis of 2-5 exons by DNA sequence analysis, mutation scanning or duplication/deletion variants of 6-10 exons, or characterization of a dynamic mutation disorder/triplet repeat by Southern blot analysis)**

ACADS (acyl-CoA dehydrogenase, C-2 to C-3 short chain) (eg, short chain acyl-CoA dehydrogenase deficiency), targeted sequence analysis (eg, exons 5 and 6)

AFF2 (AF4/FMR2 family, member 2 [FMR2]) (eg, fragile X mental retardation 2 [FRAXE]), characterization of alleles (eg, expanded size and methylation status)

AQP2 (aquaporin 2 [collecting duct]) (eg, nephrogenic diabetes insipidus), full gene sequence

ARX (aristaless related homeobox) (eg, X-linked lissencephaly with ambiguous genitalia, X-linked mental retardation), full gene sequence

AVPR2 (arginine vasopressin receptor 2) (eg, nephrogenic diabetes insipidus), full gene sequence

BBS10 (Bardet-Biedl syndrome 10) (eg, Bardet-Biedl syndrome), full gene sequence

BTD (biotinidase) (eg, biotinidase deficiency), full gene sequence

C10orf2 (chromosome 10 open reading frame 2) (eg, mitochondrial DNA depletion syndrome), full gene sequence

CAV3 (caveolin 3) (eg, CAV3-related distal myopathy, limb-girdle muscular dystrophy type 1C), full gene sequence

CD40LG (CD40 ligand) (eg, X-linked hyper IgM syndrome), full gene sequence

CDKN2A (cyclin-dependent kinase inhibitor 2A) (eg, CDKN2A-related cutaneous malignant melanoma, familial atypical mole-malignant melanoma syndrome), full gene sequence

CLRN1 (clarin 1) (eg, Usher syndrome, type 3), full gene sequence

COX6B1 (cytochrome c oxidase subunit VIb polypeptide 1) (eg, mitochondrial respiratory chain complex IV deficiency), full gene sequence

CPT2 (carnitine palmitoyltransferase 2) (eg, carnitine palmitoyltransferase II deficiency), full gene sequence

CRX (cone-rod homeobox) (eg, cone-rod dystrophy 2, Leber congenital amaurosis), full gene sequence

CSTB (cystatin B [stefin B]) (eg, Unverricht-Lundborg disease), full gene sequence

CYP1B1 (cytochrome P450, family 1, subfamily B, polypeptide 1) (eg, primary congenital glaucoma), full gene sequence

DMPK (dystrophia myotonica-protein kinase) (eg, myotonic dystrophy type 1), characterization of abnormal (eg, expanded) alleles

EGR2 (early growth response 2) (eg, Charcot-Marie-Tooth), full gene sequence

EMD (emerin) (eg, Emery-Dreifuss muscular dystrophy), duplication/deletion analysis

EPM2A (epilepsy, progressive myoclonus type 2A, Lafora disease [laforin]) (eg, progressive myoclonus epilepsy), full gene sequence

FGF23 (fibroblast growth factor 23) (eg, hypophosphatemic rickets), full gene sequence

FGFR2 (fibroblast growth factor receptor 2) (eg, craniosynostosis, Apert syndrome, Crouzon syndrome), targeted sequence analysis (eg, exons 8, 10)

FGFR3 (fibroblast growth factor receptor 3) (eg, achondroplasia, hypochondroplasia), targeted sequence analysis (eg, exons 8, 11, 12, 13)

FHL1 (four and a half LIM domains 1) (eg, Emery-Dreifuss muscular dystrophy), full gene sequence

FKRP (Fukutin related protein) (eg, congenital muscular dystrophy type 1C [MDC1C], limb-girdle muscular dystrophy [LGMD] type 2I), full gene sequence

FOXG1 (forkhead box G1) (eg, Rett syndrome), full gene sequence

FSHMD1A (facioscapulohumeral muscular dystrophy 1A) (eg, facioscapulohumeral muscular dystrophy), evaluation to detect abnormal (eg, deleted) alleles

FSHMD1A (facioscapulohumeral muscular dystrophy 1A) (eg, facioscapulohumeral muscular dystrophy), characterization of haplotype(s) (ie, chromosome 4A and 4B haplotypes)

FXN (frataxin) (eg, Friedreich ataxia), full gene sequence

GH1 (growth hormone 1) (eg, growth hormone deficiency), full gene sequence

GP1BB (glycoprotein Ib [platelet], beta polypeptide) (eg, Bernard-Soulier syndrome type B), full gene sequence

HBA1/HBA2 (alpha globin 1 and alpha globin 2) (eg, alpha thalassemia), duplication/deletion analysis

(For common deletion variants of alpha globin 1 and alpha globin 2 genes, use 81257)

HBB (hemoglobin, beta, beta-globin) (eg, thalassemia), full gene sequence

HNF1B (HNF1 homeobox B) (eg, maturity-onset diabetes of the young [MODY]), duplication/deletion analysis

HRAS (v-Ha-ras Harvey rat sarcoma viral oncogene homolog) (eg, Costello syndrome), full gene sequence

HSD3B2 (hydroxy-delta-5-steroid dehydrogenase, 3 beta- and steroid delta-isomerase 2) (eg, 3-beta-hydroxysteroid dehydrogenase type II deficiency), full gene sequence

HSD11B2 (hydroxysteroid [11-beta] dehydrogenase 2) (eg, mineralocorticoid excess syndrome), full gene sequence

HSPB1 (heat shock 27kDa protein 1) (eg, Charcot-Marie-Tooth disease), full gene sequence

INS (insulin) (eg, diabetes mellitus), full gene sequence

KCNJ1 (potassium inwardly-rectifying channel, subfamily J, member 1) (eg, Bartter syndrome), full gene sequence

KCNJ10 (potassium inwardly-rectifying channel, subfamily J, member 10) (eg, SeSAME syndrome, EAST syndrome, sensorineural hearing loss), full gene sequence

LITAF (lipopolysaccharide-induced TNF factor) (eg, Charcot-Marie-Tooth), full gene sequence

MEFV (Mediterranean fever) (eg, familial Mediterranean fever), full gene sequence

MEN1 (multiple endocrine neoplasia I) (eg, multiple endocrine neoplasia type 1, Wermer syndrome), duplication/deletion analysis

MMACHC (methylmalonic aciduria [cobalamin deficiency] cblC type, with homocystinuria) (eg, methylmalonic acidemia and homocystinuria), full gene sequence

MPV17 (MpV17 mitochondrial inner membrane protein) (eg, mitochondrial DNA depletion syndrome), duplication/deletion analysis

NDP (Norrie disease [pseudoglioma]) (eg, Norrie disease), full gene sequence

NDUFA1 (NADH dehydrogenase [ubiquinone] 1 alpha subcomplex, 1, 7.5kDa) (eg, Leigh syndrome, mitochondrial complex I deficiency), full gene sequence

NDUFAF2 (NADH dehydrogenase [ubiquinone] 1 alpha subcomplex, assembly factor 2) (eg, Leigh syndrome, mitochondrial complex I deficiency), full gene sequence

NDUFS4 (NADH dehydrogenase [ubiquinone] Fe-S protein 4, 18kDa [NADH-coenzyme Q reductase]) (eg, Leigh syndrome, mitochondrial complex I deficiency), full gene sequence

NIPA1 (non-imprinted in Prader-Willi/Angelman syndrome 1) (eg, spastic paraplegia), full gene sequence

NLGN4X (neuroligin 4, X-linked) (eg, autism spectrum disorders), duplication/deletion analysis

NPC2 (Niemann-Pick disease, type C2 [epididymal secretory protein E1]) (eg, Niemann-Pick disease type C2), full gene sequence

NR0B1 (nuclear receptor subfamily 0, group B, member 1) (eg, congenital adrenal hypoplasia), full gene sequence

PDX1 (pancreatic and duodenal homeobox 1) (eg, maturity-onset diabetes of the young [MODY]), full gene sequence

PHOX2B (paired-like homeobox 2b) (eg, congenital central hypoventilation syndrome), full gene sequence

PIK3CA (phosphatidylinositol-4,5-bisphosphate 3-kinase, catalytic subunit alpha) (eg, colorectal cancer), targeted sequence analysis (eg, exons 9 and 20)

PLP1 (proteolipid protein 1) (eg, Pelizaeus-Merzbacher disease, spastic paraplegia), duplication/deletion analysis

PQBP1 (polyglutamine binding protein 1) (eg, Renpenning syndrome), duplication/deletion analysis

PRNP (prion protein) (eg, genetic prion disease), full gene sequence

PROP1 (PROP paired-like homeobox 1) (eg, combined pituitary hormone deficiency), full gene sequence

PRPH2 (peripherin 2 [retinal degeneration, slow]) (eg, retinitis pigmentosa), full gene sequence

PRSS1 (protease, serine, 1 [trypsin 1]) (eg, hereditary pancreatitis), full gene sequence

RAF1 (v-raf-1 murine leukemia viral oncogene homolog 1) (eg, LEOPARD syndrome), targeted sequence analysis (eg, exons 7, 12, 14, 17)

RET (ret proto-oncogene) (eg, multiple endocrine neoplasia, type 2B and familial medullary thyroid carcinoma), common variants (eg, M918T, 2647_2648delinsTT, A883F)

RHO (rhodopsin) (eg, retinitis pigmentosa), full gene sequence

RP1 (retinitis pigmentosa 1) (eg, retinitis pigmentosa), full gene sequence

SCN1B (sodium channel, voltage-gated, type I, beta) (eg, Brugada syndrome), full gene sequence

SCO2 (SCO cytochrome oxidase deficient homolog 2 [SCO1L]) (eg, mitochondrial respiratory chain complex IV deficiency), full gene sequence

SDHC (succinate dehydrogenase complex, subunit C, integral membrane protein, 15kDa) (eg, hereditary paraganglioma-pheochromocytoma syndrome), duplication/deletion analysis

SDHD (succinate dehydrogenase complex, subunit D, integral membrane protein) (eg, hereditary paraganglioma), full gene sequence

SGCG (sarcoglycan, gamma [35kDa dystrophin-associated glycoprotein]) (eg, limb-girdle muscular dystrophy), duplication/deletion analysis

SH2D1A (SH2 domain containing 1A) (eg, X-linked lymphoproliferative syndrome), full gene sequence

SLC16A2 (solute carrier family 16, member 2 [thyroid hormone transporter]) (eg, specific thyroid hormone cell transporter deficiency, Allan-Herndon-Dudley syndrome), duplication/deletion analysis

SLC25A20 (solute carrier family 25 [carnitine/acylcarnitine translocase], member 20) (eg, carnitine-acylcarnitine translocase deficiency), duplication/deletion analysis

SLC25A4 (solute carrier family 25 [mitochondrial carrier; adenine nucleotide translocation], member 4) (eg, progressive external ophthalmoplegia), full gene sequence

SOD1 (superoxide dismutase 1, soluble) (eg, amyotrophic lateral sclerosis), full gene sequence

SPINK1 (serine peptidase inhibitor, Kazal type 1) (eg, hereditary pancreatitis), full gene sequence

STK11 (serine/threonine kinase 11) (eg, Peutz-Jeghers syndrome), duplication/deletion analysis

TACO1 (translational activator of mitochondrial encoded cytochrome c oxidase I) (eg, mitochondrial respiratory chain complex IV deficiency), full gene sequence

THAP1 (THAP domain containing, apoptosis associated protein 1) (eg, torsion dystonia), full gene sequence

TOR1A (torsin family 1, member A [torsin A]) (eg, torsion dystonia), full gene sequence

TP53 (tumor protein 53) (eg, tumor samples), targeted sequence analysis of 2-5 exons

TTPA (tocopherol [alpha] transfer protein) (eg, ataxia), full gene sequence

TTR (transthyretin) (eg, familial transthyretin amyloidosis), full gene sequence

TWIST1 (twist homolog 1 [Drosophila]) (eg, Saethre-Chotzen syndrome), full gene sequence

TYR (tyrosinase [oculocutaneous albinism IA]) (eg, oculocutaneous albinism IA), full gene sequence

USH1G (Usher syndrome 1G [autosomal recessive]) (eg, Usher syndrome, type 1), full gene sequence

VWF (von Willebrand factor) (eg, von Willebrand disease type 1C), targeted sequence analysis (eg, exons 26, 27, 37)

VHL (von Hippel-Lindau tumor suppressor) (eg, von Hippel-Lindau familial cancer syndrome), full gene sequence

ZEB2 (zinc finger E-box binding homeobox 2) (eg, Mowat-Wilson syndrome), duplication/deletion analysis

ZNF41 (zinc finger protein 41) (eg, X-linked mental retardation 89), full gene sequence

    🔷 0.00   🔷 0.00   **FUD** XXX   🄰 🖵

    AMA: 2016,Aug,9; 2016,Jan,13; 2015,Jan,3; 2015,Jan,16; 2014,Jan,11; 2013,Sep,3-12; 2013,Jul,11-12; 2012,May,3-10

81405 **Molecular pathology procedure, Level 6 (eg, analysis of 6-10 exons by DNA sequence analysis, mutation scanning or duplication/deletion variants of 11-25 exons, regionally targeted cytogenomic array analysis)**

ABCD1 (ATP-binding cassette, sub-family D [ALD], member 1) (eg, adrenoleukodystrophy), full gene sequence

ACADS (acyl-CoA dehydrogenase, C-2 to C-3 short chain) (eg, short chain acyl-CoA dehydrogenase deficiency), full gene sequence

ACTA2 (actin, alpha 2, smooth muscle, aorta) (eg, thoracic aortic aneurysms and aortic dissections), full gene sequence

---

ACTC1 (actin, alpha, cardiac muscle 1) (eg, familial hypertrophic cardiomyopathy), full gene sequence

ANKRD1 (ankyrin repeat domain 1) (eg, dilated cardiomyopathy), full gene sequence

APTX (aprataxin) (eg, ataxia with oculomotor apraxia 1), full gene sequence

AR (androgen receptor) (eg, androgen insensitivity syndrome), full gene sequence

ARSA (arylsulfatase A) (eg, arylsulfatase A deficiency), full gene sequence

BCKDHA (branched chain keto acid dehydrogenase E1, alpha polypeptide) (eg, maple syrup urine disease, type 1A), full gene sequence

BCS1L (BCS1-like [S. cerevisiae]) (eg, Leigh syndrome, mitochondrial complex III deficiency, GRACILE syndrome), full gene sequence

BMPR2 (bone morphogenetic protein receptor, type II [serine/threonine kinase]) (eg, heritable pulmonary arterial hypertension), duplication/deletion analysis

CASQ2 (calsequestrin 2 [cardiac muscle]) (eg, catecholaminergic polymorphic ventricular tachycardia), full gene sequence

CASR (calcium-sensing receptor) (eg, hypocalcemia), full gene sequence

CDKL5 (cyclin-dependent kinase-like 5) (eg, early infantile epileptic encephalopathy), duplication/deletion analysis

CHRNA4 (cholinergic receptor, nicotinic, alpha 4) (eg, nocturnal frontal lobe epilepsy), full gene sequence

CHRNB2 (cholinergic receptor, nicotinic, beta 2 [neuronal]) (eg, nocturnal frontal lobe epilepsy), full gene sequence

COX10 (COX10 homolog, cytochrome c oxidase assembly protein) (eg, mitochondrial respiratory chain complex IV deficiency), full gene sequence

COX15 (COX15 homolog, cytochrome c oxidase assembly protein) (eg, mitochondrial respiratory chain complex IV deficiency), full gene sequence

CYP11B1 (cytochrome P450, family 11, subfamily B, polypeptide 1) (eg, congenital adrenal hyperplasia), full gene sequence

CYP17A1 (cytochrome P450, family 17, subfamily A, polypeptide 1) (eg, congenital adrenal hyperplasia), full gene sequence

CYP21A2 (cytochrome P450, family 21, subfamily A, polypeptide2) (eg, steroid 21-hydroxylase isoform, congenital adrenal hyperplasia), full gene sequence

Cytogenomic constitutional targeted microarray analysis of chromosome 22q13 by interrogation of genomic regions for copy number and single nucleotide polymorphism (SNP) variants for chromosomal abnormalities

(When performing genome-wide cytogenomic constitutional microarray analysis, see 81228, 81229)

(Do not report analyte-specific molecular pathology procedures separately when the specific analytes are included as part of the microarray analysis of chromosome 22q13)

(Do not report 88271 when performing cytogenomic microarray analysis)

DBT (dihydrolipoamide branched chain transacylase E2) (eg, maple syrup urine disease, type 2), duplication/deletion analysis

DCX (doublecortin) (eg, X-linked lissencephaly), full gene sequence

DES (desmin) (eg, myofibrillar myopathy), full gene sequence

DFNB59 (deafness, autosomal recessive 59) (eg, autosomal recessive nonsyndromic hearing impairment), full gene sequence

DGUOK (deoxyguanosine kinase) (eg, hepatocerebral mitochondrial DNA depletion syndrome), full gene sequence

DHCR7 (7-dehydrocholesterol reductase) (eg, Smith-Lemli-Opitz syndrome), full gene sequence

EIF2B2 (eukaryotic translation initiation factor 2B, subunit 2 beta, 39kDa) (eg, leukoencephalopathy with vanishing white matter), full gene sequence

EMD (emerin) (eg, Emery-Dreifuss muscular dystrophy), full gene sequence

ENG (endoglin) (eg, hereditary hemorrhagic telangiectasia, type 1), duplication/deletion analysis

EYA1 (eyes absent homolog 1 [Drosophila]) (eg, branchio-oto-renal [BOR] spectrum disorders), duplication/deletion analysis

F9 (coagulation factor IX) (eg, hemophilia B), full gene sequence

FGFR1 (fibroblast growth factor receptor 1) (eg, Kallmann syndrome 2), full gene sequence

FH (fumarate hydratase) (eg, fumarate hydratase deficiency, hereditary leiomyomatosis with renal cell cancer), full gene sequence

FKTN (fukutin) (eg, limb-girdle muscular dystrophy [LGMD] type 2M or 2L), full gene sequence

FTSJ1 (FtsJ RNA methyltransferase homolog 1 [E. coli]) (eg, X-linked mental retardation 9), duplication/deletion analysis

GABRG2 (gamma-aminobutyric acid [GABA] A receptor, gamma 2) (eg, generalized epilepsy with febrile seizures), full gene sequence

GCH1 (GTP cyclohydrolase 1) (eg, autosomal dominant dopa-responsive dystonia), full gene sequence

GDAP1 (ganglioside-induced differentiation-associated protein 1) (eg, Charcot-Marie-Tooth disease), full gene sequence

GFAP (glial fibrillary acidic protein) (eg, Alexander disease), full gene sequence

GHR (growth hormone receptor) (eg, Laron syndrome), full gene sequence

GHRHR (growth hormone releasing hormone receptor) (eg, growth hormone deficiency), full gene sequence

GLA (galactosidase, alpha) (eg, Fabry disease), full gene sequence

HBA1/HBA2 (alpha globin 1 and alpha globin 2) (eg, thalassemia), full gene sequence

HNF1A (HNF1 homeobox A) (eg, maturity-onset diabetes of the young [MODY]), full gene sequence

HNF1B (HNF1 homeobox B) (eg, maturity-onset diabetes of the young [MODY]), full gene sequence

HTRA1 (HtrA serine peptidase 1) (eg, macular degeneration), full gene sequence

IDS (iduronate 2-sulfatase) (eg, mucopolysaccharidosis, type II), full gene sequence

IL2RG (interleukin 2 receptor, gamma) (eg, X-linked severe combined immunodeficiency), full gene sequence

ISPD (isoprenoid synthase domain containing) (eg, muscle-eye-brain disease, Walker-Warburg syndrome), full gene sequence

KRAS (Kirsten rat sarcoma viral oncogene homolog) (eg, Noonan syndrome), full gene sequence

LAMP2 (lysosomal-associated membrane protein 2) (eg, Danon disease), full gene sequence

LDLR (low density lipoprotein receptor) (eg, familial hypercholesterolemia), duplication/deletion analysis

MEN1 (multiple endocrine neoplasia I) (eg, multiple endocrine neoplasia type 1, Wermer syndrome), full gene sequence

MMAA (methylmalonic aciduria [cobalamin deficiency] type A) (eg, MMAA-related methylmalonic acidemia), full gene sequence

MMAB (methylmalonic aciduria [cobalamin deficiency] type B) (eg, MMAA-related methylmalonic acidemia), full gene sequence

MPI (mannose phosphate isomerase) (eg, congenital disorder of glycosylation 1b), full gene sequence

MPV17 (MpV17 mitochondrial inner membrane protein) (eg, mitochondrial DNA depletion syndrome), full gene sequence

---

● New Code   ▲ Revised Code   ○ Reinstated   ● New Web Release   ▲ Revised Web Release   Unlisted   Not Covered   # Resequenced

MPZ (myelin protein zero) (eg, Charcot-Marie-Tooth), full gene sequence

MTM1 (myotubularin 1) (eg, X-linked centronuclear myopathy), duplication/deletion analysis

MYL2 (myosin, light chain 2, regulatory, cardiac, slow) (eg, familial hypertrophic cardiomyopathy), full gene sequence

MYL3 (myosin, light chain 3, alkali, ventricular, skeletal, slow) (eg, familial hypertrophic cardiomyopathy), full gene sequence

MYOT (myotilin) (eg, limb-girdle muscular dystrophy), full gene sequence

NDUFS7 (NADH dehydrogenase [ubiquinone] Fe-S protein 7, 20kDa [NADH-coenzyme Q reductase]) (eg, Leigh syndrome, mitochondrial complex I deficiency), full gene sequence

NDUFS8 (NADH dehydrogenase [ubiquinone] Fe-S protein 8, 23kDa [NADH-coenzyme Q reductase]) (eg, Leigh syndrome, mitochondrial complex I deficiency), full gene sequence

NDUFV1 (NADH dehydrogenase [ubiquinone] flavoprotein 1, 51kDa) (eg, Leigh syndrome, mitochondrial complex I deficiency), full gene sequence

NEFL (neurofilament, light polypeptide) (eg, Charcot-Marie-Tooth), full gene sequence

NF2 (neurofibromin 2 [merlin]) (eg, neurofibromatosis, type 2), duplication/deletion analysis

NLGN3 (neuroligin 3) (eg, autism spectrum disorders), full gene sequence

NLGN4X (neuroligin 4, X-linked) (eg, autism spectrum disorders), full gene sequence

NPHP1 (nephronophthisis 1 [juvenile]) (eg, Joubert syndrome), deletion analysis, and duplication analysis, if performed

NPHS2 (nephrosis 2, idiopathic, steroid-resistant [podocin]) (eg, steroid-resistant nephrotic syndrome), full gene sequence

NSD1 (nuclear receptor binding SET domain protein 1) (eg, Sotos syndrome), duplication/deletion analysis

OTC (ornithine carbamoyltransferase) (eg, ornithine transcarbamylase deficiency), full gene sequence

PAFAH1B1 (platelet-activating factor acetylhydrolase 1b, regulatory subunit 1 [45kDa]) (eg, lissencephaly, Miller-Dieker syndrome), duplication/deletion analysis

PARK2 (Parkinson protein 2, E3 ubiquitin protein ligase [parkin]) (eg, Parkinson disease), duplication/deletion analysis

PCCA (propionyl CoA carboxylase, alpha polypeptide) (eg, propionic acidemia, type 1), duplication/deletion analysis

PCDH19 (protocadherin 19) (eg, epileptic encephalopathy), full gene sequence

PDHA1 (pyruvate dehydrogenase [lipoamide] alpha 1) (eg, lactic acidosis), duplication/deletion analysis

PDHB (pyruvate dehydrogenase [lipoamide] beta) (eg, lactic acidosis), full gene sequence

PINK1 (PTEN induced putative kinase 1) (eg, Parkinson disease), full gene sequence

PLP1 (proteolipid protein 1) (eg, Pelizaeus-Merzbacher disease, spastic paraplegia), full gene sequence

POU1F1 (POU class 1 homeobox 1) (eg, combined pituitary hormone deficiency), full gene sequence

PQBP1 (polyglutamine binding protein 1) (eg, Renpenning syndrome), full gene sequence

PRX (periaxin) (eg, Charcot-Marie-Tooth disease), full gene sequence

PSEN1 (presenilin 1) (eg, Alzheimer's disease), full gene sequence

RAB7A (RAB7A, member RAS oncogene family) (eg, Charcot-Marie-Tooth disease), full gene sequence

RAI1 (retinoic acid induced 1) (eg, Smith-Magenis syndrome), full gene sequence

REEP1 (receptor accessory protein 1) (eg, spastic paraplegia), full gene sequence

RET (ret proto-oncogene) (eg, multiple endocrine neoplasia, type 2A and familial medullary thyroid carcinoma), targeted sequence analysis (eg, exons 10, 11, 13-16)

RPS19 (ribosomal protein S19) (eg, Diamond-Blackfan anemia), full gene sequence

RRM2B (ribonucleotide reductase M2 B [TP53 inducible]) (eg, mitochondrial DNA depletion), full gene sequence

SCO1 (SCO cytochrome oxidase deficient homolog 1) (eg, mitochondrial respiratory chain complex IV deficiency), full gene sequence

SDHB (succinate dehydrogenase complex, subunit B, iron sulfur) (eg, hereditary paraganglioma), full gene sequence

SDHC (succinate dehydrogenase complex, subunit C, integral membrane protein, 15kDa) (eg, hereditary paraganglioma-pheochromocytoma syndrome), full gene sequence

SGCA (sarcoglycan, alpha [50kDa dystrophin-associated glycoprotein]) (eg, limb-girdle muscular dystrophy), full gene sequence

SGCB (sarcoglycan, beta [43kDa dystrophin-associated glycoprotein]) (eg, limb-girdle muscular dystrophy), full gene sequence

SGCD (sarcoglycan, delta [35kDa dystrophin-associated glycoprotein]) (eg, limb-girdle muscular dystrophy), full gene sequence

SGCE (sarcoglycan, epsilon) (eg, myoclonic dystonia), duplication/deletion analysis

SGCG (sarcoglycan, gamma [35kDa dystrophin-associated glycoprotein]) (eg, limb-girdle muscular dystrophy), full gene sequence

SHOC2 (soc-2 suppressor of clear homolog) (eg, Noonan-like syndrome with loose anagen hair), full gene sequence

SHOX (short stature homeobox) (eg, Langer mesomelic dysplasia), full gene sequence

SIL1 (SIL1 homolog, endoplasmic reticulum chaperone [S. cerevisiae]) (eg, ataxia), full gene sequence

SLC2A1 (solute carrier family 2 [facilitated glucose transporter], member 1) (eg, glucose transporter type 1 [GLUT 1] deficiency syndrome), full gene sequence

SLC16A2 (solute carrier family 16, member 2 [thyroid hormone transporter]) (eg, specific thyroid hormone cell transporter deficiency, Allan-Herndon-Dudley syndrome), full gene sequence

SLC22A5 (solute carrier family 22 [organic cation/carnitine transporter], member 5) (eg, systemic primary carnitine deficiency), full gene sequence

SLC25A20 (solute carrier family 25 [carnitine/acylcarnitine translocase], member 20) (eg, carnitine-acylcarnitine translocase deficiency), full gene sequence

SMAD4 (SMAD family member 4) (eg, hemorrhagic telangiectasia syndrome, juvenile polyposis), duplication/deletion analysis

SMN1 (survival of motor neuron 1, telomeric) (eg, spinal muscular atrophy), full gene sequence

SPAST (spastin) (eg, spastic paraplegia), duplication/deletion analysis

SPG7 (spastic paraplegia 7 [pure and complicated autosomal recessive]) (eg, spastic paraplegia), duplication/deletion analysis

SPRED1 (sprouty-related, EVH1 domain containing 1) (eg, Legius syndrome), full gene sequence

STAT3 (signal transducer and activator of transcription 3 [acute-phase response factor]) (eg, autosomal dominant hyper-IgE syndrome), targeted sequence analysis (eg, exons 12, 13, 14, 16, 17, 20, 21)

STK11 (serine/threonine kinase 11) (eg, Peutz-Jeghers syndrome), full gene sequence

SURF1 (surfeit 1) (eg, mitochondrial respiratory chain complex IV deficiency), full gene sequence

26/16 PC/TC Only   A2-Z3 ASC Payment   50 Bilateral   ♂ Male Only   ♀ Female Only   ▲ Facility RVU   ↘ Non-Facility RVU   ☐ CCI

FUD Follow-up Days   CMS: IOM (Pub 100)   A-Y OPPSI   80/80 Surg Assist Allowed / w/Doc   ↘ Lab Crosswalk   ↗ Radiology Crosswalk   ☒ CLIA

358

TARDBP (TAR DNA binding protein) (eg, amyotrophic lateral sclerosis), full gene sequence

TBX5 (T-box 5) (eg, Holt-Oram syndrome), full gene sequence

TCF4 (transcription factor 4) (eg, Pitt-Hopkins syndrome), duplication/deletion analysis

TGFBR1 (transforming growth factor, beta receptor 1) (eg, Marfan syndrome), full gene sequence

TGFBR2 (transforming growth factor, beta receptor 2) (eg, Marfan syndrome), full gene sequence

THRB (thyroid hormone receptor, beta) (eg, thyroid hormone resistance, thyroid hormone beta receptor deficiency), full gene sequence or targeted sequence analysis of >5 exons

TK2 (thymidine kinase 2, mitochondrial) (eg, mitochondrial DNA depletion syndrome), full gene sequence

TNNC1 (troponin C type 1 [slow]) (eg, hypertrophic cardiomyopathy or dilated cardiomyopathy), full gene sequence

TNNI3 (troponin 1, type 3 [cardiac]) (eg, familial hypertrophic cardiomyopathy), full gene sequence

TP53 (tumor protein 53) (eg, Li-Fraumeni syndrome, tumor samples), full gene sequence or targeted sequence analysis of >5 exons

TPM1 (tropomyosin 1 [alpha]) (eg, familial hypertrophic cardiomyopathy), full gene sequence

TSC1 (tuberous sclerosis 1) (eg, tuberous sclerosis), duplication/deletion analysis

TYMP (thymidine phosphorylase) (eg, mitochondrial DNA depletion syndrome), full gene sequence

VWF (von Willebrand factor) (eg, von Willebrand disease type 2N), targeted sequence analysis (eg, exons 18-20, 23-25)

WT1 (Wilms tumor 1) (eg, Denys-Drash syndrome, familial Wilms tumor), full gene sequence

ZEB2 (zinc finger E-box binding homeobox 2) (eg, Mowat-Wilson syndrome), full gene sequence

    📖 0.00   ⚕ 0.00   **FUD** XXX   Ⓐ 🔲

    AMA: 2016,Aug,9; 2016,Jan,13; 2015,Jan,3; 2015,Jan,16; 2014,Jan,11; 2013,Sep,3-12; 2013,Jul,11-12; 2012,May,3-10

▲   **81406**   **Molecular pathology procedure, Level 7 (eg, analysis of 11-25 exons by DNA sequence analysis, mutation scanning or duplication/deletion variants of 26-50 exons, cytogenomic array analysis for neoplasia)**

ACADVL (acyl-CoA dehydrogenase, very long chain) (eg, very long chain acyl-coenzyme A dehydrogenase deficiency), full gene sequence

ACTN4 (actinin, alpha 4) (eg, focal segmental glomerulosclerosis), full gene sequence

AFG3L2 (AFG3 ATPase family gene 3-like 2 [S. cerevisiae]) (eg, spinocerebellar ataxia), full gene sequence

AIRE (autoimmune regulator) (eg, autoimmune polyendocrinopathy syndrome type 1), full gene sequence

ALDH7A1 (aldehyde dehydrogenase 7 family, member A1) (eg, pyridoxine-dependent epilepsy), full gene sequence

ANO5 (anoctamin 5) (eg, limb-girdle muscular dystrophy), full gene sequence

APP (amyloid beta [A4] precursor protein) (eg, Alzheimer's disease), full gene sequence

ASS1 (argininosuccinate synthase 1) (eg, citrullinemia type I), full gene sequence

ATL1 (atlastin GTPase 1) (eg, spastic paraplegia), full gene sequence

ATP1A2 (ATPase, Na+/K+ transporting, alpha 2 polypeptide) (eg, familial hemiplegic migraine), full gene sequence

ATP7B (ATPase, Cu++ transporting, beta polypeptide) (eg, Wilson disease), full gene sequence

BBS1 (Bardet-Biedl syndrome 1) (eg, Bardet-Biedl syndrome), full gene sequence

BBS2 (Bardet-Biedl syndrome 2) (eg, Bardet-Biedl syndrome), full gene sequence

BCKDHB (branched-chain keto acid dehydrogenase E1, beta polypeptide) (eg, maple syrup urine disease, type 1B), full gene sequence

BEST1 (bestrophin 1) (eg, vitelliform macular dystrophy), full gene sequence

BMPR2 (bone morphogenetic protein receptor, type II [serine/threonine kinase]) (eg, heritable pulmonary arterial hypertension), full gene sequence

BRAF (B-Raf proto-oncogene, serine/threonine kinase) (eg, Noonan syndrome), full gene sequence

BSCL2 (Berardinelli-Seip congenital lipodystrophy 2 [seipin]) (eg, Berardinelli-Seip congenital lipodystrophy), full gene sequence

BTK (Bruton agammaglobulinemia tyrosine kinase) (eg, X-linked agammaglobulinemia), full gene sequence

CACNB2 (calcium channel, voltage-dependent, beta 2 subunit) (eg, Brugada syndrome), full gene sequence

CAPN3 (calpain 3) (eg, limb-girdle muscular dystrophy [LGMD] type 2A, calpainopathy), full gene sequence

CBS (cystathionine-beta-synthase) (eg, homocystinuria, cystathionine beta-synthase deficiency), full gene sequence

CDH1 (cadherin 1, type 1, E-cadherin [epithelial]) (eg, hereditary diffuse gastric cancer), full gene sequence

CDKL5 (cyclin-dependent kinase-like 5) (eg, early infantile epileptic encephalopathy), full gene sequence

CLCN1 (chloride channel 1, skeletal muscle) (eg, myotonia congenita), full gene sequence

CLCNKB (chloride channel, voltage-sensitive Kb) (eg, Bartter syndrome 3 and 4b), full gene sequence

CNTNAP2 (contactin-associated protein-like 2) (eg, Pitt-Hopkins-like syndrome 1), full gene sequence

COL6A2 (collagen, type VI, alpha 2) (eg, collagen type VI-related disorders), duplication/deletion analysis

CPT1A (carnitine palmitoyltransferase 1A [liver]) (eg, carnitine palmitoyltransferase 1A [CPT1A] deficiency), full gene sequence

CRB1 (crumbs homolog 1 [Drosophila]) (eg, Leber congenital amaurosis), full gene sequence

CREBBP (CREB binding protein) (eg, Rubinstein-Taybi syndrome), duplication/deletion analysis

Cytogenomic microarray analysis, neoplasia (eg, interrogation of copy number, and loss-of-heterozygosity via single nucleotide polymorphism [SNP]-based comparative genomic hybridization [CGH] microarray analysis)

(Do not report analyte-specific molecular pathology procedures separately when the specific analytes are included as part of the cytogenomic microarray analysis for neoplasia)

(Do not report 88271 when performing cytogenomic microarray analysis)

DBT (dihydrolipoamide branched chain transacylase E2) (eg, maple syrup urine disease, type 2), full gene sequence

DLAT (dihydrolipoamide S-acetyltransferase) (eg, pyruvate dehydrogenase E2 deficiency), full gene sequence

DLD (dihydrolipoamide dehydrogenase) (eg, maple syrup urine disease, type III), full gene sequence

DSC2 (desmocollin) (eg, arrhythmogenic right ventricular dysplasia/cardiomyopathy 11), full gene sequence

DSG2 (desmoglein 2) (eg, arrhythmogenic right ventricular dysplasia/cardiomyopathy 10), full gene sequence

DSP (desmoplakin) (eg, arrhythmogenic right ventricular dysplasia/cardiomyopathy 8), full gene sequence

EFHC1 (EF-hand domain [C-terminal] containing 1) (eg, juvenile myoclonic epilepsy), full gene sequence

EIF2B3 (eukaryotic translation initiation factor 2B, subunit 3 gamma, 58kDa) (eg, leukoencephalopathy with vanishing white matter), full gene sequence

EIF2B4 (eukaryotic translation initiation factor 2B, subunit 4 delta, 67kDa) (eg, leukoencephalopathy with vanishing white matter), full gene sequence

EIF2B5 (eukaryotic translation initiation factor 2B, subunit 5 epsilon, 82kDa) (eg, childhood ataxia with central nervous system hypomyelination/vanishing white matter), full gene sequence

ENG (endoglin) (eg, hereditary hemorrhagic telangiectasia, type 1), full gene sequence

EYA1 (eyes absent homolog 1 [Drosophila]) (eg, branchio-oto-renal [BOR] spectrum disorders), full gene sequence

F8 (coagulation factor VIII) (eg, hemophilia A), duplication/deletion analysis

FAH (fumarylacetoacetate hydrolase [fumarylacetoacetase]) (eg, tyrosinemia, type 1), full gene sequence

FASTKD2 (FAST kinase domains 2) (eg, mitochondrial respiratory chain complex IV deficiency), full gene sequence

FIG4 (FIG4 homolog, SAC1 lipid phosphatase domain containing [S. cerevisiae]) (eg, Charcot-Marie-Tooth disease), full gene sequence

FTSJ1 (FtsJ RNA methyltransferase homolog 1 [E. coli]) (eg, X-linked mental retardation 9), full gene sequence

FUS (fused in sarcoma) (eg, amyotrophic lateral sclerosis), full gene sequence

GAA (glucosidase, alpha; acid) (eg, glycogen storage disease type II [Pompe disease]), full gene sequence

GALC (galactosylceramidase) (eg, Krabbe disease), full gene sequence

GALT (galactose-1-phosphate uridylyltransferase) (eg, galactosemia), full gene sequence

GARS (glycyl-tRNA synthetase) (eg, Charcot-Marie-Tooth disease), full gene sequence

GCDH (glutaryl-CoA dehydrogenase) (eg, glutaricacidemia type 1), full gene sequence

GCK (glucokinase [hexokinase 4]) (eg, maturity-onset diabetes of the young [MODY]), full gene sequence

GLUD1 (glutamate dehydrogenase 1) (eg, familial hyperinsulinism), full gene sequence

GNE (glucosamine [UDP-N-acetyl]-2-epimerase/N-acetylmannosamine kinase) (eg, inclusion body myopathy 2 [IBM2], Nonaka myopathy), full gene sequence

GRN (granulin) (eg, frontotemporal dementia), full gene sequence

HADHA (hydroxyacyl-CoA dehydrogenase/3-ketoacyl-CoA thiolase/enoyl-CoA hydratase [trifunctional protein] alpha subunit) (eg, long chain acyl-coenzyme A dehydrogenase deficiency), full gene sequence

HADHB (hydroxyacyl-CoA dehydrogenase/3-ketoacyl-CoA thiolase/enoyl-CoA hydratase [trifunctional protein], beta subunit) (eg, trifunctional protein deficiency), full gene sequence

HEXA (hexosaminidase A, alpha polypeptide) (eg, Tay-Sachs disease), full gene sequence

HLCS (HLCS holocarboxylase synthetase) (eg, holocarboxylase synthetase deficiency), full gene sequence

HNF4A (hepatocyte nuclear factor 4, alpha) (eg, maturity-onset diabetes of the young [MODY]), full gene sequence

IDUA (iduronidase, alpha-L-) (eg, mucopolysaccharidosis type I), full gene sequence

INF2 (inverted formin, FH2 and WH2 domain containing) (eg, focal segmental glomerulosclerosis), full gene sequence

IVD (isovaleryl-CoA dehydrogenase) (eg, isovaleric acidemia), full gene sequence

JAG1 (jagged 1) (eg, Alagille syndrome), duplication/deletion analysis

JUP (junction plakoglobin) (eg, arrhythmogenic right ventricular dysplasia/cardiomyopathy 11), full gene sequence

KAL1 (Kallmann syndrome 1 sequence) (eg, Kallmann syndrome), full gene sequence

KCNH2 (potassium voltage-gated channel, subfamily H [eag-related], member 2) (eg, short QT syndrome, long QT syndrome), full gene sequence

KCNQ1 (potassium voltage-gated channel, KQT-like subfamily, member 1) (eg, short QT syndrome, long QT syndrome), full gene sequence

KCNQ2 (potassium voltage-gated channel, KQT-like subfamily, member 2) (eg, epileptic encephalopathy), full gene sequence

LDB3 (LIM domain binding 3) (eg, familial dilated cardiomyopathy, myofibrillar myopathy), full gene sequence

LDLR (low density lipoprotein receptor) (eg, familial hypercholesterolemia), full gene sequence

LEPR (leptin receptor(eg, obesity with hypogonadism), full gene sequence

LHCGR (luteinizing hormone/choriogonadotropin receptor) (eg, precocious male puberty), full gene sequence

LMNA (lamin A/C) (eg, Emery-Dreifuss muscular dystrophy [EDMD1, 2 and 3] limb-girdle muscular dystrophy [LGMD] type 1B, dilated cardiomyopathy [CMD1A], familial partial lipodystrophy [FPLD2]), full gene sequence

LRP5 (low density lipoprotein receptor-related protein 5) (eg, osteopetrosis), full gene sequence

MAP2K1 (mitogen-activated protein kinase 1) (eg, cardiofaciocutaneous syndrome), full gene sequence

MAP2K2 (mitogen-activated protein kinase 2) (eg, cardiofaciocutaneous syndrome), full gene sequence

MAPT (microtubule-associated protein tau) (eg, frontotemporal dementia), full gene sequence

MCCC1 (methylcrotonoyl-CoA carboxylase 1 [alpha]) (eg, 3-methylcrotonyl-CoA carboxylase deficiency), full gene sequence

MCCC2 (methylcrotonoyl-CoA carboxylase 2 [beta]) (eg, 3-methylcrotonyl carboxylase deficiency), full gene sequence

MFN2 (mitofusin 2) (eg, Charcot-Marie-Tooth disease), full gene sequence

MTM1 (myotubularin 1) (eg, X-linked centronuclear myopathy), full gene sequence

MUT (methylmalonyl CoA mutase) (eg, methylmalonic acidemia), full gene sequence

MUTYH (mutY homolog [E. coli]) (eg, MYH-associated polyposis), full gene sequence

NDUFS1 (NADH dehydrogenase [ubiquinone] Fe-S protein 1, 75kDa [NADH-coenzyme Q reductase]) (eg, Leigh syndrome, mitochondrial complex I deficiency), full gene sequence

NF2 (neurofibromin 2 [merlin]) (eg, neurofibromatosis, type 2), full gene sequence

NOTCH3 (notch 3) (eg, cerebral autosomal dominant arteriopathy with subcortical infarcts and leukoencephalopathy [CADASIL]), targeted sequence analysis (eg, exons 1-23)

NPC1 (Niemann-Pick disease, type C1) (eg, Niemann-Pick disease), full gene sequence

NPHP1 (nephronophthisis 1 [juvenile]) (eg, Joubert syndrome), full gene sequence

NSD1 (nuclear receptor binding SET domain protein 1) (eg, Sotos syndrome), full gene sequence

OPA1 (optic atrophy 1) (eg, optic atrophy), duplication/deletion analysis

OPTN (optineurin) (eg, amyotrophic lateral sclerosis), full gene sequence

PAFAH1B1 (platelet-activating factor acetylhydrolase 1b, regulatory subunit 1 [45kDa]) (eg, lissencephaly, Miller-Dieker syndrome), full gene sequence

PAH (phenylalanine hydroxylase) (eg, phenylketonuria), full gene sequence

PALB2 (partner and localizer of BRCA2) (eg, breast and pancreatic cancer), full gene sequence

PARK2 (Parkinson protein 2, E3 ubiquitin protein ligase [parkin]) (eg, Parkinson disease), full gene sequence

PAX2 (paired box 2) (eg, renal coloboma syndrome), full gene sequence

PC (pyruvate carboxylase) (eg, pyruvate carboxylase deficiency), full gene sequence

PCCA (propionyl CoA carboxylase, alpha polypeptide) (eg, propionic acidemia, type 1), full gene sequence

PCCB (propionyl CoA carboxylase, beta polypeptide) (eg, propionic acidemia), full gene sequence

PCDH15 (protocadherin-related 15) (eg, Usher syndrome type 1F), duplication/deletion analysis

PCSK9 (proprotein convertase subtilisin/kexin type 9) (eg familial hypercholesterolemia), full gene sequence

PDHA1 (pyruvate dehydrogenase [lipoamide] alpha 1) (eg, lactic acidosis), full gene sequence

PDHX (pyruvate dehydrogenase complex, component X) (eg, lactic acidosis), full gene sequence

PHEX (phosphate-regulating endopeptidase homolog, X-linked) (eg, hypophosphatemic rickets), full gene sequence

PKD2 (polycystic kidney disease 2 [autosomal dominant]) (eg, polycystic kidney disease), full gene sequence

PKP2 (plakophilin 2) (eg, arrhythmogenic right ventricular dysplasia/cardiomyopathy 9), full gene sequence

PNKD (eg, paroxysmal nonkinesigenic dyskinesia), full gene sequence

POLG (polymerase [DNA directed], gamma) (eg, Alpers-Huttenlocher syndrome, autosomal dominant progressive external ophthalmoplegia), full gene sequence

POMGNT1 (protein O-linked mannose beta1, 2-N acetylglucosaminyltransferase) (eg, muscle-eye-brain disease, Walker-Warburg syndrome), full gene sequence

POMT1 (protein-O-mannosyltransferase 1) (eg, limb-girdle muscular dystrophy [LGMD] type 2K, Walker-Warburg syndrome), full gene sequence

POMT2 (protein-O-mannosyltransferase 2) (eg, limb-girdle muscular dystrophy [LGMD] type 2N, Walker-Warburg syndrome), full gene sequence

PRKAG2 (protein kinase, AMP-activated, gamma 2 non-catalytic subunit) (eg, familial hypertrophic cardiomyopathy with Wolff-Parkinson-White syndrome, lethal congenital glycogen storage disease of heart), full gene sequence

PRKCG (protein kinase C, gamma) (eg, spinocerebellar ataxia), full gene sequence

PSEN2 (presenilin 2[Alzheimer's disease 4]) (eg, Alzheimer's disease), full gene sequence

PTPN11 (protein tyrosine phosphatase, non-receptor type 11) (eg, Noonan syndrome, LEOPARD syndrome), full gene sequence

PYGM (phosphorylase, glycogen, muscle) (eg, glycogen storage disease type V, McArdle disease), full gene sequence

RAF1 (v-raf-1 murine leukemia viral oncogene homolog 1) (eg, LEOPARD syndrome), full gene sequence

RET (ret proto-oncogene) (eg, Hirschsprung disease), full gene sequence

RPE65 (retinal pigment epithelium-specific protein 65kDa) (eg, retinitis pigmentosa, Leber congenital amaurosis), full gene sequence

RYR1 (ryanodine receptor 1, skeletal) (eg, malignant hyperthermia), targeted sequence analysis of exons with functionally-confirmed mutations

SCN4A (sodium channel, voltage-gated, type IV, alpha subunit) (eg, hyperkalemic periodic paralysis), full gene sequence

SCNN1A (sodium channel, nonvoltage-gated 1 alpha) (eg, pseudohypoaldosteronism), full gene sequence

SCNN1B (sodium channel, nonvoltage-gated 1, beta) (eg, Liddle syndrome, pseudohypoaldosteronism), full gene sequence

SCNN1G (sodium channel, nonvoltage-gated 1, gamma) (eg, Liddle syndrome, pseudohypoaldosteronism), full gene sequence

SDHA (succinate dehydrogenase complex, subunit A, flavoprotein [Fp]) (eg, Leigh syndrome, mitochondrial complex II deficiency), full gene sequence

SETX (senataxin) (eg, ataxia), full gene sequence

SGCE (sarcoglycan, epsilon) (eg, myoclonic dystonia), full gene sequence

SH3TC2 (SH3 domain and tetratricopeptide repeats 2) (eg, Charcot-Marie-Tooth disease), full gene sequence

SLC9A6 (solute carrier family 9 [sodium/hydrogen exchanger], member 6) (eg, Christianson syndrome), full gene sequence

SLC26A4 (solute carrier family 26, member 4) (eg, Pendred syndrome), full gene sequence

SLC37A4 (solute carrier family 37 [glucose-6-phosphate transporter], member 4) (eg, glycogen storage disease type Ib), full gene sequence

SMAD4 (SMAD family member 4) (eg, hemorrhagic telangiectasia syndrome, juvenile polyposis), full gene sequence

SOS1 (son of sevenless homolog 1) (eg, Noonan syndrome, gingival fibromatosis), full gene sequence

SPAST (spastin) (eg, spastic paraplegia), full gene sequence

SPG7 (spastic paraplegia 7 [pure and complicated autosomal recessive]) (eg, spastic paraplegia), full gene sequence

STXBP1 (syntaxin-binding protein 1) (eg, epileptic encephalopathy), full gene sequence

TAZ (tafazzin) (eg, methylglutaconic aciduria type 2, Barth syndrome), full gene sequence

TCF4 (transcription factor 4) (eg, Pitt-Hopkins syndrome), full gene sequence

TH (tyrosine hydroxylase) (eg, Segawa syndrome), full gene sequence

TMEM43 (transmembrane protein 43) (eg, arrhythmogenic right ventricular cardiomyopathy), full gene sequence

TNNT2 (troponin T, type 2 [cardiac]) (eg, familial hypertrophic cardiomyopathy), full gene sequence

TRPC6 (transient receptor potential cation channel, subfamily C, member 6) (eg, focal segmental glomerulosclerosis), full gene sequence

TSC1 (tuberous sclerosis 1) (eg, tuberous sclerosis), full gene sequence

TSC2 (tuberous sclerosis 2) (eg, tuberous sclerosis), duplication/deletion analysis

UBE3A (ubiquitin protein ligase E3A) (eg, Angelman syndrome) full gene sequence

UMOD (uromodulin) (eg, glomerulocystic kidney disease with hyperuricemia and isosthenuria), full gene sequence

VWF (von Willebrand factor) (von Willebrand disease type 2A), extended targeted sequence analysis (eg, exons 11-16, 24-26, 51, 52)

WAS (Wiskott-Aldrich syndrome [eczema-thrombocytopenia]) (eg, Wiskott-Aldrich syndrome), full gene sequence

  📁 0.00   ✂ 0.00   **FUD** XXX   A 🔲

AMA: 2016,Aug,9; 2016,Jan,13; 2015,Jan,3; 2015,Jan,16; 2014,Jan,11; 2013,Sep,3-12; 2013,Jul,11-12; 2012,May,3-10

● New Code   ▲ Revised Code   ○ Reinstated   ● New Web Release   ▲ Revised Web Release   Unlisted   Not Covered   # Resequenced

🚫 AMA Mod 51 Exempt   Ⓢ Optum Mod 51 Exempt   🚫 Mod 63 Exempt   ✎ Non-FDA Drug   ★ Telehealth   Ⓜ Maternity   🅐 Age Edit   + Add-on   **AMA:** CPT Asst

81407 **Molecular pathology procedure, Level 8 (eg, analysis of 26-50 exons by DNA sequence analysis, mutation scanning or duplication/deletion variants of >50 exons, sequence analysis of multiple genes on one platform)**

ABCC8 (ATP-binding cassette, sub-family C [CFTR/MRP], member 8) (eg, familial hyperinsulinism), full gene sequence

AGL (amylo-alpha-1, 6-glucosidase, 4-alpha-glucanotransferase) (eg, glycogen storage disease type III), full gene sequence

AHI1 (Abelson helper integration site 1) (eg, Joubert syndrome), full gene sequence

ASPM (asp [abnormal spindle] homolog, microcephaly associated [Drosophila]) (eg, primary microcephaly), full gene sequence

CACNA1A (calcium channel, voltage-dependent, P/Q type, alpha 1A subunit) (eg, familial hemiplegic migraine), full gene sequence

CHD7 (chromodomain helicase DNA binding protein 7) (eg, CHARGE syndrome), full gene sequence

COL4A4 (collagen, type IV, alpha 4) (eg, Alport syndrome), full gene sequence

COL4A5 (collagen, type IV, alpha 5) (eg, Alport syndrome), duplication/deletion analysis

COL6A1 (collagen, type VI, alpha 1) (eg, collagen type VI-related disorders), full gene sequence

COL6A2 (collagen, type VI, alpha 2) (eg, collagen type VI-related disorders), full gene sequence

COL6A3 (collagen, type VI, alpha 3) (eg, collagen type VI-related disorders), full gene sequence

CREBBP (CREB binding protein) (eg, Rubinstein-Taybi syndrome), full gene sequence

F8 (coagulation factor VIII) (eg, hemophilia A), full gene sequence

JAG1 (jagged 1) (eg, Alagille syndrome), full gene sequence

KDM5C (lysine [K]-specific demethylase 5C) (eg, X-linked mental retardation), full gene sequence

KIAA0196 (KIAA0196) (eg, spastic paraplegia), full gene sequence

L1CAM (L1 cell adhesion molecule) (eg, MASA syndrome, X-linked hydrocephaly), full gene sequence

LAMB2 (laminin, beta 2 [laminin S]) (eg, Pierson syndrome), full gene sequence

MYBPC3 (myosin binding protein C, cardiac) (eg, familial hypertrophic cardiomyopathy), full gene sequence

MYH6 (myosin, heavy chain 6, cardiac muscle, alpha) (eg, familial dilated cardiomyopathy), full gene sequence

MYH7 (myosin, heavy chain 7, cardiac muscle, beta) (eg, familial hypertrophic cardiomyopathy, Liang distal myopathy), full gene sequence

MYO7A (myosin VIIA) (eg, Usher syndrome, type 1), full gene sequence

NOTCH1 (notch 1) (eg, aortic valve disease), full gene sequence

NPHS1 (nephrosis 1, congenital, Finnish type [nephrin]) (eg, congenital Finnish nephrosis), full gene sequence

OPA1 (optic atrophy 1) (eg, optic atrophy), full gene sequence

PCDH15 (protocadherin-related 15) (eg, Usher syndrome, type 1), full gene sequence

PKD1 (polycystic kidney disease 1 [autosomal dominant]) (eg, polycystic kidney disease), full gene sequence

PLCE1 (phospholipase C, epsilon 1) (eg, nephrotic syndrome type 3), full gene sequence

SCN1A (sodium channel, voltage-gated, type 1, alpha subunit) (eg, generalized epilepsy with febrile seizures), full gene sequence

SCN5A (sodium channel, voltage-gated, type V, alpha subunit) (eg, familial dilated cardiomyopathy), full gene sequence

SLC12A1 (solute carrier family 12 [sodium/potassium/chloride transporters], member 1) (eg, Bartter syndrome), full gene sequence

SLC12A3 (solute carrier family 12 [sodium/chloride transporters], member 3) (eg, Gitelman syndrome), full gene sequence

SPG11 (spastic paraplegia 11 [autosomal recessive]) (eg, spastic paraplegia), full gene sequence

SPTBN2 (spectrin, beta, non-erythrocytic 2) (eg, spinocerebellar ataxia), full gene sequence

TMEM67 (transmembrane protein 67) (eg, Joubert syndrome), full gene sequence

TSC2 (tuberous sclerosis 2) (eg, tuberous sclerosis), full gene sequence

USH1C (Usher syndrome 1C [autosomal recessive, severe]) (eg, Usher syndrome, type 1), full gene sequence

VPS13B (vacuolar protein sorting 13 homolog B [yeast]) (eg, Cohen syndrome), duplication/deletion analysis

WDR62 (WD repeat domain 62) (eg, primary autosomal recessive microcephaly), full gene sequence

🔌 0.00   🔧 0.00   **FUD** XXX   Ⓐ🔲

AMA: 2016,Aug,9; 2016,Jan,13; 2015,Jan,3; 2015,Jan,16; 2014,Jan,11; 2013,Sep,3-12; 2013,Jul,11-12; 2012,May,3-10

81408 **Molecular pathology procedure, Level 9 (eg, analysis of >50 exons in a single gene by DNA sequence analysis)**

ABCA4 (ATP-binding cassette, sub-family A [ABC1], member 4) (eg, Stargardt disease, age-related macular degeneration), full gene sequence

ATM (ataxia telangiectasia mutated) (eg, ataxia telangiectasia), full gene sequence

CDH23 (cadherin-related 23) (eg, Usher syndrome, type 1), full gene sequence

CEP290 (centrosomal protein 290kDa) (eg, Joubert syndrome), full gene sequence

COL1A1 (collagen, type I, alpha 1) (eg, osteogenesis imperfecta, type I), full gene sequence

COL1A2 (collagen, type I, alpha 2) (eg, osteogenesis imperfecta, type I), full gene sequence

COL4A1 (collagen, type IV, alpha 1) (eg, brain small-vessel disease with hemorrhage), full gene sequence

COL4A3 (collagen, type IV, alpha 3 [Goodpasture antigen]) (eg, Alport syndrome), full gene sequence

COL4A5 (collagen, type IV, alpha 5) (eg, Alport syndrome), full gene sequence

DMD (dystrophin) (eg, Duchenne/Becker muscular dystrophy), full gene sequence

DYSF (dysferlin, limb girdle muscular dystrophy 2B [autosomal recessive]) (eg, limb-girdle muscular dystrophy), full gene sequence

FBN1 (fibrillin 1) (eg, Marfan syndrome), full gene sequence

ITPR1 (inositol 1,4,5-trisphosphate receptor, type 1) (eg, spinocerebellar ataxia), full gene sequence

LAMA2 (laminin, alpha 2) (eg, congenital muscular dystrophy), full gene sequence

LRRK2 (leucine-rich repeat kinase 2) (eg, Parkinson disease), full gene sequence

MYH11 (myosin, heavy chain 11, smooth muscle) (eg, thoracic aortic aneurysms and aortic dissections), full gene sequence

NEB (nebulin) (eg, nemaline myopathy 2), full gene sequence

NF1 (neurofibromin 1) (eg, neurofibromatosis, type 1), full gene sequence

PKHD1 (polycystic kidney and hepatic disease 1) (eg, autosomal recessive polycystic kidney disease), full gene sequence

RYR1 (ryanodine receptor 1, skeletal) (eg, malignant hyperthermia), full gene sequence

RYR2 (ryanodine receptor 2 [cardiac]) (eg, catecholaminergic polymorphic ventricular tachycardia, arrhythmogenic right ventricular dysplasia), full gene sequence or targeted sequence analysis of > 50 exons

USH2A (Usher syndrome 2A [autosomal recessive, mild]) (eg, Usher syndrome, type 2), full gene sequence

VPS13B (vacuolar protein sorting 13 homolog B [yeast]) (eg, Cohen syndrome), full gene sequence

VWF (von Willebrand factor) (eg, von Willebrand disease types 1 and 3), full gene sequence

   🔖 0.00 ⚕ 0.00 **FUD** XXX   A 🖵

   AMA: 2016,Aug,9; 2016,Jan,13; 2015,Jan,3; 2015,Jan,16; 2014,Jan,11; 2013,Sep,3-12; 2013,Jul,11-12; 2012,May,3-10

**81479**   **Unlisted molecular pathology procedure**

   🔖 0.00 ⚕ 0.00 **FUD** XXX   A

   AMA: 2016,Sep,9; 2016,Aug,9; 2016,Apr,4; 2016,Jan,13; 2015,Jan,16; 2015,Jan,3; 2014,Jan,11; 2013,Sep,3-12; 2013,Jul,11-12

81410-81479 Genomic Sequencing

81410   **Aortic dysfunction or dilation (eg, Marfan syndrome, Loeys Dietz syndrome, Ehler Danlos syndrome type IV, arterial tortuosity syndrome); genomic sequence analysis panel, must include sequencing of at least 9 genes, including *FBN1, TGFBR1, TGFBR2, COL3A1, MYH11, ACTA2, SLC2A10, SMAD3,* and *MYLK***

   🔖 0.00 ⚕ 0.00 **FUD** XXX   A 🖵

   AMA: 2016,Jan,13; 2015,Jan,3

81411   **duplication/deletion analysis panel, must include analyses for *TGFBR1, TGFBR2, MYH11,* and *COL3A1***

   🔖 0.00 ⚕ 0.00 **FUD** XXX   A 🖵

   AMA: 2016,Jan,13; 2015,Jan,3

81412   **Ashkenazi Jewish associated disorders (eg, Bloom syndrome, Canavan disease, cystic fibrosis, familial dysautonomia, Fanconi anemia group C, Gaucher disease, Tay-Sachs disease), genomic sequence analysis panel, must include sequencing of at least 9 genes, including *ASPA, BLM, CFTR, FANCC, GBA, HEXA, IKBKAP, MCOLN1,* and *SMPD1***

   🔖 0.00 ⚕ 0.00 **FUD** XXX   A 🖵

   AMA: 2016,Apr,4

● **81413**   **Cardiac ion channelopathies (eg, Brugada syndrome, long QT syndrome, short QT syndrome, catecholaminergic polymorphic ventricular tachycardia); genomic sequence analysis panel, must include sequencing of at least 10 genes, including ANK2, CASQ2, CAV3, KCNE1, KCNE2, KCNH2, KCNJ2, KCNQ1, RYR2, and SCN5A**

   EXCLUDES   *Evaluation of cardiomyopathy (81439)*

● **81414**   **duplication/deletion gene analysis panel, must include analysis of at least 2 genes, including KCNH2 and KCNQ1**

   EXCLUDES   *Evaluation of cardiomyopathy (81439)*

81415   **Exome (eg, unexplained constitutional or heritable disorder or syndrome); sequence analysis**

   🔖 0.00 ⚕ 0.00 **FUD** XXX   A 🖵

   AMA: 2016,Jan,13; 2015,Jan,3

+   **81416**   **sequence analysis, each comparator exome (eg, parents, siblings) (List separately in addition to code for primary procedure)**

   Code first (81415)

   🔖 0.00 ⚕ 0.00 **FUD** XXX   A 🖵

   AMA: 2016,Jan,13; 2015,Jan,3

81417   **re-evaluation of previously obtained exome sequence (eg, updated knowledge or unrelated condition/syndrome)**

   EXCLUDES   *Microarray assessment (81228-81229)*

           Results that are incidental

   🔖 0.00 ⚕ 0.00 **FUD** XXX   A 🖵

   AMA: 2016,Jan,13; 2015,Jan,3

81420   **Fetal chromosomal aneuploidy (eg, trisomy 21, monosomy X) genomic sequence analysis panel, circulating cell-free fetal DNA in maternal blood, must include analysis of chromosomes 13, 18, and 21**   M

   EXCLUDES   *Genome-wide microarray analysis (81228-81229)*

           Molecular cytogenetics (88271)

   🔖 0.00 ⚕ 0.00 **FUD** XXX   A 🖵

   AMA: 2016,Jan,13; 2015,Dec,18; 2015,Jan,3

● **81422**   **Fetal chromosomal microdeletion(s) genomic sequence analysis (eg, DiGeorge syndrome, Cri-du-chat syndrome), circulating cell-free fetal DNA in maternal blood**

   EXCLUDES   *Genome-wide microarray analysis (81228-81229)*

           Molecular cytogenetics (88271)

81425   **Genome (eg, unexplained constitutional or heritable disorder or syndrome); sequence analysis**

   🔖 0.00 ⚕ 0.00 **FUD** XXX   A 🖵

   AMA: 2016,Jan,13; 2015,Jan,3

+   **81426**   **sequence analysis, each comparator genome (eg, parents, siblings) (List separately in addition to code for primary procedure)**

   Code first (81425)

   🔖 0.00 ⚕ 0.00 **FUD** XXX   A 🖵

   AMA: 2016,Jan,13; 2015,Jan,3

81427   **re-evaluation of previously obtained genome sequence (eg, updated knowledge or unrelated condition/syndrome)**

   EXCLUDES   *Genome-wide microarray analysis (81228-81229)*

           Results that are incidental

   🔖 0.00 ⚕ 0.00 **FUD** XXX   A 🖵

   AMA: 2016,Jan,13; 2015,Jan,3

81430   **Hearing loss (eg, nonsyndromic hearing loss, Usher syndrome, Pendred syndrome); genomic sequence analysis panel, must include sequencing of at least 60 genes, including *CDH23, CLRN1, GJB2, GPR98, MTRNR1, MYO7A, MYO15A, PCDH15, OTOF, SLC26A4, TMC1, TMPRSS3, USH1C, USH1G, USH2A,* and *WFS1***

   🔖 0.00 ⚕ 0.00 **FUD** XXX   A 🖵

   AMA: 2016,Jan,13; 2015,Jan,3; 2012,May,3-10

81431   **duplication/deletion analysis panel, must include copy number analyses for *STRC* and *DFNB1* deletions in *GJB2* and *GJB6* genes**

   🔖 0.00 ⚕ 0.00 **FUD** XXX   A 🖵

   AMA: 2016,Jan,13; 2015,Jan,3

81432   **Hereditary breast cancer-related disorders (eg, hereditary breast cancer, hereditary ovarian cancer, hereditary endometrial cancer); genomic sequence analysis panel, must include sequencing of at least 14 genes, including *ATM, BRCA1, BRCA2, BRIP1, CDH1, MLH1, MSH2, MSH6, NBN, PALB2, PTEN, RAD51C, STK11,* and *TP53***

   🔖 0.00 ⚕ 0.00 **FUD** XXX   A 🖵

   AMA: 2016,Apr,4

81433   **duplication/deletion analysis panel, must include analyses for *BRCA1, BRCA2, MLH1, MSH2,* and *STK11***

   🔖 0.00 ⚕ 0.00 **FUD** XXX   A 🖵

   AMA: 2016,Apr,4

81434 Hereditary retinal disorders (eg, retinitis pigmentosa, Leber congenital amaurosis, cone-rod dystrophy), genomic sequence analysis panel, must include sequencing of at least 15 genes, including *ABCA4, CNGA1, CRB1, EYS, PDE6A, PDE6B, PRPF31, PRPH2, RDH12, RHO, RP1, RP2, RPE65, RPGR,* and *USH2A*

📋 0.00   ✂ 0.00   **FUD** XXX   Ⓐ 🖥

AMA: 2016,Apr,4

81435 Hereditary colon cancer disorders (eg, Lynch syndrome, PTEN hamartoma syndrome, Cowden syndrome, familial adenomatosis polyposis); genomic sequence analysis panel, must include sequencing of at least 10 genes, including *APC, BMPR1A, CDH1, MLH1, MSH2, MSH6, MUTYH, PTEN, SMAD4,* and *STK11*

📋 0.00   ✂ 0.00   **FUD** XXX   Ⓐ 🖥

AMA: 2016,Apr,4; 2016,Jan,13; 2015,Jan,3

81436 duplication/deletion analysis panel, must include analysis of at least 5 genes, including *MLH1, MSH2, EPCAM, SMAD4,* and *STK11*

📋 0.00   ✂ 0.00   **FUD** XXX   Ⓐ 🖥

AMA: 2016,Apr,4; 2016,Jan,13; 2015,Jan,3

81437 Hereditary neuroendocrine tumor disorders (eg, medullary thyroid carcinoma, parathyroid carcinoma, malignant pheochromocytoma or paraganglioma); genomic sequence analysis panel, must include sequencing of at least 6 genes, including *MAX, SDHB, SDHC, SDHD, TMEM127,* and *VHL*

📋 0.00   ✂ 0.00   **FUD** XXX   Ⓐ 🖥

AMA: 2016,Apr,4

81438 duplication/deletion analysis panel, must include analyses for *SDHB, SDHC, SDHD,* and *VHL*

📋 0.00   ✂ 0.00   **FUD** XXX   Ⓐ 🖥

AMA: 2016,Apr,4

● 81439 Inherited cardiomyopathy (eg, hypertrophic cardiomyopathy, dilated cardiomyopathy, arrhythmogenic right ventricular cardiomyopathy) genomic sequence analysis panel, must include sequencing of at least 5 genes, including DSG2, MYBPC3, MYH7, PKP2, and TTN

EXCLUDES *Genetic tests of cardiac ion channelopathies (81413-81414)*

81440 Nuclear encoded mitochondrial genes (eg, neurologic or myopathic phenotypes), genomic sequence panel, must include analysis of at least 100 genes, including *BCS1L, C10orf2, COQ2, COX10, DGUOK, MPV17, OPA1, PDSS2, POLG, POLG2, RRM2B, SCO1, SCO2, SLC25A4, SUCLA2, SUCLG1, TAZ, TK2,* and *TYMP*

📋 0.00   ✂ 0.00   **FUD** XXX   Ⓐ 🖥

AMA: 2016,Jan,13; 2015,Jan,3

81442 Noonan spectrum disorders (eg, Noonan syndrome, cardio-facio-cutaneous syndrome, Costello syndrome, LEOPARD syndrome, Noonan-like syndrome), genomic sequence analysis panel, must include sequencing of at least 12 genes, including *BRAF, CBL, HRAS, KRAS, MAP2K1, MAP2K2, NRAS, PTPN11, RAF1, RIT1, SHOC2,* and *SOS1*

📋 0.00   ✂ 0.00   **FUD** XXX   Ⓐ 🖥

AMA: 2016,Apr,4

81445 Targeted genomic sequence analysis panel, solid organ neoplasm, DNA analysis, and RNA analysis when performed, 5-50 genes (eg, *ALK, BRAF, CDKN2A, EGFR, ERBB2, KIT, KRAS, NRAS, MET, PDGFRA, PDGFRB, PGR, PIK3CA, PTEN, RET*), interrogation for sequence variants and copy number variants or rearrangements, if performed

EXCLUDES *Microarray copy number assessment (81406)*

📋 0.00   ✂ 0.00   **FUD** XXX   Ⓐ 🖥

AMA: 2016,Apr,4; 2016,Jan,13; 2015,Jan,3

81450 Targeted genomic sequence analysis panel, hematolymphoid neoplasm or disorder, DNA analysis, and RNA analysis when performed, 5-50 genes (eg, *BRAF, CEBPA, DNMT3A, EZH2, FLT3, IDH1, IDH2, JAK2, KRAS, KIT, MLL, NRAS, NPM1, NOTCH1*), interrogation for sequence variants, and copy number variants or rearrangements, or isoform expression or mRNA expression levels, if performed

EXCLUDES *Microarray copy number assessment (81406)*

📋 0.00   ✂ 0.00   **FUD** XXX   Ⓐ 🖥

AMA: 2016,Apr,4; 2016,Jan,13; 2015,Jan,3

81455 Targeted genomic sequence analysis panel, solid organ or hematolymphoid neoplasm, DNA analysis, and RNA analysis when performed, 51 or greater genes (eg, *ALK, BRAF, CDKN2A, CEBPA, DNMT3A, EGFR, ERBB2, EZH2, FLT3, IDH1, IDH2, JAK2, KIT, KRAS, MLL, NPM1, NRAS, MET, NOTCH1, PDGFRA, PDGFRB, PGR, PIK3CA, PTEN, RET*), interrogation for sequence variants and copy number variants or rearrangements, if performed

EXCLUDES *Microarray copy number assessment (81406)*

📋 0.00   ✂ 0.00   **FUD** XXX   Ⓐ 🖥

AMA: 2016,Apr,4; 2016,Jan,13; 2015,Jan,3

81460 Whole mitochondrial genome (eg, Leigh syndrome, mitochondrial encephalomyopathy, lactic acidosis, and stroke-like episodes [MELAS], myoclonic epilepsy with ragged-red fibers [MERFF], neuropathy, ataxia, and retinitis pigmentosa [NARP], Leber hereditary optic neuropathy [LHON]), genomic sequence, must include sequence analysis of entire mitochondrial genome with heteroplasmy detection

📋 0.00   ✂ 0.00   **FUD** XXX   Ⓐ 🖥

AMA: 2016,Jan,13; 2015,Jan,3

81465 Whole mitochondrial genome large deletion analysis panel (eg, Kearns-Sayre syndrome, chronic progressive external ophthalmoplegia), including heteroplasmy detection, if performed

📋 0.00   ✂ 0.00   **FUD** XXX   Ⓐ 🖥

AMA: 2016,Jan,13; 2015,Jan,3

81470 X-linked intellectual disability (XLID) (eg, syndromic and non-syndromic XLID); genomic sequence analysis panel, must include sequencing of at least 60 genes, including *ARX, ATRX, CDKL5, FGD1, FMR1, HUWE1, IL1RAPL, KDM5C, L1CAM, MECP2, MED12, MID1, OCRL, RPS6KA3,* and *SLC16A2*

Ⓐ 🖥

AMA: 2016,Jan,13; 2015,Jan,3

81471 duplication/deletion gene analysis, must include analysis of at least 60 genes, including *ARX, ATRX, CDKL5, FGD1, FMR1, HUWE1, IL1RAPL, KDM5C, L1CAM, MECP2, MED12, MID1, OCRL, RPS6KA3,* and *SLC16A2*

📋 0.00   ✂ 0.00   **FUD** XXX   Ⓐ 🖥

AMA: 2016,Jan,13; 2015,Jan,3

81479 **Resequenced code. See code following 81408.**

81490-81599 Multianalyte Assays

INCLUDES Procedures using results of multiple assay panels (eg, molecular pathology, fluorescent in situ hybridization, non-nucleic acid-based) and other patient information to perform algorithmic analysis

Required analytical services (eg, amplification, cell lysis, detection, digestion, extraction, hybridization, nucleic acid stabilization) and algorithmic analysis

EXCLUDES Genomic resequencing tests (81410-81471)

Multianalyte assays with algorithmic analyses without a Category 1 code (0001M-0004M, 0006M-0009M)

Code also procedures performed prior to cell lysis (eg, microdissection) (88380-88381)

81490 Autoimmune (rheumatoid arthritis), analysis of 12 biomarkers using immunoassays, utilizing serum, prognostic algorithm reported as a disease activity score

📋 0.00   ✂ 0.00   **FUD** XXX   Ⓠ 🖥

EXCLUDES *C-reactive protein (86140)*

26/TC PC/TC Only   N2-Z3 ASC Payment   50 Bilateral   ♂ Male Only   ♀ Female Only   📋 Facility RVU   ✂ Non-Facility RVU   🖥 CCI
FUD Follow-up Days   CMS: IOM (Pub 100)   Ⓐ-Ⓨ OPPSI   80/80 Surg Assist Allowed / w/Doc   🔲 Lab Crosswalk   🔲 Radiology Crosswalk   ❌ CLIA

364   CPT © 2016 American Medical Association. All Rights Reserved.   © 2016 Optum360, LLC

81493 **Coronary artery disease, mRNA, gene expression profiling by real-time RT-PCR of 23 genes, utilizing whole peripheral blood, algorithm reported as a risk score**
🚗 0.00   ✂ 0.00   **FUD** XXX   A ▣

81500 **Oncology (ovarian), biochemical assays of two proteins (CA-125 and HE4), utilizing serum, with menopausal status, algorithm reported as a risk score**   ♀
EXCLUDES   *Human epididymis protein 4 (HE4) (86305)*
           Immunoassay for tumor antigen, quantitative; CA 125 (86304)
🚗 0.00   ✂ 0.00   **FUD** XXX   E ▣
AMA: 2015,Jan,3; 2014,Jan,11

81503 **Oncology (ovarian), biochemical assays of five proteins (CA-125, apolipoprotein A1, beta-2 microglobulin, transferrin, and pre-albumin), utilizing serum, algorithm reported as a risk score**   ♀
EXCLUDES   *Apolipoprotein (82172)*
           Beta-2 microglobulin (82232)
           Immunoassay for tumor antigen, quantitative; CA 125 (86304)
           Prealbumin (84134)
           Transferrin (84466)
🚗 0.00   ✂ 0.00   **FUD** XXX   E ▣
AMA: 2015,Jan,3; 2014,Jan,11

81504 **Oncology (tissue of origin), microarray gene expression profiling of > 2000 genes, utilizing formalin-fixed paraffin-embedded tissue, algorithm reported as tissue similarity scores**
🚗 0.00   ✂ 0.00   **FUD** XXX   A ▣
AMA: 2015,Jan,3; 2014,Jan,11

81506 **Endocrinology (type 2 diabetes), biochemical assays of seven analytes (glucose, HbA1c, insulin, hs-CRP, adiponectin, ferritin, interleukin 2-receptor alpha), utilizing serum or plasma, algorithm reporting a risk score**
EXCLUDES   *C-reactive protein; high sensitivity (hsCRP) (86141)*
           Ferritin (82728)
           Glucose (82947)
           Hemoglobin; glycosylated (A1C) (83036)
           Immunoassay for analyte other than infectious agent antibody or infectious agent antigen (83520)
           Insulin; total (83525)
           Unlisted chemistry procedure
🚗 0.00   ✂ 0.00   **FUD** XXX   E ▣
AMA: 2015,Jan,3; 2014,Jan,11

81507 **Fetal aneuploidy (trisomy 21, 18, and 13) DNA sequence analysis of selected regions using maternal plasma, algorithm reported as a risk score for each trisomy**   ♀
EXCLUDES   *Genome-wide microarray analysis (81228-81229)*
           Molecular cytogenetics (88271)
🚗 0.00   ✂ 0.00   **FUD** XXX   A ▣
AMA: 2015,Jan,3; 2014,Jan,11

81508 **Fetal congenital abnormalities, biochemical assays of two proteins (PAPP-A, hCG [any form]), utilizing maternal serum, algorithm reported as a risk score**   ♀ +
EXCLUDES   *Gonadotropin, chorionic (hCG) (84702)*
           Pregnancy-associated plasma protein-A (PAPP-A) (84163)
🚗 0.00   ✂ 0.00   **FUD** XXX   E ▣
AMA: 2015,Jan,3; 2014,Jan,11

81509 **Fetal congenital abnormalities, biochemical assays of three proteins (PAPP-A, hCG [any form], DIA), utilizing maternal serum, algorithm reported as a risk score**   ♀
EXCLUDES   *Gonadotropin, chorionic (hCG) (84702)*
           Inhibin A (86336)
           Pregnancy-associated plasma protein-A (PAPP-A) (84163)
🚗 0.00   ✂ 0.00   **FUD** XXX   E ▣
AMA: 2015,Jan,3; 2014,Jan,11

81510 **Fetal congenital abnormalities, biochemical assays of three analytes (AFP, uE3, hCG [any form]), utilizing maternal serum, algorithm reported as a risk score**   ♀
EXCLUDES   *Alpha-fetoprotein (AFP) (82105)*
           Estriol (82677)
           Gonadotropin, chorionic (hCG) (84702)
🚗 0.00   ✂ 0.00   **FUD** XXX   E ▣
AMA: 2015,Jan,3; 2014,Jan,11

81511 **Fetal congenital abnormalities, biochemical assays of four analytes (AFP, uE3, hCG [any form], DIA) utilizing maternal serum, algorithm reported as a risk score (may include additional results from previous biochemical testing)**   ♀
EXCLUDES   *Alpha-fetoprotein (AFP) (82105)*
           Estriol (82677)
           Gonadotropin, chorionic (hCG) (84702)
           Inhibin A (86336)
🚗 0.00   ✂ 0.00   **FUD** XXX   E ▣
AMA: 2015,Jan,3; 2014,Jan,11

81512 **Fetal congenital abnormalities, biochemical assays of five analytes (AFP, uE3, total hCG, hyperglycosylated hCG, DIA) utilizing maternal serum, algorithm reported as a risk score**   ♀
EXCLUDES   *Alpha-fetoprotein (AFP) (82105)*
           Estriol (82677)
           Gonadotropin, chorionic (hCG) (84702)
           Inhibin A (86336)
🚗 0.00   ✂ 0.00   **FUD** XXX   E ▣
AMA: 2015,Jan,3; 2014,Jan,11

81519 **Oncology (breast), mRNA, gene expression profiling by real-time RT-PCR of 21 genes, utilizing formalin-fixed paraffin embedded tissue, algorithm reported as recurrence score**
🚗 0.00   ✂ 0.00   **FUD** XXX   A ▣
AMA: 2016,Jan,13; 2015,Jan,3

81525 **Oncology (colon), mRNA, gene expression profiling by real-time RT-PCR of 12 genes (7 content and 5 housekeeping), utilizing formalin-fixed paraffin-embedded tissue, algorithm reported as a recurrence score**
🚗 0.00   ✂ 0.00   **FUD** XXX   A ▣

81528 **Oncology (colorectal) screening, quantitative real-time target and signal amplification of 10 DNA markers (*KRAS* mutations, promoter methylation of *NDRG4* and *BMP3*) and fecal hemoglobin, utilizing stool, algorithm reported as a positive or negative result**
🚗 0.00   ✂ 0.00   **FUD** XXX   A ▣
EXCLUDES   *Blood, occult, by fecal hemoglobin (82274)*
           KRAS (Kirsten rat sarcoma viral oncogene homolog) (81275)

81535 **Oncology (gynecologic), live tumor cell culture and chemotherapeutic response by DAPI stain and morphology, predictive algorithm reported as a drug response score; first single drug or drug combination**
🚗 0.00   ✂ 0.00   **FUD** XXX   Q ▣

+ 81536 **each additional single drug or drug combination (List separately in addition to code for primary procedure)**
🚗 0.00   ✂ 0.00   **FUD** XXX   Q ▣
Code first (81535)

81538 **Oncology (lung), mass spectrometric 8-protein signature, including amyloid A, utilizing serum, prognostic and predictive algorithm reported as good versus poor overall survival**
🚗 0.00   ✂ 0.00   **FUD** XXX   Q ▣

● 81539 **Oncology (high-grade prostate cancer), biochemical assay of four proteins (Total PSA, Free PSA, Intact PSA, and human kallikrein-2 [hK2]), utilizing plasma or serum, prognostic algorithm reported as a probability score**

81540 Oncology (tumor of unknown origin), mRNA, gene expression profiling by real-time RT-PCR of 92 genes (87 content and 5 housekeeping) to classify tumor into main cancer type and subtype, utilizing formalin-fixed paraffin-embedded tissue, algorithm reported as a probability of a predicted main cancer type and subtype

🚑 0.00   ⚕ 0.00   **FUD** XXX   Ⓐ ▢

81545 Oncology (thyroid), gene expression analysis of 142 genes, utilizing fine needle aspirate, algorithm reported as a categorical result (eg, benign or suspicious)

🚑 0.00   ⚕ 0.00   **FUD** XXX   Ⓐ ▢

81595 Cardiology (heart transplant), mRNA, gene expression profiling by real-time quantitative PCR of 20 genes (11 content and 9 housekeeping), utilizing subfraction of peripheral blood, algorithm reported as a rejection risk score

🚑 0.00   ⚕ 0.00   **FUD** XXX   Ⓐ ▢

81599 Unlisted multianalyte assay with algorithmic analysis

    INCLUDES   MAAA services not reportable with (81490-81595, 0001M-0004M, 0006M-0009M)

🚑 0.00   ⚕ 0.00   **FUD** XXX   Ⓔ

    AMA: 2015,Jan,3; 2014,Jan,11

82009-82030 Chemistry: Acetaldehyde—Adenosine

INCLUDES   Clinical information not requested by the ordering physician
Mathematically calculated results
Quantitative analysis unless otherwise specified
Specimens from any source unless otherwise specified

EXCLUDES   Analytes from nonrequested laboratory analysis
Calculated results that represent a score or probability that was derived by algorithm
Drug testing ([80305, 80306, 80307], [80324, 80325, 80326, 80327, 80328, 80329, 80330, 80331, 80332, 80333, 80334, 80335, 80336, 80337, 80338, 80339, 80340, 80341, 80342, 80343, 80344, 80345, 80346, 80347, 80348, 80349, 80350, 80351, 80352, 80353, 80354, 80355, 80356, 80357, 80358, 80359, 80360, 80361, 80362, 80363, 80364, 80365, 80366, 80367, 80368, 80369, 80370, 80371, 80372, 80373, 80374, 80375, 80376, 80377, 83992])
Organ or disease panels (80048-80076 [80081])
Therapeutic drug assays (80150-80299 [80164, 80165, 80171])

82009 Ketone body(s) (eg, acetone, acetoacetic acid, beta-hydroxybutyrate); qualitative

🚑 0.00   ⚕ 0.00   **FUD** XXX   Ⓠ

    AMA: 2016,Jan,13; 2015,Jun,10; 2015,Apr,3; 2015,Jan,16; 2014,Jan,11; 2011,Oct,8

82010 quantitative

🚑 0.00   ⚕ 0.00   **FUD** XXX   Ⓧ Ⓠ

    AMA: 2016,Jan,13; 2015,Jun,10; 2015,Apr,3; 2015,Jan,16; 2014,Jan,11; 2011,Oct,8

82013 Acetylcholinesterase

    EXCLUDES   Acid phosphatase (84060-84066)
             Gastric acid analysis (82930)

🚑 0.00   ⚕ 0.00   **FUD** XXX   Ⓠ

    AMA: 2015,Jun,10; 2015,Apr,3; 2014,Jan,11

82016 Acylcarnitines; qualitative, each specimen

🚑 0.00   ⚕ 0.00   **FUD** XXX   Ⓠ

    AMA: 2015,Jun,10; 2015,Apr,3; 2014,Jan,11

82017 quantitative, each specimen

    EXCLUDES   Carnitine (82379)

🚑 0.00   ⚕ 0.00   **FUD** XXX   Ⓠ ▢

    AMA: 2015,Jun,10; 2015,Apr,3; 2014,Jan,11

82024 Adrenocorticotropic hormone (ACTH)

🚑 0.00   ⚕ 0.00   **FUD** XXX   Ⓠ ▢

    AMA: 2015,Jun,10; 2015,Apr,3; 2014,Jan,11

82030 Adenosine, 5-monophosphate, cyclic (cyclic AMP)

🚑 0.00   ⚕ 0.00   **FUD** XXX   Ⓠ

    AMA: 2015,Jun,10; 2015,Apr,3; 2014,Jan,11

82040-82045 Chemistry: Albumin

INCLUDES   Clinical information not requested by the ordering physician
Mathematically calculated results
Quantitative analysis unless otherwise specified
Specimens from any other sources unless otherwise specified

EXCLUDES   Analytes from nonrequested laboratory analysis
Calculated results that represent a score or probability that was derived by algorithm
Drug testing ([80305, 80306, 80307], [80324, 80325, 80326, 80327, 80328, 80329, 80330, 80331, 80332, 80333, 80334, 80335, 80336, 80337, 80338, 80339, 80340, 80341, 80342, 80343, 80344, 80345, 80346, 80347, 80348, 80349, 80350, 80351, 80352, 80353, 80354, 80355, 80356, 80357, 80358, 80359, 80360, 80361, 80362, 80363, 80364, 80365, 80366, 80367, 80368, 80369, 80370, 80371, 80372, 80373, 80374, 80375, 80376, 80377, 83992])
Organ or disease panels (80048-80076 [80081])
Therapeutic drug assays (80150-80299 [80164, 80165, 80171])

82040 Albumin; serum, plasma or whole blood

🚑 0.00   ⚕ 0.00   **FUD** XXX   Ⓧ Ⓠ

    AMA: 2016,Jan,13; 2015,Jun,10; 2015,Apr,3; 2015,Jan,16; 2014,Jan,11

82042 urine or other source, quantitative, each specimen

🚑 0.00   ⚕ 0.00   **FUD** XXX   Ⓠ

    AMA: 2015,Jun,10; 2015,Apr,3; 2014,Jan,11

82043 urine, microalbumin, quantitative

🚑 0.00   ⚕ 0.00   **FUD** XXX   Ⓧ Ⓠ ▢

    AMA: 2016,Jan,13; 2015,Jun,10; 2015,Apr,3; 2015,Jan,16; 2014,Jan,11

82044 urine, microalbumin, semiquantitative (eg, reagent strip assay)

    EXCLUDES   Prealbumin (84134)

🚑 0.00   ⚕ 0.00   **FUD** XXX   Ⓧ Ⓠ

    AMA: 2016,Jan,13; 2015,Jun,10; 2015,Apr,3; 2015,Jan,16; 2014,Jan,11; 2012,Jan,15-42; 2011,Jan,11

82045 ischemia modified

🚑 0.00   ⚕ 0.00   **FUD** XXX   Ⓠ

    AMA: 2015,Jun,10; 2015,Apr,3

82075-82107 Chemistry: Alcohol—Alpha-fetoprotein (AFP)

INCLUDES   Clinical information not requested by the ordering physician
Mathematically calculated results
Quantitative analysis unless otherwise specified
Specimens from any source unless otherwise specified

EXCLUDES   Analytes from nonrequested laboratory analysis
Calculated results that represent a score or probability that was derived by algorithm
Drug testing ([80305, 80306, 80307], [80324, 80325, 80326, 80327, 80328, 80329, 80330, 80331, 80332, 80333, 80334, 80335, 80336, 80337, 80338, 80339, 80340, 80341, 80342, 80343, 80344, 80345, 80346, 80347, 80348, 80349, 80350, 80351, 80352, 80353, 80354, 80355, 80356, 80357, 80358, 80359, 80360, 80361, 80362, 80363, 80364, 80365, 80366, 80367, 80368, 80369, 80370, 80371, 80372, 80373, 80374, 80375, 80376, 80377, 83992])
Organ or disease panels (80048-80076 [80081])
Therapeutic drug assays (80150-80299 [80164, 80165, 80171])

82075 Alcohol (ethanol), breath

🚑 0.00   **FUD** XXX   Ⓠ

    AMA: 2015,Jun,10; 2015,Apr,3

82085 Aldolase

🚑 0.00   ⚕ 0.00   **FUD** XXX   Ⓠ

    AMA: 2015,Jun,10; 2015,Apr,3

82088 Aldosterone

🚑 0.00   ⚕ 0.00   **FUD** XXX   Ⓠ ▢

    AMA: 2015,Jun,10; 2015,Apr,3

82103 Alpha-1-antitrypsin; total

🚑 0.00   ⚕ 0.00   **FUD** XXX   Ⓠ

    AMA: 2015,Jun,10; 2015,Apr,3

82104 phenotype

🚑 0.00   ⚕ 0.00   **FUD** XXX   Ⓠ

    AMA: 2015,Jun,10; 2015,Apr,3

82105 Alpha-fetoprotein (AFP); serum

🚑 0.00   ⚕ 0.00   **FUD** XXX   Ⓠ ▢

    AMA: 2015,Jun,10; 2015,Apr,3

| 26/TC PC/TC Only | A2-Z3 ASC Payment | 50 Bilateral | ♂ Male Only | ♀ Female Only | 🚑 Facility RVU | ⚕ Non-Facility RVU | ▢ CCI |
| FUD Follow-up Days | CMS: IOM (Pub 100) | A-Y OPPSI | 80/80 Surg Assist Allowed / w/Doc | | 🔬 Lab Crosswalk | Ⓧ Radiology Crosswalk | Ⓧ CLIA |

366

CPT © 2016 American Medical Association. All Rights Reserved.

© 2016 Optum360, LLC

82106	**amniotic fluid**	M
	⚕ 0.00 ⚕ 0.00 **FUD** XXX	Q M
	AMA: 2015,Jun,10; 2015,Apr,3	

82107	**AFP-L3 fraction isoform and total AFP (including ratio)**	
	⚕ 0.00 ⚕ 0.00 **FUD** XXX	Q ▢
	AMA: 2015,Jun,10; 2015,Apr,3	

82108 Chemistry: Aluminum

CMS: 100-02,11,20.2 ESRD Laboratory Services

INCLUDES Clinical information not requested by the ordering physician
Mathematically calculated results
Quantitative analysis unless otherwise specified
Specimens from any source unless otherwise specified

EXCLUDES *Analytes from nonrequested laboratory analysis*
Calculated results that represent a score or probability that was derived by algorithm
Drug testing ([80305, 80306, 80307], [80324, 80325, 80326, 80327, 80328, 80329, 80330, 80331, 80332, 80333, 80334, 80335, 80336, 80337, 80338, 80339, 80340, 80341, 80342, 80343, 80344, 80345, 80346, 80347, 80348, 80349, 80350, 80351, 80352, 80353, 80354, 80355, 80356, 80357, 80358, 80359, 80360, 80361, 80362, 80363, 80364, 80365, 80366, 80367, 80368, 80369, 80370, 80371, 80372, 80373, 80374, 80375, 80376, 80377, 83992])
Organ or disease panels (80048-80076 [80081])
Therapeutic drug assays (80150-80299 [80164, 80165, 80171])

82108	**Aluminum**	
	⚕ 0.00 ⚕ 0.00 **FUD** XXX	Q
	AMA: 2015,Jun,10; 2015,Apr,3	

82120-82261 Chemistry: Amines—Biotinidase

INCLUDES Clinical information not requested by the ordering physician
Mathematically calculated results
Quantitative analysis unless otherwise specified
Specimens from any source unless otherwise specified

EXCLUDES *Analytes from nonrequested laboratory analysis*
Calculated results that represent a score or probability that was derived by algorithm
Drug testing ([80305, 80306, 80307], [80324, 80325, 80326, 80327, 80328, 80329, 80330, 80331, 80332, 80333, 80334, 80335, 80336, 80337, 80338, 80339, 80340, 80341, 80342, 80343, 80344, 80345, 80346, 80347, 80348, 80349, 80350, 80351, 80352, 80353, 80354, 80355, 80356, 80357, 80358, 80359, 80360, 80361, 80362, 80363, 80364, 80365, 80366, 80367, 80368, 80369, 80370, 80371, 80372, 80373, 80374, 80375, 80376, 80377, 83992])
Organ or disease panels (80048-80076 [80081])
Therapeutic drug assays (80150-80299 [80164, 80165, 80171])

82120	**Amines, vaginal fluid, qualitative**	♀
	EXCLUDES *Combined pH and amines test for vaginitis (82120, 83986)*	
	⚕ 0.00 ⚕ 0.00 **FUD** XXX	X Q
	AMA: 2016,Jan,13; 2015,Jun,10; 2015,Apr,3; 2015,Jan,16; 2014,Jan,11	

82127	**Amino acids; single, qualitative, each specimen**	
	⚕ 0.00 ⚕ 0.00 **FUD** XXX	Q
	AMA: 2015,Jun,10; 2015,Apr,3	

82128	**multiple, qualitative, each specimen**	
	⚕ 0.00 ⚕ 0.00 **FUD** XXX	Q ▢
	AMA: 2015,Jun,10; 2015,Apr,3	

82131	**single, quantitative, each specimen**	
	INCLUDES Van Slyke method	
	⚕ 0.00 ⚕ 0.00 **FUD** XXX	Q ▢
	AMA: 2016,Jan,13; 2015,Jun,10; 2015,Apr,3; 2015,Jan,16; 2014,Jan,11; 2012,Jan,15-42; 2011,Jan,11	

82135	**Aminolevulinic acid, delta (ALA)**	
	⚕ 0.00 ⚕ 0.00 **FUD** XXX	Q
	AMA: 2015,Jun,10; 2015,Apr,3	

82136	**Amino acids, 2 to 5 amino acids, quantitative, each specimen**	
	⚕ 0.00 ⚕ 0.00 **FUD** XXX	Q ▢
	AMA: 2015,Jun,10; 2015,Apr,3	

82139	**Amino acids, 6 or more amino acids, quantitative, each specimen**	
	⚕ 0.00 ⚕ 0.00 **FUD** XXX	Q ▢
	AMA: 2015,Jun,10; 2015,Apr,3	

82140	**Ammonia**	
	⚕ 0.00 ⚕ 0.00 **FUD** XXX	Q
	AMA: 2015,Jun,10; 2015,Apr,3	

82143	**Amniotic fluid scan (spectrophotometric)**	M ♀
	EXCLUDES *L/S ratio (83661)*	
	⚕ 0.00 ⚕ 0.00 **FUD** XXX	Q
	AMA: 2015,Jun,10; 2015,Apr,3	

82150	**Amylase**	
	⚕ 0.00 ⚕ 0.00 **FUD** XXX	X Q
	AMA: 2015,Jun,10; 2015,Apr,3	

82154	**Androstanediol glucuronide**	
	⚕ 0.00 ⚕ 0.00 **FUD** XXX	Q
	AMA: 2016,Jan,13; 2015,Jun,10; 2015,Apr,3; 2015,Jan,16; 2014,Jan,11	

82157	**Androstenedione**	
	⚕ 0.00 ⚕ 0.00 **FUD** XXX	Q
	AMA: 2015,Jun,10; 2015,Apr,3	

82160	**Androsterone**	
	⚕ 0.00 ⚕ 0.00 **FUD** XXX	Q
	AMA: 2015,Jun,10; 2015,Apr,3	

82163	**Angiotensin II**	
	⚕ 0.00 ⚕ 0.00 **FUD** XXX	Q
	AMA: 2015,Jun,10; 2015,Apr,3	

82164	**Angiotensin I - converting enzyme (ACE)**	
	⚕ 0.00 ⚕ 0.00 **FUD** XXX	Q
	AMA: 2015,Jun,10; 2015,Apr,3	

82172	**Apolipoprotein, each**	
	⚕ 0.00 ⚕ 0.00 **FUD** XXX	Q
	AMA: 2015,Jun,10; 2015,Apr,3	

82175	**Arsenic**	
	EXCLUDES *Heavy metal screening (83015)*	
	⚕ 0.00 ⚕ 0.00 **FUD** XXX	Q
	AMA: 2015,Jun,10; 2015,Apr,3	

82180	**Ascorbic acid (Vitamin C), blood**	
	⚕ 0.00 ⚕ 0.00 **FUD** XXX	Q ▢
	AMA: 2015,Jun,10; 2015,Apr,3	

82190	**Atomic absorption spectroscopy, each analyte**	
	⚕ 0.00 ⚕ 0.00 **FUD** XXX	Q
	AMA: 2015,Jun,10; 2015,Apr,3	

82232	**Beta-2 microglobulin**	
	⚕ 0.00 ⚕ 0.00 **FUD** XXX	Q
	AMA: 2015,Jun,10; 2015,Apr,3	

82239	**Bile acids; total**	
	⚕ 0.00 ⚕ 0.00 **FUD** XXX	Q
	AMA: 2015,Jun,10; 2015,Apr,3	

82240	**cholylglycine**	
	EXCLUDES *Bile pigments, urine (81000-81005)*	
	⚕ 0.00 ⚕ 0.00 **FUD** XXX	Q
	AMA: 2015,Jun,10; 2015,Apr,3	

82247	**Bilirubin; total**	
	INCLUDES Van Den Bergh test	
	⚕ 0.00 ⚕ 0.00 **FUD** XXX	X Q
	AMA: 2016,Jan,13; 2015,Jun,10; 2015,Apr,3; 2015,Jan,16; 2014,Jan,11; 2012,Jan,15-42	

82248	**direct**	
	⚕ 0.00 ⚕ 0.00 **FUD** XXX	Q
	AMA: 2016,Jan,13; 2015,Jun,10; 2015,Apr,3; 2015,Jan,16; 2014,Jan,11; 2012,Jan,15-42	

82252	**feces, qualitative**	
	⚕ 0.00 ⚕ 0.00 **FUD** XXX	Q
	AMA: 2015,Jun,10; 2015,Apr,3	

82261	**Biotinidase, each specimen**	
	⚕ 0.00 ⚕ 0.00 **FUD** XXX	Q
	AMA: 2015,Jun,10; 2015,Apr,3	

82270-82274 Chemistry: Occult Blood

CMS: 100-04,16,70.8 CLIA Waived Tests; 100-04,18,60 Colorectal Cancer Screening

INCLUDES Clinical information not requested by the ordering physician
Mathematically calculated results
Quantitative analysis unless otherwise specified
Specimens from any source unless otherwise specified

EXCLUDES *Analytes from nonrequested laboratory analysis*
Calculated results that represent a score or probability that was derived by algorithm
Drug testing ([80305, 80306, 80307], [80324, 80325, 80326, 80327, 80328, 80329, 80330, 80331, 80332, 80333, 80334, 80335, 80336, 80337, 80338, 80339, 80340, 80341, 80342, 80343, 80344, 80345, 80346, 80347, 80348, 80349, 80350, 80351, 80352, 80353, 80354, 80355, 80356, 80357, 80358, 80359, 80360, 80361, 80362, 80363, 80364, 80365, 80366, 80367, 80368, 80369, 80370, 80371, 80372, 80373, 80374, 80375, 80376, 80377, 83992])
Organ or disease panels (80048-80076 [80081])
Therapeutic drug assays (80150-80299 [80164, 80165, 80171])

82270   Blood, occult, by peroxidase activity (eg, guaiac), qualitative; feces, consecutive collected specimens with single determination, for colorectal neoplasm screening (ie, patient was provided 3 cards or single triple card for consecutive collection)

INCLUDES Day test

🗁 0.00   ⅗ 0.00   **FUD** XXX   ☒ A ▣

AMA: 2016,Jan,13; 2015,Jun,10; 2015,Apr,3; 2015,Jan,16; 2014,Jan,11; 2012,Jan,15-42; 2011,Jan,11

82271   other sources

🗁 0.00   ⅗ 0.00   **FUD** XXX   ☒ ▣

AMA: 2015,Jun,10; 2015,Apr,3

82272   Blood, occult, by peroxidase activity (eg, guaiac), qualitative, feces, 1-3 simultaneous determinations, performed for other than colorectal neoplasm screening

🗁 0.00   ⅗ 0.00   **FUD** XXX   ☒ ▣

AMA: 2016,Jan,13; 2015,Jun,10; 2015,Apr,3; 2015,Jan,16; 2014,Jan,11; 2012,Jan,15-42; 2011,Jan,11

82274   Blood, occult, by fecal hemoglobin determination by immunoassay, qualitative, feces, 1-3 simultaneous determinations

🗁 0.00   ⅗ 0.00   **FUD** XXX   ☒ ▣ ▣

AMA: 2015,Jun,10; 2015,Apr,3

82286-82308 [82652] Chemistry: Bradykinin—Calcitonin

INCLUDES Clinical information not requested by the ordering physician
Mathematically calculated results
Quantitative analysis unless otherwise specified
Specimens from any source unless otherwise specified

EXCLUDES *Analytes from nonrequested laboratory analysis*
Calculated results that represent a score or probability that was derived by algorithm
Drug testing ([80305, 80306, 80307], [80324, 80325, 80326, 80327, 80328, 80329, 80330, 80331, 80332, 80333, 80334, 80335, 80336, 80337, 80338, 80339, 80340, 80341, 80342, 80343, 80344, 80345, 80346, 80347, 80348, 80349, 80350, 80351, 80352, 80353, 80354, 80355, 80356, 80357, 80358, 80359, 80360, 80361, 80362, 80363, 80364, 80365, 80366, 80367, 80368, 80369, 80370, 80371, 80372, 80373, 80374, 80375, 80376, 80377, 83992])
Organ or disease panels (80048-80076 [80081])
Therapeutic drug assays (80150-80299 [80164, 80165, 80171])

82286   Bradykinin

🗁 0.00   ⅗ 0.00   **FUD** XXX   ▣

AMA: 2015,Jun,10; 2015,Apr,3

82300   Cadmium

🗁 0.00   ⅗ 0.00   **FUD** XXX   ▣

AMA: 2015,Jun,10; 2015,Apr,3

82306   Vitamin D; 25 hydroxy, includes fraction(s), if performed

🗁 0.00   ⅗ 0.00   **FUD** XXX   ▣ ▣

AMA: 2015,Jun,10; 2015,Apr,3

 # 82652   1, 25 dihydroxy, includes fraction(s), if performed

🗁 0.00   ⅗ 0.00   **FUD** XXX   ▣ ▣

AMA: 2015,Jun,10; 2015,Apr,3

82308   Calcitonin

🗁 0.00   ⅗ 0.00   **FUD** XXX   ▣ ▣

AMA: 2015,Jun,10; 2015,Apr,3

82310-82373 Chemistry: Calcium, total; Carbohydrate Deficient Transferrin

INCLUDES Clinical information not requested by the ordering physician
Mathematically calculated results
Quantitative analysis unless otherwise specified
Specimens from any source unless otherwise specified

EXCLUDES *Analytes from nonrequested laboratory analysis*
Calculated results that represent a score or probability that was derived by algorithm
Drug testing ([80305, 80306, 80307], [80324, 80325, 80326, 80327, 80328, 80329, 80330, 80331, 80332, 80333, 80334, 80335, 80336, 80337, 80338, 80339, 80340, 80341, 80342, 80343, 80344, 80345, 80346, 80347, 80348, 80349, 80350, 80351, 80352, 80353, 80354, 80355, 80356, 80357, 80358, 80359, 80360, 80361, 80362, 80363, 80364, 80365, 80366, 80367, 80368, 80369, 80370, 80371, 80372, 80373, 80374, 80375, 80376, 80377, 83992])
Organ or disease panels (80048-80076 [80081])
Therapeutic drug assays (80150-80299 [80164, 80165, 80171])

82310   Calcium; total

🗁 0.00   ⅗ 0.00   **FUD** XXX   ☒ ▣

AMA: 2016,Jan,13; 2015,Jun,10; 2015,Apr,3; 2015,Jan,16; 2014,Jan,11

82330   ionized

🗁 0.00   ⅗ 0.00   **FUD** XXX   ☒ ▣

AMA: 2016,Jan,13; 2015,Jun,10; 2015,Apr,3; 2015,Jan,16; 2014,Jan,11; 2013,Apr,10-11

82331   after calcium infusion test

🗁 0.00   ⅗ 0.00   **FUD** XXX   ▣ ▣

AMA: 2015,Jun,10; 2015,Apr,3

82340   urine quantitative, timed specimen

🗁 0.00   ⅗ 0.00   **FUD** XXX   ▣

AMA: 2015,Jun,10; 2015,Apr,3

82355   Calculus; qualitative analysis

🗁 0.00   ⅗ 0.00   **FUD** XXX   ▣ ▣

AMA: 2015,Jun,10; 2015,Apr,3

82360   quantitative analysis, chemical

🗁 0.00   ⅗ 0.00   **FUD** XXX   ▣ ▣

AMA: 2015,Jun,10; 2015,Apr,3

82365   infrared spectroscopy

🗁 0.00   ⅗ 0.00   **FUD** XXX   ▣ ▣

AMA: 2015,Jun,10; 2015,Apr,3

82370   X-ray diffraction

🗁 0.00   ⅗ 0.00   **FUD** XXX   ▣ ▣

AMA: 2015,Jun,10; 2015,Apr,3

82373   Carbohydrate deficient transferrin

🗁 0.00   ⅗ 0.00   **FUD** XXX   ▣

AMA: 2015,Jun,10; 2015,Apr,3

82374 Chemistry: Carbon Dioxide

CMS: 100-02,11,20.2 ESRD Laboratory Services; 100-02,11,30.2.2 Automated Multi-Channel Chemistry (AMCC) Tests; 100-04,16,40.6.1 Automated Multi-Channel Chemistry (AMCC) Tests for ESRD Beneficiaries; 100-04,16,70.8 CLIA Waived Tests

INCLUDES Clinical information not requested by the ordering physician
Mathematically calculated results
Quantitative analysis unless otherwise specified
Specimens from any source unless otherwise specified

EXCLUDES *Analytes from nonrequested laboratory analysis*
Calculated results that represent a score or probability that was derived by algorithm
Drug testing ([80305, 80306, 80307], [80324, 80325, 80326, 80327, 80328, 80329, 80330, 80331, 80332, 80333, 80334, 80335, 80336, 80337, 80338, 80339, 80340, 80341, 80342, 80343, 80344, 80345, 80346, 80347, 80348, 80349, 80350, 80351, 80352, 80353, 80354, 80355, 80356, 80357, 80358, 80359, 80360, 80361, 80362, 80363, 80364, 80365, 80366, 80367, 80368, 80369, 80370, 80371, 80372, 80373, 80374, 80375, 80376, 80377, 83992])
Organ or disease panels (80048-80076 [80081])
Therapeutic drug assays (80150-80299 [80164, 80165, 80171])

82374   Carbon dioxide (bicarbonate)

EXCLUDES *Blood gases (82803)*

🗁 0.00   ⅗ 0.00   **FUD** XXX   ☒ ▣

AMA: 2016,Jan,13; 2015,Jun,10; 2015,Apr,3; 2015,Jan,16; 2014,Jan,11; 2013,Apr,10-11

26-TC PC/TC Only   42-Z3 ASC Payment   50 Bilateral   ♂ Male Only   ♀ Female Only   🗁 Facility RVU   ⅗ Non-Facility RVU   ▣ CCI
FUD Follow-up Days   CMS: IOM (Pub 100)   A-Y OPPSI   80/80 Surg Assist Allowed / w/Doc   Ⅎ Lab Crosswalk   ⊞ Radiology Crosswalk   ☒ CLIA

368

CPT © 2016 American Medical Association. All Rights Reserved.   © 2016 Optum360, LLC

82375-82376 Chemistry: Carboxyhemoglobin (Carbon Monoxide)

INCLUDES Clinical information not requested by the ordering physician
Mathematically calculated results
Specimens from any source unless otherwise specified

EXCLUDES *Analytes from nonrequested laboratory analysis*
Calculated results that represent a score or probability that was derived by algorithm
Drug testing ([80305, 80306, 80307], [80324, 80325, 80326, 80327, 80328, 80329, 80330, 80331, 80332, 80333, 80334, 80335, 80336, 80337, 80338, 80339, 80340, 80341, 80342, 80343, 80344, 80345, 80346, 80347, 80348, 80349, 80350, 80351, 80352, 80353, 80354, 80355, 80356, 80357, 80358, 80359, 80360, 80361, 80362, 80363, 80364, 80365, 80366, 80367, 80368, 80369, 80370, 80371, 80372, 80373, 80374, 80375, 80376, 80377, 83992])
Organ or disease panels (80048-80076 [80081])
Transcutaneous measurement of carboxyhemoglobin (88740)

82375 **Carboxyhemoglobin; quantitative**
0.00   0.00   **FUD** XXX
AMA: 2016,Jan,13; 2015,Jun,10; 2015,Apr,3; 2015,Jan,16; 2014,Jan,11

82376 **qualitative**
0.00   0.00   **FUD** XXX
AMA: 2015,Jun,10; 2015,Apr,3

82378 Chemistry: Carcinoembryonic Antigen (CEA)

CMS: 100-03,190.26 Carcinoembryonic Antigen (CEA)

INCLUDES Clinical information not requested by the ordering physician

EXCLUDES *Analytes from nonrequested laboratory analysis*
Calculated results that represent a score or probability that was derived by algorithm

82378 **Carcinoembryonic antigen (CEA)**
0.00   0.00   **FUD** XXX
AMA: 2016,Jan,13; 2015,Jun,10; 2015,Apr,3; 2015,Jan,16; 2014,Jan,11; 2012,Jan,15-42; 2011,Jan,11

82379-82415 Chemistry: Carnitine—Chloramphenicol

INCLUDES Clinical information not requested by the ordering physician
Mathematically calculated results
Quantitative analysis unless otherwise specified
Specimens from any source unless otherwise specified

EXCLUDES *Analytes from nonrequested laboratory analysis*
Calculated results that represent a score or probability that was derived by algorithm
Drug testing ([80305, 80306, 80307], [80324, 80325, 80326, 80327, 80328, 80329, 80330, 80331, 80332, 80333, 80334, 80335, 80336, 80337, 80338, 80339, 80340, 80341, 80342, 80343, 80344, 80345, 80346, 80347, 80348, 80349, 80350, 80351, 80352, 80353, 80354, 80355, 80356, 80357, 80358, 80359, 80360, 80361, 80362, 80363, 80364, 80365, 80366, 80367, 80368, 80369, 80370, 80371, 80372, 80373, 80374, 80375, 80376, 80377, 83992])
Organ or disease panels (80048-80076 [80081])
Therapeutic drug assays (80150-80299 [80164, 80165, 80171])

82379 **Carnitine (total and free), quantitative, each specimen**
EXCLUDES *Acylcarnitine (82016-82017)*
0.00   0.00   **FUD** XXX
AMA: 2015,Jun,10; 2015,Apr,3

82380 **Carotene**
0.00   0.00   **FUD** XXX
AMA: 2015,Jun,10; 2015,Apr,3

82382 **Catecholamines; total urine**
0.00   0.00   **FUD** XXX
AMA: 2015,Jun,10; 2015,Apr,3

82383 **blood**
0.00   0.00   **FUD** XXX
AMA: 2015,Jun,10; 2015,Apr,3

82384 **fractionated**
EXCLUDES *Urine metabolites (83835, 84585)*
0.00   0.00   **FUD** XXX
AMA: 2015,Jun,10; 2015,Apr,3

82387 **Cathepsin-D**
0.00   0.00   **FUD** XXX
AMA: 2015,Jun,10; 2015,Apr,3

82390 **Ceruloplasmin**
0.00   0.00   **FUD** XXX
AMA: 2015,Jun,10; 2015,Apr,3

82397 **Chemiluminescent assay**
0.00   0.00   **FUD** XXX
AMA: 2016,Jan,13; 2015,Jun,10; 2015,Apr,3; 2015,Jan,16; 2014,Jan,11

82415 **Chloramphenicol**
0.00   0.00   **FUD** XXX
AMA: 2015,Jun,10; 2015,Apr,3

82435-82438 Chemistry: Chloride

INCLUDES Clinical information not requested by the ordering physician
Mathematically calculated results
Quantitative analysis unless otherwise specified
Specimens from any source unless otherwise specified

EXCLUDES *Analytes from nonrequested laboratory analysis*
Calculated results that represent a score or probability that was derived by algorithm
Organ or disease panels (80048-80076 [80081])
Therapeutic drug assays (80150-80299 [80164, 80165, 80171])

82435 **Chloride; blood**
0.00   0.00   **FUD** XXX
AMA: 2016,Jan,13; 2015,Jun,10; 2015,Apr,3; 2015,Jan,16; 2014,Jan,11; 2013,Apr,10-11

82436 **urine**
0.00   0.00   **FUD** XXX
AMA: 2015,Jun,10; 2015,Apr,3

82438 **other source**
EXCLUDES *Sweat collections by iontophoresis (89230)*
0.00   0.00   **FUD** XXX
AMA: 2016,Jan,13; 2015,Jun,10; 2015,Apr,3; 2015,Jan,16; 2014,Jan,11

82441 Chemistry: Chlorinated Hydrocarbons

INCLUDES Clinical information not requested by the ordering physician
Mathematically calculated results
Quantitative analysis unless otherwise specified
Specimens from any source unless otherwise specified

EXCLUDES *Analytes from nonrequested laboratory analysis*
Calculated results that represent a score or probability that was derived by algorithm

82441 **Chlorinated hydrocarbons, screen**
0.00   0.00   **FUD** XXX
AMA: 2015,Jun,10; 2015,Apr,3

82465 Chemistry: Cholesterol, Total

CMS: 100-03,190.23 Lipid Testing; 100-04,16,40.6.1 Automated Multi-Channel Chemistry (AMCC) Tests for ESRD Beneficiaries; 100-04,16,70.8 CLIA Waived Tests

INCLUDES Clinical information not requested by the ordering physician
Mathematically calculated results
Quantitative analysis unless otherwise specified

EXCLUDES *Analytes from nonrequested laboratory analysis*
Calculated results that represent a score or probability that was derived by algorithm
Organ or disease panels (80048-80076 [80081])

82465 **Cholesterol, serum or whole blood, total**
EXCLUDES *High density lipoprotein (HDL) (83718)*
0.00   0.00   **FUD** XXX
AMA: 2016,Jan,13; 2015,Jun,10; 2015,Apr,3; 2015,Jan,16; 2014,Jan,11; 2012,Jan,15-42; 2011,Jan,11

82480-82507 Chemistry: Cholinesterase—Citrate

INCLUDES Clinical information not requested by the ordering physician
Mathematically calculated results
Quantitative analysis unless otherwise specified
Specimens from any source unless otherwise specified

EXCLUDES Analytes from nonrequested laboratory analysis
Calculated results that represent a score or probability that was derived by algorithm
Drug testing ([80305, 80306, 80307], [80324, 80325, 80326, 80327, 80328, 80329, 80330, 80331, 80332, 80333, 80334, 80335, 80336, 80337, 80338, 80339, 80340, 80341, 80342, 80343, 80344, 80345, 80346, 80347, 80348, 80349, 80350, 80351, 80352, 80353, 80354, 80355, 80356, 80357, 80358, 80359, 80360, 80361, 80362, 80363, 80364, 80365, 80366, 80367, 80368, 80369, 80370, 80371, 80372, 80373, 80374, 80375, 80376, 80377, 83992])
Organ or disease panels (80048-80076 [80081])
Therapeutic drug assays (80150-80299 [80164, 80165, 80171])

82480 **Cholinesterase; serum**
🚗 0.00   ⚕ 0.00   **FUD** XXX   Q
AMA: 2015,Jun,10; 2015,Apr,3

82482 **RBC**
🚗 0.00   ⚕ 0.00   **FUD** XXX   Q
AMA: 2015,Jun,10; 2015,Apr,3

82485 **Chondroitin B sulfate, quantitative**
🚗 0.00   ⚕ 0.00   **FUD** XXX   Q
AMA: 2015,Jun,10; 2015,Apr,3

82495 **Chromium**
🚗 0.00   ⚕ 0.00   **FUD** XXX   Q
AMA: 2015,Jun,10; 2015,Apr,3

82507 **Citrate**
🚗 0.00   ⚕ 0.00   **FUD** XXX   Q
AMA: 2015,Jun,10; 2015,Apr,3

82523 Chemistry: Collagen Crosslinks, Any Method

CMS: 100-03,190.19 NCD for Collagen Crosslinks, Any Method; 100-04,16,70.8 CLIA Waived Tests

INCLUDES Clinical information not requested by the ordering physician
Mathematically calculated results
Quantitative analysis unless otherwise specified
Specimens from any source unless otherwise specified

EXCLUDES Analytes from nonrequested laboratory analysis
Calculated results that represent a score or probability that was derived by algorithm
Organ or disease panels (80048-80076 [80081])
Therapeutic drug assays (80150-80299 [80164, 80165, 80171])

82523 **Collagen cross links, any method**
🚗 0.00   ⚕ 0.00   **FUD** XXX   X Q
AMA: 2015,Jun,10; 2015,Apr,3

82525-82735 Chemistry: Copper—Fluoride

INCLUDES Clinical information not requested by the ordering physician
Mathematically calculated results
Quantitative analysis unless otherwise specified
Specimens from any source unless otherwise specified

EXCLUDES Analytes from nonrequested laboratory analysis
Calculated results that represent a score or probability that was derived by algorithm
Drug testing ([80305, 80306, 80307], [80324, 80325, 80326, 80327, 80328, 80329, 80330, 80331, 80332, 80333, 80334, 80335, 80336, 80337, 80338, 80339, 80340, 80341, 80342, 80343, 80344, 80345, 80346, 80347, 80348, 80349, 80350, 80351, 80352, 80353, 80354, 80355, 80356, 80357, 80358, 80359, 80360, 80361, 80362, 80363, 80364, 80365, 80366, 80367, 80368, 80369, 80370, 80371, 80372, 80373, 80374, 80375, 80376, 80377, 83992])
Organ or disease panels (80048-80076 [80081])
Therapeutic drug assays (80150-80299 [80164, 80165, 80171])

82525 **Copper**
🚗 0.00   ⚕ 0.00   **FUD** XXX   Q
AMA: 2015,Jun,10; 2015,Apr,3

82528 **Corticosterone**
INCLUDES Porter-Silber test
🚗 0.00   ⚕ 0.00   **FUD** XXX   Q
AMA: 2015,Jun,10; 2015,Apr,3

82530 **Cortisol; free**
🚗 0.00   ⚕ 0.00   **FUD** XXX   Q 🔲
AMA: 2016,Jan,13; 2015,Jun,10; 2015,Apr,3; 2015,Jan,16; 2014,Jan,11

82533 **total**
🚗 0.00   ⚕ 0.00   **FUD** XXX   Q 🔲
AMA: 2016,Jan,13; 2015,Jun,10; 2015,Apr,3; 2015,Jan,16; 2014,Jan,11

82540 **Creatine**
🚗 0.00   ⚕ 0.00   **FUD** XXX   Q
AMA: 2015,Jun,10; 2015,Apr,3

82542 **Column chromatography, includes mass spectrometry, if performed (eg, HPLC, LC, LC/MS, LC/MS-MS, GC, GC/MS-MS, GC/MS, HPLC/MS), non-drug analyte(s) not elsewhere specified, qualitative or quantitative, each specimen**
EXCLUDES Procedure performed more than one time per specimen
🚗 0.00   ⚕ 0.00   **FUD** XXX   Q
AMA: 2016,Jan,13; 2015,Jun,10; 2015,Apr,3

82550 **Creatine kinase (CK), (CPK); total**
🚗 0.00   ⚕ 0.00   **FUD** XXX   X Q 🔲
AMA: 2016,Jan,13; 2015,Jun,10; 2015,Apr,3; 2015,Jan,16; 2014,Jan,11

82552 **isoenzymes**
🚗 0.00   ⚕ 0.00   **FUD** XXX   Q 🔲
AMA: 2016,Jan,13; 2015,Jun,10; 2015,Apr,3; 2015,Jan,16; 2014,Jan,11

82553 **MB fraction only**
🚗 0.00   ⚕ 0.00   **FUD** XXX   Q 🔲
AMA: 2016,Jan,13; 2015,Jun,10; 2015,Apr,3; 2015,Jan,16; 2014,Jan,11

82554 **isoforms**
🚗 0.00   ⚕ 0.00   **FUD** XXX   Q 🔲
AMA: 2016,Jan,13; 2015,Jun,10; 2015,Apr,3; 2015,Jan,16; 2014,Jan,11

82565 **Creatinine; blood**
🚗 0.00   ⚕ 0.00   **FUD** XXX   X Q
AMA: 2016,Jan,13; 2015,Jun,10; 2015,Apr,3; 2015,Jan,16; 2014,Jan,11; 2013,Apr,10-11

82570 **other source**
🚗 0.00   ⚕ 0.00   **FUD** XXX   X Q
AMA: 2015,Jun,10; 2015,Apr,3

82575 **clearance**
INCLUDES Holten test
🚗 0.00   ⚕ 0.00   **FUD** XXX   Q 🔲
AMA: 2015,Jun,10; 2015,Apr,3

82585 **Cryofibrinogen**
🚗 0.00   ⚕ 0.00   **FUD** XXX   Q
AMA: 2015,Jun,10; 2015,Apr,3

82595 **Cryoglobulin, qualitative or semi-quantitative (eg, cryocrit)**
EXCLUDES Quantitative, cryoglobulin (82784-82785)
🚗 0.00   ⚕ 0.00   **FUD** XXX   Q
AMA: 2015,Jun,10; 2015,Apr,3

82600 **Cyanide**
🚗 0.00   ⚕ 0.00   **FUD** XXX   Q
AMA: 2015,Jun,10; 2015,Apr,3

82607 **Cyanocobalamin (Vitamin B-12);**
🚗 0.00   ⚕ 0.00   **FUD** XXX   Q 🔲
AMA: 2015,Jun,10; 2015,Apr,3

82608 **unsaturated binding capacity**
🚗 0.00   ⚕ 0.00   **FUD** XXX   Q
AMA: 2015,Jun,10; 2015,Apr,3

82610 **Cystatin C**
🚗 0.00   ⚕ 0.00   **FUD** XXX   Q
AMA: 2016,Jan,13; 2015,Jun,10; 2015,Apr,3; 2015,Jan,16; 2014,Jan,11; 2012,Jan,15-42; 2011,Jan,11

82615 **Cystine and homocystine, urine, qualitative**
🚗 0.00   ⚕ 0.00   **FUD** XXX   Q
AMA: 2015,Jun,10; 2015,Apr,3

| 26/TC PC/TC Only | A2-Z3 ASC Payment | 50 Bilateral | ♂ Male Only | ♀ Female Only | 🚗 Facility RVU | ⚕ Non-Facility RVU | 🔲 CCI |
| FUD Follow-up Days | CMS: IOM (Pub 100) | A-Y OPPSI | 80/80 Surg Assist Allowed / w/Doc | | 🔲 Lab Crosswalk | ⚡ Radiology Crosswalk | X CLIA |

370   CPT © 2016 American Medical Association. All Rights Reserved.   © 2016 Optum360, LLC

82626   Dehydroepiandrosterone (DHEA)
> EXCLUDES   *Anabolic steroids ([80327, 80328])*
> 🚑 0.00   ⚗ 0.00   **FUD** XXX   Ⓠ
>
> **AMA:** 2016,Jan,13; 2015,Jun,10; 2015,Apr,3; 2015,Jan,16; 2014,Jan,11

82627   Dehydroepiandrosterone-sulfate (DHEA-S)
> 🚑 0.00   ⚗ 0.00   **FUD** XXX   Ⓠ
>
> **AMA:** 2016,Jan,13; 2015,Jun,10; 2015,Apr,3; 2015,Jan,16; 2014,Jan,11

82633   Desoxycorticosterone, 11-
> 🚑 0.00   ⚗ 0.00   **FUD** XXX   Ⓠ
>
> **AMA:** 2015,Jun,10; 2015,Apr,3

82634   Deoxycortisol, 11-
> 🚑 0.00   ⚗ 0.00   **FUD** XXX   Ⓠ ▢
>
> **AMA:** 2015,Jun,10; 2015,Apr,3

82638   Dibucaine number
> 🚑 0.00   ⚗ 0.00   **FUD** XXX   Ⓠ
>
> **AMA:** 2015,Jun,10; 2015,Apr,3

82652   Resequenced code, See code following 82306.

82656   Elastase, pancreatic (EL-1), fecal, qualitative or semi-quantitative
> 🚑 0.00   ⚗ 0.00   **FUD** XXX   Ⓠ
>
> **AMA:** 2016,Jan,13; 2015,Jun,10; 2015,Apr,3; 2015,Jan,16; 2014,Jan,11; 2012,Jan,15-42; 2011,Jan,11

82657   Enzyme activity in blood cells, cultured cells, or tissue, not elsewhere specified; nonradioactive substrate, each specimen
> 🚑 0.00   ⚗ 0.00   **FUD** XXX   Ⓠ
>
> **AMA:** 2015,Jun,10; 2015,Apr,3

82658   radioactive substrate, each specimen
> 🚑 0.00   ⚗ 0.00   **FUD** XXX   Ⓠ
>
> **AMA:** 2015,Jun,10; 2015,Apr,3

82664   Electrophoretic technique, not elsewhere specified
> 🚑 0.00   ⚗ 0.00   **FUD** XXX   Ⓠ
>
> **AMA:** 2015,Jun,10; 2015,Apr,3

82668   Erythropoietin
> 🚑 0.00   ⚗ 0.00   **FUD** XXX   Ⓠ
>
> **AMA:** 2015,Jun,10; 2015,Apr,3

82670   Estradiol
> 🚑 0.00   ⚗ 0.00   **FUD** XXX   Ⓠ ▢
>
> **AMA:** 2015,Jun,10; 2015,Apr,3

82671   Estrogens; fractionated
> EXCLUDES   *Estrogen receptor assay (84233)*
> 🚑 0.00   ⚗ 0.00   **FUD** XXX   Ⓠ
>
> **AMA:** 2015,Jun,10; 2015,Apr,3

82672   total
> EXCLUDES   *Estrogen receptor assay (84233)*
> 🚑 0.00   ⚗ 0.00   **FUD** XXX   Ⓠ
>
> **AMA:** 2015,Jun,10; 2015,Apr,3

82677   Estriol
> 🚑 0.00   ⚗ 0.00   **FUD** XXX   Ⓠ
>
> **AMA:** 2015,Jun,10; 2015,Apr,3

82679   Estrone
> 🚑 0.00   ⚗ 0.00   **FUD** XXX   ☒ Ⓠ
>
> **AMA:** 2015,Jun,10; 2015,Apr,3

82693   Ethylene glycol
> 🚑 0.00   ⚗ 0.00   **FUD** XXX   Ⓠ
>
> **AMA:** 2015,Jun,10; 2015,Apr,3

82696   Etiocholanolone
> EXCLUDES   *Fractionation of ketosteroids (83593)*
> 🚑 0.00   ⚗ 0.00   **FUD** XXX   Ⓠ
>
> **AMA:** 2015,Jun,10; 2015,Apr,3

82705   Fat or lipids, feces; qualitative
> 🚑 0.00   ⚗ 0.00   **FUD** XXX   Ⓠ
>
> **AMA:** 2015,Jun,10; 2015,Apr,3

82710   quantitative
> 🚑 0.00   ⚗ 0.00   **FUD** XXX   Ⓠ
>
> **AMA:** 2015,Jun,10; 2015,Apr,3

82715   Fat differential, feces, quantitative
> 🚑 0.00   ⚗ 0.00   **FUD** XXX   Ⓠ
>
> **AMA:** 2015,Jun,10; 2015,Apr,3

82725   Fatty acids, nonesterified
> 🚑 0.00   ⚗ 0.00   **FUD** XXX   Ⓠ
>
> **AMA:** 2015,Jun,10; 2015,Apr,3

82726   Very long chain fatty acids
> EXCLUDES   *Long-chain (C20-22) omega-3 fatty acids in red blood cell (RBC) membranes (0111T)*
> 🚑 0.00   ⚗ 0.00   **FUD** XXX   Ⓠ
>
> **AMA:** 2015,Jun,10; 2015,Apr,3

82728   Ferritin
> 🚑 0.00   ⚗ 0.00   **FUD** XXX   Ⓠ
>
> **AMA:** 2015,Jun,10; 2015,Apr,3

82731   Fetal fibronectin, cervicovaginal secretions, semi-quantitative   Ⓜ ♀
> 🚑 0.00   ⚗ 0.00   **FUD** XXX   Ⓠ
>
> **AMA:** 2015,Jun,10; 2015,Apr,3

82735   Fluoride
> 🚑 0.00   ⚗ 0.00   **FUD** XXX   Ⓠ
>
> **AMA:** 2015,Jun,10; 2015,Apr,3

82746-82941 Chemistry: Folic Acid—Gastrin

> INCLUDES   Clinical information not requested by the ordering physician
> Mathematically calculated results
> Quantitative analysis unless otherwise specified
> Specimens from any source unless otherwise specified
>
> EXCLUDES   *Analytes from nonrequested laboratory analysis*
> *Calculated results that represent a score or probability that was derived by algorithm*
> *Drug testing ([80305, 80306, 80307], [80324, 80325, 80326, 80327, 80328, 80329, 80330, 80331, 80332, 80333, 80334, 80335, 80336, 80337, 80338, 80339, 80340, 80341, 80342, 80343, 80344, 80345, 80346, 80347, 80348, 80349, 80350, 80351, 80352, 80353, 80354, 80355, 80356, 80357, 80358, 80359, 80360, 80361, 80362, 80363, 80364, 80365, 80366, 80367, 80368, 80369, 80370, 80371, 80372, 80373, 80374, 80375, 80376, 80377, 83992])*
> *Organ or disease panels (80048-80076 [80081])*
> *Therapeutic drug assays (80150-80299 [80164, 80165, 80171])*

82746   Folic acid; serum
> 🚑 0.00   ⚗ 0.00   **FUD** XXX   Ⓠ
>
> **AMA:** 2015,Jun,10; 2015,Apr,3

82747   RBC
> 🚑 0.00   ⚗ 0.00   **FUD** XXX   Ⓠ
>
> **AMA:** 2015,Jun,10; 2015,Apr,3

82757   Fructose, semen
> EXCLUDES   *Fructosamine (82985)*
> *Fructose, TLC screen (84375)*
> 🚑 0.00   ⚗ 0.00   **FUD** XXX   Ⓠ
>
> **AMA:** 2015,Jun,10; 2015,Apr,3

82759   Galactokinase, RBC
> 🚑 0.00   ⚗ 0.00   **FUD** XXX   Ⓠ
>
> **AMA:** 2015,Jun,10; 2015,Apr,3

82760   Galactose
> 🚑 0.00   ⚗ 0.00   **FUD** XXX   Ⓠ
>
> **AMA:** 2015,Jun,10; 2015,Apr,3

82775   Galactose-1-phosphate uridyl transferase; quantitative
> 🚑 0.00   ⚗ 0.00   **FUD** XXX   Ⓠ
>
> **AMA:** 2015,Jun,10; 2015,Apr,3

82776   screen
> 🚑 0.00   ⚗ 0.00   **FUD** XXX   Ⓠ
>
> **AMA:** 2015,Jun,10; 2015,Apr,3

82777   Galectin-3
> 🚑 0.00   ⚗ 0.00   **FUD** XXX   Ⓠ
>
> **AMA:** 2015,Jun,10; 2015,Apr,3

82784   **Gammaglobulin (immunoglobulin); IgA, IgD, IgG, IgM, each**

INCLUDES   Farr test

0.00   0.00   **FUD** XXX

AMA: 2016,Jan,13; 2015,Jun,10; 2015,Apr,3; 2015,Jan,16; 2014,Jan,11; 2012,Jan,15-42; 2011,Jan,11

82785   **IgE**

INCLUDES   Farr test

EXCLUDES   Allergen specific, IgE (86003, 86005)

0.00   0.00   **FUD** XXX

AMA: 2016,Jan,13; 2015,Jun,10; 2015,Apr,3; 2015,Jan,16; 2014,Jan,11

82787   **immunoglobulin subclasses (eg, IgG1, 2, 3, or 4), each**

EXCLUDES   Gamma-glutamyltransferase (GGT) (82977)

0.00   0.00   **FUD** XXX

AMA: 2015,Jun,10; 2015,Apr,3

82800   **Gases, blood, pH only**

0.00   0.00   **FUD** XXX

AMA: 2015,Jun,10; 2015,Apr,3

82803   **Gases, blood, any combination of pH, pCO2, pO2, CO2, HCO3 (including calculated O2 saturation);**

INCLUDES   Two or more of the listed analytes

0.00   0.00   **FUD** XXX

AMA: 2015,Jun,10; 2015,Apr,3

82805   **with O2 saturation, by direct measurement, except pulse oximetry**

0.00   0.00   **FUD** XXX

AMA: 2015,Jun,10; 2015,Apr,3

82810   **Gases, blood, O2 saturation only, by direct measurement, except pulse oximetry**

EXCLUDES   Pulse oximetry (94760)

0.00   0.00   **FUD** XXX

AMA: 2015,Jun,10; 2015,Apr,3

82820   **Hemoglobin-oxygen affinity (pO2 for 50% hemoglobin saturation with oxygen)**

0.00   0.00   **FUD** XXX

AMA: 2015,Jun,10; 2015,Apr,3

82930   **Gastric acid analysis, includes pH if performed, each specimen**

0.00   0.00   **FUD** XXX

AMA: 2016,Jan,13; 2015,Jun,10; 2015,Apr,3; 2015,Jan,16; 2014,Jan,11; 2011,Sep,3-4

82938   **Gastrin after secretin stimulation**

0.00   0.00   **FUD** XXX

AMA: 2015,Jun,10; 2015,Apr,3

82941   **Gastrin**

EXCLUDES   Qualitative column chromotography report specific analyte or (82542)

0.00   0.00   **FUD** XXX

AMA: 2015,Jun,10; 2015,Apr,3

82943-82962 Chemistry: Glucagon—Glucose Testing

CMS: 100-03,190.20 Blood Glucose Testing

INCLUDES   Clinical information not requested by the ordering physician
Mathematically calculated results
Quantitative analysis unless otherwise specified
Specimens from any source unless otherwise specified

EXCLUDES   Analytes from nonrequested laboratory analysis
Calculated results that represent a score or probability that was derived by algorithm
Organ or disease panels (80048-80076 [80081])
Therapeutic drug assays (80150-80299 [80164, 80165, 80171])
Code also glucose administration injection (96374)

82943   **Glucagon**

0.00   0.00   **FUD** XXX

AMA: 2015,Jun,10; 2015,Apr,3

82945   **Glucose, body fluid, other than blood**

0.00   0.00   **FUD** XXX

AMA: 2015,Jun,10; 2015,Apr,3

82946   **Glucagon tolerance test**

0.00   0.00   **FUD** XXX

AMA: 2015,Jun,10; 2015,Apr,3

82947   **Glucose; quantitative, blood (except reagent strip)**

0.00   0.00   **FUD** XXX

AMA: 2016,Jan,13; 2015,Jun,10; 2015,Apr,3; 2015,Jan,16; 2014,Jan,11; 2013,Apr,10-11

82948   **blood, reagent strip**

0.00   0.00   **FUD** XXX

AMA: 2016,Jan,13; 2015,Jun,10; 2015,Apr,3; 2015,Jan,16; 2014,Jan,11; 2012,Jan,15-42; 2011,Oct,8; 2011,Jan,11

82950   **post glucose dose (includes glucose)**

0.00   0.00   **FUD** XXX

AMA: 2016,Jan,13; 2015,Jun,10; 2015,Apr,3; 2015,Jan,16; 2014,Jan,11; 2012,Jan,15-42; 2011,Jan,11

82951   **tolerance test (GTT), 3 specimens (includes glucose)**

0.00   0.00   **FUD** XXX

AMA: 2016,Jan,13; 2015,Jun,10; 2015,Apr,3; 2015,Jan,16; 2014,Jan,11; 2012,Jan,15-42; 2011,Jan,11

+ **82952**   **tolerance test, each additional beyond 3 specimens (List separately in addition to code for primary procedure)**

Code first (82951)

0.00   0.00   **FUD** XXX

AMA: 2016,Jan,13; 2015,Jun,10; 2015,Apr,3; 2015,Jan,16; 2014,Jan,11; 2012,Jan,15-42; 2011,Jan,11

82955   **Glucose-6-phosphate dehydrogenase (G6PD); quantitative**

0.00   0.00   **FUD** XXX

AMA: 2015,Jun,10; 2015,Apr,3

82960   **screen**

0.00   0.00   **FUD** XXX

AMA: 2015,Jun,10; 2015,Apr,3

82962   **Glucose, blood by glucose monitoring device(s) cleared by the FDA specifically for home use**

0.00   0.00   **FUD** XXX

AMA: 2016,Jan,13; 2015,Jun,10; 2015,Apr,3; 2015,Jan,16; 2014,Jan,11; 2012,Jan,15-42; 2011,Oct,8; 2011,Jan,11

82963-83690 Chemistry: Glucosidase—Lipase

INCLUDES   Clinical information not requested by the ordering physician
Mathematically calculated results
Quantitative analysis unless otherwise specified
Specimens from any source unless otherwise specified

EXCLUDES   Analytes from nonrequested laboratory analysis
Calculated results that represent a score or probability that was derived by algorithm
Drug testing ([80305, 80306, 80307], [80324, 80325, 80326, 80327, 80328, 80329, 80330, 80331, 80332, 80333, 80334, 80335, 80336, 80337, 80338, 80339, 80340, 80341, 80342, 80343, 80344, 80345, 80346, 80347, 80348, 80349, 80350, 80351, 80352, 80353, 80354, 80355, 80356, 80357, 80358, 80359, 80360, 80361, 80362, 80363, 80364, 80365, 80366, 80367, 80368, 80369, 80370, 80371, 80372, 80373, 80374, 80375, 80376, 80377, 83992])
Organ or disease panels (80048-80076 [80081])
Therapeutic drug assays (80150-80299 [80164, 80165, 80171])

82963   **Glucosidase, beta**

0.00   0.00   **FUD** XXX

AMA: 2015,Jun,10; 2015,Apr,3

82965   **Glutamate dehydrogenase**

0.00   0.00   **FUD** XXX

AMA: 2015,Jun,10; 2015,Apr,3

82977   **Glutamyltransferase, gamma (GGT)**

0.00   0.00   **FUD** XXX

AMA: 2016,Jan,13; 2015,Jun,10; 2015,Apr,3; 2015,Jan,16; 2014,Jan,11

82978   **Glutathione**

0.00   0.00   **FUD** XXX

AMA: 2015,Jun,10; 2015,Apr,3

82979   **Glutathione reductase, RBC**

0.00   0.00   **FUD** XXX

AMA: 2015,Jun,10; 2015,Apr,3

26/TC PC/TC Only   A2-Z3 ASC Payment   50 Bilateral   ♂ Male Only   ♀ Female Only   Facility RVU   Non-Facility RVU   CCI
FUD Follow-up Days   CMS: IOM (Pub 100)   A-Y OPPSI   80/80 Surg Assist Allowed / w/Doc   Lab Crosswalk   Radiology Crosswalk   CLIA

82985	**Glycated protein**
	EXCLUDES *Gonadotropin chorionic (hCG) (84702-84703)*
	⚙ 0.00 ⚖ 0.00 **FUD** XXX ☒ Ⓠ □
	AMA: 2016,Jan,13; 2015,Jun,10; 2015,Apr,3; 2015,Jan,16; 2014,Jan,11

83001	**Gonadotropin; follicle stimulating hormone (FSH)**
	⚙ 0.00 ⚖ 0.00 **FUD** XXX ☒ Ⓠ □
	AMA: 2015,Jun,10; 2015,Apr,3

83002	**luteinizing hormone (LH)**
	EXCLUDES *Luteinizing releasing factor (LRH) (83727)*
	⚙ 0.00 ⚖ 0.00 **FUD** XXX ☒ Ⓠ □
	AMA: 2015,Jun,10; 2015,Apr,3

83003	**Growth hormone, human (HGH) (somatotropin)**
	EXCLUDES *Antibody to human growth hormone (86277)*
	⚙ 0.00 ⚖ 0.00 **FUD** XXX Ⓠ □
	AMA: 2015,Jun,10; 2015,Apr,3

83006	**Growth stimulation expressed gene 2 (ST2, Interleukin 1 receptor like-1)**
	⚙ 0.00 ⚖ 0.00 **FUD** XXX Ⓠ
	AMA: 2015,Jun,10; 2015,Apr,3

83009	**Helicobacter pylori, blood test analysis for urease activity, non-radioactive isotope (eg, C-13)**
	EXCLUDES *H. pylori, breath test analysis for urease activity (83013-83014)*
	⚙ 0.00 ⚖ 0.00 **FUD** XXX Ⓠ □
	AMA: 2015,Jun,10; 2015,Apr,3

83010	**Haptoglobin; quantitative**
	⚙ 0.00 ⚖ 0.00 **FUD** XXX Ⓠ
	AMA: 2015,Jun,10; 2015,Apr,3

83012	**phenotypes**
	⚙ 0.00 ⚖ 0.00 **FUD** XXX Ⓠ
	AMA: 2015,Jun,10; 2015,Apr,3

83013	**Helicobacter pylori; breath test analysis for urease activity, non-radioactive isotope (eg, C-13)**
	⚙ 0.00 ⚖ 0.00 **FUD** XXX Ⓠ □
	AMA: 2016,Jan,13; 2015,Jun,10; 2015,Apr,3; 2015,Jan,16; 2014,Jan,11

83014	**drug administration**
	EXCLUDES *H. pylori:*
	Blood test analysis for urease activity (83009)
	Enzyme immunoassay (87339)
	Liquid scintillation counter (78267-78268)
	Stool (87338)
	⚙ 0.00 ⚖ 0.00 **FUD** XXX Ⓠ □
	AMA: 2016,Jan,13; 2015,Jun,10; 2015,Apr,3; 2015,Jan,16; 2014,Jan,11

▲ 83015	**Heavy metal (eg, arsenic, barium, beryllium, bismuth, antimony, mercury); qualitative, any number of analytes**
	INCLUDES *Reinsch test*
	⚙ 0.00 ⚖ 0.00 **FUD** XXX Ⓠ
	AMA: 2015,Jun,10; 2015,Apr,3

▲ 83018	**quantitative, each, not elsewhere specified**
	EXCLUDES *Evaluation of a known heavy metal with a specific code*
	⚙ 0.00 ⚖ 0.00 **FUD** XXX Ⓠ
	AMA: 2015,Jun,10; 2015,Apr,3

83020	**Hemoglobin fractionation and quantitation; electrophoresis (eg, A2, S, C, and/or F)**
	⚙ 0.00 ⚖ 0.00 **FUD** XXX Ⓠ □
	AMA: 2015,Jun,10; 2015,Apr,3

83021	**chromatography (eg, A2, S, C, and/or F)**
	EXCLUDES *Analysis of glycosylated (A1c) hemoglobin by chromatography or electrophoresis without an identified hemoglobin variant (83036)*
	⚙ 0.00 ⚖ 0.00 **FUD** XXX Ⓠ □
	AMA: 2016,Jan,13; 2015,Jun,10; 2015,Apr,3; 2015,Jan,16; 2014,Jan,11

83026	**Hemoglobin; by copper sulfate method, non-automated**
	⚙ 0.00 ⚖ 0.00 **FUD** XXX ☒ Ⓠ
	AMA: 2015,Jun,10; 2015,Apr,3

83030	**F (fetal), chemical**
	⚙ 0.00 ⚖ 0.00 **FUD** XXX Ⓠ □
	AMA: 2015,Jun,10; 2015,Apr,3

83033	**F (fetal), qualitative**
	⚙ 0.00 ⚖ 0.00 **FUD** XXX Ⓠ □
	AMA: 2015,Jun,10; 2015,Apr,3

83036	**glycosylated (A1C)**
	EXCLUDES *Analysis of glycosylated (A1c) hemoglobin by chromatography or electrophoresis without an identified hemoglobin variant (83021)*
	Detection of hemoglobin, fecal, by immunoassay (82274)
	⚙ 0.00 ⚖ 0.00 **FUD** XXX ☒ Ⓠ
	AMA: 2016,Jan,13; 2015,Jun,10; 2015,Apr,3; 2015,Jan,16; 2014,Jan,11

83037	**glycosylated (A1C) by device cleared by FDA for home use**
	⚙ 0.00 ⚖ 0.00 **FUD** XXX ☒ Ⓠ □
	AMA: 2016,Jan,13; 2015,Jun,10; 2015,Apr,3; 2015,Jan,16; 2014,Jan,11; 2012,Jan,15-42; 2011,Jan,11

83045	**methemoglobin, qualitative**
	⚙ 0.00 ⚖ 0.00 **FUD** XXX Ⓠ
	AMA: 2015,Jun,10; 2015,Apr,3

83050	**methemoglobin, quantitative**
	EXCLUDES *Transcutaneous methemoglobin test (88741)*
	⚙ 0.00 ⚖ 0.00 **FUD** XXX Ⓠ □
	AMA: 2016,Jan,13; 2015,Jun,10; 2015,Apr,3; 2015,Jan,16; 2014,Jan,11

83051	**plasma**
	⚙ 0.00 ⚖ 0.00 **FUD** XXX Ⓠ
	AMA: 2015,Jun,10; 2015,Apr,3

83060	**sulfhemoglobin, quantitative**
	⚙ 0.00 ⚖ 0.00 **FUD** XXX Ⓠ
	AMA: 2015,Jun,10; 2015,Apr,3

83065	**thermolabile**
	⚙ 0.00 ⚖ 0.00 **FUD** XXX Ⓠ
	AMA: 2015,Jun,10; 2015,Apr,3

83068	**unstable, screen**
	⚙ 0.00 ⚖ 0.00 **FUD** XXX Ⓠ □
	AMA: 2015,Jun,10; 2015,Apr,3

83069	**urine**
	⚙ 0.00 ⚖ 0.00 **FUD** XXX Ⓠ
	AMA: 2015,Jun,10; 2015,Apr,3

83070	**Hemosiderin, qualitative**
	EXCLUDES *Qualitative column chromotography report specific analyte or (82542)*
	⚙ 0.00 ⚖ 0.00 **FUD** XXX Ⓠ
	AMA: 2015,Jun,10; 2015,Apr,3

83080	**b-Hexosaminidase, each assay**
	⚙ 0.00 ⚖ 0.00 **FUD** XXX Ⓠ
	AMA: 2015,Jun,10; 2015,Apr,3

83088	**Histamine**
	⚙ 0.00 ⚖ 0.00 **FUD** XXX Ⓠ
	AMA: 2015,Jun,10; 2015,Apr,3

83090	**Homocysteine**
	⚙ 0.00 ⚖ 0.00 **FUD** XXX Ⓠ □
	AMA: 2016,Jan,13; 2015,Jun,10; 2015,Apr,3; 2015,Jan,16; 2014,Jan,11; 2012,Jan,15-42; 2011,Jan,11

83150	**Homovanillic acid (HVA)**
	⚙ 0.00 ⚖ 0.00 **FUD** XXX Ⓠ
	AMA: 2015,Jun,10; 2015,Apr,3

● New Code   ▲ Revised Code   ○ Reinstated   ● New Web Release   ▲ Revised Web Release   Unlisted   Not Covered   # Resequenced
⊘ AMA Mod 51 Exempt   ⑪ Optum Mod 51 Exempt   ⑬ Mod 63 Exempt   ✗ Non-FDA Drug   ★ Telehealth   Ⓜ Maternity   Ⓐ Age Edit   + Add-on   **AMA:** CPT Asst

83491 **Hydroxycorticosteroids, 17- (17-OHCS)**
EXCLUDES Cortisol (82530, 82533)
Deoxycortisol (82634)
🚗 0.00 ⚕ 0.00 **FUD** XXX Q
AMA: 2015,Jun,10; 2015,Apr,3

83497 **Hydroxyindolacetic acid, 5-(HIAA)**
EXCLUDES Urine qualitative test (81005)
🚗 0.00 ⚕ 0.00 **FUD** XXX Q
AMA: 2015,Jun,10; 2015,Apr,3

83498 **Hydroxyprogesterone, 17-d**
🚗 0.00 ⚕ 0.00 **FUD** XXX Q ☐
AMA: 2015,Jun,10; 2015,Apr,3

83499 **Hydroxyprogesterone, 20-**
🚗 0.00 ⚕ 0.00 **FUD** XXX Q
AMA: 2015,Jun,10; 2015,Apr,3

83500 **Hydroxyproline; free**
🚗 0.00 ⚕ 0.00 **FUD** XXX Q
AMA: 2015,Jun,10; 2015,Apr,3

83505 **total**
🚗 0.00 ⚕ 0.00 **FUD** XXX Q
AMA: 2015,Jun,10; 2015,Apr,3

83516 **Immunoassay for analyte other than infectious agent antibody or infectious agent antigen; qualitative or semiquantitative, multiple step method**
🚗 0.00 ⚕ 0.00 **FUD** XXX ☒ Q ☐
AMA: 2015,Jun,10; 2015,Apr,3

83518 **qualitative or semiquantitative, single step method (eg, reagent strip)**
🚗 0.00 ⚕ 0.00 **FUD** XXX Q
AMA: 2015,Jun,10; 2015,Apr,3

83519 **quantitative, by radioimmunoassay (eg, RIA)**
🚗 0.00 ⚕ 0.00 **FUD** XXX Q ☐
AMA: 2016,Jan,13; 2015,Jun,10; 2015,Apr,3; 2015,Jan,16; 2014,Jan,11

83520 **quantitative, not otherwise specified**
🚗 0.00 ⚕ 0.00 **FUD** XXX Q ☐
AMA: 2015,Jun,10; 2015,Apr,3

83525 **Insulin; total**
EXCLUDES Proinsulin (84206)
🚗 0.00 ⚕ 0.00 **FUD** XXX Q ☐
AMA: 2015,Jun,10; 2015,Apr,3

83527 **free**
🚗 0.00 ⚕ 0.00 **FUD** XXX Q
AMA: 2016,Jan,13; 2015,Jun,10; 2015,Apr,3; 2015,Jan,16; 2014,Jan,11

83528 **Intrinsic factor**
EXCLUDES Intrinsic factor antibodies (86340)
🚗 0.00 ⚕ 0.00 **FUD** XXX Q
AMA: 2015,Jun,10; 2015,Apr,3

83540 **Iron**
🚗 0.00 ⚕ 0.00 **FUD** XXX Q
AMA: 2016,Jan,13; 2015,Jun,10; 2015,Apr,3; 2015,Jan,16; 2014,Jan,11

83550 **Iron binding capacity**
🚗 0.00 ⚕ 0.00 **FUD** XXX Q
AMA: 2015,Jun,10; 2015,Apr,3

83570 **Isocitric dehydrogenase (IDH)**
🚗 0.00 ⚕ 0.00 **FUD** XXX Q
AMA: 2015,Jun,10; 2015,Apr,3

83582 **Ketogenic steroids, fractionation**
🚗 0.00 ⚕ 0.00 **FUD** XXX Q
AMA: 2015,Jun,10; 2015,Apr,3

83586 **Ketosteroids, 17- (17-KS); total**
🚗 0.00 ⚕ 0.00 **FUD** XXX Q
AMA: 2015,Jun,10; 2015,Apr,3

83593 **fractionation**
🚗 0.00 ⚕ 0.00 **FUD** XXX Q
AMA: 2015,Jun,10; 2015,Apr,3

83605 **Lactate (lactic acid)**
🚗 0.00 ⚕ 0.00 **FUD** XXX ☒ Q
AMA: 2015,Jun,10; 2015,Apr,3

83615 **Lactate dehydrogenase (LD), (LDH);**
🚗 0.00 ⚕ 0.00 **FUD** XXX Q
AMA: 2016,Jan,13; 2015,Jun,10; 2015,Apr,3; 2015,Jan,16; 2014,Jan,11

83625 **isoenzymes, separation and quantitation**
🚗 0.00 ⚕ 0.00 **FUD** XXX Q ☐
AMA: 2016,Jan,13; 2015,Jun,10; 2015,Apr,3; 2015,Jan,16; 2014,Jan,11

83630 **Lactoferrin, fecal; qualitative**
🚗 0.00 ⚕ 0.00 **FUD** XXX Q
AMA: 2016,Jan,13; 2015,Jun,10; 2015,Apr,3; 2015,Jan,16; 2014,Jan,11

83631 **quantitative**
🚗 0.00 ⚕ 0.00 **FUD** XXX Q ☐
AMA: 2016,Jan,13; 2015,Jun,10; 2015,Apr,3; 2015,Jan,16; 2014,Jan,11; 2012,Jan,15-42; 2011,Jan,11

83632 **Lactogen, human placental (HPL) human chorionic somatomammotropin** M
🚗 0.00 ⚕ 0.00 **FUD** XXX Q
AMA: 2015,Jun,10; 2015,Apr,3

83633 **Lactose, urine, qualitative**
🚗 0.00 ⚕ 0.00 **FUD** XXX Q
AMA: 2015,Jun,10; 2015,Apr,3

83655 **Lead**
🚗 0.00 ⚕ 0.00 **FUD** XXX ☒ Q
AMA: 2015,Jun,10; 2015,Apr,3

83661 **Fetal lung maturity assessment; lecithin sphingomyelin (L/S) ratio** M
🚗 0.00 ⚕ 0.00 **FUD** XXX Q ☐
AMA: 2016,Jan,13; 2015,Jun,10; 2015,Apr,3; 2015,Jan,16; 2014,Jan,11

83662 **foam stability test** M
🚗 0.00 ⚕ 0.00 **FUD** XXX Q ☐
AMA: 2015,Jun,10; 2015,Apr,3

83663 **fluorescence polarization** M
🚗 0.00 ⚕ 0.00 **FUD** XXX Q ☐
AMA: 2015,Jun,10; 2015,Apr,3

83664 **lamellar body density** M
EXCLUDES Phosphatidylglycerol (84081)
🚗 0.00 ⚕ 0.00 **FUD** XXX Q ☐
AMA: 2015,Jun,10; 2015,Apr,3

83670 **Leucine aminopeptidase (LAP)**
🚗 0.00 ⚕ 0.00 **FUD** XXX Q
AMA: 2015,Jun,10; 2015,Apr,3

83690 **Lipase**
🚗 0.00 ⚕ 0.00 **FUD** XXX Q
AMA: 2015,Jun,10; 2015,Apr,3

83695-83727 Chemistry: Lipoprotein—Luteinizing Releasing Factor

INCLUDES Clinical information not requested by the ordering physician
Mathematically calculated results
Quantitative analysis unless otherwise specified
Specimens from any source unless otherwise specified
EXCLUDES Analytes from nonrequested laboratory analysis
Calculated results that represent a score or probability that was derived by algorithm
Organ or disease panels (80048-80076 [80081])
Therapeutic drug assays (80150-80299 [80164, 80165, 80171])

83695 **Lipoprotein (a)**
🚗 0.00 ⚕ 0.00 **FUD** XXX Q ☐
AMA: 2016,Jan,13; 2015,Jun,10; 2015,Apr,3; 2015,Jan,16; 2014,Jan,11

| 26/TC PC/TC Only | A2-Z3 ASC Payment | 50 Bilateral | ♂ Male Only | ♀ Female Only | 🚗 Facility RVU | ⚕ Non-Facility RVU | ☐ CCI |
| FUD Follow-up Days | CMS: IOM (Pub 100) | A-Y OPPSI | 80/80 Surg Assist Allowed / w/Doc | | ☒ Lab Crosswalk | ☒ Radiology Crosswalk | ☒ CLIA |

374   CPT © 2016 American Medical Association. All Rights Reserved.   © 2016 Optum360, LLC

83698	**Lipoprotein-associated phospholipase A2 (Lp-PLA2)**
	EXCLUDES Secretory type II phospholipase A2 (sPLA2-IIA) (0423T)
	0.00 0.00 **FUD** XXX [Q]
	AMA: 2015,Jun,10; 2015,Apr,3

83700	**Lipoprotein, blood; electrophoretic separation and quantitation**
	0.00 0.00 **FUD** XXX [Q] [▯]
	AMA: 2016,Jan,13; 2015,Jun,10; 2015,Apr,3; 2015,Jan,16; 2014,Jan,11

83701	**high resolution fractionation and quantitation of lipoproteins including lipoprotein subclasses when performed (eg, electrophoresis, ultracentrifugation)**
	0.00 0.00 **FUD** XXX [Q] [▯]
	AMA: 2016,Jan,13; 2015,Jun,10; 2015,Apr,3; 2015,Jan,16; 2014,Jan,11

▲ | 83704 | **quantitation of lipoprotein particle number(s) (eg, by nuclear magnetic resonance spectroscopy), includes lipoprotein particle subclass(es), when performed** |
| | 0.00   0.00   **FUD** XXX   [Q] [▯] |
| | **AMA:** 2016,Jan,13; 2015,Jun,10; 2015,Apr,3; 2015,Jan,16; 2014,Jan,11 |

83718	**Lipoprotein, direct measurement; high density cholesterol (HDL cholesterol)**
	0.00 0.00 **FUD** XXX [X] [A] [▯]
	AMA: 2016,Jan,13; 2015,Jun,10; 2015,Apr,3; 2015,Jan,16; 2014,Jan,11; 2013,Feb,3-6; 2012,Jan,15-42; 2011,Jan,11

83719	**VLDL cholesterol**
	0.00 0.00 **FUD** XXX [Q] [▯]
	AMA: 2016,Jan,13; 2015,Jun,10; 2015,Apr,3; 2015,Jan,16; 2014,Jan,11; 2013,Feb,3-6; 2012,Jan,15-42; 2011,Jan,11

83721	**LDL cholesterol**
	EXCLUDES Fractionation by high resolution electrophoresis or ultracentrifugation (83701)
	Lipoprotein particle numbers and subclasses analysis by nuclear magnetic resonance spectroscopy (83704)
	0.00 0.00 **FUD** XXX [X] [Q] [▯]
	AMA: 2016,Jan,13; 2015,Jun,10; 2015,Apr,3; 2015,Jan,16; 2014,Jan,11; 2013,Feb,3-6; 2012,Jan,15-42; 2011,Jan,11

83727	**Luteinizing releasing factor (LRH)**
	0.00 0.00 **FUD** XXX [Q]
	AMA: 2015,Jun,10; 2015,Apr,3

83735-83885 Chemistry: Magnesium—Nickel

INCLUDES Clinical information not requested by the ordering physician
Mathematically calculated results
Quantitative analysis unless otherwise specified
Specimens from any source unless otherwise specified

EXCLUDES Analytes from nonrequested laboratory analysis
Calculated results that represent a score or probability that was derived by algorithm
Organ or disease panels (80048-80076 [80081])
Therapeutic drug assays (80150-80299 [80164, 80165, 80171])

83735	**Magnesium**
	0.00 0.00 **FUD** XXX [Q]
	AMA: 2015,Jun,10; 2015,Apr,3

83775	**Malate dehydrogenase**
	0.00 0.00 **FUD** XXX [Q]
	AMA: 2015,Jun,10; 2015,Apr,3

83785	**Manganese**
	0.00 0.00 **FUD** XXX [Q]
	AMA: 2015,Jun,10; 2015,Apr,3

83789	**Mass spectrometry and tandem mass spectrometry (eg, MS, MS/MS, MALDI, MS-TOF, QTOF), non-drug analyte(s) not elsewhere specified, qualitative or quantitative, each specimen**
	EXCLUDES Procedure performed more than one time per specimen
	0.00 0.00 **FUD** XXX [Q]
	AMA: 2015,Jun,10; 2015,Apr,3

83825	**Mercury, quantitative**
	EXCLUDES Mercury screen (83015)
	0.00 0.00 **FUD** XXX [Q]
	AMA: 2015,Jun,10; 2015,Apr,3

83835	**Metanephrines**
	EXCLUDES Catecholamines (82382-82384)
	0.00 0.00 **FUD** XXX [Q]
	AMA: 2015,Jun,10; 2015,Apr,3

83857	**Methemalbumin**
	0.00 0.00 **FUD** XXX [Q]
	AMA: 2015,Jun,10; 2015,Apr,3

83861	**Microfluidic analysis utilizing an integrated collection and analysis device, tear osmolarity**
	Code also when performed on both eyes 83861 X 2
	0.00 0.00 **FUD** XXX [X] [Q] [▯]
	AMA: 2015,Jun,10; 2015,Apr,3

83864	**Mucopolysaccharides, acid, quantitative**
	0.00 0.00 **FUD** XXX [Q]
	AMA: 2015,Jun,10; 2015,Apr,3

83872	**Mucin, synovial fluid (Ropes test)**
	0.00 0.00 **FUD** XXX [Q]
	AMA: 2015,Jun,10; 2015,Apr,3

83873	**Myelin basic protein, cerebrospinal fluid**
	EXCLUDES Oligoclonal bands (83916)
	0.00 0.00 **FUD** XXX [Q]
	AMA: 2015,Jun,10; 2015,Apr,3

83874	**Myoglobin**
	0.00 0.00 **FUD** XXX [Q]
	AMA: 2016,Jan,13; 2015,Jun,10; 2015,Apr,3; 2015,Jan,16; 2014,Jan,11

83876	**Myeloperoxidase (MPO)**
	0.00 0.00 **FUD** XXX [Q] [▯]
	AMA: 2015,Jun,10; 2015,Apr,3

83880	**Natriuretic peptide**
	0.00 0.00 **FUD** XXX [X] [Q]
	AMA: 2016,Jan,13; 2015,Jun,10; 2015,Apr,3; 2015,Jan,16; 2014,Jan,11

83883	**Nephelometry, each analyte not elsewhere specified**
	0.00 0.00 **FUD** XXX [Q]
	AMA: 2015,Jun,10; 2015,Apr,3

83885	**Nickel**
	0.00 0.00 **FUD** XXX [Q]
	AMA: 2015,Jun,10; 2015,Apr,3

83915-84066 Chemistry: Nucleotidase 5'- —Phosphatase (Acid)

INCLUDES Clinical information not requested by the ordering physician
Mathematically calculated results
Quantitative analysis unless otherwise specified
Specimens from any source unless otherwise specified

EXCLUDES Analytes from nonrequested laboratory analysis
Calculated results that represent a score or probability that was derived by algorithm
Drug testing ([80305, 80306, 80307], [80324, 80325, 80326, 80327, 80328, 80329, 80330, 80331, 80332, 80333, 80334, 80335, 80336, 80337, 80338, 80339, 80340, 80341, 80342, 80343, 80344, 80345, 80346, 80347, 80348, 80349, 80350, 80351, 80352, 80353, 80354, 80355, 80356, 80357, 80358, 80359, 80360, 80361, 80362, 80363, 80364, 80365, 80366, 80367, 80368, 80369, 80370, 80371, 80372, 80373, 80374, 80375, 80376, 80377, 83992])
Organ or disease panels (80048-80076 [80081])
Therapeutic drug assays (80150-80299 [80164, 80165, 80171])

83915	**Nucleotidase 5'-**
	0.00 0.00 **FUD** XXX [Q]
	AMA: 2015,Jun,10; 2015,Apr,3

83916 Oligoclonal immune (oligoclonal bands)
🔹 0.00 ⚕ 0.00 **FUD** XXX Q ▯
AMA: 2015,Jun,10; 2015,Apr,3

83918 Organic acids; total, quantitative, each specimen
🔹 0.00 ⚕ 0.00 **FUD** XXX Q ▯
AMA: 2016,Jan,13; 2015,Jun,10; 2015,Apr,3; 2015,Jan,16; 2014,Jan,11; 2012,Jan,15-42; 2011,Jan,11

83919 qualitative, each specimen
🔹 0.00 ⚕ 0.00 **FUD** XXX Q
AMA: 2015,Jun,10; 2015,Apr,3

83921 Organic acid, single, quantitative
🔹 0.00 ⚕ 0.00 **FUD** XXX Q ▯
AMA: 2015,Jun,10; 2015,Apr,3

83930 Osmolality; blood
EXCLUDES Tear osmolarity (83861)
🔹 0.00 ⚕ 0.00 **FUD** XXX Q
AMA: 2015,Jun,10; 2015,Apr,3

83935 urine
EXCLUDES Tear osmolarity (83861)
🔹 0.00 ⚕ 0.00 **FUD** XXX Q
AMA: 2015,Jun,10; 2015,Apr,3

83937 Osteocalcin (bone g1a protein)
🔹 0.00 ⚕ 0.00 **FUD** XXX Q
AMA: 2016,Jan,13; 2015,Jun,10; 2015,Apr,3; 2015,Jan,16; 2014,Jan,11

83945 Oxalate
🔹 0.00 ⚕ 0.00 **FUD** XXX Q
AMA: 2015,Jun,10; 2015,Apr,3

83950 Oncoprotein; HER-2/neu
EXCLUDES Tissue (88342, 88365)
🔹 0.00 ⚕ 0.00 **FUD** XXX Q ▯
AMA: 2015,Jun,10; 2015,Apr,3

83951 des-gamma-carboxy-prothrombin (DCP)
🔹 0.00 ⚕ 0.00 **FUD** XXX Q ▯
AMA: 2015,Jun,10; 2015,Apr,3

83970 Parathormone (parathyroid hormone)
🔹 0.00 ⚕ 0.00 **FUD** XXX Q
AMA: 2015,Jun,10; 2015,Apr,3

83986 pH; body fluid, not otherwise specified
EXCLUDES Blood pH (82800, 82803)
🔹 0.00 ⚕ 0.00 **FUD** XXX ✖ Q
AMA: 2016,May,13; 2016,Jan,13; 2015,Jun,10; 2015,Apr,3; 2015,Jan,16; 2013,Sep,13-14

83987 exhaled breath condensate
🔹 0.00 ⚕ 0.00 **FUD** XXX Q ▯
AMA: 2015,Jun,10; 2015,Apr,3

83992 **Resequenced code. See code following 80365.**

83993 Calprotectin, fecal
🔹 0.00 ⚕ 0.00 **FUD** XXX Q
AMA: 2016,Jan,13; 2015,Jun,10; 2015,Apr,3; 2015,Jan,16; 2014,Jan,11

84030 Phenylalanine (PKU), blood
INCLUDES Guthrie test
EXCLUDES Phenylalanine-tyrosine ratio (84030, 84510)
🔹 0.00 ⚕ 0.00 **FUD** XXX Q
AMA: 2015,Jun,10; 2015,Apr,3

84035 Phenylketones, qualitative
🔹 0.00 ⚕ 0.00 **FUD** XXX Q
AMA: 2015,Jun,10; 2015,Apr,3

84060 Phosphatase, acid; total
🔹 0.00 ⚕ 0.00 **FUD** XXX Q
AMA: 2015,Jun,10; 2015,Apr,3

84061 forensic examination
🔹 0.00 ⚕ 0.00 **FUD** XXX Q
AMA: 2015,Jun,10; 2015,Apr,3

84066 prostatic
🔹 0.00 ⚕ 0.00 **FUD** XXX Q
AMA: 2015,Jun,10; 2015,Apr,3

84075-84080 Chemistry: Phosphatase (Alkaline)

CMS: 100-03,160.17 Payment for L-Dopa /Associated Inpatient Hospital Services

INCLUDES Clinical information not requested by the ordering physician
Mathematically calculated results
Quantitative analysis unless otherwise specified
Specimens from any source unless otherwise specified
EXCLUDES *Analytes from nonrequested laboratory analysis*
Calculated results that represent a score or probability that was derived by algorithm
Organ or disease panels (80048-80076 [80081])

84075 Phosphatase, alkaline;
🔹 0.00 ⚕ 0.00 **FUD** XXX ✖ Q
AMA: 2016,Jan,13; 2015,Jun,10; 2015,Apr,3; 2015,Jan,16; 2014,Jan,11

84078 heat stable (total not included)
🔹 0.00 ⚕ 0.00 **FUD** XXX Q
AMA: 2015,Jun,10; 2015,Apr,3

84080 isoenzymes
🔹 0.00 ⚕ 0.00 **FUD** XXX Q ▯
AMA: 2015,Jun,10; 2015,Apr,3

84081-84150 Chemistry: Phosphatidylglycerol—Prostaglandin

INCLUDES Clinical information not requested by the ordering physician
Mathematically calculated results
Quantitative analysis unless otherwise specified
Specimens from any source unless otherwise specified
EXCLUDES *Analytes from nonrequested laboratory analysis*
Calculated results that represent a score or probability that was derived by algorithm
Organ or disease panels (80048-80076 [80081])
Therapeutic drug assays (80150-80299 [80164, 80165, 80171])

84081 Phosphatidylglycerol
🔹 0.00 ⚕ 0.00 **FUD** XXX Q
AMA: 2015,Jun,10; 2015,Apr,3

84085 Phosphogluconate, 6-, dehydrogenase, RBC
🔹 0.00 ⚕ 0.00 **FUD** XXX Q
AMA: 2015,Jun,10; 2015,Apr,3

84087 Phosphohexose isomerase
🔹 0.00 ⚕ 0.00 **FUD** XXX Q
AMA: 2015,Jun,10; 2015,Apr,3

84100 Phosphorus inorganic (phosphate);
🔹 0.00 ⚕ 0.00 **FUD** XXX Q
AMA: 2016,Jan,13; 2015,Jun,10; 2015,Apr,3; 2015,Jan,16; 2014,Jan,11

84105 urine
🔹 0.00 ⚕ 0.00 **FUD** XXX Q
AMA: 2015,Jun,10; 2015,Apr,3

84106 Porphobilinogen, urine; qualitative
🔹 0.00 ⚕ 0.00 **FUD** XXX Q
AMA: 2015,Jun,10; 2015,Apr,3

84110 quantitative
🔹 0.00 ⚕ 0.00 **FUD** XXX Q
AMA: 2015,Jun,10; 2015,Apr,3

84112 Evaluation of cervicovaginal fluid for specific amniotic fluid protein(s) (eg, placental alpha microglobulin-1 [PAMG-1], placental protein 12 [PP12], alpha-fetoprotein), qualitative, each specimen ♀
🔹 0.00 ⚕ 0.00 **FUD** XXX Q ▯
AMA: 2015,Jun,10; 2015,Apr,3

84119 Porphyrins, urine; qualitative
🔹 0.00 ⚕ 0.00 **FUD** XXX Q
AMA: 2015,Jun,10; 2015,Apr,3

84120	**quantitation and fractionation**		
	🖧 0.00 ✑ 0.00 **FUD** XXX		Q
	AMA: 2015,Jun,10; 2015,Apr,3		

84126	**Porphyrins, feces, quantitative**		
	🖧 0.00 ✑ 0.00 **FUD** XXX		Q
	AMA: 2015,Jun,10; 2015,Apr,3		

84132	**Potassium; serum, plasma or whole blood**		
	🖧 0.00 ✑ 0.00 **FUD** XXX		☒ Q
	AMA: 2016,Jan,13; 2015,Jun,10; 2015,Apr,3; 2015,Jan,16; 2014,Jan,11; 2013,Apr,10-11		

84133	**urine**		
	🖧 0.00 ✑ 0.00 **FUD** XXX		Q
	AMA: 2015,Jun,10; 2015,Apr,3		

84134	**Prealbumin**		
	EXCLUDES Microalbumin (82043-82044)		
	🖧 0.00 ✑ 0.00 **FUD** XXX		Q
	AMA: 2015,Jun,10; 2015,Apr,3		

84135	**Pregnanediol**		♀
	🖧 0.00 ✑ 0.00 **FUD** XXX		Q
	AMA: 2015,Jun,10; 2015,Apr,3		

84138	**Pregnanetriol**		♀
	🖧 0.00 ✑ 0.00 **FUD** XXX		Q
	AMA: 2015,Jun,10; 2015,Apr,3		

84140	**Pregnenolone**		
	🖧 0.00 ✑ 0.00 **FUD** XXX		Q
	AMA: 2016,Jan,13; 2015,Jun,10; 2015,Apr,3; 2015,Jan,16; 2014,Jan,11		

84143	**17-hydroxypregnenolone**		
	🖧 0.00 ✑ 0.00 **FUD** XXX		Q
	AMA: 2016,Jan,13; 2015,Jun,10; 2015,Apr,3; 2015,Jan,16; 2014,Jan,11		

84144	**Progesterone**		
	EXCLUDES Progesterone receptor assay (84234)		
	🖧 0.00 ✑ 0.00 **FUD** XXX		Q
	AMA: 2015,Jun,10; 2015,Apr,3		

84145	**Procalcitonin (PCT)**		
	🖧 0.00 ✑ 0.00 **FUD** XXX		Q 🖵
	AMA: 2015,Jun,10; 2015,Apr,3		

84146	**Prolactin**		
	🖧 0.00 ✑ 0.00 **FUD** XXX		Q 🖵
	AMA: 2015,Jun,10; 2015,Apr,3		

84150	**Prostaglandin, each**		
	🖧 0.00 ✑ 0.00 **FUD** XXX		Q
	AMA: 2015,Jun,10; 2015,Apr,3		

84152-84154 Chemistry: Prostate Specific Antigen

CMS: 100-03,190.31 Prostate Specific Antigen (PSA); 100-03,210.1 Prostate Cancer Screening Tests

INCLUDES   Clinical information not requested by the ordering physician
Mathematically calculated results
Quantitative analysis unless otherwise specified

EXCLUDES   Analytes from nonrequested laboratory analysis
Calculated results that represent a score or probability that was derived by algorithm

84152	**Prostate specific antigen (PSA); complexed (direct measurement)**		♂
	🖧 0.00 ✑ 0.00 **FUD** XXX		Q
	AMA: 2015,Jun,10; 2015,Apr,3		

84153	**total**		♂
	🖧 0.00 ✑ 0.00 **FUD** XXX		Q
	AMA: 2016,Jan,13; 2015,Jun,10; 2015,Apr,3; 2015,Jan,16; 2014,Jan,11; 2012,Jan,15-42; 2011,Jan,11		

84154	**free**		♂
	🖧 0.00 ✑ 0.00 **FUD** XXX		Q
	AMA: 2016,Jan,13; 2015,Jun,10; 2015,Apr,3; 2015,Jan,16; 2014,Jan,11; 2012,Jan,15-42; 2011,Jan,11		

84155-84157 Chemistry: Protein, Total (Not by Refractometry)

INCLUDES   Clinical information not requested by the ordering physician
Mathematically calculated results

EXCLUDES   Analytes from nonrequested laboratory analysis
Calculated results that represent a score or probability that was derived by algorithm
Organ or disease panels (80048-80076 [80081])

84155	**Protein, total, except by refractometry; serum, plasma or whole blood**		
	🖧 0.00 ✑ 0.00 **FUD** XXX		☒ Q 🖵
	AMA: 2016,Jan,13; 2015,Jun,10; 2015,Apr,3; 2015,Jan,16; 2014,Jan,11		

84156	**urine**		
	🖧 0.00 ✑ 0.00 **FUD** XXX		Q
	AMA: 2015,Jun,10; 2015,Apr,3		

84157	**other source (eg, synovial fluid, cerebrospinal fluid)**		
	🖧 0.00 ✑ 0.00 **FUD** XXX		Q
	AMA: 2015,Jun,10; 2015,Apr,3		

84160-84432 Chemistry: Protein, Total (Refractometry)—Thyroglobulin

INCLUDES   Clinical information not requested by the ordering physician
Mathematically calculated results
Quantitative analysis unless otherwise specified
Specimens from any source unless otherwise specified

EXCLUDES   Analytes from nonrequested laboratory analysis
Calculated results that represent a score or probability that was derived by algorithm
Drug testing ([80305, 80306, 80307], [80324, 80325, 80326, 80327, 80328, 80329, 80330, 80331, 80332, 80333, 80334, 80335, 80336, 80337, 80338, 80339, 80340, 80341, 80342, 80343, 80344, 80345, 80346, 80347, 80348, 80349, 80350, 80351, 80352, 80353, 80354, 80355, 80356, 80357, 80358, 80359, 80360, 80361, 80362, 80363, 80364, 80365, 80366, 80367, 80368, 80369, 80370, 80371, 80372, 80373, 80374, 80375, 80376, 80377, 83992])
Organ or disease panels (80048-80076 [80081])
Therapeutic drug assays (80150-80299 [80164, 80165, 80171])

84160	**Protein, total, by refractometry, any source**		
	EXCLUDES Dipstick urine protein (81000-81003)		
	🖧 0.00 ✑ 0.00 **FUD** XXX		Q 🖵
	AMA: 2015,Jun,10; 2015,Apr,3		

84163	**Pregnancy-associated plasma protein-A (PAPP-A)**		♀
	🖧 0.00 ✑ 0.00 **FUD** XXX		Q
	AMA: 2015,Jun,10; 2015,Apr,3		

84165	**Protein; electrophoretic fractionation and quantitation, serum**		
	🖧 0.00 ✑ 0.00 **FUD** XXX		Q 🖵
	AMA: 2015,Jun,10; 2015,Apr,3		

84166	**electrophoretic fractionation and quantitation, other fluids with concentration (eg, urine, CSF)**		
	🖧 0.00 ✑ 0.00 **FUD** XXX		Q 🖵
	AMA: 2015,Jun,10; 2015,Apr,3		

84181	**Western Blot, with interpretation and report, blood or other body fluid**		
	🖧 0.00 ✑ 0.00 **FUD** XXX		Q 🖵
	AMA: 2015,Jun,10; 2015,Apr,3		

84182	**Western Blot, with interpretation and report, blood or other body fluid, immunological probe for band identification, each**		
	EXCLUDES Western Blot tissue testing (88371)		
	🖧 0.00 ✑ 0.00 **FUD** XXX		Q 🖵
	AMA: 2015,Jun,10; 2015,Apr,3		

84202	**Protoporphyrin, RBC; quantitative**		
	🖧 0.00 ✑ 0.00 **FUD** XXX		Q
	AMA: 2015,Jun,10; 2015,Apr,3		

84203	**screen**		
	🖧 0.00 ✑ 0.00 **FUD** XXX		Q
	AMA: 2015,Jun,10; 2015,Apr,3		

84206 **Proinsulin**
　🚜 0.00　🔧 0.00　**FUD** XXX　　Ⓠ
　AMA: 2015,Jun,10; 2015,Apr,3

84207 **Pyridoxal phosphate (Vitamin B-6)**
　🚜 0.00　🔧 0.00　**FUD** XXX　　Ⓠ🖵
　AMA: 2015,Jun,10; 2015,Apr,3

84210 **Pyruvate**
　🚜 0.00　🔧 0.00　**FUD** XXX　　Ⓠ
　AMA: 2015,Jun,10; 2015,Apr,3

84220 **Pyruvate kinase**
　🚜 0.00　🔧 0.00　**FUD** XXX　　Ⓠ
　AMA: 2015,Jun,10; 2015,Apr,3

84228 **Quinine**
　🚜 0.00　🔧 0.00　**FUD** XXX　　Ⓠ
　AMA: 2016,Jan,13; 2015,Jun,10; 2015,Apr,3

84233 **Receptor assay; estrogen**
　🚜 0.00　🔧 0.00　**FUD** XXX　　Ⓠ🖵
　AMA: 2015,Jun,10; 2015,Apr,3

84234 **progesterone**
　🚜 0.00　🔧 0.00　**FUD** XXX　　Ⓠ🖵
　AMA: 2015,Jun,10; 2015,Apr,3

84235 **endocrine, other than estrogen or progesterone (specify hormone)**
　🚜 0.00　🔧 0.00　**FUD** XXX　　Ⓠ🖵
　AMA: 2015,Jun,10; 2015,Apr,3

84238 **non-endocrine (specify receptor)**
　🚜 0.00　🔧 0.00　**FUD** XXX　　Ⓠ🖵
　AMA: 2016,Jan,13; 2015,Jun,10; 2015,Apr,3; 2015,Jan,16; 2014,Jan,11; 2012,Jan,15-42; 2011,Jan,11

84244 **Renin**
　🚜 0.00　🔧 0.00　**FUD** XXX　　Ⓠ🖵
　AMA: 2015,Jun,10; 2015,Apr,3

84252 **Riboflavin (Vitamin B-2)**
　🚜 0.00　🔧 0.00　**FUD** XXX　　Ⓠ🖵
　AMA: 2015,Jun,10; 2015,Apr,3

84255 **Selenium**
　🚜 0.00　🔧 0.00　**FUD** XXX　　Ⓠ
　AMA: 2015,Jun,10; 2015,Apr,3

84260 **Serotonin**
　EXCLUDES　*Urine metabolites (HIAA) (83497)*
　🚜 0.00　🔧 0.00　**FUD** XXX　　Ⓠ
　AMA: 2015,Jun,10; 2015,Apr,3

84270 **Sex hormone binding globulin (SHBG)**
　🚜 0.00　🔧 0.00　**FUD** XXX　　Ⓠ
　AMA: 2016,Jan,13; 2015,Jun,10; 2015,Apr,3; 2015,Jan,16; 2014,Jan,11

84275 **Sialic acid**
　🚜 0.00　🔧 0.00　**FUD** XXX　　Ⓠ
　AMA: 2015,Jun,10; 2015,Apr,3

84285 **Silica**
　🚜 0.00　🔧 0.00　**FUD** XXX　　Ⓠ
　AMA: 2015,Jun,10; 2015,Apr,3

84295 **Sodium; serum, plasma or whole blood**
　🚜 0.00　🔧 0.00　**FUD** XXX　　☒Ⓠ
　AMA: 2016,Jan,13; 2015,Jun,10; 2015,Apr,3; 2015,Jan,16; 2014,Jan,11; 2013,Apr,10-11

84300 **urine**
　🚜 0.00　🔧 0.00　**FUD** XXX　　Ⓠ
　AMA: 2015,Jun,10; 2015,Apr,3

84302 **other source**
　🚜 0.00　🔧 0.00　**FUD** XXX　　Ⓠ
　AMA: 2016,Jan,13; 2015,Jun,10; 2015,Apr,3; 2015,Jan,16; 2014,Jan,11

84305 **Somatomedin**
　🚜 0.00　🔧 0.00　**FUD** XXX　　Ⓠ
　AMA: 2016,Jan,13; 2015,Jun,10; 2015,Apr,3; 2015,Jan,16; 2014,Jan,11

84307 **Somatostatin**
　🚜 0.00　🔧 0.00　**FUD** XXX　　Ⓠ
　AMA: 2016,Jan,13; 2015,Jun,10; 2015,Apr,3; 2015,Jan,16; 2014,Jan,11

84311 **Spectrophotometry, analyte not elsewhere specified**
　🚜 0.00　🔧 0.00　**FUD** XXX　　Ⓠ
　AMA: 2015,Jun,10; 2015,Apr,3

84315 **Specific gravity (except urine)**
　EXCLUDES　*Urine specific gravity (81000-81003)*
　🚜 0.00　🔧 0.00　**FUD** XXX　　Ⓠ
　AMA: 2015,Jun,10; 2015,Apr,3

84375 **Sugars, chromatographic, TLC or paper chromatography**
　🚜 0.00　🔧 0.00　**FUD** XXX　　Ⓠ
　AMA: 2015,Jun,10; 2015,Apr,3

84376 **Sugars (mono-, di-, and oligosaccharides); single qualitative, each specimen**
　🚜 0.00　🔧 0.00　**FUD** XXX　　Ⓠ
　AMA: 2016,Jan,13; 2015,Jun,10; 2015,Apr,3; 2015,Jan,16; 2014,Jan,11

84377 **multiple qualitative, each specimen**
　🚜 0.00　🔧 0.00　**FUD** XXX　　Ⓠ🖵
　AMA: 2016,Jan,13; 2015,Jun,10; 2015,Apr,3; 2015,Jan,16; 2014,Jan,11

84378 **single quantitative, each specimen**
　🚜 0.00　🔧 0.00　**FUD** XXX　　Ⓠ🖵
　AMA: 2015,Jun,10; 2015,Apr,3

84379 **multiple quantitative, each specimen**
　🚜 0.00　🔧 0.00　**FUD** XXX　　Ⓠ🖵
　AMA: 2016,Jan,13; 2015,Jun,10; 2015,Apr,3; 2015,Jan,16; 2014,Jan,11

84392 **Sulfate, urine**
　🚜 0.00　🔧 0.00　**FUD** XXX　　Ⓠ
　AMA: 2015,Jun,10; 2015,Apr,3

84402 **Testosterone; free**
　EXCLUDES　*Anabolic steroids ([80327, 80328])*
　🚜 0.00　🔧 0.00　**FUD** XXX　　Ⓠ
　AMA: 2015,Jun,10; 2015,Apr,3

84403 **total**
　EXCLUDES　*Anabolic steroids ([80327, 80328])*
　🚜 0.00　🔧 0.00　**FUD** XXX　　Ⓠ🖵
　AMA: 2015,Jun,10; 2015,Apr,3

● **84410** **bioavailable, direct measurement (eg, differential precipitation)**

84425 **Thiamine (Vitamin B-1)**
　🚜 0.00　🔧 0.00　**FUD** XXX　　Ⓠ🖵
　AMA: 2015,Jun,10; 2015,Apr,3

84430 **Thiocyanate**
　🚜 0.00　🔧 0.00　**FUD** XXX　　Ⓠ
　AMA: 2015,Jun,10; 2015,Apr,3

84431 **Thromboxane metabolite(s), including thromboxane if performed, urine**
　Code also for determination of concurrent urine creatinine (82570)
　🚜 0.00　🔧 0.00　**FUD** XXX　　Ⓠ
　AMA: 2015,Jun,10; 2015,Apr,3

84432 **Thyroglobulin**
　EXCLUDES　*Thyroglobulin antibody (86800)*
　🚜 0.00　🔧 0.00　**FUD** XXX　　Ⓠ
　AMA: 2016,Jan,13; 2015,Jun,10; 2015,Apr,3; 2015,Jan,16; 2014,Jan,11

| 26/TC PC/TC Only | A2-Z3 ASC Payment | 50 Bilateral | ♂ Male Only | ♀ Female Only | 🚜 Facility RVU | 🔧 Non-Facility RVU | 🖵 CCI |
| FUD Follow-up Days | CMS: IOM (Pub 100) | A-Y OPPSI | 80/80 Surg Assist Allowed / w/Doc | | 🗎 Lab Crosswalk | ☒ Radiology Crosswalk | ☒ CLIA |

378　　　　CPT © 2016 American Medical Association. All Rights Reserved.　　　　© 2016 Optum360, LLC

84436-84445 Chemistry: Thyroid Tests

CMS: 100-03,190.22 Thyroid Testing

INCLUDES　Clinical information not requested by the ordering physician
Mathematically calculated results
Quantitative analysis unless otherwise specified
Specimens from any source unless otherwise specified

EXCLUDES　Analytes from nonrequested laboratory analysis
Calculated results that represent a score or probability that was derived by algorithm
Organ or disease panels (80048-80076 [80081])
Therapeutic drug assays (80150-80299 [80164, 80165, 80171])

84436　Thyroxine; total
　0.00　　0.00　**FUD** XXX
　AMA: 2016,Jan,13; 2015,Jun,10; 2015,Apr,3; 2015,Jan,16; 2014,Jan,11

84437　requiring elution (eg, neonatal)
　0.00　　0.00　**FUD** XXX
　AMA: 2015,Jun,10; 2015,Apr,3

84439　free
　0.00　　0.00　**FUD** XXX
　AMA: 2015,Jun,10; 2015,Apr,3

84442　Thyroxine binding globulin (TBG)
　0.00　　0.00　**FUD** XXX
　AMA: 2015,Jun,10; 2015,Apr,3

84443　Thyroid stimulating hormone (TSH)
　0.00　　0.00　**FUD** XXX
　AMA: 2015,Jun,10; 2015,Apr,3

84445　Thyroid stimulating immune globulins (TSI)
　0.00　　0.00　**FUD** XXX
　AMA: 2016,Jan,13; 2015,Jun,10; 2015,Apr,3; 2015,Jan,16; 2014,Jan,11

84446-84449 Chemistry: Tocopherol Alpha—Transcortin

INCLUDES　Clinical information not requested by the ordering physician
Mathematically calculated results
Quantitative analysis unless otherwise specified
Specimens from any source unless otherwise specified

EXCLUDES　Analytes from nonrequested laboratory analysis
Calculated results that represent a score or probability that was derived by algorithm
Organ or disease panels (80048-80076 [80081])
Therapeutic drug assays (80150-80299 [80164, 80165, 80171])

84446　Tocopherol alpha (Vitamin E)
　0.00　　0.00　**FUD** XXX
　AMA: 2015,Jun,10; 2015,Apr,3

84449　Transcortin (cortisol binding globulin)
　0.00　　0.00　**FUD** XXX
　AMA: 2016,Jan,13; 2015,Jun,10; 2015,Apr,3; 2015,Jan,16; 2014,Jan,11

84450-84460 Chemistry: Transferase

CMS: 100-02,11,30.2.2 Automated Multi-Channel Chemistry (AMCC) Tests; 100-03,160.17 Payment for L-Dopa /Associated Inpatient Hospital Services; 100-04,16,40.6.1 Automated Multi-Channel Chemistry (AMCC) Tests for ESRD Beneficiaries; 100-04,16,70.8 CLIA Waived Tests

INCLUDES　Clinical information not requested by the ordering physician
Mathematically calculated results
Quantitative analysis unless otherwise specified

EXCLUDES　Analytes from nonrequested laboratory analysis
Calculated results that represent a score or probability that was derived by algorithm

84450　Transferase; aspartate amino (AST) (SGOT)
　0.00　　0.00　**FUD** XXX
　AMA: 2016,Jan,13; 2015,Jun,10; 2015,Apr,3; 2015,Jan,16; 2014,Jan,11

84460　alanine amino (ALT) (SGPT)
　0.00　　0.00　**FUD** XXX
　AMA: 2016,Jan,13; 2015,Jun,10; 2015,Apr,3; 2015,Jan,16; 2014,Jan,11

84466 Chemistry: Transferrin

CMS: 100-02,11,20.2 ESRD Laboratory Services; 100-03,190.18 Serum Iron Studies

INCLUDES　Clinical information not requested by the ordering physician
Mathematically calculated results
Quantitative analysis unless otherwise specified

EXCLUDES　Analytes from nonrequested laboratory analysis
Calculated results that represent a score or probability that was derived by algorithm

84466　Transferrin
　EXCLUDES　Iron binding capacity (83550)
　0.00　　0.00　**FUD** XXX
　AMA: 2016,Jan,13; 2015,Jun,10; 2015,Apr,3; 2015,Jan,16; 2014,Jan,11

84478 Chemistry: Triglycerides

CMS: 100-02,11,30.2.2 Automated Multi-Channel Chemistry (AMCC) Tests; 100-03,190.23 Lipid Testing; 100-04,16,70.8 CLIA Waived Tests

INCLUDES　Clinical information not requested by the ordering physician
Mathematically calculated results

EXCLUDES　Analytes from nonrequested laboratory analysis
Calculated results that represent a score or probability that was derived by algorithm
Organ or disease panels (80048-80076 [80081])

84478　Triglycerides
　0.00　　0.00　**FUD** XXX
　AMA: 2016,Jan,13; 2015,Jun,10; 2015,Apr,3; 2015,Jan,16; 2014,Jan,11; 2012,Jan,15-42; 2011,Jan,11

84479-84482 Chemistry: Thyroid Hormone—Triiodothyronine

CMS: 100-03,190.22 Thyroid Testing

INCLUDES　Clinical information not requested by the ordering physician
Mathematically calculated results
Quantitative analysis unless otherwise specified
Specimens from any source unless otherwise specified

EXCLUDES　Analytes from nonrequested laboratory analysis
Calculated results that represent a score or probability that was derived by algorithm
Organ or disease panels (80048-80076 [80081])

84479　Thyroid hormone (T3 or T4) uptake or thyroid hormone binding ratio (THBR)
　0.00　　0.00　**FUD** XXX
　AMA: 2016,Jan,13; 2015,Jun,10; 2015,Apr,3; 2015,Jan,16; 2014,Jan,11

84480　Triiodothyronine T3; total (TT-3)
　0.00　　0.00　**FUD** XXX
　AMA: 2015,Jun,10; 2015,Apr,3

84481　free
　0.00　　0.00　**FUD** XXX
　AMA: 2015,Jun,10; 2015,Apr,3

84482　reverse
　0.00　　0.00　**FUD** XXX
　AMA: 2016,Jan,13; 2015,Jun,10; 2015,Apr,3; 2015,Jan,16; 2014,Jan,11

84484-84512 Chemistry: Troponin (Quantitative)—Troponin (Qualitative)

INCLUDES　Clinical information not requested by the ordering physician
Mathematically calculated results
Specimens from any source unless otherwise specified

EXCLUDES　Analytes from nonrequested laboratory analysis
Calculated results that represent a score or probability that was derived by algorithm
Organ or disease panels

84484　Troponin, quantitative
　EXCLUDES　Qualitative troponin assay (84512)
　0.00　　0.00　**FUD** XXX
　AMA: 2016,Jan,13; 2015,Jun,10; 2015,Apr,3; 2015,Jan,16; 2014,Jan,11

84485　Trypsin; duodenal fluid
　0.00　　0.00　**FUD** XXX
　AMA: 2015,Jun,10; 2015,Apr,3

84488 **feces, qualitative**
🚑 0.00   ⚕ 0.00   **FUD** XXX   Q
AMA: 2015,Jun,10; 2015,Apr,3

84490 **feces, quantitative, 24-hour collection**
🚑 0.00   ⚕ 0.00   **FUD** XXX   Q
AMA: 2015,Jun,10; 2015,Apr,3

84510 **Tyrosine**
EXCLUDES   Urate crystal identification (89060)
🚑 0.00   ⚕ 0.00   **FUD** XXX   Q
AMA: 2015,Jun,10; 2015,Apr,3

84512 **Troponin, qualitative**
EXCLUDES   Quantitative troponin assay (84484)
🚑 0.00   ⚕ 0.00   **FUD** XXX   Q
AMA: 2016,Jan,13; 2015,Jun,10; 2015,Apr,3; 2015,Jan,16; 2014,Jan,11

84520-84525 Chemistry: Urea Nitrogen (Blood)

CMS: 100-03,160.17 Payment for L-Dopa /Associated Inpatient Hospital Services
INCLUDES   Clinical information not requested by the ordering physician
Mathematically calculated results
EXCLUDES   Analytes from nonrequested laboratory analysis
Calculated results that represent a score or probability that was derived by algorithm
Organ or disease panels (80048-80076 [80081])

84520 **Urea nitrogen; quantitative**
🚑 0.00   ⚕ 0.00   **FUD** XXX   X Q
AMA: 2016,Jan,13; 2015,Jun,10; 2015,Apr,3; 2015,Jan,16; 2014,Jan,11; 2013,Apr,10-11

84525 **semiquantitative (eg, reagent strip test)**
INCLUDES   Patterson's test
🚑 0.00   ⚕ 0.00   **FUD** XXX   Q
AMA: 2016,Jan,13; 2015,Jun,10; 2015,Apr,3; 2015,Jan,16; 2014,Jan,11

84540-84630 Chemistry: Urea Nitrogen (Urine)—Zinc

INCLUDES   Clinical information not requested by the ordering physician
Mathematically calculated results
Quantitative analysis unless otherwise specified
Specimens from any source unless otherwise specified
EXCLUDES   Analytes from nonrequested laboratory analysis
Calculated results that represent a score or probability that was derived by algorithm
Organ or disease panels (80048-80076 [80081])
Therapeutic drug assays (80150-80299 [80164, 80165, 80171])

84540 **Urea nitrogen, urine**
🚑 0.00   ⚕ 0.00   **FUD** XXX   Q
AMA: 2015,Jun,10; 2015,Apr,3

84545 **Urea nitrogen, clearance**
🚑 0.00   ⚕ 0.00   **FUD** XXX   Q
AMA: 2015,Jun,10; 2015,Apr,3

84550 **Uric acid; blood**
🚑 0.00   ⚕ 0.00   **FUD** XXX   X Q
AMA: 2016,Jan,13; 2015,Jun,10; 2015,Apr,3; 2015,Jan,16; 2014,Jan,11

84560 **other source**
🚑 0.00   ⚕ 0.00   **FUD** XXX   Q
AMA: 2015,Jun,10; 2015,Apr,3

84577 **Urobilinogen, feces, quantitative**
🚑 0.00   ⚕ 0.00   **FUD** XXX   Q
AMA: 2015,Jun,10; 2015,Apr,3

84578 **Urobilinogen, urine; qualitative**
🚑 0.00   ⚕ 0.00   **FUD** XXX   Q
AMA: 2015,Jun,10; 2015,Apr,3

84580 **quantitative, timed specimen**
🚑 0.00   ⚕ 0.00   **FUD** XXX   Q ☐
AMA: 2015,Jun,10; 2015,Apr,3

84583 **semiquantitative**
🚑 0.00   ⚕ 0.00   **FUD** XXX   Q
AMA: 2015,Jun,10; 2015,Apr,3

84585 **Vanillylmandelic acid (VMA), urine**
🚑 0.00   ⚕ 0.00   **FUD** XXX   Q
AMA: 2015,Jun,10; 2015,Apr,3

84586 **Vasoactive intestinal peptide (VIP)**
🚑 0.00   ⚕ 0.00   **FUD** XXX   Q
AMA: 2016,Jan,13; 2015,Jun,10; 2015,Apr,3; 2015,Jan,16; 2014,Jan,11

84588 **Vasopressin (antidiuretic hormone, ADH)**
🚑 0.00   ⚕ 0.00   **FUD** XXX   Q
AMA: 2015,Jun,10; 2015,Apr,3

84590 **Vitamin A**
🚑 0.00   ⚕ 0.00   **FUD** XXX   Q ☐
AMA: 2015,Jun,10; 2015,Apr,3

84591 **Vitamin, not otherwise specified**
🚑 0.00   ⚕ 0.00   **FUD** XXX   Q
AMA: 2015,Jun,10; 2015,Apr,3

84597 **Vitamin K**
🚑 0.00   ⚕ 0.00   **FUD** XXX   Q ☐
AMA: 2015,Jun,10; 2015,Apr,3

84600 **Volatiles (eg, acetic anhydride, diethylether)**
EXCLUDES   Carbon tetrachloride, dichloroethane, dichloromethane (82441)
Isopropyl alcohol and methanol ([80320])
🚑 0.00   ⚕ 0.00   **FUD** XXX   Q
AMA: 2015,Jun,10; 2015,Apr,3

84620 **Xylose absorption test, blood and/or urine**
EXCLUDES   Administration (99070)
🚑 0.00   ⚕ 0.00   **FUD** XXX   Q ☐
AMA: 2015,Jun,10; 2015,Apr,3

84630 **Zinc**
🚑 0.00   ⚕ 0.00   **FUD** XXX   Q
AMA: 2015,Jun,10; 2015,Apr,3

84681-84999 Other and Unlisted Chemistry Tests

INCLUDES   Clinical information not requested by the ordering physician
Mathematically calculated results
Quantitative analysis unless otherwise specified
Specimens from any source unless otherwise specified
EXCLUDES   Analytes from nonrequested laboratory analysis
Calculated results that represent a score or probability that was derived by algorithm
Confirmational testing of a not otherwise specified drug ([80375, 80376, 80377], 80299)
Organ or disease panels (80048-80076 [80081])

84681 **C-peptide**
🚑 0.00   ⚕ 0.00   **FUD** XXX   Q ☐
AMA: 2015,Jun,10; 2015,Apr,3

84702 **Gonadotropin, chorionic (hCG); quantitative**
🚑 0.00   ⚕ 0.00   **FUD** XXX   Q ☐
AMA: 2015,Jun,10; 2015,Apr,3

84703 **qualitative**
EXCLUDES   Urine pregnancy test by visual color comparison (81025)
🚑 0.00   ⚕ 0.00   **FUD** XXX   X Q
AMA: 2015,Jun,10; 2015,Apr,3

84704 **free beta chain**
🚑 0.00   ⚕ 0.00   **FUD** XXX   Q
AMA: 2016,Jan,13; 2015,Jun,10; 2015,Apr,3; 2015,Jan,16; 2014,Jan,11; 2012,Jan,15-42; 2011,Jan,11

84830 **Ovulation tests, by visual color comparison methods for human luteinizing hormone** ♀
🚑 0.00   ⚕ 0.00   **FUD** XXX   X Q
AMA: 2016,Jan,13; 2015,Jun,10; 2015,Apr,3

84999 **Unlisted chemistry procedure**
🚑 0.00   ⚕ 0.00   **FUD** XXX   Q
AMA: 2016,Jan,13; 2015,Apr,3; 2015,Jan,16; 2014,Jan,11; 2012,Jan,15-42; 2011,Jan,11

85002 Bleeding Time Test

EXCLUDES Agglutinins (86000, 86156-86157)
Antiplasmin (85410)
Antithrombin III (85300-85301)
Blood banking procedures (86850-86999)

85002   **Bleeding time**
0.00   0.00   **FUD** XXX   Q
AMA: 2016,Jan,13; 2015,Jan,16; 2014,Jan,11

85004-85049 Blood Counts

CMS: 100-03,190.15 Blood Counts

EXCLUDES Agglutinins (86000, 86156-86157)
Antiplasmin (85410)
Antithrombin III (85300-85301)
Blood banking procedures (86850-86999)

85004   **Blood count; automated differential WBC count**
0.00   0.00   **FUD** XXX   Q ▣
AMA: 2016,Jan,13; 2015,Jan,16; 2014,Jan,11; 2012,Jan,15-42;
2011,Jan,11

85007   **blood smear, microscopic examination with manual differential WBC count**
0.00   0.00   **FUD** XXX   Q ▣
AMA: 2016,Jan,13; 2015,Jan,16; 2014,Jan,11; 2012,Jan,15-42;
2011,Jan,11

85008   **blood smear, microscopic examination without manual differential WBC count**
EXCLUDES Cell count other fluids (eg, CSF) (89050-89051)
0.00   0.00   **FUD** XXX   Q ▣
AMA: 2016,Jan,13; 2015,Jan,16; 2014,Jan,11; 2012,Jan,15-42;
2011,Jan,11

85009   **manual differential WBC count, buffy coat**
EXCLUDES Eosinophils, nasal smear (89190)
0.00   0.00   **FUD** XXX   Q ▣
AMA: 2016,Jan,13; 2015,Jan,16; 2014,Jan,11; 2012,Jan,15-42;
2011,Jan,11

85013   **spun microhematocrit**
0.00   0.00   **FUD** XXX   ✗ Q ▣
AMA: 2005,Aug,7-8; 2005,Jul,11-12

85014   **hematocrit (Hct)**
0.00   0.00   **FUD** XXX   ✗ Q ▣
AMA: 2016,Jan,13; 2015,Jan,16; 2014,Jan,11

85018   **hemoglobin (Hgb)**
EXCLUDES Immunoassay, hemoglobin, fecal (82274)
Other hemoglobin determination (83020-83069)
Transcutaneous hemoglobin measurement (88738)
0.00   0.00   **FUD** XXX   ✗ Q ▣
AMA: 2016,Jan,13; 2015,Jan,16; 2014,Jan,11

85025   **complete (CBC), automated (Hgb, Hct, RBC, WBC and platelet count) and automated differential WBC count**
0.00   0.00   **FUD** XXX   Q ▣
AMA: 2016,Jan,13; 2015,Jan,16; 2014,Jan,11; 2012,Jan,15-42;
2011,Jul,16-17; 2011,Jan,11

85027   **complete (CBC), automated (Hgb, Hct, RBC, WBC and platelet count)**
0.00   0.00   **FUD** XXX   Q ▣
AMA: 2016,Jan,13; 2015,Jan,16; 2014,Jan,11

85032   **manual cell count (erythrocyte, leukocyte, or platelet) each**
0.00   0.00   **FUD** XXX   Q ▣
AMA: 2016,Jan,13; 2015,Jan,16; 2014,Jan,11; 2012,Jan,15-42;
2011,Jan,11

85041   **red blood cell (RBC), automated**
EXCLUDES Complete blood count (85025, 85027)
0.00   0.00   **FUD** XXX   Q ▣
AMA: 2016,Jan,13; 2015,Jan,16; 2014,Jan,11

85044   **reticulocyte, manual**
0.00   0.00   **FUD** XXX   Q
AMA: 2016,Jan,13; 2015,Jan,16; 2014,Jan,11

85045   **reticulocyte, automated**
0.00   0.00   **FUD** XXX   Q ▣
AMA: 2016,Jan,13; 2015,Jan,16; 2014,Jan,11

85046   **reticulocytes, automated, including 1 or more cellular parameters (eg, reticulocyte hemoglobin content [CHr], immature reticulocyte fraction [IRF], reticulocyte volume [MRV], RNA content), direct measurement**
0.00   0.00   **FUD** XXX   Q ▣
AMA: 2005,Aug,7-8; 2005,Jul,11-12

85048   **leukocyte (WBC), automated**
0.00   0.00   **FUD** XXX   Q ▣
AMA: 2016,Jan,13; 2015,Jan,16; 2014,Jan,11

85049   **platelet, automated**
0.00   0.00   **FUD** XXX   Q ▣
AMA: 2005,Aug,7-8; 2005,Jul,11-12

85055-85705 Coagulopathy Testing

EXCLUDES Agglutinins (86000, 86156-86157)
Antiplasmin (85410)
Antithrombin III (85300-85301)
Blood banking procedures (86850-86999)

85055   **Reticulated platelet assay**
0.00   0.00   **FUD** XXX   Q
AMA: 2005,Aug,7-8; 2005,Jul,11-12

85060   **Blood smear, peripheral, interpretation by physician with written report**
0.71   0.71   **FUD** XXX   B 80
AMA: 2005,Aug,7-8; 2005,Jul,11-12

85097   **Bone marrow, smear interpretation**
EXCLUDES Bone biopsy (20220, 20225, 20240, 20245, 20250-20251)
Special stains (88312-88313)
1.42   2.54   **FUD** XXX   Q2 80
AMA: 2016,Jan,13; 2015,Jan,16; 2014,Jan,11; 2012,Jan,15-42;
2011,Jan,11

85130   **Chromogenic substrate assay**
0.00   0.00   **FUD** XXX   Q ▣
AMA: 2005,Aug,7-8; 2005,Jul,11-12

85170   **Clot retraction**
0.00   0.00   **FUD** XXX   Q ▣
AMA: 2005,Aug,7-8; 2005,Jul,11-12

85175   **Clot lysis time, whole blood dilution**
0.00   0.00   **FUD** XXX   Q ▣
AMA: 2005,Aug,7-8; 2005,Jul,11-12

85210   **Clotting; factor II, prothrombin, specific**
EXCLUDES Prothrombin time (85610-85611)
Russell viper venom time (85612-85613)
0.00   0.00   **FUD** XXX   Q ▣
AMA: 2005,Aug,7-8; 2005,Jul,11-12

85220   **factor V (AcG or proaccelerin), labile factor**
0.00   0.00   **FUD** XXX   Q ▣
AMA: 2005,Aug,7-8; 2005,Jul,11-12

85230   **factor VII (proconvertin, stable factor)**
0.00   0.00   **FUD** XXX   Q ▣
AMA: 2005,Aug,7-8; 2005,Jul,11-12

85240   **factor VIII (AHG), 1-stage**
0.00   0.00   **FUD** XXX   Q ▣
AMA: 2005,Aug,7-8; 2005,Jul,11-12

85244   **factor VIII related antigen**
0.00   0.00   **FUD** XXX   Q ▣
AMA: 2005,Aug,7-8; 2005,Jul,11-12

85245   **factor VIII, VW factor, ristocetin cofactor**
0.00   0.00   **FUD** XXX   Q ▣
AMA: 2005,Aug,7-8; 2005,Jul,11-12

85246   **factor VIII, VW factor antigen**
0.00   0.00   **FUD** XXX   Q ▣
AMA: 2005,Aug,7-8; 2005,Jul,11-12

85247 **factor VIII, von Willebrand factor, multimetric analysis**
🔧 0.00 ⚖ 0.00 **FUD** XXX   ⓠ⊡
AMA: 2005,Aug,7-8; 2005,Jul,11-12

85250 **factor IX (PTC or Christmas)**
🔧 0.00 ⚖ 0.00 **FUD** XXX   ⓠ⊡
AMA: 2005,Aug,7-8; 2005,Jul,11-12

85260 **factor X (Stuart-Prower)**
🔧 0.00 ⚖ 0.00 **FUD** XXX   ⓠ⊡
AMA: 2005,Aug,7-8; 2005,Jul,11-12

85270 **factor XI (PTA)**
🔧 0.00 ⚖ 0.00 **FUD** XXX   ⓠ⊡
AMA: 2005,Aug,7-8; 2005,Jul,11-12

85280 **factor XII (Hageman)**
🔧 0.00 ⚖ 0.00 **FUD** XXX   ⓠ⊡
AMA: 2005,Aug,7-8; 2005,Jul,11-12

85290 **factor XIII (fibrin stabilizing)**
🔧 0.00 ⚖ 0.00 **FUD** XXX   ⓠ⊡
AMA: 2005,Aug,7-8; 2005,Jul,11-12

85291 **factor XIII (fibrin stabilizing), screen solubility**
🔧 0.00 ⚖ 0.00 **FUD** XXX   ⓠ⊡
AMA: 2005,Aug,7-8; 2005,Jul,11-12

85292 **prekallikrein assay (Fletcher factor assay)**
🔧 0.00 ⚖ 0.00 **FUD** XXX   ⓠ⊡
AMA: 2005,Aug,7-8; 2005,Jul,11-12

85293 **high molecular weight kininogen assay (Fitzgerald factor assay)**
🔧 0.00 ⚖ 0.00 **FUD** XXX   ⓠ⊡
AMA: 2005,Aug,7-8; 2005,Jul,11-12

85300 **Clotting inhibitors or anticoagulants; antithrombin III, activity**
🔧 0.00 ⚖ 0.00 **FUD** XXX   ⓠ⊡
AMA: 2005,Aug,7-8; 2005,Jul,11-12

85301 **antithrombin III, antigen assay**
🔧 0.00 ⚖ 0.00 **FUD** XXX   ⓠ⊡
AMA: 2005,Aug,7-8; 2005,Jul,11-12

85302 **protein C, antigen**
🔧 0.00 ⚖ 0.00 **FUD** XXX   ⓠ⊡
AMA: 2005,Aug,7-8; 2005,Jul,11-12

85303 **protein C, activity**
🔧 0.00 ⚖ 0.00 **FUD** XXX   ⓠ⊡
AMA: 2005,Aug,7-8; 2005,Jul,11-12

85305 **protein S, total**
🔧 0.00 ⚖ 0.00 **FUD** XXX   ⓠ⊡
AMA: 2005,Jul,11-12; 2005,Aug,7-8

85306 **protein S, free**
🔧 0.00 ⚖ 0.00 **FUD** XXX   ⓠ⊡
AMA: 2005,Aug,7-8; 2005,Jul,11-12

85307 **Activated Protein C (APC) resistance assay**
🔧 0.00 ⚖ 0.00 **FUD** XXX   ⓠ⊡
AMA: 2005,Aug,7-8; 2005,Jul,11-12

85335 **Factor inhibitor test**
🔧 0.00 ⚖ 0.00 **FUD** XXX   ⓠ⊡
AMA: 2005,Aug,7-8; 2005,Jul,11-12

85337 **Thrombomodulin**
EXCLUDES *Mixing studies for inhibitors (85732)*
🔧 0.00 ⚖ 0.00 **FUD** XXX   ⓠ⊡
AMA: 2005,Aug,7-8; 2005,Jul,11-12

85345 **Coagulation time; Lee and White**
🔧 0.00 ⚖ 0.00 **FUD** XXX   ⓠ⊡
AMA: 2005,Aug,7-8; 2005,Jul,11-12

85347 **activated**
🔧 0.00 ⚖ 0.00 **FUD** XXX   ⓠ⊡
AMA: 2005,Aug,7-8; 2005,Jul,11-12

85348 **other methods**
🔧 0.00 ⚖ 0.00 **FUD** XXX   ⓠ⊡
AMA: 2005,Aug,7-8; 2005,Jul,11-12

85360 **Euglobulin lysis**
🔧 0.00 ⚖ 0.00 **FUD** XXX   ⓠ⊡
AMA: 2005,Aug,7-8; 2005,Jul,11-12

85362 **Fibrin(ogen) degradation (split) products (FDP) (FSP); agglutination slide, semiquantitative**
EXCLUDES *Immunoelectrophoresis (86320)*
🔧 0.00 ⚖ 0.00 **FUD** XXX   ⓠ⊡
AMA: 2005,Aug,7-8; 2005,Jul,11-12

85366 **paracoagulation**
🔧 0.00 ⚖ 0.00 **FUD** XXX   ⓠ⊡
AMA: 2005,Aug,7-8; 2005,Jul,11-12

85370 **quantitative**
🔧 0.00 ⚖ 0.00 **FUD** XXX   ⓠ⊡
AMA: 2005,Aug,7-8; 2005,Jul,11-12

85378 **Fibrin degradation products, D-dimer; qualitative or semiquantitative**
🔧 0.00 ⚖ 0.00 **FUD** XXX   ⓠ⊡
AMA: 2016,Jan,13; 2015,Jan,16; 2014,Jan,11

85379 **quantitative**
INCLUDES Ultrasensitive and standard sensitivity quantitative D-dimer
🔧 0.00 ⚖ 0.00 **FUD** XXX   ⓠ⊡
AMA: 2005,Aug,7-8; 2005,Jul,11-12

85380 **ultrasensitive (eg, for evaluation for venous thromboembolism), qualitative or semiquantitative**
🔧 0.00 ⚖ 0.00 **FUD** XXX   ⓠ⊡
AMA: 2016,Jan,13; 2015,Jan,16; 2014,Jan,11

85384 **Fibrinogen; activity**
🔧 0.00 ⚖ 0.00 **FUD** XXX   ⓠ⊡
AMA: 2005,Jul,11-12; 2005,Aug,7-8

85385 **antigen**
🔧 0.00 ⚖ 0.00 **FUD** XXX   ⓠ⊡
AMA: 2005,Jul,11-12; 2005,Aug,7-8

85390 **Fibrinolysins or coagulopathy screen, interpretation and report**
🔧 0.00 ⚖ 0.00 **FUD** XXX   ⓠ⊡
AMA: 2005,Jul,11-12; 2005,Aug,7-8

85396 **Coagulation/fibrinolysis assay, whole blood (eg, viscoelastic clot assessment), including use of any pharmacologic additive(s), as indicated, including interpretation and written report, per day**
🔧 0.59 ⚖ 0.59 **FUD** XXX   Ⓝ⑧⓪
AMA: 2005,Aug,7-8; 2005,Jul,11-12

85397 **Coagulation and fibrinolysis, functional activity, not otherwise specified (eg, ADAMTS-13), each analyte**
🔧 0.00 ⚖ 0.00 **FUD** XXX   ⓠ

85400 **Fibrinolytic factors and inhibitors; plasmin**
🔧 0.00 ⚖ 0.00 **FUD** XXX   ⓠ⊡
AMA: 2005,Aug,7-8; 2005,Jul,11-12

85410 **alpha-2 antiplasmin**
🔧 0.00 ⚖ 0.00 **FUD** XXX   ⓠ⊡
AMA: 2005,Aug,7-8; 2005,Jul,11-12

85415 **plasminogen activator**
🔧 0.00 ⚖ 0.00 **FUD** XXX   ⓠ⊡
AMA: 2005,Aug,7-8; 2005,Jul,11-12

85420 **plasminogen, except antigenic assay**
🔧 0.00 ⚖ 0.00 **FUD** XXX   ⓠ⊡
AMA: 2005,Aug,7-8; 2005,Jul,11-12

85421 **plasminogen, antigenic assay**
🔧 0.00 ⚖ 0.00 **FUD** XXX   ⓠ⊡
AMA: 2005,Aug,7-8; 2005,Jul,11-12

85441   **Heinz bodies; direct**
    🚗 0.00   ♙ 0.00   **FUD** XXX   Q ▢
    AMA: 2005,Aug,7-8; 2005,Jul,11-12

85445   **induced, acetyl phenylhydrazine**
    🚗 0.00   ♙ 0.00   **FUD** XXX   Q ▢
    AMA: 2005,Aug,7-8; 2005,Jul,11-12

85460   **Hemoglobin or RBCs, fetal, for fetomaternal hemorrhage; differential lysis (Kleihauer-Betke)**   Ⓜ ♀
    EXCLUDES   *Hemoglobin F (83030, 83033)*
                     Hemolysins (86940-86941)
    🚗 0.00   ♙ 0.00   **FUD** XXX   Q ▢
    AMA: 2016,Jan,13; 2015,Jan,16; 2014,Jan,11

85461   **rosette**   Ⓜ ♀
    🚗 0.00   ♙ 0.00   **FUD** XXX   Q ▢
    AMA: 2005,Jul,11-12; 2005,Aug,7-8

85475   **Hemolysin, acid**
    INCLUDES   Ham test
    EXCLUDES   *Hemolysins and agglutinins (86940-86941)*
    🚗 0.00   ♙ 0.00   **FUD** XXX   Q ▢
    AMA: 2005,Aug,7-8; 2005,Jul,11-12

85520   **Heparin assay**
    🚗 0.00   ♙ 0.00   **FUD** XXX   Q ▢
    AMA: 2005,Aug,7-8; 2005,Jul,11-12

85525   **Heparin neutralization**
    🚗 0.00   ♙ 0.00   **FUD** XXX   Q ▢
    AMA: 2005,Aug,7-8; 2005,Jul,11-12

85530   **Heparin-protamine tolerance test**
    🚗 0.00   ♙ 0.00   **FUD** XXX   Q ▢
    AMA: 2005,Aug,7-8; 2005,Jul,11-12

85536   **Iron stain, peripheral blood**
    EXCLUDES   *Iron stains on bone marrow or other tissues with physician evaluation (88313)*
    🚗 0.00   ♙ 0.00   **FUD** XXX   Q ▢
    AMA: 2005,Aug,7-8; 2005,Jul,11-12

85540   **Leukocyte alkaline phosphatase with count**
    🚗 0.00   ♙ 0.00   **FUD** XXX   Q ▢
    AMA: 2005,Aug,7-8; 2005,Jul,11-12

85547   **Mechanical fragility, RBC**
    🚗 0.00   ♙ 0.00   **FUD** XXX   Q ▢
    AMA: 2005,Aug,7-8; 2005,Jul,11-12

85549   **Muramidase**
    🚗 0.00   ♙ 0.00   **FUD** XXX   Q ▢
    AMA: 2005,Aug,7-8; 2005,Jul,11-12

85555   **Osmotic fragility, RBC; unincubated**
    🚗 0.00   ♙ 0.00   **FUD** XXX   Q ▢
    AMA: 2005,Aug,7-8; 2005,Jul,11-12

85557   **incubated**
    🚗 0.00   ♙ 0.00   **FUD** XXX   Q ▢
    AMA: 2005,Aug,7-8; 2005,Jul,11-12

85576   **Platelet, aggregation (in vitro), each agent**
    EXCLUDES   *Thromboxane metabolite(s), including thromboxane, when performed, in urine (84431)*
    🚗 0.00   ♙ 0.00   **FUD** XXX   ✖ Q ▢
    AMA: 2016,Jan,13; 2015,Jan,16; 2014,Jan,11; 2012,Jan,15-42; 2011,Jan,11

85597   **Phospholipid neutralization; platelet**
    🚗 0.00   ♙ 0.00   **FUD** XXX   Q ▢
    AMA: 2016,Jan,13; 2015,Jan,16; 2014,Jan,11; 2011,Apr,9

85598   **hexagonal phospholipid**
    🚗 0.00   ♙ 0.00   **FUD** XXX   Q ▢
    AMA: 2016,Jan,13; 2015,Jan,16; 2014,Jan,11; 2011,Apr,3-8; 2011,Apr,9

85610   **Prothrombin time;**
    🚗 0.00   ♙ 0.00   **FUD** XXX   ✖ Q ▢
    AMA: 2005,Aug,7-8; 2005,Jul,11-12

85611   **substitution, plasma fractions, each**
    🚗 0.00   ♙ 0.00   **FUD** XXX   Q ▢
    AMA: 2005,Aug,7-8; 2005,Jul,11-12

85612   **Russell viper venom time (includes venom); undiluted**
    🚗 0.00   ♙ 0.00   **FUD** XXX   Q ▢
    AMA: 2005,Aug,7-8; 2005,Jul,11-12

85613   **diluted**
    🚗 0.00   ♙ 0.00   **FUD** XXX   Q ▢
    AMA: 2005,Aug,7-8; 2005,Jul,11-12

85635   **Reptilase test**
    🚗 0.00   ♙ 0.00   **FUD** XXX   Q ▢
    AMA: 2005,Aug,7-8; 2005,Jul,11-12

85651   **Sedimentation rate, erythrocyte; non-automated**
    🚗 0.00   ♙ 0.00   **FUD** XXX   ✖ Q
    AMA: 2005,Aug,7-8; 2005,Jul,11-12

85652   **automated**
    INCLUDES   Westergren test
    🚗 0.00   ♙ 0.00   **FUD** XXX   Q ▢
    AMA: 2005,Aug,7-8; 2005,Jul,11-12

85660   **Sickling of RBC, reduction**
    EXCLUDES   *Hemoglobin electrophoresis (83020)*
    🚗 0.00   ♙ 0.00   **FUD** XXX   Q ▢
    AMA: 2005,Aug,7-8; 2005,Jul,11-12

85670   **Thrombin time; plasma**
    🚗 0.00   ♙ 0.00   **FUD** XXX   Q ▢
    AMA: 2005,Jul,11-12; 2005,Aug,7-8

85675   **titer**
    🚗 0.00   ♙ 0.00   **FUD** XXX   Q ▢
    AMA: 2005,Jul,11-12; 2005,Aug,7-8

85705   **Thromboplastin inhibition, tissue**
    EXCLUDES   *Individual clotting factors (85245-85247)*
    🚗 0.00   ♙ 0.00   **FUD** XXX   Q ▢
    AMA: 2005,Aug,7-8; 2005,Jul,11-12

85730-85732 Partial Thromboplastin Time (PTT)

    EXCLUDES   *Agglutinins (86000, 86156-86157)*
                     Antiplasmin (85410)
                     Antithrombin III (85300-85301)
                     Blood banking procedures (86850-86999)

85730   **Thromboplastin time, partial (PTT); plasma or whole blood**
    INCLUDES   Hicks-Pitney test
    🚗 0.00   ♙ 0.00   **FUD** XXX   Q ▢
    AMA: 2005,Aug,7-8; 2005,Jul,11-12

85732   **substitution, plasma fractions, each**
    🚗 0.00   ♙ 0.00   **FUD** XXX   Q ▢
    AMA: 2016,Jan,13; 2015,Jan,16; 2014,Jan,11; 2011,Apr,9

85810-85999 Blood Viscosity and Unlisted Hematology Procedures

85810   **Viscosity**
    🚗 0.00   ♙ 0.00   **FUD** XXX   Q
    AMA: 2016,Jan,13; 2015,Jan,16; 2014,Jan,11; 2012,Jan,15-42; 2011,Jan,11

85999   **Unlisted hematology and coagulation procedure**
    🚗 0.00   ♙ 0.00   **FUD** XXX   Q
    AMA: 2016,Jan,13; 2015,Jan,16; 2014,Jan,11

86000-86063 Antibody Testing

86000   **Agglutinins, febrile (eg, Brucella, Francisella, Murine typhus, Q fever, Rocky Mountain spotted fever, scrub typhus), each antigen**
    EXCLUDES   *Infectious agent antibodies (86602-86804)*
    🚗 0.00   ♙ 0.00   **FUD** XXX   Q
    AMA: 2016,Jan,13; 2015,Jan,16; 2014,Jan,11

86001 Allergen specific IgG quantitative or semiquantitative, each allergen
  🔧 0.00 ✂ 0.00 **FUD** XXX ▣ ▭
  AMA: 2005,Aug,7-8; 2005,Jul,11-12

86003 Allergen specific IgE; quantitative or semiquantitative, each allergen
  EXCLUDES Total quantitative IgE (82785)
  🔧 0.00 ✂ 0.00 **FUD** XXX ▣ ▭
  AMA: 2016,Jan,13; 2015,Jan,16; 2014,Jan,11

86005 qualitative, multiallergen screen (dipstick, paddle, or disk)
  EXCLUDES Total qualitative IgE (83518)
  🔧 0.00 ✂ 0.00 **FUD** XXX ▣
  AMA: 2016,Jan,13; 2015,Jan,16; 2014,Jan,11

86021 Antibody identification; leukocyte antibodies
  🔧 0.00 ✂ 0.00 **FUD** XXX ▣ ▭
  AMA: 2005,Jul,11-12; 2005,Aug,7-8

86022 platelet antibodies
  🔧 0.00 ✂ 0.00 **FUD** XXX ▣ ▭
  AMA: 2005,Jul,11-12; 2005,Aug,7-8

86023 platelet associated immunoglobulin assay
  🔧 0.00 ✂ 0.00 **FUD** XXX ▣ ▭
  AMA: 2005,Jul,11-12; 2005,Aug,7-8

86038 Antinuclear antibodies (ANA);
  🔧 0.00 ✂ 0.00 **FUD** XXX ▣ ▭
  AMA: 2005,Aug,7-8; 2005,Jul,11-12

86039 titer
  🔧 0.00 ✂ 0.00 **FUD** XXX ▣ ▭
  AMA: 2005,Aug,7-8; 2005,Jul,11-12

86060 Antistreptolysin 0; titer
  🔧 0.00 ✂ 0.00 **FUD** XXX ▣ ▭
  AMA: 2005,Jul,11-12; 2005,Aug,7-8

86063 screen
  🔧 0.00 ✂ 0.00 **FUD** XXX ▣
  AMA: 2005,Jul,11-12; 2005,Aug,7-8

86077-86079 Blood Bank Services

86077 Blood bank physician services; difficult cross match and/or evaluation of irregular antibody(s), interpretation and written report
  🔧 1.48 ✂ 1.60 **FUD** XXX 01 80
  AMA: 2005,Aug,7-8; 2005,Jul,11-12

86078 investigation of transfusion reaction including suspicion of transmissible disease, interpretation and written report
  🔧 1.48 ✂ 1.59 **FUD** XXX 01 80
  AMA: 2005,Aug,7-8; 2005,Jul,11-12

86079 authorization for deviation from standard blood banking procedures (eg, use of outdated blood, transfusion of Rh incompatible units), with written report
  🔧 1.46 ✂ 1.57 **FUD** XXX 01 80
  AMA: 2005,Aug,7-8; 2005,Jul,11-12

86140-86344 [86152, 86153] Diagnostic Immunology Testing

86140 C-reactive protein;
  🔧 0.00 ✂ 0.00 **FUD** XXX ▣
  AMA: 2005,Aug,7-8; 2005,Jul,11-12

86141 high sensitivity (hsCRP)
  🔧 0.00 ✂ 0.00 **FUD** XXX ▣ ▭
  AMA: 2005,Aug,7-8; 2005,Jul,11-12

86146 Beta 2 Glycoprotein I antibody, each
  🔧 0.00 ✂ 0.00 **FUD** XXX ▣
  AMA: 2005,Aug,7-8; 2005,Jul,11-12

86147 Cardiolipin (phospholipid) antibody, each Ig class
  🔧 0.00 ✂ 0.00 **FUD** XXX ▣
  AMA: 2005,Aug,7-8; 2005,Jul,11-12

\# **86152** Cell enumeration using immunologic selection and identification in fluid specimen (eg, circulating tumor cells in blood);
  🔧 0.00 ✂ 0.00 **FUD** XXX ▣ ▭
  EXCLUDES Flow cytometric immunophenotyping (88184-88189)
      Flow cytometric quantitation (86355-86357, 86359-86361, 86367)
  Code also physician interpretation/report when performed ([86153])

\# **86153** physician interpretation and report, when required
  🔧 0.00 ✂ 0.00 **FUD** 000 B ▭
  EXCLUDES Flow cytometric immunophenotyping (88184-88189)
      Flow cytometric quantitation (86355-86357, 86359-86361, 86367)
  Code first cell enumeration, when performed ([86152])

86148 Anti-phosphatidylserine (phospholipid) antibody
  EXCLUDES Antiprothrombin (phospholipid cofactor) antibody (86849)
  🔧 0.00 ✂ 0.00 **FUD** XXX ▣
  AMA: 2016,Jan,13; 2015,Jan,16; 2014,Jan,11

86152 **Resequenced code. See code following 86147.**

86153 **Resequenced code. See code before 86148.**

86155 Chemotaxis assay, specify method
  🔧 0.00 ✂ 0.00 **FUD** XXX ▣
  AMA: 2005,Aug,7-8; 2005,Jul,11-12

86156 Cold agglutinin; screen
  🔧 0.00 ✂ 0.00 **FUD** XXX ▣
  AMA: 2005,Aug,7-8; 2005,Jul,11-12

86157 titer
  🔧 0.00 ✂ 0.00 **FUD** XXX ▣ ▭
  AMA: 2005,Aug,7-8; 2005,Jul,11-12

86160 Complement; antigen, each component
  🔧 0.00 ✂ 0.00 **FUD** XXX ▣
  AMA: 2005,Aug,7-8; 2005,Jul,11-12

86161 functional activity, each component
  🔧 0.00 ✂ 0.00 **FUD** XXX ▣
  AMA: 2005,Aug,7-8; 2005,Jul,11-12

86162 total hemolytic (CH50)
  🔧 0.00 ✂ 0.00 **FUD** XXX ▣
  AMA: 2005,Aug,7-8; 2005,Jul,11-12

86171 Complement fixation tests, each antigen
  🔧 0.00 ✂ 0.00 **FUD** XXX ▣
  AMA: 2005,Aug,7-8; 2005,Jul,11-12

86185 Counterimmunoelectrophoresis, each antigen
  🔧 0.00 ✂ 0.00 **FUD** XXX ▣ ▭
  AMA: 2005,Aug,7-8; 2005,Jul,11-12

86200 Cyclic citrullinated peptide (CCP), antibody
  🔧 0.00 ✂ 0.00 **FUD** XXX ▣
  AMA: 2016,Jan,13; 2015,Jan,16; 2014,Jan,11

86215 Deoxyribonuclease, antibody
  🔧 0.00 ✂ 0.00 **FUD** XXX ▣ ▭
  AMA: 2005,Aug,7-8; 2005,Jul,11-12

86225 Deoxyribonucleic acid (DNA) antibody; native or double stranded
  EXCLUDES HIV antibody tests (86701-86703)
  🔧 0.00 ✂ 0.00 **FUD** XXX ▣ ▭
  AMA: 2005,Aug,7-8; 2005,Jul,11-12

86226 single stranded
  EXCLUDES Anti D.S, DNA, IFA, eg, using C. Lucilae (86255-86256)
  🔧 0.00 ✂ 0.00 **FUD** XXX ▣ ▭
  AMA: 2005,Aug,7-8; 2005,Jul,11-12

86235 Extractable nuclear antigen, antibody to, any method (eg, nRNP, SS-A, SS-B, Sm, RNP, Sc170, J01), each antibody
  🔧 0.00 ✂ 0.00 **FUD** XXX ▣ ▭
  AMA: 2005,Aug,7-8; 2005,Jul,11-12

86243 Fc receptor
🔲 0.00 🔲 0.00 **FUD** XXX
AMA: 2005,Aug,7-8; 2005,Jul,11-12

86255 Fluorescent noninfectious agent antibody; screen, each antibody
🔲 0.00 🔲 0.00 **FUD** XXX
AMA: 2005,Aug,9-10; 2005,Aug,7-8

86256 titer, each antibody
EXCLUDES Fluorescent technique for antigen identification in tissue (88346, [88350])
FTA (86780)
Gel (agar) diffusion tests (86331)
Indirect fluorescence (88346, [88350])
🔲 0.00 🔲 0.00 **FUD** XXX
AMA: 2005,Aug,9-10; 2005,Aug,7-8

86277 Growth hormone, human (HGH), antibody
🔲 0.00 🔲 0.00 **FUD** XXX
AMA: 2005,Aug,7-8; 2005,Jul,11-12

86280 Hemagglutination inhibition test (HAI)
EXCLUDES Antibodies to infectious agents (86602-86804)
Rubella (86762)
🔲 0.00 🔲 0.00 **FUD** XXX
AMA: 2005,Aug,7-8; 2005,Jul,11-12

86294 Immunoassay for tumor antigen, qualitative or semiquantitative (eg, bladder tumor antigen)
EXCLUDES Qualitative NMP22 protein (86386)
🔲 0.00 🔲 0.00 **FUD** XXX
AMA: 2005,Aug,7-8; 2005,Jul,11-12

86300 Immunoassay for tumor antigen, quantitative; CA 15-3 (27.29)
🔲 0.00 🔲 0.00 **FUD** XXX
AMA: 2005,Aug,7-8; 2005,Jul,11-12

86301 CA 19-9
🔲 0.00 🔲 0.00 **FUD** XXX
AMA: 2005,Aug,7-8; 2005,Jul,11-12

86304 CA 125
EXCLUDES Measurement of serum HER-2/neu oncoprotein (83950)
🔲 0.00 🔲 0.00 **FUD** XXX
AMA: 2005,Aug,7-8; 2005,Jul,11-12

86305 Human epididymis protein 4 (HE4)
🔲 0.00 🔲 0.00 **FUD** XXX

86308 Heterophile antibodies; screening
EXCLUDES Antibodies to infectious agents (86602-86804)
🔲 0.00 🔲 0.00 **FUD** XXX
AMA: 2005,Jul,11-12; 2005,Aug,7-8

86309 titer
EXCLUDES Antibodies to infectious agents (86602-86804)
🔲 0.00 🔲 0.00 **FUD** XXX
AMA: 2005,Jul,11-12; 2005,Aug,7-8

86310 titers after absorption with beef cells and guinea pig kidney
EXCLUDES Antibodies to infectious agents (86602-86804)
🔲 0.00 🔲 0.00 **FUD** XXX
AMA: 2005,Jul,11-12; 2005,Aug,7-8

86316 Immunoassay for tumor antigen, other antigen, quantitative (eg, CA 50, 72-4, 549), each
🔲 0.00 🔲 0.00 **FUD** XXX
AMA: 2016,Jan,13; 2015,Jan,16; 2014,Jan,11; 2012,Jan,15-42; 2011,Jan,11

86317 Immunoassay for infectious agent antibody, quantitative, not otherwise specified
EXCLUDES Immunoassay techniques for antigens (83516, 83518-83520, 87301-87450, 87810-87899)
Particle agglutination test (86403)
🔲 0.00 🔲 0.00 **FUD** XXX
AMA: 2005,Jul,11-12; 2005,Aug,7-8

86318 Immunoassay for infectious agent antibody, qualitative or semiquantitative, single step method (eg, reagent strip)
🔲 0.00 🔲 0.00 **FUD** XXX
AMA: 2016,Jan,13; 2015,Jan,16; 2014,Jan,11; 2012,Jan,15-42; 2011,Jan,11

86320 Immunoelectrophoresis; serum
🔲 0.00 🔲 0.00 **FUD** XXX
AMA: 2005,Jul,11-12; 2005,Aug,7-8

86325 other fluids (eg, urine, cerebrospinal fluid) with concentration
🔲 0.00 🔲 0.00 **FUD** XXX
AMA: 2005,Jul,11-12; 2005,Aug,7-8

86327 crossed (2-dimensional assay)
🔲 0.00 🔲 0.00 **FUD** XXX
AMA: 2005,Jul,11-12; 2005,Aug,7-8

86329 Immunodiffusion; not elsewhere specified
🔲 0.00 🔲 0.00 **FUD** XXX
AMA: 2016,Jan,13; 2015,Jan,16; 2014,Jan,11; 2012,Jan,15-42; 2011,Jan,11

86331 gel diffusion, qualitative (Ouchterlony), each antigen or antibody
🔲 0.00 🔲 0.00 **FUD** XXX
AMA: 2005,Aug,7-8; 2005,Jul,11-12

86332 Immune complex assay
🔲 0.00 🔲 0.00 **FUD** XXX
AMA: 2005,Aug,7-8; 2005,Jul,11-12

86334 Immunofixation electrophoresis; serum
🔲 0.00 🔲 0.00 **FUD** XXX
AMA: 2005,Jul,11-12; 2005,Aug,7-8

86335 other fluids with concentration (eg, urine, CSF)
🔲 0.00 🔲 0.00 **FUD** XXX
AMA: 2005,Jul,11-12; 2005,Aug,7-8

86336 Inhibin A
🔲 0.00 🔲 0.00 **FUD** XXX
AMA: 2005,Aug,7-8; 2005,Jul,11-12

86337 Insulin antibodies
🔲 0.00 🔲 0.00 **FUD** XXX
AMA: 2005,Aug,7-8; 2005,Jul,11-12

86340 Intrinsic factor antibodies
🔲 0.00 🔲 0.00 **FUD** XXX
AMA: 2005,Jul,11-12; 2005,Aug,7-8

86341 Islet cell antibody
🔲 0.00 🔲 0.00 **FUD** XXX
AMA: 2016,Jan,13; 2015,Jan,16; 2014,Jan,11

86343 Leukocyte histamine release test (LHR)
🔲 0.00 🔲 0.00 **FUD** XXX
AMA: 2005,Aug,7-8; 2005,Jul,11-12

86344 Leukocyte phagocytosis
🔲 0.00 🔲 0.00 **FUD** XXX
AMA: 2005,Aug,7-8; 2005,Jul,11-12

86352 Assay Cellular Function

86352 Cellular function assay involving stimulation (eg, mitogen or antigen) and detection of biomarker (eg, ATP)
🔲 0.00 🔲 0.00 **FUD** XXX

86353 Lymphocyte Mitogen Response Assay

CMS: 100-03,190.8 Lymphocyte Mitogen Response Assays

86353 Lymphocyte transformation, mitogen (phytomitogen) or antigen induced blastogenesis
EXCLUDES Cellular function assay involving stimulation and detection of biomarker (86352)
🔲 0.00 🔲 0.00 **FUD** XXX
AMA: 2005,Aug,7-8; 2005,Jul,11-12

86355-86593 Additional Diagnostic Immunology Testing

86355 **B cells, total count**

> EXCLUDES *Flow cytometry interpretation (88187-88189)*
> 🔧 0.00   ✂ 0.00   **FUD** XXX   Q 🖳
>
> AMA: 2016,Jan,13; 2015,Jan,16; 2014,Jan,11

86356 **Mononuclear cell antigen, quantitative (eg, flow cytometry), not otherwise specified, each antigen**

> EXCLUDES *Flow cytometry interpretation (88187-88189)*
> 🔧 0.00   ✂ 0.00   **FUD** XXX   Q 🖳
>
> AMA: 2016,Jan,13; 2015,Jan,16; 2014,Jan,11

86357 **Natural killer (NK) cells, total count**

> EXCLUDES *Flow cytometry interpretation (88187-88189)*
> 🔧 0.00   ✂ 0.00   **FUD** XXX   Q 🖳
>
> AMA: 2016,Jan,13; 2015,Jan,16; 2014,Jan,11

86359 **T cells; total count**

> EXCLUDES *Flow cytometry interpretation (88187-88189)*
> 🔧 0.00   ✂ 0.00   **FUD** XXX   Q 🖳
>
> AMA: 2016,Jan,13; 2015,Jan,16; 2014,Jan,11

86360 **absolute CD4 and CD8 count, including ratio**

> EXCLUDES *Flow cytometry interpretation (88187-88189)*
> 🔧 0.00   ✂ 0.00   **FUD** XXX   Q 🖳
>
> AMA: 2016,Jan,13; 2015,Jan,16; 2014,Jan,11

86361 **absolute CD4 count**

> EXCLUDES *Flow cytometry interpretation (88187-88189)*
> 🔧 0.00   ✂ 0.00   **FUD** XXX   Q 🖳
>
> AMA: 2016,Jan,13; 2015,Jan,16; 2014,Jan,11

86367 **Stem cells (ie, CD34), total count**

> EXCLUDES *Flow cytometry interpretation (88187-88189)*
> 🔧 0.00   ✂ 0.00   **FUD** XXX   Q 🖳
>
> AMA: 2016,Jan,13; 2015,Jan,16; 2014,Jan,11; 2013,Oct,3

86376 **Microsomal antibodies (eg, thyroid or liver-kidney), each**

> 🔧 0.00   ✂ 0.00   **FUD** XXX   Q 🖳
>
> AMA: 2005,Jul,11-12; 2005,Aug,7-8

86378 **Migration inhibitory factor test (MIF)**

> 🔧 0.00   ✂ 0.00   **FUD** XXX   Q 🖳
>
> AMA: 2005,Aug,7-8; 2005,Jul,11-12

86382 **Neutralization test, viral**

> 🔧 0.00   ✂ 0.00   **FUD** XXX   Q 🖳
>
> AMA: 2005,Aug,7-8; 2005,Jul,11-12

86384 **Nitroblue tetrazolium dye test (NTD)**

> 🔧 0.00   ✂ 0.00   **FUD** XXX   Q 🖳
>
> AMA: 2005,Aug,7-8; 2005,Jul,11-12

86386 **Nuclear Matrix Protein 22 (NMP22), qualitative**

> 🔧 0.00   ✂ 0.00   **FUD** XXX   ✖ Q

86403 **Particle agglutination; screen, each antibody**

> 🔧 0.00   ✂ 0.00   **FUD** XXX   Q
>
> AMA: 2005,Jul,11-12; 2005,Aug,7-8

86406 **titer, each antibody**

> 🔧 0.00   ✂ 0.00   **FUD** XXX   Q
>
> AMA: 2005,Jul,11-12; 2005,Aug,7-8

86430 **Rheumatoid factor; qualitative**

> 🔧 0.00   ✂ 0.00   **FUD** XXX   Q
>
> AMA: 2005,Aug,7-8; 2005,Jul,11-12

86431 **quantitative**

> 🔧 0.00   ✂ 0.00   **FUD** XXX   Q
>
> AMA: 2005,Aug,7-8; 2005,Jul,11-12

86480 **Tuberculosis test, cell mediated immunity antigen response measurement; gamma interferon**

> 🔧 0.00   ✂ 0.00   **FUD** XXX   Q 🖳
>
> AMA: 2016,Jan,13; 2015,Jan,16; 2014,Jan,11

86481 **enumeration of gamma interferon-producing T-cells in cell suspension**

> 🔧 0.00   ✂ 0.00   **FUD** XXX   Q 🖳
>
> AMA: 2010,Dec,7-10

86485 **Skin test; candida**

> 🔧 0.00   ✂ 0.00   **FUD** XXX   Q1 80 TC
>
> AMA: 2005,Jul,11-12; 2005,Aug,7-8

86486 **unlisted antigen, each**

> 🔧 0.14   ✂ 0.14   **FUD** XXX   Q1 80 TC
>
> AMA: 2008,Apr,5-7

86490 **coccidioidomycosis**

> 🔧 1.97   ✂ 1.97   **FUD** XXX   Q1 80 TC
>
> AMA: 2005,Aug,7-8; 2005,Jul,11-12

86510 **histoplasmosis**

> 🔧 0.17   ✂ 0.17   **FUD** XXX   Q1 80 TC
>
> AMA: 2005,Aug,7-8; 2005,Jul,11-12

86580 **tuberculosis, intradermal**

> INCLUDES Heaf test
>   Intradermal Mantoux test
> EXCLUDES *Skin test for allergy (95012-95199)*
>   *Tuberculosis test, cell mediated immunity measurement of gamma interferon antigen response (86480)*
> 🔧 0.22   ✂ 0.22   **FUD** XXX   Q1 80 TC
>
> AMA: 2005,Aug,7-8; 2005,Jul,11-12

86590 **Streptokinase, antibody**

> EXCLUDES *Antibodies to infectious agents (86602-86804)*
> 🔧 0.00   ✂ 0.00   **FUD** XXX   Q
>
> AMA: 2005,Jul,11-12; 2005,Aug,7-8

86592 **Syphilis test, non-treponemal antibody; qualitative (eg, VDRL, RPR, ART)**

> INCLUDES Wasserman test
> EXCLUDES *Antibodies to infectious agents (86602-86804)*
> 🔧 0.00   ✂ 0.00   **FUD** XXX   A
>
> AMA: 2005,Jul,11-12; 2005,Aug,7-8

86593 **quantitative**

> EXCLUDES *Antibodies to infectious agents (86602-86804)*
> 🔧 0.00   ✂ 0.00   **FUD** XXX   A
>
> AMA: 2005,Jul,11-12; 2005,Aug,7-8

86602-86698 Testing for Antibodies to Infectious Agents: Actinomyces- Histoplasma

> INCLUDES Qualitative or semiquantitative immunoassays performed by multiple-step methods for the detection of antibodies to infectious agents
> EXCLUDES *Detection of:*
>   *Antibodies other than those to infectious agents, see specific antibody or method*
>   *Infectious agent/antigen (87260-87899 [87623, 87624, 87625, 87806])*
>   *Immunoassays by single-step method (86318)*

86602 **Antibody; actinomyces**

> 🔧 0.00   ✂ 0.00   **FUD** XXX   Q
>
> AMA: 2016,Jan,13; 2015,Jan,16; 2014,Jan,11

86603 **adenovirus**

> 🔧 0.00   ✂ 0.00   **FUD** XXX   Q
>
> AMA: 2005,Jul,11-12; 2005,Aug,7-8

86606 **Aspergillus**

> 🔧 0.00   ✂ 0.00   **FUD** XXX   Q
>
> AMA: 2005,Jul,11-12; 2005,Aug,7-8

86609 **bacterium, not elsewhere specified**

> 🔧 0.00   ✂ 0.00   **FUD** XXX   Q
>
> AMA: 2005,Jul,11-12; 2005,Aug,7-8

86611 **Bartonella**

> 🔧 0.00   ✂ 0.00   **FUD** XXX   Q
>
> AMA: 2005,Jul,11-12; 2005,Aug,7-8

86612 **Blastomyces**

> 🔧 0.00   ✂ 0.00   **FUD** XXX   Q
>
> AMA: 2005,Jul,11-12; 2005,Aug,7-8

86615 **Bordetella**

> 🔧 0.00   ✂ 0.00   **FUD** XXX   Q
>
> AMA: 2005,Jul,11-12; 2005,Aug,7-8

26/TC PC/TC Only	A2-Z3 ASC Payment	50 Bilateral	♂ Male Only	♀ Female Only	🔧 Facility RVU	✂ Non-Facility RVU	🖳 CCI
FUD Follow-up Days	**CMS:** IOM (Pub 100)	A-Y OPPSI	80/80 Surg Assist Allowed / w/Doc		🔧 Lab Crosswalk	🔧 Radiology Crosswalk	✖ CLIA

86617 **Borrelia burgdorferi (Lyme disease) confirmatory test (eg, Western Blot or immunoblot)**
📷 0.00 ✂ 0.00 **FUD** XXX Q
AMA: 2005,Jul,11-12; 2005,Aug,7-8

86618 **Borrelia burgdorferi (Lyme disease)**
📷 0.00 ✂ 0.00 **FUD** XXX ☒ Q
AMA: 2005,Jul,11-12; 2005,Aug,7-8

86619 **Borrelia (relapsing fever)**
📷 0.00 ✂ 0.00 **FUD** XXX Q
AMA: 2005,Jul,11-12; 2005,Aug,7-8

86622 **Brucella**
📷 0.00 ✂ 0.00 **FUD** XXX Q
AMA: 2005,Jul,11-12; 2005,Aug,7-8

86625 **Campylobacter**
📷 0.00 ✂ 0.00 **FUD** XXX Q
AMA: 2005,Jul,11-12; 2005,Aug,7-8

86628 **Candida**
EXCLUDES Candida skin test (86485)
📷 0.00 ✂ 0.00 **FUD** XXX Q
AMA: 2005,Jul,11-12; 2005,Aug,7-8

86631 **Chlamydia**
📷 0.00 ✂ 0.00 **FUD** XXX A
AMA: 2005,Jul,11-12; 2005,Aug,7-8

86632 **Chlamydia, IgM**
EXCLUDES Chlamydia antigen (87270, 87320)
Fluorescent antibody technique (86255-86256)
📷 0.00 ✂ 0.00 **FUD** XXX A
AMA: 2005,Jul,11-12; 2005,Aug,7-8

86635 **Coccidioides**
📷 0.00 ✂ 0.00 **FUD** XXX Q
AMA: 2005,Jul,11-12; 2005,Aug,7-8

86638 **Coxiella burnetii (Q fever)**
📷 0.00 ✂ 0.00 **FUD** XXX Q
AMA: 2005,Jul,11-12; 2005,Aug,7-8

86641 **Cryptococcus**
📷 0.00 ✂ 0.00 **FUD** XXX Q
AMA: 2005,Jul,11-12; 2005,Aug,7-8

86644 **cytomegalovirus (CMV)**
📷 0.00 ✂ 0.00 **FUD** XXX Q
AMA: 2005,Jul,11-12; 2005,Aug,7-8

86645 **cytomegalovirus (CMV), IgM**
📷 0.00 ✂ 0.00 **FUD** XXX Q
AMA: 2016,Jan,13; 2015,Jan,16; 2014,Jan,11

86648 **Diphtheria**
📷 0.00 ✂ 0.00 **FUD** XXX Q
AMA: 2005,Jul,11-12; 2005,Aug,7-8

86651 **encephalitis, California (La Crosse)**
📷 0.00 ✂ 0.00 **FUD** XXX Q
AMA: 2005,Jul,11-12; 2005,Aug,7-8

86652 **encephalitis, Eastern equine**
📷 0.00 ✂ 0.00 **FUD** XXX Q
AMA: 2005,Jul,11-12; 2005,Aug,7-8

86653 **encephalitis, St. Louis**
📷 0.00 ✂ 0.00 **FUD** XXX Q
AMA: 2005,Jul,11-12; 2005,Aug,7-8

86654 **encephalitis, Western equine**
📷 0.00 ✂ 0.00 **FUD** XXX Q
AMA: 2005,Jul,11-12; 2005,Aug,7-8

86658 **enterovirus (eg, coxsackie, echo, polio)**
EXCLUDES Antibodies to:
Trichinella (86784)
Trypanosoma—see code for specific methodology
Tuberculosis (86580)
Viral—see code for specific methodology
📷 0.00 ✂ 0.00 **FUD** XXX Q
AMA: 2005,Jul,11-12; 2005,Aug,7-8

86663 **Epstein-Barr (EB) virus, early antigen (EA)**
📷 0.00 ✂ 0.00 **FUD** XXX Q
AMA: 2005,Jul,11-12; 2005,Aug,7-8

86664 **Epstein-Barr (EB) virus, nuclear antigen (EBNA)**
📷 0.00 ✂ 0.00 **FUD** XXX Q
AMA: 2005,Jul,11-12; 2005,Aug,7-8

86665 **Epstein-Barr (EB) virus, viral capsid (VCA)**
📷 0.00 ✂ 0.00 **FUD** XXX Q
AMA: 2005,Jul,11-12; 2005,Aug,7-8

86666 **Ehrlichia**
📷 0.00 ✂ 0.00 **FUD** XXX Q
AMA: 2005,Jul,11-12; 2005,Aug,7-8

86668 **Francisella tularensis**
📷 0.00 ✂ 0.00 **FUD** XXX Q
AMA: 2005,Jul,11-12; 2005,Aug,7-8

86671 **fungus, not elsewhere specified**
📷 0.00 ✂ 0.00 **FUD** XXX Q
AMA: 2005,Jul,11-12; 2005,Aug,7-8

86674 **Giardia lamblia**
📷 0.00 ✂ 0.00 **FUD** XXX Q
AMA: 2005,Jul,11-12; 2005,Aug,7-8

86677 **Helicobacter pylori**
📷 0.00 ✂ 0.00 **FUD** XXX Q
AMA: 2016,Jan,13; 2015,Jan,16; 2014,Jan,11

86682 **helminth, not elsewhere specified**
📷 0.00 ✂ 0.00 **FUD** XXX Q
AMA: 2005,Jul,11-12; 2005,Aug,7-8

86684 **Haemophilus influenza**
📷 0.00 ✂ 0.00 **FUD** XXX Q
AMA: 2005,Jul,11-12; 2005,Aug,7-8

86687 **HTLV-I**
📷 0.00 ✂ 0.00 **FUD** XXX Q
AMA: 2005,Jul,11-12; 2005,Aug,7-8

86688 **HTLV-II**
📷 0.00 ✂ 0.00 **FUD** XXX Q
AMA: 2005,Jul,11-12; 2005,Aug,7-8

86689 **HTLV or HIV antibody, confirmatory test (eg, Western Blot)**
📷 0.00 ✂ 0.00 **FUD** XXX Q
AMA: 2016,Jan,13; 2015,Jan,16; 2014,Jan,11

86692 **hepatitis, delta agent**
EXCLUDES Hepatitis delta agent, antigen (87380)
📷 0.00 ✂ 0.00 **FUD** XXX Q
AMA: 2005,Jul,11-12; 2005,Aug,7-8

86694 **herpes simplex, non-specific type test**
📷 0.00 ✂ 0.00 **FUD** XXX Q
AMA: 2005,Jul,11-12; 2005,Aug,7-8

86695 **herpes simplex, type 1**
📷 0.00 ✂ 0.00 **FUD** XXX Q
AMA: 2016,Jan,13; 2015,Jan,16; 2014,Jan,11

86696 **herpes simplex, type 2**
📷 0.00 ✂ 0.00 **FUD** XXX Q
AMA: 2005,Jul,11-12; 2005,Aug,7-8

86698 **histoplasma**
📷 0.00 ✂ 0.00 **FUD** XXX Q
AMA: 2005,Jul,11-12; 2005,Aug,7-8

86701-86703 Testing for HIV Antibodies

CMS: 100-03,190.14 Human Immunodeficiency Virus Testing (Diagnosis); 100-03,190.9 Serologic Testing for Acquired Immunodeficiency Syndrome (AIDS)

INCLUDES   Qualitative or semiquantitative immunoassays performed by multiple-step methods for the detection of antibodies to infectious agents

EXCLUDES   *Confirmatory test for HIV antibody (86689)*
HIV-1 antigen (87390)
HIV-1 antigen(s) with HIV 1 and 2 antibodies, single result (87389)
HIV-2 antigen (87391)
Immunoassays by single-step method (86318)

Code also modifier 92 for test performed using a kit or transportable instrument comprising all or part of a single-use, disposable analytical chamber

86701   **Antibody; HIV-1**
    0.00   0.00   **FUD** XXX   ☒ ⓠ
    AMA: 2016,Jan,13; 2015,Jan,16; 2014,Jan,11

86702   **HIV-2**
    0.00   0.00   **FUD** XXX   ⓠ
    AMA: 2016,Jan,13; 2015,Jan,16; 2014,Jan,11

86703   **HIV-1 and HIV-2, single result**
    0.00   0.00   **FUD** XXX   ⓠ
    AMA: 2016,Jan,13; 2015,Jan,16; 2014,Jan,11

86704-86804 Testing for Infectious Disease Antibodies: Hepatitis—Yersinia

INCLUDES   Qualitative or semiquantitative immunoassays performed by multiple-step methods for the detection of antibodies to infectious agents

EXCLUDES   *Detection of:*
   Antibodies other than those to infectious agents, see specific antibody or method
   Infectious agent/antigen (87260-87899 [87623, 87624, 87625, 87806])
   Immunoassays by single-step method (86318)

86704   **Hepatitis B core antibody (HBcAb); total**
    0.00   0.00   **FUD** XXX   ⓠ
    AMA: 2016,Jan,13; 2015,Jan,16; 2014,Jan,11

86705   **IgM antibody**
    0.00   0.00   **FUD** XXX   ⓠ
    AMA: 2016,Jan,13; 2015,Jan,16; 2014,Jan,11

86706   **Hepatitis B surface antibody (HBsAb)**
    0.00   0.00   **FUD** XXX   ⓠ
    AMA: 2005,Jul,11-12; 2005,Aug,7-8

86707   **Hepatitis Be antibody (HBeAb)**
    0.00   0.00   **FUD** XXX   ⓠ
    AMA: 2005,Jul,11-12; 2005,Aug,7-8

86708   **Hepatitis A antibody (HAAb)**
    0.00   0.00   **FUD** XXX   ⓠ
    AMA: 2016,Jan,13; 2015,Jan,16; 2014,Jan,11; 2012,Jan,15-42; 2011,Jan,11

86709   **Hepatitis A antibody (HAAb), IgM antibody**
    0.00   0.00   **FUD** XXX   ⓠ
    AMA: 2016,Jan,13; 2015,Jan,16; 2014,Jan,11; 2012,Jan,15-42; 2011,Jan,11

86710   **Antibody; influenza virus**
    0.00   0.00   **FUD** XXX   ⓠ
    AMA: 2016,Jan,13; 2015,Jan,16; 2014,Jan,11

86711   **JC (John Cunningham) virus**
    0.00   0.00   **FUD** XXX   ⓠ

86713   **Legionella**
    0.00   0.00   **FUD** XXX   ⓠ
    AMA: 2005,Jul,11-12; 2005,Aug,7-8

86717   **Leishmania**
    0.00   0.00   **FUD** XXX   ⓠ
    AMA: 2005,Jul,11-12; 2005,Aug,7-8

86720   **Leptospira**
    0.00   0.00   **FUD** XXX   ⓠ
    AMA: 2005,Jul,11-12; 2005,Aug,7-8

86723   **Listeria monocytogenes**
    0.00   0.00   **FUD** XXX   ⓠ
    AMA: 2005,Jul,11-12; 2005,Aug,7-8

86727   **lymphocytic choriomeningitis**
    0.00   0.00   **FUD** XXX   ⓠ
    AMA: 2005,Jul,11-12; 2005,Aug,7-8

86729   **lymphogranuloma venereum**
    0.00   0.00   **FUD** XXX   ⓠ
    AMA: 2005,Jul,11-12; 2005,Aug,7-8

86732   **mucormycosis**
    0.00   0.00   **FUD** XXX   ⓠ
    AMA: 2005,Jul,11-12; 2005,Aug,7-8

86735   **mumps**
    0.00   0.00   **FUD** XXX   ⓠ
    AMA: 2016,Jan,13; 2015,Jan,16; 2014,Jan,11; 2012,Jan,15-42; 2011,Jan,11

86738   **mycoplasma**
    0.00   0.00   **FUD** XXX   ⓠ
    AMA: 2005,Jul,11-12; 2005,Aug,7-8

86741   **Neisseria meningitidis**
    0.00   0.00   **FUD** XXX   ⓠ
    AMA: 2005,Jul,11-12; 2005,Aug,7-8

86744   **Nocardia**
    0.00   0.00   **FUD** XXX   ⓠ
    AMA: 2005,Jul,11-12; 2005,Aug,7-8

86747   **parvovirus**
    0.00   0.00   **FUD** XXX   ⓠ
    AMA: 2005,Jul,11-12; 2005,Aug,7-8

86750   **Plasmodium (malaria)**
    0.00   0.00   **FUD** XXX   ⓠ
    AMA: 2005,Jul,11-12; 2005,Aug,7-8

86753   **protozoa, not elsewhere specified**
    0.00   0.00   **FUD** XXX   ⓠ
    AMA: 2005,Jul,11-12; 2005,Aug,7-8

86756   **respiratory syncytial virus**
    0.00   0.00   **FUD** XXX   ⓠ
    AMA: 2005,Jul,11-12; 2005,Aug,7-8

86757   **Rickettsia**
    0.00   0.00   **FUD** XXX   ⓠ
    AMA: 2005,Jul,11-12; 2005,Aug,7-8

86759   **rotavirus**
    0.00   0.00   **FUD** XXX   ⓠ
    AMA: 2005,Jul,11-12; 2005,Aug,7-8

86762   **rubella**
    0.00   0.00   **FUD** XXX   ⓠ
    AMA: 2005,Jul,11-12; 2005,Aug,7-8

86765   **rubeola**
    0.00   0.00   **FUD** XXX   ⓠ
    AMA: 2005,Jul,11-12; 2005,Aug,7-8

86768   **Salmonella**
    0.00   0.00   **FUD** XXX   ⓠ
    AMA: 2005,Jul,11-12; 2005,Aug,7-8

86771   **Shigella**
    0.00   0.00   **FUD** XXX   ⓠ
    AMA: 2005,Jul,11-12; 2005,Aug,7-8

86774   **tetanus**
    0.00   0.00   **FUD** XXX   ⓠ
    AMA: 2005,Jul,11-12; 2005,Aug,7-8

86777   **Toxoplasma**
    0.00   0.00   **FUD** XXX   ⓠ
    AMA: 2005,Jul,11-12; 2005,Aug,7-8

86778   **Toxoplasma, IgM**
    0.00   0.00   **FUD** XXX   ⓠ
    AMA: 2005,Jul,11-12; 2005,Aug,7-8

86780   **Treponema pallidum**
    0.00   0.00   **FUD** XXX   ☒ ⓠ ▭
    EXCLUDES   *Nontreponemal antibody analysis syphilis testing (86592-86593)*

86784 **Trichinella**
🚫 0.00 ⚕ 0.00 **FUD** XXX Q
AMA: 2005,Jul,11-12; 2005,Aug,7-8

86787 **varicella-zoster**
🚫 0.00 ⚕ 0.00 **FUD** XXX Q
AMA: 2005,Jul,11-12; 2005,Aug,7-8

86788 **West Nile virus, IgM**
🚫 0.00 ⚕ 0.00 **FUD** XXX Q

86789 **West Nile virus**
🚫 0.00 ⚕ 0.00 **FUD** XXX Q

86790 **virus, not elsewhere specified**
🚫 0.00 ⚕ 0.00 **FUD** XXX Q
AMA: 2005,Jul,11-12; 2005,Aug,7-8

86793 **Yersinia**
🚫 0.00 ⚕ 0.00 **FUD** XXX Q
AMA: 2005,Jul,11-12; 2005,Aug,7-8

86800 **Thyroglobulin antibody**
EXCLUDES *Thyroglobulin (84432)*
🚫 0.00 ⚕ 0.00 **FUD** XXX Q
AMA: 2005,Jul,11-12; 2005,Aug,7-8

86803 **Hepatitis C antibody;**
🚫 0.00 ⚕ 0.00 **FUD** XXX ☒ Q ▱
AMA: 2005,Jul,11-12; 2005,Aug,7-8

86804 **confirmatory test (eg, immunoblot)**
🚫 0.00 ⚕ 0.00 **FUD** XXX Q
AMA: 2016,Jan,13; 2015,Jan,16; 2014,Jan,11

86805-86808 Pre-Transplant Antibody Cross Matching

86805 **Lymphocytotoxicity assay, visual crossmatch; with titration**
🚫 0.00 ⚕ 0.00 **FUD** XXX Q ▱
AMA: 2016,Jan,13; 2015,Jan,16; 2014,Jan,11

86806 **without titration**
🚫 0.00 ⚕ 0.00 **FUD** XXX Q
AMA: 2005,Aug,7-8; 2005,Jul,11-12

86807 **Serum screening for cytotoxic percent reactive antibody (PRA); standard method**
🚫 0.00 ⚕ 0.00 **FUD** XXX Q
AMA: 2016,Jan,13; 2015,Jan,16; 2014,Jan,11; 2012,Jan,15-42; 2011,Jan,11

86808 **quick method**
🚫 0.00 ⚕ 0.00 **FUD** XXX Q
AMA: 2016,Jan,13; 2015,Jan,16; 2014,Jan,11; 2012,Jan,15-42; 2011,Jan,11

86812-86826 Histocompatibility Testing

CMS: 100-03,110.23 Stem Cell Transplantation; 100-03,190.1 Histocompatibility Testing; 100-04,3,90.3 Stem Cell Transplantation; 100-04,3,90.3.1 Allogeneic Stem Cell Transplantation; 100-04,3,90.3.3 Billing for Allogeneic Stem Cell Transplants; 100-04,32,90 Billing for Stem Cell Transplantation

EXCLUDES *HLA typing by molecular pathology techniques (81370-81383)*

86812 **HLA typing; A, B, or C (eg, A10, B7, B27), single antigen**
🚫 0.00 ⚕ 0.00 **FUD** XXX Q
AMA: 2016,Jan,13; 2015,Jan,16; 2014,Jan,11; 2012,May,3-10; 2012,Jan,15-42; 2011,Jan,11

86813 **A, B, or C, multiple antigens**
🚫 0.00 ⚕ 0.00 **FUD** XXX Q ▱
AMA: 2016,Jan,13; 2015,Jan,16; 2014,Jan,11; 2012,May,3-10; 2012,Jan,15-42; 2011,Jan,11

86816 **DR/DQ, single antigen**
🚫 0.00 ⚕ 0.00 **FUD** XXX Q
AMA: 2016,Jan,13; 2015,Jan,16; 2014,Jan,11; 2012,May,3-10; 2012,Jan,15-42; 2011,Jan,11

86817 **DR/DQ, multiple antigens**
🚫 0.00 ⚕ 0.00 **FUD** XXX Q ▱
AMA: 2016,Jan,13; 2015,Jan,16; 2014,Jan,11; 2012,May,3-10; 2012,Jan,15-42; 2011,Jan,11

86821 **lymphocyte culture, mixed (MLC)**
🚫 0.00 ⚕ 0.00 **FUD** XXX Q
AMA: 2016,Jan,13; 2015,Jan,16; 2014,Jan,11; 2012,Jan,15-42; 2011,Jan,11

86822 **lymphocyte culture, primed (PLC)**
🚫 0.00 ⚕ 0.00 **FUD** XXX Q
AMA: 2016,Jan,13; 2015,Jan,16; 2014,Jan,11; 2012,Jan,15-42; 2011,Jan,11

86825 **Human leukocyte antigen (HLA) crossmatch, non-cytotoxic (eg, using flow cytometry); first serum sample or dilution**
🚫 0.00 ⚕ 0.00 **FUD** XXX Q ▱
INCLUDES Autologous HLA crossmatch
EXCLUDES *B cells (86355)*
Flow cytometry (88184-88189)
Lymphocytotoxicity visual crossmatch (86805-86806)
T cells (86359)

+ 86826 **each additional serum sample or sample dilution (List separately in addition to primary procedure)**
🚫 0.00 ⚕ 0.00 **FUD** XXX Q ▱
INCLUDES Autologous HLA crossmatch
EXCLUDES *B cells (86355)*
Flow cytometry (88184-88189)
Lymphocytotoxicity visual crossmatch (86805-86806)
T cells (86359)
Code first (86825)

86828-86849 HLA Antibodies

86828 **Antibody to human leukocyte antigens (HLA), solid phase assays (eg, microspheres or beads, ELISA, flow cytometry); qualitative assessment of the presence or absence of antibody(ies) to HLA Class I and Class II HLA antigens**
🚫 0.00 ⚕ 0.00 **FUD** XXX Q ▱
Code also solid phase testing of untreated and treated specimens of either class of HLA after treatment (86828-86833)

86829 **qualitative assessment of the presence or absence of antibody(ies) to HLA Class I or Class II HLA antigens**
🚫 0.00 ⚕ 0.00 **FUD** XXX Q ▱
Code also solid phase testing of untreated and treated specimens of either class of HLA after treatment (86828-86833)

86830 **antibody identification by qualitative panel using complete HLA phenotypes, HLA Class I**
🚫 0.00 ⚕ 0.00 **FUD** XXX Q ▱
Code also solid phase testing of untreated and treated specimens of either class of HLA after treatment (86828-86833)

86831 **antibody identification by qualitative panel using complete HLA phenotypes, HLA Class II**
🚫 0.00 ⚕ 0.00 **FUD** XXX Q ▱
Code also solid phase testing of untreated and treated specimens of either class of HLA after treatment (86828-86833)

86832 **high definition qualitative panel for identification of antibody specificities (eg, individual antigen per bead methodology), HLA Class I**
🚫 0.00 ⚕ 0.00 **FUD** XXX Q ▱
Code also solid phase testing of untreated and treated specimens of either class of HLA after treatment (86828-86833)

86833 **high definition qualitative panel for identification of antibody specificities (eg, individual antigen per bead methodology), HLA Class II**
🚫 0.00 ⚕ 0.00 **FUD** XXX Q ▱
Code also solid phase testing of untreated and treated specimens of either class of HLA after treatment (86828-86833)

86834 **semi-quantitative panel (eg, titer), HLA Class I**
🚫 0.00 ⚕ 0.00 **FUD** XXX Q ▱

86835 **semi-quantitative panel (eg, titer), HLA Class II**
🚫 0.00 ⚕ 0.00 **FUD** XXX Q

86849 **Unlisted immunology procedure**
🚫 0.00 ⚕ 0.00 **FUD** XXX N
AMA: 2016,Jan,13; 2015,Jan,16; 2014,Jan,11; 2012,Jan,15-42; 2011,Jan,11

86850-86999 Transfusion Services

EXCLUDES Apheresis (36511-36512)
Therapeutic phlebotomy (99195)

86850 Antibody screen, RBC, each serum technique
0.00   0.00   FUD XXX   01
AMA: 2016,Jan,13; 2015,Jan,16; 2014,Jan,11

86860 Antibody elution (RBC), each elution
0.00   0.00   FUD XXX   01
AMA: 2005,Jul,11-12; 2005,Aug,7-8

86870 Antibody identification, RBC antibodies, each panel for each serum technique
0.00   0.00   FUD XXX   02
AMA: 2016,Jan,13; 2015,Jan,16; 2014,Jan,11; 2012,Jan,15-42; 2011,Jan,11

86880 Antihuman globulin test (Coombs test); direct, each antiserum
0.00   0.00   FUD XXX   01
AMA: 2005,Aug,7-8; 2005,Jul,11-12

86885 indirect, qualitative, each reagent red cell
0.00   0.00   FUD XXX   01
AMA: 2016,Jan,13; 2015,Jan,16; 2014,Jan,11

86886 indirect, each antibody titer
EXCLUDES Indirect antihuman globulin (Coombs) test for RBC antibody identification using reagent red cell panels (86870)
Indirect antihuman globulin (Coombs) test for RBC antibody screening (86850)
0.00   0.00   FUD XXX   01
AMA: 2016,Jan,13; 2015,Jan,16; 2014,Jan,11

86890 Autologous blood or component, collection processing and storage; predeposited
0.00   0.00   FUD XXX   01
AMA: 2016,Jan,13; 2015,Jan,16; 2014,Jan,11

86891 intra- or postoperative salvage
0.00   0.00   FUD XXX   01
AMA: 2005,Aug,7-8; 2005,Jul,11-12

86900 Blood typing, serologic; ABO
0.00   0.00   FUD XXX   01
AMA: 2005,Jul,11-12; 2005,Aug,7-8

86901 Rh (D)
0.00   0.00   FUD XXX   01
AMA: 2016,Jan,13; 2015,Jan,16; 2014,Jan,11

86902 antigen testing of donor blood using reagent serum, each antigen test
Code also one time for each antigen for each unit of blood when multiple units are tested for the same antigen
0.00   0.00   FUD XXX   01
AMA: 2010,Dec,7-10

86904 antigen screening for compatible unit using patient serum, per unit screened
0.00   0.00   FUD XXX   01
AMA: 2005,Aug,7-8; 2005,Jul,11-12

86905 RBC antigens, other than ABO or Rh (D), each
0.00   0.00   FUD XXX   01
AMA: 2005,Jul,11-12; 2005,Aug,7-8

86906 Rh phenotyping, complete
EXCLUDES Use of molecular pathology procedures for human erythrocyte antigen typing (81403)
0.00   0.00   FUD XXX   01
AMA: 2005,Jul,11-12; 2005,Aug,7-8

86910 Blood typing, for paternity testing, per individual; ABO, Rh and MN
0.00   0.00   FUD XXX   E
AMA: 2005,Jul,11-12; 2005,Aug,7-8

86911 each additional antigen system
0.00   0.00   FUD XXX   E
AMA: 2005,Jul,11-12; 2005,Aug,7-8

86920 Compatibility test each unit; immediate spin technique
0.00   0.00   FUD XXX   01
AMA: 2016,Jan,13; 2015,Jan,16; 2014,Jan,11

86921 incubation technique
0.00   0.00   FUD XXX   01
AMA: 2016,Jan,13; 2015,Jan,16; 2014,Jan,11

86922 antiglobulin technique
0.00   0.00   FUD XXX   01
AMA: 2016,Jan,13; 2015,Jan,16; 2014,Jan,11

86923 electronic
EXCLUDES Other compatibility test techniques (86920-86922)
0.00   0.00   FUD XXX   01
AMA: 2016,Jan,13; 2015,Jan,16; 2014,Jan,11

86927 Fresh frozen plasma, thawing, each unit
0.00   0.00   FUD XXX   S
AMA: 2005,Aug,7-8; 2005,Jul,11-12

86930 Frozen blood, each unit; freezing (includes preparation)
0.00   0.00   FUD XXX   01
AMA: 2016,Jan,13; 2015,Jan,16; 2014,Jan,11

86931 thawing
0.00   0.00   FUD XXX   01
AMA: 2016,Jan,13; 2015,Jan,16; 2014,Jan,11

86932 freezing (includes preparation) and thawing
0.00   0.00   FUD XXX   01
AMA: 2016,Jan,13; 2015,Jan,16; 2014,Jan,11

86940 Hemolysins and agglutinins; auto, screen, each
0.00   0.00   FUD XXX   Q
AMA: 2005,Aug,7-8; 2005,Jul,11-12

86941 incubated
0.00   0.00   FUD XXX   Q
AMA: 2005,Jul,11-12; 2005,Aug,7-8

86945 Irradiation of blood product, each unit
0.00   0.00   FUD XXX   01
AMA: 2016,Jan,13; 2015,Jan,16; 2014,Jan,11; 2012,Jan,15-42; 2011,Jan,11

86950 Leukocyte transfusion
EXCLUDES Infusion allogeneic lymphocytes (38242)
Leukapheresis (36511)
0.00   0.00   FUD XXX   01
AMA: 2016,Jan,13; 2015,Jan,16; 2013,Oct,3

86960 Volume reduction of blood or blood product (eg, red blood cells or platelets), each unit
0.00   0.00   FUD XXX   01
AMA: 2016,Jan,13; 2015,Jan,16; 2014,Jan,11

86965 Pooling of platelets or other blood products
EXCLUDES Injection of platelet rich plasma (0232T)
0.00   0.00   FUD XXX   01
AMA: 2016,Jan,13; 2015,Jan,16; 2014,Jan,11

86970 Pretreatment of RBCs for use in RBC antibody detection, identification, and/or compatibility testing; incubation with chemical agents or drugs, each
0.00   0.00   FUD XXX   01
AMA: 2005,Jul,11-12; 2005,Aug,7-8

86971 incubation with enzymes, each
0.00   0.00   FUD XXX   01
AMA: 2005,Jul,11-12; 2005,Aug,7-8

86972 by density gradient separation
0.00   0.00   FUD XXX   01
AMA: 2005,Jul,11-12; 2005,Aug,7-8

86975 Pretreatment of serum for use in RBC antibody identification; incubation with drugs, each
0.00   0.00   FUD XXX   01
AMA: 2005,Jul,11-12; 2005,Aug,7-8

86976 **by dilution**
🚑 0.00 ⚕ 0.00 **FUD** XXX [01]
AMA: 2005,Jul,11-12; 2005,Aug,7-8

86977 **incubation with inhibitors, each**
🚑 0.00 ⚕ 0.00 **FUD** XXX [01]
AMA: 2005,Jul,11-12; 2005,Aug,7-8

86978 **by differential red cell absorption using patient RBCs or RBCs of known phenotype, each absorption**
🚑 0.00 ⚕ 0.00 **FUD** XXX [01]
AMA: 2005,Jul,11-12; 2005,Aug,7-8

86985 **Splitting of blood or blood products, each unit**
🚑 0.00 ⚕ 0.00 **FUD** XXX [01]
AMA: 2016,Jan,13; 2015,Jan,16; 2014,Jan,11; 2012,May,11-12

86999 **Unlisted transfusion medicine procedure**
🚑 0.00 ⚕ 0.00 **FUD** XXX [01]
AMA: 2016,Jan,13; 2015,Jan,16; 2014,Jan,11; 2012,May,11-12; 2012,Jan,15-42; 2011,Jan,11

87003-87118 Identification of Microorganisms

INCLUDES Bacteriology, mycology, parasitology, and virology
EXCLUDES *Additional tests using molecular probes, chromatography, nucleic acid resequencing, or immunologic techniques (87140-87158)*
Code also modifier 59 for multiple specimens or sites
Code also modifier 91 for repeat procedures performed on the same day

87003 **Animal inoculation, small animal, with observation and dissection**
🚑 0.00 ⚕ 0.00 **FUD** XXX [Q][□]
AMA: 2005,Aug,7-8; 2005,Jul,11-12

87015 **Concentration (any type), for infectious agents**
EXCLUDES *Direct smear for ova and parasites (87177)*
🚑 0.00 ⚕ 0.00 **FUD** XXX [Q][□]
AMA: 2005,Aug,7-8; 2005,Jul,11-12

87040 **Culture, bacterial; blood, aerobic, with isolation and presumptive identification of isolates (includes anaerobic culture, if appropriate)**
🚑 0.00 ⚕ 0.00 **FUD** XXX [Q][□]
AMA: 2016,Jan,13; 2015,Jan,16; 2014,Jan,11; 2012,Jan,15-42; 2011,Jan,11

87045 **stool, aerobic, with isolation and preliminary examination (eg, KIA, LIA), Salmonella and Shigella species**
🚑 0.00 ⚕ 0.00 **FUD** XXX [Q][□]
AMA: 2005,Aug,7-8; 2005,Jul,11-12

87046 **stool, aerobic, additional pathogens, isolation and presumptive identification of isolates, each plate**
🚑 0.00 ⚕ 0.00 **FUD** XXX [Q][□]
AMA: 2016,Jan,13; 2015,Jan,16; 2014,Jan,11

87070 **any other source except urine, blood or stool, aerobic, with isolation and presumptive identification of isolates**
EXCLUDES *Urine (87088)*
🚑 0.00 ⚕ 0.00 **FUD** XXX [Q][□]
AMA: 2016,Jan,13; 2015,Jan,16; 2014,Jan,11; 2012,Jan,15-42; 2011,Jan,11

87071 **quantitative, aerobic with isolation and presumptive identification of isolates, any source except urine, blood or stool**
EXCLUDES *Urine (87088)*
🚑 0.00 ⚕ 0.00 **FUD** XXX [Q][□]
AMA: 2016,Jan,13; 2015,Jan,16; 2014,Jan,11

87073 **quantitative, anaerobic with isolation and presumptive identification of isolates, any source except urine, blood or stool**
EXCLUDES *Definitive identification of isolates (87076, 87077)*
Typing of isolates (87140-87158)
🚑 0.00 ⚕ 0.00 **FUD** XXX [Q][□]
AMA: 2016,Jan,13; 2015,Jan,16; 2014,Jan,11

87075 **any source, except blood, anaerobic with isolation and presumptive identification of isolates**
🚑 0.00 ⚕ 0.00 **FUD** XXX [Q][□]
AMA: 2005,Aug,7-8; 2005,Jul,11-12

87076 **anaerobic isolate, additional methods required for definitive identification, each isolate**
🚑 0.00 ⚕ 0.00 **FUD** XXX [Q][□]
AMA: 2016,Jan,13; 2015,Jan,16; 2014,Jan,11

87077 **aerobic isolate, additional methods required for definitive identification, each isolate**
🚑 0.00 ⚕ 0.00 **FUD** XXX [X][Q][□]
AMA: 2016,Jan,13; 2015,Jan,16; 2014,Jan,11; 2012,Jan,15-42

87081 **Culture, presumptive, pathogenic organisms, screening only;**
🚑 0.00 ⚕ 0.00 **FUD** XXX [Q][□]
AMA: 2016,Jan,13; 2015,Jan,16; 2014,Jan,11

87084 **with colony estimation from density chart**
🚑 0.00 ⚕ 0.00 **FUD** XXX [Q][□]
AMA: 2005,Aug,7-8; 2005,Jul,11-12

87086 **Culture, bacterial; quantitative colony count, urine**
🚑 0.00 ⚕ 0.00 **FUD** XXX [Q][□]
AMA: 2016,Jan,13; 2015,Jan,16; 2014,Jan,11; 2012,Jan,15-42

87088 **with isolation and presumptive identification of each isolate, urine**
🚑 0.00 ⚕ 0.00 **FUD** XXX [Q][□]
AMA: 2016,Jan,13; 2015,Jan,16; 2014,Jan,11; 2012,Jan,15-42

87101 **Culture, fungi (mold or yeast) isolation, with presumptive identification of isolates; skin, hair, or nail**
🚑 0.00 ⚕ 0.00 **FUD** XXX [Q][□]
AMA: 2016,Jan,13; 2015,Jan,16; 2014,Jan,11; 2012,Jan,15-42; 2011,Jan,11

87102 **other source (except blood)**
🚑 0.00 ⚕ 0.00 **FUD** XXX [Q][□]
AMA: 2005,Aug,7-8; 2005,Jul,11-12

87103 **blood**
🚑 0.00 ⚕ 0.00 **FUD** XXX [Q][□]
AMA: 2005,Aug,7-8; 2005,Jul,11-12

87106 **Culture, fungi, definitive identification, each organism; yeast**
🚑 0.00 ⚕ 0.00 **FUD** XXX [Q][□]
AMA: 2005,Aug,7-8; 2005,Jul,11-12

87107 **mold**
🚑 0.00 ⚕ 0.00 **FUD** XXX [Q][□]
AMA: 2005,Aug,7-8; 2005,Jul,11-12

87109 **Culture, mycoplasma, any source**
🚑 0.00 ⚕ 0.00 **FUD** XXX [Q][□]
AMA: 2005,Aug,7-8; 2005,Jul,11-12

87110 **Culture, chlamydia, any source**
EXCLUDES *Immunofluorescence staining of shell vials (87140)*
🚑 0.00 ⚕ 0.00 **FUD** XXX [A][□]
AMA: 2005,Aug,7-8; 2005,Jul,11-12

87116 **Culture, tubercle or other acid-fast bacilli (eg, TB, AFB, mycobacteria) any source, with isolation and presumptive identification of isolates**
EXCLUDES *Concentration (87015)*
🚑 0.00 ⚕ 0.00 **FUD** XXX [Q][□]
AMA: 2005,Aug,7-8; 2005,Jul,11-12

87118 **Culture, mycobacterial, definitive identification, each isolate**
🚑 0.00 ⚕ 0.00 **FUD** XXX [Q][□]
AMA: 2005,Aug,7-8; 2005,Jul,11-12

● New Code ▲ Revised Code ○ Reinstated ● New Web Release ▲ Revised Web Release Unlisted Not Covered # Resequenced
⊘ AMA Mod 51 Exempt ⑤ Optum Mod 51 Exempt ⑥ Mod 63 Exempt ✗ Non-FDA Drug ★ Telehealth Ⓜ Maternity Ⓐ Age Edit ✚ Add-on **AMA:** CPT Asst

87140-87158 Additional Culture Typing Techniques

INCLUDES Bacteriology, mycology, parasitology, and virology
EXCLUDES *Use of molecular procedure codes as a substitute for codes in this range (81200-81408 [81161, 81162, 81287, 81288])*
Code also definitive identification
Code also modifier 59 for multiple specimens or sites
Code also modifier 91 for repeat procedures performed on the same day

87140 **Culture, typing; immunofluorescent method, each antiserum**
0.00   0.00   **FUD** XXX
AMA: 2016,Jan,13; 2015,Jan,16; 2014,Jan,11

87143 **gas liquid chromatography (GLC) or high pressure liquid chromatography (HPLC) method**
0.00   0.00   **FUD** XXX
AMA: 2005,Aug,7-8; 2005,Jul,11-12

87147 **immunologic method, other than immunofluorescence (eg, agglutination grouping), per antiserum**
0.00   0.00   **FUD** XXX
AMA: 2016,Jan,13; 2015,Jan,16; 2014,Jan,11; 2012,Jan,15-42; 2011,Jan,11

87149 **identification by nucleic acid (DNA or RNA) probe, direct probe technique, per culture or isolate, each organism probed**
0.00   0.00   **FUD** XXX
AMA: 2016,Jan,13; 2015,Jan,16; 2014,Jan,11; 2013,Sep,3-12; 2012,May,3-10

87150 **identification by nucleic acid (DNA or RNA) probe, amplified probe technique, per culture or isolate, each organism probed**
0.00   0.00   **FUD** XXX
AMA: 2016,Jan,13; 2015,Jan,16; 2014,Jan,11; 2013,Sep,3-12; 2012,May,3-10

87152 **identification by pulse field gel typing**
0.00   0.00   **FUD** XXX
AMA: 2016,Jan,13; 2015,Jan,16; 2014,Jan,11; 2013,Sep,3-12; 2012,May,3-10

87153 **identification by nucleic acid sequencing method, each isolate (eg, sequencing of the 16S rRNA gene)**
0.00   0.00   **FUD** XXX
AMA: 2016,Jan,13; 2015,Jan,16; 2013,Sep,3-12; 2012,May,3-10

87158 **other methods**
0.00   0.00   **FUD** XXX
AMA: 2016,Jan,13; 2015,Jan,16; 2014,Jan,11

87164-87255 Identification of Organism from Primary Source and Sensitivity Studies

INCLUDES Bacteriology, mycology, parasitology, and virology
EXCLUDES *Additional tests using molecular probes, chromatography, or immunologic techniques (87140-87158)*
Code also modifier 59 for multiple specimens or sites
Code also modifier 91 for repeat procedures performed on the same day

87164 **Dark field examination, any source (eg, penile, vaginal, oral, skin); includes specimen collection**
0.00   0.00   **FUD** XXX
AMA: 2005,Jul,11-12; 2005,Aug,7-8

87166 **without collection**
0.00   0.00   **FUD** XXX
AMA: 2005,Aug,7-8; 2005,Jul,11-12

87168 **Macroscopic examination; arthropod**
0.00   0.00   **FUD** XXX
AMA: 2005,Aug,7-8; 2005,Jul,11-12

87169 **parasite**
0.00   0.00   **FUD** XXX
AMA: 2005,Aug,7-8; 2005,Jul,11-12

87172 **Pinworm exam (eg, cellophane tape prep)**
0.00   0.00   **FUD** XXX
AMA: 2005,Aug,7-8; 2005,Jul,11-12

87176 **Homogenization, tissue, for culture**
0.00   0.00   **FUD** XXX
AMA: 2005,Aug,7-8; 2005,Jul,11-12

87177 **Ova and parasites, direct smears, concentration and identification**
EXCLUDES *Coccidia or microsporidia exam (87207)*
Complex special stain (trichrome, iron hematoxylin) (87209)
Concentration for infectious agents (87015)
Direct smears from primary source (87207)
Nucleic acid probes in cytologic material (88365)
0.00   0.00   **FUD** XXX
AMA: 2016,Jan,13; 2015,Jan,16; 2014,Jan,11; 2012,Jan,15-42; 2011,Jan,11

87181 **Susceptibility studies, antimicrobial agent; agar dilution method, per agent (eg, antibiotic gradient strip)**
0.00   0.00   **FUD** XXX
AMA: 2016,Jan,13; 2015,Jan,16; 2014,Jan,11

87184 **disk method, per plate (12 or fewer agents)**
0.00   0.00   **FUD** XXX
AMA: 2016,Jan,13; 2015,Jan,16; 2014,Jan,11

87185 **enzyme detection (eg, beta lactamase), per enzyme**
0.00   0.00   **FUD** XXX
AMA: 2016,Jan,13; 2015,Jan,16; 2014,Jan,11

87186 **microdilution or agar dilution (minimum inhibitory concentration [MIC] or breakpoint), each multi-antimicrobial, per plate**
0.00   0.00   **FUD** XXX
AMA: 2016,Jan,13; 2015,Jan,16; 2014,Jan,11

+ **87187** **microdilution or agar dilution, minimum lethal concentration (MLC), each plate (List separately in addition to code for primary procedure)**
Code first (87186, 87188)
0.00   0.00   **FUD** XXX
AMA: 2016,Jan,13; 2015,Jan,16; 2014,Jan,11

87188 **macrobroth dilution method, each agent**
0.00   0.00   **FUD** XXX
AMA: 2016,Jan,13; 2015,Jan,16; 2014,Jan,11

87190 **mycobacteria, proportion method, each agent**
EXCLUDES *Other mycobacterial susceptibility studies (87181, 87184, 87186, 87188)*
0.00   0.00   **FUD** XXX
AMA: 2005,Aug,7-8; 2005,Jul,11-12

87197 **Serum bactericidal titer (Schlichter test)**
0.00   0.00   **FUD** XXX
AMA: 2005,Aug,7-8; 2005,Jul,11-12

87205 **Smear, primary source with interpretation; Gram or Giemsa stain for bacteria, fungi, or cell types**
0.00   0.00   **FUD** XXX
AMA: 2016,Jan,13; 2015,Jan,16; 2014,Jan,11; 2012,Jan,15-42; 2011,Jan,11

87206 **fluorescent and/or acid fast stain for bacteria, fungi, parasites, viruses or cell types**
0.00   0.00   **FUD** XXX
AMA: 2005,Aug,7-8; 2005,Jul,11-12

87207 **special stain for inclusion bodies or parasites (eg, malaria, coccidia, microsporidia, trypanosomes, herpes viruses)**
EXCLUDES *Direct smears with concentration and identification (87177)*
Thick smear preparation (87015)
0.00   0.00   **FUD** XXX
AMA: 2016,Jan,13; 2015,Jan,16; 2014,Jan,11

87209 **complex special stain (eg, trichrome, iron hemotoxylin) for ova and parasites**
0.00   0.00   **FUD** XXX
AMA: 2016,Jan,13; 2015,Jan,16; 2014,Jan,11

87210 wet mount for infectious agents (eg, saline, India ink, KOH preps)

> EXCLUDES   KOH evaluation of skin, hair, or nails (87220)
> ⚒ 0.00   ⅀ 0.00   **FUD** XXX   ☒ ⓠ ▭
> **AMA:** 2016,May,13

87220 Tissue examination by KOH slide of samples from skin, hair, or nails for fungi or ectoparasite ova or mites (eg, scabies)

> ⚒ 0.00   ⅀ 0.00   **FUD** XXX   ⓠ ▭
> **AMA:** 2005,Aug,7-8; 2005,Jul,11-12

87230 Toxin or antitoxin assay, tissue culture (eg, Clostridium difficile toxin)

> ⚒ 0.00   ⅀ 0.00   **FUD** XXX   ⓠ ▭
> **AMA:** 2005,Aug,7-8; 2005,Jul,11-12

87250 Virus isolation; inoculation of embryonated eggs, or small animal, includes observation and dissection

> ⚒ 0.00   ⅀ 0.00   **FUD** XXX   ⓠ ▭
> **AMA:** 2005,Aug,7-8; 2005,Jul,11-12

87252 tissue culture inoculation, observation, and presumptive identification by cytopathic effect

> ⚒ 0.00   ⅀ 0.00   **FUD** XXX   ⓠ ▭
> **AMA:** 2005,Aug,7-8; 2005,Jul,11-12

87253 tissue culture, additional studies or definitive identification (eg, hemabsorption, neutralization, immunofluorescence stain), each isolate

> EXCLUDES   Electron microscopy (88348)
> Inclusion bodies in:
> Fluids (88106)
> Smears (87207-87210)
> Tissue sections (88304-88309)
> ⚒ 0.00   ⅀ 0.00   **FUD** XXX   ⓠ ▭
> **AMA:** 2005,Aug,7-8; 2005,Jul,11-12

87254 centrifuge enhanced (shell vial) technique, includes identification with immunofluorescence stain, each virus

> Code also (87252)
> ⚒ 0.00   ⅀ 0.00   **FUD** XXX   ⓠ ▭
> **AMA:** 2016,Jan,13; 2015,Jan,16; 2014,Jan,11

87255 including identification by non-immunologic method, other than by cytopathic effect (eg, virus specific enzymatic activity)

> ⚒ 0.00   ⅀ 0.00   **FUD** XXX   ⓠ ▭
> **AMA:** 2016,Jan,13; 2015,Jan,16; 2014,Jan,11

87260-87300 Fluorescence Microscopy by Organism

> INCLUDES   Primary source only
> EXCLUDES   Comparable tests on culture material (87140-87158)
> Identification of antibodies (86602-86804)
> Nonspecific agent detection (87299, 87449-87450, 87797-87799, 87899)
> Code also modifier 59 for different species or strains reported by the same code

87260 Infectious agent antigen detection by immunofluorescent technique; adenovirus

> ⚒ 0.00   ⅀ 0.00   **FUD** XXX   ⓠ ▭
> **AMA:** 2005,Jul,11-12; 2005,Aug,7-8

87265 Bordetella pertussis/parapertussis

> ⚒ 0.00   ⅀ 0.00   **FUD** XXX   ⓠ ▭
> **AMA:** 2005,Jul,11-12; 2005,Aug,7-8

87267 Enterovirus, direct fluorescent antibody (DFA)

> ⚒ 0.00   ⅀ 0.00   **FUD** XXX   ⓠ ▭
> **AMA:** 2016,Jan,13; 2015,Jan,16; 2014,Jan,11

87269 giardia

> ⚒ 0.00   ⅀ 0.00   **FUD** XXX   ⓠ ▭
> **AMA:** 2005,Jul,11-12; 2005,Aug,7-8

87270 Chlamydia trachomatis

> ⚒ 0.00   ⅀ 0.00   **FUD** XXX   Ⓐ ▭
> **AMA:** 2005,Jul,11-12; 2005,Aug,7-8

87271 Cytomegalovirus, direct fluorescent antibody (DFA)

> ⚒ 0.00   ⅀ 0.00   **FUD** XXX   ⓠ ▭
> **AMA:** 2016,Jan,13; 2015,Jan,16; 2014,Jan,11

87272 cryptosporidium

> ⚒ 0.00   ⅀ 0.00   **FUD** XXX   ⓠ ▭
> **AMA:** 2005,Jul,11-12; 2005,Aug,7-8

87273 Herpes simplex virus type 2

> ⚒ 0.00   ⅀ 0.00   **FUD** XXX   ⓠ ▭
> **AMA:** 2005,Jul,11-12; 2005,Aug,7-8

87274 Herpes simplex virus type 1

> ⚒ 0.00   ⅀ 0.00   **FUD** XXX   ⓠ ▭
> **AMA:** 2005,Jul,11-12; 2005,Aug,7-8

87275 influenza B virus

> ⚒ 0.00   ⅀ 0.00   **FUD** XXX   ⓠ ▭
> **AMA:** 2016,Jan,13; 2015,Jan,16; 2014,Jan,11

87276 influenza A virus

> ⚒ 0.00   ⅀ 0.00   **FUD** XXX   ⓠ ▭
> **AMA:** 2016,Jan,13; 2015,Jan,16; 2014,Jan,11

87277 Legionella micdadei

> ⚒ 0.00   ⅀ 0.00   **FUD** XXX   ⓠ ▭
> **AMA:** 2005,Jul,11-12; 2005,Aug,7-8

87278 Legionella pneumophila

> ⚒ 0.00   ⅀ 0.00   **FUD** XXX   ⓠ ▭
> **AMA:** 2005,Jul,11-12; 2005,Aug,7-8

87279 Parainfluenza virus, each type

> ⚒ 0.00   ⅀ 0.00   **FUD** XXX   ⓠ ▭
> **AMA:** 2005,Jul,11-12; 2005,Aug,7-8

87280 respiratory syncytial virus

> ⚒ 0.00   ⅀ 0.00   **FUD** XXX   ⓠ ▭
> **AMA:** 2005,Jul,11-12; 2005,Aug,7-8

87281 Pneumocystis carinii

> ⚒ 0.00   ⅀ 0.00   **FUD** XXX   ⓠ ▭
> **AMA:** 2005,Jul,11-12; 2005,Aug,7-8

87283 Rubeola

> ⚒ 0.00   ⅀ 0.00   **FUD** XXX   ⓠ ▭
> **AMA:** 2005,Jul,11-12; 2005,Aug,7-8

87285 Treponema pallidum

> ⚒ 0.00   ⅀ 0.00   **FUD** XXX   ⓠ ▭
> **AMA:** 2005,Jul,11-12; 2005,Aug,7-8

87290 Varicella zoster virus

> ⚒ 0.00   ⅀ 0.00   **FUD** XXX   ⓠ ▭
> **AMA:** 2005,Jul,11-12; 2005,Aug,7-8

87299 not otherwise specified, each organism

> ⚒ 0.00   ⅀ 0.00   **FUD** XXX   ⓠ ▭
> **AMA:** 2016,Jan,13; 2015,Jan,16; 2014,Jan,11

87300 Infectious agent antigen detection by immunofluorescent technique, polyvalent for multiple organisms, each polyvalent antiserum

> EXCLUDES   Physician evaluation of infectious disease agents by immunofluorescence (88346)
> ⚒ 0.00   ⅀ 0.00   **FUD** XXX   ⓠ ▭
> **AMA:** 2005,Jul,11-12; 2005,Aug,7-8

87301-87451 Enzyme Immunoassay Technique by Organism

> INCLUDES   Primary source only
> EXCLUDES   Comparable tests on culture material (87140-87158)
> Identification of antibodies (86602-86804)
> Nonspecific agent detection (87449-87450, 87797-87799, 87899)
> Code also modifier 59 for different species or strains reported by the same code

87301 Infectious agent antigen detection by immunoassay technique, (eg, enzyme immunoassay [EIA], enzyme-linked immunosorbent assay [ELISA], immunochemiluminometric assay [IMCA]) qualitative or semiquantitative, multiple-step method; adenovirus enteric types 40/41

> ⚒ 0.00   ⅀ 0.00   **FUD** XXX   ⓠ
> **AMA:** 2016,Jan,13; 2015,Jan,16; 2014,Jan,11

87305 Aspergillus

> ⚒ 0.00   ⅀ 0.00   **FUD** XXX   ⓠ

Pathology and Laboratory

87320 — 87477

87320 **Chlamydia trachomatis**
🔬 0.00 ⚗ 0.00 **FUD** XXX Ⓐ▢
AMA: 2005,Jul,11-12; 2005,Aug,7-8

87324 **Clostridium difficile toxin(s)**
🔬 0.00 ⚗ 0.00 **FUD** XXX Ⓠ▢
AMA: 2005,Jul,11-12; 2005,Aug,7-8

87327 **Cryptococcus neoformans**
EXCLUDES *Cryptococcus latex agglutination (86403)*
🔬 0.00 ⚗ 0.00 **FUD** XXX Ⓠ
AMA: 2005,Jul,11-12; 2005,Aug,7-8

87328 **cryptosporidium**
🔬 0.00 ⚗ 0.00 **FUD** XXX Ⓠ▢
AMA: 2005,Jul,11-12; 2005,Aug,7-8

87329 **giardia**
🔬 0.00 ⚗ 0.00 **FUD** XXX Ⓠ▢
AMA: 2005,Jul,11-12; 2005,Aug,7-8

87332 **cytomegalovirus**
🔬 0.00 ⚗ 0.00 **FUD** XXX Ⓠ▢
AMA: 2005,Jul,11-12; 2005,Aug,7-8

87335 **Escherichia coli O157**
EXCLUDES *Giardia antigen (87329)*
🔬 0.00 ⚗ 0.00 **FUD** XXX Ⓠ
AMA: 2005,Jul,11-12; 2005,Aug,7-8

87336 **Entamoeba histolytica dispar group**
🔬 0.00 ⚗ 0.00 **FUD** XXX Ⓠ
AMA: 2005,Jul,11-12; 2005,Aug,7-8

87337 **Entamoeba histolytica group**
🔬 0.00 ⚗ 0.00 **FUD** XXX Ⓠ
AMA: 2005,Jul,11-12; 2005,Aug,7-8

87338 **Helicobacter pylori, stool**
🔬 0.00 ⚗ 0.00 **FUD** XXX ❌Ⓠ▢
AMA: 2016,Jan,13; 2015,Jan,16; 2014,Jan,11

87339 **Helicobacter pylori**
EXCLUDES *H. pylori:*
Breath and blood by mass spectrometry (83013-83014)
Liquid scintillation counter (78267-78268)
Stool (87338)
🔬 0.00 ⚗ 0.00 **FUD** XXX Ⓠ▢
AMA: 2005,Jul,11-12; 2005,Aug,7-8

87340 **hepatitis B surface antigen (HBsAg)**
🔬 0.00 ⚗ 0.00 **FUD** XXX Ⓠ
AMA: 2016,Jan,13; 2015,Jan,16; 2014,Jan,11

87341 **hepatitis B surface antigen (HBsAg) neutralization**
🔬 0.00 ⚗ 0.00 **FUD** XXX Ⓐ
AMA: 2005,Jul,11-12; 2005,Aug,7-8

87350 **hepatitis Be antigen (HBeAg)**
🔬 0.00 ⚗ 0.00 **FUD** XXX Ⓠ▢
AMA: 2005,Jul,11-12; 2005,Aug,7-8

87380 **hepatitis, delta agent**
🔬 0.00 ⚗ 0.00 **FUD** XXX Ⓠ
AMA: 2005,Jul,11-12; 2005,Aug,7-8

87385 **Histoplasma capsulatum**
🔬 0.00 ⚗ 0.00 **FUD** XXX Ⓠ
AMA: 2005,Jul,11-12; 2005,Aug,7-8

87389 **HIV-1 antigen(s), with HIV-1 and HIV-2 antibodies, single result**
🔬 0.00 ⚗ 0.00 **FUD** XXX Ⓠ▢
Code also modifier 92 for test performed using a kit or transportable instrument that is all or in part consists of a single-use, disposable analytical chamber

87390 **HIV-1**
🔬 0.00 ⚗ 0.00 **FUD** XXX Ⓠ▢
AMA: 2005,Jul,11-12; 2005,Aug,7-8

87391 **HIV-2**
🔬 0.00 ⚗ 0.00 **FUD** XXX Ⓠ
AMA: 2005,Jul,11-12; 2005,Aug,7-8

87400 **Influenza, A or B, each**
🔬 0.00 ⚗ 0.00 **FUD** XXX Ⓠ▢
AMA: 2016,Jan,13; 2015,Jan,16; 2014,Jan,11; 2012,Jan,15-42; 2011,Jan,11

87420 **respiratory syncytial virus**
🔬 0.00 ⚗ 0.00 **FUD** XXX Ⓠ
AMA: 2005,Jul,11-12; 2005,Aug,7-8

87425 **rotavirus**
🔬 0.00 ⚗ 0.00 **FUD** XXX Ⓠ▢
AMA: 2005,Jul,11-12; 2005,Aug,7-8

87427 **Shiga-like toxin**
🔬 0.00 ⚗ 0.00 **FUD** XXX Ⓠ
AMA: 2005,Jul,11-12; 2005,Aug,7-8

87430 **Streptococcus, group A**
🔬 0.00 ⚗ 0.00 **FUD** XXX Ⓠ▢
AMA: 2016,Jan,13; 2015,Jan,16; 2012,Jan,15-42; 2011,Jan,11

87449 **Infectious agent antigen detection by immunoassay technique, (eg, enzyme immunoassay [EIA], enzyme-linked immunosorbent assay [ELISA], immunochemiluminometric assay [IMCA]), qualitative or semiquantitative; multiple-step method, not otherwise specified, each organism**
🔬 0.00 ⚗ 0.00 **FUD** XXX ❌Ⓠ▢
AMA: 2016,Jan,13; 2015,Jan,16; 2014,Jan,11; 2012,Jan,15-42; 2011,Jan,11

87450 **single step method, not otherwise specified, each organism**
🔬 0.00 ⚗ 0.00 **FUD** XXX Ⓠ
AMA: 2005,Jul,11-12; 2005,Aug,7-8

87451 **multiple step method, polyvalent for multiple organisms, each polyvalent antiserum**
🔬 0.00 ⚗ 0.00 **FUD** XXX Ⓠ
AMA: 2005,Jul,11-12; 2005,Aug,7-8

87470-87801 [87623, 87624, 87625] Detection Infectious Agent by Probe Techniques

INCLUDES Primary source only
EXCLUDES *Comparable tests on culture material (87140-87158)*
Identification of antibodies (86602-86804)
Nonspecific agent detection (87299, 87449-87450, 87797-87799, 87899)
Use of molecular procedure codes as a substitute for codes in this range (81200-81408 [81161, 81162, 81287, 81288])
Code also modifier 59 for different species or strains reported by the same code

87470 **Infectious agent detection by nucleic acid (DNA or RNA); Bartonella henselae and Bartonella quintana, direct probe technique**
🔬 0.00 ⚗ 0.00 **FUD** XXX Ⓠ▢
AMA: 2016,Jan,13; 2015,Jan,16; 2013,Sep,3-12; 2012,May,3-10

87471 **Bartonella henselae and Bartonella quintana, amplified probe technique**
🔬 0.00 ⚗ 0.00 **FUD** XXX Ⓠ▢
AMA: 2016,Jan,13; 2015,Jan,16; 2013,Sep,3-12; 2012,May,3-10

87472 **Bartonella henselae and Bartonella quintana, quantification**
🔬 0.00 ⚗ 0.00 **FUD** XXX Ⓠ▢
AMA: 2016,Jan,13; 2015,Jan,16; 2013,Sep,3-12; 2012,May,3-10

87475 **Borrelia burgdorferi, direct probe technique**
🔬 0.00 ⚗ 0.00 **FUD** XXX Ⓠ▢
AMA: 2016,Jan,13; 2015,Jan,16; 2013,Sep,3-12; 2012,May,3-10

87476 **Borrelia burgdorferi, amplified probe technique**
🔬 0.00 ⚗ 0.00 **FUD** XXX Ⓠ▢
AMA: 2016,Jan,13; 2015,Jan,16; 2013,Sep,3-12; 2012,May,3-10

87477 **Borrelia burgdorferi, quantification**
🔬 0.00 ⚗ 0.00 **FUD** XXX Ⓠ▢
AMA: 2016,Jan,13; 2015,Jan,16; 2013,Sep,3-12; 2012,May,3-10

26/TC PC/TC Only	A2-Z3 ASC Payment	50 Bilateral	♂ Male Only	♀ Female Only	🔬 Facility RVU	⚗ Non-Facility RVU	▢ CCI
FUD Follow-up Days	CMS: IOM (Pub 100)	A-Y OPPSI	80/80 Surg Assist Allowed / w/Doc		🔬 Lab Crosswalk	❌ Radiology Crosswalk	❌ CLIA

394

87480   **Candida species, direct probe technique**
   0.00   0.00   **FUD** XXX   🔲 🔲
   AMA: 2016,Jan,13; 2015,Jan,16; 2013,Sep,3-12; 2012,May,3-10

87481   **Candida species, amplified probe technique**
   0.00   0.00   **FUD** XXX   🔲 🔲
   AMA: 2016,Jan,13; 2015,Jan,16; 2013,Sep,3-12; 2012,May,3-10

87482   **Candida species, quantification**
   0.00   0.00   **FUD** XXX   🔲 🔲
   AMA: 2016,Jan,13; 2015,Jan,16; 2013,Sep,3-12; 2012,May,3-10

● **87483**   **central nervous system pathogen (eg, Neisseria meningitidis, Streptococcus pneumoniae, Listeria, Haemophilus influenzae, E. coli, Streptococcus agalactiae, enterovirus, human parechovirus, herpes simplex virus type 1 and 2, human herpesvirus 6, cytomegalovirus, varicella zoster virus, Cryptococcus), includes multiplex reverse transcription, when performed, and multiplex amplified probe technique, multiple types or subtypes, 12-25 targets**

87485   **Chlamydia pneumoniae, direct probe technique**
   0.00   0.00   **FUD** XXX   🔲 🔲
   AMA: 2016,Jan,13; 2015,Jan,16; 2013,Sep,3-12; 2012,May,3-10

87486   **Chlamydia pneumoniae, amplified probe technique**
   0.00   0.00   **FUD** XXX   🔲 🔲
   AMA: 2016,Jan,13; 2015,Jan,16; 2013,Sep,3-12; 2012,May,3-10

87487   **Chlamydia pneumoniae, quantification**
   0.00   0.00   **FUD** XXX   🔲 🔲
   AMA: 2016,Jan,13; 2015,Jan,16; 2013,Sep,3-12; 2012,May,3-10

87490   **Chlamydia trachomatis, direct probe technique**
   0.00   0.00   **FUD** XXX   🅰 🔲
   AMA: 2016,Jan,13; 2015,Jan,16; 2013,Sep,3-12; 2012,May,3-10

87491   **Chlamydia trachomatis, amplified probe technique**
   0.00   0.00   **FUD** XXX   🅰 🔲
   AMA: 2016,Jan,13; 2015,Jan,16; 2013,Sep,3-12; 2013,Jun,13; 2012,May,3-10

87492   **Chlamydia trachomatis, quantification**
   0.00   0.00   **FUD** XXX   🔲 🔲
   AMA: 2016,Jan,13; 2015,Jan,16; 2013,Sep,3-12; 2012,May,3-10

87493   **Clostridium difficile, toxin gene(s), amplified probe technique**
   0.00   0.00   **FUD** XXX   🔲 🔲
   AMA: 2016,Jan,13; 2015,Jan,16; 2014,Jan,11; 2013,Sep,3-12; 2012,May,3-10

87495   **cytomegalovirus, direct probe technique**
   0.00   0.00   **FUD** XXX   🔲 🔲
   AMA: 2016,Jan,13; 2015,Jan,16; 2013,Sep,3-12; 2012,May,3-10

87496   **cytomegalovirus, amplified probe technique**
   0.00   0.00   **FUD** XXX   🔲 🔲
   AMA: 2016,Jan,13; 2015,Jan,16; 2013,Sep,3-12; 2012,May,3-10

87497   **cytomegalovirus, quantification**
   0.00   0.00   **FUD** XXX   🔲 🔲
   AMA: 2016,Jan,13; 2015,Jan,16; 2013,Sep,3-12; 2012,May,3-10

87498   **enterovirus, amplified probe technique, includes reverse transcription when performed**
   0.00   0.00   **FUD** XXX   🔲 🔲
   AMA: 2016,Jan,13; 2015,Jan,16; 2013,Sep,3-12; 2012,May,3-10

87500   **vancomycin resistance (eg, enterococcus species van A, van B), amplified probe technique**
   0.00   0.00   **FUD** XXX   🔲 🔲
   AMA: 2016,Jan,13; 2015,Jan,16; 2014,Jan,11; 2013,Sep,3-12; 2012,May,3-10

87501   **influenza virus, includes reverse transcription, when performed, and amplified probe technique, each type or subtype**
   0.00   0.00   **FUD** XXX   🔲 🔲
   AMA: 2016,Jan,13; 2015,Jan,16; 2013,Sep,3-12; 2012,May,3-10

87502   **influenza virus, for multiple types or sub-types, includes multiplex reverse transcription, when performed, and multiplex amplified probe technique, first 2 types or sub-types**
   0.00   0.00   **FUD** XXX   ❌ 🔲 🔲
   AMA: 2016,Jan,13; 2015,Jan,16; 2013,Sep,3-12; 2012,May,3-10

+ **87503**   **influenza virus, for multiple types or sub-types, includes multiplex reverse transcription, when performed, and multiplex amplified probe technique, each additional influenza virus type or sub-type beyond 2 (List separately in addition to code for primary procedure)**
   Code first (87502)
   0.00   0.00   **FUD** XXX   🔲 🔲
   AMA: 2016,Jan,13; 2015,Jan,16; 2013,Sep,3-12; 2012,May,3-10

87505   **gastrointestinal pathogen (eg, Clostridium difficile, E. coli, Salmonella, Shigella, norovirus, Giardia), includes multiplex reverse transcription, when performed, and multiplex amplified probe technique, multiple types or subtypes, 3-5 targets**
   0.00   0.00   **FUD** XXX   🔲 🔲

87506   **gastrointestinal pathogen (eg, Clostridium difficile, E. coli, Salmonella, Shigella, norovirus, Giardia), includes multiplex reverse transcription, when performed, and multiplex amplified probe technique, multiple types or subtypes, 6-11 targets**
   0.00   0.00   **FUD** XXX   🔲 🔲

87507   **gastrointestinal pathogen (eg, Clostridium difficile, E. coli, Salmonella, Shigella, norovirus, Giardia), includes multiplex reverse transcription, when performed, and multiplex amplified probe technique, multiple types or subtypes, 12-25 targets**
   0.00   0.00   **FUD** XXX   🔲 🔲

87510   **Gardnerella vaginalis, direct probe technique**
   0.00   0.00   **FUD** XXX   🔲 🔲
   AMA: 2016,Jan,13; 2015,Jan,16; 2013,Sep,3-12; 2012,May,3-10

87511   **Gardnerella vaginalis, amplified probe technique**
   0.00   0.00   **FUD** XXX   🔲 🔲
   AMA: 2016,Jan,13; 2015,Jan,16; 2013,Sep,3-12; 2012,May,3-10

87512   **Gardnerella vaginalis, quantification**
   0.00   0.00   **FUD** XXX   🔲 🔲
   AMA: 2016,Jan,13; 2015,Jan,16; 2013,Sep,3-12; 2012,May,3-10

87515   **hepatitis B virus, direct probe technique**
   0.00   0.00   **FUD** XXX   🔲 🔲
   AMA: 2016,Jan,13; 2015,Jan,16; 2013,Sep,3-12; 2012,May,3-10

87516   **hepatitis B virus, amplified probe technique**
   0.00   0.00   **FUD** XXX   🔲 🔲
   AMA: 2016,Jan,13; 2015,Jan,16; 2013,Sep,3-12; 2012,May,3-10

87517   **hepatitis B virus, quantification**
   0.00   0.00   **FUD** XXX   🔲 🔲
   AMA: 2016,Jan,13; 2015,Jan,16; 2013,Sep,3-12; 2012,May,3-10

87520   **hepatitis C, direct probe technique**
   0.00   0.00   **FUD** XXX   🔲 🔲
   AMA: 2016,Jan,13; 2015,Jan,16; 2013,Sep,3-12; 2012,May,3-10

87521   **hepatitis C, amplified probe technique, includes reverse transcription when performed**
   0.00   0.00   **FUD** XXX   🔲 🔲
   AMA: 2016,Jan,13; 2015,Jan,16; 2013,Sep,3-12; 2012,May,3-10

87522   **hepatitis C, quantification, includes reverse transcription when performed**
   0.00   0.00   **FUD** XXX   🔲 🔲
   AMA: 2016,Jan,13; 2015,Jan,16; 2013,Sep,3-12; 2012,May,3-10

87525   **hepatitis G, direct probe technique**
   0.00   0.00   **FUD** XXX   🔲 🔲
   AMA: 2016,Jan,13; 2015,Jan,16; 2013,Sep,3-12; 2012,May,3-10

87526   **hepatitis G, amplified probe technique**
🚑 0.00   🔬 0.00   **FUD** XXX   Q ▣
AMA: 2016,Jan,13; 2015,Jan,16; 2013,Sep,3-12; 2012,May,3-10

87527   **hepatitis G, quantification**
🚑 0.00   🔬 0.00   **FUD** XXX   Q ▣
AMA: 2016,Jan,13; 2015,Jan,16; 2013,Sep,3-12; 2012,May,3-10

87528   **Herpes simplex virus, direct probe technique**
🚑 0.00   🔬 0.00   **FUD** XXX   Q ▣
AMA: 2016,Jan,13; 2015,Jan,16; 2013,Sep,3-12; 2012,May,3-10

87529   **Herpes simplex virus, amplified probe technique**
🚑 0.00   🔬 0.00   **FUD** XXX   Q ▣
AMA: 2016,Jan,13; 2015,Jan,16; 2013,Sep,3-12; 2012,May,3-10

87530   **Herpes simplex virus, quantification**
🚑 0.00   🔬 0.00   **FUD** XXX   Q ▣
AMA: 2016,Jan,13; 2015,Jan,16; 2013,Sep,3-12; 2012,May,3-10

87531   **Herpes virus-6, direct probe technique**
🚑 0.00   🔬 0.00   **FUD** XXX   Q ▣
AMA: 2016,Jan,13; 2015,Jan,16; 2013,Sep,3-12; 2012,May,3-10

87532   **Herpes virus-6, amplified probe technique**
🚑 0.00   🔬 0.00   **FUD** XXX   Q ▣
AMA: 2016,Jan,13; 2015,Jan,16; 2013,Sep,3-12; 2012,May,3-10

87533   **Herpes virus-6, quantification**
🚑 0.00   🔬 0.00   **FUD** XXX   Q ▣
AMA: 2016,Jan,13; 2015,Jan,16; 2013,Sep,3-12; 2012,May,3-10

87534   **HIV-1, direct probe technique**
🚑 0.00   🔬 0.00   **FUD** XXX   Q ▣
AMA: 2016,Jan,13; 2015,Jan,16; 2013,Sep,3-12; 2012,May,3-10

87535   **HIV-1, amplified probe technique, includes reverse transcription when performed**
🚑 0.00   🔬 0.00   **FUD** XXX   Q ▣
AMA: 2016,Jan,13; 2015,Jan,16; 2014,Jan,11; 2013,Sep,3-12; 2012,May,3-10

87536   **HIV-1, quantification, includes reverse transcription when performed**
🚑 0.00   🔬 0.00   **FUD** XXX   Q ▣
AMA: 2016,Jan,13; 2015,Jan,16; 2014,Jan,11; 2013,Sep,3-12; 2012,May,3-10; 2012,Jan,15-42

87537   **HIV-2, direct probe technique**
🚑 0.00   🔬 0.00   **FUD** XXX   Q ▣
AMA: 2016,Jan,13; 2015,Jan,16; 2013,Sep,3-12; 2012,May,3-10

87538   **HIV-2, amplified probe technique, includes reverse transcription when performed**
🚑 0.00   🔬 0.00   **FUD** XXX   Q ▣
AMA: 2016,Jan,13; 2015,Jan,16; 2013,Sep,3-12; 2012,May,3-10

87539   **HIV-2, quantification, includes reverse transcription when performed**
🚑 0.00   🔬 0.00   **FUD** XXX   Q ▣
AMA: 2016,Jan,13; 2015,Jan,16; 2013,Sep,3-12; 2012,May,3-10

\#   **87623**   **Human Papillomavirus (HPV), low-risk types (eg, 6, 11, 42, 43, 44)**
🚑 0.00   🔬 0.00   **FUD** XXX   Q ▣

\#   **87624**   **Human Papillomavirus (HPV), high-risk types (eg, 16, 18, 31, 33, 35, 39, 45, 51, 52, 56, 58, 59, 68)**
INCLUDES   Low- and high-risk types in one assay
🚑 0.00   🔬 0.00   **FUD** XXX   Q ▣
AMA: 2016,Jan,13; 2015,Oct,9

\#   **87625**   **Human Papillomavirus (HPV), types 16 and 18 only, includes type 45, if performed**
🚑 0.00   🔬 0.00   **FUD** XXX   Q ▣
AMA: 2016,Jan,13; 2015,Oct,9; 2015,Jun,10

87540   **Legionella pneumophila, direct probe technique**
🚑 0.00   🔬 0.00   **FUD** XXX   Q ▣
AMA: 2016,Jan,13; 2015,Jan,16; 2013,Sep,3-12; 2012,May,3-10

87541   **Legionella pneumophila, amplified probe technique**
🚑 0.00   🔬 0.00   **FUD** XXX   Q ▣
AMA: 2016,Jan,13; 2015,Jan,16; 2013,Sep,3-12; 2012,May,3-10

87542   **Legionella pneumophila, quantification**
🚑 0.00   🔬 0.00   **FUD** XXX   Q ▣
AMA: 2016,Jan,13; 2015,Jan,16; 2013,Sep,3-12; 2012,May,3-10

87550   **Mycobacteria species, direct probe technique**
🚑 0.00   🔬 0.00   **FUD** XXX   Q ▣
AMA: 2016,Jan,13; 2015,Jan,16; 2013,Sep,3-12; 2012,May,3-10

87551   **Mycobacteria species, amplified probe technique**
🚑 0.00   🔬 0.00   **FUD** XXX   Q ▣
AMA: 2016,Jan,13; 2015,Jan,16; 2013,Sep,3-12; 2012,May,3-10

87552   **Mycobacteria species, quantification**
🚑 0.00   🔬 0.00   **FUD** XXX   Q ▣
AMA: 2016,Jan,13; 2015,Jan,16; 2013,Sep,3-12; 2012,May,3-10

87555   **Mycobacteria tuberculosis, direct probe technique**
🚑 0.00   🔬 0.00   **FUD** XXX   Q ▣
AMA: 2016,Jan,13; 2015,Jan,16; 2013,Sep,3-12; 2012,May,3-10

87556   **Mycobacteria tuberculosis, amplified probe technique**
🚑 0.00   🔬 0.00   **FUD** XXX   Q ▣
AMA: 2016,Jan,13; 2015,Jan,16; 2013,Sep,3-12; 2012,May,3-10

87557   **Mycobacteria tuberculosis, quantification**
🚑 0.00   🔬 0.00   **FUD** XXX   Q ▣
AMA: 2016,Jan,13; 2015,Jan,16; 2013,Sep,3-12; 2012,May,3-10

87560   **Mycobacteria avium-intracellulare, direct probe technique**
🚑 0.00   🔬 0.00   **FUD** XXX   Q ▣
AMA: 2016,Jan,13; 2015,Jan,16; 2013,Sep,3-12; 2012,May,3-10

87561   **Mycobacteria avium-intracellulare, amplified probe technique**
🚑 0.00   🔬 0.00   **FUD** XXX   Q ▣
AMA: 2016,Jan,13; 2015,Jan,16; 2013,Sep,3-12; 2012,May,3-10

87562   **Mycobacteria avium-intracellulare, quantification**
🚑 0.00   🔬 0.00   **FUD** XXX   Q ▣
AMA: 2016,Jan,13; 2015,Jan,16; 2013,Sep,3-12; 2012,May,3-10

87580   **Mycoplasma pneumoniae, direct probe technique**
🚑 0.00   🔬 0.00   **FUD** XXX   Q ▣
AMA: 2016,Jan,13; 2015,Jan,16; 2013,Sep,3-12; 2012,May,3-10

87581   **Mycoplasma pneumoniae, amplified probe technique**
🚑 0.00   🔬 0.00   **FUD** XXX   Q ▣
AMA: 2016,Jan,13; 2015,Jan,16; 2013,Sep,3-12; 2012,May,3-10

87582   **Mycoplasma pneumoniae, quantification**
🚑 0.00   🔬 0.00   **FUD** XXX   Q ▣
AMA: 2016,Jan,13; 2015,Jan,16; 2013,Sep,3-12; 2012,May,3-10

87590   **Neisseria gonorrhoeae, direct probe technique**
🚑 0.00   🔬 0.00   **FUD** XXX   A ▣
AMA: 2016,Jan,13; 2015,Jan,16; 2013,Sep,3-12; 2012,May,3-10

87591   **Neisseria gonorrhoeae, amplified probe technique**
🚑 0.00   🔬 0.00   **FUD** XXX   A ▣
AMA: 2016,Jan,13; 2015,Jan,16; 2013,Sep,3-12; 2013,Jun,13; 2012,May,3-10

87592   **Neisseria gonorrhoeae, quantification**
🚑 0.00   🔬 0.00   **FUD** XXX   Q ▣
AMA: 2016,Jan,13; 2015,Jan,16; 2013,Sep,3-12; 2012,May,3-10

87623   **Resequenced code. See code following 87539.**

87624   **Resequenced code. See code following 87539.**

87625   **Resequenced code. See code before 87540.**

87631 respiratory virus (eg, adenovirus, influenza virus, coronavirus, metapneumovirus, parainfluenza virus, respiratory syncytial virus, rhinovirus), includes multiplex reverse transcription, when performed, and multiplex amplified probe technique, multiple types or subtypes, 3-5 targets

> INCLUDES Detection of multiple respiratory viruses with one test
>
> EXCLUDES Assays for typing or subtyping influenza viruses only (87501-87503)
>
> Single test for detection of multiple infectious organisms (87800-87801)

📻 0.00 ⚕ 0.00 **FUD** XXX ☒ Q 🖵

AMA: 2016,Jan,13; 2015,Jan,16; 2013,Sep,3-12

87632 respiratory virus (eg, adenovirus, influenza virus, coronavirus, metapneumovirus, parainfluenza virus, respiratory syncytial virus, rhinovirus), includes multiplex reverse transcription, when performed, and multiplex amplified probe technique, multiple types or subtypes, 6-11 targets

> INCLUDES Detection of multiple respiratory viruses with one test
>
> EXCLUDES Assays for typing or subtyping influenza viruses only (87501-87503)
>
> Single test to detect multiple infectious organisms (87800-87801)

📻 0.00 ⚕ 0.00 **FUD** XXX Q 🖵

AMA: 2016,Jan,13; 2015,Jan,16; 2013,Sep,3-12

87633 respiratory virus (eg, adenovirus, influenza virus, coronavirus, metapneumovirus, parainfluenza virus, respiratory syncytial virus, rhinovirus), includes multiplex reverse transcription, when performed, and multiplex amplified probe technique, multiple types or subtypes, 12-25 targets

> INCLUDES Detection of multiple respiratory viruses with one test
>
> EXCLUDES Assays for typing or subtyping influenza viruses only (87501-87503)
>
> Single test to detect multiple infectious organisms (87800-87801)

📻 0.00 ⚕ 0.00 **FUD** XXX Q 🖵

AMA: 2016,Jan,13; 2015,Jan,16; 2013,Sep,3-12

87640 **Staphylococcus aureus, amplified probe technique**
📻 0.00 ⚕ 0.00 **FUD** XXX Q 🖵

AMA: 2016,Jan,13; 2015,Jan,16; 2014,Jan,11; 2013,Sep,3-12; 2012,May,3-10

87641 **Staphylococcus aureus, methicillin resistant, amplified probe technique**

> EXCLUDES Assays that detect methicillin resistance and identify Staphylococcus aureus using a single nucleic acid sequence (87641)

📻 0.00 ⚕ 0.00 **FUD** XXX Q 🖵

AMA: 2016,Jan,13; 2015,Jan,16; 2014,Jan,11; 2013,Sep,3-12; 2012,May,3-10

87650 **Streptococcus, group A, direct probe technique**
📻 0.00 ⚕ 0.00 **FUD** XXX Q 🖵
AMA: 2016,Jan,13; 2015,Jan,16; 2013,Sep,3-12; 2012,May,3-10

87651 **Streptococcus, group A, amplified probe technique**
📻 0.00 ⚕ 0.00 **FUD** XXX ☒ Q 🖵
AMA: 2016,Jan,13; 2015,Jan,16; 2013,Sep,3-12; 2012,May,3-10

87652 **Streptococcus, group A, quantification**
📻 0.00 ⚕ 0.00 **FUD** XXX Q 🖵
AMA: 2016,Jan,13; 2015,Jan,16; 2013,Sep,3-12; 2012,May,3-10

87653 **Streptococcus, group B, amplified probe technique**
📻 0.00 ⚕ 0.00 **FUD** XXX Q 🖵
AMA: 2016,Jan,13; 2015,Jan,16; 2014,Jan,11; 2013,Sep,3-12; 2012,May,3-10

87660 **Trichomonas vaginalis, direct probe technique**
📻 0.00 ⚕ 0.00 **FUD** XXX Q 🖵
AMA: 2016,Jan,13; 2015,Jan,16; 2013,Sep,3-12; 2012,May,3-10

87661 **Trichomonas vaginalis, amplified probe technique**
📻 0.00 ⚕ 0.00 **FUD** XXX Q 🖵

87797 **Infectious agent detection by nucleic acid (DNA or RNA), not otherwise specified; direct probe technique, each organism**
📻 0.00 ⚕ 0.00 **FUD** XXX Q 🖵
AMA: 2016,Aug,9; 2016,Jan,13; 2015,Jan,16; 2014,Jan,11; 2013,Sep,3-12; 2012,May,3-10

87798 **amplified probe technique, each organism**
📻 0.00 ⚕ 0.00 **FUD** XXX Q 🖵
AMA: 2016,Jan,13; 2015,Jan,16; 2014,Jan,11; 2013,Sep,3-12; 2012,May,3-10

87799 **quantification, each organism**
📻 0.00 ⚕ 0.00 **FUD** XXX Q 🖵
AMA: 2016,Jan,13; 2015,Jan,16; 2013,Sep,3-12; 2012,May,3-10

87800 **Infectious agent detection by nucleic acid (DNA or RNA), multiple organisms; direct probe(s) technique**

> INCLUDES Single test to detect multiple infectious organisms
>
> EXCLUDES Detection of specific infectious agents not otherwise specified (87797-87799)
>
> Each specific organism nucleic acid detection from a primary source (87470-87660 [87623, 87624, 87625])

📻 0.00 ⚕ 0.00 **FUD** XXX A 🖵

AMA: 2016,Aug,9; 2016,Jan,13; 2015,Jan,16; 2013,Sep,3-12; 2012,May,3-10

87801 **amplified probe(s) technique**

> INCLUDES Single test to detect multiple infectious organisms
>
> EXCLUDES Detection of multiple respiratory viruses with one test (87631-87633)
>
> Detection of specific infectious agents not otherwise specified (87797-87799)
>
> Each specific organism nucleic acid detection from a primary source (87470-87660 [87623, 87624, 87625])

📻 0.00 ⚕ 0.00 **FUD** XXX Q 🖵

AMA: 2016,Jan,13; 2015,Jan,16; 2014,Jan,11; 2013,Sep,3-12; 2013,Jun,13; 2012,May,3-10

87802-87899 [87806] Detection Infectious Agent by Immunoassay with Direct Optical Observation

87802 **Infectious agent antigen detection by immunoassay with direct optical observation; Streptococcus, group B**
📻 0.00 ⚕ 0.00 **FUD** XXX Q 🖵
AMA: 2005,Aug,7-8; 2005,Jul,11-12

87803 **Clostridium difficile toxin A**
📻 0.00 ⚕ 0.00 **FUD** XXX Q 🖵
AMA: 2005,Aug,7-8; 2005,Jul,11-12

\# **87806** **HIV-1 antigen(s), with HIV-1 and HIV-2 antibodies**
📻 0.00 ⚕ 0.00 **FUD** XXX ☒ Q 🖵

87804 **Influenza**
📻 0.00 ⚕ 0.00 **FUD** XXX ☒ Q 🖵
AMA: 2016,Jan,13; 2015,Jan,16; 2014,Jan,11; 2012,Jan,15-42; 2011,Jan,11

87806 **Resequenced code. See code following 87803.**

87807 **respiratory syncytial virus**
📻 0.00 ⚕ 0.00 **FUD** XXX ☒ Q 🖵
AMA: 2005,Jul,11-12; 2005,Aug,7-8

87808 **Trichomonas vaginalis**
📻 0.00 ⚕ 0.00 **FUD** XXX ☒ Q 🖵

87809 **adenovirus**
📻 0.00 ⚕ 0.00 **FUD** XXX ☒ Q 🖵
AMA: 2016,Jan,13; 2015,Jan,16; 2014,Jan,11

87810 **Chlamydia trachomatis**
📻 0.00 ⚕ 0.00 **FUD** XXX A 🖵
AMA: 2016,Jan,13; 2015,Jan,16; 2014,Jan,11

87850	**Neisseria gonorrhoeae**

🚑 0.00   ⚕ 0.00   **FUD** XXX   [A] [🖼]

AMA: 2016,Jan,13; 2015,Jan,16; 2014,Jan,11

87880	**Streptococcus, group A**

🚑 0.00   ⚕ 0.00   **FUD** XXX   [X] [Q] [🖼]

AMA: 2016,Jan,13; 2015,Jan,16; 2014,Jan,11; 2012,Jan,15-42; 2011,Jan,11

87899	**not otherwise specified**

🚑 0.00   ⚕ 0.00   **FUD** XXX   [X] [Q] [🖼]

AMA: 2016,Jan,13; 2015,Jan,16; 2014,Jan,11; 2012,Jan,15-42; 2011,Jan,11

87900-87999 [87906, 87910, 87912] Drug Sensitivity Genotype/Phenotype

87900	**Infectious agent drug susceptibility phenotype prediction using regularly updated genotypic bioinformatics**

🚑 0.00   ⚕ 0.00   **FUD** XXX   [Q] [🖼]

AMA: 2016,Jan,13; 2015,Dec,18; 2015,Jan,16; 2014,Jan,11; 2013,Sep,3-12; 2012,May,3-10

 # 87910   Infectious agent genotype analysis by nucleic acid (DNA or RNA); cytomegalovirus

🚑 0.00   ⚕ 0.00   **FUD** XXX   [Q]

AMA: 2016,Jan,13; 2015,Jan,16

87901	**HIV-1, reverse transcriptase and protease regions**

EXCLUDES   *Infectious agent drug susceptibility phenotype prediction for HIV-1 (87900)*

🚑 0.00   ⚕ 0.00   **FUD** XXX   [Q] [🖼]

AMA: 2016,Jan,13; 2015,Jan,16; 2014,Jan,11; 2013,Sep,3-12; 2012,May,3-10

 # 87906   HIV-1, other region (eg, integrase, fusion)

🚑 0.00   ⚕ 0.00   **FUD** XXX   [Q] [🖼]

AMA: 2016,Jan,13; 2015,Jan,16

 # 87912   Hepatitis B virus

🚑 0.00   ⚕ 0.00   **FUD** XXX   [Q] [🖼]

AMA: 2016,Jan,13; 2015,Jan,16

87902	**Hepatitis C virus**

🚑 0.00   ⚕ 0.00   **FUD** XXX   [Q] [🖼]

AMA: 2016,Jan,13; 2015,Dec,18; 2015,Nov,10; 2015,Jan,16; 2014,Jan,11; 2013,Sep,3-12; 2012,May,3-10

87903	**Infectious agent phenotype analysis by nucleic acid (DNA or RNA) with drug resistance tissue culture analysis, HIV 1; first through 10 drugs tested**

🚑 0.00   ⚕ 0.00   **FUD** XXX   [Q] [🖼]

AMA: 2016,Jan,13; 2015,Jan,16; 2014,Jan,11; 2013,Sep,3-12; 2012,May,3-10

+ 87904   each additional drug tested (List separately in addition to code for primary procedure)

Code first (87903)

🚑 0.00   ⚕ 0.00   **FUD** XXX   [Q] [🖼]

AMA: 2016,Jan,13; 2015,Jan,16; 2014,Jan,11; 2013,Sep,3-12; 2012,May,3-10; 2012,Jan,15-42; 2011,Jan,11

87905	**Infectious agent enzymatic activity other than virus (eg, sialidase activity in vaginal fluid)**

🚑 0.00   ⚕ 0.00   **FUD** XXX   [X] [Q] [🖼]

EXCLUDES   *Isolation of a virus identified by a nonimmunologic method, and by noncytopathic effect (87255)*

87906	**Resequenced code. See code following 87901.**
87910	**Resequenced code. See code following 87900.**
87912	**Resequenced code. See code before 87902.**
87999	**Unlisted microbiology procedure**

🚑 0.00   ⚕ 0.00   **FUD** XXX   [N]

AMA: 2016,Jan,13; 2015,Jan,16; 2014,Jan,11

88000-88099 Autopsy Services

CMS: 100-02,15,80.1 Payment for Clinical Laboratory Services

INCLUDES   Services for physicians only

88000	**Necropsy (autopsy), gross examination only; without CNS**

🚑 0.00   ⚕ 0.00   **FUD** XXX   [E]

AMA: 2016,Jan,13; 2015,Jan,16; 2014,Jan,11

88005	**with brain**

🚑 0.00   ⚕ 0.00   **FUD** XXX   [E]

AMA: 2005,Jul,11-12; 2005,Aug,7-8

88007	**with brain and spinal cord**

🚑 0.00   ⚕ 0.00   **FUD** XXX   [E]

AMA: 2005,Jul,11-12; 2005,Aug,7-8

88012	**infant with brain** [A]

🚑 0.00   ⚕ 0.00   **FUD** XXX   [E]

AMA: 2005,Jul,11-12; 2005,Aug,7-8

88014	**stillborn or newborn with brain** [A]

🚑 0.00   ⚕ 0.00   **FUD** XXX   [E]

AMA: 2005,Jul,11-12; 2005,Aug,7-8

88016	**macerated stillborn** [A]

🚑 0.00   ⚕ 0.00   **FUD** XXX   [E]

AMA: 2005,Jul,11-12; 2005,Aug,7-8

88020	**Necropsy (autopsy), gross and microscopic; without CNS**

🚑 0.00   ⚕ 0.00   **FUD** XXX   [E]

AMA: 2005,Jul,11-12; 2005,Aug,7-8

88025	**with brain**

🚑 0.00   ⚕ 0.00   **FUD** XXX   [E]

AMA: 2005,Jul,11-12; 2005,Aug,7-8

88027	**with brain and spinal cord**

🚑 0.00   ⚕ 0.00   **FUD** XXX   [E]

AMA: 2005,Jul,11-12; 2005,Aug,7-8

88028	**infant with brain**

🚑 0.00   ⚕ 0.00   **FUD** XXX   [E]

AMA: 2005,Jul,11-12; 2005,Aug,7-8

88029	**stillborn or newborn with brain** [A]

🚑 0.00   ⚕ 0.00   **FUD** XXX   [E]

AMA: 2005,Jul,11-12; 2005,Aug,7-8

88036	**Necropsy (autopsy), limited, gross and/or microscopic; regional**

🚑 0.00   ⚕ 0.00   **FUD** XXX   [E]

AMA: 2005,Jul,11-12; 2005,Aug,7-8

88037	**single organ**

🚑 0.00   ⚕ 0.00   **FUD** XXX   [E]

AMA: 2005,Jul,11-12; 2005,Aug,7-8

88040	**Necropsy (autopsy); forensic examination**

🚑 0.00   ⚕ 0.00   **FUD** XXX   [E]

AMA: 2005,Jul,11-12; 2005,Aug,7-8

88045	**coroner's call**

🚑 0.00   ⚕ 0.00   **FUD** XXX   [E]

AMA: 2005,Jul,11-12; 2005,Aug,7-8

88099	**Unlisted necropsy (autopsy) procedure**

🚑 0.00   ⚕ 0.00   **FUD** XXX   [E]

AMA: 2016,Jan,13; 2015,Jan,16; 2014,Jan,11

88104-88140 Cytopathology: Other Than Cervical/Vaginal

88104	**Cytopathology, fluids, washings or brushings, except cervical or vaginal; smears with interpretation**

🚑 2.14   ⚕ 2.14   **FUD** XXX   [Q1] [80] [🖼]

AMA: 2016,Jan,13; 2015,Jan,16; 2014,Jan,11; 2012,Jan,15-42; 2011,Jan,11

88106	**simple filter method with interpretation**

EXCLUDES   *Cytopathology smears with interpretation (88104)*
Selective cellular enhancement (nongynecological) including filter transfer techniques (88112)

🚑 2.11   ⚕ 2.11   **FUD** XXX   [Q1] [80] [🖼]

AMA: 2016,Jan,13; 2015,Jan,16; 2014,Jan,11

88108 Cytopathology, concentration technique, smears and interpretation (eg, Saccomanno technique)

EXCLUDES Cervical or vaginal smears (88150-88155)
Gastric intubation with lavage (43754-43755)

(74340)

2.04 2.04 **FUD** XXX Q1 80 🖵

AMA: 2016,Jan,13; 2015,Jan,16; 2014,Jan,11

88112 Cytopathology, selective cellular enhancement technique with interpretation (eg, liquid based slide preparation method), except cervical or vaginal

EXCLUDES Cytopathology cellular enhancement technique (88108)

2.02 2.02 **FUD** XXX Q1 80 🖵

AMA: 2005,Aug,7-8; 2005,Jul,11-12

88120 Cytopathology, in situ hybridization (eg, FISH), urinary tract specimen with morphometric analysis, 3-5 molecular probes, each specimen; manual

EXCLUDES More than five probes (88399)
Morphometric in situ hybridization on specimens other than urinary tract (88367-88368 [88373, 88374])

17.8 17.8 **FUD** XXX Q2 80 🖵

AMA: 2010,Dec,7-10

88121 using computer-assisted technology

EXCLUDES More than five probes (88399)
Morphometric in situ hybridization on specimens other than urinary tract (88367-88368 [88373, 88374])

15.6 15.6 **FUD** XXX Q1 80 🖵

AMA: 2010,Dec,7-10

88125 Cytopathology, forensic (eg, sperm)

0.66 0.66 **FUD** XXX Q1 80 🖵

AMA: 2005,Aug,7-8; 2005,Jul,11-12

88130 Sex chromatin identification; Barr bodies

0.00 0.00 **FUD** XXX Q 🖵

AMA: 2005,Aug,7-8; 2005,Jul,11-12

88140 peripheral blood smear, polymorphonuclear drumsticks

EXCLUDES Guard stain (88313)

0.00 0.00 **FUD** XXX Q 🖵

AMA: 2016,Jan,13; 2015,Jan,16; 2014,Jan,11

88141-88155 Pap Smears

CMS: 100-03,210.2 Screening Pap Smears/Pelvic Examinations for Early Cancer Detection

88141 Cytopathology, cervical or vaginal (any reporting system), requiring interpretation by physician ♀

Code also (88142-88154, 88164-88167, 88174-88175)

0.92 0.92 **FUD** XXX N 80 26 🖵

AMA: 2016,Jan,13; 2015,Jan,16; 2014,Jan,11; 2012,Jan,15-42; 2011,Dec,14-18; 2011,May,9; 2011,Jan,11

88142 Cytopathology, cervical or vaginal (any reporting system), collected in preservative fluid, automated thin layer preparation; manual screening under physician supervision ♀

INCLUDES Bethesda or non-Bethesda method

0.00 0.00 **FUD** XXX Q 🖵

AMA: 2016,Jan,13; 2015,Jan,16; 2014,Jan,11

88143 with manual screening and rescreening under physician supervision ♀

INCLUDES Bethesda or non-Bethesda method

EXCLUDES Automated screening of automated thin layer preparation (88174-88175)

0.00 0.00 **FUD** XXX Q 🖵

AMA: 2016,Jan,13; 2015,Jan,16; 2014,Jan,11; 2012,Jan,15-42; 2011,Jan,11

88147 Cytopathology smears, cervical or vaginal; screening by automated system under physician supervision ♀

0.00 0.00 **FUD** XXX Q 🖵

AMA: 2016,Jan,13; 2015,Jan,16; 2014,Jan,11; 2012,Jan,15-42; 2011,Jan,11

88148 screening by automated system with manual rescreening under physician supervision ♀

0.00 0.00 **FUD** XXX Q 🖵

AMA: 2016,Jan,13; 2015,Jan,16; 2014,Jan,11

88150 Cytopathology, slides, cervical or vaginal; manual screening under physician supervision ♀

EXCLUDES Bethesda method Pap smears (88164-88167)

0.00 0.00 **FUD** XXX Q 🖵

AMA: 2016,Jan,13; 2015,Jan,16; 2014,Jan,11

88152 with manual screening and computer-assisted rescreening under physician supervision ♀

EXCLUDES Bethesda method Pap smears (88164-88167)

0.00 0.00 **FUD** XXX Q 🖵

AMA: 2016,Jan,13; 2015,Jan,16; 2014,Jan,11

88153 with manual screening and rescreening under physician supervision ♀

EXCLUDES Bethesda method Pap smears (88164-88167)

0.00 0.00 **FUD** XXX Q 🖵

AMA: 2016,Jan,13; 2015,Jan,16; 2014,Jan,11; 2012,Jan,15-42; 2011,Jan,11

88154 with manual screening and computer-assisted rescreening using cell selection and review under physician supervision ♀

EXCLUDES Bethesda method Pap smears (88164-88167)

0.00 0.00 **FUD** XXX Q 🖵

AMA: 2016,Jan,13; 2015,Jan,16; 2014,Jan,11

+ **88155** Cytopathology, slides, cervical or vaginal, definitive hormonal evaluation (eg, maturation index, karyopyknotic index, estrogenic index) (List separately in addition to code[s] for other technical and interpretation services) ♀

Code first (88142-88154, 88164-88167, 88174-88175)

0.00 0.00 **FUD** XXX Q 🖵

AMA: 2016,Jan,13; 2015,Jan,16; 2014,Jan,11; 2012,Jan,15-42; 2011,May,9

88160-88162 Cytopathology Smears (Other Than Pap)

88160 Cytopathology, smears, any other source; screening and interpretation

2.04 2.04 **FUD** XXX Q1 80 🖵

AMA: 2006,Dec,10-12; 2005,Jul,11-12

88161 preparation, screening and interpretation

1.83 1.83 **FUD** XXX Q1 80 🖵

AMA: 2016,Jan,13; 2015,Jan,16; 2014,Jan,11

88162 extended study involving over 5 slides and/or multiple stains

EXCLUDES Aerosol collection of sputum (89220)
Special stains (88312-88314)

2.95 2.95 **FUD** XXX Q1 80 🖵

AMA: 2005,Aug,7-8; 2005,Jul,11-12

88164-88167 Pap Smears: Bethesda System

CMS: 100-03,210.2 Screening Pap Smears/Pelvic Examinations for Early Cancer Detection

EXCLUDES Non-Bethesda method (88150-88154)

88164 Cytopathology, slides, cervical or vaginal (the Bethesda System); manual screening under physician supervision ♀

0.00 0.00 **FUD** XXX Q 🖵

AMA: 2016,Jan,13; 2015,Jan,16; 2014,Jan,11

88165 with manual screening and rescreening under physician supervision ♀

0.00 0.00 **FUD** XXX Q 🖵

AMA: 2016,Jan,13; 2015,Jan,16; 2014,Jan,11; 2012,Jan,15-42; 2011,Jan,11

88166 with manual screening and computer-assisted rescreening under physician supervision ♀

0.00 0.00 **FUD** XXX Q 🖵

AMA: 2016,Jan,13; 2015,Jan,16; 2014,Jan,11

88167 with manual screening and computer-assisted rescreening using cell selection and review under physician supervision ♀

> *EXCLUDES* *Fine needle aspiration (10021-10022)*
> 🚑 0.00 ⚕ 0.00 **FUD** XXX [Q][🖻]
> **AMA:** 2016,Jan,13; 2015,Jan,16; 2014,Jan,11

88172-88173 [88177] Cytopathology of Needle Biopsy

EXCLUDES *Fine needle aspiration (10021-10022)*

88172 Cytopathology, evaluation of fine needle aspirate; immediate cytohistologic study to determine adequacy for diagnosis, first evaluation episode, each site

> *INCLUDES* The submission of a complete set of cytologic material for evaluation regardless of the number of needle passes performed or slides prepared from each site
> *EXCLUDES* *Cytologic examination during intraoperative pathology consultation (88333-88334)*
> 🚑 1.62 ⚕ 1.62 **FUD** XXX [Q1][80][🖻]
> **AMA:** 2016,Jan,11; 2016,Jan,13; 2015,Jan,16; 2014,Jan,11; 2012,Jan,15-42; 2011,Jan,11

88173 interpretation and report

> *INCLUDES* The interpretation and report from each anatomical site no matter how many passes or evaluation episodes are performed during the aspiration
> *EXCLUDES* *Cytologic examination during intraoperative pathology consultation (88333-88334)*
> *Fine needle aspiration (10021-10022)*
> 🚑 4.34 ⚕ 4.34 **FUD** XXX [Q1][80][🖻]
> **AMA:** 2016,Jan,13; 2015,Jan,16; 2014,Jan,11; 2012,Jan,15-42; 2011,Jan,11

+ # **88177** immediate cytohistologic study to determine adequacy for diagnosis, each separate additional evaluation episode, same site (List separately in addition to code for primary procedure)

> Code also each additional immediate repeat evaluation episode(s) required from the same site (e.g., previous sample is inadequate)
> Code first (88172)
> 🚑 0.86 ⚕ 0.86 **FUD** ZZZ [N][80]
> **AMA:** 2016,Jan,11

88174-88177 Pap Smears: Automated Screening

88174 Cytopathology, cervical or vaginal (any reporting system), collected in preservative fluid, automated thin layer preparation; screening by automated system, under physician supervision ♀

> *INCLUDES* Bethesda or non-Bethesda method
> 🚑 0.00 ⚕ 0.00 **FUD** XXX [Q][🖻]
> **AMA:** 2016,Jan,13; 2015,Jan,16; 2014,Jan,11

88175 with screening by automated system and manual rescreening or review, under physician supervision ♀

> *INCLUDES* Bethesda or non-Bethesda method
> *EXCLUDES* *Manual screening (88142-88143)*
> 🚑 0.00 ⚕ 0.00 **FUD** XXX [Q][🖻]
> **AMA:** 2016,Jan,13; 2015,Jan,16; 2014,Jan,11; 2012,Jan,15-42; 2011,May,9

88177 Resequenced code, See code following 88173.

88182-88199 Cytopathology Using the Fluorescence-Activated Cell Sorter

88182 Flow cytometry, cell cycle or DNA analysis

> *EXCLUDES* *DNA ploidy analysis by morphometric technique (88358)*
> 🚑 3.16 ⚕ 3.16 **FUD** XXX [Q2][80][🖻]
> **AMA:** 2016,Jan,13; 2015,Jan,16; 2013,Oct,3

88184 Flow cytometry, cell surface, cytoplasmic, or nuclear marker, technical component only; first marker

> 🚑 2.13 ⚕ 2.13 **FUD** XXX [Q2][80][TC][🖻]
> **AMA:** 2016,Jan,13; 2015,Jan,16; 2014,Jan,11; 2013,Oct,3

+ **88185** each additional marker (List separately in addition to code for first marker)

> Code first (88184)
> 🚑 1.30 ⚕ 1.30 **FUD** ZZZ [N][80][TC][🖻]
> **AMA:** 2016,Jan,13; 2015,Jan,16; 2014,Jan,11; 2013,Oct,3; 2012,Jan,15-42; 2011,Jan,11

88187 Flow cytometry, interpretation; 2 to 8 markers

> *EXCLUDES* *Antibody assessment by flow cytometry (83516-83520, 86000-86849 [86152, 86153])*
> *Cell enumeration by immunologic selection and identification ([86152, 86153])*
> *Interpretation (86355-86357, 86359-86361, 86367)*
> 🚑 2.04 ⚕ 2.04 **FUD** XXX [B][80][26][🖻]
> **AMA:** 2016,Jan,13; 2015,Jan,16; 2014,Jan,11; 2013,Oct,3; 2012,Jan,15-42; 2011,Jan,11

88188 9 to 15 markers

> *EXCLUDES* *Antibody assessment by flow cytometry (83516-83520, 86000-86849 [86152, 86153])*
> *Cell enumeration by immunologic selection and identification ([86152, 86153])*
> *Interpretation (86355-86357, 86359-86361, 86367)*
> 🚑 2.60 ⚕ 2.60 **FUD** XXX [B][80][26][🖻]
> **AMA:** 2016,Jan,13; 2015,Jan,16; 2014,Jan,11; 2013,Oct,3; 2012,Jan,15-42; 2011,Jan,11

88189 16 or more markers

> *EXCLUDES* *Antibody assessment by flow cytometry (83516-83520, 86000-86849 [86152, 86153])*
> *Cell enumeration using immunologic selection and identification in fluid sample ([86152, 86153])*
> *Interpretation (86355-86357, 86359-86361, 86367)*
> 🚑 3.19 ⚕ 3.19 **FUD** XXX [B][80][26][🖻]
> **AMA:** 2016,Jan,13; 2015,Jan,16; 2014,Jan,11; 2013,Oct,3; 2012,Jan,15-42; 2011,Jan,11

88199 Unlisted cytopathology procedure

> *EXCLUDES* *Electron microscopy (88348)*
> 🚑 0.00 ⚕ 0.00 **FUD** XXX [Q1][80]
> **AMA:** 2016,Jan,13; 2015,Jan,16; 2014,Jan,11

88230-88299 Cytogenic Studies

CMS: 100-03,190.3 Cytogenic Studies

EXCLUDES *Acetylcholinesterase (82013)*
Alpha-fetoprotein (amniotic fluid or serum) (82105-82106)
Microdissection (88380)
Molecular pathology codes (81200-81383 [81161, 81162, 81287, 81288], 81400-81408, [81479], 81410-81471, 81500-81512, 81599)

88230 Tissue culture for non-neoplastic disorders; lymphocyte

> 🚑 0.00 ⚕ 0.00 **FUD** XXX [Q]
> **AMA:** 2016,Jan,13; 2015,Jan,16; 2014,Jan,11

88233 skin or other solid tissue biopsy

> 🚑 0.00 ⚕ 0.00 **FUD** XXX [Q]
> **AMA:** 2016,Jan,13; 2015,Jan,16; 2014,Jan,11

88235 amniotic fluid or chorionic villus cells [M]

> 🚑 0.00 ⚕ 0.00 **FUD** XXX [Q]
> **AMA:** 2016,Jan,13; 2015,Jan,16; 2014,Jan,11

88237 Tissue culture for neoplastic disorders; bone marrow, blood cells

> 🚑 0.00 ⚕ 0.00 **FUD** XXX [Q]
> **AMA:** 2016,Jan,13; 2015,Jan,16; 2014,Jan,11

88239 solid tumor

> 🚑 0.00 ⚕ 0.00 **FUD** XXX [Q]
> **AMA:** 2016,Jan,13; 2015,Jan,16; 2014,Jan,11

88240 Cryopreservation, freezing and storage of cells, each cell line

> *EXCLUDES* *Therapeutic cryopreservation and storage (38207)*
> 🚑 0.00 ⚕ 0.00 **FUD** XXX [Q][🖻]
> **AMA:** 2016,Jan,13; 2015,Jan,16; 2014,Jan,11; 2013,Oct,3

88241 Thawing and expansion of frozen cells, each aliquot

> *EXCLUDES* *Therapeutic thawing of prior harvest (38208)*
> 🚑 0.00 ⚕ 0.00 **FUD** XXX [Q][🖻]
> **AMA:** 2016,Jan,13; 2015,Jan,16; 2014,Jan,11; 2013,Oct,3

[26]/[TC] PC/TC Only · [A2-Z3] ASC Payment · [50] Bilateral · ♂ Male Only · ♀ Female Only · 🚑 Facility RVU · ⚕ Non-Facility RVU · [🖻] CCI
FUD Follow-up Days · **CMS:** IOM (Pub 100) · [A]-[Y] OPPSI · [80]/[80] Surg Assist Allowed / w/Doc · [◼] Lab Crosswalk · [◼] Radiology Crosswalk · [✕] CLIA

400
CPT © 2016 American Medical Association. All Rights Reserved.
© 2016 Optum360, LLC

88245 Chromosome analysis for breakage syndromes; baseline Sister Chromatid Exchange (SCE), 20-25 cells
🚑 0.00   ⊘ 0.00   **FUD** XXX   Q 🖵
AMA: 2016,Jan,13; 2015,Jan,16; 2014,Jan,11

88248 baseline breakage, score 50-100 cells, count 20 cells, 2 karyotypes (eg, for ataxia telangiectasia, Fanconi anemia, fragile X)
🚑 0.00   ⊘ 0.00   **FUD** XXX   Q 🖵
AMA: 2016,Jan,13; 2015,Jan,16; 2014,Jan,11

88249 score 100 cells, clastogen stress (eg, diepoxybutane, mitomycin C, ionizing radiation, UV radiation)
🚑 0.00   ⊘ 0.00   **FUD** XXX   Q 🖵
AMA: 2016,Jan,13; 2015,Jan,16; 2014,Jan,11

88261 Chromosome analysis; count 5 cells, 1 karyotype, with banding
🚑 0.00   ⊘ 0.00   **FUD** XXX   Q 🖵
AMA: 2016,Jan,13; 2015,Jan,16; 2014,Jan,11

88262 count 15-20 cells, 2 karyotypes, with banding
🚑 0.00   ⊘ 0.00   **FUD** XXX   Q 🖵
AMA: 2016,Jan,13; 2015,Jan,16; 2014,Jan,11; 2012,Jan,15-42; 2011,May,9

88263 count 45 cells for mosaicism, 2 karyotypes, with banding
🚑 0.00   ⊘ 0.00   **FUD** XXX   Q 🖵
AMA: 2016,Jan,13; 2015,Jan,16; 2014,Jan,11

88264 analyze 20-25 cells
🚑 0.00   ⊘ 0.00   **FUD** XXX   Q 🖵
AMA: 2016,Jan,13; 2015,Jan,16; 2014,Jan,11

88267 Chromosome analysis, amniotic fluid or chorionic villus, count 15 cells, 1 karyotype, with banding   M ♀
🚑 0.00   ⊘ 0.00   **FUD** XXX   Q 🖵
AMA: 2016,Jan,13; 2015,Jan,16; 2014,Jan,11

88269 Chromosome analysis, in situ for amniotic fluid cells, count cells from 6-12 colonies, 1 karyotype, with banding   M ♀
🚑 0.00   ⊘ 0.00   **FUD** XXX   Q 🖵
AMA: 2016,Jan,13; 2015,Jan,16; 2014,Jan,11

88271 Molecular cytogenetics; DNA probe, each (eg, FISH)
EXCLUDES   *Cytogenomic microarray analysis (81228-81229, 81405-81406, [81479])*
Fetal chromosome analysis using maternal blood (81420-81422)
🚑 0.00   ⊘ 0.00   **FUD** XXX   Q 🖵
AMA: 2016,Jan,13; 2015,Jan,16; 2014,Jan,11; 2013,Sep,3-12; 2012,May,3-10; 2012,Jan,15-42; 2011,Jan,11

88272 chromosomal in situ hybridization, analyze 3-5 cells (eg, for derivatives and markers)
🚑 0.00   ⊘ 0.00   **FUD** XXX   Q 🖵
AMA: 2016,Jan,13; 2015,Jan,16; 2014,Jan,11; 2013,Sep,3-12; 2012,May,3-10; 2012,Jan,15-42; 2011,Jan,11

88273 chromosomal in situ hybridization, analyze 10-30 cells (eg, for microdeletions)
🚑 0.00   ⊘ 0.00   **FUD** XXX   Q 🖵
AMA: 2016,Jan,13; 2015,Jan,16; 2014,Jan,11; 2013,Sep,3-12; 2012,May,3-10; 2012,Jan,15-42; 2011,Jan,11

88274 interphase in situ hybridization, analyze 25-99 cells
🚑 0.00   ⊘ 0.00   **FUD** XXX   Q 🖵
AMA: 2016,Jan,13; 2015,Jan,16; 2014,Jan,11; 2013,Sep,3-12; 2012,May,3-10; 2012,Jan,15-42; 2011,Jan,11

88275 interphase in situ hybridization, analyze 100-300 cells
🚑 0.00   ⊘ 0.00   **FUD** XXX   Q 🖵
AMA: 2016,Jan,13; 2015,Jan,16; 2014,Jan,11; 2013,Sep,3-12; 2012,May,3-10; 2012,Jan,15-42; 2011,Jan,11

88280 Chromosome analysis; additional karyotypes, each study
🚑 0.00   ⊘ 0.00   **FUD** XXX   Q 🖵
AMA: 2016,Jan,13; 2015,Jan,16; 2014,Jan,11

88283 additional specialized banding technique (eg, NOR, C-banding)
🚑 0.00   ⊘ 0.00   **FUD** XXX   Q 🖵
AMA: 2016,Jan,13; 2015,Jan,16; 2014,Jan,11

88285 additional cells counted, each study
🚑 0.00   ⊘ 0.00   **FUD** XXX   Q 🖵
AMA: 2016,Jan,13; 2015,Jan,16; 2014,Jan,11; 2012,Jan,15-42; 2011,May,9; 2011,Jan,11

88289 additional high resolution study
🚑 0.00   ⊘ 0.00   **FUD** XXX   Q 🖵
AMA: 2016,Jan,13; 2015,Jan,16; 2014,Jan,11

88291 Cytogenetics and molecular cytogenetics, interpretation and report
🚑 0.90   ⊘ 0.90   **FUD** XXX   M 80 26 🖵
AMA: 2016,Jan,13; 2015,Jan,16; 2014,Jan,11

88299 Unlisted cytogenetic study
🚑 0.00   ⊘ 0.00   **FUD** XXX   Q1 80
AMA: 2016,Jan,13; 2015,Jan,16; 2014,Jan,11

88300 Evaluation of Surgical Specimen: Gross Anatomy

CMS: 100-02,15,80.1 Payment for Clinical Laboratory Services

INCLUDES   Attainment, examination, and reporting
Unit of service is the specimen
EXCLUDES   *Additional procedures (88311-88365 [88341, 88350], 88399)*
Microscopic exam (88302-88309)

88300 Level I - Surgical pathology, gross examination only
🚑 0.43   ⊘ 0.43   **FUD** XXX   Q1 80
AMA: 2016,Jan,13; 2015,Jan,16; 2014,Jan,11; 2012,Jan,15-42; 2011,Dec,14-18; 2011,Jan,11

88302-88309 Evaluation of Surgical Specimens: Gross and Microscopic Anatomy

CMS: 100-02,15,80.1 Payment for Clinical Laboratory Services

INCLUDES   Attainment, examination, and reporting
Unit of service is the specimen
EXCLUDES   *Additional procedures (88311-88365 [88341, 88350], 88399)*
Mohs surgery (17311-17315)

88302 Level II - Surgical pathology, gross and microscopic examination
INCLUDES   Confirming identification and absence of disease:
Appendix, incidental
Fallopian tube, sterilization
Fingers or toes traumatic amputation
Foreskin, newborn
Hernia sac, any site
Hydrocele sac
Nerve
Skin, plastic repair
Sympathetic ganglion
Testis, castration
Vaginal mucosa, incidental
Vas deferens, sterilization
🚑 0.92   ⊘ 0.92   **FUD** XXX   Q1 80 🖵
AMA: 2016,Jan,13; 2015,Jan,16; 2014,Feb,10; 2014,Jan,11; 2012,Jan,15-42; 2011,Dec,14-18; 2011,Jan,11

88304 **Level III - Surgical pathology, gross and microscopic examination**

INCLUDES
Abortion, induced
Abscess
Anal tag
Aneurysm-atrial/ventricular
Appendix, other than incidental
Artery, atheromatous plaque
Bartholin's gland cyst
Bone fragment(s), other than pathologic fracture
Bursa/ synovial cyst
Carpal tunnel tissue
Cartilage, shavings
Cholesteatoma
Colon, colostomy stoma
Conjunctiva-biopsy/pterygium
Cornea
Diverticulum-esophagus/small intestine
Dupuytren's contracture tissue
Femoral head, other than fracture
Fissure/fistula
Foreskin, other than newborn
Gallbladder
Ganglion cyst
Hematoma
Hemorrhoids
Hydatid of Morgagni
Intervertebral disc
Joint, loose body
Meniscus
Mucocele, salivary
Neuroma-Morton's/traumatic
Pilonidal cyst/sinus
Polyps, inflammatory-nasal/sinusoidal
Skin-cyst/tag/debridement
Soft tissue, debridement
Soft tissue, lipoma
Spermatocele
Tendon/tendon sheath
Testicular appendage
Thrombus or embolus
Tonsil and/or adenoids
Varicocele
Vas deferens, other than sterilization
Vein, varicosity

🔲 1.29   ⚖ 1.29   **FUD** XXX   Q1 80 🖳

AMA: 2016,Jan,13; 2015,Jan,16; 2014,Feb,10; 2014,Jan,11; 2012,Jan,15-42; 2011,Dec,14-18; 2011,Jan,11

88305 **Level IV - Surgical pathology, gross and microscopic examination**

INCLUDES
Abortion, spontaneous/missed
Artery, biopsy
Bone exostosis
Bone marrow, biopsy
Brain/meninges, other than for tumor resection
Breast biopsy without microscopic assessment of surgical margin
Breast reduction mammoplasty
Bronchus, biopsy
Cell block, any source
Cervix, biopsy
Colon, biopsy
Duodenum, biopsy
Endocervix, curettings/biopsy
Endometrium, curettings/biopsy
Esophagus, biopsy
Extremity, amputation, traumatic
Fallopian tube, biopsy
Fallopian tube, ectopic pregnancy
Femoral head, fracture
Finger/toes, amputation, nontraumatic
Gingiva/oral mucosa, biopsy
Heart valve
Joint resection
Kidney biopsy

Larynx biopsy
Leiomyoma(s), uterine myomectomy-without uterus
Lip, biopsy/wedge resection
Lung, transbronchial biopsy
Lymph node, biopsy
Muscle, biopsy
Nasal mucosa, biopsy
Nasopharynx/oropharynx, biopsy
Nerve biopsy
Odontogenic/dental cyst
Omentum, biopsy
Ovary, biopsy/wedge resection
Ovary with or without tube, nonneoplastic
Parathyroid gland
Peritoneum, biopsy
Pituitary tumor
Placenta, other than third trimester
Pleura/pericardium-biopsy/tissue
Polyp:
  Cervical/endometrial
  Colorectal
  Stomach/small intestine
Prostate:
  Needle biopsy
  TUR
Salivary gland, biopsy
Sinus, paranasal biopsy
Skin, other than cyst/tag/debridement/plastic repair
Small intestine, biopsy
Soft tissue, other than tumor/mas/lipoma/debridement
Spleen
Stomach biopsy
Synovium
Testis, other than tumor/biopsy, castration
Thyroglossal duct/brachial cleft cyst
Tongue, biopsy
Tonsil, biopsy
Trachea biopsy
Ureter, biopsy
Urethra, biopsy
Urinary bladder, biopsy
Uterus, with or without tubes and ovaries, for prolapse
Vagina biopsy
Vulva/labial biopsy

🔲 2.07   ⚖ 2.07   **FUD** XXX   Q1 80 🖳

AMA: 2016,Jan,13; 2015,Jan,16; 2014,Feb,10; 2014,Jan,11; 2012,Jan,15-42; 2011,Dec,14-18; 2011,Jan,11

88307 **Level V - Surgical pathology, gross and microscopic examination**

INCLUDES Adrenal resection
Bone, biopsy/curettings
Bone fragment(s), pathologic fractures
Brain, biopsy
Brain meninges, tumor resection
Breast, excision of lesion, requiring microscopic evaluation of surgical margins
Breast, mastectomy-partial/simple
Cervix, conization
Colon, segmental resection, other than for tumor
Extremity, amputation, nontraumatic
Eye, enucleation
Kidney, partial/total nephrectomy
Larynx, partial/total resection
Liver
   Biopsy, needle/wedge
   Partial resection
Lung, wedge biopsy
Lymph nodes, regional resection
Mediastinum, mass
Myocardium, biopsy
Odontogenic tumor
Ovary with or without tube, neoplastic
Pancreas, biopsy
Placenta, third trimester
Prostate, except radical resection
Salivary gland
Sentinel lymph node
Small intestine, resection, other than for tumor
Soft tissue mass (except lipoma)-biopsy/simple excision
Stomach-subtotal/total resection, other than for tumor
Testis, biopsy
Thymus, tumor
Thyroid, total/lobe
Ureter, resection
Urinary bladder, TUR
Uterus, with or without tubes and ovaries, other than neoplastic/prolapse

   8.72   8.72   **FUD** XXX   Q2 80

AMA: 2016,Jan,13; 2015,Jan,16; 2014,Feb,10; 2014,Jan,11; 2012,Jan,15-42; 2011,Dec,14-18; 2011,Jan,11

88309 **Level VI - Surgical pathology, gross and microscopic examination**

INCLUDES Bone resection
Breast, mastectomy-with regional lymph nodes
Colon:
   Segmental resection for tumor
   Total resection
Esophagus, partial/total resection
Extremity, disarticulation
Fetus, with dissection
Larynx, partial/total resection-with regional lymph nodes
Lung-total/lobe/segment resection
Pancreas, total/subtotal resection
Prostate, radical resection
Small intestine, resection for tumor
Soft tissue tumor, extensive resection
Stomach, subtotal/total resection for tumor
Testis, tumor
Tongue/tonsil, resection for tumor
Urinary bladder, partial/total resection
Uterus, with or without tubes and ovaries, neoplastic
Vulva, total/subtotal resection

EXCLUDES Evaluation of fine needle aspirate (88172-88173)
     Fine needle aspiration (10021-10022)

   13.2   13.2   **FUD** XXX   Q2 80

AMA: 2016,Jan,13; 2015,Jan,16; 2014,Feb,10; 2014,Jan,11; 2012,Jan,15-42; 2011,Dec,14-18; 2011,Jan,11

88311-88399 [88341, 88350, 88364, 88373, 88374, 88377] Additional Surgical Pathology Services

CMS: 100-02,15,80.1 Payment for Clinical Laboratory Services

+ 88311 **Decalcification procedure (List separately in addition to code for surgical pathology examination)**
   Code first surgical pathology exam (88302-88309)
   0.61   0.61   **FUD** XXX   N 80

   AMA: 2016,Jan,13; 2015,Jan,16; 2014,Jan,11; 2012,Jan,15-42; 2011,Dec,14-18; 2011,Jan,11

88312 **Special stain including interpretation and report; Group I for microorganisms (eg, acid fast, methenamine silver)**
   INCLUDES Reporting one unit for each special stain performed on a surgical pathology block, cytologic sample, or hematologic smear
   2.76   2.76   **FUD** XXX   Q1 80

   AMA: 2016,Jan,13; 2015,Jan,16; 2014,Jan,11; 2012,Jan,15-42; 2011,Dec,14-18; 2011,Jan,11

88313 **Group II, all other (eg, iron, trichrome), except stain for microorganisms, stains for enzyme constituents, or immunocytochemistry and immunohistochemistry**
   INCLUDES Reporting one unit for each special stain performed on a surgical pathology block, cytologic sample, or hematologic smear
   EXCLUDES Immunocytochemistry and immunohistochemistry (88342)
   1.93   1.93   **FUD** XXX   Q1 80

   AMA: 2016,Jan,13; 2015,Jan,16; 2014,Jan,11; 2012,Jan,15-42; 2011,Dec,14-18; 2011,Jan,11

+ 88314 **histochemical stain on frozen tissue block (List separately in addition to code for primary procedure)**
   INCLUDES Reporting one unit for each special stain on each frozen surgical pathology block
   EXCLUDES Routine frozen section stain during Mohs surgery (17311-17315)
     Special stain performed on frozen tissue section specimen to identify enzyme constituents (88319)
   Code also modifier 59 for nonroutine histochemical stain on frozen section during Mohs surgery
   Code first (17311-17315, 88302-88309, 88331-88332)
   2.17   2.17   **FUD** XXX   N 80

   AMA: 2016,Jan,13; 2015,Jan,16; 2014,Jan,11; 2011,Dec,14-18

88319 **Group III, for enzyme constituents**
   INCLUDES Reporting one unit for each special stain on each frozen surgical pathology block
   EXCLUDES Detection of enzyme constituents by immunohistochemical or immunocytochemical methodology (88342)
   2.51   2.51   **FUD** XXX   Q2 80

   AMA: 2016,Jan,13; 2015,Jan,16; 2014,Jan,11; 2011,Dec,14-18

88321 **Consultation and report on referred slides prepared elsewhere**
   2.45   2.89   **FUD** XXX   Q1 80

   AMA: 2016,Jan,13; 2015,Jan,16; 2014,Jan,11; 2013,Jun,13; 2012,Jan,15-42; 2011,Dec,14-18; 2011,Jan,11

88323 **Consultation and report on referred material requiring preparation of slides**
   3.93   3.93   **FUD** XXX   Q1 80

   AMA: 2016,Jan,13; 2015,Jan,16; 2014,Jan,11; 2013,Jun,13; 2012,Jan,15-42; 2011,Dec,14-18; 2011,Jan,11

88325 **Consultation, comprehensive, with review of records and specimens, with report on referred material**
   3.86   4.88   **FUD** XXX   Q1 80

   AMA: 2016,Jan,13; 2015,Jan,16; 2014,Jan,11; 2013,Jun,13; 2012,Jan,15-42; 2011,Dec,14-18; 2011,Jan,11

88329 **Pathology consultation during surgery;**
   1.06   1.43   **FUD** XXX   Q1 80

   AMA: 2016,Jan,13; 2015,Jan,16; 2014,Feb,10; 2014,Jan,11; 2012,Jan,15-42; 2011,Dec,14-18; 2011,Jan,11

88331 first tissue block, with frozen section(s), single specimen

Code also cytologic evaluation performed at same time (88334)

🔧 2.71 ⚖ 2.71 **FUD** XXX [Q1] [80] 🖵

AMA: 2016,Jan,13; 2015,Jan,16; 2014,Feb,10; 2014,Jan,11; 2011,Dec,14-18

+ **88332** each additional tissue block with frozen section(s) (List separately in addition to code for primary procedure)

Code first (88331)

🔧 1.43 ⚖ 1.43 **FUD** XXX [N] [80] 🖵

AMA: 2016,Jan,13; 2015,Jan,16; 2014,Feb,10; 2014,Jan,11; 2011,Dec,14-18

88333 cytologic examination (eg, touch prep, squash prep), initial site

EXCLUDES Intraprocedural cytologic evaluation of fine needle aspirate (88172)

Nonintraoperative cytologic examination (88160-88162)

🔧 2.84 ⚖ 2.84 **FUD** XXX [Q2] [80] 🖵

AMA: 2016,Jan,13; 2015,Jan,16; 2014,Feb,10; 2014,Jan,11; 2012,Jan,15-42; 2011,Dec,14-18; 2011,Jan,11

+ **88334** cytologic examination (eg, touch prep, squash prep), each additional site (List separately in addition to code for primary procedure)

EXCLUDES Intraprocedural cytologic evaluation of fine needle aspirate (88172)

Nonintraoperative cytologic examination (88160-88162)

Percutaneous needle biopsy requiring intraprocedural cytologic examination (88333)

Code first (88331, 88333)

🔧 1.75 ⚖ 1.75 **FUD** XXX [N] [80] 🖵

AMA: 2016,Jan,13; 2015,Jan,16; 2014,Feb,10; 2014,Jan,11; 2011,Dec,14-18

88341 Resequenced code. See code following 88342.

88342 Immunohistochemistry or immunocytochemistry, per specimen; initial single antibody stain procedure

EXCLUDES Morphometric analysis, tumor immunohistochemistry, on same antibody (88360-88361)

Use of code more than one time for each specific antibody

🔧 3.00 ⚖ 3.00 **FUD** XXX [Q2] [80] 🖵

AMA: 2016,Jan,13; 2015,Jun,10; 2015,Jan,16; 2014,Jun,14; 2014,Jan,11; 2012,Jan,15-42; 2011,Dec,14-18; 2011,Jan,11

+ # **88341** each additional single antibody stain procedure (List separately in addition to code for primary procedure)

Code first (88342)

EXCLUDES Morphometric analysis (88360-88361)

Use of code more than one time for each specific antibody

🔧 2.52 ⚖ 2.52 **FUD** ZZZ [N] [80]

AMA: 2016,Jan,13; 2015,Jun,10

88344 each multiplex antibody stain procedure

INCLUDES Staining with multiple antibodies on the same slide

EXCLUDES Morphometric analysis, tumor immunohistochemistry, on same antibody (88360-88361)

Use of code more than one time for each specific antibody

🔧 4.86 ⚖ 4.86 **FUD** XXX [Q1] [80] 🖵

AMA: 2016,Jan,13; 2015,Jun,10

88346 Immunofluorescence, per specimen; initial single antibody stain procedure

EXCLUDES Fluorescent in situ hybridization studies (88364-88369 [88364, 88373, 88374, 88377])

Multiple immunofluorescence analysis (88399)

🔧 2.62 ⚖ 2.62 **FUD** XXX [Q2] [80] 🖵

AMA: 2016,Jan,13; 2015,Jan,16; 2014,Jan,11; 2011,Dec,14-18

+ # **88350** each additional single antibody stain procedure (List separately in addition to code for primary procedure)

🔧 2.02 ⚖ 2.02 **FUD** ZZZ [N] [80]

EXCLUDES Fluorescent in situ hybridization studies (88364-88369 [88364, 88373, 88374, 88377])

Multiple immunofluorescence analysis (88399)

Code first (88346)

88348 Electron microscopy, diagnostic

🔧 9.74 ⚖ 9.74 **FUD** XXX [Q2] [80]

AMA: 2011,Dec,14-18

88350 Resequenced code. See code following 88346.

88355 Morphometric analysis; skeletal muscle

🔧 4.42 ⚖ 4.42 **FUD** XXX [Q1] [80] 🖵

AMA: 2016,Jan,13; 2015,Jan,16; 2014,Jan,11; 2011,Dec,14-18

88356 nerve

🔧 5.78 ⚖ 5.78 **FUD** XXX [Q1] [80] 🖵

AMA: 2016,Jan,13; 2015,Jan,16; 2014,Jun,14; 2014,Jan,11; 2011,Dec,14-18

88358 tumor (eg, DNA ploidy)

EXCLUDES Special stain, Group II (88313)

🔧 2.40 ⚖ 2.40 **FUD** XXX [Q2] [80] 🖵

AMA: 2016,Jan,13; 2015,Jan,16; 2014,Jan,11; 2012,Jan,15-42; 2011,Dec,14-18; 2011,Jan,11

88360 Morphometric analysis, tumor immunohistochemistry (eg, Her-2/neu, estrogen receptor/progesterone receptor), quantitative or semiquantitative, per specimen, each single antibody stain procedure; manual

EXCLUDES Additional stain procedures unless each test is for different antibody (88341, 88342, 88344)

Morphometric analysis using in situ hybridization techniques (88367-88368 [88373, 88374])

🔧 3.40 ⚖ 3.40 **FUD** XXX [Q2] [80] 🖵

AMA: 2016,Jan,13; 2015,Jun,10; 2015,Jan,16; 2014,Jun,14; 2014,Jan,11; 2011,Dec,14-18

88361 using computer-assisted technology

EXCLUDES Additional stain procedures unless each test is for different antibody (88341, 88342, 88344)

Morphometric analysis using in situ hybridization techniques (88367-88368 [88373, 88374])

🔧 4.18 ⚖ 4.18 **FUD** XXX [Q2] [80] 🖵

AMA: 2016,Jan,13; 2015,Jun,10; 2015,Jan,16; 2014,Jun,14; 2014,Jan,11; 2011,Dec,14-18

88362 Nerve teasing preparations

🔧 7.30 ⚖ 7.30 **FUD** XXX [Q2] [80] 🖵

AMA: 2016,Jan,13; 2015,Jan,16; 2014,Jan,11; 2011,Dec,14-18

88363 Examination and selection of retrieved archival (ie, previously diagnosed) tissue(s) for molecular analysis (eg, KRAS mutational analysis)

INCLUDES Archival retrieval only

🔧 0.56 ⚖ 0.65 **FUD** XXX [Q1] [80]

AMA: 2016,Jan,13; 2015,Jan,16; 2014,Jan,11; 2011,Dec,14-18

88364 Resequenced code. See code following 88365.

88365 In situ hybridization (eg, FISH), per specimen; initial single probe stain procedure

EXCLUDES Morphometric analysis probe stain procedures with same probe (88367, [88374], 88368, [88377])

🔧 4.98 ⚖ 4.98 **FUD** XXX [Q1] [80] 🖵

AMA: 2016,Jan,13; 2015,Jan,16; 2014,Jan,11; 2013,Sep,3-12; 2012,May,3-10; 2012,Jan,15-42; 2011,Dec,14-18; 2011,Jan,11

+ # **88364** each additional single probe stain procedure (List separately in addition to code for primary procedure)

🔧 3.78 ⚖ 3.78 **FUD** ZZZ [N] [80] 🖵

Code first (88365)

88366 each multiplex probe stain procedure

🔧 7.35 ⚖ 7.35 **FUD** XXX [Q1] [80] 🖵

EXCLUDES Morphometric analysis probe stain procedures (88367, [88374], 88368, [88377])

88367 Morphometric analysis, in situ hybridization (quantitative or semi-quantitative), using computer-assisted technology, per specimen; initial single probe stain procedure

> EXCLUDES *In situ hybridization probe stain procedures for same probe (88365, 88366, 88368, [88377])*
> *Morphometric in situ hybridization evaluation of urinary tract cytologic specimens (88120-88121)*

2.99   2.99   **FUD** XXX   02 80

AMA: 2016,Jan,13; 2015,Jan,16; 2014,Jan,11; 2013,Sep,3-12; 2012,May,3-10; 2012,Jan,15-42; 2011,Dec,14-18; 2011,Jan,11

+ # 88373 each additional single probe stain procedure (List separately in addition to code for primary procedure)

2.10   2.10   **FUD** ZZZ   N 80

Code first (88367)

 # 88374 each multiplex probe stain procedure

9.66   9.66   **FUD** XXX   Q1 80

> EXCLUDES *In situ hybridization probe stain procedures for same probe (88365, 88366, 88368, [88377])*

88368 Morphometric analysis, in situ hybridization (quantitative or semi-quantitative), manual, per specimen; initial single probe stain procedure

> EXCLUDES *In situ hybridization probe stain procedures for same probe (88365, 88366-88367, [88374])*
> *Morphometric in situ hybridization evaluation of urinary tract cytologic specimens (88120-88121)*

3.20   3.20   **FUD** XXX   02 80

AMA: 2016,Jan,13; 2015,Jan,16; 2014,Jan,11; 2013,Sep,3-12; 2012,May,3-10; 2012,Jan,15-42; 2011,Dec,14-18; 2011,Jan,11

+ 88369 each additional single probe stain procedure (List separately in addition to code for primary procedure)

3.03   3.03   **FUD** ZZZ   N 80

Code first (88368)

 # 88377 each multiplex probe stain procedure

11.5   11.5   **FUD** XXX   Q1 80

> EXCLUDES *In situ hybridization probe stain procedures for same probe (88365, 88366-88367, [88374])*

88371 Protein analysis of tissue by Western Blot, with interpretation and report;

0.00   0.00   **FUD** XXX   N

AMA: 2016,Jan,13; 2015,Dec,18; 2015,Jan,16; 2014,Jan,11; 2011,Dec,14-18

88372 immunological probe for band identification, each

0.00   0.00   **FUD** XXX   N

AMA: 2016,Jan,13; 2015,Jan,16; 2014,Jan,11; 2011,Dec,14-18

88373 Resequenced code. See code following 88367.

88374 Resequenced code. See code following 88367.

88375 Optical endomicroscopic image(s), interpretation and report, real-time or referred, each endoscopic session

> EXCLUDES *Endoscopic procedures that include optical endomicroscopy (43206, 43252, 0397T)*

1.40   1.40   **FUD** XXX   B 80 26

AMA: 2016,Jan,13; 2015,Jan,16; 2013,Aug,5

88377 Resequenced code. See code following 88369.

88380 Microdissection (ie, sample preparation of microscopically identified target); laser capture

> EXCLUDES *Microdissection, manual procedure (88381)*

4.07   4.07   **FUD** XXX   N 80

AMA: 2016,Jan,13; 2015,Jan,16; 2014,Jan,11; 2013,Sep,3-12; 2012,May,3-10; 2011,Dec,14-18

88381 manual

> EXCLUDES *Microdissection, laser capture procedure (88380)*

3.30   3.30   **FUD** XXX   N 80

AMA: 2016,Jan,13; 2015,Jan,16; 2014,Jan,11; 2013,Sep,3-12; 2012,May,14-15; 2012,May,3-10; 2011,Dec,14-18

88387 Macroscopic examination, dissection, and preparation of tissue for non-microscopic analytical studies (eg, nucleic acid-based molecular studies); each tissue preparation (eg, a single lymph node)

> EXCLUDES *Pathology consultation during surgery (88329-88334, 88388)*
> *Tissue preparation for microbiologic cultures or flow cytometric studies*

1.19   1.19   **FUD** XXX   N 80

AMA: 2016,Jan,13; 2015,Jan,16; 2014,Jan,11; 2012,Jan,15-42; 2011,Dec,14-18; 2011,Jan,11

+ 88388 in conjunction with a touch imprint, intraoperative consultation, or frozen section, each tissue preparation (eg, a single lymph node) (List separately in addition to code for primary procedure)

> EXCLUDES *Tissue preparation for microbiologic cultures or flow cytometric studies*

Code first (88329-88334)

0.98   0.98   **FUD** XXX   N 80

AMA: 2016,Jan,13; 2015,Jan,16; 2014,Jan,11; 2012,Jan,15-42; 2011,Dec,14-18; 2011,Jan,11

88399 Unlisted surgical pathology procedure

0.00   0.00   **FUD** XXX   Q1 80

AMA: 2016,Jan,13; 2015,Jan,16; 2014,Jun,14; 2014,Jan,11; 2012,Jan,15-42; 2011,Jan,11

88720-88749 Transcutaneous Procedures

> EXCLUDES *Wavelength fluorescent spectroscopy of advanced glycation end products (skin) (88749)*

88720 Bilirubin, total, transcutaneous

> EXCLUDES *Transdermal oxygen saturation testing (94760-94762)*

0.00   0.00   **FUD** XXX   Q

AMA: 2016,Jan,13; 2015,Jan,16; 2014,Jan,11

88738 Hemoglobin (Hgb), quantitative, transcutaneous

> EXCLUDES *In vitro hemoglobin measurement (85018)*

0.00   0.00   **FUD** XXX   Q

AMA: 2016,Jan,13; 2015,Jan,16; 2014,Jan,11

88740 Hemoglobin, quantitative, transcutaneous, per day; carboxyhemoglobin

> EXCLUDES *In vitro carboxyhemoglobin measurement (82375)*

0.00   0.00   **FUD** XXX   Q

AMA: 2016,Jan,13; 2015,Jan,16; 2014,Jan,11

88741 methemoglobin

> EXCLUDES *In vitro quantitative methemoglobin measurement (83050)*

0.00   0.00   **FUD** XXX   Q

AMA: 2016,Jan,13; 2015,Jan,16; 2014,Jan,11

88749 Unlisted in vivo (eg, transcutaneous) laboratory service

> INCLUDES All in vivo measurements not specifically listed

0.00   0.00   **FUD** XXX   Q

AMA: 2010,Dec,7-10

89049-89240 Other Pathology Services

89049 Caffeine halothane contracture test (CHCT) for malignant hyperthermia susceptibility, including interpretation and report

1.86   7.37   **FUD** XXX   Q1 80

AMA: 2016,Jan,13; 2015,Jan,16; 2014,Jan,11; 2012,Jan,15-42; 2011,Sep,3-4; 2011,Jan,11

89050 Cell count, miscellaneous body fluids (eg, cerebrospinal fluid, joint fluid), except blood;

0.00   0.00   **FUD** XXX   Q

AMA: 2016,Jan,13; 2015,Jan,16; 2014,Jan,11; 2011,Sep,3-4

89051 with differential count

0.00   0.00   **FUD** XXX   Q

AMA: 2016,Jan,13; 2015,Jan,16; 2014,Jan,11; 2011,Sep,3-4

89055 Leukocyte assessment, fecal, qualitative or semiquantitative
🔧 0.00   📊 0.00   **FUD** XXX   [Q]
AMA: 2016,Jan,13; 2015,Jan,16; 2014,Jan,11; 2011,Sep,3-4

89060 Crystal identification by light microscopy with or without polarizing lens analysis, tissue or any body fluid (except urine)
EXCLUDES   *Crystal identification on paraffin embedded tissue*
🔧 0.00   📊 0.00   **FUD** XXX   [Q] [📋]
AMA: 2016,Jan,13; 2015,Jan,16; 2014,Jan,11; 2011,Sep,3-4

89125 Fat stain, feces, urine, or respiratory secretions
🔧 0.00   📊 0.00   **FUD** XXX   [Q] [📋]
AMA: 2016,Jan,13; 2015,Jan,16; 2014,Jan,11; 2011,Sep,3-4

89160 Meat fibers, feces
🔧 0.00   📊 0.00   **FUD** XXX   [Q] [📋]
AMA: 2016,Jan,13; 2015,Jan,16; 2014,Jan,11; 2011,Sep,3-4

89190 Nasal smear for eosinophils
🔧 0.00   📊 0.00   **FUD** XXX   [Q] [📋]
AMA: 2016,Jan,13; 2015,Jan,16; 2014,Jan,11; 2012,Jan,15-42; 2011,Sep,3-4; 2011,Jan,11

89220 Sputum, obtaining specimen, aerosol induced technique (separate procedure)
🔧 0.46   📊 0.46   **FUD** XXX   [01] [80] [TC]
AMA: 2016,Jan,13; 2015,Jan,16; 2014,Jan,11; 2011,Sep,3-4

89230 Sweat collection by iontophoresis
🔧 0.15   📊 0.15   **FUD** XXX   [01] [80] [TC] [📋]
AMA: 2016,Jan,13; 2015,Jan,16; 2014,Jan,11; 2011,Sep,3-4

89240 Unlisted miscellaneous pathology test
🔧 0.00   📊 0.00   **FUD** XXX   [01] [80]
AMA: 2016,Jan,13; 2015,Jan,16; 2014,Jan,11; 2012,Jan,15-42; 2011,Sep,3-4; 2011,Jan,11

89250-89398 Infertility Treatment Services

CMS: 100-02,1,100 Treatment for Infertility

89250 Culture of oocyte(s)/embryo(s), less than 4 days;
🔧 0.00   📊 0.00   **FUD** XXX   [01]
AMA: 2016,Jan,13; 2015,Jan,16; 2014,Jan,11; 2012,Jan,15-42; 2011,Jan,11

89251 with co-culture of oocyte(s)/embryos
EXCLUDES   *Extended culture of oocyte(s)/embryo(s) (89272)*
🔧 0.00   📊 0.00   **FUD** XXX   [02] [📋]
AMA: 2016,Jan,13; 2015,Jan,16; 2014,Jan,11; 2012,Jan,15-42; 2011,Jan,11

89253 Assisted embryo hatching, microtechniques (any method)
🔧 0.00   📊 0.00   **FUD** XXX   [01]
AMA: 2016,Jan,13; 2015,Jan,16; 2014,Jan,11; 2012,Jan,15-42; 2011,Jan,11

89254 Oocyte identification from follicular fluid
🔧 0.00   📊 0.00   **FUD** XXX   [01]
AMA: 2016,Jan,13; 2015,Jan,16; 2014,Jan,11; 2012,Jan,15-42; 2011,Jan,11

89255 Preparation of embryo for transfer (any method)
🔧 0.00   📊 0.00   **FUD** XXX   [01]
AMA: 2016,Jan,13; 2015,Jan,16; 2014,Jan,11; 2012,Jan,15-42; 2011,Jan,11

89257 Sperm identification from aspiration (other than seminal fluid)
EXCLUDES   *Semen analysis (89300-89320)*
     Sperm identification from testis tissue (89264)
🔧 0.00   📊 0.00   **FUD** XXX   [01] [📋]
AMA: 2016,Jan,13; 2015,Jan,16; 2014,Jan,11; 2012,Jan,15-42; 2011,Jan,11

89258 Cryopreservation; embryo(s)
🔧 0.00   📊 0.00   **FUD** XXX   [02]
AMA: 2016,Jan,13; 2015,Jan,16; 2014,Jan,11; 2012,Jan,15-42; 2011,Jan,11

89259 sperm
EXCLUDES   *Cryopreservation of testicular reproductive tissue (89335)*
🔧 0.00   📊 0.00   **FUD** XXX   [01]
AMA: 2016,Jan,13; 2015,Jan,16; 2014,Jan,11; 2012,Jan,15-42; 2011,Jan,11

89260 Sperm isolation; simple prep (eg, sperm wash and swim-up) for insemination or diagnosis with semen analysis
🔧 0.00   📊 0.00   **FUD** XXX   [01] [📋]
AMA: 2016,Jan,13; 2015,Jan,16; 2014,Jan,11; 2012,Jan,15-42; 2011,Jan,11

89261 complex prep (eg, Percoll gradient, albumin gradient) for insemination or diagnosis with semen analysis
EXCLUDES   *Semen analysis without sperm wash or swim-up (89320)*
🔧 0.00   📊 0.00   **FUD** XXX   [01] [📋]
AMA: 2016,Jan,13; 2015,Jan,16; 2014,Jan,11; 2012,Jan,15-42; 2011,Jan,11

89264 Sperm identification from testis tissue, fresh or cryopreserved   ♂
EXCLUDES   *Biopsy of testis (54500, 54505)*
     Semen analysis (89300-89320)
     Sperm identification from aspiration (89257)
🔧 0.00   📊 0.00   **FUD** XXX   [01] [📋]
AMA: 2016,Jan,13; 2015,Jan,16; 2014,Jan,11; 2012,Jan,15-42; 2011,Jan,11

89268 Insemination of oocytes
🔧 0.00   📊 0.00   **FUD** XXX   [01]
AMA: 2016,Jan,13; 2015,Jan,16; 2014,Jan,11; 2012,Jan,15-42; 2011,Jan,11

89272 Extended culture of oocyte(s)/embryo(s), 4-7 days
🔧 0.00   📊 0.00   **FUD** XXX   [02]
AMA: 2016,Jan,13; 2015,Jan,16; 2014,Jan,11; 2012,Jan,15-42; 2011,Jan,11

89280 Assisted oocyte fertilization, microtechnique; less than or equal to 10 oocytes
🔧 0.00   📊 0.00   **FUD** XXX   [02]
AMA: 2016,Jan,13; 2015,Jan,16; 2014,Jan,11; 2012,Jan,15-42; 2011,Jan,11

89281 greater than 10 oocytes
🔧 0.00   📊 0.00   **FUD** XXX   [01]
AMA: 2016,Jan,13; 2015,Jan,16; 2014,Jan,11; 2012,Jan,15-42; 2011,Jan,11

89290 Biopsy, oocyte polar body or embryo blastomere, microtechnique (for pre-implantation genetic diagnosis); less than or equal to 5 embryos
🔧 0.00   📊 0.00   **FUD** XXX   [01]
AMA: 2016,Jan,13; 2015,Jan,16; 2014,Jan,11; 2012,Jan,15-42; 2011,Jan,11

89291 greater than 5 embryos
🔧 0.00   📊 0.00   **FUD** XXX   [01]
AMA: 2016,Jan,13; 2015,Jan,16; 2014,Jan,11; 2012,Jan,15-42; 2011,Jan,11

89300 Semen analysis; presence and/or motility of sperm including Huhner test (post coital)   ♀
🔧 0.00   📊 0.00   **FUD** XXX   [X] [Q] [📋]
AMA: 2016,Jan,13; 2015,Jan,16; 2014,Jan,11; 2012,Jan,15-42; 2011,Jan,11

89310 motility and count (not including Huhner test)   ♂
🔧 0.00   📊 0.00   **FUD** XXX   [Q] [📋]
AMA: 2016,Jan,13; 2015,Jan,16; 2014,Jan,11; 2012,Jan,15-42; 2011,Jan,11

89320 volume, count, motility, and differential   ♂
EXCLUDES   *Skin testing (86485-86580, 95012-95199)*
🔧 0.00   📊 0.00   **FUD** XXX   [Q] [📋]
AMA: 2016,Jan,13; 2015,Jan,16; 2014,Jan,11; 2012,Jan,15-42; 2011,Jan,11

| 89321 | sperm presence and motility of sperm, if performed ♂ |

EXCLUDES Hyaluronan binding assay (HBA) (89398)
🚑 0.00   ⚕ 0.00   **FUD** XXX   ☒ Ⓠ ▭

AMA: 2016,Jan,13; 2015,Jan,16; 2014,Jan,11; 2012,Jan,15-42; 2011,Jan,11

| 89322 | volume, count, motility, and differential using strict morphologic criteria (eg, Kruger) ♂ |

🚑 0.00   ⚕ 0.00   **FUD** XXX   Ⓠ ▭

AMA: 2016,Jan,13; 2015,Jan,16; 2014,Jan,11; 2012,Jan,15-42; 2011,Jan,11

| 89325 | Sperm antibodies ♂ |

EXCLUDES Medicolegal identification of sperm (88125)
🚑 0.00   ⚕ 0.00   **FUD** XXX   Ⓠ ▭

AMA: 2016,Jan,13; 2015,Jan,16; 2014,Jan,11; 2012,Jan,15-42; 2011,Jan,11

| 89329 | Sperm evaluation; hamster penetration test ♂ |

🚑 0.00   ⚕ 0.00   **FUD** XXX   Ⓠ ▭

AMA: 2016,Jan,13; 2015,Jan,16; 2014,Jan,11; 2012,Jan,15-42; 2011,Jan,11

| 89330 | cervical mucus penetration test, with or without spinnbarkeit test ♂ |

🚑 0.00   ⚕ 0.00   **FUD** XXX   Ⓠ ▭

AMA: 2016,Jan,13; 2015,Jan,16; 2014,Jan,11; 2012,Jan,15-42; 2011,Jan,11

| 89331 | Sperm evaluation, for retrograde ejaculation, urine (sperm concentration, motility, and morphology, as indicated) ♂ |

EXCLUDES Detection of sperm in urine (81015)
Code also semen analysis on concurrent sperm specimen (89300-89322)
🚑 0.00   ⚕ 0.00   **FUD** XXX   Ⓠ ▭

AMA: 2016,Jan,13; 2015,Jan,16; 2014,Jan,11; 2012,Jan,15-42; 2011,Jan,11

| 89335 | Cryopreservation, reproductive tissue, testicular |

EXCLUDES Cryopreservation of:
    Embryo(s) (89258)
    Oocytes:
      Immature ([0357T])
      Mature (89337)
    Ovarian tissue (0058T)
    Sperm (89259)
🚑 0.00   ⚕ 0.00   **FUD** XXX   Ⓠ①

AMA: 2016,Jan,13; 2015,Jan,16; 2014,Jan,11; 2012,Jan,15-42; 2011,Jan,11

| 89337 | Cryopreservation, mature oocyte(s) ♀ |

EXCLUDES Cryopreservation of immature oocyte[s] ([0357T])
🚑 0.00   ⚕ 0.00   **FUD** XXX   Ⓠ① ▭

AMA: 2016,Jan,13; 2015,Jan,16

| 89342 | Storage (per year); embryo(s) |

🚑 0.00   ⚕ 0.00   **FUD** XXX   Ⓠ①

AMA: 2016,Jan,13; 2015,Jan,16; 2014,Jan,11; 2012,Jan,15-42; 2011,Jan,11

| 89343 | sperm/semen |

🚑 0.00   ⚕ 0.00   **FUD** XXX   Ⓠ①

AMA: 2016,Jan,13; 2015,Jan,16; 2014,Jan,11; 2012,Jan,15-42; 2011,Jan,11

| 89344 | reproductive tissue, testicular/ovarian |

🚑 0.00   ⚕ 0.00   **FUD** XXX   Ⓠ①

AMA: 2016,Jan,13; 2015,Jan,16; 2014,Jan,11; 2012,Jan,15-42; 2011,Jan,11

| 89346 | oocyte(s) |

🚑 0.00   ⚕ 0.00   **FUD** XXX   Ⓠ②

AMA: 2016,Jan,13; 2015,Jan,16; 2014,Jan,11; 2012,Jan,15-42; 2011,Jan,11

| 89352 | Thawing of cryopreserved; embryo(s) |

🚑 0.00   ⚕ 0.00   **FUD** XXX   Ⓠ①

AMA: 2016,Jan,13; 2015,Jan,16; 2014,Jan,11; 2012,Jan,15-42; 2011,Jan,11

| 89353 | sperm/semen, each aliquot |

🚑 0.00   ⚕ 0.00   **FUD** XXX   Ⓠ①

AMA: 2016,Jan,13; 2015,Jan,16; 2014,Jan,11; 2012,Jan,15-42; 2011,Jan,11

| 89354 | reproductive tissue, testicular/ovarian |

🚑 0.00   ⚕ 0.00   **FUD** XXX   Ⓠ①

AMA: 2016,Jan,13; 2015,Jan,16; 2014,Jan,11; 2012,Jan,15-42; 2011,Jan,11

| 89356 | oocytes, each aliquot |

🚑 0.00   ⚕ 0.00   **FUD** XXX   Ⓠ①

AMA: 2016,Jan,13; 2015,Jan,16; 2014,Jan,11; 2012,Jan,15-42; 2011,Jan,11

| 89398 | Unlisted reproductive medicine laboratory procedure |

🚑 0.00   ⚕ 0.00   **FUD** XXX   Ⓠ①

INCLUDES Hyaluronan binding assay (HBA)

90281-90399 Immunoglobulin Products

[INCLUDES] Immune globulin product only
Anti-infectives
Antitoxins
Isoantibodies
Monoclonal antibodies

Code also (96365-96372, 96374-96375)

90281 Immune globulin (Ig), human, for intramuscular use
[INCLUDES] Gamastan
0.00 0.00 FUD XXX [51] [E] ⚑
AMA: 2016,Jan,13; 2015,Jan,16; 2014,Jan,11; 2012,Jan,15-42; 2011,Jan,11

90283 Immune globulin (IgIV), human, for intravenous use
0.00 0.00 FUD XXX [51] [E] ⚑
AMA: 2016,Jan,13; 2015,Jan,16; 2014,Jan,11; 2012,Jan,15-42; 2011,Jan,11

90284 Immune globulin (SCIg), human, for use in subcutaneous infusions, 100 mg, each
0.00 0.00 FUD XXX [51] [E] ⚑
AMA: 2016,Jan,13; 2015,Jan,16; 2012,Jan,15-42; 2011,Jan,11

90287 Botulinum antitoxin, equine, any route
0.00 0.00 FUD XXX [51] [E] ⚑
AMA: 2016,Jan,13; 2015,Jan,16; 2014,Jan,11; 2012,Jan,15-42; 2011,Jan,11

90288 Botulism immune globulin, human, for intravenous use
0.00 0.00 FUD XXX [51] [E] ⚑
AMA: 2016,Jan,13; 2015,Jan,16; 2014,Jan,11; 2012,Jan,15-42; 2011,Jan,11

90291 Cytomegalovirus immune globulin (CMV-IgIV), human, for intravenous use
[INCLUDES] Cytogram
0.00 0.00 FUD XXX [51] [E] ⚑
AMA: 2016,Jan,13; 2015,Jan,16; 2014,Jan,11; 2012,Jan,15-42; 2011,Jan,11

90296 Diphtheria antitoxin, equine, any route
0.00 0.00 FUD XXX [51] [E] ⚑
AMA: 2016,Jan,13; 2015,Jan,16; 2014,Jan,11; 2012,Jan,15-42; 2011,Jan,11

90371 Hepatitis B immune globulin (HBIg), human, for intramuscular use
[INCLUDES] HBIG
0.00 0.00 FUD XXX [51] [K] [K2] ⚑
AMA: 2016,Jan,13; 2015,Jan,16; 2014,Jan,11; 2012,Jan,15-42; 2011,Jan,11

90375 Rabies immune globulin (RIg), human, for intramuscular and/or subcutaneous use
[INCLUDES] HyperRAB
0.00 0.00 FUD XXX [51] [K] [K2] ⚑
AMA: 2016,Jan,13; 2015,Jan,16; 2012,Jan,15-42; 2011,Jan,11

90376 Rabies immune globulin, heat-treated (RIg-HT), human, for intramuscular and/or subcutaneous use
0.00 0.00 FUD XXX [51] [K] [K2] ⚑
AMA: 2016,Jan,13; 2015,Jan,16; 2012,Jan,15-42; 2011,Jan,11

90378 Respiratory syncytial virus, monoclonal antibody, recombinant, for intramuscular use, 50 mg, each
[INCLUDES] Synagis
0.00 0.00 FUD XXX [51] [K] [K2] ⚑
AMA: 2016,Jan,13; 2015,Jan,16; 2014,Jan,11; 2012,Jan,15-42; 2011,Jan,11

90384 Rho(D) immune globulin (RhIg), human, full-dose, for intramuscular use
0.00 0.00 FUD XXX [51] [E] ⚑
AMA: 2016,Jan,13; 2015,Jan,16; 2014,Jan,11; 2012,Jan,15-42; 2011,Jan,11

90385 Rho(D) immune globulin (RhIg), human, mini-dose, for intramuscular use
0.00 0.00 FUD XXX [51] [N] [NI] ⚑
AMA: 2016,Jan,13; 2015,Jan,16; 2014,Jan,11; 2012,Jan,15-42; 2011,Jan,11

90386 Rho(D) immune globulin (RhIgIV), human, for intravenous use
0.00 0.00 FUD XXX [51] [E] ⚑
AMA: 2016,Jan,13; 2015,Jan,16; 2014,Jan,11; 2012,Jan,15-42; 2011,Jan,11

90389 Tetanus immune globulin (TIg), human, for intramuscular use
0.00 0.00 FUD XXX [51] [E] ⚑
AMA: 2016,Jan,13; 2015,Jan,16; 2014,Jan,11; 2012,Jan,15-42; 2011,Jan,11

90393 Vaccinia immune globulin, human, for intramuscular use
0.00 0.00 FUD XXX [51] [N] ⚑
AMA: 2016,Jan,13; 2015,Jan,16; 2014,Jan,11; 2012,Jan,15-42; 2011,Jan,11

90396 Varicella-zoster immune globulin, human, for intramuscular use
0.00 0.00 FUD XXX [51] [K] [K2] ⚑
AMA: 2016,Jan,13; 2015,Jan,16; 2014,Jan,11; 2012,Jan,15-42; 2011,Jan,11

90399 Unlisted immune globulin
0.00 0.00 FUD XXX [51] [E] ⚑
AMA: 2016,Jan,13; 2015,Jan,16; 2014,Jan,11; 2012,Jan,15-42; 2011,Jan,11

90460-90461 Injections Provided with Counseling

[INCLUDES] All components of influenza vaccine, report X 1 only
Combination vaccines which comprise multiple vaccine components
Components (all antigens) in vaccines to prevent disease due to specific organisms
Counseling by physician or other qualified health care professional
Multi-valent antigens or multiple antigen serotypes against single organisms are considered one component
Patient/family face-to-face counseling by doctor or qualified health care professional for patients 18 years of age and younger

[EXCLUDES] *Administration of influenza and pneumococcal vaccine for Medicare patients (G0008-G0009)*
Allergy testing (95004-95028)
Bacterial/viral/fungal skin tests (86485-86580)
Diagnostic or therapeutic injections (96365-96372, 96374-96375)
Vaccines provided without face-to-face counseling from a physician or qualified health care professional or to patients over the age of 18 (90471-90474)

Code also significant, separately identifiable E&M service when appropriate
Code also toxoid/vaccine (90476-90736 [90620, 90621, 90625, 90630, 90644, 90672, 90673, 90674])

90460 Immunization administration through 18 years of age via any route of administration, with counseling by physician or other qualified health care professional; first or only component of each vaccine or toxoid administered [A]
Code also each additional component in a vaccine (e.g., A 5-year-old receives DtaP-IPV IM administration, and MMR/Varicella vaccines SQ administration. Report initial component X 2, and additional components X 6)
0.71 0.71 FUD XXX [B] [80] ⚑
AMA: 2016,Jan,13; 2015,May,6; 2015,Apr,9; 2015,Apr,10; 2015,Jan,16; 2014,Mar,10; 2014,Jan,11; 2013,Aug,10; 2012,Jul,7; 2012,Jan,43; 2011,Mar,8; 2011,Mar,3-6

\+ **90461 each additional vaccine or toxoid component administered (List separately in addition to code for primary procedure)** [A]
Code also each additional component in a vaccine (e.g., A 5-year-old receives DtaP-IPV IM administration, and MMR/Varicella vaccines SQ administration. Report initial component X 2, and additional components X 6)
Code first the initial component in each vaccine provided (90460)
0.35 0.35 FUD ZZZ [B] [80] ⚑
AMA: 2016,Jan,13; 2015,May,6; 2015,Apr,10; 2015,Jan,16; 2014,Mar,10; 2014,Jan,11; 2013,Aug,10; 2012,Jul,7; 2012,Jan,43; 2011,Mar,8; 2011,Mar,3-6

Medicine

90471 — 90649

90471-90474 Injections and Other Routes of Administration Without Physician Counseling

CMS: 100-04,18,10.4 CWF Edits for Influenza Virus and Pneumococcal Vaccinations

EXCLUDES *Administration of influenza and pneumococcal vaccine for Medicare patients (G0008-G0009)*
Administration of vaccine with counseling (90460-90461)
Allergy testing (95004-95028)
Bacterial/viral/fungal skin tests (86485-86580)
Diagnostic or therapeutic injections (96365-96371, 96374)
Patient/family face-to-face counseling
Code also significant separately identifiable E&M service when appropriate
Code also toxoid/vaccine (90476-90736 [90620, 90621, 90625, 90630, 90644, 90672, 90673, 90674, 90750])

90471 **Immunization administration (includes percutaneous, intradermal, subcutaneous, or intramuscular injections); 1 vaccine (single or combination vaccine/toxoid)**

EXCLUDES *Intranasal/oral administration (90473)*
⚕ 0.71 ✂ 0.71 **FUD** XXX Ⓢ 80 ▢

AMA: 2016,Jan,13; 2015,May,6; 2015,Apr,9; 2015,Apr,10; 2015,Jan,16; 2014,Mar,10; 2014,Jan,11; 2013,Aug,10; 2012,Jul,7; 2012,Jan,15-42; 2011,Mar,3-6; 2011,Jan,11

+ 90472 **each additional vaccine (single or combination vaccine/toxoid) (List separately in addition to code for primary procedure)**

EXCLUDES *BCG vaccine, intravesical administration (51720, 90586)*
Immune globulin administration (96365-96371, 96374)
Immune globulin product (90281-90399)
Code first initial vaccine (90460, 90471, 90473)
⚕ 0.35 ✂ 0.35 **FUD** ZZZ Ⓝ 80 ▢

AMA: 2016,Jan,13; 2015,May,6; 2015,Apr,9; 2015,Apr,10; 2015,Jan,16; 2014,Mar,10; 2014,Jan,11; 2013,Aug,10; 2012,Jul,7; 2012,Jan,15-42; 2011,Mar,3-6; 2011,Jan,11

90473 **Immunization administration by intranasal or oral route; 1 vaccine (single or combination vaccine/toxoid)**

EXCLUDES *Administration by injection (90471)*
⚕ 0.71 ✂ 0.71 **FUD** XXX Ⓢ 80 ▢

AMA: 2016,Jan,13; 2015,May,6; 2015,Jan,16; 2014,Mar,10; 2014,Jan,11; 2013,Aug,10; 2012,Jul,7; 2011,Mar,3-6

+ 90474 **each additional vaccine (single or combination vaccine/toxoid) (List separately in addition to code for primary procedure)**

Code first initial vaccine (90460, 90471, 90473)
⚕ 0.35 ✂ 0.35 **FUD** ZZZ Ⓝ 80 ▢

AMA: 2016,Jan,13; 2015,May,6; 2015,Apr,9; 2015,Jan,16; 2014,Mar,10; 2014,Jan,11; 2013,Aug,10; 2012,Jul,7; 2011,Mar,3-6

90476-90736 [90620, 90621, 90625, 90630, 90644, 90672, 90673, 90674, 90750] Vaccination Products

INCLUDES Patient's age for coding purposes, not for product license
Vaccine product only

EXCLUDES *Coding of each component of a combination vaccine individually*
Immune globulins and administration (90281-90399, 96365-96375)
Code also administration of vaccine (90460-90474)
Code also significant separately identifiable E&M service when appropriate

90476 **Adenovirus vaccine, type 4, live, for oral use**

INCLUDES Adeno-4
⚕ 0.00 ✂ 0.00 **FUD** XXX Ⓢ Ⓝ M1 ▢

AMA: 2016,Jan,13; 2015,May,6; 2015,Jan,16; 2014,Jan,11; 2013,Aug,10; 2012,Jan,15-42; 2011,Mar,3-6; 2011,Jan,11

90477 **Adenovirus vaccine, type 7, live, for oral use**

INCLUDES Adeno-7
⚕ 0.00 ✂ 0.00 **FUD** XXX Ⓢ E ▢

AMA: 2016,Jan,13; 2015,May,6; 2015,Jan,16; 2014,Jan,11; 2013,Aug,10; 2012,Jan,15-42; 2011,Mar,3-6; 2011,Jan,11

90581 **Anthrax vaccine, for subcutaneous or intramuscular use**

INCLUDES BioThrax
⚕ 0.00 ✂ 0.00 **FUD** XXX Ⓢ Ⓝ M1 ▢

AMA: 2016,Jan,13; 2015,May,6; 2015,Jan,16; 2014,Jan,11; 2013,Aug,10; 2012,Jan,15-42; 2011,Mar,3-6; 2011,Jan,11

90585 **Bacillus Calmette-Guerin vaccine (BCG) for tuberculosis, live, for percutaneous use**

INCLUDES Mycobax
⚕ 0.00 ✂ 0.00 **FUD** XXX Ⓢ K K2 ▢

AMA: 2016,Jan,13; 2015,May,6; 2015,Jan,16; 2014,Jan,11; 2013,Aug,10; 2012,Jan,15-42; 2011,Mar,3-6; 2011,Jan,11

90586 **Bacillus Calmette-Guerin vaccine (BCG) for bladder cancer, live, for intravesical use**

INCLUDES TheraCys
TICE BCG
⚕ 0.00 ✂ 0.00 **FUD** XXX Ⓢ B ▢

AMA: 2016,Jan,13; 2015,May,6; 2015,Jan,16; 2014,Jan,11; 2013,Aug,10; 2012,Jan,15-42; 2011,Mar,3-6; 2011,Jan,11

90620 **Resequenced code. See code following 90734.**

90621 **Resequenced code. See code following 90734.**

90625 **Resequenced code. See code following 90723.**

90630 **Resequenced code. See code following 90654.**

90632 **Hepatitis A vaccine (HepA), adult dosage, for intramuscular use** Ⓐ

INCLUDES Havrix
Vaqta
⚕ 0.00 ✂ 0.00 **FUD** XXX Ⓢ Ⓝ M1 ▢

AMA: 2016,Jan,13; 2015,May,6; 2015,Jan,16; 2014,Jan,11; 2013,Aug,10; 2012,Jan,15-42; 2011,Mar,3-6; 2011,Jan,11

90633 **Hepatitis A vaccine (HepA), pediatric/adolescent dosage-2 dose schedule, for intramuscular use** Ⓐ

INCLUDES Havrix
Vaqta
⚕ 0.00 ✂ 0.00 **FUD** XXX Ⓢ Ⓝ M1 ▢

AMA: 2016,Jan,13; 2015,May,6; 2015,Jan,16; 2014,Jan,11; 2013,Aug,10; 2012,Jan,15-42; 2011,Mar,3-6; 2011,Jan,11

90634 **Hepatitis A vaccine (HepA), pediatric/adolescent dosage-3 dose schedule, for intramuscular use** Ⓐ

INCLUDES Havrix
⚕ 0.00 ✂ 0.00 **FUD** XXX Ⓢ Ⓝ M1 ▢

AMA: 2016,Jan,13; 2015,May,6; 2015,Jan,16; 2014,Jan,11; 2013,Aug,10; 2012,Jan,15-42; 2011,Mar,3-6; 2011,Jan,11

90636 **Hepatitis A and hepatitis B vaccine (HepA-HepB), adult dosage, for intramuscular use** Ⓐ

INCLUDES Twinrix
⚕ 0.00 ✂ 0.00 **FUD** XXX Ⓢ Ⓝ M1 ▢

AMA: 2016,Jan,13; 2015,May,6; 2015,Jan,16; 2014,Jan,11; 2013,Aug,10; 2012,Jan,15-42; 2011,Mar,3-6; 2011,Jan,11

90644 **Resequenced code. See code following 90732.**

90647 **Haemophilus influenzae type b vaccine (Hib), PRP-OMP conjugate, 3 dose schedule, for intramuscular use**

INCLUDES PedvaxHIB
⚕ 0.00 ✂ 0.00 **FUD** XXX Ⓢ Ⓝ M1 ▢

AMA: 2016,Jan,13; 2015,May,6; 2015,Jan,16; 2014,Jan,11; 2013,Aug,10; 2012,Jan,15-42; 2011,Mar,3-6; 2011,Jan,11

90648 **Haemophilus influenzae type b vaccine (Hib), PRP-T conjugate, 4 dose schedule, for intramuscular use**

INCLUDES ActHIB
Hiberix
⚕ 0.00 ✂ 0.00 **FUD** XXX Ⓢ Ⓝ M1 ▢

AMA: 2016,Jan,13; 2015,May,6; 2015,Jan,16; 2014,Jan,11; 2013,Aug,10; 2012,Jan,15-42; 2011,Mar,3-6; 2011,Jan,11

90649 **Human Papillomavirus vaccine, types 6, 11, 16, 18, quadrivalent (4vHPV), 3 dose schedule, for intramuscular use**

INCLUDES Gardasil
⚕ 0.00 ✂ 0.00 **FUD** XXX Ⓢ M ▢

AMA: 2016,Jan,13; 2015,May,6; 2015,Jan,16; 2014,Jan,11; 2013,Aug,10; 2012,Jan,15-42; 2011,Mar,3-6; 2011,Jan,11

90650 Human Papillomavirus vaccine, types 16, 18, bivalent (2vHPV), 3 dose schedule, for intramuscular use

[INCLUDES] Cervarix

0.00 0.00 FUD XXX [51] [M] ⚑

AMA: 2016,Jan,13; 2015,May,6; 2015,Jan,16; 2014,Jan,11; 2013,Aug,10; 2012,Jan,15-42; 2011,Mar,3-6; 2011,Jan,11

90651 Human Papillomavirus vaccine types 6, 11, 16, 18, 31, 33, 45, 52, 58, nonavalent (9vHPV), 3 dose schedule, for intramuscular use

0.00 0.00 FUD XXX [51] [E] ⚑

AMA: 2016,Jan,13; 2015,May,6; 2015,Jan,16

90653 Influenza vaccine, inactivated (IIV), subunit, adjuvanted, for intramuscular use

0.00 0.00 FUD XXX [51] [L] [L1] ⚑

AMA: 2016,Jan,13; 2015,May,6; 2015,Jan,16; 2014,Jan,11; 2013,Aug,10

90654 Influenza virus vaccine, trivalent (IIV3), split virus, preservative-free, for intradermal use

[INCLUDES] Fluzone intradermal

0.00 0.00 FUD XXX [51] [L] [L1] ⚑

AMA: 2016,Jan,13; 2015,May,6; 2015,Apr,9; 2015,Jan,16; 2014,Jan,11; 2013,Aug,10; 2012,Jan,15-42; 2011,Mar,3-6; 2011,Jan,11

\# **90630 Influenza virus vaccine, quadrivalent (IIV4), split virus, preservative free, for intradermal use**

0.00 0.00 FUD XXX [51] [L] [L1] ⚑

AMA: 2016,Jan,13; 2015,May,6; 2015,Jan,16

▲ **90655 Influenza virus vaccine, trivalent (IIV3), split virus, preservative free, 0.25 mL dosage, for intramuscular use** [A]

[INCLUDES] Afluria
Fluzone, no preservative, pediatric dose

0.00 0.00 FUD XXX [51] [L] [L1] ⚑

AMA: 2016,May,9; 2016,Jan,13; 2015,May,6; 2015,Jan,16; 2014,Jan,11; 2013,Aug,10; 2012,Jan,15-42; 2011,Mar,3-6; 2011,Jan,11

▲ **90656 Influenza virus vaccine, trivalent (IIV3), split virus, preservative free, 0.5 mL dosage, for intramuscular use** [A]

[INCLUDES] Afluria
Fluvarix
Fluvirin
Fluzone, influenza virus vaccine, no preservative

0.00 0.00 FUD XXX [51] [L] [L1] ⚑

AMA: 2016,May,9; 2016,Jan,13; 2015,May,6; 2015,Jan,16; 2014,Jan,11; 2013,Aug,10; 2012,Jan,15-42; 2011,Mar,3-6; 2011,Jan,11

▲ **90657 Influenza virus vaccine, trivalent (IIV3), split virus, 0.25 mL dosage, for intramuscular use** [A]

[INCLUDES] Afluria
Flulaval
Fluvirin
Fluzone (5 ml vial [0.25ml dose])

0.00 0.00 FUD XXX [51] [L] [L1] ⚑

AMA: 2016,May,9; 2016,Jan,13; 2015,May,6; 2015,Jan,16; 2014,Jan,11; 2013,Aug,10; 2012,Jan,15-42; 2011,Mar,3-6; 2011,Jan,11

▲ **90658 Influenza virus vaccine, trivalent (IIV3), split virus, 0.5 mL dosage, for intramuscular use** [A]

[INCLUDES] Afluria
Flulaval
Fluvirin
Fluzone

0.00 0.00 FUD XXX [51] [E] ⚑

AMA: 2016,May,9; 2016,Jan,13; 2015,May,6; 2015,Jan,16; 2014,Jan,11; 2013,Aug,10; 2012,Jan,15-42; 2011,Mar,3-6; 2011,Jan,11

90660 Influenza virus vaccine, trivalent, live (LAIV3), for intranasal use

[INCLUDES] FluMist

0.00 0.00 FUD XXX [51] [L] [L1] ⚑

AMA: 2016,Jan,13; 2015,May,6; 2015,Jan,16; 2014,Jan,11; 2013,Aug,10; 2012,Jan,15-42; 2011,Mar,3-6; 2011,Jan,11

\# **90672 Influenza virus vaccine, quadrivalent, live (LAIV4), for intranasal use**

[INCLUDES] FluMist nasal spray

0.00 0.00 FUD XXX [51] [L] [L1] ⚑

AMA: 2016,Jan,13; 2015,May,6; 2015,Jan,16; 2014,Jan,11; 2013,Aug,10

▲ **90661 Influenza virus vaccine (ccIIV3), derived from cell cultures, subunit, preservative and antibiotic free, for intramuscular use**

[INCLUDES] Flucelvax

0.00 0.00 FUD XXX [51] [L] [L1] ⚑

AMA: 2016,Jan,13; 2015,May,6; 2015,Jan,16; 2014,Jan,11; 2013,Aug,10; 2012,Jan,15-42; 2011,Mar,3-6; 2011,Jan,11

● # **90674 Influenza virus vaccine, quadrivalent (ccIIV4), derived from cell cultures, subunit, preservative and antibiotic free, 0.5 mL dosage, for intramuscular use**

0.00 0.00 FUD 000 [51]

\# **90673 Influenza virus vaccine, trivalent (RIV3), derived from recombinant DNA, hemagglutinin (HA) protein only, preservative and antibiotic free, for intramuscular use**

[INCLUDES] Flublok (single dose vial)

0.00 0.00 FUD XXX [51] [L] [L1] ⚑

AMA: 2016,Jan,13; 2015,May,6; 2015,Jan,16; 2014,Mar,10; 2014,Jan,11

90662 Influenza virus vaccine (IIV), split virus, preservative free, enhanced immunogenicity via increased antigen content, for intramuscular use

[INCLUDES] Fluzone high-dose

0.00 0.00 FUD XXX [51] [L] [L1] ⚑

AMA: 2016,Jan,13; 2015,May,6; 2015,Jan,16; 2014,Jan,11; 2013,Aug,10; 2012,Jan,15-42; 2011,Mar,3-6; 2011,Jan,11

90664 Influenza virus vaccine, live (LAIV), pandemic formulation, for intranasal use

0.00 0.00 FUD XXX [51] [E] ⚑

AMA: 2016,Jan,13; 2015,May,6; 2015,Jan,16; 2014,Jan,11; 2013,Aug,10; 2012,Jan,15-42; 2011,Mar,3-6; 2011,Jan,11

90666 Influenza virus vaccine (IIV), pandemic formulation, split virus, preservative free, for intramuscular use

0.00 0.00 FUD XXX ✗ [51] [E] ⚑

AMA: 2016,Jan,13; 2015,May,6; 2015,Jan,16; 2014,Jan,11; 2013,Aug,10; 2012,Jan,15-42; 2011,Mar,3-6; 2011,Jan,11

90667 Influenza virus vaccine (IIV), pandemic formulation, split virus, adjuvanted, for intramuscular use

0.00 0.00 FUD XXX ✗ [51] [E] ⚑

AMA: 2016,Jan,13; 2015,May,6; 2015,Jan,16; 2014,Jan,11; 2013,Aug,10; 2012,Jan,15-42; 2011,Mar,3-6; 2011,Jan,11

90668 Influenza virus vaccine (IIV), pandemic formulation, split virus, for intramuscular use

0.00 0.00 FUD XXX ✗ [51] [E] ⚑

AMA: 2016,Jan,13; 2015,May,6; 2015,Jan,16; 2014,Jan,11; 2013,Aug,10; 2012,Jan,15-42; 2011,Mar,3-6; 2011,Jan,11

90670 Pneumococcal conjugate vaccine, 13 valent (PCV13), for intramuscular use

[INCLUDES] Prevnar 13

0.00 0.00 FUD XXX [51] [L] [L1] ⚑

AMA: 2016,Jan,13; 2015,May,6; 2015,Jan,16; 2014,Jan,11; 2013,Aug,10; 2012,Jan,15-42; 2011,Mar,3-6; 2011,Mar,8; 2011,Jan,11

90672 **Resequenced code. See code following 90660.**

90673 **Resequenced code. See code following 90661.**

90674 **Resequenced code. See code following 90661.**

90675 Rabies vaccine, for intramuscular use

[INCLUDES] Imovax
RabAvert

🏢 0.00 🩺 0.00 **FUD** XXX [51] [K] [K2] ⚑

AMA: 2016,Jan,13; 2015,May,6; 2015,Jan,16; 2014,Jan,11; 2013,Aug,10; 2012,Jan,15-42; 2011,Mar,3-6; 2011,Jan,11

90676 Rabies vaccine, for intradermal use

🏢 0.00 🩺 0.00 **FUD** XXX [51] [K] [K2] ⚑

AMA: 2016,Jan,13; 2015,May,6; 2015,Jan,16; 2014,Jan,11; 2013,Aug,10; 2012,Jul,7; 2012,Jan,15-42; 2011,Mar,3-6; 2011,Jan,11

90680 Rotavirus vaccine, pentavalent (RV5), 3 dose schedule, live, for oral use

[INCLUDES] RotaTeq

🏢 0.00 🩺 0.00 **FUD** XXX [51] [N] [N1] ⚑

AMA: 2016,Jan,13; 2015,May,6; 2015,Jan,16; 2014,Jan,11; 2013,Aug,10; 2012,Jan,15-42; 2011,Mar,3-6; 2011,Jan,11

90681 Rotavirus vaccine, human, attenuated (RV1), 2 dose schedule, live, for oral use

[INCLUDES] Rotarix

🏢 0.00 🩺 0.00 **FUD** XXX [51] [E] ⚑

AMA: 2016,Jan,13; 2015,May,6; 2015,Jan,16; 2014,Jan,11; 2013,Aug,10; 2012,Jul,7; 2012,Jan,15-42; 2011,Mar,3-6; 2011,Mar,8; 2011,Jan,11

● **90682 Influenza virus vaccine, quadrivalent (RIV4), derived from recombinant DNA, hemagglutinin (HA) protein only, preservative and antibiotic free, for intramuscular use**

🏢 0.00 🩺 0.00 **FUD** 000 ⚡

▲ **90685 Influenza virus vaccine, quadrivalent (IIV4), split virus, preservative free, 0.25 mL, for intramuscular use** [A]

[INCLUDES] Fluzone Quadrivalent

🏢 0.00 🩺 0.00 **FUD** XXX [51] [L] [L1] ⚑

AMA: 2016,May,9; 2016,Jan,13; 2015,May,6; 2015,Jan,16; 2014,Mar,10; 2014,Jan,11; 2013,Aug,10

▲ **90686 Influenza virus vaccine, quadrivalent (IIV4), split virus, preservative free, 0.5 mL dosage, for intramuscular use** [A]

[INCLUDES] Fluarix Quadrivalent
Fluzone Quadrivalent

🏢 0.00 🩺 0.00 **FUD** XXX [51] [L] [L1] ⚑

AMA: 2016,May,9; 2016,Jan,13; 2015,May,6; 2015,Jan,16; 2014,Mar,10; 2014,Jan,11; 2013,Aug,10

▲ **90687 Influenza virus vaccine, quadrivalent (IIV4), split virus, 0.25 mL dosage, for intramuscular use** [A]

🏢 0.00 🩺 0.00 **FUD** XXX [51] [L] [L1] ⚑

AMA: 2016,May,9; 2016,Jan,13; 2015,May,6; 2015,Jan,16; 2014,Mar,10; 2014,Jan,11; 2013,Aug,10

▲ **90688 Influenza virus vaccine, quadrivalent (IIV4), split virus, 0.5 mL dosage, for intramuscular use** [A]

[INCLUDES] FluLaval (multidose vial)

🏢 0.00 🩺 0.00 **FUD** XXX [51] [L] [L1] ⚑

AMA: 2016,May,9; 2016,Jan,13; 2015,May,6; 2015,Jan,16; 2014,Mar,10; 2014,Jan,11; 2013,Aug,10

90690 Typhoid vaccine, live, oral

[INCLUDES] Vivotif

🏢 0.00 🩺 0.00 **FUD** XXX [51] [N] [N1] ⚑

AMA: 2016,Jan,13; 2015,May,6; 2015,Jan,16; 2014,Jan,11; 2013,Aug,10; 2012,Jan,15-42; 2011,Mar,3-6; 2011,Jan,11

90691 Typhoid vaccine, Vi capsular polysaccharide (ViCPs), for intramuscular use

[INCLUDES] Typhim Vi

🏢 0.00 🩺 0.00 **FUD** XXX [51] [N] [N1] ⚑

AMA: 2016,Jan,13; 2015,May,6; 2015,Jan,16; 2014,Jan,11; 2013,Aug,10; 2012,Jan,15-42; 2011,Mar,3-6; 2011,Jan,11

90696 Diphtheria, tetanus toxoids, acellular pertussis vaccine and inactivated poliovirus vaccine (DTaP-IPV), when administered to children 4 through 6 years of age, for intramuscular use [A]

[INCLUDES] KINRIX

🏢 0.00 🩺 0.00 **FUD** XXX [51] [N] [N1] ⚑

AMA: 2016,Jan,13; 2015,May,6; 2015,Jan,16; 2014,Jan,11; 2013,Aug,10; 2012,Jan,15-42; 2011,Mar,3-6; 2011,Jan,11

90697 Diphtheria, tetanus toxoids, acellular pertussis vaccine, inactivated poliovirus vaccine, Haemophilus influenzae type b PRP-OMP conjugate vaccine, and hepatitis B vaccine (DTaP-IPV-Hib-HepB), for intramuscular use

🏢 0.00 🩺 0.00 **FUD** XXX ⚡ [51] [E] ⚑

AMA: 2016,Jan,13; 2015,May,6; 2015,Jan,16

90698 Diphtheria, tetanus toxoids, acellular pertussis vaccine, Haemophilus influenzae type b, and inactivated poliovirus vaccine, (DTaP-IPV/Hib), for intramuscular use

[INCLUDES] Pentacel

🏢 0.00 🩺 0.00 **FUD** XXX [51] [N] [N1] ⚑

AMA: 2016,Jan,13; 2015,May,6; 2015,Jan,16; 2014,Jan,11; 2013,Aug,10; 2012,Jan,15-42; 2011,Mar,3-6; 2011,Jan,11

90700 Diphtheria, tetanus toxoids, and acellular pertussis vaccine (DTaP), when administered to individuals younger than 7 years, for intramuscular use [A]

[INCLUDES] Daptacel
Infanrix

🏢 0.00 🩺 0.00 **FUD** XXX [51] [N] [N1] ⚑

AMA: 2016,Jan,13; 2015,May,6; 2015,Jan,16; 2014,Jan,11; 2013,Aug,10; 2012,Jul,7; 2012,Jan,15-42; 2011,Mar,8; 2011,Mar,3-6; 2011,Jan,11

90702 Diphtheria and tetanus toxoids adsorbed (DT) when administered to individuals younger than 7 years, for intramuscular use [A]

[INCLUDES] Diphtheria and Tetanus Toxoids Adsorbed USP (For Pediatric Use)

🏢 0.00 🩺 0.00 **FUD** XXX [51] [N] [N1] ⚑

AMA: 2016,Jan,13; 2015,May,6; 2015,Jan,16; 2014,Jan,11; 2013,Aug,10; 2012,Jan,15-42; 2011,Mar,3-6; 2011,Jan,11

90707 Measles, mumps and rubella virus vaccine (MMR), live, for subcutaneous use

[INCLUDES] M-M-R II

🏢 0.00 🩺 0.00 **FUD** XXX [51] [N] [N1] ⚑

AMA: 2016,Jan,13; 2015,May,6; 2015,Jan,16; 2014,Jan,11; 2013,Aug,10; 2012,Jul,7; 2012,Jan,15-42; 2011,Mar,3-6; 2011,Jan,11

90710 Measles, mumps, rubella, and varicella vaccine (MMRV), live, for subcutaneous use

[INCLUDES] ProQuad

🏢 0.00 🩺 0.00 **FUD** XXX [51] [N] [N1] ⚑

AMA: 2016,Jan,13; 2015,May,6; 2015,Jan,16; 2014,Jan,11; 2013,Aug,10; 2012,Jan,15-42; 2011,Mar,3-6; 2011,Jan,11

90713 Poliovirus vaccine, inactivated (IPV), for subcutaneous or intramuscular use

[INCLUDES] IPOL

🏢 0.00 🩺 0.00 **FUD** XXX [51] [N] [N1] ⚑

AMA: 2016,Jan,13; 2015,May,6; 2015,Jan,16; 2014,Jan,11; 2013,Aug,10; 2012,Jan,15-42; 2011,Mar,8; 2011,Mar,3-6; 2011,Jan,11

90714 Tetanus and diphtheria toxoids adsorbed (Td), preservative free, when administered to individuals 7 years or older, for intramuscular use [A]

[INCLUDES] DECAVAC/TENIVAC
Tetanus-diphtheria adult

🏢 0.00 🩺 0.00 **FUD** XXX [51] [N] [N1] ⚑

AMA: 2016,Jan,13; 2015,May,6; 2015,Jan,16; 2014,Jan,11; 2013,Aug,10; 2012,Jan,15-42; 2011,Mar,3-6; 2011,Jan,11

90715 **Tetanus, diphtheria toxoids and acellular pertussis vaccine (Tdap), when administered to individuals 7 years or older, for intramuscular use** [A]

[INCLUDES] Adacel
Boostrix

🏥 0.00 🩺 0.00 FUD XXX [51] [N] [N1] ⚑

AMA: 2016,Jan,13; 2015,May,6; 2015,Jan,16; 2014,Jan,11; 2013,Aug,10; 2012,Jan,15-42; 2011,Mar,3-6; 2011,Jan,11

90716 **Varicella virus vaccine (VAR), live, for subcutaneous use**

[INCLUDES] Varivax

🏥 0.00 🩺 0.00 FUD XXX [51] [M] ⚑

AMA: 2016,Jan,13; 2015,May,6; 2015,Mar,3; 2015,Jan,16; 2014,Jan,11; 2013,Aug,10; 2012,Jan,15-42; 2011,Mar,3-6; 2011,Jan,11

90717 **Yellow fever vaccine, live, for subcutaneous use**

[INCLUDES] YF-VAX

🏥 0.00 🩺 0.00 FUD XXX [51] [N] [N1] ⚑

AMA: 2016,Jan,13; 2015,May,6; 2015,Jan,16; 2014,Jan,11; 2013,Aug,10; 2012,Jan,15-42; 2011,Mar,3-6; 2011,Jan,11

90723 **Diphtheria, tetanus toxoids, acellular pertussis vaccine, hepatitis B, and inactivated poliovirus vaccine (DTaP-HepB-IPV), for intramuscular use**

[INCLUDES] PEDIARIX

🏥 0.00 🩺 0.00 FUD XXX [51] [E] ⚑

AMA: 2016,Jan,13; 2015,May,6; 2015,Jan,16; 2014,Jan,11; 2013,Aug,10; 2012,Jan,15-42; 2011,Mar,3-6; 2011,Jan,11

\# **90625** **Cholera vaccine, live, adult dosage, 1 dose schedule, for oral use** [A]

🏥 0.00 🩺 0.00 FUD XXX [51] [E] ⚑

AMA: 2016,Jan,13

90732 **Pneumococcal polysaccharide vaccine, 23-valent (PPSV23), adult or immunosuppressed patient dosage, when administered to individuals 2 years or older, for subcutaneous or intramuscular use** [A]

[INCLUDES] Pneumovax 23

🏥 0.00 🩺 0.00 FUD XXX [51] [L] [L1] ⚑

AMA: 2016,Jan,13; 2015,May,6; 2015,Jan,16; 2014,Jan,11; 2013,Aug,10; 2012,Jan,15-42; 2011,Mar,3-6; 2011,Jan,11

▲ # **90644** **Meningococcal conjugate vaccine, serogroups C & Y and Haemophilus influenzae type b vaccine (Hib-MenCY), 4 dose schedule, when administered to children 6 weeks-18 months of age, for intramuscular use** [A]

🏥 0.00 🩺 0.00 FUD XXX [51] [E] ⚑

AMA: 2016,Jan,13; 2015,May,6; 2015,Jan,16; 2014,Jan,11; 2013,Aug,10; 2012,Jan,15-42; 2011,Mar,3-6; 2011,Jan,11

90733 **Meningococcal polysaccharide vaccine, serogroups A, C, Y, W-135, quadrivalent (MPSV4), for subcutaneous use**

[INCLUDES] Menomune-A/C/Y/W-135

🏥 0.00 🩺 0.00 FUD XXX [51] [K] [K2] ⚑

AMA: 2016,Jan,13; 2015,May,6; 2015,Jan,16; 2014,Jan,11; 2013,Aug,10; 2012,Jan,15-42; 2011,Mar,3-6; 2011,Jan,11

▲ **90734** **Meningococcal conjugate vaccine, serogroups A, C, Y and W-135, quadrivalent (MCV4 or MenACWY), for intramuscular use**

[INCLUDES] Menactra
Menveo

🏥 0.00 🩺 0.00 FUD XXX [51] [K] [K2] ⚑

AMA: 2016,Jan,13; 2015,May,6; 2015,Jan,16; 2014,Jan,11; 2013,Aug,10; 2012,Jan,15-42; 2011,Mar,3-6; 2011,Jan,11

\# **90620** **Meningococcal recombinant protein and outer membrane vesicle vaccine, serogroup B (MenB), 2 dose schedule, for intramuscular use**

🏥 0.00 🩺 0.00 FUD XXX [51] [K] [K2] ⚑

AMA: 2016,Jan,13; 2015,May,6; 2015,Jan,16

\# **90621** **Meningococcal recombinant lipoprotein vaccine, serogroup B (MenB), 3 dose schedule, for intramuscular use**

🏥 0.00 🩺 0.00 FUD XXX [51] [K] [K2] ⚑

AMA: 2016,Jan,13; 2015,May,6; 2015,Jan,16

90736 **Zoster (shingles) vaccine (HZV), live, for subcutaneous injection**

[INCLUDES] Zostavax

🏥 0.00 🩺 0.00 FUD XXX [51] [M] ⚑

AMA: 2016,Jan,13; 2015,May,6; 2015,Jan,16; 2014,Jan,11; 2013,Aug,10; 2012,Jan,15-42; 2011,Mar,3-6; 2011,Jan,11

● # **90750** **Zoster (shingles) vaccine (HZV), recombinant, sub-unit, adjuvanted, for intramuscular injection**

🏥 0.00 🩺 0.00 FUD 000 ⚡ [51]

90738 **Japanese encephalitis virus vaccine, inactivated, for intramuscular use**

[INCLUDES] Ixiaro

🏥 0.00 🩺 0.00 FUD XXX [51] [M] ⚑

AMA: 2016,Jan,13; 2015,May,6; 2015,Jan,16; 2014,Jan,11; 2013,Aug,10; 2012,Jan,15-42; 2011,Mar,3-6; 2011,Jan,11

90739 **Hepatitis B vaccine (HepB), adult dosage, 2 dose schedule, for intramuscular use**

🏥 0.00 🩺 0.00 FUD XXX ⚡ [51] [E] ⚑

AMA: 2016,Jan,13; 2015,May,6; 2015,Jan,16; 2014,Jan,11; 2013,Aug,10

90740 **Hepatitis B vaccine (HepB), dialysis or immunosuppressed patient dosage, 3 dose schedule, for intramuscular use**

[INCLUDES] Recombivax dialysis

🏥 0.00 🩺 0.00 FUD XXX [51] [F] [F4] ⚑

AMA: 2016,Jan,13; 2015,May,6; 2015,Jan,16; 2014,Jan,11; 2013,Aug,10; 2012,Jan,15-42; 2011,Mar,3-6; 2011,Jan,11

90743 **Hepatitis B vaccine (HepB), adolescent, 2 dose schedule, for intramuscular use** [A]

[INCLUDES] Energix-B
Recombivax HB

🏥 0.00 🩺 0.00 FUD XXX [51] [F] [F4] ⚑

AMA: 2016,Jan,13; 2015,May,6; 2015,Jan,16; 2014,Jan,11; 2013,Aug,10; 2012,Jan,15-42; 2011,Mar,3-6; 2011,Jan,11

90744 **Hepatitis B vaccine (HepB), pediatric/adolescent dosage, 3 dose schedule, for intramuscular use** [A]

[INCLUDES] Energix-B
Recombivax HB

🏥 0.00 🩺 0.00 FUD XXX [51] [F] [F4] ⚑

AMA: 2016,Jan,13; 2015,May,6; 2015,Jan,16; 2014,Jan,11; 2013,Aug,10; 2012,Jan,15-42; 2011,Mar,3-6; 2011,Jan,11

90746 **Hepatitis B vaccine (HepB), adult dosage, 3 dose schedule, for intramuscular use**

[INCLUDES] Energix-B
Recombivax HB

🏥 0.00 🩺 0.00 FUD XXX [51] [F] [F4] ⚑

AMA: 2016,Jan,13; 2015,May,6; 2015,Jan,16; 2014,Jan,11; 2013,Aug,10; 2012,Jan,15-42; 2011,Mar,3-6; 2011,Jan,11

90747 **Hepatitis B vaccine (HepB), dialysis or immunosuppressed patient dosage, 4 dose schedule, for intramuscular use**

[INCLUDES] Energix-B
RECOMBIVAX dialysis

🏥 0.00 🩺 0.00 FUD XXX [51] [F] [F4] ⚑

AMA: 2016,Jan,13; 2015,May,6; 2015,Jan,16; 2014,Jan,11; 2013,Aug,10; 2012,Jan,15-42; 2011,Mar,3-6; 2011,Jan,11

90748 **Hepatitis B and Haemophilus influenzae type b vaccine (Hib-HepB), for intramuscular use**

[INCLUDES] COMVAX

🏥 0.00 🩺 0.00 FUD XXX [51] [E] ⚑

AMA: 2016,Jan,13; 2015,May,6; 2015,Jan,16; 2014,Jan,11; 2013,Aug,10; 2012,Jul,7; 2012,Jan,15-42; 2011,Mar,3-6; 2011,Mar,8; 2011,Jan,11

© 2016 Optum360, LLC CPT © 2016 American Medical Association. All Rights Reserved.

Medicine

90749 — 90838

90749	Unlisted vaccine/toxoid

🔧 0.00   🔍 0.00   **FUD** XXX   Ⓢ Ⓝ Ⓜ️

AMA: 2016,Jan,13; 2015,May,6; 2015,Jan,16; 2014,Jan,11; 2012,Jan,15-42; 2011,Mar,3-6; 2011,Jan,11

90750	Resequenced code. See code following 90736.

90785 Complex Interactive Encounter

CMS: 100-02,15,160 Clinical Psychologist Services; 100-02,15,170 Clinical Social Worker (CSW) Services; 100-03,10.3 Inpatient Pain Rehabilitation Programs; 100-03,10.4 Outpatient Hospital Pain Rehabilitation Programs; 100-03,130.1 Inpatient Stays for Alcoholism Treatment; 100-04,12,100 Teaching Physician Services

INCLUDES   At least one of the following activities:

Discussion of a sentinel event demanding third-party involvement (eg, abuse or neglect reported to a state agency)

Interference by the behavior or emotional state of caregiver to understand and assist in the plan of treatment

Managing discordant communication complicating care among participating members (eg, arguing, reactivity)

Use of nonverbal communication methods (eg, toys, other devices, or translator) to eliminate communication barriers

Complicated issues of communication affecting provision of the psychiatric service

Involved communication with:

Emotionally charged or dissonant family members

Patients wanting others present during the visit (e.g., family member, translator)

Patients with impaired or undeveloped verbal skills

Patients with third parties responsible for their care (eg, parents, guardians)

Third-party involvement (eg, schools, probation and parole officers, child protective agencies)

EXCLUDES   *Adaptive behavior treatment (0364T-0367T, 0373T-0374T)*

Crisis psychotherapy (90839-90840)

+   **90785**   **Interactive complexity (List separately in addition to the code for primary procedure)**

Code first, when performed (99201-99255 [99224, 99225, 99226], 99304-99337, 99341-99350, 90791-90792, 90832-90834, 90836-90838, 90853)

🔧 0.39   🔍 0.39   **FUD** ZZZ   Ⓝ ▣

AMA: 2016,Jan,13; 2015,Jan,16; 2013,Jun,3-5; 2013,May,12

90791-90792 Psychiatric Evaluations

CMS: 100-02,15,170 Clinical Social Worker (CSW) Services; 100-02,15,270.2 Medicare Telehealth Services; 100-03,10.3 Inpatient Pain Rehabilitation Programs; 100-03,130.1 Inpatient Stays for Alcoholism Treatment; 100-03,130.2 Outpatient Hospital Services for Alcoholism; 100-04,12*Medicare Telehealth Services; 100-04,12,100 Teaching Physician Services; 100-04,12,190.7 Contractor Editing of Telehealth Claims

INCLUDES   Diagnostic assessment or reassessment without psychotherapy services

EXCLUDES   *Adaptive behavior treatment (0364T-0370T, 0373T-0374T)*

Crisis psychotherapy (90839-90840)

E&M services (99201-99337 [99224, 99225, 99226], 99341-99350, 99366-99368)

Code also interactive complexity services when applicable (90785)

90791	Psychiatric diagnostic evaluation

🔧 3.58   🔍 3.70   **FUD** XXX   ★ ⓪③ ▣

AMA: 2016,Jan,13; 2015,Jan,16; 2014,Jun,3; 2014,Jan,11; 2013,Dec,16; 2013,Jun,3-5; 2013,May,12

90792	Psychiatric diagnostic evaluation with medical services

🔧 3.97   🔍 4.09   **FUD** XXX   ★ ⓪③ ▣

AMA: 2016,Jan,13; 2015,Jan,16; 2014,Jun,3; 2014,Jan,11; 2013,Dec,16; 2013,Jun,3-5

90832-90838 Psychotherapy Services

CMS: 100-02,15,160 Clinical Psychologist Services; 100-02,15,170 Clinical Social Worker (CSW) Services; 100-03,130.1 Inpatient Stays for Alcoholism Treatment; 100-03,130.2 Outpatient Hospital Services for Alcoholism; 100-03,130.3 Chemical Aversion Therapy for Treatment of Alcoholism; 100-04,12* Medicare Telehealth Services; 100-04,12,100 Teaching Physician Services; 100-04,12,160 Clinical Psychologist Services; 100-04,12,190.7 Contractor Editing of Telehealth Claims

INCLUDES   Face-to-face time with patient (family, other informers may also be present)

Pharmacologic management in time allocated to psychotherapy service codes

Psychotherapy only (90832, 90834, 90837)

Psychotherapy with separately identifiable medical E&M services includes add-on codes (90833, 90836, 90838)

Service times of no less than 16 minutes

Services provided in all settings

Therapeutic communication to:

Ameliorate the patient's mental and behavioral symptoms

Modify behavior

Support and encourage personality growth and development

Treatment for:

Behavior disturbances

Mental illness

EXCLUDES   *Adaptive behavior treatment (0364T-0367T, 0373T-0374T)*

Crisis psychotherapy (90839-90840)

Family psychotherapy (90846-90847)

Code also interactive complexity services with the time the provider spends performing the service reflected in the time for the appropriate psychotherapy code (90785)

▲   **90832**   **Psychotherapy, 30 minutes with patient**

🔧 1.78   🔍 1.79   **FUD** XXX   ★ ⓪③ ▣

AMA: 2016,Jan,13; 2015,Oct,9; 2015,Jan,16; 2014,Aug,5; 2014,Feb,3; 2013,Aug,13; 2013,Jun,3-5; 2013,May,12; 2013,Jan,3-5

▲ +   **90833**   **Psychotherapy, 30 minutes with patient when performed with an evaluation and management service (List separately in addition to the code for primary procedure)**

Code first (99201-99255 [99224, 99225, 99226], 99304-99337, 99341-99350)

🔧 1.83   🔍 1.85   **FUD** ZZZ   ★ Ⓝ ▣

AMA: 2016,Jan,13; 2015,Oct,9; 2015,Jan,16; 2014,Aug,5; 2014,Feb,3; 2013,Aug,13; 2013,Jun,3-5; 2013,May,12; 2013,Jan,3-5

▲   **90834**   **Psychotherapy, 45 minutes with patient**

🔧 2.37   🔍 2.38   **FUD** XXX   ★ ⓪③ ▣

AMA: 2016,Jan,13; 2015,Oct,9; 2015,Jan,16; 2014,Jun,3; 2014,Feb,3; 2013,Aug,13; 2013,Jun,3-5; 2013,May,12; 2013,Jan,3-5

▲ +   **90836**   **Psychotherapy, 45 minutes with patient when performed with an evaluation and management service (List separately in addition to the code for primary procedure)**

Code first (99201-99255 [99224, 99225, 99226], 99304-99337, 99341-99350)

🔧 2.33   🔍 2.35   **FUD** ZZZ   ★ Ⓝ ▣

AMA: 2016,Jan,13; 2015,Oct,9; 2015,Jan,16; 2014,Feb,3; 2013,Aug,13; 2013,Jun,3-5; 2013,May,12; 2013,Jan,3-5

▲   **90837**   **Psychotherapy, 60 minutes with patient**

Code also prolonged service for psychotherapy performed without E&M service face-to-face with the patient lasting 90 minutes or longer (99354-99357)

🔧 3.55   🔍 3.58   **FUD** XXX   ★ ⓪③ ▣

AMA: 2016,Jan,13; 2015,Oct,9; 2015,Oct,3; 2015,Jan,16; 2014,Apr,6; 2014,Feb,3; 2013,Aug,13; 2013,Jun,3-5; 2013,May,12; 2013,Jan,3-5

▲ +   **90838**   **Psychotherapy, 60 minutes with patient when performed with an evaluation and management service (List separately in addition to the code for primary procedure)**

Code first (99201-99255 [99224, 99225, 99226], 99304-99337, 99341-99350)

🔧 3.08   🔍 3.10   **FUD** ZZZ   ★ Ⓝ ▣

AMA: 2016,Jan,13; 2015,Oct,9; 2015,Jan,16; 2014,Apr,6; 2014,Feb,3; 2013,Aug,13; 2013,Jun,3-5; 2013,May,12; 2013,Jan,3-5

26/TC PC/TC Only   A2-Z3 ASC Payment   50 Bilateral   ♂ Male Only   ♀ Female Only   🔧 Facility RVU   🔍 Non-Facility RVU   ▣ CCI

FUD Follow-up Days   CMS: IOM (Pub 100)   A-Y OPPSI   80/80 Surg Assist Allowed / w/Doc   🔲 Lab Crosswalk   🔲 Radiology Crosswalk   ❌ CLIA

414

CPT © 2016 American Medical Association. All Rights Reserved.   © 2016 Optum360, LLC

90839-90840 Services for Patients in Crisis

CMS: 100-02,15,170 Clinical Social Worker (CSW) Services; 100-03,130.1 Inpatient Stays for Alcoholism Treatment; 100-03,130.3 Chemical Aversion Therapy for Treatment of Alcoholism; 100-04,12,100 Teaching Physician Services; 100-04,12,160 Independent Psychologist Services; 100-04,12,160.1 Payment of Independent Psychologist Services; 100-04,12,170 Clinical Psychologist Services

INCLUDES 30 minutes or more of face-to-face time with the patient (for all or part of the service) and/or family providing crisis psychotherapy

All time spent exclusively with patient (for all or part of the service) and/or family, even if time is not continuous

Emergent care to a patient in severe distress (eg, life threatening or complex)

Institute interventions to minimize psychological trauma

Measures to ease the crisis and reestablish safety

Psychotherapy

EXCLUDES Adaptive behavior treatment (0364T-0367T, 0373T-0374T)

Other psychiatric services (90785-90899)

90839 **Psychotherapy for crisis; first 60 minutes**

INCLUDES First 30-74 minutes of crisis psychotherapy per day

EXCLUDES Use of code more than one time per day, even when service is not continuous on that date.

⚕ 3.71   ⚖ 3.73   **FUD** XXX   03 80 ▯

AMA: 2016,Jan,13; 2015,Oct,9; 2015,Jan,16; 2014,Aug,5; 2013,Jun,3-5

+ 90840 **each additional 30 minutes (List separately in addition to code for primary service)**

INCLUDES Up to 30 minutes of time beyond the initial 74 minutes

Code first (90839)

⚕ 1.77   ⚖ 1.78   **FUD** ZZZ   N 80 ▯

AMA: 2016,Jan,13; 2015,Oct,9; 2015,Jan,16; 2014,Aug,5; 2013,Jun,3-5

90845-90863 Additional Psychotherapy Services

CMS: 100-02,15,170 Clinical Social Worker (CSW) Services; 100-03,10.3 Inpatient Pain Rehabilitation Programs; 100-03,10.4 Outpatient Hospital Pain Rehabilitation Programs

EXCLUDES Adaptive behavior treatment (0364T-0367T, 0373T-0374T)

Analysis/programming of neurostimulators for vagus nerve stimulation therapy (95970, 95974-95975)

Crisis psychotherapy (90839-90840)

90845 **Psychoanalysis**

⚕ 2.56   ⚖ 2.57   **FUD** XXX   ★ 03 80 ▯

AMA: 2016,Jan,13; 2015,Oct,9; 2015,Jan,16; 2014,Jan,11; 2012,Jan,15-42; 2011,Jan,11

▲ 90846 **Family psychotherapy (without the patient present), 50 minutes**

EXCLUDES Adaptive behavior treatment (0368T-0371T)

Service times of less than 26 minutes

⚕ 2.87   ⚖ 2.89   **FUD** XXX   ★ 03 80 ▯

AMA: 2016,Jan,13; 2015,Oct,9; 2015,Jan,16; 2014,Jan,11; 2013,Dec,16; 2013,Jun,3-5

▲ 90847 **Family psychotherapy (conjoint psychotherapy) (with patient present), 50 minutes**

EXCLUDES Adaptive behavior treatment (0368T-0371T)

Service times of less than 26 minutes

⚕ 2.97   ⚖ 2.99   **FUD** XXX   ★ 03 80 ▯

AMA: 2016,Jan,13; 2015,Oct,9; 2015,Jan,16; 2014,Jan,11; 2013,Dec,16; 2013,Jun,3-5

90849 **Multiple-family group psychotherapy**

⚕ 0.86   ⚖ 0.96   **FUD** XXX   03 80 ▯

AMA: 2016,Jan,13; 2015,Oct,9; 2015,Jan,16; 2014,Aug,14; 2014,Jan,11

90853 **Group psychotherapy (other than of a multiple-family group)**

EXCLUDES Adaptive behavior social skills group (0372T)

Code also group psychotherapy with interactive complexity (90785)

⚕ 0.71   ⚖ 0.72   **FUD** XXX   03 80 ▯

AMA: 2016,Jan,13; 2015,Oct,9; 2015,Jan,16; 2014,Aug,14; 2014,Jun,3; 2014,Jan,11; 2013,Jun,3-5

+ 90863 **Pharmacologic management, including prescription and review of medication, when performed with psychotherapy services (List separately in addition to the code for primary procedure)**

INCLUDES Pharmacologic management in time allocated to psychotherapy service codes

Code first (90832, 90834, 90837)

⚕ 0.00   ⚖ 0.00   **FUD** XXX   ★ E ▯

AMA: 2016,Jan,13; 2015,Jan,16; 2013,Jun,3-5

90865-90870 Other Psychiatric Treatment

EXCLUDES Adaptive behavior treatment (0364T-0367T, 0373T-0374T)

Analysis/programming of neurostimulators for vagus nerve stimulation therapy (95970, 95974, 95975)

Crisis psychotherapy (90839-90840)

90865 **Narcosynthesis for psychiatric diagnostic and therapeutic purposes (eg, sodium amobarbital (Amytal) interview)**

⚕ 3.63   ⚖ 4.69   **FUD** XXX   03 80 ▯

AMA: 2016,Jan,13; 2015,Jan,16; 2014,Jan,11

90867 **Therapeutic repetitive transcranial magnetic stimulation (TMS) treatment; initial, including cortical mapping, motor threshold determination, delivery and management**

⚕ 0.00   ⚖ 0.00   **FUD** 000   S ▯

INCLUDES Evaluation E&M services related directly to:

Cortical mapping

Delivery and management of TMS services

Motor threshold determination

EXCLUDES Electromyography (95860, 95870)

Evoked potential studies (95928-95929)

Medication management

Significant, separately identifiable E&M service

Significant, separately identifiable psychotherapy service

Transcranial magnetic stimulation (TMS) motor function mapping for treatment planning, upper and lower extremity (0310T)

Transcranial magnetic stimulation (TMS), subsequent treatments (90868-90869)

Use of code more than one time for each course of treatment

90868 **subsequent delivery and management, per session**

⚕ 0.00   ⚖ 0.00   **FUD** 000   S ▯

INCLUDES E&M services related directly to:

Cortical mapping

Delivery and management of TMS services

Motor threshold determination

EXCLUDES Medication management

Significant, separately identifiable E&M service

Significant, separately identifiable psychotherapy service

Transcranial magnetic stimulation (TMS) motor function mapping for treatment planning, upper and lower extremity (0310T)

90869 **subsequent motor threshold re-determination with delivery and management**

⚕ 0.00   ⚖ 0.00   **FUD** 000   S ▯

INCLUDES E&M services related directly to:

Cortical mapping

Delivery and management of TMS services

Motor threshold determination

EXCLUDES Electromyography (95860, 95870)

Evoked potential studies (95928-95929)

Medication management

Significant, separately identifiable E&M service

Significant, separately identifiable psychotherapy service

Transcranial magnetic stimulation (TMS) motor function mapping for treatment planning, upper and lower extremity (0310T)

Transcranial magnetic stimulation (TMS), subsequent treatments (90868-90869)

● New Code   ▲ Revised Code   ○ Reinstated   ● New Web Release   ▲ Revised Web Release   Unlisted   Not Covered   # Resequenced

⊘ AMA Mod 51 Exempt   ⑤ Optum Mod 51 Exempt   ⓒ Mod 63 Exempt   ✀ Non-FDA Drug   ★ Telehealth   M Maternity   A Age Edit   + Add-on   AMA: CPT Asst

© 2016 Optum360, LLC   CPT © 2016 American Medical Association. All Rights Reserved.   **415**

90870 **Electroconvulsive therapy (includes necessary monitoring)**
🚑 3.12 ⚖ 5.00 **FUD** 000   [S] [80] [▭]
AMA: 2016,Jan,13; 2015,Jan,16; 2014,Jan,11

90875-90880 Psychiatric Therapy with Biofeedback or Hypnosis

CMS: 100-02,15,170 Clinical Social Worker (CSW) Services; 100-04,12,160 Independent Psychologist Services; 100-04,12,160.1 Payment of Independent Psychologist Services; 100-04,12,170 Clinical Psychologist Services

EXCLUDES *Adaptive behavior treatment (0364T-0367T, 0373T-0374T)*
Analysis/programming of neurostimulators for vagus nerve stimulation therapy (95970, 95974, 95975)
Crisis psychotherapy (90839-90840)

90875 **Individual psychophysiological therapy incorporating biofeedback training by any modality (face-to-face with the patient), with psychotherapy (eg, insight oriented, behavior modifying or supportive psychotherapy); 30 minutes**
🚑 1.73 ⚖ 1.73 **FUD** XXX   [E] [▭]
AMA: 2016,Jan,13; 2015,Jan,16; 2014,Jan,11; 2012,Jan,15-42; 2011,Jan,11

90876 **45 minutes**
🚑 2.74 ⚖ 3.04 **FUD** XXX   [E] [▭]
AMA: 2016,Jan,13; 2015,Jan,16; 2014,Jan,11

90880 **Hypnotherapy**
🚑 2.64 ⚖ 2.85 **FUD** XXX   [Q3] [80] [▭]
AMA: 2016,Jan,13; 2015,Jan,16; 2014,Jan,11

90882-90899 Psychiatric Services without Patient Face-to-Face Contact

CMS: 100-04,12,160 Independent Psychologist Services; 100-04,12,160.1 Payment of Independent Psychologist Services

EXCLUDES *Adaptive behavior treatment (0364T-0367T, 0373T-0374T)*
Analysis/programming of neurostimulators for vagus nerve stimulation therapy (95970, 95974, 95975)
Crisis psychotherapy (90839-90840)

90882 **Environmental intervention for medical management purposes on a psychiatric patient's behalf with agencies, employers, or institutions**
🚑 0.00 ⚖ 0.00 **FUD** XXX   [E] [▭]
AMA: 2016,Jan,13; 2015,Jan,16; 2014,Jan,11

90885 **Psychiatric evaluation of hospital records, other psychiatric reports, psychometric and/or projective tests, and other accumulated data for medical diagnostic purposes**
🚑 1.40 ⚖ 1.40 **FUD** XXX   [N] [▭]
AMA: 2016,Jan,13; 2015,Jan,16; 2014,Jan,11; 2012,Jan,15-42; 2011,Jan,11

90887 **Interpretation or explanation of results of psychiatric, other medical examinations and procedures, or other accumulated data to family or other responsible persons, or advising them how to assist patient**
EXCLUDES *Adaptive behavior treatment (0368T-0371T)*
🚑 2.14 ⚖ 2.49 **FUD** XXX   [N] [▭]
AMA: 2016,Jan,13; 2015,Jan,16; 2014,Jan,11; 2012,Jan,15-42; 2011,Jan,11

90889 **Preparation of report of patient's psychiatric status, history, treatment, or progress (other than for legal or consultative purposes) for other individuals, agencies, or insurance carriers**
🚑 0.00 ⚖ 0.00 **FUD** XXX   [N] [▭]
AMA: 2016,Jan,13; 2015,Jan,16; 2014,Jan,11

90899 **Unlisted psychiatric service or procedure**
🚑 0.00 ⚖ 0.00 **FUD** XXX   [Q3] [80]
AMA: 2016,Jan,13; 2015,Jan,16; 2014,Jan,11; 2012,Jan,15-42; 2011,Jan,11

90901-90911 Biofeedback Therapy

CMS: 100-05,5,40.7 Biofeedback Training for Urinary Incontinence

EXCLUDES *Psychophysiological therapy utilizing biofeedback training (90875-90876)*

90901 **Biofeedback training by any modality**
🚑 0.56 ⚖ 1.07 **FUD** 000   [A] [80] [▭]
AMA: 2016,Jan,13; 2015,Jan,16; 2014,Jan,11; 2012,Jan,15-42; 2011,Jan,11

90911 **Biofeedback training, perineal muscles, anorectal or urethral sphincter, including EMG and/or manometry**
EXCLUDES *Rectal sensation/tone/compliance testing (91120)*
Treatment for incontinence, pulsed magnetic neuromodulation (53899)
🚑 1.26 ⚖ 2.37 **FUD** 000   [S] [80] [▭]
AMA: 2016,Jan,13; 2015,Jan,16; 2014,Sep,13; 2014,Jan,11; 2012,Jan,15-42; 2011,Jan,11

90935-90940 Hemodialysis Services: Inpatient ESRD and Outpatient Non-ESRD

CMS: 100-02,11,20 Renal Dialysis Items and Services ; 100-04,3,100.6 Inpatient Renal Services

EXCLUDES *Attendance by physician or other qualified health care provider for a prolonged period of time (99354-99360 [99415, 99416])*
Blood specimen collection from partial/complete implantable venous access device (36591)
Declotting of cannula (36831, 36833, 36860-36861)
Hemodialysis home visit by non-physician health care professional (99512)
Thrombolytic agent declotting of implanted vascular access device/catheter (36593)
Code also significant separately identifiable E&M service not related to dialysis procedure or renal failure with modifier 25 (99201-99215, 99217-99223 [99224, 99225, 99226], 99231-99239, 99241-99245, 99281-99285, 99291-99292, 99304-99318, 99324-99337, 99341-99350, 99466-99467, 99468-99476, 99477-99480)

90935 **Hemodialysis procedure with single evaluation by a physician or other qualified health care professional**
INCLUDES All E&M services related to the patient's renal disease rendered on a day dialysis is performed
Inpatient ESRD and non-ESRD procedures
Only one evaluation of the patient related to hemodialysis procedure
Outpatient non-ESRD dialysis
🚑 2.05 ⚖ 2.05 **FUD** 000   [S] [80] [▭]
AMA: 2016,Jan,13; 2015,Jan,16; 2014,Jan,11

90937 **Hemodialysis procedure requiring repeated evaluation(s) with or without substantial revision of dialysis prescription**
INCLUDES All E&M services related to the patient's renal disease rendered on a day dialysis is performed
Inpatient ESRD and non-ESRD procedures
Outpatient non-ESRD dialysis
Re-evaluation of the patient during hemodialysis procedure
🚑 2.94 ⚖ 2.94 **FUD** 000   [B] [80] [▭]
AMA: 2016,Jan,13; 2015,Jan,16; 2014,Jan,11

90940 **Hemodialysis access flow study to determine blood flow in grafts and arteriovenous fistulae by an indicator method**
EXCLUDES *Hemodialysis access duplex scan (93990)*
🚑 0.00 ⚖ 0.00 **FUD** XXX   [N] [▭]
AMA: 2016,Jan,13; 2015,Jan,16; 2014,Jan,11; 2012,Jan,15-42; 2011,Jan,11

90945-90947 Dialysis Techniques Other Than Hemodialysis

CMS: 100-04,12,40.3 Global Surgery Review; 100-04,3,100.6 Inpatient Renal Services

INCLUDES All E&M services related to the patient's renal disease rendered on the day dialysis is performed
Procedures other than hemodialysis:
Continuous renal replacement therapies
Hemofiltration
Peritoneal dialysis
EXCLUDES *Attendance by physician or other qualified health care provider for a prolonged period of time (99354-99360 [99415, 99416])*
Hemodialysis
Tunneled intraperitoneal catheter insertion
Open (49421)
Percutaneous (49418)
Code also significant, separately identifiable E&M service not related to dialysis procedure or renal failure with modifier 25 (99201-99215, 99217-99220 [99224, 99225, 99226], 99231-99239, 99241-99245, 99281-99285, 99291-99292, 99304-99318, 99324-99337, 99341-99350, 99466-99480 [99485, 99486])

| [26]/[TC] PC/TC Only | [A2]-[Z3] ASC Payment | [50] Bilateral | ♂ Male Only | ♀ Female Only | 🚑 Facility RVU | ⚖ Non-Facility RVU | [▭] CCI |
| **FUD** Follow-up Days | **CMS:** IOM (Pub 100) | [A]-[Y] OPPSI | [80]/[80] Surg Assist Allowed / w/Doc | | [▥] Lab Crosswalk | [▤] Radiology Crosswalk | [X] CLIA |

CPT © 2016 American Medical Association. All Rights Reserved.
416
© 2016 Optum360, LLC

90945	Dialysis procedure other than hemodialysis (eg, peritoneal dialysis, hemofiltration, or other continuous renal replacement therapies), with single evaluation by a physician or other qualified health care professional

INCLUDES Only one evaluation of the patient related to the procedure

EXCLUDES *Peritoneal dialysis home infusion (99601, 99602)*

2.43   2.43   **FUD** 000   V 80

AMA: 2016,Jan,13; 2015,Jan,16; 2014,Jan,11; 2012,Jan,15-42; 2011,Jan,11

90947	Dialysis procedure other than hemodialysis (eg, peritoneal dialysis, hemofiltration, or other continuous renal replacement therapies) requiring repeated evaluations by a physician or other qualified health care professional, with or without substantial revision of dialysis prescription

EXCLUDES *Re-evaluation during a procedure*

3.51   3.51   **FUD** 000   B 80

AMA: 2016,Jan,13; 2015,Jan,16; 2014,Jan,11; 2012,Jan,15-42; 2011,Jan,11

90951-90962 End-stage Renal Disease Monthly Outpatient Services

CMS: 100-02,11,20 Renal Dialysis Items and Services ; 100-04,12,190.3.4 ESRD-Related Services as a Telehealth Service; 100-04,8,140.1 ESRD-Related Services Under the Monthly Capitation Payment

INCLUDES Establishing dialyzing cycle
Management of dialysis visits
Outpatient E&M of dialysis visits
Patient management during dialysis for a month
Telephone calls

EXCLUDES *Dialysis services provided during an inpatient hospitalization (90935-90937, 90945-90947)*
ESRD/non-ESRD dialysis services performed in an inpatient setting (90935-90937, 90945-90947)
Non-ESRD dialysis services performed in an outpatient setting (90935-90937, 90945-90947)
Non-ESRD related E&M services that cannot be performed during the dialysis session
Services provided during the time transitional care management services are being provided (99495-99496)
Services provided in the same month with chronic care management (99487-99489)

90951	End-stage renal disease (ESRD) related services monthly, for patients younger than 2 years of age to include monitoring for the adequacy of nutrition, assessment of growth and development, and counseling of parents; with 4 or more face-to-face visits by a physician or other qualified health care professional per month	A

26.6   26.6   **FUD** XXX   ★ M 80

AMA: 2016,Jan,13; 2015,Jan,16; 2014,Oct,3; 2014,Jan,11; 2013,Nov,3; 2013,Apr,3-4

90952	with 2-3 face-to-face visits by a physician or other qualified health care professional per month	A

0.00   0.00   **FUD** XXX   ★ M 80

AMA: 2016,Jan,13; 2015,Jan,16; 2014,Oct,3; 2014,Jan,11; 2013,Nov,3; 2013,Apr,3-4

90953	with 1 face-to-face visit by a physician or other qualified health care professional per month	A

0.00   0.00   **FUD** XXX   M 80

AMA: 2016,Jan,13; 2015,Jan,16; 2014,Oct,3; 2014,Jan,11; 2013,Nov,3; 2013,Apr,3-4

90954	End-stage renal disease (ESRD) related services monthly, for patients 2-11 years of age to include monitoring for the adequacy of nutrition, assessment of growth and development, and counseling of parents; with 4 or more face-to-face visits by a physician or other qualified health care professional per month	A

23.0   23.0   **FUD** XXX   ★ M 80

AMA: 2016,Jan,13; 2015,Jan,16; 2014,Oct,3; 2014,Jan,11; 2013,Nov,3; 2013,Apr,3-4

90955	with 2-3 face-to-face visits by a physician or other qualified health care professional per month	A

12.9   12.9   **FUD** XXX   ★ M 80

AMA: 2016,Jan,13; 2015,Jan,16; 2014,Oct,3; 2014,Jan,11; 2013,Nov,3; 2013,Apr,3-4

90956	with 1 face-to-face visit by a physician or other qualified health care professional per month	A

9.00   9.00   **FUD** XXX   M 80

AMA: 2016,Jan,13; 2015,Jan,16; 2014,Oct,3; 2014,Jan,11; 2013,Nov,3; 2013,Apr,3-4

90957	End-stage renal disease (ESRD) related services monthly, for patients 12-19 years of age to include monitoring for the adequacy of nutrition, assessment of growth and development, and counseling of parents; with 4 or more face-to-face visits by a physician or other qualified health care professional per month	A

18.2   18.2   **FUD** XXX   ★ M 80

AMA: 2016,Jan,13; 2015,Jan,16; 2014,Oct,3; 2014,Jan,11; 2013,Nov,3; 2013,Apr,3-4

90958	with 2-3 face-to-face visits by a physician or other qualified health care professional per month	A

12.3   12.3   **FUD** XXX   ★ M 80

AMA: 2016,Jan,13; 2015,Jan,16; 2014,Oct,3; 2014,Jan,11; 2013,Nov,3; 2013,Apr,3-4

90959	with 1 face-to-face visit by a physician or other qualified health care professional per month	A

8.37   8.37   **FUD** XXX   M 80

AMA: 2016,Jan,13; 2015,Jan,16; 2014,Oct,3; 2014,Jan,11; 2013,Nov,3; 2013,Apr,3-4

90960	End-stage renal disease (ESRD) related services monthly, for patients 20 years of age and older; with 4 or more face-to-face visits by a physician or other qualified health care professional per month	A

8.02   8.02   **FUD** XXX   ★ M 80

AMA: 2016,Jan,13; 2015,Jan,16; 2014,Oct,3; 2014,Jan,11; 2013,Nov,3; 2013,Apr,3-4

90961	with 2-3 face-to-face visits by a physician or other qualified health care professional per month	A

6.74   6.74   **FUD** XXX   ★ M 80

AMA: 2016,Jan,13; 2015,Jan,16; 2014,Oct,3; 2014,Jan,11; 2013,Nov,3; 2013,Apr,3-4

90962	with 1 face-to-face visit by a physician or other qualified health care professional per month	A

5.20   5.20   **FUD** XXX   M 80

AMA: 2016,Jan,13; 2015,Jan,16; 2014,Oct,3; 2014,Jan,11; 2013,Nov,3; 2013,Apr,3-4

90963-90966 End-stage Renal Disease Monthly Home Dialysis Services

CMS: 100-02,11,20 Renal Dialysis Items and Services ; 100-04,12,190.3.4 ESRD-Related Services as a Telehealth Service; 100-04,8,140.1 ESRD-Related Services Under the Monthly Capitation Payment; 100-04,8,140.1.1 Payment for Managing Patients on Home Dialysis

INCLUDES ESRD services for home dialysis patients
Services provided for a full month

EXCLUDES *Services provided during the time transitional care management services are being provided (99495-99496)*
Services provided in the same month with chronic care management (99487-99489)

90963	End-stage renal disease (ESRD) related services for home dialysis per full month, for patients younger than 2 years of age to include monitoring for the adequacy of nutrition, assessment of growth and development, and counseling of parents	A

15.3   15.3   **FUD** XXX   M 80

AMA: 2016,Jan,13; 2015,Jan,16; 2014,Oct,3; 2014,Jan,11; 2013,Nov,3; 2013,Apr,3-4

90964 End-stage renal disease (ESRD) related services for home dialysis per full month, for patients 2-11 years of age to include monitoring for the adequacy of nutrition, assessment of growth and development, and counseling of parents A

    📷 13.4   🔧 13.4   **FUD** XXX   M 80 🔲

    AMA: 2016,Jan,13; 2015,Jan,16; 2014,Oct,3; 2014,Jan,11; 2013,Nov,3; 2013,Apr,3-4

90965 End-stage renal disease (ESRD) related services for home dialysis per full month, for patients 12-19 years of age to include monitoring for the adequacy of nutrition, assessment of growth and development, and counseling of parents A

    📷 12.7   🔧 12.7   **FUD** XXX   M 80 🔲

    AMA: 2016,Jan,13; 2015,Jan,16; 2014,Oct,3; 2014,Jan,11; 2013,Nov,3; 2013,Apr,3-4

90966 End-stage renal disease (ESRD) related services for home dialysis per full month, for patients 20 years of age and older A

    📷 6.72   🔧 6.72   **FUD** XXX   M 80 🔲

    AMA: 2016,Jan,13; 2015,Jan,16; 2014,Oct,3; 2014,Jan,11; 2013,Nov,3; 2013,Apr,3-4

90967-90970 End-stage Renal Disease Services: Partial Month

CMS: 100-02,11,20 Renal Dialysis Items and Services

INCLUDES   ESRD services for less than a full month, such as:
    A patient who is transient, dies, recovers, or undergoes kidney transplant
    Outpatient ESRD-related services initiated prior to completion of assessment
    Patient spending part of the month as a hospital inpatient
    Services reported on a daily basis, less the days of hospitalization

EXCLUDES   *Services provided during the time transitional care management services are being provided (99495-99496)*
    Services provided in the same month with chronic care management (99487-99489)

90967 End-stage renal disease (ESRD) related services for dialysis less than a full month of service, per day; for patients younger than 2 years of age A

    📷 0.51   🔧 0.51   **FUD** XXX   M 80 🔲

    AMA: 2016,Jan,13; 2015,Jan,16; 2014,Oct,3; 2014,Jan,11; 2013,Nov,3; 2013,Apr,3-4

90968 for patients 2-11 years of age A

    📷 0.44   🔧 0.44   **FUD** XXX   M 80 🔲

    AMA: 2016,Jan,13; 2015,Jan,16; 2014,Oct,3; 2014,Jan,11; 2013,Nov,3; 2013,Apr,3-4

90969 for patients 12-19 years of age A

    📷 0.43   🔧 0.43   **FUD** XXX   M 80 🔲

    AMA: 2016,Jan,13; 2015,Jan,16; 2014,Oct,3; 2014,Jan,11; 2013,Nov,3; 2013,Apr,3-4

90970 for patients 20 years of age and older A

    📷 0.22   🔧 0.22   **FUD** XXX   M 80 🔲

    AMA: 2016,Jan,13; 2015,Jan,16; 2014,Oct,3; 2014,Jan,11; 2013,Nov,3; 2013,Apr,3-4

90989-90993 Dialysis Training Services

CMS: 100-04,3,100.6 Inpatient Renal Services

90989 Dialysis training, patient, including helper where applicable, any mode, completed course

    📷 0.00   🔧 0.00   **FUD** XXX   B 🔲

    AMA: 2016,Jan,13; 2015,Jan,16; 2014,Jan,11; 2012,Jan,15-42; 2011,Jan,11

90993 Dialysis training, patient, including helper where applicable, any mode, course not completed, per training session

    📷 0.00   🔧 0.00   **FUD** XXX   B 🔲

    AMA: 2016,Jan,13; 2015,Jan,16; 2014,Jan,11; 2012,Jan,15-42; 2011,Jan,11

90997-90999 Hemoperfusion and Unlisted Dialysis Procedures

CMS: 100-04,3,100.6 Inpatient Renal Services

90997 Hemoperfusion (eg, with activated charcoal or resin)

    📷 2.64   🔧 2.64   **FUD** 000   B 80 🔲

    AMA: 1999,Nov,1; 1997,Nov,1

90999 Unlisted dialysis procedure, inpatient or outpatient

    📷 0.00   🔧 0.00   **FUD** XXX   B 80

    AMA: 1999,Nov,1; 1997,Nov,1

91010-91022 Esophageal Manometry

91010 Esophageal motility (manometric study of the esophagus and/or gastroesophageal junction) study with interpretation and report;

    EXCLUDES   *Esophageal motility studies with high-resolution esophageal pressure topography (91299)*
    Code also for esophageal motility studies with stimulant or perfusion (91013)

    📷 4.97   🔧 4.97   **FUD** 000   S 80 🔲

    AMA: 2005,May,3-6; 1997,Nov,1

91013 with stimulation or perfusion (eg, stimulant, acid or alkali perfusion) (List separately in addition to code for primary procedure)

    📷 0.65   🔧 0.65   **FUD** ZZZ   N 80 🔲

    EXCLUDES   *Esophageal motility studies with high-resolution esophageal pressure topography (91299)*
    Use of code more than one time for each session
    Code first (91010)

91020 Gastric motility (manometric) studies

    EXCLUDES   *Gastrointestinal imaging by wireless capsule (91112)*

    📷 6.60   🔧 6.60   **FUD** 000   S 80 🔲

    AMA: 2016,Jan,13; 2015,Jan,16; 2013,Sep,13-14

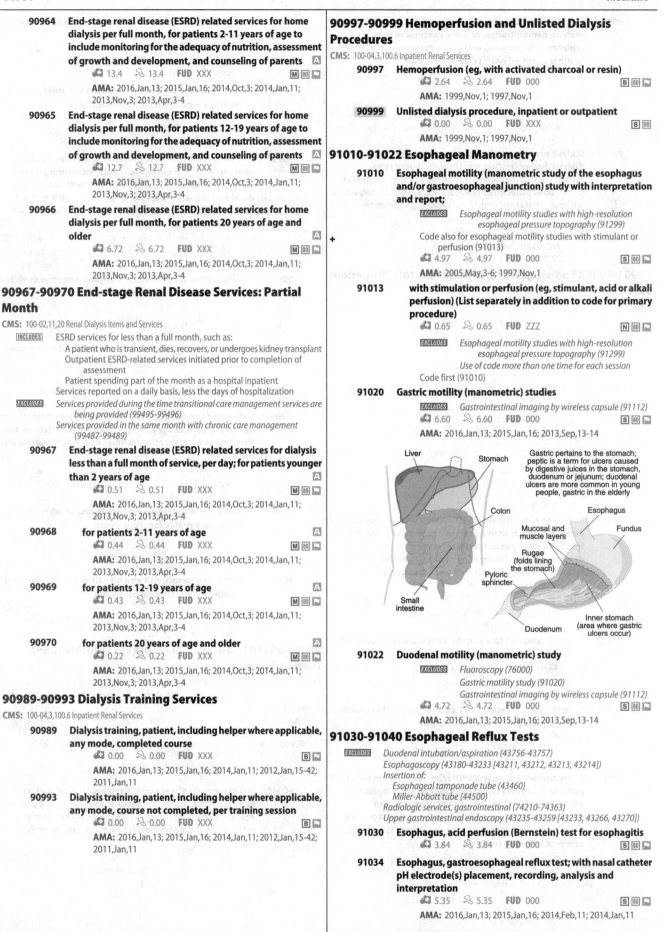

Gastric pertains to the stomach; peptic is a term for ulcers caused by digestive juices in the stomach, duodenum or jejunum; duodenal ulcers are more common in young people, gastric in the elderly

91022 Duodenal motility (manometric) study

    EXCLUDES   *Fluoroscopy (76000)*
    Gastric motility study (91020)
    Gastrointestinal imaging by wireless capsule (91112)

    📷 4.72   🔧 4.72   **FUD** 000   S 80 🔲

    AMA: 2016,Jan,13; 2015,Jan,16; 2013,Sep,13-14

91030-91040 Esophageal Reflux Tests

EXCLUDES   *Duodenal intubation/aspiration (43756-43757)*
    Esophagoscopy (43180-43233 [43211, 43212, 43213, 43214])
    Insertion of:
    Esophageal tamponade tube (43460)
    Miller-Abbott tube (44500)
    Radiologic services, gastrointestinal (74210-74363)
    Upper gastrointestinal endoscopy (43235-43259 [43233, 43266, 43270])

91030 Esophagus, acid perfusion (Bernstein) test for esophagitis

    📷 3.84   🔧 3.84   **FUD** 000   S 80 🔲

91034 Esophagus, gastroesophageal reflux test; with nasal catheter pH electrode(s) placement, recording, analysis and interpretation

    📷 5.35   🔧 5.35   **FUD** 000   S 80 🔲

    AMA: 2016,Jan,13; 2015,Jan,16; 2014,Feb,11; 2014,Jan,11

91035	with mucosal attached telemetry pH electrode placement, recording, analysis and interpretation	

INCLUDES Endoscopy only to place device

🔲 13.5   ⚖ 13.5   **FUD** 000   S 72 80 🖥

AMA: 2016,Jan,13; 2015,Jan,16; 2014,Feb,11; 2014,Jan,11

91037 Esophageal function test, gastroesophageal reflux test with nasal catheter intraluminal impedance electrode(s) placement, recording, analysis and interpretation;

🔲 4.52   ⚖ 4.52   **FUD** 000   S 80 🖥

AMA: 2005,May,3-6

91038 prolonged (greater than 1 hour, up to 24 hours)

🔲 12.6   ⚖ 12.6   **FUD** 000   S 80 🖥

AMA: 2016,Jan,13; 2015,Jan,16; 2014,Feb,11

91040 Esophageal balloon distension study, diagnostic, with provocation when performed

EXCLUDES Use of code more than one time for each session

🔲 12.2   ⚖ 12.2   **FUD** 000   S 80 🖥

AMA: 2005,May,3-6

91065 Breath Analysis

CMS: 100-03,100.5 Diagnostic Breath Analysis

EXCLUDES H. pylori breath test analysis, radioactive (C-14) or nonradioactive (C-13) (78268, 83013)

Code also each challenge administered

91065 Breath hydrogen or methane test (eg, for detection of lactase deficiency, fructose intolerance, bacterial overgrowth, or oro-cecal gastrointestinal transit)

🔲 2.20   ⚖ 2.20   **FUD** 000   S 80 🖥

AMA: 2016,Jan,13; 2015,Jan,16; 2014,Jan,11

91110-91299 Additional Gastrointestinal Diagnostic/Therapeutic Procedures

EXCLUDES Abdominal paracentesis (49082-49084)
Abdominal paracentesis with medication administration (96440, 96446)
Anoscopy (46600-46615)
Colonoscopy (45378-45393 [45388, 45390, 45398])
Duodenal intubation/aspiration (43756-43757)
Esophagoscopy (43180-43233 [43211, 43212, 43213, 43214])
Proctosigmoidoscopy (45300-45327)
Radiologic services, gastrointestinal (74210-74363)
Sigmoidoscopy (45330-45350 [45346])
Small intestine/stomal endoscopy (44360-44408 [44381, 44401])
Upper gastrointestinal endoscopy (43235-43259 [43233, 43266, 43270])

91110 Gastrointestinal tract imaging, intraluminal (eg, capsule endoscopy), esophagus through ileum, with interpretation and report

Code also modifier 52 if ileum is not visualized

EXCLUDES Imaging of colon (0355T)
Imaging of esophagus through ileum (91111)

🔲 24.8   ⚖ 24.8   **FUD** XXX   T 80 🖥

AMA: 2016,Jan,13; 2015,Jan,16; 2014,Jan,11; 2013,Sep,13-14; 2012,Jan,15-42; 2011,Jan,11

91111 Gastrointestinal tract imaging, intraluminal (eg, capsule endoscopy), esophagus with interpretation and report

EXCLUDES Imaging of colon (0355T)
Imaging of esophagus through ileum (91111)
Use of wireless capsule to measure transit times or pressure in gastrointestinal tract (91112)

🔲 20.4   ⚖ 20.4   **FUD** XXX   T 80 🖥

AMA: 2016,Jan,13; 2015,Jan,16; 2013,Sep,13-14

91112 Gastrointestinal transit and pressure measurement, stomach through colon, wireless capsule, with interpretation and report

EXCLUDES Duodenal motility study (91022)
Gastric motility studies (91020)
pH of body fluid (83986)

🔲 30.4   ⚖ 30.4   **FUD** XXX   T 80 🖥

AMA: 2016,Jan,13; 2015,Jan,16; 2013,Sep,13-14

91117 Colon motility (manometric) study, minimum 6 hours continuous recording (including provocation tests, eg, meal, intracolonic balloon distension, pharmacologic agents, if performed), with interpretation and report

EXCLUDES Anal manometry (91122)
Rectal sensation, tone and compliance testing (91120)
Use of code more than one time regardless of the number of provocations
Use of wireless capsule to measure transit times or pressure in gastrointestinal tract (91112)

🔲 3.93   ⚖ 3.93   **FUD** 000   T 80 🖥

AMA: 2016,Jan,13; 2015,Jan,16; 2013,Sep,13-14

91120 Rectal sensation, tone, and compliance test (ie, response to graded balloon distention)

EXCLUDES Anorectal manometry (91122)
Biofeedback training (90911)
Colon motility study (91117)

🔲 11.9   ⚖ 11.9   **FUD** XXX   S 80 🖥

AMA: 2016,Jan,13; 2015,Jan,16; 2014,Jan,11; 2013,Sep,13-14

91122 Anorectal manometry

EXCLUDES Colon motility study (91117)

🔲 6.41   ⚖ 6.41   **FUD** 000   T 80 🖥

AMA: 2013,Sep,13-14

91132 Electrogastrography, diagnostic, transcutaneous;

🔲 4.36   ⚖ 4.36   **FUD** XXX   S 80 🖥

91133 with provocative testing

🔲 4.85   ⚖ 4.85   **FUD** XXX   Q1 80 🖥

91200 Liver elastography, mechanically induced shear wave (eg, vibration), without imaging, with interpretation and report

🔲 0.89   ⚖ 0.89   **FUD** XXX   S NI 80 🖥

AMA: 2014,Dec,13

91299 Unlisted diagnostic gastroenterology procedure

🔲 0.00   ⚖ 0.00   **FUD** XXX   S 80

AMA: 2016,Jan,13; 2015,Jan,16; 2014,Jan,11

92002-92014 Ophthalmic Medical Services

CMS: 100-02,15,30.4 Optometrist's Services

INCLUDES Routine ophthalmoscopy
Services provided to established patients who have received professional services from the physician or other qualified health care provider or another physician or other qualified health care professional within the same group practice of the exact same specialty and subspecialty within the past three years
Services provided to new patients who have received no professional services from the physician or other qualified health care provider or another physician or other qualified health care professional within the same group practice of the exact same specialty and subspecialty within the past three years

EXCLUDES Surgical procedures on the eye/ocular adnexa (65091-68899 [67810])
Visual screening tests (99173-99174 [99177])

92002 Ophthalmological services: medical examination and evaluation with initiation of diagnostic and treatment program; intermediate, new patient

INCLUDES Evaluation of new/existing condition complicated by new diagnostic or management problem
Integrated services where medical decision making cannot be separated from examination methods
Other diagnostic procedures
Biomicroscopy
Mydriasis
Ophthalmoscopy
Tonometry
Problems not related to primary diagnosis
The following for intermediate services:
External ocular/adnexal examination
General medical observation
History

🔲 1.35   ⚖ 2.28   **FUD** XXX   V 80 🖥

AMA: 2016,Jan,13; 2015,Jan,16; 2014,Jan,11; 2012,Oct,9-11; 2012,Aug,9; 2012,Jan,15-42; 2011,Feb,6-7; 2011,Jan,11

92004 **comprehensive, new patient, 1 or more visits**

INCLUDES General evaluation of complete visual system
Integrated services where medical decision making cannot be separated from examination methods
Single service that need not be performed at one session
The following for comprehensive services:
Basic sensorimotor examination
Biomicroscopy
Dilation (cycloplegia)
External examinations
General medical observation
Gross visual fields
History
Initiation of diagnostic/treatment programs
Mydriasis
Ophthalmoscopic examinations
Other diagnostic procedures
Prescription of medication
Special diagnostic/treatment services
Tonometry
🏥 2.82   ⚕ 4.18   **FUD** XXX   V 80 💬

AMA: 2016,Jan,13; 2015,Jan,16; 2014,Jan,11; 2012,Aug,9; 2012,Jan,15-42; 2011,Feb,6-7; 2011,Jan,9-10; 2011,Jan,11

92012 **Ophthalmological services: medical examination and evaluation, with initiation or continuation of diagnostic and treatment program; intermediate, established patient**

INCLUDES Evaluation of new/existing condition complicated by new diagnostic or management problem
Integrated services where medical decision making cannot be separated from examination methods
Problems not related to primary diagnosis
The following for intermediate services:
External ocular/adnexal examination
General medical observation
History
Other diagnostic procedures:
Biomicroscopy
Mydriasis
Ophthalmoscopy
Tonometry
🏥 1.49   ⚕ 2.40   **FUD** XXX   V 80 💬

AMA: 2016,Jan,13; 2015,Jan,16; 2014,Jan,11; 2012,Aug,9; 2011,Feb,6-7

92014 **comprehensive, established patient, 1 or more visits**

INCLUDES General evaluation of complete visual system
Integrated services where medical decision making cannot be separated from examination methods
Single service that need not be performed at one session
The following for comprehensive services:
Basic sensorimotor examination
Biomicroscopy
Dilation (cycloplegia)
External examinations
General medical observation
Gross visual fields
History
Initiation of diagnostic/treatment programs
Mydriasis
Ophthalmoscopic examinations
Other diagnostic procedures
Prescription of medication
Special diagnostic/treatment services
Tonometry
🏥 2.26   ⚕ 3.48   **FUD** XXX   V 80 💬

AMA: 2016,Jan,13; 2015,Jan,16; 2014,Jan,11; 2012,Oct,9-11; 2012,Aug,9; 2012,Jan,15-42; 2011,Feb,6-7; 2011,Jan,9-10; 2011,Jan,11

92015-92145 Ophthalmic Special Services

INCLUDES Routine ophthalmoscopy
EXCLUDES *Ocular screening that is instrument-based (99174 [99177])*
Surgical procedures on the eye/ocular adnexa (65091-68899 [67810])
Code also E&M services, when performed
Code also general ophthalmological services, when performed (92002-92014)

92015 **Determination of refractive state**

INCLUDES Lens prescription
Absorptive factor
Axis
Impact resistance
Lens power
Prism
Specification of lens type:
Bifocal
Monofocal
EXCLUDES *Bilateral instrument based ocular screening (99174 [99177])*
Visual screening tests (99173-99174 [99177])
🏥 0.55   ⚕ 0.56   **FUD** XXX   E 💬

AMA: 2016,Mar,10; 2016,Jan,13; 2015,Jan,16; 2014,Jan,11; 2013,Mar,6-7; 2012,Jan,15-42; 2011,Jan,11

92018 **Ophthalmological examination and evaluation, under general anesthesia, with or without manipulation of globe for passive range of motion or other manipulation to facilitate diagnostic examination; complete**

🏥 4.11   ⚕ 4.11   **FUD** XXX   T 80 💬

AMA: 2016,Jan,13; 2015,Jan,16; 2014,Jan,11

92019 **limited**

🏥 2.03   ⚕ 2.03   **FUD** XXX   T 80 💬

AMA: 2016,Jan,13; 2015,Jan,16; 2014,Jan,11

92020 **Gonioscopy (separate procedure)**

EXCLUDES *Gonioscopy under general anesthesia (92018)*
🏥 0.59   ⚕ 0.75   **FUD** XXX   01 80 💬

AMA: 2016,Jan,13; 2015,Jan,16; 2014,Jan,11

92025 **Computerized corneal topography, unilateral or bilateral, with interpretation and report**

EXCLUDES *Corneal transplant procedures (65710-65771)*
Manual keratoscopy
🏥 1.07   ⚕ 1.07   **FUD** XXX   01 80 💬

AMA: 2016,Jan,13; 2015,Jan,16; 2014,Jan,11; 2012,Oct,9-11; 2012,Jan,15-42; 2011,Jan,11

92060 **Sensorimotor examination with multiple measurements of ocular deviation (eg, restrictive or paretic muscle with diplopia) with interpretation and report (separate procedure)**

🏥 1.83   ⚕ 1.83   **FUD** XXX   01 80 💬

AMA: 2016,Jan,13; 2015,Jan,16; 2014,Jan,11

92065 **Orthoptic and/or pleoptic training, with continuing medical direction and evaluation**

🏥 1.50   ⚕ 1.50   **FUD** XXX   01 80 💬

AMA: 2016,Jan,13; 2015,Jan,16; 2014,Jan,11; 2012,Jan,15-42; 2011,Jan,11

92071 **Fitting of contact lens for treatment of ocular surface disease**

EXCLUDES *Contact lens service for keratoconus (92072)*
Code also supply of lens with appropriate supply code or (99070)
🏥 0.95   ⚕ 1.07   **FUD** XXX   N N1 80 50 💬

AMA: 2012,Aug,9

92072 **Fitting of contact lens for management of keratoconus, initial fitting**

EXCLUDES *Contact lens service for disease of ocular surface (92071)*
Subsequent fittings (99211-99215, 92012-92014)
Code also supply of lens with appropriate supply code or (99070)
🏥 2.92   ⚕ 3.81   **FUD** XXX   N N1 80 💬

AMA: 2016,Jan,13; 2015,Jan,16; 2014,Jan,11; 2012,Aug,9

92081 Visual field examination, unilateral or bilateral, with interpretation and report; limited examination (eg, tangent screen, Autoplot, arc perimeter, or single stimulus level automated test, such as Octopus 3 or 7 equivalent)

INCLUDES Gross visual testing/confrontation testing

⏣ 0.95 ⚖ 0.95 **FUD** XXX 01 80 ▢

AMA: 2016,Jan,13; 2015,Jan,16; 2014,Jan,11; 2012,Oct,9-11; 2012,Jan,15-42; 2011,Jan,11

92082 intermediate examination (eg, at least 2 isopters on Goldmann perimeter, or semiquantitative, automated suprathreshold screening program, Humphrey suprathreshold automatic diagnostic test, Octopus program 33)

INCLUDES Gross visual testing/confrontation testing

⏣ 1.35 ⚖ 1.35 **FUD** XXX 01 80 ▢

AMA: 2016,Jan,13; 2015,Jan,16; 2014,Jan,11; 2012,Oct,9-11

92083 extended examination (eg, Goldmann visual fields with at least 3 isopters plotted and static determination within the central 30°, or quantitative, automated threshold perimetry, Octopus program G-1, 32 or 42, Humphrey visual field analyzer full threshold programs 30-2, 24-2, or 30/60-2)

INCLUDES Gross visual field testing/confrontation testing

EXCLUDES Assessment of visual field by transmission of data by patient to a surveillance center (0378T-0379T)

⏣ 1.81 ⚖ 1.81 **FUD** XXX 01 80 ▢

AMA: 2016,Jan,13; 2015,Jan,16; 2014,Jan,11; 2012,Oct,9-11

92100 Serial tonometry (separate procedure) with multiple measurements of intraocular pressure over an extended time period with interpretation and report, same day (eg, diurnal curve or medical treatment of acute elevation of intraocular pressure)

EXCLUDES Intraocular pressure monitoring for 24 hours or more (0329T)
Ocular blood flow measurements (0198T)
Single-episode tonometry (99201-99215, 92002-92004)

⏣ 0.96 ⚖ 2.25 **FUD** XXX N 80 ▢

AMA: 2016,Jan,13; 2015,Jan,16; 2014,May,5; 2014,Jan,11; 2012,Oct,9-11; 2012,Aug,9; 2012,Jan,15-42; 2011,Jan,11

92132 Scanning computerized ophthalmic diagnostic imaging, anterior segment, with interpretation and report, unilateral or bilateral

EXCLUDES Imaging of anterior segment with specular microscopy and endothelial cell analysis (92286)
Scanning computerized ophthalmic diagnostic imaging of optic nerve and retina (92133-92134)
Tear film imaging (0330T)

⏣ 0.98 ⚖ 0.98 **FUD** XXX 01 80 ▢

AMA: 2016,Jan,13; 2015,Jan,16; 2014,May,5; 2014,Jan,11; 2013,Apr,7; 2013,Mar,6-7; 2012,Oct,9-11; 2011,Feb,6-7

92133 Scanning computerized ophthalmic diagnostic imaging, posterior segment, with interpretation and report, unilateral or bilateral; optic nerve

EXCLUDES Remote imaging for retinal disease (92227-92228)
Scanning computerized ophthalmic imaging of retina at same visit (92134)

⏣ 1.24 ⚖ 1.24 **FUD** XXX 01 80 ▢

AMA: 2016,Jan,13; 2015,Jan,16; 2014,Nov,10; 2014,Jan,11; 2012,Oct,9-11; 2011,Feb,6-7

92134 retina

EXCLUDES Remote imaging for retinal disease (92227-92228)
Scanning computerized ophthalmic imaging of optic nerve at same visit (92133)

⏣ 1.27 ⚖ 1.27 **FUD** XXX 01 80 ▢

AMA: 2016,Jan,13; 2015,Jan,16; 2014,Nov,10; 2014,Jan,11; 2012,Oct,9-11; 2011,Feb,6-7

92136 Ophthalmic biometry by partial coherence interferometry with intraocular lens power calculation

EXCLUDES Tear film imaging (0330T)

⏣ 2.54 ⚖ 2.54 **FUD** XXX 01 80 ▢

AMA: 2016,Jan,13; 2015,Jan,16; 2014,May,5; 2014,Jan,11; 2012,Jan,15-42; 2011,Jan,11

~~92140~~ ~~Provocative tests for glaucoma, with interpretation and report, without tonography~~

92145 Corneal hysteresis determination, by air impulse stimulation, unilateral or bilateral, with interpretation and report

⏣ 0.43 ⚖ 0.43 **FUD** XXX 01 80 ▢

92225-92287 Other Ophthalmology Services

EXCLUDES Prescription, fitting, and/or medical supervision of ocular prosthesis adaptation by physician (99201-99215, 99241-99245, 92002-92014)

92225 Ophthalmoscopy, extended, with retinal drawing (eg, for retinal detachment, melanoma), with interpretation and report; initial

EXCLUDES Ophthalmoscopy under general anesthesia (92018)

⏣ 0.60 ⚖ 0.76 **FUD** XXX 01 80 ▢

AMA: 2016,Jan,13; 2015,Jan,16; 2014,Jan,11; 2012,Oct,9-11; 2012,Jan,15-42; 2011,Feb,6-7; 2011,Jan,11

92226 subsequent

⏣ 0.54 ⚖ 0.70 **FUD** XXX 01 80 ▢

AMA: 2016,Jan,13; 2015,Jan,16; 2014,Jan,11; 2011,Feb,6-7

92227 Remote imaging for detection of retinal disease (eg, retinopathy in a patient with diabetes) with analysis and report under physician supervision, unilateral or bilateral

EXCLUDES When services provided with E&M services as part of a single organ system or (92002-92014, 92133-92134, 92228, 92250)

⏣ 0.41 ⚖ 0.41 **FUD** XXX ★ 01 80 TC ▢

AMA: 2016,Jul,8; 2016,Jan,13; 2015,Jan,16; 2014,Jan,11; 2012,Oct,9-11; 2012,Jan,15-42; 2011,May,9; 2011,Feb,6-7

92228 Remote imaging for monitoring and management of active retinal disease (eg, diabetic retinopathy) with physician review, interpretation and report, unilateral or bilateral

EXCLUDES When services provided with E&M services as part of a single organ system or (92002-92014, 92133-92134, 92227, 92250)

⏣ 0.97 ⚖ 0.97 **FUD** XXX ★ 01 80 ▢

AMA: 2016,Jan,13; 2015,Jan,16; 2014,Jan,11; 2012,Oct,9-11; 2012,Jan,15-42; 2011,May,9; 2011,Feb,6-7

92230 Fluorescein angioscopy with interpretation and report

⏣ 0.95 ⚖ 1.64 **FUD** XXX 01 80 ▢

AMA: 2016,Jan,13; 2015,Jan,16; 2014,Jan,11; 2011,Feb,6-7

▲ **92235** Fluorescein angiography (includes multiframe imaging) with interpretation and report, unilateral or bilateral

EXCLUDES Fluorescein and indocyanine-green angiography (92242)

⏣ 3.09 ⚖ 3.09 **FUD** XXX S 80 ▢

AMA: 2016,Jan,13; 2015,Jan,16; 2014,Jan,11; 2011,Feb,6-7

▲ **92240** Indocyanine-green angiography (includes multiframe imaging) with interpretation and report, unilateral or bilateral

EXCLUDES Fluorescein and indocyanine-green angiography (92242)

⏣ 7.19 ⚖ 7.19 **FUD** XXX S 80 ▢

AMA: 2016,Jan,13; 2015,Jan,16; 2014,Jan,11; 2012,Oct,9-11; 2011,Feb,6-7

● **92242** Fluorescein angiography and indocyanine-green angiography (includes multiframe imaging) performed at the same patient encounter with interpretation and report, unilateral or bilateral

EXCLUDES Fluorescein angiography only (92235)
Indocyanine-green angiography only (92240)

● New Code ▲ Revised Code ○ Reinstated ● New Web Release ▲ Revised Web Release Unlisted Not Covered # Resequenced
⊘ AMA Mod 51 Exempt ⑤ Optum Mod 51 Exempt ⑥ Mod 63 Exempt ✗ Non-FDA Drug ★ Telehealth Ⓜ Maternity Ⓐ Age Edit + Add-on **AMA:** CPT Asst

Medicine

92250 — **92355**

92250 **Fundus photography with interpretation and report**
🗗 2.22 ⚖ 2.22 **FUD** XXX 01 80 🖵
AMA: 2016,Jul,8; 2016,Jan,13; 2015,May,9; 2015,Jan,16; 2014,Dec,16; 2014,Dec,16; 2014,Nov,10; 2014,Jan,11; 2012,Oct,9-11; 2011,Feb,6-7

92260 **Ophthalmodynamometry**
EXCLUDES *Ophthalmoscopy under general anesthesia (92018)*
🗗 0.31 ⚖ 0.52 **FUD** XXX 01 80 🖵
AMA: 2016,Jan,13; 2015,Jan,16; 2014,Jan,11; 2011,Feb,6-7

92265 **Needle oculoelectromyography, 1 or more extraocular muscles, 1 or both eyes, with interpretation and report**
🗗 2.23 ⚖ 2.23 **FUD** XXX 01 80 🖵
AMA: 2016,Jan,13; 2015,Jan,16; 2014,Jan,11; 2012,Oct,9-11

92270 **Electro-oculography with interpretation and report**
EXCLUDES *Recording of saccadic eye movements (92700)*
Vestibular function testing (92537-92538, 92540-92542, 92544-92548)
🗗 2.58 ⚖ 2.58 **FUD** XXX 01 80 🖵
AMA: 2016,Jan,13; 2015,Sep,7; 2015,Jan,16; 2014,Jan,11; 2012,Oct,9-11; 2012,Jan,15-42; 2011,Jan,11

92275 **Electroretinography with interpretation and report**
EXCLUDES *Vestibular function tests/electronystagmography (92541-92548)*
☢ (76511-76529)
🗗 4.18 ⚖ 4.18 **FUD** XXX S 80 🖵
AMA: 2016,Jan,13; 2015,Jan,16; 2014,Jan,11; 2012,Oct,9-11

92283 **Color vision examination, extended, eg, anomaloscope or equivalent**
EXCLUDES *Color vision testing with pseudoisochromatic plates (e.g., HRR, Ishihara) (92002-92004, 92012-92014, 99172)*
🗗 1.56 ⚖ 1.56 **FUD** XXX 01 80 🖵
AMA: 2016,Jan,13; 2015,Jan,16; 2014,Jan,11; 2012,Oct,9-11

92284 **Dark adaptation examination with interpretation and report**
🗗 1.73 ⚖ 1.73 **FUD** XXX 01 80 🖵
AMA: 2016,Jan,13; 2015,Jan,16; 2014,Jan,11; 2012,Oct,9-11

92285 **External ocular photography with interpretation and report for documentation of medical progress (eg, close-up photography, slit lamp photography, goniophotography, stereo-photography)**
EXCLUDES *Tear film imaging (0330T)*
🗗 0.58 ⚖ 0.58 **FUD** XXX 01 80 🖵
AMA: 2016,Jan,13; 2015,Jan,16; 2014,May,5; 2014,Jan,11; 2012,Oct,9-11; 2012,Jan,15-42; 2011,Jan,11

92286 **Anterior segment imaging with interpretation and report; with specular microscopy and endothelial cell analysis**
🗗 1.08 ⚖ 1.08 **FUD** XXX 01 80 🖵
AMA: 2016,Jan,13; 2015,Jan,16; 2014,Jan,11; 2013,Mar,6-7; 2012,Oct,9-11

92287 **with fluorescein angiography**
🗗 3.88 ⚖ 3.88 **FUD** XXX 01 80 🖵
AMA: 2016,Jan,13; 2015,Jan,16; 2014,Jan,11; 2013,Mar,6-7

92310-92326 Services Related to Contact Lenses

CMS: 100-02,15,30.4 Optometrist's Services
INCLUDES Incidental revision of lens during training period
Patient training/instruction
Specification of optical/physical characteristics:
  Curvature
  Flexibility
  Gas-permeability
  Power
  Size
EXCLUDES *Extended wear lenses follow up (92012-92014)*
General ophthalmological services
Therapeutic/surgical use of contact lens (68340, 92071-92072)

92310 **Prescription of optical and physical characteristics of and fitting of contact lens, with medical supervision of adaptation; corneal lens, both eyes, except for aphakia**
Code also modifier 52 for one eye
🗗 1.69 ⚖ 2.70 **FUD** XXX E 🖵
AMA: 2016,Jan,13; 2015,Jan,16; 2014,Jan,11; 2012,Oct,9-11

92311 **corneal lens for aphakia, 1 eye**
🗗 1.58 ⚖ 2.85 **FUD** XXX 01 80 🖵
AMA: 2016,Jan,13; 2015,Jan,16; 2014,Jan,11; 2012,Oct,9-11

92312 **corneal lens for aphakia, both eyes**
🗗 1.80 ⚖ 3.28 **FUD** XXX 01 80 🖵
AMA: 2016,Jan,13; 2015,Jan,16; 2014,Jan,11; 2012,Oct,9-11

92313 **corneoscleral lens**
🗗 1.34 ⚖ 2.73 **FUD** XXX 01 80 🖵
AMA: 2016,Jan,13; 2015,Jan,16; 2014,Jan,11; 2012,Oct,9-11

92314 **Prescription of optical and physical characteristics of contact lens, with medical supervision of adaptation and direction of fitting by independent technician; corneal lens, both eyes except for aphakia**
Code also modifier 52 for one eye
🗗 0.99 ⚖ 2.24 **FUD** XXX E 🖵
AMA: 2016,Jan,13; 2015,Jan,16; 2014,Jan,11; 2012,Oct,9-11

92315 **corneal lens for aphakia, 1 eye**
🗗 0.62 ⚖ 2.05 **FUD** XXX 01 80 🖵
AMA: 2016,Jan,13; 2015,Jan,16; 2014,Jan,11; 2012,Oct,9-11

92316 **corneal lens for aphakia, both eyes**
🗗 0.93 ⚖ 2.58 **FUD** XXX 01 80 🖵
AMA: 2016,Jan,13; 2015,Jan,16; 2014,Jan,11; 2012,Oct,9-11

92317 **corneoscleral lens**
🗗 0.63 ⚖ 2.14 **FUD** XXX 01 80 🖵
AMA: 2016,Jan,13; 2015,Jan,16; 2014,Jan,11

92325 **Modification of contact lens (separate procedure), with medical supervision of adaptation**
🗗 1.18 ⚖ 1.18 **FUD** XXX 01 80 🖵
AMA: 2016,Jan,13; 2015,Jan,16; 2014,Jan,11; 2012,Oct,9-11

92326 **Replacement of contact lens**
🗗 0.99 ⚖ 0.99 **FUD** XXX 01 80 🖵
AMA: 2016,Jan,13; 2015,Jan,16; 2014,Jan,11

92340-92499 Services Related to Eyeglasses

CMS: 100-02,15,30.4 Optometrist's Services
INCLUDES Anatomical facial characteristics measurement
Final adjustment of spectacles to visual axes/anatomical topography
Written laboratory specifications
EXCLUDES *Supply of materials*

92340 **Fitting of spectacles, except for aphakia; monofocal**
🗗 0.53 ⚖ 1.00 **FUD** XXX E 🖵
AMA: 2016,Jan,13; 2015,Jan,16; 2014,Jan,11; 2013,Mar,6-7

92341 **bifocal**
🗗 0.68 ⚖ 1.14 **FUD** XXX E 🖵
AMA: 2016,Jan,13; 2015,Jan,16; 2014,Jan,11; 2013,Mar,6-7

92342 **multifocal, other than bifocal**
🗗 0.76 ⚖ 1.23 **FUD** XXX E 🖵
AMA: 2016,Jan,13; 2015,Jan,16; 2014,Jan,11; 2013,Mar,6-7

92352 **Fitting of spectacle prosthesis for aphakia; monofocal**
🗗 0.53 ⚖ 1.14 **FUD** XXX 01 🖵
AMA: 2016,Jan,13; 2015,Jan,16; 2014,Jan,11; 2013,Mar,6-7

92353 **multifocal**
🗗 0.72 ⚖ 1.33 **FUD** XXX 01 🖵
AMA: 2016,Jan,13; 2015,Jan,16; 2014,Jan,11; 2013,Mar,6-7

92354 **Fitting of spectacle mounted low vision aid; single element system**
🗗 0.38 ⚖ 0.38 **FUD** XXX 01 🖵
AMA: 2016,Jan,13; 2015,Jan,16; 2014,Jan,11; 2013,Mar,6-7

92355 **telescopic or other compound lens system**
🗗 0.59 ⚖ 0.59 **FUD** XXX 01 🖵
AMA: 2016,Jan,13; 2015,Jan,16; 2014,Jan,11; 2013,Mar,6-7

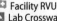

92358 **Prosthesis service for aphakia, temporary (disposable or loan, including materials)**
🚑 0.32 ⚕ 0.32 **FUD** XXX [01] 📺
AMA: 2016,Jan,13; 2015,Jan,16; 2014,Jan,11; 2013,Mar,6-7

92370 **Repair and refitting spectacles; except for aphakia**
🚑 0.46 ⚕ 0.87 **FUD** XXX [E] 📺
AMA: 2016,Jan,13; 2015,Jan,16; 2014,Jan,11; 2013,Mar,6-7

92371 **spectacle prosthesis for aphakia**
🚑 0.33 ⚕ 0.33 **FUD** XXX [01] 📺
AMA: 2016,Jan,13; 2015,Jan,16; 2014,Jan,11; 2013,Mar,6-7

92499 **Unlisted ophthalmological service or procedure**
🚑 0.00 ⚕ 0.00 **FUD** XXX [01] [80]
AMA: 2016,Jan,13; 2015,Jan,16; 2014,Jan,11

92502-92526 Special Procedures of the Ears/Nose/Throat

INCLUDES Anterior rhinoscopy, tuning fork testing, otoscopy, or removal non-impacted cerumen
Diagnostic/treatment services not generally included in an E&M service
EXCLUDES *Laryngoscopy with stroboscopy (31579)*

92502 **Otolaryngologic examination under general anesthesia**
🚑 2.77 ⚕ 2.77 **FUD** 000 [T] [80] 📺
AMA: 2016,Sep,6

92504 **Binocular microscopy (separate diagnostic procedure)**
🚑 0.27 ⚕ 0.85 **FUD** XXX [N] [80] 📺
AMA: 2016,Sep,6; 2016,Jan,13; 2015,Jan,16; 2014,Jan,11; 2013,Oct,14; 2012,Jan,15-42; 2011,Oct,10; 2011,Jan,11

92507 **Treatment of speech, language, voice, communication, and/or auditory processing disorder; individual**
EXCLUDES *Adaptive behavior treatment (0364T-0365T, 0368T-0369T)*
Auditory rehabilitation:
Postlingual hearing loss (92633)
Prelingual hearing loss (92630)
Programming of cochlear implant (92601-92604)
🚑 2.23 ⚕ 2.23 **FUD** XXX [A] [80] 📺
AMA: 2016,Sep,6; 2016,Jan,13; 2015,Jan,16; 2014,Jan,11; 2013,Oct,7

92508 **group, 2 or more individuals**
EXCLUDES *Adaptive behavior treatment (0366T-0367T, 0372T)*
Auditory rehabilitation:
Postlingual hearing loss (92633)
Prelingual hearing loss (92630)
Programming of cochlear implant (92601-92604)
🚑 0.66 ⚕ 0.66 **FUD** XXX [A] [80] 📺
AMA: 2016,Sep,6; 2016,Jan,13; 2015,Jan,16; 2014,Jun,3; 2014,Jan,11; 2013,Oct,7

92511 **Nasopharyngoscopy with endoscope (separate procedure)**
EXCLUDES *Diagnostic flexible laryngoscopy (31575)*
Transnasal esophagoscopy (43197-43198)
🚑 1.12 ⚕ 3.18 **FUD** 000 [T] [80] 📺
AMA: 2016,Sep,6

92512 **Nasal function studies (eg, rhinomanometry)**
🚑 0.82 ⚕ 1.72 **FUD** XXX [S] [80] 📺
AMA: 2016,Sep,6

92516 **Facial nerve function studies (eg, electroneuronography)**
🚑 0.66 ⚕ 1.99 **FUD** XXX [S] [80] 📺
AMA: 2016,Sep,6

92520 **Laryngeal function studies (ie, aerodynamic testing and acoustic testing)**
EXCLUDES *Other laryngeal function testing (92700)*
Swallowing/laryngeal sensory testing with flexible fiberoptic endoscope (92611-92617)
Code also modifier 52 for single test
🚑 1.18 ⚕ 2.14 **FUD** XXX [01] [80] 📺
AMA: 2016,Sep,6; 2016,Jan,13; 2015,Jan,16; 2014,Jan,11

92521 **Evaluation of speech fluency (eg, stuttering, cluttering)**
INCLUDES Ability to execute motor movements needed for speech
Comprehension of written and verbal expression
Determination of patient's ability to create and communicate expressive thought
Evaluation of the ability to produce speech sound
🚑 3.13 ⚕ 3.13 **FUD** XXX [A] [80] 📺
AMA: 2016,Sep,6; 2016,Jan,13; 2015,Jan,16; 2014,Jun,3

92522 **Evaluation of speech sound production (eg, articulation, phonological process, apraxia, dysarthria);**
INCLUDES Ability to execute motor movements needed for speech
Comprehension of written and verbal expression
Determination of patient's ability to create and communicate expressive thought
Evaluation of the ability to produce speech sound
🚑 2.61 ⚕ 2.61 **FUD** XXX [A] [80] 📺
AMA: 2016,Sep,6; 2016,Jan,13; 2015,Jan,16; 2014,Jun,3

92523 **with evaluation of language comprehension and expression (eg, receptive and expressive language)**
INCLUDES Ability to execute motor movements needed for speech
Comprehension of written and verbal expression
Determination of patient's ability to create and communicate expressive thought
Evaluation of the ability to produce speech sound
🚑 5.47 ⚕ 5.47 **FUD** XXX [A] [80] 📺
AMA: 2016,Sep,6; 2016,Jan,13; 2015,Jan,16; 2014,Jun,3

92524 **Behavioral and qualitative analysis of voice and resonance**
INCLUDES Ability to execute motor movements needed for speech
Comprehension of written and verbal expression
Determination of patient's ability to create and communicate expressive thought
Evaluation of the ability to produce speech sound
🚑 2.53 ⚕ 2.53 **FUD** XXX [A] [80] 📺
AMA: 2016,Sep,6; 2016,Jan,13; 2015,Jan,16; 2014,Jun,3

92526 **Treatment of swallowing dysfunction and/or oral function for feeding**
🚑 2.43 ⚕ 2.43 **FUD** XXX [A] [80] 📺
AMA: 2016,Sep,6

92531-92548 Vestibular Function Tests

92531 **Spontaneous nystagmus, including gaze**
EXCLUDES *When performed with E&M services (99201-99215, 99218-99223 [99224, 99225, 99226], 99231-99236, 99241-99245, 99304-99318, 99324-99337)*
🚑 0.00 ⚕ 0.00 **FUD** XXX [N] 📺
AMA: 1997,Nov,1

92532 **Positional nystagmus test**
EXCLUDES *When performed with E&M services (99201-99215, 99218-99223 [99224, 99225, 99226], 99231-99236, 99241-99245, 99304-99318, 99324-99337)*
🚑 0.00 ⚕ 0.00 **FUD** XXX [N] 📺
AMA: 2002,May,7; 1997,Nov,1

92533 **Caloric vestibular test, each irrigation (binaural, bithermal stimulation constitutes 4 tests)**
INCLUDES Barany caloric test
🚑 0.00 ⚕ 0.00 **FUD** XXX [N] 📺
AMA: 2016,Jan,13; 2015,Jan,16; 2014,Jan,11

92534 **Optokinetic nystagmus test**
🚑 0.00 ⚕ 0.00 **FUD** XXX [N] 📺
AMA: 2002,May,7; 1997,Nov,1

92537 Caloric vestibular test with recording, bilateral; bithermal (ie, one warm and one cool irrigation in each ear for a total of four irrigations)

> EXCLUDES *Electro-oculography (92270)*
> *Monothermal caloric vestibular test (92538)*
> Code also modifier 52 when only three irrigations are performed
> 🚗 1.14   ⚕ 1.14   **FUD** XXX   S 80 🖵

AMA: 2015,Sep,7

92538 monothermal (ie, one irrigation in each ear for a total of two irrigations)

> EXCLUDES *Electro-oculography (92270)*
> *Monothermal caloric vestibular test (92538)*
> Code also modifier 52 if only one irrigation is performed
> 🚗 0.58   ⚕ 0.58   **FUD** XXX   S 80 🖵

AMA: 2015,Sep,7

92540 Basic vestibular evaluation, includes spontaneous nystagmus test with eccentric gaze fixation nystagmus, with recording, positional nystagmus test, minimum of 4 positions, with recording, optokinetic nystagmus test, bidirectional foveal and peripheral stimulation, with recording, and oscillating tracking test, with recording

> EXCLUDES *Vestibular function tests (92270, 92541-92542, 92544-92545)*
> 🚗 2.87   ⚕ 2.87   **FUD** XXX   S 80 🖵

AMA: 2016,Jan,13; 2015,Sep,7

92541 Spontaneous nystagmus test, including gaze and fixation nystagmus, with recording

> EXCLUDES *Vestibular function tests (92270, 92540, 92542, 92544-92545)*
> 🚗 0.68   ⚕ 0.68   **FUD** XXX   01 80 🖵

AMA: 2016,Jan,13; 2015,Sep,7; 2015,Jan,16; 2014,Jan,11; 2012,Jan,15-42; 2011,May,9

92542 Positional nystagmus test, minimum of 4 positions, with recording

> EXCLUDES *Vestibular function tests (92270, 92540-92541, 92544-92545)*
> 🚗 0.79   ⚕ 0.79   **FUD** XXX   01 80 🖵

AMA: 2016,Jan,13; 2015,Sep,7; 2015,Jan,16; 2014,Jan,11; 2012,Jan,15-42; 2011,Jan,11

92544 Optokinetic nystagmus test, bidirectional, foveal or peripheral stimulation, with recording

> EXCLUDES *Vestibular function tests (92270, 92540-92542, 92545)*
> 🚗 0.47   ⚕ 0.47   **FUD** XXX   S 80 🖵

AMA: 2016,Jan,13; 2015,Sep,7; 2015,Jan,16; 2014,Jan,11

92545 Oscillating tracking test, with recording

> EXCLUDES *Vestibular function tests (92270, 92540-92542, 92544)*
> 🚗 0.43   ⚕ 0.43   **FUD** XXX   S 80 🖵

AMA: 2016,Jan,13; 2015,Sep,7; 2015,Jan,16; 2014,Jan,11; 2012,Jan,15-42; 2011,May,9

92546 Sinusoidal vertical axis rotational testing

> EXCLUDES *Electro-oculography (92270)*
> 🚗 2.91   ⚕ 2.91   **FUD** XXX   S 80 🖵

AMA: 2016,Jan,13; 2015,Sep,7; 2015,Jan,16; 2014,Jan,11; 2013,Jun,13; 2012,Jan,15-42; 2011,May,9; 2011,Jan,11

+ **92547** Use of vertical electrodes (List separately in addition to code for primary procedure)

> EXCLUDES *Electro-oculography (92700)*
> Code first (92540-92546)
> 🚗 0.17   ⚕ 0.17   **FUD** ZZZ   N 80 TC 🖵

AMA: 2016,Jan,13; 2015,Sep,7; 2015,Jan,16; 2014,Jan,11; 2012,Jan,15-42; 2011,Jan,11

92548 Computerized dynamic posturography

> EXCLUDES *Electro-oculography (92270)*
> 🚗 2.89   ⚕ 2.89   **FUD** XXX   01 80 🖵

AMA: 2016,Jan,13; 2015,Sep,7; 2015,Jan,16; 2014,Jan,11; 2012,Jan,15-42; 2011,May,9

92550-92597 [92558] Hearing and Speech Tests

INCLUDES Diagnostic/treatment services not generally included in a comprehensive otorhinolaryngologic evaluation or office visit
Testing of both ears
Tuning fork and whisper tests
Use of calibrated electronic equipment, recording of results, and a report with interpretation

EXCLUDES *Evaluation of speech/language/hearing problems using observation/assessment of performance (92521-92524)*

Code also modifier 52 for unilateral testing

92550 Tympanometry and reflex threshold measurements

> INCLUDES Tympanometry, acoustic reflex testing individual codes (92567-92568)
> 🚗 0.60   ⚕ 0.60   **FUD** XXX   01 80 🖵

AMA: 2016,Jan,13; 2015,Jan,16; 2014,Aug,3

92551 Screening test, pure tone, air only

> 🚗 0.34   ⚕ 0.34   **FUD** XXX   E 🖵

AMA: 2016,Jan,13; 2015,Jan,16; 2014,Aug,3

92552 Pure tone audiometry (threshold); air only

> EXCLUDES *Automated test (0208T)*
> 🚗 0.88   ⚕ 0.88   **FUD** XXX   01 80 TC 🖵

AMA: 2016,Jan,13; 2015,Jan,16; 2014,Aug,3

92553 air and bone

> EXCLUDES *Automated test (0209T)*
> 🚗 1.05   ⚕ 1.05   **FUD** XXX   01 80 TC 🖵

AMA: 2016,Jan,13; 2015,Jan,16; 2014,Aug,3; 2014,Jan,11; 2011,Mar,8

92555 Speech audiometry threshold;

> EXCLUDES *Automated test (0210T)*
> 🚗 0.66   ⚕ 0.66   **FUD** XXX   01 80 TC 🖵

AMA: 2016,Jan,13; 2015,Jan,16; 2014,Aug,3

92556 with speech recognition

> EXCLUDES *Automated test (0211T)*
> 🚗 1.05   ⚕ 1.05   **FUD** XXX   01 80 TC 🖵

AMA: 2016,Jan,13; 2015,Jan,16; 2014,Aug,3; 2014,Jan,11; 2011,Mar,8

92557 Comprehensive audiometry threshold evaluation and speech recognition (92553 and 92556 combined)

> EXCLUDES *Automated test (0208T-0212T)*
> *Evaluation/selection of hearing aid (92590-92595)*
> 🚗 0.93   ⚕ 1.06   **FUD** XXX   01 80 🖵

AMA: 2016,Jan,13; 2015,Jan,16; 2014,Aug,3; 2014,Jan,11; 2011,Mar,8

92558 Resequenced code. See code following 92586.

92559 Audiometric testing of groups

> INCLUDES For group testing, indicate tests performed
> 🚗 0.00   ⚕ 0.00   **FUD** XXX   E 🖵

AMA: 2016,Jan,13; 2015,Jan,16; 2014,Aug,3

92560 Bekesy audiometry; screening

> 🚗 0.00   ⚕ 0.00   **FUD** XXX   E 🖵

AMA: 2016,Jan,13; 2015,Jan,16; 2014,Aug,3

92561 diagnostic

> 🚗 1.07   ⚕ 1.07   **FUD** XXX   01 80 TC 🖵

AMA: 2016,Jan,13; 2015,Jan,16; 2014,Aug,3

92562 Loudness balance test, alternate binaural or monaural

> INCLUDES ABLB test
> 🚗 1.31   ⚕ 1.31   **FUD** XXX   01 80 TC 🖵

AMA: 2016,Jan,13; 2015,Jan,16; 2014,Aug,3

92563 Tone decay test

> 🚗 0.87   ⚕ 0.87   **FUD** XXX   01 80 TC 🖵

AMA: 2016,Jan,13; 2015,Jan,16; 2014,Aug,3

92564 Short increment sensitivity index (SISI)

> 🚗 0.79   ⚕ 0.79   **FUD** XXX   01 80 TC 🖵

AMA: 2016,Jan,13; 2015,Jan,16; 2014,Aug,3; 2014,Jan,11

92565 Stenger test, pure tone

> 🚗 0.45   ⚕ 0.45   **FUD** XXX   01 80 TC 🖵

AMA: 2016,Jan,13; 2015,Jan,16; 2014,Aug,3

26/TC	PC/TC Only	A2-Z3	ASC Payment	50	Bilateral	♂	Male Only	♀	Female Only	🚗	Facility RVU	⚕	Non-Facility RVU	🖵	CCI
FUD	Follow-up Days	**CMS:**	IOM (Pub 100)	A-Y	OPPSI	80/80	Surg Assist Allowed / w/Doc			📦	Lab Crosswalk	📦	Radiology Crosswalk	✖	CLIA

424

CPT © 2016 American Medical Association. All Rights Reserved.

© 2016 Optum360, LLC

92567 **Tympanometry (impedance testing)**
  🎥 0.31   ◇ 0.41   **FUD** XXX   01 80 ▣
  AMA: 2016,Jan,13; 2015,Jan,16; 2014,Aug,3; 2014,Jan,11

92568 **Acoustic reflex testing, threshold**
  🎥 0.44   ◇ 0.45   **FUD** XXX   01 80 ▣
  AMA: 2016,Jan,13; 2015,Jan,16; 2014,Aug,3; 2014,Jan,11;
  2012,Jan,15-42; 2011,Jan,11

92570 **Acoustic immittance testing, includes tympanometry (impedance testing), acoustic reflex threshold testing, and acoustic reflex decay testing**
  INCLUDES   Tympanometry, acoustic reflex testing individual codes (92567-92568)
  🎥 0.85   ◇ 0.91   **FUD** XXX   01 80 ▣
  AMA: 2016,Jan,13; 2015,Jan,16; 2014,Aug,3

92571 **Filtered speech test**
  🎥 0.77   ◇ 0.77   **FUD** XXX   01 80 TC ▣
  AMA: 2016,Jan,13; 2015,Jan,16; 2014,Aug,3; 2014,Jan,11

92572 **Staggered spondaic word test**
  🎥 1.01   ◇ 1.01   **FUD** XXX   01 80 TC ▣
  AMA: 2016,Jan,13; 2015,Jan,16; 2014,Aug,3; 2014,Jan,11

92575 **Sensorineural acuity level test**
  🎥 2.04   ◇ 2.04   **FUD** XXX   01 80 TC ▣
  AMA: 2016,Jan,13; 2015,Jan,16; 2014,Aug,3

92576 **Synthetic sentence identification test**
  🎥 1.01   ◇ 1.01   **FUD** XXX   01 80 TC ▣
  AMA: 2016,Jan,13; 2015,Jan,16; 2014,Aug,3; 2014,Jan,11

92577 **Stenger test, speech**
  🎥 0.47   ◇ 0.47   **FUD** XXX   01 80 TC ▣
  AMA: 2016,Jan,13; 2015,Jan,16; 2014,Aug,3

92579 **Visual reinforcement audiometry (VRA)**
  🎥 1.06   ◇ 1.19   **FUD** XXX   01 80 ▣
  AMA: 2016,Jan,13; 2015,Jan,16; 2014,Aug,3

92582 **Conditioning play audiometry**
  🎥 1.91   ◇ 1.91   **FUD** XXX   01 80 TC ▣
  AMA: 2016,Jan,13; 2015,Jan,16; 2014,Aug,3

92583 **Select picture audiometry**
  🎥 1.48   ◇ 1.48   **FUD** XXX   01 80 TC ▣
  AMA: 2016,Jan,13; 2015,Jan,16; 2014,Aug,3

92584 **Electrocochleography**
  🎥 2.07   ◇ 2.07   **FUD** XXX   S 80 TC ▣
  AMA: 2016,Jan,13; 2015,Jan,16; 2014,Aug,3; 2014,Jan,11;
  2012,Jan,15-42; 2011,Jul,16-17

92585 **Auditory evoked potentials for evoked response audiometry and/or testing of the central nervous system; comprehensive**
  🎥 3.83   ◇ 3.83   **FUD** XXX   S 80 ▣
  AMA: 2016,Jan,13; 2015,Jan,16; 2014,Aug,3; 2013,May,8-10

92586 **limited**
  🎥 2.41   ◇ 2.41   **FUD** XXX   S 80 TC ▣
  AMA: 2016,Jan,13; 2015,Jan,16; 2014,Aug,3

\# **92558** **Evoked otoacoustic emissions, screening (qualitative measurement of distortion product or transient evoked otoacoustic emissions), automated analysis**
  🎥 0.00   ◇ 0.00   **FUD** XXX   E ▣
  AMA: 2016,Jan,13; 2015,Jan,16; 2014,Aug,3

92587 **Distortion product evoked otoacoustic emissions; limited evaluation (to confirm the presence or absence of hearing disorder, 3-6 frequencies) or transient evoked otoacoustic emissions, with interpretation and report**
  🎥 0.61   ◇ 0.61   **FUD** XXX   S 80 ▣
  AMA: 2016,Jan,13; 2015,Jan,16; 2014,Aug,3; 2014,Jan,11

92588 **comprehensive diagnostic evaluation (quantitative analysis of outer hair cell function by cochlear mapping, minimum of 12 frequencies), with interpretation and report**
  EXCLUDES   Evaluation of central auditory function (92620-92621)
  🎥 0.93   ◇ 0.93   **FUD** XXX   S 80 ▣
  AMA: 2016,Jan,13; 2015,Jan,16; 2014,Aug,3

92590 **Hearing aid examination and selection; monaural**
  🎥 0.00   ◇ 0.00   **FUD** XXX   E ▣
  AMA: 2016,Jan,13; 2015,Jan,16; 2014,Aug,3; 2014,Jul,4

92591 **binaural**
  🎥 0.00   ◇ 0.00   **FUD** XXX   E ▣
  AMA: 2016,Jan,13; 2015,Jan,16; 2014,Aug,3

92592 **Hearing aid check; monaural**
  🎥 0.00   ◇ 0.00   **FUD** XXX   E ▣
  AMA: 2016,Jan,13; 2015,Jan,16; 2014,Aug,3

92593 **binaural**
  🎥 0.00   ◇ 0.00   **FUD** XXX   E ▣
  AMA: 2016,Jan,13; 2015,Jan,16; 2014,Aug,3

92594 **Electroacoustic evaluation for hearing aid; monaural**
  🎥 0.00   ◇ 0.00   **FUD** XXX   E ▣
  AMA: 2016,Jan,13; 2015,Jan,16; 2014,Aug,3

92595 **binaural**
  🎥 0.00   ◇ 0.00   **FUD** XXX   E ▣
  AMA: 2016,Jan,13; 2015,Jan,16; 2014,Aug,3

92596 **Ear protector attenuation measurements**
  🎥 1.19   ◇ 1.19   **FUD** XXX   01 80 TC ▣
  AMA: 2016,Jan,13; 2015,Jan,16; 2014,Aug,3

92597 **Resequenced code. See code following 92604.**

92601-92609 [92597, 92618] Services Related to Hearing and Speech Devices

INCLUDES   Diagnostic/treatment services not generally included in a comprehensive otorhinolaryngologic evaluation or office visit

92601 **Diagnostic analysis of cochlear implant, patient younger than 7 years of age; with programming**   A
  INCLUDES   Connection to cochlear implant
          Postoperative analysis/fitting of previously placed external devices
          Stimulator programming
  EXCLUDES   Cochlear implant placement (69930)
  🎥 3.40   ◇ 4.00   **FUD** XXX   S 80 ▣
  AMA: 2016,Sep,6; 2016,Jan,13; 2015,Jan,16; 2014,Jul,4;
  2014,Jan,11; 2013,Oct,7; 2012,Jan,15-42; 2011,Jul,16-17

92602 **subsequent reprogramming**   A
  INCLUDES   Internal stimulator re-programming
          Subsequent sessions for external transmitter measurements/adjustment
  EXCLUDES   Analysis with programming (92601)
          Aural rehabilitation services after a cochlear implant (92626-92627, 92630-92633)
          Cochlear implant placement (69930)
  🎥 1.96   ◇ 2.53   **FUD** XXX   S 80 ▣
  AMA: 2016,Sep,6; 2016,Jan,13; 2015,Jan,16; 2014,Jul,4;
  2014,Jan,11; 2013,Oct,7; 2012,Jan,15-42; 2011,Jan,11

92603 **Diagnostic analysis of cochlear implant, age 7 years or older; with programming**   A
  INCLUDES   Connection to cochlear implant
          Post-operative analysis/fitting of previously placed external devices
          Stimulator programming
  EXCLUDES   Cochlear implant placement (69930)
  🎥 3.47   ◇ 4.28   **FUD** XXX   S 80 ▣
  AMA: 2016,Sep,6; 2016,Jan,13; 2015,Jan,16; 2014,Jul,4;
  2014,Jan,11; 2013,Oct,7; 2012,Jan,15-42; 2011,Jul,16-17

92604 **subsequent reprogramming** Ⓐ

INCLUDES Internal stimulator re-programming
Subsequent sessions for external transmitter measurements/adjustment

EXCLUDES Analysis with programming (92603)
Cochlear implant placement (69930)

🚑 1.92 ⚕ 2.53 **FUD** XXX Ⓢ 80 ▢

AMA: 2016,Sep,6; 2016,Jan,13; 2015,Jan,16; 2014,Jul,4; 2014,Jan,11; 2013,Oct,7; 2012,Jan,15-42; 2011,Jul,16-17; 2011,Jan,11

 # 92597 **Evaluation for use and/or fitting of voice prosthetic device to supplement oral speech**

EXCLUDES Augmentative or alternative communication device services (92605, [92618], 92607-92608)

🚑 2.04 ⚕ 2.04 **FUD** XXX Ⓐ 80 ▢

AMA: 2016,Jan,13; 2015,Jan,16; 2014,Jan,11

92605 **Evaluation for prescription of non-speech-generating augmentative and alternative communication device, face-to-face with the patient; first hour**

EXCLUDES Prosthetic voice device fitting or use evaluation (92597)

🚑 2.52 ⚕ 2.63 **FUD** XXX Ⓐ ▢

AMA: 2016,Jan,13; 2015,Jan,16; 2014,Jan,11; 2013,Oct,7

+ # 92618 **each additional 30 minutes (List separately in addition to code for primary procedure)**

🚑 0.94 ⚕ 0.96 **FUD** ZZZ Ⓐ ▢

Code first (92605)

92606 **Therapeutic service(s) for the use of non-speech-generating device, including programming and modification**

🚑 2.02 ⚕ 2.35 **FUD** XXX Ⓐ ▢

AMA: 2016,Jan,13; 2015,Jan,16; 2014,Jan,11

92607 **Evaluation for prescription for speech-generating augmentative and alternative communication device, face-to-face with the patient; first hour**

EXCLUDES Evaluation for prescription of non-speech generating device (92605)
Evaluation for use/fitting of voice prosthetic (92597)

🚑 3.57 ⚕ 3.57 **FUD** XXX Ⓐ 80 ▢

AMA: 2016,Jan,13; 2015,Jan,16; 2014,Jan,11; 2013,Oct,7

+ 92608 **each additional 30 minutes (List separately in addition to code for primary procedure)**

Code first initial hour (92607)

🚑 1.49 ⚕ 1.49 **FUD** ZZZ Ⓐ 80 ▢

AMA: 2016,Jan,13; 2015,Jan,16; 2014,Jan,11; 2013,Oct,7

92609 **Therapeutic services for the use of speech-generating device, including programming and modification**

EXCLUDES Therapeutic services for use of non-speech generating device (92606)

🚑 3.12 ⚕ 3.12 **FUD** XXX Ⓐ 80 ▢

AMA: 2016,Jan,13; 2015,Jan,16; 2014,Jan,11

92610-92618 Swallowing Evaluations

92610 **Evaluation of oral and pharyngeal swallowing function**

EXCLUDES Evaluation with flexible endoscope (92612-92617)
Motion fluoroscopic evaluation of swallowing function (92611)

🚑 2.06 ⚕ 2.41 **FUD** XXX Ⓐ 80 ▢

AMA: 2016,Jan,13; 2015,Jan,16; 2014,Jan,11

92611 **Motion fluoroscopic evaluation of swallowing function by cine or video recording**

EXCLUDES Diagnostic flexible laryngoscopy (31575)
Evaluation of oral/pharyngeal swallowing function (92610)

📷 (74230)

🚑 2.46 ⚕ 2.46 **FUD** XXX Ⓐ 80 ▢

AMA: 2016,Sep,6; 2016,Jan,13; 2015,Jan,16; 2014,Jul,5; 2014,Jan,11

▲ 92612 **Flexible endoscopic evaluation of swallowing by cine or video recording;**

EXCLUDES Diagnostic flexible fiberoptic laryngoscopy (31575)
Flexible endoscopic examination/testing without cine or video recording (92700)

🚑 1.94 ⚕ 5.27 **FUD** XXX Ⓐ 80 ▢

AMA: 2016,Sep,6; 2016,Jan,13; 2015,Jan,16; 2014,Jan,11; 2012,Jan,15-42; 2011,Jan,11

▲ 92613 **interpretation and report only**

EXCLUDES Diagnostic flexible laryngoscopy (31575)
Oral/pharyngeal swallowing function examination (92610)
Swallowing function motion fluoroscopic examination (92611)

🚑 1.09 ⚕ 1.09 **FUD** XXX Ⓑ 80 ▢

AMA: 2016,Sep,6; 2016,Jan,13; 2015,Jan,16; 2014,Jan,11

▲ 92614 **Flexible endoscopic evaluation, laryngeal sensory testing by cine or video recording;**

EXCLUDES Diagnostic flexible laryngoscopy (31575)
Flexible endoscopic examination/testing without cine or video recording (92700)

🚑 1.93 ⚕ 4.13 **FUD** XXX Ⓐ 80 ▢

AMA: 2016,Sep,6; 2016,Jan,13; 2015,Jan,16; 2014,Jan,11

▲ 92615 **interpretation and report only**

EXCLUDES Diagnostic flexible laryngoscopy (31575)

🚑 0.95 ⚕ 0.96 **FUD** XXX Ⓔ 80 ▢

AMA: 2016,Sep,6; 2016,Jan,13; 2015,Jan,16; 2014,Jan,11

▲ 92616 **Flexible endoscopic evaluation of swallowing and laryngeal sensory testing by cine or video recording;**

EXCLUDES Diagnostic flexible fiberoptic laryngoscopy (31575)
Flexible endoscopic examination/testing without cine or video recording (92700)

🚑 2.88 ⚕ 5.90 **FUD** XXX Ⓐ 80 ▢

AMA: 2016,Sep,6; 2016,Jan,13; 2015,Jan,16; 2014,Jan,11

▲ 92617 **interpretation and report only**

EXCLUDES Diagnostic flexible laryngoscopy (31575)

🚑 1.19 ⚕ 1.19 **FUD** XXX Ⓔ 80 ▢

AMA: 2016,Sep,6; 2016,Jan,13; 2015,Jan,16; 2014,Jan,11

92618 **Resequenced code. See code following 92605.**

92620-92700 Diagnostic Hearing Evaluations and Rehabilitation

INCLUDES Diagnostic/treatment services not generally included in a comprehensive otorhinolaryngologic evaluation or office visit

92620 **Evaluation of central auditory function, with report; initial 60 minutes**

EXCLUDES Voice analysis (92521-92524)

🚑 2.34 ⚕ 2.66 **FUD** XXX Ⓠ1 80 ▢

AMA: 2016,Jan,13; 2015,Jan,16; 2014,Aug,3

+ 92621 **each additional 15 minutes (List separately in addition to code for primary procedure)**

EXCLUDES Voice analysis (92521-92524)

Code first (92620)

🚑 0.54 ⚕ 0.63 **FUD** ZZZ Ⓝ 80 ▢

AMA: 2016,Jan,13; 2015,Jan,16; 2014,Aug,3

92625 **Assessment of tinnitus (includes pitch, loudness matching, and masking)**

EXCLUDES Loudness test (92562)

Code also modifier 52 for unilateral procedure

🚑 1.77 ⚕ 1.98 **FUD** XXX Ⓠ1 80 ▢

AMA: 2016,Jan,13; 2015,Jan,16; 2014,Aug,3

92626 **Evaluation of auditory rehabilitation status; first hour**

INCLUDES Assessment to determine patient's proficiency in the use of remaining hearing to identify speech
Face-to-face time spent with the patient or family

🚑 2.16 ⚕ 2.53 **FUD** XXX Ⓠ1 80 ▢

AMA: 2016,Sep,6; 2016,Jan,13; 2015,Jan,16; 2014,Jul,4; 2014,May,10; 2014,Jan,11

+ 92627 each additional 15 minutes (List separately in addition to code for primary procedure)

INCLUDES Assessment to determine patient's proficiency in the use of remaining hearing to identify speech
Face-to-face time spent with the patient or family
Code first initial hour (92626)

⏣ 0.51 ⚕ 0.63 **FUD** ZZZ N 80 ▭

AMA: 2016,Sep,6; 2016,Jan,13; 2015,Jan,16; 2014,Jul,4; 2014,Jan,11

92630 Auditory rehabilitation; prelingual hearing loss

⏣ 0.00 ⚕ 0.00 **FUD** XXX E ▭

AMA: 2016,Sep,6; 2016,Jan,13; 2015,Jan,16; 2014,Jan,11; 2013,Oct,7

92633 postlingual hearing loss

⏣ 0.00 ⚕ 0.00 **FUD** XXX E ▭

AMA: 2016,Sep,6; 2016,Jan,13; 2015,Jan,16; 2014,Jan,11; 2013,Oct,7

92640 Diagnostic analysis with programming of auditory brainstem implant, per hour

⏣ 2.72 ⚕ 3.20 **FUD** XXX S 80 ▭

EXCLUDES Nonprogramming services (cardiac monitoring)

92700 Unlisted otorhinolaryngological service or procedure

INCLUDES Lombard test

⏣ 0.00 ⚕ 0.00 **FUD** XXX Q1 80 ▭

AMA: 2016,Sep,6; 2016,Jan,13; 2015,Sep,7; 2015,Sep,12; 2015,Jan,16; 2014,May,10; 2014,Jan,11; 2012,Jan,15-42; 2011,Jul,16-17; 2011,Mar,9; 2011,Jan,11

92920-92953 Emergency Cardiac Procedures

92920 Resequenced code. See code following 92998.

92921 Resequenced code. See code following 92998.

92924 Resequenced code. See code following 92998.

92925 Resequenced code. See code following 92998.

92928 Resequenced code. See code following 92998.

92929 Resequenced code. See code following 92998.

92933 Resequenced code. See code following 92998.

92934 Resequenced code. See code following 92998.

92937 Resequenced code. See code following 92998.

92938 Resequenced code. See code following 92998.

92941 Resequenced code. See code following 92998.

92943 Resequenced code. See code following 92998.

92944 Resequenced code. See code following 92998.

92950 Cardiopulmonary resuscitation (eg, in cardiac arrest)

EXCLUDES Critical care services (99291-99292)

⏣ 5.33 ⚕ 8.61 **FUD** 000 S 80 ▭

AMA: 2016,Jan,13; 2015,Jan,16; 2014,Jan,11; 2012,Oct,14; 2012,Sep,16; 2012,Jul,12-14; 2012,Jan,15-42; 2011,Jan,11

▲ **92953** Temporary transcutaneous pacing

EXCLUDES Direction of ambulance/rescue personnel by physician or other qualified health care professional (99288)

⏣ 0.32 ⚕ 0.32 **FUD** 000 Q3 80 ▭

AMA: 2016,Jan,13; 2015,Jan,16; 2014,May,4; 2014,Jan,11

92960-92961 Cardioversion

▲ **92960** Cardioversion, elective, electrical conversion of arrhythmia; external

⏣ 3.48 ⚕ 5.83 **FUD** 000 S 80 ▭

AMA: 2016,Jan,13; 2015,Jan,16; 2014,Jan,11; 2012,Jan,15-42; 2012,Jan,13-14; 2011,Jan,11

▲ **92961** internal (separate procedure)

EXCLUDES Device evaluation for implantable defibrillator/multi-lead pacemaker system (93282-93284, 93287, 93289, 93295-93296)
Electrophysiological studies (93618-93624, 93631, 93640-93642)
Intracardiac ablation (93650-93657, 93662)

⏣ 7.54 ⚕ 7.54 **FUD** 000 S ▭

AMA: 2016,Jan,13; 2015,Feb,3; 2015,Jan,16; 2014,Jan,11

92970-92979 Circulatory Assist: External/Internal

EXCLUDES Atrial septostomy, balloon (92992)
Catheter placement for use in circulatory assist devices (intra-aortic balloon pump) (33970)

92970 Cardioassist-method of circulatory assist; internal

⏣ 5.41 ⚕ 5.41 **FUD** 000 C 80 ▭

AMA: 1997,Nov,1

92971 external

⏣ 2.93 ⚕ 2.93 **FUD** 000 C 80 ▭

AMA: 1997,Nov,1

92973 Resequenced code. See code following 92998.

92974 Resequenced code. See code following 92998.

92975 Resequenced code. See code following 92998.

92977 Resequenced code. See code following 92998.

92978 Resequenced code. See code following 92998.

92979 Resequenced code. See code following 92998.

92986-92993 Percutaneous Procedures of Heart Valves and Septum

▲ **92986** Percutaneous balloon valvuloplasty; aortic valve

⏣ 38.7 ⚕ 38.7 **FUD** 090 J 80 ▭

AMA: 2016,Jan,13; 2015,Feb,3; 2015,Jan,16; 2014,Jan,11; 2013,Jan,6-8

▲ **92987** mitral valve

⏣ 39.9 ⚕ 39.9 **FUD** 090 J 80 ▭

AMA: 2016,Jan,13; 2015,Feb,3

92990 pulmonary valve

⏣ 31.5 ⚕ 31.5 **FUD** 090 J 80 ▭

AMA: 2016,Jan,13; 2015,Jul,10; 2015,Feb,3

92992 Atrial septectomy or septostomy; transvenous method, balloon (eg, Rashkind type) (includes cardiac catheterization)

⏣ 0.00 ⚕ 0.00 **FUD** 090 C 80 ▭

AMA: 2016,Jul,3; 2016,Jan,13; 2015,Jan,16; 2014,Jan,11; 2012,Jan,15-42; 2011,Jan,11

92993 blade method (Park septostomy) (includes cardiac catheterization)

⏣ 0.00 ⚕ 0.00 **FUD** 090 C 80 ▭

AMA: 2016,Jul,3; 2016,Jan,13; 2015,Jan,16; 2014,Jan,11

92997-92998 Percutaneous Angioplasty: Pulmonary Artery

92997 Percutaneous transluminal pulmonary artery balloon angioplasty; single vessel

⏣ 19.0 ⚕ 19.0 **FUD** 000 J 80 ▭

AMA: 2016,Mar,5; 2016,Jan,13; 2015,Feb,3

+ 92998 each additional vessel (List separately in addition to code for primary procedure)

Code first single vessel (92997)

⏣ 9.39 ⚕ 9.39 **FUD** ZZZ N 80 ▭

AMA: 2016,Mar,5; 2016,Jan,13; 2015,Feb,3

[92920, 92921, 92924, 92925, 92928, 92929, 92933, 92934, 92937, 92938, 92941, 92943, 92944] Intravascular Coronary Procedures

INCLUDES
Accessing the vessel
Additional procedures performed in a third branch of a major coronary artery
All procedures performed in all segments of branches of coronary arteries
    Branches of left anterior descending (diagonals), left circumflex (marginals), and right (posterior descending, posterolaterals)
    Distal, proximal, and mid segments
All procedures performed in all segments of major coronary arteries through the native vessels:
    Distal, proximal, and mid segments
    Left main, left anterior descending, left circumflex, right, and ramus intermedius arteries
All procedures performed in major coronary arteries or recognized coronary artery branches through a coronary artery bypass graft
    A sequential bypass graft with more than a single distal anastomosis as one graft
    Branching bypass grafts (eg, "Y" grafts) include a coronary vessel for the primary graft, with each branch off the primary graft making up an additional coronary vessel
    Each coronary artery bypass graft denotes a single coronary vessel
    Embolic protection devices when used
Arteriotomy closure through the access sheath
Atherectomy (eg, directional, laser, rotational)
Balloon angioplasty (eg, cryoplasty, cutting balloon, wired balloons)
Cardiac catheterization and related procedures when included in the coronary revascularization service (93454-93461, 93563-93564)
Imaging once procedure is complete
Percutaneous coronary interventions (PCI) for disease of coronary vessels, native and bypass grafts
Procedures in branches of the left main and ramus intermedius coronary arteries as they are unrecognized for purposes of individual code assignment
Radiological supervision and interpretation of intervention(s)
Reporting the most comprehensive treatment in a given vessel according to a hierarchy of intensity for the base and add-on codes:
    Add-on codes: 92944 = 92938 > 92934 > 92925 > 92929 > 92921
    Base codes (report only one): 92943 = 92941 = 92933 > 92924 > 92937 = 92928 > 92920
Revascularization achieved with a single procedure when a single lesion continues from one target vessel (major artery, branch, or bypass graft) to ...
Selective vessel catheterization
Stenting (eg, balloon expandable, bare metal, covered, drug eluting, self-expanding)
Traversing of the lesion

EXCLUDES
Application of intravascular radioelements (77770-77772)
Insertion of device for coronary intravascular brachytherapy (92974)
Reduction of septum (eg, alcohol ablation) (93799)
Code also add-on codes for procedures performed during the same session in additional recognized branches of the target vessel
Code also diagnostic angiography at the time of the interventional procedure when:
    A previous study is available, but documentation states the patient's condition has changed since the previous study or visualization of the anatomy/pathology is inadequate, or a change occurs during the procedure warranting additional evaluation of an area outside the current target area
    No previous catheter-based coronary angiography study is available, and a full diagnostic study is performed, with the decision to perform the intervention based on that study, or
Code also diagnostic angiography performed at a session separate from the interventional procedure
Code also individual base codes for treatment of a segment of a major native coronary artery and another segment of the same artery that requires treatment through a bypass graft when performed at the same time
Code also procedures for both vessels for a bifurcation lesion
Code also procedures performed in second branch of a major coronary artery
Code also treatment of arterial segment requiring access through a bypass graft

▲ # **92920** **Percutaneous transluminal coronary angioplasty; single major coronary artery or branch**
    📊 15.8   ⚖ 15.8   **FUD** 000   J 80 🖵
    AMA: 2016,Jan,13; 2015,Jan,16; 2014,Dec,6; 2013,Jan,3-5

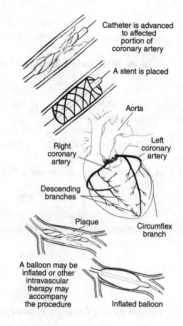

Catheter is advanced to affected portion of coronary artery
A stent is placed
Aorta
Right coronary artery
Left coronary artery
Descending branches
Plaque
Circumflex branch
A balloon may be inflated or other intravascular therapy may accompany the procedure
Inflated balloon

▲ + # **92921** **each additional branch of a major coronary artery (List separately in addition to code for primary procedure)**
    Code first (92920, 92924, 92928, 92933, 92937, 92941, 92943)
    📊 0.00   ⚖ 0.00   **FUD** ZZZ   N 🖵
    AMA: 2016,Jan,13; 2015,Jan,16; 2014,Dec,6; 2014,Sep,13; 2013,Jan,3-5

▲ # **92924** **Percutaneous transluminal coronary atherectomy, with coronary angioplasty when performed; single major coronary artery or branch**
    📊 18.8   ⚖ 18.8   **FUD** 000   J 80 🖵
    AMA: 2016,Jan,13; 2015,Jan,16; 2014,Dec,6; 2013,Jan,3-5

▲ + # **92925** **each additional branch of a major coronary artery (List separately in addition to code for primary procedure)**
    Code first (92924, 92928, 92933, 92937, 92941, 92943)
    📊 0.00   ⚖ 0.00   **FUD** ZZZ   N 🖵
    AMA: 2016,Jan,13; 2015,Jan,16; 2014,Dec,6; 2014,Sep,13; 2013,Jan,3-5

▲ # **92928** **Percutaneous transcatheter placement of intracoronary stent(s), with coronary angioplasty when performed; single major coronary artery or branch**
    📊 17.6   ⚖ 17.6   **FUD** 000   J 80 🖵
    AMA: 2016,Jan,13; 2015,Jan,16; 2014,Dec,6; 2014,Sep,13; 2014,Mar,13; 2014,Jan,3; 2013,Jan,3-5

▲ + # **92929** **each additional branch of a major coronary artery (List separately in addition to code for primary procedure)**
    Code first (92928, 92933, 92937, 92941, 92943)
    📊 0.00   ⚖ 0.00   **FUD** ZZZ   N 🖵
    AMA: 2016,Jan,13; 2015,Jan,16; 2014,Dec,6; 2014,Sep,13; 2013,Jan,3-5

▲ # **92933** **Percutaneous transluminal coronary atherectomy, with intracoronary stent, with coronary angioplasty when performed; single major coronary artery or branch**
    📊 19.7   ⚖ 19.7   **FUD** 000   J 80 🖵
    AMA: 2016,Jan,13; 2015,Jan,16; 2014,Dec,6; 2013,Jan,3-5

▲ + # 92934   **each additional branch of a major coronary artery (List separately in addition to code for primary procedure)**
Code first (92933, 92937, 92941, 92943)
🚑 0.00   ⚖ 0.00   **FUD** ZZZ   N ▭
AMA: 2016,Jan,13; 2015,Jan,16; 2014,Dec,6; 2014,Sep,13; 2013,Jan,3-5

▲ # 92937   **Percutaneous transluminal revascularization of or through coronary artery bypass graft (internal mammary, free arterial, venous), any combination of intracoronary stent, atherectomy and angioplasty, including distal protection when performed; single vessel**
🚑 17.6   ⚖ 17.6   **FUD** 000   J 80 ▭
AMA: 2016,Jan,13; 2015,Jan,16; 2014,Dec,6; 2014,Mar,13; 2013,Jan,3-5

▲ + # 92938   **each additional branch subtended by the bypass graft (List separately in addition to code for primary procedure)**
Code first (92937)
🚑 0.00   ⚖ 0.00   **FUD** ZZZ   N ▭
AMA: 2016,Jan,13; 2015,Jan,16; 2014,Dec,6; 2014,Sep,13; 2014,Mar,13; 2013,Jan,3-5

▲ # 92941   **Percutaneous transluminal revascularization of acute total/subtotal occlusion during acute myocardial infarction, coronary artery or coronary artery bypass graft, any combination of intracoronary stent, atherectomy and angioplasty, including aspiration thrombectomy when performed, single vessel**
> INCLUDES   Aspiration thrombectomy, when performed
> Embolic protection
> Rheolytic thrombectomy
> Code also mechanical thrombectomy, when performed
> Code also treatment of additional vessels, when appropriate (92920-92938, 92943-92944)
🚑 19.7   ⚖ 19.7   **FUD** 000   J 80 ▭
AMA: 2016,Jan,13; 2015,Jan,16; 2014,Dec,6; 2014,Mar,13; 2014,Jan,3; 2013,Jan,3-5

▲ # 92943   **Percutaneous transluminal revascularization of chronic total occlusion, coronary artery, coronary artery branch, or coronary artery bypass graft, any combination of intracoronary stent, atherectomy and angioplasty; single vessel**
> INCLUDES   Lack of antegrade flow with angiography and clinical criteria indicative of chronic total occlusion
🚑 19.7   ⚖ 19.7   **FUD** 000   J 80 ▭
AMA: 2016,Jan,13; 2015,Jan,16; 2014,Dec,6; 2013,Jan,3-5

▲ + # 92944   **each additional coronary artery, coronary artery branch, or bypass graft (List separately in addition to code for primary procedure)**
> EXCLUDES   Application of intravascular radioelements (77770-77772)
> Code first (92924, 92928, 92933, 92937, 92941, 92943)
🚑 0.00   ⚖ 0.00   **FUD** ZZZ   N ▭
AMA: 2016,Jan,13; 2015,Jan,16; 2014,Dec,6; 2014,Sep,13; 2013,Jan,3-5

[92973, 92974, 92975, 92977, 92978, 92979] Additional Coronary Artery Procedures

▲ + # 92973   **Percutaneous transluminal coronary thrombectomy mechanical (List separately in addition to code for primary procedure)**
> EXCLUDES   Aspiration thrombectomy
> Code first (92920, 92924, 92928, 92933, 92937, 92941, 92943, 92975, 93454-93461, 93563-93564)
🚑 5.15   ⚖ 5.15   **FUD** ZZZ   N 80 ▭
AMA: 2016,Jan,13; 2015,Jan,16; 2014,Dec,6; 2014,Jan,11; 2012,Jan,15-42; 2011,Jan,11

▲ + # 92974   **Transcatheter placement of radiation delivery device for subsequent coronary intravascular brachytherapy (List separately in addition to code for primary procedure)**
> EXCLUDES   Application of intravascular radioelements (77770-77772)
> Code first (92920, 92924, 92928, 92933, 92937, 92941, 92943, 93454-93461)
🚑 4.70   ⚖ 4.70   **FUD** ZZZ   N 80 ▭
AMA: 2016,Jan,13; 2015,Jan,16; 2014,Dec,6; 2014,Jan,11

▲ # 92975   **Thrombolysis, coronary; by intracoronary infusion, including selective coronary angiography**
> EXCLUDES   Thrombolysis, cerebral (37195)
> Thrombolysis other than coronary ([37211, 37212, 37213, 37214])
🚑 11.3   ⚖ 11.3   **FUD** 000   C 80 ▭
AMA: 1997,Nov,1; 1991,Win,1

 #   92977   **by intravenous infusion**
> EXCLUDES   Thrombolysis, cerebral (37195)
> Thrombolysis other than coronary ([37211, 37212, 37213, 37214])
🚑 1.75   ⚖ 1.75   **FUD** XXX   T 80 ▭
AMA: 1997,Nov,1; 1991,Win,1

▲ + # 92978   **Endoluminal imaging of coronary vessel or graft using intravascular ultrasound (IVUS) or optical coherence tomography (OCT) during diagnostic evaluation and/or therapeutic intervention including imaging supervision, interpretation and report; initial vessel (List separately in addition to code for primary procedure)**
Code first primary procedure (92920, 92924, 92928, 92933, 92937, 92941, 92943, 92975, 93454-93461, 93563-93564)
🚑 0.00   ⚖ 0.00   **FUD** ZZZ   N 80 ▭
AMA: 2016,Jan,13; 2015,Jan,16; 2014,Dec,6; 2014,Jan,11; 2013,Dec,16; 2012,Jan,15-42; 2011,Jan,11

▲ + # 92979   **each additional vessel (List separately in addition to code for primary procedure)**
> INCLUDES   Transducer manipulations/repositioning in the vessel examined, before and after therapeutic intervention
> EXCLUDES   Intravascular spectroscopy (0205T)
> Code first initial vessel (92978)
🚑 0.00   ⚖ 0.00   **FUD** ZZZ   N 80 ▭
AMA: 2016,Jan,13; 2015,Jan,16; 2014,Dec,6; 2014,Jan,11; 2013,Dec,16

93000-93010 Electrocardiographic Services

> INCLUDES   Specific order for the service, a separate written and signed report, and documentation of medical necessity
> EXCLUDES   Acoustic cardiography (93799)
> Echocardiography (93303-93350)
> ECG monitoring (99354-99360 [99415, 99416])
> ECG with 64 or more leads, graphic presentation, and analysis (0178T-0180T)
> Use of these codes for the review of telemetry monitoring strips

93000   **Electrocardiogram, routine ECG with at least 12 leads; with interpretation and report**
🚑 0.48   ⚖ 0.48   **FUD** XXX   M 80 ▭
AMA: 2016,Jan,13; 2015,Jan,16; 2014,Jan,11

93005   **tracing only, without interpretation and report**
🚑 0.24   ⚖ 0.24   **FUD** XXX   01 80 TC ▭
AMA: 2016,Apr,8; 2016,Jan,13; 2015,Jan,16; 2014,Jan,11

93010 interpretation and report only
🚑 0.24 🖊 0.24 **FUD** XXX ⬛B 80 26 🖵

AMA: 2016,Apr,8; 2016,Jan,13; 2015,Jan,16; 2014,Jan,11

Conduction System of the Heart

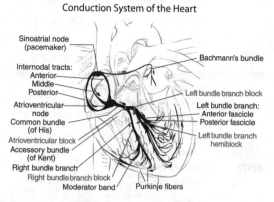

93015-93018 Stress Test

93015 Cardiovascular stress test using maximal or submaximal treadmill or bicycle exercise, continuous electrocardiographic monitoring, and/or pharmacological stress; with supervision, interpretation and report
🚑 2.15 🖊 2.15 **FUD** XXX ⬛B 80 🖵

AMA: 2016,Jan,13; 2015,Jan,16; 2014,Jan,11; 2012,Jan,15-42; 2011,Jan,11

93016 supervision only, without interpretation and report
🚑 0.63 🖊 0.63 **FUD** XXX ⬛B 80 26 🖵

AMA: 2016,Jan,13; 2015,Jan,16; 2014,Jan,11; 2012,Jan,15-42; 2011,Jan,11

93017 tracing only, without interpretation and report
🚑 1.11 🖊 1.11 **FUD** XXX 01 80 TC 🖵

AMA: 2016,Jan,13; 2015,Jan,16; 2014,Jan,11; 2012,Jan,15-42; 2011,Jan,11

93018 interpretation and report only
🚑 0.41 🖊 0.41 **FUD** XXX ⬛B 80 26 🖵

AMA: 2016,Jan,13; 2015,Jan,16; 2014,Jan,11; 2012,Jan,15-42; 2011,Jan,11

93024 Provocation Test for Coronary Vasospasm

93024 Ergonovine provocation test
🚑 3.16 🖊 3.16 **FUD** XXX 01 80 🖵

93025 Microvolt T-Wave Alternans

CMS: 100-03,20.30 Microvolt T-Wave Alternans (MTWA); 100-04,32,370 Microvolt T-wave Alternans; 100-04,32,370.1 Coding and Claims Processing for MTWA; 100-04,32,370.2 Messaging for MTWA

INCLUDES Specific order for the service, a separate written and signed report, and documentation of medical necessity

EXCLUDES ECG with 64 or more leads, graphic presentation, and analysis (0178T-0180T)
Echocardiography (93303-93350)
Use of these codes for the review of telemetry monitoring strips

93025 Microvolt T-wave alternans for assessment of ventricular arrhythmias
🚑 4.50 🖊 4.50 **FUD** XXX ⬛S 80 🖵

AMA: 2016,Jan,13; 2015,Jan,16; 2014,Jan,11

93040-93042 Rhythm Strips

INCLUDES Specific order for the service, a separate written and signed report, and documentation of medical necessity

EXCLUDES Device evaluation (93261, 93279-93289 [93260], 93291-93296, 93298-93299)
ECG with 64 or more leads, graphic presentation, and analysis (0178T-0180T)
Echocardiography (93303-93350)
Use of these codes for the review of telemetry monitoring strips

93040 Rhythm ECG, 1-3 leads; with interpretation and report
🚑 0.36 🖊 0.36 **FUD** XXX ⬛B 80 🖵

AMA: 2016,Jan,13; 2015,Jan,16; 2014,Jan,11; 2012,Nov,6-9; 2012,Aug,6-8; 2012,Jan,15-42

93041 tracing only without interpretation and report
🚑 0.16 🖊 0.16 **FUD** XXX 01 80 TC 🖵

AMA: 2016,Jan,13; 2015,Jan,16; 2014,Jan,11; 2012,Aug,6-8; 2012,Jan,15-42

93042 interpretation and report only
🚑 0.20 🖊 0.20 **FUD** XXX ⬛B 80 26 🖵

AMA: 2016,Jan,13; 2015,Jan,16; 2014,Jan,11; 2012,Aug,6-8; 2012,Jan,15-42; 2011,Oct,5-7; 2011,Jan,11

93050 Arterial Waveform Analysis

EXCLUDES Use of code with any intra-arterial diagnostic or interventional procedure

93050 Arterial pressure waveform analysis for assessment of central arterial pressures, includes obtaining waveform(s), digitization and application of nonlinear mathematical transformations to determine central arterial pressures and augmentation index, with interpretation and report, upper extremity artery, non-invasive
🚑 0.49 🖊 0.49 **FUD** XXX 01 80 🖵

93224-93227 Holter Monitor

INCLUDES Cardiac monitoring using in-person as well as remote technology for the assessment of electrocardiographic data
Up to 48 hours of recording on a continuous basis

EXCLUDES Echocardiography (93303-93355)
ECG with 64 or more leads, graphic presentation, and analysis (0178T-0180T)
Implantable patient activated cardiac event recorders (33282, 93285, 93291, 93298)
More than 48 hours of monitoring (0295T-0298T)
Code also modifier 52 when less than 12 hours of continuous recording is provided

93224 External electrocardiographic recording up to 48 hours by continuous rhythm recording and storage; includes recording, scanning analysis with report, review and interpretation by a physician or other qualified health care professional
🚑 2.57 🖊 2.57 **FUD** XXX ⬛M 80 🖵

AMA: 2016,Jan,13; 2015,Jan,16; 2014,Jan,11; 2012,Jan,15-42; 2011,Oct,5-7

93225 recording (includes connection, recording, and disconnection)
🚑 0.75 🖊 0.75 **FUD** XXX 01 80 TC 🖵

AMA: 2016,Jan,13; 2015,Jan,16; 2014,Jan,11; 2012,Jan,15-42; 2011,Oct,5-7

93226 scanning analysis with report
🚑 1.07 🖊 1.07 **FUD** XXX 01 80 TC 🖵

AMA: 2016,Jan,13; 2015,Jan,16; 2014,Jan,11; 2012,Jan,15-42; 2011,Oct,5-7

93227 review and interpretation by a physician or other qualified health care professional
🚑 0.75 🖊 0.75 **FUD** XXX ⬛M 80 26 🖵

AMA: 2016,Jan,13; 2015,Jan,16; 2014,Jan,11; 2012,Jan,15-42; 2011,Oct,5-7

93228-93229 Remote Cardiovascular Telemetry

INCLUDES Cardiac monitoring using in-person as well as remote technology for the assessment of electrocardiographic data
Mobile telemetry monitors with the capacity to:
Detect arrhythmias
Real-time data analysis for the evaluation quality of the signal
Records ECG rhythm on a continuous basis using external electrodes on the patient
Transmit a tracing at any time
Transmit data to an attended surveillance center where a technician is available to respond to device or rhythm alerts and contact the physician or qualified health care professional if needed

EXCLUDES Use of code more than one time in a 30-day period

26/TC PC/TC Only A2-Z3 ASC Payment 50 Bilateral ♂ Male Only ♀ Female Only 🚑 Facility RVU 🖊 Non-Facility RVU 🖵 CCI
FUD Follow-up Days **CMS:** IOM (Pub 100) A-Y OPPSI 80/80 Surg Assist Allowed / w/Doc 🔲 Lab Crosswalk 🔲 Radiology Crosswalk ❌ CLIA

93228 External mobile cardiovascular telemetry with electrocardiographic recording, concurrent computerized real time data analysis and greater than 24 hours of accessible ECG data storage (retrievable with query) with ECG triggered and patient selected events transmitted to a remote attended surveillance center for up to 30 days; review and interpretation with report by a physician or other qualified health care professional

> *EXCLUDES* *Review and interpretation of external ECG up to 24 hours (93224, 93227)*
>
> 🚑 0.74   ⚗ 0.74   **FUD** XXX   ★ M 80 26 ▭
>
> **AMA:** 2016,Jan,13; 2015,Jan,16; 2014,Jan,11; 2012,Jan,15-42; 2011,Oct,5-7

93229 technical support for connection and patient instructions for use, attended surveillance, analysis and transmission of daily and emergent data reports as prescribed by a physician or other qualified health care professional

> *EXCLUDES* *Cardiovascular monitors that do not perform automatic ECG triggered transmissions to an attended surveillance center (93224-93227, 93268-93272)*
> *Scanning analysis and report of external ECG up to 24 hours (93224, 93226)*
>
> 🚑 20.5   ⚗ 20.5   **FUD** XXX   ★ S 80 TC ▭
>
> **AMA:** 2016,Jan,13; 2015,Jan,16; 2014,Jan,11; 2012,Jan,15-42; 2011,Oct,5-7

93260-93272 Event Monitors

> *INCLUDES* ECG rhythm derived elements, which differ from physiologic data and include rhythm of the heart, rate, ST analysis, heart rate variability, T-wave alternans, among others
> Event monitors that:
> Record parts of ECGs in response to patient activation or an automatic detection algorithm (or both)
> Require attended surveillance
> Transmit data upon request (although not immediately when activated)
>
> *EXCLUDES* *Monitoring of cardiovascular devices (93279-93289 [93260], 93291-93296, 93298-93299)*

93260 Resequenced code. See code following 93284.

93261 Resequenced code. See code following 93289.

93268 External patient and, when performed, auto activated electrocardiographic rhythm derived event recording with symptom-related memory loop with remote download capability up to 30 days, 24-hour attended monitoring; includes transmission, review and interpretation by a physician or other qualified health care professional

> *EXCLUDES* *Implanted patient activated cardiac event recording (33282, 93285, 93291, 93298)*
>
> 🚑 5.79   ⚗ 5.79   **FUD** XXX   ★ M 80 ▭
>
> **AMA:** 2016,Jan,13; 2015,Jan,16; 2014,Jan,11; 2012,Jan,15-42; 2011,Oct,5-7

93270 recording (includes connection, recording, and disconnection)

> 🚑 0.26   ⚗ 0.26   **FUD** XXX   ★ 01 80 TC ▭
>
> **AMA:** 2016,Jan,13; 2015,Jan,16; 2014,Jan,11; 2012,Jan,15-42; 2011,Oct,5-7; 2011,Jan,11

93271 transmission and analysis

> 🚑 4.81   ⚗ 4.81   **FUD** XXX   ★ S 80 TC ▭
>
> **AMA:** 2016,Jan,13; 2015,Jan,16; 2014,Jan,11; 2012,Jan,15-42; 2011,Oct,5-7

93272 review and interpretation by a physician or other qualified health care professional

> 🚑 0.72   ⚗ 0.72   **FUD** XXX   ★ M 80 26 ▭
>
> **AMA:** 2016,Jan,13; 2015,Jan,16; 2014,Jan,11; 2012,Jan,15-42; 2011,Oct,5-7; 2011,Jan,11

93278 Signal-averaged Electrocardiography

> *EXCLUDES* *Echocardiography (93303-93355)*
> *ECG with 64 or more leads, graphic presentation, and analysis (0178T-0180T)*
> Code also modifier 26 for the interpretation and report only

93278 Signal-averaged electrocardiography (SAECG), with or without ECG

> 🚑 0.85   ⚗ 0.85   **FUD** XXX   01 80 ▭
>
> **AMA:** 2016,Jan,13; 2015,Jan,16; 2014,Jan,11; 2012,Jan,15-42; 2011,Oct,5-7

93279-93299 [93260, 93261] Monitoring of Cardiovascular Devices

> *INCLUDES* Implantable cardiovascular monitor (ICM) interrogation:
> Analysis of at least one recorded physiologic cardiovascular data element from either internal or external sensors
> Programmed parameters
> Implantable defibrillator interrogation:
> Battery
> Capture and sensing functions
> Leads
> Presence or absence of therapy for ventricular tachyarrhythmias
> Programmed parameters
> Underlying heart rhythm
> Implantable loop recorder (ILR) interrogation:
> Heart rate and rhythm during recorded episodes from both patient-initiated and device detected events
> Programmed parameters
> In-person interrogation/device evaluation (93288)
> In-person peri-procedural device evaluation/programming of device system parameters (93286)
> Interrogation evaluation of device
> Pacemaker interrogation:
> Battery
> Capture and sensing functions
> Heart rhythm
> Leads
> Programmed parameters
> Time period established by the initiation of remote monitoring or the 91st day of implantable defibrillator or pacemaker monitoring or the 31st day of ILR monitoring and extending for the succeeding 30- or 90-day period
>
> *EXCLUDES* *Evaluation of subcutaneous implantable defibrillator device (93260, 93261)*
> *Wearable device monitoring (93224-93272)*

93279 Programming device evaluation (in person) with iterative adjustment of the implantable device to test the function of the device and select optimal permanent programmed values with analysis, review and report by a physician or other qualified health care professional; single lead pacemaker system

> *EXCLUDES* *External ECG event recording up to 30 days (93268-93272)*
> *Peri-procedural and interrogation device evaluation (93286, 93288)*
> *Rhythm strips (93040-93042)*
>
> 🚑 1.40   ⚗ 1.40   **FUD** XXX   01 80 ▭
>
> **AMA:** 2016,Aug,5; 2016,May,5; 2016,Jan,13; 2015,Jan,16; 2014,Nov,5; 2014,Jul,3; 2014,Jan,11; 2013,Jul,7-9; 2013,Jun,6-8

93280 dual lead pacemaker system

> *EXCLUDES* *External ECG event recording up to 30 days (93268-93272)*
> *Peri-procedural and interrogation device evaluation (93286, 93288)*
> *Rhythm strips (93040-93042)*
>
> 🚑 1.64   ⚗ 1.64   **FUD** XXX   01 80 ▭
>
> **AMA:** 2016,Aug,5; 2016,May,5; 2016,Jan,13; 2015,Jan,16; 2014,Nov,5; 2014,Jul,3; 2014,Jan,11; 2013,Jul,7-9; 2013,Jun,6-8

93281 multiple lead pacemaker system

> *EXCLUDES* *External ECG event recording up to 30 days (93268-93272)*
> *Peri-procedural and interrogation device evaluation (93286, 93288)*
> *Rhythm strips (93040-93042)*
>
> 🚑 1.92   ⚗ 1.92   **FUD** XXX   01 80 ▭
>
> **AMA:** 2016,Aug,5; 2016,May,5; 2016,Jan,13; 2015,Jan,16; 2014,Nov,5; 2014,Jul,3; 2014,Jan,11; 2013,Jul,7-9; 2013,Jun,6-8

93282 single lead transvenous implantable defibrillator system

> EXCLUDES *Device evaluation subcutaneous lead defibrillator system (93260)*
> *External ECG event recording up to 30 days (93268-93272)*
> *Peri-procedural and interrogation device evaluation (93287, 93289)*
> *Rhythm strips (93040-93042)*
> *Wearable cardio-defibrillator system services (93745)*

🚑 1.77 ⚕ 1.77 **FUD** XXX   [01] [80] 🖥

AMA: 2016,Aug,5; 2016,Jan,13; 2015,Jan,16; 2014,Nov,5; 2014,Jul,3; 2014,Jan,11; 2013,Jul,7-9; 2013,Jun,6-8

93283 dual lead transvenous implantable defibrillator system

> EXCLUDES *External ECG event recording up to 30 days (93268-93272)*
> *Peri-procedural and interrogation device evaluation (93287, 93289)*
> *Rhythm strips (93040-93042)*

🚑 2.30 ⚕ 2.30 **FUD** XXX   [01] [80] 🖥

AMA: 2016,Aug,5; 2016,Jan,13; 2015,Jan,16; 2014,Nov,5; 2014,Jul,3; 2014,Jan,11; 2013,Jul,7-9; 2013,Jun,6-8

93284 multiple lead transvenous implantable defibrillator system

> EXCLUDES *External ECG event recording up to 30 days (93268-93272)*
> *Peri-procedural and interrogation device evaluation (93287, 93289)*
> *Rhythm strips (93040-93042)*

🚑 2.54 ⚕ 2.54 **FUD** XXX   [01] [80] 🖥

AMA: 2016,Aug,5; 2016,Jan,13; 2015,Jan,16; 2014,Nov,5; 2014,Jul,3; 2014,Jan,11; 2013,Jul,7-9; 2013,Jun,6-8

\# **93260** implantable subcutaneous lead defibrillator system

> EXCLUDES *Device evaluation (93261, 93282, 93287)*
> *External ECG event recording up to 30 days (93268-93272)*
> *Insertion/removal/replacement implantable defibrillator (33240, 33241, [33262], [33270, 33271, 33272, 33273])*
> *Rhythm strips (93040-93042)*

🚑 1.89 ⚕ 1.89 **FUD** XXX   [01] [80] 🖥

AMA: 2016,Aug,5; 2016,Jan,13; 2015,Jan,16; 2014,Nov,5

93285 implantable loop recorder system

> EXCLUDES *Device evaluation (93279-93284, 93291)*
> *External ECG event recording up to 30 days (93268-93272)*
> *Implantation of patient-activated cardiac event recorder (33282)*
> *Rhythm strips (93040-93042)*

🚑 1.19 ⚕ 1.19 **FUD** XXX   [01] [80] 🖥

AMA: 2016,Aug,5; 2016,Jan,13; 2015,Jan,16; 2014,Nov,5; 2014,Jul,3; 2014,Jan,11

93286 Peri-procedural device evaluation (in person) and programming of device system parameters before or after a surgery, procedure, or test with analysis, review and report by a physician or other qualified health care professional; single, dual, or multiple lead pacemaker system

> INCLUDES One evaluation and programming (if performed once before and once after, report as two units)
> EXCLUDES *Device evaluation (93279-93281, 93288)*
> *External ECG event recording up to 30 days (93268-93272)*
> *Rhythm strips (93040-93042)*
> *Services related to cardiac contractility modulation systems (0408T-0411T, 0414T-0415T)*
> *Subcutaneous implantable defibrillator peri-procedural device evaluation and programming (93260, 93261)*

🚑 0.77 ⚕ 0.77 **FUD** XXX   [N] [80] 🖥

AMA: 2016,Aug,5; 2016,May,5; 2016,Jan,13; 2015,Jan,16; 2014,Nov,5; 2014,Jul,3; 2014,Jan,11; 2013,Jul,7-9; 2013,Jun,6-8

93287 single, dual, or multiple lead implantable defibrillator system

> INCLUDES One evaluation and programming (if performed once before and once after, report as two units)
> EXCLUDES *Device evaluation (93282-93284, 93289)*
> *External ECG event recording up to 30 days (93268-93272)*
> *Subcutaneous implantable defibrillator peri-procedural device evaluation and programming (93260, 93261)*
> *Services related to cardiac contractility modulation systems (0408T-0411T, 0414T-0415T)*
> *Rhythm strips (93040-93042)*

🚑 1.02 ⚕ 1.02 **FUD** XXX   [N] [80] 🖥

AMA: 2016,Aug,5; 2016,May,5; 2016,Jan,13; 2015,Jan,16; 2014,Nov,5; 2014,Jul,3; 2014,Jan,11; 2013,Jul,7-9; 2013,Jun,6-8

93288 Interrogation device evaluation (in person) with analysis, review and report by a physician or other qualified health care professional, includes connection, recording and disconnection per patient encounter; single, dual, or multiple lead pacemaker system

> EXCLUDES *Device evaluation (93279-93281, 93286, 93294-93295)*
> *External ECG event recording up to 30 days (93268-93272)*
> *Rhythm strips (93040-93042)*

🚑 1.04 ⚕ 1.04 **FUD** XXX   [01] [80] 🖥

AMA: 2016,Aug,5; 2016,May,5; 2016,Jan,13; 2015,Jan,16; 2014,Nov,5; 2014,Jul,3; 2014,Jan,11; 2013,Jul,7-9; 2013,Jun,6-8

93289 single, dual, or multiple lead transvenous implantable defibrillator system, including analysis of heart rhythm derived data elements

> EXCLUDES *Monitoring physiologic cardiovascular data elements derived from an implantable defibrillator (93290)*
> EXCLUDES *Device evaluation (93261, 93282-93284, 93287, 93295-93296)*
> *External ECG event recording up to 30 days (93268-93272)*
> *Rhythm strips (93040-93042)*

🚑 1.84 ⚕ 1.84 **FUD** XXX   [01] [80] 🖥

AMA: 2016,Aug,5; 2016,May,5; 2016,Jan,13; 2015,Jan,16; 2014,Nov,5; 2014,Jul,3; 2014,Jan,11; 2013,Jul,7-9; 2013,Jun,6-8

\# **93261** implantable subcutaneous lead defibrillator system

> EXCLUDES *Device evaluation (93260, 93287, 93289)*
> *External ECG event recording up to 30 days (93268-93272)*
> *Insertion/removal/replacement implantable defibrillator (33240, 33241, [33262], [33270, 33271, 33272, 33273])*
> *Rhythm strips (93040-93042)*

🚑 1.71 ⚕ 1.71 **FUD** XXX   [01] [80] 🖥

AMA: 2016,Aug,5; 2016,Jan,13; 2015,Jan,16; 2014,Nov,5

93290 implantable cardiovascular monitor system, including analysis of 1 or more recorded physiologic cardiovascular data elements from all internal and external sensors

> EXCLUDES *Device evaluation (93297, 93299)*
> *Heart rhythm derived data (93289)*

🚑 0.88 ⚕ 0.88 **FUD** XXX   [01] [80] 🖥

AMA: 2016,Aug,5; 2016,Jan,13; 2015,Jan,16; 2014,Nov,5; 2014,Jul,3; 2014,Jan,11; 2013,Apr,10-11; 2012,Jan,15-42; 2011,Jan,11

93291 implantable loop recorder system, including heart rhythm derived data analysis

> EXCLUDES *Device evaluation (93288-93290 [93261], 93298-93299)*
> *External ECG event recording up to 30 days (93268-93272)*
> *Implantation of patient-activated cardiac event recorder (33282)*
> *Rhythm strips (93040-93042)*

🚑 1.02 ⚕ 1.02 **FUD** XXX   [01] [80] 🖥

AMA: 2016,Aug,5; 2016,Jan,13; 2015,Jan,16; 2014,Nov,5; 2014,Jul,3; 2014,Jan,11

26/TC PC/TC Only   A2-Z3 ASC Payment   50 Bilateral   ♂ Male Only   ♀ Female Only   🚑 Facility RVU   ⚕ Non-Facility RVU   🖥 CCI
FUD Follow-up Days   CMS: IOM (Pub 100)   A-Y OPPSI   80/80 Surg Assist Allowed / w/Doc   🔬 Lab Crosswalk   ☢ Radiology Crosswalk   ✖ CLIA

432

93292 **wearable defibrillator system**

> *EXCLUDES* *External ECG event recording up to 30 days (93268-93272)*
> *Rhythm strips (93040-93042)*
> *Wearable cardioverter-defibrillator system (93745)*

0.92   0.92   **FUD** XXX   [Q1] [80] [□]

AMA: 2016,Aug,5; 2016,Jan,13; 2015,Jan,16; 2014,Nov,5; 2014,Jul,3; 2014,Jan,11

93293 **Transtelephonic rhythm strip pacemaker evaluation(s) single, dual, or multiple lead pacemaker system, includes recording with and without magnet application with analysis, review and report(s) by a physician or other qualified health care professional, up to 90 days**

> *EXCLUDES* *Device evaluation (93294)*
> *External ECG event recording up to 30 days (93268-93272)*
> *Rhythm strips (93040-93042)*
> *Use of code more than one time in a 90-day period*
> *Use of code when monitoring period is less than 30 days*

1.50   1.50   **FUD** XXX   [Q1] [80] [□]

AMA: 2016,Aug,5; 2016,Jan,13; 2015,Jan,16; 2014,Nov,5; 2014,Jul,3; 2014,Jan,11

93294 **Interrogation device evaluation(s) (remote), up to 90 days; single, dual, or multiple lead pacemaker system with interim analysis, review(s) and report(s) by a physician or other qualified health care professional**

> *EXCLUDES* *Device evaluation (93288, 93293)*
> *External ECG event recording up to 30 days (93268-93272)*
> *Rhythm strips (93040-93042)*
> *Use of code more than one time in a 90-day period*
> *Use of code when monitoring period is less than 30 days*

0.96   0.96   **FUD** XXX   [M] [80] [26] [□]

AMA: 2016,Aug,5; 2016,Jan,13; 2015,Jan,16; 2014,Nov,5; 2014,Jul,3; 2014,Jan,11; 2012,Jun,3-9

93295 **single, dual, or multiple lead implantable defibrillator system with interim analysis, review(s) and report(s) by a physician or other qualified health care professional**

> *EXCLUDES* *Device evaluation (93289)*
> *External ECG event recording up to 30 days (93268-93272)*
> *Remote monitoring of physiological cardiovascular data (93297)*
> *Rhythm strips (93040-93042)*
> *Use of code more than one time in a 90-day period*
> *Use of code when monitoring period is less than 30 days*

1.91   1.91   **FUD** XXX   [M] [80] [26] [□]

AMA: 2016,Aug,5; 2016,Jan,13; 2015,Jan,16; 2014,Nov,5; 2014,Jul,3; 2014,Jan,11

93296 **single, dual, or multiple lead pacemaker system or implantable defibrillator system, remote data acquisition(s), receipt of transmissions and technician review, technical support and distribution of results**

> *EXCLUDES* *Device evaluation (93288-93289, 93299)*
> *External ECG event recording up to 30 days (93268-93272)*
> *Rhythm strips (93040-93042)*
> *Use of code more than one time in a 90-day period*
> *Use of code when monitoring period is less than 30 days*

0.73   0.73   **FUD** XXX   [Q1] [80] [TC] [□]

AMA: 2016,Aug,5; 2016,Jan,13; 2015,Jan,16; 2014,Nov,5; 2014,Jul,3; 2014,Jan,11

93297 **Interrogation device evaluation(s), (remote) up to 30 days; implantable cardiovascular monitor system, including analysis of 1 or more recorded physiologic cardiovascular data elements from all internal and external sensors, analysis, review(s) and report(s) by a physician or other qualified health care professional**

> *EXCLUDES* *Device evaluation (93290, 93298)*
> *Heart rhythm derived data (93295)*
> *Use of code more than one time in a 30-day period*
> *Use of code when monitoring period is less than 10 days*

0.75   0.75   **FUD** XXX   [M] [80] [26] [□]

AMA: 2016,Aug,5; 2016,Jan,13; 2015,Jan,16; 2014,Nov,5; 2014,Jul,3; 2014,Jan,11; 2013,Apr,10-11

93298 **implantable loop recorder system, including analysis of recorded heart rhythm data, analysis, review(s) and report(s) by a physician or other qualified health care professional**

> *EXCLUDES* *Device evaluation (93291, 93297)*
> *External ECG event recording up to 30 days (93268-93272)*
> *Implantation of patient-activated cardiac event recorder*
> *Rhythm strips (93040-93042)*
> *Use of code more than one time in a 30-day period*
> *Use of code when monitoring period is less than 10 days*

0.75   0.75   **FUD** XXX   ★ [M] [80] [26] [□]

AMA: 2016,Aug,5; 2016,Jan,13; 2015,Jan,16; 2014,Nov,5; 2014,Jul,3; 2014,Jan,11

93299 **implantable cardiovascular monitor system or implantable loop recorder system, remote data acquisition(s), receipt of transmissions and technician review, technical support and distribution of results**

> *EXCLUDES* *Device evaluation (93290-93291, 93296)*
> *External ECG event recording up to 30 days (93268-93272)*
> *Rhythm strips (93040-93042)*
> *Use of code more than one time in a 30-day period*
> *Use of code when monitoring period is less than 10 days*

0.00   0.00   **FUD** XXX   ★ [Q1] [80] [TC] [□]

AMA: 2016,Aug,5; 2016,Jan,13; 2015,Jan,16; 2014,Nov,5; 2014,Jul,3; 2014,Jan,11; 2013,Apr,10-11

93303-93355 Echocardiography

> *INCLUDES* Interpretation and report
> Obtaining ultrasonic signals from heart/great arteries
> Report of study which includes:
>   Description of recognized abnormalities
>   Documentation of all clinically relevant findings which includes obtained quantitative measurements
>   Interpretation of all information obtained
> Two-dimensional image/doppler ultrasonic signal documentation
> Ultrasound exam of:
>   Adjacent great vessels
>   Cardiac chambers/valves
>   Pericardium

> *EXCLUDES* *Contrast agents and/or drugs used for pharmacological stress Echocardiography, fetal (76825-76828)*
> *Ultrasound with thorough examination of the organ(s) or anatomic region/documentation of the image/final written report*

93303 **Transthoracic echocardiography for congenital cardiac anomalies; complete**

6.73   6.73   **FUD** XXX   [S] [80] [□]

AMA: 2016,Jan,13; 2015,May,10; 2015,Jan,16; 2014,Jan,11; 2013,Dec,14; 2013,Aug,3; 2012,Jan,15-42; 2011,Jan,11

93304 **follow-up or limited study**

4.40   4.40   **FUD** XXX   [S] [80] [□]

AMA: 2016,Jan,13; 2015,May,10; 2015,Jan,16; 2014,Jan,11; 2013,Dec,14; 2013,Aug,3

93306 Echocardiography, transthoracic, real-time with image documentation (2D), includes M-mode recording, when performed, complete, with spectral Doppler echocardiography, and with color flow Doppler echocardiography

> INCLUDES Doppler and color flow
> Two-dimensional and M-mode
> EXCLUDES *Transthoracic without spectral and color doppler (93307)*
> 🚑 6.43   🔧 6.43   **FUD** XXX   Ⓢ 80 ▣
> **AMA:** 2016,Apr,8; 2016,Jan,13; 2015,May,10; 2015,Jan,16; 2013,Aug,3

93307 Echocardiography, transthoracic, real-time with image documentation (2D), includes M-mode recording, when performed, complete, without spectral or color Doppler echocardiography

> INCLUDES Additional structures that may be viewed such as pulmonary vein or artery, pulmonic valve, inferior vena cava
> Obtaining/recording appropriate measurements
> Two-dimensional/selected M-mode exam of:
> Adjacent portions of the aorta
> Aortic/mitral/tricuspid valves
> Left/right atria
> Left/right ventricles
> Pericardium
> Using multiple views as required to obtain a complete functional/anatomic evaluation
> EXCLUDES *Doppler echocardiography (93320-93321, 93325)*
> 🚑 3.68   🔧 3.68   **FUD** XXX   Ⓢ 80 ▣
> **AMA:** 2016,Apr,8; 2016,Jan,13; 2015,May,10; 2015,Jan,16; 2014,Jan,11; 2013,Aug,3; 2012,Jan,15-42; 2011,Jan,11

93308 Echocardiography, transthoracic, real-time with image documentation (2D), includes M-mode recording, when performed, follow-up or limited study

> INCLUDES An exam that does not evaluate/document the attempt to evaluate all the structures that comprise the complete echocardiographic exam
> 🚑 3.52   🔧 3.52   **FUD** XXX   Ⓢ 80 ▣
> **AMA:** 2016,Apr,8; 2016,Jan,13; 2015,May,10; 2015,Jan,16; 2014,Jan,11; 2013,Aug,3; 2012,Mar,9-10; 2012,Jan,15-42; 2011,Jan,11

▲ **93312** Echocardiography, transesophageal, real-time with image documentation (2D) (with or without M-mode recording); including probe placement, image acquisition, interpretation and report

> EXCLUDES *Transesophageal echocardiography (93355)*
> 🚑 8.64   🔧 8.64   **FUD** XXX   Ⓢ 80 ▣
> **AMA:** 2016,Jan,13; 2015,Jan,16; 2014,Jul,8; 2014,Jan,11; 2013,Aug,3; 2012,Oct,14; 2012,Jan,15-42; 2011,Jan,11

▲ **93313** placement of transesophageal probe only

> EXCLUDES *Excludes procedure if performed by same person performing transesophageal echocardiography (93355)*
> 🚑 0.64   🔧 0.64   **FUD** XXX   Ⓢ 80 ▣
> **AMA:** 2016,Jan,13; 2015,Jan,16; 2014,Jul,8; 2014,Jan,11; 2013,Aug,3

▲ **93314** image acquisition, interpretation and report only

> EXCLUDES *Transesophageal echocardiography (93355)*
> 🚑 8.47   🔧 8.47   **FUD** XXX   Ⓝ 80 ▣
> **AMA:** 2016,Jan,13; 2015,Jan,16; 2014,Jul,8; 2014,Jan,11; 2013,Aug,3

▲ **93315** Transesophageal echocardiography for congenital cardiac anomalies; including probe placement, image acquisition, interpretation and report

> EXCLUDES *Transesophageal echocardiography (93355)*
> 🚑 0.00   🔧 0.00   **FUD** XXX   Ⓢ 80 ▣
> **AMA:** 2016,Jan,13; 2015,Jan,16; 2014,Jul,8; 2014,Jan,11; 2013,Dec,14; 2013,Aug,3

▲ **93316** placement of transesophageal probe only

> EXCLUDES *Transesophageal echocardiography (93355)*
> 🚑 1.09   🔧 1.09   **FUD** XXX   Ⓢ 80 ▣
> **AMA:** 2016,Jan,13; 2015,Jan,16; 2014,Jan,11; 2013,Dec,14; 2013,Aug,3

▲ **93317** image acquisition, interpretation and report only

> EXCLUDES *Transesophageal echocardiography (93355)*
> 🚑 0.00   🔧 0.00   **FUD** XXX   Ⓝ 80 ▣
> **AMA:** 2016,Jan,13; 2015,Jan,16; 2014,Jan,11; 2013,Dec,14; 2013,Aug,3

▲ **93318** Echocardiography, transesophageal (TEE) for monitoring purposes, including probe placement, real time 2-dimensional image acquisition and interpretation leading to ongoing (continuous) assessment of (dynamically changing) cardiac pumping function and to therapeutic measures on an immediate time basis

> EXCLUDES *Transesophageal echocardiography (93355)*
> 🚑 0.00   🔧 0.00   **FUD** XXX   Ⓢ 80 ▣
> **AMA:** 2016,Jan,13; 2015,Jan,16; 2014,Jan,11; 2013,Aug,3

+ **93320** Doppler echocardiography, pulsed wave and/or continuous wave with spectral display (List separately in addition to codes for echocardiographic imaging); complete

> EXCLUDES *Transesophageal echocardiography (93355)*
> Code first (93303-93304, 93312, 93314-93315, 93317, 93350-93351)
> 🚑 1.53   🔧 1.53   **FUD** ZZZ   Ⓝ 80 ▣
> **AMA:** 2016,Jan,13; 2015,Jan,16; 2014,Jan,11; 2013,Aug,3

+ **93321** follow-up or limited study (List separately in addition to codes for echocardiographic imaging)

> EXCLUDES *Transesophageal echocardiography (93355)*
> Code first (93303-93304, 93308, 93312, 93314-93315, 93317, 93350-93351)
> 🚑 0.77   🔧 0.77   **FUD** ZZZ   Ⓝ 80 ▣
> **AMA:** 2016,Jan,13; 2015,Jan,16; 2014,Jan,11; 2013,Aug,3

+ **93325** Doppler echocardiography color flow velocity mapping (List separately in addition to codes for echocardiography)

> EXCLUDES *Transesophageal echocardiography (93355)*
> Code first (76825-76828, 93303-93304, 93308, 93312, 93314-93315, 93317, 93350-93351)
> 🚑 0.72   🔧 0.72   **FUD** ZZZ   Ⓝ 80 ▣
> **AMA:** 2016,Jul,8; 2016,Jan,13; 2015,Jan,16; 2014,Jan,11; 2013,Aug,3

93350 Echocardiography, transthoracic, real-time with image documentation (2D), includes M-mode recording, when performed, during rest and cardiovascular stress test using treadmill, bicycle exercise and/or pharmacologically induced stress, with interpretation and report;

> EXCLUDES *Cardiovascular stress test, complete procedure (93015)*
> Code also exercise stress testing (93016-93018)
> 🚑 6.80   🔧 6.80   **FUD** XXX   Ⓢ 80 ▣
> **AMA:** 2016,Apr,8; 2016,Jan,13; 2015,Jan,16; 2014,Jul,8; 2014,Jan,11; 2013,Aug,3; 2012,Jan,15-42; 2011,Jan,11

93351 including performance of continuous electrocardiographic monitoring, with supervision by a physician or other qualified health care professional

> INCLUDES Stress echocardiogram performed with a complete cardiovascular stress test
> EXCLUDES *Cardiovascular stress test (93015-93018)*
> *Echocardiography (93350)*
> *Professional only components of complete stress test and stress echocardiogram performed in a facility by same physician, report with modifier 26*
> *Use of code for professional component (modifier 26 appended) with (93016, 93018, 93350)*
> Code also components of cardiovascular stress test when professional services not performed by same physician performing stress echocardiogram (93016-93018)
> 🚑 7.65   🔧 7.65   **FUD** XXX   Ⓢ ▣
> **AMA:** 2016,Apr,8; 2016,Jan,13; 2015,Jan,16; 2014,Jul,8; 2014,Jan,11; 2013,Aug,3; 2012,Jan,15-42; 2011,Jan,11

+ **93352** **Use of echocardiographic contrast agent during stress echocardiography (List separately in addition to code for primary procedure)**

> EXCLUDES *Use of code more than one time for each stress echocardiogram*

Code first (93350, 93351)

🚑 0.96   ⚕ 0.96   **FUD** ZZZ   M 80 ▣

AMA: 2016,Jan,13; 2015,Jan,16; 2014,Jan,11; 2013,Aug,3; 2012,Jan,15-42; 2011,Jan,11

93355 **Echocardiography, transesophageal (TEE) for guidance of a transcatheter intracardiac or great vessel(s) structural intervention(s) (eg, TAVR, transcathether pulmonary valve replacement, mitral valve repair, paravalvular regurgitation repair, left atrial appendage occlusion/closure, ventricular septal defect closure) (peri- and intra-procedural), real-time image acquisition and documentation, guidance with quantitative measurements, probe manipulation, interpretation, and report, including diagnostic transesophageal echocardiography and, when performed, administration of ultrasound contrast, Doppler, color flow, and 3D**

🚑 6.43   ⚕ 6.43   **FUD** XXX   N 80 ▣

> EXCLUDES *3D rendering (76376-76377)*
> *Doppler echocardiography (93320-93321)*
> *Transesophageal echocardiography (93312-93318)*
> *Transesophageal probe positioning by different provider (93313)*

93451-93505 Heart Catheterization

> INCLUDES Access site imaging and placement of closure device
> Catheter insertion and positioning
> Contrast injection (except as listed below)
> Imaging and insertion of closure device
> Radiology supervision and interpretation
> Roadmapping angiography

> EXCLUDES *Congenital cardiac cath procedures (93530-93533)*

Code also separately identifiable:
Aortography (93567)
Noncardiac angiography (see radiology and vascular codes)
Pulmonary angiography (93568)
Right ventricular or atrial injection (93566)

▲ **93451** **Right heart catheterization including measurement(s) of oxygen saturation and cardiac output, when performed**

> INCLUDES Cardiac output review
> Insertion catheter into 1+ right cardiac chambers or areas
> Obtaining samples for blood gas

Code also administration of medication or exercise to repeat assessment of hemodynamic measurement (93463-93464)

> EXCLUDES *Catheterization procedures that include right side of heart (93453, 93456-93457, 93460-93461)*
> *Indicator dilution studies (93561-93562)*
> *Insertion of hemodynamic monitor when done for a reason other than insertion or maintenance of hemodynamic monitoring system (0293T-0294T)*
> *Mitral valve repair (0345T)*
> *Percutaneous repair congenital interatrial defect (93580)*
> *Swan-Ganz catheter insertion (93503)*

🚑 22.2   ⚕ 22.2   **FUD** 000   ⊘ T 80 ▣

AMA: 2016,Mar,5; 2016,Jan,13; 2015,Sep,3; 2015,Jan,16; 2014,Jul,3; 2014,Jan,11; 2013,May,12; 2012,Mar,9-10; 2011,Aug,3-5; 2011,Dec,9-12

Arteries of the Heart

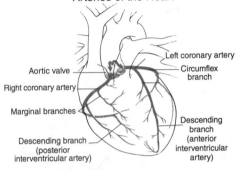

▲ **93452** **Left heart catheterization including intraprocedural injection(s) for left ventriculography, imaging supervision and interpretation, when performed**

> INCLUDES Insertion of catheter into left cardiac chambers

> EXCLUDES *Catheterization procedures that include injections for left ventriculography (93453, 93458-93461)*
> *Injection procedures (93561-93565)*
> *Insertion of hemodynamic monitor when done for a reason other than insertion or maintenance of hemodynamic monitoring system (0293T-0294T)*
> *Percutaneous repair congenital interatrial defect (93580)*
> *Services related to cardiac contractility modulation systems (0408T-0411T, 0414T-0415T)*
> *Swan-Ganz catheter insertion (93503)*

Code also administration of medication or exercise to repeat assessment of hemodynamic measurement (93463-93464)
Code also transapical or transseptal puncture (93462)

🚑 25.0   ⚕ 25.0   **FUD** 000   T 80 ▣

AMA: 2016,Jan,13; 2015,Jan,16; 2014,Jul,3; 2014,Jan,11; 2013,May,12; 2013,Jan,6-8; 2012,Mar,9-10; 2011,Aug,3-5; 2011,Dec,9-12

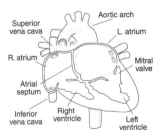

Left heart is catheterized

● New Code   ▲ Revised Code   ○ Reinstated   ● New Web Release   ▲ Revised Web Release   Unlisted   Not Covered   # Resequenced
⊘ AMA Mod 51 Exempt   ⑤ Optum Mod 51 Exempt   ⑥ Mod 63 Exempt   ✗ Non-FDA Drug   ★ Telehealth   M Maternity   A Age Edit   + Add-on   **AMA:** CPT Asst
© 2016 Optum360, LLC   CPT © 2016 American Medical Association. All Rights Reserved.

▲ 93453 Combined right and left heart catheterization including intraprocedural injection(s) for left ventriculography, imaging supervision and interpretation, when performed

INCLUDES Cardiac output review

Insertion catheter into 1+ right cardiac chambers or areas

Insertion of catheter into left cardiac chambers

Obtaining samples for blood gas

EXCLUDES *Catheterization procedures (93451-93452, 93456-93461)*

Injection procedures (93561-93565)

Insertion of hemodynamic monitor when done for a reason other than insertion or maintenance of hemodynamic monitoring system (0293T-0294T)

Mitral valve repair (0345T)

Percutaneous repair congenital interatrial defect (93580)

Services related to cardiac contractility modulation systems (0408T-0411T, 0414T-0415T)

Swan-Ganz catheter insertion (93503)

Code also administration of medication or exercise to repeat assessment of hemodynamic measurement (93463-93464)

Code also transapical or transseptal puncture (93462)

🚑 32.3 ⚕ 32.3 **FUD** 000 T 80 🖥

AMA: 2016,Mar,5; 2016,Jan,13; 2015,Sep,3; 2015,Jan,16; 2014,Jul,3; 2014,Jan,11; 2013,May,12; 2013,Jan,6-8; 2012,Mar,9-10; 2011,Aug,3-5; 2011,Dec,9-12

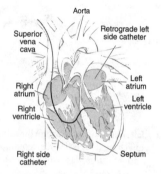

Both sides of the heart are catheterized

▲ 93454 Catheter placement in coronary artery(s) for coronary angiography, including intraprocedural injection(s) for coronary angiography, imaging supervision and interpretation;

EXCLUDES *Injection procedures (93561-93565)*

Mitral valve repair (0345T)

Swan-Ganz catheter insertion (93503)

🚑 25.4 ⚕ 25.4 **FUD** 000 T 80 🖥

AMA: 2016,Mar,5; 2016,Jan,13; 2015,Jan,16; 2014,Dec,6; 2014,Jul,3; 2014,Jan,11; 2013,May,12; 2012,Mar,9-10; 2011,Aug,3-5; 2011,Dec,9-12

▲ 93455 with catheter placement(s) in bypass graft(s) (internal mammary, free arterial, venous grafts) including intraprocedural injection(s) for bypass graft angiography

EXCLUDES *Injection procedures (93561-93565)*

Percutaneous repair congenital interatrial defect (93580)

Swan-Ganz catheter insertion (93503)

🚑 29.5 ⚕ 29.5 **FUD** 000 T 80 🖥

AMA: 2016,Mar,5; 2016,Jan,13; 2015,Jan,16; 2014,Dec,6; 2014,Jul,3; 2014,Jan,11; 2013,May,12; 2012,Mar,9-10; 2011,Aug,3-5; 2011,Dec,9-12

▲ 93456 with right heart catheterization

INCLUDES Cardiac output review

Insertion catheter into 1+ right cardiac chambers or areas

Obtaining samples for blood gas

Code also administration of medication or exercise to repeat assessment of hemodynamic measurement (93463-93464)

EXCLUDES *Injection procedures (93561-93565)*

Mitral valve repair (0345T)

Percutaneous repair congenital interatrial defect (93580)

Swan-Ganz catheter insertion (93503)

🚑 31.8 ⚕ 31.8 **FUD** 000 ⊘ T 80 🖥

AMA: 2016,Mar,5; 2016,Jan,13; 2015,Sep,3; 2015,Jan,16; 2014,Dec,6; 2014,Jul,3; 2014,Jan,11; 2013,May,12; 2012,Mar,9-10; 2011,Aug,3-5; 2011,Dec,9-12

▲ 93457 with catheter placement(s) in bypass graft(s) (internal mammary, free arterial, venous grafts) including intraprocedural injection(s) for bypass graft angiography and right heart catheterization

INCLUDES Cardiac output review

Insertion catheter into 1+ right cardiac chambers or areas

Obtaining samples for blood gas

EXCLUDES *Injection procedures (93561-93565)*

Percutaneous repair congenital interatrial defect (93580)

Swan-Ganz catheter insertion (93503)

Code also administration of medication or exercise to repeat assessment of hemodynamic measurement (93463-93464)

🚑 35.9 ⚕ 35.9 **FUD** 000 T 80 🖥

AMA: 2016,Mar,5; 2016,Jan,13; 2015,Sep,3; 2015,Jan,16; 2014,Dec,6; 2014,Jul,3; 2014,Jan,11; 2013,May,12; 2012,Mar,9-10; 2011,Aug,3-5; 2011,Dec,9-12

▲ 93458 with left heart catheterization including intraprocedural injection(s) for left ventriculography, when performed

INCLUDES Insertion of catheter into left cardiac chambers

EXCLUDES *Injection procedures (93561-93565)*

Percutaneous repair congenital interatrial defect (93580)

Services related to cardiac contractility modulation systems (0408T-0411T, 0414T-0415T)

Swan-Ganz catheter insertion (93503)

Code also administration of medication or exercise to repeat assessment of hemodynamic measurement (93463-93464)

Code also transapical or transseptal puncture (93462)

🚑 30.4 ⚕ 30.4 **FUD** 000 T 80 🖥

AMA: 2016,Mar,5; 2016,Jan,13; 2015,Sep,3; 2015,Jan,16; 2014,Dec,6; 2014,Jul,3; 2014,Jan,11; 2013,May,12; 2013,Jan,6-8; 2012,Mar,9-10; 2011,Aug,3-5; 2011,Dec,9-12

▲ 93459 with left heart catheterization including intraprocedural injection(s) for left ventriculography, when performed, catheter placement(s) in bypass graft(s) (internal mammary, free arterial, venous grafts) with bypass graft angiography

INCLUDES Insertion of catheter into left cardiac chambers

EXCLUDES *Injection procedures (93561-93565)*

Percutaneous repair congenital interatrial defect (93580)

Services related to cardiac contractility modulation systems (0408T-0411T, 0414T-0415T)

Swan-Ganz catheter insertion (93503)

Code also administration of medication or exercise to repeat assessment of hemodynamic measurement (93463-93464)

Code also transapical or transseptal puncture (93462)

🚑 33.6 ⚕ 33.6 **FUD** 000 T 80 🖥

AMA: 2016,Mar,5; 2016,Jan,13; 2015,Sep,3; 2015,Jan,16; 2014,Dec,6; 2014,Jul,3; 2014,Jan,11; 2013,May,12; 2013,Jan,6-8; 2012,Mar,9-10; 2011,Aug,3-5; 2011,Dec,9-12

▲ 93460 **with right and left heart catheterization including intraprocedural injection(s) for left ventriculography, when performed**

INCLUDES Cardiac output review
Insertion catheter into 1+ right cardiac chambers or areas
Insertion of catheter into left cardiac chambers
Obtaining samples for blood gas

EXCLUDES *Injection procedures (93561-93565)*
Percutaneous repair congenital interatrial defect (93580)
Services related to cardiac contractility modulation systems (0408T-0411T, 0414T-0415T)
Swan-Ganz catheter insertion (93503)

Code also administration of medication or exercise to repeat assessment of hemodynamic measurement (93463-93464)
Code also transapical or transseptal puncture (93462)

🚑 36.1   ⚕ 36.1   **FUD** 000   T 80 ▭

AMA: 2016,Mar,5; 2016,Jan,13; 2015,Sep,3; 2015,Jan,16; 2014,Dec,6; 2014,Jul,3; 2014,Jan,11; 2013,May,12; 2013,Jan,6-8; 2012,Mar,9-10; 2011,Aug,3-5; 2011,Dec,9-12

▲ 93461 **with right and left heart catheterization including intraprocedural injection(s) for left ventriculography, when performed, catheter placement(s) in bypass graft(s) (internal mammary, free arterial, venous grafts) with bypass graft angiography**

INCLUDES Cardiac output review
Insertion catheter into 1+ right cardiac chambers or areas
Insertion of catheter into left cardiac chambers
Obtaining samples for blood gas

EXCLUDES *Injection procedures (93561-93565)*
Mitral valve repair (0345T)
Percutaneous repair congenital interatrial defect (93580)
Services related to cardiac contractility modulation systems (0408T-0411T, 0414T-0415T)
Swan-Ganz catheter insertion (93503)

Code also administration of medication or exercise to repeat assessment of hemodynamic measurement (93463-93464)
Code also transapical or transseptal puncture (93462)

🚑 41.3   ⚕ 41.3   **FUD** 000   T 80 ▭

AMA: 2016,Mar,5; 2016,Jan,13; 2015,Sep,3; 2015,Jan,16; 2014,Dec,6; 2014,Jul,3; 2014,Jan,11; 2013,May,12; 2013,Jan,6-8; 2012,Mar,9-10; 2011,Aug,3-5; 2011,Dec,9-12

▲ + 93462 **Left heart catheterization by transseptal puncture through intact septum or by transapical puncture (List separately in addition to code for primary procedure)**

INCLUDES Insertion of catheter into left cardiac chambers

EXCLUDES *Comprehensive electrophysiologic evaluation (93656)*
Mitral valve repair (0345T)

Code first (33477, 93452-93453, 93458-93461, 93582, 93653-93654)

🚑 6.07   ⚕ 6.07   **FUD** ZZZ   N 80 ▭

AMA: 2016,Jan,13; 2015,Sep,3; 2015,Jan,16; 2014,Jul,3; 2014,Jan,11; 2013,Jun,6-8; 2013,May,12; 2012,Mar,9-10; 2011,Aug,3-5; 2011,Dec,9-12

▲ + 93463 **Pharmacologic agent administration (eg, inhaled nitric oxide, intravenous infusion of nitroprusside, dobutamine, milrinone, or other agent) including assessing hemodynamic measurements before, during, after and repeat pharmacologic agent administration, when performed (List separately in addition to code for primary procedure)**

EXCLUDES *Coronary interventional procedures (92920-92944, 92975, 92977)*
Use of code more than one time per catheterization

Code first (33477, 93451-93453, 93456-93461, 93530-93533, 93580-93581)

🚑 2.81   ⚕ 2.81   **FUD** ZZZ   N 80 ▭

AMA: 2016,Jan,13; 2015,Jan,16; 2014,Dec,6; 2014,Jul,3; 2014,Jan,11; 2012,Mar,9-10; 2011,Aug,3-5; 2011,Dec,9-12

▲ + 93464 **Physiologic exercise study (eg, bicycle or arm ergometry) including assessing hemodynamic measurements before and after (List separately in addition to code for primary procedure)**

EXCLUDES *Administration of pharmacologic agent (93463)*
Bundle of His recording (93600)
Use of code more than one time per catheterization

Code first (33477, 93451-93453, 93456-93461, 93530-93533)

🚑 7.76   ⚕ 7.76   **FUD** ZZZ   N 80 ▭

AMA: 2016,Jan,13; 2015,Jan,16; 2014,Jul,3; 2014,Jan,11; 2012,Mar,9-10; 2011,Aug,3-5; 2011,Dec,9-12

93503 **Insertion and placement of flow directed catheter (eg, Swan-Ganz) for monitoring purposes**

EXCLUDES *Diagnostic cardiac catheterization (93451-93461, 93530-93533)*
Subsequent monitoring (99356-99357)

🚑 3.70   ⚕ 3.70   **FUD** 000   ⊘ T 80 ▭

AMA: 2016,Jan,13; 2015,Jan,16; 2014,Jan,11; 2012,Jan,15-42; 2011,Aug,3-5; 2011,Dec,14-18

▲ 93505 **Endomyocardial biopsy**

EXCLUDES *Intravascular brachytherapy radionuclide insertion (77770-77772)*
Transcatheter insertion of brachytherapy delivery device (92974)

🚑 21.6   ⚕ 21.6   **FUD** 000   T 80 ▭

AMA: 2016,Jan,13; 2015,Jan,16; 2014,Jan,11; 2012,Jan,15-42; 2011,Aug,3-5; 2011,Jan,11

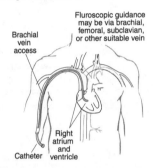

Fluroscopic guidance may be via brachial, femoral, subclavian, or other suitable vein

Brachial vein access

Right atrium and ventricle

Catheter

93530-93533 Congenital Heart Defect Catheterization

INCLUDES Access site imaging and placement of closure device
Cardiac output review
Insertion catheter into 1+ right cardiac chambers or areas
Obtaining samples for blood gas
Radiology supervision and interpretation
Roadmapping angiography

EXCLUDES *Cardiac cath on noncongenital heart (93451-93453, 93456-93461)*
Percutaneous repair congenital interatrial defect (93580)
Swan-Ganz catheter insertion (93503)

Code also (93563-93568)

▲ 93530 **Right heart catheterization, for congenital cardiac anomalies**

🚑 0.00   ⚕ 0.00   **FUD** 000   T 80 ▭

AMA: 2016,Mar,5; 2016,Jan,13; 2015,Sep,3; 2015,Jan,16; 2014,Jul,3; 2014,Jan,11; 2013,May,12; 2012,Mar,9-10; 2012,Jan,15-42; 2011,Aug,3-5; 2011,Dec,9-12; 2011,Jan,11

93531 **Combined right heart catheterization and retrograde left heart catheterization, for congenital cardiac anomalies**

🚑 0.00   ⚕ 0.00   **FUD** 000   T 80 ▭

AMA: 2016,Mar,5; 2016,Jan,13; 2015,Sep,3; 2015,Jan,16; 2014,Jul,3; 2014,Jan,11; 2012,Mar,9-10; 2011,Aug,3-5; 2011,Dec,9-12

93532 **Combined right heart catheterization and transseptal left heart catheterization through intact septum with or without retrograde left heart catheterization, for congenital cardiac anomalies**

🚑 0.00   ⚕ 0.00   **FUD** 000   T 80 ▭

AMA: 2016,Mar,5; 2016,Jan,13; 2015,Sep,3; 2015,Jan,16; 2014,Jul,3; 2014,Jan,11; 2012,Mar,9-10; 2012,Jan,15-42; 2011,Aug,3-5; 2011,Dec,9-12; 2011,Jan,11

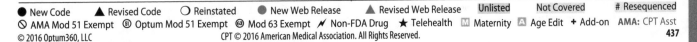

93533 Combined right heart catheterization and transseptal left heart catheterization through existing septal opening, with or without retrograde left heart catheterization, for congenital cardiac anomalies

📷 0.00 ⚕ 0.00 **FUD** 000   T 80 🖵

AMA: 2016,Mar,5; 2016,Jan,13; 2015,Sep,3; 2015,Jan,16; 2014,Jul,3; 2014,Jan,11; 2012,Mar,9-10; 2011,Aug,3-5; 2011,Dec,9-12

93561-93568 Injection Procedures

INCLUDES Catheter repositioning
Radiology supervision and interpretation
Using automatic power injector

▲ **93561** Indicator dilution studies such as dye or thermodilution, including arterial and/or venous catheterization; with cardiac output measurement (separate procedure)

EXCLUDES Cardiac output, radioisotope method (78472-78473, 78481)
Catheterization procedures (93451-93462)
Percutaneous closure patent ductus arteriosus (93582)

📷 0.00 ⚕ 0.00 **FUD** 000   N 80 🖵

AMA: 2016,Jan,13; 2015,Jan,16; 2014,Jul,3; 2014,Jan,11; 2012,Jan,15-42; 2011,Aug,3-5; 2011,Jan,11

▲ **93562** subsequent measurement of cardiac output

EXCLUDES Cardiac output, radioisotope method (78472-78473, 78481)
Catheterization procedures (93451-93462)
Percutaneous closure patent ductus arteriosus (93582)

📷 0.00 ⚕ 0.00 **FUD** 000   N 80 🖵

AMA: 2016,Jan,13; 2015,Jan,16; 2014,Jul,3; 2014,May,4; 2014,Jan,11; 2011,Aug,3-5

▲ + **93563** Injection procedure during cardiac catheterization including imaging supervision, interpretation, and report; for selective coronary angiography during congenital heart catheterization (List separately in addition to code for primary procedure)

EXCLUDES Catheterization procedures (93452-93461)
Mitral valve repair (0345T)
Code first (93530-93533)

📷 1.70 ⚕ 1.70 **FUD** ZZZ   N 80 🖵

AMA: 2016,Mar,5; 2016,Jan,13; 2015,Jan,16; 2014,Dec,6; 2014,Jan,11; 2013,Jan,6-8; 2011,Aug,3-5; 2011,Dec,9-12

▲ + **93564** for selective opacification of aortocoronary venous or arterial bypass graft(s) (eg, aortocoronary saphenous vein, free radial artery, or free mammary artery graft) to one or more coronary arteries and in situ arterial conduits (eg, internal mammary), whether native or used for bypass to one or more coronary arteries during congenital heart catheterization, when performed (List separately in addition to code for primary procedure)

EXCLUDES Catheterization procedures (93452-93461)
Mitral valve repair (0345T)
Percutaneous repair congenital interatrial defect (93580)
Code first (93530-93533)

📷 1.78 ⚕ 1.78 **FUD** ZZZ   N 80 🖵

AMA: 2016,Mar,5; 2016,Jan,13; 2015,Jan,16; 2014,Dec,6; 2014,Jan,11; 2013,Jan,6-8; 2011,Aug,3-5; 2011,Dec,9-12

▲ + **93565** for selective left ventricular or left atrial angiography (List separately in addition to code for primary procedure)

EXCLUDES Catheterization procedures (93452-93461)
Percutaneous repair congenital interatrial defect (93580)
Code first (93530-93533)

📷 1.33 ⚕ 1.33 **FUD** ZZZ   N 80 🖵

AMA: 2016,Jan,13; 2015,Jan,16; 2014,Jan,11; 2013,Jan,6-8; 2011,Aug,3-5; 2011,Dec,9-12

▲ + **93566** for selective right ventricular or right atrial angiography (List separately in addition to code for primary procedure)

EXCLUDES Percutaneous repair congenital interatrial defect (93580)
Use for right ventriculography when performed during insertion leadless pacemaker (0387T)
Code first (93451, 93453, 93456-93457, 93460-93461, 93530-93533)

📷 1.34 ⚕ 4.86 **FUD** ZZZ   N 80 🖵

AMA: 2016,Aug,5; 2016,May,5; 2016,Mar,5; 2016,Jan,13; 2015,May,3; 2015,Jan,16; 2014,Jan,11; 2013,Jan,6-8; 2011,Aug,3-5; 2011,Dec,9-12

▲ + **93567** for supravalvular aortography (List separately in addition to code for primary procedure)

EXCLUDES Abdominal aortography or non-supravalvular thoracic aortography at same time as cardiac catheterization (36221, 75600-75630)
Code first (93451-93461, 93530-93533)

📷 1.52 ⚕ 4.01 **FUD** ZZZ   N 80 🖵

AMA: 2016,Mar,5; 2016,Jan,13; 2015,Jan,16; 2014,Jan,11; 2013,Jan,6-8; 2011,Aug,3-5; 2011,Dec,9-12

▲ + **93568** for pulmonary angiography (List separately in addition to code for primary procedure)

Code first (93451, 93453, 93456-93457, 93460-93461, 93530-93533)

📷 1.37 ⚕ 4.36 **FUD** ZZZ   N 80 🖵

AMA: 2016,Mar,5; 2016,Jan,13; 2015,Jan,16; 2014,Jan,11; 2013,Jan,6-8; 2011,Aug,3-5; 2011,Dec,9-12

93571-93572 Coronary Artery Doppler Studies

INCLUDES Doppler transducer manipulations/repositioning within the vessel examined, during coronary angiography/therapeutic intervention (angioplasty)

▲ + **93571** Intravascular Doppler velocity and/or pressure derived coronary flow reserve measurement (coronary vessel or graft) during coronary angiography including pharmacologically induced stress; initial vessel (List separately in addition to code for primary procedure)

Code first (92920, 92924, 92928, 92933, 92937, 92941, 92943, 92975, 93454-93461, 93563-93564)

📷 0.00 ⚕ 0.00 **FUD** ZZZ   N 80 🖵

AMA: 2016,Jan,13; 2015,Dec,18; 2015,May,10; 2015,Jan,16; 2014,Dec,6; 2014,Jan,11; 2011,Aug,3-5

▲ + **93572** each additional vessel (List separately in addition to code for primary procedure)

Code first initial vessel (93571)

📷 0.00 ⚕ 0.00 **FUD** ZZZ   N 80 🖵

AMA: 2016,Jan,13; 2015,Dec,18; 2015,May,10; 2015,Jan,16; 2014,Dec,6; 2014,Jan,11; 2011,Aug,3-5

93580-93583 Percutaneous Repair of Congenital Heart Defects

93580 Percutaneous transcatheter closure of congenital interatrial communication (ie, Fontan fenestration, atrial septal defect) with implant

INCLUDES Injection of contrast for right heart atrial/ventricular angiograms (93564-93566)
Right heart catheterization (93451, 93453, 93456-93457, 93460-93461, 93530-93533)

EXCLUDES Bypass graft angiography (93455)
Injection of contrast for left heart atrial/ventricular angiograms (93458-93459)
Left heart catheterization (93452, 93458-93459)
Code also echocardiography, when performed (93303-93317, 93662)

📷 28.4 ⚕ 28.4 **FUD** 000   J 80 🖵

AMA: 2016,Jan,13; 2015,Jan,16; 2014,Jan,11; 2012,Jan,15-42; 2011,Jan,11

93581 Percutaneous transcatheter closure of a congenital ventricular septal defect with implant

> INCLUDES Injection of contrast for right heart atrial/ventricular angiograms (93564-93566)
> Right heart catheterization (93451, 93453, 93456-93457, 93460-93461, 93530-93533)
> EXCLUDES *Bypass graft angiography (93455)*
> *Injection of contrast for left heart atrial/ventricular angiograms (93458-93459)*
> *Left heart catheterization (93452, 93458-93459)*
> Code also echocardiography, when performed (93303-93317, 93662)

🔲 38.7 ⚖ 38.7 **FUD** 000   J 80 🖵

AMA: 2016,Jan,13; 2015,Jan,16; 2014,Jan,11; 2012,Jan,15-42; 2011,Jan,11

▲ **93582** Percutaneous transcatheter closure of patent ductus arteriosus

> INCLUDES Aorta catheter placement (36200)
> Aortography (75600-75605, 93567)
> Heart catheterization (93451-93461, 93530-93533)
> EXCLUDES *Catheterization pulmonary artery (36013-36014)*
> *Intracardiac echocardiographic services (93662)*
> *Left heart catheterization performed via transapical puncture or transseptal puncture through intact septum (93462)*
> *Ligation repair (33820, 33822, 33824)*
> *Other cardiac angiographic procedures (93563-93566, 93568)*
> *Other echocardiographic services by different provider (93315-93317)*

🔲 19.4 ⚖ 19.4 **FUD** 000   J 80 🖵

AMA: 2016,Jan,13; 2015,Jan,16; 2014,Jul,3

▲ **93583** Percutaneous transcatheter septal reduction therapy (eg, alcohol septal ablation) including temporary pacemaker insertion when performed

🔲 21.9 ⚖ 21.9 **FUD** 000   C 80 🖵

> INCLUDES Alcohol injection (93463)
> Coronary angiography during the procedure to roadmap, guide the intervention, measure the vessel, and complete the angiography (93454-93461, 93531-93533, 93563, 93563, 93565)
> Left heart catheterization (93452-93453, 93458-93461, 93531-93533)
> Temporary pacemaker insertion (33210)
> EXCLUDES *Intracardiac echocardiographic services when performed (93662)*
> *Myectomy (surgical ventriculomyotomy) to treat idiopathic hypertrophic subaortic stenosis (33416)*
> *Other echocardiographic services rendered by different provider (93312-93317)*
> Code also diagnostic cardiac catheterization procedures if the patient's condition (clinical indication) has changed since the intervention or prior study, there is no available prior catheter-based diagnostic study of the treatment zone, or the prior study is not adequate (93451, 93454-93457, 93530, 93563-93564, 93566-93568)

93590-93592 Percutaneous Repair Paravalvular Leak

> INCLUDES Access with insertion and positioning of device
> Angiography
> Fluoroscopy (76000)
> Imaging guidance
> Left heart catheterization (93452-93453, 93459-93461, 93531-93533)
> Code also diagnostic right heart catheterization and angiography performed when:
> Code also when there is no previous study and a complete diagnostic study is performed; append modifier 59
> Code also if a previous study is available, but documentation states the patient's condition has changed since the previous study; visualization is insufficient; or a change necessitates reevaluation; append modifier 59

● **93590** Percutaneous transcatheter closure of paravalvular leak; initial occlusion device, mitral valve

> INCLUDES Transseptal puncture (93462)
> Code also for transapical puncture (93462)

● **93591** initial occlusion device, aortic valve

> EXCLUDES *Transapical or transseptal puncture (93462)*

● + **93592** each additional occlusion device (List separately in addition to code for primary procedure)

🔲 0.00 ⚖ 0.00 **FUD** 000

> Code first (93590-93591)

93600-93603 Recording of Intracardiac Electrograms

> INCLUDES Unusual situations where there may be recording/pacing/attempt at arrhythmia induction from only one side of the heart
> EXCLUDES *Comprehensive electrophysiological studies (93619-93620, 93653-93654, 93656)*

93600 Bundle of His recording

🔲 0.00 ⚖ 0.00 **FUD** 000   ⊘ J 80 🖵

AMA: 2016,Jan,13; 2015,Jan,16; 2014,Apr,3; 2014,Jan,11; 2013,Jul,7-9; 2013,Jun,6-8; 2012,Jan,15-42; 2011,Jan,11

93602 Intra-atrial recording

🔲 0.00 ⚖ 0.00 **FUD** 000   ⊘ J 80 🖵

AMA: 2016,Jan,13; 2015,Jan,16; 2014,Apr,3; 2014,Jan,11; 2013,Jul,7-9; 2013,Jun,6-8; 2012,Jan,15-42; 2011,Jan,11

93603 Right ventricular recording

🔲 0.00 ⚖ 0.00 **FUD** 000   ⊘ J 80 🖵

AMA: 2016,Jan,13; 2015,Jan,16; 2014,Apr,3; 2014,Jan,11; 2013,Jul,7-9; 2013,Jun,6-8

93609-93613 Intracardiac Mapping and Pacing

▲ + **93609** Intraventricular and/or intra-atrial mapping of tachycardia site(s) with catheter manipulation to record from multiple sites to identify origin of tachycardia (List separately in addition to code for primary procedure)

> EXCLUDES *Intracardiac 3D mapping (93613)*
> *Intracardiac ablation with 3D mapping (93654)*
> Code first (93620, 93653, 93656)

🔲 0.00 ⚖ 0.00 **FUD** ZZZ   N 80 🖵

AMA: 2016,Jan,13; 2015,Jan,16; 2014,Apr,3; 2014,Jan,11; 2013,Jul,7-9; 2013,Jun,6-8

93610 Intra-atrial pacing

> INCLUDES Unusual situations where there may be recording/pacing/attempt at arrhythmia induction from only one side of the heart
> EXCLUDES *Comprehensive electrophysiological studies (93619-93620)*
> *Intracardiac ablation (93653-93654, 93656)*

🔲 0.00 ⚖ 0.00 **FUD** 000   ⊘ J 80 🖵

AMA: 2016,Jan,13; 2015,Jan,16; 2014,Apr,3; 2014,Jan,11; 2013,Jul,7-9; 2013,Jun,6-8

93612 Intraventricular pacing

> INCLUDES Unusual situations where there may be recording/pacing/attempt at arrhythmia induction from only one side of the heart
> EXCLUDES *Comprehensive electrophysiological studies (93619-93622)*
> *Intracardiac ablation (93653-93654, 93656)*

🔲 0.00 ⚖ 0.00 **FUD** 000   ⊘ J 80 🖵

AMA: 2016,Jan,13; 2015,Jan,16; 2014,Apr,3; 2014,Jan,11; 2013,Jul,7-9; 2013,Jun,6-8

▲ + **93613** Intracardiac electrophysiologic 3-dimensional mapping (List separately in addition to code for primary procedure)

> EXCLUDES *Intracardiac ablation with 3D mapping (93654)*
> *Mapping of tachycardia site (93609)*
> Code first (93620, 93653, 93656)

🔲 11.5 ⚖ 11.5 **FUD** ZZZ   N 80 🖵

AMA: 2016,Jan,13; 2015,Jan,16; 2014,Apr,3; 2014,Jan,11; 2013,Jul,7-9; 2013,Jun,6-8

93615-93616 Recording and Pacing via Esophagus

▲ **93615** Esophageal recording of atrial electrogram with or without ventricular electrogram(s);

🔲 0.00 ⚖ 0.00 **FUD** 000   ⊘ J 80 🖵

AMA: 2016,Jan,13; 2015,Jan,16; 2014,Jan,11

▲ **93616** **with pacing**
📷 0.00 ✂ 0.00 **FUD** 000 ⊘ J 80 💻
AMA: 2016,Jan,13; 2015,Jan,16; 2014,Jan,11

93618 Pacing to Produce an Arrhythmia

CMS: 100-03,20.12 Diagnostic Endocardial Electrical Stimulation (Pacing)

INCLUDES Unusual situations where there may be recording/pacing/attempt at arrhythmia induction from only one side of the heart

EXCLUDES *Comprehensive electrophysiological studies (93619-93622)*
Intracardiac ablation (93653-93654, 93656)
Intracardiac phonocardiogram (93799)

▲ **93618** **Induction of arrhythmia by electrical pacing**
📷 0.00 ✂ 0.00 **FUD** 000 ⊘ J 80 💻
AMA: 2016,Jan,13; 2015,Jan,16; 2014,Apr,3; 2014,Jan,11; 2013,Jul,7-9; 2013,Jun,6-8; 2012,Jan,15-42; 2011,Jan,11

93619-93623 Comprehensive Electrophysiological Studies

CMS: 100-03,20.12 Diagnostic Endocardial Electrical Stimulation (Pacing)

▲ **93619** **Comprehensive electrophysiologic evaluation with right atrial pacing and recording, right ventricular pacing and recording, His bundle recording, including insertion and repositioning of multiple electrode catheters, without induction or attempted induction of arrhythmia**

INCLUDES Evaluation of sinus node/atrioventricular node/His-Purkinje conduction system without arrhythmia induction

EXCLUDES *Comprehensive electrophysiological studies (93620-93622)*
Intracardiac ablation (93653-93657)
Intracardiac pacing (93610, 93612, 93618)
Recording of intracardiac electrograms (93600-93603)
📷 0.00 ✂ 0.00 **FUD** 000 J 80 💻
AMA: 2016,Jan,13; 2015,Jan,16; 2014,Apr,3; 2014,Jan,11; 2013,Jul,7-9; 2013,Jun,6-8; 2012,Nov,6-9; 2012,Jan,15-42; 2011,Jan,11

▲ **93620** **Comprehensive electrophysiologic evaluation including insertion and repositioning of multiple electrode catheters with induction or attempted induction of arrhythmia; with right atrial pacing and recording, right ventricular pacing and recording, His bundle recording**

INCLUDES Recording/pacing/attempted arrhythmia induction from one or more site(s) in the heart

EXCLUDES *Comprehensive electrophysiological study without induction/attempted induction arrhythmia (93619)*
Intracardiac ablation (93653-93657)
Intracardiac pacing (93610, 93612, 93618)
Recording of intracardiac electrograms (93600-93603)
📷 0.00 ✂ 0.00 **FUD** 000 J 80 💻
AMA: 2016,Jan,13; 2015,Jan,16; 2014,Apr,3; 2014,Jan,11; 2013,Jul,7-9; 2013,Jun,6-8; 2012,Nov,6-9; 2012,Jan,15-42; 2011,Jan,11

▲ + **93621** **with left atrial pacing and recording from coronary sinus or left atrium (List separately in addition to code for primary procedure)**

INCLUDES Recording/pacing/attempted arrhythmia induction from one or more site(s) in the heart

EXCLUDES *Intracardiac ablation (93656)*
Code first (93620, 93653-93654)
📷 0.00 ✂ 0.00 **FUD** ZZZ N 80 💻
AMA: 2016,Jan,13; 2015,Jan,16; 2014,Apr,3; 2014,Jan,11; 2013,Jul,7-9; 2013,Jun,6-8; 2012,Nov,6-9; 2012,Jan,15-42; 2011,Jan,11

▲ + **93622** **with left ventricular pacing and recording (List separately in addition to code for primary procedure)**

EXCLUDES *Intracardiac ablation (93654)*
Code first (93620, 93653, 93656)
📷 0.00 ✂ 0.00 **FUD** ZZZ N 80 💻
AMA: 2016,Jan,13; 2015,Jan,16; 2014,Apr,3; 2014,Jan,11; 2013,Jul,7-9; 2013,Jun,6-8; 2012,Nov,6-9; 2012,Jan,15-42; 2011,Jan,11

+ **93623** **Programmed stimulation and pacing after intravenous drug infusion (List separately in addition to code for primary procedure)**

INCLUDES Recording/pacing/attempted arrhythmia induction from one or more site(s) in the heart
Code first comprehensive electrophysiologic evaluation (93610, 93612, 93619-93620, 93653-93654, 93656)
📷 0.00 ✂ 0.00 **FUD** ZZZ N 80 💻
AMA: 2016,Jan,13; 2015,Jan,16; 2014,Apr,3; 2014,Jan,11; 2013,Jul,7-9; 2012,Jan,15-42; 2011,Jan,11

93624-93631 Followup and Intraoperative Electrophysiologic Studies

CMS: 100-03,20.12 Diagnostic Endocardial Electrical Stimulation (Pacing)

▲ **93624** **Electrophysiologic follow-up study with pacing and recording to test effectiveness of therapy, including induction or attempted induction of arrhythmia**

INCLUDES Recording/pacing/attempted arrhythmia induction from one or more site(s) in the heart
📷 0.00 ✂ 0.00 **FUD** 000 J 80 💻
AMA: 2016,Jan,13; 2015,Jan,16; 2014,Jan,11

93631 **Intra-operative epicardial and endocardial pacing and mapping to localize the site of tachycardia or zone of slow conduction for surgical correction**

EXCLUDES *Operative ablation of an arrhythmogenic focus or pathway by a separate provider (33250-33261)*
📷 0.00 ✂ 0.00 **FUD** 000 ⊘ N 80 💻
AMA: 2016,Jan,13; 2015,Jan,16; 2014,Jan,11

93640-93644 Electrophysiologic Studies of Cardioverter-Defibrillators

INCLUDES Recording/pacing/attempted arrhythmia induction from one or more site(s) in the heart

▲ **93640** **Electrophysiologic evaluation of single or dual chamber pacing cardioverter-defibrillator leads including defibrillation threshold evaluation (induction of arrhythmia, evaluation of sensing and pacing for arrhythmia termination) at time of initial implantation or replacement;**
📷 0.00 ✂ 0.00 **FUD** 000 N 80 💻
AMA: 2016,Jan,13; 2015,Jan,16; 2014,Jan,11; 2012,Jun,3-9

▲ **93641** **with testing of single or dual chamber pacing cardioverter-defibrillator pulse generator**

EXCLUDES *Single/dual chamber pacing cardioverter-defibrillators reprogramming/electronic analysis, subsequent/periodic (93282-93283, 93289, 93292, 93295, 93642)*
📷 0.00 ✂ 0.00 **FUD** 000 N 80 💻
AMA: 2016,Jan,13; 2015,Jan,16; 2014,Apr,3; 2014,Jan,11; 2012,Jun,3-9

▲ **93642** **Electrophysiologic evaluation of single or dual chamber transvenous pacing cardioverter-defibrillator (includes defibrillation threshold evaluation, induction of arrhythmia, evaluation of sensing and pacing for arrhythmia termination, and programming or reprogramming of sensing or therapeutic parameters)**
📷 12.1 ✂ 12.1 **FUD** 000 J 80 💻
AMA: 2016,Jan,13; 2015,Jan,16; 2014,Apr,3; 2014,Jan,11; 2013,Jul,7-9; 2013,Jun,6-8

▲ **93644** **Electrophysiologic evaluation of subcutaneous implantable defibrillator (includes defibrillation threshold evaluation, induction of arrhythmia, evaluation of sensing for arrhythmia termination, and programming or reprogramming of sensing or therapeutic parameters)**
📷 7.88 ✂ 7.88 **FUD** 000 N 80 💻

EXCLUDES *Insertion/replacement subcutaneous implantable defibrillator ([33270])*
Subcutaneous cardioverter-defibrillator electrophysiologic evaluation, subsequent/periodic (93260-93261)

26/TC PC/TC Only   A2-Z3 ASC Payment   50 Bilateral   ♂ Male Only   ♀ Female Only   📷 Facility RVU   ✂ Non-Facility RVU   💻 CCI
FUD Follow-up Days   **CMS:** IOM (Pub 100)   A-Y OPPSI   80/80 Surg Assist Allowed / w/Doc   Lab Crosswalk   Radiology Crosswalk   CLIA

440

CPT © 2016 American Medical Association. All Rights Reserved.

© 2016 Optum360, LLC

93650-93657 Intracardiac Ablation

INCLUDES Ablation services include selective delivery of cryo-energy or
radiofrequency to targeted tissue
Electrophysiologic studies performed in the same session with ablation

▲ **93650** **Intracardiac catheter ablation of atrioventricular node
function, atrioventricular conduction for creation of complete
heart block, with or without temporary pacemaker
placement**
🔪 17.5   ⚕ 17.5   **FUD** 000   [J] [80] [□]
AMA: 2016,Jan,13; 2015,Jan,16; 2014,Jan,11; 2012,May,14-15;
2012,Apr,17-18

▲ **93653** **Comprehensive electrophysiologic evaluation including
insertion and repositioning of multiple electrode catheters
with induction or attempted induction of an arrhythmia with
right atrial pacing and recording, right ventricular pacing
and recording (when necessary), and His bundle recording
(when necessary) with intracardiac catheter ablation of
arrhythmogenic focus; with treatment of supraventricular
tachycardia by ablation of fast or slow atrioventricular
pathway, accessory atrioventricular connection,
cavo-tricuspid isthmus or other single atrial focus or source
of atrial re-entry**

EXCLUDES *Comprehensive electrophysiological studies
(93619-93620)*
*Electrophysiologic evaluation pacing cardioverter
defibrillator (93642)*
*Intracardiac ablation with transseptal catheterization
(93656)*
*Intracardiac ablation with treatment ventricular
arrhythmia (93654)*
Intracardiac pacing (93610, 93612, 93618)
Recording of intracardiac electrograms (93600-93603)
🔪 24.6   ⚕ 24.6   **FUD** 000   [J] [80] [□]
AMA: 2016,Jan,13; 2015,Jan,16; 2014,Apr,3; 2013,Jul,7-9;
2013,Jun,6-8

▲ **93654** **with treatment of ventricular tachycardia or focus of
ventricular ectopy including intracardiac
electrophysiologic 3D mapping, when performed, and left
ventricular pacing and recording, when performed**

EXCLUDES *Comprehensive electrophysiological studies
(93619-93620, 93622)*
Device evaluation (93279-93284, 93286-93289)
*Electrophysiologic evaluation pacing cardioverter
defibrillator (93642)*
*Intracardiac ablation with transseptal catheterization
(93656)*
*Intracardiac ablation with treatment supraventricular
tachycardia (93653)*
Intracardiac pacing (93609-93613, 93618)
Recording of intracardiac electrograms (93600-93603)
🔪 32.8   ⚕ 32.8   **FUD** 000   [J] [80] [□]
AMA: 2016,Jan,13; 2015,Jan,16; 2014,Apr,3; 2013,Jul,7-9;
2013,Jun,6-8

▲ + **93655** **Intracardiac catheter ablation of a discrete mechanism of
arrhythmia which is distinct from the primary ablated
mechanism, including repeat diagnostic maneuvers, to treat
a spontaneous or induced arrhythmia (List separately in
addition to code for primary procedure)**
Code first (93653-93654, 93656)
🔪 12.3   ⚕ 12.3   **FUD** ZZZ   [N] [80] [□]
AMA: 2016,Jan,13; 2015,Jan,16; 2014,Apr,3; 2013,Jul,7-9;
2013,Jun,6-8

▲ **93656** **Comprehensive electrophysiologic evaluation including
transseptal catheterizations, insertion and repositioning of
multiple electrode catheters with induction or attempted
induction of an arrhythmia including left or right atrial
pacing/recording when necessary, right ventricular
pacing/recording when necessary, and His bundle recording
when necessary with intracardiac catheter ablation of atrial
fibrillation by pulmonary vein isolation**

INCLUDES His bundle recording when indicated
Left atrial pacing/recording
Right ventricular pacing/recording
EXCLUDES *Comprehensive electrophysiological studies
(93619-93621)*
Device evaluation (93279-93284, 93286-93289)
*Electrophysiologic evaluation pacing cardioverter
defibrillator (93642)*
*Intracardiac ablation with transseptal catheterization
(93656)*
*Intracardiac ablation with treatment supraventricular
tachycardia (93653)*
Intracardiac pacing (93610, 93612, 93618)
Recording of intracardiac electrograms (93600-93603)
🔪 32.8   ⚕ 32.8   **FUD** 000   [J] [80] [□]
AMA: 2016,Jan,13; 2015,Jan,16; 2014,Apr,3; 2013,Jul,7-9;
2013,Jun,6-8

▲ + **93657** **Additional linear or focal intracardiac catheter ablation of
the left or right atrium for treatment of atrial fibrillation
remaining after completion of pulmonary vein isolation (List
separately in addition to code for primary procedure)**
Code first (93656)
🔪 12.3   ⚕ 12.3   **FUD** ZZZ   [N] [80] [□]
AMA: 2016,Jan,13; 2015,Jan,16; 2014,Apr,3; 2013,Jul,7-9;
2013,Jun,6-8

93660-93662 Other Tests for Cardiac Function

93660 **Evaluation of cardiovascular function with tilt table
evaluation, with continuous ECG monitoring and intermittent
blood pressure monitoring, with or without pharmacological
intervention**

EXCLUDES *Autonomic nervous system function testing (95921,
95924, [95943])*
🔪 4.46   ⚕ 4.46   **FUD** 000   [S] [80] [□]
AMA: 2016,Jan,13; 2015,Jan,16; 2014,Jan,11; 2012,Nov,6-9

Intracardiac Echocardiography

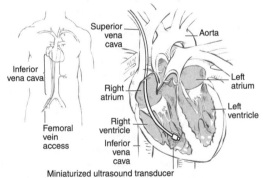

Miniaturized ultrasound transducer

+ **93662** **Intracardiac echocardiography during therapeutic/diagnostic
intervention, including imaging supervision and
interpretation (List separately in addition to code for primary
procedure)**

EXCLUDES *Internal cardioversion (92961)*
Code first (as appropriate) (92987, 93453, 93460-93462, 93532,
93580-93581, 93620-93622, 93653-93654, 93656)
🔪 0.00   ⚕ 0.00   **FUD** ZZZ   [N] [80] [□]
AMA: 2016,Jan,13; 2015,Jan,16; 2014,Jan,11; 2012,Jan,15-42;
2011,Jan,11

93668 Rehabilitation Services: Peripheral Arterial Disease

INCLUDES Monitoring:
Other cardiovascular limitations for adjustment of workload
Patient's claudication threshold
Motorized treadmill or track
Sessions lasting 45-60 minutes
Supervision by exercise physiologist/nurse
Code also appropriate E&M service, when performed

93668 Peripheral arterial disease (PAD) rehabilitation, per session
0.54   0.54   **FUD** XXX   E ▯
AMA: 2008,Mar,4-5

93701-93702 Thoracic Electrical Bioimpedance

EXCLUDES Bioelectrical impedance analysis whole body (0358T)
Indirect measurement of left ventricular filling pressure by computerized calibration of the arterial waveform response to Valsalva (93799)

93701 Bioimpedance-derived physiologic cardiovascular analysis
0.68   0.68   **FUD** XXX   Q1 80 TC ▯
AMA: 2016,Jan,13; 2015,Jan,16; 2014,Jan,11

93702 Bioimpedance spectroscopy (BIS), extracellular fluid analysis for lymphedema assessment(s)
3.05   3.05   **FUD** XXX   S 80 TC ▯

93724 Electronic Analysis of Pacemaker Function

93724 Electronic analysis of antitachycardia pacemaker system (includes electrocardiographic recording, programming of device, induction and termination of tachycardia via implanted pacemaker, and interpretation of recordings)
7.66   7.66   **FUD** 000   S 80 ▯
AMA: 2016,Jan,13; 2015,Jan,16; 2014,Jan,11

93740 Temperature Gradient Assessment

93740 Temperature gradient studies
0.23   0.23   **FUD** XXX   Q1 ▯

93745 Wearable Cardioverter-Defibrillator System Services

EXCLUDES Device evaluation (93282, 93292)

93745 Initial set-up and programming by a physician or other qualified health care professional of wearable cardioverter-defibrillator includes initial programming of system, establishing baseline electronic ECG, transmission of data to data repository, patient instruction in wearing system and patient reporting of problems or events
0.00   0.00   **FUD** XXX   S 80 ▯
AMA: 2009,Mar,5-7; 2009,Feb,3-12

93750 Ventricular Assist Device (VAD) Interrogation

CMS: 100-03,20.9 Artificial Hearts and Related Devices; 100-03,20.9.1 Ventricular Assist Devices; 100-04,32,320.1 Artificial Hearts Prior to May 1, 2008; 100-03,20.9.2 Coding for Artificial Hearts After May 1, 2008; 100-04,32,320.3 Ventricular Assist Devices; 100-04,32,320.3.1 Post-cardiotomy; 100-04,32,320.3.2 Bridge- to -Transplantation

EXCLUDES Insertion of ventricular assist device (33975-33976, 33979)
Removal/replacement ventricular assist device (33981-33983)

93750 Interrogation of ventricular assist device (VAD), in person, with physician or other qualified health care professional analysis of device parameters (eg, drivelines, alarms, power surges), review of device function (eg, flow and volume status, septum status, recovery), with programming, if performed, and report
1.32   1.58   **FUD** XXX   S 80 ▯
AMA: 2016,Jan,13; 2015,Jan,16; 2014,Jan,11

93770 Peripheral Venous Blood Pressure Assessment

CMS: 100-03,20.19 Ambulatory Blood Pressure Monitoring (20.19)

EXCLUDES Cannulization, central venous (36500, 36555-36556)

93770 Determination of venous pressure
0.23   0.23   **FUD** XXX   N ▯

93784-93790 Ambulatory Blood Pressure Monitoring

CMS: 100-03,20.19 Ambulatory Blood Pressure Monitoring (20.19); 100-04,32,10.1 Ambulatory Blood Pressure Monitoring Billing Requirements

93784 Ambulatory blood pressure monitoring, utilizing a system such as magnetic tape and/or computer disk, for 24 hours or longer; including recording, scanning analysis, interpretation and report
1.52   1.52   **FUD** XXX   B 80 ▯
AMA: 1991,Win,1

93786 recording only
0.84   0.84   **FUD** XXX   Q1 80 TC ▯

93788 scanning analysis with report
0.15   0.15   **FUD** XXX   Q1 80 TC ▯

93790 review with interpretation and report
0.53   0.53   **FUD** XXX   M 80 26 ▯

93797-93799 Cardiac Rehabilitation

CMS: 100-02,15,232 Cardiac Rehabilitation and Intensive Cardiac Rehabilitation; 100-04,32,140.2 Cardiac Rehabilitation On or After January 1, 2010; 100-04,32,140.2.1 Coding Cardiac Rehabilitation Services On or After January 1, 2010; 100-04,32,140.2.2.2 Institutional Claims for CR and ICR Services; 100-04,32,140.2.2.4 CR Services Exceeding 36 Sessions; 100-04,32,140.3 Intensive Cardiac Rehabilitation On or After January 1, 2010

93797 Physician or other qualified health care professional services for outpatient cardiac rehabilitation; without continuous ECG monitoring (per session)
0.25   0.46   **FUD** 000   S 80 ▯

93798 with continuous ECG monitoring (per session)
0.40   0.71   **FUD** 000   S 80 ▯
AMA: 2005,Nov,1-9

93799 Unlisted cardiovascular service or procedure
0.00   0.00   **FUD** XXX   S 80
AMA: 2016,May,5; 2016,Jan,13; 2015,Jan,16; 2014,Jan,11; 2013,Dec,16; 2012,Jan,15-42; 2011,Oct,5-7; 2011,Jan,11

93880-93895 Noninvasive Tests Extracranial/Intracranial Arteries

INCLUDES Patient care required to perform/supervise studies and interpret results
EXCLUDES Hand-held dopplers that do not provide a hard copy or vascular flow bidirectional analysis (See E&M codes)

93880 Duplex scan of extracranial arteries; complete bilateral study
EXCLUDES Common carotid intima-media thickness (IMT) studies (93895, 0126T)
5.76   5.76   **FUD** XXX   S 80 ▯
AMA: 2016,Jan,13; 2015,Jan,16; 2014,Jan,11

93882 unilateral or limited study
EXCLUDES Common carotid intima-media thickness (IMT) studies (93895, 0126T)
3.68   3.68   **FUD** XXX   S 80 ▯
AMA: 2016,Jan,13; 2015,Jan,16; 2014,Jan,11

93886 Transcranial Doppler study of the intracranial arteries; complete study
INCLUDES Complete transcranial doppler (TCD) study
Ultrasound evaluation of right/left anterior circulation territories and posterior circulation territory
8.00   8.00   **FUD** XXX   S 80 ▯
AMA: 2016,Jan,13; 2015,Jan,16; 2014,Jan,11

93888 limited study
INCLUDES Limited TCD study
Ultrasound examination of two or fewer of these territories (right/left anterior circulation, posterior circulation)
4.20   4.20   **FUD** XXX   S 80 ▯
AMA: 2016,Jan,13; 2015,Jan,16; 2014,Jan,11

93890 vasoreactivity study
EXCLUDES Limited TCD study (93888)
8.21   8.21   **FUD** XXX   Q1 80 ▯
AMA: 2016,Jan,13; 2015,Jan,16; 2014,Jan,11

 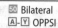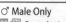

93892 **emboli detection without intravenous microbubble injection**

EXCLUDES *Limited TCD study (93888)*

9.52   9.52   **FUD** XXX   `01` `80`

AMA: 2016,Jan,13; 2015,Jan,16; 2014,Jan,11

93893 **emboli detection with intravenous microbubble injection**

EXCLUDES *Limited TCD study (93888)*

9.94   9.94   **FUD** XXX   `01` `80`

AMA: 2016,Jan,13; 2015,Jan,16; 2014,Jan,11

93895 **Quantitative carotid intima media thickness and carotid atheroma evaluation, bilateral**

0.00   0.00   **FUD** XXX   `E` `80`

EXCLUDES *Common carotid intima-media thickness (IMT) study (0126T)*

Complete and limited duplex studiies (93880, 93882)

93922-93971 Noninvasive Vascular Studies: Extremities

INCLUDES   Patient care required to perform/supervise studies and interpret results

EXCLUDES   Hand-held dopplers that do not provide a hard copy or provided vascular flow bidirectional analysis (see E&M codes)

93922 **Limited bilateral noninvasive physiologic studies of upper or lower extremity arteries, (eg, for lower extremity: ankle/brachial indices at distal posterior tibial and anterior tibial/dorsalis pedis arteries plus bidirectional, Doppler waveform recording and analysis at 1-2 levels, or ankle/brachial indices at distal posterior tibial and anterior tibial/dorsalis pedis arteries plus volume plethysmography at 1-2 levels, or ankle/brachial indices at distal posterior tibial and anterior tibial/dorsalis pedis arteries with, transcutaneous oxygen tension measurement at 1-2 levels)**

INCLUDES   Evaluation of:

Doppler analysis of bidirectional blood flow

Nonimaging physiologic recordings of pressure

Oxygen tension measurements and/or plethysmography

Lower extremity (potential levels include high thigh, low thigh, calf, ankle, metatarsal and toes) limited study includes either:

Ankle/brachial indices at distal posterior tibial and anterior tibial/dorsalis pedis arteries plus bidirectional Doppler waveform recording and analysis as 1-2 levels; OR

Ankle/brachial indices at distal posterior tibial and anterior tibial/dorsalis pedis arteries plus volume plethysmography at 1-2 levels; OR

Ankle/brachial indices at distal posterior tibial and anterior tibial/dorsalis pedis arteries with transcutaneous oxygen tension measurements at 1-2 levels

Unilateral provocative functional measurement

Unilateral study of 3 or move levels

Upper extremity (potential levels include arm, forearm, wrist, and digits) limited study includes:

Doppler-determined systolic pressures and bidirectional waveform recording with analysis at 1-2 levels; OR

Doppler-determined systolic pressures and transcutaneous oxygen tension measurements at 1-2 levels; OR

Doppler-determined systolic pressures and volume plethysmography at 1-2 levels

EXCLUDES   *Endothelial function assessment (0337T)*

Use of code more than one time for the lower extremity(s)

Use of code more than one time for the upper extremity(s)

Code also modifier 52 for unilateral study of 1-2 levels

Code also twice with modifier 59 for upper and lower extremity study

2.53   2.53   **FUD** XXX   `01` `80`

AMA: 2016,Jan,13; 2015,Jan,16; 2014,Jan,9; 2014,Jan,11; 2013,Jun,13; 2012,Jun,15-16

93923 **Complete bilateral noninvasive physiologic studies of upper or lower extremity arteries, 3 or more levels (eg, for lower extremity: ankle/brachial indices at distal posterior tibial and anterior tibial/dorsalis pedis arteries plus segmental blood pressure measurements with bidirectional Doppler waveform recording and analysis, at 3 or more levels, or ankle/brachial indices at distal posterior tibial and anterior tibial/dorsalis pedis arteries plus segmental volume plethysmography at 3 or more levels, or ankle/brachial indices at distal posterior tibial and anterior tibial/dorsalis pedis arteries plus segmental transcutaneous oxygen tension measurements at 3 or more levels), or single level study with provocative functional maneuvers (eg, measurements with postural provocative tests, or measurements with reactive hyperemia)**

INCLUDES   Evaluation of:

Doppler analysis of bidirectional blood flow

Nonimaging physiologic recordings of pressures

Oxygen tension measurements

Lower extremity:

Ankle/brachial indices at distal posterior tibial and anterior tibial/dorsalis pedis arteries plus bidirectional Doppler waveform recording and analysis at 3 or more levels; OR

Ankle/brachial indices at distal posterior tibial and anterior tibial/dorsalis pedis arteries with transcutaneous oxygen tension measurements at 3 or more levels; OR

Ankle/brachial indices at distal posterior tibial and anterior tibial/dorsalis pedis arteries plus volume plethysmography at 3 or more levels; OR

Provocative functional maneuvers and measurement at a single level

Upper extremity complete study:

Doppler-determined systolic pressures and bidirectional waveform recording with analysis at 3 or more levels; OR

Doppler-determined systolic pressures and transcutaneous oxygen tension measurements at 3 or more levels; OR

Doppler-determined systolic pressures and volume plethysmography at 3 or more levels; OR

Provocative functional maneuvers and measurement at a single level

EXCLUDES   *Endothelial function assessment (0337T)*

Unilateral study at 3 or more levels (93922)

Use of code more than one time for the lower extremity(s)

Use of code more than one time for the upper extremity(s)

Code also twice with modifier 59 for upper and lower extremity study

3.94   3.94   **FUD** XXX   `S` `80`

AMA: 2016,Jan,13; 2015,Jan,16; 2014,Jan,9; 2014,Jan,11; 2012,Jun,15-16; 2012,Jan,15-42; 2011,Jan,11

93924 **Noninvasive physiologic studies of lower extremity arteries, at rest and following treadmill stress testing, (ie, bidirectional Doppler waveform or volume plethysmography recording and analysis at rest with ankle/brachial indices immediately after and at timed intervals following performance of a standardized protocol on a motorized treadmill plus recording of time of onset of claudication or other symptoms, maximal walking time, and time to recovery) complete bilateral study**

INCLUDES   Evaluation of:

Doppler analysis of bidirectional blood flow

Non-imaging physiologic recordings of pressures

Oxygen tension measurements

Plethysmography

EXCLUDES   *Noninvasive vascular studies of extremities (93922-93923)*

Other types of exercise

4.94   4.94   **FUD** XXX   `S` `80`

AMA: 2016,Jan,13; 2015,Jan,16; 2014,Jan,9; 2014,Jan,11; 2012,Jun,15-16

93925 Duplex scan of lower extremity arteries or arterial bypass grafts; complete bilateral study
 🚑 7.40   ⚕ 7.40   **FUD** XXX   [S] [80] 🖵
 AMA: 2016,Sep,9; 2016,Jan,13; 2015,Jan,16; 2014,Jan,11

93926 unilateral or limited study
 🚑 4.36   ⚕ 4.36   **FUD** XXX   [S] [80] 🖵
 AMA: 2016,Sep,9; 2016,Jan,13; 2015,Jan,16; 2014,Jan,11

93930 Duplex scan of upper extremity arteries or arterial bypass grafts; complete bilateral study
 🚑 5.95   ⚕ 5.95   **FUD** XXX   [S] [80] 🖵
 AMA: 2016,Sep,9; 2016,Jan,13; 2015,Jan,16; 2014,Jan,11

93931 unilateral or limited study
 🚑 3.68   ⚕ 3.68   **FUD** XXX   [S] [80] 🖵
 AMA: 2016,Sep,9; 2016,Jan,13; 2015,Jan,16; 2014,Jan,11

93965 ~~Noninvasive physiologic studies of extremity veins, complete bilateral study (eg, Doppler waveform analysis with responses to compression and other maneuvers, phleborheography, impedance plethysmography)~~

93970 Duplex scan of extremity veins including responses to compression and other maneuvers; complete bilateral study
 EXCLUDES   *Endovenous ablation (36475-36476, 36478-36479)*
 🚑 5.61   ⚕ 5.61   **FUD** XXX   [S] [80] 🖵
 AMA: 2016,Sep,9; 2016,Jan,13; 2015,Jan,16; 2014,Oct,6; 2014,Jan,11; 2012,Feb,11; 2012,Jan,13-14

93971 unilateral or limited study
 EXCLUDES   *Endovenous ablation (36475-36476, 36478-36479)*
 🚑 3.43   ⚕ 3.43   **FUD** XXX   [S] [80] 🖵
 AMA: 2016,Sep,9; 2016,Jan,13; 2015,Aug,8; 2015,Jan,16; 2014,Oct,6; 2014,Jan,11; 2012,Feb,11; 2012,Jan,13-14; 2012,Jan,15-42; 2011,Apr,12; 2011,Jan,11

93975-93982 Noninvasive Vascular Studies: Abdomen/Chest/Pelvis

93975 Duplex scan of arterial inflow and venous outflow of abdominal, pelvic, scrotal contents and/or retroperitoneal organs; complete study
 🚑 8.04   ⚕ 8.04   **FUD** XXX   [S] [80] 🖵
 AMA: 2016,Aug,9; 2016,Jan,13; 2015,Mar,9; 2015,Jan,16; 2014,Jun,14; 2014,Jan,11; 2012,Jan,15-42; 2011,Jan,11

93976 limited study
 🚑 4.64   ⚕ 4.64   **FUD** XXX   [S] [80] 🖵
 AMA: 2016,Aug,9; 2016,Jan,13; 2015,Mar,9; 2015,Jan,16; 2014,Jan,11; 2012,Jan,15-42; 2011,Jan,11

93978 Duplex scan of aorta, inferior vena cava, iliac vasculature, or bypass grafts; complete study
 EXCLUDES   *Ultrasound screening for abdominal aortic aneurysm (76706)*
 🚑 5.46   ⚕ 5.46   **FUD** XXX   [S] [80] 🖵
 AMA: 2016,Jan,13; 2015,Jan,16; 2014,Jan,11

93979 unilateral or limited study
 EXCLUDES   *Ultrasound screening for abdominal aortic aneurysm (76706)*
 🚑 3.42   ⚕ 3.42   **FUD** XXX   [01] [80] 🖵
 AMA: 2016,Jan,13; 2015,Jan,16; 2014,Jun,14; 2014,Jan,11

93980 Duplex scan of arterial inflow and venous outflow of penile vessels; complete study
 🚑 3.42   ⚕ 3.42   **FUD** XXX   [S] [80] 🖵
 AMA: 2016,Jan,13; 2015,Jan,16; 2014,Jan,11

93981 follow-up or limited study
 🚑 2.08   ⚕ 2.08   **FUD** XXX   [S] [80] 🖵
 AMA: 2016,Jan,13; 2015,Jan,16; 2014,Jan,11

93982 Noninvasive physiologic study of implanted wireless pressure sensor in aneurysmal sac following endovascular repair, complete study including recording, analysis of pressure and waveform tracings, interpretation and report
 🚑 1.22   ⚕ 1.22   **FUD** XXX   [01] [80] 🖵
 EXCLUDES   *Transcatheter placement of wireless physiologic sensor in aneurysmal sac (34806)*

93990-93998 Noninvasive Vascular Studies: Hemodialysis Access

93990 Duplex scan of hemodialysis access (including arterial inflow, body of access and venous outflow)
 EXCLUDES   *Hemodialysis access flow measurement by indicator method (90940)*
 🚑 4.61   ⚕ 4.61   **FUD** XXX   [01] [80] 🖵
 AMA: 2016,Jan,13; 2015,Jan,16; 2014,Jan,11

93998 Unlisted noninvasive vascular diagnostic study
 🚑 0.00   ⚕ 0.00   **FUD** XXX   [01] [80] 🖵
 AMA: 2016,Jan,13; 2015,Jan,16; 2014,Jan,9; 2012,Oct,13; 2012,Sep,9

94002-94005 Ventilator Management Services

94002 Ventilation assist and management, initiation of pressure or volume preset ventilators for assisted or controlled breathing; hospital inpatient/observation, initial day
 EXCLUDES   *E&M services*
 🚑 2.64   ⚕ 2.64   **FUD** XXX   [Q3] [80] 🖵
 AMA: 2016,Jan,13; 2015,Jan,16; 2014,Oct,8; 2014,May,4; 2014,Jan,11; 2012,Jan,15-42; 2011,Jan,11

94003 hospital inpatient/observation, each subsequent day
 EXCLUDES   *E&M services*
 🚑 1.90   ⚕ 1.90   **FUD** XXX   [Q3] [80] 🖵
 AMA: 2016,Jan,13; 2015,Jan,16; 2014,Oct,8; 2014,May,4; 2014,Jan,11

94004 nursing facility, per day
 EXCLUDES   *E&M services*
 🚑 1.39   ⚕ 1.39   **FUD** XXX   [B] [80] 🖵
 AMA: 2016,Jan,13; 2015,Jan,16; 2014,Oct,8; 2014,Jan,11

94005 Home ventilator management care plan oversight of a patient (patient not present) in home, domiciliary or rest home (eg, assisted living) requiring review of status, review of laboratories and other studies and revision of orders and respiratory care plan (as appropriate), within a calendar month, 30 minutes or more
 Code also when a different provider reports care plan oversight in the same 30 days (99339-99340, 99374-99378)
 🚑 2.62   ⚕ 2.62   **FUD** XXX   [M] 🖵
 AMA: 2016,Jan,13; 2015,Jan,16; 2014,Oct,8; 2014,Jan,11; 2012,Jan,15-42; 2011,Jan,11

94010-94799 Respiratory Services: Diagnostic and Therapeutic

 INCLUDES   Laboratory procedure(s)
 Test results interpretation
 EXCLUDES   *Separately identifiable E&M service*

94010 Spirometry, including graphic record, total and timed vital capacity, expiratory flow rate measurement(s), with or without maximal voluntary ventilation
 INCLUDES   Measurement of expiratory airflow and volumes
 EXCLUDES   *Diffusing capacity (94729)*
 Other respiratory function services (94150, 94200, 94375, 94728)
 🚑 1.02   ⚕ 1.02   **FUD** XXX   [01] [80] 🖵
 AMA: 2016,Jan,13; 2015,Sep,9; 2015,Jan,16; 2014,Mar,11; 2014,Jan,11; 2013,Dec,12; 2012,Nov,11-12; 2012,Nov,13-14; 2012,Aug,6-8; 2012,Jan,15-42; 2011,Jan,11

▲ **94011** **Measurement of spirometric forced expiratory flows in an infant or child through 2 years of age**
📋 2.91 ⚕ 2.91 **FUD** XXX ⬜01 80 📠
AMA: 2016,Jan,13; 2015,Jan,16; 2014,Jan,11; 2013,Dec,12; 2012,Aug,6-8; 2011,Jan,11

▲ **94012** **Measurement of spirometric forced expiratory flows, before and after bronchodilator, in an infant or child through 2 years of age**
📋 4.45 ⚕ 4.45 **FUD** XXX ⬜01 80 📠
AMA: 2016,Jan,13; 2015,Jan,16; 2014,Jan,11; 2013,Dec,12; 2012,Aug,6-8; 2011,Jan,11

▲ **94013** **Measurement of lung volumes (ie, functional residual capacity [FRC], forced vital capacity [FVC], and expiratory reserve volume [ERV]) in an infant or child through 2 years of age**
📋 0.98 ⚕ 0.98 **FUD** XXX ⬜S 80 📠
AMA: 2016,Jan,13; 2015,Jan,16; 2014,Jan,11; 2013,Dec,12; 2012,Aug,6-8; 2011,Jan,11

94014 **Patient-initiated spirometric recording per 30-day period of time; includes reinforced education, transmission of spirometric tracing, data capture, analysis of transmitted data, periodic recalibration and review and interpretation by a physician or other qualified health care professional**
📋 1.59 ⚕ 1.59 **FUD** XXX ⬜01 80 📠
AMA: 2016,Jan,13; 2015,Jan,16; 2014,Jan,11; 2013,Dec,12; 2012,Aug,6-8; 2011,Jan,11

94015 **recording (includes hook-up, reinforced education, data transmission, data capture, trend analysis, and periodic recalibration)**
📋 0.87 ⚕ 0.87 **FUD** XXX ⬜01 80 TC 📠
AMA: 2016,Jan,13; 2015,Jan,16; 2014,Jan,11; 2013,Dec,12; 2012,Aug,6-8; 2011,Jan,11

94016 **review and interpretation only by a physician or other qualified health care professional**
📋 0.72 ⚕ 0.72 **FUD** XXX ⬜A 80 26 📠
AMA: 2016,Jan,13; 2015,Jan,16; 2014,Jan,11; 2013,Dec,12; 2012,Aug,6-8; 2011,Jan,11

94060 **Bronchodilation responsiveness, spirometry as in 94010, pre- and post-bronchodilator administration**
INCLUDES Spirometry performed prior to and after a bronchodilator has been administered
EXCLUDES Bronchospasm prolonged exercise test with pre- and post-spirometry (94620)
Diffusing capacity (94729)
Other respiratory function services (94150, 94200, 94375, 94640, 94728)
Code also bronchodilator supply with appropriate supply code or (99070)
📋 1.72 ⚕ 1.72 **FUD** XXX ⬜S 80 📠
AMA: 2016,Jan,13; 2015,Sep,9; 2015,Jan,16; 2014,Mar,11; 2014,Jan,11; 2013,Dec,12; 2012,Aug,6-8; 2012,Jan,15-42; 2011,Jan,11

94070 **Bronchospasm provocation evaluation, multiple spirometric determinations as in 94010, with administered agents (eg, antigen[s], cold air, methacholine)**
EXCLUDES Diffusing capacity (94729)
Inhalation treatment (diagnostic or therapeutic) (94640)
Code also antigen(s) administration with appropriate supply code or (99070)
📋 1.69 ⚕ 1.69 **FUD** XXX ⬜S 80 📠
AMA: 2016,Jan,13; 2015,Sep,9; 2015,Jan,16; 2014,Jan,11; 2013,Dec,12; 2012,Nov,11-12; 2012,Aug,6-8; 2011,Jan,11

94150 **Vital capacity, total (separate procedure)**
EXCLUDES Other respiratory function services (94010, 94060, 94728)
Thoracic gas volumes (94726-94727)
📋 0.71 ⚕ 0.71 **FUD** XXX ⬜01 📠
AMA: 2016,Jan,13; 2015,Jan,16; 2014,Mar,11; 2014,Jan,11; 2013,Dec,12; 2012,Aug,6-8; 2012,Jan,15-42; 2011,Jan,11

94200 **Maximum breathing capacity, maximal voluntary ventilation**
EXCLUDES Other respiratory function services (94010, 94060)
📋 0.71 ⚕ 0.71 **FUD** XXX ⬜01 80 📠
AMA: 2016,Jan,13; 2015,Jan,16; 2014,Mar,11; 2014,Jan,11; 2013,Dec,12; 2012,Aug,6-8; 2012,Jan,15-42; 2011,Jan,11

94250 **Expired gas collection, quantitative, single procedure (separate procedure)**
📋 0.74 ⚕ 0.74 **FUD** XXX ⬜01 80 📠
AMA: 2016,Jan,13; 2015,Dec,16; 2015,Jan,16; 2014,Jan,11; 2013,Dec,12; 2012,Aug,6-8; 2011,Jan,11

94375 **Respiratory flow volume loop**
INCLUDES Identification of obstruction patterns in central or peripheral airways (inspiratory and/or expiratory)
EXCLUDES Diffusing capacity (94729)
Other respiratory function services (94010, 94060, 94728)
📋 1.11 ⚕ 1.11 **FUD** XXX ⬜01 80 📠
AMA: 2016,Jan,13; 2015,Jan,16; 2014,Mar,11; 2014,Jan,11; 2013,Dec,12; 2012,Aug,6-8; 2011,Jan,11

94400 **Breathing response to CO2 (CO2 response curve)**
EXCLUDES Inhalation treatment (diagnostic or therapeutic) (94640)
📋 1.58 ⚕ 1.58 **FUD** XXX ⬜01 80 📠
AMA: 2016,Jan,13; 2015,Sep,9; 2015,Jan,16; 2014,Mar,11; 2014,Jan,11; 2013,Dec,12; 2012,Aug,6-8; 2012,Jan,15-42; 2011,Jan,11

94450 **Breathing response to hypoxia (hypoxia response curve)**
EXCLUDES HAST - high altitude simulation test (94452, 94453)
📋 1.93 ⚕ 1.93 **FUD** XXX ⬜01 80 📠
AMA: 2016,Jan,13; 2015,Jan,16; 2014,Jan,11; 2013,Dec,12; 2012,Aug,6-8; 2011,Jan,11

94452 **High altitude simulation test (HAST), with interpretation and report by a physician or other qualified health care professional;**
EXCLUDES HAST test with supplemental oxygen titration (94453)
Noninvasive pulse oximetry (94760-94761)
Obtaining arterial blood gases (36600)
📋 1.63 ⚕ 1.63 **FUD** XXX ⬜01 80 📠
AMA: 2016,Jan,13; 2015,Jan,16; 2014,Jan,11; 2013,Dec,12; 2012,Aug,6-8; 2011,Jan,11

94453 **with supplemental oxygen titration**
EXCLUDES HAST test without supplemental oxygen titration (94452)
Noninvasive pulse oximetry (94760-94761)
Obtaining arterial blood gases (36600)
📋 2.26 ⚕ 2.26 **FUD** XXX ⬜01 80 📠
AMA: 2016,Jan,13; 2015,Jan,16; 2014,Jan,11; 2013,Dec,12; 2012,Aug,6-8; 2011,Jan,11

94610 **Intrapulmonary surfactant administration by a physician or other qualified health care professional through endotracheal tube**
INCLUDES Reporting once per dosing episode
EXCLUDES Intubation, endotracheal (31500)
Neonatal critical care (99468-99472)
📋 1.69 ⚕ 1.69 **FUD** XXX ⊘ ⬜01 80 📠
AMA: 2016,Jan,13; 2015,Jan,16; 2014,Jan,11; 2013,Dec,12; 2012,Aug,6-8; 2012,Jan,15-42; 2011,Jan,11

94620 **Pulmonary stress testing; simple (eg, 6-minute walk test, prolonged exercise test for bronchospasm with pre- and post-spirometry and oximetry)**
📋 1.59 ⚕ 1.59 **FUD** XXX ⬜01 80 📠
AMA: 2016,Jan,13; 2015,Jan,16; 2014,Jan,11; 2013,Dec,12; 2012,Nov,13-14; 2012,Aug,6-8; 2012,Jan,15-42; 2011,Jan,11

94621 **complex (including measurements of CO2 production, O2 uptake, and electrocardiographic recordings)**
📋 4.62 ⚕ 4.62 **FUD** XXX ⬜S 80 📠
AMA: 2016,Jan,13; 2015,Jan,16; 2014,Jan,11; 2013,Dec,12; 2012,Nov,13-14; 2012,Aug,6-8; 2012,Jan,15-42; 2011,Jan,11

94640 Pressurized or nonpressurized inhalation treatment for acute airway obstruction for therapeutic purposes and/or for diagnostic purposes such as sputum induction with an aerosol generator, nebulizer, metered dose inhaler or intermittent positive pressure breathing (IPPB) device

> *EXCLUDES* 1 hour or more of continuous inhalation treatment (94644, 94645)
>
> Other respiratory function services (94060, 94070, 94400)
>
> Code also modifier 76 when more than 1 inhalation treatment is performed on the same date

🔧 0.52   ⚕ 0.52   **FUD** XXX   01 80 ▢

AMA: 2016,Jan,13; 2015,Sep,9; 2015,Jan,16; 2014,Mar,11; 2014,Jan,11; 2013,Dec,12; 2012,Aug,6-8; 2012,Jan,15-42; 2011,Jan,11

94642 Aerosol inhalation of pentamidine for pneumocystis carinii pneumonia treatment or prophylaxis

🔧 0.00   ⚕ 0.00   **FUD** XXX   01 80 ▢

AMA: 2016,Jan,13; 2015,Jan,16; 2014,Jan,11; 2013,Dec,12; 2012,Aug,6-8; 2011,Jan,11

94644 Continuous inhalation treatment with aerosol medication for acute airway obstruction; first hour

> *EXCLUDES* Services that are less than 1 hour (94640)

🔧 1.24   ⚕ 1.24   **FUD** XXX   01 80 ▢

AMA: 2016,Jan,13; 2015,Sep,9; 2015,Jan,16; 2014,Mar,11; 2014,Jan,11; 2013,Dec,12; 2012,Aug,6-8; 2011,Jan,11

+ 94645 each additional hour (List separately in addition to code for primary procedure)

> Code first initial hour (94644)

🔧 0.40   ⚕ 0.40   **FUD** XXX   N 80 ▢

AMA: 2016,Jan,13; 2015,Sep,9; 2015,Jan,16; 2014,Mar,11; 2014,Jan,11; 2013,Dec,12; 2012,Aug,6-8; 2011,Jan,11

94660 Continuous positive airway pressure ventilation (CPAP), initiation and management

🔧 1.08   ⚕ 1.79   **FUD** XXX   01 80 ▢

AMA: 2016,Jan,13; 2015,Jan,16; 2014,Oct,8; 2014,May,4; 2014,Jan,11; 2013,Dec,12; 2012,Aug,6-8; 2012,Jan,15-42; 2011,Jan,11

94662 Continuous negative pressure ventilation (CNP), initiation and management

🔧 1.06   ⚕ 1.06   **FUD** XXX   03 80 ▢

AMA: 2016,Jan,13; 2015,Jan,16; 2014,May,4; 2014,Jan,11; 2013,Dec,12; 2012,Aug,6-8; 2012,Jan,15-42; 2011,Jan,11

94664 Demonstration and/or evaluation of patient utilization of an aerosol generator, nebulizer, metered dose inhaler or IPPB device

> *INCLUDES* Reporting only one time per day of service

🔧 0.49   ⚕ 0.49   **FUD** XXX   01 80 ▢

AMA: 2016,Jan,13; 2015,Jan,16; 2014,Jan,11; 2013,Dec,12; 2012,Aug,6-8; 2012,Jan,15-42; 2011,Jan,11

94667 Manipulation chest wall, such as cupping, percussing, and vibration to facilitate lung function; initial demonstration and/or evaluation

🔧 0.74   ⚕ 0.74   **FUD** XXX   01 80 ▢

AMA: 2016,Jan,13; 2015,Sep,9; 2015,Jan,16; 2014,Mar,11; 2014,Jan,11; 2013,Dec,12; 2012,Aug,6-8; 2012,Jan,15-42; 2011,Jan,11

94668 subsequent

🔧 0.82   ⚕ 0.82   **FUD** XXX   01 80 ▢

AMA: 2016,Jan,13; 2015,Sep,9; 2015,Jan,16; 2014,Mar,11; 2014,Jan,11; 2013,Dec,12; 2012,Aug,6-8; 2012,Jan,15-42; 2011,Jan,11

94669 Mechanical chest wall oscillation to facilitate lung function, per session

> *INCLUDES* Application of an external wrap or vest to provide mechanical oscillation

🔧 0.93   ⚕ 0.93   **FUD** XXX   01 80 ▢

AMA: 2016,Jan,13; 2015,Jan,16; 2014,Jan,11; 2013,Dec,12

94680 Oxygen uptake, expired gas analysis; rest and exercise, direct, simple

🔧 1.62   ⚕ 1.62   **FUD** XXX   01 80 ▢

AMA: 2016,Jan,13; 2015,Jan,16; 2014,Jan,11; 2013,Dec,12; 2012,Aug,6-8; 2011,Jan,11

94681 including CO2 output, percentage oxygen extracted

🔧 1.49   ⚕ 1.49   **FUD** XXX   01 80 ▢

AMA: 2016,Jan,13; 2015,Jan,16; 2014,Jan,11; 2013,Dec,12; 2012,Aug,6-8; 2011,Jan,11

94690 rest, indirect (separate procedure)

> *EXCLUDES* Arterial puncture (36600)

🔧 1.41   ⚕ 1.41   **FUD** XXX   01 80 ▢

AMA: 2016,Jan,13; 2015,Jan,16; 2014,Jan,11; 2013,Dec,12; 2012,Aug,6-8; 2011,Jan,11

94726 Plethysmography for determination of lung volumes and, when performed, airway resistance

> *INCLUDES* Airway resistance
> Determination of:
>   Functional residual capacity
>   Residual volume
>   Total lung capacity
>
> *EXCLUDES* Airway resistance (94728)
> Bronchial provocation (94070)
> Diffusing capacity (94729)
> Gas dilution or washout (94727)
> Spirometry (94010, 94060)

🔧 1.49   ⚕ 1.49   **FUD** XXX   01 80 ▢

AMA: 2016,Jan,13; 2015,Jan,16; 2014,Jan,11; 2013,Dec,12; 2013,May,11; 2012,Aug,6-8; 2012,Jan,3-5

94727 Gas dilution or washout for determination of lung volumes and, when performed, distribution of ventilation and closing volumes

> *EXCLUDES* Bronchial provocation (94070)
> Diffusing capacity (94729)
> Plethysmography for lung volume/airway resistance (94726)
> Spirometry (94010, 94060)

🔧 1.19   ⚕ 1.19   **FUD** XXX   01 80 ▢

AMA: 2016,Jan,13; 2015,Jan,16; 2014,Jan,11; 2013,Dec,12; 2013,May,11; 2012,Aug,6-8; 2012,Jan,3-5

94728 Airway resistance by impulse oscillometry

> *EXCLUDES* Diffusing capacity (94729)
> Gas dilution techniques
> Other respiratory function services (94010, 94060, 94070, 94375, 94726)

🔧 1.14   ⚕ 1.14   **FUD** XXX   01 80 ▢

AMA: 2016,Jan,13; 2015,Jan,16; 2014,Mar,11; 2014,Jan,11; 2013,Dec,12; 2013,May,11; 2012,Aug,6-8; 2012,Jan,3-5

+ 94729 Diffusing capacity (eg, carbon monoxide, membrane) (List separately in addition to code for primary procedure)

> Code first (94010, 94060, 94070, 94375, 94726-94728)

🔧 1.54   ⚕ 1.54   **FUD** ZZZ   N 80 ▢

AMA: 2016,Jan,13; 2015,Jan,16; 2014,Jan,11; 2013,Dec,12; 2012,Aug,6-8; 2012,Jan,3-5

94750 Pulmonary compliance study (eg, plethysmography, volume and pressure measurements)

🔧 2.28   ⚕ 2.28   **FUD** XXX   01 80 ▢

AMA: 2016,Jan,13; 2015,Jan,16; 2014,Jan,11; 2013,Dec,12; 2012,Aug,6-8; 2011,Jan,11

94760 Noninvasive ear or pulse oximetry for oxygen saturation; single determination

> *EXCLUDES* Blood gases (82803-82810)

🔧 0.09   ⚕ 0.09   **FUD** XXX   N 80 TC ▢

AMA: 2016,Jan,13; 2015,Jan,16; 2014,May,4; 2014,Jan,11; 2013,Dec,12; 2012,Aug,6-8; 2012,Jan,15-42; 2011,Jan,11

94761 multiple determinations (eg, during exercise)

🔧 0.14   ⚕ 0.14   **FUD** XXX   N 80 TC ▢

AMA: 2016,Jan,13; 2015,Jan,16; 2014,May,4; 2014,Jan,11; 2013,Dec,12; 2012,Aug,6-8; 2012,Jan,15-42; 2011,Jan,11

 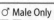 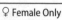 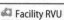 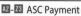

94762   **by continuous overnight monitoring (separate procedure)**
     0.69   0.69   **FUD** XXX   03 80 TC ▢
AMA: 2016,Jan,13; 2015,Jan,16; 2014,May,4; 2014,Jan,11; 2013,Dec,12; 2012,Aug,6-8; 2011,Jan,11

94770   **Carbon dioxide, expired gas determination by infrared analyzer**
> EXCLUDES   Arterial catheterization/cannulation (36620)
> Arterial puncture (36600)
> Bronchoscopy (31622-31646)
> Flow directed catheter placement (93503)
> Needle biopsy of the lung (32405)
> Orotracheal/nasotracheal intubation (31500)
> Placement of central venous catheter (36555-36556)
> Therapeutic phlebotomy (99195)
> Thoracentesis (32554-32555)
> Venipuncture (36410)

     0.21   0.21   **FUD** XXX   S 80 ▢
AMA: 2016,Jan,13; 2015,Jan,16; 2014,Mar,11; 2014,Jan,11; 2013,Dec,12; 2012,Aug,6-8; 2011,Jan,11

94772   **Circadian respiratory pattern recording (pediatric pneumogram), 12-24 hour continuous recording, infant** ▲
> EXCLUDES   Electromyograms/EEG/ECG/respiration recordings

     0.00   0.00   **FUD** XXX   S 80 ▢
AMA: 2016,Jan,13; 2015,Jan,16; 2014,Jan,11; 2013,Dec,12; 2012,Aug,6-8; 2011,Jan,11

94774   **Pediatric home apnea monitoring event recording including respiratory rate, pattern and heart rate per 30-day period of time; includes monitor attachment, download of data, review, interpretation, and preparation of a report by a physician or other qualified health care professional** ▲
> INCLUDES   Oxygen saturation monitoring
> EXCLUDES   Event monitors (93268-93272)
> Holter monitor (93224-93227)
> Pediatric home apnea services (94775-94777)
> Remote cardiovascular telemetry (93228-93229)
> Sleep testing (95805-95811 [95800, 95801])

     0.00   0.00   **FUD** YYY   B 80 ▢
AMA: 2016,Jan,13; 2015,Jan,16; 2014,Jan,11; 2013,Dec,12; 2012,Aug,6-8; 2011,Jan,11

94775   **monitor attachment only (includes hook-up, initiation of recording and disconnection)** ▲
> INCLUDES   Oxygen saturation monitoring
> EXCLUDES   Event monitors (93268-93272)
> Holter monitor (93224-93227)
> Remote cardiovascular telemetry (93228-93229)
> Sleep testing (95805-95811 [95800, 95801])

     0.00   0.00   **FUD** YYY   S 80 TC ▢
AMA: 2016,Jan,13; 2015,Jan,16; 2014,Jan,11; 2013,Dec,12; 2012,Aug,6-8; 2011,Jan,11

94776   **monitoring, download of information, receipt of transmission(s) and analyses by computer only** ▲
> INCLUDES   Oxygen saturation monitoring
> EXCLUDES   Event monitors (93268-93272)
> Holter monitor (93224-93227)
> Remote cardiovascular telemetry (93228-93229)
> Sleep testing (95805-95811 [95800, 95801])

     0.00   0.00   **FUD** YYY   S 80 TC ▢
AMA: 2016,Jan,13; 2015,Jan,16; 2014,Jan,11; 2013,Dec,12; 2012,Aug,6-8; 2011,Jan,11

94777   **review, interpretation and preparation of report only by a physician or other qualified health care professional** ▲
> INCLUDES   Oxygen saturation monitoring
> EXCLUDES   Event monitors (93268-93272)
> Holter monitor (93224-93227)
> Remote cardiovascular telemetry (93228-93229)
> Sleep testing (95805-95811 [95800, 95801])

     0.00   0.00   **FUD** YYY   B 80 26 ▢
AMA: 2016,Jan,13; 2015,Jan,16; 2014,Jan,11; 2013,Dec,12; 2012,Aug,6-8; 2011,Jan,11

94780   **Car seat/bed testing for airway integrity, neonate, with continual nursing observation and continuous recording of pulse oximetry, heart rate and respiratory rate, with interpretation and report; 60 minutes** ▲
> EXCLUDES   Pediatric and neonatal critical care services (99468-99476, 99477-99480)
> Pulse oximetry (94760-94761)
> Rhythm strips (93040-93042)
> Use of code for less than 60 minutes of service

     0.65   1.59   **FUD** XXX   Q1 ▢
AMA: 2016,Jan,13; 2015,May,10; 2015,Jan,16; 2014,Jan,11; 2013,Dec,12; 2012,Aug,6-8

+ **94781**   **each additional full 30 minutes (List separately in addition to code for primary procedure)** ▲
Code first (94780)
     0.24   0.65   **FUD** ZZZ   N ▢
AMA: 2016,Jan,13; 2015,May,10; 2015,Jan,16; 2014,Jan,11; 2013,Dec,12; 2012,Aug,6-8

94799   **Unlisted pulmonary service or procedure**
     0.00   0.00   **FUD** XXX   Q1 80
AMA: 2016,Jan,13; 2015,Dec,16; 2015,May,10; 2015,Jan,16; 2014,Jan,11; 2013,Dec,12; 2012,Nov,13-14; 2012,Aug,6-8; 2011,Jan,11

95004-95071 Allergy Tests

> EXCLUDES   Drugs administered for intractable/severe allergic reaction (eg, antihistamines, epinephrine, steroids) (96372)
> E&M services when reporting test interpretation/report
> Laboratory tests for allergies (86000-86999 [86152, 86153])

Code also medical conferences regarding use of equipment (eg, air filters, humidifiers, dehumidifiers), climate therapy, physical, occupational, and recreation therapy using appropriate E&M codes
Code also significant, separately identifiable E&M services using modifier 25, when performed (99201-99215, 99217-99223 [99224, 99225, 99226], 99231-99233, 99241-99255, 99281-99285, 99304-99318, 99324-99337, 99341-99350, 99381-99429)

95004   **Percutaneous tests (scratch, puncture, prick) with allergenic extracts, immediate type reaction, including test interpretation and report, specify number of tests**
     0.19   0.19   **FUD** XXX   Q1 80 ▢
AMA: 2016,Jan,13; 2015,Jan,16; 2014,Jan,11; 2013,Jan,9-10; 2012,Jan,15-42; 2011,Jan,11

95012   **Nitric oxide expired gas determination**
     0.54   0.54   **FUD** XXX   Q1 80 ▢
AMA: 2016,Jan,13; 2015,Jan,16; 2014,Mar,11; 2014,Jan,11; 2013,Jan,9-10; 2012,Jan,15-42; 2011,Jan,11

95017   **Allergy testing, any combination of percutaneous (scratch, puncture, prick) and intracutaneous (intradermal), sequential and incremental, with venoms, immediate type reaction, including test interpretation and report, specify number of tests**
     0.10   0.22   **FUD** XXX   Q1 80 ▢
AMA: 2016,Jan,13; 2015,Jul,9; 2015,Jan,16; 2013,Jan,9-10

95018   **Allergy testing, any combination of percutaneous (scratch, puncture, prick) and intracutaneous (intradermal), sequential and incremental, with drugs or biologicals, immediate type reaction, including test interpretation and report, specify number of tests**
     0.20   0.58   **FUD** XXX   Q1 80 ▢
AMA: 2016,Jan,13; 2015,Jul,9; 2015,Jan,16; 2013,Jan,9-10

95024 **Intracutaneous (intradermal) tests with allergenic extracts, immediate type reaction, including test interpretation and report, specify number of tests**

    📟 0.03   ✂ 0.22   **FUD** XXX   [Q1] [80] 🖵

    AMA: 2016,Jan,13; 2015,Jan,16; 2014,Jan,11; 2013,Jan,9-10; 2012,Jan,15-42; 2011,Jan,11

95027 **Intracutaneous (intradermal) tests, sequential and incremental, with allergenic extracts for airborne allergens, immediate type reaction, including test interpretation and report, specify number of tests**

    📟 0.13   ✂ 0.13   **FUD** XXX   [Q1] [80] 🖵

    AMA: 2016,Jan,13; 2015,Jan,16; 2014,Jan,11; 2013,Jan,9-10; 2012,Jan,15-42; 2011,Jan,11

95028 **Intracutaneous (intradermal) tests with allergenic extracts, delayed type reaction, including reading, specify number of tests**

    📟 0.38   ✂ 0.38   **FUD** XXX   [Q1] [80] [TC] 🖵

    AMA: 2016,Jan,13; 2015,Jan,16; 2014,Jan,11; 2013,Jan,9-10

95044 **Patch or application test(s) (specify number of tests)**

    📟 0.16   ✂ 0.16   **FUD** XXX   [Q1] [80] 🖵

    AMA: 2016,Jan,13; 2015,Jan,16; 2014,Jan,11; 2013,Jan,9-10

95052 **Photo patch test(s) (specify number of tests)**

    📟 0.19   ✂ 0.19   **FUD** XXX   [Q1] [80] 🖵

    AMA: 2016,Jan,13; 2015,Jan,16; 2014,Jan,11; 2013,Jan,9-10

95056 **Photo tests**

    📟 1.25   ✂ 1.25   **FUD** XXX   [Q1] [80] 🖵

    AMA: 2016,Jan,13; 2015,Jan,16; 2014,Jan,11; 2013,Jan,9-10

95060 **Ophthalmic mucous membrane tests**

    📟 0.99   ✂ 0.99   **FUD** XXX   [Q1] [80] [TC] 🖵

    AMA: 2016,Jan,13; 2015,Jan,16; 2014,Jan,11; 2013,Jan,9-10

95065 **Direct nasal mucous membrane test**

    📟 0.72   ✂ 0.72   **FUD** XXX   [Q1] [80] [TC] 🖵

    AMA: 2016,Jan,13; 2015,Jan,16; 2014,Jan,11; 2013,Jan,9-10

95070 **Inhalation bronchial challenge testing (not including necessary pulmonary function tests); with histamine, methacholine, or similar compounds**

    EXCLUDES   *Pulmonary function tests (94060, 94070)*

    📟 0.86   ✂ 0.86   **FUD** XXX   [S] [80] [TC] 🖵

    AMA: 2016,Jan,13; 2015,Jan,16; 2014,Jan,11; 2013,Jan,9-10; 2012,Nov,11-12

95071 **with antigens or gases, specify**

    EXCLUDES   *Pulmonary function tests (94060, 94070)*

    📟 0.99   ✂ 0.99   **FUD** XXX   [Q1] [80] [TC] 🖵

    AMA: 2016,Jan,13; 2015,Jan,16; 2014,Jan,11; 2013,Jan,9-10; 2012,Nov,11-12

95076-95079 Challenge Ingestion Testing

CMS: 100-03,110.12 Challenge Ingestion Food Testing

    INCLUDES   Assessment and monitoring for allergic reactions (eg, blood pressure, peak flow meter)

    Testing time until the test ends or to the point an E&M service is needed

    EXCLUDES   *Use of code to report testing time less than 61 minutes, such as a positive challenge resulting in ending the test (use E&M codes as appropriate)*

Code also interventions when appropriate (eg, injection of epinephrine or steroid)

95076 **Ingestion challenge test (sequential and incremental ingestion of test items, eg, food, drug or other substance); initial 120 minutes of testing**

    INCLUDES   First 120 minutes of testing time (not face-to-face time with physician)

    📟 2.08   ✂ 3.29   **FUD** XXX   [S] [80] 🖵

    AMA: 2016,Jan,13; 2015,Jan,16; 2013,Jan,9-10

+ **95079** **each additional 60 minutes of testing (List separately in addition to code for primary procedure)**

    INCLUDES   Includes each 60 minutes of additional testing time (not face-to-face time with physician)

    Code first (95076)

    📟 1.90   ✂ 2.34   **FUD** ZZZ   [N] [80] 🖵

    AMA: 2016,Jan,13; 2015,Jan,16; 2013,Jan,9-10

95115-95199 Allergy Immunotherapy

CMS: 100-03,110.9 Antigens Prepared for Sublingual Administration

    INCLUDES   Allergen immunotherapy professional services

    EXCLUDES   *Bacterial/viral/fungal extracts skin testing (86485-86580, 95028)*

    Special reports for allergy patients (99080)

    The following procedures for testing: (See Pathology/Immunology section or code:) (95199)

    Leukocyte histamine release (LHR)

    Lymphocytic transformation test (LTT)

    Mast cell degranulation test (MCDT)

    Migration inhibitory factor test (MIF)

    Nitroblue tetrazolium dye test (NTD)

    Radioallergosorbent testing (RAST)

    Rat mast cell technique (RMCT)

    Transfer factor test (TFT)

Code also significant separately identifiable E&M services, when performed

95115 **Professional services for allergen immunotherapy not including provision of allergenic extracts; single injection**

    📟 0.25   ✂ 0.25   **FUD** XXX   [S] [80] 🖵

    AMA: 2016,Jan,13; 2015,Jan,16; 2014,Jan,11; 2013,Jan,9-10

95117 **2 or more injections**

    📟 0.29   ✂ 0.29   **FUD** XXX   [S] [80] 🖵

    AMA: 2016,Jan,13; 2015,Jan,16; 2014,Jan,11; 2013,Jan,9-10; 2012,Jan,15-42; 2011,Jan,11

95120 **Professional services for allergen immunotherapy in the office or institution of the prescribing physician or other qualified health care professional, including provision of allergenic extract; single injection**

    📟 0.00   ✂ 0.00   **FUD** XXX   [E] 🖵

    AMA: 2016,Jan,13; 2015,Jan,16; 2014,Jan,11; 2013,Jan,9-10

95125 **2 or more injections**

    📟 0.00   ✂ 0.00   **FUD** XXX   [E] 🖵

    AMA: 2016,Jan,13; 2015,Jan,16; 2014,Jan,11; 2013,Jan,9-10; 2012,Jan,15-42; 2011,Jan,11

95130 **single stinging insect venom**

    📟 0.00   ✂ 0.00   **FUD** XXX   [E] 🖵

    AMA: 2016,Jan,13; 2015,Jan,16; 2014,Jan,11; 2013,Jan,9-10; 2012,Jan,15-42; 2011,Jan,11

95131 **2 stinging insect venoms**

    📟 0.00   ✂ 0.00   **FUD** XXX   [E] 🖵

    AMA: 2016,Jan,13; 2015,Jan,16; 2014,Jan,11; 2013,Jan,9-10; 2012,Jan,15-42; 2011,Jan,11

95132 **3 stinging insect venoms**

    📟 0.00   ✂ 0.00   **FUD** XXX   [E] 🖵

    AMA: 2016,Jan,13; 2015,Jan,16; 2014,Jan,11; 2013,Jan,9-10; 2012,Jan,15-42; 2011,Jan,11

95133 **4 stinging insect venoms**

    📟 0.00   ✂ 0.00   **FUD** XXX   [E] 🖵

    AMA: 2016,Jan,13; 2015,Jan,16; 2014,Jan,11; 2013,Jan,9-10; 2012,Jan,15-42; 2011,Jan,11

95134 **5 stinging insect venoms**

    📟 0.00   ✂ 0.00   **FUD** XXX   [E] 🖵

    AMA: 2016,Jan,13; 2015,Jan,16; 2014,Jan,11; 2013,Jan,9-10; 2012,Jan,15-42; 2011,Jan,11

95144 **Professional services for the supervision of preparation and provision of antigens for allergen immunotherapy, single dose vial(s) (specify number of vials)**

    INCLUDES   Single dose vial/single dose of antigen administered in one injection

    📟 0.09   ✂ 0.35   **FUD** XXX   [S] [80] 🖵

    AMA: 2016,Jan,13; 2015,Jan,16; 2014,Jan,11; 2013,Jan,9-10; 2012,Jan,15-42; 2011,Jan,11

95145 **Professional services for the supervision of preparation and provision of antigens for allergen immunotherapy (specify number of doses); single stinging insect venom**

    📟 0.09   ✂ 0.61   **FUD** XXX   [S] [80] 🖵

    AMA: 2016,Jan,13; 2015,Jan,16; 2014,Jan,11; 2013,Jan,9-10; 2012,Jan,15-42; 2011,Jan,11

| [26/TC] PC/TC Only | [A2-Z3] ASC Payment | [50] Bilateral | ♂ Male Only | ♀ Female Only | 📟 Facility RVU | ✂ Non-Facility RVU | [CCI] CCI |
| **FUD** Follow-up Days | **CMS:** IOM (Pub 100) | [A-Y] OPPSI | [80/80] Surg Assist Allowed / w/Doc | | 🖵 Lab Crosswalk | 🖵 Radiology Crosswalk | [X] CLIA |

448   CPT © 2016 American Medical Association. All Rights Reserved.   © 2016 Optum360, LLC

95146 **2 single stinging insect venoms**
    🚑 0.09   ⚕ 1.10   **FUD** XXX   S 80 ▭
    AMA: 2016,Jan,13; 2015,Jan,16; 2014,Jan,11; 2013,Jan,9-10

95147 **3 single stinging insect venoms**
    🚑 0.09   ⚕ 0.99   **FUD** XXX   S 80 ▭
    AMA: 2016,Jan,13; 2015,Jan,16; 2014,Jan,11; 2013,Jan,9-10

95148 **4 single stinging insect venoms**
    🚑 0.09   ⚕ 1.47   **FUD** XXX   S 80 ▭
    AMA: 2016,Jan,13; 2015,Jan,16; 2014,Jan,11; 2013,Jan,9-10

95149 **5 single stinging insect venoms**
    🚑 0.09   ⚕ 1.98   **FUD** XXX   S 80 ▭
    AMA: 2016,Jan,13; 2015,Jan,16; 2014,Jan,11; 2013,Jan,9-10

95165 **Professional services for the supervision of preparation and provision of antigens for allergen immunotherapy; single or multiple antigens (specify number of doses)**
    🚑 0.09   ⚕ 0.36   **FUD** XXX   S 80 ▭
    AMA: 2016,Jan,13; 2015,Jan,16; 2014,Jan,11; 2013,Jan,9-10; 2012,Jan,15-42; 2011,Jan,11

95170 **whole body extract of biting insect or other arthropod (specify number of doses)**
    INCLUDES   A dose which is the amount of antigen(s) administered in a single injection from a multiple dose vial
    🚑 0.09   ⚕ 0.27   **FUD** XXX   S 80 ▭
    AMA: 2016,Jan,13; 2015,Jan,16; 2014,Jan,11; 2013,Jan,9-10; 2012,Jan,15-42; 2011,Jan,11

95180 **Rapid desensitization procedure, each hour (eg, insulin, penicillin, equine serum)**
    🚑 2.87   ⚕ 3.78   **FUD** XXX   01 80 ▭
    AMA: 2016,Jan,13; 2015,Jan,16; 2014,Jan,11; 2013,Jan,9-10

95199 **Unlisted allergy/clinical immunologic service or procedure**
    🚑 0.00   ⚕ 0.00   **FUD** XXX   01 80
    AMA: 2016,Jan,13; 2015,Jan,16; 2014,Jan,11; 2013,Jan,9-10

95250-95251 Glucose Monitoring By Subcutaneous Device

EXCLUDES   *Physiologic data collection/interpretation (99091)*
            Use of code more than one time per month

95250 **Ambulatory continuous glucose monitoring of interstitial tissue fluid via a subcutaneous sensor for a minimum of 72 hours; sensor placement, hook-up, calibration of monitor, patient training, removal of sensor, and printout of recording**
    🚑 4.46   ⚕ 4.46   **FUD** XXX   V 80 TC ▭
    AMA: 2016,Jan,13; 2015,Jan,16; 2014,Jan,11; 2011,Jan,11

95251 **interpretation and report**
    EXCLUDES   *Implantation interstitial glucose sensor (0446T)*
    🚑 1.23   ⚕ 1.23   **FUD** XXX   B 80 26 ▭
    AMA: 2016,Jan,13; 2015,Jan,16; 2014,Jan,11

95782-95811 [95782, 95783, 95800, 95801] Sleep Studies

INCLUDES   Assessment of sleep disorders in adults and children
            Continuous and simultaneous monitoring and recording of physiological sleep parameters of 6 hours or more
            Evaluation of patient's response to therapies
            Physician:
                Interpretation
                Recording
                Report
            Recording sessions may be:
                Attended studies that include the presence of a technologist or qualified health care professional to respond to the needs of the patient or technical issues at the bedside
                Remote without the presence of a technologist or a qualified health professional
                Unattended without the presence of a technologist or qualified health care professional
            Testing parameters include:
                Actigraphy: Use of a noninvasive portable device to record gross motor movements to approximate periods of sleep and wakefulness
                Electrooculogram (EOG): Records electrical activity associated with eye movements
                Maintenance of wakefulness test (MWT): An attended study used to determine the patient's ability to stay awake
                Multiple sleep latency test (MSLT): Attended study to determine the tendency of the patient to fall asleep
                Peripheral arterial tonometry (PAT): Pulsatile volume changes in a digit are measured to determine activity in the sympathetic nervous system for respiratory analysis
                Polysomnography: An attended continuous, simultaneous recording of physiological parameters of sleep for at least 6 hours in a sleep laboratory setting that also includes four or more of the following:
                    2. Bilateral anterior tibialis EMG
                    3. Electrocardiogram (ECG)
                    1. Airflow-oral and/or nasal
                    4. Oxyhemoglobin saturation, SpO2
                    5. Respiratory effort
                Positive airway pressure (PAP): Noninvasive devices used to treat sleep-related disorders
                Respiratory airflow (ventilation): Assessment of air movement during inhalation and exhalation as measured by nasal pressure sensors and thermistor
                Respiratory analysis: Assessment of components of respiration obtained by other methods such as airflow or peripheral arterial tone
                Respiratory effort: Use of the diaphragm and/or intercostal muscle for airflow is measured using transducers to estimate thoracic and abdominal motion
                Respiratory movement: Measures the movement of the chest and abdomen during respiration
                Sleep latency: Pertains to the time it takes to get to sleep
                Sleep staging: Determination of the separate levels of sleep according to physiological measurements
                Total sleep time: Determined by the use of actigraphy and other methods
            Use of portable and in-laboratory technology
EXCLUDES   E&M services

95782 **Resequenced code. See code following 95811.**

95783 **Resequenced code. See code following 95811.**

95800 **Resequenced code. See code following 95806.**

95801 **Resequenced code. See code following 95806.**

95803 **Actigraphy testing, recording, analysis, interpretation, and report (minimum of 72 hours to 14 consecutive days of recording)**
    EXCLUDES   *Sleep studies (95806-95811 [95800, 95801])*
                Use of code more than one time in a 14-day period
    🚑 4.00   ⚕ 4.00   **FUD** XXX   01 80 ▭
    AMA: 2016,Jan,13; 2015,Jan,16; 2014,Jan,11

95805 Multiple sleep latency or maintenance of wakefulness testing, recording, analysis and interpretation of physiological measurements of sleep during multiple trials to assess sleepiness

> INCLUDES Physiological sleep parameters as measured by:
>   Frontal, central, and occipital EEG leads (3 leads)
>   Left and right EOG
>   Submental EMG lead
> EXCLUDES Polysomnography (95808-95811)
>   Sleep study, not attended (95806)
> Code also modifier 52 when less than four nap opportunities are recorded
>
> 🚗 12.0   ⚖ 12.0   **FUD** XXX   S 80 🖵
>
> **AMA:** 2016,Jan,13; 2015,Jan,16; 2014,Jan,11; 2013,Feb,14-15

95806 Sleep study, unattended, simultaneous recording of, heart rate, oxygen saturation, respiratory airflow, and respiratory effort (eg, thoracoabdominal movement)

> EXCLUDES Arterial waveform analysis (93050)
>   Event monitors (93268-93272)
>   Holter monitor (93224-93227)
>   Remote cardiovascular telemetry (93228-93229)
>   Rhythm strips (93041-93042)
>   Unattended sleep study with measurement of a minimum heart rate, oxygen saturation, and respiratory analysis (95801)
>   Unattended sleep study with measurement of heart rate, oxygen saturation, respiratory analysis, and sleep time (95800)
> Code also modifier 52 for fewer than 6 hours of recording
>
> 🚗 4.76   ⚖ 4.76   **FUD** XXX   S 80 🖵
>
> **AMA:** 2016,Jan,13; 2015,Jan,16; 2014,Jan,11; 2013,Jul,11-12; 2013,Feb,14-15; 2012,Jan,15-42; 2011,Jan,6-7; 2011,Jan,11

\# **95800** Sleep study, unattended, simultaneous recording; heart rate, oxygen saturation, respiratory analysis (eg, by airflow or peripheral arterial tone), and sleep time

> 🚗 5.04   ⚖ 5.04   **FUD** XXX   S 80 🖵
>
> **AMA:** 2016,Jan,13; 2015,Jan,16; 2014,Jan,11; 2013,Feb,14-15; 2011,Jan,6-7

\# **95801** minimum of heart rate, oxygen saturation, and respiratory analysis (eg, by airflow or peripheral arterial tone)

> 🚗 2.56   ⚖ 2.56   **FUD** XXX   01 80 🖵
>
> **AMA:** 2016,Jan,13; 2015,Jan,16; 2014,Jan,11; 2013,Feb,14-15; 2011,Jan,6-7

95807 Sleep study, simultaneous recording of ventilation, respiratory effort, ECG or heart rate, and oxygen saturation, attended by a technologist

> EXCLUDES Polysomnography (95808-95811)
>   Sleep study, not attended (95806)
> Code also modifier 52 for fewer than 6 hours of recording
>
> 🚗 13.5   ⚖ 13.5   **FUD** XXX   S 80 🖵
>
> **AMA:** 2016,Jan,13; 2015,Jan,16; 2014,Jan,11; 2013,Feb,14-15

95808 Polysomnography; any age, sleep staging with 1-3 additional parameters of sleep, attended by a technologist

> EXCLUDES Sleep study, not attended (95806)
>
> 🚗 17.8   ⚖ 17.8   **FUD** XXX   S 80 🖵
>
> **AMA:** 2016,Jan,13; 2015,Jan,16; 2014,Jan,11; 2013,Feb,14-15; 2012,Jan,15-42; 2011,Jan,11

95810 age 6 years or older, sleep staging with 4 or more additional parameters of sleep, attended by a technologist A

> EXCLUDES Sleep study, not attended (95806)
> Code also modifier 52 for fewer than 6 hours of recording
>
> 🚗 17.6   ⚖ 17.6   **FUD** XXX   S 80 🖵
>
> **AMA:** 2016,Jan,13; 2015,Jan,16; 2014,Jan,11; 2013,Feb,14-15

95811 age 6 years or older, sleep staging with 4 or more additional parameters of sleep, with initiation of continuous positive airway pressure therapy or bilevel ventilation, attended by a technologist A

> EXCLUDES Sleep study, not attended (95806)
> Code also modifier 52 for fewer than 6 hours of recording
>
> 🚗 18.5   ⚖ 18.5   **FUD** XXX   S 80 🖵
>
> **AMA:** 2016,Jan,13; 2015,Jan,16; 2014,Oct,8; 2014,Jan,11; 2013,Feb,14-15

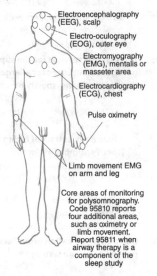

Electroencephalography (EEG), scalp
Electro-oculography (EOG), outer eye
Electromyography (EMG), mentalis or masseter area
Electrocardiography (ECG), chest
Pulse oximetry
Limb movement EMG on arm and leg

Core areas of monitoring for polysomnography. Code 95810 reports four additional areas, such as oximetry or limb movement. Report 95811 when airway therapy is a component of the sleep study.

\# **95782** younger than 6 years, sleep staging with 4 or more additional parameters of sleep, attended by a technologist A

> Code also modifier 52 for fewer than 7 hours of recording
>
> 🚗 29.0   ⚖ 29.0   **FUD** XXX   S 80 🖵
>
> **AMA:** 2016,Jan,13; 2015,Jan,16; 2014,Jan,11; 2013,Feb,14-15

\# **95783** younger than 6 years, sleep staging with 4 or more additional parameters of sleep, with initiation of continuous positive airway pressure therapy or bi-level ventilation, attended by a technologist A

> Code also modifier 52 for fewer than 7 hours of recording
>
> 🚗 30.4   ⚖ 30.4   **FUD** XXX   S 80 🖵
>
> **AMA:** 2016,Jan,13; 2015,Jan,16; 2014,Oct,8; 2014,Jan,11; 2013,Feb,14-15

95812-95830 Evaluation of Brain Activity by Electroencephalogram

> INCLUDES Only time when time is being recorded and data are being collected and does not include set-up and take-down
> EXCLUDES E&M services

95812 Electroencephalogram (EEG) extended monitoring; 41-60 minutes

> INCLUDES Hyperventilation
>   Only time when recording is taking place and data are being collected and does not include set-up and take-down
>   Photic stimulation
>   Physician interpretation
>   Recording of 41-60 minutes
>   Report
> EXCLUDES EEG digital analysis (95957)
>   EEG during nonintracranial surgery (95955)
>   EEG monitoring, 24-hour (95950-95953, 95956)
>   Wada test (95958)
> Code also modifier 26 for physician interpretation only
>
> 🚗 9.86   ⚖ 9.86   **FUD** XXX   S 80 🖵
>
> **AMA:** 2016,Jan,13; 2015,Jan,16; 2014,Jan,11; 2012,Jan,15-42; 2011,May,9; 2011,Feb,3

95813 **greater than 1 hour**

INCLUDES Hyperventilation
Only time when recording is taking place and data are being collected and does not include set-up and take-down
Photic stimulation
Physician interpretation
Recording of 61 minutes or more
Report

EXCLUDES *EEG digital analysis (95957)*
EEG during nonintracranial surgery (95955)
EEG monitoring, 24-hour (95950-95953, 95956)
Wada test (95958)

Code also modifier 26 for physician interpretation only
⏢ 11.9   ⚖ 11.9   **FUD** XXX   S 80 ▭

AMA: 2016,Jan,13; 2015,Jan,16; 2014,Jan,11; 2012,Jan,15-42; 2011,May,9; 2011,Feb,3

95816 **Electroencephalogram (EEG); including recording awake and drowsy**

INCLUDES Photic stimulation
Physician interpretation
Recording of 20-40 minutes
Report

EXCLUDES *EEG digital analysis (95957)*
EEG during nonintracranial surgery (95955)
EEG monitoring, 24-hour (95950-95953, 95956)
Wada test (95958)

Code also modifier 26 for physician interpretation only
⏢ 10.2   ⚖ 10.2   **FUD** XXX   S 80 ▭

AMA: 2016,Jan,13; 2015,Dec,16; 2015,Jan,16; 2014,Jan,11; 2012,Jan,15-42; 2011,Feb,3; 2011,Jan,11

95819 **including recording awake and asleep**

INCLUDES Hyperventilation
Photic stimulation
Physician interpretation
Recording of 20-40 minutes
Report

EXCLUDES *EEG digital analysis (95957)*
EEG during nonintracranial surgery (95955)
EEG monitoring, 24-hour (95950-95953, 95956)
Wada test (95958)

Code also modifier 26 for interpretation only
⏢ 11.7   ⚖ 11.7   **FUD** XXX   S 80 ▭

AMA: 2016,Jan,13; 2015,Dec,16; 2015,Jan,16; 2014,Jan,11; 2011,Feb,3

95822 **recording in coma or sleep only**

INCLUDES Hyperventilation
Photic stimulation
Physician interpretation
Recording of 20-40 minutes
Report

EXCLUDES *EEG digital analysis (95957)*
EEG during nonintracranial surgery (95955)
EEG monitoring, 24-hour (95950-95953, 95956)
Wada test (95958)

Code also modifier 26 for interpretation only
⏢ 10.5   ⚖ 10.5   **FUD** XXX   S 80 ▭

AMA: 2016,Jan,13; 2015,Jan,16; 2014,Dec,18; 2014,Jan,11; 2013,May,8-10; 2011,Feb,3

95824 **cerebral death evaluation only**

INCLUDES Physician interpretation
Recording
Report

EXCLUDES *EEG digital analysis (95957)*
EEG during nonintracranial surgery (95955)
EEG monitoring, 24-hour (95950-95953, 95956)
Wada test (95958)

Code also modifier 26 for physician interpretation only
⏢ 0.00   ⚖ 0.00   **FUD** XXX   S 80 ▭

AMA: 2003,Dec,4; 2001,Nov,4

95827 **all night recording**

INCLUDES Physician interpretation
Recording
Report

EXCLUDES *EEG digital analysis (95957)*
EEG during nonintracranial surgery (95955)
EEG monitoring, 24-hour (95950-95953, 95956)
Wada test (95958)

Code also modifier 26 for interpretation only
⏢ 19.7   ⚖ 19.7   **FUD** XXX   S 80 ▭

AMA: 2003,Dec,4; 2001,Nov,4

95829 **Electrocorticogram at surgery (separate procedure)**

INCLUDES Physician interpretation
Recording
Report

Code also modifier 26 for interpretation only
⏢ 53.2   ⚖ 53.2   **FUD** XXX   N 80 ▭

AMA: 2003,Dec,4; 2001,Nov,4

95830 **Insertion by physician or other qualified health care professional of sphenoidal electrodes for electroencephalographic (EEG) recording**

⏢ 2.62   ⚖ 6.95   **FUD** XXX   B 80 ▭

AMA: 2003,Dec,4; 2001,Nov,4

95831-95857 Evaluation of Muscles and Range of Motion

CMS: 100-02,15,230.4 Services By a Physical/Occupational Therapist in Private Practice

EXCLUDES *E&M services*

95831 **Muscle testing, manual (separate procedure) with report; extremity (excluding hand) or trunk**

⏢ 0.43   ⚖ 0.86   **FUD** XXX   A 80 ▭

AMA: 2016,Jan,13; 2015,Jan,16; 2014,Jan,11; 2013,Aug,7; 2012,Jan,15-42; 2011,Jan,11

95832 **hand, with or without comparison with normal side**

⏢ 0.45   ⚖ 0.83   **FUD** XXX   A 80 ▭

AMA: 2016,Jan,13; 2015,Jan,16; 2014,Jan,11; 2013,Aug,7; 2012,Jan,15-42; 2011,Jan,11

95833 **total evaluation of body, excluding hands**

⏢ 0.61   ⚖ 1.05   **FUD** XXX   A 80 ▭

AMA: 2016,Jan,13; 2015,Jan,16; 2014,Jan,11; 2013,Aug,7; 2012,Oct,14; 2012,Sep,16

95834 **total evaluation of body, including hands**

⏢ 0.89   ⚖ 1.45   **FUD** XXX   A 80 ▭

AMA: 2016,Jan,13; 2015,Jan,16; 2014,Jan,11; 2013,Aug,7

95851 **Range of motion measurements and report (separate procedure); each extremity (excluding hand) or each trunk section (spine)**

⏢ 0.22   ⚖ 0.52   **FUD** XXX   A 80 ▭

AMA: 2016,Jan,13; 2015,Jan,16; 2014,Jan,11; 2013,Aug,7; 2012,Jan,15-42; 2011,Jan,11

95852 **hand, with or without comparison with normal side**

⏢ 0.17   ⚖ 0.46   **FUD** XXX   A 80 ▭

AMA: 2016,Jan,13; 2015,Jan,16; 2014,Jan,11; 2013,Aug,7

95857 **Cholinesterase inhibitor challenge test for myasthenia gravis**

⏢ 0.84   ⚖ 1.53   **FUD** XXX   S 80 ▭

AMA: 2016,Jan,13; 2015,Jan,16; 2014,Jan,11; 2011,Feb,3

95860-95887 [95885, 95886, 95887] Evaluation of Nerve and Muscle Function: EMGs with/without Nerve Conduction Studies

INCLUDES Physician interpretation
Recording
Report

EXCLUDES E&M services

95860 **Needle electromyography; 1 extremity with or without related paraspinal areas**

INCLUDES Testing of five or more muscles per extremity

EXCLUDES Dynamic electromyography during motion analysis studies (96002-96003)

Guidance for chemodenervation (95873-95874)

🚑 3.45 ⚖ 3.45 **FUD** XXX [01] [80] 🖵

AMA: 2016,Jan,13; 2015,Mar,6; 2015,Jan,16; 2014,Jan,11; 2013,May,8-10; 2013,Mar,3-5; 2012,Feb,8; 2012,Jan,15-42; 2011,Jan,11

95861 **2 extremities with or without related paraspinal areas**

INCLUDES Testing of five or more muscles per extremity

EXCLUDES Dynamic electromyography during motion analysis studies (96002-96003)

Guidance for chemodenervation (95873-95874)

🚑 4.85 ⚖ 4.85 **FUD** XXX [01] [80] 🖵

AMA: 2016,Jan,13; 2015,Mar,6; 2015,Jan,16; 2014,Jan,11; 2013,May,8-10; 2013,Mar,3-5; 2012,Feb,8; 2012,Jan,15-42; 2011,Jan,11

95863 **3 extremities with or without related paraspinal areas**

INCLUDES Testing of five or more muscles per extremity

EXCLUDES Dynamic electromyography during motion analysis studies (96002-96003)

Guidance for chemodenervation (95873-95874)

🚑 6.02 ⚖ 6.02 **FUD** XXX [S] [80] 🖵

AMA: 2016,Jan,13; 2015,Mar,6; 2015,Jan,16; 2014,Jan,11; 2013,May,8-10; 2013,Mar,3-5; 2012,Feb,8; 2012,Jan,15-42; 2011,Jan,11

95864 **4 extremities with or without related paraspinal areas**

INCLUDES Testing of five or more muscles per extremity

EXCLUDES Dynamic electromyography during motion analysis studies (96002-96003)

Guidance for chemodenervation (95873-95874)

🚑 6.80 ⚖ 6.80 **FUD** XXX [S] [80] 🖵

AMA: 2016,Jan,13; 2015,Mar,6; 2015,Jan,16; 2014,Jan,11; 2013,May,8-10; 2013,Mar,3-5; 2012,Feb,8; 2012,Jan,15-42; 2011,Jan,11

95865 **larynx**

EXCLUDES Dynamic electromyography during motion analysis studies (96002-96003)

Guidance for chemodenervation (95873-95874)

Code also modifier 52 for unilateral procedure

🚑 4.08 ⚖ 4.08 **FUD** XXX [01] [80] 🖵

AMA: 2016,Jan,13; 2015,Mar,6; 2015,Jan,16; 2014,Jan,6; 2014,Jan,11; 2013,May,8-10; 2012,Jan,15-42; 2011,Jan,11

95866 **hemidiaphragm**

EXCLUDES Dynamic electromyography during motion analysis studies (96002-96003)

Guidance for chemodenervation (95873-95874)

🚑 3.78 ⚖ 3.78 **FUD** XXX [01] [80] 🖵

AMA: 2016,Jan,13; 2015,Mar,6; 2015,Jan,16; 2014,Jan,11; 2013,May,8-10; 2012,Jan,15-42; 2011,Jan,11

95867 **cranial nerve supplied muscle(s), unilateral**

EXCLUDES Guidance for chemodenervation (95873-95874)

🚑 2.67 ⚖ 2.67 **FUD** XXX [S] [80] 🖵

AMA: 2016,Jan,13; 2015,Mar,6; 2015,Jan,16; 2014,Jan,11; 2013,May,8-10; 2013,Mar,3-5; 2012,Feb,8; 2012,Jan,15-42; 2011,Jan,11

95868 **cranial nerve supplied muscles, bilateral**

EXCLUDES Guidance for chemodenervation (95873-95874)

🚑 3.75 ⚖ 3.75 **FUD** XXX [S] [80] 🖵

AMA: 2016,Jan,13; 2015,Mar,6; 2015,Jan,16; 2014,Jan,11; 2013,May,8-10; 2013,Mar,3-5; 2012,Feb,8; 2012,Jan,15-42; 2011,Jan,11

95869 **thoracic paraspinal muscles (excluding T1 or T12)**

EXCLUDES Dynamic electromyography during motion analysis studies (96002-96003)

Guidance for chemodenervation (95873-95874)

🚑 2.63 ⚖ 2.63 **FUD** XXX [01] [80] 🖵

AMA: 2016,Jan,13; 2015,Mar,6; 2015,Jan,16; 2014,Jan,11; 2013,May,8-10; 2013,Mar,3-5; 2012,Feb,8; 2012,Jan,15-42; 2011,Jan,11

95870 **limited study of muscles in 1 extremity or non-limb (axial) muscles (unilateral or bilateral), other than thoracic paraspinal, cranial nerve supplied muscles, or sphincters**

INCLUDES Adson test

Testing of four or less muscles per extremity

EXCLUDES Anal/urethral sphincter/detrusor/urethra/perineum musculature (51785-51792)

Complete study of extremities (95860-95864)

Dynamic electromyography during motion analysis studies (96002-96003)

Eye muscles (92265)

Guidance for chemodenervation (95873-95874)

🚑 2.63 ⚖ 2.63 **FUD** XXX [01] [80] 🖵

AMA: 2016,Jan,13; 2015,Mar,6; 2015,Jan,16; 2014,Jan,11; 2013,May,8-10; 2013,Mar,3-5; 2012,Feb,8; 2012,Jan,15-42; 2011,Jan,11

95872 **Needle electromyography using single fiber electrode, with quantitative measurement of jitter, blocking and/or fiber density, any/all sites of each muscle studied**

EXCLUDES Dynamic electromyography during motion analysis studies (96002-96003)

🚑 5.55 ⚖ 5.55 **FUD** XXX [S] [80] 🖵

AMA: 2016,Jan,13; 2015,Mar,6; 2015,Jan,16; 2014,Jan,11; 2012,Jan,15-42; 2011,Jan,11

+ # **95885** **Needle electromyography, each extremity, with related paraspinal areas, when performed, done with nerve conduction, amplitude and latency/velocity study; limited (List separately in addition to code for primary procedure)**

INCLUDES Testing of four or less muscles per extremity

EXCLUDES Dynamic electromyography during motion analysis studies (96002-96003)

Motor and sensory nerve conduction (95905)

Needle electromyography of extremities (95860-95864, 95870)

Use of code more than one time per extremity

Code also, when applicable, for a combined maximum total of four units per patient if all four extremities are tested ([95886])

Code first nerve conduction tests (95907-95913)

🚑 1.66 ⚖ 1.66 **FUD** ZZZ [N] [80] 🖵

AMA: 2016,Jan,13; 2015,Mar,6; 2015,Jan,16; 2014,Jan,11; 2013,Sep,17; 2013,May,8-10; 2013,Mar,3-5; 2012,Feb,8; 2012,Jan,15-42

+ # **95886** **complete, five or more muscles studied, innervated by three or more nerves or four or more spinal levels (List separately in addition to code for primary procedure)**

INCLUDES Testing of five or more muscles per extremity

EXCLUDES Dynamic electromyography during motion analysis studies (96002-96003)

Motor and sensory nerve conduction (95905)

Needle electromyography of extremities (95860-95864, 95870)

Use of code more than one time per extremity

Code also, when applicable, for a combined maximum total of four units per patient if all four extremities are tested ([95885])

Code first nerve conduction tests (95907-95913)

🚑 2.58 ⚖ 2.58 **FUD** ZZZ [N] [80] 🖵

AMA: 2016,Jan,13; 2015,Mar,6; 2015,Jan,16; 2014,Jan,11; 2013,Sep,17; 2013,May,8-10; 2013,Mar,3-5; 2012,Feb,8; 2012,Jan,15-42

26/TC PC/TC Only   A2-Z3 ASC Payment   50 Bilateral   ♂ Male Only   ♀ Female Only   🚑 Facility RVU   ⚖ Non-Facility RVU   🖵 CCI
FUD Follow-up Days   CMS: IOM (Pub 100)   A-Y OPPSI   80/80 Surg Assist Allowed / w/Doc   Lab Crosswalk   Radiology Crosswalk   CLIA

452   CPT © 2016 American Medical Association. All Rights Reserved.   © 2016 Optum360, LLC

+ # 95887 **Needle electromyography, non-extremity (cranial nerve supplied or axial) muscle(s) done with nerve conduction, amplitude and latency/velocity study (List separately in addition to code for primary procedure)**

INCLUDES Nerve study of unilateral cranial nerve innervated muscles

EXCLUDES *Nerve study of extra-ocular or laryngeal nerves*

EXCLUDES *Dynamic electromyography during motion analysis studies (96002-96003)*
Guidance for chemodenervation (95874)
Needle electromyography cranial nerve supplied muscles (95867-95868)
Needle electromyography except for thoracic paraspinal, cranial nerve supplied muscles, or sphincters (95870)
Use of code more than once per anatomic site

Code also modifier 50 when performed bilaterally
Code first nerve conduction tests (95907-95913)

🔧 2.29   ⚕ 2.29   **FUD** ZZZ   Ⓝ 80 ▢

AMA: 2016,Jan,13; 2015,Mar,6; 2015,Jan,16; 2014,Jan,11; 2014,Jan,8; 2013,Mar,3-5; 2012,Jul,12-14; 2012,Feb,8; 2012,Jan,15-42

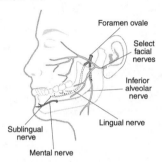

Foramen ovale
Select facial nerves
Inferior alveolar nerve
Lingual nerve
Sublingual nerve
Mental nerve

Cranial Nerves: trigeminal branches of lower face and select facial nerves

Needle EMG is performed to determine conduction, amplitude, and latency/velocity

+ 95873 **Electrical stimulation for guidance in conjunction with chemodenervation (List separately in addition to code for primary procedure)**

EXCLUDES *Chemodenervation larynx (64617)*
Needle electromyography (95860-95870)
Needle electromyography guidance for chemodenervation (95874)
Use of more than one guidance code for each code for chemodenervation

Code first chemodenervation (64612, 64615-64616, 64642-64647)

🔧 2.08   ⚕ 2.08   **FUD** ZZZ   Ⓝ 80 ▢

AMA: 2016,Jan,13; 2015,Mar,6; 2015,Jan,16; 2014,Jan,6; 2014,Jan,11; 2013,Apr,5-6; 2012,Jan,15-42; 2011,Jan,11

+ 95874 **Needle electromyography for guidance in conjunction with chemodenervation (List separately in addition to code for primary procedure)**

EXCLUDES *Chemodenervation larynx (64617)*
Needle electromyography (95860-95870)
Needle electromyography guidance for chemodenervation (95873)
Use of more than one guidance code for each code for chemodenervation

Code first chemodenervation (64612, 64615-64616, 64642-64647)

🔧 2.07   ⚕ 2.07   **FUD** ZZZ   Ⓝ 80 ▢

AMA: 2016,Jan,13; 2015,Mar,6; 2015,Jan,16; 2014,Oct,14; 2014,Jan,6; 2014,Jan,11; 2013,Apr,5-6; 2012,Jan,15-42; 2011,Jan,11

95875 **Ischemic limb exercise test with serial specimen(s) acquisition for muscle(s) metabolite(s)**

🔧 3.53   ⚕ 3.53   **FUD** XXX   Ⓢ 80 ▢

AMA: 2016,Jan,13; 2015,Mar,6; 2015,Jan,16; 2014,Jan,11; 2012,Jan,15-42; 2011,Jan,11

95885 **Resequenced code. See code following 95872.**

95886 **Resequenced code. See code following 95872.**

95887 **Resequenced code. See code before 95873.**

95905-95913 Evaluation of Nerve Function: Nerve Conduction Studies

CMS: 100-02,15,230.4 Services By a Physical/Occupational Therapist in Private Practice

INCLUDES Conduction studies of motor and sensory nerves
Reports from on-site examiner including the work product of the interpretation of results using established methodologies, calculations, comparisons to normal studies, and interpretation by physician or other qualified health care professional
Single conduction study comprising a sensory and motor conduction test with/without F or H wave testing, and all orthodromic and antidromic impulses
Total number of tests performed indicate which code is appropriate

EXCLUDES *Use of code for more than one study when multiple sites on the same nerve are tested*

Code also electromyography performed with nerve conduction studies, as appropriate ([95885, 95886, 95887])

95905 **Motor and/or sensory nerve conduction, using preconfigured electrode array(s), amplitude and latency/velocity study, each limb, includes F-wave study when performed, with interpretation and report**

INCLUDES Study with preconfigured electrodes that are customized to a specific body location

EXCLUDES *Needle electromyography ([95885, 95886])*
Nerve conduction studies (95907-95913)
Use of this code more than one time for each limb studied

🔧 1.98   ⚕ 1.98   **FUD** XXX   ⊘ 01 80 ▢

AMA: 2016,Jan,13; 2015,Jan,16; 2014,Jan,11; 2013,Mar,3-5; 2012,Feb,8

95907 **Nerve conduction studies; 1-2 studies**

🔧 2.70   ⚕ 2.70   **FUD** XXX   Ⓢ 80 ▢

AMA: 2016,Jan,13; 2015,Jan,16; 2014,Jan,11; 2013,Sep,17; 2013,May,8-10; 2013,Mar,3-5

95908 **3-4 studies**

🔧 3.35   ⚕ 3.35   **FUD** XXX   Ⓢ 80 ▢

AMA: 2016,Jan,13; 2015,Mar,6; 2015,Jan,16; 2014,Jan,11; 2013,Sep,17; 2013,May,8-10; 2013,Mar,3-5

95909 **5-6 studies**

🔧 4.08   ⚕ 4.08   **FUD** XXX   Ⓢ 80 ▢

AMA: 2016,Jan,13; 2015,Jan,16; 2014,Jan,11; 2013,Sep,17; 2013,May,8-10; 2013,Mar,3-5

95910 **7-8 studies**

🔧 5.44   ⚕ 5.44   **FUD** XXX   Ⓢ 80 ▢

AMA: 2016,Jan,13; 2015,Jan,16; 2014,Jan,11; 2013,Sep,17; 2013,May,8-10; 2013,Mar,3-5

95911 **9-10 studies**

🔧 6.57   ⚕ 6.57   **FUD** XXX   Ⓢ 80 ▢

AMA: 2016,Jan,13; 2015,Jan,16; 2014,Jan,11; 2013,Sep,17; 2013,May,8-10; 2013,Mar,3-5

95912 **11-12 studies**

🔧 7.35   ⚕ 7.35   **FUD** XXX   Ⓢ 80 ▢

AMA: 2016,Jan,13; 2015,Jan,16; 2014,Jan,11; 2013,Sep,17; 2013,May,8-10; 2013,Mar,3-5

95913 **13 or more studies**

🔧 8.41   ⚕ 8.41   **FUD** XXX   Ⓢ 80 ▢

AMA: 2016,Jan,13; 2015,Jan,16; 2014,Jan,11; 2013,Sep,17; 2013,May,8-10; 2013,Mar,3-5

[95940, 95941] Intraoperative Neurophysiological Monitoring

INCLUDES   Monitoring, testing, and data evaluation during surgical procedures by a monitoring professional dedicated only to performing the necessary testing and monitoring
Monitoring services provided by the anesthesiologist or surgeon separately

EXCLUDES   *Baseline neurophysiologic monitoring*
EEG during nonintracranial surgery (95955)
Electrocorticography (95829)
Intraoperative cortical and subcortical mapping (95961-95962)
Neurostimulator programming/analysis (95970-95975)
Time required for set-up, recording, interpretation, and removal of electrodes

Code also baseline studies (eg, EMGs, NCVs), no more than one time per operative session
Code also services provided after midnight using the date when monitoring started and the total monitoring time
Code also standby time prior to procedure (99360)
Code first (92585, 95822, 95860-95870, 95907-95913, 95925-95937 [95938, 95939])

+ #   95940   Continuous intraoperative neurophysiology monitoring in the operating room, one on one monitoring requiring personal attendance, each 15 minutes (List separately in addition to code for primary procedure)

INCLUDES   15 minute increments of monitoring service
A total of all monitoring time for procedures overlapping midnight
Based on time spent monitoring, regardless of number of tests or parameters monitored
Continuous intraoperative neurophysiologic monitoring by a dedicated monitoring professional in the operating room providing one-on-one patient care
Monitoring time may begin prior to the incision
Monitoring time that is distinct from baseline neurophysiologic study/s time or other services (eg, mapping)

EXCLUDES   *Time spent in executing or interpreting the baseline neurophysiologic study or studies*

Code also monitoring from outside of the operative room, when applicable ([95941])

🔪 0.93   ♨ 0.93   **FUD** XXX   [N] [N1] [80] ▢

AMA: 2016,Jan,13; 2015,Jan,16; 2014,Apr,10; 2014,Apr,5; 2013,May,8-10

+ #   95941   Continuous intraoperative neurophysiology monitoring, from outside the operating room (remote or nearby) or for monitoring of more than one case while in the operating room, per hour (List separately in addition to code for primary procedure)

INCLUDES   Based on time spent monitoring, regardless of number of tests or parameters monitored
Monitoring time that is distinct from baseline neurophysiologic study/s time or other services (eg, mapping)
One hour increments of monitoring service

🔪 0.00   ♨ 0.00   **FUD** XXX   [N] [N1] ▢

AMA: 2016,Jan,13; 2015,Jan,16; 2014,Dec,18; 2014,Apr,10; 2014,Apr,5; 2014,Jan,11; 2013,May,8-10; 2013,Feb,16-17

95921-95924 [95943] Evaluation of Autonomic Nervous System

INCLUDES   Physician interpretation
Recording
Report
Testing for autonomic dysfunction including site and autonomic subsystems

95921   Testing of autonomic nervous system function; cardiovagal innervation (parasympathetic function), including 2 or more of the following: heart rate response to deep breathing with recorded R-R interval, Valsalva ratio, and 30:15 ratio

INCLUDES   Display on a monitor
Minimum of two of the following elements are performed:
Cardiovascular function as indicated by a 30:15 ration (R/R interval at beat 30)/(R-R interval at beat 15)
Heart rate response to deep breathing obtained by visual quantitative analysis of recordings with patient taking 5-6 breaths per minute
Valsalva ratio (at least 2) obtained by dividing the highest heart rate by the lowest
Monitoring of heart rate by electrocardiography of rate obtained from time between two successive R waves (R-R interval)
Storage of data for waveform analysis
Testing most usually in prone position
Tilt table testing, when performed

EXCLUDES   *Autonomic nervous system testing with sympathetic adrenergic function testing (95922, 95924)*
Simultaneous measures of parasympathetic and sympathetic function ([95943])

🔪 2.44   ♨ 2.44   **FUD** XXX   [S] [80] ▢

AMA: 2016,Jan,13; 2015,Jan,16; 2014,Jan,11; 2012,Nov,6-9; 2012,Jan,15-42; 2011,Jan,11

95922   vasomotor adrenergic innervation (sympathetic adrenergic function), including beat-to-beat blood pressure and R-R interval changes during Valsalva maneuver and at least 5 minutes of passive tilt

EXCLUDES   *Autonomic nervous system testing with parasympathetic function (95921, 95924)*
Simultaneous measures of parasympathetic and sympathetic function ([95943])

🔪 2.85   ♨ 2.85   **FUD** XXX   [Q1] [80] ▢

AMA: 2016,Jan,13; 2015,Jan,16; 2014,Jan,11; 2012,Nov,6-9; 2012,Jan,15-42; 2011,Jan,11

95923   sudomotor, including 1 or more of the following: quantitative sudomotor axon reflex test (QSART), silastic sweat imprint, thermoregulatory sweat test, and changes in sympathetic skin potential

🔪 4.64   ♨ 4.64   **FUD** XXX   [Q1] [80] ▢

AMA: 2016,Jan,13; 2015,Jan,16; 2014,Jan,11; 2012,Nov,6-9; 2012,Jan,15-42; 2011,Jan,11

95924   combined parasympathetic and sympathetic adrenergic function testing with at least 5 minutes of passive tilt

INCLUDES   Tilt table testing of adrenergic and parasympathetic function

EXCLUDES   *Autonomic nervous system testing with parasympathetic function (95921-95922)*
Simultaneous measures of parasympathetic and sympathetic function ([95943])

🔪 4.21   ♨ 4.21   **FUD** XXX   [S] [80] ▢

AMA: 2016,Jan,13; 2015,Jan,16; 2012,Nov,6-9

 #   95943   Simultaneous, independent, quantitative measures of both parasympathetic function and sympathetic function, based on time-frequency analysis of heart rate variability concurrent with time-frequency analysis of continuous respiratory activity, with mean heart rate and blood pressure measures, during rest, paced (deep) breathing, Valsalva maneuvers, and head-up postural change

EXCLUDES   *Autonomic nervous system testing (95921-95922, 95924)*
Rhythm ECG (93040)

🔪 0.00   ♨ 0.00   **FUD** XXX   [S] [80] ▢

AMA: 2016,Jan,13; 2015,Jan,16; 2012,Nov,6-9

95925-95943 [95938, 95939] Neurotransmission Studies

95925 Short-latency somatosensory evoked potential study, stimulation of any/all peripheral nerves or skin sites, recording from the central nervous system; in upper limbs

EXCLUDES *Auditory evoked potentials (92585)*
Evoked potential study in both upper and lower limbs ([95938])
Evoked potential study in lower limbs (95926)
4.40 4.40 **FUD** XXX [S] [80] [⊡]
AMA: 2016,Jan,13; 2015,Jan,16; 2014,Jan,11; 2013,May,8-10; 2012,Apr,17-18

95926 in lower limbs

EXCLUDES *Auditory evoked potentials (92585)*
Evoked potential study in both upper and lower limbs ([95938])
Evoked potential study in upper limbs (95925)
3.89 3.89 **FUD** XXX [S] [80] [⊡]
AMA: 2016,Jan,13; 2015,Jan,16; 2014,Jan,11; 2013,May,8-10; 2012,Apr,17-18; 2012,Jan,15-42; 2011,Jan,11

**95938** in upper and lower limbs

EXCLUDES *Evoked potential study lower limbs and upper limbs (95925-95926)*
9.66 9.66 **FUD** XXX [S] [80] [⊡]
AMA: 2016,Jan,13; 2015,Jan,16; 2014,Jan,11; 2013,May,8-10; 2013,Feb,16-17; 2012,Apr,17-18

95927 in the trunk or head

EXCLUDES *Auditory evoked potentials (92585)*
Code also modifier 52 for unilateral test
4.02 4.02 **FUD** XXX [S] [80] [⊡]
AMA: 2016,Jan,13; 2015,Jan,16; 2014,Jan,11; 2013,May,8-10

95928 Central motor evoked potential study (transcranial motor stimulation); upper limbs

EXCLUDES *Central motor evoked potential study lower limbs (95929)*
6.35 6.35 **FUD** XXX [S] [80] [⊡]
AMA: 2016,Jan,13; 2015,Jan,16; 2013,May,8-10

95929 lower limbs

EXCLUDES *Central motor evoked potential study upper limbs (95928)*
6.40 6.40 **FUD** XXX [S] [80] [⊡]
AMA: 2016,Jan,13; 2015,Jan,16; 2014,Dec,6; 2013,May,8-10

**95939** in upper and lower limbs

EXCLUDES *Central motor evoked potential study of either lower or upper limbs (95928-95929)*
14.1 14.1 **FUD** XXX [S] [80] [⊡]
AMA: 2016,Jan,13; 2015,Jan,16; 2014,Jan,11; 2013,May,8-10; 2012,Apr,17-18

95930 Visual evoked potential (VEP) testing central nervous system, checkerboard or flash

EXCLUDES *Visual acuity screening using automated visual evoked potential devices (0333T)*
3.66 3.66 **FUD** XXX [S] [80] [⊡]
AMA: 2016,Jan,13; 2015,Jan,16; 2014,Aug,8; 2013,May,8-10

95933 Orbicularis oculi (blink) reflex, by electrodiagnostic testing
2.12 2.12 **FUD** XXX [01] [80] [⊡]
AMA: 2016,Jan,13; 2015,Jan,16; 2013,May,8-10

95937 Neuromuscular junction testing (repetitive stimulation, paired stimuli), each nerve, any 1 method
2.30 2.30 **FUD** XXX [S] [80] [⊡]
AMA: 2016,Feb,13; 2016,Jan,13; 2015,Jan,16; 2014,Jan,11; 2013,May,8-10; 2013,Mar,3-5

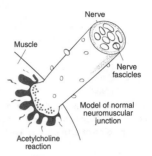

A selected neuromuscular junction is repeatedly stimulated. The test is useful to demonstrate reduced muscle action potential from fatigue

95938 Resequenced code. See code following 95926.

95939 Resequenced code. See code following 95929.

95940 Resequenced code. See code following 95913.

95941 Resequenced code. See code following 95913.

95943 Resequenced code. See code following 95924.

95950-95962 Electroencephalography For Seizure Monitoring/Intraoperative Use

EXCLUDES *E&M services*

95950 Monitoring for identification and lateralization of cerebral seizure focus, electroencephalographic (eg, 8 channel EEG) recording and interpretation, each 24 hours

INCLUDES Only time when recording is taking place and data are being collected and does not include set-up and take-down
Recording for more than 12 hours up to 24 hours
EXCLUDES *Use of code more than one time per 24-hour period*
Code also modifier 52 only when recording is 12 hours or less
9.36 9.36 **FUD** XXX [S] [80] [⊡]
AMA: 2016,Jan,13; 2015,Jan,16; 2014,Jan,11; 2011,Feb,3

95951 Monitoring for localization of cerebral seizure focus by cable or radio, 16 or more channel telemetry, combined electroencephalographic (EEG) and video recording and interpretation (eg, for presurgical localization), each 24 hours

INCLUDES Interpretations during recording with changes to care of patient
Only time when recording is taking place and data are being collected and does not include set-up and take-down
Recording for more than 12 hours up to 24 hours
EXCLUDES *Use of code more than one time per 24-hour period*
Code also modifier 52 only when recording is 12 hours or less
0.00 0.00 **FUD** XXX [S] [80] [⊡]
AMA: 2016,Jan,13; 2015,Jan,16; 2014,Dec,16; 2014,Dec,16; 2014,Jan,11; 2013,Aug,13; 2012,Jan,15-42; 2011,Feb,3; 2011,Jan,11

95953 Monitoring for localization of cerebral seizure focus by computerized portable 16 or more channel EEG, electroencephalographic (EEG) recording and interpretation, each 24 hours, unattended

> INCLUDES Only time when recording is taking place and data are being collected and does not include set-up and take-down
> Recording for more than 12 hours up to 24 hours
> EXCLUDES Use of code more than one time per 24-hour period
> Code also modifier 52 only when recording is 12 hours or less
> 11.9 11.9 **FUD** XXX S 80
>
> **AMA:** 2016,Jan,13; 2015,Jan,16; 2014,Dec,16; 2014,Dec,16; 2014,Jan,11; 2011,Feb,3

95954 Pharmacological or physical activation requiring physician or other qualified health care professional attendance during EEG recording of activation phase (eg, thiopental activation test)

> 12.7 12.7 **FUD** XXX S 80
>
> **AMA:** 2016,Jan,13; 2015,Jan,16; 2014,Jan,11

95955 Electroencephalogram (EEG) during nonintracranial surgery (eg, carotid surgery)

> 6.12 6.12 **FUD** XXX N 80
>
> **AMA:** 2016,Jan,13; 2015,Jan,16; 2014,Dec,18

95956 Monitoring for localization of cerebral seizure focus by cable or radio, 16 or more channel telemetry, electroencephalographic (EEG) recording and interpretation, each 24 hours, attended by a technologist or nurse

> INCLUDES Only time when recording is taking place and data are being collected and does not include set-up and take-down
> Recording for more than 12 hours up to 24 hours
> EXCLUDES Use of code more than one time per 24-hour period
> Code also modifier 52 only when recording is 12 hours or less
> 46.4 46.4 **FUD** XXX S 80
>
> **AMA:** 2016,Jan,13; 2015,Jan,16; 2014,Jan,11; 2011,Feb,3

95957 Digital analysis of electroencephalogram (EEG) (eg, for epileptic spike analysis)

> 8.91 8.91 **FUD** XXX N 80
>
> **AMA:** 2016,Jan,13; 2015,Jan,16; 2014,Jan,11

95958 Wada activation test for hemispheric function, including electroencephalographic (EEG) monitoring

> 16.2 16.2 **FUD** XXX S 80
>
> **AMA:** 2000,Jul,1; 1998,Nov,1

95961 Functional cortical and subcortical mapping by stimulation and/or recording of electrodes on brain surface, or of depth electrodes, to provoke seizures or identify vital brain structures; initial hour of attendance by a physician or other qualified health care professional

> INCLUDES One hour of attendance by physician or other qualified health care professional
> Code also each additional hour of attendance by physician or other qualified health care professional, when appropriate (95962)
> Code also modifier 52 for 30 minutes or less of attendance by physician or other qualified health care professional
> 8.33 8.33 **FUD** XXX S 80
>
> **AMA:** 2016,Jan,13; 2015,Jan,16; 2014,Jan,11; 2012,Jan,15-42; 2011,Feb,3; 2011,Jan,11

+ 95962 each additional hour of attendance by a physician or other qualified health care professional (List separately in addition to code for primary procedure)

> INCLUDES One hour of attendance by physician or other qualified health care professional
> Code first initial hour (95961)
> 7.42 7.42 **FUD** ZZZ N 80
>
> **AMA:** 2016,Jan,13; 2015,Jan,16; 2014,Jan,11; 2012,Jan,15-42; 2011,Feb,3; 2011,Jan,11

95965-95967 Magnetoencephalography

> INCLUDES Physician interpretation
> Recording
> Report
> EXCLUDES CT provided along with magnetoencephalography (70450-70470, 70496)
> Electroencephalography provided along with magnetoencephalography (95812-95827)
> E&M services
> MRI provided along with magnetoencephalography (70551-70553)
> Somatosensory evoked potentials/auditory evoked potentials/visual evoked potentials provided along with magnetic evoked field responses (92585, 95925, 95926, 95930)

95965 Magnetoencephalography (MEG), recording and analysis; for spontaneous brain magnetic activity (eg, epileptic cerebral cortex localization)

> 0.00 0.00 **FUD** XXX S 80
>
> **AMA:** 1997,Nov,1

95966 for evoked magnetic fields, single modality (eg, sensory, motor, language, or visual cortex localization)

> 0.00 0.00 **FUD** XXX S 80
>
> **AMA:** 1997,Nov,1

+ 95967 for evoked magnetic fields, each additional modality (eg, sensory, motor, language, or visual cortex localization) (List separately in addition to code for primary procedure)

> Code first single modality (95966)
> 0.00 0.00 **FUD** ZZZ N 80
>
> **AMA:** 1997,Nov,1

95970-95982 Evaluation of Implanted Neurostimulator

> INCLUDES Simple intraoperative or subsequent programming of neurostimulator (three or less of the following); or complex neurostimulator (three or more of the following):
> 8 or more electrode contacts
> Alternating electrode polarities
> Cycling
> Dose time
> More than 1 clinical feature
> Number of channels
> Number of programs
> Pulse amplitude
> Pulse duration
> Pulse frequency
> Rate
> Stimulation train duration
> Train spacing
> EXCLUDES E&M services
> Neurostimulator electrodes:
> Implantation (43647, 43881, 61850-61870, 63650-63655, 64553-64580)
> Revision/removal (43648, 43882, 61880, 63661-63664, 64585)
> Neurostimulator pulse generator/receiver:
> Insertion (61885, 63685, 64590)
> Revision/removal (61888, 63688, 64595)

95970 Electronic analysis of implanted neurostimulator pulse generator system (eg, rate, pulse amplitude, pulse duration, configuration of wave form, battery status, electrode selectability, output modulation, cycling, impedance and patient compliance measurements); simple or complex brain, spinal cord, or peripheral (ie, cranial nerve, peripheral nerve, sacral nerve, neuromuscular) neurostimulator pulse generator/transmitter, without reprogramming

> 0.68 1.92 **FUD** XXX 01 80
>
> **AMA:** 2016,Jul,7; 2016,Jan,13; 2015,Jan,16; 2014,Jan,11; 2012,Jan,15-42; 2011,Apr,10-11; 2011,Jan,11

95971 simple spinal cord, or peripheral (ie, peripheral nerve, sacral nerve, neuromuscular) neurostimulator pulse generator/transmitter, with intraoperative or subsequent programming

> 1.16 1.42 **FUD** XXX S 80
>
> **AMA:** 2016,Jul,7; 2016,Jan,13; 2015,Jan,16; 2014,Jan,11; 2012,Oct,14; 2012,Jan,15-42; 2011,Apr,10-11; 2011,Jan,11

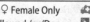 PC/TC Only
FUD Follow-up Days

A2-Z3 ASC Payment
CMS: IOM (Pub 100)

50 Bilateral
A-Y OPPSI

♂ Male Only

♀ Female Only

Facility RVU
 Lab Crosswalk

Non-Facility RVU
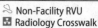 Radiology Crosswalk

CCI

80/80 Surg Assist Allowed / w/Doc

CLIA

456

CPT © 2016 American Medical Association. All Rights Reserved.

© 2016 Optum360, LLC

95972 complex spinal cord, or peripheral (ie, peripheral nerve, sacral nerve, neuromuscular) (except cranial nerve) neurostimulator pulse generator/transmitter, with intraoperative or subsequent programming

🚗 1.19 ⚕ 1.65 **FUD** XXX ⓢ 80 ▢

AMA: 2016,Jul,7; 2016,Jan,13; 2015,Jan,16; 2014,Aug,5; 2014,Jan,11; 2011,Apr,10-11; 2011,Apr,9

95974 complex cranial nerve neurostimulator pulse generator/transmitter, with intraoperative or subsequent programming, with or without nerve interface testing, first hour

Code also modifier 52 for service less than 31 minutes

🚗 4.66 ⚕ 5.89 **FUD** XXX ⓢ 80 ▢

AMA: 2016,Jul,7; 2016,Jan,13; 2015,Jan,16; 2014,Aug,5; 2014,Jan,11; 2012,Jan,15-42; 2011,Apr,10-11; 2011,Jan,11

+ 95975 complex cranial nerve neurostimulator pulse generator/transmitter, with intraoperative or subsequent programming, each additional 30 minutes after first hour (List separately in addition to code for primary procedure)

Code first initial hour (95974)

🚗 2.64 ⚕ 3.17 **FUD** ZZZ Ⓝ 80 ▢

AMA: 2016,Jul,7; 2016,Jan,13; 2015,Jan,16; 2014,Jan,11; 2012,Jan,15-42; 2011,Apr,10-11; 2011,Jan,11

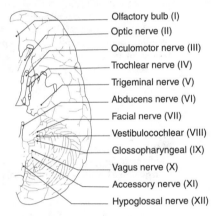

Olfactory bulb (I)
Optic nerve (II)
Oculomotor nerve (III)
Trochlear nerve (IV)
Trigeminal nerve (V)
Abducens nerve (VI)
Facial nerve (VII)
Vestibulocochlear (VIII)
Glossopharyngeal (IX)
Vagus nerve (X)
Accessory nerve (XI)
Hypoglossal nerve (XII)

Cranial nerves at base of brain

95978 Electronic analysis of implanted neurostimulator pulse generator system (eg, rate, pulse amplitude and duration, battery status, electrode selectability and polarity, impedance and patient compliance measurements), complex deep brain neurostimulator pulse generator/transmitter, with initial or subsequent programming; first hour

Code also modifier 52 for service less than 31 minutes

🚗 5.49 ⚕ 7.07 **FUD** XXX ⓢ 80 ▢

AMA: 2016,Jul,7; 2016,Jan,13; 2015,Jan,16; 2014,Aug,5; 2014,Jan,11

+ 95979 each additional 30 minutes after first hour (List separately in addition to code for primary procedure)

Code first initial hour (95978)

🚗 2.55 ⚕ 3.07 **FUD** ZZZ Ⓝ 80 ▢

AMA: 2016,Jul,7; 2016,Jan,13; 2015,Jan,16; 2014,Jan,11

95980 Electronic analysis of implanted neurostimulator pulse generator system (eg, rate, pulse amplitude and duration, configuration of wave form, battery status, electrode selectability, output modulation, cycling, impedance and patient measurements) gastric neurostimulator pulse generator/transmitter; intraoperative, with programming

INCLUDES Gastric neurostimulator of lesser curvature

EXCLUDES *Analysis, with programming when performed, of vagus nerve trunk stimulator for morbid obesity (0312T, 0317T)*

🚗 1.32 ⚕ 1.32 **FUD** XXX Ⓝ 80 ▢

AMA: 2016,Jul,7; 2016,Jan,13; 2015,Jan,16; 2014,Jan,11; 2012,Jan,15-42; 2011,Jan,11

95981 subsequent, without reprogramming

EXCLUDES *Analysis, with programming when performed, of vagus nerve trunk stimulator for morbid obesity (0312T, 0317T)*

🚗 0.51 ⚕ 0.90 **FUD** XXX Q1 80 ▢

AMA: 2016,Jul,7; 2016,Jan,13; 2015,Jan,16; 2014,Jan,11

95982 subsequent, with reprogramming

EXCLUDES *Analysis, with programming when performed, of vagus nerve trunk stimulator for morbid obesity (0312T, 0317T)*

🚗 1.04 ⚕ 1.49 **FUD** XXX Q1 80 ▢

AMA: 2016,Jul,7; 2016,Jan,13; 2015,Jan,16; 2014,Jan,11

95990-95991 Refill/Upkeep of Implanted Drug Delivery Pump to Central Nervous System

EXCLUDES *Analysis/reprogramming of implanted pump for infusion (62367-62370) E&M services*

95990 Refilling and maintenance of implantable pump or reservoir for drug delivery, spinal (intrathecal, epidural) or brain (intraventricular), includes electronic analysis of pump, when performed;

🚗 2.59 ⚕ 2.59 **FUD** XXX ⓢ 80 ▢

AMA: 2016,Jan,13; 2015,Jan,16; 2014,Jan,11; 2012,Aug,10-12; 2012,Jul,3-6; 2012,Jan,15-42; 2011,Jan,11

95991 requiring skill of a physician or other qualified health care professional

🚗 1.13 ⚕ 3.43 **FUD** XXX ⓢ 80 ▢

AMA: 2016,Jan,13; 2015,Jan,16; 2014,Jan,11; 2012,Aug,10-12; 2012,Jul,3-6

95992-95999 Other and Unlisted Neurological Procedures

95992 Canalith repositioning procedure(s) (eg, Epley maneuver, Semont maneuver), per day

EXCLUDES *Nystagmus testing (92531-92532)*

🚗 1.06 ⚕ 1.22 **FUD** XXX 🚫 Ⓐ 80 ▢

AMA: 2016,Jan,13; 2015,Jan,16; 2014,Jan,11

95999 Unlisted neurological or neuromuscular diagnostic procedure

🚗 0.00 ⚕ 0.00 **FUD** XXX Q1 80

AMA: 2016,Jan,13; 2015,Aug,8; 2015,Jan,16; 2014,Jan,11; 2012,Jan,15-42; 2011,Jan,11

96000-96004 Motion Analysis Studies

CMS: 100-02,15,230.4 Services By a Physical/Occupational Therapist in Private Practice

INCLUDES Services provided as part of major therapeutic/diagnostic decision making
Services provided in a dedicated motion analysis department capable of:
3-D kinetics/dynamic electromyography
Computerized 3-D kinematics
Videotaping from the front/back/both sides

EXCLUDES E&M services
Gait training (97116)
Needle electromyography (95860-95872 [95885, 95886, 95887])

96000 Comprehensive computer-based motion analysis by video-taping and 3D kinematics;

🚗 2.70 ⚕ 2.70 **FUD** XXX ⓢ 80 ▢

AMA: 2016,Jan,13; 2015,Jan,16; 2014,Jan,11

96001 with dynamic plantar pressure measurements during walking

  🔁 3.04 🔁 3.04 **FUD** XXX ⬜ S 80 ⬜

  AMA: 2016,Jan,13; 2015,Jan,16; 2014,Jan,11

96002 Dynamic surface electromyography, during walking or other functional activities, 1-12 muscles

  🔁 0.62 🔁 0.62 **FUD** XXX ⬜ S 80 ⬜

  AMA: 2016,Jan,13; 2015,Aug,8; 2015,Jan,16; 2014,Jan,11

96003 Dynamic fine wire electromyography, during walking or other functional activities, 1 muscle

  🔁 0.49 🔁 0.49 **FUD** XXX ⬜ Q1 80 ⬜

  AMA: 2016,Jan,13; 2015,Jan,16; 2014,Jan,11

96004 Review and interpretation by physician or other qualified health care professional of comprehensive computer-based motion analysis, dynamic plantar pressure measurements, dynamic surface electromyography during walking or other functional activities, and dynamic fine wire electromyography, with written report

  🔁 3.32 🔁 3.32 **FUD** XXX ⬜ B 80 26 ⬜

  AMA: 2016,Jan,13; 2015,Aug,8; 2015,Jan,16; 2014,Jan,11

96020 Neurofunctional Brain Testing

INCLUDES Selection/administration of testing of:
  Cognition
  Determination of validity of neurofunctional testing relative to separately interpreted functional magnetic resonance images
  Functional neuroimaging
  Language
  Memory
  Monitoring performance of testing
  Movement
  Other neurological functions
  Sensation

EXCLUDES Clinical depression treatment by repetitive transcranial magnetic stimulation (90867-90868)
  E&M services on the same date
  MRI of the brain (70554-70555)
  Neuropsychological testing on the same date (96116-96120)
  Psychological testing on the same date (96101-96103)

96020 Neurofunctional testing selection and administration during noninvasive imaging functional brain mapping, with test administered entirely by a physician or other qualified health care professional (ie, psychologist), with review of test results and report

  🔁 0.00 🔁 0.00 **FUD** XXX ⬜ N 80 ⬜

  AMA: 2016,Jan,13; 2015,Jan,16; 2014,Jan,11

96040 Genetic Counseling Services

INCLUDES Analysis for genetic risk assessment
  Counseling of patient/family
  Counseling services
  Face-to-face interviews
  Obtaining structured family genetic history
  Pedigree construction
  Review of medical data/family information
  Services provided by trained genetic counselor
  Services provided during one or more sessions
  Thirty minutes of face-to-face time and is reported one time for each 16-30 minutes of the service

EXCLUDES Education/genetic counseling by a physician or other qualified health care provider to a group (99078)
  Education/genetic counseling by a physician or other qualified health care provider to an individual; use appropriate E&M code
  Education regarding genetic risks by a nonphysician to a group (98961, 98962)
  Genetic counseling and/or risk factor reduction intervention from a physician or other qualified health care provider provided to patients without symptoms/diagnosis (99401-99412)
  Use of code when 15 minutes or less of face-to-face time is provided

96040 Medical genetics and genetic counseling services, each 30 minutes face-to-face with patient/family

  🔁 1.32 🔁 1.32 **FUD** XXX ★ B ⬜

  AMA: 2016,Jan,13; 2015,Jan,16; 2014,Jan,11

96101-96127 Cognitive Capability Assessments

CMS: 100-02,15,80.2 Psychological and Neuropsychological Tests

INCLUDES Cognitive function testing of the central nervous system

EXCLUDES Cognitive skills development (97532-97533)
  Physician conducted mini-mental status examination; use appropriate E&M code

96101 Psychological testing (includes psychodiagnostic assessment of emotionality, intellectual abilities, personality and psychopathology, eg, MMPI, Rorschach, WAIS), per hour of the psychologist's or physician's time, both face-to-face time administering tests to the patient and time interpreting these test results and preparing the report

  INCLUDES Situations when more time is needed to assimilate other clinical data sources including tests administered by a technician or computer and previously reported
  Time spent face to face, interpretation, and preparing report

  EXCLUDES Adaptive behavior services (0364T-0367T, 0373T-0374T)
  Use of code for less than 31 minutes of time

  🔁 2.24 🔁 2.25 **FUD** XXX ⬜ Q3 80 ⬜

  AMA: 2016,Sep,9; 2016,Jan,13; 2015,Aug,5; 2015,Jan,16; 2014,Jun,3; 2014,Jan,11; 2012,Jan,15-42; 2011,Oct,3-4; 2011,Jan,11

96102 Psychological testing (includes psychodiagnostic assessment of emotionality, intellectual abilities, personality and psychopathology, eg, MMPI and WAIS), with qualified health care professional interpretation and report, administered by technician, per hour of technician time, face-to-face

  EXCLUDES Adaptive behavior services (0364T-0367T, 0373T-0374T)
  Use of code for less than 31 minutes of time

  🔁 0.66 🔁 1.79 **FUD** XXX ⬜ Q3 80 ⬜

  AMA: 2016,Sep,9; 2016,Jan,13; 2015,Aug,5; 2015,Jan,16; 2014,Jan,11

96103 Psychological testing (includes psychodiagnostic assessment of emotionality, intellectual abilities, personality and psychopathology, eg, MMPI), administered by a computer, with qualified health care professional interpretation and report

  EXCLUDES Adaptive behavior services (0364T-0367T, 0373T-0374T)

  🔁 0.76 🔁 0.78 **FUD** XXX ⬜ Q1 80 ⬜

  AMA: 2016,Sep,9; 2016,Jan,13; 2015,Aug,5; 2015,Jan,16; 2014,Jan,11; 2012,Jan,15-42; 2011,Oct,10

96105 Assessment of aphasia (includes assessment of expressive and receptive speech and language function, language comprehension, speech production ability, reading, spelling, writing, eg, by Boston Diagnostic Aphasia Examination) with interpretation and report, per hour

  EXCLUDES Adaptive behavior services (0364T-0367T, 0373T-0374T)

  🔁 3.03 🔁 3.03 **FUD** XXX ⬜ A 80 ⬜

  AMA: 2016,Jan,13; 2015,Aug,5; 2015,Jan,16; 2014,Jan,11

96110 Developmental screening (eg, developmental milestone survey, speech and language delay screen), with scoring and documentation, per standardized instrument

  EXCLUDES Adaptive behavior services (0364T-0367T, 0373T-0374T)

  🔁 0.25 🔁 0.25 **FUD** XXX ⬜ E ⬜

  AMA: 2016,Jan,13; 2015,Aug,5; 2015,Jan,16; 2014,Jun,3; 2014,Jan,11

96111 Developmental testing, (includes assessment of motor, language, social, adaptive, and/or cognitive functioning by standardized developmental instruments) with interpretation and report

  EXCLUDES Adaptive behavior services (0364T-0367T, 0373T-0374T)

  🔁 3.47 🔁 3.65 **FUD** XXX ⬜ Q3 80 ⬜

  AMA: 2016,Jan,13; 2015,Aug,5; 2015,Jan,16; 2014,Jan,11

96116 Neurobehavioral status exam (clinical assessment of thinking, reasoning and judgment, eg, acquired knowledge, attention, language, memory, planning and problem solving, and visual spatial abilities), per hour of the psychologist's or physician's time, both face-to-face time with the patient and time interpreting test results and preparing the report

> INCLUDES Time spent face to face, interpretation, and preparing report
>
> EXCLUDES Adaptive behavior services (0364T-0367T, 0373T-0374T)
> Use of code for less than 31 minutes of time

🚑 2.46   🔪 2.62   **FUD** XXX   ★ 03 80 ▭

AMA: 2016,Jan,13; 2015,Aug,5; 2015,Jan,16; 2014,Jun,3; 2014,Jan,11; 2012,Jan,15-42; 2011,Oct,3-4; 2011,Jan,11

96118 Neuropsychological testing (eg, Halstead-Reitan Neuropsychological Battery, Wechsler Memory Scales and Wisconsin Card Sorting Test), per hour of the psychologist's or physician's time, both face-to-face time administering tests to the patient and time interpreting these test results and preparing the report

> INCLUDES Situations when more time is needed to assimilate other clinical data sources including tests administered by a technician or computer and previously reported
> Time spent face to face, interpretation, and preparing report
>
> EXCLUDES Adaptive behavior services (0364T-0367T, 0373T-0374T)
> Use of code for less than 31 minutes of time

🚑 2.22   🔪 2.76   **FUD** XXX   03 80 ▭

AMA: 2016,Jan,13; 2015,Aug,5; 2015,Jan,16; 2014,Jun,3; 2014,Jan,11; 2012,Jan,15-42; 2011,Oct,3-4; 2011,Jan,11

96119 Neuropsychological testing (eg, Halstead-Reitan Neuropsychological Battery, Wechsler Memory Scales and Wisconsin Card Sorting Test), with qualified health care professional interpretation and report, administered by technician, per hour of technician time, face-to-face

> EXCLUDES Adaptive behavior services (0364T-0367T, 0373T-0374T)
> Use of code for less than 31 minutes of time

🚑 0.67   🔪 2.26   **FUD** XXX   03 80 ▭

AMA: 2016,Jan,13; 2015,Aug,5; 2015,Jan,16; 2014,Jan,11

96120 Neuropsychological testing (eg, Wisconsin Card Sorting Test), administered by a computer, with qualified health care professional interpretation and report

> EXCLUDES Adaptive behavior services (0364T-0367T, 0373T-0374T)

🚑 0.74   🔪 1.36   **FUD** XXX   03 80 ▭

AMA: 2016,Jan,13; 2015,Aug,5; 2015,Jan,16; 2014,Jan,11; 2012,Jan,15-42; 2011,Jan,11

96125 Standardized cognitive performance testing (eg, Ross Information Processing Assessment) per hour of a qualified health care professional's time, both face-to-face time administering tests to the patient and time interpreting these test results and preparing the report

> INCLUDES Time spent face to face, interpretation, and preparing report
>
> EXCLUDES Adaptive behavior services (0364T-0367T, 0373T-0374T)
> Neuropsychological testing (96118-96120)
> Psychological testing (96101-96103)
> Use of code for less than 31 minutes of time

🚑 3.31   🔪 3.31   **FUD** XXX   A 80 ▭

AMA: 2016,Jan,13; 2015,Aug,5; 2015,Jan,16; 2014,Jan,11; 2012,Jan,15-42; 2011,Oct,3-4; 2011,Jan,11

96127 Brief emotional/behavioral assessment (eg, depression inventory, attention-deficit/hyperactivity disorder [ADHD] scale), with scoring and documentation, per standardized instrument

🚑 0.15   🔪 0.15   **FUD** XXX   Q1 80 TC ▭

AMA: 2016,Jan,13; 2015,Aug,5

96150-96155 Biopsychosocial Assessment/Intervention

> INCLUDES Services for patients that have primary physical illnesses/diagnoses/symptoms who may benefit from assessments/interventions that focus on the biopsychosocial factors related to the patient's health status
> Services used to identify the following factors which are important to the prevention/treatment/management of physical health problems:
> Behavioral
> Cognitive
> Emotional
> Psychological
> Social
>
> EXCLUDES Adaptive behavior services (0364T-0367T, 0373T-0374T)
> E&M services on the same date
> Preventive medicine counseling services (99401-99412)
> Psychotherapy services (90785-90899)

96150 Health and behavior assessment (eg, health-focused clinical interview, behavioral observations, psychophysiological monitoring, health-oriented questionnaires), each 15 minutes face-to-face with the patient; initial assessment

🚑 0.60   🔪 0.61   **FUD** XXX   ★ 03 80 ▭

AMA: 2016,Jan,13; 2015,Jan,16; 2014,Sep,13; 2014,Jun,3; 2014,Jan,11; 2013,May,12; 2012,Jan,15-42; 2011,Jan,11

96151 re-assessment

🚑 0.57   🔪 0.58   **FUD** XXX   ★ 03 80 ▭

AMA: 2016,Jan,13; 2015,Jan,16; 2014,Sep,13; 2014,Jun,3; 2014,Jan,11; 2013,May,12; 2012,Jan,15-42; 2011,Jan,11

96152 Health and behavior intervention, each 15 minutes, face-to-face; individual

🚑 0.55   🔪 0.56   **FUD** XXX   ★ 03 80 ▭

AMA: 2016,Jan,13; 2015,Jan,16; 2014,Sep,13; 2014,Jun,3; 2014,Jan,11; 2013,May,12; 2012,Jan,15-42; 2011,Jan,11

96153 group (2 or more patients)

🚑 0.13   🔪 0.13   **FUD** XXX   ★ 03 80 ▭

AMA: 2016,Jan,13; 2015,Jan,16; 2014,Sep,13; 2014,Jun,3; 2014,Jan,11; 2013,May,12; 2012,Jan,15-42; 2011,Jan,11

96154 family (with the patient present)

🚑 0.54   🔪 0.55   **FUD** XXX   ★ 03 80 ▭

AMA: 2016,Jan,13; 2015,Jan,16; 2014,Sep,13; 2014,Jun,3; 2014,Jan,11; 2013,May,12; 2012,Jan,15-42; 2011,Jan,11

96155 family (without the patient present)

🚑 0.64   🔪 0.64   **FUD** XXX   E ▭

AMA: 2016,Jan,13; 2015,Jan,16; 2014,Sep,13; 2014,Jun,3; 2014,Jan,11; 2013,May,12; 2012,Jan,15-42; 2011,Jan,11

96160-96161 Health Risk Assessments

● **96160** Administration of patient-focused health risk assessment instrument (eg, health hazard appraisal) with scoring and documentation, per standardized instrument

● **96161** Administration of caregiver-focused health risk assessment instrument (eg, depression inventory) for the benefit of the patient, with scoring and documentation, per standardized instrument

---

● New Code   ▲ Revised Code   ○ Reinstated   ● New Web Release   ▲ Revised Web Release   Unlisted   Not Covered   # Resequenced
⊘ AMA Mod 51 Exempt   ⑨ Optum Mod 51 Exempt   ⑥ Mod 63 Exempt   ✗ Non-FDA Drug   ★ Telehealth   M Maternity   A Age Edit   + Add-on   AMA: CPT Asst

Medicine

96360 — 96367

96360-96361 Intravenous Fluid Infusion for Hydration (Nonchemotherapy)

CMS: 100-04,4,230.2 OPPS Drug Administration

INCLUDES Administration of prepackaged fluids and electrolytes
Coding hierarchy rules for facility reporting only:
Chemotherapy services are primary to diagnostic, prophylactic, and therapeutic services
Diagnostic, prophylactic, and therapeutic services are primary to hydration services
Infusions are primary to pushes
Pushes are primary to injections
Constant observance/attendance of person administering the drug or substance
Infusion of 15 minutes or less
Direct supervision by physician or other qualified health care provider:
Direction of personnel
Minimal supervision for:
Consent
Safety oversight
Supervision of personnel
Report the initial code for the primary reason for the visit regardless of the order in which the infusions or injections are given
The following if done to facilitate the injection/infusion:
Flush at the end of infusion
Indwelling IV, subcutaneous catheter/port access
Local anesthesia
Start of IV
Supplies/tubing/syringes
Treatment plan verification
EXCLUDES *Catheter/port declotting (36593)*
Drugs/other substances
Minimal infusion to keep the vein open or during other therapeutic infusions
Services provided by physicians or other qualified health care providers in facility settings
Significant separately identifiable E&M service if performed
Use of a code for a second initial service on the same date for accessing a multi-lumen catheter, restarting an IV, or when two IV lines are needed to meet an infusion rate
Use of code for infusion for hydration that is 31 minutes or less

96360 **Intravenous infusion, hydration; initial, 31 minutes to 1 hour**

EXCLUDES *Use of code if service is performed as a concurrent infusion*

🚑 1.61   ⚕ 1.61   **FUD** XXX   S 80 ▢

AMA: 2016,Jan,13; 2015,Jan,16; 2014,May,10; 2014,Jan,11; 2013,Oct,3; 2011,Dec,3-5; 2011,Oct,3-4; 2011,May,7

+ 96361 **each additional hour (List separately in addition to code for primary procedure)**

INCLUDES Hydration infusion of more than 30 minutes beyond 1 hour
Hydration provided as a secondary or subsequent service after a different initial service via the same IV access site
Code first (96360)

🚑 0.43   ⚕ 0.43   **FUD** ZZZ   S 80 ▢

AMA: 2016,Jan,13; 2015,Jan,16; 2014,May,10; 2014,Jan,11; 2013,Oct,3; 2011,Dec,3-5; 2011,Oct,3-4; 2011,May,7

96365-96371 Infusions: Diagnostic/Preventive/Therapeutic

CMS: 100-04,4,230.2 OPPS Drug Administration

INCLUDES Administration of fluid
Administration of substances/drugs
An infusion of 16 minutes or more
Coding hierarchy rules for facility reporting:
Chemotherapy services are primary to diagnostic, prophylactic, and therapeutic services
Diagnostic, prophylactic, and therapeutic services are primary to hydration services
Infusions are primary to pushes
Pushes are primary to injections
Constant presence of health care professional administering the substance/drug
Direct supervision of physician or other qualified health care provider:
Consent
Direction of personnel
Patient assessment
Safety oversight
Supervision of personnel
The following if done to facilitate the injection/infusion:
Flush at the end of infusion
Indwelling IV, subcutaneous catheter/port access
Local anesthesia
Start of IV
Supplies/tubing/syringes
Training to assess patient and monitor vital signs
Training to prepare/dose/dispose
Treatment plan verification
EXCLUDES *Catheter/port declotting (36593)*
Services provided by physicians or other qualified health care providers in facility settings
Significant separately identifiable E&M service, when performed
Use of a code for a second initial service on the same date for accessing a multi-lumen catheter, restarting an IV, or when two IV lines are needed to meet an infusion rate
Use of code with other procedures for which IV push or infusion is an integral part of the procedure
Code also drugs/materials

96365 **Intravenous infusion, for therapy, prophylaxis, or diagnosis (specify substance or drug); initial, up to 1 hour**

Code also second initial service with modifier 59 when patient's condition or drug protocol mandates the use of two IV lines

🚑 1.95   ⚕ 1.95   **FUD** XXX   S 80 ▢

AMA: 2016,Jan,13; 2015,Jan,16; 2014,Jan,11; 2012,Jan,15-42; 2011,Dec,3-5; 2011,Oct,3-4; 2011,May,7; 2011,Jan,11

+ 96366 **each additional hour (List separately in addition to code for primary procedure)**

INCLUDES Additional hours of sequential infusion
Infusion intervals of more than 30 minutes beyond one hour
Second and subsequent infusions of the same drug or substance
Code also additional infusion, when appropriate (96367)
Code first (96365)

🚑 0.53   ⚕ 0.53   **FUD** ZZZ   S 80 ▢

AMA: 2016,Jan,13; 2015,Jan,16; 2014,Jan,11; 2012,Jan,15-42; 2011,Dec,3-5; 2011,May,7; 2011,Jan,11

+ 96367 **additional sequential infusion of a new drug/substance, up to 1 hour (List separately in addition to code for primary procedure)**

INCLUDES A secondary or subsequent service with a new drug or substance after a different initial service via the same IV access

EXCLUDES *Use of code more than one time per sequential infusion of the same mix*

Code first (96365, 96374, 96409, 96413)

🚑 0.86   ⚕ 0.86   **FUD** ZZZ   S 80 ▢

AMA: 2016,Jan,13; 2015,Jan,16; 2014,Jan,11; 2012,Jan,15-42; 2011,Dec,3-5; 2011,May,7; 2011,Jan,11

+ 96368 concurrent infusion (List separately in addition to code for primary procedure)

> **EXCLUDES** *Use of code more than one time per date of service*
> Code first (96365, 96366, 96413, 96415, 96416)
> 🚑 0.58 ⚕ 0.58 **FUD** ZZZ [N] [80] 🖵
>
> **AMA:** 2016,Jan,13; 2015,Jan,16; 2014,Jan,11; 2011,Dec,3-5; 2011,May,7

96369 Subcutaneous infusion for therapy or prophylaxis (specify substance or drug); initial, up to 1 hour, including pump set-up and establishment of subcutaneous infusion site(s)

> **EXCLUDES** *Infusions of 15 minutes or less (96372)*
> *Use of code more than one time per encounter*
> 🚑 5.42 ⚕ 5.42 **FUD** XXX [S] [80] 🖵
>
> **AMA:** 2016,Jan,13; 2015,Jan,16; 2014,Jan,11; 2011,Dec,3-5; 2011,May,7

+ 96370 each additional hour (List separately in addition to code for primary procedure)

> **INCLUDES** *Infusions of more than 30 minutes beyond one hour*
> Code first (96369)
> 🚑 0.42 ⚕ 0.42 **FUD** ZZZ [S] [80] 🖵
>
> **AMA:** 2016,Jan,13; 2015,Jan,16; 2014,Jan,11; 2011,Dec,3-5; 2011,May,7

+ 96371 additional pump set-up with establishment of new subcutaneous infusion site(s) (List separately in addition to code for primary procedure)

> **EXCLUDES** *Use of code more than one time per encounter*
> Code first (96369)
> 🚑 2.05 ⚕ 2.05 **FUD** ZZZ [N] [80] 🖵
>
> **AMA:** 2016,Jan,13; 2015,Jan,16; 2014,Jan,11; 2011,Dec,3-5; 2011,May,7

96372-96379 Injections: Diagnostic/Preventive/Therapeutic

CMS: 100-04,4,230.2 OPPS Drug Administration

INCLUDES Administration of fluid
Administration of substances/drugs
Coding hierarchy rules for facility reporting:
  Chemotherapy services are primary to diagnostic, prophylactic, and therapeutic services
  Infusions are primary to pushes
  Pushes are primary to injections
Constant presence of health care professional administering the substance/drug
Direct supervision by physician or other qualified health care provider:
  Consent
  Direction of personnel
  Patient assessment
  Safety oversight
  Supervision of personnel
Infusion of 15 minutes or less
The following if done to facilitate the injection/infusion:
  Flush at the end of infusion
  Indwelling IV, subcutaneous catheter/port access
  Local anesthesia
  Start of IV
  Supplies/tubing/syringes
Training to assess patient and monitor vital signs
Training to prepare/dose/dispose
Treatment plan verification

EXCLUDES *Catheter/port declotting (36593)*
Services provided by physicians or other qualified health care providers in facility settings
Significant separately identifiable E&M service, when performed
Use of a code for a second initial service on the same date for accessing a multi-lumen catheter, restarting an IV, or when two IV lines are needed to meet an infusion rate
Use of code with other procedures for which IV push or infusion is an integral part of the procedure

Code also drugs/materials

96372 Therapeutic, prophylactic, or diagnostic injection (specify substance or drug); subcutaneous or intramuscular

> **INCLUDES** Direct supervision by physician or other qualified health care provider when reported by the physician/other qualified health care provider. When reported by a hospital, physician/other qualified health care provider need not be present.
> Hormonal therapy injections (non-antineoplastic) (96372)
>
> **EXCLUDES** *Administration of vaccines/toxoids (90460-90474)*
> *Allergen immunotherapy injections (95115-95117)*
> *Antineoplastic hormonal injections (96402)*
> *Antineoplastic nonhormonal injections (96401)*
> *Injections administered without direct supervision by physician or other qualified health care provider (99211)*
> 🚑 0.71 ⚕ 0.71 **FUD** XXX [S] [80] 🖵
>
> **AMA:** 2016,Jan,13; 2015,Jan,16; 2014,Jan,9; 2014,Jan,11; 2013,Jan,9-10; 2012,Jan,15-42; 2011,Dec,3-5; 2011,May,7; 2011,Jan,11

96373 intra-arterial

> 🚑 0.55 ⚕ 0.55 **FUD** XXX [S] [80] 🖵
>
> **AMA:** 2016,Jan,13; 2015,Jan,16; 2014,Jan,11; 2011,Dec,3-5; 2011,May,7

96374 intravenous push, single or initial substance/drug

> Code also second initial service with modifier 59 when patient's condition or drug protocol mandates the use of two IV lines
> 🚑 1.60 ⚕ 1.60 **FUD** XXX [S] [80] 🖵
>
> **AMA:** 2016,Jan,13; 2015,Nov,3; 2015,Jan,16; 2014,Jan,11; 2013,Jun,9-11; 2013,Feb,3-6; 2011,Dec,3-5; 2011,Oct,3-4; 2011,May,7

+ 96375 each additional sequential intravenous push of a new substance/drug (List separately in addition to code for primary procedure)

> **INCLUDES** IV push of a new substance/drug provided as a secondary or subsequent service after a different initial service via same IV access site
> Code first (96365, 96374, 96409, 96413)
> 🚑 0.63 ⚕ 0.63 **FUD** ZZZ [S] [80] 🖵
>
> **AMA:** 2016,Jan,13; 2015,Nov,3; 2015,Jan,16; 2014,Jan,11; 2013,Feb,3-6; 2011,Dec,3-5; 2011,May,7

+ 96376 each additional sequential intravenous push of the same substance/drug provided in a facility (List separately in addition to code for primary procedure)

> **INCLUDES** Facilities only
> **EXCLUDES** *IV push performed within 30 minutes of a reported push of the same substance or drug*
> *Services performed by any nonfacilty provider*
> Code first (96365, 96374, 96409, 96413)
> 🚑 0.00 ⚕ 0.00 **FUD** ZZZ [N] 🖵
>
> **AMA:** 2016,Jan,13; 2015,Jan,16; 2014,Nov,14; 2014,Jan,11; 2011,Dec,3-5; 2011,May,7

● 96377 Application of on-body injector (includes cannula insertion) for timed subcutaneous injection

96379 Unlisted therapeutic, prophylactic, or diagnostic intravenous or intra-arterial injection or infusion

> 🚑 0.00 ⚕ 0.00 **FUD** XXX [S] [80]
>
> **AMA:** 2016,Jan,13; 2015,Jan,16; 2014,Jan,11; 2011,Dec,3-5; 2011,May,7

Medicine

96401 — 96416

96401-96411 Chemotherapy and Other Complex Drugs, Biologicals: Injection and IV Push

CMS: 100-03,110.2 Certain Drugs Distributed by the National Cancer Institute; 100-03,110.6 Scalp Hypothermia During Chemotherapy, to Prevent Hair Loss; 100-04,4,230.2 OPPS Drug Administration

INCLUDES   Highly complex services that require direct supervision for:
Consent
Patient assessment
Safety oversight
Supervision
More intense work and monitoring of clinical staff by physician or other qualified health care provider due to greater risk of severe patient reactions
Parenteral administration of:
Anti-neoplastic agents for noncancer diagnoses
Monoclonal antibody agents
Nonradionuclide antineoplastic drugs
Other biologic response modifiers

EXCLUDES   *Use of a code for a second initial service on the same date for accessing a multi-lumen catheter, restarting an IV, or when two IV lines are needed to meet an infusion rate*

96401   **Chemotherapy administration, subcutaneous or intramuscular; non-hormonal anti-neoplastic**

EXCLUDES   *Services performed by physicians or other qualified health care providers in facility settings*

🚑 2.10   ⚖ 2.10   **FUD** XXX   Ⓢ 80 ▭

AMA: 2016,Jan,13; 2015,Jan,16; 2014,Jan,11; 2012,Jan,15-42; 2011,Aug,9-10; 2011,Dec,3-5; 2011,Jan,11

96402   **hormonal anti-neoplastic**

EXCLUDES   *Services performed by physicians or other qualified health care providers in facility settings*

🚑 0.91   ⚖ 0.91   **FUD** XXX   Ⓢ 80 ▭

AMA: 2016,Jan,13; 2015,Jan,16; 2014,Jan,11; 2012,Jan,15-42; 2011,Aug,9-10; 2011,Dec,3-5; 2011,Jan,11

96405   **Chemotherapy administration; intralesional, up to and including 7 lesions**

🚑 0.85   ⚖ 2.31   **FUD** 000   Ⓢ ▭

AMA: 2016,Jan,13; 2015,Jan,16; 2014,Jan,11; 2012,Jan,15-42; 2011,Aug,9-10; 2011,Jan,11

96406   **intralesional, more than 7 lesions**

🚑 1.32   ⚖ 3.29   **FUD** 000   Ⓢ ▭

AMA: 2016,Jan,13; 2015,Jan,16; 2014,Jan,11; 2012,Jan,15-42; 2011,Aug,9-10; 2011,Jan,11

96409   **intravenous, push technique, single or initial substance/drug**

INCLUDES   Push technique includes:
Administration of injection directly into vessel or access line by health care professional; or
Infusion less than or equal to 15 minutes

EXCLUDES   *Insertion of arterial and venous cannula(s) for extracorpororeal circulation (36823)*
Services performed by physicians or other qualified health care providers in facility settings

Code also second initial service with modifier 59 when patient's condition or drug protocol mandates the use of two IV lines

🚑 3.12   ⚖ 3.12   **FUD** XXX   Ⓢ 80 ▭

AMA: 2016,Jan,13; 2015,Jan,16; 2014,Jan,11; 2012,Jan,15-42; 2011,Aug,9-10; 2011,Dec,3-5; 2011,May,7; 2011,Jan,11

+   96411   **intravenous, push technique, each additional substance/drug (List separately in addition to code for primary procedure)**

INCLUDES   Push technique includes:
Administration of injection directly into vessel or access line by health care professional; or
Infusion less than or equal to 15 minutes

EXCLUDES   *Insertion of arterial and venous cannula(s) for extracorpororeal circulation (36823)*
Services performed by physicians or other qualified health care providers in facility settings

Code first initial substance/drug (96409, 96413)

🚑 1.75   ⚖ 1.75   **FUD** ZZZ   Ⓢ 80 ▭

AMA: 2016,Jan,13; 2015,Jan,16; 2014,Jan,11; 2012,Jan,15-42; 2011,Aug,9-10; 2011,Dec,3-5; 2011,Jan,11

96413-96417 Chemotherapy and Complex Drugs, Biologicals: Intravenous Infusion

CMS: 100-03,110.2 Certain Drugs Distributed by the National Cancer Institute; 100-03,110.6 Scalp Hypothermia During Chemotherapy, to Prevent Hair Loss; 100-04,4,230.2 OPPS Drug Administration

INCLUDES   Highly complex services that require direct supervision for:
Consent
Patient assessment
Safety oversight
Supervision
More intense work and monitoring of clinical staff by physician or other qualified health care provider due to greater risk of severe patient reactions
Parenteral administration of:
Anti-neoplastic agents for noncancer diagnoses
Monoclonal antibody agents
Nonradionuclide antineoplastic drugs
Other biologic response modifiers
The following in the administration:
Access to IV/catheter/port
Drug preparation
Flushing at the completion of the infusion
Hydration fluid
Routine tubing/syringe/supplies
Starting the IV
Use of local anesthesia

EXCLUDES   *Administration of nonchemotherapy agents such as antibiotics/steroids/analgesics*
Declotting of catheter/port (36593)
Home infusion (99601-99602)
Insertion of arterial and venous cannula(s) for extracorpororeal circulation (36823)
Services provided by physicians or other qualified health care providers in facility settings
Use of a code for a second initial service on the same date for accessing a multi-lumen catheter, restarting an IV, or when two IV lines are needed to meet an infusion rate

Code also drug or substance
Code also significant separately identifiable E&M service, when performed

96413   **Chemotherapy administration, intravenous infusion technique; up to 1 hour, single or initial substance/drug**

INCLUDES   Push technique includes:
Administration of injection directly into vessel or access line by health care professional; or
Infusion less than or equal to 15 minutes

EXCLUDES   *Hydration administered as secondary or subsequent service via same IV access site (96361)*
Therapeutic/prophylactic/diagnostic drug infusion/injection through the same intravenous access (96366, 96367, 96375)

Code also second initial service with modifier 59 when patient's condition or drug protocol mandates the use of two IV lines

🚑 3.81   ⚖ 3.81   **FUD** XXX   Ⓢ 80 ▭

AMA: 2016,Jan,13; 2015,Jan,16; 2014,Jan,11; 2012,Jan,15-42; 2011,Aug,9-10; 2011,Dec,3-5; 2011,May,7; 2011,Jan,11

+   96415   **each additional hour (List separately in addition to code for primary procedure)**

INCLUDES   Infusion intervals of more than 30 minutes past 1-hour increments

Code first initial hour (96413)

🚑 0.80   ⚖ 0.80   **FUD** ZZZ   Ⓢ ▭

AMA: 2016,Jan,13; 2015,Jan,16; 2014,Jan,11; 2012,Jan,15-42; 2011,Aug,9-10; 2011,Dec,3-5; 2011,Jan,11

96416   **initiation of prolonged chemotherapy infusion (more than 8 hours), requiring use of a portable or implantable pump**

EXCLUDES   *Portable or implantable infusion pump/reservoir refilling/maintenance for drug delivery (96521-96523)*

🚑 3.96   ⚖ 3.96   **FUD** XXX   Ⓢ 80 ▭

AMA: 2016,Jan,13; 2015,Jan,16; 2014,Jan,11; 2012,Jan,15-42; 2011,Aug,9-10; 2011,Dec,3-5; 2011,Jan,11

+ 96417 each additional sequential infusion (different substance/drug), up to 1 hour (List separately in addition to code for primary procedure)

> INCLUDES Push technique includes:
> Administration of injection directly into vessel or access line by health care professional; or
> Infusion less than or equal to 15 minutes
> EXCLUDES *Additional hour(s) of sequential infusion (96415)*
> *Use of code more than one time per sequential infusion*
> Code first initial substance/drug (96413)
> 🔧 1.76 🔧 1.76 **FUD** ZZZ   S 80 ▣

AMA: 2016,Jan,13; 2015,Jan,16; 2014,Jan,11; 2012,Jan,15-42; 2011,Aug,9-10; 2011,Dec,3-5; 2011,Jan,11

96420-96425 Chemotherapy and Complex Drugs, Biologicals: Intra-arterial

CMS: 100-03,110.2 Certain Drugs Distributed by the National Cancer Institute; 100-03,110.6 Scalp Hypothermia During Chemotherapy, to Prevent Hair Loss; 100-04,4,230.2 OPPS Drug Administration

> INCLUDES Highly complex services that require direct supervision for:
> Consent
> Patient assessment
> Safety oversight
> Supervision
> More intense work and monitoring of clinical staff by physician or other qualified health care provider due to greater risk of severe patient reactions
> Parenteral administration of:
> Anti-neoplastic agents for noncancer diagnoses
> Monoclonal antibody agents
> Non-radionuclide antineoplastic drugs
> Other biologic response modifiers
> The following in the administration:
> Access to IV/catheter/port
> Drug preparation
> Flushing at the completion of the infusion
> Hydration fluid
> Routine tubing/syringe/supplies
> Starting the IV
> Use of local anesthesia
> EXCLUDES *Administration of non-chemotherapy agents such as antibiotics/steroids/analgesics*
> *Declotting of catheter/port (36593)*
> *Home infusion (99601-99602)*
> *Services provided by physicians or other qualified health care providers in facility settings*
> *Use of a code for a second initial service on the same date for accessing a multi-lumen catheter, restarting an IV, or when two IV lines are needed*
> Code also drug or substance
> Code also significant separately identifiable E&M service, when performed

96420 Chemotherapy administration, intra-arterial; push technique

> INCLUDES Push technique includes:
> Administration of injection directly into vessel or access line by health care professional; or
> Infusion less than or equal to 15 minutes
> Regional chemotherapy perfusion
> EXCLUDES *Insertion of arterial and venous cannula(s) for extracorpororeal circulation (36823)*
> *Placement of intra-arterial catheter*
> 🔧 2.97 🔧 2.97 **FUD** XXX   S 80 ▣

AMA: 2016,Mar,3; 2016,Jan,13; 2015,Nov,3; 2015,Jan,16; 2014,Jan,11; 2013,Nov,6; 2012,Jan,15-42; 2011,Aug,9-10; 2011,Dec,3-5; 2011,Jan,11

96422 infusion technique, up to 1 hour

> INCLUDES Push technique includes:
> Administration of injection directly into vessel or access line by health care professional; or
> Infusion less than or equal to 15 minutes
> Regional chemotherapy perfusion
> EXCLUDES *Insertion of arterial and venous cannula(s) for extracorpororeal circulation (36823)*
> *Placement of intra-arterial catheter*
> 🔧 4.78 🔧 4.78 **FUD** XXX   S 80 ▣

AMA: 2016,Mar,3; 2016,Jan,13; 2015,Nov,3; 2015,Jan,16; 2014,Jan,11; 2012,Jan,15-42; 2011,Aug,9-10; 2011,Dec,3-5; 2011,Jan,11

+ 96423 infusion technique, each additional hour (List separately in addition to code for primary procedure)

> INCLUDES Infusion intervals of more than 30 minutes past 1-hour increments
> Regional chemotherapy perfusion
> EXCLUDES *Insertion of arterial and venous cannula(s) for extracorpororeal circulation (36823)*
> *Placement of intra-arterial catheter*
> Code first initial hour (96422)
> 🔧 2.21 🔧 2.21 **FUD** ZZZ   S 80 ▣

AMA: 2016,Mar,3; 2016,Jan,13; 2015,Nov,3; 2015,Jan,16; 2014,Jan,11; 2012,Jan,15-42; 2011,Aug,9-10; 2011,Dec,3-5; 2011,Jan,11

96425 infusion technique, initiation of prolonged infusion (more than 8 hours), requiring the use of a portable or implantable pump

> INCLUDES Regional chemotherapy perfusion
> EXCLUDES *Insertion of arterial and venous cannula(s) for extracorpororeal circulation (36823)*
> *Placement of intra-arterial catheter*
> *Portable or implantable infusion pump/reservoir refilling/maintenance for drug delivery (96521-96523)*
> 🔧 5.11 🔧 5.11 **FUD** XXX   S 80 ▣

AMA: 2016,Mar,3; 2016,Jan,13; 2015,Nov,3; 2015,Jan,16; 2014,Jan,11; 2012,Jan,15-42; 2011,Aug,9-10; 2011,Dec,3-5; 2011,Jan,11

96440-96450 Chemotherapy Administration: Intrathecal/Peritoneal Cavity/Pleural Cavity

CMS: 100-03,110.2 Certain Drugs Distributed by the National Cancer Institute; 100-04,4,230.2 OPPS Drug Administration

96440 Chemotherapy administration into pleural cavity, requiring and including thoracentesis

> 🔧 4.01 🔧 23.8 **FUD** 000   S 80 ▣

AMA: 2016,Jan,13; 2015,Jan,16; 2014,Jan,11; 2012,Jan,15-42; 2011,Jan,11

96446 Chemotherapy administration into the peritoneal cavity via indwelling port or catheter

> 🔧 0.82 🔧 5.66 **FUD** XXX   S 80 ▣

AMA: 2016,Jan,13; 2015,Jan,16; 2014,Jan,11; 2012,Jan,15-42; 2011,Jan,11

96450 Chemotherapy administration, into CNS (eg, intrathecal), requiring and including spinal puncture

> EXCLUDES *Chemotherapy administration, intravesical/bladder (51720)*
> *Insertion of catheter/reservoir:*
> *Intraventricular (61210, 61215)*
> *Subarachnoid (62350-62351, 62360-62362)*
> 🔧 2.30 🔧 5.14 **FUD** 000   S 80 ▣

AMA: 2016,Jan,13; 2015,Jan,16; 2014,Jan,11; 2012,Jan,15-42; 2011,Jan,11

96521-96523 Refill/Upkeep of Drug Delivery Device

CMS: 100-04,4,230.2 OPPS Drug Administration

INCLUDES Highly complex services that require direct supervision for:
Consent
Patient assessment
Safety oversight
Supervision
Parenteral administration of:
Anti-neoplastic agents for noncancer diagnoses
Monoclonal antibody agents
Non-radionuclide antineoplastic drugs
Other biologic response modifiers
The following in the administration:
Access to IV/catheter/port
Drug preparation
Flushing at the completion of the infusion
Hydration fluid
Routine tubing/syringe/supplies
Starting the IV
Use of local anesthesia
Therapeutic drugs other than chemotherapy

EXCLUDES Administration of non-chemotherapy agents such as
antibiotics/steroids/analgesics
Blood specimen collection from completely implantable venous access device
(36591)
Declotting of catheter/port (36593)
Home infusion (99601-99602)
Services provided by physicians or other qualified health care providers in
facility settings
Code also drug or substance
Code also significant separately identifiable E&M service, when performed

96521 **Refilling and maintenance of portable pump**
🚑 3.89 ⚖ 3.89 **FUD** XXX
⬜S⬜ ⬜80⬜ ⬜
AMA: 2016,Jan,13; 2015,Jan,16; 2014,Jan,11; 2011,Dec,3-5

96522 **Refilling and maintenance of implantable pump or reservoir for drug delivery, systemic (eg, intravenous, intra-arterial)**
EXCLUDES Implantable infusion pump refilling/maintenance for
spinal/brain drug delivery (95990-95991)
🚑 3.19 ⚖ 3.19 **FUD** XXX
⬜S⬜ ⬜80⬜ ⬜
AMA: 2016,Jan,13; 2015,Jan,16; 2014,Jan,11; 2012,Aug,10-12;
2011,Dec,3-5

96523 **Irrigation of implanted venous access device for drug delivery systems**
EXCLUDES Direct supervision by physician or other qualified health
care provider in facility settings
Use of code with any other services on the same date of
service
🚑 0.70 ⚖ 0.70 **FUD** XXX
⬜Q1⬜ ⬜80⬜ ⬜
AMA: 2016,Jan,13; 2015,Jan,16; 2014,Jan,11; 2012,Jan,15-42;
2011,Dec,3-5; 2011,Jul,16-17

96542-96549 Chemotherapy Injection Into Brain

CMS: 100-04,4,230.2 OPPS Drug Administration

INCLUDES Highly complex services that require direct supervision for:
Consent
Patient assessment
Safety oversight
Supervision
Parenteral administration of:
Anti-neoplastic agents for noncancer diagnoses
Monoclonal antibody agents
Non-radionuclide antineoplastic drugs
Other biologic response modifiers
The following in the administration:
Access to IV/catheter/port
Drug preparation
Flushing at the completion of the infusion
Hydration fluid
Routine tubing/syringe/supplies
Starting the IV
Use of local anesthesia

EXCLUDES Administration of non-chemotherapy agents such as
antibiotics/steroids/analgesics
Blood specimen collection from completely implantable venous access device
(36591)
Declotting of catheter/port (36593)
Home infusion (99601-99602)
Code also drug or substance
Code also significant separately identifiable E&M service, when performed

96542 **Chemotherapy injection, subarachnoid or intraventricular via subcutaneous reservoir, single or multiple agents**
EXCLUDES Oral radioactive isotope therapy (79005)
🚑 1.20 ⚖ 3.42 **FUD** XXX
⬜S⬜ ⬜80⬜ ⬜
AMA: 2016,Jan,13; 2015,Jan,16; 2014,Jan,11

96549 **Unlisted chemotherapy procedure**
🚑 0.00 ⚖ 0.00 **FUD** XXX
⬜S⬜ ⬜80⬜
AMA: 2016,Jan,13; 2015,Jan,16; 2014,Jan,11; 2012,Jan,15-42;
2011,Jan,11

96567-96571 Destruction of Lesions: Photodynamic Therapy

EXCLUDES Ocular photodynamic therapy (67221)

96567 **Photodynamic therapy by external application of light to destroy premalignant and/or malignant lesions of the skin and adjacent mucosa (eg, lip) by activation of photosensitive drug(s), each phototherapy exposure session**
🚑 3.81 ⚖ 3.81 **FUD** XXX
⬜Q1⬜ ⬜80⬜ ⬜
AMA: 2016,Jan,13; 2015,Jan,16; 2014,Jan,11; 2012,Jan,15-42;
2011,Jan,11

+ **96570** **Photodynamic therapy by endoscopic application of light to ablate abnormal tissue via activation of photosensitive drug(s); first 30 minutes (List separately in addition to code for endoscopy or bronchoscopy procedures of lung and gastrointestinal tract)**
Code also for 38-52 minutes (96571)
Code also modifier 52 when services with report are less than
23 minutes
Code first (31641, 43229)
🚑 1.65 ⚖ 1.65 **FUD** ZZZ
⬜N⬜ ⬜
AMA: 2016,Jan,13; 2015,Jan,16; 2014,Jan,11; 2013,Apr,8-9;
2011,Oct,3-4

+ **96571** **each additional 15 minutes (List separately in addition to code for endoscopy or bronchoscopy procedures of lung and gastrointestinal tract)**
EXCLUDES 23-37 minutes of service (96570)
Code first (96570)
Code first when appropriate (31641, 43229)
🚑 0.77 ⚖ 0.77 **FUD** ZZZ
⬜N⬜ ⬜
AMA: 2016,Jan,13; 2015,Jan,16; 2014,Jan,11; 2013,Apr,8-9;
2011,Oct,3-4

96900-96999 Diagnostic/Therapeutic Skin Procedures

EXCLUDES E&M services
Injection, intralesional (11900-11901)

96900 **Actinotherapy (ultraviolet light)**
EXCLUDES Rhinophototherapy (30999)
🔬 (88160-88161)
🚑 0.58 ⚖ 0.58 **FUD** XXX
⬜Q1⬜ ⬜80⬜ ⬜
AMA: 2016,Sep,3; 2016,Jan,13; 2015,Jan,16; 2014,Jan,11;
2012,Jul,9; 2012,Jan,15-42; 2011,Jan,11

96902 **Microscopic examination of hairs plucked or clipped by the examiner (excluding hair collected by the patient) to determine telogen and anagen counts, or structural hair shaft abnormality**
🔬 (88160-88161)
🚑 0.59 ⚖ 0.61 **FUD** XXX
⬜N⬜ ⬜
AMA: 1997,Nov,1

96904 **Whole body integumentary photography, for monitoring of high risk patients with dysplastic nevus syndrome or a history of dysplastic nevi, or patients with a personal or familial history of melanoma**
🔬 (88160-88161)
🚑 1.77 ⚖ 1.77 **FUD** XXX
⬜N⬜ ⬜80⬜ ⬜
AMA: 2006,Dec,10-12

96910 **Photochemotherapy; tar and ultraviolet B (Goeckerman treatment) or petrolatum and ultraviolet B**
🔬 (88160-88161)
🚑 2.01 ⚖ 2.01 **FUD** XXX
⬜Q1⬜ ⬜80⬜ ⬜
AMA: 2016,Sep,3; 2016,Jan,13; 2015,Jan,16; 2014,Jan,11;
2012,Jul,9

96912 psoralens and ultraviolet A (PUVA)
    (88160-88161)
    2.57 2.57 **FUD** XXX [01] [80]
    AMA: 2016,Sep,3; 2016,Jan,13; 2015,Jan,16; 2014,Jan,11; 2012,Jul,9

96913 Photochemotherapy (Goeckerman and/or PUVA) for severe photoresponsive dermatoses requiring at least 4-8 hours of care under direct supervision of the physician (includes application of medication and dressings)
    (88160-88161)
    3.69 3.69 **FUD** XXX [T] [80]
    AMA: 2016,Sep,3

96920 Laser treatment for inflammatory skin disease (psoriasis); total area less than 250 sq cm
    EXCLUDES Destruction by laser of:
        Benign lesions (17110-17111)
        Cutaneous vascular proliferative lesions (17106-17108)
        Malignant lesions (17260-17286)
        Premalignant lesions (17000-17004)
    (88160-88161)
    1.90 4.39 **FUD** 000 [01]
    AMA: 2016,Sep,3; 2016,Jan,13; 2015,Jan,16; 2014,Jan,11; 2013,May,12; 2012,Jul,9; 2012,Jan,15-42; 2011,Jan,11

96921 250 sq cm to 500 sq cm
    EXCLUDES Destruction by laser of:
        Benign lesions (17110-17111)
        Cutaneous vascular proliferative lesions (17106-17108)
        Malignant lesions (17260-17286)
        Premalignant lesions (17000-17004)
    (88160-88161)
    2.15 4.83 **FUD** 000 [01]
    AMA: 2016,Sep,3; 2016,Jan,13; 2015,Jan,16; 2014,Jan,11; 2013,May,12; 2012,Jul,9; 2012,Jan,15-42; 2011,Jan,11

96922 over 500 sq cm
    EXCLUDES Destruction by laser of:
        Benign lesions (17110-17111)
        Cutaneous vascular proliferative lesions (17106-17108)
        Malignant lesions (17260-17286)
        Premalignant lesions (17000-17004)
    (88160-88161)
    3.47 6.70 **FUD** 000 [01]
    AMA: 2016,Sep,3; 2016,Jan,13; 2015,Jan,16; 2014,Jan,11; 2013,May,12; 2012,Jul,9; 2012,Jan,15-42; 2011,Jan,11

96931 Reflectance confocal microscopy (RCM) for cellular and sub-cellular imaging of skin; image acquisition and interpretation and report, first lesion
    0.00 0.00 **FUD** YYY [M] [80]
    EXCLUDES Reflectance confocal microscopy examination without generated mosaic images (96999)

96932 image acquisition only, first lesion
    0.00 0.00 **FUD** YYY [01] [80] [TC]
    EXCLUDES Reflectance confocal microscopy examination without generated mosaic images (96999)

96933 interpretation and report only, first lesion
    0.00 0.00 **FUD** YYY [B] [80] [26]
    EXCLUDES Reflectance confocal microscopy examination without generated mosaic images (96999)

+ **96934** image acquisition and interpretation and report, each additional lesion (List separately in addition to code for primary procedure)
    0.00 0.00 **FUD** YYY [N] [80]
    Code first (96931)
    EXCLUDES Reflectance confocal microscopy examination without generated mosaic images (96999)

+ **96935** image acquisition only, each additional lesion (List separately in addition to code for primary procedure)
    0.00 0.00 **FUD** YYY [N] [80] [TC]
    Code first (96932)
    EXCLUDES Reflectance confocal microscopy examination without generated mosaic images (96999)

+ **96936** interpretation and report only, each additional lesion (List separately in addition to code for primary procedure)
    0.00 0.00 **FUD** YYY [N] [80] [26]
    Code first (96933)
    EXCLUDES Reflectance confocal microscopy examination without generated mosaic images (96999)

96999 Unlisted special dermatological service or procedure
    0.00 0.00 **FUD** XXX [01] [80]
    AMA: 2016,Sep,3; 2016,Jan,13; 2015,Jan,16; 2014,Jan,11; 2013,May,12; 2012,Jul,9

97001-97006 Physical Medicine Assessments

CMS: 100-02,15,230 Practice of Physical Therapy, Occupational Therapy, and Speech-Language Pathology; 100-02,15,230.1 Practice of Physical Therapy; 100-02,15,230.4 Services By a Physical/Occupational Therapist in Private Practice; 100-03,10.3 Inpatient Pain Rehabilitation Programs; 100-03,10.4 Outpatient Hospital Pain Rehabilitation Programs; 100-03,160.17 Payment for L-Dopa /Associated Inpatient Hospital Services; 100-04,5,20.2 Reporting Units of Service

~~**97001** Physical therapy evaluation~~
    To report, see ~[97161, 97162, 97163, 97164, 97165, 97166, 97167, 97168, 97169, 97170, 97171, 97172]

~~**97002** Physical therapy re-evaluation~~
    To report, see ~[97161, 97162, 97163, 97164, 97165, 97166, 97167, 97168, 97169, 97170, 97171, 97172]

~~**97003** Occupational therapy evaluation~~
    To report, see ~[97161, 97162, 97163, 97164, 97165, 97166, 97167, 97168, 97169, 97170, 97171, 97172]

~~**97004** Occupational therapy re-evaluation~~
    To report, see ~[97161, 97162, 97163, 97164, 97165, 97166, 97167, 97168, 97169, 97170, 97171, 97172]

~~**97005** Athletic training evaluation~~
    To report, see ~[97161, 97162, 97163, 97164, 97165, 97166, 97167, 97168, 97169, 97170, 97171, 97172]

~~**97006** Athletic training re-evaluation~~
    To report, see ~[97161, 97162, 97163, 97164, 97165, 97166, 97167, 97168, 97169, 97170, 97171, 97172]

[97161, 97162, 97163, 97164] Assessment: Physical Therapy

INCLUDES Creation of care plan
Evaluation of body systems as defined in the 1997 E&M documentation guidelines:
    Cardiovascular system: Vital signs, edema of extremities
    Integumentary system: Inspection for abnormalities of skin
    Mental status: Orientation, judgment, thought processes
    Musculoskeletal system: Evaluation of gait and station, range of motion, muscle strength, height and weight
    Neuromuscular evaluation: Balance, abnormal movements

● # **97161** Physical therapy evaluation: low complexity, requiring these components: A history with no personal factors and/or comorbidities that impact the plan of care; An examination of body system(s) using standardized tests and measures addressing 1-2 elements from any of the following: body structures and functions, activity limitations, and/or participation restrictions; A clinical presentation with stable and/or uncomplicated characteristics; and Clinical decision making of low complexity using standardized patient assessment instrument and/or measurable assessment of functional outcome. Typically, 20 minutes are spent face-to-face with the patient and/or family.
    0.00 0.00 **FUD** 000

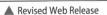

● # 97162 Physical therapy evaluation: moderate complexity, requiring these components: A history of present problem with 1-2 personal factors and/or comorbidities that impact the plan of care; An examination of body systems using standardized tests and measures in addressing a total of 3 or more elements from any of the following: body structures and functions, activity limitations, and/or participation restrictions; An evolving clinical presentation with changing characteristics; and Clinical decision making of moderate complexity using standardized patient assessment instrument and/or measurable assessment of functional outcome. Typically, 30 minutes are spent face-to-face with the patient and/or family.

🖚 0.00 🖳 0.00 **FUD** 000

● # 97163 Physical therapy evaluation: high complexity, requiring these components: A history of present problem with 3 or more personal factors and/or comorbidities that impact the plan of care; An examination of body systems using standardized tests and measures addressing a total of 4 or more elements from any of the following: body structures and functions, activity limitations, and/or participation restrictions; A clinical presentation with unstable and unpredictable characteristics; and Clinical decision making of high complexity using standardized patient assessment instrument and/or measurable assessment of functional outcome. Typically, 45 minutes are spent face-to-face with the patient and/or family.

🖚 0.00 🖳 0.00 **FUD** 000

● # 97164 Re-evaluation of physical therapy established plan of care, requiring these components: An examination including a review of history and use of standardized tests and measures is required; and Revised plan of care using a standardized patient assessment instrument and/or measurable assessment of functional outcome Typically, 20 minutes are spent face-to-face with the patient and/or family.

🖚 0.00 🖳 0.00 **FUD** 000

[97165, 97166, 97167, 97168] Assessment: Occupational Therapy

INCLUDES Creation of care plan
Evaluations as appropriate
Medical history
Occupational status
Past history of therapy

● # 97165 Occupational therapy evaluation, low complexity, requiring these components: An occupational profile and medical and therapy history, which includes a brief history including review of medical and/or therapy records relating to the presenting problem; An assessment(s) that identifies 1-3 performance deficits (ie, relating to physical, cognitive, or psychosocial skills) that result in activity limitations and/or participation restrictions; and Clinical decision making of low complexity, which includes an analysis of the occupational profile, analysis of data from problem-focused assessment(s), and consideration of a limited number of treatment options. Patient presents with no comorbidities that affect occupational performance. Modification of tasks or assistance (eg, physical or verbal) with assessment(s) is not necessary to enable completion of evaluation component. Typically, 30 minutes are spent face-to-face with the patient and/or family.

🖚 0.00 🖳 0.00 **FUD** 000

● # 97166 Occupational therapy evaluation, moderate complexity, requiring these components: An occupational profile and medical and therapy history, which includes an expanded review of medical and/or therapy records and additional review of physical, cognitive, or psychosocial history related to current functional performance; An assessment(s) that identifies 3-5 performance deficits (ie, relating to physical, cognitive, or psychosocial skills) that result in activity limitations and/or participation restrictions; and Clinical decision making of moderate analytic complexity, which includes an analysis of the occupational profile, analysis of data from detailed assessment(s), and consideration of several treatment options. Patient may present with comorbidities that affect occupational performance. Minimal to moderate modification of tasks or assistance (eg, physical or verbal) with assessment(s) is necessary to enable patient to complete evaluation component. Typically, 45 minutes are spent face-to-face with the patient and/or family.

🖚 0.00 🖳 0.00 **FUD** 000

● # 97167 Occupational therapy evaluation, high complexity, requiring these components: An occupational profile and medical and therapy history, which includes review of medical and/or therapy records and extensive additional review of physical, cognitive, or psychosocial history related to current functional performance; An assessment(s) that identifies 5 or more performance deficits (ie, relating to physical, cognitive, or psychosocial skills) that result in activity limitations and/or participation restrictions; and Clinical decision making of high analytic complexity, which includes an analysis of the patient profile, analysis of data from comprehensive assessment(s), and consideration of multiple treatment options. Patient presents with comorbidities that affect occupational performance. Significant modification of tasks or assistance (eg, physical or verbal) with assessment(s) is necessary to enable patient to complete evaluation component. Typically, 60 minutes are spent face-to-face with the patient and/or family.

🖚 0.00 🖳 0.00 **FUD** 000

● # 97168 Re-evaluation of occupational therapy established plan of care, requiring these components: An assessment of changes in patient functional or medical status with revised plan of care; An update to the initial occupational profile to reflect changes in condition or environment that affect future interventions and/or goals; and A revised plan of care. A formal reevaluation is performed when there is a documented change in functional status or a significant change to the plan of care is required. Typically, 30 minutes are spent face-to-face with the patient and/or family.

🖚 0.00 🖳 0.00 **FUD** 000

[97169, 97170, 97171, 97172] Assessment: Athletic Training

INCLUDES Creation of care plan
Evaluation of body systems as defined in the 1997 E&M documentation guidelines:
Cardiovascular system: Vital signs, edema of extremities
Integumentary system: Inspection for abnormalities of skin
Musculoskeletal system: Evaluation of gait and station, range of motion, muscle strength, height and weight
Neuromuscular evaluation: Balance, abnormal movements

● # 97169 Athletic training evaluation, low complexity, requiring these components: A history and physical activity profile with no comorbidities that affect physical activity; An examination of affected body area and other symptomatic or related systems addressing 1-2 elements from any of the following: body structures, physical activity, and/or participation deficiencies; and Clinical decision making of low complexity using standardized patient assessment instrument and/or measurable assessment of functional outcome. Typically, 15 minutes are spent face-to-face with the patient and/or family.

🖚 0.00 🖳 0.00 **FUD** 000

● # **97170** **Athletic training evaluation, moderate complexity, requiring these components: A medical history and physical activity profile with 1-2 comorbidities that affect physical activity; An examination of affected body area and other symptomatic or related systems addressing a total of 3 or more elements from any of the following: body structures, physical activity, and/or participation deficiencies; and Clinical decision making of moderate complexity using standardized patient assessment instrument and/or measurable assessment of functional outcome. Typically, 30 minutes are spent face-to-face with the patient and/or family.**
🏥 0.00 ⚕ 0.00 FUD 000

● # **97171** **Athletic training evaluation, high complexity, requiring these components: A medical history and physical activity profile, with 3 or more comorbidities that affect physical activity; A comprehensive examination of body systems using standardized tests and measures addressing a total of 4 or more elements from any of the following: body structures, physical activity, and/or participation deficiencies; Clinical presentation with unstable and unpredictable characteristics; and Clinical decision making of high complexity using standardized patient assessment instrument and/or measurable assessment of functional outcome. Typically, 45 minutes are spent face-to-face with the patient and/or family.**
🏥 0.00 ⚕ 0.00 FUD 000

● # **97172** **Re-evaluation of athletic training established plan of care requiring these components: An assessment of patient's current functional status when there is a documented change; and A revised plan of care using a standardized patient assessment instrument and/or measurable assessment of functional outcome with an update in management options, goals, and interventions. Typically, 20 minutes are spent face-to-face with the patient and/or family.**
🏥 0.00 ⚕ 0.00 FUD 000

97010-97028 Physical Therapy Treatment Modalities: Supervised

CMS: 100-02,15,230 Practice of Physical Therapy, Occupational Therapy, and Speech-Language Pathology; 100-02,15,230.1 Practice of Physical Therapy; 100-02,15,230.2 Practice of Occupational Therapy; 100-02,15,230.4 Services By a Physical/Occupational Therapist in Private Practice; 100-03,10.3 Inpatient Pain Rehabilitation Programs; 100-03,10.4 Outpatient Hospital Pain Rehabilitation Programs; 100-03,160.17 Payment for L-Dopa /Associated Inpatient Hospital Services; 100-04,5,10 Part B Outpatient Rehabilitation and Comprehensive Outpatient Rehabilitation Facility (CORF) Services - General; 100-04,5,10.2 Financial Limitation for Outpatient Rehabilitation Services; 100-04,5,20.2 Reporting Units of Service

[INCLUDES] Adding incremental intervals of treatment time for the same visit to calculate the total service time

[EXCLUDES] *Direct patient contact by the provider*
Electromyography (95860-95872 [95885, 95886, 95887])
EMG biofeedback training (90901)
Muscle and range of motion tests (95831-95857)
Nerve conduction studies (95905-95913)
Transcutaneous nerve stimulation (TNS) (64550)

97010 **Application of a modality to 1 or more areas; hot or cold packs**
🏥 0.17 ⚕ 0.17 FUD XXX [51] [A] ⚑
AMA: 2016,Jun,8; 2016,Jan,13; 2015,Jan,16; 2014,Jan,11; 2012,Jan,15-42; 2011,Jan,11

97012 **traction, mechanical**
🏥 0.45 ⚕ 0.45 FUD XXX [51] [A] [80] ⚑
AMA: 2016,Jun,8; 2016,Jan,13; 2015,Jan,16; 2014,Jan,11; 2012,Jan,15-42; 2011,Jan,11

97014 **electrical stimulation (unattended)**
[EXCLUDES] *Acupuncture with electrical stimulation (97813, 97814)*
🏥 0.45 ⚕ 0.45 FUD XXX [51] [E] ⚑
AMA: 2016,Jan,13; 2015,Jan,16; 2014,Jan,11; 2012,Jan,15-42; 2011,Aug,6-7; 2011,Jan,11

97016 **vasopneumatic devices**
🏥 0.54 ⚕ 0.54 FUD XXX [51] [A] [80] ⚑
AMA: 2016,Jan,13; 2015,Jan,16; 2014,Jan,11; 2012,Jan,15-42; 2011,Jan,11

97018 **paraffin bath**
🏥 0.31 ⚕ 0.31 FUD XXX [51] [A] [80] ⚑
AMA: 2016,Jan,13; 2015,Jan,16; 2014,Jan,11; 2012,Jan,15-42; 2011,Jan,11

97022 **whirlpool**
🏥 0.66 ⚕ 0.66 FUD XXX [51] [A] [80] ⚑
AMA: 2016,Jan,13; 2015,Jan,16; 2014,Jan,11; 2012,Jan,15-42; 2011,Jan,11

97024 **diathermy (eg, microwave)**
🏥 0.18 ⚕ 0.18 FUD XXX [51] [A] [80] ⚑
AMA: 2016,Jan,13; 2015,Jan,16; 2014,Jan,11; 2012,Jan,15-42; 2011,Jan,11

97026 **infrared**
🏥 0.17 ⚕ 0.17 FUD XXX [51] [A] [80] ⚑
AMA: 2016,Jan,13; 2015,Jan,16; 2014,Jan,11; 2012,Jan,15-42; 2011,Jan,11

97028 **ultraviolet**
🏥 0.21 ⚕ 0.21 FUD XXX [51] [A] [80] ⚑
AMA: 2016,Jan,13; 2015,Jan,16; 2014,Jan,11; 2012,Jan,15-42; 2011,Jan,11

97032-97039 Physical Therapy Treatment Modalities: Constant Attendance

CMS: 100-02,15,230 Practice of Physical Therapy, Occupational Therapy, and Speech-Language Pathology; 100-02,15,230.1 Practice of Physical Therapy; 100-02,15,230.2 Practice of Occupational Therapy; 100-02,15,230.4 Services By a Physical/Occupational Therapist in Private Practice; 100-03,10.3 Inpatient Pain Rehabilitation Programs; 100-03,10.4 Outpatient Hospital Pain Rehabilitation Programs; 100-03,160.17 Payment for L-Dopa /Associated Inpatient Hospital Services; 100-04,5,10 Part B Outpatient Rehabilitation and Comprehensive Outpatient Rehabilitation Facility (CORF) Services - General; 100-04,5,20.2 Reporting Units of Service

[INCLUDES] Adding incremental intervals of treatment time for the same visit to calculate the total service time
Direct patient contact by the provider

[EXCLUDES] *Electromyography (95860-95872 [95885, 95886, 95887])*
EMG biofeedback training (90901)
Muscle and range of motion tests (95831-95857)
Nerve conduction studies (95905-95913)
Transcutaneous nerve stimulation (TNS) (64550)

97032 **Application of a modality to 1 or more areas; electrical stimulation (manual), each 15 minutes**
[EXCLUDES] *Transcutaneous electrical modulation pain reprocessing (TEMPR) (scrambler therapy) (0278T)*
🏥 0.54 ⚕ 0.54 FUD XXX [51] [A] [80] ⚑
AMA: 2016,Jan,13; 2015,Jan,16; 2014,Jan,11; 2012,Jan,15-42; 2011,Jan,11

97033 **iontophoresis, each 15 minutes**
🏥 0.74 ⚕ 0.74 FUD XXX [51] [A] [80] ⚑
AMA: 2016,Jan,13; 2015,Jan,16; 2014,Jan,11

97034 **contrast baths, each 15 minutes**
🏥 0.51 ⚕ 0.51 FUD XXX [51] [A] [80] ⚑
AMA: 2016,Jan,13; 2015,Jan,16; 2014,Jan,11

97035 **ultrasound, each 15 minutes**
🏥 0.36 ⚕ 0.36 FUD XXX [51] [A] [80] ⚑
AMA: 2016,Jan,13; 2015,Jan,16; 2014,Jan,11; 2012,Jan,15-42; 2011,Jan,11

97036 **Hubbard tank, each 15 minutes**
🏥 0.93 ⚕ 0.93 FUD XXX [51] [A] [80] ⚑
AMA: 2016,Jan,13; 2015,Jan,16; 2014,Jan,11

97039 **Unlisted modality (specify type and time if constant attendance)**
🏥 0.00 ⚕ 0.00 FUD XXX [A] [80] ⚑
AMA: 2016,Jun,8; 2016,Jan,13; 2015,Jan,16; 2014,Jan,11; 2012,Jan,15-42; 2011,Jan,11

97110-97546 Other Therapeutic Techniques With Direct Patient Contact

CMS: 100-02,15,230 Practice of Physical Therapy, Occupational Therapy, and Speech-Language Pathology; 100-02,15,230.1 Practice of Physical Therapy; 100-02,15,230.2 Practice of Occupational Therapy; 100-02,15,230.4 Services By a Physical/Occupational Therapist in Private Practice; 100-03,10.3 Inpatient Pain Rehabilitation Programs; 100-03,10.4 Outpatient Hospital Pain Rehabilitation Programs; 100-04,5,10 Part B Outpatient Rehabilitation and Comprehensive Outpatient Rehabilitation Facility (CORF) Services - General; 100-04,5,10.2 Financial Limitation for Outpatient Rehabilitation Services; 100-04,5,20.2 Reporting Units of Service

[INCLUDES] Application of clinical skills/services to improve function
Direct patient contact by the provider

[EXCLUDES] *Electromyography (95860-95872 [95885, 95886, 95887])*
EMG biofeedback training (90901)
Muscle and range of motion tests (95831-95857)
Nerve conduction studies (95905-95913)
Transcutaneous nerve stimulation (TNS) (64550)

97110 **Therapeutic procedure, 1 or more areas, each 15 minutes; therapeutic exercises to develop strength and endurance, range of motion and flexibility**
🏢 0.91 🩺 0.91 **FUD** XXX [51] [A] [80] ⚑
AMA: 2016,Jun,8; 2016,Jan,13; 2015,Jan,16; 2014,Aug,5; 2014,Mar,13; 2014,Jan,11; 2012,Mar,9-10; 2012,Jan,15-42; 2011,Jan,11

97112 **neuromuscular reeducation of movement, balance, coordination, kinesthetic sense, posture, and/or proprioception for sitting and/or standing activities**
🏢 0.95 🩺 0.95 **FUD** XXX [51] [A] [80] ⚑
AMA: 2016,Jan,13; 2015,Jan,16; 2014,Mar,13; 2014,Jan,11; 2012,Mar,9-10; 2012,Jan,15-42; 2011,Jan,11

97113 **aquatic therapy with therapeutic exercises**
🏢 1.21 🩺 1.21 **FUD** XXX [51] [A] [80] ⚑
AMA: 2016,Jan,13; 2015,Jan,16; 2014,Mar,13; 2014,Jan,11; 2012,Jan,15-42; 2011,Jan,11

97116 **gait training (includes stair climbing)**
[EXCLUDES] *Comprehensive gait/motion analysis (96000-96003)*
🏢 0.80 🩺 0.80 **FUD** XXX [51] [A] [80] ⚑
AMA: 2016,Jan,13; 2015,Jan,16; 2014,Mar,13; 2014,Jan,11; 2012,Jan,15-42; 2011,Jan,11

97124 **massage, including effleurage, petrissage and/or tapotement (stroking, compression, percussion)**
[EXCLUDES] *Myofascial release (97140)*
🏢 0.74 🩺 0.74 **FUD** XXX [51] [A] [80] ⚑
AMA: 2016,Jun,8; 2016,Jan,13; 2015,Jan,16; 2014,Mar,13; 2014,Jan,11; 2012,Jan,15-42; 2011,Jan,11

97139 **Unlisted therapeutic procedure (specify)**
🏢 0.00 🩺 0.00 **FUD** XXX [A] [80] ⚑
AMA: 2016,Jan,13; 2015,Jan,16; 2014,Mar,13; 2014,Jan,11; 2012,Jan,15-42; 2011,Jan,11

97140 **Manual therapy techniques (eg, mobilization/ manipulation, manual lymphatic drainage, manual traction), 1 or more regions, each 15 minutes**
🏢 0.84 🩺 0.84 **FUD** XXX [51] [A] [80] ⚑
AMA: 2016,Sep,9; 2016,Aug,3; 2016,Jan,13; 2015,Mar,9; 2015,Jan,16; 2014,Mar,13; 2014,Jan,11; 2012,Jan,15-42; 2011,Jan,11

97150 **Therapeutic procedure(s), group (2 or more individuals)**
[INCLUDES] Constant attendance by the physician/therapist
Reporting this procedure for each member of group
[EXCLUDES] *Adaptive behavior services (0366T-0367T, 0372T)*
Osteopathic manipulative treatment (98925-98929)
🏢 0.49 🩺 0.49 **FUD** XXX [51] [A] [80] ⚑
AMA: 2016,Jan,13; 2015,Jan,16; 2014,Mar,13; 2014,Jan,11; 2012,Jan,15-42; 2011,Jan,11

97161 **Resequenced code. See code before 97010.**

97162 **Resequenced code. See code before 97010.**

97163 **Resequenced code. See code before 97010.**

97164 **Resequenced code. See code before 97010.**

97165 **Resequenced code. See code before 97010.**

97166 **Resequenced code. See code before 97010.**

97167 **Resequenced code. See code before 97010.**

97168 **Resequenced code. See code before 97010.**

97169 **Resequenced code. See code before 97010.**

97170 **Resequenced code. See code before 97010.**

97171 **Resequenced code. See code before 97010.**

97172 **Resequenced code. See code before 97010.**

97530 **Therapeutic activities, direct (one-on-one) patient contact (use of dynamic activities to improve functional performance), each 15 minutes**
🏢 0.98 🩺 0.98 **FUD** XXX [51] [A] [80] ⚑
AMA: 2016,Jan,13; 2015,Jan,16; 2014,Mar,13; 2014,Jan,11; 2012,Jan,15-42; 2011,Jan,11

97532 **Development of cognitive skills to improve attention, memory, problem solving (includes compensatory training), direct (one-on-one) patient contact, each 15 minutes**
🏢 0.75 🩺 0.75 **FUD** XXX [51] [A] [80] ⚑
AMA: 2016,Aug,9; 2016,Jan,13; 2015,Jan,16; 2014,Mar,13; 2014,Jan,11

97533 **Sensory integrative techniques to enhance sensory processing and promote adaptive responses to environmental demands, direct (one-on-one) patient contact, each 15 minutes**
🏢 0.82 🩺 0.82 **FUD** XXX [51] [A] [80] ⚑
AMA: 2016,Jan,13; 2015,Jan,16; 2014,Mar,13; 2014,Jan,11

97535 **Self-care/home management training (eg, activities of daily living (ADL) and compensatory training, meal preparation, safety procedures, and instructions in use of assistive technology devices/adaptive equipment) direct one-on-one contact, each 15 minutes**
🏢 0.99 🩺 0.99 **FUD** XXX [51] [A] [80] ⚑
AMA: 2016,Aug,3; 2016,Jan,13; 2015,Jun,10; 2015,Mar,9; 2015,Jan,16; 2014,Mar,13; 2014,Jan,11; 2012,Jan,15-42; 2011,Jan,11

97537 **Community/work reintegration training (eg, shopping, transportation, money management, avocational activities and/or work environment/modification analysis, work task analysis, use of assistive technology device/adaptive equipment), direct one-on-one contact, each 15 minutes**
[EXCLUDES] *Wheelchair management/propulsion training (97542)*
🏢 0.85 🩺 0.85 **FUD** XXX [51] [A] [80] ⚑
AMA: 2016,Jan,13; 2015,Jan,16; 2014,Mar,13; 2014,Jan,11

97542 **Wheelchair management (eg, assessment, fitting, training), each 15 minutes**
🏢 0.87 🩺 0.87 **FUD** XXX [51] [A] [80] ⚑
AMA: 2016,Jan,13; 2015,Jun,10; 2015,Jan,16; 2014,Mar,13; 2014,Jan,11

97545 **Work hardening/conditioning; initial 2 hours**
🏢 0.00 🩺 0.00 **FUD** XXX [51] [A] [80] ⚑
AMA: 2016,Jan,13; 2015,Jan,16; 2014,Mar,13; 2014,Jan,11; 2012,Jan,15-42; 2011,Jan,11

\+ **97546** **each additional hour (List separately in addition to code for primary procedure)**
Code first initial 2 hours (97545)
🏢 0.00 🩺 0.00 **FUD** ZZZ [51] [A] [80] ⚑
AMA: 2016,Jan,13; 2015,Jan,16; 2014,Mar,13; 2014,Jan,11; 2012,Jan,15-42; 2011,Jan,11

97597-97610 Treatment of Wounds

CMS: 100-02,15,230.4 Services By a Physical/Occupational Therapist in Private Practice; 100-03,270.3 Blood-derived Products for Chronic Nonhealing Wounds; 100-04,4,200.9 Billing for "Sometimes Therapy" Services that May be Paid as Non-Therapy Services; 100-04,5,10 Part B Outpatient Rehabilitation and Comprehensive Outpatient Rehabilitation Facility (CORF) Services - General

INCLUDES Direct patient contact
Removing devitalized/necrotic tissue and promoting healing
EXCLUDES Burn wound debridement (16020-16030)

97597 Debridement (eg, high pressure waterjet with/without suction, sharp selective debridement with scissors, scalpel and forceps), open wound, (eg, fibrin, devitalized epidermis and/or dermis, exudate, debris, biofilm), including topical application(s), wound assessment, use of a whirlpool, when performed and instruction(s) for ongoing care, per session, total wound(s) surface area; first 20 sq cm or less

    🔧 0.66   ⚕ 2.12   **FUD** 000   ⑨ Ⓣ 80 🖵

    AMA: 2016,Aug,9; 2016,Jan,13; 2015,Jan,16; 2014,Jun,11; 2014,Jan,11; 2012,Oct,3-8; 2012,Mar,3; 2012,Jan,15-42; 2012,Jan,6-10; 2011,Sep,11-12; 2011,May,3-5; 2011,Jan,11

Wound may be washed, addressed with scissors, and/or tweezers and scalpel

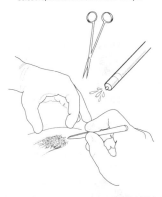

+ 97598 each additional 20 sq cm, or part thereof (List separately in addition to code for primary procedure)
Code first (97597)

    🔧 0.31   ⚕ 0.69   **FUD** ZZZ   ⑨ Ⓝ 80 🖵

    AMA: 2016,Aug,9; 2016,Jan,13; 2015,Jan,16; 2014,Jun,11; 2014,Jan,11; 2012,Mar,3; 2012,Jan,15-42; 2012,Jan,6-10; 2011,Sep,11-12; 2011,May,3-5

▲ 97602 Removal of devitalized tissue from wound(s), non-selective debridement, without anesthesia (eg, wet-to-moist dressings, enzymatic, abrasion, larval therapy), including topical application(s), wound assessment, and instruction(s) for ongoing care, per session

    🔧 0.00   ⚕ 0.00   **FUD** XXX   ⑨ 01 🖵

    AMA: 2016,Jan,13; 2015,Jan,16; 2014,Jun,11; 2014,Jan,11; 2012,Dec,12; 2012,Mar,3; 2012,Jan,6-10; 2012,Jan,15-42; 2011,Aug,6-7; 2011,May,3-5; 2011,Jan,11

97605 Negative pressure wound therapy (eg, vacuum assisted drainage collection), utilizing durable medical equipment (DME), including topical application(s), wound assessment, and instruction(s) for ongoing care, per session; total wound(s) surface area less than or equal to 50 square centimeters

    EXCLUDES *Negative pressure wound therapy using disposable medical equipment (97607-97608)*

    🔧 0.71   ⚕ 1.16   **FUD** XXX   ⑨ 01 80 🖵

    AMA: 2016,Feb,13; 2016,Jan,13; 2015,Jan,16; 2014,Nov,8; 2014,Jan,11; 2012,Jan,15-42; 2011,May,3-5; 2011,Jan,11

97606 total wound(s) surface area greater than 50 square centimeters

    EXCLUDES *Negative pressure wound therapy using disposable medical equipment (97607-97608)*

    🔧 0.77   ⚕ 1.37   **FUD** XXX   ⑨ 01 80 🖵

    AMA: 2016,Feb,13; 2016,Jan,13; 2015,Jan,16; 2014,Nov,8; 2014,Jan,11; 2012,Jan,15-42; 2011,May,3-5; 2011,Jan,11

97607 Negative pressure wound therapy, (eg, vacuum assisted drainage collection), utilizing disposable, non-durable medical equipment including provision of exudate management collection system, topical application(s), wound assessment, and instructions for ongoing care, per session; total wound(s) surface area less than or equal to 50 square centimeters

    EXCLUDES *Negative pressure wound therapy using durable medical equipment (97605-97606)*

    🔧 0.00   ⚕ 0.00   **FUD** XXX   ⑨ Ⓣ 80 🖵

    AMA: 2016,Jan,13; 2015,Jan,16; 2014,Nov,8

97608 total wound(s) surface area greater than 50 square centimeters

    EXCLUDES *Negative pressure wound therapy using durable medical equipment (97605-97606)*

    🔧 0.00   ⚕ 0.00   **FUD** XXX   ⑨ Ⓣ 80 🖵

    AMA: 2016,Jan,13; 2015,Jan,16; 2014,Nov,8

97610 Low frequency, non-contact, non-thermal ultrasound, including topical application(s), when performed, wound assessment, and instruction(s) for ongoing care, per day

    🔧 0.45   ⚕ 3.37   **FUD** XXX   ⑨ 01 80 🖵

    AMA: 2016,Jan,13; 2015,Jan,16; 2014,Jun,11

97750-97799 Assessments and Training

CMS: 100-02,15,230.1 Practice of Physical Therapy; 100-02,15,230.2 Practice of Occupational Therapy; 100-02,15,230.4 Services By a Physical/Occupational Therapist in Private Practice; 100-04,5,10 Part B Outpatient Rehabilitation and Comprehensive Outpatient Rehabilitation Facility (CORF) Services - General

97750 Physical performance test or measurement (eg, musculoskeletal, functional capacity), with written report, each 15 minutes

    INCLUDES Direct patient contact
    EXCLUDES *Muscle/range of motion testing and electromyography/nerve velocity determination (95831-95857, 95860-95872, [95885, 95886, 95887], 95907-95913)*

    🔧 0.93   ⚕ 0.93   **FUD** XXX   ⑨ Ⓐ 80 🖵

    AMA: 2016,Jan,13; 2015,Jan,16; 2014,Jan,11; 2013,Aug,7; 2012,Jan,15-42; 2011,Jan,11

97755 Assistive technology assessment (eg, to restore, augment or compensate for existing function, optimize functional tasks and/or maximize environmental accessibility), direct one-on-one contact, with written report, each 15 minutes

    INCLUDES Direct patient contact
    EXCLUDES *Augmentative/alternative communication device (92605, 92607)*
    Muscle/range of motion testing and electromyography/nerve velocity determination (95831-95857, 95860-95872, [95885, 95886, 95887], 95907-95913)

    🔧 1.01   ⚕ 1.01   **FUD** XXX   ⑨ Ⓐ 80 🖵

    AMA: 1996,Sep,7; 1995,Sum,5

97760 Orthotic(s) management and training (including assessment and fitting when not otherwise reported), upper extremity(s), lower extremity(s) and/or trunk, each 15 minutes

    EXCLUDES *Gait training, if performed on the same extremity (97116)*

    🔧 1.07   ⚕ 1.07   **FUD** XXX   ⑨ Ⓐ 80 🖵

    AMA: 2016,Jan,13; 2015,Jan,16; 2014,Jan,11

97761 Prosthetic training, upper and/or lower extremity(s), each 15 minutes

    🔧 0.93   ⚕ 0.93   **FUD** XXX   ⑨ Ⓐ 80 🖵

    AMA: 2016,Jan,13; 2015,Jan,16; 2014,Jan,11; 2012,Jan,15-42; 2011,Jan,11

97762 Checkout for orthotic/prosthetic use, established patient, each 15 minutes

    🔧 1.34   ⚕ 1.34   **FUD** XXX   ⑨ Ⓐ 80 🖵

    AMA: 2016,Jan,13; 2015,Jan,16; 2014,Jan,11

97799 Unlisted physical medicine/rehabilitation service or procedure

    0.00   0.00   **FUD** XXX   A 80

    AMA: 2016,Jan,13; 2015,Jan,16; 2014,Jan,11

97802-97804 Medical Nutrition Therapy Services

CMS: 100-02,15,270.2 Medicare Telehealth Services; 100-03,180.1 Medical Nutrition Therapy; 100-04,12* Medicare Telehealth Services; 100-04,12,190.7 Contractor Editing of Telehealth Claims; 100-04,4,300 Medical Nutrition Therapy Services; 100-04,4,300.6 CWF Edits for MNT/DSMT; 100-04,9,182 Medical Nutrition Therapy (MNT) Services

EXCLUDES *Medical nutrition therapy assessment/intervention provided by physician or other qualified health care provider; use appropriate E&M codes*

97802 Medical nutrition therapy; initial assessment and intervention, individual, face-to-face with the patient, each 15 minutes

    0.92   0.98   **FUD** XXX   ★ A 80

    AMA: 2016,Jan,13; 2015,Jan,16; 2014,Jan,11

97803 re-assessment and intervention, individual, face-to-face with the patient, each 15 minutes

    0.78   0.85   **FUD** XXX   ★ A 80

    AMA: 2016,Jan,13; 2015,Jan,16; 2014,Jan,11

97804 group (2 or more individual(s)), each 30 minutes

    0.43   0.45   **FUD** XXX   ★ A 80

    AMA: 2016,Jan,13; 2015,Jan,16; 2014,Jan,11

97810-97814 Acupuncture

CMS: 100-02,15,230.4 Services By a Physical/Occupational Therapist in Private Practice; 100-03,10.3 Inpatient Pain Rehabilitation Programs; 100-03,10.4 Outpatient Hospital Pain Rehabilitation Programs; 100-03,30.3 Acupuncture; 100-03,30.3.1 Acupuncture for Fibromyalgia; 100-03,30.3.2 Acupuncture for Osteoarthritis

INCLUDES 15 minute increments of face-to-face contact with the patient
Reporting only one code for each 15 minute increment
Code also significant separately identifiable E&M service using modifier 25, when performed

97810 Acupuncture, 1 or more needles; without electrical stimulation, initial 15 minutes of personal one-on-one contact with the patient

    EXCLUDES *Treatment with electrical stimulation (97813-97814)*

    0.87   1.03   **FUD** XXX   E

    AMA: 2016,Jan,13; 2015,Jan,16; 2014,Jan,11; 2012,Jan,15-42; 2011,Jan,11

+ **97811** without electrical stimulation, each additional 15 minutes of personal one-on-one contact with the patient, with re-insertion of needle(s) (List separately in addition to code for primary procedure)

    EXCLUDES *Treatment with electrical stimulation (97813-97814)*
    Code first initial 15 minutes (97810)

    0.72   0.77   **FUD** ZZZ   E

    AMA: 2016,Jan,13; 2015,Jan,16; 2014,Jan,11

97813 with electrical stimulation, initial 15 minutes of personal one-on-one contact with the patient

    EXCLUDES *Treatment without electrical stimulation (97813-97814)*

    0.94   1.10   **FUD** XXX   E

    AMA: 2016,Jan,13; 2015,Jan,16; 2014,Jan,11

+ **97814** with electrical stimulation, each additional 15 minutes of personal one-on-one contact with the patient, with re-insertion of needle(s) (List separately in addition to code for primary procedure)

    EXCLUDES *Treatment without electrical stimulation (97813-97814)*
    Code first initial 15 minutes (97813)

    0.79   0.87   **FUD** ZZZ   E

    AMA: 2016,Jan,13; 2015,Jan,16; 2014,Jan,11

98925-98929 Osteopathic Manipulation

CMS: 100-03,150.1 Manipulation

INCLUDES Physician applied manual treatment done to eliminate/alleviate somatic dysfunction and related disorders using a variety of techniques
The following body regions:
    Abdomen/visceral region
    Cervical region
    Head region
    Lower extremities
    Lumbar region
    Pelvic region
    Rib cage region
    Sacral region
    Thoracic region
    Upper extremities
Code also significant separately identifiable E&M service using modifier 25, when performed

98925 Osteopathic manipulative treatment (OMT); 1-2 body regions involved

    0.67   0.89   **FUD** 000   Q1 80

    AMA: 2016,Jan,13; 2015,Jan,16; 2014,Jan,11; 2012,Jan,15-42; 2011,Jan,11

98926 3-4 body regions involved

    1.02   1.29   **FUD** 000   Q1 80

    AMA: 2016,Jan,13; 2015,Jan,16; 2014,Jan,11; 2012,Jan,15-42; 2011,Jan,11

98927 5-6 body regions involved

    1.34   1.67   **FUD** 000   Q1 80

    AMA: 2016,Jan,13; 2015,Jan,16; 2014,Jan,11; 2012,Jan,15-42; 2011,Jan,11

98928 7-8 body regions involved

    1.69   2.05   **FUD** 000   Q1 80

    AMA: 2016,Jan,13; 2015,Jan,16; 2014,Jan,11; 2012,May,14-15; 2012,Jan,15-42; 2011,Jan,11

98929 9-10 body regions involved

    2.03   2.45   **FUD** 000   Q1 80

    AMA: 2016,Jan,13; 2015,Jan,16; 2014,Jan,11; 2012,Jan,15-42; 2011,Jan,11

98940-98943 Chiropractic Manipulation

CMS: 100-01,5,70.6 Chiropractors; 100-02,15,240 Chiropractic Services - General; 100-02,15,240.1.3 Necessity for Treatment; 100-02,15,30.5 Chiropractor's Services; 100-03,150.1 Manipulation

INCLUDES Form of manual treatment performed to influence joint/neurophysical function
The following five extraspinal regions:
    Abdomen
    Head, including temporomandibular joint, excluding atlanto-occipital region
    Lower extremities
    Rib cage, not including costotransverse/costovertebral joints
    Upper extremities
The following five spinal regions:
    Cervical region (atlanto-occipital joint)
    Lumbar region
    Pelvic region (sacro-iliac joint)
    Sacral region
    Thoracic region (costovertebral/costotransverse joints)
Code also significant separately identifiable E&M service using modifier 25 when performed

98940 Chiropractic manipulative treatment (CMT); spinal, 1-2 regions

    0.64   0.80   **FUD** 000   Q1 80

    AMA: 2016,Jan,13; 2015,Jan,16; 2014,Jan,11; 2013,Dec,14; 2012,Jan,15-42; 2011,Jan,11

98941 spinal, 3-4 regions

    0.98   1.15   **FUD** 000   Q1 80

    AMA: 2016,Jan,13; 2015,Jan,16; 2014,Jan,11; 2013,Dec,14; 2012,Jan,15-42; 2011,Jan,11

98942 spinal, 5 regions

    1.32   1.50   **FUD** 000   Q1 80

    AMA: 2016,Jan,13; 2015,Jan,16; 2014,Jan,11; 2013,Dec,14; 2012,Jan,15-42; 2011,Jan,11

98943 **extraspinal, 1 or more regions**
0.67 0.77 **FUD** XXX E ▢

AMA: 2016,Jan,13; 2015,Jan,16; 2014,Jan,11; 2013,Dec,14; 2012,Jan,15-42; 2011,Jan,11

98960-98962 Self-Management Training

INCLUDES Education/training services:
Prescribed by a physician or other qualified health care professional
Provided by a qualified nonphysician health care provider
Standardized curriculum that may be modified as necessary for:
Clinical needs
Cultural norms
Health literacy
Teaching the patient how to manage the illness/delay the comorbidity(s)

EXCLUDES Genetic counseling education services (96040, 98961-98962)
Health/behavior assessment (96150-96155)
Medical nutrition therapy (97802-97804)
The following services:
Counseling/education to a group (99078)
Counseling/education to individuals (99201-99215, 99217-99223 [99224, 99225, 99226], 99231-99233, 99241-99255, 99281-99285, 99304-99318, 99324-99337, 99341-99350, 99401-99429)
Counseling/risk factor reduction without symptoms/established disease (99401-99412)

98960 **Education and training for patient self-management by a qualified, nonphysician health care professional using a standardized curriculum, face-to-face with the patient (could include caregiver/family) each 30 minutes; individual patient**
0.79 0.79 **FUD** XXX ★ E ▢

AMA: 2016,Jan,13; 2015,Jan,16; 2014,Oct,3; 2014,Jan,11; 2013,Nov,3; 2013,Apr,3-4

98961 **2-4 patients**
INCLUDES Group education regarding genetic risks
0.38 0.38 **FUD** XXX ★ E ▢

AMA: 2016,Jan,13; 2015,Jan,16; 2014,Oct,3; 2014,Jan,11; 2013,Nov,3; 2013,Apr,3-4

98962 **5-8 patients**
INCLUDES Group education regarding genetic risks
0.28 0.28 **FUD** XXX ★ E ▢

AMA: 2016,Jan,13; 2015,Jan,16; 2014,Oct,3; 2014,Jan,11; 2013,Nov,3; 2013,Apr,3-4

98966-98968 Nonphysician Telephone Services

INCLUDES Assessment and management services provided by telephone by a qualified health care professional
Episode of care initiated by an established patient or his/her guardian

EXCLUDES Call initiated by the qualified health care professional
Calls during the postoperative period of a procedure
Decision to see the patient at the next available urgent care appointment
Decision to see the patient within 24 hours of the call
Patient management services during same time frame as (99487-99489, 99495-99496)
Telephone services provided by a physician (99441-99443)
Telephone services that are considered a part of a previous or subsequent service
Use of codes if same codes billed within the past seven days

98966 **Telephone assessment and management service provided by a qualified nonphysician health care professional to an established patient, parent, or guardian not originating from a related assessment and management service provided within the previous 7 days nor leading to an assessment and management service or procedure within the next 24 hours or soonest available appointment; 5-10 minutes of medical discussion**
0.36 0.39 **FUD** XXX E ▢

AMA: 2016,Jan,13; 2015,Jan,16; 2014,Oct,3; 2014,Jan,11; 2013,Oct,11; 2013,Nov,3; 2013,Apr,3-4

98967 **11-20 minutes of medical discussion**
0.72 0.76 **FUD** XXX E ▢

AMA: 2016,Jan,13; 2015,Jan,16; 2014,Oct,3; 2014,Jan,11; 2013,Oct,11; 2013,Nov,3; 2013,Apr,3-4

98968 **21-30 minutes of medical discussion**
1.08 1.11 **FUD** XXX E ▢

AMA: 2016,Jan,13; 2015,Jan,16; 2014,Oct,3; 2014,Jan,11; 2013,Oct,11; 2013,Nov,3; 2013,Apr,3-4

98969 Nonphysician Online Service

INCLUDES On-line assessment and management service provided by a qualified health care professional
Timely reply to the patient as well as:
Ordering laboratory services
Permanent record of the service; either hard copy or electronic
Providing a prescription
Related telephone calls

EXCLUDES Anticoagulant management (99363-99364)
On-line evaluation service:
Provided during the postoperative period of a procedure
Provided more than once in a seven day period
Related to a service provided in the previous seven days
Patient management services during same time frame as (99487-99489, 99495-99496)

98969 **Online assessment and management service provided by a qualified nonphysician health care professional to an established patient or guardian, not originating from a related assessment and management service provided within the previous 7 days, using the Internet or similar electronic communications network**
0.00 0.00 **FUD** XXX E ▢

AMA: 2016,Jan,13; 2015,Jan,16; 2014,Oct,3; 2014,Jan,11; 2013,Oct,11; 2013,Nov,3; 2013,Apr,3-4

99000-99091 Supplemental Services and Supplies

INCLUDES Supplemental reporting for services adjunct to the basic service provided

99000 **Handling and/or conveyance of specimen for transfer from the office to a laboratory**
0.00 0.00 **FUD** XXX E ▢

AMA: 2016,Jan,13; 2015,Jan,16; 2014,Jan,11; 2012,Jan,15-42; 2011,Jan,11

99001 **Handling and/or conveyance of specimen for transfer from the patient in other than an office to a laboratory (distance may be indicated)**
0.00 0.00 **FUD** XXX E ▢

AMA: 2016,Jan,13; 2015,Jan,16; 2014,Jan,11; 2012,Jan,15-42; 2011,Jan,11

99002 **Handling, conveyance, and/or any other service in connection with the implementation of an order involving devices (eg, designing, fitting, packaging, handling, delivery or mailing) when devices such as orthotics, protectives, prosthetics are fabricated by an outside laboratory or shop but which items have been designed, and are to be fitted and adjusted by the attending physician or other qualified health care professional**
EXCLUDES Venous blood routine collection (36415)
0.00 0.00 **FUD** XXX B ▢

AMA: 2016,Jan,13; 2015,Jan,16; 2014,Jan,11; 2012,Jan,15-42; 2011,Jan,11

99024 **Postoperative follow-up visit, normally included in the surgical package, to indicate that an evaluation and management service was performed during a postoperative period for a reason(s) related to the original procedure**
0.00 0.00 **FUD** XXX B ▢

AMA: 2016,Jan,13; 2015,Mar,3; 2015,Jan,16; 2014,Jan,11; 2012,Jan,15-42; 2011,Jan,11

99026 **Hospital mandated on call service; in-hospital, each hour**
EXCLUDES Physician stand-by services with prolonged physician attendance (99360)
Time spent providing procedures or services that may be separately reported
0.00 0.00 **FUD** XXX E ▢

AMA: 2016,Jan,13; 2015,Jan,16; 2014,Jan,11; 2012,Jan,15-42; 2011,Jan,11

99027 **out-of-hospital, each hour**

> *EXCLUDES* *Physician stand-by services with prolonged physician attendance (99360)*
> *Time spent providing procedures or services that may be separately reported*

🚑 0.00   ⚕ 0.00   **FUD** XXX   E 🔲

AMA: 2016,Jan,13; 2015,Jan,16; 2014,Jan,11; 2012,Jan,15-42; 2011,Jan,11

99050 **Services provided in the office at times other than regularly scheduled office hours, or days when the office is normally closed (eg, holidays, Saturday or Sunday), in addition to basic service**

> Code also more than one adjunct code per encounter when appropriate
> Code first basic service provided

🚑 0.00   ⚕ 0.00   **FUD** XXX   SI B 🔲

AMA: 2016,Jan,13; 2015,Jan,16; 2014,Jan,11; 2012,Jan,15-42; 2011,Jan,11

99051 **Service(s) provided in the office during regularly scheduled evening, weekend, or holiday office hours, in addition to basic service**

> Code also more than one adjunct code per encounter when appropriate
> Code first basic service provided

🚑 0.00   ⚕ 0.00   **FUD** XXX   SI B 🔲

AMA: 2016,Jan,13; 2015,Jan,16; 2014,Jan,11; 2012,Jan,15-42; 2011,Jan,11

99053 **Service(s) provided between 10:00 PM and 8:00 AM at 24-hour facility, in addition to basic service**

> Code also more than one adjunct code per encounter when appropriate
> Code first basic service provided

🚑 0.00   ⚕ 0.00   **FUD** XXX   SI B 🔲

AMA: 2016,Jan,13; 2015,Jan,16; 2014,Jan,11; 2012,Jan,15-42; 2011,Jan,11

99056 **Service(s) typically provided in the office, provided out of the office at request of patient, in addition to basic service**

> Code also more than one adjunct code per encounter when appropriate
> Code first basic service provided

🚑 0.00   ⚕ 0.00   **FUD** XXX   SI B 🔲

AMA: 2016,Jan,13; 2015,Jan,16; 2014,Jan,11; 2012,Jan,15-42; 2011,Jan,11

99058 **Service(s) provided on an emergency basis in the office, which disrupts other scheduled office services, in addition to basic service**

> Code also more than one adjunct code per encounter when appropriate
> Code first basic service provided

🚑 0.00   ⚕ 0.00   **FUD** XXX   SI B 🔲

AMA: 2016,Jan,13; 2015,Jan,16; 2014,Jan,11; 2012,Jan,15-42; 2011,Jan,11

99060 **Service(s) provided on an emergency basis, out of the office, which disrupts other scheduled office services, in addition to basic service**

> Code also more than one adjunct code per encounter when appropriate
> Code first basic service provided

🚑 0.00   ⚕ 0.00   **FUD** XXX   SI B 🔲

AMA: 2016,Jan,13; 2015,Jan,16; 2014,Jan,11; 2012,Jan,15-42; 2011,Jan,11

99070 **Supplies and materials (except spectacles), provided by the physician or other qualified health care professional over and above those usually included with the office visit or other services rendered (list drugs, trays, supplies, or materials provided)**

> *EXCLUDES* *Spectacles supply*

🚑 0.00   ⚕ 0.00   **FUD** XXX   B 🔲

AMA: 2016,Jan,13; 2015,Jan,16; 2014,Mar,11; 2014,Jan,11; 2013,Dec,12; 2013,Mar,6-7; 2012,Nov,11-12; 2012,Aug,9; 2012,Apr,10; 2012,Jan,15-42; 2011,Jan,11

99071 **Educational supplies, such as books, tapes, and pamphlets, for the patient's education at cost to physician or other qualified health care professional**

🚑 0.00   ⚕ 0.00   **FUD** XXX   B 🔲

AMA: 2016,Jan,13; 2015,Jan,16; 2014,Oct,3; 2014,Jan,11; 2013,Nov,3; 2013,Apr,3-4; 2012,Jan,15-42; 2011,Jan,11

99075 **Medical testimony**

🚑 0.00   ⚕ 0.00   **FUD** XXX   E 🔲

AMA: 2016,Jan,13; 2015,Jan,16; 2014,Jan,11; 2012,Jan,15-42; 2011,Jan,11

99078 **Physician or other qualified health care professional qualified by education, training, licensure/regulation (when applicable) educational services rendered to patients in a group setting (eg, prenatal, obesity, or diabetic instructions)**

🚑 0.00   ⚕ 0.00   **FUD** XXX   N 🔲

AMA: 2016,Jan,13; 2015,Jan,16; 2014,Oct,3; 2014,Jan,11; 2013,Nov,3; 2013,Apr,3-4; 2012,Jan,15-42; 2011,Jan,11

99080 **Special reports such as insurance forms, more than the information conveyed in the usual medical communications or standard reporting form**

> *EXCLUDES* *Completion of workmen's compensation forms (99455-99456)*

🚑 0.00   ⚕ 0.00   **FUD** XXX   B 🔲

AMA: 2016,Jan,13; 2015,Jan,16; 2014,Oct,3; 2014,Jan,11; 2013,Nov,3; 2013,Apr,3-4; 2012,Jan,15-42; 2011,Jan,11

99082 **Unusual travel (eg, transportation and escort of patient)**

🚑 0.00   ⚕ 0.00   **FUD** XXX   B 80 🔲

AMA: 2016,Jan,13; 2015,Jan,16; 2014,Jan,11; 2012,Jan,15-42; 2011,Jan,11

99090 **Analysis of clinical data stored in computers (eg, ECGs, blood pressures, hematologic data)**

> *EXCLUDES* *Collection/interpretation by health care professional/physician of physiologic data stored/transmitted by patient or caregiver (99091)*
> *Use of this code when a more specific CPT code exists for cardiographic services, glucose monitoring, or musculoskeletal function testing (93227, 93272, 95250, 97750, 0206T)*

🚑 0.00   ⚕ 0.00   **FUD** XXX   B 🔲

AMA: 2016,Jan,13; 2015,Jan,16; 2014,Oct,3; 2014,May,4; 2014,Jan,11; 2013,Nov,3; 2013,Apr,3-4; 2012,Jan,15-42; 2011,Jan,11

99091 **Collection and interpretation of physiologic data (eg, ECG, blood pressure, glucose monitoring) digitally stored and/or transmitted by the patient and/or caregiver to the physician or other qualified health care professional, qualified by education, training, licensure/regulation (when applicable) requiring a minimum of 30 minutes of time**

🚑 1.59   ⚕ 1.59   **FUD** XXX   N 🔲

AMA: 2016,Jan,13; 2015,Jan,16; 2014,Oct,3; 2014,Jan,11; 2013,Nov,3; 2013,Apr,3-4; 2012,Jan,15-42; 2011,Jan,11

99100-99140 Modifying Factors for Anesthesia Services

CMS: 100-04,12,140.3 Payment for Qualified Nonphysician Anesthetists; 100-04,12,140.3.3 Billing Modifiers; 100-04,12,140.3.4 General Billing Instructions; 100-04,12,140.4.1 Anesthesiologist/Qualified Nonphysican Anesthetist; 100-04,12,140.4.2 Anesthetist and Anesthesiologist in a Single Procedure; 100-04,12,140.4.4 Conversion Factors for Anesthesia Services; 100-04,4,250.3.2 Anesthesia in a Hospital Outpatient Setting

Code first primary anesthesia procedure

+ **99100** **Anesthesia for patient of extreme age, younger than 1 year and older than 70 (List separately in addition to code for primary anesthesia procedure)** A

> *EXCLUDES* *Anesthesia services for infants one year old or less at the time of surgery (00326, 00561, 00834, 00836)*

🚑 0.00   ⚕ 0.00   **FUD** ZZZ   B 🔲

AMA: 2016,Jan,13; 2015,Jan,16; 2014,Jan,11

+ **99116** **Anesthesia complicated by utilization of total body hypothermia (List separately in addition to code for primary anesthesia procedure)**

> EXCLUDES *Anesthesia for procedures on heart/pericardial sac/great vessels of chest with pump oxygenator (00561)*
>
> 🔲 0.00   ✂ 0.00   **FUD** ZZZ   B ▣
>
> **AMA:** 2016,Jan,13; 2015,Jan,16; 2014,Jan,11

+ **99135** **Anesthesia complicated by utilization of controlled hypotension (List separately in addition to code for primary anesthesia procedure)**

> EXCLUDES *Anesthesia for procedures on heart/pericardial sac/great vessels of chest with pump oxygenator (00561)*
>
> 🔲 0.00   ✂ 0.00   **FUD** ZZZ   B ▣
>
> **AMA:** 2016,Jan,13; 2015,Jan,16; 2014,Jan,11

+ **99140** **Anesthesia complicated by emergency conditions (specify) (List separately in addition to code for primary anesthesia procedure)**

> INCLUDES *Conditions where postponement of treatment could be dangerous to life or health*
>
> 🔲 0.00   ✂ 0.00   **FUD** ZZZ   B ▣
>
> **AMA:** 2016,Jan,13; 2015,Jan,16; 2014,Jan,11; 2012,Jan,15-42; 2011,Jan,11

99143-99150 Moderate Sedation Services

99143 ~~Moderate sedation services (other than those services described by codes 00100-01999) provided by the same physician or other qualified health care professional performing the diagnostic or therapeutic service that the sedation supports, requiring the presence of an independent trained observer to assist in the monitoring of the patient's level of consciousness and physiological status; younger than 5 years of age, first 30 minutes intra-service time~~

> To report, see ~99151-99153

99144 ~~age 5 years or older, first 30 minutes intra-service time~~

> To report, see ~99151-99153

99145 ~~each additional 15 minutes intra-service time (List separately in addition to code for primary service)~~

> To report, see ~99151-99153

99148 ~~Moderate sedation services (other than those services described by codes 00100-01999), provided by a physician or other qualified health care professional other than the health care professional performing the diagnostic or therapeutic service that the sedation supports; younger than 5 years of age, first 30 minutes intra-service time~~

> To report, see ~99155-99157

99149 ~~age 5 years or older, first 30 minutes intra-service time~~

> To report, see ~99155-99157

99150 ~~each additional 15 minutes intra-service time (List separately in addition to code for primary service)~~

> To report, see ~99155-99157

99151-99157 Moderate Sedation Services

> INCLUDES Intraservice work that begins with administration of the sedation drugs and ends when the procedure is over
> Monitoring of:
>   Patient response to the drugs
>   Vital signs
> Ordering and providing the drug to the patient (first and subsequent)
> Pre- and postservice procedures

● **99151** **Moderate sedation services provided by the same physician or other qualified health care professional performing the diagnostic or therapeutic service that the sedation supports, requiring the presence of an independent trained observer to assist in the monitoring of the patient's level of consciousness and physiological status; initial 15 minutes of intraservice time, patient younger than 5 years of age**

> 🔲 0.00   ✂ 0.00   **FUD** 000   ⊘
>
> INCLUDES First 15 minutes of intraservice time for patients under age 5
> Services provided to patients by same provider of the service for which moderate sedation is necessary with monitoring by a trained observer

● **99152** **initial 15 minutes of intraservice time, patient age 5 years or older**

> 🔲 0.00   ✂ 0.00   **FUD** 000   ⊘
>
> INCLUDES First 15 minutes of intraservice time for patients age 5 and over
> Services provided to patients by same provider of the service for which moderate sedation is necessary with monitoring by a trained observer

● + **99153** **each additional 15 minutes intraservice time (List separately in addition to code for primary service)**

> 🔲 0.00   ✂ 0.00   **FUD** 000
>
> INCLUDES Services provided to patients by same provider of the service for which moderate sedation is necessary with monitoring by a trained observer
>
> EXCLUDES *Services provided to patients by a physician/other qualified health care professional other than the provider rendering the service*
>
> Code first (99151-99152)

● **99155** **Moderate sedation services provided by a physician or other qualified health care professional other than the physician or other qualified health care professional performing the diagnostic or therapeutic service that the sedation supports; initial 15 minutes of intraservice time, patient younger than 5 years of age**

> INCLUDES First 15 minutes of intraservice time for patients under age 5
> Services provided to patients by a physician/other qualified health care professional other than the provider rendering the service for which moderate sedation is necessary

● **99156** **initial 15 minutes of intraservice time, patient age 5 years or older**

> INCLUDES First 15 minutes of intraservice time for patients age 5 and over
> Services provided to patients by a physician/other qualified health care professional other than the provider rendering the service for which moderate sedation is necessary

● + **99157** **each additional 15 minutes intraservice time (List separately in addition to code for primary service)**

> 🔲 0.00   ✂ 0.00   **FUD** 000
>
> INCLUDES Each subsequent 15 minutes of services
> Services provided to patients by a physician/other qualified health care professional other than the provider rendering the service for which moderate sedation is necessary
>
> EXCLUDES *Services provided to patients by same provider of the service for which moderate sedation is necessary with monitoring by a trained observer (99151-99152)*
>
> Code first (99155-99156)

99170 Specialized Examination of Child

> EXCLUDES *Moderate sedation (99151-99157)*

99170 **Anogenital examination, magnified, in childhood for suspected trauma, including image recording when performed**   A

> 🔲 2.53   ✂ 4.90   **FUD** 000   T ▣
>
> **AMA:** 2016,Jan,13; 2015,Jan,16; 2014,Sep,7; 2014,Jan,11

● New Code   ▲ Revised Code   ○ Reinstated   ● New Web Release   ▲ Revised Web Release   Unlisted   Not Covered   # Resequenced
⊘ AMA Mod 51 Exempt   ⑨ Optum Mod 51 Exempt   ⊛ Mod 63 Exempt   ⁄ Non-FDA Drug   ★ Telehealth   M Maternity   A Age Edit   + Add-on   AMA: CPT Asst

99172-99173 Visual Acuity Screening Tests

INCLUDES Graduated visual acuity stimuli that allow a quantitative determination/estimation of visual acuity

99172 **Visual function screening, automated or semi-automated bilateral quantitative determination of visual acuity, ocular alignment, color vision by pseudoisochromatic plates, and field of vision (may include all or some screening of the determination[s] for contrast sensitivity, vision under glare)**

EXCLUDES General ophthalmological or E&M services
Screening for visual acuity, amblyogenic factors (99173, 99174 [99177])

⏴ 0.00 ⏴ 0.00 **FUD** XXX   E ▣

AMA: 2016,Jan,13; 2015,Jan,16; 2014,Jan,11; 2012,Jan,15-42; 2011,Jan,11

99173 **Screening test of visual acuity, quantitative, bilateral**

EXCLUDES Screening for visual function, amblyogenic factors (99172, 99174, [99177])

⏴ 0.09 ⏴ 0.09 **FUD** XXX   E ▣

AMA: 2016,Jan,13; 2015,Jan,16; 2014,Jan,11

99174 [99177] Screening For Amblyogenic Factors

EXCLUDES General ophthalmological services (92002-92014)
Screening for visual acuity (99172-99173)

99174 **Instrument-based ocular screening (eg, photoscreening, automated-refraction), bilateral; with remote analysis and report**

EXCLUDES Ocular screening on-site analysis ([99177])

⏴ 0.00 ⏴ 0.00 **FUD** XXX   E ▣

AMA: 2016,Mar,10; 2016,Jan,13; 2015,Jan,16; 2014,Jan,11; 2013,Mar,6-7

**99177** **with on-site analysis**

EXCLUDES Remote ocular screening (99174)

⏴ 0.00 ⏴ 0.00 **FUD** XXX   E ▣

AMA: 2016,Mar,10

99175-99177 Drug Administration to Induce Vomiting

EXCLUDES Diagnostic gastric lavage (43754-43755)
Diagnostic gastric intubation (43754-43755)

99175 **Ipecac or similar administration for individual emesis and continued observation until stomach adequately emptied of poison**

⏴ 0.48 ⏴ 0.48 **FUD** XXX   N 80 ▣

AMA: 1997,Nov,1

99177 **Resequenced code. See code following 99174.**

99183-99184 Hyperbaric Oxygen Therapy

CMS: 100-03,20.29 Hyperbaric Oxygen Therapy; 100-04,32,30.1 HBO Therapy for Lower Extremity Diabetic Wounds

EXCLUDES E&M services, when performed
Other procedures such as wound debridement, when performed

99183 **Physician or other qualified health care professional attendance and supervision of hyperbaric oxygen therapy, per session**

⏴ 3.13 ⏴ 3.13 **FUD** XXX   B 80 26 ▣

AMA: 2016,Jan,13; 2015,Jan,16; 2014,Jan,11; 2012,Jan,15-42; 2011,Jan,11

99184 **Initiation of selective head or total body hypothermia in the critically ill neonate, includes appropriate patient selection by review of clinical, imaging and laboratory data, confirmation of esophageal temperature probe location, evaluation of amplitude EEG, supervision of controlled hypothermia, and assessment of patient tolerance of cooling**   A

EXCLUDES Use of code more than one time per hospitalization

⏴ 6.49 ⏴ 6.49 **FUD** XXX   C 80 ▣

AMA: 2016,Jan,13; 2015,Oct,8

99188 Topical Fluoride Application

99188 **Application of topical fluoride varnish by a physician or other qualified health care professional**

⏴ 0.00 ⏴ 0.00 **FUD** XXX   E 80 ▣

99190-99192 Assemble and Manage Pump with Oxygenator/Heat Exchange

99190 **Assembly and operation of pump with oxygenator or heat exchanger (with or without ECG and/or pressure monitoring); each hour**

⏴ 0.00 ⏴ 0.00 **FUD** XXX   C ▣

AMA: 1997,Nov,1

99191 **45 minutes**

⏴ 0.00 ⏴ 0.00 **FUD** XXX   C ▣

AMA: 1997,Nov,1

99192 **30 minutes**

⏴ 0.00 ⏴ 0.00 **FUD** XXX   C ▣

AMA: 1997,Nov,1

99195-99199 Therapeutic Phlebotomy and Unlisted Procedures

99195 **Phlebotomy, therapeutic (separate procedure)**

⏴ 2.82 ⏴ 2.82 **FUD** XXX   Q1 80 ▣

AMA: 2016,Jan,13; 2015,Jan,16; 2014,Jan,11; 2012,Jan,15-42; 2011,Jan,11

99199 **Unlisted special service, procedure or report**

⏴ 0.00 ⏴ 0.00 **FUD** XXX   B 80

AMA: 2016,Jan,13; 2015,Jan,16; 2014,Jan,11; 2012,Oct,13; 2012,Sep,9; 2012,Jun,15-16

99500-99602 Home Visit By Non-Physician Professionals

INCLUDES Services performed by non-physician providers
Services provided in patient's:
  Assisted living apartment
  Custodial care facility
  Group home
  Non-traditional private home
  Residence
  School

EXCLUDES Home visits performed by physicians (99341-99350)
Other services/procedures provided by physicians to patients at home
Code also home visit E&M codes if health care provider is authorized to use (99341-99350)
Code also significant separately identifiable E&M service, when performed

99500 **Home visit for prenatal monitoring and assessment to include fetal heart rate, non-stress test, uterine monitoring, and gestational diabetes monitoring**   M ♀

⏴ 0.00 ⏴ 0.00 **FUD** XXX   E ▣

AMA: 2016,Jan,13; 2015,Jan,16; 2014,Jan,11; 2012,Jan,15-42; 2011,Jan,11

99501 **Home visit for postnatal assessment and follow-up care**   M ♀

⏴ 0.00 ⏴ 0.00 **FUD** XXX   E ▣

AMA: 2016,Jan,13; 2015,Jan,16; 2014,Jan,11

99502 **Home visit for newborn care and assessment**   A

⏴ 0.00 ⏴ 0.00 **FUD** XXX   E ▣

AMA: 2016,Jan,13; 2015,Jan,16; 2014,Jan,11

99503 **Home visit for respiratory therapy care (eg, bronchodilator, oxygen therapy, respiratory assessment, apnea evaluation)**

⏴ 0.00 ⏴ 0.00 **FUD** XXX   E ▣

AMA: 2016,Jan,13; 2015,Jan,16; 2014,Jan,11

99504 **Home visit for mechanical ventilation care**

⏴ 0.00 ⏴ 0.00 **FUD** XXX   E ▣

AMA: 2016,Jan,13; 2015,Jan,16; 2014,Jan,11

99505 **Home visit for stoma care and maintenance including colostomy and cystostomy**

⏴ 0.00 ⏴ 0.00 **FUD** XXX   E ▣

AMA: 2016,Jan,13; 2015,Jan,16; 2014,Jan,11

99506 Home visit for intramuscular injections
⚙ 0.00 ⚗ 0.00 **FUD** XXX E ▭
AMA: 2016,Jan,13; 2015,Jan,16; 2014,Jan,11

99507 Home visit for care and maintenance of catheter(s) (eg, urinary, drainage, and enteral)
⚙ 0.00 ⚗ 0.00 **FUD** XXX E ▭
AMA: 2016,Jan,13; 2015,Jan,16; 2014,Jan,11

99509 Home visit for assistance with activities of daily living and personal care
EXCLUDES *Medical nutrition therapy/assessment home services (97802-97804)*
Self-care/home management training (97535)
Speech therapy home services (92507-92508)
⚙ 0.00 ⚗ 0.00 **FUD** XXX E ▭
AMA: 2016,Jan,13; 2015,Jan,16; 2014,Jan,11

99510 Home visit for individual, family, or marriage counseling
⚙ 0.00 ⚗ 0.00 **FUD** XXX E ▭
AMA: 2016,Jan,13; 2015,Jan,16; 2014,Jan,11

99511 Home visit for fecal impaction management and enema administration
⚙ 0.00 ⚗ 0.00 **FUD** XXX E ▭
AMA: 2016,Jan,13; 2015,Jan,16; 2014,Jan,11

99512 Home visit for hemodialysis
EXCLUDES *Peritoneal dialysis home infusion (99601-99602)*
⚙ 0.00 ⚗ 0.00 **FUD** XXX E ▭
AMA: 2016,Jan,13; 2015,Jan,16; 2014,Jan,11

99600 Unlisted home visit service or procedure
⚙ 0.00 ⚗ 0.00 **FUD** XXX E ▭
AMA: 2016,Jan,13; 2015,Jan,16; 2014,Jan,11; 2012,Jan,15-42; 2011,Jan,11

99601 Home infusion/specialty drug administration, per visit (up to 2 hours);
⚙ 0.00 ⚗ 0.00 **FUD** XXX E ▭
AMA: 2005,Nov,1-9; 2003,Oct,7

+ **99602** each additional hour (List separately in addition to code for primary procedure)
Code first (99601)
⚙ 0.00 ⚗ 0.00 **FUD** XXX E ▭
AMA: 2005,Nov,1-9; 2003,Oct,7

99605-99607 Medication Management By Pharmacist

INCLUDES Direct (face-to-face) assessment and intervention by a pharmacist for the purpose of:
Managing medication complications and/or interactions
Maximizing the patient's response to drug therapy
Documenting the following required elements:
Advice given regarding improvement of treatment compliance and outcomes
Profile of medications (prescription and nonprescription)
Review of applicable patient history
EXCLUDES *Routine tasks associated with dispensing and related activities (e.g., providing product information)*

99605 Medication therapy management service(s) provided by a pharmacist, individual, face-to-face with patient, with assessment and intervention if provided; initial 15 minutes, new patient
⚙ 0.00 ⚗ 0.00 **FUD** XXX E ▭
AMA: 2016,Jan,13; 2015,Jan,16; 2014,Oct,3; 2014,Jan,11; 2013,Nov,3; 2013,Apr,3-4; 2012,Jan,15-42

99606 initial 15 minutes, established patient
⚙ 0.00 ⚗ 0.00 **FUD** XXX E ▭
AMA: 2016,Jan,13; 2015,Jan,16; 2014,Oct,3; 2014,Jan,11; 2013,Nov,3; 2013,Apr,3-4; 2012,Jan,15-42

+ **99607** each additional 15 minutes (List separately in addition to code for primary service)
Code first (99605, 99606)
⚙ 0.00 ⚗ 0.00 **FUD** XXX E ▭
AMA: 2016,Jan,13; 2015,Jan,16; 2014,Oct,3; 2014,Jan,11; 2013,Nov,3; 2013,Apr,3-4; 2012,Jan,15-42; 2011,Jan,11

● New Code ▲ Revised Code ○ Reinstated ● New Web Release ▲ Revised Web Release Unlisted Not Covered # Resequenced
⊘ AMA Mod 51 Exempt ⑤ Optum Mod 51 Exempt ⑥³ Mod 63 Exempt ⁄ Non-FDA Drug ★ Telehealth M Maternity A Age Edit + Add-on **AMA:** CPT Asst

Evaluation and Management (E/M) Services Guidelines

In addition to the information presented in the Introduction, several other items unique to this section are defined or identified here.

Classification of Evaluation and Management (E/M) Services

The E/M section is divided into broad categories such as office visits, hospital visits, and consultations. Most of the categories are further divided into two or more subcategories of E/M services. For example, there are two subcategories of office visits (new patient and established patient) and there are two subcategories of hospital visits (initial and subsequent). The subcategories of E/M services are further classified into levels of E/M services that are identified by specific codes. This classification is important because the nature of work varies by type of service, place of service, and the patient's status.

The basic format of the levels of E/M services is the same for most categories. First, a unique code number is listed. Second, the place and/or type of service is specified, eg, office consultation. Third, the content of the service is defined, eg, comprehensive history and comprehensive examination. (See "Levels of E/M Services," for details on the content of E/M services.) Fourth, the nature of the presenting problem(s) usually associated with a given level is described. Fifth, the time typically required to provide the service is specified. (A detailed discussion of time is provided separately.)

Definitions of Commonly Used Terms

Certain key words and phrases are used throughout the E/M section. The following definitions are intended to reduce the potential for differing interpretations and to increase the consistency of reporting by physicians in differing specialties. E/M services may also be reported by other qualified health care professionals who are authorized to perform such services within the scope of their practice.

New and Established Patient

Solely for the purposes of distinguishing between new and established patients, professional services are those face-to-face services rendered by physicians and other qualified health care professionals who may report E/M services with a specific CPT® code or codes. A new patient is one who has not received any professional services from the physician/qualified health care professional or another physician/qualified health care professional of the exact same specialty and subspecialty who belongs to the same group practice, within the past three years.

An established patient is one who has received professional services from the physician/qualified health care professional or another physician/qualified health care professional of the exact same specialty and subspecialty who belongs to the same group practice, within the past three years. See the decision tree at right.

When a physician/qualified health care professional is on call or covering for another physician/qualified health care professional, the patient's encounter is classified as it would have been by the physician/qualified health care professional who is not available. When advanced practice nurses and physician assistants are working with physicians, they are considered as working in the exact same specialty and exact same subspecialties as the physician.

No distinction is made between new and established patients in the emergency department. E/M services in the emergency department category may be reported for any new or established patient who presents for treatment in the emergency department.

The decision tree in the next column is provided to aid in determining whether to report the E/M service provided as a new or an established patient encounter.

Chief Complaint

A chief complaint is a concise statement describing the symptom, problem, condition, diagnosis, or other factor that is the reason for the encounter, usually stated in the patient's words.

Concurrent Care and Transfer of Care

Concurrent care is the provision of similar services (e.g., hospital visits) to the same patient by more than one physician or other qualified health care professional on the same day. When concurrent care is provided, no special reporting is required. Transfer of care is the process whereby a physician or other qualified health care professional who is managing some or all of a patient's problems relinquishes this responsibility to another physician or other qualified health care professional who explicitly agrees to accept this responsibility and who, from the initial encounter, is not providing consultative services. The physician or other qualified health care professional transferring care is then no longer providing care for these problems though he or she may continue providing care for other conditions when appropriate. Consultation codes should not be reported by the physician or other qualified health care professional who has agreed to accept transfer of care before an initial evaluation, but they are appropriate to report if the decision to accept transfer of care cannot be made until after the initial consultation evaluation, regardless of site of service.

Decision Tree for New vs Established Patients

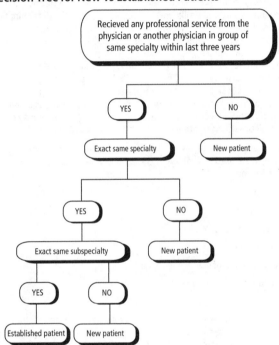

Counseling

Counseling is a discussion with a patient and/or family concerning one or more of the following areas:

- Diagnostic results, impressions, and/or recommended diagnostic studies

- Prognosis

- Risks and benefits of management (treatment) options

- Instructions for management (treatment) and/or follow-up

- Importance of compliance with chosen management (treatment) options

- Risk factor reduction

- Patient and family education
  (For psychotherapy, see 90832–90834, 90836–90840)

Family History

A review of medical events in the patient's family that includes significant information about:

- The health status or cause of death of parents, siblings, and children

- Specific diseases related to problems identified in the Chief Complaint or History of the Present Illness, and/or System Review

- Diseases of family members that may be hereditary or place the patient at risk

History of Present Illness

A chronological description of the development of the patient's present illness from the first sign and/or symptom to the present. This includes a description of location, quality, severity, timing, context, modifying factors, and associated signs and symptoms significantly related to the presenting problem(s).

Levels of E/M Services

Within each category or subcategory of E/M service, there are three to five levels of E/M services available for reporting purposes. Levels of E/M services are not interchangeable among the different categories or subcategories of service. For example, the first level of E/M services in the subcategory of office visit, new patient, does not have the same definition as the first level of E/M services in the subcategory of office visit, established patient.

The levels of E/M services include examinations, evaluations, treatments, conferences with or concerning patients, preventive pediatric and adult health supervision, and similar medical services, such as the determination of the need and/or location for appropriate care. Medical screening includes the history, examination, and medical decision-making required to determine the need and/or location for appropriate care and treatment of the patient (eg, office and other outpatient setting, emergency department, nursing facility). The levels of E/M services encompass the wide variations in skill, effort, time, responsibility, and medical knowledge required for the prevention or diagnosis and treatment of illness or injury and the promotion of optimal health. Each level of E/M services may be used by all physicians or other qualified health care professionals.

The descriptors for the levels of E/M services recognize seven components, six of which are used in defining the levels of E/M services. These components are:

- History
- Examination
- Medical decision making
- Counseling
- Coordination of care
- Nature of presenting problem
- Time

The first three of these components (history, examination, and medical decision making) are considered the key components in selecting a level of E/M services. (See "Determine the Extent of History Obtained.")

The next three components (counseling, coordination of care, and the nature of the presenting problem) are considered contributory factors in the majority of encounters. Although the first two of these contributory factors are important E/M services, it is not required that these services be provided at every patient encounter.

Coordination of care with other physicians, other qualified health care professionals, or agencies without a patient encounter on that day is reported using the case management codes.

The final component, time, is discussed in detail below.

Any specifically identifiable procedure (ie, identified with a specific CPT code) performed on or subsequent to the date of initial or subsequent E/M services should be reported separately.

The actual performance and/or interpretation of diagnostic tests/studies ordered during a patient encounter are not included in the levels of E/M services. Physician performance of diagnostic tests/studies for which specific CPT codes are available may be reported separately, in addition to the appropriate E/M code. The physician's interpretation of the results of diagnostic tests/studies (ie, professional component) with preparation of a separate distinctly identifiable signed written report may also be reported separately, using the appropriate CPT code with modifier 26 appended.

The physician or other health care professional may need to indicate that on the day a procedure or service identified by a CPT code was performed, the patient's condition required a significant separately identifiable E/M service above and beyond other services provided or beyond the usual preservice and postservice care associated with the procedure that was performed. The E/M service may be caused or prompted by the symptoms or condition for which the procedure and/or service was provided. This circumstance may be reported by adding modifier 25 to the appropriate level of E/M service. As such, different diagnoses are not required for reporting of the procedure and the E/M services on the same date.

Nature of Presenting Problem

A presenting problem is a disease, condition, illness, injury, symptom, sign, finding, complaint, or other reason for encounter, with or without a diagnosis being established at the time of the encounter. The E/M codes recognize five types of presenting problems that are defined as follows:

Minimal: A problem that may not require the presence of the physician or other qualified health care professional, but service is provided under the physician's or other qualified health care professional's supervision.

Self-limited or minor: A problem that runs a definite and prescribed course, is transient in nature, and is not likely to permanently alter health status OR has a good prognosis with management/compliance.

Low severity: A problem where the risk of morbidity without treatment is low; there is little to no risk of mortality without treatment; full recovery without functional impairment is expected.

Moderate severity: A problem where the risk of morbidity without treatment is moderate; there is moderate risk of mortality without treatment; uncertain prognosis OR increased probability of prolonged functional impairment.

High severity: A problem where the risk of morbidity without treatment is high to extreme; there is a moderate to high risk of mortality without treatment OR high probability of severe, prolonged functional impairment.

Past History

A review of the patient's past experiences with illnesses, injuries, and treatments that includes significant information about:

- Prior major illnesses and injuries
- Prior operations
- Prior hospitalizations
- Current medications
- Allergies (eg, drug, food)
- Age appropriate immunization status
- Age appropriate feeding/dietary status

Social History

An age appropriate review of past and current activities that includes significant information about:

- Marital status and/or living arrangements
- Current employment
- Occupational history
- Military history
- Use of drugs, alcohol, and tobacco
- Level of education
- Sexual history
- Other relevant social factors

System Review (Review of Systems)

An inventory of body systems obtained through a series of questions seeking to identify signs and/or symptoms that the patient may be experiencing or has experienced. For the purposes of the CPT codebook the following elements of a system review have been identified:

- Constitutional symptoms (fever, weight loss, etc)
- Eyes
- Ears, nose, mouth, throat

- Cardiovascular
- Respiratory
- Gastrointestinal
- Genitourinary
- Musculoskeletal
- Integumentary (skin and/or breast)
- Neurological
- Psychiatric
- Endocrine
- Hematologic/lymphatic
- Allergic/immunologic

The review of systems helps define the problem, clarify the differential diagnosis, identify needed testing, or serves as baseline data on other systems that might be affected by any possible management options.

Time

The inclusion of time in the definitions of levels of E/M services has been implicit in prior editions of the CPT codebook. The inclusion of time as an explicit factor beginning in *CPT 1992* is done to assist in selecting the most appropriate level of E/M services. It should be recognized that the specific times expressed in the visit code descriptors are averages and, therefore, represent a range of times that may be higher or lower depending on actual clinical circumstances.

Time is not a descriptive component for the emergency department levels of E/M services because emergency department services are typically provided on a variable intensity basis, often involving multiple encounters with several patients over an extended period of time. Therefore, it is often difficult to provide accurate estimates of the time spent face-to-face with the patient.

Studies to establish levels of E/M services employed surveys of practicing physicians to obtain data on the amount of time and work associated with typical E/M services. Since "work" is not easily quantifiable, the codes must rely on other objective, verifiable measures that correlate with physicians' estimates of their "work." It has been demonstrated that estimations of intraservice time, both within and across specialties, is a variable that is predictive of the "work" of E/M services. This same research has shown there is a strong relationship between intraservice time and total time for E/M services. Intraservice time, rather than total time, was chosen for inclusion with the codes because of its relative ease of measurement and because of its direct correlation with measurements of the total amount of time and work associated with typical E/M services.

Intraservice times are defined as face-to-face time for office and other outpatient visits and as unit/floor time for hospital and other inpatient visits. This distinction is necessary because most of the work of typical office visits takes place during the face-to-face time with the patient, while most of the work of typical hospital visits takes place during the time spent on the patient's floor or unit. When prolonged time occurs in either the office or the inpatient areas, the appropriate add-on code should be reported.

Face-to-face time (office and other outpatient visits and office consultations): For coding purposes, face-to-face time for these services is defined as only that time spent face-to-face with the patient and/or family. This includes the time spent performing such tasks as obtaining a history, performing an examination, and counseling the patient.

Time is also spent doing work before or after the face-to-face time with the patient, performing such tasks as reviewing records and tests, arranging for further services, and communicating further with other professionals and the patient through written reports and telephone contact.

This non-face-to-face time for office services—also called pre- and postencounter time—is not included in the time component described in the E/M codes. However, the pre- and post-non-face-to-face work associated with an encounter was included in calculating the total work of typical services in physician surveys.

Thus, the face-to-face time associated with the services described by any E/M code is a valid proxy for the total work done before, during, and after the visit.

Unit/floor time (hospital observation services, inpatient hospital care, initial inpatient hospital consultations, nursing facility): For reporting purposes, intraservice time for these services is defined as unit/floor time, which includes the time present on the patient's hospital unit and at the bedside rendering services for that patient. This includes the time to establish and/or review the patient's chart, examine the patient, write notes, and communicate with other professionals and the patient's family.

In the hospital, pre- and post-time includes time spent off the patient's floor performing such tasks as reviewing pathology and radiology findings in another part of the hospital.

This pre- and postvisit time is not included in the time component described in these codes. However, the pre- and postwork performed during the time spent off the floor or unit was included in calculating the total work of typical services in physician surveys.

Thus, the unit/floor time associated with the services described by any code is a valid proxy for the total work done before, during, and after the visit.

Unlisted Service

An E/M service may be provided that is not listed in this section of the CPT codebook. When reporting such a service, the appropriate unlisted code may be used to indicate the service, identifying it by "Special Report," as discussed in the following paragraph. The "Unlisted Services" and accompanying codes for the E/M section are as follows:

99429	**Unlisted preventive medicine service**
99499	**Unlisted evaluation and management service**

Special Report

An unlisted service or one that is unusual, variable, or new may require a special report demonstrating the medical appropriateness of the service. Pertinent information should include an adequate definition or description of the nature, extent, and need for the procedure and the time, effort, and equipment necessary to provide the service. Additional items that may be included are complexity of symptoms, final diagnosis, pertinent physical findings, diagnostic and therapeutic procedures, concurrent problems, and follow-up care.

Instructions for Selecting a Level of E/M Service

Review the Reporting Instructions for the Selected Category or Subcategory

Most of the categories and many of the subcategories of service have special guidelines or instructions unique to that category or subcategory. Where these are indicated, eg, "Inpatient Hospital Care," special instructions will be presented preceding the levels of E/M services.

Review the Level of E/M Service Descriptors and Examples in the Selected Category or Subcategory

The descriptors for the levels of E/M services recognize seven components, six of which are used in defining the levels of E/M services. These components are:

- History
- Examination
- Medical decision making
- Counseling
- Coordination of care
- Nature of presenting problem
- Time

The first three of these components (ie, history, examination, and medical decision making) should be considered the key components in selecting the level of E/M services. An exception to this rule is in the case of visits that consist predominantly of counseling or coordination of care.

The nature of the presenting problem and time are provided in some levels to assist the physician in determining the appropriate level of E/M service.

Determine the Extent of History Obtained

The extent of the history is dependent upon clinical judgment and on the nature of the presenting problem(s). The levels of E/M services recognize four types of history that are defined as follows:

Problem focused: Chief complaint; brief history of present illness or problem.

Expanded problem focused: Chief complaint; brief history of present illness; problem pertinent system review.

Detailed: Chief complaint; extended history of present illness; problem pertinent system review extended to include a review of a limited number of additional systems; pertinent past, family, and/or social history directly related to the patient's problems.

Comprehensive: Chief complaint; extended history of present illness; review of systems that is directly related to the problem(s) identified in the history of the present illness plus a review of all additional body systems; complete past, family, and social history.

The comprehensive history obtained as part of the preventive medicine E/M service is not problem-oriented and does not involve a chief complaint or present illness. It does, however, include a comprehensive system review and comprehensive or interval past, family, and social history as well as a comprehensive assessment/history of pertinent risk factors.

Determine the Extent of Examination Performed

The extent of the examination performed is dependent on clinical judgment and on the nature of the presenting problem(s). The levels of E/M services recognize four types of examination that are defined as follows:

Problem focused: A limited examination of the affected body area or organ system.

Expanded problem focused: A limited examination of the affected body area or organ system and other symptomatic or related organ system(s).

Detailed: An extended examination of the affected body area(s) and other symptomatic or related organ system(s).

Comprehensive: A general multisystem examination or a complete examination of a single organ system. Note: The comprehensive examination performed as part of the preventive medicine E/M service is multisystem, but its extent is based on age and risk factors identified.

For the purposes of these CPT definitions, the following body areas are recognized:

- Head, including the face
- Neck
- Chest, including breasts and axilla
- Abdomen
- Genitalia, groin, buttocks
- Back
- Each extremity

For the purposes of these CPT definitions, the following organ systems are recognized:

- Eyes
- Ears, nose, mouth, and throat
- Cardiovascular
- Respiratory
- Gastrointestinal
- Genitourinary
- Musculoskeletal
- Skin
- Neurologic
- Psychiatric
- Hematologic/lymphatic/immunologic

Determine the Complexity of Medical Decision Making

Medical decision making refers to the complexity of establishing a diagnosis and/or selecting a management option as measured by:

- The number of possible diagnoses and/or the number of management options that must be considered
- The amount and/or complexity of medical records, diagnostic tests, and/or other information that must be obtained, reviewed, and analyzed
- The risk of significant complications, morbidity, and/or mortality, as well as comorbidities associated with the patient's presenting problem(s), the diagnostic procedure(s), and/or the possible management options

Four types of medical decision making are recognized: straightforward, low complexity, moderate complexity, and high complexity. To qualify for a given type of decision making, two of the three elements in Table 1 must be met or exceeded.

Comorbidities and underlying diseases, in and of themselves, are not considered in selecting a level of E/M services unless their presence significantly increases the complexity of the medical decision making.

Select the Appropriate Level of E/M Services Based on the Following

For the following categories/subcategories, all of the key components, ie, history, examination, and medical decision making, must meet or exceed the stated requirements to qualify for a particular level of E/M service: office, new patient; hospital observation services; initial hospital care; office consultations; initial inpatient consultations; emergency department services; initial nursing facility care; domiciliary care, new patient; and home, new patient.

For the following categories/subcategories, two of the three key components (ie, history, examination, and medical decision making) must meet or exceed the stated requirements to qualify for a particular level of E/M services: office, established patient; subsequent hospital care; subsequent nursing facility care; domiciliary care, established patient; and home, established patient.

When counseling and/or coordination of care dominates (more than 50 percent) the encounter with the patient and/or family (face-to-face time in the office or other outpatient setting or floor/unit time in the hospital or nursing facility), then time shall be considered the key or controlling factor to qualify for a particular level of E/M services. This includes time spent with parties who have assumed responsibility for the care of the patient or decision making whether or not they are family members (e.g., foster parents, person acting in loco parentis, legal guardian). The extent of counseling and/or coordination of care must be documented in the medical record.

CONSULTATION CODES AND MEDICARE REIMBURSEMENT

The Centers for Medicare and Medicaid Services (CMS) no longer provides benefits for CPT consultation codes. CMS has, however, redistributed the value of the consultation codes across the other E/M codes for services which are covered by Medicare. CMS has retained codes 99241 - 99251 in the Medicare Physician Fee Schedule for those private payers that use this data for reimbursement. Note that private payers may choose to follow

CMS or CPT guidelines, and the use of consultation codes should be verified with individual payers.

Table 1

Complexity of Medical Decision Making

Number of Diagnoses or Management Options	Amount and/or Complexity of Data to Be Reviewed	Risk of Complications and/or Morbidity or Mortality	Type of Decision Making
minimal	minimal or none	minimal	straightforward
limited	limited	low	low complexity
multiple	moderate	moderate	moderate complexity
extensive	extensive	high	high complexity

99201-99215 Outpatient and Other Visits

CMS: 100-02,15,270.2 Medicare Telehealth Services; 100-04,11,40.1.3 Independent Attending Physician Services; 100-04,12* Medicare Telehealth Services; 100-04,12,100.1.1 Teaching Physicians E/M Services; 100-04,12,190.7 Contractor Editing of Telehealth Claims; 100-04,12,230 Primary Care Incentive Payment Program; 100-04,12,230.1 Definition of Primary Care Practitioners and Services; 100-04,12,230.2 Coordination with Other Payments; 100-04,12,230.3 Claims Processing and Payment; 100-04,12,30.6.10 Consultation Services; 100-04,12,30.6.15.1 Prolonged Services With Direct Face-to-Face Patient Contact Service (Codes 99354 - 99357); 100-04,12,30.6.4 Services Furnished Incident to Physician's Service; 100-04,12,30.6.7 Payment for Office or Other Outpatient E&M Visits; 100-04,12,40.3 Global Surgery Review; 100-04,18,80.2 Contractor Billing Requirements; 100-04,32,130.1 Billing and Payment of External counterpulsation (ECP)

INCLUDES Established patients: received prior professional services from the physician or qualified health care professional or another physician or qualified health care professional in the practice of the exact same specialty and subspecialty in the previous three years (99211-99215)
New patients: have not received professional services from the physician or qualified health care professional or any other physician or qualified health care professional in the same practice in the exact same specialty and subspecialty in the previous three years (99201-99205)
Office visits
Outpatient services (including services prior to a formal admission to a facility)

EXCLUDES Services provided in:
Emergency department (99281-99285)
Hospital observation (99217-99220 [99224, 99225, 99226])
Hospital observation or inpatient with same day admission and discharge (99234-99236)

99201 Office or other outpatient visit for the evaluation and management of a new patient, which requires these 3 key components: A problem focused history; A problem focused examination; Straightforward medical decision making. Counseling and/or coordination of care with other physicians, other qualified health care professionals, or agencies are provided consistent with the nature of the problem(s) and the patient's and/or family's needs. Usually, the presenting problem(s) are self limited or minor. Typically, 10 minutes are spent face-to-face with the patient and/or family.
0.75 1.23 **FUD** XXX ★ B 80
AMA: 2016,Sep,6; 2016,Mar,10; 2016,Jan,13; 2016,Jan,7; 2015,Dec,3; 2015,Oct,3; 2015,Jan,16; 2015,Jan,12; 2014,Nov,14; 2014,Oct,3; 2014,Oct,8; 2014,Aug,3; 2014,Jan,11; 2013,Aug,13; 2013,Jun,3-5; 2013,Jan,9-10; 2012,Aug,3-5; 2012,Apr,10; 2012,Jan,15-42; 2012,Jan,3-5; 2011,Jun,3-7; 2011,Feb,6-7; 2011,Jan,11; 2011,Jan,3-5

99202 Office or other outpatient visit for the evaluation and management of a new patient, which requires these 3 key components: An expanded problem focused history; An expanded problem focused examination; Straightforward medical decision making. Counseling and/or coordination of care with other physicians, other qualified health care professionals, or agencies are provided consistent with the nature of the problem(s) and the patient's and/or family's needs. Usually, the presenting problem(s) are of low to moderate severity. Typically, 20 minutes are spent face-to-face with the patient and/or family.
1.42 2.10 **FUD** XXX ★ B 80
AMA: 2016,Sep,6; 2016,Mar,10; 2016,Jan,13; 2016,Jan,7; 2015,Dec,3; 2015,Oct,3; 2015,Jan,12; 2015,Jan,16; 2014,Nov,14; 2014,Oct,3; 2014,Oct,8; 2014,Aug,3; 2014,Jan,11; 2013,Aug,13; 2013,Jun,3-5; 2013,Jan,9-10; 2012,Aug,3-5; 2012,Apr,10; 2012,Jan,3-5; 2012,Jan,15-42; 2011,Jun,3-7; 2011,Feb,6-7; 2011,Jan,11; 2011,Jan,3-5

99203 Office or other outpatient visit for the evaluation and management of a new patient, which requires these 3 key components: A detailed history; A detailed examination; Medical decision making of low complexity. Counseling and/or coordination of care with other physicians, other qualified health care professionals, or agencies are provided consistent with the nature of the problem(s) and the patient's and/or family's needs. Usually, the presenting problem(s) are of moderate severity. Typically, 30 minutes are spent face-to-face with the patient and/or family.
2.17 3.04 **FUD** XXX ★ B 80
AMA: 2016,Sep,6; 2016,Mar,10; 2016,Jan,13; 2016,Jan,7; 2015,Dec,3; 2015,Oct,3; 2015,Jan,12; 2015,Jan,16; 2014,Nov,14; 2014,Oct,3; 2014,Oct,8; 2014,Aug,3; 2014,Jan,11; 2013,Aug,13; 2013,Jun,3-5; 2013,Jan,9-10; 2012,Aug,3-5; 2012,Apr,10; 2012,Jan,3-5; 2012,Jan,15-42; 2011,Jun,3-7; 2011,Feb,6-7; 2011,Jan,11; 2011,Jan,3-5

99204 Office or other outpatient visit for the evaluation and management of a new patient, which requires these 3 key components: A comprehensive history; A comprehensive examination; Medical decision making of moderate complexity. Counseling and/or coordination of care with other physicians, other qualified health care professionals, or agencies are provided consistent with the nature of the problem(s) and the patient's and/or family's needs. Usually, the presenting problem(s) are of moderate to high severity. Typically, 45 minutes are spent face-to-face with the patient and/or family.
3.67 4.64 **FUD** XXX ★ B 80
AMA: 2016,Sep,6; 2016,Mar,10; 2016,Jan,13; 2016,Jan,7; 2015,Dec,3; 2015,Oct,3; 2015,Jan,12; 2015,Jan,16; 2014,Nov,14; 2014,Oct,8; 2014,Oct,3; 2014,Aug,3; 2014,Jan,11; 2013,Aug,13; 2013,Jun,3-5; 2013,Jan,9-10; 2012,Aug,3-5; 2012,Apr,10; 2012,Jan,3-5; 2012,Jan,15-42; 2011,Jun,3-7; 2011,Feb,6-7; 2011,Jan,3-5; 2011,Jan,11

99205 Office or other outpatient visit for the evaluation and management of a new patient, which requires these 3 key components: A comprehensive history; A comprehensive examination; Medical decision making of high complexity. Counseling and/or coordination of care with other physicians, other qualified health care professionals, or agencies are provided consistent with the nature of the problem(s) and the patient's and/or family's needs. Usually, the presenting problem(s) are of moderate to high severity. Typically, 60 minutes are spent face-to-face with the patient and/or family.
4.77 5.82 **FUD** XXX ★ B 80
AMA: 2016,Sep,6; 2016,Mar,10; 2016,Jan,13; 2016,Jan,7; 2015,Dec,3; 2015,Oct,3; 2015,Jan,12; 2015,Jan,16; 2014,Nov,14; 2014,Oct,8; 2014,Oct,3; 2014,Aug,3; 2014,Jan,11; 2013,Aug,13; 2013,Jun,3-5; 2013,Jan,9-10; 2012,Aug,3-5; 2012,Apr,10; 2012,Jan,3-5; 2012,Jan,15-42; 2011,Jun,3-7; 2011,Feb,6-7; 2011,Jan,3-5; 2011,Jan,11

99211 Office or other outpatient visit for the evaluation and management of an established patient, that may not require the presence of a physician or other qualified health care professional. Usually, the presenting problem(s) are minimal. Typically, 5 minutes are spent performing or supervising these services.
0.26 0.56 **FUD** XXX B 80
AMA: 2016,Sep,6; 2016,Mar,10; 2016,Jan,13; 2016,Jan,7; 2015,Dec,3; 2015,Oct,3; 2015,Jan,16; 2015,Jan,12; 2014,Nov,14; 2014,Oct,8; 2014,Oct,3; 2014,Aug,3; 2014,Mar,13; 2014,Jan,11; 2013,Nov,3; 2013,Aug,13; 2013,Jun,3-5; 2013,Mar,13; 2013,Jan,9-10; 2012,Aug,3-5; 2012,Apr,10; 2012,Jan,15-42; 2012,Jan,3-5; 2011,Feb,6-7; 2011,Jan,11; 2011,Jan,3-5

99212 Office or other outpatient visit for the evaluation and management of an established patient, which requires at least 2 of these 3 key components: A problem focused history; A problem focused examination; Straightforward medical decision making. Counseling and/or coordination of care with other physicians, other qualified health care professionals, or agencies are provided consistent with the nature of the problem(s) and the patient's and/or family's needs. Usually, the presenting problem(s) are self limited or minor. Typically, 10 minutes are spent face-to-face with the patient and/or family.

⚕ 0.71 ⚖ 1.22 **FUD** XXX ★ B 80 ▣

AMA: 2016,Sep,6; 2016,Mar,10; 2016,Jan,13; 2016,Jan,7; 2015,Dec,3; 2015,Oct,3; 2015,Jan,16; 2015,Jan,12; 2014,Nov,14; 2014,Oct,8; 2014,Oct,3; 2014,Aug,3; 2014,Jan,11; 2013,Nov,3; 2013,Aug,13; 2013,Jun,3-5; 2013,Mar,13; 2013,Jan,9-10; 2012,Aug,3-5; 2012,Apr,10; 2012,Mar,4-7; 2012,Jan,15-42; 2012,Jan,3-5; 2011,Jun,3-7; 2011,Feb,6-7; 2011,Jan,11; 2011,Jan,3-5

99213 Office or other outpatient visit for the evaluation and management of an established patient, which requires at least 2 of these 3 key components: An expanded problem focused history; An expanded problem focused examination; Medical decision making of low complexity. Counseling and coordination of care with other physicians, other qualified health care professionals, or agencies are provided consistent with the nature of the problem(s) and the patient's and/or family's needs. Usually, the presenting problem(s) are of low to moderate severity. Typically, 15 minutes are spent face-to-face with the patient and/or family.

⚕ 1.44 ⚖ 2.05 **FUD** XXX ★ B 80 ▣

AMA: 2016,Sep,6; 2016,Mar,10; 2016,Jan,7; 2016,Jan,13; 2015,Dec,3; 2015,Oct,3; 2015,Jan,16; 2015,Jan,12; 2014,Nov,14; 2014,Oct,3; 2014,Oct,8; 2014,Aug,3; 2014,Jan,11; 2013,Nov,3; 2013,Aug,13; 2013,Jun,3-5; 2013,Mar,13; 2013,Jan,9-10; 2012,Aug,3-5; 2012,Mar,4-7; 2012,Apr,10; 2012,Jan,15-42; 2012,Jan,3-5; 2011,Jun,3-7; 2011,Feb,6-7; 2011,Jan,3-5; 2011,Jan,11

99214 Office or other outpatient visit for the evaluation and management of an established patient, which requires at least 2 of these 3 key components: A detailed history; A detailed examination; Medical decision making of moderate complexity. Counseling and/or coordination of care with other physicians, other qualified health care professionals, or agencies are provided consistent with the nature of the problem(s) and the patient's and/or family's needs. Usually, the presenting problem(s) are of moderate to high severity. Typically, 25 minutes are spent face-to-face with the patient and/or family.

⚕ 2.21 ⚖ 3.02 **FUD** XXX ★ B 80 ▣

AMA: 2016,Sep,6; 2016,Mar,10; 2016,Jan,7; 2016,Jan,13; 2015,Dec,3; 2015,Oct,3; 2015,Jan,16; 2015,Jan,12; 2014,Nov,14; 2014,Oct,3; 2014,Oct,8; 2014,Aug,3; 2014,Jan,11; 2013,Nov,3; 2013,Aug,13; 2013,Jun,3-5; 2013,Mar,13; 2013,Jan,9-10; 2012,Aug,3-5; 2012,Mar,4-7; 2012,Apr,10; 2012,Jan,15-42; 2012,Jan,3-5; 2011,Jun,3-7; 2011,Feb,6-7; 2011,Jan,3-5; 2011,Jan,11

99215 Office or other outpatient visit for the evaluation and management of an established patient, which requires at least 2 of these 3 key components: A comprehensive history; A comprehensive examination; Medical decision making of high complexity. Counseling and/or coordination of care with other physicians, other qualified health care professionals, or agencies are provided consistent with the nature of the problem(s) and the patient's and/or family's needs. Usually, the presenting problem(s) are of moderate to high severity. Typically, 40 minutes are spent face-to-face with the patient and/or family.

⚕ 3.13 ⚖ 4.07 **FUD** XXX ★ B 80 ▣

AMA: 2016,Sep,6; 2016,Mar,10; 2016,Jan,7; 2016,Jan,13; 2015,Dec,3; 2015,Oct,3; 2015,Jan,16; 2015,Jan,12; 2014,Nov,14; 2014,Oct,3; 2014,Oct,8; 2014,Aug,3; 2014,Jan,11; 2013,Nov,3; 2013,Aug,13; 2013,Jun,3-5; 2013,Mar,13; 2013,Jan,9-10; 2012,Aug,3-5; 2012,Apr,10; 2012,Jan,15-42; 2012,Jan,3-5; 2011,Jun,3-7; 2011,Feb,6-7; 2011,Jan,3-5; 2011,Jan,11

99217-99220 Facility Observation Visits: Initial and Discharge

CMS: 100-04,11,40.1.3 Independent Attending Physician Services; 100-04,12,100.1.1 Teaching Physicians E/M Services; 100-04,12,30.6.4 Services Furnished Incident to Physician's Service; 100-04,12,30.6.8 Payment for Hospital Observation Services; 100-04,12,40.3 Global Surgery Review; 100-04,32,130.1 Billing and Payment of External counterpulsation (ECP)

INCLUDES   Services provided on the same date in other settings or departments associated with the observation status admission (99201-99215, 99281-99285, 99304-99318, 99324-99337, 99341-99350, 99381-99429)

Services provided to new and established patients admitted to a hospital specifically for observation (not required to be a designated area of the hospital)

EXCLUDES   *Services provided by physicians or another qualified health care professional other than the admitting physician ([99224, 99225, 99226], 99241-99245)*

Services provided to a patient admitted and discharged from observation status on the same date (99234-99236)

Services provided to a patient admitted to the hospital following observation status (99221-99223)

Services provided to a patient discharged from inpatient care (99238-99239)

99217 Observation care discharge day management (This code is to be utilized to report all services provided to a patient on discharge from "observation status" if the discharge is on other than the initial date of "observation status." To report services to a patient designated as "observation status" or "inpatient status" and discharged on the same date, use the codes for Observation or Inpatient Care Services [including Admission and Discharge Services, 99234-99236 as appropriate.])

INCLUDES   Discussing the observation admission with the patient
Final patient evaluation:
Discharge instructions
Sign off on discharge medical records

⚕ 2.05 ⚖ 2.05 **FUD** XXX B 80 ▣

AMA: 2016,Jan,7; 2016,Jan,13; 2015,Dec,3; 2015,Jan,16; 2014,Nov,14; 2014,Oct,8; 2014,Jan,11; 2013,Jun,3-5; 2013,Jan,9-10; 2012,Jul,10-11; 2011,Jun,3-7; 2011,Feb,6-7

99218 Initial observation care, per day, for the evaluation and management of a patient which requires these 3 key components: A detailed or comprehensive history; A detailed or comprehensive examination; and Medical decision making that is straightforward or of low complexity. Counseling and/or coordination of care with other physicians, other qualified health care professionals, or agencies are provided consistent with the nature of the problem(s) and the patient's and/or family's needs. Usually, the problem(s) requiring admission to "observation status" are of low severity. Typically, 30 minutes are spent at the bedside and on the patient's hospital floor or unit.

🛏 2.81   ⚕ 2.81   **FUD** XXX   B 80 🖵

AMA: 2016,Jan,7; 2016,Jan,13; 2015,Dec,3; 2015,Jul,3; 2015,Mar,3; 2015,Jan,16; 2014,Nov,14; 2014,Oct,8; 2014,Jan,11; 2013,Aug,13; 2013,Jun,3-5; 2013,Jan,9-10; 2012,Aug,3-5; 2012,Jul,10-11; 2012,Jan,15-42; 2011,Jun,3-7; 2011,Feb,6-7; 2011,Jan,11

99219 Initial observation care, per day, for the evaluation and management of a patient, which requires these 3 key components: A comprehensive history; A comprehensive examination; and Medical decision making of moderate complexity. Counseling and/or coordination of care with other physicians, other qualified health care professionals, or agencies are provided consistent with the nature of the problem(s) and the patient's and/or family's needs. Usually, the problem(s) requiring admission to "observation status" are of moderate severity. Typically, 50 minutes are spent at the bedside and on the patient's hospital floor or unit.

🛏 3.82   ⚕ 3.82   **FUD** XXX   B 80 🖵

AMA: 2016,Jan,7; 2016,Jan,13; 2015,Dec,3; 2015,Jul,3; 2015,Jan,16; 2014,Nov,14; 2014,Oct,8; 2014,Jan,11; 2013,Aug,13; 2013,Jun,3-5; 2013,Jan,9-10; 2012,Aug,3-5; 2012,Jul,10-11; 2012,Jan,15-42; 2011,Jun,3-7; 2011,Feb,6-7; 2011,Jan,11

99220 Initial observation care, per day, for the evaluation and management of a patient, which requires these 3 key components: A comprehensive history; A comprehensive examination; and Medical decision making of high complexity. Counseling and/or coordination of care with other physicians, other qualified health care professionals, or agencies are provided consistent with the nature of the problem(s) and the patient's and/or family's needs. Usually, the problem(s) requiring admission to "observation status" are of high severity. Typically, 70 minutes are spent at the bedside and on the patient's hospital floor or unit.

🛏 5.22   ⚕ 5.22   **FUD** XXX   B 80 🖵

AMA: 2016,Jan,7; 2016,Jan,13; 2015,Dec,3; 2015,Jul,3; 2015,Jan,16; 2014,Nov,14; 2014,Oct,8; 2014,Jan,11; 2013,Aug,13; 2013,Jun,3-5; 2013,Jan,9-10; 2012,Aug,3-5; 2012,Jul,10-11; 2012,Jan,15-42; 2011,Jun,3-7; 2011,Feb,6-7; 2011,Jan,11

[99224, 99225, 99226] Facility Observation Visits: Subsequent

CMS: 100-04,11,40.1.3 Independent Attending Physician Services; 100-04,12,100.1.1 Teaching Physicians E/M Services; 100-04,12,30.6.4 Services Furnished Incident to Physician's Service; 100-04,12,30.6.8 Payment for Hospital Observation Services; 100-04,12,30.6.9.1 Initial Hospital Care and Observation or Inpatient Care Services

INCLUDES   Changes in patient's status (e.g., physical condition, history; response to medical management)
Medical record review
Review of diagnostic test results
Services provided on the same date in other settings or departments associated with the observation status admission (99201-99215, 99281-99285, 99304-99318, 99324-99337, 99341-99350, 99381-99429)

EXCLUDES   *Observation admission and discharge on the same day (99234-99236)*

\#   **99224** Subsequent observation care, per day, for the evaluation and management of a patient, which requires at least 2 of these 3 key components: Problem focused interval history; Problem focused examination; Medical decision making that is straightforward or of low complexity. Counseling and/or coordination of care with other physicians, other qualified health care professionals, or agencies are provided consistent with the nature of the problem(s) and the patient's and/or family's needs. Usually, the patient is stable, recovering, or improving. Typically, 15 minutes are spent at the bedside and on the patient's hospital floor or unit.

🛏 1.12   ⚕ 1.12   **FUD** XXX   B 80 🖵

AMA: 2016,Jan,7; 2016,Jan,13; 2015,Dec,3; 2015,Jan,16; 2014,Nov,14; 2014,Oct,8; 2014,Jan,11; 2013,Aug,13; 2013,Jun,3-5; 2013,Jan,9-10; 2012,Aug,3-5; 2012,Jul,10-11; 2011,Aug,11; 2011,Jun,3-7; 2011,Feb,6-7

\#   **99225** Subsequent observation care, per day, for the evaluation and management of a patient, which requires at least 2 of these 3 key components: An expanded problem focused interval history; An expanded problem focused examination; Medical decision making of moderate complexity. Counseling and/or coordination of care with other physicians, other qualified health care professionals, or agencies are provided consistent with the nature of the problem(s) and the patient's and/or family's needs. Usually, the patient is responding inadequately to therapy or has developed a minor complication. Typically, 25 minutes are spent at the bedside and on the patient's hospital floor or unit.

🛏 2.05   ⚕ 2.05   **FUD** XXX   B 80 🖵

AMA: 2016,Jan,7; 2016,Jan,13; 2015,Dec,3; 2015,Jan,16; 2014,Nov,14; 2014,Oct,8; 2014,Jan,11; 2013,Aug,13; 2013,Jun,3-5; 2013,Jan,9-10; 2012,Aug,3-5; 2012,Jul,10-11; 2011,Aug,11; 2011,Jun,3-7; 2011,Feb,6-7

\#   **99226** Subsequent observation care, per day, for the evaluation and management of a patient, which requires at least 2 of these 3 key components: A detailed interval history; A detailed examination; Medical decision making of high complexity. Counseling and/or coordination of care with other physicians, other qualified health care professionals, or agencies are provided consistent with the nature of the problem(s) and the patient's and/or family's needs. Usually, the patient is unstable or has developed a significant complication or a significant new problem. Typically, 35 minutes are spent at the bedside and on the patient's hospital floor or unit.

🛏 2.96   ⚕ 2.96   **FUD** XXX   B 80 🖵

AMA: 2016,Jan,7; 2016,Jan,13; 2015,Dec,3; 2015,Jan,16; 2014,Nov,14; 2014,Oct,8; 2014,Jan,11; 2013,Aug,13; 2013,Jun,3-5; 2013,Jan,9-10; 2012,Aug,3-5; 2012,Jul,10-11; 2011,Aug,11; 2011,Jun,3-7; 2011,Feb,6-7

99221-99233 Inpatient Hospital Visits: Initial and Subsequent

CMS: 100-04,11,40.1.3 Independent Attending Physician Services; 100-04,12,100.1.1 Teaching Physicians E/M Services; 100-04,12,30.6.10 Consultation Services; 100-04,12,30.6.15.1 Prolonged Services With Direct Face-to-Face Patient Contact Service (Codes 99354 - 99357); 100-04,12,30.6.4 Services Furnished Incident to Physician's Service; 100-04,12,30.6.9 Payment for Inpatient Hospital Visits - General

INCLUDES   Initial physician services provided to the patient in the hospital or "partial" hospital settings (99221-99223)
Services provided on the date of admission in other settings or departments associated with an observation status admission (99201-99215, 99281-99285, 99304-99318, 99324-99337, 99341-99350, 99381-99397)
Services provided to a new or established patient

EXCLUDES   *Inpatient admission and discharge on the same date (99234-99236)*
Inpatient E&M services provided by other than the admitting physician

99221 Initial hospital care, per day, for the evaluation and management of a patient, which requires these 3 key components: A detailed or comprehensive history; A detailed or comprehensive examination; and Medical decision making that is straightforward or of low complexity. Counseling and/or coordination of care with other physicians, other qualified health care professionals, or agencies are provided consistent with the nature of the problem(s) and the patient's and/or family's needs. Usually, the problem(s) requiring admission are of low severity. Typically, 30 minutes are spent at the bedside and on the patient's hospital floor or unit.

🚑 2.86   ⚖ 2.86   **FUD** XXX   B 80 🖵

AMA: 2016,Mar,10; 2016,Jan,7; 2016,Jan,13; 2015,Dec,3; 2015,Dec,18; 2015,Jul,3; 2015,Jan,16; 2014,Nov,14; 2014,Oct,8; 2014,Jan,11; 2013,Aug,13; 2013,Jun,3-5; 2013,Jan,9-10; 2012,Aug,3-5; 2012,Jul,10-11; 2012,Jul,12-14; 2012,Jan,15-42; 2011,Jun,3-7; 2011,Feb,6-7; 2011,Jan,11

99222 Initial hospital care, per day, for the evaluation and management of a patient, which requires these 3 key components: A comprehensive history; A comprehensive examination; and Medical decision making of moderate complexity. Counseling and/or coordination of care with other physicians, other qualified health care professionals, or agencies are provided consistent with the nature of the problem(s) and the patient's and/or family's needs. Usually, the problem(s) requiring admission are of moderate severity. Typically, 50 minutes are spent at the bedside and on the patient's hospital floor or unit.

🚑 3.86   ⚖ 3.86   **FUD** XXX   B 80 🖵

AMA: 2016,Mar,10; 2016,Jan,13; 2016,Jan,7; 2015,Dec,3; 2015,Dec,18; 2015,Jul,3; 2015,Mar,3; 2015,Jan,16; 2014,Nov,14; 2014,Oct,8; 2014,Jan,11; 2013,Aug,13; 2013,Jun,3-5; 2013,Jan,9-10; 2012,Aug,3-5; 2012,Jul,10-11; 2012,Jul,12-14; 2012,Jan,15-42; 2011,Jun,3-7; 2011,Feb,6-7; 2011,Jan,11

99223 Initial hospital care, per day, for the evaluation and management of a patient, which requires these 3 key components: A comprehensive history; A comprehensive examination; and Medical decision making of high complexity. Counseling and/or coordination of care with other physicians, other qualified health care professionals, or agencies are provided consistent with the nature of the problem(s) and the patient's and/or family's needs. Usually, the problem(s) requiring admission are of high severity. Typically, 70 minutes are spent at the bedside and on the patient's hospital floor or unit.

🚑 5.71   ⚖ 5.71   **FUD** XXX   B 80 🖵

AMA: 2016,Mar,10; 2016,Jan,13; 2016,Jan,7; 2015,Dec,3; 2015,Dec,18; 2015,Jul,3; 2015,Jan,16; 2014,Nov,14; 2014,Oct,8; 2014,Jan,11; 2013,Aug,13; 2013,Jun,3-5; 2013,Jan,9-10; 2012,Aug,3-5; 2012,Jul,10-11; 2012,Jul,12-14; 2012,Jan,15-42; 2011,Jun,3-7; 2011,Feb,6-7; 2011,Jan,11

99224 Resequenced code. See code following 99220.

99225 Resequenced code. See code following 99220.

99226 Resequenced code. See code before 99221.

99231 Subsequent hospital care, per day, for the evaluation and management of a patient, which requires at least 2 of these 3 key components: A problem focused interval history; A problem focused examination; Medical decision making that is straightforward or of low complexity. Counseling and/or coordination of care with other physicians, other qualified health care professionals, or agencies are provided consistent with the nature of the problem(s) and the patient's and/or family's needs. Usually, the patient is stable, recovering or improving. Typically, 15 minutes are spent at the bedside and on the patient's hospital floor or unit.

🚑 1.11   ⚖ 1.11   **FUD** XXX   B 80 🖵

AMA: 2016,Jan,7; 2016,Jan,13; 2015,Dec,3; 2015,Jul,3; 2015,Jan,16; 2014,Nov,14; 2014,Oct,8; 2014,May,4; 2014,Jan,11; 2013,Sep,17; 2013,Aug,13; 2013,Jun,3-5; 2013,Jan,9-10; 2012,Aug,3-5; 2012,Jul,12-14; 2012,Jan,15-42; 2011,Aug,11; 2011,Jun,3-7; 2011,Feb,6-7; 2011,Jan,11

99232 Subsequent hospital care, per day, for the evaluation and management of a patient, which requires at least 2 of these 3 key components: An expanded problem focused interval history; An expanded problem focused examination; Medical decision making of moderate complexity. Counseling and/or coordination of care with other physicians, other qualified health care professionals, or agencies are provided consistent with the nature of the problem(s) and the patient's and/or family's needs. Usually, the patient is responding inadequately to therapy or has developed a minor complication. Typically, 25 minutes are spent at the bedside and on the patient's hospital floor or unit.

🚑 2.03   ⚖ 2.03   **FUD** XXX   ★ B 80 🖵

AMA: 2016,Jan,7; 2016,Jan,13; 2015,Dec,3; 2015,Jul,3; 2015,Jan,16; 2014,Nov,14; 2014,Oct,8; 2014,Jan,11; 2013,Aug,13; 2013,Jun,3-5; 2013,Jan,9-10; 2012,Aug,3-5; 2012,Jul,12-14; 2012,Jan,15-42; 2011,Aug,11; 2011,Jun,3-7; 2011,Feb,6-7; 2011,Jan,11

99233 Subsequent hospital care, per day, for the evaluation and management of a patient, which requires at least 2 of these 3 key components: A detailed interval history; A detailed examination; Medical decision making of high complexity. Counseling and/or coordination of care with other physicians, other qualified health care professionals, or agencies are provided consistent with the nature of the problem(s) and the patient's and/or family's needs. Usually, the patient is unstable or has developed a significant complication or a significant new problem. Typically, 35 minutes are spent at the bedside and on the patient's hospital floor or unit.

🚑 2.93   ⚖ 2.93   **FUD** XXX   ★ B 80 🖵

AMA: 2016,Jan,7; 2016,Jan,13; 2015,Dec,3; 2015,Jul,3; 2015,Jan,16; 2014,Nov,14; 2014,Oct,8; 2014,May,4; 2014,Jan,11; 2013,Aug,13; 2013,Jun,3-5; 2013,Jan,9-10; 2012,Aug,3-5; 2012,Jul,12-14; 2012,Jan,15-42; 2011,Aug,11; 2011,Jun,3-7; 2011,Feb,6-7; 2011,Jan,11

99234-99236 Observation/Inpatient Visits: Admitted/Discharged on Same Date

CMS: 100-04,11,40.1.3 Independent Attending Physician Services; 100-04,12,100.1.1 Teaching Physicians E/M Services; 100-04,12,30.6.4 Services Furnished Incident to Physician's Service; 100-04,12,30.6.8 Payment for Hospital Observation Services; 100-04,12,30.6.9 Swing Bed Visits; 100-04,12,30.6.9.1 Initial Hospital Care and Observation or Inpatient Care Services; 100-04,12,30.6.9.2 Hospital Discharge Management; 100-04,12,40.3 Global Surgery Review

INCLUDES   Admission and discharge services on the same date in an observation or inpatient setting
All services provided by admitting physician or other qualified health care professional on same date of service, even when initiated in another setting (e.g., emergency department, nursing facility, office)

EXCLUDES   *Services provided to patients admitted to observation and discharged on a different date (99217-99220, [99224, 99225, 99226])*

99234   **Observation or inpatient hospital care, for the evaluation and management of a patient including admission and discharge on the same date, which requires these 3 key components: A detailed or comprehensive history; A detailed or comprehensive examination; and Medical decision making that is straightforward or of low complexity. Counseling and/or coordination of care with other physicians, other qualified health care professionals, or agencies are provided consistent with the nature of the problem(s) and the patient's and/or family's needs. Usually the presenting problem(s) requiring admission are of low severity. Typically, 40 minutes are spent at the bedside and on the patient's hospital floor or unit.**

   ⚕ 3.77   ⚕ 3.77   **FUD** XXX   Ⓑ 80 ▣

   AMA: 2016,Jan,13; 2015,Jul,3; 2015,Jan,16; 2014,Oct,8; 2014,Jan,11; 2013,Jun,3-5; 2012,Jul,10-11; 2012,Jan,15-42; 2011,Jun,3-7; 2011,Feb,6-7; 2011,Jan,11

99235   **Observation or inpatient hospital care, for the evaluation and management of a patient including admission and discharge on the same date, which requires these 3 key components: A comprehensive history; A comprehensive examination; and Medical decision making of moderate complexity. Counseling and/or coordination of care with other physicians, other qualified health care professionals, or agencies are provided consistent with the nature of the problem(s) and the patient's and/or family's needs. Usually the presenting problem(s) requiring admission are of moderate severity. Typically, 50 minutes are spent at the bedside and on the patient's hospital floor or unit.**

   ⚕ 4.76   ⚕ 4.76   **FUD** XXX   Ⓑ 80 ▣

   AMA: 2016,Jan,13; 2015,Jul,3; 2015,Jan,16; 2014,Oct,8; 2014,Jan,11; 2013,Jun,3-5; 2012,Jul,10-11; 2012,Jan,15-42; 2011,Jun,3-7; 2011,Feb,6-7; 2011,Jan,11

99236   **Observation or inpatient hospital care, for the evaluation and management of a patient including admission and discharge on the same date, which requires these 3 key components: A comprehensive history; A comprehensive examination; and Medical decision making of high complexity. Counseling and/or coordination of care with other physicians, other qualified health care professionals, or agencies are provided consistent with the nature of the problem(s) and the patient's and/or family's needs. Usually the presenting problem(s) requiring admission are of high severity. Typically, 55 minutes are spent at the bedside and on the patient's hospital floor or unit.**

   ⚕ 6.13   ⚕ 6.13   **FUD** XXX   Ⓑ 80 ▣

   AMA: 2016,Jan,13; 2015,Jul,3; 2015,Jan,16; 2014,Oct,8; 2014,Jan,11; 2013,Jun,3-5; 2012,Jul,10-11; 2012,Jan,15-42; 2011,Jun,3-7; 2011,Feb,6-7; 2011,Jan,11

99238-99239 Inpatient Hospital Discharge Services

CMS: 100-04,11,40.1.3 Independent Attending Physician Services; 100-04,12,100.1.1 Teaching Physicians E/M Services; 100-04,12,30.6.4 Services Furnished Incident to Physician's Service; 100-04,12,30.6.9 Payment for Inpatient Hospital Visits - General; 100-04,12,30.6.9.1 Initial Hospital Care and Observation or Inpatient Care Services; 100-04,12,30.6.9.2 Subsequent Hospital Visit and Discharge Management; 100-04,12,40.3 Global Surgery Review

INCLUDES   All services on discharge day when discharge and admission are not the same day
Discharge instructions
Final patient evaluation
Final preparation of the patient's medical records
Provision of prescriptions/referrals, as needed
Review of the inpatient admission

EXCLUDES   *Admission/discharge on same date (99234-99236)*
Discharge from observation (99217)
Discharge from nursing facility (99315-99316)
Healthy newborn evaluated and discharged on same date (99463)
Services provided by other than attending physician or other qualified health care professional on date of discharge (99231-99233)

99238   **Hospital discharge day management; 30 minutes or less**

   ⚕ 2.04   ⚕ 2.04   **FUD** XXX   Ⓑ 80 ▣

   AMA: 2016,Jan,13; 2015,Jan,16; 2014,Oct,8; 2014,Jan,11; 2013,Aug,13; 2013,Jun,3-5; 2012,Jul,12-14; 2012,Jul,10-11; 2012,Jan,15-42; 2011,Jul,16-17; 2011,Feb,6-7; 2011,Jan,11

99239   **more than 30 minutes**

   ⚕ 3.02   ⚕ 3.02   **FUD** XXX   Ⓑ 80 ▣

   AMA: 2016,Jan,13; 2015,Jan,16; 2014,Oct,8; 2014,Jan,11; 2013,Aug,13; 2013,Jun,3-5; 2012,Jul,12-14; 2012,Jan,15-42; 2011,Jul,16-17; 2011,Feb,6-7; 2011,Jan,11

99241-99245 Consultations: Office and Outpatient

CMS: 100-02,15,270.2 Medicare Telehealth Services; 100-04,11,40.1.3 Independent Attending Physician Services; 100-04,12* Medicare Telehealth Services; 100-04,12,190.7 Contractor Editing of Telehealth Claims; 100-04,12,30.6.10 Consultation Services; 100-04,12,30.6.15.1 Prolonged Services With Direct Face-to-Face Patient Contact Service (Codes 99354 - 99357); 100-04,12,30.6.4 Services Furnished Incident to Physician's Service; 100-04,12,30.6.9.1 Initial Hospital Care and Observation or Inpatient Care Services; 100-04,12,40.3 Global Surgery Review; 100-04,32,130.1 Billing and Payment of External counterpulsation (ECP); 100-04,4,160 Clinic and Emergency Visits Under OPPS

INCLUDES   A third-party mandated consultation
All outpatient consultations provided in the office, outpatient or other ambulatory facility, domiciliary/rest home, emergency department, patient's home, and hospital observation
Documentation of a request for a consultation from an appropriate source
Documentation of the need for consultation in the patient's medical record
One consultation per consultant
Provision by a physician or qualified nonphysician practitioner whose advice, opinion, recommendation, suggestion, direction, or counsel, etc., is requested for evaluating/treating a patient since that individual's expertise in a specific medical area is beyond the scope of knowledge of the requesting physician
Provision of a written report of findings/recommendations from the consultant to the referring physician

EXCLUDES   *Another appropriately requested and documented consultation pertaining to the same/new problem; repeat use of consultation codes*
Any distinctly recognizable procedure/service provided on or following the consultation
Assumption of care (all or partial); report subsequent codes as appropriate for the place of service (99211-99215, 99334-99337, 99347-99350)
Consultation prompted by the patient/family; report codes for office, domiciliary/rest home, or home visits instead (99201-99215, 99324-99337, 99341-99350)
Services provided to Medicare patients; E&M code as appropriate for the place of service or HCPCS code (99221-99223, 99231-99233, G0406-G0408, G0425-G0427)

99241   **Office consultation for a new or established patient, which requires these 3 key components: A problem focused history; A problem focused examination; and Straightforward medical decision making. Counseling and/or coordination of care with other physicians, other qualified health care professionals, or agencies are provided consistent with the nature of the problem(s) and the patient's and/or family's needs. Usually, the presenting problem(s) are self limited or minor. Typically, 15 minutes are spent face-to-face with the patient and/or family.**

   ⚕ 0.92   ⚕ 1.34   **FUD** XXX   ★ Ⓔ ▣

   AMA: 2016,Sep,6; 2016,Jan,13; 2016,Jan,7; 2015,Jan,12; 2015, Jan,16; 2014,Nov,14; 2014,Oct,8; 2014,Sep,13; 2014,Aug,3; 2014, Jan,11; 2013,Jun,3-5; 2013,Jan,9-10; 2012,Aug,3-5; 2012,Apr,10; 2012,Jan,15-42; 2011,Jun,3-7; 2011,Feb,6-7; 2011,Jan,11

26/TC PC/TC Only   A2-Z3 ASC Payment   50 Bilateral   ♂ Male Only   ♀ Female Only   ⚕ Facility RVU   ⚕ Non-Facility RVU   ▢ CCI
FUD Follow-up Days   **CMS:** IOM (Pub 100)   A-Y OPPSI   80/80 Surg Assist Allowed / w/Doc   ▣ Lab Crosswalk   ▣ Radiology Crosswalk   ✖ CLIA

486   CPT © 2016 American Medical Association. All Rights Reserved.   © 2016 Optum360, LLC

99242 Office consultation for a new or established patient, which requires these 3 key components: An expanded problem focused history; An expanded problem focused examination; and Straightforward medical decision making. Counseling and/or coordination of care with other physicians, other qualified health care professionals, or agencies are provided consistent with the nature of the problem(s) and the patient's and/or family's needs. Usually, the presenting problem(s) are of low severity. Typically, 30 minutes are spent face-to-face with the patient and/or family.

🔧 1.93 ⚖ 2.52 **FUD** XXX ★Ⓔ☐

AMA: 2016,Sep,6; 2016,Jan,13; 2016,Jan,7; 2015,Jan,12; 2015,Jan,16; 2014,Nov,14; 2014,Oct,8; 2014,Sep,13; 2014,Aug,3; 2014,Jan,11; 2013,Jun,3-5; 2013,Jan,9-10; 2012,Aug,3-5; 2012,Apr,10; 2012,Jan,15-42; 2011,Jun,3-7; 2011,Feb,6-7; 2011,Jan,11

99243 Office consultation for a new or established patient, which requires these 3 key components: A detailed history; A detailed examination; and Medical decision making of low complexity. Counseling and/or coordination of care with other physicians, other qualified health care professionals, or agencies are provided consistent with the nature of the problem(s) and the patient's and/or family's needs. Usually, the presenting problem(s) are of moderate severity. Typically, 40 minutes are spent face-to-face with the patient and/or family.

🔧 2.70 ⚖ 3.45 **FUD** XXX ★Ⓔ☐

AMA: 2016,Sep,6; 2016,Jan,13; 2016,Jan,7; 2015,Jan,12; 2015,Jan,16; 2014,Nov,14; 2014,Oct,8; 2014,Sep,13; 2014,Aug,3; 2014,Jan,11; 2013,Jun,3-5; 2013,Jan,9-10; 2012,Aug,3-5; 2012,Apr,10; 2012,Jan,15-42; 2011,Jun,3-7; 2011,Feb,6-7; 2011,Jan,11

99244 Office consultation for a new or established patient, which requires these 3 key components: A comprehensive history; A comprehensive examination; and Medical decision making of moderate complexity. Counseling and/or coordination of care with other physicians, other qualified health care professionals, or agencies are provided consistent with the nature of the problem(s) and the patient's and/or family's needs. Usually, the presenting problem(s) are of moderate to high severity. Typically, 60 minutes are spent face-to-face with the patient and/or family.

🔧 4.34 ⚖ 5.16 **FUD** XXX ★Ⓔ☐

AMA: 2016,Sep,6; 2016,Jan,13; 2016,Jan,7; 2015,Jan,12; 2015,Jan,16; 2014,Nov,14; 2014,Oct,8; 2014,Sep,13; 2014,Aug,3; 2014,Jan,11; 2013,Aug,12; 2013,Jun,3-5; 2013,Jan,9-10; 2012,Aug,3-5; 2012,Apr,10; 2012,Jan,15-42; 2011,Jun,3-7; 2011,Feb,6-7; 2011,Jan,11

99245 Office consultation for a new or established patient, which requires these 3 key components: A comprehensive history; A comprehensive examination; and Medical decision making of high complexity. Counseling and/or coordination of care with other physicians, other qualified health care professionals, or agencies are provided consistent with the nature of the problem(s) and the patient's and/or family's needs. Usually, the presenting problem(s) are of moderate to high severity. Typically, 80 minutes are spent face-to-face with the patient and/or family.

🔧 5.37 ⚖ 6.29 **FUD** XXX ★Ⓔ☐

AMA: 2016,Sep,6; 2016,Jan,13; 2016,Jan,7; 2015,Jan,12; 2015,Jan,16; 2014,Nov,14; 2014,Oct,8; 2014,Sep,13; 2014,Aug,3; 2014,Jan,11; 2013,Jun,3-5; 2013,Jan,9-10; 2012,Aug,3-5; 2012,Apr,10; 2012,Jan,15-42; 2011,Jun,3-7; 2011,Feb,6-7; 2011,Jan,11

99251-99255 Consultations: Inpatient

CMS: 100-04,11,40.1.3 Independent Attending Physician Services; 100-04,12* Medicare Telehealth Services; 100-04,12,190.7 Contractor Editing of Telehealth Claims; 100-04,12,30.6.10 Consultation Services; 100-04,12,30.6.15.1 Prolonged Services With Direct Face-to-Face Patient Contact Service (Codes 99354 - 99357); 100-04,12,30.6.4 Services Furnished Incident to Physician's Service; 100-04,12,30.6.9.1 Initial Hospital Care and Observation or Inpatient Care Services; 100-04,12,40.3 Global Surgery Review

INCLUDES A third-party mandated consultation
All inpatient consultations include services provided in the hospital inpatient or partial hospital settings and nursing facilities
Consultation services provided outpatient for the same inpatient hospitalization (99241-99245)
Documentation of a request for a consultation from an appropriate source
Documentation of the need for consultation in the patient's medical record
One consultation by consultant per admission
Provision by a physician or qualified nonphysician practitioner whose advice, opinion, recommendation, suggestion, direction, or counsel, etc. is requested for evaluating/treating a patient since that individual's expertise in a specific medical area is beyond the scope of knowledge of the requesting physician
Provision of a written report of findings/recommendations from the consultant to the referring physician

EXCLUDES *Another appropriately requested and documented consultation pertaining to the same/new problem: repeat use of consultation codes*
Any distinctly recognizable procedure/service provided on or following the consultation
Assumption of care (all or partial): report subsequent codes as appropriate for the place of service (99231-99233, 99307-99310)
Consultation prompted by the patient/family: report codes for office, domiciliary/rest home, or home visits instead (99201-99215, 99324-99337, 99341-99350)
Services provided to Medicare patients; E&M code as appropriate for the place of service or HCPCS code (99201-99215, 99221-99223, 99231-99233, G0406-G0408, G0425-G0427)

99251 Inpatient consultation for a new or established patient, which requires these 3 key components: A problem focused history; A problem focused examination; and Straightforward medical decision making. Counseling and/or coordination of care with other physicians, other qualified health care professionals, or agencies are provided consistent with the nature of the problem(s) and the patient's and/or family's needs. Usually, the presenting problem(s) are self limited or minor. Typically, 20 minutes are spent at the bedside and on the patient's hospital floor or unit.

🔧 1.38 ⚖ 1.38 **FUD** XXX ★Ⓔ☐

AMA: 2016,Jan,7; 2016,Jan,13; 2015,Jan,16; 2014,Nov,14; 2014,Oct,8; 2014,Jan,11; 2013,Jun,3-5; 2013,Jan,9-10; 2012,Aug,3-5; 2012,Jan,15-42; 2011,Feb,6-7; 2011,Jan,11

99252 Inpatient consultation for a new or established patient, which requires these 3 key components: An expanded problem focused history; An expanded problem focused examination; and Straightforward medical decision making. Counseling and/or coordination of care with other physicians, other qualified health care professionals, or agencies are provided consistent with the nature of the problem(s) and the patient's and/or family's needs. Usually, the presenting problem(s) are of low severity. Typically, 40 minutes are spent at the bedside and on the patient's hospital floor or unit.

🔧 2.11 ⚖ 2.11 **FUD** XXX ★Ⓔ☐

AMA: 2016,Jan,7; 2016,Jan,13; 2015,Jan,16; 2014,Nov,14; 2014,Oct,8; 2014,Jan,11; 2013,Jun,3-5; 2013,Jan,9-10; 2012,Aug,3-5; 2012,Jan,15-42; 2011,Feb,6-7; 2011,Jan,11

99253 Inpatient consultation for a new or established patient, which requires these 3 key components: A detailed history; A detailed examination; and Medical decision making of low complexity. Counseling and/or coordination of care with other physicians, other qualified health care professionals, or agencies are provided consistent with the nature of the problem(s) and the patient's and/or family's needs. Usually, the presenting problem(s) are of moderate severity. Typically, 55 minutes are spent at the bedside and on the patient's hospital floor or unit.

    3.24   3.24 **FUD** XXX   ★ E ▢

    AMA: 2016,Jan,7; 2016,Jan,13; 2015,Jan,16; 2014,Nov,14; 2014,Oct,8; 2014,Jan,11; 2013,Jun,3-5; 2013,Jan,9-10; 2012,Aug,3-5; 2012,Jan,15-42; 2011,Feb,6-7; 2011,Jan,11

99254 Inpatient consultation for a new or established patient, which requires these 3 key components: A comprehensive history; A comprehensive examination; and Medical decision making of moderate complexity. Counseling and/or coordination of care with other physicians, other qualified health care professionals, or agencies are provided consistent with the nature of the problem(s) and the patient's and/or family's needs. Usually, the presenting problem(s) are of moderate to high severity. Typically, 80 minutes are spent at the bedside and on the patient's hospital floor or unit.

    4.71   4.71 **FUD** XXX   ★ E ▢

    AMA: 2016,Jan,7; 2016,Jan,13; 2015,Jan,16; 2014,Nov,14; 2014,Oct,8; 2014,Jan,11; 2013,Jun,3-5; 2013,Jan,9-10; 2012,Aug,3-5; 2012,Jan,15-42; 2011,Feb,6-7; 2011,Jan,11

99255 Inpatient consultation for a new or established patient, which requires these 3 key components: A comprehensive history; A comprehensive examination; and Medical decision making of high complexity. Counseling and/or coordination of care with other physicians, other qualified health care professionals, or agencies are provided consistent with the nature of the problem(s) and the patient's and/or family's needs. Usually, the presenting problem(s) are of moderate to high severity. Typically, 110 minutes are spent at the bedside and on the patient's hospital floor or unit.

    5.68   5.68 **FUD** XXX   ★ E ▢

    AMA: 2016,Jan,7; 2016,Jan,13; 2015,Jan,16; 2014,Nov,14; 2014,Oct,8; 2014,Jan,11; 2013,Jun,3-5; 2013,Jan,9-10; 2012,Aug,3-5; 2012,Jan,15-42; 2011,Feb,6-7; 2011,Jan,11

99281-99288 Emergency Department Visits

CMS: 100-04,11,40.1.3 Independent Attending Physician Services; 100-04,12,30.6.11 Emergency Department Visits; 100-04,4,160 Clinic and Emergency Visits Under OPPS

    INCLUDES Any amount of time spent with the patient, which usually involves a series of encounters while the patient is in the emergency department
    Care provided to new and established patients

    EXCLUDES Critical care services (99291-99292)
    Observation services (99217-99220, 99234-99236)

99281 Emergency department visit for the evaluation and management of a patient, which requires these 3 key components: A problem focused history; A problem focused examination; and Straightforward medical decision making. Counseling and/or coordination of care with other physicians, other qualified health care professionals, or agencies are provided consistent with the nature of the problem(s) and the patient's and/or family's needs. Usually, the presenting problem(s) are self limited or minor.

    0.60   0.60 **FUD** XXX   J 80 ▢

    AMA: 2016,Jan,13; 2016,Jan,7; 2015,Jan,12; 2015,Jan,16; 2014,Nov,14; 2014,Oct,8; 2014,Jan,11; 2013,Jun,3-5; 2013,Jan,9-10; 2012,Jan,15-42; 2011,Feb,6-7; 2011,Jan,11

99282 Emergency department visit for the evaluation and management of a patient, which requires these 3 key components: An expanded problem focused history; An expanded problem focused examination; and Medical decision making of low complexity. Counseling and/or coordination of care with other physicians, other qualified health care professionals, or agencies are provided consistent with the nature of the problem(s) and the patient's and/or family's needs. Usually, the presenting problem(s) are of low to moderate severity.

    1.17   1.17 **FUD** XXX   J 80 ▢

    AMA: 2016,Jan,7; 2016,Jan,13; 2015,Jan,12; 2015,Jan,16; 2014,Nov,14; 2014,Oct,8; 2014,Jan,11; 2013,Jun,3-5; 2013,Jan,9-10; 2012,Jan,15-42; 2011,Feb,6-7; 2011,Jan,11

99283 Emergency department visit for the evaluation and management of a patient, which requires these 3 key components: An expanded problem focused history; An expanded problem focused examination; and Medical decision making of moderate complexity. Counseling and/or coordination of care with other physicians, other qualified health care professionals, or agencies are provided consistent with the nature of the problem(s) and the patient's and/or family's needs. Usually, the presenting problem(s) are of moderate severity.

    1.75   1.75 **FUD** XXX   J 80 ▢

    AMA: 2016,Jan,13; 2016,Jan,7; 2015,Jan,12; 2015,Jan,16; 2014,Nov,14; 2014,Oct,8; 2014,Jan,11; 2013,Jun,3-5; 2013,Jan,9-10; 2012,Jan,15-42; 2011,Feb,6-7; 2011,Jan,11

99284 Emergency department visit for the evaluation and management of a patient, which requires these 3 key components: A detailed history; A detailed examination; and Medical decision making of moderate complexity. Counseling and/or coordination of care with other physicians, other qualified health care professionals, or agencies are provided consistent with the nature of the problem(s) and the patient's and/or family's needs. Usually, the presenting problem(s) are of high severity, and require urgent evaluation by the physician, or other qualified health care professionals but do not pose an immediate significant threat to life or physiologic function.

    3.32   3.32 **FUD** XXX   J 80 ▢

    AMA: 2016,Jan,13; 2016,Jan,7; 2015,Jan,12; 2015,Jan,16; 2014,Nov,14; 2014,Oct,8; 2014,Jan,11; 2013,Jun,3-5; 2013,Jan,9-10; 2012,Jan,15-42; 2011,Feb,6-7; 2011,Jan,11

99285 Emergency department visit for the evaluation and management of a patient, which requires these 3 key components within the constraints imposed by the urgency of the patient's clinical condition and/or mental status: A comprehensive history; A comprehensive examination; and Medical decision making of high complexity. Counseling and/or coordination of care with other physicians, other qualified health care professionals, or agencies are provided consistent with the nature of the problem(s) and the patient's and/or family's needs. Usually, the presenting problem(s) are of high severity and pose an immediate significant threat to life or physiologic function.

    4.90   4.90 **FUD** XXX   J 80 ▢

    AMA: 2016,Jan,13; 2016,Jan,7; 2015,Jan,12; 2015,Jan,16; 2014,Nov,14; 2014,Oct,8; 2014,Jan,11; 2013,Jun,3-5; 2013,Jan,9-10; 2012,Jan,15-42; 2011,Feb,6-7; 2011,Jan,11

| 26/TC PC/TC Only | A2-Z3 ASC Payment | 50 Bilateral | ♂ Male Only | ♀ Female Only | Facility RVU | Non-Facility RVU | CCI |
| FUD Follow-up Days | CMS: IOM (Pub 100) | A-Y OPPSI | 80/80 Surg Assist Allowed / w/Doc | | Lab Crosswalk | Radiology Crosswalk | CLIA |

488   CPT © 2016 American Medical Association. All Rights Reserved.   © 2016 Optum360, LLC

99288 **Physician or other qualified health care professional direction of emergency medical systems (EMS) emergency care, advanced life support**

INCLUDES Management provided by an emergency/intensive care based physician or other qualified health care professional via voice contact to ambulance/rescue staff for services such as heart monitoring and drug administration

🔲 0.00 ⚕ 0.00 **FUD** XXX B 🖥

AMA: 2016,Jan,13; 2015,Jan,16; 2014,Oct,8; 2014,Jan,11; 2013,May,6-7; 2011,Feb,6-7

99291-99292 Critical Care Visits: Patients 72 Months of Age and Older

CMS: 100-04,11,40.1.3 Independent Attending Physician Services; 100-04,12,30.6.4 Services Furnished Incident to Physician's Service; 100-04,12,30.6.9 Swing Bed Visits; 100-04,12,40.3 Global Surgery Review; 100-04,4,160 Clinic and Emergency Visits Under OPPS; 100-04,4,160.1 Critical Care Services

INCLUDES 30 minutes or more of direct care provided by the physician or other qualified health care professional to a critically ill or injured patient, regardless of the location
All activities performed outside of the unit or off the floor
All time spent exclusively with patient/family/caregivers on the nursing unit or elsewhere
Outpatient critical care provided to neonates and pediatric patients up through 71 months of age
Physician or other qualified health care professional presence during interfacility transfer for critically ill/injured patients over 24 months of age
Professional services for interpretation of:
Blood gases
Chest films (71010, 71015, 71020)
Measurement of cardiac output (93561-93562)
Other computer stored information (99090)
Pulse oximetry (94760-94762)
Professional services for:
Gastric intubation (43752-43753)
Transcutaneous pacing, temporary (92953)
Venous access, arterial puncture (36000, 36410, 36415, 36591, 36600)
Ventilation assistance and management, includes CPAP, CNP (94002-94004, 94660, 94662)

EXCLUDES All services that are less than 30 minutes; report appropriate E&M code
Critical care services provided via remote real-time interactive videoconferencing (0188T, 0189T)
Inpatient critical care services provided to child 2 through 5 years of age (99475-99476)
Inpatient critical care services provided to infants 29 days through 24 months of age (99471-99472)
Inpatient critical care services provided to neonates that are age 28 days or less (99468-99469)
Other procedures not listed as included performed by the physician or other qualified health care professional rendering critical care
Patients who are not critically ill but in the critical care department (report appropriate E&M code)
Physician or other qualified health care professional presence during interfacility transfer for critically ill/injured patients under 24 months of age (99466-99467)
Supervisory services of control physician during interfacility transfer for critically ill/injured patients under 24 months of age ([99485, 99486])

99291 **Critical care, evaluation and management of the critically ill or critically injured patient; first 30-74 minutes**

🔲 6.31 ⚕ 7.75 **FUD** XXX J 80 🖥

AMA: 2016,Aug,9; 2016,May,3; 2016,Jan,13; 2015,Jul,3; 2015,Feb,10; 2015,Jan,16; 2014,Oct,8; 2014,Oct,14; 2014,Aug,5; 2014,May,4; 2014,Jan,11; 2013,May,6-7; 2013,Feb,16-17; 2012,Oct,14; 2012,Sep,16; 2012,Jul,12-14; 2012,Jan,15-42; 2011,Aug,9-10; 2011,Sep,3-4; 2011,Feb,6-7; 2011,Jan,11

+ **99292** **each additional 30 minutes (List separately in addition to code for primary service)**

Code first (99291)
🔲 3.16 ⚕ 3.46 **FUD** ZZZ N 80 🖥

AMA: 2016,Aug,9; 2016,May,3; 2016,Jan,13; 2015,Jul,3; 2015,Feb,10; 2015,Jan,16; 2014,Oct,14; 2014,Oct,8; 2014,Aug,5; 2014,May,4; 2014,Jan,11; 2013,May,6-7; 2013,Feb,16-17; 2012,Jan,15-42; 2011,Aug,9-10; 2011,Sep,3-4; 2011,Feb,6-7; 2011,Jan,11

99304-99310 Nursing Facility Visits

CMS: 100-04,11,40.1.3 Independent Attending Physician Services; 100-04,12,230 Primary Care Incentive Payment Program; 100-04,12,230.1 Definition of Primary Care Practitioners and Services; 100-04,12,230.2 Coordination with Other Payments; 100-04,12,230.3 Claims Processing and Payment; 100-04,12,30.6.10 Consultation Services; 100-04,12,30.6.13 Nursing Facility Visits; 100-04,12,30.6.15.1 Prolonged Services With Direct Face-to-Face Patient Contact Service (Codes 99354 - 99357); 100-04,12,30.6.4 Services Furnished Incident to Physician's Service; 100-04,12,30.6.9 Swing Bed Visits

INCLUDES All E&M services provided by the admitting physician on the date of nursing facility admission in other locations (e.g., office, emergency department)
Initial care, subsequent care, discharge, and yearly assessments
Initial services include patient assessment and physician participation in developing a plan of care (99304-99306)
Services provided in a psychiatric residential treatment center
Services provided to new and established patients in a nursing facility (skilled, intermediate, and long-term care facilities)
Subsequent services include physician review of medical records, reassessment, and review of test results (99307-99310)

EXCLUDES Care plan oversight services (99379-99380)
Code also hospital discharge services on the same date of admission or readmission to the nursing home (99217, 99234-99236, 99238-99239)

99304 **Initial nursing facility care, per day, for the evaluation and management of a patient, which requires these 3 key components: A detailed or comprehensive history; A detailed or comprehensive examination; and Medical decision making that is straightforward or of low complexity. Counseling and/or coordination of care with other physicians, other qualified health care professionals, or agencies are provided consistent with the nature of the problem(s) and the patient's and/or family's needs. Usually, the problem(s) requiring admission are of low severity. Typically, 25 minutes are spent at the bedside and on the patient's facility floor or unit.**

🔲 2.58 ⚕ 2.58 **FUD** XXX B 80 🖥

AMA: 2016,Jan,7; 2016,Jan,13; 2015,Jan,16; 2014,Nov,14; 2014,Oct,8; 2014,Jan,11; 2013,Jun,3-5; 2013,Jan,9-10; 2012,Aug,3-5; 2012,Jul,12-14; 2012,Jan,3-5; 2011,Jun,3-7; 2011,Feb,6-7; 2011,Jan,3-5

99305 **Initial nursing facility care, per day, for the evaluation and management of a patient, which requires these 3 key components: A comprehensive history; A comprehensive examination; and Medical decision making of moderate complexity. Counseling and/or coordination of care with other physicians, other qualified health care professionals, or agencies are provided consistent with the nature of the problem(s) and the patient's and/or family's needs. Usually, the problem(s) requiring admission are of moderate severity. Typically, 35 minutes are spent at the bedside and on the patient's facility floor or unit.**

🔲 3.67 ⚕ 3.67 **FUD** XXX B 80 🖥

AMA: 2016,Jan,7; 2016,Jan,13; 2015,Jan,16; 2014,Nov,14; 2014,Oct,8; 2014,Jan,11; 2013,Jun,3-5; 2013,Jan,9-10; 2012,Aug,3-5; 2012,Jul,12-14; 2012,Jan,3-5; 2011,Jun,3-7; 2011,Feb,6-7; 2011,Jan,3-5

99306 **Initial nursing facility care, per day, for the evaluation and management of a patient, which requires these 3 key components: A comprehensive history; A comprehensive examination; and Medical decision making of high complexity. Counseling and/or coordination of care with other physicians, other qualified health care professionals, or agencies are provided consistent with the nature of the problem(s) and the patient's and/or family's needs. Usually, the problem(s) requiring admission are of high severity. Typically, 45 minutes are spent at the bedside and on the patient's facility floor or unit.**

🔲 4.68 ⚕ 4.68 **FUD** XXX B 80 🖥

AMA: 2016,Jan,7; 2016,Jan,13; 2015,Jan,16; 2014,Nov,14; 2014,Oct,8; 2014,Jan,11; 2013,Jun,3-5; 2013,Jan,9-10; 2012,Aug,3-5; 2012,Jul,12-14; 2012,Jan,3-5; 2011,Jun,3-7; 2011,Feb,6-7; 2011,Jan,3-5

99307 Subsequent nursing facility care, per day, for the evaluation and management of a patient, which requires at least 2 of these 3 key components: A problem focused interval history; A problem focused examination; Straightforward medical decision making. Counseling and/or coordination of care with other physicians, other qualified health care professionals, or agencies are provided consistent with the nature of the problem(s) and the patient's and/or family's needs. Usually, the patient is stable, recovering, or improving. Typically, 10 minutes are spent at the bedside and on the patient's facility floor or unit.

    🚑 1.26   ⚕ 1.26   **FUD** XXX   ★ B 80 ▣

    AMA: 2016,Jan,13; 2016,Jan,7; 2015,Jan,16; 2014,Nov,14; 2014,Oct,8; 2014,Jan,11; 2013,Jun,3-5; 2013,Jan,9-10; 2012,Aug,3-5; 2012,Jul,12-14; 2012,Jan,3-5; 2012,Jan,15-42; 2011,Feb,6-7; 2011,Jan,3-5; 2011,Jan,11

99308 Subsequent nursing facility care, per day, for the evaluation and management of a patient, which requires at least 2 of these 3 key components: An expanded problem focused interval history; An expanded problem focused examination; Medical decision making of low complexity. Counseling and/or coordination of care with other physicians, other qualified health care professionals, or agencies are provided consistent with the nature of the problem(s) and the patient's and/or family's needs. Usually, the patient is responding inadequately to therapy or has developed a minor complication. Typically, 15 minutes are spent at the bedside and on the patient's facility floor or unit.

    🚑 1.95   ⚕ 1.95   **FUD** XXX   ★ B 80 ▣

    AMA: 2016,Jan,7; 2016,Jan,13; 2015,Jan,16; 2014,Nov,14; 2014,Oct,8; 2014,Jan,11; 2013,Jun,3-5; 2013,Jan,9-10; 2012,Aug,3-5; 2012,Jul,12-14; 2012,Jan,3-5; 2011,Feb,6-7; 2011,Jan,3-5

99309 Subsequent nursing facility care, per day, for the evaluation and management of a patient, which requires at least 2 of these 3 key components: A detailed interval history; A detailed examination; Medical decision making of moderate complexity. Counseling and/or coordination of care with other physicians, other qualified health care professionals, or agencies are provided consistent with the nature of the problem(s) and the patient's and/or family's needs. Usually, the patient has developed a significant complication or a significant new problem. Typically, 25 minutes are spent at the bedside and on the patient's facility floor or unit.

    🚑 2.57   ⚕ 2.57   **FUD** XXX   ★ B 80 ▣

    AMA: 2016,Jan,7; 2016,Jan,13; 2015,Jan,16; 2014,Nov,14; 2014,Oct,8; 2014,Jan,11; 2013,Jun,3-5; 2013,Jan,9-10; 2012,Aug,3-5; 2012,Jul,12-14; 2012,Jan,3-5; 2011,Feb,6-7; 2011,Jan,3-5

99310 Subsequent nursing facility care, per day, for the evaluation and management of a patient, which requires at least 2 of these 3 key components: A comprehensive interval history; A comprehensive examination; Medical decision making of high complexity. Counseling and/or coordination of care with other physicians, other qualified health care professionals, or agencies are provided consistent with the nature of the problem(s) and the patient's and/or family's needs. The patient may be unstable or may have developed a significant new problem requiring immediate physician attention. Typically, 35 minutes are spent at the bedside and on the patient's facility floor or unit.

    🚑 3.82   ⚕ 3.82   **FUD** XXX   ★ B 80 ▣

    AMA: 2016,Jan,13; 2016,Jan,7; 2015,Jan,16; 2014,Nov,14; 2014,Oct,8; 2014,Jan,11; 2013,Jun,3-5; 2013,Jan,9-10; 2012,Aug,3-5; 2012,Jul,12-14; 2012,Jan,3-5; 2012,Jan,15-42; 2011,Feb,6-7; 2011,Jan,3-5; 2011,Jan,11

99315-99316 Nursing Home Discharge

CMS: 100-04,11,40.1.3 Independent Attending Physician Services; 100-04,12,230 Primary Care Incentive Payment Program; 100-04,12,230.1 Definition of Primary Care Practitioners and Services; 100-04,12,230.2 Coordination with Other Payments; 100-04,12,230.3 Claims Processing and Payment; 100-04,12,30.6.13 Nursing Facility Visits; 100-04,12,30.6.4 Services Furnished Incident to Physician's Service; 100-04,12,40.3 Global Surgery Review

INCLUDES Discharge services include all time spent by the physician or other qualified health care professional for:
Completion of discharge records
Discharge instructions for patient and caregivers
Discussion regarding the stay in the facility
Final patient examination
Provide prescriptions and referrals as appropriate

99315 Nursing facility discharge day management; 30 minutes or less

    🚑 2.06   ⚕ 2.06   **FUD** XXX   B 80 ▣

    AMA: 2016,Jan,13; 2016,Jan,7; 2015,Jan,16; 2014,Nov,14; 2014,Oct,8; 2014,Jan,11; 2013,Jun,3-5; 2013,Jan,9-10; 2012,Jul,12-14; 2012,Jan,3-5; 2012,Jan,15-42; 2011,Feb,6-7; 2011,Jan,11; 2011,Jan,3-5

99316 more than 30 minutes

    🚑 2.98   ⚕ 2.98   **FUD** XXX   B 80 ▣

    AMA: 2016,Jan,13; 2016,Jan,7; 2015,Jan,16; 2014,Nov,14; 2014,Oct,8; 2014,Jan,11; 2013,Jun,3-5; 2013,Jan,9-10; 2012,Jul,12-14; 2012,Jan,3-5; 2012,Jan,15-42; 2011,Feb,6-7; 2011,Jan,11; 2011,Jan,3-5

99318 Annual Nursing Home Assessment

CMS: 100-04,12,230 Primary Care Incentive Payment Program; 100-04,12,230.1 Definition of Primary Care Practitioners and Services; 100-04,12,230.2 Coordination with Other Payments; 100-04,12,230.3 Claims Processing and Payment; 100-04,12,30.6.13 Nursing Facility Visits; 100-04,12,30.6.15.1 Prolonged Services With Direct Face-to-Face Patient Contact Service (Codes 99354 - 99357); 100-04,12,30.6.4 Services Furnished Incident to Physician's Service; 100-04,12,30.6.9 Swing Bed Visits

INCLUDES Includes nursing facility visits on same date of service as (99304-99316)

99318 Evaluation and management of a patient involving an annual nursing facility assessment, which requires these 3 key components: A detailed interval history; A comprehensive examination; and Medical decision making that is of low to moderate complexity. Counseling and/or coordination of care with other physicians, other qualified health care professionals, or agencies are provided consistent with the nature of the problem(s) and the patient's and/or family's needs. Usually, the patient is stable, recovering, or improving. Typically, 30 minutes are spent at the bedside and on the patient's facility floor or unit.

    🚑 2.70   ⚕ 2.70   **FUD** XXX   B 80 ▣

    AMA: 2016,Jan,7; 2016,Jan,13; 2015,Jan,16; 2014,Nov,14; 2014,Oct,8; 2014,Jan,11; 2013,Jun,3-5; 2013,Jan,9-10; 2012,Jan,3-5; 2011,Feb,6-7; 2011,Jan,3-5

99324-99337 Domiciliary Care, Rest Home, Assisted Living Visits

CMS: 100-04,11,40.1.3 Independent Attending Physician Services; 100-04,12,230 Primary Care Incentive Payment Program; 100-04,12,230.1 Definition of Primary Care Practitioners and Services; 100-04,12,230.2 Coordination with Other Payments; 100-04,12,230.3 Claims Processing and Payment; 100-04,12,30.6.14 Domiciliary Care, Rest Home, Assisted Living Visits; 100-04,12,30.6.15.1 Prolonged Services With Direct Face-to-Face Patient Contact Service (Codes 99354 - 99357); 100-04,12,30.6.4 Services Furnished Incident to Physician's Service

INCLUDES E&M services for patients residing in assisted living, domiciliary care, and rest homes where medical care is not included
Services provided to new patients or established patients (99324-99328, 99334-99337)

EXCLUDES *Care plan oversight services provided to a patient in a rest home under the care of a home health agency (99374-99375)*
Care plan oversight services provided to a patient under the care of a hospice agency (99377-99378)

99324 Domiciliary or rest home visit for the evaluation and management of a new patient, which requires these 3 key components: A problem focused history; A problem focused examination; and Straightforward medical decision making. Counseling and/or coordination of care with other physicians, other qualified health care professionals, or agencies are provided consistent with the nature of the problem(s) and the patient's and/or family's needs. Usually, the presenting problem(s) are of low severity. Typically, 20 minutes are spent with the patient and/or family or caregiver.

🔧 1.56   ⚖ 1.56   **FUD** XXX   B 80 ▣

AMA: 2016,Jan,13; 2016,Jan,7; 2015,Jan,16; 2014,Nov,14; 2014,Oct,8; 2014,Oct,3; 2014,Jan,11; 2013,Jun,3-5; 2013,Jan,9-10; 2012,Aug,3-5; 2012,Apr,10; 2012,Jan,3-5; 2011,Feb,6-7; 2011,Jan,3-5

99325 Domiciliary or rest home visit for the evaluation and management of a new patient, which requires these 3 key components: An expanded problem focused history; An expanded problem focused examination; and Medical decision making of low complexity. Counseling and/or coordination of care with other physicians, other qualified health care professionals, or agencies are provided consistent with the nature of the problem(s) and the patient's and/or family's needs. Usually, the presenting problem(s) are of moderate severity. Typically, 30 minutes are spent with the patient and/or family or caregiver.

🔧 2.27   ⚖ 2.27   **FUD** XXX   B 80 ▣

AMA: 2016,Jan,13; 2016,Jan,7; 2015,Jan,16; 2014,Nov,14; 2014,Oct,8; 2014,Oct,3; 2014,Jan,11; 2013,Jun,3-5; 2013,Jan,9-10; 2012,Aug,3-5; 2012,Apr,10; 2012,Jan,3-5; 2011,Feb,6-7; 2011,Jan,3-5

99326 Domiciliary or rest home visit for the evaluation and management of a new patient, which requires these 3 key components: A detailed history; A detailed examination; and Medical decision making of moderate complexity. Counseling and/or coordination of care with other physicians, other qualified health care professionals, or agencies are provided consistent with the nature of the problem(s) and the patient's and/or family's needs. Usually, the presenting problem(s) are of moderate to high severity. Typically, 45 minutes are spent with the patient and/or family or caregiver.

🔧 3.92   ⚖ 3.92   **FUD** XXX   B 80 ▣

AMA: 2016,Jan,13; 2016,Jan,7; 2015,Jan,16; 2014,Nov,14; 2014,Oct,8; 2014,Oct,3; 2014,Jan,11; 2013,Jun,3-5; 2013,Jan,9-10; 2012,Aug,3-5; 2012,Apr,10; 2012,Jan,3-5; 2011,Feb,6-7; 2011,Jan,3-5

99327 Domiciliary or rest home visit for the evaluation and management of a new patient, which requires these 3 key components: A comprehensive history; A comprehensive examination; and Medical decision making of moderate complexity. Counseling and/or coordination of care with other physicians, other qualified health care professionals, or agencies are provided consistent with the nature of the problem(s) and the patient's and/or family's needs. Usually, the presenting problem(s) are of high severity. Typically, 60 minutes are spent with the patient and/or family or caregiver.

🔧 5.23   ⚖ 5.23   **FUD** XXX   B 80 ▣

AMA: 2016,Jan,13; 2016,Jan,7; 2015,Jan,16; 2014,Nov,14; 2014,Oct,8; 2014,Oct,3; 2014,Jan,11; 2013,Jun,3-5; 2013,Jan,9-10; 2012,Aug,3-5; 2012,Apr,10; 2012,Jan,3-5; 2011,Feb,6-7; 2011,Jan,3-5

99328 Domiciliary or rest home visit for the evaluation and management of a new patient, which requires these 3 key components: A comprehensive history; A comprehensive examination; and Medical decision making of high complexity. Counseling and/or coordination of care with other physicians, other qualified health care professionals, or agencies are provided consistent with the nature of the problem(s) and the patient's and/or family's needs. Usually, the patient is unstable or has developed a significant new problem requiring immediate physician attention. Typically, 75 minutes are spent with the patient and/or family or caregiver.

🔧 6.11   ⚖ 6.11   **FUD** XXX   B 80 ▣

AMA: 2016,Jan,13; 2016,Jan,7; 2015,Jan,16; 2014,Nov,14; 2014,Oct,8; 2014,Oct,3; 2014,Jan,11; 2013,Jun,3-5; 2013,Jan,9-10; 2012,Aug,3-5; 2012,Apr,10; 2012,Jan,3-5; 2011,Feb,6-7; 2011,Jan,3-5

99334 Domiciliary or rest home visit for the evaluation and management of an established patient, which requires at least 2 of these 3 key components: A problem focused interval history; A problem focused examination; Straightforward medical decision making. Counseling and/or coordination of care with other physicians, other qualified health care professionals, or agencies are provided consistent with the nature of the problem(s) and the patient's and/or family's needs. Usually, the presenting problem(s) are self-limited or minor. Typically, 15 minutes are spent with the patient and/or family or caregiver.

🔧 1.70   ⚖ 1.70   **FUD** XXX   B 80 ▣

AMA: 2016,Jan,13; 2016,Jan,7; 2015,Jan,16; 2014,Nov,14; 2014,Oct,8; 2014,Oct,3; 2014,Jan,11; 2013,Nov,3; 2013,Jun,3-5; 2013,Jan,9-10; 2012,Aug,3-5; 2012,Apr,10; 2012,Jan,3-5; 2011,Feb,6-7; 2011,Jan,3-5

99335 Domiciliary or rest home visit for the evaluation and management of an established patient, which requires at least 2 of these 3 key components: An expanded problem focused interval history; An expanded problem focused examination; Medical decision making of low complexity. Counseling and/or coordination of care with other physicians, other qualified health care professionals, or agencies are provided consistent with the nature of the problem(s) and the patient's and/or family's needs. Usually, the presenting problem(s) are of low to moderate severity. Typically, 25 minutes are spent with the patient and/or family or caregiver.

🔧 2.68   ⚖ 2.68   **FUD** XXX   B 80 ▣

AMA: 2016,Jan,13; 2016,Jan,7; 2015,Jan,16; 2014,Nov,14; 2014,Oct,8; 2014,Oct,3; 2014,Jan,11; 2013,Nov,3; 2013,Jun,3-5; 2013,Jan,9-10; 2012,Aug,3-5; 2012,Apr,10; 2012,Jan,3-5; 2011,Feb,6-7; 2011,Jan,3-5

99336 Domiciliary or rest home visit for the evaluation and management of an established patient, which requires at least 2 of these 3 key components: A detailed interval history; A detailed examination; Medical decision making of moderate complexity. Counseling and/or coordination of care with other physicians, other qualified health care professionals, or agencies are provided consistent with the nature of the problem(s) and the patient's and/or family's needs. Usually, the presenting problem(s) are of moderate to high severity. Typically, 40 minutes are spent with the patient and/or family or caregiver.

🔧 3.79   ⚖ 3.79   **FUD** XXX   B 80 ▣

AMA: 2016,Jan,13; 2016,Jan,7; 2015,Jan,16; 2014,Nov,14; 2014,Oct,8; 2014,Oct,3; 2014,Jan,11; 2013,Nov,3; 2013,Jun,3-5; 2013,Jan,9-10; 2012,Aug,3-5; 2012,Apr,10; 2012,Jan,3-5; 2011,Feb,6-7; 2011,Jan,3-5

99337 Domiciliary or rest home visit for the evaluation and management of an established patient, which requires at least 2 of these 3 key components: A comprehensive interval history; A comprehensive examination; Medical decision making of moderate to high complexity. Counseling and/or coordination of care with other physicians, other qualified health care professionals, or agencies are provided consistent with the nature of the problem(s) and the patient's and/or family's needs. Usually, the presenting problem(s) are of moderate to high severity. The patient may be unstable or may have developed a significant new problem requiring immediate physician attention. Typically, 60 minutes are spent with the patient and/or family or caregiver.

🚑 5.43   ⚕ 5.43   **FUD** XXX   Ⓑ 80 ▭

AMA: 2016,Jan,13; 2016,Jan,7; 2015,Jan,16; 2014,Nov,14; 2014,Oct,8; 2014,Oct,3; 2014,Jan,11; 2013,Nov,3; 2013,Jun,3-5; 2013,Jan,9-10; 2012,Aug,3-5; 2012,Apr,10; 2012,Jan,3-5; 2011,Feb,6-7; 2011,Jan,3-5

99339-99340 Care Plan Oversight: Rest Home, Domiciliary Care, Assisted Living, and Home

CMS: 100-04,12,180 Payment of Care Plan Oversight (CPO); 100-04,12,180.1 Billing for Care Plan Oversight (CPO); 100-04,12,230 Primary Care Incentive Payment Program; 100-04,12,230.1 Definition of Primary Care Practitioners and Services; 100-04,12,230.2 Coordination with Other Payments; 100-04,12,230.3 Claims Processing and Payment; 100-04,12,30.6.14 Domiciliary Care, Rest Home, Assisted Living Visits; 100-04,12,30.6.4 Services Furnished Incident to Physician's Service

INCLUDES   Care plan oversight for patients residing in assisted living, domiciliary care, private residences, and rest homes
Patient management services during same time frame as (99441-99444, 99487-99489, 99495-99496, 98966-98969) and related E&M services provided within 24 hours of patient management call

EXCLUDES   *Care plan oversight services furnished under a home health agency, nursing facility, or hospice (99374-99380)*

99339 Individual physician supervision of a patient (patient not present) in home, domiciliary or rest home (eg, assisted living facility) requiring complex and multidisciplinary care modalities involving regular physician development and/or revision of care plans, review of subsequent reports of patient status, review of related laboratory and other studies, communication (including telephone calls) for purposes of assessment or care decisions with health care professional(s), family member(s), surrogate decision maker(s) (eg, legal guardian) and/or key caregiver(s) involved in patient's care, integration of new information into the medical treatment plan and/or adjustment of medical therapy, within a calendar month; 15-29 minutes

🚑 2.18   ⚕ 2.18   **FUD** XXX   Ⓑ ▭

AMA: 2016,Jan,13; 2015,Jan,16; 2014,Oct,8; 2014,Oct,3; 2014,Jan,11; 2013,Nov,3; 2013,Sep,15-16; 2013,Jun,3-5; 2013,Apr,3-4; 2012,Jan,3-5; 2012,Jan,15-42; 2011,Feb,6-7; 2011,Jan,11

99340 30 minutes or more

🚑 3.06   ⚕ 3.06   **FUD** XXX   Ⓑ ▭

AMA: 2016,Jan,13; 2015,Jan,16; 2014,Oct,8; 2014,Oct,3; 2014,Jan,11; 2013,Nov,3; 2013,Sep,15-16; 2013,Jun,3-5; 2013,Apr,3-4; 2012,Jan,3-5; 2012,Jan,15-42; 2011,Feb,6-7; 2011,Jan,11

99341-99350 Home Visits

CMS: 100-04,11,40.1.3 Independent Attending Physician Services; 100-04,12,230 Primary Care Incentive Payment Program; 100-04,12,230.1 Definition of Primary Care Practitioners and Services; 100-04,12,230.2 Coordination with Other Payments; 100-04,12,230.3 Claims Processing and Payment; 100-04,12,30.6.14 Domiciliary Care, Rest Home, Assisted Living Visits; 100-04,12,30.6.14.1 Home Visits; 100-04,12,30.6.15.1 Prolonged Services With Direct Face-to-Face Patient Contact Service (Codes 99354 - 99357); 100-04,12,30.6.4 Services Furnished Incident to Physician's Service; 100-04,12,40.3 Global Surgery Review

INCLUDES   Services for a new patient or an established patient (99341-99345, 99347-99350)
Services provided to a patient in a private home

EXCLUDES   *Services provided to patients under home health agency or hospice care (99374-99378)*

99341 Home visit for the evaluation and management of a new patient, which requires these 3 key components: A problem focused history; A problem focused examination; and Straightforward medical decision making. Counseling and/or coordination of care with other physicians, other qualified health care professionals, or agencies are provided consistent with the nature of the problem(s) and the patient's and/or family's needs. Usually, the presenting problem(s) are of low severity. Typically, 20 minutes are spent face-to-face with the patient and/or family.

🚑 1.55   ⚕ 1.55   **FUD** XXX   Ⓑ 80 ▭

AMA: 2016,Jan,7; 2016,Jan,13; 2015,Jan,16; 2014,Nov,14; 2014,Oct,3; 2014,Oct,8; 2014,Jan,11; 2013,Jun,3-5; 2013,Jan,9-10; 2012,Aug,3-5; 2012,Apr,10; 2012,Jan,3-5; 2011,Feb,6-7; 2011,Jan,3-5

99342 Home visit for the evaluation and management of a new patient, which requires these 3 key components: An expanded problem focused history; An expanded problem focused examination; and Medical decision making of low complexity. Counseling and/or coordination of care with other physicians, other qualified health care professionals, or agencies are provided consistent with the nature of the problem(s) and the patient's and/or family's needs. Usually, the presenting problem(s) are of moderate severity. Typically, 30 minutes are spent face-to-face with the patient and/or family.

🚑 2.23   ⚕ 2.23   **FUD** XXX   Ⓑ 80 ▭

AMA: 2016,Jan,7; 2016,Jan,13; 2015,Jan,16; 2014,Nov,14; 2014,Oct,3; 2014,Oct,8; 2014,Jan,11; 2013,Jun,3-5; 2013,Jan,9-10; 2012,Aug,3-5; 2012,Apr,10; 2012,Jan,3-5; 2011,Feb,6-7; 2011,Jan,3-5

99343 Home visit for the evaluation and management of a new patient, which requires these 3 key components: A detailed history; A detailed examination; and Medical decision making of moderate complexity. Counseling and/or coordination of care with other physicians, other qualified health care professionals, or agencies are provided consistent with the nature of the problem(s) and the patient's and/or family's needs. Usually, the presenting problem(s) are of moderate to high severity. Typically, 45 minutes are spent face-to-face with the patient and/or family.

🚑 3.66   ⚕ 3.66   **FUD** XXX   Ⓑ 80 ▭

AMA: 2016,Jan,7; 2016,Jan,13; 2015,Jan,16; 2014,Nov,14; 2014,Oct,3; 2014,Oct,8; 2014,Jan,11; 2013,Jun,3-5; 2013,Jan,9-10; 2012,Aug,3-5; 2012,Apr,10; 2012,Jan,3-5; 2011,Feb,6-7; 2011,Jan,3-5

99344 Home visit for the evaluation and management of a new patient, which requires these 3 key components: A comprehensive history; A comprehensive examination; and Medical decision making of moderate complexity. Counseling and/or coordination of care with other physicians, other qualified health care professionals, or agencies are provided consistent with the nature of the problem(s) and the patient's and/or family's needs. Usually, the presenting problem(s) are of high severity. Typically, 60 minutes are spent face-to-face with the patient and/or family.

🚑 5.13   ⚕ 5.13   **FUD** XXX   Ⓑ 80 ▭

AMA: 2016,Jan,13; 2016,Jan,7; 2015,Jan,16; 2014,Nov,14; 2014,Oct,8; 2014,Oct,3; 2014,Jan,11; 2013,Jun,3-5; 2013,Jan,9-10; 2012,Aug,3-5; 2012,Apr,10; 2012,Jan,3-5; 2011,Feb,6-7; 2011,Jan,3-5

99345 Home visit for the evaluation and management of a new patient, which requires these 3 key components: A comprehensive history; A comprehensive examination; and Medical decision making of high complexity. Counseling and/or coordination of care with other physicians, other qualified health care professionals, or agencies are provided consistent with the nature of the problem(s) and the patient's and/or family's needs. Usually, the patient is unstable or has developed a significant new problem requiring immediate physician attention. Typically, 75 minutes are spent face-to-face with the patient and/or family.

📋 6.22   ✂ 6.22   **FUD** XXX   Ⓑ 80 ▣

AMA: 2016,Jan,13; 2016,Jan,7; 2015,Jan,16; 2014,Nov,14; 2014,Oct,8; 2014,Oct,3; 2014,Jan,11; 2013,Jun,3-5; 2013,Jan,9-10; 2012,Aug,3-5; 2012,Apr,10; 2012,Jan,3-5; 2011,Feb,6-7; 2011,Jan,3-5

99347 Home visit for the evaluation and management of an established patient, which requires at least 2 of these 3 key components: A problem focused interval history; A problem focused examination; Straightforward medical decision making. Counseling and/or coordination of care with other physicians, other qualified health care professionals, or agencies are provided consistent with the nature of the problem(s) and the patient's and/or family's needs. Usually, the presenting problem(s) are self limited or minor. Typically, 15 minutes are spent face-to-face with the patient and/or family.

📋 1.56   ✂ 1.56   **FUD** XXX   Ⓑ 80 ▣

AMA: 2016,Jan,13; 2016,Jan,7; 2015,Jan,16; 2014,Nov,14; 2014,Oct,8; 2014,Oct,3; 2014,Jan,11; 2013,Nov,3; 2013,Jun,3-5; 2013,Jan,9-10; 2012,Aug,3-5; 2012,Apr,10; 2012,Jan,3-5; 2011,Feb,6-7; 2011,Jan,3-5

99348 Home visit for the evaluation and management of an established patient, which requires at least 2 of these 3 key components: An expanded problem focused interval history; An expanded problem focused examination; Medical decision making of low complexity. Counseling and/or coordination of care with other physicians, other qualified health care professionals, or agencies are provided consistent with the nature of the problem(s) and the patient's and/or family's needs. Usually, the presenting problem(s) are of low to moderate severity. Typically, 25 minutes are spent face-to-face with the patient and/or family.

📋 2.37   ✂ 2.37   **FUD** XXX   Ⓑ 80 ▣

AMA: 2016,Jan,13; 2016,Jan,7; 2015,Jan,16; 2014,Nov,14; 2014,Oct,8; 2014,Oct,3; 2014,Jan,11; 2013,Nov,3; 2013,Jun,3-5; 2013,Jan,9-10; 2012,Aug,3-5; 2012,Apr,10; 2012,Jan,3-5; 2011,Feb,6-7; 2011,Jan,3-5

99349 Home visit for the evaluation and management of an established patient, which requires at least 2 of these 3 key components: A detailed interval history; A detailed examination; Medical decision making of moderate complexity. Counseling and/or coordination of care with other physicians, other qualified health care professionals, or agencies are provided consistent with the nature of the problem(s) and the patient's and/or family's needs. Usually, the presenting problem(s) are moderate to high severity. Typically, 40 minutes are spent face-to-face with the patient and/or family.

📋 3.61   ✂ 3.61   **FUD** XXX   Ⓑ 80 ▣

AMA: 2016,Jan,13; 2016,Jan,7; 2015,Jan,16; 2014,Nov,14; 2014,Oct,8; 2014,Oct,3; 2014,Jan,11; 2013,Nov,3; 2013,Jun,3-5; 2013,Jan,9-10; 2012,Aug,3-5; 2012,Apr,10; 2012,Jan,3-5; 2011,Feb,6-7; 2011,Jan,3-5

99350 Home visit for the evaluation and management of an established patient, which requires at least 2 of these 3 key components: A comprehensive interval history; A comprehensive examination; Medical decision making of moderate to high complexity. Counseling and/or coordination of care with other physicians, other qualified health care professionals, or agencies are provided consistent with the nature of the problem(s) and the patient's and/or family's needs. Usually, the presenting problem(s) are of moderate to high severity. The patient may be unstable or may have developed a significant new problem requiring immediate physician attention. Typically, 60 minutes are spent face-to-face with the patient and/or family.

📋 5.01   ✂ 5.01   **FUD** XXX   Ⓑ 80 ▣

AMA: 2016,Jan,13; 2016,Jan,7; 2015,Jan,16; 2014,Nov,14; 2014,Oct,8; 2014,Oct,3; 2014,Jan,11; 2013,Nov,3; 2013,Jun,3-5; 2013,Jan,9-10; 2012,Aug,3-5; 2012,Apr,10; 2012,Jan,3-5; 2011,Feb,6-7; 2011,Jan,3-5

99354-99357 Prolonged Services Direct Contact

CMS: 100-04,11,40.1.3 Independent Attending Physician Services; 100-04,12,30.6.15.1 Prolonged Services With Direct Face-to-Face Patient Contact Service (Codes 99354 - 99357); 100-04,12,30.6.4 Services Furnished Incident to Physician's Service

INCLUDES Personal contact with the patient by the physician or other qualified health professional
Services extending beyond the customary service provided in the inpatient or outpatient setting
Time spent providing additional indirect contact services on the floor or unit of the hospital or nursing facility during the same session as the direct contact
Time spent providing prolonged services on a date of service, even when the time is not continuous

EXCLUDES *Services less than 30 minutes, less than 15 minutes after the first hour, or after the final 30 minutes*
Services provided independent of the date of personal contact with the patient (99358-99359)

Code first E&M service code, as appropriate

+ 99354 Prolonged evaluation and management or psychotherapy service(s) (beyond the typical service time of the primary procedure) in the office or other outpatient setting requiring direct patient contact beyond the usual service; first hour (List separately in addition to code for office or other outpatient Evaluation and Management or psychotherapy service)

EXCLUDES *Prolonged service provided by clinical staff under supervision ([99415, 99416])*
Use of code more than one time per date of service
Code first (99201-99215, 99241-99245, 99324-99337, 99341-99350, 90837)

📋 2.62   ✂ 2.82   **FUD** ZZZ   ★ N 80 ▣

AMA: 2016,Jan,13; 2015,Oct,3; 2015,Oct,9; 2015,Jan,16; 2014,Oct,8; 2014,Jun,14; 2014,Apr,6; 2014,Jan,11; 2013,Oct,11; 2013,Jun,3-5; 2013,May,12; 2012,Aug,3-5; 2012,Apr,10

+ 99355 each additional 30 minutes (List separately in addition to code for prolonged service)

EXCLUDES *Prolonged service provided by clinical staff under supervision ([99415, 99416])*
Code first (99354)

📋 2.54   ✂ 2.74   **FUD** ZZZ   ★ N 80 ▣

AMA: 2016,Jan,13; 2015,Oct,3; 2015,Oct,9; 2015,Jan,16; 2014,Oct,8; 2014,Jun,14; 2014,Apr,6; 2014,Jan,11; 2013,Oct,11; 2013,Jun,3-5; 2013,May,12; 2012,Aug,3-5; 2012,Apr,10

+ 99356 Prolonged service in the inpatient or observation setting, requiring unit/floor time beyond the usual service; first hour (List separately in addition to code for inpatient Evaluation and Management service)

EXCLUDES *Use of code more than one time per date of service*
Code first (99218-99223 [99224, 99225, 99226], 99231-99236, 99251-99255, 99304-99310, 90837)

📋 2.59   ✂ 2.59   **FUD** ZZZ   Ⓒ 80 ▣

AMA: 2016,Jan,13; 2015,Oct,3; 2015,Oct,9; 2015,Jan,16; 2014,Oct,8; 2014,Jun,14; 2014,Apr,6; 2014,Jan,11; 2013,Oct,11; 2013,Jun,3-5; 2013,May,12; 2012,Aug,3-5; 2012,Jul,10-11; 2011,Aug,11; 2011,Jun,3-7

+ 99357 each additional 30 minutes (List separately in addition to code for prolonged service)
Code first (99356)
🚑 2.57 ⚕ 2.57 **FUD** ZZZ C 80 ▭
AMA: 2016,Jan,13; 2015,Oct,3; 2015,Oct,9; 2015,Jan,16; 2014,Oct,8; 2014,Jun,14; 2014,Apr,6; 2014,Jan,11; 2013,Oct,11; 2013,Jun,3-5; 2013,May,12; 2012,Aug,3-5; 2012,Jul,10-11; 2011,Aug,11; 2011,Jun,3-7

99358-99359 Prolonged Services Indirect Contact

CMS: 100-04,11,40.1.3 Independent Attending Physician Services; 100-04,12,30.6.15.2 Prolonged Services Without Face to Face Service; 100-04,12,30.6.4 Services Furnished Incident to Physician's Service

INCLUDES Services extending beyond the customary service
Time spent providing indirect contact services by the physician or other qualified health care professional in relation to patient management where face-to-face services have or will occur on a different date
Time spent providing prolonged services performed on a date of service (which may be other than the date of the primary service) that are not continuous

EXCLUDES Anticoagulation services (99363-99364)
Any additional unit or floor time in the hospital or nursing facility during the same evaluation and management session
Care plan oversight (99339-99340, 99374-99380)
Online medical services (99444)
Other indirect services that have a more specific code and no upper time limit in the code
Patient management services during same time frame as (99487-99489, 99495-99496)
Services less than 30 minutes, less than 15 minutes after the first hour, or after the final 30 minutes
Time spent in medical team conference (99366-99368)
Use of code more than one time per date of service
Code also E&M or other services provided

99358 Prolonged evaluation and management service before and/or after direct patient care; first hour
EXCLUDES Use of code more than one time per date of service
🚑 3.06 ⚕ 3.06 **FUD** XXX N ▭
AMA: 2016,Jan,13; 2015,Jan,16; 2014,Oct,3; 2014,Oct,8; 2014,Jan,11; 2013,Oct,11; 2013,Nov,3; 2013,Apr,3-4; 2012,Aug,3-5

+ 99359 each additional 30 minutes (List separately in addition to code for prolonged service)
Code first (99358)
🚑 1.48 ⚕ 1.48 **FUD** ZZZ N ▭
AMA: 2016,Jan,13; 2015,Jan,16; 2014,Oct,3; 2014,Oct,8; 2014,Jan,11; 2013,Oct,11; 2013,Nov,3; 2013,Apr,3-4; 2012,Aug,3-5

[99415, 99416] Prolonged Clinical Staff Services Under Supervision

INCLUDES Time spent by clinical staff providing prolonged face-to-face services extending beyond the customary service under the supervision of a physician or other qualified health professional
Time spent by clinical staff providing prolonged services on a date of service, even when the time is not continuous

EXCLUDES Prolonged service provided by physician or other qualified health care professional (99354-99357)
Services less than 45 minutes
Services provided to more than two patients at the same time
Code also E&M or other services provided

+ # 99415 Prolonged clinical staff service (the service beyond the typical service time) during an evaluation and management service in the office or outpatient setting, direct patient contact with physician supervision; first hour (List separately in addition to code for outpatient Evaluation and Management service)
EXCLUDES Use of code more than one time per date of service
Code first (99201-99215)
🚑 0.25 ⚕ 0.25 **FUD** XXX N 80 TC ▭
AMA: 2016,Mar,8; 2016,Feb,13; 2016,Jan,13; 2015,Oct,3

+ # 99416 each additional 30 minutes (List separately in addition to code for prolonged service)
EXCLUDES Services less than 30 minutes, less than 15 minutes after the first hour, or after the final 30 minutes
Code first ([99415])
🚑 0.14 ⚕ 0.14 **FUD** XXX N 80 TC ▭
AMA: 2016,Mar,8; 2016,Feb,13; 2016,Jan,13; 2015,Oct,3

99360 Standby Services

CMS: 100-04,12,30.6.15.3 Standby Services; 100-04,12,30.6.4 Services Furnished Incident to Physician's Service

INCLUDES Services requested by physician or qualified health care professional that involve no direct patient contact
Total standby time for the day

EXCLUDES Delivery attendance (99464)
Less than 30 minutes of standby time
On-call services mandated by the hospital (99026-99027)
Code also as appropriate (99460, 99465)

99360 Standby service, requiring prolonged attendance, each 30 minutes (eg, operative standby, standby for frozen section, for cesarean/high risk delivery, for monitoring EEG)
🚑 1.73 ⚕ 1.73 **FUD** XXX B ▭
AMA: 2016,Jan,13; 2015,Jan,16; 2014,Oct,8; 2014,Apr,5; 2014,Jan,11; 2013,May,8-10; 2012,Jan,15-42; 2011,Feb,3; 2011,Jan,11

99363-99364 Supervision of Warfarin Therapy

CMS: 100-03,190.11 Home PT/INR Monitoring for Anticoagulation Management; 100-04,32,60.4.1 Anticoagulation Management: Covered Diagnosis Codes

INCLUDES Services provided on an outpatient basis only
Supervision of therapy with warfarin: ordering, dosage adjustments, analysis of International Normalized Ration (INR) tests, patient discussion

EXCLUDES E&M services (99217-99239 [99224, 99225, 99226], 99291-99292, 99304-99318, 99471-99476, 99477-99480)
Initial services provided/continued in the hospital or in observation: new period of subsequent therapy starts with discharge (99364)
Patient management services during same time frame as (99487-99489, 99495-99496)
Services provided for less than 60 uninterrupted days
Services that fail to meet the required criteria (e.g., at least 8 INR tests/initial 90 days; 3 INR tests/each following 90 days)
Warfarin therapy supervision accomplished online or via telephone contact (99441-99444, 98966-98969)

99363 Anticoagulant management for an outpatient taking warfarin, physician review and interpretation of International Normalized Ratio (INR) testing, patient instructions, dosage adjustment (as needed), and ordering of additional tests; initial 90 days of therapy (must include a minimum of 8 INR measurements)
🚑 2.38 ⚕ 3.58 **FUD** XXX B ▭
AMA: 2016,Jan,13; 2015,Jan,16; 2014,Oct,8; 2014,Oct,3; 2014,Jan,11; 2013,Nov,3; 2013,Apr,3-4

99364 each subsequent 90 days of therapy (must include a minimum of 3 INR measurements)
🚑 0.91 ⚕ 1.22 **FUD** XXX B ▭
AMA: 2016,Jan,13; 2015,Jan,16; 2014,Oct,8; 2014,Oct,3; 2014,Jan,11; 2013,Nov,3; 2013,Apr,3-4

99366-99368 Interdisciplinary Conferences

CMS: 100-04,11,40.1.3 Independent Attending Physician Services

INCLUDES Documentation of participation, contribution, and recommendations of the conference
Face-to-face participation by minimum of three qualified people from different specialties or disciplines
Only participants who have performed face-to-face evaluations or direct treatment to the patient within the previous 60 days
Start of the review of an individual patient and ends at conclusion of review

EXCLUDES *Conferences of less than 30 minutes (not reportable)*
More than one individual from the same specialty at the same encounter
Patient management services during same time frame as (99487-99489, 99495-99496)
Time spent record keeping or writing a report

99366 **Medical team conference with interdisciplinary team of health care professionals, face-to-face with patient and/or family, 30 minutes or more, participation by nonphysician qualified health care professional**

INCLUDES Team conferences of 30 minutes or more
EXCLUDES *Team conferences by a physician with patient or family present, see appropriate evaluation and management service code*

⚙ 1.18   ⚖ 1.21   **FUD** XXX   N ▢

AMA: 2016,Jan,13; 2015,Jan,16; 2014,Oct,8; 2014,Oct,3; 2014,Jun,3; 2014,Jan,11; 2013,Nov,3; 2013,Apr,3-4; 2012,Jan,15-42; 2011,Jan,11

99367 **Medical team conference with interdisciplinary team of health care professionals, patient and/or family not present, 30 minutes or more; participation by physician**

INCLUDES Team conferences of 30 minutes or more
⚙ 1.59   ⚖ 1.59   **FUD** XXX   N ▢

AMA: 2016,Jan,13; 2015,Jan,16; 2014,Oct,8; 2014,Jun,3; 2014,Jan,11; 2013,Nov,3; 2013,Apr,3-4

99368 **participation by nonphysician qualified health care professional**

INCLUDES Team conferences of 30 minutes or more
⚙ 1.04   ⚖ 1.04   **FUD** XXX   N ▢

AMA: 2016,Jan,13; 2015,Jan,16; 2014,Oct,8; 2014,Oct,3; 2014,Jun,3; 2014,Jan,11; 2013,Nov,3; 2013,Apr,3-4; 2012,Jan,15-42; 2011,Jan,11

99374-99380 Care Plan Oversight: Patient Under Care of HHA, Hospice, or Nursing Facility

CMS: 100-04,11,40.1.3 Independent Attending Physician Services; 100-04,12,180 Payment of Care Plan Oversight (CPO); 100-04,12,180.1 Billing for Care Plan Oversight (CPO); 100-04,12,30.6.4 Services Furnished Incident to Physician's Service

INCLUDES Analysis of reports, diagnostic tests, treatment plans
Discussions with other health care providers, outside of the practice, involved in the patient's care
Establishment of and revisions to care plans within a 30-day period
Payment to one physician per month for covered care plan oversight services (must be the same one who signed the plan of care)

EXCLUDES *Care plan oversight services provided in a hospice agency (99377-99378)*
Care plan oversight services provided in assisted living, domiciliary care, or private residence, not under care of a home health agency or hospice (99339-99340)
Patient management services during same time frame as (99441-99444, 99487-99498, 99495-99496, 98966-98969)
Routine postoperative care provided during a global surgery period
Time discussing treatment with patient and/or caregivers

Code also office/outpatient visits, hospital, home, nursing facility, domiciliary, or non-face-to-face services

99374 **Supervision of a patient under care of home health agency (patient not present) in home, domiciliary or equivalent environment (eg, Alzheimer's facility) requiring complex and multidisciplinary care modalities involving regular development and/or revision of care plans by that individual, review of subsequent reports of patient status, review of related laboratory and other studies, communication (including telephone calls) for purposes of assessment or care decisions with health care professional(s), family member(s), surrogate decision maker(s) (eg, legal guardian) and/or key caregiver(s) involved in patient's care, integration of new information into the medical treatment plan and/or adjustment of medical therapy, within a calendar month; 15-29 minutes**

⚙ 1.59   ⚖ 1.97   **FUD** XXX   B ▢

AMA: 2016,Jan,13; 2015,Jan,16; 2014,Oct,8; 2014,Oct,3; 2014,Jan,11; 2013,Nov,3; 2013,Sep,15-16; 2013,Jul,11-12; 2013,Apr,3-4

99375 **30 minutes or more**

⚙ 2.49   ⚖ 2.95   **FUD** XXX   E ▢

AMA: 2016,Jan,13; 2015,Jan,16; 2014,Oct,8; 2014,Oct,3; 2014,Jan,11; 2013,Nov,3; 2013,Sep,15-16; 2013,Jul,11-12; 2013,Apr,3-4

99377 **Supervision of a hospice patient (patient not present) requiring complex and multidisciplinary care modalities involving regular development and/or revision of care plans by that individual, review of subsequent reports of patient status, review of related laboratory and other studies, communication (including telephone calls) for purposes of assessment or care decisions with health care professional(s), family member(s), surrogate decision maker(s) (eg, legal guardian) and/or key caregiver(s) involved in patient's care, integration of new information into the medical treatment plan and/or adjustment of medical therapy, within a calendar month; 15-29 minutes**

⚙ 1.59   ⚖ 1.97   **FUD** XXX   B ▢

AMA: 2016,Jan,13; 2015,Jan,16; 2014,Oct,8; 2014,Oct,3; 2014,Jan,11; 2013,Nov,3; 2013,Sep,15-16; 2013,Jul,11-12; 2013,Apr,3-4

99378 **30 minutes or more**

⚙ 2.49   ⚖ 2.95   **FUD** XXX   E ▢

AMA: 2016,Jan,13; 2015,Jan,16; 2014,Oct,8; 2014,Oct,3; 2014,Jan,11; 2013,Nov,3; 2013,Sep,15-16; 2013,Jul,11-12; 2013,Apr,3-4

99379 **Supervision of a nursing facility patient (patient not present) requiring complex and multidisciplinary care modalities involving regular development and/or revision of care plans by that individual, review of subsequent reports of patient status, review of related laboratory and other studies, communication (including telephone calls) for purposes of assessment or care decisions with health care professional(s), family member(s), surrogate decision maker(s) (eg, legal guardian) and/or key caregiver(s) involved in patient's care, integration of new information into the medical treatment plan and/or adjustment of medical therapy, within a calendar month; 15-29 minutes**

⚙ 1.59   ⚖ 1.97   **FUD** XXX   B ▢

AMA: 2016,Jan,13; 2015,Jan,16; 2014,Oct,8; 2014,Oct,3; 2014,Jan,11; 2013,Nov,3; 2013,Sep,15-16; 2013,Jul,11-12; 2013,Apr,3-4

99380 **30 minutes or more**

⚙ 2.49   ⚖ 2.95   **FUD** XXX   B ▢

AMA: 2016,Jan,13; 2015,Jan,16; 2014,Oct,8; 2014,Oct,3; 2014,Jan,11; 2013,Nov,3; 2013,Sep,15-16; 2013,Jul,11-12; 2013,Apr,3-4

99381-99397 Preventive Medicine Visits

CMS: 100-04,11,40.1.3 Independent Attending Physician Services; 100-04,12,30.6.2 Medically Necessary and Preventive Medicine Service on Same Date; 100-04,12,30.6.4 Services Furnished Incident to Physician's Service

INCLUDES Care of a small problem or preexisting condition that requires no extra work
New patients or established patients (99381-99387, 99391-99397)
Regular preventive care (e.g., well-child exams) for all age groups

EXCLUDES Behavioral change interventions (99406-99409)
Counseling/risk factor reduction interventions not provided with a preventive medical examination (99401-99412)
Diagnostic tests and other procedures

Code also immunization administration and product (90460-90461, 90471-90474, 90476-90750 [90620, 90621, 90625, 90630, 90644, 90672, 90673, 90674])
Code also significant, separately identifiable E&M service on the same date for substantial problems requiring additional work using modifier 25 and (99201-99215)

99381 Initial comprehensive preventive medicine evaluation and management of an individual including an age and gender appropriate history, examination, counseling/anticipatory guidance/risk factor reduction interventions, and the ordering of laboratory/diagnostic procedures, new patient; infant (age younger than 1 year) A
🚑 2.16 ⚕ 3.10 **FUD** XXX E 🔲
AMA: 2016,Mar,8; 2016,Jan,13; 2015,Jan,16; 2014,Oct,8; 2014,Jan,11; 2013,Jan,9-10; 2012,Jan,15-42; 2011,Jan,11

99382 early childhood (age 1 through 4 years) A
🚑 2.30 ⚕ 3.24 **FUD** XXX E 🔲
AMA: 2016,Mar,8; 2016,Jan,13; 2015,Jan,16; 2014,Oct,8; 2014,Jan,11; 2013,Jan,9-10

99383 late childhood (age 5 through 11 years) A
🚑 2.45 ⚕ 3.38 **FUD** XXX E 🔲
AMA: 2016,Mar,8; 2016,Jan,13; 2015,Jan,16; 2014,Oct,8; 2014,Jan,11; 2013,Jan,9-10

99384 adolescent (age 12 through 17 years) A
🚑 2.88 ⚕ 3.82 **FUD** XXX E 🔲
AMA: 2016,Mar,8; 2016,Jan,13; 2015,Jan,16; 2015,Jan,12; 2014,Oct,8; 2014,Jan,11; 2013,Jan,9-10

99385 18-39 years A
🚑 2.76 ⚕ 3.69 **FUD** XXX E 🔲
AMA: 2016,Mar,8; 2016,Jan,13; 2015,Jan,16; 2015,Jan,12; 2014,Oct,8; 2014,Jan,11; 2013,Jan,9-10

99386 40-64 years A
🚑 3.36 ⚕ 4.29 **FUD** XXX E 🔲
AMA: 2016,Mar,8; 2016,Jan,13; 2015,Jan,16; 2015,Jan,12; 2014,Oct,8; 2014,Jan,11; 2013,Jan,9-10

99387 65 years and older A
🚑 3.61 ⚕ 4.65 **FUD** XXX E 🔲
AMA: 2016,Mar,8; 2016,Jan,13; 2015,Jan,16; 2014,Oct,8; 2014,Jan,11; 2013,Jan,9-10

99391 Periodic comprehensive preventive medicine reevaluation and management of an individual including an age and gender appropriate history, examination, counseling/anticipatory guidance/risk factor reduction interventions, and the ordering of laboratory/diagnostic procedures, established patient; infant (age younger than 1 year) A
🚑 1.97 ⚕ 2.79 **FUD** XXX E 🔲
AMA: 2016,Mar,8; 2016,Jan,13; 2015,Jan,16; 2014,Oct,8; 2014,Jan,11; 2013,Jan,9-10

99392 early childhood (age 1 through 4 years) A
🚑 2.16 ⚕ 2.98 **FUD** XXX E 🔲
AMA: 2016,Mar,8; 2016,Jan,13; 2015,Jan,16; 2014,Oct,8; 2014,Jan,11; 2013,Jan,9-10

99393 late childhood (age 5 through 11 years) A
🚑 2.16 ⚕ 2.97 **FUD** XXX E 🔲
AMA: 2016,Mar,8; 2016,Jan,13; 2015,Jan,16; 2014,Oct,8; 2014,Jan,11; 2013,Jan,9-10

99394 adolescent (age 12 through 17 years) A
🚑 2.45 ⚕ 3.26 **FUD** XXX E 🔲
AMA: 2016,Mar,8; 2016,Jan,13; 2015,Jan,16; 2015,Jan,12; 2014,Oct,8; 2014,Jan,11; 2013,Jan,9-10

99395 18-39 years A
🚑 2.52 ⚕ 3.33 **FUD** XXX E 🔲
AMA: 2016,Mar,8; 2016,Jan,13; 2015,Jan,16; 2015,Jan,12; 2014,Oct,8; 2014,Jan,11; 2013,Jan,9-10

99396 40-64 years A
🚑 2.74 ⚕ 3.55 **FUD** XXX E 🔲
AMA: 2016,Mar,8; 2016,Jan,13; 2015,Jan,16; 2015,Jan,12; 2014,Oct,8; 2014,Jan,11; 2013,Jan,9-10; 2012,Mar,4-7

99397 65 years and older A
🚑 2.88 ⚕ 3.82 **FUD** XXX E 🔲
AMA: 2016,Mar,8; 2016,Jan,13; 2015,Jan,16; 2014,Oct,8; 2014,Jan,11; 2013,Jan,9-10; 2012,Jan,15-42; 2011,Jan,11

99401-99416 Counseling Services: Risk Factor and Behavioral Change Modification

INCLUDES Face-to-face services for new and established patients based on time increments of 15 to 60 minutes
Health and behavioral services provided on the same day (96150-96155)
Issues such as a healthy diet, exercise, alcohol and drug abuse
Services provided by a physician or other qualified healthcare professional for the purpose of promoting health and reducing illness and injury

EXCLUDES Counseling and risk factor reduction interventions included in preventive medicine services (99381-99397)
Counseling services provided to patient groups with existing symptoms or illness (99078)

Code also significant, separately identifiable E&M services when performed and append modifier 25 to that service

99401 Preventive medicine counseling and/or risk factor reduction intervention(s) provided to an individual (separate procedure); approximately 15 minutes
🚑 0.69 ⚕ 1.02 **FUD** XXX E 🔲
AMA: 2016,Mar,8; 2016,Jan,13; 2015,Jan,16; 2014,Oct,8; 2014,Aug,5; 2014,Jan,11; 2013,Jan,9-10

99402 approximately 30 minutes
🚑 1.41 ⚕ 1.74 **FUD** XXX E 🔲
AMA: 2016,Mar,8; 2016,Jan,13; 2015,Jan,16; 2014,Oct,8; 2014,Aug,5; 2014,Jan,11; 2013,Jan,9-10

99403 approximately 45 minutes
🚑 2.11 ⚕ 2.43 **FUD** XXX E 🔲
AMA: 2016,Mar,8; 2016,Jan,13; 2015,Jan,16; 2014,Oct,8; 2014,Aug,5; 2014,Jan,11; 2013,Jan,9-10

99404 approximately 60 minutes
🚑 2.82 ⚕ 3.14 **FUD** XXX E 🔲
AMA: 2016,Mar,8; 2016,Jan,13; 2015,Jan,16; 2014,Oct,8; 2014,Aug,5; 2014,Jan,11; 2013,Jan,9-10

99406 Smoking and tobacco use cessation counseling visit; intermediate, greater than 3 minutes up to 10 minutes
🚑 0.35 ⚕ 0.40 **FUD** XXX ★ S 80 🔲
AMA: 2016,Mar,8; 2016,Jan,13; 2015,Jan,16; 2014,Oct,8; 2014,Jan,11; 2013,Jan,9-10; 2012,Jan,15-42; 2011,Jan,11

99407 intensive, greater than 10 minutes
INCLUDES Time duration of (99406)
🚑 0.73 ⚕ 0.78 **FUD** XXX ★ S 80 🔲
AMA: 2016,Mar,8; 2016,Jan,13; 2015,Jan,16; 2014,Oct,8; 2014,Jan,11; 2013,Jan,9-10; 2012,Jan,15-42; 2011,Jan,11

99408 Alcohol and/or substance (other than tobacco) abuse structured screening (eg, AUDIT, DAST), and brief intervention (SBI) services; 15 to 30 minutes
INCLUDES Health risk assessment (96160-96161)
Only initial screening and brief intervention
Services of 15 minutes or more
🚑 0.94 ⚕ 0.99 **FUD** XXX ★ E 🔲
AMA: 2016,Mar,8; 2016,Jan,13; 2015,Jan,16; 2014,Oct,8; 2014,Jan,11; 2013,Jan,9-10

99409 greater than 30 minutes

INCLUDES Health risk assessment (96160-96161)
Only initial screening and brief intervention
Time duration of (99408)

1.88   1.93   **FUD** XXX   ★ E 🖵

AMA: 2016,Mar,8; 2016,Jan,13; 2015,Jan,16; 2014,Oct,8;
2014,Jan,11; 2013,Jan,9-10

99411 **Preventive medicine counseling and/or risk factor reduction intervention(s) provided to individuals in a group setting (separate procedure); approximately 30 minutes**

0.22   0.46   **FUD** XXX   E 🖵

AMA: 2016,Mar,8; 2016,Jan,13; 2015,Jan,16; 2014,Oct,8;
2014,Jan,11; 2013,Jan,9-10

99412 **approximately 60 minutes**

0.36   0.60   **FUD** XXX   E 🖵

AMA: 2016,Mar,8; 2016,Jan,13; 2015,Jan,16; 2014,Oct,8;
2014,Jan,11; 2013,Jan,9-10

99415 **Resequenced code. See code following 99359.**

99416 **Resequenced code. See code following 99359.**

99420-99429 Health Risk Assessment

CMS: 100-04,11,40.1.3 Independent Attending Physician Services

99420 ~~Administration and interpretation of health risk assessment instrument (eg, health hazard appraisal)~~

To report, see ~96160-96161

99429 **Unlisted preventive medicine service**

0.00   0.00   **FUD** XXX   E 🖵

AMA: 2016,Mar,8; 2016,Jan,13; 2015,Jan,16; 2014,Oct,8;
2014,Jan,11; 2013,Jan,9-10

99441-99443 Telephone Calls for Patient Management

CMS: 100-04,11,40.1.3 Independent Attending Physician Services

INCLUDES Episodes of care initiated by an established patient or the patient or
guardian of an established patient
Non-face-to-face E&M services provided by a physician or other health
care provider qualified to report E&M services
Related E&M services provided within:
Postoperative period of a completed procedure
Seven days prior to the service

EXCLUDES Patient management services during same time frame as (99339-99340,
99363-99364, 99374-99380, 99487-99489, 99495-99496)
Services provided by a qualified nonphysician health care professional unable
to report E&M codes (98966-98968)

99441 **Telephone evaluation and management service by a physician or other qualified health care professional who may report evaluation and management services provided to an established patient, parent, or guardian not originating from a related E/M service provided within the previous 7 days nor leading to an E/M service or procedure within the next 24 hours or soonest available appointment; 5-10 minutes of medical discussion**

0.36   0.39   **FUD** XXX   E 🖵

AMA: 2016,Jan,13; 2015,Jan,16; 2014,Oct,8; 2014,Oct,3;
2014,Jan,11; 2013,Oct,11; 2013,Nov,3; 2013,Apr,3-4

99442 **11-20 minutes of medical discussion**

0.72   0.76   **FUD** XXX   E 🖵

AMA: 2016,Jan,13; 2015,Jan,16; 2014,Oct,8; 2014,Oct,3;
2014,Jan,11; 2013,Oct,11; 2013,Nov,3; 2013,Apr,3-4

99443 **21-30 minutes of medical discussion**

1.08   1.11   **FUD** XXX   E 🖵

AMA: 2016,Jan,13; 2015,Jan,16; 2014,Oct,8; 2014,Oct,3;
2014,Jan,11; 2013,Oct,11; 2013,Nov,3; 2013,Apr,3-4

99444 Online Patient Management Services

CMS: 100-04,11,40.1.3 Independent Attending Physician Services

INCLUDES All related communications such as related phone calls, prescription and
lab orders
Permanent electronic or hardcopy storage
Physician evaluation and management services provided via the internet
in response to a patient's on-line inquiry
Physician's personal timely response
Related E&M services provided within:
Postoperative period of a completed procedure
Seven days prior to the service

EXCLUDES Online medical evaluation by a qualified nonphysician health care professional
(98969)
Patient management services during same time frame as (99339-99340,
99363-99364, 99374-99380, 99487-99489, 99495-99496)

99444 **Online evaluation and management service provided by a physician or other qualified health care professional who may report evaluation and management services provided to an established patient or guardian, not originating from a related E/M service provided within the previous 7 days, using the Internet or similar electronic communications network**

0.00   0.00   **FUD** XXX   E 🖵

AMA: 2016,Jan,13; 2015,Jan,16; 2014,Oct,8; 2014,Oct,3;
2014,Jan,11; 2013,Oct,11; 2013,Nov,3; 2013,Apr,3-4;
2012,Nov,13-14

99446-99449 Online and Telephone Consultative Services

CMS: 100-04,11,40.1.3 Independent Attending Physician Services

INCLUDES Multiple telephone and/or internet contact needed to complete the
consultation (e.g., test result(s) follow-up)
New or established patient with new problem or exacerbation of existing
problem and not seen within the last 14 days
Review of pertinent lab, imaging and/or pathology studies, medical records,
medications reported only once within a 7 day period

EXCLUDES Any service less than 5 minutes
Communication with family with or without the patient present (99441-99444,
98966-98969)
Online services
Physician to patient (99444)
Qualified health care professional to patient (98969)
Requesting physician's time 30 minutes over the typical E&M service and
patient is not on-site (99358-99359)
Requesting physician's time 30 minutes over the typical E&M service and
patient is on-site (99354-99357)
Telephone services
Physician to patient (99441-99443)
Qualified health care professional to patient (98966-98968)
Transfer of care only

99446 **Interprofessional telephone/Internet assessment and management service provided by a consultative physician including a verbal and written report to the patient's treating/requesting physician or other qualified health care professional; 5-10 minutes of medical consultative discussion and review**

0.00   0.00   **FUD** XXX   E 🖵

AMA: 2016,Jan,13; 2015,Jan,16; 2014,Oct,8; 2014,Jun,14;
2013,Oct,11

99447 **11-20 minutes of medical consultative discussion and review**

0.00   0.00   **FUD** XXX   E 🖵

AMA: 2016,Jan,13; 2015,Jan,16; 2014,Oct,8; 2014,Jun,14;
2013,Oct,11

99448 **21-30 minutes of medical consultative discussion and review**

0.00   0.00   **FUD** XXX   E 🖵

AMA: 2016,Jan,13; 2015,Jan,16; 2014,Oct,8; 2014,Jun,14;
2013,Oct,11

99449 **31 minutes or more of medical consultative discussion and review**

0.00   0.00   **FUD** XXX   E 🖵

AMA: 2016,Jan,13; 2015,Jan,16; 2014,Oct,8; 2014,Jun,14;
2013,Oct,11

99450-99456 Life/Disability Insurance Eligibility Visits

CMS: 100-04,12,30.6.4 Services Furnished Incident to Physician's Service

INCLUDES Assessment services for insurance eligibility and work-related disability without medical management of the patient's illness/injury
Services provided to new/established patients at any site of service

EXCLUDES Any additional E&M services or procedures performed on the same date of service: report with appropriate code

99450 Basic life and/or disability examination that includes: Measurement of height, weight, and blood pressure; Completion of a medical history following a life insurance pro forma; Collection of blood sample and/or urinalysis complying with "chain of custody" protocols; and Completion of necessary documentation/certificates.
🚑 0.00 ⚕ 0.00 **FUD** XXX E

AMA: 2016,Jan,13; 2015,Jan,16; 2014,Oct,8; 2014,Jan,11

99455 Work related or medical disability examination by the treating physician that includes: Completion of a medical history commensurate with the patient's condition; Performance of an examination commensurate with the patient's condition; Formulation of a diagnosis, assessment of capabilities and stability, and calculation of impairment; Development of future medical treatment plan; and Completion of necessary documentation/certificates and report.
INCLUDES Special reports (99080)
🚑 0.00 ⚕ 0.00 **FUD** XXX B 80

AMA: 2016,Jan,13; 2015,Jan,16; 2014,Oct,8; 2014,Jan,11; 2013,Aug,13

99456 Work related or medical disability examination by other than the treating physician that includes: Completion of a medical history commensurate with the patient's condition; Performance of an examination commensurate with the patient's condition; Formulation of a diagnosis, assessment of capabilities and stability, and calculation of impairment; Development of future medical treatment plan; and Completion of necessary documentation/certificates and report.
INCLUDES Special reports (99080)
🚑 0.00 ⚕ 0.00 **FUD** XXX B 80

AMA: 2016,Jan,13; 2015,Jan,16; 2014,Oct,8; 2014,Jan,11; 2013,Aug,13

99460-99463 Evaluation and Management Services for Age 28 Days or Less

CMS: 100-04,12,30.6.4 Services Furnished Incident to Physician's Service

INCLUDES Family consultation
Healthy newborn history and physical
Medical record documentation
Ordering of diagnostic test and treatments
Services provided to healthy newborns age 28 days or less

EXCLUDES Neonatal intensive and critical care services (99466-99469 [99485, 99486], 99477-99480)
Newborn follow up services in an office or outpatient setting (99201-99215, 99381, 99391)
Newborn hospital discharge services if provided on a date subsequent to the admission date (99238-99239)
Nonroutine neonatal inpatient evaluation and management services (99221-99233)
Code also circumcision (54150)
Code also attendance at delivery (99464)
Code also emergency resuscitation services (99465)

99460 Initial hospital or birthing center care, per day, for evaluation and management of normal newborn infant A
🚑 2.72 ⚕ 2.72 **FUD** XXX V 80

AMA: 2016,Jan,13; 2015,Jan,16; 2014,Oct,8; 2014,Jan,11

99461 Initial care, per day, for evaluation and management of normal newborn infant seen in other than hospital or birthing center A
🚑 1.78 ⚕ 2.58 **FUD** XXX M 80

AMA: 2016,Jan,13; 2015,Jan,16; 2014,Oct,8; 2014,Jan,11

99462 Subsequent hospital care, per day, for evaluation and management of normal newborn A
🚑 1.18 ⚕ 1.18 **FUD** XXX C 80

AMA: 2016,Jan,13; 2015,Jan,16; 2014,Oct,8; 2014,Jan,11

99463 Initial hospital or birthing center care, per day, for evaluation and management of normal newborn infant admitted and discharged on the same date A
🚑 3.36 ⚕ 3.36 **FUD** XXX V 80

AMA: 2016,Jan,13; 2015,Jan,16; 2014,Oct,8; 2014,Jan,11

99464-99465 Newborn Delivery Attendance/Resuscitation

CMS: 100-04,12,30.6.4 Services Furnished Incident to Physician's Service

99464 Attendance at delivery (when requested by the delivering physician or other qualified health care professional) and initial stabilization of newborn A
EXCLUDES Resuscitation at delivery (99465)
🚑 2.02 ⚕ 2.02 **FUD** XXX N 80

AMA: 2016,Jan,13; 2015,Jan,16; 2014,Oct,8; 2014,Jan,11

99465 Delivery/birthing room resuscitation, provision of positive pressure ventilation and/or chest compressions in the presence of acute inadequate ventilation and/or cardiac output A
EXCLUDES Attendance at delivery (99464)
Code also any necessary procedures performed as part of the resuscitation
🚑 4.31 ⚕ 4.31 **FUD** XXX S 80

AMA: 2016,Jan,13; 2015,Jan,16; 2014,Oct,8; 2014,Jan,11

99466-99467 Critical Care Transport Age 24 Months or Younger

CMS: 100-04,12,30.6.4 Services Furnished Incident to Physician's Service

INCLUDES Face-to-face care starting when the physician assumes responsibility of the patient at the referring facility until the receiving facility accepts the patient
Physician presence during interfacility transfer of critically ill/injured patient 24 months of age or less
Services provided by the physician during transport:
Blood gases
Chest x-rays (71010, 71015, 71020)
Data stored in computers (e.g., ECGs, blood pressures, hematologic data) (99090)
Gastric intubation (43752-43753)
Interpretation of cardiac output measurements (93562)
Pulse oximetry (94760-94762)
Routine monitoring:
Heart rate
Respiratory rate
Temporary transcutaneous pacing (92953)
Vascular access procedures (36000, 36400, 36405-36406, 36415, 36591, 36600)
Ventilatory management (94002-94003, 94660, 94662)

EXCLUDES Neonatal hypothermia (99184)
Patient critical care transport services with personal contact with patient of less than 30 minutes
Physician directed emergency care via two-way voice communication with transporting staff (99288, [99485, 99486])
Services less than 30 minutes in duration (see E&M codes)
Services of the physician directing transport (control physician) ([99485, 99486])
Code also any services not designated as included in the critical care transport service

99466 Critical care face-to-face services, during an interfacility transport of critically ill or critically injured pediatric patient, 24 months of age or younger; first 30-74 minutes of hands-on care during transport A
🚑 6.50 ⚕ 6.50 **FUD** XXX N 80

AMA: 2016,Jan,13; 2015,Jan,16; 2014,Oct,8; 2014,Jan,11; 2013,May,6-7; 2011,Sep,3-4

+ **99467** each additional 30 minutes (List separately in addition to code for primary service) A
Code first (99466)
🚑 3.29 ⚕ 3.29 **FUD** ZZZ N 80

AMA: 2016,Jan,13; 2015,Jan,16; 2014,Oct,8; 2014,Jan,11; 2013,May,6-7; 2011,Sep,3-4

26/TC PC/TC Only A2-Z3 ASC Payment 50 Bilateral ♂ Male Only ♀ Female Only 🚑 Facility RVU ⚕ Non-Facility RVU CCI
FUD Follow-up Days CMS: IOM (Pub 100) A-Y OPPSI 80/80 Surg Assist Allowed / w/Doc ⚕ Lab Crosswalk Radiology Crosswalk CLIA

[99485, 99486] Critical Care Transport Supervision Age 24 Months or Younger

INCLUDES Advice for treatment to the transport team from the control physician
Non face-to-face care starts with first contact by the control physician with the transport team and ends when patient responsibility is assumed by the receiving facility

EXCLUDES *Emergency systems physician direction for pediatric patient older than 24 months (99288)*
Services provided by transport team
Services less than 15 minutes
Services performed by control physician for the same time period
Services performed by same physician providing critical care transport (99466-99467)

\# **99485** **Supervision by a control physician of interfacility transport care of the critically ill or critically injured pediatric patient, 24 months of age or younger, includes two-way communication with transport team before transport, at the referring facility and during the transport, including data interpretation and report; first 30 minutes** [A]

🚑 2.16   ⚕ 2.16   **FUD** XXX   [B] [▭]

AMA: 2016,Jan,13; 2015,Jan,16; 2014,Oct,8; 2013,May,6-7

+ \# **99486** **each additional 30 minutes (List separately in addition to code for primary procedure)** [A]

Code first ([99485])

🚑 1.88   ⚕ 1.88   **FUD** XXX   [B] [▭]

AMA: 2016,Jan,13; 2015,Jan,16; 2014,Oct,8; 2013,May,6-7

99468-99476 Critical Care Age 5 Years or Younger

CMS: 100-04,12,30.6.4 Services Furnished Incident to Physician's Service

INCLUDES All services included in codes 99291-99292 as well as the following which may be reported by facilities only:
Administration of blood/blood components (36430, 36440)
Administration of intravenous fluids (96360-96361)
Administration of surfactant (94610)
Bladder aspiration, suprapubic (51100)
Bladder catheterization (51701, 51702)
Car seat evaluation (94780-94781)
Catheterization umbilical artery (36660)
Catheterization umbilical vein (36510)
Central venous catheter, centrally inserted (36555)
Endotracheal intubation (31500)
Lumbar puncture (62270)
Oral or nasogastric tube placement (43752)
Pulmonary function testing, performed at the bedside (94375)
Pulse or ear oximetry (94760-94762)
Vascular access, arteries (36140, 36620)
Vascular access, venous (36400-36406, 36420, 36600)
Ventilatory management (94002-94004, 94660)
Initial and subsequent care provided to a critically ill infant or child
Other hospital care or intensive care services by same group or individual done on same day that patient was transferred to initial neonatal/pediatric critical care
Readmission to critical unit on same day or during the same stay (subsequent care)

EXCLUDES *Critical care services for patients 6 years of age or older (99291-99292)*
Critical care services provided by a second physician or physician of a different specialty (99291-99292)
Neonatal hypothermia (99184)
Remote critical care (0188T-0189T)
Services performed by individual in another group receiving a patient transferred to a lower level of care (99231-99233, 99478-99480)
Services performed by individual transferring a patient to a lower level of care (99231-99233, 99291-99292)
Services performed by same or different individual in same group on same day (99291-99292)
Services performed by transferring individual prior to transfer of patient to an individual in a different group (99221-99233, 99291-99292, 99460-99462, 99477-99480)
Code also normal newborn care if done on same day by same group or individual that provides critical care. Report modifier 25 with initial critical care code (99460-99462)

99468 **Initial inpatient neonatal critical care, per day, for the evaluation and management of a critically ill neonate, 28 days of age or younger** [A]

🚑 26.6   ⚕ 26.6   **FUD** XXX   [C] [80] [▭]

AMA: 2016,May,3; 2016,Jan,13; 2015,Oct,8; 2015,Jul,3; 2015,Feb,10; 2015,Jan,16; 2014,Oct,8; 2014,May,4; 2014,Jan,11; 2012,Aug,6-8

99469 **Subsequent inpatient neonatal critical care, per day, for the evaluation and management of a critically ill neonate, 28 days of age or younger** [A]

🚑 11.2   ⚕ 11.2   **FUD** XXX   [C] [80] [▭]

AMA: 2016,May,3; 2016,Jan,13; 2015,Oct,8; 2015,Jul,3; 2015,Feb,10; 2015,Jan,16; 2014,Oct,8; 2014,May,4; 2014,Jan,11; 2012,Aug,6-8

99471 **Initial inpatient pediatric critical care, per day, for the evaluation and management of a critically ill infant or young child, 29 days through 24 months of age** [A]

🚑 24.7   ⚕ 24.7   **FUD** XXX   [C] [80] [▭]

AMA: 2016,May,3; 2016,Jan,13; 2015,Jul,3; 2015,Feb,10; 2015,Jan,16; 2014,Oct,8; 2014,Jan,11; 2012,Aug,6-8

99472 **Subsequent inpatient pediatric critical care, per day, for the evaluation and management of a critically ill infant or young child, 29 days through 24 months of age** [A]

🚑 11.5   ⚕ 11.5   **FUD** XXX   [C] [80] [▭]

AMA: 2016,May,3; 2016,Jan,13; 2015,Jul,3; 2015,Feb,10; 2015,Jan,16; 2014,Oct,8; 2014,Jan,11; 2012,Aug,6-8

99475 **Initial inpatient pediatric critical care, per day, for the evaluation and management of a critically ill infant or young child, 2 through 5 years of age** [A]

🚑 16.2   ⚕ 16.2   **FUD** XXX   [C] [80] [▭]

AMA: 2016,May,3; 2016,Jan,13; 2015,Jul,3; 2015,Feb,10; 2015,Jan,16; 2014,Oct,8; 2014,Jan,11

99476 **Subsequent inpatient pediatric critical care, per day, for the evaluation and management of a critically ill infant or young child, 2 through 5 years of age** [A]

🚑 9.79   ⚕ 9.79   **FUD** XXX   [C] [80] [▭]

AMA: 2016,May,3; 2016,Jan,13; 2015,Jul,3; 2015,Feb,10; 2015,Jan,16; 2014,Oct,8; 2014,Jan,11

99477-99486 Initial Inpatient Neonatal Intensive Care and Other Services

INCLUDES All services included in codes 99291-99292 as well as the following that may be reported by facilities only:
Adjustments to enteral and/or parenteral nutrition
Airway and ventilator management (31500, 94002-94004, 94375, 94610, 94660)
Bladder catheterization (51701-51702)
Blood transfusion (36430, 36440)
Car seat evaluation (94780-94781)
Constant and/or frequent monitoring of vital signs
Continuous observation by the healthcare team
Heat maintenance
Intensive cardiac or respiratory monitoring
Oral or nasogastric tube insertion (43752)
Oxygen saturation (94760-94762)
Spinal puncture (62270)
Suprapubic catheterization (51100)
Vascular access procedures (36000, 36140, 36400, 36405-36406, 36420, 36510, 36555, 36600, 36620, 36660)

EXCLUDES *Critical care services for patient transferred after initial or subsequent intensive care is provided (99291-99292)*
Initial day intensive care provided by transferring individual same day neonate/infant transferred to a lower level of care (99477)
Inpatient neonatal/pediatric critical care services received on same day (99468-99476)
Necessary resuscitation services done as part of delivery care prior to admission
Neonatal hypothermia (99184)
Services provided by receiving individual when patient is transferred for critical care (99468-99476)
Services for receiving provider when patient improves after the initial day and is transferred to a lower level of care (99231-99233, 99478-99480)
Subsequent care of a sick neonate, under 28 days of age, more than 5000 grams, not requiring critical or intensive care services (99231-99233)
Code also care provided by receiving individual when patient is transferred to an individual in different group (99231-99233, 99462)
Code also initial neonatal intensive care service when physician or other qualified health care professional is present for delivery and/or neonate requires resuscitation (99464-99465); append modifier 25 to (99477)

● New Code   ▲ Revised Code   ○ Reinstated   ● New Web Release   ▲ Revised Web Release   Unlisted   Not Covered   \# Resequenced
⊘ AMA Mod 51 Exempt   ⑪ Optum Mod 51 Exempt   ⊕ Mod 63 Exempt   ∥ Non-FDA Drug   ★ Telehealth   [M] Maternity   [A] Age Edit   + Add-on   **AMA:** CPT Asst

99477 Initial hospital care, per day, for the evaluation and management of the neonate, 28 days of age or younger, who requires intensive observation, frequent interventions, and other intensive care services   A

> *EXCLUDES*   *Initiation of care of a critically ill neonate (99468)*
> *Initiation of inpatient care of a normal newborn (99460)*

   10.0   10.0   **FUD** XXX   C 80

AMA: 2016,Jan,13; 2015,Jul,3; 2015,Jan,16; 2014,Oct,8; 2014,Jan,11; 2012,Aug,6-8

99478 Subsequent intensive care, per day, for the evaluation and management of the recovering very low birth weight infant (present body weight less than 1500 grams)   A

   3.86   3.86   **FUD** XXX   C 80

AMA: 2016,Jan,13; 2015,Jul,3; 2015,Jan,16; 2014,Oct,8; 2014,Jan,11; 2012,Aug,6-8

99479 Subsequent intensive care, per day, for the evaluation and management of the recovering low birth weight infant (present body weight of 1500-2500 grams)   A

   3.52   3.52   **FUD** XXX   C 80

AMA: 2016,Jan,13; 2015,Jul,3; 2015,Jan,16; 2014,Oct,8; 2014,Jan,11; 2012,Aug,6-8

99480 Subsequent intensive care, per day, for the evaluation and management of the recovering infant (present body weight of 2501-5000 grams)   A

   3.37   3.37   **FUD** XXX   C 80

AMA: 2016,Jan,13; 2015,Jul,3; 2015,Jan,16; 2014,Oct,8; 2014,Jan,11; 2012,Aug,6-8

99485 Resequenced code. See code following 99467.

99486 Resequenced code. See code following 99467.

[99490] Coordination of Services for Chronic Care

INCLUDES   Case management services provided to patients that:
Have two or more conditions anticipated to endure more than 12 months or until the patient's death
Require at least 20 minutes of staff time monthly
Risk is high that conditions will result in decompensation, deterioration, or death
Patient management services during same time frame as (99339-99340, 99358-99359, 99363-99364, 99366-99368, 99374-99380, 99441-99444, 99495-99496, 90951-90970, 98960-98962, 98966-98969, 99071, 99078, 99080, 99090-99091, 99605-99607)
Services performed during a postoperative surgical period

 # 99490 Chronic care management services, at least 20 minutes of clinical staff time directed by a physician or other qualified health care professional, per calendar month, with the following required elements: multiple (two or more) chronic conditions expected to last at least 12 months, or until the death of the patient; chronic conditions place the patient at significant risk of death, acute exacerbation/decompensation, or functional decline; comprehensive care plan established, implemented, revised, or monitored.

   0.88   1.14   **FUD** XXX   V

AMA: 2016,Jan,13; 2015,Feb,3; 2015,Jan,16; 2014,Oct,3

99487-99490 Coordination of Complex Services for Chronic Care

INCLUDES   All clinical non-face-to-face time with patient, family, and caregivers
Only services given by physician or other qualified health caregiver who has the role of care coordination for the patient for the month
Patient management services during same time frame as (99339-99340, 99358-99359, 99363-99364, 99366-99368, 99374-99380, 99441-99444, 99495-99496, 90951-90970, 98960-98962, 98966-98969, 99071, 99078, 99080, 99090-99091, 99605-99607)
Services provided to patients in a rest home, domiciliary, assisted living facility, or at home that include:
Caregiver education to family or patient, addressing independent living and self-management
Communication with patient and all caregivers and professionals regarding care
Determining which community and health resources would benefit the patient
Developing and maintaining a care plan
Health outcomes data and registry documentation
Providing communication with home health and other patient utilized services
Support for treatment and medication adherence
The facilitation of services and care
Services that address activities of daily living, psychosocial, and medical needs

99487 Complex chronic care management services, with the following required elements: multiple (two or more) chronic conditions expected to last at least 12 months, or until the death of the patient, chronic conditions place the patient at significant risk of death, acute exacerbation/decompensation, or functional decline, establishment or substantial revision of a comprehensive care plan, moderate or high complexity medical decision making; 60 minutes of clinical staff time directed by a physician or other qualified health care professional, per calendar month

> *INCLUDES*   Clinical services, 60 to 74 minutes, during a calendar month

   0.00   0.00   **FUD** XXX   N 80

AMA: 2016,Jan,13; 2015,Jan,16; 2014,Oct,8; 2014,Oct,3; 2014,Jun,3; 2014,Feb,3; 2014,Jan,11; 2013,Nov,3; 2013,Sep,15-16; 2013,Apr,3-4; 2013,Jan,3-5

+ 99489 each additional 30 minutes of clinical staff time directed by a physician or other qualified health care professional, per calendar month (List separately in addition to code for primary procedure)

> *EXCLUDES*   *Clinical services less than 30 minutes beyond the initial 60 minutes of care, per calendar month*

Code first (99487)

   0.00   0.00   **FUD** ZZZ   N 80

AMA: 2016,Jan,13; 2015,Jan,16; 2014,Oct,8; 2014,Oct,3; 2014,Jun,3; 2014,Jan,11; 2013,Nov,3; 2013,Sep,15-16; 2013,Apr,3-4; 2013,Jan,3-5

99490 Resequenced code. See code before 99487.

26/TC PC/TC Only   A2-Z3 ASC Payment   50 Bilateral   ♂ Male Only   ♀ Female Only   Facility RVU   Non-Facility RVU   CCI
FUD Follow-up Days   **CMS:** IOM (Pub 100)   A-Y OPPSI   80/80 Surg Assist Allowed / w/Doc   Lab Crosswalk   Radiology Crosswalk   CLIA
500

99495-99496 Management of Transitional Care Services

CMS: 100-02,15,270.2 Medicare Telehealth Services; 100-04,12* Medicare Telehealth Services

INCLUDES First interaction (face-to-face, by telephone, or electronic) with patient or his/her caregiver and must be done within 2 working days of discharge

Initial face-to-face; must be done within code time frame and include medication management

New or established patient with moderate to high complexity medical decision making needs during care transitions

Patient management services during same time frame as (99339-99340, 99358-99359, 99363-99364, 99366-99368, 99374-99380, 99441-99444, 99487-99489, 90951-90970, 98960-98962, 98966-98969, 99071, 99078, 99080, 99090-99091, 99605-99607)

Services from discharge day up to 29 days post discharge

Subsequent discharge within 30 days

Without face-to-face patient care given by physician or other qualified health care professional includes:

Arrangement of follow-up and referrals with community resources and providers

Contacting qualified health care professionals for specific problems of patient

Discharge information review

Need for follow-up care review based on tests and treatments

Patient, family, and caregiver education

Without face-to-face patient care given by staff under the guidance of physician or other qualified health care professional includes:

Caregiver education to family or patient, addressing independent living and self-management

Communication with patient and all caregivers and professionals regarding care

Determining which community and health resources would benefit the patient

Providing communication with home health and other patient utilized services

Support for treatment and medication adherence

The facilitation of services and care

EXCLUDES *E&M services after the first face-to-face visit*

99495 **Transitional Care Management Services with the following required elements: Communication (direct contact, telephone, electronic) with the patient and/or caregiver within 2 business days of discharge Medical decision making of at least moderate complexity during the service period Face-to-face visit, within 14 calendar days of discharge**

🚑 3.11   ⚕ 4.62   **FUD** XXX   ★ V 80 ▣

AMA: 2016,Jan,13; 2015,Jan,16; 2014,Oct,8; 2014,Oct,3; 2014,Mar,13; 2014,Jan,11; 2013,Nov,3; 2013,Dec,11; 2013,Sep,15-16; 2013,Aug,13; 2013,Jul,11-12; 2013,Apr,3-4; 2013,Jan,3-5

99496 **Transitional Care Management Services with the following required elements: Communication (direct contact, telephone, electronic) with the patient and/or caregiver within 2 business days of discharge Medical decision making of high complexity during the service period Face-to-face visit, within 7 calendar days of discharge**

🚑 4.50   ⚕ 6.51   **FUD** XXX   ★ V 80 ▣

AMA: 2016,Jan,13; 2015,Jan,16; 2014,Oct,8; 2014,Oct,3; 2014,Mar,13; 2014,Jan,11; 2013,Nov,3; 2013,Sep,15-16; 2013,Aug,13; 2013,Jul,11-12; 2013,Apr,3-4; 2013,Jan,3-5

99497-99498 Advance Directive Guidance

CMS: 100-02,15,280.5.1 Advance Care Planning with an Annual Wellness Visit; 100-04,18,140.8 Advance Care Planning with an Annual Wellness Visit (AWV)

EXCLUDES *Critical care services (99291-99292, 99468-99469, 99471-99472, 99475-99476, 99477-99480)*

Treatment/management for an active problem (see appropriate E&M service)

99497 **Advance care planning including the explanation and discussion of advance directives such as standard forms (with completion of such forms, when performed), by the physician or other qualified health care professional; first 30 minutes, face-to-face with the patient, family member(s), and/or surrogate**

🚑 2.22   ⚕ 2.40   **FUD** XXX   01 80 ▣

AMA: 2016,Feb,7; 2016,Jan,13; 2015,Jan,16; 2014,Dec,11

+ **99498** **each additional 30 minutes (List separately in addition to code for primary procedure)**

Code first (99497)

🚑 2.08   ⚕ 2.09   **FUD** ZZZ   N 80 ▣

AMA: 2016,Feb,7; 2016,Jan,13; 2015,Jan,16; 2014,Dec,11

99499 Unlisted Evaluation and Management Services

CMS: 100-04,12,30.6.10 Consultation Services; 100-04,12,30.6.4 Services Furnished Incident to Physician's Service; 100-04,12,30.6.9.1 Initial Hospital Care and Observation or Inpatient Care Services

99499 **Unlisted evaluation and management service**

🚑 0.00   ⚕ 0.00   **FUD** XXX   B 80

AMA: 2016,Jan,13; 2015,Jan,16; 2014,Oct,8; 2014,Jan,11; 2012,Nov,13-14; 2012,Jul,10-11; 2012,Apr,10; 2012,Jan,15-42; 2011,May,7; 2011,Jan,11

0001F-0015F Quality Measures with Multiple Components

INCLUDES   Several measures grouped within a single code descriptor to make possible reporting for clinical conditions when all of the components have been met

0001F   **Heart failure assessed (includes assessment of all the following components) (CAD): Blood pressure measured (2000F) Level of activity assessed (1003F) Clinical symptoms of volume overload (excess) assessed (1004F) Weight, recorded (2001F) Clinical signs of volume overload (excess) assessed (2002F)**

INCLUDES   Blood pressure measured (2000F)
Clinical signs of volume overload (excess) assessed (2002F)
Clinical symptoms of volume overload (excess) assessed (1004F)
Level of activity assessed (1003F)
Weight recorded (2001F)

⚐ 0.00   ⚒ 0.00   **FUD** XXX   E

AMA: 2016,Jan,13; 2015,Jan,16; 2014,Jan,11

0005F   **Osteoarthritis assessed (OA) Includes assessment of all the following components: Osteoarthritis symptoms and functional status assessed (1006F) Use of anti-inflammatory or over-the-counter (OTC) analgesic medications assessed (1007F) Initial examination of the involved joint(s) (includes visual inspection, palpation, range of motion) (2004F)**

INCLUDES   Initial examination of the involved joint(s) (includes visual inspection/palpation/range of motion) (2004F)
Osteoarthritis symptoms and functional status assessed (1006F)
Use of anti-inflammatory or over-the-counter (OTC) analgesic medications assessed (1007F)

⚐ 0.00   ⚒ 0.00   **FUD** XXX   E

AMA: 2005,Oct,1-5

0012F   **Community-acquired bacterial pneumonia assessment (includes all of the following components) (CAP): Co-morbid conditions assessed (1026F) Vital signs recorded (2010F) Mental status assessed (2014F) Hydration status assessed (2018F)**

⚐ 0.00   ⚒ 0.00   **FUD** XXX   E

INCLUDES   Co-morbid conditions assessed (1026F)
Hydration status assessed (2018F)
Mental status assessed (2014F)
Vital signs recorded (2010F)

0014F   **Comprehensive preoperative assessment performed for cataract surgery with intraocular lens (IOL) placement (includes assessment of all of the following components) (EC): Dilated fundus evaluation performed within 12 months prior to cataract surgery (2020F) Pre-surgical (cataract) axial length, corneal power measurement and method of intraocular lens power calculation documented (must be performed within 12 months prior to surgery) (3073F) Preoperative assessment of functional or medical indication(s) for surgery prior to the cataract surgery with intraocular lens placement (must be performed within 12 months prior to cataract surgery) (3325F)**

INCLUDES   Evaluation of dilated fundus done within 12 months prior to surgery (2020F)
Preoperative assessment of functional or medical indications done within 12 months prior to surgery (3325F)
Presurgical measurement of axial length, corneal power, and IOL power calculation performed within 12 months prior to surgery (3073F)

⚐ 0.00   ⚒ 0.00   **FUD** XXX   E

AMA: 2008,Mar,8-12

0015F   **Melanoma follow up completed (includes assessment of all of the following components) (ML): History obtained regarding new or changing moles (1050F) Complete physical skin exam performed (2029F) Patient counseled to perform a monthly self skin examination (5005F)**

INCLUDES   Complete physical skin exam (2029F)
Counseling to perform monthly skin self-examination (5005F)
History obtained of new or changing moles (1050F)

⚐ 0.00   ⚒ 0.00   **FUD** XXX   E

AMA: 2008,Mar,8-12

0500F-0584F Care Provided According to Prevailing Guidelines

INCLUDES   Measures of utilization or patient care provided for certain clinical purposes

0500F   **Initial prenatal care visit (report at first prenatal encounter with health care professional providing obstetrical care. Report also date of visit and, in a separate field, the date of the last menstrual period [LMP]) (Prenatal)**   M ♀

⚐ 0.00   ⚒ 0.00   **FUD** XXX   E

AMA: 2016,Jan,13; 2015,Jan,16; 2014,Jan,11

0501F   **Prenatal flow sheet documented in medical record by first prenatal visit (documentation includes at minimum blood pressure, weight, urine protein, uterine size, fetal heart tones, and estimated date of delivery). Report also: date of visit and, in a separate field, the date of the last menstrual period [LMP] (Note: If reporting 0501F Prenatal flow sheet, it is not necessary to report 0500F Initial prenatal care visit) (Prenatal)**   M ♀

⚐ 0.00   ⚒ 0.00   **FUD** XXX   E

AMA: 2004,Nov,1

0502F   **Subsequent prenatal care visit (Prenatal) [Excludes: patients who are seen for a condition unrelated to pregnancy or prenatal care (eg, an upper respiratory infection; patients seen for consultation only, not for continuing care)]**   M ♀

EXCLUDES   Patients seen for an unrelated pregnancy/prenatal care condition (e.g., upper respiratory infection; patients seen for consultation only, not for continuing care)

⚐ 0.00   ⚒ 0.00   **FUD** XXX   E

AMA: 2004,Nov,1

0503F   **Postpartum care visit (Prenatal)**   M ♀

⚐ 0.00   ⚒ 0.00   **FUD** XXX   E

AMA: 2004,Nov,1

0505F   **Hemodialysis plan of care documented (ESRD, P-ESRD)**

⚐ 0.00   ⚒ 0.00   **FUD** XXX   E

AMA: 2008,Mar,8-12

0507F   **Peritoneal dialysis plan of care documented (ESRD)**

⚐ 0.00   ⚒ 0.00   **FUD** XXX   E

AMA: 2008,Mar,8-12

0509F   **Urinary incontinence plan of care documented (GER)**

⚐ 0.00   ⚒ 0.00   **FUD** XXX   M

0513F   **Elevated blood pressure plan of care documented (CKD)**

⚐ 0.00   ⚒ 0.00   **FUD** XXX   M

AMA: 2008,Mar,8-12

0514F   **Plan of care for elevated hemoglobin level documented for patient receiving Erythropoiesis-Stimulating Agent therapy (ESA) (CKD)**

⚐ 0.00   ⚒ 0.00   **FUD** XXX   E

AMA: 2008,Mar,8-12

0516F   **Anemia plan of care documented (ESRD)**

⚐ 0.00   ⚒ 0.00   **FUD** XXX   E

AMA: 2008,Mar,8-12

0517F   **Glaucoma plan of care documented (EC)**

⚐ 0.00   ⚒ 0.00   **FUD** XXX   M

AMA: 2008,Mar,8-12

0518F Falls plan of care documented (GER)
  0.00   0.00   FUD XXX   M
  AMA: 2008,Mar,8-12

0519F Planned chemotherapy regimen, including at a minimum: drug(s) prescribed, dose, and duration, documented prior to initiation of a new treatment regimen (ONC)
  0.00   0.00   FUD XXX   E
  AMA: 2008,Mar,8-12

0520F Radiation dose limits to normal tissues established prior to the initiation of a course of 3D conformal radiation for a minimum of 2 tissue/organ (ONC)
  0.00   0.00   FUD XXX   M
  AMA: 2008,Mar,8-12

0521F Plan of care to address pain documented (COA) (ONC)
  0.00   0.00   FUD XXX   M
  AMA: 2008,Mar,8-12

0525F Initial visit for episode (BkP)
  0.00   0.00   FUD XXX   E
  AMA: 2008,Mar,8-12

0526F Subsequent visit for episode (BkP)
  0.00   0.00   FUD XXX   M
  AMA: 2008,Mar,8-12

0528F Recommended follow-up interval for repeat colonoscopy of at least 10 years documented in colonoscopy report (End/Polyp)
  0.00   0.00   FUD XXX   M

0529F Interval of 3 or more years since patient's last colonoscopy, documented (End/Polyp)
  0.00   0.00   FUD XXX   M

0535F Dyspnea management plan of care, documented (Pall Cr)
  0.00   0.00   FUD XXX   E

0540F Glucorticoid Management Plan Documented (RA)
  0.00   0.00   FUD XXX   M

0545F Plan for follow-up care for major depressive disorder, documented (MDD ADOL)
  0.00   0.00   FUD XXX   E

0550F Cytopathology report on routine nongynecologic specimen finalized within two working days of accession date (PATH)
  0.00   0.00   FUD XXX   E

0551F Cytopathology report on nongynecologic specimen with documentation that the specimen was non-routine (PATH)
  0.00   0.00   FUD XXX   E

0555F Symptom management plan of care documented (HF)
  0.00   0.00   FUD XXX   E

0556F Plan of care to achieve lipid control documented (CAD)
  0.00   0.00   FUD XXX   E

0557F Plan of care to manage anginal symptoms documented (CAD)
  0.00   0.00   FUD XXX   M

0575F HIV RNA control plan of care, documented (HIV)
  0.00   0.00   FUD XXX   E

0580F Multidisciplinary care plan developed or updated (ALS)
  0.00   0.00   FUD XXX   E

0581F Patient transferred directly from anesthetizing location to critical care unit (Peri2)
  0.00   0.00   FUD XXX   M

0582F Patient not transferred directly from anesthetizing location to critical care unit (Peri2)
  0.00   0.00   FUD XXX   E

0583F Transfer of care checklist used (Peri2)
  0.00   0.00   FUD XXX   M

0584F Transfer of care checklist not used (Peri2)
  0.00   0.00   FUD XXX   E

1000F-1505F Elements of History/Review of Systems

INCLUDES Measures for specific aspects of patient history or review of systems

1000F Tobacco use assessed (CAD, CAP, COPD, PV) (DM)
  0.00   0.00   FUD XXX   E
  AMA: 2016,Jan,13; 2015,Jan,16; 2014,Jan,11

1002F Anginal symptoms and level of activity assessed (NMA-No Measure Associated)
  0.00   0.00   FUD XXX   E
  AMA: 2004,Nov,1

1003F Level of activity assessed (NMA-No Measure Associated)
  0.00   0.00   FUD XXX   E
  AMA: 2006,Dec,10-12

1004F Clinical symptoms of volume overload (excess) assessed (NMA-No Measure Associated)
  0.00   0.00   FUD XXX   E
  AMA: 2006,Dec,10-12

1005F Asthma symptoms evaluated (includes documentation of numeric frequency of symptoms or patient completion of an asthma assessment tool/survey/questionnaire) (NMA-No Measure Associated)
  0.00   0.00   FUD XXX   E

1006F Osteoarthritis symptoms and functional status assessed (may include the use of a standardized scale or the completion of an assessment questionnaire, such as the SF-36, AAOS Hip & Knee Questionnaire) (OA) [Instructions: Report when osteoarthritis is addressed during the patient encounter]
  0.00   0.00   FUD XXX   M

INCLUDES Osteoarthritis when it is addressed during the patient encounter

1007F Use of anti-inflammatory or analgesic over-the-counter (OTC) medications for symptom relief assessed (OA)
  0.00   0.00   FUD XXX   E

1008F Gastrointestinal and renal risk factors assessed for patients on prescribed or OTC non-steroidal anti-inflammatory drug (NSAID) (OA)
  0.00   0.00   FUD XXX   E

1010F Severity of angina assessed by level of activity (CAD)
  0.00   0.00   FUD XXX   M

1011F Angina present (CAD)
  0.00   0.00   FUD XXX   M

1012F Angina absent (CAD)
  0.00   0.00   FUD XXX   M

1015F Chronic obstructive pulmonary disease (COPD) symptoms assessed (Includes assessment of at least 1 of the following: dyspnea, cough/sputum, wheezing), or respiratory symptom assessment tool completed (COPD)
  0.00   0.00   FUD XXX   E

1018F Dyspnea assessed, not present (COPD)
  0.00   0.00   FUD XXX   E

1019F Dyspnea assessed, present (COPD)
  0.00   0.00   FUD XXX   E

1022F Pneumococcus immunization status assessed (CAP, COPD)
  0.00   0.00   FUD XXX   E
  AMA: 2010,Jul,3-5; 2008,Mar,8-12

1026F Co-morbid conditions assessed (eg, includes assessment for presence or absence of: malignancy, liver disease, congestive heart failure, cerebrovascular disease, renal disease, chronic obstructive pulmonary disease, asthma, diabetes, other co-morbid conditions) (CAP)
  0.00   0.00   FUD XXX   E

1030F Influenza immunization status assessed (CAP)
  0.00   0.00   FUD XXX   E
  AMA: 2008,Mar,8-12

1031F Smoking status and exposure to second hand smoke in the home assessed (Asthma)
🚗 0.00   ♦ 0.00   **FUD** XXX   [E]

1032F Current tobacco smoker or currently exposed to secondhand smoke (Asthma)
🚗 0.00   ♦ 0.00   **FUD** XXX   [E]

1033F Current tobacco non-smoker and not currently exposed to secondhand smoke (Asthma)
🚗 0.00   ♦ 0.00   **FUD** XXX   [E]

1034F Current tobacco smoker (CAD, CAP, COPD, PV) (DM)
🚗 0.00   ♦ 0.00   **FUD** XXX   [E]
AMA: 2008,Mar,8-12

1035F Current smokeless tobacco user (eg, chew, snuff) (PV)
🚗 0.00   ♦ 0.00   **FUD** XXX   [E]
AMA: 2008,Mar,8-12

1036F Current tobacco non-user (CAD, CAP, COPD, PV) (DM) (IBD)
🚗 0.00   ♦ 0.00   **FUD** XXX   [M]
AMA: 2008,Mar,8-12

1038F Persistent asthma (mild, moderate or severe) (Asthma)
🚗 0.00   ♦ 0.00   **FUD** XXX   [M]
AMA: 2016,Jan,13; 2015,Jan,16; 2014,Jan,11

1039F Intermittent asthma (Asthma)
🚗 0.00   ♦ 0.00   **FUD** XXX   [M]
AMA: 2016,Jan,13; 2015,Jan,16; 2014,Jan,11

1040F DSM-5 criteria for major depressive disorder documented at the initial evaluation (MDD, MDD ADOL)
🚗 0.00   ♦ 0.00   **FUD** XXX   [E]
AMA: 2008,Mar,8-12

1050F History obtained regarding new or changing moles (ML)
🚗 0.00   ♦ 0.00   **FUD** XXX   [E]
AMA: 2008,Mar,8-12

1052F Type, anatomic location, and activity all assessed (IBD)
🚗 0.00   ♦ 0.00   **FUD** XXX   [E]

1055F Visual functional status assessed (EC)
🚗 0.00   ♦ 0.00   **FUD** XXX   [E]

1060F Documentation of permanent or persistent or paroxysmal atrial fibrillation (STR)
🚗 0.00   ♦ 0.00   **FUD** XXX   [E]

1061F Documentation of absence of permanent and persistent and paroxysmal atrial fibrillation (STR)
🚗 0.00   ♦ 0.00   **FUD** XXX   [E]

1065F Ischemic stroke symptom onset of less than 3 hours prior to arrival (STR)
🚗 0.00   ♦ 0.00   **FUD** XXX   [E]

1066F Ischemic stroke symptom onset greater than or equal to 3 hours prior to arrival (STR)
🚗 0.00   ♦ 0.00   **FUD** XXX   [E]

1070F Alarm symptoms (involuntary weight loss, dysphagia, or gastrointestinal bleeding) assessed; none present (GERD)
🚗 0.00   ♦ 0.00   **FUD** XXX   [E]

1071F 1 or more present (GERD)
🚗 0.00   ♦ 0.00   **FUD** XXX   [E]

1090F Presence or absence of urinary incontinence assessed (GER)
🚗 0.00   ♦ 0.00   **FUD** XXX   [M]

1091F Urinary incontinence characterized (eg, frequency, volume, timing, type of symptoms, how bothersome) (GER)
🚗 0.00   ♦ 0.00   **FUD** XXX   [E]

1100F Patient screened for future fall risk; documentation of 2 or more falls in the past year or any fall with injury in the past year (GER)
🚗 0.00   ♦ 0.00   **FUD** XXX   [M]
AMA: 2008,Mar,8-12

1101F documentation of no falls in the past year or only 1 fall without injury in the past year (GER)
🚗 0.00   ♦ 0.00   **FUD** XXX   [M]
AMA: 2008,Mar,8-12

1110F Patient discharged from an inpatient facility (eg, hospital, skilled nursing facility, or rehabilitation facility) within the last 60 days (GER)
🚗 0.00   ♦ 0.00   **FUD** XXX   [E]

1111F Discharge medications reconciled with the current medication list in outpatient medical record (COA) (GER)
🚗 0.00   ♦ 0.00   **FUD** XXX   [M]

1116F Auricular or periauricular pain assessed (AOE)
🚗 0.00   ♦ 0.00   **FUD** XXX   [E]
AMA: 2008,Mar,8-12

1118F GERD symptoms assessed after 12 months of therapy (GERD)
🚗 0.00   ♦ 0.00   **FUD** XXX   [E]
AMA: 2008,Mar,8-12

1119F Initial evaluation for condition (HEP C)(EPI, DSP)
🚗 0.00   ♦ 0.00   **FUD** XXX   [E]
AMA: 2008,Mar,8-12

1121F Subsequent evaluation for condition (HEP C)(EPI)
🚗 0.00   ♦ 0.00   **FUD** XXX   [E]
AMA: 2008,Mar,8-12

1123F Advance Care Planning discussed and documented advance care plan or surrogate decision maker documented in the medical record (DEM) (GER, Pall Cr)
🚗 0.00   ♦ 0.00   **FUD** XXX   [M]
AMA: 2008,Mar,8-12

1124F Advance Care Planning discussed and documented in the medical record, patient did not wish or was not able to name a surrogate decision maker or provide an advance care plan (DEM) (GER, Pall Cr)
🚗 0.00   ♦ 0.00   **FUD** XXX   [M]
AMA: 2008,Mar,8-12

1125F Pain severity quantified; pain present (COA) (ONC)
🚗 0.00   ♦ 0.00   **FUD** XXX   [M]
AMA: 2008,Mar,8-12

1126F no pain present (COA) (ONC)
🚗 0.00   ♦ 0.00   **FUD** XXX   [M]
AMA: 2008,Mar,8-12

1127F New episode for condition (NMA-No Measure Associated)
🚗 0.00   ♦ 0.00   **FUD** XXX   [E]
AMA: 2008,Mar,8-12

1128F Subsequent episode for condition (NMA-No Measure Associated)
🚗 0.00   ♦ 0.00   **FUD** XXX   [E]
AMA: 2008,Mar,8-12

1130F Back pain and function assessed, including all of the following: Pain assessment and functional status and patient history, including notation of presence or absence of "red flags" (warning signs) and assessment of prior treatment and response, and employment status (BkP)
🚗 0.00   ♦ 0.00   **FUD** XXX   [E]
AMA: 2008,Mar,8-12

1134F Episode of back pain lasting 6 weeks or less (BkP)
🚗 0.00   ♦ 0.00   **FUD** XXX   [E]
AMA: 2008,Mar,8-12

1135F Episode of back pain lasting longer than 6 weeks (BkP)
🚗 0.00   ♦ 0.00   **FUD** XXX   [E]
AMA: 2008,Mar,8-12

1136F Episode of back pain lasting 12 weeks or less (BkP)
🚗 0.00   ♦ 0.00   **FUD** XXX   [E]
AMA: 2008,Mar,8-12

1137F Episode of back pain lasting longer than 12 weeks (BkP)
0.00   0.00   FUD XXX   E
AMA: 2008,Mar,8-12

1150F Documentation that a patient has a substantial risk of death within 1 year (Pall Cr)
0.00   0.00   FUD XXX   E

1151F Documentation that a patient does not have a substantial risk of death within one year (Pall Cr)
0.00   0.00   FUD XXX   E

1152F Documentation of advanced disease diagnosis, goals of care prioritize comfort (Pall Cr)
0.00   0.00   FUD XXX   E

1153F Documentation of advanced disease diagnosis, goals of care do not prioritize comfort (Pall Cr)
0.00   0.00   FUD XXX   E

1157F Advance care plan or similar legal document present in the medical record (COA)
0.00   0.00   FUD XXX   E

1158F Advance care planning discussion documented in the medical record (COA)
0.00   0.00   FUD XXX   M

1159F Medication list documented in medical record (COA)
0.00   0.00   FUD XXX   E

1160F Review of all medications by a prescribing practitioner or clinical pharmacist (such as, prescriptions, OTCs, herbal therapies and supplements) documented in the medical record (COA)
0.00   0.00   FUD XXX   E

1170F Functional status assessed (COA) (RA)
0.00   0.00   FUD XXX   M

1175F Functional status for dementia assessed and results reviewed (DEM)
0.00   0.00   FUD XXX   M

1180F All specified thromboembolic risk factors assessed (AFIB)
0.00   0.00   FUD XXX   E

1181F Neuropsychiatric symptoms assessed and results reviewed (DEM)
0.00   0.00   FUD XXX   M

1182F Neuropsychiatric symptoms, one or more present (DEM)
0.00   0.00   FUD XXX   E

1183F Neuropsychiatric symptoms, absent (DEM)
0.00   0.00   FUD XXX   E

1200F Seizure type(s) and current seizure frequency(ies) documented (EPI)
0.00   0.00   FUD XXX   E

1205F Etiology of epilepsy or epilepsy syndrome(s) reviewed and documented (EPI)
0.00   0.00   FUD XXX   E

1220F Patient screened for depression (SUD)
0.00   0.00   FUD XXX   E

1400F Parkinson's disease diagnosis reviewed (Prkns)
0.00   0.00   FUD XXX   M

1450F Symptoms improved or remained consistent with treatment goals since last assessment (HF)
0.00   0.00   FUD XXX   E

1451F Symptoms demonstrated clinically important deterioration since last assessment (HF)
0.00   0.00   FUD XXX   E

1460F Qualifying cardiac event/diagnosis in previous 12 months (CAD)
0.00   0.00   FUD XXX   M

1461F No qualifying cardiac event/diagnosis in previous 12 months (CAD)
0.00   0.00   FUD XXX   M

1490F Dementia severity classified, mild (DEM)
0.00   0.00   FUD XXX   M

1491F Dementia severity classified, moderate (DEM)
0.00   0.00   FUD XXX   M

1493F Dementia severity classified, severe (DEM)
0.00   0.00   FUD XXX   M

1494F Cognition assessed and reviewed (DEM)
0.00   0.00   FUD XXX   M

1500F Symptoms and signs of distal symmetric polyneuropathy reviewed and documented (DSP)
0.00   0.00   FUD XXX   E

1501F Not initial evaluation for condition (DSP)
0.00   0.00   FUD XXX   E

1502F Patient queried about pain and pain interference with function using a valid and reliable instrument (DSP)
0.00   0.00   FUD XXX   E

1503F Patient queried about symptoms of respiratory insufficiency (ALS)
0.00   0.00   FUD XXX   E

1504F Patient has respiratory insufficiency (ALS)
0.00   0.00   FUD XXX   E

1505F Patient does not have respiratory insufficiency (ALS)
0.00   0.00   FUD XXX   E

2000F-2060F Elements of Examination

INCLUDES   Components of clinical assessment or physical exam

2000F Blood pressure measured (CKD)(DM)
0.00   0.00   FUD XXX   M
AMA: 2016,Jan,13; 2015,Jan,16; 2014,Jan,11

2001F Weight recorded (PAG)
0.00   0.00   FUD XXX   E
AMA: 2006,Dec,10-12

2002F Clinical signs of volume overload (excess) assessed (NMA-No Measure Associated)
0.00   0.00   FUD XXX   E
AMA: 2006,Dec,10-12

2004F Initial examination of the involved joint(s) (includes visual inspection, palpation, range of motion) (OA) [Instructions: Report only for initial osteoarthritis visit or for visits for new joint involvement]
INCLUDES   Visits for initial osteoarthritis examination or new joint involvement
0.00   0.00   FUD XXX   E
AMA: 2004,Feb,3; 2003,Aug,1

2010F Vital signs (temperature, pulse, respiratory rate, and blood pressure) documented and reviewed (CAP) (EM)
0.00   0.00   FUD XXX   E

2014F Mental status assessed (CAP) (EM)
0.00   0.00   FUD XXX   E

2015F Asthma impairment assessed (Asthma)
0.00   0.00   FUD XXX   E

2016F Asthma risk assessed (Asthma)
0.00   0.00   FUD XXX   E

2018F Hydration status assessed (normal/mildly dehydrated/severely dehydrated) (CAP)
0.00   0.00   FUD XXX   E

2019F Dilated macular exam performed, including documentation of the presence or absence of macular thickening or hemorrhage and the level of macular degeneration severity (EC)
0.00   0.00   FUD XXX   M

2020F Dilated fundus evaluation performed within 12 months prior to cataract surgery (EC)
📷 0.00   🔧 0.00   **FUD** XXX   E
AMA: 2008,Mar,8-12

2021F Dilated macular or fundus exam performed, including documentation of the presence or absence of macular edema and level of severity of retinopathy (EC)
📷 0.00   🔧 0.00   **FUD** XXX   E

2022F Dilated retinal eye exam with interpretation by an ophthalmologist or optometrist documented and reviewed (DM)
📷 0.00   🔧 0.00   **FUD** XXX   M
AMA: 2008,Mar,8-12

2024F 7 standard field stereoscopic photos with interpretation by an ophthalmologist or optometrist documented and reviewed (DM)
📷 0.00   🔧 0.00   **FUD** XXX   M
AMA: 2008,Mar,8-12

2026F Eye imaging validated to match diagnosis from 7 standard field stereoscopic photos results documented and reviewed (DM)
📷 0.00   🔧 0.00   **FUD** XXX   M
AMA: 2008,Mar,8-12

2027F Optic nerve head evaluation performed (EC)
📷 0.00   🔧 0.00   **FUD** XXX   M

2028F Foot examination performed (includes examination through visual inspection, sensory exam with monofilament, and pulse exam - report when any of the 3 components are completed) (DM)
📷 0.00   🔧 0.00   **FUD** XXX   E

2029F Complete physical skin exam performed (ML)
📷 0.00   🔧 0.00   **FUD** XXX   E
AMA: 2008,Mar,8-12

2030F Hydration status documented, normally hydrated (PAG)
📷 0.00   🔧 0.00   **FUD** XXX   E

2031F Hydration status documented, dehydrated (PAG)
📷 0.00   🔧 0.00   **FUD** XXX   E

2035F Tympanic membrane mobility assessed with pneumatic otoscopy or tympanometry (OME)
📷 0.00   🔧 0.00   **FUD** XXX   E
AMA: 2008,Mar,8-12

2040F Physical examination on the date of the initial visit for low back pain performed, in accordance with specifications (BkP)
📷 0.00   🔧 0.00   **FUD** XXX   E
AMA: 2008,Mar,8-12

2044F Documentation of mental health assessment prior to intervention (back surgery or epidural steroid injection) or for back pain episode lasting longer than 6 weeks (BkP)
📷 0.00   🔧 0.00   **FUD** XXX   E
AMA: 2008,Mar,8-12

2050F Wound characteristics including size and nature of wound base tissue and amount of drainage prior to debridement documented (CWC)
📷 0.00   🔧 0.00   **FUD** XXX   E

2060F Patient interviewed directly on or before date of diagnosis of major depressive disorder (MDD ADOL)
📷 0.00   🔧 0.00   **FUD** XXX   E

3006F-3776F Findings from Diagnostic or Screening Tests

INCLUDES   Results and medical decision making with regards to ordered tests:
Clinical laboratory tests
Other examination procedures
Radiological examinations

3006F Chest X-ray results documented and reviewed (CAP)
📷 0.00   🔧 0.00   **FUD** XXX   E
AMA: 2016,Jan,13; 2015,Jan,16; 2014,Jan,11

3008F Body Mass Index (BMI), documented (PV)
📷 0.00   🔧 0.00   **FUD** XXX   E

3011F Lipid panel results documented and reviewed (must include total cholesterol, HDL-C, triglycerides and calculated LDL-C) (CAD)
📷 0.00   🔧 0.00   **FUD** XXX   E

3014F Screening mammography results documented and reviewed (PV)
📷 0.00   🔧 0.00   **FUD** XXX   M
AMA: 2008,Mar,8-12

3015F Cervical cancer screening results documented and reviewed (PV)
📷 0.00   🔧 0.00   **FUD** XXX   ♀   E

3016F Patient screened for unhealthy alcohol use using a systematic screening method (PV) (DSP)
📷 0.00   🔧 0.00   **FUD** XXX   E

3017F Colorectal cancer screening results documented and reviewed (PV)
📷 0.00   🔧 0.00   **FUD** XXX   M
AMA: 2008,Mar,8-12

3018F Pre-procedure risk assessment and depth of insertion and quality of the bowel prep and complete description of polyp(s) found, including location of each polyp, size, number and gross morphology and recommendations for follow-up in final colonoscopy report documented (End/Polyp)
📷 0.00   🔧 0.00   **FUD** XXX   E

3019F Left ventricular ejection fraction (LVEF) assessment planned post discharge (HF)
📷 0.00   🔧 0.00   **FUD** XXX   E

3020F Left ventricular function (LVF) assessment (eg, echocardiography, nuclear test, or ventriculography) documented in the medical record (Includes quantitative or qualitative assessment results) (NMA-No Measure Associated)
📷 0.00   🔧 0.00   **FUD** XXX   E
AMA: 2006,Dec,10-12

3021F Left ventricular ejection fraction (LVEF) less than 40% or documentation of moderately or severely depressed left ventricular systolic function (CAD, HF)
📷 0.00   🔧 0.00   **FUD** XXX   M

3022F Left ventricular ejection fraction (LVEF) greater than or equal to 40% or documentation as normal or mildly depressed left ventricular systolic function (CAD, HF)
📷 0.00   🔧 0.00   **FUD** XXX   M

3023F Spirometry results documented and reviewed (COPD)
📷 0.00   🔧 0.00   **FUD** XXX   M

3025F Spirometry test results demonstrate FEV1/FVC less than 70% with COPD symptoms (eg, dyspnea, cough/sputum, wheezing) (CAP, COPD)
📷 0.00   🔧 0.00   **FUD** XXX   E

3027F Spirometry test results demonstrate FEV1/FVC greater than or equal to 70% or patient does not have COPD symptoms (COPD)
📷 0.00   🔧 0.00   **FUD** XXX   E

3028F Oxygen saturation results documented and reviewed (includes assessment through pulse oximetry or arterial blood gas measurement) (CAP, COPD) (EM)
📷 0.00   🔧 0.00   **FUD** XXX   E

3035F Oxygen saturation less than or equal to 88% or a PaO2 less than or equal to 55 mm Hg (COPD)
📷 0.00   🔧 0.00   **FUD** XXX   E

● New Code   ▲ Revised Code   ○ Reinstated   ● New Web Release   ▲ Revised Web Release   Unlisted   Not Covered   # Resequenced
⊘ AMA Mod 51 Exempt   ⑤ Optum Mod 51 Exempt   ⑥ Mod 63 Exempt   ✎ Non-FDA Drug   ★ Telehealth   Ⓜ Maternity   Ⓐ Age Edit   + Add-on   **AMA:** CPT Asst
CPT © 2016 American Medical Association. All Rights Reserved.

3037F Oxygen saturation greater than 88% or PaO2 greater than 55 mm Hg (COPD)
  ⚙ 0.00   ⚖ 0.00   **FUD** XXX   E

3038F Pulmonary function test performed within 12 months prior to surgery (Lung/Esop Cx)
  ⚙ 0.00   ⚖ 0.00   **FUD** XXX   E

3040F Functional expiratory volume (FEV1) less than 40% of predicted value (COPD)
  ⚙ 0.00   ⚖ 0.00   **FUD** XXX   E

3042F Functional expiratory volume (FEV1) greater than or equal to 40% of predicted value (COPD)
  ⚙ 0.00   ⚖ 0.00   **FUD** XXX   E

3044F Most recent hemoglobin A1c (HbA1c) level less than 7.0% (DM)
  ⚙ 0.00   ⚖ 0.00   **FUD** XXX   M

3045F Most recent hemoglobin A1c (HbA1c) level 7.0-9.0% (DM)
  ⚙ 0.00   ⚖ 0.00   **FUD** XXX   M

3046F Most recent hemoglobin A1c level greater than 9.0% (DM)
  ⚙ 0.00   ⚖ 0.00   **FUD** XXX   M
  EXCLUDES   Levels of hemoglobin A1c less than or equal to 9.0% (3044F-3045F)

3048F Most recent LDL-C less than 100 mg/dL (CAD) (DM)
  ⚙ 0.00   ⚖ 0.00   **FUD** XXX   E

3049F Most recent LDL-C 100-129 mg/dL (CAD) (DM)
  ⚙ 0.00   ⚖ 0.00   **FUD** XXX   E

3050F Most recent LDL-C greater than or equal to 130 mg/dL (CAD) (DM)
  ⚙ 0.00   ⚖ 0.00   **FUD** XXX   E

3055F Left ventricular ejection fraction (LVEF) less than or equal to 35% (HF)
  ⚙ 0.00   ⚖ 0.00   **FUD** XXX   E

3056F Left ventricular ejection fraction (LVEF) greater than 35% or no LVEF result available (HF)
  ⚙ 0.00   ⚖ 0.00   **FUD** XXX   E

3060F Positive microalbuminuria test result documented and reviewed (DM)
  ⚙ 0.00   ⚖ 0.00   **FUD** XXX   M

3061F Negative microalbuminuria test result documented and reviewed (DM)
  ⚙ 0.00   ⚖ 0.00   **FUD** XXX   M

3062F Positive macroalbuminuria test result documented and reviewed (DM)
  ⚙ 0.00   ⚖ 0.00   **FUD** XXX   M

3066F Documentation of treatment for nephropathy (eg, patient receiving dialysis, patient being treated for ESRD, CRF, ARF, or renal insufficiency, any visit to a nephrologist) (DM)
  ⚙ 0.00   ⚖ 0.00   **FUD** XXX   M

3072F Low risk for retinopathy (no evidence of retinopathy in the prior year) (DM)
  ⚙ 0.00   ⚖ 0.00   **FUD** XXX   M
  AMA: 2008,Mar,8-12

3073F Pre-surgical (cataract) axial length, corneal power measurement and method of intraocular lens power calculation documented within 12 months prior to surgery (EC)
  ⚙ 0.00   ⚖ 0.00   **FUD** XXX   E
  AMA: 2008,Mar,8-12

3074F Most recent systolic blood pressure less than 130 mm Hg (DM), (HTN, CKD, CAD)
  ⚙ 0.00   ⚖ 0.00   **FUD** XXX   E
  AMA: 2008,Mar,8-12

3075F Most recent systolic blood pressure 130-139 mm Hg (DM) (HTN, CKD, CAD)
  ⚙ 0.00   ⚖ 0.00   **FUD** XXX   E
  AMA: 2008,Mar,8-12

3077F Most recent systolic blood pressure greater than or equal to 140 mm Hg (HTN, CKD, CAD) (DM)
  ⚙ 0.00   ⚖ 0.00   **FUD** XXX   E
  AMA: 2008,Mar,8-12

3078F Most recent diastolic blood pressure less than 80 mm Hg (HTN, CKD, CAD) (DM)
  ⚙ 0.00   ⚖ 0.00   **FUD** XXX   E
  AMA: 2008,Mar,8-12

3079F Most recent diastolic blood pressure 80-89 mm Hg (HTN, CKD, CAD) (DM)
  ⚙ 0.00   ⚖ 0.00   **FUD** XXX   E
  AMA: 2008,Mar,8-12

3080F Most recent diastolic blood pressure greater than or equal to 90 mm Hg (HTN, CKD, CAD) (DM)
  ⚙ 0.00   ⚖ 0.00   **FUD** XXX   E
  AMA: 2008,Mar,8-12

3082F Kt/V less than 1.2 (Clearance of urea [Kt]/volume [V]) (ESRD, P-ESRD)
  ⚙ 0.00   ⚖ 0.00   **FUD** XXX   E
  AMA: 2008,Mar,8-12

3083F Kt/V equal to or greater than 1.2 and less than 1.7 (Clearance of urea [Kt]/volume [V]) (ESRD, P-ESRD)
  ⚙ 0.00   ⚖ 0.00   **FUD** XXX   E
  AMA: 2008,Mar,8-12

3084F Kt/V greater than or equal to 1.7 (Clearance of urea [Kt]/volume [V]) (ESRD, P-ESRD)
  ⚙ 0.00   ⚖ 0.00   **FUD** XXX   E
  AMA: 2008,Mar,8-12

3085F Suicide risk assessed (MDD, MDD ADOL)
  ⚙ 0.00   ⚖ 0.00   **FUD** XXX   E

3088F Major depressive disorder, mild (MDD)
  ⚙ 0.00   ⚖ 0.00   **FUD** XXX   E

3089F Major depressive disorder, moderate (MDD)
  ⚙ 0.00   ⚖ 0.00   **FUD** XXX   E

3090F Major depressive disorder, severe without psychotic features (MDD)
  ⚙ 0.00   ⚖ 0.00   **FUD** XXX   E

3091F Major depressive disorder, severe with psychotic features (MDD)
  ⚙ 0.00   ⚖ 0.00   **FUD** XXX   E

3092F Major depressive disorder, in remission (MDD)
  ⚙ 0.00   ⚖ 0.00   **FUD** XXX   E

3093F Documentation of new diagnosis of initial or recurrent episode of major depressive disorder (MDD)
  ⚙ 0.00   ⚖ 0.00   **FUD** XXX   E
  AMA: 2008,Mar,8-12

3095F Central dual-energy X-ray absorptiometry (DXA) results documented (OP)(IBD)
  ⚙ 0.00   ⚖ 0.00   **FUD** XXX   M

3096F Central dual-energy X-ray absorptiometry (DXA) ordered (OP)(IBD)
  ⚙ 0.00   ⚖ 0.00   **FUD** XXX   E

3100F Carotid imaging study report (includes direct or indirect reference to measurements of distal internal carotid diameter as the denominator for stenosis measurement) (STR, RAD)
  ⚙ 0.00   ⚖ 0.00   **FUD** XXX   M
  AMA: 2008,Mar,8-12

3110F Documentation in final CT or MRI report of presence or absence of hemorrhage and mass lesion and acute infarction (STR)
📢 0.00 ⚕ 0.00 **FUD** XXX   E

3111F CT or MRI of the brain performed in the hospital within 24 hours of arrival or performed in an outpatient imaging center, to confirm initial diagnosis of stroke, TIA or intracranial hemorrhage (STR)
📢 0.00 ⚕ 0.00 **FUD** XXX   E

3112F CT or MRI of the brain performed greater than 24 hours after arrival to the hospital or performed in an outpatient imaging center for purpose other than confirmation of initial diagnosis of stroke, TIA, or intracranial hemorrhage (STR)
📢 0.00 ⚕ 0.00 **FUD** XXX   E

3115F Quantitative results of an evaluation of current level of activity and clinical symptoms (HF)
📢 0.00 ⚕ 0.00 **FUD** XXX   E

3117F Heart failure disease specific structured assessment tool completed (HF)
📢 0.00 ⚕ 0.00 **FUD** XXX   E

3118F New York Heart Association (NYHA) Class documented (HF)
📢 0.00 ⚕ 0.00 **FUD** XXX   E

3119F No evaluation of level of activity or clinical symptoms (HF)
📢 0.00 ⚕ 0.00 **FUD** XXX   E

3120F 12-Lead ECG Performed (EM)
📢 0.00 ⚕ 0.00 **FUD** XXX   M

3126F Esophageal biopsy report with a statement about dysplasia (present, absent, or indefinite, and if present, contains appropriate grading) (PATH)
📢 0.00 ⚕ 0.00 **FUD** XXX   M

3130F Upper gastrointestinal endoscopy performed (GERD)
📢 0.00 ⚕ 0.00 **FUD** XXX   E

3132F Documentation of referral for upper gastrointestinal endoscopy (GERD)
📢 0.00 ⚕ 0.00 **FUD** XXX   E

3140F Upper gastrointestinal endoscopy report indicates suspicion of Barrett's esophagus (GERD)
📢 0.00 ⚕ 0.00 **FUD** XXX   E

3141F Upper gastrointestinal endoscopy report indicates no suspicion of Barrett's esophagus (GERD)
📢 0.00 ⚕ 0.00 **FUD** XXX   E

3142F Barium swallow test ordered (GERD)
📢 0.00 ⚕ 0.00 **FUD** XXX   E

    INCLUDES   Documentation of barium swallow test

3150F Forceps esophageal biopsy performed (GERD)
📢 0.00 ⚕ 0.00 **FUD** XXX   E

3155F Cytogenetic testing performed on bone marrow at time of diagnosis or prior to initiating treatment (HEM)
📢 0.00 ⚕ 0.00 **FUD** XXX   M
AMA: 2008,Mar,8-12

3160F Documentation of iron stores prior to initiating erythropoietin therapy (HEM)
📢 0.00 ⚕ 0.00 **FUD** XXX   M
AMA: 2008,Mar,8-12

3170F Flow cytometry studies performed at time of diagnosis or prior to initiating treatment (HEM)
📢 0.00 ⚕ 0.00 **FUD** XXX   M
AMA: 2008,Mar,8-12

3200F Barium swallow test not ordered (GERD)
📢 0.00 ⚕ 0.00 **FUD** XXX   E

3210F Group A Strep Test Performed (PHAR)
📢 0.00 ⚕ 0.00 **FUD** XXX   M
AMA: 2008,Mar,8-12

3215F Patient has documented immunity to Hepatitis A (HEP-C)
📢 0.00 ⚕ 0.00 **FUD** XXX   M
AMA: 2008,Mar,8-12

3216F Patient has documented immunity to Hepatitis B (HEP-C)(IBD)
📢 0.00 ⚕ 0.00 **FUD** XXX   E
AMA: 2008,Mar,8-12

3218F RNA testing for Hepatitis C documented as performed within 6 months prior to initiation of antiviral treatment for Hepatitis C (HEP-C)
📢 0.00 ⚕ 0.00 **FUD** XXX   E
AMA: 2008,Mar,8-12

3220F Hepatitis C quantitative RNA testing documented as performed at 12 weeks from initiation of antiviral treatment (HEP-C)
📢 0.00 ⚕ 0.00 **FUD** XXX   E
AMA: 2008,Mar,8-12

3230F Documentation that hearing test was performed within 6 months prior to tympanostomy tube insertion (OME)
📢 0.00 ⚕ 0.00 **FUD** XXX   E
AMA: 2008,Mar,8-12

3250F Specimen site other than anatomic location of primary tumor (PATH)
📢 0.00 ⚕ 0.00 **FUD** XXX   M

3260F pT category (primary tumor), pN category (regional lymph nodes), and histologic grade documented in pathology report (PATH)
📢 0.00 ⚕ 0.00 **FUD** XXX   M
AMA: 2008,Mar,8-12

3265F Ribonucleic acid (RNA) testing for Hepatitis C viremia ordered or results documented (HEP C)
📢 0.00 ⚕ 0.00 **FUD** XXX   E
AMA: 2008,Mar,8-12

3266F Hepatitis C genotype testing documented as performed prior to initiation of antiviral treatment for Hepatitis C (HEP C)
📢 0.00 ⚕ 0.00 **FUD** XXX   E
AMA: 2008,Mar,8-12

3267F Pathology report includes pT category, pN category, Gleason score, and statement about margin status (PATH)
📢 0.00 ⚕ 0.00 **FUD** XXX   M

3268F Prostate-specific antigen (PSA), and primary tumor (T) stage, and Gleason score documented prior to initiation of treatment (PRCA)
📢 0.00 ⚕ 0.00 **FUD** XXX   E
AMA: 2008,Mar,8-12

3269F Bone scan performed prior to initiation of treatment or at any time since diagnosis of prostate cancer (PRCA)
📢 0.00 ⚕ 0.00 **FUD** XXX   M
AMA: 2008,Mar,8-12

3270F Bone scan not performed prior to initiation of treatment nor at any time since diagnosis of prostate cancer (PRCA)
📢 0.00 ⚕ 0.00 **FUD** XXX   M
AMA: 2008,Mar,8-12

3271F Low risk of recurrence, prostate cancer (PRCA)
📢 0.00 ⚕ 0.00 **FUD** XXX   M
AMA: 2008,Mar,8-12

3272F Intermediate risk of recurrence, prostate cancer (PRCA)
📢 0.00 ⚕ 0.00 **FUD** XXX   E
AMA: 2008,Mar,8-12

3273F High risk of recurrence, prostate cancer (PRCA)
📢 0.00 ⚕ 0.00 **FUD** XXX   E
AMA: 2008,Mar,8-12

● New Code   ▲ Revised Code   ○ Reinstated   ● New Web Release   ▲ Revised Web Release   Unlisted   Not Covered   # Resequenced
⊘ AMA Mod 51 Exempt   ⑪ Optum Mod 51 Exempt   ⑥³ Mod 63 Exempt   ✗ Non-FDA Drug   ★ Telehealth   M Maternity   A Age Edit   + Add-on   **AMA:** CPT Asst

3274F Prostate cancer risk of recurrence not determined or neither low, intermediate nor high (PRCA)
0.00   0.00   **FUD** XXX   E
AMA: 2008,Mar,8-12

3278F Serum levels of calcium, phosphorus, intact Parathyroid Hormone (PTH) and lipid profile ordered (CKD)
0.00   0.00   **FUD** XXX   E
AMA: 2008,Mar,8-12

3279F Hemoglobin level greater than or equal to 13 g/dL (CKD, ESRD)
0.00   0.00   **FUD** XXX   E
AMA: 2008,Mar,8-12

3280F Hemoglobin level 11 g/dL to 12.9 g/dL (CKD, ESRD)
0.00   0.00   **FUD** XXX   E
AMA: 2008,Mar,8-12

3281F Hemoglobin level less than 11 g/dL (CKD, ESRD)
0.00   0.00   **FUD** XXX   E
AMA: 2008,Mar,8-12

3284F Intraocular pressure (IOP) reduced by a value of greater than or equal to 15% from the pre-intervention level (EC)
0.00   0.00   **FUD** XXX   M
AMA: 2008,Mar,8-12

3285F Intraocular pressure (IOP) reduced by a value less than 15% from the pre-intervention level (EC)
0.00   0.00   **FUD** XXX   M
AMA: 2008,Mar,8-12

3288F Falls risk assessment documented (GER)
0.00   0.00   **FUD** XXX   M
AMA: 2008,Mar,8-12

3290F Patient is D (Rh) negative and unsensitized (Pre-Cr)
0.00   0.00   **FUD** XXX   E
AMA: 2008,Mar,8-12

3291F Patient is D (Rh) positive or sensitized (Pre-Cr)
0.00   0.00   **FUD** XXX   E
AMA: 2008,Mar,8-12

3292F HIV testing ordered or documented and reviewed during the first or second prenatal visit (Pre-Cr)
0.00   0.00   **FUD** XXX   E

3293F ABO and Rh blood typing documented as performed (Pre-Cr)
0.00   0.00   **FUD** XXX   E

3294F Group B Streptococcus (GBS) screening documented as performed during week 35-37 gestation (Pre-Cr)
0.00   0.00   **FUD** XXX   E

3300F American Joint Committee on Cancer (AJCC) stage documented and reviewed (ONC)
0.00   0.00   **FUD** XXX   M
AMA: 2008,Mar,8-12

3301F Cancer stage documented in medical record as metastatic and reviewed (ONC)
EXCLUDES   *Cancer staging measures (3321F-3390F)*
0.00   0.00   **FUD** XXX   M
AMA: 2008,Mar,8-12

3315F Estrogen receptor (ER) or progesterone receptor (PR) positive breast cancer (ONC)
0.00   0.00   **FUD** XXX   M
AMA: 2008,Mar,8-12

3316F Estrogen receptor (ER) and progesterone receptor (PR) negative breast cancer (ONC)
0.00   0.00   **FUD** XXX   M
AMA: 2008,Mar,8-12

3317F Pathology report confirming malignancy documented in the medical record and reviewed prior to the initiation of chemotherapy (ONC)
0.00   0.00   **FUD** XXX   E
AMA: 2008,Mar,8-12

3318F Pathology report confirming malignancy documented in the medical record and reviewed prior to the initiation of radiation therapy (ONC)
0.00   0.00   **FUD** XXX   E
AMA: 2008,Mar,8-12

3319F 1 of the following diagnostic imaging studies ordered: chest x-ray, CT, Ultrasound, MRI, PET, or nuclear medicine scans (ML)
0.00   0.00   **FUD** XXX   M
AMA: 2008,Mar,8-12

3320F None of the following diagnostic imaging studies ordered: chest X-ray, CT, Ultrasound, MRI, PET, or nuclear medicine scans (ML)
0.00   0.00   **FUD** XXX   M
AMA: 2008,Mar,8-12

3321F AJCC Cancer Stage 0 or IA Melanoma, documented (ML)
0.00   0.00   **FUD** XXX   M

3322F Melanoma greater than AJCC Stage 0 or IA (ML)
0.00   0.00   **FUD** XXX   M

3323F Clinical tumor, node and metastases (TNM) staging documented and reviewed prior to surgery (Lung/Esop Cx)
0.00   0.00   **FUD** XXX   E

3324F MRI or CT scan ordered, reviewed or requested (EPI)
0.00   0.00   **FUD** XXX   E

3325F Preoperative assessment of functional or medical indication(s) for surgery prior to the cataract surgery with intraocular lens placement (must be performed within 12 months prior to cataract surgery) (EC)
0.00   0.00   **FUD** XXX   E
AMA: 2008,Mar,8-12

3328F Performance status documented and reviewed within 2 weeks prior to surgery (Lung/Esop Cx)
0.00   0.00   **FUD** XXX   E

3330F Imaging study ordered (BkP)
0.00   0.00   **FUD** XXX   E
AMA: 2008,Mar,8-12

3331F Imaging study not ordered (BkP)
0.00   0.00   **FUD** XXX   E
AMA: 2008,Mar,8-12

3340F Mammogram assessment category of "incomplete: need additional imaging evaluation" documented (RAD)
0.00   0.00   **FUD** XXX   M
AMA: 2008,Mar,8-12

3341F Mammogram assessment category of "negative," documented (RAD)
0.00   0.00   **FUD** XXX   M
AMA: 2008,Mar,8-12

3342F Mammogram assessment category of "benign," documented (RAD)
0.00   0.00   **FUD** XXX   M
AMA: 2008,Mar,8-12

3343F Mammogram assessment category of "probably benign," documented (RAD)
0.00   0.00   **FUD** XXX   M
AMA: 2008,Mar,8-12

3344F Mammogram assessment category of "suspicious," documented (RAD)
0.00   0.00   **FUD** XXX   M
AMA: 2008,Mar,8-12

3345F Mammogram assessment category of "highly suggestive of malignancy," documented (RAD)
  📖 0.00   🔧 0.00   **FUD** XXX   Ⓜ
  AMA: 2008,Mar,8-12

3350F Mammogram assessment category of "known biopsy proven malignancy," documented (RAD)
  📖 0.00   🔧 0.00   **FUD** XXX   Ⓜ
  AMA: 2008,Mar,8-12

3351F Negative screen for depressive symptoms as categorized by using a standardized depression screening/assessment tool (MDD)
  📖 0.00   🔧 0.00   **FUD** XXX   Ⓔ

3352F No significant depressive symptoms as categorized by using a standardized depression assessment tool (MDD)
  📖 0.00   🔧 0.00   **FUD** XXX   Ⓔ

3353F Mild to moderate depressive symptoms as categorized by using a standardized depression screening/assessment tool (MDD)
  📖 0.00   🔧 0.00   **FUD** XXX   Ⓔ

3354F Clinically significant depressive symptoms as categorized by using a standardized depression screening/assessment tool (MDD)
  📖 0.00   🔧 0.00   **FUD** XXX   Ⓔ

3370F AJCC Breast Cancer Stage 0 documented (ONC)
  📖 0.00   🔧 0.00   **FUD** XXX   Ⓜ

3372F AJCC Breast Cancer Stage I: T1mic, T1a or T1b (tumor size ≤ 1 cm) documented (ONC)
  📖 0.00   🔧 0.00   **FUD** XXX   Ⓜ

3374F AJCC Breast Cancer Stage I: T1c (tumor size > 1 cm to 2 cm) documented (ONC)
  📖 0.00   🔧 0.00   **FUD** XXX   Ⓜ

3376F AJCC Breast Cancer Stage II documented (ONC)
  📖 0.00   🔧 0.00   **FUD** XXX   Ⓜ

3378F AJCC Breast Cancer Stage III documented (ONC)
  📖 0.00   🔧 0.00   **FUD** XXX   Ⓜ

3380F AJCC Breast Cancer Stage IV documented (ONC)
  📖 0.00   🔧 0.00   **FUD** XXX   Ⓜ

3382F AJCC colon cancer, Stage 0 documented (ONC)
  📖 0.00   🔧 0.00   **FUD** XXX   Ⓜ

3384F AJCC colon cancer, Stage I documented (ONC)
  📖 0.00   🔧 0.00   **FUD** XXX   Ⓜ

3386F AJCC colon cancer, Stage II documented (ONC)
  📖 0.00   🔧 0.00   **FUD** XXX   Ⓜ

3388F AJCC colon cancer, Stage III documented (ONC)
  📖 0.00   🔧 0.00   **FUD** XXX   Ⓜ

3390F AJCC colon cancer, Stage IV documented (ONC)
  📖 0.00   🔧 0.00   **FUD** XXX   Ⓜ

3394F Quantitative HER2 immunohistochemistry (IHC) evaluation of breast cancer consistent with the scoring system defined in the ASCO/CAP guidelines (PATH)
  📖 0.00   🔧 0.00   **FUD** XXX   Ⓜ

3395F Quantitative non-HER2 immunohistochemistry (IHC) evaluation of breast cancer (eg, testing for estrogen or progesterone receptors [ER/PR]) performed (PATH)
  📖 0.00   🔧 0.00   **FUD** XXX   Ⓜ

3450F Dyspnea screened, no dyspnea or mild dyspnea (Pall Cr)
  📖 0.00   🔧 0.00   **FUD** XXX   Ⓔ

3451F Dyspnea screened, moderate or severe dyspnea (Pall Cr)
  📖 0.00   🔧 0.00   **FUD** XXX   Ⓔ

3452F Dyspnea not screened (Pall Cr)
  📖 0.00   🔧 0.00   **FUD** XXX   Ⓔ

3455F TB screening performed and results interpreted within six months prior to initiation of first-time biologic disease modifying anti-rheumatic drug therapy for RA (RA)
  📖 0.00   🔧 0.00   **FUD** XXX   Ⓜ

3470F Rheumatoid arthritis (RA) disease activity, low (RA)
  📖 0.00   🔧 0.00   **FUD** XXX   Ⓜ

3471F Rheumatoid arthritis (RA) disease activity, moderate (RA)
  📖 0.00   🔧 0.00   **FUD** XXX   Ⓜ

3472F Rheumatoid arthritis (RA) disease activity, high (RA)
  📖 0.00   🔧 0.00   **FUD** XXX   Ⓜ

3475F Disease prognosis for rheumatoid arthritis assessed, poor prognosis documented (RA)
  📖 0.00   🔧 0.00   **FUD** XXX   Ⓜ

3476F Disease prognosis for rheumatoid arthritis assessed, good prognosis documented (RA)
  📖 0.00   🔧 0.00   **FUD** XXX   Ⓜ

3490F History of AIDS-defining condition (HIV)
  📖 0.00   🔧 0.00   **FUD** XXX   Ⓔ

3491F HIV indeterminate (infants of undetermined HIV status born of HIV-infected mothers) (HIV)
  📖 0.00   🔧 0.00   **FUD** XXX   Ⓔ

3492F History of nadir CD4+ cell count <350 cells/mm3 (HIV)
  📖 0.00   🔧 0.00   **FUD** XXX   Ⓔ

3493F No history of nadir CD4+ cell count <350 cells/mm3 and no history of AIDS-defining condition (HIV)
  📖 0.00   🔧 0.00   **FUD** XXX   Ⓔ

3494F CD4+ cell count <200 cells/mm3 (HIV)
  📖 0.00   🔧 0.00   **FUD** XXX   Ⓜ

3495F CD4+ cell count 200 - 499 cells/mm3 (HIV)
  📖 0.00   🔧 0.00   **FUD** XXX   Ⓜ

3496F CD4+ cell count ≥ 500 cells/mm3 (HIV)
  📖 0.00   🔧 0.00   **FUD** XXX   Ⓜ

3497F CD4+ cell percentage <15% (HIV)
  📖 0.00   🔧 0.00   **FUD** XXX   Ⓔ

3498F CD4+ cell percentage ≥ 15% (HIV)
  📖 0.00   🔧 0.00   **FUD** XXX   Ⓔ

3500F CD4+ cell count or CD4+ cell percentage documented as performed (HIV)
  📖 0.00   🔧 0.00   **FUD** XXX   Ⓔ

3502F HIV RNA viral load below limits of quantification (HIV)
  📖 0.00   🔧 0.00   **FUD** XXX   Ⓔ

3503F HIV RNA viral load not below limits of quantification (HIV)
  📖 0.00   🔧 0.00   **FUD** XXX   Ⓔ

3510F Documentation that tuberculosis (TB) screening test performed and results interpreted (HIV) (IBD)
  📖 0.00   🔧 0.00   **FUD** XXX   Ⓜ

3511F Chlamydia and gonorrhea screenings documented as performed (HIV)
  📖 0.00   🔧 0.00   **FUD** XXX   Ⓔ

3512F Syphilis screening documented as performed (HIV)
  📖 0.00   🔧 0.00   **FUD** XXX   Ⓔ

3513F Hepatitis B screening documented as performed (HIV)
  📖 0.00   🔧 0.00   **FUD** XXX   Ⓔ

3514F Hepatitis C screening documented as performed (HIV)
  📖 0.00   🔧 0.00   **FUD** XXX   Ⓔ

3515F Patient has documented immunity to Hepatitis C (HIV)
  📖 0.00   🔧 0.00   **FUD** XXX   Ⓔ

3517F Hepatitis B Virus (HBV) status assessed and results interpreted within one year prior to receiving a first course of anti-TNF (tumor necrosis factor) therapy (IBD)
  📖 0.00   🔧 0.00   **FUD** XXX   Ⓜ

● New Code   ▲ Revised Code   ○ Reinstated   ● New Web Release   ▲ Revised Web Release   Unlisted   Not Covered   # Resequenced
⊘ AMA Mod 51 Exempt   ⑤ Optum Mod 51 Exempt   ⑥⑨ Mod 63 Exempt   ⚡ Non-FDA Drug   ★ Telehealth   Ⓜ Maternity   Ⓐ Age Edit   + Add-on   **AMA:** CPT Asst

3520F Clostridium difficile testing performed (IBD)
📷 0.00 ⚕ 0.00 **FUD** XXX
E

3550F Low risk for thromboembolism (AFIB)
📷 0.00 ⚕ 0.00 **FUD** XXX
E

3551F Intermediate risk for thromboembolism (AFIB)
📷 0.00 ⚕ 0.00 **FUD** XXX
E

3552F High risk for thromboembolism (AFIB)
📷 0.00 ⚕ 0.00 **FUD** XXX
E

3555F Patient had International Normalized Ratio (INR) measurement performed (AFIB)
📷 0.00 ⚕ 0.00 **FUD** XXX
E
AMA: 2010,Jul,3-5

3570F Final report for bone scintigraphy study includes correlation with existing relevant imaging studies (eg, X-ray, MRI, CT) corresponding to the same anatomical region in question (NUC_MED)
📷 0.00 ⚕ 0.00 **FUD** XXX
M

3572F Patient considered to be potentially at risk for fracture in a weight-bearing site (NUC_MED)
📷 0.00 ⚕ 0.00 **FUD** XXX
E

3573F Patient not considered to be potentially at risk for fracture in a weight-bearing site (NUC_MED)
📷 0.00 ⚕ 0.00 **FUD** XXX
E

3650F Electroencephalogram (EEG) ordered, reviewed or requested (EPI)
📷 0.00 ⚕ 0.00 **FUD** XXX
E

3700F Psychiatric disorders or disturbances assessed (Prkns)
📷 0.00 ⚕ 0.00 **FUD** XXX
M

3720F Cognitive impairment or dysfunction assessed (Prkns)
📷 0.00 ⚕ 0.00 **FUD** XXX
M

3725F Screening for depression performed (DEM)
📷 0.00 ⚕ 0.00 **FUD** XXX
M

3750F Patient not receiving dose of corticosteroids greater than or equal to 10mg/day for 60 or greater consecutive days (IBD)
📷 0.00 ⚕ 0.00 **FUD** XXX
E

3751F Electrodiagnostic studies for distal symmetric polyneuropathy conducted (or requested), documented, and reviewed within 6 months of initial evaluation for condition (DSP)
📷 0.00 ⚕ 0.00 **FUD** XXX
E

3752F Electrodiagnostic studies for distal symmetric polyneuropathy not conducted (or requested), documented, or reviewed within 6 months of initial evaluation for condition (DSP)
📷 0.00 ⚕ 0.00 **FUD** XXX
E

3753F Patient has clear clinical symptoms and signs that are highly suggestive of neuropathy AND cannot be attributed to another condition, AND has an obvious cause for the neuropathy (DSP)
📷 0.00 ⚕ 0.00 **FUD** XXX
E

3754F Screening tests for diabetes mellitus reviewed, requested, or ordered (DSP)
📷 0.00 ⚕ 0.00 **FUD** XXX
E

3755F Cognitive and behavioral impairment screening performed (ALS)
📷 0.00 ⚕ 0.00 **FUD** XXX
E

3756F Patient has pseudobulbar affect, sialorrhea, or ALS-related symptoms (ALS)
📷 0.00 ⚕ 0.00 **FUD** XXX
E

3757F Patient does not have pseudobulbar affect, sialorrhea, or ALS-related symptoms (ALS)
📷 0.00 ⚕ 0.00 **FUD** XXX
E

3758F Patient referred for pulmonary function testing or peak cough expiratory flow (ALS)
📷 0.00 ⚕ 0.00 **FUD** XXX
E

3759F Patient screened for dysphagia, weight loss, and impaired nutrition, and results documented (ALS)
📷 0.00 ⚕ 0.00 **FUD** XXX
E

3760F Patient exhibits dysphagia, weight loss, or impaired nutrition (ALS)
📷 0.00 ⚕ 0.00 **FUD** XXX
E

3761F Patient does not exhibit dysphagia, weight loss, or impaired nutrition (ALS)
📷 0.00 ⚕ 0.00 **FUD** XXX
E

3762F Patient is dysarthric (ALS)
📷 0.00 ⚕ 0.00 **FUD** XXX
E

3763F Patient is not dysarthric (ALS)
📷 0.00 ⚕ 0.00 **FUD** XXX
E

3775F Adenoma(s) or other neoplasm detected during screening colonoscopy (SCADR)
📷 0.00 ⚕ 0.00 **FUD** XXX
M

3776F Adenoma(s) or other neoplasm not detected during screening colonoscopy (SCADR)
📷 0.00 ⚕ 0.00 **FUD** XXX
M

4000F-4563F Therapies Provided (Includes Preventive Services)

INCLUDES Behavioral/pharmacologic/procedural therapies
Preventive services including patient education/counseling

4000F Tobacco use cessation intervention, counseling (COPD, CAP, CAD, Asthma) (DM) (PV)
📷 0.00 ⚕ 0.00 **FUD** XXX
E
AMA: 2016,Jan,13; 2015,Jan,16; 2014,Jan,11

4001F Tobacco use cessation intervention, pharmacologic therapy (COPD, CAD, CAP, PV, Asthma) (DM) (PV)
📷 0.00 ⚕ 0.00 **FUD** XXX
E
AMA: 2008,Mar,8-12; 2004,Nov,1

4003F Patient education, written/oral, appropriate for patients with heart failure, performed (NMA-No Measure Associated)
📷 0.00 ⚕ 0.00 **FUD** XXX
E
AMA: 2004,Nov,1

4004F Patient screened for tobacco use and received tobacco cessation intervention (counseling, pharmacotherapy, or both), if identified as a tobacco user (PV, CAD)
📷 0.00 ⚕ 0.00 **FUD** XXX
M

4005F Pharmacologic therapy (other than minerals/vitamins) for osteoporosis prescribed (OP) (IBD)
📷 0.00 ⚕ 0.00 **FUD** XXX
M

4008F Beta-blocker therapy prescribed or currently being taken (CAD,HF)
📷 0.00 ⚕ 0.00 **FUD** XXX
M

4010F Angiotensin Converting Enzyme (ACE) Inhibitor or Angiotensin Receptor Blocker (ARB) therapy prescribed or currently being taken (CAD, CKD, HF) (DM)
📷 0.00 ⚕ 0.00 **FUD** XXX
M

4011F Oral antiplatelet therapy prescribed (CAD)
📷 0.00 ⚕ 0.00 **FUD** XXX
E
AMA: 2004,Nov,1

4012F Warfarin therapy prescribed (NMA-No Measure Associated)
📷 0.00 ⚕ 0.00 **FUD** XXX
E

4013F Statin therapy prescribed or currently being taken (CAD)
📷 0.00 ⚕ 0.00 **FUD** XXX
E

4014F Written discharge instructions provided to heart failure patients discharged home (Instructions include all of the following components: activity level, diet, discharge medications, follow-up appointment, weight monitoring, what to do if symptoms worsen) (NMA-No Measure Associated)
📷 0.00 ⚕ 0.00 **FUD** XXX
E

4015F　Persistent asthma, preferred long term control medication or an acceptable alternative treatment, prescribed (NMA-No Measure Associated)

　　　　🔢 0.00　　✂ 0.00　　**FUD** XXX　　　　　E

　　　　EXCLUDES　Use of code with modifier 1P
　　　　Code also modifier 2P for patient reasons for not prescribing

4016F　Anti-inflammatory/analgesic agent prescribed (OA) (Use for prescribed or continued medication[s], including over-the-counter medication[s])

　　　　🔢 0.00　　✂ 0.00　　**FUD** XXX　　　　　E

　　　　INCLUDES　Over-the-counter medication(s)
　　　　Prescribed/continued medication(s)

4017F　Gastrointestinal prophylaxis for NSAID use prescribed (OA)

　　　　🔢 0.00　　✂ 0.00　　**FUD** XXX　　　　　E

4018F　Therapeutic exercise for the involved joint(s) instructed or physical or occupational therapy prescribed (OA)

　　　　🔢 0.00　　✂ 0.00　　**FUD** XXX　　　　　E

4019F　Documentation of receipt of counseling on exercise and either both calcium and vitamin D use or counseling regarding both calcium and vitamin D use (OP)

　　　　🔢 0.00　　✂ 0.00　　**FUD** XXX　　　　　E

4025F　Inhaled bronchodilator prescribed (COPD)

　　　　🔢 0.00　　✂ 0.00　　**FUD** XXX　　　　　M

4030F　Long-term oxygen therapy prescribed (more than 15 hours per day) (COPD)

　　　　🔢 0.00　　✂ 0.00　　**FUD** XXX　　　　　E

4033F　Pulmonary rehabilitation exercise training recommended (COPD)

　　　　🔢 0.00　　✂ 0.00　　**FUD** XXX　　　　　E

　　　　Code also dyspnea assessed, present (1019F)

4035F　Influenza immunization recommended (COPD) (IBD)

　　　　🔢 0.00　　✂ 0.00　　**FUD** XXX　　　　　E

　　　　AMA: 2008,Mar,8-12

4037F　Influenza immunization ordered or administered (COPD, PV, CKD, ESRD)(IBD)

　　　　🔢 0.00　　✂ 0.00　　**FUD** XXX　　　　　E

　　　　AMA: 2008,Mar,8-12

4040F　Pneumococcal vaccine administered or previously received (COPD) (PV), (IBD)

　　　　🔢 0.00　　✂ 0.00　　**FUD** XXX　　　　　M

　　　　AMA: 2008,Mar,8-12

4041F　Documentation of order for cefazolin OR cefuroxime for antimicrobial prophylaxis (PERI 2)

　　　　🔢 0.00　　✂ 0.00　　**FUD** XXX　　　　　E

4042F　Documentation that prophylactic antibiotics were neither given within 4 hours prior to surgical incision nor given intraoperatively (PERI 2)

　　　　🔢 0.00　　✂ 0.00　　**FUD** XXX　　　　　M

4043F　Documentation that an order was given to discontinue prophylactic antibiotics within 48 hours of surgical end time, cardiac procedures (PERI 2)

　　　　🔢 0.00　　✂ 0.00　　**FUD** XXX　　　　　E

4044F　Documentation that an order was given for venous thromboembolism (VTE) prophylaxis to be given within 24 hours prior to incision time or 24 hours after surgery end time (PERI 2)

　　　　🔢 0.00　　✂ 0.00　　**FUD** XXX　　　　　M

4045F　Appropriate empiric antibiotic prescribed (CAP), (EM)

　　　　🔢 0.00　　✂ 0.00　　**FUD** XXX　　　　　E

4046F　Documentation that prophylactic antibiotics were given within 4 hours prior to surgical incision or given intraoperatively (PERI 2)

　　　　🔢 0.00　　✂ 0.00　　**FUD** XXX　　　　　M

4047F　Documentation of order for prophylactic parenteral antibiotics to be given within 1 hour (if fluoroquinolone or vancomycin, 2 hours) prior to surgical incision (or start of procedure when no incision is required) (PERI 2)

　　　　🔢 0.00　　✂ 0.00　　**FUD** XXX　　　　　E

4048F　Documentation that administration of prophylactic parenteral antibiotic was initiated within 1 hour (if fluoroquinolone or vancomycin, 2 hours) prior to surgical incision (or start of procedure when no incision is required) as ordered (PERI 2)

　　　　🔢 0.00　　✂ 0.00　　**FUD** XXX　　　　　E

4049F　Documentation that order was given to discontinue prophylactic antibiotics within 24 hours of surgical end time, non-cardiac procedure (PERI 2)

　　　　🔢 0.00　　✂ 0.00　　**FUD** XXX　　　　　M

4050F　Hypertension plan of care documented as appropriate (NMA-No Measure Associated)

　　　　🔢 0.00　　✂ 0.00　　**FUD** XXX　　　　　E

4051F　Referred for an arteriovenous (AV) fistula (ESRD, CKD)

　　　　🔢 0.00　　✂ 0.00　　**FUD** XXX　　　　　E

　　　　AMA: 2008,Mar,8-12

4052F　Hemodialysis via functioning arteriovenous (AV) fistula (ESRD)

　　　　🔢 0.00　　✂ 0.00　　**FUD** XXX　　　　　E

　　　　AMA: 2008,Mar,8-12

4053F　Hemodialysis via functioning arteriovenous (AV) graft (ESRD)

　　　　🔢 0.00　　✂ 0.00　　**FUD** XXX　　　　　E

　　　　AMA: 2008,Mar,8-12

4054F　Hemodialysis via catheter (ESRD)

　　　　🔢 0.00　　✂ 0.00　　**FUD** XXX　　　　　E

　　　　AMA: 2008,Mar,8-12

4055F　Patient receiving peritoneal dialysis (ESRD)

　　　　🔢 0.00　　✂ 0.00　　**FUD** XXX　　　　　E

　　　　AMA: 2008,Mar,8-12

4056F　Appropriate oral rehydration solution recommended (PAG)

　　　　🔢 0.00　　✂ 0.00　　**FUD** XXX　　　　　E

4058F　Pediatric gastroenteritis education provided to caregiver (PAG)

　　　　🔢 0.00　　✂ 0.00　　**FUD** XXX　　　　　E

4060F　Psychotherapy services provided (MDD, MDD ADOL)

　　　　🔢 0.00　　✂ 0.00　　**FUD** XXX　　　　　E

4062F　Patient referral for psychotherapy documented (MDD, MDD ADOL)

　　　　🔢 0.00　　✂ 0.00　　**FUD** XXX　　　　　E

4063F　Antidepressant pharmacotherapy considered and not prescribed (MDD ADOL)

　　　　🔢 0.00　　✂ 0.00　　**FUD** XXX　　　　　E

4064F　Antidepressant pharmacotherapy prescribed (MDD, MDD ADOL)

　　　　🔢 0.00　　✂ 0.00　　**FUD** XXX　　　　　E

4065F　Antipsychotic pharmacotherapy prescribed (MDD)

　　　　🔢 0.00　　✂ 0.00　　**FUD** XXX　　　　　E

4066F　Electroconvulsive therapy (ECT) provided (MDD)

　　　　🔢 0.00　　✂ 0.00　　**FUD** XXX　　　　　E

4067F　Patient referral for electroconvulsive therapy (ECT) documented (MDD)

　　　　🔢 0.00　　✂ 0.00　　**FUD** XXX　　　　　E

4069F　Venous thromboembolism (VTE) prophylaxis received (IBD)

　　　　🔢 0.00　　✂ 0.00　　**FUD** XXX　　　　　E

4070F Deep vein thrombosis (DVT) prophylaxis received by end of hospital day 2 (STR)
📁 0.00   ⅄ 0.00   **FUD** XXX   E

4073F Oral antiplatelet therapy prescribed at discharge (STR)
📁 0.00   ⅄ 0.00   **FUD** XXX   E

4075F Anticoagulant therapy prescribed at discharge (STR)
📁 0.00   ⅄ 0.00   **FUD** XXX   E

4077F Documentation that tissue plasminogen activator (t-PA) administration was considered (STR)
📁 0.00   ⅄ 0.00   **FUD** XXX   E

4079F Documentation that rehabilitation services were considered (STR)
📁 0.00   ⅄ 0.00   **FUD** XXX   E

4084F Aspirin received within 24 hours before emergency department arrival or during emergency department stay (EM)
📁 0.00   ⅄ 0.00   **FUD** XXX   E

4086F Aspirin or clopidogrel prescribed or currently being taken (CAD)
📁 0.00   ⅄ 0.00   **FUD** XXX   M

4090F Patient receiving erythropoietin therapy (HEM)
📁 0.00   ⅄ 0.00   **FUD** XXX   M
AMA: 2008,Mar,8-12

4095F Patient not receiving erythropoietin therapy (HEM)
📁 0.00   ⅄ 0.00   **FUD** XXX   E
AMA: 2008,Mar,8-12

4100F Bisphosphonate therapy, intravenous, ordered or received (HEM)
📁 0.00   ⅄ 0.00   **FUD** XXX   M
AMA: 2008,Mar,8-12

4110F Internal mammary artery graft performed for primary, isolated coronary artery bypass graft procedure (CABG)
📁 0.00   ⅄ 0.00   **FUD** XXX   M

4115F Beta blocker administered within 24 hours prior to surgical incision (CABG)
📁 0.00   ⅄ 0.00   **FUD** XXX   M

4120F Antibiotic prescribed or dispensed (URI, PHAR), (A-BRONCH)
📁 0.00   ⅄ 0.00   **FUD** XXX   M
AMA: 2008,Mar,8-12

4124F Antibiotic neither prescribed nor dispensed (URI, PHAR), (A-BRONCH)
📁 0.00   ⅄ 0.00   **FUD** XXX   M
AMA: 2008,Mar,8-12

4130F Topical preparations (including OTC) prescribed for acute otitis externa (AOE)
📁 0.00   ⅄ 0.00   **FUD** XXX   M
AMA: 2010,Jan,6-7; 2008,Mar,8-12

4131F Systemic antimicrobial therapy prescribed (AOE)
📁 0.00   ⅄ 0.00   **FUD** XXX   M
AMA: 2008,Mar,8-12

4132F Systemic antimicrobial therapy not prescribed (AOE)
📁 0.00   ⅄ 0.00   **FUD** XXX   M
AMA: 2008,Mar,8-12

4133F Antihistamines or decongestants prescribed or recommended (OME)
📁 0.00   ⅄ 0.00   **FUD** XXX   E
AMA: 2008,Mar,8-12

4134F Antihistamines or decongestants neither prescribed nor recommended (OME)
📁 0.00   ⅄ 0.00   **FUD** XXX   E
AMA: 2008,Mar,8-12

4135F Systemic corticosteroids prescribed (OME)
📁 0.00   ⅄ 0.00   **FUD** XXX   E
AMA: 2008,Mar,8-12

4136F Systemic corticosteroids not prescribed (OME)
📁 0.00   ⅄ 0.00   **FUD** XXX   E
AMA: 2008,Mar,8-12

4140F Inhaled corticosteroids prescribed (Asthma)
📁 0.00   ⅄ 0.00   **FUD** XXX   M

4142F Corticosteroid sparing therapy prescribed (IBD)
📁 0.00   ⅄ 0.00   **FUD** XXX   M

4144F Alternative long-term control medication prescribed (Asthma)
📁 0.00   ⅄ 0.00   **FUD** XXX   M

4145F Two or more anti-hypertensive agents prescribed or currently being taken (CAD, HTN)
📁 0.00   ⅄ 0.00   **FUD** XXX   E

4148F Hepatitis A vaccine injection administered or previously received (HEP-C)
📁 0.00   ⅄ 0.00   **FUD** XXX   M

4149F Hepatitis B vaccine injection administered or previously received (HEP-C, HIV) (IBD)
📁 0.00   ⅄ 0.00   **FUD** XXX   E

4150F Patient receiving antiviral treatment for Hepatitis C (HEP-C)
📁 0.00   ⅄ 0.00   **FUD** XXX   E
AMA: 2008,Mar,8-12

▲ **4151F** Patient did not start or is not receiving antiviral treatment for Hepatitis C during the measurement period (HEP-C)
📁 0.00   ⅄ 0.00   **FUD** XXX   M
AMA: 2008,Mar,8-12

4153F Combination peginterferon and ribavirin therapy prescribed (HEP-C)
📁 0.00   ⅄ 0.00   **FUD** XXX   E
AMA: 2008,Mar,8-12

4155F Hepatitis A vaccine series previously received (HEP-C)
📁 0.00   ⅄ 0.00   **FUD** XXX   E
AMA: 2008,Mar,8-12

4157F Hepatitis B vaccine series previously received (HEP-C)
📁 0.00   ⅄ 0.00   **FUD** XXX   E
AMA: 2008,Mar,8-12

4158F Patient counseled about risks of alcohol use (HEP-C)
📁 0.00   ⅄ 0.00   **FUD** XXX   E
AMA: 2008,Mar,8-12

4159F Counseling regarding contraception received prior to initiation of antiviral treatment (HEP-C)
📁 0.00   ⅄ 0.00   **FUD** XXX   E
AMA: 2008,Mar,8-12

4163F Patient counseling at a minimum on all of the following treatment options for clinically localized prostate cancer: active surveillance, and interstitial prostate brachytherapy, and external beam radiotherapy, and radical prostatectomy, provided prior to initiation of treatment (PRCA)
📁 0.00   ⅄ 0.00   **FUD** XXX   E
AMA: 2008,Mar,8-12

4164F Adjuvant (ie, in combination with external beam radiotherapy to the prostate for prostate cancer) hormonal therapy (gonadotropin-releasing hormone [GnRH] agonist or antagonist) prescribed/administered (PRCA)
📁 0.00   ⅄ 0.00   **FUD** XXX   M
AMA: 2008,Mar,8-12

4165F 3-dimensional conformal radiotherapy (3D-CRT) or intensity modulated radiation therapy (IMRT) received (PRCA)
📁 0.00   ⅄ 0.00   **FUD** XXX   E
AMA: 2008,Mar,8-12

26/TC PC/TC Only   A2-Z3 ASC Payment   50 Bilateral   ♂ Male Only   ♀ Female Only   📁 Facility RVU   ⅄ Non-Facility RVU   CCI
FUD Follow-up Days   CMS: IOM (Pub 100)   A-Y OPPSI   80/80 Surg Assist Allowed / w/Doc   📋 Lab Crosswalk   ⚡ Radiology Crosswalk   CLIA

4167F   Head of bed elevation (30-45 degrees) on first ventilator day ordered (CRIT)
　　　🚑 0.00　⚕ 0.00　**FUD** XXX　　　　　　　E
　　　AMA: 2008,Mar,8-12

4168F   Patient receiving care in the intensive care unit (ICU) and receiving mechanical ventilation, 24 hours or less (CRIT)
　　　🚑 0.00　⚕ 0.00　**FUD** XXX　　　　　　　E
　　　AMA: 2008,Mar,8-12

4169F   Patient either not receiving care in the intensive care unit (ICU) OR not receiving mechanical ventilation OR receiving mechanical ventilation greater than 24 hours (CRIT)
　　　🚑 0.00　⚕ 0.00　**FUD** XXX　　　　　　　E
　　　AMA: 2008,Mar,8-12

4171F   Patient receiving erythropoiesis-stimulating agents (ESA) therapy (CKD)
　　　🚑 0.00　⚕ 0.00　**FUD** XXX　　　　　　　E
　　　AMA: 2008,Mar,8-12

4172F   Patient not receiving erythropoiesis-stimulating agents (ESA) therapy (CKD)
　　　🚑 0.00　⚕ 0.00　**FUD** XXX　　　　　　　E
　　　AMA: 2008,Mar,8-12

4174F   Counseling about the potential impact of glaucoma on visual functioning and quality of life, and importance of treatment adherence provided to patient and/or caregiver(s) (EC)
　　　🚑 0.00　⚕ 0.00　**FUD** XXX　　　　　　　E
　　　AMA: 2008,Mar,8-12

4175F   Best-corrected visual acuity of 20/40 or better (distance or near) achieved within the 90 days following cataract surgery (EC)
　　　🚑 0.00　⚕ 0.00　**FUD** XXX　　　　　　　M
　　　AMA: 2008,Mar,8-12

4176F   Counseling about value of protection from UV light and lack of proven efficacy of nutritional supplements in prevention or progression of cataract development provided to patient and/or caregiver(s) (NMA-No Measure Associated)
　　　🚑 0.00　⚕ 0.00　**FUD** XXX　　　　　　　E

4177F   Counseling about the benefits and/or risks of the Age-Related Eye Disease Study (AREDS) formulation for preventing progression of age-related macular degeneration (AMD) provided to patient and/or caregiver(s) (EC)
　　　🚑 0.00　⚕ 0.00　**FUD** XXX　　　　　　　M
　　　AMA: 2008,Mar,8-12

4178F   Anti-D immune globulin received between 26 and 30 weeks gestation (Pre-Cr)　　　　　　　　　　　　　　　M
　　　🚑 0.00　⚕ 0.00　**FUD** XXX　　　　　　　E
　　　AMA: 2008,Mar,8-12

4179F   Tamoxifen or aromatase inhibitor (AI) prescribed (ONC)
　　　🚑 0.00　⚕ 0.00　**FUD** XXX　　　　　　　M
　　　AMA: 2008,Mar,8-12

4180F   Adjuvant chemotherapy referred, prescribed, or previously received for Stage III colon cancer (ONC)
　　　🚑 0.00　⚕ 0.00　**FUD** XXX　　　　　　　E
　　　AMA: 2008,Mar,8-12

4181F   Conformal radiation therapy received (NMA-No Measure Associated)
　　　🚑 0.00　⚕ 0.00　**FUD** XXX　　　　　　　E

4182F   Conformal radiation therapy not received (NMA-No Measure Associated)
　　　🚑 0.00　⚕ 0.00　**FUD** XXX　　　　　　　E

4185F   Continuous (12-months) therapy with proton pump inhibitor (PPI) or histamine H2 receptor antagonist (H2RA) received (GERD)
　　　🚑 0.00　⚕ 0.00　**FUD** XXX　　　　　　　E
　　　AMA: 2008,Mar,8-12

4186F   No continuous (12-months) therapy with either proton pump inhibitor (PPI) or histamine H2 receptor antagonist (H2RA) received (GERD)
　　　🚑 0.00　⚕ 0.00　**FUD** XXX　　　　　　　E
　　　AMA: 2008,Mar,8-12

4187F   Disease modifying anti-rheumatic drug therapy prescribed or dispensed (RA)
　　　🚑 0.00　⚕ 0.00　**FUD** XXX　　　　　　　M

4188F   Appropriate angiotensin converting enzyme (ACE)/angiotensin receptor blockers (ARB) therapeutic monitoring test ordered or performed (AM)
　　　🚑 0.00　⚕ 0.00　**FUD** XXX　　　　　　　E

4189F   Appropriate digoxin therapeutic monitoring test ordered or performed (AM)
　　　🚑 0.00　⚕ 0.00　**FUD** XXX　　　　　　　E
　　　AMA: 2008,Mar,8-12

4190F   Appropriate diuretic therapeutic monitoring test ordered or performed (AM)
　　　🚑 0.00　⚕ 0.00　**FUD** XXX　　　　　　　E
　　　AMA: 2008,Mar,8-12

4191F   Appropriate anticonvulsant therapeutic monitoring test ordered or performed (AM)
　　　🚑 0.00　⚕ 0.00　**FUD** XXX　　　　　　　E
　　　AMA: 2008,Mar,8-12

4192F   Patient not receiving glucocorticoid therapy (RA)
　　　🚑 0.00　⚕ 0.00　**FUD** XXX　　　　　　　M

4193F   Patient receiving <10 mg daily prednisone (or equivalent), or RA activity is worsening, or glucocorticoid use is for less than 6 months (RA)
　　　　　　　　　　　　　　　　　　　　　　　M

4194F   Patient receiving ≥10 mg daily prednisone (or equivalent) for longer than 6 months, and improvement or no change in disease activity (RA)
　　　🚑 0.00　⚕ 0.00　**FUD** XXX　　　　　　　M

4195F   Patient receiving first-time biologic disease modifying anti-rheumatic drug therapy for rheumatoid arthritis (RA)
　　　🚑 0.00　⚕ 0.00　**FUD** XXX　　　　　　　M

4196F   Patient not receiving first-time biologic disease modifying anti-rheumatic drug therapy for rheumatoid arthritis (RA)
　　　🚑 0.00　⚕ 0.00　**FUD** XXX　　　　　　　M

4200F   External beam radiotherapy as primary therapy to prostate with or without nodal irradiation (PRCA)
　　　🚑 0.00　⚕ 0.00　**FUD** XXX　　　　　　　E
　　　AMA: 2008,Mar,8-12

4201F   External beam radiotherapy with or without nodal irradiation as adjuvant or salvage therapy for prostate cancer patient (PRCA)
　　　🚑 0.00　⚕ 0.00　**FUD** XXX　　　　　　　E
　　　AMA: 2008,Mar,8-12

4210F   Angiotensin converting enzyme (ACE) or angiotensin receptor blockers (ARB) medication therapy for 6 months or more (MM)
　　　🚑 0.00　⚕ 0.00　**FUD** XXX　　　　　　　E
　　　AMA: 2008,Mar,8-12

4220F   Digoxin medication therapy for 6 months or more (MM)
　　　🚑 0.00　⚕ 0.00　**FUD** XXX　　　　　　　E
　　　AMA: 2008,Mar,8-12

4221F   Diuretic medication therapy for 6 months or more (MM)
　　　🚑 0.00　⚕ 0.00　**FUD** XXX　　　　　　　E
　　　AMA: 2008,Mar,8-12

4230F   Anticonvulsant medication therapy for 6 months or more (MM)
　　　🚑 0.00　⚕ 0.00　**FUD** XXX　　　　　　　E
　　　AMA: 2008,Mar,8-12

● New Code　▲ Revised Code　○ Reinstated　● New Web Release　▲ Revised Web Release　Unlisted　Not Covered　# Resequenced
⊘ AMA Mod 51 Exempt　⑪ Optum Mod 51 Exempt　⑥³ Mod 63 Exempt　✎ Non-FDA Drug　★ Telehealth　Ⓜ Maternity　🅰 Age Edit　+ Add-on　**AMA:** CPT Asst

4240F Instruction in therapeutic exercise with follow-up provided to patients during episode of back pain lasting longer than 12 weeks (BkP)

🔲 0.00   🔲 0.00   **FUD** XXX   E

AMA: 2008,Mar,8-12

4242F Counseling for supervised exercise program provided to patients during episode of back pain lasting longer than 12 weeks (BkP)

🔲 0.00   🔲 0.00   **FUD** XXX   E

AMA: 2008,Mar,8-12

4245F Patient counseled during the initial visit to maintain or resume normal activities (BkP)

🔲 0.00   🔲 0.00   **FUD** XXX   E

AMA: 2008,Mar,8-12

4248F Patient counseled during the initial visit for an episode of back pain against bed rest lasting 4 days or longer (BkP)

🔲 0.00   🔲 0.00   **FUD** XXX   E

AMA: 2008,Mar,8-12

4250F Active warming used intraoperatively for the purpose of maintaining normothermia, or at least 1 body temperature equal to or greater than 36 degrees Centigrade (or 96.8 degrees Fahrenheit) recorded within the 30 minutes immediately before or the 15 minutes immediately after anesthesia end time (CRIT)

🔲 0.00   🔲 0.00   **FUD** XXX   E

AMA: 2008,Mar,8-12

4255F Duration of general or neuraxial anesthesia 60 minutes or longer, as documented in the anesthesia record (CRIT) (Peri2)

🔲 0.00   🔲 0.00   **FUD** XXX   M

4256F Duration of general or neuraxial anesthesia less than 60 minutes, as documented in the anesthesia record (CRIT) (Peri2)

🔲 0.00   🔲 0.00   **FUD** XXX   E

4260F Wound surface culture technique used (CWC)

🔲 0.00   🔲 0.00   **FUD** XXX   E

4261F Technique other than surface culture of the wound exudate used (eg, Levine/deep swab technique, semi-quantitative or quantitative swab technique) or wound surface culture technique not used (CWC)

🔲 0.00   🔲 0.00   **FUD** XXX   E

4265F Use of wet to dry dressings prescribed or recommended (CWC)

🔲 0.00   🔲 0.00   **FUD** XXX   E

4266F Use of wet to dry dressings neither prescribed nor recommended (CWC)

🔲 0.00   🔲 0.00   **FUD** XXX   E

4267F Compression therapy prescribed (CWC)

🔲 0.00   🔲 0.00   **FUD** XXX   E

4268F Patient education regarding the need for long term compression therapy including interval replacement of compression stockings received (CWC)

🔲 0.00   🔲 0.00   **FUD** XXX   E

4269F Appropriate method of offloading (pressure relief) prescribed (CWC)

🔲 0.00   🔲 0.00   **FUD** XXX   E

4270F Patient receiving potent antiretroviral therapy for 6 months or longer (HIV)

🔲 0.00   🔲 0.00   **FUD** XXX   E

4271F Patient receiving potent antiretroviral therapy for less than 6 months or not receiving potent antiretroviral therapy (HIV)

🔲 0.00   🔲 0.00   **FUD** XXX   E

4274F Influenza immunization administered or previously received (HIV) (P-ESRD)

🔲 0.00   🔲 0.00   **FUD** XXX   E

4276F Potent antiretroviral therapy prescribed (HIV)

🔲 0.00   🔲 0.00   **FUD** XXX   E

4279F Pneumocystis jiroveci pneumonia prophylaxis prescribed (HIV)

🔲 0.00   🔲 0.00   **FUD** XXX   E

4280F Pneumocystis jiroveci pneumonia prophylaxis prescribed within 3 months of low CD4+ cell count or percentage (HIV)

🔲 0.00   🔲 0.00   **FUD** XXX   E

4290F Patient screened for injection drug use (HIV)

🔲 0.00   🔲 0.00   **FUD** XXX   E

4293F Patient screened for high-risk sexual behavior (HIV)

🔲 0.00   🔲 0.00   **FUD** XXX   E

4300F Patient receiving warfarin therapy for nonvalvular atrial fibrillation or atrial flutter (AFIB)

🔲 0.00   🔲 0.00   **FUD** XXX   E

4301F Patient not receiving warfarin therapy for nonvalvular atrial fibrillation or atrial flutter (AFIB)

🔲 0.00   🔲 0.00   **FUD** XXX   E

4305F Patient education regarding appropriate foot care and daily inspection of the feet received (CWC)

🔲 0.00   🔲 0.00   **FUD** XXX   E

4306F Patient counseled regarding psychosocial and pharmacologic treatment options for opioid addiction (SUD)

🔲 0.00   🔲 0.00   **FUD** XXX   E

4320F Patient counseled regarding psychosocial and pharmacologic treatment options for alcohol dependence (SUD)

🔲 0.00   🔲 0.00   **FUD** XXX   E

4322F Caregiver provided with education and referred to additional resources for support (DEM)

🔲 0.00   🔲 0.00   **FUD** XXX   M

4324F Patient (or caregiver) queried about Parkinson's disease medication related motor complications (Prkns)

🔲 0.00   🔲 0.00   **FUD** XXX   E

4325F Medical and surgical treatment options reviewed with patient (or caregiver) (Prkns)

🔲 0.00   🔲 0.00   **FUD** XXX   M

4326F Patient (or caregiver) queried about symptoms of autonomic dysfunction (Prkns)

🔲 0.00   🔲 0.00   **FUD** XXX   E

4328F Patient (or caregiver) queried about sleep disturbances (Prkns)

🔲 0.00   🔲 0.00   **FUD** XXX   M

4330F Counseling about epilepsy specific safety issues provided to patient (or caregiver(s)) (EPI)

🔲 0.00   🔲 0.00   **FUD** XXX   E

4340F Counseling for women of childbearing potential with epilepsy (EPI)

🔲 0.00   🔲 0.00   **FUD** XXX   M

4350F Counseling provided on symptom management, end of life decisions, and palliation (DEM)

🔲 0.00   🔲 0.00   **FUD** XXX   E

4400F Rehabilitative therapy options discussed with patient (or caregiver) (Prkns)

🔲 0.00   🔲 0.00   **FUD** XXX   M

4450F Self-care education provided to patient (HF)

🔲 0.00   🔲 0.00   **FUD** XXX   E

4470F Implantable cardioverter-defibrillator (ICD) counseling provided (HF)

🔲 0.00   🔲 0.00   **FUD** XXX   E

4480F Patient receiving ACE inhibitor/ARB therapy and beta-blocker therapy for 3 months or longer (HF)
🔲 0.00   ⚕ 0.00   **FUD** XXX   E

4481F Patient receiving ACE inhibitor/ARB therapy and beta-blocker therapy for less than 3 months or patient not receiving ACE inhibitor/ARB therapy and beta-blocker therapy (HF)
🔲 0.00   ⚕ 0.00   **FUD** XXX   E

4500F Referred to an outpatient cardiac rehabilitation program (CAD)
🔲 0.00   ⚕ 0.00   **FUD** XXX   M

4510F Previous cardiac rehabilitation for qualifying cardiac event completed (CAD)
🔲 0.00   ⚕ 0.00   **FUD** XXX   M

4525F Neuropsychiatric intervention ordered (DEM)
🔲 0.00   ⚕ 0.00   **FUD** XXX   M

4526F Neuropsychiatric intervention received (DEM)
🔲 0.00   ⚕ 0.00   **FUD** XXX   M

4540F Disease modifying pharmacotherapy discussed (ALS)
🔲 0.00   ⚕ 0.00   **FUD** XXX   E

4541F Patient offered treatment for pseudobulbar affect, sialorrhea, or ALS-related symptoms (ALS)
🔲 0.00   ⚕ 0.00   **FUD** XXX   E

4550F Options for noninvasive respiratory support discussed with patient (ALS)
🔲 0.00   ⚕ 0.00   **FUD** XXX   E

4551F Nutritional support offered (ALS)
🔲 0.00   ⚕ 0.00   **FUD** XXX   E

4552F Patient offered referral to a speech language pathologist (ALS)
🔲 0.00   ⚕ 0.00   **FUD** XXX   E

4553F Patient offered assistance in planning for end of life issues (ALS)
🔲 0.00   ⚕ 0.00   **FUD** XXX   E

4554F Patient received inhalational anesthetic agent (Peri2)
🔲 0.00   ⚕ 0.00   **FUD** XXX   M

4555F Patient did not receive inhalational anesthetic agent (Peri2)
🔲 0.00   ⚕ 0.00   **FUD** XXX   E

4556F Patient exhibits 3 or more risk factors for post-operative nausea and vomiting (Peri2)
🔲 0.00   ⚕ 0.00   **FUD** XXX   M

4557F Patient does not exhibit 3 or more risk factors for post-operative nausea and vomiting (Peri2)
🔲 0.00   ⚕ 0.00   **FUD** XXX   E

4558F Patient received at least 2 prophylactic pharmacologic anti-emetic agents of different classes preoperatively and intraoperatively (Peri2)
🔲 0.00   ⚕ 0.00   **FUD** XXX   M

4559F At least 1 body temperature measurement equal to or greater than 35.5 degrees Celsius (or 95.9 degrees Fahrenheit) recorded within the 30 minutes immediately before or the 15 minutes immediately after anesthesia end time (Peri2)
🔲 0.00   ⚕ 0.00   **FUD** XXX   M

4560F Anesthesia technique did not involve general or neuraxial anesthesia (Peri2)
🔲 0.00   ⚕ 0.00   **FUD** XXX   E

4561F Patient has a coronary artery stent (Peri2)
🔲 0.00   ⚕ 0.00   **FUD** XXX   E

4562F Patient does not have a coronary artery stent (Peri2)
🔲 0.00   ⚕ 0.00   **FUD** XXX   E

4563F Patient received aspirin within 24 hours prior to anesthesia start time (Peri2)
🔲 0.00   ⚕ 0.00   **FUD** XXX   E

5005F-5250F Results Conveyed and Documented

INCLUDES   Patient's:
    Functional status
    Morbidity/mortality
    Satisfaction/experience with care
    Review/communication of test results to patients

5005F Patient counseled on self-examination for new or changing moles (ML)
🔲 0.00   ⚕ 0.00   **FUD** XXX   E
AMA: 2008,Mar,8-12

5010F Findings of dilated macular or fundus exam communicated to the physician or other qualified health care professional managing the diabetes care (EC)
🔲 0.00   ⚕ 0.00   **FUD** XXX   M

5015F Documentation of communication that a fracture occurred and that the patient was or should be tested or treated for osteoporosis (OP)
🔲 0.00   ⚕ 0.00   **FUD** XXX   M

5020F Treatment summary report communicated to physician(s) or other qualified health care professional(s) managing continuing care and to the patient within 1 month of completing treatment (ONC)
🔲 0.00   ⚕ 0.00   **FUD** XXX   E
AMA: 2008,Mar,8-12

5050F Treatment plan communicated to provider(s) managing continuing care within 1 month of diagnosis (ML)
🔲 0.00   ⚕ 0.00   **FUD** XXX   M
AMA: 2008,Mar,8-12

5060F Findings from diagnostic mammogram communicated to practice managing patient's on-going care within 3 business days of exam interpretation (RAD)
🔲 0.00   ⚕ 0.00   **FUD** XXX   E N1
AMA: 2008,Mar,8-12

5062F Findings from diagnostic mammogram communicated to the patient within 5 days of exam interpretation (RAD)
🔲 0.00   ⚕ 0.00   **FUD** XXX   E
AMA: 2008,Mar,8-12

5100F Potential risk for fracture communicated to the referring physician or other qualified health care professional within 24 hours of completion of the imaging study (NUC_MED)
🔲 0.00   ⚕ 0.00   **FUD** XXX   E

5200F Consideration of referral for a neurological evaluation of appropriateness for surgical therapy for intractable epilepsy within the past 3 years (EPI)
🔲 0.00   ⚕ 0.00   **FUD** XXX   E

5250F Asthma discharge plan provided to patient (Asthma)
🔲 0.00   ⚕ 0.00   **FUD** XXX   E

6005F-6150F Elements Related to Patient Safety Processes

INCLUDES   Patient safety practices

6005F Rationale (eg, severity of illness and safety) for level of care (eg, home, hospital) documented (CAP)
🔲 0.00   ⚕ 0.00   **FUD** XXX   E
AMA: 2016,Jan,13; 2015,Jan,16; 2014,Jan,11

6010F Dysphagia screening conducted prior to order for or receipt of any foods, fluids, or medication by mouth (STR)
🔲 0.00   ⚕ 0.00   **FUD** XXX   E

6015F Patient receiving or eligible to receive foods, fluids, or medication by mouth (STR)
🔲 0.00   ⚕ 0.00   **FUD** XXX   E

6020F NPO (nothing by mouth) ordered (STR)
🔲 0.00   ⚕ 0.00   **FUD** XXX   E

● New Code   ▲ Revised Code   ○ Reinstated   ● New Web Release   ▲ Revised Web Release   Unlisted   Not Covered   # Resequenced
⊘ AMA Mod 51 Exempt   ⑤ Optum Mod 51 Exempt   ⊚ Mod 63 Exempt   ⁄ Non-FDA Drug   ★ Telehealth   M Maternity   A Age Edit   + Add-on   **AMA:** CPT Asst

6030F All elements of maximal sterile barrier technique, hand hygiene, skin preparation and, if ultrasound is used, **sterile ultrasound techniques followed (CRIT)**
🚑 0.00 ⚐ 0.00 **FUD** XXX   M
AMA: 2008,Mar,8-12

6040F Use of appropriate radiation dose reduction devices OR manual techniques for appropriate moderation of exposure, documented (RAD)
🚑 0.00 ⚐ 0.00 **FUD** XXX   E

6045F Radiation exposure or exposure time in final report for procedure using fluoroscopy, documented (RAD)
🚑 0.00 ⚐ 0.00 **FUD** XXX   E
AMA: 2008,Mar,8-12

6070F Patient queried and counseled about anti-epileptic drug (AED) side effects (EPI)
🚑 0.00 ⚐ 0.00 **FUD** XXX   E

6080F Patient (or caregiver) queried about falls (Prkns, DSP)
🚑 0.00 ⚐ 0.00 **FUD** XXX   E

6090F Patient (or caregiver) counseled about safety issues appropriate to patient's stage of disease (Prkns)
🚑 0.00 ⚐ 0.00 **FUD** XXX   E

6100F Timeout to verify correct patient, correct site, and correct procedure, documented (PATH)
🚑 0.00 ⚐ 0.00 **FUD** XXX   E

6101F Safety counseling for dementia provided (DEM)
🚑 0.00 ⚐ 0.00 **FUD** XXX   M

6102F Safety counseling for dementia ordered (DEM)
🚑 0.00 ⚐ 0.00 **FUD** XXX   M

6110F Counseling provided regarding risks of driving and the alternatives to driving (DEM)
🚑 0.00 ⚐ 0.00 **FUD** XXX   M

6150F Patient not receiving a first course of anti-TNF (tumor necrosis factor) therapy (IBD)
🚑 0.00 ⚐ 0.00 **FUD** XXX   E

7010F-7025F Recall/Reminder System in Place

INCLUDES Capabilities of the provider
Measures that address the setting or system of care provided

7010F Patient information entered into a recall system that includes: target date for the next exam specified and a process to follow up with patients regarding missed or unscheduled appointments (ML)
🚑 0.00 ⚐ 0.00 **FUD** XXX   M
AMA: 2008,Mar,8-12

7020F Mammogram assessment category (eg, Mammography Quality Standards Act [MQSA], Breast Imaging Reporting and Data System [BI-RADS], or FDA approved equivalent categories) entered into an internal database to allow for analysis of abnormal interpretation (recall) rate (RAD)
🚑 0.00 ⚐ 0.00 **FUD** XXX   E
AMA: 2008,Mar,8-12

7025F Patient information entered into a reminder system with a target due date for the next mammogram (RAD)
🚑 0.00 ⚐ 0.00 **FUD** XXX   M
AMA: 2008,Mar,8-12

9001F-9007F No Measure Associated

INCLUDES Aspects of care not associated with measures at the current time

9001F Aortic aneurysm less than 5.0 cm maximum diameter on centerline formatted CT or minor diameter on axial formatted CT (NMA-No Measure Associated)
🚑 0.00 ⚐ 0.00 **FUD** XXX   E

9002F Aortic aneurysm 5.0 - 5.4 cm maximum diameter on centerline formatted CT or minor diameter on axial formatted CT (NMA-No Measure Associated)
🚑 0.00 ⚐ 0.00 **FUD** XXX   E

9003F Aortic aneurysm 5.5 - 5.9 cm maximum diameter on centerline formatted CT or minor diameter on axial formatted CT (NMA-No Measure Associated)
🚑 0.00 ⚐ 0.00 **FUD** XXX   M

9004F Aortic aneurysm 6.0 cm or greater maximum diameter on centerline formatted CT or minor diameter on axial formatted CT (NMA-No Measure Associated)
🚑 0.00 ⚐ 0.00 **FUD** XXX   M

9005F Asymptomatic carotid stenosis: No history of any transient ischemic attack or stroke in any carotid or vertebrobasilar territory (NMA-No Measure Associated)
🚑 0.00 ⚐ 0.00 **FUD** XXX   E

9006F Symptomatic carotid stenosis: Ipsilateral carotid territory TIA or stroke less than 120 days prior to procedure (NMA-No Measure Associated)
🚑 0.00 ⚐ 0.00 **FUD** XXX   M

9007F Other carotid stenosis: Ipsilateral TIA or stroke 120 days or greater prior to procedure or any prior contralateral carotid territory or vertebrobasilar TIA or stroke (NMA-No Measure Associated)
🚑 0.00 ⚐ 0.00 **FUD** XXX   M

0019T-0042T

0019T ~~Extracorporeal shock wave involving musculoskeletal system, not otherwise specified, low energy~~

     To report, see ~20999

0042T Cerebral perfusion analysis using computed tomography with contrast administration, including post-processing of parametric maps with determination of cerebral blood flow, cerebral blood volume, and mean transit time

     0.00   0.00   **FUD** XXX   N 80

     AMA: 2003,Nov,5

0051T-0053T

0051T Implantation of a total replacement heart system (artificial heart) with recipient cardiectomy

     EXCLUDES   *Ventricular assist device implant (33975-33976)*

     0.00   0.00   **FUD** XXX   C 80

     AMA: 2004,Jun,7; 2003,Aug,1

0052T Replacement or repair of thoracic unit of a total replacement heart system (artificial heart)

     EXCLUDES   *Exchange or repair of other artificial heart components (0053T)*

     0.00   0.00   **FUD** XXX   C 80

     AMA: 2016,Jan,13; 2015,Jan,16; 2014,Jan,11

0053T Replacement or repair of implantable component or components of total replacement heart system (artificial heart), excluding thoracic unit

     EXCLUDES   *Exchange or repair of thoracic unit of artificial heart (0052T)*

     0.00   0.00   **FUD** XXX   C 80

     AMA: 2004,Jun,7; 2003,Aug,1

0054T-0055T

+ 0054T Computer-assisted musculoskeletal surgical navigational orthopedic procedure, with image-guidance based on fluoroscopic images (List separately in addition to code for primary procedure)

     Code first primary procedure

     0.00   0.00   **FUD** XXX   N 80

     AMA: 2016,Jan,13; 2015,Jan,16; 2014,Jan,11; 2012,Jan,15-42; 2011,Jan,11

+ 0055T Computer-assisted musculoskeletal surgical navigational orthopedic procedure, with image-guidance based on CT/MRI images (List separately in addition to code for primary procedure)

     INCLUDES   Performance of both CT and MRI in same session (1 unit)

     Code first primary procedure

     0.00   0.00   **FUD** XXX   N 80

     AMA: 2016,Jan,13; 2015,Jan,16; 2014,Jan,11; 2012,Jan,15-42; 2011,Jan,11

0058T [0357T]

     EXCLUDES   *Cryopreservation of:*
         Embryos (89258)
         Oocyte(s), mature (89337)
         Sperm (89259)
         Testicular reproductive tissue (89335)

0058T Cryopreservation; reproductive tissue, ovarian

     0.00   0.00   **FUD** XXX   Q1 80

     AMA: 2004,Apr,1; 2004,Jun,7

 # 0357T immature oocyte(s)   ♀

     0.00   0.00   **FUD** XXX   Q1 80

0071T-0072T

     EXCLUDES   *Insertion bladder catheter (51702)*
         MRI guidance for parenchymal tissue ablation (77022)

0071T Focused ultrasound ablation of uterine leiomyomata, including MR guidance; total leiomyomata volume less than 200 cc of tissue   ♀

     0.00   0.00   **FUD** XXX   T 80

     AMA: 2005,Mar,1-6; 2005,Dec,3-6

0072T total leiomyomata volume greater or equal to 200 cc of tissue   ♀

     0.00   0.00   **FUD** XXX   T 80

     AMA: 2005,Mar,1-6; 2005,Dec,3-6

0075T-0076T

0075T Transcatheter placement of extracranial vertebral artery stent(s), including radiologic supervision and interpretation, open or percutaneous; initial vessel

     INCLUDES   All diagnostic services for stenting
         Ipsilateral extracranial vertebral selective catheterization when confirming the need for stenting

     EXCLUDES   *Selective catheterization and imaging when stenting is not required (report only selective catheterization codes)*

+   0.00   0.00   **FUD** XXX   C 80

     AMA: 2016,Jan,13; 2015,Jan,16; 2014,Mar,8

0076T each additional vessel (List separately in addition to code for primary procedure)

     Code first (0075T)

     0.00   0.00   **FUD** XXX   C 80

     AMA: 2016,Jan,13; 2015,Jan,16; 2014,Mar,8

0085T

0085T Breath test for heart transplant rejection

     0.00   0.00   **FUD** XXX   E

     AMA: 2005,May,7-12

0095T-0098T

     INCLUDES   Fluoroscopy

+ 0095T Removal of total disc arthroplasty (artificial disc), anterior approach, each additional interspace, cervical (List separately in addition to code for primary procedure)

     EXCLUDES   *Lumbar disc (0164T)*
         Revision of total disc arthroplasty, cervical (22861)
         Revision of total disc arthroplasty, lumbar (22862)

     Code first (22864)

     0.00   0.00   **FUD** XXX   C 80

     AMA: 2006,Feb,1-6; 2005,Jun,6-8

+ 0098T Revision including replacement of total disc arthroplasty (artificial disc), anterior approach, each additional interspace, cervical (List separately in addition to code for primary procedure)

     EXCLUDES   *Application of intervertebral biomechanical device(s) at the same level (22853-22854, [22859])*
         Removal of total disc arthroplasty (0095T)
         Spinal cord decompression (63001-63048)

     Code first (22861)

     0.00   0.00   **FUD** XXX   C 80

     AMA: 2006,Feb,1-6; 2005,Jun,6-8

0100T-0159T

0100T Placement of a subconjunctival retinal prosthesis receiver and pulse generator, and implantation of intra-ocular retinal electrode array, with vitrectomy

     0.00   0.00   **FUD** XXX   T 62 80

     AMA: 2016,Jan,13; 2015,Jan,16; 2014,Jan,11; 2012,Jan,15-42

0101T Extracorporeal shock wave involving musculoskeletal system, not otherwise specified, high energy

     EXCLUDES   *Extracorporeal shock wave therapy for healing of integumentary system wounds (0299T-0300T)*

     0.00   0.00   **FUD** XXX   T 62 80

     AMA: 2016,Jan,13; 2015,Jan,16; 2014,Jan,11; 2012,Jan,15-42

● New Code   ▲ Revised Code   ○ Reinstated   ● New Web Release   ▲ Revised Web Release   Unlisted   Not Covered   # Resequenced
⊘ AMA Mod 51 Exempt   Ⓢ Optum Mod 51 Exempt   63 Mod 63 Exempt   ✗ Non-FDA Drug   ★ Telehealth   Ⓜ Maternity   ▲ Age Edit   + Add-on   **AMA:** CPT Asst

0102T Extracorporeal shock wave, high energy, performed by a physician, requiring anesthesia other than local, involving lateral humeral epicondyle
  📷 0.00 ⚕ 0.00 **FUD** XXX [T] [62] [80] 📋
  AMA: 2016,Jan,13; 2015,Jan,16; 2014,Jan,11; 2012,Jan,15-42

0106T Quantitative sensory testing (QST), testing and interpretation per extremity; using touch pressure stimuli to assess large diameter sensation
  📷 0.00 ⚕ 0.00 **FUD** XXX [01] [80] 📋
  AMA: 2016,Jan,13; 2015,Jan,16; 2014,Jan,11; 2012,Jan,15-42; 2011,May,9

0107T using vibration stimuli to assess large diameter fiber sensation
  📷 0.00 ⚕ 0.00 **FUD** XXX [01] [80] 📋
  AMA: 2016,Jan,13; 2015,Jan,16; 2014,Jan,11; 2011,May,9

0108T using cooling stimuli to assess small nerve fiber sensation and hyperalgesia
  📷 0.00 ⚕ 0.00 **FUD** XXX [01] [80] 📋
  AMA: 2016,Jan,13; 2015,Jan,16; 2014,Jan,11; 2011,May,9

0109T using heat-pain stimuli to assess small nerve fiber sensation and hyperalgesia
  📷 0.00 ⚕ 0.00 **FUD** XXX [01] [80] 📋
  AMA: 2016,Jan,13; 2015,Jan,16; 2014,Jan,11; 2011,May,9

0110T using other stimuli to assess sensation
  📷 0.00 ⚕ 0.00 **FUD** XXX [01] [80] 📋
  AMA: 2016,Jan,13; 2015,Jan,16; 2014,Jan,11; 2011,May,9

0111T Long-chain (C20-22) omega-3 fatty acids in red blood cell (RBC) membranes
  EXCLUDES Very long chain fatty acids (82726)
  📷 0.00 ⚕ 0.00 **FUD** XXX [A] 📋
  AMA: 2016,Jan,13; 2015,Jan,16; 2014,Jan,11

0126T Common carotid intima-media thickness (IMT) study for evaluation of atherosclerotic burden or coronary heart disease risk factor assessment
  EXCLUDES Duplex scan extracranial arteries (93880-93882)
  Evaluation carotid intima media and atheroma (93895)
  📷 0.00 ⚕ 0.00 **FUD** XXX [01] [80] 📋
  AMA: 2016,Jan,13; 2015,Jan,16; 2014,Jan,11

+ **0159T** Computer-aided detection, including computer algorithm analysis of MRI image data for lesion detection/characterization, pharmacokinetic analysis, with further physician review for interpretation, breast MRI (List separately in addition to code for primary procedure)
  EXCLUDES 3D rendering (76376-76377)
  Code first (77058-77059)
  📷 0.00 ⚕ 0.00 **FUD** ZZZ [N] [80] 📋
  AMA: 2016,Jan,13; 2015,Jan,16; 2014,Jan,11

0163T-0165T

CMS: 100-03,150.10 Lumbar Artificial Disc Replacement (LADR)
  INCLUDES Fluoroscopy
  EXCLUDES Application of intervertebral biomechanical device(s) at the same level (22853-22854, [22859])
  Cervical disc procedures (22856)
  Decompression (63001-63048)
  Exploration retroperitoneal area at same level (49010)

+ **0163T** Total disc arthroplasty (artificial disc), anterior approach, including discectomy to prepare interspace (other than for decompression), each additional interspace, lumbar (List separately in addition to code for primary procedure)
  Code first (22857)
  📷 0.00 ⚕ 0.00 **FUD** YYY [C] [80] 📋
  AMA: 2016,Jan,13; 2015,Jan,16; 2014,Jan,11

+ **0164T** Removal of total disc arthroplasty, (artificial disc), anterior approach, each additional interspace, lumbar (List separately in addition to code for primary procedure)
  Code first (22865)
  📷 0.00 ⚕ 0.00 **FUD** YYY [C] [80] 📋
  AMA: 2016,Jan,13; 2015,Jan,16; 2014,Jan,11

+ **0165T** Revision including replacement of total disc arthroplasty (artificial disc), anterior approach, each additional interspace, lumbar (List separately in addition to code for primary procedure)
  Code first (22862)
  📷 0.00 ⚕ 0.00 **FUD** YYY [C] [80] 📋
  AMA: 2016,Jan,13; 2015,Jan,16; 2014,Jan,11

0169T-0175T

0169T ~~Stereotactic placement of infusion catheter(s) in the brain for delivery of therapeutic agent(s), including computerized stereotactic planning and burr hole(s)~~
  To report, see ~64999

0171T ~~Insertion of posterior spinous process distraction device (including necessary removal of bone or ligament for insertion and imaging guidance), lumbar; single level~~
  To report, see ~22867, 22869

0172T ~~each additional level (List separately in addition to code for primary procedure)~~
  To report, see ~22868, 22870

+ **0174T** Computer-aided detection (CAD) (computer algorithm analysis of digital image data for lesion detection) with further physician review for interpretation and report, with or without digitization of film radiographic images, chest radiograph(s), performed concurrent with primary interpretation (List separately in addition to code for primary procedure)
  Code first (71010, 71020-71022, 71030)
  📷 0.00 ⚕ 0.00 **FUD** XXX [N] [80] 📋
  AMA: 2007,Jul,6-10; 2007,Mar,7-8

0175T Computer-aided detection (CAD) (computer algorithm analysis of digital image data for lesion detection) with further physician review for interpretation and report, with or without digitization of film radiographic images, chest radiograph(s), performed remote from primary interpretation
  INCLUDES Chest x-rays (71010, 71020-71022, 71030)
  📷 0.00 ⚕ 0.00 **FUD** XXX [N] [80] 📋
  AMA: 2007,Jul,6-10; 2007,Mar,7-8

0178T-0180T

  EXCLUDES Separately performed 12-lead electrocardiogram (93000-93010)

0178T Electrocardiogram, 64 leads or greater, with graphic presentation and analysis; with interpretation and report
  📷 0.00 ⚕ 0.00 **FUD** XXX [B] [80] 📋

0179T tracing and graphics only, without interpretation and report
  📷 0.00 ⚕ 0.00 **FUD** XXX [01] [80] [TC] 📋

0180T interpretation and report only
  📷 0.00 ⚕ 0.00 **FUD** XXX [B] [80] [26] 📋

0184T

0184T Excision of rectal tumor, transanal endoscopic microsurgical approach (ie, TEMS), including muscularis propria (ie, full thickness)
  INCLUDES Operating microscope (66990)
  Sigmoidoscopy (45300-45327)
  EXCLUDES Nonendoscopic excision of rectal tumor (45160, 45171-45172)
  📷 0.00 ⚕ 0.00 **FUD** XXX [J] [80] 📋
  AMA: 2016,Feb,12; 2016,Jan,13; 2015,Jan,16; 2014,Jan,11

0188T-0189T

INCLUDES
30 minutes or more of direct medical care by a physician(s) or other qualified health care professional(s) to a critically ill or critically injured patient from an off-site location

Additional on-site critical care services when a critically ill or injured patient requires critical care resources not available on-site

Other critical care services provided during the same time period by provider or other individual (99291-99292, 99468-99476)

Real time ability to:
Document the remote care services in the medical record
Enter orders electronically
Evaluate patients with high fidelity audio/video capabilities
Observe patient monitors, infusion pumps, ventilators
Talk to patients and family members
Videoconference with the health care team on-site in the patient's room

Real-time access to the patient's:
Clinical laboratory test results
Diagnostic test results
Medical records
Radiographic images

Review and/or interpretation of all diagnostic information

Time spent with the patient, family, or surrogate decision makers to obtain a medical history, review the patient's condition/prognosis, or discuss treatment options from the remote site

EXCLUDES
Time spent away from the remote site without real-time capabilities
Time spent for services that do not directly contribute to patient treatment

0188T **Remote real-time interactive video-conferenced critical care, evaluation and management of the critically ill or critically injured patient; first 30-74 minutes**

INCLUDES
First 30 to 74 minutes of remote critical care each day
Remote critical care less than 30 minutes total duration

🔲 0.00   ⚕ 0.00   **FUD** XXX   ★ M ▭

AMA: 2016,May,3; 2016,Jan,13; 2015,Jan,16; 2014,Jan,11; 2012,Jan,15-42; 2011,Aug,9-10

+ **0189T** **each additional 30 minutes (List separately in addition to code for primary service)**

INCLUDES
Up to 30 minutes each beyond the first 74 minutes
Code first (0188T)

🔲 0.00   ⚕ 0.00   **FUD** XXX   ★ M ▭

AMA: 2016,May,3; 2016,Jan,13; 2015,Jan,16; 2014,Jan,11; 2012,Jan,15-42; 2011,Aug,9-10

0190T-0191T [0253T, 0376T]

+ **0190T** **Placement of intraocular radiation source applicator (List separately in addition to primary procedure)**

EXCLUDES
Insertion of brachytherapy source by radiation oncologist (see Clinical Brachytherapy Section)
Code also brachytherapy source
Code first (67036)

🔲 0.00   ⚕ 0.00   **FUD** XXX   N 80 ▭

AMA: 2008,Jan,6-7

0191T **Insertion of anterior segment aqueous drainage device, without extraocular reservoir, internal approach, into the trabecular meshwork; initial insertion**

🔲 0.00   ⚕ 0.00   **FUD** XXX   J 62 80 ▭

AMA: 2016,Jan,13; 2015,Jan,16; 2014,Jan,11; 2012,Dec,12

+ # **0376T** **each additional device insertion (List separately in addition to code for primary procedure)**

🔲 0.00   ⚕ 0.00   **FUD** XXX   N U1 80 ▭

Code first (0191T)

0253T **Insertion of anterior segment aqueous drainage device, without extraocular reservoir, internal approach, into the suprachoroidal space**

🔲 0.00   ⚕ 0.00   **FUD** YYY   J 62 80 ▭

EXCLUDES
Insertion aqueous drainage device, external approach (66183)

0195T-0196T

INCLUDES
Application of intervertebral biomechanical device(s) at the same level (22853-22854, [22859])
Computed tomography (76380, 76497, 77011-77012)
Epidurography (72275)
Fluoroscopy (76000, 76496, 77002-77003)
Grafts (20930-20938)
Instrumentation (22840, 22845)
Lumbar arthrodesis (22558)
Pelvic fixation (22848)

0195T **Arthrodesis, pre-sacral interbody technique, disc space preparation, discectomy, without instrumentation, with image guidance, includes bone graft when performed; L5-S1 interspace**

🔲 0.00   ⚕ 0.00   **FUD** XXX   C 80 ▭

AMA: 2016,Jan,13; 2015,Jan,16; 2013,Jul,3-5; 2012,Apr,14-16

+ **0196T** **L4-L5 interspace (List separately in addition to code for primary procedure)**

Code first (0195T)

🔲 0.00   ⚕ 0.00   **FUD** XXX   C 80 ▭

AMA: 2016,Jan,13; 2015,Jan,16; 2013,Jul,3-5; 2012,Apr,14-16

0198T

0198T **Measurement of ocular blood flow by repetitive intraocular pressure sampling, with interpretation and report**

🔲 0.00   ⚕ 0.00   **FUD** XXX   91 80 ▭

AMA: 2016,Jan,13; 2015,Jan,16; 2014,Jan,11; 2012,Aug,9; 2012,Jan,15-42; 2011,Mar,9

0200T-0201T

INCLUDES
Deep bone biopsy (20225)

▲ **0200T** **Percutaneous sacral augmentation (sacroplasty), unilateral injection(s), including the use of a balloon or mechanical device, when used, 1 or more needles, includes imaging guidance and bone biopsy, when performed**

🔲 0.00   ⚕ 0.00   **FUD** XXX   T 62 80 50 ▭

AMA: 2016,Jan,13; 2015,Dec,18; 2015,Apr,8; 2015,Jan,8

▲ **0201T** **Percutaneous sacral augmentation (sacroplasty), bilateral injections, including the use of a balloon or mechanical device, when used, 2 or more needles, includes imaging guidance and bone biopsy, when performed**

🔲 0.00   ⚕ 0.00   **FUD** XXX   T 62 80 ▭

AMA: 2016,Jan,13; 2015,Dec,18; 2015,Apr,8; 2015,Jan,8

0202T-0207T

0202T **Posterior vertebral joint(s) arthroplasty (eg, facet joint[s] replacement), including facetectomy, laminectomy, foraminotomy, and vertebral column fixation, injection of bone cement, when performed, including fluoroscopy, single level, lumbar spine**

🔲 0.00   ⚕ 0.00   **FUD** XXX   C 80 ▭

INCLUDES
Instrumentation (22840, 22853-22854, [22859])
Laminectomy (63005, 63012, 63017, 63047)
Laminotomy (63030, 63042)
Lumbar arthroplasty (22857)
Percutaneous lumbar vertebral augmentation (22514)
Percutaneous vertebroplasty (22511)
Spinal cord decompression (63056)

+ **0205T** **Intravascular catheter-based coronary vessel or graft spectroscopy (eg, infrared) during diagnostic evaluation and/or therapeutic intervention including imaging supervision, interpretation, and report, each vessel (List separately in addition to code for primary procedure)**

🔲 0.00   ⚕ 0.00   **FUD** ZZZ   N 80 ▭

Code first (92920, 92924, 92928, 92933, 92937, 92941, 92943, 92975, 93454-93461, 93563-93564)

Category III Codes *(side tab)*

0206T — 0231T *(side tab)*

0206T Computerized database analysis of multiple cycles of digitized cardiac electrical data from two or more ECG leads, including transmission to a remote center, application of multiple nonlinear mathematical transformations, with coronary artery obstruction severity assessment

🖻 0.00   ⚖ 0.00   **FUD** XXX   [01] [80] [TC] [□]

Code also 12-lead ECG when performed (93000-93010)

0207T Evacuation of meibomian glands, automated, using heat and intermittent pressure, unilateral

🖻 0.00   ⚖ 0.00   **FUD** XXX   [01] [80] [□]

AMA: 2016,Jan,13; 2015,Jan,16; 2014,May,5

0208T-0212T

EXCLUDES Manual audiometric testing by a qualified health care professional, using audiometers (92551-92557)

0208T Pure tone audiometry (threshold), automated; air only

🖻 0.00   ⚖ 0.00   **FUD** XXX   [01] [80] [TC] [□]

AMA: 2016,Jan,13; 2015,Jan,16; 2014,Aug,3

0209T air and bone

🖻 0.00   ⚖ 0.00   **FUD** XXX   [01] [80] [TC] [□]

AMA: 2016,Jan,13; 2015,Jan,16; 2014,Aug,3; 2014,Jan,11; 2011,Mar,8

0210T Speech audiometry threshold, automated;

🖻 0.00   ⚖ 0.00   **FUD** XXX   [01] [80] [TC] [□]

AMA: 2014,Aug,3

0211T with speech recognition

🖻 0.00   ⚖ 0.00   **FUD** XXX   [01] [80] [TC] [□]

AMA: 2016,Jan,13; 2015,Jan,16; 2014,Aug,3; 2014,Jan,11; 2011,Mar,8

0212T Comprehensive audiometry threshold evaluation and speech recognition (0209T, 0211T combined), automated

🖻 0.00   ⚖ 0.00   **FUD** XXX   [01] [80] [TC] [□]

AMA: 2016,Jan,13; 2015,Jan,16; 2014,Aug,3; 2014,Jan,11; 2011,Mar,8

0213T-0215T

0213T Injection(s), diagnostic or therapeutic agent, paravertebral facet (zygapophyseal) joint (or nerves innervating that joint) with ultrasound guidance, cervical or thoracic; single level

🖻 0.00   ⚖ 0.00   **FUD** XXX   [T] [R2] [80] [50] [□]

AMA: 2016,Jan,13; 2015,Jan,16; 2014,Jan,11; 2011,Jul,14; 2011,Feb,4-5

+ **0214T** second level (List separately in addition to code for primary procedure)

Code first (0213T)

🖻 0.00   ⚖ 0.00   **FUD** ZZZ   [N] [80] [50] [□]

AMA: 2016,Jan,13; 2015,Jan,16; 2014,Jan,11; 2011,Jul,14; 2011,Feb,4-5

+ **0215T** third and any additional level(s) (List separately in addition to code for primary procedure)

EXCLUDES Use of code more than one time per date of service

Code first (0213T-0214T)

🖻 0.00   ⚖ 0.00   **FUD** ZZZ   [N] [80] [50] [□]

AMA: 2016,Jan,13; 2015,Jan,16; 2014,Jan,11; 2011,Jul,14; 2011,Feb,4-5

0216T-0218T

EXCLUDES Injection with CT or fluoroscopic guidance (64490-64495)

0216T Injection(s), diagnostic or therapeutic agent, paravertebral facet (zygapophyseal) joint (or nerves innervating that joint) with ultrasound guidance, lumbar or sacral; single level

🖻 0.00   ⚖ 0.00   **FUD** XXX   [T] [R2] [80] [50] [□]

AMA: 2016,Jan,13; 2015,Jan,16; 2014,Jan,11; 2011,Jul,14; 2011,Feb,4-5

+ **0217T** second level (List separately in addition to code for primary procedure)

Code first (0216T)

🖻 0.00   ⚖ 0.00   **FUD** ZZZ   [N] [80] [50] [□]

AMA: 2016,Jan,13; 2015,Jan,16; 2014,Jan,11; 2011,Jul,14; 2011,Feb,4-5

+ **0218T** third and any additional level(s) (List separately in addition to code for primary procedure)

EXCLUDES Use of code more than one time per date of service

Code first (0216T, 0217T)

🖻 0.00   ⚖ 0.00   **FUD** ZZZ   [N] [80] [50] [□]

AMA: 2016,Jan,13; 2015,Jan,16; 2014,Jan,11; 2011,Jul,14; 2011,Feb,4-5

0219T-0222T

INCLUDES Allografts at same level (20930-20931)
Application of intervertebral biomechanical device(s) at the same level (22853-22854, [22859])
Arthrodesis at same level (22600-22614)
Instrumentation at same level (22840)
Radiologic services

0219T Placement of a posterior intrafacet implant(s), unilateral or bilateral, including imaging and placement of bone graft(s) or synthetic device(s), single level; cervical

🖻 0.00   ⚖ 0.00   **FUD** XXX   [C] [80] [□]

AMA: 2016,Jan,13; 2015,Jan,16; 2014,Jan,11; 2012,Jun,10-11; 2012,Jan,15-42; 2011,Jul,16-17

0220T thoracic

🖻 0.00   ⚖ 0.00   **FUD** XXX   [C] [80] [□]

AMA: 2016,Jan,13; 2015,Jan,16; 2014,Jan,11; 2012,Jun,10-11; 2012,Jan,15-42; 2011,Jul,16-17

0221T lumbar

🖻 0.00   ⚖ 0.00   **FUD** XXX   [T] [80] [□]

AMA: 2016,Jan,13; 2015,Jan,16; 2014,Jan,11; 2012,Jun,10-11; 2012,Jan,15-42; 2011,Jul,16-17

+ **0222T** each additional vertebral segment (List separately in addition to code for primary procedure)

Code first (0219T-0221T)

🖻 0.00   ⚖ 0.00   **FUD** ZZZ   [N] [80] [□]

AMA: 2016,Jan,13; 2015,Jan,16; 2014,Jan,11; 2012,Jun,10-11; 2012,Jan,15-42; 2011,Jul,16-17

0228T-0232T

0228T Injection(s), anesthetic agent and/or steroid, transforaminal epidural, with ultrasound guidance, cervical or thoracic; single level

🖻 0.00   ⚖ 0.00   **FUD** XXX   [T] [62] [50] [□]

AMA: 2016,Jan,13; 2015,Jan,16; 2014,Jan,11; 2012,Jan,15-42; 2011,Jul,16-17; 2011,Feb,4-5

+ **0229T** each additional level (List separately in addition to code for primary procedure)

Code first (0228T)

🖻 0.00   ⚖ 0.00   **FUD** XXX   [N] [50] [□]

AMA: 2016,Jan,13; 2015,Jan,16; 2014,Jan,11; 2012,Jan,15-42; 2011,Jul,16-17; 2011,Feb,4-5

0230T Injection(s), anesthetic agent and/or steroid, transforaminal epidural, with ultrasound guidance, lumbar or sacral; single level

🖻 0.00   ⚖ 0.00   **FUD** XXX   [T] [62] [50] [□]

AMA: 2016,Jan,13; 2015,Jan,16; 2014,Jan,11; 2012,Jan,15-42; 2011,Jul,16-17; 2011,Feb,4-5

+ **0231T** each additional level (List separately in addition to code for primary procedure)

INCLUDES Ultrasound guidance (76942, 76998-76999)

EXCLUDES Injection performed with CT or fluoroscopic guidance (64479-64484)

Code first (0230T)

🖻 0.00   ⚖ 0.00   **FUD** XXX   [N] [50] [□]

AMA: 2016,Jan,13; 2015,Jan,16; 2014,Jan,11; 2012,Jan,15-42; 2011,Jul,16-17; 2011,Feb,4-5

CPT © 2016 American Medical Association. All Rights Reserved.   © 2016 Optum360, LLC

0232T **Injection(s), platelet rich plasma, any site, including image guidance, harvesting and preparation when performed**

INCLUDES Arthrocentesis (20600-20610)
Imaging guidance (76942, 77002, 77012, 77021)
Injections (20550-20551)
Platelet/blood product pooling (86965)
Tissue grafts (20926)

EXCLUDES Aspiration of bone marrow for grafting, biopsy, harvesting for transplant (38220-38221, 38230)

🔲 0.00 🔲 0.00 **FUD** XXX 🔲🔲

AMA: 2016,Jan,13; 2015,Jan,16; 2014,Jan,11; 2012,Oct,14; 2012,May,11-12

0234T-0238T

INCLUDES Atherectomy by any technique in arteries above the inguinal ligaments
Radiology supervision and interpretation

EXCLUDES Accessing and catheterization of the vessel
Atherectomy performed below the inguinal ligaments (37225, 37227, 37229, 37231, 37233, 37235)
Closure of the arteriotomy by any technique
Negotiating the lesion
Other interventions to the same or different vessels
Protection from embolism

0234T **Transluminal peripheral atherectomy, open or percutaneous, including radiological supervision and interpretation; renal artery**

🔲 0.00 🔲 0.00 **FUD** YYY 🔲🔲🔲

AMA: 2016,Jan,13; 2015,Jan,16; 2014,Jan,11; 2011,Jul,3-11

0235T **visceral artery (except renal), each vessel**

🔲 0.00 🔲 0.00 **FUD** YYY 🔲🔲🔲

AMA: 2016,Jan,13; 2015,Jan,16; 2014,Jan,11; 2011,Jul,3-11

0236T **abdominal aorta**

🔲 0.00 🔲 0.00 **FUD** YYY 🔲🔲🔲

AMA: 2016,Jan,13; 2015,Jan,16; 2014,Jan,11; 2011,Jul,3-11

0237T **brachiocephalic trunk and branches, each vessel**

🔲 0.00 🔲 0.00 **FUD** YYY 🔲🔲🔲

AMA: 2016,Jan,13; 2015,Jan,16; 2014,Jan,11; 2011,Jul,3-11

0238T **iliac artery, each vessel**

🔲 0.00 🔲 0.00 **FUD** YYY 🔲🔲🔲🔲

AMA: 2016,Jan,13; 2015,Jan,16; 2014,Jan,11; 2011,Jul,3-11

0249T-0255T

0249T **Ligation, hemorrhoidal vascular bundle(s), including ultrasound guidance**

INCLUDES Ultrasound guidance (76870, 76872, 76998)

EXCLUDES Anoscopy (46600)
Hemorrhoidectomy (46221, [46945, 46946], 46250-46262)
Placement seton (46020)

🔲 0.00 🔲 0.00 **FUD** YYY 🔲🔲🔲🔲

AMA: 2016,Jan,13; 2015,Mar,9

0253T **Resequenced code, See code following 0191T.**

0254T **Endovascular repair of iliac artery bifurcation (eg, aneurysm, pseudoaneurysm, arteriovenous malformation, trauma) using bifurcated endoprosthesis from the common iliac artery into both the external and internal iliac artery, unilateral;**

🔲 (0255T)

🔲 0.00 🔲 0.00 **FUD** YYY 🔲🔲🔲

AMA: 2016,Jan,13; 2015,Jan,16; 2014,Jan,11; 2013,Dec,8

0255T **radiological supervision and interpretation**

🔲 0.00 🔲 0.00 **FUD** YYY 🔲🔲🔲

AMA: 2016,Jan,13; 2015,Jan,16; 2014,Jan,11; 2013,Dec,8

0263T-0265T

EXCLUDES Bone marrow and stem cell services (38204-38242 [38243])

0263T **Intramuscular autologous bone marrow cell therapy, with preparation of harvested cells, multiple injections, one leg, including ultrasound guidance, if performed; complete procedure including unilateral or bilateral bone marrow harvest**

🔲 0.00 🔲 0.00 **FUD** XXX 🔲🔲🔲🔲

INCLUDES Duplex scan (93925-93926)
Ultrasonic guidance (76942)

0264T **complete procedure excluding bone marrow harvest**

🔲 0.00 🔲 0.00 **FUD** XXX 🔲🔲🔲🔲

INCLUDES Bone marrow harvest only (0265T)
Duplex scan (93925-93926)
Ultrasonic guidance (76942)

0265T **unilateral or bilateral bone marrow harvest only for intramuscular autologous bone marrow cell therapy**

🔲 0.00 🔲 0.00 **FUD** XXX 🔲🔲🔲🔲

EXCLUDES Complete procedure (0263T-0264T)

0266T-0273T

0266T **Implantation or replacement of carotid sinus baroreflex activation device; total system (includes generator placement, unilateral or bilateral lead placement, intra-operative interrogation, programming, and repositioning, when performed)**

🔲 0.00 🔲 0.00 **FUD** YYY 🔲🔲🔲

INCLUDES Components of complete procedure (0267T-0268T)

0267T **lead only, unilateral (includes intra-operative interrogation, programming, and repositioning, when performed)**

🔲 0.00 🔲 0.00 **FUD** YYY 🔲🔲🔲

EXCLUDES Complete procedure (0266T)
Device interrogation (0272T-0273T)
Removal/revision device or components (0269T-0271T)

0268T **pulse generator only (includes intra-operative interrogation, programming, and repositioning, when performed)**

🔲 0.00 🔲 0.00 **FUD** YYY 🔲🔲🔲

EXCLUDES Complete procedure (0266T)
Device interrogation (0272T-0273T)
Removal/revision device or components (0269T-0271T)

0269T **Revision or removal of carotid sinus baroreflex activation device; total system (includes generator placement, unilateral or bilateral lead placement, intra-operative interrogation, programming, and repositioning, when performed)**

🔲 0.00 🔲 0.00 **FUD** XXX 🔲🔲🔲🔲

EXCLUDES Device interrogation (0272T-0273T)
Implantation/replacement device and/or components (0266T-0268T)
Removal/revision components of device (0270T-0271T)

0270T **lead only, unilateral (includes intra-operative interrogation, programming, and repositioning, when performed)**

🔲 0.00 🔲 0.00 **FUD** XXX 🔲🔲🔲🔲

EXCLUDES Device interrogation (0272T-0273T)
Implantation/replacement device and/or components (0266T-0268T)
Removal/revision device or components (0269T-0271T)

0271T **pulse generator only (includes intra-operative interrogation, programming, and repositioning, when performed)**

🔲 0.00 🔲 0.00 **FUD** XXX 🔲🔲🔲🔲

EXCLUDES Device interrogation (0272T-0273T)
Implantation/replacement device or components (0266T-0268T)
Removal/revision device or components (0269T-0271T)

Category III Codes (sidebar)

0272T — 0296T (sidebar)

0272T Interrogation device evaluation (in person), carotid sinus baroreflex activation system, including telemetric iterative communication with the implantable device to monitor device diagnostics and programmed therapy values, with interpretation and report (eg, battery status, lead impedance, pulse amplitude, pulse width, therapy frequency, pathway mode, burst mode, therapy start/stop times each day);

🖭 0.00   ⅄ 0.00   **FUD** XXX   S 80 ▣

EXCLUDES   Device interrogation with programming (0273T)
Implantation/replacement device or components (0266T-0268T)
Removal/revision device or components (0269T-0271T)

0273T with programming

🖭 0.00   ⅄ 0.00   **FUD** XXX   S 80 ▣

EXCLUDES   Device interrogation without programming (0272T)
Implantation/replacement device or components (0266T-0268T)
Removal/revision device or components (0269T-0271T)

0274T-0275T

EXCLUDES   Laminotomy/hemilaminectomy by open and endoscopically assisted approach (63020-63035)
Percutaneous decompression of nucleus pulposus of intervertebral disc by needle-based technique (62287)

▲ **0274T** Percutaneous laminotomy/laminectomy (interlaminar approach) for decompression of neural elements, (with or without ligamentous resection, discectomy, facetectomy and/or foraminotomy), any method, under indirect image guidance (eg, fluoroscopic, CT), single or multiple levels, unilateral or bilateral; cervical or thoracic

🖭 0.00   ⅄ 0.00   **FUD** YYY   J G2 80 ▣

AMA: 2016,Jan,13; 2015,Jan,16; 2014,Jan,11; 2012,Jul,3-6; 2012,Jan,13-14

▲ **0275T** lumbar

🖭 0.00   ⅄ 0.00   **FUD** XXX   J G2 ▣

AMA: 2016,Jan,13; 2015,Jan,16; 2014,Jan,11; 2012,Jul,3-6; 2012,Jan,13-14

0278T-0281T

0278T Transcutaneous electrical modulation pain reprocessing (eg, scrambler therapy), each treatment session (includes placement of electrodes)

🖭 0.00   ⅄ 0.00   **FUD** XXX   Q1 80 ▣

~~0281T~~ ~~Percutaneous transcatheter closure of the left atrial appendage with implant, including fluoroscopy, transseptal puncture, catheter placement(s), left atrial angiography, left atrial appendage angiography, radiological supervision and interpretation~~

To report, see ~33340

0282T-0285T

~~0282T~~ ~~Percutaneous or open implantation of neurostimulator electrode array(s), subcutaneous (peripheral subcutaneous field stimulation), including imaging guidance, when performed, cervical, thoracic or lumbar; for trial, including removal at the conclusion of trial period~~

To report, see ~64999

~~0283T~~ ~~permanent, with implantation of a pulse generator~~

To report, see ~64999

~~0284T~~ ~~Revision or removal of pulse generator or electrodes, including imaging guidance, when performed, including addition of new electrodes, when performed~~

To report, see ~64999

~~0285T~~ ~~Electronic analysis of implanted peripheral subcutaneous field stimulation pulse generator, with reprogramming when performed~~

To report, see ~64999

0286T-0287T

~~0286T~~ ~~Near-infrared spectroscopy studies of lower extremity wounds (eg, for oxyhemoglobin measurement)~~

To report, see ~76499

~~0287T~~ ~~Near-infrared guidance for vascular access requiring real-time digital visualization of subcutaneous vasculature for evaluation of potential access sites and vessel patency~~

0288T

~~0288T~~ ~~Anoscopy, with delivery of thermal energy to the muscle of the anal canal (eg, for fecal incontinence)~~

To report, see ~46999

0289T-0290T

Code first (65710, 65730, 65750, 65755)

~~0289T~~ ~~Corneal incisions in the donor cornea created using a laser, in preparation for penetrating or lamellar keratoplasty (List separately in addition to code for primary procedure)~~

+ **0290T** Corneal incisions in the recipient cornea created using a laser, in preparation for penetrating or lamellar keratoplasty (List separately in addition to code for primary procedure)

🖭 0.00   ⅄ 0.00   **FUD** ZZZ   N 80 ▣

AMA: 2016,Jan,13; 2015,Jan,16; 2014,Jan,11; 2012,Aug,9

0291T-0292T

~~0291T~~ ~~Intravascular optical coherence tomography (coronary native vessel or graft) during diagnostic evaluation and/or therapeutic intervention, including imaging supervision, interpretation, and report; initial vessel (List separately in addition to primary procedure)~~

To report, see ~[92978, 92979]

~~0292T~~ ~~each additional vessel (List separately in addition to primary procedure)~~

To report, see ~[92978, 92979]

0293T-0294T

EXCLUDES   Intracardiac echocardiography during procedure (93662)
Left heart catheterization with transseptal puncture (93462)
Code also when performed for separate clinical reason other than calibration or placement of left atrial hemodynamic monitoring system (33202-33249, 93451-93453) (33202-33249 [33221, 33227, 33228, 33229, 33230, 33231, 33262, 33263, 33264], 93451-93453)

▲ **0293T** Insertion of left atrial hemodynamic monitor; complete system, includes implanted communication module and pressure sensor lead in left atrium including transseptal access, radiological supervision and interpretation, and associated injection procedures, when performed

🖭 0.00   ⅄ 0.00   **FUD** XXX   C 80 ▣

▲ + **0294T** pressure sensor lead at time of insertion of pacing cardioverter-defibrillator pulse generator including radiological supervision and interpretation and associated injection procedures, when performed (List separately in addition to code for primary procedure)

🖭 0.00   ⅄ 0.00   **FUD** ZZZ   C 80 ▣

Code first (33230-33231, 33240, [33262, 33263, 33264], 33249)

0295T-0298T

EXCLUDES   External echocardiograph monitoring up to 48 hours
External electrocardiographic monitoring (93260-93272)
Mobile cardiovascular telemetry with echocardiograph recording (93228-93229)

0295T External electrocardiographic recording for more than 48 hours up to 21 days by continuous rhythm recording and storage; includes recording, scanning analysis with report, review and interpretation

🖭 0.00   ⅄ 0.00   **FUD** XXX   M 80 ▣

AMA: 2016,Jan,13; 2015,Jan,16; 2014,Jan,11; 2013,Feb,16-17

0296T recording (includes connection and initial recording)

🖭 0.00   ⅄ 0.00   **FUD** XXX   Q1 80 ▣

AMA: 2016,Jan,13; 2015,Jan,16; 2014,Jan,11; 2013,Feb,16-17

0297T	scanning analysis with report	

📷 0.00   ✂ 0.00   **FUD** XXX   01 80 📶

AMA: 2016,Jan,13; 2015,Jan,16; 2014,Jan,11; 2013,Feb,16-17

0298T	review and interpretation

📷 0.00   ✂ 0.00   **FUD** XXX   M 80 📶

AMA: 2016,Jan,13; 2015,Jan,16; 2014,Jan,11; 2013,Feb,16-17

0299T-0300T

EXCLUDES   *High energy extracorporeal shock wave for musculoskeletal system (28890, 0101T-0102T)*

Code first (0299T)

0299T	Extracorporeal shock wave for integumentary wound healing, high energy, including topical application and dressing care; initial wound

📷 0.00   ✂ 0.00   **FUD** XXX   T R2 80 📶

+	0300T	each additional wound (List separately in addition to code for primary procedure)

📷 0.00   ✂ 0.00   **FUD** ZZZ   N 80 📶

0301T

EXCLUDES   *Hyperthermia (77600-77615)*
         Ultrasound procedures of breast (76641-76642, 76942, 76998)

▲	0301T	Destruction/reduction of malignant breast tumor with externally applied focused microwave, including interstitial placement of disposable catheter with combined temperature monitoring probe and microwave focusing sensocatheter under ultrasound thermotherapy guidance

📷 0.00   ✂ 0.00   **FUD** XXX   T G2 80 📶

0302T-0304T

EXCLUDES   *Electrocardiographic services (93000-93010)*

▲	0302T	Insertion or removal and replacement of intracardiac ischemia monitoring system including imaging supervision and interpretation when performed and intra-operative interrogation and programming when performed; complete system (includes device and electrode)

📷 0.00   ✂ 0.00   **FUD** YYY   J J8 📶

▲	0303T	electrode only

📷 0.00   ✂ 0.00   **FUD** YYY   J J8 📶

▲	0304T	device only

📷 0.00   ✂ 0.00   **FUD** YYY   J J8 📶

0305T-0307T

0305T	Programming device evaluation (in person) of intracardiac ischemia monitoring system with iterative adjustment of programmed values, with analysis, review, and report

📷 0.00   ✂ 0.00   **FUD** XXX   01 80 📶

EXCLUDES   *Electrocardiographic services (93000-93010)*
         Intracardiac ischemia monitoring system (0302T-0304T, 0306T)

0306T	Interrogation device evaluation (in person) of intracardiac ischemia monitoring system with analysis, review, and report

📷 0.00   ✂ 0.00   **FUD** XXX   01 80 📶

EXCLUDES   *Electrocardiographic services (93000-93010)*
         Intracardiac ischemia monitoring system (0302T-0305T)

▲	0307T	Removal of intracardiac ischemia monitoring device

📷 0.00   ✂ 0.00   **FUD** YYY   02 G2 📶

0308T-0310T

▲	0308T	Insertion of ocular telescope prosthesis including removal of crystalline lens or intraocular lens prosthesis

INCLUDES   Injection procedures (66020, 66030)
         Iridectomy when performed (66600-66635, 66761)
         Operating microscope (69990)
         Repositioning of intraocular lens (66825)

EXCLUDES   *Cataract extraction (66982-66986)*

📷 0.00   ✂ 0.00   **FUD** YYY   J J8 50 📶

AMA: 2016,Jan,13; 2015,Jan,16; 2014,Jan,11; 2013,Mar,6-7

+	0309T	Arthrodesis, pre-sacral interbody technique, including disc space preparation, discectomy, with posterior instrumentation, with image guidance, includes bone graft, when performed, lumbar, L4-L5 interspace (List separately in addition to code for primary procedure)

📷 0.00   ✂ 0.00   **FUD** ZZZ   C 80 📶

INCLUDES   Bone graft (20930-20938)
         Imaging guidance (77002-77003, 77011-77012)
         Instrumentation (22840)

Code first (22586)

0310T	Motor function mapping using non-invasive navigated transcranial magnetic stimulation (nTMS) for therapeutic treatment planning, upper and lower extremity

📷 0.00   ✂ 0.00   **FUD** XXX   S 80 📶

INCLUDES   Electromyography (95860-95870)
         Evoked potential studies (95928-95929)

0312T-0317T

EXCLUDES   *Analysis and/or programming (or reprogramming) of vagus nerve stimulator (95970, 95974-95975)*
         Implantation, replacement, removal, and/or revision of vagus nerve neurostimulator (electrode array and/or pulse generator) for stimulation of vagus nerve other than at the esophagogastric junction (64568-64570)

0312T	Vagus nerve blocking therapy (morbid obesity); laparoscopic implantation of neurostimulator electrode array, anterior and posterior vagal trunks adjacent to esophagogastric junction (EGJ), with implantation of pulse generator, includes programming

📷 0.00   ✂ 0.00   **FUD** XXX   J 80 📶

AMA: 2016,Jan,13; 2015,Jan,16; 2013,Jan,11-12

0313T	laparoscopic revision or replacement of vagal trunk neurostimulator electrode array, including connection to existing pulse generator

📷 0.00   ✂ 0.00   **FUD** XXX   T G2 80 📶

AMA: 2016,Jan,13; 2015,Jan,16; 2013,Jan,11-12

0314T	laparoscopic removal of vagal trunk neurostimulator electrode array and pulse generator

📷 0.00   ✂ 0.00   **FUD** XXX   02 G2 80 📶

AMA: 2016,Jan,13; 2015,Jan,16; 2013,Jan,11-12

0315T	removal of pulse generator

EXCLUDES   *Removal with replacement pulse generator (0316T)*

📷 0.00   ✂ 0.00   **FUD** XXX   02 G2 80 📶

AMA: 2016,Jan,13; 2015,Jan,16; 2013,Jan,11-12

0316T	replacement of pulse generator

EXCLUDES   *Removal without replacement pulse generator (0315T)*

📷 0.00   ✂ 0.00   **FUD** XXX   J J8 80 📶

AMA: 2016,Jan,13; 2015,Jan,16; 2013,Jan,11-12

0317T	neurostimulator pulse generator electronic analysis, includes reprogramming when performed

📷 0.00   ✂ 0.00   **FUD** XXX   01 80 📶

AMA: 2016,Jan,13; 2015,Jan,16; 2013,Jan,11-12

0329T-0330T

0329T	Monitoring of intraocular pressure for 24 hours or longer, unilateral or bilateral, with interpretation and report

📷 0.00   ✂ 0.00   **FUD** YYY   E 📶

AMA: 2016,Jan,13; 2015,Jan,16; 2014,May,5

0330T	Tear film imaging, unilateral or bilateral, with interpretation and report

📷 0.00   ✂ 0.00   **FUD** YYY   01 📶

AMA: 2016,Jan,13; 2015,Jan,16; 2014,May,5

0331T-0332T

EXCLUDES   *Myocardial infarction avid imaging (78466, 78468, 78469)*

0331T	Myocardial sympathetic innervation imaging, planar qualitative and quantitative assessment;

📷 0.00   ✂ 0.00   **FUD** YYY   S Z2 📶

AMA: 2016,Jan,13; 2015,Jan,16; 2014,Jun,14

0332T **with tomographic SPECT**
0.00 0.00 FUD YYY [S] [Z2]
AMA: 2016,Jan,13; 2015,Jan,16; 2014,Jun,14

0333T-0337T

▲ 0333T **Visual evoked potential, screening of visual acuity, automated, with report**
[EXCLUDES] *Visual evoked potential testing for glaucoma (0464T)*
0.00 0.00 FUD YYY [E]
AMA: 2016,Jan,13; 2015,Jan,16; 2014,Aug,8

▲ 0335T **Extra-osseous subtalar joint implant for talotarsal stabilization**
0.00 0.00 FUD YYY [T] [G2]

~~0336T~~ **~~Laparoscopy, surgical, ablation of uterine fibroid(s), including intraoperative ultrasound guidance and monitoring, radiofrequency~~**
To report, see ~58674

0337T **Endothelial function assessment, using peripheral vascular response to reactive hyperemia, non-invasive (eg, brachial artery ultrasound, peripheral artery tonometry), unilateral or bilateral**
0.00 0.00 FUD YYY [Q1]
[EXCLUDES] *Noninvasive vascular studies extremities (93922-93923)*

0338T-0339T

[INCLUDES] Selective catheter placement renal arteries (36251-36254)

0338T **Transcatheter renal sympathetic denervation, percutaneous approach including arterial puncture, selective catheter placement(s) renal artery(ies), fluoroscopy, contrast injection(s), intraprocedural roadmapping and radiological supervision and interpretation, including pressure gradient measurements, flush aortogram and diagnostic renal angiography when performed; unilateral**
0.00 0.00 FUD YYY [J] [G2]

0339T **bilateral**
0.00 0.00 FUD YYY [J] [G2]

0340T-0342T

▲ 0340T **Ablation, pulmonary tumor(s), including pleura or chest wall when involved by tumor extension, percutaneous, cryoablation, unilateral, includes imaging guidance**
0.00 0.00 FUD YYY [T] [G2]
[INCLUDES] Imaging guidance (76940, 77013, 77022)

0341T **Quantitative pupillometry with interpretation and report, unilateral or bilateral**
0.00 0.00 FUD YYY [N]

0342T **Therapeutic apheresis with selective HDL delipidation and plasma reinfusion**
0.00 0.00 FUD YYY [S] [G2]

0345T-0347T

0345T **Transcatheter mitral valve repair percutaneous approach via the coronary sinus**
[EXCLUDES] *Cardiac catheterization procedures integral to valve procedure (93451-93454, 93456-93461, 93563-93564)*
Repair of mitral valve including transseptal puncture (33418-33419)
0.00 0.00 FUD YYY [C]
AMA: 2016,Jan,13; 2015,Sep,3

\+ 0346T **Ultrasound, elastography (List separately in addition to code for primary procedure)**
0.00 0.00 FUD YYY [N]
Code first (76536, 76604, 76641-76642, 76700, 76705, 76770, 76775, 76830, 76856-76857, 76870, 76872, 76881-76882)

0347T **Placement of interstitial device(s) in bone for radiostereometric analysis (RSA)**
0.00 0.00 FUD YYY [Q1]
AMA: 2016,Jan,13; 2015,Jun,8

0348T-0350T

0348T **Radiologic examination, radiostereometric analysis (RSA); spine, (includes cervical, thoracic and lumbosacral, when performed)**
0.00 0.00 FUD YYY [Q1]
AMA: 2016,Jan,13; 2015,Jun,8

0349T **upper extremity(ies), (includes shoulder, elbow, and wrist, when performed)**
0.00 0.00 FUD YYY [Q1]
AMA: 2016,Jan,13; 2015,Jun,8

0350T **lower extremity(ies), (includes hip, proximal femur, knee, and ankle, when performed)**
0.00 0.00 FUD YYY [Q1]
AMA: 2016,Jan,13; 2015,Jun,8

0351T-0354T

0351T **Optical coherence tomography of breast or axillary lymph node, excised tissue, each specimen; real-time intraoperative**
[INCLUDES] Interpretation and report (0352T)
0.00 0.00 FUD YYY [N]
AMA: 2016,Jan,13; 2015,Apr,6

0352T **interpretation and report, real-time or referred**
0.00 0.00 FUD YYY [B]
AMA: 2016,Jan,13; 2015,Apr,6

0353T **Optical coherence tomography of breast, surgical cavity; real-time intraoperative**
[INCLUDES] Interpretation and report (0354T)
[EXCLUDES] *Use of code more than one time per session*
0.00 0.00 FUD YYY [N]
AMA: 2016,Jan,13; 2015,Apr,6

0354T **interpretation and report, real time or referred**
0.00 0.00 FUD YYY [B]
AMA: 2016,Jan,13; 2015,Apr,6

0355T-0358T

0355T **Gastrointestinal tract imaging, intraluminal (eg, capsule endoscopy), colon, with interpretation and report**
0.00 0.00 FUD YYY [T]
[INCLUDES] Includes distal ileum imaging when performed
[EXCLUDES] *Capsule endoscopy esophagus only (91111)*
Capsule endoscopy esophagus through ileum (91110)

0356T **Insertion of drug-eluting implant (including punctal dilation and implant removal when performed) into lacrimal canaliculus, each**
0.00 0.00 FUD YYY [Q1]
[EXCLUDES] *Drug-eluting ocular insert (0444T-0445T)*

0357T **Resequenced code. See code following 0058T.**

0358T **Bioelectrical impedance analysis whole body composition assessment, with interpretation and report**
0.00 0.00 FUD YYY [Q1]

0359T

INCLUDES Adaptive behavior evaluation by physician/other qualified health care professional with assistance of technician(s)

EXCLUDES Evaluation for occupational therapy ([97165, 97166, 97167, 97168])
The following services when provided on the same date of service:
Assessment/evaluation/testing of cognitive function (96101-96125)
Psychiatric services (90785-90899)
Behavior/health assessment (96150-96155)

0359T **Behavior identification assessment, by the physician or other qualified health care professional, face-to-face with patient and caregiver(s), includes administration of standardized and non-standardized tests, detailed behavioral history, patient observation and caregiver interview, interpretation of test results, discussion of findings and recommendations with the primary guardian(s)/caregiver(s), and preparation of report**

🚑 0.00   ✂ 0.00   **FUD** YYY   V 🖵

AMA: 2016,Jan,13; 2015,Jan,16; 2014,Jun,3

0360T-0363T

INCLUDES Follow-up assessments
Provided to patients with destructive behaviors
Only the time of one technician when more than one is in attendance
Time reported during one day only

EXCLUDES The following services when provided on the same date of service:
Assessment/evaluation/testing of cognitive function (96101-96125)
Behavior/health assessment (96150-96155)
Psychiatric services (90785-90899)

0360T **Observational behavioral follow-up assessment, includes physician or other qualified health care professional direction with interpretation and report, administered by one technician; first 30 minutes of technician time, face-to-face with the patient**

INCLUDES Time based on face-to-face time provided by one technician and not the collective time of several technicians

EXCLUDES Less than 16 minutes of face-to-face technician time

🚑 0.00   ✂ 0.00   **FUD** YYY   V 🖵

AMA: 2016,Jan,13; 2015,Jan,16; 2014,Jun,3

+ **0361T** **each additional 30 minutes of technician time, face-to-face with the patient (List separately in addition to code for primary service)**

Code first (0360T)

🚑 0.00   ✂ 0.00   **FUD** ZZZ   N 🖵

AMA: 2016,Jan,13; 2015,Jan,16; 2014,Jun,3

0362T **Exposure behavioral follow-up assessment, includes physician or other qualified health care professional direction with interpretation and report, administered by physician or other qualified health care professional with the assistance of one or more technicians; first 30 minutes of technician(s) time, face-to-face with the patient**

INCLUDES Time based on face-to-face time provided by one technician and not the collective time of several technicians

🚑 0.00   ✂ 0.00   **FUD** YYY   V 🖵

AMA: 2016,Jan,13; 2015,Jan,16; 2014,Jun,3

+ **0363T** **each additional 30 minutes of technician(s) time, face-to-face with the patient (List separately in addition to code for primary procedure)**

🚑 0.00   ✂ 0.00   **FUD** ZZZ   N 🖵

AMA: 2016,Jan,13; 2015,Jan,16; 2014,Jun,3

0364T-0372T

0364T **Adaptive behavior treatment by protocol, administered by technician, face-to-face with one patient; first 30 minutes of technician time**

EXCLUDES Assessment/evaluation/testing of cognitive function (96101-96125)
Cognitive skills development (97532)
Psychiatric services (90785-90899)
Treatment of speech language disorder (92507)

🚑 0.00   ✂ 0.00   **FUD** YYY   S 🖵

AMA: 2016,Sep,6; 2016,Jan,13; 2015,Jan,16; 2014,Jun,3

+ **0365T** **each additional 30 minutes of technician time (List separately in addition to code for primary procedure)**

EXCLUDES Assessment/evaluation/testing of cognitive function (96101-96125)
Cognitive skills development (97532)
Psychiatric services (90785-90899)
Treatment of speech language disorder, individual (92507)

Code first (0364T)

🚑 0.00   ✂ 0.00   **FUD** ZZZ   N 🖵

AMA: 2016,Sep,6; 2016,Jan,13; 2015,Jan,16; 2014,Jun,3

0366T **Group adaptive behavior treatment by protocol, administered by technician, face-to-face with two or more patients; first 30 minutes of technician time**

EXCLUDES Assessment/evaluation/testing of cognitive function (96101-96125)
Cognitive skills development (97532)
Groups comprising more than eight patients
Psychiatric services (90785-90899)
Therapeutic procedures (97150)
Treatment of speech language disorder, group (92508)

🚑 0.00   ✂ 0.00   **FUD** YYY   S 🖵

AMA: 2016,Sep,6; 2016,Jan,13; 2015,Jan,16; 2014,Jun,3

+ **0367T** **each additional 30 minutes of technician time (List separately in addition to code for primary procedure)**

EXCLUDES Assessment/evaluation/testing of cognitive function (96101-96125)
Cognitive skills development (97532)
Groups comprising more than eight patients
Psychiatric services (90785-90899)
Therapeutic procedures (97150)
Treatment of speech language disorder, group (92508)

Code first (0366T)

🚑 0.00   ✂ 0.00   **FUD** ZZZ   N 🖵

AMA: 2016,Sep,6; 2016,Jan,13; 2015,Jan,16; 2014,Jun,3

0368T **Adaptive behavior treatment with protocol modification administered by physician or other qualified health care professional with one patient; first 30 minutes of patient face-to-face time**

EXCLUDES Cognitive skills development (97532)
Explanation/interpretation psychiatric and other services (90887)
Family psychotherapy (90846-90847)
Psychiatric diagnostic evaluation (90791-90792)
Treatment of speech language disorder, individual (92507)

🚑 0.00   ✂ 0.00   **FUD** YYY   S 🖵

AMA: 2016,Sep,6; 2016,Jan,13; 2015,Jan,16; 2014,Jun,3

+ **0369T** **each additional 30 minutes of patient face-to-face time (List separately in addition to code for primary procedure)**

EXCLUDES Cognitive skills development (97532)
Explanation/interpretation psychiatric and other services (90887)
Family psychotherapy (90846-90847)
Psychiatric diagnostic evaluation (90791-90792)
Treatment of speech language disorder, individual (92507)

Code first (0368T)

🚑 0.00   ✂ 0.00   **FUD** ZZZ   N 🖵

AMA: 2016,Sep,6; 2016,Jan,13; 2015,Jan,16; 2014,Jun,3

0370T **Family adaptive behavior treatment guidance, administered by physician or other qualified health care professional (without the patient present)**

EXCLUDES Cognitive skills development (97532)
Explanation/interpretation psychiatric and other services (90887)
Family psychotherapy (90846-90847)
Psychiatric diagnostic evaluation (90791-90792)

🚑 0.00   ✂ 0.00   **FUD** YYY   S 🖵

AMA: 2016,Jan,13; 2015,Jan,16; 2014,Jun,3

0371T Multiple-family group adaptive behavior treatment guidance, administered by physician or other qualified health care professional (without the patient present)

EXCLUDES Explanation/interpretation psychiatric and other services (90887)
Family psychotherapy (90846-90847)
Groups comprising more than families of eight patients
Psychiatric diagnostic evaluation (90791-90792)

0.00 0.00 **FUD** YYY [S] [⌷]

AMA: 2016,Jan,13; 2015,Jan,16; 2014,Jun,3

0372T Adaptive behavior treatment social skills group, administered by physician or other qualified health care professional face-to-face with multiple patients

EXCLUDES Groups comprising more than families of eight patients
Group psychotherapy (90853)
Therapeutic procedures (97150)
Treatment of speech language disorder, group (92508)

0.00 0.00 **FUD** YYY [S] [⌷]

AMA: 2016,Sep,6; 2016,Jan,13; 2015,Jan,16; 2014,Jun,3

0373T-0374T

EXCLUDES Assessment/evaluation/testing of cognitive function (96101-96125)
Psychiatric services (90785-90899)

0373T Exposure adaptive behavior treatment with protocol modification requiring two or more technicians for severe maladaptive behavior(s); first 60 minutes of technicians' time, face-to-face with patient

0.00 0.00 **FUD** YYY [S] [⌷]

AMA: 2016,Jan,13; 2015,Jan,16; 2014,Jun,3

+ **0374T** each additional 30 minutes of technicians' time face-to-face with patient (List separately in addition to code for primary procedure)

Code first (0373T)

0.00 0.00 **FUD** ZZZ [N] [⌷]

AMA: 2014,Jun,3

0375T

0375T Total disc arthroplasty (artificial disc), anterior approach, including discectomy with end plate preparation (includes osteophytectomy for nerve root or spinal cord decompression and microdissection), cervical, three or more levels

EXCLUDES Procedures performed at same level with (22853-22854, [22859], 22856, [22858])

0.00 0.00 **FUD** XXX [C] [80] [⌷]

AMA: 2016,Jan,13; 2015,Apr,7

0376T-0377T

0376T Resequenced code. See code following 0191T.

0377T Anoscopy with directed submucosal injection of bulking agent for fecal incontinence

0.00 0.00 **FUD** XXX [T] [G2] [80] [⌷]

INCLUDES Diagnostic anoscopy (46600)

0378T-0380T

0378T Visual field assessment, with concurrent real time data analysis and accessible data storage with patient initiated data transmitted to a remote surveillance center for up to 30 days; review and interpretation with report by a physician or other qualified health care professional

0.00 0.00 **FUD** XXX [B] [80] [⌷]

AMA: 2016,Jan,13; 2015,Jan,10

0379T technical support and patient instructions, surveillance, analysis and transmission of daily and emergent data reports as prescribed by a physician or other qualified health care professional

0.00 0.00 **FUD** XXX [Q1] [80] [⌷]

AMA: 2016,Jan,13; 2015,Jan,10

0380T Computer-aided animation and analysis of time series retinal images for the monitoring of disease progression, unilateral or bilateral, with interpretation and report

0.00 0.00 **FUD** XXX [Q1] [80] [⌷]

AMA: 2016,Feb,12

0381T-0386T

0381T External heart rate and 3-axis accelerometer data recording up to 14 days to assess changes in heart rate and to monitor motion analysis for the purposes of diagnosing nocturnal epilepsy seizure events; includes report, scanning analysis with report, review and interpretation by a physician or other qualified health care professional

0.00 0.00 **FUD** XXX [M] [80] [⌷]

EXCLUDES External heart rate and data recording for 15 days or more (0383T-0386T)

0382T review and interpretation only

0.00 0.00 **FUD** XXX [M] [80] [⌷]

EXCLUDES External heart rate and data recording for 15 days or more (0383T-0386T)

0383T External heart rate and 3-axis accelerometer data recording from 15 to 30 days to assess changes in heart rate and to monitor motion analysis for the purposes of diagnosing nocturnal epilepsy seizure events; includes report, scanning analysis with report, review and interpretation by a physician or other qualified health care professional

0.00 0.00 **FUD** XXX [M] [80] [⌷]

EXCLUDES External heart rate and data recording for 14 days or less (0381T-0382T)
External heart rate and data recording for 30 days or more (0385T-0386T)

0384T review and interpretation only

0.00 0.00 **FUD** XXX [M] [80] [⌷]

EXCLUDES External heart rate and data recording for 14 days or less (0381T-0382T)
External heart rate and data recording for 30 days or more (0385T-0386T)

0385T External heart rate and 3-axis accelerometer data recording more than 30 days to assess changes in heart rate and to monitor motion analysis for the purposes of diagnosing nocturnal epilepsy seizure events; includes report, scanning analysis with report, review and interpretation by a physician or other qualified health care professional

0.00 0.00 **FUD** XXX [M] [80] [⌷]

EXCLUDES External heart rate and data recording for 30 days or less (0381T-0384T)

0386T review and interpretation only

0.00 0.00 **FUD** XXX [M] [80] [⌷]

EXCLUDES External heart rate and data recording for 30 days or less (0381T-0384T)

0387T-0391T

0387T Transcatheter insertion or replacement of permanent leadless pacemaker, ventricular

INCLUDES Device evaluation (0389T-0391T)
Fluoroscopy (76000)
Lead removal when replacement performed (0388T)
Right ventriculography (93566)
Venography, femoral (75820)

EXCLUDES Procedures related to pacemaker systems with leads (33202-33203, 33206-33222 [33221], 33224-33226)

0.00 0.00 **FUD** XXX [J] [J8] [80] [⌷]

AMA: 2016,Aug,5; 2016,May,5; 2016,Jan,13; 2015,May,3; 2015,Jan,16; 2014,Dec,16; 2014,Dec,16

0388T Transcatheter removal of permanent leadless pacemaker, ventricular

> INCLUDES Fluoroscopy (76000)
> Right ventriculography (93566)
> Venography, femoral (75820)
> EXCLUDES *Insertion or replacement of device (0387T)*
> *Procedures related to removal of pacemaker systems with leads (33233-33238 [33227, 33228, 33229])*
> 0.00 0.00 **FUD** XXX T 62 80

AMA: 2016,Aug,5; 2016,May,5; 2016,Jan,13; 2015,May,3; 2015,Jan,16; 2014,Dec,16; 2014,Dec,16

0389T Programming device evaluation (in person) with iterative adjustment of the implantable device to test the function of the device and select optimal permanent programmed values with analysis, review and report, leadless pacemaker system

> EXCLUDES *Device evaluation (0390T-0391T)*
> *Insertion or replacement of device (0387T)*
> *Procedures to program pacemaker systems with leads (93279-93281)*
> 0.00 0.00 **FUD** XXX Q1 80

AMA: 2016,Aug,5; 2016,May,5; 2016,Jan,13; 2015,May,3; 2015,Jan,16; 2014,Dec,16; 2014,Dec,16

0390T Peri-procedural device evaluation (in person) and programming of device system parameters before or after a surgery, procedure or test with analysis, review and report, leadless pacemaker system

> EXCLUDES *Device evaluation (0389T, 0391T)*
> *Insertion or replacement of device (0387T)*
> *Procedures for peri-procedural evaluation and programming of pacemaker systems with leads (93286-93287)*
> 0.00 0.00 **FUD** XXX N 80

AMA: 2016,Aug,5; 2016,May,5; 2016,Jan,13; 2015,May,3; 2015,Jan,16; 2014,Dec,16; 2014,Dec,16

0391T Interrogation device evaluation (in person) with analysis, review and report, includes connection, recording and disconnection per patient encounter, leadless pacemaker system

> EXCLUDES *Device evaluation (0389T-0390T)*
> *Insertion or replacement of device (0387T)*
> *Procedures for interrogation device evaluation of pacemaker systems with leads (93288-93289)*
> 0.00 0.00 **FUD** XXX Q1 80

AMA: 2016,Aug,5; 2016,May,5; 2016,Jan,13; 2015,May,3

0392T-0393T

0392T ~~Laparoscopy, surgical, esophageal sphincter augmentation procedure, placement of sphincter augmentation device (ie, magnetic band)~~

> To report, see ~43284

0393T ~~Removal of esophageal sphincter augmentation device~~

> To report, see ~43285

0394T-0395T

> EXCLUDES *Radiation oncology procedures (77261-77263, 77300, 77306-77307, 77316-77318, 77332-77334, 77336, 77427-77499, 77761-77772, 77778, 77789)*

0394T High dose rate electronic brachytherapy, skin surface application, per fraction, includes basic dosimetry, when performed

> 0.00 0.00 **FUD** XXX S Z2 80
> EXCLUDES *Superficial non-brachytherapy radiation (77401)*

0395T High dose rate electronic brachytherapy, interstitial or intracavitary treatment, per fraction, includes basic dosimetry, when performed

> 0.00 0.00 **FUD** XXX S Z2 80
> EXCLUDES *High dose rate skin surface application (0394T)*

0396T-0399T

+ 0396T Intra-operative use of kinetic balance sensor for implant stability during knee replacement arthroplasty (List separately in addition to code for primary procedure)

> 0.00 0.00 **FUD** XXX N 80
> Code first (27445-27447, 27486-27488)

▲ + 0397T Endoscopic retrograde cholangiopancreatography (ERCP), with optical endomicroscopy (List separately in addition to code for primary procedure)

> 0.00 0.00 **FUD** XXX N 80
> INCLUDES Optical endomicroscopic image(s) (88375)
> EXCLUDES *Use of code more than one time per operative session*
> Code first (43260-43270 [43274, 43275, 43276, 43277, 43278])

0398T Magnetic resonance image guided high intensity focused ultrasound (MRgFUS), stereotactic ablation lesion, intracranial for movement disorder including stereotactic navigation and frame placement when performed

> 0.00 0.00 **FUD** XXX E 80
> INCLUDES Application stereotactic headframe (61800)
> Stereotactic computer-assisted navigation (61781)

+ 0399T Myocardial strain imaging (quantitative assessment of myocardial mechanics using image-based analysis of local myocardial dynamics) (List separately in addition to code for primary procedure)

> 0.00 0.00 **FUD** XXX N 80
> EXCLUDES *Use of code more than one time per session*
> Code first (93303-93312, 93314-93315, 93317, 93350-93351, 93355)

0400T-0401T

0400T Multi-spectral digital skin lesion analysis of clinically atypical cutaneous pigmented lesions for detection of melanomas and high risk melanocytic atypia; one to five lesions

> 0.00 0.00 **FUD** XXX N 80

0401T six or more lesions

> 0.00 0.00 **FUD** XXX N 80
> INCLUDES Treatment of one to five lesions (0400T)

0402T-0405T

0402T Collagen cross-linking of cornea (including removal of the corneal epithelium and intraoperative pachymetry when performed)

> INCLUDES Corneal epithelium removal (65435)
> Corneal pachymetry (76514)
> Operating microscope (69990)
> 0.00 0.00 **FUD** XXX T R2 80
> **AMA:** 2016,Feb,12

0403T Preventive behavior change, intensive program of prevention of diabetes using a standardized diabetes prevention program curriculum, provided to individuals in a group setting, minimum 60 minutes, per day

> 0.00 0.00 **FUD** XXX E 80
> **AMA:** 2015,Aug,4

0404T Transcervical uterine fibroid(s) ablation with ultrasound guidance, radiofrequency ♀

> 0.00 0.00 **FUD** XXX J 80

0405T Oversight of the care of an extracorporeal liver assist system patient requiring review of status, review of laboratories and other studies, and revision of orders and liver assist care plan (as appropriate), within a calendar month, 30 minutes or more of non-face-to-face time

> 0.00 0.00 **FUD** XXX B 80

0406T-0407T

INCLUDES Sinus procedures when performed on the same side (31200-31205, 31231, 31237, 31240, 31254-31255, 31288, 31290)

0406T **Nasal endoscopy, surgical, ethmoid sinus, placement of drug eluting implant;**
0.00 0.00 **FUD** XXX [N] [80] [CCI]
AMA: 2016,Feb,10

0407T **with biopsy, polypectomy or debridement**
EXCLUDES Endoscopy of sinus when performed on the same side (0406T)
0.00 0.00 **FUD** XXX [N] [80] [CCI]
AMA: 2016,Feb,10

0408T-0418T

● **0408T** **Insertion or replacement of permanent cardiac contractility modulation system, including contractility evaluation when performed, and programming of sensing and therapeutic parameters; pulse generator with transvenous electrodes**
0.00 0.00 **FUD** XXX [J] [J8] [80] [CCI]
INCLUDES Device evaluation (93286-93287, 0415T, 0417T-0418T)
Insertion or replacement of entire system
EXCLUDES Cardiac catheterization (93452-93453, 93458-93461)
Code also removal of each electrode when pulse generator and electrodes are removed and replaced (0410T-0411T)

● **0409T** **pulse generator only**
0.00 0.00 **FUD** XXX [J] [J8] [80] [CCI]
INCLUDES Device evaluation (93286-93287, 0415T, 0417T-0418T)
EXCLUDES Cardiac catheterization (93452-93453, 93458-93461)

● **0410T** **atrial electrode only**
0.00 0.00 **FUD** XXX [J] [J8] [80] [CCI]
INCLUDES Device evaluation (93286-93287, 0415T, 0417T-0418T)
Each atrial electrode inserted or replaced
EXCLUDES Cardiac catheterization (93452-93453, 93458-93461)

● **0411T** **ventricular electrode only**
0.00 0.00 **FUD** XXX [J] [J8] [80] [CCI]
INCLUDES Device evaluation (93286-93287, 0415T, 0417T-0418T)
Each ventricular electrode inserted or replaced
EXCLUDES Cardiac catheterization (93452-93453, 93458-93461)
Insertion or replacement of complete CCM system (0408T)

● **0412T** **Removal of permanent cardiac contractility modulation system; pulse generator only**
0.00 0.00 **FUD** XXX [02] [G2] [80] [CCI]
EXCLUDES Device evaluation (0417T-0418T)
Insertion or replacement of complete CCM system (0408T)

● **0413T** **transvenous electrode (atrial or ventricular)**
0.00 0.00 **FUD** XXX [02] [G2] [80] [CCI]
INCLUDES Each electrode removed
EXCLUDES Device evaluation (0417T-0418T)
Insertion or replacement of complete CCM system (0408T)
Code also removal and replacement of electrode(s), as appropriate (0410T-0411T)
Code also removal of pulse generator when leads also removed (0412T)

● **0414T** **Removal and replacement of permanent cardiac contractility modulation system pulse generator only**
0.00 0.00 **FUD** XXX [J] [J8] [80] [CCI]
EXCLUDES Cardiac catheterization (93452-93453, 93458-93461)
Device evaluation (93286-93287, 0417T-0418T)
Code also replacement of pulse generator when leads also removed and replaced (0408T, 0412T-0413T)

● **0415T** **Repositioning of previously implanted cardiac contractility modulation transvenous electrode, (atrial or ventricular lead)**
0.00 0.00 **FUD** XXX [T] [G2] [80] [CCI]
EXCLUDES Cardiac catheterization (93452-93453, 93458-93461)
Device evaluation (93286-93287, 0417T-0418T)
Insertion/replacement entire system or components (0408T-0411T)

● **0416T** **Relocation of skin pocket for implanted cardiac contractility modulation pulse generator**
0.00 0.00 **FUD** XXX [T] [G2] [80] [CCI]

● **0417T** **Programming device evaluation (in person) with iterative adjustment of the implantable device to test the function of the device and select optimal permanent programmed values with analysis, including review and report, implantable cardiac contractility modulation system**
0.00 0.00 **FUD** XXX [Q1] [80] [CCI]
EXCLUDES Insertion/replacement/removal/repositioning of device or components (0408T-0415T, 0418T)

● **0418T** **Interrogation device evaluation (in person) with analysis, review and report, includes connection, recording and disconnection per patient encounter, implantable cardiac contractility modulation system**
0.00 0.00 **FUD** XXX [Q1] [80] [CCI]
EXCLUDES Insertion/replacement/removal/repositioning of device or components (0408T-0415T, 0417T)

0419T-0420T

EXCLUDES Neurofibroma excision (64792)
Use of code more than one time per session

● **0419T** **Destruction of neurofibroma, extensive (cutaneous, dermal extending into subcutaneous); face, head and neck, greater than 50 neurofibromas**
0.00 0.00 **FUD** XXX [T] [R2] [80] [CCI]
AMA: 2016,Apr,3

● **0420T** **trunk and extremities, extensive, greater than 100 neurofibromas**
0.00 0.00 **FUD** XXX [T] [R2] [80] [CCI]
AMA: 2016,Apr,3

0421T-0423T

● **0421T** **Transurethral waterjet ablation of prostate, including control of post-operative bleeding, including ultrasound guidance, complete (vasectomy, meatotomy, cystourethroscopy, urethral calibration and/or dilation, and internal urethrotomy are included when performed)** ♂
0.00 0.00 **FUD** XXX [E] [80] [CCI]
EXCLUDES Transrectal ultrasound (76872)
Transurethral prostate resection (52500, 52630)

● **0422T** **Tactile breast imaging by computer-aided tactile sensors, unilateral or bilateral**
0.00 0.00 **FUD** XXX [Q1] [Z2] [80] [CCI]

● **0423T** **Secretory type II phospholipase A2 (sPLA2-IIA)**
0.00 0.00 **FUD** XXX [A]
EXCLUDES Lipoprotein-associated phospholipase A2 [LpPLA2] (83698)

0424T-0436T

INCLUDES Phrenic nerve stimulation system includes:
Pulse generator
Sensing lead (placed in azygos vein)
Stimulation lead (placed into right brachiocephalic vein or left periocardiophrenic vein)

● **0424T** **Insertion or replacement of neurostimulator system for treatment of central sleep apnea; complete system (transvenous placement of right or left stimulation lead, sensing lead, implantable pulse generator)**
0.00 0.00 **FUD** XXX [J] [80] [CCI]
INCLUDES Device evaluation (0434T-0436T)
Insertion/replacement system components (0424T-0427T)
Repositioning of leads (0432T-0433T)
Code also when pulse generator and all leads are removed and replaced (0428T-0430T)

0425T sensing lead only
🚑 0.00 ⚬ 0.00 **FUD** XXX   J 80 ▭
EXCLUDES Device evaluation (0434T-0436T)
Insertion/replacement complete system (0424T)
Repositioning of leads (0432T-0433T)

0426T stimulation lead only
🚑 0.00 ⚬ 0.00 **FUD** XXX   J 80 ▭
EXCLUDES Device evaluation (0434T-0436T)
Insertion/replacement complete system (0424T)
Repositioning of leads (0432T-0433T)

0427T pulse generator only
🚑 0.00 ⚬ 0.00 **FUD** XXX   J 80 ▭
EXCLUDES Device evaluation (0434T-0436T)
Insertion/replacement complete system (0424T)
Repositioning of leads (0432T-0433T)

0428T Removal of neurostimulator system for treatment of central sleep apnea; pulse generator only
🚑 0.00 ⚬ 0.00 **FUD** XXX   Q2 80 ▭
EXCLUDES Device evaluation (0434T-0436T)
Removal with replacement of pulse generator and all leads (0424T, 0429T-0430T)
Repositioning of leads (0432T-0433T)
Code also when a lead is removed (0429T-0430T)

0429T sensing lead only
🚑 0.00 ⚬ 0.00 **FUD** XXX   Q2 80 ▭
INCLUDES Removal of one sensing lead
EXCLUDES Device evaluation (0434T-0436T)

0430T stimulation lead only
INCLUDES Removal of one stimulation lead
EXCLUDES Device evaluation (0434T-0436T)
🚑 0.00 ⚬ 0.00 **FUD** XXX   Q2 80 ▭
AMA: 2015,Aug,4

0431T Removal and replacement of neurostimulator system for treatment of central sleep apnea, pulse generator only
🚑 0.00 ⚬ 0.00 **FUD** XXX   J 80 ▭
EXCLUDES Device evaluation (0434T-0436T)
Removal with replacement of pulse generator and all leads (0424T, 0428T-0430T)
Replacement or removal of generator and all three leads (0424T, 0428T-0430T)

0432T Repositioning of neurostimulator system for treatment of central sleep apnea; stimulation lead only
🚑 0.00 ⚬ 0.00 **FUD** XXX   T 80 ▭
EXCLUDES Device evaluation (0434T-0436T)
Insertion/replacement complete system or components (0424T-0427T)

0433T sensing lead only
🚑 0.00 ⚬ 0.00 **FUD** XXX   T 80 ▭
EXCLUDES Device evaluation (0434T-0436T)
Insertion/replacement complete system or components (0424T-0427T)

0434T Interrogation device evaluation implanted neurostimulator pulse generator system for central sleep apnea
🚑 0.00 ⚬ 0.00 **FUD** XXX   S 80 ▭
EXCLUDES Insertion/replacement complete system or components (0424T-0427T)
Removal system or components (0428T-0431T)
Repositioning leads (0432T-0433T)

0435T Programming device evaluation of implanted neurostimulator pulse generator system for central sleep apnea; single session
🚑 0.00 ⚬ 0.00 **FUD** XXX   S 80 ▭
EXCLUDES Device evaluation (0436T)
Insertion/replacement complete system or components (0424T-0427T)
Removal system or components (0428T-0431T)
Repositioning leads (0432T-0433T)

0436T during sleep study
🚑 0.00 ⚬ 0.00 **FUD** XXX   S 80 ▭
EXCLUDES Device evaluation (0435T)
Insertion/replacement complete system or components (0424T-0427T)
Removal system or components (0428T-0431T)
Repositioning leads (0432T-0433T)
Use of code more than one time for each sleep study

0437T-0439T

● + **0437T** Implantation of non-biologic or synthetic implant (eg, polypropylene) for fascial reinforcement of the abdominal wall (List separately in addition to code for primary procedure)
🚑 0.00 ⚬ 0.00 **FUD** ZZZ   N 80 ▭
EXCLUDES Implantation mesh, other material for repair incisional or ventral hernia (49560-49561, 49565-49566, 49568)
Insertion mesh, other material for closure of wound caused by necrotizing soft tissue infection (11004-11006, 49568)

● **0438T** Transperineal placement of biodegradable material, peri-prostatic (via needle), single or multiple, includes image guidance
🚑 0.00 ⚬ 0.00 **FUD** YYY   T G2 80 ▭
INCLUDES Ultrasonic guidance (76942)

● + **0439T** Myocardial contrast perfusion echocardiography, at rest or with stress, for assessment of myocardial ischemia or viability (List separately in addition to code for primary procedure)
Code first (93306-93308, 93350-93351)
🚑 0.00 ⚬ 0.00 **FUD** ZZZ   N 80 ▭
AMA: 2016,Apr,8

0440T-0442T

● **0440T** Ablation, percutaneous, cryoablation, includes imaging guidance; upper extremity distal/peripheral nerve
🚑 0.00 ⚬ 0.00 **FUD** YYY   J G2 80 ▭

● **0441T** lower extremity distal/peripheral nerve
🚑 0.00 ⚬ 0.00 **FUD** YYY   J G2 80 ▭

● **0442T** nerve plexus or other truncal nerve (eg, brachial plexus, pudendal nerve)
🚑 0.00 ⚬ 0.00 **FUD** YYY   J G2 80 ▭

0443T

● + **0443T** Real-time spectral analysis of prostate tissue by fluorescence spectroscopy, including imaging guidance (List separately in addition to code for primary procedure)
🚑 0.00 ⚬ 0.00 **FUD** ZZZ   T G2 80 ▭
EXCLUDES Use of code more than one time for each session
Code also (55700)

0444T-0445T

EXCLUDES Insertion/removal drug-eluting stent into canaliculus

● **0444T** Initial placement of a drug-eluting ocular insert under one or more eyelids, including fitting, training, and insertion, unilateral or bilateral
🚑 0.00 ⚬ 0.00 **FUD** YYY   N 80 ▭

● **0445T** Subsequent placement of a drug-eluting ocular insert under one or more eyelids, including re-training, and removal of existing insert, unilateral or bilateral
🚑 0.00 ⚬ 0.00 **FUD** YYY   N 80 ▭

0446T-0448T

EXCLUDES Placement non-implantable interstitial glucose sensor without pocket (95250)

● **0446T** Creation of subcutaneous pocket with insertion of implantable interstitial glucose sensor, including system activation and patient training
EXCLUDES Interpretation/report of ambulatory glucose monitoring of interstitial tissue (95251)
Removal interstitial glucose sensor (0447T-0448T)

Category III Codes

0447T — 0461T

● **0447T** Removal of implantable interstitial glucose sensor from subcutaneous pocket via incision

● **0448T** Removal of implantable interstitial glucose sensor with creation of subcutaneous pocket at different anatomic site and insertion of new implantable sensor, including system activation

> EXCLUDES Initial insertion of sensor (0446T)
> Removal of sensor (0447T)

0449T-0450T

> EXCLUDES Removal by internal approach of aqueous drainage device without extraocular reservoir in subconjunctival space (92499)

● **0449T** Insertion of aqueous drainage device, without extraocular reservoir, internal approach, into the subconjunctival space; initial device

● + **0450T** each additional device (List separately in addition to code for primary procedure)
> 🔧 0.00   ✂ 0.00   **FUD** 000
> Code first (0449T)

0451T-0463T

> INCLUDES Access procedures (36000-36010)
> Catheterization of vessel (36200-36228)
> Diagnostic angiography (75600-75774)
> Imaging guidance (76000-76001, 76936-76937, 77001-77002, 77011-77012, 77021)
> Injection procedures (93561-93572)
> Radiological supervision and interpretation
> EXCLUDES Cardiac catheterization (93451-93533)

● **0451T** Insertion or replacement of a permanently implantable aortic counterpulsation ventricular assist system, endovascular approach, and programming of sensing and therapeutic parameters; complete system (counterpulsation device, vascular graft, implantable vascular hemostatic seal, mechano-electrical skin interface and subcutaneous electrodes)
> EXCLUDES Aortic counterpulsation ventricular assist system procedures (0452T-0458T)
> Insertion intra-aortic balloon assist device (33967, 33970, 33973)
> Insertion/replacement extracorporeal ventricular assist device (33975-33976, 33981)
> Insertion/replacement intracorporeal ventricular assist device (33979, 33982-33983)
> Insertion ventricular assist device (33990-33991)

● **0452T** aortic counterpulsation device and vascular hemostatic seal
> EXCLUDES Insertion intra-aortic balloon assist device (33973)
> Insertion intracorporeal ventricular assist device (33979, 33982-33983)
> Insertion/replacement counterpulsation ventricular assist system procedures (0451T)
> Insertion ventricular assist device (33990-33991)
> Removal counterpulsation ventricular assist system (0455T-0456T)

● **0453T** mechano-electrical skin interface
> EXCLUDES Insertion intra-aortic balloon assist device (33973)
> Insertion intracorporeal ventricular assist device (33979, 33982-33983)
> Insertion/replacement counterpulsation ventricular assist system procedures (0451T)
> Insertion ventricular assist device (33990-33991)
> Removal counterpulsation ventricular assist system (0455T, 0457T)

● **0454T** subcutaneous electrode
> INCLUDES Each electrode inserted or replaced
> EXCLUDES Insertion intra-aortic balloon assist device (33973, 33982-33983)
> Insertion/replacement counterpulsation ventricular assist system (0451T)
> Insertion/replacement intracorporeal ventricular assist device (33979, 33982-33983)
> Insertion ventricular assist device (33990-33991)
> Removal device or component (0455T, 0458T)

● **0455T** Removal of permanently implantable aortic counterpulsation ventricular assist system; complete system (aortic counterpulsation device, vascular hemostatic seal, mechano-electrical skin interface and electrodes)
> EXCLUDES Insertion/replacement system or component (0451T-0454T)
> Removal:
> Extracorporeal ventricular assist device (33977-33978)
> Intra-aortic balloon assist device (33968, 33971, 33974)
> Intracorporeal ventricular assist device (33980)
> Percutaneous ventricular assist device (33992)
> System or component (0456T-0458T)

● **0456T** aortic counterpulsation device and vascular hemostatic seal
> EXCLUDES Insertion/replacement system or component (0451T-0452T)
> Removal:
> Aortic counterpulsation ventricular assist system (0455T)
> Intra-aortic balloon assist device (33974)
> Intracorporeal ventricular assist device (33980)
> Percutaneous ventricular assist device (33992)

● **0457T** mechano-electrical skin interface
> EXCLUDES Insertion/replacement system or component (0451T, 0453T)
> Removal:
> Aortic counterpulsation ventricular assist system (0455T)
> Intra-aortic balloon assist device (33974)
> Intracorporeal ventricular assist device (33980)
> Percutaneous ventricular assist device (33992)

● **0458T** subcutaneous electrode
> INCLUDES Each electrode removed
> EXCLUDES Insertion/replacement system or component (0451T, 0454T)
> Removal:
> Aortic counterpulsation ventricular assist system (0455T)
> Intra-aortic balloon assist device (33974)
> Intracorporeal ventricular assist device (33980)
> Percutaneous ventricular assist device (33992)

● **0459T** Relocation of skin pocket with replacement of implanted aortic counterpulsation ventricular assist device, mechano-electrical skin interface and electrodes
> EXCLUDES Repositioning percutaneous ventricular assist device (33993)

● **0460T** Repositioning of previously implanted aortic counterpulsation ventricular assist device; subcutaneous electrode
> INCLUDES Reporting for repositioning of each electrode
> EXCLUDES Insertion/replacement system or component (0451T, 0454T)
> Repositioning of percutaneous ventricular assist device (33993)

● **0461T** aortic counterpulsation device
> EXCLUDES Repositioning of percutaneous ventricular assist device (33993)

● **0462T** **Programming device evaluation (in person) with iterative adjustment of the implantable mechano-electrical skin interface and/or external driver to test the function of the device and select optimal permanent programmed values with analysis, including review and report, implantable aortic counterpulsation ventricular assist system, per day**

> EXCLUDES Device evaluation (0463T)
> Insertion/replacement system or component (0451T-0454T)
> Relocation of pocket (0459T)
> Removal system or component (0455T-0458T)
> Repositioning device (0460T-0461T)

● **0463T** **Interrogation device evaluation (in person) with analysis, review and report, includes connection, recording and disconnection per patient encounter, implantable aortic counterpulsation ventricular assist system, per day**

> EXCLUDES Device evaluation (0462T)
> Insertion/replacement system or component (0451T-0454T)
> Relocation of pocket (0459T)
> Removal system or component (0455T-0458T)
> Repositioning device (0460T-0461T)

0464T-0465T

● **0464T** **Visual evoked potential, testing for glaucoma, with interpretation and report**

> EXCLUDES Visual evoked potential visual acuity screening (0333T)

● **0465T** **Suprachoroidal injection of a pharmacologic agent (does not include supply of medication)**

> EXCLUDES Intravitreal implantation or injection (67025-67028)

0466T-0468T

> EXCLUDES Replacement/revision cranial nerve neurostimulator electrode array (64569)

● + **0466T** **Insertion of chest wall respiratory sensor electrode or electrode array, including connection to pulse generator (List separately in addition to code for primary procedure)**

> ⚙ 0.00   ✂ 0.00   **FUD** 000
>
> EXCLUDES Revision/removal chest wall respiratory sensor electrode or array (0467T-0468T)
> Code first (64568)

● **0467T** **Revision or replacement of chest wall respiratory sensor electrode or electrode array, including connection to existing pulse generator**

> EXCLUDES Insertion/removal chest wall respiratory sensor electrode or array (0466T, 0468T)
> Replacement/revision cranial neurostimulator electrode array (64569)

● **0468T** **Removal of chest wall respiratory sensor electrode or electrode array**

> EXCLUDES Insertion/removal chest wall respiratory sensor electrode or array (0466T-0467T)
> Removal cranial neurostimulator electrode array (64570)

Appendix A — Modifiers

CPT Modifiers

A modifier is a two-position alpha or numeric code appended to a CPT® code to clarify the services being billed. Modifiers provide a means by which a service can be altered without changing the procedure code. They add more information, such as the anatomical site, to the code. In addition, they help to eliminate the appearance of duplicate billing and unbundling. Modifiers are used to increase accuracy in reimbursement, coding consistency, editing, and to capture payment data.

22 Increased Procedural Services: When the work required to provide a service is substantially greater than typically required, it may be identified by adding modifier 22 to the usual procedure code. Documentation must support the substantial additional work and the reason for the additional work (ie, increased intensity, time, technical difficulty of procedure, severity of patient's condition, physical and mental effort required).
Note: This modifier should not be appended to an E/M service.

23 Unusual Anesthesia: Occasionally, a procedure, which usually requires either no anesthesia or local anesthesia, because of unusual circumstances must be done under general anesthesia. This circumstance may be reported by adding modifier 23 to the procedure code of the basic service.

24 Unrelated Evaluation and Management Service by the Same Physician or Other Qualified Health Care Professional During a Postoperative Period: The physician or other qualified health care professional may need to indicate that an evaluation and management service was performed during a postoperative period for a reason(s) unrelated to the original procedure. This circumstance may be reported by adding modifier 24 to the appropriate level of E/M service.

25 Significant, Separately Identifiable Evaluation and Management Service by the Same Physician or Other Qualified Health Care Professional on the Same Day of the Procedure or Other Service: It may be necessary to indicate that on the day a procedure or service identified by a CPT code was performed, the patient's condition required a significant, separately identifiable E/M service above and beyond the other service provided or beyond the usual preoperative and postoperative care associated with the procedure that was performed. A significant, separately identifiable E/M service is defined or substantiated by documentation that satisfies the relevant criteria for the respective E/M service to be reported (see Evaluation and Management Services Guidelines for instructions on determining level of E/M service). The E/M service may be prompted by the symptom or condition for which the procedure and/or service was provided. As such, different diagnoses are not required for reporting of the E/M services on the same date. This circumstance may be reported by adding modifier 25 to the appropriate level of E/M service.
Note: This modifier is not used to report an E/M service that resulted in a decision to perform surgery. See modifier 57. For significant, separately identifiable non-E/M services, see modifier 59.

26 Professional Component: Certain procedures are a combination of a physician or other qualified health care professional component and a technical component. When the physician or other qualified health care professional component is reported separately, the service may be identified by adding modifier 26 to the usual procedure number.

32 Mandated Services: Services related to mandated consultation and/or related services (eg, third-party payer, governmental, legislative or regulatory requirement) may be identified by adding modifier 32 to the basic procedure.

33 Preventive Services: When the primary purpose of the service is the delivery of an evidence-based service in accordance with a U.S. Preventive Services Task Force A or B rating in effect and other preventive services identified in preventive services mandates (legislative or regulatory), the service may be identified by adding 33 to the procedure. For separately reported services specifically identified as preventive, the modifier should not be used.

47 Anesthesia by Surgeon: Regional or general anesthesia provided by the surgeon may be reported by adding modifier 47 to the basic service. (This does not include local anesthesia.)
Note: Modifier 47 would not be used as a modifier for the anesthesia procedures 00100-01999.

50 Bilateral Procedure: Unless otherwise identified in the listings, bilateral procedures that are performed at the same session should be identified by adding modifier 50 to the appropriate 5-digit code.

51 Multiple Procedures: When multiple procedures, other than E/M services, Physical Medicine and Rehabilitation services or provision of supplies (e.g., vaccines), are performed at the same session by the same individual, the primary procedure or service may be reported as listed. The additional procedure(s) or service(s) may be identified by appending modifier 51 to the additional procedure or service code(s).
Note: This modifier should not be appended to designated "add-on" codes.

52 Reduced Services: Under certain circumstances a service or procedure is partially reduced or eliminated at the discretion of the physician or other qualified health care professional. Under these circumstances the service provided can be identified by its usual procedure number and the addition of modifier 52, signifying that the service is reduced. This provides a means of reporting reduced services without disturbing the identification of the basic service.
Note: For hospital outpatient reporting of a previously scheduled procedure/service that is partially reduced or cancelled as a result of extenuating circumstances or those that threaten the well-being of the patient prior to or after administration of anesthesia, see modifiers 73 and 74 (see modifiers approved for ASC hospital outpatient use).

53 Discontinued Procedure: Under certain circumstances, the physician or other qualified health care professional may elect to terminate a surgical or diagnostic procedure. Due to extenuating circumstances or those that threaten the well being of the patient, it may be necessary to indicate that a surgical or diagnostic procedure was started but discontinued. This circumstance may be reported by adding modifier 53 to the code reported by the physician for the discontinued procedure.
Note: This modifier is not used to report the elective cancellation of a procedure prior to the patient's anesthesia induction and/or surgical preparation in the operating suite. For outpatient hospital/ambulatory surgery center (ASC) reporting of a previously scheduled procedure/service that is partially reduced or cancelled as a result of extenuating circumstances or those that threaten the well being of the patient prior to or after administration of anesthesia, see modifiers 73 and 74 (see modifiers approved for ASC hospital outpatient use).

54 Surgical Care Only: When 1 physician or other qualified health care professional performs a surgical procedure and another provides preoperative and/or postoperative management, surgical services may be identified by adding modifier 54 to the usual procedure number.

55 Postoperative Management Only: When 1 physician or other qualified health care professional performed the postoperative management and another performed the surgical procedure, the postoperative component may be identified by adding modifier 55 to the usual procedure number.

56 Preoperative Management Only: When 1 physician or other qualified health care professional performed the preoperative care and evaluation and another performed the surgical procedure, the preoperative component may be identified by adding modifier 56 to the usual procedure number.

57 Decision for Surgery: An evaluation and management service that resulted in the initial decision to perform the surgery may be identified by adding modifier 57 to the appropriate level of E/M service.

58   Staged or Related Procedure or Service by the Same Physician or Other Qualified Health Care Professional During the Postoperative Period: It may be necessary to indicate that the performance of a procedure or service during the postoperative period was (a) planned or anticipated (staged); (b) more extensive than the original procedure; or (c) for therapy following a surgical procedure. This circumstance may be reported by adding modifier 58 to the staged or related procedure.
Note: For treatment of a problem that requires a return to the operating or procedure room (eg, unanticipated clinical condition), see modifier 78.

59   Distinct Procedural Service: Under certain circumstances, it may be necessary to indicate that a procedure or service was distinct or independent from other non-E/M services performed on the same day. Modifier 59 is used to identify procedures/services, other than E/M services, that are not normally reported together but are appropriate under the circumstances. Documentation must support a different session, different procedure or surgery, different site or organ system, separate incision/excision, separate lesion, or separate injury (or area of injury in extensive injuries) not ordinarily encountered or performed on the same day by the same individual. However, when another already established modifier is appropriate it should be used rather than modifier 59. Only if no more descriptive modifier is available and the use of modifier 59 best explains the circumstances, should modifier 59 be used.
Note: Modifier 59 should not be appended to an E/M service. To report a separate and distinct E/M service with a non-E/M service performed on the same date, see modifier 25. See also "Level II (HCPCS/National) Modifiers."

62   Two Surgeons: When 2 surgeons work together as primary surgeons performing distinct part(s) of a procedure, each surgeon should report his/her distinct operative work by adding modifier 62 to the procedure code and any associated add-on code(s) for that procedure as long as both surgeons continue to work together as primary surgeons. Each surgeon should report the cosurgery once using the same procedure code. If additional procedure(s) (including add-on procedure[s]) are performed during the same surgical session, separate code(s) may also be reported with modifier 62 added.
Note: If a cosurgeon acts as an assistant in the performance of additional procedure(s), other than those reported with the modifier 62, during the same surgical session, those services may be reported using separate procedure code(s) with modifier 80 or modifier 82 added, as appropriate.

63   Procedure Performed on Infants less than 4 kg: Procedures performed on neonates and infants up to a present body weight of 4 kg may involve significantly increased complexity and physician or other qualified health care professional work commonly associated with these patients. This circumstance may be reported by adding modifier 63 to the procedure number.
Note: Unless otherwise designated, this modifier may only be appended to procedures/services listed in the 20005-69990 code series. Modifier 63 should not be appended to any CPT codes listed in the Evaluation and Management Services, Anesthesia, Radiology, Pathology/Laboratory, or Medicine sections.

66   Surgical Team: Under some circumstances, highly complex procedures (requiring the concomitant services of several physicians or other qualified health care professionals, often of different specialties, plus other highly skilled, specially trained personnel, various types of complex equipment) are carried out under the "surgical team" concept. Such circumstances may be identified by each participating individual with the addition of modifier 66 to the basic procedure number used for reporting services.

76   Repeat Procedure or Service by Same Physician or Other Qualified Health Care Professional: It may be necessary to indicate that a procedure or service was repeated by the same physician or other qualified health care professional subsequent to the original procedure or service. This circumstance may be reported by adding modifier 76 to the repeated procedure or service.
Note: This modifier should not be appended to an E/M service.

77   Repeat Procedure by Another Physician or Other Qualified Health Care Professional: It may be necessary to indicate that a basic procedure or service was repeated by another physician or other qualified health care professional subsequent to the original procedure or service. This circumstance may be reported by adding modifier 77 to the repeated procedure or service.
Note: This modifier should not be appended to an E/M service.

78   Unplanned Return to the Operating/Procedure Room by the Same Physician or Other Qualified Health Care Professional Following Initial Procedure for a Related Procedure During the Postoperative Period: It may be necessary to indicate that another procedure was performed during the postoperative period of the initial procedure (unplanned procedure following initial procedure). When this procedure is related to the first, and requires the use of an operating/procedure room, it may be reported by adding modifier 78 to the related procedure. (For repeat procedures, see modifier 76.)

79   Unrelated Procedure or Service by the Same Physician or Other Qualified Health Care Professional During the Postoperative Period: The individual may need to indicate that the performance of a procedure or service during the postoperative period was unrelated to the original procedure. This circumstance may be reported by using modifier 79. (For repeat procedures on the same day, see modifier 76.)

80   Assistant Surgeon: Surgical assistant services may be identified by adding modifier 80 to the usual procedure number(s).

81   Minimum Assistant Surgeon: Minimum surgical assistant services are identified by adding modifier 81 to the usual procedure number.

82   Assistant Surgeon (when qualified resident surgeon not available): The unavailability of a qualified resident surgeon is a prerequisite for use of modifier 82 appended to the usual procedure code number(s).

90   Reference (Outside) Laboratory: When laboratory procedures are performed by a party other than the treating or reporting physician or other qualified health care professional, the procedure may be identified by adding modifier 90 to the usual procedure number.

91   Repeat Clinical Diagnostic Laboratory Test: In the course of treatment of the patient, it may be necessary to repeat the same laboratory test on the same day to obtain subsequent (multiple) test results. Under these circumstances, the laboratory test performed can be identified by its usual procedure number and the addition of modifier 91.
Note: This modifier may not be used when tests are rerun to confirm initial results; due to testing problems with specimens or equipment; or for any other reason when a normal, one-time, reportable result is all that is required. This modifier may not be used when another code(s) describes a series of test results (eg, glucose tolerance tests, evocative/suppression testing). This modifier may only be used for a laboratory test(s) performed more than once on the same day on the same patient.

92   Alternative Laboratory Platform Testing: When laboratory testing is being performed using a kit or transportable instrument that wholly or in part consists of a single use, disposable analytical chamber, the service may be identified by adding modifier 92 to the usual laboratory procedure code (HIV testing 86701-86703, and 87389). The test does not require permanent dedicated space, hence by its design may be hand carried or transported to the vicinity of the patient for immediate testing at that site, although location of the testing is not in itself determinative of the use of this modifier.

95 **Synchronous Telemedicine Service Rendered Via a Real-Time Interactive Audio and Video Telecommunications System:** Synchronous telemedicine service is defined as a **real-time** interaction between a physician or other qualified health care professional and a patient who is located at a distant site from the physician or other qualified health care professional. The totality of the communication of information exchanged between the physician or other qualified health care professional and patient during the course of the synchronous telemedicine service must be of an amount and nature that would be sufficient to meet the key components and/or requirements of the same service when rendered via a face-to-face interaction. Modifier 95 may only be appended to the services listed in Appendix F. Appendix F is the list of CPT codes for services that are typically performed face-to-face, but may be rendered via real-time (synchronous) interactive audio and video telecommunications system.

99 **Multiple Modifiers:** Under certain circumstances 2 or more modifiers may be necessary to completely delineate a service. In such situations, modifier 99 should be added to the basic procedure and other applicable modifiers may be listed as part of the description of the service.

Anesthesia Physical Status Modifiers

All anesthesia services are reported by use of the five-digit anesthesia procedure code with the appropriate physical status modifier appended.

Under certain circumstances, when other modifier(s) are appropriate, they should be reported in addition to the physical status modifier.

P1 A normal healthy patient

P2 A patient with mild systemic disease

P3 A patient with severe systemic disease

P4 A patient with severe systemic disease that is a constant threat to life

P5 A moribund patient who is not expected to survive without the operation

P6 A declared brain-dead patient whose organs are being removed for donor purposes

Modifiers Approved for Ambulatory Surgery Center (ASC) Hospital Outpatient Use

CPT Level I Modifiers

25 **Significant, Separately Identifiable Evaluation and Management Service by the Same Physician or Other Qualified Health Care Professional on the Same Day of the Procedure or Other Service:** It may be necessary to indicate that on the day a procedure or service identified by a CPT code was performed, the patient's condition required a significant, separately identifiable E/M service above and beyond the other service provided or beyond the usual preoperative and postoperative care associated with the procedure that was performed. A significant, separately identifiable E/M service is defined or substantiated by documentation that satisfies the relevant criteria for the respective E/M service to be reported (see Evaluation and Management Services Guidelines for instructions on determining level of E/M service). The E/M service may be prompted by the symptom or condition for which the procedure and/or service was provided. As such, different diagnoses are not required for reporting of the E/M services on the same date. This circumstance may be reported by adding modifier 25 to the appropriate level of E/M service.
Note: This modifier is not used to report an E/M service that resulted in a decision to perform surgery. See modifier 57. For significant, separately identifiable non-E/M services, see modifier 59.

27 **Multiple Outpatient Hospital E/M Encounters on the Same Date:** For hospital outpatient reporting purposes, utilization of hospital resources related to separate and distinct E/M encounters performed in multiple outpatient hospital settings on the same date may be reported by adding modifier 27 to each appropriate level outpatient and/or emergency department E/M code(s). This modifier provides a means of reporting circumstances involving evaluation and management services provided by a physician(s) in more than one (multiple) outpatient hospital setting(s) (eg, hospital emergency department, clinic).
Note: This modifier is not to be used for physician reporting of multiple E/M services performed by the same physician on the same date. For physician reporting of all outpatient evaluation and management services provided by the same physician on the same date and performed in multiple outpatient settings (eg, hospital emergency department, clinic), see Evaluation and Management, Emergency Department, or Preventive Medicine Services codes.

50 **Bilateral Procedure:** Unless otherwise identified in the listings, bilateral procedures that are performed at the same session should be identified by adding modifier 50 to the appropriate 5-digit code.

52 **Reduced Services:** Under certain circumstances a service or procedure is partially reduced or eliminated at the discretion of the physician or other qualified health care professional. Under these circumstances the service provided can be identified by its usual procedure number and the addition of modifier 52, signifying that the service is reduced. This provides a means of reporting reduced services without disturbing the identification of the basic service.
Note: For hospital outpatient reporting of a previously scheduled procedure/service that is partially reduced or cancelled as a result of extenuating circumstances or those that threaten the well-being of the patient prior to or after administration of anesthesia, see modifiers 73 and 74 (see modifiers approved for ASC hospital outpatient use).

58 **Staged or Related Procedure or Service by the Same Physician or Other Qualified Health Care Professional During the Postoperative Period:** It may be necessary to indicate that the performance of a procedure or service during the postoperative period was (a) planned or anticipated (staged); (b) more extensive than the original procedure; or (c) for therapy following a surgical procedure. This circumstance may be reported by adding modifier 58 to the staged or related procedure.
Note: For treatment of a problem that requires a return to the operating or procedure room (eg, unanticipated clinical condition), see modifier 78.

59 **Distinct Procedural Service:** Under certain circumstances, it may be necessary to indicate that a procedure or service was distinct or independent from other non-E/M services performed on the same day. Modifier 59 is used to identify procedures/services, other than E/M services, that are not normally reported together but are appropriate under the circumstances. Documentation must support a different session, different procedure or surgery, different site or organ system, separate incision/excision, separate lesion, or separate injury (or area of injury in extensive injuries) not ordinarily encountered or performed on the same day by the same individual. However, when another already established modifier is appropriate it should be used rather than modifier 59. Only if no more descriptive modifier is available and the use of modifier 59 best explains the circumstances, should modifier 59 be used.
Note: Modifier 59 should not be appended to an E/M service. To report a separate and distinct E/M service with a non-E/M service performed on the same date, see modifier 25. See also "Level II (HCPCS/National) Modifiers."

73 **Discontinued Out-Patient Hospital/Ambulatory Surgery Center (ASC) Procedure Prior to the Administration of Anesthesia:** Due to extenuating circumstances or those that threaten the well being of the patient, the physician may cancel a surgical or diagnostic procedure subsequent to the patient's surgical preparation (including sedation when provided, and being taken to the room where the procedure is to be performed), but prior to the administration of anesthesia (local, regional block(s), or general). Under these circumstances, the intended service that is prepared for but cancelled can be reported by its usual procedure number and the addition of modifier 73.
Note: The elective cancellation of a service prior to the administration of anesthesia and/or surgical preparation of the patient should not be reported. For physician reporting of a discontinued procedure, see modifier 53.

74 **Discontinued Out-Patient Hospital/Ambulatory Surgery Center (ASC) Procedure After Administration of Anesthesia:** Due to extenuating circumstances or those that threaten the well being of the patient, the physician may terminate a surgical or diagnostic procedure after the administration of anesthesia (local, regional block(s), general) or after the procedure was started (incision made, intubation started, scope inserted, etc.). Under these circumstances, the procedure started but terminated can be reported by its usual procedure number and the addition of modifier 74.
Note: The elective cancellation of a service prior to the administration of anesthesia and/or surgical preparation of the patient should not be reported. For physician reporting of a discontinued procedure, see modifier 53.

76 **Repeat Procedure or Service by Same Physician or Other Qualified Health Care Professional:** It may be necessary to indicate that a procedure or service was repeated by the same physician or other qualified health care professional subsequent to the original procedure or service. This circumstance may be reported by adding modifier 76 to the repeated procedure or service.
Note: This modifier should not be appended to an E/M service.

77 **Repeat Procedure by Another Physician or Other Qualified Health Care Professional:** It may be necessary to indicate that a basic procedure or service was repeated by another physician or other qualified health care professional subsequent to the original procedure or service. This circumstance may be reported by adding modifier 77 to the repeated procedure or service.
Note: This modifier should not be appended to an E/M service.

78 **Unplanned Return to the Operating/Procedure Room by the Same Physician or Other Qualified Health Care Professional Following Initial Procedure for a Related Procedure During the Postoperative Period:** It may be necessary to indicate that another procedure was performed during the postoperative period of the initial procedure (unplanned procedure following initial procedure). When this procedure is related to the first, and requires the use of an operating/procedure room, it may be reported by adding modifier 78 to the related procedure. (For repeat procedures, see modifier 76.)

79 **Unrelated Procedure or Service by the Same Physician During the Postoperative Period:** The individual may need to indicate that the performance of a procedure or service during the postoperative period was unrelated to the original procedure. This circumstance may be reported by using modifier 79. (For repeat procedures on the same day, see modifier 76.)

91 **Repeat Clinical Diagnostic Laboratory Test:** In the course of treatment of the patient, it may be necessary to repeat the same laboratory test on the same day to obtain subsequent (multiple) test results. Under these circumstances, the laboratory test performed can be identified by its usual procedure number and the addition of modifier 91.
Note: This modifier may not be used when tests are rerun to confirm initial results; due to testing problems with specimens or equipment; or for any other reason when a normal, one-time, reportable result is all that is required. This modifier may not be used when another code(s) describe a series of test results (eg, glucose tolerance tests, evocative/suppression testing). This modifier may only be used for a laboratory test(s) performed more than once on the same day on the same patient.

Level II (HCPCS/National) Modifiers

The HCPCS Level II modifiers included here are those most commonly used when coding procedures. See your 2017 HCPCS Level II book for a complete listing

Anatomical Modifiers

E1 Upper left, eyelid
E2 Lower left, eyelid
E3 Upper right, eyelid
E4 Lower right, eyelid
F1 Left hand, second digit
F2 Left hand, third digit
F3 Left hand, fourth digit
F4 Left hand, fifth digit
F5 Right hand, thumb
F6 Right hand, second digit
F7 Right hand, third digit
F8 Right hand, fourth digit
F9 Right hand, fifth digit
FA Left hand, thumb
LT Left side (used to identify procedures performed on the left side of the body)
RT Right side (used to identify procedures performed on the right side of the body)
T1 Left foot, second digit
T2 Left foot, third digit
T3 Left foot, fourth digit
T4 Left foot, fifth digit
T5 Right foot, great toe
T6 Right foot, second digit
T7 Right foot, third digit
T8 Right foot, fourth digit
T9 Right foot, fifth digit
TA Left foot, great toe

Anesthesia Modifiers

AA Anesthesia services performed personally by anesthesiologist
AD Medical supervision by a physician: more than four concurrent anesthesia procedures
G8 Monitored anesthesia care (MAC) for deep complex, complicated, or markedly invasive surgical procedure
G9 Monitored anesthesia care for patient who has history of severe cardiopulmonary condition
P1 A normal healthy patient
P2 A patient with mild systemic disease
P3 A patient with severe systemic disease
P4 A patient with severe systemic disease that is a constant threat to life
P5 A moribund patient who is not expected to survive without the operation
P6 A declared brain-dead patient whose organs are being removed for donor purposes
QK Medical direction of two, three, or four concurrent anesthesia procedures involving qualified individuals
QS Monitored anesthesia care service
QX CRNA service: with medical direction by a physician
QY Medical direction of one certified registered nurse anesthetist (CRNA) by an anesthesiologist
QZ CRNA service: without medical direction by a physician

Coronary Artery Modifiers

LC   Left circumflex coronary artery

LD   Left anterior descending coronary artery

LM   Left main coronary artery

RC   Right coronary artery

RI   Ramus intermedius coronary artery

Ophthalmology Modifiers

AP   Determination of refractive state was not performed in the course of diagnostic ophthalmological examination

LS   FDA-monitored intraocular lens implant

PL   Progressive addition lenses

VP   Aphakic patient

Other Modifiers

AE   Registered dietician

AF   Specialty physician

AG   Primary physician

AH   Clinical psychologist

AI   Principal physician of record

AJ   Clinical social worker

AK   Nonparticipating physician

AM   Physician, team member service

AO   Alternate payment method declined by provider of service

AQ   Physician providing a service in an unlisted health professional shortage area (HPSA)

AR   Physician provider services in a physician scarcity area

AS   Physician assistant, nurse practitioner, or clinical nurse specialist services for assistant at surgery

AT   Acute treatment (this modifier should be used when reporting service 98940, 98941, 98942)

CA   Procedure payable only in the inpatient setting when performed emergently on an outpatient who expires prior to admission

CB   Service ordered by a renal dialysis facility (RDF) physician as part of the ESRD beneficiary's dialysis benefit, is not part of the composite rate, and is separately reimbursable

CC   Procedure code change (use 'CC' when the procedure code submitted was changed either for administrative reasons or because an incorrect code was filed)

CG   Policy criteria applied

CP   Adjunctive service related to a procedure assigned to a comprehensive ambulatory payment classification (c-APC) procedure, but reported on a different claim

CR   Catastrophe/disaster related

CS   Item or service related, in whole or in part, to an illness, injury, or condition that was caused by or exacerbated by the effects, direct or indirect, of the 2010 oil spill in the gulf of Mexico, including but not limited to subsequent clean up activities

CT   Computed tomography services furnished using equipment that does not meet each of the attributes of the national electrical manufacturers association (NEMA) xr-29-2013 standard

EA   Erythropoetic stimulating agent (ESA) administered to treat anemia due to anticancer chemotherapy

EB   Erythropoetic stimulating agent (ESA) administered to treat anemia due to anticancer radiotherapy

EC   Erythropoetic stimulating agent (ESA) administered to treat anemia not due to anticancer radiotherapy or anticancer chemotherapy

EP   Service provided as part of Medicaid early periodic screening diagnosis and treatment (EPSDT) program

ET   Emergency services

EX   Expatriate beneficiary

EY   No physician or other licensed health care provider order for this item or service

FP   Service provided as part of family planning program

FX   X-ray taken using film

G7   Pregnancy resulted from rape or incest or pregnancy certified by physician as life threatening

GA   Waiver of liability statement issued as required by payer policy, individual case

GB   Claim being resubmitted for payment because it is no longer covered under a global payment demonstration

GC   This service has been performed in part by a resident under the direction of a teaching physician

GD   Units of service exceeds medically unlikely edit value and represents reasonable and necessary services

GE   This service has been performed by a resident without the presence of a teaching physician under the primary care exception

GF   Non-physician (e.g. nurse practitioner (NP), certified registered nurse anesthetist (CRNA), certified registered nurse (CRN), clinical nurse specialist (CNS), physician assistant (PA)) services in a critical access hospital

GG   Performance and payment of a screening mammogram and diagnostic mammogram on the same patient, same day

GH   Diagnostic mammogram converted from screening mammogram on same day

GJ   Opt out physician or practitioner emergency or urgent service

GK   Reasonable and necessary item/service associated with GA or GZ modifier

GN   Service delivered under an outpatient speech-language pathology plan of care

GO   Service delivered an outpatient occupational therapy plan of care

GP   Service delivered under an outpatient physical therapy plan of care

GQ   Via asynchronous telecommunications system

GR   This service was performed in whole or in part by a resident in a department of veterans affairs medical center or clinic, supervised in accordance with VA policy

GT   Via interactive audio and video telecommunication systems

GU   Waiver of liability statement issued as required by payer policy, routine notice

GV   Attending physician not employed or paid under arrangement by the patient's hospice provider

GW   Service not related to the hospice patient's terminal condition

GX   Notice of liability issued, voluntary under payer policy

GY   Item or service statutorily excluded, does not meet the definition of any Medicare benefit or for non-Medicare insurers, is not a contract benefit

GZ   Item or service expected to be denied as not reasonable and necessary

H9   Court-ordered

HA   Child/adolescent program

HB   Adult program, nongeriatric

HC   Adult program, geriatric

HD   Pregnant/parenting women's program

HE   Mental health program

HF   Substance abuse program

HG   Opioid addiction treatment program

HH   Integrated mental health/substance abuse program

HI   Integrated mental health and mental retardation/developmental disabilities program

HJ   Employee assistance program

HK   Specialized mental health programs for high-risk populations

HL   Intern

HM   Less than bachelor degree level

HN   Bachelors degree level

HO   Masters degree level

HP   Doctoral level

HQ Group setting

HR Family/couple with client present

HS Family/couple without client present

HT Multi-disciplinary team

HU Funded by child welfare agency

HV Funded state addictions agency

HW Funded by state mental health agency

HX Funded by county/local agency

HY Funded by juvenile justice agency

HZ Funded by criminal justice agency

LR Laboratory round trip

M2 Medicare secondary payer (MSP)

PA Surgical or other invasive procedure on wrong body part

PB Surgical or other invasive procedure on wrong patient

PC Wrong surgery or other invasive procedure on patient

PD Diagnostic or related nondiagnostic item or service provided in a wholly owned or operated entity to a patient who is admitted as an inpatient within 3 days

PI Positron emission tomography (PET) or PET/computed tomography (CT) to inform the initial treatment strategy of tumors that are biopsy proven or strongly suspected of being cancerous based on other diagnostic testing

PM Post-mortem

PN Non-excepted service provided at an off-campus, outpatient, provider-based department of a hospital

PO Excepted service provided at an off-campus, outpatient, provider-based department of a hospital

PS Positron emission tomography (PET) or PET/computed tomography (CT) to inform the subsequent treatment strategy of cancerous tumor when the beneficiary's treating physician determines that the PET study is needed to inform subsequent anti-tumor strategy

PT Colorectal cancer screening test; converted to diagnostic test or other procedure

Q0 Investigational clinical service provided in a clinical research study that is in an approved clinical research study

Q1 Routine clinical service provided in a clinical research study that is in an approved clinical research study

Q2 Demonstration procedure/service

Q4 Service for ordering/referring physician qualifies as a service exemption

Q5 Service furnished by a substitute physician under a reciprocal billing arrangement

Q6 Service furnished by a locum tenens physician

Q7 One Class A finding

Q8 Two Class B findings

Q9 One Class B and 2 Class C findings

QC Single channel monitoring

QD Recording and storage in solid state memory by a digital recorder

QJ Services/items provided to a prisoner or patient in state or local custody, however the state or local government, as applicable, meets the requirements in 42 CFR 411.4 (B)

QN Ambulance service furnished directly by a provider of services

QP Documentation is on file showing that the laboratory test(s) was ordered individually or ordered as a CPT-recognized panel other than automated profile codes

QT Recording and storage on tape by an analog tape recorder

QW CLIA waived test

RE Furnished in full compliance with FDA-mandated risk evaluation and mitigation strategy (REMS)

SA Nurse practitioner rendering service in collaboration with a physician

SB Nurse Midwife

SC Medically necessary service or supply

SD Services provided by registered nurse with specialized, highly technical home infusion training

SE State and/or federally funded programs/services

SF Second opinion ordered by a professional review organization (PRO) per section 9401, P.L.99-272 (100% reimbursement - no Medicare deductible or coinsurance)

SG Ambulatory surgical center (ASC) facility service

SH Second concurrently administered infusion therapy

SJ Third or more concurrently administered infusion therapy

SK Member of high risk population (use only with codes for immunization)

SL State supplied vaccine

SM Second surgical opinion

SN Third surgical opinion

SQ Item ordered by home health

SS Home infusion services provided in the infusion suite of the IV therapy provider

ST Related to trauma or injury

SU Procedure performed in physician's office (to denote use of facility and equipment)

SW Services provided by a certified diabetic educator

SY Persons who are in close contact with member of high-risk population (use only with codes for immunization)

TC Technical component. Under certain circumstances, a charge may be made for the technical component alone. Under those circumstances the technical component charge is identified by adding modifier 'TC' to the usual procedure number. Technical component charges are institutional charges and not billed separately by physicians. However, portable x-ray suppliers only bill for technical component and should utilize modifier TC. The charge data from portable x-ray suppliers will then be used to build customary and prevailing profiles.

TD RN

TE LPN/LVN

TF Intermediate level of care

TG Complex/high level of care

TH Obstetrical treatment/services, prenatal or postpartum

TJ Program group, child and/or adolescent

TK Extra patient or passenger, nonambulance

TL Early intervention/individualized family service plan (IFSP)

TM Individualized education program (IEP)

TN Rural/outside providers' customary service area

TR School-based individualized education program (IEP) services provided outside the public school district responsible for the student

TS Follow-up service

TT Individualized service provided to more than one patient in same setting

TU Special payment rate, overtime

TV Special payment rates, holidays/weekends

U1 Medicaid level of care 1, as defined by each state

U2 Medicaid level of care 2, as defined by each state

U3 Medicaid level of care 3, as defined by each state

U4 Medicaid level of care 4, as defined by each state

U5 Medicaid level of care 5, as defined by each state

U6 Medicaid level of care 6, as defined by each state

U7 Medicaid level of care 7, as defined by each state

U8 Medicaid level of care 8, as defined by each state

U9 Medicaid level of care 9, as defined by each state

UA Medicaid level of care 10, as defined by each state

UB Medicaid level of care 11, as defined by each state

UC Medicaid level of care 12, as defined by each state

UD Medicaid level of care 13, as defined by each state

UF Services provided in the morning

UG Services provided in the afternoon

UH Services provided in the evening

UJ Services provided at night

UK Services provided on behalf of the client to someone other than the client (collateral relationship)

UN Two patients served

UP Three patients served

UQ Four patients served

UR Five patients served

US Six or more patients served

V1 Demonstration modifier 1

V2 Demonstration modifier 2

V3 Demonstration modifier 3

V5 Vascular catheter (alone or with any other vascular access)

V6 Arteriovenous graft (or other vascular access not including a vascular catheter)

V7 Arteriovenous fistula only (in use with 2 needles)

* **XE** Separate encounter, a service that Is distinct because it occurred during a separate encounter

* **XP** Separate practitioner, a service that is distinct because it was performed by a different practitioner

* **XS** Separate structure, a service that is distinct because it was performed on a separate organ/structure

* **XU** Unusual non-overlapping service, the use of a service that is distinct because it does not overlap usual components of the main service

ZA Novartis/Sandoz

ZB Pfizer/Hospira

* CMS instituted additional HCPCS modifiers to define explicit subsets of modifier 59 Distinct Procedural Service.

Category II Modifiers

1P Performance measure exclusion modifier due to medical reasons

Includes:

- Not indicated (absence of organ/limb, already received/performed, other)
- Contraindicated (patient allergic history, potential adverse drug interaction, other)
- Other medical reasons

2P Performance measure exclusion modifier due to patient reasons

Includes:

- Patient declined
- Economic, social, or religious reasons
- Other patient reasons

3P Performance measure exclusion modifier due to system reasons

Includes:

- Resources to perform the services not available (eg, equipment, supplies)
- Insurance coverage or payer-related limitations
- Other reasons attributable to health care delivery system

8P Performance measure reporting modifier - action not performed, reason not otherwise specified

Dental Modifiers

AZ Physician providing a service in a dental health professional shortage area for the purpose of an electronic health record incentive payment

DA Oral health assessment by a licensed health professional other than a dentist

ET Emergency services (dental procedures performed in emergency situations should show the modifier ET)

ESRD Modifiers

AY Item or service furnished to an ESRD patient that is not for the treatment of ESRD

CD AMCC test has been ordered by an ESRD facility or MCP physician that is a part of the composite rate and is not separately billable

CE AMCC test has been ordered by an ESRD facility or MCP physician that is a composite rate test but is beyond the normal frequency covered under the rate and is separately reimbursable based on medically necessary

CF AMCC test has been ordered by an ESRD facility or MCP physician that is not part of the composite rate and is separately billable

ED Hematocrit level has exceeded 39% (or hemoglobin level has exceeded 13.0 G/dl) for 3 or more consecutive billing cycles immediately prior to and including the current cycle

EE Hematocrit level has not exceeded 39% (or hemoglobin level has not exceeded 13.0 G/dl) for 3 or more consecutive billing cycles immediately prior to and including the current cycle

EJ Subsequent claims for a defined course of therapy, e.g., EPO, sodium hyaluronate, infliximab

EM Emergency reserve supply (for ESRD benefit only)

G1 Most recent URR reading of less than 60

G2 Most recent URR reading of 60 to 64.9

G3 Most recent URR reading of 65 to 69.9

G4 Most recent URR reading of 70 to 74.9

G5 Most recent URR reading of 75 or greater

G6 ESRD patient for whom less than 6 dialysis sessions have been provided in a month

GS Dosage of EPO or darbepoietin alfa has been reduced and maintained in response to hematocrit or hemoglobin level

JE Administered via dialysate

Q3 Live kidney donor surgery and related services

Appendix B — New, Changed and Deleted Codes

New Codes

22853 Insertion of interbody biomechanical device(s) (eg, synthetic cage, mesh) with integral anterior instrumentation for device anchoring (eg, screws, flanges), when performed, to intervertebral disc space in conjunction with interbody arthrodesis, each interspace (List separately in addition to code for primary procedure)

22854 Insertion of intervertebral biomechanical device(s) (eg, synthetic cage, mesh) with integral anterior instrumentation for device anchoring (eg, screws, flanges), when performed, to vertebral corpectomy(ies) (vertebral body resection, partial or complete) defect, in conjunction with interbody arthrodesis, each contiguous defect (List separately in addition to code for primary procedure)

22859 Insertion of intervertebral biomechanical device(s) (eg, synthetic cage, mesh, methylmethacrylate) to intervertebral disc space or vertebral body defect without interbody arthrodesis, each contiguous defect (List separately in addition to code for primary procedure)

22867 Insertion of interlaminar/interspinous process stabilization/distraction device, without fusion, including image guidance when performed, with open decompression, lumbar; single level

22868 Insertion of interlaminar/interspinous process stabilization/distraction device, without fusion, including image guidance when performed, with open decompression, lumbar; second level (List separately in addition to code for primary procedure)

22869 Insertion of interlaminar/interspinous process stabilization/distraction device, without open decompression or fusion, including image guidance when performed, lumbar; single level

22870 Insertion of interlaminar/interspinous process stabilization/distraction device, without open decompression or fusion, including image guidance when performed, lumbar; second level (List separately in addition to code for primary procedure)

27197 Closed treatment of posterior pelvic ring fracture(s), dislocation(s), diastasis or subluxation of the ilium, sacroiliac joint, and/or sacrum, with or without anterior pelvic ring fracture(s) and/or dislocation(s) of the pubic symphysis and/or superior/inferior rami, unilateral or bilateral; without manipulation

27198 Closed treatment of posterior pelvic ring fracture(s), dislocation(s), diastasis or subluxation of the ilium, sacroiliac joint, and/or sacrum, with or without anterior pelvic ring fracture(s) and/or dislocation(s) of the pubic symphysis and/or superior/inferior rami, unilateral or bilateral; with manipulation, requiring more than local anesthesia (ie, general anesthesia, moderate sedation, spinal/epidural)

28291 Hallux rigidus correction with cheilectomy, debridement and capsular release of the first metatarsophalangeal joint; with implant

28295 Correction, hallux valgus (bunionectomy), with sesamoidectomy, when performed; with proximal metatarsal osteotomy, any method

31551 Laryngoplasty; for laryngeal stenosis, with graft, without indwelling stent placement, younger than 12 years of age

31552 Laryngoplasty; for laryngeal stenosis, with graft, without indwelling stent placement, age 12 years or older

31553 Laryngoplasty; for laryngeal stenosis, with graft, with indwelling stent placement, younger than 12 years of age

31554 Laryngoplasty; for laryngeal stenosis, with graft, with indwelling stent placement, age 12 years or older

31572 Laryngoscopy, flexible; with ablation or destruction of lesion(s) with laser, unilateral

31573 Laryngoscopy, flexible; with therapeutic injection(s) (eg, chemodenervation agent or corticosteroid, injected percutaneous, transoral, or via endoscope channel), unilateral

31574 Laryngoscopy, flexible; with injection(s) for augmentation (eg, percutaneous, transoral), unilateral

31591 Laryngoplasty, medialization, unilateral

31592 Cricotracheal resection

33340 Percutaneous transcatheter closure of the left atrial appendage with endocardial implant, including fluoroscopy, transseptal puncture, catheter placement(s), left atrial angiography, left atrial appendage angiography, when performed, and radiological supervision and interpretation

33390 Valvuloplasty, aortic valve, open, with cardiopulmonary bypass; simple (ie, valvotomy, debridement, debulking, and/or simple commissural resuspension)

33391 Valvuloplasty, aortic valve, open, with cardiopulmonary bypass; complex (eg, leaflet extension, leaflet resection, leaflet reconstruction, or annuloplasty)

36456 Partial exchange transfusion, blood, plasma or crystalloid necessitating the skill of a physician or other qualified health care professional, newborn

36473 Endovenous ablation therapy of incompetent vein, extremity, inclusive of all imaging guidance and monitoring, percutaneous, mechanochemical; first vein treated

36474 Endovenous ablation therapy of incompetent vein, extremity, inclusive of all imaging guidance and monitoring, percutaneous, mechanochemical; subsequent vein(s) treated in a single extremity, each through separate access sites (List separately in addition to code for primary procedure)

36901 Introduction of needle(s) and/or catheter(s), dialysis circuit, with diagnostic angiography of the dialysis circuit, including all direct puncture(s) and catheter placement(s), injection(s) of contrast, all necessary imaging from the arterial anastomosis and adjacent artery through entire venous outflow including the inferior or superior vena cava, fluoroscopic guidance, radiological supervision and interpretation and image documentation and report;

36902 Introduction of needle(s) and/or catheter(s), dialysis circuit, with diagnostic angiography of the dialysis circuit, including all direct puncture(s) and catheter placement(s), injection(s) of contrast, all necessary imaging from the arterial anastomosis and adjacent artery through entire venous outflow including the inferior or superior vena cava, fluoroscopic guidance, radiological supervision and interpretation and image documentation and report; with transluminal balloon angioplasty, peripheral dialysis segment, including all imaging and radiological supervision and interpretation necessary to perform the angioplasty

36903 Introduction of needle(s) and/or catheter(s), dialysis circuit, with diagnostic angiography of the dialysis circuit, including all direct puncture(s) and catheter placement(s), injection(s) of contrast, all necessary imaging from the arterial anastomosis and adjacent artery through entire venous outflow including the inferior or superior vena cava, fluoroscopic guidance, radiological supervision and interpretation and image documentation and report; with transcatheter placement of intravascular stent(s), peripheral dialysis segment, including all imaging and radiological supervision and interpretation necessary to perform the stenting, and all angioplasty within the peripheral dialysis segment

36904 Percutaneous transluminal mechanical thrombectomy and/or infusion for thrombolysis, dialysis circuit, any method, including all imaging and radiological supervision and interpretation, diagnostic angiography, fluoroscopic guidance, catheter placement(s), and intraprocedural pharmacological thrombolytic injection(s);

36905 Percutaneous transluminal mechanical thrombectomy and/or infusion for thrombolysis, dialysis circuit, any method, including all imaging and radiological supervision and interpretation, diagnostic angiography, fluoroscopic guidance, catheter placement(s), and intraprocedural pharmacological thrombolytic injection(s); with transluminal balloon angioplasty, peripheral dialysis segment, including all imaging and radiological supervision and interpretation necessary to perform the angioplasty

36906 Percutaneous transluminal mechanical thrombectomy and/or infusion for thrombolysis, dialysis circuit, any method, including all imaging and radiological supervision and interpretation, diagnostic angiography, fluoroscopic guidance, catheter placement(s), and intraprocedural pharmacological thrombolytic injection(s); with transcatheter placement of intravascular stent(s), peripheral dialysis segment, including all imaging and radiological supervision and interpretation necessary to perform the stenting, and all angioplasty within the peripheral dialysis circuit

36907 Transluminal balloon angioplasty, central dialysis segment, performed through dialysis circuit, including all imaging and radiological supervision and interpretation required to perform the angioplasty (List separately in addition to code for primary procedure)

36908 Transcatheter placement of intravascular stent(s), central dialysis segment, performed through dialysis circuit, including all imaging radiological supervision and interpretation required to perform the stenting, and all angioplasty in the central dialysis segment (List separately in addition to code for primary procedure)

36909 Dialysis circuit permanent vascular embolization or occlusion (including main circuit or any accessory veins), endovascular, including all imaging and radiological supervision and interpretation necessary to complete the intervention (List separately in addition to code for primary procedure)

37246 Transluminal balloon angioplasty (except lower extremity artery(ies) for occlusive disease, intracranial, coronary, pulmonary, or dialysis circuit), open or percutaneous, including all imaging and radiological supervision and interpretation necessary to perform the angioplasty within the same artery; initial artery

37247 Transluminal balloon angioplasty (except lower extremity artery(ies) for occlusive disease, intracranial, coronary, pulmonary, or dialysis circuit), open or percutaneous, including all imaging and radiological supervision and interpretation necessary to perform the angioplasty within the same artery; each additional artery (List separately in addition to code for primary procedure)

37248 Transluminal balloon angioplasty (except dialysis circuit), open or percutaneous, including all imaging and radiological supervision and interpretation necessary to perform the angioplasty within the same vein; initial vein

37249 Transluminal balloon angioplasty (except dialysis circuit), open or percutaneous, including all imaging and radiological supervision and interpretation necessary to perform the angioplasty within the same vein; each additional vein (List separately in addition to code for primary procedure)

43284 Laparoscopy, surgical, esophageal sphincter augmentation procedure, placement of sphincter augmentation device (ie, magnetic band), including cruroplasty when performed

43285 Removal of esophageal sphincter augmentation device

58674 Laparoscopy, surgical, ablation of uterine fibroid(s) including intraoperative ultrasound guidance and monitoring, radiofrequency

62320 Injection(s), of diagnostic or therapeutic substance(s) (eg, anesthetic, antispasmodic, opioid, steroid, other solution), not including neurolytic substances, including needle or catheter placement, interlaminar epidural or subarachnoid, cervical or thoracic; without imaging guidance

62321 Injection(s), of diagnostic or therapeutic substance(s) (eg, anesthetic, antispasmodic, opioid, steroid, other solution), not including neurolytic substances, including needle or catheter placement, interlaminar epidural or subarachnoid, cervical or thoracic; with imaging guidance (ie, fluoroscopy or CT)

62322 Injection(s), of diagnostic or therapeutic substance(s) (eg, anesthetic, antispasmodic, opioid, steroid, other solution), not including neurolytic substances, including needle or catheter placement, interlaminar epidural or subarachnoid, lumbar or sacral (caudal); without imaging guidance

62323 Injection(s), of diagnostic or therapeutic substance(s) (eg, anesthetic, antispasmodic, opioid, steroid, other solution), not including neurolytic substances, including needle or catheter placement, interlaminar epidural or subarachnoid, lumbar or sacral (caudal); with imaging guidance (ie, fluoroscopy or CT)

62324 Injection(s), including indwelling catheter placement, continuous infusion or intermittent bolus, of diagnostic or therapeutic substance(s) (eg, anesthetic, antispasmodic, opioid, steroid, other solution), not including neurolytic substances, interlaminar epidural or subarachnoid, cervical or thoracic; without imaging guidance

62325 Injection(s), including indwelling catheter placement, continuous infusion or intermittent bolus, of diagnostic or therapeutic substance(s) (eg, anesthetic, antispasmodic, opioid, steroid, other solution), not including neurolytic substances, interlaminar epidural or subarachnoid, cervical or thoracic; with imaging guidance (ie, fluoroscopy or CT)

62326 Injection(s), including indwelling catheter placement, continuous infusion or intermittent bolus, of diagnostic or therapeutic substance(s) (eg, anesthetic, antispasmodic, opioid, steroid, other solution), not including neurolytic substances, interlaminar epidural or subarachnoid, lumbar or sacral (caudal); without imaging guidance

62327 Injection(s), including indwelling catheter placement, continuous infusion or intermittent bolus, of diagnostic or therapeutic substance(s) (eg, anesthetic, antispasmodic, opioid, steroid, other solution), not including neurolytic substances, interlaminar epidural or subarachnoid, lumbar or sacral (caudal); with imaging guidance (ie, fluoroscopy or CT)

62380 Endoscopic decompression of spinal cord, nerve root(s), including laminotomy, partial facetectomy, foraminotomy, discectomy and/or excision of herniated intervertebral disc, 1 interspace, lumbar

76706 Ultrasound, abdominal aorta, real time with image documentation, screening study for abdominal aortic aneurysm (AAA)

77065 Diagnostic mammography, including computer-aided detection (CAD) when performed; unilateral

77066 Diagnostic mammography, including computer-aided detection (CAD) when performed; bilateral

77067 Screening mammography, bilateral (2-view study of each breast), including computer-aided detection (CAD) when performed

80305 Drug test(s), presumptive, any number of drug classes, any number of devices or procedures (eg, immunoassay); capable of being read by direct optical observation only (eg, dipsticks, cups, cards, cartridges) includes sample validation when performed, per date of service

80306 Drug test(s), presumptive, any number of drug classes, any number of devices or procedures (eg, immunoassay); read by instrument assisted direct optical observation (eg, dipsticks, cups, cards, cartridges), includes sample validation when performed, per date of service

80307 Drug test(s), presumptive, any number of drug classes, any number of devices or procedures, by instrument chemistry analyzers (eg, utilizing immunoassay [eg, EIA, ELISA, EMIT, FPIA, IA, KIMS, RIA]), chromatography (eg, GC, HPLC), and mass spectrometry either with or without chromatography, (eg, DART, DESI, GC-MS, GC-MS/MS, LC-MS, LC-MS/MS, LDTD, MALDI, TOF) includes sample validation when performed, per date of service

81327 SEPT9 (Septin9) (eg, colorectal cancer) methylation analysis

81413 Cardiac ion channelopathies (eg, Brugada syndrome, long QT syndrome, short QT syndrome, catecholaminergic polymorphic ventricular tachycardia); genomic sequence analysis panel, must include sequencing of at least 10 genes, including ANK2, CASQ2, CAV3, KCNE1, KCNE2, KCNH2, KCNJ2, KCNQ1, RYR2, and SCN5A

81414　Cardiac ion channelopathies (eg, Brugada syndrome, long QT syndrome, short QT syndrome, catecholaminergic polymorphic ventricular tachycardia); duplication/deletion gene analysis panel, must include analysis of at least 2 genes, including KCNH2 and KCNQ1

81422　Fetal chromosomal microdeletion(s) genomic sequence analysis (eg, DiGeorge syndrome, Cri-du-chat syndrome), circulating cell-free fetal DNA in maternal blood

81439　Inherited cardiomyopathy (eg, hypertrophic cardiomyopathy, dilated cardiomyopathy, arrhythmogenic right ventricular cardiomyopathy) genomic sequence analysis panel, must include sequencing of at least 5 genes, including DSG2, MYBPC3, MYH7, PKP2, and TTN

81539　Oncology (high-grade prostate cancer), biochemical assay of four proteins (Total PSA, Free PSA, Intact PSA, and human kallikrein-2 [hK2]), utilizing plasma or serum, prognostic algorithm reported as a probability score

84410　Testosterone; bioavailable, direct measurement (eg, differential precipitation)

87483　Infectious agent detection by nucleic acid (DNA or RNA); central nervous system pathogen (eg, Neisseria meningitidis, Streptococcus pneumoniae, Listeria, Haemophilus influenzae, E. coli, Streptococcus agalactiae, enterovirus, human parechovirus, herpes simplex virus type 1 and 2, human herpesvirus 6, cytomegalovirus, varicella zoster virus, Cryptococcus), includes multiplex reverse transcription, when performed, and multiplex amplified probe technique, multiple types or subtypes, 12-25 targets

90674　Influenza virus vaccine, quadrivalent (ccIIV4), derived from cell cultures, subunit, preservative and antibiotic free, 0.5 mL dosage, for intramuscular use

92242　Fluorescein angiography and indocyanine-green angiography (includes multiframe imaging) performed at the same patient encounter with interpretation and report, unilateral or bilateral

93590　Percutaneous transcatheter closure of paravalvular leak; initial occlusion device, mitral valve

93591　Percutaneous transcatheter closure of paravalvular leak; initial occlusion device, aortic valve

93592　Percutaneous transcatheter closure of paravalvular leak; each additional occlusion device (List separately in addition to code for primary procedure)

96160　Administration of patient-focused health risk assessment instrument (eg, health hazard appraisal) with scoring and documentation, per standardized instrument

96161　Administration of caregiver-focused health risk assessment instrument (eg, depression inventory) for the benefit of the patient, with scoring and documentation, per standardized instrument

96377　Application of on-body injector (includes cannula insertion) for timed subcutaneous injection

97161　Physical therapy evaluation: low complexity, requiring these components: A history with no personal factors and/or comorbidities that impact the plan of care; An examination of body system(s) using standardized tests and measures addressing 1-2 elements from any of the following: body structures and functions, activity limitations, and/or participation restrictions; A clinical presentation with stable and/or uncomplicated characteristics; and Clinical decision making of low complexity using standardized patient assessment instrument and/or measurable assessment of functional outcome. Typically, 20 minutes are spent face-to-face with the patient and/or family.

97162　Physical therapy evaluation: moderate complexity, requiring these components: A history of present problem with 1-2 personal factors and/or comorbidities that impact the plan of care; An examination of body systems using standardized tests and measures in addressing a total of 3 or more elements from any of the following: body structures and functions, activity limitations, and/or participation restrictions; An evolving clinical presentation with changing characteristics; and Clinical decision making of moderate complexity using standardized patient assessment instrument and/or measurable assessment of functional outcome. Typically, 30 minutes are spent face-to-face with the patient and/or family.

97163　Physical therapy evaluation: high complexity, requiring these components: A history of present problem with 3 or more personal factors and/or comorbidities that impact the plan of care; An examination of body systems using standardized tests and measures addressing a total of 4 or more elements from any of the following: body structures and functions, activity limitations, and/or participation restrictions; A clinical presentation with unstable and unpredictable characteristics; and Clinical decision making of high complexity using standardized patient assessment instrument and/or measurable assessment of functional outcome. Typically, 45 minutes are spent face-to-face with the patient and/or family.

97164　Re-evaluation of physical therapy established plan of care, requiring these components: An examination including a review of history and use of standardized tests and measures is required; and Revised plan of care using a standardized patient assessment instrument and/or measurable assessment of functional outcome Typically, 20 minutes are spent face-to-face with the patient and/or family.

97165　Occupational therapy evaluation, low complexity, requiring these components: An occupational profile and medical and therapy history, which includes a brief history including review of medical and/or therapy records relating to the presenting problem; An assessment(s) that identifies 1-3 performance deficits (ie, relating to physical, cognitive, or psychosocial skills) that result in activity limitations and/or participation restrictions; and Clinical decision making of low complexity, which includes an analysis of the occupational profile, analysis of data from problem-focused assessment(s), and consideration of a limited number of treatment options. Patient presents with no comorbidities that affect occupational performance. Modification of tasks or assistance (eg, physical or verbal) with assessment(s) is not necessary to enable completion of evaluation component. Typically, 30 minutes are spent face-to-face with the patient and/or family.

97166　Occupational therapy evaluation, moderate complexity, requiring these components: An occupational profile and medical and therapy history, which includes an expanded review of medical and/or therapy records and additional review of physical, cognitive, or psychosocial history related to current functional performance; An assessment(s) that identifies 3-5 performance deficits (ie, relating to physical, cognitive, or psychosocial skills) that result in activity limitations and/or participation restrictions; and Clinical decision making of moderate analytic complexity, which includes an analysis of the occupational profile, analysis of data from detailed assessment(s), and consideration of several treatment options. Patient may present with comorbidities that affect occupational performance. Minimal to moderate modification of tasks or assistance (eg, physical or verbal) with assessment(s) is necessary to enable patient to complete evaluation component. Typically, 45 minutes are spent face-to-face with the patient and/or family.

97167　Occupational therapy evaluation, high complexity, requiring these components: An occupational profile and medical and therapy history, which includes review of medical and/or therapy records and extensive additional review of physical, cognitive, or psychosocial history related to current functional performance; An assessment(s) that identifies 5 or more performance deficits (ie, relating to physical, cognitive, or psychosocial skills) that result in activity limitations and/or participation restrictions; and Clinical decision making of high analytic complexity, which includes an analysis of the patient profile, analysis of data from comprehensive assessment(s), and consideration of multiple treatment options. Patient presents with comorbidities that affect occupational performance. Significant modification of tasks or assistance (eg, physical or verbal) with assessment(s) is necessary to enable patient to complete evaluation component. Typically, 60 minutes are spent face-to-face with the patient and/or family.

97168　Re-evaluation of occupational therapy established plan of care, requiring these components: An assessment of changes in patient functional or medical status with revised plan of care; An update to the initial occupational profile to reflect changes in condition or environment that affect future interventions and/or goals; and A revised plan of care. A formal reevaluation is performed when there is a documented change in functional status or a significant change to the plan of care is required. Typically, 30 minutes are spent face-to-face with the patient and/or family.

97169 Athletic training evaluation, low complexity, requiring these components: A history and physical activity profile with no comorbidities that affect physical activity; An examination of affected body area and other symptomatic or related systems addressing 1-2 elements from any of the following: body structures, physical activity, and/or participation deficiencies; and Clinical decision making of low complexity using standardized patient assessment instrument and/or measurable assessment of functional outcome. Typically, 15 minutes are spent face-to-face with the patient and/or family.

97170 Athletic training evaluation, moderate complexity, requiring these components: A medical history and physical activity profile with 1-2 comorbidities that affect physical activity; An examination of affected body area and other symptomatic or related systems addressing a total of 3 or more elements from any of the following: body structures, physical activity, and/or participation deficiencies; and Clinical decision making of moderate complexity using standardized patient assessment instrument and/or measurable assessment of functional outcome. Typically, 30 minutes are spent face-to-face with the patient and/or family.

97171 Athletic training evaluation, high complexity, requiring these components: A medical history and physical activity profile, with 3 or more comorbidities that affect physical activity; A comprehensive examination of body systems using standardized tests and measures addressing a total of 4 or more elements from any of the following: body structures, physical activity, and/or participation deficiencies; Clinical presentation with unstable and unpredictable characteristics; and Clinical decision making of high complexity using standardized patient assessment instrument and/or measurable assessment of functional outcome. Typically, 45 minutes are spent face-to-face with the patient and/or family.

97172 Re-evaluation of athletic training established plan of care requiring these components: An assessment of patient's current functional status when there is a documented change; and A revised plan of care using a standardized patient assessment instrument and/or measurable assessment of functional outcome with an update in management options, goals, and interventions. Typically, 20 minutes are spent face-to-face with the patient and/or family.

99151 Moderate sedation services provided by the same physician or other qualified health care professional performing the diagnostic or therapeutic service that the sedation supports, requiring the presence of an independent trained observer to assist in the monitoring of the patient's level of consciousness and physiological status; initial 15 minutes of intraservice time, patient younger than 5 years of age

99152 Moderate sedation services provided by the same physician or other qualified health care professional performing the diagnostic or therapeutic service that the sedation supports, requiring the presence of an independent trained observer to assist in the monitoring of the patient's level of consciousness and physiological status; initial 15 minutes of intraservice time, patient age 5 years or older

99153 Moderate sedation services provided by the same physician or other qualified health care professional performing the diagnostic or therapeutic service that the sedation supports, requiring the presence of an independent trained observer to assist in the monitoring of the patient's level of consciousness and physiological status; each additional 15 minutes intraservice time (List separately in addition to code for primary service)

99155 Moderate sedation services provided by a physician or other qualified health care professional other than the physician or other qualified health care professional performing the diagnostic or therapeutic service that the sedation supports; initial 15 minutes of intraservice time, patient younger than 5 years of age

99156 Moderate sedation services provided by a physician or other qualified health care professional other than the physician or other qualified health care professional performing the diagnostic or therapeutic service that the sedation supports; initial 15 minutes of intraservice time, patient age 5 years or older

99157 Moderate sedation services provided by a physician or other qualified health care professional other than the physician or other qualified health care professional performing the diagnostic or therapeutic service that the sedation supports; each additional 15 minutes intraservice time (List separately in addition to code for primary service)

0437T Implantation of non-biologic or synthetic implant (eg, polypropylene) for fascial reinforcement of the abdominal wall (List separately in addition to code for primary procedure)

0438T Transperineal placement of biodegradable material, peri-prostatic (via needle), single or multiple, includes image guidance

0439T Myocardial contrast perfusion echocardiography, at rest or with stress, for assessment of myocardial ischemia or viability (List separately in addition to code for primary procedure)

0440T Ablation, percutaneous, cryoablation, includes imaging guidance; upper extremity distal/peripheral nerve

0441T Ablation, percutaneous, cryoablation, includes imaging guidance; lower extremity distal/peripheral nerve

0442T Ablation, percutaneous, cryoablation, includes imaging guidance; nerve plexus or other truncal nerve (eg, brachial plexus, pudendal nerve)

0443T Real-time spectral analysis of prostate tissue by fluorescence spectroscopy, including imaging guidance (List separately in addition to code for primary procedure)

0444T Initial placement of a drug-eluting ocular insert under one or more eyelids, including fitting, training, and insertion, unilateral or bilateral

0445T Subsequent placement of a drug-eluting ocular insert under one or more eyelids, including re-training, and removal of existing insert, unilateral or bilateral

0446T Creation of subcutaneous pocket with insertion of implantable interstitial glucose sensor, including system activation and patient training

0447T Removal of implantable interstitial glucose sensor from subcutaneous pocket via incision

0448T Removal of implantable interstitial glucose sensor with creation of subcutaneous pocket at different anatomic site and insertion of new implantable sensor, including system activation

0449T Insertion of aqueous drainage device, without extraocular reservoir, internal approach, into the subconjunctival space; initial device

0450T Insertion of aqueous drainage device, without extraocular reservoir, internal approach, into the subconjunctival space; each additional device (List separately in addition to code for primary procedure)

0451T Insertion or replacement of a permanently implantable aortic counterpulsation ventricular assist system, endovascular approach, and programming of sensing and therapeutic parameters; complete system (counterpulsation device, vascular graft, implantable vascular hemostatic seal, mechano-electrical skin interface and subcutaneous electrodes)

0452T Insertion or replacement of a permanently implantable aortic counterpulsation ventricular assist system, endovascular approach, and programming of sensing and therapeutic parameters; aortic counterpulsation device and vascular hemostatic seal

0453T Insertion or replacement of a permanently implantable aortic counterpulsation ventricular assist system, endovascular approach, and programming of sensing and therapeutic parameters; mechano-electrical skin interface

0454T Insertion or replacement of a permanently implantable aortic counterpulsation ventricular assist system, endovascular approach, and programming of sensing and therapeutic parameters; subcutaneous electrode

0455T Removal of permanently implantable aortic counterpulsation ventricular assist system; complete system (aortic counterpulsation device, vascular hemostatic seal, mechano-electrical skin interface and electrodes)

0456T Removal of permanently implantable aortic counterpulsation ventricular assist system; aortic counterpulsation device and vascular hemostatic seal

0457T   Removal of permanently implantable aortic counterpulsation ventricular assist system; mechano-electrical skin interface

0458T   Removal of permanently implantable aortic counterpulsation ventricular assist system; subcutaneous electrode

0459T   Relocation of skin pocket with replacement of implanted aortic counterpulsation ventricular assist device, mechano-electrical skin interface and electrodes

0460T   Repositioning of previously implanted aortic counterpulsation ventricular assist device; subcutaneous electrode

0461T   Repositioning of previously implanted aortic counterpulsation ventricular assist device; aortic counterpulsation device

0462T   Programming device evaluation (in person) with iterative adjustment of the implantable mechano-electrical skin interface and/or external driver to test the function of the device and select optimal permanent programmed values with analysis, including review and report, implantable aortic counterpulsation ventricular assist system, per day

0463T   Interrogation device evaluation (in person) with analysis, review and report, includes connection, recording and disconnection per patient encounter, implantable aortic counterpulsation ventricular assist system, per day

Changed Codes

20240   Biopsy, bone, open; superficial (eg, ~~ilium~~ sternum, spinous process, rib, ~~sternum~~ patella, ~~spinous~~ olecranon process, calcaneus, tarsal,~~ribs~~ metatarsal, ~~trochanter of femur~~ carpal, metacarpal, phalanx)

20245   deep (eg,~~humerus~~ humeral shaft, ischium, ~~femur~~ femoral shaft)

28289   Hallux rigidus correction with cheilectomy, debridement and capsular release of the first metatarsophalangeal joint; without implant

28292   Correction, hallux valgus bunion(bunionectomy), with sesamoidectomy, ~~or without~~ when performed; ~~Keller McBride~~ with resection of proximal phalanx base, ~~or Mayo type procedure~~ when performed, any method

28296   with distal metatarsal osteotomy, ~~(eg, Mitchell, Chevron, or concentric type procedures)~~any method

28297   ~~Lapidus-type procedure~~ with first metatarsal and medial cuneiform joint arthrodesis, any method

28298   ~~by~~ with proximal phalanx osteotomy, any method

28299   ~~by~~ with double osteotomy, any method

31575   Laryngoscopy, flexible ~~fiberoptic~~; diagnostic

31576   with biopsy(ies)

31577   with removal of foreign body(s)

31578   Laryngoscopy, flexible; with removal of lesion(s), non-laser

31579   Laryngoscopy, flexible or rigid ~~fiberoptic~~telescopic, with stroboscopy

31580   Laryngoplasty; for laryngeal web, ~~2-stage~~with indwelling keel ~~insertion or removal~~ or stent insertion

31584

31587   Laryngoplasty, cricoid split, without graft placement

33405   Replacement, aortic valve, open, with cardiopulmonary bypass; with prosthetic valve other than homograft or stentless valve

33406   with allograft valve (freehand)

33410   with stentless tissue valve

36476   Endovenous ablation therapy of incompetent vein, extremity, inclusive of all imaging guidance and monitoring, percutaneous, radiofrequency; ~~second and~~subsequent vein(s) treated in a single extremity, each through separate access sites (List separately in addition to code for primary procedure)

36479   ~~second and~~ subsequent vein(s) treated in a single extremity, each through separate access sites (List separately in addition to code for primary procedure)

47538   Placement of stent(s) into a bile duct, percutaneous, including diagnostic cholangiography, imaging guidance (eg, fluoroscopy and/or ultrasound), balloon dilation, catheter exchange(s) and catheter removal(s) when performed, and all associated radiological supervision and interpretation; ~~each stent~~ existing access

47539   new access, without placement of separate biliary drainage catheter

47540   new access, with placement of separate biliary drainage catheter (eg, external or internal-external)

62287   Decompression procedure, percutaneous, of nucleus pulposus of intervertebral disc, any method utilizing needle based technique to remove disc material under fluoroscopic imaging or other form of indirect visualization, ~~with the use of an endoscope~~ with discography and/or epidural injection(s) at the treated level(s), when performed, single or multiple levels, lumbar

67101   Repair of retinal detachment, ~~1 or more sessions~~ including drainage of subretinal fluid when performed; cryotherapy or diathermy, including drainage of subretinal fluid, when performed

67105   photocoagulation, including drainage of subretinal fluid, when performed

77002   Fluoroscopic guidance for needle placement (eg, biopsy, aspiration, injection, localization device) (List separately in addition to code for primary procedure)

77003   Fluoroscopic guidance and localization of needle or catheter tip for spine or paraspinous diagnostic or therapeutic injection procedures (epidural or subarachnoid) (List separately in addition to code for primary procedure)

81401   Molecular pathology procedure, Level 2 (eg, 2-10 SNPs, 1 methylated variant, or 1 somatic variant [typically using nonsequencing target variant analysis], or detection of a dynamic mutation disorder/triplet repeat) *SEPT9 (septin9)* ~~(eg, colon cancer, methylation analysis~~

81403   Molecular pathology procedure, Level 4 (eg, analysis of single exon by DNA sequence analysis, analysis of >10 amplicons using multiplex PCR in 2 or more independent reactions, mutation scanning or duplication/deletion variants of 2-5 exons) Known familial variant not otherwise specified, for gene listed in Tier 1 or Tier 2, or identified during a genomic sequencing procedure, DNA sequence analysis, each variant exon

81406   Molecular pathology procedure, Level 7 (eg, analysis of 11-25 exons by DNA sequence analysis, mutation scanning or duplication/deletion variants of 26-50 exons, cytogenomic array analysis for neoplasia) ~~Do not report 81406 for KCNH2 full gene sequence in conjunction with 81280~~ ~~Do not report 81406 for KCNQ1 full gene sequence in conjunction with 81280~~

83015   Heavy metal (eg, arsenic, barium, beryllium, bismuth, antimony, mercury); ~~screen~~ qualitative, any number of analytes

83018   quantitative, each, not elsewhere specified

83704   Lipoprotein, blood; quantitation of lipoprotein particle ~~subclasses~~ number(s) (eg, by nuclear magnetic resonance spectroscopy), includes lipoprotein particle subclass(es), when performed

90655   Influenza virus vaccine, trivalent (IIV3), split virus, preservative free, ~~when administered to children 6-35 months of age~~ 0.25 mL dosage, for intramuscular use

90656   Influenza virus vaccine, trivalent (IIV3), split virus, preservative free, ~~when administered to individuals 3 years and older~~ 0.5 mL dosage, for intramuscular use

90657   Influenza virus vaccine, trivalent (IIV3), split virus, ~~when administered to children 6-35 months of age~~ 0.25 mL dosage, for intramuscular use

90658   Influenza virus vaccine, trivalent (IIV3), split virus, ~~when administered to individuals 3 years and older~~ 0.5 mL dosage, for intramuscular use

90661   Influenza virus vaccine, trivalent (ccIIV3), derived from cell cultures, subunit, preservative and antibiotic free, 0.5 mL dosage, for intramuscular use

90685   Influenza virus vaccine, quadrivalent (IIV4), split virus, preservative free, ~~when administered to children 6-35 months of age~~ 0.25 mL, for intramuscular use

90686 Influenza virus vaccine, quadrivalent (IIV4), split virus, when administered to individuals 3 years and older preservative free, 0.5 mL dosage, for intramuscular use

90687 Influenza virus vaccine, quadrivalent (IIV4), split virus, when administered to children 6-35 months of age 0.25 mL dosage, for intramuscular use

90688 Influenza virus vaccine, quadrivalent (IIV4), split virus, when administered to individuals 3 years and older 0.5 mL dosage, for intramuscular use

90644 Meningococcal conjugate vaccine, serogroups C & Y and Haemophilus influenzae type b vaccine (Hib-MenCY), 4 dose schedule, when administered to children 2-6 weeks-18 months of age, for intramuscular use

90734 Meningococcal conjugate vaccine, serogroups A, C, Y and W-135, quadrivalent (MenACWY)(MCV4 or MenACWY), for intramuscular use

90832 Psychotherapy, 30 minutes with patient and/or family member

90833 Psychotherapy, 30 minutes with patient and/or family member when performed with an evaluation and management service (List separately in addition to the code for primary procedure)

90834 Psychotherapy, 45 minutes with patient and/or family member

90836 Psychotherapy, 45 minutes with patient and/or family member when performed with an evaluation and management service (List separately in addition to the code for primary procedure)

90837 Psychotherapy, 60 minutes with patient and/or family member

90838 Psychotherapy, 60 minutes with patient and/or family member when performed with an evaluation and management service (List separately in addition to the code for primary procedure)

90846 Family psychotherapy (without the patient present), 50 minutes

90847 Family psychotherapy (conjoint psychotherapy) (with patient present), 50 minutes

92235 Fluorescein angiography (includes multiframe imaging) with interpretation and report, unilateral or bilateral

92240 Indocyanine-green angiography (includes multiframe imaging) with interpretation and report, unilateral or bilateral

92612 Flexible fiberoptic endoscopic evaluation of swallowing by cine or video recording;

92613 interpretation and report only

92614 Flexible fiberoptic endoscopic evaluation, laryngeal sensory testing by cine or video recording;

92615 interpretation and report only

92616 Flexible fiberoptic endoscopic evaluation of swallowing and laryngeal sensory testing by cine or video recording;

92617 interpretation and report only

92978 Intravascular ultrasound Endoluminal imaging of coronary vessel or graft using intravascular ultrasound (IVUS) or optical coherence tomography (OCT) during diagnostic evaluation and/or therapeutic intervention including imaging supervision, interpretation and report; initial vessel (List separately in addition to code for primary procedure)

92979 each additional vessel (List separately in addition to code for primary procedure)

97602 Removal of devitalized tissue from wound(s), non-selective debridement, without anesthesia (eg, wet-to-moist dressings, enzymatic, abrasion, larval therapy), including topical application(s), wound assessment, and instruction(s) for ongoing care, per session

4151F Patient did not start or is not receiving antiviral treatment for Hepatitis C during the measurement period (HEP-C)

0274T Percutaneous laminotomy/laminectomy (interlaminar approach) for decompression of neural elements, (with or without ligamentous resection, discectomy, facetectomy and/or foraminotomy), any method, under indirect image guidance (eg, fluoroscopic, CT), with or without the use of an endoscope single or multiple levels, unilateral or bilateral; cervical or thoracic

0275T lumbar

Deleted Codes

11752	21495	22305	22851	27193	27194	28290
28293	28294	31582	31588	33400	33401	33403
35450	35452	35458	35460	35471	35472	35475
35476	36147	36148	36870	62310	62311	62318
62319	75791	75962	75964	75966	75968	75978
77051	77052	77055	77056	77057	80300	80301
80302	80303	80304	81280	81281	81282	92140
93965	97001	97002	97003	97004	97005	97006
99143	99144	99145	99148	99149	99150	99420
0019T	0169T	0171T	0172T	0281T	0282T	0283T
0284T	0285T	0286T	0287T	0288T	0289T	0291T
0292T	0336T	0392T	0393T	0010M		

Web Release New and Changed Codes

Codes indicated as "Web Release" codes indicate CPT codes that are in *Current Procedural Coding Expert* for the current year, but will not be in the AMA CPT book until the following year. This can also include those codes designated by the AMA as new or revised for 2017 but that actually appeared in the 2016 Optum360 book. These codes will have the appropriate new or changed icon appended to match the CPT code book, however. See the complete list below:

New codes and changes to codes in the 2017 *Current Procedural Coding Expert* that will not appear in the CPT code book until 2018 are indicated with the following icons: ● ▲ These icons will be green in the body of the book.

New or revised codes not in the CPT code book for 2017 include:

0333T Visual evoked potential, screening of visual acuity, automated, with report

0464T Visual evoked potential, testing for glaucoma, with interpretation and report

0465T Suprachoroidal injection of a pharmacologic agent (does not include supply of medication)

0466T Insertion of chest wall respiratory sensor electrode or electrode array, including connection to pulse generator (List separately in addition to code for primary procedure)

0467T Revision or replacement of chest wall respiratory sensor electrode or electrode array, including connection to existing pulse generator

0468T Removal of chest wall respiratory sensor electrode or electrode array

90682 Influenza virus vaccine, quadrivalent (RIV4), derived from recombinant DNA, hemagglutinin (HA) protein only, preservative and antibiotic free, for intramuscular use

90750 Zoster (shingles) vaccine (HZV), recombinant, sub-unit, adjuvanted, for intramuscular injection

Codes that were new to *Current Procedural Coding Expert* for 2016 and are now in the 2017 CPT code book include:

0408T Insertion or replacement of permanent cardiac contractility modulation system, including contractility evaluation when performed, and programming of sensing and therapeutic parameters; pulse generator with transvenous electrodes

0409T Insertion or replacement of permanent cardiac contractility modulation system, including contractility evaluation when performed, and programming of sensing and therapeutic parameters; pulse generator only

0410T Insertion or replacement of permanent cardiac contractility modulation system, including contractility evaluation when performed, and programming of sensing and therapeutic parameters; atrial electrode only

0411T Insertion or replacement of permanent cardiac contractility modulation system, including contractility evaluation when performed, and programming of sensing and therapeutic parameters; ventricular electrode only

0412T Removal of permanent cardiac contractility modulation system; pulse generator only

0413T Removal of permanent cardiac contractility modulation system; transvenous electrode (atrial or ventricular)

0414T Removal and replacement of permanent cardiac contractility modulation system pulse generator only

0415T Repositioning of previously implanted cardiac contractility modulation transvenous electrode, (atrial or ventricular lead)

0416T Relocation of skin pocket for implanted cardiac contractility modulation pulse generator

0417T Programming device evaluation (in person) with iterative adjustment of the implantable device to test the function of the device and select optimal permanent programmed values with analysis, including review and report, implantable cardiac contractility modulation system

0418T Interrogation device evaluation (in person) with analysis, review and report, includes connection, recording and disconnection per patient encounter, implantable cardiac contractility modulation system

0419T Destruction of neurofibroma, extensive (cutaneous, dermal extending into subcutaneous); face, head and neck, greater than 50 neurofibromas

0420T Destruction of neurofibroma, extensive (cutaneous, dermal extending into subcutaneous); trunk and extremities, extensive, greater than 100 neurofibromas

0421T Transurethral waterjet ablation of prostate, including control of post-operative bleeding, including ultrasound guidance, complete (vasectomy, meatotomy, cystourethroscopy, urethral calibration and/or dilation, and internal urethrotomy are included when performed)

0422T Tactile breast imaging by computer-aided tactile sensors, unilateral or bilateral

0423T Secretory type II phospholipase A2 (sPLA2-IIA)

0424T Insertion or replacement of neurostimulator system for treatment of central sleep apnea; complete system (transvenous placement of right or left stimulation lead, sensing lead, implantable pulse generator)

0425T Insertion or replacement of neurostimulator system for treatment of central sleep apnea; sensing lead only

0426T Insertion or replacement of neurostimulator system for treatment of central sleep apnea; stimulation lead only

0427T Insertion or replacement of neurostimulator system for treatment of central sleep apnea; pulse generator only

0428T Removal of neurostimulator system for treatment of central sleep apnea; pulse generator only

0429T Removal of neurostimulator system for treatment of central sleep apnea; sensing lead only

0430T Removal of neurostimulator system for treatment of central sleep apnea; stimulation lead only

0431T Removal and replacement of neurostimulator system for treatment of central sleep apnea, pulse generator only

0432T Repositioning of neurostimulator system for treatment of central sleep apnea; stimulation lead only

0433T Repositioning of neurostimulator system for treatment of central sleep apnea; sensing lead only

0434T Interrogation device evaluation implanted neurostimulator pulse generator system for central sleep apnea

0435T Programming device evaluation of implanted neurostimulator pulse generator system for central sleep apnea; single session

0436T Programming device evaluation of implanted neurostimulator pulse generator system for central sleep apnea; during sleep study

AMA Icon Only Changes

Codes for which the only revision for 2017 was the deletion of the moderate sedation icon:

0200T	0201T	0293T	0294T	0301T	0302T	0303T
0304T	0307T	0308T	0335T	0340T	0397T	10030
19298	20982	20983	22510	22511	22512	22513
22514	22515	22526	22527	31615	31622	31623
31624	31625	31626	31627	31628	31629	31632
31633	31634	31635	31645	31646	31647	31648
31649	31651	31652	31653	31654	31660	31661
31725	32405	32550	32551	32553	33010	33011
33206	33207	33208	33210	33211	33212	33213
33214	33216	33217	33218	33220	33221	33222
33223	33227	33228	33229	33230	33231	33233
33234	33235	33240	33241	33244	33249	33262
33263	33264	33282	33284	33990	33991	33992
33993	36010	36140	36200	36221	36222	36223
36224	36225	36226	36227	36228	36245	36246
36247	36248	36251	36252	36253	36254	36481
36555	36557	36558	36560	36561	36563	36565
36566	36568	36570	36571	36576	36578	36581
36582	36583	36585	36590	37183	37184	37185
37186	37187	37188	37191	37193	37197	37211
37212	37213	37214	37215	37216	37218	37220
37221	37222	37223	37224	37225	37226	37227
37228	37229	37230	37231	37232	37233	37234
37235	37236	37237	37238	37239	37241	37242
37243	37244	37252	37253	43200	43201	43202
43204	43205	43206	43211	43212	43213	43214
43215	43216	43217	43220	43226	43227	43229
43231	43232	43233	43235	43236	43237	43238
43239	43240	43241	43242	43243	43244	43245
43246	43247	43248	43249	43250	43251	43252
43253	43254	43255	43257	43259	43260	43261
43262	43263	43264	43265	43266	43270	43273
43274	43275	43276	43277	43278	43453	44360
44361	44363	44364	44365	44366	44369	44370
44372	44373	44376	44377	44378	44379	44380
44381	44382	44384	44385	44386	44388	44389
44390	44391	44392	44394	44401	44402	44403
44404	44405	44406	44407	44408	44500	45303
45305	45307	45308	45309	45315	45317	45320
45321	45327	45332	45333	45334	45335	45337
45338	45340	45341	45342	45346	45347	45349
45350	45378	45379	45380	45381	45382	45384
45385	45386	45388	45389	45390	45391	45392
45393	45398	47000	47382	47383	47532	47533
47534	47535	47536	47541	47542	47533	47544
49405	49406	49407	49411	49418	49440	49441
49442	49446	50200	50382	50384	50385	50386
50387	50430	50432	50433	50434	50592	50593
50606	50693	50694	50695	50705	50706	57155
66720	69300	77371	77600	77605	77610	77615
92920	92921	92924	92925	92928	92929	92933
92934	92937	92938	92941	92943	92944	92953
92960	92961	92973	92974	92975	92986	92987
93312	93313	93314	93315	93316	93317	93318
93451	93452	93453	93454	93455	93456	93457
93458	93459	93460	93461	93462	93463	93464
93505	93530	93561	93562	93563	93564	93565
93566	93567	93568	93571	93572	93582	93583
93609	93613	93615	93616	93618	93619	93620
93621	93622	93624	93640	93641	93642	93644
93650	93653	93654	93655	93656	93657	94011
94012	94013					

Appendix C: Evaluation and Management Extended Guidelines

This appendix provides an overview of evaluation and management (E/M) services, tables that identify the documentation elements associated with each code, and the federal documentation guidelines with emphasis on the 1997 exam guidelines. This set of guidelines represent the most complete discussion of the elements of the currently accepted versions. The 1997 version identifies both general multi-system physical examinations and single-system examinations, but providers may also use the original 1995 version of the E/M guidelines; both are currently supported by the Centers for Medicare and Medicaid Services (CMS) for audit purposes.

The levels of E/M services define the wide variations in skill, effort, and time and are required for preventing and/or diagnosing and treating illness or injury, and promoting optimal health. These codes are intended to represent physician work, and because much of this work involves the amount of training, experience, expertise, and knowledge that a provider may employ when treating a given patient, the true indications of the level of this work may be difficult to recognize without some explanation.

At first glance, selecting an E/M code may appear to be difficult, but the system of coding clinical visits may be mastered once the requirements for code selection are learned and used.

Providers

The AMA advises coders that while a particular service or procedure may be assigned to a specific section, the service or procedure itself is not limited to use only by that specialty group (see paragraphs 2 and 3 under "Instructions for Use of the CPT® Codebook" on page xii of the CPT Book). Additionally, the procedures and services listed throughout the book are for use by any qualified physician or other qualified health care professional or entity (e.g., hospitals, laboratories, or home health agencies).

The use of the phrase "physician or other qualified health care professional" (OQHCP) was adopted to identify a health care provider other than a physician. This type of provider is further described in CPT as an individual "qualified by education, training, licensure/regulation (when applicable), and facility privileging (when applicable)." State licensure guidelines determine the scope of practice and a qualified health care professional must practice within these guidelines, even if more restrictive than the CPT guidelines. The qualified health care professional may report services independently or under incident-to guidelines. The professionals within this definition are separate from "clinical staff" and are able to practice independently. CPT defines clinical staff as "a person who works under the supervision of a physician or other qualified health care professional and who is allowed, by law, regulation, and facility policy to perform or assist in the performance of a specified professional service, but who does not individually report that professional service." Keep in mind that there may be other policies or guidance that can affect who may report a specific service.

Types of E/M Services

When approaching E/M, the first choice that a provider must make is what type of code to use. The following tables outline the E/M codes for different levels of care for:

- Office or other outpatient services—new patient
- Office or other outpatient services—established patient
- Hospital observation services—initial care, subsequent, and discharge
- Hospital inpatient services—initial care, subsequent, and discharge
- Observation or inpatient care (including admission and discharge services)
- Consultations—office or other outpatient
- Consultations—inpatient
- Emergency department services
- Critical care
- Nursing facility—initial services
- Nursing facility—subsequent services

- Nursing facility—discharge and annual assessment
- Domiciliary, rest home, or custodial care—new patient
- Domiciliary, rest home, or custodial care—established patient
- Home services—new patient
- Home services—established patient
- Newborn care services
- Neonatal and pediatric interfacility transport
- Neonatal and pediatric critical care—inpatient
- Neonate and infant intensive care services—initial and continuing

The specifics of the code components that determine code selection are listed in the table and discussed in the next section. Before a level of service is decided upon, the correct type of service is identified.

A new patient is a patient who has not received any face-to-face professional services from the physician or other qualified health care provider within the past three years. An established patient is a patient who has received face-to-face professional services from the physician or other qualified health care provider within the past three years. In the case of group practices, if a physician or other qualified health care provider of the exact same specialty or subspecialty has seen the patient within three years, the patient is considered established.

If a physician or other qualified health care provider is on call or covering for another physician or other qualified health care provider, the patient's encounter is classified as it would have been by the physician or other qualified health care provider who is not available. Thus, a locum tenens physician or other qualified health care provider who sees a patient on behalf of the patient's attending physician or other qualified health care provider may not bill a new patient code unless the attending physician or other qualified health care provider has not seen the patient for any problem within three years.

Office or other outpatient services are E/M services provided in the physician or other qualified health care provider's office, the outpatient area, or other ambulatory facility. Until the patient is admitted to a health care facility, he/she is considered to be an outpatient. Hospital observation services are E/M services provided to patients who are designated or admitted as "observation status" in a hospital.

Codes 99218-99220 are used to indicate initial observation care. These codes include the initiation of the observation status, supervision of patient care including writing orders, and the performance of periodic reassessments. These codes are used only by the provider "admitting" the patient for observation.

Codes 99234-99236 are used to indicate evaluation and management services to a patient who is admitted to and discharged from observation status or hospital inpatient on the same day. If the patient is admitted as an inpatient from observation on the same day, use the appropriate level of Initial Hospital Care (99221-99223).

Code 99217 indicates discharge from observation status. It includes the final physical examination of the patient, instructions, and preparation of the discharge records. It should not be used when admission and discharge are on the same date of service. As mentioned above, report codes 99234-99236 to appropriately describe same day observation services.

If a patient is in observation longer than one day, subsequent observation care codes 99224-99226 should be reported. If the patient is discharged on the second day, observation discharge code 99217 should be reported. If the patient status is changed to inpatient on a subsequent date, the appropriate inpatient code, 99221-99233, should be reported.

Initial hospital care is defined as E/M services provided during the first hospital inpatient encounter with the patient by the admitting provider. (If a physician other than the admitting physician performs the initial inpatient encounter, refer to consultations or subsequent hospital care in the CPT book.) Subsequent hospital care includes all follow-up encounters with the patient by all physicians or other qualified health care providers.

As there may only be one admitting physician, HCPCS Level II modifier AI Principal physician of record, should be appended to the initial hospital care code by the attending physician or other qualified health care provider.

A consultation is the provision of a physician or other qualified health care provider's opinion or advice about a patient for a specific problem at the request of another physician or other appropriate source. CPT also states that a consultation may be performed when a physician or other qualified health care provider is determining whether to accept the transfer of patient care at the request of another physician or appropriate source. An office or other outpatient consultation is a consultation provided in the consultant's office, in the emergency department, or in an outpatient or other ambulatory facility including hospital observation services, home services, domiciliary, rest home, or custodial care. An inpatient consultation is a consultation provided in the hospital or partial hospital nursing facility setting. Report only one inpatient consultation by a consultant for each admission to the hospital or nursing facility.

If a consultant participates in the patient's management after the opinion or advice is provided, use codes for subsequent hospital or observation care or for office or other outpatient services (established patient), as appropriate.

Under CMS guidelines, the inpatient and office/outpatient consultation codes contained in the CPT manual are not covered services.

All outpatient consultation services will be reported for Medicare using the appropriate new or established evaluation and management (E/M) codes.

Inpatient consultation services for the initial encounter should be reported by the physician providing the service using initial hospital care codes 99221–99223, and subsequent inpatient care codes 99231–99233.

Codes 99487, 99489, and 99490 are used to report evaluation and management services for chronic care management. These codes represent management and support services provided by clinical staff, under the direction of a physician or other qualified health care professional, to patients residing at home or in a domiciliary, rest home, or assisted living facility. The qualified provider oversees the management and/or coordination of services for all medical conditions, psychosocial needs, and activities of daily living. These codes are reported only once per calendar month and have specific time-based thresholds.

Codes 99497-99498 are used to report the discussion and explanation of advanced directives by a physician or other qualified health care professional. These codes represent a face-to-face service between the provider and a patient, family member, or surrogate. These codes are time-based codes and, since no active management of the problem(s) is undertaken during this time, may be reported on the same day as another E/M service.

Beginning in 2017, certain codes that CPT considers appropriate telehealth services are identified with the ★ icon and reported with modifier 95 Synchronous telemedicine service rendered via a real-time interactive audio and video telecommunications system. Medicare recognizes certain CPT and HCPCS Level II G codes as telehealth services reported with modifier GT. Check with individual payers for telehealth modifier guidance.

Office or Other Outpatient Services—New Patient

E/M Code	History[1]	Exam[1]	Medical Decision Making[1]	Problem Severity	Coordination of Care; Counseling	Time Spent Face-to-Face (avg.)
99201	Problem-focused	Problem-focused	Straight-forward	Minor or self-limited	Consistent with problem(s) and patient's needs	10 min.
99202	Expanded problem-focused	Expanded problem-focused	Straight-forward	Low to moderate	Consistent with problem(s) and patient's needs	20 min.
99203	Detailed	Detailed	Low complexity	Moderate	Consistent with problem(s) and patient's needs	30 min.
99204	Comprehensive	Comprehensive	Moderate complexity	Moderate to high	Consistent with problem(s) and patient's needs	45 min.
99205	Comprehensive	Comprehensive	High complexity	Moderate to high	Consistent with problem(s) and patient's needs	60 min.

1 Key component. For new patients, all three components (history, exam, and medical decision making) are crucial for selecting the correct code.

Office or Other Outpatient Services—Established Patient[1]

E/M Code	History[2]	Exam[2]	Medical Decision Making[2]	Problem Severity	Coordination of Care; Counseling	Time Spent Face-to-Face (avg.)
99211	—	—	Physician supervision, but presence not required	Minimal	Consistent with problem(s) and patient's needs	5 min.
99212	Problem-focused	Problem-focused	Straight-forward	Minor or self-limited	Consistent with problem(s) and patient's needs	10 min.
99213	Expanded problem-focused	Expanded problem-focused	Low complexity	Low to moderate	Consistent with problem(s) and patient's needs	15 min.
99214	Detailed	Detailed	Moderate complexity	Moderate to high	Consistent with problem(s) and patient's needs	25 min.
99215	Comprehensive	Comprehensive	High complexity	Moderate to high	Consistent with problem(s) and patient's needs	40 min.

1 Includes follow-up, periodic reevaluation, and evaluation and management of new problems.
2 Key component. For established patients, at least two of the three components (history, exam, and medical decision making) are needed to select the correct code.

Hospital Observation Services

E/M Code	History[1]	Exam[1]	Medical Decision Making[1]	Problem Severity	Coordination of Care; Counseling	Time Spent Bedside and on Unit/Floor (avg.)
99217	Observation care discharge day management					
99218	Detailed or comprehensive	Detailed or comprehensive	Straight-forward or low complexity	Low	Consistent with problem(s) and patient's needs	30 min.
99219	Comprehensive	Comprehensive	Moderate complexity	Moderate	Consistent with problem(s) and patient's needs	50 min.
99220	Comprehensive	Comprehensive	High complexity	High	Consistent with problem(s) and patient's needs	70 min.

1 Key component. All three components (history, exam, and medical decision making) are crucial for selecting the correct code.

Subsequent Hospital Observation Services[1]

E/M Code[2]	History[3]	Exam[3]	Medical Decision Making[3]	Problem Severity	Coordination of Care; Counseling	Time Spent Bedside and on Unit/Floor (avg.)
99224	Problem-focused interval	Problem-focused	Straight-forward or low complexity	Stable, recovering, or improving	Consistent with problem(s) and patient's needs	15 min.
99225	Expanded problem-focused interval	Expanded problem-focused	Moderate complexity	Inadequate response to treatment; minor complications	Consistent with problem(s) and patient's needs	25 min.
99226	Detailed interval	Detailed	High complexity	Unstable; significant new problem or significant complication	Consistent with problem(s) and patient's needs	35 min.

1 All subsequent levels of service include reviewing the medical record, diagnostic studies, and changes in the patient's status, such as history, physical condition, and response to treatment since the last assessment.
2 These codes are resequenced in CPT and are printed following codes 99217-99220.
3 Key component. For subsequent care, at least two of the three components (history, exam, and medical decision making) are needed to select the correct code.

Hospital Inpatient Services—Initial Care[1]

E/M Code	History[2]	Exam[2]	Medical Decision Making[2]	Problem Severity	Coordination of Care; Counseling	Time Spent Bedside and on Unit/Floor (avg.)
99221	Detailed or comprehensive	Detailed or comprehensive	Straight-forward or low complexity	Low	Consistent with problem(s) and patient's needs	30 min.
99222	Comprehensive	Comprehensive	Moderate complexity	Moderate	Consistent with problem(s) and patient's needs	50 min.
99223	Comprehensive	Comprehensive	High complexity	High	Consistent with problem(s) and patient's needs	70 min.

1 The admitting physician should append modifier AI, Principal physician of record, for Medicare patients
2 Key component. For initial care, all three components (history, exam, and medical decision making) are crucial for selecting the correct code.

Hospital Inpatient Services—Subsequent Care[1]

E/M Code	History[2]	Exam[2]	Medical Decision Making[2]	Problem Severity	Coordination of Care; Counseling	Time Spent Bedside and on Unit/Floor (avg.)
99231	Problem-focused interval	Problem-focused	Straight-forward or low complexity	Stable, recovering or Improving	Consistent with problem(s) and patient's needs	15 min.
99232	Expanded problem-focused interval	Expanded problem-focused	Moderate complexity	Inadequate response to treatment; minor complications	Consistent with problem(s) and patient's needs	25 min.
99233	Detailed interval	Detailed	High complexity	Unstable; significant new problem or significant complication	Consistent with problem(s) and patient's needs	35 min.
99238	Hospital discharge day management					30 min. or less
99239	Hospital discharge day management					> 30 min.

1 All subsequent levels of service include reviewing the medical record, diagnostic studies, and changes in the patient's status, such as history, physical condition, and response to treatment since the last assessment.
2 Key component. For subsequent care, at least two of the three components (history, exam, and medical decision making) are needed to select the correct code.

Observation or Inpatient Care Services (Including Admission and Discharge Services)

E/M Code	History[1]	Exam[1]	Medical Decision Making[1]	Problem Severity	Coordination of Care; Counseling	Time
99234	Detailed or comprehensive	Detailed or comprehensive	Straight-forward or low complexity	Low	Consistent with problem(s) and patient's needs	40 min.
99235	Comprehensive	Comprehensive	Moderate	Moderate	Consistent with problem(s) and patient's needs	50 min.
99236	Comprehensive	Comprehensive	High	High	Consistent with problem(s) and patient's needs	55 min.

1 Key component. All three components (history, exam, and medical decision making) are crucial for selecting the correct code.

Consultations—Office or Other Outpatient

E/M Code	History[1]	Exam[1]	Medical Decision Making[1]	Problem Severity	Coordination of Care; Counseling	Time Spent Face-to-Face (avg.)
99241	Problem-focused	Problem-focused	Straight-forward	Minor or self-limited	Consistent with problem(s) and patient's needs	15 min.
99242	Expanded problem-focused	Expanded problem-focused	Straight-forward	Low	Consistent with problem(s) and patient's needs	30 min.
99243	Detailed	Detailed	Low complexity	Moderate	Consistent with problem(s) and patient's needs	40 min.
99244	Comprehensive	Comprehensive	Moderate complexity	Moderate to high	Consistent with problem(s) and patient's needs	60 min.
99245	Comprehensive	Comprehensive	High complexity	Moderate to high	Consistent with problem(s) and patient's needs	80 min.

1 Key component. For office or other outpatient consultations, all three components (history, exam, and medical decision making) are crucial for selecting the correct code.

Consultations—Inpatient[1]

E/M Code	History[2]	Exam[2]	Medical Decision Making[2]	Problem Severity	Coordination of Care; Counseling	Time Spent Bedside and on Unit/Floor (avg.)
99251	Problem-focused	Problem-focused	Straight-forward	Minor or self-limited	Consistent with problem(s) and patient's needs	20 min.
99252	Expanded problem-focused	Expanded problem-focused	Straight-forward	Low	Consistent with problem(s) and patient's needs	40 min.
99253	Detailed	Detailed	Low complexity	Moderate	Consistent with problem(s) and patient's needs	55 min.
99254	Comprehensive	Comprehensive	Moderate complexity	Moderate to high	Consistent with problem(s) and patient's needs	80 min.
99255	Comprehensive	Comprehensive	High complexity	Moderate to high	Consistent with problem(s) and patient's needs	110 min.

1 These codes are used for hospital inpatients, residents of nursing facilities or patients in a partial hospital setting.

2 Key component. For initial inpatient consultations, all three components (history, exam, and medical decision making) are crucial for selecting the correct code.

Emergency Department Services, New or Established Patient

E/M Code	History[1]	Exam[1]	Medical Decision Making[1]	Problem Severity[3]	Coordination of Care; Counseling	Time Spent[2] Face-to-Face (avg.)
99281	Problem-focused	Problem-focused	Straight-forward	Minor or self-limited	Consistent with problem(s) and patient's needs	N/A
99282	Expanded problem-focused	Expanded problem-focused	Low complexity	Low to moderate	Consistent with problem(s) and patient's needs	N/A
99283	Expanded problem-focused	Expanded problem-focused	Moderate complexity	Moderate	Consistent with problem(s) and patient's needs	N/A
99284	Detailed	Detailed	Moderate complexity	High; requires urgent evaluation	Consistent with problem(s) and patient's needs	N/A
99285	Comprehensive	Comprehensive	High complexity	High; poses immediate/ significant threat to life or physiologic function	Consistent with problem(s) and patient's needs	N/A
99288[4]			High complexity			N/A

1 Key component. For emergency department services, all three components (history, exam, and medical decision making) are crucial for selecting the correct code and must be adequately documented in the medical record to substantiate the level of service reported.
2 Typical times have not been established for this category of services.
3 NOTE: The severity of the patient's problem, while taken into consideration when evaluating and treating the patient, does not automatically determine the level of E/M service unless the medical record documentation reflects the severity of the patient's illness, injury, or condition in the details of the history, physical examination, and medical decision making process. Federal auditors will "downcode" the level of E/M service despite the nature of the patient's problem when the documentation does not support the E/M code reported.
4 Code 99288 is used to report two-way communication with emergency medical services personnel in the field.

Critical Care

E/M Code	Patient Status	Physician Attendance	Time[1]
99291	Critically ill or critically injured	Constant	First 30–74 minutes
99292	Critically ill or critically injured	Constant	Each additional 30 minutes beyond the first 74 minutes

1 Per the guidelines for time in *CPT 2016 page xv,* "A unit of time is attained when the mid-point is passed. For example, an hour is attained when 31 minutes have elapsed (more than midway between zero and 60 minutes)."

Nursing Facility Services—Initial Nursing Facility Care[1]

E/M Code	History[1]	Exam[1]	Medical Decision Making[1]	Problem Severity	Coordination of Care; Counseling
99304	Detailed or comprehensive	Detailed or comprehensive	Straight-forward or low complexity	Low	25 min.
99305	Comprehensive	Comprehensive	Moderate complexity	Moderate	35 min.
99306	Comprehensive	Comprehensive	High complexity	High	45 min.

1 These services must be performed by the physician. See CPT Corrections Document – CPT 2013 page 3 or guidelines CPT 2016 page 26.
2 Key component. For new patients, all three components (history, exam, and medical decision making) are crucial for selecting the correct code.

 © 2016 Optum360, LLC

Nursing Facility Services—Subsequent Nursing Facility Care

E/M Code	History[1]	Exam[1]	Medical Decision Making[2]	Problem Severity	Coordination of Care; Counseling
99307	Problem-focused interval	Problem-focused	Straight-forward	Stable, recovering or improving	10 min.
99308	Expanded problem-focused interval	Expanded problem-focused	Low complexity	Responding inadequately or has developed a minor complication	15 min.
99309	Detailed interval	Detailed	Moderate complexity	Significant complication or a significant new problem	25 min.
99310	Comprehensive interval	Comprehensive	High complexity	Developed a significant new problem requiring immediate attention	35 min.

1 Key component. For established patients, at least two of the three components (history, exam, and medical decision making) are needed for selecting the correct code.

Nursing Facility Discharge and Annual Assessment

E/M Code	History[1]	Exam[1]	Medical Decision Making[1]	Problem Severity	Time Spent Bedside and on Unit/Floor (avg.)
99315	Nursing facility discharge day management				30 min. or less
99316	Nursing facility discharge day management				more than 30 min.
99318	Detailed interval	Comprehensive	Low to moderate complexity	Stable, recovering or improving	30 min.

1 Key component. For annual nursing facility assessment, all three components (history, exam, and medical decision making) are crucial for selecting the correct code.

Domiciliary, Rest Home (e.g., Boarding Home) or Custodial Care Services—New Patient

E/M Code	History[1]	Exam[1]	Medical Decision Making[1]	Problem Severity	Coordination of Care; Counseling	Time Spent Face-to-Face (avg.)
99324	Problem-focused	Problem-focused	Straight-forward	Low	Consistent with problem(s) and patient's needs	20 min.
99325	Expanded problem-focused	Expanded problem-focused	Low complexity	Moderate	Consistent with problem(s) and patient's needs	30 min.
99326	Detailed	Detailed	Moderate complexity	Moderate to high	Consistent with problem(s) and patient's needs	45 min.
99327	Comprehensive	Comprehensive	Moderate complexity	High	Consistent with problem(s) and patient's needs	60 min.
99328	Comprehensive	Comprehensive	High complexity	Unstable or developed a new problem requiring immediate physician attention	Consistent with problem(s) and patient's needs	75 min.

1 Key component. For new patients, all three components (history, exam, and medical decision making) are crucial for selecting the correct code and must be adequately documented in the medical record to substantiate the level of service reported.

Domiciliary, Rest Home (e.g., Boarding Home) or Custodial Care Services— Established Patient

E/M Code	History[1]	Exam[1]	Medical Decision Making[1]	Problem Severity	Coordination of Care; Counseling	Time Spent Face-to-Face (avg.)
99334	Problem-focused interval	Problem-focused	Straight-forward	Minor or self-limited	Consistent with problem(s) and patient's needs	15 min.
99335	Expanded problem-focused interval	Expanded problem-focused	Low complexity	Low to moderate	Consistent with problem(s) and patient's needs	25 min.
99336	Detailed interval	Detailed	Moderate complexity	Moderate to high	Consistent with problem(s) and patient's needs	40 min.
99337	Comprehensive interval	Comprehensive	Moderate to high complexity	Moderate to high	Consistent with problem(s) and patient's needs	60 min.

1 Key component. For established patients, at least two of the three components (history, exam, and medical decision making) are needed for selecting the correct code.

Domiciliary, Rest Home (e.g., Assisted Living Facility), or Home Care Plan Oversight Services

E/M Code	Intent of Service	Presence of Patient	Time
99339	Individual physician supervision of a patient (patient not present) in home, domiciliary or rest home (e.g., assisted living facility) requiring complex and multidisciplinary care modalities involving regular physician development and/or revision of care plans, review of subsequent reports of patient status, review of related laboratory and other studies, communication (including telephone calls) for purposes of assessment or care decisions with health care professional(s), family member(s), surrogate decision maker(s) (e.g., legal guardian) and/or key caregiver(s) involved in patient's care, integration of new information into the medical treatment plan and/or adjustment of medical therapy, within a calendar month	Patient not present	15–29 min.
99340	Same as 99339	Patient not present	30 min. or more

Home Services—New Patient

E/M Code	History[1]	Exam[1]	Medical Decision Making[1]	Problem Severity	Coordination of Care; Counseling	Time Spent Face-to-Face (avg.)
99341	Problem-focused	Problem-focused	Straight-forward complexity	Low	Consistent with problem(s) and patient's needs	20 min.
99342	Expanded problem-focused	Expanded problem-focused	Low complexity	Moderate	Consistent with problem(s) and patient's needs	30 min.
99343	Detailed	Detailed	Moderate complexity	Moderate to high	Consistent with problem(s) and patient's needs	45 min.
99344	Comprehensive	Comprehensive	Moderate complexity	High	Consistent with problem(s) and patient's needs	60 min.
99345	Comprehensive	Comprehensive	High complexity	Usually the patient has developed a significant new problem requiring immediate physician attention	Consistent with problem(s) and patient's needs	75 min.

1 Key component. For new patients, all three components (history, exam, and medical decision making) are crucial for selecting the correct code and must be adequately documented in the medical record to substantiate the level of service reported.

© 2016 Optum360, LLC

Home Services—Established Patient

E/M Code	History[1]	Exam[1]	Medical Decision Making[1]	Problem Severity	Coordination of Care; Counseling	Time Spent Face-to-Face (avg.)
99347	Problem-focused interval	Problem-focused	Straight-forward	Minor or self-limited	Consistent with problem(s) and patient's needs	15 min.
99348	Expanded problem-focused interval	Expanded problem-focused	Low complexity	Low to moderate	Consistent with problem(s) and patient's needs	25 min.
99349	Detailed interval	Detailed	Moderate complexity	Moderate to high	Consistent with problem(s) and patient's needs	40 min.
99350	Comprehensive interval	Comprehensive	Moderate to high complexity	Moderate to high Usually the patient has developed a significant new problem requiring immediate physician attention	Consistent with problem(s) and patient's needs	60 min.

1 Key component. For established patients, at least two of the three components (history, exam, and medical decision making) are needed for selecting the correct code.

Newborn Care Services

E/M Code	Patient Status	Type of Visit
99460	Normal newborn	Inpatient initial inpatient hospital or birthing center per day
99461	Normal newborn	Inpatient initial treatment not in hospital or birthing center per day
99462	Normal newborn	Inpatient subsequent per day
99463	Normal newborn	Inpatient initial inpatient and discharge in hospital or birthing center per day
99464	Unstable newborn	Attendance at delivery
99465	High-risk newborn at delivery	Resuscitation, ventilation, and cardiac treatment

Neonatal and Pediatric Interfacility Transportation

E/M Code	Patient Status	Type of Visit
99466	Critically ill or injured infant or young child, to 24 months	Face-to-face transportation from one facility to another, initial 30-74 minutes
99467	Critically ill or injured infant or young child, to 24 months	Face-to-face transportation from one facility to another, each additional 30 minutes
99485[1]	Critically ill or injured infant or young child, to 24 months	Supervision of patient transport from one facility to another, initial 30 minutes
99486[1]	Critically ill or injured infant or young child, to 24 months	Supervision of patient transport from one facility to another, each additional 30 minutes

1 These codes are resequenced in CPT and are printed following codes 99466-99467.

Inpatient Neonatal and Pediatric Critical Care

E/M Code	Patient Status	Type of Visit
99468[1]	Critically ill neonate, aged 28 days or less	Inpatient initial per day
99469[2]	Critically ill neonate, aged 28 days or less	Inpatient subsequent per day
99471	Critically ill infant or young child, aged 29 days to 24 months	Inpatient initial per day
99472	Critically ill infant or young child, aged 29 days to 24 months	Inpatient subsequent per day
99475	Critically ill infant or young child, 2 to 5 years[3]	Inpatient initial per day
99476	Critically ill infant or young child, 2 to 5 years	Inpatient subsequent per day

1 Codes 99468, 99471, and 99475 may be reported only once per admission.
2 Codes 99469, 99472, and 99476 may be reported only once per day and by only one provider.
3 See 99291-99292 for patients 6 years of age and older.

Neonate and Infant Initial and Continuing Intensive Care Services

E/M Code	Patient Status	Type of Visit
99477	Neonate, aged 28 days or less	Inpatient initial per day
99478	Infant with present body weight of less than 1500 grams, no longer critically ill	Inpatient subsequent per day
99479	Infant with present body weight of 1500-2500 grams, no longer critically ill	Inpatient subsequent per day
99480	Infant with present body weight of 2501-5000 grams, no longer critically ill	Inpatient subsequent per day

Levels of E/M Services

Confusion may be experienced when first approaching E/M due to the way that each description of a code component or element seems to have another layer of description beneath. The three key components—history, exam, and decision making—are each comprised of elements that combine to create varying levels of that component.

For example, an expanded problem-focused history includes the chief complaint, a brief history of the present illness, and a system review focusing on the patient's problems. The level of exam is not made up of different elements but rather distinguished by the extent of exam across body areas or organ systems.

The single largest source of confusion are the "labels" or names applied to the varying degrees of history, exam, and decision-making. Terms such as expanded problem-focused, detailed, and comprehensive are somewhat meaningless unless they are defined. The lack of definition in CPT guidelines relative to these terms is precisely what caused the first set of federal guidelines to be developed in 1995 and again in 1997.

Documentation Guidelines for Evaluation and Management Services

Both versions of the federal guidelines go well beyond CPT guidelines in defining specific code requirements. The current version of the CPT guidelines does not explain the number of history of present illness (HPI) elements or the specific number of organ systems or body areas to be examined as they are in the federal guidelines. Adherence to some version of the guidelines is required when billing E/M to federal payers, but at this time, the CPT guidelines do not incorporate this level of detail into the code definitions. Although that could be interpreted to mean that non-governmental payers have a lesser documentation standard, it is best to adopt one set of the federal versions for all payer types for both consistency and ease of use.

The 1997 guidelines supply a great amount of detail relative to history and exam and will give the provider clear direction to follow when documenting elements. With that stated, the 1995 guidelines are equally valid and place a lesser documentation burden on the provider in regards to the physical exam.

The 1995 guidelines ask only for a notation of "normal" on systems with normal findings. The only narrative required is for abnormal findings. The 1997 version calls for much greater detail, or an "elemental" or "bullet-point" approach to organ systems, although a notation of normal is sufficient when addressing the elements within a system. The 1997 version works well in a template or electronic health record (EHR) format for recording E/M services.

The 1997 version did produce the single system specialty exam guidelines. When reviewing the complete guidelines listed below, note the differences between exam requirements in the 1995 and 1997 versions.

A Comparison of 1995 and 1997 Exam Guidelines

There are four types of exams indicated in the levels of E/M codes. Although the descriptors or labels are the same under 1995 and 1997 guidelines, the degree of detail required is different. The remaining content on this topic references the 1997 general multi-system speciality examination, at the end of this chapter.

The levels under each set of guidelines are:

1995 Exam Guidelines:

Problem focused:	One body area or system
Expanded problem focused:	Two to seven body areas or organ systems
Detailed:	Two to seven body areas or organ systems
Comprehensive:	Eight or more organ systems or a complete single-system examination

1997 Exam Guidelines:

Problem-focused:	Perform and document examination of one to five bullet point elements in one or more organ systems/body areas from the general multi-system examination

OR

	Perform or document examination of one to five bullet point elements from one of the 10 single-organ-system examinations, shaded or unshaded boxes

Expanded problem-focused:	Perform and document examination of at least six bullet point elements in one or more organ systems from the general multi-system examination

OR

	Perform and document examination of at least six bullet point elements from one of the 10 single-organ-system examinations, shaded or unshaded boxes

Detailed:	Perform and document examination of at least six organ systems or body areas, including at least two bullet point elements for each organ system or body area from the general multi-system examination

OR

	Perform and document examination of at least 12 bullet point elements in two or more organ systems or body areas from the general multisystem examination

OR

	Perform and document examination of at least 12 bullet elements from one of the single-organ-system examinations, shaded or unshaded boxes

Comprehensive:	Perform and document examination of at least nine organ systems or body areas, with all bullet elements for each organ system or body area (unless specific instructions are expected to limit examination content with at least two bullet elements for each organ system or body area) from the general multi-system examination

OR

Perform and document examination of all bullet point elements from one of the 10 single-organ system examinations with documentation of every element in shaded boxes and at least one element in each unshaded box from the single-organ-system examination.

The Documentation Guidelines

The following guidelines were developed jointly by the American Medical Association (AMA) and the Centers for Medicare and Medicaid Services (CMS). Their mutual goal was to provide physicians and claims reviewers with advice about preparing or reviewing documentation for Evaluation and Management (E/M) services.

I.   Introduction

What is Documentation and Why Is It Important?

Medical record documentation is required to record pertinent facts, findings, and observations about an individual's health history, including past and present illnesses, examinations, tests, treatments, and outcomes. The medical record chronologically documents the care of the patient and is an important element contributing to high quality care. The medical record facilitates:

- The ability of the physician and other health care professionals to evaluate and plan the patient's immediate treatment and to monitor his/her health care over time
- Communication and continuity of care among physicians and other health care professionals involved in the patient's care
- Accurate and timely claims review and payment
- Appropriate utilization review and quality of care evaluations
- Collection of data that may be useful for research and education

An appropriately documented medical record can reduce many of the problems associated with claims processing and may serve as a legal document to verify the care provided, if necessary.

What Do Payers Want and Why?

Because payers have a contractual obligation to enrollees, they may require reasonable documentation that services are consistent with the insurance coverage provided. They may request information to validate:

- The site of service
- The medical necessity and appropriateness of the diagnostic and/or therapeutic services provided
- Services provided have been accurately reported

II.   General Principles of Medical Record Documentation

The principles of documentation listed below are applicable to all types of medical and surgical services in all settings. For Evaluation and Management (E/M) services, the nature and amount of physician work and documentation varies by type of service, place of service, and the patient's status. The general principles listed below may be modified to account for these variable circumstances in providing E/M services.

- The medical record should be complete and legible
- The documentation of each patient encounter should include:
  - A reason for the encounter and relevant history, physical examination findings, and prior diagnostic test results
  - Assessment, clinical impression, or diagnosis
  - Plan for care
  - Date and legible identity of the practitioner
- If not documented, the rationale for ordering diagnostic and other ancillary services should be easily inferred
- Past and present diagnoses should be accessible to the treating and/or consulting physician
- Appropriate health risk factors should be identified
- The patient's progress, response to, and changes in treatment and revision of diagnosis should be documented
- The CPT and ICD-9-CM codes reported on the health insurance claim form or billing statement should be supported by the documentation in the medical record

III.   Documentation of E/M Services 1995 and 1997

The following information provides definitions and documentation guidelines for the three key components of E/M services and for visits that consist predominately of counseling or coordination of care. The three key components—history, examination, and medical decision making—appear in the descriptors for office and other outpatient services, hospital observation services, hospital inpatient services, consultations, emergency department services, nursing facility services, domiciliary care services, and home services. While some of the text of the CPT guidelines has been repeated in this document, the reader should refer to CMS or CPT for the complete descriptors for E/M services and instructions for selecting a level of service. Documentation guidelines are identified by the symbol DG.

The descriptors for the levels of E/M services recognize seven components that are used in defining the levels of E/M services. These components are:

- History
- Examination
- Medical decision making
- Counseling
- Coordination of care
- Nature of presenting problem
- Time

The first three of these components (i.e., history, examination, and medical decision making) are the key components in selecting the level of E/M services. In the case of visits that consist predominately of counseling or coordination of care, time is the key or controlling factor to qualify for a particular level of E/M service.

Because the level of E/M service is dependent on two or three key components, performance and documentation of one component (e.g., examination) at the highest level does not necessarily mean that the encounter in its entirety qualifies for the highest level of E/M service.

These Documentation Guidelines for E/M services reflect the needs of the typical adult population. For certain groups of patients, the recorded information may vary slightly from that described here. Specifically, the medical records of infants, children, adolescents, and pregnant women may have additional or modified information, as appropriate, recorded in each history and examination area.

As an example, newborn records may include under history of the present illness (HPI) the details of the mother's pregnancy and the infant's status at birth; social history will focus on family structure; and family history will focus on congenital anomalies and hereditary disorders in the family. In addition, the content of a pediatric examination will vary with the age and development of the child. Although not specifically defined in these documentation guidelines, these patient group variations on history and examination are appropriate.

A.   Documentation of History

The levels of E/M services are based on four types of history (Problem Focused, Expanded Problem Focused, Detailed, and Comprehensive). Each type of history includes some or all of the following elements:

- Chief complaint (CC)
- History of present illness (HPI)
- Review of systems (ROS)
- Past, family, and/or social history (PFSH)

The extent of history of present illness, review of systems, and past, family, and/or social history that is obtained and documented is dependent upon clinical judgment and the nature of the presenting problem.

The chart below shows the progression of the elements required for each type of history. To qualify for a given type of history all three elements in the table must be met. (A chief complaint is indicated at all levels.)

- DG: The CC, ROS, and PFSH may be listed as separate elements of history or they may be included in the description of the history of present illness

- DG: A ROS and/or a PFSH obtained during an earlier encounter does not need to be re-recorded if there is evidence that the physician reviewed and updated the previous information. This may occur when a physician updates his/her own record or in an institutional setting or group practice where many physicians use a common record. The review and update may be documented by:

    – Describing any new ROS and/or PFSH information or noting there has been no change in the information

    – Noting the date and location of the earlier ROS and/or PFSH

- DG: The ROS and/or PFSH may be recorded by ancillary staff or on a form completed by the patient. To document that the physician reviewed the information, there must be a notation supplementing or confirming the information recorded by others

- DG: If the physician is unable to obtain a history from the patient or other source, the record should describe the patient's condition or other circumstance that precludes obtaining a history

Definitions and specific documentation guidelines for each of the elements of history are listed below.

Chief Complaint (CC)

The CC is a concise statement describing the symptom, problem, condition, diagnosis, physician recommended return, or other factor that is the reason for the encounter, usually stated in the patient's words.

- DG: The medical record should clearly reflect the chief complaint

History of Present Illness (HPI)

The HPI is a chronological description of the development of the patient's present illness from the first sign and/or symptom or from the previous encounter to the present. It includes the following elements:

- Location
- Quality
- Severity
- Duration
- Timing
- Context
- Modifying factors
- Associated signs and symptoms

Brief and extended HPIs are distinguished by the amount of detail needed to accurately characterize the clinical problem.

A brief HPI consists of one to three elements of the HPI.

- DG: The medical record should describe one to three elements of the present illness (HPI)

An extended HPI consists of at least four elements of the HPI or the status of at least three chronic or inactive conditions.

- DG: The medical record should describe at least four elements of the present illness (HPI) or the status of at least three chronic or inactive conditions

Beginning with services performed on or after September 10, 2013, CMS has stated that physicians and other qualified health care professionals will be able to use the 1997 guidelines for an extended history of present illness (HPI) in combination with other elements from the 1995 documentation guidelines to document a particular level of evaluation and management service.

History of Present Illness	Review of systems (ROS)	PFSH	Type of History
Brief	N/A	N/A	Problem-focused
Brief	Problem Pertinent	N/A	Expanded Problem-Focused
Extended	Extended	Pertinent	Detailed
Extended	Complete	Complete	Comprehensive

Review of Systems (ROS)

A ROS is an inventory of body systems obtained through a series of questions seeking to identify signs and/or symptoms that the patient may be experiencing or has experienced. For purposes of ROS, the following systems are recognized:

- Constitutional symptoms (e.g., fever, weight loss)
- Eyes
- Ears, nose, mouth, throat
- Cardiovascular
- Respiratory
- Gastrointestinal
- Genitourinary
- Musculoskeletal
- Integumentary (skin and/or breast)
- Neurological
- Psychiatric
- Endocrine
- Hematologic/lymphatic
- Allergic/immunologic

A problem pertinent ROS inquires about the system directly related to the problem identified in the HPI.

- DG: The patient's positive responses and pertinent negatives for the system related to the problem should be documented

An extended ROS inquires about the system directly related to the problem identified in the HPI and a limited number of additional systems.

- DG: The patient's positive responses and pertinent negatives for two to nine systems should be documented

A complete ROS inquires about the system directly related to the problem identified in the HPI plus all additional body systems.

- DG: At least 10 organ systems must be reviewed. Those systems with positive or pertinent negative responses must be individually documented. For the remaining systems, a notation indicating all other systems are negative is permissible. In the absence of such a notation, at least 10 systems must be individually documented

Past, Family, and/or Social History (PFSH)

The PFSH consists of a review of three areas:

- Past history (the patient's past experiences with illnesses, operations, injuries, and treatment)
- Family history (a review of medical events in the patient's family, including diseases that may be hereditary or place the patient at risk)
- Social history (an age appropriate review of past and current activities)

For certain categories of E/M services that include only an interval history, it is not necessary to record information about the PFSH. Those categories are subsequent hospital care, follow-up inpatient consultations, and subsequent nursing facility care.

A pertinent PFSH is a review of the history area directly related to the problem identified in the HPI.

- DG: At least one specific item from any of the three history areas must be documented for a pertinent PFSH

A complete PFSH is a review of two or all three of the PFSH history areas, depending on the category of the E/M service. A review of all three history areas is required for services that by their nature include a comprehensive assessment or reassessment of the patient. A review of two of the three history areas is sufficient for other services.

- DG: A least one specific item from two of the three history areas must be documented for a complete PFSH for the following categories of E/M services: office or other outpatient services, established patient; emergency department; domiciliary care, established patient; and home care, established patient

- DG: At least one specific item from each of the three history areas must be documented for a complete PFSH for the following categories of E/M services: office or other outpatient services, new patient; hospital observation services; hospital inpatient services, initial care; consultations; comprehensive nursing facility assessments; domiciliary care, new patient; and home care, new patient

B.   *Documentation of Examination 1997 Guidelines*

The levels of E/M services are based on four types of examination:

- **Problem Focused:** A limited examination of the affected body area or organ system
- **Expanded Problem Focused:** A limited examination of the affected body area or organ system and any other symptomatic or related body area or organ system
- **Detailed:** An extended examination of the affected body area or organ system and any other symptomatic or related body area or organ system
- **Comprehensive:** A general multi-system examination or complete examination of a single organ system and other symptomatic or related body area or organ system

These types of examinations have been defined for general multi-system and the following single organ systems:

- Cardiovascular
- Ears, nose, mouth, and throat
- Eyes
- Genitourinary (Female)
- Genitourinary (Male)
- Hematologic/lymphatic/immunologic
- Musculoskeletal
- Neurological
- Psychiatric
- Respiratory
- Skin

Any physician regardless of specialty may perform a general multi-system examination or any of the single organ system examinations. The type (general multi-system or single organ system) and content of examination are selected by the examining physician and are based upon clinical judgment, the patient's history, and the nature of the presenting problem.

The content and documentation requirements for each type and level of examination are summarized below and described in detail in a table found later on in this document. In the table, organ systems and body areas recognized by CPT for purposes of describing examinations are shown in the left column. The content, or individual elements, of the examination pertaining to that body area or organ system are identified by bullets (•) in the right column.

Parenthetical examples "(e.g., ...)," have been used for clarification and to provide guidance regarding documentation. Documentation for each

element must satisfy any numeric requirements (such as "Measurement of any three of the following seven...") included in the description of the element. Elements with multiple components but with no specific numeric requirement (such as "Examination of liver and spleen") require documentation of at least one component. It is possible for a given examination to be expanded beyond what is defined here. When that occurs, findings related to the additional systems and/or areas should be documented.

- DG: Specific abnormal and relevant negative findings from the examination of the affected or symptomatic body area or organ system should be documented. A notation of "abnormal" without elaboration is insufficient

- DG: Abnormal or unexpected findings from the examination of any asymptomatic body area or organ system should be described

- DG: A brief statement or notation indicating "negative" or "normal" is sufficient to document normal findings related to an unaffected areas or asymptomatic organ system

General Multi-System Examinations

General multi-system examinations are described in detail later in this document. To qualify for a given level of multi-system examination, the following content and documentation requirements should be met:

- **Problem Focused Examination:** It should include performance and documentation of one to five elements identified by a bullet (•) in one or more organ systems or body areas
- **Expanded Problem Focused Examination:** It should include performance and documentation of at least six elements identified by a bullet (•) in one or more organ systems or body areas
- **Detailed Examination:** It should include at least six organ systems or body areas. For each system/area selected, performance and documentation of at least two elements identified by a bullet (•) is expected. Alternatively, a detailed examination may include performance and documentation of at least 12 elements identified by a bullet (•) in two or more organ systems or body areas
- **Comprehensive Examination:** It should include at least nine organ systems or body areas. For each system/area selected, all elements of the examination identified by a bullet (•) should be performed, unless specific directions limit the content of the examination. For each area/system, documentation of at least two elements identified by a bullet (•) is expected

Single Organ System Examinations

The single organ system examinations recognized by CMS include eyes; ears, nose, mouth, and throat; cardiovascular; respiratory; genitourinary (male and female); musculoskeletal; neurologic; hematologic, lymphatic, and immunologic; skin; and psychiatric. Note that for each specific single organ examination type, the performance and documentation of the stated number of elements, identified by a bullet (•) should be included, whether in a box with a shaded or unshaded border. The following content and documentation requirements must be met to qualify for a given level:

- **Problem Focused Examination:** one to five elements
- **Expanded Problem Focused Examination:** at least six elements
- **Detailed Examination:** at least 12 elements (other than eye and psychiatric examinations)
- **Comprehensive Examination:** all elements (Documentation of every element in a box with a shaded border and at least one element in a box with an unshaded border is expected)

Content and Documentation Requirements

General Multisystem Examination 1997

System/Body Area	Elements of Examination
Constitutional	• Measurement of any three of the following seven vital signs: 1) sitting or standing blood pressure, 2) supine blood pressure, 3) pulse rate and regularity, 4) respiration, 5) temperature, 6) height, 7) weight (May be measured and recorded by ancillary staff). • General appearance of patient (e.g., development, nutrition, body habitus, deformities attention to grooming)
Eyes	• Inspection of conjunctivae and lids • Examination of pupils and irises (e.g., reaction to light and accommodation, size and symmetry) • Ophthalmoscopic examination of optic discs (e.g., size, C/D ratio, appearance) and posterior segments (e.g., vessel changes, exudates, hemorrhages)
Ears, nose, mouth, and throat	• External inspection of ears and nose (e.g., overall appearance, scars, lesions, masses) • Otoscopic examination of external auditory canals and tympanic membranes • Assessment of hearing (e.g., whispered voice, finger rub, tuning fork) • Inspection of nasal mucosa, septum and turbinates • Inspection of lips, teeth and gums • Examination of oropharynx: oral mucosa, salivary glands, hard and soft palates, tongue, tonsils and posterior pharynx
Neck	• Examination of neck (e.g., masses, overall appearance, symmetry, tracheal position, crepitus) • Examination of thyroid (e.g., enlargement, tenderness, mass)
Respiratory	• Assessment of respiratory effort (e.g., intercostal retractions, use of accessory muscles, diaphragmatic movement) • Percussion of chest (e.g., dullness, flatness, hyperresonance) • Palpation of chest (e.g., tactile fremitus) • Auscultation of lungs (e.g., breath sounds, adventitious sounds, rubs)
Cardiovascular	• Palpation of heart (e.g., location, size, thrills) • Auscultation of heart with notation of abnormal sounds and murmurs • Examination of: 　— carotid arteries (e.g., pulse amplitude, bruits) 　— abdominal aorta (e.g., size, bruits) 　— femoral arteries (e.g., pulse amplitude, bruits) 　— pedal pulses (e.g., pulse amplitude) 　— extremities for edema and/or varicosities
Chest (Breasts)	• Inspection of breasts (e.g., symmetry, nipple discharge) • Palpation of breasts and axillae (e.g., masses or lumps, tenderness)
Gastrointestinal (Abdomen)	• Examination of abdomen with notation of presence of masses or tenderness • Examination of liver and spleen • Examination for presence or absence of hernia • Examination (when indicated) of anus, perineum and rectum, including sphincter tone, presence of hemorrhoids, rectal masses • Obtain stool sample for occult blood test when indicated
Genitourinary	**Male:** • Examination of the scrotal contents (e.g., hydrocele, spermatocele, tenderness of cord, testicular mass) • Examination of the penis • Digital rectal examination of prostate gland (e.g., size, symmetry, nodularity tenderness) **Female**: • Pelvic examination (with or without specimen collection for smears and cultures), including: 　— examination of external genitalia (e.g., general appearance, hair distribution, lesions) and vagina (e.g., general appearance, estrogen effect, discharge, lesions, pelvic support, cystocele, rectocele) 　— examination of urethra (e.g., masses, tenderness, scarring) 　— examination of bladder (e.g., fullness, masses, tenderness) • Cervix (e.g., general appearance, lesions, discharge) • Uterus (e.g., size, contour, position, mobility, tenderness, consistency, descent or support) • Adnexa/parametria (e.g., masses, tenderness)
Lymphatic	Palpation of lymph nodes in **two or more** areas: • Neck • Groin • Axillae • Other

© 2016 Optum360, LLC

System/Body Area	Elements of Examination
Musculoskeletal	• Examination of gait and station *(if circled, add to total at bottom of column to the left) • Inspection and/or palpation of digits and nails (e.g., clubbing, cyanosis, inflammatory conditions, petechiae, ischemia, infections, nodes) *(if circled, add to total at bottom of column to the left) Examination of joints, bones and muscles of **one or more of the following six** areas: 1) head and neck; 2) spine, ribs, and pelvis; 3) right upper extremity; 4) left upper extremity; 5) right lower extremity; and 6) left lower extremity. The examination of a given area includes: • Inspection and/or palpation with notation of presence of any misalignment, asymmetry, crepitation, defects, tenderness, masses, effusions • Assessment of range of motion with notation of any pain, crepitation or contracture • Assessment of stability with notation of any dislocation (luxation), subluxation, or laxity • Assessment of muscle strength and tone (e.g., flaccid, cog wheel, spastic) with notation of any atrophy or abnormal movements
Skin	• Inspection of skin and subcutaneous tissue (e.g., rashes, lesions, ulcers) • Palpation of skin and subcutaneous tissue (e.g., induration, subcutaneous nodules, tightening)
Neurologic	• Test cranial nerves with notation of any deficits • Examination of deep tendon reflexes with notation of pathological reflexes (e.g., Babinski) • Examination of sensation (e.g., by touch, pin, vibration, proprioception)
Psychiatric	• Description of patient's judgment and insight • Brief assessment of mental status including: — Orientation to time, place and person — Recent and remote memory — Mood and affect (e.g., depression, anxiety, agitation)

Content and Documentation Requirements

Level of exam	Perform and document
Problem focused	**One to five** elements identified by a bullet.
Expanded problem focused	**At least six** elements identified by a bullet.
Detailed	**At least 12** elements identified by a bullet, whether in a box with a shaded or unshaded border
Comprehensive	Performance of **all** elements identified by a bullet; whether in a box or with a shaded or unshaded box. Documentation of every element in each with a shaded border and at least one element in a box with un shaded border is expected

Number of Diagnoses or Management Options	Amount and/or Complexity of Data to be Reviewed	Risk of Complications and/or Morbidity or Mortality	Type of Decision Making
Minimal	Minimal or None	Minimal	Straightforward
Limited	Limited	Low	Low Complexity
Multiple	Moderate	Moderate	Moderate Complexity
Extensive	Extensive	High	High Complexity

C. Documentation of the Complexity of Medical Decision Making 1995 and 1997

The levels of E/M services recognize four types of medical decision-making (straightforward, low complexity, moderate complexity, and high complexity). Medical decision-making refers to the complexity of establishing a diagnosis and/or selecting a management option as measured by:

• The number of possible diagnoses and/or the number of management options that must be considered

• The amount and/or complexity of medical records, diagnostic tests, and/or other information that must be obtained, reviewed, and analyzed

• The risk of significant complications, morbidity, and/or mortality, as well as comorbidities, associated with the patient's presenting problem, the diagnostic procedure, and/or the possible management options

The following chart shows the progression of the elements required for each level of medical decision-making. To qualify for a given type of decision-making, two of the three elements in the table must be either met or exceeded.

Each of the elements of medical decision-making is described below.

Number of Diagnoses or Management Options

The number of possible diagnoses and/or the number of management options that must be considered is based on the number and types of

problems addressed during the encounter, the complexity of establishing a diagnosis, and the management decisions that are made by the physician.

Generally, decision making with respect to a diagnosed problem is easier than that for an identified but undiagnosed problem. The number and type of diagnostic tests employed may be an indicator of the number of possible diagnoses. Problems that are improving or resolving are less complex than those that are worsening or failing to change as expected. The need to seek advice from others is another indicator of complexity of diagnostic or management problems.

• DG: For each encounter, an assessment, clinical impression, or diagnosis should be documented. It may be explicitly stated or implied in documented decisions regarding management plans and/or further evaluation

— For a presenting problem with an established diagnosis, the record should reflect whether the problem is: a) improved, well controlled, resolving, or resolved; or b) inadequately controlled, worsening, or failing to change as expected

— For a presenting problem without an established diagnosis, the assessment or clinical impression may be stated in the form of a differential diagnosis or as a "possible," "probable," or "rule-out" (R/O) diagnosis

• DG:	The initiation of, or changes in, treatment should be documented. Treatment includes a wide range of management options including patient instructions, nursing instructions, therapies, and medications
• DG:	If referrals are made, consultations requested, or advice sought, the record should indicate to whom or where the referral or consultation is made or from whom the advice is requested

Amount and/or Complexity of Data to be Reviewed

The amount and complexity of data to be reviewed is based on the types of diagnostic testing ordered or reviewed. A decision to obtain and review old medical records and/or obtain history from sources other than the patient increases the amount and complexity of data to be reviewed.

Discussion of contradictory or unexpected test results with the physician who performed or interpreted the test is an indication of the complexity of data being reviewed. On occasion, the physician who ordered a test may personally review the image, tracing, or specimen to supplement information from the physician who prepared the test report or interpretation; this is another indication of the complexity of data being reviewed.

• DG:	If a diagnostic service (test or procedure) is ordered, planned, scheduled, or performed at the time of the E/M encounter, the type of service (e.g., lab or x-ray) should be documented
• DG:	The review of lab, radiology, and/or other diagnostic tests should be documented. A simple notation such as WBC elevated" or "chest x-ray unremarkable" is acceptable. Alternatively, the review may be documented by initialing and dating the report containing the test results
• DG:	A decision to obtain old records or a decision to obtain additional history from the family, caretaker, or other source to supplement that obtained from the patient should be documented
• DG:	Relevant findings from the review of old records and/or the receipt of additional history from the family, caretaker, or other source to supplement that obtained from the patient should be documented. If there is no relevant information beyond that already obtained, that fact should be documented. A notation of "old records reviewed" or "additional history obtained from family" without elaboration is insufficient

• DG:	The results of discussion of laboratory, radiology, or other diagnostic tests with the physician who performed or interpreted the study should be documented
• DG:	The direct visualization and independent interpretation of an image, tracing, or specimen previously or subsequently interpreted by another physician should be documented

Risk of Significant Complications, Morbidity, and/or Mortality

The risk of significant complications, morbidity, and/or mortality is based on the risks associated with the presenting problem, the diagnostic procedure, and the possible management options.

• DG:	Comorbidities/underlying disease or other factors that increase the complexity of medical decision making by increasing the risk of complications, morbidity, and/or mortality should be documented
• DG:	If a surgical or invasive diagnostic procedure is ordered, planned, or scheduled at the time of the E/M encounter, the type of procedure (e.g., laparoscopy) should be documented
• DG:	If a surgical or invasive diagnostic procedure is performed at the time of the E/M encounter, the specific procedure should be documented
• DG:	The referral for or decision to perform a surgical or invasive diagnostic procedure on an urgent basis should be documented or implied

The following Table of Risk may be used to help determine whether the risk of significant complications, morbidity, and/or mortality is minimal, low, moderate, or high. Because the determination of risk is complex and not readily quantifiable, the table includes common clinical examples rather than absolute measures of risk. The assessment of risk of the presenting problem is based on the risk related to the disease process anticipated between the present encounter and the next one. The assessment of risk of selecting diagnostic procedures and management options is based on the risk during and immediately following any procedures or treatment. The highest level of risk in any one category (presenting problem, diagnostic procedure, or management options) determines the overall risk.

Table of Risk

Level of Risk	Presenting Problem(s)	Diagnostic Procedure(s) Ordered	Management Options Selected
Minimal	One self-limited or minor problem (e.g., cold, insect bite, tinea corporis)	Laboratory test requiring veinpuncture Chest x-rays EKG/EEG Urinalysis Ultrasound (e.g., echocardiography) KOH prep	Rest Gargles Elastic bandages Superficial dressings
Low	Two or more self-limited or minor problems One stable chronic illness (e.g., well controlled hypertension, non-insulin dependent diabetes, cataract, BPH) Acute, uncomplicated illness or injury (e.g., cystitis, allergic rhinitis, simple sprain)	Physiologic tests not under stress (e.g., pulmonary function tests) Non-cardiovascular imaging studies with contrast (e.g., barium enema) Superficial needle biopsies Clinical laboratory tests requiring arterial puncture Skin biopsies	Over-the-counter drugs Minor surgery with no identified risk factors Physical therapy Occupational therapy IV fluids without additives
Moderate	One or more chronic illnesses with mild exacerbation, progression or side effects of treatment Two or more stable chronic illnesses Undiagnosed new problem with uncertain prognosis (e.g., lump in breast) Acute illness with systemic symptoms (e.g., pyelonephritis, pneumonitis, colitis) Acute complicated injury (e.g., head injury with brief loss of consciousness)	Physiologic tests not under stress (e.g., cardiac stress test, fetal contraction stress test) Diagnostic endoscopies with no identified risk factors Deep needle or incisional biopsy Cardiovascular imaging studies with contrast and no identified risk factors (e.g., arteriogram, cardiac catheterization) Obtain fluid from body cavity (e.g., lumbar puncture, thoracentesis, culdocentesis)	Minor surgery with identified risk factors Effective major surgery (open, percutaneous or endoscopic) with no identified risk factors Prescription drug management Therapeutic nuclear medicine IV fluids with additives Closed treatment of fracture or dislocation without manipulation
High	One or more chronic illnesses with severe exacerbation, progression or side effects of treatment Acute/chronic illnesses that may pose a threat to life or bodily function (e.g., multiple trauma, acute MI, pulmonary embolus, severe respiratory distress, progressive severe rheumatoid arthritis, psychiatric illness with potential threat to self or others, peritonitis, acute renal failure An abrupt change in neurologic status (e.g., seizure, TIA, weakness or sensory loss)	Cardiovascular imaging studies with contrast with identified risk factors Cardiac electrophysiological tests Diagnostic endoscopies with identified risk factors Discography	Elective major surgery (open, percutaneous or endoscopic) with identified risk factors Emergency major surgery (open, percutaneous or endoscopic) Parenteral controlled substances Drug therapy requiring intensive monitoring for toxicity Decision not to resuscitate or to de-escalate care because of poor prognosis

D. Documentation of an Encounter Dominated by Counseling or Coordination of Care

In the case where counseling and/or coordination of care dominates (more than 50 percent) the physician/patient and/or family encounter (face-to-face time in the office or other outpatient setting or floor-unit time in the hospital or nursing facility), time is considered the key or controlling factor to qualify for a particular level of E/M service.

- DG: If the physician elects to report the level of service based on counseling and/or coordination of care, the total length of time of the encounter (face-to-face or floor time, as appropriate) should be documented and the record should describe the counseling and/or activities to coordinate care

Appendix D — Crosswalk of Deleted Codes

The deleted code crosswalk is meant to be used as a reference tool to find active codes that could be used in place of the deleted code. This will not always be an exact match. Please review the code descriptions and guidelines before selecting a code.

Code	Cross reference
11752	To report, see 26236, 28124, 28160
21495	To report, see 31584
22305	To report, see appropriate E&M codes
22851	To report, see 22853-22854, [22859]
27193	To report, see 27197
27194	To report, see 27198
28290	To report, see 28292
28293	To report, see 28291
28294	To report, see 28899
31582	To report, see [31551, 31552, 31553, 31554]
31588	To report, see 31599
33400	To report, see 33990-33991
33401	To report, see 33390-33391
33403	To report, see 33390-33391
35450	To report, see 36902, 36905, 36907, [37246, 37247, 37248, 37249]
35452	To report, see 36902, 36905, 36907, [37246, 37247, 37248, 37249]
35458	To report, see 36902, 36905, 36907, [37246, 37247, 37248, 37249]
35460	To report, see 36902, 36905, 36907, [37246, 37247, 37248, 37249]
35471	To report, see 36902, 36905, 36907, [37246, 37247, 37248, 37249]
35472	To report, see 36902, 36905, 36907, [37246, 37247, 37248, 37249]
35475	To report, see 36902, 36905, 36907, [37246, 37247, 37248, 37249]
35476	To report, see 36902, 36905, 36907, [37246, 37247, 37248, 37249]
36147	To report, see 36901-36906
36148	To report, see 36901-36906
36870	To report, see 36904-36906
62310	To report, see 62320-62321

Code	Cross reference
62311	To report, see 62322-62323
62318	To report, see 62324-62325
62319	To report, see 62326-62327
75791	To report, see 36901-36906
75962	To report, see 36902, 36905, [37246, 37247]
75964	To report, see 36902, 36905, [37246, 37247]
75966	To report, see 36902, 36905, [37246, 37247]
75968	To report, see 36902, 36905, [37246, 37247]
75978	To report, see 36902, 36905, 36907, [37248], [37249]
77051	To report, see 77065-77066
77052	To report, see 77067
77055	To report, see 77065
77056	To report, see 77066
77057	To report, see 77067
80300	To report, see [80305, 80306]
80301	To report, see [80307]
80302	To report, see [80307]
80303	To report, see [80307]
80304	To report, see [80307]
97001	To report, see [97161, 97162, 97163, 97164, 97165, 97166, 97167, 97168, 97169, 97170, 97171, 97172]
97002	To report, see [97161, 97162, 97163, 97164, 97165, 97166, 97167, 97168, 97169, 97170, 97171, 97172]
97003	To report, see [97161, 97162, 97163, 97164, 97165, 97166, 97167, 97168, 97169, 97170, 97171, 97172]

Code	Cross reference
97004	To report, see [97161, 97162, 97163, 97164, 97165, 97166, 97167, 97168, 97169, 97170, 97171, 97172]
97005	To report, see [97161, 97162, 97163, 97164, 97165, 97166, 97167, 97168, 97169, 97170, 97171, 97172]
97006	To report, see [97161, 97162, 97163, 97164, 97165, 97166, 97167, 97168, 97169, 97170, 97171, 97172]
99143	To report, see 99151-99153
99144	To report, see 99151-99153
99145	To report, see 99151-99153
99148	To report, see 99155-99157
99149	To report, see 99155-99157
99150	To report, see 99155-99157
99420	To report, see 96160-96161
0010M	To report, see 81539
0019T	To report, see 20999
0169T	To report, see 64999
0171T	To report, see 22867, 22869
0172T	To report, see 22868, 22870
0281T	To report, see 33340
0282T	To report, see 64999
0283T	To report, see 64999
0284T	To report, see 64999
0285T	To report, see 64999
0286T	To report, see 76499
0288T	To report, see 46999
0291T	To report, see [92978, 92979]
0292T	To report, see [92978, 92979]
0336T	To report, see 58674
0392T	To report, see 43284
0393T	To report, see 43285

Appendix E — Resequenced Codes

Code	Description	Reference
11045	Debridement, subcutaneous tissue (includes epidermis and dermis, if performed); each additional 20 sq cm, or part thereof (List separately in addition to code for primary procedure)	See code following 11042.
11046	Debridement, muscle and/or fascia (includes epidermis, dermis, and subcutaneous tissue, if performed); each additional 20 sq cm, or part thereof (List separately in addition to code for primary procedure)	See code following 11043.
21552	Excision, tumor, soft tissue of neck or anterior thorax, subcutaneous; 3 cm or greater	See code following 21555.
21554	Excision, tumor, soft tissue of neck or anterior thorax, subfascial (eg, intramuscular); 5 cm or greater	See code following 21556.
22858	Total disc arthroplasty (artificial disc), anterior approach, including discectomy with end plate preparation (includes osteophytectomy for nerve root or spinal cord decompression and microdissection); second level, cervical (List separately in addition to code for primary procedure)	See code following 22856.
22859	Insertion of intervertebral biomechanical device(s) (eg, synthetic cage, mesh, methylmethacrylate) to intervertebral disc space or vertebral body defect without interbody arthrodesis, each contiguous defect (List separately in addition to code for primary procedure)	See code following 22854.
23071	Excision, tumor, soft tissue of shoulder area, subcutaneous; 3 cm or greater	See code following 23075.
23073	Excision, tumor, soft tissue of shoulder area, subfascial (eg, intramuscular); 5 cm or greater	See code following 23076.
24071	Excision, tumor, soft tissue of upper arm or elbow area, subcutaneous; 3 cm or greater	See code following 24075.
24073	Excision, tumor, soft tissue of upper arm or elbow area, subfascial (eg, intramuscular); 5 cm or greater	See code following 24076.
25071	Excision, tumor, soft tissue of forearm and/or wrist area, subcutaneous; 3 cm or greater	See code following 25075.
25073	Excision, tumor, soft tissue of forearm and/or wrist area, subfascial (eg, intramuscular); 3 cm or greater	See code following 25076.
26111	Excision, tumor or vascular malformation, soft tissue of hand or finger, subcutaneous; 1.5 cm or greater	See code following 26115.
26113	Excision, tumor, soft tissue, or vascular malformation, of hand or finger, subfascial (eg, intramuscular); 1.5 cm or greater	See code following 26116.
27043	Excision, tumor, soft tissue of pelvis and hip area, subcutaneous; 3 cm or greater	See code following 27047.
27045	Excision, tumor, soft tissue of pelvis and hip area, subfascial (eg, intramuscular); 5 cm or greater	See code following 27048.
27059	Radical resection of tumor (eg, sarcoma), soft tissue of pelvis and hip area; 5 cm or greater	See code following 27049.
27329	Radical resection of tumor (eg, sarcoma), soft tissue of thigh or knee area; less than 5 cm	See code following 27360.
27337	Excision, tumor, soft tissue of thigh or knee area, subcutaneous; 3 cm or greater	See code following 27327.
27339	Excision, tumor, soft tissue of thigh or knee area, subfascial (eg, intramuscular); 5 cm or greater	See code following 27328.
27632	Excision, tumor, soft tissue of leg or ankle area, subcutaneous; 3 cm or greater	See code following 27618.
27634	Excision, tumor, soft tissue of leg or ankle area, subfascial (eg, intramuscular); 5 cm or greater	See code following 27619.
28039	Excision, tumor, soft tissue of foot or toe, subcutaneous; 1.5 cm or greater	See code following 28043.
28041	Excision, tumor, soft tissue of foot or toe, subfascial (eg, intramuscular); 1.5 cm or greater	See code following 28045.
28295	Correction, hallux valgus (bunionectomy), with sesamoidectomy, when performed; with proximal metatarsal osteotomy, any method	See code following 28296.
29914	Arthroscopy, hip, surgical; with femoroplasty (ie, treatment of cam lesion)	See code following 29863.
29915	Arthroscopy, hip, surgical; with acetabuloplasty (ie, treatment of pincer lesion)	See code following 29863.
29916	Arthroscopy, hip, surgical; with labral repair	See code before 29866.
31551	Laryngoplasty; for laryngeal stenosis, with graft, without indwelling stent placement, younger than 12 years of age	See code following 31580.
31552	Laryngoplasty; for laryngeal stenosis, with graft, without indwelling stent placement, age 12 years or older	See code following 31580.
31553	Laryngoplasty; for laryngeal stenosis, with graft, with indwelling stent placement, younger than 12 years of age	See code following 31580.
31554	Laryngoplasty; for laryngeal stenosis, with graft, with indwelling stent placement, age 12 years or older	See code following 31580.
31572	Laryngoscopy, flexible; with ablation or destruction of lesion(s) with laser, unilateral	See code following 31578.
31573	Laryngoscopy, flexible; with therapeutic injection(s) (eg, chemodenervation agent or corticosteroid, injected percutaneous, transoral, or via endoscope channel), unilateral	See code following 31578.
31574	Laryngoscopy, flexible; with injection(s) for augmentation (eg, percutaneous, transoral), unilateral	See code following 31578.
31651	Bronchoscopy, rigid or flexible, including fluoroscopic guidance, when performed; with balloon occlusion, when performed, assessment of air leak, airway sizing, and insertion of bronchial valve(s), each additional lobe (List separately in addition to code for primary procedure[s])	See code following 31647.
33221	Insertion of pacemaker pulse generator only; with existing multiple leads	See code following 33213.
33227	Removal of permanent pacemaker pulse generator with replacement of pacemaker pulse generator; single lead system	See code following 33233.
33228	Removal of permanent pacemaker pulse generator with replacement of pacemaker pulse generator; dual lead system	See code following 33233.
33229	Removal of permanent pacemaker pulse generator with replacement of pacemaker pulse generator; multiple lead system	See code before 33234.
33230	Insertion of implantable defibrillator pulse generator only; with existing dual leads	See code following 33240.
33231	Insertion of implantable defibrillator pulse generator only; with existing multiple leads	See code before 33241.

Code	Description	Reference
33262	Removal of implantable defibrillator pulse generator with replacement of implantable defibrillator pulse generator; single lead system	See code following 33241.
33263	Removal of implantable defibrillator pulse generator with replacement of implantable defibrillator pulse generator; dual lead system	See code following 33241.
33264	Removal of implantable defibrillator pulse generator with replacement of implantable defibrillator pulse generator; multiple lead system	See code before 33243.
33270	Insertion or replacement of permanent subcutaneous implantable defibrillator system, with subcutaneous electrode, including defibrillation threshold evaluation, induction of arrhythmia, evaluation of sensing for arrhythmia termination, and programming or reprogramming of sensing or therapeutic parameters, when performed	See code following 33249.
33271	Insertion of subcutaneous implantable defibrillator electrode	See code following 33249.
33272	Removal of subcutaneous implantable defibrillator electrode	See code following 33249.
33273	Repositioning of previously implanted subcutaneous implantable defibrillator electrode	See code following 33249.
33962	Extracorporeal membrane oxygenation (ECMO)/extracorporeal life support (ECLS) provided by physician; reposition peripheral (arterial and/or venous) cannula(e), open, 6 years and older (includes fluoroscopic guidance, when performed)	See code following 33959.
33963	Extracorporeal membrane oxygenation (ECMO)/extracorporeal life support (ECLS) provided by physician; reposition of central cannula(e) by sternotomy or thoracotomy, birth through 5 years of age (includes fluoroscopic guidance, when performed)	See code following 33959.
33964	Extracorporeal membrane oxygenation (ECMO)/extracorporeal life support (ECLS) provided by physician; reposition central cannula(e) by sternotomy or thoracotomy, 6 years and older (includes fluoroscopic guidance, when performed)	See code following 33959.
33965	Extracorporeal membrane oxygenation (ECMO)/extracorporeal life support (ECLS) provided by physician; removal of peripheral (arterial and/or venous) cannula(e), percutaneous, birth through 5 years of age	See code following 33959.
33966	Extracorporeal membrane oxygenation (ECMO)/extracorporeal life support (ECLS) provided by physician; removal of peripheral (arterial and/or venous) cannula(e), percutaneous, 6 years and older	See code following 33959.
33969	Extracorporeal membrane oxygenation (ECMO)/extracorporeal life support (ECLS) provided by physician; removal of peripheral (arterial and/or venous) cannula(e), open, birth through 5 years of age	See code following 33959.
33984	Extracorporeal membrane oxygenation (ECMO)/extracorporeal life support (ECLS) provided by physician; removal of peripheral (arterial and/or venous) cannula(e), open, 6 years and older	See code following 33959.
33985	Extracorporeal membrane oxygenation (ECMO)/extracorporeal life support (ECLS) provided by physician; removal of central cannula(e) by sternotomy or thoracotomy, birth through 5 years of age	See code following 33959.
33986	Extracorporeal membrane oxygenation (ECMO)/extracorporeal life support (ECLS) provided by physician; removal of central cannula(e) by sternotomy or thoracotomy, 6 years and older	See code following 33959.
33987	Arterial exposure with creation of graft conduit (eg, chimney graft) to facilitate arterial perfusion for ECMO/ECLS (List separately in addition to code for primary procedure)	See code following 33959.
33988	Insertion of left heart vent by thoracic incision (eg, sternotomy, thoracotomy) for ECMO/ECLS	See code following 33959.
33989	Removal of left heart vent by thoracic incision (eg, sternotomy, thoracotomy) for ECMO/ECLS	See code following 33959.
37211	Transcatheter therapy, arterial infusion for thrombolysis other than coronary, any method, including radiological supervision and interpretation, initial treatment day	See code following 37200.
37212	Transcatheter therapy, venous infusion for thrombolysis, any method, including radiological supervision and interpretation, initial treatment day	See code following 37200.
37213	Transcatheter therapy, arterial or venous infusion for thrombolysis other than coronary, any method, including radiological supervision and interpretation, continued treatment on subsequent day during course of thrombolytic therapy, including follow-up catheter contrast injection, position change, or exchange, when performed;	See code following 37200.
37214	Transcatheter therapy, arterial or venous infusion for thrombolysis other than coronary, any method, including radiological supervision and interpretation, continued treatment on subsequent day during course of thrombolytic therapy, including follow-up catheter contrast injection, position change, or exchange, when performed; cessation of thrombolysis including removal of catheter and vessel closure by any method	See code following 37200.
37246	Transluminal balloon angioplasty (except lower extremity artery(ies) for occlusive disease, intracranial, coronary, pulmonary, or dialysis circuit), open or percutaneous, including all imaging and radiological supervision and interpretation necessary to perform the angioplasty within the same artery; initial artery	See code following 37235.
37247	Transluminal balloon angioplasty (except lower extremity artery(ies) for occlusive disease, intracranial, coronary, pulmonary, or dialysis circuit), open or percutaneous, including all imaging and radiological supervision and interpretation necessary to perform the angioplasty within the same artery; each additional artery (List separately in addition to code for primary procedure)	See code following 37235.
37248	Transluminal balloon angioplasty (except dialysis circuit), open or percutaneous, including all imaging and radiological supervision and interpretation necessary to perform the angioplasty within the same vein; initial vein	See code following 37235.
37249	Transluminal balloon angioplasty (except dialysis circuit), open or percutaneous, including all imaging and radiological supervision and interpretation necessary to perform the angioplasty within the same vein; each additional vein (List separately in addition to code for primary procedure)	See code following 37235.
38243	Hematopoietic progenitor cell (HPC); HPC boost	See code following 38241.
42310	Esophagogastroduodenoscopy, flexible, transoral; with esophagogastric fundoplasty, partial or complete, includes duodenoscopy when performed	See coded following 43259.

Code	Description	Reference
43211	Esophagoscopy, flexible, transoral; with endoscopic mucosal resection	See code following 43217.
43212	Esophagoscopy, flexible, transoral; with placement of endoscopic stent (includes pre- and post-dilation and guide wire passage, when performed)	See code following 43217.
43213	Esophagoscopy, flexible, transoral; with dilation of esophagus, by balloon or dilator, retrograde (includes fluoroscopic guidance, when performed)	See code following 43220.
43214	Esophagoscopy, flexible, transoral; with dilation of esophagus with balloon (30 mm diameter or larger) (includes fluoroscopic guidance, when performed)	See code following 43220.
43233	Esophagogastroduodenoscopy, flexible, transoral; with dilation of esophagus with balloon (30 mm diameter or larger) (includes fluoroscopic guidance, when performed)	See code following 43249.
43266	Esophagogastroduodenoscopy, flexible, transoral; with placement of endoscopic stent (includes pre- and post-dilation and guide wire passage, when performed)	See code following 43255.
43270	Esophagogastroduodenoscopy, flexible, transoral; with ablation of tumor(s), polyp(s), or other lesion(s) (includes pre- and post-dilation and guide wire passage, when performed)	See code following 43257.
43274	Endoscopic retrograde cholangiopancreatography (ERCP); with placement of endoscopic stent into biliary or pancreatic duct, including pre- and post-dilation and guide wire passage, when performed, including sphincterotomy, when performed, each stent	See code following 43265.
43275	Endoscopic retrograde cholangiopancreatography (ERCP); with removal of foreign body(s) or stent(s) from biliary/pancreatic duct(s)	See code following 43265.
43276	Endoscopic retrograde cholangiopancreatography (ERCP); with removal and exchange of stent(s), biliary or pancreatic duct, including pre- and post-dilation and guide wire passage, when performed, including sphincterotomy, when performed, each stent exchanged	See code following 43265.
43277	Endoscopic retrograde cholangiopancreatography (ERCP); with trans-endoscopic balloon dilation of biliary/pancreatic duct(s) or of ampulla (sphincteroplasty), including sphincterotomy, when performed, each duct	See code before 43273.
43278	Endoscopic retrograde cholangiopancreatography (ERCP); with ablation of tumor(s), polyp(s), or other lesion(s), including pre- and post-dilation and guide wire passage, when performed	See code before 43273.
44381	Ileoscopy, through stoma; with transendoscopic balloon dilation	See code following 44382.
44401	Colonoscopy through stoma; with ablation of tumor(s), polyp(s), or other lesion(s) (includes pre-and post-dilation and guide wire passage, when performed)	See code following 44392.
45346	Sigmoidoscopy, flexible; with ablation of tumor(s), polyp(s), or other lesion(s) (includes pre- and post-dilation and guide wire passage, when performed)	See code following 45338.
45388	Colonoscopy, flexible; with ablation of tumor(s), polyp(s), or other lesion(s) (includes pre- and post-dilation and guide wire passage, when performed)	See code following 45382.
45390	Colonoscopy, flexible; with endoscopic mucosal resection	See code following 45392.
45398	Colonoscopy, flexible; with band ligation(s) (eg, hemorrhoids)	See code following 45393.
45399	Unlisted procedure, colon	See code before 45990.
46220	Excision of single external papilla or tag, anus	See code before 46230.
46320	Excision of thrombosed hemorrhoid, external	See code following 46230.
46945	Hemorrhoidectomy, internal, by ligation other than rubber band; single hemorrhoid column/group	See code following 46221.
46946	Hemorrhoidectomy, internal, by ligation other than rubber band; 2 or more hemorrhoid columns/groups	See code following 46221.
46947	Hemorrhoidopexy (eg, for prolapsing internal hemorrhoids) by stapling	See code following 46762.
50430	Injection procedure for antegrade nephrostogram and/or ureterogram, complete diagnostic procedure including imaging guidance (eg, ultrasound and fluoroscopy) and all associated radiological supervision and interpretation; new access	See code following 43259
50431	Injection procedure for antegrade nephrostogram and/or ureterogram, complete diagnostic procedure including imaging guidance (eg, ultrasound and fluoroscopy) and all associated radiological supervision and interpretation; existing access	See code following 43259.
50432	Placement of nephrostomy catheter, percutaneous, including diagnostic nephrostogram and/or ureterogram when performed, imaging guidance (eg, ultrasound and/or fluoroscopy) and all associated radiological supervision and interpretation	See code following 43259.
50433	Placement of nephroureteral catheter, percutaneous, including diagnostic nephrostogram and/or ureterogram when performed, imaging guidance (eg, ultrasound and/or fluoroscopy) and all associated radiological supervision and interpretation, new access	See code following 43259.
50434	Convert nephrostomy catheter to nephroureteral catheter, percutaneous, including diagnostic nephrostogram and/or ureterogram when performed, imaging guidance (eg, ultrasound and/or fluoroscopy) and all associated radiological supervision and interpretation, via pre-existing nephrostomy tract	See code following 43259.
50435	Exchange nephrostomy catheter, percutaneous, including diagnostic nephrostogram and/or ureterogram when performed, imaging guidance (eg, ultrasound and/or fluoroscopy) and all associated radiological supervision and interpretation	See code following 43259.
51797	Voiding pressure studies, intra-abdominal (ie, rectal, gastric, intraperitoneal) (List separately in addition to code for primary procedure)	See code following 51729.
52356	Cystourethroscopy, with ureteroscopy and/or pyeloscopy; with lithotripsy including insertion of indwelling ureteral stent (eg, Gibbons or double-J type)	See code following 52353.
64461	Paravertebral block (PVB) (paraspinous block), thoracic; single injection site (includes imaging guidance, when performed)	See code following 64484.

Code	Description	Reference
64462	Paravertebral block (PVB) (paraspinous block), thoracic; second and any additional injection site(s) (includes imaging guidance, when performed) (List separately in addition to code for primary procedure)	See code following 64484.
64463	Paravertebral block (PVB) (paraspinous block), thoracic; continuous infusion by catheter (includes imaging guidance, when performed)	See code following 64484.
64633	Destruction by neurolytic agent, paravertebral facet joint nerve(s), with imaging guidance (fluoroscopy or CT); cervical or thoracic, single facet joint	See code following 64620.
64634	Destruction by neurolytic agent, paravertebral facet joint nerve(s), with imaging guidance (fluoroscopy or CT); cervical or thoracic, each additional facet joint (List separately in addition to code for primary procedure)	See code following 64620.
64635	Destruction by neurolytic agent, paravertebral facet joint nerve(s), with imaging guidance (fluoroscopy or CT); lumbar or sacral, single facet joint	See code following 64620.
64636	Destruction by neurolytic agent, paravertebral facet joint nerve(s), with imaging guidance (fluoroscopy or CT); lumbar or sacral, each additional facet joint (List separately in addition to code for primary procedure)	See code before 64630.
67810	Incisional biopsy of eyelid skin including lid margin	See code following 67715.
77085	Dual-energy X-ray absorptiometry (DXA), bone density study, 1 or more sites; axial skeleton (eg, hips, pelvis, spine), including vertebral fracture assessment	See code following 77081.
77086	Vertebral fracture assessment via dual-energy X-ray absorptiometry (DXA)	See code before 77084.
77295	3-dimensional radiotherapy plan, including dose-volume histograms	See code before 77300.
77385	Intensity modulated radiation treatment delivery (IMRT), includes guidance and tracking, when performed; simple	See code following 77417.
77386	Intensity modulated radiation treatment delivery (IMRT), includes guidance and tracking, when performed; complex	See code following 77417.
77387	Guidance for localization of target volume for delivery of radiation treatment delivery, includes intrafraction tracking, when performed	See code following 77417.
77424	Intraoperative radiation treatment delivery, x-ray, single treatment session	See code before 77422.
77425	Intraoperative radiation treatment delivery, electrons, single treatment session	See code before 77422.
80081	Obstetric panel (includes HIV testing)	See code following 80055.
80164	Valproic acid (dipropylacetic acid); total	See code following 80201.
80165	Valproic acid (dipropylacetic acid); free	See code following 80201.
80171	Gabapentin, whole blood, serum, or plasma	See code following 80169.
80305	Drug test(s), presumptive, any number of drug classes, any number of devices or procedures (eg, immunoassay); capable of being read by direct optical observation only (eg, dipsticks, cups, cards, cartridges) includes sample validation when performed, per date of service	See code before 80150.
80306	Drug test(s), presumptive, any number of drug classes, any number of devices or procedures (eg, immunoassay); read by instrument assisted direct optical observation (eg, dipsticks, cups, cards, cartridges), includes sample validation when performed, per date of service	See code before 80150.
80307	Drug test(s), presumptive, any number of drug classes, any number of devices or procedures, by instrument chemistry analyzers (eg, utilizing immunoassay [eg, EIA, ELISA, EMIT, FPIA, IA, KIMS, RIA]), chromatography (eg, GC, HPLC), and mass spectrometry either with or without chromatography, (eg, DART, DESI, GC-MS, GC-MS/MS, LC-MS, LC-MS/MS, LDTD, MALDI, TOF) includes sample validation when performed, per date of service	See code before 80150.
80320	Alcohols	See code before 80150.
80321	Alcohol biomarkers; 1 or 2	See code before 80150.
80322	Alcohol biomarkers; 3 or more	See code before 80150.
80323	Alkaloids, not otherwise specified	See code before 80150.
80324	Amphetamines; 1 or 2	See code before 80150.
80325	Amphetamines; 3 or 4	See code before 80150.
80326	Amphetamines; 5 or more	See code before 80150.
80327	Anabolic steroids; 1 or 2	See code before 80150.
80328	Anabolic steroids; 3 or more	See code before 80150.
80329	Analgesics, non-opioid; 1 or 2	See code before 80150.
80330	Analgesics, non-opioid; 3-5	See code before 80150.
80331	Analgesics, non-opioid; 6 or more	See code before 80150.
80332	Antidepressants, serotonergic class; 1 or 2	See code before 80150.
80333	Antidepressants, serotonergic class; 3-5	See code before 80150.
80334	Antidepressants, serotonergic class; 6 or more	See code before 80150.
80335	Antidepressants, tricyclic and other cyclicals; 1 or 2	See code before 80150.
80336	Antidepressants, tricyclic and other cyclicals; 3-5	See code before 80150.
80337	Antidepressants, tricyclic and other cyclicals; 6 or more	See code before 80150.
80338	Antidepressants, not otherwise specified	See code before 80150.
80339	Antiepileptics, not otherwise specified; 1-3	See code before 80150.
80340	Antiepileptics, not otherwise specified; 4-6	See code before 80150.
80341	Antiepileptics, not otherwise specified; 7 or more	See code before 80150.

Code	Description	Reference
80342	Antipsychotics, not otherwise specified; 1-3	See code before 80150.
80343	Antipsychotics, not otherwise specified; 4-6	See code before 80150.
80344	Antipsychotics, not otherwise specified; 7 or more	See code before 80150.
80345	Barbiturates	See code before 80150.
80346	Benzodiazepines; 1-12	See code before 80150.
80347	Benzodiazepines; 13 or more	See code before 80150.
80348	Buprenorphine	See code before 80150.
80349	Cannabinoids, natural	See code before 80150.
80350	Cannabinoids, synthetic; 1-3	See code before 80150.
80351	Cannabinoids, synthetic; 4-6	See code before 80150.
80352	Cannabinoids, synthetic; 7 or more	See code before 80150.
80353	Cocaine	See code before 80150.
80354	Fentanyl	See code before 80150.
80355	Gabapentin, non-blood	See code before 80150.
80356	Heroin metabolite	See code before 80150.
80357	Ketamine and norketamine	See code before 80150.
80358	Methadone	See code before 80150.
80359	Methylenedioxyamphetamines (MDA, MDEA, MDMA)	See code before 80150.
80360	Methylphenidate	See code before 80150.
80361	Opiates, 1 or more	See code before 80150.
80362	Opioids and opiate analogs; 1 or 2	See code before 80150.
80363	Opioids and opiate analogs; 3 or 4	See code before 80150.
80364	Opioids and opiate analogs; 5 or more	See code before 80150.
80365	Oxycodone	See code following 80364.
80366	Pregabalin	See code following 83992.
80367	Propoxyphene	See code following 80366.
80368	Sedative hypnotics (non-benzodiazepines)	See code following 80367.
80369	Skeletal muscle relaxants; 1 or 2	See code following 80368.
80370	Skeletal muscle relaxants; 3 or more	See code following 80369.
80371	Stimulants, synthetic	See code following 80370.
80372	Tapentadol	See code following 80371.
80373	Tramadol	See code following 80372.
80374	Stereoisomer (enantiomer) analysis, single drug class	See code following 80373.
80375	Drug(s) or substance(s), definitive, qualitative or quantitative, not otherwise specified; 1-3	See code following 80374.
80376	Drug(s) or substance(s), definitive, qualitative or quantitative, not otherwise specified; 4-6	See code following 80375.
80377	Drug(s) or substance(s), definitive, qualitative or quantitative, not otherwise specified; 7 or more	See code following 80376.
81161	DMD (dystrophin) (eg, Duchenne/Becker muscular dystrophy) deletion analysis, and duplication analysis, if performed	See code following 81229.
81162	BRCA1, BRCA2 (breast cancer 1 and 2) (eg, hereditary breast and ovarian cancer) gene analysis; full sequence analysis and full duplication/deletion analysis	See code following 81211.
81287	MGMT (O-6-methylguanine-DNA methyltransferase) (eg, glioblastoma multiforme), methylation analysis	See code following 81290.
81288	MLH1 (mutL homolog 1, colon cancer, nonpolyposis type 2) (eg, hereditary non-polyposis colorectal cancer, Lynch syndrome) gene analysis; promoter methylation analysis	See code following 81292.
81479	Unlisted molecular pathology procedure	See code following 81408.
82652	Vitamin D; 1, 25 dihydroxy, includes fraction(s), if performed	See code following 82306.
83992	Phencyclidine (PCP)	See code following 80365.
86152	Cell enumeration using immunologic selection and identification in fluid specimen (eg, circulating tumor cells in blood);	See code following 86147.
86153	Cell enumeration using immunologic selection and identification in fluid specimen (eg, circulating tumor cells in blood); physician interpretation and report, when required	See code before 86148.
87623	Infectious agent detection by nucleic acid (DNA or RNA); Human Papillomavirus (HPV), low-risk types (eg, 6, 11, 42, 43, 44)	See code following 87539.
87624	Infectious agent detection by nucleic acid (DNA or RNA); Human Papillomavirus (HPV), high-risk types (eg, 16, 18, 31, 33, 35, 39, 45, 51, 52, 56, 58, 59, 68)	See code following 87539.
87625	Infectious agent detection by nucleic acid (DNA or RNA); Human Papillomavirus (HPV), types 16 and 18 only, includes type 45, if performed	See code before 87540.
87806	Infectious agent antigen detection by immunoassay with direct optical observation; HIV-1 antigen(s), with HIV-1 and HIV-2 antibodies	See code following 87803.
87906	Infectious agent genotype analysis by nucleic acid (DNA or RNA); HIV-1, other region (eg, integrase, fusion)	See code following 87901.
87910	Infectious agent genotype analysis by nucleic acid (DNA or RNA); cytomegalovirus	See code following 87900.
87912	Infectious agent genotype analysis by nucleic acid (DNA or RNA); Hepatitis B virus	See code before 87902.

Code	Description	Reference
88177	Cytopathology, evaluation of fine needle aspirate; immediate cytohistologic study to determine adequacy for diagnosis, each separate additional evaluation episode, same site (List separately in addition to code for primary procedure)	See code following 88173.
88341	Immunohistochemistry or immunocytochemistry, per specimen; each additional single antibody stain procedure (List separately in addition to code for primary procedure)	See code following 88342.
88350	Immunofluorescence, per specimen; each additional single antibody stain procedure (List separately in addition to code for primary procedure)	See code following 88346.
88364	In situ hybridization (eg, FISH), per specimen; each additional single probe stain procedure (List separately in addition to code for primary procedure)	See code following 88365.
88373	Morphometric analysis, in situ hybridization (quantitative or semi-quantitative), using computer-assisted technology, per specimen; each additional single probe stain procedure (List separately in addition to code for primary procedure)	See code following 88367.
88374	Morphometric analysis, in situ hybridization (quantitative or semi-quantitative), using computer-assisted technology, per specimen; each multiplex probe stain procedure	See code following 88367.
88377	Morphometric analysis, in situ hybridization (quantitative or semi-quantitative), manual, per specimen; each multiplex probe stain procedure	See code following 88369.
90620	Meningococcal recombinant protein and outer membrane vesicle vaccine, serogroup B (MenB), 2 dose schedule, for intramuscular use	See code following 90734.
90621	Meningococcal recombinant lipoprotein vaccine, serogroup B (MenB), 3 dose schedule, for intramuscular use	See code following 90734.
90625	Cholera vaccine, live, adult dosage, 1 dose schedule, for oral use	See code following 90723.
90630	Influenza virus vaccine, quadrivalent (IIV4), split virus, preservative free, for intradermal use	See code following 90654.
90644	Meningococcal conjugate vaccine, serogroups C & Y and Haemophilus influenzae type b vaccine (Hib-MenCY), 4 dose schedule, when administered to children 6 weeks-18 months of age, for intramuscular use	See code following 90732.
90672	Influenza virus vaccine, quadrivalent, live, for intranasal use	See code following 90660.
90673	Influenza virus vaccine, trivalent, derived from recombinant DNA (RIV3), hemagglutinin (HA) protein only, preservative and antibiotic free, for intramuscular use	See code following 90661.
90674	Influenza virus vaccine, quadrivalent (ccIIV4), derived from cell cultures, subunit, preservative and antibiotic free, 0.5 mL dosage, for intramuscular use	See code following 90661.
90750	Zoster (shingles) vaccine (HZV), recombinant, sub-unit, adjuvanted, for intramuscular injection	See code following 90736.
92558	Evoked otoacoustic emissions, screening (qualitative measurement of distortion product or transient evoked otoacoustic emissions), automated analysis	See code following 92586.
92597	Evaluation for use and/or fitting of voice prosthetic device to supplement oral speech	See code following 92604.
92618	Evaluation for prescription of non-speech-generating augmentative and alternative communication device, face-to-face with the patient; each additional 30 minutes (List separately in addition to code for primary procedure)	See code following 92605.
92920	Percutaneous transluminal coronary angioplasty; single major coronary artery or branch	See code following 92998.
92921	Percutaneous transluminal coronary angioplasty; each additional branch of a major coronary artery (List separately in addition to code for primary procedure)	See code following 92998.
92924	Percutaneous transluminal coronary atherectomy, with coronary angioplasty when performed; single major coronary artery or branch	See code following 92998.
92925	Percutaneous transluminal coronary atherectomy, with coronary angioplasty when performed; each additional branch of a major coronary artery (List separately in addition to code for primary procedure)	See code following 92998.
92928	Percutaneous transcatheter placement of intracoronary stent(s), with coronary angioplasty when performed; single major coronary artery or branch	See code following 92998.
92929	Percutaneous transcatheter placement of intracoronary stent(s), with coronary angioplasty when performed; each additional branch of a major coronary artery (List separately in addition to code for primary procedure)	See code following 92998.
92933	Percutaneous transluminal coronary atherectomy, with intracoronary stent, with coronary angioplasty when performed; single major coronary artery or branch	See code following 92998.
92934	Percutaneous transluminal coronary atherectomy, with intracoronary stent, with coronary angioplasty when performed; each additional branch of a major coronary artery (List separately in addition to code for primary procedure)	See code following 92998.
92937	Percutaneous transluminal revascularization of or through coronary artery bypass graft (internal mammary, free arterial, venous), any combination of intracoronary stent, atherectomy and angioplasty, including distal protection when performed; single vessel	See code following 92998.
92938	Percutaneous transluminal revascularization of or through coronary artery bypass graft (internal mammary, free arterial, venous), any combination of intracoronary stent, atherectomy and angioplasty, including distal protection when performed; each additional branch subtended by the bypass graft (List separately in addition to code for primary procedure)	See code following 92998.
92941	Percutaneous transluminal revascularization of acute total/subtotal occlusion during acute myocardial infarction, coronary artery or coronary artery bypass graft, any combination of intracoronary stent, atherectomy and angioplasty, including aspiration thrombectomy when performed, single vessel	See code following 92998.
92943	Percutaneous transluminal revascularization of chronic total occlusion, coronary artery, coronary artery branch, or coronary artery bypass graft, any combination of intracoronary stent, atherectomy and angioplasty; single vessel	See code following 92998.

Code	Description	Reference
92944	Percutaneous transluminal revascularization of chronic total occlusion, coronary artery, coronary artery branch, or coronary artery bypass graft, any combination of intracoronary stent, atherectomy and angioplasty; each additional coronary artery, coronary artery branch, or bypass graft (List separately in addition to code for primary procedure)	See code following 92998.
92973	Percutaneous transluminal coronary thrombectomy mechanical (List separately in addition to code for primary procedure)	See code following 92998.
92974	Transcatheter placement of radiation delivery device for subsequent coronary intravascular brachytherapy (List separately in addition to code for primary procedure)	See code following 92998.
92975	Thrombolysis, coronary; by intracoronary infusion, including selective coronary angiography	See code following 92998.
92977	Thrombolysis, coronary; by intravenous infusion	See code following 92998.
92978	Endoluminal imaging of coronary vessel or graft using intravascular ultrasound (IVUS) or optical coherence tomography (OCT) during diagnostic evaluation and/or therapeutic intervention including imaging supervision, interpretation and report; initial vessel (List separately in addition to code for primary procedure)	See code following 92998.
92979	Endoluminal imaging of coronary vessel or graft using intravascular ultrasound (IVUS) or optical coherence tomography (OCT) during diagnostic evaluation and/or therapeutic intervention including imaging supervision, interpretation and report; each additional vessel (List separately in addition to code for primary procedure)	See code following 92998.
93260	Programming device evaluation (in person) with iterative adjustment of the implantable device to test the function of the device and select optimal permanent programmed values with analysis, review and report by a physician or other qualified health care professional; implantable subcutaneous lead defibrillator system	See code following 93284.
93261	Interrogation device evaluation (in person) with analysis, review and report by a physician or other qualified health care professional, includes connection, recording and disconnection per patient encounter; implantable subcutaneous lead defibrillator system	See code following 93289.
95782	Polysomnography; younger than 6 years, sleep staging with 4 or more additional parameters of sleep, attended by a technologist	See code following 95811.
95783	Polysomnography; younger than 6 years, sleep staging with 4 or more additional parameters of sleep, with initiation of continuous positive airway pressure therapy or bi-level ventilation, attended by a technologist	See code following 95811.
95800	Sleep study, unattended, simultaneous recording; heart rate, oxygen saturation, respiratory analysis (eg, by airflow or peripheral arterial tone), and sleep time	See code following 95806.
95801	Sleep study, unattended, simultaneous recording; minimum of heart rate, oxygen saturation, and respiratory analysis (eg, by airflow or peripheral arterial tone)	See code following 95806.
95885	Needle electromyography, each extremity, with related paraspinal areas, when performed, done with nerve conduction, amplitude and latency/velocity study; limited (List separately in addition to code for primary procedure)	See code following 95872.
95886	Needle electromyography, each extremity, with related paraspinal areas, when performed, done with nerve conduction, amplitude and latency/velocity study; complete, five or more muscles studied, innervated by three or more nerves or four or more spinal levels (List separately in addition to code for primary procedure)	See code following 95872.
95887	Needle electromyography, non-extremity (cranial nerve supplied or axial) muscle(s) done with nerve conduction, amplitude and latency/velocity study (List separately in addition to code for primary procedure)	See code before 95873.
95938	Short-latency somatosensory evoked potential study, stimulation of any/all peripheral nerves or skin sites, recording from the central nervous system; in upper and lower limbs	See code following 95926.
95939	Central motor evoked potential study (transcranial motor stimulation); in upper and lower limbs	See code following 95929.
95940	Continuous intraoperative neurophysiology monitoring in the operating room, one on one monitoring requiring personal attendance, each 15 minutes (List separately in addition to code for primary procedure)	See code following 95913.
95941	Continuous intraoperative neurophysiology monitoring, from outside the operating room (remote or nearby) or for monitoring of more than one case while in the operating room, per hour (List separately in addition to code for primary procedure)	See code following 95913.
95943	Simultaneous, independent, quantitative measures of both parasympathetic function and sympathetic function, based on time-frequency analysis of heart rate variability concurrent with time-frequency analysis of continuous respiratory activity, with mean heart rate and blood pressure measures, during rest, paced (deep) breathing, Valsalva maneuvers, and head-up postural change	See code following 95924.
97161	Physical therapy evaluation: low complexity, requiring these components: A history with no personal factors and/or comorbidities that impact the plan of care; An examination of body system(s) using standardized tests and measures addressing 1-2 elements from any of the following: body structures and functions, activity limitations, and/or participation restrictions; A clinical presentation with stable and/or uncomplicated characteristics; and Clinical decision making of low complexity using standardized patient assessment instrument and/or measurable assessment of functional outcome. Typically, 20 minutes are spent face-to-face with the patient and/or family.	See code before 97010.
97162	Physical therapy evaluation: moderate complexity, requiring these components: A history of present problem with 1-2 personal factors and/or comorbidities that impact the plan of care; An examination of body systems using standardized tests and measures in addressing a total of 3 or more elements from any of the following: body structures and functions, activity limitations, and/or participation restrictions; An evolving clinical presentation with changing characteristics; and Clinical decision making of moderate complexity using standardized patient assessment instrument and/or measurable assessment of functional outcome. Typically, 30 minutes are spent face-to-face with the patient and/or family.	See code before 97010.

Code	Description	Reference
97163	Physical therapy evaluation: high complexity, requiring these components: A history of present problem with 3 or more personal factors and/or comorbidities that impact the plan of care; An examination of body systems using standardized tests and measures addressing a total of 4 or more elements from any of the following: body structures and functions, activity limitations, and/or participation restrictions; A clinical presentation with unstable and unpredictable characteristics; and Clinical decision making of high complexity using standardized patient assessment instrument and/or measurable assessment of functional outcome. Typically, 45 minutes are spent face-to-face with the patient and/or family.	See code before 97010.
97164	Re-evaluation of physical therapy established plan of care, requiring these components: An examination including a review of history and use of standardized tests and measures is required; and revised plan of care using a standardized patient assessment instrument and/or measurable assessment of functional outcome Typically, 20 minutes are spent face-to-face with the patient and/or family.	See code before 97010.
97165	Occupational therapy evaluation, low complexity, requiring these components: An occupational profile and medical and therapy history, which includes a brief history including review of medical and/or therapy records relating to the presenting problem; An assessment(s) that identifies 1-3 performance deficits (ie, relating to physical, cognitive, or psychosocial skills) that result in activity limitations and/or participation restrictions; and Clinical decision making of low complexity, which includes an analysis of the occupational profile, analysis of data from problem-focused assessment(s), and consideration of a limited number of treatment options. Patient presents with no comorbidities that affect occupational performance. Modification of tasks or assistance (eg, physical or verbal) with assessment(s) is not necessary to enable completion of evaluation component. Typically, 30 minutes are spent face-to-face with the patient and/or family.	See code before 97010.
97166	Occupational therapy evaluation, moderate complexity, requiring these components: An occupational profile and medical and therapy history, which includes an expanded review of medical and/or therapy records and additional review of physical, cognitive, or psychosocial history related to current functional performance; An assessment(s) that identifies 3-5 performance deficits (ie, relating to physical, cognitive, or psychosocial skills) that result in activity limitations and/or participation restrictions; and Clinical decision making of moderate analytic complexity, which includes an analysis of the occupational profile, analysis of data from detailed assessment(s), and consideration of several treatment options. Patient may present with comorbidities that affect occupational performance. Minimal to moderate modification of tasks or assistance (eg, physical or verbal) with assessment(s) is necessary to enable patient to complete evaluation component. Typically, 45 minutes are spent face-to-face with the patient and/or family.	See code before 97010.
97167	Occupational therapy evaluation, high complexity, requiring these components: An occupational profile and medical and therapy history, which includes review of medical and/or therapy records and extensive additional review of physical, cognitive, or psychosocial history related to current functional performance; An assessment(s) that identifies 5 or more performance deficits (ie, relating to physical, cognitive, or psychosocial skills) that result in activity limitations and/or participation restrictions; and Clinical decision making of high analytic complexity, which includes an analysis of the patient profile, analysis of data from comprehensive assessment(s), and consideration of multiple treatment options. Patient presents with comorbidities that affect occupational performance. Significant modification of tasks or assistance (eg, physical or verbal) with assessment(s) is necessary to enable patient to complete evaluation component. Typically, 60 minutes are spent face-to-face with the patient and/or family.	See code before 97010.
97168	Re-evaluation of occupational therapy established plan of care, requiring these components: An assessment of changes in patient functional or medical status with revised plan of care; An update to the initial occupational profile to reflect changes in condition or environment that affect future interventions and/or goals; and A revised plan of care. A formal reevaluation is performed when there is a documented change in functional status or a significant change to the plan of care is required. Typically, 30 minutes are spent face-to-face with the patient and/or family.	See code before 97010.
97169	Athletic training evaluation, low complexity, requiring these components: A history and physical activity profile with no comorbidities that affect physical activity; An examination of affected body area and other symptomatic or related systems addressing 1-2 elements from any of the following: body structures, physical activity, and/or participation deficiencies; and Clinical decision making of low complexity using standardized patient assessment instrument and/or measurable assessment of functional outcome. Typically, 15 minutes are spent face-to-face with the patient and/or family.	See code before 97010.
97170	Athletic training evaluation, moderate complexity, requiring these components: A medical history and physical activity profile with 1-2 comorbidities that affect physical activity; An examination of affected body area and other symptomatic or related systems addressing a total of 3 or more elements from any of the following: body structures, physical activity, and/or participation deficiencies; and Clinical decision making of moderate complexity using standardized patient assessment instrument and/or measurable assessment of functional outcome. Typically, 30 minutes are spent face-to-face with the patient and/or family.	See code before 97010.
97171	Athletic training evaluation, high complexity, requiring these components: A medical history and physical activity profile, with 3 or more comorbidities that affect physical activity; A comprehensive examination of body systems using standardized tests and measures addressing a total of 4 or more elements from any of the following: body structures, physical activity, and/or participation deficiencies; Clinical presentation with unstable and unpredictable characteristics; and Clinical decision making of high complexity using standardized patient assessment instrument and/or measurable assessment of functional outcome. Typically, 45 minutes are spent face-to-face with the patient and/or family.	See code before 97010.
97172	Re-evaluation of athletic training established plan of care requiring these components: An assessment of patient's current functional status when there is a documented change; and A revised plan of care using a standardized patient assessment instrument and/or measurable assessment of functional outcome with an update in management options, goals, and interventions. Typically, 20 minutes are spent face-to-face with the patient and/or family.	See code before 97010.
99177	Instrument-based ocular screening (eg, photoscreening, automated-refraction), bilateral; with on-site analysis	See code following 99174.

Code	Description	Reference
99224	Subsequent observation care, per day, for the evaluation and management of a patient, which requires at least 2 of these 3 key components: Problem focused interval history; Problem focused examination; Medical decision making that is straightforward or of low complexity. Counseling and/or coordination of care with other physicians, other qualified health care professionals, or agencies are provided consistent with the nature of the problem(s) and the patient's and/or family's needs. Usually, the patient is stable, recovering, or improving. Typically, 15 minutes are spent at the bedside and on the patient's hospital floor or unit.	See code following 99220.
99225	Subsequent observation care, per day, for the evaluation and management of a patient, which requires at least 2 of these 3 key components: An expanded problem focused interval history; An expanded problem focused examination; Medical decision making of moderate complexity. Counseling and/or coordination of care with other physicians, other qualified health care professionals, or agencies are provided consistent with the nature of the problem(s) and the patient's and/or family's needs. Usually, the patient is responding inadequately to therapy or has developed a minor complication. Typically, 25 minutes are spent at the bedside and on the patient's hospital floor or unit.	See code following 99220.
99226	Subsequent observation care, per day, for the evaluation and management of a patient, which requires at least 2 of these 3 key components: A detailed interval history; A detailed examination; Medical decision making of high complexity. Counseling and/or coordination of care with other physicians, other qualified health care professionals, or agencies are provided consistent with the nature of the problem(s) and the patient's and/or family's needs. Usually, the patient is unstable or has developed a significant complication or a significant new problem. Typically, 35 minutes are spent at the bedside and on the patient's hospital floor or unit.	See code before 99221.
99415	Prolonged clinical staff service (the service beyond the typical service time) during an evaluation and management service in the office or outpatient setting, direct patient contact with physician supervision; first hour (List separately in addition to code for outpatient Evaluation and Management service)	See code following 99359.
99416	Prolonged clinical staff service (the service beyond the typical service time) during an evaluation and management service in the office or outpatient setting, direct patient contact with physician supervision; each additional 30 minutes (List separately in addition to code for prolonged service)	See code following 99359.
99485	Supervision by a control physician of interfacility transport care of the critically ill or critically injured pediatric patient, 24 months of age or younger, includes two-way communication with transport team before transport, at the referring facility and during the transport, including data interpretation and report; first 30 minutes	See code following 99467.
99486	Supervision by a control physician of interfacility transport care of the critically ill or critically injured pediatric patient, 24 months of age or younger, includes two-way communication with transport team before transport, at the referring facility and during the transport, including data interpretation and report; each additional 30 minutes (List separately in addition to code for primary procedure)	See code following 99467.
99490	Chronic care management services, at least 20 minutes of clinical staff time directed by a physician or other qualified health care professional, per calendar month, with the following required elements: multiple (two or more) chronic conditions expected to last at least 12 months, or until the death of the patient; chronic conditions place the patient at significant risk of death, acute exacerbation/decompensation, or functional decline; comprehensive care plan established, implemented, revised, or monitored.	See code before 99487.
0253T	Insertion of anterior segment aqueous drainage device, without extraocular reservoir, internal approach, into the suprachoroidal space	See code following 0191T.
0357T	Cryopreservation; immature oocyte(s)	See code following 0058T.
0376T	Insertion of anterior segment aqueous drainage device, without extraocular reservoir, internal approach, into the trabecular meshwork; each additional device insertion (List separately in addition to code for primary procedure)	See code following 0191T.

Appendix F — Add-on Codes, Modifier 51 Exempt, Optum Modifier 51 Exempt, Modifier 63 Exempt, and Modifier 95 Telemedicine Services

Codes specified as add-on, exempt from modifier 51 and 63, and modifier 95 (telemedicine services) are listed. The lists are designed to be read left to right rather than vertically.

99116	99135	99140	99153	99157	99292	99354
99355	99356	99357	99359	99415	99416	99467
99486	99489	99498	99602	99607		

Add-on Codes

0054T	0055T	0076T	0095T	0098T	0159T	0163T
0164T	0165T	0174T	0189T	0190T	01953	01968
01969	0196T	0205T	0214T	0215T	0217T	0218T
0222T	0229T	0231T	0290T	0294T	0300T	0309T
0346T	0361T	0363T	0365T	0367T	0369T	0374T
0376T	0396T	0397T	0399T	0437T	0439T	0443T
0450T	0466T	10036	11001	11008	11045	11046
11047	11101	11201	11732	11922	13102	13122
13133	13153	14302	15003	15005	15101	15111
15116	15121	15131	15136	15151	15152	15156
15157	15201	15221	15241	15261	15272	15274
15276	15278	15777	15787	15847	16036	17003
17312	17314	17315	19001	19082	19084	19086
19126	19282	19284	19286	19288	19297	20930
20931	20936	20937	20938	20985	22103	22116
22208	22216	22226	22328	22512	22515	22527
22534	22552	22585	22614	22632	22634	22840
22841	22842	22843	22844	22845	22846	22847
22848	22853	22854	22858	22859	22868	22870
26125	26861	26863	27358	27692	29826	31627
31632	31633	31637	31649	31651	31654	32501
32506	32507	32667	32668	32674	33141	33225
33257	33258	33259	33367	33368	33369	33419
33508	33517	33518	33519	33521	33522	33523
33530	33572	33768	33884	33924	33987	34806
34808	34813	34826	35306	35390	35400	35500
35572	35600	35681	35682	35683	35685	35686
35697	35700	36218	36227	36228	36248	36474
36476	36479	36907	36908	36909	37185	37186
37222	37223	37232	37233	37234	37235	37237
37239	37247	37249	37252	37253	38102	38746
38747	38900	43273	43283	43338	43635	44015
44121	44128	44139	44203	44213	44701	44955
47001	47542	47543	47544	47550	48400	49326
49327	49412	49435	49568	49905	50606	50705
50706	51797	52442	56606	57267	58110	58611
59525	60512	61316	61517	61610	61611	61612
61641	61642	61651	61781	61782	61783	61797
61799	61800	61864	61868	62148	62160	63035
63043	63044	63048	63057	63066	63076	63078
63082	63086	63088	63091	63103	63295	63308
63621	64462	64480	64484	64491	64492	64494
64495	64634	64636	64643	64645	64727	64778
64783	64787	64832	64837	64859	64872	64874
64876	64901	64902	65757	66990	67225	67320
67331	67332	67334	67335	67340	69990	74301
74713	75565	75774	76125	76802	76810	76812
76814	76937	77001	77002	77003	77063	77293
78020	78496	78730	81266	81416	81426	81536
82952	86826	87187	87503	87904	88155	88177
88185	88311	88314	88332	88334	88341	88350
88364	88369	88373	88388	90461	90472	90474
90785	90833	90836	90838	90840	90863	91013
92547	92608	92618	92621	92627	92921	92925
92929	92934	92938	92944	92973	92974	92978
92979	92998	93320	93321	93325	93352	93462
93463	93464	93563	93564	93565	93566	93567
93568	93571	93572	93592	93609	93613	93621
93622	93623	93655	93657	93662	94645	94729
94781	95079	95873	95874	95885	95886	95887
95940	95941	95962	95967	95975	95979	96361
96366	96367	96368	96370	96371	96375	96376
96411	96415	96417	96423	96570	96571	96934
96935	96936	97546	97598	97811	97814	99100

AMA Modifer 51 Exempt Codes

17004	20697	20974	20975	31500	36620	44500
61107	93451	93456	93503	93600	93602	93603
93610	93612	93615	93616	93618	93631	94610
95905	95992	99151	99152			

Modifier 63 Exempt Codes

30540	30545	31520	33470	33502	33503	33505
33506	33610	33611	33619	33647	33670	33690
33694	33730	33732	33735	33736	33750	33755
33762	33778	33786	33922	33946	33947	33948
33949	36415	36420	36450	36460	36510	36660
39503	43313	43314	43520	43831	44055	44126
44127	44128	46070	46705	46715	46716	46730
46735	46740	46742	46744	47700	47701	49215
49491	49492	49495	49496	49600	49605	49606
49610	49611	53025	54000	54150	54160	63700
63702	63704	63706	65820			

Optum Modifier 51 Exempt Codes

90281	90283	90284	90287	90288	90291	90296
90371	90375	90376	90378	90384	90385	90386
90389	90393	90396	90399	90476	90477	90581
90585	90586	90620	90621	90625	90630	90632
90633	90634	90636	90644	90647	90648	90649
90650	90651	90653	90654	90655	90656	90657
90658	90660	90661	90662	90664	90666	90667
90668	90670	90672	90673	90674	90675	90676
90680	90681	90685	90686	90687	90688	90690
90691	90696	90697	90698	90700	90702	90707
90710	90713	90714	90715	90716	90717	90723
90732	90733	90734	90736	90738	90739	90740
90743	90744	90746	90747	90748	90749	90750
97010	97012	97014	97016	97018	97022	97024
97026	97028	97032	97033	97034	97035	97036
97110	97112	97113	97116	97124	97140	97150
97530	97532	97533	97535	97537	97542	97545
97546	97597	97598	97602	97605	97606	97607
97608	97610	97750	97755	97760	97761	97762
99050	99051	99053	99056	99058	99060	

Telemedicine Services Codes

The codes on the following list may be used to report telemedicine services when modifier 95 Synchronous Telemedicine Service Rendered via a Real-Time Interactive Audio and Visual Telecommunications System, is appended.

0188T	0189T	90791	90792	90832	90833	90834
90836	90837	90838	90845	90846	90847	90863
90951	90952	90954	90955	90957	90958	90960
90961	92227	92228	93228	93229	93268	93270
93271	93272	93298	93299	96040	96116	96150
96151	96152	96153	96154	97802	97803	97804
98960	98961	98962	99201	99202	99203	99204
99205	99212	99213	99214	99215	99231	99232
99233	*99241	*99242	*99243	*99244	*99245	*99251
*99252	*99253	*99254	*99255	99307	99308	99309
99310	99354	99355	99406	99407	99408	99409
99495	99496					

* Consultations are noncovered by Medicare

Appendix G — Medicare Internet-only Manuals (IOMs)

The Centers for Medicare and Medicaid Services restructured its paper-based manual system as a web-based system on October 1, 2003. Called the online CMS manual system, it combines all of the various program instructions into internet-only manuals (IOMs), which are used by all CMS programs and contractors. In many instances, the references from the online manuals in appendix G contain a mention of the old paper manuals from which the current information was obtained when the manuals were converted. This information is shown in the header of the text, in the following format, when applicable, as A3-3101, HO-210, and B3-2049. Complete versions of all of the manuals can be found at https://www.cms.gov/Regulations-and-Guidance/Guidance/Manuals/Internet-Only-Manuals-IOMs.html.

Effective with implementation of the IOMs, the former method of publishing program memoranda (PMs) to communicate program instructions was replaced by the following four templates:

- One-time notification
- Manual revisions
- Business requirements
- Confidential requirements

The web-based system has been organized by functional area (e.g., eligibility, entitlement, claims processing, benefit policy, program integrity) in an effort to eliminate redundancy within the manuals, simplify updating, and make CMS program instructions available more quickly. The web-based system contains the functional areas included below:

Pub. 100	Introduction
Pub. 100-01	Medicare General Information, Eligibility, and Entitlement Manual
Pub. 100-02	Medicare Benefit Policy Manual
Pub. 100-03	Medicare National Coverage Determinations (NCD) Manual
Pub. 100-04	Medicare Claims Processing Manual
Pub. 100-05	Medicare Secondary Payer Manual
Pub. 100-06	Medicare Financial Management Manual
Pub. 100-07	State Operations Manual
Pub. 100-08	Medicare Program Integrity Manual
Pub. 100-09	Medicare Contractor Beneficiary and Provider Communications Manual
Pub. 100-10	Quality Improvement Organization Manual
Pub. 100-11	Programs of All-Inclusive Care for the Elderly (PACE) Manual
Pub. 100-12	State Medicaid Manual (under development)
Pub. 100-13	Medicaid State Children's Health Insurance Program (under development)
Pub. 100-14	Medicare ESRD Network Organizations Manual
Pub. 100-15	Medicaid Integrity Program (MIP)
Pub. 100-16	Medicare Managed Care Manual
Pub. 100-17	CMS/Business Partners Systems Security Manual
Pub. 100-18	Medicare Prescription Drug Benefit Manual
Pub. 100-19	Demonstrations
Pub. 100-20	One-Time Notification
Pub. 100-21	Recurring Update Notification
Pub. 100-22	Medicare Quality Reporting Incentive Programs Manual
Pub. 100-24	State Buy-In Manual
Pub. 100-25	Information Security Acceptable Risk Safeguards Manual

A brief description of the Medicare manuals primarily used for *CPC Expert* follows:

The *National Coverage Determinations Manual* (NCD), is organized according to categories such as diagnostic services, supplies, and medical procedures. The table of contents lists each category and subject within that category. Revision transmittals identify any new or background material, recap the changes, and provide an effective date for the change.

When complete, the manual will contain two chapters. Chapter 1 currently includes a description of CMS's national coverage determinations. When available, chapter 2 will contain a list of HCPCS codes related to each coverage determination. The manual is organized in accordance with CPT category sequences.

The *Medicare Benefit Policy Manual* contains Medicare general coverage instructions that are not national coverage determinations. As a general rule, in the past these instructions have been found in chapter II of the *Medicare Carriers Manual,* the *Medicare Intermediary Manual*, other provider manuals, and program memoranda.

The *Medicare Claims Processing Manual* contains instructions for processing claims for contractors and providers.

The *Medicare Program Integrity Manual* communicates the priorities and standards for the Medicare integrity programs.

Medicare IOM references

100-01, 3, 20.5

Blood Deductibles (Part A and Part B)

Program payment may not be made for the first 3 pints of whole blood or equivalent units of packed red cells received under Part A and Part B combined in a calendar year. However, blood processing (e.g., administration, storage) is not subject to the deductible.

The blood deductibles are in addition to any other applicable deductible and coinsurance amounts for which the patient is responsible.

The deductible applies only to the first 3 pints of blood furnished in a calendar year, even if more than one provider furnished blood.

100-01, 5, 70.6

Chiropractors

A. General

A licensed chiropractor who meets uniform minimum standards (see subsection C) is a physician for specified services. Coverage extends only to treatment by means of manual manipulation of the spine to correct a subluxation demonstrated by X-ray, provided such treatment is legal in the State where performed. All other services furnished or ordered by chiropractors are not covered. An X-ray obtained by a chiropractor for his or her own diagnostic purposes before commencing treatment may suffice for claims documentation purposes. This means that if a chiropractor orders, takes, or interprets an X-ray to demonstrate a subluxation of the spine, the X-ray can be used for claims processing purposes. However, there is no coverage or payment for these services or for any other diagnostic or therapeutic service ordered or furnished by the chiropractor. In addition, in performing manual manipulation of the spine, some chiropractors use manual devices that are hand-held with the thrust of the force of the device being controlled manually. While such manual manipulation may be covered, there is no separate payment permitted for use of this device.

B. Licensure and Authorization to Practice

A chiropractor must be licensed or legally authorized to furnish chiropractic services by the State or jurisdiction in which the services are furnished.

C. Uniform Minimum Standards

I. Prior to July 1, 1974, Chiropractors licensed or authorized to practice prior to July 1, 1974, and those individuals who commenced their studies in a chiropractic college before that date must meet all of the following minimum standards to render payable services under the program:

   a. Preliminary education equal to the requirements for graduation from an accredited high school or other secondary school;

   b. Graduation from a college of chiropractic approved by the State's chiropractic examiners that included the completion of a course of study covering a period of not less than 3 school years of 6 months each year in actual continuous attendance covering adequate course of study in the subjects of anatomy, physiology, symptomatology and diagnosis, hygiene and sanitation, chemistry, histology, pathology, and principles and practice of chiropractic, including clinical instruction in vertebral palpation, nerve tracing and adjusting; and

c. Passage of an examination prescribed by the State's chiropractic examiners covering the subjects listed in subsection b.

2. After June 30, 1974 - Individuals commencing their studies in a chiropractic college after June 30, 1974, must meet all of the following additional requirements:

a. Satisfactory completion of 2 years of pre-chiropractic study at the college level;

b. Satisfactory completion of a 4-year course of 8 months each year (instead of a 3-year course of 6 months each year) at a college or school of chiropractic that includes not less than 4,000 hours in the scientific and chiropractic courses specified in subsection1.b, plus courses in the use and effect of X-ray and chiropractic analysis; and

c. The practitioner must be over 21 years of age.

100-02, 1, 90
Termination of Pregnancy
B3-4276.1,.2

Effective for services furnished on or after October 1, 1998, Medicare will cover abortions procedures in the following situations:

1. If the pregnancy is the result of an act or rape or incest; or

2. In the case where a woman suffers from a physical disorder, physical injury, or physical illness, including a life-endangering physical condition caused by the pregnancy itself that would, as certified by a physician, place the woman in danger of death unless an abortion is performed.

NOTE: The "G7" modifier must be used with the following CPT codes in order for these services to be covered when the pregnancy resulted from rape or incest, or the pregnancy is certified by a physician as life threatening to the mother:

59840, 59841, 59850, 59851, 59852, 59855, 59856, 59857, 59866

100-02, 1, 100
Treatment for Infertility
A3-3101.13

Effective for services rendered on or after January 15, 1980, reasonable and necessary services associated with treatment for infertility are covered under Medicare. Like pregnancy (see Sec. 80 above), infertility is a condition sufficiently at variance with the usual state of health to make it appropriate for a person who normally would be expected to be fertile to seek medical consultation and treatment. Contractors should coordinate with QIOs to see that utilization guidelines are established for this treatment if inappropriate utilization or abuse is suspected.

100-02, 11, 20
Renal Dialysis Items and Services

Medicare provides payment under the ESRD PPS for all renal dialysis services for outpatient maintenance dialysis when they are furnished to Medicare ESRD patients for the treatment of ESRD by a Medicare certified ESRD facility or a special purpose dialysis facility. Renal dialysis services are the items and services included under the composite rate and the ESRD-related items and services that were separately paid as of December 31, 2010 that were used for the treatment of ESRD.

Renal dialysis services are furnished in various settings including hospital outpatient ESRD facilities, independent ESRD facilities, or in the patient's home. Renal dialysis items and services furnished at ESRD facilities differ according to the types of patients being treated, the types of equipment and supplies used, the preferences of the treating physician, and the capability and makeup of the staff. Although not all facilities provide an identical range of services, the most common elements of dialysis treatment include:

- Laboratory Tests;
- Drugs and Biologicals;
- Equipment and supplies - dialysis machine use and maintenance;
- Personnel services;
- Administrative services;
- Overhead costs;
- Monitoring access and related declotting or referring the patient, and
- Direct nursing services include registered nurses, licensed practical nurses, technicians, social workers, and dietitians.

100-02, 11, 20.2
Laboratory Services

All laboratory services furnished to individuals for the treatment of ESRD are included in the ESRD PPS as Part B services and are not paid separately as of January 1, 2011. The laboratory services include but are not limited to:

- Laboratory tests included under the composite rate as of December 31, 2010 (discussed below); and
- Former separately billable Part B laboratory tests that were billed by ESRD facilities and independent laboratories for ESRD patients.

Composite rate laboratory tests are listed in §20.2.E of this chapter. More information regarding composite rate laboratory tests can be found in Pub. 100-4, Medicare Claims Processing Manual, chapter 8, §50.1, §60.1, and §80. As discussed below, composite rate laboratory services should not be reported on claims.

The distinction of what is considered to be a renal dialysis laboratory test is a clinical decision determined by the ESRD patient's ordering practitioner. If a laboratory test is ordered for the treatment of ESRD, then the laboratory test is not paid separately.

Payment for all renal dialysis laboratory tests furnished under the ESRD PPS is made directly to the ESRD facility responsible for the patient's care. The ESRD facility must furnish the laboratory tests directly or under arrangement and report renal dialysis laboratory tests on the ESRD facility claim (with the exception of composite rate laboratory services).

An ESRD facility must report renal dialysis laboratory services on its claims in order for the laboratory tests to be included in the outlier payment calculation. Renal dialysis laboratory services that were or would have been paid separately under Medicare Part B prior to January 1, 2011, are priced for the outlier payment calculation using the Clinical Laboratory Fee Schedule. Further information regarding the outlier policy can be found in §60.D of this chapter.

Certain laboratory services will be subject to Part B consolidated billing requirements and will no longer be separately payable when provided to ESRD beneficiaries by providers other than the renal dialysis facility. The list below includes the renal dialysis laboratory tests that are routinely performed for the treatment of ESRD. Payment for the laboratory tests identified on this list is included in the ESRD PPS. The laboratory tests listed in the table are used to enforce consolidated billing edits to ensure that payment is not made for renal dialysis laboratory tests outside of the ESRD PPS. The list of renal dialysis laboratory tests is not an all-inclusive list. If any laboratory test is ordered for the treatment of ESRD, then the laboratory test is considered to be included in the ESRD PPS and is the responsibility of the ESRD facility. Additional renal dialysis laboratory tests may be added through administrative issuances in the future.

LABS SUBJECT TO ESRD CONSOLIDATED BILLING

CPT/ HCPCS	Short Description
80047	Basic Metabolic Panel (Calcium, ionized)
80048	Basic Metabolic Panel (Calcium, total)
80051	Electrolyte Panel
80053	Comprehensive Metabolic Panel
80061	Lipid Panel
80069	Renal Function Panel
80076	Hepatic Function Panel
82040	Assay of serum albumin
82108	Assay of aluminum
82306	Vitamin d, 25 hydroxy
82310	Assay of calcium
82330	Assay of calcium, Ionized
82374	Assay, blood carbon dioxide
82379	Assay of carnitine
82435	Assay of blood chloride
82565	Assay of creatinine
82570	Assay of urine creatinine
82575	Creatinine clearance test
82607	Vitamin B-12
82652	Vit d 1, 25-dihydroxy
82668	Assay of erythropoietin
82728	Assay of ferritin
82746	Blood folic acid serum
83540	Assay of iron
83550	Iron binding test
83735	Assay of magnesium
83970	Assay of parathormone
84075	Assay alkaline phosphatase
84100	Assay of phosphorus
84132	Assay of serum potassium
84134	Assay of prealbumin

CPT/ HCPCS	Short Description
84155	Assay of protein, serum
84157	Assay of protein by other source
84295	Assay of serum sodium
84466	Assay of transferrin
84520	Assay of urea nitrogen
84540	Assay of urine/urea-n
84545	Urea-N clearance test
85014	Hematocrit
85018	Hemoglobin
85025	Complete (cbc), automated (HgB, Hct, RBC, WBC, and Platelet count) and automated differential WBC count.
85027	Complete (cbc), automated (HgB, Hct, RBC, WBC, and Platelet count)
85041	Automated rbc count
85044	Manual reticulocyte count
85045	Automated reticulocyte count
85046	Reticyte/hgb concentrate
85048	Automated leukocyte count
86704	Hep b core antibody, total
86705	Hep b core antibody, igm
86706	Hep b surface antibody
87040	Blood culture for bacteria
87070	Culture, bacteria, other
87071	Culture bacteri aerobic othr
87073	Culture bacteria anaerobic
87075	Cultr bacteria, except blood
87076	Culture anaerobe ident, each
87077	Culture aerobic identify
87081	Culture screen only
87340	Hepatitis b surface ag, eia
G0306	CBC/diff wbc w/o platelet
G0307	CBC without platelet

A. Automated Multi-Channel Chemistry (AMCC) Tests

During the ESRD PPS transition period (see §70 of this chapter) ESRD facilities are required to report the renal dialysis AMCC tests with the appropriate modifiers (CD, CE, or CF) on their claims for purposes of applying the 50/50 rule under the composite rate portion of the blended payment. Refer to §70.B of this chapter for additional information regarding the composite rate portion of the blended payment during the transition.

The 50/50 rule is necessary for those ESRD facilities that chose to go through the transition period. If the 50/50 rule allows for separate payment, then the laboratory tests are priced using the clinical laboratory fee schedule. Information regarding the 50/50 rule can be found in §20.2.E of this chapter and in Pub. 100-4, Medicare Claims Processing Manual, chapter 16, §40.6.

NOTE: An ESRD facility billing a renal dialysis AMCC test must use the CF modifier when the AMCC is not in the composite rate but is a renal dialysis service. AMCC tests that are furnished to individuals for reasons other than for the treatment of ESRD should be billed with the AY modifier to Medicare directly by the entity furnishing the service with the AY modifier.

B. Laboratory Services Furnished for Reasons Other Than for the Treatment of ESRD

1. Independent Laboratory

A patient's physician or practitioner may order a laboratory test that is included on the list of items and services subject to consolidated billing edits for reasons other than for the treatment of ESRD. When this occurs, the patient's physician or practitioner should notify the independent laboratory or the ESRD facility (with the appropriate clinical laboratory certification in accordance with the Clinical Laboratory Improvement Act) that furnished the laboratory service that the test is not a renal dialysis service and that entity may bill Medicare separately using the AY modifier. The AY modifier serves as an attestation that the item or service is medically necessary for the patient but is not being used for the treatment of ESRD.

2. Hospital-Based Laboratory

Hospital outpatient clinical laboratories furnishing renal dialysis laboratory tests to ESRD patients for reasons other than for the treatment of ESRD may submit a claim for separate payment using the AY modifier. The AY modifier serves as an attestation that the item or service is medically necessary for the patient but is not being used for the treatment of ESRD.

C. Laboratory Services Performed in Emergency Rooms or Emergency Departments

In an emergency room or emergency department, the ordering physician or practitioner may not know at the time the laboratory test is being ordered, if it is being ordered as a renal dialysis service. Consequently, emergency rooms or emergency departments are not required to append an AY modifier to these laboratory tests when submitting claims with dates of service on or after January 1, 2012.

When a renal dialysis laboratory service is furnished to an ESRD patient in an emergency room or emergency department on a different date of service, hospitals can append an ET modifier to the laboratory tests furnished to ESRD patients to indicate that the laboratory test was furnished in conjunction with the emergency visit. Appending the ET modifier indicates that the laboratory service being furnished on a day other than the emergency visit is related to the emergency visit and at the time the ordering physician was unable to determine if the test was ordered for reasons of treating the patient's ESRD.

Allowing laboratory testing to bypass consolidated billing edits in the emergency room or department does not mean that ESRD facilities should send patients to other settings for routine laboratory testing for the purpose of not assuming financial responsibility of renal dialysis items and services. For additional information regarding laboratory services furnished in a variety of settings, see Pub. 100-4, Medicare Claims Processing Manual, chapter 16, §30.3 and §40.6.

D. Hepatitis B Laboratory Services for Transient Patients

Laboratory testing for hepatitis B is a renal dialysis service. Effective January 1, 2011, hepatitis B testing is included in the ESRD PPS and therefore cannot be billed separately to Medicare.

The Conditions for Coverage for ESRD facilities require routine hepatitis B testing (42 CFR §494.30(a)(1)). The ESRD facility is responsible for the payment of the laboratory test, regardless of frequency. If an ESRD patient wishes to travel, the patient's home ESRD facility should have systems in place for communicating hepatitis B test results to the destination ESRD facility.

E. Laboratory Services Included Under Composite Rate

Prior to the implementation of the ESRD PPS, the costs of certain ESRD laboratory services furnished for outpatient maintenance dialysis by either the ESRD facility's staff or an independent laboratory, were included in the composite rate calculations. Therefore, payment for all of these laboratory tests was included in the ESRD facility's composite rate and the tests could not have been billed separately to the Medicare program.

All laboratory services that were included under the composite rate are included under the ESRD PPS unless otherwise specified. Payments for these laboratory tests are included in the ESRD PPS and are not paid separately under the composite rate portion of the blended payment and are not eligible for outlier payments. Therefore, composite rate laboratory services should not be reported on the claim. Laboratory tests included in the composite payment rate are identified below.

1. Routinely Covered Tests Paid Under Composite Rate

The tests listed below are usually performed for dialysis patients and were routinely covered at the frequency specified in the absence of indications to the contrary, (i.e., no documentation of medical necessity was required other than knowledge of the patient's status as an ESRD beneficiary). When any of these tests were performed at a frequency greater than that specified, the additional tests were separately billable and were covered only if they were medically justified by accompanying documentation. A diagnosis of ESRD alone was not sufficient medical evidence to warrant coverage of the additional tests. The nature of the illness or injury (diagnosis, complaint, or symptom) requiring the performance of the test(s) must have been present, along with ICD diagnosis coding, on the claim for payment.

a. Hemodialysis, IPD, CCPD, and Hemofiltration

  – Per Treatment - All hematocrit, hemoglobin, and clotting time tests furnished incident to dialysis treatments;

  – Weekly - Prothrombin time for patients on anticoagulant therapy and Serum Creatinine;

  – Weekly or Thirteen Per Quarter - BUN;

  – Monthly - Serum Calcium, Serum Potassium, Serum Chloride, CBC, Serum Bicarbonate, Serum Phosphorous, Total Protein, Serum Albumin, Alkaline Phosphatase, aspartate amino transferase (AST) (SGOT) and LDH; and

  – Automated Multi-Channel Chemistry (AMCC) - If an automated battery of tests, such as the SMA-12, is performed and contains most of the tests listed in one of the weekly or monthly categories, it is not necessary to separately identify any tests in the battery that are not listed. Further information concerning automated tests and the "50 percent rule" can be found below and in Pub. 100-4, Medicare Claims Processing Manual, chapter 16, §40.6.1.

b. CAPD

  – Monthly – BUN, Creatinine, Sodium, Potassium, CO2, Calcium, Magnesium, Phosphate, Total Protein, Albumin, Alkaline Phosphatase, LDH, AST, SGOT, HCT, Hbg, and Dialysate Protein.

Under the ESRD PPS, frequency requirements do not apply for the purpose of payment. However, laboratory tests should be ordered as necessary and should not be restricted because of financial reasons.

2. Separately Billable Tests Under the Composite Rate

The following list identifies certain separately billable laboratory tests that were covered routinely and without documentation of medical necessity other than knowledge of the patient's status as an ESRD beneficiary, when furnished at specified frequencies. If they were performed at a frequency greater than that specified, they were covered only if accompanied by medical documentation. A diagnosis of ESRD alone was not sufficient documentation. The medical necessity of the test(s), the nature of the illness or injury (diagnosis, complaint or symptom) requiring the performance of the test(s) must have been furnished on claims using the ICD diagnosis coding system.

— Separately Billable Tests for Hemodialysis, IPD, CCPD, and Hemofiltration

Serum Aluminum - one every 3 months

Serum Ferritin - one every 3 months

— Separately Billable Tests for CAPD

WBC, RBC, and Platelet count – One every 3 months

Residual renal function and 24 hour urine volume – One every 6 months

Under the ESRD PPS frequency requirements do not apply for the purpose of payment. However, laboratory tests should be ordered as necessary and should not be restricted because of financial reasons.

3. **Automated Multi-Channel Chemistry (AMCC) Tests Under the Composite Rate**

Clinical diagnostic laboratory tests that comprise the AMCC (listed in Appendix A and B) could be considered to be composite rate and non-composite rate laboratory services. Composite rate payment was paid by the A/B MAC (A). To determine if separate payment was allowed for non-composite rate tests for a particular date of service, 50 percent or more of the covered tests must be non-composite rate tests. This policy also applies to the composite rate portion of the blended payment during the transition. Beginning January 1, 2014, the 50 percent rule will no longer apply and no separate payment will be made under the composite rate portion of the blended payment.

Medicare applied the following to AMCC tests for ESRD beneficiaries:

— Payment was the lowest rate for services performed by the same provider, for the same beneficiary, for the same date of service.

— The A/B MAC identified, for a particular date of service, the AMCC tests ordered that were included in the composite rate and those that were not included. The composite rate tests were defined for Hemodialysis, IPD, CCPD, and Hemofiltration (see Appendix A) and for CAPD (see Appendix B).

— If 50 percent or more of the covered tests were included under the composite rate payment, then all submitted tests were included within the composite payment. In this case, no separate payment in addition to the composite rate was made for any of the separately billable tests.

— If less than 50 percent of the covered tests were composite rate tests, all AMCC tests submitted for that Date of Service (DOS) were separately payable.

— A non-composite rate test was defined as any test separately payable outside of the composite rate or beyond the normal frequency covered under the composite rate that was reasonable and necessary.

Three pricing modifiers identify the different payment situations for ESRD AMCC tests. The physician who ordered the tests was responsible for identifying the appropriate modifier when ordering the tests.

— CD - AMCC test had been ordered by an ESRD facility or Medicare capitation payment (MCP) physician that was part of the composite rate and was not separately billable

— CE - AMCC test had been ordered by an ESRD facility or MCP physician that was a composite rate test but was beyond the normal frequency covered under the rate and was separately reimbursable based on medical necessity

— CF - AMCC test had been ordered by an ESRD facility or MCP physician that was not part of the composite rate and was separately billable

The ESRD clinical diagnostic laboratory tests identified with modifiers "CD", "CE" or "CF" may not have been billed as organ or disease panels. Effective October 1, 2003, all ESRD clinical diagnostic laboratory tests must be billed individually. See Pub. 100-4, Medicare Claims Processing Manual, chapter 16, §40.6.1, for additional billing and payment instructions as well as examples of the 50/50 rule.

For ESRD dialysis patients, CPT code 82330 Calcium; ionized shall be included in the calculation for the 50/50 rule (Pub. 100-4, Medicare Claims Processing Manual, chapter 16, §40.6.1). When CPT code 82330 is billed as a substitute for CPT code 82310, Calcium; total, it shall be billed with modifier CD or CE. When CPT code 82330 is billed in addition to CPT 82310, it shall be billed with CF modifier.

100-02, 15, 20.1

Physician Expense for Surgery, Childbirth, and Treatment for Infertility

B3-2005.I

A. Surgery and Childbirth

Skilled medical management is covered throughout the events of pregnancy, beginning with diagnosis, continuing through delivery and ending after the necessary postnatal care. Similarly, in the event of termination of pregnancy, regardless of whether terminated spontaneously or for therapeutic reasons (i.e., where the life of the mother would be endangered if the fetus were brought to term), the need for skilled medical management and/or medical services is equally important as in those cases carried to full term. After the infant is delivered and is a

separate individual, items and services furnished to the infant are not covered on the basis of the mother's eligibility.

Most surgeons and obstetricians bill patients an all-inclusive package charge intended to cover all services associated with the surgical procedure or delivery of the child. All expenses for surgical and obstetrical care, including preoperative/prenatal examinations and tests and post-operative/postnatal services, are considered incurred on the date of surgery or delivery, as appropriate. This policy applies whether the physician bills on a package charge basis, or itemizes the bill separately for these items.

Occasionally, a physician's bill may include charges for additional services not directly related to the surgical procedure or the delivery. Such charges are considered incurred on the date the additional services are furnished.

The above policy applies only where the charges are imposed by one physician or by a clinic on behalf of a group of physicians. Where more than one physician imposes charges for surgical or obstetrical services, all preoperative/prenatal and post-operative/postnatal services performed by the physician who performed the surgery or delivery are considered incurred on the date of the surgery or delivery. Expenses for services rendered by other physicians are considered incurred on the date they were performed.

B. Treatment for Infertility

Reasonable and necessary services associated with treatment for infertility are covered under Medicare. Infertility is a condition sufficiently at variance with the usual state of health to make it appropriate for a person who normally is expected to be fertile to seek medical consultation and treatment.

100-02, 15, 30.4

Optometrist's Services

B3-2020.25

Effective April 1, 1987, a doctor of optometry is considered a physician with respect to all services the optometrist is authorized to perform under State law or regulation. To be covered under Medicare, the services must be medically reasonable and necessary for the diagnosis or treatment of illness or injury, and must meet all applicable coverage requirements. See the Medicare Benefit Policy Manual, Chapter 16, "General Exclusions from Coverage," for exclusions from coverage that apply to vision care services, and the Medicare Claims Processing Manual, Chapter 12, "Physician/Practitioner Billing," for information dealing with payment for items and services furnished by optometrists.

A. FDA Monitored Studies of Intraocular Lenses

Special coverage rules apply to situations in which an ophthalmologist is involved in a Food and Drug Administration (FDA) monitored study of the safety and efficacy of an investigational Intraocular Lens (IOL). The investigation process for IOLs is unique in that there is a core period and an adjunct period. The core study is a traditional, well-controlled clinical investigation with full record keeping and reporting requirements. The adjunct study is essentially an extended distribution phase for lenses in which only limited safety data are compiled. Depending on the lens being evaluated, the adjunct study may be an extension of the core study or may be the only type of investigation to which the lens may be subject.

All eye care services related to the investigation of the IOL must be provided by the investigator (i.e., the implanting ophthalmologist) or another practitioner (including a doctor of optometry) who provides services at the direction or under the supervision of the investigator and who has an agreement with the investigator that information on the patient is given to the investigator so that he or she may report on the patient to the IOL manufacturer. Eye care services furnished by anyone other than the investigator (or a practitioner who assists the investigator, as described in the preceding paragraph) are not covered during the period the IOL is being investigated, unless the services are not related to the investigation.

B. Concurrent Care

Where more than one practitioner furnishes concurrent care, services furnished to a beneficiary by both an ophthalmologist and another physician (including an optometrist) may be recognized for payment if it is determined that each practitioner's services were reasonable and necessary. (See Sec.30.E.)

100-02, 15, 30.5

Chiropractor's Services

B3-2020.26

A chiropractor must be licensed or legally authorized to furnish chiropractic services by the State or jurisdiction in which the services are furnished. In addition, a licensed chiropractor must meet the following uniform minimum standards to be considered a physician for Medicare coverage. Coverage extends only to treatment by means of manual manipulation of the spine to correct a subluxation provided such treatment is legal in the State where performed. All other services furnished or ordered by chiropractors are not covered. If a chiropractor orders, takes, or interprets an x-ray or other diagnostic procedure to demonstrate a subluxation of the spine, the x-ray can be used for documentation. However, there is no coverage or payment for these services or for any other diagnostic or therapeutic service ordered or furnished by the chiropractor. For detailed information on using x-rays to determine subluxation, see Sec.240.1.2. In addition, in performing manual manipulation of the spine, some chiropractors use manual devices that are hand-held with the thrust of the force of the device being controlled manually. While such manual manipulation may be covered, there is no separate payment permitted for use of this device.

A. Uniform Minimum Standards

Prior to July 1, 1974

Chiropractors licensed or authorized to practice prior to July 1, 1974, and those individuals who commenced their studies in a chiropractic college before that date must meet all of the following three minimum standards to render payable services under the program:

- Preliminary education equal to the requirements for graduation from an accredited high school or other secondary school;

- Graduation from a college of chiropractic approved by the State's chiropractic examiners that included the completion of a course of study covering a period of not less than 3 school years of 6 months each year in actual continuous attendance covering adequate course of study in the subjects of anatomy, physiology, symptomatology and diagnosis, hygiene and sanitation, chemistry, histology, pathology, and principles and practice of chiropractic, including clinical instruction in vertebral palpation, nerve tracing, and adjusting; and

- Passage of an examination prescribed by the State's chiropractic examiners covering the subjects listed above.

After June 30, 1974

Individuals commencing their studies in a chiropractic college after June 30, 1974, must meet all of the above three standards and all of the following additional requirements:

- Satisfactory completion of 2 years of pre-chiropractic study at the college level;

- Satisfactory completion of a 4-year course of 8 months each year (instead of a 3-year course of 6 months each year) at a college or school of chiropractic that includes not less than 4,000 hours in the scientific and chiropractic courses specified in the second bullet under "Prior to July 1, 1974" above, plus courses in the use and effect of x-ray and chiropractic analysis; and

- The practitioner must be over 21 years of age.

B. Maintenance Therapy

Under the Medicare program, Chiropractic maintenance therapy is not considered to be medically reasonable or necessary, and is therefore not payable. Maintenance therapy is defined as a treatment plan that seeks to prevent disease, promote health, and prolong and enhance the quality of life; or therapy that is performed to maintain or prevent deterioration of a chronic condition. When further clinical improvement cannot reasonably be expected from continuous ongoing care, and the chiropractic treatment becomes supportive rather than corrective in nature, the treatment is then considered maintenance therapy. For information on how to indicate on a claim a treatment is or is not maintenance, see Sec.240.1.3.

100-02, 15, 50.4.4.2

Immunizations

Vaccinations or inoculations are excluded as immunizations unless they are directly related to the treatment of an injury or direct exposure to a disease or condition, such as anti-rabies treatment, tetanus antitoxin or booster vaccine, botulin antitoxin, antivenin sera, or immune globulin. In the absence of injury or direct exposure, preventive immunization (vaccination or inoculation) against such diseases as smallpox, polio, diphtheria, etc., is not covered. However, pneumococcal, hepatitis B, and influenza virus vaccines are exceptions to this rule. (See items A, B, and C below.) In cases where a vaccination or inoculation is excluded from coverage, related charges are also not covered.

A. Pneumococcal Pneumonia Vaccinations

1. Background and History of Coverage:

   Section 1861(s)(10)(A) of the Social Security Act and regulations at 42 CFR 410.57 authorize Medicare coverage under Part B for pneumococcal vaccine and its administration.

   For services furnished on or after May 1, 1981 through September 18, 2014, the Medicare Part B program covered pneumococcal pneumonia vaccine and its administration when furnished in compliance with any applicable State law by any provider of services or any entity or individual with a supplier number. Coverage included an initial vaccine administered only to persons at high risk of serious pneumococcal disease (including all people 65 and older; immunocompetent adults at increased risk of pneumococcal disease or its complications because of chronic illness; and individuals with compromised immune systems), with revaccination administered only to persons at highest risk of serious pneumococcal infection and those likely to have a rapid decline in pneumococcal antibody levels, provided that at least 5 years had passed since the previous dose of pneumococcal vaccine.

   Those administering the vaccine did not require the patient to present an immunization record prior to administering the pneumococcal vaccine, nor were they compelled to review the patient's complete medical record if it was not available, relying on the patient's verbal history to determine prior vaccination status.

   Effective July 1, 2000, Medicare no longer required for coverage purposes that a doctor of medicine or osteopathy order the vaccine. Therefore, a beneficiary could receive the vaccine upon request without a physician's order and without physician supervision.

2. Coverage Requirements:

   Effective for claims with dates of service on and after September 19, 2014, an initial pneumococcal vaccine may be administered to all Medicare beneficiaries who have never received a pneumococcal vaccination under Medicare Part B. A different, second pneumococcal vaccine may be administered 1 year after the first vaccine was administered (i.e., 11 full months have passed following the month in which the last pneumococcal vaccine was administered).

   Those administering the vaccine should not require the patient to present an immunization record prior to administering the pneumococcal vaccine, nor should they feel compelled to review the patient's complete medical record if it is not available. Instead, provided that the patient is competent, it is acceptable to rely on the patient's verbal history to determine prior vaccination status.

   Medicare does not require for coverage purposes that a doctor of medicine or osteopathy order the vaccine. Therefore, the beneficiary may receive the vaccine upon request without a physician's order and without physician supervision.

B. Hepatitis B Vaccine

Effective for services furnished on or after September 1, 1984, P.L. 98-369 provides coverage under Part B for hepatitis B vaccine and its administration, furnished to a Medicare beneficiary who is at high or intermediate risk of contracting hepatitis B. High-risk groups currently identified include (see exception below):

- ESRD patients;

- Hemophiliacs who receive Factor VIII or IX concentrates;

- Clients of institutions for the mentally retarded;

- Persons who live in the same household as a Hepatitis B Virus (HBV) carrier;

- Homosexual men;

- Illicit injectable drug abusers; and

- Persons diagnosed with diabetes mellitus.

Intermediate risk groups currently identified include:

- Staff in institutions for the mentally retarded; and

- Workers in health care professions who have frequent contact with blood or blood-derived body fluids during routine work.

EXCEPTION: Persons in both of the above-listed groups in paragraph B, would not be considered at high or intermediate risk of contracting hepatitis B, however, if there were laboratory evidence positive for antibodies to hepatitis B. (ESRD patients are routinely tested for hepatitis B antibodies as part of their continuing monitoring and therapy.)

For Medicare program purposes, the vaccine may be administered upon the order of a doctor of medicine or osteopathy, by a doctor of medicine or osteopathy, or by home health agencies, skilled nursing facilities, ESRD facilities, hospital outpatient departments, and persons recognized under the incident to physicians' services provision of law.

A charge separate from the ESRD composite rate will be recognized and paid for administration of the vaccine to ESRD patients.

C. Influenza Virus Vaccine

Effective for services furnished on or after May 1, 1993, the Medicare Part B program covers influenza virus vaccine and its administration when furnished in compliance with any applicable State law by any provider of services or any entity or individual with a supplier number. Typically, these vaccines are administered once a flu season. Medicare does not require, for coverage purposes, that a doctor of medicine or osteopathy order the vaccine. Therefore, the beneficiary may receive the vaccine upon request without a physician's order and without physician supervision.

100-02, 15, 80.1

Clinical Laboratory Services

Section 1833 and 1861 of the Act provides for payment of clinical laboratory services under Medicare Part B. Clinical laboratory services involve the biological, microbiological, serological, chemical, immunohematological, hematological, biophysical, cytological, pathological, or other examination of materials derived from the human body for the diagnosis, prevention, or treatment of a disease or assessment of a medical condition. Laboratory services must meet all applicable requirements of the Clinical Laboratory Improvement Amendments of 1988 (CLIA), as set forth at 42 CFR part 493. Section 1862(a)(1)(A) of the Act provides that Medicare payment may not be made for services that are not reasonable and necessary. Clinical laboratory services must be ordered and used promptly by the physician who is treating the beneficiary as described in 42 CFR 410.32(a), or by a qualified nonphysician practitioner, as described in 42 CFR 410.32(a)(3).

See section 80.6 of this manual for related physician ordering instructions.

See the Medicare Claims Processing Manual Chapter 16 for related claims processing instructions.

100-02, 15, 80.2

Psychological Tests and Neuropsychological Tests

Medicare Part B coverage of psychological tests and neuropsychological tests is authorized under section 1861(s)(3) of the Social Security Act. Payment for psychological and neuropsychological tests is authorized under section 1842(b)(2)(A) of the Social Security Act. The payment amounts for the new psychological and neuropsychological tests (CPT codes 96102, 96103, 96119 and 96120) that are effective January 1, 2006, and are billed for tests administered by a technician or a computer reflect a site of service payment differential for the facility and non-facility settings.

Additionally, there is no authorization for payment for diagnostic tests when performed on an "incident to" basis.

Under the diagnostic tests provision, all diagnostic tests are assigned a certain level of supervision. Generally, regulations governing the diagnostic tests provision require that only physicians can provide the assigned level of supervision for diagnostic tests.

However, there is a regulatory exception to the supervision requirement for diagnostic psychological and neuropsychological tests in terms of who can provide the supervision.

That is, regulations allow a clinical psychologist (CP) or a physician to perform the general supervision assigned to diagnostic psychological and neuropsychological tests.

In addition, nonphysician practitioners such as nurse practitioners (NPs), clinical nurse specialists (CNSs) and physician assistants (PAs) who personally perform diagnostic psychological and neuropsychological tests are excluded from having to perform these tests under the general supervision of a physician or a CP. Rather, NPs and CNSs must perform such tests under the requirements of their respective benefit instead of the requirements for diagnostic psychological and neuropsychological tests. Accordingly, NPs and CNSs must perform tests in collaboration (as defined under Medicare law at section 1861(aa)(6) of the Act) with a physician. PAs perform tests under the general supervision of a physician as required for services furnished under the PA benefit.

Furthermore, physical therapists (PTs), occupational therapists (OTs) and speech language pathologists (SLPs) are authorized to bill three test codes as "sometimes therapy" codes. Specifically, CPT codes 96105, 96110 and 96111 may be performed by these therapists. However, when PTs, OTs and SLPs perform these three tests, they must be performed under the general supervision of a physician or a CP.

Who May Bill for Diagnostic Psychological and Neuropsychological Tests CPs - see qualifications under chapter 15, section 160 of the Benefits Policy Manual, Pub. 100-2.
- NPs -to the extent authorized under State scope of practice. See qualifications under chapter 15, section 200 of the Benefits Policy Manual, Pub. 100-2.
- CNSs -to the extent authorized under State scope of practice. See qualifications under chapter 15, section 210 of the Benefits Policy Manual, Pub. 100-2.
- PAs - to the extent authorized under State scope of practice. See qualifications under chapter 15, section 190 of the Benefits Policy Manual, Pub. 100-2.
- Independently Practicing Psychologists (IPPs) PTs, OTs and SLPs - see qualifications under chapter 15, sections 220-230.6 of the Benefits Policy Manual, Pub. 100-2.

Psychological and neuropsychological tests performed by a psychologist (who is not a CP) practicing independently of an institution, agency, or physician's office are covered when a physician orders such tests. An IPP is any psychologist who is licensed or certified to practice psychology in the State or jurisdiction where furnishing services or, if the jurisdiction does not issue licenses, if provided by any practicing psychologist. (It is CMS' understanding that all States, the District of Columbia, and Puerto Rico license psychologists, but that some trust territories do not. Examples of psychologists, other than CPs, whose psychological and neuropsychological tests are covered under the diagnostic tests provision include, but are not limited to, educational psychologists and counseling psychologists.)

The carrier must secure from the appropriate State agency a current listing of psychologists holding the required credentials to determine whether the tests of a particular IPP are covered under Part B in States that have statutory licensure or certification. In States or territories that lack statutory licensing or certification, the carrier checks individual qualifications before provider numbers are issued. Possible reference sources are the national directory of membership of the American Psychological Association, which provides data about the educational background of individuals and indicates which members are board-certified, the records and directories of the State or territorial psychological association, and the National Register of Health Service Providers. If qualification is dependent on a doctoral degree from a currently accredited program, the carrier verifies the date of accreditation of the school involved, since such accreditation is not retroactive. If the listed reference sources do not provide enough information (e.g., the psychologist is not a member of one of these sources), the carrier contacts the psychologist personally for the required information. Generally, carriers maintain a continuing list of psychologists whose qualifications have been verified.

NOTE: When diagnostic psychological tests are performed by a psychologist who is not practicing independently, but is on the staff of an institution, agency, or clinic, that entity bills for the psychological tests.

The carrier considers psychologists as practicing independently when:
- They render services on their own responsibility, free of the administrative and professional control of an employer such as a physician, institution or agency;
- The persons they treat are their own patients; and
- They have the right to bill directly, collect and retain the fee for their services.

A psychologist practicing in an office located in an institution may be considered an independently practicing psychologist when both of the following conditions exist:

- The office is confined to a separately-identified part of the facility which is used solely as the psychologist's office and cannot be construed as extending throughout the entire institution; and
- The psychologist conducts a private practice, i.e., services are rendered to patients from outside the institution as well as to institutional patients.

Payment for Diagnostic Psychological and Neuropsychological Tests
Expenses for diagnostic psychological and neuropsychological tests are not subject to the outpatient mental health treatment limitation, that is, the payment limitation on treatment services for mental, psychoneurotic and personality disorders as authorized under Section 1833(c) of the Act. The payment amount for the new psychological and neuropsychological tests (CPT codes 96102, 96103, 96119 and 96120) that are billed for tests performed by a technician or a computer reflect a site of service payment differential for the facility and non-facility settings. CPs, NPs, CNSs and PAs are required by law to accept assigned payment for psychological and neuropsychological tests. However, while IPPs are not required by law to accept assigned payment for these tests, they must report the name and address of the physician who ordered the test on the claim form when billing for tests.

CPT Codes for Diagnostic Psychological and Neuropsychological Tests
The range of CPT codes used to report psychological and neuropsychological tests is 96101-96120. CPT codes 96101, 96102, 96103, 96105, 96110, and 96111 are appropriate for use when billing for psychological tests. CPT codes 96116, 96118, 96119 and 96120 are appropriate for use when billing for neuropsychological tests.

All of the tests under this CPT code range 96101-96120 are indicated as active codes under the physician fee schedule database and are covered if medically necessary.

Payment and Billing Guidelines for Psychological and Neuropsychological Tests
The technician and computer CPT codes for psychological and neuropsychological tests include practice expense, malpractice expense and professional work relative value units.

Accordingly, CPT psychological test code 96101 should not be paid when billed for the same tests or services performed under psychological test codes 96102 or 96103. CPT neuropsychological test code 96118 should not be paid when billed for the same tests or services performed under neuropsychological test codes 96119 or 96120. However, CPT codes 96101 and 96118 can be paid separately on the rare occasion when billed on the same date of service for different and separate tests from 96102, 96103, 96119 and 96120.

Under the physician fee schedule, there is no payment for services performed by students or trainees. Accordingly, Medicare does not pay for services represented by CPT codes 96102 and 96119 when performed by a student or a trainee. However, the presence of a student or a trainee while the test is being administered does not prevent a physician, CP, IPP, NP, CNS or PA from performing and being paid for the psychological test under 96102 or the neuropsychological test under 96119.

100-02, 15, 80.5.5

Frequency Standards
Medicare pays for a screening BMM once every 2 years (at least 23 months have passed since the month the last covered BMM was performed).

When medically necessary, Medicare may pay for more frequent BMMs. Examples include, but are not limited to, the following medical circumstances:

- Monitoring beneficiaries on long-term glucocorticoid (steroid) therapy of more than 3 months.
- Confirming baseline BMMs to permit monitoring of beneficiaries in the future.

100-02, 15, 150.1

Treatment of Temporomandibular Joint (TMJ) Syndrome
There are a wide variety of conditions that can be characterized as TMJ, and an equally wide variety of methods for treating these conditions. Many of the procedures fall within the Medicare program's statutory exclusion that prohibits payment for items and services that have not been demonstrated to be reasonable and necessary for the diagnosis and treatment of illness or injury (§1862(a)(1) of the Act). Other services and appliances used to treat TMJ fall within the Medicare program's statutory exclusion at 1862(a)(12), which prohibits payment "for services in connection with the care, treatment, filling, removal, or replacement of teeth or structures directly supporting teeth...." For these reasons, a diagnosis of TMJ on a claim is insufficient. The actual condition or symptom must be determined.

100-02, 15, 160

Clinical Psychologist Services

A. Clinical Psychologist (CP) Defined
To qualify as a clinical psychologist (CP), a practitioner must meet the following requirements: Hold a doctoral degree in psychology; Be licensed or certified, on the basis of the doctoral degree in psychology, by the State in which he or she practices, at the independent practice level of psychology to furnish diagnostic, assessment, preventive, and therapeutic services directly to individuals.

B. Qualified Clinical Psychologist Services Defined

Effective July 1, 1990, the diagnostic and therapeutic services of CPs and services and supplies furnished incident to such services are covered as the services furnished by a physician or as incident to physician's services are covered. However, the CP must be legally authorized to perform the services under applicable licensure laws of the State in which they are furnished.

C. Types of Clinical Psychologist Services

That May Be Covered Diagnostic and therapeutic services that the CP is legally authorized to perform in accordance with State law and/or regulation. Carriers pay all qualified CPs based on the physician fee schedule for the diagnostic and therapeutic services. (Psychological tests by practitioners who do not meet the requirements for a CP may be covered under the provisions for diagnostic tests as described in Sec. 80.2.

Services and supplies furnished incident to a CP's services are covered if the requirements that apply to services incident to a physician's services, as described in Sec.60 are met. These services must be:

- Mental health services that are commonly furnished in CPs' offices;
- An integral, although incidental, part of professional services performed by the CP;
- Performed under the direct personal supervision of the CP; i.e., the CP must be physically present and immediately available;
- Furnished without charge or included in the CP's bill; and
- Performed by an employee of the CP (or an employee of the legal entity that employs the supervising CP) under the common law control test of the Act, as set forth in 20 CFR 404.1007 and Sec.RS 2101.020 of the Retirement and Survivors Insurance part of the Social Security Program Operations Manual System.
- Diagnostic psychological testing services when furnished under the general supervision of a CP.

Carriers are required to familiarize themselves with appropriate State laws and/or regulations governing a CP's scope of practice.

D. Noncovered Services

The services of CPs are not covered if the service is otherwise excluded from Medicare coverage even though a clinical psychologist is authorized by State law to perform them.

For example, Sec.1862(a)(1)(A) of the Act excludes from coverage services that are not "reasonable and necessary for the diagnosis or treatment of an illness or injury or to improve the functioning of a malformed body member." Therefore, even though the services are authorized by State law, the services of a CP that are determined to be not reasonable and necessary are not covered. Additionally, any therapeutic services that are billed by CPs under CPT psychotherapy codes that include medical evaluation and management services are not covered.

E. Requirement for Consultation

When applying for a Medicare provider number, a CP must submit to the carrier a signed Medicare provider/supplier enrollment form that indicates an agreement to the effect that, contingent upon the patient's consent, the CP will attempt to consult with the patient's attending or primary care physician in accordance with accepted professional ethical norms, taking into consideration patient confidentiality.

If the patient assents to the consultation, the CP must attempt to consult with the patient's physician within a reasonable time after receiving the consent. If the CP's attempts to consult directly with the physician are not successful, the CP must notify the physician within a reasonable time that he or she is furnishing services to the patient. Additionally, the CP must document, in the patient's medical record, the date the patient consented or declined consent to consultations, the date of consultation, or, if attempts to consult did not succeed, that date and manner of notification to the physician.

The only exception to the consultation requirement for CPs is in cases where the patient's primary care or attending physician refers the patient to the CP. Also, neither a CP nor a primary care nor attending physician may bill Medicare or the patient for this required consultation.

F. Outpatient Mental Health Services Limitation

All covered therapeutic services furnished by qualified CPs are subject to the outpatient mental health services limitation in Pub 100-1, Medicare General Information, Eligibility, and Entitlement Manual, Chapter 3, "Deductibles, Coinsurance Amounts, and Payment Limitations," Sec.30, (i.e., only 62 1/2 percent of expenses for these services are considered incurred expenses for Medicare purposes). The limitation does not apply to diagnostic services.

G. Assignment Requirement Assignment iSec. required.

100-02, 15, 170

Clinical Social Worker (CSW) Services

B3-2152

See the Medicare Claims Processing Manual Chapter 12, Physician/Nonphysician Practitioners, §150, "Clinical Social Worker Services," for payment requirements.

A. Clinical Social Worker Defined

Section 1861(hh) of the Act defines a "clinical social worker" as an individual who:

- Possesses a master's or doctor's degree in social work;
- Has performed at least two years of supervised clinical social work; and

- Is licensed or certified as a clinical social worker by the State in which the services are performed; or
- In the case of an individual in a State that does not provide for licensure or certification, has completed at least 2 years or 3,000 hours of post master's degree supervised clinical social work practice under the supervision of a master's level social worker in an appropriate setting such as a hospital, SNF, or clinic.

B. Clinical Social Worker Services Defined

Section 1861(hh)(2) of the Act defines "clinical social worker services" as those services that the CSW is legally authorized to perform under State law (or the State regulatory mechanism provided by State law) of the State in which such services are performed for the diagnosis and treatment of mental illnesses. Services furnished to an inpatient of a hospital or an inpatient of a SNF that the SNF is required to provide as a requirement for participation are not included. The services that are covered are those that are otherwise covered if furnished by a physician or as incident to a physician's professional service.

C. Covered Services

Coverage is limited to the services a CSW is legally authorized to perform in accordance with State law (or State regulatory mechanism established by State law). The services of a CSW may be covered under Part B if they are:

- The type of services that are otherwise covered if furnished by a physician, or as incident to a physician's service. (See §30 for a description of physicians' services and §70 of Pub 100-1, the Medicare General Information, Eligibility, and Entitlement Manual, Chapter 5, for the definition of a physician.);
- Performed by a person who meets the definition of a CSW (See subsection A.); and
- Not otherwise excluded from coverage. Carriers should become familiar with the State law or regulatory mechanism governing a CSW's scope of practice in their service area.

D. Noncovered Services

Services of a CSW are not covered when furnished to inpatients of a hospital or to inpatients of a SNF if the services furnished in the SNF are those that the SNF is required to furnish as a condition of participation in Medicare. In addition, CSW services are not covered if they are otherwise excluded from Medicare coverage even though a CSW is authorized by State law to perform them. For example, the Medicare law excludes from coverage services that are not "reasonable and necessary for the diagnosis or treatment of an illness or injury or to improve the functioning of a malformed body member."

E. Outpatient Mental Health Services Limitation

All covered therapeutic services furnished by qualified CSWs are subject to the outpatient psychiatric services limitation in Pub 100-1, Medicare General Information, Eligibility, and Entitlement Manual, Chapter 3, "Deductibles, Coinsurance Amounts, and Payment Limitations," §30, (i.e., only 62 1/2 percent of expenses for these services are considered incurred expenses for Medicare purposes). The limitation does not apply to diagnostic services.

F. Assignment Requirement

Assignment is required.

100-02, 15, 180

Nurse-Midwife (CNM) Services

B3-2154

A. General

Effective on or after July 1, 1988, the services provided by a certified nurse-midwife or incident to the certified nurse-midwife's services are covered. Payment is made under assignment only. See the Medicare Claims Processing Manual, Chapter 12, "Physician and Nonphysician Practitioners," §130, for payment methodology for nurse midwife services.

B. Certified Nurse-Midwife Defined

A certified nurse-midwife is a registered nurse who has successfully completed a program of study and clinical experience in nurse-midwifery, meeting guidelines prescribed by the Secretary, or who has been certified by an organization recognized by the Secretary. The Secretary has recognized certification by the American College of Nurse-Midwives and State qualifying requirements in those States that specify a program of education and clinical experience for nurse-midwives for these purposes. A nurse-midwife must:

- Be currently licensed to practice in the State as a registered professional nurse; and
- Meet one of the following requirements:
    1. Be legally authorized under State law or regulations to practice as a nurse-midwife and have completed a program of study and clinical experience for nurse-midwives, as specified by the State; or
    2. If the State does not specify a program of study and clinical experience that nurse-midwives must complete to practice in that State, the nurse-midwife must:
        a. Be currently certified as a nurse-midwife by the American College of Nurse-Midwives;
        b. Have satisfactorily completed a formal education program (of at least one academic year) that, upon completion, qualifies the nurse to take

the certification examination offered by the American College of Nurse-Midwives; or

c. Have successfully completed a formal education program for preparing registered nurses to furnish gynecological and obstetrical care to women during pregnancy, delivery, and the postpartum period, and care to normal newborns, and have practiced as a nurse-midwife for a total of 12 months during any 18-month period from August 8, 1976, to July 16, 1982.

C. Covered Services

1. General - Effective January 1, 1988, through December 31, 1993, the coverage of nurse-midwife services was restricted to the maternity cycle. The maternity cycle is a period that includes pregnancy, labor, and the immediate postpartum period.

   Beginning with services furnished on or after January 1, 1994, coverage is no longer limited to the maternity cycle. Coverage is available for services furnished by a nurse-midwife that he or she is legally authorized to perform in the State in which the services are furnished and that would otherwise be covered if furnished by a physician, including obstetrical and gynecological services.

2. Incident To- Services and supplies furnished incident to a nurse midwife's service are covered if they would have been covered when furnished incident to the services of a doctor of medicine or osteopathy, as described in §60.

D. Noncovered Services

The services of nurse-midwives are not covered if they are otherwise excluded from Medicare coverage even though a nurse-midwife is authorized by State law to perform them. For example, the Medicare program excludes from coverage routine physical checkups and services that are not reasonable and necessary for the diagnosis or treatment of an illness or injury or to improve the functioning of a malformed body member. Coverage of service to the newborn continues only to the point that the newborn is or would normally be treated medically as a separate individual. Items and services furnished the newborn from that point are not covered on the basis of the mother's eligibility.

E. Relationship With Physician

Most States have licensure and other requirements applicable to nurse-midwives. For example, some require that the nurse-midwife have an arrangement with a physician for the referral of the patient in the event a problem develops that requires medical attention. Others may require that the nurse-midwife function under the general supervision of a physician. Although these and similar State requirements must be met in order for the nurse-midwife to provide Medicare covered care, they have no effect on the nurse-midwife's right to personally bill for and receive direct Medicare payment. That is, billing does not have to flow through a physician or facility. See §60.2 for coverage of services performed by nurse-midwives incident to the service of physicians.

F. Place of Service

There is no restriction on place of service. Therefore, nurse-midwife services are covered if provided in the nurse-midwife's office, in the patient's home, or in a hospital or other facility, such as a clinic or birthing center owned or operated by a nurse-midwife.

G. Assignment Requirement

Assignment is required.

100-02, 15, 220

Coverage of Outpatient Rehabilitation Therapy Services (Physical Therapy, Occupational Therapy, and Speech-Language Pathology Services) Under Medical Insurance

A comprehensive knowledge of the policies that apply to therapy services cannot be obtained through manuals alone. The most definitive policies are Local Coverage Determinations found at the Medicare Coverage Database www.cms.hhs.gov/mcd. A list of Medicare contractors is found at the CMS Web site. Specific questions about all Medicare policies should be addressed to the contractors through the contact information supplied on their Web sites. General Medicare questions may be addressed to the Medicare regional offices http://www.cms.hhs.gov/RegionalOffices/.

A. Definitions

The following defines terms used in this section and §230:

ACTIVE PARTICIPATION of the clinician in treatment means that the clinician personally furnishes in its entirety at least 1 billable service on at least 1 day of treatment.

ASSESSMENT is separate from evaluation, and is included in services or procedures, (it is not separately payable). The term assessment as used in Medicare manuals related to therapy services is distinguished from language in Current Procedural Terminology (CPT) codes that specify assessment, e.g., 97755, Assistive Technology Assessment, which may be payable). Assessments shall be provided only by clinicians, because assessment requires professional skill to gather data by observation and patient inquiry and may include limited objective testing and measurement to make clinical judgments regarding the patient's condition(s). Assessment determines, e.g., changes in the patient's status since the last visit/treatment day and whether the planned procedure or service should be modified. Based on these assessment data, the professional may make judgments about progress toward goals and/or determine that a more complete evaluation or re-evaluation (see definitions below) is indicated. Routine weekly

assessments of expected progression in accordance with the plan are not payable as re-evaluations.

CERTIFICATION is the physician's/nonphysician practitioner's (NPP) approval of the plan of care. Certification requires a dated signature on the plan of care or some other document that indicates approval of the plan of care.

The CLINICIAN is a term used in this manual and in Pub 100-4, chapter 5, section 10 or section 20, to refer to only a physician, nonphysician practitioner or a therapist (but not to an assistant, aide or any other personnel) providing a service within their scope of practice and consistent with state and local law. Clinicians make clinical judgments and are responsible for all services they are permitted to supervise. Services that require the skills of a therapist, may be appropriately furnished by clinicians, that is, by or under the supervision of qualified physicians/NPPs when their scope of practice, state and local laws allow it and their personal professional training is judged by Medicare contractors as sufficient to provide to the beneficiary skills equivalent to a therapist for that service.

COMPLEXITIES are complicating factors that may influence treatment, e.g., they may influence the type, frequency, intensity and/or duration of treatment. Complexities may be represented by diagnoses (ICD codes), by patient factors such as age, severity, acuity, multiple conditions, and motivation, or by the patient's social circumstances such as the support of a significant other or the availability of transportation to therapy.

A DATE may be in any form (written, stamped or electronic). The date may be added to the record in any manner and at any time, as long as the dates are accurate. If they are different, refer to both the date a service was performed and the date the entry to the record was made. For example, if a physician certifies a plan and fails to date it, staff may add "Received Date" in writing or with a stamp. The received date is valid for certification/re-certification purposes. Also, if the physician faxes the referral, certification, or re-certification and forgets to date it, the date that prints out on the fax is valid. If services provided on one date are documented on another date, both dates should be documented.

The EPISODE of Outpatient Therapy – For the purposes of therapy policy, an outpatient therapy episode is defined as the period of time, in calendar days, from the first day the patient is under the care of the clinician (e.g., for evaluation or treatment) for the current condition(s) being treated by one therapy discipline (PT, or OT, or SLP) until the last date of service for that discipline in that setting.

During the episode, the beneficiary may be treated for more than one condition; including conditions with an onset after the episode has begun. For example, a beneficiary receiving PT for a hip fracture who, after the initial treatment session, develops low back pain would also be treated under a PT plan of care for rehabilitation of low back pain. That plan may be modified from the initial plan, or it may be a separate plan specific to the low back pain, but treatment for both conditions concurrently would be considered the same episode of PT treatment. If that same patient developed a swallowing problem during intubation for the hip surgery, the first day of treatment by the SLP would be a new episode of SLP care.

EVALUATION is a separately payable comprehensive service provided by a clinician, as defined above, that requires professional skills to make clinical judgments about conditions for which services are indicated based on objective measurements and subjective evaluations of patient performance and functional abilities. Evaluation is warranted e.g., for a new diagnosis or when a condition is treated in a new setting. These evaluative judgments are essential to development of the plan of care, including goals and the selection of interventions.

FUNCTIONAL REPORTING, which is required on claims for all outpatient therapy services pursuant to 42CFR410.59, 410.60, and 410.62, uses nonpayable G-codes and related modifiers to convey information about the patient's functional status at specified points during therapy. (See Pub 100-4, chapter 5, section 10.6)

RE-EVALUATION provides additional objective information not included in other documentation. Re-evaluation is separately payable and is periodically indicated during an episode of care when the professional assessment of a clinician indicates a significant improvement, or decline, or change in the patient's condition or functional status that was not anticipated in the plan of care. Although some state regulations and state practice acts require re-evaluation at specific times, for Medicare payment, reevaluations must also meet Medicare coverage guidelines. The decision to provide a reevaluation shall be made by a clinician.

INTERVAL of certified treatment (certification interval) consists of 90 calendar days or less, based on an individual's needs. A physician/NPP may certify a plan of care for an interval length that is less than 90 days. There may be more than one certification interval in an episode of care. The certification interval is not the same as a Progress Report period.

MAINTENANCE PROGRAM (MP) means a program established by a therapist that consists of activities and/or mechanisms that will assist a beneficiary in maximizing or maintaining the progress he or she has made during therapy or to prevent or slow further deterioration due to a disease or illness.

NONPHYSICIAN PRACTITIONERS (NPP) means physician assistants, clinical nurse specialists, and nurse practitioners, who may, if state and local laws permit it, and when appropriate rules are followed, provide, certify or supervise therapy services.

PHYSICIAN with respect to outpatient rehabilitation therapy services means a doctor of medicine, osteopathy (including an osteopathic practitioner), podiatric medicine, or optometry (for low vision rehabilitation only). Chiropractors and doctors of dental surgery or dental medicine are not considered physicians for therapy services and may neither refer patients for rehabilitation therapy services nor establish therapy plans of care.

PATIENT, client, resident, and beneficiary are terms used interchangeably to indicate enrolled recipients of Medicare covered services.

PROVIDERS of services are defined in §1861(u) of the Act, 42CFR400.202 and 42CFR485 Subpart H as participating hospitals, critical access hospitals (CAH), skilled nursing facilities (SNF), comprehensive outpatient rehabilitation facilities (CORF), home health agencies (HHA), hospices, participating clinics, rehabilitation agencies or outpatient rehabilitation facilities (ORF). Providers are also defined as public health agencies with agreements only to furnish outpatient therapy services, or community mental health centers with agreements only to furnish partial hospitalization services. To qualify as providers of services, these providers must meet certain conditions enumerated in the law and enter into an agreement with the Secretary in which they agree not to charge any beneficiary for covered services for which the program will pay and to refund any erroneous collections made. Note that the word PROVIDER in sections 220 and 230 is not used to mean a person who provides a service, but is used as in the statute to mean a facility or agency such as rehabilitation agency or home health agency.

QUALIFIED PROFESSIONAL means a physical therapist, occupational therapist, speech-language pathologist, physician, nurse practitioner, clinical nurse specialist, or physician's assistant, who is licensed or certified by the state to furnish therapy services, and who also may appropriately furnish therapy services under Medicare policies. Qualified professional may also include a physical therapist assistant (PTA) or an occupational therapy assistant (OTA) when furnishing services under the supervision of a qualified therapist, who is working within the state scope of practice in the state in which the services are furnished. Assistants are limited in the services they may furnish (see section 230.1 and 230.2) and may not supervise other therapy caregivers.

QUALIFIED PERSONNEL means staff (auxiliary personnel) who have been educated and trained as therapists and qualify to furnish therapy services only under direct supervision incident to a physician or NPP. See §230.5 of this chapter. Qualified personnel may or may not be licensed as therapists but meet all of the requirements for therapists with the exception of licensure.

SIGNATURE means a legible identifier of any type acceptable according to policies in Pub. 100-08, Medicare Program Integrity Manual, chapter 3, §3.3.2.4 concerning signatures.

SUPERVISION LEVELS for outpatient rehabilitation therapy services are the same as those for diagnostic tests defined in 42CFR410.32. Depending on the setting, the levels include personal supervision (in the room), direct supervision (in the office suite), and general supervision (physician/NPP is available but not necessarily on the premises).

SUPPLIERS of therapy services include individual practitioners such as physicians, NPPs, physical therapists and occupational therapists who have Medicare provider numbers. Regulatory references on physical therapists in private practice (PTPPs) and occupational therapists in private practice (OTPPs) are at 42CFR410.60 (C)(1), 485.701-729, and 486.150-163.

THERAPIST refers only to qualified physical therapists, occupational therapists and speech-language pathologists, as defined in §230. Qualifications that define therapists are in §§230.1, 230.2, and 230.3. Skills of a therapist are defined by the scope of practice for therapists in the state).

THERAPY (or outpatient rehabilitation services) includes only outpatient physical therapy (PT), occupational therapy (OT) and speech-language pathology (SLP) services paid using the Medicare Physician Fee Schedule or the same services when provided in hospitals that are exempt from the hospital Outpatient Prospective Payment System and paid on a reasonable cost basis, including critical access hospitals.

Therapy services referred to in this chapter are those skilled services furnished according to the standards and conditions in CMS manuals, (e.g., in this chapter and in Pub. 100-4, Medicare Claims Processing Manual, chapter 5), within their scope of practice by qualified professionals or qualified personnel, as defined in this section, represented by procedures found in the American Medical Association's "Current Procedural Terminology (CPT)." A list of CPT (HCPCS) codes is provided in Pub. 100-4, chapter 5, §20, and in Local Coverage Determinations developed by contractors.

TREATMENT DAY means a single calendar day on which treatment, evaluation and/or reevaluation is provided. There could be multiple visits, treatment sessions/encounters on a treatment day.

VISITS OR TREATMENT SESSIONS begin at the time the patient enters the treatment area (of a building, office, or clinic) and continue until all services (e.g., activities, procedures, services) have been completed for that session and the patient leaves that area to participate in a non-therapy activity. It is likely that not all minutes in the visits/treatment sessions are billable (e.g., rest periods). There may be two treatment sessions in a day, for example, in the morning and afternoon. When there are two visits/ treatment sessions in a day, plans of care indicate treatment amount of twice a day.

B. References

Paper Manuals. The following manuals, now outdated, were resources for the Internet Only Manuals:

- Part A Medicare Intermediary Manual, (Pub. 13)
- Part B Medicare Carrier Manual, (Pub. 14)
- Hospital Manual, (Pub. 10)
- Outpatient Physical Therapy/CORF Manual, (Pub. 9)

Regulation and Statute. The information in this section is based in part on the following current references:

- 42CFR refers to Title 42, Code of Federal Regulation (CFR).
- The Act refers to the Social Security Act.

Internet Only Manuals. Current Policies that concern providers and suppliers of therapy services are located in many places throughout CMS Manuals. Sites that may be of interest include:

- Pub.100-1 GENERAL INFORMATION, ELIGIBILITY, AND ENTITLEMENT
  — Chapter 1- General Overview
    – 10.1 - Hospital Insurance (Part A) for Inpatient Hospital, Hospice, Home Health and SNF Services - A Brief Description
    – 10.2 - Home Health Services
    – 10.3 - Supplementary Medical Insurance (Part B) - A Brief Description
    – 20.2 - Discrimination Prohibited
- Pub. 100-2, MEDICARE BENEFIT POLICY MANUAL
  — Ch 6 - Hospital Services Covered Under Part B
    – 10 - Medical and Other Health Services Furnished to Inpatients of Participating Hospitals
    – 20 - Outpatient Hospital Services
    – 20.2 - Outpatient Defined
    – 20.4.1 - Diagnostic Services Defined
    – 70 - Outpatient Hospital Psychiatric Services
  — Ch 8 - Coverage of Extended Care (SNF) Services Under Hospital Insurance
    – 30.4. - Direct Skilled Rehabilitation Services to Patients
    – 40 - Physician Certification and Recertification for Extended Care Services
    – 50.3 - Physical Therapy, Speech-Language Pathology, and Occupational Therapy Furnished by the Skilled Nursing Facility or by Others Under Arrangements with the Facility and Under Its Supervision
    – 70.3 - Inpatient Physical Therapy, Occupational Therapy, and Speech Pathology Services
  — Ch 12 - Comprehensive Outpatient Rehabilitation Facility (CORF) Coverage
    – 10 - Comprehensive Outpatient Rehabilitation Facility (CORF) Services Provided by Medicare
    – 20 - Required and Optional CORF Services
    – 20.1 - Required Services
    – 20.2 - Optional CORF Services
    – 30 - Rules for Provision of Services
    – 30.1 - Rules for Payment of CORF Services
    – 40 - Specific CORF Services
    – 40.1 - Physicians' Services
    – 40.2 - Physical Therapy Services
    – 40.3 - Occupational Therapy Services
    – 40.4 – Speech Language Pathology Services
- Pub. 100-3 MEDICARE NATIONAL COVERAGE DETERMINATIONS MANUAL
  — Part 1
    – 20.10 - Cardiac Rehabilitation Programs
    – 30.1 - Biofeedback Therapy
    – 30.1.1 - Biofeedback Therapy for the Treatment of Urinary Incontinence
    – 50.1 – Speech Generating Devices
    – 50.2 - Electronic Speech Aids
    – 50.4 - Tracheostomy Speaking Valve
  — Part 2
    – 150.2 - Osteogenic Stimulator
    – 160.7 - Electrical Nerve Stimulators
    – 160.12 - Neuromuscular Electrical Stimulation (NMES)
    – 160.13 - Supplies Used in the Delivery of Transcutaneous Electrical Nerve Stimulation (TENS) and Neuromuscular Electrical Stimulation (NMES)
    – 160.17 - L-Dopa
  — Part 3

- 170.1 - Institutional and Home Care Patient Education Programs
- 170.2 - Melodic Intonation Therapy
- 170.3 - Speech Pathology Services for the Treatment of Dysphagia
- 180 – Nutrition
— Part 4
- 230.8 - Non-implantable Pelvic Flood Electrical Stimulator
- 240.7 - Postural Drainage Procedures and Pulmonary Exercises
- 270.1 -Electrical Stimulation (ES) and Electromagnetic Therapy for the Treatment of Wounds
- 270.4 - Treatment of Decubitus Ulcers
- 280.3 - Mobility Assisted Equipment (MAE)
- 280.4 - Seat Lift
- 280.13 - Transcutaneous Electrical Nerve Stimulators (TENS)
- 290.1 - Home Health Visits to A Blind Diabetic
- Pub. 100-08 PROGRAM INTEGRITY MANUAL
  — Chapter 3 - Verifying Potential Errors and Taking Corrective Actions
    - 3.4.1.1 - Linking LCD and NCD ID Numbers to Edits
  — Chapter 13 - Local Coverage Determinations
    - 13.5.1 - Reasonable and Necessary Provisions in LCDs

Specific policies may differ by setting. Other policies concerning therapy services are found in other manuals. When a therapy service policy is specific to a setting, it takes precedence over these general outpatient policies. For special rules on:

- CORFs - See chapter 12 of this manual and also Pub. 100-4, chapter 5;
- SNF - See chapter 8 of this manual and also Pub. 100-4, chapter 6, for SNF claims/billing;
- HHA - See chapter 7 of this manual, and Pub. 100-4, chapter 10;
- GROUP THERAPY AND STUDENTS - See Pub. 100-2, chapter 15, §230;
- ARRANGEMENTS - Pub. 100-1, chapter 5, §10.3;
- COVERAGE is described in the Medicare Program Integrity Manual, Pub. 100-08, chapter 13, §13.5.1; and
- THERAPY CAPS - See Pub. 100-4, chapter 5, §10.2, for a complete description of this financial limitation.

C. General

Therapy services are a covered benefit in §§1861(g), 1861(p), and 1861(ll) of the Act. Therapy services may also be provided incident to the services of a physician/NPP under §§1861(s)(2) and 1862(a)(20) of the Act.

Covered therapy services are furnished by providers, by others under arrangements with and under the supervision of providers, or furnished by suppliers (e.g., physicians, NPP, enrolled therapists), who meet the requirements in Medicare manuals for therapy services.

Where a prospective payment system (PPS) applies, therapy services are paid when services conform to the requirements of that PPS. Reimbursement for therapy provided to Part A inpatients of hospitals or residents of SNFs in covered stays is included in the respective PPS rates.

Payment for therapy provided by an HHA under a plan of treatment is included in the home health PPS rate. Therapy may be billed by an HHA on bill type 34x if there are no home health services billed under a home health plan of care at the same time (e.g., the patient is not homebound), and there is a valid therapy plan of treatment.

In addition to the requirements described in this chapter, the services must be furnished in accordance with health and safety requirements set forth in regulations at 42CFR484, and 42CFR485.

When therapy services may be furnished appropriately in a community pool by a clinician in a physical therapist or occupational therapist private practice, physician office, outpatient hospital, or outpatient SNF, the practice/office or provider shall rent or lease the pool, or a specific portion of the pool. The use of that part of the pool during specified times shall be restricted to the patients of that practice or provider. The written agreement to rent or lease the pool shall be available for review on request. When part of the pool is rented or leased, the agreement shall describe the part of the pool that is used exclusively by the patients of that practice/office or provider and the times that exclusive use applies. Other providers, including rehabilitation agencies (previously referred to as OPTs and ORFs) and CORFs, are subject to the requirements outlined in the respective State Operations Manual regarding rented or leased community pools.

100-02, 15, 230

Practice of Physical Therapy, Occupational Therapy, and Speech-Language Pathology

A. Group Therapy Services.

Contractors pay for outpatient physical therapy services (which includes outpatient speech-language pathology services) and outpatient occupational therapy services provided simultaneously to two or more individuals by a practitioner as group therapy services (97150). The individuals can be, but need not be performing the same activity. The physician or therapist involved in group therapy services must be in constant attendance, but one-on-one patient contact is not required.

B. Therapy Students

1. General

   Only the services of the therapist can be billed and paid under Medicare Part B. The services performed by a student are not reimbursed even if provided under "line of sight" supervision of the therapist; however, the presence of the student "in the room" does not make the service unbillable. Pay for the direct (one-to-one) patient contact services of the physician or therapist provided to Medicare Part B patients. Group therapy services performed by a therapist or physician may be billed when a student is also present "in the room".

   EXAMPLES:

   Therapists may bill and be paid for the provision of services in the following scenarios:

   — The qualified practitioner is present and in the room for the entire session. The student participates in the delivery of services when the qualified practitioner is directing the service, making the skilled judgment, and is responsible for the assessment and treatment.

   — The qualified practitioner is present in the room guiding the student in service delivery when the therapy student and the therapy assistant student are participating in the provision of services, and the practitioner is not engaged in treating another patient or doing other tasks at the same time.

   — The qualified practitioner is responsible for the services and as such, signs all documentation. (A student may, of course, also sign but it is not necessary since the Part B payment is for the clinician's service, not for the student's services).

2. Therapy Assistants as Clinical Instructors

   Physical therapist assistants and occupational therapy assistants are not precluded from serving as clinical instructors for therapy students, while providing services within their scope of work and performed under the direction and supervision of a licensed physical or occupational therapist to a Medicare beneficiary.

3. Services Provided Under Part A and Part B

   The payment methodologies for Part A and B therapy services rendered by a student are different. Under the MPFS (Medicare Part B), Medicare pays for services provided by physicians and practitioners that are specifically authorized by statute. Students do not meet the definition of practitioners under Medicare Part B. Under SNF PPS, payments are based upon the case mix or Resource Utilization Group (RUG) category that describes the patient. In the rehabilitation groups, the number of therapy minutes delivered to the patient determines the RUG category. Payment levels for each category are based upon the costs of caring for patients in each group rather than providing pecific payment for each therapy service as is done in Medicare Part B.

100-02, 15, 230.1

Practice of Physical Therapy

A. General

Physical therapy services are those services provided within the scope of practice of physical therapists and necessary for the diagnosis and treatment of impairments, functional limitations, disabilities or changes in physical function and health status. (See Pub. 100-3, the Medicare National Coverage Determinations Manual, for specific conditions or services.) For descriptions of aquatic therapy in a community center pool see section 220C of this chapter.

B. Qualified Physical Therapist Defined

Reference: 42CFR484.4

The new personnel qualifications for physical therapists were discussed in the 2008 Physician Fee Schedule. See the Federal Register of November 27, 2007, for the full text. See also the correction notice for this rule, published in the Federal Register on January 15, 2008.

The regulation provides that a qualified physical therapist (PT) is a person who is licensed, if applicable, as a PT by the state in which he or she is practicing unless licensure does not apply, has graduated from an accredited PT education program and passed a national examination approved by the state in which PT services are provided.

The phrase, "by the state in which practicing" includes any authorization to practice provided by the same state in which the service is provided, including temporary licensure, regardless of the location of the entity billing the services. The curriculum accreditation is provided by the Commission on Accreditation in Physical Therapy Education (CAPTE) or, for those who graduated before CAPTE, curriculum approval was provided by the American Physical Therapy Association (APTA). For internationally educated PTs, curricula are approved by a credentials evaluation organization either approved by the APTA or identified in 8 CFR 212.15(e) as it relates to PTs. For example, in 2007, 8 CFR 212.15(e) approved the credentials evaluation provided by the Federation of State Boards of Physical Therapy (FSBPT) and the Foreign Credentialing Commission on Physical Therapy (FCCPT). The requirements above apply to all PTs effective January 1, 2010, if they have not met any of the following requirements prior to January 1, 2010.

Physical therapists whose current license was obtained on or prior to December 31, 2009, qualify to provide PT services to Medicare beneficiaries if they:

- graduated from a CAPTE approved program in PT on or before December 31, 2009 (examination is not required); or,

- graduated on or before December 31, 2009, from a PT program outside the U.S. that is determined to be substantially equivalent to a U.S. program by a credentials evaluating organization approved by either the APTA or identified in 8 CFR 212.15(e) and also passed an examination for PTs approved by the state in which practicing.

Or, PTs whose current license was obtained before January 1, 2008, may meet the requirements in place on that date (i.e., graduation from a curriculum approved by either the APTA, the Committee on Allied Health Education and Accreditation of the American Medical Association, or both).

Or, PTs meet the requirements who are currently licensed and were licensed or qualified as a PT on or before December 31, 1977, and had 2 years appropriate experience as a PT, and passed a proficiency examination conducted, approved, or sponsored by the U.S. Public Health Service.

Or, PTs meet the requirements if they are currently licensed and before January 1, 1966, they were:

— admitted to membership by the APTA; or

— admitted to registration by the American Registry of Physical Therapists; or

— graduated from a 4-year PT curriculum approved by a State Department of Education; or

— licensed or registered and prior to January 1, 1970, they had 15 years of fulltime experience in PT under the order and direction of attending and referring doctors of medicine or osteopathy.

Or, PTs meet requirements if they are currently licensed and they were trained outside the U.S. before January 1, 2008, and after 1928 graduated from a PT curriculum approved in the country in which the curriculum was located, if that country had an organization that was a member of the World Confederation for Physical Therapy, and that PT qualified as a member of the organization.

For outpatient PT services that are provided incident to the services of physicians/NPPs, the requirement for PT licensure does not apply; all other personnel qualifications do apply. The qualified personnel providing PT services incident to the services of a physician/NPP must be trained in an accredited PT curriculum. For example, a person who, on or before December 31, 2009, graduated from a PT curriculum accredited by CAPTE, but who has not passed the national examination or obtained a license, could provide Medicare outpatient PT therapy services incident to the services of a physician/NPP if the physician assumes responsibility for the services according to the incident to policies. On or after January 1, 2010, although licensure does not apply, both education and examination requirements that are effective January 1, 2010, apply to qualified personnel who provide PT services incident to the services of a physician/NPP.

C. Services of Physical Therapy Support Personnel
Reference: 42CFR 484.4

Personnel Qualifications. The new personnel qualifications for physical therapist assistants (PTA) were discussed in the 2008 Physician Fee Schedule. See the Federal Register of November 27, 2007, for the full text. See also the correction notice for this rule, published in the Federal Register on January 15, 2008.

The regulation provides that a qualified PTA is a person who is licensed as a PTA unless licensure does not apply, is registered or certified, if applicable, as a PTA by the state in which practicing, and graduated from an approved curriculum for PTAs, and passed a national examination for PTAs. The phrase, "by the state in which practicing" includes any authorization to practice provided by the same state in which the service is provided, including temporary licensure, regardless of the location or the entity billing for the services. Approval for the curriculum is provided by CAPTE or, if internationally or military trained PTAs apply, approval will be through a credentialing body for the curriculum for PTAs identified by either the American Physical Therapy Association or identified in 8 CFR 212.15(e). A national examination for PTAs is, for example the one furnished by the Federation of State Boards of Physical Therapy. These requirements above apply to all PTAs effective January 1, 2010, if they have not met any of the following requirements prior to January 1, 2010.

Those PTAs also qualify who, on or before December 31, 2009, are licensed, registered or certified as a PTA and met one of the two following requirements:

1. Is licensed or otherwise regulated in the state in which practicing; or

2. In states that have no licensure or other regulations, or where licensure does not apply, PTAs have:

   — graduated on or before December 31, 2009, from a 2-year college-level program approved by the APTA or CAPTE; and

   — effective January 1, 2010, those PTAs must have both graduated from a CAPTE approved curriculum and passed a national examination for PTAs; or

   — PTAs may also qualify if they are licensed, registered or certified as a PTA, if applicable and meet requirements in effect before January 1, 2008, that is,

     – they have graduated before January 1, 2008, from a 2 year college level program approved by the APTA; or

     – on or before December 31, 1977, they were licensed or qualified as a PTA and passed a proficiency examination conducted, approved, or sponsored by the U.S. Public Health Service.

Services. The services of PTAs used when providing covered therapy benefits are included as part of the covered service. These services are billed by the supervising physical therapist. PTAs may not provide evaluation services, make clinical judgments or decisions or take responsibility for the service. They act at the direction and under the supervision of the treating physical therapist and in accordance with state laws.

A physical therapist must supervise PTAs. The level and frequency of supervision differs by setting (and by state or local law). General supervision is required for PTAs in all settings except private practice (which requires direct supervision) unless state practice requirements are more stringent, in which case state or local requirements must be followed. See specific settings for details. For example, in clinics, rehabilitation services, either on or off the organization's premises, those services are supervised by a qualified physical therapist who makes an onsite supervisory visit at least once every 30 days or more frequently if required by state or local laws or regulation.

The services of a PTA shall not be billed as services incident to a physician/NPP's service, because they do not meet the qualifications of a therapist.

The cost of supplies (e.g., theraband, hand putty, electrodes) used in furnishing covered therapy care is included in the payment for the HCPCS codes billed by the physical therapist, and are, therefore, not separately billable. Separate coverage and billing provisions apply to items that meet the definition of brace in Sec.130.

Services provided by aides, even if under the supervision of a therapist, are not therapy services and are not covered by Medicare. Although an aide may help the therapist by providing unskilled services, those services that are unskilled are not covered by Medicare and shall be denied as not reasonable and necessary if they are billed as therapy services.

D. Application of Medicare Guidelines to PT Services
This subsection will be used in the future to illustrate the application of the above guidelines to some of the physical therapy modalities and procedures utilized in the treatment of patients.

100-02, 15, 230.2

Practice of Occupational Therapy

230.2 - Practice of Occupational Therapy (Rev. 88, Issued: 05-07-08, Effective: 01-01-08, Implementation: 06-09-08)

A. General
Occupational therapy services are those services provided within the scope of practice of occupational therapists and necessary for the diagnosis and treatment of impairments, functional disabilities or changes in physical function and health status. (See Pub. 100- 03, the Medicare National Coverage Determinations Manual, for specific conditions or services.)

Occupational therapy is medically prescribed treatment concerned with improving or restoring functions which have been impaired by illness or injury or, where function has been permanently lost or reduced by illness or injury, to improve the individual's ability to perform those tasks required for independent functioning. Such therapy may involve:

- The evaluation, and reevaluation as required, of a patient's level of function by administering diagnostic and prognostic tests;

- The selection and teaching of task-oriented therapeutic activities designed to restore physical function; e.g., use of woodworking activities on an inclined table to restore shoulder, elbow, and wrist range of motion lost as a result of burns;

- The planning, implementing, and supervising of individualized therapeutic activity programs as part of an overall "active treatment" program for a patient with a diagnosed psychiatric illness; e.g., the use of sewing activities which require following a pattern to reduce confusion and restore reality orientation in a schizophrenic patient;

- The planning and implementing of therapeutic tasks and activities to restore sensoryintegrative function; e.g., providing motor and tactile activities to increase sensory input and improve response for a stroke patient with functional loss resulting in a distorted body image;

- The teaching of compensatory technique to improve the level of independence in the activities of daily living, for example:

  — Teaching a patient who has lost the use of an arm how to pare potatoes and chop vegetables with one hand;

  — Teaching an upper extremity amputee how to functionally utilize a prosthesis;

  — Teaching a stroke patient new techniques to enable the patient to perform feeding, dressing, and other activities as independently as possible; or

  — Teaching a patient with a hip fracture/hip replacement techniques of standing tolerance and balance to enable the patient to perform such functional activities as dressing and homemaking tasks.

The designing, fabricating, and fitting of orthotics and self-help devices; e.g., making a hand splint for a patient with rheumatoid arthritis to maintain the hand in a functional position or constructing a device which would enable an individual to hold a utensil and feed independently; or Vocational and prevocational assessment and training, subject to the limitations specified in item B below.

Only a qualified occupational therapist has the knowledge, training, and experience required to evaluate and, as necessary, reevaluate a patient's level of function, determine whether an occupational therapy program could reasonably be expected to improve, restore, or compensate for lost function and, where appropriate, recommend to the physician/NPP a plan of treatment.

B. Qualified Occupational Therapist Defined

Reference: 42CFR484.4 The new personnel qualifications for occupational therapists (OT) were discussed in the 2008 Physician Fee Schedule. See the Federal Register of November 27, 2007, for the full text. See also the correction notice for this rule, published in the Federal Register on January 15, 2008.

The regulation provides that a qualified OT is an individual who is licensed, if licensure applies, or otherwise regulated, if applicable, as an OT by the state in which practicing, and graduated from an accredited education program for OTs, and is eligible to take or has passed the examination for OTs administered by the National Board for Certification in Occupational Therapy, Inc. (NBCOT). The phrase, "by the state in which practicing" includes any authorization to practice provided by the same state in which the service is provided, including temporary licensure, regardless of the location of the entity billing the services. The education program for U.S. trained OTs is accredited by the Accreditation Council for Occupational Therapy Education (ACOTE). The requirements above apply to all OTs effective January 1, 2010, if they have not met any of the following requirements prior to January 1, 2010.

The OTs may also qualify if on or before December 31, 2009:

- they are licensed or otherwise regulated as an OT in the state in which practicing (regardless of the qualifications they met to obtain that licensure or regulation); or
- when licensure or other regulation does not apply, OTs have graduated from an OT education program accredited by ACOTE and are eligible to take, or have successfully completed the NBCOT examination for OTs.

Also, those OTs who met the Medicare requirements for OTs that were in 42CFR484.4 prior to January 1, 2008, qualify to provide OT services for Medicare beneficiaries if:

- on or before January 1, 2008, they graduated an OT program approved jointly by the American Medical Association and the AOTA, or
- they are eligible for the National Registration Examination of AOTA or the National Board for Certification in OT.

Also, they qualify who on or before December 31, 1977, had 2 years of appropriate experience as an occupational therapist, and had achieved a satisfactory grade on a proficiency examination conducted, approved, or sponsored by the U.S. Public Health Service.

Those educated outside the U.S. may meet the same qualifications for domestic trained OTs. For example, they qualify if they were licensed or otherwise regulated by the state in which practicing on or before December 31, 2009. Or they are qualified if they:

- graduated from an OT education program accredited as substantially equivalent to a U.S. OT education program by ACOTE, the World Federation of Occupational Therapists, or a credentialing body approved by AOTA; and
- passed the NBCOT examination for OT; and
- Effective January 1, 2010, are licensed or otherwise regulated, if applicable as an OT by the state in which practicing.

For outpatient OT services that are provided incident to the services of physicians/NPPs, the requirement for OT licensure does not apply; all other personnel qualifications do apply. The qualified personnel providing OT services incident to the services of a physician/NPP must be trained in an accredited OT curriculum. For example, a person who, on or before December 31, 2009, graduated from an OT curriculum accredited by ACOTE and is eligible to take or has successfully completed the entry-level certification examination for OTs developed and administered by NBCOT, could provide Medicare outpatient OT services incident to the services of a physician/NPP if the physician assumes responsibility for the services according to the incident to policies. On or after January 1, 2010, although licensure does not apply, both education and examination requirements that are effective January 1, 2010, apply to qualified personnel who provide OT services incident to the services of a physician/NPP.

C. Services of Occupational Therapy Support Personnel

Reference: 42CFR 484.4

The new personnel qualifications for occupational therapy assistants were discussed in the 2008 Physician Fee Schedule. See the Federal Register of November 27, 2007, for the full text. See also the correction notice for this rule, published in the Federal Register on January 15, 2008.

The regulation provides that an occupational therapy assistant is a person who is licensed, unless licensure does not apply, or otherwise regulated, if applicable, as an OTA by the state in which practicing, and graduated from an OTA education program accredited by ACOTE and is eligible to take or has successfully completed the NBCOT examination for OTAs. The phrase, "by the state in which practicing" includes any authorization to practice provided by the same state in which the service is provided, including temporary licensure, regardless of the location of the entity billing the services.

If the requirements above are not met, an OTA may qualify if, on or before December 31, 2009, the OTA is licensed or otherwise regulated as an OTA, if applicable, by the state in which practicing, or meets any qualifications defined by the state in which practicing.

Or, where licensure or other state regulation does not apply, OTAs may qualify if they have, on or before December 31, 2009:

- completed certification requirements to practice as an OTA established by a credentialing organization approved by AOTA; and
- after January 1, 2010, they have also completed an education program accredited by ACOTE and passed the NBCOT examination for OTAs.

OTAs who qualified under the policies in effect prior to January 1, 2008, continue to qualify to provide OT directed and supervised OTA services to Medicare beneficiaries.

Therefore, OTAs qualify who after December 31, 1977, and on or before December 31, 2007:

- completed certification requirements to practice as an OTA established by a credentialing organization approved by AOTA; or
- completed the requirements to practice as an OTA applicable in the state in which practicing.

Those OTAs who were educated outside the U.S. may meet the same requirements as domestically trained OTAs. Or, if educated outside the U.S. on or after January 1, 2008, they must have graduated from an OTA program accredited as substantially equivalent to OTA entry level education in the U.S. by ACOTE, its successor organization, or the World Federation of Occupational Therapists or a credentialing body approved by AOTA. In addition, they must have passed an exam for OTAs administered by NBCOT.

Services. The services of OTAs used when providing covered therapy benefits are included as part of the covered service. These services are billed by the supervising occupational therapist. OTAs may not provide evaluation services, make clinical judgments or decisions or take responsibility for the service. They act at the direction and under the supervision of the treating occupational therapist and in accordance with state laws.

An occupational therapist must supervise OTAs. The level and frequency of supervision differs by setting (and by state or local law). General supervision is required for OTAs in all settings except private practice (which requires direct supervision) unless state practice requirements are more stringent, in which case state or local requirements must be followed. See specific settings for details. For example, in clinics, rehabilitation agencies, and public health agencies, 42CFR485.713 indicates that when an OTA provides services, either on or off the organization's premises, those services are supervised by a qualified occupational therapist who makes an onsite supervisory visit at least once every 30 days or more frequently if required by state or local laws or regulation.

The services of an OTA shall not be billed as services incident to a physician/NPP's service, because they do not meet the qualifications of a therapist.

The cost of supplies (e.g., looms, ceramic tiles, or leather) used in furnishing covered therapy care is included in the payment for the HCPCS codes billed by the occupational therapist and are, therefore, not separately billable. Separate coverage and billing provisions apply to items that meet the definition of brace in Sec.130 of this manual.

Services provided by aides, even if under the supervision of a therapist, are not therapy services in the outpatient setting and are not covered by Medicare. Although an aide may help the therapist by providing unskilled services, those services that are unskilled are not covered by Medicare and shall be denied as not reasonable and necessary if they are billed as therapy services.

D. Application of Medicare Guidelines to Occupational Therapy Services

Occupational therapy may be required for a patient with a specific diagnosed psychiatric illness. If such services are required, they are covered assuming the coverage criteria are met. However, where an individual's motivational needs are not related to a specific diagnosed psychiatric illness, the meeting of such needs does not usually require an individualized therapeutic program. Such needs can be met through general activity programs or the efforts of other professional personnel involved in the care of the patient. Patient motivation is an appropriate and inherent function of all health disciplines, which is interwoven with other functions performed by such personnel for the patient. Accordingly, since the special skills of an occupational therapist are not required, an occupational therapy program for individuals who do not have a specific diagnosed psychiatric illness is not to be considered reasonable and necessary for the treatment of an illness or injury. Services furnished under such a program are not covered.

Occupational therapy may include vocational and prevocational assessment and training. When services provided by an occupational therapist are related solely to specific employment opportunities, work skills, or work settings, they are not reasonable or necessary for the diagnosis or treatment of an illness or injury and are not covered. However, carriers and intermediaries exercise care in applying this exclusion, because the assessment of level of function and the teaching of compensatory techniques to improve the level of function, especially in activities of daily living, are services which occupational therapists provide for both vocational and nonvocational purposes. For example, an assessment of sitting and standing tolerance might be nonvocational for a mother of young children or a retired individual living alone, but could also be a vocational test for a sales clerk. Training an amputee in the use of prosthesis for telephoning is necessary for everyday activities as well as for employment purposes. Major changes in life style may be mandatory for an individual with a substantial disability. The techniques of adjustment cannot be considered exclusively vocational or nonvocational.

100-02, 15, 230.4

Services Furnished by a Therapist in Private Practice

A. General

See section 220 of this chapter for definitions. Therapist refers only to a qualified physical therapist, occupational therapist or speech-language pathologist. TPP refers to therapists in private practice (qualified physical therapists, occupational therapists and speech-language pathologists).

In order to qualify to bill Medicare directly as a therapist, each individual must be enrolled as a private practitioner and employed in one of the following practice types: an unincorporated solo practice, unincorporated partnership, unincorporated group practice, physician/NPP group or groups that are not professional corporations, if allowed by state and local law. Physician/NPP group practices may employ TPP if state and local law permits this employee relationship.

For purposes of this provision, a physician/NPP group practice is defined as one or more physicians/NPPs enrolled with Medicare who may bill as one entity. For further details on issues concerning enrollment, see the provider enrollment Web site at www.cms.hhs.gov/MedicareProviderSupEnroll and Pub. 100-08, Medicare Program Integrity Manual, chapter15, section 15.4.4.9.

Private practice also includes therapists who are practicing therapy as employees of another supplier, of a professional corporation or other incorporated therapy practice. Private practice does not include individuals when they are working as employees of an institutional provider.

Services should be furnished in the therapist's or group's office or in the patient's home. The office is defined as the location(s) where the practice is operated, in the state(s) where the therapist (and practice, if applicable) is legally authorized to furnish services, during the hours that the therapist engages in the practice at that location. If services are furnished in a private practice office space, that space shall be owned, leased, or rented by the practice and used for the exclusive purpose of operating the practice. For descriptions of aquatic therapy in a community center pool see section 220C of this chapter.

Therapists in private practice must be approved as meeting certain requirements, but do not execute a formal provider agreement with the Secretary.

If therapists who have their own Medicare National Provider Identifier (NPI) are employed by therapist groups, physician/NPP groups, or groups that are not professional organizations, the requirement that therapy space be owned, leased, or rented may be satisfied by the group that employs the therapist. Each therapist employed by a group should enroll as a TPP.

When therapists with a Medicare NPI provide services in the physician's/NPP's office in which they are employed, and bill using their NPI for each therapy service, then the direct supervision requirement for enrolled staff apply.

When the therapist who has a Medicare NPI is employed in a physician's/NPP's office the services are ordinarily billed as services of the therapist, with the therapist identified on the claim as the supplier of services. However, services of the therapist who has a Medicare NPI may also be billed by the physician/NPP as services incident to the physician's/NPP's service. (See §230.5 for rules related to therapy services incident to a physician.) In that case, the physician/NPP is the supplier of service, the NPI of the supervising physician/NPP is reported on the claim with the service and all the rules for both therapy services and incident to services (§230.5) must be followed.

B. Private Practice Defined

Reference: Federal Register November, 1998, pages 58863-58869; 42CFR 410.38(b), 42CFR410.59, 42CFR410.60, 42CFR410.62

The contractor considers a therapist to be in private practice if the therapist maintains office space at his or her own expense and furnishes services only in that space or the patient's home. Or, a therapist is employed by another supplier and furnishes services in facilities provided at the expense of that supplier.

The therapist need not be in full-time private practice but must be engaged in private practice on a regular basis; i.e., the therapist is recognized as a private practitioner and for that purpose has access to the necessary equipment to provide an adequate program of therapy.

The therapy services must be provided either by or under the direct supervision of the TPP. Each TPP should be enrolled as a Medicare provider. If a therapist is not enrolled, the services of that therapist must be directly supervised by an enrolled therapist. Direct supervision requires that the supervising private practice therapist be present in the office suite at the time the service is performed. These direct supervision requirements apply only in the private practice setting and only for therapists and their assistants. In other outpatient settings, supervision rules differ. The services of support personnel must be included in the therapist's bill. The supporting personnel, including other therapists, must be W-2 or 1099 employees of the TPP or other qualified employer.

Coverage of outpatient therapy under Part B includes the services of a qualified TPP when furnished in the therapist's office or at the beneficiary's home. For this purpose, "home" includes an institution that is used as a home, but not a hospital, CAH or SNF, (Federal Register Nov. 2, 1998, pg 58869).

C. Assignment

Reference: Nov. 2, 1998 Federal Register, pg. 58863

See also Pub. 100-4 chapter 1, §30.2.

When physicians, NPPs, or TPPs obtain provider numbers, they have the option of accepting assignment (participating) or not accepting assignment

(nonparticipating). In contrast, providers, such as outpatient hospitals, SNFs, rehabilitation agencies, and CORFs, do not have the option. For these providers, assignment is mandatory.

If physicians/NPPs, or TPPs accept assignment (are participating), they must accept the Medicare Physician Fee Schedule amount as payment. Medicare pays 80% and the patient is responsible for 20%. In contrast, if they do not accept assignment, Medicare will only pay 95% of the fee schedule amount. However, when these services are not furnished on an assignment-related basis, the limiting charge applies. (See §1848(g)(2)(c) of the Act.)

NOTE: Services furnished by a therapist in the therapist's office under arrangements with hospitals in rural communities and public health agencies (or services provided in the beneficiary's home under arrangements with a provider of outpatient physical or occupational therapy services) are not covered under this provision. See section 230.6.

100-02, 15, 232

Cardiac Rehabilitation (CR) and Intensive Cardiac Rehabilitation (ICR) Services Furnished On or After January 1, 2010

Cardiac rehabilitation (CR) services mean a physician-supervised program that furnishes physician prescribed exercise, cardiac risk factor modification, including education, counseling, and behavioral intervention; psychosocial assessment, outcomes assessment, and other items/services as determined by the Secretary under certain conditions. Intensive cardiac rehabilitation (ICR) services mean a physician-supervised program that furnishes the same items/services under the same conditions as a CR program but must also demonstrate, as shown in peer-reviewed published research, that it improves patients' cardiovascular disease through specific outcome measurements described in 42 CFR 410.49(c). Effective January 1, 2010, Medicare Part B pays for CR/ICR programs and related items/services if specific criteria is met by the Medicare beneficiary, the CR/ICR program itself, the setting in which is it administered, and the physician administering the program, as outlined below:

CR/ICR Program Beneficiary Requirements:

Medicare covers CR/ICR program services for beneficiaries who have experienced one or more of the following:

- Acute myocardial infarction within the preceding 12 months;
- Coronary artery bypass surgery;
- Current stable angina pectoris;
- Heart valve repair or replacement;
- Percutaneous transluminal coronary angioplasty (PTCA) or coronary stenting;
- Heart or heart-lung transplant.

For cardiac rehabilitation only: Stable, chronic heart failure defined as patients with left ventricular ejection fraction of 35% or less and New York Heart Association (NYHA) class II to IV symptoms despite being on optimal heart failure therapy for at least 6 weeks. (Effective February 18, 2014.)

CR/ICR Program Component Requirements:

- Physician-prescribed exercise. This physical activity includes aerobic exercise combined with other types of exercise (i.e., strengthening, stretching) as determined to be appropriate for individual patients by a physician each day CR/ICR items/services are furnished.
- Cardiac risk factor modification. This includes education, counseling, and behavioral intervention, tailored to the patients' individual needs.
- Psychosocial assessment. This assessment means an evaluation of an individual's mental and emotional functioning as it relates to the individual's rehabilitation. It should include: (1) an assessment of those aspects of the individual's family and home situation that affects the individual's rehabilitation treatment and, (2) a psychosocial evaluation of the individual's response to, and rate of progress under, the treatment plan.
- Outcomes assessment. These should include: (i) minimally, assessments from the commencement and conclusion of CR/ICR, based on patient-centered outcomes which must be measured by the physician immediately at the beginning and end of the program, and, (ii) objective clinical measures of the effectiveness of the CR/ICR program for the individual patient, including exercise performance and self-reported measures of exertion and behavior.
- Individualized treatment plan. This plan should be written and tailored to each individual patient and include (i) a description of the individual's diagnosis; (ii) the type, amount, frequency, and duration of the CR/ICR items/services furnished; and (iii) the goals set for the individual under the plan. The individualized treatment plan must be established, reviewed, and signed by a physician every 30 days.

As specified at 42 CFR 410.49(f)(1), CR sessions are limited to a maximum of 2 1-hour sessions per day for up to 36 sessions over up to 36 weeks with the option for an additional 36 sessions over an extended period of time if approved by the contractor under section 1862(a)(1)(A) of the Act. ICR sessions are limited to 72 1-hour sessions (as defined in section 1848(b)(5) of the Act), up to 6 sessions per day, over a period of up to 18 weeks.

CR/ICR Program Setting Requirements:

CR/ICR services must be furnished in a physician's office or a hospital outpatient setting (for ICR, the hospital outpatient setting must provide ICR using an approved

ICR program). All settings must have a physician immediately available and accessible for medical consultations and emergencies at all times when items/services are being furnished under the program. This provision is satisfied if the physician meets the requirements for direct supervision of physician office services as specified at 42 CFR 410.26, and for hospital outpatient services as specified at 42 CFR 410.27.

ICR Program Approval Requirements:

All prospective ICR programs must be approved through the national coverage determination (NCD) process. To be approved as an ICR program, it must demonstrate through peer-reviewed, published research that it has accomplished one or more of the following for its patients: (i) positively affected the progression of coronary heart disease, (ii) reduced the need for coronary bypass surgery, or, (iii) reduced the need for percutaneous coronary interventions.

An ICR program must also demonstrate through peer-reviewed, published research that it accomplished a statistically significant reduction in five or more of the following measures for patients from their levels before CR services to after CR services: (i) low density lipoprotein, (ii) triglycerides, (iii) body mass index, (iv) systolic blood pressure, (v) diastolic blood pressure, and (vi) the need for cholesterol, blood pressure, and diabetes medications.

A list of approved ICR programs, identified through the NCD process, will be posted to the CMS Web site and listed in the Federal Register.

Once an ICR program is approved through the NCD process, all prospective ICR sites wishing to furnish ICR items/services via an approved ICR program may enroll with their local contractor to become an ICR program supplier using the designated forms as specified at 42 CFR 424.510, and report specialty code 31 to be identified as an enrolled ICR supplier. For purposes of appealing an adverse determination concerning site approval, an ICR site is considered a supplier (or prospective supplier) as defined in 42 CFR 498.2.

CR/ICR Program Physician Requirements:

Physicians responsible for CR/ICR programs are identified as medical directors who oversee or supervise the CR/ICR program at a particular site. The medical director, in consultation with staff, is involved in directing the progress of individuals in the program. The medical director, as well as physicians acting as the supervising physician, must possess all of the following: (1) expertise in the management of individuals with cardiac pathophysiology, (2) cardiopulmonary training in basic life support or advanced cardiac life support, and (3) licensed to practice medicine in the state in which the CR/ICR program is offered. Direct physician supervision may be provided by a supervising physician or the medical director.

(See Pub. 100-3, Medicare National Coverage Determinations Manual, Chapter 1, Part 1, section 20.10.1, Pub. 100-4, Medicare Claims Processing Manual, Chapter 32, section 140, Pub. 100-08, Medicare Program Integrity Manual, Chapter 15, section 15.4.2.8, for specific claims processing, coding, and billing requirements for CR/ICR program services.)

100-02, 15, 240

Chiropractic Services - General

B3-2250, B3-4118

The term "physician" under Part B includes a chiropractor who meets the specified qualifying requirements set forth in Sec.30.5 but only for treatment by means of manual manipulation of the spine to correct a subluxation.

Effective for claims with dates of services on or after January 1, 2000, an x-ray is not required to demonstrate the subluxation.

Implementation of the chiropractic benefit requires an appreciation of the differences between chiropractic theory and experience and traditional medicine due to fundamental differences regarding etiology and theories of the pathogenesis of disease. Judgments about the reasonableness of chiropractic treatment must be based on the application of chiropractic principles. So that Medicare beneficiaries receive equitable adjudication of claims based on such principles and are not deprived of the benefits intended by the law, carriers may use chiropractic consultation in carrier review of Medicare chiropractic claims.

Payment is based on the physician fee schedule and made to the beneficiary or, on assignment, to the chiropractor.

A. Verification of Chiropractor's Qualifications

Carriers must establish a reference file of chiropractors eligible for payment as physicians under the criteria in Sec.30.1. They pay only chiropractors on file. Information needed to establish such files is furnished by the CMS RO.

The RO is notified by the appropriate State agency which chiropractors are licensed and whether each meets the national uniform standards.

100-02, 15, 240.1.3

Necessity for Treatment

The patient must have a significant health problem in the form of a neuromusculoskeletal condition necessitating treatment, and the manipulative services rendered must have a direct therapeutic relationship to the patient's condition and provide reasonable expectation of recovery or improvement of function. The patient must have a subluxation of the spine as demonstrated by x-ray or physical exam, as described above.

Most spinal joint problems fall into the following categories:

- Acute subluxation-A patient's condition is considered acute when the patient is being treated for a new injury, identified by x-ray or physical exam as specified above. The result of chiropractic manipulation is expected to be an improvement in, or arrest of progression, of the patient's condition.

- Chronic subluxation-A patient's condition is considered chronic when it is not expected to significantly improve or be resolved with further treatment (as is the case with an acute condition), but where the continued therapy can be expected to result in some functional improvement. Once the clinical status has remained stable for a given condition, without expectation of additional objective clinical improvements, further manipulative treatment is considered maintenance therapy and is not covered.

For Medicare purposes, a chiropractor must place an AT modifier on a claim when providing active/corrective treatment to treat acute or chronic subluxation. However the presence of the AT modifier may not in all instances indicate that the service is reasonable and necessary. As always, contractors may deny if appropriate after medical review.

A. Maintenance Therapy

Maintenance therapy includes services that seek to prevent disease, promote health and prolong and enhance the quality of life, or maintain or prevent deterioration of a chronic condition. When further clinical improvement cannot reasonably be expected from continuous ongoing care, and the chiropractic treatment becomes supportive rather than corrective in nature, the treatment is then considered maintenance therapy. The AT modifier must not be placed on the claim when maintenance therapy has been provided. Claims without the AT modifier will be considered as maintenance therapy and denied. Chiropractors who give or receive from beneficiaries an ABN shall follow the instructions in Pub. 100-4, Medicare Claims Processing Manual, chapter 23, section 20.9.1.1 and include a GA (or in rare instances a GZ) modifier on the claim.

B. Contraindications

Dynamic thrust is the therapeutic force or maneuver delivered by the physician during manipulation in the anatomic region of involvement. A relative contraindication is a condition that adds significant risk of injury to the patient from dynamic thrust, but does not rule out the use of dynamic thrust. The doctor should discuss this risk with the patient and record this in the chart. The following are relative contraindications to dynamic thrust:

- Articular hyper mobility and circumstances where the stability of the joint is uncertain;

- Severe demineralization of bone;

- Benign bone tumors (spine);

- Bleeding disorders and anticoagulant therapy; and

- Radiculopathy with progressive neurological signs.

- Dynamic thrust is absolutely contraindicated near the site of demonstrated subluxation and proposed manipulation in the following:

- Acute arthropathies characterized by acute inflammation and ligamentous laxity and anatomic subluxation or dislocation; including acute rheumatoid arthritis and ankylosing spondylitis;

- Acute fractures and dislocations or healed fractures and dislocations with signs of instability;

- An unstable os odontoideum;

- Malignancies that involve the vertebral column;

- Infection of bones or joints of the vertebral column;

- Signs and symptoms of myelopathy or cauda equina syndrome;

- For cervical spinal manipulations, vertebrobasilar insufficiency syndrome; and

- A significant major artery aneurysm near the proposed manipulation.

100-02, 15, 280.5.1

Advance Care Planning (ACP) Furnished as an Optional Element with an Annual Wellness Visit (AWV) Upon Agreement with the Patient

(Rev. 216 Issued: 12-22-15, Effective: 01-01-16, Implementation: 01-04-16)

Beginning in CY 2016, CMS will treat an AWV and voluntary ACP that are furnished on the same day and by the same provider as a preventive service. Voluntary ACP services, upon agreement with the patient, will be an optional element of the AWV. (See section 1861(hhh)(2)(G) of the Act.) When ACP services are furnished as a part of an AWV, according to sections 1833(a)(1) and 1833(b)(10) of the Act, the coinsurance and deductible are waived.

Voluntary advance care planning means the face-to-face service between a physician (or other qualified health care professional) and the patient discussing advance directives, with or without completing relevant legal forms. An advance directive is a document appointing an agent and/or recording the wishes of a patient pertaining to his/her medical treatment at a future time should he/she lack decisional capacity at that time.

See Pub. 100-04, Medicare Claims Processing Manual, chapter 18, section 140.8 for claims processing and billing instructions.

100-02, 15, 290
Foot Care

A. Treatment of Subluxation of Foot

Subluxations of the foot are defined as partial dislocations or displacements of joint surfaces, tendons ligaments, or muscles of the foot. Surgical or nonsurgical treatments undertaken for the sole purpose of correcting a subluxated structure in the foot as an isolated entity are not covered.

However, medical or surgical treatment of subluxation of the ankle joint (talo-crural joint) is covered. In addition, reasonable and necessary medical or surgical services, diagnosis, or treatment for medical conditions that have resulted from or are associated with partial displacement of structures is covered. For example, if a patient has osteoarthritis that has resulted in a partial displacement of joints in the foot, and the primary treatment is for the osteoarthritis, coverage is provided.

B. Exclusions from Coverage

The following foot care services are generally excluded from coverage under both Part A and Part B. (See Sec. 290.F and Sec. 290.G for instructions on applying foot care exclusions.)

1. Treatment of Flat Foot

   The term "flat foot" is defined as a condition in which one or more arches of the foot have flattened out. Services or devices directed toward the care or correction of such conditions, including the prescription of supportive devices, are not covered.

2. Routine Foot Care

   Except as provided above, routine foot care is excluded from coverage. Services that normally are considered routine and not covered by Medicare include the following:

   — The cutting or removal of corns and calluses;

   — The trimming, cutting, clipping, or debriding of nails; and

   — Other hygienic and preventive maintenance care, such as cleaning and soaking the feet, the use of skin creams to maintain skin tone of either ambulatory or bedfast patients, and any other service performed in the absence of localized illness, injury, or symptoms involving the foot.

3. Supportive Devices for Feet Orthopedic shoes and other supportive devices for the feet generally are not covered.

   However, this exclusion does not apply to such a shoe if it is an integral part of a leg brace, and its expense is included as part of the cost of the brace. Also, this exclusion does not apply to therapeutic shoes furnished to diabetics.

C. Exceptions to Routine Foot Care Exclusion

1. Necessary and Integral Part of Otherwise Covered Services

   In certain circumstances, services ordinarily considered to be routine may be covered if they are performed as a necessary and integral part of otherwise covered services, such as diagnosis and treatment of ulcers, wounds, or infections.

2. Treatment of Warts on Foot

   The treatment of warts (including plantar warts) on the foot is covered to the same extent as services provided for the treatment of warts located elsewhere on the body.

3. Presence of Systemic Condition

   The presence of a systemic condition such as metabolic, neurologic, or peripheral vascular disease may require scrupulous foot care by a professional that in the absence of such condition(s) would be considered routine (and, therefore, excluded from coverage). Accordingly, foot care that would otherwise be considered routine may be covered when systemic condition(s) result in severe circulatory embarrassment or areas of diminished sensation in the individual's legs or feet. (See subsection A.)

   In these instances, certain foot care procedures that otherwise are considered routine (e.g., cutting or removing corns and calluses, or trimming, cutting, clipping, or debriding nails) may pose a hazard when performed by a nonprofessional person on patients with such systemic conditions. (See Sec.290.G for procedural instructions.)

4. Mycotic Nails

   In the absence of a systemic condition, treatment of mycotic nails may be covered.

   The treatment of mycotic nails for an ambulatory patient is covered only when the physician attending the patient's mycotic condition documents that (1) there is clinical evidence of mycosis of the toenail, and (2) the patient has marked limitation of ambulation, pain, or secondary infection resulting from the thickening and dystrophy of the infected toenail plate.

   The treatment of mycotic nails for a nonambulatory patient is covered only when the physician attending the patient's mycotic condition documents that (1) there is clinical evidence of mycosis of the toenail, and (2) the patient suffers from pain or secondary infection resulting from the thickening and dystrophy of the infected toenail plate.

   For the purpose of these requirements, documentation means any written information that is required by the carrier in order for services to be covered. Thus, the information submitted with claims must be substantiated by information found in the patient's medical record. Any information, including that contained in a form letter, used for documentation purposes is subject to carrier verification in order to ensure that the information adequately justifies coverage of the treatment of mycotic nails.

D. Systemic Conditions That Might Justify Coverage

Although not intended as a comprehensive list, the following metabolic, neurologic, and peripheral vascular diseases (with synonyms in parentheses) most commonly represent the underlying conditions that might justify coverage for routine foot care.

Diabetes mellitus *

Arteriosclerosis obliterans (A.S.O., arteriosclerosis of the extremities, occlusive peripheral arteriosclerosis)

Buerger's disease (thromboangiitis obliterans)

Chronic thrombophlebitis *

Peripheral neuropathies involving the feet -

— Associated with malnutrition and vitamin deficiency *

   – Malnutrition (general, pellagra)

   – Alcoholism

   – Malabsorption (celiac disease, tropical sprue)

   – Pernicious anemia Associated with carcinoma *

— Associated with diabetes mellitus *

— Associated with drugs and toxins *

— Associated with multiple sclerosis *

— Associated with uremia (chronic renal disease) *

— Associated with traumatic injury

— Associated with leprosy or neurosyphilis

— Associated with hereditary disorders

   – Hereditary sensory radicular neuropathy

   – Angiokeratoma corporis diffusum (Fabry's)

   – Amyloid neuropathy

When the patient's condition is one of those designated by an asterisk (*), routine procedures are covered only if the patient is under the active care of a doctor of medicine or osteopathy who documents the condition.

E. Supportive Devices for Feet Orthopedic shoes and other supportive devices for the feet generally are not covered.

However, this exclusion does not apply to such a shoe if it is an integral part of a leg brace, and its expense is included as part of the cost of the brace. Also, this exclusion does not apply to therapeutic shoes furnished to diabetics.

F. Presumption of Coverage

In evaluating whether the routine services can be reimbursed, a presumption of coverage may be made where the evidence available discloses certain physical and/or clinical findings consistent with the diagnosis and indicative of severe peripheral involvement.

For purposes of applying this presumption the following findings are pertinent:

Class A Findings

Nontraumatic amputation of foot or integral skeletal portion thereof.

Class B Findings

Absent posterior tibial pulse;

Advanced trophic changes as: hair growth (decrease or absence) nail changes (thickening) pigmentary changes (discoloration) skin texture (thin, shiny) skin color (rubor or redness) (Three required); and

Absent dorsalis pedis pulse.

Class C Findings

Claudication;

Temperature changes (e.g., cold feet);

Edema;

Paresthesias (abnormal spontaneous sensations in the feet); and

Burning.

The presumption of coverage may be applied when the physician rendering the routine foot care has identified:

1. A Class A finding;

2. Two of the Class B findings; or

3. One Class B and two Class C findings.

Cases evidencing findings falling short of these alternatives may involve podiatric treatment that may constitute covered care and should be reviewed by the intermediary's medical staff and developed as necessary.

For purposes of applying the coverage presumption where the routine services have been rendered by a podiatrist, the contractor may deem the active care requirement met if the claim or other evidence available discloses that the patient has seen an M.D. or D.O. for treatment and/or evaluation of the complicating disease process during the 6-month period prior to the rendition of the routine-type services. The intermediary may also accept the podiatrist's statement that the diagnosing and treating M.D. or D.O. also concurs with the podiatrist's findings as to the severity of the peripheral involvement indicated.

Services ordinarily considered routine might also be covered if they are performed as a necessary and integral part of otherwise covered services, such as diagnosis and treatment of diabetic ulcers, wounds, and infections.

G. Application of Foot Care Exclusions to Physician's Services

The exclusion of foot care is determined by the nature of the service. Thus, payment for an excluded service should be denied whether performed by a podiatrist, osteopath, or a doctor of medicine, and without regard to the difficulty or complexity of the procedure.

When an itemized bill shows both covered services and noncovered services not integrally related to the covered service, the portion of charges attributable to the noncovered services should be denied. (For example, if an itemized bill shows surgery for an ingrown toenail and also removal of calluses not necessary for the performance of toe surgery, any additional charge attributable to removal of the calluses should be denied.) In reviewing claims involving foot care, the carrier should be alert to the following exceptional situations:

1. Payment may be made for incidental noncovered services performed as a necessary and integral part of, and secondary to, a covered procedure. For example, if trimming of toenails is required for application of a cast to a fractured foot, the carrier need not allocate and deny a portion of the charge for the trimming of the nails. However, a separately itemized charge for such excluded service should be disallowed. When the primary procedure is covered the administration of anesthesia necessary for the performance of such procedure is also covered.

2. Payment may be made for initial diagnostic services performed in connection with a specific symptom or complaint if it seems likely that its treatment would be covered even though the resulting diagnosis may be one requiring only noncovered care.

The name of the M.D. or D.O. who diagnosed the complicating condition must be submitted with the claim. In those cases, where active care is required, the approximate date the beneficiary was last seen by such physician must also be indicated.

NOTE: Section 939 of P.L. 96-499 removed "warts" from the routine foot care exclusion effective July 1, 1981.

Relatively few claims for routine-type care are anticipated considering the severity of conditions contemplated as the basis for this exception. Claims for this type of foot care should not be paid in the absence of convincing evidence that nonprofessional performance of the service would have been hazardous for the beneficiary because of an underlying systemic disease. The mere statement of a diagnosis such as those mentioned in Sec.D above does not of itself indicate the severity of the condition. Where development is indicated to verify diagnosis and/or severity the carrier should follow existing claims processing practices, which may include review of carrier's history and medical consultation as well as physician contacts.

The rules in Sec.290.F concerning presumption of coverage also apply.

Codes and policies for routine foot care and supportive devices for the feet are not exclusively for the use of podiatrists. These codes must be used to report foot care services regardless of the specialty of the physician who furnishes the services. Carriers must instruct physicians to use the most appropriate code available when billing for routine foot care.

100-02, 16, 10

General Exclusions From Coverage

A3-3150, HO-260, HHA-232, B3-2300

No payment can be made under either the hospital insurance or supplementary medicalinsurance program for certain items and services, when the following conditions exist:

- Not reasonable and necessary (§20);
- No legal obligation to pay for or provide (§40);
- Paid for by a governmental entity (§50);
- Not provided within United States (§60);
- Resulting from war (§70);
- Personal comfort (§80);
- Routine services and appliances (§90);
- Custodial care (§110);
- Cosmetic surgery (§120);
- Charges by immediate relatives or members of household (§130);
- Dental services (§140);
- Paid or expected to be paid under workers' compensation (§150);
- Nonphysician services provided to a hospital inpatient that were not provided directly or arranged for by the hospital (§170);
- Services Related to and Required as a Result of Services Which are not Covered Under Medicare (§180);
- Excluded foot care services and supportive devices for feet (§30); or

- Excluded investigational devices (See Chapter 14, §30).

100-02, 16, 100

Hearing Aids and Auditory Implants

Section 1862(a)(7) of the Social Security Act states that no payment may be made under part A or part B for any expenses incurred for items or services "where such expenses are for . . . hearing aids or examinations therefore. . . ." This policy is further reiterated at 42 CFR 411.15(d) which specifically states that "hearing aids or examination for the purpose of prescribing, fitting, or changing hearing aids" are excluded from coverage.

Hearing aids are amplifying devices that compensate for impaired hearing. Hearing aids include air conduction devices that provide acoustic energy to the cochlea via stimulation of the tympanic membrane with amplified sound. They also include bone conduction devices that provide mechanical energy to the cochlea via stimulation of the scalp with amplified mechanical vibration or by direct contact with the tympanic membrane or middle ear ossicles.

Certain devices that produce perception of sound by replacing the function of the middle ear, cochlea or auditory nerve are payable by Medicare as prosthetic devices. These devices are indicated only when hearing aids are medically inappropriate or cannot be utilized due to congenital malformations, chronic disease, severe sensorineural hearing loss or surgery. The following are prosthetic devices:

- Cochlear implants and auditory brainstem implants, i.e., devices that replace the function of cochlear structures or auditory nerve and provide electrical energy to auditory nerve fibers and other neural tissue via implanted electrode arrays.

- Osseointegrated implants, i.e., devices implanted in the skull that replace the function of the middle ear and provide mechanical energy to the cochlea via a mechanical transducer.

Medicare contractors deny payment for an item or service that is associated with any hearing aid as defined above. See Sec.180 for policy for the medically necessary treatment of complications of implantable hearing aids, such as medically necessary removals of implantable hearing aids due to infection.

100-02, 16, 120

Cosmetic Surgery

A3-3160, HO-260.11, B3-2329

Cosmetic surgery or expenses incurred in connection with such surgery is not covered. Cosmetic surgery includes any surgical procedure directed at improving appearance, except when required for the prompt (i.e., as soon as medically feasible) repair of accidental injury or for the improvement of the functioning of a malformed body member. For example, this exclusion does not apply to surgery in connection with treatment of severe burns or repair of the face following a serious automobile accident, or to surgery for therapeutic purposes which coincidentally also serves some cosmetic purpose.

100-02, 16, 180

Services Related to and Required as a Result of Services Which Are Not Covered Under Medicare

B3-2300.1, A3-3101.14, HO-210.12

Medical and hospital services are sometimes required to treat a condition that arises as a result of services that are not covered because they are determined to be not reasonable and necessary or because they are excluded from coverage for other reasons. Services "related to" noncovered services (e.g., cosmetic surgery, noncovered organ transplants, noncovered artificial organ implants, etc.), including services related to follow-up care and complications of noncovered services which require treatment during a hospital stay in which the noncovered service was performed, are not covered services under Medicare. Services "not related to" noncovered services are covered under Medicare. Following are examples of services "related to" and "not related to" noncovered services while the beneficiary is an inpatient:

- A beneficiary was hospitalized for a noncovered service and broke a leg while in the hospital. Services related to care of the broken leg during this stay is a clear example of "not related to" services and are covered under Medicare.

- A beneficiary was admitted to the hospital for covered services, but during the course of hospitalization became a candidate for a noncovered transplant or implant and actually received the transplant or implant during that hospital stay. When the original admission was entirely unrelated to the diagnosis that led to a recommendation for a noncovered transplant or implant, the services related to the admitting condition would be covered.

- A beneficiary was admitted to the hospital for covered services related to a condition which ultimately led to identification of a need for transplant and receipt of a transplant during the same hospital stay. If, on the basis of the nature of the services and a comparison of the date they are received with the date on which the beneficiary is identified as a transplant candidate, the services could reasonably be attributed to preparation for the noncovered transplant, the services would be "related to" noncovered services and would also be noncovered.

Following is an example of services received subsequent to a noncovered inpatient stay:

- After a beneficiary has been discharged from the hospital stay in which the beneficiary received noncovered services, medical and hospital services required to treat a condition or complication that arises as a result of the prior noncovered services may be covered when they are reasonable and necessary in all other respects. Thus, coverage could be provided for subsequent inpatient stays or outpatient treatment ordinarily covered by Medicare, even if the need for treatment arose because of a previous noncovered procedure. Some examples of services that may be found to be covered under this policy are the reversal of intestinal bypass surgery for obesity, repair of complications from transsexual surgery or from cosmetic surgery, removal of a noncovered bladder stimulator, or treatment of any infection at the surgical site of a noncovered transplant that occurred following discharge from the hospital.

However, any subsequent services that could be expected to have been incorporated into a global fee are considered to have been paid in the global fee, and may not be paid again. Thus, where a patient undergoes cosmetic surgery and the treatment regimen calls for a series of postoperative visits to the surgeon for evaluating the patient's progress, these visits are not paid.

100-03, 10.2

NCD for Transcutaneous Electrical Nerve Stimulation (TENS) for Acute Post-Operative Pain (10.2)

Indications and Limitations of Coverage

The use of Transcutaneous Electrical Nerve Stimulation (TENS) for the relief of acute post-operative pain is covered under Medicare. TENS may be covered whether used as an adjunct to the use of drugs, or as an alternative to drugs, in the treatment of acute pain resulting from surgery.

TENS devices, whether durable or disposable, may be used in furnishing this service. When used for the purpose of treating acute post-operative pain, TENS devices are considered supplies. As such they may be hospital supplies furnished inpatients covered under Part A, or supplies incident to a physician's service when furnished in connection with surgery done on an outpatient basis, and covered under Part B.

It is expected that TENS, when used for acute post-operative pain, will be necessary for relatively short periods of time, usually 30 days or less. In cases when TENS is used for longer periods, Medicare Administrative Contractors should attempt to ascertain whether TENS is no longer being used for acute pain but rather for chronic pain, in which case the TENS device may be covered as durable medical equipment as described in §160.27.

Cross-references:

Medicare Benefit Policy Manual, Chapter 1, "Inpatient Hospital Services," §40;

Medicare Benefit Policy Manual, Chapter 2, "Hospital Services Covered Under Part B," §§20, 20.4, and 80; Medicare Benefit Policy Manual, Chapter 15, "Covered Medical and other Health Services, §110."

100-03, 10.3

NCD for Inpatient Hospital Pain Rehabilitation Programs (10.3)

Since pain rehabilitation programs of a lesser scope than that described above would raise a question as to whether the program could be provided in a less intensive setting than on an inpatient hospital basis, carefully evaluate such programs to determine whether the program does, in fact, necessitate a hospital level of care. Some pain rehabilitation programs may utilize services and devices which are excluded from coverage, e.g., acupuncture (see 35-8), biofeedback (see 35-27), dorsal column stimulator (see 65-8), and family counseling services (see 35-l4). In determining whether the scope of a pain program does necessitate inpatient hospital care, evaluate only those services and devices which are covered. Although diagnostic tests may be an appropriate part of pain rehabilitation programs, such tests would be covered in an individual case only where they can be reasonably related to a patient's illness, complaint, symptom, or injury and where they do not represent an unnecessary duplication of tests previously performed.

An inpatient program of 4 weeks' duration is generally required to modify pain behavior. After this period it would be expected that any additional rehabilitation services which might be required could be effectively provided on an outpatient basis under an outpatient pain rehabilitation program (see 10.4 of the NCD Manual) or other outpatient program. The first 7-l0 days of such an inpatient program constitute, in effect, an evaluation period. If a patient is unable to adjust to the program within this period, it is generally concluded that it is unlikely that the program will be effective and the patient is discharged from the program. On occasions a program longer than 4 weeks may be required in a particular case. In such a case there should be documentation to substantiate that inpatient care beyond a 4-week period was reasonable and necessary. Similarly, where it appears that a patient participating in a program is being granted frequent outside passes, a question would exist as to whether an inpatient program is reasonable and necessary for the treatment of the patient's condition.

An inpatient hospital stay for the purpose of participating in a pain rehabilitation program would be covered as reasonable and necessary to the treatment of a patient's condition where the pain is attributable to a physical cause, the usual methods of treatment have not been successful in alleviating it, and a significant loss of ability to function independently has resulted from the pain. Chronic pain patients often have psychological problems which accompany or stem from the physical pain and it is appropriate to include psychological treatment in the multidisciplinary approach. However, patients whose pain symptoms result from a mental condition, rather than from any physical cause, generally cannot be succesfully treated in a pain rehabilitation program.

100-03, 10.4

NCD for Outpatient Hospital Pain Rehabilitation Programs (10.4)

Coverage of services furnished under outpatient hospital pain rehabilitation programs, including services furnished in group settings under individualized plans of treatment, is available if the patient's pain is attributable to a physical cause, the usual methods of treatment have not been successful in alleviating it, and a significant loss of ability by the patient to function independently has resulted from the pain. If a patient meets these conditions and the program provides services of the types discussed in §10.3, the services provided under the program may be covered. Non-covered services (e.g., vocational counseling, meals for outpatients, or acupuncture) continue to be excluded from coverage, and A/B Medicare Administrative Contractors would not be precluded from finding, in the case of particular patients, that the pain rehabilitation program is not reasonable and necessary under §1862(a)(1) of the Social Security Act for the treatment of their conditions.

100-03, 10.5

NCD for Autogenous Epidural Blood Graft (10.5)

Autogenous epidural blood grafts are considered a safe and effective remedy for severe headaches that may occur after performance of spinal anesthesia, spinal taps or myelograms, and are covered.

100-03, 10.6

NCD for Anesthesia in Cardiac Pacemaker Surgery (10.6)

The use of general or monitored anesthesia during transvenous cardiac pacemaker surgery may be reasonable and necessary and therefore covered under Medicare only if adequate documentation of medical necessity is provided on a case-by-case basis. The Medicare Adminstrative Contractor obtains advice from its medical consultants or from appropriate specialty physicians or groups in its locality regarding the adequacy of documentation before deciding whether a particular claim should be covered.

A second type of pacemaker surgery that is sometimes performed involves the use of the thoracic method of implantation which requires open surgery. Where the thoracic method is employed, general anesthesia is always used and should not require special medical documentation.

100-03, 20.2

NCD for Extracranial-Intracranial (EC-IC) Arterial Bypass Surgery (20.2)

Extracranial-Intracranial (EC-IC) arterial bypass surgery is not a covered procedure when it is performed as a treatment for ischemic cerebrovascular disease of the carotid or middle cerebral arteries which includes the treatment or prevention of strokes. The premise that this procedure which bypasses narrowed arterial segments, improves the blood supply to the brain and reduces the risk of having a stroke has not been demonstrated to be any more effective than no surgical intervention. Accordingly, EC-IC arterial bypass surgery is not considered reasonable and necessary within the meaning of §1862(a)(1) of the Act when it is performed as a treatment for ischemic cerebrovascular disease of the carotid or middle cerebral arteries.

100-03, 20.12

NCD for Diagnostic Endocardial Electrical Stimulation (Pacing) (20.12)

Diagnostic endocardial electrical stimulation (EES), also called programmed electrical stimulation of the heart, is covered under Medicare when used for patients with severe cardiac arrhythmias.

100-03, 20.19

NCD for Ambulatory Blood Pressure Monitoring (20.19)

ABPM must be performed for at least 24 hours to meet coverage criteria.

ABPM is only covered for those patients with suspected white coat hypertension. Suspected white coat hypertension is defined as

1) office blood pressure > 140/90 mm Hg on at least three separate clinic/office visits with two separate measurements made at each visit;

2) at least two documented blood pressure measurements taken outside the office which are < 140/90 mm Hg; and

3) no evidence of end-organ damage.

The information obtained by ABPM is necessary in order to determine the appropriate management of the patient. ABPM is not covered for any other uses. In the rare circumstance that ABPM needs to be performed more than once in a patient, the qualifying criteria described above must be met for each subsequent ABPM test.

For those patients that undergo ABPM and have an ambulatory blood pressure of < 135/85 with no evidence of end-organ damage, it is likely that their cardiovascular risk is similar to that of normotensives. They should be followed over time. Patients for which ABPM demonstrates a blood pressure of > 135/85 may be at increased cardiovascular risk, and a physician may wish to consider antihypertensive therapy.

100-03, 20.26

NCD for Partial Ventriculectomy (20.26)

Since the mortality rate is high and there are no published scientific articles or clinical studies regarding partial ventriculectomy, this procedure cannot be considered reasonable and necessary within the meaning of Sec.1862(a)(1) of the Act. Therefore, partial ventriculectomy is not covered by Medicare.

100-03, 20.28

NCD for Therapeutic Embolization (20.28)

Therapeutic embolization is covered when done for hemorrhage, and for other conditions amenable to treatment by the procedure, when reasonable and necessary for the individual patient. Renal embolization for the treatment of renal adenocarcinoma continues to be covered, effective December 15, 1978, as one type of therapeutic embolization, to:

- Reduce tumor vascularity preoperatively;
- Reduce tumor bulk in inoperable cases; or
- Palliate specific symptoms.

100-03, 20.29

NCD for Hyperbaric Oxygen Therapy (20.29)

A. Covered Conditions

Program reimbursement for HBO therapy will be limited to that which is administered in a chamber (including the one man unit) and is limited to the following conditions:

1. Acute carbon monoxide intoxication,
2. Decompression illness,
3. Gas embolism,
4. Gas gangrene,
5. Acute traumatic peripheral ischemia. HBO therapy is a valuable adjunctive treatment to be used in combination with accepted standard therapeutic measures when loss of function, limb, or life is threatened.
6. Crush injuries and suturing of severed limbs. As in the previous conditions, HBO therapy would be an adjunctive treatment when loss of function, limb, or life is threatened.
7. Progressive necrotizing infections (necrotizing fasciitis),
8. Acute peripheral arterial insufficiency,
9. Preparation and preservation of compromised skin grafts (not for primary management of wounds),
10. Chronic refractory osteomyelitis, unresponsive to conventional medical and surgical management,
11. Osteoradionecrosis as an adjunct to conventional treatment,
12. Soft tissue radionecrosis as an adjunct to conventional treatment,
13. Cyanide poisoning,
14. Actinomycosis, only as an adjunct to conventional therapy when the disease process is refractory to antibiotics and surgical treatment,
14. Diabetic wounds of the lower extremities in patients who meet the following three criteria:
    a. Patient has type I or type II diabetes and has a lower extremity wound that is due to diabetes;
    b. Patient has a wound classified as Wagner grade III or higher; and
    c. Patient has failed an adequate course of standard wound therapy.

The use of HBO therapy is covered as adjunctive therapy only after there are no measurable signs of healing for at least 30 -days of treatment with standard wound therapy and must be used in addition to standard wound care. Standard wound care in patients with diabetic wounds includes: assessment of a patient's vascular status and correction of any vascular problems in the affected limb if possible, optimization of nutritional status, optimization of glucose control, debridement by any means to remove devitalized tissue, maintenance of a clean, moist bed of granulation tissue with appropriate moist dressings, appropriate off-loading, and necessary treatment to resolve any infection that might be present. Failure to respond to standard wound care occurs when there are no measurable signs of healing for at least 30 consecutive days. Wounds must be evaluated at least every 30 days during administration of HBO therapy. Continued treatment with HBO therapy is not covered if measurable signs of healing have not been demonstrated within any 30-day period of treatment.

B. Noncovered Conditions

All other indications not specified under Sec.270.4(A) are not covered under the Medicare program. No program payment may be made for any conditions other than those listed in Sec. 270.4(A).

No program payment may be made for HBO in the treatment of the following conditions:

1. Cutaneous, decubitus, and stasis ulcers.
2. Chronic peripheral vascular insufficiency.
3. Anaerobic septicemia and infection other than clostridial.
4. Skin burns (thermal).
5. Senility.
6. Myocardial infarction.
7. Cardiogenic shock.
8. Sickle cell anemia.
9. Acute thermal and chemical pulmonary damage, i.e., smoke inhalation with pulmonary insufficiency.
10. Acute or chronic cerebral vascular insufficiency.
11. Hepatic necrosis.
12. Aerobic septicemia.
13. Nonvascular causes of chronic brain syndrome (Pick's disease, Alzheimer's disease, Korsakoff's disease).
14. Tetanus.
15. Systemic aerobic infection.
16. Organ transplantation.
17. Organ storage.
18. Pulmonary emphysema.
19. Exceptional blood loss anemia.
20. Multiple Sclerosis.
21. Arthritic Diseases.
22. Acute cerebral edema.

C. Topical Application of Oxygen

This method of administering oxygen does not meet the definition of HBO therapy as stated above. Also, its clinical efficacy has not been established. Therefore, no Medicare reimbursement may be made for the topical application of oxygen.

100-03, 20.30

NCD for Microvolt T-Wave Alternans (MTWA) (20.30)

B. Nationally Covered Indications

Microvolt T-wave Alternans diagnostic testing is covered for the evaluation of patients at risk for SCD, only when the spectral analysis method is used.

C. Nationally Non-Covered Indications

Microvolt T-wave Alternans diagnostic test is non-covered for the evaluation of patients at risk for SCD if measurement is not performed employing the spectral analysis.

D. Other

N/A

100-03, 20.32

Transcatheter Aortic Valve Replacement (TAVR)

A. General

Transcatheter aortic valve replacement (TAVR - also known as TAVI or transcatheter aortic valve implantation) is used in the treatment of aortic stenosis. A bioprosthetic valve is inserted percutaneously using a catheter and implanted in the orifice of the aortic valve.

B. Nationally Covered Indications

The Centers for Medicare & Medicaid Services (CMS) covers transcatheter aortic valve replacement (TAVR) under Coverage with Evidence Development (CED) with the following conditions:

A. TAVR is covered for the treatment of symptomatic aortic valve stenosis when furnished according to a Food and Drug Administration (FDA)-approved indication and when all of the following conditions are met:

1. The procedure is furnished with a complete aortic valve and implantation system that has received FDA premarket approval (PMA) for that system's FDA approved indication.

2. Two cardiac surgeons have independently examined the patient face-to-face and evaluated the patient's suitability for open aortic valve replacement (AVR) surgery; and both surgeons have documented the rationale for their clinical judgment and the rationale is available to the heart team.

3. The patient (preoperatively and postoperatively) is under the care of a heart team: a cohesive, multi-disciplinary, team of medical professionals. The heart team concept embodies collaboration and dedication across medical specialties to offer optimal patient-centered care.

    TAVR must be furnished in a hospital with the appropriate infrastructure that includes but is not limited to:

a. On-site heart valve surgery program,

b. Cardiac catheterization lab or hybrid operating room/catheterization lab equipped with a fixed radiographic imaging system with flat-panel fluoroscopy, offering quality imaging,

c. Non-invasive imaging such as echocardiography, vascular ultrasound, computed tomography (CT) and magnetic resonance (MR),

d. Sufficient space, in a sterile environment, to accommodate necessary equipment for cases with and without complications,

e. Post-procedure intensive care facility with personnel experienced in managing patients who have undergone open-heart valve procedures,

f. Appropriate volume requirements per the applicable qualifications below.

There are two sets of qualifications; the first set outlined below is for hospital programs and heart teams without previous TAVR experience and the second set is for those with TAVR experience.

Qualifications to begin a TAVR program for hospitals without TAVR experience:

The hospital program must have the following:

a. ≥ 50 total AVRs in the previous year prior to TAVR, including = 10 high-risk patients, and;

b. ≥ 2 physicians with cardiac surgery privileges, and;

c. ≥ 1000 catheterizations per year, including = 400 percutaneous coronary interventions (PCIs) per year.

Qualifications to begin a TAVR program for heart teams without TAVR experience:

The heart team must include:

a. Cardiovascular surgeon with:

i. ≥ 100 career AVRs including 10 high-risk patients; or,

ii. ≥ 25 AVRs in one year; or,

iii. ≥ 50 AVRs in 2 years; and which include at least 20 AVRs in the last year prior to TAVR initiation; and,

b. Interventional cardiologist with:

i. Professional experience with 100 structural heart disease procedures lifetime; or,

ii. 30 left-sided structural procedures per year of which 60% should be balloon aortic valvuloplasty (BAV). Atrial septal defect and patent foramen ovale closure are not considered left-sided procedures; and,

c. Additional members of the heart team such as echocardiographers, imaging specialists, heart failure specialists, cardiac anesthesiologists, intensivists, nurses, and social workers; and,

d. Device-specific training as required by the manufacturer.

Qualifications for hospital programs with TAVR experience:

The hospital program must maintain the following:

a. ≥ 20 AVRs per year or = 40 AVRs every 2 years; and,

b. ≥ 2 physicians with cardiac surgery privileges; and,

c. ≥ 1000 catheterizations per year, including = 400 percutaneous coronary interventions (PCIs) per year.

Qualifications for heart teams with TAVR experience:

The heart team must include:

a. cardiovascular surgeon and an interventional cardiologist whose combined experience maintains the following:

i. ≥ 20 TAVR procedures in the prior year, or,

ii. ≥ 40 TAVR procedures in the prior 2 years; and,

b. Additional members of the heart team such as echocardiographers, imaging specialists, heart failure specialists, cardiac anesthesiologists, intensivists, nurses, and social workers.

4. The heart team's interventional cardiologist(s) and cardiac surgeon(s) must jointly participate in the intra-operative technical aspects of TAVR.

5. The heart team and hospital are participating in a prospective, national, audited registry that: 1) consecutively enrolls TAVR patients; 2) accepts all manufactured devices; 3) follows the patient for at least one year; and, 4) complies with relevant regulations relating to protecting human research subjects, including 45 CFR Part 46 and 21 CFR Parts 50 & 56. The following outcomes must be tracked by the registry; and the registry must be designed to permit identification and analysis of patient, practitioner and facility level variables that predict each of these outcomes:

i. Stroke;

ii. All cause mortality;

iii. Transient Ischemic Attacks (TIAs);

iv. Major vascular events;

v. Acute kidney injury;

vi. Repeat aortic valve procedures;

vii. Quality of Life (QoL).

The registry should collect all data necessary and have a written executable analysis plan in place to address the following questions (to appropriately address some questions, Medicare claims or other outside data may be necessary):

– When performed outside a controlled clinical study, how do outcomes and adverse events compare to the pivotal clinical studies?

– How do outcomes and adverse events in subpopulations compare to patients in the pivotal clinical studies?

– What is the long term (≥ 5 year) durability of the device?

– What are the long term (≥ 5 year) outcomes and adverse events?

– How do the demographics of registry patients compare to the pivotal studies?

Consistent with section 1142 of the Act, the Agency for Healthcare Research and Quality (AHRQ) supports clinical research studies that CMS determines meet the above-listed standards and address the above-listed research questions.

B. TAVR is covered for uses that are not expressly listed as an FDA-approved indication when performed within a clinical study that fulfills all of the following.

1. The heart team's interventional cardiologist(s) and cardiac surgeon(s) must jointly participate in the intra-operative technical aspects of TAVR.

2. As a fully-described, written part of its protocol, the clinical research study must critically evaluate not only each patient's quality of life pre- and post-TAVR (minimum of 1 year), but must also address at least one of the following questions: § What is the incidence of stroke?

– What is the rate of all cause mortality?

– What is the incidence of transient ischemic attacks (TIAs)?

– What is the incidence of major vascular events?

– What is the incidence of acute kidney injury?

– What is the incidence of repeat aortic valve procedures?

3. The clinical study must adhere to the following standards of scientific integrity and relevance to the Medicare population:

a. The principal purpose of the research study is to test whether a particular intervention potentially improves the participants' health outcomes.

b. The research study is well supported by available scientific and medical information or it is intended to clarify or establish the health outcomes of interventions already in common clinical use.

c. The research study does not unjustifiably duplicate existing studies.

d. The research study design is appropriate to answer the research question being asked in the study.

e. The research study is sponsored by an organization or individual capable of executing the proposed study successfully.

f. The research study is in compliance with all applicable Federal regulations concerning the protection of human subjects found in the Code of Federal Regulations (CFR) at 45 CFR Part 46. If a study is regulated by the Food and Drug Administration (FDA), it also must be in compliance with 21 CFR Parts 50 and 56. In particular, the informed consent includes a straightforward explanation of the reported increased risks of stroke and vascular complications that have been published for TAVR.

g. All aspects of the research study are conducted according to appropriate standards of scientific integrity (see http://www.icmje.org).

h. The research study has a written protocol that clearly addresses, or incorporates by reference, the standards listed as Medicare coverage requirements.

i. The clinical research study is not designed to exclusively test toxicity or disease pathophysiology in healthy individuals. Trials of all medical technologies measuring therapeutic outcomes as one of the objectives meet this standard only if the disease or condition being studied is life threatening as defined in 21 CFR §312.81(a) and the patient has no other viable treatment options.

j. The clinical research study is registered on the www.ClinicalTrials.gov website by the principal sponsor/investigator prior to the enrollment of the first study subject.

k. The research study protocol specifies the method and timing of public release of all pre-specified outcomes to be measured including release of outcomes if outcomes are negative or study is terminated early. The results must be made public within 24 months of the end of data collection. If a report is planned to be published in a peer reviewed journal, then that initial release may be an abstract that meets the requirements of the International Committee of Medical Journal Editors (http://www.icmje.org). However a full report of the outcomes must be made public no later than three (3) years after the end of data collection.

l. The research study protocol must explicitly discuss subpopulations affected by the treatment under investigation, particularly traditionally underrepresented groups in clinical studies, how the inclusion and exclusion criteria affect enrollment of these populations, and a plan for the retention and reporting of said populations on the trial. If the inclusion and exclusion criteria are expected to have a negative effect on the recruitment or retention of underrepresented populations, the protocol must discuss why these criteria are necessary.

m. The research study protocol explicitly discusses how the results are or are not expected to be generalizable to the Medicare population to infer whether Medicare patients may benefit from the intervention. Separate discussions in the protocol may be necessary for populations eligible for Medicare due to age, disability or Medicaid eligibility. Consistent with section 1142 of the Act, AHRQ supports clinical research studies that CMS determines meet the above-listed standards and address the above-listed research questions.

4. The principal investigator must submit the complete study protocol, identify the relevant CMS research question(s) that will be addressed, and cite the location of the detailed analysis plan for those questions in the protocol, plus provide a statement addressing how the study satisfies each of the standards of scientific integrity (a. through m. listed above), as well as the investigator's contact information, to the address below. The information will be reviewed, and approved studies will be identified on the CMS Website.

> Director, Coverage and Analysis Group
> Re: TAVR CED
> Centers for Medicare & Medicaid Services (CMS)
> 7500 Security Blvd., Mail Stop S3-02-01
> Baltimore, MD 21244-1850

C. Nationally Non-Covered Indications
TAVR is not covered for patients in whom existing co-morbidities would preclude the expected benefit from correction of the aortic stenosis.

D.
NA

(This NCD last reviewed May 2012.)

100-03, 20.34

Percutaneous Left Atrial Appendage Closure (LAAC)
(Rev. 192, Issued: 05-06-16, Effective: 02-08-16, Implementation: 10-03-16)

A. General
Patients with atrial fibrillation (AF), an irregular heartbeat, are at an increased risk of stroke. The left atrial appendage (LAA) is a tubular structure that opens into the left atrium and has been shown to be one potential source for blood clots that can cause strokes. While thinning the blood with anticoagulant medications has been proven to prevent strokes, percutaneous LAA closure (LAAC) has been studied as a non-pharmacologic alternative for patients with AF.

B. Nationally Covered Indications
The Centers for Medicare & Medicaid Services (CMS) covers percutaneous LAAC for non-valvular atrial fibrillation (NVAF) through Coverage with Evidence Development (CED) with the following conditions:

a. LAAC devices are covered when the device has received Food and Drug Administration (FDA) Premarket Approval (PMA) for that device's FDA-approved indication and meet all of the conditions specified below:

The patient must have:

- A CHADS2 score ≥ 2 (Congestive heart failure, Hypertension, Age >75, Diabetes, Stroke/transient ischemia attack/thromboembolism) or CHA2DS2-VASc score ≥ 3 (Congestive heart failure, Hypertension, Age ≥ 65, Diabetes, Stroke/transient ischemia attack/thromboembolism, Vascular disease, Sex category)

- A formal shared decision making interaction with an independent non-interventional physician using an evidence-based decision tool on oral anticoagulation in patients with NVAF prior to LAAC. Additionally, the shared decision making interaction must be documented in the medical record.

- A suitability for short-term warfarin but deemed unable to take long-term oral anticoagulation following the conclusion of shared decision making, as LAAC is only covered as a second line therapy to oral anticoagulants. The patient (preoperatively and postoperatively) is under the care of a cohesive, multidisciplinary team (MDT) of medical professionals. The procedure must be furnished in a hospital with an established structural heart disease (SHD) and/or electrophysiology (EP) program.

The procedure must be performed by an interventional cardiologist(s), electrophysiologist(s), or cardiovascular surgeon (s) that meet the following criteria:

- Has received training prescribed by the manufacturer on the safe and effective use of the device prior to performing LAAC; and,

- Has performed ≥ 25 interventional cardiac procedures that involve transeptal puncture through an intact septum; and,

- Continues to perform ≥ 25 interventional cardiac procedures that involve transeptal puncture through an intact septum, of which at least 12 are LAAC, over a 2-year period.

The patient is enrolled in, and the MDT and hospital must participate in, a prospective, national, audited registry that: 1) consecutively enrolls LAAC patients, and, 2) tracks the following annual outcomes for each patient for a period of at least 4 years from the time of the LAAC:

- Operator-specific complications
- Device-specific complications including device thrombosis
- Stroke, adjudicated, by type
- Transient Ischemic Attack (TIA)
- Systemic embolism
- Death
- Major bleeding, by site and severity

The registry must be designed to permit identification and analysis of patient, practitioner, and facility level factors that predict patient risk for these outcomes. The registry must collect all data necessary to conduct analyses adjusted for relevant confounders, and have a written executable analysis plan in place to address the following questions:

- How do the outcomes listed above compare to outcomes in the pivotal clinical trials in the short term (≤12 months) and in the long term (≥ 4 years)?
- What is the long term (≥ 4 year) durability of the device?
- What are the short term (≤12 months) and the long term (≥4 years) device-specific complications including device thromboses?

To appropriately address some of these questions, Medicare claims or other outside data may be necessary.

Registries must be reviewed and approved by CMS. Potential registry sponsors must submit all registry documentation to CMS for approval, including the written executable analysis plan and auditing plan. CMS will review the qualifications of candidate registries to ensure that the approved registry follows standard data collection practices, and collects data necessary to evaluate the patient outcomes specified above. The registry's national clinical trial number must be recorded on the claim.

Consistent with section 1142 of the Social Security Act (the Act), the Agency for Healthcare Research and Quality (AHRQ) supports clinical research studies that CMS determines address the above-listed research questions and the a-m criteria listed in Section c. of this decision.

All approved registries will be posted on the CED website located at: https://www.cms.gov/Medicare/Coverage/Coverage-with-Evidence-Development/index.html.

b. LAAC is covered for NVAF patients not included in Section a. of this decision when performed within an FDA-approved randomized controlled trial (RCT) if such trials meet the criteria established below:

As a fully-described written part of its protocol, the RCT must critically answer, in comparison to optimal medical therapy, the following questions:

- As a primary endpoint, what is the true incidence of ischemic stroke and systemic embolism?
- As a secondary endpoint, what is cardiovascular mortality and all-cause mortality?

FDA-approved RCTs must be reviewed and approved by CMS. Consistent with section 1142 of the Act, AHRQ supports clinical research studies that CMS determines address the above-listed research questions and the a-m criteria listed in Section c. of this decision.

The principal investigator must submit the complete study protocol, identify the relevant CMS research question(s) that will be addressed, and cite the location of the detailed analysis plan for those questions in the protocol, plus provide a statement addressing how the study satisfies each of the standards of scientific integrity a. through m. listed in section c. of this decision, as well as the investigator's contact information, to the address below.

Director, Coverage and Analysis Group Re: LAAC CED Centers for Medicare & Medicaid Services 7500 Security Blvd., Mail Stop S3-02-01 Baltimore, MD 21244-1850

c. All clinical studies, RCTs and registries submitted for review must adhere to the following standards of scientific integrity and relevance to the Medicare population:

a. The principal purpose of the study is to test whether the item or service meaningfully improves health outcomes of affected beneficiaries who are represented by the enrolled subjects.

b. The rationale for the study is well supported by available scientific and medical evidence.

c. The study results are not anticipated to unjustifiably duplicate existing knowledge.

d. The study design is methodologically appropriate and the anticipated number of enrolled subjects is sufficient to answer the research question(s) being asked in the National Coverage Determination.

e. The study is sponsored by an organization or individual capable of completing it successfully.

f. The research study is in compliance with all applicable Federal regulations concerning the protection of human subjects found in the Code of Federal Regulations (CFR) at 45 CFR Part 46. If a study is regulated by the FDA, it is also in compliance with 21 CFR Parts 50 and 56. In addition, to further enhance the protection of human subjects in studies conducted under CED, the study must provide and obtain meaningful informed consent from patients regarding the risks associated with the study items and/or services, and the use and eventual disposition of the collected data.

g. All aspects of the study are conducted according to appropriate standards of scientific integrity.

h. The study has a written protocol that clearly demonstrates adherence to the standards listed here as Medicare requirements.

i. The study is not designed to exclusively test toxicity or disease pathophysiology in healthy individuals. Such studies may meet this requirement only if the disease or condition being studied is life threatening as defined in 21 CFR §312.81(a) and the patient has no other viable treatment options.

j. The clinical research studies and registries are registered on the www.ClinicalTrials.gov website by the principal sponsor/investigator prior to the enrollment of the first study subject. Registries are also registered in the AHRQ Registry of Patient Registries (RoPR).

k. The research study protocol specifies the method and timing of public release of all prespecified outcomes to be measured including release of outcomes if outcomes are negative or study is terminated early. The results must be made public within 12 months of the study's primary completion date, which is the date the final subject had final data collection for the primary endpoint, even if the trial does not achieve its primary aim. The results must include number started/completed, summary results for primary and secondary outcome measures, statistical analyses, and adverse events. Final results must be reported in a publicly accessibly manner; either in a peer-reviewed scientific journal (in print or on-line), in an on-line publicly accessible registry dedicated to the dissemination of clinical trial information such as ClinicalTrials.gov, or in journals willing to publish in abbreviated format (e.g., for studies with negative or incomplete results).

l. The study protocol must explicitly discuss beneficiary subpopulations affected by the item or service under investigation, particularly traditionally underrepresented groups in clinical studies, how the inclusion and exclusion criteria effect enrollment of these populations, and a plan for the retention and reporting of said populations in the trial. If the inclusion and exclusion criteria are expected to have a negative effect on the recruitment or retention of underrepresented populations, the protocol must discuss why these criteria are necessary.

m. The study protocol explicitly discusses how the results are or are not expected to be generalizable to affected beneficiary subpopulations. Separate discussions in the protocol may be necessary for populations eligible for Medicare due to age, disability, or Medicaid eligibility.

C. Nationally Non-Covered Indications

LAAC is non-covered for the treatment of NVAF when not furnished under CED according to the above-noted criteria.

(This NCD last reviewed February 2016.)

100-03, 20.9

Artificial Hearts and Related Devices (Various Effective Dates Below)

A. General

An artificial heart is a biventricular replacement device which requires removal of a substantial part of the native heart, including both ventricles. Removal of this device is not compatible with life, unless the patient has a heart transplant.

B. Nationally Covered Indications

1. Bridge-to-transplant (BTT) (effective for services performed on or after May 1, 2008)

   An artificial heart for bridge-to-transplantation (BTT) is covered when performed under coverage with evidence development (CED) when a clinical study meets all of the criteria listed below. The clinical study must address at least one of the following questions:

   — Were there unique circumstances such as expertise available in a particular facility or an unusual combination of conditions in particular patients that affected their outcomes?

   — What will be the average time to device failure when the device is made available to larger numbers of patients?

   — Do results adequately give a reasonable indication of the full range of outcomes (both positive and negative) that might be expected from more widespread use?

The clinical study must meet all of the criteria stated in Section D of this policy. The above information should be mailed to: Director, Coverage and Analysis Group, Centers for Medicare & Medicaid Services (CMS), Re: Artificial Heart, Mailstop S3-02-01, 7500 Security Blvd, Baltimore, MD 21244-1850.

Clinical studies that are determined by CMS to meet the above requirements will be listed on the CMS Web site at: http://www.cms.gov/Medicare/Coverage/Coverage-with-Evidence-Development /Artificial-Hearts.html.

2. Destination therapy (DT) (effective for services performed on or after May 1, 2008)

   An artificial heart for destination therapy (DT) is covered when performed under CED when a clinical study meets all of the criteria listed below. The clinical study must address at least one of the following questions:

   — Were there unique circumstances such as expertise available in a particular facility or an unusual combination of conditions in particular patients that affected their outcomes?

   — What will be the average time to device failure when the device is made available to larger numbers of patients?

   — Do results adequately give a reasonable indication of the full range of outcomes (both positive and negative) that might be expected from more widespread use?

The clinical study must meet all of the criteria stated in Section D of this policy. The above information should be mailed to: Director, Coverage and Analysis Group, Centers for Medicare & Medicaid Services, Re: Artificial Heart, Mailstop S3-02-01, 7500 Security Blvd, Baltimore, MD 21244-1850.

Clinical studies that are determined by CMS to meet the above requirements will be listed on the CMS Web site at: http://www.cms.gov/Medicare/Coverage/Coverage-with-Evidence-Development/Ar tificial-Hearts.html.

C. Nationally Non-Covered Indications

All other indications for the use of artificial hearts not otherwise listed remain non-covered, except in the context of Category B investigational device exemption clinical trials (42 CFR 405) or as a routine cost in clinical trials defined under section 310.1 of the National Coverage Determinations (NCD) Manual.

D. Other

Clinical study criteria:

- The study must be reviewed and approved by the Food and Drug Administration (FDA).

- The principal purpose of the research study is to test whether a particular intervention potentially improves the participants' health outcomes.

- The research study is well supported by available scientific and medical information, or it is intended to clarify or establish the health outcomes of interventions already in common clinical use.

- The research study does not unjustifiably duplicate existing studies.

- The research study design is appropriate to answer the research question being asked in the study.

- The research study is sponsored by an organization or individual capable of executing the proposed study successfully.

- The research study is in compliance with all applicable Federal regulations concerning the protection of human subjects found at 45 CFR Part 46. If a study is FDA-regulated it also must be in compliance with 21 CFR Parts 50 and 56.

- All aspects of the research study are conducted according to appropriate standards of scientific integrity (see http://www.icmje.org).

- The research study has a written protocol that clearly addresses, or incorporates by reference, the standards listed here as Medicare requirements for CED.

- The clinical research study is not designed to exclusively test toxicity or disease pathophysiology in healthy individuals. Trials of all medical technologies measuring therapeutic outcomes as one of the objectives meet this standard only if the disease or condition being studied is life threatening as defined in 21 CFR §312.81(a) and the patient has no other viable treatment options.

- The clinical research study is registered on the www.ClinicalTrials.gov Web site by the principal sponsor/investigator as demonstrated by having a Clinicaltrials.gov Identifier.

- The research study protocol specifies the method and timing of public release of all pre-specified outcomes to be measured including release of outcomes if outcomes are negative or study is terminated early. The results must be made public within 24 months of the end of data collection. If a report is planned to be published in a peer-reviewed journal, then that initial release may be an abstract that meets the requirements of the International Committee of Medical Journal Editors (ICMJE) (http://www.icmje.org). However a full report of the outcomes must be made public no later than three (3) years after the end of data collection.

- The research study protocol must explicitly discuss subpopulations affected by the treatment under investigation, particularly traditionally under-represented groups in clinical studies, how the inclusion and exclusion criteria effect enrollment of these populations, and a plan for the retention and reporting of said populations in the trial. If the inclusion and exclusion criteria are expected to have a negative effect on the recruitment or retention of under-represented populations, the protocol must discuss why these criteria are necessary.

- The research study protocol explicitly discusses how the results are or are not expected to be generalizable to the Medicare population to infer whether Medicare patients may benefit from the intervention. Separate discussions in the protocol may be necessary for populations eligible for Medicare due to age, disability, or Medicaid eligibility.

Consistent with section 1142 of the Social Security Act (the Act), the Agency for Healthcare Research and Quality (AHRQ) supports clinical research studies that CMS determines meet the above-listed standards and address the above-listed research questions.

The principal investigator of an artificial heart clinical study seeking Medicare payment should submit the following documentation to CMS and should expect to be notified when the CMS review is complete:

- Complete study protocol (must be dated or identified with a version number);
- Protocol summary;
- Statement that the submitted protocol version has been agreed upon by the FDA;
- Statement that the above study standards are met;
- Statement that the study addresses at least one of the above questions related to artificial hearts;
- Complete contact information (phone number, email address, and mailing address); and,
- Clinicaltrials.gov Identifier.

100-03, 20.9.1

Ventricular Assist Devices (Various Effective Dates Below)

A. General

A ventricular assist device (VAD) is surgically attached to one or both intact ventricles and is used to assist or augment the ability of a damaged or weakened native heart to pump blood. Improvement in the performance of the native heart may allow the device to be removed.

B. Nationally Covered Indications

1. Post-cardiotomy (effective for services performed on or after October 18, 1993) Post-cardiotomy is the period following open-heart surgery. VADs used for support of blood circulation post-cardiotomy are covered only if they have received approval from the Food and Drug Administration (FDA) for that purpose, and the VADs are used according to the FDA-approved labeling instructions.

2. Bridge-to-Transplant (effective for services performed on or after January 22, 1996)

   The VADs used for bridge to transplant are covered only if they have received approval from the FDA for that purpose, and the VADs are used according to FDA-approved labeling instructions. All of the following criteria must be fulfilled in order for Medicare coverage to be provided for a VAD used as a bridge to transplant:

   — The patient is approved for heart transplantation by a Medicare-approved heart transplant center and is active on the Organ Procurement and Transplantation Network (OPTN) heart transplant waitlist.

   — The implanting site, if different than the Medicare-approved transplant center, must receive written permission from the Medicare-approved transplant center under which the patient is listed prior to implantation of the VAD.

3. Destination Therapy (DT) (effective for services performed on or after October 1, 2003)

   Destination therapy (DT) is for patients that require mechanical cardiac support. The VADs used for DT are covered only if they have received approval from the FDA for that purpose.

   Patient Selection (effective November 9, 2010):

   The VADs are covered for patients who have chronic end-stage heart failure (New York Heart Association Class IV end-stage left ventricular failure) who are not candidates for heart transplantation at the time of VAD implant, and meet the following conditions:Have failed to respond to optimal medical management (including beta-blockers and ACE inhibitors if tolerated) for 45 of the last 60 days, or have been balloon pump-dependent for 7 days, or IV inotrope-dependent for 14 days; and,

   — Have a left ventricular ejection fraction (LVEF) <25%; and,

   — Have demonstrated functional limitation with a peak oxygen consumption of =14 ml/kg/min unless balloon pump- or inotrope-dependent or physically unable to perform the test. Facility Criteria (effective October 30, 2013):

   Facilities currently credentialed by the Joint Commission for placement of VADs as DT may continue as Medicare-approved facilities until October 30, 2014. At the conclusion of this transition period, these facilities must be in compliance with the following criteria as determined by a credentialing organization. As of the effective date, new facilities must meet the following criteria as a condition of coverage of this procedure as DT under section 1862(a)(1)(A) of the Social Security Act (the Act):

Beneficiaries receiving VADs for DT must be managed by an explicitly identified cohesive, multidisciplinary team of medical professionals with the appropriate qualifications, training, and experience. The team embodies collaboration and dedication across medical specialties to offer optimal patient-centered care. Collectively, the team must ensure that patients and caregivers have the knowledge and support necessary to participate in shared decision making and to provide appropriate informed consent. The team members must be based at the facility and must include individuals with experience working with patients before and after placement of a VAD.

The team must include, at a minimum:

- At least one physician with cardiothoracic surgery privileges and individual experience implanting at least 10 durable, intracorporeal, left VADs as BTT or DT over the course of the previous 36 months with activity in the last year.
- At least one cardiologist trained in advanced heart failure with clinical competence in medical and device-based management including VADs, and clinical competence in the management of patients before and after heart transplant.
- A VAD program coordinator.
- A social worker.
- A palliative care specialist. Facilities must be credentialed by an organization approved by the Centers for Medicare & Medicaid Services.

C. Nationally Non-Covered Indications

All other indications for the use of VADs not otherwise listed remain non-covered, except in the context of Category B investigational device exemption clinical trials (42 CFR 405) or as a routine cost in clinical trials defined under section 310.1 of the National Coverage Determinations (NCD) Manual.

D. Other

This policy does not address coverage of VADs for right ventricular support, biventricular support, use in beneficiaries under the age of 18, use in beneficiaries with complex congenital heart disease, or use in beneficiaries with acute heart failure without a history of chronic heart failure. Coverage under section 1862(a)(1)(A) of the Act for VADs in these situations will be made by local Medicare Administrative Contractors within their respective jurisdictions.

100-03, 30.3

NCD for Acupuncture (30.3)

Although acupuncture has been used for thousands of years in China and for decades in parts of Europe, it is a new agent of unknown use and efficacy in the United States. Even in those areas of the world where it has been widely used, its mechanism is not known. Three units of the National Institutes of Health, the National Institute of General Medical Sciences, National Institute of Neurological Diseases and Stroke, and Fogarty International Center have been designed to assess and identify specific opportunities and needs for research attending the use of acupuncture for surgical anesthesia and relief of chronic pain. Until the pending scientific assessment of the technique has been completed and its efficacy has been established, Medicare reimbursement for acupuncture, as an anesthetic or as an analgesic or for other therapeutic purposes, may not be made. Accordingly, acupuncture is not considered reasonable and necessary within the meaning of §1862(a)(1) of the Act.

100-03, 30.3.1

NCD for Acupuncture for Fibromyalgia (30.3.1)

General

Although acupuncture has been used for thousands of years in China and for decades in parts of Europe, it is still a relatively new agent of unknown use and efficacy in the United States. Even in those areas of the world where it has been widely used, its mechanism is not known. Three units of the National Institutes of Health, the National Institute of General Medical Sciences, National Institute of Neurological Diseases and Stroke, and Fogarty International Center were designated to assess and identify specific opportunities and needs for research attending the use of acupuncture for surgical anesthesia and relief of chronic pain. Following thorough review, and pending completion of the scientific assessment and efficacy of the technique, CMS initially issued a national noncoverage determination for acupuncture in May 1980.

Nationally Covered Indications

Not applicable.

Nationally Noncovered Indications

After careful reconsideration of its initial noncoverage determination for acupuncture, CMS concludes that there is no convincing evidence for the use of acupuncture for pain relief in patients with fibromyalgia. Study design flaws presently prohibit assessing acupuncture's utility for improving health outcomes. Accordingly, CMS determines that acupuncture is not considered reasonable and necessary for the treatment of fibromyalgia within the meaning of §1862(a)(1) of the Social Security Act, and the national noncoverage determination for acupuncture continues.

(This NCD last reviewed April 2004.)

100-03, 30.3.2

NCD for Acupuncture for Osteoarthritis (30.3.2)

General

Although acupuncture has been used for thousands of years in China and for decades in parts of Europe, it is still a relatively new agent of unknown use and efficacy in the United States. Even in those areas of the world where it has been widely used, its mechanism is not known. Three units of the National Institutes of Health, the National Institute of General Medical Sciences, National Institute of Neurological Diseases and Stroke, and Fogarty International Center were designated to assess and identify specific opportunities and needs for research attending the use of acupuncture for surgical anesthesia and relief of chronic pain. Following thorough review, and pending completion of the scientific assessment and efficacy of the technique, CMS initially issued a national noncoverage determination for acupuncture in May 1980.

Nationally Covered Indications

Not applicable.

Nationally Noncovered Indications

After careful reconsideration of its initial noncoverage determination for acupuncture, CMS concludes that there is no convincing evidence for the use of acupuncture for pain relief in patients with osteoarthritis. Study design flaws presently prohibit assessing acupuncture's utility for improving health outcomes. Accordingly, CMS determines that acupuncture is not considered reasonable and necessary for the treatment of osteoarthritis within the meaning of §1862(a)(1) of the Social Security Act, and the national noncoverage determination for acupuncture continues.

(This NCD last reviewed April 2004.)

100-03, 80.7

NCD for Refractive Keratoplasty (80.7)

The correction of common refractive errors by eyeglasses, contact lenses or other prosthetic devices is specifically excluded from coverage. The use of radial keratotomy and/or keratoplasty for the purpose of refractive error compensation is considered a substitute or alternative to eye glasses or contact lenses, which are specifically excluded by Sec.1862(a)(7) of the Act (except in certain cases in connection with cataract surgery). In addition, many in the medical community consider such procedures cosmetic surgery, which is excluded by section Sec.1862(a)(10) of the Act. Therefore, radial keratotomy and keratoplasty to treat refractive defects are not covered.

Keratoplasty that treats specific lesions of the cornea, such as phototherapeutic keratectomy that removes scar tissue from the visual field, deals with an abnormality of the eye and is not cosmetic surgery. Such cases may be covered under Sec.1862(a)(1)(A) of the Act.

The use of lasers to treat ophthalmic disease constitutes opthalmalogic surgery. Coverage is restricted to practitioners who have completed an approved training program in ophthalmologic surgery.

100-03, 80.10

NCD for Phaco-Emulsification procedure - cataract extraction (80.10)

In view of recommendations of authoritative sources in the field of ophthalmology, the subject technique is viewed as an accepted procedure for removal of cataracts. Accordingly, program reimbursement may be made for necessary services furnished in connection with cataract extraction utilizing the phaco-emulsification procedure.

100-03, 80.12

NCD for Intraocular Lenses (IOLs) (80.12)

Intraocular lens implantation services, as well as the lens itself, may be covered if reasonable and necessary for the individual. Implantation services may include hospital, surgical, and other medical services, including pre-implantation ultrasound (A-scan) eye measurement of one or both eyes.

100-03, 100.1

100.1 - Bariatric Surgery for Treatment of Co-Morbid Conditions Related to Morbid Obesity

Please note, sections 40.5, 100.8, 100.11, and 100.14 have been removed from the National Coverage Determination (NCD) Manual and incorporated into NCD 100.1.

A. General

Obesity may be caused by medical conditions such as hypothyroidism, Cushing's disease, and hypothalamic lesions, or can aggravate a number of cardiac and respiratory diseases as well as diabetes and hypertension. Non-surgical services in connection with the treatment of obesity are covered when such services are an integral and necessary part of a course of treatment for one of these medical conditions.

In addition, supplemented fasting is a type of very low calorie weight reduction regimen used to achieve rapid weight loss. The reduced calorie intake is supplemented by a mixture of protein, carbohydrates, vitamins, and minerals. Serious questions exist about the safety of prolonged adherence for 2 months or more to a very low calorie weight reduction regimen as a general treatment for obesity, because of instances of cardiopathology and sudden death, as well as possible loss of body protein.

Bariatric surgery procedures are performed to treat comorbid conditions associated with morbid obesity. Two types of surgical procedures are employed. Malabsorptive procedures divert food from the stomach to a lower part of the digestive tract where the normal mixing of digestive fluids and absorption of nutrients cannot occur. Restrictive procedures restrict the size of the stomach and decrease intake. Surgery can combine both types of procedures.

The following are descriptions of bariatric surgery procedures:

1. Roux-en-Y Gastric Bypass (RYGBP)

   The RYGBP achieves weight loss by gastric restriction and malabsorption. Reduction of the stomach to a small gastric pouch (30 cc) results in feelings of satiety following even small meals. This small pouch is connected to a segment of the jejunum, bypassing the duodenum and very proximal small intestine, thereby reducing absorption. RYGBP procedures can be open or laparoscopic.

2. Biliopancreatic Diversion with Duodenal Switch (BPD/DS) or Gastric Reduction Duodenal Switch (BPD/GRDS)

   The BPD achieves weight loss by gastric restriction and malabsorption. The stomach is partially resected, but the remaining capacity is generous compared to that achieved with RYGBP. As such, patients eat relatively normal-sized meals and do not need to restrict intake radically, since the most proximal areas of the small intestine (i.e., the duodenum and jejunum) are bypassed, and substantial malabsorption occurs. The partial BPD/DS or BPD/GRDS is a variant of the BPD procedure. It involves resection of the greater curvature of the stomach, preservation of the pyloric sphincter, and transection of the duodenum above the ampulla of Vater with a duodeno-ileal anastomosis and a lower ileo-ileal anastomosis. BPD/DS or BPD/GRDS procedures can be open or laparoscopic.

3. Adjustable Gastric Banding (AGB)

   The AGB achieves weight loss by gastric restriction only. A band creating a gastric pouch with a capacity of approximately 15 to 30 cc's encircles the uppermost portion of the stomach. The band is an inflatable doughnut-shaped balloon, the diameter of which can be adjusted in the clinic by adding or removing saline via a port that is positioned beneath the skin. The bands are adjustable, allowing the size of the gastric outlet to be modified as needed, depending on the rate of a patient's weight loss. AGB procedures are laparoscopic only.

4. Sleeve Gastrectomy

   Sleeve gastrectomy is a 70%-80% greater curvature gastrectomy (sleeve resection of the stomach) with continuity of the gastric lesser curve being maintained while simultaneously reducing stomach volume. In the past, sleeve gastrectomy was the first step in a two-stage procedure when performing RYGBP, but more recently has been offered as a stand-alone surgery. Sleeve gastrectomy procedures can be open or laparoscopic.

5. Vertical Gastric Banding (VGB)

   The VGB achieves weight loss by gastric restriction only. The upper part of the stomach is stapled, creating a narrow gastric inlet or pouch that remains connected with the remainder of the stomach. In addition, a non-adjustable band is placed around this new inlet in an attempt to prevent future enlargement of the stoma (opening). As a result, patients experience a sense of fullness after eating small meals. Weight loss from this procedure results entirely from eating less. VGB procedures are essentially no longer performed.

B. Nationally Covered Indications

Effective for services performed on and after February 21, 2006, Open and laparoscopic Roux-en-Y gastric bypass (RYGBP), open and laparoscopic Biliopancreatic Diversion with Duodenal Switch (BPD/DS) or Gastric Reduction Duodenal Switch (BPD/GRDS), and laparoscopic adjustable gastric banding (LAGB) are covered for Medicare beneficiaries who have a body-mass index = 35, have at least one co-morbidity related to obesity, and have been previously unsuccessful with medical treatment for obesity.

Effective for dates of service on and after February 21, 2006, these procedures are only covered when performed at facilities that are: (1) certified by the American College of Surgeons as a Level 1 Bariatric Surgery Center (program standards and requirements in effect on February 15, 2006); or (2) certified by the American Society for Bariatric Surgery as a Bariatric Surgery Center of Excellence (program standards and requirements in effect on February 15, 2006). Effective for dates of service on and after September 24, 2013, facilities are no longer required to be certified.

Effective for services performed on and after February 12, 2009, the Centers for Medicare & Medicaid Services (CMS) determines that Type 2 diabetes mellitus is a co-morbidity for purposes of this NCD.

A list of approved facilities and their approval dates are listed and maintained on the CMS Coverage Web site at http://www.cms.gov/Medicare/Medicare-General-Information/MedicareApprovedFacilitie/Bariatric-Surgery.html , and published in the Federal Register for services provided up to and including date of service September 23, 2013.

C. Nationally Non-Covered Indications

Treatments for obesity alone remain non-covered.

Supplemented fasting is not covered under the Medicare program as a general treatment for obesity (see section D. below for discretionary local coverage).

The following bariatric surgery procedures are non-covered for all Medicare beneficiaries:

- Open adjustable gastric banding;
- Open sleeve gastrectomy;
- Laparoscopic sleeve gastrectomy (prior to June 27, 2012);
- Open and laparoscopic vertical banded gastroplasty;
- Intestinal bypass surgery; and,
- Gastric balloon for treatment of obesity.

D. Other

Effective for services performed on and after June 27, 2012, Medicare Administrative Contractors (MACs) acting within their respective jurisdictions may determine coverage of stand-alone laparoscopic sleeve gastrectomy (LSG) for the treatment of co-morbid conditions related to obesity in Medicare beneficiaries only when all of the following conditions a.-c. are satisfied.

a. The beneficiary has a body-mass index (BMI) = 35 kg/m2,

b. The beneficiary has at least one co-morbidity related to obesity, and,

c. The beneficiary has been previously unsuccessful with medical treatment for obesity.

The determination of coverage for any bariatric surgery procedures that are not specifically identified in an NCD as covered or non-covered, for Medicare beneficiaries who have a body-mass index = 35, have at least one co-morbidity related to obesity, and have been previously unsuccessful with medical treatment for obesity, is left to the local MACs.

Where weight loss is necessary before surgery in order to ameliorate the complications posed by obesity when it coexists with pathological conditions such as cardiac and respiratory diseases, diabetes, or hypertension (and other more conservative techniques to achieve this end are not regarded as appropriate), supplemented fasting with adequate monitoring of the patient is eligible for coverage on a case-by-case basis or pursuant to a local coverage determination. The risks associated with the achievement of rapid weight loss must be carefully balanced against the risk posed by the condition requiring surgical treatment.

100-03, 100.5

NCD for Diagnostic Breath Analyses (100.5)

The Following Breath Test is Covered:

- Lactose breath hydrogen to detect lactose malabsorption.

The Following Breath Tests are Excluded from Coverage;

- Lactulose breath hydrogen for diagnosing small bowel bacterial overgrowth and measuring small bowel transit time.
- CO_2 for diagnosing bile acid malabsorption.
- CO_2 for diagnosing fat malabsorption.

100-03, 100.13

NCD for Laparoscopic Cholecystectomy (100.13)

Laparoscopic cholecystectomy is a covered surgical procedure in which a diseased gall bladder is removed through the use of instruments introduced via cannulae, with vision of the operative field maintained by use of a high-resolution television camera-monitor system (video laparoscope). For inpatient claims, use ICD-9-CM code 51.23, Laparoscopic cholecystectomy. For all other claims, use CPT codes 49310 for laparoscopy, surgical; cholecystectomy (any method), and 49311 for laparoscopy, surgical: cholecystectomy with cholangiography.

100-03, 110.1

NCD for Hyperthermia for Treatment of Cancer (110.1)

Local hyperthermia is covered under Medicare when used in connection with radiation therapy for the treatment of primary or metastatic cutaneous or subcutaneous superficial malignancies. It is not covered when used alone or in connection with chemotherapy.

100-03, 110.2

NCD for Certain Drugs Distributed by the National Cancer Institute (110.2)

Under its Cancer Therapy Evaluation, the Division of Cancer Treatment of the National Cancer Institute (NCI), in cooperation with the Food and Drug Administration, approves and distributes certain drugs for use in treating terminally ill cancer patients. One group of these drugs, designated as Group C drugs, unlike other drugs distributed by the NCI, is not limited to use in clinical trials for the purpose of testing their efficacy. Drugs are classified as Group C drugs only if there is sufficient evidence demonstrating their efficacy within a tumor type and that they can be safely administered.

A physician is eligible to receive Group C drugs from the Divison of Cancer Treatment only if the following requirements are met:

- A physician must be registered with the NCI as an investigator by having completed an FD-Form 1573;
- A written request for the drug, indicating the disease to be treated, must be submitted to the NCI;
- The use of the drug must be limited to indications outlined in the NCI's guidelines; and
- All adverse reactions must be reported to the Investigational Drug Branch of the Division of Cancer Treatment.

In view of these NCI controls on distribution and use of Group C drugs, A/B Medicare Adminstrative Contractors (MACs) may assume, in the absence of evidence to the contrary, that a Group C drug and the related hospital stay are covered if all other applicable coverage requirements are satisfied.

If there is reason to question coverage in a particular case, the matter should be resolved with the assistance of the Quality Improvement Organization (QIO), or if there is none, the assistance of the MAC's medical consultants.

Information regarding those drugs which are classified as Group C drugs may be obtained from:

Chief, Investigational Drug Branch
Cancer Therapy Evaluation Program
Executive Plaza North, Suite 7134
National Cancer Institute
Rockville, Maryland 20852-7426

100-03, 110.4

Extracorporeal Photopheresis

A. General

Extracorporeal photopheresis is a medical procedure in which a patient's white blood cells are exposed first to a drug called 8-methoxypsoralen (8-MOP) and then to ultraviolet A (UVA) light. The procedure starts with the removal of the patient's blood, which is centrifuged to isolate the white blood cells. The drug is typically administered directly to the white blood cells after they have been removed from the patient (referred to as ex vivo administration) but the drug can alternatively be administered directly to the patient before the white blood cells are withdrawn. After UVA light exposure, the treated white blood cells are then re-infused into the patient.

B. Nationally Covered Indications

The Centers for Medicare & Medicaid Services (CMS) has determined that extracorporeal photopheresis is reasonable and necessary under §1862(a)(1)(A) of the Social Security Act (the Act) under the following circumstances:

1. Effective April 8, 1988, Medicare provides coverage for:

    Palliative treatment of skin manifestations of cutaneous T-cell lymphoma that has not responded to other therapy.

2. Effective December 19, 2006, Medicare also provides coverage for:

    Patients with acute cardiac allograft rejection whose disease is refractory to standard immunosuppressive drug treatment; and,

    Patients with chronic graft versus host disease whose disease is refractory to standard immunosuppressive drug treatment.

3. Effective April 30, 2012, Medicare also provides coverage for:

    Extracorporeal photopheresis for the treatment of bronchiolitis obliterans syndrome (BOS) following lung allograft transplantation only when extracorporeal photopheresis is provided under a clinical research study that meets the following conditions:

    The clinical research study meets the requirements specified below to assess the effect of extracorporeal photopheresis for the treatment of BOS following lung allograft transplantation. The clinical study must address one or more aspects of the following question:

    Prospectively, do Medicare beneficiaries who have received lung allografts, developed BOS refractory to standard immunosuppressive therapy, and received extracorporeal photopheresis , experience improved patient-centered health outcomes as indicated by:

    a. improved forced expiratory volume in one second (FEV1);

    b. improved survival after transplant; and/or,

    c. improved quality of life?

        The required clinical study must adhere to the following standards of scientific integrity and relevance to the Medicare population:

    a. The principal purpose of the research study is to test whether extracorporeal photopheresis potentially improves the participants' health outcomes.

    b. The research study is well supported by available scientific and medical information or it is intended to clarify or establish the health outcomes of interventions already in common clinical use.

    c. The research study does not unjustifiably duplicate existing studies.

d. The research study design is appropriate to answer the research question being asked in the study.

e. The research study is sponsored by an organization or individual capable of successfully executing the proposed study.

f. The research study is in compliance with all applicable Federal regulations concerning the protection of human subjects found at 45 CFR Part 46. If a study is regulated by the Food and Drug Administration (FDA), it must also be in compliance with 21 CFR parts 50 and 56.

g. All aspects of the research study are conducted according to appropriate standards of scientific integrity (see http://www.icmje.org).

h. The research study has a written protocol that clearly addresses, or incorporates by reference, the standards listed here as Medicare requirements for coverage with evidence development.

i. The clinical research study is not designed to exclusively test toxicity or disease pathophysiology in healthy individuals. Trials of all medical technologies measuring therapeutic outcomes as one of the objectives meet this standard only if the disease or condition being studied is life threatening as defined in 21 CFR § 312.81(a) and the patient has no other viable treatment options.

j. The clinical research study is registered on the ClinicalTrials.gov website by the principal sponsor/investigator prior to the enrollment of the first study subject.

k. The research study protocol specifies the method and timing of public release of all prespecified outcomes to be measured including release of outcomes if outcomes are negative or study is terminated early. The results must be made public within 24 months of the end of data collection. If a report is planned to be published in a peer-reviewed journal, then that initial release may be an abstract that meets the requirements of the International Committee of Medical Journal Editors (http://www.icmje.org).

l. The research study protocol must explicitly discuss subpopulations affected by the treatment under investigation, particularly traditionally underrepresented groups in clinical studies, how the inclusion and exclusion criteria effect enrollment of these populations, and a plan for the retention and reporting of said populations on the trial. If the inclusion and exclusion criteria are expected to have a negative effect on the recruitment or retention of underrepresented populations, the protocol must discuss why these criteria are necessary.

m. The research study protocol explicitly discusses how the results are or are not expected to be generalizable to the Medicare population to infer whether Medicare patients may benefit from the intervention. Separate discussions in the protocol may be necessary for populations eligible for Medicare due to age, disability or Medicaid eligibility.

Consistent with section 1142 of the Act, the Agency for Healthcare Research and Quality supports clinical research studies that CMS determines meet the above-listed standards and address the above-listed research questions.

Any clinical study under which there is coverage of extracorporeal photopheresis for this indication pursuant to this national coverage determination (NCD) must be approved by April 30, 2014. If there are no approved clinical studies on this date, this NCD will expire and coverage of extracorporeal photopheresis for BOS will revert to the coverage policy in effect prior to the issuance of the final decision memorandum for this NCD.

C. Nationally Non-Covered Indications

All other indications for extracorporeal photopheresis not otherwise indicated above as covered remain non-covered.

D. Other

Claims processing instructions can be found in chapter 32, section 190 of the Medicare Claims Processing Manual.

(This NCD last reviewed April 2012.)

100-03, 110.6

NCD for Scalp Hypothermia During Chemotherapy, to Prevent Hair Loss (110.6)

While ice-filled bags or bandages or other devices used for scalp hypothermia during chemotherapy may be covered as supplies of the kind commonly furnished without a separate charge, no separate charge for them would be recognized.

100-03, 110.7

NCD for Blood Transfusions (110.7)

B. Policy Governing Transfusions

For Medicare coverage purposes, it is important to distinguish between a transfusion itself and preoperative blood services; e.g., collection, processing, storage. Medically necessary transfusion of blood, regardless of the type, may generally be a covered service under both Part A and Part B of Medicare. Coverage does not make a distinction between the transfusion of homologous, autologous, or donor-directed blood. With respect to the coverage of the services associated with the preoperative

collection, processing, and storage of autologous and donor-directed blood, the following policies apply.

1. Hospital Part A and B Coverage and Payment

Under Sec.1862(a)(14) of the Act, non-physician services furnished to hospital patients are covered and paid for as hospital services. As provided in Sec.1886 of the Act, under the prospective [payment system (PPS), the diganosis related group (DRG) payment to the hospital includes all covered blood and blood processing expenses, whether or not the blood is eventually used.

Under its provider agreement, a hospital is required to furnish or arrange for all covered services furnished to hospital patients. medicare payment is made to the hospital, under PPS or cost reimbursement, for covered inpatient services, and it is intended to reflect payment for all costs of furnishing those services.

2. Nonhospital Part B Coverage

Under Part B, to be eligible for separate coverage, a service must fit the definition of one of the services authorized by Sec.1832 of the Act. These services are defined in 42 CFR 410.10 and do not include a separate category for a supplier's services associated with blood donation services, either autologous or donor-directed. That is, the collection, processing, and storage of blood for later transfusion into the beneficiary is not recognized as a separate service under Part B. Therefore, there is no avenue through which a blood supplier can receive direct payment under Part B for blood donation services.

C. Perioperative Blood Salvage

When the perioperative blood salvage process is used in surgery on a hospital patient, payment made to the hospital (under PPS or through cost reimbursement) for the procedure in which that process is used is intended to encompass payment for all costs relating to that process.

100-03, 110.8

NCD for Blood Platelet Transfusions (110.8)

Blood platelet transplants are safe and effective for the correction of thrombocytopenia and other blood defects. It is covered under Medicare when treatment is reasonable and necessary for the individual patient.

100-03, 110.8.1

NCD for Stem Cell Transplantation (110.8.1)

Indications and Limitations of Coverage

1. Allogeneic Hematopoietic Stem Cell Transplantation (HSCT)

Allogeneic hematopoietic stem cell transplantation (HSCT) is a procedure in which a portion of a healthy donor's stem cell or bone marrow is obtained and prepared for intravenous infusion.

a. Nationally Covered Indications

The following uses of allogeneic HSCT are covered under Medicare:

i. Effective for services performed on or after August 1, 1978, for the treatment of leukemia, leukemia in remission, or aplastic anemia when it is reasonable and necessary,

ii. Effective for services performed on or after June 3, 1985, for the treatment of severe combined immunodeficiency disease (SCID) and for the treatment of Wiskott-Aldrich syndrome.

iii. Effective for services performed on or after August 4, 2010, for the treatment of Myelodysplastic Syndromes (MDS) pursuant to Coverage with Evidence Development (CED) in the context of a Medicare-approved, prospective clinical study.

The MDS refers to a group of diverse blood disorders in which the bone marrow does not produce enough healthy, functioning blood cells. These disorders are varied with regard to clinical characteristics, cytologic and pathologic features, and cytogenetics. The abnormal production of blood cells in the bone marrow leads to low blood cell counts, referred to as cytopenias, which are a hallmark feature of MDS along with a dysplastic and hypercellular-appearing bone marrow.

Medicare payment for these beneficiaries will be restricted to patients enrolled in an approved clinical study. In accordance with the Stem Cell Therapeutic and Research Act of 2005 (US Public Law 109-129) a standard dataset is collected for all allogeneic transplant patients in the United States by the Center for International Blood and Marrow Transplant Research. The elements in this dataset, comprised of two mandatory forms plus one additional form, encompass the information we require for a study under CED.

A prospective clinical study seeking Medicare payment for treating a beneficiary with allogeneic HSCT for MDS pursuant to CED must meet one or more aspects of the following questions:

— Prospectively, compared to Medicare beneficiaries with MDS who do not receive HSCT, do Medicare beneficiaries with MDS who receive HSCT have improved outcomes as indicated by:

– Relapse-free mortality,

– progression free survival,

– relapse, and

— overall survival?

— Prospectively, in Medicare beneficiaries with MDS who receive HSCT, how do International Prognostic Scoring System (IPSS) score, patient age, cytopenias and comorbidities predict the following outcomes:

– Relapse-free mortality,

– progression free survival,

– relapse, and

– overall survival?

— Prospectively, in Medicare beneficiaries with MDS who receive HSCT, what treatment facility characteristics predict meaningful clinical improvement in the following outcomes:

– Relapse-free mortality,

– progression free survival,

– relapse, and

– overall survival?

In addition, the clinical study must adhere to the following standards of scientific integrity and relevance to the Medicare population:

a. The principal purpose of the research study is to test whether a particular intervention potentially improves the participants' health outcomes.

b. The research study is well supported by available scientific and medical information or it is intended to clarify or establish the health outcomes of interventions already in common clinical use.

c. The research study does not unjustifiably duplicate existing studies.

d. The research study design is appropriate to answer the research question being asked in the study.

e. The research study is sponsored by an organization or individual capable of executing the proposed study successfully.

f. The research study is in compliance with all applicable Federal regulations concerning the protection of human subjects found at 45 CFR Part 46.

g. All aspects of the research study are conducted according to appropriate standards of scientific integrity (see http://www.icmje.org).

h. The research study has a written protocol that clearly addresses, or incorporates by reference, the standards listed here as Medicare requirements for CED coverage.

i. The clinical research study is not designed to exclusively test toxicity or disease pathophysiology in healthy individuals. Trials of all medical technologies measuring therapeutic outcomes as one of the objectives meet this standard only if the disease or condition being studied is life threatening as defined in 21 CFR §312.81(a) and the patient has no other viable treatment options.

j. The clinical research study is registered on the ClinicalTrials.gov Web site by the principal sponsor/investigator prior to the enrollment of the first study subject.

k. The research study protocol specifies the method and timing of public release of all pre-specified outcomes to be measured including release of outcomes if outcomes are negative or study is terminated early. The results must be made public within 24 months of the end of data collection. If a report is planned to be published in a peer-reviewed journal, then that initial release may be an abstract that meets the requirements of the International Committee of Medical Journal Editors (http://www.icmje.org). However a full report of the outcomes must be made public no later than 3 years after the end of data collection.

l. The research study protocol must explicitly discuss subpopulations affected by the treatment under investigation, particularly traditionally underrepresented groups in clinical studies, how the inclusion and exclusion criteria effect enrollment of these populations, and a plan for the retention and reporting of said populations on the trial. If the inclusion and exclusion criteria are expected to have a negative effect on the recruitment or retention of underrepresented populations, the protocol must discuss why these criteria are necessary.

m. The research study protocol explicitly discusses how the results are or are not expected to be generalizable to the Medicare population to infer whether Medicare patients may benefit from the intervention. Separate discussions in the protocol may be necessary for populations eligible for Medicare due to age, disability or Medicaid eligibility.

Consistent with section 1142 of the Social Security Act, the Agency for Health Research and Quality (AHRQ) supports clinical research studies that CMS determines meet the above-listed standards and address the above-listed research questions.

The clinical research study should also have the following features:

— It should be a prospective, longitudinal study with clinical information from the period before HSCT and short- and long-term follow-up information.

— Outcomes should be measured and compared among pre-specified subgroups within the cohort.

— The study should be powered to make inferences in subgroup analyses.

— Risk stratification methods should be used to control for selection bias. Data elements to be used in risk stratification models should include:

Patient selection:

— Patient Age at diagnosis of MDS and at transplantation

— Date of onset of MDS

— Disease classification (specific MDS subtype at diagnosis prior to preparative/conditioning regimen using World Health Organization (WHO) classifications). Include presence/absence of refractory cytopenias

— Comorbid conditions

— IPSS score (and WHO-adapted Prognostic Scoring System (WPSS) score, if applicable) at diagnosis and prior to transplantation

— Score immediately prior to transplantation and one year post-transplantation

— Disease assessment at diagnosis at start of preparative regimen and last assessment prior to preparative regimen Subtype of MDS (refractory anemia with or without blasts, degree of blasts, etc.)

— Type of preparative/conditioning regimen administered (myeloabalative, non-myeloablative, reduced–intensity conditioning)

— Donor type

— Cell Source

— IPSS Score at diagnosis

Facilities must submit the required transplant essential data to the Stem Cell Therapeutics Outcomes Database.

b. Nationally Non-Covered Indications

Effective for services performed on or after May 24, 1996, allogeneic HSCT is not covered as treatment for multiple myeloma.

2. Autologous Stem Cell Transplantation (AuSCT)

Autologous stem cell transplantation (AuSCT) is a technique for restoring stem cells using the patient's own previously stored cells.

a. Nationally Covered Indications

i. Effective for services performed on or after April 28, 1989, AuSCT is considered reasonable and necessary under §I862(a)(1)(A) of the Social Security Act (the Act) for the following conditions and is covered under Medicare for patients with:

• Acute leukemia in remission who have a high probability of relapse and who have no human leucocyte antigens (HLA)-matched;

• Resistant non-Hodgkin's lymphomas or those presenting with poor prognostic features following an initial response;

• Recurrent or refractory neuroblastoma; or

• Advanced Hodgkin's disease who have failed conventional therapy and have no HLA-matched donor.

ii. Effective October 1, 2000, single AuSCT is only covered for Durie-Salmon Stage II or III patients that fit the following requirements:

• Newly diagnosed or responsive multiple myeloma. This includes those patients with previously untreated disease, those with at least a partial response to prior chemotherapy (defined as a 50% decrease either in measurable paraprotein [serum and/or urine] or in bone marrow infiltration, sustained for at least 1 month), and those in responsive relapse; and,

• Adequate cardiac, renal, pulmonary, and hepatic function.

iii. Effective for services performed on or after March 15, 2005, when recognized clinical risk factors are employed to select patients for transplantation, high dose melphalan (HDM) together with AuSCT is reasonable and necessary for Medicare beneficiaries of any age group with primary amyloid light chain (AL) amyloidosis who meet the following criteria:

• Amyloid deposition in 2 or fewer organs; and,

• Cardiac left ventricular ejection fraction (EF) greater than 45%.

b. Nationally Non-Covered Indications

Insufficient data exist to establish definite conclusions regarding the efficacy of AuSCT for the following conditions:

– Acute leukemia not in remission;

– Chronic granulocytic leukemia;

– Solid tumors (other than neuroblastoma);

– Up to October 1, 2000, multiple myeloma;

– Tandem transplantation (multiple rounds of AuSCT) for patients with multiple myeloma;

– Effective October 1, 2000, non primary AL amyloidosis; and,

– Effective October 1, 2000, thru March 14, 2005, primary AL amyloidosis for Medicare beneficiaries age 64 or older.

In these cases, AuSCT is not considered reasonable and necessary within the meaning of §I862(a)(1)(A) of the Act and is not covered under Medicare.

B. Other

All other indications for stem cell transplantation not otherwise noted above as covered or non-covered nationally remain at Medicare Administrative Contractor discretion.

100-03, 110.9

NCD for Antigens Prepared for Sublingual Administration (110.9)

For antigens provided to patients on or after November 17, 1996, Medicare does not cover such antigens if they are to be administered sublingually, i.e., by placing drops under the patient's tongue. This kind of allergy therapy has not been proven to be safe and effective. Antigens are covered only if they are administered by injection.

100-03, 110.12

NCD for Challenge Ingestion Food Testing (110.12)

This procedure is covered when it is used on an outpatient basis if it is reasonable and necessary for the individual patient.

Challenge ingestion food testing has not been proven to be effective in the diagnosis of rheumatoid arthritis, depression, or respiratory disorders. Accordingly, its use in the diagnosis of these conditions is not reasonable and necessary within the meaning of section 1862(a)(1) of the Medicare law, and no program payment is made for this procedure when it is so used.

100-03, 110.14

NCD for Apheresis (Therapeutic Pheresis) (110.14)

B. Indications

Apheresis is covered for the following indications:

- Plasma exchange for acquired myasthenia gravis;
- Leukapheresis in the treatment of leukemia
- Plasmapheresis in the treatment of primary macroglobulinemia (Waldenstrom);
- Treatment of hyperglobulinemias, including (but not limited to) multiple myelomas, cryoglobulinemia and hyperviscosity syndromes;
- Plasmapheresis or plasma exchange as a last resort treatment of thrombotic thrombocytopenic purpura (TTP);
- Plasmapheresis or plasma exchange in the last resort treatment of life threatening rheumatoid vasculitis;
- Plasma perfusion of charcoal filters for treatment of pruritus of cholestatic liver disease;
- Plasma exchange in the treatment of Goodpasture's Syndrome;
- Plasma exchange in the treatment of glomerulonephritis associated with antiglomerular basement membrane antibodies and advancing renal failure or pulmonary hemorrhage;
- Treatment of chronic relapsing polyneuropathy for patients with severe or life threatening symptoms who have failed to respond to conventional therapy;
- Treatment of life threatening scleroderma and polymyositis when the patient is unresponsive to conventional therapy;
- Treatment of Guillain-Barre Syndrome; and
- Treatment of last resort for life threatening systemic lupus erythematosus (SLE) when conventional therapy has failed to prevent clinical deterioration.

C. Settings

Apheresis is covered only when performed in a hospital setting (either inpatient or outpatient). or in a nonhospital setting. e.g. physician directed clinic when the following conditions are met:

- A physician (or a number of physicians) is present to perform medical services and to respond to medical emergencies at all times during patient care hours;
- Each patient is under the care of a physician; and
- All nonphysician services are furnished under the direct, personal supervision of a physician.

100-03, 110.16

NCD for Nonselective (Random) Transfusions and Living Related Donor Specific Transfusions (DST) in Kidney Transplantation (110.16)

These pretransplant transfusions are covered under Medicare without a specific limitation on the number of transfusions, subject to the normal Medicare blood deductible provisions. Where blood is given directly to the transplant patient; e.g., in the case of donor specific transfusions, the blood is considered replaced for purposes of the blood deductible provisions.

100-03, 110.23

Stem Cell Transplantation (Formerly 110.8.1) (Various Effective Dates Below)

(Rev. 193, Issued; 07-01-16, Effective: 01-27-16, Implementation: 10-03-16)

A. General

Stem cell transplantation is a process in which stem cells are harvested from either a patient's (autologous) or donor's (allogeneic) bone marrow or peripheral blood for intravenous infusion. Autologous stem cell transplantation (AuSCT) is a technique for restoring stem cells using the patient's own previously stored cells. AuSCT must be used to effect hematopoietic reconstitution following severely myelotoxic doses of chemotherapy (HDCT) and/or radiotherapy used to treat various malignancies. Allogeneic hematopoietic stem cell transplantation (HSCT) is a procedure in which a portion of a healthy donor's stem cell or bone marrow is obtained and prepared for intravenous infusion. Allogeneic HSCT may be used to restore function in recipients having an inherited or acquired deficiency or defect. Hematopoietic stem cells are multi-potent stem cells that give rise to all the blood cell types; these stem cells form blood and immune cells. A hematopoietic stem cell is a cell isolated from blood or bone marrow that can renew itself, differentiate to a variety of specialized cells, can mobilize out of the bone marrow into circulating blood, and can undergo programmed cell death, called apoptosis - a process by which cells that are unneeded or detrimental will self-destruct.

The Centers for Medicare & Medicaid Services (CMS) is clarifying that bone marrow and peripheral blood stem cell transplantation is a process which includes mobilization, harvesting, and transplant of bone marrow or peripheral blood stem cells and the administration of high dose chemotherapy or radiotherapy prior to the actual transplant. When bone marrow or peripheral blood stem cell transplantation is covered, all necessary steps are included in coverage. When bone marrow or peripheral blood stem cell transplantation is non-covered, none of the steps are covered.

B. Nationally Covered Indications

I. Allogeneic Hematopoietic Stem Cell Transplantation (HSCT)

a) Effective for services performed on or after August 1, 1978, for the treatment of leukemia, leukemia in remission, or aplastic anemia when it is reasonable and necessary,

b) Effective for services performed on or after June 3, 1985, for the treatment of severe combined immunodeficiency disease (SCID) and for the treatment of Wiskott-Aldrich syndrome.

c) Effective for services performed on or after August 4, 2010, for the treatment of Myelodysplastic Syndromes (MDS) pursuant to Coverage with Evidence Development (CED) in the context of a Medicare-approved, prospective clinical study.

MDS refers to a group of diverse blood disorders in which the bone marrow does not produce enough healthy, functioning blood cells. These disorders are varied with regard to clinical characteristics, cytologic and pathologic features, and cytogenetics. The abnormal production of blood cells in the bone marrow leads to low blood cell counts, referred to as cytopenias, which are a hallmark feature of MDS along with a dysplastic and hypercellular-appearing bone marrow

Medicare payment for these beneficiaries will be restricted to patients enrolled in an approved clinical study. In accordance with the Stem Cell Therapeutic and Research Act of 2005 (US Public Law 109-129) a standard dataset is collected for all allogeneic transplant patients in the United States by the Center for International Blood and Marrow Transplant Research. The elements in this dataset, comprised of two mandatory forms plus one additional form, encompass the information we require for a study under CED.

A prospective clinical study seeking Medicare payment for treating a beneficiary with allogeneic HSCT for MDS pursuant to CED must meet one or more aspects of the following questions:

1. Prospectively, compared to Medicare beneficiaries with MDS who do not receive HSCT, do Medicare beneficiaries with MDS who receive HSCT have improved outcomes as indicated by:
- Relapse-free mortality,
- progression free survival,
- relapse, and
- overall survival?

2. Prospectively, in Medicare beneficiaries with MDS who receive HSCT, how do International Prognostic Scoring System (IPSS) scores, patient age, cytopenias, and comorbidities predict the following outcomes:
- Relapse-free mortality,
- progression free survival,
- relapse, and
- overall survival?

3. Prospectively, in Medicare beneficiaries with MDS who receive HSCT, what treatment facility characteristics predict meaningful clinical improvement in the following outcomes:
- Relapse-free mortality,
- progression free survival,

- relapse, and
- overall survival?

In addition, the clinical study must adhere to the following standards of scientific integrity and relevance to the Medicare population:

a. The principal purpose of the research study is to test whether a particular intervention potentially improves the participants' health outcomes.

b. The research study is well supported by available scientific and medical information or it is intended to clarify or establish the health outcomes of interventions already in common clinical use.

c. The research study does not unjustifiably duplicate existing studies.

d. The research study design is appropriate to answer the research question being asked in the study.

e. The research study is sponsored by an organization or individual capable of executing the proposed study successfully.

f. The research study is in compliance with all applicable Federal regulations concerning the protection of human subjects found at 45 CFR Part 46. If a study is regulated by the Food and Drug Administration (FDA), it must be in compliance with 21 CFR parts 50 and 56.

g. All aspects of the research study are conducted according to appropriate standards of scientific integrity (see http://www.icmje.org).

h. The research study has a written protocol that clearly addresses, or incorporates by reference, the standards listed here as Medicare requirements for CED coverage.

i. The clinical research study is not designed to exclusively test toxicity or disease pathophysiology in healthy individuals. Trials of all medical technologies measuring therapeutic outcomes as one of the objectives meet this standard only if the disease or condition being studied is life threatening as defined in 21 CFR §312.81(a) and the patient has no other viable treatment options.

j. The clinical research study is registered on the ClinicalTrials.gov Web site by the principal sponsor/investigator prior to the enrollment of the first study subject.

k. The research study protocol specifies the method and timing of public release of all pre-specified outcomes to be measured including release of outcomes if outcomes are negative or study is terminated early. The results must be made public within 24 months of the end of data collection. If a report is planned to be published in a peer-reviewed journal, then that initial release may be an abstract that meets the requirements of the International Committee of Medical Journal Editors (http://www.icmje.org). However a full report of the outcomes must be made public no later than 3 years after the end of data collection.

l. The research study protocol must explicitly discuss subpopulations affected by the treatment under investigation, particularly traditionally underrepresented groups in clinical studies, how the inclusion and exclusion criteria effect enrollment of these populations, and a plan for the retention and reporting of said populations on the trial. If the inclusion and exclusion criteria are expected to have a negative effect on the recruitment or retention of underrepresented populations, the protocol must discuss why these criteria are necessary.

m. The research study protocol explicitly discusses how the results are or are not expected to be generalizable to the Medicare population to infer whether Medicare patients may benefit from the intervention. Separate discussions in the protocol may be necessary for populations eligible for Medicare due to age, disability or Medicaid eligibility.

Consistent with section 1142 of the Social Security Act, the Agency for Health Research and Quality (AHRQ) supports clinical research studies that CMS determines meet the above-listed standards and address the above-listed research questions.

The clinical research study should also have the following features:

- It should be a prospective, longitudinal study with clinical information from the period before HSCT and short- and long-term follow-up information.

- Outcomes should be measured and compared among pre-specified subgroups within the cohort.

- The study should be powered to make inferences in subgroup analyses.

- Risk stratification methods should be used to control for selection bias. Data elements to be used in risk stratification models should include:

Patient selection:

  – Patient Age at diagnosis of MDS and at transplantation

  – Date of onset of MDS

  – Disease classification (specific MDS subtype at diagnosis prior to preparative/conditioning regimen using World Health Organization (WHO) classifications). Include presence/absence of refractory cytopenias

  – Comorbid conditions

  – IPSS score (and WHO-adapted Prognostic Scoring System (WPSS) score, if applicable) at diagnosis and prior to transplantation

  – Score immediately prior to transplantation and one year post-transplantation

  – Disease assessment at diagnosis at start of preparative regimen and last assessment prior to preparative regimen Subtype of MDS (refractory anemia with or without blasts, degree of blasts, etc.)

  – Type of preparative/conditioning regimen administered (myeloabalative, non-myeloablative, reduced–intensity conditioning)

  – Donor type

  – Cell Source

Facilities must submit the required transplant essential data to the Stem Cell Therapeutics Outcomes Database.

d) Effective for claims with dates of service on or after January 27, 2016, allogeneic HSCT for multiple myeloma is covered by Medicare only for beneficiaries with Durie-Salmon Stage II or III multiple myeloma, or International Staging System (ISS) Stage II or Stage III multiple myeloma, and participating in an approved prospective clinical study that meets the criteria below. There must be appropriate statistical techniques to control for selection bias and confounding by age, duration of diagnosis, disease classification, International Myeloma Working Group (IMWG) classification, ISS stage, comorbid conditions, type of preparative/conditioning regimen, graft vs. host disease (GVHD) prophylaxis, donor type and cell source.

A prospective clinical study seeking Medicare coverage for allogeneic HSCT for multiple myeloma pursuant to CED must address the following question:

Compared to patients who do not receive allogeneic HSCT, do Medicare beneficiaries with multiple myeloma who receive allogeneic HSCT have improved outcomes as indicated by:

  – Graft vs. host disease (acute and chronic);

  – Other transplant-related adverse events;

  – Overall survival; and

  – (optional) Quality of life?

All CMS-approved clinical studies and registries must adhere to the below listed standards of scientific integrity and relevance to the Medicare population as listed in section g.

e) Effective for claims with dates of service on or after January 27, 2016, allogeneic HSCT for myelofibrosis (MF) is covered by Medicare only for beneficiaries with Dynamic International Prognostic Scoring System (DIPSSplus) intermediate-2 or High primary or secondary MF and participating in an approved prospective clinical study. All Medicare approved studies must use appropriate statistical techniques in the analysis to control for selection bias and potential confounding by age, duration of diagnosis, disease classification, DIPSSplus score, comorbid conditions, type of preparative/conditioning regimen, graft vs. host disease (GVHD) prophylaxis, donor type and cell source.

A prospective clinical study seeking Medicare coverage for allogeneic HSCT for myelofibrosis pursuant to Coverage with Evidence Development (CED) must address the following question:

Compared to patients who do not receive allogeneic HSCT, do Medicare beneficiaries with MF who receive allogeneic HSCT transplantation have improved outcomes as indicated by:

  – Graft vs. host disease (acute and chronic);

  – Other transplant-related adverse events;

  – Overall survival; and

  – (optional) Quality of life?

All CMS-approved clinical studies and registries must adhere to the below listed standards of scientific integrity and relevance to the Medicare population as listed in section g.

f) Effective for claims with dates of service on or after January 27, 2016, allogeneic HSCT for sickle cell disease (SCD) is covered by Medicare only for beneficiaries with severe, symptomatic SCD who participate in an approved prospective clinical study.

A prospective clinical study seeking Medicare coverage for allogeneic HSCT for sickle cell disease pursuant to Coverage with Evidence Development (CED) must address the following question:

Compared to patients who do not receive allogeneic HSCT, do Medicare beneficiaries with SCD who receive allogeneic HSCT have improved outcomes as indicated by:

  – Graft vs. host disease (acute and chronic),

  – Other transplant-related adverse events;

  – Overall survival; and

  – (optional) Quality of life?

All CMS-approved clinical studies and registries must adhere to the below listed standards of scientific integrity and relevance to the Medicare population listed in section g:

g) All CMS-approved clinical studies and registries in sections d, e and f must adhere to the below listed standards of scientific integrity and relevance to the Medicare population:

a. The principal purpose of the study is to test whether the item or service meaningfully improves health outcomes of affected beneficiaries who are represented by the enrolled subjects.

b. The rationale for the study is well supported by available scientific and medical evidence.

c. The study results are not anticipated to unjustifiably duplicate existing knowledge.

d. The study design is methodologically appropriate and the anticipated number of enrolled subjects is sufficient to answer the research question(s) being asked in the National Coverage Determination.

e. The study is sponsored by an organization or individual capable of completing it successfully.

f. The research study is in compliance with all applicable Federal regulations concerning the protection of human subjects found in the Code of Federal Regulations (CFR) at 45 CFR Part 46. If a study is regulated by the Food and Drug Administration (FDA), it is also in compliance with 21 CFR Parts 50 and 56. In addition, to further enhance the protection of human subjects in studies conducted under CED, the study must provide and obtain meaningful informed consent from patients regarding the risks associated with the study items and/or services, and the use and eventual disposition of the collected data.

g. All aspects of the study are conducted according to appropriate standards of scientific integrity.

h. The study has a written protocol that clearly demonstrates adherence to the standards listed here as Medicare requirements.

i. The study is not designed to exclusively test toxicity or disease pathophysiology in healthy individuals. Such studies may meet this requirement only if the disease or condition being studied is life threatening as defined in 21 CFR §312.81(a) and the patient has no other viable treatment options.

j. The clinical research studies and registries are registered on the www.ClinicalTrials.gov website by the principal sponsor/investigator prior to the enrollment of the first study subject. Registries are also registered in the Agency for Healthcare Quality (AHRQ) Registry of Patient Registries (RoPR).

k. The research study protocol specifies the method and timing of public release of all prespecified outcomes to be measured including release of outcomes if outcomes are negative or study is terminated early. The results must be made public within 12 months of the study's primary completion date, which is the date the final subject had final data collection for the primary endpoint, even if the trial does not achieve its primary aim. The results must include number started/completed, summary results for primary and secondary outcome measures, statistical analyses, and adverse events. Final results must be reported in a publicly accessible manner; either in a peer-reviewed scientific journal (in print or on-line), in an on-line publicly accessible registry dedicated to the dissemination of clinical trial information such as ClinicalTrials.gov, or in journals willing to publish in abbreviated format (e.g., for studies with negative or inconclusive results).

l. The study protocol must explicitly discuss beneficiary subpopulations affected by the item or service under investigation, particularly traditionally underrepresented groups in clinical studies, how the inclusion and exclusion criteria effect enrollment of these populations, and a plan for the retention and reporting of said populations in the trial. If the inclusion and exclusion criteria are expected to have a negative effect on the recruitment or retention of underrepresented populations, the protocol must discuss why these criteria are necessary.

m. The study protocol explicitly discusses how the results are or are not expected to be generalizable to affected beneficiary subpopulations. Separate discussions in the protocol may be necessary for populations eligible for Medicare due to age, disability or Medicaid eligibility.

Consistent with section 1142 of the Act, the Agency for Healthcare Research and Quality (AHRQ) supports clinical research studies that CMS determines meet the above-listed standards and address the above-listed research questions.

II. Autologous Stem Cell Transplantation (AuSCT)

a) Effective for services performed on or after April 28, 1989, AuSCT is considered reasonable and necessary under §l862(a)(1)(A) of the Act for the following conditions and is covered under Medicare for patients with:

1. Acute leukemia in remission who have a high probability of relapse and who have no human leucocyte antigens (HLA)-matched;

2. Resistant non-Hodgkin's lymphomas or those presenting with poor prognostic features following an initial response;

3. Recurrent or refractory neuroblastoma; or,

4. Advanced Hodgkin's disease who have failed conventional therapy and have no HLA-matched donor.

b) Effective October 1, 2000, single AuSCT is only covered for Durie-Salmon Stage II or III patients that fit the following requirements:

– Newly diagnosed or responsive multiple myeloma. This includes those patients with previously untreated disease, those with at least a partial response to prior chemotherapy (defined as a 50% decrease either in measurable paraprotein [serum and/or urine] or in bone marrow infiltration, sustained for at least 1 month), and those in responsive relapse; and

– Adequate cardiac, renal, pulmonary, and hepatic function.

c) Effective for services performed on or after March 15, 2005, when recognized clinical risk factors are employed to select patients for transplantation, high dose melphalan (HDM) together with AuSCT is reasonable and necessary for Medicare beneficiaries of any age group with primary amyloid light chain (AL) amyloidosis who meet the following criteria:

– Amyloid deposition in 2 or fewer organs; and,

– Cardiac left ventricular ejection fraction (EF) greater than 45%.

C. Nationally Non-Covered Indications

I. Allogeneic Hematopoietic Stem Cell Transplantation (HSCT)

Effective for claims with dates of service on or after May 24, 1996, through January 26, 2016, allogeneic HSCT is not covered as treatment for multiple myeloma.

II. Autologous Stem Cell Transplantation (AuSCT)

Insufficient data exist to establish definite conclusions regarding the efficacy of AuSCT for the following conditions:

a) Acute leukemia not in remission;

b) Chronic granulocytic leukemia;

c) Solid tumors (other than neuroblastoma);

d) Up to October 1, 2000, multiple myeloma;

e) Tandem transplantation (multiple rounds of AuSCT) for patients with multiple myeloma;

f) Effective October 1, 2000, non primary AL amyloidosis; and,

g) Effective October 1, 2000, through March 14, 2005, primary AL amyloidosis for Medicare beneficiaries age 64 or older.

In these cases, AuSCT is not considered reasonable and necessary within the meaning of §l862(a)(1)(A) of the Act and is not covered under Medicare.

D. Other

All other indications for stem cell transplantation not otherwise noted above as covered or non-covered remain at local Medicare Administrative Contractor discretion.

(This NCD last reviewed January 2016.)

100-03, 130.1

NCD for Inpatient Hospital Stays for Treatment of Alcoholism (130.1)

A. Inpatient Hospital Stay for Alcohol Detoxification
Many hospitals provide detoxification services during the more acute stages of alcoholism or alcohol withdrawal. When the high probability or occurrence of medical complications (e.g., delirium, confusion, trauma, or unconsciousness) during detoxification for acute alcoholism or alcohol withdrawal necessitates the constant availability of physicians and/or complex medical equipment found only in the hospital setting, inpatient hospital care during this period is considered reasonable and necessary and is therefore covered under the program. Generally, detoxification can be accomplished within two to three days with an occasional need for up to five days where the patient's condition dictates. This limit (five days) may be extended in an individual case where there is a need for a longer period for detoxification for a particular patient.

In such cases, however, there should be documentation by a physician which substantiates that a longer period of detoxification was reasonable and necessary. When the detoxification needs of an individual no longer require an inpatient hospital setting, coverage should be denied on the basis that inpatient hospital care is not reasonable and necessary as required by §1862(a)(l) of the Social Security Act (the Act). Following detoxification a patient may be transferred to an inpatient rehabilitation unit or discharged to a residential treatment program or outpatient treatment setting.

B. Inpatient Hospital Stay for Alcohol Rehabilitation
Hospitals may also provide structured inpatient alcohol rehabilitation programs to the chronic alcoholic. These programs are composed primarily of coordinated educational and psychotherapeutic services provided on a group basis. Depending on the subject matter, a series of lectures, discussions, films, and group therapy sessions are led by either physicians, psychologists, or alcoholism counselors from the hospital or various outside organizations. In addition, individual psychotherapy and

family counseling (see §70.1) may be provided in selected cases. These programs are conducted under the supervision and direction of a physician. Patients may directly enter an inpatient hospital rehabilitation program after having undergone detoxification in the same hospital or in another hospital or may enter an inpatient hospital rehabilitation program without prior hospitalization for detoxification.

Alcohol rehabilitation can be provided in a variety of settings other than the hospital setting. In order for an inpatient hospital stay for alcohol rehabilitation to be covered under Medicare it must be medically necessary for the care to be provided in the inpatient hospital setting rather than in a less costly facility or on an outpatient basis. Inpatient hospital care for receipt of an alcohol rehabilitation program would generally be medically necessary where either (I) there is documentation by the physician that recent alcohol rehabilitation services in a less intensive setting or on an outpatient basis have proven unsuccessful and, as a consequence, the patient requires the supervision and intensity of services which can only be found in the controlled environment of the hospital, or (2) only the hospital environment can assure the medical management or control of the patient's concomitant conditions during the course of alcohol rehabilitation. (However, a patient's concomitant condition may make the use of certain alcohol treatment modalities medically inappropriate.)

In addition, the "active treatment" criteria (see the Medicare Benefit Policy Manual, Chapter 2, "Inpatient Psychiatric Hospital Services," §20) should be applied to psychiatric care in the general hospital as well as to psychiatric care in a psychiatric hospital. Since alcoholism is classifiable as a psychiatric condition the "active treatment" criteria must also be met in order for alcohol rehabilitation services to be covered under Medicare. (Thus, it is the combined need for "active treatment" and for covered care which can only be provided in the inpatient hospital setting, rather than the fact that rehabilitation immediately follows a period of detoxification which provides the basis for coverage of inpatient hospital alcohol rehabilitation programs.)

Generally 16-19 days of rehabilitation services are sufficient to bring a patient to a point where care could be continued in other than an inpatient hospital setting. An inpatient hospital stay for alcohol rehabilitation may be extended beyond this limit in an individual case where a longer period of alcohol rehabilitation is medically necessary. In such cases, however, there should be documentation by a physician which substantiates the need for such care. Where the rehabilitation needs of an individual no longer require an inpatient hospital setting, coverage should be denied on the basis that inpatient hospital care is not reasonable and necessary as required by §1862 (a)(I) of the Act.

Subsequent admissions to the inpatient hospital setting for alcohol rehabilitation follow-up, reinforcement, or "recap" treatments are considered to be readmissions (rather than an extension of the original stay) and must meet the requirements of this section for coverage under Medicare. Prior admissions to the inpatient hospital setting - either in the same hospital or in a different hospital - may be an indication that the "active treatment" requirements are not met (i.e., there is no reasonable expectation of improvement) and the stay should not be covered. Accordingly, there should be documentation to establish that "readmission" to the hospital setting for alcohol rehabilitation services can reasonably be expected to result in improvement of the patient's condition. For example, the documentation should indicate what changes in the patient's medical condition, social or emotional status, or treatment plan make improvement likely, or why the patient's initial hospital treatment was not sufficient.

C. Combined Alcohol Detoxification/Rehabilitation Programs

Medicare Administrative Contractors (MACs) should apply the guidelines in A. and B. above to both phases of a combined inpatient hospital alcohol detoxification/rehabilitation program. Not all patients who require the inpatient hospital setting for detoxification also need the inpatient hospital setting for rehabilitation. (See §130.1 for coverage of outpatient hospital alcohol rehabilitation services.) Where the inpatient hospital setting is medically necessary for both alcohol detoxification and rehabilitation, generally a 3-week period is reasonable and necessary to bring the patient to the point where care can be continued in other than an inpatient hospital setting.

Decisions regarding reasonableness and necessity of treatment, the need for an inpatient hospital level of care, and length of treatment should be made by A/B MAC (A) based on accepted medical practice with the advice of their medical consultant. (In hospitals under PSRO review, PSRO determinations of medical necessity of services and appropriateness of the level of care at which services are provided are binding on A/B MAC (A) for purposes of adjudicating claims for payment.)

100-03, 130.2

NCD for Outpatient Hospital Services for Treatment of Alcoholism (130.2)

Coverage is available for both diagnostic and therapeutic services furnished for the treatment of alcoholism by the hospital to outpatients subject to the same rules applicable to outpatient hospital services in general. While there is no coverage for day hospitalization programs, per se, individual services which meet the requirements in the Medicare Benefit Policy Manual, Chapter 6, Sec.20 may be covered. (Meals, transportation and recreational and social activities do not fall within the scope of covered outpatient hospital services under Medicare.)

All services must be reasonable and necessary for diagnosis or treatment of the patient's condition (see the Medicare Benefit Policy Manual, chapter 16 Sec.20). Thus, educational services and family counseling would only be covered where they are directly related to treatment of the patient's condition. The frequency of treatment and period of time over which it occurs must also be reasonable and necessary.

100-03, 130.3

NCD for Chemical AversionTherapy for Treatment of Alcoholism (130.3)

Chemical aversion therapy is a behavior modification technique that is used in the treatment of alcoholism. Chemical aversion therapy facilitates alcohol abstinence through the development of conditioned aversions to the taste, smell, and sight of alcohol beverages. This is accomplished by repeatedly pairing alcohol with unpleasant symptoms (e.g., nausea) which have been induced by one of several chemical agents. While a number of drugs have been employed in chemical aversion therapy, the three most commonly used are emetine, apomorphine, and lithium. None of the drugs being used, however, have yet been approved by the Food and Drug Administration specifically for use in chemical aversion therapy for alcoholism. Accordingly, when these drugs are being employed in conjunction with this therapy, patients undergoing this treatment need to be kept under medical observation.

Available evidence indicates that chemical aversion therapy may be an effective component of certain alcoholism treatment programs, particularly as part of multi-modality treatment programs which include other behavioral techniques and therapies, such as psychotherapy. Based on this evidence, the Centers for Medicare & Medicaid Services' medical consultants have recommended that chemical aversion therapy be covered under Medicare. However, since chemical aversion therapy is a demanding therapy which may not be appropriate for all Medicare beneficiaries needing treatment for alcoholism, a physician should certify to the appropriateness of chemical aversion therapy in the individual case. Therefore, if chemical aversion therapy for treatment of alcoholism is determined to be reasonable and necessary for an individual patient, it is covered under Medicare.

When it is medically necessary for a patient to receive chemical aversion therapy as a hospital inpatient, coverage for care in that setting is available. (See §130.1 regarding coverage of multi-modality treatment programs.) Follow-up treatments for chemical aversion therapy can generally be provided on an outpatient basis. Thus, where a patient is admitted as an inpatient for receipt of chemical aversion therapy, there must be documentation by the physician of the need in the individual case for the inpatient hospital admission.

Decisions regarding reasonableness and necessity of treatment and the need for an inpatient hospital level of care should be made by the A/B MAC (A) based on accepted medical practice with the advice of their medical consultant. (In hospitals under Quality Improvement Organization (QIO) review, QIO determinations of medical necessity of services and appropriateness of the level of care at which services are provided are binding on the A/B MAC (A) for purposes of adjudicating claims for payment.)

100-03, 140.1

NCD for Abortion (140.1)

Abortions are not covered Medicare procedures except:

1. If the pregnancy is the result of an act of rape or incest; or

2. In the case where a woman suffers from a physical disorder, physical injury, or physical illness, including a life-endangering physical condition caused by or arising from the pregnancy itself, that would, as certified by a physician, place the woman in danger of death unless an abortion is performed.

100-03, 140.2

NCD for Breast Reconstruction Following Mastectomy (140.2)

Reconstruction of the affected and the contralateral unaffected breast following a medically necessary mastectomy is considered a relatively safe and effective noncosmetic procedure. Accordingly, program payment may be made for breast reconstruction surgery following removal of a breast for any medical reason.

Program payment may not be made for breast reconstruction for cosmetic reasons. (Cosmetic surgery is excluded from coverage under Sec.I862(a)(I0) of the Social Security Act.)

100-03, 140.5

NCD for Laser Procedures (140.5)

Medicare recognizes the use of lasers for many medical indications. Procedures performed with lasers are sometimes used in place of more conventional techniques. In the absence of a specific noncoverage instruction, and where a laser has been approved for marketing by the Food and Drug Administration, Medicare Administrative Contractor may use to determine whether a procedure performed with a laser is reasonable and necessary and, therefore, covered.

The determination of coverage for a procedure performed using a laser is made on the basis that the use of lasers to alter, revise, or destroy tissue is a surgical procedure. Therefore, coverage of laser procedures is restricted to practitioners with training in the surgical management of the disease or condition being treated.

100-03, 150.1

NCD for Manipulation (150.1)

Manipulation of the Rib Cage.--Manual manipulation of the rib cage contributes to the treatment of respiratory conditions such as bronchitis, emphysema, and asthma as part of a regimen which includes other elements of therapy, and is covered only under such circumstances.

Manipulation of the Head.--Manipulation of the occipitocervical or temporomandibular regions of the head when indicated for conditions affecting those portions of the head and neck is a covered service.

100-03, 150.2

NCD for Osteogenic Stimulators (150.2)

Electrical Osteogenic Stimulators

B. Nationally Covered Indications
1. Noninvasive Stimulator.

   The noninvasive stimulator device is covered only for the following indications:

   — Nonunion of long bone fractures;

   — Failed fusion, where a minimum of nine months has elapsed since the last surgery;

   — Congenital pseudarthroses; and

   — Effective July 1, 1996, as an adjunct to spinal fusion surgery for patients at high risk of pseudarthrosis due to previously failed spinal fusion at the same site or for those undergoing multiple level fusion. A multiple level fusion involves 3 or more vertebrae (e.g., L3-L5, L4-S1, etc).

   — Effective September 15, 1980, nonunion of long bone fractures is considered to exist only after 6 or more months have elapsed without healing of the fracture.

   — Effective April 1, 2000, nonunion of long bone fractures is considered to exist only when serial radiographs have confirmed that fracture healing has ceased for 3 or more months prior to starting treatment with the electrical osteogenic stimulator. Serial radiographs must include a minimum of 2 sets of radiographs, each including multiple views of the fracture site, separated by a minimum of 90 days.

2. Invasive (Implantable) Stimulator.

   The invasive stimulator device is covered only for the following indications:

   — Nonunion of long bone fractures

   — Effective July 1, 1996, as an adjunct to spinal fusion surgery for patients at high risk of pseudarthrosis due to previously failed spinal fusion at the same site or for those undergoing multiple level fusion. A multiple level fusion involves 3 or more vertebrae (e.g., L3-5, L4-S1, etc.).

   — Effective September 15, 1980, nonunion of long bone fractures is considered to exist only after 6 or more months have elapsed without healing of the fracture.

   — Effective April 1, 2000, non union of long bone fractures is considered to exist only when serial radiographs have confirmed that fracture healing has ceased for 3 or more months prior to starting treatment with the electrical osteogenic stimulator. Serial radiographs must include a minimum of 2 sets of radiographs, each including multiple views of the fracture site, separated by a minimum of 90 days.

   — Effective for services performed on or after January 1, 2001, ultrasonic osteogenic stimulators are covered as medically reasonable and necessary for the treatment of non-union fractures. In demonstrating nonunion of fractures, we would expect:

     – A minimum of two sets of radiographs obtained prior to starting treatment with the osteogenic stimulator, separated by a minimum of 90 days. Each radiograph must include multiple views of the fracture site accompanied with a written interpretation by a physician stating that there has been no clinically significant evidence of fracture healing between the two sets of radiographs.

     – Indications that the patient failed at least one surgical intervention for the treatment of the fracture.

   — Effective April 27, 2005, upon the recommendation of the ultrasound stimulation for nonunion fracture healing, CMS determins that the evidence is adequate to condlude that noninvasive ultrasound stimulation for the treatment of nonunion bone fractures prior to surfical intervention is reasonable and necessary. In demonstrating non-union fracturs, CMS expects:

     – A minimum of 2 sets of radiographs, obtained prior to starting treating with the osteogenic stimulator, separated by a minimum of 90 days. Each radiograph set must include multiple views of the fracture site accompanied with a written interpretation by a physician stating that there has been no clinically significant evidence of fracture healing between the 2 sets of radiographs.

C. Nationally Non-Covered Indications
Nonunion fractures of the skull, vertebrae and those that are tumor-related are excluded from coverage.

Ultrasonic osteogenic stimulators may not be used concurrently with other non-invasive osteogenic devices.

Ultrasonic osteogenic stimulators for fresh fractures and delayed unions remain non-covered.

(This NCD last reviewed June 2005)

100-03, 150.7

NCD for Prolotherapy, Joint Sclerotherapy, and Ligamentous Injections with Sclerosing Agents (150.7)

The medical effectiveness of the above therapies has not been verified by scientifically controlled studies. Accordingly, reimbursement for these modalities should be denied on the ground that they are not reasonable and necessary as required by Sec.1862(a)(1) of the Act.

100-03, 150.10

NCD for Lumbar Artificial Disc Replacement (LADR) (150.10)

A. General
The lumbar artificial disc replacement (LADR) is a surgical procedure on the lumbar spine that involves complete removal of the damaged or diseased lumbar intervertebral disc and implantation of an artificial disc. The procedure may be done as an alternative to lumbar spinal fusion and is intended to reduce pain, increase movement at the site of surgery and restore intervertebral disc height. The Food and Drug Administration has approved the use of LADR for spine arthroplasty in skeletally mature patients with degenerative or discogenic disc disease at one level for L3 to S1.

B. Nationally Covered Indications
N/A

C. Nationally Non-Covered Indications
Effective for services performed from May 16, 2006 through August 13, 2007, the Centers for Medicare and Medicaid Services (CMS) has found that LADR with the ChariteTM lumbar artificial disc is not reasonable and necessary for the Medicare population over 60 years of age; therefore, LADR with the ChariteTM lumbar artificial disc is non-covered for Medicare beneficiaries over 60 years of age.

Effective for services performed on or after August 14, 2007, CMS has found that LADR is not reasonable and necessary for the Medicare population over 60 years of age; therefore, LADR is non-covered for Medicare beneficiaries over 60 years of age.

D. Other
For Medicare beneficiaries 60 years of age and younger, there is no national coverage determination for LADR, leaving such determinations to continue to be made by the local Medicare Administrative Contractors.

For dates of service May 16, 2006 through August 13, 2007, Medicare coverage under the investigational device exemption (IDE) for LADR with a disc other than the ChariteTM lumbar disc in eligible clinical trials is not impacted.

100-03, 160.8

NCD for Electroencephalographic (EEG) Monitoring During Surgical Procedures Involving the Cerebral Vasculature (160.8)
CIM 35-57

Electroencephalographic (EEG) monitoring is a safe and reliable technique for the assessment of gross cerebral blood flow during general anesthesia and is covered under Medicare. Very characteristic changes in the EEG occur when cerebral perfusion is inadequate for cerebral function. EEG monitoring as an indirect measure of cerebral perfusion requires the expertise of an electroencephalographer, a neurologist trained in EEG, or an advanced EEG technician for its proper interpretation.

The EEG monitoring may be covered routinely in carotid endarterectomies and in other neurological procedures where cerebral perfusion could be reduced. Such other procedures might include aneurysm surgery where hypotensive anesthesia is used or other cerebral vascular procedures where cerebral blood flow may be interrupted.

100-03, 160.17

NCD for L-DOPA (160.17)

A. Part A Payment for L-Dopa and Associated Inpatient Hospital Services
A hospital stay and related ancillary services for the administration of L-Dopa are covered if medically required for this purpose. Whether a drug represents an allowable inpatient hospital cost during such stay depends on whether it meets the definition of a drug in Sec.1861(t) of the Act; i.e., on its inclusion in the compendia named in the Act or approval by the hospital's pharmacy and drug therapeutics (P&DT) or equivalent committee. (Levodopa (L-Dopa) has been favorably evaluated for the treatment of Parkinsonism by A.M.A. Drug Evaluations, First Edition 1971, the replacement compendia for "New Drugs.")

Inpatient hospital services are frequently not required in many cases when L-Dopa therapy is initiated. Therefore, determine the medical need for inpatient hospital services on the basis of medical facts in the individual case. It is not necessary to hospitalize the typical, well-functioning, ambulatory Parkinsonian patient who has no concurrent disease at the start of L-Dopa treatment. It is reasonable to provide inpatient hospital services for Parkinsonian patients with concurrent diseases, particularly of the cardiovascular, gastrointestinal, and neuropsychiatric systems. Although many patients require hospitalization for a period of under 2 weeks, a 4-week period of inpatient care is not unreasonable.

Laboratory tests in connection with the administration of L-Dopa - The tests medically warranted in connection with the achievement of optimal dosage and the control of the side effects of L-Dopa include a complete blood count, liver function tests such as SGOT, SGPT, and/or alkaline phosphatase, BUN or creatinine and urinalysis, blood sugar, and electrocardiogram.

Whether or not the patient is hospitalized, laboratory tests in certain cases are reasonable at weekly intervals although some physicians prefer to perform the tests much less frequently.

Physical therapy furnished in connection with administration of L-Dopa - Where, following administration of the drug, the patient experiences a reduction of rigidity which permits the reestablishment of a restorative goal for him/her, physical therapy services required to enable him/her to achieve this goal are payable provided they require the skills of a qualified physical therapist and are furnished by or under the supervision of such a therapist. However, once the individual's restoration potential has been achieved, the services required to maintain him/her at this level do not generally require the skills of a qualified physical therapist. In such situations, the role of the therapist is to evaluate the patient's needs in consultation with his/her physician and design a program of exercise appropriate to the capacity and tolerance of the patient and treatment objectives of the physician, leaving to others the actual carrying out of the program. While the evaluative services rendered by a qualified physical therapist are payable as physical therapy, services furnished by others in connection with the carrying out of the maintenance program established by the therapist are not.

B. Part A Reimbursement for L-Dopa Therapy in SNFs

Initiation of L-Dopa therapy can be appropriately carried out in the SNF setting, applying the same guidelines used for initiation of L-Dopa therapy in the hospital, including the types of patients who should be covered for inpatient services, the role of physical therapy, and the use of laboratory tests. (See subsection A.) Where inpatient care is required and L-Dopa therapy is initiated in the SNF, limit the stay to a maximum of 4 weeks; but in many cases the need may be no longer than 1 or 2 weeks, depending upon the patient's condition. However, where L-Dopa therapy is begun in the hospital and the patient is transferred to an SNF for continuation of the therapy, a combined length of stay in hospital and SNF of no longer than 4 weeks is reasonable (i.e., 1 week hospital stay followed by 3 weeks SNF stay; or 2 weeks hospital stay followed by 2 weeks SNF stay; etc.). Medical need must be demonstrated in cases where the combined length of stay in hospital and SNF is longer than 4 weeks. The choice of hospital or SNF, and the decision regarding the relative length of time spent in each, should be left to the medical judgment of the treating physician.

C. L-Dopa Coverage Under Part B

Part B reimbursement may not be made for the drug L-Dopa since it is a self-administrable drug. However, physician services rendered in connection with its administration and control of its side effects are covered if determined to be reasonable and necessary. Initiation of L-Dopa therapy on an outpatient basis is possible in most cases. Visit frequency ranging from every week to every 2 or 3 months is acceptable. However, after half a year of therapy, visits more frequent than every month would usually not be reasonable.

100-03, 180.1

NCD for Medical Nutrition Therapy (180.1)

Effective October 1, 2002, basic coverage of MNT for the first year a beneficiary receives MNT with either a diagnosis of renal disease or diabetes as defined at 42 CFR Sec.410.130 is 3 hours. Also effective October 1, 2002, basic coverage in subsequent years for renal disease or diabetes is 2 hours. The dietitian/nutritionist may choose how many units are performed per day as long as all of the other requirements in this NCD and 42 CFR Secs.410.130-410.134 are met. Pursuant to the exception at 42 CFR Sec.410.132(b)(5), additional hours are considered to be medically necessary and covered if the treating physician determines that there is a change in medical condition, diagnosis, or treatment regimen that requires a change in MNT and orders additional hours during that episode of care.

Effective October 1, 2002, if the treating physician determines that receipt of both MNT and DSMT is medically necessary in the same episode of care, Medicare will cover both DSMT and MNT initial and subsequent years without decreasing either benefit as long as DSMT and MNT are not provided on the same date of service. The dietitian/nutritionist may choose how many units are performed per day as long as all of the other requirements in the NCD and 42 CFR Secs.410.130-410.134 are met. Pursuant to the exception at 42 CFR 410.132(b)(5), additional hours are considered to be medically necessary and covered if the treating physician determines that there is a change in medical condition, diagnosis, or treatment regimen that requires a change in MNT and orders additional hours during that episode of care.

100-03, 190.1

NCD for Histocompatibility Testing (190.1)

This testing is safe and effective when it is performed on patients:

- In preparation for a kidney transplant;
- In preparation for bone marrow transplantation;
- In preparation for blood platelet transfusions (particularly where multiple infusions are involved); or
- Who are suspected of having ankylosing spondylitis.

This testing is covered under Medicare when used for any of the indications listed in A, B, and C and if it is reasonable and necessary for the patient.

It is covered for ankylosing spondylitis in cases where other methods of diagnosis would not be appropriate or have yielded inconclusive results. Request documentation supporting the medical necessity of the test from the physician in all cases where ankylosing spondylitis is indicated as the reason for the test.

100-03, 190.8

NCD for Lymphocyte Mitogen Response Assays (190.8)

It is a covered test under Medicare when it is medically necessary to assess lymphocytic function in diagnosed immunodeficiency diseases and to monitor immunotherapy.

It is not covered when it is used to monitor the treatment of cancer, because its use for that purpose is experimental.

100-03, 190.9

NCD for Serologic Testing for Acquired Immunodeficiency Syndrome (AIDS) (190.9)

These tests may be covered when performed to help determine a diagnosis for symptomatic patients. They are not covered when furnished as part of a screening program for asymptomatic persons.

Note: Two enzyme-linked immunosorbent assay (ELISA) tests that were conducted on the same specimen must both be positive before Medicare will cover the Western blot test.

100-03, 190.11

NCD for Home Prothrombin Time International Normalized Ratio (INR) Monitoring for Anticoagulation Management (190.11)

A. General

Use of the International Normalized Ratio (INR) or prothrombin time (PT) - standard measurement for reporting the blood's clotting time) - allows physicians to determine the level of anticoagulation in a patient independent of the laboratory reagents used. The INR is the ratio of the patient's PT (extrinsic or tissue-factor dependent coagulation pathway) compared to the mean PT for a group of normal individuals. Maintaining patients within his/her prescribed therapeutic range minimizes adverse events associated with inadequate or excessive anticoagulation such as serious bleeding or thromboembolic events. Patient self-testing and self-management through the use of a home INR monitor may be used to improve the time in therapeutic rate (TTR) for select groups of patients. Increased TTR leads to improved clinical outcomes and reductions in thromboembolic and hemorrhagic events.

Warfarin (also prescribed under other trade names, e.g., Coumadin(R)) is a self-administered, oral anticoagulant (blood thinner) medication that affects the vitamin K- dependent clotting factors II, VII, IX and X. It is widely used for various medical conditions, and has a narrow therapeutic index, meaning it is a drug with less than a 2-fold difference between median lethal dose and median effective dose. For this reason, since October 4, 2006, it falls under the category of a Food and Drug dministration (FDA) "black-box" drug whose dosage must be closely monitored to avoid serious complications. A PT/INR monitoring system is a portable testing device that includes a finger-stick and an FDA-cleared meter that measures the time it takes for a person's blood plasma to clot.

B. Nationally Covered Indications

For services furnished on or after March 19, 2008, Medicare will cover the use of home PT/INR monitoring for chronic, oral anticoagulation management for patients with mechanical heart valves, chronic atrial fibrillation, or venous thromboembolism (inclusive of deep venous thrombosis and pulmonary embolism) on warfarin. The monitor and the home testing must be prescribed by a treating physician as provided at 42 CFR 410.32(a), and all of the following requirements must be met:

1. The patient must have been anticoagulated for at least 3 months prior to use of the home INR device; and,

2. The patient must undergo a face-to-face educational program on anticoagulation anagement and must have demonstrated the correct use of the device prior to its use in the home; and,

3. The patient continues to correctly use the device in the context of the management of the anticoagulation therapy following the initiation of home monitoring; and,

4. Self-testing with the device should not occur more frequently than once a week.

C. Nationally Non-Covered Indications

N/A

D. Other

1. All other indications for home PT/INR monitoring not indicated as nationally covered above remain at local Medicare contractor discretion.

2. This national coverage determination (NCD) is distinct from, and makes no changes to, the PT clinical laboratory NCD at section 190.17 of Publication 100-3 of the NCD Manual.

100-03, 190.14

NCD for Human Immunodeficiency Virus (HIV) Testing (Diagnosis) (190.14)

Indications and Limitations of Coverage

Indications

Diagnostic testing to establish HIV infection may be indicated when there is a strong clinical suspicion supported by one or more of the following clinical findings:

- The patient has a documented, otherwise unexplained, AIDS-defining or AIDS-associated opportunistic infection.

- The patient has another documented sexually transmitted disease which identifies significant risk of exposure to HIV and the potential for an early or subclinical infection.

- The patient has documented acute or chronic hepatitis B or C infection that identifies a significant risk of exposure to HIV and the potential for an early or subclinical infection.

- The patient has a documented AIDS-defining or AIDS-associated neoplasm.

- The patient has a documented AIDS-associated neurologic disorder or otherwise unexplained dementia.

- The patient has another documented AIDS-defining clinical condition, or a history of other severe, recurrent, or persistent conditions which suggest an underlying immune deficiency (for example, cutaneous or mucosal disorders).

- The patient has otherwise unexplained generalized signs and symptoms suggestive of a chronic process with an underlying immune deficiency (for example, fever, weight loss, malaise, fatigue, chronic diarrhea, failure to thrive, chronic cough, hemoptysis, shortness of breath, or lymphadenopathy).

- The patient has otherwise unexplained laboratory evidence of a chronic disease process with an underlying immune deficiency (for example, anemia, leukopenia, pancytopenia, lymphopenia, or low CD4+ lymphocyte count).

- The patient has signs and symptoms of acute retroviral syndrome with fever, malaise, lymphadenopathy, and skin rash.

- The patient has documented exposure to blood or body fluids known to be capable of transmitting HIV (for example, needlesticks and other significant blood exposures) and antiviral therapy is initiated or anticipated to be initiated.

- The patient is undergoing treatment for rape. (HIV testing is a part of the rape treatment protocol.)

Limitations

HIV antibody testing in the United States is usually performed using HIV-1 or HIV-½ combination tests. HIV-2 testing is indicated if clinical circumstances suggest HIV-2 is likely (that is, compatible clinical findings and HIV-1 test negative). HIV-2 testing may also be indicated in areas of the country where there is greater prevalence of HIV-2 infections.

The Western Blot test should be performed only after documentation that the initial EIA tests are repeatedly positive or equivocal on a single sample.

- The HIV antigen tests currently have no defined diagnostic usage.

- Direct viral RNA detection may be performed in those situations where serologic testing does not establish a diagnosis but strong clinical suspicion persists (for example, acute retroviral syndrome, nonspecific serologic evidence of HIV, or perinatal HIV infection).

- If initial serologic tests confirm an HIV infection, repeat testing is not indicated.

- If initial serologic tests are HIV EIA negative and there is no indication for confirmation of infection by viral RNA detection, the interval prior to retesting is 3-6 months.

- Testing for evidence of HIV infection using serologic methods may be medically appropriate in situations where there is a risk of exposure to HIV. However, in the absence of a documented AIDS defining or HIV- associated disease, an HIV associated sign or symptom, or documented exposure to a known HIV-infected source, the testing is considered by Medicare to be screening and thus is not covered by Medicare (for example, history of multiple blood component transfusions, exposure to blood or body fluids not resulting in consideration of therapy, history of transplant, history of illicit drug use, multiple sexual partners, same-sex encounters, prostitution, or contact with prostitutes).

- The CPT Editorial Panel has issued a number of codes for infectious agent detection by direct antigen or nucleic acid probe techniques that have not yet been developed or are only being used on an investigational basis. Laboratory providers are advised to remain current on FDA-approval status for these tests.

100-03, 190.15

NCD for Blood Counts (190.15)

Indications

Indications for a CBC or hemogram include red cell, platelet, and white cell disorders. Examples of these indications are enumerated individually below.

1. Indications for a CBC generally include the evaluation of bone marrow dysfunction as a result of neoplasms, therapeutic agents, exposure to toxic substances, or pregnancy. The CBC is also useful in assessing peripheral destruction of blood cells, suspected bone marrow failure or bone marrow infiltrate, suspected myeloproliferative, myelodysplastic, or lymphoproliferative processes, and immune disorders.

2. Indications for hemogram or CBC related to red cell (RBC) parameters of the hemogram include signs, symptoms, test results, illness, or disease that can be associated with anemia or other red blood cell disorder (e.g., pallor, weakness, fatigue, weight loss, bleeding, acute injury associated with blood loss or suspected blood loss, abnormal menstrual bleeding, hematuria, hematemesis, hematochezia, positive fecal occult blood test, malnutrition, vitamin deficiency, malabsorption, neuropathy, known malignancy, presence of acute or chronic disease that may have associated anemia, coagulation or hemostatic disorders, postural dizziness, syncope, abdominal pain, change in bowel habits, chronic marrow hypoplasia or decreased RBC production, tachycardia, systolic heart murmur, congestive heart failure, dyspnea, angina, nailbed deformities, growth retardation, jaundice, hepatomegaly, splenomegaly, lymphadenopathy, ulcers on the lower extremities).

3. Indications for hemogram or CBC related to red cell (RBC) parameters of the hemogram include signs, symptoms, test results, illness, or disease that can be associated with polycythemia (for example, fever, chills, ruddy skin, conjunctival redness, cough, wheezing, cyanosis, clubbing of the fingers, orthopnea, heart murmur, headache, vague cognitive changes including memory changes, sleep apnea, weakness, pruritus, dizziness, excessive sweating, visual symptoms, weight loss, massive obesity, gastrointestinal bleeding, paresthesias, dyspnea, joint symptoms, epigastric distress, pain and erythema of the fingers or toes, venous or arterial thrombosis, thromboembolism, myocardial infarction, stroke, transient ischemic attacks, congenital heart disease, chronic obstructive pulmonary disease, increased erythropoietin production associated with neoplastic, renal or hepatic disorders, androgen or diuretic use, splenomegaly, hepatomegaly, diastolic hypertension.)

4. Specific indications for CBC with differential count related to the WBC include signs, symptoms, test results, illness, or disease associated with leukemia, infections or inflammatory processes, suspected bone marrow failure or bone marrow infiltrate, suspected myeloproliferative, myelodysplastic or lymphoproliferative disorder, use of drugs that may cause leukopenia, and immune disorders (e.g., fever, chills, sweats, shock, fatigue, malaise, tachycardia, tachypnea, heart murmur, seizures, alterations of consciousness, mengismus, pain such as headache, abdominal pain, arthralgia, odynophagia, or dysuria, redness or swelling of skin, soft tissue bone, or joint, ulcers of the skin or mucous membranes, gangrene, mucous membrane discharge, bleeding, thrombosis, respiratory failure, pulmonary infiltrate, jaundice, diarrhea, vomiting, hepatomegaly, splenomegaly, lymphadenopathy, opportunistic infection such as oral candidiasis.)

5. Specific indications for CBC related to the platelet count include signs, symptoms, test results, illness, or disease associated with increased or decreased platelet production and destruction, or platelet dysfunction (e.g., gastrointestinal bleeding, genitourinary tract bleeding, bilateral epistaxis, thrombosis, ecchymosis, purpura, jaundice, petechiae, fever, heparin therapy, suspected DIC, shock, pre-eclampsia, neonate with maternal ITP, massive transfusion, recent platelet transfusion, cardiopulmonary bypass, hemolytic uremic syndrome, renal diseases, lymphadenopathy, hepatomegaly, splenomegaly, hypersplenism, neurologic abnormalities, viral or other infection, myeloproliferative, myelodysplastic, or lymphoproliferative disorder, thrombosis, exposure to toxic agents, excessive alcohol ingestion, autoimmune disorders (SLE, RA and other).

6. Indications for hemogram or CBC related to red cell (RBC) parameters of the hemogram include, in addition to those already listed, thalassemia, suspected hemoglobinopathy, lead poisoning, arsenic poisoning, and spherocytosis.

7. Specific indications for CBC with differential count related to the WBC include, in addition to those already listed, storage diseases; mucopolysaccharidoses, and use of drugs that cause leukocytosis such as G-CSF or GM-CSF.

8. Specific indications for CBC related to platelet count include, in addition to those already listed, May-Hegglin syndrome and Wiskott-Aldrich syndrome.

Limitations

1. Testing of patients who are asymptomatic, or who do not have a condition that could be expected to result in a hematological abnormality, is screening and is not a covered service.

2. In some circumstances it may be appropriate to perform only a hemoglobin or hematocrit to assess the oxygen carrying capacity of the blood. When the ordering provider requests only a hemoglobin or hematocrit, the remaining components of the CBC are not covered.

3. When a blood count is performed for an end-stage renal disease (ESRD) patient, and is billed outside the ESRD rate, documentation of the medical necessity for the blood count must be submitted with the claim.

4. In some patients presenting with certain signs, symptoms or diseases, a single CBC may be appropriate. Repeat testing may not be indicated unless abnormal results are found, or unless there is a change in clinical condition. If repeat testing is performed, a more descriptive diagnosis code (e.g., anemia) should be reported to support medical necessity. However, repeat testing may be indicated where results are normal in patients with conditions where there is a continued risk for the development of hematologic abnormality.

100-03, 190.18

Serum Iron Studies

Indications:

1. Ferritin (82728), iron (83540) and either iron binding capacity (83550) or transferrin (84466) are useful in the differential diagnosis of iron deficiency, anemia, and for iron overload conditions.

   a. The following presentations are examples that may support the use of these studies for evaluating iron deficiency:

   – Certain abnormal blood count values (i.e., decreased mean corpuscular volume (MCV), decreased hemoglobin/hematocrit when the MCV is low or normal, or increased red cell distribution width (RDW) and low or normal MCV);

   – Abnormal appetite (pica);

   – Acute or chronic gastrointestinal blood loss;

   – Hematuria;

   – Menorrhagia;

   – Malabsorption;

   – Status post-gastrectomy;

   – Status post-gastrojejunostomy;

   – Malnutrition;

   – Preoperative autologous blood collection(s);

   – Malignant, chronic inflammatory and infectious conditions associated with anemia which may present in a similar manner to iron deficiency anemia;

   – Following a significant surgical procedure where blood loss had occurred and had not been repaired with adequate iron replacement.

   b. The following presentations are examples that may support the use of these studies for evaluating iron overload:

   – Chronic Hepatitis;

   – Diabetes;

   – Hyperpigmentation of skin;

   – Arthropathy;

   – Cirrhosis;

   – Hypogonadism;

   – Hypopituitarism;

   – Impaired porphyrin metabolism;

   – Heart failure;

   – Multiple transfusions;

   – Sideroblastic anemia;

   – Thalassemia major;

   – Cardiomyopathy, cardiac dysrhythmias and conduction disturbances.

2. Follow-up testing may be appropriate to monitor response to therapy, e.g., oral or parenteral iron, ascorbic acid, and erythropoietin.

3. Iron studies may be appropriate in patients after treatment for other nutritional deficiency anemias, such as folate and vitamin B12, because iron deficiency may not be revealed until such a nutritional deficiency is treated.

4. Serum ferritin may be appropriate for monitoring iron status in patients with chronic renal disease with or without dialysis.

5. Serum iron may also be indicated for evaluation of toxic effects of iron and other metals (e.g., nickel, cadmium, aluminum, lead) whether due to accidental, intentional exposure or metabolic causes.

Limitations:

1. Iron studies should be used to diagnose and manage iron deficiency or iron overload states. These tests are not to be used solely to assess acute phase reactants where disease management will be unchanged. For example, infections and malignancies are associated with elevations in acute phase reactants such as ferritin, and decreases in serum iron concentration, but iron studies would only be medically necessary if results of iron studies might alter the management of the primary diagnosis or might warrant direct treatment of an iron disorder or condition.

2. If a normal serum ferritin level is documented, repeat testing would not ordinarily be medically necessary unless there is a change in the patient's condition, and ferritin assessment is needed for the ongoing management of the patient. For example, a patient presents with new onset insulin-dependent diabetes mellitus and has a serum ferritin level performed for the suspicion of hemochromatosis. If the ferritin level is normal, the repeat ferritin for diabetes mellitus would not be medically necessary.

3. When an End Stage Renal Disease (ESRD) patient is tested for ferritin, testing more frequently than every three months (the frequency authorized by 3167.3, Fiscal Intermediary manual) requires documentation of medical necessity [e.g.,

other than "Chronic Renal Failure" (ICD-9-CM 585) or "Renal Failure, Unspecified" (ICD-9-CM 586)].

4. It is ordinarily not necessary to measure both transferrin and TIBC at the same time because TIBC is an indirect measure of transferrin. When transferrin is ordered as part of the nutritional assessment for evaluating malnutrition, it is not necessary to order other iron studies unless iron deficiency or iron overload is suspected as well.

5. It is not ordinarily necessary to measure both iron/TIBC (or transferrin) and ferritin in initial patient testing. If clinically indicated after evaluation of the initial iron studies, it may be appropriate to perform additional iron studies either on the initial specimen or on a subsequently obtained specimen. After a diagnosis of iron deficiency or iron overload is established, either iron/TIBC (or transferrin) or ferritin may be medically necessary for monitoring, but not both.

6. It would not ordinarily be considered medically necessary to do a ferritin as a preoperative test except in the presence of anemia or recent autologous blood collections prior to the surgery.

100-03, 190.19

Collagen Crosslinks, Any Method

Indications:

Generally speaking, collagen crosslink testing is useful mostly in "fast losers" of bone. The age when these bone markers can help direct therapy is often pre-Medicare. By the time a fast loser of bone reaches age 65, she will most likely have been stabilized by appropriate therapy or have lost so much bone mass that further testing is useless. Coverage for bone marker assays may be established, however, for younger Medicare beneficiaries and for those men and women who might become fast losers because of some other therapy such as glucocorticoids. Safeguards should be incorporated to prevent excessive use of tests in patients for whom they have no clinical relevance.

Collagen crosslinks testing is used to:

• Identify individuals with elevated bone resorption, who have osteoporosis in whom response to treatment is being monitored;

• Predict response (as assessed by bone mass measurements) to FDA approved antiresorptive therapy in postmenopausal women; and

• Assess response to treatment of patients with osteoporosis, Paget's disease of the bone, or risk for osteoporosis where treatment may include FDA approved antiresorptive agents, anti-estrogens or selective estrogen receptor moderators.

Limitations:

Because of significant specimen to specimen collagen crosslink physiologic variability (15-20%), current recommendations for appropriate utilization include: one or two base-line assays from specified urine collections on separate days; followed by a repeat assay about three months after starting anti-resorptive therapy; followed by a repeat assay in 12 months after the three-month assay; and thereafter not more than annually, unless there is a change in therapy in which circumstance an additional test may be indicated three months after the initiation of new therapy.

Some collagen crosslink assays may not be appropriate for use in some disorders, according to FDA labeling restrictions.

Note: Scroll down for links to the quarterly Covered Code Lists (including narrative).

100-03, 190.20

NCD for Blood Glucose Testing (190.20)

Indications:

Blood glucose values are often necessary for the management of patients with diabetes mellitus, where hyperglycemia and hypoglycemia are often present. They are also critical in the determination of control of blood glucose levels in the patient with impaired fasting glucose (FPG 110-125 mg/dL), the patient with insulin resistance syndrome and/or carbohydrate intolerance (excessive rise in glucose following ingestion of glucose or glucose sources of food), in the patient with a hypoglycemia disorder such as nesidioblastosis or insulinoma, and in patients with a catabolic or malnutrition state. In addition to those conditions already listed, glucose testing may be medically necessary in patients with tuberculosis, unexplained chronic or recurrent infections, alcoholism, coronary artery disease (especially in women), or unexplained skin conditions (including pruritus, local skin infections, ulceration and gangrene without an established cause).

Many medical conditions may be a consequence of a sustained elevated or depressed glucose level. These include comas, seizures or epilepsy, confusion, abnormal hunger, abnormal weight loss or gain, and loss of sensation. Evaluation of glucose may also be indicated in patients on medications known to affect carbohydrate metabolism.

Effective January 1, 2005, the Medicare law expanded coverage to diabetic screening services. Some forms of blood glucode testing covered under this national coverage determination may be covered for screening purposes subject to specified frequencies. See 42 CFR 410.18 and section 90, chapter 18 of the Claims Processing Manual, for a full description of this screening benefit.

Limitations:

Frequent home blood glucose testing by diabetic patients should be encouraged. In stable, non-hospitalized patients who are unable or unwilling to do home monitoring, it may be reasonable and necessary to measure quantitative blood glucose up to four times annually.

Depending upon the age of the patient, type of diabetes, degree of control, complications of diabetes, and other co-morbid conditions, more frequent testing than four times annually may be reasonable and necessary.

In some patients presenting with nonspecific signs, symptoms, or diseases not normally associated with disturbances in glucose metabolism, a single blood glucose test may be medically necessary. Repeat testing may not be indicated unless abnormal results are found or unless there is a change in clinical condition. If repeat testing is performed, a specific diagnosis code (e.g., diabetes) should be reported to support medical necessity. However, repeat testing may be indicated where results are normal in patients with conditions where there is a confirmed continuing risk of glucose metabolism abnormality (e.g., monitoring glucocorticoid therapy).

100-03, 190.22

NCD for Thyroid Testing (190.22)

Indications

Thyroid function tests are used to define hyper function, euthyroidism, or hypofunction of thyroid disease. Thyroid testing may be reasonable and necessary to:

- Distinguish between primary and secondary hypothyroidism;
- Confirm or rule out primary hypothyroidism;
- Monitor thyroid hormone levels (for example, patients with goiter, thyroid nodules, or thyroid cancer);
- Monitor drug therapy in patients with primary hypothyroidism;
- Confirm or rule out primary hyperthyroidism; and
- Monitor therapy in patients with hyperthyroidism.

Thyroid function testing may be medically necessary in patients with disease or neoplasm of the thyroid and other endocrine glands. Thyroid function testing may also be medically necessary in patients with metabolic disorders; malnutrition; hyperlipidemia; certain types of anemia; psychosis and non-psychotic personality disorders; unexplained depression; ophthalmologic disorders; various cardiac arrhythmias; disorders of menstruation; skin conditions; myalgias; and a wide array of signs and symptoms, including alterations in consciousness; malaise; hypothermia; symptoms of the nervous and musculoskeletal system; skin and integumentary system; nutrition and metabolism; cardiovascular; and gastrointestinal system.

It may be medically necessary to do follow-up thyroid testing in patients with a personal history of malignant neoplasm of the endocrine system and in patients on long-term thyroid drug therapy.

Limitations

Testing may be covered up to two times a year in clinically stable patients; more frequent testing may be reasonable and necessary for patients whose thyroid therapy has been altered or in whom symptoms or signs of hyperthyroidism or hypothyroidism are noted.

100-03, 190.23

NCD for Lipid Testing (190.23)

Indications and Limitations of Coverage

Indications

The medical community recognizes lipid testing as appropriate for evaluating atherosclerotic cardiovascular disease. Conditions in which lipid testing may be indicated include:

- Assessment of patients with atherosclerotic cardiovascular disease.
- Evaluation of primary dyslipidemia.
- Any form of atherosclerotic disease, or any disease leading to the formation of atherosclerotic disease.
- Diagnostic evaluation of diseases associated with altered lipid metabolism, such as: nephrotic syndrome, pancreatitis, hepatic disease, and hypo and hyperthyroidism.
- Secondary dyslipidemia, including diabetes mellitus, disorders of gastrointestinal absorption, chronic renal failure.
- Signs or symptoms of dyslipidemias, such as skin lesions.
- As follow-up to the initial screen for coronary heart disease (total cholesterol + HDL cholesterol) when total cholesterol is determined to be high (>240 mg/dL), or borderline-high (200-240 mg/dL) plus two or more coronary heart disease risk factors, or an HDL cholesterol, <35 mg/dl.

To monitor the progress of patients on anti-lipid dietary management and pharmacologic therapy for the treatment of elevated blood lipid disorders, total cholesterol, HDL cholesterol and LDL cholesterol may be used. Triglycerides may be obtained if this lipid fraction is also elevated or if the patient is put on drugs (for example, thiazide diuretics, beta blockers, estrogens, glucocorticoids, and tamoxifen) which may raise the triglyceride level.

When monitoring long term anti-lipid dietary or pharmacologic therapy and when following patients with borderline high total or LDL cholesterol levels, it may be reasonable to perform the lipid panel annually. A lipid panel at a yearly interval will usually be adequate while measurement of the serum total cholesterol or a measured LDL should suffice for interim visits if the patient does not have hypertriglyceridemia.

Any one component of the panel or a measured LDL may be reasonable and necessary up to six times the first year for monitoring dietary or pharmacologic therapy. More frequent total cholesterol HDL cholesterol, LDL cholesterol and triglyceride testing may be indicated for marked elevations or for changes to anti-lipid therapy due to inadequate initial patient response to dietary or pharmacologic therapy. The LDL cholesterol or total cholesterol may be measured three times yearly after treatment goals have been achieved.

Electrophoretic or other quantitation of lipoproteins may be indicated if the patient has a primary disorder of lipoid metabolism.

Effective January 1, 2005, the Medicare law expanded coverage to cardiovascular screening services. Several of the procedures included in this NCD may be covered for screening purposes subject to specified frequencies. See 42 CFR 410.17 and section 100, chapter 18, of the Claims Processing Manual, for a full description of this benefit.

Limitations

Lipid panel and hepatic panel testing may be used for patients with severe psoriasis which has not responded to conventional therapy and for which the retinoid etretinate has been prescribed and who have developed hyperlipidemia or hepatic toxicity. Specific examples include erythrodermia and generalized pustular type and psoriasis associated with arthritis.

Routine screening and prophylactic testing for lipid disorder are not covered by Medicare. While lipid screening may be medically appropriate, Medicare by statute does not pay for it. Lipid testing in asymptomatic individuals is considered to be screening regardless of the presence of other risk factors such as family history, tobacco use, etc.

Once a diagnosis is established, one or several specific tests are usually adequate for monitoring the course of the disease. Less specific diagnoses (for example, other chest pain) alone do not support medical necessity of these tests.

When monitoring long term anti-lipid dietary or pharmacologic therapy and when following patients with borderline high total or LDL cholesterol levels, it is reasonable to perform the lipid panel annually. A lipid panel at a yearly interval will usually be adequate while measurement of the serum total cholesterol or a measured LDL should suffice for interim visits if the patient does not have hypertriglyceridemia.

Any one component of the panel or a measured LDL may be medically necessary up to six times the first year for monitoring dietary or pharmacologic therapy. More frequent total cholesterol HDL cholesterol, LDL cholesterol and triglyceride testing may be indicated for marked elevations or for changes to anti-lipid therapy due to inadequate initial patient response to dietary or pharmacologic therapy. The LDL cholesterol or total cholesterol may be measured three times yearly after treatment goals have been achieved.

If no dietary or pharmacological therapy is advised, monitoring is not necessary.

When evaluating non-specific chronic abnormalities of the liver (for example, elevations of transaminase, alkaline phosphatase, abnormal imaging studies, etc.), a lipid panel would generally not be indicated more than twice per year.

100-03, 190.26

NCD for Carcinoembryonic Antigen (CEA)

Carcinoembryonic antigen (CEA) is a protein polysaccharide found in some carcinomas. It is effective as a biochemical marker for monitoring the response of certain malignancies to therapy.

Indications

CEA may be medically necessary for follow-up of patients with colorectal carcinoma. It would however only be medically necessary at treatment decision-making points. In some clinical situations (e.g. adenocarcinoma of the lung, small cell carcinoma of the lung, and some gastrointestinal carcinomas) when a more specific marker is not expressed by the tumor, CEA may be a medically necessary alternative marker for monitoring. Preoperative CEA may also be helpful in determining the post-operative adequacy of surgical resection and subsequent medical management. In general, a single tumor marker will suffice in following patients with colorectal carcinoma or other malignancies that express such tumor markers.

In following patients who have had treatment for colorectal carcinoma, ASCO guideline suggests that if resection of liver metastasis would be indicated, it is recommended that post-operative CEA testing be performed every two to three months in patients with initial stage II or stage III disease for at least two years after diagnosis.

For patients with metastatic solid tumors which express CEA, CEA may be measured at the start of the treatment and with subsequent treatment cycles to assess the tumor's response to therapy.

Limitations:

Serum CEA determinations are generally not indicated more frequently than once per chemotherapy treatment cycle for patients with metastatic solid tumors which express CEA or every two months post-surgical treatment for patients who have had colorectal carcinoma. However, it may be proper to order the test more frequently in certain situations, for example, when there has been a significant change from prior CEA level or a significant change in patient status which could reflect disease progression or recurrence.

Testing with a diagnosis of an in situ carcinoma is not reasonably done more frequently than once, unless the result is abnormal, in which case the test may be repeated once.

100-03, 190.3

NCD for Cytogenetic Studies (190.3)

Medicare covers these tests when they are reasonable and necessary for the diagnosis or treatment of the following conditions:

- Genetic disorders (e.g., mongolism) in a fetus (See Medicare Benefit Policy Manual, Chapter 15, "Covered medical and Other health Services," Sec. 20.1)

- Failure of sexual development;

- Chronic myelogenous leukemia;

- Acute leukemias lymphoid (FAB L1-L3), myeloid (FAB M0-M7), and unclassified; or

- Mylodysplasia

100-03, 190.31

NCD for Prostate Specific Antigen (PSA) (190.31)

Indications:

PSA is of proven value in differentiating benign from malignant disease in men with lower urinary tract signs and symptoms (e.g., hematuria, slow urine stream, hesitancy, urgency, frequency, nocturia and incontinence) as well as with patients with palpably abnormal prostate glands on physician exam, and in patients with other laboratory or imaging studies that suggest the possibility of a malignant prostate disorder. PSA is also a marker used to follow the progress of prostate cancer once a diagnosis has been established, such as in detecting metastatic or persistent disease in patients who may require additional treatment. PSA testing may also be useful in the differential diagnosis of men presenting with as yet undiagnosed disseminated metastatic disease.

Limitations:

Generally, for patients with lower urinary tract signs or symptoms, the test is performed only once per year unless there is a change in the patient's medical condition.

Testing with a diagnosis of in situ carcinoma is not reasonably done more frequently than once, unless the result is abnormal, in which case the test may be repeated once.

100-03, 210.1

NCD for Prostate Cancer Screening Tests (210.1)

Indications and Limitations of Coverage

CIM 50-55

Covered

A. General

Section 4103 of the Balanced Budget Act of 1997 provides for coverage of certain prostate cancer screening tests subject to certain coverage, frequency, and payment limitations. Medicare will cover prostate cancer screening tests/procedures for the early detection of prostate cancer. Coverage of prostate cancer screening tests includes the following procedures furnished to an individual for the early detection of prostate cancer:

- Screening digital rectal examination; and

- Screening prostate specific antigen blood test

B. Screening Digital Rectal Examinations

Screening digital rectal examinations are covered at a frequency of once every 12 months for men who have attained age 50 (at least 11 months have passed following the month in which the last Medicare-covered screening digital rectal examination was performed). Screening digital rectal examination means a clinical examination of an individual's prostate for nodules or other abnormalities of the prostate. This screening must be performed by a doctor of medicine or osteopathy (as defined in §1861(r)(1) of the Act), or by a physician assistant, nurse practitioner, clinical nurse specialist, or certified nurse midwife (as defined in §1861(aa) and §1861(gg) of the Act) who is authorized under State law to perform the examination, fully knowledgeable about the beneficiary's medical condition, and would be responsible for using the results of any examination performed in the overall management of the beneficiary's specific medical problem.

C. Screening Prostate Specific Antigen Tests

Screening prostate specific antigen tests are covered at a frequency of once every 12 months for men who have attained age 50 (at least 11 months have passed following the month in which the last Medicare-covered screening prostate specific antigen test was performed). Screening prostate specific antigen tests (PSA) means a test to detect the marker for adenocarcinoma of prostate. PSA is a reliable immunocytochemical marker for primary and metastatic adenocarcinoma of prostate. This screening must be ordered by the beneficiary's physician or by the beneficiary's physician assistant, nurse practitioner, clinical nurse specialist, or certified nurse midwife (the term "attending physician"; is defined in §1861(r)(1) of the Act to mean a doctor of medicine or osteopathy and the terms ";physician assistant, nurse practitioner, clinical nurse specialist, or certified nurse midwife"; are defined in §1861(aa) and §1861(gg) of the Act) who is fully knowledgeable about the beneficiary's medical condition, and who would be responsible for using the results of any examination (test) performed in the overall management of the beneficiary's specific medical problem.

100-03, 210.2

NCD for Screening Pap Smears and Pelvic Examinations for Early Detection of Cervical or Vaginal Cancer (210.2)

Screening Pap Smear

A screening pap smear and related medically necessary services provided to a woman for the early detection of cervical cancer (including collection of the sample of cells and a physician's interpretation of the test results) and pelvic examination (including clinical breast examination) are covered under Medicare Part B when ordered by a physician (or authorized practitioner) under one of the following conditions:

- She has not had such a test during the preceding two years or is a woman of childbearing age (Â§1861(nn) of the Social Security Act (the Act).

- There is evidence (on the basis of her medical history or other findings) that she is at high risk of developing cervical cancer and her physician (or authorized practitioner) recommends that she have the test performed more frequently than every two years.

High risk factors for cervical and vaginal cancer are:

- Early onset of sexual activity (under 16 years of age)

- Multiple sexual partners (five or more in a lifetime)

- History of sexually transmitted disease (including HIV infection)

- Fewer than three negative or any pap smears within the previous seven years; and

- DES (diethylstilbestrol) - exposed daughters of women who took DES during pregnancy.

NOTE: Claims for pap smears must indicate the beneficiary's low or high risk status by including the appropriate diagnosis code on the line item (Item 24E of the Form CMS-1500).

Definitions

A woman as described in Â§1861(nn) of the Act is a woman who is of childbearing age and has had a pap smear test during any of the preceding 3 years that indicated the presence of cervical or vaginal cancer or other abnormality, or is at high risk of developing cervical or vaginal cancer.

A woman of childbearing age is one who is premenopausal and has been determined by a physician or other qualified practitioner to be of childbearing age, based upon the medical history or other findings.

Other qualified practitioner, as defined in 42 CFR 410.56(a) includes a certified nurse midwife (as defined in Â§1861(gg) of the Act), or a physician assistant, nurse practitioner, or clinical nurse specialist (as defined in Â§1861(aa) of the Act) who is authorized under State law to perform the examination.

Screening Pelvic Examination

Section 4102 of the Balanced Budget Act of 1997 provides for coverage of screening pelvic examinations (including a clinical breast examination) for all female beneficiaries, subject to certain frequency and other limitations. A screening pelvic examination (including a clinical breast examination) should include at least seven of the following eleven elements:

- Inspection and palpation of breasts for masses or lumps, tenderness, symmetry, or nipple discharge.

- Digital rectal examination including sphincter tone, presence of hemorrhoids, and rectal masses. Pelvic examination (with or without specimen collection for smears and cultures) including:

- External genitalia (for example, general appearance, hair distribution, or lesions).

- Urethral meatus (for example, size, location, lesions, or prolapse).

- Urethra (for example, masses, tenderness, or scarring).

- Bladder (for example, fullness, masses, or tenderness).

- Vagina (for example, general appearance, estrogen effect, discharge lesions, pelvic support, cystocele, or rectocele).

- Cervix (for example, general appearance, lesions, or discharge).

- Uterus (for example, size, contour, position, mobility, tenderness, consistency, descent, or support).

- Adnexa/parametria (for example, masses, tenderness, organomegaly, or nodularity).

- Anus and perineum.

This description is from Documentation Guidelines for Evaluation and Management Services, published in May 1997 and was developed by the Centers for Medicare & Medicaid Services and the American Medical Association.

100-03, 210.2.1

Screening for Cervical Cancer with Human Papillomavirus (HPV) Testing (Effective July 9, 2015)

(Rev. 189, Issued: 02-05-16, Effective: 07-05-16; Implementation: 03-07-16 - for non-shared MAC edits; 07-05-16 - CWF analysis and design; 10-03-16 - CWF Coding, Testing and Implementation, MCS, and FISS Implementation; 01-03-17 - Requirement BR9434.04.8.2)

A. General

Medicare covers a screening pelvic examination and Pap test for all female beneficiaries at 12 or 24 month intervals, based on specific risk factors. See 42 C.F.R. §410.56; Medicare National Coverage Determinations Manual, §210.2.1 Current Medicare coverage does not include the HPV testing. Pursuant to §1861(ddd) of the Social Security Act, the Secretary may add coverage of "additional preventive services" if certain statutory requirements are met.

B. Nationally Covered Indications

Effective for services performed on or after July 9, 2015, CMS has determined that the evidence is sufficient to add Human Papillomavirus (HPV) testing once every five years as an additional preventive service benefit under the Medicare program for asymptomatic beneficiaries aged 30 to 65 years in conjunction with the Pap smear test. CMS will cover screening for cervical cancer with the appropriate U.S. Food and Drug Administration (FDA) approved/cleared laboratory tests, used consistent with FDA approved labeling and in compliance with the Clinical Laboratory Improvement Act (CLIA) regulations.

C. Nationally Non-Covered Indications

Unless specifically covered in this NCD, any other NCD, by statute or regulation, preventive services are non-covered by Medicare.

D. Other

(This NCD last reviewed July 2015.)

100-03, 220.6.9

NCD for PET (FDG) for Refractory Seizures (220.6.9)

Beginning July 1, 2001, Medicare covers FDG PET for pre-surgical evaluation for the purpose of localization of a focus of refractory seizure activity.

Limitations: Covered only for pre-surgical evaluation.

Documentation that these conditions are met should be maintained by the referring physician in the beneficiary's medical record, as is normal business practice.

(This NCD last reviewed June 2001.)

100-03, 220.6.17

NCD for Positron Emission Tomography (FDG) for Oncologic Conditions (220.6.17)

A. General

FDG (2-[F18] fluoro-2-deoxy-D-glucose) Positron Emission Tomography (PET) is a minimally-invasive diagnostic imaging procedure used to evaluate glucose metabolism in normal tissue as well as in diseased tissues in conditions such as cancer, ischemic heart disease, and some neurologic disorders. FDG is an injected radionuclide (or radiopharmaceutical) that emits sub-atomic particles, known as positrons, as it decays. FDG PET uses a positron camera (tomograph) to measure the decay of FDG. The rate of FDG decay provides biochemical information on glucose metabolism in the tissue being studied. As malignancies can cause abnormalities of metabolism and blood flow, FDG PET evaluation may indicate the probable presence or absence of a malignancy based upon observed differences in biologic activity compared to adjacent tissues.

The Centers for Medicare and Medicaid Services (CMS) was asked by the National Oncologic PET Registry (NOPR) to reconsider section 220.6 of the National Coverage Determinations (NCD) Manual to end the prospective data collection requirements under Coverage with Evidence Development (CED) across all oncologic indications of FDG PET imaging. The CMS received public input indicating that the current coverage framework of prospective data collection under CED be ended for all oncologic uses of FDG PET imaging.

1. Framework

   Effective for claims with dates of service on and after June 11, 2013, CMS is adopting a coverage framework that ends the prospective data collection requirements by NOPR under CED for all oncologic uses of FDG PET imaging. CMS is making this change for all NCDs that address coverage of FDG PET for oncologic uses addressed in this decision. This decision does not change coverage for any use of PET imaging using radiopharmaceuticals NaF-18 (fluorine-18 labeled sodium fluoride), ammonia N-13, or rubidium-82 (Rb-82).

2. Initial Anti-Tumor Treatment Strategy

   CMS continues to believe that the evidence is adequate to determine that the results of FDG PET imaging are useful in determining the appropriate initial anti-tumor treatment strategy for beneficiaries with suspected cancer and improve health outcomes and thus are reasonable and necessary under §1862(a)(1)(A) of the Social Security Act (the Act).

   Therefore, CMS continues to nationally cover one FDG PET study for beneficiaries who have cancers that are biopsy proven or strongly suspected based on other diagnostic testing when the beneficiary's treating physician determines that the FDG PET study is needed to determine the location and/or extent of the tumor for the following therapeutic purposes related to the initial anti-tumor treatment strategy:

   — To determine whether or not the beneficiary is an appropriate candidate for an invasive diagnostic or therapeutic procedure; or

   — To determine the optimal anatomic location for an invasive procedure; or

— To determine the anatomic extent of tumor when the recommended antitumor treatment reasonably depends on the extent of the tumor.

See the table at the end of this section for a synopsis of all nationally covered and noncovered oncologic uses of FDG PET imaging.

B.1. Initial Anti-Tumor Treatment Strategy Nationally Covered Indications

a. CMS continues to nationally cover FDG PET imaging for the initial anti-tumor treatment strategy for male and female breast cancer only when used in staging distant metastasis.

b. CMS continues to nationally cover FDG PET to determine initial anti-tumor treatment strategy for melanoma other than for the evaluation of regional lymph nodes.

c. CMS continues to nationally cover FDG PET imaging for the detection of pre-treatment metastasis (i.e., staging) in newly diagnosed cervical cancers following conventional imaging.

C.1. Initial Anti-Tumor Treatment Strategy Nationally Non-Covered Indications

a. CMS continues to nationally non-cover initial anti-tumor treatment strategy in Medicare beneficiaries who have adenocarcinoma of the prostate.

b. CMS continues to nationally non-cover FDG PET imaging for diagnosis of breast cancer and initial staging of axillary nodes.

c. CMS continues to nationally non-cover FDG PET imaging for initial anti-tumor treatment strategy for the evaluation of regional lymph nodes in melanoma.

d. CMS continues to nationally non-cover FDG PET imaging for the diagnosis of cervical cancer related to initial anti-tumor treatment strategy.

3. Subsequent Anti-Tumor Treatment Strategy

B.2. Subsequent Anti-Tumor Treatment Strategy Nationally Covered Indications

Three FDG PET scans are nationally covered when used to guide subsequent management of anti-tumor treatment strategy after completion of initial anti-cancer therapy. Coverage of more than three FDG PET scans to guide subsequent management of anti-tumor treatment strategy after completion of initial anti-cancer therapy shall be determined by the local Medicare Administrative Contractors.

4. Synopsis of Coverage of FDG PET for Oncologic Conditions

Effective for claims with dates of service on and after June 11, 2013, the chart below summarizes national FDG PET coverage for oncologic conditions:

FDG PET for Cancers Tumor Type	Initial Treatment Strategy (formerly "diagnosis" & "staging")	Subsequent Treatment Strategy (formerly "restaging" & "monitoring response to treatment"
Colorectal	Cover	Cover
Esophagus	Cover	Cover
Head & Neck (not Thyroid, CNS)	Cover	Cover
Lymphoma	Cover	Cover
Non-Small Cell Lung	Cover	Cover
Ovary	Cover	Cover
Brain	Cover	Cover
Cervix	Cover w/exception*	Cover
Small Cell Lung	Cover	Cover
Soft Tissue Sarcoma	Cover	Cover
Pancreas	Cover	Cover
Testes	Cover	Cover
Prostate	Non-cover	Cover
Thyroid	Cover	Cover
Breast (male and female)	Cover w/exception*	Cover
Melanoma	Cover w/exception*	Cover
All Other Solid Tumors	Cover	Cover
Myeloma	Cover	Cover
All other cancers not listed	Cover	Cover

* Cervix: Nationally non-covered for the initial diagnosis of cervical cancer related to initial anti-tumor treatment strategy. All other indications for initial anti-tumor treatment strategy for cervical cancer are nationally covered.

* Breast: Nationally non-covered for initial diagnosis and/or staging of axillary lymph nodes. Nationally covered for initial staging of metastatic disease. All other indications for initial anti-tumor treatment strategy for breast cancer are nationally covered.

* Melanoma: Nationally non-covered for initial staging of regional lymph nodes. All other indications for initial anti-tumor treatment strategy for melanoma are nationally covered.

D. Other
N/A

100-03, 220.6.19

Positron Emission Tomography NaF-18 (NaF-18 PET) to Identify Bone Metastasis of Cancer (Effective February 26, 2010)

A. General

Positron Emission Tomography (PET) is a non-invasive, diagnostic imaging procedure that assesses the level of metabolic activity and perfusion in various organ systems of the body. A positron camera (tomograph) is used to produce cross-sectional tomographic images, which are obtained from positron-emitting radioactive tracer substances (radiopharmaceuticals) such as F-18 sodium fluoride. NaF-18 PET has been recognized as an excellent technique for imaging areas of altered osteogenic activity in bone. The clinical value of detecting and assessing the initial extent of metastatic cancer in bone is attested by a number of professional guidelines for oncology. Imaging to detect bone metastases is also recommended when a patient, following completion of initial treatment, is symptomatic with bone pain suspicious for metastases from a known primary tumor.

B. Nationally Covered Indications

Effective February 26, 2010, the Centers for Medicare & Medicaid Services (CMS) will cover NaF-18 PET imaging when the beneficiary's treating physician determines that the NaF-18 PET study is needed to inform to inform the initial antitumor treatment strategy or to guide subsequent antitumor treatment strategy after the completion of initial treatment, and when the beneficiary is enrolled in, and the NaF-18 PET provider is participating in, the following type of prospective clinical study:

A NaF-18 PET clinical study that is designed to collect additional information at the time of the scan to assist in initial antitumor treatment planning or to guide subsequent treatment strategy by the identification, location and quantification of bone metastases in beneficiaries in whom bone metastases are strongly suspected based on clinical symptoms or the results of other diagnostic studies. Qualifying clinical studies must ensure that specific hypotheses are addressed; appropriate data elements are collected; hospitals and providers are qualified to provide the PET scan and interpret the results; participating hospitals and providers accurately report data on all enrolled patients not included in other qualifying trials through adequate auditing mechanisms; and all patient confidentiality, privacy, and other Federal laws must be followed.

The clinical studies for which Medicare will provide coverage must answer one or more of the following questions:

Prospectively, in Medicare beneficiaries whose treating physician determines that the NaF-18 PET study results are needed to inform the initial antitumor treatment strategy or to guide subsequent antitumor treatment strategy after the completion of initial treatment, does the addition of NaF-18 PET imaging lead to:

- A change in patient management to more appropriate palliative care; or
- A change in patient management to more appropriate curative care; or
- Improved quality of life; or Improved survival?

The study must adhere to the following standards of scientific integrity and relevance to the Medicare population:

a. The principal purpose of the research study is to test whether a particular intervention potentially improves the participants' health outcomes.

b. The research study is well-supported by available scientific and medical information or it is intended to clarify or establish the health outcomes of interventions already in common clinical use.

c. The research study does not unjustifiably duplicate existing studies.

d. The research study design is appropriate to answer the research question being asked in the study.

e. The research study is sponsored by an organization or individual capable of executing the proposed study successfully.

f. The research study is in compliance with all applicable Federal regulations concerning the protection of human subjects found in the Code of Federal Regulations (CFR) at 45 CFR Part 46. If a study is regulated by the Food and Drug Administration (FDA), it also must be in compliance with 21 CFR Parts 50 and 56.

g. All aspects of the research study are conducted according to the appropriate standards of scientific integrity.

h. The research study has a written protocol that clearly addresses, or incorporates by reference, the Medicare standards.

i. The clinical research study is not designed to exclusively test toxicity or disease pathophysiology in healthy individuals. Trials of all medical technologies measuring therapeutic outcomes as one of the objectives meet this standard only if the disease or condition being studied is life-threatening as defined in 21 CFR Sec.312.81(a) and the patient has no other viable treatment options.

j. The clinical research study is registered on the www.ClinicalTrials.gov Web site by the principal sponsor/investigator prior to the enrollment of the first study subject.

k. The research study protocol specifies the method and timing of public release of all pre-specified outcomes to be measured including release of outcomes if outcomes are negative or study is terminated early. The results must be made public within 24 months of the end of data collection. If a report is planned to be

published in a peer-reviewed journal, then that initial release may be an abstract that meets the requirements of the International Committee of Medical Journal Editors. However, a full report of the outcomes must be made public no later than three (3) years after the end of data collection.

l. The research study protocol must explicitly discuss subpopulations affected by the treatment under investigation, particularly traditionally underrepresented groups in clinical studies, how the inclusion and exclusion criteria affect enrollment of these populations, and a plan for the retention and reporting of said populations on the trial. If the inclusion and exclusion criteria are expected to have a negative effect on the recruitment or retention of underrepresented populations, the protocol must discuss why these criteria are necessary.

m. The research study protocol explicitly discusses how the results are or are not expected to be generalizable to the Medicare population to infer whether Medicare patients may benefit from the intervention. Separate discussions in the protocol may be necessary for populations eligible for Medicare due to age, disability or Medicaid eligibility.

Consistent with section 1142 of the Social Security Act (the Act), the Agency for Healthcare Research and Quality (AHRQ) supports clinical research studies that the Centers for Medicare and Medicaid Services (CMS) determines meet the above-listed standards and address the above-listed research questions.

C. Nationally Non-Covered Indications

Effective February 26, 2010, CMS determines that the evidence is not sufficient to determine that the results of NaF-18 PET imaging to identify bone metastases improve health outcomes of beneficiaries with cancer and is not reasonable and necessary under Sec.1862(a)(1)(A) of the Act unless it is to inform initial antitumor treatment strategy or to guide subsequent antitumor treatment strategy after completion of initial treatment, and then only under CED. All other uses and clinical indications of NaF-18 PET are nationally non-covered.

D. Other

The only radiopharmaceutical diagnostic imaging agents covered by Medicare for PET cancer imaging are 2-[F-18] Fluoro-D-Glucose (FDG) and NaF-18 (sodium fluoride-18). All other PET radiopharmaceutical diagnostic imaging agents are non-covered for this indication.

(This NCD was last reviewed in February 2010.)

100-03, 220.13

NCD for Percutaneous Image-Guided Breast Biopsy (220.13)

Percutaneous image-guided breast biopsy is a method of obtaining a breast biopsy through a percutaneous incision by employing image guidance systems. Image guidance systems may be either ultrasound or stereotactic.

The Breast Imaging Reporting and Data System (or BIRADS system) employed by the American College of Radiology provides a standardized lexicon with which radiologists may report their interpretation of a mammogram. The BIRADS grading of mammograms is as follows: Grade I-Negative, Grade II-Benign finding, Grade III-Probably benign, Grade IV-Suspicious abnormality, and Grade V-Highly suggestive of malignant neoplasm.

A. Non-Palpable Breast Lesions

Effective January 1, 2003, Medicare covers percutaneous image-guided breast biopsy using stereotactic or ultrasound imaging for a radiographic abnormality that is non-palpable and is graded as a BIRADS III, IV, or V.

B. Palpable Breast Lesions

Effective January 1, 2003, Medicare covers percutaneous image guided breast biopsy using stereotactic or ultrasound imaging for palpable lesions that are difficult to biopsy using palpation alone. Medicare Administrative Contractors have the discretion to decide what types of palpable lesions are difficult to biopsy using palpation.

100-03, 230.1

NCD for Treatment of Kidney Stones (230.1)

In addition to the traditional surgical/endoscopic techniques for the treatment of kidney stones, the following lithotripsy techniques are also covered for services rendered on or after March 15, 1985.

Extracorporeal Shock Wave Lithotripsy.--Extracorporeal Shock Wave Lithotripsy (ESWL) is a non-invasive method of treating kidney stones using a device called a lithotriptor. The lithotriptor uses shock waves generated outside of the body to break up upper urinary tract stones. It focuses the shock waves specifically on stones under X-ray visualization, pulverizing them by repeated shocks. ESWL is covered under Medicare for use in the treatment of upper urinary tract kidney stones.

Percutaneous Lithotripsy.--Percutaneous lithotripsy (or nephrolithotomy) is an invasive method of treating kidney stones by using ultrasound, electrohydraulic or mechanical lithotripsy. A probe is inserted through an incision in the skin directly over the kidney and applied to the stone. A form of lithotripsy is then used to fragment the stone. Mechanical or electrohydraulic lithotripsy may be used as an alternative or adjunct to ultrasonic lithotripsy. Percutaneous lithotripsy of kidney stones by ultrasound or by the related techniques of electrohydraulic or mechanical lithotripsy is covered under Medicare.

The following is covered for services rendered on or after January 16, 1988.

Transurethral Ureteroscopic Lithotripsy.--Transurethral ureteroscopic lithotripsy is a method of fragmenting and removing ureteral and renal stones through a cystoscope. The cystoscope is inserted through the urethra into the bladder. Catheters are passed through the scope into the opening where the ureters enter the bladder. Instruments passed through this opening into the ureters are used to manipulate and ultimately disintegrate stones, using either mechanical crushing, transcystoscopic electrohydraulic shock waves, ultrasound or laser. Transurethral ureteroscopic lithotripsy for the treatment of urinary tract stones of the kidney or ureter is covered under Medicare.

100-03, 230.3

NCD for Sterilization (230.3)

A. Nationally Covered Conditions

Payment may be made only where sterilization is a necessary part of the treatment of an illness or injury, e.g., removal of a uterus because of a tumor, removal of diseased ovaries.

Sterilization of a mentally challenged beneficiary is covered if it is a necessary part of the treatment of an illness or injury (bilateral oophorectomy or bilateral orchidectomy in a case of cancer of the prostate. The Medicare Administrative Contractor denies claims when the pathological evidence of the necessity to perform any such procedures to treat an illness or injury is absent; and

Monitor such surgeries closely and obtain the information needed to determine whether in fact the surgery was performed as a means of treating an illness or injury or only to achieve sterilization.

B. Nationally Non-Covered Conditions

- Elective hysterectomy, tubal ligation, and vasectomy, if the primary indication for these procedures is sterilization;

- A sterilization that is performed because a physician believes another pregnancy would endanger the overall general health of the woman is not considered to be reasonable and necessary for the diagnosis or treatment of illness or injury within the meaning of §1862(a)(1) of the Social Security Act. The same conclusion would apply where the sterilization is performed only as a measure to prevent the possible development of, or effect on, a mental condition should the individual become pregnant; and sterilization of a mentally retarded person where the purpose is to prevent conception, rather than the treatment of an illness or injury.

100-03, 230.4

NCD for Diagnosis and Treatment of Impotence (230.4)

Program payment may be made for diagnosis and treatment of sexual impotence. Impotence is a failure of a body part for which the diagnosis, and frequently the treatment, require medical expertise. Depending on the cause of the condition, treatment may be surgical; e.g., implantation of a penile prosthesis, or nonsurgical; e.g., medical or psychotherapeutic treatment. Since causes and, therefore, appropriate treatment vary, if abuse is suspected it may be necessary to request documentation of appropriateness in individual cases. If treatment is furnished to patients (other than hospital inpatients) in connection with a mental condition, apply the psychiatric service limitation described in the Medicare General Information, Eligibility, and Entitlement Manual, Chapter 3.

100-03, 230.10

NCD for Incontinence Control Devices (230.10)

A - Mechanical/Hydraulic Incontinence Control Devices

Mechanical/hydraulic incontinence control devices are accepted as safe and effective in the management of urinary incontinence in patients with permanent anatomic and neurologic dysfunctions of the bladder. This class of devices achieves control of urination by compression of the urethra. The materials used and the success rate may vary somewhat from device to device. Such a device is covered when its use is reasonable and necessary for the individual patient.

B - Collagen Implant

A collagen implant, which is injected into the submucosal tissues of the urethra and/or the bladder neck and into tissues adjacent to the urethra, is a prosthetic device used in the treatment of stress urinary incontinence resulting from intrinsic sphincter deficiency (ISD). ISD is a cause of stress urinary incontinence in which the urethral sphincter is unable to contract and generate sufficient resistance in the bladder, especially during stress maneuvers.

Prior to collagen implant therapy, a skin test for collagen sensitivity must be administered and evaluated over a 4 week period.

In male patients, the evaluation must include a complete history and physical examination and a simple cystometrogram to determine that the bladder fills and stores properly. The patient then is asked to stand upright with a full bladder and to cough or otherwise exert abdominal pressure on his bladder. If the patient leaks, the diagnosis of ISD is established.

In female patients, the evaluation must include a complete history and physical examination (including a pelvic exam) and a simple cystometrogram to rule out abnormalities of bladder compliance and abnormalities of urethral support. Following that determination, an abdominal leak point pressure (ALLP) test is performed. Leak point pressure, stated in cm H2O, is defined as the intra-abdominal pressure at which leakage occurs from the bladder (around a catheter) when the

bladder has been filled with a minimum of 150 cc fluid. If the patient has an ALLP of less than 100 cm H_2O, the diagnosis of ISD is established.

To use a collagen implant, physicians must have urology training in the use of a cystoscope and must complete a collagen implant training program.

Coverage of a collagen implant, and the procedure to inject it, is limited to the following types of patients with stress urinary incontinence due to ISD:

- Male or female patients with congenital sphincter weakness secondary to conditions such as myelomeningocele or epispadias;

- Male or female patients with acquired sphincter weakness secondary to spinal cord lesions;

- Male patients following trauma, including prostatectomy and/or radiation; and

- Female patients without urethral hypermobility and with abdominal leak point pressures of 100 cm H2O or less.

Patients whose incontinence does not improve with 5 injection procedures (5 separate treatment sessions) are considered treatment failures, and no further treatment of urinary incontinence by collagen implant is covered. Patients who have a reoccurrence of incontinence following successful treatment with collagen implants in the past (e.g., 6-12 months previously) may benefit from additional treatment sessions. Coverage of additional sessions may be allowed but must be supported by medical justification.

100-03, 260.1

Adult Liver Transplantation

A. General

Liver transplantation, which is in situ replacement of a patient's liver with a donor liver, in certain circumstances, may be an accepted treatment for patients with end-stage liver disease due to a variety of causes. The procedure is used in selected patients as a treatment for malignancies, including primary liver tumors and certain metastatic tumors, which are typically rare but lethal with very limited treatment options. It has also been used in the treatment of patients with extrahepatic perihilar malignancies. Examples of malignancies include extrahepatic unresectable cholangiocarcinoma (CCA), liver metastases due to a neuroendocrine tumor (NET), and, hemangioendothelioma (HAE). Despite potential short- and long-term complications, transplantation may offer the only chance of cure for selected patients while providing meaningful palliation for some others.

B. Nationally Covered Indications

Effective July 15, 1996, adult liver transplantation when performed on beneficiaries with end- stage liver disease other than hepatitis B or malignancies is covered under Medicare when performed in a facility which is approved by the Centers for Medicare & Medicaid Services (CMS) as meeting institutional coverage criteria.

Effective December 10, 1999, adult liver transplantation when performed on beneficiaries with end-stage liver disease other than malignancies is covered under Medicare when performed in a facility which is approved by CMS as meeting institutional coverage criteria.

Effective September 1, 2001, Medicare covers adult liver transplantation for hepatocellular carcinoma when the following conditions are met:

- The patient is not a candidate for subtotal liver resection;

- The patient's tumor(s) is less than or equal to 5 cm in diameter;

- There is no macrovascular involvement;

- There is no identifiable extrahepatic spread of tumor to surrounding lymph nodes, lungs, abdominal organs or bone; and,

- The transplant is furnished in a facility that is approved by CMS as meeting institutional coverage criteria for liver transplants (see 65 FR 15006).

Effective June 21, 2012, Medicare Adminstrative Contractors acting within their respective jurisdictions may determine coverage of adult liver transplantation for the following malignancies: (1) extrahepatic unresectable cholangiocarcinoma (CCA); (2) liver metastases due to a neuroendocrine tumor (NET); and, (3) hemangioendothelioma (HAE).

1. Follow-Up Care

   Follow-up care or re-transplantation required as a result of a covered liver transplant is covered, provided such services are otherwise reasonable and necessary. Follow-up care is also covered for patients who have been discharged from a hospital after receiving non-covered liver transplant. Coverage for follow-up care is for items and services that are reasonable and necessary as determined by Medicare guidelines.

2. Immunosuppressive Drugs

   See the Medicare Benefit Policy Manual, Chapter 15, "Covered Medical and Other Health Services," §50.5.1 and the Medicare Claims Processing Manual, Chapter 17, "Drugs and Biologicals," §80.3.

C. Nationally Non-Covered Indications

Adult liver transplantation for other malignancies remains excluded from coverage.

D. Other

Coverage of adult liver transplantation is effective as of the date of the facility's approval, but for applications received before July 13, 1991, can be effective as early as March 8, 1990. (See 56 FR 15006 dated April 12, 1991.)

(This NCD last reviewed June 2012.)

100-03, 260.2

NCD for Pediatric Liver Transplantation (260.2)

Liver transplantation is covered for children (under age 18) with extrahepatic biliary atresia or any other form of end stage liver disease, except that coverage is not provided for children with a malignancy extending beyond the margins of the liver or those with persistent viremia.

Liver transplantation is covered for Medicare beneficiaries when performed in a pediatric hospital that performs pediatric liver transplants if the hospital submits an application which CMS approves documenting that:

- The hospital's pediatric liver transplant program is operated jointly by the hospital and another facility that has been found by CMS to meet the institutional coverage criteria in the "Federal Register" notice of April 12, 1991;

- The unified program shares the same transplant surgeons and quality assurance program (including oversight committee, patient protocol, and patient selection criteria); and

- The hospital is able to provide the specialized facilities, services, and personnel that are required by pediatric liver transplant patients.

100-03, 260.3

NCD for Pancreas Transplants (260.3)

B. Nationally Covered Indications

Effective for services performed on or after July 1, 1999, whole organ pancreas transplantation is nationally covered by Medicare when performed simultaneous with or after a kidney transplant. If the pancreas transplant occurs after the kidney transplant, immunosuppressive therapy begins with the date of discharge from the inpatient stay for the pancreas transplant.

Effective for services performed on or after April 26, 2006, pancreas transplants alone (PA) are reasonable and necessary for Medicare beneficiaries in the following limited circumstances:

1. PA will be limited to those facilities that are Medicare-approved for kidney transplantation. (Approved centers can be found at http://www.cms.hhs.gov/ESRDGeneralInformation/02_Data.asp#TopOfPage

2. Patients must have a diagnosis of type I diabetes:

   — Patient with diabetes must be beta cell autoantibody positive; or

   — Patient must demonstrate insulinopenia defined as a fasting C-peptide level that is less than or equal to 110% of the lower limit of normal of the laboratory's measurement method. Fasting C-peptide levels will only be considered valid with a concurrently obtained fasting glucose <225 mg/dL;

3. Patients must have a history of medically-uncontrollable labile (brittle) insulin-dependent diabetes mellitus with documented recurrent, severe, acutely life-threatening metabolic complications that require hospitalization. Aforementioned complications include frequent hypoglycemia unawareness or recurring severe ketoacidosis, or recurring severe hypoglycemic attacks;

4. Patients must have been optimally and intensively managed by an endocrinologist for at least 12 months with the most medically-recognized advanced insulin formulations and delivery systems;

5. Patients must have the emotional and mental capacity to understand the significant risks associated with surgery and to effectively manage the lifelong need for immunosuppression; and,

6. Patients must otherwise be a suitable candidate for transplantation.

C. Nationally Non-Covered Indications

The following procedure is not considered reasonable and necessary within the meaning of section 1862(a)(1)(A) of the Social Security Act:

1. Transplantation of partial pancreatic tissue or islet cells (except in the context of a clinical trial (see section 260.3.1 of the National Coverage Determinations Manual).

D. Other

Not applicable.

(This NCD last reviewed April 2006.)

100-03, 260.5

NCD for Intestinal and Multi-Visceral Transplantation (260.5)

A. General

Medicare covers intestinal and multi-visceral transplantation for the purpose of restoring intestinal function in patients with irreversible intestinal failure. Intestinal failure is defined as the loss of absorptive capacity of the small bowel secondary to severe primary gastrointestinal disease or surgically induced short bowel syndrome. It may be associated with both mortality and profound morbidity. Multi-visceral transplantation includes organs in the digestive system (stomach, duodenum, pancreas, liver and intestine).

The evidence supports the fact that aged patients generally do not survive as well as younger patients receiving intestinal transplantation. Nonetheless, some older

patients who are free from other contraindications have received the procedure and are progressing well, as evidenced by the United Network for Organ Sharing (UNOS) data. Thus, it is not appropriate to include specific exclusions from coverage, such as an age limitation, in the national coverage policy.

B. Nationally Covered Indications

Effective for services performed on or after April 1, 2001, this procedure is covered only when performed for patients who have failed total parenteral nutrition (TPN) and only when performed in centers that meet approval criteria.

1. Failed TPN

   The TPN delivers nutrients intravenously, avoiding the need for absorption through the small bowel. TPN failure includes the following:

   — Impending or overt liver failure due to TPN induced liver injury. The clinical manifestations include elevated serum bilirubin and/or liver enzymes, splenomegaly, thrombocytopenia, gastroesophageal varices, coagulopathy, stomal bleeding or hepatic fibrosis/cirrhosis.

   — Thrombosis of the major central venous channels; jugular, subclavian, and femoral veins. Thrombosis of two or more of these vessels is considered a life threatening complication and failure of TPN therapy. The sequelae of central venous thrombosis are lack of access for TPN infusion, fatal sepsis due to infected thrombi, pulmonary embolism, Superior Vena Cava syndrome, or chronic venous insufficiency.

   — Frequent line infection and sepsis. The development of two or more episodes of systemic sepsis secondary to line infection per year that requires hospitalization indicates failure of TPN therapy. A single episode of line related fungemia, septic shock and/or Acute Respiratory Distress Syndrome are considered indicators of TPN failure.

   — Frequent episodes of severe dehydration despite intravenous fluid supplement in addition to TPN. Under certain medical conditions such as secretory diarrhea and non-constructable gastrointestinal tract, the loss of the gastrointestinal and pancreatobiliary secretions exceeds the maximum intravenous infusion rates that can be tolerated by the cardiopulmonary system. Frequent episodes of dehydration are deleterious to all body organs particularly kidneys and the central nervous system with the development of multiple kidney stones, renal failure, and permanent brain damage.

2. Approved Transplant Facilities

   Intestinal transplantation is covered by Medicare if performed in an approved facility. The criteria for approval of centers will be based on a volume of 10 intestinal transplants per year with a 1-year actuarial survival of 65 percent using the Kaplan-Meier technique.

C. Nationally Non-covered Indications

All other indications remain non-covered.

D. Other

NA.

(This NCD last reviewed May 2006.)

100-03, 260.9

NCD for Heart Transplants (260.9)

A. General

Cardiac transplantation is covered under Medicare when performed in a facility which is approved by Medicare as meeting institutional coverage criteria. (See CMS Ruling 87-1.)

B. Exceptions

In certain limited cases, exceptions to the criteria may be warranted if there is justification and if the facility ensures our objectives of safety and efficacy. Under no circumstances will exceptions be made for facilities whose transplant programs have been in existence for less than two years, and applications from consortia will not be approved.

Although consortium arrangements will not be approved for payment of Medicare heart transplants, consideration will be given to applications from heart transplant facilities that consist of more than one hospital where all of the following conditions exist:

- The hospitals are under the common control or have a formal affiliation arrangement with each other under the auspices of an organization such as a university or a legally-constituted medical research institute; and

- The hospitals share resources by routinely using the same personnel or services in their transplant programs. The sharing of resources must be supported by the submission of operative notes or other information that documents the routine use of the same personnel and services in all of the individual hospitals. At a minimum, shared resources means:

- The individual members of the transplant team, consisting of the cardiac transplant surgeons, cardiologists and pathologists, must practice in all the hospitals and it can be documented that they otherwise function as members of the transplant team;

- The same organ procurement organization, immunology, and tissue-typing services must be used by all the hospitals;

- The hospitals submit, in the manner required (Kaplan-Meier method) their individual and pooled experience and survival data; and

- The hospitals otherwise meet the remaining Medicare criteria for heart transplant facilities; that is, the criteria regarding patient selection, patient management, program commitment, etc.

C. Pediatric Hospitals

Cardiac transplantation is covered for Medicare beneficiaries when performed in a pediatric hospital that performs pediatric heart transplants if the hospital submits an application which CMS approves as documenting that:

- The hospital's pediatric heart transplant program is operated jointly by the hospital and another facility that has been found by CMS to meet the institutional coverage criteria in CMS Ruling 87-1;

- The unified program shares the same transplant surgeons and quality assurance program (including oversight committee, patient protocol, and patient selection criteria); and

- The hospital is able to provide the specialized facilities, services, and personnel that are required by pediatric heart transplant patients.

D. Follow-Up Care

Follow-up care required as a result of a covered heart transplant is covered, provided such services are otherwise reasonable and necessary. Follow-up care is also covered for patients who have been discharged from a hospital after receiving a noncovered heart transplant. Coverage for follow-up care would be for items and services that are reasonable and necessary, as determined by Medicare guidelines. (See the Medicare Benefit Policy Manual, Chapter 16, "General Exclusions from Coverage," Sec.180.)

E. Immunosuppressive Drugs

See the Medicare Claims Processing Manual, Chapter 17, "Drugs and Biologicals," Sec.80.3.1, and Chapter 8, "Outpatient ESRD Hospital, Independent Facility, and Physician/Supplier Claims," Sec.120.1.

F. Artificial Hearts

Medicare does not cover the use of artificial hearts as a permanent replacement for a human heart or as a temporary life-support system until a human heart becomes available for transplant (often referred to as a "bridge to transplant"). Medicare does cover a ventricular assist device (VAD) when used in conjunction with specific criteria listed in Sec.20.9 of the NCD Manual.

100-03, 270.3

NCD for Blood-Derived Products for Chronic Non-Healing Wounds (270.3)

A. General

Wound healing is a dynamic, interactive process that involves multiple cells and proteins. There are three progressive stages of normal wound healing, and the typical wound healing duration is about 4 weeks. While cutaneous wounds are a disruption of the normal, anatomic structure and function of the skin, subcutaneous wounds involve tissue below the skin's surface. Wounds are categorized as either acute, in where the normal wound healing stages are not yet completed but it is presumed they will be, resulting in orderly and timely wound repair, or chronic, in where a wound has failed to progress through the normal wound healing stages and repair itself within a sufficient time period.

Platelet-rich plasma (PRP) is produced in an autologous or homologous manner. Autologous PRP is comprised of blood from the patient who will ultimately receive the PRP. Alternatively, homologous PRP is derived from blood from multiple donors.

Blood is donated by the patient and centrifuged to produce an autologous gel for treatment of chronic, non-healing cutaneous wounds that persists for 30 days or longer and fail to properly complete the healing process. Autologous blood derived products for chronic, non-healing wounds includes both: (1) platelet derived growth factor (PDGF) products (such as Procuren), and (2) PRP (such as AutoloGel).

The PRP is different from previous products in that it contains whole cells including white cells, red cells, plasma, platelets, fibrinogen, stem cells, macrophages, and fibroblasts.

The PRP is used by physicians in clinical settings in treating chronic, non-healing wounds, open, cutaneous wounds, soft tissue, and bone. Alternatively, PDGF does not contain cells and was previously marketed as a product to be used by patients at home.

B. Nationally Covered Indications

Effective August 2, 2012, upon reconsideration, The Centers for Medicare and Medicaid Services (CMS) has determined that platelet-rich plasma (PRP) – an autologous blood-derived product, will be covered only for the treatment of chronic non-healing diabetic, venous and/or pressure wounds and only when the following conditions are met:

The patient is enrolled in a clinical trial that addresses the following questions using validated and reliable methods of evaluation. Clinical study applications for coverage pursuant to this National coverage Determination (NCD) must be received by August 2, 2014.

The clinical research study must meet the requirements specified below to assess the effect of PRP for the treatment of chronic non-healing diabetic, venous and/or pressure wounds. The clinical study must address:

Prospectively, do Medicare beneficiaries that have chronic non-healing diabetic, venous and/or pressure wounds who receive well-defined optimal usual care along with PRP therapy, experience clinically significant health outcomes compared to patients who receive well-defined optimal usual care for chronic non-healing diabetic, venous and/or pressure wounds as indicated by addressing at least one of the following:

a. Complete wound healing?

b. Ability to return to previous function and resumption of normal activities?

c. Reduction of wound size or healing trajectory which results in the patient's ability to return to previous function and resumption of normal activities?

The required clinical trial of PRP must adhere to the following standards of scientific integrity and relevance to the Medicare population:

a. The principal purpose of the CLINICAL STUDY is to test whether PRP improves the participants' health outcomes.

b. The CLINICAL STUDY is well supported by available scientific and medical information or it is intended to clarify or establish the health outcomes of interventions already in common clinical use.

c. The CLINICAL STUDY does not unjustifiably duplicate existing studies.

d. The CLINICAL STUDY design is appropriate to answer the research question being asked in the study.

e. The CLINICAL STUDY is sponsored by an organization or individual capable of executing the proposed study successfully.

f. The CLINICAL STUDY is in compliance with all applicable Federal regulations concerning the protection of human subjects found at 45 CFR Part 46.

g. All aspects of the CLINICAL STUDY are conducted according to appropriate standards of scientific integrity set by the International Committee of Medical Journal Editors (http://www.icmje.org).

h. The CLINICAL STUDY has a written protocol that clearly addresses, or incorporates by reference, the standards listed here as Medicare requirements for coverage with evidence development (CED).

i. The CLINICAL STUDY is not designed to exclusively test toxicity or disease pathophysiology in healthy individuals. Trials of all medical technologies measuring therapeutic outcomes as one of the objectives meet this standard only if the disease or condition being studied is life threatening as defined in 21 CFR §312.81(a) and the patient has no other viable treatment options.

j. The CLINICAL STUDY is registered on the ClinicalTrials.gov website by the principal sponsor/investigator prior to the enrollment of the first study subject.

k. The CLINICAL STUDY protocol specifies the method and timing of public release of all pre-specified outcomes to be measured including release of outcomes if outcomes are negative or study is terminated early. The results must be made public within 24 months of the end of data collection. If a report is planned to be published in a peer reviewed journal, then that initial release may be an abstract that meets the requirements of the International Committee of Medical Journal Editors (http://www.icmje.org). However a full report of the outcomes must be made public no later than three (3) years after the end of data collection.

l. The CLINICAL STUDY protocol must explicitly discuss subpopulations affected by the treatment under investigation, particularly traditionally underrepresented groups in clinical studies, how the inclusion and exclusion criteria effect enrollment of these populations, and a plan for the retention and reporting of said populations on the trial. If the inclusion and exclusion criteria are expected to have a negative effect on the recruitment or retention of underrepresented populations, the protocol must discuss why these criteria are necessary.

m. The CLINICAL STUDY protocol explicitly discusses how the results are or are not expected to be generalizable to the Medicare population to infer whether Medicare patients may benefit from the intervention. Separate discussions in the protocol may be necessary for populations eligible for Medicare due to age, disability or Medicaid eligibility. Consistent with §1142 of the Social Security Act (the Act), the Agency for Healthcare Research and Quality (AHRQ) supports clinical research studies that CMS determines meet the above-listed standards and address the above-listed research questions.

Any clinical study undertaken pursuant to this NCD must be approved no later than August 2, 2014. If there are no approved clinical studies on or before August 2, 2014, this CED will expire. Any clinical study approved will adhere to the timeframe designated in the approved clinical study protocol.

C. Nationally Non-Covered Indications

1. Effective December 28, 1992, the Centers for Medicare & Medicaid Services (CMS) issued a national non-coverage determination for platelet-derived wound-healing formulas intended to treat patients with chronic, non-healing wounds. This decision was based on a lack of sufficient published data to determine safety and efficacy, and a public health service technology assessment.

100-04, 3, 90.1

Kidney Transplant - General

A3-3612, HO-E414

A major treatment for patients with ESRD is kidney transplantation. This involves removing a kidney, usually from a living relative of the patient or from an unrelated person who has died, and surgically placing the kidney into the patient. After the beneficiary receives a kidney transplant, Medicare pays the transplant hospital for the transplant and appropriate standard acquisition charges. Special provisions apply to payment. For the list of approved Medicare certified transplant facilities, refer to the following Web site:

http://www.cms.hhs.gov/CertificationandComplianc/20_Transplant.asp#TopOfPage

A transplant hospital may acquire cadaver kidneys by:

- Excising kidneys from cadavers in its own hospital; and
- Arrangements with a freestanding organ procurement organization (OPO) that provides cadaver kidneys to any transplant hospital or by a hospital based OPO.

A transplant hospital that is also a certified organ procurement organization may acquire cadaver kidneys by:

- Having its organ procurement team excise kidneys from cadavers in other hospitals;
- Arrangements with participating community hospitals, whether they excise kidneys on a regular or irregular basis; and
- Arrangements with an organ procurement organization that services the transplant hospital as a member of a network.

When the transplant hospital also excises the cadaver kidney, the cost of the procedure is included in its kidney acquisition costs and is considered in arriving at its standard cadaver kidney acquisition charge. When the transplant hospital excises a kidney to provide another hospital, it may use its standard cadaver kidney acquisition charge or its standard detailed departmental charges to bill that hospital.

When the excising hospital is not a transplant hospital, it bills its customary charges for services used in excising the cadaver kidney to the transplant hospital or organ procurement agency.

If the transplanting hospital's organ procurement team excises the cadaver kidney at another hospital, the cost of operating such a team is included in the transplanting hospital's kidney acquisition costs, along with the reasonable charges billed by the other hospital of its services.

100-04, 3, 90.1.1

The Standard Kidney Acquisition Charge

There are two basic standard charges that must be developed by transplant hospitals from costs expected to be incurred in the acquisition of kidneys:

- The standard charge for acquiring a live donor kidney; and
- The standard charge for acquiring a cadaver kidney.

The standard charge is not a charge representing the acquisition cost of a specific kidney; rather, it is a charge that reflects the average cost associated with each type of kidney acquisition.

When the transplant hospital bills the program for the transplant, it shows its standard kidney acquisition charge on revenue code 081X. Kidney acquisition charges are not considered for the IPPS outlier calculation.

Acquisition services are billed from the excising hospital to the transplant hospital. A billing form is not submitted from the excising hospital to the FI. The transplant hospital keeps an itemized statement that identifies the services furnished, the charges, the person receiving the service (donor/recipient), and whether this is a potential transplant donor or recipient. These charges are reflected in the transplant hospital's kidney acquisition costcenter and are used in determining the hospital's standard charge for acquiring a live donor's kidney or a cadaver's kidney. The standard charge is not a charge representing the acquisition cost of a specific kidney. Rather, it is a charge that reflects the average cost associated with each type of kidney acquisition. Also, it is an all-inclusive charge for all services required in acquisition of a kidney, i.e., tissue typing, post-operative evaluation.

A. Billing For Blood And Tissue Typing of the Transplant Recipient Whether or Not Medicare Entitlement Is Established

Tissue typing and pre-transplant evaluation can be reflected only through the kidney acquisition charge of the hospital where the transplant will take place. The transplant hospital includes in its kidney acquisition cost center the reasonable charges it pays to the independent laboratory or other hospital which typed the potential transplant recipient, either before or after his entitlement. It also includes reasonable charges paid for physician tissue typing services, applicable to live donors and recipients (during the preentitlement period and after entitlement, but prior to hospital admission for transplantation).

B. Billing for Blood and Tissue Typing and Other Pre-Transplant Evaluation of Live Donors

The entitlement date of the beneficiary who will receive the transplant is not a consideration in reimbursing for the services to donors, since no bill is submitted directly to Medicare. All charges for services to donors prior to admission into the hospital for excision are "billed" indirectly to Medicare through the live donor acquisition charge of transplanting hospitals.

C. Billing Donor And Recipient Pre-Transplant Services (Performed by Transplant Hospitals or Other Providers) to the Kidney Acquisition Cost Center

The transplant hospital prepares an itemized statement of the services rendered for submittal to its cost accounting department. Regular Medicare billing forms are not necessary for this purpose, since no bills are submitted to the A/B MAC (A) at this point.

The itemized statement should contain information that identifies the person receiving the service (donor/recipient), the health care insurance number, the service rendered and the charge for the service, as well as a statement as to whether this is a potential transplant donor or recipient. If it is a potential donor, the provider must identify the prospective recipient.

EXAMPLE:

Mary Jones
Health care insurance number
200 Adams St.
Anywhere, MS

Transplant donor evaluation services for recipient:

John Jones
Health care insurance number
200 Adams St.
Anywhere, MS

Services performed in a hospital other than the potential transplant hospital or by an independent laboratory are billed by that facility to the potential transplant hospital. This holds true regardless of where in the United States the service is performed. For example, if the donor services are performed in a Florida hospital and the transplant is to take place in a California hospital, the Florida hospital bills the California hospital (as described in above). The Florida hospital is paid by the California hospital, which recoups the monies through the kidney acquisition cost center.

D. Billing for Cadaveric Donor Services

Normally, various tests are performed to determine the type and suitability of a cadaver kidney. Such tests may be performed by the excising hospital (which may also be a transplant hospital) or an independent laboratory. When the excising-only hospital performs the tests, it includes the related charges on its bill to the transplant hospital or to the organ procurement agency. When the tests are performed by the transplant hospital, it uses the related costs in establishing the standard charge for acquiring the cadaver kidney. The transplant hospital includes the costs and charges in the appropriate departments for final cost settlement purposes. When the tests are performed by an independent laboratory for the excising-only hospital or the transplant hospital, the laboratory bills the hospital that engages its services or the organ procurement agency. The excising-only hospital includes such charges in its charges to the transplant hospital, which then includes the charges in developing its standard charge for acquiring the cadaver kidney. It is the transplant hospitals' responsibility to assure that the independent laboratory does not bill both hospitals. The cost of these services cannot be billed directly to the program, since such tests and other procedures performed on a cadaver are not identifiable to a specific patient.

E. Billing For Physicians' Services Prior to Transplantation

Physicians' services applicable to kidney excisions involving live donors and recipients (during the pre-entitlement period and after entitlement, but prior to entrance into the hospital for transplantation) as well as all physicians' services applicable to cadavers are considered Part A hospital services (kidney acquisition costs).

F. Billing for Physicians' Services After Transplantation

All physicians' services rendered to the living donor and all physicians' services rendered to the transplant recipient are billed to the Medicare program in the same manner as all Medicare Part B services are billed. All donor physicians' services must be billed to the account of the recipient (i.e., the recipient's Medicare number).

G. Billing For Physicians' Renal Transplantation Services

To ensure proper payment when submitting a Part B bill for the renal surgeon's services to the recipient, the appropriate HCPCS codes must be submitted, including HCPCS codes for concurrent surgery, as applicable.

The bill must include all living donor physicians' services, e.g., Revenue Center code 081X.

100-04, 3, 90.1.2

Billing for Kidney Transplant and Acquisition Services

Applicable standard kidney acquisition charges are identified separately by revenue code 0811 (Living Donor Kidney Acquisition) or 0812 (Cadaver Donor Kidney Acquisition). Where interim bills are submitted, the standard acquisition charge appears on the billing form for the period during which the transplant took place. This charge is in addition to the hospital's charges for services rendered directly to the Medicare recipient.

The contractor deducts kidney acquisition charges for PPS hospitals for processing through Pricer. These costs, incurred by approved kidney transplant hospitals, are not included in the kidney transplant prospective payment. They are paid on a reasonable cost basis. Interim payment is paid as a "pass through" item. (See the Provider Reimbursement Manual, Part 1, §2802 B.8.) The contractor includes kidney acquisition charges under the appropriate revenue code in CWF.

Bill Review Procedures

The Medicare Code Editor (MCE) creates a Limited Coverage edit for kidney transplant procedure codes. Where these procedure codes are identified by MCE, the contractor checks the provider number to determine if the provider is an approved transplant center, and checks the effective approval date. The contractor shall also determine if the facility is certified for adults and/or pediatric transplants dependent upon the patient's age. If payment is appropriate (i.e., the center is approved and the service is on or after the approval date) it overrides the limited coverage edit.

100-04, 3, 90.2

Heart Transplants

Cardiac transplantation is covered under Medicare when performed in a facility which is approved by Medicare as meeting institutional coverage criteria. On April 6, 1987, CMS Ruling 87-1, "Criteria for Medicare Coverage of Heart Transplants" was published in the "Federal Register." For Medicare coverage purposes, heart transplants are medically reasonable and necessary when performed in facilities that meet these criteria. If a hospital wishes to bill Medicare for heart transplants, it must submit an application and documentation, showing its ongoing compliance with each criterion.

If a contractor has any questions concerning the effective or approval dates of its hospitals, it should contact its RO.

For a complete list of approved transplant centers, visit:

http://www.cms.hhs.gov/CertificationandComplianc/20_Transplant.asp#TopOfPage

A. Effective Dates

The effective date of coverage for heart transplants performed at facilities applying after July 6, 1987, is the date the facility receives approval as a heart transplant facility. Coverage is effective for discharges October 17, 1986 for facilities that would have qualified and that applied by July 6, 1987. All transplant hospitals will be recertified under the final rule, Federal Register / Vol. 72, No. 61 / Friday, March 30, 2007, / Rules and Regulations.

The CMS informs each hospital of its effective date in an approval letter.

B. Drugs

Medicare Part B covers immunosuppressive drugs following a covered transplant in an approved facility.

C. Noncovered Transplants

Medicare will not cover transplants or re-transplants in facilities that have not been approved as meeting the facility criteria. If a beneficiary is admitted for and receives a heart transplant from a hospital that is not approved, physicians' services, and inpatient services associated with the transplantation procedure are not covered.

If a beneficiary received a heart transplant from a hospital while it was not an approved facility and later requires services as a result of the noncovered transplant, the services are covered when they are reasonable and necessary in all other respects.

D. Charges for Heart Acquisition Services

The excising hospital bills the OPO, who in turn bills the transplant (implant) hospital for applicable services. It should not submit a bill to its contractor. The transplant hospital must keep an itemized statement that identifies the services rendered, the charges, the person receiving the service (donor/recipient), and whether this person is a potential transplant donor or recipient. These charges are reflected in the transplant hospital's heart acquisition cost center and are used in determining its standard charge for acquiring a donor's heart. The standard charge is not a charge representing the acquisition cost of a specific heart; rather, it reflects the average cost associated with each type of heart acquisition. Also, it is an all inclusive charge for all services required in acquisition of a heart, i.e., tissue typing, post-operative evaluation, etc.

E. Bill Review Procedures

The contractor takes the following actions to process heart transplant bills. It may accomplish them manually or modify its MCE and Grouper interface programs to handle the processing.

1. MCE Interface

   The MCE creates a Limited Coverage edit for heart transplant procedure codes. Where these procedure codes are identified by MCE, the contractor checks the provider number to determine if the provider is an approved transplant center, and checks the effective approval date. The contractor shall also determine if the facility is certified for adults and/or pediatric transplants dependent upon the patient's age. If payment is appropriate (i.e., the center is approved and the service is on or after the approval date) it overrides the limited coverage edit.

2. Handling Heart Transplant Billings From Nonapproved Hospitals

   Where a heart transplant and covered services are provided by a nonapproved hospital, the bill data processed through Grouper and Pricer must exclude transplant procedure codes and related charges.

100-04, 3, 90.3

Stem Cell Transplantation

(Rev. 3556, Issued: 07-01-16; Effective: 1-27-16; Implementation: 10-3-16)

A. General

Stem cell transplantation is a process in which stem cells are harvested from either a patient's (autologous) or donor's (allogeneic) bone marrow or peripheral blood for intravenous infusion. Autologous stem cell transplantation (AuSCT) is a technique for restoring stem cells using the patient's own previously stored cells. AuSCT must be used to effect hematopoietic reconstitution following severely myelotoxic doses of chemotherapy (HDCT) and/or radiotherapy used to treat various malignancies. Allogeneic hematopoietic stem cell transplantation (HSCT) is a procedure in which a portion of a healthy donor's stem cell or bone marrow is obtained and prepared for intravenous infusion. Allogeneic HSCT may be used to restore function in recipients having an inherited or acquired deficiency or defect. Hematopoietic stem cells are multi-potent stem cells that give rise to all the blood cell types; these stem cells form blood and immune cells. A hematopoietic stem cell is a cell isolated from blood or bone marrow that can renew itself, differentiate to a variety of specialized cells, can mobilize out of the bone marrow into circulating blood, and can undergo programmed cell death, called apoptosis - a process by which cells that are unneeded or detrimental will self-destruct.

The Centers for Medicare & Medicaid Services (CMS) is clarifying that bone marrow and peripheral blood stem cell transplantation is a process which includes mobilization, harvesting, and transplant of bone marrow or peripheral blood stem cells and the administration of high dose chemotherapy or radiotherapy prior to the actual transplant. When bone marrow or peripheral blood stem cell transplantation is covered, all necessary steps are included in coverage. When bone marrow or peripheral blood stem cell transplantation is non-covered, none of the steps are covered.

Allogeneic and autologous stem cell transplants are covered under Medicare for specific diagnoses. Effective October 1, 1990, these cases were assigned to MS-DRG 009, Bone Marrow Transplant.

The A/B MAC (A)'s Medicare Code Editor (MCE) will edit stem cell transplant procedure codes against diagnosis codes to determine which cases meet specified coverage criteria. Cases with a diagnosis code for a covered condition will pass (as covered) the MCE noncovered procedure edit. When a stem cell transplant case is selected for review based on the random selection of beneficiaries, the QIO will review the case on a post-payment basis to assure proper coverage decisions.

Bone marrow transplant codes that are reported with an ICD-9-CM that is "not otherwise specified" are returned to the hospital for a more specific procedure code. ICD-10-PCS codes are more precise and clearly identify autologous and nonautologous stem cells.

The A/B MAC (A) may choose to review if data analysis deems it a priority.

B. Nationally Covered Indications

I. Allogeneic Hematopoietic Stem Cell Transplantation (HSCT)

   a. General

   Allogeneic stem cell transplantation (ICD-9-CM Procedure Codes 41.02, 41.03, 41.05, and 41.08,; ICD-10-PCS codes 30230G1, 30230Y1, 30233G1, 30233Y1, 30240G1, 30240Y1, 30243G1, 30243Y1, 30250G1, 30250Y1, 30253G1, 30253Y1, 30260G1, 30260Y1, 30263G1, and 30263Y1) is a procedure in which a portion of a healthy donor's stem cells are obtained and prepared for intravenous infusion to restore normal hematopoietic function in recipients having an inherited or acquired hematopoietic deficiency or defect. See Pub. 100-03, National Coverage Determinations (NCD) Manual, chapter 1, section 110.23, for further information about this policy, and Pub. 100-04, CPM, chapter 32, section 90, for information on coding.

   Expenses incurred by a donor are a covered benefit to the recipient/beneficiary but, except for physician services, are not paid separately. Services to the donor include physician services, hospital care in connection with screening the stem cell, and ordinary follow-up care.

   b. Covered Conditions

      i. Effective for services performed on or after August 1, 1978: For the treatment of leukemia, leukemia in remission, or aplastic anemia when it is reasonable and necessary;

      ii. Effective for services performed on or after June 3, 1985: For the treatment of severe combined immunodeficiency disease (SCID), and for the treatment of Wiskott-Aldrich syndrome;

      iii. Effective for services performed on or after August 4, 2010: For the treatment of Myelodysplastic Syndromes (MDS) pursuant to Coverage with Evidence Development (CED) in the context of a Medicare-approved, prospective clinical study.

      iv. Effective for claims with dates of service on or after January 27, 2016:

   1. Allogeneic HSCT for multiple myeloma is covered by Medicare only for beneficiaries with Durie-Salmon Stage II or III multiple myeloma, or International Staging System (ISS) Stage II or Stage III multiple myeloma, and participating in an approved prospective clinical study.

   2. Allogeneic HSCT for myelofibrosis (MF) is covered by Medicare only for beneficiaries with Dynamic International Prognostic Scoring System (DIPSSplus) intermediate-2 or High primary or secondary MF and participating in an approved prospective clinical study.

   3. Allogeneic HSCT for sickle cell disease (SCD) is covered by Medicare only for beneficiaries with severe, symptomatic SCD who participate in an approved prospective clinical study.

II. Autologous Stem Cell Transplantation (AuSCT)

a. General

Autologous stem cell transplantation (ICD-9-CM Procedure Codes 41.01, 41.04, 41.07, and 41.09; ICD-10-PCS codes 30230AZ, 30230G0, 30230Y0, 30233G0, 30233Y0, 30240G0, 30240Y0, 30243G0, 30243Y0, 30250G0, 30250Y0, 30253G0, 30253Y0, 30260G0, 30260Y0, 30263G0, and 30263Y0) is a technique for restoring stem cells using the patient's own previously stored cells. AuSCT must be used to effect hematopoietic reconstitution following severely myelotoxic doses of chemotherapy (high dose chemotherapy (HDCT)) and/or radiotherapy used to treat various malignancies. Refer to Pub. 100-03, NCD Manual, chapter 1, section 110.23, for further information about this policy, and Pub. 100-04, CPM, chapter 32, section 90, for information on coding.

b. Covered Conditions

1. Effective for services performed on or after April 28, 1989: Acute leukemia in remission who have a high probability of relapse and who have no human leucocyte antigens (HLA)-matched; Resistant non-Hodgkin's lymphomas or those presenting with poor prognostic features following an initial response; Recurrent or refractory neuroblastoma; or, Advanced Hodgkin's disease who have failed conventional therapy and have no HLA-matched donor.

2. Effective for services performed on or after October 1, 2000: Single AuSCT is only covered for Durie-Salmon Stage II or III patients that fit the following requirements:

   - Newly diagnosed or responsive multiple myeloma. This includes those patients with previously untreated disease, those with at least a partial response to prior chemotherapy (defined as a 50% decrease either in measurable paraprotein [serum and/or urine] or in bone marrow infiltration, sustained for at least 1 month), and those in responsive relapse; and

   - Adequate cardiac, renal, pulmonary, and hepatic function.

3. Effective for services performed on or after March 15, 2005: When recognized clinical risk factors are employed to select patients for transplantation, high dose melphalan (HDM) together with AuSCT is reasonable and necessary for Medicare beneficiaries of any age group with primary amyloid light chain (AL) amyloidosis who meet the following criteria:

   - Amyloid deposition in 2 or fewer organs; and,

   - Cardiac left ventricular ejection fraction (EF) greater than 45%.

C. Nationally Non-Covered Indications

I. Allogeneic Hematopoietic Stem Cell Transplantation (HSCT)

Effective for claims with dates of service on or after May 24, 1996, through January 26, 2016, allogeneic HSCT is not covered as treatment for multiple myeloma. Refer to Pub. 100-03, NCD Manual, chapter 1, section 110.23, for further information about this policy, and Pub. 100-04, CPM, chapter 32, section 90, for information on coding.

II. Autologous Stem Cell Transplantation (AuSCT)

Insufficient data exist to establish definite conclusions regarding the efficacy of AuSCT for the following conditions:

a) Acute leukemia not in remission;

b) Chronic granulocytic leukemia;

c) Solid tumors (other than neuroblastoma); Up to October 1, 2000, multiple myeloma;

e) Tandem transplantation (multiple rounds of AuSCT) for patients with multiple myeloma;

f) Effective October 1, 2000, non primary AL amyloidosis; and,

g) Effective October 1, 2000, through March 14, 2005, primary AL amyloidosis for Medicare beneficiaries age 64 or older. In these cases, AuSCT is not considered reasonable and necessary within the meaning of §1862(a)(1)(A) of the Act and is not covered under Medicare. Refer to Pub. 100-03, NCD Manual, chapter 1, section 110.23, for further information about this policy, and Pub. 100-04, CPM, chapter 32, section 90, for information on coding.

D. Other

All other indications for stem cell transplantation not otherwise noted above as covered or non-covered remain at local Medicare Administrative Contractor discretion.

100-04, 3, 90.3.1

Allogeneic Stem Cell Transplantation

Rev. 3556, Issued: 07-01-16; Effective: 1-27-16; Implementation: 10-3-16

A. Billing for Allogeneic Stem Cell Transplants

1. Definition of Acquisition Charges for Allogeneic Stem Cell Transplants

Acquisition charges for allogeneic stem cell transplants include, but are not limited to, charges for the costs of the following services:

- National Marrow Donor Program fees, if applicable, for stem cells from an unrelated donor;

- Tissue typing of donor and recipient;

- Donor evaluation;

- Physician pre-admission/pre-procedure donor evaluation services;

- Costs associated with harvesting procedure (e.g., general routine and special care services, procedure/operating room and other ancillary services, apheresis services, etc.);

- Post-operative/post-procedure evaluation of donor; and

- Preparation and processing of stem cells.

Payment for these acquisition services is included in the MS-DRG payment for the allogeneic stem cell transplant when the transplant occurs in the inpatient setting, and in the OPPS APC payment for the allogeneic stem cell transplant when the transplant occurs in the outpatient setting. The Medicare contractor does not make separate payment for these acquisition services, because hospitals may bill and receive payment only for services provided to the Medicare beneficiary who is the recipient of the stem cell transplant and whose illness is being treated with the stem cell transplant. Unlike the acquisition costs of solid organs for transplant (e.g., hearts and kidneys), which are paid on a reasonable cost basis, acquisition costs for allogeneic stem cells are included in prospective payment.

Acquisition charges for stem cell transplants apply only to allogeneic transplants, for which stem cells are obtained from a donor (other than the recipient himself or herself). Acquisition charges do not apply to autologous transplants (transplanted stem cells are obtained from the recipient himself or herself), because autologous transplants involve services provided to the beneficiary only (and not to a donor), for which the hospital may bill and receive payment (see Pub. 100-04, chapter 4, §231.10 and paragraph B of this section for information regarding billing for autologous stem cell transplants).

2. Billing for Acquisition Services

The hospital bills and shows acquisition charges for allogeneic stem cell transplants based on the status of the patient (i.e., inpatient or outpatient) when the transplant is furnished. See Pub. 100-04, chapter 4, §231.11 for instructions regarding billing for acquisition services for allogeneic stem cell transplants that are performed in the outpatient setting.

When the allogeneic stem cell transplant occurs in the inpatient setting, the hospital identifies stem cell acquisition charges for allogeneic bone marrow/stem cell transplants separately by using revenue code 0819 (Other Organ Acquisition). Revenue code 0819 charges should include all services required to acquire stem cells from a donor, as defined above.

On the recipient's transplant bill, the hospital reports the acquisition charges, cost report days, and utilization days for the donor's hospital stay (if applicable) and/or charges for other encounters in which the stem cells were obtained from the donor. The donor is covered for medically necessary inpatient hospital days of care or outpatient care provided in connection with the allogeneic stem cell transplant under Part A. Expenses incurred for complications are paid only if they are directly and immediately attributable to the stem cell donation procedure. The hospital reports the acquisition charges on the billing form for the recipient, as described in the first paragraph of this section. It does not charge the donor's days of care against the recipient's utilization record. For cost reporting purposes, it includes the covered donor days and charges as Medicare days and charges.

The transplant hospital keeps an itemized statement that identifies the services furnished, the charges, the person receiving the service (donor/recipient), and whether this is a potential transplant donor or recipient. These charges will be reflected in the transplant hospital's stem cell/bone marrow acquisition cost center. For allogeneic stem cell acquisition services in cases that do not result in transplant, due to death of the intended recipient or other causes, hospitals include the costs associated with the acquisition services on the Medicare cost report.

The hospital shows charges for the transplant itself in revenue center code 0362 or another appropriate cost center. Selection of the cost center is up to the hospital.

B. Billing for Autologous Stem Cell Transplants

The hospital bills and shows all charges for autologous stem cell harvesting, processing, and transplant procedures based on the status of the patient (i.e., inpatient or outpatient) when the services are furnished. It shows charges for the actual transplant, in revenue center code 0362 or another appropriate cost center. ICD-9-CM or ICD-10-PCS codes are used to identify inpatient procedures.

The HCPCS codes describing autologous stem cell harvesting procedures may be billed and are separately payable under the OPPS when provided in the hospital outpatient setting of care. Autologous harvesting procedures are distinct from the acquisition services described in Pub. 100-04, chapter 4, §231.11 and section A. above for allogeneic stem cell transplants, which include services provided when stem cells are obtained from a donor and not from the patient undergoing the stem cell transplant. The HCPCS codes describing autologous stem cell processing procedures also may be billed and are separately payable under the OPPS when provided to hospital outpatients.

Payment for autologous stem cell harvesting procedures performed in the hospital inpatient setting of care, with transplant also occurring in the inpatient setting of care, is included in the MS-DRG payment for the autologous stem cell transplant.

100-04, 3, 90.3.2

Autologous Stem Cell Transplantation (AuSCT)

Autologous Stem Cell Transplantation (AuSCT)

A. General

Autologous stem cell transplantation (AuSCT) (ICD-9-CM procedure code 41.01, 41.04, 41.07, and 41.09 and CPT-4 code 38241) is a technique for restoring stem cells using the patient's own previously stored cells. AuSCT must be used to effect hematopoietic reconstitution following severely myelotoxic doses of chemotherapy (high dose chemotherapy (HDCT)) and/or radiotherapy used to treat various malignancies.

If ICD-9-CM is applicable, use the following Procedure Codes and Descriptions

ICD-9-CM Code	Description
41.01	Autologous bone marrow transplant without purging
41.04	Autologous hematopoietic stem cell transplant without purging
41.07	Autologous hematopoietic stem cell transplant with purging
41.09	Autologous bone marrow transplant with purging

If ICD-10-PCS is applicable, use the following Procedure Codes and Descriptions

ICD-10-PCS Code	Description
30230AZ	Transfusion of Embryonic Stem Cells into Peripheral Vein, Open Approach
30230G0	Transfusion of Autologous Bone Marrow into Peripheral Vein, Open Approach
30230Y0	Transfusion of Autologous Hematopoietic Stem Cells into Peripheral Vein, Open Approach
30233G0	Transfusion of Autologous Bone Marrow into Peripheral Vein, Percutaneous Approach
30233Y0	Transfusion of Autologous Hematopoietic Stem Cells into Peripheral Vein, Percutaneous Approach
30240G0	Transfusion of Autologous Bone Marrow into Central Vein, Open Approach
30240Y0	Transfusion of Autologous Hematopoietic Stem Cells into Central Vein, Open Approach
30243G0	Transfusion of Autologous Bone Marrow into Central Vein, Percutaneous Approach
30243Y0	Transfusion of Autologous Hematopoietic Stem Cells into Central Vein, Percutaneous Approach
30250G0	Transfusion of Autologous Bone Marrow into Peripheral Artery, Open Approach
30250Y0	Transfusion of Autologous Hematopoietic Stem Cells into Peripheral Artery, Open Approach
30253G0	Transfusion of Autologous Bone Marrow into Peripheral Artery, Percutaneous Approach
30253Y0	Transfusion of Autologous Hematopoietic Stem Cells into Peripheral Artery, Percutaneous Approach
30260G0	Transfusion of Autologous Bone Marrow into Central Artery, Open Approach
30260Y0	Transfusion of Autologous Hematopoietic Stem Cells into Central Artery, Open Approach
30263G0	Transfusion of Autologous Bone Marrow into Central Artery, Percutaneous Approach
30263Y0	Transfusion of Autologous Hematopoietic Stem Cells into Central Artery, Percutaneous Approach

B. Covered Conditions

1. Effective for services performed on or after April 28, 1989:

For acute leukemia in remission for patients who have a high probability of relapse and who have no human leucocyte antigens (HLA)-matched the following diagnosis codes are reported:

If ICD-9-CM is applicable, use the following Diagnosis Codes and Descriptions

Diagnosis Code	Description
204.01	Lymphoid leukemia, acute, in remission
205.01	Myeloid leukemia, acute, in remission
206.01	Monocytic leukemia, acute, in remission
207.01	Acute erythremia and erythroleukemia, in remission
208.01	Leukemia of unspecified cell type, acute, in remission

If ICD-10-CM is applicable, use the following Diagnosis Codes and Descriptions

Diagnosis Code	Description
C91.01	Acute lymphoblastic leukemia, in remission
C92.01	Acute myeloblastic leukemia, in remission
C92.41	Acute promyelocytic leukemia, in remission
C92.51	Acute myelomonocytic leukemia, in remission
C92.61	Acute myeloid leukemia with 11q23-abnormality in remission

Diagnosis Code	Description
C92.A1	Acute myeloid leukemia with multilineage dysplasia, in remission
C93.01	Acute monoblastic/monocytic leukemia, in remission
C94.01	Acute erythroid leukemia, in remission
C94.21	Acute megakaryoblastic leukemia, in remission
C94.41	Acute parmyelosis with myelofibrosis, in remission
C95.01	Acute leukemia of unspecified cell type, in remission

For resistant non-Hodgkin's lymphomas (or those presenting with poor prognostic features following an initial response the following diagnosis codes are reported:

If ICD-9-CM is applicable, use the following code ranges:
200.00 - 200.08,

200.10 - 00.18,

200.20 - 200.28,

200.80 - 200.88,

202.00 - 202.08,

202.80 - 202.88, and

202.90 - 202.98.

If ICD-10-CM is applicable use the following code ranges:
C82.00 - C85.29,

C85.80 - C86.6,

C96.4, and

C96.Z - C96.9.

For recurrent or refractory neuroblastoma (see ICD-9-CM Neoplasm by site, malignant for the appropriate diagnosis code)

If ICD-10-CM is applicable the following ranges are reported:

C00 - C96, and

D00 - D09 Resistant non-Hodgkin's lymphomas

For advanced Hodgkin's disease patients who have failed conventional therapy and have no HLA-matched donor the following diagnosis codes are reported:

If ICD-9-CM is applicable, 201.00-201.98.

If ICD-10-CM is applicable, C81.00 – C81.99.

2. Effective for services performed on or after October 1, 2000:

Durie-Salmon Stage II or III that fit the following requirement are covered: Newly diagnosed or responsive multiple myeloma (if ICD-9-CM is applicable, diagnosis codes 203.00 and 238.6, and, if ICD-10-CM is applicable, diagnosis codes C90.00 and D47.Z9). This includes those patients with previously untreated disease, those with at least a partial response to prior chemotherapy (defined as a 50% decrease either in measurable paraprotein [serum and/or urine] or in bone marrow infiltration, sustained for at least 1 month), and those in responsive relapse, and adequate cardiac, renal, pulmonary, and hepatic function.

3. Effective for Services On or After March 15, 2005

Effective for services performed on or after March 15, 2005 when recognized clinical risk factors are employed to select patients for transplantation, high-dose melphalan (HDM), together with AuSCT, in treating Medicare beneficiaries of any age group with primary amyloid light-chain (AL) amyloidosis who meet the following criteria:

Amyloid deposition in 2 or fewer organs; and,

Cardiac left ventricular ejection fraction (EF) of 45% or greater.

C. Noncovered Conditions

Insufficient data exist to establish definite conclusions regarding the efficacy of autologous stem cell transplantation for the following conditions:

*   Acute leukemia not in remission:
    — If ICD-9-CM is applicable, diagnosis codes 204.00, 205.00, 206.00, 207.00 and 208.00 are noncovered;
    — If ICD-10-CM is applicable, diagnosis codes C91.00, C92.00, C92.40, C92.50, C92.60, C92.A0, C93.00, C94.00, and C95.00 are noncovered.
*   Chronic granulocytic leukemia:
    — If ICD-9-CM is applicable, diagnosis codes 205.10 and 205.11;
    — If ICD-10-CM is applicable, diagnosis codes C92.10 and C92.11.
*   Solid tumors (other than neuroblastoma):
    — If ICD-9-CM is applicable, diagnosis codes 140.0-199.1;
    — If ICD-10-CM is applicable, diagnosis codes C00.0 - C80.2 and D00.0 - D09.9. Multiple myeloma (ICD-9-CM codes 203.00 and 238.6), through September 30, 2000.
*   Tandem transplantation (multiple rounds of autologous stem cell transplantation) for patients with multiple myeloma
    — If ICD-9-CM is applicable, diagnosis codes 203.00 and 238.6 and,

— If ICD-10-CM is applicable, diagnosis codes C90.00 and D47.Z9)

- Non-primary (AL) amyloidosis,

  — If ICD-9-CM is applicable, diagnosis code 277.3. Effective October 1, 2000; ICD-9-CM code 277.3 was expanded to codes 277.30, 277.31, and 277.39 effective October 1, 2006.

  — If ICD-10-CM is applicable, diagnosis codes are E85.0 – E85.9. or

- Primary (AL) amyloidosis

  — If ICD-9-CM is applicable, diagnosis codes 277.30, 277.31, and 277.39 and for Medicare beneficiaries age 64 or older, effective October 1, 2000, through March 14, 2005.

  — If ICD-10-CM is applicable, diagnosis codes are E85.0 - E85.9.

NOTE: Coverage for conditions other than these specifically designated as covered or non-covered is left to the discretion of the A/B MAC (A).

100-04, 3, 90.3.3

Billing for Stem Cell Transplantation

A. Billing for Allogeneic Stem Cell Transplants
1. Definition of Acquisition Charges for Allogeneic Stem Cell Transplants

   Acquisition charges for allogeneic stem cell transplants include, but are not limited to, charges for the costs of the following services:

   — National Marrow Donor Program fees, if applicable, for stem cells from an unrelated donor;

   — Tissue typing of donor and recipient;

   — Donor evaluation;

   — Physician pre-admission/pre-procedure donor evaluation services;

   — Costs associated with harvesting procedure (e.g., general routine and special care services, procedure/operating room and other ancillary services, apheresis services, etc.);

   — Post-operative/post-procedure evaluation of donor; and

   — Preparation and processing of stem cells.

   Payment for these acquisition services is included in the MS-DRG payment for the allogeneic stem cell transplant when the transplant occurs in the inpatient setting, and in the OPPS APC payment for the allogeneic stem cell transplant when the transplant occurs in the outpatient setting. The Medicare contractor does not make separate payment for these acquisition services, because hospitals may bill and receive payment only for services provided to the Medicare beneficiary who is the recipient of the stem cell transplant and whose illness is being treated with the stem cell transplant. Unlike the acquisition costs of solid organs for transplant (e.g., hearts and kidneys), which are paid on a reasonable cost basis, acquisition costs for allogeneic stem cells are included in prospective payment.

   Acquisition charges for stem cell transplants apply only to allogeneic transplants, for which stem cells are obtained from a donor (other than the recipient himself or herself). Acquisition charges do not apply to autologous transplants (transplanted stem cells are obtained from the recipient himself or herself), because autologous transplants involve services provided to the beneficiary only (and not to a donor), for which the hospital may bill and receive payment (see Pub. 100-4, chapter 4, §231.10 and paragraph B of this section for information regarding billing for autologous stem cell transplants).

2. Billing for Acquisition Services

   The hospital bills and shows acquisition charges for allogeneic stem cell transplants based on the status of the patient (i.e., inpatient or outpatient) when the transplant is furnished. See Pub. 100-4, chapter 4, §231.11 for instructions regarding billing for acquisition services for allogeneic stem cell transplants that are performed in the outpatient setting.

   When the allogeneic stem cell transplant occurs in the inpatient setting, the hospital identifies stem cell acquisition charges for allogeneic bone marrow/stem cell transplants separately in FL 42 of Form CMS-1450 (or electronic equivalent) by using revenue code 0819 (Other Organ Acquisition). Revenue code 0819 charges should include all services required to acquire stem cells from a donor, as defined above.

   On the recipient's transplant bill, the hospital reports the acquisition charges, cost report days, and utilization days for the donor's hospital stay (if applicable) and/or charges for other encounters in which the stem cells were obtained from the donor. The donor is covered for medically necessary inpatient hospital days of care or outpatient care provided in connection with the allogeneic stem cell transplant under Part A. Expenses incurred for complications are paid only if they are directly and immediately attributable to the stem cell donation procedure. The hospital reports the acquisition charges on the billing form for the recipient, as described in the first paragraph of this section. It does not charge the donor's days of care against the recipient's utilization record. For cost reporting purposes, it includes the covered donor days and charges as Medicare days and charges.

   The transplant hospital keeps an itemized statement that identifies the services furnished, the charges, the person receiving the service (donor/recipient), and whether this is a potential transplant donor or recipient. These charges will be reflected in the transplant hospital's stem cell/bone marrow acquisition cost

center. For allogeneic stem cell acquisition services in cases that do not result in transplant, due to death of the intended recipient or other causes, hospitals include the costs associated with the acquisition services on the Medicare cost report.

The hospital shows charges for the transplant itself in revenue center code 0362 or another appropriate cost center. Selection of the cost center is up to the hospital.

B. Billing for Autologous Stem Cell Transplants
The hospital bills and shows all charges for autologous stem cell harvesting, processing, and transplant procedures based on the status of the patient (i.e., inpatient or outpatient) when the services are furnished. It shows charges for the actual transplant, described by the appropriate ICD-9-CM procedure or CPT codes, in revenue center code 0362 or another appropriate cost center. ICD-9-CM or ICD-10-PCS codes are used to identify inpatient procedures.

The CPT codes describing autologous stem cell harvesting procedures may be billed and are separately payable under the OPPS when provided in the hospital outpatient setting of care. Autologous harvesting procedures are distinct from the acquisition services described in Pub. 100-4, chapter 4, §231.11 and section A. above for allogeneic stem cell transplants, which include services provided when stem cells are obtained from a donor and not from the patient undergoing the stem cell transplant. The CPT codes describing autologous stem cell processing procedures also may be billed and are separately payable under the OPPS when provided to hospital outpatients.

Payment for autologous stem cell harvesting procedures performed in the hospital inpatient setting of care, with transplant also occurring in the inpatient setting of care, is included in the MS-DRG payment for the autologous stem cell transplant.

100-04, 3, 90.4

Liver Transplants

A. Background
For Medicare coverage purposes, liver transplants are considered medically reasonable and necessary for specified conditions when performed in facilities that meet specific criteria. Coverage guidelines may be found in Publication 100-3, Section 260.1.

Effective for claims with dates of service June 21, 2012 and later, contractors may, at their discretion cover adult liver transplantation for patients with extrahepatic unresectable cholangiocarcinoma (CCA), (2) liver metastases due to a neuroendocrine tumor (NET) or (3) hemangioendothelimo (HAE) when furnished in an approved Liver Transplant Center (below). All other nationally non-covered malignancies continue to remain nationally non-covered.

To review the current list of approved Liver Transplant Centers, see http://www.cms.hhs.gov/CertificationandComplianc/20_Transplant.asp#TopOfPage

100-04, 3, 90.4.1

Standard Liver Acquisition Charge
A3-3615.1, A3-3615.3

Each transplant facility must develop a standard charge for acquiring a cadaver liver from costs it expects to incur in the acquisition of livers.

This standard charge is not a charge that represents the acquisition cost of a specific liver. Rather, it is a charge that reflects the average cost associated with a liver acquisition.

Services associated with liver acquisition are billed from the organ procurement organization or, in some cases, the excising hospital to the transplant hospital. The excising hospital does not submit a billing form to the FI. The transplant hospital keeps an itemized statement that identifies the services furnished, the charges, the person receiving the service (donor/recipient), and the potential transplant donor. These charges are reflected in the transplant hospital's liver acquisition cost center and are used in determining the hospital's standard charge for acquiring a cadaver's liver. The standard charge is not a charge representing the acquisition cost of a specific liver. Rather, it is a charge that reflects the average cost associated with liver acquisition. Also, it is an all inclusive charge for all services required in acquisition of a liver, e.g., tissue typing, transportation of organ, and surgeons' retrieval fees.

100-04, 3, 90.4.2

Billing for Liver Transplant and Acquisition Services
The inpatient claim is completed in accordance with instructions in chapter 25 for the beneficiary who receives a covered liver transplant. Applicable standard liver acquisition charges are identified separately in FL 42 by revenue code 0817 (Donor-Liver). Where interim bills are submitted, the standard acquisition charge appears on the billing form for the period during which the transplant took place. This charge is in addition to the hospital's charge for services furnished directly to the Medicare recipient.

The contractor deducts liver acquisition charges for IPPS hospitals prior to processing through Pricer. Costs of liver acquisition incurred by approved liver transplant facilities are not included in prospective payment DRG 480 (Liver Transplant). They are paid on a reasonable cost basis. This item is a "pass-through" cost for which interim payments are made. (See the Provider Reimbursement Manual, Part 1, §2802

B.8.) The contractor includes liver acquisition charges under revenue code 0817 in the HUIP record that it sends to CWF and the QIO.

A. Bill Review Procedures

The contractor takes the following actions to process liver transplant bills.

1. Operative Report

   The contractor requires the operative report with all claims for liver transplants, or sends a development request to the hospital for each liver transplant with a diagnosis code for a covered condition.

2. MCE Interface

   The MCE contains a limited coverage edit for liver transplant procedures using ICD-9-CM code 50.59 if ICD-9 is applicable, and, if ICD-10 is applicable, using ICD-10-PCS codes 0FY00Z0, 0FY00Z1, and 0FY00Z2.

   Where a liver transplant procedure code is identified by the MCE, the contractor shall check the provider number and effective date to determine if the provider is an approved liver transplant facility at the time of the transplant, and the contractor shall also determine if the facility is certified for adults and/or pediatric transplants dependent upon the patient's age. If yes, the claim is suspended for review of the operative report to determine whether the beneficiary has at least one of the covered conditions when the diagnosis code is for a covered condition. If payment is appropriate (i.e., the facility is approved, the service is furnished on or after the approval date, and the beneficiary has a covered condition), the contractor sends the claim to Grouper and Pricer.

   If none of the diagnoses codes are for a covered condition, or if the provider is not an approved liver transplant facility, the contractor denies the claim.

   NOTE: Some noncovered conditions are included in the covered diagnostic codes. (The diagnostic codes are broader than the covered conditions. Do not pay for noncovered conditions.

3. Grouper

   If the bill shows a discharge date before March 8, 1990, the liver transplant procedure is not covered. If the discharge date is March 8, 1990 or later, the contractor processes the bill through Grouper and Pricer. If the discharge date is after March 7, 1990, and before October 1, 1990, Grouper assigned CMS DRG 191 or 192. The contractor sent the bill to Pricer with review code 08. Pricer would then overlay CMS DRG 191 or 192 with CMS DRG 480 and the weights and thresholds for CMS DRG 480 to price the bill. If the discharge date is after September 30, 1990, Grouper assigns CMS DRG 480 and Pricer is able to price without using review code 08. If the discharge date is after September 30, 2007, Grouper assigns MS-DRG 005 or 006 (Liver transplant with MCC or Intestinal Transplant or Liver transplant without MCC, respectively) and Pricer is able to price without using review code 08.

4. Liver Transplant Billing From Non-approved Hospitals

   Where a liver transplant and covered services are provided by a non-approved hospital, the bill data processed through Grouper and Pricer must exclude transplant procedure codes and related charges.

   When CMS approves a hospital to furnish liver transplant services, it informs the hospital of the effective date in the approval letter. The contractor will receive a copy of the letter.

100-04, 3, 90.5

Pancreas Transplants Kidney Transplants

(Rev. 3481, Issued: 03-18-16, Effective: 06-20-16, Implementation: 06-20-16)

A. Background

Effective July 1, 1999, Medicare covered pancreas transplantation when performed simultaneously with or following a kidney transplant if ICD-9 is applicable, ICD-9-CM procedure code 55.69. If ICD-10 is applicable, the following ICD-10-PCS codes will be used:

   0TY00Z0,

   0TY00Z1,

   0TY00Z2,

   0TY10Z0.

   0TY10Z1, and

   0TY10Z2.

Pancreas transplantation is performed to induce an insulin independent, euglycemic state in diabetic patients. The procedure is generally limited to those patients with severe secondary complications of diabetes including kidney failure. However, pancreas transplantation is sometimes performed on patients with labile diabetes and hypoglycemic unawareness.

Medicare has had a policy of not covering pancreas transplantation. The Office of Health Technology Assessment performed an assessment on pancreas-kidney transplantation in 1994. They found reasonable graft survival outcomes for patients receiving either simultaneous pancreas-kidney (SPK) transplantation or pancreas after kidney (PAK) transplantation. For a list of facilities approved to perform SPK or PAK, refer to the following Web site: https://www.cms.gov/Medicare/

Provider-Enrollment-and-Certification/CertificationandComplianc/downloads/ApprovedTransplantPrograms.pdf

B. Billing for Pancreas Transplants

There are no special provisions related to managed care participants. Managed care plans are required to provide all Medicare covered services. Medicare does not restrict which hospitals or physicians may perform pancreas transplantation.

The transplant procedure and revenue code 0360 for the operating room are paid under these codes. Procedures must be reported using the current ICD-9-CM procedure codes for pancreas and kidney transplants. Providers must place at least one of the following transplant procedure codes on the claim:

If ICD-9 Is Applicable

   52.80   Transplant of pancreas

   52.82   Homotransplant of pancreas

The Medicare Code Editor (MCE) has been updated to include 52.80 and 52.82 as limited coverage procedures. The contractor must determine if the facility is approved for the transplant and certified for either pediatric or adult transplants dependent upon the age of the patient.

Effective October 1, 2000, ICD-9-CM code 52.83 was moved in the MCE to non-covered. The contractor must override any deny edit on claims that came in with 52.82 prior to October 1, 2000 and adjust, as 52.82 is the correct code.

If the discharge date is July 1, 1999, or later: the contractor processes the bill through Grouper and Pricer.

If ICD-10 is applicable, the following procedure codes (ICD-10-PCS) are:

   0FYG0Z0 Transplantation of Pancreas, Allogeneic, Open Approach

   0FYG0Z1 Transplantation of Pancreas, Syngeneic, Open Approach

Pancreas transplantation is reasonable and necessary for the following diagnosis codes. However, since this is not an all-inclusive list, the contractor is permitted to determine if any additional diagnosis codes will be covered for this procedure.

If ICD-9-CM is applicable, Diabetes Diagnosis Codes and Descriptions

ICD-9-CM Code	Description
250.00	Diabetes mellitus without mention of complication, type II (non-insulin dependent) (NIDDM) (adult onset) or unspecified type, not stated as uncontrolled.
250.01	Diabetes mellitus without mention of complication, type I (insulin dependent) (IDDM) (juvenile), not stated as uncontrolled.
250.02	Diabetes mellitus without mention of complication, type II (non-insulin dependent) (NIDDM) (adult onset) or unspecified type, uncontrolled.
250.03	Diabetes mellitus without mention of complication, type I (insulin dependent) (IDDM) (juvenile), uncontrolled.
250.1X	Diabetes with ketoacidosis
250.2X	Diabetes with hyperosmolarity
250.3X	Diabetes with coma
250.4X	Diabetes with renal manifestations
250.5X	Diabetes with ophthalmic manifestations
250.6X	Diabetes with neurological manifestations
250.7X	Diabetes with peripheral circulatory disorders
250.8X	Diabetes with other specified manifestations
250.9X	Diabetes with unspecified complication

NOTE: X=0-3

If ICD-10-CM is applicable, the diagnosis codes are: E10.10 - E10.9

Hypertensive Renal Diagnosis Codes and Descriptions if ICD-9-CM is applicable :

ICD-9-CM Code	Description
403.01	Malignant hypertensive renal disease, with renal failure
403.11	Benign hypertensive renal disease, with renal failure
403.91	Unspecified hypertensive renal disease, with renal failure
404.02	Malignant hypertensive heart and renal disease, with renal failure
404.03	Malignant hypertensive heart and renal disease, with congestive heart failure or renal failure
404.12	Benign hypertensive heart and renal disease, with renal failure
404.13	Benign hypertensive heart and renal disease, with congestive heart failure or renal failure
404.92	Unspecified hypertensive heart and renal disease, with renal failure
404.93	Unspecified hypertensive heart and renal disease, with congestive heart failure or renal failure
585.1–585.6, 585.9	Chronic Renal Failure Code

If ICD-10-CM is applicable, diagnosis codes and descriptions are:

ICD-10-CM code	Description
I12.0	Hypertensive chronic kidney disease with stage 5 chronic kidney disease or end stage renal disease
I13.11	Hypertensive heart and chronic kidney disease without heart failure, with stage 5 chronic kidney disease, or end stage renal disease
I13.2	Hypertensive heart and chronic kidney disease with heart failure and with stage 5 chronic kidney disease, or end stage renal disease
N18.1	Chronic kidney disease, stage 1
N18.2	Chronic kidney disease, stage 2 (mild)
N18.3	Chronic kidney disease, stage 3 (moderate)
N18.4	Chronic kidney disease, stage 4 (severe)
N18.5	Chronic kidney disease, stage 5
N18.6	End stage renal disease
N18.9	Chronic kidney disease, unspecified

NOTE: If a patient had a kidney transplant that was successful, the patient no longer has chronic kidney failure, therefore it would be inappropriate for the provider to bill ICD-9-CM codes 585.1 - 585.6, 585.9 or, if ICD-10-CM is applicable, the diagnosis codes N18.1 - N18.9 on such a patient. In these cases one of the following codes should be present on the claim or in the beneficiary's history.

The provider uses the following ICD-9-CM status codes only when a kidney transplant was performed before the pancreas transplant and ICD-9 is applicable:

ICD-9-CM code	Description
V42.0	Organ or tissue replaced by transplant kidney
V43.89	Organ tissue replaced by other means, kidney or pancreas

If ICD-10-CM is applicable, the following ICD-10-CM status codes will be used:

ICD-10-CM code	Description
Z48.22	Encounter for aftercare following kidney transplant
Z94.0	Kidney transplant status

NOTE: If a kidney and pancreas transplants are performed simultaneously, the claim should contain a diabetes diagnosis code and a renal failure code or one of the hypertensive renal failure diagnosis codes. The claim should also contain two transplant procedure codes. If the claim is for a pancreas transplant only, the claim should contain a diabetes diagnosis code and a status code to indicate a previous kidney transplant. If the status code is not on the claim for the pancreas transplant, the contractor will search the beneficiary's claim history for a status code indicating a prior kidney transplant.

C. Drugs
If the pancreas transplant occurs after the kidney transplant, immunosuppressive therapy will begin with the date of discharge from the inpatient stay for the pancreas transplant.

D. Charges for Pancreas Acquisition Services
A separate organ acquisition cost center has been established for pancreas transplantation. The Medicare cost report will include a separate line to account for pancreas transplantation costs. The 42 CFR 412.2(e)(4) was changed to include pancreas in the list of organ acquisition costs that are paid on a reasonable cost basis.

Acquisition costs for pancreas transplantation as well as kidney transplants will occur in Revenue Center 081X. The contractor overrides any claims that suspend due to repetition of revenue code 081X on the same claim if the patient had a simultaneous kidney/pancreas transplant. It pays for acquisition costs for both kidney and pancreas organs if transplants are performed simultaneously. It will not pay for more than two organ acquisitions on the same claim.

E. Medicare Summary Notices (MSN) and Remittance Advice Messages
If the provider submits a claim for simultaneous pancreas kidney transplantation or pancreas transplantation following a kidney transplant, and omits one of the appropriate diagnosis/procedure codes, the contractor shall reject the claim.

The following reflects the remittance advice messages and associated codes that will appear when rejecting/denying claims under this policy. This CARC/RARC combination is compliant with CAQH CORE Business Scenario 3.

　Group Code: CO

　CARC: B15

　RARC: N/A

　MSN: 16.32

If no evidence of a prior kidney transplant is presented, then the contractor shall deny the claim.

The following reflects the remittance advice messages and associated codes that will appear when rejecting/denying claims under this policy. This CARC/RARC combination is compliant with CAQH CORE Business Scenario 3.

　Group Code: CO

　CARC: 50

　RARC: MA126

　MSN: 15.4

100-04, 3, 90.5.1

Pancreas Transplants Alone (PA)

Rev.3481, Issued: 03-18-16. Effective: 06-20-16, Implementation: 06-20-16

A. General
Pancreas transplantation is performed to induce an insulin-independent, euglycemic state in diabetic patients. The procedure is generally limited to those patients with severe secondary complications of diabetes, including kidney failure. However, pancreas transplantation is sometimes performed on patients

with labile diabetes and hypoglycemic unawareness. Medicare has had a long-standing policy of not covering pancreas transplantation, as the safety and effectiveness of the procedure had not been demonstrated. The Office of Health Technology Assessment performed an assessment of pancreas-kidney transplantation in 1994. It found reasonable graft survival outcomes for patients receiving either simultaneous pancreas-kidney transplantation or pancreas-after-kidney transplantation.

B. Nationally Covered Indications
CMS determines that whole organ pancreas transplantation will be nationally covered by Medicare when performed simultaneous with or after a kidney transplant. If the pancreas transplant occurs after the kidney transplant, immunosuppressive therapy will begin with the date of discharge from the inpatient stay for the pancreas transplant.

C. Billing and Claims Processing
Contractors shall pay for Pancreas Transplantation Alone (PA) effective for services on or after April 26, 2006 when performed in those facilities that are Medicare-approved for kidney transplantation. Approved facilities are located at the following address: https://www.cms.gov/Medicare/Provider-Enrollment-and-Certification/Certification andComplianc/downloads/ApprovedTransplantPrograms.pdf

Contractors who receive claims for PA services that were performed in an unapproved facility, should reject such claims. The following reflects the remittance advice messages and associated codes that will appear when rejecting/denying claims under this policy. This CARC/RARC combination is compliant with CAQH CORE Business Scenario 3.

Group Code: CO

CARC: 58

RARC: N/A

MSN: 16.2.

Payment will be made for a PA service performed in an approved facility, and which meets the coverage guidelines mentioned above for beneficiaries with type I diabetes.

All-Inclusive List of Covered Diagnosis Codes for PA if ICD-9-CM is applicable

(NOTE: "X" = 1 and 3 only)

ICD-9-CM code	Description
250.0X	Diabetes mellitus without mention of complication, type I (insulin dependent) (IDDM) (juvenile), not stated as uncontrolled.
250.1X	Diabetes with ketoacidosis
250.2X	Diabetes with hyperosmolarity
250.3X	Diabetes with coma
250.4X	Diabetes with renal manifestations
250.5X	Diabetes with ophthalmic manifestations
250.6X	Diabetes with neurological manifestations
250.7X	Diabetes with peripheral circulatory disorders
250.8X	Diabetes with other specified manifestations
250.9X	Diabetes with unspecified complication

If ICD-10-CM is applicable, the provider uses the following range of ICD-10-CM codes:
E10.10 – E10.9.

Procedure Codes

If ICD-9 CM is applicable
52.80 - Transplant of pancreas

52.82 - Homotransplant of pancreas

If ICD-10 is applicable, the provider uses the following ICD-10-PCS codes:
0FYG0Z0 Transplantation of Pancreas, Allogeneic, Open Approach

0FYG0Z1 Transplantation of Pancreas, Syngeneic, Open Approach

Contractors who receive claims for PA that are not billed using the covered diagnosis/procedure codes listed above shall reject such claims. The MCE edits to ensure that the transplant is covered based on the diagnosis. The MCE also considers ICD-9-CM codes 52.80 and 52.82 and ICD-10-PCS codes ØFYGØZØ and ØFYGØZ1 as limited coverage dependent upon whether the facility is approved to perform the transplant and is certified for the age of the patient.

The following reflects the remittance advice messages and associated codes that will appear when rejecting/denying claims under this policy. This CARC/RARC combination is compliant with CAQH CORE Business Scenario 3.

> Group Code: CO
>
> CARC: 50
>
> RARC: N/A
>
> MSN: 15.4

Contractors shall hold the provider liable for denied\rejected claims unless the hospital issues a Hospital Issued Notice of Non-coverage (HINN) or a physician issues an Advanced Beneficiary Notice (ABN) for Part-B for physician services.

D. Charges for Pancreas Alone Acquisition Services

A separate organ acquisition cost center has been established for pancreas transplantation. The Medicare cost report will include a separate line to account for pancreas transplantation costs. The 42 CFR 412.2(e)(4) was changed to include PA in the list of organ acquisition costs that are paid on a reasonable cost basis.

Acquisition costs for PA transplantation are billed in Revenue Code 081X. The contractor removes acquisition charges prior to sending the claims to Pricer so such charges are not included in the outlier calculation.

100-04, 3, 90.6

Intestinal and Multi-Visceral Transplants

(Rev. 3481, Issued: 03-18-16. Effective: 06-20-16, Implementation: 06-20-16)

A. Background

Effective for services on or after April 1, 2001, Medicare covers intestinal and multi-visceral transplantation for the purpose of restoring intestinal function in patients with irreversible intestinal failure. Intestinal failure is defined as the loss of absorptive capacity of the small bowel secondary to severe primary gastrointestinal disease or surgically induced short bowel syndrome. Intestinal failure prevents oral nutrition and may be associated with both mortality and profound morbidity. Multi-Visceral transplantation includes organs in the digestive system (stomach, duodenum, liver, and intestine). See §260.5 of the National Coverage Determinations Manual for further information.

B. Approved Transplant Facilities

Medicare will cover intestinal transplantation if performed in an approved facility. The approved facilities are located at: https://www.cms.gov/Medicare/Provider-Enrollment-and-Certification/Certification andComplianc/downloads/ApprovedTransplantPrograms.pdf

C. Billing

If ICD-9-CM is applicable, ICD-9-CM procedure code 46.97 is effective for discharges on or after April 1, 2001. If ICD-10 is applicable, the ICD-10-PCS procedure codes are ØDY8ØZØ, ØDY8ØZ1, ØDY8ØZ2, ØDYEØZØ, ØDYEØZ1, and ØDYEØZ2. The Medicare Code Editor (MCE) lists these codes as limited coverage procedures. The contractor shall override the MCE when this procedure code is listed and the coverage criteria are met in an approved transplant facility, and also determine if the facility is certified for adults and/or pediatric transplants dependent upon the patient's age.

For these procedures where the provider is approved as transplant facility and certified for the adult and/or pediatric population, and the service is performed on or after the transplant approval date, the contractor must suspend the claim for clerical review of the operative report to determine whether the beneficiary has at least one of the covered conditions listed when the diagnosis code is for a covered condition.

This review is not part of the contractor's medical review workload. Instead, the contractor should complete this review as part of its claims processing workload.

If ICD-9-CM is applicable, charges for ICD-9-CM procedure code 46.97, and, if ICD-10 is applicable, the ICD-10-PCS procedure codes ØDY8ØZØ, ØDY8ØZ1, ØDY8ØZ2, ØDYEØZØ, ØDYEØZ1, or ØDYEØZ2 should be billed under revenue code 0360, Operating Room Services.

For discharge dates on or after October 1, 2001, acquisition charges are billed under revenue code 081X, Organ Acquisition. For discharge dates between April 1, 2001, and September 30, 2001, hospitals were to report the acquisition charges on the claim, but there was no interim pass-through payment made for these costs.

Bill the procedure used to obtain the donor's organ on the same claim, using appropriate ICD procedure codes.

The 11X bill type should be used when billing for intestinal transplants.

Immunosuppressive therapy for intestinal transplantation is covered and should be billed consistent with other organ transplants under the current rules.

If ICD-9-CM is applicable, there is no specific ICD-9-CM diagnosis code for intestinal failure. Diagnosis codes exist to capture the causes of intestinal failure. Some examples of intestinal failure include but are not limited to the following conditions and their associated ICD-9-CM codes:

- Volvulus 560.2,

- Volvulus gastroschisis 756.79, other [congenital] anomalies of abdominal wall,

- Volvulus gastroschisis 569.89, other specified disorders of intestine,

- Necrotizing enterocolitis 777.5, necrotizing enterocolitis in fetus or newborn,

- Necrotizing enterocolitis 014.8, other tuberculosis of intestines, peritoneum, and mesenteric,

- Necrotizing enterocolitis and splanchnic vascular thrombosis 557.0, acute vascular insufficiency of intestine,

- Inflammatory bowel disease 569.9, unspecified disorder of intestine,

- Radiation enteritis 777.5, necrotizing enterocolitis in fetus or newborn, and

- Radiation enteritis 558.1.

If ICD-10-CM is applicable, some diagnosis codes that may be used for intestinal failure are:

- Volvulus K56.2,

- Enteroptosis K63.4,

- Other specified diseases of intestine K63.89,

- Other specified diseases of the digestive system K92.89,

- Postsurgical malabsorption, not elsewhere classified K91.2,

- Other congenital malformations of abdominal wall Q79.59,

- Necrotizing enterocolitis in newborn, unspecified P77.9,

- Stage 1 necrotizing enterocolitis in newborn P77.1,

- Stage 2 necrotizing enterocolitis in newborn P77.2, and

- Stage 3 necrotizing enterocolitis in newborn P77.3

D. Acquisition Costs

A separate organ acquisition cost center was established for acquisition costs incurred on or after October 1, 2001. The Medicare Cost Report will include a separate line to account for these transplantation costs.

For intestinal and multi-visceral transplants performed between April 1, 2001, and October 1, 2001, the DRG payment was payment in full for all hospital services related to this procedure.

E. Medicare Summary Notices (MSN), Remittance Advice Messages, and Notice of Utilization Notices (NOU)

If an intestinal transplant is billed by an unapproved facility after April 1, 2001, the contractor shall deny the claim.

The following reflects the remittance advice messages and associated codes that will appear when rejecting/denying claims under this policy. This CARC/RARC combination is compliant with CAQH CORE Business Scenario 3.

> Group Code: CO
>
> CARC: 171
>
> RARC: N/A

MSN: 21.6 or 21.18 or 16.2

100-04, 3, 100.1

Billing for Abortion Services

(Rev. 3481, Issued: 03-18-16. Effective: 06-20-16, Implementation: 06-20-16)

Effective October 1, 1998, abortions are not covered under the Medicare program except for instances where the pregnancy is a result of an act of rape or incest; or the woman suffers from a physical disorder, physical injury, or physical illness, including a life endangering physical condition caused by the pregnancy itself that would, as certified by a physician, place the woman in danger of death unless an abortion is performed.

A. "G" Modifier

The "G7" modifier is defined as "the pregnancy resulted from rape or incest, or pregnancy certified by physician as life threatening."

Beginning July 1, 1999, providers should bill for abortion services using the new Modifier G7. This modifier can be used on claims with dates of services October 1, 1998, and after. CWF will be able to recognize the modifier beginning July 1, 1999.

B. A/B MAC (A) Billing Instructions

1. Hospital Inpatient Billing

   Hospitals use bill type 11X. Medicare will pay only when one of the following condition codes is reported:

Condition Code	Description
AA	Abortion Performed due to Rape
AB	Abortion Performed due to Incest
AD	Abortion Performed due to life endangering physical condition

With one of the following:

If ICD-9-CM Is Applicable:

- an appropriate ICD principal diagnosis code that will group to DRG 770 (Abortion W D&C, Aspiration Curettage Or Hysterotomy) or

- an appropriate ICD principal diagnosis code and one of the following ICD-9-CM operating room procedure that will group to DRG 779 (Abortion W/O D&C):69.01, 69.02, 69.51, 74.91.

If ICD-10-CM is applicable, one of the following ICD-10-PCS codes are used:

ICD-10-PCS code	Description
10A07ZZ	Abortion of Products of Conception, Via Natural or Artificial Opening
10A08ZZ	Abortion of Products of Conception, Via Natural or Artificial Opening Endoscopic
10D17ZZ	Extraction of Products of Conception, Retained, Via Natural or Artificial Opening
10D18ZZ	Extraction of Products of Conception, Retained, Via Natural or Artificial Opening Endoscopic
10A07ZZ	Abortion of Products of Conception, Via Natural or Artificial Opening
10A08ZZ	Abortion of Products of Conception, Via Natural or Artificial Opening Endoscopic
10A00ZZ	Abortion of Products of Conception, Open Approach
10A03ZZ	Abortion of Products of Conception, Percutaneous Approach
10A04ZZ	Abortion of Products of Conception, Percutaneous Endoscopic Approach

Providers must use ICD-9-CM codes 69.01 and 69.02 if ICD-9-CM is applicable, or, if ICD-10-CM is applicable, the related 1CD-10-PCS codes to describe exactly the procedure or service performed.

The A/B MAC (A) must manually review claims with the above ICD-9-CM/ICD-10-PCS procedure codes to verify that all of the above conditions are met.

2. Outpatient Billing

Hospitals will use bill type 13X and 85X. Medicare will pay only if one of the following CPT codes is used with the "G7" modifier.

59840	59851	59856	59841	59852
59857	59850	59855	59866	

C. Common Working File (CWF) Edits

For hospital outpatient claims, CWF will bypass its edits for a managed care beneficiary who is having an abortion outside their plan and the claim is submitted with the "G7" modifier and one of the above CPT codes.

For hospital inpatient claims, CWF will bypass its edits for a managed care beneficiary who is having an abortion outside their plan and the claim is submitted with one of the above inpatient procedure codes.

D. Medicare Summary Notices (MSN)/Explanation of Your Medicare Benefits Remittance Advice Message

If a claim is submitted with one of the above CPT procedure codes but no "G7" modifier, the claim is denied.

The following reflects the remittance advice messages and associated codes that will appear when rejecting/denying claims under this policy. This CARC/RARC combination is compliant with CAQH CORE Business Scenario 3.

Group Code: CO

CARC: 272

RARC: N/A

MSN: 21.21

100-04, 3, 100.6

Inpatient Renal Services

HO-E400

Section 405.103I of Subpart J of Regulation 5 stipulates that only approved hospitals may bill for ESRD services. Hence, to allow hospitals to bill and be reimbursed for inpatient dialysis services furnished under arrangements, both facilities participating in the arrangement must meet the conditions of 405.2120 and 405.2160 of Subpart U of Regulation 5. In order for renal dialysis facilities to have a written arrangement with each other to provide inpatient dialysis care both facilities must meet the minimum utilization rate requirement, i.e., two dialysis stations with a performance capacity of at least four dialysis treatments per week.

Dialysis may be billed by an SNF as a service if: (a) it is provided by a hospital with which the facility has a transfer agreement in effect, and that hospital is approved to provide staff-assisted dialysis for the Medicare program; or (b) it is furnished directly by an SNF meeting all nonhospital maintenance dialysis facility requirements, including minimum utilization requirements. (See 1861(h)(6), 1861(h)(7), title XVIII.)

100-04, 4, 20.6.12

Use of HCPCS Modifier – CT

(Rev. 3425, Issued: 12-18-15, Effective: 01-01-16, Implementation: 01-04-16)

Effective January 1, 2016, the definition of modifier – CT is "Computed tomography services furnished using equipment that does not meet each of the attributes of the National Electrical Manufacturers Association (NEMA) XR-29-2013 standard." This modifier is required to be reported on claims for computed tomography (CT) scans described by applicable HCPCS codes that are furnished on non-NEMA Standard XR-29-2013-compliant equipment. The applicable CT services are identified by HCPCS codes 70450 through 70498; 71250 through 71275; 72125 through 72133; 72191 through 72194; 73200 through 73206; 73700 through 73706; 74150 through 74178; 74261 through 74263; and 75571 through 75574 (and any succeeding codes).

This modifier should not be reported with codes that describe CT scans not listed above.

100-04, 4, 160

Clinic and Emergency Visits

CMS has acknowledged from the beginning of the OPPS that CMS believes that CPT Evaluation and Management (E/M) codes were designed to reflect the activities of physicians and do not describe well the range and mix of services provided by hospitals during visits of clinic and emergency department patients. While awaiting the development of a national set of facility-specific codes and guidelines, providers should continue to apply their current internal guidelines to the existing CPT codes. Each hospital's internal guidelines should follow the intent of the CPT code descriptors, in that the guidelines should be designed to reasonably relate the intensity of hospital resources to the different levels of effort represented by the codes. Hospitals should ensure that their guidelines accurately reflect resource distinctions between the five levels of codes.

Effective January 1, 2007, CMS is distinguishing between two types of emergency departments: Type A emergency departments and Type B emergency departments.

A Type A emergency department is defined as an emergency department that is available 24 hours a day, 7 days a week and is either licensed by the State in which it is located under applicable State law as an emergency room or emergency department or it is held out to the public (by name, posted signs, advertising, or other means) as a place that provides care for emergency medical conditions on an urgent basis without requiring a previously scheduled appointment.

A Type B emergency department is defined as an emergency department that meets the definition of a "dedicated emergency department" as defined in 42 CFR 489.24 under the EMTALA regulations. It must meet at least one of the following requirements: (1) It is licensed by the State in which it is located under applicable State law as an emergency room or emergency department; (2) It is held out to the public (by name, posted signs, advertising, or other means) as a place that provides care for emergency medical conditions on an urgent basis without requiring a previously scheduled appointment; or (3) During the calendar year immediately preceding the calendar year in which a determination under 42 CFR 489.24 is being made, based on a representative sample of patient visits that occurred during that calendar year, it provides at least one-third of all of its outpatient visits for the treatment of emergency medical conditions on an urgent basis without requiring a previously scheduled appointment.

Hospitals must bill for visits provided in Type A emergency departments using CPT emergency department E/M codes. Hospitals must bill for visits provided in Type B emergency departments using the G-codes that describe visits provided in Type B emergency departments.

Hospitals that will be billing the new Type B ED visit codes may need to update their internal guidelines to report these codes.

Emergency department and clinic visits are paid in some cases separately and in other cases as part of a composite APC payment. See section 10.2.1 of this chapter for further details.

100-04, 4, 200.1

Billing for Corneal Tissue

(Rev. 3425, Issued: 12-18-15, Effective: 01-01-16, Implementation: 01-04-16)

Corneal tissue will be paid on a cost basis, not under OPPS, only when it is used in a corneal transplant procedure described by one of the following CPT codes: 65710, 65730, 65750, 65755, 65756, 65765, 65767, and any successor code or new code describing a new type of corneal transplant procedure that uses eye banked corneal tissue. In all other procedures cornea tissue is packaged. To receive cost based reimbursement hospitals must bill charges for corneal tissue using HCPCS code V2785.

100-04, 4, 200.3.1

Billing Instructions for IMRT Planning and Delivery

(Rev. 3557, Issued; 07-01-16; Effective: 07-01-16; Implementation: 07-05-16)

Payment for the services identified by CPT codes 77014, 77280, 77285, 77290, 77295, 77306 through 77321, 77331, and 77370 are included in the APC payment for CPT code 77301 (IMRT planning). These codes should not be reported in addition to CPT code 77301 when provided prior to or as part of the development of the IMRT plan.

100-04, 4, 200.3.2

Billing for Multi-Source Photon (Cobalt 60-Based) Stereotactic Radiosurgery (SRS) Planning and Delivery

(Rev. 3741, Issued: 02-26-16, Effective: 04-01-16, Implementation: 04-04-16)

Effective for services furnished on or after January 1, 2014, hospitals must report SRS planning and delivery services using only the CPT codes that accurately describe the service furnished. For the delivery services, hospitals must report CPT code 77371, 77372, or 77373.

CPT Code	Long Descriptor
77371	Radiation treatment delivery, stereotactic radiosurgery (srs), complete course of treatment of cranial lesion(s) consisting of 1 session; multi-source cobalt 60 based
77372	Radiation treatment delivery, stereotactic radiosurgery (srs), complete course of treatment of cranial lesion(s) consisting of 1 session; linear accelerator based
77373	Stereotactic body radiation therapy, treatment delivery, per fraction to 1 or more lesions, including image guidance, entire course not to exceed 5 fractions

As instructed in the CY 2014 OPPS/ASC final rule, CPT code 77371 is to be used only for single session cranial SRS cases performed with a Cobalt-60 device, and CPT code 77372 is to be used only for single session cranial SRS cases performed with a linac-based device. The term "cranial" means that the pathological lesion(s) that are the target of the radiation is located in the patient's cranium or head. The term "single session" means that the entire intracranial lesion(s) that comprise the patient's diagnosis are treated in their entirety during a single treatment session on a single day. CPT code 77372 is never to be used for the first fraction or any other fraction of a fractionated SRS treatment. CPT code 77372 is to be used only for single session cranial linac-based SRS treatment. Fractionated SRS treatment is any SRS delivery service requiring more than a single session of SRS treatment for a cranial lesion, up to a total of no more than five fractions, and one to five sessions (but no more than five) for non-cranial lesions. CPT code 77373 is to be used for any fraction (including the first fraction) in any series of fractionated treatments, regardless of the anatomical location of the lesion or lesions being radiated. Fractionated cranial SRS is any cranial SRS that exceeds one treatment session and fractionated non-cranial SRS is any non-cranial SRS, regardless of the number of fractions but never more than five. Therefore, CPT code 77373 is the exclusive code (and the use of no other SRS treatment delivery code is permitted) for any and all fractionated SRS treatment services delivered anywhere in the body, including, but not limited to, the cranium or head. 77372 is not to be used for the first fraction of a fractionated cranial SRS treatment series and must only be used in cranial SRS when there is a single treatment session to treat the patient's entire condition.

In addition, for the planning services, hospitals must report the specific CPT code that accurately describes the service provided. The planning services may include but are not limited to CPT code 77290, 77295, 77300, 77334, or 77370.

CPT Code	Long Descriptor
77290	Therapeutic radiology simulation-aided field setting; complex
77295	Therapeutic radiology simulation-aided field setting; 3-dimensional
77300	Basic radiation dosimetry calculation, central axis depth dose calculation, tdf, nsd, gap calculation, off axis factor, tissue inhomogeneity factors, calculation of non-ionizing radiation surface and depth dose, as required during course of treatment, only when prescribed by the treating physician
77334	Treatment devices, design and construction; complex (irregular blocks, special shields, compensators, wedges, molds or casts)
77370	Special medical radiation physics consultation

Effective for cranial single session stereotactic radiosurgery procedures (CPT code 77371 or 77372) furnished on or after January 1, 2016 until December 31, 2017, costs for certain adjunctive services (e.g., planning and preparation) are not factored into the APC payment rate for APC 5627 (Level 7 Radiation Therapy). Rather, the ten planning and preparation codes listed in table below, will be paid according to their assigned status indicator when furnished 30 days prior or 30 days post SRS treatment delivery.

In addition, hospitals must report modifier "CP" (Adjunctive service related to a procedure assigned to a comprehensive ambulatory payment classification [C-APC] procedure) on TOB 13X claims for any other services (excluding the ten codes in table below) that are adjunctive or related to SRS treatment but billed on a different claim and within either 30 days prior or 30 days after the date of service for either CPT code 77371 (Radiation treatment delivery, stereotactic radiosurgery, complete course of treatment cranial lesion(s) consisting of 1 session; multi-source Cobalt 60-based) or CPT code 77372 (Linear accelerator based). The "CP" modifier need not be reported with the ten planning and preparation CPT codes table below. Adjunctive/related services include but are not necessarily limited to imaging, clinical treatment planning/preparation, and consultations. Any service related to the SRS delivery should have the CP modifier appended. We would not expect the "CP" modifier to be

reported with services such as chemotherapy administration as this is considered to be a distinct service that is not directly adjunctive, integral, or dependent on delivery of SRS treatment.

Excluded Planning and Preparation CPT Codes

CPT Code	CY 2016 Short Descriptor	CY 2016 Status Indicator
70551	Mri brain stem w/o dye	Q3
70552	Mri brain stem w/dye	Q3
70553	Mri brain stem w/o & w/dye	Q3
77011	Ct scan for localization	N
77014	Ct scan for therapy guide	N
77280	Set radiation therapy field	S
77285	Set radiation therapy field	S
77290	Set radiation therapy field	S
77295	3-d radiotherapy plan	S
77336	Radiation physics consult	S

100-04, 4, 231.10

Billing for Autologous Stem Cell Transplants

(Rev.3556, Issued: 07-01-2016; Effective: 1-27-16; Implementation: 10-3-16)

The hospital bills and shows all charges for autologous stem cell harvesting, processing, and transplant procedures based on the status of the patient (i.e., inpatient or outpatient) when the services are furnished. It shows charges for the actual transplant, described by the appropriate ICD procedure or CPT codes in Revenue Center 0362 (Operating Room Services; Organ Transplant, Other than Kidney) or another appropriate cost center.

The CPT codes describing autologous stem cell harvesting procedures may be billed and are separately payable under the Outpatient Prospective Payment System (OPPS) when provided in the hospital outpatient setting of care. Autologous harvesting procedures are distinct from the acquisition services described in Pub. 100-04, Chapter 3, §90.3.1 and §231.11 of this chapter for allogeneic stem cell transplants, which include services provided when stem cells are obtained from a donor and not from the patient undergoing the stem cell transplant.

The CPT codes describing autologous stem cell processing procedures also may be billed and are separately payable under the OPPS when provided to hospital outpatients.

100-04, 4, 231.11

Billing for Allogeneic Stem Cell Transplants

(Rev.3556, Issued: 07-01-2016; Effective: 1-27-16; Implementation: 10-3-16)

1. Definition of Acquisition Charges for Allogeneic Stem Cell Transplants

Acquisition charges for allogeneic stem cell transplants include, but are not limited to, charges for the costs of the following services:

- National Marrow Donor Program fees, if applicable, for stem cells from an unrelated donor;
- Tissue typing of donor and recipient;
- Donor evaluation;
- Physician pre-procedure donor evaluation services;
- Costs associated with harvesting procedure (e.g., general routine and special care services, procedure/operating room and other ancillary services, apheresis services, etc.);
- Post-operative/post-procedure evaluation of donor; and
- Preparation and processing of stem cells.

Payment for these acquisition services is included in the OPPS APC payment for the allogeneic stem cell transplant when the transplant occurs in the hospital outpatient setting, and in the MS-DRG payment for the allogeneic stem cell transplant when the transplant occurs in the inpatient setting. The Medicare contractor does not make separate payment for these acquisition services, because hospitals may bill and receive payment only for services provided to the Medicare beneficiary who is the recipient of the stem cell transplant and whose illness is being treated with the stem cell transplant. Unlike the acquisition costs of solid organs for transplant (e.g., hearts and kidneys), which are paid on a reasonable cost basis, acquisition costs for allogeneic stem cells are included in prospective payment. Recurring update notifications describing changes to and billing instructions for various payment policies implemented in the OPPS are issues annually.

Acquisition charges for stem cell transplants apply only to allogeneic transplants, for which stem cells are obtained from a donor (other than the recipient himself or herself). Acquisition charges do not apply to autologous transplants (transplanted stem cells are obtained from the recipient himself or herself), because autologous transplants involve services provided to the beneficiary only (and not to a donor), for which the hospital may bill and receive payment (see Pub. 100-04, chapter 3, §90.3.1 and §231.10 of this chapter for information regarding billing for autologous stem cell transplants).

2. Billing for Acquisition Services

The hospital bills and shows acquisition charges for allogeneic stem cell transplants based on the status of the patient (i.e., inpatient or outpatient) when the transplant is furnished. See Pub. 100-04, chapter 3, §90.3.1 for instructions regarding billing for acquisition services for allogeneic stem cell transplants that are performed in the inpatient setting.

When the allogeneic stem cell transplant occurs in the outpatient setting, the hospital identifies stem cell acquisition charges for allogeneic bone marrow/stem cell transplants separately in FL 42 of Form CMS-1450 (or electronic equivalent) by using revenue code 0819 (Other Organ Acquisition). Revenue code 0819 charges should include all services required to acquire stem cells from a donor, as defined above, and should be reported on the same date of service as the transplant procedure in order to be appropriately packaged for payment purposes.

The transplant hospital keeps an itemized statement that identifies the services furnished, the charges, the person receiving the service (donor/recipient), and whether this is a potential transplant donor or recipient. These charges will be reflected in the transplant hospital's stem cell/bone marrow acquisition cost center. For allogeneic stem cell acquisition services in cases that do not result in transplant, due to death of the intended recipient or other causes, hospitals include the costs associated with the acquisition services on the Medicare cost report.

In the case of an allogeneic transplant in the hospital outpatient setting, the hospital reports the transplant itself with the appropriate CPT code, and a charge under revenue center code 0362 or another appropriate cost center. Selection of the cost center is up to the hospital.

100-04, 4, 250.16

Multiple Procedure Payment Reduction (MPPR) on Certain Diagnostic Imaging Procedures Rendered by Physicians

(Rev. 3578, Issued: 08-05 Effective: 01-01-17, Implementation: 01-03-17)

Diagnostic imaging procedures rendered by a physician that has reassigned their billing rights to a Method II CAH are payable by Medicare when the procedures are eligible and billed on type of bill 85x with revenue code (RC) 096x, 097x and/or 098x.

The MPPR on diagnostic imaging applies when multiple services are furnished by the same physician to the same patient in the same session on the same day. Full payment is made for each service with the highest payment under the MPFS. Effective for dates of services on or after January 1, 2012, payment is made at 75 percent for each subsequent service; and effective for dates of services on or after January 1, 2017, payment is made at 95 percent for each subsequent service.

100-04, 4, 290.5.3

Billing and Payment for Observation Services Furnished Beginning January 1, 2016

(Rev. 3425, Issued: 12-18-15, Effective: 01-01-16, Implementation: 01-04-16)

Observation services are reported using HCPCS code G0378 (Hospital observation service, per hour). Beginning January 1, 2008, HCPCS code G0378 for hourly observation services is assigned status indicator N, signifying that its payment is always packaged. No separate payment is made for observation services reported with HCPCS code G0378, and APC 0339 is deleted as of January 1, 2008. In most circumstances, observation services are supportive and ancillary to the other services provided to a patient. Beginning January 1, 2016, in certain circumstances when observation services are billed in conjunction with a clinic visit, Type A emergency department visit (Level 1 through 5), Type B emergency department visit (Level 1 through 5), critical care services, or a direct referral as an integral part of a patient's extended encounter of care, comprehensive payment may be made for all services on the claim including, the entire extended care encounter through comprehensive APC 8011 (Comprehensive Observation Services) when certain criteria are met. For information about comprehensive APCs, see §10.2.3 (Comprehensive APCs) of this chapter.

There is no limitation on diagnosis for payment of APC 8011; however, comprehensive APC payment will not be made when observation services are reported in association with a surgical procedure (T status procedure) or the hours of observation care reported are less than 8. The I/OCE evaluates every claim received to determine if payment through a comprehensive APC is appropriate. If payment through a comprehensive APC is inappropriate, the I/OCE, in conjunction with the Pricer, determines the appropriate status indicator, APC, and payment for every code on a claim.

All of the following requirements must be met in order for a hospital to receive a comprehensive APC payment through the Comprehensive Observation Services APC (APC 8011):

1. Observation Time

a. Observation time must be documented in the medical record.

b. Hospital billing for observation services begins at the clock time documented in the patient's medical record, which coincides with the time that observation services are initiated in accordance with a physician's order for observation services.

c. A beneficiary's time receiving observation services (and hospital billing) ends when all clinical or medical interventions have been completed, including follow-up care furnished by hospital staff and physicians that may take place

after a physician has ordered the patient be released or admitted as an inpatient.

d. The number of units reported with HCPCS code G0378 must equal or exceed 8 hours.

2. Additional Hospital Services

a. The claim for observation services must include one of the following services in addition to the reported observation services. The additional services listed below must have a line item date of service on the same day or the day before the date reported for observation:

- A Type A or B emergency department visit (CPT codes 99281 through 99285 or HCPCS codes G0380 through G0384); or

- A clinic visit (HCPCS code G0463); or

- Critical care (CPT code 99291); or

- Direct referral for observation care reported with HCPCS code G0379 (APC 5013) must be reported on the same date of service as the date reported for observation services.

b. No procedure with a T status indicator or a J1 status indicator can be reported on the claim.

3. Physician Evaluation

a. The beneficiary must be in the care of a physician during the period of observation, as documented in the medical record by outpatient registration, discharge, and other appropriate progress notes that are timed, written, and signed by the physician.

b. The medical record must include documentation that the physician explicitly assessed patient risk to determine that the beneficiary would benefit from observation care.

Criteria 1 and 3 related to observation care beginning and ending time and physician evaluation apply regardless of whether the hospital believes that the criteria will be met for payment of the extended encounter through the Comprehensive Observation Services APC (APC 8011).

Only visits, critical care and observation services that are billed on a 13X bill type may be considered for a comprehensive APC payment through the Comprehensive Observation Services APC (APC 8011).

Non-repetitive services provided on the same day as either direct referral for observation care or observation services must be reported on the same claim because the OCE claim-by-claim logic cannot function properly unless all services related to the episode of observation care, including hospital clinic visits, emergency department visits, critical care services, and T status procedures, are reported on the same claim. Additional guidance can be found in chapter 1, section 50.2.2 of this manual.

If a claim for services provided during an extended assessment and management encounter including observation care does not meet all of the requirements listed above, then the usual APC logic will apply to separately payable items and services on the claim; the special logic for direct admission will apply, and payment for the observation care will be packaged into payments for other separately payable services provided to the beneficiary in the same encounter.

100-04, 5, 10

Part B Outpatient Rehabilitation and Comprehensive Outpatient Rehabilitation Facility (CORF) Services - General

(Rev. 3454, Issued: 02-04-16, Effective: 07-01-16, Implementation: 07-05-16)

Language in this section is defined or described in Pub. 100-02, chapter 15, sections 220 and 230.

Section §1834(k)(5) to the Social Security Act (the Act), requires that all claims for outpatient rehabilitation services and comprehensive outpatient rehabilitation facility (CORF) services, be reported using a uniform coding system. The CMS chose HCPCS (Healthcare Common Procedure Coding System) as the coding system to be used for the reporting of these services. This coding requirement is effective for all claims for outpatient rehabilitation services and CORF services submitted on or after April 1, 1998.

The Act also requires payment under a prospective payment system for outpatient rehabilitation services including CORF services. Effective for claims with dates of service on or after January 1, 1999, the Medicare Physician Fee Schedule (MPFS) became the method of payment for outpatient therapy services furnished by:

- Comprehensive outpatient rehabilitation facilities (CORFs);

- Outpatient physical therapy providers (OPTs), also known as rehabilitation agencies;

- Hospitals (to outpatients and inpatients who are not in a covered Part A stay);

- Skilled nursing facilities (SNFs) (to residents not in a covered Part A stay and to nonresidents who receive outpatient rehabilitation services from the SNF); and

- Home health agencies (HHAs) (to individuals who are not homebound or otherwise are not receiving services under a home health plan of care (POC)).

NOTE: No provider or supplier other than the SNF will be paid for therapy services during the time the beneficiary is in a covered SNF Part A stay. For information regarding SNF consolidated billing see chapter 6, section 10 of this manual.

Similarly, under the HH prospective payment system, HHAs are responsible to provide, either directly or under arrangements, all outpatient rehabilitation therapy services to beneficiaries receiving services under a home health POC. No other provider or supplier will be paid for these services during the time the beneficiary is in a covered Part A stay. For information regarding HH consolidated billing see chapter10, section 20 of this manual.

Section 143 of the Medicare Improvements for Patients and Provider's Act of 2008 (MIPPA) authorizes the Centers for Medicare & Medicaid Services (CMS) to enroll speech-language pathologists (SLP) as suppliers of Medicare services and for SLPs to begin billing Medicare for outpatient speech-language pathology services furnished in private practice beginning July 1, 2009. Enrollment will allow SLPs in private practice to bill Medicare and receive direct payment for their services. Previously, the Medicare program could only pay SLP services if an institution, physician or nonphysician practitioner billed them.

In Chapter 23, as part of the CY 2009 Medicare Physician Fee Schedule Database, the descriptor for PC/TC indicator "7", as applied to certain HCPCS/CPT codes, is described as specific to the services of privately practicing therapists. Payment may not be made if the service is provided to either a hospital outpatient or a hospital inpatient by a physical therapist, occupational therapist, or speech-language pathologist in private practice.

The MPFS is used as a method of payment for outpatient rehabilitation services furnished under arrangement with any of these providers.

In addition, the MPFS is used as the payment system for CORF services identified by the HCPCS codes in §20. Assignment is mandatory.

Services that are paid subject to the MPFS are adjusted based on the applicable payment locality. Rehabilitation agencies and CORFs with service locations in different payment localities shall follow the instructions for multiple service locations in chapter 1, section 170.1.1.

The Medicare allowed charge for the services is the lower of the actual charge or the MPFS amount. The Medicare payment for the services is 80 percent of the allowed charge after the Part B deductible is met. Coinsurance is made at 20 percent of the lower of the actual charge or the MPFS amount. The general coinsurance rule (20 percent of the actual charges) does not apply when making payment under the MPFS. This is a final payment.

The MPFS does not apply to outpatient rehabilitation services furnished by critical access hospitals (CAHs) or hospitals in Maryland. CAHs are to be paid on a reasonable cost basis. Maryland hospitals are paid under the Maryland All-Payer Model.

Contractors process outpatient rehabilitation claims from hospitals, including CAHs, SNFs, HHAs, CORFs, outpatient rehabilitation agencies, and outpatient physical therapy providers for which they have received a tie in notice from the Regional Office (RO). These provider types submit their claims to the contractors using the ASC X12 837 institutional claim format or the CMS-1450 paper form when permissible. Contractors also process claims from physicians, certain nonphysician practitioners (NPPs), therapists in private practices (TPPs), (which are limited to physical and occupational therapists, and speech-language pathologists in private practices), and physician-directed clinics that bill for services furnished incident to a physician's service (see Pub. 100-02, Medicare Benefit Policy Manual, chapter 15, for a definition of "incident to"). These provider types submit their claims to the contractor using the ASC X 12 837 professional claim format or the CMS-1500 paper form when permissible.

There are different fee rates for nonfacility and facility services. Chapter 23 describes the differences in these two rates. (See fields 28 and 29 of the record therein described). Facility rates apply to professional services performed in a facility other than the professional's office. Nonfacility rates apply when the service is performed in the professional's office. The nonfacility rate (that is paid when the provider performs the services in its own facility) accommodates overhead and indirect expenses the provider incurs by operating its own facility. Thus it is somewhat higher than the facility rate.

Contractors pay the nonfacility rate on institutional claims for services performed in the provider's facility. Contractors may pay professional claims using the facility or nonfacility rate depending upon where the service is performed (place of service on the claim), and the provider specialty.

Contractors pay the codes in §20 under the MPFS on professional claims regardless of whether they may be considered rehabilitation services. However, contractors must use this list for institutional claims to determine whether to pay under outpatient rehabilitation rules or whether payment rules for other types of service may apply, e.g., OPPS for hospitals, reasonable costs for CAHs.

Note that because a service is considered an outpatient rehabilitation service does not automatically imply payment for that service. Additional criteria, including coverage, plan of care and physician certification must also be met. These criteria are described in Pub. 100-02, Medicare Benefit Policy Manual, chapters 1 and 15.

Payment for rehabilitation services provided to Part A inpatients of hospitals or SNFs is included in the respective PPS rate. Also, for SNFs (but not hospitals), if the beneficiary has Part B, but not Part A coverage (e.g., Part A benefits are exhausted), the SNF must bill for any rehabilitation service.

Payment for rehabilitation therapy services provided by home health agencies under a home health plan of care is included in the home health PPS rate. HHAs may submit bill type 34X and be paid under the MPFS if there are no home health services billed under a home health plan of care at the same time, and there is a valid rehabilitation POC (e.g., the patient is not homebound).

An institutional employer (other than a SNF) of the TPPs, or physician performing outpatient services, (e.g., hospital, CORF, etc.), or a clinic billing on behalf of the physician or therapist may bill the contractor on a professional claim.

The MPFS is the basis of payment for outpatient rehabilitation services furnished by TPPs, physicians, and certain nonphysician practitioners or for diagnostic tests provided incident to the services of such physicians or nonphysician practitioners. (See Pub. 100-02, Medicare Benefit Policy Manual, Chapter 15, for a definition of "incident to, therapist, therapy and related instructions.") Such services are billed to the contractor on the professional claim format. Assignment is mandatory.

The following table identifies the provider and supplier types, and identifies which claim format they may use to submit claims for outpatient therapy services to the contractor.

"Provider/Supplier Service" Type	Format	Bill Type	Comment
Inpatient SNF Part A	Institutional	21X	Included in PPS
Inpatient hospital Part B	Institutional	12X	Hospital may obtain services under arrangements and bill, or rendering provider may bill.
Inpatient SNF Part B (audiology tests are not included)	Institutional	22X	SNF must provide and bill, or obtain under arrangements and bill.
Outpatient hospital	Institutional	13X	Hospital may provide and bill or obtain under arrangements and bill.
Outpatient SNF	Institutional	23X	SNF must provide and bill or obtain under arrangements and bill.
HHA billing for services not rendered under a Part A or Part B home health plan of care, but rendered under a therapy plan of care.	Institutional	34X	Service not under home health plan of care.
Outpatient physical therapy providers (OPTs), also known as rehabilitation agencies	Institutional	74X	Paid MPFS for outpatient rehabilitation services.
Comprehensive Outpatient Rehabilitation Facility (CORF)	Institutional	75X	Paid MPFS for outpatient rehabilitation services and all other services except drugs. Drugs are paid 95% of the AWP.
Physician, NPPs, TPPs, (therapy services in hospital or SNF)	Professional	See Chapter 26 for place of service coding.	Payment may not be made for therapy services to Part A inpatients of hospitals or SNFs, or for Part B SNF residents. NOTE: Payment may be made to physicians and NPPs for their professional services defined as "sometimes therapy" (not part of a therapy plan) in certain situations; for example, when furnished to a beneficiary registered as an outpatient of a hospital.
Physician/NPP/TPPs office, or patient's home	Professional	See Chapter 26 for place of service coding.	Paid via MPFS.
Critical Access Hospital - inpatient Part B	Institutional	12X	Rehabilitation services are paid at cost.
Critical Access Hospital – outpatient Part B	Institutional	85X	Rehabilitation services are paid at cost.

For a list of the outpatient rehabilitation HCPCS codes see §20.

If a contractor receives an institutional claim for one of these HCPCS codes with dates of service on or after July 1, 2003, that does not appear on the supplemental file it currently uses to pay the therapy claims, it contacts its professional claims area to obtain the non-facility price in order to pay the claim.

NOTE: The list of codes in §20 contains commonly utilized codes for outpatient rehabilitation services. Contractors may consider other codes on institutional claims for payment under the MPFS as outpatient rehabilitation services to the extent that such codes are determined to be medically reasonable and necessary and could be performed within the scope of practice of the therapist providing the service.

100-04, 8, 140.1

Payment for ESRD-Related Services Under the Monthly Capitation Payment (Center Based Patients)

Physicians and practitioners managing center based patients on dialysis are paid a monthly rate for most outpatient dialysis-related physician services furnished to a Medicare ESRD beneficiary. The payment amount varies based on the number of visits provided within each month and the age of the ESRD beneficiary. Under this methodology, separate codes are billed for providing one visit per month, two to three visits per month and four or more visits per month. The lowest payment amount applies when a physician provides one visit per month; a higher payment is provided for two to three visits per month. To receive the highest payment amount, a physician or practitioner would have to provide at least four ESRD-related visits per month. The MCP is reported once per month for services performed in an outpatient setting that are related to the patients' ESRD.

The physician or practitioner who provides the complete assessment, establishes the patient's plan of care, and provides the ongoing management is the physician or practitioner who submits the bill for the monthly service.

    a. Month defined.

For purposes of billing for physician and practitioner ESRD related services, the term 'month' means a calendar month. The first month the beneficiary begins dialysis treatments is the date the dialysis treatments begin through the end of the calendar month. Thereafter, the term 'month' refers to a calendar month.

    b. Determination of the age of beneficiary.

The beneficiary's age at the end of the month is the age of the patient for determining the appropriate age related ESRD-related services code.

    c. Qualifying Visits Under the MCP

- General policy.

Visits must be furnished face-to-face by a physician, clinical nurse specialist, nurse practitioner, or physician's assistant.

- Visits furnished by another physician or practitioner (who is not the MCP physician or practitioner).

The MCP physician or practitioner may use other physicians or qualified nonphysician practitioners to provide some of the visits during the month. The MCP physician or practitioner does not have to be present when these other physicians or practitioners provide visits. In this instance, the rules are consistent with the requirements for hospital split/shared evaluation and management visits. The non-MCP physician or practitioner must be a partner, an employee of the same group practice, or an employee of the MCP physician or practitioner. For example, the physician or practitioner furnishing visits under the MCP may be either a W-2 employee or 1099 independent contractor.

When another physician is used to furnish some of the visits during the month, the physician who provides the complete assessment, establishes the patient's plan of care, and provides the ongoing management should bill for the MCP service.

If the nonphysician practitioner is the practitioner who performs the complete assessment and establishes the plan of care, then the MCP service should be billed under the PIN of the clinical nurse specialist, nurse practitioner, or physician assistant.

- Residents, interns and fellows.

Patient visits by residents, interns and fellows enrolled in an approved Medicare graduate medical education (GME) program may be counted towards the MCP visits if the teaching MCP physician is present during the visit.

- Patients designated/admitted as hospital observation status.

ESRD-related visits furnished to patients in hospital observation status that occur on or after January 1, 2005, should be counted for purposes of billing the MCP codes. Visits furnished to patients in hospital observation status are included when submitting MCP claims for ESRD-related services.

- ESRD-related visits furnished to beneficiaries residing in a SNF.

ESRD-related visits furnished to beneficiaries residing in a SNF should be counted for purposes of billing the MCP codes.

- SNF residents admitted as an inpatient.

Inpatient visits are not counted for purposes of the MCP service. If the beneficiary residing in a SNF is admitted to the hospital as an inpatient, the appropriate inpatient visit code should be billed.

- ESRD Related Visits as a Telehealth Service

ESRD-related services with 2 or 3 visits per month and ESRD-related services with 4 or more visits per month may be furnished as a telehealth service. However, at least one visit per month is required in person to examine the vascular access site. A clinical examination of the vascular access site must be furnished face-to-face (not as a telehealth service) by a physician, nurse practitioner or physician's assistant. For more information on how ESRD-related visits may be furnished as a Medicare telehealth service and for general Medicare telehealth policy see Pub. 100-2, Medicare Benefit Policy manual, chapter 15, section 270. For claims processing instructions see Pub. 100-4, Medicare Claims Processing manual chapter 12, section 190.

100-04, 8, 140.1.1

Payment for Managing Patients on Home Dialysis

Physicians and practitioners managing ESRD patients who dialyze at home are paid a single monthly rate based on the age of the beneficiary. The MCP physician (or practitioner) must furnish at least one face-to-face patient visit per month for the home dialysis MCP service. Documentation by the MCP physician (or practitioner) should support at least one face-to-face encounter per month with the home dialysis patient. Medicare contractors may waive the requirement for a monthly face-to-face visit for the home dialysis MCP service on a case by case basis, for example, when the nephrologist's notes indicate that the physician actively and adequately managed the care of the home dialysis patient throughout the month. The management of home dialysis patients who remain a home dialysis patient the entire month should be coded using the ESRD-related services for home dialysis patients HCPCS codes.

When another physician is used to furnish some of the visits during the month, the physician who provides the complete assessment, establishes the patient's plan of care, and provides the ongoing management should bill for the MCP service.

If the nonphysician practitioner is the practitioner who performs the complete assessment and establishes the plan of care, then the MCP service should be billed under the PIN of the clinical nurse specialist, nurse practitioner, or physician assistant.

Residents, interns and fellows. Patient visits by residents, interns and fellows enrolled in an approved Medicare graduate medical education (GME) program may be counted towards the MCP visits if the teaching MCP physician is present during the visit.

    a. Month defined.

For purposes of billing for physician and practitioner ESRD related services, the term 'month' means a calendar month. The first month the beneficiary begins dialysis treatments is the date the dialysis treatments begin through the end of the calendar month. Thereafter, the term 'month' refers to a calendar month.

    b. Qualifying Visits under the MCP

- General policy.

Visits must be furnished face-to-face by a physician, clinical nurse specialist, nurse practitioner, or physician's assistant.

- Visits furnished by another physician or practitioner (who is not the MCP physician or practitioner).

The MCP physician or practitioner may use other physicians or qualified nonphysician practitioners to provide the visit(s) during the month. The MCP physician or practitioner does not have to be present when these other physicians or practitioners provide visit(s). The non-MCP physician or practitioner must be a partner, an employee of the same group practice, or an employee of the MCP physician or practitioner. For example, the physician or practitioner furnishing visits under the MCP may be either a W-2 employee or 1099 independent contractor.

When another physician is used to furnish some of the visits during the month, the physician who provides the complete assessment, establishes the patient's plan of care, and provides the ongoing management should bill for the MCP service.

If the nonphysician practitioner is the practitioner who performs the complete assessment and establishes the plan of care, then the MCP service should be billed under the PIN of the clinical nurse specialist, nurse practitioner, or physician assistant.

- Residents, interns and fellows.

Patient visits by residents, interns and fellows enrolled in an approved Medicare graduate medical education (GME) program may be counted towards the MCP visits if the teaching MCP physician is present during the visit.

100-04, 9, 182

Medical Nutrition Therapy (MNT) Services

A - FQHCs

Previously, MNT type services were considered incident to services under the FQHC benefit, if all relevant program requirements were met. Therefore, separate all-inclusive encounter rate payment could not be made for the provision of MNT services. With passage of DRA, effective January 1, 2006, FQHCs are eligible for a separate payment under Part B for these services provided they meet all program requirements. Payment is made at the all-inclusive encounter rate to the FQHC. This payment can be in addition to payment for any other qualifying visit on the same date of service as the beneficiary received qualifying MNT services.

For FQHCs to qualify for a separate visit payment for MNT services, the services must be a one-on-one face-to-face encounter. Group sessions don't constitute a billable visit for any FQHC services. Rather, the cost of group sessions is included in the calculation of the all-inclusive FQHC visit rate. To receive payment for MNT services, the MNT services must be billed on TOB 73X with the appropriate individual MNT HCPCS code (codes 97802, 97803, or G0270) and with the appropriate site of service revenue code in the 052X revenue code series. This payment can be in addition to payment for any other qualifying visit on the same date of service as the beneficiary received qualifying MNT services as long as the claim for MNT services contain the appropriate coding specified above.

NOTE: MNT is not a qualifying visit on the same day that DSMT is provided.

Additional information on MNT can be found in Chapter 4, section 300 of this manual.

Group services (HCPCS 97804 or G0271) do not meet the criteria for a separate qualifying encounter. All line items billed on TOB 73x with HCPCS code 97804 or G0271 will be denied.

B - RHCs

Separate payment to RHCs for these practitioners/services continues to be precluded as these services are not within the scope of Medicare-covered RHC benefits. All line items billed on TOB 71x with HCPCS codes for MNT services will be denied.

100-04, 11, 40.1.3

Independent Attending Physician Services

When hospice coverage is elected, the beneficiary waives all rights to Medicare Part B payments for professional services that are related to the treatment and management of his/her terminal illness during any period his/her hospice benefit election is in force, except for professional services of an independent attending physician, who is not an employee of the designated hospice nor receives compensation from the hospice for those services. For purposes of administering the hospice benefit provisions, an "attending physician" means an individual who:

- Is a doctor of medicine or osteopathy or

- A nurse practitioner (for professional services related to the terminal illness that are furnished on or after December 8, 2003); and

- Is identified by the individual, at the time he/she elects hospice coverage, as having the most significant role in the determination and delivery of their medical care.

Hospices should reiterate with patients that they must not see independent physicians for care related to their terminal illness other than their independent attending physician unless the hospice arranges it.

Even though a beneficiary elects hospice coverage, he/she may designate and use an independent attending physician, who is not employed by nor receives compensation from the hospice for professional services furnished, in addition to the services of hospice-employed physicians. The professional services of an independent attending physician, who may be a nurse practitioner as defined in Chapter 9, that are reasonable and necessary for the treatment and management of a hospice patient's terminal illness are not considered Medicare Part A hospice services.

Where the service is related to the hospice patient's terminal illness but was furnished by someone other than the designated "attending physician" [or a physician substituting for the attending physician]) the physician or other provider must look to the hospice for payment.

Professional services related to the hospice patient's terminal condition that were furnished by an independent attending physician, who may be a nurse practitioner, are billed to the Medicare contractor through Medicare Part B. When the independent attending physician furnishes a terminal illness related service that includes both a professional and technical component (e.g., x-rays), he/she bills the professional component of such services to the Medicare contractor on a professional claim and looks to the hospice for payment for the technical component. Likewise, the independent attending physician, who may be a nurse practitioner, would look to the hospice for payment for terminal illness related services furnished that have no professional component (e.g., clinical lab tests). The remainder of this section explains this in greater detail.

When a Medicare beneficiary elects hospice coverage he/she may designate an attending physician, who may be a nurse practitioner, not employed by the hospice, in addition to receiving care from hospice-employed physicians. The professional services of a non-hospice affiliated attending physician for the treatment and management of a hospice patient's terminal illness are not considered Medicare Part A "hospice services." These independent attending physician services are billed through Medicare Part B to the Medicare contractor, provided they were not furnished under a payment arrangement with the hospice. The independent attending physician codes services with the GV modifier "Attending physician not employed or paid under agreement by the patient's hospice provider" when billing his/her professional services furnished for the treatment and management of a hospice patient's terminal condition. The Medicare contractor makes payment to the independent attending physician or beneficiary, as appropriate, based on the payment and deductible rules applicable to each covered service.

Payments for the services of an independent attending physician are not counted in determining whether the hospice cap amount has been exceeded because Part B services provided by an independent attending physician are not part of the hospice's care.

Services provided by an independent attending physician who may be a nurse practitioner must be coordinated with any direct care services provided by hospice physicians.

Only the direct professional services of an independent attending physician, who may be a nurse practitioner, to a patient may be billed; the costs for services such as lab or x-rays are not to be included in the bill.

If another physician covers for a hospice patient's designated attending physician, the services of the substituting physician are billed by the designated attending physician under the reciprocal or locum tenens billing instructions. In such instances, the attending physician bills using the GV modifier in conjunction with either the Q5 or Q6 modifier.

When services related to a hospice patient's terminal condition are furnished under a payment arrangement with the hospice by the designated attending physician who may be a nurse practitioner (i.e., by a non-independent physician/nurse practitioner), the physician must look to the hospice for payment. In this situation the physicians' services are Part A hospice services and are billed by the hospice to its Medicare contractor.

Medicare contractors must process and pay for covered, medically necessary Part B services that physicians furnish to patients after their hospice benefits are revoked even if the patient remains under the care of the hospice. Such services are billed without the GV or GW modifiers. Make payment based on applicable Medicare payment and deductible rules for each covered service even if the beneficiary continues to be treated by the hospice after hospice benefits are revoked.

The CWF response contains the periods of hospice entitlement. This information is a permanent part of the notice and is furnished on all CWF replies and automatic notices. Medicare contractor use the CWF reply for validating dates of hospice coverage and to research, examine and adjudicate services coded with the GV or GW modifiers.

100-04, 12, 20.4.7

Services That Do Not Meet the National Electrical Manufacturers Association (NEMA) Standard XR-29-2013

(Rev. 3402, Issued: 11-06-15, Effective: 01-01-16, Implementation: 01-04-16)

Section 218(a) of the Protecting Access to Medicare Act of 2014 (PAMA) is titled "Quality Incentives To Promote Patient Safety and Public Health in Computed Tomography Diagnostic Imaging." It amends the Social Security Act (SSA) by reducing payment for the technical component (and the technical component of the global fee) of the Physician Fee Schedule service (5 percent in 2016 and 15 percent in 2017 and subsequent years) for computed tomography (CT) services identified by CPT codes 70450-70498, 71250-71275, 72125-72133, 72191-72194, 73200-73206, 73700-73706,

74150-74178, 74261-74263, and 75571-75574 furnished using equipment that does not meet each of the attributes of the National Electrical Manufacturers Association (NEMA) Standard XR-29-2013, entitled "Standard Attributes on CT Equipment Related to Dose Optimization and Management."

The statutory provision requires that information be provided and attested to by a supplier and a hospital outpatient department that indicates whether an applicable CT service was furnished that was not consistent with the NEMA CT equipment standard, and that such information may be included on a claim and may be a modifier. The statutory provision also provides that such information shall be verified, as appropriate, as part of the periodic accreditation of suppliers under SSA section 1834(e) and hospitals under SSA section 1865(a). Any reduced expenditures resulting from this provision are not budget neutral. To implement this provision, CMS created modifier "CT" (Computed tomography services furnished using equipment that does not meet each of the attributes of the National Electrical Manufacturers Association (NEMA) XR-29-2013 standard).

Beginning in 2016, claims for CT scans described by above-listed CPT codes (and any successor codes) that are furnished on non-NEMA Standard XR-29-2013-compliant CT scans must include modifier "CT" that will result in the applicable payment reduction.

A list of codes subject to the CT modifier will be maintained in the web supporting files for the annual rule.

Beginning January 1, 2016, a payment reduction of 5 percent applies to the technical component (and the technical component of the global fee) for Computed Tomography (CT) services furnished using equipment that is inconsistent with the CT equipment standard and for which payment is made under the physician fee schedule. This payment reduction becomes 15 percent beginning January 1, 2017, and after.

100-04, 12, 30.1

Digestive System

B3-15100

A. Upper Gastrointestinal Endoscopy Including Endoscopic Ultrasound (EUS) (Code 43259)

If the person performing the original diagnostic endoscopy has access to the EUS and the clinical situation requires an EUS, the EUS may be done at the same time. The procedure, diagnostic and EUS, is reported under the same code, CPT 43259. This code conforms to CPT guidelines for the indented codes. The service represented by the indented code, in this case code 43259 for EUS, includes the service represented by the unintended code preceding the list of indented codes. Therefore, when a diagnostic examination of the upper gastrointestinal tract "including esophagus, stomach, and either the duodenum or jejunum as appropriate," includes the use of endoscopic ultrasonography, the service is reported by a single code, namely 43259.

Interpretation, whether by a radiologist or endoscopist, is reported under CPT code 76975-26. These codes may both be reported on the same day.

B. Incomplete Colonoscopies (Codes 45330 and 45378)

An incomplete colonoscopy, e.g., the inability to extend beyond the splenic flexure, is billed and paid using colonoscopy code 45378 with modifier "-53." The Medicare physician fee schedule database has specific values for code 45378-53. These values are the same as for code 45330, sigmoidoscopy, as failure to extend beyond the splenic flexure means that a sigmoidoscopy rather than a colonoscopy has been performed.

However, code 45378-53 should be used when an incomplete colonoscopy has been done because other MPFSDB indicators are different for codes 45378 and 45330.

100-04, 12, 30.6.2

Billing for Medically Necessary Visit on Same Occasion as Preventive Medicine Service

See Chapter 18 for payment for covered preventive services.

When a physician furnishes a Medicare beneficiary a covered visit at the same place and on the same occasion as a noncovered preventive medicine service (CPT codes 99381- 99397), consider the covered visit to be provided in lieu of a part of the preventive medicine service of equal value to the visit. A preventive medicine service (CPT codes 99381-99397) is a noncovered service. The physician may charge the beneficiary, as a charge for the noncovered remainder of the service, the amount by which the physician's current established charge for the preventive medicine service exceeds his/her current established charge for the covered visit. Pay for the covered visit based on the lesser of the fee schedule amount or the physician's actual charge for the visit. The physician is not required to give the beneficiary written advance notice of noncoverage of the part of the visit that constitutes a routine preventive visit. However, the physician is responsible for notifying the patient in advance of his/her liability for the charges for services that are not medically necessary to treat the illness or injury.

There could be covered and noncovered procedures performed during this encounter (e.g., screening x-ray, EKG, lab tests.). These are considered individually. Those procedures which are for screening for asymptomatic conditions are considered noncovered and, therefore, no payment is made. Those procedures ordered to diagnose or monitor a symptom, medical condition, or treatment are evaluated for medical necessity and, if covered, are paid.

100-04, 12, 30.6.4

Evaluation and Management (E/M) Services Furnished Incident to Physician's Service by Nonphysician Practitioners

When evaluation and management services are furnished incident to a physician's service by a nonphysician practitioner, the physician may bill the CPT code that describes the evaluation and management service furnished.

When evaluation and management services are furnished incident to a physician's service by a nonphysician employee of the physician, not as part of a physician service, the physician bills code 99211 for the service.

A physician is not precluded from billing under the "incident to" provision for services provided by employees whose services cannot be paid for directly under the Medicare program. Employees of the physician may provide services incident to the physician's service, but the physician alone is permitted to bill Medicare.

Services provided by employees as "incident to" are covered when they meet all the requirements for incident to and are medically necessary for the individual needs of the patient.

100-04, 12, 30.6.7

Payment for Office or Other Outpatient Evaluation and Management (E/M) Visits

A. Definition of New Patient for Selection of E/M Visit Code

Interpret the phrase "new patient" to mean a patient who has not received any professional services, i.e., E/M service or other face-to-face service (e.g., surgical procedure) from the physician or physician group practice (same physician specialty) within the previous 3 years. For example, if a professional component of a previous procedure is billed in a 3 year time period, e.g., a lab interpretation is billed and no E/M service or other face-to-face service with the patient is performed, then this patient remains a new patient for the initial visit. An interpretation of a diagnostic test, reading an x-ray or EKG etc., in the absence of an E/M service or other face-to-face service with the patient does not affect the designation of a new patient.

B. Office/Outpatient E/M Visits Provided on Same Day for Unrelated Problems

As for all other E/M services except where specifically noted, carriers may not pay two E/M office visits billed by a physician (or physician of the same specialty from the same group practice) for the same beneficiary on the same day unless the physician documents that the visits were for unrelated problems in the office or outpatient setting which could not be provided during the same encounter (e.g., office visit for

blood pressure medication evaluation, followed five hours later by a visit for evaluation of leg pain following an accident).

C. Office/Outpatient or Emergency Department E/M Visit on Day of Admission to Nursing Facility

Carriers may not pay a physician for an emergency department visit or an office visit and a comprehensive nursing facility assessment on the same day. Bundle E/M visits on the same date provided in sites other than the nursing facility into the initial nursing facility care code when performed on the same date as the nursing facility admission by the same physician.

D. Drug Administration Services and E/M Visits Billed on Same Day of Service

Carriers must advise physicians that CPT code 99211 cannot be paid if it is billed with a drug administration service such as a chemotherapy or nonchemotherapy drug infusion code (effective January 1, 2004). This drug administration policy was expanded in the Physician Fee Schedule Final Rule, November 15, 2004, to also include a therapeutic or diagnostic injection code (effective January 1, 2005). Therefore, when a medically necessary, significant and separately identifiable E/M service (which meets a higher complexity level than CPT code 99211) is performed, in addition to one of these drug administration services, the appropriate E/M CPT code should be reported with modifier -25. Documentation should support the level of E/M service billed. For an E/M service provided on the same day, a different diagnosis is not required.

100-04, 12, 30.6.8

Payment for Hospital Observation Services and Observation or Inpatient Care Services (Including Admission and Discharge Services)

A. Who May Bill Observation Care Codes

Observation care is a well-defined set of specific, clinically appropriate services, which include ongoing short term treatment, assessment, and reassessment, that are furnished while a decision is being made regarding whether patients will require further treatment as hospital inpatients or if they are able to be discharged from the hospital. Observation services are commonly ordered for patients who present to the emergency department and who then require a significant period of treatment or monitoring in order to make a decision concerning their admission or discharge.

In only rare and exceptional cases do reasonable and necessary outpatient observation services span more than 48 hours. In the majority of cases, the decision whether to discharge a patient from the hospital following resolution of the reason for the observation care or to admit the patient as an inpatient can be made in less than 48 hours, usually in less than 24 hours.

Contractors pay for initial observation care billed by only the physician who ordered hospital outpatient observation services and was responsible for the patient during his/her observation care. A physician who does not have inpatient admitting privileges but who is authorized to furnish hospital outpatient observation services may bill these codes.

For a physician to bill observation care codes, there must be a medical observation record for the patient which contains dated and timed physician's orders regarding the observation services the patient is to receive, nursing notes, and progress notes prepared by the physician while the patient received observation services. This record must be in addition to any record prepared as a result of an emergency department or outpatient clinic encounter.

Payment for an initial observation care code is for all the care rendered by the ordering physician on the date the patient's observation services began. All other physicians who furnish consultations or additional evaluations or services while the patient is receiving hospital outpatient observation services must bill the appropriate outpatient service codes.

For example, if an internist orders observation services and asks another physician to additionally evaluate the patient, only the internist may bill the initial and subsequent observation care codes. The other physician who evaluates the patient must bill the new or established office or other outpatient visit codes as appropriate.

For information regarding hospital billing of observation services, see Chapter 4, §290.

B. Physician Billing for Observation Care Following Initiation of Observation Services

Similar to initial observation codes, payment for a subsequent observation care code is for all the care rendered by the treating physician on the day(s) other than the initial or discharge date. All other physicians who furnish consultations or additional evaluations or services while the patient is receiving hospital outpatient observation services must bill the appropriate outpatient service codes.

When a patient receives observation care for less than 8 hours on the same calendar date, the Initial Observation Care, from CPT code range 99218 – 99220, shall be reported by the physician. The Observation Care Discharge Service, CPT code 99217, shall not be reported for this scenario.

When a patient is admitted for observation care and then is discharged on a different calendar date, the physician shall report Initial Observation Care, from CPT code range 99218 – 99220, and CPT observation care discharge CPT code 99217. On the rare occasion when a patient remains in observation care for 3 days, the physician shall report an initial observation care code (99218-99220) for the first day of observation care, a subsequent observation care code (99224-99226) for the second day of observation care, and an observation care discharge CPT code 99217 for the observation care on the discharge date. When observation care continues beyond 3 days, the physician shall report a subsequent observation care code (99224-99226) for each day between the first day of observation care and the discharge date.

When a patient receives observation care for a minimum of 8 hours, but less than 24 hours, and is discharged on the same calendar date, Observation or Inpatient Care Services (Including Admission and Discharge Services) from CPT code range 99234 – 99236 shall be reported. The observation discharge, CPT code 99217, cannot also be reported for this scenario.

C. Documentation Requirements for Billing Observation or Inpatient Care Services (Including Admission and Discharge Services)
The physician shall satisfy the E/M documentation guidelines for furnishing observation care or inpatient hospital care. In addition to meeting the documentation requirements for history, examination, and medical decision making, documentation in the medical record shall include:

- Documentation stating the stay for observation care or inpatient hospital care involves 8 hours, but less than 24 hours;
- Documentation identifying the billing physician was present and personally performed the services; and
- Documentation identifying the order for observation services, progress notes, and discharge notes were written by the billing physician.

In the rare circumstance when a patient receives observation services for more than 2 calendar dates, the physician shall bill observation services furnished on day(s) other than the initial or discharge date using subsequent observation care codes. The physician may not use the subsequent hospital care codes since the patient is not an inpatient of the hospital.

D. Admission to Inpatient Status Following Observation Care
If the same physician who ordered hospital outpatient observation services also admits the patient to inpatient status before the end of the date on which the patient began receiving hospital outpatient observation services, pay only an initial hospital visit for the evaluation and management services provided on that date. Medicare payment for the initial hospital visit includes all services provided to the patient on the date of admission by that physician, regardless of the site of service. The physician may not bill an initial or subsequent observation care code for services on the date that he or she admits the patient to inpatient status. If the patient is admitted to inpatient status from hospital outpatient observation care subsequent to the date of initiation of observation services, the physician must bill an initial hospital visit for the services provided on that date. The physician may not bill the hospital observation discharge management code (code 99217) or an outpatient/office visit for the care provided while the patient received hospital outpatient observation services on the date of admission to inpatient status.

E. Hospital Observation Services During Global Surgical Period
The global surgical fee includes payment for hospital observation (codes 99217, 99218, 99219, 99220, 99224, 99225, 99226, 99234, 99235, and 99236) services unless the criteria for use of CPT modifiers "-24," "-25," or "-57" are met. Contractors must pay for these services in addition to the global surgical fee only if both of the following requirements are met:

- The hospital observation service meets the criteria needed to justify billing it with CPT modifiers "-24," "-25," or "-57" (decision for major surgery); and
- The hospital observation service furnished by the surgeon meets all of the criteria for the hospital observation code billed.

Examples of the decision for surgery during a hospital observation period are:

- An emergency department physician orders hospital outpatient observation services for a patient with a head injury. A neurosurgeon is called in to evaluate the need for surgery while the patient is receiving observation services and decides that the patient requires surgery. The surgeon would bill a new or established office or other outpatient visit code as appropriate with the "-57" modifier to indicate that the decision for surgery was made during the evaluation. The surgeon must bill the office or other outpatient visit code because the patient receiving hospital outpatient observation services is not an inpatient of the hospital. Only the physician who ordered hospital outpatient observation services may bill for observation care.
- A neurosurgeon orders hospital outpatient observation services for a patient with a head injury. During the observation period, the surgeon makes the decision for surgery. The surgeon would bill the appropriate level of hospital observation code with the "-57" modifier to indicate that the decision for surgery was made while the surgeon was providing hospital observation care.

Examples of hospital observation services during the postoperative period of a surgery are:

- A surgeon orders hospital outpatient observation services for a patient with abdominal pain from a kidney stone on the 80th day following a TURP (performed by that surgeon). The surgeon decides that the patient does not require surgery. The surgeon would bill the observation code with CPT modifier "-24" and documentation to support that the observation services are unrelated to the surgery.
- A surgeon orders hospital outpatient observation services for a patient with abdominal pain on the 80th day following a TURP (performed by that surgeon). While the patient is receiving hospital outpatient observation services, the surgeon decides that the patient requires kidney surgery. The surgeon would bill the observation code with HCPCS modifier "-57" to indicate that the decision for

surgery was made while the patient was receiving hospital outpatient observation services. The subsequent surgical procedure would be reported with modifier "-79."

- A surgeon orders hospital outpatient observation services for a patient with abdominal pain on the 20th day following a resection of the colon (performed by that surgeon). The surgeon determines that the patient requires no further colon surgery and discharges the patient. The surgeon may not bill for the observation services furnished during the global period because they were related to the previous surgery.

An example of a billable hospital observation service on the same day as a procedure is when a physician repairs a laceration of the scalp in the emergency department for a patient with a head injury and then subsequently orders hospital outpatient observation services for that patient. The physician would bill the observation code with a CPT modifier 25 and the procedure code.

100-04, 12, 30.6.9
Payment for Inpatient Hospital Visits - General

A. Hospital Visit and Critical Care on Same Day
When a hospital inpatient or office/outpatient evaluation and management service (E/M) are furnished on a calendar date at which time the patient does not require critical care and the patient subsequently requires critical care both the critical Care Services (CPT codes 99291 and 99292) and the previous E/M service may be paid on the same date of service. Hospital emergency department services are not paid for the same date as critical care services when provided by the same physician to the same patient.

During critical care management of a patient those services that do not meet the level of critical care shall be reported using an inpatient hospital care service with CPT Subsequent Hospital Care using a code from CPT code range 99231 – 99233.

Both Initial Hospital Care (CPT codes 99221 – 99223) and Subsequent Hospital Care codes are "per diem" services and may be reported only once per day by the same physician or physicians of the same specialty from the same group practice.

Physicians and qualified nonphysician practitioners (NPPs) are advised to retain documentation for discretionary contractor review should claims be questioned for both hospital care and critical care claims. The retained documentation shall support claims for critical care when the same physician or physicians of the same specialty in a group practice report critical care services for the same patient on the same calendar date as other E/M services.

B. Two Hospital Visits Same Day
Contractors pay a physician for only one hospital visit per day for the same patient, whether the problems seen during the encounters are related or not. The inpatient hospital visit descriptors contain the phrase "per day" which means that the code and the payment established for the code represent all services provided on that date. The physician should select a code that reflects all services provided during the date of the service.

C. Hospital Visits Same Day But by Different Physicians
In a hospital inpatient situation involving one physician covering for another, if physician A sees the patient in the morning and physician B, who is covering for A, sees the same patient in the evening, contractors do not pay physician B for the second visit. The hospital visit descriptors include the phrase "per day" meaning care for the day.

If the physicians are each responsible for a different aspect of the patient's care, pay both visits if the physicians are in different specialties and the visits are billed with different diagnoses. There are circumstances where concurrent care may be billed by physicians of the same specialty.

D. Visits to Patients in Swing Beds
If the inpatient care is being billed by the hospital as inpatient hospital care, the hospital care codes apply. If the inpatient care is being billed by the hospital as nursing facility care, then the nursing facility codes apply.

100-04, 12, 30.6.9.1
Payment for Initial Hospital Care Services and Observation or Inpatient Care Services (Including Admission and Discharge Services)

A. Initial Hospital Care From Emergency Room
Contractors pay for an initial hospital care service if a physician sees a patient in the emergency room and decides to admit the person to the hospital. They do not pay for both E/M services. Also, they do not pay for an emergency department visit by the same physician on the same date of service. When the patient is admitted to the hospital via another site of service (e.g., hospital emergency department, physician's office, nursing facility), all services provided by the physician in conjunction with that admission are considered part of the initial hospital care when performed on the same date as the admission.

B. Initial Hospital Care on Day Following Visit
Contractors pay both visits if a patient is seen in the office on one date and admitted to the hospital on the next date, even if fewer than 24 hours has elapsed between the visit and the admission.

C. Initial Hospital Care and Discharge on Same Day

When the patient is admitted to inpatient hospital care for less than 8 hours on the same date, then Initial Hospital Care, from CPT code range 99221 – 99223, shall be reported by the physician. The Hospital Discharge Day Management service, CPT codes 99238 or 99239, shall not be reported for this scenario.

When a patient is admitted to inpatient initial hospital care and then discharged on a different calendar date, the physician shall report an Initial Hospital Care from CPT code range 99221 – 99223 and a Hospital Discharge Day Management service, CPT code 99238 or 99239.

When a patient has been admitted to inpatient hospital care for a minimum of 8 hours but less than 24 hours and discharged on the same calendar date, Observation or Inpatient Hospital Care Services (Including Admission and Discharge Services), from CPT code range 99234 – 99236, shall be reported.

D. Documentation Requirements for Billing Observation or Inpatient Care Services (Including Admission and Discharge Services)

The physician shall satisfy the E/M documentation guidelines for admission to and discharge from inpatient observation or hospital care. In addition to meeting the documentation requirements for history, examination and medical decision making documentation in the medical record shall include:

- Documentation stating the stay for hospital treatment or observation care status involves 8 hours but less than 24 hours;
- Documentation identifying the billing physician was present and personally performed the services; and
- Documentation identifying the admission and discharge notes were written by the billing physician.

E. Physician Services Involving Transfer From One Hospital to Another; Transfer Within Facility to Prospective Payment System (PPS) Exempt Unit of Hospital; Transfer From One Facility to Another Separate Entity Under Same Ownership and/or Part of Same Complex; or Transfer From One Department to Another Within Single Facility

Physicians may bill both the hospital discharge management code and an initial hospital care code when the discharge and admission do not occur on the same day if the transfer is between:

- Different hospitals;
- Different facilities under common ownership which do not have merged records; or
- Between the acute care hospital and a PPS exempt unit within the same hospital when there are no merged records.

In all other transfer circumstances, the physician should bill only the appropriate level of subsequent hospital care for the date of transfer.

F. Initial Hospital Care Service History and Physical That Is Less Than Comprehensive

When a physician performs a visit that meets the definition of a Level 5 office visit several days prior to an admission and on the day of admission performs less than a comprehensive history and physical, he or she should report the office visit that reflects the services furnished and also report the lowest level initial hospital care code (i.e., code 99221) for the initial hospital admission. Contractors pay the office visit as billed and the Level 1 initial hospital care code.

Physicians who provide an initial visit to a patient during inpatient hospital care that meets the minimum key component work and/or medical necessity requirements shall report an initial hospital care code (99221-99223). The principal physician of record shall append modifier "-AI" (Principal Physician of Record) to the claim for the initial hospital care code. This modifier will identify the physician who oversees the patient's care from all other physicians who may be furnishing specialty care.

Physicians may bill initial hospital care service codes (99221-99223), for services that were reported with CPT consultation codes (99241 – 99255) prior to January 1, 2010, when the furnished service and documentation meet the minimum key component work and/or medical necessity requirements. Physicians must meet all the requirements of the initial hospital care codes, including "a detailed or comprehensive history" and "a detailed or comprehensive examination" to report CPT code 99221, which are greater than the requirements for consultation codes 99251 and 99252.

Subsequent hospital care CPT codes 99231 and 99232, respectively, require "a problem focused interval history" and "an expanded problem focused interval history." An E/M service that could be described by CPT consultation code 99251 or 99252 could potentially meet the component work and medical necessity requirements to report 99231 or 99232. Physicians may report a subsequent hospital care CPT code for services that were reported as CPT consultation codes (99241 – 99255) prior to January 1, 2010, where the medical record appropriately demonstrates that the work and medical necessity requirements are met for reporting a subsequent hospital care code (under the level selected), even though the reported code is for the provider's first E/M service to the inpatient during the hospital stay.

Reporting CPT code 99499 (Unlisted evaluation and management service) should be limited to cases where there is no other specific E/M code payable by Medicare that describes that service.

Reporting CPT code 99499 requires submission of medical records and contractor manual medical review of the service prior to payment. Contractors shall expect reporting under these circumstances to be unusual.

G. Initial Hospital Care Visits by Two Different M.D.s or D.O.s When They Are Involved in Same Admission

In the inpatient hospital setting all physicians (and qualified nonphysician practitioners where permitted) who perform an initial evaluation may bill the initial hospital care codes (99221 – 99223) or nursing facility care codes (99304 – 99306). Contractors consider only one M.D. or D.O. to be the principal physician of record (sometimes referred to as the admitting physician.) The principal physician of record is identified in Medicare as the physician who oversees the patient's care from other physicians who may be furnishing specialty care. Only the principal physician of record shall append modifier "-AI" (Principal Physician of Record) in addition to the E/M code. Follow-up visits in the facility setting shall be billed as subsequent hospital care visits and subsequent nursing facility care visits.

100-04, 12, 30.6.9.2

Subsequent Hospital Visit and Hospital Discharge Day Management

A. Subsequent Hospital Visits During the Global Surgery Period

(Refer to Secs.40-40.4 on global surgery) The Medicare physician fee schedule payment amount for surgical procedures includes all services (e.g., evaluation and management visits) that are part of the global surgery payment; therefore, contractors shall not pay more than that amount when a bill is fragmented for staged procedures.

B. Hospital Discharge Day Management Service Hospital Discharge Day

Management Services, CPT code 99238 or 99239 is a face-to-face evaluation and management (E/M) service between the attending physician and the patient. The E/M discharge day management visit shall be reported for the date of the actual visit by the physician or qualified nonphysician practitioner even if the patient is discharged from the facility on a different calendar date. Only one hospital discharge day management service is payable per patient per hospital stay.

Only the attending physician of record reports the discharge day management service. Physicians or qualified nonphysician practitioners, other than the attending physician, who have been managing concurrent health care problems not primarily managed by the attending physician, and who are not acting on behalf of the attending physician, shall use Subsequent Hospital Care (CPT code range 99231 - 99233) for a final visit.

Medicare pays for the paperwork of patient discharge day management through the pre- and post- service work of an E/M service.

C. Subsequent Hospital Visit and Discharge Management on Same Day

Pay only the hospital discharge management code on the day of discharge (unless it is also the day of admission, in which case, refer to Sec.30.6.9.1 C for the policy on Observation or Inpatient Care Services (Including Admission and Discharge Services CPT Codes 99234 - 99236). Contractors do not pay both a subsequent hospital visit in addition to hospital discharge day management service on the same day by the same physician. Instruct physicians that they may not bill for both a hospital visit and hospital discharge management for the same date of service.

D. Hospital Discharge Management (CPT Codes 99238 and 99239) and Nursing Facility Admission Code When Patient Is Discharged From Hospital and Admitted to Nursing Facility on Same Day

Contractors pay the hospital discharge code (codes 99238 or 99239) in addition to a nursing facility admission code when they are billed by the same physician with the same date of service.

If a surgeon is admitting the patient to the nursing facility due to a condition that is not as a result of the surgery during the postoperative period of a service with the global surgical period, he/she bills for the nursing facility admission and care with a modifier "-24" and provides documentation that the service is unrelated to the surgery (e.g., return of an elderly patient to the nursing facility in which he/she has resided for five years following discharge from the hospital for cholecystectomy).

Contractors do not pay for a nursing facility admission by a surgeon in the postoperative period of a procedure with a global surgical period if the patient's admission to the nursing facility is to receive post operative care related to the surgery (e.g., admission to a nursing facility to receive physical therapy following a hip replacement). Payment for the nursing facility admission and subsequent nursing facility services are included in the global fee and cannot be paid separately.

E. Hospital Discharge Management and Death Pronouncement

Only the physician who personally performs the pronouncement of death shall bill for the face-to-face Hospital Discharge Day Management Service, CPT code 99238 or 99239. The date of the pronouncement shall reflect the calendar date of service on the day it was performed even if the paperwork is delayed to a subsequent date.

100-04, 12, 30.6.10

Consultation Services

Consultation Services versus Other Evaluation and Management (E/M) Visits

Effective January 1, 2010, the consultation codes are no longer recognized for Medicare Part B payment. Physicians shall code patient evaluation and management visits with E/M codes that represent where the visit occurs and that identify the complexity of the visit performed.

In the inpatient hospital setting and the nursing facility setting, physicians (and qualified nonphysician practitioners where permitted) may bill the most appropriate initial hospital care code (99221-99223), subsequent hospital care code (99231 and

99232), initial nursing facility care code (99304-99306), or subsequent nursing facility care code (99307-99310) that reflects the services the physician or practitioner furnished. Subsequent hospital care codes could potentially meet the component work and medical necessity requirements to be reported for an E/M service that could be described by CPT consultation code 99251 or 99252. Contractors shall not find fault in cases where the medical record appropriately demonstrates that the work and medical necessity requirements are met for reporting a subsequent hospital care code (under the level selected), even though the reported code is for the provider's first E/M service to the inpatient during the hospital stay. Unlisted evaluation and management service (code 99499) shall only be reported for consultation services when an E/M service that could be described by codes 99251 or 99252 is furnished, and there is no other specific E/M code payable by Medicare that describes that service. Reporting code 99499 requires submission of medical records and contractor manual review of the service prior to payment. CMS expects reporting under these circumstances to be unusual. T he principal physician of record is identified in Medicare as the physician who oversees the patient's care from other physicians who may be furnishing specialty care. The principal physician of record shall append modifier "-AI" (Principal Physician of Record), in addition to the E/M code. Follow-up visits in the facility setting shall be billed as subsequent hospital care visits and subsequent nursing facility care visits.

In the CAH setting, those CAHs that use method II shall bill the appropriate new or established visit code for those physician and non-physician practitioners who have reassigned their billing rights, depending on the relationship status between the physician and patient.

In the office or other outpatient setting where an evaluation is performed, physicians and qualified nonphysician practitioners shall use the CPT codes (99201 – 99215) depending on the complexity of the visit and whether the patient is a new or established patient to that physician. All physicians and qualified nonphysician practitioners shall follow the E/M documentation guidelines for all E/M services. These rules are applicable for Medicare secondary payer claims as well as for claims in which Medicare is the primary payer.

100-04, 12, 30.6.11

Emergency Department Visits

A. Use of Emergency Department Codes by Physicians Not Assigned to Emergency Department

Any physician seeing a patient registered in the emergency department may use emergency department visit codes (for services matching the code description). It is not required that the physician be assigned to the emergency department.

B. Use of Emergency Department Codes In Office

Emergency department coding is not appropriate if the site of service is an office or outpatient setting or any sight of service other than an emergency department. The emergency department codes should only be used if the patient is seen in the emergency department and the services described by the HCPCS code definition are provided. The emergency department is defined as an organized hospital-based facility for the provision of unscheduled or episodic services to patients who present for immediate medical attention.

C. Use of Emergency Department Codes to Bill Nonemergency Services

Services in the emergency department may not be emergencies. However the codes (99281 - 99288) are payable if the described services are provided.

However, if the physician asks the patient to meet him or her in the emergency department as an alternative to the physician's office and the patient is not registered as a patient in the emergency department, the physician should bill the appropriate office/outpatient visit codes. Normally a lower level emergency department code would be reported for a nonemergency condition.

D. Emergency Department or Office/Outpatient Visits on Same Day As Nursing Facility Admission

Emergency department visit provided on the same day as a comprehensive nursing facility assessment are not paid. Payment for evaluation and management services on the same date provided in sites other than the nursing facility are included in the payment for initial nursing facility care when performed on the same date as the nursing facility admission.

E. Physician Billing for Emergency Department Services Provided to Patient by Both Patient's Personal Physician and Emergency Department Physician

If a physician advises his/her own patient to go to an emergency department (ED) of a hospital for care and the physician subsequently is asked by the ED physician to come to the hospital to evaluate the patient and to advise the ED physician as to whether the patient should be admitted to the hospital or be sent home, the physicians should bill as follows:

If the patient is admitted to the hospital by the patient's personal physician, then the patient's regular physician should bill only the appropriate level of the initial hospital care (codes 99221 - 99223) because all evaluation and management services provided by that physician in conjunction with that admission are considered part of the initial hospital care when performed on the same date as the admission. The ED physician who saw the patient in the emergency department should bill the appropriate level of the ED codes.

If the ED physician, based on the advice of the patient's personal physician who came to the emergency department to see the patient, sends the patient home, then the ED physician should bill the appropriate level of emergency department service. The patient's personal physician should also bill the level of emergency department code

that describes the service he or she provided in the emergency department. If the patient's personal physician does not come to the hospital to see the patient, but only advises the emergency department physician by telephone, then the patient's personal physician may not bill.

F. Emergency Department Physician Requests Another Physician to See the Patient in Emergency Department or Office/Outpatient Setting

If the emergency department physician requests that another physician evaluate a given patient, the other physician should bill an emergency department visit code. If the patient is admitted to the hospital by the second physician performing the evaluation, he or she should bill an initial hospital care code and not an emergency department visit code.

100-04, 12, 30.6.13

Nursing Facility Services

A. Visits to Perform the Initial Comprehensive Assessment and Annual Assessments

The distinction made between the delegation of physician visits and tasks in a skilled nursing facility (SNF) and in a nursing facility (NF) is based on the Medicare Statute. Section 1819 (b) (6) (A) of the Social Security Act (the Act) governs SNFs while section 1919 (b) (6) (A) of the Act governs NFs. For further information refer to Medlearn Matters article number SE0418 at www.cms.hhs.gov/medlearn/matters.

The federally mandated visits in a SNF and NF must be performed by the physician except as otherwise permitted (42 CFR 483.40 (c) (4) and (f)). The principal physician of record must append the modifier "-AI", (Principal Physician of Record), to the initial nursing facility care code. This modifier will identify the physician who oversees the patient's care from other physicians who may be furnishing specialty care. All other physicians or qualified NPPs who perform an initial evaluation in the NF or SNF may bill the initial nursing facility care code. The initial federally mandated visit is defined in S&C-04-08 (see www.cms.hhs.gov/medlearn/matters) as the initial comprehensive visit during which the physician completes a thorough assessment, develops a plan of care, and writes or verifies admitting orders for the nursing facility resident. For Survey and Certification requirements, a visit must occur no later than 30 days after admission.

Further, per the Long Term Care regulations at 42 CFR 483.40 (c) (4) and (e) (2), in a SNF the physician may not delegate a task that the physician must personally perform. Therefore, as stated in S&C-04-08 the physician may not delegate the initial federally mandated comprehensive visit in a SNF.

The only exception, as to who performs the initial visit, relates to the NF setting. In the NF setting, a qualified NPP (i.e., a nurse practitioner (NP), physician assistant (PA), or a clinical nurse specialist (CNS)), who is not employed by the facility, may perform the initial visit when the State law permits. The evaluation and management (E/M) visit shall be within the State scope of practice and licensure requirements where the E/M visit is performed and the requirements for physician collaboration and physician supervision shall be met.

Under Medicare Part B payment policy, other medically necessary E/M visits may be performed and reported prior to and after the initial visit, if the medical needs of the patient require an E/M visit. A qualified NPP may perform medically necessary E/M visits prior to and after the initial visit if all the requirements for collaboration, general physician supervision, licensure, and billing are met.

The CPT Nursing Facility Services codes shall be used with place of service (POS) 31 (SNF) if the patient is in a Part A SNF stay. They shall be used with POS 32 (nursing facility) if the patient does not have Part A SNF benefits or if the patient is in a NF or in a non-covered SNF stay (e.g., there was no preceding 3-day hospital stay). The CPT Nursing Facility code definition also includes POS 54 (Intermediate Care Facility/Mentally Retarded) and POS 56 (Psychiatric Residential Treatment Center). For further guidance on POS codes and associated CPT codes refer to §30.6.14.

Effective January 1, 2006, the Initial Nursing Facility Care codes 99301– 99303 are deleted.

Beginning January 1, 2006, the new CPT codes, Initial Nursing Facility Care, per day, (99304 – 99306) shall be used to report the initial federally mandated visit. Only a physician may report these codes for an initial federally mandated visit performed in a SNF or NF (with the exception of the qualified NPP in the NF setting who is not employed by the facility and when State law permits, as explained above).

A readmission to a SNF or NF shall have the same payment policy requirements as an initial admission in both the SNF and NF settings.

A physician who is employed by the SNF/NF may perform the E/M visits and bill independently to Medicare Part B for payment. An NPP who is employed by the SNF or NF may perform and bill Medicare Part B directly for those services where it is permitted as discussed above. The employer of the PA shall always report the visits performed by the PA. A physician, NP or CNS has the option to bill Medicare directly or to reassign payment for his/her professional service to the facility.

As with all E/M visits for Medicare Part B payment policy, the E/M documentation guidelines apply.

Medically Necessary Visits

Qualified NPPs may perform medically necessary E/M visits prior to and after the physician's initial federally mandated visit in both the SNF and NF. Medically necessary E/M visits for the diagnosis or treatment of an illness or injury or to improve the functioning of a malformed body member are payable under the physician fee schedule under Medicare Part B. A physician or NPP may bill the most appropriate initial nursing facility care code (CPT codes 99304-99306) or subsequent nursing facility care code (CPT codes 99307-99310), even if the E/M service is provided prior to the initial federally mandated visit.

SNF Setting--Place of Service Code 31

Following the initial federally mandated visit by the physician, the physician may delegate alternate federally mandated physician visits to a qualified NPP who meets collaboration and physician supervision requirements and is licensed as such by the State and performing within the scope of practice in that State.

NF Setting--Place of Service Code 32

Per the regulations at 42 CFR 483.40 (f), a qualified NPP, who meets the collaboration and physician supervision requirements, the State scope of practice and licensure requirements, and who is not employed by the NF, may at the option of the State, perform the initial federally mandated visit in a NF, and may perform any other federally mandated physician visit in a NF in addition to performing other medically necessary E/M visits.

Questions pertaining to writing orders or certification and recertification issues in the SNF and NF settings shall be addressed to the appropriate State Survey and Certification Agency departments for clarification.

B. Visits to Comply With Federal Regulations (42 CFR 483.40 (c) (1)) in the SNF and NF

Payment is made under the physician fee schedule by Medicare Part B for federally mandated visits. Following the initial federally mandated visit by the physician or qualified NPP where permitted, payment shall be made for federally mandated visits that monitor and evaluate residents at least once every 30 days for the first 90 days after admission and at least once every 60 days thereafter.

Effective January 1, 2006, the Subsequent Nursing Facility Care, per day, codes 99311– 99313 are deleted.

Beginning January 1, 2006, the new CPT codes, Subsequent Nursing Facility Care, per day, (99307 – 99310) shall be used to report federally mandated physician E/M visits and medically necessary E/M visits.

Carriers shall not pay for more than one E/M visit performed by the physician or qualified NPP for the same patient on the same date of service. The Nursing Facility Services codes represent a "per day" service.

The federally mandated E/M visit may serve also as a medically necessary E/M visit if the situation arises (i.e., the patient has health problems that need attention on the day the scheduled mandated physician E/M visit occurs). The physician/qualified NPP shall bill only one E/M visit.

Beginning January 1, 2006, the new CPT code, Other Nursing Facility Service (99318), may be used to report an annual nursing facility assessment visit on the required schedule of visits on an annual basis. For Medicare Part B payment policy, an annual nursing facility assessment visit code may substitute as meeting one of the federally mandated physician visits if the code requirements for CPT code 99318 are fully met and in lieu of reporting a Subsequent Nursing Facility Care, per day, service (codes 99307 – 99310). It shall not be performed in addition to the required number of federally mandated physician visits. The new CPT annual assessment code does not represent a new benefit service for Medicare Part B physician services.

Qualified NPPs, whether employed or not by the SNF, may perform alternating federally mandated physician visits, at the option of the physician, after the initial federally mandated visit by the physician in a SNF.

Qualified NPPs in the NF setting, who are not employed by the NF and who are working in collaboration with a physician, may perform federally mandated physician visits, at the option of the State.

Medicare Part B payment policy does not pay for additional E/M visits that may be required by State law for a facility admission or for other additional visits to satisfy facility or other administrative purposes. E/M visits, prior to and after the initial federally mandated physician visit, that are reasonable and medically necessary to meet the medical needs of the individual patient (unrelated to any State requirement or administrative purpose) are payable under Medicare Part B.

C. Visits by Qualified Nonphysician Practitioners

All E/M visits shall be within the State scope of practice and licensure requirements where the visit is performed and all the requirements for physician collaboration and physician supervision shall be met when performed and reported by qualified NPPs. General physician supervision and employer billing requirements shall be met for PA services in addition to the PA meeting the State scope of practice and licensure requirements where the E/M visit is performed.

Medically Necessary Visits

Qualified NPPs may perform medically necessary E/M visits prior to and after the physician's initial visit in both the SNF and NF. Medically necessary E/M visits for the diagnosis or treatment of an illness or injury or to improve the functioning of a malformed body member are payable under the physician fee schedule under Medicare Part B. A physician or NPP may bill the most appropriate initial nursing facility care code (CPT codes 99304-99306) or subsequent nursing facility care code (CPT codes 99307-99310), even if the E/M service is provided prior to the initial federally mandated visit.

SNF Setting--Place of Service Code 31

Following the initial federally mandated visit by the physician, the physician may delegate alternate federally mandated physician visits to a qualified NPP who meets collaboration and physician supervision requirements and is licensed as such by the State and performing within the scope of practice in that State.

NF Setting--Place of Service Code 32

Per the regulations at 42 CFR 483.40 (f), a qualified NPP, who meets the collaboration and physician supervision requirements, the State scope of practice and licensure requirements, and who is not employed by the NF, may at the option of the State, perform the initial federally mandated visit in a NF, and may perform any other federally mandated physician visit in a NF in addition to performing other medically necessary E/M visits.

Questions pertaining to writing orders or certification and recertification issues in the SNF and NF settings shall be addressed to the appropriate State Survey and Certification Agency departments for clarification.

D. Medically Complex Care

Payment is made for E/M visits to patients in a SNF who are receiving services for medically complex care upon discharge from an acute care facility when the visits are reasonable and medically necessary and documented in the medical record. Physicians and qualified NPPs shall report initial nursing facility care codes for their first visit with the patient. The principal physician of record must append the modifier "-AI" (Principal Physician of Record), to the initial nursing facility care code when billed to identify the physician who oversees the patient's care from other physicians who may be furnishing specialty care. Follow-up visits shall be billed as subsequent nursing facility care visits.

E. Incident to Services

Where a physician establishes an office in a SNF/NF, the "incident to" services and requirements are confined to this discrete part of the facility designated as his/her office. "Incident to" E/M visits, provided in a facility setting, are not payable under the Physician Fee Schedule for Medicare Part B. Thus, visits performed outside the designated "office" area in the SNF/NF would be subject to the coverage and payment rules applicable to the SNF/NF setting and shall not be reported using the CPT codes for office or other outpatient visits or use place of service code 11.

F. Use of the Prolonged Services Codes and Other Time-Related Services

Beginning January 1, 2008, typical/average time units for E/M visits in the SNF/NF settings are reestablished. Medically necessary prolonged services for E/M visits (codes 99356 and 99357) in a SNF or NF may be billed with the Nursing Facility Services in the code ranges (99304 – 99306, 99307 – 99310 and 99318).

Counseling and Coordination of Care Visits

With the reestablishment of typical/average time units, medically necessary E/M visits for counseling and coordination of care, for Nursing Facility Services in the code ranges (99304 – 99306, 99307 – 99310 and 99318) that are time-based services, may be billed with the appropriate prolonged services codes (99356 and 99357).

G. Multiple Visits

The complexity level of an E/M visit and the CPT code billed must be a covered and medically necessary visit for each patient (refer to §§1862 (a)(1)(A) of the Act). Claims for an unreasonable number of daily E/M visits by the same physician to multiple patients at a facility within a 24-hour period may result in medical review to determine medical necessity for the visits. The E/M visit (Nursing Facility Services) represents a "per day" service per patient as defined by the CPT code. The medical record must be personally documented by the physician or qualified NPP who performed the E/M visit and the documentation shall support the specific level of E/M visit to each individual patient.

H. Split/Shared E/M Visit

A split/shared E/M visit cannot be reported in the SNF/NF setting. A split/shared E/M visit is defined by Medicare Part B payment policy as a medically necessary encounter with a patient where the physician and a qualified NPP each personally perform a substantive portion of an E/M visit face-to-face with the same patient on the same date of service. A substantive portion of an E/M visit involves all or some portion of the history, exam or medical decision making key components of an E/M service. The physician and the qualified NPP must be in the same group practice or be employed by the same employer. The split/shared E/M visit applies only to selected E/M visits and settings (i.e., hospital inpatient, hospital outpatient, hospital observation, emergency department, hospital discharge, office and non facility clinic visits, and prolonged visits associated with these E/M visit codes). The split/shared E/M policy does not apply to critical care services or procedures.

I. SNF/NF Discharge Day Management Service

Medicare Part B payment policy requires a face-to-face visit with the patient provided by the physician or the qualified NPP to meet the SNF/NF discharge day management service as defined by the CPT code. The E/M discharge day management visit shall be reported for the date of the actual visit by the physician or qualified NPP even if the patient is discharged from the facility on a different calendar date. The CPT codes 99315 – 99316 shall be reported for this visit. The Discharge Day Management Service may be reported using CPT code 99315 or 99316, depending on the code requirement, for a patient who has expired, but only if the physician or qualified NPP personally performed the death pronouncement.

100-04, 12, 30.6.14

Home Care and Domiciliary Care Visits

Physician Visits to Patients Residing in Various Places of Service

The American Medical Association's Current Procedural Terminology (CPT) 2006 new patient codes 99324 - 99328 and established patient codes 99334 - 99337(new codes beginning January 2006), for Domiciliary, Rest Home (e.g., Boarding Home), or Custodial Care Services, are used to report evaluation and management (E/M) services to residents residing in a facility which provides room, board, and other personal assistance services, generally on a long-term basis. These CPT codes are used to report E/M services in facilities assigned places of service (POS) codes 13 (Assisted Living Facility), 14 (Group Home), 33 (Custodial Care Facility) and 55 (Residential Substance Abuse Facility). Assisted living facilities may also be known as adult living facilities.

Physicians and qualified nonphysician practitioners (NPPs) furnishing E/M services to residents in a living arrangement described by one of the POS listed above must use the level of service code in the CPT code range 99324 - 99337 to report the service they provide. The CPT codes 99321 - 99333 for Domiciliary, Rest Home (e.g., Boarding Home), or Custodial Care Services are deleted beginning January, 2006.

Beginning in 2006, reasonable and medically necessary, face-to-face, prolonged services, represented by CPT codes 99354 - 99355, may be reported with the appropriate companion E/M codes when a physician or qualified NPP, provides a prolonged service involving direct (face-to-face) patient contact that is beyond the usual E/M visit service for a Domiciliary, Rest Home (e.g., Boarding Home) or Custodial Care Service. All the requirements for prolonged services at Sec.30.6.15.1 must be met.

The CPT codes 99341 through 99350, Home Services codes, are used to report E/M services furnished to a patient residing in his or her own private residence (e.g., private home, apartment, town home) and not residing in any type of congregate/shared facility living arrangement including assisted living facilities and group homes. The Home Services codes apply only to the specific 2-digit POS 12 (Home). Home Services codes may not be used for billing E/M services provided in settings other than in the private residence of an individual as described above.

Beginning in 2006, E/M services provided to patients residing in a Skilled Nursing Facility (SNF) or a Nursing Facility (NF) must be reported using the appropriate CPT level of service code within the range identified for Initial Nursing Facility Care (new CPT codes 99304 - 99306) and Subsequent Nursing Facility Care (new CPT codes 99307 - 99310). Use the CPT code, Other Nursing Facility Services (new CPT code 99318), for an annual nursing facility assessment. Use CPT codes 99315 - 99316 for SNF/NF discharge services. The CPT codes 99301 - 99303 and 99311 - 99313 are deleted beginning January, 2006. The Home Services codes should not be used for these places of service.

The CPT SNF/NF code definition includes intermediate care facilities (ICFs) and long term care facilities (LTCFs). These codes are limited to the specific 2-digit POS 31 (SNF), 32 (Nursing Facility), 54 (Intermediate Care Facility/Mentally Retarded) and 56 (Psychiatric Residential Treatment Center).

The CPT nursing facility codes should be used with POS 31 (SNF) if the patient is in a Part A SNF stay and POS 32 (nursing facility) if the patient does not have Part A SNF benefits. There is no longer a different payment amount for a Part A or Part B benefit period in these POS settings.

100-04, 12, 30.6.14.1

Home Services
B3-15515, B3-15066

A. Requirement for Physician Presence
Home services codes 99341-99350 are paid when they are billed to report evaluation and management services provided in a private residence. A home visit cannot be billed by a physician unless the physician was actually present in the beneficiary's home.

B. Homebound Status
Under the home health benefit the beneficiary must be confined to the home for services to be covered. For home services provided by a physician using these codes, the beneficiary does not need to be confined to the home. The medical record must document the medical necessity of the home visit made in lieu of an office or outpatient visit.

C. Fee Schedule Payment for Services to Homebound
Patients under General Supervision Payment may be made in some medically underserved areas where there is a lack of medical personnel and home health services for injections, EKGs, and venipunctures that are performed for homebound patients under general physician supervision by nurses and paramedical employees of physicians or physician-directed clinics. Section 10 provides additional information on the provision of services to homebound Medicare patients.

100-04, 12, 30.6.15.1

Prolonged Services With Direct Face-to-Face Patient Contact Service

A. Definition
Prolonged physician services (CPT code 99354) in the office or other outpatient setting with direct face-to-face patient contact which require 1 hour beyond the usual service are payable when billed on the same day by the same physician or qualified nonphysician practitioner (NPP) as the companion evaluation and management codes. The time for usual service refers to the typical/average time units associated with the companion evaluation and management service as noted in the CPT code. Each additional 30 minutes of direct face-to-face patient contact following the first hour of prolonged services may be reported by CPT code 99355.

Prolonged physician services (code 99356) in the inpatient setting, with direct face-to-face patient contact which require 1 hour beyond the usual service are payable when they are billed on the same day by the same physician or qualified NPP as the companion evaluation and management codes. Each additional 30 minutes of

direct face-to-face patient contact following the first hour of prolonged services may be reported by CPT code 99357.

Prolonged service of less than 30 minutes total duration on a given date is not separately reported because the work involved is included in the total work of the evaluation and management codes.

Code 99355 or 99357 may be used to report each additional 30 minutes beyond the first hour of prolonged services, based on the place of service. These codes may be used to report the final 15 – 30 minutes of prolonged service on a given date, if not otherwise billed. Prolonged service of less than 15 minutes beyond the first hour or less than 15 minutes beyond the final 30 minutes is not reported separately.

B. Required Companion Codes
- The companion evaluation and management codes for 99354 are the Office or Other Outpatient visit codes (99201 - 99205, 99212 – 99215), the Domiciliary, Rest Home, or Custodial Care Services codes (99324 – 99328, 99334 – 99337), the Home Services codes (99341 - 99345, 99347 – 99350);
- The companion codes for 99355 are 99354 and one of the evaluation and management codes required for 99354 to be used;
- The companion evaluation and management codes for 99356 are the Initial Hospital Care codes and Subsequent Hospital Care codes (99221 - 99223, 99231 – 99233); Nursing Facility Services codes (99304 -99318); or
- The companion codes for 99357 are 99356 and one of the evaluation and management codes required for 99356 to be used.

Prolonged services codes 99354 – 99357 are not paid unless they are accompanied by the companion codes as indicated.

C. Requirement for Physician Presence
Physicians may count only the duration of direct face-to-face contact between the physician and the patient (whether the service was continuous or not) beyond the typical/average time of the visit code billed to determine whether prolonged services can be billed and to determine the prolonged services codes that are allowable. In the case of prolonged office services, time spent by office staff with the patient, or time the patient remains unaccompanied in the office cannot be billed. In the case of prolonged hospital services, time spent reviewing charts or discussion of a patient with house medical staff and not with direct face-to-face contact with the patient, or waiting for test results, for changes in the patient's condition, for end of a therapy, or for use of facilities cannot be billed as prolonged services.

D. Documentation
Documentation is not required to accompany the bill for prolonged services unless the physician has been selected for medical review. Documentation is required in the medical record about the duration and content of the medically necessary evaluation and management service and prolonged services billed. The medical record must be appropriately and sufficiently documented by the physician or qualified NPP to show that the physician or qualified NPP personally furnished the direct face-to-face time with the patient specified in the CPT code definitions. The start and end times of the visit shall be documented in the medical record along with the date of service.

E. Use of the Codes
Prolonged services codes can be billed only if the total duration of the physician or qualified NPP direct face-to-face service (including the visit) equals or exceeds the threshold time for the evaluation and management service the physician or qualified NPP provided (typical/average time associated with the CPT E/M code plus 30 minutes). If the total duration of direct face-to-face time does not equal or exceed the threshold time for the level of evaluation and management service the physician or qualified NPP provided, the physician or qualified NPP may not bill for prolonged services.

F. Threshold Times for Codes 99354 and 99355 (Office or Other Outpatient Setting)
If the total direct face-to-face time equals or exceeds the threshold time for code 99354, but is less than the threshold time for code 99355, the physician should bill the evaluation and management visit code and code 99354. No more than one unit of 99354 is acceptable. If the total direct face-to-face time equals or exceeds the threshold time for code 99355 by no more than 29 minutes, the physician should bill the visit code 99354 and one unit of code 99355. One additional unit of code 99355 is billed for each additional increment of 30 minutes extended duration. Contractors use the following threshold times to determine if the prolonged services codes 99354 and/or 99355 can be billed with the office or other outpatient settings including domiciliary, rest home, or custodial care services and home services codes.

Threshold Time for Prolonged Visit Codes 99354 and/or 99355 Billed with Office/Outpatient Code

Code	Typical Time for Code	Threshold Time to Bill Code 99354	Threshold Time to Bill Codes 99354 and 99355
99201	10	40	85
99202	20	50	95
99203	30	60	105
99204	45	75	120
99205	60	90	135
99212	10	40	85
99213	15	45	90
99214	25	55	100

Code	Typical Time for Code	Threshold Time to Bill Code 99354	Threshold Time to Bill Codes 99354 and 99355
99215	40	70	115
99324	20	50	95
99325	30	60	105
99326	45	75	120
99327	60	90	135
99328	75	105	150
99334	15	45	90
99335	25	55	100
99336	40	70	115
99337	60	90	135
99341	20	50	95
99342	30	60	105
99343	45	75	120
99344	60	90	135
99345	75	105	150
99347	15	45	90
99348	25	55	100
99349	40	70	115
99350	60	90	135

G. Threshold Times for Codes 99356 and 99357

(Inpatient Setting) If the total direct face-to-face time equals or exceeds the threshold time for code 99356, but is less than the threshold time for code 99357, the physician should bill the visit and code 99356. Contractors do not accept more than one unit of code 99356. If the total direct face-to-face time equals or exceeds the threshold time for code 99356 by no more than 29 minutes, the physician bills the visit code 99356 and one unit of code 99357. One additional unit of code 99357 is billed for each additional increment of 30 minutes extended duration. Contractors use the following threshold times to determine if the prolonged services codes 99356 and/or 99357 can be billed with the inpatient setting codes.

Threshold Time for Prolonged Visit Codes 99356 and/or 99357 Billed with Inpatient Setting Codes Code

Code	Typical Time for Code	Threshold Time to Bill Code 99356	Threshold Time to Bill Codes 99356 and 99357
99221	30	60	105
99222	50	80	125
99223	70	100	145
99231	15	45	90
99232	25	55	100
99233	35	65	110
99304	25	55	100
99305	35	65	110
99306	45	75	120
99307	10	40	85
99308	15	45	90
99309	25	55	100
99310	35	65	110
99318	30	60	10

Add 30 minutes to the threshold time for billing codes 99356 and 99357 to get the threshold time for billing code 99356 and two units of 99357.

H. Prolonged Services Associated With Evaluation and Management Services Based on Counseling and/or Coordination of Care (Time-Based)

When an evaluation and management service is dominated by counseling and/or coordination of care (the counseling and/or coordination of care represents more than 50% of the total time with the patient) in a face-to-face encounter between the physician or qualified NPP and the patient in the office/clinic or the floor time (in the scenario of an inpatient service), then the evaluation and management code is selected based on the typical/average time associated with the code levels. The time approximation must meet or exceed the specific CPT code billed (determined by the typical/average time associated with the evaluation and management code) and should not be "rounded" to the next higher level.

In those evaluation and management services in which the code level is selected based on time, prolonged services may only be reported with the highest code level in that family of codes as the companion code.

I. Examples of Billable Prolonged Services

EXAMPLE 1

A physician performed a visit that met the definition of an office visit code 99213 and the total duration of the direct face-to-face services (including the visit) was 65 minutes. The physician bills code 99213 and one unit of code 99354.

EXAMPLE 2

A physician performed a visit that met the definition of a domiciliary, rest home care visit code 99327 and the total duration of the direct face-to-face contact (including the visit) was 140 minutes. The physician bills codes 99327, 99354, and one unit of code 99355.

EXAMPLE 3

A physician performed an office visit to an established patient that was predominantly counseling, spending 75 minutes (direct face-to-face) with the patient. The physician should report CPT code 99215 and one unit of code 99354.

J. Examples of Nonbillable Prolonged Services

EXAMPLE 1

A physician performed a visit that met the definition of visit code 99212 and the total duration of the direct face-to-face contact (including the visit) was 35 minutes. The physician cannot bill prolonged services because the total duration of direct face-to-face service did not meet the threshold time for billing prolonged services.

EXAMPLE 2

A physician performed a visit that met the definition of code 99213 and, while the patient was in the office receiving treatment for 4 hours, the total duration of the direct face-to-face service of the physician was 40 minutes. The physician cannot bill prolonged services because the total duration of direct face-to-face service did not meet the threshold time for billing prolonged services.

EXAMPLE 3

A physician provided a subsequent office visit that was predominantly counseling, spending 60 minutes (face-to-face) with the patient. The physician cannot code 99214, which has a typical time of 25 minutes, and one unit of code 99354. The physician must bill the highest level code in the code family (99215 which has 40 minutes typical/average time units associated with it). The additional time spent beyond this code is 20 minutes and does not meet the threshold time for billing prolonged services.

100-04, 12, 30.6.15.2

Prolonged Services Without Face to Face Service

Contractors may not pay prolonged services codes 99358 and 99359, which do not require any direct patient face-to-face contact (e.g., telephone calls). Payment for these services is included in the payment for direct face-to-face services that physicians bill. The physician cannot bill the patient for these services since they are Medicare covered services and payment is included in the payment for other billable services.

100-04, 12, 30.6.15.3

Physician Standby Service

Standby services are not payable to physicians. Physicians may not bill Medicare or beneficiaries for standby services. Payment for standby services is included in the Part A payment to the facility. Such services are a part of hospital costs to provide quality care.

If hospitals pay physicians for standby services, such services are part of hospital costs to provide quality care.

100-04, 12, 40.3

Claims Review for Global Surgeries

A. Relationship to Correct Coding Initiative (CCI)

The CCI policy and computer edits allow A/B MACs (B) to detect instances of fragmented billing for certain intra-operative services and other services furnished on the same day as the surgery that are considered to be components of the surgical procedure and, therefore, included in the global surgical fee. When both correct coding and global surgery edits apply to the same claim, A/B MACs (B) first apply the correct coding edits, then, apply the global surgery edits to the correctly coded services.

B. Prepayment Edits to Detect Separate Billing of Services Included in the Global Package

In addition to the correct coding edits, A/B MACs (B) must be capable of detecting certain other services included in the payment for a major or minor surgery or for an endoscopy. On a prepayment basis, A/B MACs (B) identify the services that meet the following conditions:

- Preoperative services that are submitted on the same claim or on a subsequent claim as a surgical procedure; or

- Same day or postoperative services that are submitted on the same claim or on a subsequent claim as a surgical procedure or endoscopy;

   and -

- Services that were furnished within the prescribed global period of the surgical procedure;

- Services that are billed without modifier "-78," "-79," "-24," "25," or "-57" or are billed with modifier "-24" but without the required documentation; and

- Services that are billed with the same provider or group number as the surgical procedure or endoscopy. Also, edit for any visits billed separately during the postoperative period without modifier "-24" by a physician who billed for the postoperative care only with modifier "-55."

A/B MACs (B) use the following evaluation and management codes in establishing edits for visits included in the global package. CPT codes 99241, 99242, 99243, 99244, 99245, 99251, 99252, 99253, 99254, 99255, 99271, 99272, 99273, 99274, and 99275 have been transferred from the excluded category and are now included in the global surgery edits.

Evaluation and Management Codes for A/B MAC (B) Edits

92012	92014	99211	99212	99213	99214	99215
99217	99218	99219	99220	99221	99222	99223
99231	99232	99233	99234	99235	99236	99238
99239	99241	99242	99243	99244	99245	99251
99252	99253	99254	99255	99261	99262	99263
99271	99272	99273	99274	99275	99291	99292
99301	99302	99303	99311	99312	99313	99315
99316	99331	99332	99333	99347	99348	99349
99350	99374	99375	99377	99378		

NOTE: In order for codes 99291 or 99292 to be paid for services furnished during the preoperative or postoperative period, modifier "-25" or "-24," respectively, must be used to indicate that the critical care was unrelated to the specific anatomic injury or general surgical procedure performed.

If a surgeon is admitting a patient to a nursing facility for a condition not related to the global surgical procedure, the physician should bill for the nursing facility admission and care with a "-24" modifier and appropriate documentation. If a surgeon is admitting a patient to a nursing facility and the patient's admission to that facility relates to the global surgical procedure, the nursing facility admission and any services related to the global surgical procedure are included in the global surgery fee.

C. Exclusions from Prepayment Edits

A/B MACs (B) exclude the following services from the prepayment audit process and allow separate payment if all usual requirements are met:

- Services listed in §40.1.B; and
- Services billed with the modifier "-25," "-57," "-58," "-78," or "-79."

Exceptions

See §§40.2.A.8, 40.2.A.9, and 40.4.A for instances where prepayment review is required for modifier "-25." In addition, prepayment review is necessary for CPT codes 90935, 90937, 90945, and 90947 when a visit and modifier "-25" are billed with these services.

Exclude the following codes from the prepayment edits required in §40.3.B.

92002	92004	99201	99202	99203	99204	99205
99281	99282	99283	99284	99285	99321	99322
99323	99341	99342	99343	99344	99345	

100-04, 12, 40.7

Claims for Bilateral Surgeries

B3-4827, B3-15040

A. General

Bilateral surgeries are procedures performed on both sides of the body during the same operative session or on the same day.

The terminology for some procedure codes includes the terms "bilateral" (e.g., code 27395; Lengthening of the hamstring tendon; multiple, bilateral.) or "unilateral or bilateral" (e.g., code 52290; cystourethroscopy; with ureteral meatotomy, unilateral or bilateral). The payment adjustment rules for bilateral surgeries do not apply to procedures identified by CPT as "bilateral" or "unilateral or bilateral" since the fee schedule reflects any additional work required for bilateral surgeries.

Field 22 of the MFSDB indicates whether the payment adjustment rules apply to a surgical procedure.

B. Billing Instructions for Bilateral Surgeries

If a procedure is not identified by its terminology as a bilateral procedure (or unilateral or bilateral), physicians must report the procedure with modifier "-50." They report such procedures as a single line item. (NOTE: This differs from the CPT coding guidelines which indicate that bilateral procedures should be billed as two line items.)

If a procedure is identified by the terminology as bilateral (or unilateral or bilateral), as in codes 27395 and 52290, physicians do not report the procedure with modifier "-50."

C. Claims Processing System Requirements

Carriers must be able to:

1. Identify bilateral surgeries by the presence on the claim form or electronic submission of the "-50" modifier or of the same code on separate lines reported once with modifier "-LT" and once with modifier "-RT";

2. Access Field 34 or 35 of the MFSDB to determine the Medicare payment amount;

3. Access Field 22 of the MFSDB:

   — If Field 22 contains an indicator of "0," "2," or "3," the payment adjustment rules for bilateral surgeries do not apply. Base payment on the lower of the billed amount or 100 percent of the fee schedule amount (Field 34 or 35) unless other payment adjustment rules apply.

   NOTE: Some codes which have a bilateral indicator of "0" in the MFSDB may be performed more than once on a given day. These are services that would never be considered bilateral and thus should not be billed with modifier "-50." Where such a code is billed on multiple line tems or with more than 1 in the units field and carriers have determined that the code may be reported more than once, bypass the "0" bilateral indicator and refer to the multiple surgery field for pricing;

   — If Field 22 contains an indicator of "1," the standard adjustment rules apply. Base payment on the lower of the billed amount or 150 percent of the fee schedule amount (Field 34 or 35). (Multiply the payment amount in Field 34 or 35 for the surgery by 150 percent and round to the nearest cent.)

4. Apply the requirements 40 - 40.4 on global surgeries to bilateral surgeries; and

5. Retain the "-50" modifier in history for any bilateral surgeries paid at the adjusted amount.

   (NOTE: The "-50" modifier is not retained for surgeries which are bilateral by definition such as code 27395.)

100-04, 12, 40.8

Claims for Co-Surgeons and Team Surgeons

B3-4828, B3-15046

A. General

Under some circumstances, the individual skills of two or more surgeons are required to perform surgery on the same patient during the same operative session. This may be required because of the complex nature of the procedure(s) and/or the patient's condition.

In these cases, the additional physicians are not acting as assistants-at-surgery.

B. Billing Instructions

The following billing procedures apply when billing for a surgical procedure or procedures that required the use of two surgeons or a team of surgeons:

- If two surgeons (each in a different specialty) are required to perform a specific procedure, each surgeon bills for the procedure with a modifier "-62. " Co-surgery also refers to surgical procedures involving two surgeons performing the parts of the procedure simultaneously, i.e., heart transplant or bilateral knee replacements. Documentation of the medical necessity for two surgeons is required for certain services identified in the MFSDB. (See 40.8.C.5.);

- If a team of surgeons (more than 2 surgeons of different specialties) is required to perform a specific procedure, each surgeon bills for the procedure with a modifier "-66." Field 25 of the MFSDB identifies certain services submitted with a "-66" modifier which must be sufficiently documented to establish that a team was medically necessary. All claims for team surgeons must contain sufficient information to allow pricing "by report."

- If surgeons of different specialties are each performing a different procedure (with specific CPT codes), neither co-surgery nor multiple surgery rules apply (even if the procedures are performed through the same incision). If one of the surgeons performs multiple procedures, the multiple procedure rules apply to that surgeon's services. (See 40.6 for multiple surgery payment rules.)

For co-surgeons (modifier 62), the fee schedule amount applicable to the payment for each co-surgeon is 62.5 percent of the global surgery fee schedule amount. Team surgery (modifier 66) is paid for on a "By Report" basis.

C. Claims Processing System Requirements

Carriers must be able to:

1. Identify a surgical procedure performed by two surgeons or a team of surgeons by the presence on the claim form or electronic submission of the "-62" or "-66" modifier;

2. Access Field 34 or 35 of the MFSDB to determine the fee schedule payment amount for the surgery;

3. Access Field 24 or 25, as appropriate, of the MFSDB. These fields provide guidance on whether two or team surgeons are generally required for the surgical procedure;

4. If the surgery is billed with a "-62" or "-66" modifier and Field 24 or 25 contains an indicator of "0," payment adjustment rules for two or team surgeons do not apply:

   — Carriers pay the first bill submitted, and base payment on the lower of the billed amount or 100 percent of the fee schedule amount (Field 34 or 35) unless other payment adjustment rules apply;

   — Carriers deny bills received subsequently from other physicians and use the appropriate MSN message in 40.8.D. As these are medical necessity denials, the instructions in the Program Integrity Manual regarding denial of unassigned claims for medical necessity are applied;

5. If the surgery is billed with a "-62" modifier and Field 24 contains an indicator of "1," suspend the claim for manual review of any documentation submitted with the claim. If the documentation supports the need for co-surgeons, base payment for each physician on the lower of the billed amount or 62.5 percent of the fee schedule amount (Field 34 or 35);

6. If the surgery is billed with a "-62" modifier and Field 24 contains an indicator of "2," payment rules for two surgeons apply. Carriers base payment for each physician on the lower of the billed amount or 62.5 percent of the fee schedule amount (Field 34 or 35);

7. If the surgery is billed with a "-66" modifier and Field 25 contains an indicator of "1," carriers suspend the claim for manual review. If carriers determine that team surgeons were medically necessary, each physician is paid on a "by report" basis;

8. If the surgery is billed with a "-66" modifier and Field 25 contains an indicator of "2," carriers pay "by report";

NOTE: A Medicare fee may have been established for some surgical procedures that are billed with the "-66" modifier. In these cases, all physicians on the team must agree on the percentage of the Medicare payment amount each is to receive.

If carriers receive a bill with a "-66" modifier after carriers have paid one surgeon the full Medicare payment amount (on a bill without the modifier), deny the subsequent claim.

9. Apply the rules global surgical packages to each of the physicians participating in a co- or team surgery; and

10. Retain the "-62" and "-66" modifiers in history for any co- or team surgeries.

D. Beneficiary Liability on Denied Claims for Assistant, Co- surgeon and Team Surgeons

MSN message 23.10 which states "Medicare does not pay for a surgical assistant for this kind of surgery," was established for denial of claims for assistant surgeons. Where such payment is denied because the procedure is subject to the statutory restriction against payment for assistants-at-surgery. Carriers include the following statement in the MSN:

"You cannot be charged for this service." (Unnumbered add-on message.)

Carriers use Group Code CO on the remittance advice to the physician to signify that the beneficiary may not be billed for the denied service and that the physician could be subject to penalties if a bill is issued to the beneficiary.

If Field 23 of the MFSDB contains an indicator of "0" or "1" (assistant-at-surgery may not be paid) for procedures CMS has determined that an assistant surgeon is not generally medically necessary.

For those procedures with an indicator of "0," the limitation on liability provisions described in Chapter 30 apply to assigned claims. Therefore, carriers include the appropriate limitation of liability language from Chapter 21. For unassigned claims, apply the rules in the Program Integrity Manual concerning denial for medical necessity.

Where payment may not be made for a co- or team surgeon, use the following MSN message (MSN message number 15.13):

Medicare does not pay for team surgeons for this procedure.

Where payment may not be made for a two surgeons, use the following MSN message (MSN message number 15.12):

Medicare does not pay for two surgeons for this procedure.

Also see limitation of liability remittance notice REF remark codes M25, M26, and M27.

Use the following message on the remittance notice:

Multiple physicians/assistants are not covered in this case. (Reason code 54.)

100-04, 12, 100

Teaching Physician Services

Definitions

For purposes of this section, the following definitions apply.

Resident -An individual who participates in an approved graduate medical education (GME) program or a physician who is not in an approved GME program but who is authorized to practice only in a hospital setting. The term includes interns and fellows in GME programs recognized as approved for purposes of direct GME payments made by the FI. Receiving a staff or faculty appointment or participating in a fellowship does not by itself alter the status of "resident". Additionally, this status remains unaffected regardless of whether a hospital includes the physician in its full time equivalency count of residents.

Student- An individual who participates in an accredited educational program (e.g., a medical school) that is not an approved GME program. A student is never considered to be an intern or a resident. Medicare does not pay for any service furnished by a student. See 100.1.1B for a discussion concerning E/M service documentation performed by students.

Teaching Physician -A physician (other than another resident) who involves residents in the care of his or her patients.

Direct Medical and Surgical Services -Services to individual beneficiaries that are either personally furnished by a physician or furnished by a resident under the supervision of a physician in a teaching hospital making the reasonable cost election for physician services furnished in teaching hospitals. All payments for such services are made by the FI for the hospital.

Teaching Hospital -A hospital engaged in an approved GME residency program in medicine, osteopathy, dentistry, or podiatry.

Teaching Setting -Any provider, hospital-based provider, or nonprovider setting in which Medicare payment for the services of residents is made by the FI under the direct graduate medical education payment methodology or freestanding SNF or HHA in which such payments are made on a reasonable cost basis.

Critical or Key Portion- That part (or parts) of a service that the teaching physician determines is (are) a critical or key portion(s). For purposes of this section, these terms are interchangeable.

Documentation- Notes recorded in the patient's medical records by a resident, and/or teaching physician or others as outlined in the specific situations below regarding the service furnished. Documentation may be dictated and typed or hand-written, or computer-generated and typed or handwritten. Documentation must be dated and include a legible signature or identity. Pursuant to 42 CFR 415.172 (b), documentation must identify, at a minimum, the service furnished, the participation of the teaching physician in providing the service, and whether the teaching physician was physically present. In the context of an electronic medical record, the term 'macro' means a command in a computer or dictation application that automatically generates predetermined text that is not edited by the user.

When using an electronic medical record, it is acceptable for the teaching physician to use a macro as the required personal documentation if the teaching physician adds it personally in a secured (password protected) system. In addition to the teaching physician's macro, either the resident or the teaching physician must provide customized information that is sufficient to support a medical necessity determination. The note in the electronic medical record must sufficiently describe the specific services furnished to the specific patient on the specific date. It is insufficient documentation if both the resident and the teaching physician use macros only.

Physically Present- The teaching physician is located in the same room (or partitioned or curtained area, if the room is subdivided to accommodate multiple patients) as the patient and/or performs a face-to-face service.

100-04, 12, 100.1.1

Evaluation and Management (E/M) Services

A. General Documentation Instructions and Common Scenarios

Evaluation and Management (E/M) Services -- For a given encounter, the selection of the appropriate level of E/M service should be determined according to the code definitions in the American Medical Association's Current Procedural Terminology (CPT) and any applicable documentation guidelines.

For purposes of payment, E/M services billed by teaching physicians require that they personally document at least the following:

*   That they performed the service or were physically present during the key or critical portions of the service when performed by the resident; and

*   The participation of the teaching physician in the management of the patient.

When assigning codes to services billed by teaching physicians, reviewers will combine the documentation of both the resident and the teaching physician.

Documentation by the resident of the presence and participation of the teaching physician is not sufficient to establish the presence and participation of the teaching physician.

On medical review, the combined entries into the medical record by the teaching physician and the resident constitute the documentation for the service and together must support the medical necessity of the service.

Following are four common scenarios for teaching physicians providing E/M services:

Scenario 1:

The teaching physician personally performs all the required elements of an E/M service without a resident. In this scenario the resident may or may not have performed the E/M service independently.

In the absence of a note by a resident, the teaching physician must document as he/she would document an E/M service in a nonteaching setting.

Where a resident has written notes, the teaching physician's note may reference the resident's note. The teaching physician must document that he/she performed the critical or key portion(s) of the service, and that he/she was directly involved in the management of the patient. For payment, the composite of the teaching physician's entry and the resident's entry together must support the medical necessity of the billed service and the level of the service billed by the teaching physician.

Scenario 2:

The resident performs the elements required for an E/M service in the presence of, or jointly with, the teaching physician and the resident documents the service. In this case, the teaching physician must document that he/she was present during the performance of the critical or key portion(s) of the service and that he/she was directly involved in the management of the patient. The teaching physician's note should reference the resident's note. For payment, the composite of the teaching physician's entry and the resident's entry together must support the medical necessity and the level of the service billed by the teaching physician.

Scenario 3:

The resident performs some or all of the required elements of the service in the absence of the teaching physician and documents his/her service. The teaching physician independently performs the critical or key portion(s) of the service with or without the resident present and, as appropriate, discusses the case with the resident. In this instance, the teaching physician must document that he/she personally saw the patient, personally performed critical or key portions of the service, and participated in the management of the patient. The teaching physician's note should reference the resident's note. For payment, the composite of the teaching physician's entry and the resident's entry together must support the medical necessity of the billed service and the level of the service billed by the teaching physician.

Scenario 4:

When a medical resident admits a patient to a hospital late at night and the teaching physician does not see the patient until later, including the next calendar day:

- The teaching physician must document that he/she personally saw the patient and participated in the management of the patient. The teaching physician may reference the resident's note in lieu of re-documenting the history of present illness, exam, medical decision-making, review of systems and/or past family/social history provided that the patient's condition has not changed, and the teaching physician agrees with the resident's note.

- The teaching physician's note must reflect changes in the patient's condition and clinical course that require that the resident's note be amended with further information to address the patient's condition and course at the time the patient is seen personally by the teaching physician.

- The teaching physician's bill must reflect the date of service he/she saw the patient and his/her personal work of obtaining a history, performing a physical, and participating in medical decision-making regardless of whether the combination of the teaching physician's and resident's documentation satisfies criteria for a higher level of service. For payment, the composite of the teaching physician's entry and the resident's entry together must support the medical necessity of the billed service and the level of the service billed by the teaching physician.

Following are examples of minimally acceptable documentation for each of these scenarios:

Scenario 1:

Admitting Note: "I performed a history and physical examination of the patient and discussed his management with the resident. I reviewed the resident's note and agree with the documented findings and plan of care."

Follow-up Visit: "Hospital Day #3. I saw and evaluated the patient. I agree with the findings and the plan of care as documented in the resident's note."

Follow-up Visit: "Hospital Day #5. I saw and examined the patient. I agree with the resident's note except the heart murmur is louder, so I will obtain an echo to evaluate."

(NOTE: In this scenario if there are no resident notes, the teaching physician must document as he/she would document an E/M service in a non-teaching setting.)

Scenario 2:

Initial or Follow-up Visit: "I was present with the resident during the history and exam. I discussed the case with the resident and agree with the findings and plan as documented in the resident's note."

Follow-up Visit: "I saw the patient with the resident and agree with the resident's findings and plan."

Scenarios 3 and 4:

Initial Visit: "I saw and evaluated the patient. I reviewed the resident's note and agree, except that picture is more consistent with pericarditis than myocardial ischemia. Will begin NSAIDs."

Initial or Follow-up Visit: "I saw and evaluated the patient. Discussed with resident and agree with resident's findings and plan as documented in the resident's note."

Follow-up Visit: "See resident's note for details. I saw and evaluated the patient and agree with the resident's finding and plans as written."

Follow-up Visit: "I saw and evaluated the patient. Agree with resident's note but lower extremities are weaker, now 3/5; MRI of L/S Spine today."

Following are examples of unacceptable documentation:

- "Agree with above." followed by legible countersignature or identity;

- "Rounded, Reviewed, Agree." followed by legible countersignature or identity;

- "Discussed with resident. Agree." followed by legible countersignature or identity;

- "Seen and agree." followed by legible countersignature or identity;

- "Patient seen and evaluated." followed by legible countersignature or identity; and

- A legible countersignature or identity alone.

Such documentation is not acceptable, because the documentation does not make it possible to determine whether the teaching physician was present, evaluated the patient, and/or had any involvement with the plan of care.

B. E/M Service Documentation Provided By Students

Any contribution and participation of a student to the performance of a billable service (other than the review of systems and/or past family/social history which are not separately billable, but are taken as part of an E/M service) must be performed in the physical presence of a teaching physician or physical presence of a resident in a service meeting the requirements set forth in this section for teaching physician billing.

Students may document services in the medical record. However, the documentation of an E/M service by a student that may be referred to by the teaching physician is limited to documentation related to the review of systems and/or past family/social history. The teaching physician may not refer to a student's documentation of physical exam findings or medical decision making in his or her personal note. If the medical student documents E/M services, the teaching physician must verify and redocument the history of present illness as well as perform and redocument the physical exam and medical decision making activities of the service.

C. Exception for E/M Services Furnished in Certain Primary Care Centers

Teaching physicians providing E/M services with a GME program granted a primary care exception may bill Medicare for lower and mid-level E/M services provided by residents. For the E/M codes listed below, teaching physicians may submit claims for services furnished by residents in the absence of a teaching physician:

New Patient	Established Patient
99201	99211
99202	99212
99203	99213

Effective January 1, 2005, the following code is included under the primary care exception: HCPCS code G0402 (Initial preventive physical examination; face-to-face visit services limited to new beneficiary during the first 12 months of Medicare enrollment).

Effective January 1, 2011, the following codes are included under the primary care exception: HCPCS codes G0438 (Annual wellness visit, including personal preventive plan service, first visit) and G0439 (Annual wellness visit, including personal preventive plan service, subsequent visit).

If a service other than those listed above needs to be furnished, then the general teaching physician policy set forth in §100.1 applies. For this exception to apply, a center must attest in writing that all the following conditions are met for a particular residency program. Prior approval is not necessary, but centers exercising the primary care exception must maintain records demonstrating that they qualify for the exception.

The services must be furnished in a center located in the outpatient department of a hospital or another ambulatory care entity in which the time spent by residents in patient care activities is included in determining direct GME payments to a teaching hospital by the hospital's FI. This requirement is not met when the resident is assigned to a physician's office away from the center or makes home visits. In the case of a nonhospital entity, verify with the FI that the entity meets the requirements of a written agreement between the hospital and the entity set forth at 42 CFR 413.78(e)(3)(ii).

Under this exception, residents providing the billable patient care service without the physical presence of a teaching physician must have completed at least 6 months of a GME approved residency program. Centers must maintain information under the provisions at 42 CFR 413.79(a)(6).

Teaching physicians submitting claims under this exception may not supervise more than four residents at any given time and must direct the care from such proximity as to constitute immediate availability. Teaching physicians may include residents with less than 6 months in a GME approved residency program in the mix of four residents under the teaching physician's supervision. However, the teaching physician must be physically present for the critical or key portions of services furnished by the residents with less than 6 months in a GME approved residency program. That is, the primary care exception does not apply in the case of residents with less than 6 months in a GME approved residency program.

Teaching physicians submitting claims under this exception must:

- Not have other responsibilities (including the supervision of other personnel) at the time the service was provided by the resident;

- Have the primary medical responsibility for patients cared for by the residents;

- Ensure that the care provided was reasonable and necessary;

- Review the care provided by the resident during or immediately after each visit. This must include a review of the patient's medical history, the resident's findings on physical examination, the patient's diagnosis, and treatment plan (i.e., record of tests and therapies); and

- Document the extent of his/her own participation in the review and direction of the services furnished to each patient.

Patients under this exception should consider the center to be their primary location for health care services. The residents must be expected to generally provide care to the same group of established patients during their residency training. The types of services furnished by residents under this exception include:

- Acute care for undifferentiated problems or chronic care for ongoing conditions including chronic mental illness;

- Coordination of care furnished by other physicians and providers; and,

- Comprehensive care not limited by organ system or diagnosis.

Residency programs most likely qualifying for this exception include family practice, general internal medicine, geriatric medicine, pediatrics, and obstetrics/gynecology.

Certain GME programs in psychiatry may qualify in special situations such as when the program furnishes comprehensive care for chronically mentally ill patients. These would be centers in which the range of services the residents are trained to furnish, and actually do furnish, include comprehensive medical care as well as psychiatric care. For example, antibiotics are being prescribed as well as psychotropic drugs.

100-04, 12, 140.1

Qualified Nonphysician Anesthetists

For payment purposes, qualified nonphysician anesthetists include both CRNAs and AAs. Thus, the term qualified nonphysician anesthetist will be used to refer to both CRNAs and AAs unless it is necessary to separately discuss these provider groups.

An AA is a person who:

- Is permitted by State law to administer anesthesia; and who
- Has successfully completed a six-year program for AAs of which two years consist of specialized academic and clinical training in anesthesia.

In contrast, a CRNA is a registered nurse who is licensed by the State in which the nurse practices and who:

- Is currently certified by the Council on Certification of Nurse Anesthetists or the Council on Recertification of Nurse Anesthetists, or
- Has graduated within the past 18 months from a nurse anesthesia program that meets the standards of the Council of Accreditation of Nurse Anesthesia Educational Programs and is awaiting initial certification.

100-04, 12, 140.3

Anesthesia Fee Schedule Payment for Qualified Nonphysician Anesthetists

Pay for the services of a qualified nonphysician anesthetist only on an assignment basis. The assignment agreed to by the qualified nonphysician anesthetist is binding upon any other person or entity claiming payment for the service. Except for deductible and coinsurance amounts, any person who knowingly and willfully presents or causes to be presented to a Medicare beneficiary a bill or request for payment for services of a qualified nonphysician anesthetist for which payment may be made on an assignment-related basis is subject to civil monetary penalties.

Services furnished by qualified nonphysician anesthetists are subject to the Part B deductible and coinsurance. If the Part B deductible has been satisfied, the fee schedule for anesthesia services prior to January 1, 1996, is the least of 80 percent of:

- The actual charge;
- The applicable CRNA conversion factor multiplied by the sum of allowable base and time units; or
- The applicable locality participating anesthesiologist's conversion factor multiplied by the sum of allowable base and time units.

For services furnished on or after January 1, 1996, the fee schedule for anesthesia services furnished by qualified nonphysician anesthetists is the least of 80 percent of:

- The actual charge;
- The applicable locality anesthesia conversion factor multiplied by the sum of allowable base and time units.

100-04, 12, 140.3.3

Billing Modifiers

The following modifiers are used when billing for anesthesia services:

- QX - Qualified nonphysician anesthetist with medical direction by a physician.
- QZ - CRNA without medical direction by a physician.
- QS - Monitored anesthesiology care services (can be billed by a qualified nonphysician anesthetist or a physician).
- QY - Medical direction of one qualified nonphysician anesthetist by an anesthesiologist. This modifier is effective for anesthesia services furnished by a qualified nonphysician anesthetist on or after January 1, 1998.

100-04, 12, 140.3.4

General Billing Instructions

Claims for reimbursement for qualified nonphysician anesthetist services should be completed in accord with existing billing instructions for anesthesiologists with the following additions.

- If an employer-physician furnishes concurrent medical direction for a procedure involving CRNAs and the medical direction service is unassigned, the physician should bill on an assigned basis on a separate claim for the qualified nonphysician anesthetist service. If the physician is participating or takes assignment, both services should be billed on one claim but as separate line items.
- All claims forms must have the provider billing number of the CRNA, AA and/or the employer of the qualified nonphysician anesthetist performing the service in

either block 24.H of the Form CMS-1500 and/or block 31 as applicable. Verify that the billing number is valid before making payment.

Payments should be calculated in accordance with Medicare payment rules in §140.3. Contractors must institute all necessary payment edits to assure that duplicate payments are not made to physicians for CRNA or AA services or to a CRNA or AA directly for bills submitted on their behalf by qualified billers.

CRNAs are identified on the provider file by specialty code 43. AAs are identified on the provider file by specialty code 32.

100-04, 12, 140.4.1

An Anesthesiologist and Qualified Nonphysician Anesthetist Work Together

Contractors will distribute educational releases and use other established means to ensure that anesthesiologists understand the requirements for medical direction of qualified nonphysician anesthetists.

Contractors will perform reviews of payments for anesthesiology services to identify situations in which an excessive number of concurrent anesthesiology services may have been performed. They will use peer practice and their experience in developing review criteria. They will also periodically review a sample of claims for medical direction of four or fewer concurrent anesthesia procedures. During this process physicians may be requested to submit documentation of the names of procedures performed and the names of the anesthetists directed.

Physicians who cannot supply the necessary documentation for the sample claims must submit documentation with all subsequent claims before payment will be made.

100-04, 12, 140.4.2

Qualified Nonphysician Anesthetist and an Anesthesiologist in a Single Anesthesia Procedure

Where a single anesthesia procedure involves both a physician medical direction service and the service of the medically directed qualified nonphysician anesthetist, and the service is furnished on or after January 1, 1998, the payment amount for the service of each is 50 percent of the allowance otherwise recognized had the service been furnished by the anesthesiologist alone. The modifier to be used for current procedure identification is QX.

Beginning on or after January 1, 1998, where the qualified nonphysician anesthetist and the anesthesiologist are involved in a single anesthesia case, and the physician is performing medical direction, the service is billed in accordance with the following procedures:

- For the single medically directed service, the physician will use the modifier "QY" (MEDICAL DIRECTION OF ONE QUALIFIED NONPHYSICIAN ANESTHETIST BY AN ANESTHESIOLOGIST). This modifier is effective for claims for dates of service on or after January 1, 1998, and
- For the anesthesia service furnished by the medically directed qualified nonphysician anesthetist, the qualified nonphysician anesthetist will use the current modifier "QX."

In unusual circumstances when it is medically necessary for both the CRNA and the anesthesiologist to be completely and fully involved during a procedure, full payment for the services of each provider is allowed. The physician would report using the "AA" modifier and the CRNA would use "QZ," or the modifier for a nonmedically directed case.

Documentation must be submitted by each provider to support payment of the full fee.

100-04, 12, 140.4.3

Payment for Medical or Surgical Services Furnished by CRNAs

Payment shall be made for reasonable and necessary medical or surgical services furnished by CRNAs if they are legally authorized to perform these services in the state in which services are furnished. Payment is determined under the physician fee schedule on the basis of the national physician fee schedule conversion factor, the geographic adjustment factor, and the resource-based relative value units for the medical or surgical service.

100-04, 12, 140.4.4

Conversion Factors for Anesthesia Services of Qualified Nonphysician Anesthetists Furnished on or After January 1, 1992

Conversion factors used to determine fee schedule payments for anesthesia services furnished by qualified nonphysician anesthetists on or after January 1, 1992, are determined based on a statutory methodology.

For example, for anesthesia services furnished by a medically directed qualified nonphysician anesthetist in 1994, the medically directed allowance is 60 percent of the allowance that would be recognized for the anesthesia service if the physician personally performed the service without an assistant, i.e., alone. For subsequent years, the medically directed allowance is the following percent of the personally performed allowance.

Services furnished in 1995	57.5 percent

Services furnished in 1996	55.0 percent
Services furnished in 1997	52.5 percent
Services furnished in 1998 and after	50.0 percent

100-04, 12, 160

Independent Psychologist Services

B3-2150, B3-2070.2 See the Medicare Benefit Policy Manual, Chapter 15, for coverage requirements.

There are a number of types of psychologists. Educational psychologists engage in identifying and treating education-related issues. In contrast, counseling psychologists provide services that include a broader realm including phobias, familial issues, etc.

Psychometrists are psychologists who have been trained to administer and interpret tests.

However, clinical psychologists are defined as a provider of diagnostic and therapeutic services. Because of the differences in services provided, services provided by psychologists who do not provide clinical services are subject to different billing guidelines. One service often provided by nonclinical psychologist is diagnostic testing.

NOTE: Diagnostic psychological testing services performed by persons who meet these requirements are covered as other diagnostic tests. When, however, the psychologist is not practicing independently, but is on the staff of an institution, agency, or clinic, that entity bills for the diagnostic services.

Expenses for such testing are not subject to the payment limitation on treatment for mental, psychoneurotic, and personality disorders. Independent psychologists are not required by law to accept assignment when performing psychological tests. However, regardless of whether the psychologist accepts assignment, he or she must report on the claim form the name and address of the physician who ordered the test.

100-04, 12, 160.1

Payment

Diagnostic testing services are not subject to the outpatient mental health limitation. Refer to §210, below, for a discussion of the outpatient mental health limitation. The diagnostic testing services performed by a psychologist (who is not a clinical psychologist) practicing independently of an institution, agency, or physician's office are covered as other diagnostic tests if a physician orders such testing. Medicare covers this type of testing as an outpatient service if furnished by any psychologist who is licensed or certified to practice psychology in the State or jurisdiction where he or she is furnishing services or, if the jurisdiction does not issue licenses, if provided by any practicing psychologist. (It is CMS' understanding that all States, the District of Columbia, and Puerto Ricolicense psychologists, but that some trust territories do not. Examples of psychologists, other than clinical psychologists, whose services are covered under this provision include, but are not limited to, educational psychologists and counseling psychologists.)

To determine whether the diagnostic psychological testing services of a particular independent psychologist are covered under Part B in States which have statutory licensure or certification, carriers must secure from the appropriate State agency a current listing of psychologists holding the required credentials. In States or territories which lack statutory licensing and certification, carriers must check individual qualifications as claims are submitted. Possible reference sources are the national directory of membership of the American Psychological Association, which provides data about the educational background of individuals and indicates which members are board-certified, and records and directories of the State or territorial psychological association. If qualification is dependent on a doctoral degree from a currently accredited program, carriers must verify the date of accreditation of the school involved, since such accreditation is not retroactive. If the reference sources listed above do not provide enough information (e.g., the psychologist is not a member of the association), carriers must contact the psychologist personally for the required information. Carriers may wish to maintain a continuing list of psychologists whose qualifications have been verified.

Medicare excludes expenses for diagnostic testing from the payment limitation on treatment for mental/psychoneurotic/personality disorders.

Carriers must identify the independent psychologist's choice whether or not to accept assignment when performing psychological tests.

Carriers must accept an independent psychologist claim only if the psychologist reports the name/UPIN of the physician who ordered a test.

Carriers pay nonparticipating independent psychologists at 95 percent of the physician fee schedule allowed amount.

Carriers pay participating independent psychologists at 100 percent of the physician fee schedule allowed amount. Independent psychologists are identified on the provider file by specialty code 62 and provider type 35.

100-04, 12, 170

Clinical Psychologist Services

B3-2150 See Medicare Benefit Policy Manual, Chapter 15, for general coverage requirements.

Direct payment may be made under Part B for professional services. However, services furnished incident to the professional services of CPs to hospital patients remain bundled.

Therefore, payment must continue to be made to the hospital (by the FI) for such "incident to" services.

100-04, 12, 180

Care Plan Oversight Services

The Medicare Benefit Policy Manual, Chapter 15, contains requirements for coverage for medical and other health services including those of physicians and non-physician practitioners.

Care plan oversight (CPO) is the physician supervision of a patient receiving complex and/or multidisciplinary care as part of Medicare-covered services provided by a participating home health agency or Medicare approved hospice.

CPO services require complex or multidisciplinary care modalities involving:

- Regular physician development and/or revision of care plans;
- Review of subsequent reports of patient status;
- Review of related laboratory and other studies;
- Communication with other health professionals not employed in the same practice who are involved in the patient's care;
- Integration of new information into the medical treatment plan; and/or
- Adjustment of medical therapy.

The CPO services require recurrent physician supervision of a patient involving 30 or more minutes of the physician's time per month. Services not countable toward the 30 minutes threshold that must be provided in order to bill for CPO include, but are not limited to:

- Time associated with discussions with the patient, his or her family or friends to adjust medication or treatment;
- Time spent by staff getting or filing charts;
- Travel time; and/or Physician's time spent telephoning prescriptions into the pharmacist unless the telephone conversation involves discussions of pharmaceutical therapies.

Implicit in the concept of CPO is the expectation that the physician has coordinated an aspect of the patient's care with the home health agency or hospice during the month for which CPO services were billed. The physician who bills for CPO must be the same physician who signs the plan of care.

Nurse practitioners, physician assistants, and clinical nurse specialists, practicing within the scope of State law, may bill for care plan oversight. These non-physician practitioners must have been providing ongoing care for the beneficiary through evaluation and management services. These non-physician practitioners may not bill for CPO if they have been involved only with the delivery of the Medicare-covered home health or hospice service.

A. Home Health CPO

Non-physician practitioners can perform CPO only if the physician signing the plan of care provides regular ongoing care under the same plan of care as does the NPP billing for CPO and either:

- The physician and NPP are part of the same group practice; or
- If the NPP is a nurse practitioner or clinical nurse specialist, the physician signing the plan of care also has a collaborative agreement with the NPP; or
- If the NPP is a physician assistant, the physician signing the plan of care is also the physician who provides general supervision of physician assistant services for the practice.

Billing may be made for care plan oversight services furnished by an NPP when:

- The NPP providing the care plan oversight has seen and examined the patient;
- The NPP providing care plan oversight is not functioning as a consultant whose participation is limited to a single medical condition rather than multidisciplinary coordination of care; and
- The NPP providing care plan oversight integrates his or her care with that of the physician who signed the plan of care.

NPPs may not certify the beneficiary for home health care.

B. Hospice CPO

The attending physician or nurse practitioner (who has been designated as the attending physician) may bill for hospice CPO when they are acting as an "attending physician".

An "attending physician" is one who has been identified by the individual, at the time he/she elects hospice coverage, as having the most significant role in the determination and delivery of their medical care. They are not employed nor paid by the hospice. The care plan oversight services are billed using Form CMS-1500 or electronic equivalent.

For additional information on hospice CPO, see Chapter 11, 40.1.3.1 of this manual.

100-04, 12, 180.1

Care Plan Oversight Billing Requirements

A. Codes for Which Separate Payment May Be Made

Effective January 1, 1995, separate payment may be made for CPO oversight services for 30 minutes or more if the requirements specified in the Medicare Benefits Policy Manual, Chapter 15 are met.

Providers billing for CPO must submit the claim with no other services billed on that claim and may bill only after the end of the month in which the CPO services were rendered. CPO services may not be billed across calendar months and should be submitted (and paid) only for one unit of service.

Physicians may bill and be paid separately for CPO services only if all the criteria in the Medicare Benefit Policy Manual, Chapter 15 are met.

B. Physician Certification and Recertification of Home Health Plans of Care

Effective 2001, two new HCPCS codes for the certification and recertification and development of plans of care for Medicare-covered home health services were created.

See the Medicare General Information, Eligibility, and Entitlement Manual, Pub. 100-1, Chapter 4, "Physician Certification and Recertification of Services," 10-60, and the Medicare Benefit Policy Manual, Pub. 100-2, Chapter 7, "Home Health Services", 30.

The home health agency certification code can be billed only when the patient has not received Medicare-covered home health services for at least 60 days. The home health agency recertification code is used after a patient has received services for at least 60 days (or one certification period) when the physician signs the certification after the initial certification period. The home health agency recertification code will be reported only once every 60 days, except in the rare situation when the patient starts a new episode before 60 days elapses and requires a new plan of care to start a new episode.

C. Provider Number of Home Health Agency (HHA) or Hospice

For claims for CPO submitted on or after January 1, 1997, physicians must enter on the Medicare claim form the 6-character Medicare provider number of the HHA or hospice providing Medicare-covered services to the beneficiary for the period during which CPO services was furnished and for which the physician signed the plan of care. Physicians are responsible for obtaining the HHA or hospice Medicare provider numbers.

Additionally, physicians should provide their UPIN to the HHA or hospice furnishing services to their patient.

NOTE: There is currently no place on the HIPAA standard ASC X12N 837 professional format to specifically include the HHA or hospice provider number required for a care plan oversight claim. For this reason, the requirement to include the HHA or hospice provider number on a care plan oversight claim is temporarily waived until a new version of this electronic standard format is adopted under HIPAA and includes a place to provide the HHA and hospice provider numbers for care plan oversight claims.

100-04, 12, 190.3

List of Medicare Telehealth Services

(Rev. 3476, Issued: 03-11-16, Effective: 01-01-15, Effective: 04-11-16)

The use of a telecommunications system may substitute for an in-person encounter for professional consultations, office visits, office psychiatry services, and a limited number of other physician fee schedule (PFS) services. The various services and corresponding current procedure terminology (CPT) or Healthcare Common Procedure Coding System (HCPCS) codes are listed on the CMS website at www.cms.gov/Medicare/Medicare-General-Information/Telehealth/.

NOTE: Beginning January 1, 2010, CMS eliminated the use of all consultation codes, except for inpatient telehealth consultation G-codes. CMS no longer recognizes office/outpatient or inpatient consultation CPT codes for payment of office/outpatient or inpatient visits. Instead, physicians and practitioners are instructed to bill a new or established patient office/outpatient visit CPT code or appropriate hospital or nursing facility care code, as appropriate to the particular patient, for all office/outpatient or inpatient visits.

100-04, 12, 190.3.4

Payment for ESRD-Related Services as a Telehealth Service

(Rev. 3476, Issued: 03-11-16, Effective: 01-01-15, Effective: 04-11-16)

The ESRD-related services included in the monthly capitation payment (MCP) with 2 or 3 visits per month and ESRD-related services with 4 or more visits per month may be paid as Medicare telehealth services. However, at least 1 visit must be furnished face-to-face "hands on" to examine the vascular access site by a physician, clinical nurse specialist, nurse practitioner, or physician assistant. An interactive audio and video telecommunications system may be used for providing additional visits required under the 2-to-3 visit MCP and the 4-or-more visit MCP. The medical record must indicate that at least one of the visits was furnished face-to-face "hands on" by a physician, clinical nurse specialist, nurse practitioner, or physician assistant.

The MCP physician, for example, the physician or practitioner who is responsible for the complete monthly assessment of the patient and establishes the patient's plan of care, may use other physicians and practitioners to furnish ESRD-related visits

through an interactive audio and video telecommunications system. The non-MCP physician or practitioner must have a relationship with the billing physician or practitioner such as a partner, employees of the same group practice or an employee of the MCP physician, for example, the non MCP physician or practitioner is either a W-2 employee or 1099 independent contractor. However, the physician or practitioner who is responsible for the complete monthly assessment and establishes the ESRD beneficiary's plan of care should bill for the MCP in any given month.

Clinical Criteria

The visit, including a clinical examination of the vascular access site, must be conducted face-to-face "hands on" by a physician, clinical nurse specialist, nurse practitioner or physician's assistant. For additional visits, the physician or practitioner at the distant site is required, at a minimum, to use an interactive audio and video telecommunications system that allows the physician or practitioner to provide medical management services for a maintenance dialysis beneficiary. For example, an ESRD-related visit conducted via telecommunications system must permit the physician or practitioner at the distant site to perform an assessment of whether the dialysis is working effectively and whether the patient is tolerating the procedure well (physiologically and psychologically). During this assessment, the physician or practitioner at the distant site must be able to determine whether alteration in any aspect of the beneficiary's prescription is indicated, due to such changes as the estimate of the patient's dry weight.

100-04, 12, 190.3.5

Payment for Subsequent Hospital Care Services and Subsequent Nursing Facility Care Services as Telehealth Services

(Rev. 3476, Issued: 03-11-16, Effective: 01-01-15, Effective: 04-11-16)

Subsequent hospital care services are limited to one telehealth visit every 3 days. The frequency limit of the benefit is not intended to apply to consulting physicians or practitioners, who should continue to report initial or follow-up inpatient telehealth consultations using the applicable HCPCS G-codes.

Similarly, subsequent nursing facility care services are limited to one telehealth visit every 30 days. Furthermore, subsequent nursing facility care services reported for a Federally-mandated periodic visit under 42 CFR 483.40(c) may not be furnished through telehealth. The frequency limit of the benefit is not intended to apply to consulting physicians or practitioners, who should continue to report initial or follow-up inpatient telehealth consultations using the applicable HCPCS G-codes.

Inpatient telehealth consultations are furnished to beneficiaries in hospitals or skilled nursing facilities via telehealth at the request of the physician of record, the attending physician, or another appropriate source. The physician or practitioner who furnishes the initial inpatient consultation via telehealth cannot be the physician or practitioner of record or the attending physician or practitioner, and the initial inpatient telehealth consultation would be distinct from the care provided by the physician or practitioner of record or the attending physician or practitioner. Counseling and coordination of care with other providers or agencies is included as well, consistent with the nature of the problem(s) and the patient's needs. Initial and follow-up inpatient telehealth consultations are subject to the criteria for inpatient telehealth consultation services, as described in section 190.3 of this chapter.

100-04, 12, 190.3.6

Payment for Diabetes Self-Management Training (DSMT) as a Telehealth Service

(Rev. 3476, Issued: 03-11-16, Effective: 01-01-15, Effective: 04-11-16)

Individual and group DSMT services may be paid as a Medicare telehealth service; however, at least 1 hour of the 10 hour benefit in the year following the initial DSMT service must be furnished in-person to allow for effective injection training. The injection training may be furnished through either individual or group DSMT services. By reporting the –GT or –GQ modifier with HCPCS code G0108 (Diabetes outpatient self-management training services, individual, per 30 minutes) or G0109 (Diabetes outpatient self-management training services, group session (2 or more), per 30 minutes), the distant site practitioner certifies that the beneficiary has received or will receive 1 hour of in-person DSMT services for purposes of injection training during the year following the initial DSMT service.

As specified in 42 CFR 410.141(e) and stated in Pub. 100-02, Medicare Benefit Policy Manual, chapter 15, section 300.2, individual DSMT services may be furnished by a physician, individual, or entity that furnishes other services for which direct Medicare payment may be made and that submits necessary documentation to, and is accredited by, an accreditation organization approved by CMS. However, consistent with the statutory requirements of section 1834(m)(1) of the Act, as provided in 42 CFR 410.78(b)(1) and (b)(2) and stated in section 190.6 of this chapter, Medicare telehealth services, including individual DSMT services furnished as a telehealth service, could only be furnished by a licensed PA, NP, CNS, CNM , clinical psychologist, clinical social worker, or registered dietitian or nutrition professional.

100-04, 12, 190.5

Originating Site Facility Fee Payment Methodology

(Rev. 3476, Issued: 03-11-16, Effective: 01-01-15, Effective: 04-11-16)

1. Originating site defined

The term originating site means the location of an eligible Medicare beneficiary at the time the service being furnished via a telecommunications system occurs. For asynchronous, store and forward telecommunications technologies, an originating site is only a Federal telemedicine demonstration program conducted in Alaska or Hawaii.

2. Facility fee for originating site

The originating site facility fee is a separately billable Part B payment. The contractor pays it outside of other payment methodologies. This fee is subject to post payment verification.

For telehealth services furnished from October 1, 2001, through December 31, 2002, the originating site facility fee was the lesser of $20 or the actual charge. For services furnished on or after January 1 of each subsequent year, the originating site facility fee is updated by the Medicare Economic Index. The updated fee is included in the Medicare Physician Fee Schedule (MPFS) Final Rule, which is published by November 1 prior to the start of the calendar year for which it is effective. The updated fee for each calendar year is also issued annually in a Recurring Update Notification instruction for January of each year.

3. Payment amount:

The originating site facility fee is a separately billable Part B payment. The payment amount to the originating site is the lesser of 80 percent of the actual charge or 80 percent of the originating site facility fee, except CAHs. The beneficiary is responsible for any unmet deductible amount and Medicare coinsurance.

The originating site facility fee payment methodology for each type of facility is clarified below.

Hospital outpatient department. When the originating site is a hospital outpatient department, payment for the originating site facility fee must be made as described above and not under the OPPS. Payment is not based on the OPPS payment methodology.

Hospital inpatient. For hospital inpatients, payment for the originating site facility fee must be made outside the diagnostic related group (DRG) payment, since this is a Part B benefit, similar to other services paid separately from the DRG payment, (e.g., hemophilia blood clotting factor).

Critical access hospitals. When the originating site is a critical access hospital, make payment separately from the cost-based reimbursement methodology. For CAH's, the payment amount is 80 percent of the originating site facility fee.

Federally qualified health centers (FQHCs) and rural health clinics (RHCs). The originating site facility fee for telehealth services is not an FQHC or RHC service. When an FQHC or RHC serves as the originating site, the originating site facility fee must be paid separately from the center or clinic all-inclusive rate.

Physicians' and practitioners' offices. When the originating site is a physician's or practitioner's office, the payment amount, in accordance with the law, is the lesser of 80 percent of the actual charge or 80 percent of the originating site facility fee, regardless of geographic location. The A/B MAC (B) shall not apply the geographic practice cost index (GPCI) to the originating site facility fee. This fee is statutorily set and is not subject to the geographic payment adjustments authorized under the MPFS.

Hospital-based or critical access-hospital based renal dialysis center (or their satellites). When a hospital-based or critical access hospital-based renal dialysis center (or their satellites) serves as the originating site, the originating site facility fee is covered in addition to any composite rate or MCP amount.

Skilled nursing facility (SNF). The originating site facility fee is outside the SNF prospective payment system bundle and, as such, is not subject to SNF consolidated billing. The originating site facility fee is a separately billable Part B payment.

Community Mental Health Center (CMHC). The originating site facility fee is not a partial hospitalization service. The originating site facility fee does not count towards the number of services used to determine payment for partial hospitalization services. The originating site facility fee is not bundled in the per diem payment for partial hospitalization. The originating site facility fee is a separately billable Part B payment.

To receive the originating facility site fee, the provider submits claims with HCPCS code "Q3014, telehealth originating site facility fee"; short description "telehealth facility fee." The type of service for the telehealth originating site facility fee is "9, other items and services." For A/B MAC (B) processed claims, the "office" place of service (code 11) is the only payable setting for code Q3014. There is no participation payment differential for code Q3014. Deductible and coinsurance rules apply to Q3014. By submitting Q3014 HCPCS code, the originating site authenticates they are located in either a rural HPSA or non-MSA county.

This benefit may be billed on bill types 12X, 13X, 22X, 23X, 71X, 72X, 73X, 76X, and 85X. Unless otherwise applicable, report the originating site facility fee under revenue code 078X and include HCPCS code "Q3014, telehealth originating site facility fee."

Hospitals and critical access hospitals bill their A/B/MAC (A) for the originating site facility fee. Telehealth bills originating in inpatient hospitals must be submitted on a 12X TOB using the date of discharge as the line item date of service.

Independent and provider-based RHCs and FQHCs bill the appropriate A/B/MAC (A) using the RHC or FQHC bill type and billing number. HCPCS code Q3014 is the only non-RHC/FQHC service that is billed using the clinic/center bill type and provider number. All RHCs and FQHCs must use revenue code 078X when billing for the originating site facility fee. For all other non-RHC/FQHC services, provider based RHCs and FQHCs must bill using the base provider's bill type and billing number.

Independent RHCs and FQHCs must bill the A/B MAC (B) for all other non-RHC/FQHC services. If an RHC/FQHC visit occurs on the same day as a telehealth service, the RHC/FQHC serving as an originating site must bill for HCPCS code Q3014 telehealth originating site facility fee on a separate revenue line from the RHC/FQHC visit using revenue code 078X.

Hospital-based or CAH-based renal dialysis centers (including satellites) bill their A/B/MAC (A) for the originating site facility fee. Telehealth bills originating in renal dialysis centers must be submitted on a 72X TOB. All hospital-based or CAH-based renal dialysis centers (including satellites) must use revenue code 078X when billing for the originating site facility fee. The renal dialysis center serving as an originating site must bill for HCPCS code Q3014, telehealth originating site facility fee, on a separate revenue line from any other services provided to the beneficiary.

Skilled nursing facilities (SNFs) bill their A/B/MAC (A) for the originating site facility fee. Telehealth bills originating in SNFs must be submitted on TOB 22X or 23X. For SNF inpatients in a covered Part A stay, the originating site facility fee must be submitted on a 22X TOB. All SNFs must use revenue code 078X when billing for the originating site facility fee. The SNF serving as an originating site must bill for HCPCS code Q3014, telehealth originating site facility fee, on a separate revenue line from any other services provided to the beneficiary.

Community mental health centers (CMHCs) bill their A/B/MAC (A) for the originating site facility fee. Telehealth bills originating in CMHCs must be submitted on a 76X TOB. All CMHCs must use revenue code 078X when billing for the originating site facility fee. The CMHC serving as an originating site must bill for HCPCS code Q3014, telehealth originating site facility fee, on a separate revenue line from any other services provided to the beneficiary. Note that Q3014 does not count towards the number of services used to determine per diem payments for partial hospitalization services.

The beneficiary is responsible for any unmet deductible amount and Medicare coinsurance.

100-04, 12, 190.6

Payment Methodology for Physician/Practitioner at the Distant Site

(Rev. 3476, Issued: 03-11-16, Effective: 01-01-15, Effective: 04-11-16)

1. Distant Site Defined

The term "distant site" means the site where the physician or practitioner, providing the professional service, is located at the time the service is provided via a telecommunications system.

2. Payment Amount (professional fee)

The payment amount for the professional service provided via a telecommunications system by the physician or practitioner at the distant site is equal to the current fee schedule amount for the service provided. Payment for an office visit, consultation, individual psychotherapy or pharmacologic management via a telecommunications system should be made at the same amount as when these services are furnished without the use of a telecommunications system. For Medicare payment to occur, the service must be within a practitioner's scope of practice under State law. The beneficiary is responsible for any unmet deductible amount and applicable coinsurance.

3. Medicare Practitioners Who May Receive Payment at the Distant Site (i.e., at a site other than where beneficiary is)

As a condition of Medicare Part B payment for telehealth services, the physician or practitioner at the distant site must be licensed to provide the service under state law. When the physician or practitioner at the distant site is licensed under state law to provide a covered telehealth service (i.e., professional consultation, office and other outpatient visits, individual psychotherapy, and pharmacologic management) then he or she may bill for and receive payment for this service when delivered via a telecommunications system.

If the physician or practitioner at the distant site is located in a CAH that has elected Method II, and the physician or practitioner has reassigned his/her benefits to the CAH, the CAH bills its regular A/B/MAC (A) for the professional services provided at the distant site via a telecommunications system, in any of the revenue codes 096x, 097x or 098x. All requirements for billing distant site telehealth services apply.

4. Medicare Practitioners Who May Bill for Covered Telehealth Services are Listed Below (subject to State law)

- Physician
- Nurse practitioner
- Physician assistant
- Nurse-midwife
- Clinical nurse specialist
- Clinical psychologist*
- Clinical social worker*
- Registered dietitian or nutrition professional
- Certified registered nurse anesthetist

*Clinical psychologists and clinical social workers cannot bill for psychotherapy services that include medical evaluation and management services under Medicare. These practitioners may not bill or receive payment for the following CPT codes: 90805, 90807, and 90809.

100-04, 12, 190.7

A/B MAC (B) Editing of Telehealth Claims

(Rev. 997, Issued: 07-07-06; Effective: 01-01-06; Implementation: 08-07-06)

Medicare telehealth services (as listed in section 190.3) are billed with either the "GT" or "GQ" modifier. The A/B MAC (B) shall approve covered telehealth services if the physician or practitioner is licensed under State law to provide the service. A/B MACs (B) must familiarize themselves with licensure provisions of States for which they process claims and disallow telehealth services furnished by physicians or practitioners who are not authorized to furnish the applicable telehealth service under State law. For example, if a nurse practitioner is not licensed to provide individual psychotherapy under State law, he or she would not be permitted to receive payment for individual psychotherapy under Medicare. The A/B MAC (B) shall install edits to ensure that only properly licensed physicians and practitioners are paid for covered telehealth services.

If an A/B MAC (B) receives claims for professional telehealth services coded with the "GQ" modifier (representing "via asynchronous telecommunications system"), it shall approve/pay for these services only if the physician or practitioner is affiliated with a Federal telemedicine demonstration conducted in Alaska or Hawaii. The A/B MAC (B) may require the physician or practitioner at the distant site to document his or her participation in a Federal telemedicine demonstration program conducted in Alaska or Hawaii prior to paying for telehealth services provided via asynchronous, store and forward technologies.

If a n A/B MAC (B) denies telehealth services because the physician or practitioner may not bill for them, the A/B MAC (B) uses MSN message 21.18: "This item or service is not covered when performed or ordered by this practitioner." The A/B MAC (B) uses remittance advice message 52 when denying the claim based upon MSN message 21.18.

If a service is billed with one of the telehealth modifiers and the procedure code is not designated as a covered telehealth service, the A/B MAC (B) denies the service using MSN message 9.4: "This item or service was denied because information required to make payment was incorrect." The remittance advice message depends on what is incorrect, e.g., B18 if procedure code or modifier is incorrect, 125 for submission billing errors, 4-12 for difference inconsistencies. The A/B MAC (B) uses B18 as the explanation for the denial of the claim.

The only claims from institutional facilities that A/B MACs (A) shall pay for telehealth services at the distant site, except for MNT services, are for physician or practitioner services when the distant site is located in a CAH that has elected Method II, and the physician or practitioner has reassigned his/her benefits to the CAH. The CAH bills its regular A/B MAC (A) for the professional services provided at the distant site via a telecommunications system, in any of the revenue codes 096x, 097x or 098x. All requirements for billing distant site telehealth services apply.

Claims from hospitals or CAHs for MNT services are submitted to the hospital's or CAH's regular A/B MAC (A). Payment is based on the non-facility amount on the Medicare Physician Fee Schedule for the particular HCPCS codes.

100-04, 12, 230

Primary Care Incentive Payment Program (PCIP)

Section 5501(a) of the Affordable Care Act revises Section 1833 of the Social Security Act (the Act) by adding a new paragraph, (x), "Incentive Payments for Primary Care Services." Section 1833(x) of the Act states that in the case of primary care services furnished on or after January 1, 2011, and before January 1, 2016, there shall be a 10 percent incentive payment for such services under Part B when furnished by a primary care practitioner.

Information regarding Primary Care Incentive Payment Program (PCIP) payments made to critical access hospitals (CAHs) paid under the optional method can be found in Pub. 100-4, Chapter 4, §250.12 of this manual.

100-04, 12, 230.1

Definition of Primary Care Practitioners and Primary Care Services

Primary care practitioners are defined as:

1. A physician who has a primary specialty designation of family medicine, internal medicine, geriatric medicine, or pediatric medicine for whom primary care services accounted for at least 60 percent of the allowed charges under Part B for the practitioner in a prior period as determined appropriate by the Secretary; or

2. A nurse practitioner, clinical nurse specialist, or physician assistant for whom primary care services accounted for at least 60 percent of the allowed charges under Part B for the practitioner in a prior period as determined appropriate by the Secretary.

Primary care services are defined as HCPCS Codes:

1. 99201 through 99215 for new and established patient office or outpatient evaluation and management (E/M) visits;

2. 99304 through 99340 for initial, subsequent, discharge, and other nursing facility E/M services; new and established patient domiciliary, rest home or custodial care E/M services; and domiciliary, rest home or home care plan oversight services; and

3. 99341 through 99350 for new and established patient home E/M visits.

Practitioner Identification

Eligible practitioners will be identified on claims by the National Provider Identifier (NPI) number of the rendering practitioner. If the claim is submitted by a practitioner's group practice, the rendering practitioner's NPI must be included on the line-item for the primary care service and reflect an eligible HCPCS as identified. In order to be eligible for the PCIP, physician assistants, clinical nurse specialists, and nurse practitioners must be billing for their services under their own NPI and not furnishing services incident to physicians' services. Regardless of the specialty area in which they may be practicing, the specific nonphysician practitioners are eligible for the PCIP based on their profession and historical percentage of allowed charges as primary care services that equals or exceeds the 60 percent threshold.

Beginning in calendar year (CY) 2011, primary care practitioners will be identified based on their primary specialty of enrollment in Medicare and percentage of allowed charges for primary care services that equals or exceeds the 60 percent threshold from Medicare claims data 2 years prior to the bonus payment year.

Eligible practitioners for PCIP payments in a given calendar year (CY) will be listed by eligible NPI in the Primary Care Incentive Payment Program Eligibility File, available after January 31, of the payment year on their Medicare contractor's website. Practitioners should contact their contractor with any questions regarding their eligibility for the PCIP.

100-04, 12, 230.2

Coordination with Other Payments

Section 5501(a)(3) of the Affordable Care Act provides payment under the PCIP as an additional payment amount for specified primary care services without regard to any additional payment for the service under Section 1833(m) of the Act. Therefore, an eligible primary care physician furnishing a primary care service in a health professional shortage area (HPSA) may receive both a HPSA physician bonus payment (as described in the Medicare Claims Processing Manual, Pub. 100-4, Chapter 12, §90.4) under the HPSA physician bonus program and a PCIP incentive payment under the new program beginning in CY 2011.

100-04, 12, 230.3

Claims Processing and Payment

A. General Overview

Incentive payments will be made on a quarterly basis and shall be equal to 10 percent of the amount paid for such services under the Medicare Physician Fee Schedule (PFS) for those services furnished during the bonus payment year. For information on PCIP payments to CAHs paid under the optional method, see the Medicare Claims Processing Manual, Pub. 100-4, Chapter 4, §250.12.

On an annual basis Medicare contractors shall receive a Primary Care Incentive Payment Program Eligibility File that they shall post to their website. The file will list the NPIs of all practitioners who are eligible to receive PCIP payments for the upcoming CY.

B. Method of Payment

- Calculate and pay qualifying primary care practitioners an additional 10 percent incentive payment;

- Calculate the payment based on the amount actually paid for the services, not the Medicare approved amounts;

- Combine the PCIP incentive payments, when appropriate, with other incentive payments, including the HPSA physician bonus payment, and the HPSA Surgical Incentive Payment Program (HSIP) payment;

- Provide a special remittance form that is forwarded with the incentive payment so that physicians and practitioners can identify which type of incentive payment (HPSA physician and/or PCIP) was paid for which services;

- Practitioners should contact their contractor with any questions regarding PCIP payments.

C. Changes for Contractor Systems

The Medicare Carrier System, (MCS), Common Working File (CWF) and the National Claims History (NCH) shall be modified to accept a new PCIP indicator on the claim line. Once the type of incentive payment has been identified by the shared systems, the shared system shall modify their systems to set the indicator on the claim line as follows:

    1 = HPSA;

    2 = PSA;

    3 = HPSA and PSA;

    4 = HSIP;

    5 = HPSA and HSIP;

    6 = PCIP;

    7 = HPSA and PCIP; and

    Space = Not Applicable.

The contractor shared system shall send the HIGLAS 810 invoice for incentive payment invoices, including the new PCIP payment. The contractor shall also combine the provider's HPSA physician bonus, physician scarcity (PSA) bonus (if it should become available at a later date), HSIP payment and/or PCIP payment invoice per provider. The contractor shall receive the HIGLAS 835 payment file from HIGLAS showing a single incentive payment per provider

100-04, 13, 30.1.3.1

A/B MAC (A) Payment for Low Osmolar Contrast Material (LOCM) (Radiology)

The LOCM is paid on a reasonable cost basis when rendered by a SNF to its Part B patients (in addition to payment for the radiology procedure) when it is used in one of the situations listed below.

The following HCPCS are used when billing for LOCM.

HCPCS Code	Description (January 1. 1994, and later)
A4644	Supply of low osmolar contrast material (100-199 mgs of iodine);
A4645	Supply of low osmolar contrast material (200-299 mgs of iodine); or
A4646	Supply of low osmolar contrast material (300-399 mgs of iodine).

When billing for LOCM, SNFs use revenue code 0636. If the SNF charge for the radiology procedure includes a charge for contrast material, the SNF must adjust the charge for the radiology procedure to exclude any amount for the contrast material.

NOTE: LOCM is never billed with revenue code 0255 or as part of the radiology procedure.

The A/B MAC (A) will edit for the intrathecal procedure codes and the following codes to determine if payment for LOCM is to be made. If an intrathecal procedure code is not present, or one of the ICD codes is not present to indicate that a required medical condition is met, the A/B MAC (A) will deny payment for LOCM. In these instances, LOCM is not covered and should not be billed to Medicare.

When LOCM Is Separately Billable and Related Coding Requirements

* In all intrathecal injections. HCPCS codes that indicate intrathecal injections are:

  70010, 70015, 72240, 72255, 72265, 72270, 72285, 72295

  One of these must be included on the claim; or

* In intravenous and intra-arterial injections only when certain medical conditions are present in an outpatient. The SNF must verify the existence of at least one of the following medical conditions, and report the applicable diagnosis code(s) either as a principal diagnosis code or other diagnosis codes on the claim:

  — A history of previous adverse reaction to contrast material. The applicable ICD-9-CM codes are V14.8 and V14.9. The applicable ICD-10-CM codes are Z88.8 and Z88.9. The conditions which should not be considered adverse reactions are a sensation of heat, flushing, or a single episode of nausea or vomiting. If the adverse reaction occurs on that visit with the induction of contrast material, codes describing hives, urticaria, etc. should also be present, as well as a code describing the external cause of injury and poisoning, ICD-9-CM code E947.8. The applicable ICD-10 CM codes are: T50.8X5A Adverse effect of diagnostic agents, initial encounter, T50.8X5S Adverse effect of diagnostic agents, sequela , T50.995A Adverse effect of other drugs, medicaments and biological substances, initial encounter, or T50.995S Adverse effect of other drugs, medicaments and biological substances, sequela;

  — A history or condition of asthma or allergy. The applicable ICD-9-CM codes are V07.1, V14.0 through V14.9, V15.0, 493.00, 493.01, 493.10, 493.11, 493.20, 493.21, 493.90, 493.91, 495.0, 495.1, 495.2, 495.3, 495.4, 495.5, 495.6, 495.7, 495.8, 495.9, 995.0, 995.1, 995.2, and 995.3. The applicable ICD-10-CM codes are in the table below:

ICD-10-CM Codes

J44.0	J44.9	J45.20	J45.22	J45.30	J45.32	J45.40
J45.42	J45.50	J45.52	J45.902	J45.909	J45.998	J67.0
J67.1	JJ67.2	J67.3	J67.4	J67.5	J67.6	J67.7
J67.8	J67.9	J96.00	J96.01	J96.02	J96.90	J96.91
J96.92	T36.0X5A	T36.1X5A	T36.2X5A	T36.3X5A	T36.4X5A	T36.5X5A
T36.6X5A	T36.7X5A	T36.8X5A	T36.95XA	T37.0X5A	T37.1X5A	T37.2X5A
T37.3X5A	T37.8X5A	T37.95XA	T38.0X5A	T38.1X5A	T38.2X5A	T38.3X5A
T38.4X5A	T38.6X5A	T38.7X5A	T38.805A	T38.815A	T38.895A	T38.905A
T38.995A	T39.015A	T39.095A	T39.1X5A	T39.2X5A	T39.2X5A	T39.315A
T39.395A	T39.4X5A	T39.8X5A	T39.95XA	T40.0X5A	T40.1X5A	T40.2X5A
T40.3X5A	T40.4X5A	T40.5X5A	T40.605A	T40.695A	T40.7X5A	T40.8X5A
T40.905A	T40.995A	T41.0X5A	T41.1X5A	T41.205A	T41.295A	T41.3X5A
T41.4X5A	T41.X5A	T41.5X5A	T42.0X5A	T42.1X5A	T42.2X5A	T42.3X5A
T42.4X5A	T42.5X5A	T42.6X5A	427.5XA	428.X5A	T43.015A	T43.025A
T43.1X5A	T43.205A	T43.215A	T43.225A	T43.295A	T43.3X5A	T43.4X5A
T43.505A	T43.595A	T43.605A	T43.615A	T43.625A	T43.635A	T43.695A
T43.8X5A	T43.95XA	T44.0X5A	T44.1X5A	T44.2X5A	T44.3X5A	T44.6X5A
T44.7X5A	T44.8X5A	T44.905A	T44.995A	T45.0X5A	T45.1X5A	T45.2X5A
T45.3X5A	T45.4X5A	T45.515A	T45.525A	T45.605A	T45.615A	T45.625A

T45.695A	T45.7X5A	T45.8X5A	T45.95XA	T46.0X5A	T46.1X5A	T46.2X5A
T46.3X5A	T46.4X5A	T46.5X5A	T46.6X5A	T46.7X5A	T46.8X5A	T46.905A
T46.995A	T47.0X5A	T47.1X5A	T47.2X5A	T47.3X5A	T47.4X5A	T47.5X5A
T47.6X5A	T47.7X5A	T47.8X5A	T47.95XA	T48.0X5A	T48.1X5A	T48.205A
T48.295A	T48.3X5A	T48.4X5A	T48.5X5A	T48.6X5A	T48.905A	T48.995A
T49.0X5A	T49.1X5A	T49.2X5A	T49.3X5A	T49.4X5A	T49.5X5A	T49.6X5A
T49.6X5A	T47.X5A9	T49.8X5A	T49.95XA	T50.0X5A	T50.1X5A	T50.2X5A
T50.3X5A	T50.4X5A	T50.5X5A	T50.6X5A	T50.7X5A	T50.8X5A	T50.905a
T50.995A	T50.A15A	T50.A25A	T50.A95A	T50.B15A	T50.B95A	T50.Z15A
T50.Z95A	T78.2XXA	T78.3XXA	T78.40XA	T78.41XA	T88.52XA	T88.59XA
T88.6XXA	Z51.89	Z88.0	Z88.1	Z88.2	Z88.3	Z88.4
Z88.5	Z88.6	Z88.7	Z88.8	Z88.9	Z91.010	

— Significant cardiac dysfunction including recent or imminent cardiac decompensation, severe arrhythmia, unstable angina pectoris, recent myocardial infarction, and pulmonary hypertension. The applicable ICD-9-CM codes are:

ICD-9-CM

402.00	402.01	402.10	402.11	402.90	402.91	404.00
404.01	404.02	404.03	404.10	404.11	404.12	404.13
404.90	404.91	404.92	404.93	410.00	410.01	410.02
410.10	410.11	410.12	410.20	410.21	410.22	410.30
410.31	410.32	410.40	410.41	410.42	410.50	410.51
410.52	410.60	410.61	410.62	410.70	410.71	410.72
410.80	410.81	410.82	410.90	410.91	410.92	411.1
415.0	416.0	416.1	416.8	416.9	420.0	420.90
420.91	420.99	424.90	424.91	424.99	427.0	427.1
427.2	427.31	427.32	427.41	427.42	427.5	427.60
427.61	427.69	427.81	427.89	427.9	428.0	428.1
428.9	429.0	429.1	429.2	429.3	429.4	429.5
429.6	429.71	429.79	429.81	429.82	429.89	429.9
785.50	785.51	785.59				

— The applicable ICD-10-CM codes are in the table below:

ICD-10-CM Codes

A18.84	I11.0	I11.9	I13.0	I13.10	I13.11	I13.2
I20.0	I21.01	I21.02	I21.09	I21.11	I21.19	I21.21
I21.29	I21.3	I21.4	I22.1	I22.2	I22.8	I23.0
I23.1	I23.2	I23.3	I23.4	I23.5	I23.6	I23.7
I23.8	I25.10	I25.110	I25.700	I25.710	I25.720	I25.730
I25.750	I25.760	I25.790	I26.01	I26.02	I26.09	I27.0
I27.1	I27.2	I27.81	I27.89	I27.9	I30.0	I30.1
I30.8	I30.9	I32	I38	I39	I46.2	I46.8
I46.9	I47.0	I471	I472	I47.9	I48.0	I48.1
I48.1	I48.2	I48.3	I48.4	I48.91	I48.92	I49.01
I49.02	I49.1	I49.2	I49.3	I49.40	I49.49	I49.5
I49.8	I49.9	I50.1	I50.20	I50.21	I50.22	I50.23
I50.30	I50.31	I50.32	I50.33	I50.40	I50.41	I50.42
I50.43	I50.9	I51	I51.0	I51.1	I51.2	I51.3
I51.4	I51.5	I51.7	I51.89	I51.9	I52	I97.0
I97.110	I97.111	I97.120	I97.121	I97.130	I97.131	I97.190
I97.191	M32.11	M32.12	R00.1	R57.0	R57.8	R57.9

— Generalized severe debilitation. The applicable ICD-9-CM codes are: 203.00, 203.01, all codes for diabetes mellitus, 518.81, 585, 586, 799.3, 799.4, and V46.1. The applicable ICD-10-CM codes are: J96.850, J96.00 through J96.02, J96.90 through J96.91, N18.1 through N19, R53.81, R64, and Z99.11 through Z99.12. Or

— Sickle Cell disease. The applicable ICD-9-CM codes are 282.4, 282.60, 282.61, 282.62, 282.63, and 282.69. The applicable ICD-10-CM codes are D56.0 through D56.3, D56.5 through D56.9, D57.00 through D57.1, D57.20, D57.411 through D57.419, and D57.811 through D57.819.

100-04, 13, 40.1.1

Magnetic Resonance Angiography (MRA) Coverage Summary

Section 1861(s)(2)(C) of the Social Security Act provides for coverage of diagnostic testing. Coverage of magnetic resonance angiography (MRA) of the head and neck, and MRA of the peripheral vessels of the lower extremities is limited as described in Publication (Pub.) 100-3, the Medicare National Coverage Determinations (NCD) Manual. This instruction has been revised as of July 1, 2003, based on a determination that coverage is reasonable and necessary in additional circumstances. Under that instruction, MRA is generally covered only to the extent that it is used as a substitute for contrast angiography, except to the extent that there are documented circumstances consistent with that instruction that demonstrates the medical necessity of both tests. Prior to June 3, 2010, there was no coverage of MRA outside of the indications and circumstances described in that instruction.

Effective for claims with dates of service on or after June 3, 2010, contractors have the discretion to cover or not cover all indications of MRA (and magnetic resonance imaging (MRI)) that are not specifically nationally covered or nationally non-covered as stated in section 220.2 of the NCD Manual.

Because the status codes for HCPCS codes 71555, 71555-TC, 71555-26, 74185, 74185-TC, and 74185-26 were changed in the Medicare Physician Fee Schedule Database from 'N' to 'R' on April 1, 1998, any MRA claims with those HCPCS codes with dates of service between April 1, 1998, and June 30, 1999, are to be processed according to the contractor's discretionary authority to determine payment in the absence of national policy.

Effective for claims with dates of service on or after February 24, 201l, Medicare will provide coverage for MRIs for beneficiaries with implanted cardiac pacemakers or implantable cardioverter defibrillators if the beneficiary is enrolled in an approved clinical study under the Coverage with Study Participation form of Coverage with Evidence Development that meets specific criteria per Pub. 100-3, the NCD Manual, chapter 1, section 220.2.C.1

100-04, 13, 40.1.2

HCPCS Coding Requirements

Providers must report HCPCS codes when submitting claims for MRA of the chest, abdomen, head, neck or peripheral vessels of lower extremities. The following HCPCS codes should be used to report these services:

MRA of head	70544, 70544-26, 70544-TC
MRA of head	70545, 70545-26, 70545-TC
MRA of head	70546, 70546-26, 70546-TC
MRA of neck	70547, 70547-26, 70547-TC
MRA of neck	70548, 70548-26, 70548-TC
MRA of neck	70549, 70549-26, 70549-TC
MRA of chest	71555, 71555-26, 71555-TC
MRA of pelvis	72198, 72198-26, 72198-TC
MRA of abdomen (dates of service on or after July 1, 2003) – see below.	74185, 74185-26, 74185-TC
MRA of peripheral vessels of lower extremities	73725, 73725-26, 73725-TC

100-04, 13, 60

Positron Emission Tomography (PET) Scans - General Information

Positron emission tomography (PET) is a noninvasive imaging procedure that assesses perfusion and the level of metabolic activity in various organ systems of the human body. A positron camera (tomograph) is used to produce cross-sectional tomographic images which are obtained by detecting radioactivity from a radioactive tracer substance radiopharmaceutical) that emits a radioactive tracer substance (radiopharmaceutical FDG) such as 2 -[F-18] flouro-D-glucose FDG, that is administered intravenously to the patient.

The Medicare National Coverage Determinations (NCD) Manual, Chapter 1, Sec.220.6, contains additional coverage instructions to indicate the conditions under which a PET scan is performed.

A. Definitions

For all uses of PET, excluding Rubidium 82 for perfusion of the heart, myocardial viability and refractory seizures, the following definitions apply:

- **Diagnosis:** PET is covered only in clinical situations in which the PET results may assist in avoiding an invasive diagnostic procedure, or in which the PET results may assist in determining the optimal anatomical location to perform an invasive diagnostic procedure. In general, for most solid tumors, a tissue diagnosis is made prior to the performance of PET scanning. PET scans following a tissue diagnosis are generally performed for the purpose of staging, rather than diagnosis. Therefore, the use of PET in the diagnosis of lymphoma, esophageal and colorectal cancers, as well as in melanoma, should be rare. PET is not covered for other diagnostic uses, and is not covered for screening (testing of patients without specific signs and symptoms of disease).

- **Staging:** PET is covered in clinical situations in which (1) (a) the stage of the cancer remains in doubt after completion of a standard diagnostic workup, including conventional imaging (computed tomography, magnetic resonance imaging, or ultrasound) or, (b) the use of PET would also be considered reasonable and necessary if it could potentially replace one or more conventional imaging studies when it is expected that conventional study information is insufficient for the clinical management of the patient and, (2) clinical management of the patient would differ depending on the stage of the cancer identified.

NOTE: Effective for services on or after April 3, 2009, the terms "diagnosis" and "staging" will be replaced with "Initial Treatment Strategy." For further information on this new term, refer to Pub. 100-3, NCD Manual, section 220.6.17.

- **Restaging:** PET will be covered for restaging: (1) after the completion of treatment for the purpose of detecting residual disease, (2) for detecting suspected recurrence, or metastasis, (3) to determine the extent of a known recurrence, or (4) if it could potentially replace one or more conventional imaging studies when it is expected that conventional study information is to determine the extent of a known recurrence, or if study information is insufficient for the clinical management of the patient. Restaging applies to testing after a course of treatment is completed and is covered subject to the conditions above.

- **Monitoring:** Use of PET to monitor tumor response to treatment during the planned course of therapy (i.e., when a change in therapy is anticipated).

NOTE: Effective for services on or after April 3, 2009, the terms "restaging" and "monitoring" will be replaced with "Subsequent Treatment Strategy." For further information on this new term, refer to Pub. 100-3, NCD Manual, section 220.6.17.

B. Limitations

For staging and restaging: PET is covered in either/or both of the following circumstances:

- The stage of the cancer remains in doubt after completion of a standard diagnostic workup, including conventional imaging (computed tomography, magnetic resonance imaging, or ultrasound); and/or

- The clinical management of the patient would differ depending on the stage of the cancer identified. PET will be covered for restaging after the completion of treatment for the purpose of detecting residual disease, for detecting suspected recurrence, or to determine the extent of a known recurrence. Use of PET would also be considered reasonable and necessary if it could potentially replace one or more conventional imaging studies when it is expected that conventional study information is insufficient for the clinical management of the patient.

The PET is not covered for other diagnostic uses, and is not covered for screening (testing of patients without specific symptoms). Use of PET to monitor tumor response during the planned course of therapy (i.e. when no change in therapy is being contemplated) is not covered.

100-04, 13, 60.13

Billing Requirements for PET Scans for Specific Indications of Cervical Cancer for Services Performed on or After January 28, 2005

Contractors shall accept claims for these services with the appropriate CPT code listed in section 60.3.1. Refer to Pub. 100-3, section 220.6.17, for complete coverage guidelines for this new PET oncology indication. The implementation date for these CPT codes will be April 18, 2005. Also see section 60.17, of this chapter for further claims processing instructions for cervical cancer indications.

100-04, 13, 60.15

Billing Requirements for CMS - Approved Clinical Trials and Coverage With Evidence Development Claims for PET Scans for Neurodegenerative Diseases, Previously Specified Cancer Indications, and All Other Cancer Indications Not Previously Specified

A/B MACs (A and B)

Effective for services on or after January 28, 2005, contractors shall accept and pay for claims for Positron Emission Tomography (PET) scans for lung cancer, esophageal cancer, colorectal cancer, lymphoma, melanoma, head & neck cancer, breast cancer, thyroid cancer, soft tissue sarcoma, brain cancer, ovarian cancer, pancreatic cancer, small cell lung cancer, and testicular cancer, as well as for neurodegenerative diseases and all other cancer indications not previously mentioned in this chapter, if these scans were performed as part of a Centers for Medicare & Medicaid (CMS)-approved clinical trial. (See Pub. 100-3, National Coverage Determinations (NCD) Manual, sections 220.6.13 and 220.6.17.)

Contractors shall also be aware that PET scans for all cancers not previously specified at Pub. 100-3, NCD Manual, section 220.6.17, remain nationally non-covered unless performed in conjunction with a CMS-approved clinical trial.

Effective for dates of service on or after June 11, 2013, Medicare has ended the coverage with evidence development (CED) requirement for FDG (2-[F18] fluoro-2-deoxy-D-glucose) PET and PET/computed tomography (CT) and PET/magnetic resonance imaging (MRI) for all oncologic indications contained in section 220.6.17 of the NCD Manual. Modifier -Q0 (Investigational clinical service provided in a clinical research study that is in an approved clinical research study) or -Q1 (routine clinical service

provided in a clinical research study that is in an approved clinical research study) is no longer mandatory for these services when performed on or after June 11, 2013.

A/B MACs (B) Only

A/B MACs (B) shall pay claims for PET scans for beneficiaries participating in a CMS-approved clinical trial submitted with an appropriate current procedural terminology (CPT) code from section 60.3.1 of this chapter and modifier Q0/Q1 for services performed on or after January 1, 2008, through June 10, 2013. (NOTE: Modifier QR (Item or service provided in a Medicare specified study) and QA (FDA investigational device exemption) were replaced by modifier Q0 effective January 1, 2008.) Modifier QV (item or service provided as routine care in a Medicare qualifying clinical trial) was replaced by modifier Q1 effective January 1, 2008.) Beginning with services performed on or after June 11, 2013, modifier Q0/Q1 is no longer required for PET FDG services.

A/B MACs (A) Only

In order to pay claims for PET scans on behalf of beneficiaries participating in a CMS-approved clinical trial, A/B MACs (A) require providers to submit claims with, if ICD-9-CM is applicable, ICD-9 code V70.7; if ICD-10-CM is applicable, ICD-10 code Z00.6 in the primary/secondary diagnosis position using the ASC X12 837 institutional claim format or on Form CMS-1450, with the appropriate principal diagnosis code and an appropriate CPT code from section 60.3.1. Effective for PET scan claims for dates of service on or after January 28, 2005, through December 31, 2007, A/B MACs (A) shall accept claims with the QR, QV, or QA modifier on other than inpatient claims. Effective for services on or after January 1, 2008, through June 10, 2013, modifier Q0 replaced the-QR and QA modifier, modifier Q1 replaced the QV modifier. Modifier Q0/Q1 is no longer required for services performed on or after June 11, 2013.

100-04, 13, 60.16

Billing and Coverage Changes for PET Scans

A. Summary of Changes

Effective for services on or after April 3, 2009, Medicare will not cover the use of FDG PET imaging to determine initial treatment strategy in patients with adenocarcinoma of the prostate.

Medicare will also not cover FDG PET imaging for subsequent treatment strategy for tumor types other than breast, cervical, colorectal, esophagus, head and neck (non-CNS/thyroid), lymphoma, melanoma, myeloma, non-small cell lung, and ovarian, unless the FDG PET is provided under the coverage with evidence development (CED) paradigm (billed with modifier -Q0/-Q1, see section 60.15 of this chapter).

Medicare will cover FDG PET imaging for initial treatment strategy for myeloma.

Effective for services performed on or after June 11, 2013, Medicare has ended the CED requirement for FDG PET and PET/CT and PET/MRI for all oncologic indications contained in section 220.6.17 of the NCD Manual. Effective for services on or after June 11, 2013, the Q0/Q1 modifier is no longer required.

Beginning with services performed on or after June 11, 2013, contractors shall pay for up to three (3) FDG PET scans when used to guide subsequent management of anti-tumor treatment strategy (modifier PS) after completion of initial anti-cancer therapy (modifier PI) for the exact same cancer diagnosis.

Coverage of any additional FDG PET scans (that is, beyond 3) used to guide subsequent management of anti-tumor treatment strategy after completion of initial anti-tumor therapy for the same cancer diagnosis will be determined by the A/B MACs (A or B). Claims will include the KX modifier indicating the coverage criteria is met for coverage of four or more FDG PET scans for subsequent treatment strategy for the same cancer diagnosis under this NCD.

A different cancer diagnosis whether submitted with a PI or a PS modifier will begin the count of one initial and three subsequent FDG PET scans not requiring the KX modifier and four or more FDG PET scans for subsequent treatment strategy for the same cancer diagnosis requiring the KX modifier.

NOTE: The presence or absence of an initial treatment strategy claim in a beneficiary's record does not impact the frequency criteria for subsequent treatment strategy claims for the same cancer diagnosis.

NOTE: Providers please refer to the following link for a list of appropriate diagnosis codes,
http://cms.gov/medicare/coverage/determinationprocess/downloads/petforsolidtumorsoncologicdxcodesattachment_NCD220_6_17.pdf

For further information regarding the changes in coverage, refer to Pub.100-3, NCD Manual, section 220.6.17.

B. Modifiers for PET Scans

Effective for claims with dates of service on or after April 3, 2009, the following modifiers have been created for use to inform for the initial treatment strategy of biopsy-proven or strongly suspected tumors or subsequent treatment strategy of cancerous tumors:

PI Positron Emission Tomography (PET) or PET/Computed Tomography (CT) to inform the initial treatment strategy of tumors that are biopsy proven or strongly suspected of being cancerous based on other diagnostic testing.

Short descriptor: PET tumor init tx strat

PS Positron Emission Tomography (PET) or PET/Computed Tomography (CT) to inform the subsequent treatment strategy of cancerous tumors when the beneficiary's treatment physician determines that the PET study is needed to inform subsequent anti-tumor strategy.

Short descriptor: PS - PET tumor subsq tx strategy

C. Billing for A/B MACs (A and B)

Effective for claims with dates of service on or after April 3, 2009, contractors shall accept FDG PET claims billed to inform initial treatment strategy with the following CPT codes AND modifier PI: 78608, 78811, 78812, 78813, 78814, 78815, 78816.

Effective for claims with dates of service on or after April 3, 2009, contractors shall accept FDG PET claims with modifier PS for the subsequent treatment strategy for solid tumors using a CPT code above AND a cancer diagnosis code.

Contractors shall also accept FDG PET claims billed to inform initial treatment strategy or subsequent treatment strategy when performed under CED with one of the PET or PET/CT CPT codes above AND modifier PI OR modifier PS AND a cancer diagnosis code AND modifier Q0/Q1. Effective for services performed on or after June 11, 2013, the CED requirement has ended and modifier Q0/Q1, along with condition code 30 (institutional claims only), or ICD-9 code V70.7, (both institutional and practitioner claims) are no longer required.

D. Medicare Summary Notices, Remittance Advice Remark Codes, and Claim Adjustment Reason Codes

Effective for dates of service on or after April 3, 2009, contractors shall return as unprocessable/return to provider claims that do not include the PI modifier with one of the PET/PET/CT CPT codes listed in subsection C. above when billing for the initial treatment strategy for solid tumors in accordance with Pub.100-3, NCD Manual, section 220.6.17.

In addition, contractors shall return as unprocessable/return to provider claims that do not include the PS modifier with one of the CPT codes listed in subsection C. above when billing for the subsequent treatment strategy for solid tumors in accordance with Pub.100-3, NCD Manual, section 220.6.17.

The following messages apply:

- Claim Adjustment Reason Code (CARC) 4 - The procedure code is inconsistent with the modifier used or a required modifier is missing.
- Remittance Advice Remark Code (RARC) MA-130 - Your claim contains incomplete and/or invalid information, and no appeal rights are afforded because the claim is unprocessable. Submit a new claim with the complete/correct information.
- RARC M16 - Alert: See our Web site, mailings, or bulletins for more details concerning this policy/procedure/decision.

Effective for claims with dates of service on or after April 3, 2009, through June 10, 2013, contractors shall return as unprocessable/return to provider FDG PET claims billed to inform initial treatment strategy or subsequent treatment strategy when performed under CED without one of the PET/PET/CT CPT codes listed in subsection C. above AND modifier PI OR modifier PS AND a cancer diagnosis code AND modifier Q0/Q1.

The following messages apply to return as unprocessable claims:

- CARC 4 - The procedure code is inconsistent with the modifier used or a required modifier is missing.
- RARC MA-130 - Your claim contains incomplete and/or invalid information, and no appeal rights are afforded because the claim is unprocessable. Submit a new claim with the complete/correct information.
- RARC M16 - Alert: See our Web site, mailings, or bulletins for more details concerning this policy/procedure/decision.

Effective April 3, 2009, contractors shall deny claims with ICD-9/ICD-10 diagnosis code 185/C61 for FDG PET imaging for the initial treatment strategy of patients with adenocarcinoma of the prostate.

For dates of service prior to June 11, 2013, contractors shall also deny claims for FDG PET imaging for subsequent treatment strategy for tumor types other than breast, cervical, colorectal, esophagus, head and neck (non-CNS/thyroid), lymphoma, melanoma, myeloma, non-small cell lung, and ovarian, unless the FDG PET is provided under CED (submitted with the Q0/Q1 modifier) and use the following messages:

- Medicare Summary Notice 15.4 - Medicare does not support the need for this service or item
- CARC 50 - These are non-covered services because this is not deemed a 'medical necessity' by the payer.
- Contractors shall use Group Code CO (Contractual Obligation)

If the service is submitted with a GA modifier indicating there is a signed Advance Beneficiary Notice (ABN) on file, the liability falls to the beneficiary. However, if the service is submitted with a GZ modifier indicating no ABN was provided, the liability falls to the provider.

Effective for dates of service on or after June 11, 2013, contractors shall use the following messages when denying claims in excess of three for PET FDG scans for subsequent treatment strategy when the KX modifier is not included, identified by CPT codes 78608, 78811, 78812, 78813, 78814, 78815, or 78816, modifier PS, HCPCS A9552, and the same cancer diagnosis code.

- CARC 96: "Non-Covered Charge(s). Note: Refer to the 835 Healthcare Policy Identification Segment (loop 2110 Service Payment Information REF), if present."
- RARC N435: "Exceeds number/frequency approved/allowed within time period without support documentation."
- MSN 23.17: "Medicare won't cover these services because they are not considered medically necessary."

Spanish Version: "Medicare no cubrirá estos servicios porque no son considerados necesarios por razones médicas."

Contractors shall use Group Code PR assigning financial liability to the beneficiary, if a claim is received with a GA modifier indicating a signed ABN is on file.

Contractors shall use Group Code CO assigning financial liability to the provider, if a claim is received with a GZ modifier indicating no signed ABN is on file.

100-04, 13, 60.17

Billing and Coverage Changes for PET Scans for Cervical Cancer Effective for Services on or After November 10, 2009

A. Billing Changes for A/B MACs (A and B)
Effective for claims with dates of service on or after November 10, 2009, contractors shall accept FDG PET oncologic claims billed to inform initial treatment strategy; specifically for staging in beneficiaries who have biopsy-proven cervical cancer when the beneficiary's treating physician determines the FDG PET study is needed to determine the location and/or extent of the tumor as specified in Pub. 100-3, section 220.6.17.

EXCEPTION: CMS continues to non-cover FDG PET for initial diagnosis of cervical cancer related to initial treatment strategy.

NOTE: Effective for claims with dates of service on and after November 10, 2009, the –Q0 modifier is no longer necessary for FDG PET for cervical cancer.

B. Medicare Summary Notices, Remittance Advice Remark Codes, and Claim Adjustment Reason Codes
Additionally, contractors shall return as unprocessable /return to provider for FDG PET for cervical cancer for initial treatment strategy billed without the following: one of the PET/PET/ CT CPT codes listed in 60.16 C above AND modifier –PI AND a cervical cancer diagnosis code.

Use the following messages:

- Claim Adjustment Reason Code 4 – the procedure code is inconsistent with the modifier used or a required modifier is missing.

- Remittance Advice Remark Code MA-130 - Your claim contains incomplete and/or invalid information, and no appeal rights are afforded because the claim is unprocessable. Submit a new claim with the complete/correct information.

- Remittance Advice Remark Code M16 - Alert: See our Web site, mailings, or bulletins for more details concerning this policy/procedure/decision.

100-04, 13, 60.18

Billing and Coverage Changes for PET (NaF-18) Scans to Identify Bone Metastasis of Cancer Effective for Claims With Dates of Services on or After February 26, 2010

Billing and Coverage Changes for PET (NaF-18) Scans to Identify Bone Metastasis of Cancer Effective for Claims With Dates of Services on or After February 26, 2010

A. Billing Changes for A/B MACs (A and B)
Effective for claims with dates of service on and after February 26, 2010, contractors shall pay for NaF-18 PET oncologic claims to inform of initial treatment strategy (PI) or subsequent treatment strategy (PS) for suspected or biopsy proven bone metastasis ONLY in the context of a clinical study and as specified in Pub. 100-3, section 220.6. All other claims for NaF-18 PET oncology claims remain non-covered.

B. Medicare Summary Notices, Remittance Advice Remark Codes, and Claim Adjustment Reason Codes
Effective for claims with dates of service on or after February 26, 2010, contractors shall return as unprocessable NaF-18 PET oncologic claims billed with modifier TC or globally (for A/B MACs (A) modifier TC or globally does not apply) and HCPCS A9580 to inform the initial treatment strategy or subsequent treatment strategy for bone metastasis that do not include ALL of the following:

- PI or –PS modifier AND
- PET or PET/CT CPT code (78811, 78812, 78813, 78814, 78815, 78816) AND
- Cancer diagnosis code AND
- Q0 modifier – Investigational clinical service provided in a clinical research study, are present on the claim.

NOTE: For institutional claims, continue to include ICD-9 diagnosis code V70.7 or ICD-10 diagnosis code Z00.6 and condition code 30 to denote a clinical study.

Use the following messages:

- Claim Adjustment Reason Code 4 – The procedure code is inconsistent with the modifier used or a required modifier is missing. Note: Refer to the 835 Healthcare Policy Identification Segment (loop 2110 Service Payment Information REF), if present.

- Remittance Advice Remark Code MA-130 - Your claim contains incomplete and/or invalid information, and no appeal rights are afforded because the claim is unprocessable. Submit a new claim with the complete/correct information.

- Remittance Advice Remark Code M16 - Alert: See our Web site, mailings, or bulletins for more details concerning this policy/procedure/decision.

- Claim Adjustment Reason Code 167 – This (these) diagnosis(es) is (are) not covered.

Effective for claims with dates of service on or after February 26, 2010, contractors shall accept PET oncologic claims billed with modifier 26 and modifier KX to inform the initial treatment strategy or strategy or subsequent treatment strategy for bone metastasis that include the following:

- PI or –PS modifier AND
- PET or PET/CT CPT code (78811, 78812, 78813, 78814, 78815, 78816) AND
- Cancer diagnosis code AND
- Q0 modifier – Investigational clinical service provided in a clinical research study, are present on the claim.

NOTE: If modifier KX is present on the professional component service, Contractors shall process the service as PET NaF-18 rather than PET with FDG.

Contractors shall also return as unprocessable NaF-18 PET oncologic professional component claims (i.e., claims billed with modifiers 26 and KX) to inform the initial treatment strategy or strategy or subsequent treatment strategy for bone metastasis billed with HCPCS A9580 and use the following message:

Claim Adjustment Reason Code 97 – The benefit for this service is included in the payment/allowance for another service/procedure that has already been adjudicated.

NOTE: Refer to the 835 Healthcare Policy identification Segment (loop 2110 Service Payment Information REF), if present.

100-04, 13, 60.2

Use of Gamma Cameras and Full Ring and Partial Ring PET Scanners for PET Scans

See the Medicare NCD Manual, Section 220.6, concerning 2-[F-18] Fluoro-D-Glucose (FDG) PET scanners and details about coverage.

On July 1, 2001, HCPCS codes G0210 - G0230 were added to allow billing for all currently covered indications for FDG PET. Although the codes do not indicate the type of PET scanner, these codes were used until January 1, 2002, by providers to bill for services in a manner consistent with the coverage policy.

Effective January 1, 2002, HCPCS codes G0210 - G0230 were updated with new descriptors to properly reflect the type of PET scanner used. In addition, four new HCPCS codes became effective for dates of service on and after January 1, 2002, (G0231, G0232, G0233, G0234) for covered conditions that may be billed if a gamma camera is used for the PET scan. For services performed from January 1, 2002, through January 27, 2005, providers should bill using the revised HCPCS codes G0210 - G0234.

Beginning January 28, 2005 providers should bill using the appropriate CPT code.

100-04, 13, 60.3

PET Scan Qualifying Conditions and HCPCS Code Chart
Below is a summary of all covered PET scan conditions, with effective dates.

NOTE: The G codes below except those a # can be used to bill for PET Scan services through January 27, 2005. Effective for dates of service on or after January 28, 2005, providers must bill for PET Scan services using the appropriate CPT codes. See section 60.3.1. The G codes with a # can continue to be used for billing after January 28, 2005 and these remain non-covered by Medicare. (NOTE: PET Scanners must be FDA-approved.)

Conditions	Coverage Effective Date	**** HCPCS/CPT
*Myocardial perfusion imaging (following previous PET G0030-G0047) single study, rest or stress (exercise and/or pharmacologic)	3/14/95	G0030
*Myocardial perfusion imaging (following previous PET G0030-G0047) multiple studies, rest or stress (exercise and/or pharmacologic)	3/14/95	G0031
*Myocardial perfusion imaging (following rest SPECT, 78464); single study, rest or stress (exercise and/or pharmacologic)	3/14/95	G0032
*Myocardial perfusion imaging (following rest SPECT 78464); multiple studies, rest or stress (exercise and/or pharmacologic)	3/14/95	G0033
*Myocardial perfusion (following stress SPECT 78465); single study, rest or stress (exercise and/or pharmacologic)	3/14/95	G0034
*Myocardial Perfusion Imaging (following stress SPECT 78465); multiple studies, rest or stress (exercise and/or pharmacologic)	3/14/95	G0035
*Myocardial Perfusion Imaging (following coronary angiography 93510-93529); single study, rest or stress (exercise and/or pharmacologic)	3/14/95	G0036
*Myocardial Perfusion Imaging, (following coronary angiography), 93510-93529); multiple studies, rest or stress (exercise and/or pharmacologic)	3/14/95	G0037
*Myocardial Perfusion Imaging (following stress planar myocardial perfusion, 78460); single study, rest or stress (exercise and/or pharmacologic)	3/14/95	G0038

Conditions	Coverage Effective Date	****HCPCS/CPT
*Myocardial Perfusion Imaging (following stress planar myocardial perfusion, 78460); multiple studies, rest or stress (exercise and/or pharmacologic)	3/14/95	G0039
*Myocardial Perfusion Imaging (following stress echocardiogram 93350); single study, rest or stress (exercise and/or pharmacologic)	3/14/95	G0040
*Myocardial Perfusion Imaging (following stress echocardiogram, 93350); multiple studies, rest or stress (exercise and/or pharmacologic)	3/14/95	G0041
*Myocardial Perfusion Imaging (following stress nuclear ventriculogram 78481 or 78483); single study, rest or stress (exercise and/or pharmacologic)	3/14/95	G0042
*Myocardial Perfusion Imaging (following stress nuclear ventriculogram 78481 or 78483); multiple studies, rest or stress (exercise and/or pharmacologic)	3/14/95	G0043
*Myocardial Perfusion Imaging (following stress ECG, 93000); single study, rest or stress (exercise and/or pharmacologic)	3/14/95	G0044
*Myocardial perfusion (following stress ECG, 93000), multiple studies; rest or stress (exercise and/or pharmacologic)	3/14/95	G0045
*Myocardial perfusion (following stress ECG, 93015), single study; rest or stress (exercise and/or pharmacologic)	3/14/95	G0046
*Myocardial perfusion (following stress ECG, 93015); multiple studies, rest or stress (exercise and/or pharmacologic)	3/14/95	G0047
PET imaging regional or whole body; single pulmonary nodule	1/1/98	G0125
Lung cancer, non-small cell (PET imaging whole body) Diagnosis, Initial Staging, Restaging	7/1/01	G0210 G0211 G0212
Colorectal cancer (PET imaging whole body) Diagnosis, Initial Staging, Restaging	7/1/01	G0213 G0214 G0215
Melanoma (PET imaging whole body) Diagnosis, Initial Staging, Restaging	7/1/01	G0216 G0217 G0218
Melanoma for non-covered indications	7/1/01	#G0219
Lymphoma (PET imaging whole body) Diagnosis, Initial Staging, Restaging	7/1/01	G0220 G0221 G0222
Head and neck cancer; excluding thyroid and CNS cancers (PET imaging whole body or regional) Diagnosis, Initial Staging, Restaging	7/1/01	G0223 G0224 G0225
Esophageal cancer (PET imaging whole body) Diagnosis, Initial Staging, Restaging	7/1/01	G0226 G0227 G0228
Metabolic brain imaging for pre-surgical evaluation of refractory seizures	7/1/01	G0229
Metabolic assessment for myocardial viability following inconclusive SPECT study	7/1/01	G0230
Recurrence of colorectal or colorectal metastatic cancer (PET whole body, gamma cameras only)	1/1/02	G0231
Staging and characterization of lymphoma (PET whole body, gamma cameras only)	1/1/02	G0232
Recurrence of melanoma or melanoma metastatic cancer (PET whole body, gamma cameras only)	1/1/02	G0233
Regional or whole body, for solitary pulmonary nodule following CT, or for initial staging of nonsmall cell lung cancer (gamma cameras only)	1/1/02	G0234
Non-Covered Service PET imaging, any site not otherwise specified	1/28/05	#G0235

Conditions	Coverage Effective Date	****HCPCS/CPT
Non-Covered Service Initial diagnosis of breast cancer and/or surgical planning for breast cancer (e.g., initial staging of axillary lymph nodes), not covered (full- and partialring PET scanners only)	10/1/02	#G0252
Breast cancer, staging/restaging of local regional recurrence or distant metastases, i.e., staging/restaging after or prior to course of treatment (full- and partial-ring PET scanners only)	10/1/02	G0253
Breast cancer, evaluation of responses to treatment, performed during course of treatment (full- and partial-ring PET scanners only)	10/1/02	G0254
Myocardial imaging, positron emission tomography (PET), metabolic evaluation	10/1/02	78459
Restaging or previously treated thyroid cancer of follicular cell origin following negative I-131 whole body scan (full- and partial-ring PET scanner only)	10/1/03	G0296
Tracer Rubidium**82 (Supply of Radiopharmaceutical Diagnostic Imaging Agent) (This is only billed through Outpatient Perspective Payment System, OPPS.) (Carriers must use HCPCS Code A4641.)	10/1/03	Q3000
Supply of Radiopharmaceutical Diagnostic Imaging Agent, Ammonia N-13	01/1/04	A9526
PET imaging, brain imaging for the differential diagnosis of Alzheimer's disease with aberrant features vs. fronto-temporal dementia	09/15/04	Appropriate CPT Code from section 60.3.1
PET Cervical Cancer Staging as adjunct to conventional imaging, other staging, diagnosis, restaging, monitoring	1/28/05	Appropriate CPT Code from section 60.3.1

*   NOTE: Carriers must report A4641 for the tracer Rubidium 82 when used with PET scan codes G0030 through G0047 for services performed on or before January 27, 2005

**   NOTE: Not FDG PET

***   NOTE: For dates of service October 1, 2003, through December 31, 2003, use temporary code Q4078 for billing this radiopharmaceutical.

100-04, 13, 60.3.1

Appropriate CPT Codes Effective for PET Scans for Services Performed on or After January 28, 2005

NOTE: All PET scan services require the use of a radiopharmaceutical diagnostic imaging agent (tracer). The applicable tracer code should be billed when billing for a PET scan service. See section 60.3.2 below for applicable tracer codes.

CPT Code	Description
78459	Myocardial imaging, positron emission tomography (PET), metabolic evaluation
78491	Myocardial imaging, positron emission tomography (PET), perfusion, single study at rest or stress
78492	Myocardial imaging, positron emission tomography (PET), perfusion, multiple studies at rest and/or stress
78608	Brain imaging, positron emission tomography (PET); metabolic evaluation
78811	Tumor imaging, positron emission tomography (PET); limited area (eg, chest, head/neck)
78812	Tumor imaging, positron emission tomography (PET); skull base to mid-thigh
78813	Tumor imaging, positron emission tomography (PET); whole body
78814	Tumor imaging, positron emission tomography (PET) with concurrently acquired computed tomography (CT) for attenuation correction and anatomical localization; limited area (eg, chest, head/neck)
78815	Tumor imaging, positron emission tomography (PET) with concurrently acquired computed tomography (CT) for attenuation correction and anatomical localization; skull base to mid-thigh
78816	Tumor imaging, positron emission tomography (PET) with concurrently acquired computed tomography (CT) for attenuation correction and anatomical localization; whole body

100-04, 13, 60.3.2

Tracer Codes Required for PET Scans

The following tracer codes are applicable only to CPT 78491 and 78492. They can not be reported with any other code.

Institutional providers billing the fiscal intermediary

HCPCS	Description
*A9555	Rubidium Rb-82, Diagnostic, Per study dose, Up To 60 Millicuries
* Q3000 (Deleted effective 12/31/05)	Supply of Radiopharmaceutical Diagnostic Imaging Agent, Rubidium Rb-82, per dose
A9526	Nitrogen N-13 Ammonia, Diagnostic, Per study dose, Up To 40 Millicuries

* NOTE: For claims with dates of service prior to 1/01/06, providers report Q3000 for supply of radiopharmaceutical diagnostic imaging agent, Rubidium Rb-82. For claims with dates of service 1/01/06 and later, providers report A9555 for radiopharmaceutical diagnostic imaging agent, Rubidium Rb-82 in place of Q3000.

Physicians / practitioners billing the carrier:

*A4641	Supply of Radiopharmaceutical Diagnostic Imaging Agent, Not Otherwise Classified
A9526	Nitrogen N-13 Ammonia, Diagnostic, Per study dose, Up To 40 Millicuries
A9555	Rubidium Rb-82, Diagnostic, Per study dose, Up To 60 Millicuries

* NOTE: Effective January 1, 2008, tracer code A4641 is not applicable for PET Scans.

The following tracer codes are applicable only to CPT 78459, 78608, 78811-78816. They can not be reported with any other code:

Institutional providers billing the fiscal intermediary:

* A9552	Fluorodeoxyglucose F18, FDG, Diagnostic, Per study dose, Up to 45 Millicuries
* C1775 (Deleted effective 12/31/05)	Supply of Radiopharmaceutical Diagnostic Imaging Agent, Fluorodeoxyglucose F18, (2-Deoxy-2-18F Fluoro-D-Glucose), Per dose (4-40 Mci/Ml)
**A4641	Supply of Radiopharmaceutical Diagnostic Imaging Agent, Not Otherwise Classified
A9580	Sodium Fluoride F-18, Diagnostic, per study dose, up to 30 Millicuries

* NOTE: For claims with dates of service prior to 1/01/06, OPPS hospitals report C1775 for supply of radiopharmaceutical diagnostic imaging agent, Fluorodeoxyglucose F18. For claims with dates of service January 1, 2006 and later, providers report A9552 for radiopharmaceutical diagnostic imaging agent, Fluorodeoxyglucose F18 in place of C1775.
** NOTE: Effective January 1, 2008, tracer code A4641 is not applicable for PET Scans.
*** NOTE: Effective for claims with dates of service February 26, 2010 and later, tracer code A9580 is applicable for PET Scans.

Physicians / practitioners billing the carrier:

A9552	Fluorodeoxyglucose F18, FDG, Diagnostic, Per study dose, Up to 45 Millicuries
*A4641	Supply of Radiopharmaceutical Diagnostic Imaging Agent, Not Otherwise Classified
A9580	Sodium Fluoride F-18, Diagnostic, per study dose, up to 30 Millicuries

* NOTE: Effective January 1, 2008, tracer code A4641 is not applicable for PET Scans.
*** NOTE: Effective for claims with dates of service February 26, 2010 and later, tracer code A9580 is applicable for PET Scans.

Positron Emission Tomography Reference Table

CPT	Short Descriptor	Tracer/ Code	or	Tracer/ Code	Comment
78459	Myocardial imaging, positron emission tomography (PET), metabolic imaging	FDG A9552	--	--	N/A
78491	Myocardial imaging, positron emission tomography (PET), perfusion; single study at rest or stress	N-13 A9526	or	Rb-82 A9555	N/A
78492	Myocardial imaging, positron emission tomography (PET), perfusion; multiple studies at rest and/or stress	N-13 A9526	or	Rb-82 A9555	N/A
78608	Brain imaging, positron emission tomography (PET); metabolic evaluation	FDG A9552	--	--	Covered indications: Alzheimer's disease/dementias, intractable seizures. Note: This code is also covered for dedicated PET brain tumor imaging.
78609	Brain imaging, positron emission tomography (PET); perfusion evaluation	--	--	--	Nationally noncovered
78811	Positron emission tomography (PET) imaging; limited area (e.g, chest, head/neck)	FDG A9552	or	NaF-18 A9580	NaF-18 PET is covered only to identify bone metastasis of cancer.
78812	Positron emission tomography (PET) imaging, skull base to mid-thigh	FDG A9552	or	NaF-18 A9580	NaF-18 PET is covered only to identify bone metastasis of cancer.
78813	Positron emission tomography (PET) imaging, whole body	FDG A9552	or	NaF-18 A9580	NaF-18 PET is covered only to identify bone metastasis of cancer.
78814	PET/CT imaging, limited area (e.g., chest, head/neck)	FDG A9552	or	NaF-18 A9580	NaF-18 PET is covered only to identify bone metastasis of cancer.
78815	PET/CT imaging skull base to mid-thigh	FDG A9552	or	NaF-18 A9580	NaF-18 PET is covered only to identify bone metastasis of cancer.
78816	PET/CT imaging, whole body	FDG A9552	or	NaF-18 A9580	NaF-18 PET is covered only to identify bone metastasis of cancer.

100-04, 13, 70.3

Radiation Treatment Delivery (CPT 77401 - 77417)

Carriers pay for these TC services on a daily basis under CPT codes 77401-77416 for radiation treatment delivery. They do not use local codes and RVUs in paying for the TC of radiation oncology services. Multiple treatment sessions on the same day are payable as long as there has been a distinct break in therapy services, and the individual sessions are of the character usually furnished on different days. Carriers pay for CPT code 77417 (Therapeutic radiology port film(s)) on a weekly (five fractions) basis.

100-04, 13, 70.4

Clinical Brachytherapy (CPT Codes 77750 - 77799)

Carriers must apply the bundled services policy to procedures in this family of codes other than CPT code 77776. For procedures furnished in settings in which TC payments are made, carriers must pay separately for the expendable source associated with these procedures under CPT code 79900 except in the case of remote after-loading high intensity brachytherapy procedures (CPT codes 77781-77784). In the four codes cited, the expendable source is included in the RVUs for the TC of the procedures.

100-04, 13, 70.5

Radiation Physics Services (CPT Codes 77300 - 77399)

Carriers pay for the PC and TC of CPT codes 77300-77334 and 77399 on the same basis as they pay for radiologic services generally. For professional component billings in all settings, carriers presume that the radiologist participated in the provision of the service, e.g., reviewed/validated the physicist's calculation. CPT codes 77336 and 77370 are technical services only codes that are payable by carriers in settings in which only technical component is are payable.

100-04, 13, 80.1

Physician Presence

Radiologic supervision and interpretation (S&I) codes are used to describe the personal supervision of the performance of the radiologic portion of a procedure by one or more physicians and the interpretation of the findings. In order to bill for the supervision aspect of the procedure, the physician must be present during its performance. This kind of personal supervision of the performance of the procedure is a service to an individual beneficiary and differs from the type of general supervision of the radiologic procedures performed in a hospital for which FIs pay the costs as physician services to the hospital. The interpretation of the procedure may be performed later by another physician. In situations in which a cardiologist, for example, bills for the supervision (the "S") of the S&I code, and a radiologist bills for the interpretation (the "I") of the code, both physicians should use a "-52" modifier indicating a reduced service, e.g., only one of supervision and/or interpretation. Payment for the fragmented S&I code is no more than if a single physician furnished both aspects of the procedure.

100-04, 13, 80.2

Multiple Procedure Reduction

Carriers make no multiple procedure reductions in the S&I or primary non-radiologic codes in these types of procedures, or in any procedure codes for which the descriptor and RVUs reflect a multiple service reduction. For additional procedure codes that do not reflect such a reduction, carriers apply the multiple procedure reductions.

100-04, 16, 40.6.1

Automated Multi-Channel Chemistry (AMCC) Tests for ESRD Beneficiaries

Instructions for Services Provided on and After January 1, 2011

Section 153b of the MIPPA requires that all ESRD-related laboratory tests must be reported by the ESRD facility whether provided directly or under arrangements with an independent laboratory. When laboratory services are billed by providers other than the ESRD facility and the laboratory test furnished is designated as a laboratory test that is included in the ESRD PPS (ESRD-related), the claim will be rejected or denied. In the event that an ESRD-related laboratory test was furnished to an ESRD beneficiary for reasons other than for the treatment of ESRD, the provider may submit a claim for separate payment using modifier AY. The AY modifier serves as an attestation that the item or service is medically necessary for the dialysis patient but is not being used for the treatment of ESRD. The items and services subject to consolidated billing located on the CMS website includes the list of ESRD-related laboratory tests that are routinely performed for the treatment of ESRD.

For services provided on or after January 1, 2011, the 50/50 rule no longer applies to independent laboratory claims for AMCC tests furnished to ESRD beneficiaries. The 50/50 rule modifiers (CD, CE, and CF) are no longer required for independent laboratories effective for dates of service on and after January 1, 2011. However, for services provided between January 1, 2011 and March 31, 2015, the 50/50 rule modifiers are still required for use by ESRD facilities that are receiving the transitional blended payment amount (the transition ends in CY 2014). For services provided on or after April 1, 2015, the 50/50 rule modifiers are no longer required for use by ESRD facilities.

Effective for dates of service on and after January 1, 2012, contractors shall allow organ disease panel codes (i.e., HCPCS codes 80047, 80048, 80051, 80053, 80061, 80069, and 80076) to be billed by independent laboratories for AMCC panel tests furnished to ESRD eligible beneficiaries if:

- The beneficiary is not receiving dialysis treatment for any reason (e.g., post-transplant beneficiaries), or
- The test is not related to the treatment of ESRD, in which case the supplier would append modifier "AY".

Contractors shall make payment for organ disease panels according to the Clinical Laboratory Fee Schedule and shall apply the normal ESRD PPS editing rules for independent laboratory claims. The aforementioned organ disease panel codes were added to the list of bundled ESRD PPS laboratory tests in January 2012.

Effective for dates of service on and after April 1, 2015, contractors shall allow organ disease panel codes (i.e., HCPCS codes 80047, 80048, 80051, 80053, 80061, 80069, and 80076) to be billed by ESRD facilities for AMCC panel tests furnished to ESRD eligible beneficiaries if:

- These codes best describe the laboratory services provided to the beneficiary, which are paid under the ESRD PPS, or
- The test is not related to the treatment of ESRD, in which case the ESRD facility would append modifier "AY" and the service may be paid separately from the ESRD PPS.

Instructions for Services Provided Prior to January 1, 2011

For claims with dates of service prior to January 1, 2011, Medicare will apply the following rules to Automated Multi-Channel Chemistry (AMCC) tests for ESRD beneficiaries:

- Payment is at the lowest rate for tests performed by the same provider, for the same beneficiary, for the same date of service.
- The facility/laboratory must identify, for a particular date of service, the AMCC tests ordered that are included in the composite rate and those that are not included. See Publication 100-2, Chapter 11, Section 30.2.2 for the chart detailing the composite rate tests for Hemodialysis, Intermittent Peritoneal Dialysis (IPD), Continuous Cycling Peritoneal Dialysis (CCPD), and Hemofiltration as well as a second chart detailing the composite rate tests for Continuous Ambulatory Peritoneal Dialysis (CAPD).
- If 50 percent or more of the covered tests are included under the composite rate payment, then all submitted tests are included within the composite payment. In this case, no separate payment in addition to the composite rate is made for any of the separately billable tests.
- If less than 50 percent of the covered tests are composite rate tests, all AMCC tests submitted for that Date of Service (DOS) for that beneficiary are separately payable.
- A noncomposite rate test is defined as any test separately payable outside of the composite rate or beyond the normal frequency covered under the composite rate that is reasonable and necessary.
- For carrier processed claims, all chemistries ordered for beneficiaries with chronic dialysis for ESRD must be billed individually and must be rejected when billed as a panel.

(See §100.6UH for details regarding pricing modifiers.)

Implementation of this Policy:

ESRD facilities when ordering an ESRD-related AMCC must specify for each test within the AMCC whether the test:

a. Is part of the composite rate and not separately payable;

b. Is a composite rate test but is, on the date of the order, beyond the frequency covered under the composite rate and thus separately payable; or

c. Is not part of the ESRD composite rate and thus separately payable.

Laboratories must:

a. Identify which tests, if any, are not included within the ESRD facility composite rate payment

b. Identify which tests ordered for chronic dialysis for ESRD as follows:

   1) Modifier CD: AMCC Test has been ordered by an ESRD facility or MCP physician that is part of the composite rate and is not separately billable.

   2) Modifier CE: AMCC Test has been ordered by an ESRD facility or MCP physician that is a composite rate test but is beyond the normal frequency covered under the rate and is separately reimbursable based on medical necessity.

   3) Modifier CF: AMCC Test has been ordered by an ESRD facility or MCP physician that is not part of the composite rate and is separately billable.

c. Bill all tests ordered for a chronic dialysis ESRD beneficiary individually and not as a panel.

The shared system must calculate the number of AMCC tests provided for any given date of service. Sum all AMCC tests with a CD modifier and divide the sum of all tests with a CD, CE, and CF modifier for the same beneficiary and provider for any given date of service.

If the result of the calculation for a date of service is 50 percent or greater, do not pay for the tests.

If the result of the calculation for a date of service is less than 50 percent, pay for all of the tests.

For FI processed claims, all tests for a date of service must be billed on the monthly ESRD bill. Providers that submit claims to a FI must send in an adjustment if they identify additional tests that have not been billed.

Carrier standard systems shall adjust the previous claim when the incoming claim for a date of service is compared to a claim on history and the action is adjust payment. Carrier standard systems shall spread the payment amount over each line item on both claims (the claim on history and the incoming claim).

The organ and disease oriented panels (80048, 80051, 80053, and 80076) are subject to the 50 percent rule. However, clinical diagnostic laboratories shall not bill these services as panels, they must be billed individually. Laboratory tests that are not covered under the composite rate and that are furnished to CAPD end stage renal disease (ESRD) patients dialyzing at home are billed in the same way as any other test furnished home patients.

FI Business Requirements for ESRD Reimbursement of AMCC Tests:

Requirement #	Requirements	Responsibility
1.1	The FI shared system must RTP a claim for AMCC tests when a claim for that date of service has already been submitted.	Shared system

Requirement #	Requirements	Responsibility
1.2	Based upon the presence of the CD, CE and CF payment modifiers, identify the AMCC tests ordered that are included and not included in the composite rate payment.	Shared System
1.3	Based upon the determination of requirement 1.2, if 50 percent or more of the covered tests are included under the composite rate, no separate payment is made.	Shared System
1.4	Based upon the determination of requirement 1.2, if less than 50 percent are covered tests included under the composite rate, all AMCC tests for that date of service are payable.	Shared System
1.5	Effective for claims with dates of service on or after January 1, 2006, include any line items with a modifier 91 used in conjunction with the "CD," "CE," or "CF" modifier in the calculation of the 50/50 rule.	Shared System
1.6	FIs must return any claims for additional tests for any date of service within the billing period when the provider has already submitted a claim. Instruct the provider to adjust the first claim.	FI or Shared System
1.7	After the calculation of the 50/50 rule, services used to determine the payment amount may never exceed 22. Effective for claims with dates of service on or after January 1, 2006, accept all valid line items submitted for the date of service and pay a maximum of the ATP 22 rate.	Shared System

Carrier Business Requirements for ESRD Reimbursement of AMCC Tests:

Requirement #	Requirements	Responsibility
1	The standard systems shall calculate payment at the lowest rate for these automated tests even if reported on separate claims for services performed by the same provider, for the same beneficiary, for the same date of service.	Standard Systems
2	Standard Systems shall identify the AMCC tests ordered that are included and are not included in the composite rate payment based upon the presence of the "CD," "CE" and "CF" modifiers.	Standard Systems
3	Based upon the determination of requirement 2 if 50 percent or more of the covered services are included under the composite rate payment, Standard Systems shall indicate that no separate payment is provided for the services submitted for that date of service.	Standard Systems
4	Based upon the determination of requirement 2 if less than 50 percent are covered services included under the composite rate, Standard Systems shall indicate that all AMCC tests for that date of service are payable under the 50/50 rule.	Standard Systems
5	Effective for claims with dates of service on or after January 1, 2006, include any line items with a modifier 91 used in conjunction with the "CD," "CE," or "CF" modifier in the calculation of the 50/50 rule.	Standard Systems
6	Standard Systems shall adjust the previous claim when the incoming claim is compared to the claim on history and the action is to deny the previous claim. Spread the payment amount over each line item on both claims (the adjusted claim and the incoming claim).	Standard Systems
7	Standard Systems shall spread the adjustment across the incoming claim unless the adjusted amount would exceed the submitted amount of the services on the claim.	Standard System
8	After the calculation of the 50/50 rule, services used to determine the payment amount may never exceed 22. Accept all valid line items for the date of service and pay a maximum of the ATP 22 rate.	Standard Systems

Examples of the Application of the 50/50 Rule

The following examples are to illustrate how claims should be paid. The percentages in the action section represent the number of composite rate tests over the total tests. If this percentage is 50 percent or greater, no payment should be made for the claim.

Example 1:
Provider Name: Jones Hospital
DOS 2/1/02

Claim/Services
82040 Mod CD
82310 Mod CD
82374 Mod CD
82435 Mod CD
82947 Mod CF
84295 Mod CF
82040 Mod CD (Returned as duplicate)
84075 Mod CE
82310 Mod CE
84155 Mod CE

ACTION: 9 services total, 2 non-composite rate tests, 3 composite rate tests beyond the frequency, 4 composite rate tests; 4/9 = 44.4%<50% pay at ATP 09

Example 2:
Provider Name: Bon Secours Renal Facility
DOS 2/15/02

Claim/Services
82040 Mod CE and Mod 91
84450 Mod CE
82310 Mod CE
82247 Mod CF
82465 No modifier present
82565 Mod CE
84550 Mod CF
82040 Mod CD
84075 Mod CE
82435 Mod CE
82550 Mod CF
82947 Mod CF
82977 Mod CF

ACTION: 12 services total, 5 non-composite rate tests, 6 composite rate tests beyond the frequency, 1 composite rate test; 1/12 = 8.3%<50% pay at ATP 12

Example 3:
Provider Name: Sinai Hospital Renal Facility
DOS 4/02/02

Claim/Services
82565 Mod CD
83615 Mod CD
82247 Mod CF
82248 Mod CF
82040 Mod CD
84450 Mod CD
82565 Mod CE

100-04, 16, 70.8

Certificate of Waiver

Effective September 1, 1992, all laboratory testing sites (except as provided in 42 CFR 493.3(b)) must have either a CLIA certificate of waiver, certificate for provider-performed microscopy procedures, certificate of registration, certificate of compliance, or certificate of accreditation to legally perform clinical laboratory testing on specimens from individuals in the United States.

The Food and Drug Administration approves CLIA waived tests on a flow basis. The CMS identifies CLIA waived tests by providing an updated list of waived tests to the Medicare contractors on a quarterly basis via a Recurring Update Notification. To be recognized as a waived test, some CLIA waived tests have unique HCPCS procedure codes and some must have a QW modifier included with the HCPCS code.

For a list of specific HCPCS codes subject to CLIA see

http://www.cms.hhs.gov/CLIA/downloads/waivetbl.pdf

100-04, 18, 10.2.2.1

FI Payment for Pneumococcal Pneumonia Virus, Influenza Virus, and Hepatitis B Virus Vaccines and Their Administration
Payment for Vaccines

Payment for all of these vaccines is on a reasonable cost basis for hospitals, home health agencies (HHAs), skilled nursing facilities (SNFs), critical access hospitals (CAHs), and hospital-based renal dialysis facilities (RDFs). Payment for comprehensive outpatient rehabilitation facilities (CORFs), Indian Health Service hospitals (IHS), IHS CAHs and independent RDFs is based on 95 percent of the average wholesale price (AWP). Section 10.2.4 of this chapter contains information on payment of these vaccines when provided by RDFs or hospices. See §10.2.2.2 for payment to independent and provider-based Rural Health Centers and Federally Qualified Health Clinics.

Payment for these vaccines is as follows:

Facility	Type of Bill	Payment
Hospitals, other than Indian Health Service (IHS) Hospitals and Critical Access Hospitals (CAHs)	12x, 13x	Reasonable cost
IHS Hospitals	12x, 13x, 83x	95% of AWP
IHS CAHs	85x	95% of AWP
CAHs Method I and Method II	85x	Reasonable cost
Skilled Nursing Facilities	22x, 23x	Reasonable cost
Home Health Agencies	34x	Reasonable cost
Comprehensive Outpatient Rehabilitation Facilities	75x	95% of the AWP
Independent Renal Dialysis Facilities	72x	95% of the AWP
Hospital-based Renal Dialysis Facilities	72x	Reasonable cost

Payment for Vaccine Administration

Payment for the administration of Influenza Virus and PPV vaccines is as follows:

Facility	Type of Bill	Payment
Hospitals, other than IHS Hospitals and CAHs	12x, 13x	Outpatient Prospective Payment System (OPPS) for hospitals subject to OPPS Reasonable cost for hospitals not subject to OPPS
IHS Hospitals	12x, 13x, 83x	MPFS as indicated in guidelines below.
IHS CAHs	85x	MPFS as indicated in guidelines below.
CAHs Method I and II	85x	Reasonable cost
Skilled Nursing Facilities	22x, 23x	MPFS as indicated in the guidelines below
Home Health Agencies	34x	OPPS
Comprehensive Outpatient Rehabilitation Facilities	75x	MPFS as indicated in the guidelines below
Independent RDFs	72x	MPFS as indicated in the guidelines below
Hospital-based RDFs	72x	Reasonable cost

Guidelines for pricing PPV and Influenza vaccine administration under the MPFS.

Make reimbursement based on the rate in the MPFS associated with the CPT code 90782 or 90471 as follows:

HCPCS code	Effective prior to March 1, 2003	Effective on and after March 1, 2003
G0008	90782	90471
G0009	90782	90471

See §10.2.2.2 for payment to independent and provider based Rural Health Centers and Federally Qualified Health Clinics.

Payment for the administration of Hepatitis B vaccine is as follows:

Facility	Type of Bill	Payment
Hospitals other than IHS hospitals and CAHs	12x, 13x	Outpatient Prospective Payment System (OPPS) for hospitals subject to OPPS Reasonable cost for hospitals not subject to OPPS
IHS Hospitals	12x, 13x, 83x	MPFS as indicated in the guidelines below
CAHs Method I and II	85x	Reasonable cost
IHS CAHs	85x	MPFS as indicated in guidelines below.
Skilled Nursing Facilities	22x, 23x	MPFS as indicated in the chart below
Home Health Agencies	34x	OPPS
Comprehensive Outpatient Rehabilitation Facilities	75x	MPFS as indicated in the guidelines below
Independent RDFs	72x	MPFS as indicated in the chart below

Facility	Type of Bill	Payment
Hospital-based RDFs	72x	Reasonable cost

Guidelines for pricing Hepatitis B vaccine administration under the MPFS.

Make reimbursement based on the rate in the MPFS associated with the CPT code 90782 or 90471 as follows:

HCPCS code	Effective prior to March 1, 2003	Effective on and after March 1, 2003
G0010	90782	90471

See §10.2.2.2 for payment to independent and provider based Rural Health Centers and Federally Qualified Health Clinics.

100-04, 18, 10.4

CWF Edits

In order to prevent duplicate payments for influenza virus and pneumococcal vaccination claims by the local contractor/AB MAC and the centralized billing contractor, effective for claims received on or after July 1, 2002, CWF has implemented a number of edits.

NOTE: 90659 was discontinued December 31, 2003.

CWF returns information in Trailer 13 information from the history claim. The following fields are returned to the contractor:

- Trailer Code;
- Contractor Number;
- Document Control Number;
- First Service Date;
- Last Service Date;
- Provider, Physician, Supplier Number;
- Claim Type; Procedure code;
- Alert Code (where applicable); and,
- More history (where applicable.)

100-04, 18, 10.4.1

CWF Edits on A/B MAC (A) Claims

(Rev. 3429, Issued: 12-22-15; Effective: 08-01-15; Implementation: 12-11-15 for requirement 9357.8; April 4, 2016 for all other requirements)

In order to prevent duplicate payment by the same A/B MAC (A), CWF edits by line item on the A/B MAC (A) number, the beneficiary Health Insurance Claim (HIC) number, and the date of service, the influenza virus procedure codes 90630, 90653, 90654, 90655, 90656, 90657, 90660, 90661, 90662, 90672, 90673, 90685, 90686, 90687, or 90688 and the pneumococcal procedure codes 90669, 90670, or 90732, and the administration codes G0008 or G0009.

If CWF receives a claim with either HCPCS codes 90630, 90653, 90654, 90655, 90656, 90657, 90660, 90661, 90662, 90672, 90673, 90685, 90686, 90687, or 90688 and it already has on record a claim with the same HIC number, same A/B MAC (A) number, same date of service, and any one of those HCPCS codes, the second claim submitted to CWF rejects.

If CWF receives a claim with HCPCS codes 90669, 90670, or 90732 and it already has on record a claim with the same HIC number, same A/B MAC (A) number, same date of service, and the same HCPCS code, the second claim submitted to CWF rejects when all four items match.

If CWF receives a claim with HCPCS administration codes G0008 or G0009 and it already has on record a claim with the same HIC number, same A/B MAC (A) number, same date of service, and same procedure code, CWF rejects the second claim submitted when all four items match.

CWF returns to the A/B MAC a reject code "7262" for this edit. A/B MACs (A) must deny the second claim and use the same messages they currently use for the denial of duplicate claims.

100-04, 18, 10.4.2

CWF Edits on A/B MAC (B) Claims

(Rev. 3429, Issued: 12-22-15; Effective: 08-01-15; Implementation: 12-11-15 for requirement 9357.8; April 4, 2016 for all other requirements)

In order to prevent duplicate payment by the same A/B MAC (B), CWF will edit by line item on the A/B MAC (B) number, the HIC number, the date of service, the influenza virus procedure codes 90630, 90653, 90654, 90655, 90656, 90657, 90660, 90661, 90662, 90672, 90673, 90685, 90686, 90687, or 90688; the pneumococcal procedure codes 90669, 90670, or 90732; and the administration code G0008 or G0009.

If CWF receives a claim with either HCPCS codes 90630, 90653, 90654, 90655, 90656, 90657, 90660, 90661, 90662, 90672, 90673, 90685, 90686, 90687, or 90688 and it already has on record a claim with the same HIC number, same A/B MAC (B) number, same date of service, and any one of those HCPCS codes, the second claim submitted to CWF will reject.

If CWF receives a claim with HCPCS codes 90669, 90670, or 90732 and it already has on record a claim with the same HIC number, same A/B MAC (B) number, same date of service, and the same HCPCS code, the second claim submitted to CWF will reject when all four items match.

If CWF receives a claim with HCPCS administration codes G0008 or G0009 and it already has on record a claim with the same HIC number, same A/B MAC (B) number, same date of service, and same procedure code, CWF will reject the second claim submitted.

CWF will return to the A/B MAC (B) a specific reject code for this edit. A/B MACs (B) must deny the second claim and use the same messages they currently use for the denial of duplicate claims.

In order to prevent duplicate payment by the centralized billing contractor and local A/B MAC (B), CWF will edit by line item for carrier number, same HIC number, same date of service, the influenza virus procedure codes 90630, 90653, 90654, 90655, 90656, 90657, 90660, 90661, 90662, 90672, 90673, 90685, 90686, 90687, or 90688; the pneumococcal procedure codes 90669, 90670, or 90732; and the administration code G0008 or G0009.

If CWF receives a claim with either HCPCS codes 90630, 90653, 90654, 90655, 90656, 90657, 90660, 90661, 90662, 90672, 90673, 90685, 90686, 90687, or 90688 and it already has on record a claim with a different A/B MAC (B) number, but same HIC number, same date of service, and any one of those same HCPCS codes, the second claim submitted to CWF will reject.

If CWF receives a claim with HCPCS codes 90669, 90670, or 90732 and it already has on record a claim with the same HIC number, different A/B MAC (B) number, same date of service, and the same HCPCS code, the second claim submitted to CWF will reject.

If CWF receives a claim with HCPCS administration codes G0008 or G0009 and it already has on record a claim with a different A/B MAC (B) number, but the same HIC number, same date of service, and same procedure code, CWF will reject the second claim submitted.

CWF will return a specific reject code for this edit. A/B MACs (B) must deny the second claim. For the second edit, the reject code should automatically trigger the following Medicare Summary Notice (MSN) and Remittance Advice (RA) messages.

MSN: 7.2 – "This is a duplicate of a claim processed by another contractor. You should receive a Medicare Summary Notice from them."

Claim adjustment reason code 18 – duplicate claim or service

100-04, 18, 10.4.3

CWF Crossover Edits A/B MAC (B) Claims

(Rev. 3429, Issued: 12-22-15; Effective: 08-01-15; Implementation: 12-11-15 for requirement 9357.8; April 4, 2016 for all other requirements)

When CWF receives a claim from the A/B MAC (B), it will review Part B outpatient claims history to verify that a duplicate claim has not already been posted.

CWF will edit on the beneficiary HIC number; the date of service; the influenza virus procedure codes 90630, 90653, 90654, 90655, 90656, 90657, 90660, 90661, 90662, 90672, 90673, 90685, 90686, 90687, or 90688; the pneumococcal procedure codes 90669, 90670, or 90732; and the administration code G0008 or G0009.

CWF will return a specific reject code for this edit. Contractors must deny the second claim and use the same messages they currently use for the denial of duplicate claims.

100-04, 18, 60

Colorectal Cancer Screening

(Rev. 3436, Issued: 12-30-15, Effective: 10-09-14, Implementation: 09-08-15 for non-shared MAC edits; 01-04-16 - For all shared system changes.)

See the Medicare Benefit Policy Manual, Chapter 15, and the Medicare National Coverage Determinations (NCD) Manual, Chapter 1, Section 210.3 for Medicare Part B coverage requirements and effective dates of colorectal cancer screening services.

Effective for services furnished on or after January 1, 1998, payment may be made for colorectal cancer screening for the early detection of cancer. For screening colonoscopy services (one of the types of services included in this benefit) prior to July 2001, coverage was limited to high-risk individuals. For services July 1, 2001, and later screening colonoscopies are covered for individuals not at high risk.

The following services are considered colorectal cancer screening services:

- Fecal-occult blood test (FOBT),1-3 simultaneous determinations (guaiac-based);
- Flexible sigmoidoscopy;
- Colonoscopy; and,
- Barium enema

Effective for services on or after January 1, 2004, payment may be made for the following colorectal cancer screening service as an alternative for the guaiac-based FOBT, 1-3 simultaneous determinations:

- Fecal-occult blood test, immunoassay, 1-3 simultaneous determinations

Effective for claims with dates of service on or after October 9, 2014, payment may be made for colorectal cancer screening using the Cologuard™ multitarget stool DNA (sDNA) test:

G0464 (Colorectal cancer screening; stool-based DNA and fecal occult hemoglobin (e.g., KRAS, NDRG4 and BMP3).

100-04, 18, 80.2

A/B Medicare Administrative Contractor (MAC) (B) Billing Requirements

Effective for dates of service on and after January 1, 2005, through December 31, 2008, contractors shall recognize the HCPCS codes G0344, G0366, G0367, and G0368 shown above in §80.1 for an IPPE. The type of service (TOS) for each of these codes is as follows:

G0344: TOS = 1

G0366: TOS = 5

G0367: TOS = 5

G0368: TOS = 5

Contractors shall pay physicians or qualified nonphysician practitioners for only one IPPE performed not later than 6 months after the date the individual's first coverage begins under Medicare Part B, but only if that coverage period begins on or after January 1, 2005.

Effective for dates of service on and after January 1, 2009, contractors shall recognize the HCPCS codes G0402, G0403, G0404, and G0405 shown above in §80.1 for an IPPE. The TOS for each of these codes is as follows:

G0402: TOS = 1

G0403: TOS = 5

G0404: TOS = 5

G0405: TOS = 5

Under the MIPPA of 2008, contractors shall pay physicians or qualified nonphysician practitioners for only one IPPE performed not later than 12 months after the date the individual's first coverage begins under Medicare Part B only if that coverage period begins on or after January 1, 2009.

Contractors shall allow payment for a medically necessary Evaluation and Management (E/M) service at the same visit as the IPPE when it is clinically appropriate. Physicians and qualified nonphysician practitioners shall use CPT codes 99201-99215 to report an E/M with CPT modifier 25 to indicate that the E/M is a significant, separately identifiable service from the IPPE code reported (G0344 or G0402, whichever applies based on the date the IPPE is performed). Refer to chapter 12, § 30.6.1.1, of this manual for the physician/practitioner billing correct coding and payment policy regarding E/M services.

If the EKG performed as a component of the IPPE is not performed by the primary physician or qualified NPP during the IPPE visit, another physician or entity may perform and/or interpret the EKG. The referring physician or qualified NPP needs to make sure that the performing physician or entity bills the appropriate G code for the screening EKG, and not a CPT code in the 93000 series. **Both the IPPE and the EKG should be billed in order for the beneficiary to receive the complete IPPE service.** Effective for dates of service on and after January 1, 2009, the screening EKG is optional and is no longer a mandated service of an IPPE if performed as a result of a referral from an IPPE.

Should the same physician or NPP need to perform an additional medically necessary EKG in the 93000 series on the same day as the IPPE, report the appropriate EKG CPT code(s) with modifier 59, indicating that the EKG is a distinct procedural service.

Physicians or qualified nonphysician practitioners shall bill the contractor the appropriate HCPCS codes for IPPE on the Form CMS-1500 claim or an approved electronic format. The HCPCS codes for an IPPE and screening EKG are paid under the Medicare Physician Fee Schedule (MPFS).

See §1.3 of this chapter for waiver of cost sharing requirements of coinsurance, copayment and deductible for furnished preventive services available in Medicare.

100-04, 18, 140.8

Advance Care Planning (ACP) as an Optional Element of an Annual Wellness Visit (AWV)

(Rev. 3428 Issued: 12-22-15, Effective: 01-01-16, Implementation: 01-04-16)

For services furnished on or after January 1, 2016, Advance Care Planning (ACP) is treated as a preventive service when furnished with an AWV. The Medicare coinsurance and Part B deductible are waived for ACP when furnished as an optional element of an AWV.

The codes for the optional ACP services furnished as part of an AWV are 99497 (Advance care planning including the explanation and discussion of advance directives such as standard forms (with completion of such forms, when performed), by the physician or other qualified health professional; first 30 minutes, face-to-face with the patient, family member(s) and/or surrogate;) and an add-on code 99498 (each additional 30 minutes (List separately in addition to code for primary procedure)). When ACP services are provided as a part of an AWV, practitioners would report CPT code 99497 (and add-on CPT code 99498 when applicable) for the ACP services in addition to either of the AWV codes (G0438 or G0439).

The deductible and coinsurance for ACP will only be waived when billed with modifier 33 on the same day and on the same claim as an AWV (code G0438 or G0439), and must also be furnished by the same provider. Waiver of the deductible and coinsurance for ACP is limited to once per year. Payment for an AWV is limited to once per year. If the AWV billed with ACP is denied for exceeding the once per year limit, the deductible and coinsurance will be applied to the ACP.

Also see Pub. 100-02, *Medicare Benefit Policy Manual*, chapter 15, section 280.5.1 for more information.

100-04, 32, 10.1

Ambulatory Blood Pressure Monitoring (ABPM) Billing Requirements

A. Coding Applicable to A/B MACs (A and B)

Effective April 1, 2002, a National Coverage Decision was made to allow for Medicare coverage of ABPM for those beneficiaries with suspected "white coat hypertension" (WCH). ABPM involves the use of a non-invasive device, which is used to measure blood pressure in 24-hour cycles. These 24-hour measurements are stored in the device and are later interpreted by a physician. Suspected "WCH" is defined as: (1) Clinic/office blood pressure >140/90 mm Hg on at least three separate clinic/office visits with two separate measurements made at each visit; (2) At least two documented separate blood pressure measurements taken outside the clinic/office which are < 140/90 mm Hg; and (3) No evidence of end-organ damage. ABPM is not covered for any other uses. Coverage policy can be found in Medicare National Coverage Determinations Manual, Chapter 1, Part 1, §20.19. (http://www.cms.hhs.gov/manuals/103_cov_determ/ncd103index.asp).

The ABPM must be performed for at least 24 hours to meet coverage criteria. Payment is not allowed for institutionalized beneficiaries, such as those receiving Medicare covered skilled nursing in a facility. In the rare circumstance that ABPM needs to be performed more than once for a beneficiary, the qualifying criteria described above must be met for each subsequent ABPM test.

Effective dates for applicable Common Procedure Coding System (HCPCS) codes for ABPM for suspected WCH and their covered effective dates are as follows:

HCPCS	Definition	Effective Date
93784	ABPM, utilizing a system such as magnetic tape and/or computer disk, for 24 hours or longer; including recording, scanning analysis, interpretation and report.	04/01/2002
93786	ABPM, utilizing a system such as magnetic tape and/or computer disk, for 24 hours or longer; recording only.	04/01/2002
93788	ABPM, utilizing a system such as magnetic tape and/or computer disk, for 24 hours or longer; scanning analysis with report.	01/01/2004
93790	ABPM, utilizing a system such as magnetic tape and/or computer disk, for 24 hours or longer; physician review with interpretation and report.	04/01/2002

In addition, one of the following diagnosis codes must be present:

	Diagnosis Code	Description
If ICD-9-CM is applicable	796.2	Elevated blood pressure reading without diagnosis of hypertension.
If ICD-10-CM is applicable	R03.0	Elevated blood pressure reading without diagnosis of hypertension

B. A/B MAC (A) Billing Instructions

The applicable types of bills acceptable when billing for ABPM services are 13X, 23X, 71X, 73X, 75X, and 85X. Chapter 25 of this manual provides general billing instructions that must be followed for bills submitted to A/B MACs (A). The A/B MACs (A) pay for hospital outpatient ABPM services billed on a 13X type of bill with HCPCS 93786 and/or 93788 as follows: (1) Outpatient Prospective Payment System (OPPS) hospitals pay based on the Ambulatory Payment Classification (APC); (2) non-OPPS hospitals (Indian Health Services Hospitals, Hospitals that provide Part B services only, and hospitals located in American Samoa, Guam, Saipan and the Virgin Islands) pay based on reasonable cost, except for Maryland Hospitals which are paid based on a percentage of cost. Effective 4/1/06, type of bill 14X is for non-patient laboratory specimens and is no longer applicable for ABPM.

The A/B MACs (A) pay for comprehensive outpatient rehabilitation facility (CORF) ABPM services billed on a 75x type of bill with HCPCS code 93786 and/or 93788 based on the Medicare Physician Fee Schedule (MPFS) amount for that HCPCS code.

The A/B MACs (A) pay for ABPM services for critical access hospitals (CAHs) billed on a 85x type of bill as follows: (1) for CAHs that elected the Standard Method and billed HCPCS code 93786 and/or 93788, pay based on reasonable cost for that HCPCS code; and (2) for CAHs that elected the Optional Method and billed any combination of HCPCS codes 93786, 93788 and 93790 pay based on reasonable cost for HCPCS 93786 and 93788 and pay 115% of the MPFS amount for HCPCS 93790.

The A/B MACs (A) pay for ABPM services for skilled nursing facility (SNF) outpatients billed on a 23x type of bill with HCPCS code 93786 and/or 93788, based on the MPFS.

The A/B MACs (A) accept independent and provider-based rural health clinic (RHC) bills for visits under the all-inclusive rate when the RHC bills on a 71x type of bill with revenue code 052x for providing the professional component of ABPM services. The A/B MACs (A) should not make a separate payment to a RHC for the professional component of ABPM services in addition to the all-inclusive rate. RHCs are not required to use ABPM HCPCS codes for professional services covered under the all-inclusive rate.

The A/B MACs (A) accept free-standing and provider-based federally qualified health center (FQHC) bills for visits under the all-inclusive rate when the FQHC bills on a 73x type of bill with revenue code 052x for providing the professional component of ABPM services.

The A/B MACs (A) should not make a separate payment to a FQHC for the professional component of ABPM services in addition to the all-inclusive rate. FQHCs are not required to use ABPM HCPCS codes for professional services covered under the all-inclusive rate.

The A/B MACs (A) pay provider-based RHCs/FQHCs for the technical component of ABPM services when billed under the base provider's number using the above requirements for that particular base provider type, i.e., a OPPS hospital based RHC would be paid for the ABPM technical component services under the OPPS using the APC for code 93786 and/or 93788 when billed on a 13x type of bill.

Independent and free-standing RHC/FQHC practitioners are only paid for providing the technical component of ABPM services when billed to the A/B MAC (B) following the MAC's instructions.

C. A/B MAC (B) Claims

A/B MACs (B) pay for ABPM services billed with ICD-9-CM diagnosis code 796.2 (if ICD-9 is applicable) or, if ICD-10 is applicable, ICD-10-CM diagnosis code R03.0 and HCPCS codes 93784 or for any combination of 93786, 93788 and 93790, based on the MPFS for the specific HCPCS code billed.

D. Coinsurance and Deductible

The A/B MACs (A and B) shall apply coinsurance and deductible to payments for ABPM services except for services billed to the A/B MAC (A) by FQHCs. For FQHCs only co-insurance applies.

100-04, 32, 30.1

Billing Requirements for HBO Therapy for the Treatment of Diabetic Wounds of the Lower Extremities

Hyperbaric Oxygen Therapy is a modality in which the entire body is exposed to oxygen under increased atmospheric pressure. Effective April 1, 2003, a National Coverage Decision expanded the use of HBO therapy to include coverage for the treatment of diabetic wounds of the lower extremities. For specific coverage criteria for HBO Therapy, refer to the National Coverage Determinations Manual, Chapter 1, section 20.29.

NOTE: Topical application of oxygen does not meet the definition of HBO therapy as stated above. Also, its clinical efficacy has not been established. Therefore, no Medicare reimbursement may be made for the topical application of oxygen.

I. Billing Requirements for A/B MACs (A)

Claims for HBO therapy should be submitted using the ASC X12 837 institutional claim format or, in rare cases, on Form CMS-1450.

a. Applicable Bill Types

The applicable hospital bill types are 11X, 13X and 85X.

b. Procedural Coding

99183– Physician attendance and supervision of hyperbaric oxygen therapy, per session.

C1300 – Hyperbaric oxygen under pressure, full body chamber, per 30-minute interval.

NOTE: Code C1300 is not available for use other than in a hospital outpatient department. In skilled nursing facilities (SNFs), HBO therapy is part of the SNF PPS payment for beneficiaries in covered Part A stays.

For hospital inpatients and critical access hospitals (CAHs) not electing Method I, HBO therapy is reported under revenue code 940 without any HCPCS code. For inpatient services, if ICD-9-is applicable, show ICD-9-CM procedure code 93.59. If ICD-10 is applicable, show ICD-10-PCS code 5A05121.

For CAHs electing Method I, HBO therapy is reported under revenue code 940 along with HCPCS code 99183.

c. Payment Requirements for A/B MACs (A)

Payment is as follows:

A/B MAC (A) payment is allowed for HBO therapy for diabetic wounds of the lower extremities when performed as a physician service in a hospital outpatient setting and for inpatients. Payment is allowed for claims with valid diagnosis codes as shown above with dates of service on or after April 1, 2003. Those claims with invalid codes should be denied as not medically necessary.

For hospitals, payment will be based upon the Ambulatory Payment Classification (APC) or the inpatient Diagnosis Related Group (DRG). Deductible and coinsurance apply.

Payment to Critical Access Hospitals (electing Method I) is made under cost reimbursement. For Critical Access Hospitals electing Method II, the technical component is paid under cost reimbursement and the professional component is paid under the Physician Fee Schedule.

II. A/B MAC (B) Billing Requirements

Claims for this service should be submitted using the ASC X12 837 professional claim format or Form CMS-1500.

The following HCPCS code applies:

99183 – Physician attendance and supervision of hyperbaric oxygen therapy, per session.

a. Payment Requirements for A/B MACs (B)

Payment and pricing information will occur through updates to the Medicare Physician Fee Schedule Database (MPFSDB). Pay for this service on the basis of the MPFSDB. Deductible and coinsurance apply. Claims from physicians or other practitioners where assignment was not taken, are subject to the Medicare limiting charge.

III. Medicare Summary Notices (MSNs)

Use the following MSN Messages where appropriate:

In situations where the claim is being denied on the basis that the condition does not meet our coverage requirements, use one of the following MSN Messages:

"Medicare does not pay for this item or service for this condition." (MSN Message 16.48)

The Spanish version of the MSN message should read:

"Medicare no paga por este articulo o servicio para esta afeccion."

In situations where, based on the above utilization policy, medical review of the claim results in a determination that the service is not medically necessary, use the following MSN message:

"The information provided does not support the need for this service or item." (MSN Message 15.4)

The Spanish version of the MSN message should read:

"La informacion proporcionada no confirma la necesidad para este servicio o articulo."

IV. Remittance Advice Notices

Use appropriate existing remittance advice remark codes and claim adjustment reason codes at the line level to express the specific reason if you deny payment for HBO therapy for the treatment of diabetic wounds of lower extremities.

100-04, 32, 60.4.1

Allowable Covered Diagnosis Codes

Allowable Covered Diagnosis Codes

For services furnished on or after July 1, 2002, the applicable ICD-9-CM diagnosis code for this benefit is V43.3, organ or tissue replaced by other means; heart valve.

For services furnished on or after March 19, 2008, the applicable ICD-9-CM diagnosis codes for this benefit are:

- V43.3 (organ or tissue replaced by other means; heart valve),
- 289.81 (primary hypercoagulable state),
- 451.0-451.9 (includes 451.11, 451.19, 451.2, 451.80-451.84, 451.89) (phlebitis & thrombophlebitis),
- 453.0-453.3 (other venous embolism & thrombosis),
- 453.40-453.49 (includes 453.40-453.42, 453.8-453.9) (venous embolism and thrombosis of the deep vessels of the lower extremity, and other specified veins/unspecified sites)
- 415.11-415.12, 415.19 (pulmonary embolism & infarction) or,
- 427.31 (atrial fibrillation (established) (paroxysmal)).

For services furnished on or after the implementation of ICD-10 the applicable ICD-10-CM diagnosis codes for this benefit are:

Heart Valve Replacement
- Z95.2 - Presence of prosthetic heart valve

Primary Hypercoagulable State

ICD-10-CM	Code Description
D68.51	Activated protein C resistance
D68.52	Prothrombin gene mutation
D68.59	Other primary thrombophilia
D68.61	Antiphospholipid syndrome
D68.62	Lupus anticoagulant syndrome

Phlebitis & Thrombophlebitis

ICD-10-CM	Code Description
I80.00	Phlebitis and thrombophlebitis of superficial vessels of unspecified lower extremity
I80.01	Phlebitis and thrombophlebitis of superficial vessels of right lower extremity
I80.02	Phlebitis and thrombophlebitis of superficial vessels of left lower extremity
I80.03	Phlebitis and thrombophlebitis of superficial vessels of lower extremities, bilateral
I80.10	Phlebitis and thrombophlebitis of unspecified femoral vein
I80.11	Phlebitis and thrombophlebitis of right femoral vein
I80.12	Phlebitis and thrombophlebitis of left femoral vein
I80.13	Phlebitis and thrombophlebitis of femoral vein, bilateral
I80.201	Phlebitis and thrombophlebitis of unspecified deep vessels of right lower extremity
I80.202	Phlebitis and thrombophlebitis of unspecified deep vessels of left lower extremity
I80.203	Phlebitis and thrombophlebitis of unspecified deep vessels of lower extremities, bilateral
I80.209	Phlebitis and thrombophlebitis of unspecified deep vessels of unspecified lower extremity
I80.221	Phlebitis and thrombophlebitis of right popliteal vein
I80.222	Phlebitis and thrombophlebitis of left popliteal vein
I80.223	Phlebitis and thrombophlebitis of popliteal vein, bilateral
I80.229	Phlebitis and thrombophlebitis of unspecified popliteal vein
I80.231	Phlebitis and thrombophlebitis of right tibial vein
I80.232	Phlebitis and thrombophlebitis of left tibial vein
I80.233	Phlebitis and thrombophlebitis of tibial vein, bilateral
I80.239	Phlebitis and thrombophlebitis of unspecified tibial vein
I80.291	Phlebitis and thrombophlebitis of other deep vessels of right lower extremity
I80.292	Phlebitis and thrombophlebitis of other deep vessels of left lower extremity
I80.293	Phlebitis and thrombophlebitis of other deep vessels of lower extremity, bilateral
I80.299	Phlebitis and thrombophlebitis of other deep vessels of unspecified lower extremity
I80.3	Phlebitis and thrombophlebitis of lower extremities, unspecified
I80.211	Phlebitis and thrombophlebitis of right iliac vein
I80.212	Phlebitis and thrombophlebitis of left iliac vein
I80.213	Phlebitis and thrombophlebitis of iliac vein, bilateral
I80.219	Phlebitis and thrombophlebitis of unspecified iliac vein
I80.8	Phlebitis and thrombophlebitis of other sites
I80.9	Phlebitis and thrombophlebitis of unspecified site

Other Venous Embolism & Thrombosis

ICD-10-CM	Code Description
I82.0	Budd- Chiari syndrome
I82.1	Thrombophlebitis migrans
I82.211	Chronic embolism and thrombosis of superior vena cava
I82.220	Acute embolism and thrombosis of inferior vena cava
I82.221	Chronic embolism and thrombosis of inferior vena cava
I82.291	Chronic embolism and thrombosis of other thoracic veins
I82.3	Embolism and thrombosis of renal vein

Venous Embolism and thrombosis of the deep vessels of the lower extremity, and other specified veins/unspecified sites

ICD-10-CM	Code Description
I82.401	Acute embolism and thrombosis of unspecified deep veins of right lower extremity
I82.402	Acute embolism and thrombosis of unspecified deep veins of left lower extremity
I82.403	Acute embolism and thrombosis of unspecified deep veins of lower extremity, bilateral
I82.409	Acute embolism and thrombosis of unspecified deep veins of unspecified lower extremity
I82.411	Acute embolism and thrombosis of right femoral vein
I82.412	Acute embolism and thrombosis of left femoral vein
I82.413	Acute embolism and thrombosis of femoral vein, bilateral
I82.419	Acute embolism and thrombosis of unspecified femoral vein
I82.421	Acute embolism and thrombosis of right iliac vein
I82.422	Acute embolism and thrombosis of left iliac vein
I82.423	Acute embolism and thrombosis of iliac vein, bilateral
I82.429	Acute embolism and thrombosis of unspecified iliac vein

ICD-10-CM	Code Description
I82.431	Acute embolism and thrombosis of right popliteal vein
I82.432	Acute embolism and thrombosis of left popliteal vein
I82.433	Acute embolism and thrombosis of popliteal vein, bilateral
I82.439	Acute embolism and thrombosis of unspecified popliteal vein
I82.4Y1	Acute embolism and thrombosis of unspecified deep veins of right proximal lower extremity
I82.4Y2	Acute embolism and thrombosis of unspecified deep veins of left proximal lower extremity
I82.4Y3	Acute embolism and thrombosis of unspecified deep veins of proximal lower extremity, bilateral
I82.4Y9	Acute embolism and thrombosis of unspecified deep veins of unspecified proximal lower extremity
I82.441	Acute embolism and thrombosis of right tibial vein
I82.442	Acute embolism and thrombosis of left tibial vein
I82.443	Acute embolism and thrombosis of tibial vein, bilateral
I82.449	Acute embolism and thrombosis of unspecified tibial vein
I82.491	Acute embolism and thrombosis of other specified deep vein of right lower extremity
I82.492	Acute embolism and thrombosis of other specified deep vein of left lower extremity
I82.493	Acute embolism and thrombosis of other specified deep vein of lower extremity, bilateral
I82.499	Acute embolism and thrombosis of other specified deep vein of unspecified lower extremity
I82.4Z1	Acute embolism and thrombosis of unspecified deep veins of right distal lower extremity
I82.4Z2	Acute embolism and thrombosis of unspecified deep veins of left distal lower extremity
I82.4Z3	Acute embolism and thrombosis of unspecified deep veins of distal lower extremity, bilateral
I82.4Z9	Acute embolism and thrombosis of unspecified deep veins of unspecified distal lower extremity
I82.501	Chronic embolism and thrombosis of unspecified deep veins of right lower extremity
I82.502	Chronic embolism and thrombosis of unspecified deep veins of left lower extremity
I82.503	Chronic embolism and thrombosis of unspecified deep veins of lower extremity, bilateral
I82.509	Chronic embolism and thrombosis of unspecified deep veins of unspecified lower extremity
I82.591	Chronic embolism and thrombosis of other specified deep vein of right lower extremity
I82.592	Chronic embolism and thrombosis of other specified deep vein of left lower extremity
I82.593	Chronic embolism and thrombosis of other specified deep vein of lower extremity, bilateral
I82.599	Chronic embolism and thrombosis of other specified deep vein of unspecified lower extremity
I82.511	Chronic embolism and thrombosis of right femoral vein
I82.512	Chronic embolism and thrombosis of left femoral vein
I82.513	Chronic embolism and thrombosis of femoral vein, bilateral
I82.519	Chronic embolism and thrombosis of unspecified femoral vein
I82.521	Chronic embolism and thrombosis of right iliac vein
I82.522	Chronic embolism and thrombosis of left iliac vein
I82.523	Chronic embolism and thrombosis of iliac vein, bilateral
I82.529	Chronic embolism and thrombosis of unspecified iliac vein
I82.531	Chronic embolism and thrombosis of right popliteal vein
I82.532	Chronic embolism and thrombosis of left popliteal vein
I82.533	Chronic embolism and thrombosis of popliteal vein, bilateral
I82.539	Chronic embolism and thrombosis of unspecified popliteal vein
I82.5Y1	Chronic embolism and thrombosis of unspecified deep veins of right proximal lower extremity
I82.5Y2	Chronic embolism and thrombosis of unspecified deep veins of left proximal lower extremity
I82.5Y3	Chronic embolism and thrombosis of unspecified deep veins of proximal lower extremity, bilateral
I82.5Y9	Chronic embolism and thrombosis of unspecified deep veins of unspecified proximal lower extremity
I82.541	Chronic embolism and thrombosis of right tibial vein
I82.542	Chronic embolism and thrombosis of left tibial vein

ICD-10-CM	Code Description
I82.543	Chronic embolism and thrombosis of tibial vein, bilateral
I82.549	Chronic embolism and thrombosis of unspecified tibial vein
I82.5Z1	Chronic embolism and thrombosis of unspecified deep veins of right distal lower extremity
I82.5Z2	Chronic embolism and thrombosis of unspecified deep veins of left distal lower extremity
I82.5Z3	Chronic embolism and thrombosis of unspecified deep veins of distal lower extremity, bilateral
I82.5Z9	Chronic embolism and thrombosis of unspecified deep veins of unspecified distal lower extremity
I82.611	Acute embolism and thrombosis of superficial veins of right upper extremity
I82.612	Acute embolism and thrombosis of superficial veins of left upper extremity
I82.613	Acute embolism and thrombosis of superficial veins of upper extremity, bilateral
I82.619	Acute embolism and thrombosis of superficial veins of unspecified upper extremity
I82.621	Acute embolism and thrombosis of deep veins of right upper extremity
I82.622	Acute embolism and thrombosis of deep veins of left upper extremity
I82.623	Acute embolism and thrombosis of deep veins of upper extremity, bilateral
I82.629	Acute embolism and thrombosis of deep veins of unspecified upper extremity
I82.601	Acute embolism and thrombosis of unspecified veins of right upper extremity
I82.602	Acute embolism and thrombosis of unspecified veins of left upper extremity
I82.603	Acute embolism and thrombosis of unspecified veins of upper extremity, bilateral
I82.609	Acute embolism and thrombosis of unspecified veins of unspecified upper extremity
I82.A11	Acute embolism and thrombosis of right axillary vein
I82.A12	Acute embolism and thrombosis of left axillary vein
I82.A13	Acute embolism and thrombosis of axillary vein, bilateral
I82.A19	Acute embolism and thrombosis of unspecified axillary vein
I82.A21	Chronic embolism and thrombosis of right axillary vein
I82.A22	Chronic embolism and thrombosis of left axillary vein
I82.A23	Chronic embolism and thrombosis of axillary vein, bilateral
I82.A29	Chronic embolism and thrombosis of unspecified axillary vein
I82.B11	Acute embolism and thrombosis of right subclavian vein
I82.B12	Acute embolism and thrombosis of left subclavian vein
I82.B13	Acute embolism and thrombosis of subclavian vein, bilateral
I82.B19	Acute embolism and thrombosis of unspecified subclavian vein
I82.B21	Chronic embolism and thrombosis of right subclavian vein
I82.B22	Chronic embolism and thrombosis of left subclavian vein
I82.B23	Chronic embolism and thrombosis of subclavian vein, bilateral
I82.B29	Chronic embolism and thrombosis of unspecified subclavian vein
I82.C11	Acute embolism and thrombosis of right internal jugular vein
I82.C12	Acute embolism and thrombosis of left internal jugular vein
I82.C13	Acute embolism and thrombosis of internal jugular vein, bilateral
I82.C19	Acute embolism and thrombosis of unspecified internal jugular vein
I82.C21	Chronic embolism and thrombosis of right internal jugular vein
I82.C22	Chronic embolism and thrombosis of left internal jugular vein
I82.C23	Chronic embolism and thrombosis of internal jugular vein, bilateral
I82.C29	Chronic embolism and thrombosis of unspecified internal jugular vein
I82.210	Acute embolism and thrombosis of superior vena cava
I82.290	Acute embolism and thrombosis of other thoracic veins
I82.701	Chronic embolism and thrombosis of unspecified veins of right upper extremity
I82.702	Chronic embolism and thrombosis of unspecified veins of left upper extremity
I82.703	Chronic embolism and thrombosis of unspecified veins of upper extremity, bilateral
I82.709	Chronic embolism and thrombosis of unspecified veins of unspecified upper extremity
I82.711	Chronic embolism and thrombosis of superficial veins of right upper extremity

ICD-10-CM	Code Description
I82.712	Chronic embolism and thrombosis of superficial veins of left upper extremity
I82.713	Chronic embolism and thrombosis of superficial veins of upper extremity, bilateral
I82.719	Chronic embolism and thrombosis of superficial veins of unspecified upper extremity
I82.721	Chronic embolism and thrombosis of deep veins of right upper extremity
I82.722	Chronic embolism and thrombosis of deep veins of left upper extremity
I82.723	Chronic embolism and thrombosis of deep veins of upper extremity, bilateral
I82.729	Chronic embolism and thrombosis of deep veins of unspecified upper extremity
I82.811	Embolism and thrombosis of superficial veins of right lower extremities
I82.812	Embolism and thrombosis of superficial veins of left lower extremities
I82.813	Embolism and thrombosis of superficial veins of lower extremities, bilateral
I82.819	Embolism and thrombosis of superficial veins of unspecified lower extremities
I82.890	Acute embolism and thrombosis of other specified veins
I82.891	Chronic embolism and thrombosis of other specified veins
I82.90	Acute embolism and thrombosis of unspecified vein
I82.91	Chronic embolism and thrombosis of unspecified vein

Pulmonary Embolism & Infarction

ICD-10-CM	Code Description
I26.90	Septic pulmonary embolism without acute cor pulmonale
I26.99	Other pulmonary embolism without acute cor pulmonale
I26.01	Septic pulmonary embolism with acute cor pulmonale
I26.90	Septic pulmonary embolism without acute cor pulmonale
I26.09	Other pulmonary embolism with acute cor pulmonale
I26.99	Other pulmonary embolism without acute cor pulmonale

Atrial Fibrillation

ICD-10-CM	Code Description
I48.0	Paroxysmal atrial fibrillation
I48.2	Chronic atrial fibrillation
I48	-91 Unspecified atrial fibrillation Other
I23.6	Thrombosis of atrium, auricular appendage, and ventricle as current complications following acute myocardial infarction
I27.82	Chronic pulmonary embolism
I67.6	Nonpyogenic thrombosis of intracranial venous system
O22.50	Cerebral venous thrombosis in pregnancy, unspecified trimester
O22.51	Cerebral venous thrombosis in pregnancy, first trimester
O22.52	Cerebral venous thrombosis in pregnancy, second trimester
O22.53	Cerebral venous thrombosis in pregnancy, third trimester
O87.3	Cerebral venous thrombosis in the puerperium
Z79.01	Long term (current) use of anticoagulants

Coverage policy can be found in Pub. 100-3, Medicare National Coverage Determinations Manual, Chapter 1, section 190.11 PT/INR. (http://www.cms.hhs.gov/manuals/103_cov_determ/ncd103index.asp

100-04, 32, 60.5.2

Applicable Diagnosis Codes for A/B Macs

For services furnished on or after July 1, 2002, the applicable ICD-9-CM diagnosis code for this benefit is V43.3, organ or tissue replaced by other means; heart valve.

For services furnished on or after March 19, 2008, the applicable ICD-9-CM diagnosis codes for this benefit are:

- V43.3 (organ or tissue replaced by other means; heart valve),
- 289.81 (primary hypercoagulable state),
- 451.0-451.9 (includes 451.11, 451.19, 451.2, 451.80-451.84, 451.89) (phlebitis & thrombophlebitis),
- 453.0-453.3 (other venous embolism & thrombosis),
- 453.40-453.49 (includes 453.40-453.42, 453.8-453.9) (venous embolism and thrombosis of the deep vessels of the lower extremity, and other specified veins/unspecified sites)

- 415.11-415.12, 415.19 (pulmonary embolism & infarction) or,
- 427.31 (atrial fibrillation (established) (paroxysmal)).

For services furnished on or after implementation of ICD-10 the applicable ICD-10-CM diagnosis codes for this benefit are:

Heart Valve Replacement
- Z95.2 - Presence of prosthetic heart valve

Primary Hypercoagulable State

ICD-10-CM	Code Description
D68.51	Activated protein C resistance
D68.52	Prothrombin gene mutation
D68.59	Other primary thrombophilia
D68.61	Antiphospholipid syndrome
D68.62	Lupus anticoagulant syndrome

Phlebitis & Thrombophlebitis

ICD-10-CM	Code Description
I80.00	Phlebitis and thrombophlebitis of superficial vessels of unspecified lower extremity
I80.01	Phlebitis and thrombophlebitis of superficial vessels of right lower extremity
I80.02	Phlebitis and thrombophlebitis of superficial vessels of left lower extremity
I80.03	Phlebitis and thrombophlebitis of superficial vessels of lower extremities, bilateral
I80.10	Phlebitis and thrombophlebitis of unspecified femoral vein
I80.11	Phlebitis and thrombophlebitis of right femoral vein
I80.12	Phlebitis and thrombophlebitis of left femoral vein
I80.13	Phlebitis and thrombophlebitis of femoral vein, bilateral
I80.201	Phlebitis and thrombophlebitis of unspecified deep vessels of right lower extremity
I80.202	Phlebitis and thrombophlebitis of unspecified deep vessels of left lower extremity
I80.203	Phlebitis and thrombophlebitis of unspecified deep vessels of lower extremities, bilateral
I80.209	Phlebitis and thrombophlebitis of unspecified deep vessels of unspecified lower extremity
I80.221	Phlebitis and thrombophlebitis of right popliteal vein
I80.222	Phlebitis and thrombophlebitis of left popliteal vein
I80.223	Phlebitis and thrombophlebitis of popliteal vein, bilateral
I80.229	Phlebitis and thrombophlebitis of unspecified popliteal vein
I80.231	Phlebitis and thrombophlebitis of right tibial vein
I80.232	Phlebitis and thrombophlebitis of left tibial vein
I80.233	Phlebitis and thrombophlebitis of tibial vein, bilateral
I80.239	Phlebitis and thrombophlebitis of unspecified tibial vein
I80.291	Phlebitis and thrombophlebitis of other deep vessels of right lower extremity
I80.292	Phlebitis and thrombophlebitis of other deep vessels of left lower extremity
I80.293	Phlebitis and thrombophlebitis of other deep vessels of lower extremity, bilateral
I80.299	Phlebitis and thrombophlebitis of other deep vessels of unspecified lower extremity
I80.3	Phlebitis and thrombophlebitis of lower extremities, unspecified
I80.211	Phlebitis and thrombophlebitis of right iliac vein
I80.212	Phlebitis and thrombophlebitis of left iliac vein
I80.213	Phlebitis and thrombophlebitis of iliac vein, bilateral
I80.219	Phlebitis and thrombophlebitis of unspecified iliac vein
I80.8	Phlebitis and thrombophlebitis of other sites
I80.9	Phlebitis and thrombophlebitis of unspecified site

Other Venous Embolism & Thrombosis

ICD-10-CM	Code Description
I82.0	Budd- Chiari syndrome
I82.1	Thrombophlebitis migrans
I82.211	Chronic embolism and thrombosis of superior vena cava
I82220	Acute embolism and thrombosis of inferior vena cava
I82.221	Chronic embolism and thrombosis of inferior vena cava
I82.291	Chronic embolism and thrombosis of other thoracic veins
I82.3	Embolism and thrombosis of renal vein

Venous Embolism and thrombosis of the deep vessels of the lower extremity, and other specified veins/unspecified sites

ICD-10-CM	Code Description
I82.4Ø1	Acute embolism and thrombosis of unspecified deep veins of right lower extremity
I82.4Ø2	Acute embolism and thrombosis of unspecified deep veins of left lower extremity
I82.4Ø3	Acute embolism and thrombosis of unspecified deep veins of lower extremity, bilateral
I82. 4Ø9	Acute embolism and thrombosis of unspecified deep veins of unspecified lower extremity
I82.411	Acute embolism and thrombosis of right femoral vein
I82.412	Acute embolism and thrombosis of left femoral vein
I82.413	Acute embolism and thrombosis of femoral vein, bilateral
I82.419	Acute embolism and thrombosis of unspecified femoral vein
I82.421	Acute embolism and thrombosis of right iliac vein
I82.422	Acute embolism and thrombosis of left iliac vein
I82.423	Acute embolism and thrombosis of iliac vein, bilateral
I82.429	Acute embolism and thrombosis of unspecified iliac vein
I82.431	Acute embolism and thrombosis of right popliteal vein
I82.432	Acute embolism and thrombosis of left popliteal vein
I82.433	Acute embolism and thrombosis of popliteal vein, bilateral
I82.439	Acute embolism and thrombosis of unspecified popliteal vein
I82.4Y1	Acute embolism and thrombosis of unspecified deep veins of right proximal lower extremity
I82.4Y2	Acute embolism and thrombosis of unspecified deep veins of left proximal lower extremity
I82.4Y3	Acute embolism and thrombosis of unspecified deep veins of proximal lower extremity, bilateral
I82.4Y9	Acute embolism and thrombosis of unspecified deep veins of unspecified proximal lower extremity
I82.441	Acute embolism and thrombosis of right tibial vein
I82.442	Acute embolism and thrombosis of left tibial vein
I82.443	Acute embolism and thrombosis of tibial vein, bilateral
I82.449	Acute embolism and thrombosis of unspecified tibial vein
I82.491	Acute embolism and thrombosis of other specified deep vein of right lower extremity
I82.492	Acute embolism and thrombosis of other specified deep vein of left lower extremity
I82.493	Acute embolism and thrombosis of other specified deep vein of lower extremity, bilateral
I82.499	Acute embolism and thrombosis of other specified deep vein of unspecified lower extremity
I82.4Z1	Acute embolism and thrombosis of unspecified deep veins of right distal lower extremity
I82.4Z2	Acute embolism and thrombosis of unspecified deep veins of left distal lower extremity
I82.4Z3	Acute embolism and thrombosis of unspecified deep veins of distal lower extremity, bilateral
I82.4Z9	Acute embolism and thrombosis of unspecified deep veins of unspecified distal lower extremity
I82.5Ø1	Chronic embolism and thrombosis of unspecified deep veins of right lower extremity
I82.5Ø2	Chronic embolism and thrombosis of unspecified deep veins of left lower extremity
I82.5Ø3	Chronic embolism and thrombosis of unspecified deep veins of lower extremity, bilateral
I82.5Ø9	Chronic embolism and thrombosis of unspecified deep veins of unspecified lower extremity
I82.591	Chronic embolism and thrombosis of other specified deep vein of right lower extremity
I82.592	Chronic embolism and thrombosis of other specified deep vein of left lower extremity
I82.593	Chronic embolism and thrombosis of other specified deep vein of lower extremity, bilateral
I82.599	Chronic embolism and thrombosis of other specified deep vein of unspecified lower extremity
I82.511	Chronic embolism and thrombosis of right femoral vein
I82.512	Chronic embolism and thrombosis of left femoral vein
I82.513	Chronic embolism and thrombosis of femoral vein, bilateral
I82.519	Chronic embolism and thrombosis of unspecified femoral vein
I82.521	Chronic embolism and thrombosis of right iliac vein

ICD-10-CM	Code Description
I82.522	Chronic embolism and thrombosis of left iliac vein
I82.523	Chronic embolism and thrombosis of iliac vein, bilateral
I82.529	Chronic embolism and thrombosis of unspecified iliac vein
I82.531	Chronic embolism and thrombosis of right popliteal vein
I82.532	Chronic embolism and thrombosis of left popliteal vein
I82.533	Chronic embolism and thrombosis of popliteal vein, bilateral
I82.539	Chronic embolism and thrombosis of unspecified popliteal vein
I82.5Y1	Chronic embolism and thrombosis of unspecified deep veins of right proximal lower extremity
I82.5Y2	Chronic embolism and thrombosis of unspecified deep veins of left proximal lower extremity
I82.5Y3	Chronic embolism and thrombosis of unspecified deep veins of proximal lower extremity, bilateral
I82.5Y9	Chronic embolism and thrombosis of unspecified deep veins of unspecified proximal lower extremity
I82.541	Chronic embolism and thrombosis of right tibial vein
I82.42	Chronic embolism and thrombosis of left tibial vein
I82.543	Chronic embolism and thrombosis of tibial vein, bilateral
I82.549	Chronic embolism and thrombosis of unspecified tibial vein
I82.5Z1	Chronic embolism and thrombosis of unspecified deep veins of right distal lower extremity
I82.5Z2	Chronic embolism and thrombosis of unspecified deep veins of left distal lower extremity
I82.5Z3	Chronic embolism and thrombosis of unspecified deep veins of distal lower extremity, bilateral
I82.5Z9	Chronic embolism and thrombosis of unspecified deep veins of unspecified distal lower extremity
I82.611	Acute embolism and thrombosis of superficial veins of right upper extremity
I82.612	Acute embolism and thrombosis of superficial veins of left upper extremity
I82.613	Acute embolism and thrombosis of superficial veins of upper extremity, bilateral
I82.619	Acute embolism and thrombosis of superficial veins of unspecified upper extremity
I82.621	Acute embolism and thrombosis of deep veins of right upper extremity
I82.622	Acute embolism and thrombosis of deep veins of left upper extremity
I82.623	Acute embolism and thrombosis of deep veins of upper extremity, bilateral
I82.629	Acute embolism and thrombosis of deep veins of unspecified upper extremity
I82.6Ø1	Acute embolism and thrombosis of unspecified veins of right upper extremity
I82.6Ø2	Acute embolism and thrombosis of unspecified veins of left upper extremity
I82.6Ø3	Acute embolism and thrombosis of unspecified veins of upper extremity, bilateral
I82.6Ø9	Acute embolism and thrombosis of unspecified veins of unspecified upper extremity
I82.A11	Acute embolism and thrombosis of right axillary vein
I82.A12	Acute embolism and thrombosis of left axillary vein
I82.A13	Acute embolism and thrombosis of axillary vein, bilateral
I82.A19	Acute embolism and thrombosis of unspecified axillary vein
I82.A21	Chronic embolism and thrombosis of right axillary vein
I82.A22	Chronic embolism and thrombosis of left axillary vein
I82.A23	Chronic embolism and thrombosis of axillary vein, bilateral
I82.A29	Chronic embolism and thrombosis of unspecified axillary vein
I82.B11	Acute embolism and thrombosis of right subclavian vein
I82.B12	Acute embolism and thrombosis of left subclavian vein
I82.B13	Acute embolism and thrombosis of subclavian vein, bilateral
I82.B19	Acute embolism and thrombosis of unspecified subclavian vein
I82.B21	Chronic embolism and thrombosis of right subclavian vein
I82.B22	Chronic embolism and thrombosis of left subclavian vein
I82.B23	Chronic embolism and thrombosis of subclavian vein, bilateral
I82.B29	Chronic embolism and thrombosis of unspecified subclavian vein
I82.C11	Acute embolism and thrombosis of right internal jugular vein
I82.C12	Acute embolism and thrombosis of left internal jugular vein
I82.C13	Acute embolism and thrombosis of internal jugular vein, bilateral

ICD-10-CM	Code Description
I82.C19	Acute embolism and thrombosis of unspecified internal jugular vein
I82.C21	Chronic embolism and thrombosis of right internal jugular vein
I82.C22	Chronic embolism and thrombosis of left internal jugular vein
I82.C23	Chronic embolism and thrombosis of internal jugular vein, bilateral
I82.C29	Chronic embolism and thrombosis of unspecified internal jugular vein
I82.210	Acute embolism and thrombosis of superior vena cava
I82.290	Acute embolism and thrombosis of other thoracic veins
I82.701	Chronic embolism and thrombosis of unspecified veins of right upper extremity
I82.702	Chronic embolism and thrombosis of unspecified veins of left upper extremity
I82.703	Chronic embolism and thrombosis of unspecified veins of upper extremity, bilateral
I82.709	Chronic embolism and thrombosis of unspecified veins of unspecified upper extremity
I82.711	Chronic embolism and thrombosis of superficial veins of right upper extremity
I82.712	Chronic embolism and thrombosis of superficial veins of left upper extremity
I82.713	Chronic embolism and thrombosis of superficial veins of upper extremity, bilateral
I82.719	Chronic embolism and thrombosis of superficial veins of unspecified upper extremity
I82.721	Chronic embolism and thrombosis of deep veins of right upper extremity
I82.722	Chronic embolism and thrombosis of deep veins of left upper extremity
I82.723	Chronic embolism and thrombosis of deep veins of upper extremity, bilateral
I82.729	Chronic embolism and thrombosis of deep veins of unspecified upper extremity
I82.811	Embolism and thrombosis of superficial veins of right lower extremities
I82.812	Embolism and thrombosis of superficial veins of left lower extremities
I82.813	Embolism and thrombosis of superficial veins of lower extremities, bilateral
I82.819	Embolism and thrombosis of superficial veins of unspecified lower extremities
I82.890	Acute embolism and thrombosis of other specified veins
I82.891	Chronic embolism and thrombosis of other specified veins
I82.90	Acute embolism and thrombosis of unspecified vein
I82.91	Chronic embolism and thrombosis of unspecified vein

Pulmonary Embolism & Infarction

ICD-10-CM	Code Description
I26.01	Septic pulmonary embolism with acute cor pulmonale
I26.90	Septic pulmonary embolism without acute cor pulmonale
I26.09	Other pulmonary embolism with acute cor pulmonale
I26.99	Other pulmonary embolism without acute cor pulmonale

Atrial Fibrillation

ICD-10-CM	Code Description
I48.0	Paroxysmal atrial fibrillation
I48.2	Chronic atrial fibrillation
I48.	-91 Unspecified atrial fibrillation Other
I23.6	Thrombosis of atrium, auricular appendage, and ventricle as current complications following acute myocardial infarction
I27.82	Chronic pulmonary embolism
I67.6	Nonpyogenic thrombosis of intracranial venous system
O22.50	Cerebral venous thrombosis in pregnancy, unspecified trimester
O22.51	Cerebral venous thrombosis in pregnancy, first trimester
O22.52	Cerebral venous thrombosis in pregnancy, second trimester
O22.53	Cerebral venous thrombosis in pregnancy, third trimester
O87.3	Cerebral venous thrombosis in the puerperium
Z79.01	Long term (current) use of anticoagulants
Z86.718	Personal history of other venous thrombosis and embolism
Z95.4	Presence of other heart

Coverage policy can be found in Pub. 100-3, Medicare National Coverage Determinations Manual, Chapter 1, section 190.11 PT/INR. (http://www.cms.hhs.gov/manuals/103_cov_determ/ncd103index.asp

100-04, 32, 80.8

CWF Utilization Edits

Edit 1

Should CWF receive a claim from an FI for G0245 or G0246 and a second claim from a contractor for either G0245 or G0246 (or vice versa) and they are different dates of service and less than 6 months apart, the second claim will reject. CWF will edit to allow G0245 or G0246 to be paid no more than every 6 months for a particular beneficiary, regardless of who furnished the service. If G0245 has been paid, regardless of whether it was posted as a facility or professional claim, it must be 6 months before G0245 can be paid again or G0246 can be paid. If G0246 has been paid, regardless of whether it was posted as a facility or professional claim, it must be 6 months before G0246 can be paid again or G0245 can be paid. CWF will not impose limits on how many times each code can be paid for a beneficiary as long as there has been 6 months between each service.

The CWF will return a specific reject code for this edit to the contractors and FIs that will be identified in the CWF documentation. Based on the CWF reject code, the contractors and FIs must deny the claims and return the following messages:

> MSN 18.4 -- This service is being denied because it has not been __ months since your last examination of this kind (NOTE: Insert 6 as the appropriate number of months.)

> RA claim adjustment reason code 96 - Non-covered charges, along with remark code M86 - Service denied because payment already made for same/similar procedure within set time frame.

Edit 2

The CWF will edit to allow G0247 to pay only if either G0245 or G0246 has been submitted and accepted as payable on the same date of service. CWF will return a specific reject code for this edit to the contractors and FIs that will be identified in the CWF documentation. Based on this reject code, contractors and FIs will deny the claims and return the following messages:

> MSN 21.21 - This service was denied because Medicare only covers this service under certain circumstances.

> RA claim adjustment reason code 107 - The related or qualifying claim/service was not identified on this claim.

Edit 3

Once a beneficiary's condition has progressed to the point where routine foot care becomes a covered service, payment will no longer be made for LOPS evaluation and management services. Those services would be considered to be included in the regular exams and treatments afforded to the beneficiary on a routine basis. The physician or provider must then just bill the routine foot care codes, per Pub 100-2, Chapter 15, Sec. 290.

The CWF will edit to reject LOPS codes G0245, G0246, and/or G0247 when on the beneficiary's record it shows that one of the following routine foot care codes were billed and paid within the prior 6 months: 11055, 11056, 11057, 11719, 11720, and/or 11721.

The CWF will return a specific reject code for this edit to the contractors and FIs that will be identified in the CWF documentation. Based on the CWF reject code, the contractors and FIs must deny the claims and return the following messages:

> MSN 21.21 - This service was denied because Medicare only covers this service under certain circumstances.

> The RA claim adjustment reason code 96 - Non-covered charges, along with remark code M86 - Service denied because payment already made for same/similar procedure within set time frame.

100-04, 32, 90

Stem Cell Transplantation

Rev.3556, Issued: 07-01-2016; Effective: 1-27-16; Implementation: 10-3-16

A. General

Stem cell transplantation is a process in which stem cells are harvested from either a patient's (autologous) or donor's (allogeneic) bone marrow or peripheral blood for intravenous infusion.

Allogeneic and autologous stem cell transplants are covered under Medicare for specific diagnoses. See Pub. 100-03, National Coverage Determinations Manual, section 110.23, for a complete description of covered and noncovered conditions. For Part A hospital inpatient claims processing instructions, refer to Pub. 100-04, Chapter 3, section 90. The following sections contain claims processing instructions for all other claims.

B. Nationally Covered Indications

I.   Allogeneic Hematopoietic Stem Cell Transplantation (HSCT)

HCPCS Code 38240

ICD-9-CM Procedure Codes 41.02, 41.03, 41.05, and 41.08

ICD-10-PCS Procedure Codes 30230G1, 30230Y1, 30233G1, 30233Y1, 30240G1, 30240Y1, 30243G1, 30243Y1, 30250G1, 30250Y1, 30253G1, 30253Y1, 30260G1, 30260Y1, 30263G1, and 30263Y1

> a.   Effective for services performed on or after August 1, 1978:

i. For the treatment of leukemia, leukemia in remission (ICD-9-CM codes 204.00 through 208.91; see table below for ICD-10-CM codes)

ICD-10	Description
C91.01	Acute lymphoblastic leukemia, in remission
C91.11	Chronic lymphocytic leukemia of B-cell type in remission
C91.31	Prolymphocytic leukemia of B-cell type, in remission
C91.51	Adult T-cell lymphoma/leukemia (HTLV-1-associated), in remission
C91.61	Prolymphocytic leukemia of T-cell type, in remission
C91.91	Lymphoid leukemia, unspecified, in remission
C91.A1	Mature B-cell leukemia Burkitt-type, in remission
C91.Z1	Other lymphoid leukemia, in remission
C92.01	Acute myeloblastic leukemia, in remission
C92.11	Chronic myeloid leukemia, BCR/ABL-positive, in remission
C92.21	Atypical chronic myeloid leukemia, BCR/ABL-negative, in remission
C92.31	Myeloid sarcoma, in remission
C92.41	Acute promyelocytic leukemia, in remission
C92.51	Acute myelomonocytic leukemia, in remission
C92.61	Acute myeloid leukemia with 11q23-abnormality in remission
C92.91	Myeloid leukemia, unspecified in remission
C92.A1	Acute myeloid leukemia with multilineage dysplasia, in remission
C92.Z1	Other myeloid leukemia, in remission
C93.01	Acute monoblastic/monocytic leukemia, in remission
C93.11	Chronic myelomonocytic leukemia, in remission
C93.31	Juvenile myelomonocytic leukemia, in remission
C93.91	Monocytic leukemia, unspecified in remission
C93.Z1	Other monocytic leukemia, in remission
C94.01	Acute erythroid leukemia, in remission
C94.21	Acute megakaryoblastic leukemia, in remission
C94.31	Mast cell leukemia, in remission
C94.81	Other specified leukemias, in remission
C95.01	Acute leukemia of unspecified cell type, in remission
C95.11	Chronic leukemia of unspecified cell type, in remission
C95.91	Leukemia, unspecified, in remission
D45	Polycythemia vera

ii. For the treatment of aplastic anemia (ICD-9-CM codes 284.0 through 284.9; see table below for ICD-10-CM codes)

ICD-10	Description
D60.0	Chronic acquired pure red cell aplasia
D60.1	Transient acquired pure red cell aplasia
D60.8	Other acquired pure red cell aplasias
D60.9	Acquired pure red cell aplasia, unspecified
D61.01	Constitutional (pure) red blood cell aplasia
D61.09	Other constitutional aplastic anemia
D61.1	Drug-induced aplastic anemia
D61.2	Aplastic anemia due to other external agents

ICD-10	Description
D61.3	Idiopathic aplastic anemia
D61.810	Antineoplastic chemotherapy induced pancytopenia
D61.811	Other drug-induced pancytopenia
D61.818	Other pancytopenia
D61.82	Myelophthisis
D61.89	Other specified aplastic anemias and other bone marrow failure syndromes
D61.9	Aplastic anemia, unspecified

b. Effective for services performed on or after June 3, 1985:

   i. For the treatment of severe combined immunodeficiency disease (SCID) (ICD-9-CM code 279.2; ICD-10-CM codes D81.0, D81.1, D81.2, D81.6, D81.7, D81.89, and D81.9). ii. For the treatment of Wiskott-Aldrich syndrome (ICD-9-CM code 279.12; ICD-10-CM code D82.0)

c. Effective for services performed on or after August 4, 2010: For the treatment of Myelodysplastic Syndromes (MDS) (ICD-9-CM codes 238.72, 238.73, 238.74, 238.75 and ICD-10-CM codes D46.B, D46.C, D46.0, D46.1, D46.20, D46.21, D46.22, D46.4, D46.9, D46.Z) pursuant to Coverage with Evidence Development (CED) in the context of a Medicare-approved, prospective clinical study. Refer to Pub. 100-03, NCD Manual, chapter 1, section 110.23, for further information about this policy. See section F below for billing instructions.

d. Effective for services performed on or after January 27, 2016:

   i. Allogeneic HSCT for multiple myeloma (ICD-10-CM codes C90.00, C90.01, and C90.02) is covered by Medicare only for beneficiaries with Durie-Salmon Stage II or III multiple myeloma, or International Staging System (ISS) Stage II or Stage III multiple myeloma, and participating in an approved prospective clinical study. Refer to Pub. 100-03, NCD Manual, chapter 1, section 110.23, for further information about this policy. See section F below for billing instructions.

   ii. Allogeneic HSCT for myelofibrosis (MF) (ICD-10-CM codes C94.40, C94.41, C94.42, D47.4, and D75.81) is covered by Medicare only for beneficiaries with Dynamic International Prognostic Scoring System (DIPSSplus) intermediate-2 or High primary or secondary MF and participating in an approved prospective clinical study. Refer to Pub. 100-03, NCD Manual, chapter 1, section 110.23, for further information about this policy. See section F below for billing instructions.

   iii. Allogeneic HSCT for sickle cell disease (SCD) (ICD-10-CM codes D57.00, D57.01, D57.02, D57.1, D57.20, D57.211, D57.212, D57.219, D57.40, D57.411, D57.412, D57.419, D57.80, D57.811, D57.812, and D57.819) is covered by Medicare only for beneficiaries with severe, symptomatic SCD who participate in an approved prospective clinical study. Refer to Pub. 100-03, NCD Manual, chapter 1, section 110.23, for further information about this policy. See section F below for billing instructions.

II. Autologous Stem Cell Transplantation (AuSCT)

HCPCS Code 38241

ICD-9-CM Procedure Codes 41.01, 41.04, 41.07, and 41.09;

ICD-10-PCS Procedure Codes 30230AZ, 30230G0, 30230Y0, 30233G0, 30233Y0, 30240G0, 30240Y0, 30243G0, 30243Y0, 30250G0, 30250Y0, 30253G0, 30253Y0, 30260G0, 30260Y0, 30263G0, and 30263Y0

a. Effective for services performed on or after April 28, 1989: Acute leukemia in remission who have a high probability of relapse and who have no human leucocyte antigens (HLA)-matched (ICD-9-CM codes 204.01, 205.01, 206.01, 207.01, 208.01; ICD-10-CM diagnosis codes C91.01, C92.01, C92.41, C92.51, C92.61, C92.A1, C93.01, C94.01, C94.21, C94.41, C95.01); Resistant non-Hodgkin's lymphomas or those presenting with poor prognostic features following an initial response (ICD-9-CM codes 200.00 - 200.08, 200.10-200.18, 200.20-200.28, 200.80-200.88, 202.00-202.08, 202.80-202.88 or 202.90-202.98; ICD-10-CM diagnosis codes C82.00-C85.29, C85.80-C86.6, C96.4, and C96.Z-C96.9); Recurrent or refractory neuroblastoma (see ICD-9-CM codes Neoplasm by site, malignant for the appropriate diagnosis code; if ICD-10-CM is applicable the following ranges are reported: C00 - C96, and D00 - D09 Resistant non-Hodgkin's lymphomas); or, Advanced Hodgkin's disease who have failed conventional therapy and have no HLA-matched donor (ICD-9-CM codes 201.00 - 201.98; ICD-10-CM codes C81.00 - C81.99).

b. Effective for services performed on or after October 1, 2000: Single AuSCT is only covered for Durie-Salmon Stage II or III multiple myeloma patients (ICD-9-CM codes 203.00 or 238.6; ICD-10-CM codes C90.00, C90.01, C90.02 and D47.Z9) that fit the following requirements:

   • Newly diagnosed or responsive multiple myeloma. This includes those patients with previously untreated disease, those with at least a partial response to prior chemotherapy (defined as a 50% decrease either in measurable paraprotein [serum and/or urine] or in bone marrow infiltration, sustained for at least 1 month), and those in responsive relapse; and • Adequate cardiac, renal, pulmonary, and hepatic function.

c. Effective for services performed on or after March 15, 2005: When recognized clinical risk factors are employed to select patients for transplantation, high dose melphalan (HDM) together with AuSCT is reasonable and necessary for Medicare beneficiaries of any age group with primary amyloid light chain (AL) amyloidosis (ICD-9-CM code 277.3 or 277.39) who meet the following criteria:

- Amyloid deposition in 2 or fewer organs; and,
- Cardiac left ventricular ejection fraction (EF) greater than 45%.

ICD-9-CM code	Description	ICD-10-CM code	Description
277.30	Amyloidosis, unspecified	E85.9	Amyloidosis, unspecified
277.39	Other amyloidosis	E85.8	Other amyloidosis
		E85.4	Organ-limited amyloidosis

As the ICD-9-CM codes 277.3, and 277.39 for amyloidosis do not differentiate between primary and non-primary, A/B MACs (B) should perform prepay reviews on all claims with a diagnosis of ICD-9-CM code 277.3 to determine whether payment is appropriate.

If ICD-10-CM is applicable, as the applicable ICD-10 CM codes E85.4, E85.8, and E85.9 for amyloidosis do not differentiate between primary and non-primary, A/B MACs (B) should perform prepay reviews on all claims with a diagnosis of ICD-10-CM code E85.4, E85.8, and E85.9 to determine whether payment is appropriate.

C. Nationally Non-Covered Indications

I.　Allogeneic Hematopoietic Stem Cell Transplantation (HSCT)

Effective for claims with dates of service on or after May 24, 1996, through January 27, 2016, allogeneic HSCT is not covered as treatment for multiple myeloma (if ICD-9-CM is applicable, ICD-9-CM code 203.00 and 203.01; or if ICD-10-CM is applicable, ICD-10-CMcodes C90.00, C90.01, C90.02 and D47.Z9).

II.　Autologous Stem Cell Transplantation (AuSCT)

AuSCT is not considered reasonable and necessary within the meaning of §I862(a)(1)(A) of the Act and is not covered under Medicare for the following conditions:

a) Acute leukemia not in remission (if ICD-9-CM is applicable, ICD-9-CM codes 204.00, 205.00, 206.00, 207.00 and 208.00; or if ICD-10-CM is applicable, ICD-10-CM codes C91.00, C92.00, C93.00, C94.00, andC95.00)

b) Chronic granulocytic leukemia (if ICD-9-CM is applicable, ICD-9-CM codes 205.10 and 205.11; or if ICD-10-CM is applicable, ICD-10-CM codes C92.10 andC92.11);

c) Solid tumors (other than neuroblastoma) (if ICD-9-CM is applicable, ICD-9-CM codes 140.0 through 199.1; or if ICD-10-CM is applicable, ICD-10-CM codesC00.0 – C80.2 and D00.0 – D09.9);

d) Up to October 1, 2000, multiple myeloma (if ICD-9-CM is applicable, ICD-9-CM code 203.00 and 203.01; or if ICD-10-CM is applicable, ICD-10-CM codes C90.00, C90.01, C90.02 and D47.Z9);

e) Tandem transplantation (multiple rounds of AuSCT) for patients with multiple myeloma (if ICD-9-CM is applicable, ICD-9-CM code 203.00 and 203.01; or if ICD-10-CM is applicable, ICD-10-CM codes C90.00, C90.01, C90.02 and D47.Z9);

f) Effective October 1, 2000, non-primary AL amyloidosis (see table below for applicable ICD codes); and,

g) Effective October 1, 2000, through March 14, 2005, primary AL amyloidosis for Medicare beneficiaries age 64 or older (see table below for applicable ICD codes).

ICD-9-CM codes	Description	ICD-10-CM codes	Description
277.30	Amyloidosis, unspecified	E85.9	Amyloidosis, unspecified
277.31	Familial Mediterranean fever	E85.0	Non-neuropathic heredofamilial amyloidosis
277.39	Other amyloidosis	E85.8	Other amyloidosis
		E85.1	Neuropathic heredofamilial amyloidosis
		E85.2	Heredofamilial amyloidosis, unspecified
		E85.3	Secondary systemic amyloidosis
		E85.4	Organ-limited amyloidosis

As the ICD-9-CM code 277.3 and 277.39 for amyloidosis do not differentiate between primary and non-primary, A/B MACs (B) should perform prepay reviews on all claims with a diagnosis of ICD-9-CM code 277.3 and 277.39 to determine whether payment is appropriate.

If ICD-10-CM is applicable, as the applicable ICD-10 CM codes E85.4, E85.8, and E85.9 for amyloidosis do not differentiate between primary and non-primary, A/B MACs (B) should perform prepay reviews on all claims with a diagnosis of ICD-10-CM code E85.4, E85.8, and E85.9 to determine whether payment is appropriate.

D. Other

All other indications for stem cell transplantation not otherwise noted above as covered or non-covered remain at local Medicare Administrative Contractor discretion.

E. Suggested MSN and RA Messages

The contractor shall use an appropriate MSN and RA message such as the following:

MSN - 15.4, The information provided does not support the need for this service or item;

RA - 150, Payment adjusted because the payer deems the information submitted does not support this level of service.

F. Clinical Trials for Allogeneic Hematopoietic Stem Cell Transplantation (HSCT) for Myelodysplastic Syndrome (MDS), Multiple Myeloma, Myelofibrosis (MF), and for Sickle Cell Disease (SCD)

I.　Background

Effective for services performed on or after August 4, 2010, contractors shall pay for claims for allogeneic HSCT for the treatment of Myelodysplastic Syndromes (MDS) pursuant to Coverage with Evidence Development (CED) in the context of a Medicare-approved, prospective clinical study.

Effective for services performed on or after January 27, 2016, contractors shall pay for claims for allogeneic HSCT for the treatment of multiple myeloma, myelofibrosis (MF), and for sickle cell disease (SCD) pursuant to CED, in the context of a Medicare-approved, prospective clinical study.

Refer to Pub.100-03, National Coverage Determinations Manual, Chapter 1, section 110.23, for more information about this policy, and Pub. 100-04, Medicare Claims Processing Manual, Chapter 3, section 90.3, for information on inpatient billing of this CED.

II.　Adjudication Requirements Payable Conditions. For claims with dates of service on and after August 4, 2010, contractors shall pay for claims for allogeneic HSCT for MDS when the service was provided pursuant to a Medicare-approved clinical study under CED; these services are paid only in the inpatient setting (Type of Bill (TOB) 11X), as outpatient Part B (TOB 13X), and in Method II critical access hospitals (TOB 85X).

Contractors shall require the following coding in order to pay for these claims:

- Existing Medicare-approved clinical trial coding conventions, as required in Pub. 100-04, Medicare Claims Processing Manual, Chapter 32, section 69, and inpatient billing requirements regarding acquisition of stem cells in Pub. 100-04, Medicare Claims Processing Manual, Chapter 3, section 90.3.1.
- If ICD-9-CM is applicable, for Inpatient Hospital Claims: ICD-9-CM procedure codes 41.02, 41.03, 41.05, and 41.08 or,
- If ICD-10-CM is applicable, ICD-10-PCS, procedure codes 30230G1, 30230Y1, 30233G1, 30233Y1, 30240G1, 30240Y1, 30243G1, 30243Y1, 30250G1,30250Y1, 30253G1, 30253Y1, 30260G1, 30260Y1, 30263G1, and 30263Y1
- If Outpatient Hospital or Professional Claims: HCPCS procedure code 38240
- If ICD-9-CM is applicable, ICD-9-CM diagnosis codes 238.72, 238.73, 238.74, 238.75 or,
- If ICD-10-CM is applicable, ICD-10-CM codes D46.A, D46.B, D46.C, D46.0, D46.1, D46.20, D46.21, D46.22, D46.4, D46.9, D46.Z,
- Professional claims only: place of service codes 19, 21, or 22.

Payable Conditions. For claims with dates of service on and after January 27, 2016, contractors shall pay for claims for allogeneic HSCT for multiple myeloma, myelofibrosis (MF), and for sickle cell disease (SCD) when the service was provided pursuant to a Medicare-approved clinical study under CED; these services are paid only in the inpatient setting (Type of Bill (TOB) 11X), as outpatient Part B (TOB 13X), and in Method II critical access hospitals (TOB 85X).

Contractors shall require the following coding in order to pay for these claims:

- Existing Medicare-approved clinical trial coding conventions, as required in Pub. 100-04, Medicare Claims Processing Manual, Chapter 32, section 69, and inpatient billing requirements regarding acquisition of stem cells in Pub. 100-04, Medicare Claims Processing Manual, Chapter 3, section 90.3.1.
- ICD-10-PCS codes 30230G1, 30230Y1, 30233G1, 30233Y1, 30240G1, 30240Y1, 30243G1, 30243Y1, 30250G1, 30250Y1, 30253G1, 30253Y1, 30260G1, 30260Y1, 30263G1, and 30263Y1
- If Outpatient Hospital or Professional Claims: HCPCS procedure code 38240
- ICD-10-CM diagnosis codes C90.00, C90.01, C90.02, C94.40, C94.41, C94.42, D47.4, D75.81, D57.00, D57.01, D57.02, D57.1, D57.20, D57.211, D57.212, D57.219, D57.40, D57.411, D57.412, D57.419, D57.80, D57.811, D57.812, and D57.819
- Professional claims only: place of service codes 19, 21, or 22.

Denials. Contractors shall deny claims failing to meet any of the above criteria. In addition, contractors shall apply the following requirements:

- Providers shall issue a hospital issued notice of non-coverage (HINN) or advance beneficiary notice (ABN) to the beneficiary if the services performed are not provided in accordance with CED.

- Contractors shall deny claims that do not meet the criteria for coverage with the following messages:

CARC 50 - These are non-covered services because this is not deemed a 'medical necessity' by the payer.

NOTE: Refer to the 835 Healthcare Policy Identification Segment (loop 2110 Service Payment Information REF), if present.

RARC N386 - This decision was based on a National Coverage Determination (NCD). An NCD provides a coverage determination as to whether a particular item or service is covered. A copy of this policy is available at http:www.cms.hhs.gov/mcd/search.asp. If you do not have web access, you may contact the contractor to request a copy of the NCD.

Group Code – Patient Responsibility (PR) if HINN/ABN issued, otherwise Contractual Obligation (CO)

MSN 16.77 – This service/item was not covered because it was not provided as part of a qualifying trial/study. (Este servicio/artículo no fue cubierto porque no estaba incluido como parte de un ensayo clínico/estudio calificado.)

MSN 15.20 – The following policies [NCD 110.23] were used when we made this decision. (Las siguientes políticas [NCD 110.23] fueron utilizadas cuando se tomó esta decisión.)

100-04, 32, 90.2

HCPCS and Diagnosis Coding

Allogeneic Stem Cell Transplantation

- Effective for services performed on or after August 1, 1978:

  - For the treatment of leukemia or leukemia in remission, providers shall use ICD-9-CM codes 204.00 through 208.91 and HCPCS code 38240.

  - For the treatment of aplastic anemia, providers shall use ICD-9-CM codes 284.0 through 284.9 and HCPCS code 38240.

- Effective for services performed on or after June 3, 1985:

  - For the treatment of severe combined immunodeficiency disease, providers shall use ICD-9-CM code 279.2 and HCPCS code 38240.

  - For the treatment of Wiskott-Aldrich syndrome, providers shall use ICD-9-CM code 279.12 and HCPCS code 38240.

- Effective for services performed on or after May 24, 1996:

  - Allogeneic stem cell transplantation, HCPCS code 38240 is not covered as treatment for the diagnosis of multiple myeloma ICD-9-CM codes 203.00 or 203.01.

Autologous Stem Cell Transplantation.--Is covered under the following circumstances effective for services performed on or after April 28, 1989:

- For the treatment of patients with acute leukemia in remission who have a high probability of relapse and who have no human leucocyte antigens (HLA) matched, providers shall use ICD-9-CM code 204.01 lymphoid; ICD-9-CM code 205.01 myeloid; ICD-9-CM code 206.01 monocytic; or ICD-9-CM code 207.01 acute erythremia and erythroleukemia; or ICD-9-CM code 208.01 unspecified cell type and HCPCS code 38241.

- For the treatment of resistant non-Hodgkin's lymphomas for those patients presenting with poor prognostic features following an initial response, providers shall use ICD-9-CM codes 200.00 - 200.08, 200.10-200.18, 200.20-200.28, 200.80-200.88, 202.00-202.08, 202.80-202.88 or 202.90-202.98 and HCPCS code 38241.

- For the treatment of recurrent or refractory neuroblastoma, providers shall use ICD-9-CM codes Neoplasm by site, malignant, the appropriate HCPCS code and HCPCS code 38241.

- For the treatment of advanced Hodgkin's disease for patients who have failed conventional therapy and have no HLA-matched donor, providers shall use ICD-9-CM codes 201.00 - 201.98 and HCPCS code 38241.

Autologous Stem Cell Transplantation.--Is covered under the following circumstances effective for services furnished on or after October 1, 2000:

- For the treatment of multiple myeloma (only for beneficiaries who are less than age 78, have Durie-Salmon stage II or III newly diagnosed or responsive multiple myeloma, and have adequate cardiac, renal, pulmonary and hepatic functioning), providers shall use ICD- 9-CM code 203.00 or 238.6 and HCPCS code 38241.

- For the treatment of recurrent or refractory neuroblastoma, providers shall use appropriate code (see ICD-9-CM neoplasm by site, malignant) and HCPCS code 38241.

- Effective for services performed on or after March 15, 2005, when recognized clinical risk factors are employed to select patients for transplantation, high-dose melphalan (HDM) together with autologous stem cell transplantation (HDM/AuSCT) is reasonable and necessary for Medicare beneficiaries of any age

group for the treatment of primary amyloid light chain (AL) amyloidosis, ICD-9-CM code 277.3 who meet the following criteria:

- Amyloid deposition in 2 or fewer organs; and,

- Cardiac left ventricular ejection fraction (EF) greater than 45%.

100-04, 32, 90.2.1

HCPCS and Diagnosis Coding for Stem Cell Transplantation - ICD-10-CM Applicable

ICD-10 is applicable to services on and after the implementation of ICD-.

For services provided use the appropriate code from the ICD-10 CM codes in the table below. See §90.2 for a list of covered conditions.

ICD-10	Description
C91.01	Acute lymphoblastic leukemia, in remission
C91.11	Chronic lymphocytic leukemia of B-cell type in remission
C91.31	Prolymphocytic leukemia of B-cell type, in remission
C91.51	Adult T-cell lymphoma/leukemia (HTLV-1-associated), in remission
C91.61	Prolymphocytic leukemia of T-cell type, in remission
C91.91	Lymphoid leukemia, unspecified, in remission
C91.A1	Mature B-cell leukemia Burkitt-type, in remission
C91.Z1	Other lymphoid leukemia, in remission
C92.01	Acute myeloblastic leukemia, in remission
C92.11	Chronic myeloid leukemia, BCR/ABL-positive, in remission
C92.21	Atypical chronic myeloid leukemia, BCR/ABL-negative, in remission
C92.31	Myeloid sarcoma, in remission
C92.41	Acute promyelocytic leukemia, in remission
C92.51	Acute myelomonocytic leukemia, in remission
C92.61	Acute myeloid leukemia with 11q23-abnormality in remission
C92.91	Myeloid leukemia, unspecified in remission
C92.A1	Acute myeloid leukemia with multilineage dysplasia, in remission
C92.Z1	Other myeloid leukemia, in remission
C93.01	Acute monoblastic/monocytic leukemia, in remission
C93.11	Chronic myelomonocytic leukemia, in remission
C93.31	Juvenile myelomonocytic leukemia, in remission
C93.91	Monocytic leukemia, unspecified in remission
C93.91	Monocytic leukemia, unspecified in remission
C93.Z1	Other monocytic leukemia, in remission
C94.01	Acute erythroid leukemia, in remission
C94.21	Acute megakaryoblastic leukemia, in remission
C94.31	Mast cell leukemia, in remission
C94.81	Other specified leukemias, in remission
C95.01	Acute leukemia of unspecified cell type, in remission
C95.11	Chronic leukemia of unspecified cell type, in remission
C95.91	Leukemia, unspecified, in remission
D45	Polycythemia vera
D61.01	Constitutional (pure) red blood cell aplasia
D61.09	Other constitutional aplastic anemia
D82.0	Wiskott-Aldrich syndrome
D81.0	Severe combined immunodeficiency [SCID] with reticular dysgenesis
D81.1	Severe combined immunodeficiency [SCID] with low T- and B-cell numbers
D81.2	Severe combined immunodeficiency [SCID] with low or normal B-cell numbers
D81.6	Major histocompatibility complex class I deficiency
D81.7	Major histocompatibility complex class II deficiency
D81.89	Other combined immunodeficiencies
D81.9	Combined immunodeficiency, unspecified
D81.2	Severe combined immunodeficiency [SCID] with low or normal B-cell numbers
D81.6	Major histocompatibility complex class I deficiency
D60.0	Chronic acquired pure red cell aplasia
D60.1	Transient acquired pure red cell aplasia
D60.8	Other acquired pure red cell aplasias
D60.9	Acquired pure red cell aplasia, unspecified
D61.01	Constitutional (pure) red blood cell aplasia
D61.09	Other constitutional aplastic anemia
D61.1	Drug-induced aplastic anemia
D61.2	Aplastic anemia due to other external agents

ICD-10	Description
D61.3	Idiopathic aplastic anemia
D61.810	Antineoplastic chemotherapy induced pancytopenia
D61.811	Other drug-induced pancytopenia
D61.818	Other pancytopenia
D61.82	Myelophthisis
D61.89	Other specified aplastic anemias and other bone marrow failure syndromes
D61.9	Aplastic anemia, unspecified

- If ICD-10-CM is applicable, the following ranges of ICD-10-CM codes are also covered for AuSCT: Resistant non-Hodgkin's lymphomas, ICD-10-CM diagnosis codes C82.00-C85.29, C85.80-C86.6, C96.4, and C96.Z-C96.9.
- Tandem transplantation (multiple rounds of autologous stem cell transplantation) for patients with multiple myeloma, ICD-10-CM codes C90.00 and D47.Z9

NOTE: The following conditions are not covered:

- Acute leukemia not in remission
- Chronic granulocytic leukemia
- Solid tumors (other than neuroblastoma)
- Multiple myeloma
- For Medicare beneficiaries age 64 or older, all forms of amyloidosis, primary and non-primary
- Non-primary amyloidosis

Also coverage for conditions other than those specifically designated as covered in §90.2 or specifically designated as non-covered in this section or in §90.3 will be at the discretion of the individual contractor.

100-04, 32, 90.3

Non-Covered Conditions

Autologous stem cell transplantation is not covered for the following conditions:

- Acute leukemia not in remission (If ICD-9-CM is applicable, ICD-9-CM codes 204.00, 205.00, 206.00, 207.00 and 208.00) or (If ICD-10-CM is applicable, ICD-10-CM codes C91.00, C92.00, C93.00, C94.00, and C95.00)
- Chronic granulocytic leukemia (ICD-9-CM codes 205.10 and 205.11 if ICD-9-CM is applicable) or (if ICD-10-CM is applicable, ICD-10-CM codes C92.10 and C92.11);
- Solid tumors (other than neuroblastoma) (ICD-9-CM codes 140.0 through 199.1 if ICD-9-CM is applicable or if ICD-10-CM is applicable, ICD-10-CM codes C00.0 – C80.2 and D00.0 – D09.9.)
- Effective for services rendered on or after May 24, 1996 through September 30, 2000, multiple myeloma (ICD-9-CM code 203.00 and 203.01 if ICD-9-CM is applicable or if ICD-10-CM is applicable, ICD-10-CM codes C90.00 and D47.Z9);
- Effective for services on or after October 1, 2000, through March 14, 2005, for Medicare beneficiaries age 64 or older, all forms of amyloidosis, primary and non-primary
- Effective for services on or after 10/01/00, for all Medicare beneficiaries, non-primary amyloidosis

ICD-9-CM	Description	ICD-10-CM	Description
277.30	Amyloidosis, unspecified	E85.9	Amyloidosis, unspecified
277.31	Familial Mediterranean fever	E85.0	Non-neuropathic heredofamilial amyloidosis
277.39	Other amyloidosis	E85.1	Neuropathic heredofamilial amyloidosis
277.39	Other amyloidosis	E85.2	Heredofamilial amyloidosis, unspecified
277.39	Other amyloidosis	E85.3	Secondary systemic amyloidosis
277.39	Other amyloidosis	E85.4	Organ-limited amyloidosis
277.39	Other amyloidosis	E85.8	Other amyloidosis

NOTE: Coverage for conditions other than those specifically designated as covered in 90.2 or 90.2.1 or specifically designated as non-covered in this section will be at the discretion of the individual A/B MAC (B).

100-04, 32, 90.4

Edits

NOTE: Coverage for conditions other than those specifically designated as covered in 80.2 or specifically designated as non-covered in this section will be at the discretion of the individual A/B MAC (B).

Appropriate diagnosis to procedure code edits should be implemented for the non-covered conditions and services in 90.2 90.2.1, and 90.3 as applicable.

As the ICD-9-CM code 277.3 for amyloidosis does not differentiate between primary and non-primary, A/B MACs (B) should perform prepay reviews on all claims with a diagnosis of ICD-9-CM code 277.3 and a HCPCS procedure code of 38241 to determine whether payment is appropriate.

If ICD-10-CM is applicable, the applicable ICD-10 CM codes are: E85.0, E85.1, E85.2, E85.3, E85.4, E85.8, and E85.9.

100-04, 32, 90.6

Clinical Trials for Allogeneic Hematopoietic Stem Cell Transplantation (HSCT) for Myelodysplastic Syndrome (MDS)

A. Background

Myelodysplastic Syndrome (MDS) refers to a group of diverse blood disorders in which the bone marrow does not produce enough healthy, functioning blood cells. These disorders are varied with regard to clinical characteristics, cytologic and pathologic features, and cytogenetics.

On August 4, 2010, the Centers for Medicare & Medicaid Services (CMS) issued a national coverage determination (NCD) stating that CMS believes that the evidence does not demonstrate that the use of allogeneic hematopoietic stem cell transplantation (HSCT) improves health outcomes in Medicare beneficiaries with MDS. Therefore, allogeneic HSCT for MDS is not reasonable and necessary under §1862(a)(1)(A) of the Social Security Act (the Act). However, allogeneic HSCT for MDS is reasonable and necessary under §1862(a)(1)(E) of the Act and therefore covered by Medicare ONLY if provided pursuant to a Medicare-approved clinical study under Coverage with Evidence Development (CED). Refer to Pub.100-3, NCD Manual, Chapter 1, section 110.8.1, for more information about this policy, and Pub. 100-4, MCP Manual, Chapter 3, section 90.3.1, for information on CED.

B. Adjudication Requirements

Payable Conditions. For claims with dates of service on and after August 4, 2010, contractors shall pay for claims for HSCT for MDS when the service was provided pursuant to a Medicare-approved clinical study under CED; these services are paid only in the inpatient setting (Type of Bill (TOB) 11X), as outpatient Part B (TOB 13X), and in Method II critical access hospitals (TOB 85X). Contractors shall require the following coding in order to pay for these claims:

- Existing Medicare-approved clinical trial coding conventions, as required in Pub. 100-4, MCP Manual, Chapter 32, section 69, and inpatient billing requirements regarding acquisition of stem cells in Pub. 100-4, MCP Manual, Chapter 3, section 90.3.3.
- If ICD-9-CM is applicable, for Inpatient Hospital Claims: ICD-9-CM procedure codes 41.02, 41.03, 41.05, and 41.08 or,
- If ICD-10-CM is applicable, ICD-10-PCS, procedure codes 30230G1, 30230Y1, 3023G1, 30233Y1, 30240G1, 30240Y1, 30243G1, 30243Y1, 30250G1,30250Y1, 30253G1, 30253Y1, 30260G1, 30260Y1, 30263G1, and 30263Y1
- If Outpatient Hospital or Professional Claims: HCPCS procedure code 38240
- If ICD-9-CM is applicable, ICD-9-CM diagnosis code 238.75 or If ICD-10-CM is applicable, ICD-10-CM diagnosis codes D46.9, D46.Z, or Z00.6 Professional claims only: place of service codes 21 or 22.

Denials. Contractors shall deny claims failing to meet any of the above criteria. In addition, contractors shall apply the following requirements:

- Providers shall issue a hospital issued notice of non-coverage (HINN) or advance beneficiary notice (ABN) to the beneficiary if the services performed are not provided in accordance with CED.
- Contractors shall deny claims that do not meet the criteria for coverage with the following messages:

   CARC 50 - These are non-covered services because this is not deemed a 'medical necessity' by the payer.

   NOTE: Refer to the 835 Healthcare Policy Identification Segment (loop 2110 Service Payment Information REF), if present.

   RARC N386 - This decision was based on a National Coverage Determination (NCD). An NCD provides a coverage determination as to whether a particular item or service is covered. A copy of this policy is available at http://www.cms.hhs.gov/mcd/search.asp. If you do not have web access, you may contact the contractor to request a copy of the NCD.

   Group Code – Patient Responsibility (PR) if HINN/ABN issued, otherwise Contractual Obligation (CO)

   MSN 16.77 – This service/item was not covered because it was not provided as part of a qualifying trial/study. (Este servicio/artículo no fue cubierto porque no estaba incluido como parte de un ensayo clínico/estudio calificado.)

100-04, 32, 120.2

Coding and General Billing Requirements

Physicians and hospitals must report one of the following Current Procedural Terminology (CPT) codes on the claim:

   66982   Extracapsular cataract removal with insertion of intraocular lens prosthesis (one stage procedure), manual or mechanical technique (e.g., irrigation and aspiration or phacoemulsification), complex requiring devices or techniques not generally used in routine cataract surgery (e.g., iris expansion device, suture support for intraocular lens, or primary posterior capsulorrhexis) or performed on patients in the amblyogenic development stage.

66983   Intracapsular cataract with insertion of intraocular lens prosthesis (one stage procedure)

66984   Extracapsular cataract removal with insertion of intraocular lens prosthesis (one stage procedure), manual or mechanical technique (e.g., irrigation and aspiration or phacoemulsification)

66985   Insertion of intraocular lens prosthesis (secondary implant), not associated with concurrent cataract extraction

66986   Exchange of intraocular lens

In addition, physicians inserting a P-C IOL or A-C IOL in an office setting may bill code V2632 (posterior chamber intraocular lens) for the IOL. Medicare will make payment for the lens based on reasonable cost for a conventional IOL. Place of Service (POS) = 11.

Effective for dates of service on and after January 1, 2006, physician, hospitals and ASCs may also bill the non-covered charges related to the P-C function of the IOL using HCPCS code V2788. Effective for dates of service on and after January 22, 2007 through January 1, 2008, non-covered charges related to A-C function of the IOL can be billed using HCPCS code V2788. The type of service indicator for the non-covered billed charges is Q. (The type of service is applied by the Medicare carrier and not the provider). Effective for A-C IOL insertion services on or after January 1, 2008, physicians, hospitals and ASCs should use V2787 rather than V2788 to report any additional charges that accrue.

When denying the non-payable charges submitted with V2787 or V2788, contractors shall use an appropriate Medical Summary Notice (MSN) such as 16.10 (Medicare does not pay for this item or service) and an appropriate claim adjustment reason code such as 96 (non-covered charges) for claims submitted with the non-payable charges.

Hospitals and physicians may use the proper CPT code(s) to bill Medicare for evaluation and management services usually associated with services following cataract extraction surgery, if appropriate.

A - Applicable Bill Types
The hospital applicable bill types are 12X, 13X, 83X and 85X.

B - Other Special Requirements for Hospitals
Hospitals shall continue to pay CAHs method 2 claims under current payment methodologies for conditional IOLs.

100-04, 32, 130.1

Billing and Payment Requirements

Effective for dates of service on or after January 1, 2000, use HCPCS code G0166 (External counterpulsation, per session) to report ECP services. The codes for external cardiac assist (92971), ECG rhythm strip and report (93040 or 93041), pulse oximetry (94760 or 94761) and plethysmography (93922 or 93923) or other monitoring tests for examining the effects of this treatment are not clinically necessary with this service and should not be paid on the same day, unless they occur in a clinical setting not connected with the delivery of the ECP. Daily evaluation and management service, e.g., 99201-99205, 99211-99215, 99217-99220, 99241-99245, cannot be billed with the ECP treatments. Any evaluation and management service must be justified with adequate documentation of the medical necessity of the visit. Deductible and coinsurance apply.

100-04, 32, 140.2

Cardiac Rehabilitation Program Services Furnished On or After January 1, 2010

As specified at 42 CFR 410.49, Medicare covers cardiac rehabilitation items and services for patients who have experienced one or more of the following:

- An acute myocardial infarction within the preceding 12 months; or
- A coronary artery bypass surgery; or
- Current stable angina pectoris; or
- Heart valve repair or replacement; or
- Percutaneous transluminal coronary angioplasty (PTCA) or coronary stenting; or
- A heart or heart-lung transplant or;
- Stable, chronic heart failure defined as patients with left ventricular ejection fraction of 35% or less and New York Heart Association (NYHA) class II to IV symptoms despite being on optimal heart failure therapy for at least 6 weeks (effective February 18, 2014).

Cardiac rehabilitation programs must include the following components:

- Physician-prescribed exercise each day cardiac rehabilitation items and services are furnished;
- Cardiac risk factor modification, including education, counseling, and behavioral intervention at least once during the program, tailored to patients' individual needs;

- Psychosocial assessment;
- Outcomes assessment; and
- An individualized treatment plan detailing how components are utilized for each patient.

Cardiac rehabilitation items and services must be furnished in a physician's office or a hospital outpatient setting. All settings must have a physician immediately available and accessible for medical consultations and emergencies at all times items and services are being furnished under the program. This provision is satisfied if the physician meets the requirements for the direct supervision of physician's office services as specified at 42 CFR 410.26 and for hospital outpatient therapeutic services as specified at 42 CFR 410.27.

As specified at 42 CFR 410.49(f)(1), cardiac rehabilitation program sessions are limited to a maximum of 2 1-hour sessions per day for up to 36 sessions over up to 36 weeks, with the option for an additional 36 sessions over an extended period of time if approved by the Medicare contractor.

100-04, 32, 140.2.1

Coding Requirements for Cardiac Rehabilitation Services Furnished On or After January 1, 2010

The following are the applicable CPT codes for cardiac rehabilitation services: 93797 - Physician services for outpatient cardiac rehabilitation; without continuous ECG monitoring (per session) and 93798 - Physician services for outpatient cardiac rehabilitation; with continuous ECG monitoring (per session) Effective for dates of service on or after January 1, 2010, hospitals and practitioners may report a maximum of 2 1-hour sessions per day. In order to report one session of cardiac rehabilitation services in a day, the duration of treatment must be at least 31 minutes. Two sessions of cardiac rehabilitation services may only be reported in the same day if the duration of treatment is at least 91 minutes. In other words, the first session would account for 60 minutes and the second session would account for at least 31 minutes if two sessions are reported. If several shorter periods of cardiac rehabilitation services are furnished on a given day, the minutes of service during those periods must be added together for reporting in 1-hour session increments.

Example: If the patient receives 20 minutes of cardiac rehabilitation services in the day, no cardiac rehabilitation session may be reported because less than 31 minutes of services were furnished.

Example: If a patient receives 20 minutes of cardiac rehabilitation services in the morning and 35 minutes of cardiac rehabilitation services in the afternoon of a single day, the hospital or practitioner would report 1 session of cardiac rehabilitation services under 1 unit of the appropriate CPT code for the total duration of 55 minutes of cardiac rehabilitation services on that day.

Example: If the patient receives 70 minutes of cardiac rehabilitation services in the morning and 25 minutes of cardiac rehabilitation services in the afternoon of a single day, the hospital or practitioner would report two sessions of cardiac rehabilitation services under the appropriate CPT code(s) because the total duration of cardiac rehabilitation services on that day of 95 minutes exceeds 90 minutes.

Example: If the patient receives 70 minutes of cardiac rehabilitation services in the morning and 85 minutes of cardiac rehabilitation services in the afternoon of a single day, the hospital or practitioner would report two sessions of cardiac rehabilitation services under the appropriate CPT code(s) for the total duration of cardiac rehabilitation services of 155 minutes. A maximum of two sessions per day may be reported, regardless of the total duration of cardiac rehabilitation services.

100-04, 32, 140.2.2.2

Requirements for CR and ICR Services on Institutional Claims

Effective for claims with dates of service on and after January 1, 2010, contractors shall pay for CR and ICR services when submitted on Types of Bill (TOBs) 13X and 85X only. All other TOBs shall be denied.

The following messages shall be used when contractors deny CR and ICR claims for TOBs 13X and 85X:

Claim Adjustment Reason Code (CARC) 171 – Payment is denied when performed/billed by this type of provider in this type of facility.

Remittance Advice Remark Code (RARC) N428 - Service/procedure not covered when performed in this place of service.

Medicare Summary Notice (MSN) 21.25 - This service was denied because Medicare only covers this service in certain settings.

Group Code PR (Patient Responsibility) – Where a claim is received with the GA modifier indicating that a signed ABN is on file.

Group Code CO (Contractor Responsibility) – Where a claim is received with the GZ modifier indicating that no signed ABN is on file.

100-04, 32, 140.2.2.4

Edits for CR Services Exceeding 36 Sessions

Effective for claims with dates of service on or after January 1, 2010, contractors shall deny all claims with HCPCS 93797 and 93798 (both professional and institutional claims) that exceed 36 CR sessions when a KX modifier is not included on the claim line.

The following messages shall be used when contractors deny CR claims that exceed 36 sessions, when a KX modifier is not included on the claim line:

Claim Adjustment Reason Code (CARC) 119 – Benefit maximum for this period or occurrence has been reached.

RARC N435 - Exceeds number/frequency approved/allowed within time period without support documentation.

MSN 23.17- Medicare won't cover these services because they are not considered medically necessary.

Spanish Version - Medicare no cubrirá estos servicios porque no son considerados necesarios por razones médicas.

Group Code PR (Patient Responsibility) – Where a claim is received with the GA modifier indicating that a signed ABN is on file.

Group Code CO (Contractor Responsibility) – Where a claim is received with the GZ modifier indicating that no signed ABN is on file.

Contractors shall not research and adjust CR claims paid for more than 36 sessions processed prior to the implementation of CWF edits. However, contractors may adjust claims brought to their attention.

100-04, 32, 140.3

Intensive Cardiac Rehabilitation Program Services Furnished On or After January 1, 2010

As specified at 42 CFR 410.49, Medicare covers intensive cardiac rehabilitation items and services for patients who have experienced one or more of the following:

- An acute myocardial infarction within the preceding 12 months; or
- A coronary artery bypass surgery; or
- Current stable angina pectoris; or
- Heart valve repair or replacement; or
- Percutaneous transluminal coronary angioplasty (PTCA) or coronary stenting; or
- A heart or heart-lung transplant or;
- A stable, chronic heart failure defined as patients with left ventricular ejection fraction of 35% or less and New York Heart Association (NYHA) class II to IV symptoms despite being on optimal heart failure therapy for at least 6 weeks (effective February 18, 2014).

Intensive cardiac rehabilitation programs must include the following components:

- Physician-prescribed exercise each day cardiac rehabilitation items and services are furnished;
- Cardiac risk factor modification, including education, counseling, and behavioral intervention at least once during the program, tailored to patients' individual needs;
- Psychosocial assessment;
- Outcomes assessment; and
- An individualized treatment plan detailing how components are utilized for each patient.

Intensive cardiac rehabilitation programs must be approved by Medicare. In order to be approved, a program must demonstrate through peer-reviewed published research that it has accomplished one or more of the following for its patients:

- Positively affected the progression of coronary heart disease;
- Reduced the need for coronary bypass surgery; and
- Reduced the need for percutaneous coronary interventions.

An intensive cardiac rehabilitation program must also demonstrate through peer-reviewed published research that it accomplished a statistically significant reduction in 5 or more of the following measures for patients from their levels before cardiac rehabilitation services to after cardiac rehabilitation services:

- Low density lipoprotein;
- Triglycerides;
- Body mass index;
- Systolic blood pressure;
- Diastolic blood pressure; and
- The need for cholesterol, blood pressure, and diabetes medications.

Intensive cardiac rehabilitation items and services must be furnished in a physician's office or a hospital outpatient setting. All settings must have a physician immediately available and accessible for medical consultations and emergencies at all times items and services are being furnished under the program. This provision is satisfied if the physician meets the requirements for direct supervision of physician office services as specified at 42 CFR 410.26 and for hospital outpatient therapeutic services as specified at 42 CFR 410.27.

As specified at 42 CFR 410.49(f)(2), intensive cardiac rehabilitation program sessions are limited to 72 1-hour sessions, up to 6 sessions per day, over a period of up to 18 weeks.

100-04, 32, 150.1

Bariatric Surgery for Treatment of Co-Morbid Conditions Related to Morbid Obesity

Effective for services on or after February 21, 2006, Medicare has determined that the following bariatric surgery procedures are reasonable and necessary under certain conditions for the treatment of morbid obesity. The patient must have a body-mass index (BMI) =35, have at least one co-morbidity related to obesity, and have been previously unsuccessful with medical treatment for obesity. This medical information must be documented in the patient's medical record. In addition, the procedure must be performed at an approved facility. A list of approved facilities may be found at http://www.cms.gov/Medicare/Medicare-General-Information/MedicareApprovedFacilitie/Bariatric-Surgery.html

Effective for services performed on and after February 12, 2009, Medicare has determined that Type 2 diabetes mellitus is a co-morbidity for purposes of processing bariatric surgery claims.

Effective for dates of service on and after September 24, 2013, the Centers for Medicare & Medicaid Services (CMS) has removed the certified facility requirements for Bariatric Surgery for Treatment of Co-Morbid Conditions Related to Morbid Obesity.

Please note the additional national coverage determinations related to bariatric surgery will be consolidated and subsumed into Publication 100-3, Chapter 1, section 100.1. These include sections 40.5, 100.8, 100.11 and 100.14.

- Open Roux-en-Y gastric bypass (RYGBP)
- Laparoscopic Roux-en-Y gastric bypass (RYGBP)
- Laparoscopic adjustable gastric banding (LAGB)
- Open biliopancreatic diversion with duodenal switch (BPD/DS) or gastric reduction duodenal switch (BPD/GRDS)
- Laparoscopic biliopancreatic diversion with duodenal switch (BPD/DS) or gastric reduction duodenal switch (BPD/GRDS)
- Laparoscopic sleeve gastrectomy (LSG) (Effective June 27, 2012, covered at Medicare Administrative Contractor (MAC) discretion.

100-04, 32, 150.2

HCPCS Procedure Codes for Bariatric Surgery

A. Covered HCPCS Procedure Codes

For services on or after February 21, 2006, the following HCPCS procedure codes are covered for bariatric surgery:

43770 Laparoscopy, surgical, gastric restrictive procedure; placement of adjustable gastric band (gastric band and subcutaneous port components).

43644 Laparoscopy, surgical, gastric restrictive procedure; with gastric bypass and Roux-en-Y gastroenterostomy (roux limb 150 cm or less).

43645 Laparoscopy with gastric bypass and small intestine reconstruction to limit absorption. (Do not report 43645 in conjunction with 49320, 43847.)

43845 Gastric restrictive procedure with partial gastrectomy, pylorus-preserving duodenoileostomy and ileoieostomy (50 to 100 cm common channel) to limit absorption (biliopancreatic diversion with duodenal switch).

43846 Gastric restrictive procedure, with gastric bypass for morbid obesity; with short limb (150 cm or less Roux-en-Y gastroenterostomy. (For greater than 150 cm, use 43847.) (For laparoscopic procedure, use 43644.)

43847 With small intestine reconstruction to limit absorption.

43775 Laparoscopy, surgical, gastric restrictive procedure; longitudinal gastrectomy (i.e., sleeve gastrectomy) (Effective June 27, 2012, covered at contractor's discretion.)

B. Noncovered HCPCS Procedure Codes

For services on or after February 21, 2006, the following HCPCS procedure codes are non-covered for bariatric surgery:

43842 Gastric restrictive procedure, without gastric bypass, for morbid obesity; vertical banded gastroplasty.

NOC code 43999 used to bill for:

Laparoscopic vertical banded gastroplasty

Open sleeve gastrectomy

Laparoscopic sleeve gastrectomy (for contractor non-covered instances)

Open adjustable gastric banding

100-04, 32, 150.5

ICD Diagnosis Codes for BMI Greater Than or Equal to 35

The following ICD-9 diagnosis codes identify BMI >=35 :

V85.35 - Body Mass Index 35.0-35.9, adult

V85.36 - Body Mass Index 36.0-36.9, adult

V85.37 - Body Mass Index 37.0-37.9, adult

V85.38 - Body Mass Index 38.0-38.9, adult

V85.39 - Body Mass Index 39.0-39.9, adult

V85.41 - Body Mass Index 40.0-44.9, adult

V85.42 - Body Mass Index 45.0-49.9, adult

V85.43 - Body Mass Index 50.0-59.9, adult

V85.44 - Body Mass Index 60.0-69.9, adult

V85.45 - Body Mass Index 70.0 and over, adult

The following ICD-10 diagnosis codes identify BMI >=35:

Z6835 - Body Mass Index 35.0-35.9, adult

Z6836 - Body Mass Index 36.0-36.9, adult.

Z6837 - Body Mass Index 37.0-37.9, adult

Z6838 - Body Mass Index 38.0-38.9, adult

Z6839 - Body Mass Index 39.0-39.9, adult

Z6841 - Body Mass Index 40.0-44.9, adult

Z6842 - Body Mass Index 45.0-49.9, adult

Z6843 - Body Mass Index 50.0-59.9, adult

Z6844 - Body Mass Index 60.0-69.9, adult

Z6845 - Body Mass Index 70.0 and over, adult

100-04, 32, 150.6

Claims Guidance for Payment

Covered Bariatric Surgery Procedures for Treatment of Co-Morbid Conditions Related to Morbid Obesity

Contractors shall process covered bariatric surgery claims as follows:

1. Identify bariatric surgery claims.

   Contractors identify inpatient bariatric surgery claims by the presence of ICD-9/ICD-10 diagnosis code 278.01/E66.01as the primary diagnosis (for morbid obesity) and one of the covered ICD-9/ICD-10 procedure codes listed in §150.3.

   Contractors identify practitioner bariatric surgery claims by the presence of ICD-9/ICD-10 diagnosis code 278.01/E66.01 as the primary diagnosis (for morbid obesity) and one of the covered HCPCS procedure codes listed in §150.2.

2. Perform facility certification validation for all bariatric surgery claims on a pre-pay basis up to and including date of service September 23, 2013.

   A list of approved facilities are found at the link noted in section 150.1, section A, above.

3. Review bariatric surgery claims data and determine whether a pre- or post-pay sample of bariatric surgery claims need further review to assure that the beneficiary has a BMI =35 (V85.35-V85.45/Z68.35-Z68.45) (see ICD-10 equivalents above in section 150.5), and at least one co-morbidity related to obesity

   The A/B MAC medical director may define the appropriate method for addressing the obesity-related co-morbid requirement.

   Effective for dates of service on and after September 24, 2013, CMS has removed the certified facility requirements for Bariatric Surgery for Treatment of Co-Morbid Conditions Related to Morbid Obesity.

NOTE: If ICD-9/ICD-10 diagnosis code 278.01/E66.01 is present, but a covered procedure code (listed in §150.2 or §150.3) is/are not present, the claim is not for bariatric surgery and should be processed under normal procedures.

100-04, 32, 161

Intracranial Percutaneous Transluminal Angioplasty (PTA) With Stenting

A. Background

In the past, PTA to treat obstructive lesions of the cerebral arteries was non-covered by Medicare because the safety and efficacy of the procedure had not been established. This national coverage determination (NCD) meant that the procedure was also non-covered for beneficiaries participating in Food and Drug Administration (FDA)-approved investigational device exemption (IDE) clinical trials.

B. Policy

On February 9, 2006, a request for reconsideration of this NCD initiated a national coverage analysis. CMS reviewed the evidence and determined that intracranial PTA with stenting is reasonable and necessary under §1862(a)(1)(A) of the Social Security Act for the treatment of cerebral vessels (as specified in The National Coverage Determinations Manual, Chapter 1, part 1, section 20.7) only when furnished in accordance with FDA-approved protocols governing Category B IDE clinical trials. All other indications for intracranial PTA with stenting remain non-covered.

C. Billing

Providers of covered intracranial PTA with stenting shall use Category B IDE billing requirements, as listed above in section 68.4. In addition to these requirements,

providers must bill the appropriate procedure and diagnosis codes for the date of service to receive payment. That is, under Part A, providers must bill intracranial PTA using ICD-9-CM procedure codes 00.62 and 00.65, if ICD-9-CM is applicable, or, if ICD-10-PCS is applicable, ICD-10-PCS procedure codes 037G34Z, 037G3DZ, 037G3ZZ, 037G44Z, 037G4DZ, 037G4ZZ, 03CG3ZZ, 057L3DZ, 057L4DZ and 05CL3ZZ. ICD-9-CM diagnosis code 437.0 or ICD-10-CM diagnosis code 167.2applies, depending on the date of service.

Under Part B, providers must bill HCPCS procedure code 37799. If ICD-9-CM is applicable ICD-9-CM diagnosis code 437.0 or if ICD-10-CM is applicable,ICD-10-CM diagnosis code 167.2 applies.

NOTE: ICD- codes are subject to modification. Providers must always ensure they are using the latest and most appropriate codes.

100-04, 32, 190

Billing Requirements for Extracorporeal Photopheresis

Effective for dates of services on and after December 19, 2006, Medicare has expanded coverage for extracorporeal photopheresis for patients with acute cardiac allograft rejection whose disease is refractory to standard immunosuppreive drug treatment and patients with chronic graft versus host disease whose disease is refractory to standard immunosuppreive drug treatment. (See Pub. 100-3, chapter 1, section 110.4, for complete coverage guidelines).

Effective for claims with dates of service on or after April 30, 2012, CMS has expanded coverage for extracorporeal photopheresis for the treatment of BOS following lung allograft transplantation only when extracorporeal photopheresis is provided under a clinical research study that meets specific requirements to assess the effect of extracorporeal photopheresis for the treatment of BOS following lung allograft transplantation. Further coverage criteria is outlined in Publication 100-3, Section 110.4 of the NCD.

100-04, 32, 190.2

Healthcare Common Procedural Coding System (HCPCS), Applicable Diagnosis Codes and Procedure Code

The following HCPCS procedure code is used for billing extracorporeal photopheresis:

- 36522 - Photopheresis, extracorporeal

The following are the applicable ICD-9-CM diagnosis codes for the new expanded coverage:

- 996.83 - Complications of transplanted heart, or,

- 996.85 - Complications of transplanted bone marrow, or,

- 996.88 – Complications of transplanted organ, stem cell

Effective for services for BOS following lung allograft transplantation the following is a list of applicable ICD-9-CM diagnosis codes:

- 996.84 – Complications of transplanted lung

- 491.9 - Unspecified chronic bronchitis

- 491.20 – Obstructive chronic bronchitis without exacerbation

- 491.21 – Obstructive chronic bronchitis with (acute) exacerbation

- 496 – Chronic airway obstruction, not elsewhere classified

The following is the applicable ICD-9-CM procedure code for the new expanded coverage:

- 99.88 - Therapeutic photopheresis

NOTE: Contractors shall edit for an appropriate oncological and autoimmune disorder diagnosis for payment of extracorporeal photopheresis according to the NCD.

Effective for claims with dates of service on or after April 30, 2012, in addition to HCPCS 36522, the following ICD-9-CM codes are applicable for extracorporeal photopheresis for the treatment of BOS following lung allograft transplantation only when extracorporeal photopheresis is provided under a clinical research study as outlined in Section 190 above:

A reference listing of ICD-9 CM and ICD-10-CM coding and descriptions is listed V70.7 below:

ICD9	Long Description	ICD10	ICD10 Description
491.20	Obstructive chronic	J44.9	Chronic obstructive bronchitis without exacerbation pulmonary disease, unspecified
491.21	Obstructive chronic bronchitis with (acute) exacerbation	J44.1	Chronic obstructive pulmonary disease with (acute) exacerbation
491.9	Unspecified chronic bronchitis	J42	Unspecified chronic bronchitis
496	Chronic airway obstruction, not elsewhere classified	J44.9	Chronic obstructive pulmonary disease, unspecified
996.84	Complications of transplanted lung	T86.810	Lung transplant rejection

ICD9	Long Description	ICD10	ICD10 Description
996.84	Complications of transplanted lung	T86.811	Lung transplant failure
996.84	Complications of transplanted lung	T86.812	Lung transplant infection (not recommended for extracorporeal photopheresis coverage)
996.84	Complications of transplanted lung	T86.818	Other complications of lung transplant
996.84	Complications of transplanted lung	T86.819	Unspecified complication of lung transplant
996.88	Complications of Transplanted organ, Stem cell	T86.5	Complications of Stem Cell Transplant
V70.7	Examination of participant in clinical trial	Z00.6	Encounter for examination for normal comparison and control in clinical research program (needed for CED)

Contractors must also report modifier Q0 - (investigational clinical service provided in a clinical research study that is in an approved research study) or Q1 (routine clinical service provided in a clinical research study that is in an approved clinical research study) as appropriate on these claims. Contractors must use diagnosis code V70.7/Z00.6 and condition code 30 (A/B MAC (A) only), along with value code D4 and the 8-digit clinical identifier number (A/MACs only) for these claims.

100-04, 32, 190.3

Medicare Summary Notices (MSNs), Remittance Advice Remark Codes (RAs) and Claim Adjustment Reason Code

Contractors shall continue to use the appropriate existing messages that they have in place when denying claims submitted that do not meet the Medicare coverage criteria for extracorporeal photopheresis.

Contractors shall deny claims when the service is not rendered to an inpatient or outpatient of a hospital, including critical access hospitals (CAHs) using the following codes:

- Claim Adjustment Reason code: 58 – "Claim/service denied/reduced because treatment was deemed by payer to have been rendered in an inappropriate or invalid place of service."
- MSN 16.2 - "This service cannot be paid when provided in this location/facility." Spanish translation: "Este servicio no se puede pagar cuando es suministrado en esta sitio/facilidad." (Include either MSN 36.1 or 36.2 dependant on liablity.)
- RA MA 30 - "Missing/incomplete/invalid type of bill." (FIs and A/MACs only)
- Group Code - CO (Contractual Obligations) or PR (Patient Responsibility) dependant on liability. Contractors shall return to provider/ return as unprocessable claims for BOS containing HCPCS procedure code 36522 along with one of the following ICD-9-CM diagnosis codes: 996.84, 491.9, 491.20, 491.21, and 496 but is missing Diagnosis code V70.7 (as secondary diagnosis, Institutional only), Condition code 30 Institutional claims only), Clinical trial modifier Q0. Use the following messages:
  — CARC 4 – The procedure code is inconsistent with the modifier used or a required modifier is missing. Note: Refer to the 835 Healthcare Policy Identification Segment (loop 2110 Service Payment Information REF), if present.
  — RARC MA 130 – Your claim contains incomplete and/or invalid information, and no appeal rights are afforded because the claim is unprocessable. Please submit a new claim with the complete/correct information.
  — RARC M16 – Alert: Please see our web site, mailings, or bulletins for more details concerning this policy/procedure/decision.

100-04, 32, 220.1

220.1 - General

Effective for services on or after September 29, 2008, the Center for Medicare & Medicaid Services (CMS) made the decision that Thermal Intradiscal Procedures (TIPS) are not reasonable and necessary for the treatment of low back pain. Therefore, TIPs are non-covered. Refer to Pub.100-3, Medicare National Coverage Determination (NCD) Manual Chapter 1, Part 2, Section 150.11, for further information on the NCD.

100-04, 32, 290.1.1

Coding Requirements for TAVR Services Furnished on or After January 1, 2013

Beginning January 1, 2013, the following are the applicable Current Procedural Terminology (CPT) codes for TAVR:

- 33361 Transcatheter aortic valve replacement (TAVR/TAVI) with prosthetic valve; percutaneous femoral artery approach
- 33362 Transcatheter aortic valve replacement (TAVR/TAVI) with prosthetic valve; open femoral approach

- 33363 Transcatheter aortic valve replacement (TAVR/TAVI) with prosthetic valve; open axillary artery approach
- 33364 Transcatheter aortic valve replacement (TAVR/TAVI) with prosthetic valve; open iliac artery approach
- 3336 Transcatheter aortic valve replacement (TAVR/TAVI) with prosthetic valve; transaortic approach (e.g., median sternotomy, mediastinotomy)
- 0318T Transcatheter aortic valve replacement (TAVR/TAVI) with prosthetic valve; transapical approach (e.g., left thoracotomy)

Beginning January 1, 2014, temporary CPT code 0318T above is retired. TAVR claims with dates of service on and after January 1, 2014 shall instead use permanent CPT code:

- 33366 Transcatheter aortic valve replacement (TAVR/TAVI) with prosthetic valve; transapical exposure (e.g., left thoracotomy)

100-04, 32, 290.2

Claims Processing Requirements for TAVR Services on Professional Claims

Place of Service (POS) Professional Claims

Effective for claims with dates of service on and after May 1, 2012, place of service (POS) code 21 shall be used for TAVR services. All other POS codes shall be denied.

The following messages shall be used when Medicare contractors deny TAVR claims for POS:

Claim Adjustment Reason Code (CARC) 58: "Treatment was deemed by the payer to have been rendered in an inappropriate or invalid place of service. NOTE: Refer to the 835 Healthcare Policy Identification Segment (loop 2110 Service Payment Information REF), if present."

Remittance advice remark code (RARC) N428: "Not covered when performed in this place of service."

Medicare Summary Notice (MSN) 21.25: "This service was denied because Medicare only covers this service in certain settings."

Spanish Version: "El servicio fue denegado porque Medicare solamente lo cubre en ciertas situaciones."

Professional Claims Modifier -62

For TAVR claims processed on or after July 1, 2013, contractors shall pay claim lines with 0256T, 0257T, 0258T, 0259T, 33361, 33362, 33363, 33364, 33365 & 0318T only when billed with modifier -62. Claim lines billed without modifier -62 shall be returned as unprocessable.

Beginning January 1, 2014, temporary CPT code 0318T above is retired. TAVR claims with dates of service on and after January 1, 2014 shall instead use permanent CPT code 33366.

The following messages shall be used when Medicare contractors return TAVR claims billed without modifier -62 as unprocessable:

CARC 4: "The procedure code is inconsistent with the modifier used or a required modifier is missing. Note: Refer to the 835 Healthcare Policy Identification Segment (loop 2110 Service Payment Information REF), if present."

RARC N29: "Missing documentation/orders/notes/summary/report/chart."

RARC MA130: "Your claim contains incomplete and/or invalid information, and no appeal rights are afforded because the claim is unprocessable. Please submit a new claim with the complete/correct information."

Professional Claims Modifier -Q0

For claims processed on or after July 1, 2013, contractors shall pay TAVR claim lines for 0256T, 0257T, 0258T, 0259T, 33361, 33362, 33363, 33364, 33365 & 0318T when billed with modifier -Q0. Claim lines billed without modifier -Q0 shall be returned as unprocessable.

Beginning January 1, 2014, temporary CPT code 0318T above is retired. TAVR claims with dates of service on and after January 1, 2014 shall instead use permanent CPT code 33366.

The following messages shall be used when Medicare contractors return TAVR claims billed without modifier -Q0 as unprocessable:

CARC 4: "The procedure code is inconsistent with the modifier used or a required modifier is missing. Note: Refer to the 835 Healthcare Policy Identification Segment (loop 2110 Service Payment Information REF), if present."

RARC N29: "Missing documentation/orders/notes/summary/report/chart."

RARC MA130: "Your claim contains incomplete and/or invalid information, and no appeal rights are afforded because the claim is unprocessable. Please submit a new claim with the complete/correct information."

For claims processed on or after July 1, 2013, contractors shall pay TAVR claim lines for 0256T, 0257T, 0258T, 0259T, 33361, 33362, 33363, 33364, 33365 & 0318T when billed with diagnosis code V70.7 (ICD-10=Z00.6). Claim lines billed without diagnosis code V70.7 (ICD-10=Z00.6) shall be returned as unprocessable.

Beginning January 1, 2014, temporary CPT code 0318T above is retired. TAVR claims with dates of service on and after January 1, 2014 shall instead use permanent CPT code 33366.

The following messages shall be used when Medicare contractors return TAVR claims billed without diagnosis code V70.7 (ICD-10=Z00.6) as unprocessable:

CARC 16: "Claim/service lacks information which is needed for adjudication. At least one Remark Code must be provided (may be comprised of either the NCPDP Reject Reason Code, or Remittance Advice Remark Code that is not an ALERT)."

RARC M76: "Missing/incomplete/invalid diagnosis or condition"

RARC MA130: "Your claim contains incomplete and/or invalid information, and no appeal rights are afforded because the claim is unprocessable. Please submit a new claim with the complete/correct information."

Professional Claims 8-digit ClinicalTrials.gov Identifier Number

For claims processed on or after July 1, 2013, contractors shall pay TAVR claim lines for 0256T, 0257T, 0258T, 0259T, 33361, 33362, 33363, 33364, 33365 & 0318T when billed with the numeric, 8-digit clinicaltrials.gov identifier number preceded by the two alpha characters "CT" when placed in Field 19 of paper Form CMS-1500, or when entered without the "CT" prefix in the electronic 837P in Loop 2300REF02(REF01=P4). Claim lines billed without an 8-digit clinicaltrials.gov identifier number shall be returned as unprocessable.

Beginning January 1, 2014, temporary CPT code 0318T above is retired. TAVR claims with dates of service on and after January 1, 2014 shall instead use permanent CPT code 33366.

The following messages shall be used when Medicare contractors return TAVR claims billed without an 8-digit clinicaltrials.gov identifier number as unprocessable:

CARC 16: "Claim/service lacks information which is needed for adjudication. At least one Remark Code must be provided (may be comprised of either NCPDP Reject Reason Code, or Remittance Advice Remark Code that is not an ALERT)."

RARC MA50: "Missing/incomplete/invalid Investigational Device Exemption number for FDA-approved clinical trial services."

RARC MA130: "Your claim contains incomplete and/or invalid information, and no appeal rights are afforded because the claim is unprocessable. Please submit a new claim with the complete/correct information."

NOTE: Clinicaltrials.gov identifier numbers for TAVR are listed on our website:

(http://www.cms.gov/Medicare/Coverage/Coverage-with-Evidence-Development/Transcatheter-Aortic-Valve-Replacement-TAVR-.html)

290.3 - Claims Processing Requirements for TAVR Services on Inpatient Hospital Claims

(Rev.2827. Issued: 11-29-13, Effective: 01-01-14, Implementation: 01-06-14)

Inpatient hospitals shall bill for TAVR on an 11X TOB effective for discharges on or after May 1, 2012. Refer to Section 69 of this chapter for further guidance on billing under CED.

Inpatient hospital discharges for TAVR shall be covered when billed with:

- V70.7 and Condition Code 30.
- An 8-digit clinicaltrials.gov identifier number listed on the CMS website (effective July 1, 2013)

Inpatient hospital discharges for TAVR shall be rejected when billed without:

- V70.7 and Condition Code 30.
- An 8-digit clinicaltrials.gov identifier number listed on the CMS website (effective July 1, 2013)

Claims billed by hospitals not participating in the trial/registry shall be rejected with the following messages:

CARC: 50 -These are non-covered services because this is not deemed a "medical necessity" by the payer.

RARC N386 - This decision was based on a National Coverage Determination (NCD). An NCD provides a coverage determination as to whether a particular item or service is covered. A copy of this policy is available at http://www.cms.hhs.gov/mcd/ search.asp. If you do not have web access, you may contact the contractor to request a copy of the NCD.

Group Code –Contractual Obligation (CO)

MSN 16.77 – This service/item was not covered because it was not provided as part of a qualifying trial/study. (Este servicio/artículo no fue cubierto porque no estaba incluido como parte de un ensayo clínico/estudio calificado.)

100-04, 32, 290.3

Claims Processing Requirements for TAVR Services on Inpatient Hospital Claims

Inpatient hospitals shall bill for TAVR on an 11X TOB effective for discharges on or after May 1, 2012. Refer to Section 69 of this chapter for further guidance on billing under CED.

Inpatient hospital discharges for TAVR shall be covered when billed with:

- V70.7 and Condition Code 30.
- An 8-digit clinicaltrials.gov identifier number listed on the CMS website (effective July 1, 2013)

Inpatient hospital discharges for TAVR shall be rejected when billed without:

- V70.7 and Condition Code 30.
- An 8-digit clinicaltrials.gov identifier number listed on the CMS website (effective July 1, 2013)

Claims billed by hospitals not participating in the trial/registry shall be rejected with the following messages:

CARC: 50 -These are non-covered services because this is not deemed a "medical necessity" by the payer.

RARC N386 - This decision was based on a National Coverage Determination (NCD). An NCD provides a coverage determination as to whether a particular item or service is covered. A copy of this policy is available at http://www.cms.hhs.gov/mcd/ search.asp. If you do not have web access, you may contact the contractor to request a copy of the NCD.

Group Code –Contractual Obligation (CO)

MSN 16.77 – This service/item was not covered because it was not provided as part of a qualifying trial/study. (Este servicio/artículo no fue cubierto porque no estaba incluido como parte de un ensayo clínico/estudio calificado.)

100-04, 32, 290.4

Claims Processing Requirements for TAVR Services for Medicare Advantage (MA) Plan Participants

MA plans are responsible for payment of TAVR services for MA plan participants. Medicare coverage for TAVR is included under section 310.1 of the NCD Manual (Routine Costs in Clinical Trials).

100-04, 32, 320.1

Coding Requirements for Artificial Hearts Furnished Before May 1, 2008

Effective for discharges before May 1, 2008, Medicare does not cover the use of artificial hearts, either as a permanent replacement for a human heart or as a temporary life-support system until a human heart becomes available for transplant (often referred to a "bridge to transplant").

100-04, 32, 320.2

Coding Requirements for Artificial Hearts Furnished On or After May 1, 2008

Effective for discharges on or after May 1, 2008, the use of artificial hearts will be covered by Medicare under Coverage with Evidence Development (CED) when beneficiaries are enrolled in a clinical study that meets all of the criteria listed in IOM Pub. 100-3, Medicare NCD Manual, section 20.9.

Claims Coding

For claims with dates of service on or after May 1, 2008, artificial hearts in the context of an approved clinical study for a Category A IDE, refer to section 69 in this manual for more detail on CED billing. Appropriate ICD-10 diagnosis and procedure codes are included below:

ICD-10 Diagnosis Code	Definition	Discharges Effective
I09.81	Rheumatic heart failure	On or After ICD-10 Implementation
I11.0	Hypertensive heart disease with heart failure	
I13.0	Hypertensive heart and chronic kidney disease with heart failure and stage 1 through stage 4 chronic kidney disease, or unspecified chronic kidney disease	
I13.2	Hypertensive heart and chronic kidney disease with heart failure and with stage 5 chronic kidney disease, or end stage renal disease	
I20.0	Unstable angina	
I21.01	ST elevation (STEMI) myocardial infarction involving left main coronary artery	

ICD-10 Diagnosis Code	Definition	Discharges Effective
I21.Ø2	ST elevation (STEMI) myocardial infarction involving left anterior descending coronary artery	On or After ICD-10 Implementation
I21.Ø9	ST elevation (STEMI) myocardial infarction involving other coronary artery of anterior wall	
I21.11	ST elevation (STEMI) myocardial infarction involving right coronary artery	
I21.19	ST elevation (STEMI) myocardial infarction involving other coronary artery of inferior wall	
I21.21	ST elevation (STEMI) myocardial infarction involving left circumflex coronary artery	
I21.29	ST elevation (STEMI) myocardial infarction involving other sites	
I21.3	ST elevation (STEMI) myocardial infarction of unspecified site	
I21.4	Non-ST elevation (NSTEMI) myocardial infarction	
I22.Ø	Subsequent ST elevation (STEMI) myocardial infarction of anterior wall	
I22.1	Subsequent ST elevation (STEMI) myocardial infarction of inferior wall	
I22.2	Subsequent non-ST elevation (NSTEMI) myocardial infarction	
I22.8	Subsequent ST elevation (STEMI) myocardial infarction of other sites	
I22.9	Subsequent ST elevation (STEMI) myocardial infarction of unspecified site	
I24.Ø	Acute coronary thrombosis not resulting in myocardial infarction	
I24.1	Dressler's syndrome	
I24.8	Other forms of acute ischemic heart disease	
I24.9	Acute ischemic heart disease, unspecified	
I25.1Ø	Atherosclerotic heart disease of native coronary artery without angina pectoris	
I25.11Ø	Atherosclerotic heart disease of native coronary artery with unstable angina pectoris	
I25.111	Atherosclerotic heart disease of native coronary artery with angina pectoris with documented spasm	
I25.118	Atherosclerotic heart disease of native coronary artery with other forms of angina pectoris	
I25.119	Atherosclerotic heart disease of native coronary artery with unspecified angina pectoris	
I25.5	Ischemic cardiomyopathy	
I25.6	Silent myocardial ischemia	
I25.7ØØ	Atherosclerosis of coronary artery bypass graft(s), unspecified, with unstable angina pectoris	
I25.7Ø1	Atherosclerosis of coronary artery bypass graft(s), unspecified, with angina pectoris with documented spasm	
I25.7Ø8	Atherosclerosis of coronary artery bypass graft(s), unspecified, with other forms of angina pectoris	
I25.7Ø9	Atherosclerosis of coronary artery bypass graft(s), unspecified, with unspecified angina pectoris	
I25.71Ø	Atherosclerosis of autologous vein coronary artery bypass graft(s) with unstable angina pectoris	
I25.711	Atherosclerosis of autologous vein coronary artery bypass graft(s) with angina pectoris with documented spasm	
I25.718	Atherosclerosis of autologous vein coronary artery bypass graft(s) with other forms of angina pectoris	
I25.719	Atherosclerosis of autologous vein coronary artery bypass graft(s) with unspecified angina pectoris	
I25.72Ø	Atherosclerosis of autologous artery coronary artery bypass graft(s) with unstable angina pectoris	

ICD-10 Diagnosis Code	Definition	Discharges Effective
I25.721	Atherosclerosis of autologous artery coronary artery bypass graft(s) with angina pectoris with documented spasm	On or After ICD-10 Implementation
I25.728	Atherosclerosis of autologous artery coronary artery bypass graft(s) with other forms of angina pectoris	
I25.729	Atherosclerosis of autologous artery coronary artery bypass graft(s) with unspecified angina pectoris	
I25.73Ø	Atherosclerosis of nonautologous biological coronary artery bypass graft(s) with unstable angina pectoris	
I25.731	Atherosclerosis of nonautologous biological coronary artery bypass graft(s) with angina pectoris with documented spasm	
I25.738	Atherosclerosis of nonautologous biological coronary artery bypass graft(s) with other forms of angina pectoris	
I25.739	Atherosclerosis of nonautologous biological coronary artery bypass graft(s) with unspecified angina pectoris	
I25.75Ø	Atherosclerosis of native coronary artery of transplanted heart with unstable angina	
I25.751	Atherosclerosis of native coronary artery of transplanted heart with angina pectoris with documented spasm	
I25.758	Atherosclerosis of native coronary artery of transplanted heart with other forms of angina pectoris	
I25.759	Atherosclerosis of native coronary artery of transplanted heart with unspecified angina pectoris	
I25.76Ø	Atherosclerosis of bypass graft of coronary artery of transplanted heart with unstable angina	
I25.761	Atherosclerosis of bypass graft of coronary artery of transplanted heart with angina pectoris with documented spasm	
I25.768	Atherosclerosis of bypass graft of coronary artery of transplanted heart with other forms of angina pectoris	
I25.769	Atherosclerosis of bypass graft of coronary artery of transplanted heart with unspecified angina pectoris	
I25.79Ø	Atherosclerosis of other coronary artery bypass graft(s) with unstable angina pectoris	
I25.791	Atherosclerosis of other coronary artery bypass graft(s) with angina pectoris with documented spasm	
I25.798	Atherosclerosis of other coronary artery bypass graft(s) with other forms of angina pectoris	
I25.799	Atherosclerosis of other coronary artery bypass graft(s) with unspecified angina pectoris	
I25.81Ø	Atherosclerosis of coronary artery bypass graft(s) without angina pectoris	
I25.811	Atherosclerosis of native coronary artery of transplanted heart without angina pectoris	
I25.812	Atherosclerosis of bypass graft of coronary artery of transplanted heart without angina pectoris	
I25.89	Other forms of chronic ischemic heart disease	
I25.9	Chronic ischemic heart disease, unspecified	
I34.Ø	Nonrheumatic mitral (valve) insufficiency	
I34.1	Nonrheumatic mitral (valve) prolapse	
I34.2	Nonrheumatic mitral (valve) stenosis	
I34.8	Other nonrheumatic mitral valve disorders	
I34.9	Nonrheumatic mitral valve disorder, unspecified	
I35.Ø	Nonrheumatic aortic (valve) stenosis	
I35.1	Nonrheumatic aortic (valve) insufficiency	
I35.2	Nonrheumatic aortic (valve) stenosis with insufficiency	
I35.8	Other nonrheumatic aortic valve disorders	

ICD-10 Diagnosis Code	Definition	Discharges Effective
I35.9	Nonrheumatic aortic valve disorder, unspecified	On or After ICD-10 Implementation
I36.0	Nonrheumatic tricuspid (valve) stenosis	
I36.1	Nonrheumatic tricuspid (valve) insufficiency	
I36.2	Nonrheumatic tricuspid (valve) stenosis with insufficiency	
I36.8	Other nonrheumatic tricuspid valve disorders	
I36.9	Nonrheumatic tricuspid valve disorder, unspecified	
I37.0	Nonrheumatic pulmonary valve stenosis	
I37.1	Nonrheumatic pulmonary valve insufficiency	
I37.2	Nonrheumatic pulmonary valve stenosis with insufficiency	
I37.8	Other nonrheumatic pulmonary valve disorders	
I37.9	Nonrheumatic pulmonary valve disorder, unspecified	
I38	Endocarditis, valve unspecified	
I39	Endocarditis and heart valve disorders in diseases classified elsewhere	
I42.0	Dilated cardiomyopathy	
I42.2	Other hypertrophic cardiomyopathy	
I42.3	Endomyocardial (eosinophilic) disease	
I42.4	Endocardial fibroelastosis	
I42.5	Other restrictive cardiomyopathy	
I42.6	Alcoholic cardiomyopathy	
I42.7	Cardiomyopathy due to drug and external agent	
I42.8	Other cardiomyopathies	
I42.9	Cardiomyopathy, unspecified	
I43	Cardiomyopathy in diseases classified elsewhere	
I46.2	Cardiac arrest due to underlying cardiac condition	
I46.8	Cardiac arrest due to other underlying condition	
I46.9	Cardiac arrest, cause unspecified	
I47.0	Re-entry ventricular arrhythmia	
I47.1	Supraventricular tachycardia	
I47.2	Ventricular tachycardia	
I47.9	Paroxysmal tachycardia, unspecified	
I48.0	Atrial fibrillation	
I48.1	Atrial flutter	
I49.01	Ventricular fibrillation	
I49.02	Ventricular flutter	
I49.1	Atrial premature depolarization	
I49.2	Junctional premature depolarization	
I49.3	Ventricular premature depolarization	
I49.40	Unspecified premature depolarization	
I49.49	Other premature depolarization	
I49.5	Sick sinus syndrome	
I49.8	Other specified cardiac arrhythmias	
I49.9	Cardiac arrhythmia, unspecified	
I50.1	Left ventricular failure	
I50.20	Unspecified systolic (congestive) heart failure	
I50.21	Acute systolic (congestive) heart failure	
I50.22	Chronic systolic (congestive) heart failure	
I50.23	Acute on chronic systolic (congestive) heart failure	
I50.30	Unspecified diastolic (congestive) heart failure	
I50.31	Acute diastolic (congestive) heart failure	
I50.32	Chronic diastolic (congestive) heart failure	
I50.33	Acute on chronic diastolic (congestive) heart failure	
I50.40	Unspecified combined systolic (congestive) and diastolic (congestive) heart failure	

ICD-10 Diagnosis Code	Definition	Discharges Effective
I50.41	Acute combined systolic (congestive) and diastolic (congestive) heart failure	On or After ICD-10 Implementation
I50.42	Chronic combined systolic (congestive) and diastolic (congestive) heart failure	
I50.43	Acute on chronic combined systolic (congestive) and diastolic (congestive) heart failure	
I50.9	Heart failure, unspecified	
I51.4	Myocarditis, unspecified	
I51.9	Heart disease, unspecified	
I52	Other heart disorders in diseases classified elsewhere	
I97.0	Postcardiotomy syndrome	
I97.110	Postprocedural cardiac insufficiency following cardiac surgery	
I97.111	Postprocedural cardiac insufficiency following other surgery	
I97.120	Postprocedural cardiac arrest following cardiac surgery	
I97.121	Postprocedural cardiac arrest following other surgery	
I97.130	Postprocedural heart failure following cardiac surgery	
I97.131	Postprocedural heart failure following other surgery	
I97.190	Other postprocedural cardiac functional disturbances following cardiac surgery	
I97.191	Other postprocedural cardiac functional disturbances following other surgery	
I97.710	Intraoperative cardiac arrest during cardiac surgery	
I97.711	Intraoperative cardiac arrest during other surgery	
I97.790	Other intraoperative cardiac functional disturbances during cardiac surgery	
I97.791	Other intraoperative cardiac functional disturbances during other surgery	
I97.88	Other intraoperative complications of the circulatory system, not elsewhere classified	
I97.89	Other postprocedural complications and disorders of the circulatory system, not elsewhere classified	
M32.11	Endocarditis in systemic lupus erythematosus	
O90.89	Other complications of the puerperium, not elsewhere classified	
Q20.0	Common arterial trunk	
Q20.1	Double outlet right ventricle	
Q20.2	Double outlet left ventricle	
Q20.3	Discordant ventriculoarterial connection	
Q20.4	Double inlet ventricle	
Q20.5	Discordant atrioventricular connection	
Q20.6	Isomerism of atrial appendages	
Q20.8	Other congenital malformations of cardiac chambers and connections	
Q20.9	Congenital malformation of cardiac chambers and connections, unspecified	
Q21.0	Ventricular septal defect	
Q21.1	Atrial septal defect	
Q21.2	Atrioventricular septal defect	
Q21.3	Tetralogy of Fallot	
Q21.4	Aortopulmonary septal defect	
Q21.8	Other congenital malformations of cardiac septa	
Q21.9	Congenital malformation of cardiac septum, unspecified	
Q22.0	Pulmonary valve atresia	
Q22.1	Congenital pulmonary valve stenosis	
Q22.2	Congenital pulmonary valve insufficiency	
Q22.3	Other congenital malformations of pulmonary valve	

ICD-10 Diagnosis Code	Definition	Discharges Effective
Q22.4	Congenital tricuspid stenosis	On or After ICD-10 Implementation
Q22.5	Ebstein's anomaly	
Q22.6	Hypoplastic right heart syndrome	
Q22.8	Other congenital malformations of tricuspid valve	
Q22.9	Congenital malformation of tricuspid valve, unspecified	
Q23.0	Congenital stenosis of aortic valve	
Q23.1	Congenital insufficiency of aortic valve	
Q23.2	Congenital mitral stenosis	
Q23.3	Congenital mitral insufficiency	
Q23.4	Hypoplastic left heart syndrome	
Q23.8	Other congenital malformations of aortic and mitral valves	
Q23.9	Congenital malformation of aortic and mitral valves, unspecified	
Q24.0	Dextrocardia	
Q24.1	Levocardia	
Q24.2	Cor triatriatum	
Q24.3	Pulmonary infundibular stenosis	
Q24.4	Congenital subaortic stenosis	
Q24.5	Malformation of coronary vessels	
Q24.6	Congenital heart block	
Q24.8	Other specified congenital malformations of heart	
Q24.9	Congenital malformation of heart, unspecified	
R00.1	Bradycardia, unspecified	
R57.0	Cardiogenic shock	
T82.221A	Breakdown (mechanical) of biological heart valve graft, initial encounter	
T82.222A	Displacement of biological heart valve graft, initial encounter	
T82.223A	Leakage of biological heart valve graft, initial encounter	
T82.228A	Other mechanical complication of biological heart valve graft, initial encounter	
T82.512A	Breakdown (mechanical) of artificial heart, initial encounter	
T82.514A	Breakdown (mechanical) of infusion catheter, initial encounter	
T82.518A	Breakdown (mechanical) of other cardiac and vascular devices and implants, initial encounter	
T82.519A	Breakdown (mechanical) of unspecified cardiac and vascular devices and implants, initial encounter	
T82.522A	Displacement of artificial heart, initial encounter	
T82.524A	Displacement of infusion catheter, initial encounter	
T82.528A	Displacement of other cardiac and vascular devices and implants, initial encounter	
T82.529A	Displacement of unspecified cardiac and vascular devices and implants, initial encounter	
T82.532A	Leakage of artificial heart, initial encounter	
T82.534A	Leakage of infusion catheter, initial encounter	
T82.538A	Leakage of other cardiac and vascular devices and implants, initial encounter	
T82.539A	Leakage of unspecified cardiac and vascular devices and implants, initial encounter	
T82.592A	Other mechanical complication of artificial heart, initial encounter	
T82.594A	Other mechanical complication of infusion catheter, initial encounter	
T82.598A	Other mechanical complication of other cardiac and vascular devices and implants, initial encounter	
T82.599A	Other mechanical complication of unspecified cardiac and vascular devices and implants, initial encounter	
T86.20	Unspecified complication of heart transplant	

ICD-10 Diagnosis Code	Definition	Discharges Effective
T86.21	Heart transplant rejection	On or After ICD-10 Implementation
T86.22	Heart transplant failure	
T86.23	Heart transplant infection	
T86.290	Cardiac allograft vasculopathy	
T86.298	Other complications of heart transplant	
T86.30	Unspecified complication of heart-lung transplant	
T86.31	Heart-lung transplant rejection	
T86.32	Heart-lung transplant failure	
T86.33	Heart-lung transplant infection	
T86.39	Other complications of heart-lung transplant	
Z48.21	Encounter for aftercare following heart transplant	
Z48.280	Encounter for aftercare following heart-lung transplant	
Z94.1	Heart transplant status	
Z94.3	Heart and lungs transplant status	
Z95.9	Presence of cardiac and vascular implant and graft, unspecified	
Q24.0	Dextrocardia	
Q24.1	Levocardia	
Q24.2	Cor triatriatum	
Q24.3	Pulmonary infundibular stenosis	
Q24.4	Congenital subaortic stenosis	
Q24.5	Malformation of coronary vessels	
Q24.6	Congenital heart block	
Q24.8	Other specified congenital malformations of heart	
Q24.9	Congenital malformation of heart, unspecified	
R00.1	Bradycardia, unspecified	
R57.0	Cardiogenic shock	
T82.221A	Breakdown (mechanical) of biological heart valve graft, initial encounter	
T82.222A	Displacement of biological heart valve graft, initial encounter	
T82.223A	Leakage of biological heart valve graft, initial encounter	
T82.228A	Other mechanical complication of biological heart valve graft, initial encounter	
T82.512A	Breakdown (mechanical) of artificial heart, initial encounter	
T82.514A	Breakdown (mechanical) of infusion catheter, initial encounter	
T82.518A	Breakdown (mechanical) of other cardiac and vascular devices and implants, initial encounter	
T82.519A	Breakdown (mechanical) of unspecified cardiac and vascular devices and implants, initial encounter	
T82.522A	Displacement of artificial heart, initial encounter	
T82.524A	Displacement of infusion catheter, initial encounter	
T82.528A	Displacement of other cardiac and vascular devices and implants, initial encounter	
T82.529A	Displacement of unspecified cardiac and vascular devices and implants, initial encounter	
T82.532A	Leakage of artificial heart, initial encounter	
T82.534A	Leakage of infusion catheter, initial encounter	
T82.538A	Leakage of other cardiac and vascular devices and implants, initial encounter	
T82.539A	Leakage of unspecified cardiac and vascular devices and implants, initial encounter	
T82.592A	Other mechanical complication of artificial heart, initial encounter	
T82.594A	Other mechanical complication of infusion catheter, initial encounter	
T82.598A	Other mechanical complication of other cardiac and vascular devices and implants, initial encounter	

ICD-10 Diagnosis Code	Definition	Discharges Effective
T82.599A	Other mechanical complication of unspecified cardiac and vascular devices and implants, initial encounter	On or After ICD-10 Implementation
T86.20	Unspecified complication of heart transplant	
T86.21	Heart transplant rejection	
T86.22	Heart transplant failure	
T86.23	Heart transplant infection	
T86.290	Cardiac allograft vasculopathy	
T86.298	Other complications of heart transplant	
T86.30	Unspecified complication of heart-lung transplant	
T86.31	Heart-lung transplant rejection	
T86.32	Heart-lung transplant failure	
T86.33	Heart-lung transplant infection	
T86.39	Other complications of heart-lung transplant	
Z48.21	Encounter for aftercare following heart transplant	
Z48.280	Encounter for aftercare following heart-lung transplant	
Z94.1	Heart transplant status	
Z94.3	Heart and lungs transplant status	
Z95.9	Presence of cardiac and vascular implant and graft, unspecified	
02RK0JZ	Replacement of Right Ventricle with Synthetic Substitute, Open Approach	
02RL0JZ	Revision of Synthetic Substitute in Heart, Open Approach	
02WA0JZ	Revision of Synthetic Substitute in Heart, Open Approach	

NOTE: Total artificial heart is reported with a "cluster" of 2 codes for open replacement with synthetic substitute of the right and left ventricles- 02RK0JZ + 02RL0JZ

100-04, 32, 320.3

Ventricular Assist Devices

Medicare may cover a Ventricular Assist Device (VAD). A VAD is used to assist a damaged or weakened heart in pumping blood. VADs are used as a bridge to a heart transplant, for support of blood circulation post-cardiotomy or destination therapy. Refer to the IOM Pub. 100-3, NCD Manual, section 20.9.1 for coverage criteria.

100-04, 32, 320.3.1

Post-cardiotomy

Post-cardiotomy is the period following open-heart surgery. VADs used for support of blood circulation post-cardiotomy are covered only if they have received approval from the Food and Drug Administration (FDA) for that purpose, and the VADs are used according to the FDA-approved labeling instructions

100-04, 32, 320.3.2

Bridge- to -Transplantation (BTT)

Coverage for BTT is restricted to patients listed for heart transplantation. The Centers for Medicare & Medicaid Services (CMS) has clearly identified that the patient must be active on the waitlist maintained by the Organ Procurement and Transplantation Network. CMS has also removed the general time requirement that patients receive a transplant as soon as medically reasonable.

100-04, 32, 370

Microvolt T-wave Alternans (MTWA)

On March 21, 2006, the Centers for Medicare & Medicaid Services (CMS) began national coverage of microvolt T-wave Alternans (MTWA) diagnostic testing when it was performed using only the spectral analysis (SA) method for the evaluation of patients at risk for sudden cardiac death (SCD) from ventricular arrhythmias and patients who may be candidates for Medicare coverage of the placement of an implantable cardiac defibrillator (ICD).

Effective for claims with dates of service on and after January 13, 2015, Medicare Administrative Contractors (MACs) may determine coverage of MTWA diagnostic testing when it is performed using methods of analysis other than SA for the evaluation of patients at risk for SCD from ventricular arrhythmias. Further information can be found at Publication 100-3, section 20.30, of the National Coverage Determinations Manual.

100-04, 32, 370.1

Coding and Claims Processing for MTWA

Effective for claims with dates of service on and after March 21, 2006, MACs shall accept CPT 93025 (MTWA for assessment of ventricular arrhythmias) for MTWA diagnostic testing for the evaluation of patients at risk for SCD with the SA method of analysis only. All other methods of analysis for MTWA are non-covered.

Effective for claims with dates of service on and after January 13, 2015, MACs shall at their discretion determine coverage for CPT 93025 for MTWA diagnostic testing for the evaluation of patients at risk for SCD with methods of analysis other than SA. The –KX modifier shall be used as an attestation by the practitioner and/or provider of the service that documentation is on file verifying the MTWA was performed using a method of analysis other than SA for the evaluation of patients at risk for SCD from ventricular arrhythmias and that all other NCD criteria was met.

NOTE: The –KX modifier is NOT required on MTWA claims for the evaluation of patients at risk for SCD if the SA analysis method is used.

NOTE: This diagnosis code list/translation was approved by CMS/Coverage. It may or may not be a complete list of covered indications/diagnosis codes that are covered but should serve as a finite starting point.

As this policy indicates, individual A/B MACs within their respective jurisdictions have the discretion to make coverage determinations they deem reasonable and necessary under section 1862(a)1)(A) of the Social Security Act. Therefore, A/B MACs may have additional covered diagnosis codes in their individual policies where contractor discretion is appropriate.

ICD-9 Codes

410.11	Acute myocardial infarction of other anterior wall, initial episode of care
410.11	Acute myocardial infarction of other anterior wall, initial episode of care
410.01	Acute myocardial infarction of anterolateral wall, initial episode of care
410.11	Acute myocardial infarction of other anterior wall, initial episode of care
410.31	Acute myocardial infarction of inferoposterior wall, initial episode of care
410.21	Acute myocardial infarction of inferolateral wall, initial episode of care
410.41	Acute myocardial infarction of other inferior wall, initial episode of care
410.81	Acute myocardial infarction of other specified sites, initial episode of care
410.51	Acute myocardial infarction of other lateral wall, initial episode of care
410.61	True posterior wall infarction, initial episode of care
410.81	Acute myocardial infarction of other specified sites, initial episode of care
410.91	Acute myocardial infarction of unspecified site, initial episode of care
410.71	Subendocardial infarction, initial episode of care
410.01	Acute myocardial infarction of anterolateral wall, initial episode of care
410.11	Acute myocardial infarction of other anterior wall, initial episode of care
410.21	Acute myocardial infarction of inferolateral wall, initial episode of care
410.31	Acute myocardial infarction of inferoposterior wall, initial episode of care
410.41	Acute myocardial infarction of other inferior wall, initial episode of care
410.71	Subendocardial infarction, initial episode of care
410.51	Acute myocardial infarction of other lateral wall, initial episode of care
410.61	True posterior wall infarction, initial episode of care
410.81	Acute myocardial infarction of other specified sites, initial episode of care
410.91	Acute myocardial infarction of unspecified site, initial episode of care
411.89	Other acute and subacute forms of ischemic heart disease, other
411.89	Other acute and subacute forms of ischemic heart disease, other
427.1	Paroxysmal ventricular tachycardia
427.1	Paroxysmal ventricular tachycardia
427.41	Ventricular fibrillation
427.42	Ventricular flutter
780.2	Syncope and collapse
V45.89	Other postprocedural status

ICD- 10 Codes

I21.01	ST elevation (STEMI) myocardial infarction involving left main coronary artery
I21.02	ST elevation (STEMI) myocardial infarction involving left anterior descending coron
I21.09	ST elevation (STEMI) myocardial infarction involving other coronary artery of anteri
I21.09	ST elevation (STEMI) myocardial infarction involving other coronary artery of anteri
I21.11	ST elevation (STEMI) myocardial infarction involving right coronary artery

I21.19	ST elevation (STEMI) myocardial infarction involving other coronary artery of inferi
I21.19	ST elevation (STEMI) myocardial infarction involving other coronary artery of inferi
I21.21	ST elevation (STEMI) myocardial infarction involving left circumflex coronary artery
I21.29	ST elevation (STEMI) myocardial infarction involving other sites
I21.29	ST elevation (STEMI) myocardial infarction involving other sites
I21.29	ST elevation (STEMI) myocardial infarction involving other sites
I21.3	ST elevation (STEMI) myocardial infarction of unspecified site
I21.4	Non-ST elevation (NSTEMI) myocardial infarction
I22.0	Subsequent ST elevation (STEMI) myocardial infarction of anterior wall
I22.0	Subsequent ST elevation (STEMI) myocardial infarction of anterior wall
I22.1	Subsequent ST elevation (STEMI) myocardial infarction of inferior wall
I22.1	Subsequent ST elevation (STEMI) myocardial infarction of inferior wall
I22.1	Subsequent ST elevation (STEMI) myocardial infarction of inferior wall
I22.2	Subsequent non-ST elevation (NSTEMI) myocardial infarction
I22.8	Subsequent ST elevation (STEMI) myocardial infarction of other sites
I22.8	Subsequent ST elevation (STEMI) myocardial infarction of other sites
I22.8	Subsequent ST elevation (STEMI) myocardial infarction of other sites
I22.9	Subsequent ST elevation (STEMI) myocardial infarction of unspecified site
I24.8	Other forms of acute ischemic heart disease
I24.9	Acute ischemic heart disease, unspecified
I47.0	Re-entry ventricular arrhythmia
I47.2	Ventricular tachycardia
I49.01	Ventricular fibrillation
I49.02	Ventricular flutter
R55	Syncope and collapse
Z98.89	Other specified postprocedural states

100-04, 32, 370.2

Messaging for MTWA

Effective for claims with dates of service on and after January 13, 2015, MACs shall deny claims for MTWA CPT 93025 with methods of analysis other than SA without modifier -KX using the following messages:

CARC 4: "The procedure code is inconsistent with the modifier used or a required modifier is missing. Note: Refer to the 835 Healthcare Policy Identification Segment (loop 2110 Service Payment Information REF), if present."

RARC N657 – This should be billed with the appropriate code for these services.

Group Code: CO (Contractual Obligation) assigning financial liability to the provider

MSN 15.20 - The following policies [NCD 20.30] were used when we made this decision

Spanish Equivalent - 15.20 - Las siguientes políticas [NCD 20.30] fueron utilizadas cuando se tomó esta decisión.

100-05, 10.3.2

Exceptions Process

(Rev. 3367 Issued: 10-07-2015, Effective: 01-01-2016, Implementation: 01-04-2016)

An exception may be made when the patient's condition is justified by documentation indicating that the beneficiary requires continued skilled therapy, i.e., therapy beyond the amount payable under the therapy cap, to achieve their prior functional status or maximum expected functional status within a reasonable amount of time.

No special documentation is submitted to the contractor for exceptions. The clinician is responsible for consulting guidance in the Medicare manuals and in the professional literature to determine if the beneficiary may qualify for the exception because documentation justifies medically necessary services above the caps. The clinician's opinion is not binding on the Medicare contractor who makes the final determination concerning whether the claim is payable.

Documentation justifying the services shall be submitted in response to any Additional Documentation Request (ADR) for claims that are selected for medical review. Follow the documentation requirements in Pub. 100-02, chapter 15, section 220.3. If medical records are requested for review, clinicians may include, at their discretion, a summary that specifically addresses the justification for therapy cap exception.

In making a decision about whether to utilize the exception, clinicians shall consider, for example, whether services are appropriate to--

The patient's condition, including the diagnosis, complexities, and severity;

The services provided, including their type, frequency, and duration;

The interaction of current active conditions and complexities that directly and significantly influence the treatment such that it causes services to exceed caps.

In addition, the following should be considered before using the exception process:

1. Exceptions for Evaluation Services

Evaluation. The CMS will except therapy evaluations from caps after the therapy caps are reached when evaluation is necessary, e.g., to determine if the current status of the beneficiary requires therapy services. For example, the following CPT codes for evaluation procedures may be appropriate:

92521, 92522, 92523, 92524, 92597, 92607, 92608, 92610, 92611, 92612, 92614, 92616, 96105, 96125, 97001, 97002, 97003, 97004.

These codes will continue to be reported as outpatient therapy procedures as listed in the Annual Therapy Update for the current year at: http://www.cms.gov/TherapyServices/05_Annual_Therapy_Update.asp#TopOfPage.

They are not diagnostic tests. Definitions of evaluations and documentation are found in Pub. 100-02, chapter 15, sections 220 and 230.

Other Services. There are a number of sources that suggest the amount of certain services that may be typical, either per service, per episode, per condition, or per discipline. For example, see the CSC - Therapy Cap Report, 3/21/2008, and CSC – Therapy Edits Tables 4/14/2008 at www.cms.hhs.gov/TherapyServices (Studies and Reports), or more recent utilization reports. Professional literature and guidelines from professional associations also provide a basis on which to estimate whether the type, frequency, and intensity of services are appropriate to an individual. Clinicians and contractors should utilize available evidence related to the patient's condition to justify provision of medically necessary services to individual beneficiaries, especially when they exceed caps. Contractors shall not limit medically necessary services that are justified by scientific research applicable to the beneficiary. Neither contractors nor clinicians shall utilize professional literature and scientific reports to justify payment for continued services after an individual's goals have been met earlier than is typical. Conversely, professional literature and scientific reports shall not be used as justification to deny payment to patients whose needs are greater than is typical or when the patient's condition is not represented by the literature.

2. Exceptions for Medically Necessary Services

Clinicians may utilize the process for exception for any diagnosis or condition for which they can justify services exceeding the cap. Regardless of the diagnosis or condition, the patient must also meet other requirements for coverage.

Bill the most relevant diagnosis. As always, when billing for therapy services, the diagnosis code that best relates to the reason for the treatment shall be on the claim, unless there is a compelling reason to report another diagnosis code. For example, when a patient with diabetes is being treated with therapy for gait training due to amputation, the preferred diagnosis is abnormality of gait (which characterizes the treatment). Where it is possible in accordance with State and local laws and the contractors' local coverage determinations, avoid using vague or general diagnoses. When a claim includes several types of services, or where the physician/NPP must supply the diagnosis, it may not be possible to use the most relevant therapy diagnosis code in the primary position. In that case, the relevant diagnosis code should, if possible, be on the claim in another position.

Codes representing the medical condition that caused the treatment are used when there is no code representing the treatment. Complicating conditions are preferably used in non-primary positions on the claim and are billed in the primary position only in the rare circumstance that there is no more relevant code.

The condition or complexity that caused treatment to exceed caps must be related to the therapy goals and must either be the condition that is being treated or a complexity that directly and significantly impacts the rate of recovery of the condition being treated such that it is appropriate to exceed the caps. Documentation for an exception should indicate how the complexity (or combination of complexities) directly and significantly affects treatment for a therapy condition.

If the contractor has determined that certain codes do not characterize patients who require medically necessary services, providers/suppliers may not use those codes, but must utilize a billable diagnosis code allowed by their contractor to describe the patient's condition. Contractors shall not apply therapy caps to services based on the patient's condition, but only on the medical necessity of the service for the condition. If a service would be payable before the cap is reached and is still medically necessary after the cap is reached, that service is excepted.

Contact your contractor for interpretation if you are not sure that a service is applicable for exception.

It is very important to recognize that most conditions would not ordinarily result in services exceeding the cap. Use the KX modifier only in cases where the condition of the individual patient is such that services are APPROPRIATELY provided in an episode that exceeds the cap. Routine use of the KX modifier for all patients with these conditions will likely show up on data analysis as aberrant and invite inquiry. Be sure that documentation is sufficiently detailed to support the use of the modifier.

In justifying exceptions for therapy caps, clinicians and contractors should not only consider the medical diagnoses and medical complications that might directly and significantly influence the amount of treatment required. Other variables (such as the availability of a caregiver at home) that affect appropriate treatment shall also be considered. Factors that influence the need for treatment should be supportable by published research, clinical guidelines from professional sources, and/or clinical or common sense. See Pub. 100-02, chapter 15, section 220.3 for information related to documentation of the evaluation, and section 220.2 on medical necessity for some factors that complicate treatment.

NOTE: The patient's lack of access to outpatient hospital therapy services alone, when outpatient hospital therapy services are excluded from the limitation, does not justify excepted services. Residents of skilled nursing facilities prevented by consolidated billing from accessing hospital services, debilitated patients for whom transportation to the hospital is a physical hardship, or lack of therapy services at

hospitals in the beneficiary's county may or may not qualify as justification for continued services above the caps. The patient's condition and complexities might justify extended services, but their location does not. For dates of service on or after October 1, 2012, therapy services furnished in an outpatient hospital are not excluded from the limitation.

Appendix H — Physician Quality Reporting System (PQRS)

The Centers for Medicare and Medicare Services (CMS) released the final rule on October 14, 2016, with regards to the Medicare Access and CHIP Reauthorization Act (MACRA), legislation that represents widespread changes for physician payment for services. This legislation replaces the current Medicare Part B sustainable growth rate (SGR) reimbursement formula with a new value-based reimbursement system called the Quality Payment Program (QPP).

The QPP comprises two tracks:

*   The Merit-based Incentive Payment System (MIPS)

*   Advanced Alternative Payment Models (Advanced APMs).

MIPS utilizes the existing quality and value reporting systems—Physician Quality Reporting System (PQRS), Medicare Meaningful Use (MU), and Value-Based Modifier (VBM) programs—to define the following performance categories:

*   Quality (60 percent for 2017)

*   Advancing Care Information (previously called Meaningful Use) (25 percent for 2017)

*   Clinical Practice Improvement Activities (CPIA) (15 percent for 2017)

*   Resource Use (0 percent for 2017)

Based on the score received, an eligible provider may obtain a composite performance score (CPS) of up to 100 points from these weighted performance categories. This performance score then defines the payment adjustments in the second calendar year after the year the score is obtained. For instance, the score obtained for the 2017 performance year is linked to payment for Medicare Part B services in 2019.

Providers may also choose to participate in Advanced Alternative Payment Models. These providers would not be subject to MIPS payment adjustments and would also be eligible for a 5 percent Medicare Part B incentive payment. To be eligible to participate in an Advanced Alternative Payment Model, providers would need to meet a threshold of a minimum number of patients and other specific requirements.

Even though the MIPS has origins in the PQRS program, CMS will increase and revise existing measures and develop new measures consistent with MIPS. Payment adjustments for PQRS will terminate with the implementation of MIPS payment effective January 1, 2019. Due to the multiple changes anticipated in the coming year due to regulatory changes, the appendix on the Physician Quality Reporting System (PQRS) will no longer be included in this publication. For 2016 diagnostic and procedure information, see www.OptumCoding.com/Product/Updates/PQRS16.

Appendix I — Medically Unlikely Edits (MUEs)

The Centers for Medicare & Medicaid Services (CMS) began to publish many of the edits used in the medically unlikely edits (MUE) program for the first time effective October 2008. What follows below is a list of the published CPT codes that have MUEs assigned to them and the number of units allowed with each code. CMS publishes the updates on a quarterly basis. Not all MUEs will be published, however. MUEs intended to detect and discourage any questionable payments will not be published as the agency feels the efficacy of these edits would be compromised. CMS added another component to the MUEs—the MUE Adjudication Indicator (MAI). The appropriate MAI can be found in parentheses following the MUE in this table and specify the maximum units of service (UOS) for a CPT/HCPCS code for the service. The MAI designates whether the UOS edit is applied to the line or claim.

The three MAIs are defined as follows:

MAI 1 (Line Edit) This MAI will continue to be adjudicated as the line edit on the claim and is auto-adjudicated by the contractor.

MAI 2 (Date of Service Edit, Policy) This MAI is considered to be the "absolute date of service edit" and is based on policy. The total unit of services (UOS) for that CPT code and that date of service (DOS) are combined for this edit. Medicare contractors are required to review all claims for the same patient, same date of service, and same provider.

MAI 3 (Date of Service Edit: Clinical) This MAI is also a date-of-service edit but is based upon clinical standards. The review takes current and previously submitted claims for the same patient, same date of service, and same provider into account. When medical necessity is clearly documented, the edit may be bypassed or the claim resubmitted.

The quarterly updates are published on the CMS website at http://www.cms.gov/NationalCorrectCodInitEd/08_MUE.asp.

Professional

CPT	MUE	CPT	MUE	CPT	MUE	CPT	MUE	CPT	MUE	CPT	MUE	CPT	MUE	CPT	MUE
0001M	1(1)	0179T	1(3)	0253T	1(3)	0305T	1(3)	0366T	1(2)	0407T	2(2)	10030	2(3)	11307	3(3)
0002M	1(1)	0180T	1(3)	0254T	2(2)	0306T	1(3)	0367T	1(1)	0408T	1(3)	10035	1(2)	11308	4(3)
0003M	1(1)	0184T	1(3)	0255T	2(2)	0307T	1(3)	0368T	1(2)	0409T	1(3)	10036	2(1)	11310	4(3)
0006M	1(2)	0190T	2(2)	0263T	1(3)	0308T	1(3)	0369T	1(1)	0410T	1(3)	10040	1(2)	11311	4(3)
0007M	1(2)	0191T	2(2)	0264T	1(3)	0309T	1(3)	0370T	1(3)	0411T	1(3)	10060	1(2)	11312	3(3)
0008M	1(3)	0195T	1(2)	0265T	1(3)	0310T	1(3)	0371T	1(3)	0412T	1(2)	10061	1(2)	11313	3(3)
0019T	1(3)	0196T	1(2)	0266T	1(2)	0312T	1(3)	0372T	1(3)	0413T	1(3)	10080	1(3)	11400	3(3)
0042T	1(3)	0198T	2(2)	0267T	1(3)	0313T	1(3)	0373T	1(2)	0414T	1(2)	10081	1(3)	11401	3(3)
0051T	1(2)	01996	1(2)	0268T	1(3)	0314T	1(3)	0374T	1(1)	0415T	1(3)	10120	3(3)	11402	3(3)
0052T	1(2)	0200T	1(2)	0269T	1(2)	0315T	1(3)	0375T	1(2)	0416T	1(3)	10121	2(3)	11403	2(3)
0053T	1(2)	0201T	1(2)	0270T	1(3)	0316T	1(3)	0376T	2(3)	0417T	1(3)	10140	2(3)	11404	2(3)
0054T	1(3)	0202T	1(3)	0271T	1(3)	0317T	1(3)	0377T	1(2)	0418T	1(3)	10160	3(3)	11406	2(3)
0055T	1(3)	0205T	3(3)	0272T	1(3)	0329T	1(2)	0378T	1(2)	0419T	1(2)	10180	2(3)	11420	3(3)
0058T	1(2)	0206T	1(3)	0273T	1(3)	0330T	1(2)	0379T	1(2)	0420T	1(2)	11000	1(2)	11421	3(3)
0071T	1(2)	0207T	2(2)	0274T	1(2)	0331T	1(3)	0380T	1(2)	0421T	1(2)	11001	1(3)	11422	3(3)
0072T	1(2)	0208T	1(3)	0275T	1(2)	0332T	1(3)	0381T	1(2)	0422T	1(3)	11004	1(2)	11423	2(3)
0075T	1(2)	0209T	1(3)	0278T	1(3)	0333T	1(2)	0382T	1(2)	0423T	1(3)	11005	1(2)	11424	2(3)
0076T	1(2)	0210T	1(3)	0281T	1(2)	0335T	2(2)	0383T	1(2)	0424T	1(3)	11006	1(2)	11426	2(3)
0095T	1(3)	0211T	1(3)	0282T	1(3)	0336T	1(3)	0384T	1(2)	0425T	1(3)	11008	1(2)	11440	4(3)
0098T	2(3)	0212T	1(3)	0283T	1(3)	0337T	1(3)	0385T	1(2)	0426T	1(3)	11010	2(3)	11441	3(3)
0100T	2(2)	0213T	1(2)	0284T	1(3)	0338T	1(2)	0386T	1(2)	0427T	1(3)	11011	2(3)	11442	3(3)
0101T	1(3)	0214T	1(2)	0285T	1(3)	0339T	1(2)	0387T	1(3)	0428T	1(2)	11012	2(3)	11443	2(3)
0102T	2(2)	0215T	1(2)	0286T	1(2)	0347T	1(3)	0388T	1(3)	0429T	1(2)	11042	1(2)	11444	2(3)
0106T	4(2)	0216T	1(2)	0287T	1(3)	0348T	1(3)	0389T	1(3)	0430T	1(2)	11043	1(2)	11446	2(3)
0107T	4(2)	0217T	1(2)	0288T	1(2)	0349T	1(3)	0390T	1(3)	0431T	1(2)	11044	1(2)	11450	1(2)
0108T	4(2)	0218T	1(2)	0289T	2(2)	0350T	1(3)	0391T	1(3)	0432T	1(3)	11045	12(3)	11451	1(2)
0109T	4(2)	0219T	1(2)	0290T	1(3)	0351T	5(3)	0392T	1(2)	0433T	1(3)	11046	10(3)	11462	1(2)
0110T	4(2)	0220T	1(2)	0291T	1(2)	0352T	5(3)	0393T	1(2)	0434T	1(3)	11047	10(3)	11463	1(2)
0111T	1(3)	0221T	1(2)	0292T	1(3)	0353T	2(3)	0394T	2(3)	0435T	1(3)	11055	1(2)	11470	3(2)
0126T	1(3)	0222T	1(3)	0293T	1(2)	0354T	2(3)	0395T	2(3)	0436T	1(3)	11056	1(2)	11471	2(3)
0159T	2(2)	0228T	1(2)	0294T	1(3)	0355T	1(2)	0396T	2(2)	0437T	1(3)	11057	1(2)	11600	2(3)
0163T	1(3)	0229T	2(3)	0295T	1(2)	0356T	4(2)	0397T	1(3)	0438T	1(2)	11100	1(2)	11601	2(3)
0164T	4(2)	0230T	1(2)	0296T	1(2)	0357T	1(2)	0398T	1(3)	0439T	1(3)	11101	6(3)	11602	3(3)
0165T	4(2)	0231T	2(3)	0297T	1(2)	0358T	1(2)	0399T	1(3)	0440T	3(1)	11200	1(2)	11603	2(3)
0169T	1(3)	0232T	1(3)	0298T	1(2)	0359T	1(2)	0400T	1(2)	0441T	3(1)	11201	0(3)	11604	2(3)
0171T	1(2)	0234T	2(2)	0299T	1(2)	0360T	1(2)	0401T	1(2)	0442T	3(1)	11300	5(3)	11606	2(3)
0172T	2(3)	0235T	2(3)	0300T	1(3)	0361T	3(3)	0402T	2(2)	0443T	1(2)	11301	6(3)	11620	2(3)
0174T	1(3)	0236T	1(2)	0301T	1(2)	0362T	1(2)	0403T	1(2)	0444T	1(2)	11302	4(3)	11621	2(3)
0175T	1(3)	0237T	2(3)	0302T	1(3)	0363T	3(3)	0404T	1(2)	0445T	1(2)	11303	3(3)	11622	2(3)
0178T	1(3)	0238T	2(3)	0303T	1(3)	0364T	1(2)	0405T	1(2)	10021	4(3)	11305	4(3)	11623	2(3)
		0249T	1(2)	0304T	1(3)	0365T	1(1)	0406T	2(2)	10022	4(3)	11306	4(3)	11624	2(3)

CPT	MUE	CPT	MUE	CPT	MUE	CPT	MUE	CPT	MUE	CPT	MUE	CPT	MUE	CPT	MUE
11626	2(3)	12047	1(2)	15272	3(3)	15851	1(2)	17360	1(2)	20101	2(3)	20938	1(2)	21141	1(2)
11640	2(3)	12051	1(2)	15273	1(2)	15852	1(3)	17380	1(3)	20102	3(3)	20950	2(3)	21142	1(2)
11641	2(3)	12052	1(2)	15274	60(1)	15860	1(3)	19000	2(3)	20103	4(3)	20955	1(3)	21143	1(2)
11642	3(3)	12053	1(2)	15275	1(2)	15876	1(2)	19001	5(3)	20150	2(3)	20956	1(3)	21145	1(2)
11643	2(3)	12054	1(2)	15276	3(2)	15877	1(2)	19020	2(3)	20200	2(3)	20957	1(3)	21146	1(2)
11644	2(3)	12055	1(2)	15277	1(2)	15878	1(2)	19030	1(2)	20205	4(3)	20962	1(3)	21147	1(2)
11646	2(3)	12056	1(2)	15278	15(1)	15879	1(2)	19081	1(2)	20206	3(3)	20969	2(3)	21150	1(2)
11719	1(2)	12057	1(2)	15570	2(3)	15920	1(3)	19082	2(3)	20220	4(3)	20970	1(3)	21151	1(2)
11720	1(2)	13100	1(2)	15572	2(3)	15922	1(3)	19083	1(2)	20225	4(3)	20972	2(3)	21154	1(2)
11721	1(2)	13101	1(2)	15574	2(3)	15931	1(3)	19084	2(3)	20240	4(3)	20973	1(2)	21155	1(2)
11730	1(2)	13102	9(3)	15576	2(3)	15933	1(3)	19085	1(2)	20245	4(3)	20974	1(3)	21159	1(2)
11732	9(3)	13120	1(2)	15600	2(3)	15934	1(3)	19086	2(3)	20250	3(3)	20975	1(3)	21160	1(2)
11740	3(3)	13121	1(2)	15610	2(3)	15935	1(3)	19100	4(3)	20251	3(3)	20979	1(3)	21172	1(3)
11750	6(3)	13122	9(3)	15620	2(3)	15936	1(3)	19101	3(3)	20500	2(3)	20982	1(2)	21175	1(2)
11752	3(3)	13131	1(2)	15630	2(3)	15937	1(3)	19105	2(3)	20501	2(3)	20983	1(2)	21179	1(2)
11755	4(3)	13132	1(2)	15650	1(3)	15940	2(3)	19110	1(3)	20520	4(3)	20985	2(3)	21180	1(2)
11760	4(3)	13133	7(3)	15731	1(3)	15941	2(3)	19112	2(3)	20525	4(3)	21010	1(2)	21181	1(3)
11762	2(3)	13151	1(2)	15732	3(3)	15944	2(3)	19120	1(2)	20526	1(2)	21011	4(3)	21182	1(2)
11765	4(3)	13152	1(2)	15734	4(3)	15945	2(3)	19125	1(2)	20527	2(3)	21012	3(3)	21183	1(2)
11770	1(3)	13153	2(3)	15736	2(3)	15946	2(3)	19126	3(3)	20550	5(3)	21013	4(3)	21184	1(2)
11771	1(3)	13160	2(3)	15738	4(3)	15950	2(3)	19260	2(3)	20551	5(3)	21014	3(3)	21188	1(2)
11772	1(3)	14000	2(3)	15740	3(3)	15951	2(3)	19271	1(3)	20552	1(2)	21015	1(3)	21193	1(2)
11900	1(2)	14001	2(3)	15750	2(3)	15952	2(3)	19272	1(3)	20553	1(2)	21016	2(3)	21194	1(2)
11901	1(2)	14020	4(3)	15756	2(3)	15953	2(3)	19281	1(2)	20555	1(3)	21025	2(3)	21195	1(2)
11920	1(2)	14021	3(3)	15757	2(3)	15956	2(3)	19282	2(3)	20600	6(3)	21026	2(3)	21196	1(2)
11921	1(2)	14040	4(3)	15758	2(3)	15958	2(3)	19283	1(2)	20604	4(3)	21029	1(3)	21198	1(3)
11922	1(3)	14041	3(3)	15760	2(3)	16000	1(2)	19284	2(3)	20605	4(3)	21030	1(3)	21199	1(2)
11950	1(2)	14060	4(3)	15770	2(3)	16020	1(3)	19285	1(2)	20606	4(3)	21031	2(3)	21206	1(3)
11951	1(2)	14061	2(3)	15775	1(2)	16025	1(3)	19286	2(3)	20610	4(3)	21032	1(3)	21208	1(3)
11952	1(2)	14301	2(3)	15776	1(2)	16030	1(3)	19287	1(2)	20611	4(3)	21034	1(3)	21209	1(3)
11954	1(3)	14302	8(3)	15777	1(3)	16035	1(2)	19288	2(3)	20612	2(3)	21040	2(3)	21210	2(3)
11960	2(3)	14350	2(3)	15780	1(2)	16036	8(3)	19296	1(3)	20615	1(3)	21044	1(3)	21215	2(3)
11970	2(3)	15002	1(2)	15781	1(3)	17000	1(2)	19297	2(3)	20650	4(3)	21045	1(3)	21230	2(3)
11971	2(3)	15003	60(3)	15782	1(3)	17003	13(2)	19298	1(2)	20660	1(2)	21046	2(3)	21235	2(3)
11976	1(2)	15004	1(2)	15783	1(3)	17004	1(2)	19300	1(2)	20661	1(2)	21047	2(3)	21240	1(2)
11980	1(2)	15005	19(3)	15786	1(2)	17106	1(2)	19301	1(2)	20662	1(2)	21048	2(3)	21242	1(2)
11981	1(3)	15040	1(2)	15787	2(3)	17107	1(2)	19302	1(2)	20663	1(2)	21049	1(3)	21243	1(2)
11982	1(3)	15050	1(3)	15788	1(2)	17108	1(2)	19303	1(2)	20664	1(2)	21050	1(2)	21244	1(2)
11983	1(3)	15100	1(2)	15789	1(3)	17110	1(2)	19304	1(2)	20665	1(2)	21060	1(2)	21245	2(2)
12001	1(2)	15101	40(3)	15792	1(3)	17111	1(2)	19305	1(2)	20670	3(3)	21070	1(2)	21246	2(2)
12002	1(2)	15110	1(2)	15793	1(3)	17250	4(3)	19306	1(2)	20680	3(3)	21073	1(2)	21247	1(2)
12004	1(2)	15111	5(3)	15819	1(2)	17260	7(3)	19307	1(2)	20690	2(3)	21076	1(2)	21248	2(3)
12005	1(2)	15115	1(2)	15820	1(2)	17261	7(3)	19316	1(2)	20692	2(3)	21077	1(2)	21249	2(3)
12006	1(2)	15116	2(3)	15821	1(2)	17262	6(3)	19318	1(2)	20693	2(3)	21079	1(2)	21255	1(2)
12007	1(2)	15120	1(2)	15822	1(2)	17263	5(3)	19324	1(2)	20694	2(3)	21080	1(2)	21256	1(2)
12011	1(2)	15121	8(3)	15823	1(2)	17264	3(3)	19325	1(2)	20696	2(3)	21081	1(2)	21260	1(2)
12013	1(2)	15130	1(2)	15824	1(2)	17266	2(3)	19328	1(2)	20697	4(3)	21082	1(2)	21261	1(2)
12014	1(2)	15131	2(3)	15825	1(2)	17270	6(3)	19330	1(2)	20802	1(2)	21083	1(2)	21263	1(2)
12015	1(2)	15135	1(2)	15826	1(2)	17271	4(3)	19340	1(2)	20805	1(2)	21084	1(2)	21267	1(2)
12016	1(2)	15136	1(3)	15828	1(2)	17272	5(3)	19342	1(2)	20808	1(2)	21085	1(3)	21268	1(2)
12017	1(2)	15150	1(2)	15829	1(2)	17273	4(3)	19350	1(2)	20816	3(3)	21086	1(2)	21270	1(2)
12018	1(2)	15151	1(2)	15830	1(2)	17274	4(3)	19355	1(2)	20822	3(3)	21087	1(2)	21275	1(2)
12020	2(3)	15152	5(1)	15832	1(2)	17276	3(3)	19357	1(2)	20824	1(2)	21088	1(2)	21280	1(2)
12021	3(3)	15155	1(2)	15833	1(2)	17280	6(3)	19361	1(2)	20827	1(2)	21100	1(2)	21282	1(2)
12031	1(2)	15156	1(2)	15834	1(2)	17281	6(3)	19364	1(2)	20838	1(2)	21110	2(3)	21295	1(2)
12032	1(2)	15157	1(3)	15835	1(3)	17282	5(3)	19366	1(2)	20900	2(3)	21116	1(2)	21296	1(2)
12034	1(2)	15200	1(2)	15836	1(2)	17283	4(3)	19367	1(2)	20902	2(3)	21120	1(2)	21310	1(2)
12035	1(2)	15201	9(3)	15837	2(3)	17284	3(3)	19368	1(2)	20910	1(3)	21121	1(2)	21315	1(2)
12036	1(2)	15220	1(2)	15838	1(2)	17286	3(3)	19369	1(2)	20912	1(3)	21122	1(2)	21320	1(2)
12037	1(2)	15221	9(3)	15839	2(3)	17311	4(3)	19370	1(2)	20920	1(3)	21123	1(2)	21325	1(2)
12041	1(2)	15240	1(2)	15840	1(3)	17312	6(3)	19371	1(2)	20922	1(3)	21125	2(2)	21330	1(2)
12042	1(2)	15241	9(3)	15841	2(3)	17313	3(3)	19380	1(2)	20924	2(3)	21127	2(3)	21335	1(2)
12044	1(2)	15260	1(2)	15842	2(3)	17314	4(3)	19396	1(2)	20926	2(3)	21137	1(2)	21336	1(2)
12045	1(2)	15261	6(3)	15845	2(3)	17315	15(3)	20005	4(3)	20931	1(2)	21138	1(2)	21337	1(2)
12046	1(2)	15271	1(2)	15847	1(2)	17340	1(2)	20100	2(3)	20937	1(2)	21139	1(2)	21338	1(2)

CPT	MUE	CPT	MUE	CPT	MUE	CPT	MUE	CPT	MUE	CPT	MUE	CPT	MUE	CPT	MUE
21339	1(2)	21685	1(2)	22554	1(2)	23100	1(2)	23552	1(2)	24305	4(3)	24802	1(2)	25280	9(3)
21340	1(2)	21700	1(2)	22556	1(2)	23101	2(2)	23570	1(2)	24310	3(3)	24900	1(2)	25290	12(3)
21343	1(2)	21705	1(2)	22558	1(2)	23105	1(2)	23575	1(2)	24320	2(3)	24920	1(2)	25295	9(3)
21344	1(2)	21720	1(3)	22585	7(3)	23106	1(2)	23585	1(2)	24330	1(3)	24925	1(2)	25300	1(2)
21345	1(2)	21725	1(3)	22586	1(2)	23107	1(2)	23600	1(2)	24331	1(3)	24930	1(2)	25301	1(2)
21346	1(2)	21740	1(2)	22590	1(2)	23120	1(2)	23605	1(2)	24332	1(2)	24931	1(2)	25310	5(3)
21347	1(2)	21742	1(2)	22595	1(2)	23125	1(2)	23615	1(2)	24340	1(2)	24935	1(2)	25312	5(3)
21348	1(2)	21743	1(2)	22600	1(2)	23130	1(2)	23616	1(2)	24341	2(3)	24940	1(2)	25315	1(3)
21355	1(2)	21750	1(2)	22610	1(2)	23140	1(3)	23620	1(2)	24342	2(3)	25000	2(3)	25316	1(3)
21356	1(2)	21811	1(2)	22612	1(2)	23145	1(3)	23625	1(2)	24343	1(2)	25001	1(3)	25320	1(2)
21360	1(2)	21812	1(2)	22614	13(3)	23146	1(3)	23630	1(2)	24344	1(2)	25020	1(2)	25332	1(2)
21365	1(2)	21813	1(2)	22630	1(2)	23150	1(3)	23650	1(2)	24345	1(2)	25023	1(2)	25335	1(2)
21366	1(2)	21820	1(2)	22632	4(2)	23155	1(3)	23655	1(2)	24346	1(2)	25024	1(2)	25337	1(2)
21385	1(2)	21825	1(2)	22633	1(2)	23156	1(3)	23660	1(2)	24357	2(3)	25025	1(2)	25350	1(3)
21386	1(2)	21920	3(3)	22634	4(2)	23170	1(3)	23665	1(2)	24358	2(3)	25028	4(3)	25355	1(3)
21387	1(2)	21925	3(3)	22800	1(2)	23172	1(3)	23670	1(2)	24359	2(3)	25031	2(3)	25360	1(3)
21390	1(2)	21930	5(3)	22802	1(2)	23174	1(3)	23675	1(2)	24360	1(2)	25035	2(3)	25365	1(3)
21395	1(2)	21931	3(3)	22804	1(2)	23180	1(3)	23680	1(2)	24361	1(2)	25040	1(3)	25370	1(2)
21400	1(2)	21932	4(3)	22808	1(2)	23182	1(3)	23700	1(2)	24362	1(2)	25065	3(3)	25375	1(2)
21401	1(2)	21933	3(3)	22810	1(2)	23184	1(3)	23800	1(2)	24363	1(2)	25066	2(3)	25390	1(2)
21406	1(2)	21935	1(3)	22812	1(2)	23190	1(3)	23802	1(2)	24365	1(2)	25071	3(3)	25391	1(2)
21407	1(2)	21936	1(3)	22818	1(2)	23195	1(2)	23900	1(2)	24366	1(2)	25073	3(3)	25392	1(2)
21408	1(2)	22010	2(3)	22819	1(2)	23200	1(3)	23920	1(2)	24370	1(2)	25075	6(3)	25393	1(2)
21421	1(2)	22015	2(3)	22830	1(2)	23210	1(3)	23921	1(2)	24371	1(2)	25076	5(3)	25394	1(3)
21422	1(2)	22100	1(2)	22840	1(2)	23220	1(3)	23930	2(3)	24400	1(3)	25077	1(3)	25400	1(2)
21423	1(2)	22101	1(2)	22842	1(3)	23330	2(3)	23931	2(3)	24410	1(2)	25078	1(3)	25405	1(2)
21431	1(2)	22102	1(2)	22843	1(3)	23333	1(3)	23935	2(3)	24420	1(2)	25085	1(2)	25415	1(2)
21432	1(2)	22103	3(3)	22844	1(3)	23334	1(3)	24000	1(2)	24430	1(3)	25100	1(2)	25420	1(2)
21433	1(2)	22110	1(2)	22845	1(3)	23335	1(2)	24006	1(2)	24435	1(3)	25101	1(2)	25425	1(2)
21435	1(2)	22112	1(2)	22846	1(3)	23350	1(2)	24065	2(3)	24470	1(2)	25105	1(2)	25426	1(2)
21436	1(2)	22114	1(2)	22847	1(3)	23395	1(2)	24066	2(3)	24495	1(2)	25107	1(2)	25430	1(3)
21440	2(2)	22116	3(3)	22848	1(2)	23397	1(3)	24071	3(3)	24498	1(2)	25109	4(3)	25431	1(3)
21445	2(2)	22206	1(2)	22849	1(2)	23400	1(2)	24073	3(3)	24500	1(2)	25110	3(3)	25440	1(2)
21450	1(2)	22207	1(2)	22850	1(2)	23405	2(3)	24075	5(3)	24505	1(2)	25111	1(3)	25441	1(2)
21451	1(2)	22208	6(3)	22851	5(3)	23406	1(3)	24076	4(3)	24515	1(2)	25112	1(3)	25442	1(2)
21452	1(2)	22210	1(2)	22852	1(2)	23410	1(2)	24077	1(3)	24516	1(2)	25115	1(3)	25443	1(2)
21453	1(2)	22212	1(2)	22855	1(2)	23412	1(2)	24079	1(3)	24530	1(2)	25116	1(3)	25444	1(2)
21454	1(2)	22214	1(2)	22856	1(2)	23415	1(2)	24100	1(2)	24535	1(2)	25118	5(3)	25445	1(2)
21461	1(2)	22216	6(3)	22857	1(2)	23420	1(2)	24101	1(2)	24538	1(2)	25119	1(2)	25446	1(2)
21462	1(2)	22220	1(2)	22858	1(2)	23430	1(2)	24102	1(2)	24545	1(2)	25120	1(3)	25447	4(3)
21465	1(2)	22222	1(2)	22861	1(2)	23440	1(2)	24105	1(2)	24546	1(2)	25125	1(3)	25449	1(2)
21470	1(2)	22224	1(2)	22862	1(2)	23450	1(2)	24110	1(3)	24560	1(3)	25126	1(3)	25450	1(2)
21480	1(2)	22226	4(3)	22864	1(2)	23455	1(2)	24115	1(3)	24565	1(3)	25130	1(3)	25455	1(2)
21485	1(2)	22305	1(2)	22865	1(2)	23460	1(2)	24116	1(3)	24566	1(3)	25135	1(3)	25490	1(2)
21490	1(2)	22310	1(2)	22900	3(3)	23462	1(2)	24120	1(3)	24575	1(3)	25136	1(3)	25491	1(2)
21495	1(2)	22315	1(2)	22901	2(3)	23465	1(2)	24125	1(3)	24576	1(3)	25145	1(3)	25492	1(2)
21497	1(2)	22318	1(2)	22902	4(3)	23466	1(2)	24126	1(3)	24577	1(3)	25150	1(3)	25500	1(2)
21501	3(3)	22319	1(2)	22903	3(3)	23470	1(2)	24130	1(2)	24579	1(3)	25151	1(3)	25505	1(2)
21502	1(3)	22325	1(2)	22904	1(3)	23472	1(2)	24134	1(3)	24582	1(3)	25170	1(3)	25515	1(2)
21510	1(3)	22326	1(2)	22905	1(3)	23473	1(2)	24136	1(3)	24586	1(3)	25210	2(1)	25520	1(2)
21550	3(3)	22327	1(2)	23000	1(2)	23474	1(2)	24138	1(3)	24587	1(2)	25215	1(2)	25525	1(2)
21552	4(3)	22328	6(3)	23020	1(2)	23480	1(2)	24140	1(3)	24600	1(2)	25230	1(2)	25526	1(2)
21554	2(3)	22505	1(2)	23030	2(3)	23485	1(2)	24145	1(3)	24605	1(2)	25240	1(2)	25530	1(2)
21555	4(3)	22510	1(2)	23031	1(3)	23490	1(2)	24147	1(2)	24615	1(2)	25246	1(2)	25535	1(2)
21556	3(3)	22511	1(2)	23035	1(3)	23491	1(2)	24149	1(2)	24620	1(2)	25248	3(3)	25545	1(2)
21557	1(3)	22512	5(3)	23040	1(2)	23500	1(2)	24150	1(3)	24635	1(2)	25250	1(2)	25560	1(2)
21558	1(3)	22513	1(2)	23044	1(3)	23505	1(2)	24152	1(3)	24640	1(2)	25251	1(2)	25565	1(2)
21600	5(3)	22514	1(2)	23065	2(3)	23515	1(2)	24155	1(2)	24650	1(2)	25259	1(2)	25574	1(2)
21610	1(3)	22515	5(3)	23066	2(3)	23520	1(2)	24160	1(2)	24655	1(2)	25260	9(3)	25575	1(2)
21615	1(2)	22532	1(2)	23071	2(3)	23525	1(2)	24164	1(2)	24665	1(2)	25263	4(3)	25600	1(2)
21616	1(2)	22533	1(2)	23073	2(3)	23530	1(2)	24200	3(3)	24666	1(2)	25265	4(3)	25605	1(2)
21620	1(2)	22534	3(3)	23075	3(3)	23532	1(2)	24201	3(3)	24670	1(2)	25270	8(3)	25606	1(2)
21627	1(2)	22548	1(2)	23076	2(3)	23540	1(2)	24220	1(2)	24675	1(2)	25272	4(3)	25607	1(2)
21630	1(2)	22551	1(2)	23077	1(3)	23545	1(2)	24300	1(2)	24685	1(2)	25274	4(3)	25608	1(2)
21632	1(2)	22552	5(3)	23078	1(3)	23550	1(2)	24301	2(3)	24800	1(2)	25275	2(3)	25609	1(2)

Appendix I — Medically Unlikely Edits (MUEs) — Professional

CPT	MUE	CPT	MUE	CPT	MUE	CPT	MUE	CPT	MUE	CPT	MUE	CPT	MUE	CPT	MUE
25622	1(2)	26145	6(3)	26502	3(3)	26770	3(3)	27100	1(2)	27284	1(2)	27429	1(2)	27570	1(2)
25624	1(2)	26160	5(3)	26508	1(2)	26775	4(3)	27105	1(3)	27286	1(2)	27430	1(2)	27580	1(2)
25628	1(2)	26170	5(3)	26510	4(3)	26776	4(3)	27110	1(2)	27290	1(2)	27435	1(2)	27590	1(2)
25630	1(3)	26180	4(3)	26516	1(2)	26785	3(3)	27111	1(2)	27295	1(2)	27437	1(2)	27591	1(2)
25635	1(3)	26185	1(3)	26517	1(2)	26820	1(2)	27120	1(2)	27301	3(3)	27438	1(2)	27592	1(2)
25645	1(3)	26200	2(3)	26518	1(2)	26841	1(2)	27122	1(2)	27303	2(3)	27440	1(2)	27594	1(2)
25650	1(2)	26205	1(3)	26520	4(3)	26842	1(2)	27125	1(2)	27305	1(2)	27441	1(2)	27596	1(2)
25651	1(2)	26210	2(3)	26525	4(3)	26843	2(3)	27130	1(2)	27306	1(2)	27442	1(2)	27598	1(2)
25652	1(2)	26215	2(3)	26530	4(3)	26844	2(3)	27132	1(2)	27307	1(2)	27443	1(2)	27600	1(2)
25660	1(2)	26230	2(3)	26531	4(3)	26850	5(3)	27134	1(2)	27310	1(2)	27445	1(2)	27601	1(2)
25670	1(2)	26235	2(3)	26535	4(3)	26852	2(3)	27137	1(2)	27323	2(3)	27446	1(2)	27602	1(2)
25671	1(2)	26236	2(3)	26536	4(3)	26860	1(2)	27138	1(2)	27324	3(3)	27447	1(2)	27603	2(3)
25675	1(2)	26250	2(3)	26540	4(3)	26861	4(3)	27140	1(2)	27325	1(2)	27448	1(3)	27604	2(3)
25676	1(2)	26260	1(3)	26541	4(3)	26862	1(2)	27146	1(3)	27326	1(2)	27450	1(3)	27605	1(2)
25680	1(2)	26262	1(3)	26542	4(3)	26863	3(3)	27147	1(3)	27327	5(3)	27454	1(3)	27606	1(2)
25685	1(2)	26320	4(3)	26545	4(3)	26910	4(3)	27151	1(3)	27328	4(3)	27455	1(3)	27607	2(3)
25690	1(2)	26340	4(3)	26546	2(3)	26951	8(3)	27156	1(3)	27329	1(3)	27457	1(3)	27610	1(2)
25695	1(2)	26341	2(3)	26548	3(3)	26952	5(3)	27158	1(2)	27330	1(2)	27465	1(2)	27612	1(2)
25800	1(2)	26350	6(3)	26550	1(2)	26990	2(3)	27161	1(2)	27331	1(2)	27466	1(2)	27613	4(3)
25805	1(2)	26352	2(3)	26551	1(2)	26991	1(3)	27165	1(2)	27332	1(2)	27468	1(2)	27614	3(3)
25810	1(2)	26356	4(3)	26553	1(3)	26992	2(3)	27170	1(2)	27333	1(2)	27470	1(2)	27615	1(3)
25820	1(2)	26357	2(3)	26554	1(3)	27000	1(3)	27175	1(2)	27334	1(2)	27472	1(2)	27616	1(3)
25825	1(2)	26358	2(3)	26555	2(3)	27001	1(3)	27176	1(2)	27335	1(2)	27475	1(2)	27618	4(3)
25830	1(2)	26370	3(3)	26556	2(3)	27003	1(2)	27177	1(2)	27337	4(3)	27477	1(2)	27619	4(3)
25900	1(2)	26372	1(3)	26560	2(3)	27005	1(2)	27178	1(2)	27339	4(3)	27479	1(2)	27620	1(2)
25905	1(2)	26373	2(3)	26561	2(3)	27006	1(2)	27179	1(2)	27340	1(2)	27485	1(2)	27625	1(2)
25907	1(2)	26390	2(3)	26562	2(3)	27025	1(3)	27181	1(2)	27345	1(2)	27486	1(2)	27626	1(2)
25909	1(2)	26392	2(3)	26565	3(3)	27027	1(2)	27185	1(2)	27347	1(2)	27487	1(2)	27630	2(3)
25915	1(2)	26410	4(3)	26567	3(3)	27030	1(2)	27187	1(2)	27350	1(2)	27488	1(2)	27632	4(3)
25920	1(2)	26412	3(3)	26568	2(3)	27033	1(2)	27193	1(2)	27355	1(3)	27495	1(2)	27634	2(3)
25922	1(2)	26415	2(3)	26580	1(2)	27035	1(2)	27194	1(2)	27356	1(3)	27496	1(2)	27635	1(3)
25924	1(2)	26416	2(3)	26587	2(3)	27036	1(2)	27200	1(2)	27357	1(3)	27497	1(2)	27637	1(3)
25927	1(2)	26418	4(3)	26590	2(3)	27040	2(3)	27202	1(2)	27358	1(3)	27498	1(2)	27638	1(3)
25929	1(2)	26420	4(3)	26591	4(3)	27041	3(3)	27220	1(2)	27360	2(3)	27499	1(2)	27640	1(3)
25931	1(2)	26426	4(3)	26593	9(3)	27043	3(3)	27222	1(2)	27364	1(3)	27500	1(2)	27641	1(3)
26010	2(3)	26428	2(3)	26596	1(3)	27045	3(3)	27226	1(2)	27365	1(3)	27501	1(2)	27645	1(3)
26011	3(3)	26432	2(3)	26600	2(3)	27047	4(3)	27227	1(2)	27370	1(2)	27502	1(2)	27646	1(3)
26020	4(3)	26433	2(3)	26605	3(3)	27048	2(3)	27228	1(2)	27372	2(3)	27503	1(2)	27647	1(3)
26025	1(2)	26434	2(3)	26607	2(3)	27049	1(3)	27230	1(2)	27380	2(2)	27506	1(2)	27648	1(2)
26030	1(2)	26437	4(3)	26608	5(3)	27050	1(2)	27232	1(2)	27381	2(2)	27507	1(2)	27650	1(2)
26034	2(3)	26440	6(3)	26615	4(3)	27052	1(2)	27235	1(2)	27385	2(3)	27508	1(2)	27652	1(2)
26035	1(3)	26442	5(3)	26641	1(2)	27054	1(2)	27236	1(2)	27386	2(3)	27509	1(2)	27654	1(2)
26037	1(3)	26445	5(3)	26645	1(2)	27057	1(2)	27238	1(2)	27390	1(2)	27510	1(2)	27656	1(3)
26040	1(2)	26449	5(3)	26650	1(2)	27059	1(3)	27240	1(2)	27391	1(2)	27511	1(2)	27658	2(3)
26045	1(2)	26450	6(3)	26665	1(2)	27060	1(2)	27244	1(2)	27392	1(2)	27513	1(2)	27659	2(3)
26055	5(3)	26455	6(3)	26670	2(3)	27062	1(2)	27245	1(2)	27393	1(2)	27514	1(2)	27664	2(3)
26060	5(3)	26460	4(3)	26675	1(3)	27065	1(3)	27246	1(2)	27394	1(2)	27516	1(2)	27665	2(3)
26070	2(3)	26471	4(3)	26676	3(3)	27066	1(3)	27248	1(2)	27395	1(2)	27517	1(2)	27675	1(2)
26075	4(3)	26474	4(3)	26685	3(3)	27067	1(3)	27250	1(2)	27396	1(2)	27519	1(2)	27676	1(2)
26080	4(3)	26476	4(3)	26686	3(3)	27070	1(3)	27252	1(2)	27397	1(2)	27520	1(2)	27680	3(3)
26100	1(3)	26477	4(3)	26700	3(3)	27071	1(3)	27253	1(2)	27400	1(2)	27524	1(2)	27681	1(2)
26105	2(3)	26478	6(3)	26705	3(3)	27075	1(3)	27254	1(2)	27403	1(3)	27530	1(2)	27685	2(3)
26110	3(3)	26479	4(3)	26706	4(3)	27076	1(2)	27256	1(2)	27405	2(2)	27532	1(2)	27686	3(3)
26111	4(3)	26480	4(3)	26715	4(3)	27077	1(2)	27257	1(2)	27407	2(2)	27535	1(2)	27687	1(2)
26113	4(3)	26483	4(3)	26720	4(3)	27078	1(2)	27258	1(2)	27409	1(2)	27536	1(2)	27690	2(3)
26115	4(3)	26485	4(3)	26725	4(3)	27080	1(2)	27259	1(2)	27412	1(2)	27538	1(2)	27691	2(3)
26116	2(3)	26489	3(3)	26727	4(3)	27086	1(3)	27265	1(2)	27415	1(2)	27540	1(2)	27692	4(3)
26117	2(3)	26490	3(3)	26735	4(3)	27087	1(3)	27266	1(2)	27416	1(2)	27550	1(2)	27695	1(2)
26118	1(3)	26492	2(3)	26740	3(3)	27090	1(1)	27267	1(2)	27418	1(2)	27552	1(2)	27696	1(2)
26121	1(2)	26494	1(3)	26742	3(3)	27091	1(1)	27268	1(2)	27420	1(2)	27556	1(2)	27698	2(2)
26123	1(2)	26496	1(3)	26746	3(3)	27093	1(1)	27269	1(2)	27422	1(2)	27557	1(2)	27700	1(2)
26125	4(3)	26497	2(3)	26750	3(3)	27095	1(1)	27275	2(2)	27424	1(2)	27558	1(2)	27702	1(2)
26130	1(3)	26498	1(3)	26755	3(3)	27096	1(1)	27279	1(2)	27425	1(2)	27560	1(2)	27703	1(2)
26135	4(3)	26499	2(3)	26756	3(3)	27097	1(3)	27280	1(2)	27427	1(2)	27562	1(2)	27704	1(2)
26140	3(3)	26500	4(3)	26765	5(3)	27098	1(2)	27282	1(2)	27428	1(2)	27566	1(2)	27705	1(3)

CPT	MUE	CPT	MUE	CPT	MUE	CPT	MUE	CPT	MUE	CPT	MUE	CPT	MUE	CPT	MUE
27707	1(3)	27894	1(2)	28220	1(2)	28485	5(3)	29200	1(2)	29856	1(2)	30410	1(2)	31294	1(2)
27709	1(3)	28001	2(3)	28222	1(2)	28490	1(2)	29240	1(2)	29860	1(2)	30420	1(2)	31295	1(2)
27712	1(2)	28002	3(3)	28225	1(2)	28495	1(2)	29260	1(3)	29861	1(2)	30430	1(2)	31296	1(2)
27715	1(2)	28003	2(3)	28226	1(2)	28496	1(2)	29280	2(3)	29862	1(2)	30435	1(2)	31297	1(2)
27720	1(2)	28005	3(3)	28230	1(2)	28505	1(2)	29305	1(3)	29863	1(2)	30450	1(2)	31300	1(2)
27722	1(2)	28008	2(3)	28232	6(3)	28510	4(3)	29325	1(3)	29866	1(2)	30460	1(2)	31320	1(2)
27724	1(2)	28010	4(1)	28234	6(3)	28515	4(3)	29345	1(3)	29867	1(2)	30462	1(2)	31360	1(2)
27725	1(2)	28011	4(1)	28238	1(2)	28525	4(3)	29355	1(3)	29868	1(3)	30465	1(2)	31365	1(2)
27726	1(2)	28020	2(3)	28240	1(2)	28530	1(2)	29358	1(3)	29870	1(2)	30520	1(2)	31367	1(2)
27727	1(2)	28022	4(3)	28250	1(2)	28531	1(2)	29365	1(3)	29871	1(2)	30540	1(2)	31368	1(2)
27730	1(2)	28024	4(3)	28260	1(2)	28540	1(3)	29405	1(3)	29873	1(2)	30545	1(2)	31370	1(2)
27732	1(2)	28035	1(2)	28261	1(3)	28545	1(3)	29425	1(3)	29874	1(2)	30560	1(2)	31375	1(2)
27734	1(2)	28039	3(3)	28262	1(2)	28546	1(3)	29435	1(3)	29875	1(2)	30580	2(3)	31380	1(2)
27740	1(2)	28041	3(3)	28264	1(2)	28555	1(3)	29440	1(2)	29876	1(2)	30600	1(3)	31382	1(2)
27742	1(2)	28043	4(3)	28270	6(3)	28570	1(2)	29445	1(3)	29877	1(2)	30620	1(2)	31390	1(2)
27745	1(2)	28045	4(3)	28272	6(3)	28575	1(2)	29450	1(3)	29879	1(2)	30630	1(2)	31395	1(2)
27750	1(2)	28046	1(3)	28280	1(2)	28576	1(2)	29505	1(2)	29880	1(2)	30801	1(2)	31400	1(3)
27752	1(2)	28047	1(3)	28285	4(3)	28585	1(3)	29515	1(2)	29881	1(2)	30802	1(2)	31420	1(2)
27756	1(2)	28050	2(3)	28286	1(2)	28600	2(3)	29520	1(2)	29882	1(2)	30901	1(3)	31500	2(3)
27758	1(2)	28052	2(3)	28288	5(3)	28605	2(3)	29530	1(2)	29883	1(2)	30903	1(3)	31502	1(3)
27759	1(2)	28054	2(3)	28289	1(2)	28606	3(3)	29540	1(2)	29884	1(2)	30905	1(2)	31505	1(3)
27760	1(2)	28055	1(3)	28290	1(2)	28615	5(3)	29550	1(2)	29885	1(2)	30906	1(3)	31510	1(2)
27762	1(2)	28060	1(2)	28292	1(2)	28630	2(3)	29580	1(2)	29886	1(2)	30915	1(3)	31511	1(3)
27766	1(2)	28062	1(2)	28293	1(2)	28635	2(3)	29581	1(2)	29887	1(2)	30920	1(3)	31512	1(3)
27767	1(2)	28070	2(3)	28294	1(2)	28636	4(3)	29582	1(2)	29888	1(2)	30930	1(2)	31513	1(3)
27768	1(2)	28072	4(3)	28296	1(2)	28645	4(3)	29583	1(2)	29889	1(2)	31000	1(2)	31515	1(3)
27769	1(2)	28080	4(3)	28297	1(2)	28660	4(3)	29584	1(2)	29891	1(2)	31002	1(2)	31520	1(3)
27780	1(2)	28086	2(3)	28298	1(2)	28665	4(3)	29700	2(3)	29892	1(2)	31020	1(2)	31525	1(3)
27781	1(2)	28088	2(3)	28299	1(2)	28666	4(3)	29705	1(3)	29893	1(2)	31030	1(2)	31526	1(3)
27784	1(2)	28090	2(3)	28300	1(2)	28675	4(3)	29710	1(2)	29894	1(2)	31032	1(2)	31527	1(2)
27786	1(2)	28092	2(3)	28302	1(2)	28705	1(2)	29720	1(2)	29895	1(2)	31040	1(2)	31528	1(2)
27788	1(2)	28100	1(3)	28304	1(3)	28715	1(2)	29730	1(3)	29897	1(2)	31050	1(2)	31529	1(3)
27792	1(2)	28102	1(3)	28305	1(3)	28725	1(2)	29740	1(3)	29898	1(2)	31051	1(2)	31530	1(3)
27808	1(2)	28103	1(3)	28306	1(2)	28730	1(2)	29750	1(3)	29899	1(2)	31070	1(2)	31531	1(3)
27810	1(2)	28104	2(3)	28307	1(2)	28735	1(2)	29800	1(2)	29900	2(3)	31075	1(2)	31535	1(3)
27814	1(2)	28106	1(3)	28308	4(3)	28737	1(2)	29804	1(2)	29901	2(3)	31080	1(2)	31536	1(3)
27816	1(2)	28107	1(3)	28309	1(2)	28740	5(3)	29805	1(2)	29902	2(3)	31081	1(2)	31540	1(3)
27818	1(2)	28108	2(3)	28310	1(2)	28750	1(2)	29806	1(2)	29904	1(2)	31084	1(2)	31541	1(3)
27822	1(2)	28110	1(2)	28312	4(3)	28755	1(2)	29807	1(2)	29905	1(2)	31085	1(2)	31545	1(2)
27823	1(2)	28111	1(2)	28313	4(3)	28760	1(2)	29819	1(2)	29906	1(2)	31086	1(2)	31546	1(2)
27824	1(2)	28112	4(3)	28315	1(2)	28800	1(2)	29820	1(2)	29907	1(2)	31087	1(2)	31560	1(2)
27825	1(3)	28113	1(2)	28320	1(2)	28805	1(2)	29821	1(2)	29914	1(2)	31090	1(2)	31561	1(2)
27826	1(2)	28114	1(2)	28322	2(3)	28810	6(3)	29822	1(2)	29915	1(2)	31200	1(2)	31570	1(2)
27827	1(2)	28116	1(2)	28340	2(3)	28820	6(3)	29823	1(2)	29916	1(2)	31201	1(2)	31571	1(2)
27828	1(2)	28118	1(2)	28341	2(3)	28825	10(2)	29824	1(2)	30000	1(3)	31205	1(2)	31575	1(3)
27829	1(2)	28119	1(2)	28344	1(2)	28890	1(2)	29825	1(2)	30020	1(3)	31225	1(2)	31576	1(3)
27830	1(2)	28120	2(3)	28345	2(3)	29000	1(3)	29826	1(2)	30100	2(3)	31230	1(2)	31577	1(3)
27831	1(2)	28122	4(3)	28360	1(2)	29010	1(3)	29827	1(2)	30110	1(2)	31231	1(2)	31578	1(3)
27832	1(2)	28124	4(3)	28400	1(2)	29015	1(3)	29828	1(2)	30115	1(2)	31233	1(2)	31579	1(2)
27840	1(2)	28126	4(3)	28405	1(2)	29035	1(3)	29830	1(2)	30117	2(3)	31235	1(2)	31580	1(2)
27842	1(2)	28130	1(2)	28406	1(2)	29040	1(3)	29834	1(2)	30118	1(3)	31237	1(2)	31582	1(2)
27846	1(2)	28140	4(3)	28415	1(2)	29044	1(3)	29835	1(2)	30120	1(2)	31238	1(3)	31584	1(2)
27848	1(2)	28150	4(3)	28420	1(2)	29046	1(3)	29836	1(2)	30124	2(3)	31239	1(2)	31587	1(2)
27860	1(2)	28153	6(3)	28430	1(2)	29049	1(3)	29837	1(2)	30125	1(3)	31254	1(2)	31588	1(2)
27870	1(2)	28160	5(3)	28435	1(2)	29055	1(3)	29838	1(2)	30130	1(2)	31255	1(2)	31590	1(2)
27871	1(3)	28171	1(3)	28436	1(2)	29058	1(3)	29840	1(2)	30140	1(2)	31256	1(2)	31595	1(2)
27880	1(2)	28173	2(3)	28445	1(2)	29065	1(3)	29843	1(2)	30150	1(2)	31267	1(2)	31600	1(2)
27881	1(2)	28175	2(3)	28446	1(2)	29075	1(3)	29844	1(2)	30160	1(2)	31276	1(2)	31601	1(2)
27882	1(2)	28190	3(3)	28450	2(3)	29085	1(3)	29845	1(2)	30200	1(2)	31287	1(2)	31603	1(2)
27884	1(2)	28192	2(3)	28455	3(3)	29086	2(3)	29846	1(2)	30210	1(3)	31288	1(2)	31605	1(2)
27886	1(2)	28193	2(3)	28456	2(3)	29105	1(2)	29847	1(2)	30220	1(2)	31290	1(2)	31610	1(2)
27888	1(2)	28200	4(3)	28465	3(3)	29125	1(2)	29848	1(2)	30300	1(3)	31291	1(2)	31611	1(2)
27889	1(2)	28202	2(3)	28470	2(3)	29126	1(2)	29850	1(2)	30310	1(3)	31292	1(2)	31612	1(3)
27892	1(2)	28208	4(3)	28475	5(3)	29130	3(3)	29851	1(2)	30320	1(3)	31293	1(2)	31613	1(2)
27893	1(2)	28210	2(3)	28476	4(3)	29131	2(3)	29855	1(2)	30400	1(2)			31614	1(2)

CPT	MUE	CPT	MUE	CPT	MUE	CPT	MUE	CPT	MUE	CPT	MUE	CPT	MUE	CPT	MUE
31615	1(3)	32200	2(3)	32800	1(3)	33244	1(2)	33465	1(2)	33690	1(2)	33917	1(2)	34451	1(3)
31622	1(3)	32215	1(2)	32810	1(3)	33249	1(3)	33468	1(2)	33692	1(2)	33920	1(2)	34471	1(2)
31623	1(3)	32220	1(2)	32815	1(3)	33250	1(2)	33470	1(2)	33694	1(2)	33922	1(2)	34490	1(2)
31624	1(3)	32225	1(2)	32820	1(2)	33251	1(2)	33471	1(2)	33697	1(2)	33924	1(2)	34501	1(2)
31625	1(2)	32310	1(3)	32850	1(2)	33254	1(2)	33474	1(2)	33702	1(2)	33925	1(2)	34502	1(2)
31626	1(2)	32320	1(3)	32851	1(2)	33255	1(2)	33475	1(2)	33710	1(2)	33926	1(2)	34510	2(3)
31627	1(3)	32400	2(3)	32852	1(2)	33256	1(2)	33476	1(2)	33720	1(2)	33930	1(2)	34520	1(3)
31628	1(2)	32405	2(3)	32853	1(2)	33257	1(2)	33477	1(2)	33722	1(3)	33933	1(2)	34530	1(2)
31629	1(2)	32440	1(2)	32854	1(2)	33258	1(2)	33478	1(2)	33724	1(2)	33935	1(2)	34800	1(2)
31630	1(3)	32442	1(2)	32855	1(2)	33259	1(2)	33496	1(3)	33726	1(2)	33940	1(2)	34802	1(2)
31631	1(2)	32445	1(2)	32856	1(2)	33261	1(2)	33500	1(3)	33730	1(2)	33944	1(2)	34803	1(2)
31632	2(3)	32480	1(2)	32900	1(2)	33262	1(3)	33501	1(3)	33732	1(2)	33945	1(2)	34804	1(2)
31633	2(3)	32482	1(2)	32905	1(2)	33263	1(3)	33502	1(3)	33735	1(2)	33946	1(2)	34805	1(2)
31634	1(3)	32484	2(3)	32906	1(2)	33264	1(3)	33503	1(3)	33736	1(2)	33947	1(2)	34806	1(2)
31635	1(3)	32486	1(3)	32940	1(3)	33265	1(2)	33504	1(3)	33737	1(2)	33948	1(2)	34808	1(3)
31636	1(2)	32488	1(2)	32960	1(2)	33266	1(2)	33505	1(3)	33750	1(3)	33949	1(2)	34812	1(2)
31637	2(3)	32491	1(2)	32997	1(2)	33270	1(3)	33506	1(3)	33755	1(2)	33951	1(1)	34813	1(2)
31638	1(3)	32501	1(3)	32998	1(2)	33271	1(3)	33507	1(3)	33762	1(2)	33952	1(1)	34820	1(2)
31640	1(3)	32503	1(2)	33010	1(2)	33272	1(3)	33508	1(2)	33764	1(3)	33953	1(1)	34825	1(2)
31641	1(3)	32504	1(2)	33011	1(3)	33273	1(3)	33510	1(2)	33766	1(2)	33954	1(1)	34826	4(3)
31643	1(2)	32505	1(2)	33015	1(3)	33282	1(2)	33511	1(2)	33767	1(2)	33955	1(3)	34830	1(2)
31645	1(2)	32506	3(3)	33020	1(3)	33284	1(2)	33512	1(2)	33768	1(2)	33956	1(3)	34831	1(2)
31646	2(3)	32507	2(3)	33025	1(2)	33300	1(3)	33513	1(2)	33770	1(2)	33957	1(3)	34832	1(2)
31647	1(2)	32540	1(3)	33030	1(2)	33305	1(3)	33514	1(2)	33771	1(2)	33958	1(3)	34833	1(2)
31648	1(2)	32550	2(3)	33031	1(2)	33310	1(2)	33516	1(2)	33774	1(2)	33959	1(3)	34834	1(2)
31649	2(3)	32551	2(3)	33050	1(2)	33315	1(2)	33517	1(2)	33775	1(2)	33962	1(3)	34839	1(2)
31651	3(3)	32552	2(2)	33120	1(3)	33320	1(3)	33518	1(2)	33776	1(2)	33963	1(3)	34841	1(2)
31652	1(3)	32553	1(2)	33130	1(3)	33321	1(3)	33519	1(2)	33777	1(2)	33964	1(2)	34842	1(2)
31653	1(3)	32554	2(3)	33140	1(2)	33322	1(3)	33521	1(2)	33778	1(2)	33965	1(3)	34843	1(2)
31654	1(3)	32555	2(3)	33141	1(2)	33330	1(3)	33522	1(2)	33779	1(2)	33966	1(3)	34844	1(2)
31660	1(2)	32556	2(3)	33202	1(2)	33335	1(3)	33523	1(2)	33780	1(2)	33967	1(3)	34845	1(2)
31661	1(2)	32557	2(3)	33203	1(2)	33361	1(2)	33530	1(2)	33781	1(2)	33968	1(3)	34846	1(2)
31717	1(3)	32560	1(3)	33206	1(3)	33362	1(2)	33533	1(2)	33782	1(2)	33969	1(3)	34847	1(2)
31720	1(3)	32561	1(2)	33207	1(3)	33363	1(2)	33534	1(2)	33783	1(2)	33970	1(3)	34848	1(2)
31725	1(3)	32562	1(2)	33208	1(3)	33364	1(2)	33535	1(2)	33786	1(2)	33971	1(3)	34900	1(2)
31730	1(3)	32601	1(3)	33210	1(3)	33365	1(2)	33536	1(2)	33788	1(2)	33973	1(3)	35001	1(2)
31750	1(2)	32604	1(3)	33211	1(3)	33366	1(2)	33542	1(2)	33800	1(2)	33974	1(3)	35002	1(2)
31755	1(2)	32606	1(3)	33212	1(3)	33367	1(2)	33545	1(2)	33802	1(3)	33975	1(3)	35005	1(2)
31760	1(2)	32607	1(3)	33213	1(3)	33368	1(2)	33548	1(2)	33803	1(3)	33976	1(3)	35011	1(2)
31766	1(2)	32608	1(3)	33214	1(3)	33369	1(2)	33572	3(2)	33813	1(2)	33977	1(3)	35013	1(2)
31770	2(3)	32609	1(3)	33215	2(3)	33400	1(2)	33600	1(3)	33814	1(2)	33978	1(3)	35021	1(2)
31775	1(3)	32650	1(2)	33216	1(3)	33401	1(2)	33602	1(3)	33820	1(2)	33979	1(3)	35022	1(2)
31780	1(2)	32651	1(2)	33217	1(3)	33403	1(2)	33606	1(2)	33822	1(2)	33980	1(3)	35045	2(3)
31781	1(2)	32652	1(2)	33218	1(3)	33404	1(2)	33608	1(2)	33824	1(2)	33981	1(3)	35081	1(2)
31785	1(3)	32653	1(3)	33220	1(3)	33405	1(2)	33610	1(2)	33840	1(2)	33982	1(3)	35082	1(2)
31786	1(3)	32654	1(3)	33221	1(3)	33406	1(2)	33611	1(2)	33845	1(2)	33983	1(3)	35091	1(2)
31800	1(3)	32655	1(3)	33222	1(3)	33410	1(2)	33612	1(2)	33851	1(2)	33984	1(3)	35092	1(2)
31805	1(3)	32656	1(2)	33223	1(3)	33411	1(2)	33615	1(2)	33852	1(2)	33985	1(3)	35102	1(2)
31820	1(2)	32658	1(3)	33224	1(3)	33412	1(2)	33617	1(2)	33853	1(2)	33986	1(3)	35103	1(2)
31825	1(2)	32659	1(2)	33225	1(3)	33413	1(2)	33619	1(2)	33860	1(2)	33987	1(3)	35111	1(2)
31830	1(2)	32661	1(3)	33226	1(3)	33414	1(2)	33620	1(2)	33863	1(2)	33988	1(3)	35112	1(2)
32035	1(2)	32662	1(3)	33227	1(3)	33415	1(2)	33621	1(3)	33864	1(2)	33989	1(3)	35121	1(3)
32036	1(3)	32663	1(3)	33228	1(3)	33416	1(2)	33622	1(2)	33870	1(2)	33990	1(3)	35122	1(3)
32096	1(3)	32664	1(2)	33229	1(3)	33417	1(2)	33641	1(2)	33875	1(2)	33991	1(3)	35131	1(2)
32097	1(3)	32665	1(2)	33230	1(3)	33418	1(3)	33645	1(2)	33877	1(2)	33992	1(2)	35132	1(2)
32098	1(2)	32666	1(3)	33231	1(3)	33419	1(3)	33647	1(2)	33880	1(2)	33993	1(3)	35141	1(2)
32100	1(3)	32667	3(3)	33233	1(2)	33420	1(2)	33660	1(2)	33881	1(2)	34001	1(3)	35142	1(2)
32110	1(3)	32668	2(3)	33234	1(2)	33422	1(2)	33665	1(2)	33883	1(2)	34051	1(3)	35151	1(2)
32120	1(3)	32669	2(3)	33235	1(2)	33425	1(2)	33670	1(2)	33884	2(3)	34101	1(3)	35152	1(2)
32124	1(3)	32670	1(2)	33236	1(2)	33426	1(2)	33675	1(2)	33886	1(2)	34111	2(3)	35180	2(3)
32140	1(3)	32671	1(2)	33237	1(2)	33427	1(2)	33676	1(2)	33889	1(2)	34151	2(3)	35182	2(3)
32141	1(3)	32672	1(3)	33238	1(2)	33430	1(2)	33677	1(2)	33891	1(2)	34201	1(3)	35184	2(3)
32150	1(3)	32673	1(2)	33240	1(3)	33460	1(2)	33681	1(2)	33910	1(3)	34203	1(2)	35188	2(3)
32151	1(3)	32674	1(2)	33241	1(2)	33463	1(2)	33684	1(2)	33915	1(3)	34401	1(3)	35189	1(3)
32160	1(3)	32701	1(2)	33243	1(2)	33464	1(2)	33688	1(2)	33916	1(3)	34421	1(3)	35190	2(3)

CPT	MUE	CPT	MUE	CPT	MUE	CPT	MUE	CPT	MUE	CPT	MUE	CPT	MUE	CPT	MUE
35201	2(3)	35537	1(3)	35879	2(3)	36479	2(3)	36870	2(3)	37660	1(2)	38765	1(2)	41018	2(3)
35206	2(3)	35538	1(3)	35881	2(3)	36481	1(3)	37140	1(2)	37700	1(2)	38770	1(2)	41019	1(2)
35207	3(3)	35539	1(3)	35883	1(3)	36500	4(3)	37145	1(3)	37718	1(2)	38780	1(2)	41100	3(3)
35211	3(3)	35540	1(3)	35884	1(3)	36510	1(3)	37160	1(3)	37722	1(2)	38790	1(2)	41105	3(3)
35216	2(3)	35556	1(3)	35901	1(3)	36511	1(3)	37180	1(2)	37735	1(2)	38792	1(3)	41108	2(3)
35221	3(3)	35558	1(3)	35903	2(3)	36512	1(3)	37181	1(2)	37760	1(2)	38794	1(2)	41110	2(3)
35226	3(3)	35560	1(3)	35905	1(3)	36513	1(3)	37182	1(2)	37761	1(2)	38900	1(3)	41112	2(3)
35231	2(3)	35563	1(3)	35907	1(3)	36514	1(3)	37183	1(2)	37765	1(2)	39000	1(2)	41113	2(3)
35236	2(3)	35565	1(3)	36000	4(3)	36515	1(3)	37184	1(2)	37766	1(2)	39010	1(2)	41114	2(3)
35241	2(3)	35566	1(3)	36002	2(3)	36516	1(3)	37185	2(3)	37780	1(2)	39200	1(2)	41115	1(2)
35246	2(3)	35570	1(3)	36005	2(3)	36522	1(3)	37186	2(3)	37785	1(2)	39220	1(2)	41116	2(3)
35251	2(3)	35571	2(3)	36010	2(3)	36555	2(3)	37187	1(3)	37788	1(2)	39401	1(3)	41120	1(2)
35256	2(3)	35572	2(3)	36011	4(3)	36556	2(3)	37188	1(3)	37790	1(2)	39402	1(3)	41130	1(2)
35261	1(3)	35583	1(2)	36012	4(3)	36557	2(3)	37191	1(3)	38100	1(2)	39501	1(3)	41135	1(2)
35266	2(3)	35585	2(3)	36013	2(3)	36558	2(3)	37192	1(3)	38101	1(3)	39503	1(2)	41140	1(2)
35271	2(3)	35587	2(2)	36014	2(3)	36560	2(3)	37193	1(3)	38102	1(2)	39540	1(2)	41145	1(2)
35276	2(3)	35600	2(3)	36015	4(3)	36561	2(3)	37195	1(3)	38115	1(3)	39541	1(2)	41150	1(2)
35281	2(3)	35601	1(3)	36100	2(3)	36563	1(3)	37197	2(3)	38120	1(2)	39545	1(2)	41153	1(2)
35286	2(3)	35606	1(3)	36120	2(3)	36565	1(3)	37200	2(3)	38200	1(3)	39560	1(3)	41155	1(2)
35301	2(3)	35612	1(3)	36140	3(3)	36566	1(3)	37211	1(2)	38205	1(3)	39561	1(3)	41250	2(3)
35302	1(2)	35616	1(3)	36147	2(3)	36568	2(3)	37212	1(2)	38206	1(3)	40490	3(3)	41251	2(3)
35303	1(2)	35621	1(3)	36148	1(3)	36569	2(3)	37213	1(2)	38208	0(3)	40500	2(3)	41252	2(3)
35304	1(2)	35623	1(3)	36160	2(3)	36570	2(3)	37214	1(2)	38209	0(3)	40510	2(3)	41500	1(2)
35305	1(2)	35626	3(3)	36200	2(3)	36571	2(3)	37215	1(2)	38210	0(3)	40520	2(3)	41510	1(2)
35306	2(3)	35631	4(3)	36215	6(3)	36575	2(3)	37217	1(2)	38211	0(3)	40525	2(3)	41512	1(2)
35311	1(2)	35632	1(3)	36216	4(3)	36576	2(3)	37218	1(2)	38212	0(3)	40527	2(3)	41520	1(3)
35321	1(2)	35633	1(3)	36217	2(3)	36578	2(3)	37220	2(2)	38213	0(3)	40530	2(3)	41530	1(3)
35331	1(2)	35634	1(3)	36218	6(3)	36580	2(3)	37221	2(2)	38214	0(3)	40650	2(3)	41800	2(3)
35341	3(3)	35636	1(3)	36221	1(3)	36581	2(3)	37222	2(3)	38215	0(3)	40652	2(3)	41805	3(3)
35351	1(3)	35637	1(3)	36222	1(3)	36582	2(3)	37223	2(3)	38220	1(3)	40654	2(3)	41806	3(3)
35355	1(2)	35638	1(3)	36223	1(3)	36583	2(3)	37224	2(2)	38221	1(3)	40700	1(2)	41820	4(2)
35361	1(2)	35642	1(3)	36224	1(3)	36584	2(3)	37225	2(2)	38230	1(2)	40701	1(2)	41821	2(3)
35363	1(2)	35645	1(3)	36225	1(3)	36585	2(3)	37226	2(2)	38232	1(2)	40702	1(2)	41822	1(2)
35371	1(2)	35646	1(3)	36226	1(3)	36589	2(3)	37227	2(2)	38240	1(3)	40720	1(2)	41823	1(2)
35372	1(2)	35647	1(3)	36227	1(3)	36590	2(3)	37228	2(2)	38241	1(2)	40761	1(2)	41825	2(3)
35390	1(3)	35650	1(3)	36228	4(3)	36591	2(3)	37229	2(2)	38242	1(2)	40800	2(3)	41826	2(3)
35400	1(3)	35654	1(3)	36245	6(3)	36592	1(3)	37230	2(2)	38243	1(3)	40801	2(3)	41827	2(3)
35450	2(3)	35656	1(3)	36246	4(3)	36593	2(3)	37231	2(2)	38300	1(3)	40804	2(3)	41828	4(2)
35452	1(2)	35661	1(3)	36247	3(3)	36595	2(3)	37232	2(3)	38305	1(3)	40805	2(3)	41830	2(3)
35458	2(3)	35663	1(3)	36248	6(3)	36596	2(3)	37233	2(3)	38308	1(3)	40806	2(2)	41850	2(3)
35460	2(3)	35665	1(3)	36251	1(3)	36597	2(3)	37234	2(3)	38380	1(2)	40808	4(3)	41870	2(3)
35471	3(3)	35666	2(3)	36252	1(3)	36598	2(3)	37235	2(3)	38381	1(2)	40810	4(3)	41872	4(2)
35472	1(2)	35671	2(3)	36253	1(3)	36600	4(3)	37236	1(2)	38382	1(2)	40812	4(3)	41874	4(2)
35475	4(3)	35681	1(3)	36254	1(3)	36620	3(3)	37237	2(3)	38500	2(3)	40814	4(3)	42000	1(3)
35476	5(3)	35682	1(2)	36260	1(2)	36625	2(3)	37238	1(2)	38505	3(3)	40816	2(3)	42100	3(3)
35500	2(3)	35683	1(2)	36261	1(2)	36640	1(3)	37239	2(3)	38510	1(2)	40818	2(3)	42104	3(3)
35501	1(3)	35685	2(3)	36262	1(2)	36660	1(3)	37241	2(3)	38520	1(2)	40819	2(2)	42106	2(3)
35506	1(3)	35686	1(3)	36400	1(3)	36680	1(3)	37242	2(3)	38525	1(2)	40820	5(3)	42107	2(3)
35508	1(3)	35691	1(3)	36405	1(3)	36800	1(3)	37243	1(3)	38530	1(2)	40830	2(3)	42120	1(2)
35509	1(3)	35693	1(3)	36406	1(3)	36810	1(3)	37244	2(3)	38542	1(2)	40831	2(3)	42140	1(2)
35510	1(3)	35694	1(3)	36410	3(3)	36815	1(3)	37252	1(3)	38550	1(3)	40840	1(2)	42145	1(2)
35511	1(3)	35695	1(3)	36415	4(3)	36818	1(3)	37253	3(1)	38555	1(3)	40842	1(2)	42160	2(3)
35512	1(3)	35697	2(3)	36420	2(3)	36819	1(3)	37500	1(3)	38562	1(2)	40843	1(2)	42180	1(3)
35515	1(3)	35700	2(3)	36425	2(3)	36820	1(3)	37565	1(2)	38564	1(2)	40844	1(2)	42182	1(3)
35516	1(3)	35701	1(2)	36430	1(2)	36821	2(3)	37600	1(3)	38570	1(2)	40845	1(3)	42200	1(2)
35518	1(3)	35721	1(2)	36440	1(3)	36823	1(3)	37605	1(3)	38571	1(2)	41000	2(3)	42205	1(2)
35521	1(3)	35741	1(2)	36450	1(3)	36825	1(3)	37606	1(3)	38572	1(2)	41005	2(3)	42210	1(2)
35522	1(3)	35761	2(3)	36455	1(3)	36830	2(3)	37607	1(3)	38700	1(2)	41006	2(3)	42215	1(2)
35523	1(3)	35800	2(3)	36460	2(3)	36831	1(3)	37609	1(2)	38720	1(2)	41007	2(3)	42220	1(2)
35525	1(3)	35820	2(3)	36468	1(3)	36832	2(3)	37615	2(3)	38724	1(2)	41008	2(3)	42225	1(2)
35526	1(3)	35840	2(3)	36470	1(3)	36833	1(3)	37616	1(3)	38740	1(2)	41009	2(3)	42226	1(2)
35531	2(3)	35860	2(3)	36471	1(2)	36835	1(3)	37617	3(3)	38745	1(2)	41010	1(2)	42227	1(2)
35533	1(3)	35870	1(3)	36475	1(3)	36838	1(3)	37618	2(3)	38746	1(2)	41015	2(3)	42235	1(2)
35535	1(3)	35875	2(3)	36476	2(3)	36860	2(3)	37619	4(3)	38747	1(2)	41016	2(3)	42260	1(3)
35536	1(3)	35876	2(3)	36478	1(3)	36861	2(3)	37650	1(2)	38760	1(2)	41017	2(3)	42280	1(2)

CPT	MUE	CPT	MUE	CPT	MUE	CPT	MUE	CPT	MUE	CPT	MUE	CPT	MUE	CPT	MUE
42281	1(2)	43020	1(2)	43252	1(2)	43520	1(2)	44050	1(2)	44370	1(2)	45116	1(2)	45560	1(2)
42300	2(3)	43030	1(2)	43253	1(3)	43605	1(2)	44055	1(2)	44372	1(2)	45119	1(2)	45562	1(2)
42305	2(3)	43045	1(2)	43254	1(3)	43610	2(3)	44100	1(2)	44373	1(2)	45120	1(2)	45563	1(2)
42310	2(3)	43100	1(3)	43255	2(3)	43611	2(3)	44110	1(2)	44376	1(3)	45121	1(2)	45800	1(3)
42320	2(3)	43101	1(3)	43257	1(2)	43620	1(2)	44111	1(2)	44377	1(2)	45123	1(2)	45805	1(3)
42330	2(3)	43107	1(2)	43259	1(3)	43621	1(2)	44120	1(2)	44378	1(3)	45126	1(2)	45820	1(3)
42335	2(2)	43108	1(2)	43260	1(3)	43622	1(2)	44121	4(3)	44379	1(2)	45130	1(2)	45825	1(3)
42340	1(2)	43112	1(2)	43261	1(2)	43631	1(2)	44125	1(2)	44380	1(3)	45135	1(2)	45900	1(2)
42400	2(3)	43113	1(2)	43262	2(2)	43632	1(2)	44126	1(2)	44381	1(3)	45136	1(2)	45905	1(2)
42405	2(3)	43116	1(2)	43263	1(2)	43633	1(2)	44127	1(2)	44382	1(2)	45150	1(2)	45910	1(2)
42408	1(3)	43117	1(2)	43264	1(2)	43634	1(2)	44128	2(3)	44384	1(3)	45160	1(3)	45915	1(2)
42409	1(3)	43118	1(2)	43265	1(2)	43635	1(2)	44130	3(3)	44385	1(3)	45171	2(3)	45990	1(2)
42410	1(2)	43121	1(2)	43266	1(3)	43640	1(2)	44132	1(2)	44386	1(2)	45172	2(3)	46020	2(3)
42415	1(2)	43122	1(2)	43270	1(3)	43641	1(2)	44133	1(2)	44388	1(3)	45190	1(3)	46030	1(3)
42420	1(2)	43123	1(2)	43273	1(2)	43644	1(2)	44135	1(2)	44389	1(2)	45300	1(3)	46040	2(3)
42425	1(2)	43124	1(2)	43274	2(3)	43645	1(2)	44136	1(2)	44390	1(3)	45303	1(3)	46045	2(3)
42426	1(2)	43130	1(3)	43275	1(3)	43647	1(2)	44137	1(2)	44391	1(3)	45305	1(2)	46050	2(3)
42440	1(2)	43135	1(3)	43276	2(3)	43648	1(2)	44139	1(2)	44392	1(2)	45307	1(3)	46060	2(3)
42450	2(3)	43180	1(2)	43277	3(3)	43651	1(2)	44140	2(3)	44394	1(2)	45308	1(2)	46070	1(2)
42500	2(3)	43191	1(3)	43278	1(3)	43652	1(2)	44141	1(3)	44401	1(2)	45309	1(2)	46080	1(2)
42505	2(3)	43192	1(3)	43279	1(2)	43653	1(2)	44143	1(2)	44402	1(3)	45315	1(2)	46083	2(3)
42507	1(2)	43193	1(3)	43280	1(2)	43752	2(3)	44144	1(3)	44403	1(3)	45317	1(3)	46200	1(3)
42509	1(2)	43194	1(3)	43281	1(2)	43753	1(2)	44145	1(2)	44404	1(2)	45320	1(2)	46220	1(2)
42510	1(2)	43195	1(3)	43282	1(2)	43754	1(3)	44146	1(2)	44405	1(3)	45321	1(2)	46221	1(2)
42550	2(3)	43196	1(3)	43283	1(2)	43755	1(3)	44147	1(3)	44406	1(3)	45327	1(2)	46230	1(2)
42600	2(3)	43197	1(3)	43300	1(2)	43756	1(2)	44150	1(2)	44407	1(2)	45330	1(3)	46250	1(2)
42650	2(3)	43198	1(3)	43305	1(2)	43757	1(2)	44151	1(2)	44408	1(3)	45331	1(2)	46255	1(2)
42660	2(3)	43200	1(3)	43310	1(2)	43760	2(3)	44155	1(2)	44500	1(3)	45332	1(3)	46257	1(2)
42665	2(3)	43201	1(2)	43312	1(2)	43761	2(3)	44156	1(2)	44602	1(2)	45333	1(2)	46258	1(2)
42700	2(3)	43202	1(2)	43313	1(2)	43770	1(2)	44157	1(2)	44603	1(2)	45334	1(3)	46260	1(2)
42720	1(3)	43204	1(2)	43314	1(2)	43771	1(2)	44158	1(2)	44604	1(2)	45335	1(2)	46261	1(2)
42725	1(3)	43205	1(2)	43320	1(2)	43772	1(2)	44160	1(2)	44605	1(2)	45337	1(2)	46262	1(2)
42800	3(3)	43206	1(2)	43325	1(2)	43773	1(2)	44180	1(2)	44615	4(3)	45338	1(2)	46270	1(3)
42804	3(3)	43210	1(2)	43327	1(2)	43774	1(2)	44186	1(2)	44620	2(3)	45340	1(2)	46275	1(3)
42806	1(3)	43211	1(3)	43328	1(2)	43775	1(2)	44187	1(3)	44625	1(3)	45341	1(2)	46280	1(2)
42808	2(3)	43212	1(3)	43330	1(2)	43800	1(2)	44188	1(3)	44626	1(3)	45342	1(2)	46285	1(3)
42809	1(3)	43213	1(2)	43331	1(2)	43810	1(2)	44202	1(2)	44640	2(3)	45346	1(2)	46288	1(3)
42810	1(3)	43214	1(3)	43332	1(2)	43820	1(2)	44203	2(3)	44650	2(3)	45347	1(3)	46320	2(3)
42815	1(3)	43215	1(3)	43333	1(2)	43825	1(2)	44204	2(3)	44660	1(3)	45349	1(3)	46500	1(2)
42820	1(2)	43216	1(2)	43334	1(2)	43830	1(2)	44205	1(2)	44661	1(3)	45350	1(3)	46505	1(2)
42821	1(2)	43217	1(2)	43335	1(2)	43831	1(2)	44206	1(2)	44680	1(3)	45378	1(3)	46600	1(3)
42825	1(2)	43220	1(3)	43336	1(2)	43832	1(2)	44207	1(2)	44700	1(2)	45379	1(3)	46601	1(3)
42826	1(2)	43226	1(3)	43337	1(2)	43840	2(3)	44208	1(2)	44701	1(2)	45380	1(2)	46604	1(2)
42830	1(2)	43227	1(3)	43338	1(2)	43843	1(2)	44210	1(2)	44705	1(3)	45381	1(2)	46606	1(2)
42831	1(2)	43229	1(3)	43340	1(2)	43845	1(2)	44211	1(2)	44715	1(2)	45382	1(3)	46607	1(2)
42835	1(2)	43231	1(2)	43341	1(2)	43846	1(2)	44212	1(2)	44720	2(3)	45384	1(2)	46608	1(3)
42836	1(2)	43232	1(2)	43351	1(2)	43847	1(2)	44213	1(2)	44721	2(3)	45385	1(2)	46610	1(2)
42842	1(3)	43233	1(3)	43352	1(2)	43848	1(2)	44227	1(3)	44800	1(3)	45386	1(2)	46611	1(2)
42844	1(3)	43235	1(3)	43360	1(2)	43850	1(2)	44300	1(3)	44820	1(3)	45388	1(2)	46612	1(2)
42845	1(3)	43236	1(2)	43361	1(2)	43855	1(2)	44310	2(3)	44850	1(3)	45389	1(3)	46614	1(3)
42860	1(3)	43237	1(2)	43400	1(2)	43860	1(2)	44312	1(2)	44900	1(2)	45390	1(3)	46615	1(3)
42870	1(3)	43238	1(2)	43401	1(2)	43865	1(2)	44314	1(2)	44950	1(2)	45391	1(2)	46700	1(2)
42890	1(3)	43239	1(2)	43405	1(2)	43870	1(2)	44316	1(2)	44955	1(2)	45392	1(2)	46705	1(2)
42892	1(3)	43240	1(2)	43410	1(3)	43880	1(3)	44320	1(2)	44960	1(2)	45393	1(3)	46706	1(3)
42894	1(3)	43241	1(3)	43415	1(3)	43881	1(3)	44322	1(2)	44970	1(2)	45395	1(2)	46707	1(3)
42900	1(3)	43242	1(2)	43420	1(3)	43882	1(3)	44340	1(2)	45000	1(3)	45397	1(2)	46710	1(3)
42950	1(2)	43243	1(2)	43425	1(3)	43886	1(2)	44345	1(2)	45005	1(3)	45398	1(2)	46712	1(3)
42953	1(3)	43244	1(2)	43450	1(3)	43887	1(2)	44346	1(2)	45020	1(3)	45400	1(2)	46715	1(3)
42955	1(2)	43245	1(2)	43453	1(3)	43888	1(2)	44360	1(3)	45100	2(3)	45402	1(2)	46716	1(2)
42960	1(3)	43246	1(2)	43460	1(3)	44005	1(2)	44361	1(2)	45108	1(2)	45500	1(2)	46730	1(2)
42961	1(3)	43247	1(2)	43496	1(3)	44010	1(2)	44363	1(3)	45110	1(2)	45505	1(2)	46735	1(2)
42962	1(3)	43248	1(3)	43500	1(2)	44015	1(2)	44364	1(2)	45111	1(2)	45520	1(2)	46740	1(2)
42970	1(3)	43249	1(3)	43501	1(3)	44020	2(3)	44365	1(2)	45112	1(2)	45540	1(2)	46742	1(2)
42971	1(3)	43250	1(2)	43502	1(2)	44021	1(3)	44366	1(3)	45113	1(2)	45541	1(2)	46744	1(2)
42972	1(3)	43251	1(2)	43510	1(2)	44025	1(3)	44369	1(2)	45114	1(2)	45550	1(2)	46746	1(2)

CPT	MUE	CPT	MUE	CPT	MUE	CPT	MUE	CPT	MUE	CPT	MUE	CPT	MUE	CPT	MUE
46748	1(2)	47540	2(1)	48556	1(2)	49520	1(2)	50323	1(2)	50686	2(3)	51555	1(2)	52276	1(2)
46750	1(2)	47541	1(3)	49000	1(2)	49521	1(2)	50325	1(2)	50688	2(3)	51565	1(2)	52277	1(2)
46751	1(2)	47542	2(3)	49002	1(3)	49525	1(2)	50327	1(3)	50690	2(3)	51570	1(2)	52281	1(2)
46753	1(2)	47543	1(3)	49010	1(3)	49540	1(2)	50328	1(3)	50693	2(3)	51575	1(2)	52282	1(2)
46754	1(3)	47544	1(3)	49020	2(3)	49550	1(2)	50329	1(3)	50694	2(3)	51580	1(2)	52283	1(2)
46760	1(2)	47550	1(3)	49040	2(3)	49553	1(2)	50340	1(2)	50695	2(3)	51585	1(2)	52285	1(2)
46761	1(2)	47552	1(3)	49060	2(3)	49555	1(2)	50360	1(2)	50700	1(2)	51590	1(2)	52287	1(2)
46762	1(2)	47553	1(2)	49062	1(3)	49557	1(2)	50365	1(2)	50705	2(3)	51595	1(2)	52290	1(2)
46900	1(2)	47554	1(3)	49082	1(3)	49560	2(3)	50370	1(2)	50706	2(3)	51596	1(2)	52300	1(2)
46910	1(2)	47555	1(2)	49083	2(3)	49561	2(3)	50380	1(2)	50715	1(2)	51597	1(2)	52301	1(2)
46916	1(2)	47556	1(2)	49084	1(3)	49565	2(3)	50382	1(3)	50722	1(2)	51600	1(3)	52305	1(2)
46917	1(2)	47562	1(2)	49180	2(3)	49566	2(3)	50384	1(3)	50725	1(3)	51605	1(3)	52310	1(3)
46922	1(2)	47563	1(2)	49185	2(3)	49568	2(3)	50385	1(3)	50727	1(3)	51610	1(3)	52315	2(3)
46924	1(2)	47564	1(2)	49203	1(2)	49570	1(3)	50386	1(3)	50728	1(3)	51700	1(3)	52317	1(3)
46930	1(2)	47570	1(2)	49204	1(2)	49572	1(3)	50387	1(3)	50740	1(2)	51701	2(3)	52318	1(3)
46940	1(2)	47600	1(2)	49205	1(2)	49580	1(2)	50389	1(3)	50750	1(2)	51702	2(3)	52320	1(2)
46942	1(3)	47605	1(2)	49215	1(2)	49582	1(2)	50390	2(3)	50760	1(2)	51703	2(3)	52325	1(3)
46945	1(2)	47610	1(2)	49220	1(2)	49585	1(2)	50391	1(3)	50770	1(2)	51705	1(3)	52327	1(2)
46946	1(2)	47612	1(2)	49250	1(2)	49587	1(2)	50395	1(2)	50780	1(2)	51710	1(3)	52330	1(2)
46947	1(2)	47620	1(2)	49255	1(2)	49590	1(2)	50396	1(3)	50782	1(2)	51715	1(2)	52332	1(2)
47000	3(3)	47700	1(2)	49320	1(3)	49600	1(2)	50400	1(2)	50783	1(2)	51720	1(3)	52334	1(2)
47001	3(3)	47701	1(2)	49321	1(2)	49605	1(2)	50405	1(2)	50785	1(2)	51725	1(3)	52341	1(2)
47010	3(3)	47711	1(2)	49322	1(2)	49606	1(2)	50430	2(3)	50800	1(2)	51726	1(3)	52342	1(2)
47015	1(2)	47712	1(2)	49323	1(2)	49610	1(2)	50431	2(3)	50810	1(3)	51727	1(3)	52343	1(2)
47100	3(3)	47715	1(2)	49324	1(2)	49611	1(2)	50432	2(3)	50815	1(2)	51728	1(3)	52344	1(2)
47120	2(3)	47720	1(2)	49325	1(2)	49650	1(2)	50433	2(3)	50820	1(2)	51729	1(3)	52345	1(2)
47122	1(2)	47721	1(2)	49326	1(2)	49651	1(2)	50434	2(3)	50825	1(3)	51736	1(3)	52346	1(2)
47125	1(2)	47740	1(2)	49327	1(2)	49652	2(3)	50435	2(3)	50830	1(3)	51741	1(3)	52351	1(3)
47130	1(2)	47741	1(2)	49400	1(3)	49653	2(3)	50500	1(3)	50840	1(2)	51784	1(3)	52352	1(2)
47133	1(2)	47760	1(2)	49402	1(3)	49654	2(3)	50520	1(3)	50845	1(2)	51785	1(3)	52353	1(2)
47135	1(2)	47765	1(2)	49405	2(3)	49655	2(3)	50525	1(3)	50860	1(2)	51792	1(3)	52354	1(3)
47140	1(2)	47780	1(2)	49406	2(3)	49656	2(3)	50526	1(3)	50900	1(3)	51797	1(3)	52355	1(3)
47141	1(2)	47785	1(2)	49407	1(3)	49657	2(3)	50540	1(2)	50920	2(3)	51798	1(3)	52356	1(2)
47142	1(2)	47800	1(2)	49411	1(2)	49900	1(3)	50541	1(2)	50930	2(3)	51800	1(2)	52400	1(2)
47143	1(2)	47801	1(3)	49412	1(2)	49904	1(3)	50542	1(2)	50940	1(2)	51820	1(2)	52402	1(2)
47144	1(2)	47802	1(2)	49418	1(3)	49905	1(3)	50543	1(2)	50945	1(2)	51840	1(2)	52441	1(2)
47145	1(2)	47900	1(2)	49419	1(2)	49906	1(3)	50544	1(2)	50947	1(2)	51841	1(2)	52442	5(1)
47146	3(3)	48000	1(2)	49421	1(2)	50010	1(2)	50545	1(2)	50948	1(2)	51845	1(2)	52450	1(2)
47147	2(3)	48001	1(2)	49422	1(2)	50020	1(3)	50546	1(2)	50951	1(3)	51860	1(3)	52500	1(2)
47300	2(3)	48020	1(3)	49423	2(3)	50040	1(2)	50547	1(2)	50953	1(3)	51865	1(3)	52601	1(2)
47350	1(3)	48100	1(3)	49424	3(3)	50045	1(2)	50548	1(2)	50955	1(2)	51880	1(2)	52630	1(2)
47360	1(3)	48102	1(3)	49425	1(2)	50060	1(2)	50551	1(3)	50957	1(2)	51900	1(3)	52640	1(2)
47361	1(3)	48105	1(2)	49426	1(3)	50065	1(2)	50553	1(3)	50961	1(2)	51920	1(3)	52647	1(2)
47362	1(3)	48120	1(3)	49427	1(3)	50070	1(2)	50555	1(2)	50970	1(3)	51925	1(2)	52648	1(2)
47370	1(2)	48140	1(2)	49428	1(2)	50075	1(2)	50557	1(2)	50972	1(3)	51940	1(2)	52649	1(2)
47371	1(2)	48145	1(2)	49429	1(2)	50080	1(2)	50561	1(2)	50974	1(2)	51960	1(2)	52700	1(3)
47380	1(2)	48146	1(2)	49435	1(2)	50081	1(2)	50562	1(3)	50976	1(2)	51980	1(2)	53000	1(2)
47381	1(2)	48148	1(2)	49436	1(3)	50100	1(2)	50570	1(3)	50980	1(2)	51990	1(2)	53010	1(2)
47382	1(2)	48150	1(2)	49440	1(3)	50120	1(2)	50572	1(3)	51020	1(2)	51992	1(2)	53020	1(2)
47383	1(2)	48152	1(2)	49441	1(3)	50125	1(2)	50574	1(2)	51030	1(2)	52000	1(3)	53025	1(2)
47400	1(3)	48153	1(2)	49442	1(3)	50130	1(2)	50575	1(2)	51040	1(3)	52001	1(3)	53040	1(3)
47420	1(2)	48154	1(2)	49446	1(2)	50135	1(2)	50576	1(2)	51045	2(3)	52005	2(3)	53060	1(3)
47425	1(2)	48155	1(2)	49450	1(3)	50200	1(3)	50580	1(2)	51050	1(3)	52007	1(2)	53080	1(3)
47460	1(2)	48400	1(3)	49451	1(3)	50205	1(3)	50590	1(2)	51060	1(3)	52010	1(2)	53085	1(3)
47480	1(2)	48500	1(3)	49452	1(3)	50220	1(2)	50592	1(2)	51065	1(3)	52204	1(2)	53200	1(3)
47490	1(2)	48510	1(3)	49460	1(3)	50225	1(2)	50593	1(2)	51080	1(3)	52214	1(2)	53210	1(2)
47531	2(3)	48520	1(3)	49465	1(3)	50230	1(2)	50600	1(3)	51100	1(3)	52224	1(2)	53215	1(2)
47532	1(3)	48540	1(3)	49491	1(2)	50234	1(2)	50605	1(3)	51101	1(3)	52234	1(2)	53220	1(3)
47533	1(3)	48545	1(3)	49492	1(2)	50236	1(2)	50606	2(3)	51102	1(3)	52235	1(2)	53230	1(3)
47534	1(3)	48547	1(2)	49495	1(2)	50240	1(2)	50610	1(2)	51500	1(2)	52240	1(2)	53235	1(3)
47535	1(3)	48548	1(2)	49496	1(2)	50250	1(2)	50620	1(2)	51520	1(2)	52250	1(2)	53240	1(3)
47536	1(3)	48550	1(2)	49500	1(2)	50280	1(2)	50630	1(2)	51525	1(2)	52260	1(2)	53250	1(3)
47537	1(3)	48551	1(2)	49501	1(2)	50290	1(3)	50650	1(2)	51530	1(2)	52265	1(2)	53260	1(2)
47538	2(1)	48552	2(3)	49505	1(2)	50300	1(2)	50660	1(3)	51535	1(2)	52270	1(2)	53265	1(3)
47539	2(1)	48554	1(2)	49507	1(2)	50320	1(2)	50684	1(3)	51550	1(2)	52275	1(2)	53270	1(2)

CPT	MUE	CPT	MUE	CPT	MUE	CPT	MUE	CPT	MUE	CPT	MUE	CPT	MUE	CPT	MUE
53275	1(2)	54230	1(3)	54861	1(2)	56632	1(2)	57320	1(3)	58345	1(3)	58956	1(2)	59866	1(2)
53400	1(2)	54231	1(3)	54865	1(3)	56633	1(2)	57330	1(3)	58346	1(2)	58957	1(2)	59870	1(2)
53405	1(2)	54235	1(3)	54900	1(2)	56634	1(2)	57335	1(2)	58350	1(2)	58958	1(2)	59871	1(2)
53410	1(2)	54240	1(2)	54901	1(2)	56637	1(2)	57400	1(2)	58353	1(3)	58960	1(2)	60000	1(3)
53415	1(2)	54250	1(3)	55000	1(3)	56640	1(2)	57410	1(2)	58356	1(3)	58970	1(3)	60100	3(3)
53420	1(2)	54300	1(2)	55040	1(2)	56700	1(2)	57415	1(3)	58400	1(3)	58974	1(3)	60200	2(3)
53425	1(2)	54304	1(2)	55041	1(2)	56740	1(3)	57420	1(3)	58410	1(3)	58976	2(3)	60210	1(2)
53430	1(2)	54308	1(2)	55060	1(2)	56800	1(2)	57421	1(3)	58520	1(2)	59000	1(3)	60212	1(2)
53431	1(2)	54312	1(2)	55100	2(3)	56805	1(2)	57423	1(2)	58540	1(2)	59001	1(3)	60220	1(3)
53440	1(2)	54316	1(2)	55110	1(2)	56810	1(2)	57425	1(2)	58541	1(3)	59012	1(3)	60225	1(2)
53442	1(2)	54318	1(2)	55120	1(3)	56820	1(2)	57426	1(2)	58542	1(3)	59015	1(3)	60240	1(2)
53444	1(3)	54322	1(2)	55150	1(2)	56821	1(2)	57452	1(3)	58543	1(3)	59020	2(3)	60252	1(2)
53445	1(2)	54324	1(2)	55175	1(2)	57000	1(3)	57454	1(3)	58544	1(2)	59025	3(3)	60254	1(2)
53446	1(2)	54326	1(2)	55180	1(2)	57010	1(3)	57455	1(3)	58545	1(2)	59030	4(3)	60260	1(2)
53447	1(2)	54328	1(2)	55200	1(2)	57020	1(3)	57456	1(3)	58546	1(2)	59050	1(3)	60270	1(2)
53448	1(2)	54332	1(2)	55250	1(2)	57022	1(3)	57460	1(3)	58548	1(2)	59051	1(3)	60271	1(2)
53449	1(2)	54336	1(2)	55300	1(2)	57023	1(3)	57461	1(3)	58550	1(3)	59070	2(3)	60280	1(3)
53450	1(2)	54340	1(2)	55400	1(2)	57061	1(2)	57500	1(3)	58552	1(3)	59072	2(3)	60281	1(3)
53460	1(2)	54344	1(2)	55450	1(2)	57065	1(2)	57505	1(3)	58553	1(3)	59074	1(3)	60300	2(3)
53500	1(2)	54348	1(2)	55500	1(2)	57100	3(3)	57510	1(3)	58554	1(2)	59076	1(3)	60500	1(2)
53502	1(3)	54352	1(2)	55520	1(2)	57105	2(3)	57511	1(3)	58555	1(3)	59100	1(2)	60502	1(3)
53505	1(3)	54360	1(2)	55530	1(2)	57106	1(2)	57513	1(3)	58558	1(3)	59120	1(3)	60505	1(3)
53510	1(3)	54380	1(2)	55535	1(2)	57107	1(2)	57520	1(3)	58559	1(3)	59121	1(3)	60512	1(3)
53515	1(3)	54385	1(2)	55540	1(2)	57109	1(2)	57522	1(3)	58560	1(3)	59130	1(3)	60520	1(2)
53520	1(3)	54390	1(2)	55550	1(2)	57110	1(2)	57530	1(3)	58561	1(3)	59135	1(3)	60521	1(2)
53600	1(3)	54400	1(2)	55600	1(2)	57111	1(2)	57531	1(2)	58562	1(3)	59136	1(3)	60522	1(3)
53601	1(3)	54401	1(2)	55605	1(2)	57112	1(2)	57540	1(2)	58563	1(3)	59140	1(2)	60540	1(2)
53605	1(3)	54405	1(2)	55650	1(2)	57120	1(2)	57545	1(3)	58565	1(2)	59150	1(3)	60545	1(2)
53620	1(2)	54406	1(2)	55680	1(3)	57130	1(2)	57550	1(3)	58570	1(3)	59151	1(3)	60600	1(3)
53621	1(3)	54408	1(2)	55700	1(2)	57135	2(3)	57555	1(2)	58571	1(2)	59160	1(2)	60605	1(3)
53660	1(2)	54410	1(2)	55705	1(2)	57150	1(3)	57556	1(2)	58572	1(3)	59200	1(3)	60650	1(2)
53661	1(3)	54411	1(2)	55706	1(2)	57155	1(3)	57558	1(3)	58573	1(2)	59300	1(2)	61000	1(2)
53665	1(3)	54415	1(2)	55720	1(3)	57156	1(3)	57700	1(3)	58600	1(2)	59320	1(2)	61001	1(2)
53850	1(2)	54416	1(2)	55725	1(3)	57160	1(2)	57720	1(3)	58605	1(2)	59325	1(2)	61020	2(3)
53852	1(2)	54417	1(2)	55801	1(2)	57170	1(2)	57800	1(3)	58611	1(2)	59350	1(2)	61026	2(3)
53855	1(2)	54420	1(2)	55810	1(2)	57180	1(3)	58100	1(3)	58615	1(2)	59400	1(2)	61050	1(3)
53860	1(2)	54430	1(2)	55812	1(2)	57200	1(3)	58110	1(3)	58660	1(2)	59409	2(3)	61055	1(3)
54000	1(2)	54435	1(2)	55815	1(2)	57210	1(3)	58120	1(3)	58661	1(2)	59410	1(2)	61070	2(3)
54001	1(2)	54437	1(2)	55821	1(2)	57220	1(2)	58140	1(3)	58662	1(2)	59412	1(3)	61105	1(3)
54015	1(3)	54438	1(2)	55831	1(2)	57230	1(2)	58145	1(3)	58670	1(2)	59414	1(3)	61107	1(3)
54050	1(2)	54440	1(2)	55840	1(2)	57240	1(2)	58146	1(3)	58671	1(2)	59425	1(2)	61108	1(3)
54055	1(2)	54450	1(2)	55842	1(2)	57250	1(2)	58150	1(3)	58672	1(2)	59426	1(2)	61120	1(3)
54056	1(2)	54500	1(3)	55845	1(2)	57260	1(2)	58152	1(2)	58673	1(2)	59430	1(2)	61140	1(3)
54057	1(2)	54505	1(3)	55860	1(2)	57265	1(2)	58180	1(3)	58700	1(2)	59510	1(2)	61150	1(3)
54060	1(2)	54512	1(3)	55862	1(2)	57267	2(3)	58200	1(2)	58720	1(2)	59514	1(3)	61151	1(3)
54065	1(2)	54520	1(2)	55865	1(2)	57268	1(2)	58210	1(2)	58740	1(2)	59515	1(2)	61154	1(3)
54100	2(3)	54522	1(2)	55866	1(2)	57270	1(2)	58240	1(2)	58750	1(2)	59525	1(2)	61156	1(3)
54105	2(3)	54530	1(2)	55870	1(2)	57280	1(2)	58260	1(3)	58752	1(2)	59610	1(2)	61210	1(3)
54110	1(2)	54535	1(2)	55873	1(2)	57282	1(2)	58262	1(3)	58760	1(2)	59612	2(3)	61215	1(3)
54111	1(2)	54550	1(2)	55875	1(2)	57283	1(2)	58263	1(2)	58770	1(2)	59614	1(2)	61250	1(3)
54112	1(3)	54560	1(2)	55876	1(2)	57284	1(2)	58267	1(2)	58800	1(2)	59618	1(2)	61253	1(3)
54115	1(3)	54600	1(2)	55920	1(2)	57285	1(2)	58270	1(2)	58805	1(2)	59620	1(2)	61304	1(3)
54120	1(2)	54620	1(2)	56405	2(3)	57287	1(2)	58275	1(2)	58820	1(3)	59622	1(2)	61305	1(3)
54125	1(2)	54640	1(2)	56420	1(3)	57288	1(2)	58280	1(2)	58822	1(3)	59812	1(2)	61312	2(3)
54130	1(2)	54650	1(2)	56440	1(3)	57289	1(2)	58285	1(3)	58825	1(2)	59820	1(2)	61313	2(3)
54135	1(2)	54660	1(2)	56441	1(2)	57291	1(2)	58290	1(3)	58900	1(2)	59821	1(2)	61314	2(3)
54150	1(2)	54670	1(3)	56442	1(2)	57292	1(2)	58291	1(2)	58920	1(2)	59830	1(2)	61315	1(3)
54160	1(2)	54680	1(2)	56501	1(2)	57295	1(2)	58292	1(2)	58925	1(3)	59840	1(2)	61316	1(3)
54161	1(2)	54690	1(2)	56515	1(2)	57296	1(2)	58293	1(2)	58940	1(2)	59841	1(2)	61320	2(3)
54162	1(2)	54692	1(2)	56605	1(2)	57300	1(3)	58294	1(2)	58943	1(2)	59850	1(2)	61321	1(3)
54163	1(2)	54700	1(3)	56606	6(3)	57305	1(3)	58301	1(3)	58950	1(2)	59851	1(2)	61322	1(3)
54164	1(2)	54800	1(2)	56620	1(2)	57307	1(3)	58321	1(2)	58951	1(2)	59852	1(2)	61323	1(3)
54200	1(2)	54830	1(2)	56625	1(2)	57308	1(3)	58322	1(2)	58952	1(2)	59855	1(2)	61330	1(2)
54205	1(2)	54840	1(2)	56630	1(2)	57310	1(3)	58323	1(3)	58953	1(2)	59856	1(2)	61332	1(2)
54220	1(3)	54860	1(2)	56631	1(2)	57311	1(3)	58340	1(3)	58954	1(2)	59857	1(2)	61333	1(2)

CPT	MUE	CPT	MUE	CPT	MUE	CPT	MUE	CPT	MUE	CPT	MUE	CPT	MUE
61340	1(2)	61600	1(3)	62005	1(3)	62365	1(2)	63266	1(3)	64425	1(3)	64643	3(2)	64858	1(2)
61343	1(2)	61601	1(3)	62010	1(3)	62367	1(3)	63267	1(3)	64430	1(3)	64644	1(2)	64859	2(3)
61345	1(3)	61605	1(3)	62100	1(3)	62368	1(3)	63268	1(3)	64435	1(3)	64645	3(2)	64861	1(2)
61450	1(3)	61606	1(3)	62115	1(2)	62369	1(3)	63270	1(3)	64445	1(3)	64646	1(2)	64862	1(2)
61458	1(2)	61607	1(3)	62117	1(2)	62370	1(3)	63271	1(3)	64446	1(2)	64647	1(2)	64864	2(3)
61460	1(2)	61608	1(3)	62120	1(2)	63001	1(2)	63272	1(3)	64447	1(3)	64650	1(2)	64865	1(3)
61480	1(2)	61610	1(3)	62121	1(2)	63003	1(2)	63273	1(3)	64448	1(2)	64653	1(2)	64866	1(3)
61500	1(3)	61611	1(3)	62140	1(3)	63005	1(2)	63275	1(3)	64449	1(2)	64680	1(2)	64868	1(3)
61501	1(3)	61612	1(3)	62141	1(3)	63011	1(2)	63276	1(3)	64450	10(3)	64681	1(2)	64872	1(3)
61510	1(3)	61613	1(3)	62142	2(3)	63012	1(2)	63277	1(3)	64455	1(2)	64702	2(3)	64874	1(3)
61512	1(3)	61615	1(3)	62143	2(3)	63015	1(2)	63278	1(3)	64461	1(2)	64704	4(3)	64876	1(3)
61514	2(3)	61616	1(3)	62145	2(3)	63016	1(2)	63280	1(3)	64462	1(2)	64708	3(3)	64885	1(3)
61516	1(3)	61618	2(3)	62146	2(3)	63017	1(2)	63281	1(3)	64463	1(3)	64712	1(2)	64886	1(3)
61517	1(3)	61619	2(3)	62147	1(3)	63020	1(2)	63282	1(3)	64479	1(2)	64713	1(2)	64890	2(3)
61518	1(3)	61623	2(3)	62148	1(3)	63030	1(2)	63283	1(3)	64480	4(3)	64714	1(2)	64891	2(3)
61519	1(3)	61624	2(3)	62160	1(3)	63035	4(3)	63285	1(3)	64483	1(2)	64716	2(3)	64892	2(3)
61520	1(3)	61626	2(3)	62161	1(3)	63040	1(2)	63286	1(3)	64484	4(3)	64718	1(2)	64893	2(3)
61521	1(3)	61630	1(3)	62162	1(3)	63042	1(2)	63287	1(3)	64486	1(3)	64719	1(2)	64895	2(3)
61522	1(3)	61635	2(3)	62163	1(3)	63043	4(3)	63290	1(3)	64487	1(2)	64721	1(2)	64896	2(3)
61524	2(3)	61645	3(2)	62164	1(3)	63044	4(2)	63295	1(2)	64488	1(3)	64722	4(3)	64897	2(3)
61526	1(3)	61650	1(2)	62165	1(2)	63045	1(2)	63300	1(2)	64489	1(2)	64726	2(3)	64898	2(3)
61530	1(3)	61651	2(2)	62180	1(3)	63046	1(2)	63301	1(2)	64490	1(2)	64727	2(3)	64901	2(3)
61531	1(2)	61680	1(3)	62190	1(3)	63047	1(2)	63302	1(2)	64491	1(2)	64732	1(2)	64902	1(3)
61533	2(3)	61682	1(3)	62192	1(3)	63048	5(3)	63303	1(2)	64492	1(2)	64734	1(2)	64905	1(3)
61534	1(3)	61684	1(3)	62194	1(3)	63050	1(2)	63304	1(2)	64493	1(2)	64736	1(2)	64907	1(3)
61535	2(3)	61686	1(3)	62200	1(2)	63051	1(2)	63305	1(2)	64494	1(2)	64738	1(2)	64910	3(3)
61536	1(3)	61690	1(3)	62201	1(2)	63055	1(2)	63306	1(2)	64495	1(2)	64740	1(2)	64911	2(3)
61537	1(3)	61692	1(3)	62220	1(3)	63056	1(2)	63307	1(2)	64505	1(3)	64742	1(2)	65091	1(2)
61538	1(2)	61697	2(3)	62223	1(3)	63057	3(3)	63308	3(3)	64508	1(3)	64744	1(2)	65093	1(2)
61539	1(3)	61698	1(3)	62225	2(3)	63064	1(2)	63600	2(3)	64510	1(3)	64746	1(2)	65101	1(2)
61540	1(3)	61700	2(3)	62230	2(3)	63066	1(3)	63610	1(3)	64517	1(3)	64755	1(2)	65103	1(2)
61541	1(2)	61702	1(3)	62252	2(3)	63075	1(2)	63615	1(3)	64520	1(3)	64760	1(2)	65105	1(2)
61543	1(2)	61703	1(3)	62256	1(3)	63076	3(3)	63620	1(2)	64530	1(3)	64763	1(2)	65110	1(2)
61544	1(3)	61705	1(3)	62258	1(3)	63077	1(2)	63621	2(2)	64550	1(3)	64766	1(2)	65112	1(2)
61545	1(2)	61708	1(3)	62263	1(2)	63078	3(3)	63650	2(3)	64553	1(3)	64771	2(3)	65114	1(2)
61546	1(2)	61710	1(3)	62264	1(2)	63081	1(2)	63655	1(3)	64555	2(3)	64772	2(3)	65125	1(2)
61548	1(2)	61711	1(3)	62267	2(3)	63082	6(2)	63661	1(2)	64561	1(3)	64774	2(3)	65130	1(2)
61550	1(2)	61720	1(3)	62268	1(3)	63085	1(2)	63662	1(2)	64565	2(3)	64776	1(2)	65135	1(2)
61552	1(2)	61735	1(3)	62269	2(3)	63086	2(3)	63663	1(3)	64566	1(3)	64778	1(3)	65140	1(2)
61556	1(3)	61750	2(3)	62270	2(3)	63087	1(2)	63664	1(3)	64568	1(3)	64782	2(2)	65150	1(2)
61557	1(2)	61751	2(3)	62272	1(3)	63088	4(3)	63685	1(3)	64569	1(3)	64783	2(3)	65155	1(2)
61558	1(3)	61760	1(2)	62273	2(3)	63090	1(2)	63688	1(3)	64570	1(3)	64784	3(3)	65175	1(2)
61559	1(3)	61770	1(2)	62280	1(3)	63091	3(3)	63700	1(3)	64575	2(3)	64786	1(3)	65205	1(3)
61563	2(3)	61781	1(3)	62281	1(3)	63101	1(2)	63702	1(3)	64580	2(3)	64787	4(3)	65210	1(3)
61564	1(2)	61782	1(3)	62282	1(3)	63102	1(2)	63704	1(3)	64581	2(3)	64788	5(3)	65220	1(3)
61566	1(3)	61783	1(3)	62284	1(3)	63103	3(3)	63706	1(3)	64585	2(3)	64790	1(3)	65222	1(3)
61567	1(2)	61790	1(2)	62287	1(2)	63170	1(3)	63707	1(3)	64590	1(3)	64792	2(3)	65235	1(3)
61570	1(3)	61791	1(2)	62290	5(2)	63172	1(3)	63709	1(3)	64595	1(3)	64795	2(3)	65260	1(3)
61571	1(3)	61796	1(2)	62291	4(3)	63173	1(3)	63710	1(3)	64600	2(3)	64802	1(2)	65265	1(3)
61575	1(2)	61797	4(3)	62292	1(2)	63180	1(2)	63740	1(3)	64605	1(2)	64804	1(2)	65270	1(3)
61576	1(2)	61798	1(2)	62294	1(3)	63182	1(2)	63741	1(3)	64610	1(2)	64809	1(2)	65272	1(3)
61580	1(2)	61799	4(3)	62302	1(3)	63185	1(2)	63744	1(3)	64611	1(2)	64818	1(2)	65273	1(3)
61581	1(2)	61800	1(2)	62303	1(3)	63190	1(2)	63746	1(2)	64612	1(2)	64820	4(3)	65275	1(3)
61582	1(2)	61850	1(3)	62304	1(3)	63191	1(2)	64400	4(3)	64615	1(2)	64821	1(2)	65280	1(3)
61583	1(2)	61860	1(3)	62305	1(3)	63194	1(2)	64402	1(3)	64616	1(2)	64822	1(2)	65285	1(3)
61584	1(2)	61863	1(2)	62310	1(3)	63195	1(2)	64405	1(3)	64617	1(2)	64823	1(2)	65286	1(3)
61585	1(3)	61864	1(3)	62311	1(3)	63196	1(2)	64408	1(3)	64620	5(3)	64831	1(2)	65290	1(3)
61586	1(3)	61867	1(2)	62318	1(3)	63197	1(2)	64410	1(3)	64630	1(3)	64832	3(3)	65400	1(3)
61590	1(2)	61868	2(3)	62319	1(3)	63198	1(2)	64413	1(3)	64632	1(2)	64834	1(2)	65410	1(3)
61591	1(2)	61870	1(3)	62350	1(3)	63199	1(2)	64415	1(3)	64633	1(2)	64835	1(2)	65420	1(2)
61592	1(2)	61880	1(2)	62351	1(3)	63200	1(2)	64416	1(2)	64634	4(3)	64836	1(2)	65426	1(2)
61595	1(2)	61885	2(3)	62355	1(3)	63250	1(3)	64417	1(3)	64635	1(2)	64837	2(3)	65430	1(2)
61596	1(2)	61886	1(3)	62360	1(2)	63251	1(3)	64418	1(3)	64636	4(2)	64840	1(2)	65435	1(2)
61597	1(2)	61888	1(3)	62361	1(2)	63252	1(3)	64420	3(3)	64640	5(3)	64856	2(3)	65436	1(2)
61598	1(3)	62000	1(3)	62362	1(2)	63265	1(3)	64421	3(3)	64642	1(2)	64857	2(3)	65450	1(3)

CPT	MUE	CPT	MUE	CPT	MUE	CPT	MUE	CPT	MUE	CPT	MUE	CPT	MUE	CPT	MUE
65600	1(2)	66820	1(2)	67346	1(3)	68100	1(3)	69433	1(2)	70010	1(3)	71015	2(3)	72198	1(3)
65710	1(2)	66821	1(2)	67400	1(2)	68110	1(3)	69436	1(2)	70015	1(3)	71020	4(3)	72200	2(3)
65730	1(2)	66825	1(2)	67405	1(2)	68115	1(3)	69440	1(2)	70030	2(2)	71021	1(3)	72202	1(3)
65750	1(2)	66830	1(2)	67412	1(2)	68130	1(3)	69450	1(2)	70100	2(3)	71022	1(3)	72220	1(3)
65755	1(2)	66840	1(2)	67413	1(2)	68135	1(3)	69501	1(3)	70110	2(3)	71023	1(3)	72240	1(2)
65756	1(2)	66850	1(2)	67414	1(2)	68200	1(3)	69502	1(2)	70120	1(3)	71030	1(3)	72255	1(2)
65757	1(3)	66852	1(2)	67415	1(3)	68320	1(2)	69505	1(2)	70130	1(3)	71034	1(3)	72265	1(2)
65770	1(2)	66920	1(2)	67420	1(2)	68325	1(2)	69511	1(2)	70134	1(3)	71035	3(3)	72270	1(2)
65772	1(2)	66930	1(2)	67430	1(2)	68326	2(2)	69530	1(2)	70140	2(3)	71100	2(3)	72275	3(3)
65775	1(2)	66940	1(2)	67440	1(2)	68328	2(2)	69535	1(2)	70150	1(3)	71101	2(3)	72285	4(3)
65778	1(2)	66982	1(2)	67445	1(2)	68330	1(3)	69540	1(3)	70160	1(3)	71110	1(3)	72295	5(3)
65779	1(2)	66983	1(2)	67450	1(2)	68335	1(3)	69550	1(3)	70170	2(2)	71111	1(3)	73000	2(3)
65780	1(2)	66984	1(2)	67500	1(3)	68340	1(3)	69552	1(2)	70190	1(2)	71120	1(3)	73010	2(3)
65781	1(2)	66985	1(2)	67505	1(3)	68360	1(3)	69554	1(2)	70200	2(3)	71130	1(3)	73020	2(3)
65782	1(2)	66986	1(2)	67515	1(3)	68362	1(3)	69601	1(2)	70210	1(3)	71250	2(3)	73030	4(3)
65785	2(2)	66990	1(3)	67550	1(2)	68371	1(3)	69602	1(2)	70220	1(3)	71260	2(3)	73040	2(2)
65800	1(2)	67005	1(2)	67560	1(2)	68400	1(2)	69603	1(2)	70240	1(2)	71270	1(3)	73050	1(3)
65810	1(2)	67010	1(2)	67570	1(2)	68420	1(2)	69604	1(2)	70250	2(3)	71275	1(3)	73060	2(3)
65815	1(3)	67015	1(2)	67700	2(3)	68440	2(2)	69605	1(2)	70260	1(3)	71550	1(3)	73070	2(3)
65820	1(2)	67025	1(2)	67710	1(2)	68500	1(2)	69610	1(2)	70300	1(3)	71551	1(3)	73080	2(3)
65850	1(2)	67027	1(2)	67715	1(3)	68505	1(2)	69620	1(2)	70310	1(3)	71552	1(3)	73085	2(2)
65855	1(2)	67028	1(3)	67800	1(2)	68510	1(2)	69631	1(2)	70320	1(3)	71555	1(3)	73090	2(3)
65860	1(2)	67030	1(2)	67801	1(2)	68520	1(2)	69632	1(3)	70328	1(3)	72020	4(3)	73092	2(3)
65865	1(2)	67031	1(2)	67805	1(2)	68525	1(2)	69633	1(2)	70330	1(3)	72040	3(3)	73100	2(3)
65870	1(2)	67036	1(2)	67808	1(2)	68530	1(2)	69635	1(3)	70332	2(3)	72050	1(3)	73110	3(3)
65875	1(2)	67039	1(2)	67810	2(3)	68540	1(2)	69636	1(3)	70336	1(3)	72052	1(3)	73115	2(2)
65880	1(2)	67040	1(2)	67820	1(2)	68550	1(2)	69637	1(3)	70350	1(3)	72070	1(3)	73120	3(3)
65900	1(3)	67041	1(2)	67825	1(2)	68700	1(2)	69641	1(2)	70355	1(3)	72072	1(3)	73130	3(3)
65920	1(2)	67042	1(2)	67830	1(2)	68705	2(2)	69642	1(2)	70360	2(3)	72074	1(3)	73140	3(3)
65930	1(3)	67043	1(2)	67835	1(2)	68720	1(2)	69643	1(2)	70370	1(3)	72080	1(3)	73200	2(3)
66020	1(3)	67101	1(2)	67840	4(3)	68745	1(2)	69644	1(2)	70371	1(2)	72081	1(3)	73201	2(3)
66030	1(3)	67105	1(2)	67850	3(3)	68750	1(2)	69645	1(2)	70380	2(3)	72082	1(3)	73202	2(3)
66130	1(3)	67107	1(2)	67875	1(2)	68760	4(2)	69646	1(2)	70390	2(3)	72083	1(3)	73206	2(3)
66150	1(2)	67108	1(2)	67880	1(2)	68761	4(2)	69650	1(2)	70450	3(3)	72084	1(3)	73218	2(3)
66155	1(2)	67110	1(2)	67882	1(2)	68770	1(3)	69660	1(2)	70460	1(3)	72100	2(3)	73219	2(3)
66160	1(2)	67113	1(2)	67900	1(2)	68801	4(2)	69661	1(2)	70470	2(3)	72110	1(3)	73220	2(3)
66170	1(2)	67115	1(1)	67901	1(2)	68810	1(2)	69662	1(2)	70480	1(3)	72114	1(3)	73221	2(3)
66172	1(2)	67120	1(2)	67902	1(2)	68811	1(2)	69666	1(2)	70481	1(3)	72120	1(3)	73222	2(3)
66174	1(2)	67121	1(2)	67903	1(2)	68815	1(2)	69667	1(2)	70482	1(3)	72125	1(3)	73223	2(3)
66175	1(2)	67141	1(2)	67904	1(2)	68816	1(2)	69670	1(2)	70486	1(3)	72126	1(3)	73501	2(3)
66179	1(2)	67145	1(2)	67906	1(2)	68840	1(2)	69676	1(2)	70487	1(3)	72127	1(3)	73502	2(3)
66180	1(2)	67208	1(2)	67908	1(2)	68850	1(3)	69700	1(3)	70488	1(3)	72128	1(3)	73503	2(3)
66183	1(3)	67210	1(2)	67909	1(2)	69000	1(3)	69711	1(2)	70490	1(3)	72129	1(3)	73521	2(3)
66184	1(2)	67218	1(2)	67911	4(2)	69005	1(3)	69714	1(2)	70491	1(3)	72130	1(3)	73522	2(3)
66185	1(3)	67220	1(2)	67912	1(2)	69020	1(3)	69715	1(3)	70492	1(3)	72131	1(3)	73523	2(3)
66220	1(2)	67221	1(2)	67914	1(3)	69100	3(3)	69717	1(2)	70496	2(3)	72132	1(3)	73525	2(2)
66225	1(2)	67225	1(2)	67915	1(3)	69105	1(3)	69718	1(2)	70498	2(3)	72133	1(3)	73551	2(3)
66250	1(2)	67227	1(2)	67916	1(3)	69110	1(2)	69720	1(2)	70540	1(3)	72141	1(3)	73552	2(3)
66500	1(2)	67228	1(2)	67917	1(3)	69120	1(3)	69725	1(2)	70542	1(3)	72142	1(3)	73560	4(3)
66505	1(2)	67229	1(2)	67921	1(3)	69140	1(2)	69740	1(2)	70543	1(3)	72146	1(3)	73562	4(3)
66600	1(2)	67250	1(2)	67922	1(3)	69145	1(3)	69745	1(2)	70544	2(3)	72147	1(3)	73564	4(3)
66605	1(2)	67255	1(2)	67923	1(3)	69150	1(3)	69801	1(3)	70545	1(3)	72148	1(3)	73565	1(3)
66625	1(2)	67311	1(2)	67924	1(3)	69155	1(3)	69805	1(3)	70546	1(3)	72149	1(3)	73580	2(2)
66630	1(2)	67312	1(2)	67930	2(3)	69200	1(2)	69806	1(3)	70547	1(3)	72156	1(3)	73590	3(3)
66635	1(2)	67314	1(2)	67935	2(3)	69205	1(3)	69820	1(2)	70548	1(3)	72157	1(3)	73592	2(3)
66680	1(2)	67316	1(2)	67938	2(3)	69209	2(2)	69840	1(3)	70549	1(3)	72158	1(3)	73600	3(3)
66682	1(2)	67318	1(2)	67950	2(2)	69210	1(2)	69905	1(2)	70551	2(3)	72170	2(3)	73610	3(3)
66700	1(2)	67320	2(3)	67961	4(2)	69220	1(2)	69910	1(2)	70552	2(3)	72190	1(3)	73615	2(2)
66710	1(2)	67331	1(2)	67966	4(2)	69222	1(2)	69915	1(3)	70553	2(3)	72191	1(3)	73620	3(3)
66711	1(2)	67332	1(2)	67971	1(3)	69300	1(2)	69930	1(2)	70554	1(3)	72192	1(3)	73630	3(3)
66720	1(2)	67334	1(2)	67973	1(3)	69310	1(2)	69950	1(2)	70555	1(3)	72193	1(3)	73650	2(3)
66740	1(2)	67335	1(2)	67974	1(3)	69320	1(2)	69955	1(2)	70557	1(3)	72194	1(3)	73660	2(3)
66761	1(2)	67340	2(2)	67975	1(3)	69420	1(2)	69960	1(2)	70558	1(3)	72195	1(3)	73700	2(3)
66762	1(2)	67343	1(2)	68020	1(3)	69421	1(2)	69970	1(3)	70559	1(3)	72196	1(3)	73701	2(3)
66770	1(3)	67345	1(3)	68040	1(2)	69424	1(2)	69990	1(3)	71010	6(3)	72197	1(3)	73702	2(3)

CPT	MUE	CPT	MUE	CPT	MUE	CPT	MUE	CPT	MUE	CPT	MUE	CPT	MUE	CPT	MUE
73706	2(3)	74710	1(3)	75957	1(2)	76857	1(3)	77306	1(3)	78104	1(2)	78496	1(3)	80159	2(3)
73718	2(3)	74712	1(3)	75958	2(3)	76870	1(2)	77307	1(3)	78110	1(2)	78579	1(3)	80162	2(3)
73719	2(3)	74713	2(3)	75959	1(2)	76872	1(3)	77316	1(3)	78111	1(2)	78580	1(3)	80163	2(3)
73720	2(3)	74740	1(3)	75962	1(1)	76873	1(2)	77317	1(3)	78120	1(2)	78582	1(3)	80164	2(3)
73721	3(3)	74742	2(2)	75964	2(3)	76881	2(3)	77318	1(3)	78121	1(2)	78597	1(3)	80165	2(3)
73722	2(3)	74775	1(2)	75966	1(1)	76882	2(3)	77321	1(2)	78122	1(2)	78598	1(3)	80168	2(3)
73723	2(3)	75557	1(3)	75968	2(3)	76885	1(2)	77331	3(3)	78130	1(2)	78600	1(3)	80169	1(3)
73725	2(3)	75559	1(3)	75970	1(3)	76886	1(2)	77332	4(3)	78135	1(3)	78601	1(3)	80170	2(3)
74000	4(3)	75561	1(3)	75978	3(3)	76930	1(3)	77333	2(3)	78140	1(3)	78605	1(3)	80171	1(3)
74010	2(3)	75563	1(3)	75984	2(3)	76932	1(2)	77334	10(3)	78185	1(2)	78606	1(3)	80173	2(3)
74020	2(3)	75565	1(3)	75989	2(3)	76936	1(3)	77336	1(2)	78190	1(2)	78607	1(3)	80175	1(3)
74022	2(3)	75571	1(3)	76000	3(3)	76937	2(3)	77338	1(3)	78191	1(2)	78608	1(3)	80176	1(3)
74150	1(3)	75572	1(3)	76001	1(3)	76940	1(3)	77370	1(3)	78195	1(2)	78610	1(3)	80177	1(3)
74160	1(3)	75573	1(3)	76010	2(3)	76941	3(3)	77371	1(2)	78201	1(3)	78630	1(3)	80178	2(3)
74170	1(3)	75574	1(3)	76080	3(3)	76942	1(3)	77372	1(2)	78202	1(3)	78635	1(3)	80180	1(3)
74174	1(3)	75600	1(3)	76098	3(3)	76945	1(3)	77373	1(3)	78205	1(3)	78645	1(3)	80183	1(3)
74175	1(3)	75605	1(3)	76100	2(3)	76946	1(3)	77401	1(2)	78206	1(3)	78647	1(3)	80184	2(3)
74176	2(3)	75625	1(3)	76101	1(3)	76948	1(2)	77402	2(3)	78215	1(3)	78650	1(3)	80185	2(3)
74177	2(3)	75630	1(3)	76102	1(3)	76965	2(3)	77407	2(3)	78216	1(3)	78660	1(2)	80186	2(3)
74178	1(3)	75635	1(3)	76120	1(3)	76970	2(3)	77412	2(3)	78226	1(3)	78700	1(3)	80188	2(3)
74181	1(3)	75658	1(3)	76125	1(3)	76975	1(3)	77417	1(2)	78227	1(3)	78701	1(3)	80190	2(3)
74182	1(3)	75705	13(3)	76376	2(3)	76977	1(2)	77422	1(3)	78230	1(3)	78707	1(2)	80192	2(3)
74183	1(3)	75710	2(3)	76377	2(3)	76998	1(3)	77423	1(3)	78231	1(3)	78708	1(3)	80194	2(3)
74185	1(3)	75716	1(3)	76380	2(3)	77001	2(3)	77424	1(2)	78232	1(3)	78709	1(2)	80195	2(3)
74190	1(3)	75726	3(3)	76506	1(2)	77002	1(3)	77425	1(3)	78258	1(2)	78710	1(3)	80197	2(3)
74210	1(3)	75731	1(3)	76510	2(2)	77003	1(3)	77427	1(2)	78261	1(2)	78725	1(3)	80198	2(3)
74220	1(3)	75733	1(3)	76511	2(2)	77011	1(3)	77431	1(2)	78262	1(2)	78730	1(2)	80199	1(3)
74230	1(3)	75736	2(3)	76512	2(2)	77012	1(3)	77432	1(2)	78264	1(2)	78740	1(2)	80200	2(3)
74235	1(3)	75741	1(3)	76513	2(2)	77013	1(3)	77435	1(2)	78265	1(2)	78761	1(2)	80201	2(3)
74240	2(3)	75743	1(3)	76514	1(2)	77014	2(3)	77469	1(2)	78266	1(2)	78800	1(2)	80202	2(3)
74241	1(3)	75746	1(3)	76516	1(2)	77021	1(3)	77470	1(2)	78267	1(2)	78801	1(2)	80203	1(3)
74245	1(3)	75756	2(3)	76519	2(2)	77022	1(3)	77520	1(3)	78268	1(2)	78802	1(2)	80299	3(3)
74246	1(3)	75774	7(3)	76529	2(2)	77051	2(3)	77522	1(3)	78270	1(2)	78803	1(2)	80400	1(3)
74247	1(3)	75791	1(3)	76536	1(3)	77052	1(2)	77523	1(3)	78271	1(2)	78804	1(2)	80402	1(3)
74249	1(3)	75801	1(3)	76604	1(3)	77053	2(2)	77525	1(3)	78272	1(2)	78805	1(3)	80406	1(3)
74250	1(3)	75803	1(3)	76641	2(2)	77054	2(2)	77600	1(3)	78278	2(3)	78806	1(2)	80408	1(3)
74251	1(3)	75805	1(2)	76642	2(2)	77055	1(3)	77605	1(3)	78282	1(2)	78807	1(3)	80410	1(3)
74260	1(2)	75807	1(2)	76700	1(3)	77056	1(3)	77610	1(3)	78290	1(3)	78808	1(2)	80412	1(3)
74261	1(2)	75809	1(3)	76705	2(3)	77057	1(2)	77615	1(3)	78291	1(3)	78811	1(2)	80414	1(3)
74262	1(2)	75810	1(3)	76770	1(3)	77058	1(2)	77620	1(3)	78300	1(2)	78812	1(2)	80415	1(3)
74270	1(3)	75820	2(3)	76775	2(3)	77059	1(2)	77750	1(3)	78305	1(2)	78813	1(2)	80416	1(3)
74280	1(3)	75822	1(3)	76776	2(3)	77063	1(2)	77761	1(3)	78306	1(2)	78814	1(2)	80417	1(3)
74283	1(3)	75825	1(3)	76800	1(3)	77071	1(3)	77762	1(3)	78315	1(2)	78815	1(2)	80418	1(3)
74290	1(3)	75827	1(3)	76801	1(2)	77072	1(2)	77763	1(3)	78320	1(2)	78816	1(2)	80420	1(2)
74300	1(3)	75831	1(3)	76802	2(3)	77073	1(2)	77767	2(3)	78414	1(2)	79005	1(3)	80422	1(3)
74301	1(3)	75833	1(3)	76805	1(2)	77074	1(2)	77768	2(3)	78428	1(3)	79101	1(3)	80424	1(3)
74328	1(3)	75840	1(3)	76810	2(3)	77075	1(2)	77770	2(3)	78445	1(3)	79200	1(3)	80426	1(3)
74329	1(3)	75842	1(3)	76811	1(2)	77076	1(2)	77771	2(3)	78451	1(2)	79300	1(3)	80428	1(3)
74330	1(3)	75860	2(3)	76812	2(3)	77077	1(2)	77772	2(3)	78452	1(2)	79403	1(3)	80430	1(3)
74340	1(3)	75870	1(3)	76813	1(2)	77078	1(2)	77778	1(3)	78453	1(2)	79440	1(3)	80432	1(3)
74355	1(3)	75872	1(3)	76814	2(3)	77080	1(2)	77789	2(3)	78454	1(2)	79445	1(3)	80434	1(3)
74360	1(3)	75880	1(3)	76815	1(2)	77081	1(2)	77790	1(3)	78456	1(2)	80047	2(3)	80435	1(3)
74363	2(3)	75885	1(3)	76816	3(3)	77084	1(2)	78012	1(3)	78457	1(2)	80048	2(3)	80436	1(3)
74400	1(3)	75887	1(3)	76817	1(3)	77085	1(2)	78013	1(3)	78458	1(2)	80051	2(3)	80438	1(3)
74410	1(3)	75889	1(3)	76818	3(3)	77086	1(2)	78014	1(2)	78459	1(2)	80053	1(3)	80439	1(3)
74415	1(3)	75891	1(3)	76819	3(3)	77261	1(3)	78015	1(3)	78466	1(2)	80061	1(3)	80500	1(3)
74420	2(3)	75893	2(3)	76820	3(3)	77262	1(3)	78016	1(3)	78468	1(2)	80069	1(3)	80502	1(3)
74425	2(3)	75894	2(3)	76821	3(3)	77263	1(3)	78018	1(2)	78469	1(2)	80074	1(2)	81000	2(3)
74430	1(3)	75898	2(3)	76825	3(3)	77280	2(3)	78020	1(3)	78472	1(2)	80076	1(3)	81001	2(3)
74440	1(2)	75901	1(3)	76826	3(3)	77285	1(3)	78070	1(3)	78473	1(2)	80081	1(2)	81002	2(3)
74445	1(2)	75902	2(3)	76827	3(3)	77290	1(3)	78071	1(3)	78481	1(2)	80150	2(3)	81003	2(3)
74450	1(3)	75952	1(2)	76828	3(3)	77293	1(3)	78072	1(3)	78483	1(2)	80155	1(3)	81005	2(3)
74455	1(3)	75953	4(3)	76830	1(3)	77295	1(3)	78075	1(2)	78491	1(3)	80156	2(3)	81007	1(3)
74470	2(2)	75954	2(3)	76831	1(3)	77300	10(3)	78102	1(2)	78492	1(2)	80157	2(3)	81015	2(3)
74485	2(3)	75956	1(2)	76856	1(3)	77301	1(3)	78103	1(2)	78494	1(3)	80158	2(1)	81020	1(3)

CPT	MUE	CPT	MUE	CPT	MUE	CPT	MUE	CPT	MUE	CPT	MUE	CPT	MUE	CPT	MUE
81025	1(3)	81281	1(3)	81410	1(3)	82104	1(2)	82465	1(3)	82805	2(1)	83550	1(3)	84075	2(3)
81050	2(3)	81282	1(3)	81411	1(3)	82105	1(3)	82480	2(3)	82810	2(3)	83570	1(3)	84078	1(2)
81161	1(3)	81287	1(3)	81412	1(2)	82106	2(3)	82482	1(3)	82820	1(3)	83582	1(3)	84080	1(3)
81162	1(2)	81288	1(3)	81415	1(1)	82107	1(3)	82485	1(3)	82930	1(1)	83586	1(3)	84081	1(3)
81170	1(2)	81290	1(3)	81416	2(1)	82108	1(3)	82495	1(3)	82938	1(3)	83593	1(3)	84085	1(2)
81200	1(2)	81291	1(3)	81417	1(1)	82120	1(3)	82507	1(3)	82941	1(3)	83605	3(1)	84087	1(3)
81201	1(2)	81292	1(2)	81420	1(3)	82127	1(3)	82523	1(3)	82943	1(3)	83615	2(3)	84100	2(3)
81202	1(3)	81293	1(3)	81425	1(1)	82128	2(3)	82525	2(3)	82945	4(3)	83625	1(3)	84105	1(3)
81203	1(3)	81294	1(3)	81426	2(1)	82131	2(3)	82528	1(3)	82946	1(2)	83630	1(3)	84106	1(2)
81205	1(3)	81295	1(2)	81427	1(1)	82135	1(3)	82530	4(3)	82947	5(3)	83631	1(3)	84110	1(3)
81206	1(3)	81296	1(3)	81430	1(2)	82136	2(3)	82533	5(3)	82950	3(3)	83632	1(3)	84112	1(3)
81207	1(3)	81297	1(3)	81431	1(2)	82139	2(3)	82540	1(3)	82951	1(2)	83633	1(3)	84119	1(2)
81208	1(3)	81298	1(2)	81432	1(2)	82140	2(3)	82542	6(3)	82952	3(3)	83655	2(3)	84120	1(3)
81209	1(3)	81299	1(3)	81433	1(2)	82143	2(3)	82550	3(3)	82955	1(2)	83661	3(3)	84126	1(3)
81210	1(3)	81300	1(3)	81434	1(2)	82150	2(3)	82552	3(3)	82960	1(2)	83662	4(3)	84132	2(3)
81211	1(2)	81301	1(3)	81435	1(2)	82154	1(3)	82553	3(3)	82963	1(3)	83663	3(3)	84133	2(3)
81212	1(2)	81302	1(3)	81436	1(2)	82157	1(3)	82554	1(3)	82965	1(3)	83664	3(3)	84134	1(3)
81213	1(2)	81303	1(3)	81437	1(2)	82160	1(3)	82565	2(1)	82977	1(3)	83670	1(3)	84135	1(3)
81214	1(2)	81304	1(3)	81438	1(2)	82163	1(3)	82570	3(3)	82978	1(3)	83690	2(3)	84138	1(3)
81215	1(2)	81310	1(3)	81440	1(2)	82164	1(3)	82575	1(3)	82979	1(3)	83695	1(3)	84140	1(3)
81216	1(2)	81311	1(3)	81442	1(2)	82172	3(3)	82585	1(2)	82985	1(3)	83698	1(3)	84143	2(3)
81217	1(2)	81313	1(3)	81445	1(2)	82175	2(3)	82595	1(3)	83001	1(3)	83700	1(2)	84144	1(3)
81218	1(3)	81314	1(3)	81450	1(2)	82180	1(2)	82600	1(3)	83002	1(3)	83701	1(3)	84145	1(3)
81219	1(3)	81315	1(3)	81455	1(2)	82190	2(3)	82607	1(2)	83003	5(3)	83704	1(3)	84146	3(3)
81220	1(3)	81316	1(2)	81460	1(2)	82232	2(3)	82608	1(2)	83006	1(2)	83718	1(3)	84150	2(3)
81221	1(3)	81317	1(3)	81465	1(2)	82239	1(3)	82610	1(3)	83009	1(3)	83719	1(3)	84152	1(2)
81222	1(3)	81318	1(3)	81470	1(2)	82240	1(3)	82615	1(3)	83010	1(3)	83721	1(3)	84153	1(2)
81223	1(2)	81319	1(2)	81471	1(2)	82247	2(3)	82626	1(3)	83012	1(2)	83727	1(3)	84154	1(2)
81224	1(3)	81321	1(3)	81490	1(2)	82248	2(3)	82627	1(3)	83013	1(3)	83735	4(3)	84155	1(3)
81225	1(3)	81322	1(3)	81493	1(2)	82252	1(3)	82633	1(3)	83014	1(2)	83775	1(3)	84156	1(3)
81226	1(3)	81323	1(3)	81500	1(3)	82261	1(3)	82634	1(3)	83015	1(2)	83785	1(3)	84157	2(3)
81227	1(3)	81324	1(3)	81503	1(3)	82270	1(3)	82638	1(3)	83018	4(3)	83789	4(3)	84160	2(3)
81228	1(3)	81325	1(3)	81504	1(3)	82271	1(3)	82652	1(2)	83020	2(3)	83825	2(3)	84163	1(3)
81229	1(3)	81326	1(3)	81506	1(3)	82272	1(3)	82656	1(3)	83021	2(3)	83835	2(3)	84165	1(2)
81235	1(3)	81330	1(3)	81507	1(3)	82274	1(3)	82657	3(3)	83026	1(3)	83857	1(3)	84166	2(3)
81240	1(2)	81331	1(3)	81508	1(3)	82286	1(3)	82658	2(3)	83030	1(3)	83861	2(2)	84181	3(3)
81241	1(2)	81332	1(3)	81509	1(3)	82300	1(3)	82664	2(3)	83033	1(3)	83864	1(2)	84182	6(3)
81242	1(3)	81340	1(3)	81510	1(3)	82306	1(2)	82668	1(3)	83036	1(2)	83872	2(3)	84202	1(2)
81243	1(3)	81341	1(3)	81511	1(3)	82308	1(3)	82670	2(3)	83037	1(2)	83873	1(3)	84203	1(2)
81244	1(3)	81342	1(3)	81512	1(3)	82310	2(3)	82671	1(3)	83045	1(3)	83874	2(3)	84206	1(2)
81245	1(3)	81350	1(3)	81519	1(2)	82330	2(3)	82672	1(3)	83050	1(3)	83876	1(3)	84207	1(2)
81246	1(3)	81355	1(3)	81525	1(3)	82331	1(3)	82677	1(3)	83051	1(3)	83880	1(3)	84210	1(3)
81250	1(3)	81370	1(2)	81528	1(3)	82340	1(3)	82679	1(3)	83060	1(3)	83883	6(3)	84220	1(3)
81251	1(3)	81371	1(2)	81535	1(3)	82355	2(3)	82693	2(3)	83065	1(2)	83885	2(3)	84228	1(3)
81252	1(3)	81372	1(2)	81536	3(1)	82360	2(3)	82696	1(3)	83068	1(2)	83915	1(3)	84233	1(3)
81253	1(3)	81373	2(2)	81538	1(2)	82365	2(3)	82705	1(3)	83069	1(3)	83916	2(3)	84234	1(3)
81254	1(3)	81374	1(3)	81540	1(3)	82370	2(3)	82710	1(3)	83070	1(2)	83918	2(3)	84235	1(3)
81255	1(3)	81375	1(2)	81545	1(3)	82373	1(3)	82715	3(3)	83080	2(3)	83919	1(3)	84238	3(3)
81256	1(2)	81376	5(3)	81595	1(2)	82374	2(1)	82725	1(3)	83088	1(3)	83921	2(3)	84244	2(3)
81257	1(2)	81377	2(3)	82009	1(3)	82375	1(3)	82726	1(3)	83090	2(3)	83930	2(3)	84252	1(2)
81260	1(3)	81378	1(2)	82010	1(3)	82376	1(1)	82728	1(3)	83150	1(3)	83935	2(3)	84255	2(3)
81261	1(3)	81379	1(2)	82013	1(3)	82378	1(3)	82731	1(3)	83491	1(3)	83937	1(3)	84260	1(3)
81262	1(3)	81380	2(2)	82016	1(3)	82379	1(3)	82735	1(3)	83497	1(3)	83945	2(3)	84270	1(3)
81263	1(3)	81381	3(3)	82017	1(3)	82380	1(3)	82746	1(2)	83498	2(3)	83950	1(2)	84275	1(3)
81264	1(3)	81382	6(3)	82024	4(3)	82382	1(2)	82747	1(2)	83499	1(3)	83951	1(2)	84285	1(3)
81265	1(3)	81383	2(3)	82030	1(3)	82383	1(3)	82757	1(2)	83500	1(3)	83970	2(3)	84295	3(1)
81266	2(3)	81400	2(3)	82040	1(3)	82384	2(3)	82759	1(3)	83505	1(3)	83986	2(3)	84300	2(3)
81267	1(3)	81401	2(3)	82042	2(3)	82387	1(3)	82760	1(3)	83516	4(3)	83987	1(3)	84302	1(1)
81268	4(3)	81402	1(3)	82043	1(3)	82390	1(2)	82775	1(3)	83518	1(3)	83992	2(3)	84305	1(3)
81270	1(2)	81403	4(3)	82044	1(3)	82397	3(3)	82776	1(2)	83519	5(3)	83993	1(3)	84307	1(3)
81272	1(3)	81404	5(3)	82045	1(3)	82415	1(3)	82777	1(3)	83520	8(3)	84030	1(2)	84311	2(3)
81273	1(3)	81405	2(3)	82075	2(3)	82435	2(1)	82784	6(3)	83525	4(3)	84035	1(2)	84315	1(3)
81275	1(3)	81406	1(3)	82085	1(3)	82436	1(3)	82785	1(3)	83527	1(3)	84060	1(3)	84375	1(3)
81276	1(3)	81407	1(3)	82088	2(3)	82438	1(3)	82787	4(3)	83528	1(3)	84061	1(3)	84376	1(3)
81280	1(3)	81408	2(3)	82103	1(3)	82441	1(2)	82800	1(1)	83540	2(3)	84066	1(3)	84377	1(3)

CPT	MUE	CPT	MUE	CPT	MUE	CPT	MUE	CPT	MUE	CPT	MUE	CPT	MUE	CPT	MUE
84378	2(3)	85032	1(3)	85530	1(3)	86304	1(2)	86641	2(3)	86788	2(3)	87045	3(3)	87276	1(3)
84379	1(3)	85041	1(3)	85536	1(2)	86305	1(2)	86644	2(3)	86789	2(3)	87046	6(3)	87277	1(3)
84392	1(3)	85044	1(2)	85540	1(2)	86308	1(2)	86645	1(3)	86790	4(3)	87070	3(1)	87278	1(3)
84402	1(3)	85045	1(2)	85547	1(2)	86309	1(2)	86648	2(3)	86793	2(3)	87071	4(3)	87279	1(3)
84403	2(3)	85046	1(2)	85549	1(3)	86310	1(2)	86651	2(3)	86800	1(3)	87073	3(3)	87280	1(3)
84425	1(2)	85048	2(3)	85555	1(2)	86316	2(3)	86652	2(3)	86803	1(3)	87075	6(3)	87281	1(3)
84430	1(3)	85049	2(3)	85557	1(2)	86317	6(1)	86653	2(3)	86804	1(2)	87076	6(3)	87283	1(3)
84431	1(3)	85055	1(3)	85576	7(3)	86318	2(3)	86654	2(3)	86805	2(3)	87077	10(3)	87285	1(3)
84432	1(2)	85060	1(3)	85597	1(3)	86320	1(2)	86658	12(3)	86807	2(3)	87081	6(3)	87290	1(3)
84436	1(2)	85097	2(3)	85598	1(3)	86325	2(3)	86663	2(3)	86808	1(3)	87084	1(3)	87299	1(3)
84437	1(2)	85130	1(3)	85610	4(3)	86327	1(3)	86664	2(3)	86812	1(2)	87086	3(3)	87300	2(3)
84439	1(2)	85170	1(3)	85611	2(3)	86329	3(3)	86665	2(3)	86813	1(2)	87088	6(3)	87301	1(3)
84442	1(2)	85175	1(3)	85612	1(3)	86331	12(3)	86666	4(3)	86816	1(2)	87101	4(3)	87305	1(3)
84443	4(2)	85210	2(3)	85613	1(3)	86332	1(3)	86668	2(3)	86817	1(2)	87102	4(3)	87320	1(3)
84445	1(2)	85220	2(3)	85635	1(3)	86334	1(2)	86671	3(3)	86821	1(3)	87103	2(3)	87324	2(3)
84446	1(2)	85230	2(3)	85651	1(2)	86335	2(3)	86674	3(3)	86822	1(3)	87106	4(3)	87327	1(3)
84449	1(3)	85240	2(3)	85652	1(2)	86336	1(3)	86677	3(3)	86825	1(3)	87107	4(3)	87328	2(3)
84450	1(3)	85244	1(3)	85660	1(2)	86337	1(2)	86682	2(3)	86826	2(3)	87109	2(3)	87329	2(3)
84460	1(3)	85245	2(3)	85670	2(3)	86340	1(2)	86684	2(3)	86828	1(3)	87110	2(3)	87332	1(3)
84466	1(3)	85246	2(3)	85675	1(3)	86341	1(3)	86687	1(3)	86829	1(3)	87116	2(1)	87335	1(3)
84478	1(3)	85247	2(3)	85705	1(3)	86343	1(3)	86688	1(3)	86830	2(3)	87118	3(3)	87336	1(3)
84479	1(2)	85250	2(3)	85730	4(3)	86344	1(2)	86689	2(3)	86831	2(3)	87140	3(3)	87337	1(3)
84480	1(2)	85260	2(3)	85732	4(3)	86352	1(3)	86692	2(3)	86832	2(3)	87143	2(3)	87338	1(1)
84481	1(2)	85270	2(3)	85810	2(3)	86353	7(3)	86694	2(3)	86833	1(3)	87149	4(3)	87339	1(3)
84482	1(2)	85280	2(3)	86000	6(3)	86355	1(2)	86695	2(3)	86834	1(3)	87150	12(3)	87340	1(2)
84484	2(3)	85290	2(3)	86001	20(1)	86356	7(3)	86696	2(3)	86835	1(3)	87152	1(3)	87341	1(2)
84485	1(3)	85291	1(3)	86005	2(3)	86357	1(2)	86698	3(3)	86850	3(3)	87153	3(3)	87350	1(2)
84488	1(3)	85292	1(3)	86021	1(2)	86359	1(2)	86701	1(3)	86860	2(3)	87158	1(1)	87380	1(2)
84490	1(2)	85293	1(3)	86022	1(2)	86360	1(2)	86702	2(3)	86870	2(3)	87164	2(3)	87385	2(3)
84510	1(3)	85300	2(3)	86023	3(3)	86361	1(2)	86703	1(2)	86880	4(3)	87166	2(3)	87389	1(3)
84512	1(3)	85301	1(3)	86038	1(3)	86367	1(3)	86704	1(2)	86885	2(3)	87168	2(3)	87390	1(3)
84520	4(1)	85302	1(3)	86039	1(3)	86376	2(3)	86705	1(2)	86886	3(1)	87169	2(3)	87391	1(3)
84525	1(3)	85303	2(3)	86060	1(3)	86378	1(3)	86706	2(3)	86890	1(1)	87172	1(3)	87400	2(3)
84540	2(3)	85305	2(3)	86063	1(3)	86382	3(3)	86707	1(3)	86891	1(1)	87176	2(3)	87420	1(3)
84545	1(3)	85306	2(3)	86077	1(2)	86384	1(3)	86708	1(2)	86900	1(3)	87177	3(3)	87425	1(3)
84550	1(3)	85307	2(3)	86078	1(3)	86386	1(2)	86709	1(2)	86901	1(3)	87181	12(3)	87427	2(3)
84560	2(3)	85335	2(3)	86079	1(3)	86406	2(3)	86710	4(3)	86902	6(3)	87184	8(3)	87430	1(3)
84577	1(3)	85337	1(3)	86140	1(2)	86430	2(3)	86711	2(3)	86904	2(1)	87185	4(3)	87449	3(3)
84578	1(3)	85345	1(3)	86141	1(2)	86431	2(3)	86713	3(3)	86905	8(3)	87186	12(3)	87450	2(3)
84580	1(3)	85347	5(3)	86146	3(3)	86480	1(3)	86717	8(3)	86906	1(2)	87187	3(3)	87451	2(3)
84583	1(3)	85348	1(3)	86147	4(3)	86481	1(3)	86720	2(3)	86920	9(3)	87188	6(3)	87470	1(3)
84585	1(2)	85360	1(3)	86148	3(3)	86485	1(2)	86723	2(3)	86921	2(1)	87190	9(3)	87471	1(3)
84586	1(2)	85362	2(3)	86152	1(3)	86486	2(3)	86727	2(3)	86922	5(3)	87197	1(3)	87472	1(3)
84588	1(3)	85366	1(3)	86153	1(3)	86490	1(2)	86729	0(2)	86923	10(3)	87205	3(1)	87475	1(3)
84590	1(2)	85370	1(3)	86155	1(3)	86510	1(2)	86732	2(3)	86927	2(1)	87206	6(3)	87476	1(3)
84591	1(3)	85378	1(3)	86156	1(2)	86580	1(2)	86735	2(3)	86930	0(3)	87207	3(3)	87477	1(3)
84597	1(3)	85379	2(3)	86157	1(2)	86590	1(3)	86738	2(3)	86931	1(3)	87209	4(3)	87480	1(3)
84600	2(3)	85380	1(3)	86160	4(3)	86592	2(3)	86741	2(3)	86932	2(1)	87210	4(3)	87481	1(1)
84620	1(2)	85384	2(3)	86161	2(3)	86593	2(3)	86744	2(3)	86940	1(3)	87220	3(3)	87482	1(3)
84630	2(3)	85385	1(3)	86162	1(2)	86602	3(3)	86747	2(3)	86941	1(3)	87230	3(3)	87485	1(3)
84681	1(3)	85390	3(3)	86171	2(3)	86603	2(3)	86750	4(3)	86945	2(3)	87250	1(3)	87486	1(3)
84702	2(3)	85396	1(2)	86185	1(3)	86609	14(3)	86753	3(3)	86950	1(3)	87252	2(3)	87487	1(3)
84703	1(3)	85397	3(3)	86200	1(3)	86611	4(3)	86756	2(3)	86960	1(3)	87253	2(3)	87490	1(3)
84704	1(3)	85400	1(3)	86215	1(3)	86612	2(3)	86757	6(3)	86965	1(3)	87254	7(3)	87491	2(3)
84830	1(2)	85410	1(3)	86225	1(3)	86615	6(3)	86759	2(3)	86970	1(1)	87255	2(3)	87492	1(3)
85002	1(3)	85415	2(3)	86226	1(3)	86617	2(3)	86762	2(3)	86971	1(3)	87260	1(3)	87493	2(3)
85004	1(3)	85420	2(3)	86235	10(3)	86618	2(3)	86765	2(3)	86972	1(3)	87265	1(3)	87495	1(3)
85007	1(3)	85421	1(3)	86243	1(3)	86619	2(3)	86768	5(3)	86975	1(3)	87267	1(3)	87496	1(3)
85008	1(3)	85441	1(2)	86255	5(3)	86622	2(3)	86771	2(3)	86976	1(3)	87269	1(3)	87497	2(3)
85009	1(3)	85445	1(2)	86256	9(3)	86625	1(3)	86774	2(3)	86977	1(3)	87270	1(3)	87498	1(3)
85013	1(3)	85460	1(3)	86277	1(3)	86628	3(3)	86777	2(3)	86978	1(3)	87271	1(3)	87500	1(3)
85014	2(3)	85461	1(2)	86280	1(3)	86631	6(3)	86778	2(3)	86985	1(1)	87272	1(3)	87501	1(3)
85018	2(3)	85475	1(3)	86294	1(3)	86632	3(3)	86780	2(3)	87003	1(3)	87273	1(3)	87502	1(3)
85025	2(3)	85520	1(3)	86300	2(3)	86635	4(3)	86784	1(3)	87015	4(3)	87274	1(3)	87503	1(3)
85027	2(3)	85525	2(3)	86301	1(2)	86638	6(3)	86787	2(3)	87040	2(1)	87275	1(3)	87505	1(2)

CPT	MUE	CPT	MUE	CPT	MUE	CPT	MUE	CPT	MUE	CPT	MUE	CPT	MUE	CPT	MUE
87506	1(2)	87804	3(3)	88262	2(3)	88741	1(2)	90585	1(2)	90785	1(3)	91040	1(2)	92504	1(3)
87507	1(3)	87806	1(3)	88263	1(3)	89049	1(3)	90586	1(2)	90791	1(3)	91065	2(2)	92507	1(3)
87510	1(3)	87807	2(3)	88264	2(3)	89050	2(3)	90620	1(2)	90792	1(3)	91110	1(2)	92508	1(3)
87511	1(3)	87808	1(3)	88267	2(3)	89051	2(3)	90621	1(2)	90832	1(3)	91111	1(2)	92511	1(3)
87512	1(3)	87809	2(3)	88269	2(3)	89055	2(3)	90625	1(2)	90833	1(3)	91112	1(3)	92512	1(2)
87515	1(3)	87810	2(3)	88271	16(3)	89060	2(3)	90630	1(2)	90834	1(3)	91117	1(2)	92516	1(3)
87516	1(3)	87850	1(3)	88272	12(3)	89125	2(3)	90632	1(2)	90836	1(3)	91120	1(2)	92520	1(2)
87517	1(3)	87880	2(3)	88273	3(3)	89160	1(3)	90633	1(2)	90837	1(3)	91122	1(2)	92521	1(2)
87520	1(3)	87899	4(3)	88274	5(3)	89190	1(3)	90634	1(2)	90838	1(3)	91132	1(3)	92522	1(2)
87521	1(3)	87900	1(2)	88275	12(3)	89220	1(3)	90636	1(2)	90839	1(2)	91133	1(3)	92523	1(2)
87522	1(3)	87901	1(2)	88280	8(3)	89230	1(2)	90644	1(2)	90840	3(3)	91200	1(3)	92524	1(2)
87525	1(3)	87902	1(2)	88283	5(3)	89250	1(2)	90647	1(2)	90845	1(2)	92002	1(2)	92526	1(2)
87526	1(3)	87903	1(2)	88285	10(3)	89251	1(2)	90648	1(2)	90846	1(3)	92004	1(2)	92531	0(3)
87527	1(3)	87904	14(3)	88289	1(3)	89253	1(3)	90649	1(2)	90847	1(3)	92012	1(3)	92532	0(3)
87528	1(3)	87905	2(3)	88291	1(1)	89254	1(3)	90650	1(2)	90849	1(3)	92014	1(3)	92534	0(3)
87529	2(3)	87906	2(3)	88300	4(3)	89255	1(3)	90651	1(2)	90853	1(3)	92018	1(2)	92537	1(2)
87530	2(3)	87910	1(3)	88302	4(3)	89257	1(3)	90653	1(2)	90863	1(3)	92019	1(2)	92538	1(2)
87531	1(3)	87912	1(3)	88304	5(3)	89258	1(2)	90654	1(2)	90865	1(3)	92020	1(2)	92540	1(3)
87532	1(3)	88104	5(3)	88305	16(3)	89259	1(2)	90655	1(2)	90867	1(2)	92025	1(2)	92541	1(3)
87533	1(3)	88106	5(3)	88307	8(3)	89260	1(2)	90656	1(2)	90868	1(3)	92060	1(2)	92542	1(3)
87534	1(3)	88108	6(3)	88309	3(3)	89261	1(2)	90657	1(2)	90869	1(3)	92065	1(2)	92544	1(3)
87535	1(3)	88112	6(3)	88311	4(3)	89264	1(3)	90658	1(2)	90870	2(3)	92071	2(2)	92545	1(3)
87536	1(3)	88120	2(3)	88312	9(3)	89268	1(2)	90660	1(2)	90880	1(3)	92072	1(2)	92546	1(3)
87537	1(3)	88121	2(3)	88313	8(3)	89272	1(2)	90661	1(2)	90885	0(3)	92081	1(2)	92547	1(3)
87538	1(3)	88125	1(3)	88314	6(3)	89280	1(2)	90662	1(2)	90887	0(3)	92082	1(2)	92548	1(3)
87539	1(3)	88130	1(2)	88319	11(3)	89281	1(2)	90664	1(2)	90889	0(3)	92083	1(2)	92550	1(2)
87540	1(3)	88140	1(2)	88321	1(2)	89290	1(2)	90666	1(2)	90901	1(3)	92100	1(2)	92552	1(2)
87541	1(3)	88141	1(3)	88323	1(2)	89291	1(2)	90667	1(2)	90911	1(3)	92132	1(2)	92553	1(2)
87542	1(3)	88142	1(3)	88325	1(2)	89300	1(2)	90668	1(2)	90935	1(3)	92133	1(2)	92555	1(2)
87550	1(3)	88143	1(3)	88329	2(3)	89310	1(2)	90670	1(2)	90937	1(3)	92134	1(2)	92556	1(2)
87551	2(3)	88147	1(3)	88331	11(3)	89320	1(2)	90672	1(2)	90940	1(3)	92136	2(2)	92557	1(2)
87552	1(3)	88148	1(3)	88332	13(3)	89321	1(2)	90673	1(2)	90945	1(3)	92140	1(2)	92558	0(3)
87555	1(1)	88150	1(3)	88333	4(3)	89322	1(2)	90675	1(2)	90947	1(3)	92145	1(2)	92561	1(2)
87556	1(1)	88152	1(3)	88334	5(3)	89325	1(2)	90676	1(2)	90951	1(2)	92225	2(2)	92562	1(2)
87557	1(3)	88153	1(3)	88342	3(3)	89329	1(2)	90680	1(2)	90952	1(2)	92226	2(2)	92563	1(2)
87560	1(3)	88154	1(3)	88344	1(1)	89330	1(2)	90681	1(2)	90953	1(2)	92227	1(2)	92564	1(2)
87561	1(3)	88155	1(3)	88346	2(1)	89331	1(2)	90685	1(2)	90954	1(2)	92228	1(2)	92565	1(2)
87562	1(3)	88160	4(3)	88348	1(3)	89335	1(3)	90686	1(2)	90955	1(2)	92230	2(2)	92567	1(2)
87580	1(3)	88161	4(3)	88350	4(1)	89337	1(2)	90687	1(2)	90956	1(2)	92235	2(2)	92568	1(2)
87581	1(3)	88162	3(3)	88355	1(3)	89342	1(2)	90688	1(2)	90957	1(2)	92240	2(2)	92570	1(2)
87582	1(3)	88164	1(3)	88356	1(1)	89343	1(2)	90690	1(2)	90958	1(2)	92250	1(2)	92571	1(2)
87590	1(3)	88165	1(3)	88358	2(3)	89344	1(2)	90691	1(2)	90959	1(2)	92260	1(2)	92572	1(2)
87591	2(3)	88166	1(3)	88360	6(3)	89346	1(2)	90696	1(2)	90960	1(2)	92265	1(2)	92575	1(2)
87592	1(3)	88167	1(3)	88361	6(3)	89352	1(2)	90697	1(2)	90961	1(2)	92270	1(2)	92576	1(2)
87623	1(2)	88172	5(3)	88362	1(3)	89353	1(3)	90698	1(2)	90962	1(2)	92275	1(2)	92577	1(2)
87624	1(2)	88173	5(3)	88363	2(3)	89354	1(3)	90700	1(2)	90963	1(2)	92283	1(2)	92579	1(2)
87625	1(2)	88174	1(3)	88364	3(3)	89356	2(3)	90702	1(2)	90964	1(2)	92284	1(2)	92582	1(2)
87631	1(3)	88175	1(3)	88365	4(3)	90284	0(3)	90707	1(2)	90965	1(2)	92285	1(2)	92583	1(2)
87632	1(3)	88177	6(3)	88366	2(3)	90296	1(2)	90710	1(2)	90966	1(2)	92286	1(2)	92584	1(2)
87633	1(3)	88182	2(3)	88367	2(1)	90371	10(3)	90713	1(2)	90967	1(2)	92287	1(2)	92585	1(2)
87640	1(3)	88184	2(3)	88368	2(1)	90375	20(3)	90714	1(2)	90968	1(2)	92311	1(2)	92586	1(2)
87641	1(3)	88187	2(3)	88369	3(1)	90376	20(3)	90715	1(2)	90969	1(2)	92312	1(2)	92587	1(2)
87650	1(3)	88188	2(3)	88371	1(3)	90378	4(3)	90716	1(2)	90970	1(2)	92313	1(3)	92588	1(2)
87651	1(3)	88189	2(3)	88372	1(3)	90385	1(2)	90717	1(2)	90989	1(2)	92315	1(2)	92596	1(2)
87652	1(3)	88230	2(3)	88373	3(1)	90393	1(2)	90732	1(2)	90993	1(3)	92316	1(2)	92597	1(3)
87653	1(3)	88233	2(3)	88374	5(3)	90396	1(2)	90733	1(2)	90997	1(3)	92317	1(3)	92601	1(3)
87660	1(3)	88235	2(3)	88375	1(3)	90460	6(3)	90734	1(2)	91010	1(2)	92325	1(3)	92602	1(3)
87661	1(1)	88237	4(3)	88377	5(3)	90461	5(3)	90736	1(2)	91013	1(3)	92326	2(3)	92603	1(3)
87797	3(3)	88239	3(3)	88380	1(1)	90471	1(2)	90738	1(2)	91020	1(2)	92352	0(3)	92604	1(3)
87798	13(3)	88240	1(3)	88381	1(1)	90472	4(3)	90739	1(2)	91022	1(2)	92353	0(3)	92605	0(3)
87799	3(3)	88241	3(3)	88387	2(3)	90473	1(2)	90740	1(2)	91030	1(2)	92354	0(3)	92607	1(3)
87800	2(3)	88245	1(2)	88388	1(3)	90474	1(3)	90743	1(2)	91034	1(2)	92355	0(3)	92608	4(3)
87801	3(3)	88248	1(2)	88720	1(3)	90476	1(2)	90744	1(2)	91035	1(2)	92358	0(3)	92609	1(3)
87802	2(3)	88249	1(2)	88738	1(3)	90477	1(2)	90746	1(2)	91037	1(2)	92371	0(3)	92610	1(2)
87803	3(3)	88261	2(3)	88740	1(2)	90581	1(2)	90747	1(2)	91038	1(2)	92502	1(3)	92611	1(3)

CPT	MUE	CPT	MUE	CPT	MUE	CPT	MUE	CPT	MUE	CPT	MUE	CPT	MUE	CPT	MUE
92612	1(3)	93261	1(3)	93533	1(3)	93923	1(1)	94776	1(2)	95866	1(3)	96003	1(3)	96920	1(2)
92613	1(2)	93268	1(2)	93561	1(3)	93924	1(2)	94777	1(2)	95867	1(3)	96004	1(2)	96921	1(2)
92614	1(3)	93270	1(2)	93562	1(3)	93925	1(3)	94780	1(2)	95868	1(3)	96020	1(2)	96922	1(2)
92615	1(2)	93271	1(2)	93563	1(3)	93926	1(3)	94781	2(3)	95869	1(3)	96040	4(3)	96931	1(2)
92616	1(3)	93272	1(2)	93564	1(3)	93930	1(3)	95004	80(1)	95870	4(3)	96101	8(3)	96932	1(2)
92617	1(2)	93278	1(3)	93565	1(3)	93931	1(3)	95012	2(3)	95872	4(3)	96102	4(3)	96933	1(2)
92618	1(3)	93279	1(3)	93566	1(3)	93965	1(3)	95017	27(1)	95873	1(2)	96103	1(2)	96934	4(1)
92620	1(2)	93280	1(3)	93567	1(3)	93970	1(3)	95018	19(3)	95874	1(2)	96105	3(3)	96935	4(1)
92621	4(3)	93281	1(3)	93568	1(3)	93971	1(3)	95024	40(1)	95875	2(3)	96110	2(3)	96936	4(1)
92625	1(2)	93282	1(3)	93571	1(3)	93975	1(3)	95027	90(1)	95885	4(2)	96111	1(3)	97001	1(3)
92626	1(2)	93283	1(3)	93572	2(3)	93976	1(3)	95028	30(1)	95886	4(2)	96116	4(3)	97002	1(3)
92627	6(3)	93284	1(3)	93580	1(3)	93978	1(3)	95044	80(1)	95887	1(2)	96118	8(3)	97003	1(3)
92640	1(3)	93285	1(3)	93581	1(3)	93979	1(3)	95052	20(1)	95905	2(3)	96119	6(3)	97004	1(3)
92920	3(3)	93286	2(3)	93582	1(2)	93980	1(3)	95056	1(2)	95907	1(2)	96120	1(2)	97010	0(3)
92921	6(2)	93287	2(3)	93583	1(2)	93981	1(3)	95060	1(2)	95908	1(2)	96125	2(3)	97012	1(3)
92924	2(3)	93288	1(3)	93600	1(3)	93982	1(3)	95065	1(3)	95909	1(2)	96127	2(1)	97014	0(3)
92925	6(2)	93289	1(3)	93602	1(3)	93990	2(3)	95070	1(3)	95910	1(2)	96150	8(3)	97016	1(3)
92928	3(3)	93290	1(3)	93603	1(3)	94002	1(2)	95071	1(2)	95911	1(2)	96151	6(3)	97018	1(3)
92929	6(2)	93291	1(3)	93609	1(3)	94003	1(2)	95076	1(2)	95912	1(2)	96152	6(3)	97022	1(3)
92933	2(3)	93292	1(3)	93610	1(3)	94004	1(2)	95079	2(3)	95913	1(2)	96153	8(3)	97024	1(3)
92934	6(2)	93293	1(2)	93612	1(3)	94010	1(3)	95115	1(2)	95921	1(3)	96154	8(3)	97026	1(3)
92937	2(3)	93294	1(2)	93613	1(3)	94011	1(3)	95117	1(2)	95922	1(3)	96360	1(1)	97028	1(3)
92938	6(3)	93295	1(2)	93615	1(3)	94012	1(3)	95144	30(3)	95923	1(3)	96361	8(3)	97032	4(3)
92941	1(3)	93296	1(2)	93616	1(3)	94013	1(3)	95145	10(3)	95924	1(3)	96365	1(1)	97033	4(3)
92943	2(3)	93297	1(2)	93618	1(3)	94014	1(2)	95146	10(3)	95925	1(3)	96366	8(3)	97034	2(3)
92944	3(3)	93298	1(2)	93619	1(3)	94015	1(2)	95147	10(3)	95926	1(3)	96367	4(3)	97035	2(3)
92950	2(3)	93299	1(2)	93620	1(3)	94016	1(2)	95148	10(3)	95927	1(3)	96368	1(2)	97036	3(3)
92953	2(3)	93303	1(3)	93621	1(3)	94060	1(3)	95149	10(3)	95928	1(3)	96369	1(2)	97110	6(3)
92960	2(3)	93304	1(3)	93622	1(3)	94070	1(2)	95165	30(3)	95929	1(3)	96370	3(3)	97112	4(3)
92961	1(3)	93306	1(3)	93623	1(3)	94150	0(3)	95170	10(3)	95930	1(3)	96371	1(3)	97113	6(3)
92970	1(3)	93307	1(3)	93624	1(3)	94200	1(3)	95180	6(3)	95933	1(3)	96372	4(3)	97116	4(3)
92971	1(3)	93308	1(3)	93631	1(3)	94250	1(3)	95250	1(2)	95937	4(3)	96373	2(3)	97124	4(3)
92973	2(3)	93312	1(3)	93640	1(3)	94375	1(3)	95251	1(2)	95938	1(3)	96374	1(3)	97140	6(3)
92974	1(3)	93313	1(3)	93641	1(2)	94400	1(3)	95782	1(2)	95939	1(3)	96375	6(3)	97150	1(3)
92975	1(3)	93314	1(3)	93642	1(3)	94450	1(3)	95783	1(2)	95940	32(3)	96376	0(3)	97530	6(3)
92977	1(3)	93315	1(3)	93644	1(2)	94452	1(2)	95800	1(2)	95943	1(3)	96401	3(3)	97532	8(3)
92978	1(3)	93316	1(3)	93650	1(2)	94453	1(2)	95801	1(2)	95950	1(2)	96402	2(3)	97533	4(3)
92979	2(3)	93317	1(3)	93653	1(3)	94610	2(3)	95803	1(2)	95951	1(2)	96405	1(2)	97535	8(3)
92986	1(2)	93318	1(3)	93654	1(3)	94620	1(3)	95805	1(2)	95953	1(2)	96406	1(2)	97537	8(3)
92987	1(2)	93320	1(3)	93655	2(3)	94621	1(3)	95806	1(2)	95954	1(3)	96409	1(3)	97542	8(3)
92990	1(2)	93321	1(3)	93656	1(3)	94640	4(3)	95807	1(2)	95955	1(3)	96411	3(3)	97545	1(2)
92992	1(2)	93325	1(3)	93657	1(3)	94642	1(3)	95808	1(2)	95956	1(2)	96413	1(3)	97546	2(3)
92993	1(2)	93350	1(2)	93660	1(3)	94644	1(2)	95810	1(2)	95957	1(3)	96415	8(3)	97597	1(3)
92997	1(2)	93351	1(2)	93662	1(3)	94645	2(3)	95811	1(2)	95958	1(3)	96416	1(3)	97598	8(3)
92998	2(3)	93352	1(3)	93701	1(2)	94660	1(2)	95812	1(3)	95961	1(2)	96417	3(3)	97602	0(3)
93000	3(3)	93355	1(3)	93702	1(2)	94662	1(2)	95813	1(3)	95962	5(3)	96420	1(3)	97605	1(3)
93005	3(3)	93451	1(3)	93724	1(3)	94664	1(3)	95816	1(3)	95965	1(3)	96422	2(3)	97606	1(3)
93010	5(3)	93452	1(3)	93740	0(3)	94667	1(2)	95819	1(3)	95966	1(3)	96423	1(3)	97607	1(3)
93015	1(3)	93453	1(3)	93745	1(2)	94668	2(3)	95822	1(3)	95967	3(3)	96425	1(3)	97608	1(3)
93016	1(3)	93454	1(3)	93750	4(3)	94669	4(3)	95824	1(3)	95970	1(3)	96440	1(3)	97610	1(2)
93017	1(3)	93455	1(3)	93770	0(3)	94680	1(3)	95827	1(3)	95971	1(3)	96446	1(3)	97750	8(3)
93018	1(3)	93456	1(3)	93784	1(2)	94681	1(3)	95829	1(3)	95972	1(2)	96450	1(3)	97755	8(3)
93024	1(3)	93457	1(3)	93786	1(2)	94690	1(3)	95830	1(3)	95974	1(2)	96521	2(3)	97760	6(3)
93025	1(2)	93458	1(3)	93788	1(2)	94726	1(3)	95831	5(2)	95975	2(3)	96522	1(3)	97761	6(3)
93040	3(3)	93459	1(3)	93790	1(2)	94727	1(3)	95832	1(3)	95978	1(2)	96523	1(3)	97762	4(3)
93041	2(3)	93460	1(3)	93797	2(2)	94728	1(3)	95833	1(3)	95979	6(3)	96542	1(3)	97802	8(3)
93042	3(3)	93461	1(3)	93798	2(2)	94729	1(3)	95834	1(3)	95980	1(3)	96567	1(3)	97803	8(3)
93050	1(3)	93462	1(3)	93880	1(3)	94750	1(3)	95851	3(3)	95981	1(3)	96570	1(2)	97804	6(3)
93224	1(2)	93463	1(3)	93882	1(3)	94760	1(3)	95852	1(3)	95982	1(3)	96571	2(3)	98925	1(2)
93225	1(2)	93464	1(3)	93886	1(3)	94761	1(2)	95857	1(2)	95990	1(3)	96900	1(3)	98926	1(2)
93226	1(2)	93503	2(3)	93888	1(3)	94762	1(2)	95860	1(3)	95991	1(3)	96902	0(3)	98927	1(2)
93227	1(2)	93505	1(2)	93890	1(3)	94770	1(3)	95861	1(3)	95992	1(2)	96904	1(2)	98928	1(2)
93228	1(2)	93530	1(3)	93892	1(3)	94772	1(2)	95863	1(3)	96000	1(2)	96910	1(3)	98929	1(2)
93229	1(2)	93531	1(3)	93893	1(3)	94774	1(2)	95864	1(3)	96001	1(2)	96912	1(3)	98940	1(2)
93260	1(2)	93532	1(3)	93922	1(1)	94775	1(2)	95865	1(3)	96002	1(3)	96913	1(3)	98941	1(2)

Appendix I — Medically Unlikely Edits (MUEs) — Professional

CPT	MUE	CPT	MUE	CPT	MUE	CPT	MUE	CPT	MUE	CPT	MUE	CPT	MUE	CPT	MUE
98942	1(2)	99284	1(3)	99478	1(2)	A4470	1(1)	A7037	0(3)	A9564	20(3)	C1830	2(3)	C8932	1(3)
99002	0(3)	99285	1(3)	99479	1(2)	A4480	1(1)	A7039	0(3)	A9566	1(3)	C1840	1(3)	C8933	1(3)
99024	0(3)	99288	0(3)	99480	1(2)	A4555	0(3)	A7040	2(1)	A9567	2(3)	C1841	1(3)	C8957	2(3)
99050	0(3)	99291	1(2)	99485	1(3)	A4557	2(1)	A7041	2(1)	A9568	0(3)	C1882	1(3)	C9113	0(3)
99051	0(3)	99292	8(3)	99486	4(1)	A4561	1(1)	A7044	0(3)	A9569	1(3)	C1886	1(3)	C9121	0(3)
99053	0(3)	99304	1(2)	99487	1(2)	A4562	1(1)	A7047	0(3)	A9570	1(3)	C1900	1(3)	C9132	5500(3)
99056	0(3)	99305	1(2)	99490	1(2)	A4565	2(3)	A7048	10(3)	A9571	1(3)	C2613	2(1)	C9248	1(3)
99058	0(3)	99306	1(2)	99495	1(2)	A4602	0(3)	A7501	0(3)	A9572	1(3)	C2616	1(3)	C9250	1(3)
99060	0(3)	99307	1(2)	99496	1(2)	A4606	0(3)	A7504	0(3)	A9575	200(3)	C2619	1(3)	C9254	0(3)
99070	0(3)	99308	1(2)	99497	1(2)	A4611	0(3)	A7507	0(3)	A9576	40(3)	C2620	1(3)	C9257	5(3)
99071	0(3)	99309	1(2)	99498	3(3)	A4614	1(1)	A7520	0(3)	A9577	50(3)	C2621	1(3)	C9275	1(3)
99078	0(3)	99310	1(2)	99605	0(2)	A4625	30(3)	A7524	0(3)	A9578	50(3)	C2622	1(3)	C9285	2(3)
99080	0(3)	99315	1(2)	99606	0(3)	A4633	0(3)	A7527	0(3)	A9579	100(3)	C2623	3(1)	C9290	266(3)
99082	1(1)	99316	1(2)	99607	0(3)	A4635	0(3)	A9272	0(1)	A9580	1(3)	C2624	1(3)	C9293	700(3)
99090	0(3)	99318	1(2)	A0021	0(3)	A4638	0(3)	A9284	0(3)	A9581	20(3)	C2626	1(3)	C9349	54(1)
99091	0(3)	99324	1(2)	A0080	0(3)	A4640	0(3)	A9500	3(3)	A9582	1(3)	C2631	1(3)	C9352	3(3)
99100	1(3)	99325	1(2)	A0090	0(3)	A4642	1(3)	A9501	1(3)	A9583	18(3)	C2634	24(3)	C9353	4(3)
99116	0(3)	99326	1(2)	A0100	0(3)	A4648	5(3)	A9502	3(3)	A9584	1(3)	C2635	124(3)	C9354	300(3)
99135	0(3)	99327	1(2)	A0110	0(3)	A4650	3(1)	A9503	1(3)	A9585	300(3)	C2636	600(3)	C9355	3(3)
99140	0(3)	99328	1(2)	A0120	0(3)	A5056	90(3)	A9504	1(3)	A9586	1(3)	C2637	0(3)	C9356	125(3)
99143	2(3)	99334	1(3)	A0130	0(3)	A5057	90(3)	A9505	4(3)	A9599	1(3)	C2638	150(3)	C9358	800(3)
99144	2(3)	99335	1(3)	A0140	0(3)	A5120	150(3)	A9507	1(3)	A9600	7(3)	C2639	150(3)	C9359	30(3)
99145	9(3)	99336	1(3)	A0160	0(3)	A5500	0(3)	A9508	2(3)	A9604	1(3)	C2640	150(3)	C9360	300(3)
99148	2(3)	99337	1(3)	A0170	0(3)	A5501	0(3)	A9509	5(3)	A9606	203(3)	C2641	150(3)	C9361	10(3)
99149	2(3)	99341	1(2)	A0180	0(3)	A5503	0(3)	A9510	1(3)	A9700	2(3)	C2642	120(3)	C9362	60(3)
99150	6(3)	99342	1(2)	A0190	0(3)	A5504	0(3)	A9512	30(3)	B4081	0(3)	C2643	120(3)	C9363	500(3)
99170	1(3)	99343	1(2)	A0200	0(3)	A5505	0(3)	A9516	4(3)	B4082	0(3)	C2644	500(1)	C9364	600(3)
99175	1(3)	99344	1(2)	A0210	0(3)	A5506	0(3)	A9517	200(3)	B4083	0(3)	C2645	6912(1)	C9447	1(3)
99177	1(2)	99345	1(2)	A0225	0(3)	A5507	0(3)	A9520	1(3)	B4087	0(3)	C5271	1(2)	C9460	100(1)
99183	1(3)	99347	1(3)	A0380	0(3)	A5508	0(3)	A9521	2(3)	B4088	0(3)	C5272	3(2)	C9497	1(3)
99184	1(2)	99348	1(3)	A0382	0(3)	A5510	0(3)	A9524	10(3)	B4149	0(3)	C5273	1(2)	C9600	3(3)
99191	1(3)	99349	1(3)	A0384	0(3)	A5512	0(3)	A9526	2(3)	B4153	0(3)	C5274	35(3)	C9601	2(3)
99192	1(3)	99350	1(3)	A0390	0(3)	A5513	0(3)	A9527	195(3)	B4157	0(3)	C5275	1(2)	C9602	2(3)
99195	2(3)	99354	1(2)	A0392	0(3)	A6501	2(1)	A9528	10(3)	B4160	0(3)	C5276	3(2)	C9603	2(3)
99201	1(2)	99355	4(3)	A0394	0(3)	A6502	2(1)	A9529	10(3)	B4164	0(3)	C5277	1(2)	C9604	2(3)
99202	1(2)	99356	1(2)	A0396	0(3)	A6503	2(1)	A9530	200(3)	B4168	0(3)	C5278	15(3)	C9605	2(3)
99203	1(2)	99357	4(3)	A0398	0(3)	A6504	4(1)	A9531	100(3)	B4172	0(3)	C8900	1(3)	C9606	1(3)
99204	1(2)	99366	0(3)	A0420	0(3)	A6505	4(1)	A9532	10(3)	B4176	0(3)	C8901	1(3)	C9607	1(2)
99205	1(2)	99367	0(3)	A0422	0(3)	A6506	4(1)	A9536	1(3)	B4178	0(3)	C8902	1(3)	C9608	2(3)
99211	1(3)	99368	0(3)	A0424	0(3)	A6507	4(1)	A9537	1(3)	B4180	0(3)	C8903	1(3)	C9725	1(3)
99212	2(3)	99406	1(2)	A0425	250(1)	A6508	4(1)	A9538	1(3)	B4189	0(3)	C8904	1(3)	C9727	1(2)
99213	2(3)	99407	1(2)	A0426	2(3)	A6509	2(1)	A9539	2(3)	B4199	0(3)	C8905	1(3)	C9728	1(2)
99214	2(3)	99415	1(2)	A0427	2(3)	A6510	2(1)	A9540	2(3)	B5000	0(3)	C8906	1(3)	C9733	1(3)
99215	1(3)	99416	2(1)	A0428	4(3)	A6511	2(1)	A9541	1(3)	B5100	0(3)	C8907	1(3)	C9734	1(3)
99217	1(2)	99446	1(2)	A0429	2(3)	A6513	0(3)	A9542	1(3)	B5200	0(3)	C8908	1(3)	C9739	1(2)
99218	1(2)	99447	1(2)	A0430	1(3)	A6531	0(3)	A9543	1(3)	C1716	4(3)	C8909	1(3)	C9740	1(2)
99219	1(2)	99448	1(2)	A0431	1(3)	A6532	0(3)	A9544	1(3)	C1717	10(3)	C8910	1(3)	C9741	1(3)
99220	1(2)	99449	1(2)	A0432	1(3)	A6545	0(3)	A9545	1(3)	C1719	99(3)	C8911	1(3)	C9742	1(2)
99221	1(3)	99455	1(3)	A0433	1(3)	A7000	0(3)	A9546	1(3)	C1721	1(3)	C8912	1(3)	E0100	0(3)
99222	1(3)	99456	1(3)	A0434	2(3)	A7003	0(3)	A9547	2(3)	C1722	1(3)	C8913	1(3)	E0105	0(3)
99223	1(3)	99460	1(2)	A0435	999(3)	A7005	0(3)	A9548	2(3)	C1749	1(3)	C8914	1(3)	E0110	0(3)
99224	1(2)	99461	1(2)	A0436	300(3)	A7006	0(3)	A9550	1(3)	C1764	1(3)	C8918	1(3)	E0111	0(3)
99225	1(2)	99462	1(2)	A0888	0(3)	A7013	0(3)	A9551	1(3)	C1767	2(3)	C8919	1(3)	E0112	0(3)
99226	1(2)	99463	1(2)	A0998	0(3)	A7014	0(3)	A9552	1(3)	C1771	1(3)	C8920	1(3)	E0113	0(3)
99231	1(3)	99464	1(2)	A4221	0(3)	A7016	0(3)	A9553	1(3)	C1772	1(3)	C8921	1(3)	E0114	0(3)
99232	1(3)	99465	1(2)	A4235	2(1)	A7017	0(3)	A9554	1(3)	C1776	10(3)	C8922	1(3)	E0116	0(3)
99233	1(3)	99466	1(2)	A4253	0(3)	A7020	0(3)	A9555	2(3)	C1778	4(3)	C8923	1(3)	E0117	0(3)
99234	1(3)	99467	4(3)	A4255	0(3)	A7025	0(3)	A9556	10(3)	C1782	1(3)	C8924	1(3)	E0118	0(3)
99235	1(3)	99468	1(2)	A4257	0(3)	A7026	0(3)	A9557	2(3)	C1785	1(3)	C8925	1(3)	E0130	0(3)
99236	1(3)	99469	1(2)	A4258	0(3)	A7027	0(3)	A9558	7(3)	C1786	1(3)	C8926	1(3)	E0135	0(3)
99238	1(2)	99471	1(2)	A4259	0(3)	A7028	0(3)	A9559	1(1)	C1813	1(3)	C8927	1(3)	E0140	0(3)
99239	1(2)	99472	1(2)	A4301	1(2)	A7029	0(3)	A9560	2(3)	C1815	1(3)	C8928	1(2)	E0141	0(3)
99281	1(3)	99475	1(2)	A4337	0(3)	A7032	0(3)	A9561	1(3)	C1817	1(3)	C8929	1(3)	E0143	0(3)
99282	1(3)	99476	1(2)	A4356	1(1)	A7035	0(3)	A9562	2(3)	C1820	2(3)	C8930	1(2)	E0144	0(3)
99283	1(3)	99477	1(2)	A4459	0(3)	A7036	0(3)	A9563	10(3)	C1822	1(3)	C8931	1(3)	E0147	0(3)

Appendix I — Medically Unlikely Edits (MUEs) — Professional

CPT	MUE	CPT	MUE	CPT	MUE	CPT	MUE	CPT	MUE	CPT	MUE	CPT	MUE	CPT	MUE
E0148	0(3)	E0260	0(3)	E0482	0(3)	E0676	1(3)	E0952	0(3)	E1100	0(3)	E1590	0(3)	E2226	0(3)
E0149	0(3)	E0261	0(3)	E0483	0(3)	E0691	0(3)	E0955	0(3)	E1110	0(3)	E1592	0(3)	E2227	0(3)
E0153	0(3)	E0265	0(3)	E0484	0(3)	E0692	0(3)	E0956	0(3)	E1130	0(3)	E1594	0(3)	E2228	0(3)
E0154	0(3)	E0266	0(3)	E0485	0(3)	E0693	0(3)	E0957	0(3)	E1140	0(3)	E1600	0(3)	E2231	0(3)
E0155	0(3)	E0270	0(3)	E0486	0(3)	E0694	0(3)	E0958	0(3)	E1150	0(3)	E1610	0(3)	E2291	1(2)
E0156	0(3)	E0271	0(3)	E0487	0(3)	E0700	0(3)	E0959	0(3)	E1160	0(3)	E1615	0(3)	E2292	1(2)
E0157	0(3)	E0272	0(3)	E0500	0(3)	E0705	0(3)	E0960	0(3)	E1161	0(3)	E1620	0(3)	E2293	1(2)
E0158	0(3)	E0273	0(3)	E0550	0(3)	E0710	0(3)	E0961	0(3)	E1170	0(3)	E1625	0(3)	E2294	1(2)
E0159	2(2)	E0274	0(3)	E0555	0(3)	E0720	0(3)	E0966	0(3)	E1171	0(3)	E1630	0(3)	E2295	0(3)
E0160	0(3)	E0275	0(3)	E0560	0(3)	E0730	0(3)	E0967	0(3)	E1172	0(3)	E1632	0(3)	E2300	0(3)
E0161	0(3)	E0276	0(3)	E0561	0(3)	E0731	0(3)	E0968	0(3)	E1180	0(3)	E1634	0(3)	E2301	0(3)
E0162	0(3)	E0277	0(3)	E0562	0(3)	E0740	0(3)	E0970	0(3)	E1190	0(3)	E1635	0(3)	E2310	0(3)
E0163	0(3)	E0280	0(3)	E0565	0(3)	E0744	0(3)	E0971	0(3)	E1195	0(3)	E1636	0(3)	E2311	0(3)
E0165	0(3)	E0290	0(3)	E0570	0(3)	E0745	0(3)	E0973	0(3)	E1200	0(3)	E1637	0(3)	E2312	0(3)
E0167	0(3)	E0291	0(3)	E0572	0(3)	E0746	1(3)	E0974	0(3)	E1220	0(3)	E1639	0(3)	E2313	0(3)
E0168	0(3)	E0292	0(3)	E0574	0(3)	E0747	0(3)	E0978	0(3)	E1221	0(3)	E1700	0(3)	E2321	0(3)
E0170	0(3)	E0293	0(3)	E0575	0(3)	E0748	0(3)	E0981	0(3)	E1222	0(3)	E1701	0(3)	E2322	0(3)
E0171	0(3)	E0294	0(3)	E0580	0(3)	E0749	1(3)	E0982	0(3)	E1223	0(3)	E1702	0(3)	E2323	0(3)
E0172	0(3)	E0295	0(3)	E0585	0(3)	E0755	0(3)	E0983	0(3)	E1224	0(3)	E1800	0(3)	E2324	0(3)
E0175	0(3)	E0296	0(3)	E0600	0(3)	E0760	0(3)	E0984	0(3)	E1225	0(3)	E1801	0(3)	E2325	0(3)
E0181	0(3)	E0297	0(3)	E0601	0(3)	E0761	0(3)	E0985	0(3)	E1226	0(3)	E1802	0(3)	E2326	0(3)
E0182	0(3)	E0300	0(3)	E0602	0(3)	E0762	0(3)	E0986	0(3)	E1228	0(3)	E1805	0(3)	E2327	0(3)
E0184	0(3)	E0301	0(3)	E0603	0(3)	E0764	0(3)	E0988	0(3)	E1229	0(3)	E1806	0(3)	E2328	0(3)
E0185	0(3)	E0302	0(3)	E0604	0(3)	E0765	0(3)	E0990	0(3)	E1230	0(3)	E1810	0(3)	E2329	0(3)
E0186	0(3)	E0303	0(3)	E0605	0(3)	E0766	0(3)	E0992	0(3)	E1231	0(3)	E1811	0(3)	E2330	0(3)
E0187	0(3)	E0304	0(3)	E0606	0(3)	E0769	0(3)	E0994	0(3)	E1232	0(3)	E1812	0(3)	E2331	0(3)
E0188	0(3)	E0305	0(3)	E0607	0(3)	E0770	1(3)	E0995	0(3)	E1233	0(3)	E1815	0(3)	E2340	0(3)
E0189	0(3)	E0310	0(3)	E0610	0(3)	E0776	0(3)	E1002	0(3)	E1234	0(3)	E1816	0(3)	E2341	0(3)
E0190	0(3)	E0315	0(3)	E0615	0(3)	E0779	0(3)	E1003	0(3)	E1235	0(3)	E1818	0(3)	E2342	0(3)
E0191	0(3)	E0316	0(3)	E0616	1(2)	E0780	0(3)	E1004	0(3)	E1236	0(3)	E1820	0(3)	E2343	0(3)
E0193	0(3)	E0325	0(3)	E0617	0(3)	E0781	1(2)	E1005	0(3)	E1237	0(3)	E1821	0(3)	E2351	0(3)
E0194	0(3)	E0326	0(3)	E0618	0(3)	E0782	1(2)	E1006	0(3)	E1238	0(3)	E1825	0(3)	E2358	0(3)
E0196	0(3)	E0328	0(3)	E0619	0(3)	E0783	1(2)	E1007	0(3)	E1240	0(3)	E1830	0(3)	E2359	0(3)
E0197	0(3)	E0329	0(3)	E0620	0(3)	E0784	0(3)	E1008	0(3)	E1250	0(3)	E1831	0(3)	E2361	0(3)
E0198	0(3)	E0350	0(3)	E0621	0(3)	E0785	1(2)	E1009	0(3)	E1260	0(3)	E1840	0(3)	E2363	0(3)
E0199	0(3)	E0352	0(3)	E0625	0(3)	E0786	1(2)	E1010	0(3)	E1270	0(3)	E1841	0(3)	E2365	0(3)
E0200	0(3)	E0370	0(3)	E0627	0(3)	E0791	0(3)	E1011	0(3)	E1280	0(3)	E1902	0(3)	E2366	0(3)
E0202	0(3)	E0371	0(3)	E0628	0(3)	E0830	0(3)	E1012	0(3)	E1285	0(3)	E2000	0(3)	E2367	0(3)
E0203	0(3)	E0372	0(3)	E0629	0(3)	E0840	0(3)	E1014	0(3)	E1290	0(3)	E2100	0(3)	E2368	0(3)
E0205	0(3)	E0373	0(3)	E0630	0(3)	E0849	0(3)	E1015	0(3)	E1295	0(3)	E2101	0(3)	E2369	0(3)
E0210	0(3)	E0424	0(3)	E0635	0(3)	E0850	0(3)	E1016	0(3)	E1300	0(3)	E2120	0(3)	E2370	0(3)
E0215	0(3)	E0425	0(3)	E0636	0(3)	E0855	0(3)	E1017	0(3)	E1310	0(3)	E2201	0(3)	E2371	0(3)
E0217	0(3)	E0430	0(3)	E0637	0(3)	E0856	0(3)	E1018	0(3)	E1352	0(3)	E2202	0(3)	E2373	0(3)
E0218	0(3)	E0431	0(3)	E0638	0(3)	E0860	0(3)	E1020	0(3)	E1353	0(3)	E2203	0(3)	E2374	0(3)
E0221	0(3)	E0434	0(3)	E0639	0(3)	E0870	0(3)	E1028	0(3)	E1354	0(3)	E2204	0(3)	E2375	0(3)
E0225	0(3)	E0435	0(3)	E0640	0(3)	E0880	0(3)	E1029	0(3)	E1355	0(3)	E2205	0(3)	E2376	0(3)
E0231	0(3)	E0439	0(3)	E0641	0(3)	E0890	0(3)	E1030	0(3)	E1356	0(3)	E2206	0(3)	E2377	0(3)
E0232	0(3)	E0440	0(3)	E0642	0(3)	E0900	0(3)	E1031	0(3)	E1357	0(3)	E2207	0(3)	E2378	0(3)
E0235	0(3)	E0441	0(3)	E0650	0(3)	E0910	0(3)	E1035	0(3)	E1358	0(3)	E2208	0(3)	E2381	0(3)
E0236	0(3)	E0442	0(3)	E0651	0(3)	E0911	0(3)	E1037	0(3)	E1372	0(3)	E2209	0(3)	E2382	0(3)
E0239	0(3)	E0443	0(3)	E0652	0(3)	E0912	0(3)	E1038	0(3)	E1390	0(3)	E2210	0(3)	E2383	0(3)
E0240	0(3)	E0444	0(3)	E0655	0(3)	E0920	0(3)	E1039	0(3)	E1391	0(3)	E2211	0(3)	E2384	0(3)
E0241	0(3)	E0445	0(3)	E0656	0(3)	E0930	0(3)	E1050	0(3)	E1392	0(3)	E2212	0(3)	E2385	0(3)
E0242	0(3)	E0446	0(3)	E0657	0(3)	E0935	0(3)	E1060	0(3)	E1405	0(3)	E2213	0(3)	E2386	0(3)
E0243	0(3)	E0455	0(3)	E0660	0(3)	E0936	0(3)	E1070	0(3)	E1406	0(3)	E2214	0(3)	E2387	0(3)
E0244	0(3)	E0457	0(3)	E0665	0(3)	E0940	0(3)	E1083	0(3)	E1500	0(3)	E2215	0(3)	E2388	0(3)
E0245	0(3)	E0459	0(3)	E0666	0(3)	E0941	0(3)	E1084	0(3)	E1510	0(3)	E2216	0(3)	E2389	0(3)
E0246	0(3)	E0462	0(3)	E0667	0(3)	E0942	0(3)	E1085	0(3)	E1520	0(3)	E2217	0(3)	E2390	0(3)
E0247	0(3)	E0465	0(3)	E0668	0(3)	E0944	0(3)	E1086	0(3)	E1530	0(3)	E2218	0(3)	E2391	0(3)
E0248	0(3)	E0466	0(3)	E0669	0(3)	E0945	0(3)	E1087	0(3)	E1540	0(3)	E2219	0(3)	E2392	0(3)
E0249	0(3)	E0470	0(3)	E0670	0(3)	E0946	0(3)	E1088	0(3)	E1550	0(3)	E2220	0(3)	E2394	0(3)
E0250	0(3)	E0471	0(3)	E0671	0(3)	E0947	0(3)	E1089	0(3)	E1560	0(3)	E2221	0(3)	E2395	0(3)
E0251	0(3)	E0472	0(3)	E0672	0(3)	E0948	0(3)	E1090	0(3)	E1570	0(3)	E2222	0(3)	E2396	0(3)
E0255	0(3)	E0480	0(3)	E0673	0(3)	E0950	0(3)	E1092	0(3)	E1575	0(3)	E2224	0(3)	E2397	0(3)
E0256	0(3)	E0481	0(3)	E0675	0(3)	E0951	0(3)	E1093	0(3)	E1580	0(3)	E2225	0(3)	E2402	0(3)

CPT	MUE	CPT	MUE	CPT	MUE	CPT	MUE	CPT	MUE	CPT	MUE	CPT	MUE	CPT	MUE
E2500	0(3)	G0148	1(3)	G0403	1(2)	G6012	2(3)	J0515	3(3)	J0881	500(3)	J1460	10(2)	J1953	300(3)
E2502	0(3)	G0166	2(3)	G0404	1(2)	G6013	2(3)	J0520	0(3)	J0882	200(3)	J1556	300(3)	J1955	11(3)
E2504	0(3)	G0168	2(3)	G0405	1(2)	G6014	2(3)	J0558	24(3)	J0885	60(1)	J1557	300(3)	J1956	4(3)
E2506	0(3)	G0175	1(3)	G0406	1(3)	G6015	2(3)	J0561	24(3)	J0887	360(1)	J1559	375(1)	J1960	0(3)
E2508	0(3)	G0177	0(3)	G0407	1(3)	G6016	2(3)	J0571	0(3)	J0888	360(1)	J1560	1(2)	J1980	2(3)
E2510	0(3)	G0179	1(2)	G0408	1(3)	G6017	2(3)	J0572	0(3)	J0890	0(2)	J1561	300(3)	J1990	0(3)
E2511	0(3)	G0180	1(2)	G0410	1(3)	G9143	1(2)	J0573	0(3)	J0894	100(3)	J1562	375(1)	J2001	60(3)
E2512	0(3)	G0181	1(2)	G0411	1(3)	G9156	1(2)	J0574	0(3)	J0895	12(3)	J1566	300(1)	J2010	10(3)
E2601	0(3)	G0182	1(2)	G0412	1(2)	G9157	1(2)	J0575	0(3)	J0897	120(3)	J1568	300(3)	J2020	6(3)
E2602	0(3)	G0186	1(2)	G0413	1(2)	G9187	1(3)	J0583	250(3)	J0945	4(3)	J1569	300(3)	J2060	4(3)
E2603	0(3)	G0202	1(2)	G0414	1(2)	G9480	1(3)	J0585	600(3)	J1000	1(3)	J1570	4(3)	J2150	8(3)
E2604	0(3)	G0204	2(3)	G0415	1(2)	J0120	1(3)	J0586	300(3)	J1020	8(3)	J1571	20(3)	J2170	8(3)
E2605	0(3)	G0206	2(3)	G0416	1(2)	J0129	100(3)	J0587	300(3)	J1030	8(3)	J1572	300(3)	J2175	4(3)
E2606	0(3)	G0235	1(3)	G0420	2(3)	J0130	6(3)	J0588	600(3)	J1040	4(3)	J1575	900(1)	J2180	0(3)
E2607	0(3)	G0237	8(3)	G0421	4(3)	J0131	400(3)	J0592	6(3)	J1050	1000(3)	J1580	9(3)	J2185	30(3)
E2608	0(3)	G0238	8(3)	G0422	6(2)	J0132	12(3)	J0594	320(3)	J1071	400(3)	J1590	0(3)	J2210	1(3)
E2609	0(3)	G0239	1(3)	G0423	6(2)	J0133	1200(3)	J0595	8(3)	J1094	0(3)	J1595	1(3)	J2212	240(3)
E2611	0(3)	G0245	1(2)	G0424	2(2)	J0135	8(3)	J0596	840(3)	J1100	120(3)	J1599	300(3)	J2248	150(3)
E2612	0(3)	G0246	1(2)	G0425	1(3)	J0153	180(3)	J0597	250(3)	J1110	3(3)	J1600	2(3)	J2250	22(3)
E2613	0(3)	G0247	1(2)	G0426	1(3)	J0171	20(3)	J0598	100(3)	J1120	2(3)	J1602	300(3)	J2260	4(3)
E2614	0(3)	G0248	1(2)	G0427	1(3)	J0178	4(3)	J0600	3(3)	J1160	2(3)	J1610	2(3)	J2265	400(3)
E2615	0(3)	G0249	3(3)	G0429	1(2)	J0180	150(3)	J0610	15(3)	J1162	1(3)	J1620	0(3)	J2270	9(3)
E2616	0(3)	G0250	1(2)	G0432	1(2)	J0190	0(3)	J0620	1(3)	J1165	50(3)	J1626	30(3)	J2274	250(3)
E2617	0(3)	G0257	0(3)	G0433	1(2)	J0200	0(3)	J0630	1(3)	J1170	350(3)	J1630	5(3)	J2278	999(3)
E2619	0(3)	G0259	2(3)	G0435	1(2)	J0202	12(3)	J0636	100(3)	J1180	2(3)	J1631	9(3)	J2280	4(3)
E2620	0(3)	G0260	2(3)	G0436	1(2)	J0205	0(3)	J0637	20(3)	J1190	8(3)	J1640	626(3)	J2300	4(3)
E2621	0(3)	G0268	1(2)	G0437	1(2)	J0207	4(3)	J0638	180(3)	J1200	8(3)	J1642	40(3)	J2310	4(3)
E2622	0(3)	G0270	8(3)	G0438	1(2)	J0210	4(3)	J0640	24(3)	J1205	4(3)	J1644	40(3)	J2315	380(3)
E2623	0(3)	G0271	4(3)	G0439	1(2)	J0215	30(3)	J0641	1200(3)	J1212	1(3)	J1645	10(3)	J2320	4(3)
E2624	0(3)	G0277	5(3)	G0442	1(2)	J0220	1(3)	J0670	10(3)	J1230	3(3)	J1650	30(3)	J2323	300(3)
E2625	0(3)	G0278	1(2)	G0443	1(2)	J0221	300(3)	J0690	12(3)	J1240	6(3)	J1652	20(3)	J2325	0(3)
E2626	0(3)	G0281	1(3)	G0444	1(2)	J0256	3500(3)	J0692	12(3)	J1245	6(3)	J1655	0(3)	J2353	60(3)
E2627	0(3)	G0283	1(3)	G0445	1(2)	J0257	1400(3)	J0694	8(3)	J1250	2(3)	J1670	1(3)	J2354	60(3)
E2628	0(3)	G0288	1(2)	G0446	1(3)	J0270	32(3)	J0695	60(3)	J1260	2(3)	J1675	0(3)	J2355	2(3)
E2629	0(3)	G0289	1(2)	G0448	1(3)	J0275	1(3)	J0696	16(3)	J1265	20(3)	J1700	0(3)	J2357	90(3)
E2630	0(3)	G0293	1(2)	G0452	6(3)	J0278	15(3)	J0697	4(3)	J1267	150(3)	J1710	0(3)	J2358	405(3)
E2631	0(3)	G0294	1(2)	G0453	40(3)	J0280	7(3)	J0698	10(3)	J1270	8(3)	J1720	10(3)	J2360	2(3)
E2632	0(3)	G0296	1(2)	G0454	1(2)	J0282	5(3)	J0702	18(3)	J1290	30(3)	J1725	250(3)	J2370	2(3)
E2633	0(3)	G0297	1(2)	G0455	1(2)	J0285	5(3)	J0706	1(3)	J1300	120(3)	J1730	0(3)	J2400	4(3)
G0008	1(2)	G0302	1(2)	G0458	1(3)	J0287	20(3)	J0710	0(3)	J1320	0(3)	J1740	3(3)	J2405	64(3)
G0009	1(2)	G0303	1(2)	G0459	1(3)	J0288	0(3)	J0712	120(3)	J1322	220(1)	J1741	8(3)	J2407	120(3)
G0010	1(3)	G0304	1(2)	G0460	1(3)	J0289	50(3)	J0713	12(3)	J1324	108(3)	J1742	2(3)	J2410	2(3)
G0027	1(2)	G0305	1(2)	G0463	0(3)	J0290	24(3)	J0714	4(1)	J1325	1(3)	J1743	66(3)	J2425	125(3)
G0101	1(2)	G0306	1(3)	G0472	1(2)	J0295	12(3)	J0715	0(3)	J1327	1(3)	J1744	30(3)	J2426	819(3)
G0102	1(2)	G0307	1(3)	G0475	1(2)	J0300	8(3)	J0716	4(1)	J1330	1(3)	J1745	150(3)	J2430	3(3)
G0103	1(2)	G0328	1(2)	G0476	1(2)	J0330	10(3)	J0717	400(3)	J1335	2(3)	J1750	45(3)	J2440	4(3)
G0104	1(2)	G0329	1(3)	G0477	1(2)	J0348	200(3)	J0720	15(3)	J1364	2(3)	J1756	500(3)	J2460	0(3)
G0105	1(2)	G0333	0(3)	G0478	1(2)	J0350	0(3)	J0725	10(3)	J1380	4(3)	J1786	900(3)	J2469	10(3)
G0106	1(2)	G0337	1(2)	G0479	1(2)	J0360	2(3)	J0735	50(3)	J1410	4(3)	J1790	2(3)	J2501	2(3)
G0108	6(3)	G0339	1(2)	G0480	1(2)	J0364	6(3)	J0740	2(3)	J1430	10(3)	J1800	6(3)	J2502	60(1)
G0109	12(3)	G0340	2(3)	G0481	1(2)	J0365	0(3)	J0743	16(3)	J1435	1(3)	J1810	0(3)	J2503	2(3)
G0117	1(2)	G0341	1(2)	G0482	1(2)	J0380	1(3)	J0744	6(3)	J1436	0(3)	J1815	8(3)	J2504	15(3)
G0118	1(2)	G0342	1(2)	G0483	1(2)	J0390	0(3)	J0745	2(3)	J1438	2(3)	J1817	0(3)	J2505	1(3)
G0120	1(2)	G0343	1(2)	G3001	1(2)	J0395	0(3)	J0760	4(3)	J1439	750(3)	J1830	1(3)	J2507	8(3)
G0121	1(2)	G0364	2(3)	G6001	1(2)	J0400	39(3)	J0770	5(3)	J1442	3360(3)	J1833	372(3)	J2510	4(3)
G0123	1(3)	G0365	2(3)	G6002	2(3)	J0401	400(3)	J0775	180(3)	J1443	1(3)	J1835	0(3)	J2513	1(3)
G0124	1(3)	G0372	1(2)	G6003	2(3)	J0456	4(3)	J0780	4(3)	J1447	960(3)	J1840	3(3)	J2515	1(3)
G0127	1(2)	G0379	0(3)	G6004	2(3)	J0461	200(3)	J0795	100(3)	J1450	4(3)	J1850	4(3)	J2540	75(3)
G0128	1(3)	G0389	1(2)	G6005	2(3)	J0470	2(3)	J0800	3(3)	J1451	1(3)	J1885	8(3)	J2543	16(3)
G0130	1(2)	G0396	1(2)	G6006	2(3)	J0475	8(3)	J0833	3(3)	J1452	0(3)	J1890	0(3)	J2545	1(3)
G0141	1(3)	G0397	1(2)	G6007	2(3)	J0476	2(3)	J0834	3(3)	J1453	150(3)	J1930	120(3)	J2547	600(3)
G0143	1(3)	G0398	1(2)	G6008	2(3)	J0480	1(3)	J0840	6(3)	J1455	18(3)	J1931	760(3)	J2550	3(3)
G0144	1(3)	G0399	1(2)	G6009	2(3)	J0485	1500(3)	J0850	9(3)	J1457	500(3)	J1940	6(3)	J2560	1(3)
G0145	1(3)	G0400	1(2)	G6010	2(3)	J0490	160(3)	J0875	300(3)	J1458	100(3)	J1945	0(3)	J2562	48(3)
G0147	1(3)	G0402	1(2)	G6011	2(3)	J0500	4(3)	J0878	1500(3)	J1459	300(1)	J1950	12(3)	J2590	3(3)

CPT	MUE	CPT	MUE	CPT	MUE	CPT	MUE	CPT	MUE	CPT	MUE	CPT	MUE	CPT	MUE
J2597	45(3)	J3301	16(3)	J7195	6000(1)	J7628	0(3)	J9041	35(3)	J9307	80(3)	K0672	0(3)	K0884	0(3)
J2650	0(3)	J3302	0(3)	J7196	175(3)	J7629	0(3)	J9042	200(3)	J9308	300(3)	K0730	0(3)	K0885	0(3)
J2670	0(3)	J3303	24(3)	J7197	6300(1)	J7631	4(3)	J9043	60(3)	J9310	12(3)	K0733	0(3)	K0886	0(3)
J2675	1(3)	J3305	0(3)	J7198	6000(1)	J7632	0(3)	J9045	22(3)	J9315	40(3)	K0738	0(3)	K0890	0(3)
J2680	4(3)	J3310	0(3)	J7200	20000(1)	J7633	0(3)	J9047	120(3)	J9320	4(3)	K0743	0(3)	K0891	0(3)
J2690	4(3)	J3315	6(3)	J7201	9000(1)	J7634	0(3)	J9050	6(3)	J9328	400(3)	K0744	0(3)	K0898	1(2)
J2700	48(3)	J3320	0(3)	J7205	9750(1)	J7635	0(3)	J9055	120(3)	J9330	50(3)	K0745	0(3)	K0900	0(3)
J2704	80(3)	J3350	0(3)	J7297	1(3)	J7636	0(3)	J9060	24(3)	J9340	4(3)	K0746	0(3)	K0901	0(3)
J2710	2(3)	J3355	1(3)	J7298	1(3)	J7637	0(3)	J9065	20(3)	J9351	120(3)	K0800	0(3)	K0902	0(3)
J2720	5(3)	J3357	90(3)	J7301	0(3)	J7638	0(3)	J9070	55(3)	J9354	600(3)	K0801	0(3)	L0112	0(3)
J2724	4000(3)	J3360	6(3)	J7308	3(3)	J7639	3(3)	J9098	5(3)	J9355	100(3)	K0802	0(3)	L0113	0(3)
J2725	0(3)	J3364	0(3)	J7309	1(3)	J7640	0(3)	J9100	120(3)	J9357	4(3)	K0806	0(3)	L0120	0(3)
J2730	2(3)	J3365	0(3)	J7310	2(2)	J7641	0(3)	J9120	5(3)	J9360	45(3)	K0807	0(3)	L0130	0(3)
J2760	2(3)	J3370	12(3)	J7311	1(3)	J7642	0(3)	J9130	24(3)	J9370	4(3)	K0808	0(3)	L0140	0(3)
J2765	10(3)	J3380	300(3)	J7312	14(3)	J7643	0(3)	J9150	12(3)	J9371	5(3)	K0812	0(3)	L0150	0(3)
J2770	6(3)	J3385	92(3)	J7313	19(1)	J7644	3(3)	J9151	10(3)	J9390	36(3)	K0813	0(3)	L0160	0(3)
J2778	10(3)	J3396	150(3)	J7315	2(3)	J7645	0(3)	J9155	240(3)	J9395	20(3)	K0814	0(3)	L0170	0(3)
J2780	16(3)	J3400	0(3)	J7316	4(2)	J7647	0(3)	J9160	7(3)	J9400	600(3)	K0815	0(3)	L0172	0(3)
J2783	60(3)	J3410	8(3)	J7321	2(2)	J7648	0(3)	J9165	0(3)	J9600	4(3)	K0816	0(3)	L0174	0(3)
J2785	4(3)	J3411	4(3)	J7323	2(2)	J7649	0(3)	J9171	240(3)	K0001	0(3)	K0820	0(3)	L0180	0(3)
J2788	1(3)	J3415	6(3)	J7324	2(2)	J7650	0(3)	J9175	10(3)	K0002	0(3)	K0821	0(3)	L0190	0(3)
J2791	50(3)	J3420	1(3)	J7325	96(3)	J7657	0(3)	J9178	150(3)	K0003	0(3)	K0822	0(3)	L0200	0(3)
J2793	320(3)	J3430	25(3)	J7326	2(2)	J7658	0(3)	J9179	50(3)	K0004	0(3)	K0823	0(3)	L0220	0(3)
J2794	100(3)	J3465	40(3)	J7327	2(2)	J7659	0(3)	J9185	2(3)	K0005	0(3)	K0824	0(3)	L0450	0(3)
J2795	200(3)	J3470	3(3)	J7328	336(3)	J7660	0(3)	J9190	20(3)	K0006	0(3)	K0825	0(3)	L0452	0(3)
J2796	150(3)	J3471	999(2)	J7330	1(3)	J7665	127(2)	J9200	5(3)	K0007	0(3)	K0826	0(3)	L0454	0(3)
J2800	3(3)	J3472	2(3)	J7336	1120(3)	J7667	0(3)	J9201	20(3)	K0009	0(3)	K0827	0(3)	L0455	0(3)
J2805	3(3)	J3473	450(3)	J7340	100(3)	J7668	0(3)	J9202	3(3)	K0015	0(3)	K0828	0(3)	L0456	0(3)
J2810	5(3)	J3475	20(3)	J7500	0(3)	J7669	0(3)	J9206	42(3)	K0017	0(3)	K0829	0(3)	L0457	0(3)
J2820	15(3)	J3480	40(3)	J7501	1(3)	J7670	0(3)	J9207	90(3)	K0018	0(3)	K0830	0(3)	L0458	0(3)
J2850	16(3)	J3485	160(3)	J7502	0(3)	J7676	0(3)	J9208	15(3)	K0019	0(3)	K0831	0(3)	L0460	0(3)
J2860	170(3)	J3486	4(3)	J7504	15(3)	J7680	0(3)	J9209	55(3)	K0020	0(3)	K0835	0(3)	L0462	0(3)
J2910	0(3)	J3489	5(3)	J7505	1(3)	J7681	0(3)	J9211	6(3)	K0037	0(3)	K0836	0(3)	L0464	0(3)
J2916	20(3)	J3520	0(3)	J7507	0(3)	J7682	2(3)	J9212	0(3)	K0038	0(3)	K0837	0(3)	L0466	0(3)
J2920	25(3)	J3530	0(3)	J7508	0(3)	J7683	0(3)	J9213	12(3)	K0039	0(3)	K0838	0(3)	L0467	0(3)
J2930	25(3)	J7030	5(3)	J7509	0(3)	J7684	0(3)	J9214	100(3)	K0040	0(3)	K0839	0(3)	L0468	0(3)
J2940	0(3)	J7040	6(3)	J7510	0(3)	J7685	0(3)	J9215	0(3)	K0041	0(3)	K0840	0(3)	L0469	0(3)
J2941	8(3)	J7042	6(3)	J7511	9(3)	J7686	1(3)	J9216	2(3)	K0042	0(3)	K0841	0(3)	L0470	0(3)
J2950	0(3)	J7050	10(3)	J7512	0(3)	J8501	0(3)	J9217	6(3)	K0043	0(3)	K0842	0(3)	L0472	0(3)
J2993	2(3)	J7060	10(3)	J7513	6(3)	J8510	0(3)	J9218	1(3)	K0044	0(3)	K0843	0(3)	L0480	0(3)
J2995	0(3)	J7070	4(3)	J7515	0(3)	J8520	0(3)	J9219	1(3)	K0045	0(3)	K0848	0(3)	L0482	0(3)
J2997	8(3)	J7100	2(3)	J7516	1(3)	J8521	0(3)	J9225	1(3)	K0046	0(3)	K0849	0(3)	L0484	0(3)
J3000	2(3)	J7110	2(3)	J7517	0(3)	J8530	0(3)	J9226	1(3)	K0047	0(3)	K0850	0(3)	L0486	0(3)
J3010	100(3)	J7120	4(3)	J7518	0(3)	J8540	0(3)	J9228	1100(3)	K0050	0(3)	K0851	0(3)	L0488	0(3)
J3030	1(3)	J7121	4(3)	J7520	0(3)	J8560	0(3)	J9230	5(3)	K0051	0(3)	K0852	0(3)	L0490	0(3)
J3060	900(3)	J7131	500(3)	J7525	2(3)	J8562	0(3)	J9245	9(3)	K0052	0(3)	K0853	0(3)	L0491	0(3)
J3070	3(3)	J7178	7700(1)	J7527	0(3)	J8600	0(3)	J9250	25(3)	K0053	0(3)	K0854	0(3)	L0492	0(3)
J3090	200(3)	J7180	6000(1)	J7604	0(3)	J8610	0(3)	J9260	20(3)	K0056	0(3)	K0855	0(3)	L0621	0(3)
J3095	150(3)	J7181	3850(1)	J7605	2(3)	J8650	0(3)	J9261	80(3)	K0065	0(3)	K0856	0(3)	L0622	0(3)
J3101	50(3)	J7182	22000(1)	J7606	2(3)	J8655	0(3)	J9262	700(3)	K0069	0(3)	K0857	0(3)	L0623	0(3)
J3105	2(3)	J7183	15000(1)	J7607	0(3)	J8700	0(3)	J9263	700(3)	K0070	0(3)	K0858	0(3)	L0624	0(3)
J3110	2(3)	J7185	4000(1)	J7608	3(3)	J8705	0(3)	J9266	2(3)	K0071	0(3)	K0859	0(3)	L0625	0(3)
J3121	400(3)	J7186	8000(1)	J7609	0(3)	J9000	20(3)	J9267	750(3)	K0072	0(3)	K0860	0(3)	L0626	0(3)
J3145	750(3)	J7187	7500(1)	J7610	0(3)	J9015	1(3)	J9268	1(3)	K0073	0(3)	K0861	0(3)	L0627	0(3)
J3230	2(3)	J7188	22000(1)	J7611	10(3)	J9017	30(3)	J9270	0(3)	K0077	0(3)	K0862	0(3)	L0628	0(3)
J3240	1(3)	J7189	13000(1)	J7612	10(3)	J9019	60(3)	J9271	300(3)	K0105	0(3)	K0863	0(3)	L0629	0(3)
J3243	150(3)	J7190	30000(1)	J7613	10(3)	J9020	0(3)	J9280	12(3)	K0195	0(3)	K0864	0(3)	L0630	0(3)
J3246	1(3)	J7191	0(3)	J7614	10(3)	J9025	300(3)	J9293	8(3)	K0455	0(3)	K0868	0(3)	L0631	0(3)
J3250	2(3)	J7192	22000(1)	J7615	0(3)	J9027	100(3)	J9299	440(3)	K0462	0(3)	K0869	0(3)	L0632	0(3)
J3260	8(3)	J7193	4000(1)	J7620	6(3)	J9031	1(3)	J9300	0(3)	K0602	0(3)	K0870	0(3)	L0633	0(3)
J3262	800(3)	J7194	9000(1)	J7622	0(3)	J9032	300(3)	J9301	100(3)	K0605	0(3)	K0871	0(3)	L0634	0(3)
J3265	0(3)			J7624	0(3)	J9033	300(3)	J9302	200(3)	K0606	0(3)	K0877	0(3)	L0635	0(3)
J3280	0(3)			J7626	2(3)	J9035	180(3)	J9303	100(3)	K0607	0(3)	K0878	0(3)	L0636	0(3)
J3285	1(3)			J7627	0(3)	J9039	35(3)	J9305	150(3)	K0608	0(3)	K0879	0(3)	L0637	0(3)
J3300	160(3)					J9040	4(3)	J9306	840(3)	K0609	0(3)	K0880	0(3)	L0638	0(3)

CPT	MUE	CPT	MUE	CPT	MUE	CPT	MUE	CPT	MUE	CPT	MUE	CPT	MUE	CPT	MUE
L0639	0(3)	L1690	0(3)	L2132	0(3)	L2680	0(3)	L3480	0(3)	L3960	0(3)	L5400	0(3)	L5673	0(3)
L0640	0(3)	L1700	0(3)	L2134	0(3)	L2750	0(3)	L3485	0(3)	L3961	0(3)	L5410	0(3)	L5676	0(3)
L0641	0(3)	L1710	0(3)	L2136	0(3)	L2755	0(3)	L3500	0(3)	L3962	0(3)	L5420	0(3)	L5677	0(3)
L0642	0(3)	L1720	0(3)	L2180	0(3)	L2760	0(3)	L3510	0(3)	L3967	0(3)	L5430	0(3)	L5678	0(3)
L0643	0(3)	L1730	0(3)	L2182	0(3)	L2768	0(3)	L3520	0(3)	L3971	0(3)	L5450	0(3)	L5679	0(3)
L0648	0(3)	L1755	0(3)	L2184	0(3)	L2780	0(3)	L3530	0(3)	L3973	0(3)	L5460	0(3)	L5680	0(3)
L0649	0(3)	L1810	0(3)	L2186	0(3)	L2785	0(3)	L3540	0(3)	L3975	0(3)	L5500	0(3)	L5681	0(3)
L0650	0(3)	L1812	0(3)	L2188	0(3)	L2795	0(3)	L3550	0(3)	L3976	0(3)	L5505	0(3)	L5682	0(3)
L0651	0(3)	L1820	0(3)	L2190	0(3)	L2800	0(3)	L3560	0(3)	L3977	0(3)	L5510	0(3)	L5683	0(3)
L0700	0(3)	L1830	0(3)	L2192	0(3)	L2810	0(3)	L3570	0(3)	L3978	0(3)	L5520	0(3)	L5684	0(3)
L0710	0(3)	L1831	0(3)	L2200	0(3)	L2820	0(3)	L3580	0(3)	L3980	0(3)	L5530	0(3)	L5685	0(3)
L0810	0(3)	L1832	0(3)	L2210	0(3)	L2830	0(3)	L3590	0(3)	L3981	0(3)	L5535	0(3)	L5686	0(3)
L0820	0(3)	L1833	0(3)	L2220	0(3)	L3000	0(3)	L3595	0(3)	L3982	0(3)	L5540	0(3)	L5688	0(3)
L0830	0(3)	L1834	0(3)	L2230	0(3)	L3001	0(3)	L3600	0(3)	L3984	0(3)	L5560	0(3)	L5690	0(3)
L0859	0(3)	L1836	0(3)	L2232	0(3)	L3002	0(3)	L3610	0(3)	L4000	0(3)	L5570	0(3)	L5692	0(3)
L0861	0(3)	L1840	0(3)	L2240	0(3)	L3003	0(3)	L3620	0(3)	L4002	0(3)	L5580	0(3)	L5694	0(3)
L0970	0(3)	L1843	0(3)	L2250	0(3)	L3010	0(3)	L3630	0(3)	L4010	0(3)	L5585	0(3)	L5695	0(3)
L0972	0(3)	L1844	0(3)	L2260	0(3)	L3020	0(3)	L3640	0(3)	L4020	0(3)	L5590	0(3)	L5696	0(3)
L0974	0(3)	L1845	0(3)	L2265	0(3)	L3030	0(3)	L3650	0(3)	L4030	0(3)	L5595	0(3)	L5697	0(3)
L0976	0(3)	L1846	0(3)	L2270	0(3)	L3031	0(3)	L3660	0(3)	L4040	0(3)	L5600	0(3)	L5698	0(3)
L0978	0(3)	L1847	0(3)	L2275	0(3)	L3040	0(3)	L3670	0(3)	L4045	0(3)	L5610	0(3)	L5699	0(3)
L0980	0(3)	L1848	0(3)	L2280	0(3)	L3050	0(3)	L3671	0(3)	L4050	0(3)	L5611	0(3)	L5700	0(3)
L0982	0(3)	L1850	0(3)	L2300	0(3)	L3060	0(3)	L3674	0(3)	L4055	0(3)	L5613	0(3)	L5701	0(3)
L0984	0(3)	L1860	0(3)	L2310	0(3)	L3070	0(3)	L3675	0(3)	L4060	0(3)	L5614	0(3)	L5702	0(3)
L1000	0(3)	L1900	0(3)	L2320	0(3)	L3080	0(3)	L3677	0(3)	L4070	0(3)	L5616	0(3)	L5703	0(3)
L1001	0(3)	L1902	0(3)	L2330	0(3)	L3090	0(3)	L3678	0(3)	L4080	0(3)	L5617	0(3)	L5704	0(3)
L1005	0(3)	L1904	0(3)	L2335	0(3)	L3100	0(3)	L3702	0(3)	L4090	0(3)	L5618	0(3)	L5705	0(3)
L1010	0(3)	L1906	0(3)	L2340	0(3)	L3140	0(3)	L3710	0(3)	L4100	0(3)	L5620	0(3)	L5706	0(3)
L1020	0(3)	L1907	0(3)	L2350	0(3)	L3150	0(3)	L3720	0(3)	L4110	0(3)	L5622	0(3)	L5707	0(3)
L1025	0(3)	L1910	0(3)	L2360	0(3)	L3160	0(3)	L3730	0(3)	L4130	0(3)	L5624	0(3)	L5710	0(3)
L1030	0(3)	L1920	0(3)	L2370	0(3)	L3170	0(3)	L3740	0(3)	L4205	0(3)	L5626	0(3)	L5711	0(3)
L1040	0(3)	L1930	0(3)	L2375	0(3)	L3215	0(3)	L3760	0(3)	L4210	0(3)	L5628	0(3)	L5712	0(3)
L1050	0(3)	L1932	0(3)	L2380	0(3)	L3216	0(3)	L3762	0(3)	L4350	0(3)	L5629	0(3)	L5714	0(3)
L1060	0(3)	L1940	0(3)	L2385	0(3)	L3217	0(3)	L3763	0(3)	L4360	0(3)	L5630	0(3)	L5716	0(3)
L1070	0(3)	L1945	0(3)	L2387	0(3)	L3219	0(3)	L3764	0(3)	L4361	0(3)	L5631	0(3)	L5718	0(3)
L1080	0(3)	L1950	0(3)	L2390	0(3)	L3221	0(3)	L3765	0(3)	L4370	0(3)	L5632	0(3)	L5722	0(3)
L1085	0(3)	L1951	0(3)	L2395	0(3)	L3222	0(3)	L3766	0(3)	L4386	0(3)	L5634	0(3)	L5724	0(3)
L1090	0(3)	L1960	0(3)	L2397	0(3)	L3224	0(3)	L3806	0(3)	L4387	0(3)	L5636	0(3)	L5726	0(3)
L1100	0(3)	L1970	0(3)	L2405	0(3)	L3225	0(3)	L3807	0(3)	L4392	0(3)	L5637	0(3)	L5728	0(3)
L1110	0(3)	L1971	0(3)	L2415	0(3)	L3230	0(3)	L3808	0(3)	L4394	0(3)	L5638	0(3)	L5780	0(3)
L1120	0(3)	L1980	0(3)	L2425	0(3)	L3250	0(3)	L3809	0(3)	L4396	0(3)	L5639	0(3)	L5781	0(3)
L1200	0(3)	L1990	0(3)	L2430	0(3)	L3251	0(3)	L3900	0(3)	L4397	0(3)	L5640	0(3)	L5782	0(3)
L1210	0(3)	L2000	0(3)	L2492	0(3)	L3252	0(3)	L3901	0(3)	L4398	0(3)	L5642	0(3)	L5785	0(3)
L1220	0(3)	L2005	0(3)	L2500	0(3)	L3253	0(3)	L3904	0(3)	L4631	0(3)	L5643	0(3)	L5790	0(3)
L1230	0(3)	L2010	0(3)	L2510	0(3)	L3300	0(3)	L3905	0(3)	L5000	0(3)	L5644	0(3)	L5795	0(3)
L1240	0(3)	L2020	0(3)	L2520	0(3)	L3310	0(3)	L3906	0(3)	L5010	0(3)	L5645	0(3)	L5810	0(3)
L1250	0(3)	L2030	0(3)	L2525	0(3)	L3330	0(3)	L3908	0(3)	L5020	0(3)	L5646	0(3)	L5811	0(3)
L1260	0(3)	L2034	0(3)	L2526	0(3)	L3332	0(3)	L3912	0(3)	L5050	0(3)	L5647	0(3)	L5812	0(3)
L1270	0(3)	L2035	0(3)	L2530	0(3)	L3334	0(3)	L3913	0(3)	L5060	0(3)	L5648	0(3)	L5814	0(3)
L1280	0(3)	L2036	0(3)	L2540	0(3)	L3340	0(3)	L3915	0(3)	L5100	0(3)	L5649	0(3)	L5816	0(3)
L1290	0(3)	L2037	0(3)	L2550	0(3)	L3350	0(3)	L3916	0(3)	L5105	0(3)	L5650	0(3)	L5818	0(3)
L1300	0(3)	L2038	0(3)	L2570	0(3)	L3360	0(3)	L3917	0(3)	L5150	0(3)	L5651	0(3)	L5822	0(3)
L1310	0(3)	L2040	0(3)	L2580	0(3)	L3370	0(3)	L3918	0(3)	L5160	0(3)	L5652	0(3)	L5824	0(3)
L1499	1(3)	L2050	0(3)	L2600	0(3)	L3380	0(3)	L3919	0(3)	L5200	0(3)	L5653	0(3)	L5826	0(3)
L1600	0(3)	L2060	0(3)	L2610	0(3)	L3390	0(3)	L3921	0(3)	L5210	0(3)	L5654	0(3)	L5828	0(3)
L1610	0(3)	L2070	0(3)	L2620	0(3)	L3400	0(3)	L3923	0(3)	L5220	0(3)	L5655	0(3)	L5830	0(3)
L1620	0(3)	L2080	0(3)	L2622	0(3)	L3410	0(3)	L3924	0(3)	L5230	0(3)	L5656	0(3)	L5840	0(3)
L1630	0(3)	L2090	0(3)	L2624	0(3)	L3420	0(3)	L3925	0(3)	L5250	0(3)	L5658	0(3)	L5845	0(3)
L1640	0(3)	L2106	0(3)	L2627	0(3)	L3430	0(3)	L3927	0(3)	L5270	0(3)	L5661	0(3)	L5848	0(3)
L1650	0(3)	L2108	0(3)	L2628	0(3)	L3440	0(3)	L3929	0(3)	L5280	0(3)	L5665	0(3)	L5850	0(3)
L1652	0(3)	L2112	0(3)	L2630	0(3)	L3450	0(3)	L3930	0(3)	L5301	0(3)	L5666	0(3)	L5855	0(3)
L1660	0(3)	L2114	0(3)	L2640	0(3)	L3455	0(3)	L3931	0(3)	L5312	0(3)	L5668	0(3)	L5856	0(3)
L1680	0(3)	L2116	0(3)	L2650	0(3)	L3460	0(3)	L3933	0(3)	L5321	0(3)	L5670	0(3)	L5857	0(3)
L1685	0(3)	L2126	0(3)	L2660	0(3)	L3465	0(3)	L3935	0(3)	L5331	0(3)	L5671	0(3)	L5858	0(3)
L1686	0(3)	L2128	0(3)	L2670	0(3)	L3470	0(3)	L3956	0(3)	L5341	0(3)	L5672	0(3)	L5859	0(3)

CPT	MUE	CPT	MUE	CPT	MUE	CPT	MUE	CPT	MUE	CPT	MUE	CPT	MUE	CPT	MUE
L5910	0(3)	L6600	0(3)	L6880	0(3)	L8043	0(3)	L8687	1(1)	Q0114	1(1)	Q2043	1(1)	Q4151	24(1)
L5920	0(3)	L6605	0(3)	L6881	0(3)	L8044	0(3)	L8688	1(1)	Q0115	1(1)	Q2049	14(3)	Q4152	24(1)
L5925	0(3)	L6610	0(3)	L6882	0(3)	L8045	0(3)	L8689	1(1)	Q0138	510(3)	Q2050	14(3)	Q4153	6(1)
L5930	0(3)	L6611	0(3)	L6883	0(3)	L8046	0(3)	L8690	2(2)	Q0139	510(3)	Q2052	1(3)	Q4154	36(1)
L5940	0(3)	L6615	0(3)	L6884	0(3)	L8047	0(3)	L8691	1(3)	Q0144	0(3)	Q3014	1(3)	Q4155	100(1)
L5950	0(3)	L6616	0(3)	L6885	0(3)	L8048	1(3)	L8692	0(3)	Q0161	0(3)	Q3027	30(3)	Q4156	49(1)
L5960	0(3)	L6620	0(3)	L6890	0(3)	L8049	0(3)	L8693	1(3)	Q0162	0(3)	Q3028	0(3)	Q4157	24(1)
L5961	0(3)	L6621	0(3)	L6895	0(3)	L8300	0(3)	L8695	1(1)	Q0163	0(3)	Q4001	1(1)	Q4158	70(1)
L5962	0(3)	L6623	0(3)	L6900	0(3)	L8310	0(3)	L8696	1(3)	Q0164	0(3)	Q4002	1(1)	Q4159	7(1)
L5964	0(3)	L6624	0(3)	L6905	0(3)	L8320	0(3)	P2028	1(3)	Q0166	0(3)	Q4003	2(1)	Q4160	36(1)
L5966	0(3)	L6625	0(3)	L6910	0(3)	L8330	0(3)	P2029	1(3)	Q0167	0(3)	Q4004	2(1)	Q4161	42(1)
L5968	0(3)	L6628	0(3)	L6915	0(3)	L8400	0(3)	P2033	1(3)	Q0169	0(3)	Q4025	1(1)	Q4162	4(1)
L5969	0(3)	L6629	0(3)	L6920	0(3)	L8410	0(3)	P2038	1(3)	Q0173	0(3)	Q4026	1(1)	Q4163	32(1)
L5970	0(3)	L6630	0(3)	L6925	0(3)	L8415	0(3)	P3000	1(3)	Q0174	0(3)	Q4027	1(1)	Q4164	400(1)
L5971	0(3)	L6632	0(3)	L6930	0(3)	L8417	0(3)	P3001	1(3)	Q0175	0(3)	Q4028	1(1)	Q4165	100(1)
L5972	0(3)	L6635	0(3)	L6935	0(3)	L8420	0(3)	P9010	2(3)	Q0177	0(3)	Q4074	3(3)	Q5101	3360(3)
L5974	0(3)	L6637	0(3)	L6940	0(3)	L8430	0(3)	P9011	2(3)	Q0180	0(3)	Q4081	100(3)	Q9950	5(3)
L5975	0(3)	L6638	0(3)	L6945	0(3)	L8435	0(3)	P9012	8(3)	Q0478	1(1)	Q4101	88(3)	Q9951	0(3)
L5976	0(3)	L6640	0(3)	L6950	0(3)	L8440	0(3)	P9016	3(3)	Q0479	1(1)	Q4102	21(3)	Q9953	10(3)
L5978	0(3)	L6641	0(3)	L6955	0(3)	L8460	0(3)	P9017	2(3)	Q0480	1(1)	Q4103	0(3)	Q9954	18(3)
L5979	0(3)	L6642	0(3)	L6960	0(3)	L8465	0(3)	P9019	2(3)	Q0481	1(2)	Q4104	50(3)	Q9955	10(2)
L5980	0(3)	L6645	0(3)	L6965	0(3)	L8470	0(3)	P9020	2(3)	Q0482	1(1)	Q4105	250(3)	Q9956	9(3)
L5981	0(3)	L6646	0(3)	L6970	0(3)	L8480	0(3)	P9021	3(3)	Q0483	1(1)	Q4106	76(3)	Q9957	3(3)
L5982	0(3)	L6647	0(3)	L6975	0(3)	L8485	0(3)	P9022	2(3)	Q0484	1(1)	Q4107	50(3)	Q9958	300(3)
L5984	0(3)	L6648	0(3)	L7007	0(3)	L8500	0(3)	P9023	2(3)	Q0485	1(1)	Q4108	250(3)	Q9959	0(3)
L5985	0(3)	L6650	0(3)	L7008	0(3)	L8501	0(3)	P9031	12(3)	Q0486	1(1)	Q4110	250(3)	Q9960	250(3)
L5986	0(3)	L6655	0(3)	L7009	0(3)	L8507	0(3)	P9032	12(3)	Q0487	1(1)	Q4111	56(3)	Q9961	200(3)
L5987	0(3)	L6660	0(3)	L7040	0(3)	L8509	1(1)	P9033	12(3)	Q0488	1(1)	Q4112	2(3)	Q9962	150(3)
L5988	0(3)	L6665	0(3)	L7045	0(3)	L8510	0(3)	P9034	2(3)	Q0489	1(1)	Q4113	4(3)	Q9963	240(3)
L5990	0(3)	L6670	0(3)	L7170	0(3)	L8511	1(1)	P9035	2(3)	Q0490	1(1)	Q4114	6(3)	Q9964	0(3)
L6000	0(3)	L6672	0(3)	L7180	0(3)	L8514	1(1)	P9036	2(3)	Q0491	1(1)	Q4115	240(3)	Q9966	250(3)
L6010	0(3)	L6675	0(3)	L7181	0(3)	L8515	1(1)	P9037	2(3)	Q0492	1(1)	Q4116	192(3)	Q9967	300(3)
L6020	0(3)	L6676	0(3)	L7185	0(3)	L8600	2(1)	P9038	2(3)	Q0493	1(1)	Q4117	200(3)	Q9969	3(1)
L6026	0(3)	L6677	0(3)	L7186	0(3)	L8604	3(3)	P9039	2(3)	Q0494	1(1)	Q4118	1000(3)	Q9980	50(3)
L6050	0(3)	L6680	0(3)	L7190	0(3)	L8605	4(3)	P9040	3(3)	Q0495	1(1)	Q4119	150(3)	R0070	2(3)
L6055	0(3)	L6682	0(3)	L7191	0(3)	L8606	5(3)	P9041	5(3)	Q0497	2(1)	Q4120	50(3)	R0075	2(3)
L6100	0(3)	L6684	0(3)	L7259	0(3)	L8607	20(3)	P9043	5(3)	Q0498	1(1)	Q4121	78(3)	V2020	0(3)
L6110	0(3)	L6686	0(3)	L7360	0(3)	L8609	1(1)	P9044	10(3)	Q0499	1(1)	Q4122	96(3)	V2025	0(3)
L6120	0(3)	L6687	0(3)	L7362	0(3)	L8610	2(1)	P9045	20(3)	Q0501	1(1)	Q4123	160(3)	V2100	0(3)
L6130	0(3)	L6688	0(3)	L7364	0(3)	L8612	2(1)	P9046	25(3)	Q0502	1(1)	Q4124	140(3)	V2101	0(3)
L6200	0(3)	L6689	0(3)	L7366	0(3)	L8613	2(1)	P9047	20(3)	Q0503	3(1)	Q4125	28(3)	V2102	0(3)
L6205	0(3)	L6690	0(3)	L7367	0(3)	L8614	2(1)	P9048	1(3)	Q0504	1(1)	Q4126	32(3)	V2103	0(3)
L6250	0(3)	L6691	0(3)	L7368	0(3)	L8615	2(1)	P9050	1(3)	Q0506	8(3)	Q4127	100(3)	V2104	0(3)
L6300	0(3)	L6692	0(3)	L7400	0(3)	L8616	2(1)	P9051	2(3)	Q0507	1(3)	Q4128	128(3)	V2105	0(3)
L6310	0(3)	L6693	0(3)	L7401	0(3)	L8617	2(1)	P9052	2(3)	Q0508	1(3)	Q4129	81(3)	V2106	0(3)
L6320	0(3)	L6694	0(3)	L7402	0(3)	L8618	2(1)	P9053	2(3)	Q0509	1(3)	Q4130	100(3)	V2107	0(3)
L6350	0(3)	L6695	0(3)	L7403	0(3)	L8619	2(1)	P9054	2(3)	Q0510	0(3)	Q4131	60(3)	V2108	0(3)
L6360	0(3)	L6696	0(3)	L7404	0(3)	L8621	600(3)	P9055	2(3)	Q0511	0(3)	Q4132	50(3)	V2109	0(3)
L6370	0(3)	L6697	0(3)	L7405	0(3)	L8622	2(1)	P9056	2(3)	Q0512	0(3)	Q4133	113(3)	V2110	0(3)
L6380	0(3)	L6698	0(3)	L7510	4(3)	L8627	2(2)	P9057	2(3)	Q0513	0(3)	Q4134	160(3)	V2111	0(3)
L6382	0(3)	L6703	0(3)	L7900	0(3)	L8628	2(2)	P9058	2(3)	Q0514	0(3)	Q4135	900(3)	V2112	0(3)
L6384	0(3)	L6704	0(3)	L7902	0(3)	L8629	2(2)	P9059	2(3)	Q0515	0(3)	Q4136	900(3)	V2113	0(3)
L6386	0(3)	L6706	0(3)	L8000	0(3)	L8631	4(1)	P9060	2(3)	Q1004	2(1)	Q4137	32(1)	V2114	0(3)
L6388	0(3)	L6707	0(3)	L8001	0(3)	L8641	4(1)	P9070	2(1)	Q1005	2(1)	Q4138	32(1)	V2115	0(3)
L6400	0(3)	L6708	0(3)	L8002	0(3)	L8642	2(1)	P9071	2(1)	Q2004	1(3)	Q4139	2(3)	V2118	0(3)
L6450	0(3)	L6709	0(3)	L8015	0(3)	L8658	4(1)	P9072	2(1)	Q2009	100(3)	Q4140	32(1)	V2121	0(3)
L6500	0(3)	L6711	0(3)	L8020	0(3)	L8659	4(1)	P9603	300(3)	Q2017	12(3)	Q4141	25(1)	V2199	2(3)
L6550	0(3)	L6712	0(3)	L8030	0(3)	L8670	4(1)	P9604	2(3)	Q2026	45(3)	Q4142	600(1)	V2200	0(3)
L6570	0(3)	L6713	0(3)	L8031	0(3)	L8679	3(3)	P9612	1(3)	Q2028	1470(3)	Q4143	96(1)	V2201	0(3)
L6580	0(3)	L6714	0(3)	L8032	0(3)	L8681	1(3)	P9615	1(3)	Q2034	1(1)	Q4145	160(1)	V2202	0(3)
L6582	0(3)	L6715	0(3)	L8035	0(3)	L8682	2(1)	Q0035	1(1)	Q2035	1(2)	Q4146	50(1)	V2203	0(3)
L6584	0(3)	L6721	0(3)	L8039	0(3)	L8683	1(1)	Q0091	1(1)	Q2036	1(2)	Q4147	150(1)	V2204	0(3)
L6586	0(3)	L6722	0(3)	L8040	0(3)	L8684	1(1)	Q0111	2(1)	Q2037	1(2)	Q4148	18(1)	V2205	0(3)
L6588	0(3)	L6805	0(3)	L8041	0(3)	L8685	1(1)	Q0112	3(1)	Q2038	1(2)	Q4149	10(1)	V2206	0(3)
L6590	0(3)	L6810	0(3)	L8042	0(3)	L8686	2(1)	Q0113	2(1)	Q2039	1(2)	Q4150	32(1)	V2207	0(3)

CPT	MUE	CPT	MUE	CPT	MUE	CPT	MUE	CPT	MUE	CPT	MUE	CPT	MUE	CPT	MUE
V2208	0(3)	V2300	0(3)	V2313	0(3)	V2502	0(3)	V2600	0(3)	V2700	0(3)	V2762	0(3)	V5011	0(1)
V2209	0(3)	V2301	0(3)	V2314	0(3)	V2503	0(3)	V2610	0(3)	V2702	0(3)	V2770	0(3)	V5274	0(3)
V2210	0(3)	V2302	0(3)	V2315	0(3)	V2510	0(3)	V2615	0(3)	V2710	0(3)	V2780	0(3)	V5281	0(3)
V2211	0(3)	V2303	0(3)	V2318	0(3)	V2511	0(3)	V2623	0(3)	V2715	0(3)	V2781	0(3)	V5282	0(3)
V2212	0(3)	V2304	0(3)	V2319	0(3)	V2512	0(3)	V2624	0(3)	V2718	0(3)	V2782	0(3)	V5284	0(3)
V2213	0(3)	V2305	0(3)	V2320	0(3)	V2513	0(3)	V2625	0(3)	V2730	0(3)	V2783	0(3)	V5285	0(3)
V2214	0(3)	V2306	0(3)	V2321	0(3)	V2520	2(1)	V2626	0(3)	V2744	0(3)	V2784	0(3)	V5286	0(3)
V2215	0(3)	V2307	0(3)	V2399	0(3)	V2521	2(1)	V2627	0(3)	V2745	0(3)	V2785	2(1)	V5287	0(3)
V2218	0(3)	V2308	0(3)	V2410	0(3)	V2522	2(1)	V2628	0(3)	V2750	0(3)	V2786	0(3)	V5288	0(3)
V2219	0(3)	V2309	0(3)	V2430	0(3)	V2523	2(1)	V2629	0(3)	V2755	0(3)	V2790	1(1)	V5289	0(3)
V2220	0(3)	V2310	0(3)	V2499	2(3)	V2530	0(3)	V2630	2(1)	V2756	0(3)	V2797	0(3)		
V2221	0(3)	V2311	0(3)	V2500	0(3)	V2531	0(3)	V2631	2(1)	V2760	0(3)	V5008	0(1)		
V2299	0(3)	V2312	0(3)	V2501	0(3)	V2599	2(3)	V2632	2(1)	V2761	0(3)	V5010	0(1)		

OPPS

CPT	MUE	CPT	MUE	CPT	MUE	CPT	MUE	CPT	MUE	CPT	MUE	CPT	MUE	CPT	MUE
0001M	1(1)	0216T	1(2)	0310T	1(3)	0394T	2(3)	10140	2(3)	11603	2(3)	12034	1(2)	15157	1(3)
0002M	1(1)	0217T	1(2)	0312T	1(3)	0395T	2(3)	10160	3(3)	11604	2(3)	12035	1(2)	15200	1(2)
0003M	1(1)	0218T	1(2)	0313T	1(3)	0396T	2(2)	10180	2(3)	11606	2(3)	12036	1(2)	15201	9(3)
0006M	1(2)	0219T	1(2)	0314T	1(3)	0397T	1(3)	11000	1(2)	11620	2(3)	12037	1(2)	15220	1(2)
0007M	1(2)	0220T	1(2)	0315T	1(3)	0398T	1(3)	11001	1(3)	11621	2(3)	12041	1(2)	15221	9(3)
0008M	1(3)	0221T	1(2)	0316T	1(3)	0399T	1(3)	11004	1(2)	11622	2(3)	12042	1(2)	15240	1(2)
0019T	1(3)	0222T	1(3)	0317T	1(3)	0400T	1(2)	11005	1(2)	11623	2(3)	12044	1(2)	15241	9(3)
0042T	1(3)	0228T	1(3)	0329T	1(2)	0401T	1(2)	11006	1(2)	11624	2(3)	12045	1(2)	15260	1(2)
0051T	1(2)	0229T	2(3)	0330T	1(3)	0402T	2(2)	11008	1(2)	11626	2(3)	12046	1(2)	15261	6(3)
0052T	1(2)	0230T	1(3)	0331T	1(3)	0403T	2(3)	11010	2(3)	11640	2(3)	12047	1(2)	15271	1(2)
0053T	1(2)	0231T	2(3)	0332T	1(3)	0404T	1(2)	11011	2(3)	11641	2(3)	12051	1(2)	15272	3(3)
0054T	1(3)	0232T	1(3)	0333T	1(2)	0405T	1(2)	11012	2(3)	11642	3(3)	12052	1(2)	15273	1(2)
0055T	1(3)	0234T	2(2)	0335T	2(2)	0406T	2(2)	11042	1(2)	11643	2(3)	12053	1(2)	15274	60(1)
0058T	1(2)	0235T	2(3)	0336T	1(3)	0407T	2(2)	11043	1(2)	11644	2(3)	12054	1(2)	15275	1(2)
0071T	1(2)	0236T	1(2)	0337T	1(3)	0408T	1(3)	11044	1(2)	11646	2(3)	12055	1(2)	15276	3(2)
0072T	1(2)	0237T	2(3)	0338T	1(2)	0409T	1(3)	11045	12(3)	11719	1(2)	12056	1(2)	15277	1(2)
0075T	1(2)	0238T	2(3)	0339T	1(2)	0410T	1(3)	11046	10(3)	11720	1(2)	12057	1(2)	15278	15(1)
0076T	1(2)	0249T	1(2)	0347T	1(3)	0411T	1(3)	11047	10(3)	11721	1(2)	13100	1(2)	15570	2(3)
0095T	1(3)	0253T	1(3)	0348T	1(3)	0412T	1(2)	11055	1(2)	11730	1(2)	13101	1(2)	15572	2(3)
0098T	2(3)	0254T	2(2)	0349T	1(3)	0413T	1(3)	11056	1(2)	11732	9(3)	13102	9(3)	15574	2(3)
0100T	2(2)	0255T	2(2)	0350T	1(3)	0414T	1(2)	11057	1(2)	11740	3(3)	13120	1(2)	15576	2(3)
0101T	1(3)	0263T	1(3)	0351T	5(3)	0415T	1(3)	11100	1(2)	11750	6(3)	13121	1(2)	15600	2(3)
0102T	2(2)	0264T	1(3)	0352T	5(3)	0416T	1(3)	11101	6(3)	11752	3(3)	13122	9(3)	15610	2(3)
0106T	4(2)	0265T	1(3)	0353T	2(3)	0417T	1(3)	11200	1(2)	11755	4(3)	13131	1(2)	15620	2(3)
0107T	4(2)	0266T	1(2)	0354T	2(3)	0418T	1(3)	11201	0(3)	11760	4(3)	13132	1(2)	15630	2(3)
0108T	4(2)	0267T	1(3)	0355T	1(2)	0419T	1(2)	11300	5(3)	11762	2(3)	13133	7(3)	15650	1(3)
0109T	4(2)	0268T	1(3)	0356T	4(2)	0420T	1(2)	11301	6(3)	11765	4(3)	13151	1(2)	15731	1(3)
0110T	4(2)	0269T	1(2)	0357T	1(2)	0421T	1(2)	11302	4(3)	11770	1(3)	13152	1(2)	15732	3(3)
0111T	1(3)	0270T	1(3)	0358T	1(2)	0422T	1(3)	11303	3(3)	11771	1(3)	13153	2(3)	15734	4(3)
0126T	1(3)	0271T	1(3)	0359T	1(2)	0423T	1(3)	11305	4(3)	11772	1(3)	13160	2(3)	15736	2(3)
0159T	2(2)	0272T	1(3)	0360T	1(2)	0424T	1(3)	11306	4(3)	11900	1(2)	14000	2(3)	15738	4(3)
0163T	1(3)	0273T	1(3)	0361T	3(3)	0425T	1(3)	11307	3(3)	11901	1(2)	14001	2(3)	15740	3(3)
0164T	4(2)	0274T	1(2)	0362T	1(2)	0426T	1(3)	11308	4(3)	11920	1(2)	14020	4(3)	15750	2(3)
0165T	4(2)	0275T	1(2)	0363T	3(3)	0427T	1(3)	11310	4(3)	11921	1(2)	14021	3(3)	15756	2(3)
0169T	1(3)	0278T	1(3)	0364T	1(2)	0428T	1(2)	11311	4(3)	11922	1(3)	14040	4(3)	15757	2(3)
0171T	1(2)	0281T	1(2)	0365T	1(1)	0429T	1(2)	11312	3(3)	11950	1(2)	14041	3(3)	15758	2(3)
0172T	2(3)	0282T	1(3)	0366T	1(2)	0430T	1(2)	11313	3(3)	11951	1(2)	14060	4(3)	15760	2(3)
0174T	1(3)	0283T	1(3)	0367T	1(1)	0431T	1(2)	11400	3(3)	11952	1(2)	14061	2(3)	15770	2(3)
0175T	1(3)	0284T	1(3)	0368T	1(2)	0432T	1(3)	11401	3(3)	11954	1(3)	14301	2(3)	15775	1(2)
0178T	1(3)	0285T	1(3)	0369T	1(1)	0433T	1(3)	11402	3(3)	11960	2(3)	14302	8(3)	15776	1(2)
0179T	1(3)	0286T	1(2)	0370T	1(3)	0434T	1(3)	11403	2(3)	11970	2(3)	14350	2(3)	15777	1(3)
0180T	1(3)	0287T	1(3)	0371T	1(3)	0435T	1(3)	11404	2(3)	11971	2(3)	15002	1(2)	15780	1(2)
0184T	1(3)	0288T	1(2)	0372T	1(3)	0436T	1(3)	11406	2(3)	11976	1(2)	15003	60(3)	15781	1(3)
0190T	2(2)	0289T	2(2)	0373T	1(2)	0437T	1(3)	11420	3(3)	11980	1(2)	15004	1(2)	15782	1(3)
0191T	2(2)	0290T	1(3)	0374T	1(1)	0438T	1(2)	11421	3(3)	11981	1(3)	15005	19(3)	15783	1(3)
0195T	1(2)	0291T	1(2)	0375T	1(2)	0439T	1(3)	11422	3(3)	11982	1(3)	15040	1(2)	15786	1(2)
0196T	1(2)	0292T	1(3)	0376T	2(3)	0440T	3(1)	11423	2(3)	11983	1(3)	15050	1(3)	15787	2(3)
0198T	2(2)	0293T	1(2)	0377T	1(2)	0441T	3(1)	11424	2(3)	12001	1(2)	15100	1(2)	15788	1(2)
01996	1(2)	0294T	1(3)	0378T	1(2)	0442T	3(1)	11426	2(3)	12002	1(2)	15101	40(3)	15789	1(2)
0200T	1(2)	0295T	1(2)	0379T	1(2)	0443T	1(2)	11440	4(3)	12004	1(2)	15110	1(2)	15792	1(3)
0201T	1(2)	0296T	1(2)	0380T	1(2)	0444T	1(2)	11441	3(3)	12005	1(2)	15111	5(3)	15793	1(3)
0202T	1(3)	0297T	1(2)	0381T	1(2)	0445T	1(2)	11442	3(3)	12006	1(2)	15115	1(2)	15819	1(2)
0205T	3(3)	0298T	1(2)	0382T	1(2)	10021	4(3)	11443	2(3)	12007	1(2)	15116	2(3)	15820	1(2)
0206T	1(3)	0299T	1(2)	0383T	1(2)	10022	4(3)	11444	2(3)	12011	1(2)	15120	1(2)	15821	1(2)
0207T	2(2)	0300T	1(3)	0384T	1(2)	10030	2(3)	11446	2(3)	12013	1(2)	15121	8(3)	15822	1(2)
0208T	1(3)	0301T	1(3)	0385T	1(2)	10035	1(2)	11450	1(2)	12014	1(2)	15130	1(2)	15823	1(2)
0209T	1(3)	0302T	1(3)	0386T	1(2)	10036	2(1)	11451	1(2)	12015	1(2)	15131	2(3)	15824	1(2)
0210T	1(3)	0303T	1(3)	0387T	1(3)	10040	1(2)	11462	1(2)	12016	1(2)	15135	1(2)	15825	1(2)
0211T	1(3)	0304T	1(3)	0388T	1(3)	10060	1(2)	11463	1(2)	12017	1(2)	15136	1(3)	15826	1(2)
0212T	1(3)	0305T	1(3)	0389T	1(3)	10061	1(2)	11470	3(2)	12018	1(2)	15150	1(2)	15828	1(2)
0213T	1(2)	0306T	1(3)	0390T	1(3)	10080	1(3)	11471	2(3)	12020	2(3)	15151	1(2)	15829	1(2)
0214T	1(2)	0307T	1(3)	0391T	1(3)	10081	1(3)	11600	2(3)	12021	3(3)	15152	5(1)	15830	1(2)
0215T	1(2)	0308T	1(3)	0392T	1(2)	10120	3(3)	11601	2(3)	12031	1(2)	15155	1(2)	15832	1(2)
		0309T	1(3)	0393T	1(2)	10121	2(3)	11602	3(3)	12032	1(2)	15156	1(2)	15833	1(2)

CPT	MUE	CPT	MUE	CPT	MUE	CPT	MUE	CPT	MUE	CPT	MUE	CPT	MUE	CPT	MUE
15834	1(2)	17281	6(3)	19364	1(2)	20838	1(2)	21110	2(3)	21295	1(2)	21556	3(3)	22511	1(2)
15835	1(3)	17282	5(3)	19366	1(2)	20900	2(3)	21116	1(2)	21296	1(2)	21557	1(3)	22512	5(3)
15836	1(2)	17283	4(3)	19367	1(2)	20902	2(3)	21120	1(2)	21310	1(2)	21558	1(3)	22513	1(2)
15837	2(3)	17284	3(3)	19368	1(2)	20910	1(3)	21121	1(2)	21315	1(2)	21600	5(3)	22514	1(2)
15838	1(2)	17286	3(3)	19369	1(2)	20912	1(3)	21122	1(2)	21320	1(2)	21610	1(3)	22515	5(3)
15839	2(3)	17311	4(3)	19370	1(2)	20920	1(3)	21123	1(2)	21325	1(2)	21615	1(2)	22532	1(2)
15840	1(3)	17312	6(3)	19371	1(2)	20922	1(3)	21125	2(2)	21330	1(2)	21616	1(2)	22533	1(2)
15841	2(3)	17313	3(3)	19380	1(2)	20924	2(3)	21127	2(3)	21335	1(2)	21620	1(2)	22534	3(3)
15842	2(3)	17314	4(3)	19396	1(2)	20926	2(3)	21137	1(2)	21336	1(2)	21627	1(2)	22548	1(2)
15845	2(3)	17315	15(3)	20005	4(3)	20931	1(2)	21138	1(2)	21337	1(2)	21630	1(2)	22551	1(2)
15847	1(2)	17340	1(2)	20100	2(3)	20937	1(2)	21139	1(2)	21338	1(2)	21632	1(2)	22552	5(3)
15851	1(2)	17360	1(2)	20101	2(3)	20938	1(2)	21141	1(2)	21339	1(2)	21685	1(2)	22554	1(2)
15852	1(3)	17380	1(3)	20102	3(3)	20950	2(3)	21142	1(2)	21340	1(2)	21700	1(2)	22556	1(2)
15860	1(3)	19000	2(3)	20103	4(3)	20955	1(3)	21143	1(2)	21343	1(2)	21705	1(2)	22558	1(2)
15876	1(2)	19001	5(3)	20150	2(3)	20956	1(3)	21145	1(2)	21344	1(2)	21720	1(3)	22585	7(3)
15877	1(2)	19020	2(3)	20200	2(3)	20957	1(3)	21146	1(2)	21345	1(2)	21725	1(3)	22586	1(2)
15878	1(2)	19030	1(2)	20205	4(3)	20962	1(3)	21147	1(2)	21346	1(2)	21740	1(2)	22590	1(2)
15879	1(2)	19081	1(2)	20206	3(3)	20969	2(3)	21150	1(2)	21347	1(2)	21742	1(2)	22595	1(2)
15920	1(3)	19082	2(3)	20220	4(3)	20970	1(3)	21151	1(2)	21348	1(2)	21743	1(2)	22600	1(2)
15922	1(3)	19083	1(2)	20225	4(3)	20972	2(3)	21154	1(2)	21355	1(2)	21750	1(2)	22610	1(2)
15931	1(3)	19084	2(3)	20240	4(3)	20973	1(2)	21155	1(2)	21356	1(2)	21811	1(2)	22612	1(2)
15933	1(3)	19085	1(2)	20245	4(3)	20974	1(3)	21159	1(2)	21360	1(2)	21812	1(2)	22614	13(3)
15934	1(3)	19086	2(3)	20250	3(3)	20975	1(3)	21160	1(2)	21365	1(2)	21813	1(2)	22630	1(2)
15935	1(3)	19100	4(3)	20251	3(3)	20979	1(3)	21172	1(3)	21366	1(2)	21820	1(2)	22632	4(2)
15936	1(3)	19101	3(3)	20500	2(3)	20982	1(2)	21175	1(2)	21385	1(2)	21825	1(2)	22633	1(2)
15937	1(3)	19105	2(3)	20501	2(3)	20983	1(2)	21179	1(2)	21386	1(2)	21920	3(3)	22634	4(2)
15940	2(3)	19110	1(3)	20520	4(3)	20985	2(3)	21180	1(2)	21387	1(2)	21925	3(3)	22800	1(2)
15941	2(3)	19112	2(3)	20525	4(3)	21010	1(2)	21181	1(3)	21390	1(2)	21930	5(3)	22802	1(2)
15944	2(3)	19120	1(2)	20526	1(2)	21011	4(3)	21182	1(2)	21395	1(2)	21931	3(3)	22804	1(2)
15945	2(3)	19125	1(2)	20527	2(3)	21012	3(3)	21183	1(2)	21400	1(2)	21932	4(3)	22808	1(2)
15946	2(3)	19126	3(3)	20550	5(3)	21013	4(3)	21184	1(2)	21401	1(2)	21933	3(3)	22810	1(2)
15950	2(3)	19260	2(3)	20551	5(3)	21014	3(3)	21188	1(2)	21406	1(2)	21935	1(3)	22812	1(2)
15951	2(3)	19271	1(3)	20552	1(2)	21015	1(3)	21193	1(2)	21407	1(2)	21936	1(3)	22818	1(2)
15952	2(3)	19272	1(3)	20553	1(2)	21016	2(3)	21194	1(2)	21408	1(2)	22010	2(3)	22819	1(2)
15953	2(3)	19281	1(2)	20555	1(3)	21025	2(3)	21195	1(2)	21421	1(2)	22015	2(3)	22830	1(2)
15956	2(3)	19282	2(3)	20600	6(3)	21026	2(3)	21196	1(2)	21422	1(2)	22100	1(2)	22840	1(2)
15958	2(3)	19283	1(2)	20604	4(3)	21029	1(3)	21198	1(3)	21423	1(2)	22101	1(2)	22842	1(3)
16000	1(2)	19284	2(3)	20605	4(3)	21030	1(3)	21199	1(2)	21431	1(2)	22102	1(2)	22843	1(3)
16020	1(3)	19285	1(2)	20606	4(3)	21031	2(3)	21206	1(3)	21432	1(2)	22103	3(3)	22844	1(3)
16025	1(3)	19286	2(3)	20610	4(3)	21032	1(3)	21208	1(3)	21433	1(2)	22110	1(2)	22845	1(3)
16030	1(3)	19287	1(2)	20611	4(3)	21034	1(3)	21209	1(3)	21435	1(2)	22112	1(2)	22846	1(3)
16035	1(2)	19288	2(3)	20612	2(3)	21040	2(3)	21210	2(3)	21436	1(2)	22114	1(2)	22847	1(3)
16036	8(3)	19296	1(3)	20615	1(3)	21044	1(3)	21215	2(3)	21440	2(2)	22116	3(3)	22848	1(2)
17000	1(2)	19297	2(3)	20650	4(3)	21045	1(3)	21230	2(3)	21445	2(2)	22206	1(2)	22849	1(2)
17003	13(2)	19298	1(2)	20660	1(2)	21046	2(3)	21235	2(3)	21450	1(2)	22207	1(2)	22850	1(2)
17004	1(2)	19300	1(2)	20661	1(2)	21047	2(3)	21240	1(2)	21451	1(2)	22208	6(3)	22851	5(3)
17106	1(2)	19301	1(2)	20662	1(2)	21048	2(3)	21242	1(2)	21452	1(2)	22210	1(2)	22852	1(2)
17107	1(2)	19302	1(2)	20663	1(2)	21049	1(3)	21243	1(2)	21453	1(2)	22212	1(2)	22855	1(2)
17108	1(2)	19303	1(2)	20664	1(2)	21050	1(2)	21244	1(2)	21454	1(2)	22214	1(2)	22856	1(2)
17110	1(2)	19304	1(2)	20665	1(2)	21060	1(2)	21245	2(2)	21461	1(2)	22216	6(3)	22857	1(2)
17111	1(2)	19305	1(2)	20670	3(3)	21070	1(2)	21246	2(2)	21462	1(2)	22220	1(2)	22858	1(2)
17250	4(3)	19306	1(2)	20680	3(3)	21073	1(2)	21247	1(2)	21465	1(2)	22222	1(2)	22861	1(2)
17260	7(3)	19307	1(2)	20690	2(3)	21076	1(2)	21248	2(3)	21470	1(2)	22224	1(2)	22862	1(2)
17261	7(3)	19316	1(2)	20692	2(3)	21077	1(2)	21249	2(3)	21480	1(2)	22226	4(3)	22864	1(2)
17262	6(3)	19318	1(2)	20693	2(3)	21079	1(2)	21255	1(2)	21485	1(2)	22305	1(2)	22865	1(2)
17263	5(3)	19324	1(2)	20694	2(3)	21080	1(2)	21256	1(2)	21490	1(2)	22310	1(2)	22900	3(3)
17264	3(3)	19325	1(2)	20696	2(3)	21081	1(2)	21260	1(2)	21495	1(2)	22315	1(2)	22901	2(3)
17266	2(3)	19328	1(2)	20697	4(3)	21082	1(2)	21261	1(2)	21497	1(2)	22318	1(2)	22902	4(3)
17270	6(3)	19330	1(2)	20802	1(2)	21083	1(2)	21263	1(2)	21501	3(3)	22319	1(2)	22903	3(3)
17271	4(3)	19340	1(2)	20805	1(2)	21084	1(2)	21267	1(2)	21502	1(3)	22325	1(2)	22904	1(3)
17272	5(3)	19342	1(2)	20808	1(2)	21085	1(3)	21268	1(2)	21510	1(3)	22326	1(2)	22905	1(3)
17273	4(3)	19350	1(2)	20816	3(3)	21086	1(2)	21270	1(2)	21550	3(3)	22327	1(2)	23000	1(2)
17274	4(3)	19355	1(2)	20822	3(3)	21087	1(2)	21275	1(2)	21552	4(3)	22328	6(3)	23020	1(2)
17276	3(3)	19357	1(2)	20824	1(2)	21088	1(2)	21280	1(2)	21554	2(3)	22505	1(2)	23030	2(3)
17280	6(3)	19361	1(2)	20827	1(2)	21100	1(2)	21282	1(2)	21555	4(3)	22510	1(2)	23031	1(3)

CPT	MUE	CPT	MUE	CPT	MUE	CPT	MUE	CPT	MUE	CPT	MUE	CPT	MUE	CPT	MUE
23035	1(3)	23491	1(2)	24149	1(2)	24620	1(2)	25248	3(3)	25545	1(2)	26113	4(3)	26483	4(3)
23040	1(2)	23500	1(2)	24150	1(3)	24635	1(2)	25250	1(2)	25560	1(2)	26115	4(3)	26485	4(3)
23044	1(3)	23505	1(2)	24152	1(3)	24640	1(2)	25251	1(2)	25565	1(2)	26116	2(3)	26489	3(3)
23065	2(3)	23515	1(2)	24155	1(2)	24650	1(2)	25259	1(2)	25574	1(2)	26117	2(3)	26490	3(3)
23066	2(3)	23520	1(2)	24160	1(2)	24655	1(2)	25260	9(3)	25575	1(2)	26118	1(3)	26492	2(3)
23071	2(3)	23525	1(2)	24164	1(2)	24665	1(2)	25263	4(3)	25600	1(2)	26121	1(2)	26494	1(3)
23073	2(3)	23530	1(2)	24200	3(3)	24666	1(2)	25265	4(3)	25605	1(2)	26123	1(2)	26496	1(3)
23075	3(3)	23532	1(2)	24201	3(3)	24670	1(2)	25270	8(3)	25606	1(2)	26125	4(3)	26497	2(3)
23076	2(3)	23540	1(2)	24220	1(2)	24675	1(2)	25272	4(3)	25607	1(2)	26130	1(3)	26498	1(3)
23077	1(3)	23545	1(2)	24300	1(2)	24685	1(2)	25274	4(3)	25608	1(2)	26135	4(3)	26499	2(3)
23078	1(3)	23550	1(2)	24301	2(3)	24800	1(2)	25275	2(3)	25609	1(2)	26140	3(3)	26500	4(3)
23100	1(2)	23552	1(2)	24305	4(3)	24802	1(2)	25280	9(3)	25622	1(2)	26145	6(3)	26502	3(3)
23101	2(2)	23570	1(2)	24310	3(3)	24900	1(2)	25290	12(3)	25624	1(2)	26160	5(3)	26508	1(2)
23105	1(2)	23575	1(2)	24320	2(3)	24920	1(2)	25295	9(3)	25628	1(2)	26170	5(3)	26510	4(3)
23106	1(2)	23585	1(2)	24330	1(3)	24925	1(2)	25300	1(2)	25630	1(3)	26180	4(3)	26516	1(2)
23107	1(2)	23600	1(2)	24331	1(3)	24930	1(2)	25301	1(2)	25635	1(3)	26185	1(3)	26517	1(2)
23120	1(2)	23605	1(2)	24332	1(2)	24931	1(2)	25310	5(3)	25645	1(3)	26200	2(3)	26518	1(2)
23125	1(2)	23615	1(2)	24340	1(2)	24935	1(2)	25312	5(3)	25650	1(2)	26205	1(3)	26520	4(3)
23130	1(2)	23616	1(2)	24341	2(3)	24940	1(2)	25315	1(3)	25651	1(2)	26210	2(3)	26525	4(3)
23140	1(3)	23620	1(2)	24342	2(3)	25000	2(3)	25316	1(3)	25652	1(2)	26215	2(3)	26530	4(3)
23145	1(3)	23625	1(2)	24343	1(2)	25001	1(3)	25320	1(2)	25660	1(2)	26230	2(3)	26531	4(3)
23146	1(3)	23630	1(2)	24344	1(2)	25020	1(2)	25332	1(2)	25670	1(2)	26235	2(3)	26535	4(3)
23150	1(3)	23650	1(2)	24345	1(2)	25023	1(2)	25335	1(2)	25671	1(2)	26236	2(3)	26536	4(3)
23155	1(3)	23655	1(2)	24346	1(2)	25024	1(2)	25337	1(2)	25675	1(2)	26250	2(3)	26540	4(3)
23156	1(3)	23660	1(2)	24357	2(3)	25025	1(2)	25350	1(3)	25676	1(2)	26260	1(3)	26541	4(3)
23170	1(3)	23665	1(2)	24358	2(3)	25028	4(3)	25355	1(3)	25680	1(2)	26262	1(3)	26542	4(3)
23172	1(3)	23670	1(2)	24359	2(3)	25031	2(3)	25360	1(3)	25685	1(2)	26320	4(3)	26545	4(3)
23174	1(3)	23675	1(2)	24360	1(2)	25035	2(3)	25365	1(3)	25690	1(2)	26340	4(3)	26546	2(3)
23180	1(3)	23680	1(2)	24361	1(2)	25040	1(3)	25370	1(2)	25695	1(2)	26341	2(3)	26548	3(3)
23182	1(3)	23700	1(2)	24362	1(2)	25065	3(3)	25375	1(2)	25800	1(2)	26350	6(3)	26550	1(2)
23184	1(3)	23800	1(2)	24363	1(2)	25066	2(3)	25390	1(2)	25805	1(2)	26352	2(3)	26551	1(2)
23190	1(3)	23802	1(2)	24365	1(2)	25071	3(3)	25391	1(2)	25810	1(2)	26356	4(3)	26553	1(3)
23195	1(2)	23900	1(2)	24366	1(2)	25073	3(3)	25392	1(2)	25820	1(2)	26357	2(3)	26554	1(3)
23200	1(3)	23920	1(2)	24370	1(2)	25075	6(3)	25393	1(2)	25825	1(2)	26358	2(3)	26555	2(3)
23210	1(3)	23921	1(2)	24371	1(2)	25076	5(3)	25394	1(3)	25830	1(2)	26370	3(3)	26556	2(3)
23220	1(3)	23930	2(3)	24400	1(3)	25077	1(3)	25400	1(2)	25900	1(2)	26372	1(3)	26560	2(3)
23330	2(3)	23931	2(3)	24410	1(2)	25078	1(3)	25405	1(2)	25905	1(2)	26373	2(3)	26561	2(3)
23333	1(3)	23935	2(3)	24420	1(2)	25085	1(2)	25415	1(2)	25907	1(2)	26390	2(3)	26562	2(3)
23334	1(2)	24000	1(2)	24430	1(3)	25100	1(2)	25420	1(2)	25909	1(2)	26392	2(3)	26565	3(3)
23335	1(2)	24006	1(2)	24435	1(3)	25101	1(2)	25425	1(2)	25915	1(2)	26410	4(3)	26567	3(3)
23350	1(2)	24065	2(3)	24470	1(2)	25105	1(2)	25426	1(2)	25920	1(2)	26412	3(3)	26568	2(3)
23395	1(2)	24066	2(3)	24495	1(2)	25107	1(2)	25430	1(3)	25922	1(2)	26415	2(3)	26580	1(2)
23397	1(3)	24071	3(3)	24498	1(2)	25109	4(3)	25431	1(3)	25924	1(2)	26416	2(3)	26587	2(3)
23400	1(2)	24073	3(3)	24500	1(2)	25110	3(3)	25440	1(2)	25927	1(2)	26418	4(3)	26590	2(3)
23405	2(3)	24075	5(3)	24505	1(2)	25111	1(3)	25441	1(2)	25929	1(2)	26420	4(3)	26591	4(3)
23406	1(3)	24076	4(3)	24515	1(2)	25112	1(3)	25442	1(2)	25931	1(2)	26426	4(3)	26593	9(3)
23410	1(2)	24077	1(3)	24516	1(2)	25115	1(3)	25443	1(2)	26010	2(3)	26428	2(3)	26596	1(3)
23412	1(2)	24079	1(3)	24530	1(2)	25116	1(3)	25444	1(2)	26011	3(3)	26432	2(3)	26600	2(3)
23415	1(2)	24100	1(2)	24535	1(2)	25118	5(3)	25445	1(2)	26020	4(3)	26433	2(3)	26605	3(3)
23420	1(2)	24101	1(2)	24538	1(2)	25119	1(2)	25446	1(2)	26025	1(2)	26434	2(3)	26607	2(3)
23430	1(2)	24102	1(2)	24545	1(2)	25120	1(3)	25447	4(3)	26030	1(2)	26437	4(3)	26608	5(3)
23440	1(2)	24105	1(2)	24546	1(2)	25125	1(3)	25449	1(2)	26034	2(3)	26440	6(3)	26615	4(3)
23450	1(2)	24110	1(3)	24560	1(3)	25126	1(3)	25450	1(2)	26035	1(3)	26442	5(3)	26641	1(2)
23455	1(2)	24115	1(3)	24565	1(3)	25130	1(3)	25455	1(2)	26037	1(3)	26445	5(3)	26645	1(2)
23460	1(2)	24116	1(3)	24566	1(3)	25135	1(3)	25490	1(2)	26040	1(3)	26449	1(3)	26650	1(2)
23462	1(2)	24120	1(3)	24575	1(3)	25136	1(3)	25491	1(2)	26045	1(2)	26450	6(3)	26665	1(2)
23465	1(2)	24125	1(3)	24576	1(3)	25145	1(3)	25492	1(2)	26055	5(3)	26455	6(3)	26670	2(3)
23466	1(2)	24126	1(3)	24577	1(3)	25150	1(3)	25500	1(2)	26060	5(3)	26460	4(3)	26675	1(3)
23470	1(2)	24130	1(2)	24579	1(3)	25151	1(3)	25505	1(2)	26070	2(3)	26471	4(3)	26676	3(3)
23472	1(2)	24134	1(3)	24582	1(3)	25170	1(3)	25515	1(2)	26075	4(3)	26474	4(3)	26685	3(3)
23473	1(2)	24136	1(3)	24586	1(3)	25210	2(1)	25520	1(2)	26080	4(3)	26476	4(3)	26686	3(3)
23474	1(2)	24138	1(3)	24587	1(2)	25215	1(2)	25525	1(2)	26100	1(3)	26477	4(3)	26700	3(3)
23480	1(2)	24140	1(3)	24600	1(2)	25230	1(2)	25526	1(2)	26105	2(3)	26478	6(3)	26705	3(3)
23485	1(2)	24145	1(3)	24605	1(2)	25240	1(2)	25530	1(2)	26110	3(3)	26479	4(3)	26706	4(3)
23490	1(2)	24147	1(2)	24615	1(2)	25246	1(2)	25535	1(2)	26111	4(3)	26480	4(3)	26715	4(3)

CPT	MUE	CPT	MUE	CPT	MUE	CPT	MUE	CPT	MUE	CPT	MUE	CPT	MUE	CPT	MUE
26720	4(3)	27078	1(2)	27258	1(2)	27409	1(2)	27536	1(2)	27690	2(3)	27870	1(2)	28160	5(3)
26725	4(3)	27080	1(2)	27259	1(2)	27412	1(2)	27538	1(2)	27691	2(3)	27871	1(3)	28171	1(3)
26727	4(3)	27086	1(3)	27265	1(2)	27415	1(2)	27540	1(2)	27692	4(3)	27880	1(2)	28173	2(3)
26735	4(3)	27087	1(3)	27266	1(2)	27416	1(2)	27550	1(2)	27695	1(2)	27881	1(2)	28175	2(3)
26740	3(3)	27090	1(1)	27267	1(2)	27418	1(2)	27552	1(2)	27696	1(2)	27882	1(2)	28190	3(3)
26742	3(3)	27091	1(1)	27268	1(2)	27420	1(2)	27556	1(2)	27698	2(2)	27884	1(2)	28192	2(3)
26746	3(3)	27093	1(1)	27269	1(2)	27422	1(2)	27557	1(2)	27700	1(2)	27886	1(2)	28193	2(3)
26750	3(3)	27095	1(1)	27275	2(2)	27424	1(2)	27558	1(2)	27702	1(2)	27888	1(2)	28200	4(3)
26755	3(3)	27096	1(1)	27279	1(2)	27425	1(2)	27560	1(2)	27703	1(2)	27889	1(2)	28202	2(3)
26756	3(3)	27097	1(3)	27280	1(2)	27427	1(2)	27562	1(2)	27704	1(2)	27892	1(2)	28208	4(3)
26765	5(3)	27098	1(2)	27282	1(2)	27428	1(2)	27566	1(2)	27705	1(3)	27893	1(2)	28210	2(3)
26770	3(3)	27100	1(2)	27284	1(2)	27429	1(2)	27570	1(2)	27707	1(3)	27894	1(2)	28220	1(2)
26775	4(3)	27105	1(3)	27286	1(2)	27430	1(2)	27580	1(2)	27709	1(3)	28001	2(3)	28222	1(2)
26776	4(3)	27110	1(2)	27290	1(2)	27435	1(2)	27590	1(2)	27712	1(2)	28002	3(3)	28225	1(2)
26785	3(3)	27111	1(2)	27295	1(2)	27437	1(2)	27591	1(2)	27715	1(2)	28003	2(3)	28226	1(2)
26820	1(2)	27120	1(2)	27301	3(3)	27438	1(2)	27592	1(2)	27720	1(2)	28005	3(3)	28230	1(2)
26841	1(2)	27122	1(2)	27303	2(3)	27440	1(2)	27594	1(2)	27722	1(2)	28008	2(3)	28232	6(3)
26842	1(2)	27125	1(2)	27305	1(2)	27441	1(2)	27596	1(2)	27724	1(2)	28010	4(1)	28234	6(3)
26843	2(3)	27130	1(2)	27306	1(2)	27442	1(2)	27598	1(2)	27725	1(2)	28011	4(1)	28238	1(2)
26844	2(3)	27132	1(2)	27307	1(2)	27443	1(2)	27600	1(2)	27726	1(2)	28020	2(3)	28240	1(2)
26850	5(3)	27134	1(2)	27310	1(2)	27445	1(2)	27601	1(2)	27727	1(2)	28022	4(3)	28250	1(2)
26852	2(3)	27137	1(2)	27323	2(3)	27446	1(2)	27602	1(2)	27730	1(2)	28024	4(3)	28260	1(2)
26860	1(2)	27138	1(2)	27324	3(3)	27447	1(2)	27603	2(3)	27732	1(2)	28035	1(2)	28261	1(3)
26861	4(3)	27140	1(2)	27325	1(2)	27448	1(3)	27604	2(3)	27734	1(2)	28039	3(3)	28262	1(2)
26862	1(2)	27146	1(3)	27326	1(2)	27450	1(3)	27605	1(2)	27740	1(2)	28041	3(3)	28264	1(2)
26863	3(3)	27147	1(3)	27327	5(3)	27454	1(2)	27606	1(2)	27742	1(2)	28043	4(3)	28270	6(3)
26910	4(3)	27151	1(3)	27328	4(3)	27455	1(3)	27607	2(3)	27745	1(2)	28045	4(3)	28272	6(3)
26951	8(3)	27156	1(2)	27329	1(3)	27457	1(3)	27610	1(2)	27750	1(2)	28046	1(3)	28280	1(2)
26952	5(3)	27158	1(2)	27330	1(2)	27465	1(2)	27612	1(2)	27752	1(2)	28047	1(3)	28285	4(3)
26990	2(3)	27161	1(2)	27331	1(2)	27466	1(2)	27613	4(3)	27756	1(2)	28050	2(3)	28286	1(2)
26991	1(3)	27165	1(2)	27332	1(2)	27468	1(2)	27614	3(3)	27758	1(2)	28052	2(3)	28288	5(3)
26992	2(3)	27170	1(2)	27333	1(2)	27470	1(2)	27615	1(3)	27759	1(2)	28054	2(3)	28289	1(2)
27000	1(3)	27175	1(2)	27334	1(2)	27472	1(2)	27616	1(3)	27760	1(2)	28055	1(3)	28290	1(2)
27001	1(3)	27176	1(2)	27335	1(2)	27475	1(2)	27618	4(3)	27762	1(2)	28060	1(2)	28292	1(2)
27003	1(2)	27177	1(2)	27337	4(3)	27477	1(2)	27619	4(3)	27766	1(2)	28062	1(2)	28293	1(2)
27005	1(2)	27178	1(2)	27339	4(3)	27479	1(2)	27620	1(2)	27767	1(2)	28070	2(3)	28294	1(2)
27006	1(2)	27179	1(2)	27340	1(2)	27485	1(2)	27625	1(2)	27768	1(2)	28072	4(3)	28296	1(2)
27025	1(3)	27181	1(2)	27345	1(2)	27486	1(2)	27626	1(2)	27769	1(2)	28080	4(3)	28297	1(2)
27027	1(2)	27185	1(2)	27347	1(2)	27487	1(2)	27630	2(3)	27780	1(2)	28086	2(3)	28298	1(2)
27030	1(2)	27187	1(2)	27350	1(2)	27488	1(2)	27632	4(3)	27781	1(2)	28088	2(3)	28299	1(2)
27033	1(2)	27193	1(2)	27355	1(3)	27495	1(2)	27634	2(3)	27784	1(2)	28090	2(3)	28300	1(2)
27035	1(2)	27194	1(2)	27356	1(3)	27496	1(2)	27635	1(3)	27786	1(2)	28092	2(3)	28302	1(2)
27036	1(2)	27200	1(2)	27357	1(3)	27497	1(2)	27637	1(3)	27788	1(2)	28100	1(3)	28304	1(3)
27040	2(3)	27202	1(2)	27358	1(3)	27498	1(2)	27638	1(3)	27792	1(2)	28102	1(3)	28305	1(3)
27041	3(3)	27220	1(2)	27360	2(3)	27499	1(2)	27640	1(3)	27808	1(2)	28103	1(3)	28306	1(2)
27043	3(3)	27222	1(2)	27364	1(3)	27500	1(2)	27641	1(3)	27810	1(2)	28104	2(3)	28307	1(2)
27045	3(3)	27226	1(2)	27365	1(3)	27501	1(2)	27645	1(3)	27814	1(2)	28106	1(3)	28308	4(3)
27047	4(3)	27227	1(2)	27370	1(2)	27502	1(2)	27646	1(3)	27816	1(2)	28107	1(3)	28309	1(2)
27048	2(3)	27228	1(2)	27372	2(3)	27503	1(2)	27647	1(3)	27818	1(2)	28108	2(3)	28310	1(2)
27049	1(3)	27230	1(2)	27380	1(2)	27506	1(2)	27648	1(2)	27822	1(2)	28110	1(2)	28312	4(3)
27050	1(2)	27232	1(2)	27381	2(2)	27507	1(2)	27650	1(2)	27823	1(2)	28111	1(2)	28313	4(3)
27052	1(2)	27235	1(2)	27385	2(3)	27508	1(2)	27652	1(2)	27824	1(2)	28112	4(3)	28315	1(2)
27054	1(2)	27236	1(2)	27386	2(3)	27509	1(2)	27654	1(2)	27825	1(2)	28113	1(2)	28320	1(2)
27057	1(2)	27238	1(2)	27390	1(2)	27510	1(2)	27656	1(3)	27826	1(2)	28114	1(2)	28322	2(3)
27059	1(3)	27240	1(2)	27391	1(2)	27511	1(2)	27658	2(3)	27827	1(2)	28116	1(2)	28340	2(3)
27060	1(2)	27244	1(2)	27392	1(2)	27513	1(2)	27659	2(3)	27828	1(2)	28118	1(2)	28341	2(3)
27062	1(2)	27245	1(2)	27393	1(2)	27514	1(2)	27664	2(3)	27829	1(2)	28119	1(2)	28344	1(2)
27065	1(3)	27246	1(2)	27394	1(2)	27516	1(2)	27665	2(3)	27830	1(2)	28120	2(3)	28345	2(3)
27066	1(3)	27248	1(2)	27395	1(2)	27517	1(2)	27675	1(2)	27831	1(2)	28122	4(3)	28360	1(2)
27067	1(3)	27250	1(2)	27396	1(2)	27519	1(2)	27676	1(2)	27832	1(2)	28124	4(3)	28400	1(2)
27070	1(3)	27252	1(2)	27397	1(2)	27520	1(2)	27680	3(3)	27840	1(2)	28126	4(3)	28405	1(2)
27071	1(3)	27253	1(2)	27400	1(2)	27524	1(2)	27681	1(2)	27842	1(2)	28130	1(2)	28406	1(2)
27075	1(3)	27254	1(2)	27403	1(3)	27530	1(2)	27685	2(3)	27846	1(2)	28140	4(3)	28415	1(2)
27076	1(2)	27256	1(2)	27405	2(2)	27532	1(2)	27686	3(3)	27848	1(2)	28150	4(3)	28420	1(2)
27077	1(2)	27257	1(2)	27407	2(2)	27535	1(2)	27687	1(2)	27860	1(2)	28153	6(3)	28430	1(2)

CPT	MUE	CPT	MUE	CPT	MUE	CPT	MUE	CPT	MUE	CPT	MUE	CPT	MUE
28435	1(2)	29055	1(3)	29838	1(2)	30130	1(2)	31254	1(2)	31590	1(2)	32097	1(3)
28436	1(2)	29058	1(3)	29840	1(2)	30140	1(2)	31255	1(2)	31595	1(2)	32098	1(2)
28445	1(2)	29065	1(3)	29843	1(2)	30150	1(2)	31256	1(2)	31600	1(2)	32100	1(3)
28446	1(2)	29075	1(3)	29844	1(2)	30160	1(2)	31267	1(2)	31601	1(2)	32110	1(3)
28450	2(3)	29085	1(3)	29845	1(2)	30200	1(2)	31276	1(2)	31603	1(2)	32120	1(3)
28455	3(3)	29086	2(3)	29846	1(2)	30210	1(3)	31287	1(2)	31605	1(2)	32124	1(3)
28456	2(3)	29105	1(2)	29847	1(2)	30220	1(2)	31288	1(2)	31610	1(2)	32140	1(3)
28465	3(3)	29125	1(2)	29848	1(2)	30300	1(3)	31290	1(2)	31611	1(2)	32141	1(3)
28470	2(3)	29126	1(2)	29850	1(2)	30310	1(3)	31291	1(2)	31612	1(3)	32150	1(3)
28475	5(3)	29130	3(3)	29851	1(2)	30320	1(3)	31292	1(2)	31613	1(2)	32151	1(3)
28476	4(3)	29131	2(3)	29855	1(2)	30400	1(2)	31293	1(2)	31614	1(2)	32160	1(3)
28485	5(3)	29200	1(2)	29856	1(2)	30410	1(2)	31294	1(2)	31615	1(3)	32200	2(3)
28490	1(2)	29240	1(2)	29860	1(2)	30420	1(2)	31295	1(2)	31622	1(3)	32215	1(2)
28495	1(2)	29260	1(3)	29861	1(2)	30430	1(2)	31296	1(2)	31623	1(3)	32220	1(2)
28496	1(2)	29280	2(3)	29862	1(2)	30435	1(2)	31297	1(2)	31624	1(3)	32225	1(2)
28505	1(2)	29305	1(3)	29863	1(2)	30450	1(2)	31300	1(2)	31625	1(2)	32310	1(3)
28510	4(3)	29325	1(3)	29866	1(2)	30460	1(2)	31320	1(2)	31626	1(2)	32320	1(3)
28515	4(3)	29345	1(3)	29867	1(2)	30462	1(2)	31360	1(2)	31627	1(3)	32400	2(3)
28525	4(3)	29355	1(3)	29868	1(3)	30465	1(2)	31365	1(2)	31628	1(2)	32405	2(3)
28530	1(2)	29358	1(3)	29870	1(2)	30520	1(2)	31367	1(2)	31629	1(2)	32440	1(2)
28531	1(2)	29365	1(3)	29871	1(2)	30540	1(2)	31368	1(2)	31630	1(3)	32442	1(2)
28540	1(3)	29405	1(3)	29873	1(2)	30545	1(2)	31370	1(2)	31631	1(2)	32445	1(2)
28545	1(3)	29425	1(3)	29874	1(2)	30560	1(2)	31375	1(2)	31632	2(3)	32480	1(2)
28546	1(3)	29435	1(3)	29875	1(2)	30580	2(3)	31380	1(2)	31633	2(3)	32482	1(2)
28555	1(3)	29440	1(2)	29876	1(2)	30600	1(3)	31382	1(2)	31634	1(3)	32484	2(3)
28570	1(2)	29445	1(3)	29877	1(2)	30620	1(2)	31390	1(2)	31635	1(3)	32486	1(3)
28575	1(2)	29450	1(3)	29879	1(2)	30630	1(2)	31395	1(2)	31636	1(2)	32488	1(2)
28576	1(2)	29505	1(2)	29880	1(2)	30801	1(2)	31400	1(3)	31637	2(3)	32491	1(2)
28585	1(3)	29515	1(2)	29881	1(2)	30802	1(2)	31420	1(2)	31638	1(3)	32501	1(3)
28600	2(3)	29520	1(2)	29882	1(2)	30901	1(3)	31500	2(3)	31640	1(3)	32503	1(2)
28605	2(3)	29530	1(2)	29883	1(2)	30903	1(3)	31502	1(3)	31641	1(3)	32504	1(2)
28606	3(3)	29540	1(2)	29884	1(2)	30905	1(2)	31505	1(3)	31643	1(2)	32505	1(2)
28615	5(3)	29550	1(2)	29885	1(2)	30906	1(3)	31510	1(2)	31645	1(2)	32506	3(3)
28630	2(3)	29580	1(2)	29886	1(2)	30915	1(3)	31511	1(3)	31646	2(3)	32507	2(3)
28635	2(3)	29581	1(2)	29887	1(2)	30920	1(3)	31512	1(3)	31647	1(2)	32540	1(3)
28636	4(3)	29582	1(2)	29888	1(2)	30930	1(2)	31513	1(3)	31648	1(2)	32550	2(3)
28645	4(3)	29583	1(2)	29889	1(2)	31000	1(2)	31515	1(3)	31649	2(3)	32551	2(3)
28660	4(3)	29584	1(2)	29891	1(2)	31002	1(2)	31520	1(3)	31651	3(3)	32552	2(2)
28665	4(3)	29700	2(3)	29892	1(2)	31020	1(2)	31525	1(3)	31652	1(3)	32553	1(2)
28666	4(3)	29705	1(3)	29893	1(2)	31030	1(2)	31526	1(3)	31653	1(3)	32554	2(3)
28675	4(3)	29710	1(2)	29894	1(2)	31032	1(2)	31527	1(2)	31654	1(3)	32555	2(3)
28705	1(2)	29720	1(2)	29895	1(2)	31040	1(2)	31528	1(2)	31660	1(2)	32556	2(3)
28715	1(2)	29730	1(3)	29897	1(2)	31050	1(2)	31529	1(3)	31661	1(2)	32557	2(3)
28725	1(2)	29740	1(3)	29898	1(2)	31051	1(2)	31530	1(3)	31717	1(3)	32560	1(3)
28730	1(2)	29750	1(3)	29899	1(2)	31070	1(2)	31531	1(3)	31720	1(3)	32561	1(2)
28735	1(2)	29800	1(2)	29900	2(3)	31075	1(2)	31535	1(3)	31725	1(3)	32562	1(2)
28737	1(2)	29804	1(2)	29901	2(3)	31080	1(2)	31536	1(3)	31730	1(3)	32601	1(3)
28740	5(3)	29805	1(2)	29902	2(3)	31081	1(2)	31540	1(3)	31750	1(2)	32604	1(3)
28750	1(2)	29806	1(2)	29904	1(2)	31084	1(2)	31541	1(3)	31755	1(2)	32606	1(3)
28755	1(2)	29807	1(2)	29905	1(2)	31085	1(2)	31545	1(2)	31760	1(2)	32607	1(3)
28760	1(2)	29819	1(2)	29906	1(2)	31086	1(2)	31546	1(2)	31766	1(2)	32608	1(3)
28800	1(2)	29820	1(2)	29907	1(2)	31087	1(2)	31560	1(2)	31770	2(3)	32609	1(3)
28805	1(2)	29821	1(2)	29914	1(2)	31090	1(2)	31561	1(2)	31775	1(3)	32650	1(2)
28810	6(3)	29822	1(2)	29915	1(2)	31200	1(2)	31570	1(2)	31780	1(2)	32651	1(2)
28820	6(3)	29823	1(2)	29916	1(2)	31201	1(2)	31571	1(2)	31781	1(2)	32652	1(2)
28825	10(2)	29824	1(2)	30000	1(3)	31205	1(2)	31575	1(3)	31785	1(3)	32653	1(3)
28890	1(2)	29825	1(2)	30020	1(3)	31225	1(2)	31576	1(3)	31786	1(3)	32654	1(3)
29000	1(3)	29826	1(2)	30100	2(3)	31230	1(2)	31577	1(3)	31800	1(3)	32655	1(3)
29010	1(3)	29827	1(2)	30110	1(2)	31231	1(2)	31578	1(3)	31805	1(3)	32656	1(2)
29015	1(3)	29828	1(2)	30115	1(2)	31233	1(2)	31579	1(3)	31820	1(2)	32658	1(3)
29035	1(3)	29830	1(2)	30117	2(3)	31235	1(2)	31580	1(2)	31825	1(2)	32659	1(2)
29040	1(3)	29834	1(2)	30118	1(3)	31237	1(2)	31582	1(2)	31830	1(2)	32661	1(3)
29044	1(3)	29835	1(2)	30120	1(2)	31238	1(3)	31584	1(2)	32035	1(2)	32662	1(3)
29046	1(3)	29836	1(2)	30124	2(3)	31239	1(2)	31587	1(2)	32036	1(3)	32663	1(3)
29049	1(3)	29837	1(2)	30125	1(3)	31240	1(2)	31588	1(2)	32096	1(3)	32664	1(2)
												32665	1(2)
												32666	1(3)
												32667	3(3)
												32668	2(3)
												32669	2(3)
												32670	1(2)
												32671	1(2)
												32672	1(3)
												32673	1(2)
												32674	1(2)
												32701	1(2)
												32800	1(3)
												32810	1(3)
												32815	1(3)
												32820	1(2)
												32850	1(2)
												32851	1(2)
												32852	1(2)
												32853	1(2)
												32854	1(2)
												32855	1(2)
												32856	1(2)
												32900	1(2)
												32905	1(2)
												32906	1(2)
												32940	1(3)
												32960	1(2)
												32997	1(2)
												32998	1(2)
												33010	1(2)
												33011	1(3)
												33015	1(3)
												33020	1(3)
												33025	1(2)
												33030	1(2)
												33031	1(2)
												33050	1(2)
												33120	1(3)
												33130	1(3)
												33140	1(2)
												33141	1(2)
												33202	1(2)
												33203	1(2)
												33206	1(3)
												33207	1(3)
												33208	1(3)
												33210	1(3)
												33211	1(3)
												33212	1(3)
												33213	1(3)
												33214	1(3)
												33215	2(3)
												33216	1(3)
												33217	1(3)
												33218	1(3)
												33220	1(3)
												33221	1(3)
												33222	1(3)
												33223	1(3)
												33224	1(3)
												33225	1(3)
												33226	1(3)
												33227	1(3)
												33228	1(3)
												33229	1(3)

CPT	MUE	CPT	MUE	CPT	MUE	CPT	MUE	CPT	MUE	CPT	MUE	CPT	MUE	CPT	MUE
33230	1(3)	33418	1(3)	33645	1(2)	33877	1(2)	33992	1(2)	35132	1(2)	35516	1(3)	35701	1(2)
33231	1(3)	33419	1(3)	33647	1(2)	33880	1(2)	33993	1(3)	35141	1(2)	35518	1(3)	35721	1(2)
33233	1(2)	33420	1(2)	33660	1(2)	33881	1(2)	34001	1(3)	35142	1(2)	35521	1(3)	35741	1(2)
33234	1(2)	33422	1(2)	33665	1(2)	33883	1(2)	34051	1(3)	35151	1(2)	35522	1(3)	35761	2(3)
33235	1(2)	33425	1(2)	33670	1(2)	33884	2(3)	34101	1(3)	35152	1(2)	35523	1(3)	35800	2(3)
33236	1(2)	33426	1(2)	33675	1(2)	33886	1(2)	34111	2(3)	35180	2(3)	35525	1(3)	35820	2(3)
33237	1(2)	33427	1(2)	33676	1(2)	33889	1(2)	34151	2(3)	35182	2(3)	35526	1(3)	35840	2(3)
33238	1(2)	33430	1(2)	33677	1(2)	33891	1(2)	34201	1(3)	35184	2(3)	35531	2(3)	35860	2(3)
33240	1(3)	33460	1(2)	33681	1(2)	33910	1(3)	34203	1(2)	35188	2(3)	35533	1(3)	35870	1(3)
33241	1(2)	33463	1(2)	33684	1(2)	33915	1(3)	34401	1(3)	35189	1(3)	35535	1(3)	35875	2(3)
33243	1(2)	33464	1(2)	33688	1(2)	33916	1(3)	34421	1(3)	35190	2(3)	35536	1(3)	35876	2(3)
33244	1(2)	33465	1(2)	33690	1(2)	33917	1(2)	34451	1(3)	35201	2(3)	35537	1(3)	35879	2(3)
33249	1(3)	33468	1(2)	33692	1(2)	33920	1(2)	34471	1(2)	35206	2(3)	35538	1(3)	35881	2(3)
33250	1(2)	33470	1(2)	33694	1(2)	33922	1(2)	34490	1(2)	35207	3(3)	35539	1(3)	35883	1(3)
33251	1(2)	33471	1(2)	33697	1(2)	33924	1(2)	34501	1(2)	35211	3(3)	35540	1(3)	35884	1(3)
33254	1(2)	33474	1(2)	33702	1(2)	33925	1(2)	34502	1(2)	35216	2(3)	35556	1(3)	35901	1(3)
33255	1(2)	33475	1(2)	33710	1(2)	33926	1(2)	34510	2(3)	35221	3(3)	35558	1(3)	35903	2(3)
33256	1(2)	33476	1(2)	33720	1(2)	33930	1(2)	34520	1(3)	35226	3(3)	35560	1(3)	35905	1(3)
33257	1(2)	33477	1(2)	33722	1(3)	33933	1(2)	34530	1(2)	35231	2(3)	35563	1(3)	35907	1(3)
33258	1(2)	33478	1(2)	33724	1(2)	33935	1(2)	34800	1(2)	35236	2(3)	35565	1(3)	36000	4(3)
33259	1(2)	33496	1(3)	33726	1(2)	33940	1(2)	34802	1(2)	35241	2(3)	35566	1(3)	36002	2(3)
33261	1(2)	33500	1(3)	33730	1(2)	33944	1(2)	34803	1(2)	35246	2(3)	35570	1(3)	36005	2(3)
33262	1(3)	33501	1(3)	33732	1(2)	33945	1(2)	34804	1(2)	35251	2(3)	35571	2(3)	36010	2(3)
33263	1(3)	33502	1(3)	33735	1(2)	33946	1(2)	34805	1(2)	35256	2(3)	35572	2(3)	36011	4(3)
33264	1(3)	33503	1(3)	33736	1(2)	33947	1(2)	34806	1(2)	35261	1(3)	35583	1(2)	36012	4(3)
33265	1(2)	33504	1(3)	33737	1(2)	33948	1(2)	34808	1(3)	35266	2(3)	35585	2(3)	36013	2(3)
33266	1(2)	33505	1(3)	33750	1(3)	33949	1(2)	34812	1(2)	35271	2(3)	35587	2(2)	36014	2(3)
33270	1(3)	33506	1(3)	33755	1(2)	33951	1(1)	34813	1(2)	35276	2(3)	35600	2(3)	36015	4(3)
33271	1(3)	33507	1(3)	33762	1(2)	33952	1(1)	34820	1(2)	35281	2(3)	35601	1(3)	36100	2(3)
33272	1(3)	33508	1(2)	33764	1(3)	33953	1(1)	34825	1(2)	35286	2(3)	35606	1(3)	36120	2(3)
33273	1(3)	33510	1(2)	33766	1(2)	33954	1(1)	34826	4(3)	35301	2(3)	35612	1(3)	36140	3(3)
33282	1(2)	33511	1(2)	33767	1(2)	33955	1(3)	34830	1(2)	35302	1(2)	35616	1(3)	36147	2(3)
33284	1(2)	33512	1(2)	33768	1(2)	33956	1(3)	34831	1(2)	35303	1(2)	35621	1(3)	36148	1(3)
33300	1(3)	33513	1(2)	33770	1(2)	33957	1(3)	34832	1(2)	35304	1(2)	35623	1(3)	36160	2(3)
33305	1(3)	33514	1(2)	33771	1(2)	33958	1(3)	34833	1(2)	35305	1(2)	35626	3(3)	36200	2(3)
33310	1(2)	33516	1(2)	33774	1(2)	33959	1(3)	34834	1(2)	35306	2(3)	35631	4(3)	36215	6(3)
33315	1(2)	33517	1(2)	33775	1(2)	33962	1(3)	34839	1(2)	35311	1(2)	35632	1(3)	36216	4(3)
33320	1(3)	33518	1(2)	33776	1(2)	33963	1(3)	34841	1(2)	35321	1(2)	35633	1(3)	36217	2(3)
33321	1(3)	33519	1(2)	33777	1(2)	33964	1(3)	34842	1(2)	35331	1(2)	35634	1(3)	36218	6(3)
33322	1(3)	33521	1(2)	33778	1(2)	33965	1(3)	34843	1(2)	35341	3(3)	35636	1(3)	36221	1(3)
33330	1(3)	33522	1(2)	33779	1(2)	33966	1(3)	34844	1(2)	35351	1(3)	35637	1(3)	36222	1(3)
33335	1(3)	33523	1(2)	33780	1(2)	33967	1(3)	34845	1(2)	35355	1(2)	35638	1(3)	36223	1(3)
33361	1(2)	33530	1(2)	33781	1(2)	33968	1(3)	34846	1(2)	35361	1(2)	35642	1(3)	36224	1(3)
33362	1(2)	33533	1(2)	33782	1(2)	33969	1(3)	34847	1(2)	35363	1(2)	35645	1(3)	36225	1(3)
33363	1(2)	33534	1(2)	33783	1(2)	33970	1(3)	34848	1(2)	35371	1(2)	35646	1(3)	36226	1(3)
33364	1(2)	33535	1(2)	33786	1(2)	33971	1(3)	34900	1(2)	35372	1(2)	35647	1(3)	36227	1(3)
33365	1(2)	33536	1(2)	33788	1(2)	33973	1(3)	35001	1(2)	35390	1(3)	35650	1(3)	36228	4(3)
33366	1(2)	33542	1(2)	33800	1(2)	33974	1(3)	35002	1(2)	35400	1(3)	35654	1(3)	36245	6(3)
33367	1(2)	33545	1(2)	33802	1(3)	33975	1(3)	35005	1(2)	35450	2(3)	35656	1(3)	36246	4(3)
33368	1(2)	33548	1(2)	33803	1(3)	33976	1(3)	35011	1(2)	35452	1(2)	35661	1(3)	36247	3(3)
33369	1(2)	33572	3(2)	33813	1(2)	33977	1(3)	35013	1(2)	35458	2(3)	35663	1(3)	36248	6(3)
33400	1(2)	33600	1(3)	33814	1(2)	33978	1(3)	35021	1(2)	35460	2(3)	35665	1(3)	36251	1(3)
33401	1(2)	33602	1(3)	33820	1(2)	33979	1(3)	35022	1(2)	35471	3(3)	35666	2(3)	36252	1(3)
33403	1(2)	33606	1(2)	33822	1(2)	33980	1(3)	35045	2(3)	35472	1(2)	35671	2(3)	36253	1(3)
33404	1(2)	33608	1(2)	33824	1(2)	33981	1(3)	35081	1(2)	35475	4(3)	35681	1(3)	36254	1(3)
33405	1(2)	33610	1(2)	33840	1(2)	33982	1(3)	35082	1(2)	35476	5(3)	35682	1(2)	36260	1(2)
33406	1(2)	33611	1(2)	33845	1(2)	33983	1(3)	35091	1(2)	35500	2(3)	35683	1(2)	36261	1(2)
33410	1(2)	33612	1(2)	33851	1(2)	33984	1(3)	35092	1(2)	35501	1(3)	35685	2(3)	36262	1(2)
33411	1(2)	33615	1(2)	33852	1(2)	33985	1(3)	35102	1(2)	35506	1(3)	35686	1(3)	36400	1(3)
33412	1(2)	33617	1(2)	33853	1(2)	33986	1(3)	35103	1(2)	35508	1(3)	35691	1(3)	36405	1(3)
33413	1(2)	33619	1(2)	33860	1(2)	33987	1(3)	35111	1(2)	35509	1(3)	35693	1(3)	36406	1(3)
33414	1(2)	33620	1(2)	33863	1(2)	33988	1(3)	35112	1(2)	35510	1(3)	35694	1(3)	36410	3(3)
33415	1(2)	33621	1(3)	33864	1(2)	33989	1(3)	35121	1(3)	35511	1(3)	35695	1(3)	36415	4(3)
33416	1(2)	33622	1(3)	33870	1(2)	33990	1(3)	35122	1(3)	35512	1(3)	35697	2(3)	36420	2(3)
33417	1(2)	33641	1(2)	33875	1(2)	33991	1(3)	35131	1(2)	35515	1(3)	35700	2(3)	36425	2(3)

CPT	MUE	CPT	MUE	CPT	MUE	CPT	MUE	CPT	MUE	CPT	MUE	CPT	MUE	CPT	MUE
36430	1(2)	36821	2(3)	37600	1(3)	38570	1(2)	40845	1(3)	42200	1(2)	42894	1(3)	43241	1(3)
36440	1(3)	36823	1(3)	37605	1(3)	38571	1(3)	41000	2(3)	42205	1(2)	42900	1(3)	43242	1(2)
36450	1(3)	36825	1(3)	37606	1(3)	38572	1(2)	41005	2(3)	42210	1(2)	42950	1(2)	43243	1(2)
36455	1(3)	36830	2(3)	37607	1(3)	38700	1(2)	41006	2(3)	42215	1(2)	42953	1(3)	43244	1(2)
36460	2(3)	36831	1(3)	37609	1(2)	38720	1(2)	41007	2(3)	42220	1(2)	42955	1(2)	43245	1(2)
36468	1(3)	36832	2(3)	37615	2(3)	38724	1(2)	41008	2(3)	42225	1(2)	42960	1(3)	43246	1(2)
36470	1(3)	36833	1(3)	37616	1(3)	38740	1(2)	41009	2(3)	42226	1(2)	42961	1(3)	43247	1(2)
36471	1(2)	36835	1(3)	37617	3(3)	38745	1(2)	41010	1(2)	42227	1(2)	42962	1(3)	43248	1(3)
36475	1(3)	36838	1(3)	37618	2(3)	38746	1(2)	41015	2(3)	42235	1(2)	42970	1(3)	43249	1(3)
36476	2(3)	36860	2(3)	37619	1(2)	38747	1(2)	41016	2(3)	42260	1(3)	42971	1(3)	43250	1(2)
36478	1(3)	36861	2(3)	37650	1(2)	38760	1(2)	41017	2(3)	42280	1(2)	42972	1(3)	43251	1(2)
36479	2(3)	36870	2(3)	37660	1(2)	38765	1(2)	41018	2(3)	42281	1(2)	43020	1(2)	43252	1(2)
36481	1(3)	37140	1(2)	37700	1(2)	38770	1(2)	41019	1(2)	42300	2(3)	43030	1(2)	43253	1(3)
36500	4(3)	37145	1(3)	37718	1(2)	38780	1(2)	41100	3(3)	42305	2(3)	43045	1(2)	43254	1(3)
36510	1(3)	37160	1(3)	37722	1(2)	38790	1(2)	41105	3(3)	42310	2(3)	43100	1(3)	43255	2(3)
36511	1(3)	37180	1(2)	37735	1(2)	38792	1(3)	41108	2(3)	42320	2(3)	43101	1(3)	43257	1(2)
36512	1(3)	37181	1(2)	37760	1(2)	38794	1(2)	41110	2(3)	42330	2(3)	43107	1(2)	43259	1(2)
36513	1(3)	37182	1(2)	37761	1(2)	38900	1(3)	41112	2(3)	42335	2(2)	43108	1(2)	43260	1(3)
36514	1(3)	37183	1(2)	37765	1(2)	39000	1(2)	41113	2(3)	42340	1(2)	43112	1(2)	43261	1(2)
36515	1(3)	37184	1(2)	37766	1(2)	39010	1(2)	41114	2(3)	42400	2(3)	43113	1(2)	43262	2(2)
36516	1(3)	37185	2(3)	37780	1(2)	39200	1(2)	41115	1(2)	42405	2(3)	43116	1(2)	43263	1(2)
36522	1(3)	37186	2(3)	37785	1(2)	39220	1(2)	41116	2(3)	42408	1(3)	43117	1(2)	43264	1(2)
36555	2(3)	37187	1(3)	37788	1(2)	39401	1(3)	41120	1(2)	42409	1(3)	43118	1(2)	43265	1(2)
36556	2(3)	37188	1(3)	37790	1(2)	39402	1(3)	41130	1(2)	42410	1(2)	43121	1(2)	43266	1(3)
36557	2(3)	37191	1(3)	38100	1(2)	39501	1(3)	41135	1(2)	42415	1(2)	43122	1(2)	43270	1(3)
36558	2(3)	37192	1(3)	38101	1(3)	39503	1(2)	41140	1(2)	42420	1(2)	43123	1(2)	43273	1(2)
36560	2(3)	37193	1(3)	38102	1(2)	39540	1(2)	41145	1(2)	42425	1(2)	43124	1(2)	43274	2(3)
36561	2(3)	37195	1(3)	38115	1(3)	39541	1(2)	41150	1(2)	42426	1(2)	43130	1(3)	43275	1(3)
36563	1(3)	37197	2(3)	38120	1(2)	39545	1(2)	41153	1(2)	42440	1(2)	43135	1(3)	43276	2(3)
36565	1(3)	37200	2(3)	38200	1(3)	39560	1(3)	41155	1(2)	42450	2(3)	43180	1(2)	43277	3(3)
36566	1(3)	37211	1(2)	38205	1(3)	39561	1(3)	41250	2(3)	42500	2(3)	43191	1(3)	43278	1(3)
36568	2(3)	37212	1(2)	38206	1(3)	40490	3(3)	41251	2(3)	42505	2(3)	43192	1(3)	43279	1(2)
36569	2(3)	37213	1(2)	38208	0(3)	40500	2(3)	41252	2(3)	42507	1(2)	43193	1(3)	43280	1(2)
36570	2(3)	37214	1(2)	38209	0(3)	40510	2(3)	41500	1(2)	42509	1(2)	43194	1(3)	43281	1(2)
36571	2(3)	37215	1(2)	38210	0(3)	40520	2(3)	41510	1(2)	42510	1(2)	43195	1(3)	43282	1(2)
36575	2(3)	37217	1(2)	38211	0(3)	40525	2(3)	41512	1(2)	42550	2(3)	43196	1(3)	43283	1(2)
36576	2(3)	37218	1(2)	38212	0(3)	40527	2(3)	41520	1(3)	42600	2(3)	43197	1(3)	43300	1(2)
36578	2(3)	37220	2(2)	38213	0(3)	40530	2(3)	41530	1(3)	42650	2(3)	43198	1(3)	43305	1(2)
36580	2(3)	37221	2(2)	38214	0(3)	40650	2(3)	41800	2(3)	42660	2(3)	43200	1(3)	43310	1(2)
36581	2(3)	37222	2(3)	38215	0(3)	40652	2(3)	41805	3(3)	42665	2(3)	43201	1(2)	43312	1(2)
36582	2(3)	37223	2(3)	38220	1(3)	40654	2(3)	41806	3(3)	42700	2(3)	43202	1(2)	43313	1(2)
36583	2(2)	37224	2(2)	38221	1(3)	40700	1(2)	41820	4(2)	42720	1(3)	43204	1(2)	43314	1(2)
36584	2(3)	37225	2(2)	38230	1(2)	40701	1(2)	41821	2(3)	42725	1(3)	43205	1(2)	43320	1(2)
36585	2(3)	37226	2(2)	38232	1(2)	40702	1(2)	41822	1(2)	42800	3(3)	43206	1(2)	43325	1(2)
36589	2(3)	37227	2(2)	38240	1(3)	40720	1(2)	41823	1(2)	42804	3(3)	43210	1(2)	43327	1(2)
36590	2(3)	37228	2(2)	38241	1(2)	40761	1(2)	41825	2(3)	42806	1(3)	43211	1(3)	43328	1(2)
36591	2(3)	37229	2(2)	38242	1(2)	40800	2(3)	41826	2(3)	42808	2(3)	43212	1(3)	43330	1(2)
36592	1(3)	37230	2(2)	38243	1(3)	40801	2(3)	41827	2(3)	42809	1(3)	43213	1(2)	43331	1(2)
36593	2(3)	37231	2(2)	38300	1(3)	40804	2(3)	41828	4(2)	42810	1(3)	43214	1(3)	43332	1(2)
36595	2(3)	37232	2(3)	38305	1(3)	40805	2(3)	41830	2(3)	42815	1(3)	43215	1(3)	43333	1(2)
36596	2(3)	37233	2(3)	38308	1(3)	40806	2(2)	41850	2(3)	42820	1(2)	43216	1(2)	43334	1(2)
36597	2(3)	37234	2(3)	38380	1(2)	40808	4(3)	41870	2(3)	42821	1(2)	43217	1(2)	43335	1(2)
36598	2(3)	37235	2(3)	38381	1(2)	40810	4(3)	41872	4(2)	42825	1(2)	43220	1(3)	43336	1(2)
36600	4(3)	37236	1(2)	38382	1(2)	40812	4(3)	41874	4(2)	42826	1(2)	43226	1(3)	43337	1(2)
36620	3(3)	37237	2(3)	38500	2(3)	40814	4(3)	42000	1(3)	42830	1(2)	43227	1(3)	43338	1(2)
36625	2(3)	37238	1(2)	38505	3(3)	40816	2(3)	42100	3(3)	42831	1(2)	43229	1(3)	43340	1(2)
36640	1(3)	37239	2(3)	38510	1(2)	40818	2(3)	42104	3(3)	42835	1(2)	43231	1(2)	43341	1(2)
36660	1(3)	37241	2(3)	38520	1(2)	40819	2(2)	42106	2(3)	42836	1(2)	43232	1(2)	43351	1(2)
36680	1(3)	37242	2(3)	38525	1(2)	40820	5(3)	42107	2(3)	42842	1(3)	43233	1(3)	43352	1(2)
36800	1(3)	37243	1(3)	38530	1(2)	40830	2(3)	42120	1(2)	42844	1(3)	43235	1(3)	43360	1(2)
36810	1(3)	37244	2(3)	38542	1(2)	40831	2(3)	42140	1(2)	42845	1(3)	43236	1(2)	43361	1(2)
36815	1(3)	37252	1(3)	38550	1(3)	40840	1(2)	42145	1(2)	42860	1(3)	43237	1(2)	43400	1(2)
36818	1(3)	37253	3(1)	38555	1(3)	40842	1(2)	42160	2(3)	42870	1(3)	43238	1(2)	43401	1(2)
36819	1(3)	37500	1(3)	38562	1(2)	40843	1(2)	42180	1(3)	42890	1(2)	43239	1(2)	43405	1(2)
36820	1(3)	37565	1(2)	38564	1(2)	40844	1(2)	42182	1(3)	42892	1(3)	43240	1(2)	43410	1(3)

CPT	MUE	CPT	MUE	CPT	MUE	CPT	MUE	CPT	MUE	CPT	MUE	CPT	MUE	CPT	MUE
43415	1(3)	43881	1(3)	44322	1(2)	44970	1(2)	45395	1(2)	46707	1(3)	47480	1(2)	48500	1(3)
43420	1(3)	43882	1(3)	44340	1(2)	45000	1(3)	45397	1(2)	46710	1(3)	47490	1(2)	48510	1(3)
43425	1(3)	43886	1(2)	44345	1(2)	45005	1(3)	45398	1(2)	46712	1(3)	47531	2(3)	48520	1(3)
43450	1(3)	43887	1(2)	44346	1(2)	45020	1(3)	45400	1(2)	46715	1(2)	47532	1(3)	48540	1(3)
43453	1(3)	43888	1(2)	44360	1(3)	45100	2(3)	45402	1(2)	46716	1(2)	47533	1(3)	48545	1(3)
43460	1(3)	44005	1(2)	44361	1(2)	45108	1(2)	45500	1(2)	46730	1(2)	47534	1(3)	48547	1(2)
43496	1(3)	44010	1(2)	44363	1(3)	45110	1(2)	45505	1(2)	46735	1(2)	47535	1(3)	48548	1(2)
43500	1(2)	44015	1(2)	44364	1(2)	45111	1(2)	45520	1(2)	46740	1(2)	47536	1(3)	48550	1(2)
43501	1(3)	44020	2(3)	44365	1(2)	45112	1(2)	45540	1(2)	46742	1(2)	47537	1(3)	48551	1(2)
43502	1(2)	44021	1(3)	44366	1(3)	45113	1(2)	45541	1(2)	46744	1(2)	47538	2(1)	48552	2(3)
43510	1(2)	44025	1(3)	44369	1(2)	45114	1(2)	45550	1(2)	46746	1(2)	47539	2(1)	48554	1(2)
43520	1(2)	44050	1(2)	44370	1(2)	45116	1(2)	45560	1(2)	46748	1(2)	47540	2(1)	48556	1(2)
43605	1(2)	44055	1(2)	44372	1(2)	45119	1(2)	45562	1(2)	46750	1(2)	47541	1(3)	49000	1(2)
43610	2(3)	44100	1(2)	44373	1(2)	45120	1(2)	45563	1(2)	46751	1(2)	47542	2(3)	49002	1(3)
43611	2(3)	44110	1(2)	44376	1(3)	45121	1(2)	45800	1(3)	46753	1(2)	47543	1(3)	49010	1(3)
43620	1(2)	44111	1(2)	44377	1(2)	45123	1(2)	45805	1(3)	46754	1(3)	47544	1(3)	49020	2(3)
43621	1(2)	44120	1(2)	44378	1(3)	45126	1(2)	45820	1(3)	46760	1(2)	47550	1(3)	49040	2(3)
43622	1(2)	44121	4(3)	44379	1(2)	45130	1(2)	45825	1(3)	46761	1(2)	47552	1(3)	49060	2(3)
43631	1(2)	44125	1(2)	44380	1(3)	45135	1(2)	45900	1(2)	46762	1(2)	47553	1(2)	49062	1(3)
43632	1(2)	44126	1(2)	44381	1(3)	45136	1(2)	45905	1(2)	46900	1(2)	47554	1(3)	49082	1(3)
43633	1(2)	44127	1(2)	44382	1(2)	45150	1(2)	45910	1(2)	46910	1(2)	47555	1(2)	49083	2(3)
43634	1(2)	44128	2(3)	44384	1(3)	45160	1(3)	45915	1(2)	46916	1(2)	47556	1(2)	49084	1(3)
43635	1(2)	44130	3(3)	44385	1(3)	45171	2(3)	45990	1(2)	46917	1(2)	47562	1(2)	49180	2(3)
43640	1(2)	44132	1(2)	44386	1(2)	45172	2(3)	46020	2(3)	46922	1(2)	47563	1(2)	49185	2(3)
43641	1(2)	44133	1(2)	44388	1(3)	45190	1(3)	46030	1(3)	46924	1(2)	47564	1(2)	49203	1(2)
43644	1(2)	44135	1(2)	44389	1(2)	45300	1(3)	46040	2(3)	46930	1(2)	47570	1(2)	49204	1(2)
43645	1(2)	44136	1(2)	44390	1(3)	45303	1(3)	46045	2(3)	46940	1(2)	47600	1(2)	49205	1(2)
43647	1(2)	44137	1(2)	44391	1(3)	45305	1(2)	46050	2(3)	46942	1(3)	47605	1(2)	49215	1(2)
43648	1(2)	44139	1(2)	44392	1(2)	45307	1(3)	46060	2(3)	46945	1(2)	47610	1(2)	49220	1(2)
43651	1(2)	44140	2(3)	44394	1(2)	45308	1(2)	46070	1(2)	46946	1(2)	47612	1(2)	49250	1(2)
43652	1(2)	44141	1(3)	44401	1(2)	45309	1(2)	46080	1(2)	46947	1(2)	47620	1(2)	49255	1(2)
43653	1(2)	44143	1(2)	44402	1(3)	45315	1(2)	46083	2(3)	47000	3(3)	47700	1(2)	49320	1(3)
43752	2(3)	44144	1(3)	44403	1(3)	45317	1(3)	46200	1(3)	47001	3(3)	47701	1(2)	49321	1(2)
43753	1(3)	44145	1(2)	44404	1(3)	45320	1(2)	46220	1(2)	47010	3(3)	47711	1(2)	49322	1(2)
43754	1(3)	44146	1(2)	44405	1(3)	45321	1(2)	46221	1(2)	47015	1(2)	47712	1(2)	49323	1(2)
43755	1(3)	44147	1(3)	44406	1(3)	45327	1(2)	46230	1(2)	47100	3(3)	47715	1(2)	49324	1(2)
43756	1(2)	44150	1(2)	44407	1(2)	45330	1(3)	46250	1(2)	47120	2(3)	47720	1(2)	49325	1(2)
43757	1(2)	44151	1(2)	44408	1(3)	45331	1(2)	46255	1(2)	47122	1(2)	47721	1(2)	49326	1(2)
43760	2(3)	44155	1(2)	44500	1(3)	45332	1(3)	46257	1(2)	47125	1(2)	47740	1(2)	49327	1(2)
43761	2(3)	44156	1(2)	44602	1(2)	45333	1(2)	46258	1(2)	47130	1(2)	47741	1(2)	49400	1(3)
43770	1(2)	44157	1(2)	44603	1(2)	45334	1(3)	46260	1(2)	47133	1(2)	47760	1(2)	49402	1(3)
43771	1(2)	44158	1(2)	44604	1(2)	45335	1(2)	46261	1(2)	47135	1(2)	47765	1(2)	49405	2(3)
43772	1(2)	44160	1(2)	44605	1(2)	45337	1(2)	46262	1(2)	47140	1(2)	47780	1(2)	49406	2(3)
43773	1(2)	44180	1(2)	44615	4(3)	45338	1(2)	46270	1(3)	47141	1(2)	47785	1(2)	49407	1(3)
43774	1(2)	44186	1(2)	44620	2(3)	45340	1(2)	46275	1(3)	47142	1(2)	47800	1(2)	49411	1(2)
43775	1(2)	44187	1(3)	44625	1(3)	45341	1(2)	46280	1(2)	47143	1(2)	47801	1(3)	49412	1(2)
43800	1(2)	44188	1(3)	44626	1(3)	45342	1(2)	46285	1(3)	47144	1(2)	47802	1(2)	49418	1(3)
43810	1(2)	44202	1(2)	44640	2(3)	45346	1(2)	46288	1(3)	47145	1(2)	47900	1(2)	49419	1(2)
43820	1(2)	44203	2(3)	44650	2(3)	45347	1(3)	46320	2(3)	47146	3(3)	48000	1(2)	49421	1(2)
43825	1(2)	44204	2(3)	44660	1(3)	45349	1(3)	46500	1(2)	47147	2(3)	48001	1(2)	49422	1(2)
43830	1(2)	44205	1(2)	44661	1(3)	45350	1(2)	46505	1(2)	47300	2(3)	48020	1(3)	49423	2(3)
43831	1(2)	44206	1(2)	44680	1(3)	45378	1(3)	46600	1(3)	47350	1(3)	48100	1(3)	49424	3(3)
43832	1(2)	44207	1(2)	44700	1(2)	45379	1(3)	46601	1(3)	47360	1(3)	48102	1(3)	49425	1(2)
43840	2(3)	44208	1(2)	44701	1(3)	45380	1(2)	46604	1(2)	47361	1(3)	48105	1(3)	49426	1(3)
43843	1(2)	44210	1(2)	44705	1(3)	45381	1(3)	46606	1(2)	47362	1(3)	48120	1(3)	49427	1(3)
43845	1(2)	44211	1(2)	44715	1(2)	45382	1(3)	46607	1(2)	47370	1(2)	48140	1(3)	49428	1(2)
43846	1(2)	44212	1(2)	44720	2(3)	45384	1(2)	46608	1(3)	47371	1(2)	48145	1(2)	49429	1(2)
43847	1(2)	44213	1(2)	44721	2(3)	45385	1(2)	46610	1(2)	47380	1(2)	48146	1(2)	49435	1(2)
43848	1(2)	44227	1(3)	44800	1(3)	45386	1(2)	46611	1(2)	47381	1(2)	48148	1(2)	49436	1(2)
43850	1(2)	44300	1(3)	44820	1(3)	45388	1(2)	46612	1(2)	47382	1(2)	48150	1(2)	49440	1(3)
43855	1(2)	44310	2(3)	44850	1(3)	45389	1(3)	46614	1(3)	47383	1(2)	48152	1(2)	49441	1(3)
43860	1(2)	44312	1(2)	44900	1(3)	45390	1(3)	46615	1(2)	47400	1(3)	48153	1(2)	49442	1(3)
43865	1(2)	44314	1(2)	44950	1(3)	45391	1(2)	46700	1(2)	47420	1(2)	48154	1(2)	49446	1(2)
43870	1(2)	44316	1(2)	44955	1(2)	45392	1(2)	46705	1(2)	47425	1(2)	48155	1(2)	49450	1(3)
43880	1(3)	44320	1(2)	44960	1(2)	45393	1(3)	46706	1(3)	47460	1(2)	48400	1(3)	49451	1(3)

CPT	MUE	CPT	MUE	CPT	MUE	CPT	MUE	CPT	MUE	CPT	MUE	CPT	MUE	CPT	MUE
49452	1(3)	50220	1(2)	50592	1(2)	51065	1(3)	52204	1(2)	53200	1(3)	54130	1(2)	54650	1(2)
49460	1(3)	50225	1(2)	50593	1(2)	51080	1(3)	52214	1(2)	53210	1(2)	54135	1(2)	54660	1(2)
49465	1(3)	50230	1(2)	50600	1(3)	51100	1(3)	52224	1(2)	53215	1(2)	54150	1(2)	54670	1(3)
49491	1(2)	50234	1(2)	50605	1(3)	51101	1(3)	52234	1(2)	53220	1(3)	54160	1(2)	54680	1(2)
49492	1(2)	50236	1(2)	50606	2(3)	51102	1(3)	52235	1(2)	53230	1(3)	54161	1(2)	54690	1(2)
49495	1(2)	50240	1(2)	50610	1(2)	51500	1(2)	52240	1(2)	53235	1(3)	54162	1(2)	54692	1(2)
49496	1(2)	50250	1(3)	50620	1(2)	51520	1(2)	52250	1(2)	53240	1(3)	54163	1(2)	54700	1(3)
49500	1(2)	50280	1(2)	50630	1(2)	51525	1(2)	52260	1(2)	53250	1(3)	54164	1(2)	54800	1(2)
49501	1(2)	50290	1(3)	50650	1(2)	51530	1(2)	52265	1(2)	53260	1(2)	54200	1(2)	54830	1(2)
49505	1(2)	50300	1(2)	50660	1(3)	51535	1(2)	52270	1(2)	53265	1(3)	54205	1(2)	54840	1(2)
49507	1(2)	50320	1(2)	50684	1(3)	51550	1(2)	52275	1(2)	53270	1(2)	54220	1(3)	54860	1(2)
49520	1(2)	50323	1(2)	50686	2(3)	51555	1(2)	52276	1(2)	53275	1(2)	54230	1(3)	54861	1(2)
49521	1(2)	50325	1(2)	50688	2(3)	51565	1(2)	52277	1(2)	53400	1(2)	54231	1(3)	54865	1(3)
49525	1(2)	50327	1(3)	50690	2(3)	51570	1(2)	52281	1(2)	53405	1(2)	54235	1(3)	54900	1(2)
49540	1(2)	50328	1(3)	50693	2(3)	51575	1(2)	52282	1(2)	53410	1(2)	54240	1(2)	54901	1(2)
49550	1(2)	50329	1(3)	50694	2(3)	51580	1(2)	52283	1(2)	53415	1(2)	54250	1(2)	55000	1(3)
49553	1(2)	50340	1(2)	50695	2(3)	51585	1(2)	52285	1(2)	53420	1(2)	54300	1(2)	55040	1(2)
49555	1(2)	50360	1(2)	50700	1(2)	51590	1(2)	52287	1(2)	53425	1(2)	54304	1(2)	55041	1(2)
49557	1(2)	50365	1(2)	50705	2(3)	51595	1(2)	52290	1(2)	53430	1(2)	54308	1(2)	55060	1(2)
49560	2(3)	50370	1(2)	50706	2(3)	51596	1(2)	52300	1(2)	53431	1(2)	54312	1(2)	55100	2(3)
49561	2(3)	50380	1(2)	50715	1(2)	51597	1(2)	52301	1(2)	53440	1(2)	54316	1(2)	55110	1(2)
49565	2(3)	50382	1(3)	50722	1(2)	51600	1(3)	52305	1(2)	53442	1(2)	54318	1(2)	55120	1(3)
49566	2(3)	50384	1(3)	50725	1(3)	51605	1(3)	52310	1(3)	53444	1(3)	54322	1(2)	55150	1(2)
49568	2(3)	50385	1(3)	50727	1(3)	51610	1(3)	52315	2(3)	53445	1(2)	54324	1(2)	55175	1(2)
49570	1(3)	50386	1(3)	50728	1(3)	51700	1(3)	52317	1(3)	53446	1(2)	54326	1(2)	55180	1(2)
49572	1(3)	50387	1(3)	50740	1(2)	51701	2(3)	52318	1(3)	53447	1(2)	54328	1(2)	55200	1(2)
49580	1(2)	50389	1(3)	50750	1(2)	51702	2(3)	52320	1(2)	53448	1(2)	54332	1(2)	55250	1(2)
49582	1(2)	50390	2(3)	50760	1(2)	51703	2(3)	52325	1(3)	53449	1(2)	54336	1(2)	55300	1(2)
49585	1(2)	50391	1(3)	50770	1(2)	51705	1(3)	52327	1(2)	53450	1(2)	54340	1(2)	55400	1(2)
49587	1(2)	50395	1(2)	50780	1(2)	51710	1(3)	52330	1(2)	53460	1(2)	54344	1(2)	55450	1(2)
49590	1(2)	50396	1(3)	50782	1(2)	51715	1(2)	52332	1(2)	53500	1(2)	54348	1(2)	55500	1(2)
49600	1(2)	50400	1(2)	50783	1(2)	51720	1(3)	52334	1(2)	53502	1(3)	54352	1(2)	55520	1(2)
49605	1(2)	50405	1(2)	50785	1(2)	51725	1(3)	52341	1(2)	53505	1(3)	54360	1(2)	55530	1(2)
49606	1(2)	50430	2(3)	50800	1(2)	51726	1(3)	52342	1(2)	53510	1(3)	54380	1(2)	55535	1(2)
49610	1(2)	50431	2(3)	50810	1(3)	51727	1(3)	52343	1(2)	53515	1(3)	54385	1(2)	55540	1(2)
49611	1(2)	50432	2(3)	50815	1(2)	51728	1(3)	52344	1(2)	53520	1(3)	54390	1(2)	55550	1(2)
49650	1(2)	50433	2(3)	50820	1(2)	51729	1(3)	52345	1(2)	53600	1(3)	54400	1(2)	55600	1(2)
49651	1(2)	50434	2(3)	50825	1(3)	51736	1(3)	52346	1(2)	53601	1(3)	54401	1(2)	55605	1(2)
49652	2(3)	50435	2(3)	50830	1(3)	51741	1(3)	52351	1(3)	53605	1(3)	54405	1(2)	55650	1(2)
49653	2(3)	50500	1(3)	50840	1(2)	51784	1(3)	52352	1(2)	53620	1(2)	54406	1(2)	55680	1(3)
49654	2(3)	50520	1(3)	50845	1(2)	51785	1(3)	52353	1(2)	53621	1(3)	54408	1(2)	55700	1(2)
49655	2(3)	50525	1(3)	50860	1(2)	51792	1(3)	52354	1(3)	53660	1(2)	54410	1(2)	55705	1(2)
49656	2(3)	50526	1(3)	50900	1(3)	51797	1(3)	52355	1(3)	53661	1(3)	54411	1(2)	55706	1(2)
49657	2(3)	50540	1(2)	50920	2(3)	51798	1(3)	52356	1(2)	53665	1(3)	54415	1(2)	55720	1(3)
49900	1(3)	50541	1(2)	50930	2(3)	51800	1(2)	52400	1(2)	53850	1(2)	54416	1(2)	55725	1(3)
49904	1(3)	50542	1(2)	50940	1(2)	51820	1(2)	52402	1(2)	53852	1(2)	54417	1(2)	55801	1(2)
49905	1(3)	50543	1(2)	50945	1(2)	51840	1(2)	52441	1(2)	53855	1(2)	54420	1(2)	55810	1(2)
49906	1(3)	50544	1(2)	50947	1(2)	51841	1(2)	52442	5(1)	53860	1(2)	54430	1(2)	55812	1(2)
50010	1(2)	50545	1(2)	50948	1(2)	51845	1(2)	52450	1(2)	54000	1(2)	54435	1(2)	55815	1(2)
50020	1(3)	50546	1(2)	50951	1(3)	51860	1(3)	52500	1(2)	54001	1(2)	54437	1(2)	55821	1(2)
50040	1(2)	50547	1(2)	50953	1(3)	51865	1(3)	52601	1(2)	54015	1(3)	54438	1(2)	55831	1(2)
50045	1(2)	50548	1(2)	50955	1(2)	51880	1(2)	52630	1(2)	54050	1(2)	54440	1(2)	55840	1(2)
50060	1(2)	50551	1(3)	50957	1(2)	51900	1(3)	52640	1(2)	54055	1(2)	54450	1(2)	55842	1(2)
50065	1(2)	50553	1(3)	50961	1(2)	51920	1(3)	52647	1(2)	54056	1(2)	54500	1(3)	55845	1(2)
50070	1(2)	50555	1(2)	50970	1(3)	51925	1(2)	52648	1(2)	54057	1(2)	54505	1(3)	55860	1(2)
50075	1(2)	50557	1(2)	50972	1(3)	51940	1(2)	52649	1(2)	54060	1(2)	54512	1(3)	55862	1(2)
50080	1(2)	50561	1(2)	50974	1(2)	51960	1(2)	52700	1(3)	54065	1(2)	54520	1(2)	55865	1(2)
50081	1(2)	50562	1(3)	50976	1(2)	51980	1(2)	53000	1(2)	54100	2(3)	54522	1(2)	55866	1(2)
50100	1(2)	50570	1(3)	50980	1(2)	51990	1(2)	53010	1(2)	54105	2(3)	54530	1(2)	55870	1(2)
50120	1(2)	50572	1(3)	51020	1(2)	51992	1(2)	53020	1(2)	54110	1(2)	54535	1(2)	55873	1(2)
50125	1(2)	50574	1(2)	51030	1(2)	52000	1(3)	53025	1(2)	54111	1(2)	54550	1(2)	55875	1(2)
50130	1(2)	50575	1(2)	51040	1(3)	52001	1(3)	53040	1(3)	54112	1(3)	54560	1(2)	55876	1(2)
50135	1(2)	50576	1(2)	51045	2(3)	52005	2(3)	53060	1(3)	54115	1(3)	54600	1(2)	55920	1(2)
50200	1(3)	50580	1(2)	51050	1(3)	52007	1(2)	53080	1(3)	54120	1(2)	54620	1(2)	56405	2(3)
50205	1(3)	50590	1(2)	51060	1(3)	52010	1(2)	53085	1(3)	54125	1(2)	54640	1(2)	56420	1(3)

CPT	MUE	CPT	MUE	CPT	MUE	CPT	MUE	CPT	MUE	CPT	MUE	CPT	MUE	CPT	MUE
56440	1(3)	57289	1(2)	58285	1(3)	58825	1(2)	59820	1(2)	61313	2(3)	61583	1(2)	61860	1(3)
56441	1(2)	57291	1(2)	58290	1(3)	58900	1(2)	59821	1(2)	61314	2(3)	61584	1(2)	61863	1(2)
56442	1(2)	57292	1(2)	58291	1(2)	58920	1(2)	59830	1(2)	61315	1(3)	61585	1(2)	61864	1(3)
56501	1(2)	57295	1(2)	58292	1(2)	58925	1(3)	59840	1(2)	61316	1(3)	61586	1(3)	61867	1(2)
56515	1(2)	57296	1(2)	58293	1(2)	58940	1(2)	59841	1(2)	61320	2(3)	61590	1(2)	61868	2(3)
56605	1(2)	57300	1(3)	58294	1(2)	58943	1(2)	59850	1(2)	61321	1(3)	61591	1(2)	61870	1(3)
56606	6(3)	57305	1(3)	58301	1(3)	58950	1(2)	59851	1(2)	61322	1(3)	61592	1(2)	61880	1(2)
56620	1(2)	57307	1(3)	58321	1(2)	58951	1(2)	59852	1(2)	61323	1(3)	61595	1(2)	61885	2(3)
56625	1(2)	57308	1(3)	58322	1(2)	58952	1(2)	59855	1(2)	61330	1(2)	61596	1(2)	61886	1(3)
56630	1(2)	57310	1(3)	58323	1(3)	58953	1(2)	59856	1(2)	61332	1(2)	61597	1(2)	61888	1(3)
56631	1(2)	57311	1(3)	58340	1(3)	58954	1(2)	59857	1(2)	61333	1(2)	61598	1(3)	62000	1(3)
56632	1(2)	57320	1(3)	58345	1(2)	58956	1(2)	59866	1(2)	61340	1(2)	61600	1(3)	62005	1(3)
56633	1(2)	57330	1(3)	58346	1(2)	58957	1(2)	59870	1(2)	61343	1(2)	61601	1(3)	62010	1(3)
56634	1(2)	57335	1(2)	58350	1(2)	58958	1(2)	59871	1(2)	61345	1(3)	61605	1(3)	62100	1(3)
56637	1(2)	57400	1(2)	58353	1(3)	58960	1(2)	60000	1(3)	61450	1(3)	61606	1(3)	62115	1(2)
56640	1(2)	57410	1(2)	58356	1(3)	58970	1(3)	60100	3(3)	61458	1(2)	61607	1(3)	62117	1(2)
56700	1(2)	57415	1(3)	58400	1(3)	58974	1(3)	60200	2(3)	61460	1(2)	61608	1(3)	62120	1(2)
56740	1(3)	57420	1(3)	58410	1(2)	58976	2(3)	60210	1(2)	61480	1(2)	61610	1(3)	62121	1(2)
56800	1(2)	57421	1(3)	58520	1(2)	59000	1(3)	60212	1(2)	61500	1(3)	61611	1(3)	62140	1(3)
56805	1(2)	57423	1(2)	58540	1(3)	59001	1(3)	60220	1(3)	61501	1(3)	61612	1(3)	62141	1(3)
56810	1(2)	57425	1(2)	58541	1(3)	59012	1(3)	60225	1(2)	61510	1(3)	61613	1(3)	62142	2(3)
56820	1(2)	57426	1(2)	58542	1(2)	59015	1(3)	60240	1(2)	61512	1(3)	61615	1(3)	62143	2(3)
56821	1(2)	57452	1(3)	58543	1(3)	59020	2(3)	60252	1(2)	61514	2(3)	61616	1(3)	62145	2(3)
57000	1(3)	57454	1(3)	58544	1(2)	59025	3(3)	60254	1(2)	61516	1(3)	61618	2(3)	62146	2(3)
57010	1(3)	57455	1(3)	58545	1(2)	59030	4(3)	60260	1(2)	61517	1(3)	61619	2(3)	62147	1(3)
57020	1(3)	57456	1(3)	58546	1(2)	59050	1(3)	60270	1(2)	61518	1(3)	61623	2(3)	62148	1(3)
57022	1(3)	57460	1(3)	58548	1(2)	59051	1(3)	60271	1(2)	61519	1(3)	61624	2(3)	62160	1(3)
57023	1(3)	57461	1(3)	58550	1(3)	59070	2(3)	60280	1(3)	61520	1(3)	61626	2(3)	62161	1(3)
57061	1(2)	57500	1(3)	58552	1(3)	59072	2(3)	60281	1(3)	61521	1(3)	61630	1(3)	62162	1(3)
57065	1(2)	57505	1(3)	58553	1(3)	59074	1(3)	60300	2(3)	61522	1(3)	61635	2(3)	62163	1(3)
57100	3(3)	57510	1(3)	58554	1(2)	59076	1(3)	60500	1(2)	61524	2(3)	61645	3(2)	62164	1(3)
57105	2(3)	57511	1(3)	58555	1(3)	59100	1(2)	60502	1(3)	61526	1(3)	61650	1(2)	62165	1(2)
57106	1(2)	57513	1(3)	58558	1(3)	59120	1(3)	60505	1(3)	61530	1(3)	61651	2(2)	62180	1(3)
57107	1(2)	57520	1(3)	58559	1(3)	59121	1(3)	60512	1(3)	61531	1(2)	61680	1(3)	62190	1(3)
57109	1(2)	57522	1(3)	58560	1(3)	59130	1(3)	60520	1(2)	61533	2(3)	61682	1(3)	62192	1(3)
57110	1(2)	57530	1(3)	58561	1(3)	59135	1(3)	60521	1(2)	61534	1(3)	61684	1(3)	62194	1(3)
57111	1(2)	57531	1(2)	58562	1(3)	59136	1(3)	60522	1(2)	61535	2(3)	61686	1(3)	62200	1(2)
57112	1(2)	57540	1(2)	58563	1(3)	59140	1(2)	60540	1(2)	61536	1(3)	61690	1(3)	62201	1(2)
57120	1(2)	57545	1(3)	58565	1(2)	59150	1(3)	60545	1(2)	61537	1(3)	61692	1(3)	62220	1(3)
57130	1(2)	57550	1(3)	58570	1(3)	59151	1(3)	60600	1(3)	61538	1(2)	61697	2(3)	62223	1(3)
57135	2(3)	57555	1(2)	58571	1(2)	59160	1(2)	60605	1(3)	61539	1(3)	61698	1(3)	62225	2(3)
57150	1(3)	57556	1(2)	58572	1(3)	59200	1(3)	60650	1(2)	61540	1(3)	61700	2(3)	62230	2(3)
57155	1(3)	57558	1(3)	58573	1(2)	59300	1(2)	61000	1(2)	61541	1(2)	61702	1(3)	62252	2(3)
57156	1(3)	57700	1(3)	58600	1(2)	59320	1(2)	61001	1(2)	61543	1(2)	61703	1(3)	62256	1(3)
57160	1(2)	57720	1(3)	58605	1(2)	59325	1(2)	61020	2(3)	61544	1(3)	61705	1(3)	62258	1(3)
57170	1(2)	57800	1(3)	58611	1(2)	59350	1(2)	61026	2(3)	61545	1(2)	61708	1(3)	62263	1(2)
57180	1(3)	58100	1(3)	58615	1(2)	59400	1(2)	61050	1(3)	61546	1(2)	61710	1(3)	62264	1(2)
57200	1(3)	58110	1(3)	58660	1(2)	59409	2(3)	61055	1(3)	61548	1(2)	61711	1(3)	62267	2(3)
57210	1(3)	58120	1(3)	58661	1(2)	59410	1(2)	61070	2(3)	61550	1(2)	61720	1(3)	62268	1(3)
57220	1(2)	58140	1(3)	58662	1(2)	59412	1(3)	61105	1(3)	61552	1(2)	61735	1(3)	62269	2(3)
57230	1(2)	58145	1(3)	58670	1(2)	59414	1(3)	61107	1(3)	61556	1(3)	61750	2(3)	62270	2(3)
57240	1(2)	58146	1(3)	58671	1(2)	59425	1(2)	61108	1(3)	61557	1(2)	61751	2(3)	62272	1(3)
57250	1(2)	58150	1(3)	58672	1(2)	59426	1(2)	61120	1(3)	61558	1(3)	61760	1(2)	62273	2(3)
57260	1(2)	58152	1(2)	58673	1(2)	59430	1(2)	61140	1(3)	61559	1(3)	61770	1(2)	62280	1(3)
57265	1(2)	58180	1(3)	58700	1(2)	59510	1(2)	61150	1(3)	61563	2(3)	61781	1(3)	62281	1(3)
57267	2(3)	58200	1(2)	58720	1(2)	59514	1(3)	61151	1(3)	61564	1(2)	61782	1(3)	62282	1(3)
57268	1(2)	58210	1(2)	58740	1(2)	59515	1(2)	61154	1(3)	61566	1(3)	61783	1(3)	62284	1(3)
57270	1(2)	58240	1(2)	58750	1(2)	59525	1(2)	61156	1(3)	61567	1(2)	61790	1(2)	62287	1(2)
57280	1(2)	58260	1(3)	58752	1(2)	59610	1(2)	61210	1(3)	61570	1(3)	61791	1(2)	62290	5(2)
57282	1(2)	58262	1(3)	58760	1(2)	59612	2(3)	61215	1(3)	61571	1(3)	61796	1(2)	62291	4(3)
57283	1(2)	58263	1(2)	58770	1(2)	59614	1(2)	61250	1(3)	61575	1(2)	61797	4(3)	62292	1(2)
57284	1(2)	58267	1(2)	58800	1(2)	59618	1(2)	61253	1(3)	61576	1(2)	61798	1(2)	62294	1(3)
57285	1(2)	58270	1(2)	58805	1(2)	59620	1(2)	61304	1(3)	61580	1(2)	61799	4(3)	62302	1(3)
57287	1(2)	58275	1(2)	58820	1(3)	59622	1(2)	61305	1(3)	61581	1(2)	61800	1(2)	62303	1(3)
57288	1(2)	58280	1(2)	58822	1(3)	59812	1(2)	61312	2(3)	61582	1(2)	61850	1(3)	62304	1(3)

CPT	MUE	CPT	MUE	CPT	MUE	CPT	MUE	CPT	MUE	CPT	MUE	CPT	MUE	CPT	MUE
62305	1(3)	63194	1(2)	64402	1(3)	64616	1(2)	64822	1(2)	65285	1(3)	66635	1(2)	67314	1(2)
62310	1(3)	63195	1(2)	64405	1(3)	64617	1(2)	64823	1(2)	65286	1(3)	66680	1(2)	67316	1(2)
62311	1(3)	63196	1(2)	64408	1(3)	64620	5(3)	64831	1(2)	65290	1(3)	66682	1(2)	67318	1(2)
62318	1(3)	63197	1(2)	64410	1(3)	64630	1(3)	64832	3(3)	65400	1(3)	66700	1(2)	67320	2(3)
62319	1(3)	63198	1(2)	64413	1(3)	64632	1(2)	64834	1(2)	65410	1(3)	66710	1(2)	67331	1(2)
62350	1(3)	63199	1(2)	64415	1(3)	64633	1(2)	64835	1(2)	65420	1(2)	66711	1(2)	67332	1(2)
62351	1(3)	63200	1(2)	64416	1(2)	64634	4(3)	64836	1(2)	65426	1(2)	66720	1(2)	67334	1(2)
62355	1(3)	63250	1(3)	64417	1(3)	64635	1(2)	64837	2(3)	65430	1(2)	66740	1(2)	67335	1(2)
62360	1(2)	63251	1(3)	64418	1(3)	64636	4(2)	64840	1(2)	65435	1(2)	66761	1(2)	67340	2(2)
62361	1(2)	63252	1(3)	64420	3(3)	64640	5(3)	64856	2(3)	65436	1(2)	66762	1(2)	67343	1(2)
62362	1(2)	63265	1(3)	64421	3(3)	64642	1(2)	64857	2(3)	65450	1(3)	66770	1(3)	67345	1(3)
62365	1(2)	63266	1(3)	64425	1(3)	64643	3(2)	64858	1(2)	65600	1(2)	66820	1(2)	67346	1(3)
62367	1(3)	63267	1(3)	64430	1(3)	64644	1(2)	64859	2(3)	65710	1(2)	66821	1(2)	67400	1(2)
62368	1(3)	63268	1(3)	64435	1(3)	64645	3(2)	64861	1(2)	65730	1(2)	66825	1(2)	67405	1(2)
62369	1(3)	63270	1(3)	64445	1(3)	64646	1(2)	64862	1(2)	65750	1(2)	66830	1(2)	67412	1(2)
62370	1(3)	63271	1(3)	64446	1(2)	64647	1(2)	64864	2(3)	65755	1(2)	66840	1(2)	67413	1(2)
63001	1(2)	63272	1(3)	64447	1(3)	64650	1(2)	64865	1(3)	65756	1(2)	66850	1(2)	67414	1(2)
63003	1(2)	63273	1(3)	64448	1(2)	64653	1(2)	64866	1(3)	65757	1(3)	66852	1(2)	67415	1(3)
63005	1(2)	63275	1(3)	64449	1(2)	64680	1(2)	64868	1(3)	65770	1(2)	66920	1(2)	67420	1(2)
63011	1(2)	63276	1(3)	64450	10(3)	64681	1(2)	64872	1(3)	65772	1(2)	66930	1(2)	67430	1(2)
63012	1(2)	63277	1(3)	64455	1(2)	64702	2(3)	64874	1(3)	65775	1(2)	66940	1(2)	67440	1(2)
63015	1(2)	63278	1(3)	64461	1(2)	64704	4(3)	64876	1(3)	65778	1(2)	66982	1(2)	67445	1(2)
63016	1(2)	63280	1(3)	64462	1(2)	64708	3(3)	64885	1(3)	65779	1(2)	66983	1(2)	67450	1(2)
63017	1(2)	63281	1(3)	64463	1(3)	64712	1(2)	64886	1(3)	65780	1(2)	66984	1(2)	67500	1(3)
63020	1(2)	63282	1(3)	64479	1(2)	64713	1(2)	64890	2(3)	65781	1(2)	66985	1(2)	67505	1(3)
63030	1(2)	63283	1(3)	64480	4(3)	64714	1(2)	64891	2(3)	65782	1(2)	66986	1(2)	67515	1(3)
63035	4(3)	63285	1(3)	64483	1(2)	64716	2(3)	64892	2(3)	65785	2(2)	66990	1(3)	67550	1(2)
63040	1(2)	63286	1(3)	64484	4(3)	64718	1(2)	64893	2(3)	65800	1(2)	67005	1(2)	67560	1(2)
63042	1(2)	63287	1(3)	64486	1(3)	64719	1(2)	64895	2(3)	65810	1(2)	67010	1(2)	67570	1(2)
63043	4(3)	63290	1(3)	64487	1(2)	64721	1(2)	64896	2(3)	65815	1(3)	67015	1(2)	67700	2(3)
63044	4(2)	63295	1(2)	64488	1(3)	64722	4(3)	64897	2(3)	65820	1(2)	67025	1(2)	67710	1(2)
63045	1(2)	63300	1(2)	64489	1(2)	64726	2(3)	64898	2(3)	65850	1(2)	67027	1(2)	67715	1(3)
63046	1(2)	63301	1(2)	64490	1(2)	64727	2(3)	64901	2(3)	65855	1(2)	67028	1(3)	67800	1(2)
63047	1(2)	63302	1(2)	64491	1(2)	64732	1(2)	64902	1(3)	65860	1(2)	67030	1(2)	67801	1(2)
63048	5(3)	63303	1(2)	64492	1(2)	64734	1(2)	64905	1(3)	65865	1(2)	67031	1(2)	67805	1(2)
63050	1(2)	63304	1(2)	64493	1(2)	64736	1(2)	64907	1(3)	65870	1(2)	67036	1(2)	67808	1(2)
63051	1(2)	63305	1(2)	64494	1(2)	64738	1(2)	64910	3(3)	65875	1(2)	67039	1(2)	67810	2(3)
63055	1(2)	63306	1(2)	64495	1(2)	64740	1(2)	64911	2(3)	65880	1(2)	67040	1(2)	67820	1(2)
63056	1(2)	63307	1(2)	64505	1(3)	64742	1(2)	65091	1(2)	65900	1(3)	67041	1(2)	67825	1(2)
63057	3(3)	63308	3(3)	64508	1(3)	64744	1(2)	65093	1(2)	65920	1(2)	67042	1(2)	67830	1(2)
63064	1(2)	63600	2(3)	64510	1(3)	64746	1(2)	65101	1(2)	65930	1(3)	67043	1(2)	67835	1(2)
63066	1(3)	63610	1(3)	64517	1(3)	64755	1(2)	65103	1(2)	66020	1(3)	67101	1(2)	67840	4(3)
63075	1(2)	63615	1(3)	64520	1(3)	64760	1(2)	65105	1(2)	66030	1(3)	67105	1(2)	67850	3(3)
63076	3(3)	63620	1(2)	64530	1(3)	64763	1(2)	65110	1(2)	66130	1(3)	67107	1(2)	67875	1(2)
63077	1(2)	63621	2(2)	64550	1(3)	64766	1(2)	65112	1(2)	66150	1(2)	67108	1(2)	67880	1(2)
63078	3(3)	63650	2(3)	64553	1(3)	64771	2(3)	65114	1(2)	66155	1(2)	67110	1(2)	67882	1(2)
63081	1(2)	63655	1(3)	64555	2(3)	64772	2(3)	65125	1(2)	66160	1(2)	67113	1(2)	67900	1(2)
63082	6(2)	63661	1(2)	64561	1(3)	64774	2(3)	65130	1(2)	66170	1(2)	67115	1(1)	67901	1(2)
63085	1(2)	63662	1(2)	64565	2(3)	64776	1(2)	65135	1(2)	66172	1(2)	67120	1(2)	67902	1(2)
63086	2(3)	63663	1(3)	64566	1(3)	64778	1(3)	65140	1(2)	66174	1(2)	67121	1(2)	67903	1(2)
63087	1(2)	63664	1(3)	64568	1(3)	64782	2(2)	65150	1(2)	66175	1(2)	67141	1(2)	67904	1(2)
63088	4(3)	63685	1(3)	64569	1(3)	64783	2(3)	65155	1(2)	66179	1(2)	67145	1(2)	67906	1(2)
63090	1(2)	63688	1(3)	64570	1(3)	64784	3(3)	65175	1(2)	66180	1(2)	67208	1(2)	67908	1(2)
63091	3(3)	63700	1(3)	64575	2(3)	64786	1(3)	65205	1(3)	66183	1(3)	67210	1(2)	67909	1(2)
63101	1(2)	63702	1(3)	64580	2(3)	64787	4(3)	65210	1(3)	66184	1(2)	67218	1(2)	67911	4(2)
63102	1(2)	63704	1(3)	64581	2(3)	64788	5(3)	65220	1(3)	66185	1(3)	67220	1(2)	67912	1(2)
63103	3(3)	63706	1(3)	64585	2(3)	64790	1(3)	65222	1(3)	66220	1(2)	67221	1(2)	67914	1(3)
63170	1(3)	63707	1(3)	64590	1(3)	64792	2(3)	65235	1(3)	66225	1(2)	67225	1(2)	67915	1(3)
63172	1(3)	63709	1(3)	64595	1(3)	64795	2(3)	65260	1(3)	66250	1(2)	67227	1(2)	67916	1(3)
63173	1(3)	63710	1(3)	64600	2(3)	64802	1(2)	65265	1(3)	66500	1(2)	67228	1(2)	67917	1(3)
63180	1(2)	63740	1(3)	64605	1(2)	64804	1(2)	65270	1(2)	66505	1(2)	67229	1(2)	67921	1(3)
63182	1(2)	63741	1(3)	64610	1(2)	64809	1(2)	65272	1(3)	66600	1(2)	67250	1(2)	67922	1(3)
63185	1(2)	63744	1(3)	64611	1(2)	64818	1(2)	65273	1(3)	66605	1(2)	67255	1(2)	67923	1(3)
63190	1(2)	63746	1(2)	64612	1(2)	64820	4(3)	65275	1(3)	66625	1(2)	67311	1(2)	67924	1(3)
63191	1(2)	64400	4(3)	64615	1(2)	64821	1(2)	65280	1(3)	66630	1(2)	67312	1(2)	67930	2(3)

CPT	MUE	CPT	MUE	CPT	MUE	CPT	MUE	CPT	MUE	CPT	MUE	CPT	MUE	CPT	MUE
67935	2(3)	69205	1(3)	69820	1(2)	70548	1(3)	72157	1(3)	73592	2(3)	74410	1(3)	75889	1(3)
67938	2(3)	69209	2(2)	69840	1(3)	70549	1(3)	72158	1(3)	73600	3(3)	74415	1(3)	75891	1(3)
67950	2(2)	69210	1(2)	69905	1(2)	70551	2(3)	72170	2(3)	73610	3(3)	74420	2(3)	75893	2(3)
67961	4(2)	69220	1(2)	69910	1(2)	70552	2(3)	72190	1(3)	73615	2(2)	74425	2(3)	75894	2(3)
67966	4(2)	69222	1(2)	69915	1(3)	70553	2(3)	72191	1(3)	73620	3(3)	74430	1(3)	75898	2(3)
67971	1(2)	69300	1(2)	69930	1(2)	70554	1(3)	72192	1(3)	73630	3(3)	74440	1(2)	75901	1(3)
67973	1(2)	69310	1(2)	69950	1(2)	70555	1(3)	72193	1(3)	73650	2(3)	74445	1(2)	75902	2(3)
67974	1(2)	69320	1(2)	69955	1(2)	70557	1(3)	72194	1(3)	73660	2(3)	74450	1(3)	75952	1(2)
67975	1(2)	69420	1(2)	69960	1(2)	70558	1(3)	72195	1(3)	73700	2(3)	74455	1(3)	75953	4(3)
68020	1(3)	69421	1(2)	69970	1(3)	70559	1(3)	72196	1(3)	73701	2(3)	74470	2(2)	75954	2(3)
68040	1(3)	69424	1(2)	69990	1(3)	71010	6(3)	72197	1(3)	73702	2(3)	74485	2(3)	75956	1(2)
68100	1(3)	69433	1(2)	70010	1(3)	71015	2(3)	72198	1(3)	73706	2(3)	74710	1(3)	75957	1(2)
68110	1(3)	69436	1(2)	70015	1(3)	71020	4(3)	72200	2(3)	73718	2(3)	74712	1(3)	75958	2(3)
68115	1(3)	69440	1(2)	70030	2(2)	71021	1(3)	72202	1(3)	73719	2(3)	74713	2(3)	75959	1(2)
68130	1(3)	69450	1(2)	70100	2(3)	71022	1(3)	72220	1(3)	73720	2(3)	74740	1(3)	75962	1(1)
68135	1(3)	69501	1(3)	70110	2(3)	71023	1(3)	72240	1(2)	73721	3(3)	74742	2(2)	75964	2(3)
68200	1(3)	69502	1(2)	70120	1(3)	71030	1(3)	72255	1(2)	73722	2(3)	74775	1(2)	75966	1(1)
68320	1(2)	69505	1(2)	70130	1(3)	71034	1(3)	72265	1(2)	73723	2(3)	75557	1(3)	75968	2(3)
68325	1(2)	69511	1(2)	70134	1(3)	71035	3(3)	72270	1(2)	73725	2(3)	75559	1(3)	75970	1(3)
68326	2(2)	69530	1(2)	70140	2(3)	71100	2(3)	72275	3(3)	74000	4(3)	75561	1(3)	75978	3(3)
68328	2(2)	69535	1(2)	70150	1(3)	71101	2(3)	72285	4(3)	74010	2(3)	75563	1(3)	75984	2(3)
68330	1(3)	69540	1(3)	70160	1(3)	71110	1(3)	72295	5(3)	74020	2(3)	75565	1(3)	75989	2(3)
68335	1(3)	69550	1(3)	70170	2(2)	71111	1(3)	73000	2(3)	74022	2(3)	75571	1(3)	76000	3(3)
68340	1(3)	69552	1(2)	70190	1(2)	71120	1(3)	73010	2(3)	74150	1(3)	75572	1(3)	76001	1(3)
68360	1(3)	69554	1(2)	70200	2(3)	71130	1(3)	73020	2(3)	74160	1(3)	75573	1(3)	76010	2(3)
68362	1(3)	69601	1(2)	70210	1(3)	71250	2(3)	73030	4(3)	74170	1(3)	75574	1(3)	76080	3(3)
68371	1(3)	69602	1(2)	70220	1(3)	71260	2(3)	73040	2(2)	74174	1(3)	75600	1(3)	76098	3(3)
68400	1(2)	69603	1(2)	70240	1(2)	71270	1(3)	73050	1(3)	74175	1(3)	75605	1(3)	76100	2(3)
68420	1(2)	69604	1(2)	70250	2(3)	71275	1(3)	73060	2(3)	74176	2(3)	75625	1(3)	76101	1(3)
68440	2(2)	69605	1(2)	70260	1(3)	71550	1(3)	73070	2(3)	74177	2(3)	75630	1(3)	76102	1(3)
68500	1(2)	69610	1(2)	70300	1(3)	71551	1(3)	73080	2(3)	74178	1(3)	75635	1(3)	76120	1(3)
68505	1(2)	69620	1(2)	70310	1(3)	71552	1(3)	73085	2(2)	74181	1(3)	75658	1(3)	76125	1(3)
68510	1(2)	69631	1(2)	70320	1(3)	71555	1(3)	73090	2(3)	74182	1(3)	75705	13(3)	76376	2(3)
68520	1(2)	69632	1(3)	70328	1(3)	72020	4(3)	73092	2(3)	74183	1(3)	75710	2(3)	76377	2(3)
68525	1(2)	69633	1(2)	70330	1(3)	72040	3(3)	73100	2(3)	74185	1(3)	75716	1(3)	76380	2(3)
68530	1(2)	69635	1(3)	70332	2(3)	72050	1(3)	73110	3(3)	74190	1(3)	75726	3(3)	76506	1(2)
68540	1(2)	69636	1(3)	70336	1(3)	72052	1(3)	73115	2(3)	74210	1(3)	75731	1(3)	76510	2(2)
68550	1(2)	69637	1(3)	70350	1(3)	72070	1(3)	73120	3(3)	74220	1(3)	75733	1(3)	76511	2(2)
68700	1(2)	69641	1(2)	70355	1(3)	72072	1(3)	73130	3(3)	74230	1(3)	75736	2(3)	76512	2(2)
68705	2(2)	69642	1(2)	70360	2(3)	72074	1(3)	73140	3(3)	74235	1(3)	75741	1(3)	76513	2(2)
68720	1(2)	69643	1(2)	70370	1(3)	72080	1(3)	73200	2(3)	74240	2(3)	75743	1(3)	76514	1(2)
68745	1(3)	69644	1(2)	70371	1(2)	72081	1(3)	73201	2(3)	74241	1(3)	75746	1(3)	76516	1(2)
68750	1(2)	69645	1(2)	70380	2(3)	72082	1(3)	73202	2(3)	74245	1(3)	75756	2(3)	76519	2(2)
68760	4(2)	69646	1(2)	70390	2(3)	72083	1(3)	73206	2(3)	74246	1(3)	75774	7(3)	76529	2(2)
68761	4(2)	69650	1(2)	70450	3(3)	72084	1(3)	73218	2(3)	74247	1(3)	75791	1(3)	76536	1(3)
68770	1(3)	69660	1(2)	70460	1(3)	72100	2(3)	73219	2(3)	74249	1(3)	75801	1(3)	76604	1(3)
68801	4(2)	69661	1(2)	70470	2(3)	72110	1(3)	73220	2(3)	74250	1(3)	75803	1(3)	76641	2(2)
68810	1(2)	69662	1(2)	70480	1(3)	72114	1(3)	73221	2(3)	74251	1(3)	75805	1(2)	76642	2(2)
68811	1(2)	69666	1(2)	70481	1(3)	72120	1(3)	73222	2(3)	74260	1(2)	75807	1(2)	76700	1(3)
68815	1(2)	69667	1(2)	70482	1(3)	72125	1(3)	73223	2(3)	74261	1(2)	75809	1(3)	76705	2(3)
68816	1(2)	69670	1(2)	70486	1(3)	72126	1(3)	73501	2(3)	74262	1(2)	75810	1(3)	76770	1(3)
68840	1(2)	69676	1(2)	70487	1(3)	72127	1(3)	73502	2(3)	74270	1(3)	75820	2(3)	76775	2(3)
68850	1(3)	69700	1(3)	70488	1(3)	72128	1(3)	73503	2(3)	74280	1(3)	75822	1(3)	76776	2(3)
69000	1(3)	69711	1(2)	70490	1(3)	72129	1(3)	73521	2(3)	74283	1(3)	75825	1(3)	76800	1(3)
69005	1(3)	69714	1(2)	70491	1(3)	72130	1(3)	73522	2(3)	74290	1(3)	75827	1(3)	76801	1(2)
69020	1(3)	69715	1(3)	70492	1(3)	72131	1(3)	73523	2(3)	74300	1(3)	75831	1(3)	76802	2(3)
69100	3(3)	69717	1(2)	70496	2(3)	72132	1(3)	73525	2(2)	74301	1(3)	75833	1(3)	76805	1(2)
69105	1(3)	69718	1(2)	70498	2(3)	72133	1(3)	73551	2(3)	74328	1(3)	75840	1(3)	76810	2(3)
69110	1(2)	69720	1(2)	70540	1(3)	72141	1(3)	73552	2(3)	74329	1(3)	75842	1(3)	76811	1(2)
69120	1(3)	69725	1(2)	70542	1(3)	72142	1(3)	73560	4(3)	74330	1(3)	75860	2(3)	76812	2(3)
69140	1(2)	69740	1(2)	70543	1(3)	72146	1(3)	73562	4(3)	74340	1(3)	75870	1(3)	76813	1(2)
69145	1(3)	69745	1(2)	70544	2(3)	72147	1(3)	73564	4(3)	74355	1(3)	75872	1(3)	76814	2(3)
69150	1(3)	69801	1(3)	70545	1(3)	72148	1(3)	73565	1(3)	74360	1(3)	75880	1(3)	76815	1(2)
69155	1(3)	69805	1(3)	70546	1(3)	72149	1(3)	73580	2(3)	74363	2(3)	75885	1(3)	76816	3(3)
69200	1(2)	69806	1(3)	70547	1(3)	72156	1(3)	73590	3(3)	74400	1(3)	75887	1(3)	76817	1(3)

CPT	MUE	CPT	MUE	CPT	MUE	CPT	MUE	CPT	MUE	CPT	MUE	CPT	MUE	CPT	MUE
76818	3(3)	77086	1(2)	78014	1(2)	78459	1(3)	80053	1(3)	80439	1(3)	81264	1(3)	81382	6(3)
76819	3(3)	77261	1(3)	78015	1(3)	78466	1(3)	80061	1(3)	80500	1(3)	81265	1(3)	81383	2(3)
76820	3(3)	77262	1(3)	78016	1(3)	78468	1(3)	80069	1(3)	80502	1(3)	81266	2(3)	81400	2(3)
76821	3(3)	77263	1(3)	78018	1(2)	78469	1(3)	80074	1(2)	81000	2(3)	81267	1(3)	81401	2(3)
76825	3(3)	77280	2(3)	78020	1(3)	78472	1(2)	80076	1(3)	81001	2(3)	81268	4(3)	81402	1(3)
76826	3(3)	77285	1(3)	78070	1(2)	78473	1(2)	80081	1(2)	81002	2(3)	81270	1(2)	81403	4(3)
76827	3(3)	77290	1(3)	78071	1(3)	78481	1(2)	80150	2(3)	81003	2(3)	81272	1(3)	81404	5(3)
76828	3(3)	77293	1(3)	78072	1(3)	78483	1(2)	80155	1(3)	81005	2(3)	81273	1(3)	81405	2(3)
76830	1(3)	77295	1(3)	78075	1(2)	78491	1(3)	80156	2(3)	81007	1(3)	81275	1(3)	81406	2(3)
76831	1(3)	77300	10(3)	78102	1(2)	78492	1(2)	80157	2(3)	81015	2(3)	81276	1(3)	81407	1(3)
76856	1(3)	77301	1(3)	78103	1(2)	78494	1(3)	80158	2(1)	81020	1(3)	81280	1(3)	81408	2(3)
76857	1(3)	77306	1(3)	78104	1(2)	78496	1(3)	80159	2(3)	81025	1(3)	81281	1(3)	81410	1(3)
76870	1(2)	77307	1(3)	78110	1(2)	78579	1(3)	80162	2(3)	81050	2(3)	81282	1(3)	81411	1(3)
76872	1(3)	77316	1(3)	78111	1(2)	78580	1(3)	80163	2(3)	81161	1(3)	81287	1(3)	81412	1(2)
76873	1(2)	77317	1(3)	78120	1(2)	78582	1(3)	80164	2(3)	81162	1(2)	81288	1(3)	81415	1(1)
76881	2(3)	77318	1(3)	78121	1(2)	78597	1(3)	80165	2(3)	81170	1(2)	81290	1(3)	81416	2(1)
76882	2(3)	77321	1(2)	78122	1(2)	78598	1(3)	80168	2(3)	81200	1(3)	81291	1(3)	81417	1(1)
76885	1(2)	77331	3(3)	78130	1(2)	78600	1(3)	80169	1(3)	81201	1(3)	81292	1(2)	81420	1(3)
76886	1(2)	77332	4(3)	78135	1(3)	78601	1(3)	80170	2(3)	81202	1(3)	81293	1(3)	81425	1(1)
76930	1(3)	77333	2(3)	78140	1(3)	78605	1(3)	80171	1(3)	81203	1(3)	81294	1(3)	81426	2(1)
76932	1(2)	77334	10(3)	78185	1(2)	78606	1(3)	80173	2(3)	81205	1(3)	81295	1(2)	81427	1(1)
76936	1(3)	77336	1(2)	78190	1(2)	78607	1(3)	80175	1(3)	81206	1(3)	81296	1(3)	81430	1(2)
76937	2(3)	77338	1(3)	78191	1(2)	78608	1(3)	80176	1(3)	81207	1(3)	81297	1(3)	81431	1(2)
76940	1(3)	77370	1(3)	78195	1(2)	78610	1(3)	80177	1(3)	81208	1(3)	81298	1(2)	81432	1(2)
76941	3(3)	77371	1(2)	78201	1(3)	78630	1(3)	80178	2(3)	81209	1(3)	81299	1(3)	81433	1(2)
76942	1(3)	77372	1(2)	78202	1(3)	78635	1(3)	80180	1(3)	81210	1(3)	81300	1(3)	81434	1(2)
76945	1(3)	77373	1(3)	78205	1(3)	78645	1(3)	80183	1(3)	81211	1(2)	81301	1(3)	81435	1(2)
76946	1(3)	77401	1(2)	78206	1(3)	78647	1(3)	80184	2(3)	81212	1(2)	81302	1(3)	81436	1(2)
76948	1(2)	77402	2(3)	78215	1(3)	78650	1(3)	80185	2(3)	81213	1(2)	81303	1(3)	81437	1(2)
76965	2(3)	77407	2(3)	78216	1(3)	78660	1(2)	80186	2(3)	81214	1(2)	81304	1(3)	81438	1(2)
76970	2(3)	77412	2(3)	78226	1(3)	78700	1(3)	80188	2(3)	81215	1(2)	81310	1(3)	81440	1(2)
76975	1(3)	77417	1(2)	78227	1(3)	78701	1(3)	80190	2(3)	81216	1(2)	81311	1(3)	81442	1(2)
76977	1(2)	77422	1(3)	78230	1(3)	78707	1(2)	80192	2(3)	81217	1(2)	81313	1(3)	81445	1(2)
76998	1(3)	77423	1(3)	78231	1(3)	78708	1(2)	80194	2(3)	81218	1(3)	81314	1(3)	81450	1(2)
77001	2(3)	77424	1(2)	78232	1(3)	78709	1(2)	80195	2(3)	81219	1(3)	81315	1(3)	81455	1(2)
77002	1(3)	77425	1(3)	78258	1(2)	78710	1(3)	80197	2(3)	81220	1(3)	81316	1(2)	81460	1(2)
77003	1(3)	77427	1(2)	78261	1(2)	78725	1(3)	80198	2(3)	81221	1(3)	81317	1(3)	81465	1(2)
77011	1(3)	77431	1(2)	78262	1(2)	78730	1(2)	80199	1(3)	81222	1(3)	81318	1(3)	81470	1(2)
77012	1(3)	77432	1(2)	78264	1(2)	78740	1(2)	80200	2(3)	81223	1(2)	81319	1(2)	81471	1(2)
77013	1(3)	77435	1(2)	78265	1(2)	78761	1(2)	80201	2(3)	81224	1(3)	81321	1(3)	81490	1(2)
77014	2(3)	77469	1(2)	78266	1(2)	78800	1(2)	80202	2(3)	81225	1(3)	81322	1(3)	81493	1(2)
77021	1(3)	77470	1(2)	78267	1(2)	78801	1(3)	80203	1(3)	81226	1(3)	81323	1(3)	81500	1(3)
77022	1(3)	77520	1(3)	78268	1(2)	78802	1(2)	80299	3(3)	81227	1(3)	81324	1(3)	81503	1(3)
77051	2(3)	77522	1(3)	78270	1(2)	78803	1(2)	80400	1(3)	81228	1(3)	81325	1(3)	81504	1(3)
77052	1(2)	77523	1(3)	78271	1(2)	78804	1(2)	80402	1(3)	81229	1(3)	81326	1(3)	81506	1(3)
77053	2(2)	77525	1(3)	78272	1(2)	78805	1(3)	80406	1(3)	81235	1(3)	81330	1(3)	81507	1(3)
77054	2(2)	77600	1(3)	78278	2(3)	78806	1(2)	80408	1(3)	81240	1(2)	81331	1(3)	81508	1(3)
77055	1(3)	77605	1(3)	78282	1(2)	78807	1(3)	80410	1(3)	81241	1(2)	81332	1(3)	81509	1(3)
77056	1(3)	77610	1(3)	78290	1(3)	78808	1(2)	80412	1(3)	81242	1(3)	81340	1(3)	81510	1(3)
77057	1(2)	77615	1(3)	78291	1(3)	78811	1(2)	80414	1(3)	81243	1(3)	81341	1(3)	81511	1(3)
77058	1(2)	77620	1(3)	78300	1(2)	78812	1(2)	80415	1(3)	81244	1(3)	81342	1(3)	81512	1(3)
77059	1(2)	77750	1(3)	78305	1(2)	78813	1(2)	80416	1(3)	81245	1(3)	81350	1(3)	81519	1(2)
77063	1(2)	77761	1(3)	78306	1(2)	78814	1(2)	80417	1(3)	81246	1(3)	81355	1(3)	81525	1(3)
77071	1(3)	77762	1(3)	78315	1(2)	78815	1(2)	80418	1(3)	81250	1(3)	81370	1(2)	81528	1(3)
77072	1(2)	77763	1(3)	78320	1(2)	78816	1(2)	80420	1(2)	81251	1(3)	81371	1(2)	81535	1(3)
77073	1(2)	77767	2(3)	78414	1(2)	79005	1(3)	80422	1(3)	81252	1(3)	81372	1(2)	81536	3(1)
77074	1(2)	77768	2(3)	78428	1(3)	79101	1(3)	80424	1(3)	81253	1(3)	81373	2(3)	81538	1(2)
77075	1(2)	77770	2(3)	78445	1(3)	79200	1(3)	80426	1(3)	81254	1(3)	81374	1(3)	81540	1(3)
77076	1(2)	77771	2(3)	78451	1(2)	79300	1(3)	80428	1(3)	81255	1(3)	81375	1(2)	81545	1(3)
77077	1(2)	77772	2(3)	78452	1(2)	79403	1(3)	80430	1(3)	81256	1(2)	81376	5(3)	81595	1(2)
77078	1(2)	77778	1(3)	78453	1(2)	79440	1(3)	80432	1(3)	81257	1(2)	81377	2(3)	82009	1(3)
77080	1(2)	77789	2(3)	78454	1(2)	79445	1(3)	80434	1(3)	81260	1(3)	81378	1(3)	82010	1(3)
77081	1(2)	77790	1(3)	78456	1(3)	80047	2(3)	80435	1(3)	81261	1(3)	81379	1(2)	82013	1(3)
77084	1(2)	78012	1(3)	78457	1(3)	80048	2(3)	80436	1(3)	81262	1(3)	81380	2(2)	82016	1(3)
77085	1(2)	78013	1(3)	78458	1(2)	80051	2(3)	80438	1(3)	81263	1(3)	81381	3(3)	82017	1(3)

CPT	MUE	CPT	MUE	CPT	MUE	CPT	MUE	CPT	MUE	CPT	MUE	CPT	MUE	CPT	MUE
82024	4(3)	82382	1(2)	82747	1(2)	83499	1(3)	83951	1(2)	84285	1(3)	84830	1(2)	85410	1(3)
82030	1(3)	82383	1(3)	82757	1(2)	83500	1(3)	83970	2(3)	84295	3(1)	85002	1(3)	85415	2(3)
82040	1(3)	82384	2(3)	82759	1(3)	83505	1(3)	83986	2(3)	84300	2(3)	85004	1(3)	85420	2(3)
82042	2(3)	82387	1(3)	82760	1(3)	83516	4(3)	83987	1(3)	84302	1(1)	85007	1(3)	85421	1(3)
82043	1(3)	82390	1(2)	82775	1(3)	83518	1(3)	83992	2(3)	84305	1(3)	85008	1(3)	85441	1(2)
82044	1(3)	82397	3(3)	82776	1(2)	83519	5(3)	83993	1(3)	84307	1(3)	85009	1(3)	85445	1(2)
82045	1(3)	82415	1(3)	82777	1(3)	83520	8(3)	84030	1(2)	84311	2(3)	85013	1(3)	85460	1(3)
82075	2(3)	82435	2(1)	82784	6(3)	83525	4(3)	84035	1(2)	84315	1(3)	85014	2(3)	85461	1(2)
82085	1(3)	82436	1(3)	82785	1(3)	83527	1(3)	84060	1(3)	84375	1(3)	85018	2(3)	85475	1(3)
82088	2(3)	82438	1(3)	82787	4(3)	83528	1(3)	84061	1(3)	84376	1(3)	85025	2(3)	85520	1(3)
82103	1(3)	82441	1(2)	82800	1(1)	83540	2(3)	84066	1(3)	84377	1(3)	85027	2(3)	85525	2(3)
82104	1(2)	82465	1(3)	82805	2(1)	83550	1(3)	84075	2(3)	84378	2(3)	85032	1(3)	85530	1(3)
82105	1(3)	82480	2(3)	82810	2(3)	83570	1(3)	84078	1(2)	84379	1(3)	85041	1(3)	85536	1(2)
82106	2(3)	82482	1(3)	82820	1(3)	83582	1(3)	84080	1(3)	84392	1(3)	85044	1(3)	85540	1(2)
82107	1(3)	82485	1(3)	82930	1(1)	83586	1(3)	84081	1(3)	84402	1(3)	85045	1(2)	85547	1(2)
82108	1(3)	82495	1(3)	82938	1(3)	83593	1(3)	84085	1(2)	84403	2(3)	85046	1(2)	85549	1(3)
82120	1(3)	82507	1(3)	82941	1(3)	83605	3(1)	84087	1(3)	84425	1(2)	85048	2(3)	85555	1(2)
82127	1(3)	82523	1(3)	82943	1(3)	83615	2(3)	84100	2(3)	84430	1(3)	85049	2(3)	85557	1(2)
82128	2(3)	82525	2(3)	82945	4(3)	83625	1(3)	84105	1(2)	84431	1(3)	85055	1(3)	85576	7(3)
82131	2(3)	82528	1(3)	82946	1(2)	83630	1(3)	84106	1(2)	84432	1(2)	85060	1(3)	85597	1(3)
82135	1(3)	82530	4(3)	82947	5(3)	83631	1(3)	84110	1(3)	84436	1(2)	85097	2(3)	85598	1(3)
82136	2(3)	82533	5(3)	82950	3(3)	83632	1(3)	84112	1(3)	84437	1(2)	85130	1(3)	85610	4(3)
82139	2(3)	82540	1(3)	82951	1(2)	83633	1(3)	84119	1(2)	84439	1(2)	85170	1(3)	85611	2(3)
82140	2(3)	82542	6(3)	82952	3(3)	83655	2(3)	84120	1(3)	84442	1(2)	85175	1(3)	85612	1(3)
82143	2(3)	82550	3(3)	82955	1(2)	83661	3(3)	84126	1(3)	84443	4(2)	85210	2(3)	85613	1(3)
82150	2(3)	82552	3(3)	82960	1(2)	83662	4(3)	84132	2(3)	84445	1(2)	85220	2(3)	85635	1(3)
82154	1(3)	82553	3(3)	82963	1(3)	83663	3(3)	84133	2(3)	84446	1(2)	85230	2(3)	85651	1(2)
82157	1(3)	82554	1(3)	82965	1(3)	83664	3(3)	84134	1(3)	84449	1(3)	85240	2(3)	85652	1(2)
82160	1(3)	82565	2(1)	82977	1(3)	83670	1(3)	84135	1(3)	84450	1(3)	85244	1(3)	85660	1(2)
82163	1(3)	82570	3(3)	82978	1(3)	83690	2(3)	84138	1(3)	84460	1(3)	85245	2(3)	85670	2(3)
82164	1(3)	82575	1(3)	82979	1(3)	83695	1(3)	84140	1(3)	84466	1(3)	85246	2(3)	85675	1(3)
82172	3(3)	82585	1(2)	82985	1(3)	83698	1(3)	84143	2(3)	84478	1(3)	85247	2(3)	85705	1(3)
82175	2(3)	82595	1(3)	83001	1(3)	83700	1(2)	84144	1(3)	84479	1(2)	85250	2(3)	85730	4(3)
82180	1(2)	82600	1(3)	83002	1(3)	83701	1(3)	84145	1(3)	84480	1(2)	85260	2(3)	85732	4(3)
82190	2(3)	82607	1(2)	83003	5(3)	83704	1(3)	84146	3(3)	84481	1(2)	85270	2(3)	85810	2(3)
82232	2(3)	82608	1(2)	83006	1(2)	83718	1(3)	84150	2(3)	84482	1(2)	85280	2(3)	86000	6(3)
82239	1(3)	82610	1(3)	83009	1(3)	83719	1(3)	84152	1(2)	84484	2(3)	85290	2(3)	86001	20(1)
82240	1(3)	82615	1(3)	83010	1(3)	83721	1(3)	84153	1(2)	84485	1(3)	85291	1(3)	86005	2(3)
82247	2(3)	82626	1(3)	83012	1(2)	83727	1(3)	84154	1(2)	84488	1(3)	85292	1(3)	86021	1(2)
82248	2(3)	82627	1(3)	83013	1(3)	83735	4(3)	84155	1(3)	84490	1(2)	85293	1(3)	86022	1(2)
82252	1(3)	82633	1(3)	83014	1(2)	83775	1(3)	84156	1(3)	84510	1(3)	85300	2(3)	86023	3(3)
82261	1(3)	82634	1(3)	83015	1(2)	83785	1(3)	84157	2(3)	84512	1(3)	85301	1(3)	86038	1(3)
82270	1(3)	82638	1(3)	83018	4(3)	83789	4(3)	84160	2(3)	84520	4(1)	85302	1(3)	86039	1(3)
82271	1(3)	82652	1(2)	83020	2(3)	83825	2(3)	84163	1(3)	84525	1(3)	85303	2(3)	86060	1(3)
82272	1(3)	82656	1(3)	83021	2(3)	83835	2(3)	84165	1(2)	84540	2(3)	85305	2(3)	86063	1(3)
82274	1(3)	82657	3(3)	83026	1(3)	83857	1(3)	84166	2(3)	84545	1(3)	85306	2(3)	86077	1(2)
82286	1(3)	82658	2(3)	83030	1(3)	83861	2(2)	84181	3(3)	84550	1(3)	85307	2(3)	86078	1(3)
82300	1(3)	82664	2(3)	83033	1(3)	83864	1(2)	84182	6(3)	84560	2(3)	85335	2(3)	86079	1(3)
82306	1(2)	82668	1(3)	83036	1(2)	83872	2(3)	84202	1(2)	84577	1(3)	85337	1(3)	86140	1(2)
82308	1(3)	82670	2(3)	83037	1(2)	83873	1(3)	84203	1(2)	84578	1(3)	85345	1(3)	86141	1(2)
82310	2(3)	82671	1(3)	83045	1(3)	83874	2(3)	84206	1(2)	84580	1(3)	85347	5(3)	86146	3(3)
82330	2(3)	82672	1(3)	83050	1(3)	83876	1(3)	84207	1(2)	84583	1(3)	85348	1(3)	86147	4(3)
82331	1(3)	82677	1(3)	83051	1(3)	83880	1(3)	84210	1(3)	84585	1(2)	85360	1(3)	86148	3(3)
82340	1(3)	82679	1(3)	83060	1(3)	83883	6(3)	84220	1(3)	84586	1(3)	85362	2(3)	86152	1(3)
82355	2(3)	82693	2(3)	83065	1(2)	83885	2(3)	84228	1(3)	84588	1(3)	85366	1(3)	86153	1(3)
82360	2(3)	82696	1(3)	83068	1(2)	83915	1(3)	84233	1(3)	84590	1(2)	85370	1(3)	86155	1(3)
82365	2(3)	82705	1(3)	83069	1(3)	83916	2(3)	84234	1(3)	84591	1(3)	85378	1(3)	86156	1(2)
82370	2(3)	82710	1(3)	83070	1(2)	83918	2(3)	84235	1(3)	84597	1(3)	85379	2(3)	86157	1(2)
82373	1(3)	82715	3(3)	83080	2(3)	83919	1(3)	84238	3(3)	84600	2(3)	85380	1(3)	86160	4(3)
82374	2(1)	82725	1(3)	83088	1(3)	83921	2(3)	84244	2(3)	84620	1(2)	85384	2(3)	86161	2(3)
82375	1(3)	82726	1(3)	83090	2(3)	83930	2(3)	84252	1(2)	84630	2(3)	85385	1(3)	86162	1(2)
82376	1(1)	82728	1(3)	83150	1(3)	83935	2(3)	84255	2(3)	84681	1(3)	85390	3(3)	86171	2(3)
82378	1(3)	82731	1(3)	83491	1(3)	83937	1(3)	84260	1(3)	84702	2(3)	85396	1(2)	86185	1(3)
82379	1(3)	82735	1(3)	83497	1(3)	83945	2(3)	84270	1(3)	84703	1(3)	85397	3(3)	86200	1(3)
82380	1(3)	82746	1(2)	83498	2(3)	83950	1(2)	84275	1(3)	84704	1(3)	85400	1(3)	86215	1(3)

CPT	MUE	CPT	MUE	CPT	MUE	CPT	MUE	CPT	MUE	CPT	MUE	CPT	MUE	CPT	MUE
86225	1(3)	86615	6(3)	86759	2(3)	86970	1(1)	87255	2(3)	87492	1(3)	87652	1(3)	88230	2(3)
86226	1(3)	86617	2(3)	86762	2(3)	86971	1(3)	87260	1(3)	87493	2(3)	87653	1(3)	88233	2(3)
86235	10(3)	86618	2(3)	86765	2(3)	86972	1(3)	87265	1(3)	87495	1(3)	87660	1(3)	88235	2(3)
86243	1(3)	86619	2(3)	86768	5(3)	86975	1(3)	87267	1(3)	87496	1(3)	87661	1(1)	88237	4(3)
86255	5(3)	86622	2(3)	86771	2(3)	86976	1(3)	87269	1(3)	87497	2(3)	87797	3(3)	88239	3(3)
86256	9(3)	86625	1(3)	86774	2(3)	86977	1(3)	87270	1(3)	87498	1(3)	87798	13(3)	88240	1(3)
86277	1(3)	86628	3(3)	86777	2(3)	86978	1(1)	87271	1(3)	87500	1(3)	87799	3(3)	88241	3(3)
86280	1(3)	86631	6(3)	86778	2(3)	86985	1(1)	87272	1(3)	87501	1(3)	87800	2(3)	88245	1(2)
86294	1(3)	86632	3(3)	86780	2(3)	87003	1(3)	87273	1(3)	87502	1(3)	87801	3(3)	88248	1(2)
86300	2(3)	86635	4(3)	86784	1(3)	87015	4(3)	87274	1(3)	87503	1(3)	87802	2(3)	88249	1(2)
86301	1(2)	86638	6(3)	86787	2(3)	87040	2(1)	87275	1(3)	87505	1(2)	87803	3(3)	88261	2(3)
86304	1(2)	86641	2(3)	86788	2(3)	87045	3(3)	87276	1(3)	87506	1(2)	87804	3(3)	88262	2(3)
86305	1(2)	86644	2(3)	86789	2(3)	87046	6(3)	87277	1(3)	87507	1(3)	87806	1(2)	88263	1(3)
86308	1(2)	86645	1(3)	86790	4(3)	87070	3(1)	87278	1(3)	87510	1(3)	87807	2(3)	88264	2(3)
86309	1(2)	86648	2(3)	86793	2(3)	87071	4(3)	87279	1(3)	87511	1(3)	87808	1(3)	88267	2(3)
86310	1(2)	86651	2(3)	86800	1(3)	87073	3(3)	87280	1(3)	87512	1(3)	87809	2(3)	88269	2(3)
86316	2(3)	86652	2(3)	86803	1(3)	87075	6(3)	87281	1(3)	87515	1(3)	87810	2(3)	88271	16(3)
86317	6(1)	86653	2(3)	86804	1(2)	87076	6(3)	87283	1(3)	87516	1(3)	87850	1(3)	88272	12(3)
86318	2(3)	86654	2(3)	86805	2(3)	87077	10(3)	87285	1(3)	87517	1(3)	87880	2(3)	88273	3(3)
86320	1(2)	86658	12(3)	86807	2(3)	87081	6(3)	87290	1(3)	87520	1(3)	87899	4(3)	88274	5(3)
86325	2(3)	86663	2(3)	86808	1(3)	87084	1(3)	87299	1(3)	87521	1(3)	87900	1(2)	88275	12(3)
86327	1(3)	86664	2(3)	86812	1(2)	87086	3(3)	87300	2(3)	87522	1(3)	87901	1(2)	88280	8(3)
86329	3(3)	86665	2(3)	86813	1(2)	87088	6(3)	87301	1(3)	87525	1(3)	87902	1(2)	88283	5(3)
86331	12(3)	86666	4(3)	86816	1(2)	87101	4(3)	87305	1(3)	87526	1(3)	87903	1(2)	88285	10(3)
86332	1(3)	86668	2(3)	86817	1(2)	87102	4(3)	87320	1(3)	87527	1(3)	87904	14(3)	88289	1(3)
86334	1(2)	86671	3(3)	86821	1(3)	87103	2(3)	87324	2(3)	87528	1(3)	87905	2(3)	88291	1(1)
86335	2(3)	86674	3(3)	86822	1(3)	87106	4(3)	87327	1(3)	87529	2(3)	87906	2(3)	88300	4(3)
86336	1(3)	86677	3(3)	86825	1(3)	87107	4(3)	87328	2(3)	87530	2(3)	87910	1(3)	88302	4(3)
86337	1(2)	86682	2(3)	86826	2(3)	87109	2(3)	87329	2(3)	87531	1(3)	87912	1(3)	88304	5(3)
86340	1(2)	86684	2(3)	86828	1(3)	87110	2(3)	87332	1(3)	87532	1(3)	88104	5(3)	88305	16(3)
86341	1(3)	86687	1(3)	86829	1(3)	87116	2(1)	87335	1(3)	87533	1(3)	88106	5(3)	88307	8(3)
86343	1(3)	86688	1(3)	86830	2(3)	87118	3(3)	87336	1(3)	87534	1(3)	88108	6(3)	88309	3(3)
86344	1(2)	86689	2(3)	86831	2(3)	87140	3(3)	87337	1(3)	87535	1(3)	88112	6(3)	88311	4(3)
86352	1(3)	86692	2(3)	86832	2(3)	87143	2(3)	87338	1(1)	87536	1(3)	88120	2(3)	88312	9(3)
86353	7(3)	86694	2(3)	86833	1(3)	87149	4(3)	87339	1(3)	87537	1(3)	88121	2(3)	88313	8(3)
86355	1(2)	86695	2(3)	86834	1(3)	87150	12(3)	87340	1(2)	87538	1(3)	88125	1(3)	88314	6(3)
86356	7(3)	86696	2(3)	86835	1(3)	87152	1(3)	87341	1(2)	87539	1(3)	88130	1(2)	88319	11(3)
86357	1(2)	86698	3(3)	86850	3(3)	87153	3(3)	87350	1(2)	87540	1(3)	88140	1(2)	88321	1(2)
86359	1(2)	86701	1(3)	86860	2(3)	87158	1(1)	87380	1(2)	87541	1(3)	88141	1(3)	88323	1(2)
86360	1(2)	86702	2(3)	86870	2(3)	87164	2(3)	87385	2(3)	87542	1(3)	88142	1(3)	88325	1(2)
86361	1(2)	86703	1(2)	86880	4(3)	87166	2(3)	87389	1(3)	87550	1(3)	88143	1(3)	88329	2(3)
86367	1(3)	86704	1(2)	86885	2(3)	87168	2(3)	87390	1(3)	87551	2(3)	88147	1(3)	88331	11(3)
86376	2(3)	86705	1(2)	86886	3(3)	87169	2(3)	87391	1(3)	87552	1(3)	88148	1(3)	88332	13(3)
86378	1(3)	86706	2(3)	86890	1(1)	87172	1(3)	87400	2(3)	87555	1(1)	88150	1(3)	88333	4(3)
86382	3(3)	86707	1(3)	86891	1(1)	87176	2(3)	87420	1(3)	87556	1(1)	88152	1(3)	88334	5(3)
86384	1(3)	86708	1(2)	86900	1(3)	87177	3(3)	87425	1(3)	87557	1(3)	88153	1(3)	88342	3(3)
86386	1(2)	86709	1(2)	86901	1(3)	87181	12(3)	87427	2(3)	87560	1(3)	88154	1(3)	88344	1(1)
86406	2(3)	86710	4(3)	86902	6(3)	87184	8(3)	87430	1(3)	87561	1(3)	88155	1(3)	88346	2(1)
86430	2(3)	86711	2(1)	86904	2(1)	87185	4(3)	87449	3(3)	87562	1(3)	88160	4(3)	88348	1(3)
86431	2(3)	86713	3(3)	86905	8(3)	87186	12(3)	87450	2(3)	87580	1(3)	88161	4(3)	88350	4(1)
86480	1(3)	86717	8(3)	86906	1(2)	87187	3(3)	87451	2(3)	87581	1(3)	88162	3(3)	88355	1(3)
86481	1(3)	86720	2(3)	86920	9(3)	87188	6(3)	87470	1(3)	87582	1(3)	88164	1(3)	88356	1(1)
86485	1(2)	86723	2(3)	86921	2(1)	87190	9(3)	87471	1(3)	87590	1(3)	88165	1(3)	88358	2(3)
86486	2(3)	86727	2(3)	86922	5(3)	87197	1(3)	87472	1(3)	87591	2(3)	88166	1(3)	88360	6(3)
86490	1(2)	86729	0(2)	86923	10(3)	87205	3(1)	87475	1(3)	87592	1(3)	88167	1(3)	88361	6(3)
86510	1(2)	86732	2(3)	86927	2(1)	87206	6(3)	87476	1(3)	87623	1(2)	88172	5(3)	88362	1(3)
86580	1(2)	86735	2(3)	86930	0(3)	87207	3(3)	87477	1(3)	87624	1(2)	88173	5(3)	88363	2(3)
86590	1(3)	86738	2(3)	86931	1(3)	87209	4(3)	87480	1(3)	87625	1(2)	88174	1(3)	88364	3(3)
86592	2(3)	86741	2(3)	86932	2(1)	87210	4(3)	87481	1(1)	87631	1(3)	88175	1(3)	88365	4(3)
86593	2(3)	86744	2(3)	86940	1(3)	87220	3(3)	87482	1(3)	87632	1(3)	88177	6(3)	88366	2(3)
86602	3(3)	86747	2(3)	86941	1(3)	87230	3(3)	87485	1(3)	87633	1(3)	88182	2(3)	88367	2(1)
86603	2(3)	86750	4(3)	86945	2(3)	87250	1(3)	87486	1(3)	87640	1(3)	88184	2(3)	88368	2(1)
86609	14(3)	86753	3(3)	86950	1(3)	87252	2(3)	87487	1(3)	87641	1(3)	88187	2(3)	88369	3(1)
86611	4(3)	86756	2(3)	86960	1(3)	87253	2(3)	87490	1(3)	87650	1(3)	88188	2(3)	88371	1(3)
86612	2(3)	86757	6(3)	86965	1(3)	87254	7(3)	87491	2(3)	87651	1(3)	88189	2(3)	88372	1(3)

CPT	MUE	CPT	MUE	CPT	MUE	CPT	MUE	CPT	MUE	CPT	MUE	CPT	MUE	CPT	MUE
88373	3(1)	90393	1(2)	90732	1(2)	90993	1(3)	92316	1(2)	92597	1(3)	93040	3(3)	93459	1(3)
88374	5(3)	90396	1(2)	90733	1(2)	90997	1(3)	92317	1(3)	92601	1(3)	93041	2(3)	93460	1(3)
88375	1(3)	90460	6(3)	90734	1(2)	91010	1(2)	92325	1(3)	92602	1(3)	93042	3(3)	93461	1(3)
88377	5(3)	90461	5(3)	90736	1(2)	91013	1(3)	92326	2(2)	92603	1(3)	93050	1(3)	93462	1(3)
88380	1(1)	90471	1(2)	90738	1(2)	91020	1(2)	92352	0(3)	92604	1(3)	93224	1(2)	93463	1(3)
88381	1(1)	90472	4(3)	90739	1(2)	91022	1(2)	92353	0(3)	92605	0(3)	93225	1(2)	93464	1(3)
88387	2(3)	90473	1(2)	90740	1(2)	91030	1(2)	92354	0(3)	92607	1(3)	93226	1(2)	93503	2(3)
88388	1(3)	90474	1(3)	90743	1(2)	91034	1(2)	92355	0(3)	92608	4(3)	93227	1(2)	93505	1(2)
88720	1(3)	90476	1(2)	90744	1(2)	91035	1(2)	92358	0(3)	92609	1(3)	93228	1(2)	93530	1(3)
88738	1(3)	90477	1(2)	90746	1(2)	91037	1(2)	92371	0(3)	92610	1(2)	93229	1(2)	93531	1(3)
88740	1(2)	90581	1(2)	90747	1(2)	91038	1(2)	92502	1(3)	92611	1(3)	93260	1(2)	93532	1(3)
88741	1(2)	90585	1(2)	90785	1(3)	91040	1(2)	92504	1(3)	92612	1(3)	93261	1(3)	93533	1(3)
89049	1(3)	90586	1(2)	90791	1(3)	91065	2(2)	92507	1(3)	92613	1(2)	93268	1(2)	93561	1(3)
89050	2(3)	90620	1(2)	90792	1(3)	91110	1(2)	92508	1(3)	92614	1(3)	93270	1(2)	93562	1(3)
89051	2(3)	90621	1(2)	90832	1(3)	91111	1(2)	92511	1(3)	92615	1(2)	93271	1(2)	93563	1(3)
89055	2(3)	90625	1(2)	90833	1(3)	91112	1(3)	92512	1(2)	92616	1(3)	93272	1(2)	93564	1(3)
89060	2(3)	90630	1(2)	90834	1(3)	91117	1(2)	92516	1(3)	92617	1(2)	93278	1(3)	93565	1(3)
89125	2(3)	90632	1(2)	90836	1(3)	91120	1(2)	92520	1(2)	92618	1(3)	93279	1(3)	93566	1(3)
89160	1(3)	90633	1(2)	90837	1(3)	91122	1(2)	92521	1(2)	92620	1(2)	93280	1(3)	93567	1(3)
89190	1(3)	90634	1(2)	90838	1(3)	91132	1(3)	92522	1(2)	92621	4(3)	93281	1(3)	93568	1(3)
89220	1(3)	90636	1(2)	90839	1(2)	91133	1(3)	92523	1(2)	92625	1(2)	93282	1(3)	93571	1(3)
89230	1(2)	90644	1(2)	90840	3(3)	91200	1(3)	92524	1(2)	92626	1(2)	93283	1(3)	93572	2(3)
89250	1(2)	90647	1(2)	90845	1(2)	92002	1(2)	92526	1(2)	92627	6(3)	93284	1(3)	93580	1(3)
89251	1(2)	90648	1(2)	90846	1(3)	92004	1(2)	92531	0(3)	92640	1(3)	93285	1(3)	93581	1(3)
89253	1(3)	90649	1(2)	90847	1(3)	92012	1(3)	92532	0(3)	92920	3(3)	93286	2(3)	93582	1(2)
89254	1(3)	90650	1(2)	90849	1(3)	92014	1(3)	92534	0(3)	92921	6(2)	93287	2(3)	93583	1(2)
89255	1(3)	90651	1(2)	90853	1(3)	92018	1(2)	92537	1(2)	92924	2(3)	93288	1(3)	93600	1(3)
89257	1(3)	90653	1(2)	90863	1(3)	92019	1(2)	92538	1(2)	92925	6(2)	93289	1(3)	93602	1(3)
89258	1(2)	90654	1(2)	90865	1(3)	92020	1(2)	92540	1(3)	92928	3(3)	93290	1(3)	93603	1(3)
89259	1(2)	90655	1(2)	90867	1(2)	92025	1(2)	92541	1(3)	92929	6(2)	93291	1(3)	93609	1(3)
89260	1(2)	90656	1(2)	90868	1(3)	92060	1(2)	92542	1(3)	92933	2(3)	93292	1(3)	93610	1(3)
89261	1(2)	90657	1(2)	90869	1(3)	92065	1(2)	92544	1(3)	92934	6(2)	93293	1(2)	93612	1(3)
89264	1(3)	90658	1(2)	90870	2(3)	92071	2(2)	92545	1(3)	92937	2(3)	93294	1(2)	93613	1(3)
89268	1(2)	90660	1(2)	90880	1(3)	92072	1(2)	92546	1(3)	92938	6(3)	93295	1(2)	93615	1(3)
89272	1(2)	90661	1(2)	90885	0(3)	92081	1(2)	92547	1(3)	92941	1(3)	93296	1(2)	93616	1(3)
89280	1(2)	90662	1(2)	90887	0(3)	92082	1(2)	92548	1(3)	92943	2(3)	93297	1(2)	93618	1(3)
89281	1(2)	90664	1(2)	90889	0(3)	92083	1(2)	92550	1(2)	92944	3(3)	93298	1(2)	93619	1(3)
89290	1(2)	90666	1(2)	90901	1(3)	92100	1(2)	92552	1(2)	92950	2(3)	93299	1(2)	93620	1(3)
89291	1(2)	90667	1(2)	90911	1(3)	92132	1(2)	92553	1(2)	92953	2(3)	93303	1(3)	93621	1(3)
89300	1(2)	90668	1(2)	90935	1(3)	92133	1(2)	92555	1(2)	92960	2(3)	93304	1(3)	93622	1(3)
89310	1(2)	90670	1(2)	90937	1(3)	92134	1(2)	92556	1(2)	92961	1(3)	93306	1(3)	93623	1(3)
89320	1(2)	90672	1(2)	90940	1(3)	92136	2(2)	92557	1(2)	92970	1(3)	93307	1(3)	93624	1(3)
89321	1(2)	90673	1(2)	90945	1(3)	92140	1(2)	92558	0(3)	92971	1(3)	93308	1(3)	93631	1(3)
89322	1(2)	90675	1(2)	90947	1(3)	92145	1(2)	92561	1(2)	92973	2(3)	93312	1(3)	93640	1(3)
89325	1(2)	90676	1(2)	90951	1(2)	92225	2(2)	92562	1(2)	92974	1(3)	93313	1(3)	93641	1(2)
89329	1(2)	90680	1(2)	90952	1(2)	92226	2(2)	92563	1(2)	92975	1(3)	93314	1(3)	93642	1(3)
89330	1(2)	90681	1(2)	90953	1(2)	92227	1(2)	92564	1(2)	92977	1(3)	93315	1(3)	93644	1(2)
89331	1(2)	90685	1(2)	90954	1(2)	92228	1(2)	92565	1(2)	92978	1(3)	93316	1(3)	93650	1(2)
89335	1(3)	90686	1(2)	90955	1(2)	92230	2(2)	92567	1(2)	92979	2(3)	93317	1(3)	93653	1(3)
89337	1(2)	90687	1(2)	90956	1(2)	92235	2(2)	92568	1(2)	92986	1(2)	93318	1(3)	93654	1(3)
89342	1(2)	90688	1(2)	90957	1(2)	92240	2(2)	92570	1(2)	92987	1(2)	93320	1(3)	93655	2(3)
89343	1(2)	90690	1(2)	90958	1(2)	92250	1(2)	92571	1(2)	92990	1(2)	93321	1(3)	93656	1(3)
89344	1(2)	90691	1(2)	90959	1(2)	92260	1(2)	92572	1(2)	92992	1(2)	93325	1(3)	93657	1(3)
89346	1(2)	90696	1(2)	90960	1(2)	92265	1(2)	92575	1(2)	92993	1(2)	93350	1(2)	93660	1(3)
89352	1(2)	90697	1(2)	90961	1(2)	92270	1(2)	92576	1(2)	92997	1(2)	93351	1(2)	93662	1(3)
89353	1(3)	90698	1(2)	90962	1(2)	92275	1(2)	92577	1(2)	92998	2(3)	93352	1(3)	93701	1(2)
89354	1(3)	90700	1(2)	90963	1(2)	92283	1(2)	92579	1(2)	93000	3(3)	93355	1(3)	93702	1(2)
89356	2(3)	90702	1(2)	90964	1(2)	92284	1(2)	92582	1(2)	93005	3(3)	93451	1(3)	93724	1(3)
90284	0(3)	90707	1(2)	90965	1(2)	92285	1(2)	92583	1(2)	93010	5(3)	93452	1(3)	93740	0(3)
90296	1(2)	90710	1(2)	90966	1(2)	92286	1(2)	92584	1(2)	93015	1(3)	93453	1(3)	93745	1(2)
90371	10(3)	90713	1(2)	90967	1(2)	92287	1(2)	92585	1(2)	93016	1(3)	93454	1(3)	93750	4(3)
90375	20(3)	90714	1(2)	90968	1(2)	92311	1(2)	92586	1(2)	93017	1(3)	93455	1(3)	93770	0(3)
90376	20(3)	90715	1(2)	90969	1(2)	92312	1(2)	92587	1(2)	93018	1(3)	93456	1(3)	93784	1(2)
90378	4(3)	90716	1(2)	90970	1(2)	92313	1(3)	92588	1(2)	93024	1(3)	93457	1(3)	93786	1(2)
90385	1(2)	90717	1(2)	90989	1(2)	92315	1(2)	92596	1(2)	93025	1(2)	93458	1(3)	93788	1(2)

CPT	MUE	CPT	MUE	CPT	MUE	CPT	MUE	CPT	MUE	CPT	MUE	CPT	MUE	CPT	MUE
93790	1(2)	94727	1(3)	95832	1(3)	95978	1(2)	96523	1(3)	97762	4(3)	99231	1(3)	99464	1(2)
93797	2(2)	94728	1(3)	95833	1(3)	95979	6(3)	96542	1(3)	97802	8(3)	99232	1(3)	99465	1(2)
93798	2(2)	94729	1(3)	95834	1(3)	95980	1(3)	96567	1(3)	97803	8(3)	99233	1(3)	99466	1(2)
93880	1(3)	94750	1(3)	95851	3(3)	95981	1(3)	96570	1(2)	97804	6(3)	99234	1(3)	99467	4(3)
93882	1(3)	94760	1(3)	95852	1(3)	95982	1(3)	96571	2(3)	98925	1(2)	99235	1(3)	99468	1(2)
93886	1(3)	94761	1(2)	95857	1(2)	95990	1(3)	96900	1(3)	98926	1(2)	99236	1(3)	99469	1(2)
93888	1(3)	94762	1(2)	95860	1(3)	95991	1(3)	96902	0(3)	98927	1(2)	99238	1(2)	99471	1(2)
93890	1(3)	94770	1(3)	95861	1(3)	95992	1(2)	96904	1(2)	98928	1(2)	99239	1(2)	99472	1(2)
93892	1(3)	94772	1(2)	95863	1(3)	96000	1(2)	96910	1(3)	98929	1(2)	99281	1(3)	99475	1(2)
93893	1(3)	94774	1(2)	95864	1(3)	96001	1(2)	96912	1(3)	98940	1(2)	99282	1(3)	99476	1(2)
93922	1(1)	94775	1(2)	95865	1(3)	96002	1(3)	96913	1(3)	98941	1(2)	99283	1(3)	99477	1(2)
93923	1(1)	94776	1(2)	95866	1(3)	96003	1(3)	96920	1(2)	98942	1(2)	99284	1(3)	99478	1(2)
93924	1(2)	94777	1(2)	95867	1(3)	96004	1(2)	96921	1(2)	99002	0(3)	99285	1(3)	99479	1(2)
93925	1(3)	94780	1(2)	95868	1(3)	96020	1(2)	96922	1(2)	99024	0(3)	99288	0(3)	99480	1(2)
93926	1(3)	94781	2(3)	95869	1(3)	96040	4(3)	96931	1(2)	99050	0(3)	99291	1(2)	99485	1(3)
93930	1(3)	95004	80(1)	95870	4(3)	96101	8(3)	96932	1(2)	99051	0(3)	99292	8(3)	99486	4(1)
93931	1(3)	95012	2(3)	95872	4(3)	96102	4(3)	96933	1(2)	99053	0(3)	99304	1(2)	99487	1(2)
93965	1(3)	95017	27(1)	95873	1(2)	96103	1(2)	96934	4(1)	99056	0(3)	99305	1(2)	99490	1(2)
93970	1(3)	95018	19(3)	95874	1(2)	96105	3(3)	96935	4(1)	99058	0(3)	99306	1(2)	99495	1(2)
93971	1(3)	95024	40(1)	95875	2(3)	96110	2(3)	96936	4(1)	99060	0(3)	99307	1(2)	99496	1(2)
93975	1(3)	95027	90(1)	95885	4(2)	96111	1(3)	97001	1(3)	99070	0(3)	99308	1(2)	99497	1(2)
93976	1(3)	95028	30(1)	95886	4(2)	96116	4(3)	97002	1(3)	99071	0(3)	99309	1(2)	99498	3(3)
93978	1(3)	95044	80(1)	95887	1(2)	96118	8(3)	97003	1(3)	99078	0(3)	99310	1(2)	99605	0(2)
93979	1(3)	95052	20(1)	95905	2(3)	96119	6(3)	97004	1(3)	99080	0(3)	99315	1(2)	99606	0(3)
93980	1(3)	95056	1(2)	95907	1(2)	96120	1(2)	97010	0(3)	99082	1(1)	99316	1(2)	99607	0(3)
93981	1(3)	95060	1(2)	95908	1(2)	96125	2(3)	97012	1(3)	99090	0(3)	99318	1(2)	A0021	0(3)
93982	1(3)	95065	1(3)	95909	1(2)	96127	2(1)	97014	0(3)	99091	0(3)	99324	1(2)	A0080	0(3)
93990	2(3)	95070	1(3)	95910	1(2)	96150	8(3)	97016	1(3)	99100	1(3)	99325	1(2)	A0090	0(3)
94002	1(2)	95071	1(2)	95911	1(2)	96151	6(3)	97018	1(3)	99116	0(3)	99326	1(2)	A0100	0(3)
94003	1(2)	95076	1(2)	95912	1(2)	96152	6(3)	97022	1(3)	99135	0(3)	99327	1(2)	A0110	0(3)
94004	1(2)	95079	2(3)	95913	1(2)	96153	8(3)	97024	1(3)	99140	0(3)	99328	1(2)	A0120	0(3)
94010	1(3)	95115	1(2)	95921	1(3)	96154	8(3)	97026	1(3)	99143	2(3)	99334	1(3)	A0130	0(3)
94011	1(3)	95117	1(2)	95922	1(3)	96360	1(1)	97028	1(3)	99144	2(3)	99335	1(3)	A0140	0(3)
94012	1(3)	95144	30(3)	95923	1(3)	96361	8(3)	97032	4(3)	99145	9(3)	99336	1(3)	A0160	0(3)
94013	1(3)	95145	10(3)	95924	1(3)	96365	1(1)	97033	4(3)	99148	2(3)	99337	1(3)	A0170	0(3)
94014	1(2)	95146	10(3)	95925	1(3)	96366	8(3)	97034	2(3)	99149	2(3)	99341	1(2)	A0180	0(3)
94015	1(2)	95147	10(3)	95926	1(3)	96367	4(3)	97035	2(3)	99150	6(3)	99342	1(2)	A0190	0(3)
94016	1(2)	95148	10(3)	95927	1(3)	96368	1(2)	97036	3(3)	99170	1(3)	99343	1(2)	A0200	0(3)
94060	1(3)	95149	10(3)	95928	1(3)	96369	1(2)	97110	6(3)	99175	1(3)	99344	1(2)	A0210	0(3)
94070	1(2)	95165	30(3)	95929	1(3)	96370	3(3)	97112	4(3)	99177	1(2)	99345	1(2)	A0225	0(3)
94150	0(3)	95170	10(3)	95930	1(3)	96371	1(3)	97113	6(3)	99183	1(3)	99347	1(3)	A0380	0(3)
94200	1(3)	95180	6(3)	95933	1(3)	96372	4(3)	97116	4(3)	99184	1(2)	99348	1(3)	A0382	0(3)
94250	1(3)	95250	1(2)	95937	4(3)	96373	2(3)	97124	4(3)	99191	1(3)	99349	1(3)	A0384	0(3)
94375	1(3)	95251	1(2)	95938	1(3)	96374	1(3)	97140	6(3)	99192	1(3)	99350	1(3)	A0390	0(3)
94400	1(3)	95782	1(2)	95939	1(3)	96375	6(3)	97150	1(3)	99195	2(3)	99354	1(2)	A0392	0(3)
94450	1(3)	95783	1(2)	95940	32(3)	96376	0(3)	97530	6(3)	99201	1(2)	99355	4(3)	A0394	0(3)
94452	1(2)	95800	1(2)	95943	1(3)	96401	3(3)	97532	8(3)	99202	1(2)	99356	1(2)	A0396	0(3)
94453	1(2)	95801	1(2)	95950	1(2)	96402	2(3)	97533	4(3)	99203	1(2)	99357	4(3)	A0398	0(3)
94610	2(3)	95803	1(2)	95951	1(2)	96405	1(2)	97535	8(3)	99204	1(2)	99366	0(3)	A0420	0(3)
94620	1(3)	95805	1(2)	95953	1(2)	96406	1(2)	97537	8(3)	99205	1(2)	99367	0(3)	A0422	0(3)
94621	1(3)	95806	1(2)	95954	1(3)	96409	1(3)	97542	8(3)	99211	1(3)	99368	0(3)	A0424	0(3)
94640	4(3)	95807	1(2)	95955	1(3)	96411	3(3)	97545	1(2)	99212	2(3)	99406	1(2)	A0425	250(1)
94642	1(3)	95808	1(2)	95956	1(3)	96413	1(3)	97546	2(3)	99213	2(3)	99407	1(2)	A0426	2(3)
94644	1(2)	95810	1(2)	95957	1(3)	96415	8(3)	97597	1(3)	99214	2(3)	99415	1(2)	A0427	2(3)
94645	2(3)	95811	1(2)	95958	1(3)	96416	1(3)	97598	8(3)	99215	1(3)	99416	2(1)	A0428	4(3)
94660	1(2)	95812	1(3)	95961	1(2)	96417	3(3)	97602	0(3)	99217	1(2)	99446	1(2)	A0429	2(3)
94662	1(2)	95813	1(3)	95962	5(3)	96420	1(3)	97605	1(3)	99218	1(2)	99447	1(2)	A0430	1(3)
94664	1(3)	95816	1(3)	95965	1(3)	96422	2(3)	97606	1(3)	99219	1(2)	99448	1(2)	A0431	1(3)
94667	1(2)	95819	1(3)	95966	1(3)	96423	1(3)	97607	1(3)	99220	1(2)	99449	1(2)	A0432	1(3)
94668	2(3)	95822	1(3)	95967	3(3)	96425	1(3)	97608	1(3)	99221	1(3)	99455	1(3)	A0433	1(3)
94669	4(3)	95824	1(3)	95970	1(3)	96440	1(3)	97610	1(2)	99222	1(3)	99456	1(3)	A0434	2(3)
94680	1(3)	95827	1(2)	95971	1(3)	96446	1(3)	97750	8(3)	99223	1(3)	99460	1(2)	A0435	999(3)
94681	1(3)	95829	1(3)	95972	1(2)	96450	1(3)	97755	8(3)	99224	1(2)	99461	1(2)	A0436	300(3)
94690	1(3)	95830	1(3)	95974	1(2)	96521	2(3)	97760	6(3)	99225	1(2)	99462	1(2)	A0888	0(3)
94726	1(3)	95831	5(2)	95975	2(3)	96522	1(3)	97761	6(3)	99226	1(2)	99463	1(2)	A0998	0(3)

CPT © 2016 American Medical Association. All Rights Reserved.

CPT	MUE	CPT	MUE	CPT	MUE	CPT	MUE	CPT	MUE	CPT	MUE	CPT	MUE	CPT	MUE
A4221	0(3)	A7016	0(3)	A9553	1(3)	C1772	1(3)	C8921	1(3)	E0114	0(3)	E0243	0(3)	E0455	0(3)
A4235	2(1)	A7017	0(3)	A9554	1(3)	C1776	10(3)	C8922	1(3)	E0116	0(3)	E0244	0(3)	E0457	0(3)
A4253	0(3)	A7020	0(3)	A9555	2(3)	C1778	4(3)	C8923	1(3)	E0117	0(3)	E0245	0(3)	E0459	0(3)
A4255	0(3)	A7025	0(3)	A9556	10(3)	C1782	1(3)	C8924	1(3)	E0118	0(3)	E0246	0(3)	E0462	0(3)
A4257	0(3)	A7026	0(3)	A9557	2(3)	C1785	1(3)	C8925	1(3)	E0130	0(3)	E0247	0(3)	E0465	0(3)
A4258	0(3)	A7027	0(3)	A9558	7(3)	C1786	1(3)	C8926	1(3)	E0135	0(3)	E0248	0(3)	E0466	0(3)
A4259	0(3)	A7028	0(3)	A9559	1(1)	C1813	1(3)	C8927	1(3)	E0140	0(3)	E0249	0(3)	E0470	0(3)
A4301	1(2)	A7029	0(3)	A9560	2(3)	C1815	1(3)	C8928	1(2)	E0141	0(3)	E0250	0(3)	E0471	0(3)
A4337	0(3)	A7032	0(3)	A9561	1(3)	C1817	1(3)	C8929	1(3)	E0143	0(3)	E0251	0(3)	E0472	0(3)
A4356	1(1)	A7035	0(3)	A9562	2(3)	C1820	2(3)	C8930	1(2)	E0144	0(3)	E0255	0(3)	E0480	0(3)
A4459	0(3)	A7036	0(3)	A9563	10(3)	C1822	1(3)	C8931	1(3)	E0147	0(3)	E0256	0(3)	E0481	0(3)
A4470	1(1)	A7037	0(3)	A9564	20(3)	C1830	2(3)	C8932	1(3)	E0148	0(3)	E0260	0(3)	E0482	0(3)
A4480	1(1)	A7039	0(3)	A9566	1(3)	C1840	1(3)	C8933	1(3)	E0149	0(3)	E0261	0(3)	E0483	0(3)
A4555	0(3)	A7040	2(1)	A9567	2(3)	C1841	1(3)	C8957	2(3)	E0153	0(3)	E0265	0(3)	E0484	0(3)
A4557	2(1)	A7041	2(1)	A9568	0(3)	C1882	1(3)	C9113	0(3)	E0154	0(3)	E0266	0(3)	E0485	0(3)
A4561	1(1)	A7044	0(3)	A9569	1(3)	C1886	1(3)	C9121	0(3)	E0155	0(3)	E0270	0(3)	E0486	0(3)
A4562	1(1)	A7047	0(3)	A9570	1(3)	C1900	1(3)	C9132	5500(3)	E0156	0(3)	E0271	0(3)	E0487	0(3)
A4565	2(3)	A7048	10(3)	A9571	1(3)	C2613	2(1)	C9248	0(3)	E0157	0(3)	E0272	0(3)	E0500	0(3)
A4602	0(3)	A7501	0(3)	A9572	1(3)	C2616	1(3)	C9250	1(3)	E0158	0(3)	E0273	0(3)	E0550	0(3)
A4606	0(3)	A7504	0(3)	A9575	200(3)	C2619	1(3)	C9254	0(3)	E0159	2(2)	E0274	0(3)	E0555	0(3)
A4611	0(3)	A7507	0(3)	A9576	40(3)	C2620	1(3)	C9257	5(3)	E0160	0(3)	E0275	0(3)	E0560	0(3)
A4614	1(1)	A7520	0(3)	A9577	50(3)	C2621	1(3)	C9275	1(3)	E0161	0(3)	E0276	0(3)	E0561	0(3)
A4625	30(3)	A7524	0(3)	A9578	50(3)	C2622	1(3)	C9285	2(3)	E0162	0(3)	E0277	0(3)	E0562	0(3)
A4633	0(3)	A7527	0(3)	A9579	100(3)	C2623	3(1)	C9290	266(3)	E0163	0(3)	E0280	0(3)	E0565	0(3)
A4635	0(3)	A9272	0(1)	A9580	1(3)	C2624	1(3)	C9293	700(3)	E0165	0(3)	E0290	0(3)	E0570	0(3)
A4638	0(3)	A9284	0(3)	A9581	20(3)	C2626	1(3)	C9349	54(1)	E0167	0(3)	E0291	0(3)	E0572	0(3)
A4640	0(3)	A9500	3(3)	A9582	1(3)	C2631	1(3)	C9352	3(3)	E0168	0(3)	E0292	0(3)	E0574	0(3)
A4642	1(3)	A9501	1(3)	A9583	18(3)	C2634	24(3)	C9353	4(3)	E0170	0(3)	E0293	0(3)	E0575	0(3)
A4648	5(3)	A9502	3(3)	A9584	1(3)	C2635	124(3)	C9354	300(3)	E0171	0(3)	E0294	0(3)	E0580	0(3)
A4650	3(1)	A9503	1(3)	A9585	300(3)	C2636	600(3)	C9355	3(3)	E0172	0(3)	E0295	0(3)	E0585	0(3)
A5056	90(3)	A9504	1(3)	A9586	1(3)	C2637	0(3)	C9356	125(3)	E0175	0(3)	E0296	0(3)	E0600	0(3)
A5057	90(3)	A9505	4(3)	A9599	1(3)	C2638	150(3)	C9358	800(3)	E0181	0(3)	E0297	0(3)	E0601	0(3)
A5120	150(3)	A9507	1(3)	A9600	7(3)	C2639	150(3)	C9359	30(3)	E0182	0(3)	E0300	0(3)	E0602	0(3)
A5500	0(3)	A9508	2(3)	A9604	1(3)	C2640	150(3)	C9360	300(3)	E0184	0(3)	E0301	0(3)	E0603	0(3)
A5501	0(3)	A9509	5(3)	A9606	203(3)	C2641	150(3)	C9361	10(3)	E0185	0(3)	E0302	0(3)	E0604	0(3)
A5503	0(3)	A9510	1(3)	A9700	2(3)	C2642	120(3)	C9362	60(3)	E0186	0(3)	E0303	0(3)	E0605	0(3)
A5504	0(3)	A9512	30(3)	B4081	0(3)	C2643	120(3)	C9363	500(3)	E0187	0(3)	E0304	0(3)	E0606	0(3)
A5505	0(3)	A9516	4(3)	B4082	0(3)	C2644	500(1)	C9364	600(3)	E0188	0(3)	E0305	0(3)	E0607	0(3)
A5506	0(3)	A9517	200(3)	B4083	0(3)	C2645	6912(1)	C9447	1(3)	E0189	0(3)	E0310	0(3)	E0610	0(3)
A5507	0(3)	A9520	1(3)	B4087	0(3)	C5271	1(2)	C9460	100(1)	E0190	0(3)	E0315	0(3)	E0615	0(3)
A5508	0(3)	A9521	2(3)	B4088	0(3)	C5272	3(2)	C9497	1(3)	E0191	0(3)	E0316	0(3)	E0616	1(2)
A5510	0(3)	A9524	10(3)	B4149	0(3)	C5273	1(2)	C9600	3(3)	E0193	0(3)	E0325	0(3)	E0617	0(3)
A5512	0(3)	A9526	2(3)	B4153	0(3)	C5274	35(3)	C9601	2(3)	E0194	0(3)	E0326	0(3)	E0618	0(3)
A5513	0(3)	A9527	195(3)	B4157	0(3)	C5275	1(2)	C9602	2(3)	E0196	0(3)	E0328	0(3)	E0619	0(3)
A6501	2(1)	A9528	10(3)	B4160	0(3)	C5276	3(2)	C9603	2(3)	E0197	0(3)	E0329	0(3)	E0620	0(3)
A6502	2(1)	A9529	10(3)	B4164	0(3)	C5277	1(2)	C9604	2(3)	E0198	0(3)	E0350	0(3)	E0621	0(3)
A6503	2(1)	A9530	200(3)	B4168	0(3)	C5278	15(3)	C9605	2(3)	E0199	0(3)	E0352	0(3)	E0625	0(3)
A6504	4(1)	A9531	100(3)	B4172	0(3)	C8900	1(3)	C9606	1(3)	E0200	0(3)	E0370	0(3)	E0627	0(3)
A6505	4(1)	A9532	10(3)	B4176	0(3)	C8901	1(3)	C9607	1(2)	E0202	0(3)	E0371	0(3)	E0628	0(3)
A6506	4(1)	A9536	1(3)	B4178	0(3)	C8902	1(3)	C9608	2(3)	E0203	0(3)	E0372	0(3)	E0629	0(3)
A6507	4(1)	A9537	1(3)	B4180	0(3)	C8903	1(3)	C9725	1(3)	E0205	0(3)	E0373	0(3)	E0630	0(3)
A6508	4(1)	A9538	1(3)	B4189	0(3)	C8904	1(3)	C9727	1(2)	E0210	0(3)	E0424	0(3)	E0635	0(3)
A6509	2(1)	A9539	2(3)	B4199	0(3)	C8905	1(3)	C9728	1(2)	E0215	0(3)	E0425	0(3)	E0636	0(3)
A6510	2(1)	A9540	2(3)	B5000	0(3)	C8906	1(3)	C9733	1(3)	E0217	0(3)	E0430	0(3)	E0637	0(3)
A6511	2(1)	A9541	1(3)	B5100	0(3)	C8907	1(3)	C9734	1(3)	E0218	0(3)	E0431	0(3)	E0638	0(3)
A6513	0(3)	A9542	1(3)	B5200	0(3)	C8908	1(3)	C9739	1(2)	E0221	0(3)	E0434	0(3)	E0639	0(3)
A6531	0(3)	A9543	1(3)	C1716	4(3)	C8909	1(3)	C9740	1(2)	E0225	0(3)	E0435	0(3)	E0640	0(3)
A6532	0(3)	A9544	1(3)	C1717	10(3)	C8910	1(3)	C9741	1(3)	E0231	0(3)	E0439	0(3)	E0641	0(3)
A6545	0(3)	A9545	1(3)	C1719	99(3)	C8911	1(3)	C9742	1(2)	E0232	0(3)	E0440	0(3)	E0642	0(3)
A7000	0(3)	A9546	1(3)	C1721	1(3)	C8912	1(3)	E0100	0(3)	E0235	0(3)	E0441	0(3)	E0650	0(3)
A7003	0(3)	A9547	2(3)	C1722	1(3)	C8913	1(3)	E0105	0(3)	E0236	0(3)	E0442	0(3)	E0651	0(3)
A7005	0(3)	A9548	2(3)	C1749	1(3)	C8914	1(3)	E0110	0(3)	E0239	0(3)	E0443	0(3)	E0652	0(3)
A7006	0(3)	A9550	1(3)	C1764	1(3)	C8918	1(3)	E0111	0(3)	E0240	0(3)	E0444	0(3)	E0655	0(3)
A7013	0(3)	A9551	1(3)	C1767	2(3)	C8919	1(3)	E0112	0(3)	E0241	0(3)	E0445	0(3)	E0656	0(3)
A7014	0(3)	A9552	1(3)	C1771	1(3)	C8920	1(3)	E0113	0(3)	E0242	0(3)	E0446	0(3)	E0657	0(3)

CPT	MUE	CPT	MUE	CPT	MUE	CPT	MUE	CPT	MUE	CPT	MUE	CPT	MUE	CPT	MUE
E0660	0(3)	E0936	0(3)	E1070	0(3)	E1406	0(3)	E2214	0(3)	E2387	0(3)	G0121	1(2)	G0364	2(3)
E0665	0(3)	E0940	0(3)	E1083	0(3)	E1500	0(3)	E2215	0(3)	E2388	0(3)	G0123	1(3)	G0365	2(3)
E0666	0(3)	E0941	0(3)	E1084	0(3)	E1510	0(3)	E2216	0(3)	E2389	0(3)	G0124	1(3)	G0372	1(2)
E0667	0(3)	E0942	0(3)	E1085	0(3)	E1520	0(3)	E2217	0(3)	E2390	0(3)	G0127	1(2)	G0379	0(3)
E0668	0(3)	E0944	0(3)	E1086	0(3)	E1530	0(3)	E2218	0(3)	E2391	0(3)	G0128	1(3)	G0389	1(2)
E0669	0(3)	E0945	0(3)	E1087	0(3)	E1540	0(3)	E2219	0(3)	E2392	0(3)	G0130	1(2)	G0396	1(2)
E0670	0(3)	E0946	0(3)	E1088	0(3)	E1550	0(3)	E2220	0(3)	E2394	0(3)	G0141	1(3)	G0397	1(2)
E0671	0(3)	E0947	0(3)	E1089	0(3)	E1560	0(3)	E2221	0(3)	E2395	0(3)	G0143	1(3)	G0398	1(2)
E0672	0(3)	E0948	0(3)	E1090	0(3)	E1570	0(3)	E2222	0(3)	E2396	0(3)	G0144	1(3)	G0399	1(2)
E0673	0(3)	E0950	0(3)	E1092	0(3)	E1575	0(3)	E2224	0(3)	E2397	0(3)	G0145	1(3)	G0400	1(2)
E0675	0(3)	E0951	0(3)	E1093	0(3)	E1580	0(3)	E2225	0(3)	E2402	0(3)	G0147	1(3)	G0402	1(2)
E0676	1(3)	E0952	0(3)	E1100	0(3)	E1590	0(3)	E2226	0(3)	E2500	0(3)	G0148	1(3)	G0403	1(2)
E0691	0(3)	E0955	0(3)	E1110	0(3)	E1592	0(3)	E2227	0(3)	E2502	0(3)	G0166	2(3)	G0404	1(2)
E0692	0(3)	E0956	0(3)	E1130	0(3)	E1594	0(3)	E2228	0(3)	E2504	0(3)	G0168	2(3)	G0405	1(2)
E0693	0(3)	E0957	0(3)	E1140	0(3)	E1600	0(3)	E2231	0(3)	E2506	0(3)	G0175	1(3)	G0406	1(3)
E0694	0(3)	E0958	0(3)	E1150	0(3)	E1610	0(3)	E2291	1(2)	E2508	0(3)	G0177	0(3)	G0407	1(3)
E0700	0(3)	E0959	0(3)	E1160	0(3)	E1615	0(3)	E2292	1(2)	E2510	0(3)	G0179	1(2)	G0408	1(3)
E0705	0(3)	E0960	0(3)	E1161	0(3)	E1620	0(3)	E2293	1(2)	E2511	0(3)	G0180	1(2)	G0410	1(3)
E0710	0(3)	E0961	0(3)	E1170	0(3)	E1625	0(3)	E2294	1(2)	E2512	0(3)	G0181	1(2)	G0411	1(3)
E0720	0(3)	E0966	0(3)	E1171	0(3)	E1630	0(3)	E2295	0(3)	E2601	0(3)	G0182	1(2)	G0412	1(2)
E0730	0(3)	E0967	0(3)	E1172	0(3)	E1632	0(3)	E2300	0(3)	E2602	0(3)	G0186	1(2)	G0413	1(2)
E0731	0(3)	E0968	0(3)	E1180	0(3)	E1634	0(3)	E2301	0(3)	E2603	0(3)	G0202	1(2)	G0414	1(2)
E0740	0(3)	E0970	0(3)	E1190	0(3)	E1635	0(3)	E2310	0(3)	E2604	0(3)	G0204	2(3)	G0415	1(2)
E0744	0(3)	E0971	0(3)	E1195	0(3)	E1636	0(3)	E2311	0(3)	E2605	0(3)	G0206	2(3)	G0416	1(2)
E0745	0(3)	E0973	0(3)	E1200	0(3)	E1637	0(3)	E2312	0(3)	E2606	0(3)	G0235	1(3)	G0420	2(3)
E0746	1(3)	E0974	0(3)	E1220	0(3)	E1639	0(3)	E2313	0(3)	E2607	0(3)	G0237	8(3)	G0421	4(3)
E0747	0(3)	E0978	0(3)	E1221	0(3)	E1700	0(3)	E2321	0(3)	E2608	0(3)	G0238	8(3)	G0422	6(2)
E0748	0(3)	E0981	0(3)	E1222	0(3)	E1701	0(3)	E2322	0(3)	E2609	0(3)	G0239	1(3)	G0423	6(2)
E0749	1(3)	E0982	0(3)	E1223	0(3)	E1702	0(3)	E2323	0(3)	E2611	0(3)	G0245	1(2)	G0424	2(2)
E0755	0(3)	E0983	0(3)	E1224	0(3)	E1800	0(3)	E2324	0(3)	E2612	0(3)	G0246	1(2)	G0425	1(3)
E0760	0(3)	E0984	0(3)	E1225	0(3)	E1801	0(3)	E2325	0(3)	E2613	0(3)	G0247	1(2)	G0426	1(3)
E0761	0(3)	E0985	0(3)	E1226	0(3)	E1802	0(3)	E2326	0(3)	E2614	0(3)	G0248	1(2)	G0427	1(3)
E0762	0(3)	E0986	0(3)	E1228	0(3)	E1805	0(3)	E2327	0(3)	E2615	0(3)	G0249	3(3)	G0429	1(2)
E0764	0(3)	E0988	0(3)	E1229	0(3)	E1806	0(3)	E2328	0(3)	E2616	0(3)	G0250	1(2)	G0432	1(2)
E0765	0(3)	E0990	0(3)	E1230	0(3)	E1810	0(3)	E2329	0(3)	E2617	0(3)	G0257	0(3)	G0433	1(2)
E0766	0(3)	E0992	0(3)	E1231	0(3)	E1811	0(3)	E2330	0(3)	E2619	0(3)	G0259	2(3)	G0435	1(2)
E0769	0(3)	E0994	0(3)	E1232	0(3)	E1812	0(3)	E2331	0(3)	E2620	0(3)	G0260	2(3)	G0436	1(2)
E0770	1(3)	E0995	0(3)	E1233	0(3)	E1815	0(3)	E2340	0(3)	E2621	0(3)	G0268	1(2)	G0437	1(2)
E0776	0(3)	E1002	0(3)	E1234	0(3)	E1816	0(3)	E2341	0(3)	E2622	0(3)	G0270	8(3)	G0438	1(2)
E0779	0(3)	E1003	0(3)	E1235	0(3)	E1818	0(3)	E2342	0(3)	E2623	0(3)	G0271	4(3)	G0439	1(2)
E0780	0(3)	E1004	0(3)	E1236	0(3)	E1820	0(3)	E2343	0(3)	E2624	0(3)	G0277	5(3)	G0442	1(2)
E0781	1(2)	E1005	0(3)	E1237	0(3)	E1821	0(3)	E2351	0(3)	E2625	0(3)	G0278	1(2)	G0443	1(2)
E0782	1(2)	E1006	0(3)	E1238	0(3)	E1825	0(3)	E2358	0(3)	E2626	0(3)	G0281	1(3)	G0444	1(2)
E0783	1(2)	E1007	0(3)	E1240	0(3)	E1830	0(3)	E2359	0(3)	E2627	0(3)	G0283	1(3)	G0445	1(2)
E0784	0(3)	E1008	0(3)	E1250	0(3)	E1831	0(3)	E2361	0(3)	E2628	0(3)	G0288	1(2)	G0446	1(3)
E0785	1(2)	E1009	0(3)	E1260	0(3)	E1840	0(3)	E2363	0(3)	E2629	0(3)	G0289	1(2)	G0448	1(3)
E0786	1(2)	E1010	0(3)	E1270	0(3)	E1841	0(3)	E2365	0(3)	E2630	0(3)	G0293	1(2)	G0452	6(3)
E0791	0(3)	E1011	0(3)	E1280	0(3)	E1902	0(3)	E2366	0(3)	E2631	0(3)	G0294	1(2)	G0453	40(3)
E0830	0(3)	E1012	0(3)	E1285	0(3)	E2000	0(3)	E2367	0(3)	E2632	0(3)	G0296	1(2)	G0454	1(2)
E0840	0(3)	E1014	0(3)	E1290	0(3)	E2100	0(3)	E2368	0(3)	E2633	0(3)	G0297	1(2)	G0455	1(2)
E0849	0(3)	E1015	0(3)	E1295	0(3)	E2101	0(3)	E2369	0(3)	G0008	1(2)	G0302	1(2)	G0458	1(3)
E0850	0(3)	E1016	0(3)	E1300	0(3)	E2120	0(3)	E2370	0(3)	G0009	1(2)	G0303	1(2)	G0459	1(3)
E0855	0(3)	E1017	0(3)	E1310	0(3)	E2201	0(3)	E2371	0(3)	G0010	1(3)	G0304	1(2)	G0460	1(3)
E0856	0(3)	E1018	0(3)	E1352	0(3)	E2202	0(3)	E2373	0(3)	G0027	1(2)	G0305	1(2)	G0463	0(3)
E0860	0(3)	E1020	0(3)	E1353	0(3)	E2203	0(3)	E2374	0(3)	G0101	1(2)	G0306	1(3)	G0472	1(2)
E0870	0(3)	E1028	0(3)	E1354	0(3)	E2204	0(3)	E2375	0(3)	G0102	1(2)	G0307	1(3)	G0475	1(2)
E0880	0(3)	E1029	0(3)	E1355	0(3)	E2205	0(3)	E2376	0(3)	G0103	1(2)	G0328	1(2)	G0476	1(2)
E0890	0(3)	E1030	0(3)	E1356	0(3)	E2206	0(3)	E2377	0(3)	G0104	1(2)	G0329	1(3)	G0477	1(2)
E0900	0(3)	E1031	0(3)	E1357	0(3)	E2207	0(3)	E2378	0(3)	G0105	1(2)	G0333	0(3)	G0478	1(2)
E0910	0(3)	E1035	0(3)	E1358	0(3)	E2208	0(3)	E2381	0(3)	G0106	1(2)	G0337	1(2)	G0479	1(2)
E0911	0(3)	E1037	0(3)	E1372	0(3)	E2209	0(3)	E2382	0(3)	G0108	6(3)	G0339	1(2)	G0480	1(2)
E0912	0(3)	E1038	0(3)	E1390	0(3)	E2210	0(3)	E2383	0(3)	G0109	12(3)	G0340	2(3)	G0481	1(2)
E0920	0(3)	E1039	0(3)	E1391	0(3)	E2211	0(3)	E2384	0(3)	G0117	1(2)	G0341	1(2)	G0482	1(2)
E0930	0(3)	E1050	0(3)	E1392	0(3)	E2212	0(3)	E2385	0(3)	G0118	1(2)	G0342	1(2)	G0483	1(2)
E0935	0(3)	E1060	0(3)	E1405	0(3)	E2213	0(3)	E2386	0(3)	G0120	1(2)	G0343	1(2)	G3001	1(2)

CPT	MUE	CPT	MUE	CPT	MUE	CPT	MUE	CPT	MUE	CPT	MUE	CPT	MUE	CPT	MUE
G6001	1(2)	J0400	39(3)	J0770	5(3)	J1442	3360(3)	J1833	372(3)	J2510	4(3)	J3230	2(3)	J7188	22000(1)
G6002	2(3)	J0401	400(3)	J0775	180(3)	J1443	1(3)	J1835	0(3)	J2513	1(3)	J3240	1(3)	J7189	13000(1)
G6003	2(3)	J0456	4(3)	J0780	4(3)	J1447	960(3)	J1840	3(3)	J2515	1(3)	J3243	150(3)	J7190	30000(1)
G6004	2(3)	J0461	200(3)	J0795	100(3)	J1450	4(3)	J1850	4(3)	J2540	75(3)	J3246	1(3)	J7191	0(3)
G6005	2(3)	J0470	2(3)	J0800	3(3)	J1451	1(3)	J1885	8(3)	J2543	16(3)	J3250	2(3)	J7192	22000(1)
G6006	2(3)	J0475	8(3)	J0833	3(3)	J1452	0(3)	J1890	0(3)	J2545	1(3)	J3260	8(3)	J7193	4000(1)
G6007	2(3)	J0476	2(3)	J0834	3(3)	J1453	150(3)	J1930	120(3)	J2547	600(3)	J3262	800(3)	J7194	9000(1)
G6008	2(3)	J0480	1(3)	J0840	6(3)	J1455	18(3)	J1931	760(3)	J2550	3(3)	J3265	0(3)	J7195	6000(1)
G6009	2(3)	J0485	1500(3)	J0850	9(3)	J1457	500(3)	J1940	6(3)	J2560	1(3)	J3280	0(3)	J7196	175(3)
G6010	2(3)	J0490	160(3)	J0875	300(3)	J1458	100(3)	J1945	0(3)	J2562	48(3)	J3285	1(3)	J7197	6300(1)
G6011	2(3)	J0500	4(3)	J0878	1500(3)	J1459	300(1)	J1950	12(3)	J2590	3(3)	J3300	160(3)	J7198	6000(1)
G6012	2(3)	J0515	3(3)	J0881	500(3)	J1460	10(2)	J1953	300(3)	J2597	45(3)	J3301	16(3)	J7200	20000(1)
G6013	2(3)	J0520	0(3)	J0882	200(3)	J1556	300(3)	J1955	11(3)	J2650	0(3)	J3302	0(3)	J7201	9000(1)
G6014	2(3)	J0558	24(3)	J0885	60(1)	J1557	300(3)	J1956	4(3)	J2670	0(3)	J3303	24(3)	J7205	9750(1)
G6015	2(3)	J0561	24(3)	J0887	360(1)	J1559	375(1)	J1960	0(3)	J2675	1(3)	J3305	0(3)	J7297	1(3)
G6016	2(3)	J0571	0(3)	J0888	360(1)	J1560	1(2)	J1980	2(3)	J2680	4(3)	J3310	0(3)	J7298	1(3)
G6017	2(3)	J0572	0(3)	J0890	0(2)	J1561	300(3)	J1990	0(3)	J2690	4(3)	J3315	6(3)	J7301	0(3)
G9143	1(2)	J0573	0(3)	J0894	100(3)	J1562	375(1)	J2001	60(3)	J2700	48(3)	J3320	0(3)	J7308	3(3)
G9156	1(2)	J0574	0(3)	J0895	12(3)	J1566	300(1)	J2010	10(3)	J2704	80(3)	J3350	0(3)	J7309	1(3)
G9157	1(2)	J0575	0(3)	J0897	120(3)	J1568	300(3)	J2020	6(3)	J2710	2(3)	J3355	1(3)	J7310	2(2)
G9187	1(3)	J0583	250(3)	J0945	4(3)	J1569	300(3)	J2060	4(3)	J2720	5(3)	J3357	90(3)	J7311	1(3)
G9480	1(3)	J0585	600(3)	J1000	1(3)	J1570	4(3)	J2150	8(3)	J2724	4000(3)	J3360	6(3)	J7312	14(3)
J0120	1(3)	J0586	300(3)	J1020	8(3)	J1571	20(3)	J2170	8(3)	J2725	0(3)	J3364	0(3)	J7313	19(1)
J0129	100(3)	J0587	300(3)	J1030	8(3)	J1572	300(3)	J2175	4(3)	J2730	2(3)	J3365	0(3)	J7315	2(3)
J0130	6(3)	J0588	600(3)	J1040	4(3)	J1575	900(1)	J2180	0(3)	J2760	2(3)	J3370	12(3)	J7316	4(2)
J0131	400(3)	J0592	6(3)	J1050	1000(3)	J1580	9(3)	J2185	30(3)	J2765	10(3)	J3380	300(3)	J7321	2(2)
J0132	12(3)	J0594	320(3)	J1071	400(3)	J1590	0(3)	J2210	1(3)	J2770	6(3)	J3385	92(3)	J7323	2(2)
J0133	1200(3)	J0595	8(3)	J1094	0(3)	J1595	1(3)	J2212	240(3)	J2778	10(3)	J3396	150(3)	J7324	2(2)
J0135	8(3)	J0596	840(3)	J1100	120(3)	J1599	300(3)	J2248	150(3)	J2780	16(3)	J3400	0(3)	J7325	96(3)
J0153	180(3)	J0597	250(3)	J1110	3(3)	J1600	2(3)	J2250	22(3)	J2783	60(3)	J3410	8(3)	J7326	2(2)
J0171	20(3)	J0598	100(3)	J1120	2(3)	J1602	300(3)	J2260	4(3)	J2785	4(3)	J3411	4(3)	J7327	2(2)
J0178	4(3)	J0600	3(3)	J1160	2(3)	J1610	2(3)	J2265	400(3)	J2788	1(3)	J3415	6(3)	J7328	336(3)
J0180	150(3)	J0610	15(3)	J1162	1(3)	J1620	0(3)	J2270	9(3)	J2791	50(3)	J3420	1(3)	J7330	1(3)
J0190	0(3)	J0620	1(3)	J1165	50(3)	J1626	30(3)	J2274	250(3)	J2793	320(3)	J3430	25(3)	J7336	1120(3)
J0200	0(3)	J0630	1(3)	J1170	350(3)	J1630	5(3)	J2278	999(3)	J2794	100(3)	J3465	40(3)	J7340	100(3)
J0202	12(3)	J0636	100(3)	J1180	2(3)	J1631	9(3)	J2280	4(3)	J2795	200(3)	J3470	3(3)	J7500	0(3)
J0205	0(3)	J0637	20(3)	J1190	8(3)	J1640	626(3)	J2300	4(3)	J2796	150(3)	J3471	999(2)	J7501	1(3)
J0207	4(3)	J0638	180(3)	J1200	8(3)	J1642	40(3)	J2310	4(3)	J2800	3(3)	J3472	2(3)	J7502	0(3)
J0210	4(3)	J0640	24(3)	J1205	4(3)	J1644	40(3)	J2315	380(3)	J2805	3(3)	J3473	450(3)	J7504	15(3)
J0215	30(3)	J0641	1200(3)	J1212	1(3)	J1645	10(3)	J2320	4(3)	J2810	5(3)	J3475	20(3)	J7505	1(3)
J0220	1(3)	J0670	10(3)	J1230	3(3)	J1650	30(3)	J2323	300(3)	J2820	15(3)	J3480	40(3)	J7507	0(3)
J0221	300(3)	J0690	12(3)	J1240	6(3)	J1652	20(3)	J2325	0(3)	J2850	16(3)	J3485	160(3)	J7508	0(3)
J0256	3500(3)	J0692	12(3)	J1245	6(3)	J1655	0(3)	J2353	60(3)	J2860	170(3)	J3486	4(3)	J7509	0(3)
J0257	1400(3)	J0694	8(3)	J1250	2(3)	J1670	1(3)	J2354	60(3)	J2910	0(3)	J3489	5(3)	J7510	0(3)
J0270	32(3)	J0695	60(3)	J1260	2(3)	J1675	0(3)	J2355	2(3)	J2916	20(3)	J3520	0(3)	J7511	9(3)
J0275	1(3)	J0696	16(3)	J1265	20(3)	J1700	0(3)	J2357	90(3)	J2920	25(3)	J3530	0(3)	J7512	0(3)
J0278	15(3)	J0697	4(3)	J1267	150(3)	J1710	0(3)	J2358	405(3)	J2930	25(3)	J7030	5(3)	J7513	6(3)
J0280	7(3)	J0698	10(3)	J1270	8(3)	J1720	10(3)	J2360	2(3)	J2940	0(3)	J7040	6(3)	J7515	0(3)
J0282	5(3)	J0702	18(3)	J1290	30(3)	J1725	250(3)	J2370	2(3)	J2941	8(3)	J7042	6(3)	J7516	1(3)
J0285	5(3)	J0706	1(3)	J1300	120(3)	J1730	0(3)	J2400	4(3)	J2950	0(3)	J7050	10(3)	J7517	0(3)
J0287	20(3)	J0710	0(3)	J1320	0(3)	J1740	3(3)	J2405	64(3)	J2993	2(3)	J7060	10(3)	J7518	0(3)
J0288	0(3)	J0712	120(3)	J1322	220(1)	J1741	8(3)	J2407	120(3)	J2995	0(3)	J7070	4(3)	J7520	0(3)
J0289	50(3)	J0713	12(3)	J1324	108(3)	J1742	2(3)	J2410	2(3)	J2997	8(3)	J7100	2(3)	J7525	2(3)
J0290	24(3)	J0714	4(1)	J1325	1(3)	J1743	66(3)	J2425	125(3)	J3000	2(3)	J7110	2(3)	J7527	0(3)
J0295	12(3)	J0715	0(3)	J1327	1(3)	J1744	30(3)	J2426	819(3)	J3010	100(3)	J7120	4(3)	J7604	0(3)
J0300	8(3)	J0716	4(1)	J1330	1(3)	J1745	150(3)	J2430	3(3)	J3030	1(3)	J7121	4(3)	J7605	2(3)
J0330	10(3)	J0717	400(3)	J1335	2(3)	J1750	45(3)	J2440	4(3)	J3060	900(3)	J7131	500(3)	J7606	2(3)
J0348	200(3)	J0720	15(3)	J1364	2(3)	J1756	500(3)	J2460	0(3)	J3070	3(3)	J7178	7700(1)	J7607	0(3)
J0350	0(3)	J0725	10(3)	J1380	4(3)	J1786	900(3)	J2469	10(3)	J3090	200(3)	J7180	6000(1)	J7608	3(3)
J0360	2(3)	J0735	50(3)	J1410	4(3)	J1790	2(3)	J2501	2(3)	J3095	150(3)	J7181	3850(1)	J7609	0(3)
J0364	6(3)	J0740	2(3)	J1430	10(3)	J1800	6(3)	J2502	60(1)	J3101	50(3)	J7182	22000(1)	J7610	0(3)
J0365	0(3)	J0743	16(3)	J1435	1(3)	J1810	0(3)	J2503	2(3)	J3105	2(3)	J7183	15000(1)	J7611	10(3)
J0380	1(3)	J0744	6(3)	J1436	0(3)	J1815	8(3)	J2504	15(3)	J3110	2(3)	J7185	4000(1)	J7612	10(3)
J0390	0(3)	J0745	2(3)	J1438	2(3)	J1817	0(3)	J2505	1(3)	J3121	400(3)	J7186	8000(1)	J7613	10(3)
J0395	0(3)	J0760	4(3)	J1439	750(3)	J1830	1(3)	J2507	8(3)	J3145	750(3)	J7187	7500(1)	J7614	10(3)

CPT	MUE	CPT	MUE	CPT	MUE	CPT	MUE	CPT	MUE	CPT	MUE	CPT	MUE	CPT	MUE
J7615	0(3)	J9031	1(3)	J9300	0(3)	K0602	0(3)	K0870	0(3)	L0633	0(3)	L1650	0(3)	L2108	0(3)
J7620	6(3)	J9032	300(3)	J9301	100(3)	K0605	0(3)	K0871	0(3)	L0634	0(3)	L1652	0(3)	L2112	0(3)
J7622	0(3)	J9033	300(3)	J9302	200(3)	K0606	0(3)	K0877	0(3)	L0635	0(3)	L1660	0(3)	L2114	0(3)
J7624	0(3)	J9035	180(3)	J9303	100(3)	K0607	0(3)	K0878	0(3)	L0636	0(3)	L1680	0(3)	L2116	0(3)
J7626	2(3)	J9039	35(3)	J9305	150(3)	K0608	0(3)	K0879	0(3)	L0637	0(3)	L1685	0(3)	L2126	0(3)
J7627	0(3)	J9040	4(3)	J9306	840(3)	K0609	0(3)	K0880	0(3)	L0638	0(3)	L1686	0(3)	L2128	0(3)
J7628	0(3)	J9041	35(3)	J9307	80(3)	K0672	0(3)	K0884	0(3)	L0639	0(3)	L1690	0(3)	L2132	0(3)
J7629	0(3)	J9042	200(3)	J9308	300(3)	K0730	0(3)	K0885	0(3)	L0640	0(3)	L1700	0(3)	L2134	0(3)
J7631	4(3)	J9043	60(3)	J9310	12(3)	K0733	0(3)	K0886	0(3)	L0641	0(3)	L1710	0(3)	L2136	0(3)
J7632	0(3)	J9045	22(3)	J9315	40(3)	K0738	0(3)	K0890	0(3)	L0642	0(3)	L1720	0(3)	L2180	0(3)
J7633	0(3)	J9047	120(3)	J9320	4(3)	K0743	0(3)	K0891	0(3)	L0643	0(3)	L1730	0(3)	L2182	0(3)
J7634	0(3)	J9050	6(3)	J9328	400(3)	K0744	0(3)	K0898	1(2)	L0648	0(3)	L1755	0(3)	L2184	0(3)
J7635	0(3)	J9055	120(3)	J9330	50(3)	K0745	0(3)	K0900	0(3)	L0649	0(3)	L1810	0(3)	L2186	0(3)
J7636	0(3)	J9060	24(3)	J9340	4(3)	K0746	0(3)	K0901	0(3)	L0650	0(3)	L1812	0(3)	L2188	0(3)
J7637	0(3)	J9065	20(3)	J9351	120(3)	K0800	0(3)	K0902	0(3)	L0651	0(3)	L1820	0(3)	L2190	0(3)
J7638	0(3)	J9070	55(3)	J9354	600(3)	K0801	0(3)	L0112	0(3)	L0700	0(3)	L1830	0(3)	L2192	0(3)
J7639	3(3)	J9098	5(3)	J9355	100(3)	K0802	0(3)	L0113	0(3)	L0710	0(3)	L1831	0(3)	L2200	0(3)
J7640	0(3)	J9100	120(3)	J9357	4(3)	K0806	0(3)	L0120	0(3)	L0810	0(3)	L1832	0(3)	L2210	0(3)
J7641	0(3)	J9120	5(3)	J9360	45(3)	K0807	0(3)	L0130	0(3)	L0820	0(3)	L1833	0(3)	L2220	0(3)
J7642	0(3)	J9130	24(3)	J9370	4(3)	K0808	0(3)	L0140	0(3)	L0830	0(3)	L1834	0(3)	L2230	0(3)
J7643	0(3)	J9150	12(3)	J9371	5(3)	K0812	0(3)	L0150	0(3)	L0859	0(3)	L1836	0(3)	L2232	0(3)
J7644	3(3)	J9151	10(3)	J9390	36(3)	K0813	0(3)	L0160	0(3)	L0861	0(3)	L1840	0(3)	L2240	0(3)
J7645	0(3)	J9155	240(3)	J9395	20(3)	K0814	0(3)	L0170	0(3)	L0970	0(3)	L1843	0(3)	L2250	0(3)
J7647	0(3)	J9160	7(3)	J9400	600(3)	K0815	0(3)	L0172	0(3)	L0972	0(3)	L1844	0(3)	L2260	0(3)
J7648	0(3)	J9165	0(3)	J9600	4(3)	K0816	0(3)	L0174	0(3)	L0974	0(3)	L1845	0(3)	L2265	0(3)
J7649	0(3)	J9171	240(3)	K0001	0(3)	K0820	0(3)	L0180	0(3)	L0976	0(3)	L1846	0(3)	L2270	0(3)
J7650	0(3)	J9175	10(3)	K0002	0(3)	K0821	0(3)	L0190	0(3)	L0978	0(3)	L1847	0(3)	L2275	0(3)
J7657	0(3)	J9178	150(3)	K0003	0(3)	K0822	0(3)	L0200	0(3)	L0980	0(3)	L1848	0(3)	L2280	0(3)
J7658	0(3)	J9179	50(3)	K0004	0(3)	K0823	0(3)	L0220	0(3)	L0982	0(3)	L1850	0(3)	L2300	0(3)
J7659	0(3)	J9185	2(3)	K0005	0(3)	K0824	0(3)	L0450	0(3)	L0984	0(3)	L1860	0(3)	L2310	0(3)
J7660	0(3)	J9190	20(3)	K0006	0(3)	K0825	0(3)	L0452	0(3)	L1000	0(3)	L1900	0(3)	L2320	0(3)
J7665	127(2)	J9200	5(3)	K0007	0(3)	K0826	0(3)	L0454	0(3)	L1001	0(3)	L1902	0(3)	L2330	0(3)
J7667	0(3)	J9201	20(3)	K0009	0(3)	K0827	0(3)	L0455	0(3)	L1005	0(3)	L1904	0(3)	L2335	0(3)
J7668	0(3)	J9202	3(3)	K0015	0(3)	K0828	0(3)	L0456	0(3)	L1010	0(3)	L1906	0(3)	L2340	0(3)
J7669	0(3)	J9206	42(3)	K0017	0(3)	K0829	0(3)	L0457	0(3)	L1020	0(3)	L1907	0(3)	L2350	0(3)
J7670	0(3)	J9207	90(3)	K0018	0(3)	K0830	0(3)	L0458	0(3)	L1025	0(3)	L1910	0(3)	L2360	0(3)
J7676	0(3)	J9208	15(3)	K0019	0(3)	K0831	0(3)	L0460	0(3)	L1030	0(3)	L1920	0(3)	L2370	0(3)
J7680	0(3)	J9209	55(3)	K0020	0(3)	K0835	0(3)	L0462	0(3)	L1040	0(3)	L1930	0(3)	L2375	0(3)
J7681	0(3)	J9211	6(3)	K0037	0(3)	K0836	0(3)	L0464	0(3)	L1050	0(3)	L1932	0(3)	L2380	0(3)
J7682	2(3)	J9212	0(3)	K0038	0(3)	K0837	0(3)	L0466	0(3)	L1060	0(3)	L1940	0(3)	L2385	0(3)
J7683	0(3)	J9213	12(3)	K0039	0(3)	K0838	0(3)	L0467	0(3)	L1070	0(3)	L1945	0(3)	L2387	0(3)
J7684	0(3)	J9214	100(3)	K0040	0(3)	K0839	0(3)	L0468	0(3)	L1080	0(3)	L1950	0(3)	L2390	0(3)
J7685	0(3)	J9215	0(3)	K0041	0(3)	K0840	0(3)	L0469	0(3)	L1085	0(3)	L1951	0(3)	L2395	0(3)
J7686	1(3)	J9216	2(3)	K0042	0(3)	K0841	0(3)	L0470	0(3)	L1090	0(3)	L1960	0(3)	L2397	0(3)
J8501	0(3)	J9217	6(3)	K0043	0(3)	K0842	0(3)	L0472	0(3)	L1100	0(3)	L1970	0(3)	L2405	0(3)
J8510	0(3)	J9218	1(3)	K0044	0(3)	K0843	0(3)	L0480	0(3)	L1110	0(3)	L1971	0(3)	L2415	0(3)
J8520	0(3)	J9219	1(3)	K0045	0(3)	K0848	0(3)	L0482	0(3)	L1120	0(3)	L1980	0(3)	L2425	0(3)
J8521	0(3)	J9225	1(3)	K0046	0(3)	K0849	0(3)	L0484	0(3)	L1200	0(3)	L1990	0(3)	L2430	0(3)
J8530	0(3)	J9226	1(3)	K0047	0(3)	K0850	0(3)	L0486	0(3)	L1210	0(3)	L2000	0(3)	L2492	0(3)
J8540	0(3)	J9228	1100(3)	K0050	0(3)	K0851	0(3)	L0488	0(3)	L1220	0(3)	L2005	0(3)	L2500	0(3)
J8560	0(3)	J9230	5(3)	K0051	0(3)	K0852	0(3)	L0490	0(3)	L1230	0(3)	L2010	0(3)	L2510	0(3)
J8562	0(3)	J9245	9(3)	K0052	0(3)	K0853	0(3)	L0491	0(3)	L1240	0(3)	L2020	0(3)	L2520	0(3)
J8600	0(3)	J9250	25(3)	K0053	0(3)	K0854	0(3)	L0492	0(3)	L1250	0(3)	L2030	0(3)	L2525	0(3)
J8610	0(3)	J9260	20(3)	K0056	0(3)	K0855	0(3)	L0621	0(3)	L1260	0(3)	L2034	0(3)	L2526	0(3)
J8650	0(3)	J9261	80(3)	K0065	0(3)	K0856	0(3)	L0622	0(3)	L1270	0(3)	L2035	0(3)	L2530	0(3)
J8655	0(3)	J9262	700(3)	K0069	0(3)	K0857	0(3)	L0623	0(3)	L1280	0(3)	L2036	0(3)	L2540	0(3)
J8700	0(3)	J9263	700(3)	K0070	0(3)	K0858	0(3)	L0624	0(3)	L1290	0(3)	L2037	0(3)	L2550	0(3)
J8705	0(3)	J9266	2(3)	K0071	0(3)	K0859	0(3)	L0625	0(3)	L1300	0(3)	L2038	0(3)	L2570	0(3)
J9000	20(3)	J9267	750(3)	K0072	0(3)	K0860	0(3)	L0626	0(3)	L1310	0(3)	L2040	0(3)	L2580	0(3)
J9015	1(3)	J9268	1(3)	K0073	0(3)	K0861	0(3)	L0627	0(3)	L1499	1(3)	L2050	0(3)	L2600	0(3)
J9017	30(3)	J9270	0(3)	K0077	0(3)	K0862	0(3)	L0628	0(3)	L1600	0(3)	L2060	0(3)	L2610	0(3)
J9019	60(3)	J9271	300(3)	K0105	0(3)	K0863	0(3)	L0629	0(3)	L1610	0(3)	L2070	0(3)	L2620	0(3)
J9020	0(3)	J9280	12(3)	K0195	0(3)	K0864	0(3)	L0630	0(3)	L1620	0(3)	L2080	0(3)	L2622	0(3)
J9025	300(3)	J9293	8(3)	K0455	0(3)	K0868	0(3)	L0631	0(3)	L1630	0(3)	L2090	0(3)	L2624	0(3)
J9027	100(3)	J9299	440(3)	K0462	0(3)	K0869	0(3)	L0632	0(3)	L1640	0(3)	L2106	0(3)	L2627	0(3)

CPT	MUE	CPT	MUE	CPT	MUE	CPT	MUE	CPT	MUE	CPT	MUE	CPT	MUE	CPT	MUE
L2628	0(3)	L3440	0(3)	L3929	0(3)	L5280	0(3)	L5665	0(3)	L5850	0(3)	L6580	0(3)	L6714	0(3)
L2630	0(3)	L3450	0(3)	L3930	0(3)	L5301	0(3)	L5666	0(3)	L5855	0(3)	L6582	0(3)	L6715	0(3)
L2640	0(3)	L3455	0(3)	L3931	0(3)	L5312	0(3)	L5668	0(3)	L5856	0(3)	L6584	0(3)	L6721	0(3)
L2650	0(3)	L3460	0(3)	L3933	0(3)	L5321	0(3)	L5670	0(3)	L5857	0(3)	L6586	0(3)	L6722	0(3)
L2660	0(3)	L3465	0(3)	L3935	0(3)	L5331	0(3)	L5671	0(3)	L5858	0(3)	L6588	0(3)	L6805	0(3)
L2670	0(3)	L3470	0(3)	L3956	0(3)	L5341	0(3)	L5672	0(3)	L5859	0(3)	L6590	0(3)	L6810	0(3)
L2680	0(3)	L3480	0(3)	L3960	0(3)	L5400	0(3)	L5673	0(3)	L5910	0(3)	L6600	0(3)	L6880	0(3)
L2750	0(3)	L3485	0(3)	L3961	0(3)	L5410	0(3)	L5676	0(3)	L5920	0(3)	L6605	0(3)	L6881	0(3)
L2755	0(3)	L3500	0(3)	L3962	0(3)	L5420	0(3)	L5677	0(3)	L5925	0(3)	L6610	0(3)	L6882	0(3)
L2760	0(3)	L3510	0(3)	L3967	0(3)	L5430	0(3)	L5678	0(3)	L5930	0(3)	L6611	0(3)	L6883	0(3)
L2768	0(3)	L3520	0(3)	L3971	0(3)	L5450	0(3)	L5679	0(3)	L5940	0(3)	L6615	0(3)	L6884	0(3)
L2780	0(3)	L3530	0(3)	L3973	0(3)	L5460	0(3)	L5680	0(3)	L5950	0(3)	L6616	0(3)	L6885	0(3)
L2785	0(3)	L3540	0(3)	L3975	0(3)	L5500	0(3)	L5681	0(3)	L5960	0(3)	L6620	0(3)	L6890	0(3)
L2795	0(3)	L3550	0(3)	L3976	0(3)	L5505	0(3)	L5682	0(3)	L5961	0(3)	L6621	0(3)	L6895	0(3)
L2800	0(3)	L3560	0(3)	L3977	0(3)	L5510	0(3)	L5683	0(3)	L5962	0(3)	L6623	0(3)	L6900	0(3)
L2810	0(3)	L3570	0(3)	L3978	0(3)	L5520	0(3)	L5684	0(3)	L5964	0(3)	L6624	0(3)	L6905	0(3)
L2820	0(3)	L3580	0(3)	L3980	0(3)	L5530	0(3)	L5685	0(3)	L5966	0(3)	L6625	0(3)	L6910	0(3)
L2830	0(3)	L3590	0(3)	L3981	0(3)	L5535	0(3)	L5686	0(3)	L5968	0(3)	L6628	0(3)	L6915	0(3)
L3000	0(3)	L3595	0(3)	L3982	0(3)	L5540	0(3)	L5688	0(3)	L5969	0(3)	L6629	0(3)	L6920	0(3)
L3001	0(3)	L3600	0(3)	L3984	0(3)	L5560	0(3)	L5690	0(3)	L5970	0(3)	L6630	0(3)	L6925	0(3)
L3002	0(3)	L3610	0(3)	L4000	0(3)	L5570	0(3)	L5692	0(3)	L5971	0(3)	L6632	0(3)	L6930	0(3)
L3003	0(3)	L3620	0(3)	L4002	0(3)	L5580	0(3)	L5694	0(3)	L5972	0(3)	L6635	0(3)	L6935	0(3)
L3010	0(3)	L3630	0(3)	L4010	0(3)	L5585	0(3)	L5695	0(3)	L5974	0(3)	L6637	0(3)	L6940	0(3)
L3020	0(3)	L3640	0(3)	L4020	0(3)	L5590	0(3)	L5696	0(3)	L5975	0(3)	L6638	0(3)	L6945	0(3)
L3030	0(3)	L3650	0(3)	L4030	0(3)	L5595	0(3)	L5697	0(3)	L5976	0(3)	L6640	0(3)	L6950	0(3)
L3031	0(3)	L3660	0(3)	L4040	0(3)	L5600	0(3)	L5698	0(3)	L5978	0(3)	L6641	0(3)	L6955	0(3)
L3040	0(3)	L3670	0(3)	L4045	0(3)	L5610	0(3)	L5699	0(3)	L5979	0(3)	L6642	0(3)	L6960	0(3)
L3050	0(3)	L3671	0(3)	L4050	0(3)	L5611	0(3)	L5700	0(3)	L5980	0(3)	L6645	0(3)	L6965	0(3)
L3060	0(3)	L3674	0(3)	L4055	0(3)	L5613	0(3)	L5701	0(3)	L5981	0(3)	L6646	0(3)	L6970	0(3)
L3070	0(3)	L3675	0(3)	L4060	0(3)	L5614	0(3)	L5702	0(3)	L5982	0(3)	L6647	0(3)	L6975	0(3)
L3080	0(3)	L3677	0(3)	L4070	0(3)	L5616	0(3)	L5703	0(3)	L5984	0(3)	L6648	0(3)	L7007	0(3)
L3090	0(3)	L3678	0(3)	L4080	0(3)	L5617	0(3)	L5704	0(3)	L5985	0(3)	L6650	0(3)	L7008	0(3)
L3100	0(3)	L3702	0(3)	L4090	0(3)	L5618	0(3)	L5705	0(3)	L5986	0(3)	L6655	0(3)	L7009	0(3)
L3140	0(3)	L3710	0(3)	L4100	0(3)	L5620	0(3)	L5706	0(3)	L5987	0(3)	L6660	0(3)	L7040	0(3)
L3150	0(3)	L3720	0(3)	L4110	0(3)	L5622	0(3)	L5707	0(3)	L5988	0(3)	L6665	0(3)	L7045	0(3)
L3160	0(3)	L3730	0(3)	L4130	0(3)	L5624	0(3)	L5710	0(3)	L5990	0(3)	L6670	0(3)	L7170	0(3)
L3170	0(3)	L3740	0(3)	L4205	0(3)	L5626	0(3)	L5711	0(3)	L6000	0(3)	L6672	0(3)	L7180	0(3)
L3215	0(3)	L3760	0(3)	L4210	0(3)	L5628	0(3)	L5712	0(3)	L6010	0(3)	L6675	0(3)	L7181	0(3)
L3216	0(3)	L3762	0(3)	L4350	0(3)	L5629	0(3)	L5714	0(3)	L6020	0(3)	L6676	0(3)	L7185	0(3)
L3217	0(3)	L3763	0(3)	L4360	0(3)	L5630	0(3)	L5716	0(3)	L6026	0(3)	L6677	0(3)	L7186	0(3)
L3219	0(3)	L3764	0(3)	L4361	0(3)	L5631	0(3)	L5718	0(3)	L6050	0(3)	L6680	0(3)	L7190	0(3)
L3221	0(3)	L3765	0(3)	L4370	0(3)	L5632	0(3)	L5722	0(3)	L6055	0(3)	L6682	0(3)	L7191	0(3)
L3222	0(3)	L3766	0(3)	L4386	0(3)	L5634	0(3)	L5724	0(3)	L6100	0(3)	L6684	0(3)	L7259	0(3)
L3224	0(3)	L3806	0(3)	L4387	0(3)	L5636	0(3)	L5726	0(3)	L6110	0(3)	L6686	0(3)	L7360	0(3)
L3225	0(3)	L3807	0(3)	L4392	0(3)	L5637	0(3)	L5728	0(3)	L6120	0(3)	L6687	0(3)	L7362	0(3)
L3230	0(3)	L3808	0(3)	L4394	0(3)	L5638	0(3)	L5780	0(3)	L6130	0(3)	L6688	0(3)	L7364	0(3)
L3250	0(3)	L3809	0(3)	L4396	0(3)	L5639	0(3)	L5781	0(3)	L6200	0(3)	L6689	0(3)	L7366	0(3)
L3251	0(3)	L3900	0(3)	L4397	0(3)	L5640	0(3)	L5782	0(3)	L6205	0(3)	L6690	0(3)	L7367	0(3)
L3252	0(3)	L3901	0(3)	L4398	0(3)	L5642	0(3)	L5785	0(3)	L6250	0(3)	L6691	0(3)	L7368	0(3)
L3253	0(3)	L3904	0(3)	L4631	0(3)	L5643	0(3)	L5790	0(3)	L6300	0(3)	L6692	0(3)	L7400	0(3)
L3300	0(3)	L3905	0(3)	L5000	0(3)	L5644	0(3)	L5795	0(3)	L6310	0(3)	L6693	0(3)	L7401	0(3)
L3310	0(3)	L3906	0(3)	L5010	0(3)	L5645	0(3)	L5810	0(3)	L6320	0(3)	L6694	0(3)	L7402	0(3)
L3330	0(3)	L3908	0(3)	L5020	0(3)	L5646	0(3)	L5811	0(3)	L6350	0(3)	L6695	0(3)	L7403	0(3)
L3332	0(3)	L3912	0(3)	L5050	0(3)	L5647	0(3)	L5812	0(3)	L6360	0(3)	L6696	0(3)	L7404	0(3)
L3334	0(3)	L3913	0(3)	L5060	0(3)	L5648	0(3)	L5814	0(3)	L6370	0(3)	L6697	0(3)	L7405	0(3)
L3340	0(3)	L3915	0(3)	L5100	0(3)	L5649	0(3)	L5816	0(3)	L6380	0(3)	L6698	0(3)	L7510	4(3)
L3350	0(3)	L3916	0(3)	L5105	0(3)	L5650	0(3)	L5818	0(3)	L6382	0(3)	L6703	0(3)	L7900	0(3)
L3360	0(3)	L3917	0(3)	L5150	0(3)	L5651	0(3)	L5822	0(3)	L6384	0(3)	L6704	0(3)	L7902	0(3)
L3370	0(3)	L3918	0(3)	L5160	0(3)	L5652	0(3)	L5824	0(3)	L6386	0(3)	L6706	0(3)	L8000	0(3)
L3380	0(3)	L3919	0(3)	L5200	0(3)	L5653	0(3)	L5826	0(3)	L6388	0(3)	L6707	0(3)	L8001	0(3)
L3390	0(3)	L3921	0(3)	L5210	0(3)	L5654	0(3)	L5828	0(3)	L6400	0(3)	L6708	0(3)	L8002	0(3)
L3400	0(3)	L3923	0(3)	L5220	0(3)	L5655	0(3)	L5830	0(3)	L6450	0(3)	L6709	0(3)	L8015	0(3)
L3410	0(3)	L3924	0(3)	L5230	0(3)	L5656	0(3)	L5840	0(3)	L6500	0(3)	L6711	0(3)	L8020	0(3)
L3420	0(3)	L3925	0(3)	L5250	0(3)	L5658	0(3)	L5845	0(3)	L6550	0(3)	L6712	0(3)	L8030	0(3)
L3430	0(3)	L3927	0(3)	L5270	0(3)	L5661	0(3)	L5848	0(3)	L6570	0(3)	L6713	0(3)	L8031	0(3)

CPT	MUE	CPT	MUE	CPT	MUE	CPT	MUE	CPT	MUE	CPT	MUE	CPT	MUE	CPT	MUE
L8032	0(3)	L8622	2(1)	P9044	10(3)	Q0487	1(1)	Q4074	3(3)	Q4155	100(1)	V2201	0(3)	V2522	2(1)
L8035	0(3)	L8627	2(2)	P9045	20(3)	Q0488	1(1)	Q4081	100(3)	Q4156	49(1)	V2202	0(3)	V2523	2(1)
L8039	0(3)	L8628	2(2)	P9046	25(3)	Q0489	1(1)	Q4101	88(3)	Q4157	24(1)	V2203	0(3)	V2530	0(3)
L8040	0(3)	L8629	2(2)	P9047	20(3)	Q0490	1(1)	Q4102	21(3)	Q4158	70(1)	V2204	0(3)	V2531	0(3)
L8041	0(3)	L8631	4(1)	P9048	1(3)	Q0491	1(1)	Q4103	0(3)	Q4159	7(1)	V2205	0(3)	V2599	2(3)
L8042	0(3)	L8641	4(1)	P9050	1(3)	Q0492	1(1)	Q4104	50(3)	Q4160	36(1)	V2206	0(3)	V2600	0(3)
L8043	0(3)	L8642	2(1)	P9051	2(3)	Q0493	1(1)	Q4105	250(3)	Q4161	42(1)	V2207	0(3)	V2610	0(3)
L8044	0(3)	L8658	4(1)	P9052	2(3)	Q0494	1(1)	Q4106	76(3)	Q4162	4(1)	V2208	0(3)	V2615	0(3)
L8045	0(3)	L8659	4(1)	P9053	2(3)	Q0495	1(1)	Q4107	50(3)	Q4163	32(1)	V2209	0(3)	V2623	0(3)
L8046	0(3)	L8670	4(1)	P9054	2(3)	Q0497	2(1)	Q4108	250(3)	Q4164	400(1)	V2210	0(3)	V2624	0(3)
L8047	0(3)	L8679	3(3)	P9055	2(3)	Q0498	1(1)	Q4110	250(3)	Q4165	100(1)	V2211	0(3)	V2625	0(3)
L8048	1(3)	L8681	1(1)	P9056	2(3)	Q0499	1(1)	Q4111	56(3)	Q5101	3360(3)	V2212	0(3)	V2626	0(3)
L8049	0(3)	L8682	2(1)	P9057	2(3)	Q0501	1(1)	Q4112	2(3)	Q9950	5(3)	V2213	0(3)	V2627	0(3)
L8300	0(3)	L8683	1(1)	P9058	2(3)	Q0502	1(1)	Q4113	4(3)	Q9951	0(3)	V2214	0(3)	V2628	0(3)
L8310	0(3)	L8684	1(1)	P9059	2(3)	Q0503	3(1)	Q4114	6(3)	Q9953	10(3)	V2215	0(3)	V2629	0(3)
L8320	0(3)	L8685	1(1)	P9060	2(3)	Q0504	1(1)	Q4115	240(3)	Q9954	18(3)	V2218	0(3)	V2630	2(1)
L8330	0(3)	L8686	2(1)	P9070	2(1)	Q0506	8(3)	Q4116	192(3)	Q9955	10(2)	V2219	0(3)	V2631	2(1)
L8400	0(3)	L8687	1(1)	P9071	2(1)	Q0507	1(3)	Q4117	200(3)	Q9956	9(3)	V2220	0(3)	V2632	2(1)
L8410	0(3)	L8688	1(1)	P9072	2(1)	Q0508	1(3)	Q4118	1000(3)	Q9957	3(3)	V2221	0(3)	V2700	0(3)
L8415	0(3)	L8689	1(1)	P9603	300(3)	Q0509	1(3)	Q4119	150(3)	Q9958	300(3)	V2299	0(3)	V2702	0(3)
L8417	0(3)	L8690	2(2)	P9604	2(3)	Q0510	0(3)	Q4120	50(3)	Q9959	0(3)	V2300	0(3)	V2710	0(3)
L8420	0(3)	L8691	1(3)	P9612	1(3)	Q0511	0(3)	Q4121	78(3)	Q9960	250(3)	V2301	0(3)	V2715	0(3)
L8430	0(3)	L8692	0(3)	P9615	1(3)	Q0512	0(3)	Q4122	96(3)	Q9961	200(3)	V2302	0(3)	V2718	0(3)
L8435	0(3)	L8693	1(3)	Q0035	1(1)	Q0513	0(3)	Q4123	160(3)	Q9962	150(3)	V2303	0(3)	V2730	0(3)
L8440	0(3)	L8695	1(1)	Q0091	1(1)	Q0514	0(3)	Q4124	140(3)	Q9963	240(3)	V2304	0(3)	V2744	0(3)
L8460	0(3)	L8696	1(3)	Q0111	2(1)	Q0515	0(3)	Q4125	28(3)	Q9964	0(3)	V2305	0(3)	V2745	0(3)
L8465	0(3)	P2028	1(3)	Q0112	3(1)	Q1004	2(1)	Q4126	32(3)	Q9966	250(3)	V2306	0(3)	V2750	0(3)
L8470	0(3)	P2029	1(3)	Q0113	2(1)	Q1005	2(1)	Q4127	100(3)	Q9967	300(3)	V2307	0(3)	V2755	0(3)
L8480	0(3)	P2033	1(3)	Q0114	1(1)	Q2004	1(3)	Q4128	128(3)	Q9969	3(1)	V2308	0(3)	V2756	0(3)
L8485	0(3)	P2038	1(3)	Q0115	1(1)	Q2009	100(3)	Q4129	81(3)	Q9980	50(3)	V2309	0(3)	V2760	0(3)
L8500	0(3)	P3000	1(3)	Q0138	510(3)	Q2017	12(3)	Q4130	100(3)	R0070	2(3)	V2310	0(3)	V2761	0(3)
L8501	0(3)	P3001	1(3)	Q0139	510(3)	Q2026	45(3)	Q4131	60(3)	R0075	2(3)	V2311	0(3)	V2762	0(3)
L8507	0(3)	P9010	2(3)	Q0144	0(3)	Q2028	1470(3)	Q4132	50(3)	V2020	0(3)	V2312	0(3)	V2770	0(3)
L8509	1(1)	P9011	2(3)	Q0161	0(3)	Q2034	1(1)	Q4133	113(3)	V2025	0(3)	V2313	0(3)	V2780	0(3)
L8510	0(3)	P9012	8(3)	Q0162	0(3)	Q2035	1(2)	Q4134	160(3)	V2100	0(3)	V2314	0(3)	V2781	0(3)
L8511	1(1)	P9016	3(3)	Q0163	0(3)	Q2036	1(2)	Q4135	900(3)	V2101	0(3)	V2315	0(3)	V2782	0(3)
L8514	1(1)	P9017	2(3)	Q0164	0(3)	Q2037	1(2)	Q4136	900(3)	V2102	0(3)	V2318	0(3)	V2783	0(3)
L8515	1(1)	P9019	2(3)	Q0166	0(3)	Q2038	1(2)	Q4137	32(1)	V2103	0(3)	V2319	0(3)	V2784	0(3)
L8600	2(1)	P9020	2(3)	Q0167	0(3)	Q2039	1(2)	Q4138	32(1)	V2104	0(3)	V2320	0(3)	V2785	2(1)
L8604	3(3)	P9021	3(3)	Q0169	0(3)	Q2043	1(1)	Q4139	2(3)	V2105	0(3)	V2321	0(3)	V2786	0(3)
L8605	4(3)	P9022	2(3)	Q0173	0(3)	Q2049	14(3)	Q4140	32(1)	V2106	0(3)	V2399	0(3)	V2790	1(1)
L8606	5(3)	P9023	2(3)	Q0174	0(3)	Q2050	14(3)	Q4141	25(1)	V2107	0(3)	V2410	0(3)	V2797	0(3)
L8607	20(3)	P9031	12(3)	Q0175	0(3)	Q2052	1(3)	Q4142	600(1)	V2108	0(3)	V2430	0(3)	V5008	0(1)
L8609	1(1)	P9032	12(3)	Q0177	0(3)	Q3014	1(3)	Q4143	96(1)	V2109	0(3)	V2499	2(3)	V5010	0(1)
L8610	2(1)	P9033	12(3)	Q0180	0(3)	Q3027	30(3)	Q4145	160(1)	V2110	0(3)	V2500	0(3)	V5011	0(1)
L8612	2(1)	P9034	2(3)	Q0478	1(1)	Q3028	0(3)	Q4146	50(1)	V2111	0(3)	V2501	0(3)	V5274	0(3)
L8613	2(1)	P9035	2(3)	Q0479	1(1)	Q4001	1(1)	Q4147	150(1)	V2112	0(3)	V2502	0(3)	V5281	0(3)
L8614	2(1)	P9036	2(3)	Q0480	1(1)	Q4002	1(1)	Q4148	18(1)	V2113	0(3)	V2503	0(3)	V5282	0(3)
L8615	2(1)	P9037	2(3)	Q0481	1(2)	Q4003	2(1)	Q4149	10(1)	V2114	0(3)	V2510	0(3)	V5284	0(3)
L8616	2(1)	P9038	2(3)	Q0482	1(1)	Q4004	2(1)	Q4150	32(1)	V2115	0(3)	V2511	0(3)	V5285	0(3)
L8617	2(1)	P9039	2(3)	Q0483	1(1)	Q4025	1(1)	Q4151	24(1)	V2118	0(3)	V2512	0(3)	V5286	0(3)
L8618	2(1)	P9040	3(3)	Q0484	1(1)	Q4026	1(1)	Q4152	24(1)	V2121	0(3)	V2513	0(3)	V5287	0(3)
L8619	2(1)	P9041	5(3)	Q0485	1(1)	Q4027	1(1)	Q4153	6(1)	V2199	2(3)	V2520	2(1)	V5288	0(3)
L8621	600(3)	P9043	5(3)	Q0486	1(1)	Q4028	1(1)	Q4154	36(1)	V2200	0(3)	V2521	2(1)	V5289	0(3)

Appendix J — Inpatient Only Procedures

Inpatient Only Procedures—This appendix identifies services with the status indicator C. Medicare will not pay an OPPS hospital or ASC when they are performed on a Medicare patient as an outpatient. Physicians should refer to this list when scheduling Medicare patients for surgical procedures. CMS updates this list quarterly.

00176	Anesth pharyngeal surgery	01404 Anesth amputation at knee	20805 Replant forearm complete
00192	Anesth facial bone surgery	01442 Anesth knee artery surg	20808 Replantation hand complete
00211	Anesth cran surg hematoma	01444 Anesth knee artery repair	20816 Replantation digit complete
00214	Anesth skull drainage	01486 Anesth ankle replacement	20824 Replantation thumb complete
00215	Anesth skull repair/fract	01502 Anesth lwr leg embolectomy	20827 Replantation thumb complete
00474	Anesth surgery of rib	01634 Anesth shoulder joint amput	20838 Replantation foot complete
0051T	Implant total heart system	01636 Anesth forequarter amput	20955 Fibula bone graft microvasc
00524	Anesth chest drainage	01638 Anesth shoulder replacement	20956 Iliac bone graft microvasc
0052T	Replace thrc unit hrt syst	0163T Lumb artif diskectomy addl	20957 Mt bone graft microvasc
0053T	Replace implantable hrt syst	0164T Remove lumb artif disc addl	20962 Other bone graft microvasc
00540	Anesth chest surgery	01652 Anesth shoulder vessel surg	20969 Bone/skin graft microvasc
00542	Anesthesia removal pleura	01654 Anesth shoulder vessel surg	20970 Bone/skin graft iliac crest
00546	Anesth lung chest wall surg	01656 Anesth arm-leg vessel surg	21045 Extensive jaw surgery
00560	Anesth heart surg w/o pump	0165T Revise lumb artif disc addl	21141 Lefort i-1 piece w/o graft
00561	Anesth heart surg <1 yr	0169T Place stereo cath brain	21142 Lefort i-2 piece w/o graft
00562	Anesth hrt surg w/pmp age 1+	01756 Anesth radical humerus surg	21143 Lefort i-3/> piece w/o graft
00567	Anesth CABG w/pump	0195T Prescrl fuse w/o instr l5/s1	21145 Lefort i-1 piece w/ graft
00580	Anesth heart/lung transplnt	0196T Prescrl fuse w/o instr l4/l5	21146 Lefort i-2 piece w/ graft
00604	Anesth sitting procedure	01990 Support for organ donor	21147 Lefort i-3/> piece w/ graft
00632	Anesth removal of nerves	0202T Post vert arthrplst 1 lumbar	21151 Lefort ii w/bone grafts
00670	Anesth spine cord surgery	0219T Plmt post facet implt cerv	21154 Lefort iii w/o lefort i
0075T	Perq stent/chest vert art	0220T Plmt post facet implt thor	21155 Lefort iii w/ lefort i
0076T	S&i stent/chest vert art	0235T Trluml perip athrc visceral	21159 Lefort iii w/fhdw/o lefort i
00792	Anesth hemorr/excise liver	0254T Evasc rpr iliac art bifur	21160 Lefort iii w/fhd w/ lefort i
00794	Anesth pancreas removal	0255T Evasc rpr iliac art bifr s&i	21179 Reconstruct entire forehead
00796	Anesth for liver transplant	0266T Implt/rpl crtd sns dev total	21180 Reconstruct entire forehead
00802	Anesth fat layer removal	0281T Laa closure w/implant	21182 Reconstruct cranial bone
00844	Anesth pelvis surgery	0293T Ins lt atrl press monitor	21183 Reconstruct cranial bone
00846	Anesth hysterectomy	0294T Ins lt atrl mont pres lead	21184 Reconstruct cranial bone
00848	Anesth pelvic organ surg	0309T Prescrl fuse w/ instr l4/l5	21188 Reconstruction of midface
00864	Anesth removal of bladder	0345T Transcath mtral vlve repair	21194 Reconst lwr jaw w/graft
00865	Anesth removal of prostate	0375T Total disc arthrp ant appr	21196 Reconst lwr jaw w/fixation
00866	Anesth removal of adrenal	11004 Debride genitalia & perineum	21247 Reconstruct lower jaw bone
00868	Anesth kidney transplant	11005 Debride abdom wall	21255 Reconstruct lower jaw bone
00882	Anesth major vein ligation	11006 Debride genit/per/abdom wall	21268 Revise eye sockets
00904	Anesth perineal surgery	11008 Remove mesh from abd wall	21343 Open tx dprsd front sinus fx
00908	Anesth removal of prostate	15756 Free myo/skin flap microvasc	21344 Open tx compl front sinus fx
00932	Anesth amputation of penis	15757 Free skin flap microvasc	21347 Opn tx nasomax fx multple
00934	Anesth penis nodes removal	15758 Free fascial flap microvasc	21348 Opn tx nasomax fx w/graft
00936	Anesth penis nodes removal	16036 Escharotomy addl incision	21366 Opn tx complx malar w/grft
00944	Anesth vaginal hysterectomy	19271 Revision of chest wall	21422 Treat mouth roof fracture
0095T	Rmvl artific disc addl crvcl	19272 Extensive chest wall surgery	21423 Treat mouth roof fracture
0098T	Rev artific disc addl	19305 Mast radical	21431 Treat craniofacial fracture
01140	Anesth amputation at pelvis	19306 Mast rad urban type	21432 Treat craniofacial fracture
01150	Anesth pelvic tumor surgery	19361 Breast reconstr w/lat flap	21433 Treat craniofacial fracture
01212	Anesth hip disarticulation	19364 Breast reconstruction	21435 Treat craniofacial fracture
01214	Anesth hip arthroplasty	19367 Breast reconstruction	21436 Treat craniofacial fracture
01232	Anesth amputation of femur	19368 Breast reconstruction	21510 Drainage of bone lesion
01234	Anesth radical femur surg	19369 Breast reconstruction	21615 Removal of rib
01272	Anesth femoral artery surg	20661 Application of head brace	21616 Removal of rib and nerves
01274	Anesth femoral embolectomy	20664 Application of halo	21620 Partial removal of sternum
01402	Anesth knee arthroplasty	20802 Replantation arm complete	21627 Sternal debridement

21630	Extensive sternum surgery	22848	Insert pelv fixation device	27151	Incision of hip bones
21632	Extensive sternum surgery	22849	Reinsert spinal fixation	27156	Revision of hip bones
21705	Revision of neck muscle/rib	22850	Remove spine fixation device	27158	Revision of pelvis
21740	Reconstruction of sternum	22852	Remove spine fixation device	27161	Incision of neck of femur
21750	Repair of sternum separation	22855	Remove spine fixation device	27165	Incision/fixation of femur
21825	Treat sternum fracture	22857	Lumbar artif diskectomy	27170	Repair/graft femur head/neck
22010	I&d p-spine c/t/cerv-thor	22861	Revise cerv artific disc	27175	Treat slipped epiphysis
22015	I&d abscess p-spine l/s/ls	22862	Revise lumbar artif disc	27176	Treat slipped epiphysis
22110	Remove part of neck vertebra	22864	Remove cerv artif disc	27177	Treat slipped epiphysis
22112	Remove part thorax vertebra	22865	Remove lumb artif disc	27178	Treat slipped epiphysis
22114	Remove part lumbar vertebra	23200	Resect clavicle tumor	27181	Treat slipped epiphysis
22116	Remove extra spine segment	23210	Resect scapula tumor	27185	Revision of femur epiphysis
22206	Incis spine 3 column thorac	23220	Resect prox humerus tumor	27187	Reinforce hip bones
22207	Incis spine 3 column lumbar	23335	Shoulder prosthesis removal	27222	Treat hip socket fracture
22208	Incis spine 3 column adl seg	23472	Reconstruct shoulder joint	27226	Treat hip wall fracture
22210	Incis 1 vertebral seg cerv	23474	Revis reconst shoulder joint	27227	Treat hip fracture(s)
22212	Incis 1 vertebral seg thorac	23900	Amputation of arm & girdle	27228	Treat hip fracture(s)
22214	Incis 1 vertebral seg lumbar	23920	Amputation at shoulder joint	27232	Treat thigh fracture
22216	Incis addl spine segment	24900	Amputation of upper arm	27236	Treat thigh fracture
22220	Incis w/discectomy cervical	24920	Amputation of upper arm	27240	Treat thigh fracture
22222	Incis w/discectomy thoracic	24930	Amputation follow-up surgery	27244	Treat thigh fracture
22224	Incis w/discectomy lumbar	24931	Amputate upper arm & implant	27245	Treat thigh fracture
22226	Revise extra spine segment	24940	Revision of upper arm	27248	Treat thigh fracture
22318	Treat odontoid fx w/o graft	25900	Amputation of forearm	27253	Treat hip dislocation
22319	Treat odontoid fx w/graft	25905	Amputation of forearm	27254	Treat hip dislocation
22325	Treat spine fracture	25915	Amputation of forearm	27258	Treat hip dislocation
22326	Treat neck spine fracture	25920	Amputate hand at wrist	27259	Treat hip dislocation
22327	Treat thorax spine fracture	25924	Amputation follow-up surgery	27268	Cltx thigh fx w/mnpj
22328	Treat each add spine fx	25927	Amputation of hand	27269	Optx thigh fx
22532	Lat thorax spine fusion	26551	Great toe-hand transfer	27280	Fusion of sacroiliac joint
22533	Lat lumbar spine fusion	26553	Single transfer toe-hand	27282	Fusion of pubic bones
22534	Lat thor/lumb addl seg	26554	Double transfer toe-hand	27284	Fusion of hip joint
22548	Neck spine fusion	26556	Toe joint transfer	27286	Fusion of hip joint
22556	Thorax spine fusion	26992	Drainage of bone lesion	27290	Amputation of leg at hip
22558	Lumbar spine fusion	27005	Incision of hip tendon	27295	Amputation of leg at hip
22586	Prescrl fuse w/ instr l5-s1	27025	Incision of hip/thigh fascia	27303	Drainage of bone lesion
22590	Spine & skull spinal fusion	27030	Drainage of hip joint	27365	Resect femur/knee tumor
22595	Neck spinal fusion	27036	Excision of hip joint/muscle	27445	Revision of knee joint
22600	Neck spine fusion	27054	Removal of hip joint lining	27447	Total knee arthroplasty
22610	Thorax spine fusion	27070	Part remove hip bone super	27448	Incision of thigh
22630	Lumbar spine fusion	27071	Part removal hip bone deep	27450	Incision of thigh
22632	Spine fusion extra segment	27075	Resect hip tumor	27454	Realignment of thigh bone
22633	Lumbar spine fusion combined	27076	Resect hip tum incl acetabul	27455	Realignment of knee
22634	Spine fusion extra segment	27077	Resect hip tum w/innom bone	27457	Realignment of knee
22800	Post fusion </6 vert seg	27078	Rsect hip tum incl femur	27465	Shortening of thigh bone
22802	Post fusion 7-12 vert seg	27090	Removal of hip prosthesis	27466	Lengthening of thigh bone
22804	Post fusion 13/> vert seg	27091	Removal of hip prosthesis	27468	Shorten/lengthen thighs
22808	Ant fusion 2-3 vert seg	27120	Reconstruction of hip socket	27470	Repair of thigh
22810	Ant fusion 4-7 vert seg	27122	Reconstruction of hip socket	27472	Repair/graft of thigh
22812	Ant fusion 8/> vert seg	27125	Partial hip replacement	27486	Revise/replace knee joint
22818	Kyphectomy 1-2 segments	27130	Total hip arthroplasty	27487	Revise/replace knee joint
22819	Kyphectomy 3 or more	27132	Total hip arthroplasty	27488	Removal of knee prosthesis
22830	Exploration of spinal fusion	27134	Revise hip joint replacement	27495	Reinforce thigh
22841	Insert spine fixation device	27137	Revise hip joint replacement	27506	Treatment of thigh fracture
22843	Insert spine fixation device	27138	Revise hip joint replacement	27507	Treatment of thigh fracture
22844	Insert spine fixation device	27140	Transplant femur ridge	27511	Treatment of thigh fracture
22846	Insert spine fixation device	27146	Incision of hip bone	27513	Treatment of thigh fracture
22847	Insert spine fixation device	27147	Revision of hip bone	27514	Treatment of thigh fracture

27519	Treat thigh fx growth plate	32110	Explore/repair chest	32851	Lung transplant single
27535	Treat knee fracture	32120	Re-exploration of chest	32852	Lung transplant with bypass
27536	Treat knee fracture	32124	Explore chest free adhesions	32853	Lung transplant double
27540	Treat knee fracture	32140	Removal of lung lesion(s)	32854	Lung transplant with bypass
27556	Treat knee dislocation	32141	Remove/treat lung lesions	32855	Prepare donor lung single
27557	Treat knee dislocation	32150	Removal of lung lesion(s)	32856	Prepare donor lung double
27558	Treat knee dislocation	32151	Remove lung foreign body	32900	Removal of rib(s)
27580	Fusion of knee	32160	Open chest heart massage	32905	Revise & repair chest wall
27590	Amputate leg at thigh	32200	Drain open lung lesion	32906	Revise & repair chest wall
27591	Amputate leg at thigh	32215	Treat chest lining	32940	Revision of lung
27592	Amputate leg at thigh	32220	Release of lung	32997	Total lung lavage
27596	Amputation follow-up surgery	32225	Partial release of lung	33015	Incision of heart sac
27598	Amputate lower leg at knee	32310	Removal of chest lining	33020	Incision of heart sac
27645	Resect tibia tumor	32320	Free/remove chest lining	33025	Incision of heart sac
27646	Resect fibula tumor	32440	Remove lung pneumonectomy	33030	Partial removal of heart sac
27702	Reconstruct ankle joint	32442	Sleeve pneumonectomy	33031	Partial removal of heart sac
27703	Reconstruction ankle joint	32445	Removal of lung extrapleural	33050	Resect heart sac lesion
27712	Realignment of lower leg	32480	Partial removal of lung	33120	Removal of heart lesion
27715	Revision of lower leg	32482	Bilobectomy	33130	Removal of heart lesion
27724	Repair/graft of tibia	32484	Segmentectomy	33140	Heart revascularize (tmr)
27725	Repair of lower leg	32486	Sleeve lobectomy	33141	Heart tmr w/other procedure
27727	Repair of lower leg	32488	Completion pneumonectomy	33202	Insert epicard eltrd open
27880	Amputation of lower leg	32491	Lung volume reduction	33203	Insert epicard eltrd endo
27881	Amputation of lower leg	32501	Repair bronchus add-on	33236	Remove electrode/thoracotomy
27882	Amputation of lower leg	32503	Resect apical lung tumor	33237	Remove electrode/thoracotomy
27886	Amputation follow-up surgery	32504	Resect apical lung tum/chest	33238	Remove electrode/thoracotomy
27888	Amputation of foot at ankle	32505	Wedge resect of lung initial	33243	Remove eltrd/thoracotomy
28800	Amputation of midfoot	32506	Wedge resect of lung add-on	33250	Ablate heart dysrhythm focus
31225	Removal of upper jaw	32507	Wedge resect of lung diag	33251	Ablate heart dysrhythm focus
31230	Removal of upper jaw	32540	Removal of lung lesion	33254	Ablate atria lmtd
31290	Nasal/sinus endoscopy surg	32650	Thoracoscopy w/pleurodesis	33255	Ablate atria w/o bypass ext
31291	Nasal/sinus endoscopy surg	32651	Thoracoscopy remove cortex	33256	Ablate atria w/bypass exten
31360	Removal of larynx	32652	Thoracoscopy rem totl cortex	33257	Ablate atria lmtd add-on
31365	Removal of larynx	32653	Thoracoscopy remov fb/fibrin	33258	Ablate atria x10sv add-on
31367	Partial removal of larynx	32654	Thoracoscopy contrl bleeding	33259	Ablate atria w/bypass add-on
31368	Partial removal of larynx	32655	Thoracoscopy resect bullae	33261	Ablate heart dysrhythm focus
31370	Partial removal of larynx	32656	Thoracoscopy w/pleurectomy	33265	Ablate atria lmtd endo
31375	Partial removal of larynx	32658	Thoracoscopy w/sac fb remove	33266	Ablate atria x10sv endo
31380	Partial removal of larynx	32659	Thoracoscopy w/sac drainage	33300	Repair of heart wound
31382	Partial removal of larynx	32661	Thoracoscopy w/pericard exc	33305	Repair of heart wound
31390	Removal of larynx & pharynx	32662	Thoracoscopy w/mediast exc	33310	Exploratory heart surgery
31395	Reconstruct larynx & pharynx	32663	Thoracoscopy w/lobectomy	33315	Exploratory heart surgery
31725	Clearance of airways	32664	Thoracoscopy w/ th nrv exc	33320	Repair major blood vessel(s)
31760	Repair of windpipe	32665	Thoracoscop w/esoph musc exc	33321	Repair major vessel
31766	Reconstruction of windpipe	32666	Thoracoscopy w/wedge resect	33322	Repair major blood vessel(s)
31770	Repair/graft of bronchus	32667	Thoracoscopy w/w resect addl	33330	Insert major vessel graft
31775	Reconstruct bronchus	32668	Thoracoscopy w/w resect diag	33335	Insert major vessel graft
31780	Reconstruct windpipe	32669	Thoracoscopy remove segment	33361	Replace aortic valve perq
31781	Reconstruct windpipe	32670	Thoracoscopy bilobectomy	33362	Replace aortic valve open
31786	Remove windpipe lesion	32671	Thoracoscopy pneumonectomy	33363	Replace aortic valve open
31800	Repair of windpipe injury	32672	Thoracoscopy for lvrs	33364	Replace aortic valve open
31805	Repair of windpipe injury	32673	Thoracoscopy w/thymus resect	33365	Replace aortic valve open
32035	Thoracostomy w/rib resection	32674	Thoracoscopy lymph node exc	33366	Trcath replace aortic valve
32036	Thoracostomy w/flap drainage	32800	Repair lung hernia	33367	Replace aortic valve w/byp
32096	Open wedge/bx lung infiltr	32810	Close chest after drainage	33368	Replace aortic valve w/byp
32097	Open wedge/bx lung nodule	32815	Close bronchial fistula	33369	Replace aortic valve w/byp
32098	Open biopsy of lung pleura	32820	Reconstruct injured chest	33400	Repair of aortic valve
32100	Exploration of chest	32850	Donor pneumonectomy	33401	Valvuloplasty open

33403 Valvuloplasty w/cp bypass	33545 Repair of heart damage	33780 Repair great vessels defect
33404 Prepare heart-aorta conduit	33548 Restore/remodel ventricle	33781 Repair great vessels defect
33405 Replacement of aortic valve	33572 Open coronary endarterectomy	33782 Nikaidoh proc
33406 Replacement of aortic valve	33600 Closure of valve	33783 Nikaidoh proc w/ostia implt
33410 Replacement of aortic valve	33602 Closure of valve	33786 Repair arterial trunk
33411 Replacement of aortic valve	33606 Anastomosis/artery-aorta	33788 Revision of pulmonary artery
33412 Replacement of aortic valve	33608 Repair anomaly w/conduit	33800 Aortic suspension
33413 Replacement of aortic valve	33610 Repair by enlargement	33802 Repair vessel defect
33414 Repair of aortic valve	33611 Repair double ventricle	33803 Repair vessel defect
33415 Revision subvalvular tissue	33612 Repair double ventricle	33813 Repair septal defect
33416 Revise ventricle muscle	33615 Repair modified fontan	33814 Repair septal defect
33417 Repair of aortic valve	33617 Repair single ventricle	33820 Revise major vessel
33418 Repair tcat mitral valve	33619 Repair single ventricle	33822 Revise major vessel
33420 Revision of mitral valve	33620 Apply r&l pulm art bands	33824 Revise major vessel
33422 Revision of mitral valve	33621 Transthor cath for stent	33840 Remove aorta constriction
33425 Repair of mitral valve	33622 Redo compl cardiac anomaly	33845 Remove aorta constriction
33426 Repair of mitral valve	33641 Repair heart septum defect	33851 Remove aorta constriction
33427 Repair of mitral valve	33645 Revision of heart veins	33852 Repair septal defect
33430 Replacement of mitral valve	33647 Repair heart septum defects	33853 Repair septal defect
33460 Revision of tricuspid valve	33660 Repair of heart defects	33860 Ascending aortic graft
33463 Valvuloplasty tricuspid	33665 Repair of heart defects	33863 Ascending aortic graft
33464 Valvuloplasty tricuspid	33670 Repair of heart chambers	33864 Ascending aortic graft
33465 Replace tricuspid valve	33675 Close mult vsd	33870 Transverse aortic arch graft
33468 Revision of tricuspid valve	33676 Close mult vsd w/resection	33875 Thoracic aortic graft
33470 Revision of pulmonary valve	33677 Cl mult vsd w/rem pul band	33877 Thoracoabdominal graft
33471 Valvotomy pulmonary valve	33681 Repair heart septum defect	33880 Endovasc taa repr incl subcl
33474 Revision of pulmonary valve	33684 Repair heart septum defect	33881 Endovasc taa repr w/o subcl
33475 Replacement pulmonary valve	33688 Repair heart septum defect	33883 Insert endovasc prosth taa
33476 Revision of heart chamber	33690 Reinforce pulmonary artery	33884 Endovasc prosth taa add-on
33477 Implant tcat pulm vlv perq	33692 Repair of heart defects	33886 Endovasc prosth delayed
33478 Revision of heart chamber	33694 Repair of heart defects	33889 Artery transpose/endovas taa
33496 Repair prosth valve clot	33697 Repair of heart defects	33891 Car-car bp grft/endovas taa
33500 Repair heart vessel fistula	33702 Repair of heart defects	33910 Remove lung artery emboli
33501 Repair heart vessel fistula	33710 Repair of heart defects	33915 Remove lung artery emboli
33502 Coronary artery correction	33720 Repair of heart defect	33916 Surgery of great vessel
33503 Coronary artery graft	33722 Repair of heart defect	33917 Repair pulmonary artery
33504 Coronary artery graft	33724 Repair venous anomaly	33920 Repair pulmonary atresia
33505 Repair artery w/tunnel	33726 Repair pul venous stenosis	33922 Transect pulmonary artery
33506 Repair artery translocation	33730 Repair heart-vein defect(s)	33924 Remove pulmonary shunt
33507 Repair art intramural	33732 Repair heart-vein defect	33925 Rpr pul art unifocal w/o cpb
33510 Cabg vein single	33735 Revision of heart chamber	33926 Repr pul art unifocal w/cpb
33511 Cabg vein two	33736 Revision of heart chamber	33930 Removal of donor heart/lung
33512 Cabg vein three	33737 Revision of heart chamber	33933 Prepare donor heart/lung
33513 Cabg vein four	33750 Major vessel shunt	33935 Transplantation heart/lung
33514 Cabg vein five	33755 Major vessel shunt	33940 Removal of donor heart
33516 Cabg vein six or more	33762 Major vessel shunt	33944 Prepare donor heart
33517 Cabg artery-vein single	33764 Major vessel shunt & graft	33945 Transplantation of heart
33518 Cabg artery-vein two	33766 Major vessel shunt	33946 Ecmo/ecls initiation venous
33519 Cabg artery-vein three	33767 Major vessel shunt	33947 Ecmo/ecls initiation artery
33521 Cabg artery-vein four	33768 Cavopulmonary shunting	33948 Ecmo/ecls daily mgmt-venous
33522 Cabg artery-vein five	33770 Repair great vessels defect	33949 Ecmo/ecls daily mgmt artery
33523 Cabg art-vein six or more	33771 Repair great vessels defect	33951 Ecmo/ecls insj prph cannula
33530 Coronary artery bypass/reop	33774 Repair great vessels defect	33952 Ecmo/ecls insj prph cannula
33533 Cabg arterial single	33775 Repair great vessels defect	33953 Ecmo/ecls insj prph cannula
33534 Cabg arterial two	33776 Repair great vessels defect	33954 Ecmo/ecls insj prph cannula
33535 Cabg arterial three	33777 Repair great vessels defect	33955 Ecmo/ecls insj ctr cannula
33536 Cabg arterial four or more	33778 Repair great vessels defect	33956 Ecmo/ecls insj ctr cannula
33542 Removal of heart lesion	33779 Repair great vessels defect	33957 Ecmo/ecls repos perph cnula

33958 Ecmo/ecls repos perph cnula	34843 Endovasc visc aorta 3 graft	35452 Repair arterial blockage
33959 Ecmo/ecls repos perph cnula	34844 Endovasc visc aorta 4 graft	35501 Art byp grft ipsilat carotid
33962 Ecmo/ecls repos perph cnula	34845 Visc & infraren abd 1 prosth	35506 Art byp grft subclav-carotid
33963 Ecmo/ecls repos perph cnula	34846 Visc & infraren abd 2 prosth	35508 Art byp grft carotid-vertbrl
33964 Ecmo/ecls repos perph cnula	34847 Visc & infraren abd 3 prosth	35509 Art byp grft contral carotid
33965 Ecmo/ecls rmvl perph cannula	34848 Visc & infraren abd 4+ prost	35510 Art byp grft carotid-brchial
33966 Ecmo/ecls rmvl prph cannula	34900 Endovasc iliac repr w/graft	35511 Art byp grft subclav-subclav
33967 Insert i-aort percut device	35001 Repair defect of artery	35512 Art byp grft subclav-brchial
33968 Remove aortic assist device	35002 Repair artery rupture neck	35515 Art byp grft subclav-vertbrl
33969 Ecmo/ecls rmvl perph cannula	35005 Repair defect of artery	35516 Art byp grft subclav-axilary
33970 Aortic circulation assist	35013 Repair artery rupture arm	35518 Art byp grft axillary-axilry
33971 Aortic circulation assist	35021 Repair defect of artery	35521 Art byp grft axill-femoral
33973 Insert balloon device	35022 Repair artery rupture chest	35522 Art byp grft axill-brachial
33974 Remove intra-aortic balloon	35081 Repair defect of artery	35523 Art byp grft brchl-ulnr-rdl
33975 Implant ventricular device	35082 Repair artery rupture aorta	35525 Art byp grft brachial-brchl
33976 Implant ventricular device	35091 Repair defect of artery	35526 Art byp grft aor/carot/innom
33977 Remove ventricular device	35092 Repair artery rupture aorta	35531 Art byp grft aorcel/aormesen
33978 Remove ventricular device	35102 Repair defect of artery	35533 Art byp grft axill/fem/fem
33979 Insert intracorporeal device	35103 Repair artery rupture aorta	35535 Art byp grft hepatorenal
33980 Remove intracorporeal device	35111 Repair defect of artery	35536 Art byp grft splenorenal
33981 Replace vad pump ext	35112 Repair artery rupture spleen	35537 Art byp grft aortoiliac
33982 Replace vad intra w/o bp	35121 Repair defect of artery	35538 Art byp grft aortobi-iliac
33983 Replace vad intra w/bp	35122 Repair artery rupture belly	35539 Art byp grft aortofemoral
33984 Ecmo/ecls rmvl prph cannula	35131 Repair defect of artery	35540 Art byp grft aortbifemoral
33985 Ecmo/ecls rmvl ctr cannula	35132 Repair artery rupture groin	35556 Art byp grft fem-popliteal
33986 Ecmo/ecls rmvl ctr cannula	35141 Repair defect of artery	35558 Art byp grft fem-femoral
33987 Artery expos/graft artery	35142 Repair artery rupture thigh	35560 Art byp grft aortorenal
33988 Insertion of left heart vent	35151 Repair defect of artery	35563 Art byp grft ilioiliac
33989 Removal of left heart vent	35152 Repair ruptd popliteal art	35565 Art byp grft iliofemoral
33990 Insert vad artery access	35182 Repair blood vessel lesion	35566 Art byp fem-ant-post tib/prl
33991 Insert vad art&vein access	35189 Repair blood vessel lesion	35570 Art byp tibial-tib/peroneal
33992 Remove vad different session	35211 Repair blood vessel lesion	35571 Art byp pop-tibl-prl-other
33993 Reposition vad diff session	35216 Repair blood vessel lesion	35583 Vein byp grft fem-popliteal
34001 Removal of artery clot	35221 Repair blood vessel lesion	35585 Vein byp fem-tibial peroneal
34051 Removal of artery clot	35241 Repair blood vessel lesion	35587 Vein byp pop-tibl peroneal
34151 Removal of artery clot	35246 Repair blood vessel lesion	35600 Harvest art for cabg add-on
34401 Removal of vein clot	35251 Repair blood vessel lesion	35601 Art byp common ipsi carotid
34451 Removal of vein clot	35271 Repair blood vessel lesion	35606 Art byp carotid-subclavian
34502 Reconstruct vena cava	35276 Repair blood vessel lesion	35612 Art byp subclav-subclavian
34800 Endovas aaa repr w/sm tube	35281 Repair blood vessel lesion	35616 Art byp subclav-axillary
34802 Endovas aaa repr w/2-p part	35301 Rechanneling of artery	35621 Art byp axillary-femoral
34803 Endovas aaa repr w/3-p part	35302 Rechanneling of artery	35623 Art byp axillary-pop-tibial
34804 Endovas aaa repr w/1-p part	35303 Rechanneling of artery	35626 Art byp aorsubcl/carot/innom
34805 Endovas aaa repr w/long tube	35304 Rechanneling of artery	35631 Art byp aor-celiac-msn-renal
34806 Aneurysm press sensor add-on	35305 Rechanneling of artery	35632 Art byp ilio-celiac
34808 Endovas iliac a device addon	35306 Rechanneling of artery	35633 Art byp ilio-mesenteric
34812 Xpose for endoprosth femorl	35311 Rechanneling of artery	35634 Art byp iliorenal
34813 Femoral endovas graft add-on	35331 Rechanneling of artery	35636 Art byp spenorenal
34820 Xpose for endoprosth iliac	35341 Rechanneling of artery	35637 Art byp aortoiliac
34825 Endovasc extend prosth init	35351 Rechanneling of artery	35638 Art byp aortobi-iliac
34826 Endovasc exten prosth addl	35355 Rechanneling of artery	35642 Art byp carotid-vertebral
34830 Open aortic tube prosth repr	35361 Rechanneling of artery	35645 Art byp subclav-vertebrl
34831 Open aortoiliac prosth repr	35363 Rechanneling of artery	35646 Art byp aortobifemoral
34832 Open aortofemor prosth repr	35371 Rechanneling of artery	35647 Art byp aortofemoral
34833 Xpose for endoprosth iliac	35372 Rechanneling of artery	35650 Art byp axillary-axillary
34834 Xpose endoprosth brachial	35390 Reoperation carotid add-on	35654 Art byp axill-fem-femoral
34841 Endovasc visc aorta 1 graft	35400 Angioscopy	35656 Art byp femoral-popliteal
34842 Endovasc visc aorta 2 graft	35450 Repair arterial blockage	35661 Art byp femoral-femoral

35663 Art byp ilioiliac	39499 Chest procedure	43338 Esoph lengthening
35665 Art byp iliofemoral	39501 Repair diaphragm laceration	43340 Fuse esophagus & intestine
35666 Art byp fem-ant-post tib/prl	39503 Repair of diaphragm hernia	43341 Fuse esophagus & intestine
35671 Art byp pop-tibl-prl-other	39540 Repair of diaphragm hernia	43351 Surgical opening esophagus
35681 Composite byp grft pros&vein	39541 Repair of diaphragm hernia	43352 Surgical opening esophagus
35682 Composite byp grft 2 veins	39545 Revision of diaphragm	43360 Gastrointestinal repair
35683 Composite byp grft 3/> segmt	39560 Resect diaphragm simple	43361 Gastrointestinal repair
35691 Art trnsposj vertbrl carotid	39561 Resect diaphragm complex	43400 Ligate esophagus veins
35693 Art trnsposj subclavian	39599 Diaphragm surgery procedure	43401 Esophagus surgery for veins
35694 Art trnsposj subclav carotid	41130 Partial removal of tongue	43405 Ligate/staple esophagus
35695 Art trnsposj carotid subclav	41135 Tongue and neck surgery	43410 Repair esophagus wound
35697 Reimplant artery each	41140 Removal of tongue	43415 Repair esophagus wound
35700 Reoperation bypass graft	41145 Tongue removal neck surgery	43425 Repair esophagus opening
35701 Exploration carotid artery	41150 Tongue mouth jaw surgery	43460 Pressure treatment esophagus
35721 Exploration femoral artery	41153 Tongue mouth neck surgery	43496 Free jejunum flap microvasc
35741 Exploration popliteal artery	41155 Tongue jaw & neck surgery	43500 Surgical opening of stomach
35800 Explore neck vessels	42426 Excise parotid gland/lesion	43501 Surgical repair of stomach
35820 Explore chest vessels	42845 Extensive surgery of throat	43502 Surgical repair of stomach
35840 Explore abdominal vessels	42894 Revision of pharyngeal walls	43520 Incision of pyloric muscle
35870 Repair vessel graft defect	42953 Repair throat esophagus	43605 Biopsy of stomach
35901 Excision graft neck	42961 Control throat bleeding	43610 Excision of stomach lesion
35905 Excision graft thorax	42971 Control nose/throat bleeding	43611 Excision of stomach lesion
35907 Excision graft abdomen	43045 Incision of esophagus	43620 Removal of stomach
36660 Insertion catheter artery	43100 Excision of esophagus lesion	43621 Removal of stomach
36823 Insertion of cannula(s)	43101 Excision of esophagus lesion	43622 Removal of stomach
37140 Revision of circulation	43107 Removal of esophagus	43631 Removal of stomach partial
37145 Revision of circulation	43108 Removal of esophagus	43632 Removal of stomach partial
37160 Revision of circulation	43112 Removal of esophagus	43633 Removal of stomach partial
37180 Revision of circulation	43113 Removal of esophagus	43634 Removal of stomach partial
37181 Splice spleen/kidney veins	43116 Partial removal of esophagus	43635 Removal of stomach partial
37182 Insert hepatic shunt (tips)	43117 Partial removal of esophagus	43640 Vagotomy & pylorus repair
37215 Transcath stent cca w/eps	43118 Partial removal of esophagus	43641 Vagotomy & pylorus repair
37217 Stent placemt retro carotid	43121 Partial removal of esophagus	43644 Lap gastric bypass/roux-en-y
37218 Stent placemt ante carotid	43122 Partial removal of esophagus	43645 Lap gastr bypass incl smll i
37616 Ligation of chest artery	43123 Partial removal of esophagus	43771 Lap revise gastr adj device
37617 Ligation of abdomen artery	43124 Removal of esophagus	43772 Lap rmvl gastr adj device
37618 Ligation of extremity artery	43135 Removal of esophagus pouch	43773 Lap replace gastr adj device
37660 Revision of major vein	43279 Lap myotomy heller	43774 Lap rmvl gastr adj all parts
37788 Revascularization penis	43282 Lap paraesoph her rpr w/mesh	43775 Lap sleeve gastrectomy
38100 Removal of spleen total	43283 Lap esoph lengthening	43800 Reconstruction of pylorus
38101 Removal of spleen partial	43300 Repair of esophagus	43810 Fusion of stomach and bowel
38102 Removal of spleen total	43305 Repair esophagus and fistula	43820 Fusion of stomach and bowel
38115 Repair of ruptured spleen	43310 Repair of esophagus	43825 Fusion of stomach and bowel
38380 Thoracic duct procedure	43312 Repair esophagus and fistula	43832 Place gastrostomy tube
38381 Thoracic duct procedure	43313 Esophagoplasty congenital	43840 Repair of stomach lesion
38382 Thoracic duct procedure	43314 Tracheo-esophagoplasty cong	43843 Gastroplasty w/o v-band
38562 Removal pelvic lymph nodes	43320 Fuse esophagus & stomach	43845 Gastroplasty duodenal switch
38564 Removal abdomen lymph nodes	43325 Revise esophagus & stomach	43846 Gastric bypass for obesity
38724 Removal of lymph nodes neck	43327 Esoph fundoplasty lap	43847 Gastric bypass incl small i
38746 Remove thoracic lymph nodes	43328 Esoph fundoplasty thor	43848 Revision gastroplasty
38747 Remove abdominal lymph nodes	43330 Esophagomyotomy abdominal	43850 Revise stomach-bowel fusion
38765 Remove groin lymph nodes	43331 Esophagomyotomy thoracic	43855 Revise stomach-bowel fusion
38770 Remove pelvis lymph nodes	43332 Transab esoph hiat hern rpr	43860 Revise stomach-bowel fusion
38780 Remove abdomen lymph nodes	43333 Transab esoph hiat hern rpr	43865 Revise stomach-bowel fusion
39000 Exploration of chest	43334 Transthor diaphrag hern rpr	43880 Repair stomach-bowel fistula
39010 Exploration of chest	43335 Transthor diaphrag hern rpr	43881 Impl/redo electrd antrum
39200 Resect mediastinal cyst	43336 Thorabd diaphr hern repair	43882 Revise/remove electrd antrum
39220 Resect mediastinal tumor	43337 Thorabd diaphr hern repair	44005 Freeing of bowel adhesion

44010 Incision of small bowel	44602 Suture small intestine	46744 Repair of cloacal anomaly
44015 Insert needle cath bowel	44603 Suture small intestine	46746 Repair of cloacal anomaly
44020 Explore small intestine	44604 Suture large intestine	46748 Repair of cloacal anomaly
44021 Decompress small bowel	44605 Repair of bowel lesion	46751 Repair of anal sphincter
44025 Incision of large bowel	44615 Intestinal stricturoplasty	47010 Open drainage liver lesion
44050 Reduce bowel obstruction	44620 Repair bowel opening	47015 Inject/aspirate liver cyst
44055 Correct malrotation of bowel	44625 Repair bowel opening	47100 Wedge biopsy of liver
44110 Excise intestine lesion(s)	44626 Repair bowel opening	47120 Partial removal of liver
44111 Excision of bowel lesion(s)	44640 Repair bowel-skin fistula	47122 Extensive removal of liver
44120 Removal of small intestine	44650 Repair bowel fistula	47125 Partial removal of liver
44121 Removal of small intestine	44660 Repair bowel-bladder fistula	47130 Partial removal of liver
44125 Removal of small intestine	44661 Repair bowel-bladder fistula	47133 Removal of donor liver
44126 Enterectomy w/o taper cong	44680 Surgical revision intestine	47135 Transplantation of liver
44127 Enterectomy w/taper cong	44700 Suspend bowel w/prosthesis	47140 Partial removal donor liver
44128 Enterectomy cong add-on	44715 Prepare donor intestine	47141 Partial removal donor liver
44130 Bowel to bowel fusion	44720 Prep donor intestine/venous	47142 Partial removal donor liver
44132 Enterectomy cadaver donor	44721 Prep donor intestine/artery	47143 Prep donor liver whole
44133 Enterectomy live donor	44800 Excision of bowel pouch	47144 Prep donor liver 3-segment
44135 Intestine transplnt cadaver	44820 Excision of mesentery lesion	47145 Prep donor liver lobe split
44136 Intestine transplant live	44850 Repair of mesentery	47146 Prep donor liver/venous
44137 Remove intestinal allograft	44899 Bowel surgery procedure	47147 Prep donor liver/arterial
44139 Mobilization of colon	44900 Drain appendix abscess open	47300 Surgery for liver lesion
44140 Partial removal of colon	44960 Appendectomy	47350 Repair liver wound
44141 Partial removal of colon	45110 Removal of rectum	47360 Repair liver wound
44143 Partial removal of colon	45111 Partial removal of rectum	47361 Repair liver wound
44144 Partial removal of colon	45112 Removal of rectum	47362 Repair liver wound
44145 Partial removal of colon	45113 Partial proctectomy	47380 Open ablate liver tumor rf
44146 Partial removal of colon	45114 Partial removal of rectum	47381 Open ablate liver tumor cryo
44147 Partial removal of colon	45116 Partial removal of rectum	47400 Incision of liver duct
44150 Removal of colon	45119 Remove rectum w/reservoir	47420 Incision of bile duct
44151 Removal of colon/ileostomy	45120 Removal of rectum	47425 Incision of bile duct
44155 Removal of colon/ileostomy	45121 Removal of rectum and colon	47460 Incise bile duct sphincter
44156 Removal of colon/ileostomy	45123 Partial proctectomy	47480 Incision of gallbladder
44157 Colectomy w/ileoanal anast	45126 Pelvic exenteration	47550 Bile duct endoscopy add-on
44158 Colectomy w/neo-rectum pouch	45130 Excision of rectal prolapse	47570 Laparo cholecystoenterostomy
44160 Removal of colon	45135 Excision of rectal prolapse	47600 Removal of gallbladder
44187 Lap ileo/jejuno-stomy	45136 Excise ileoanal reservoir	47605 Removal of gallbladder
44188 Lap colostomy	45395 Lap removal of rectum	47610 Removal of gallbladder
44202 Lap enterectomy	45397 Lap remove rectum w/pouch	47612 Removal of gallbladder
44203 Lap resect s/intestine addl	45400 Laparoscopic proc	47620 Removal of gallbladder
44204 Laparo partial colectomy	45402 Lap proctopexy w/sig resect	47700 Exploration of bile ducts
44205 Lap colectomy part w/ileum	45540 Correct rectal prolapse	47701 Bile duct revision
44206 Lap part colectomy w/stoma	45550 Repair rectum/remove sigmoid	47711 Excision of bile duct tumor
44207 L colectomy/coloproctostomy	45562 Exploration/repair of rectum	47712 Excision of bile duct tumor
44208 L colectomy/coloproctostomy	45563 Exploration/repair of rectum	47715 Excision of bile duct cyst
44210 Laparo total proctocolectomy	45800 Repair rect/bladder fistula	47720 Fuse gallbladder & bowel
44211 Lap colectomy w/proctectomy	45805 Repair fistula w/colostomy	47721 Fuse upper gi structures
44212 Laparo total proctocolectomy	45820 Repair rectourethral fistula	47740 Fuse gallbladder & bowel
44213 Lap mobil splenic fl add-on	45825 Repair fistula w/colostomy	47741 Fuse gallbladder & bowel
44227 Lap close enterostomy	46705 Repair of anal stricture	47760 Fuse bile ducts and bowel
44300 Open bowel to skin	46710 Repr per/vag pouch sngl proc	47765 Fuse liver ducts & bowel
44310 Ileostomy/jejunostomy	46712 Repr per/vag pouch dbl proc	47780 Fuse bile ducts and bowel
44314 Revision of ileostomy	46715 Rep perf anoper fistu	47785 Fuse bile ducts and bowel
44316 Devise bowel pouch	46716 Rep perf anoper/vestib fistu	47800 Reconstruction of bile ducts
44320 Colostomy	46730 Construction of absent anus	47801 Placement bile duct support
44322 Colostomy with biopsies	46735 Construction of absent anus	47802 Fuse liver duct & intestine
44345 Revision of colostomy	46740 Construction of absent anus	47900 Suture bile duct injury
44346 Revision of colostomy	46742 Repair of imperforated anus	48000 Drainage of abdomen

48001 Placement of drain pancreas	50120 Exploration of kidney	50810 Fusion of ureter & bowel
48020 Removal of pancreatic stone	50125 Explore and drain kidney	50815 Urine shunt to intestine
48100 Biopsy of pancreas open	50130 Removal of kidney stone	50820 Construct bowel bladder
48105 Resect/debride pancreas	50135 Exploration of kidney	50825 Construct bowel bladder
48120 Removal of pancreas lesion	50205 Renal biopsy open	50830 Revise urine flow
48140 Partial removal of pancreas	50220 Remove kidney open	50840 Replace ureter by bowel
48145 Partial removal of pancreas	50225 Removal kidney open complex	50845 Appendico-vesicostomy
48146 Pancreatectomy	50230 Removal kidney open radical	50860 Transplant ureter to skin
48148 Removal of pancreatic duct	50234 Removal of kidney & ureter	50900 Repair of ureter
48150 Partial removal of pancreas	50236 Removal of kidney & ureter	50920 Closure ureter/skin fistula
48152 Pancreatectomy	50240 Partial removal of kidney	50930 Closure ureter/bowel fistula
48153 Pancreatectomy	50250 Cryoablate renal mass open	50940 Release of ureter
48154 Pancreatectomy	50280 Removal of kidney lesion	51525 Removal of bladder lesion
48155 Removal of pancreas	50290 Removal of kidney lesion	51530 Removal of bladder lesion
48400 Injection intraop add-on	50300 Remove cadaver donor kidney	51550 Partial removal of bladder
48500 Surgery of pancreatic cyst	50320 Remove kidney living donor	51555 Partial removal of bladder
48510 Drain pancreatic pseudocyst	50323 Prep cadaver renal allograft	51565 Revise bladder & ureter(s)
48520 Fuse pancreas cyst and bowel	50325 Prep donor renal graft	51570 Removal of bladder
48540 Fuse pancreas cyst and bowel	50327 Prep renal graft/venous	51575 Removal of bladder & nodes
48545 Pancreatorrhaphy	50328 Prep renal graft/arterial	51580 Remove bladder/revise tract
48547 Duodenal exclusion	50329 Prep renal graft/ureteral	51585 Removal of bladder & nodes
48548 Fuse pancreas and bowel	50340 Removal of kidney	51590 Remove bladder/revise tract
48551 Prep donor pancreas	50360 Transplantation of kidney	51595 Remove bladder/revise tract
48552 Prep donor pancreas/venous	50365 Transplantation of kidney	51596 Remove bladder/create pouch
48554 Transpl allograft pancreas	50370 Remove transplanted kidney	51597 Removal of pelvic structures
48556 Removal allograft pancreas	50380 Reimplantation of kidney	51800 Revision of bladder/urethra
49000 Exploration of abdomen	50400 Revision of kidney/ureter	51820 Revision of urinary tract
49002 Reopening of abdomen	50405 Revision of kidney/ureter	51840 Attach bladder/urethra
49010 Exploration behind abdomen	50500 Repair of kidney wound	51841 Attach bladder/urethra
49020 Drainage abdom abscess open	50520 Close kidney-skin fistula	51865 Repair of bladder wound
49040 Drain open abdom abscess	50525 Close nephrovisceral fistula	51900 Repair bladder/vagina lesion
49060 Drain open retroperi abscess	50526 Close nephrovisceral fistula	51920 Close bladder-uterus fistula
49062 Drain to peritoneal cavity	50540 Revision of horseshoe kidney	51925 Hysterectomy/bladder repair
49203 Exc abd tum 5 cm or less	50545 Laparo radical nephrectomy	51940 Correction of bladder defect
49204 Exc abd tum over 5 cm	50546 Laparoscopic nephrectomy	51960 Revision of bladder & bowel
49205 Exc abd tum over 10 cm	50547 Laparo removal donor kidney	51980 Construct bladder opening
49215 Excise sacral spine tumor	50548 Laparo remove w/ureter	53415 Reconstruction of urethra
49220 Multiple surgery abdomen	50600 Exploration of ureter	53448 Remov/replc ur sphinctr comp
49255 Removal of omentum	50605 Insert ureteral support	54125 Removal of penis
49412 Ins device for rt guide open	50610 Removal of ureter stone	54130 Remove penis & nodes
49425 Insert abdomen-venous drain	50620 Removal of ureter stone	54135 Remove penis & nodes
49428 Ligation of shunt	50630 Removal of ureter stone	54390 Repair penis and bladder
49605 Repair umbilical lesion	50650 Removal of ureter	54430 Revision of penis
49606 Repair umbilical lesion	50660 Removal of ureter	54438 Replantation of penis
49610 Repair umbilical lesion	50700 Revision of ureter	55605 Incise sperm duct pouch
49611 Repair umbilical lesion	50715 Release of ureter	55650 Remove sperm duct pouch
49900 Repair of abdominal wall	50722 Release of ureter	55801 Removal of prostate
49904 Omental flap extra-abdom	50725 Release/revise ureter	55810 Extensive prostate surgery
49905 Omental flap intra-abdom	50728 Revise ureter	55812 Extensive prostate surgery
49906 Free omental flap microvasc	50740 Fusion of ureter & kidney	55815 Extensive prostate surgery
50010 Exploration of kidney	50750 Fusion of ureter & kidney	55821 Removal of prostate
50040 Drainage of kidney	50760 Fusion of ureters	55831 Removal of prostate
50045 Exploration of kidney	50770 Splicing of ureters	55840 Extensive prostate surgery
50060 Removal of kidney stone	50780 Reimplant ureter in bladder	55842 Extensive prostate surgery
50065 Incision of kidney	50782 Reimplant ureter in bladder	55845 Extensive prostate surgery
50070 Incision of kidney	50783 Reimplant ureter in bladder	55862 Extensive prostate surgery
50075 Removal of kidney stone	50785 Reimplant ureter in bladder	55865 Extensive prostate surgery
50100 Revise kidney blood vessels	50800 Implant ureter in bowel	55866 Laparo radical prostatectomy

56630 Extensive vulva surgery	58960 Exploration of abdomen	61458 Incise skull for brain wound
56631 Extensive vulva surgery	59120 Treat ectopic pregnancy	61460 Incise skull for surgery
56632 Extensive vulva surgery	59121 Treat ectopic pregnancy	61480 Incise skull for surgery
56633 Extensive vulva surgery	59130 Treat ectopic pregnancy	61500 Removal of skull lesion
56634 Extensive vulva surgery	59135 Treat ectopic pregnancy	61501 Remove infected skull bone
56637 Extensive vulva surgery	59136 Treat ectopic pregnancy	61510 Removal of brain lesion
56640 Extensive vulva surgery	59140 Treat ectopic pregnancy	61512 Remove brain lining lesion
57110 Remove vagina wall complete	59325 Revision of cervix	61514 Removal of brain abscess
57111 Remove vagina tissue compl	59350 Repair of uterus	61516 Removal of brain lesion
57112 Vaginectomy w/nodes compl	59514 Cesarean delivery only	61517 Implt brain chemotx add-on
57270 Repair of bowel pouch	59525 Remove uterus after cesarean	61518 Removal of brain lesion
57280 Suspension of vagina	59620 Attempted vbac delivery only	61519 Remove brain lining lesion
57296 Revise vag graft open abd	59830 Treat uterus infection	61520 Removal of brain lesion
57305 Repair rectum-vagina fistula	59850 Abortion	61521 Removal of brain lesion
57307 Fistula repair & colostomy	59851 Abortion	61522 Removal of brain abscess
57308 Fistula repair transperine	59852 Abortion	61524 Removal of brain lesion
57311 Repair urethrovaginal lesion	59855 Abortion	61526 Removal of brain lesion
57531 Removal of cervix radical	59856 Abortion	61530 Removal of brain lesion
57540 Removal of residual cervix	59857 Abortion	61531 Implant brain electrodes
57545 Remove cervix/repair pelvis	60254 Extensive thyroid surgery	61533 Implant brain electrodes
58140 Myomectomy abdom method	60270 Removal of thyroid	61534 Removal of brain lesion
58146 Myomectomy abdom complex	60505 Explore parathyroid glands	61535 Remove brain electrodes
58150 Total hysterectomy	60521 Removal of thymus gland	61536 Removal of brain lesion
58152 Total hysterectomy	60522 Removal of thymus gland	61537 Removal of brain tissue
58180 Partial hysterectomy	60540 Explore adrenal gland	61538 Removal of brain tissue
58200 Extensive hysterectomy	60545 Explore adrenal gland	61539 Removal of brain tissue
58210 Extensive hysterectomy	60600 Remove carotid body lesion	61540 Removal of brain tissue
58240 Removal of pelvis contents	60605 Remove carotid body lesion	61541 Incision of brain tissue
58267 Vag hyst w/urinary repair	60650 Laparoscopy adrenalectomy	61543 Removal of brain tissue
58275 Hysterectomy/revise vagina	61105 Twist drill hole	61544 Remove & treat brain lesion
58280 Hysterectomy/revise vagina	61107 Drill skull for implantation	61545 Excision of brain tumor
58285 Extensive hysterectomy	61108 Drill skull for drainage	61546 Removal of pituitary gland
58293 Vag hyst w/uro repair compl	61120 Burr hole for puncture	61548 Removal of pituitary gland
58400 Suspension of uterus	61140 Pierce skull for biopsy	61550 Release of skull seams
58410 Suspension of uterus	61150 Pierce skull for drainage	61552 Release of skull seams
58520 Repair of ruptured uterus	61151 Pierce skull for drainage	61556 Incise skull/sutures
58540 Revision of uterus	61154 Pierce skull & remove clot	61557 Incise skull/sutures
58548 Lap radical hyst	61156 Pierce skull for drainage	61558 Excision of skull/sutures
58605 Division of fallopian tube	61210 Pierce skull implant device	61559 Excision of skull/sutures
58611 Ligate oviduct(s) add-on	61250 Pierce skull & explore	61563 Excision of skull tumor
58700 Removal of fallopian tube	61253 Pierce skull & explore	61564 Excision of skull tumor
58720 Removal of ovary/tube(s)	61304 Open skull for exploration	61566 Removal of brain tissue
58740 Adhesiolysis tube ovary	61305 Open skull for exploration	61567 Incision of brain tissue
58750 Repair oviduct	61312 Open skull for drainage	61570 Remove foreign body brain
58752 Revise ovarian tube(s)	61313 Open skull for drainage	61571 Incise skull for brain wound
58760 Fimbrioplasty	61314 Open skull for drainage	61575 Skull base/brainstem surgery
58822 Drain ovary abscess percut	61315 Open skull for drainage	61576 Skull base/brainstem surgery
58825 Transposition ovary(s)	61316 Implt cran bone flap to abdo	61580 Craniofacial approach skull
58940 Removal of ovary(s)	61320 Open skull for drainage	61581 Craniofacial approach skull
58943 Removal of ovary(s)	61321 Open skull for drainage	61582 Craniofacial approach skull
58950 Resect ovarian malignancy	61322 Decompressive craniotomy	61583 Craniofacial approach skull
58951 Resect ovarian malignancy	61323 Decompressive lobectomy	61584 Orbitocranial approach/skull
58952 Resect ovarian malignancy	61332 Explore/biopsy eye socket	61585 Orbitocranial approach/skull
58953 Tah rad dissect for debulk	61333 Explore orbit/remove lesion	61586 Resect nasopharynx skull
58954 Tah rad debulk/lymph remove	61340 Subtemporal decompression	61590 Infratemporal approach/skull
58956 Bso omentectomy w/tah	61343 Incise skull (press relief)	61591 Infratemporal approach/skull
58957 Resect recurrent gyn mal	61345 Relieve cranial pressure	61592 Orbitocranial approach/skull
58958 Resect recur gyn mal w/lym	61450 Incise skull for surgery	61595 Transtemporal approach/skull

61596 Transcochlear approach/skull	62143 Replace skull plate/flap	63272 Excise intrspinl lesion lmbr
61597 Transcondylar approach/skull	62145 Repair of skull & brain	63273 Excise intrspinl lesion scrl
61598 Transpetrosal approach/skull	62146 Repair of skull with graft	63275 Bx/exc xdrl spine lesn crvl
61600 Resect/excise cranial lesion	62147 Repair of skull with graft	63276 Bx/exc xdrl spine lesn thrc
61601 Resect/excise cranial lesion	62148 Retr bone flap to fix skull	63277 Bx/exc xdrl spine lesn lmbr
61605 Resect/excise cranial lesion	62161 Dissect brain w/scope	63278 Bx/exc xdrl spine lesn scrl
61606 Resect/excise cranial lesion	62162 Remove colloid cyst w/scope	63280 Bx/exc idrl spine lesn crvl
61607 Resect/excise cranial lesion	62163 Zneuroendoscopy w/fb removal	63281 Bx/exc idrl spine lesn thrc
61608 Resect/excise cranial lesion	62164 Remove brain tumor w/scope	63282 Bx/exc idrl spine lesn lmbr
61610 Transect artery sinus	62165 Remove pituit tumor w/scope	63283 Bx/exc idrl spine lesn scrl
61611 Transect artery sinus	62180 Establish brain cavity shunt	63285 Bx/exc idrl imed lesn cervl
61612 Transect artery sinus	62190 Establish brain cavity shunt	63286 Bx/exc idrl imed lesn thrc
61613 Remove aneurysm sinus	62192 Establish brain cavity shunt	63287 Bx/exc idrl imed lesn thrlmb
61615 Resect/excise lesion skull	62200 Establish brain cavity shunt	63290 Bx/exc xdrl/idrl lsn any lvl
61616 Resect/excise lesion skull	62201 Brain cavity shunt w/scope	63295 Repair laminectomy defect
61618 Repair dura	62220 Establish brain cavity shunt	63300 Remove vert xdrl body crvcl
61619 Repair dura	62223 Establish brain cavity shunt	63301 Remove vert xdrl body thrc
61624 Transcath occlusion cns	62256 Remove brain cavity shunt	63302 Remove vert xdrl body thrlmb
61630 Intracranial angioplasty	62258 Replace brain cavity shunt	63303 Remov vert xdrl bdy lmbr/sac
61635 Intracran angioplsty w/stent	63050 Cervical laminoplsty 2/> seg	63304 Remove vert idrl body crvcl
61650 Evasc prlng admn rx agnt 1st	63051 C-laminoplasty w/graft/plate	63305 Remove vert idrl body thrc
61651 Evasc prlng admn rx agnt add	63077 Spine disk surgery thorax	63306 Remov vert idrl bdy thrclmbr
61680 Intracranial vessel surgery	63078 Spine disk surgery thorax	63307 Remov vert idrl bdy lmbr/sac
61682 Intracranial vessel surgery	63081 Remove vert body dcmprn crvl	63308 Remove vertebral body add-on
61684 Intracranial vessel surgery	63082 Remove vertebral body add-on	63700 Repair of spinal herniation
61686 Intracranial vessel surgery	63085 Remove vert body dcmprn thrc	63702 Repair of spinal herniation
61690 Intracranial vessel surgery	63086 Remove vertebral body add-on	63704 Repair of spinal herniation
61692 Intracranial vessel surgery	63087 Remov vertbr dcmprn thrclmbr	63706 Repair of spinal herniation
61697 Brain aneurysm repr complx	63088 Remove vertebral body add-on	63707 Repair spinal fluid leakage
61698 Brain aneurysm repr complx	63090 Remove vert body dcmprn lmbr	63709 Repair spinal fluid leakage
61700 Brain aneurysm repr simple	63091 Remove vertebral body add-on	63710 Graft repair of spine defect
61702 Inner skull vessel surgery	63101 Remove vert body dcmprn thrc	63740 Install spinal shunt
61703 Clamp neck artery	63102 Remove vert body dcmprn lmbr	64755 Incision of stomach nerves
61705 Revise circulation to head	63103 Remove vertebral body add-on	64760 Incision of vagus nerve
61708 Revise circulation to head	63170 Incise spinal cord tract(s)	64809 Remove sympathetic nerves
61710 Revise circulation to head	63172 Drainage of spinal cyst	64818 Remove sympathetic nerves
61711 Fusion of skull arteries	63173 Drainage of spinal cyst	64866 Fusion of facial/other nerve
61735 Incise skull/brain surgery	63180 Revise spinal cord ligaments	64868 Fusion of facial/other nerve
61750 Incise skull/brain biopsy	63182 Revise spinal cord ligaments	65273 Repair of eye wound
61751 Brain biopsy w/ct/mr guide	63185 Incise spine nrv half segmnt	69155 Extensive ear/neck surgery
61760 Implant brain electrodes	63190 Incise spine nrv >2 segmnts	69535 Remove part of temporal bone
61850 Implant neuroelectrodes	63191 Incise spine accessory nerve	69554 Remove ear lesion
61860 Implant neuroelectrodes	63194 Incise spine & cord cervical	69950 Incise inner ear nerve
61863 Implant neuroelectrode	63195 Incise spine & cord thoracic	75952 Endovasc repair abdom aorta
61864 Implant neuroelectrde addl	63196 Incise spine&cord 2 trx crvl	75953 Abdom aneurysm endovas rpr
61867 Implant neuroelectrode	63197 Incise spine&cord 2 trx thrc	75954 Iliac aneurysm endovas rpr
61868 Implant neuroelectrde addl	63198 Incise spin&cord 2 stgs crvl	75956 Xray endovasc thor ao repr
61870 Implant neuroelectrodes	63199 Incise spin&cord 2 stgs thrc	75957 Xray endovasc thor ao repr
62005 Treat skull fracture	63200 Release spinal cord lumbar	75958 Xray place prox ext thor ao
62010 Treatment of head injury	63250 Revise spinal cord vsls crvl	75959 Xray place dist ext thor ao
62100 Repair brain fluid leakage	63251 Revise spinal cord vsls thrc	92970 Cardioassist internal
62115 Reduction of skull defect	63252 Revise spine cord vsl thrlmb	92971 Cardioassist external
62117 Reduction of skull defect	63265 Excise intraspinl lesion crv	92975 Dissolve clot heart vessel
62120 Repair skull cavity lesion	63266 Excise intrspinl lesion thrc	92992 Revision of heart chamber
62121 Incise skull repair	63267 Excise intrspinl lesion lmbr	92993 Revision of heart chamber
62140 Repair of skull defect	63268 Excise intrspinl lesion scrl	93583 Perq transcath septal reduxn
62141 Repair of skull defect	63270 Excise intrspinl lesion crvl	99184 Hypothermia ill neonate
62142 Remove skull plate/flap	63271 Excise intrspinl lesion thrc	99190 Special pump services

99191	Special pump services
99192	Special pump services
99356	Prolonged service inpatient
99357	Prolonged service inpatient
99462	Sbsq nb em per day hosp
99468	Neonate crit care initial
99469	Neonate crit care subsq
99471	Ped critical care initial

99472	Ped critical care subsq
99475	Ped crit care age 2-5 init
99476	Ped crit care age 2-5 subsq
99477	Init day hosp neonate care
99478	Ic lbw inf < 1500 gm subsq
99479	Ic lbw inf 1500-2500 g subsq
99480	Ic inf pbw 2501-5000 g subsq
G0341	Percutaneous islet celltrans

G0342	Laparoscopy islet cell trans
G0343	Laparotomy islet cell transp
G0412	Open tx iliac spine uni/bil
G0414	Pelvic ring fx treat int fix
G0415	Open tx post pelvic fxcture

Appendix K — Place of Service and Type of Service

Place-of-Service Codes for Professional Claims

Listed below are place of service codes and descriptions. These codes should be used on professional claims to specify the entity where service(s) were rendered. Check with individual payers (e.g., Medicare, Medicaid, other private insurance) for reimbursement policies regarding these codes. To comment on a code(s) or description(s), please send your request to posinfo@cms.gov.

01 Pharmacy — A facility or location where drugs and other medically related items and services are sold, dispensed, or otherwise provided directly to patients.

02 Unassigned — N/A

03 School — A facility whose primary purpose is education.

04 Homeless shelter — A facility or location whose primary purpose is to provide temporary housing to homeless individuals (e.g., emergency shelters, individual or family shelters).

05 Indian Health Service freestanding facility — A facility or location, owned and operated by the Indian Health Service, which provides diagnostic, therapeutic (surgical and non-surgical), and rehabilitation services to American Indians and Alaska natives who do not require hospitalization.

06 Indian Health Service provider-based facility — A facility or location, owned and operated by the Indian Health Service, which provides diagnostic, therapeutic (surgical and nonsurgical), and rehabilitation services rendered by, or under the supervision of, physicians to American Indians and Alaska natives admitted as inpatients or outpatients.

07 Tribal 638 freestanding facility — A facility or location owned and operated by a federally recognized American Indian or Alaska native tribe or tribal organization under a 638 agreement, which provides diagnostic, therapeutic (surgical and nonsurgical), and rehabilitation services to tribal members who do not require hospitalization.

08 Tribal 638 provider-based Facility — A facility or location owned and operated by a federally recognized American Indian or Alaska native tribe or tribal organization under a 638 agreement, which provides diagnostic, therapeutic (surgical and nonsurgical), and rehabilitation services to tribal members admitted as inpatients or outpatients.

09 Prison/correctional facility — A prison, jail, reformatory, work farm, detention center, or any other similar facility maintained by either federal, state or local authorities for the purpose of confinement or rehabilitation of adult or juvenile criminal offenders.

10 Unassigned — N/A

11 Office — Location, other than a hospital, skilled nursing facility (SNF), military treatment facility, community health center, State or local public health clinic, or intermediate care facility (ICF), where the health professional routinely provides health examinations, diagnosis, and treatment of illness or injury on an ambulatory basis.

12 Home — Location, other than a hospital or other facility, where the patient receives care in a private residence.

13 Assisted living facility — Congregate residential facility with self-contained living units providing assessment of each resident's needs and on-site support 24 hours a day, 7 days a week, with the capacity to deliver or arrange for services including some health care and other services.

14 Group home — A residence, with shared living areas, where clients receive supervision and other services such as social and/or behavioral services, custodial service, and minimal services (e.g., medication administration).

15 Mobile unit — A facility/unit that moves from place-to-place equipped to provide preventive, screening, diagnostic, and/or treatment services.

16 Temporary lodging — A short-term accommodation such as a hotel, campground, hostel, cruise ship or resort where the patient receives care, and which is not identified by any other POS code.

17 Walk-in retail health clinic — A walk-in health clinic, other than an office, urgent care facility, pharmacy, or independent clinic and not described by any other place of service code, that is located within a retail operation and provides preventive and primary care services on an ambulatory basis.

18 Place of employment/ worksite — A location, not described by any other POS code, owned or operated by a public or private entity where the patient is employed, and where a health professional provides on-going or episodic occupational medical, therapeutic or rehabilitative services to the individual.

19 Off campus-outpatient hospital — A portion of an off-campus hospital provider based department which provides diagnostic, therapeutic (both surgical and nonsurgical), and rehabilitation services to sick or injured persons who do not require hospitalization or institutionalization.

20 Urgent care facility — Location, distinct from a hospital emergency room, an office, or a clinic, whose purpose is to diagnose and treat illness or injury for unscheduled, ambulatory patients seeking immediate medical attention.

21	Inpatient hospital	A facility, other than psychiatric, which primarily provides diagnostic, therapeutic (both surgical and nonsurgical), and rehabilitation services by, or under, the supervision of physicians to patients admitted for a variety of medical conditions.
22	On campus-outpatient hospital	A portion of a hospital's main campus which provides diagnostic, therapeutic (both surgical and nonsurgical), and rehabilitation services to sick or injured persons who do not require hospitalization or institutionalization.
23	Emergency room—hospital	A portion of a hospital where emergency diagnosis and treatment of illness or injury is provided.
24	Ambulatory surgical center	A freestanding facility, other than a physician's office, where surgical and diagnostic services are provided on an ambulatory basis.
25	Birthing center	A facility, other than a hospital's maternity facilities or a physician's office, which provides a setting for labor, delivery, and immediate post-partum care as well as immediate care of new born infants.
26	Military treatment facility	A medical facility operated by one or more of the uniformed services. Military treatment facility (MTF) also refers to certain former U.S. Public Health Service (USPHS) facilities now designated as uniformed service treatment facilities (USTF).
27-30	Unassigned	N/A
31	Skilled nursing facility	A facility which primarily provides inpatient skilled nursing care and related services to patients who require medical, nursing, or rehabilitative services but does not provide the level of care or treatment available in a hospital.
32	Nursing facility	A facility which primarily provides to residents skilled nursing care and related services for the rehabilitation of injured, disabled, or sick persons, or, on a regular basis, health-related care services above the level of custodial care to other than mentally retarded individuals.
33	Custodial care facility	A facility which provides room, board, and other personal assistance services, generally on a long-term basis, and which does not include a medical component.
34	Hospice	A facility, other than a patient's home, in which palliative and supportive care for terminally ill patients and their families are provided.
35-40	Unassigned	N/A
41	Ambulance—land	A land vehicle specifically designed, equipped and staffed for lifesaving and transporting the sick or injured.
42	Ambulance—air or water	An air or water vehicle specifically designed, equipped and staffed for lifesaving and transporting the sick or injured.
43-48	Unassigned	N/A

49	Independent clinic	A location, not part of a hospital and not described by any other place-of-service code, that is organized and operated to provide preventive, diagnostic, therapeutic, rehabilitative, or palliative services to outpatients only.
50	Federally qualified health center	A facility located in a medically underserved area that provides Medicare beneficiaries preventive primary medical care under the general direction of a physician.
51	Inpatient psychiatric facility	A facility that provides inpatient psychiatric services for the diagnosis and treatment of mental illness on a 24-hour basis, by or under the supervision of a physician.
52	Psychiatric facility-partial hospitalization	A facility for the diagnosis and treatment of mental illness that provides a planned therapeutic program for patients who do not require full time hospitalization, but who need broader programs than are possible from outpatient visits to a hospital-based or hospital-affiliated facility.
53	Community mental health center	A facility that provides the following services: outpatient services, including specialized outpatient services for children, the elderly, individuals who are chronically ill, and residents of the CMHC's mental health services area who have been discharged from inpatient treatment at a mental health facility; 24 hour a day emergency care services; day treatment, other partial hospitalization services, or psychosocial rehabilitation services; screening for patients being considered for admission to state mental health facilities to determine the appropriateness of such admission; and consultation and education services.
54	Intermediate care facility/individuals with intellectual disabilities	A facility which primarily provides health-related care and services above the level of custodial care to individuals with Intellectual Disabilities but does not provide the level of care or treatment available in a hospital or SNF.
55	Residential substance abuse treatment facility	A facility which provides treatment for substance (alcohol and drug) abuse to live-in residents who do not require acute medical care. Services include individual and group therapy and counseling, family counseling, laboratory tests, drugs and supplies, psychological testing, and room and board.
56	Psychiatric residential treatment center	A facility or distinct part of a facility for psychiatric care which provides a total 24-hour therapeutically planned and professionally staffed group living and learning environment.
57	Non-residential substance abuse treatment facility	A location which provides treatment for substance (alcohol and drug) abuse on an ambulatory basis. Services include individual and group therapy and counseling, family counseling, laboratory tests, drugs and supplies, and psychological testing.
58-59	Unassigned	N/A

60	Mass immunization center	A location where providers administer pneumococcal pneumonia and influenza virus vaccinations and submit these services as electronic media claims, paper claims, or using the roster billing method. This generally takes place in a mass immunization setting, such as, a public health center, pharmacy, or mall but may include a physician office setting.
61	Comprehensive inpatient rehabilitation facility	A facility that provides comprehensive rehabilitation services under the supervision of a physician to inpatients with physical disabilities. Services include physical therapy, occupational therapy, speech pathology, social or psychological services, and orthotics and prosthetics services.
62	Comprehensive outpatient rehabilitation facility	A facility that provides comprehensive rehabilitation services under the supervision of a physician to outpatients with physical disabilities. Services include physical therapy, occupational therapy, and speech pathology services.
63-64	Unassigned	N/A
65	End-stage renal disease treatment facility	A facility other than a hospital, which provides dialysis treatment, maintenance, and/or training to patients or caregivers on an ambulatory or home-care basis.
66-70	Unassigned	N/A
71	State or local public health clinic	A facility maintained by either state or local health departments that provides ambulatory primary medical care under the general direction of a physician.
72	Rural health clinic	A certified facility which is located in a rural medically underserved area that provides ambulatory primary medical care under the general direction of a physician.
73-80	Unassigned	N/A
81	Independent laboratory	A laboratory certified to perform diagnostic and/or clinical tests independent of an institution or a physician's office.
82-98	Unassigned	N/A
99	Other place of service	Other place of service not identified above.

Type of Service

Common Working File Type of Service (TOS) Indicators

For submitting a claim to the Common Working File (CWF), use the following table to assign the proper TOS. Some procedures may have more than one applicable TOS. CWF will reject alerts on codes with incorrect TOS designations. CWF will produce alerts on codes with incorrect TOS designations.

The only exceptions to this annual update are:

- Surgical services billed for dates of service through December 31, 2007, containing the ASC facility service modifier SG must be reported as TOS F. Effective for services on or after January 1, 2008, the SG modifier is no longer applicable for Medicare services. ASC providers should discontinue applying the SG modifier on ASC facility claims. The indicator F does not appear in the TOS table because its use depends upon claims submitted with POS 24 (ASC facility) from an ASC (specialty 49). This became effective for dates of service January 1, 2008, or after.

- Surgical services billed with an assistant-at-surgery modifier (80-82, AS,) must be reported with TOS 8. The 8 indicator does not appear on the TOS table because its use is dependent upon the use of the appropriate modifier. (See Pub. 100-4 *Medicare Claims Processing*

Manual, chapter 12, "Physician/Practitioner Billing," for instructions on when assistant-at-surgery is allowable.)

- Psychiatric treatment services that are subject to the outpatient mental health treatment limitation should be reported with TOS T.

- TOS H appears in the list of descriptors. However, it does not appear in the table. In CWF, "H" is used only as an indicator for hospice. The contractor should not submit TOS H to CWF at this time.

- For outpatient services, when a transfusion medicine code appears on a claim that also contains a blood product, the service is paid under reasonable charge at 80 percent; coinsurance and deductible apply. When transfusion medicine codes are paid under the clinical laboratory fee schedule they are paid at 100 percent; coinsurance and deductible do not apply.

Note: For injection codes with more than one possible TOS designation, use the following guidelines when assigning the TOS:

When the choice is L or 1:

- Use TOS L when the drug is used related to ESRD; or

- Use TOS 1 when the drug is not related to ESRD and is administered in the office.

When the choice is G or 1:

- Use TOS G when the drug is an immunosuppressive drug; or

- Use TOS 1 when the drug is used for other than immunosuppression.

When the choice is P or 1:

- Use TOS P if the drug is administered through durable medical equipment (DME); or

- Use TOS 1 if the drug is administered in the office.

The place of service or diagnosis may be considered when determining the appropriate TOS. The descriptors for each of the TOS codes listed in the annual HCPCS update are:

0	Whole blood
1	Medical care
2	Surgery
3	Consultation
4	Diagnostic radiology
5	Diagnostic laboratory
6	Therapeutic radiology
7	Anesthesia
8	Assistant at surgery
9	Other medical items or services
A	Used DME
D	Ambulance
E	Enteral/parenteral nutrients/supplies
F	Ambulatory surgical center (facility usage for surgical services)
G	Immunosuppressive drugs
J	Diabetic shoes
K	Hearing items and services
L	ESRD supplies
M	Monthly capitation payment for dialysis
N	Kidney donor
P	Lump sum purchase of DME, prosthetics, orthotics
Q	Vision items or services
R	Rental of DME
S	Surgical dressings or other medical supplies
U	Occupational therapy
V	Pneumococcal/flu vaccine
W	Physical therapy

Berenson-Eggers Type of Service (BETOS) Codes

The BETOS coding system was developed primarily for analyzing the growth in Medicare expenditures. The coding system covers all HCPCS codes; assigns a HCPCS code to only one BETOS code; consists of readily understood clinical categories (as opposed to statistical or financial categories); consists of categories that permit objective assignment; is stable over time; and is relatively immune to minor changes in technology or practice patterns.

BETOS Codes and Descriptions:

1. Evaluation and Management
1. M1A   Office visits—new
2. M1B   Office visits—established
3. M2A   Hospital visit—initial
4. M2B   Hospital visit—subsequent
5. M2C   Hospital visit—critical care
6. M3   Emergency room visit
7. M4A   Home visit
8. M4B   Nursing home visit
9. M5A   Specialist—pathology
10. M5B   Specialist—psychiatry
11. M5C   Specialist—ophthalmology
12. M5D   Specialist—other
13. M6   Consultations

2. Procedures
1. P0   Anesthesia
2. P1A   Major procedure—breast
3. P1B   Major procedure—colectomy
4. P1C   Major procedure—cholecystectomy
5. P1D   Major procedure—TURP
6. P1E   Major procedure—hysterectomy
7. P1F   Major procedure—explor/decompr/excis disc
8. P1G   Major procedure—other
9. P2A   Major procedure, cardiovascular—CABG
10. P2B   Major procedure, cardiovascular—aneurysm repair
11. P2C   Major procedure, cardiovascular—thromboendarterectomy
12. P2D   Major procedure, cardiovascular—coronary angioplasty (PTCA)
13. P2E   Major procedure, cardiovascular—pacemaker insertion
14. P2F   Major procedure, cardiovascular—other
15. P3A   Major procedure, orthopedic—hip fracture repair
16. P3B   Major procedure, orthopedic—hip replacement
17. P3C   Major procedure, orthopedic—knee replacement
18. P3D   Major procedure, orthopedic—other
19. P4A   Eye procedure—corneal transplant
20. P4B   Eye procedure—cataract removal/lens insertion
21. P4C   Eye procedure—retinal detachment
22. P4D   Eye procedure—treatment of retinal lesions
23. P4E   Eye procedure—other
24. P5A   Ambulatory procedures—skin
25. P5B   Ambulatory procedures—musculoskeletal
26. P5C   Ambulatory procedures—inguinal hernia repair
27. P5D   Ambulatory procedures—lithotripsy
28. P5E   Ambulatory procedures—other
29. P6A   Minor procedures—skin
30. P6B   Minor procedures—musculoskeletal
31. P6C   Minor procedures—other (Medicare fee schedule)
32. P6D   Minor procedures—other (non-Medicare fee schedule)
33. P7A   Oncology—radiation therapy
34. P7B   Oncology—other
35. P8A   Endoscopy—arthroscopy
36. P8B   Endoscopy—upper gastrointestinal
37. P8C   Endoscopy—sigmoidoscopy
38. P8D   Endoscopy—colonoscopy
39. P8E   Endoscopy—cystoscopy
40. P8F   Endoscopy—bronchoscopy
41. P8G   Endoscopy—laparoscopic cholecystectomy
42. P8H   Endoscopy—laryngoscopy
43. P8I   Endoscopy—other
44. P9A   Dialysis services (Medicare fee schedule)
45. P9B   Dialysis services (non-Medicare fee schedule)

3. Imaging
1. I1A   Standard imaging—chest
2. I1B   Standard imaging—musculoskeletal
3. I1C   Standard imaging—breast
4. I1D   Standard imaging—contrast gastrointestinal
5. I1E   Standard imaging—nuclear medicine
6. I1F   Standard imaging—other
7. I2A   Advanced imaging—CAT/CT/CTA; brain/head/neck
8. I2B   Advanced imaging—CAT/CT/CTA; other
9. I2C   Advanced imaging—MRI/MRA; brain/head/neck
10. I2D   Advanced imaging—MRI/MRA; other
11. I3A   Echography/ultrasonography—eye
12. I3B   Echography/ultrasonography—abdomen/pelvis
13. I3C   Echography/ultrasonography—heart
14. I3D   Echography/ultrasonography—carotid arteries
15. I3E   Echography/ultrasonography—prostate, transrectal
16. I3F   Echography/ultrasonography—other
17. I4A   Imaging/procedure—heart, including cardiac catheterization
18. I4B   Imaging/procedure—other

4. Tests
1. T1A   Lab tests—routine venipuncture (non-Medicare fee schedule)
2. T1B   Lab tests—automated general profiles
3. T1C   Lab tests—urinalysis
4. T1D   Lab tests—blood counts
5. T1E   Lab tests—glucose
6. T1F   Lab tests—bacterial cultures
7. T1G   Lab tests—other (Medicare fee schedule)
8. T1H   Lab tests—other (non-Medicare fee schedule)
9. T2A   Other tests—electrocardiograms
10. T2B   Other tests—cardiovascular stress tests
11. T2C   Other tests—EKG monitoring
12. T2D   Other tests—other

5. Durable Medical Equipment
1. D1A   Medical/surgical supplies
1. D1B   Hospital beds
1. D1C   Oxygen and supplies
1. D1D   Wheelchairs
1. D1E   Other DME
1. D1F   Prosthetic/orthotic devices
1. D1G   Drugs administered through DME

6. Other
1. O1A   Ambulance
2. O1B   Chiropractic
3. O1C   Enteral and parenteral
4. O1D   Chemotherapy
5. O1E   Other drugs
6. O1F   Hearing and speech services
7. O1G   Immunizations/vaccinations

7. Exceptions/Unclassified
1. Y1   Other—Medicare fee schedule
2. Y2   Other—Non-Medicare fee schedule
3. Z1   Local codes
4. Z2   Undefined codes

Appendix L — Multianalyte Assays with Algorithmic Analyses

The following is a list of administrative codes for multianalyte assays with algorithmic analysis (MAAA) procedures that are usually exclusive to one single clinical laboratory or manufacturer. These tests use the results from several different assays, including molecular pathology assays, fluorescent in situ hybridization assays, and nonnucleic acid-based assays (e.g., proteins, polypeptides, lipids, and carbohydrates) to perform an algorithmic analysis that is reported as a numeric score or probability. Although the laboratory report may list results of individual component tests of the MAAAs, these assays are not separately reportable.

The following list includes the proprietary name and clinical laboratory/manufacturer, an alphanumeric code, and the code descriptor.

The format for the code descriptor usually includes:

- Type of disease (e.g., oncology, autoimmune, tissue rejection)
- Chemical(s) analyzed (e.g., DNA, RNA, protein, antibody)
- Number of markers (e.g., number of genes, number of proteins)
- Methodology(s) (e.g., microarray, real-time [RT]-PCR, in situ hybridization [ISH], enzyme linked immunosorbent assays [ELISA])
- Number of functional domains (when indicated)
- Type of specimen (e.g., blood, fresh tissue, formalin-fixed paraffin embedded)
- Type of algorithm result (e.g., prognostic, diagnostic)
- Report (e.g., probability index, risk score)

MAAA procedures with a Category I code are noted on the following list and can also be found in code range 81500–81599 in the pathology and laboratory chapter. If a specific MAAA test does not have a Category I code, it is denoted with a four-digit number and the letter M. Use code 81599 if an MAAA test is not included on the following list or in the Category I codes. The codes on the list are exclusive to the assays identified by proprietary name. Report code 81599 also when an analysis is performed that may possibly fall within a specific descriptor but the proprietary name is not included in the list. The list does not contain all MAAA procedures.

Proprietary Name/Clinical Laboratory/Manufacturer	Code	Descriptor
Administrative Codes for Multianalyte Assays with Algorithmic Analyses (MAAA)		
HCV FibroSURE™, LabCorp FibroTest™, Quest Diagnostics/BioPredictive	▲ 0001M	Infectious disease, HCV, six biochemical assays (ALT, A2-macroglobulin, apolipoprotein A-1, total bilirubin, GGT, and haptoglobin) utilizing serum, prognostic algorithm reported as scores for fibrosis and necroinflammatory activity in liver
ASH FibroSURE™, LabCorp	0002M	Liver disease, 10 biochemical assays (ALT, A2-macroglobulin, apolipoprotein A-1, total bilirubin, GGT, haptoglobin, AST, glucose, total cholesterol, and triglycerides) utilizing serum, prognostic algorithm reported as quantitative scores for fibrosis, steatosis, and alcoholic steatohepatitis (ASH)
NASH FibroSURE™, LabCorp	0003M	Liver disease, 10 biochemical assays (ALT, A2-macroglobulin, apolipoprotein A-1, total bilirubin, GGT, haptoglobin, AST, glucose, total cholesterol, and triglycerides) utilizing serum, prognostic algorithm reported as quantitative scores for fibrosis, steatosis, and nonalcoholic steatohepatitis (NASH)
ScoliScore™ Transgenomic	0004M	Scoliosis, DNA analysis of 53 single nucleotide polymorphisms (SNPs), using saliva, prognostic algorithm reported as a risk score
HeproDX™, GoPath Laboratories, LLC	0006M	Oncology (hepatic), mRNA expression levels of 161 genes, utilizing fresh hepatocellular carcinoma tumor tissue, with alpha-fetoprotein level, algorithm reported as a risk classifier
NETest (Wren Laboratories, LLC)	0007M	Oncology (gastrointestinal neuroendocrine tumors), real-time PCR expression analysis of 51 genes, utilizing whole peripheral blood, algorithm reported as a nomogram of tumor disease index
Prosigna Breast Cancer Assay (NanoString Technologies)	0008M	Oncology (breast), mRNA analysis of 58 genes using hybrid capture, on formalin-fixed paraffin-embedded (FFPE) tissue, prognostic algorithm reported as a risk score
VisibiliT™ test, Sequenom Center for Molecular Medicine, LLC	0009M	Fetal aneuploidy (trisomy 21, and 18) DNA sequence analysis of selected regions using maternal plasma, algorithm reported as a risk score for each trisomy
	~~0010M~~ To report, see 81539	
Category I Codes for Multianalyte Assays with Algorithmic Analyses (MAAA)		
Vectra® DA, Crescendo Bioscience, Inc	81490	Autoimmune (rheumatoid arthritis), analysis of 12 biomarkers using immunoassays, utilizing serum, prognostic algorithm reported as a disease activity score (Do not report 81490 with 86140)
Corus® CAD, CardioDx, Inc.	81493	Coronary artery disease, mRNA, gene expression profiling by real-time RT-PCR of 23 genes, utilizing whole peripheral blood, algorithm reported as a risk score
Risk of Ovarian Malignancy Algorithm (ROMA)™, Fujirebio Diagnostics	81500	Oncology (ovarian), biochemical assays of two proteins (CA-125 and HE4), utilizing serum, with menopausal status, algorithm reported as a risk score
OVA1™, Vermillion, Inc.	81503	Oncology (ovarian), biochemical assays of five proteins (CA-125, apolipoprotein A1, beta-2 microglobulin, transferrin, and pre-albumin), utilizing serum, algorithm reported as a risk score

Proprietary Name/Clinical Laboratory/Manufacturer	Code	Descriptor
Pathwork® Tissue of Origin Test, Pathwork Diagnostics	81504	Oncology (tissue of origin), microarray gene expression profiling of >2000 genes, utilizing formalin-fixed paraffin embedded tissue, algorithm reported as tissue similarity scores
PreDx Diabetes Risk Score™, Tethys Clinical Laboratory	81506	Endocrinology (type 2 diabetes), biochemical assays of seven analytes (glucose, HbA1c, insulin, hs-CRP, adiponectin, ferritin, interleukin 2-receptor alpha), utilizing serum or plasma, algorithm reporting a risk score
Harmony™ Prenatal Test, Ariosa Diagnostics	81507	Fetal aneuploidy (trisomy 21, 18, and 13) DNA sequence analysis of selected regions using maternal plasma, algorithm reported as a risk score for each trisomy
No proprietary name and clinical laboratory or manufacturer. Maternal serum screening procedures are performed by many labs and are not exclusive to a single facility.	81508	Fetal congenital abnormalities, biochemical assays of two proteins (PAPP-A, hCG [any form]), utilizing maternal serum, algorithm reported as a risk score
	81509	Fetal congenital abnormalities, biochemical assays of three proteins (PAPP-A, hCG [any form], DIA), utilizing maternal serum, algorithm reported as a risk score
	81510	Fetal congenital abnormalities, biochemical assays of three analytes (AFP, uE3, hCG (any form)), utilizing maternal serum, algorithm reported as a risk score
	81511	Fetal congenital abnormalities, biochemical assays of four analytes (AFP, uE3, hCG (any form), DIA) utilizing maternal serum, algorithm reported as a risk score (may include additional results from previous biochemical testing)
	81512	Fetal congenital abnormalities, biochemical assays of five analytes (AFP, uE3, total hCG, hyperglycosylated hCG, DIA) utilizing maternal serum, algorithm reported as a risk score
Oncotype DX® (Genomic Health)	81519	Oncology (breast), mRNA, gene expression profiling by real-time RT-PCR of 21 genes, utilizing formalin-fixed paraffin embedded tissue, algorithm reported as recurrence score
Oncotype DX® Colon Cancer Assay, Genomic Health	81525	Oncology (colon), mRNA, gene expression profiling by real-time RT-PCR of 12 genes (7 content and 5 housekeeping), utilizing formalin-fixed paraffin-embedded tissue, algorithm reported as a recurrence score
Cologuard™, Exact Sciences, Inc.	81528	Oncology (colorectal) screening, quantitative real-time target and signal amplification of 10 DNA markers (KRAS mutations, promoter methylation of NDRG4 and BMP3) and fecal hemoglobin, utilizing stool, algorithm reported as a positive or negative result (Do not report 81528 with 81275, 82274)
ChemoFX®, Helomics, Corp.	81535	Oncology (gynecologic), live tumor cell culture and chemotherapeutic response by DAPI stain and morphology, predictive algorithm reported as a drug response score; first single drug or drug combination
ChemoFX®, Helomics, Corp.	+ 81536	Oncology (gynecologic), live tumor cell culture and chemotherapeutic response by DAPI stain and morphology, predictive algorithm reported as a drug response score; each additional single drug or drug combination (List separately in addition to code for primary procedure) (Code first 81535)
VeriStrat, Biodesix, Inc.	81538	Oncology (lung), mass spectrometric 8-protein signature, including amyloid A, utilizing serum, prognostic and predictive algorithm reported as good versus poor overall survival
4Kscore test, OPKO Health Inc.	81539	Oncology (high-grade prostate cancer), biochemical assay of four proteins (Total PSA, Free PSA, Intact PSA, and human kallikrein-2 [hK2]), utilizing plasma or serum, prognostic algorithm reported as a probability score
CancerTYPE ID, bioTheranostics, Inc.	81540	Oncology (tumor of unknown origin), mRNA, gene expression profiling by real-time RT-PCR of 92 genes (87 content and 5 housekeeping) to classify tumor into main cancer type and subtype, utilizing formalin-fixed paraffin-embedded tissue, algorithm reported as a probability of a predicted main cancer type and subtype
Afirma® Gene Expression Classifier, Veracyte, Inc.	81545	Oncology (thyroid), gene expression analysis of 142 genes, utilizing fine needle aspirate, algorithm reported as a categorical result (eg, benign or suspicious)
AlloMap®, CareDx, Inc	81595	Cardiology (heart transplant, mRNA gene expression profiling by real-time qualitative PCR of 20 genes (11 content and 9 housekeeping), utilizing subfraction of peripheral blood, algorithm reported as a rejection risk score
	81599	Unlisted multianalyte assay with algorithmic analysis

Appendix M — Glossary

-centesis. Puncture, as with a needle, trocar, or aspirator; often done for withdrawing fluid from a cavity.

-ectomy. Excision, removal.

-orrhaphy. Suturing.

-ostomy. Indicates a surgically created artificial opening.

-otomy. Making an incision or opening.

-plasty. Indicates surgically formed or molded.

abdominal lymphadenectomy. Surgical removal of the abdominal lymph nodes grouping, with or without para-aortic and vena cava nodes.

ablation. Removal or destruction of a body part or tissue or its function. Ablation may be performed by surgical means, hormones, drugs, radiofrequency, heat, chemical application, or other methods.

abnormal alleles. Form of gene that includes disease-related variations.

absorbable sutures. Strands prepared from collagen or a synthetic polymer and capable of being absorbed by tissue over time. Examples include surgical gut and collagen sutures; or synthetics like polydioxanone (PDS), polyglactin 910 (Vicryl), poliglecaprone 25 (Monocryl), polyglyconate (Maxon), and polyglycolic acid (Dexon).

acetabuloplasty. Surgical repair or reconstruction of the large cup-shaped socket in the hipbone (acetabulum) with which the head of the femur articulates.

Achilles tendon. Tendon attached to the back of the heel bone (calcaneus) that flexes the foot downward.

acromioclavicular joint. Junction between the clavicle and the scapula. The acromion is the projection from the back of the scapula that forms the highest point of the shoulder and connects with the clavicle. Trauma or injury to the acromioclavicular joint is often referred to as a dislocation of the shoulder. This is not correct, however, as a dislocation of the shoulder is a disruption of the glenohumeral joint.

acromionectomy. Surgical treatment for acromioclavicular arthritis in which the distal portion of the acromion process is removed.

acromioplasty. Repair of the part of the shoulder blade that connects to the deltoid muscles and clavicle.

actigraphy. Science of monitoring activity levels, particularly during sleep. In most cases, the patient wears a wristband that records motion while sleeping. The data are recorded, analyzed, and interpreted to study sleep/wake patterns and circadian rhythms.

air conduction. Transportation of sound from the air, through the external auditory canal, to the tympanic membrane and ossicular chain. Air conduction hearing is tested by presenting an acoustic stimulus through earphones or a loudspeaker to the ear.

air puff device. Instrument that measures intraocular pressure by evaluating the force of a reflected amount of air blown against the cornea.

alleles. Form of gene usually arising from a mutation responsible for a hereditary variation.

allogeneic collection. Collection of blood or blood components from one person for the use of another. Allogeneic collection was formerly termed homologous collection.

allograft. Graft from one individual to another of the same species.

amniocentesis. Surgical puncture through the abdominal wall, with a specialized needle and under ultrasonic guidance, into the interior of the pregnant uterus and directly into the amniotic sac to collect fluid for diagnostic analysis or therapeutic reduction of fluid levels.

anastomosis. Surgically created connection between ducts, blood vessels, or bowel segments to allow flow from one to the other.

anesthesia time. Time period factored into anesthesia procedures beginning with the anesthesiologist preparing the patient for surgery and ending when the patient is turned over to the recovery department.

Angelman syndrome. Early childhood emergence of a pattern of interrupted development, stiff, jerky gait, absence or impairment of speech, excessive laughter, and seizures.

angioplasty. Reconstruction or repair of a diseased or damaged blood vessel.

annuloplasty. Surgical plication of weakened tissue of the heart, to improve its muscular function. Annuli are thick, fibrous rings and one is found surrounding each of the cardiac chambers. The atrial and ventricular muscle fibers attach to the annuli. In annuloplasty, weakened annuli may be surgically plicated, or tucked, to improve muscular functions.

anorectal anometry. Measurement of pressure generated by anal sphincter to diagnose incontinence.

anterior chamber lenses. Lenses inserted into the anterior chamber following intracapsular cataract extraction.

applanation tonometer. Instrument that measures intraocular pressure by recording the force required to flatten an area of the cornea.

appropriateness of care. Proper setting of medical care that best meets the patient's care or diagnosis, as defined by a health care plan or other legal entity.

aqueous humor. Fluid within the anterior and posterior chambers of the eye that is continually replenished as it diffuses out into the blood. When the flow of aqueous is blocked, a build-up of fluid in the eye causes increased intraocular pressure and leads to glaucoma and blindness.

arteriogram. Radiograph of arteries.

arteriovenous fistula. Connecting passage between an artery and a vein.

arteriovenous malformation. Connecting passage between an artery and a vein.

arthrotomy. Surgical incision into a joint that may include exploration, drainage, or removal of a foreign body.

ASA. 1) Acetylsalicylic acid. Synonym(s): aspirin. 2) American Society of Anesthesiologists. National organization for anesthesiology that maintains and publishes the guidelines and relative values for anesthesia coding.

aspirate. To withdraw fluid or air from a body cavity by suction.

assay. Chemical analysis of a substance to establish the presence and strength of its components. A therapeutic drug assay is used to determine if a drug is within the expected therapeutic range for a patient.

atrial septal defect. Cardiac anomaly consisting of a patent opening in the atrial septum due to a fusion failure, classified as ostium secundum type, ostium primum defect, or endocardial cushion defect.

attended surveillance. Ability of a technician at a remote surveillance center or location to respond immediately to patient transmissions regarding rhythm or device alerts as they are produced and received at the remote location. These transmissions may originate from wearable or implanted therapy or monitoring devices.

auricle. External ear, which is a single elastic cartilage covered in skin and normal adnexal features (hair follicles, sweat glands, and sebaceous glands), shaped to channel sound waves into the acoustic meatus.

autogenous transplant. Tissue, such as bone, that is harvested from the patient and used for transplantation back into the same patient.

autograft. Any tissue harvested from one anatomical site of a person and grafted to another anatomical site of the same person. Most commonly, blood vessels, skin, tendons, fascia, and bone are used as autografts.

AVF. Arteriovenous fistula.

AVM. Arteriovenous malformation. Clusters of abnormal blood vessels that grow in the brain comprised of a blood vessel "nidus" or nest through which arteries and veins connect directly without going through the capillaries. As time passes, the nidus may enlarge resulting in the formation of a mass that may bleed. AVMs are more prone to bleeding in patients ages 10 to 55. Once older than age 55, the possibility of bleeding is reduced dramatically.

backbench preparation. Procedures performed on a donor organ following procurement to prepare the organ for transplant into the recipient. Excess fat and other tissue may be removed, the organ may be perfused, and vital arteries may be sized, repaired, or modified to fit the patient. These procedures are done on a back table in the operating room before transplantation can begin.

Bartholin's gland. Mucous-producing gland found in the vestibular bulbs on either side of the vaginal orifice and connected to the mucosal membrane at the opening by a duct.

Bartholin's gland abscess. Pocket of pus and surrounding cellulitis caused by infection of the Bartholin's gland and causing localized swelling and pain in the posterior labia majora that may extend into the lower vagina.

basic value. Relative weighted value based upon the usual anesthesia services and the relative work or cost of the specific anesthesia service assigned to each anesthesia-specific procedure code.

Berman locator. Small, sensitive tool used to detect the location of a metallic foreign body in the eye.

bifurcated. Having two branches or divisions, such as the left pulmonary veins that split off from the left atrium to carry oxygenated blood away from the heart.

Billroth's operation. Anastomosis of the stomach to the duodenum or jejunum.

bioprosthetic heart valve. Replacement cardiac valve made of biological tissue. Allograft, xenograft or engineered tissue.

biopsy. Tissue or fluid removed for diagnostic purposes through analysis of the cells in the biopsy material.

Blalock-Hanlon procedure. Atrial septectomy procedure to allow free mixing of the blood from the right and left atria.

Blalock-Taussig procedure. Anastomosis of the left subclavian artery to the left pulmonary artery or the right subclavian artery to the right pulmonary artery in order to shunt some of the blood flow from the systemic to the pulmonary circulation.

blepharochalasis. Loss of elasticity and relaxation of skin of the eyelid, thickened or indurated skin on the eyelid associated with recurrent episodes of edema, and intracellular atrophy.

blepharoplasty. Plastic surgery of the eyelids to remove excess fat and redundant skin weighting down the lid. The eyelid is pulled tight and sutured to support sagging muscles.

blepharoptosis. Droop or displacement of the upper eyelid, caused by paralysis, muscle problems, or outside mechanical forces.

blepharorrhaphy. Suture of a portion or all of the opposing eyelids to shorten the palpebral fissure or close it entirely.

bone conduction. Transportation of sound through the bones of the skull to the inner ear.

bone mass measurement. Radiologic or radioisotopic procedure or other procedure approved by the FDA for identifying bone mass, detecting bone loss, or determining bone quality. The procedure includes a physician's interpretation of the results. Qualifying individuals must be an estrogen-deficient woman at clinical risk for osteoporosis with vertebral abnormalities.

brachytherapy. Form of radiation therapy in which radioactive pellets or seeds are implanted directly into the tissue being treated to deliver their dose of radiation in a more directed fashion. Brachytherapy provides radiation to the prescribed body area while minimizing exposure to normal tissue.

breakpoint. Point at which a chromosome breaks.

Bristow procedure. Anterior capsulorrhaphy prevents chronic separation of the shoulder. In this procedure, the bone block is affixed to the anterior glenoid rim with a screw.

buccal mucosa. Tissue from the mucous membrane on the inside of the cheek.

bundle of His. Bundle of modified cardiac fibers that begins at the atrioventricular node and passes through the right atrioventricular fibrous ring to the interventricular septum, where it divides into two branches. Bundle of His recordings are taken for intracardiac electrograms.

Caldwell-Luc operation. Intraoral antrostomy approach into the maxillary sinus for the removal of tooth roots or tissue, or for packing the sinus to reduce zygomatic fractures by creating a window above the teeth in the canine fossa area.

canthorrhaphy. Suturing of the palpebral fissure, the juncture between the eyelids, at either end of the eye.

canthotomy. Horizontal incision at the canthus (junction of upper and lower eyelids) to divide the outer canthus and enlarge lid margin separation.

cardio-. Relating to the heart.

cardiopulmonary bypass. Venous blood is diverted to a heart-lung machine, which mechanically pumps and oxygenates the blood temporarily so the heart can be bypassed while an open procedure on the heart or coronary arteries is performed. During bypass, the lungs are deflated and immobile.

cardioverter-defibrillator. Device that uses both low energy cardioversion or defibrillating shocks and antitachycardia pacing to treat ventricular tachycardia or ventricular fibrillation.

care plan oversight services. Physician's ongoing review and revision of a patient's care plan involving complex or multidisciplinary care modalities.

case management services. Physician case management is a process of involving direct patient care as well as coordinating and controlling access to the patient or initiating and/or supervising other necessary health care services.

cataract extraction. Surgical removal of the cataract or cloudy lens. Anterior chamber lenses are inserted in conjunction with intracapsular cataract extraction and posterior chamber lenses are inserted in conjunction with extracapsular cataract extraction.

catheter. Flexible tube inserted into an area of the body for introducing or withdrawing fluid.

Centers for Medicare and Medicaid Services. Federal agency that oversees the administration of the public health programs such as Medicare, Medicaid, and State Children's Insurance Program.

certified nurse midwife. Registered nurse who has successfully completed a program of study and clinical experience or has been certified by a recognized organization for the care of pregnant or delivering patients.

CFR. Code of Federal Regulations.

CHAMPUS. Civilian Health and Medical Program of the Uniformed Services. See Tricare.

CHAMPVA. Civilian Health and Medical Program of the Department of Veterans Affairs.

chemodenervation. Chemical destruction of nerves. A substance, for example, Botox, is used to temporarily inhibit the transfer of chemicals at the presynaptic membrane, blocking the neuromuscular junctions.

chemoembolization. Administration of chemotherapeutic agents directly to a tumor in combination with the percutaneous administration of an occlusive substance into a vessel to deprive the tumor of its blood supply. This ensures a prolonged level of therapy directed at the tumor. Chemoembolization is primarily being used for cancers of the liver and endocrine system.

chemosurgery. Application of chemical agents to destroy tissue, originally referring to the in situ chemical fixation of premalignant or malignant lesions to facilitate surgical excision.

Chiari osteotomy. Top of the femur is altered to correct a dislocated hip caused by congenital conditions or cerebral palsy. Plate and screws are often used.

chimera. Organ or anatomic structure consisting of tissues of diverse genetic constitution.

choanal atresia. Congenital, membranous, or bony closure of one or both posterior nostrils due to failure of the embryonic bucconasal membrane to rupture and open up the nasal passageway.

chondromalacia. Condition in which the articular cartilage softens, seen in various body sites but most often in the patella, and may be congenital or acquired.

chorionic villus sampling. Aspiration of a placental sample through a catheter, under ultrasonic guidance. The specialized needle is placed transvaginally through the cervix or transabdominally into the uterine cavity.

chronic pain management services. Distinct services frequently performed by anesthesiologists who have additional training in pain management procedures. Pain management services include initial and subsequent evaluation and management (E/M) services, trigger point injections, spine and spinal cord injections, and nerve blocks.

cineplastic amputation. Amputation in which muscles and tendons of the remaining portion of the extremity are arranged so that they may be utilized for motor functions. Following this type of amputation, a specially constructed prosthetic device allows the individual to execute more complex movements because the muscles and tendons are able to communicate independent movements to the device.

circadian. Relating to a cyclic, 24-hour period.

clinical social worker. Individual who possesses a master's or doctor's degree in social work and, after obtaining the degree, has performed at least two years of supervised clinical social work. A clinical social worker must be licensed by the state or, in the case of states without licensure, must completed at least two years or 3,000 hours of post-master's degree supervised clinical social work practice under the supervision of a master's level social worker.

clinical staff. Someone who works for, or under, the direction of a physician or qualified health care professional and does not bill services separately. The person may be licensed or regulated to help the physician perform specific duties.

clonal. Originating from one cell.

CMS. Centers for Medicare and Medicaid Services. Federal agency that administers the public health programs.

CO2 laser. Carbon dioxide laser that emits an invisible beam and vaporizes water-rich tissue. The vapor is suctioned from the site.

codons. Series of three adjoining bases in one polynucleotide chain of a DNA or RNA molecule that provides the codes for a specific amino acid.

cognitive. Being aware by drawing from knowledge, such as judgment, reason, perception, and memory.

colostomy. Artificial surgical opening anywhere along the length of the colon to the skin surface for the diversion of feces.

commissurotomy. Surgical division or disruption of any two parts that are joined to form a commissure in order to increase the opening. The procedure most often refers to opening the adherent leaflet bands of fibrous tissue in a stenosed mitral valve.

common variants. Nucleotide sequence differences associated with abnormal gene function. Tests are usually performed in a single series of laboratory testing (in a single, typically multiplex, assay arrangement or using more than one assay to include all variants to be examined). Variants are representative of a mutation that mainly causes a single disease, such as cystic fibrosis. Other uncommon variants could provide additional information. Tests may be performed based on society recommendations and guidelines.

community mental health center. Facility providing outpatient mental health day treatment, assessments, and education as appropriate to community members.

computerized corneal topography. Digital imaging and analysis by computer of the shape of the corneal.

conjunctiva. Mucous membrane lining of the eyelids and covering of the exposed, anterior sclera.

conjunctivodacryocystostomy. Surgical connection of the lacrimal sac directly to the conjunctival sac.

conjunctivorhinostomy. Correction of an obstruction of the lacrimal canal achieved by suturing the posterior flaps and removing any lacrimal obstruction, preserving the conjunctiva.

constitutional. Cells containing genetic code that may be passed down to future generations. May also be referred to as germline.

consultation. Advice or opinion regarding diagnosis and treatment or determination to accept transfer of care of a patient rendered by a medical professional at the request of the primary care provider.

continuous positive airway pressure device. Pressurized device used to maintain the patient's airway for spontaneous or mechanically aided breathing. Often used for patients with mild to moderate sleep apnea.

core needle biopsy. Large-bore biopsy needle inserted into a mass and a core of tissue is removed for diagnostic study.

corpectomy. Removal of the body of a bone, such as a vertebra.

costochondral. Pertaining to the ribs and the scapula.

CPT. Current Procedural Terminology. Definitive procedural coding system developed by the American Medical Association that lists descriptive terms and identifying codes to provide a uniform language that describes medical, surgical, and diagnostic services for nationwide communication among physicians, patients, and third parties, used to report professional and outpatient services.

craniosynostosis. Congenital condition in which one or more of the cranial sutures fuse prematurely, creating a deformed or aberrant head shape.

craterization. Excision of a portion of bone creating a crater-like depression to facilitate drainage from infected areas of bone.

cricoid. Circular cartilage around the trachea.

CRNA. Certified registered nurse anesthetist. Nurse trained and specializing in the administration of anesthesia.

cryolathe. Tool used for reshaping a button of corneal tissue.

cryosurgery. Application of intense cold, usually produced using liquid nitrogen, to locally freeze diseased or unwanted tissue and induce tissue necrosis without causing harm to adjacent tissue.

CT. Computed tomography.

cutdown. Small, incised opening in the skin to expose a blood vessel, especially over a vein (venous cutdown) to allow venipuncture and permit a needle or cannula to be inserted for the withdrawal of blood or administration of fluids.

cytogenetic studies. Procedures in CPT that are related to the branch of genetics that studies cellular (cyto) structure and function as it relates to heredity (genetics). White blood cells, specifically T-lymphocytes, are the most commonly used specimen for chromosome analysis.

cytogenomic. Chromosomic evaluation using molecular methods.

dacryocystotome. Instrument used for incising the lacrimal duct strictures.

debride. To remove all foreign objects and devitalized or infected tissue from a burn or wound to prevent infection and promote healing.

definitive drug testing. Drug tests used to further analyze or confirm the presence or absence of specific drugs or classes of drugs used by the patient. These tests are able to provide more conclusive information regarding the concentration of the drug and their metabolites. May be used for medical, workplace, or legal purposes.

definitive identification. Identification of microorganisms using additional tests to specify the genus or species (e.g., slide cultures or biochemical panels).

dentoalveolar structure. Area of alveolar bone surrounding the teeth and adjacent tissue.

Department of Health and Human Services. Cabinet department that oversees the operating divisions of the federal government responsible for health and welfare. HHS oversees the Centers for Medicare and Medicaid Services, Food and Drug Administration, Public Health Service, and other such entities.

Department of Justice. Attorneys from the DOJ and the United States Attorney's Office have, under the memorandum of understanding, the same direct access to contractor data and records as the OIG and the Federal Bureau of Investigation (FBI). DOJ is responsible for prosecution of fraud and civil or criminal cases presented.

dermis. Skin layer found under the epidermis that contains a papillary upper layer and the deep reticular layer of collagen, vascular bed, and nerves.

dermis graft. Skin graft that has been separated from the epidermal tissue and the underlying subcutaneous fat, used primarily as a substitute for fascia grafts in plastic surgery.

desensitization. 1) Administration of extracts of allergens periodically to build immunity in the patient. 2) Application of medication to decrease the symptoms, usually pain, associated with a dental condition or disease.

destruction. Ablation or eradication of a structure or tissue.

diabetes outpatient self-management training services. Educational and training services furnished by a certified provider in an outpatient setting. The physician managing the individual's diabetic condition must certify that the services are needed under a comprehensive plan of care and provide the patient with the skills and knowledge necessary for therapeutic program compliance (including skills related to the self-administration of injectable drugs). The provider must meet applicable standards established by the National Diabetes Advisory or be recognized by an organization that represents individuals with diabetes as meeting standards for furnishing the services.

diagnostic procedures. Procedure performed on a patient to obtain information to assess the medical condition of the patient or to identify a disease and to determine the nature and severity of an illness or injury.

dialysis. Artificial filtering of the blood to remove contaminating waste elements and restore normal balance.

diaphragm. 1) Muscular wall separating the thorax and its structures from the abdomen. 2) Flexible disk inserted into the vagina and against the cervix as a method of birth control.

diaphysectomy. Surgical removal of a portion of the shaft of a long bone, often done to facilitate drainage from infected bone.

diathermy. Applying heat to body tissues by various methods for therapeutic treatment or surgical purposes to coagulate and seal tissue.

dilation. Artificial increase in the diameter of an opening or lumen made by medication or by instrumentation.

dissect. Cut apart or separate tissue for surgical purposes or for visual or microscopic study.

DNA. Deoxyribonucleic acid. Chemical containing the genetic information necessary to produce and propagate living organisms. Molecules are comprised of two twisting paired strands, called a double helix.

DNA marker. Specific gene sequence within a chromosome indicating the inheritance of a certain trait.

dorsal. Pertaining to the back or posterior aspect.

drugs and biologicals. Drugs and biologicals included - or approved for inclusion - in the United States Pharmacopoeia, the National Formulary, the United States Homeopathic Pharmacopoeia, in New Drugs or Accepted Dental Remedies, or approved by the pharmacy and drug therapeutics committee of the medical staff of the hospital. Also included are medically accepted and FDA approved drugs used in an anticancer chemotherapeutic regimen. The carrier determines medical acceptance based on supportive clinical evidence.

dual-lead device. Implantable cardiac device (pacemaker or implantable cardioverter-defibrillator [ICD]) in which pacing and sensing components are placed in only two chambers of the heart.

duplex scan. Noninvasive vascular diagnostic technique that uses ultrasonic scanning to identify the pattern and direction of blood flow within arteries or veins displayed in real time images. Duplex scanning combines B-mode two-dimensional pictures of the vessel structure with spectra and/or color flow Doppler mapping or imaging of the blood as it moves through the vessels.

duplication/deletion (DUP/DEL). Term used in molecular testing which examines genomic regions to determine if there are extra chromosomes (duplication) or missing chromosomes (deletions). Normal gene dosage is two copies per cell except for the sex chromosomes which have one per cell.

DuToit staple capsulorrhaphy. Reattachment of the capsule of the shoulder and glenoid labrum to the glenoid lip using staples to anchor the avulsed capsule and glenoid labrum.

Dx. Diagnosis.

DXA. Dual energy x-ray absorptiometry. Radiological technique for bone density measurement using a two-dimensional projection system in which two x-ray beams with different levels of energy are pulsed alternately and the results are given in two scores, reported as standard deviations from peak bone mass density.

dynamic mutation. Unstable or changing polynucleotides resulting in repeats related to genes that can undergo disease-producing increases or decreases in the repeats that differ within tissues or over generations.

ECMO. Extracorporeal membrane oxygenation.

ectropion. Drooping of the lower eyelid away from the eye or outward turning or eversion of the edge of the eyelid, exposing the palpebral conjunctiva and causing irritation.

Eden-Hybinette procedure. Anterior shoulder repair using an anterior bone block to augment the bony anterior glenoid lip.

EDTA. Drug used to inhibit damage to the cornea by collagenase. EDTA is especially effective in alkali burns as it neutralizes soluble alkali, including lye.

effusion. Escape of fluid from within a body cavity.

electrocardiographic rhythm derived. Analysis of data obtained from readings of the heart's electrical activation, including heart rate and rhythm, variability of heart rate, ST analysis, and T-wave alternans. Other data may also be assessed when warranted.

electrocautery. Division or cutting of tissue using high-frequency electrical current to produce heat, which destroys cells.

electrode array. Electronic device containing more than one contact whose function can be adjusted during programming services. Electrodes are specialized for a particular electrochemical reaction that acts as a medium between a body surface and another instrument.

electromyography. Test that measures muscle response to nerve stimulation determining if muscle weakness is present and if it is related to the muscles themselves or a problem with the nerves that supply the muscles.

electrooculogram (EOG). Record of electrical activity associated with eye movements.

electrophysiologic studies. Electrical stimulation and monitoring to diagnose heart conduction abnormalities that predispose patients to bradyarrhythmias and to determine a patient's chance for developing ventricular and supraventricular tachyarrhythmias.

embolization. Placement of a clotting agent, such as a coil, plastic particles, gel, foam, etc., into an area of hemorrhage to stop the bleeding or to block blood flow to a problem area, such as an aneurysm or a tumor.

emergency. Serious medical condition or symptom (including severe pain) resulting from injury, sickness, or mental illness that arises suddenly and requires immediate care and treatment, generally received within 24 hours of onset, to avoid jeopardy to the life, limb, or health of a covered person.

empyema. Accumulation of pus within the respiratory, or pleural, cavity.

EMTALA. Emergency Medical Treatment and Active Labor Act.

end-stage renal disease. Chronic, advanced kidney disease requiring renal dialysis or a kidney transplant to prevent imminent death.

endarterectomy. Removal of the thickened, endothelial lining of a diseased or damaged artery.

endomicroscopy. Diagnostic technology that allows for the examination of tissue at the cellular level during endoscopy. The technology decreases the need for biopsy with histological examination for some types of lesions.

endovascular embolization. Procedure whereby vessels are occluded by a variety of therapeutic substances for the treatment of abnormal blood vessels by inhibiting the flow of blood to a tumor, arteriovenous malformations, lymphatic malformation, and to prevent or stop hemorrhage.

entropion. Inversion of the eyelid, turning the edge in toward the eyeball and causing irritation from contact of the lashes with the surface of the eye.

enucleation. Removal of a growth or organ cleanly so as to extract it in one piece.

epidermis. Outermost, nonvascular layer of skin that contains four to five differentiated layers depending on its body location: stratum corneum, lucidum, granulosum, spinosum, and basale.

epiphysiodesis. Surgical fusion of an epiphysis performed to prematurely stop further bone growth.

escharotomy. Surgical incision into the scab or crust resulting from a severe burn in order to relieve constriction and allow blood flow to the distal unburned tissue.

established patient. 1) Patient who has received professional services in a face-to-face setting within the last three years from the same physician/qualified health care professional or another physician/qualified health care professional of the exact same specialty and subspecialty who belongs to the same group practice. 2) For OPPS hospitals, patient who has been registered as an inpatient or outpatient in a hospital's provider-based clinic or emergency department within the past three years.

evacuation. Removal or purging of waste material.

evaluation and management codes. Assessment and management of a patient's health care.

evaluation and management service components. Key components of history, examination, and medical decision making that are key to selecting the correct E/M codes. Other non-key components include counseling, coordination of care, nature of presenting problem, and time.

event recorder. Portable, ambulatory heart monitor worn by the patient that makes electrocardiographic recordings of the length and frequency of aberrant cardiac rhythm to help diagnose heart conditions and to assess pacemaker functioning or programming.

exenteration. Surgical removal of the entire contents of a body cavity, such as the pelvis or orbit.

exon. One of multiple nucleic acid sequences used to encode information for a gene polypeptide or protein. Exons are separated from other exons by non-protein-coding sequences known as introns.

extended care services. Items and services provided to an inpatient of a skilled nursing facility, including nursing care, physical or occupational therapy, speech pathology, drugs and supplies, and medical social services.

external electrical capacitor device. External electrical stimulation device designed to promote bone healing. This device may also promote neural regeneration, revascularization, epiphyseal growth, and ligament maturation.

external pulsating electromagnetic field. External stimulation device designed to promote bone healing. This device may also promote neural regeneration, revascularization, epiphyseal growth, and ligament maturation.

extracorporeal. Located or taking place outside the body.

Eyre-Brook capsulorrhaphy. Reattachment of the capsule of the shoulder and glenoid labrum to the glenoid lip.

False Claims Act. Governs civil actions for filing false claims. Liability under this act pertains to any person who knowingly presents or causes to be presented a false or fraudulent claim to the government for payment or approval.

fascia. Fibrous sheet or band of tissue that envelops organs, muscles, and groupings of muscles.

fasciectomy. Excision of fascia or strips of fascial tissue.

fasciotomy. Incision or transection of fascial tissue.

fat graft. Graft composed of fatty tissue completely freed from surrounding tissue that is used primarily to fill in depressions.

FDA. Food and Drug Administration. Federal agency responsible for protecting public health by substantiating the safety, efficacy, and security of human and veterinary drugs, biological products, medical devices, national food supply, cosmetics, and items that give off radiation.

filtered speech test. Test most commonly used to identify central auditory dysfunction in which the patient is presented monosyllabic words that are low pass filtered, allowing only the parts of each word below a certain pitch to be presented. A score is given on the number of correct responses. This may be a subset of a standard battery of tests provided during a single encounter.

fissure. Deep furrow, groove, or cleft in tissue structures.

fistulization. Creation of a communication between two structures that were not previously connected.

flexor digitorum profundus tendon. Tendon originating in the proximal forearm and extending to the index finger and wrist. A thickened FDP sheath, usually caused by age, illness, or injury, can fill the carpal canal and lead to impingement of the median nerve.

fluoroscopy. Radiology technique that allows visual examination of part of the body or a function of an organ using a device that projects an x-ray image on a fluorescent screen.

focal length. Distance between the object in focus and the lens.

focused medical review. Process of targeting and directing medical review efforts on Medicare claims where the greatest risk of inappropriate program payment exists. The goal is to reduce the number of noncovered claims or unnecessary services. CMS analyzes national data such as internal billing, utilization, and payment data and provides its findings to the FI. Local medical review policies are developed identifying aberrances, abuse, and overutilized services. Providers are responsible for knowing national Medicare coverage and billing guidelines and local medical review policies, and for determining whether the services provided to Medicare beneficiaries are covered by Medicare.

fragile X syndrome. Intellectual disabilities, enlarged testes, big jaw, high forehead, and long ears in males. In females, fragile X presents with mild intellectual disabilities and heterozygous sexual structures. In some families, males have shown no symptoms but carry the gene.

free flap. Tissue that is completely detached from the donor site and transplanted to the recipient site, receiving its blood supply from capillary ingrowth at the recipient site.

free microvascular flap. Tissue that is completely detached from the donor site following careful dissection and preservation of the blood vessels, then attached to the recipient site with the transferred blood vessels anastomosed to the vessels in the recipient bed.

fulguration. Destruction of living tissue by using sparks from a high-frequency electric current.

gas tamponade. Absorbable gas may be injected to force the retina against the choroid. Common gases include room air, short-acting sulfahexafluoride, intermediate-acting perfluoroethane, or long-acting perfluorooctane.

Gaucher disease. Genetic metabolic disorder in which fat deposits may accumulate in the spleen, liver, lungs, bone marrow, and brain.

gene. Basic unit of heredity that contains nucleic acid. Genes are arranged in different and unique sequences or strings that determine the gene's function. Human genes usually include multiple protein coding regions such as exons separated by introns which are nonprotein coding sections.

genome. Complete set of DNA of an organism. Each cell in the human body is comprised of a complete copy of the approximately three billion DNA base pairs that constitute the human genome.

HCPCS. Healthcare Common Procedure Coding System.

HCPCS Level I. Healthcare Common Procedure Coding System Level I. Numeric coding system used by physicians, facility outpatient departments, and ambulatory surgery centers (ASC) to code ambulatory, laboratory, radiology, and other diagnostic services for Medicare billing. This coding system contains only the American Medical Association's Physicians' Current Procedural Terminology (CPT) codes. The AMA updates codes annually.

HCPCS Level II. Healthcare Common Procedure Coding System Level II. National coding system, developed by CMS, that contains alphanumeric codes for physician and nonphysician services not included in the CPT coding system. HCPCS Level II covers such things as ambulance services, durable medical equipment, and orthotic and prosthetic devices.

HCPCS modifiers. Two-character code (AA-ZZ) that identifies circumstances that alter or enhance the description of a service or supply. They are recognized by carriers nationally and are updated annually by CMS.

Hct. Hematocrit.

health care provider. Entity that administers diagnostic and therapeutic services.

hemilaminectomy. Excision of a portion of the vertebral lamina.

hemodialysis. Cleansing of wastes and contaminating elements from the blood by virtue of different diffusion rates through a semipermeable membrane, which separates blood from a filtration solution that diffuses other elements out of the blood. The blood is slowly filtered extracorporeally through special dialysis equipment and returned to the body. Synonym(s): renal dialysis.

hemodialysis. Cleansing of wastes and contaminating elements from the blood by virtue of different diffusion rates through a semipermeable membrane, which separates blood from a filtration solution that diffuses other elements out of the blood.

hemoperitoneum. Effusion of blood into the peritoneal cavity, the space between the continuous membrane lining the abdominopelvic walls and encasing the visceral organs.

heterograft. Surgical graft of tissue from one animal species to a different animal species. A common type of heterograft is porcine (pig) tissue, used for temporary wound closure.

heterotopic transplant. Tissue transplanted from a different anatomical site for usage as is natural for that tissue, for example, buccal mucosa to a conjunctival site.

HGNC. HUGO gene nomenclature committee.

HGVS. Human genome variation society.

Hickman catheter. Central venous catheter used for long-term delivery of medications, such as antibiotics, nutritional substances, or chemotherapeutic agents.

HLA. Human leukocyte antigen.

home health services. Services furnished to patients in their homes under the care of physicians. These services include part-time or intermittent skilled nursing care, physical therapy, medical social services, medical supplies, and some rehabilitation equipment. Home health supplies and services must be prescribed by a physician, and the beneficiary must be confined at home in order for Medicare to pay the benefits in full.

homograft. Graft from one individual to another of the same species.

hospice care. Items and services provided to a terminally ill individual by a hospice program under a written plan established and periodically reviewed by the individual's attending physician and by the medical director: Nursing care provided by or under the supervision of a registered professional nurse; Physical or occupational therapy or speech-language pathology services; Medical social services under the direction of a physician; Services of a home health aide who has successfully completed a training program; Medical supplies (including drugs and biologicals) and the use of medical appliances; Physicians' services; Short-term inpatient care (including both respite care and procedures necessary for pain control and acute and chronic symptom management) in an inpatient facility on an intermittent basis and not consecutively over longer than five days; Counseling (including dietary counseling) with respect to care of the terminally ill individual and adjustment to his death; Any item or service which is specified in the plan and for which payment may be made.

hospital. Institution that provides, under the supervision of physicians, diagnostic, therapeutic, and rehabilitation services for medical diagnosis, treatment, and care of patients. Hospitals receiving federal funds must maintain clinical records on all patients, provide 24-hour nursing services, and have a discharge planning process in place. The term "hospital" also includes religious nonmedical health care institutions and facilities of 50 beds or less located in rural areas.

HUGO. Human genome organization

IA. Intra-arterial.

ICD. Implantable cardioverter defibrillator.

ICD-10-CM. International Classification of Diseases, 10th Revision, Clinical Modification. Clinical modification of the alphanumeric classification of diseases used by the World Health Organization, already in use in much of the world, and used for mortality reporting in the United States. The implementation date for ICD-10-CM diagnostic coding system to replace ICD-9-CM in the United States was October 1, 2015.

ICD-10-PCS. International Classification of Diseases, 10th Revision, Procedure Coding System. Beginning October 1, 2015, inpatient hospital services and surgical procedures must be coded using ICD-10-PCS codes, replacing ICD-9-CM, Volume 3 for procedures.

ICM. Implantable cardiovascular monitor.

ileostomy. Artificial surgical opening that brings the end of the ileum out through the abdominal wall to the skin surface for the diversion of feces through a stoma.

iliopsoas tendon. Fibrous tissue that connects muscle to bone in the pelvic region, common to the iliacus and psoas major.

ILR. Implantable loop recorder.

IM. 1) Infectious mononucleosis. 2) Internal medicine. 3) Intramuscular.

immunotherapy. Therapeutic use of serum or gamma globulin.

implant. Material or device inserted or placed within the body for therapeutic, reconstructive, or diagnostic purposes.

implantable cardiovascular monitor. Implantable electronic device that stores cardiovascular physiologic data such as intracardiac pressure waveforms collected from internal sensors or data such as weight and blood pressure collected from external sensors. The information stored in these devices is used as an aid in managing patients with heart failure and other cardiac conditions that are non-rhythm related. The data may be transmitted via local telemetry or remotely to a surveillance technician or an internet-based file server.

implantable cardioverter-defibrillator. Implantable electronic cardiac device used to control rhythm abnormalities such as tachycardia, fibrillation, or bradycardia by producing high- or low-energy stimulation and pacemaker functions. It may also have the capability to provide the functions of an implantable loop recorder or implantable cardiovascular monitor.

implantable loop recorder. Implantable electronic cardiac device that constantly monitors and records electrocardiographic rhythm. It may be triggered by the patient when a symptomatic episode occurs or activated automatically by rapid or slow heart rates. This may be the sole purpose of the device or it may be a component of another cardiac device, such as a pacemaker or implantable cardioverter-defibrillator. The data can be transmitted via local telemetry or remotely to a surveillance technician or an internet-based file server.

implantable venous access device. Catheter implanted for continuous access to the venous system for long-term parenteral feeding or for the administration of fluids or medications.

IMRT. Intensity modulated radiation therapy. External beam radiation therapy delivery using computer planning to specify the target dose and to modulate the radiation intensity, usually as a treatment for a malignancy. The delivery system approaches the patient from multiple angles, minimizing damage to normal tissue.

in situ. Located in the natural position or contained within the origin site, not spread into neighboring tissue.

incontinence. Inability to control urination or defecation.

infundibulectomy. Excision of the anterosuperior portion of the right ventricle of the heart.

internal direct current stimulator. Electrostimulation device placed directly into the surgical site designed to promote bone regeneration by encouraging cellular healing response in bone and ligaments.

interrogation device evaluation. Assessment of an implantable cardiac device (pacemaker, cardioverter-defibrillator, cardiovascular monitor, or loop recorder) in which collected data about the patient's heart rate and rhythm, battery and pulse generator function, and any leads or sensors present, are retrieved and evaluated. Determinations regarding device programming and appropriate treatment settings are made based on the findings. CPT provides required components for evaluation of the various types of devices.

intramedullary implants. Nail, rod, or pin placed into the intramedullary canal at the fracture site. Intramedullary implants not only provide a method of aligning the fracture, they also act as a splint and may reduce fracture pain. Implants may be rigid or flexible. Rigid implants are preferred for prophylactic treatment of diseased bone, while flexible implants are preferred for traumatic injuries.

intraocular lens. Artificial lens implanted into the eye to replace a damaged natural lens or cataract.

intravenous. Within a vein or veins.

introducer. Instrument, such as a catheter, needle, or tube, through which another instrument or device is introduced into the body.

intron. Nonprotein section of a gene that separates exons in human genes. Contains vital sequences that allow splicing of exons to produce a functional protein from a gene. Sometimes referred to as intervening sequences (IVS).

IP. 1) Interphalangeal. 2) Intraperitoneal.

irrigation. To wash out or cleanse a body cavity, wound, or tissue with water or other fluid.

Kayser-Fleischer ring. Condition found in Wilson's disease in which deposits of copper cause a pigmented ring around the cornea's outer border in the deep epithelial layers.

keratoprosthesis. Surgical procedure in which the physician creates a new anterior chamber with a plastic optical implant to replace a severely damaged cornea that cannot be repaired.

keratotomy. Surgical incision of the cornea.

krypton laser. Laser light energy that uses ionized krypton by electric current as the active source, has a radiation beam between the visible yellow-red spectrum, and is effective in photocoagulation of retinal bleeding, macular lesions, and vessel aberrations of the choroid.

lacrimal. Tear-producing gland or ducts that provides lubrication and flushing of the eyes and nasal cavities.

lacrimal punctum. Opening of the lacrimal papilla of the eyelid through which tears flow to the canaliculi to the lacrimal sac.

lacrimotome. Knife for cutting the lacrimal sac or duct.

lacrimotomy. Incision of the lacrimal sac or duct.

laparotomy. Incision through the flank or abdomen for therapeutic or diagnostic purposes.

laryngoscopy. Examination of the hypopharynx, larynx, and tongue base with an endoscope.

larynx. Musculocartilaginous structure between the trachea and the pharynx that functions as the valve preventing food and other particles from entering the respiratory tract, as well as the voice mechanism. Also called the voicebox, the larynx is composed of three single cartilages: cricoid, epiglottis, and thyroid; and three paired cartilages: arytenoid, corniculate, and cuneiform.

laser surgery. Use of concentrated, sharply defined light beams to cut, cauterize, coagulate, seal, or vaporize tissue.

LEEP. Loop electrode excision procedure. Biopsy specimen or cone shaped wedge of cervical tissue is removed using a hot cautery wire loop with an electrical current running through it.

levonorgestrel. Drug inhibiting ovulation and preventing sperm from penetrating cervical mucus. It is delivered subcutaneously in polysiloxone capsules. The capsules can be effective for up to five years, and provide a cumulative pregnancy rate of less than 2 percent. The capsules are not biodegradable, and therefore must be removed. Removal is more difficult than insertion of levonorgestrel capsules because fibrosis develops around the capsules. Normal hormonal activity and a return to fertility begins immediately upon removal.

ligament. Band or sheet of fibrous tissue that connects the articular surfaces of bones or supports visceral organs.

ligation. Tying off a blood vessel or duct with a suture or a soft, thin wire.

lymphadenectomy. Dissection of lymph nodes free from the vessels and removal for examination by frozen section in a separate procedure to detect early-stage metastases.

lysis. Destruction, breakdown, dissolution, or decomposition of cells or substances by a specific catalyzing agent.

Magnuson-Stack procedure. Treatment for recurrent anterior dislocation of the shoulder that involves tightening and realigning the subscapularis tendon.

maintenance of wakefulness test. Attended study determining the patient's ability to stay awake.

Manchester operation. Preservation of the uterus following prolapse by amputating the vaginal portion of the cervix, shortening the cardinal ligaments, and performing a colpoperineorrhaphy posteriorly.

mapping. Multidimensional depiction of a tachycardia that identifies its site of origin and its electrical conduction pathway after tachycardia has been induced. The recording is made from multiple catheter sites within the heart, obtaining electrograms simultaneously or sequentially.

marsupialization. Creation of a pouch in surgical treatment of a cyst in which one wall is resected and the remaining cut edges are sutured to adjacent tissue creating an open pouch of the previously enclosed cyst.

mastectomy. Surgical removal of one or both breasts.

McDonald procedure. Polyester tape is placed around the cervix with a running stitch to assist in the prevention of pre-term delivery. Tape is removed at term for vaginal delivery.

MCP. Metacarpophalangeal.

medial. Middle or midline.

mediastinotomy. Incision into the mediastinum for purposes of exploration, foreign body removal, drainage, or biopsy.

medical review. Review by a Medicare administrative contractor, carrier, and/or quality improvement organization (QIO) of services and items provided by physicians, other health care practitioners, and providers of health care services under Medicare. The review determines if the items and services are reasonable and necessary and meet Medicare coverage requirements, whether the quality meets professionally recognized standards of health care, and whether the services are medically appropriate in an inpatient, outpatient, or other setting as supported by documentation.

Medicare contractor. Medicare Part A fiscal intermediary, Medicare Part B carrier, Medicare administrative contractor (MAC), or a durable medical equipment Medicare administrative contractor (DME MAC).

Medicare physician fee schedule. List of payments Medicare allows by procedure or service. Payments may vary through geographic adjustments. The MPFS is based on the resource-based relative value scale (RBRVS). A national total relative value unit (RVU) is given to each procedure (HCPCS Level I CPT, Level II national codes). Each total RVU has three components: physician work, practice expense, and malpractice insurance.

metabolite. Chemical compound resulting from the natural process of metabolism. In drug testing, the metabolite of the drug may endure in a higher concentration or for a longer duration than the initial "parent" drug.

methylation. Mechanism used to regulate genes and protect DNA from some types of cleavage.

microarray. Small surface onto which multiple specific nucleic acid sequences can be attached to be used for analysis. Microarray may also be known as a gene chip or DNA chip. Tests can be run on the sequences for any variants that may be present.

mitral valve. Valve with two cusps that is between the left atrium and left ventricle of the heart.

moderate sedation. Medically controlled state of depressed consciousness, with or without analgesia, while maintaining the patient's airway, protective reflexes, and ability to respond to stimulation or verbal commands.

Mohs micrographic surgery. Special technique used to treat complex or ill-defined skin cancer and requires a single physician to provide two distinct services. The first service is surgical and involves the destruction of the lesion by a combination of chemosurgery and excision. The second service is that of a pathologist and includes mapping, color coding of specimens, microscopic examination of specimens, and complete histopathologic preparation.

monitored anesthesia care. Sedation, with or without analgesia, used to achieve a medically controlled state of depressed consciousness while maintaining the patient's airway, protective reflexes, and ability to respond to stimulation or verbal commands. In dental conscious sedation, the patient is rendered free of fear, apprehension, and anxiety through the use of pharmacological agents.

monoclonal. Relating to a single clone of cells.

multiple sleep latency test (MSLT). Attended study to determine the tendency of the patient to fall asleep.

multiple-lead device. Implantable cardiac device (pacemaker or implantable cardioverter-defibrillator [ICD]) in which pacing and sensing components are placed in at least three chambers of the heart.

Mustard procedure. Corrective measure for transposition of great vessels involves an intra-atrial baffle made of pericardial tissue or synthetic material. The baffle is secured between pulmonary veins and mitral valve and between mitral and tricuspid valves. The baffle directs systemic venous flow into the left ventricle and lungs and pulmonary venous flow into the right ventricle and aorta.

mutation. Alteration in gene function that results in changes to a gene or chromosome. Can cause deficits or disease that can be inherited, can have beneficial effects, or result in no noticeable change.

mutation scanning. Process normally used on multiple polymerase chain reaction (PCR) amplicons to determine DNA sequence variants by differences in characteristics compared to normal. Specific DNA variants can then be studied further.

myotomy. Surgical cutting of a muscle to gain access to underlying tissues or for therapeutic reasons.

myringotomy. Incision in the eardrum done to prevent spontaneous rupture precipitated by fluid pressure build-up behind the tympanic membrane and to prevent stagnant infection and erosion of the ossicles.

nasal polyp. Fleshy outgrowth projecting from the mucous membrane of the nose or nasal sinus cavity that may obstruct ventilation or affect the sense of smell.

nasal sinus. Air-filled cavities in the cranial bones lined with mucous membrane and continuous with the nasal cavity, draining fluids through the nose.

nasogastric tube. Long, hollow, cylindrical catheter made of soft rubber or plastic that is inserted through the nose down into the stomach, and is used for feeding, instilling medication, or withdrawing gastric contents.

nasolacrimal punctum. Opening of the lacrimal duct near the nose.

nasopharynx. Membranous passage above the level of the soft palate.

Nd:YAG laser. Laser light energy that uses an yttrium, aluminum, and garnet crystal doped with neodymium ions as the active source, has a radiation beam nearing the infrared spectrum, and is effective in photocoagulation, photoablation, cataract extraction, and lysis of vitreous strands.

nebulizer. Latin for mist, a device that converts liquid into a fine spray and is commonly used to deliver medicine to the upper respiratory, bronchial, and lung areas.

nerve conduction study. Diagnostic test performed to assess muscle or nerve damage. Nerves are stimulated with electric shocks along the course of the muscle. Sensors are utilized to measure and record nerve functions, including conduction and velocity.

neurectomy. Excision of all or a portion of a nerve.

neuromuscular junction. Nerve synapse at the meeting point between the terminal end of a nerve (motor neuron) and a muscle fiber.

neuropsychological testing. Evaluation of a patient's behavioral abilities wherein a physician or other health care professional administers a series of tests in thinking, reasoning, and judgment.

new patient. Patient who is receiving face-to-face care from a provider/qualified health care professional or another physician/qualified health care professional of the exact same specialty and subspecialty who belongs to the same group practice for the first time in three years. For OPPS hospitals, a patient who has not been registered as an inpatient or outpatient, including off-campus provider based clinic or emergency department, within the past three years.

Niemann-Pick syndrome. Accumulation of phospholipid in histiocytes in the bone marrow, liver, lymph nodes, and spleen, cerebral involvement, and red macular spots similar to Tay-Sachs disease. Most commonly found in Jewish infants.

Nissen fundoplasty. Surgical repair technique that involves the fundus of the stomach being wrapped around the lower end of the esophagus to treat reflux esophagitis.

nonabsorbable sutures. Strands of natural or synthetic material that resist absorption into living tissue and are removed once healing is under way. Nonabsorbable sutures are commonly used to close skin wounds and repair tendons or collagenous tissue.

obturator. Prosthesis used to close an acquired or congenital opening in the palate that aids in speech and chewing.

obturator nerve. Lumbar plexus nerve with anterior and posterior divisions that innervate the adductor muscles (e.g., adductor longus, adductor brevis) of the leg and the skin over the medial area of the thigh or a sacral plexus nerve with anterior and posterior divisions that innervate the superior gemellus muscles.

occult blood test. Chemical or microscopic test to determine the presence of blood in a specimen.

ocular implant. Implant inside muscular cone.

oophorectomy. Surgical removal of all or part of one or both ovaries, either as open procedure or laparoscopically. Menstruation and childbearing ability continues when one ovary is removed.

orthosis. Derived from a Greek word meaning "to make straight," it is an artificial appliance that supports, aligns, or corrects an anatomical deformity or improves the use of a moveable body part. Unlike a prosthesis, an orthotic device is always functional in nature.

osteo-. Having to do with bone.

osteogenesis stimulator. Device used to stimulate the growth of bone by electrical impulses or ultrasound.

osteotomy. Surgical cutting of a bone.

ostomy. Artificial (surgical) opening in the body used for drainage or for delivery of medications or nutrients.

pacemaker. Implantable cardiac device that controls the heart's rhythm and maintains regular beats by artificial electric discharges. This device consists of the pulse generator with a battery and the electrodes, or leads, which are placed in single or dual chambers of the heart, usually transvenously.

palmaris longus tendon. Tendon located in the hand that flexes the wrist joint.

paratenon graft. Graft composed of the fatty tissue found between a tendon and its sheath.

passive mobilization. Pressure, movement, or pulling of a limb or body part utilizing an apparatus or device.

pedicle flap. Full-thickness skin and subcutaneous tissue for grafting that remains partially attached to the donor site by a pedicle or stem in which the blood vessels supplying the flap remain intact.

Pemberton osteotomy. Osteotomy is performed to position triradiate cartilage as a hinge for rotating the acetabular roof in cases of dysplasia of the hip in children.

penetrance. Being formed by, or pertaining to, a single clone.

percutaneous intradiscal electrothermal annuloplasty. Procedure corrects tears in the vertebral annulus by applying heat to the collagen disc walls percutaneously through a catheter. The heat contracts and thickens the wall, which may contract and close any annular tears.

percutaneous skeletal fixation. Treatment that is neither open nor closed and the injury site is not directly visualized. Fixation devices (pins, screws) are placed through the skin to stabilize the dislocation using x-ray guidance.

pericardium. Thin and slippery case in which the heart lies that is lined with fluid so that the heart is free to pulse and move as it beats.

peripheral arterial tonometry (PAT). Pulsatile volume changes in a digit are measured to determine activity in the sympathetic nervous system for respiratory analysis.

peritoneal. Space between the lining of the abdominal wall, or parietal peritoneum, and the surface layer of the abdominal organs, or visceral peritoneum. It contains a thin, watery fluid that keeps the peritoneal surfaces moist.

peritoneal dialysis. Dialysis that filters waste from blood inside the body using the peritoneum, the natural lining of the abdomen, as the semipermeable membrane across which ultrafiltration is accomplished. A special catheter is inserted into the abdomen and a dialysis solution is drained into the abdomen. This solution extracts fluids and wastes, which are then discarded when the fluid is drained. Various forms of peritoneal dialysis include CAPD, CCPD, and NIDP.

peritoneal effusion. Persistent escape of fluid within the peritoneal cavity.

pessary. Device placed in the vagina to support and reposition a prolapsing or retropositioned uterus, rectum, or vagina.

phenotype. Physical expression of a trait or characteristic as determined by an individual's genetic makeup or genotype.

photocoagulation. Application of an intense laser beam of light to disrupt tissue and condense protein material to a residual mass, used especially for treating ocular conditions.

physical status modifiers. Alphanumeric modifier used to identify the patient's health status as it affects the work related to providing the anesthesia service.

physical therapy modality. Therapeutic agent or regimen applied or used to provide appropriate treatment of the musculoskeletal system.

physician. Legally authorized practitioners including a doctor of medicine or osteopathy, a doctor of dental surgery or of dental medicine, a doctor of podiatric medicine, a doctor of optometry, and a chiropractor only with respect to treatment by means of manual manipulation of the spine (to correct a subluxation).

PICC. Peripherally inserted central catheter. PICC is inserted into one of the large veins of the arm and threaded through the vein until the tip sits in a large vein just above the heart.

PKR. Photorefractive therapy. Procedure involving the removal of the surface layer of the cornea (epithelium) by gentle scraping and use of a computer-controlled excimer laser to reshape the stroma.

pleurodesis. Injection of a sclerosing agent into the pleural space for creating adhesions between the parietal and the visceral pleura to treat a collapsed lung caused by air trapped in the pleural cavity, or severe cases of pleural effusion.

plication. Surgical technique involving folding, tucking, or pleating to reduce the size of a hollow structure or organ.

polyclonal. Containing one or more cells.

polymorphism. Genetic variation in the same species that does not harm the gene function or create disease.

polypeptide. Chain of amino acids held together by covalent bonds. Proteins are made up of amino acids.

polysomnography. Test involving monitoring of respiratory, cardiac, muscle, brain, and ocular function during sleep.

Potts-Smith-Gibson procedure. Side-to-side anastomosis of the aorta and left pulmonary artery creating a shunt that enlarges as the child grows.

Prader-Willi syndrome. Rounded face, almond-shaped eyes, strabismus, low forehead, hypogonadism, hypotonia, intellectual disabilities, and an insatiable appetite.

presumptive drug testing. Drug screening tests to identify the presence or absence of drugs in a patient's system. Tests are usually able to identify low concentrations of the drug. These tests may be used for medical, workplace, or legal purposes.

presumptive identification. Identification of microorganisms using media growth, colony morphology, gram stains, or up to three specific tests (e.g., catalase, indole, oxidase, urease).

professional component. Portion of a charge for health care services that represents the physician's (or other practitioner's) work in providing the service, including interpretation and report of the procedure. This component of the service usually is charged for and billed separately from the inpatient hospital charges.

profunda. Denotes a part of a structure that is deeper from the surface of the body than the rest of the structure.

prolonged physician services. Extended pre- or post-service care provided to a patient whose condition requires services beyond the usual.

prostate. Male gland surrounding the bladder neck and urethra that secretes a substance into the seminal fluid.

prosthetic. Device that replaces all or part of an internal body organ or body part, or that replaces part of the function of a permanently inoperable or malfunctioning internal body organ or body part.

provider of services. Institution, individual, or organization that provides health care.

proximal. Located closest to a specified reference point, usually the midline or trunk.

psychiatric hospital. Specialized institution that provides, under the supervision of physicians, services for the diagnosis and treatment of mentally ill persons.

pterygium. Benign, wedge-shaped, conjunctival thickening that advances from the inner corner of the eye toward the cornea.

pterygomaxillary fossa. Wide depression on the external surface of the maxilla above and to the side of the canine tooth socket.

pulmonary artery banding. Surgical constriction of the pulmonary artery to prevent irreversible pulmonary vascular obstructive changes and overflow into the left ventricle.

Putti-Platt procedure. Realignment of the subscapularis tendon to treat recurrent anterior dislocation, thereby partially eliminating external rotation. The anterior capsule is also tightened and reinforced.

pyloroplasty. Enlargement and reconstruction of the lower portion of the stomach opening into the duodenum performed after vagotomy to speed gastric emptying and treat duodenal ulcers.

qualified health care professional. Educated, licensed or certified, and regulated professional operating under a specified scope of practice to provide patient services that are separate and distinct from other clinical staff. Services may be billed independently or under the facility's services.

RAC. Recovery audit contractor. National program using CMS-affiliated contractors to review claims prior to payment as well as for payments on claims already processed, including overpayments and underpayments.

radiation therapy simulation. Radiation therapy simulation. Procedure by which the specific body area to be treated with radiation is defined and marked. A CT scan is performed to define the body contours and these images are used to create a plan customized treatment for the patient, targeting the area to be treated while sparing adjacent tissue. The center of the area to be treated is marked and an immobilization device (e.g., cradle, mold) is created to make sure the patient is in the same position each time for treatment. Complexity of treatment depends on the number of treatment areas and the use of tools to isolate the area of treatment.

radioactive substances. Materials used in the diagnosis and treatment of disease that emit high-speed particles and energy-containing rays.

radiology services. Services that include diagnostic and therapeutic radiology, nuclear medicine, CT scan procedures, magnetic resonance imaging services, ultrasound, and other imaging procedures.

radiotherapy afterloading. Part of the radiation therapy process in which the chemotherapy agent is actually instilled into the tumor area subsequent to surgery and placement of an expandable catheter into the void remaining after tumor excision. The specialized catheter remains in place and the patient may come in for multiple treatments with radioisotope placed to treat the margin of tissue surrounding the excision. After the radiotherapy is completed, the patient returns to have the catheter emptied and removed. This is a new therapy in breast cancer treatment.

Rashkind procedure. Transvenous balloon atrial septectomy or septostomy performed by cardiac catheterization. A balloon catheter is inserted into the heart either to create or enlarge an opening in the interatrial septal wall.

respiratory airflow (ventilation). Assessment of air movement during inhalation and exhalation as measured by nasal pressure sensors and thermistor.

respiratory analysis. Assessment of components of respiration obtained by other methods such as airflow or peripheral arterial tone.

respiratory effort. Measurement of diaphragm and/or intercostal muscle for airflow using transducers to estimate thoracic and abdominal motion.

respiratory movement. Measurement of chest and abdomen movement during respiration.

ribbons. In oncology, small plastic tubes containing radioactive sources for interstitial placement that may be cut into specific lengths tailored to the size of the area receiving ionizing radiation treatment.

Ridell sinusotomy. Frontal sinus tissue is destroyed to eliminate tumors.

RNA. Ribonucleic acid.

rural health clinic. Clinic in an area where there is a shortage of health services staffed by a nurse practitioner, physician assistant, or certified nurse midwife under physician direction that provides routine diagnostic services, including clinical laboratory services, drugs, and biologicals and that has prompt access to additional diagnostic services from facilities meeting federal requirements.

Salter osteotomy. Innominate bone of the hip is cut, removed, and repositioned to repair a congenital dislocation, subluxation, or deformity.

saucerization. Creation of a shallow, saucer-like depression in the bone to facilitate drainage of infected areas.

Schiotz tonometer. Instrument that measures intraocular pressure by recording the depth of an indentation on the cornea by a plunger of known weight.

screening mammography. Radiologic images taken of the female breast for the early detection of breast cancer.

screening pap smear. Diagnostic laboratory test consisting of a routine exfoliative cytology test (Papanicolaou test) provided to a woman for the early detection of cervical or vaginal cancer. The exam includes a clinical breast examination and a physician's interpretation of the results.

seeds. Small (1 mm or less) sources of radioactive material that are permanently placed directly into tumors.

Senning procedure. Flaps of intra-atrial septum and right atrial wall are used to create two interatrial channels to divert the systemic and pulmonary venous circulation.

sensitivity tests. Number of methods of applying selective suspected allergens to the skin or mucous.

sensorineural conduction. Transportation of sound from the cochlea to the acoustic nerve and central auditory pathway to the brain.

sentinel lymph node. First node to which lymph drainage and metastasis from a cancer can occur.

separate procedures. Services commonly carried out as a fundamental part of a total service and, as such, do not usually warrant separate identification. These services are identified in CPT with the parenthetical phrase (separate procedure) at the end of the description and are payable only when performed alone.

septectomy. 1) Surgical removal of all or part of the nasal septum. 2) Submucosal resection of the nasal septum.

Shirodkar procedure. Treatment of an incompetent cervical os by placing nonabsorbent suture material in purse-string sutures as a cerclage to support the cervix.

short tandem repeat (STR). Short sequences of a DNA pattern that are repeated. Can be used as genetic markers for human identity testing.

sialodochoplasty. Surgical repair of a salivary gland duct.

single-lead device. Implantable cardiac device (pacemaker or implantable cardioverter-defibrillator [ICD]) in which pacing and sensing components are placed in only one chamber of the heart.

single-nucleotide polymorphism (SNP). Single nucleotide (A, T, C, or G that is different in a DNA sequence. This difference occurs at a significant frequency in the population.

sinus of Valsalva. Any of three sinuses corresponding to the individual cusps of the aortic valve, located in the most proximal part of the aorta just above the cusps. These structures are contained within the pericardium and appear as distinct but subtle outpouchings or dilations of the aortic wall between each of the semilunar cusps of the valve.

sleep apnea. Intermittent cessation of breathing during sleep that may cause hypoxemia and pulmonary arterial hypertension.

sleep latency. Time period between lying down in bed and the onset of sleep.

sleep staging. Determination of the separate levels of sleep according to physiological measurements.

somatic. 1) Pertaining to the body or trunk. 2) In genetics acquired or occurring after birth.

speculoscopy. Viewing the cervix utilizing a magnifier and a special wavelength of light, allowing detection of abnormalities that may not be discovered on a routine Pap smear.

speech-language pathology services. Speech, language, and related function assessment and rehabilitation service furnished by a qualified speech-language pathologist. Audiology services include hearing and balance assessment services furnished by a qualified audiologist. A qualified speech pathologist and audiologist must have a master's or doctoral degree in their respective fields and be licensed to serve in the state. Speech pathologists and audiologists practicing in states without licensure must complete 350 hours of supervised clinical work and perform at least nine months of supervised full-time service after earning their degrees.

sphincteroplasty. Surgical repair done to correct, augment, or improve the muscular function of a sphincter, such as the anus or intestines.

spirometry. Measurement of the lungs' breathing capacity.

splint. Brace or support. 1) dynamic splint: brace that permits movement of an anatomical structure such as a hand, wrist, foot, or other part of the body after surgery or injury. 2) static splint: brace that prevents movement and maintains support and position for an anatomical structure after surgery or injury.

stent. Tube to provide support in a body cavity or lumen.

stereotactic radiosurgery. Delivery of externally-generated ionizing radiation to specific targets for destruction or inactivation. Most often utilized in the treatment of brain or spinal tumors, high-resolution stereotactic imaging is used to identify the target and then deliver the treatment. Computer-assisted planning may also be employed. Simple and complex cranial lesions and spinal lesions are typically treated in a single planning and treatment session, although a maximum of five sessions may be required. No incision is made for stereotactic radiosurgery procedures.

stereotaxis. Three-dimensional method for precisely locating structures.

Stoffel rhizotomy. Nerve roots are sectioned to relieve pain or spastic paralysis.

strabismus. Misalignment of the eyes due to an imbalance in extraocular muscles.

surgical package. Normal, uncomplicated performance of specific surgical services, with the assumption that, on average, all surgical procedures of a given type are similar with respect to skill level, duration, and length of normal follow-up care.

symblepharopterygium. Adhesion in which the eyelid is adhered to the eyeball by a band that resembles a pterygium.

sympathectomy. Surgical interruption or transection of a sympathetic nervous system pathway.

tarso-. 1) Relating to the foot. 2) Relating to the margin of the eyelid.

tarsocheiloplasty. Plastic operation upon the edge of the eyelid for the treatment of trichiasis.

tarsorrhaphy. Suture of a portion or all of the opposing eyelids together for the purpose of shortening the palpebral fissure or closing it entirely.

technical component. Portion of a health care service that identifies the provision of the equipment, supplies, technical personnel, and costs attendant to the performance of the procedure other than the professional services.

tendon. Fibrous tissue that connects muscle to bone, consisting primarily of collagen and containing little vasculature.

tendon allograft. Allografts are tissues obtained from another individual of the same species. Tendon allografts are usually obtained from cadavers and frozen or freeze dried for later use in soft tissue repairs where the physician elects not to obtain an autogenous graft (a graft obtained from the individual on whom the surgery is being performed).

tendon suture material. Tendons are composed of fibrous tissue consisting primarily of collagen and containing few cells or blood vessels. This tissue heals more slowly than tissues with more vascularization. Because of this, tendons are usually repaired with nonabsorbable suture material. Examples include surgical silk, surgical cotton, linen, stainless steel, surgical nylon, polyester fiber, polybutester (Novafil), polyethylene (Dermalene), and polypropylene (Prolene, Surilene).

tendon transplant. Replacement of a tendon with another tendon.

tenon's capsule. Connective tissue that forms the capsule enclosing the posterior eyeball, extending from the conjunctival fornix and continuous with the muscular fascia of the eye.

tenonectomy. Excision of a portion of a tendon to make it shorter.

tenotomy. Cutting into a tendon.

TENS. Transcutaneous electrical nerve stimulator. TENS is applied by placing electrode pads over the area to be stimulated and connecting the electrodes to a transmitter box, which sends a current through the skin to sensory nerve fibers to help decrease pain in that nerve distribution.

tensilon. Edrophonium chloride. Agent used for evaluation and treatment of myasthenia gravis.

terminally ill. Individual whose medical prognosis for life expectancy is six months or less.

tetralogy of Fallot. Specific combination of congenital cardiac defects: obstruction of the right ventricular outflow tract with pulmonary stenosis, interventricular septal defect, malposition of the aorta, overriding the interventricular septum and receiving blood from both the venous and arterial systems, and enlargement of the right ventricle.

therapeutic services. Services performed for treatment of a specific diagnosis. These services include performance of the procedure, various incidental elements, and normal, related follow-up care.

thoracentesis. Surgical puncture of the chest cavity with a specialized needle or hollow tubing to aspirate fluid from within the pleural space for diagnostic or therapeutic reasons.

thoracic lymphadenectomy. Procedure to cut out the lymph nodes near the lungs, around the heart, and behind the trachea.

thoracostomy. Creation of an opening in the chest wall for drainage.

thyroglossal duct. Embryonic duct at the front of the neck, which becomes the pyramidal lobe of the thyroid gland with obliteration of the remaining duct, but may form a cyst or sinus in adulthood if it persists.

total disc arthroplasty with artificial disc. Removal of an intravertebral disc and its replacement with an implant. The implant is an artificial disc consisting of two metal plates with a weight-bearing surface of polyethylene between the plates. The plates are anchored to the vertebral immediately above and below the affected disc.

total shoulder replacement. Prosthetic replacement of the entire shoulder joint, including the humeral head and the glenoid fossa.

trabeculae carneae cordis. Bands of muscular tissue that line the walls of the ventricles in the heart.

trabeculectomy. Surgical incision between the anterior portion of the eye and the canal of Schlemm to drain the aqueous humor.

tracheostomy. Formation of a tracheal opening on the neck surface with tube insertion to allow for respiration in cases of obstruction or decreased patency. A tracheostomy may be planned or performed on an emergency basis for temporary or long-term use.

tracheotomy. Formation of a tracheal opening on the neck surface with tube insertion to allow for respiration in cases of obstruction or decreased patency. A tracheotomy may be planned or performed on an emergency basis for temporary or long-term use.

traction. Drawing out or holding tension on an area by applying a direct therapeutic pulling force.

transcranial magnetic stimulation. Application of electromagnetic energy to the brain through a coil placed on the scalp. The procedure stimulates cortical neurons and is intended to activate and normalize their processes.

transcription. Process by which messenger RNA is synthesized from a DNA template resulting in the transfer of genetic information from the DNA molecule to the messenger RNA.

translocation. Disconnection of all or part of a chromosome that reattaches to another position in the DNA sequence of the same or another chromosome. Often results in a reciprocal exchange of DNA sequences between two differently numbered chromosomes. May or may not result in a clinically significant loss of DNA.

trephine. 1) Specialized round saw for cutting circular holes in bone, especially the skull. 2) Instrument that removes small disc-shaped buttons of corneal tissue for transplanting.

tricuspid atresia. Congenital absence of the valve that may occur with other defects, such as atrial septal defect, pulmonary atresia, and transposition of great vessels.

turbinates. Scroll or shell-shaped elevations from the wall of the nasal cavity, the inferior turbinate being a separate bone, while the superior and middle turbinates are of the ethmoid bone.

tympanic membrane. Thin, sensitive membrane across the entrance to the middle ear that vibrates in response to sound waves, allowing the waves to be transmitted via the ossicular chain to the internal ear.

tympanoplasty. Surgical repair of the structures of the middle ear, including the eardrum and the three small bones, or ossicles.

unlisted procedure. Procedural descriptions used when the overall procedure and outcome of the procedure are not adequately described by an existing procedure code. Such codes are used as a last resort and only when there is not a more appropriate procedure code.

ureterorrhaphy. Surgical repair using sutures to close an open wound or injury of the ureter.

vagotomy. Division of the vagus nerves, interrupting impulses resulting in lower gastric acid production and hastening gastric emptying. Used in the treatment of chronic gastric, pyloric, and duodenal ulcers that can cause severe pain and difficulties in eating and sleeping.

variant. Nucleotide deviation from the normal sequence of a region. Variations are usually either substitutions or deletions. Substitution variations are the result of one nucleotide taking the place of another. A deletion occurs when one or more nucleotides are left out. In some cases, several in a reasonably close proximity on the same chromosome in a DNA strand. These variations result in amino acid changes in the protein made by the gene. However, the term variant does not itself imply a functional change. Intron variations are usually described in one of two ways: 1) the changed nucleotide is defined by a plus or a minus sign indicating the position relative to the first or last nucleotide to the intron, or 2) the second variant description is indicated relative to the last nucleotide of the preceding exon or first nucleotide of the following exon.

vascular family. Group of vessels (family) that branch from the aorta or vena cava. At each branching, the vascular order increases by one. The first order vessel is the primary branch off the aorta or vena cava. The second order vessel branches from the first order, the third order branches from the second order, and any further branching is beyond the third order. For example, for the inferior vena cava, the common iliac artery is a first order vessel. The internal and external iliac arteries are second order vessels, as they each originate from the first order common iliac artery. The external iliac artery extends directly from the common iliac artery and the internal iliac artery bifurcates from the common iliac artery. A third order vessel from the external iliac artery is the inferior epigastric artery and a third order vessel from the internal iliac artery is the obturator artery. Note orders are not always identical bilaterally (e.g., the left common carotid artery is a first order and the right common carotid is a second order. Synonym(s): vascular origins and distributions.

vasectomy. Surgical procedure involving the removal of all or part of the vas deferens, usually performed for sterilization or in conjunction with a prostatectomy.

vena cava interruption. Procedure that places a filter device, called an umbrella or sieve, within the large vein returning deoxygenated blood to the heart to prevent pulmonary embolism caused by clots.

ventricular assist device. Temporary measure used to support the heart by substituting for left and/or right heart function. The device replaces the work of the left and/or right ventricle when a patient has a damaged or weakened heart. A left ventricular assist device (VAD) helps the heart pump blood through the rest of the body. A right VAD helps the heart pump blood to the lungs to become oxygenated again. Catheters are inserted to circulate the blood through external tubing to a pump machine located outside of the body and back to the correct artery.

ventricular septal defect. Congenital cardiac anomaly resulting in a continual opening in the septum between the ventricles that, in severe cases, causes oxygenated blood to flow back into the lungs, resulting in pulmonary hypertension.

vertebral interspace. Non-bony space between two adjacent vertebral bodies that contains the cushioning intervertebral disk.

volar. Palm of the hand (palmar) or sole of the foot (plantar).

Waterston procedure. Type of aortopulmonary shunting done to increase pulmonary blood flow. The ascending aorta is anastomosed to the right pulmonary artery.

Wharton's ducts. Salivary ducts below the mandible.

wick catheter. Device used to monitor interstitial fluid pressure, and sometimes used intraoperatively during fasciotomy procedures to evaluate the effectiveness of the decompression.

wound closure. Closure or repair of a wound created surgically or due to trauma (e.g., laceration). The closure technique depends on the type, site, and depth of the defect. Consideration is also given to cosmetic and functional outcome. A single layer closure involves approximation of the edges of the wound. The second type of closure involves closing the one or more deeper layers of tissue prior to skin closure. The most complex type of closure may include techniques such as debridement or undermining, which involves manipulation of tissue around the wound to allow the skin to cover the wound. The AMA CPT® book defines these as Simple, Intermediate and Complex repair.

xenograft. Tissue that is nonhuman and harvested from one species and grafted to another. Pigskin is the most common xenograft for human skin and is applied to a wound as a temporary closure until a permanent option is performed.

z-plasty. Plastic surgery technique used primarily to release tension or elongate contracted scar tissue in which a Z-shaped incision is made with the middle line of the Z crossing the area of greatest tension. The triangular flaps are then rotated so that they cross the incision line in the opposite direction, creating a reversed Z.

ZPIC. Zone Program Integrity Contractor. CMS contractor that replaced the existing Program Safeguard Contractors (PSC). Contractors are responsible for ensuring the integrity of all Medicare-related claims under Parts A and B (hospital, skilled nursing, home health, provider, and durable medical equipment claims), Part C (Medicare Advantage health plans), Part D (prescription drug plans), and coordination of Medicare-Medicaid data matches (Medi-Medi).

Appendix N — Listing of Sensory, Motor, and Mixed Nerves

This list contains the sensory, motor, and mixed nerves assigned to each nerve conduction study to improve coding accuracy. Each nerve makes up one single unit of service.

Motor Nerves Assigned to Codes 95900 and 95907-95913

I. Upper extremity, cervical plexus, and brachial plexus motor nerves
   A. Axillary motor nerve to the deltoid
   B. Long thoracic motor nerve to the serratus anterior
   C. Median nerve
      1. Median motor nerve to the abductor pollicis brevis
      2. Median motor nerve, anterior interosseous branch, to the flexor pollicis longus
      3. Median motor nerve, anterior interosseous branch, to the pronator quadratus
      4. Median motor nerve to the first lumbrical
      5. Median motor nerve to the second lumbrical
   D. Musculocutaneous motor nerve to the biceps brachii
   E. Radial nerve
      1. Radial motor nerve to the extensor carpi ulnaris
      2. Radial motor nerve to the extensor digitorum communis
      3. Radial motor nerve to the extensor indicis proprius
      4. Radial motor nerve to the brachioradialis
   F. Suprascapular nerve
      1. Suprascapular motor nerve to the supraspinatus
      2. Suprascapular motor nerve to the infraspinatus
   G. Thoracodorsal motor nerve to the latissimus dorsi
   H. Ulnar nerve
      1. Ulnar motor nerve to the abductor digiti minimi
      2. Ulnar motor nerve to the palmar interosseous
      3. Ulnar motor nerve to the first dorsal interosseous
      4. Ulnar motor nerve to the flexor carpi ulnaris
   I. Other
II. Lower extremity motor nerves
   A. Femoral motor nerve to the quadriceps
      1. Femoral motor nerve to vastus medialis
      2. Femoral motor nerve to vastus lateralis
      3. Femoral motor nerve to vastus intermedialis
      4. Femoral motor nerve to rectus femoris
   B. Ilioinguinal motor nerve
   C. Peroneal (fibular) nerve
      1. Peroneal motor nerve to the extensor digitorum brevis
      2. Peroneal motor nerve to the peroneus brevis
      3. Peroneal motor nerve to the peroneus longus
      4. Peroneal motor nerve to the tibialis anterior
   D. Plantar motor nerve
   E. Sciatic nerve
   F. Tibial nerve
      1. Tibial motor nerve, inferior calcaneal branch, to the abductor digiti minimi
      2. Tibial motor nerve, medial plantar branch, to the abductor hallucis
      3. Tibial motor nerve, lateral plantar branch, to the flexor digiti minimi brevis
   G. Other
III. Cranial nerves and trunk
   A. Cranial nerve VII (facial motor nerve)
      1. Facial nerve to the frontalis
      2. Facial nerve to the nasalis
      3. Facial nerve to the orbicularis oculi
      4. Facial nerve to the orbicularis oris
   B. Cranial nerve XI (spinal accessory motor nerve)
   C. Cranial nerve XII (hypoglossal motor nerve)
   D. Intercostal motor nerve
   E. Phrenic motor nerve to the diaphragm
   F. Recurrent laryngeal nerve
   G. Other
IV. Nerve Roots
   A. Cervical nerve root stimulation
      1. Cervical level 5 (C5)
      2. Cervical level 6 (C6)
      3. Cervical level 7 (C7)
      4. Cervical level 8 (C8)
   B. Thoracic nerve root stimulation
      1. Thoracic level 1 (T1)
      2. Thoracic level 2 (T2)
      3. Thoracic level 3 (T3)
      4. Thoracic level 4 (T4)
      5. Thoracic level 5 (T5)
      6. Thoracic level 6 (T6)
      7. Thoracic level 7 (T7)
      8. Thoracic level 8 (T8)
      9. Thoracic level 9 (T9)
      10. Thoracic level 10 (T10)
      11. Thoracic level 11 (T11)
      12. Thoracic level 12 (T12)
   C. Lumbar nerve root stimulation
      1. Lumbar level 1 (L1)
      2. Lumbar level 2 (L2)
      3. Lumbar level 3 (L3)
      4. Lumbar level 4 (L4)
      5. Lumbar level 5 (L5)
   D. Sacral nerve root stimulation
      1. Sacral level 1 (S1)

2. Sacral level 2 (S2)

3. Sacral level 3 (S3)

4. Sacral level 4 (S4)

Sensory and Mixed Nerves Assigned to Codes 95907–95913

I. Upper extremity sensory and mixed nerves

　A. Lateral antebrachial cutaneous sensory nerve

　B. Medial antebrachial cutaneous sensory nerve

　C. Medial brachial cutaneous sensory nerve

　D. Median nerve

　　1. Median sensory nerve to the first digit

　　2. Median sensory nerve to the second digit

　　3. Median sensory nerve to the third digit

　　4. Median sensory nerve to the fourth digit

　　5. Median palmar cutaneous sensory nerve

　　6. Median palmar mixed nerve

　E. Posterior antebrachial cutaneous sensory nerve

　F. Radial sensory nerve

　　1. Radial sensory nerve to the base of the thumb

　　2. Radial sensory nerve to digit 1

　G. Ulnar nerve

　　1. Ulnar dorsal cutaneous sensory nerve

　　2. Ulnar sensory nerve to the fourth digit

　　3. Ulnar sensory nerve to the fifth digit

　　4. Ulnar palmar mixed nerve

　H. Intercostal sensory nerve

　I. Other

II. Lower extremity sensory and mixed nerves

　A. Lateral femoral cutaneous sensory nerve

　B. Medical calcaneal sensory nerve

　C. Medial femoral cutaneous sensory nerve

　D. Peroneal nerve

　　1. Deep peroneal sensory nerve

　　2. Superficial peroneal sensory nerve, medial dorsal cutaneous branch

　　3. Superficial peroneal sensory nerve, intermediate dorsal cutaneous branch

　E. Posterior femoral cutaneous sensory nerve

　F. Saphenous nerve

　　1. Saphenous sensory nerve (distal technique)

　　2. Saphenous sensory nerve (proximal technique)

　G. Sural nerve

　　1. Sural sensory nerve, lateral dorsal cutaneous branch

　　2. Sural sensory nerve

　H. Tibial sensory nerve (digital nerve to toe 1)

　I. Tibial sensory nerve (medial plantar nerve)

　J. Tibial sensory nerve (lateral plantar nerve)

　K. Other

III. Head and trunk sensory nerves

　A. Dorsal nerve of the penis

　B. Greater auricular nerve

　C. Ophthalmic branch of the trigeminal nerve

　D. Pudendal sensory nerve

　E. Suprascapular sensory nerves

　F. Other

In the following table, the reasonable maximum number of studies per diagnostic category is listed that allows for a physician or other qualified health care professional to obtain a diagnosis for 90 percent of patients with that same final diagnosis. The numbers denote the suggested number of studies, although the decision is up to the provider.

Type of Study/Maximum Number of Studies

Indication	Limbs Studied by Needle EMG (95860–95864, 95867–95870, 95885–95887)	Nerve Conduction Studies (Total nerves studied, 95907-95913)	Neuromuscular Junction Testing (Repetitive Stimulation 95937)
Carpal Tunnel (Unilateral)	1	7	—
Carpal Tunnel (Bilateral)	2	10	—
Radiculopathy	2	7	—
Mononeuropathy	1	8	—
Polyneuropathy/Mononeuropathy Multiplex	3	10	—
Myopathy	2	4	2
Motor Neuronopathy (e.g., ALS)	4	6	2
Plexopathy	2	12	—
Neuromuscular Junction	2	4	3
Tarsal Tunnel Syndrome (Unilateral)	1	8	—
Tarsal Tunnel Syndrome (Bilateral)	2	11	—
Weakness, Fatigue, Cramps, or Twitching (Focal)	2	7	2
Weakness, Fatigue, Cramps, or Twitching (General)	4	8	2
Pain, Numbness, or Tingling (Unilateral)	1	9	—
Pain, Numbness, or Tingling (Bilateral)	2	12	—

Appendix N — Listing of Sensory, Motor, and Mixed Nerves

Appendix O — Vascular Families

This table assumes that the starting point is aortic catheterization. This categorization would not be accurate if, for instance, a femoral or carotid artery were catheterized with the blood's flow. The names of the arteries appearing in bold face type in the following table indicate those arteries that are most often the subject of arteriographic procedures.

First Order	Second Order Branch	Third Order Branch	Beyond Third Order Branches

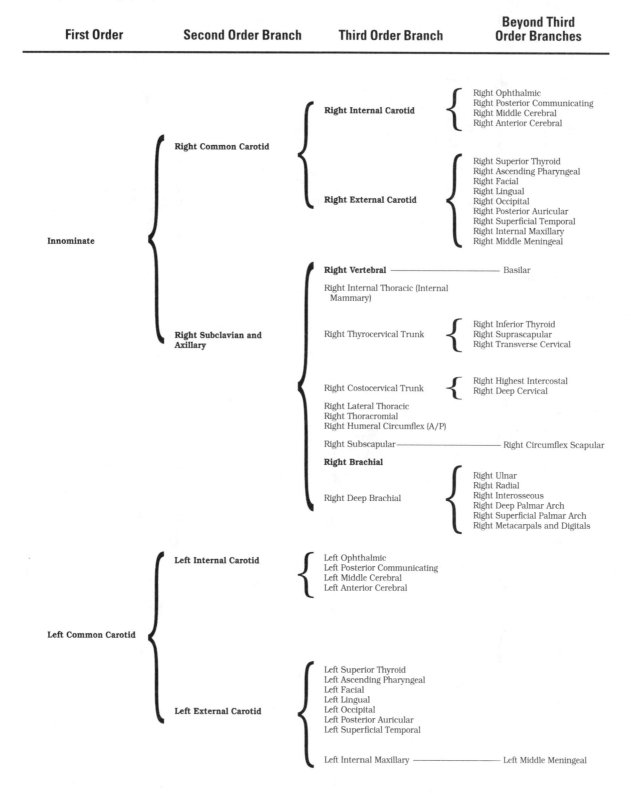

Innominate

Right Common Carotid

Right Internal Carotid
- Right Ophthalmic
- Right Posterior Communicating
- Right Middle Cerebral
- Right Anterior Cerebral

Right External Carotid
- Right Superior Thyroid
- Right Ascending Pharyngeal
- Right Facial
- Right Lingual
- Right Occipital
- Right Posterior Auricular
- Right Superficial Temporal
- Right Internal Maxillary
- Right Middle Meningeal

Right Subclavian and Axillary

Right Vertebral ———— Basilar

Right Internal Thoracic (Internal Mammary)

Right Thyrocervical Trunk
- Right Inferior Thyroid
- Right Suprascapular
- Right Transverse Cervical

Right Costocervical Trunk
- Right Highest Intercostal
- Right Deep Cervical

Right Lateral Thoracic
Right Thoracromial
Right Humeral Circumflex (A/P)

Right Subscapular ———— Right Circumflex Scapular

Right Brachial

Right Deep Brachial
- Right Ulnar
- Right Radial
- Right Interosseous
- Right Deep Palmar Arch
- Right Superficial Palmar Arch
- Right Metacarpals and Digitals

Left Common Carotid

Left Internal Carotid
- Left Ophthalmic
- Left Posterior Communicating
- Left Middle Cerebral
- Left Anterior Cerebral

Left External Carotid
- Left Superior Thyroid
- Left Ascending Pharyngeal
- Left Facial
- Left Lingual
- Left Occipital
- Left Posterior Auricular
- Left Superficial Temporal

Left Internal Maxillary ———— Left Middle Meningeal

Appendix O — Vascular Families

First Order	Second Order Branch	Third Order Branch	Beyond Third Order Branches

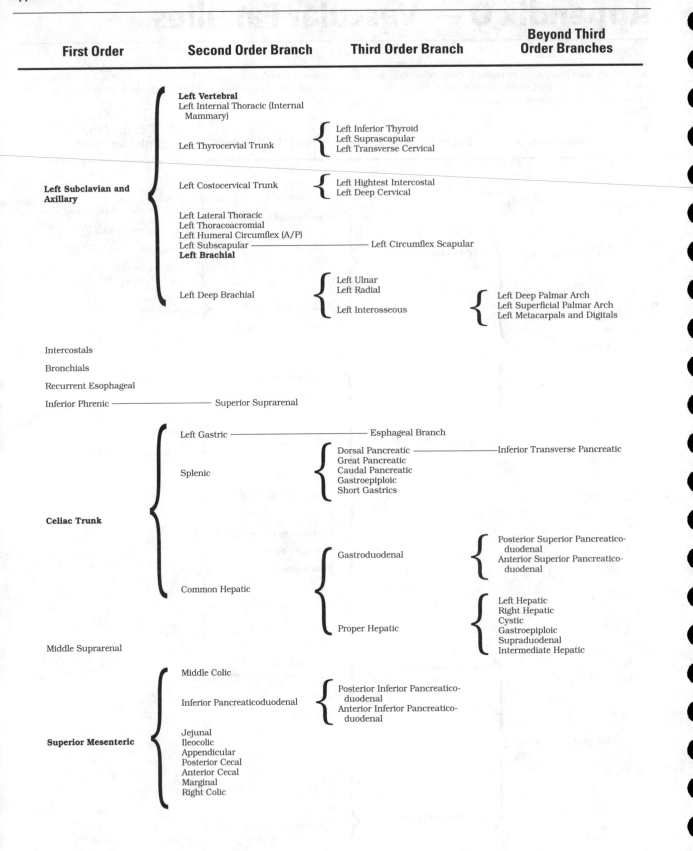

Left Subclavian and Axillary

- **Left Vertebral**
- Left Internal Thoracic (Internal Mammary)
- Left Thyrocervial Trunk
  - Left Inferior Thyroid
  - Left Suprascapular
  - Left Transverse Cervical
- Left Costocervical Trunk
  - Left Hightest Intercostal
  - Left Deep Cervical
- Left Lateral Thoracic
- Left Thoracoacromial
- Left Humeral Circumflex (A/P)
- Left Subscapular —— Left Circumflex Scapular
- **Left Brachial**
- Left Deep Brachial
  - Left Ulnar
  - Left Radial
  - Left Interosseous
    - Left Deep Palmar Arch
    - Left Superficial Palmar Arch
    - Left Metacarpals and Digitals

Intercostals

Bronchials

Recurrent Esophageal

Inferior Phrenic —————————— Superior Suprarenal

Celiac Trunk

- Left Gastric ———————————— Esphageal Branch
- Splenic
  - Dorsal Pancreatic ———————— Inferior Transverse Pancreatic
  - Great Pancreatic
  - Caudal Pancreatic
  - Gastroepiploic
  - Short Gastrics
- Common Hepatic
  - Gastroduodenal
    - Posterior Superior Pancreatico-duodenal
    - Anterior Superior Pancreatico-duodenal
  - Proper Hepatic
    - Left Hepatic
    - Right Hepatic
    - Cystic
    - Gastroepiploic
    - Supraduodenal
    - Intermediate Hepatic

Middle Suprarenal

Superior Mesenteric

- Middle Colic
- Inferior Pancreaticoduodenal
  - Posterior Inferior Pancreatico-duodenal
  - Anterior Inferior Pancreatico-duodenal
- Jejunal
- Ileocolic
- Appendicular
- Posterior Cecal
- Anterior Cecal
- Marginal
- Right Colic

First Order	Second Order Branch	Third Order Branch	Beyond Third Order Branches

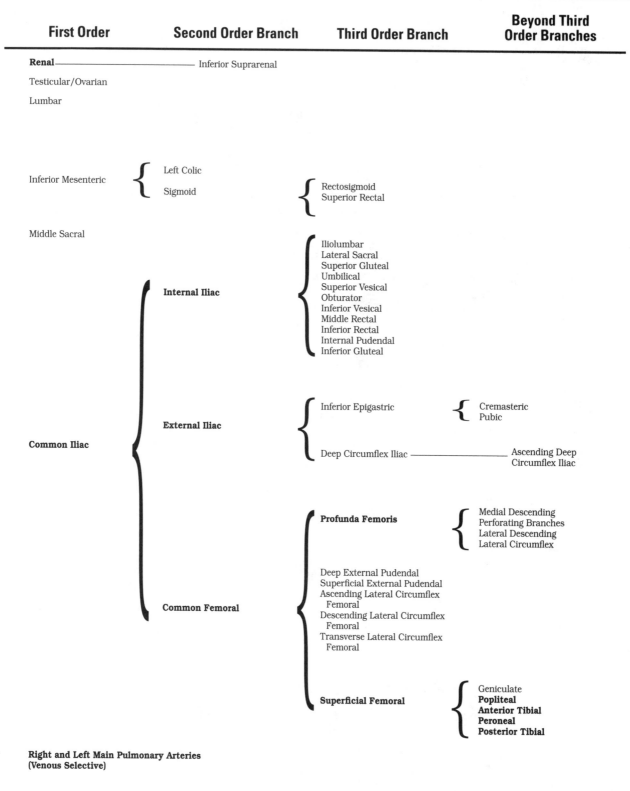

Renal —————————————————— Inferior Suprarenal

Testicular/Ovarian

Lumbar

Inferior Mesenteric { Left Colic / Sigmoid

{ Rectosigmoid / Superior Rectal

Middle Sacral

Internal Iliac { Iliolumbar / Lateral Sacral / Superior Gluteal / Umbilical / Superior Vesical / Obturator / Inferior Vesical / Middle Rectal / Inferior Rectal / Internal Pudendal / Inferior Gluteal

External Iliac { Inferior Epigastric { Cremasteric / Pubic

Deep Circumflex Iliac ——————————— Ascending Deep Circumflex Iliac

Common Iliac

Profunda Femoris { Medial Descending / Perforating Branches / Lateral Descending / Lateral Circumflex

Common Femoral { Deep External Pudendal / Superficial External Pudendal / Ascending Lateral Circumflex Femoral / Descending Lateral Circumflex Femoral / Transverse Lateral Circumflex Femoral

Superficial Femoral { Geniculate / **Popliteal** / **Anterior Tibial** / **Peroneal** / **Posterior Tibial**

**Right and Left Main Pulmonary Arteries
(Venous Selective)**

Reference: Kadir S. *Atlas of Normal and Variant Angiographic Anatomy.* Philadelphia, Pa: WB Saunders Co; 1991

Appendix P — Interventional Radiology Illustrations

Normal Aortic Arch and Branch Anatomy—Transfemoral Approach

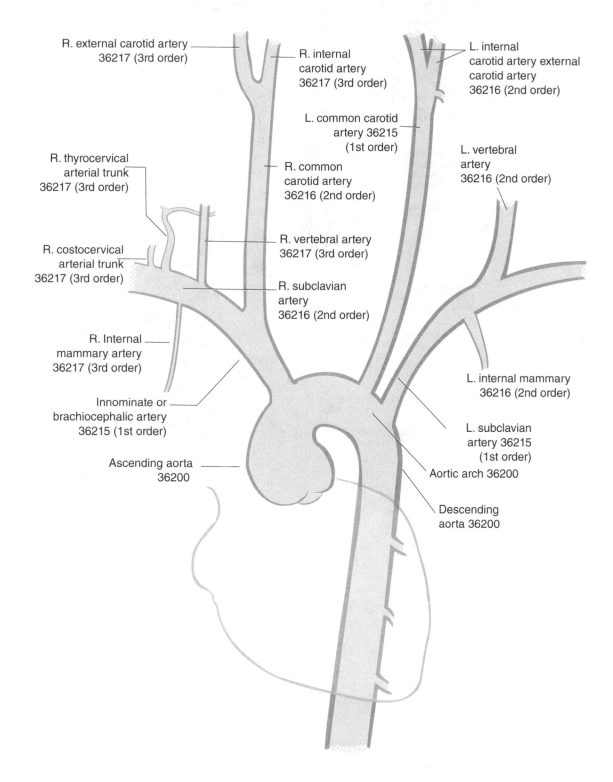

R. external carotid artery
36217 (3rd order)

R. internal
carotid artery
36217 (3rd order)

L. internal
carotid artery external
carotid artery
36216 (2nd order)

L. common carotid
artery 36215
(1st order)

R. common
carotid artery
36216 (2nd order)

L. vertebral
artery
36216 (2nd order)

R. thyrocervical
arterial trunk
36217 (3rd order)

R. vertebral artery
36217 (3rd order)

R. costocervical
arterial trunk
36217 (3rd order)

R. subclavian
artery
36216 (2nd order)

R. Internal
mammary artery
36217 (3rd order)

L. internal mammary
36216 (2nd order)

Innominate or
brachiocephalic artery
36215 (1st order)

L. subclavian
artery 36215
(1st order)

Aortic arch 36200

Ascending aorta
36200

Descending
aorta 36200

Superior and Inferior Mesenteric Arteries and Branches

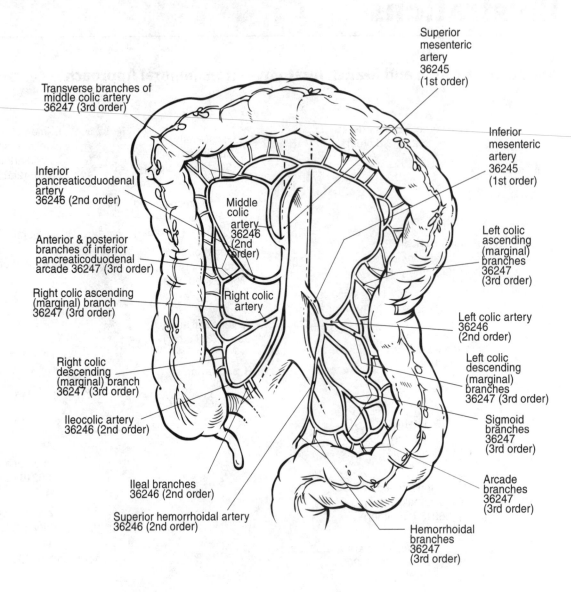

Transverse branches of
middle colic artery
36247 (3rd order)

Inferior
pancreaticoduodenal
artery
36246 (2nd order)

Anterior & posterior
branches of inferior
pancreaticoduodenal
arcade 36247 (3rd order)

Right colic ascending
(marginal) branch
36247 (3rd order)

Right colic
descending
(marginal) branch
36247 (3rd order)

Ileocolic artery
36246 (2nd order)

Ileal branches
36246 (2nd order)

Superior hemorrhoidal artery
36246 (2nd order)

Middle
colic
artery
36246
(2nd
order)

Right colic
artery

Superior
mesenteric
artery
36245
(1st order)

Inferior
mesenteric
artery
36245
(1st order)

Left colic
ascending
(marginal)
branches
36247
(3rd order)

Left colic artery
36246
(2nd order)

Left colic
descending
(marginal)
branches
36247 (3rd order)

Sigmoid
branches
36247
(3rd order)

Arcade
branches
36247
(3rd order)

Hemorrhoidal
branches
36247
(3rd order)

Portal System

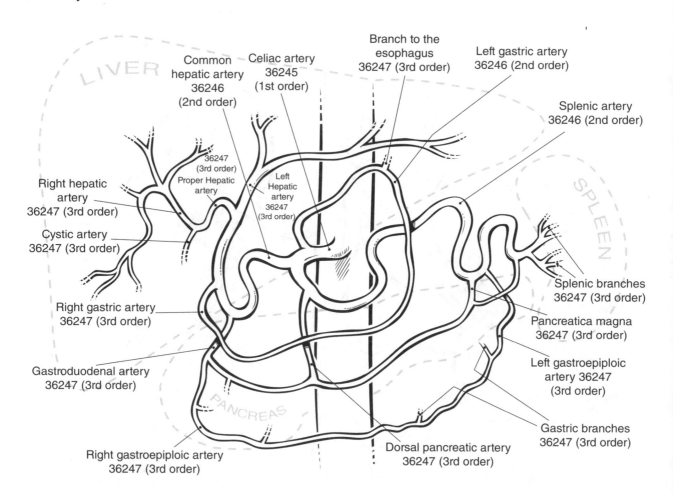

Appendix P — Interventional Radiology Illustrations

Renal Artery Anatomy—Femoral Approach

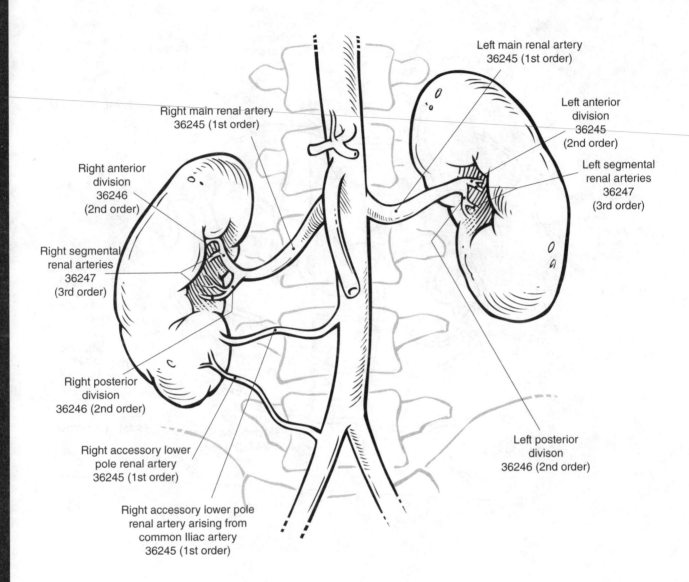

Left main renal artery
36245 (1st order)

Right main renal artery
36245 (1st order)

Left anterior
division
36245
(2nd order)

Right anterior
division
36246
(2nd order)

Left segmental
renal arteries
36247
(3rd order)

Right segmental
renal arteries
36247
(3rd order)

Right posterior
division
36246 (2nd order)

Left posterior
divison
36246 (2nd order)

Right accessory lower
pole renal artery
36245 (1st order)

Right accessory lower pole
renal artery arising from
common Iliac artery
36245 (1st order)

Upper Extremity Arterial Anatomy—Transfemoral or Contralateral Approach

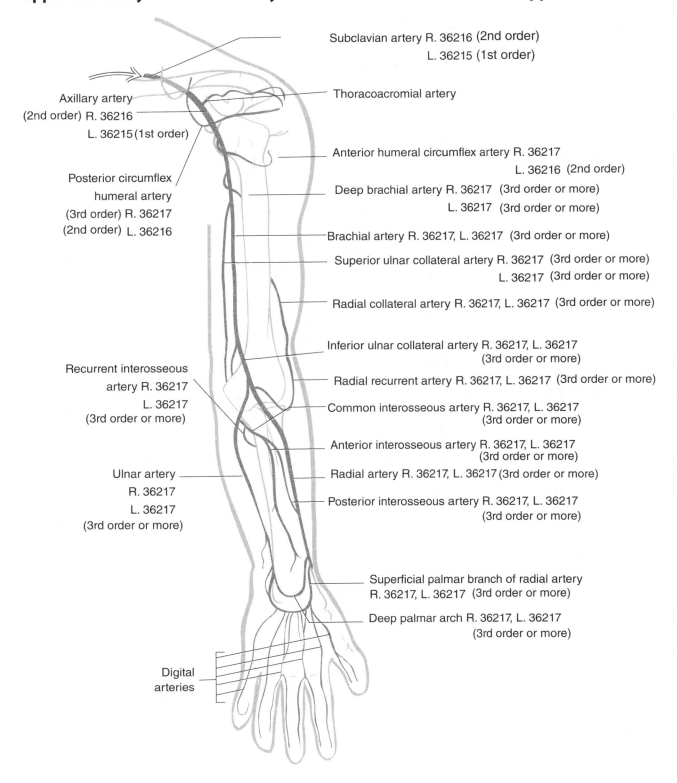

Subclavian artery R. 36216 (2nd order)

L. 36215 (1st order)

Axillary artery
(2nd order) R. 36216

L. 36215 (1st order)

Thoracoacromial artery

Posterior circumflex
humeral artery
(3rd order) R. 36217
(2nd order) L. 36216

Anterior humeral circumflex artery R. 36217

L. 36216 (2nd order)

Deep brachial artery R. 36217 (3rd order or more)

L. 36217 (3rd order or more)

Brachial artery R. 36217, L. 36217 (3rd order or more)

Superior ulnar collateral artery R. 36217 (3rd order or more)

L. 36217 (3rd order or more)

Radial collateral artery R. 36217, L. 36217 (3rd order or more)

Inferior ulnar collateral artery R. 36217, L. 36217
(3rd order or more)

Recurrent interosseous
artery R. 36217

L. 36217
(3rd order or more)

Radial recurrent artery R. 36217, L. 36217 (3rd order or more)

Common interosseous artery R. 36217, L. 36217
(3rd order or more)

Anterior interosseous artery R. 36217, L. 36217
(3rd order or more)

Radial artery R. 36217, L. 36217 (3rd order or more)

Ulnar artery
R. 36217
L. 36217
(3rd order or more)

Posterior interosseous artery R. 36217, L. 36217
(3rd order or more)

Superficial palmar branch of radial artery
R. 36217, L. 36217 (3rd order or more)

Deep palmar arch R. 36217, L. 36217
(3rd order or more)

Digital
arteries

Lower Extremity Arterial Anatomy—Contralateral, Axillary or Brachial Approach

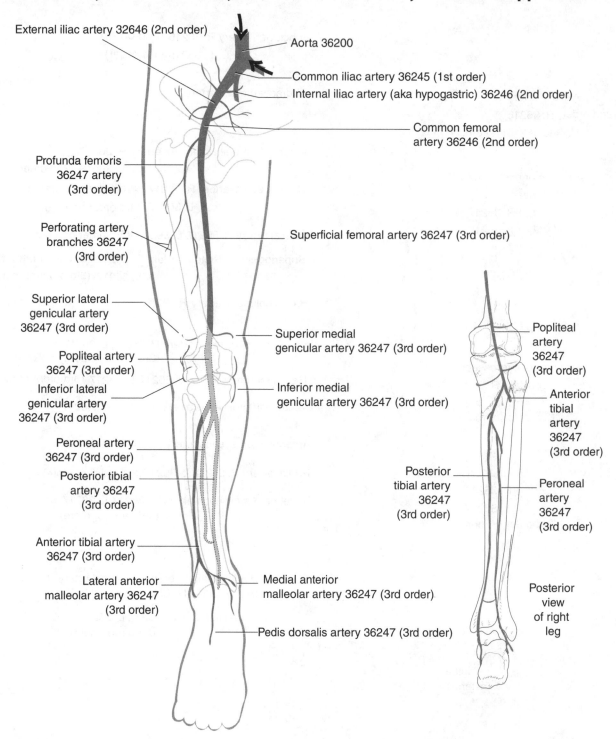

External iliac artery 32646 (2nd order)

Aorta 36200

Common iliac artery 36245 (1st order)

Internal iliac artery (aka hypogastric) 36246 (2nd order)

Common femoral artery 36246 (2nd order)

Profunda femoris 36247 artery (3rd order)

Perforating artery branches 36247 (3rd order)

Superficial femoral artery 36247 (3rd order)

Superior lateral genicular artery 36247 (3rd order)

Superior medial genicular artery 36247 (3rd order)

Popliteal artery 36247 (3rd order)

Inferior lateral genicular artery 36247 (3rd order)

Inferior medial genicular artery 36247 (3rd order)

Peroneal artery 36247 (3rd order)

Posterior tibial artery 36247 (3rd order)

Anterior tibial artery 36247 (3rd order)

Lateral anterior malleolar artery 36247 (3rd order)

Medial anterior malleolar artery 36247 (3rd order)

Pedis dorsalis artery 36247 (3rd order)

Popliteal artery 36247 (3rd order)

Anterior tibial artery 36247 (3rd order)

Posterior tibial artery 36247 (3rd order)

Peroneal artery 36247 (3rd order)

Posterior view of right leg

Portal System

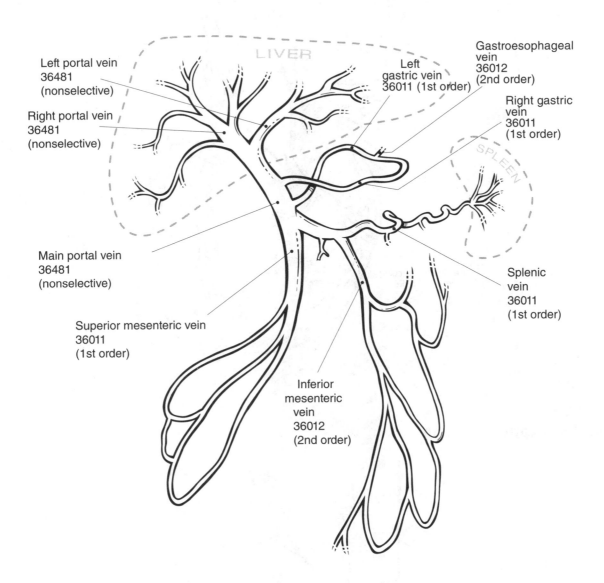

Left portal vein
36481
(nonselective)

Right portal vein
36481
(nonselective)

Main portal vein
36481
(nonselective)

Superior mesenteric vein
36011
(1st order)

Left
gastric vein
36011 (1st order)

Gastroesophageal
vein
36012
(2nd order)

Right gastric
vein
36011
(1st order)

Splenic
vein
36011
(1st order)

Inferior
mesenteric
vein
36012
(2nd order)

LIVER

SPLEEN

Coronary Arteries Anterior View

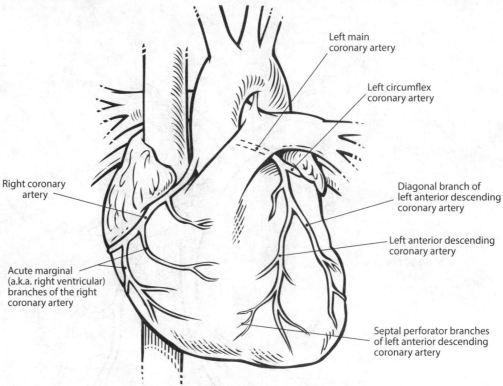

Left main coronary artery

Left circumflex coronary artery

Right coronary artery

Diagonal branch of left anterior descending coronary artery

Left anterior descending coronary artery

Acute marginal (a.k.a. right ventricular) branches of the right coronary artery

Septal perforator branches of left anterior descending coronary artery

Left Heart Catheterization

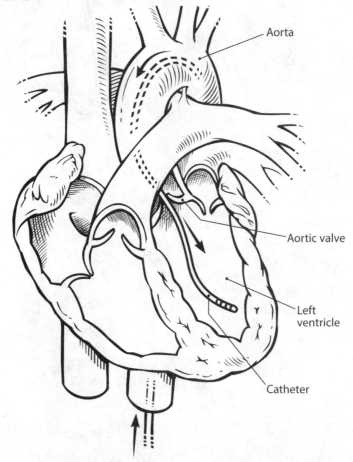

Aorta

Aortic valve

Left ventricle

Catheter

Heart Conduction System

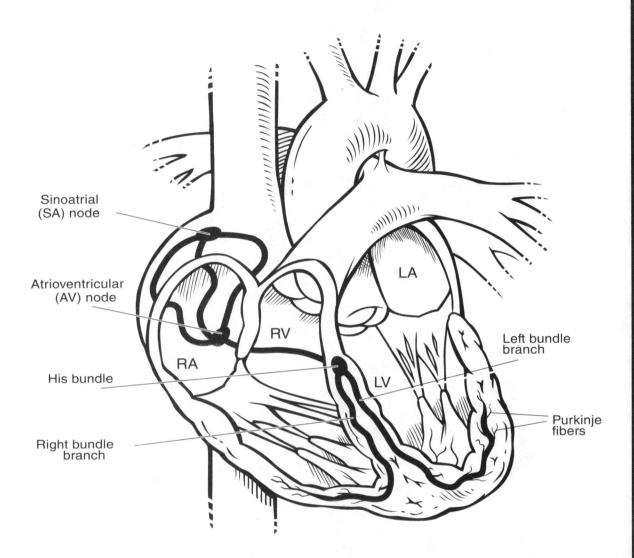

Sinoatrial (SA) node

Atrioventricular (AV) node

His bundle

Right bundle branch

RA

RV

LA

LV

Left bundle branch

Purkinje fibers

Notes